BRIEF CONTENTS OF VOLUME 2

PART II: Psychosocial Modules

MODULE 22	Addiction	1519
MODULE 23	Cognition	1575
MODULE 24	Culture and Diversity	1629
MODULE 25	Development	1647
MODULE 26	Family	1707
MODULE 27	Grief and Loss	1741
MODULE 28	Mood and Affect	1775
MODULE 29	Self	1831
MODULE 30	Spirituality	1871
MODULE 31	Stress and Coping	1895
MODULE 32	Violence	1953

PART III: Reproduction Module

| MODULE 33 | Reproduction | 2011 |

PART IV: Nursing Domain

MODULE 34	Assessment	2269
MODULE 35	Caring Interventions	2301
MODULE 36	Clinical Decision Making	2315
MODULE 37	Collaboration	2375
MODULE 38	Communication	2397
MODULE 39	Managing Care	2455
MODULE 40	Professional Behaviors	2479
MODULE 41	Teaching and Learning	2499

PART V: Healthcare Domain

MODULE 42	Accountability	2535
MODULE 43	Advocacy	2555
MODULE 44	Ethics	2563
MODULE 45	Evidence-Based Practice	2583
MODULE 46	Healthcare Systems	2595
MODULE 47	Health Policy	2619
MODULE 48	Informatics	2631
MODULE 49	Legal Issues	2653
MODULE 50	Quality Improvement	2681
MODULE 51	Safety	2695

Appendix A: NANDA-Approved Nursing Diagnoses 2012–2014

Glossary

Combined Index, Volumes 1 and 2

Available online at nursing.pearsonhighered.com and within the interactive e-text:

Appendix B: Diagnostic Values and Laboratory Tests

D0579070

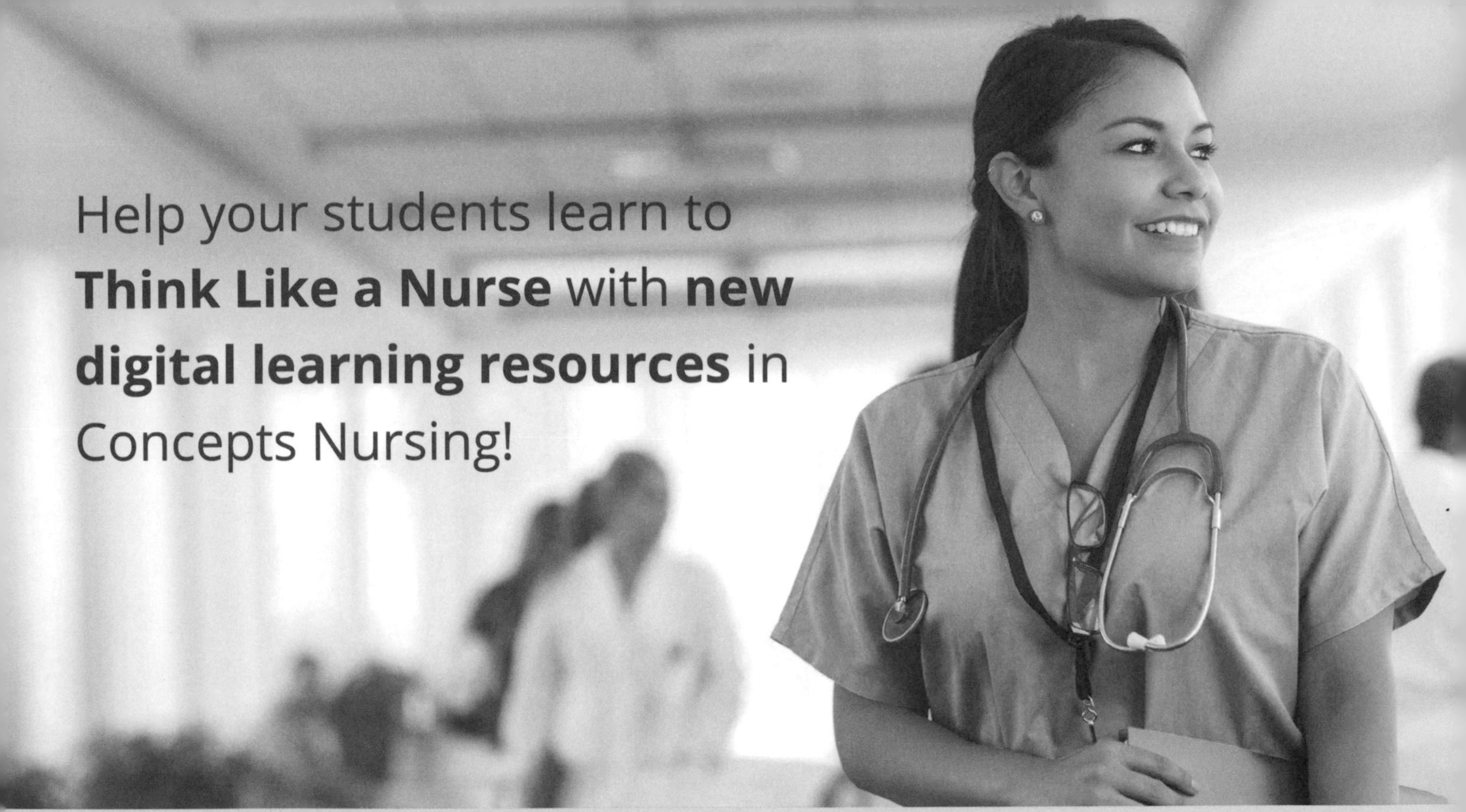

Help your students learn to **Think Like a Nurse** with **new digital learning resources** in Concepts Nursing!

MyNursingLab®

MyNursingLab's personalized learning path helps students master and retain course information more quickly so they can focus on higher-level decision-making skills.

NEW! Clinical Decision-Making Cases in MyNursingLab provide opportunities for students to practice analyzing information and make important decisions at key moments in patient care scenarios.

Learn more at mynursinglab.com

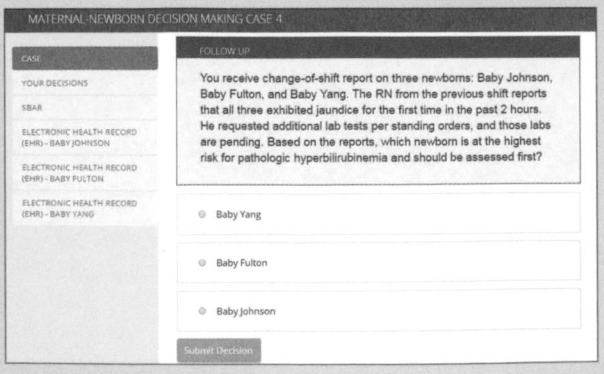

NEW! Concepts Connection in Nursing

The Concepts Connections in Nursing app helps students make important connections between concepts in nursing and exemplars or alterations. Understanding these key concepts and the connections between them enables students to focus on the critical thinking and decision-making skills necessary for successful clinical practice. Now available on both the Apple App Store and Google Play.

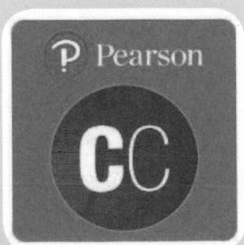

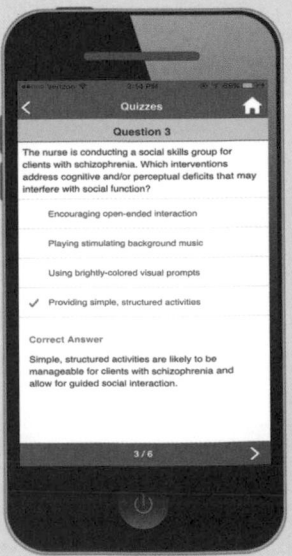

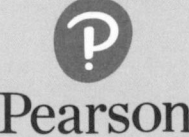

Pearson

VOLUME 2

NURSING
A Concept-Based Approach to Learning
SECOND EDITION

PEARSON

Boston   Columbus   Indianapolis   New York   San Francisco   Hoboken
Amsterdam   Cape Town   Dubai   London   Madrid   Milan   Munich   Paris   Montreal   Toronto
Delhi   Mexico City   Sao Paulo   Sydney   Hong Kong   Seoul   Singapore   Taipei   Tokyo

Publisher: Julie Alexander
Executive Editor: Kelly Trakalo
Development Editors: Laura S. Horowitz and Adelaide R. McCulloch
Program Manager: Melissa Bashe
Editorial Assistants: Erin Rafferty and Kevin Wilson
Director of Marketing: David Gesell
Senior Marketing Manager: Phoenix Harvey
Marketing Specialist: Michael Sirinides
Director, Product Management Services: Etain O'Dea
Project Management Team Lead: Patrick Walsh
Project Manager: Maria Reyes
Manufacturing Manager: Maura Zaldivar-Garcia
Art Director/Cover and Interior Design: Mary Siener
Cover Art: Aaron Craven/Vetta/Getty Images
Lead Digital Project Manager: Karen Bretz
Full-Service Project Management: Kelly Ricci
Composition: Aptara®, Inc.
Printer/Binder: CSCCommunications/Kendallville
Cover Printer: Lehigh-Phoenix Color/Hagerstown

Many of the designations by manufacturers and sellers to distinguish their products are claimed as trademarks. Where those designations appear in this book, and the publisher was aware of a trademark claim, the designations have been printed in initial caps or all caps.

A note about nursing diagnoses: Nursing diagnoses in this text are taken from *Nursing Diagnoses—Definitions and Classification 2012–2014*. Copyright © 2012, 1994–2012 by NANDA International. Used by arrangement with John Wiley & Sons Limited. In order to make safe and effective judgments using NANDA-I nursing diagnoses it is essential that nurses refer to the definitions and defining characteristics of the diagnoses listed in this work.

Library of Congress Cataloging-in-Publication Data
Nursing (Pearson : 2015)
  Nursing : a concept-based approach to learning.—Second edition.
    p. ; cm.
  Includes bibliographical references and index.
  ISBN-13: 978-0-13-517153-0 (v. 2)
  ISBN-10: 0-13-517153-9 (v. 2)
  I. Title.
  [DNLM: 1. Nursing.   2. Nursing Care. WY 100.1]
  RT40
  610.73—dc23
                2013045274

1 17

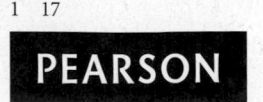

ISBN 13: 978-0-13-517153-0

ISBN 10:   0-13-517153-9

ACKNOWLEDGMENTS

We would like to extend our heartfelt thanks to more than 80 of our colleagues from schools of nursing across the country who have given their time generously during the past few years to help us create this concept-based learning package. The talented faculty on our Concepts Advisory Panel, and all of the Contributors and Reviewers helped us to develop this second version through contributions and answering a myriad of questions right up to the time of publication. *Nursing: A Concept-Based Approach to Learning*, Second Edition, has benefited immeasurably from their efforts, insights, suggestions, objections, encouragement, and inspiration, as well as from their vast experience as faculty and practicing nurses.

We would like to thank the editorial team, especially Julie Alexander, Publisher, for her continual support throughout this process; Kim Norbuta, the editor that started us off and Kelly Trakalo, the Executive Editor who came in at the end. Kevin Wilson and Erin Rafferty, editorial assistants, for helping to keep all the balls in the air; Melissa Bashe for keeping us organized and most of all Laura Horowitz and Addy McCulloch, development editors, for their dedication and attention to detail that promoted an excellent outcome once again. Many thanks to the Pearson production team of Maria Reyes and Patrick Walsh, and to Kelly Ricci and the Aptara team for producing this book with precision. Finally, a special thanks to the design team, led by Mary Siener, for the thoughtful and integrated design of our concepts solution.

CONCEPTS ADVISORY PANEL

Janet B. Arthurs, EdD, MSN, RNC
Gaston College
Dallas, NC

Colleen Coletta Burgess, EdD, PMHCNS-BC, MSN, RN
Cabarrus College
Concord, NC

Michelle Byrne, PhD, RN, CNOR, CNE
University of West Georgia
Carrollton, GA

Barbara Callahan, MEd, RN, NCC, CHSE
Lenoir Community College
Kinston, NC

Karen Carlson, PhD, RN
University of New Mexico
Albuquerque, NM

Linda K. Daley, PhD, RN, ANEF
The Ohio State University
Columbus, OH

Kathy Magorian, EdD, RN
University of South Dakota
Vermillion, SD

Pamela Phillips, PhD, RN
Blue Ridge Community College
Flat Rock, NC

T. Kim Rodehorst, PhD, RN
University of Nebraska Medical Center
Scottsbluff, NE

Susan Wilhelm, PhD, RNC
University of Nebraska Medical Center
Omaha, NE

CONTRIBUTORS

Barbara Hope Arnoldussen, MBA, BSN, RN, CPHQ
International Technological University
San Jose, CA

Cynthia D. Booher, MSN, CNRN, RN
Guilford Technical Community College
Jamestown, NC

Colleen Coletta Burgess, EdD, PMHCNS-BC, MSN, RN
Cabarrus College
Concord, NC

Michelle Byrne, PhD, CNOR, CNE, RN
University of West Georgia
Carrollton, GA

Barbara Callahan, MEd, RN, NCC, CHSE
Lenoir Community College
Kinston, NC

Patricia Caudle, DNSc, CNM, FNP-BC
Frontier Nursing University
Hyden, KY

Amy Mitchell Corbitt, MSN, RN
ECPI University
Newport News, VA

Deborah Duchesneau, FNP-BC, MSN, BSN, BACS
Carolina East Internal Medicine
Pollocksville, NC

Brigette Dupuch-Knudsen, MS, RN, CNOR
University of North Georgia
Northside Hospital
Atlanta, GA

Carolyn Gersch, MSN, CNE, RN
Kettering College
Kettering, OH

Camella G. Marcom, MSN, RN
Vance-Granville Community College
Henderson, NC

Jeanne Marie Papa, MBE, MSN, ACNP-BC, CCRN
Neumann University
Aston, PA

Cynthia A. Parkman, PhD, RN
National University
San Diego, CA

Carole Rae-Reed, PhD, RN, APN, PMHCNS
The Richard Stockton College of New Jersey
Galloway, NJ

Amanda C. Reichert, MS(NEd), MS, RN
Georgia Gwinnett College
Lawrenceville, GA

T. Kim Rodehorst, PhD, RN
University of Nebraska Medical Center
Scottsbluff, NE

Barbara Sittner, PhD, RN, APRN-CNS
Bryan College of Health Sciences
Lincoln, NE

Margaret M. Slusser, PhD, RN
The Richard Stockton College of New Jersey
Galloway, NJ

Sharon Souter, PhD, CNE, RN
University of Mary Hardin-Baylor
Belton, TX

Sharon L. Stewart, RN, CPHQ
Baltimore, MD

Susan Wilhelm, PhD, RNC
University of Nebraska Medical Center
Omaha, NE

REVIEWERS

The following reviewers gave valuable feedback on drafts of the modules:

Linda Alfieri, MSN, CNE
Cayuga Community College
Auburn, NY

Jacqueline Bencker, BSN, RN, CNOR
St. Mary Medical Center
Langhorne, PA

Lorraine Buchanan, MSN, RN
University of Kansas School of Nursing
Kansas City, KS

Cara Busenhart, MSN, APRN, CNM
University of Kansas School of Nursing
Kansas City, KS

Michelle Byrne, PhD, RN, CNE, CNOR
University of North Georgia
Dahlonega, GA

Karen Carlson, PhD, RN
University of New Mexico
Albuquerque, NM

Rachel Choudhury, MSN, RN, CNE
Chamberlain College of Nursing
Columbus, Ohio

Marilyn Cox, MSN, RN, CDE, BC-ADM
Children's Medical Center Dallas
Dallas, TX

Ann Crawford, PhD, MSN, BSN
University of Mary Hardin-Baylor
Belton, TX

Judy Flowers, MSN, MEd, RN
Catawba Valley Community College
Hickory, NC

J. Kaye Fuson, BSN, RN
Davidson County Community College
Mocksville, NC

Lance Hadley, DNP, MSN, BSN
West Texas A&M University
Canyon, TX

Robin Harris, MSN, MSEd, BSN, RN
College of The Albemarle
Elizabeth City, NC

Fairuz Lutz, MSN, BSN, RN
Wesley College
Dover, DE

Kathy Magorian, EdD, MSN, RN
University of South Dakota
Vermillion, SD

Steven A. Marinos, MSN, RN
Johnston Community College
Smithfield, NC

Sue Ellen Miller, MSN, RN, CNE
Forsyth Technical Community College
Winston-Salem, NC

Geri Neuberger, EdD, APRN-CNS
University of Kansas School of Nursing
Kansas City, KS

Martha Olson, MSN, RN
University of Nebraska Medical Center
Omaha, NE

Karen Panunto, EdD, MSN, RN, APN
Wesley College
Dover, DE

Pamela Phillips, PhD, RN
Blue Ridge Community College
Flat Rock, NC

Theresa Pietsch, PhD, RN, CRRN, CNE
Neumann University
Aston, PA

Sharon Rappold, MSN, RN, BC
Wharton County Junior College
Wharton, TX

Jean Robley, MSN, PHN, BSN
Alexandria Technical and Community College
Alexandria, MN

Judith Rolph, MSN, RN
MassBay Community College
Framingham, MA

T. Kim Rodehorst, PhD, RN
University of Nebraska Medical Center
Scottsbluff, NE

Dana K. Samson, MSN, RN
University of Nebraska Medical Center
Omaha, NE

Patricia Sharpnack, DNP, RN, CNE, NEA-BC
Ursuline College
Pepper Pike, OH

Debbie Stevenson, MSN, BSN, RN
Lincoln Technical Institute
Fern Park, FL

Ferquita Stokes, MSN-Ed, BSN, RN
Herzing University
Orlando, FL

Karen Tarnow, PhD, RN
University of Kansas School of Nursing
Kansas City, KS

Gerry Walker, DHEd, MSN, BSN, RN
Park University
Parkville, MO

Arthur West, MPA, MSN, BSN, CCRN, ADN
Southeastern Community College
Whiteville, NC

Jackie Williams, PhD, MEd, MSN, BSN
Georgia Perimeter College
Clarkston, GA

FIRST EDITION ADVISORS AND CONTRIBUTORS

Charlotte Blackwell, MSEd, BSN, RN
Wake Technical Community College

Carol Hardin Boles, MSN, RN
Surry Community College

Catherine Borysewicz, MSN, RN, BC, CNE
Carolinas College of Health Sciences

Colleen Burgess, EdD, MSN, RN, APRN, BC
Catawba Valley Community College

Barbara Callahan, MEd, BSN, RN, NCC
Lenoir Community College

Sheryl Cornelius, MSN, RN
Mitchell Community College

Rachelle Denney, MSNC, RN, BSN
Fayetteville Technical Community College

Cathy L. H. Franklin-Griffin, PhD, RN
Surry Community College

Delia Frederick, MSNEd, RN
Southwestern Community College

Martha Freeze, MSN, ACNSBC
Rowan Cabarrus Community College

Robin Harris, MSED, BSN, RN
College of the Albemarle

Barbara Knopp, MSN, RN
North Carolina Board of Nursing

June Martin, MSN, RN
Forsyth Technical Community College

Debra S. McKinney, MSN, MBA/HCM, RN
University of Phoenix Online

Katherine K. Phillips, MSN, RN
Guilford Technical Community College

Camille Reese, EdD, MSN, RNC
Mitchell Community College

Linda Smith, MSN, RN
Johnston Community College

Marilyn Springle, MSN, RN, FNPBC
Carteret Community College

Renee Taylor, BSN, RN
Robeson Community College

Kathy Williford, MSN, RN
NEWH Nursing Consortium

Linda Wright, MSN, RN
Western Piedmont Community College

PREFACE

Nursing: A Concept-Based Approach to Learning, Second Edition, represents the cutting edge in nursing education. This uniquely integrated solution provides students with a consistent design of content and assessment that specifically supports a concept-based curriculum. Available as a fully integrated digital experience or in print format, this solution meets the needs of today's nursing student.

The goal of this program is to help students learn the essential knowledge they will need for client care.

▶ CONTENT ORGANIZATION

Fifty-one concepts have been chosen in three domains. Some nursing programs will use this program in its entirety, others will choose some concepts and supplement with additional materials. To learn more about how to develop a concept-based program, see the *Faculty Guide to Concept-Based Learning* and *Student Guide to Concept-Based Learning* at nursing.pearsonhighered.com.

The content is organized as shown in the following chart:

DOMAIN	COMPETENCIES
Individual Parts I, II, and III of text	Developmentally appropriate client-centered care, collaboration, cultural competence, evidence-based practice, assessment, and communication
Nursing Part IV of text	Professional behavior, assessment, communication, clinical decision making, and other National League for Nursing Accreditation Committee (NLNAC) competencies for graduates of associate degree programs
Healthcare Part V of text	Quality improvement, evidence-based practice, informatics, and other elements essential to nursing within the healthcare system

Within each domain, the curriculum presents information that is critical to the practice of nursing. Each domain is divided into modules that include a concept and its essential exemplars. Within the individual domain, the concept model delineates human systems of functioning, first describing the normal process of each system and then presenting common alterations from normal that are related to the system. These alterations are referred to as *exemplars*. For example, in the module on Oxygenation, the normal process of ventilation and gas exchange is presented in The Concept of Oxygenation, followed by five frequently seen alterations, or exemplars: Acute Respiratory Distress Syndrome, Asthma, Chronic Obstructive Pulmonary Disease, Respiratory Syncytial Virus/Bronchiolitis, and Sudden Infant Death Syndrome. The information is provided in such a way that students will be able to apply information learned to other alterations in oxygenation in addition to those presented in the curriculum.

Further, the individual domain presents each concept with the underlying premise that no one concept functions without input from various other concepts. As such, this model provides opportunities for students to link concepts and their interactions together. For example, how does the concept of oxygenation link to the concept of perfusion? To the concept of cognition?

The curriculum addresses traditional therapies and treatments as well as newer complementary and alternative therapies. It provides information about diagnostic testing, assessment interviews, case studies and discussion questions, as well as critical thinking questions to promote linking of concepts, which helps students understand that all of the concepts are integrated.

▶ NEW TO THE SECOND EDITION

The Second Edition reflects feedback from users of the First Edition and extensive discussion and work by the Concepts Advisory Panel. It has been significantly updated and rewritten and reflects a consistent approach to learning.

Three New Concepts!
- *Digestion*
- *Nutrition*
- *Perioperative Care*

13 New Exemplars!
- Gastroesophageal Reflux Disease, Hepatitis, Malabsorption Disorders, Pancreatitis, and Pyloric Stenosis (within the Digestion Module)
- Diabetes in Children (within the Metabolism Module)
- Adjustment Disorder with Depressed Mood (within the Mood and Affect Module)
- Nursing Plan of Care and Prioritizing Care (supporting the Clinical Decision Making Module)
- Groups and Group Communication (within the Communication Module)
- Just Culture (within the Legal Module)
- Safety Considerations Across the Life Span and Workplace Safety (within the Safety Module)

- *New! Concepts Related To . . .* tables appear in each module to clearly show how concepts can be integrated.
- *New! Case Studies.* Each module contains one to four multipart longitudinal case studies.

■ *New! Community-Based Care feature.* These special boxes show how nurses can help clients manage their care in the community.

▶ ADDITIONAL RESOURCES

eText. For a fully integrated experience, the eText version of the content contains interactive self-assessments and links to additional content and multimedia. The highlighting, notes, search tools, and more provide a completely interactive experience. Look for these icons:

 MiniModules and Charts. These online features provide additional content on enrichment topics such as anatomy and physiology, additional Nursing Care Plans, and extra case studies to supplement student learning.

 Videos, animations and narrated lectures are placed throughout the content to help students understand key topics and concepts.

 NCLEX® Review. Learners can access the practice NCLEX® style questions that are an extension of their textbook experience.

 Relate and Reflect. Critical thinking questions link together concepts and exemplars. Case Studies provide practical nursing situations with critical thinking questions.

MyNursingLab. Specifically created to support a concept-based approach, this assessment tool provides a guided learning path proven to help students synthesize vast amounts of information. Each concept is broken into a series of short lessons and each lesson contains a pretest, personalized study tools, and a post-test. Robust reporting tools help students and instructors gauge progress.

Clinical Nursing Skills: A Concept-Based Approach. This companion skills book has been specifically designed to meet the needs of a concept-based curriculum.

The Neighborhood 2.0. Created by Dr. Jean Giddens in response to a need within a concept-based curriculum, The Neighborhood 2.0 is a virtual community of characters that engages students and provides a rich foundation of information that supports concepts and exemplars.

Instructor Resources

Annotated Instructor's eText. The instructors version of the eText contains detailed outlines and suggestions for classroom and clinical activities. Use the whiteboard feature to bring content into your classroom! Icons visible only to the instructor include:

 Learning Outcomes. This icon provides a link to where in the concept the learning outcome is met.

 Lecture Outlines. This icon provides a link to an outline that educators can use to frame their lectures.

 Activities. Individual, group and clinical activity suggestions are provided to enhance learning.

 The Neighborhood 2.0. The Neighborhood is an online virtual community that helps students bridge the gap between lecture and clinical experience for a deeper understanding of the entire context of patient care. Students get to know the unfolding nature of health and illness of all these characters with text, photos, video clips and medical records. Cases from The Neighborhood are presented in various concepts and exemplars.

Class Preparation Resources. This resource provides instructors with a searchable database of activities, lecture PowerPoints, Clicker Questions, Images, and more!

ClassMaster. This online wizard maps course topics, concepts, and exemplars, to corresponding activities, resources, and reading assignments.

Test Bank. The test bank consists of NCLEX®-style questions with complete rationales for correct and incorrect answers. Available in a variety of formats.

FEATURES

▶ CONSISTENT STRUCTURE!

Each module is consistently formatted and color-coded to promote learning.

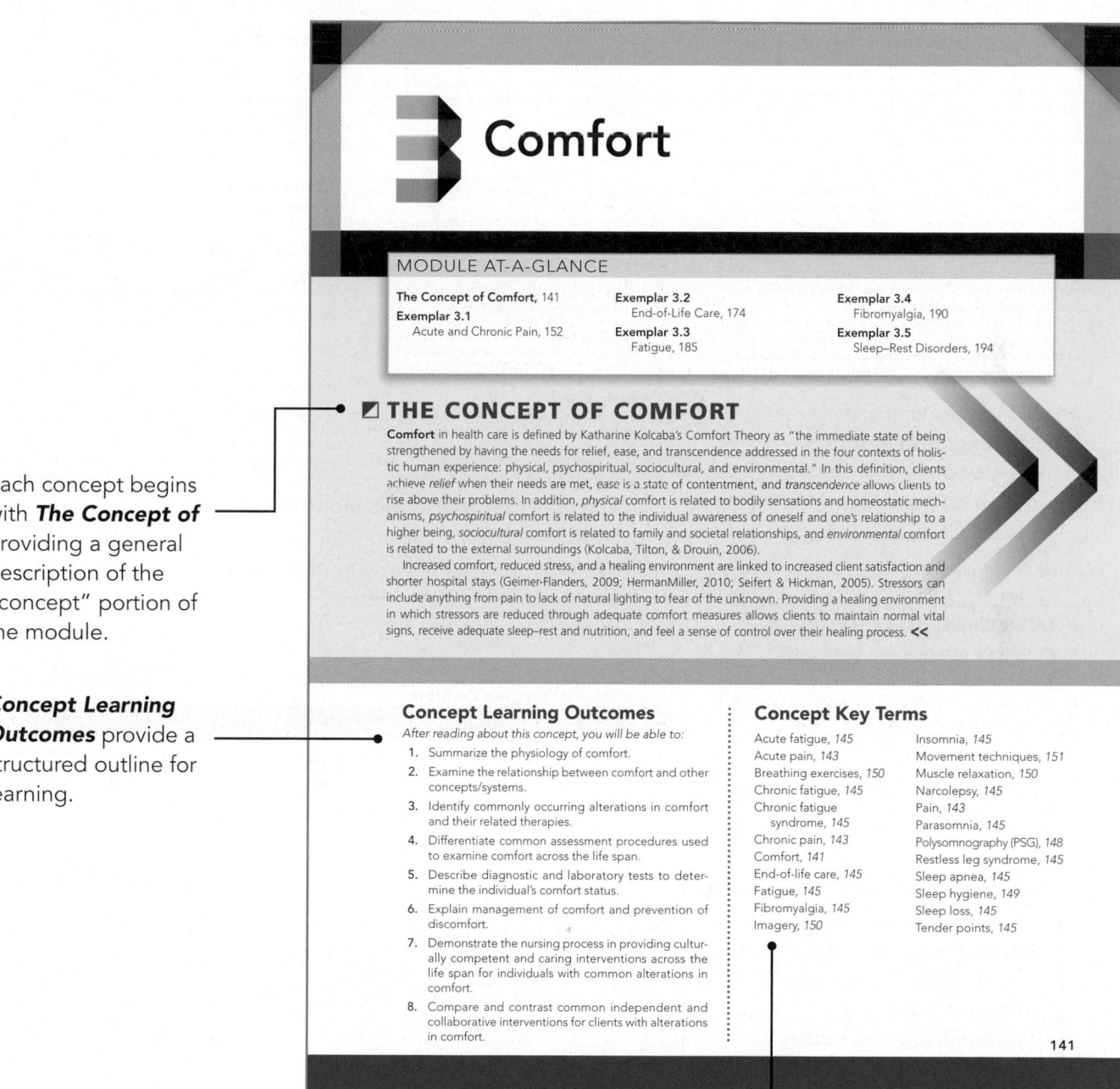

3 Comfort

MODULE AT-A-GLANCE

The Concept of Comfort, 141

Exemplar 3.1
  Acute and Chronic Pain, 152

Exemplar 3.2
  End-of-Life Care, 174

Exemplar 3.3
  Fatigue, 185

Exemplar 3.4
  Fibromyalgia, 190

Exemplar 3.5
  Sleep–Rest Disorders, 194

◤ THE CONCEPT OF COMFORT

Comfort in health care is defined by Katharine Kolcaba's Comfort Theory as "the immediate state of being strengthened by having the needs for relief, ease, and transcendence addressed in the four contexts of holistic human experience: physical, psychospiritual, sociocultural, and environmental." In this definition, clients achieve *relief* when their needs are met, *ease* is a state of contentment, and *transcendence* allows clients to rise above their problems. In addition, *physical* comfort is related to bodily sensations and homeostatic mechanisms, *psychospiritual* comfort is related to the individual awareness of oneself and one's relationship to a higher being, *sociocultural* comfort is related to family and societal relationships, and *environmental* comfort is related to the external surroundings (Kolcaba, Tilton, & Drouin, 2006).

Increased comfort, reduced stress, and a healing environment are linked to increased client satisfaction and shorter hospital stays (Geimer-Flanders, 2009; HermanMiller, 2010; Seifert & Hickman, 2005). Stressors can include anything from pain to lack of natural lighting to fear of the unknown. Providing a healing environment in which stressors are reduced through adequate comfort measures allows clients to maintain normal vital signs, receive adequate sleep–rest and nutrition, and feel a sense of control over their healing process. ≪

Concept Learning Outcomes

After reading about this concept, you will be able to:

1. Summarize the physiology of comfort.
2. Examine the relationship between comfort and other concepts/systems.
3. Identify commonly occurring alterations in comfort and their related therapies.
4. Differentiate common assessment procedures used to examine comfort across the life span.
5. Describe diagnostic and laboratory tests to determine the individual's comfort status.
6. Explain management of comfort and prevention of discomfort.
7. Demonstrate the nursing process in providing culturally competent and caring interventions across the life span for individuals with common alterations in comfort.
8. Compare and contrast common independent and collaborative interventions for clients with alterations in comfort.

Concept Key Terms

Acute fatigue, *145*
Acute pain, *143*
Breathing exercises, *150*
Chronic fatigue, *145*
Chronic fatigue
  syndrome, *145*
Chronic pain, *143*
Comfort, *141*
End-of-life care, *145*
Fatigue, *145*
Fibromyalgia, *145*
Imagery, *150*

Insomnia, *145*
Movement techniques, *151*
Muscle relaxation, *150*
Narcolepsy, *145*
Pain, *143*
Parasomnia, *145*
Polysomnography (PSG), *148*
Restless leg syndrome, *145*
Sleep apnea, *145*
Sleep hygiene, *149*
Sleep loss, *145*
Tender points, *145*

141

Each concept begins with **The Concept of** providing a general description of the "concept" portion of the module.

Concept Learning Outcomes provide a structured outline for learning.

Concept Key Terms list provides a study tool for learning new vocabulary specific to the concept. Page numbers are included for easy reference.

Normal Presentation and Alterations to the Concept: Across the Lifespan!

▶ NORMAL PRESENTATION OF COMFORT

Comfort is a relative feeling based on expectations and past experiences. Therefore, a "normal" level of comfort may be different for every client. However, there are some elements of comfort that are common to all individuals.

Physiology Review

An individual experiences comfort when each level of Maslow's hierarchy of needs is fulfilled (Figure 3–1 ●). The most basic physiological needs of oxygen, shelter, food, water, and sleep are met, and the individual feels safe and free from anxiety, fear, and pain. The individual who experiences true comfort senses love and belonging from family and friends. For individuals seeking health care, comfort also includes participating in a healthy nurse–client relationship. In addition, individuals experience comfort in the areas of self-esteem and self-actualization by giving and receiving respect, feeling confident, and accepting reality.

Because comfort is subjective, the nurse should aim to understand what is "comfortable" or "normal" for the client. Some clients have difficulty articulating this or have such a high tolerance for discomfort that it is difficult to determine an appropriate baseline. For example, a woman who has worked for the Peace Corps in Africa for several years may be unperturbed by an extra day's stay in the hospital, but an Olympic athlete might find the extra day of confinement and rest intolerable.

Signs of comfort can sometimes be determined from client assessment for sympathetic nervous system responses such as heart and respiratory rate, blood pressure, and body and skin temperature. However, "normal" vital signs are not always reli-

> Each concept begins with an overview of the **Normal Presentation** including a review of physiology and genetic and lifespan considerations.

▶ ALTERATIONS TO COMFORT

Very few people meet the criteria for comfort stated by Kolcaba. What aspects of discomfort are most commonly encountered by nurses? This chapter focuses on five common sources of discomfort: pain, end-of-life care, fatigue, fibromyalgia, and sleep–rest disorders. Read Concepts Related to Comfort to see how Comfort is interrelated with other concepts.

Alterations and Manifestations

Pain, fatigue, and sleep–rest disorders are basic alterations in comfort caused by disease, illness, or injury; fibromyalgia is a classic example of a disease characterized by these three types of discomfort. Discomfort is also a reality at the end of life, and nurses must provide comfort for clients and families during end-of-life care. These alterations in comfort will be summarized here and explored in depth in the exemplar sections (also see the Alterations and Therapies feature).

> **Alterations** to the concept include prevalence, genetic considerations, and nonmodifiable risk factors.

> **Alterations and Therapies** summarize commonly seen alterations and possible treatments.

Lifespan Considerations Comfort

Infants/Toddlers

- Infants verbalize discomfort by crying. Ask the parents for descriptions of the infant's manifestations of pain, including suspected location and how the pain influences eating, sleeping, and behavior.
- Discomfort in otherwise healthy infants may be related to milk components. Bottle-fed infants may need a specialized formula. For breastfed infants, the mother's diet may need to be modified.
- Infants and toddlers should be comforted by being held, rocking, murmuring soothing words, and rubbing or patting the torso or extremities.
- Many pain medications have no dosing instructions for children under 2 years old. Warn parents to follow physician's orders for all medications given to infants and toddlers.

Children

- Involve the child in describing any discomfort, but also ask the parent(s) or guardian about the child's behaviors related to discomfort.
- Before performing any procedures or tests, explain the procedure to the child to help decrease anxiety. When possible, it may also help to demonstrate the procedure on the parent before performing the procedure on the child.
- Depending on age and personality, children may be comforted by being held, hugging, holding hands, or receiving a treat like a sucker, sticker, or small toy.
- If you must perform a painful procedure such as an injection, engage the parent in the child's care by asking the parent to offer comfort or distraction.

Adolescents

- Adolescents may respond to treatment and comfort better if you interact with them as adults rather than as children.
- Some adolescents may reject any offer of comfort.

Adults

- If diagnosed with a chronic or fatal disease, adults may find comfort in knowledge. Take the time to describe the disease and what to expect for tests, medications, and other interventions, and to answer any questions they have.
- Comfort is a subjective experience, so listen carefully when the client is describing any feelings of discomfort, and care for the client accordingly.

Pregnant Women

- Pregnant women, especially first-time mothers, may be very anxious about their health and the health of their baby. Take time to explain the expected growth and development of the fetus and expected maternal changes. Answer any questions.
- Provide tips about self-care, physical activity, and sleeping positions that will help ease discomfort. Encourage adequate nutrition, hydration, and sleep–rest.

Older Adults

- Older adults are more likely to suffer from chronic conditions such as diabetes, chronic pain, heart disease, cancer, and arthritis. Provide a safe and comfortable environment for regular appointments, and foster a healthy nurse–client relationship to promote comfort.
- Explain procedures and medications at each visit; some older adult clients have memory deficits. Provide written instructions and explanations. Provide assistance with movement as needed, especially for clients with chronic pain or arthritis.

End of Life

- Provide adequate pain relief with pharmacologic agents as ordered.
- Promote psychosocial comfort by offering to arrange a visit from a spiritual leader and/or loved ones.
- Facilitate referrals for grief counseling for the family and other loved ones.
- Honor the client's and family's decisions about end-of-life care.

> **Lifespan Considerations** highlight concept considerations specific to infants, children, adolescents, pregnancy, and older adults.

Alterations and Therapies Comfort

ALTERATION	DESCRIPTION/ DEFINITION	MANIFESTATIONS	INTERVENTIONS AND THERAPIES
Acute pain	Pain of varying severity, location, and etiology that lasts fewer than 6 months.	■ Elevated blood pressure ■ Increased heart rate ■ Nausea and vomiting ■ Sweating ■ Rapid/shallow respirations ■ Anxiety ■ Decreased function in activities of daily living	Pharmacologic pain management: ■ Opioid analgesics ■ Nonsteroidal anti-inflammatory drugs (NSAIDs) ■ Nonopioid analgesics Nonpharmacologic therapy: ■ Massage ■ Diversionary therapies (music, involvement in hobbies, aroma therapy) ■ Application of heat and cold
Chronic pain	Pain of varying severity, location, and etiology that lasts 6 months or more (even if intermittent).	■ Depression ■ Irritability ■ Impaired mobility and/or activity ■ Sleep disturbance	Pharmacologic pain management: ■ Nonopioid analgesics ■ Antidepressants ■ NSAIDs ■ Muscle relaxants ■ Opioid analgesics Nonpharmacologic therapy: ■ Guided imagery ■ Massage ■ Nerve stimulation units ■ Chiropractic interventions ■ Physical therapy ■ Relaxation techniques ■ Positioning
End-of-life care	Care that takes place when death is imminent	■ Loss of muscle tone ■ Slowing of circulation ■ Change in respirations ■ Sensory impairments ■ Impaired metabolic processes	■ Palliative or aggressive care as chosen by client and family ■ Maintenance of comfort ■ Maintenance of hygiene ■ Psychosocial support for client and family
Fatigue	Lack of energy or motivation with or without drowsiness	■ Tiredness ■ Depression ■ Anxiety ■ Irritability ■ Decreased cognition	Pharmacologic therapy: ■ Sleeping aids ■ Stimulants ■ Antidepressants ■ Pain management Nonpharmacologic therapy: ■ Improved sleep hygiene

Concepts Related to Comfort

Promotion of comfort is an integral part of nursing care. The exemplars included in this module explore several common manifestations of discomfort, including pain, fatigue, and sleep–rest disorders. However, alterations in comfort are not limited to these specific manifestations. The concept of comfort is interrelated to numerous other physiological and psychosocial concepts. For example, one of the classic symptoms of inflammation is pain. Therefore, nurses can offer comfort to clients with inflammation by administering pain medications as ordered and providing nonpharmacologic comfort measures such as cold therapy. Clients with pain, especially joint pain, lower back pain, or trauma pain, often experience decreased mobility. Nursing interventions for these clients may include ambulation assistance and hygiene care. Impaired tissue integrity is a common cause of discomfort and can

also lead to more serious complications, such as infection. Comfort measures may include assessing the client for infection, providing hygiene care for the wound, and assisting with repositioning for immobile clients.

Promotion of comfort includes both physical and psychosocial wellness. Individuals suffering grief over a lost loved one or lost personal health may need emotional comfort in the form of therapeutic communication or referrals to support groups. Comfort care is also closely tied to ethical issues for many clients, such as individuals with drug addiction who need opioid treatment for severe pain or the family deciding about withdrawing or withholding of life-sustaining treatments for a client at the end of life. The relationship between comfort and the concepts of inflammation, mobility, tissue integrity, grief and loss, and ethics are summarized in the following table.

CONCEPT	RELATIONSHIP TO COMFORT	NURSING IMPLICATIONS
Inflammation		
■ Assessment interview: Inflammation ■ Independent interventions and therapies	Inflammation → pain.	■ Assess pain in clients with inflammation; provide pharmacologic treatments as ordered. ■ Offer comfort measures such as ice or heat; promote adequate sleep and rest.
Mobility		
■ Mobility assessment ■ Assessment interview: Mobility	↓ mobility is often caused by pain, injury, or disease.	■ Assist with ambulation and activities of daily living; encourage adequate sleep and rest. ■ Offer pharmacologic treatments as ordered.
Tissue Integrity		
■ Integumentary assessment ■ Pressure ulcers	↓ tissue integrity = ↑ risk for pain, inflammation, and infection.	■ Assess for skin breakdown; promote mobility. ■ Assist with repositioning as needed; monitor for signs and symptoms of infection.
Grief and Loss		
■ Assessment interview: Grief and loss	Loss or expected loss of a loved one is emotionally distressing.	■ Use therapeutic communication techniques; encourage expression of emotions; facilitate referrals to counselors and support groups.
Ethics		
	Physicians may be reluctant to prescribe opioids based on race, ethnicity, or history of addiction.	■ Advocate for the provision of adequate pain relief to all clients; provide culturally sensitive care; offer nonpharmacologic comfort measures to all clients.

▶ INTERVENTIONS AND THERAPIES

For the client experiencing alterations in comfort, initial interventions are directed at identifying the source of the discomfort. For clients with physical pain, while pain relief is a priority, masking the pain through analgesic administration can make identifying the underlying cause much more difficult. For this reason, especially until the cause of the client's discomfort is identified, interventions to promote comfort may focus on nonpharmacologic measures. These include simple interventions such as applying heat or cold as

Independent

Promotion of comfort includes teaching clients about lifestyle changes that can help decrease their symptoms of pain, depression, or fatigue. Three basic independent categories of teaching include sleep hygiene, psychosocial well-being, and relaxation therapy.

Collaborative

For the client experiencing discomfort, collaborative therapies include both pharmacologic and nonpharmacologic interventions. Pharmacologic interventions involve the administration of medications, examples of which are listed in the Medications feature. Nonpharmacologic therapies may be either alternative therapies, which are used instead of pharmacologic therapies, or complementary therapies, which are used in addition to pharmacologic therapies. Common nonpharmacologic therapies, such as acupuncture and herbal supplements, are discussed in the specific exemplars.

Medications Sleep

CLASSIFICATION AND DRUG EXAMPLES	MECHANISM OF ACTION	NURSING CONSIDERATIONS
Hypnotics/Sedatives ■ Benzodiazepines ■ Nonbenzodiazepines *Drug examples:* Temazepam, zolpidem, eszopiclone	Produces CNS depression by acting on the limbic, thalamic, and hypothalamic regions of the CNS (benzodiazepines). Interacts with GABA receptor (nonbenzodiazepines).	Monitor older adults for paradoxical reaction. Do not use in depressed, suicidal, or pregnant clients. Tolerance and addiction may result from benzodiazepine use; slowly taper dosage when discontinuing therapy; drugs should not be used for more than 4–6 months.

Complementary and Alternative Therapy Herbal Supplements for Sleep Disorders

Herbal supplements may be an alternative for individuals who do not tolerate pharmacologic therapy because of side effects. Two herbs that are traditionally used to aid sleep are valerian (*Valeriana officinalis*) and chamomile (*Matricaria recutita*). Valerian usually has to be taken for 2 or 3 weeks before it produces an effect, and clinical trials have not proven its effectiveness. Possible side effects of valerian include indigestion, headache, palpitations, and dizziness. Chamomile, often taken as a tea, has a soothing effect that may induce sleep and decrease restlessness, although this effect has not been proven in clinical studies. It is safe for both adults and

children except individuals who are allergic to ragweed or daisies.

Melatonin is a sleep hormone produced by the pineal gland. Synthetic melatonin is sold in many pharmacies and health food stores and may be taken to regulate sleep patterns. It is often helpful for sleep disturbances related to shift work or jet lag. It has been proven effective in treating sleep disorders in children with autism (Rossignol & Frye, 2011) and children with ADHD (Hoebert et al., 2009). It may also be helpful for older adults with insomnia when combined with magnesium and zinc supplements (Rondanelli et al., 2011).

New! Concepts Related to feature helps you understand how concepts are integrated, how a client with an alteration in one concept will likely have alterations in other concepts as well.

Interventions and Therapies sections divide therapies into *Independent* (those nurses can perform on their own) and *Collaborative* (those done with primary care providers or other members of the healthcare team)

Medication boxes provide specific drug information and nursing considerations.

Complementary and Alternative Therapy boxes provide additional information on herbal and other nonpharmacologic therapies.

Clinical Reasoning, Client-Focused Nursing Care, and Evidence-Based Practice

New! Three to Four Case Studies in each module in Parts IV and V, the Nursing and Healthcare Domains, apply the content to the clinical setting. Each case study includes a set of Critical Thinking Questions.

CASE STUDY \\ A

Caroline Nava is a 28-year-old nursing student enrolled in her final clinical rotation and due to graduate in 2 months. She is working on a surgical unit managing care for five individuals. Having completed her charting, she leaves the nursing unit 2 hours late. She is exhausted from a particularly busy clinical day and returns home. Just as she sits down to enjoy a little relaxation time, she remembers that she failed to obtain information from the chart of a new postoperative client. Earlier today, her instructor asked Caroline to report back to her about this individual's laboratory results by the end of the day. The client returned to the unit late from postanesthesia care, as Caroline was ready to leave.

Caroline begins to panic and is uncertain about what she is going to do. Suddenly, she remembers that her friend Joan McIntyre, another student, is in clinical on the same unit until late that evening. Caroline calls Joan and asks her for a favor. She explains to Joan that she is in a bind and has to call her nursing instructor with the information as soon as possible. Caroline asks Joan to take a picture with her cell phone of the laboratory results in the client's chart and to send her the picture. Joan is glad to be able to help her friend and successfully sends the information to Caroline. Caroline is able to contact her instructor with the necessary information about her client.

Critical Thinking Questions

1. Do you believe Caroline handled the situation ethically? Support your answer.
2. If you were Joan, what would you have done in this situation?

CASE STUDY \\ B

Mary Reynolds, who is a nurse of the baby-boomer generation, disagrees with Ashley Maloney, a new graduate, about how Ms. Maloney handled a situation with a client's family. You overhear Ms. Reynolds telling a friend of hers that she hopes that Ms. Maloney never takes care of her or her family. You are on break, and Ms. Reynolds repeats to you her story about Ms. Maloney. She informs you that Ms. Maloney "ignored the family" sitting at the bedside and that the family complained to her. Ms. Reynolds apologized for Ms. Maloney and told the family, "She is a problem. Thanks for telling me. I will take care of it for you." The family rewards Ms. Reynolds by writing a supportive note to the nurse manager about her and also detailing their perception of how Ms. Maloney dealt with their family.

Critical Thinking Questions

1. On the basis of your knowledge of formation of professional behavior and bullying, how might you respond to Ms. Reynolds?
2. Using what you have learned about communication, frame a respectful confrontation of Ms. Reynolds.
3. If you were the nurse manager, how would you handle this situation while applying a provision of the ANA Code of Ethics?

REFLECT Case Study

Cheryl Goodwin is a nurse executive who is widely respected for her rapport with nurse educators. She is the dean of a nursing college and is a doctoral-prepared nurse who maintains a small private practice. She is active in state organizations and willing to help both faculty and students. A hospital administrator calls Ms. Goodwin in for a private meeting. In the course of the meeting, Ms. Goodwin is told that a faculty member in the nursing college has committed an act of abuse and neglect toward a client in the hospital. The Chief Nurse Executive (CNE) of the hospital, who is also at the meeting, informs Ms. Goodwin that the faculty member is no longer permitted to practice at that hospital.

Upon questioning the faculty member involved, Ms. Goodwin discovers that the individual did in fact commit the offenses willfully as reported by the CNE. Ms. Goodwin informs this faculty member that his actions created dire consequences for the client involved and that his position at the college is terminated. He had been on probation for bullying and maltreatment of students before this incident.

The college administration permits the nursing faculty member to resign his position. He begins a campaign to attack the dean, Ms. Goodwin. This nurse accuses her of making a number of false accusations. Friends rally around the dismissed employee, as he has taught at the college for a number of years. He has been known for covering for and doing favors for other faculty members for extra cash, such as picking up an extra clinical day, and for granting favors to the faculty members who reported to him. As a senior faculty member, he also coordinated clinical rotations and scheduling.

Ms. Goodwin is not at liberty to discuss the incident that led to this faculty member's resignation. The other faculty members are not aware of the consequences suffered by the client and family. The hospital has requested that the situation remain confidential as the family has not been notified of the abuse. Faculty members who have known Ms. Goodwin for many years begin questioning her motives and labeling her as "sick." They talk behind her back and do not invite her to nursing functions that she has always attended. They bully any faculty member who associates with her. Ms. Goodwin acquires another position and leaves a position that she loved.

1. How would you describe the behaviors and actions of the faculty members in the scenario?
2. What recourse does Ms. Goodwin have?
3. Why do you suppose the faculty members who had a prior satisfactory relationship with Ms. Goodwin did not support her? Do you believe they did the right thing? How and why might they have handled the situation differently?

▶ PREVENTION

Prevention of discomfort begins with the client. Personal preferences, lifestyle habits, and culture are all factors in the development of chronic diseases and other contributors to discomfort, and only the client can change behaviors that increase the risk of discomfort. However, nurses provide essential client education that can encourage clients to change their behaviors to decrease the risk of developing a chronic disease or experiencing an acute illness or injury.

Lifestyle habits that predispose individuals to chronic health alterations, such as poor nutrition, smoking, excessive alcohol consumption, and poor sleep hygiene, all increase an individual's risk for experiencing discomfort. Poor nutrition can include both overeating and undernutrition. Eating a healthy diet in combination with good sleep hygiene can help prevent the development of many chronic diseases that lead to symptoms of discomfort.

Smoking, alcohol consumption, and illicit drug use can also lead to alterations in comfort. Because nicotine, alcohol, and illicit drugs are addictive, quitting drug use is associated with withdrawal symptoms. Emotional withdrawal symptoms include anxiety, irritability, insomnia, and depression. Physical withdrawal symptoms include sweating, palpitations, nausea, and difficulty breathing.

Other lifestyle habits that may lead to discomfort are working at a job that requires heavy lifting, long hours, or repetitive movement, which increases the risk of injury and fatigue. Participation in physical activities such as team sports or extreme sports also increases susceptibility to injury and consequent discomfort.

Sections on *Prevention* and *Assessment* cover modifiable risk factors, screenings, nursing assessments, and diagnostic tests.

▶ ASSESSMENT

The nursing assessment should explore not only the client's level of discomfort but also the degree to which discomfort is affecting the client's daily life. Some clients may not even realize the extent to which discomfort is impacting their lifestyle and overall well-being.

Comfort Assessment

ASSESSMENT/METHOD	NORMAL FINDINGS	ABNORMAL FINDINGS	LIFESPAN OR DEVELOPMENTAL CONSIDERATIONS
Interview Client History			
Client description of symptoms. Pain scale. Depression assessment.	The client should report no signs or symptoms of discomfort.	■ Client reports mild to severe pain. ■ Client reports disrupted sleep patterns. ■ Client reports or displays signs of nausea or vomiting. ■ Client reports lack of appetite or ravenous appetite. ■ Client reports lack of motivation, feelings of despair, or feelings of anxiety.	■ Look for nonverbal signs of discomfort such as crying, shielding an injured area, lack of affect, or withdrawal in nonverbal children and mentally impaired clients. ■ Signs of depression and anxiety in children may indicate abuse, and assessment of the child in the absence of the parent(s) may be warranted. ■ Gastrointestinal discomfort can be a physiological response to disease or it can be a side effect of medication. Check client history for current medications and known drug allergies. ■ Depression and anxiety can be primary or secondary conditions. Be sure to assess the depressed or anxious client for symptoms of chronic conditions.
Physical Assessment			
Vital signs. Visual inspection. Polysomnography (PSG) for identification of suspected sleep disorders. Blood and urine analysis.	Client should have normal vital signs, and no obvious external injuries or infections. Results of all clinical tests should be within normal limits.	■ Severe pain may be accompanied by sympathetic nervous system findings such as increased heart rate, sweating, and nausea. ■ PSG indicates abnormal REM/NREM cycles or severe apnea (Mayo Clinic, 2011a). ■ Client appears depressed, nervous, or confused. ■ Abnormal blood and urine analysis may indicate illness or malnutrition.	■ Children may be fearful of physical assessment. To promote com... the dur... ■ Take ical adu asse

Assessment and **Assessment Interview** features summarize normal and abnormal findings and questions to ask the client.

Assessment Interview Discomfort (Pain, Depression, Anxiety, Appetite, Sleep Disorder)

Current Problem
■ When did your discomfort start?
■ How would you describe your discomfort?
■ On a scale of 0 to 10, with 0 meaning no pain and 10 meaning the worst pain you can imagine, how would you rate your current pain intensity?
■ Which activities make the discomfort better or worse?
■ How long have you had this discomfort?
■ How does this discomfort affect your activities of daily living?
■ What do you do to alleviate your discomfort?
■ Are you currently taking any medications to alleviate your discomfort?
■ Does your discomfort affect your sleep pattern or your mood?
■ Does your discomfort affect your appetite?
■ Does eating or drinking make your discomfort better or worse?
■ Do you feel that your discomfort is related to another disease or condition?
■ Do you feel sad frequently?

■ Do you have trouble motivating yourself to participate in daily activities?
■ Have you had thoughts of suicide?
■ Have you had any changes in daily habits that increased your symptoms of discomfort?

Client History
■ Have you had this discomfort in the past?
■ How often does this symptom of discomfort occur?
■ Have you taken medications for this problem in the past?
■ Have you had past experiences that affect the way you view this discomfort?

Lifestyle
■ Do you drink alcohol? If so, how much? Do you feel this contributes to your symptoms?
■ Do you smoke? If so, how much? Do you feel this contributes to your symptoms?
■ Do you exercise? Is your condition related to your participation in physical activity?
■ Describe your average daily food and drink intake. Do you feel that your diet contributes to your symptoms?

Evidence-Based Practice Overcoming Barriers to Adequate Pain Management

Problem

Pain is a major reason that clients seek health care and take medications, and it accounts for a substantial portion of lost work productivity and disability. However, clients in pain are often underdiagnosed and undertreated, especially racial and ethnic minorities, people of lower socioeconomic status, women, children, older adults, military veterans, surgery and cancer clients, and people at the end of life (IOM, 2011).

Evidence

Pain management remains ineffective due to attitudes and educational deficits of healthcare providers and clients and limitations of pharmacologic agents. Attitudes of healthcare providers can be influenced by both medical evidence and clients' psychosocial influences. In particular, providers are more likely to suggest clients are feigning pain in the absence of medical evidence, and they are less likely to take clients' report of pain into account, if psychosocial influences are present (De Ruddere et al., 2013). Methods of pain management also need to be improved. Using multiple pain medications with different mechanisms of action and side effects will improve efficacy in relieving pain and decrease the incidence of adverse reactions compared to single drug therapies (Sinatra, 2010). In addition, compared to no intervention, physical and psychosocial nonpharmacologic interventions for pain can significantly improve clients' pain level (Park & Hughes, 2012).

Implications

Healthcare professionals need to have a better understanding of pain and pain management. The perception of pain involves both physiological and psychosocial aspects, and pain management should include adequate pharmacologic interventions as well as complementary nonpharmacologic methods to reduce physiological pain and increase psycho-

social well-being. Education for healthcare providers should include training programs that offer standardized information about pain, guidelines related to caring for clients in pain, and experience in caring for clients in pain (IOM, 2011). Education should also include information about the proper use of opioids. Opioids, which are the most effective pain medications, are often underprescribed because of prejudices, misconceptions, and fears about their use (Notcutt & Gibbs, 2010). All healthcare providers should be encouraged to keep their knowledge current by participating in continuing education courses, and certification examinations should assess providers' knowledge about pain (IOM, 2011).

Critical Thinking Application

1. Do you have any biases that may hinder your ability to provide adequate pain management for clients? Think about a variety of situations that may present opportunities for bias, including caring for clients of different cultures, clients with drug addiction, young children and older adults, and clients at the end of life.
2. You are caring for a 72-year-old woman with osteoarthritis who is receiving inadequate pain control. How will you act as an advocate to provide better pain management for your client?
3. You are caring for a 19-year-old male who is a known gang member. During a recent altercation, he sustained a stab wound. He is sleeping restlessly and moaning. It is time for his next dose of opioids, but your nurse manager tells you to give him only half the prescribed dose because he is probably a drug addict and you don't want to feed his addiction. What should you do?
4. What are three ways in which you can stay up-to-date on current pain management nursing standards?

Evidence-Based Practice features demonstrate how research informs practice.

Pathophysiology and Etiology sections occur in most exemplars and include risk factors and prevention.

▶ PATHOPHYSIOLOGY AND ETIOLOGY

Pain is triggered by the peripheral nervous system, which lies outside the brain and spinal cord. There are two types of neurons in the peripheral nervous system: sensory and motor neurons. **Nociceptors**, or sensory receptors that respond to pain, send a signal along the sensory neurons to the spinal cord, where the signal is transmitted to the brain for interpretation. The brain then sends a signal back to the site of pain via motor neurons, causing the body to respond to the painful stimuli. This process happens so rapidly that the individual may reflexively withdraw from the painful stimuli even before becoming aware of the pain.

Nociceptors (**Figure 3–3 ●**) are specialized pain receptors that are present on all body tissues, with the exception of the brain. Skin and muscles contain many nociceptors, whereas internal organs have relatively few nociceptors. Categories of pain stimuli include biological, chemical, electrical, mechanical, and thermal (**Table 3–1 ●**). The duration of exposure and magnitude of the stimuli determine the intensity of the pain response.

In addition to being stimulated by external factors, cellular injury can trigger the local release of biochemicals that stimulate nociceptors, including prostaglandins, serotonin, bradykinin, and hydrogen ions. These mediators act on ion channels and G protein–coupled receptors to directly or indirectly initiate a pain impulse (Fein, 2012).

Multisystem Effects of Leukemia

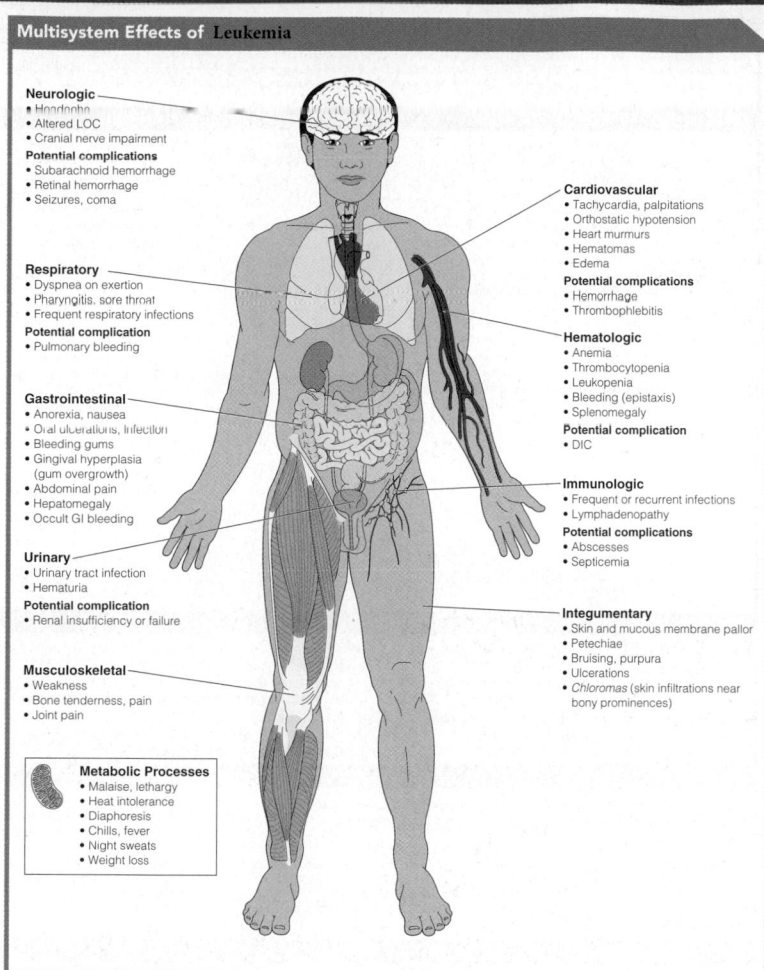

Neurologic
- Headache
- Altered LOC
- Cranial nerve impairment

Potential complications
- Subarachnoid hemorrhage
- Retinal hemorrhage
- Seizures, coma

Respiratory
- Dyspnea on exertion
- Pharyngitis, sore throat
- Frequent respiratory infections

Potential complication
- Pulmonary bleeding

Gastrointestinal
- Anorexia, nausea
- Oral ulcerations, infection
- Bleeding gums
- Gingival hyperplasia (gum overgrowth)
- Abdominal pain
- Hepatomegaly
- Occult GI bleeding

Urinary
- Urinary tract infection
- Hematuria

Potential complication
- Renal insufficiency or failure

Musculoskeletal
- Weakness
- Bone tenderness, pain
- Joint pain

Metabolic Processes
- Malaise, lethargy
- Heat intolerance
- Diaphoresis
- Chills, fever
- Night sweats
- Weight loss

Cardiovascular
- Tachycardia, palpitations
- Orthostatic hypotension
- Heart murmurs
- Hematomas
- Edema

Potential complications
- Hemorrhage
- Thrombophlebitis

Hematologic
- Anemia
- Thrombocytopenia
- Leukopenia
- Bleeding (epistaxis)
- Splenomegaly

Potential complication
- DIC

Immunologic
- Frequent or recurrent infections
- Lymphadenopathy

Potential complications
- Abscesses
- Septicemia

Integumentary
- Skin and mucous membrane pallor
- Petechiae
- Bruising, purpura
- Ulcerations
- *Chloromas* (skin infiltrations near bony prominences)

Multisystem Effects features show how certain alterations affect many body systems.

▶ COLLABORATION

In order to treat pain effectively, nurses collaborate with other healthcare providers. Pharmacologic therapies are nonopioids, NSAIDs, opioids, and coanalgesics. Nonpharmacologic therapies include nerve blocks, spinal cord stimulation, physical therapy, and nutritional supplements, among others. For clients with severe chronic pain, pain clinics offer the expertise needed to discover the right combination of treatments to provide consistent pain relief.

Diagnostic Tests

While laboratory and diagnostic tests may be performed to determine the cause of pain, no laboratory tests are available to directly measure a client's pain level. Instead, pain scales such as a faces pain scale or a numeric pain scale are available to help gauge a client's pain level. Changes in vital signs can also be an indication of pain, although these changes are also seen with other conditions. In addition, the body releases stress hormones in response to pain, which may be detected by blood tests. The most prevalent stress hormones are cortisol and catecholamines.

Surgery

Depending upon the pain's etiology, surgery may be a viable treatment option. For example, surgical repair of a bone fracture may be the first major step toward alleviating severe pain. Recovery from surgery often brings about its own pain, but that pain is usually short-lived compared to the pain that would result from not performing the surgery. In addition, clients may

---

Collaboration sections cover diagnostic tests, pharmacologic, and nonpharmacologic therapies used to address the alteration.

Client Teaching Sleep Hygiene

Fatigue is often the result of inadequate sleep. Nurses should promote and teach good sleep hygiene to all clients with fatigue, sleep–rest disorders, and acute and chronic illnesses that could cause fatigue. Good sleep hygiene includes

- Practicing bedtime rituals that are calming, such as reading, taking a bath, praying, and listening to music.
- Maintaining a restful environment that is free of distractions (e.g., lights and noise), is a comfortable temperature, and has appropriate ventilation.
- Wearing loose-fitting sleepwear.
- Using clean and dry linens.
- Sleeping in a position that aids in muscle relaxation and supports injured areas.

- Scheduling medications to promote sleep (i.e., taking medications that cause alertness in the morning and medications that cause drowsiness at night).
- Avoiding naps during the day.
- Avoiding stimulants such as caffeine and alcohol, especially in the evening; also avoiding heavy meals late in the evening.
- Using the bed for sleep, not other activities such as watching TV.
- Setting consistent times for sleeping and waking, and allowing adequate hours for sleep.
- Exercising in the morning or afternoon rather than the evening.

Client Teaching, Community-Based Care, and *Safety Alerts* broaden the scope of content and provide necessary nursing information.

Community-Based Care Managing Chronic Pain at Home

Clients with chronic pain have to live at home and care for themselves in spite of their pain. Teaching clients and their family how to administer drugs, watch for side effects, and perform nonpharmacologic interventions will help enhance both the clients' and the caregivers' lives. See **Table 3–6 ●** for an overview of medications used for the management of chronic pain. Discussions should include the following topics:

- Describe the drugs to be taken, including dose, frequency, route of administration, side effects, and potential drug, food, or herbal interactions.
- Discuss the importance of taking drugs around the clock rather than prn.

- Dispel any myths or misconceptions about opioid analgesics, including teaching clients that the risk of addiction is very low when pain medications are taken as prescribed.
- Help clients and their family choose appropriate nonpharmacologic interventions to decrease pain, and teach them how to perform the interventions correctly.
- Teach clients and their family the importance of adequate sleep and rest and not overusing the area in pain.
- Provide information about community resources, including support groups, pain clinics, and the American Pain Society.

SAFETY ALERT
Studies have shown that taking short breaks can reduce fatigue and improve performance. Nurses should be vigilant about taking adequate breaks (i.e., 10 minutes every 2 hours, 30 minutes for meals, free of client care responsibilities) to prevent fatigue and errors that may occur because of fatigue (Rogers, 2008).

SAFETY ALERT
All clients on opioids should be monitored for sedation and respiratory depression during the first 24 hours (especially after surgery), during the peak effect, after increasing or decreasing a dose, before additional doses of opioids are given, or when changing opioids or routes of administration. If the respiratory rate falls below 8–10/min, the client should be aroused and naloxone therapy should be considered (Jarzyna et al., 2011).

NURSING PROCESS

Current studies estimate that 43% of American adults—or approximately 100 million Americans—suffer from chronic pain. This presents an economic burden of $560–$635 billion per year in both healthcare costs and lost work productivity. Because of the overwhelming prevalence of pain, nurses are constantly caring for clients in pain.

Uncontrolled pain can lead to comorbidities such as depression, sleep disturbances, and obesity; changes in the nervous system's response to painful stimuli; accelerated disease progression; and increased length of hospital stay. Proper application of the nursing process provides information needed for appropriate care, attainable and measurable client goals for pain management, effective nursing interventions for pain relief, and evaluation of the client's pain level for potential revision of the nursing care plan.

Assessment

Unless a client's physiological needs require priority attention (e.g., severe burns, complex fracture, gunshot wound), all clients should be asked whether they are experiencing pain. Many clients do not voluntarily complain about pain even when pain is present, and persistent pain can contribute to a poor prognosis.

Client Interview

The client interview should begin with eliciting a description of the client's pain. Ask questions about

- *Location.* "Where does it hurt?"
- *Intensity.* "On a scale of 0 to 10, with 0 representing no pain and 10 representing the worst possible pain, how would you rate the intensity of your pain now?"

Nursing Process sections within each exemplar cover assessment, diagnosis, planning, implementation, and evaluation of clients with a particular alteration.

Nursing Care Plans focusing on one client with an alteration are provided with many exemplars.

NURSING CARE PLAN A Client With Chronic Pain

James Grier, age 28, visits the pain clinic with chronic low back pain. He states that he worked in a warehouse three years ago and injured his back while lifting heavy boxes. Although he was treated for the initial injury, he has had chronic back pain since then. During severe flare-ups, he can barely move, and he misses work approximately five days per month because of his back pain.

ASSESSMENT	DIAGNOSIS	PLANNING
■ In an interview with Kenneth Hill, RN, regarding his pain, Mr. Grier rates his pain as a 7 on a scale of 0–10. Flare-ups usually last about a week before his pain is controlled to a 5. Mr. Grier describes his constant pain as a dull ache, but it throbs during flare-ups with sharp piercing sensations during movement. Nothing seems to relieve the pain except lying completely still, although the pain keeps him from falling asleep. He is currently taking ibuprofen as needed, which is usually 400 mg q4h. In the past, he has taken Vicodin, 5–10 mg q4–6h, with moderate success, although it gives him slight nausea and drowsiness. ■ Upon observation, Mr. Hill notes that Mr. Grier has no obvious external sources of pain, but he does have beads of sweat on his forehead. Mr. Hill also notices that Mr. Grier grimaces and holds his breath during movement, and his movements are very slow. A physical assessment indicates a pulse of 92bpm, respiratory rate of 20/min with shallow breaths, blood pressure of 130/84 mmHg, and temperature of 100.8°F.	● *Chronic Pain* related to lower back pain as evidenced by behavioral and sympathetic reactions and the client's report. ● *Impaired Physical Mobility* related to severe lower back pain as evidenced by slow movements and grimacing during movement. ● *Disturbed Sleep Pattern* related to lower back pain as evidenced by client's report. ● *Readiness for Enhanced Knowledge* about pain management. ● *Fear* about potential job loss. (NANDA-I © 2012)	■ After 3 days on the pain medication, the client will report a decrease in pain intensity from a 7 to a 3 or 4 on the numerical scale. ■ The client will report increased physical mobility with no increase in pain intensity over baseline during movement. ■ The client will demonstrate an understanding of good sleep hygiene and will report receiving adequate sleep. ■ The client will demonstrate knowledge about nonpharmacologic methods of pain relief. ■ The client will choose three methods of nonpharmacologic pain relief to implement. ■ The client will report decreased pain as a result of nonpharmacologic therapies. ■ The client will report a decrease in lost workdays as a result of lower back pain.

IMPLEMENTATION

- Consult with a physician about opioid and nonopioid analgesic therapies for Mr. Grier.
- Teach Mr. Grier the importance of taking pain medications around the clock.
- Teach Mr. Grier about nonpharmacologic interventions, including heat, distractions, acupuncture, massage, and mild exercise.
- Encourage Mr. Grier to talk about his pain, and validate his pain experience.
- Provide Mr. Grier with contact information for the pain clinic and encourage him to call the clinic if his prescribed therapies are ineffective.
- Encourage Mr. Grier to set regular follow up appointments to help manage his pain effectively over time.

EVALUATION

Four days after Mr. Grier's appointment, Mr. Hill calls Mr. Grier to assess his pain. Mr. Grier reports that he has been taking his pain medications as prescribed. He is applying heat to his back for 30 minutes three times a day, and he is performing strengthening exercises for his back. When the pain is most severe, he listens to music to help distract him from the pain. Mr. Grier reports that with this new therapy, his pain is now a 4 on a scale of 0–10.

One month after his appointment, Mr. Grier returns to the pain clinic for a follow up appointment. He reports that his pain has been a 2 or 3 for the past week, and he has missed only one day of work in the past month. He continues to take the nonopioid analgesics as instructed and performs strengthening exercises three times a week. His boss has noticed an increase in his work productivity. To maintain pain control without opioids, Mr. Hill recommends alternating acetaminophen and ibuprofen and adding a monthly back massage to Mr. Grier's therapeutic regimen.

CRITICAL THINKING

1. Mr. Grier asks you why he needs to continue the strengthening exercises and include back massages in his therapy. What do you tell him?
2. If Mr. Grier reports excessive nausea in response to his opioid medication, what suggestions will you give him to decrease his nausea and provide comfort?
3. How would you adapt this care plan to a client with knee pain instead of back pain?

Relating Concepts and Exemplars: Practical Applications

REVIEW The Concept of Comfort

RELATE Link the Concepts

Linking the concept of comfort with the concept of elimination:
1. How can you help clients with "embarrassing" symptoms such as bowel incontinence feel more comfortable talking about their condition?
2. Describe comfort measures for a client who requires catheterization for treatment of urinary retention.

Linking the concept of comfort with the concept of violence:
3. Explain the psychosocial considerations related to promoting comfort during the care and assessment of a rape victim.
4. When assessing a child who is believed to have been abused, what comfort measures can be used to reduce the child's anxiety and promote trust?

READY Go to Companion Skills Manual

REFER Go to Pearson Student Nursing Resources
nursing.pearsonhighered.com
- Additional review materials

REFLECT Case Study \\ Part 3
Ms. Daves has been visiting her primary care provider as recommended for follow up care. Six months after beginning treatment with milnacipran (Savella), Ms. Daves returns for a

regular checkup. As you review her chart, you note that Ms. Daves's physician confirmed the ED physician's diagnoses of fibromyalgia. Upon assessment, Ms. Daves's vital signs are normal, and her pain intensity is a 3 on a scale of 0–10. She also reports that she is sleeping better at night, although she occasionally has insomnia even though the pain is manageable. When you ask how Savella is working for her, she says that it has helped her pain and stiffness but her mouth has been really dry since she started taking it and she sometimes has slight nausea.

Clinical Reasoning Questions Level I
1. What suggestions can you giv[e] her dry mouth and nausea?
2. What further assessment shou[ld] mine the cause of Ms. Daves's [pain]?
3. Can you suggest other therapie[s] pain even further?

Clinical Reasoning Questions Lev[el]
4. What nursing interventions ca[n] vent future flare-ups of Ms. Da[ves]
5. What information should you gi[ve] (Savella) and drug-drug interact[ion]
6. What coping techniques wou[ld] she deals with fibromyalgia?

New! Each **Concept** section ends with a Review section that includes critical thinking questions that link concepts together, a list of additional resources, and Part 3 of the longitudinal case study.

Each **Exemplar** section ends with a similar Review section. Critical thinking questions link together concepts and exemplars. Case Studies provide practical nursing situations with critical thinking questions. Additional resources are also listed.

REVIEW Acute and Chronic Pain

RELATE Link the Concepts and Exemplars

Linking the exemplar of acute and chronic pain with the concept of culture and diversity:
1. When you are caring for a client who appears to be in pain but denies it, how might understanding of the client's culture help you interpret the dichotomy between body language and reported pain?
2. How might interpretations and interventions for pain differ among cultures?

Linking the exemplar of acute and chronic pain with the concept of stress and coping:
3. What alterations in stress and coping would you anticipate when a client experiences chronic pain?
4. When caring for a mother with acute pain over the past few weeks, the client relates she has just not had the energy to deal with her children. How is pain impacting this mother's ability to cope with her children's needs?

READY Go to Companion Skills Manual

REFER Go to Pearson Student Nursing Resources
nursing.pearsonhighered.com
- Additional review material
- Chart: Printable pain management flow sheet
- Minimodule: Neonates and Pain

REFLECT Case Study
Mr. Backwater is a 48-year-old Cherokee Indian. His history includes nicotine abuse, lung cancer, arthritis in both knees, and headaches. Mr. Backwater has trouble breathing, especially after exertion. During a routine checkup, the nurse's assessment reveals that Mr. Backwater is experiencing severe pain in his right side when inhaling, and he has painful mouth sores as a result of his chemotherapy treatment. Between the chemotherapy and the mouth sores, Mr. Backwater is losing weight because of inadequate food intake.

1. What cultural influences do you need to consider when assessing Mr. Backwater's pain?
2. Should Mr. Backwater's history of nicotine abuse influence which pharmacologic agents are prescribed for his pain? Why or why not? How can you advocate for Mr. Backwater if inadequate pain medications are prescribed?
3. What cultural practices can you recommend as nonpharmacologic therapy for Mr. Backwater's pain?

TO THE INSTRUCTOR

▶ INTRODUCTION

Nursing education is evolving. As the nursing profession has developed to encompass a variety of roles at all levels of society, including direct client care, advocacy, and leadership at the local, state, and national levels, nursing education is changing to help nursing students prepare to enter a more robust, demanding, and rewarding profession. Societal forces that have created the climate for transforming nursing education include, but are not limited to, the global economy, technological advances, and changes in healthcare delivery systems. Tried and true teaching methods now seem antiquated as faculty compete for students' attention with a variety of new and engaging sources of information and entertainment. In addition, the overwhelming discovery of new knowledge in the "information age" has resulted in nursing students feeling overwhelmed by the quantity of knowledge and skills they must gain in order to become practicing nurses.

University and college nursing programs across the United States have begun evaluating how their programs can meet the needs of today's nursing students. Many are moving to the model of concept-based learning in an effort to meet the challenges facing nursing students and nurses today. This model provides the impetus for educators to transition away from traditional methods of faculty-centered teaching and passive learning toward active, focused, participative, and collaborative teaching and learning. *Nursing: A Concept-Based Approach to Learning,* Second Edition, is designed to assist nursing faculty to provide students with a broader perspective while promoting a deeper understanding of content in a focused, participative, and collaborative learning environment.

▶ WHAT IS CONCEPT-BASED LEARNING?

Concept-based learning is a paradigm for learning that classifies essential content into categories that have common relevant features, reinforces those concepts by teaching exemplars, and then encourages learners to determine whether each concept does or does not apply to a given situation. The goal is to teach the concepts well enough that students can recognize them in any context. Concept-based learning is more student centered and student directed than traditional education models. Students are expected to delve into the content and learn how to access information independently. In concept-based learning, the instructor is more of a facilitator of learning than an expert imparting knowledge to students.

Using this approach involves drawing attention to conceptual lenses, that is, to concepts that force students to think at the integration level and relate topics to broader contexts. *Nursing: A Concept-Based Approach to Learning,* Second Edition, uses the individual client as a conceptual lens, focusing on human systems functioning and providing examples of common deviations from health across the life span, and then making links to how concepts are related and interrelated. Professional behavior and healthcare system concepts are interwoven with the human system concepts to guide care decisions and delivery systems for individuals, families, and communities.

With the conceptual lens of the individual client across the life span identified, essential concepts have been selected that reflect critical areas of nursing practice. These concepts are the "big ideas" that reflect different aspects of the conceptual lens. Generalizations, or central ideas of enduring understanding, are derived from the concepts and assist the learner to apply the concept. Generalizations coupled with learning outcomes clarify what students should be able to do when they complete the unit of instruction and help guide all other activities. Exemplars have been selected based on incidence, prevalence, or broad applicability to other concepts (see below). Topics, processes, and skills reflect content that is needed to complete the performance outcome. As a result, faculty and learners keep reflecting back on the "big ideas" and performance outcomes to increase understanding of the whole, and then the part, and then back to the whole again.

The benefit of concept-based learning is that organized and sequenced conceptual structures create stable and usable bodies of knowledge that promote independent and critical thinking. This in turn promotes the higher-order thinking necessary to meet the demands of our constantly changing world. As students become more actively engaged in learning rather than simply memorizing facts, they begin to see patterns and to use those patterns to think about the facts they learn. For example, when a student is involved in a clinical simulation centered around a child who has respiratory distress, the student has the opportunity to auscultate abnormal breath sounds, inspect the chest to see retractions and rapid breathing, observe the child with cyanosis, and see an oxygen saturation level that is below normal, while also thinking about developmental issues, the effects of stress, and the safety of the child. Through multiple ways of learning (e.g., clinical experience, discussion of case studies with peers), these patterns become a part of the student's learning repertoire, which is based on a full experience rather than memorization of facts. An added benefit of connecting essential facts to a broader context is that it helps learners retain information. The facts become more meaningful when students can relate them to their own lives and experiences. A concept-process approach also helps students make connections between other related subject areas. *A goal in this type of learning is to build a conceptual understanding of nursing that will be transferable to future knowledge and developments in a variety of related client-care situations.*

A concept-based approach also helps students develop critical thinking skills and integrate new knowledge with what they have already learned to attain a level of constructed knowledge. As learners progress to higher levels of knowing, then the higher level critical thinking/clinical reasoning skills can be added, including (1) assumptions about a healthcare situation that must be questioned, and (2) evidence utilization to determine the outcome including empirical data, expert opinions, professional standards, and personal experiences. Implications, the highest level of critical thinking/clinical reasoning skills, are best applied with real-world situations or simulations. This skill is related to the constructed, conceptual knowing level in which the learner integrates all aspects of the healthcare situation.

In summary, a conceptual approach to teaching provides nursing students with a deeper understanding of their field that is transferable to a broader spectrum of both current and future practice.

▶ BASIS FOR SELECTION OF CONCEPTS AND EXEMPLARS

Nursing: A Concept-Based Approach to Learning examines the professional requirements of nursing care through the lens of the human life span, and categorizes content into three domains: the individual domain, the nursing domain, and the healthcare domain. Within each of these domains, content is organized into modules, which include the concept and specific exemplars that contain relevant critical or essential content that illustrates the concept.

For the First Edition, faculty advisors from the state of North Carolina identified concepts and exemplars based on a number of national initiatives, feedback from clinical partners, and other considerations. Prior to developing the Second Edition, a Concepts Advisory Panel consisting of nursing faculty from throughout the country, representing both two- and four-year programs, was selected to guide the revision. They reviewed the First Edition text, studied feedback from faculty using the text as well as those representing programs not using the text, and identified workplace trends and national priorities to develop a new template and modify and select the concepts and exemplars for *Nursing: A Concept-Based Approach to Learning,* Second Edition.

Like its predecessor, this Second Edition takes into consideration the need for nurses to practice safe, effective care within today's healthcare environments, and the need for nursing students to be "floor ready" when they graduate. To that extent, concepts and exemplars included in this text have their basis in a number of national initiatives and identified priorities, including:

- Reports from the Institute of Medicine, including *Crossing the Quality Chasm: A New Health System for the 21st Century* (2001)

- *Healthy People 2020*
- Prevalence rates determined by the Centers for Disease Control and Prevention, the National Institutes of Health, the American Psychiatric Association, and other government and professional organizations
- Priorities, standards of practice, and codes of behavior established by the American Nurses Association, the National Council of State Boards of Nursing, the American Association of Colleges of Nursing, the National League for Nursing, and other professional nursing organizations
- Federal legislation that impacts healthcare providers and agencies, such as the Health Insurance Portability and Accountability Act, and federal agencies that administer federal regulations, such as the Centers for Medicare and Medicaid Services and the Occupational Safety and Health Administration
- QSEN and KSA competencies
- NCLEX-RN examination priorities
- Workplace expectations and requirements.

▶ ORGANIZATION OF MATERIAL

Nursing: A Concept-Based Approach to Learning, Second Edition, offers 51 concepts and their exemplars organized into modules.

Parts I, II, and III: The Individual Domain

All of the concepts related to the holistic individual, family, and community are presented in the modules in Parts I, II, and III, which encompass the Individual Domain. These modules address the biological, physical, cognitive, and psychosocial processes and their alterations that most frequently bring the individual into contact with the nursing and healthcare domains. Each concept within the individual domain addresses the impact of that concept on individuals across the life span, inclusive of cultural, gender, and developmental considerations. Part I includes the biological and physical concepts (e.g., Acid–Base Balance and Elimination). Part II includes the primarily psychosocial concepts (e.g., Family and Mood and Affect). Part III is devoted to the concept of Reproduction.

Part IV: The Nursing Domain

Part IV, the Nursing Domain, contains concepts related to competencies for graduates of nursing programs such as Assessment, Clinical Decision Making, Collaboration, and Professional Behaviors.

Part V: The Healthcare Domain

Part V, the Healthcare Domain, contains such IOM and QSEN competencies as Evidence-Based Practice, Informatics, and Safety, as well as additional elements essential to nursing, including Advocacy, Ethics, and Legal Issues.

▶ CONCLUSION

Written by nurses, and based on a strong foundation of adult learning, this concept-based curriculum provides a focal point to direct learning through concepts, examples of alterations via exemplars, faculty and student activities, and collaborative group exercises. In addition to input from the Concepts Advisory Panel and content written by nurses, academicians from across the United States provided peer reviews of the concepts and exemplars.

This curriculum provides many opportunities for student nurses to learn collaboratively through skill development, case studies and discussions, group examination of resources and technology, and student–faculty interactions. By working together, faculty and students will become partners in learning, promoting greater acquisition of knowledge and understanding, and greater skill development—all of which will produce the most successful, empathetic, informed, and skilled graduates of nursing programs.

TO THE STUDENT

▶ CONCEPT-BASED LEARNING

The practice of nursing occurs in complex environments. Nurses must be able to take the knowledge they have learned in school and in practice and transfer it to new situations. Nurses must become lifelong learners to stay current with new disorders, new treatments, and evidence-based practice. To help you achieve these goals, your school or instructor has chosen a new way to help you learn to be a nurse. You will be taking a concept-based approach to learning. Concept-based learning is a student-centered approach to learning. Students participate actively in the learning environment, assuming responsibility for their own knowledge as they learn to integrate concepts, apply information, and use clinical reasoning to provide client-centered care. So instead of memorizing 3,000 alterations to the body systems in a lecture-driven platform as is done in traditional programs, you are going to learn more in-depth knowledge of selected alterations, using critical thinking skills so that you will be able to transfer your knowledge to new situations and client presentations.

You will learn:

- 51 concepts that affect all ages (such as Oxygenation, Mobility, Communication, and Safety)
- 235 exemplars (that is, disorders or examples) of those concepts that cover the life span
- How to integrate your knowledge of the 51 concepts in order to provide care for clients of all ages
- How to learn on your own to evaluate and use evidence and to stay current with new standards so you can take excellent care of your clients.

▶ THE MODULES

Each of the 51 concepts is combined with its exemplars in a module. As examples, consider the modules on Oxygenation and Communication. See the section on Features starting on page vii for samples of these sections and features.

The Concept of Oxygenation

The beginning section of the module on Oxygenation is *The Concept of Oxygenation*, and in this section you will learn about

- *Normal Oxygenation*. What does normal oxygenation look like and sound like in a client? What are the genetic and lifespan considerations for normal oxygenation?

- *Alterations to Oxygenation* and how they manifest in clients such as a decreased level of oxygen in the blood (hypoxemia), breathing too fast (tachypnea), and shortness of breath (dyspnea).
- The relationship of oxygenation to other concepts in a feature called *Concepts Related to Oxygenation.* For example, if a client has altered oxygenation, she may also have altered Acid–Base Balance, altered Cognition, and altered Perfusion.
- *Prevention* of poor oxygenation in your clients.
- *Assessment* of oxygenation in a client including taking a history and performing a physical assessment.
- *Interventions and Therapies* used to help the client with altered oxygenation. These are divided into *Independent* therapies (those you can do on your own such as elevating the head of the client's bed to allow him to breathe more easily) and *Collaborative* (those that need orders from a physician, such as medication, or are performed by other members of the healthcare team, such as a respiratory therapist).

In addition, a three-part *Case Study* of a client with altered oxygenation helps you see how nursing care is provided.

The Oxygenation Exemplars

After you have learned about The Concept of Oxygenation, you'll move on to study the oxygenation *Exemplars.* There are five exemplars for Oxygenation: Acute Respiratory Distress Syndrome (ARDS), Asthma, Chronic Obstructive Pulmonary Disease (COPD), Respiratory Syncytial Virus (RSV)/Bronchiolitis, and Sudden Infant Death Syndrome (SIDS). These five exemplars were chosen for a variety of reasons:

- Some are very common (asthma, COPD) and you will likely see them often in practice.
- Some (ARDS, asthma, COPD) have been identified by national standards or organizations (e.g., the Institute of Medicine, *Healthy People 2020,* The Joint Commission) as priorities to be addressed.
- They cover the life span: Asthma is seen at all ages, SIDS occurs in infants, COPD is a disorder primarily seen in older adults, and RSV is seen in both infants/toddlers and older adults.
- Some are treated mostly in the doctor's office or at home (asthma), and others are treated almost exclusively in hospitals (ARDS).

Once you learn about these exemplars in detail, you will be able to apply that knowledge to care for clients with other disorders that include alterations in oxygenation.

The Concept of Communication

The Concept of Communication starts with a description of the communication process and then covers modes of communication (verbal, nonverbal, electronic, and written). The next topic is factors that influence the communication process such as development, gender, and sociocultural characteristics, including features to help you communicate with children, teens, and older adults. The next main topic is barriers to communication (such as being defensive), and the final section is on types of communicators (aggressive, passive, and assertive) with special emphasis on how to be an assertive communicator. Other features include the following.

- The *Concepts Related to Communication* feature shows how Communication is integrated with Oxygenation, Grief and Loss, Safety, and Advocacy.
- A *Nursing Process* section shows you how communication is an integral part of the nursing process.
- Two *Case Studies* help you see communication in action and prompt you to think about how you would communicate in those situations.

The Communication Exemplars

The module on Communication has four exemplars:

- *Groups and Group Communications* covers different types of groups, their functions, and how groups communicate with an emphasis on healthcare groups such as teams, task forces, and therapy groups.
- *Therapeutic Communication* covers therapeutic communication techniques (such as empathizing, attentive listening, and confronting), barriers to communication, the phases of and development of therapeutic relationships, and communicating with children and families.
- *Documentation* covers the purposes of documentation, various documentation methods and systems, the legal and ethical considerations in documentation, how to document nursing activities, facility-specific documentation, and general guidelines for recording.
- *Reporting* covers the topic of communicating specific information to a person or group of people including handoff communication, telephone reports, care plan conferences, and nursing rounds.

▶ INTEGRATING THE CONCEPTS

As mentioned above, the body works as a unified whole. A disturbance in one part of the body impacts the entire individual. That is, a client who has altered Oxygenation will most likely have additional alterations that impact care. For example, a client with chronic obstructive pulmonary disease (COPD) may have altered Cognition, because his brain is not getting enough oxygen. He may have issues with Safety because he is using supplemental oxygen (which is flammable) at home, and he still wants to smoke. He may have altered Fluids and Electrolytes because he is not drinking enough because his Mobility is limited

and he has trouble getting to the kitchen and does not want to have to get up too often to urinate. And his nurse may have difficulty with Communication because his Cognition is altered.

To help you integrate the concepts, the *Concepts Related to …* feature gives examples of other concepts that are often altered when the concept being studied is altered. The end of each concept and each exemplar has a *Review* section that contains sets of questions designed to help you think through the links that exist with other concepts and exemplars. These questions promote deep thinking, which you need for nursing practice. For example, in the review section for *The Concept of Oxygenation,* the linking questions are:

Linking the concept of oxygenation with the concept of infection:

1. Why would alterations in oxygenation lead to an increased risk of certain infections?
2. What are some ways to decrease the risk of infections that are caused by alterations in oxygenation?

Linking the concept of oxygenation with the concept of mobility:

3. How might alterations in oxygenation affect mobility?
4. What are some nursing interventions that can decrease the risk of altered mobility for clients with alterations in oxygenation?

Linking the concept of oxygenation with the concept of perfusion:

5. How are the concepts of oxygenation and perfusion related?
6. What disease processes related to oxygenation can affect the body's ability to perfuse adequately?

Linking the concept of oxygenation with the concept of cognition:

7. How might an alteration in oxygenation impact an individual's orientation?
8. How might lack of oxygenation to the brain be detected?

And in the *Review* section for the exemplar on *Therapeutic Communication* in the module on Communication, the linking questions are:

Linking the exemplar of therapeutic communication with the concept of advocacy:

1. How do strong therapeutic communication skills contribute to the nurse's role as a client advocate?
2. How do strong therapeutic communication skills contribute to the nurse's ability to work within groups to advocate for clients?

Linking the exemplar of therapeutic communication with the concept of teaching and learning:

3. The nurse is preparing to teach a client who is newly diagnosed with diabetes about self-care. Describe the three phases of the therapeutic relationship as it applies to the client teaching plan.
4. While teaching the client with diabetes, the nurse accidentally creates a barrier to the therapeutic relationship by misspeaking. What should the nurse do next?

And most important of all, your instructors will coach you in learning to integrate the concepts, and eventually, you will learn to do so on your own.

Even though the concepts in this book are integrated, you will learn them one at a time. The order in which you learn them may depend on the region where you live, your school's curriculum, and the clients you serve. If your instructor chooses to teach Oxygenation as your first concept, you would need to know a little bit about Acid–Base Balance, Cellular Regulation, Cognition, Comfort, Infection, Mobility, and Perfusion just to understand the Concepts Related to Oxygenation feature and to answer the linking questions in the Review section. You can do this in several ways:

■ Use the knowledge you already have. Think about the anatomy and physiology of the cardiovascular system to remember how Perfusion might affect Oxygenation. Think about the older adults in your life to consider how Mobility might affect Oxygenation.

■ You can read ahead: If you have a linking question about a concept you have not yet studied in class, read that module, or at least skim the Normal Presentation section to help you remember what you already know about the concept in question.

■ You should research the topics on your own and revisit the content often. The more exposure you have to the content, the deeper your learning will be.

We hope you enjoy *Nursing: A Concept-Based Approach to Learning,* Second Edition.

CONTENTS

Part II Psychosocial Modules   **1517**

MODULE 22 Addiction   **1519**
The Concept of Addiction   1519
Exemplar 22.1   Alcohol Abuse   1534
Exemplar 22.2   Nicotine Addiction   1545
Exemplar 22.3   Prenatal Substance Exposure   1551
Exemplar 22.4   Substance Abuse   1560

MODULE 23 Cognition   **1575**
The Concept of Cognition   1575
Exemplar 23.1   Alzheimer Disease   1594
Exemplar 23.2   Confusion   1605
Exemplar 23.3   Schizophrenia   1610

MODULE 24 Culture and Diversity   **1629**
The Concept of Culture and Diversity   1629

MODULE 25 Development   **1647**
The Concept of Development   1647
Exemplar 25.1   Attention-Deficit/Hyperactivity
   Disorder   1680
Exemplar 25.2   Autism Spectrum Disorder   1688
Exemplar 25.3   Cerebral Palsy   1695
Exemplar 25.4   Failure to Thrive   1701

MODULE 26 Family   **1707**
The Concept of Family   1707
Exemplar 26.1   Family Health Promotion   1724
Exemplar 26.2   Family Response to Health
   Alterations   1730

MODULE 27 Grief and Loss   **1741**
The Concept of Grief and Loss   1741
Exemplar 27.1   Children's Response to Loss   1751
Exemplar 27.2   Death and Dying   1757
Exemplar 27.3   Older Adult's Response
   to Loss   1763
Exemplar 27.4   Perinatal Loss   1767

MODULE 28 Mood and Affect   **1775**
The Concept of Mood and Affect   1775
Exemplar 28.1   Depression   1798
Exemplar 28.2   Adjustment Disorder With
   Depressed Mood   1805
Exemplar 28.3   Bipolar Disorders   1808
Exemplar 28.4   Postpartum Depression   1816

MODULE 29 Self   **1831**
The Concept of Self   1831
Exemplar 29.1   Feeding and Eating Disorders   1843
Exemplar 29.2   Personality Disorders   1852

MODULE 30 Spirituality   **1871**
The Concept of Spirituality   1871
Exemplar 30.1   Morality   1878
Exemplar 30.2   Religion   1883
Exemplar 30.3   Spiritual Distress   1890

MODULE 31 Stress and Coping   **1895**
The Concept of Stress and Coping   1895
Exemplar 31.1   Anxiety Disorders   1917
Exemplar 31.2   Crisis   1927
Exemplar 31.3   Obsessive-Compulsive
   Disorder   1934
Exemplar 31.4   Phobias   1939
Exemplar 31.5   Posttraumatic Stress Disorder   1945

MODULE 32 Violence   **1953**
The Concept of Violence   1953
Exemplar 32.1   Abuse   1964
Exemplar 32.2   Assault and Homicide   1975
Exemplar 32.3   Rape and Rape-Trauma
   Syndrome   1983
Exemplar 32.4   Suicide   1990
Exemplar 32.5   Unintentional Injury:
   Motor Vehicle Crashes   1998

Part III Reproduction Module   **2009**

MODULE 33 Reproduction   **2011**
The Concept of Reproduction   2011
Exemplar 33.1   Antepartum Care   2067
Exemplar 33.2   Intrapartum Care   2112
Exemplar 33.3   Postpartum Care   2170
Exemplar 33.4   Newborn Care   2191
Exemplar 33.5   Prematurity   2249

Part IV Nursing Domain   **2267**

MODULE 34 Assessment   **2269**
The Concept of Assessment   2269
Exemplar 34.1   Holistic Health
   Assessment Across the Life Span   2285

xxii Contents

MODULE 35 Caring Interventions **2301**

The Concept of Caring Interventions 2301

MODULE 36 Clinical Decision Making **2315**

The Concept of Clinical Decision Making 2315

Exemplar 36.1 The Nursing Process 2328

Exemplar 36.2 The Nursing Plan of Care 2354

Exemplar 36.3 Prioritizing Care 2363

MODULE 37 Collaboration **2375**

The Concept of Collaboration 2375

Exemplar 37.1 Case Management 2382

Exemplar 37.2 Conflict Resolution 2387

Exemplar 37.3 Interdisciplinary Teams 2391

MODULE 38 Communication **2397**

The Concept of Communication 2397

Exemplar 38.1 Groups and Group
Communication 2418

Exemplar 38.2 Therapeutic Communication 2424

Exemplar 38.3 Documentation 2438

Exemplar 38.4 Reporting 2450

MODULE 39 Managing Care **2455**

The Concept of Managing Care 2455

Exemplar 39.1 Care Coordination 2460

Exemplar 39.2 Cost-Effective Care 2462

Exemplar 39.3 Delegation 2466

Exemplar 39.4 Management Principles 2474

MODULE 40 Professional Behaviors **2479**

The Concept of Professional Behaviors 2479

Exemplar 40.1 Commitment to Profession 2486

Exemplar 40.2 Leadership Principles 2489

Exemplar 40.3 Work Ethic 2491

MODULE 41 Teaching and Learning **2499**

The Concept of Teaching and Learning 2499

Exemplar 41.1 Client/Consumer Education 2509

Exemplar 41.2 Mentoring 2524

Exemplar 41.3 Staff Development 2528

Part V Healthcare Domain **2533**

MODULE 42 Accountability **2535**

The Concept of Accountability 2535

Exemplar 42.1 Competence 2543

Exemplar 42.2 Professional Development 2545

MODULE 43 Advocacy **2555**

The Concept of Advocacy 2555

MODULE 44 Ethics **2563**

The Concept of Ethics 2563

Exemplar 44.1 Ethical Dilemmas 2571

Exemplar 44.2 Patient Rights 2578

MODULE 45 Evidence-Based Practice **2583**

The Concept of Evidence-Based Practice 2583

MODULE 46 Healthcare Systems **2595**

The Concept of Healthcare Systems 2595

Exemplar 46.1 Access to Health Care 2603

Exemplar 46.2 Allocation of Resources 2607

Exemplar 46.3 Emergency Preparedness 2608

MODULE 47 Health Policy **2619**

The Concept of Health Policy 2619

Exemplar 47.1 Regulatory Agencies 2621

Exemplar 47.2 Accrediting Bodies 2624

Exemplar 47.3 Professional Organizations 2625

Exemplar 47.4 Types of Reimbursement 2627

MODULE 48 Informatics **2631**

The Concept of Informatics 2631

Exemplar 48.1 Clinical Decision Support
Systems 2644

Exemplar 48.2 Individual Information
at Point of Care 2646

MODULE 49 Legal Issues **2653**

The Concept of Legal Issues 2653

Exemplar 49.1 Nurse Practice Acts 2663

Exemplar 49.2 Advance Directives 2667

Exemplar 49.3 Health Insurance Portability
and Accountability Act 2670

Exemplar 49.4 Just Culture 2672

Exemplar 49.5 Mandatory Reporting 2674

Exemplar 49.6 Risk Management 2676

MODULE 50 Quality Improvement **2681**

The Concept of Quality Improvement 2681

MODULE 51 Safety **2695**

The Concept of Safety 2695

Exemplar 51.1 Safety Considerations Across
the Life Span 2708

Exemplar 51.2 Workplace Safety 2715

Appendix A: NANDA-Approved Nursing
Diagnoses 2012–2014 A-1

Glossary G-1

Combined Index I-1

Available online at nursing.pearsonhighered.com and
within the interactive e-text:

Appendix B: Diagnostic Values and Laboratory Tests

Part II
Psychosocial Modules

Part II consists of the psychosocial modules within the individual domain. Each module presents a concept that directly relates to sociological or psychological domains that impact client health and well-being—such as cognition, family, and stress and coping—and selected alterations of that concept presented as exemplars. In the concept of cognition, for example, exemplars include Alzheimer disease, confusion, and schizophrenia. Each module addresses the impact of that concept and selected alterations on individuals across the life span, inclusive of cultural, gender, and developmental considerations.

Module 22 Addiction 1519
Module 23 Cognition 1575
Module 24 Culture and Diversity 1629
Module 25 Development 1647
Module 26 Family 1707
Module 27 Grief and Loss 1741
Module 28 Mood and Affect 1775
Module 29 Self 1831
Module 30 Spirituality 1871
Module 31 Stress and Coping 1895
Module 32 Violence 1953

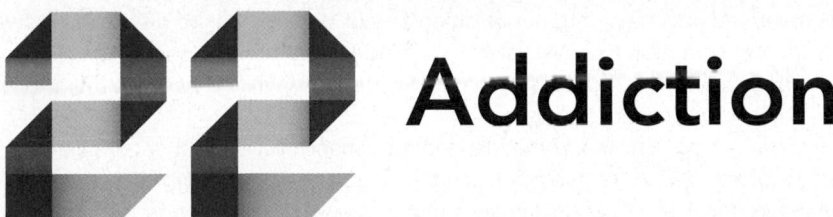

22 Addiction

MODULE AT-A-GLANCE

The Concept of Addiction, 1519

Exemplar 22.1
Alcohol Abuse, 1534

Exemplar 22.2
Nicotine Addiction, 1545

Exemplar 22.3
Prenatal Substance Exposure, 1551

Exemplar 22.4
Substance Abuse, 1560

◢ THE CONCEPT OF ADDICTION

Addiction is defined as a psychological or physical need for a substance (such as alcohol) or process (such as gambling) to the extent that the individual will risk negative consequences in an attempt to meet the need. Many individuals use substances recreationally to modify mood or behavior. There are, however, wide sociocultural variations in the acceptability of chemical use. Alcohol, caffeine, and tobacco are legal substances, but the social acceptability of their use varies. Some prescription medications such as narcotics, sedatives, and stimulants are used illegally. The general population considers recreational use of illicit substances to be socially unacceptable. Other illegal drugs include marijuana/hashish, cocaine (including crack), heroin, hallucinogens, and inhalants. An individual may abuse any of these substances to the point of becoming addicted and unable to stop, despite dangerous, often life-threatening consequences.

(continued on next page)

Concept Learning Outcomes

After reading about this concept, you will be able to:

1. Summarize the physiological and psychological processes that contribute to addiction.
2. Examine the relationship between addiction and other concepts/systems.
3. Identify commonly occurring addictions and their related therapies.
4. Differentiate assessments of addictions across the life span.
5. Describe diagnostic and laboratory tests to determine an individual's addiction status.
6. Explain prevention and management of addictions.
7. Demonstrate the nursing process in providing culturally competent and caring interventions across the life span for individuals with addictions.
8. Compare and contrast common independent and collaborative interventions for addiction.

Concept Key Terms

Abstinence, 1525
Addiction, 1519
Behavioral therapy, 1529
Binge drinking, 1521
Boundaries, 1524
Codependence, 1525
Contingency
  contracts, 1529
Co-occurring
  disorders, 1525
Delirium tremens
  (DTs), 1525
Dependence, 1520
Enabling behavior, 1525
Extinction, 1529

Family therapy, 1532
Group therapy, 1530
Here-and-now
  concept, 1530
Intervention, 1529
Milieu therapy, 1530
Process addictions, 1520
Punishment, 1529
Recovery, 1528
Reinforcement, 1529
Sobriety, 1525
Social microcosm, 1530
Token economies, 1530
Tolerance, 1520

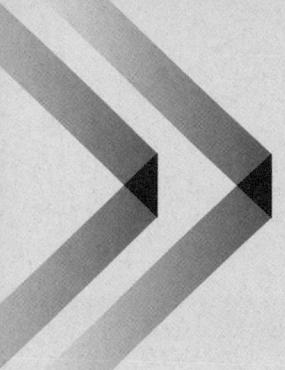

Other forms of addiction, often referred to as **process addictions**, include workaholism, gambling, shopping, cutting, pornography, spending and indebtedness, Internet or other type of gaming, eating disorders, and sexual addictions. Process addictions involve compulsive behaviors that serve to reduce anxiety. Some clinicians believe that these behaviors are more closely linked to an obsessive-compulsive disorder, while others see them as addictions resulting from a decreased ability to experience pleasure.

The etiology of addiction is multifaceted. Childhood trauma, genetic variabilities, and other considerations are thought to play a role. Regardless of the reasons or etiology behind addiction, it can have grave consequences for both individuals and those who care for them. Nurses can play a role in prevention, education, and treatment of substance abuse and addiction. **<<**

▶ NORMAL PRESENTATION

Addiction needs to be differentiated from dependence. **Dependence** is a physiological need for a substance that the client cannot control, and that results in withdrawal symptoms if the substance (most often a chemical) is withheld. Dependence on a substance also results in the user developing a physiological **tolerance** for the substance, requiring use of greater quantities to achieve the same effect. Addiction includes the physiological process of dependence, but also includes a psychological need that causes addicts to seek the substance to which they are addicted—at any cost. Addicts may neglect their children, their work, or other responsibilities to meet their physiological and psychological needs.

Physiology and Psychology of Addiction

Various factors help explain why one person becomes addicted while another does not. The biopsychosocial model theorized by psychiatrist George L. Engel has been generally accepted as the most comprehensive theory for the process of addiction. Clinicians use his model as a foundation to link biological, genetic, psychological, emotional, and sociocultural factors contributing to the development of addiction.

Biological factors were first identified by E. Morton Jellinek in his disease model of alcoholism. He hypothesized that addiction to alcohol had a biochemical basis and identified specific phases of the disease (Jellinek, 1946). Expanding on Jellinek's early work, researchers implicated low levels of dopamine and serotonin in the development of alcohol dependence (Czermak et al., 2004; Nellissery et al., 2003). More recent clinical studies have continued to confirm this finding (Cosgrove, 2010; Kash, 2012). Dopamine and dopamine receptor sites are intricately involved in the complex workings between the nervous system and abusive substances. Any drug's ability to have an impact on the biochemical mechanism of the brain must be able to do so at a receptor site or at a number of receptor sites (**Figure 22–1 ●**). Most abused substances mimic or block the brain's most important neurotransmitters at their respective receptor sites. For example, heroin and other opiates mimic natural opiate-like neurotransmitters such as endorphin,

enkephalin, and dynorphin. In contrast, cocaine and other stimulants block the reuptake of dopamine, serotonin, and norepinephrine (Stuart, 2008).

Neurobiological research into addiction postulates that addiction is the result of an increase in focus on a particular addictive behavior with a corresponding gradual loss of interest in other activities. The mesolimbic dopaminergic system is believed to play an important role in the search for rewarding stimuli, with a resulting increase in dopamine when the stimulus is received. Particular areas in the brain define something as pleasure. When these areas are stimulated as a result of addiction, the substance or behavior takes on an increased level of need.

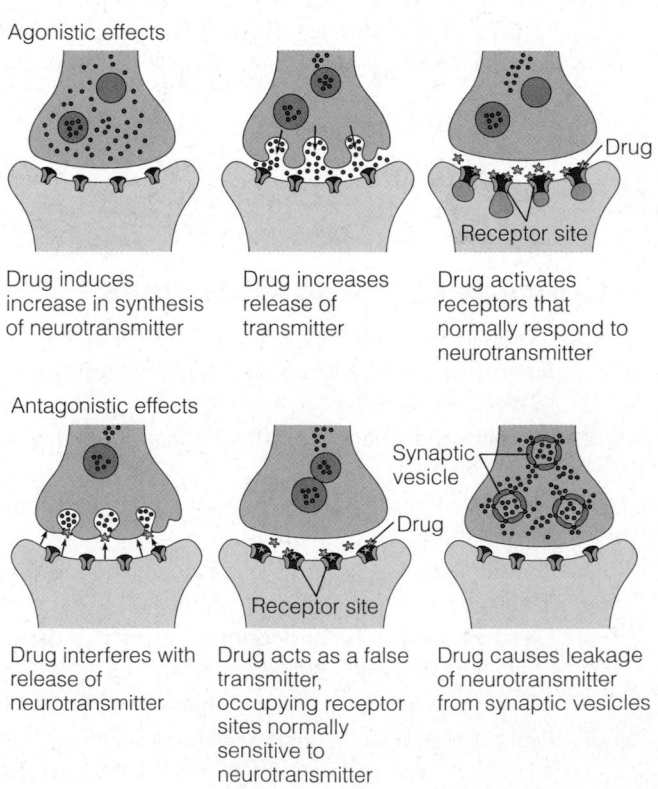

Agonistic effects

Drug induces increase in synthesis of neurotransmitter

Drug increases release of transmitter

Drug activates receptors that normally respond to neurotransmitter

Antagonistic effects

Drug interferes with release of neurotransmitter

Drug acts as a false transmitter, occupying receptor sites normally sensitive to neurotransmitter

Drug causes leakage of neurotransmitter from synaptic vesicles

Figure 22–1 ● Action of abused substances at brain receptor sites.

Genetic factors include an apparent hereditary factor that affects alcohol use and dependence. A link has been found between addiction and impulse control, although it is not fully understood. Addiction is strongly linked to the dopaminergic system of the brain's reward system. The speed with which someone becomes addicted depends on the substance, the frequency of use, the means of ingestion, the intensity of the high the person obtains, and the person's genetic and psychological susceptibility. Adequate proof exists that addiction is, at least in part, genetically moderated.

Researchers are using case-control studies and genome-wide association studies to map genes that contribute to the genetically complex disorder of alcohol dependence. Researchers are also using animal studies to identify genetic regions or individual genes involved in different aspects of alcoholism. This work has led to the identification of several genes that seem to influence the risk for alcohol dependence (Foroud & Phillips, 2012).

Psychological factors of substance abuse are examined in psychoanalytical, behavioral, and family system theories. Psychoanalytical theorists view substance abuse as a fixation at the oral stage of development, whereas behavioral theorists see addiction as a learned maladaptive behavior. Family system theory focuses on a dysfunctional pattern of family relationships throughout several generations.

No addictive personality type has been identified; however, several common factors seem to exist among alcoholics and drug users. Many substance abusers have experienced sexual or physical abuse in their childhood and, as a result, experience anxiety, low self-esteem, and difficulty expressing emotions. A link also exists between substance abuse and psychiatric disorders such as depression, anxiety, and antisocial and dependent personalities. The habit of using a substance becomes a form of self-medication to cope with day-to-day problems and develops into an addiction over time.

Emotional factors are considered in the pleasure model, proposed by Nils Bejerot, which views addiction as an emotional fixation acquired through learning that is aimed at obtaining pleasure and avoiding discomfort. If the pleasure (euphoria) that results is sufficiently strong, it induces repetition and overcomes the person's natural drive, resulting in addiction. This model is the basis of zero tolerance for drugs as a prevention strategy.

Sociocultural factors are thought to play a strong role in the development of and tolerance for an addiction. Sociocultural factors often influence individuals' decisions as to when, what, and how they use substances. The way drugs are processed, the degree of acceptance or rejection of drug use, and an individual's financial resources influence what substance is used, how much is used, and what peer pressure the individual will face in his or her culture as the abuse becomes evident.

As stated earlier, substance abuse is a multifaceted problem. A clear example of this can be seen in the risks for substance abuse among adolescents (**Box 22–1** ●).

Sociocultural factors such as personality and religion/spirituality appear to play a part in the risk profile for developing alcoholism. People taking personality tests who scored low in agreeableness and conscientiousness had higher alcohol use. Also, people who scored high in neuroticism had higher alco-

---

Box 22–1   Risk for Substance Abuse Among Adolescents

Drug use often starts in adolescence. Brain circuits involving reward and memory are still developing and may increase the adolescent's risk for developing substance abuse. Sociological factors are known to play a role. Research indicates a high correlation among substance use and childhood and adolescent trauma (National Child Traumatic Stress Network, 2008). Therapist Peter Bernstein (2013) states "The vast majority of people with substance abuse problems have a traumatic past" (p. 16). Peer pressure, ease of access, and the stresses of school and family may also increase adolescent vulnerability. Rebellion from parental or religious values also may increase the risk for substance abuse. Psychological factors, including a need for immediate gratification and the insecurity and low self-esteem associated with adolescence, play a role as adolescents find pleasure or decreased levels of anxiety and inhibition with substance use. A study of teenagers portrayed in movies found that one in five actors drank alcohol, negative consequences were rarely filmed, and seldom did a character refuse an invitation to drink or use drugs (Stern & Morr, 2013).

Substance abuse in adolescence is a serious issue. According to the *Results from the 2011 National Survey on Drug Use and Health*, 10.1% of 12- to 17-year-olds reported using illicit drugs (Substance Abuse and Mental Health Services Administration [SAMHSA], 2012a). Use and abuse of substances are associated with risk behaviors, injuries, violence, and greater risk of acquiring a sexually transmitted infection (Centers for Disease Control and Prevention [CDC], 2012).

---

hol use. On the other hand, interest in religion/spirituality practices was correlated with lower alcohol use (Haber, Koenig, & Jacob, 2011).

Recent research has looked at the association of sexual orientation and substance use. It found that lesbian and bisexual women are at greater risk for alcohol and drug use disorders. On the other hand, gay and bisexual men are at greater risk for illicit drug use. Affiliation with the gay culture and HIV status are correlated with increased substance abuse (Green & Feinstein, 2012).

Many factors place an individual at risk for substance use, abuse, and dependence. No single cause can explain why one individual develops a pattern of drug use and another person does not.

Lifespan Considerations

Children encounter dramatic physical, emotional, and lifestyle changes as they move from adolescence into young adulthood. Developmental transitions, such as puberty and increasing independence, have been associated with alcohol use. Research shows that many adolescents start to drink at very young ages. According to data from the 2012 Monitoring the Future study (Johnston et al., 2013), an annual survey of U.S. adolescents, over half (54%) of 12th graders and more than one seventh (13%) of 8th graders report having been drunk at least once in their life. In 2012, one quarter (24%) of 12th graders reported **binge drinking** (having five or more drinks in a row at least once in the prior 2 weeks). Added to the statistics about drinking, the survey discovered that 1 in 15 (6.5%) high school seniors is a daily, or near-daily, marijuana user. As far as legal cigarettes, 1 in 6 (16%) 8th graders has tried smoking, and nearly 1 in 20 (5%) is currently smoking. By 12th grade, more than a third (40%) have tried smoking, and nearly 1 in 6 (17%) is currently smoking.

The brain continues to develop well into the twenties, during which time it continues to establish important communication connections and further refines its function. This lengthy developmental period may help explain some of the risk-taking behavior that is characteristic of adolescence. For some adolescents, thrill-seeking might include experimenting with alcohol and drugs. Developmental changes also offer a possible physiological explanation for why teens act impulsively, often not recognizing that their risky behaviors have consequences.

The number of middle-aged adults who abuse alcohol, prescription medications, and illicit drugs is growing. Substance abuse among people 50 years old and older is expected to more than double by 2020 (Wu & Blazer, 2011). A survey by the Hanley Center, a Florida-based drug and alcohol treatment and recovery facility, found that 40% of its alumni reported that the onset of their substance abuse occurred after age 48 (Singer, 2012).

Although genetic predisposition continues to be a major factor in the development of addiction, many other reasons have been suggested for the increasing substance abuse in this population. Substance use seems to buffer the pain of developmental and situational stressors such as the empty-nest syndrome, divorce, unemployment, retirement, health setbacks, and the death of a parent or spouse. Depression may be one of the biggest precursors to addiction, especially between the ages of 45 and 60. The abuse of substances, especially of alcohol and prescription drugs, among adults ages 60 and older is one of the fastest growing health problems facing the United States (National Institute on Aging, 2012).

Substance abuse in older adults is believed to be underestimated, underidentified, underdiagnosed, and undertreated. Until relatively recently, alcohol and prescription drug misuse, which affects a growing number of older adults, was not discussed in either the substance abuse or the gerontological literature. For example, alcohol use disorders affect 1% to 3% of older adults. But researchers believe that might still be an underestimate (Caputo et al., 2012).

Insufficient knowledge, limited research data, and hurried office visits are cited as causes for why healthcare providers often overlook substance abuse and misuse in this population. Diagnosis is often difficult because symptoms of substance abuse in older individuals sometimes mimic symptoms of other medical and behavioral disorders common among older adults, such as diabetes, dementia, and depression. Additionally, many older adults do not seek treatment for substance abuse because they do not feel they need it (Wu & Blazer, 2011).

▶ ALTERATIONS FROM NORMAL

Addiction can take many different forms, some of which are discussed later in this module.

Addiction to nicotine, which is considered by some to be one of the most highly addictive substances, may lead to multiple

health problems. Some of these include cancers of the lungs, bladder, and colon; heart disease; premature aging; and hypertension. Substance abuse is increasing in the United States and impacts the drug user, the user's family, and society as a whole. In 2011, an estimated 22.5 million Americans ages 12 or older were current (past month) illicit drug users, meaning they had used an illicit drug during the month prior to the survey interview (**Figure 22–2 ●**). This estimate represents 8.7% of the population ages 12 or older.

Substance abuse has a high rate of morbidity with both physical and mental illness (see the Concepts Related to Addiction feature). Imaging scans, chest x-rays, and blood tests show the damaging effects of drug abuse throughout the body. For example, tests show that tobacco smoke causes cancer of the mouth, throat, larynx, blood, lungs, stomach, pancreas, kidney, bladder, and cervix. Some drugs of abuse, such as inhalants, are toxic to nerve cells and may damage or destroy them either in the brain or the peripheral nervous system.

Medical illnesses can be promoted or exacerbated by neglect of one's health and lack of preventive health care. Immunity is often compromised by malnutrition, poor hygiene, and risky behaviors related to addiction. Some infectious diseases, such as hepatitis A, B, and C, HIV and AIDS, and tuberculosis, are transmitted by substance abuse, either directly or indirectly. The central nervous system (CNS) is probably the body system most profoundly affected by the effects of acute and chronic alcohol use. The adverse CNS effects are seen in manifestations of substance dependance, tolerance, craving, and withdrawal. Chronic alcohol use can also lead to varying degrees of dementia or organic brain disease. Wernicke syndrome and Korsakoff psychosis are two such syndromes that are tied to alcoholism. Addiction behaviors affect the mental health and physical health of the addicted client as well as the client's family.

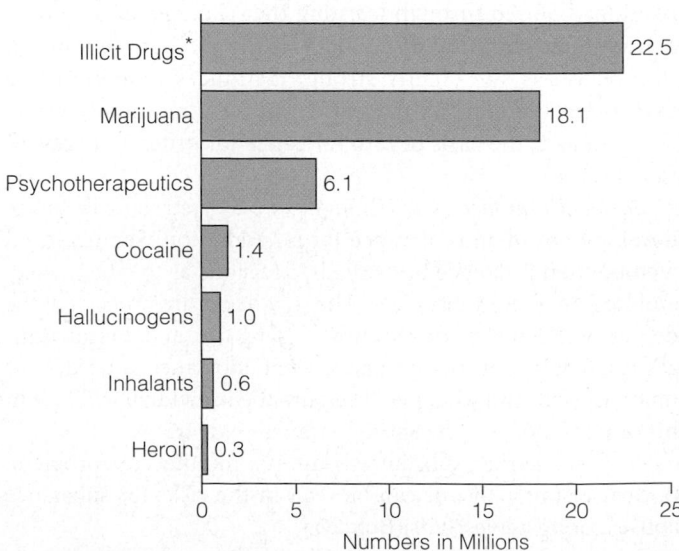

Figure 22–2 ● Past month illicit drug use among individuals ages 12 or older, 2011.

*Illicit drugs include marijuana/hashish, cocaine (including crack), heroin, hallucinogens, inhalants, or prescription-type psychotherapeutics used nonmedically.

Concepts Related to **Addiction**

Addiction interrupts family processes, resulting in rigid boundaries and a closed family system. Family members take on the shame of addiction, keeping it secret from those outside the family and going to great lengths to protect or enable the family member who is addicted. Abuse of substances affects an individual's nutritional status, decreasing intake of healthy nutrients as well as decreasing the body's ability to synthesize antibodies due to lack of appropriate intake. Substance use also impacts cognitive ability, including slowing reaction times, decreasing inhibitions, and impairing judgment and memory. Individuals often use substances as a method of coping, replacing healthy coping mechanisms with unhealthy ones.

CONCEPT	RELATIONSHIP TO ADDICTION	NURSING IMPLICATIONS
Family		
■ Interrupted family processes ■ Closed family system ■ Rigid boundaries	↑ Substance use and abuse of family member → ↑ Family secrecy → ↑ Family isolation → ↓ Supportive resources available	■ Determine family understanding of substance abuse and addiction. ■ Communicate clearly, honestly, openly, and without judgment. ■ Anticipate involving the entire family in all aspects of the treatment process.
Nutrition		
■ Poor nutritional status	↓ Nutritional status → ↓ Body's ability to synthesize antibodies	■ Be alert to signs/symptoms of malnutrition and opportunistic infections. ■ Anticipate the need for a nutritional assessment, balanced diet, vitamin and mineral supplements. ■ Provide discharge planning that promotes client's ability to meet nutritional needs.
Cognition		
	↓ B_1 (thiamine) in the brain can cause changes in cognition, specifically confusion ↓ Memory, judgment, reaction times, cognitive ability	■ Assess for Wernicke encephalopathy, Korsakoff psychosis, and dementia. ■ Provide for client safety. ■ Anticipate provision of thiamine therapy.
Stress and Coping		
■ ↑ Anxiety	↑ Ego defense mechanisms to ↓ anxiety ■ Denial ■ Minimization ■ Rationalization ■ Projection	■ Assess for use of ego defense mechanisms. ■ Assist client in gaining insight into defensive coping patterns. ■ Provide safe and nonjudgmental environment. ■ Anticipate need for an interprofessional healthcare team collaboration in treatment planning.
Safety		
	↑ in risk-taking behaviors leads to ↑ in risk for injury, violence, and HIV.	■ Assess for risk behaviors, including driving under the influence, unprotected sex, sharing needles. ■ Provide education related to safety. ■ Anticipate denial, family interference, or enabling.

Alterations and Manifestations

Substance abusers have a higher incidence of mental health disorders than the general population. Researchers have estimated that more than 40% of individuals treated for substance abuse present with at least one current independent mood disorder (Pettinati & Dundon, 2011).

The depression that may be a part of the addiction process itself must be differentiated from a diagnosable Axis I mental health disorder. Because drug abuse and addiction—both of which are mental disorders—often co-occur with other mental illnesses, clients presenting with one condition should be assessed for the other(s). And when these problems co-occur, treatment should address both (or all), including the use of medications as appropriate.

Individuals who abuse substances commonly present with numerous social problems. Educational backgrounds vary. Many high-functioning addicts may appear to have intact employment, relationship, and family situations. Others may be unemployed or underemployed, lacking job skills or work experience. Some are homeless, have been incarcerated, and face significant barriers in accessing safe and affordable housing.

Substance abuse can have particularly devastating consequences for families, because it increases the family members' risk for social isolation and decreases their access to social supports that can be helpful to those experiencing addiction and their families. Typically, defensive coping mechanisms (particularly denial) arise as family members find themselves unable to cope with the addiction in a healthy way. Substance abuse can also interfere with normal family processes, from day-to-day activities related to parenting to long-term changes such as role reversals, with older children taking on caregiving responsibilities.

Addiction within the family is often cloaked in secrecy and shame and is very disruptive to the family as a whole. The individual who is addicted is unable to control her substance use (or, the case

of process addiction, excessive, compulsive behavior) and will use any means necessary to satisfy her need for the substance. Family members, in an effort to protect the family and the addicted member from discovery, often become very closed to the outside world.

Often, the term **boundaries** is used when talking about interpersonal relationships and addiction. While such boundaries are not physical ones like those seen in property boundaries, they do represent a type of relationship safety zone around a family and its members. Children and parents in healthy relationships have boundaries that are usually dictated by their role in the family. For example, the parent takes care of the children, the co-habiting adult couple has an intimate personal and physical relationship, and the child is a friend to peers and other children. Normally, boundaries around families are flexible, allowing members to interact with those outside of the family and with the community as needed and desired. Clear boundaries keep people safe within functional relationships. When addiction is present in a family, these boundaries often become rigid and inflexible. These boundaries do not let information about the family needs or requests for needed assistance "out" and do not allow input or assistance from those outside of the family.

In these families, the nonaddicted members are often seen as enablers, inadvertent supporters of the addicts' behaviors.

Alterations and Therapies **Addictions**

ALTERATION	DESCRIPTION	TREATMENT
Nicotine addiction	Addiction to nicotine can result from smoking tobacco in the form of cigarettes, cigars, or pipes as well as from chewing tobacco.	■ Medications (e.g., nicotine gum, Chantix, nicotine nasal spray) ■ Behavior therapy ■ Support groups
Alcohol addiction	Chronic use of alcohol can lead to addiction resulting in delirium tremens (DTs) if alcohol is not consumed.	■ Medications (e.g., Antabuse) ■ Behavioral therapy ■ Support groups ■ 12-step program (e.g., Alcoholics Anonymous [AA]) ■ Detoxification ■ Milieu therapy ■ Family therapy
Substance addiction	Substance addiction may include abuse of heroin, cocaine, marijuana, crack, narcotics, barbiturates, inhalants, or any chemical substance that leads to addiction.	■ Behavior therapy ■ Support groups ■ Detoxification ■ Pharmacologic therapy, which may be required to minimize complications from withdrawal ■ Removal of peers providing substance ■ Milieu therapy ■ 12-step programs (e.g., Narcotics Anonymous [NA]) ■ Family therapy
Process addictions (sex, gambling, shopping, work)	Process addictions are those behaviors compulsively performed to reduce anxiety; they are considered by some to be a form of obsessive-compulsive disorder.	■ Psychotherapy ■ Behavior therapy ■ Milieu therapy ■ Support groups ■ 12-step programs (e.g., Gambler's Anonymous) ■ Family therapy

Enabling behavior is any action an individual takes that consciously or unconsciously facilitates substance dependence. Examples of enabling include family members making excuses to employers or teachers or discontinuing their own social relationships with friends or neighbors in order to preserve the "healthy image" of the family in the community. In families where addiction is present, communication is poor within and outside of the family system. Isolation results in an escalating cycle of addiction and dysfunction for the entire family. It is important for healthcare providers to recognize that shame and fear often lead to this isolation. A nonjudgmental approach to assessment and intervention, coupled with empathy and respect, is essential when working with those who are addicted to substances and their families. Substance abuse sometimes correlates with a history of abuse, particularly domestic and sexual abuse, economic instability, criminal behavior, and educational upheaval. Addiction is a family disease and should be viewed and treated within the context of the family.

The Language of Addiction and Recovery

The process of addiction and recovery has its own vocabulary. These terms are used by professionals from all aspects of health care who work with substance-abusing clients and their families. Many of these terms are appropriate regardless of the substance or process being abused. See **Table 22–1** ● for a list of some of these terms and their definitions.

Effects of Addiction on Families

As discussed earlier, substance abuse is a family problem. It alters both family problems and behaviors of individual family members. The longer the addiction continues, the further

entrenched family members become in behaviors that further the addiction, such as denial and enabling. This codependency, in which the behaviors of the addict and those of the family revolve around the addiction and their shared behaviors in service of the addiction, harms the family. Children may carry these behaviors into adulthood, taking on specific characteristics beyond the family relationship. Characteristics of codependent individuals are described in **Box 22–2** ●. A number of support networks and groups, including Adult Children of Alcoholics and Al-Anon, exist to help family members learn about and recover from the effects of addiction.

Children growing up in a household with a parent who is addicted to drugs or alcohol face a number of challenges. Parents often neglect their responsibilities for drugs, alcohol, or other behaviors, up to and including diverting household funds to pay for their addiction. Parents may disappear for hours or days at a time, and even when at home, they may become both emotionally and physically unavailable to their children. Parental judgment becomes impaired, and in some cases, children are exposed to criminal activity.

Because of the secrecy and shame associated with substance abuse, children of addicts do not generally talk about their own feelings, needs, and wants; some do not feel at all. Typically, these children are expected to be in control of their behavior and feelings at all times and are expected to be perfect and never make mistakes.

While some children growing up in families with an addicted member have obvious and apparent problems, others cope quite well. Children's alleged coping styles are widely discussed, but efforts to verify these behavior patterns have generally been unsuccessful. One common coping strategy that children may adopt focuses on the family roles they may

TABLE 22–1 Terminology Associated With Substance Abuse

TERM	DEFINITION
Abstinence	Voluntarily going without drugs or alcohol
Codependence	A cluster of maladaptive behaviors exhibited by significant others of a substance-abusing individual that serves to enable and protect the abuse at the expense of living a full and satisfying life
Co-occurring disorders	Concurrent diagnosis of a substance use disorder and a psychiatric disorder; one disorder can precede and cause the other, such as the theorized relationship between alcoholism and depression
Cross-tolerance	Tolerance to one drug conferring tolerance to another drug
Delirium tremens (DTs)	A medical emergency usually occurring 3–5 days following alcohol withdrawal and lasting 2–3 days; characterized by paranoia, disorientation, delusions, visual hallucinations, elevated vital signs, vomiting, diarrhea, and diaphoresis; also known as alcohol withdrawal delirium
Detoxification	The process of helping an addicted individual safely through withdrawal; commonly referred to as detox
Dual diagnosis	The coexistence of substance abuse/dependence and a psychiatric disorder in one individual (used interchangeably with dual disorder and co-occurring disorders)
Korsakoff psychosis	Secondary dementia caused by thiamine (B_1) deficiency that may be associated with chronic alcoholism; characterized by progressive cognitive deterioration, confabulation, peripheral neuropathy, and myopathy
Physical dependence	A state in which withdrawal syndrome will occur if drug use is discontinued
Polysubstance abuse	The simultaneous use of many substances
Psychological dependence	An intensive, subjective need for a particular psychoactive drug
Sobriety	The state of habitual refrain from using alcohol or drugs
Tolerance	A state in which a particular dose elicits a smaller response than it formerly did; with increased tolerance, the individual needs higher and higher doses to obtain the desired response
Withdrawal syndrome	A constellation of signs and symptoms that occurs in physically dependent individuals when they discontinue drug use

Box 22–2 Characteristics of Codependent Individuals

- Have low self-esteem.
- Have an exaggerated sense of responsibility for others' actions.
- Feel guilty when they assert themselves.
- Deny that they have a problem; think the problem is someone else or the situation.
- Tend to become hurt when their efforts aren't recognized.
- Have a tendency to become obsessed with other people's problems.
- Do more than their share of work all of the time; have trouble saying "no" to anyone.
- Need approval and recognition.
- Fear being abandoned or alone.
- Have difficulty identifying their feelings.
- Have difficulty adjusting to change.
- Struggle with intimacy and boundaries.
- Have poor communication skills.
- Have difficulty making decisions.
- Experience painful emotions.
- Offer advice whether it has been asked for or not.
- Feel like a victim.
- Use manipulation, share, or guilt to control others' behavior.

Sources: Based on Mental Health America. (2013). *Co-dependency.* Retrieved from http://www.mentalhealthamerica.net/go/codependency; Lancer, D. (2012). *Symptoms of codependency.* Retrieved from http://psychcentral.com/lib/2012/symptoms-of-codependency/; Recovery Connection. (2012). *Top ten indicators that you suffer from codependency.* Retrieved from http://www.recoveryconnection.org/top-ten-indicators-that-you-suffer-from-codependency.

assume. In dysfunctional families, these self-designated roles can serve to keep the family balanced. A familiar typology of roles that children adopt includes the *family hero*, the *lost child*, the family *mascot*, and the *scapegoat* (National Council on Alcoholism and Drug Abuse, 2009). The common denominator to these roles is that each in its own way is an attempt to cope and survive. The danger is that children may get frozen in these childhood roles for life. Growing up without mature adult role models, these children may deny the stresses of their dysfunctional families and this denial may become a frequent defense mechanism as they proceed through life. Some grow up to repeat the family pattern by becoming addicted themselves or marrying an addicted person.

Prevalence

Substance abuse in the United States is so common that very few people are unaffected by it.

- In 2011, an estimated 22.5 million Americans ages 12 or older (8.7% of the population) had used an illicit drug or abused a psychotherapeutic medication in the past month (National Institute on Drug Abuse [NIDA], 2012b).
- Abuse of tobacco, alcohol, and illicit drugs is costly; in the United States, the costs related to crime, lost work productivity, and health care are estimated to be $600 billion annually (NIDA, 2013c).
- In 2009, 4.8 million Americans ages 12 or older abused cocaine in any form, and 1.0 million abused crack at least once in the year prior to the survey (NIDA, 2011a).

- In 2011, an estimated 18.1 million people used marijuana (an increase of 5.8% since 2007) (NIDA, 2012b).
- In 2008 there were 114,000 first-time users of heroin ages 12 and older (NIDA, 2010b).
- The Drug Abuse Warning Network (DAWN) estimated that 4.5 million drug-related visits were made to emergency departments (EDs) in general-purpose hospitals, and that drug-related ED visits have increased by more than 80% since 2004 (SAMHSA, 2011).

These statistics only scratch the surface of the number of people dealing with addiction. These figures in combination with figures related to process addictions demonstrate the need for nurses to understand, recognize, and be able to screen clients for past and present addictions and behaviors.

CASE STUDY \\ PART 1

Paul is the 19-year-old son of Mark and Susan John. The Johns have been married for 20 years. Mrs. Johns is a full-time, stay-at-home mom. Paul's dad is a corporate attorney who has always been somewhat demanding of his wife and children. He drinks alcohol daily but has always been employed and has maintained a middle-class lifestyle for his family. Paul has two younger sisters: Mara, the younger of the two, has been treated for anorexia since the age of 12. His 15-year-old sister, Jess, is doing well in high school. Paul did well in high school where he played varsity soccer and did fairly well academically.

Paul has just returned home from his first full year at college. His mother is concerned because he doesn't seem like his old self; he shows no interest in his old friends or in getting a summer job. On the other hand, he seems secretive and has left the house on many occasions claiming that he has new friends who "get it." He is very short tempered with his sisters, constantly irritable and discontent. He is very evasive when asked about his grades or any college activities. He has noticeable weight loss and appears unkempt. His father is intolerant of his behavior. His mother is concerned and has arranged to accompany him on a visit to his primary care provider. She is hoping to find out what his problem is so it can be treated before his father becomes angrier with him and his behavior. You are the nurse who is assessing Paul.

Clinical Reasoning Questions Level I

1. Describe the elements of the interview/assessment environment that you should consider before beginning Paul's client assessment.
2. What questions would be appropriate in assessing Paul's physiological, emotional, and psychological status?
3. What elements of the family history might indicate a potential for substance use or abuse in Paul?

Clinical Reasoning Questions Level II

4. If substance abuse is suspected, how should you proceed to address any ego defense mechanisms displayed?
5. What diagnostic measures might be needed based on your assessment?
6. If depression is suspected, what further assessments would you perform?

▶ PREVENTION

Prevention efforts related to substance abuse generally revolve around education. Federal initiatives include prevention efforts by the Substance Abuse and Mental Health Services Administration (SAMHSA) and other federal organizations. Community and local initiatives, often sponsored as collaborations among law enforcement and local health and mental health professionals, may be developed to target needs in a specific community. At the individual level, nurses and other healthcare professionals assess clients' risk for substance abuse and provide education related to prevention, especially related to using healthy coping mechanisms and obtaining appropriate treatment for existing mental health disorders, such as depression.

Stay Current: SAMHSA offers a registry of evidence-based prevention and treatment programs at **http://nrepp.samhsa.gov**.

▶ ASSESSMENT

A trusting nurse–client relationship, along with the nurse's ethical obligation to maintain confidentiality, may help the client share information more freely. By including family members in the assessment process, nurses may uncover addictions the client is hiding. Nurses must help clients understand the importance of full disclosure of any addictions to protect them from potential treatment complications, such as administration of a narcotic to someone with a narcotic addiction. All too often clients fail to admit addiction until permanent damage has already

Assessment Interview Crisis

Individual Assessment

1. What is the most significant stress/problem occurring in your life right now?
2. Has this problem increased the frequency of substance use? (Quantify change in frequency or amount of substance used.)
3. Is your addiction behavior causing or contributing to the problem?
4. Who is the problem, or your addiction behavior, impacting? You? Your family? Your employer? The community?
5. How long has this been a problem?
6. Is this a temporary or permanent problem?
7. What does this problem mean to you?
8. What are the factors that cause this problem to continue?
9. Would the problem resolve if you stopped abusing the substance?
10. Have you had similar stresses/problems in the past?
11. What other stresses do you have in your life?
12. How are you managing your usual life roles (partner, parent, homemaker, worker, student, etc.)?
13. In what way has your life changed as a result of this problem?
14. Are you feeling as though you want to harm yourself or others?
15. Describe how you have managed problems in the past.
16. What have you done to try to solve the problem so far?
17. What happened when you tried this?
18. Describe possible resources (e.g., family, friends, employer, teacher; financial, spiritual).
19. Are you interested in abstaining from substance abuse? Are you considering a rehabilitation program?
20. What are your expectations and hopes concerning this problem?
21. What is the most you hope for when this problem is resolved?
22. What is the least you will settle for to resolve this problem?
23. What part of the overall problem is most important to deal with first?

Family Assessment

1. How do you perceive the current problem and the client's addiction behavior?
2. In what way has the problem and the client's addiction behavior affected your roles in the family?
3. How has your lifestyle changed since this problem began?
4. Describe communication within the family before this current problem.
5. Describe communication within the family since the problem began.
6. How does the family typically manage problems?
7. What has the family done to try and solve the problem so far?
8. What has the family done to try to stop the addiction behavior?
9. What happened when you tried this?
10. How well do you believe the family is coping at this time?
11. Describe possible resources (e.g., extended family, friends; financial).
12. What are your expectations and hopes concerning this problem and the client's addiction behavior?
13. Which part of the overall problem is most important to deal with first?
14. Can the problem be resolved without resolution of the addiction behavior?

Community Assessment

1. What are the special demands of the client's community?
2. What are the living conditions of the neighborhood?
3. Are recreational centers available?
4. Are affordable child care services available?
5. Is there a community mental health center?
6. What support groups are available in the community?
7. Is there a rehabilitation center to help the client resolve addiction behavior issues?
8. Are there any possible funding resources?

occurred. The nurse's responsibility is to recognize clues while complications are still preventable.

Nursing Assessment

The nursing history plays an important role in determining potential addictive behavior. Clients may feel shame, contempt, or embarrassment about revealing their addiction. In addition, fear of legal reprisal may cause the client to be reluctant to share information if the addiction is to an illegal substance.

Clients also may need to be assessed regarding the extent of crisis they are facing in their lives as the result of their addiction behaviors, particularly if a crisis event or behavior motivates them to seek health care. The Assessment Interview feature provides a general crisis assessment that can be used in any problem-solving situation. It is of particular use for the client whose crisis is the result of addiction behavior.

Physical Assessment

Physical assessment findings depend on the nature of the addiction. Clients with an addiction to self-inflicted wounding, called *cutting*, may have many unexplained lacerations, often located in areas that are covered by clothing. Clients addicted to narcotics may demonstrate symptoms described in the exemplar on Substance Abuse later in this module. When performing a physical assessment, nurses must be alert for symptoms that are abnormal or not within expected boundaries and assess client explanations for inconsistencies. Unless the client comes to the provider under the influence or is referred by an employer, the physical examination may provide the first indications that an addiction is involved.

Diagnostic Tests

Diagnostic tests required for clients with addiction will be ordered based on the type of addiction they display. Specific diagnostic tests will be ordered for each type of addiction and may include:

- Serum drug levels
- Toxicology testing
- Chest x-ray for inhaled substances
- Organ biopsies related to damage caused by substance
- Urine, saliva, and serum testing for substance metabolites
- Hair testing to determine substance use within a period of 90 days.

CASE STUDY \\ PART 2

Paul is admitted to the emergency department (ED) at 2 a.m. on a Sunday morning in August as the result of a motor vehicle crash. His speech is slurred and his gate is ataxic. He is bleeding from a laceration on his left forehead and he is complaining that his left arm is extremely painful and "falling off." A decision is made to admit Paul to the trauma unit. His father, as next of kin, is notified of the admission. His father states, "I knew this would happen. Let him rot." Paul becomes combative as you attempt to assess his state of consciousness and physical injuries.

Clinical Reasoning Questions Level I

1. You suspect substance use. What are your immediate concerns?
2. How will you promote Paul's cooperation with your assessment and eventual treatment?
3. What specific diagnostic tests will be appropriate related to both his suspected substance use and his physical injuries?

Clinical Reasoning Questions Level II

4. *Refer to the module on Legal Issues:* Are you able to begin assessment and treatment of Paul without consent from next-of-kin? What are the legal implications in this situation?
5. Paul's mother arrives in the ED. She is very upset and demanding to see him. Will you involve Paul's mother in his care? Why or why not?

▶ INTERVENTIONS AND THERAPIES

Nurses may use a number of independent and collaborative caring interventions with clients who are addicted or who exhibit addiction behaviors. **Recovery** is generally defined as a state of voluntary sobriety in which the individual maintains personal health and functions normally within society without the use of the addictive substance or behavior. The goal of all interventions is to move the client toward treatment and into recovery. For the addict, recovery is a lifelong process. Nurses must remember that no single intervention is sufficient to ensure permanent recovery, which requires substantial and continual work on the part of the addict. All interventions, even pharmacologic therapies, have one thing in common: They begin with successful communication.

Independent

Nursing interventions for clients with addictive behaviors primarily focus around nursing care for any specific presenting symptoms, developing and maintaining the therapeutic nurse–client relationship (including establishing and maintaining appropriate boundaries), and promoting healthy client communication and coping skills. See the module on Stress and Coping for a discussion about defense mechanisms and nursing interventions to help clients develop healthy coping skills.

COMMUNICATION Respect, empathy, and caring are essential components of caring for those with addictions. When nurses care for the client with an addiction, whether it is a substance or a process addiction, establishing a therapeutic nurse–client relationship involves the use of therapeutic communication, which places the client at the center of all communication. This is critical for two reasons: (a) Many clients with addictions have poor communication skills and rely on their addictive behaviors to avoid communicating with others, and (b) clients with addictions are experienced at hiding their addictions and avoiding the addiction as the topic of discussion. Although therapeutic communication is discussed in detail in the exemplar on Therapeutic Communication in the module on Communication, it is important here to discuss aspects of communication that greatly benefit the client with an addiction and family members.

Many clients with addictions or addictive behaviors need assistance with verbal and nonverbal communication. It is important for nurses to encourage clients to use facial expressions, eye contact, posture, gestures, and interpersonal distance to enhance communication. They should keep in mind that nonverbal communication is culturally determined and teach within those cultural expectations. Nurses can give examples of how being aware of nonverbal communication helps build relationships. Finally, nurses should ask clients to demonstrate a thought or feeling (e.g., happiness, anger) without using words. The goal is to increase clients' awareness of his nonverbal communication and that of others.

Conversation is another social skill. Nurses should discuss volume, tone, and rate of speech and model taking turns speaking and not interrupting. They should have clients practice skills such as initiating conversations, asking questions, making appropriate self-disclosures, and ending conversations gracefully. Assertiveness training is appropriate for clients who are either passive or aggressive in their style of relating to others. Assertive people are able to say no to unreasonable demands and to activities in which they do not want to participate. They are able to express positive and negative feelings in an appropriate manner and accept constructive criticism and praise from other people. Assertiveness may be inappropriate in some cultures, especially those in which children and teens are not allowed to disagree with parents or those in which women are expected to be obedient and submissive to men.

Collaborative

Treatment for addiction may be determined by level of severity and how the individual comes to seek treatment. Some clients are adjudicated to treatment by the judicial system. Clients with severe impairment of function may be involuntarily admitted or may be admitted for medical care associated with an injury. These are some of the many factors that influence individual client plans of care.

In some cases, individuals seek care after being persuaded they need care through a process of confrontation called **intervention**. The goal of intervention is to prevent the addict from denying the problem and force her to face the negative aspects of behavior and enroll in treatment, typically in a residential treatment facility. In *family intervention* the family enlists the help of a professional clinician to conduct the intervention with the participation of the family. The clinician and family confront the individual together, with family members stating how the individual's addiction affects the family.

Regardless of the timing of the intervention, the family should make preparations in advance for the addict to enter rehabilitation immediately after the meeting, if the individual agrees to seek help. Waiting hours or days can result in a change of mind as the addict's withdrawal or addiction symptoms escalate.

Frequently individuals come to treatment because the cycle of addiction results in a deteriorating ability of the client to manage life skills and events, often resulting in a crisis situation. It is not atypical for crises associated with addiction to result in legal ramifications for a client. Some situations in which clients may encounter the legal system as a result of their addiction include impaired driving citations and vehicle crashes, child custody disputes, separation and divorce, and violent encoun-

ters. It is during these crisis situations when addicts are most likely to be motivated to seek help to treat their addiction and turn their lives around. The inability to maintain emotional equilibrium is an important feature of a crisis. The state of disequilibrium usually lasts 4–6 weeks. Typically, the high level of anxiety during this short period forces the individual to do one of the following:

- Adapt and return to the previous level of addiction.
- Develop more constructive coping skills and seek help for the addiction.
- Decompensate to a lower level of functioning.

During this time, people are most receptive to professional intervention. A thorough assessment of support and previous coping behaviors includes an evaluation of the client's self-destructive feelings and behavior. Treatment options include individual behavioral therapy, milieu therapy, group therapy, self-help groups, and family therapy all of which are described below. If the level of impairment caused by the addiction is severe, or if there is considerable threat to client safety, inpatient intervention may be necessary.

BEHAVIORAL THERAPY   In **behavioral therapy**, clients learn techniques to modify or change their addictive behaviors. Behavioral therapy is based on the principle that all behavior has specific consequences. Behavior is changed by conditioning—a process of reinforcement, punishment, and extinction.

Consequences that lead to an increase in a particular behavior are referred to as **reinforcement**. *Positive reinforcement* provides a reward for the desired behavior, such as the pleasant sensation, or high, that comes from the use of a substance. *Negative reinforcement* removes a negative stimulus to increase the chances that the desired behavior will occur. An example of negative reinforcement is when the family of an addict refuses to support the behavior that results from use of the substance. Consequences that lead to a decrease in undesirable behavior are referred to as **punishment**. *Positive punishment* is the addition of a negative consequence if the undesirable behavior occurs; for example, the addict who drives under the influence is jailed or fined. *Negative punishment* is the removal of a positive reward if the undesirable behavior occurs; for example, the addict who does not show up for work loses his job. **Extinction** refers to the progressive weakening of an undesirable behavior through repeated nonreinforcement of the behavior. For example, family members may choose to ignore negative attention-seeking behaviors such as making statements like "You're just trying to control my life." If the addict begins to see that these types of angry, provoking statements no longer elicit a response, he will (hopefully) be forced to find more appropriate ways to seek attention.

Most behavioral therapists believe that reinforcement is more desirable than punishment. There is no doubt that punishment is effective and sometimes necessary when the behavior is dangerous. But behavior changed through reinforcement is a more desirable clinical outcome than behavior changed through punishment. **Contingency contracts** may be an effective reinforcement process. These contracts operate by "if-then" rules. If the client performs a targeted response, such as abstinence from the addictive behavior (gambling, drug use, cutting, etc.), then the client receives desired reinforcers. Contingency contracts are only as effective as the rewards chosen (e.g., food treats, activities, or privileges). What one person considers a reward, another person may not. When a client is first learning the targeted behavior, rewards are given immediately, along with verbal praise and specific feedback. An example is "Good job. You admitted you have a problem. Here is the reward we talked about."

Token economies are formalized programs of contingency contracts. They are established for all members of a group and are often used with groups of addicts in treatment programs. The three parts of a token economy are as follows:

1. Identify behaviors that everyone in the group is expected to demonstrate.
2. Specify token rewards for doing those behaviors (e.g., if you face the problems you caused your family as a result of your addiction, you will receive 10 tokens); inappropriate behaviors are also identified for which tokens may be lost.
3. Establish rules for redeeming tokens: what types of activities or privileges may be swapped for tokens, how many tokens each one costs, and when and where tokens are swapped.

Behavioral therapy is well suited to treating addiction behavior because the client must alter familiar coping mechanisms and find means of reducing anxiety other than resorting to the source of the addiction. Nurses are in an ideal position to evaluate client response to treatment. Because they spend a great deal of time with clients, nurses can see developing patterns of behavioral change.

MILIEU THERAPY   The successful recovery environment involves creating a surrounding for the addict that will support behavior changes, teach new coping measures, and help the client move from addiction to an addiction-free life. This is often referred to as **milieu therapy**. In its earliest conception, *milieu* described a scientifically planned community. Research efforts focused on defining the types of environments that would be most therapeutic for the client facing addiction.

A. M. Kraft (1966) defined the idea of milieu more precisely as a therapeutic community in which the entire social structure of the unit or residence is designed to be part of the helping process. Kraft's idea of a therapeutic community emphasized the social and interpersonal interactions that become the therapeutic tools influencing change in client behavior. This view differed somewhat from the pure idea of milieu therapy, in which the emphasis was on "manipulation" of the environment to effect therapeutic change. The concepts inherent in milieu therapy are provided in residential substance abuse treatment programs, where individuals are provided interdisciplinary care. In addition to a thorough, focused assessment related to substance abuse, they receive a complete medical assessment. Individual and group therapy, family therapy, self-help groups, and other forms of intervention, including pharmacologic therapy, may be offered in different combinations based on client needs.

Hildegard Peplau (1952), the mother of psychiatric nursing theory, described the roles of the nurse in the therapeutic milieu. Peplau also described the *therapeutic use of self*, that is, using one's personhood to provide psychiatric nursing care. Within the nurse–client relationship, nurses use their personalities, beliefs, values, feelings, cognitions, and perceptions as they implement holistic nursing practice.

Milieu therapy has certain basic goals, whether the setting is a group home, a community center, a day program, or an inpatient unit. These goals include an emphasis on:

- Clients as responsible people
- Group and social interaction
- Client rights to choose and participate in a variety of treatments
- Informality of relationships with healthcare professionals.

Milieu therapy also includes clear communication, a safe environment, an activity schedule with therapeutic goals, and a support network. The overall goal behind all of these components is to support the changes in the client's behavior necessary to free the client from addiction. Within this environment, the nurse plays a pivotal role by modeling and teaching desirable behaviors. Often, the nurse is the member of the client's psychiatric team who spends the most time with, and around, the client. The nurse's observations of, and interactions with, the client provide information and opportunities critical to understanding the client's addiction behavior and to helping the client determine a successful path to recovery.

GROUP THERAPY   Therapeutic groups provide support to the members as they work through their problems. **Group therapy** is a beneficial experience in which the group members help each other with psychological, cognitive, behavioral, and spiritual dysfunctions through a process of change, aided by a professional group therapist.

Groups can be held in an inpatient unit, an outpatient clinic, a community mental health center, or a variety of other settings. Ballinger and Yalom (1995) identified mechanisms of change within a group and called them *curative factors* of group therapy. These factors provide a rationale for a variety of group interventions. **Table 22–2 ●** describes the curative factors.

Ballinger and Yalom (1995) also identified two concepts basic to group therapy: the group as a social microcosm and the here-and-now concept. The term **social microcosm** refers to the concept that group members eventually behave in the therapy group the same way they behave with families and friends. The group becomes a living example of how each member relates to others outside the group. The therapist's task is to help members recognize dysfunctional ways of relating to others. As group members interact with one another and discuss this process, individuals engage in self-reflection, leading to affective, behavioral, cognitive, and spiritual changes.

The **here-and-now concept** refers to the present moment of group experience. Although the past and the future have some importance, changes can be made only in the present. People who get stuck in the past ruminate over what was and what might have been. Others spend a great deal of time worrying about the future. The therapist's task is to keep the focus in the present by discussing what happens and why it happens.

Nurses function as group therapists in many different settings, establishing the type of group that is appropriate for the

TABLE 22–2   Curative Factors of Group Therapy

FACTOR	DESCRIPTION
Instillation of hope	As clients observe other members further along in the therapeutic process, they begin to feel a sense of hope for themselves.
Universality	Through interaction with other group members, clients realize they are not alone in their problems or pain.
Imparting of information	Teaching and suggestions usually come from the group leader but may also be generated by the group members.
Altruism	Through the group process, clients recognize that they have something to give to the other group members.
Corrective recapitulation of the primary family group	Many clients have a history of dysfunctional family relationships. The therapy group is often like a family, and clients can learn more functional patterns of communication, interaction, and behavior.
Development of socializing techniques	Development of social skills takes place in groups. Group members give feedback about maladaptive social behavior. Clients learn more appropriate ways of socializing with others.
Imitative behavior	Clients often model their behavior after the leader or other group members. This trial process enables them to discover what behaviors work well for them as individuals.
Interpersonal learning	Through the group process, clients learn the positive benefits of good interpersonal relationships. Emotional healing takes place through this process.
Existential factors	The group provides opportunities for clients to explore the meaning of their life and their place in the world.
Catharsis	Clients learn how to express their own feelings in a goal-directed way, speak openly about what is bothering them, and express strong feelings about other members in a responsible way.
Group cohesiveness	Cohesiveness occurs when members feel a sense of belonging.

Source: Adapted from Yalom, I. D., & Leszcz, M. (2005). *The theory and practice of group psychotherapy* (5th ed.). New York, NY: Basic Books.

desired outcomes. A single nurse may lead groups, or two cotherapists may share leadership. Initially, the members are strangers, and the leader, as the unifying force, helps the members relate to one another. Some of the important tasks of the group leader include (Ballinger & Yalom, 1995):

- Encouraging members to remain in the group
- Helping the group develop a sense of cohesiveness
- Establishing a code of behavior and norms with the group.

Group therapy can be effective with children and adolescents who may be addicts or the children of addicts. In working with young children, the size of the group is usually limited to five. Age and attention span determine the duration of the group session. Group therapy with children is usually activity oriented and may include daily goal setting, art projects, music or movement therapy, or play therapy.

Because adolescents can reason and talk about their behavior, thoughts, and feelings, group therapy with adolescents is a verbal process rather than the activity process used with children. Peers are very important in teenagers' lives, providing support, feedback, and information. As a result, group therapy with adolescents is often more productive than individual sessions.

There is often a parallel group for the parents of children and adolescents so that the entire family can receive treatment simultaneously. Such a group enables the parents to support each other, learn growth and developmental stages, gain an awareness of their contribution to family dynamics, increase parenting skills, and explore their own needs and problems.

Support Groups   Nurses frequently refer clients and their families to support groups, which are very important for mental health clients. In this type of group, members share their thoughts and feelings and help one another examine issues and concerns. The characteristics of support groups include the following:

- Clients define their own needs.
- Members have equal power.
- Groups may or may not be autonomous from mental health professionals.
- Attendance is voluntary.
- Groups may be responsive to a special population (e.g., a bilingual population); those with eating disorders; or those defined by racial, gender, or sexual identity.

Support groups function to educate community members; to help family and friends support the individual; and to act as a crisis support, a source of referrals, and an advocate to help people get their needs met through the healthcare system. Because people with addictions typically have a very restricted social network, often comprising others with similar addictions, it is important to help clients form a healthier base of support. This helps prevent recidivism into the addictive behavior they are seeking to resolve. As a result, the interpersonal contact of support groups is vitally important. These groups contribute to an increased self-esteem, a sense of identity, increased dignity, and improved self-responsibility.

Twelve-Step Programs   In the United States, an estimated 3.5 million people attend 12-step programs annually. Twelve-step programs are support groups that offer a spiritual plan for recovery. They include Al-Anon, Narcotics Anonymous, Cocaine Anonymous, Adult Children of Alcoholics, Emotions Anonymous, Gamblers Anonymous, Overeaters Anonymous, and Sex Addicts Anonymous.

The 12-step program consists of prescribed beliefs, values, and behaviors. The sequential plan for recovery is stated in 12

Box 22–3   The 12 Steps of Alcoholics Anonymous

WE

1. Admitted we were powerless over alcohol, that our lives had become unmanageable.
2. Came to believe that a Power greater than ourselves could restore us to sanity.
3. Made a decision to turn our will and our lives over to the care of God as we understood Him.
4. Made a searching and fearless moral inventory of ourselves.
5. Admitted to God, to ourselves, and to another human being the exact nature of our wrongs.
6. Were entirely ready to have God remove all these defects of character.
7. Humbly asked Him to remove our shortcomings.

8. Made a list of all persons we had harmed and became willing to make amends to them all.
9. Made direct amends to such people wherever possible, except when to do so would injure them or others.
10. Continued to take personal inventory and when we were wrong promptly admitted it.
11. Sought through prayer and meditation to improve our conscious contact with God as we understood Him, praying only for knowledge of His will for us and the power to carry that out.
12. Having had a spiritual awakening as the result of these steps, we tried to carry this message to alcoholics and to practice these principles in all our affairs.

Source: The Twelve Steps are reprinted with permission of Alcoholics Anonymous World Services, Inc. (A.A.W.S.). Permission to reprint the Twelve Steps does not mean that A.A.W.S. has reviewed or approves the contents of this publication, or that A.A.W.S. necessarily agrees with the views expressed herein. A.A. is a program of recovery from alcoholism only—use of the Twelve Steps in connection with programs and activities which are patterned after A.A., but which address other problems, or in any other non-A.A. context, does not imply otherwise.

---

steps, as described in **Box 22–3** ●. Step work is considered to be a lifelong process and is usually accomplished with the aid of a sponsor. Twelve-step fellowship includes the activities of the organization, such as helping others, building relationships among members, and sharing joys and hardships.

The only requirement for membership is the sincere desire to change the target behavior. Any interested person can attend open meetings. Closed meetings are reserved for members only. Some 12-step groups cater to demographic subsets such as women, men, adolescents, gays and lesbians, and nurses.

FAMILY THERAPY   Family therapy is a specialized area of study, and becoming a family therapist requires extensive preparation. In **family therapy**, the family system is treated as a unit and the focus is on family dynamics. The goals are to help families cope, improve their communication and interpersonal skills, establish boundaries, and moderate family cohesion and flexibility. Families strive to maintain balance and harmony. When an addicted member causes the balance to shift, families must use their internal and external resources to adapt. Competent families seem to adapt more efficiently than dysfunctional families.

Family therapy is recommended when the nurse or family determines that the family system is impaired because of the presence of a psychosocial problem or addiction in one or more family members. Schools, courts, and healthcare providers may identify impairment of family functioning. For family therapy to be successful, all family members must believe that they are part of the problem-solving and decision-making processes and that their personal welfare is always considered. Some advanced practice nurses provide home-based family therapy. This allows the nurse-therapist to observe the family in the natural setting of the home. Comfort with their environment encourages family members to participate. Direct observation illuminates family dynamics rather quickly and can effectively guide nursing interventions.

Family therapists help family members look at a number of issues. They assess the family hierarchy, which defines power relationships among the members. They identify subsystems—groups of people within the family who join together to perform various functions—such as the parental or sibling subsystem. Therapists identify and discuss boundaries, which define the degree of emotional closeness among family members and subsystems.

The overall goals of family therapy are to:

- Teach parents better parenting and nurturing skills.
- Reinstate generational boundaries in the family hierarchy.
- Improve family communication.
- Teach the family how to problem solve.

Although most nurses are not family therapists, this is not to say that nurses in the mental healthcare system do not intervene with families. Nurses in both inpatient and outpatient settings are likely to have a great deal of contact with their clients' families. Family members interact with nurses in a variety of situations, most of which are informal. When nurses work informally with families, they assess for a number of factors, including:

- Relationships among individual members of the family
- Roles that various members of the family assume
- Family communication patterns
- Achievement of the family's developmental tasks
- Normal coping strategies that the family uses
- Past and current efforts to cope with addiction
- Family support systems
- Sociocultural norms and values of the family
- Personal goals for each family member.

Disagreements and conflicts in family relationships are normal. The problem in families with an addictive member is not that they disagree, but that they do not know how to resolve their differences. Families dealing with a member's addiction often become so involved in dysfunctional behavior that they start to see this behavior as normal. Teaching families general principles for resolving conflict is a helpful nursing intervention. **Box 22–4** ● lists eight steps for resolving family disagreements.

PHARMACOLOGIC THERAPY   Pharmacologic therapies are available to treat and prevent symptoms of withdrawal and to treat overdose. Treating symptoms of withdrawal may involve reducing physiological cravings for the drug of choice, but it may

Box 22-4 Eight Steps Used to Resolve Family Disagreements

1. *Stay calm.* When people are calm, they think more clearly. People have difficulty remaining calm when they call each other names, become sarcastic, or drag up past injustices. Do not try to solve problems when members are angry.

2. *Express commitment to the relationship.* Arguments often leave people feeling like enemies rather than members of a caring family unit. It is important to defuse that by saying, "I love you. Let's work together to solve this problem."

3. *Identify areas of agreement or success.* Teach people to look for similarities in their viewpoints or to find positive characteristics in the other person. Family members often get stuck on arguing about one small point and overlook the fact that they agree on many other points.

4. *Identify the specific problem.* It is difficult to resolve problems when arguments keep escalating with the addition of more problems.

5. *Express the desired outcome.* Family members should clearly state what they want to happen so that everybody is clear about each other's goals.

6. *Listen carefully to the other person's concerns.* Each person needs to hear what the other person is saying. If necessary, have family members repeat the essence of what they heard to show that they understand. Problems cannot be solved if individuals are planning what they are going to say next, rather than listening carefully to what someone is saying to them.

7. *Seek solutions that benefit the relationship.* Teach family members to brainstorm possible solutions and to look for ways to compromise and meet everyone's needs.

8. *Assess the outcome.* Teach family members to analyze the solution before it is implemented. Does everyone feel respected and heard? Is everyone at least partially satisfied with the solution? If so, the conflict has probably been resolved successfully.

Medications **Addictions**

CLASSIFICATION AND DRUG EXAMPLES	MECHANISMS OF ACTION	NURSING CONSIDERATIONS
Opioid Antagonists *Drug example:* naloxone	Used to treat a narcotic overdose, these drugs block narcotic receptor sites and quickly reverse the effect of the narcotic if administered via IV therapy.	▪ Monitor client condition, including respiratory rate, and anticipate the need for pain management as narcotic effects are reversed.
Acetaldehyde Dehydrogenase Inhibitors *Drug example:* ▪ disulfiram	Inhibit the enzyme that metabolizes alcohol, causing the client to become violently ill if alcohol is consumed while taking this medication. Symptoms include shortness of breath, headache, nausea, and vomiting.	▪ Teach client to avoid all alcohol, including that found in substances such as mouthwash, liquid medications, and food. Use of this medication requires a client who is highly motivated. Assess client's motivational level to quit drinking.
Antiseizure Drugs *Drug examples:* ▪ phenytoin ▪ carbamazepine ▪ valproic acid	Raise the threshold of cerebral excitation, reducing the likelihood and severity of seizure activity that can occur as the result of withdrawal from substances such as sedatives and hypnotics.	▪ Implement seizure precautions to maintain client safety. If a seizure occurs, place a pillow under the client's head and time the seizure, noting client behavior during and after the event.
Nicotine Replacement Therapy *Drug examples:* ▪ nicotine patch ▪ nicotine gum ▪ nicotine lozenge ▪ nicotine nasal spray ▪ nicotine inhaler	Supplies the body with nicotine to support smoking cessation therapy.	▪ Client support is an important element of smoking cessation, and clients benefit from behavior modification teaching in addition to pharmacotherapy.
Antidepressants *Drug examples:* ▪ bupropion ▪ hydrochloride	Some antidepressants have been shown to reduce the craving for nicotine and support smoking cessation programs. Can also be administered to reduce depression occurring as the result of substance withdrawal.	▪ Monitor and question clients about thoughts of suicide. ▪ Assess for drug side effects, including drowsiness, insomnia, and blurred vision. ▪ Teach client about self-administration of medications and symptoms to report.
Nicotine Acetylcholine Receptor Agonists *Drug example:* ▪ varenicline	Stimulates nicotine receptors more weakly than nicotine itself does, reducing cravings for and decreasing the pleasurable effects of tobacco.	▪ Assess for nicotine withdrawal symptoms such as depression, agitation, and exacerbation of preexisting mental health disorders. ▪ Suicide and suicidal ideation have been associated with use of varenicline. Assess clients for thoughts of suicide or changes in mood and affect.

also involve reducing anxiety to prevent the client from feeding the addiction or to prevent dangerous symptoms associated with sudden withdrawal from powerful substances such as sedatives and hypnotics. A number of pharmacologic therapies are available. Many of these, however, have multiple drug interactions and should be used with caution. For example, disulfiram should never be used during pregnancy and should be used with caution in clients taking phenytoin. See the Medications feature.

> **SAFETY ALERT**
> Drugs of abuse alter the brain's structure and function, resulting in changes that persist long after drug use has ceased. This may explain why drug abusers are at risk for relapse even after long periods of abstinence and despite the potentially devastating consequences (NIDA, 2012a).

REVIEW The Concept of Addiction

RELATE Link the Concepts

Linking the concept of addiction with the concept of family:

1. In a family with rigid boundaries—those in which rules and roles remain fixed under all circumstances—what approach(s) might be optimal for gaining trust in and building a therapeutic relationship?

2. Considering the many treatment options for those with addictions, design a comprehensive treatment plan to meet the needs of a family such as the one that we have been exploring through our case study, the Johns family.

Linking the concept of addiction with the concept of immunity:

3. Dietary support is an essential component of recovery. Describe the diagnostic assessment for deficiencies in the B-complex vitamins, particularly thiamin, folate, and B_{12}, and the fat-soluble vitamins, A, D, and E.

4. Why are individuals with addictions prone to opportunistic infection?

READY Go to Companion Skills Manual

REFER Go to Pearson Nursing Student Resources nursing.pearsonhighered.com

- Additional review materials

REFLECT Case Study \\ Part 3

Reread Parts 1 and 2 of the Case Study.

It is 36 hours post-ED admission and Paul is being transferred from the trauma unit to a semiprivate room on a general medical-surgical unit. The scalp laceration is healing; there is no evidence of head injury. Paul's right humerus was fractured in the crash and a cast applied following a closed reduction. Laboratory studies revealed a blood alcohol level of 0.28 on admission. Paul now appears mildly anxious, and has a mild visible tremor of his hands. He is being prepared for discharge tomorrow. Admission to a substance abuse treatment program is being considered.

Clinical Reasoning Questions Level I

1. List at least three nursing diagnoses that would apply to Paul.

2. What members of the interprofessional (IP) healthcare team should be involved in Paul's care and discharge planning? Delineate the role of each team member.

3. Consider the impact of Paul's addiction on him and on his entire family.

4. Can Paul be treated independently of his family?

5. Give some specific examples of how family involvement could be planned by members of the IP team.

Clinical Reasoning Questions Level II

6. Identify comprehensive, measurable long-term treatment goals for Paul and his family.

7. Discuss inpatient, outpatient, and community treatment options for Paul and his family. Consider the advantages and disadvantages of each.

8. Consider the impact of cognition (both Paul's and his family's) in Paul's long-term treatment plan.

9. What lifestyle changes may be necessary for Paul and his family?

EXEMPLAR 22.1 Alcohol Abuse

EXEMPLAR KEY TERMS
Alcohol dependence, *1535*
Alcohol poisoning, *1539*
Alcohol withdrawal delirium, *1538*
Alcohol withdrawal syndrome, *1538*
Alcoholism, *1535*
Binge drinking, *1535*
Blackouts, *1538*
Confabulation, *1536*
Craving, *1536*
Korsakoff psychosis, *1536*
Phenotypes, *1536*
Polysubstance abuse, *1540*
Wernicke encephalopathy, *1536*

EXEMPLAR LEARNING OUTCOMES
After reading about this exemplar, you will be able to:

1. Describe the pathophysiology, psychopathology, etiology, clinical manifestations, and direct and indirect causes of alcohol abuse.

2. Identify risk factors associated with alcohol abuse.

3. Illustrate the nursing process in providing culturally competent care across the life span for individuals who abuse alcohol.

4. Formulate priority nursing diagnoses appropriate for an individual who abuses alcohol.

5. Summarize therapies used by interdisciplinary teams in the collaborative care of an individual who abuses alcohol.

6. Plan evidence-based care for an individual who abuses alcohol and his or her family in collaboration with other members of the healthcare team.

7. Evaluate expected outcomes for an individual who abuses alcohol.

▶ OVERVIEW

Alcohol includes liquor, beer, and wine. While much of society uses the use of nicotine and drugs as inappropriate, use of alcohol is still socially acceptable and often encouraged. Alcohol is frequently offered at weddings and other family events, beer is the favorite drink at sports venues across the country, and many grocery stores and restaurants now offer weekly or monthly wine tastings. The availability of alcohol may be the primary reason it is so widely abused. A recent estimate of the economic costs of alcohol abuse in the United States is $235 billion (NIDA, 2013c).

These costs result from losses in workplace productivity, healthcare expenses for problems caused by excessive drinking, law enforcement and other criminal justice expenses related to excessive alcohol consumption, and motor vehicle crash costs from impaired driving (6% of the total cost) (NIDA, 2013c).

Alcohol is the most commonly used and abused substance in the United States.

In 2011, slightly more than half (51.8%) of Americans ages 12 or older reported being current drinkers of alcohol. This translates to an estimated 133.4 million current drinkers (SAMHSA, 2012a). In 1992, the Joint Committee of the National Council on Alcoholism and Drug Dependence and the American Society of Addiction Medicine defined **alcoholism** as a "primary, chronic disease with genetic, psychosocial, and environmental factors influencing its development and manifestations" (Morse & Flavin, 1992). It is characterized by the behaviors discussed in the Concept section of this module: inability to control the primary addictive behavior (drinking), fixation with the drug and continued use of it regardless of consequences, and impaired thought processes.

The *pattern of dependence* on alcohol varies from person to person. Some people have a regular daily intake of large amounts of alcohol. Others restrict their use to heavy drinking on weekends or days off from work, often drinking copious amounts in a single session, a type of alcoholism known as **binge drinking**. Some people abstain for long periods of time and then begin their drinking patterns again. At times, people with alcohol dependence can drink with control; at other times, they cannot control the drinking behavior. As the course of alcoholism continues, addiction behaviors appear with increasing frequency. These may include starting the day off with a drink, sneaking drinks throughout the day, gulping alcoholic drinks, shifting from one alcoholic beverage to another, and hiding bottles at work and at home. An individual with alcoholism may give up hobbies and other interests in order to have more time to drink (Liska, 2008).

🔅 **Stay Current:** *Visit the Web site of the National Institute on Alcohol Abuse and Alcoholism to see current research on alcohol dependence:* **www.niaaa.nih.gov/publications/journals-and-reports/alcohol-research**.

▶ PATHOPHYSIOLOGY AND ETIOLOGY

Alcohol is a CNS depressant; as such, it acts on neurotransmitters in the brain, such as gamma-aminobutyric acid (GABA). GABA, the most prevalent inhibitory neurotransmitter in the brain, has a major role in decreasing neuronal excitability. Alcohol creates an additive effect with GABA, further inhibiting arousal and depressing the autonomic nervous system. Alcohol decreases glutamate activity, a major excitatory neurotransmitter. This may explain why cross-tolerance effects occur when alcohol and other CNS depressants are used in combination (Varcarolis & Halter, 2009, p. 408). When taken together, alcohol and other CNS depressants (e.g., benzodiazepines and barbiturates) can lead to respiratory depression and death.

Alcohol is absorbed in the mouth, stomach, and digestive tract. The liver metabolizes approximately 95% of the ingested alcohol; the rest is excreted via the skin, kidney, and lungs. Generally, an individual can break down approximately 1 ounce of whiskey every 90 minutes. Factors such as body mass, food intake, and liver function can affect the rate of alcohol absorption.

Mood and substance use disorders commonly co-occur (Pettinati, O'Brien, & Dundon, 2013). *Dual diagnosis* and *dual disorder* are older terms used to describe an individual who has both a diagnosis of substance abuse and a psychiatric illness. For example, a depressed individual may use self-medication in the form of alcohol to treat the depression, or someone with alcoholism may become depressed. Research has found that medications for managing mood symptoms can be effective in people with substance dependence. Interestingly, in most studies, medications for managing mood symptoms did not impact the substance use disorder. But a recent clinical study did find that combining one medication for depression with another for alcohol dependence reduced both the depression and the drinking simultaneously (Pettinati et al., 2013).

Epidemiology

Alcoholism, also referred to as **alcohol dependence** or alcohol use disorder, is a major health problem, one that is responsible for 100,000 deaths annually in the United States (APA, 2013). Two thirds of the nation's adult population consumes alcohol regularly. An estimated 18 million Americans have an alcohol use disorder or alcohol abuse (National Institute on Alcohol Abuse and Alcoholism, 2013).

Although the legal drinking age in all 50 states is 21, there were an estimated 9.7 million underage (ages 12 to 20) drinkers in 2011, including 6.1 million binge drinkers and 1.7 million heavy drinkers (SAMHSA, 2012a). During 2011, the rate of ED visits involving alcohol (with or without other drugs) for those ages 20 and younger was 215.8 visits per 100,000 population with the majority of those visits involving alcohol only (134.6 visits per 100,000 population) (SAMHSA, 2011).

In 2011, an estimated 11.1% of individuals ages 12 or older reported that they drove under the influence of alcohol at least once during the past year; this estimate corresponds to 28.6 million individuals (SAMHSA, 2012a).

Risk Factors

Understanding the complexity of identifying risk factors for substance dependence can best be demonstrated by using an example of one ethnic/racial group in the United States. Addiction is a primary source of health issues for Native Americans. Different tribes have different rates of alcohol and drug use, but overall population studies have shown that half of the risk of substance dependence for Native Americans comes from genetic influences.

The first genetic influence on addiction is related to **phenotypes**, which are observable individual characteristics. Researchers found an overlap in the gene location for addiction and for the body mass index (BMI). This suggests that combination could produce a "disorder of consumption." Second, Native Americans do not have genes that alter alcohol-metabolizing enzymes, but they do lack protective variants found in other groups. Third, Native Americans' genes are associated with risk factors of drug sensitivity or tolerance. To produce the final picture, specific environmental factors weigh in: trauma exposure, early onset of use of substances, and environmental hardship. All of those factors combine to produce an elevated risk for addiction (Ehlers & Gizer, 2013).

A longitudinal study following over 800 fifth-grade students for more than 20 years found demographic characteristics that were associated with higher rates of substance misuse. Those with less education after high school and those who did not marry by age 30 had the highest rates of substance misuse. Becoming parents was associated with lower rates of substance misuse for both men and women. For successful prevention efforts, attention should be directed to the finding that the patterns of substance misuse were consistent and already observed by age 18 (Oesterle, Hawkins, & Hill, 2011).

Another area that has received much research attention is that of the children of alcoholics (COAs). One study looked at the interaction of the influence of drinking peers and genetic variations. The effect was different for men than for women. Investigators could correlate a specific genetic variation of male children with having drinking peers, which increased the men's risk of alcoholism from the teenage to mature adult years. This same type of correlation was only true for younger women. They concluded that the risk for COAs would have to take into account genetic influences, peer affiliation, age, and gender differences (Chassin et al., 2012).

Another study contrasted the lifestyles of COAs with those who did not have that history. The COAs' families had higher unemployment rates. Even after controlling for their lower socioeconomic status, compared to the controls, the COAs had significantly more mental health difficulties and a higher rate of substance use. Unhealthy lifestyle habits (e.g., lack of exercise, eating fast food, and other poor food choices) were significantly more prevalent for COAs than for the controls. Female COAs reported more emotional and somatic symptoms than male COAs (Serec et al., 2012).

▶ CLINICAL MANIFESTATIONS

When used in moderation, certain types of alcohol can have positive physiological effects by decreasing coronary artery disease and protecting against stroke. However, when consumed in excess, alcohol can lead to **craving** (a strong desire or urge to

use alcohol), can severely diminish one's ability to function, and can ultimately lead to life-threatening conditions (APA, 2013). Chronic use of alcohol can cause severe neurological and psychiatric disorders. Severe damage to the liver occurs with chronic alcohol abuse, and that damage can progress from fatty liver to other liver diseases such as hepatitis and cirrhosis. Chronic alcoholism is the major cause of fatal cirrhosis. Chronic abuse of alcohol also can cause damaging effects to many other systems. These effects include myocardial disease, erosive gastritis, acute and chronic pancreatitis, sexual dysfunction, and an increased risk of breast cancer.

Malnutrition is another serious complication of chronic alcoholism; thiamine (B_1) deficiency in particular can result in neurological impairments. Thiamine depletion is thought to cause the Wernicke-Korsakoff syndrome observed in individuals with chronic alcoholism (Stuart, 2008). Severe cognitive impairment is a principal feature of Wernicke encephalopathy and Korsakoff psychosis. **Wernicke encephalopathy** is characterized by ataxia (lack of coordination), abnormal eye movements, and confusion. About 80% of people with Wernicke encephalopathy also develop **Korsakoff psychosis**, characterized by intact intellectual functioning but an inability to retrieve events from long-term memory or retain new information. **Confabulation**, making up information to fill in memory blanks, develops in an individual's attempt to protect self-esteem when confronted with memory loss. Although Wernicke encephalopathy and Korsakoff psychosis are sometimes considered to be two distinct disorders, they are actually different phases of the same disease, commonly called Wernicke-Korsakoff syndrome. Wernicke encephalopathy indicates the acute stage of the illness, whereas Korsakoff psychosis indicates the chronic stage.

Although alcohol is a CNS depressant, it actually disrupts sleep, thus altering the sleep cycle, decreasing the quality of sleep, intensifying obstructive sleep apnea, and reducing total sleeping time. Heavy drinkers have a higher mortality rate, and many fatalities occur from alcohol-related accidents.

Blood alcohol levels (BALs) are highly predictive of CNS effects. At 0.10%, ataxia and dysarthria occur. From 0.20% to 0.25%, the person is unable to sit or stand upright without support. Between 0.3% and 0.4%, slipping into a coma is possible. Toxic levels in excess of 0.5% can cause death. Note that an individual with chronic alcoholism might have BALs in these ranges, but not have the same consequences, due to their developed tolerance to the effect of drinking (McNeece & DiNitto, 2012). In the United States, the legal level of intoxication is 0.08%.

Chronic consumption of alcohol not only produces tolerance, but it creates cross-tolerance to general anesthetics, barbiturates, benzodiazepines, and other CNS depressants. If alcohol is withdrawn abruptly, the brain becomes overly excited because previously inhibited receptors are no longer inhibited. This hyperexcitability manifests clinically as anxiety, tachycardia, hypertension, diaphoresis, nausea, vomiting, tremors, sleeplessness, and irritability. Severe manifestations of alcohol withdrawal include seizures, convulsions, and DTs. Complications of DTs include respiratory failure, aspiration pneumonitis, and cardiac arrhythmias.

Clinical Manifestations and Therapies **Alcohol Abuse**

ETIOLOGY	CLINICAL MANIFESTATIONS	CLINICAL THERAPIES
DTs as a result of sudden withdrawal of alcohol	■ Confusion ■ Disorientation ■ Agitation ■ Severe autonomic instability ■ Perceptual disturbances ■ Hallucinations (primarily visual but may be tactile) ■ Tremors of extremities ■ Anxiety, panic, and paranoia	■ Prescribe benzodiazepines. ■ Reduce stimuli, but keep well lit to minimize visual misinterpretations. ■ If present, treat with antiseizure medications.
Cirrhosis of the liver resulting from damage done by chronic alcoholism	■ Spider angiomata ■ Palmar erythema ■ Muehrcke nails, Terry nails, or clubbing ■ Hypertrophic osteoarthropathy ■ Dupuytren contracture ■ Gynecomastia ■ Hypogonadism ■ Hepatomegaly ■ Ascites ■ Splenomegaly ■ Jaundice ■ Asterixis ■ Weakness, fatigue, anorexia, weight loss	■ Explain that cirrhosis cannot be reversed, but abstaining from alcohol can delay or prevent further damage. ■ Emphasize abstaining from alcohol. ■ Stop any medications that are potentially damaging to the liver, such as acetaminophen. ■ Consider abdominocentesis to reduce ascites. ■ Monitor ammonia levels. ■ Prevent complications such as esophageal varices, hepatic encephalopathy, and hepatorenal syndrome. ■ Monitor for delayed coagulation times and apply pressure to punctures for 10 minutes.
Assaultive behaviors	■ Sexual assault in adolescent and young adult is commonly related to alcohol use. ■ Because of the release of inhibitions, control of emotions such as anger is reduced. ■ Access to weapons increases the risk of assaultive behavior becoming homicide. ■ Spousal or child abuse has strong link to alcohol ingestion.	■ Promote sobriety. ■ Encourage management classes. ■ Provide crisis intervention for family members who have been assaulted. ■ Provide follow-up counseling to reduce posttraumatic stress response.
Esophageal varices, which may result from portal hypertension due to cirrhosis	■ Hematemesis ranging from mild to severe ■ Heartburn ■ Black or tarry stools ■ Decreased urination secondary to hypotension ■ Light-headedness ■ Shock ■ Weight loss ■ Weakness, fatigue, jaundice ■ Pruritus of hands and feet ■ Edema of lower extremity ■ Mental confusion	■ Encourage abstinence from alcohol. ■ Perform emergency surgery to stop bleeding involving removal of part of the esophagus or cauterization of varicosities. ■ Perform therapeutic endoscopy. ■ Monitor intake and output. ■ Take vital signs frequently during bleeding episodes to monitor for shock. ■ Administer fluids via IV therapy. ■ Administer beta-blockers if necessary to reduce incidence of bleeding.

(continued on next page)

Clinical Manifestations and Therapies Alcohol Abuse (continued)

ETIOLOGY	CLINICAL MANIFESTATIONS	CLINICAL THERAPIES
Gastritis	■ Esophageal reflux ■ Decreased appetite ■ Recurrent diarrhea	■ Provide foods that will not exacerbate GI symptoms while meeting nutritional requirements. ■ Teach client to remain upright for 3–4 hours following meals, eat small frequent meals, and avoid gas-producing foods. ■ Antidiarrheals, antacids, and H_2 blockers may be appropriate medications to reduce symptoms.
Wernicke encephalopathy	■ Ataxia ■ Abnormal eye movements ■ Mental confusion ■ Short-term memory loss	■ Provide for client safety. ■ Place clocks and calendars to reduce mental confusion. ■ Assess cognition and document findings. ■ Administer IV or IM thiamine. ■ Avoid glucose administration until after thiamine administration. ■ Hydrate client.

Multisystem Effects

Alcohol is a chemical irritant that has a direct toxic effect on many organ systems, as described in **Table 22–3** ●.

Blackouts, a fairly early sign of alcoholism, are a form of amnesia about events that occurred during the drinking period. An individual with alcoholism may carry out conversations and elaborate activities with no loss of consciousness but have no memory of those activities the next day. This may be explained by the toxic effects of alcohol on glutamate transmission necessary for memory storage. A more advanced CNS problem is Wernicke-Korsakoff syndrome, described previously.

Dementia occurs five times more often in older adults with alcoholism than in nondrinkers. On the plus side, prevention of drinking relapse in older adults with alcoholism is often better than that of younger clients. More than 20% of treated older alcohol-dependent individuals remain abstinent after 4 years (Caputo et al., 2012).

Withdrawal

Alcohol withdrawal syndrome typically begins about 6–8 hours after an individual with alcoholism's last drink. Early symptoms include irritability, anxiety, insomnia, tremors, sweating, and mild tachycardia. In rare cases, the person may experience grand mal seizures or intermittent visual, tactile, or auditory hallucinations. Symptoms of withdrawal usually peak during the second day of abstinence and are likely to show significant improvement by the fourth or fifth day.

Alcohol withdrawal delirium, sometimes referred to as delirium tremens (DTs), usually occurs on days 2 and 3 but may appear as late as 14 days after the last drink. The person experiences

TABLE 22–3 Physiological Complications From Alcohol Dependence

BODY SYSTEMS	TOXIC EFFECTS
Gastrointestinal	Esophageal reflux, esophagitis, esophageal varices, gastritis, decreased appetite, malabsorption, recurrent diarrhea, acute or chronic pancreatitis (75% of cases related to alcohol abuse)
Liver	Hepatomegaly, fatty liver, alcoholic hepatitis, cirrhosis, cancer, elevated gamma-glutamyl transpeptidase results
Cardiovascular	Hypertension, cardiomyopathy, arrhythmias, increased risk for stroke, coronary artery disease, sudden cardiac death
Respiratory	Pneumonia, bronchitis, tuberculosis
Hematological	Bone marrow depression, anemia, leukopenia, blood clotting abnormalities
Neurological	Seizures, peripheral neuropathy, optic neuropathy, Wernicke encephalopathy, Korsakoff syndrome, alcoholic dementia, impaired cognitive function, labile moods, sleep disturbances
Endocrine	Hyperglycemia, decreased thyroid function
Reproductive	Erectile problems, decreased testosterone, decreased sex drive, menstrual irregularities
Nutritional	Thiamine deficiency, folic acid deficiency, vitamin A deficiency, magnesium deficiency, zinc deficiency

Source: American Psychiatric Association. (2013). *Diagnostic and statistical manual of mental disorders* (5th ed.). Washington, DC: Author; Dunphy, L. M., & Winland-Brown, J. E. (2001). *The art and science of advanced practice nursing.* Philadelphia, PA: F. A. Davis; Naegle, M. A., & D'Avanzo, C. E. (2001). *Addictions and substance abuse: Strategies for advanced practice nursing.* Upper Saddle River, NJ: Prentice Hall.

confusion, disorientation, hallucinations, tachycardia, hypertension or hypotension, extreme tremors, agitation, diaphoresis, and fever. Death may result from cardiovascular collapse or hyperthermia. With intensive care and advanced pharmacology, the mortality rate has dropped from 35% to 5% (Burns, 2013).

Overdose

Signs of alcohol intoxication include nausea, vomiting, lack of coordination, slurred speech, staggering, disorientation, irritability, short attention span, loud and frequent talking, poor judgment, lack of inhibition, labile emotions, and (for some) violent behavior. Alcohol intoxication may result in accidents or falls that cause contusions, sprains, fractures, and facial or head trauma. High BALs may result in unconsciousness, coma, respiratory depression, and death.

Alcohol poisoning is a toxic condition that results from excessive consumption of large amounts of alcohol in a very short period of time. Advanced states of intoxication and alcohol poisoning are critical situations in the ED and necessitate careful triage and monitoring to prevent death or permanent disability.

▶ COLLABORATION

When caring for a client who abuses alcohol, the nurse must work as a collaborative member of a team that may include physicians, psychologists, counselors, nutritionists, and assistive personnel who share the collaborative goal of helping the client achieve sobriety. The treatment team also may include a recovering alcoholic or a sponsor. A sponsor is a successfully recovering alcoholic, usually with several years of sobriety, who provides peer counseling and support, often taking the client to AA 12-step meetings.

Diagnostic Tests

The simplest method of detecting blood alcohol content is by using a Breathalyzer. BALs are the main biological measures for assessment purposes. Knowledge of the symptoms associated with a range of BALs is helpful in ascertaining level of intoxication, level of tolerance, and whether the person accurately reported recent drinking. At 0.10% (after 5–6 drinks in 1–2 hours), voluntary motor action becomes clumsy, resulting in ataxia and dysarthria. The degree of impairment varies with gender, weight, and food ingestion. Small women who drink alcohol on an empty stomach achieve intoxication more quickly than large males who have eaten a full meal. At 0.20% to 0.25% (after 10–12 drinks in 2–4 hours), function of the motor area in the brain is depressed, causing an inability to remain upright (McNeece & DiNitto, 2012). A level above 0.10% without associated behavioral symptoms indicates the presence of tolerance. High tolerance is a sign of physical dependence.

Assessing for withdrawal symptoms is important when the BAL is high. Medications given for treatment of withdrawal from alcohol are usually not started until the BAL is below a set norm (usually below 0.10%) unless withdrawal symptoms become severe. Measurement of BAL may be repeated several times, several hours apart, to determine the body's metabolism of alcohol and at a time it is safe to give the client medication to minimize the withdrawal symptoms.

Treatment of Withdrawal

All CNS depressants, including alcohol, benzodiazepines, and barbiturates, have a potentially dangerous progression of withdrawal. Alcohol and the entire class of CNS depressants share the same withdrawal syndrome. Treatment of severe withdrawal during detoxification is mostly symptomatic through acetaminophen, vitamins, and medications to minimize discomfort.

In managing alcohol withdrawal, the goal is to minimize adverse outcomes such as client discomfort, seizures, delirium tremens, and mortality and to avoid the adverse effects of withdrawal medications, such as excess sedation. Close monitoring is essential to ensure protection of the client. Critical care monitoring may be indicated to manage alcohol withdrawal delirium, particularly when very high doses of benzodiazepines are needed or when significant concurrent medical conditions are present. Medications such as benzodiazepines are a first-line therapy, used to minimize the discomfort associated with alcohol withdrawal and to prevent serious adverse effects, particularly seizures (Manasco et al., 2012).

Two contrasting treatment approaches are fixed-schedule dosing and a symptom-triggered approach. The Clinical Institute Withdrawal Assessment for Alcohol—Revised (CIWA-Ar) scale is currently recommended as the best scale to assess the severity of symptoms of acute alcohol withdrawal (Manasco et al., 2012). Triage nurses can use that scale to determine the need for inpatient hospital admission, such as when the CIWA-Ar score is 10 or more points. However, recent research indicates that the CIWA-Ar scale may underestimate the severity of alcohol withdrawal syndrome in certain ethnic groups, such as Native Americans (Rappaport et al., 2013).

Two unique medications used to treat alcoholism are disulfiram (Antabuse) and naltrexone (ReVia, Depade). Disulfiram is a form of aversion therapy that prevents the breakdown of alcohol, causing physical illness (intense vomiting) if taken while drinking alcohol. All forms of alcohol, including over-the-counter cough and cold preparations, must be avoided. Naltrexone can help reduce the craving for alcohol by blocking the pathways to the brain that trigger a feeling of pleasure when alcohol and other narcotics are used. Because naltrexone blocks opiate receptors, clients should avoid taking any narcotics, such as codeine, morphine, or heroin, while on naltrexone. Clients also should discontinue all narcotics 7–10 days before starting on naltrexone. It also is recommended that clients wear a medical alert bracelet stating that they are on naltrexone, in case of emergency medical treatment. Clients taking disulfiram or naltrexone must also participate in psychosocial treatments such as AA meetings, individual counseling, or group therapy because the desire to "take a break" from treatment can overcome the client's motivation to continue taking the medication. AA meetings and therapy provide support and reinforce clients' efforts to continue treatment. Peer connections made through AA can be especially motivating.

Complementary and Alternative Therapy

Electroencephalograph (EEG) biofeedback, also called *neurotherapy*, has been found to provide some benefit in the treatment of alcoholism (Fontaine, 2010). Many people who are addicted to alcohol and other addicts also have found yoga to be helpful in the recovery process. Both neurotherapy and yoga may provide calming effects on the centers of the brain involved in anxiety and impulse control. Yoga involves maintaining control over one's body and using deep breathing techniques and is frequently hailed as an effective stress reliever.

◼ NURSING PROCESS

Nurses may interact with clients experiencing alcohol abuse or dependence in a variety of settings. The most common setting is an alcohol abuse treatment program where clients are hospitalized for an average of 10–15 days for detoxification and inpatient therapy. These clients may be voluntarily admitted, but many are court ordered to undergo treatment after charges of DUI or alcohol-related child abuse.

Clients with alcohol abuse or dependence have impaired senses and increased risk-taking behaviors, which can lead to injuries from falls and accidents requiring medical attention. Therefore, hospital EDs as well as medical and surgical units are places where nurses encounter these clients. Occupational nurses and community health nurses also interact with clients who abuse alcohol through employee assistance programs and community health departments. Urgent care centers, pain clinics, and ambulatory care centers are other settings in which clients with alcohol abuse disorders frequently appear for minor health problems associated with chronic disorders related to alcohol abuse or dependence.

In caring for a client who is intoxicated, the focus of nursing care is to maintain the client's safety until the alcohol in the client's system has been metabolized. While under the influence of alcohol, the client is not considered mentally competent to make decisions and may not sign a consent form or agree to treatment until his or her BAL decreases to normal limits as defined by state law.

Nursing care of the client with alcohol abuse or dependence is challenging and requires a nonjudgmental atmosphere that promotes trust and respect. Efforts at promoting health are aimed at preventing alcohol use among children and adolescents and reducing the risks among adults. Adolescence is the most common phase for the first experience with drugs (Stuart, 2008), partly due to the vulnerability of teenagers, who can be quick to succumb to peer pressure. Healthy lifestyles, parental support, stress management, good nutrition, and information about ways to steer clear of peer pressure are important topics for the nurse to provide in school programs.

Nurses have a responsibility to educate their clients about the physiological effects of alcohol on the body, as well as about ways to manage stress and anxiety. Nurses must encourage and support periods of abstinence while assisting clients to make major changes in lifestyles, habits, relationships, and coping methods.

Assessment

A thorough history of the client's past alcohol use is important to ascertain the possibility of tolerance, physical dependence, or withdrawal syndrome. The following questions are helpful in eliciting a pattern of substance use behavior:

- How many substances has the client used simultaneously (**polysubstance abuse**: the simultaneous use of many substances) in the past?

- How often, how much, and when did the client first use alcohol?
- Is there a history of blackouts, delirium, or seizures?
- Is there a history of withdrawal syndrome, overdoses, and complications from previous alcohol use?
- Has the client ever been treated in an alcohol abuse clinic?
- Has the client ever been arrested for DUI or charged with any criminal offense while using alcohol?
- Is there a family history of alcohol use?

The client's medical history is another important area for assessment and should include the existence of any concomitant physical or mental condition (e.g., HIV, hepatitis, cirrhosis, esophageal varices, pancreatitis, gastritis, Wernicke-Korsakoff syndrome, depression, schizophrenia, anxiety, or personality disorder). Information about prescribed and over-the-counter medications as well as any allergies or sensitivity to drugs is vital. A brief overview of the client's current mental status also is significant:

- Is there a history of abuse (physical or sexual) or family violence?
- Has the client ever tried to commit suicide?
- Is the client currently having suicidal or homicidal ideation?

Information about the client's level of stress and other psychosocial concerns can help in assessing problems with alcohol use, as follows:

- Has the client's alcohol use affected his or her ability to hold a job?
- Has the client's alcohol use affected relationships with spouse, family, friends, or coworkers?
- How does the client usually cope with stress?
- Does the client have a support system that helps in time of need?
- How does the client spend his or her leisure time?

Several screening tools such as the Michigan Alcohol Screening Test (MAST) (Pokorny, Miller, & Kaplan, 1972) and the Brief Drug Abuse Screening Test (B-DAST) (Skinner, 1982) may help the nurse determine the degree of severity of alcohol abuse or dependence. The following screening tools provide a nonjudgmental, brief, and easy method for ascertaining patterns of substance abuse behaviors:

- ***Michigan Alcohol Screening Test (MAST) Brief Version*** is a 10-question self-administered questionnaire that takes 10–15 minutes to complete. An answer of yes to three or more questions indicates a potentially dangerous pattern of alcohol abuse.
- ***The CAGE questionnaire*** (Ewing, 1984) is useful when the client may not recognize that he or she has an alcohol problem or is uncomfortable acknowledging it. This questionnaire is designed to be a self-report of drinking behavior, or it may be administered by a professional. One affirmative response raises concern and indicates the need for further discussion and follow-up. Two or more yes answers signify a problem with alcohol that may require treatment.

A nonthreatening question such as "How much alcohol do you drink?" is preferable to the judgmental question "You don't drink too much alcohol, do you?" Open-ended questions that elicit more than a simple yes or no answer help to determine the direction of future counseling. The professional should use therapeutic communication techniques to establish trust prior to the assessment process.

Nurses working in medical-surgical units, psychiatric units, and special alcohol abuse units routinely care for clients experiencing acute alcohol withdrawal. Several assessment tools are available to determine the severity of withdrawal symptoms and indicate the need for pharmacologic treatment to manage withdrawal symptoms. An example of a withdrawal assessment tool is the Clinical Institute Withdrawal Assessment for Alcohol—Revised (CIWA-Ar) scale discussed earlier (Sullivan et al., 1989) (**Figure 22–3 ●**). This assessment is used widely in clinical and research settings for initial assessment and ongoing monitoring of alcohol withdrawal signs and symptoms.

The CIWA-Ar scale is a validated 10-item assessment tool that can be used to monitor and medicate clients going through alcohol withdrawal. The CIWA-Ar assesses for several alcohol withdrawal symptoms (e.g., high blood pressure, rapid pulse and respirations, tremors, insomnia, irritability, sweating, and convulsions) and results in a score that is used to direct the administration of benzodiazepines or other drugs to relieve associated symptoms of withdrawal and to prevent seizures. A score of 8 points or fewer corresponds to mild withdrawal symptoms. Scores of 9–15 points indicate moderate withdrawal, whereas a score of 15 or greater denotes severe withdrawal and an increased risk of DTs and seizures.

Diagnosis

Nursing diagnoses are individualized to specific client needs. Primary diagnoses may include:

- *Risk for Injury*
- *Risk for Violence*
- *Ineffective Denial*
- *Ineffective Coping*
- *Imbalanced Nutrition: Less Than Body Requirements*
- *Chronic or Situational Low Self-Esteem*
- *Deficient Knowledge*
- *Disturbed Sensory Perception*
- *Disturbed Thought Processes.*

(NANDA-I © 2012)

Planning

Goals for client care depend on client needs. The client who denies a problem with alcohol will have far different needs than the client experiencing withdrawal, participating in an alcohol abuse program, or facing serious complications from years of abuse. Possible goals may include the following:

- The client will admit alcohol is controlling his or her life.
- The client will agree to enter an alcohol treatment facility.
- The client will experience no complications (or no further complications) as a result of alcohol abuse or alcohol withdrawal.
- The client will obtain optimal nutritional status.
- The client will remain sober.
- The client will participate in support groups such as AA after discharge from treatment facility.

Implementation

Caring interventions are based on the client's need, diagnoses chosen, and goals set for care. The following interventions are organized by nursing diagnosis.

Promote Safety

- Assess the client's level of disorientation to determine specific risks to safety. Knowledge of the client's level of cognitive functioning is essential to the development of an appropriate plan of care.
- Obtain a drug history as well as urine and blood samples for laboratory analysis of substance content. Subjective history often is not accurate, and knowledge regarding substance use is important for accurate assessment.
- Place the client in a quiet private room to decrease excessive stimuli, but do not leave the client alone if excessive hyperactivity or suicidal ideation is present. Excessive stimuli can increase the client's agitation.
- Frequently orient the client to reality and the environment, ensuring that potentially harmful objects are stored outside the client's access. The client may harm self or others if disoriented and confused.
- Monitor vital signs every 15 minutes until stable. Assess blood alcohol level and for signs of intoxication or withdrawal. The most reliable information about withdrawal symptoms comes from BAL and vital signs; they provide information about the need for medication during detoxification.

Promote Participation in Treatment

- Be genuine, honest, and respectful of the client. Keep all promises and convey an attitude of acceptance. The development of a nonjudgmental, therapeutic nurse–client relationship is essential to gain the client's trust.
- Identify maladaptive behaviors or situations that have occurred in the client's life and discuss how the use of alcohol may have been a contributing factor. The first step in combating denial is for the client to recognize the relationship between alcohol use and personal problems.
- Do not accept the use of defense mechanisms such as rationalization or projection as the client attempts to blame others or make excuses for his or her behavior. Use confrontation with care to avoid placing the client on the defensive. Confrontation interferes with the client's ability to use denial.
- Encourage client participation in therapeutic group activities such as AA meetings with other people who are experiencing or have experienced similar problems. Clients often are more accepting of peer feedback than feedback from authority figures.

Promote Healthy Coping Skills

- Establish a trusting relationship. Trust is essential to the nurse–client relationship.
- Set limits on manipulative behavior and maintain consistency in responses. The client with an alcohol dependence problem is unable to set limits and must begin to accept responsibility without being manipulative.

Clinical Institute Withdrawal Assessment of Alcohol Scale, Revised (CIWA-Ar)

Patient:_____ Date: _____ Time: _____ (24 hour clock, midnight = 00:00)

Pulse or heart rate, taken for one minute:_____ Blood pressure:_____

NAUSEA AND VOMITING -- Ask "Do you feel sick to your stomach? Have you vomited?" Observation.
0 no nausea and no vomiting
1 mild nausea with no vomiting
2
3
4 intermittent nausea with dry heaves
5
6
7 constant nausea, frequent dry heaves and vomiting

TREMOR -- Arms extended and fingers spread apart.
Observation.
0 no tremor
1 not visible, but can be felt fingertip to fingertip
2
3
4 moderate, with patient's arms extended
5
6
7 severe, even with arms not extended

PAROXYSMAL SWEATS -- Observation.
0 no sweat visible
1 barely perceptible sweating, palms moist
2
3
4 beads of sweat obvious on forehead
5
6
7 drenching sweats

ANXIETY -- Ask "Do you feel nervous?" Observation.
0 no anxiety, at ease
1 mild anxious
2
3
4 moderately anxious, or guarded, so anxiety is inferred
5
6
7 equivalent to acute panic states as seen in severe delirium or acute schizophrenic reactions

AGITATION -- Observation.
0 normal activity
1 somewhat more than normal activity
2
3
4 moderately fidgety and restless
5
6
7 paces back and forth during most of the interview, or constantly thrashes about

TACTILE DISTURBANCES -- Ask "Have you any itching, pins and needles sensations, any burning, any numbness, or do you feel bugs crawling on or under your skin?" Observation.
0 none
1 very mild itching, pins and needles, burning or numbness
2 mild itching, pins and needles, burning or numbness
3 moderate itching, pins and needles, burning or numbness
4 moderately severe hallucinations
5 severe hallucinations
6 extremely severe hallucinations
7 continuous hallucinations

AUDITORY DISTURBANCES -- Ask "Are you more aware of sounds around you? Are they harsh? Do they frighten you? Are you hearing anything that is disturbing to you? Are you hearing things you know are not there?" Observation.
0 not present
1 very mild harshness or ability to frighten
2 mild harshness or ability to frighten
3 moderate harshness or ability to frighten
4 moderately severe hallucinations
5 severe hallucinations
6 extremely severe hallucinations
7 continuous hallucinations

VISUAL DISTURBANCES -- Ask "Does the light appear to be too bright? Is its color different? Does it hurt your eyes? Are you seeing anything that is disturbing to you? Are you seeing things you know are not there?" Observation.
0 not present
1 very mild sensitivity
2 mild sensitivity
3 moderate sensitivity
4 moderately severe hallucinations
5 severe hallucinations
6 extremely severe hallucinations
7 continuous hallucinations

HEADACHE, FULLNESS IN HEAD -- Ask "Does your head feel different? Does it feel like there is a band around your head?" Do not rate for dizziness or lightheadedness. Otherwise, rate severity.
0 not present
1 very mild
2 mild
3 moderate
4 moderately severe
5 severe
6 very severe
7 extremely severe

ORIENTATION AND CLOUDING OF SENSORIUM -- Ask "What day is this? Where are you? Who am I?"
0 oriented and can do serial additions
1 cannot do serial additions or is uncertain about date
2 disoriented for date by no more than 2 calendar days
3 disoriented for date by more than 2 calendar days
4 disoriented for place/or person

Total **CIWA-Ar** Score _____
Rater's Initials _____
Maximum Possible Score 67

The CIWA-Ar is not copyrighted and may be reproduced freely. This assessment for monitoring withdrawal symptoms requires approximately 5 minutes to administer. The maximum score is 67 (see instrument). Patients scoring less than 10 do not usually need additional medication for withdrawal.

Sullivan, J.T.; Sykora, K.; Schneiderman, J.; Naranjo, C.A.; and Sellers, E.M. Assessment of alcohol withdrawal: The revised Clinical Institute Withdrawal Assessment for Alcohol scale (**CIWA-Ar**). *British Journal of Addiction* 84:1353–1357, 1989.

Figure 22–3 ● Assessment tool for alcohol withdrawal.

- Encourage the client to verbalize feelings, fears, or anxieties. Use attentive listening and validate the client's feelings with observations or statements that acknowledge these feelings. Verbalization of feelings helps the client develop insight into behaviors and long-standing problems.

- Explore methods of dealing with stressful situations other than resorting to alcohol use. Provide encouragement for changing to a healthier lifestyle. Teach healthy coping mechanisms (e.g., physical exercise, progressive muscle relaxation, deep breathing exercises, meditation, and imagery). The client needs to know how to adapt to stress without resorting to alcohol use.

Promote Adequate Nutrition

- Administer vitamins and dietary supplements as ordered by the physician. Vitamin B_1 (thiamine) is necessary to prevent complications from chronic alcoholism (e.g., Wernicke syndrome).

- Monitor lab work (e.g., total albumin, complete blood count, urinalysis, electrolytes, and liver enzymes) and report significant changes to the physician. Objective laboratory tests provide necessary information to determine the extent of malnourishment.

- Collaborate with a dietitian to determine the number of calories needed to provide adequate nutrition and a realistic weight. Document intake, output, and calorie count. Weigh the client daily if condition warrants. Weight loss or gain is important assessment information for inclusion in the plan of care.

- Teach the importance of adequate nutrition by explaining the Food Guide Pyramid and relating the physical effects of malnutrition on body systems. The client may have inadequate knowledge of proper nutritional habits.

Promote Healthy Self-Esteem

- Spend time with the client and convey an attitude of acceptance. Encourage the client to accept responsibility for his or her behaviors and feelings. An attitude of acceptance enhances self-worth.

- Encourage the client to focus on strengths and accomplishments rather than weaknesses and failures. Minimize attention to negative ruminations.

- Encourage participation in therapeutic group activities. Offer recognition and positive feedback for actual achievements. Success and recognition increase self-esteem.

- Teach assertiveness techniques and effective communication techniques such as the use of "I feel" rather than "You make me feel" statements. Previous patterns of communication may have been aggressive and accusatory, causing barriers to interpersonal relationships.

Provide Client Education

- Assess the client's level of knowledge and readiness to learn the effects of alcohol on the body. Baseline assessment is required to develop appropriate teaching material.

- Develop a teaching plan that includes measurable objectives. Include significant others if possible. Lifestyle changes often affect all family members.

- Begin teaching with simple concepts and progress to more complex issues. Use interactive teaching strategies and written materials appropriate to the client's educational level. Include information on the physiological effects of alcohol, the propensity for physical and psychological dependence, and risks to the fetus if the client is pregnant. Active participation and handouts enhance retention of important concepts.

Promote Client Safety During Withdrawal

- Observe the client for withdrawal symptoms. Monitor vital signs. Provide adequate nutrition and hydration. Take seizure precautions. These actions provide supportive physical care during detoxification.

- Assess the client's level of orientation frequently. Orient and reassure the client of safety in the presence of hallucinations, delusions, or illusions. The client may be frightened.

- Explain all interventions before approaching the client. Avoid loud noises and talk softly to the client. Decrease external stimuli by dimming lights. Excessive stimuli increase agitation.

- Administer medications according to the detoxification schedule. Benzodiazepines help minimize the discomfort of withdrawal symptoms.

- Give positive reinforcement when thinking and behavior are appropriate or when the client recognizes that delusions are not based in reality. Alcohol can interfere with the client's perception of reality.

- Use simple step-by-step instructions and face-to-face interaction when communicating with the client. The client may be confused or disoriented.

- Express reasonable doubt if the client relays suspicious or paranoid beliefs. Reinforce accurate perception of people or situations. It is important to communicate that you do not share the false belief as reality.

- Do not argue with the client experiencing delusions or hallucinations. Convey acceptance that the client believes a situation to be true, but that you do not see or hear what is not there. Arguing with the client or denying the belief serves no useful purpose because it does not eliminate the delusions.

- Talk to the client about real events and real people. Respond to feelings and reassure the client about being safe from harm. Discussions that focus on the delusions may aggravate the condition. Verbalization of feelings in a nonthreatening environment may help the client develop insight.

The community provides many options for treating alcohol abuse, including a mixture of individual, group, and family therapy. Medical detoxification can occur in hospitals, psychiatric units, special alcohol abuse units, clinics, and outpatient settings. Less restrictive environments include residential rehabilitation programs, halfway houses, and partial hospitalization programs. These programs provide structured environments for the recovering alcohol abuser while the individual maintains a viable presence in the community. In addition, clients can obtain vocational counseling, become involved in self-help groups such as AA, and receive health education.

SAFETY ALERT

Clients are at highest risk for relapse within the first few months of stopping use of alcohol. An acronym that can assist the client in recognizing behaviors that lead to relapse is HALT:

Hungry
Angry
Lonely
Tired.

Nurses should emphasize the importance of a balanced diet, adequate sleep, healthy recreational activities, and a caring support system to prevent relapse.

Evaluation

The client is evaluated on the ability to meet goals set during the planning stage of the nursing process. Potential expected outcomes include the following:

- The client controls anxiety to a tolerable level.
- The client displays new coping mechanisms and reduces or eliminates the use of withdrawal.
- The client experiences no complications and no new complications as a result of alcohol use or withdrawal.
- The client accepts responsibility for how his or her behavior impacts the family unit.

NURSING CARE PLAN   A Client Experiencing Withdrawal From Alcohol

George Russell, age 58, fell at home and broke his arm. His wife took him to the emergency department where an open reduction internal fixation of his right wrist was performed under general anesthetic in the operating room. He was admitted to the postoperative unit for observation following surgery because he required large amounts of anesthesia during the procedure.

Mr. Russell has a ruddy complexion and looks older than his stated age. He discloses that he was laid off from his factory job 2 years ago and has been working odd jobs until last week, when he was hired by a local assembly plant. His father was a recovering alcoholic, and his 30-year-old son has been treated for alcohol abuse in the past. Mr. Russell states that he knows alcoholism runs in the family, but he believes that he has his drinking under control. However, he cannot remember the events that led up to his fall and how he might have broken his arm.

ASSESSMENT

During the nursing assessment, Mr. Russell is hesitant to provide information and refuses to make eye contact. Prior to his operation, a BAL was drawn because the ED nurse detected alcohol on his breath. His BAL was 0.40%, which is five times the legal limit for intoxication. His vital signs are within the upper limits of normal, but he is confused and disoriented with slurred speech and a slight tremor of the hands. He is 6 feet tall and weighs 140 pounds. His total albumin is 2.9 mg, and he has elevated liver enzymes. His wife states that he rarely eats the meals she prepares because he is usually drinking and has no appetite for food.

DIAGNOSES

- *Ineffective Individual Coping* related to possible hereditary factor and personal vulnerability
- *Risk for Injury* related to aggressive behavior, unsteady gait, and impaired motor responses
- *Ineffective Denial* related to inability to recognize maladaptive behaviors caused by substance use
- *Imbalanced Nutrition: Less Than Body Requirements* related to anorexia manifested by decreased weight and low serum protein levels

(NANDA-I © 2012)

PLANNING

- The client will express his true feelings associated with using alcohol as a method of coping with stressful situations.
- The client will identify three adaptive coping mechanisms he can use as alternatives to alcohol in response to stress.
- The client will verbalize the negative effects of alcohol and agree to seek professional help with his drinking.
- The client will be free of injury as evidenced by steady gait and absence of subsequent falls.
- The client will gain 1 pound (0.45 kilogram) per week without evidence of increased fluid retention. Serum albumin levels will return to normal range.

IMPLEMENTATION

- Establish a trusting relationship with the client and spend time with him discussing his feelings, fears, and anxieties.
- Consult with a physician regarding a schedule for medications during detoxification and observe the client for signs of withdrawal syndrome.
- Explain the effects of alcohol abuse on the body and emphasize that prognosis is closely associated with abstinence.
- Teach a relaxation technique that the client believes is useful.

- Provide community resource information about self-help groups and, if the client is receptive, a list of meeting times and phone numbers.
- Consult with a dietitian to determine the number of calories needed to provide adequate nutrition and a realistic weight. Document intake, output, and calorie count.
- Consult with a physician to begin vitamin B_1 (thiamine) and dietary supplements.

EVALUATION

Mr. Russell is discharged from the postoperative unit without complications. He successfully undergoes detoxification and contacts the employee assistance program at his new place of employment. He is on medical leave while his arm completely heals and now attends AA meetings 5 days a week. He reports that he enjoys taking long walks with his wife in the warm weather and that his appetite has returned. He has gained 10 pounds in the past 6 weeks and feels better physically than he has in many years.

CRITICAL THINKING

1. *Explain why, during the initial nursing assessment, it would be important to ask questions about Mr. Russell's medication history and his use of other medications.*
2. *Mr. Russell asks you to explain the risks of taking disulfiram (Antabuse). What should you tell him?*
3. *Develop a care plan for Mr. Russell for the nursing diagnosis of* Imbalanced Nutrition: Less Than Body Requirements. *Why is this care plan necessary?*

REVIEW Alcohol Abuse

RELATE Link the Concepts and Exemplars

Linking the exemplar of alcohol abuse with the concept of comfort:

1. Why might the client who has detoxified from alcohol have trouble sleeping?

2. What nursing care might you provide to improve the client's ability to sleep?

Linking the exemplar of alcohol abuse with the concept of infection:

3. What pathophysiology would increase the risk for infection in the client who chronically abuses alcohol?

4. What nursing care would you provide this client to reduce the risk of infection?

Linking the exemplar of alcohol abuse with the concept of legal issues:

5. The nurse, working in an ED, admits a client accompanied by a police officer who requests that a serum BAL be drawn and tested for use in a court case related to the client's driving while intoxicated. What are the client's legal rights, and what legal obligations does the nurse have regarding this client's rights of privacy?

Linking the exemplar of alcohol abuse with the concept of safety:

6. The nurse is caring for a client who was brought to the ED with a BAL of 0.32%. The client is somnolent, is speaking in incomplete sentences that are garbled and difficult to understand, and has a laceration on his forehead. He is admitted to the acute care facility for observation. How will you assess this client's neurological status to determine whether there is an alteration in level of consciousness reflecting a brain injury or alcohol intoxication?

READY Go to Companion Skills Manual

REFER Go to Pearson Nursing Student Resources
nursing.pearsonhighered.com

- Additional review materials

REFLECT Case Study

Candy Collins, a 46-year-old wife and mother of two, comes to her physician's office seeking help for alcohol abuse. She says her husband has threatened to leave her and take her children with him if she doesn't stop. The nurse determines that Mrs. Collins drinks at least five or six alcoholic beverages daily, usually starting after dinner, although sometimes she begins drinking after the children leave for school. The nurse learns Mrs. Collins's behavior began 5 years ago, shortly after her youngest child began preschool. She denies having blackouts, although she reports occasionally waking in the morning with no memory of the night before.

1. What other data would you want to collect from Mrs. Collins related to her abuse of alcohol?

2. What treatment would you anticipate as appropriate for this client?

3. What teaching would you provide both Mrs. Collins and her husband?

EXEMPLAR 22.2 Nicotine Addiction

EXEMPLAR KEY TERMS
Nicotine, *1545*
Nicotine replacement therapy (NRT), *1547*

EXEMPLAR LEARNING OUTCOMES
After reading about this exemplar, you will be able to:

1. Describe the pathophysiology, etiology, clinical manifestations, and direct and indirect causes of nicotine addiction.

2. Identify risk factors associated with nicotine addiction.

3. Illustrate the nursing process in providing culturally competent care across the life span for individuals with nicotine addiction.

4. Formulate priority nursing diagnoses appropriate for an individual with nicotine addiction.

5. Summarize therapies used by interdisciplinary teams in the collaborative care of an individual with nicotine addiction.

6. Plan evidence-based care for an individual with nicotine addiction and his or her family in collaboration with other members of the healthcare team.

7. Evaluate expected outcomes for an individual with nicotine addiction.

▶ OVERVIEW

Cigarette smoking is the single most preventable cause of disease and death in the United States. The CDC (2013c) estimates that 443,000 deaths each year are attributable to cigarette smoking. This estimate does not include clients exposed to secondhand smoke or clients who consume nicotine by using chewing tobacco. The history of smoking can be dated to as early as 5000 B.C. and is recorded in many historical records. Nicotine use was considered not only socially acceptable, but also desirable until the dangers became evident in the late 1950s and 1960s. Since that time, the U.S. government, healthcare providers, and anyone invested in promoting healthy lifestyles have worked to make nicotine use socially unacceptable and to help adolescents make better choices than their parents and grandparents did.

Nicotine, a highly addictive chemical found in tobacco, enters the body via the lungs (cigarettes, pipes, and cigars) and oral mucous membranes (chewing tobacco as well as smoking). Although smoking is legal, it has become increasingly socially unacceptable, as evidence of the danger of both smoking and breathing in others' secondhand smoke has been demonstrated. Burning of tobacco releases the active substances in the plant, making it available for absorption via the lungs into the bloodstream.

Commercial tobacco contains over 4,000 chemicals, including nicotine, arsenic, and hydrogen cyanide (**Table 22-4 ●**). Cancer-causing agents in commercial tobacco include nitrosamines, cadmium, benzopyrene, polonium-210,

TABLE 22–4 Common Chemicals Found in Tobacco and Their Effect

CHEMICAL	EFFECT
Benzene	Is a carcinogen associated with leukemia.
Formaldehyde	Causes cancer, respiratory, skin, and GI problems.
Ammonia	Frees nicotine, turning it into a gas to be absorbed through the lungs or oral mucosa into the bloodstream.
Acetone	This simple ketone, also found in nail polish remover, can be irritating to the tissues and is a CNS depressant.
Tar	Is deposited in the lungs from cigarette smoke, reducing elasticity of the alveoli and slowing air exchange.
Nicotine	Is one of the most addictive substances known to humans.
Carbon monoxide	Is a poisonous gas that is rapidly fatal.

nickel, diberiz acidine, urethane, and toluidine. As a result of the combination of chemicals entering the bloodstream, smoking has profound effects on virtually every organ system, ranging from hypertension due to vasoconstriction to suppression of the immune system.

▶ PATHOPHYSIOLOGY AND ETIOLOGY

Nicotine is a psychoactive substance found in tobacco. In low doses, nicotine stimulates nicotinic receptors in the brain to release dopamine (a precursor to norepinephrine) and epinephrine, causing vasoconstriction. This increases the heart rate, blood pressure, and peripheral vascular resistance, increasing the heart's workload. GI effects include an increase in gastric acid secretion, an increase in the tone and motility of GI smooth muscle, nausea, and increased risk of vomiting.

In the CNS, nicotine occupies the receptors for acetylcholine in both dopamine and serotonin neural pathways. This causes the release of dopamine and norepinephrine. Initially, nicotine increases mental alertness, and cognitive ability, but eventually it depresses those responses (Kneisl & Trigoboff, 2013).

Smokers can develop tolerance to nausea and dizziness, which may be experienced with initial use of nicotine, but not to the cardiovascular effects. Furthermore, because of the

Focus on Diversity and Culture
Smoking

Smoking is acceptable in a number of cultures. For example, in some cultures it is used as part of a ritual to communicate peace, spirituality, and communication. Formal Native American ceremonies, for example, often involve the use of a peace pipe, or calumet. Despite the known health risks of tobacco use, the nurse may need to respect the client's cultural view of smoking as an important ritual.

vasoconstriction, tissue oxygenation can be impaired in areas where vessels are already narrowed by atherosclerosis.

Smokers often have more difficulty falling asleep than nonsmokers do because nicotine acts as a stimulant. Smokers are usually easily aroused and often describe themselves as light sleepers. By refraining from smoking after the evening meal, the person usually sleeps better; moreover, many former smokers report that their sleeping patterns improve once they stop smoking.

Nicotine dependence results from chronic use. Research suggests that dopaminergic processes have a role in regulating the reinforcing effects of nicotine, making cessation difficult (Kneisl & Trigoboff, 2013). Withdrawal symptoms include craving, nervousness, restlessness, irritability, impatience, increased hostility, insomnia, impaired concentration, increased appetite, and weight gain. Gradual reduction in nicotine use seems to prolong suffering. Chronic health problems from smoking have been well established in the form of cancer, heart disease, emphysema, hypertension, and death (Kneisl & Trigoboff, 2013).

Epidemiology

Approximately one in five U.S. adults smokes cigarettes, and certain subpopulations have a higher prevalence of smoking. Cigarette smoking is the number one cause of preventable disease and death worldwide. Smoking-related diseases claim over 393,000 American lives each year (American Lung Association, 2013). Smoking is the most common form of recreational drug use, practiced by more than 1 billion people in the majority of human societies. According to a 2012 Surgeon General's report, *Preventing Tobacco Use Among Youth and Young Adults* (2012), more than 80% of adult smokers began smoking by 18 years of age with 99% of them lighting up by age 26.

Smoking harms nearly every organ in the body, and is a main cause of lung cancer and chronic obstructive pulmonary disease (COPD, including chronic bronchitis and emphysema). It is also a cause of coronary heart disease, stroke, and a host of other cancers and diseases (American Lung Association, 2013). More women in the United States die from lung cancer than any other type of cancer, and cigarette smoking causes most cases. Smoking also causes cancers of the esophagus, larynx, mouth, throat, kidney, bladder, pancreas, stomach, uterine cervix, and acute myeloid leukemia. Graves disease, infertility, early menopause, dysmenorrhea, impotence, osteoporosis, and degenerative disc disease have also been associated with smoking. Other less serious consequences include discolored teeth and fingernails, premature aging and wrinkling, bad breath, reduced sense of smell and taste, strong smell of smoke clinging to hair and clothing, and gum disease. Smoking during pregnancy has been associated with preterm labor, spontaneous abortion, low-birth-weight infants, sudden infant death syndrome (SIDS), and learning disorders (Albrecht et al., 2011; Zhang & Wang, 2013).

Nonsmokers who are exposed to secondhand smoke at home or work increase their lung cancer risk by 20%–30%. Concentrations of many cancer-causing and toxic chemicals are higher in secondhand smoke than in the smoke inhaled by smokers (CDC, 2013b). Secondhand smoke presents a number of dangers, particularly to children of smokers. According to the CDC:

- Infant children of mothers who smoke are more likely to die from SIDS than children born to nonsmoking mothers.
- Exposure to secondhand smoke causes asthmatic children to have more frequent and severe attacks.
- Children exposed to secondhand smoke are at increased risk for respiratory symptoms and otitis media.
- Mothers who smoke and mothers who are exposed to secondhand smoke are more likely to have lower-birth-weight babies (CDC, 2013c).

Risk Factors

Some of the most common factors that influence people to smoke are emotions, social pressure, alcohol use, lack of education, and age. People of lower socioeconomic status are more likely to smoke than those of higher socioeconomic status, partially because smoking is more socially acceptable in groups with fewer resources. Furthermore, quitting smoking is less successful in lower socioeconomic groups because they lack high-quality health education, lack support for quitting, and are exposed to smoking more often.

Prevention

Smoking and smokeless tobacco use are initiated and established primarily during adolescence. Adolescents and young adults are uniquely susceptible to social and environmental influences to use tobacco, and tobacco companies spend billions of dollars on cigarette and smokeless tobacco marketing. The Surgeon General's 2012 report provides evidence that coordinated, high-impact interventions including mass media campaigns, price increases, and community-level changes protecting people from secondhand smoke are effective in reducing the initiation and prevalence of smoking among youth.

National, state, and local program activities that have reduced and prevented youth tobacco use in the past have included combinations of the following:

- Counteradvertising mass-media campaigns (i.e., TV and radio commercials, posters, and other media messages targeted toward youth to counter pro-tobacco marketing)
- Comprehensive school-based tobacco-use prevention policies and programs (e.g., tobacco-free campuses)
- Community interventions that reduce tobacco advertising, promotions, and commercial availability of tobacco products
- Higher costs for tobacco products through increased excise taxes.

▶ CLINICAL MANIFESTATIONS

Clinical manifestations of nicotine use are usually nonexistent in the early stages of use and are seen only when a complication such as COPD, cancer, or heart disease occurs. People who smoke for many years often have deep voices secondary to trauma to the vocal cords caused by the heat of the smoke and the chronic cough they often develop. See the exemplar on Lung Cancer in the module on Cellular Regulation, for manifestations of cancers associated with nicotine use; the exemplar on Chronic Obstructive Pulmonary Disease in the module on Oxygenation, for the impact of smoking on lung function; and the exemplars on Coronary Artery Disease and Peripheral Vascular Disease in the module on Perfusion, for information related to heart disease and peripheral vascular disease.

▶ COLLABORATION

As with any addiction, the treatment process is a collaborative one. Nicotine addicts benefit from the support of family and friends, especially during times when they would usually be smoking or using tobacco. Although pharmacologic therapies are available over the counter, it is important for the client to discuss treatment with healthcare providers to minimize symptoms of withdrawal and prevent interactions with prescribed medications. Some clients may seek complementary therapies and support groups to help them quit smoking.

Nicotine Replacement Therapy

Nicotine replacement therapy (NRT) helps relieve some of the physiological effects of withdrawal, including cravings, for clients trying to quit smoking or using tobacco. NRT transdermal patches and gums are available over the counter; nicotine inhalers and nasal sprays are available by prescription only. Use of these nicotine substitution products is not without complications. They do not treat underlying psychological needs or address addictive behaviors associated with tobacco use. They also come with contraindications and warnings. Nurses should provide information about theses contraindications and warnings to clients considering NRT. Nurses also should encourage clients to use nicotine therapy in combination with a smoking cessation program that will help them address the psychological issues related to nicotine abuse.

Smoking Cessation Programs

Smoking cessation programs provide peer support, group therapy, and behavior therapy modifications that can help clients who smoke to quit smoking. The Web sites of the U.S. Surgeon General, the CDC, the American Heart Association, and the American Lung Association all provide information about smoking cessation programs and other means of quitting smoking.

Complementary Therapy

A number of complementary therapies have been advocated as tools for quitting smoking, hypnotherapy and acupuncture among them. Generally speaking, any therapy that helps reduce client anxiety levels, such as yoga and massage, will lower the likelihood that the client will want to use nicotine to alleviate anxiety.

There is conflicting evidence about the success of hypnotherapy as a smoking cessation tool. As with any type of therapy, the qualifications and experience of the therapist have an effect on the success of the therapy. To increase the likelihood of success, nurses should encourage clients who are considering hypnotherapy also to participate in more traditional cessation programs.

Clinical Manifestations and Therapies **Nicotine Addiction**

ETIOLOGY	CLINICAL MANIFESTATIONS	CLINICAL THERAPIES
Carcinogens are in commercial cigarettes, cigars, and pipes.	■ Lung cancer ■ Stomach cancer ■ Bladder cancer ■ Oral cancers ■ Laryngeal cancers	■ Chemotherapy ■ Radiation therapy ■ Supportive care ■ Pain management
Smoke, chemicals, and heat from smoke irritate and damage tissues in the respiratory system.	■ Chronic cough ■ COPD ■ Increased mucus production ■ Chronic hypercapnia	■ Bronchodilators ■ Expectorants ■ Oxygen therapy ■ Coughing and deep breathing ■ Positioning ■ Smoking cessation
Damaging effects of second-hand smoke put those around the smoker at risk.	■ Children at increased risk for upper respiratory tract infections, otitis media ■ Everyone exposed to smoke at risk for cancer secondary to exposure to carcinogens	■ Stop smoking. ■ Avoid exposing others to smoke, especially in confined areas with poor ventilation.
External exposure to smoke affects cellular regeneration.	■ Wrinkles in the skin ■ Premature aging ■ Yellowing of fingernails and fingers	■ Stop smoking. ■ Smoke in well-ventilated area and hold cigarette or cigar so smoke does not pass over fingers.
Smell of smoke is prevalent.	■ Reduced sense of smell ■ Hair, skin, and clothing smelling of smoke	■ Stopping smoking is best. ■ Smoke in well-ventilated area.
Nicotine and other chemicals make smoking very addictive.	■ High level of recidivism when attempting to quit smoking	Provide multiple layers of support when a client chooses to quit, including: ■ Nicotine replacement ■ Pharmacologic therapy ■ Group and individual support ■ Motivational strategies.

■ NURSING PROCESS

Nurses may interact with clients addicted to nicotine in a variety of settings ranging from acute care to outpatient centers. Nurses often note the smell of smoke on a nicotine user and can implement a plan of care aimed at helping the client make healthier lifestyle choices. Because of the high rate of smoking among clients with mental health disorders, psychiatric facilities are a common place to meet clients with nicotine addictions. It is not uncommon for clients to have addictions to multiple substances, and nurses should assess for other substance abuse problems. A nonjudgmental approach is important when caring for clients addicted to nicotine. Health promotion efforts are directed toward education about making healthy life choices and strategies to support the client in abstaining from nicotine. Through school programs, nurses can provide adolescents with ways to avoid peer pressure, thereby preventing nicotine use.

Assessment

When assessing clients who use nicotine, it is important to assess for amount and frequency of use, length of time nicotine has been used, and the presence of any symptoms indicating possible complications such as a chronic cough, shortness of breath, hypertension, chest pain, or unexpected symptoms. A comprehensive approach to the assessment of substance use is essential to ensure adequate and appropriate intervention. Three important areas to assess are a history of the client's past substance use, medical and psychiatric history, and the presence of psychosocial concerns. Ask questions in a nonthreatening, matter-of-fact manner, phrased so as not to imply wrongdoing. Open-ended questions that elicit more than a simple yes or no answer help to determine the direction of future counseling (**Box 22–5** ●). Part of every assessment of individuals who abuse nicotine should be to determine their willingness and motivation to consider abstinence.

Box 22-5 Examples of Open-Ended Questions for Assessment of Nicotine Addiction

- On average, how long have you used nicotine-containing products?
- On a typical day, how many cigarettes (cigars or pipes) do you smoke (or how much tobacco do you chew)?
- When did you last smoke or use tobacco?
- What kinds of problems has nicotine use caused for you and your family, friends, finances, and health? How much money do you think you spend on smoking or tobacco use?
- Tell me about any attempts you've made to quit using nicotine. How long did you quit? What made you return to nicotine use?
- How do you feel about the idea of being nicotine-free? Do you want help to quit now?

- How does the client usually cope with stress?
- Does the client have a support system that helps in time of need?
- How does the client spend leisure time?

The client's medical history is another important area for assessment and should include the existence of any concomitant physical or mental condition. Ask about prescribed and over-the-counter medications as well as any allergies or sensitivity to drugs. A brief overview of the client's current mental status also is significant. Questions to ask may include the following:

- How often do you feel sad or depressed?
- Do you have any other family members who use nicotine or other drugs? If so, how much or how often?
- Have you ever thought about hurting yourself? Someone else?

Address Psychosocial Issues

Information about the client's level of stress and other psychosocial concerns can help in the assessment of substance use problems.

- Has the client's nicotine use affected his or her ability to hold or find a job?
- Has the client's nicotine use affected relationships with spouse, family, friends, or coworkers?

Diagnosis

Every client is unique, and the choice of the nursing diagnosis will depend on the type of complications the client may be experiencing as a result of nicotine use. The needs of a client being treated for lung cancer or heart disease after years of smoking will differ from the needs of the adolescent client who may not yet be experiencing adverse effects from the newly begun habit. Possible nursing diagnoses include the following:

- *Risk for Injury*
- *Ineffective Denial*
- *Ineffective Coping*
- *Ineffective Airway Clearance*
- *Anxiety.*

(NANDA-I © 2012)

Planning

When designing the plan of care, the nurse must put the client's needs, and no other expectations, at the forefront of the plan. If the client has no motivation to make healthier life choices, the nurse must respect the choices the client makes. Goals for client care may include the following:

- The client will verbalize the negative effects, both short term and cumulative, associated with smoking.
- The client will voice strategies for support with quitting if/when the client is ready to stop smoking.

Evidence-Based Practice Adolescents and Their Control of Tobacco Use

Problem

In 2011, young adults ages 18–25 had the highest rate of current use of a tobacco product (39.5%) compared with youths ages 12–17 and adults ages 26 or older. Young adults had the highest usage rates of each of the specific tobacco products as well. In 2011, the rates of past month use among young adults were 33.5% for cigarettes, 10.9% for cigars, 5.4% for smokeless tobacco, and 1.9% for pipe tobacco (SAMHSA, 2012a).

Evidence

Researchers (Sussman, Black, & Rohrbach, 2010; Sussman et al., 2013) examined the effectiveness of different types, or modalities, of tobacco-use prevention programs designed to decrease incidence and prevalence of tobacco use among youth. The preventive strategies were varied and included policy regulations such as tax increases, warning labels, limits on access, smoke-free policies, and restrictions on marketing; mass media programming; school-based classroom education; family involvement; and involvement of medical, social and political community agents. It was suggested that the most effective means of prevention might involve a careful selection of pro-

gram type combinations. Careful coordination of combination programs may be the means to maximize effectiveness.

Implications

Importantly, for future research and practice, examination of tobacco use prevention as a complex system may be needed to maximize effects from combinations of modalities of prevention programming. Future studies will need to more systematically consider and uncover the combination rules and related incremental effects underlying efficacious multipronged community-based programming.

Critical Thinking Application

1. You are caring for a 12-year-old girl who tells you that she smokes cigarettes occasionally and believes it makes her more popular with her older friends. She admits that she knows that smoking is supposed to be bad for you, but she doesn't see the harm in smoking a few cigarettes every day. How do you respond?
2. Do you think nurses and other healthcare professionals should quit smoking? Why or why not?

- The client will identify three activities that can aid in avoiding nicotine use.
- The client will not experience complications as a result of nicotine use.

Implementation

The nurse's role regarding smoking is to (a) serve as a role model by not smoking, (b) provide educational information regarding the dangers of smoking, (c) help make smoking socially unacceptable (e.g., by posting no-smoking signs in client lounges and offices), and (d) suggest resources such as hypnosis, lifestyle training, and behavior modification to clients who want to stop smoking. Nurses also can promote health related to tobacco by being aware of marketing efforts that target young adults. The tobacco industry has developed very effective campaigns to encourage smoking among young adults by advertising and sponsoring entertainment events. Nurses also need to be aware of research that shows that risk factors for young adult smokers include perceiving that teenage smoking is useful or widespread, as well as being around people smoking, engaging in binge drinking, and seeing ads in bars and clubs (Ling, Neilands, & Glantz, 2009).

Evaluation

Clients are evaluated based on the goals created during the planning stage. Expected outcomes may include the following:

- The client describes feelings regarding nicotine use, abstinence, and methods of coping without the use of nicotine.
- The client verbalizes negative effects on his or her own life and the lives of loved ones as a result of nicotine use.
- The client is free of injury or complications resulting from nicotine use.
- The client describes strategies that will be or can be useful when beginning a program to quit smoking.

NURSING CARE PLAN   A Client Addicted to Nicotine

Ronald Kohler, age 32, began smoking when he was a junior in high school. His parents tried to discourage his smoking, but they never actually forbade it in their home because both of them smoked and believed it would be hypocritical to hold him to different standards than they practiced. Mr. Kohler says now he wishes his parents had told him all of the negatives and enforced a strict no-smoking rule because, he says, "It would have been easier not to start than it is to quit." Recently, during an annual health exam required by his employer, the physician pointed out early pulmonary changes associated with emphysema. Mr. Kohler denies any symptoms other than a productive cough in the morning upon awakening. Mr. Kohler lives with his wife and two daughters, 8 and 5 years of age. His wife strictly forbids smoking in the house and wishes her children did not see their father smoking for fear that they will eventually smoke as adults because of the poor role model he portrays.

ASSESSMENT	DIAGNOSES	PLANNING
During the nursing assessment, Mr. Kohler's vital signs are T 37°C (98.6°F, oral), P 80 bpm, R 16/min, BP 138/86 mmHg. Breath sounds are clear and equal except for mild crackles in the lowest part of the lung bases. He has an intermittent moist, often productive cough, and his oxygen saturation is 91%. Peak flow readings are 480 mL, but he has no baseline for comparison purposes. When questioned, he reports that he has smoked 1 pack of filtered low-tar cigarettes a day on most days but when under stress, he may smoke as much as 2 packs (or 50 cigarettes) per day. He has tried quitting twice, but both times he lasted less than 24 hours before smoking again. He says he knows he should quit for his girls, his wife would be much happier if he didn't smell like cigarettes when he got close to her, and it would be better for his health, but he reports he is just not interested in quitting because he enjoys the habit and finds that it calms him during times of stress.	■ *Risk for Injury* related to damage to his cardiorespiratory system from cigarette smoke ■ *Ineffective Denial* related to inability to recognize maladaptive behaviors related to smoking (NANDA-I © 2012)	■ The client will express his true feelings associated with using nicotine as a method of coping with stressful situations. ■ The client will identify three adaptive coping mechanisms he can use as alternatives to nicotine use in response to stress. ■ The client will verbalize the negative effects of smoking and agree to consider smoking cessation. ■ The client will be free of injury as evidenced by normal cardiorespiratory function on assessment.

IMPLEMENTATION

- Establish a trusting relationship with the client and spend time with him discussing his feelings, fears, and anxieties.
- Explain the effects of nicotine abuse on the body and emphasize that a good prognosis is closely associated with abstinence.
- Teach a relaxation technique that the client believes he can use instead of nicotine during times of stress.

- Provide community resource information about self-help groups and, if client is receptive, a list of meeting times and phone numbers.
- Consult with a physician regarding possible use of Chantix (varenicline) if the client chooses that method of smoking cessation.

NURSING CARE PLAN   *(continued)*

EVALUATION

Mr. Kohler opts not to quit smoking at this visit but returns in 3 months and is diagnosed with left lower lobe pneumonia and relates that his oldest daughter told him, "Dad, if you loved us, you'd quit smoking because you'd want to be around to walk us down the aisle and meet your grandchildren." He says it made him think about how silly lighting a "stick on fire" was in comparison to that, and he would like to discuss quitting at this visit.

CRITICAL THINKING

1. *Explain why it would be important during the initial nursing assessment to include questions about Mr. Kohler's medication history and his use of other medications.*
2. *Mr. Kohler asks you to explain the risks of taking Chantix (varenicline). What do you tell him?*
3. *Based on his first visit to the center, develop a care plan for Mr. Kohler for the nursing diagnosis of ineffective denial. Why is this care plan necessary?*

◢ REVIEW   Nicotine Addiction

RELATE Link the Concepts and Exemplars

Linking the exemplar of nicotine addiction with the concept of oxygenation:

1. Describe the pathophysiology of the respiratory system and the ability of the alveoli to oxygenate the tissues when a client smokes.
2. While caring for a client who is known to have smoked for more than 30 years, how would you amend your nursing plan of care as related to oxygenation?

Linking the exemplar of nicotine addiction with the concept of grief and loss:

3. The nurse is caring for a client with terminal lung cancer and is talking with the family. The client's daughter says, "If Dad wanted to stay around and be with us, he wouldn't have made the choice to smoke." How would you respond to this statement and help the family members deal with their anger over the client's lifestyle choices?
4. Why might a client with acute COPD who continues to smoke be denied a lung transplant? How can you help this client (and family) deal with the grief and loss they experience as a result of this decision?

READY Go to Companion Skills Manual

REFER Go to Pearson Nursing Student Resources
nursing.pearsonhighered.com

- Additional review materials

REFLECT Case Study

Mr. W., a 50-year-old professional man, has pneumonia and is currently being treated with antibiotics. He smokes two packs of cigarettes a day. Since this bout of pneumonia, he voices concern about his smoking and wonders if he should try to quit again. He states, "I've tried everything and nothing works. The longest I last is about 1 month." He admits to being 30 pounds overweight and states that his wife and he have started walking 30 minutes every evening. His wife also has started making low-fat meals. He is concerned that if he quits smoking, he will gain more weight.

1. What information or knowledge is important for the nurse to remember when assisting a client to advance to the next stage of change?
2. Each contact between a nurse and a client is an opportunity for health promotion. Based on the knowledge or key concepts listed above, what question(s) would you ask Mr. W.?
3. In which state of change is Mr. W. relating to his cigarette smoking? What strategies could you, the nurse, consider?

◢ EXEMPLAR 22.3   Prenatal Substance Exposure

EXEMPLAR KEY TERMS
Club drugs, *1554*
Cocaine, *1553*
Crack, *1553*
Epigenetic, *1554*
Fetal alcohol spectrum disorder/fetal alcohol syndrome, *1552*
Heroin, *1554*
Neonatal abstinence syndrome (NAS), *1554*
Teratogen, *1552*

EXEMPLAR LEARNING OUTCOMES
After reading about this exemplar, you will be able to:

1. Describe the pathophysiology, etiology, clinical manifestations, and direct and indirect effects of prenatal substance use on both the mother and the fetus.

2. Identify risk factors associated with prenatal substance use.
3. Illustrate the nursing process in providing culturally competent care across the life span for individuals who abuse substances during pregnancy.
4. Formulate priority nursing diagnoses appropriate for an individual who abuses substances during pregnancy and for her newborn.
5. Summarize therapies used by interdisciplinary teams in the collaborative care of women who abuse substances during pregnancy, their newborns, and their family members.
6. Plan evidence-based care for women who abuse substances during pregnancy, their newborns, and their family members in collaboration with other members of the healthcare team.
7. Evaluate expected outcomes for women who abuse substances during pregnancy, their newborns, and their family members.

▶ OVERVIEW

The rate of addiction in women during pregnancy has increased during the past 30 years. The result is that about 225,000 infants every year are born exposed to in utero illicit substances. Their neonatal care needs to be specialized to treat symptoms. The best approach to address this public health issue is a combination of routine screening of and educating women in their childbearing years (Keegan et al., 2010).

During pregnancy, the fetus is exposed to most of what the mother consumes, uses, or inhales. Any chemical that has the potential to harm the fetus is known as a **teratogen** and can include pesticides, viruses, and medications. If the mother uses or abuses substances, the fetus can experience life-changing alterations ranging from developmental delays to death. Drugs that are commonly misused include tobacco, alcohol, cocaine, marijuana, amphetamines, barbiturates, hallucinogens, club drugs, heroin, and other narcotics. Polysubstance use, which involves multiple substances such as alcohol, tobacco, and illicit drugs, contributes to the risks that a pregnant woman faces.

Drug use during pregnancy, particularly in the first trimester, may adversely affect the health of the woman and the growth and development of the fetus. Unfortunately, prenatal drug use may be the most frequently missed diagnosis in all of maternity care. Physicians and nurses may fail to ask women about drug and alcohol use because of their own lack of knowledge, discomfort, or biases. Often women who are abusing substances wait until late in pregnancy to seek health care. Moreover, such women who do seek early prenatal care may not voluntarily reveal an addiction. Caregivers should ask direct, nonjudgmental questions and be alert for a history or physical signs that suggest substance abuse.

Providing effective prenatal care to women who are chemically dependent presents many challenges for clinicians. However, pregnancy represents a period in most women's lives when they recognize the need for and are receptive to caring interventions.

Table 22–5 ● identifies common addictive drugs and their effects on the fetus or newborn.

▶ PATHOPHYSIOLOGY AND ETIOLOGY

The substance used, the amount of chemical consumed, and the period of gestation when the fetus is exposed all play an important role in determining the effects on the fetus. The greatest potential for gross abnormalities in the fetus occurs during the first trimester of pregnancy, when fetal organs are first developing. The classic period of teratogenesis in a woman with a 28-day cycle extends from day 31 after the last menstrual period (17 days after fertilization) to day 71 (54 days after fertilization) (Niebyl & Simpson, 2012). Many factors influence teratogenic effects, including the specific type of teratogen and the dose, the stage of embryonic development, and the genetic sensitivity of the mother and fetus. Understanding the risks and providing care for the pregnant woman who abuses substances require an understanding of the effects of the chemical in the body.

Substances Commonly Abused During Pregnancy

Client teaching ideally begins before pregnancy with any woman of childbearing age. When assessing the woman, nurses should determine if any substances are currently used that could potentially harm the fetus. If the client admits to substance use, the nurse can focus care on providing strategies to help her make healthier choices with the long-term goal of healthier children.

CAFFEINE Caffeine from several dietary sources, including coffee, teas, colas and chocolate, crosses the placenta and enters the fetal bloodstream. This fact has prompted clinical studies to look at a potential problematic relationship between caffeine consumption and fetal development. However, multiple studies have not shown a definitive correlation. For example, Morgan, Koren, and Bozzo (2013) describe the difficulty of predicting the risk of miscarriage, but state that most data do not suggest an increased risk of pregnancy complications or fetal development problems. However, current medical advice suggests limiting the amount of caffeine consumption per day to a moderate amount, less than 200 mg daily (American College of Obstetricians and Gynecologists [ACOG], 2010).

ALCOHOL Over half of women of childbearing age drink alcohol (Keegan et al., 2010). Alcohol is a CNS depressant and a potent teratogen. Birth defects related to fetal alcohol exposure can occur in the first 3–8 weeks of gestation, often before the woman even knows she is pregnant. Alcohol use among pregnant women tends to decrease by trimester.

The effects of alcohol on the fetus may result in a group of signs known as **fetal alcohol spectrum disorders**, also referred to as **fetal alcohol syndrome**. The spectrum of disorders has characteristic physical and mental abnormalities that vary in severity and combination. Characterized by growth retardation, facial anomalies, and CNS dysfunction of varying severity, fetal alcohol syndrome is the most common preventable cause of mental retardation in the United States. Pregnant women who have more than three drinks per week have an increased risk for miscarriage. Mothers-to-be who have five or more drinks per week increase their risk for intrauterine death by two to three times that of women who are nondrinkers (Wisner et al., 2012). There is no definitive answer to how much alcohol a woman can safely consume during pregnancy. Consequently, the expectant woman should avoid alcohol completely. The opinions of the CDC, the U.S. Surgeon General, ACOG, and the American Academy of Pediatrics agree: Even low levels of alcohol cannot be recommended (Uscher, 2012).

Chronic abuse of alcohol can undermine maternal health by causing malnutrition (especially folic acid and thiamine deficiencies), bone marrow suppression, increased incidence of infections, and liver disease. As a result of alcohol dependence, a woman may have withdrawal seizures in the intrapartum period as early as 12–48 hours after she stops drinking. DTs may occur in the postpartum period, and the newborn may suffer withdrawal syndrome. The nursing staff in the maternal newborn unit must be aware of the manifestations of alcohol abuse so they can prepare for the client's special needs. The care regimen includes sedation to decrease irritability and tremors,

TABLE 22–5 Possible Effects of Selected Drugs of Abuse/Addiction on Fetus and Newborn

MATERNAL DRUG	EFFECT ON FETUS/NEWBORN
Depressants	
Alcohol	Mental retardation, microcephaly, midfacial hypoplasia, cardiac anomalies, intrauterine growth restriction (IUGR), potential teratogenic effects, fetal alcohol spectrum disorder (FASD) or fetal alcohol syndrome (FAS)
Narcotics	
Heroin	Withdrawal symptoms, convulsions, intrauterine growth restriction (IUGR), tremors, irritability, sneezing, vomiting, fever, diarrhea, and abnormal respiratory function
Methadone	Fetal distress, meconium aspiration; with abrupt termination of the drug, severe withdrawal symptoms, preterm labor, rapid labor, abruption
Barbiturates	
Phenobarbital	Withdrawal symptoms Fetal growth restriction
"T's and Blues" (combination of the following)	
Talwin (narcotic)	Safe for use in pregnancy; depresses respiration if taken close to time of birth
Amytal (barbiturate)	See barbiturates
Tranquilizers	
Phenothiazine derivatives	Withdrawal, extrapyramidal dysfunction, delayed respiratory onset, hyperbilirubinemia, hypotonia or hyperactivity, decreased platelet count
Diazepam (Valium)	Hypotonia, hypothermia, low Apgar score, respiratory depression, poor sucking reflex, cleft lip
Antianxiety Drugs	
Lithium	Congenital anomalies
Stimulant: Amphetamines	
Amphetamine sulfate (Benzedrine)	Generalized arthritis, learning disabilities, poor motor coordination, transposition of the great vessels, cleft palate
Dextroamphetamine sulfate (Dexedrine)	Congenital heart defects, biliary atresia, limb reduction defects
Cocaine	Cerebral infarctions, microcephaly, learning disabilities, poor state organization, decreased interactive behavior, CNS anomalies, cardiac anomalies, genitourinary anomalies, sudden infant death syndrome (SIDS)
Nicotine (half to one pack cigarettes/day)	Spontaneous abortion, placental abruption, small for gestational age (SGA), small head circumference, decreased length, SIDS, attention-deficit/hyperactivity disorder (ADHD) in school-age children
Stimulant: Psychotropics	
PCP ("angel dust")	Withdrawal symptoms Behavioral and developmental abnormalities
LSD	Chromosomal breakage
Marijuana	IUGR

seizure precautions, intravenous (IV) fluid therapy for hydration, and preparation for an addicted newborn. Although high doses of sedatives and analgesics may be necessary for the woman, caution is advised because these medications can cause fetal depression.

Breastfeeding generally is not contraindicated if the mother drinks alcohol, although alcohol is excreted in breast milk. Excessive alcohol consumption may intoxicate the infant and inhibit the maternal letdown reflex. Discharge planning for the mother with an alcohol addiction and her newborn needs to be coordinated with the social services department of the hospital.

COCAINE AND CRACK **Cocaine** is a powerful stimulant of natural origin that acts at the nerve terminals to prevent the reuptake of dopamine and norepinephrine, which in turn results in vasoconstriction, tachycardia, and hypertension. Placental vasoconstriction decreases blood flow to the fetus. The onset of cocaine effects occurs rapidly, but the euphoria lasts only about 30 minutes. Euphoria and excitement are usually followed by irritability, depression, pessimism, fatigue, and a strong desire for more cocaine. This pattern often leads the user to take repeated doses to sustain the effect. Cocaine metabolites may be present in the urine of a pregnant woman for as long as 4–7 days after use.

Cocaine can be taken by IV injection or by snorting the powdered form. **Crack**, a form of freebase cocaine that is made up of baking soda, water, and cocaine mixed into a paste and microwaved to form a rock, can be smoked. Smoking crack leads to a quicker, more intense high because the drug is absorbed through the large surface area of the lungs.

Cocaine crosses into breast milk and may cause symptoms in the breastfeeding infant, including extreme irritability, vomiting, diarrhea, dilated pupils, and apnea. Also both the dose and contaminants are often unknown. Thus, women who continue to use cocaine after childbirth should avoid breastfeeding, since the risks outweigh the benefits (Behnke & Smith, 2013).

MARIJUANA Perhaps not surprisingly, marijuana is the most widely used illicit drug among women, both pregnant and nonpregnant (SAMHSA, 2012a). The prevalence of marijuana use in society raises many concerns about its effects on the fetus. Research on marijuana use in pregnancy is difficult, however, because it is an illegal drug. Unreliability of reporting, lack of a representative population, inability to determine strength or composition of the marijuana used (including the presence of herbicides), and concurrent use of other drugs are major factors complicating research efforts. In general, maternal marijuana use has not been correlated with fetal growth restriction. To date, there is no strong evidence that marijuana has teratogenic effects on the fetus. Neonatal abstinence symptoms have not been observed in such infants. However, prenatal marijuana use is associated with the newborn's increased startles and tremors. Similar to breastfeeding advice for cocaine, the risks to the infant of maternal cannabis use are considered to outweigh the benefits of breastfeeding (Behnke & Smith, 2013).

PHENCYCLIDINE (PCP) PCP is a popular hallucinogen that can be smoked, taken orally, or injected intravenously. The drug causes confusion, delirium, and hallucinations with possible feelings of euphoria. The greatest risk for the pregnant woman is overdose or psychotic response. Signs of overdose include hypertension, hyperthermia, diaphoresis, and possible coma, which may jeopardize fetal well-being.

MDMA (ECSTASY) MDMA (3,4-methylenedioxymethamphetamine) is a mood- and perception-altering drug that is chemically similar to hallucinogens and stimulants (NIDA, 2012b). Better known as Ecstasy, it is the most commonly used **club drug**, so-called due to popularity among adolescents and young adults who frequent dance clubs and "raves." Other club drugs include flunitrazepam (Rohypnol), gamma hydroxybutyrate (GHB), and ketamine hydrochloride. PCP and LSD are sometimes classified as club drugs as well.

MDMA is the third most widely used illicit drug in the United States after marijuana and amphetamines. MDMA is taken by mouth, usually as a tablet. It produces euphoria and feelings of empathy for others. Originally it was widely perceived as a "safe" drug. However, current research has demonstrated that recreational MDMA users have memory dysfunctions characterized by verbal learning and recall deficits (Bosch et al., 2013).

Little is known about the effects of MDMA on fetuses. A decade of research using rats suggests that prenatal use of MDMA may be associated with long-term impaired memory and learning in the child. Adult rats prenatally exposed to MDMA display persistent deficits in working memory and attention. Investigators have found both structural changes in their noradrenergic system and functional alterations in their norepinephrine neurotransmission (Thompson et al., 2012).

HEROIN **Heroin** is an illicit CNS depressant narcotic that alters perception and produces euphoria. It is an addictive drug that is generally administered intravenously. Pregnancy in women who use heroin is considered a high risk because of the increased incidence of poor nutrition, iron deficiency anemia, and preeclampsia. Women addicted to heroin also have a higher incidence of sexually transmitted infections, because many rely on prostitution to support their drug habit.

Problematic outcomes for the baby can be up to six times higher for those born to mothers who use opiates (Keegan et al., 2010). The fetus of a woman addicted to heroin is at increased risk for IUGR, meconium aspiration, and hypoxia. The newborn frequently shows signs of heroin addiction such as restlessness; a shrill, high-pitched cry; irritability; fist sucking; vomiting; and seizures. Signs of withdrawal usually appear within 72 hours and may last for several days.

The newborn may exhibit poor consolability for 3 months or more. These behaviors may interfere with successful maternal attachment and increase the risk for parenting problems or abuse in an already high-risk mother.

METHADONE Methadone is the most commonly used therapy for nonpregnant women dependent on opioids such as heroin. Methadone blocks withdrawal symptoms, and reduces or eliminates the craving for narcotics.

In the situation of a pregnant woman who is opioid dependent, a different medication might be preferred, to reduce **neonatal abstinence syndrome (NAS)**. NAS is a combination of neonatal signs and symptoms caused by withdrawal of gestational opioid exposure. Buprenorphine is suggested as the alternative treatment to methadone during pregnancy (Jansson & Velez, 2012). Fetal monitoring has shown that buprenorphine caused less fetal cardiac and movement suppression than methadone (Jones, Finnegan, & Kaltenbach, 2012).

The motivating therapeutic goal is to use a therapy that helps the mother recover from illicit drug abuse, to optimize her health and that of her baby. Choices should be made on an individual basis, taking into account:

- Opioid dependence history
- Previous and current treatment experiences
- Medical circumstances
- Treatment preferences (Jones et al., 2012).

TOBACCO The latest statistics on the prevalence rate of pregnant women smokers and quitters comes from the 2008 Pregnancy Risk Assessment and Monitoring System (PRAMS) data from 29 states. About one in eight women (13%) smoked during their last trimester. However, on the positive side, almost half (45%) of the previously smoking women quit during their pregnancy. Women of childbearing age who smoke cigarettes face three obstacles to giving birth to a full-term infant. First, they have greater difficulty conceiving. Second, they are more likely to miscarry than nonsmoking women. Third, they more often go into early labor and give birth prematurely (CDC, 2013d).

The development of their fetus in utero is also affected. Prenatal smoke exposure has been linked with reduced birth weight and increased risks for diseases and behavioral disorders. **Epigenetic** studies that focus on the development of the zygote and fetus in utero have found that maternal smoking during pregnancy alters fetal DNA and microRNA (Knopik et al., 2012).

Box 22–6 Risk Factors for Substance Abuse

COMMUNITY

1. Availability of drugs
2. Community laws and norms favorable toward drug use
3. Transitions and mobility
4. Low neighborhood attachment and community disorganization
5. Extreme economic deprivation

FAMILY

6. Family history of the problem behavior
7. Family management problems
8. Family conflict
9. Favorable parental attitudes and involvement in the problem behavior

INDIVIDUAL/PEER

10. Alienation and rebelliousness
11. Friends who engage in the problem behavior
12. Favorable attitudes toward the problem behavior
13. Early initiation of the problem behavior
14. Constitutional factors

SCHOOL

15. Early and persistent antisocial behavior
16. Academic failure beginning in late elementary school
17. Lack of commitment to school.

Source: The Whatcom County Health Department (2009). Retrieved from http://www.co.whatcom.wa.us/health/human/substance_abuse/riskfactors.jsp.

Epidemiology

In general, the rate of illicit drug use among pregnant women is significantly less than the rate among nonpregnant women. Specifically, approximately 5% of pregnant women ages 15–44 report having used an illicit drug in the past month as compared with 10% of nonpregnant women (SAMHSA, 2012a). However, illicit drug usage varies significantly by race and by age, with higher rates among women ages 18–25 than among women ages 26–44. Rates are highest among American Indians and Alaskan Natives (13.4%) and lowest among Asians (3.8%). Rates are 10% among Blacks, 8.7% among Whites, 8.4% among Hispanics, and 11.0% among Native Hawaiians or Other Pacific Islanders (SAMHSA, 2012a). Among pregnant women ages 15–44, 9.4% reported current alcohol use, 2.6% reported binge drinking, and 0.4% reported heavy drinking (SAMHSA, 2012a).

Risk Factors

The Whatcom County Health Department in Washington State cites 17 identified risk factors for substance abuse, which are outlined in **Box 22–6** ●. While these risk factors for substance abuse apply to all clients, they can be of particular assistance to the nurse in trying to evaluate a pregnant woman's risk for substance abuse.

To provide information for caregivers and clients, the U.S. Food and Drug Administration (FDA) has developed the following classification system for all medications administered during pregnancy. This system can be used to help determine the risk of prenatal substance exposure from use of legal medications whether they are abused or prescribed by a physician.

■ *Category A.* Controlled studies in women have demonstrated no associated fetal risk. Few drugs fall into this category.

■ *Category B.* Animal studies show no risk. There have been no controlled studies in women in particular, but controlled human studies have failed to demonstrate a risk. The penicillins fall into this category.

■ *Category C.* Either (a) no adequate animal or human studies are available or (b) animal studies show teratogenic effects but no controlled studies in women are available. Many drugs fall into this category. The lack of information makes this problematic for caregivers. Epinephrine, beta-blockers, and zidovudine (a drug used to decrease perinatal transmission of HIV) fall into this category.

■ *Category D.* Evidence of human fetal risk exists, but the benefits of the drug in certain situations are thought to outweigh the risks. Examples of drugs in this category include tetracycline, vincristine, lithium, and hydrochlorothiazide.

■ *Category X.* The demonstrated fetal risks clearly outweigh any possible benefit. Examples of drugs in this category include isotretinoin (Accutane), an acne medication, which can cause multiple CNS, facial, and cardiovascular anomalies.

Prevention

Interprofessional statewide programs are needed to help prevent poor birth outcomes by ensuring that babies are born to women who decrease or eliminate alcohol, tobacco, and other drug use during pregnancy. Community and provider-wide efforts, such as the ones being provided through the Prenatal Substance Use Prevention Program, a three-tier prevention program administered by the Indiana State Department of Health, are needed to:

1. Identify high-risk, pregnant women who are chemically dependent; provide perinatal addiction education; promote abstinence; and provide referrals to treatment services and follow-up.
2. Provide public education on the hazards to a fetus when alcohol, tobacco, and other drugs are used during pregnancy.
3. Facilitate training and education for professionals and paraprofessionals who do not provide substance abuse treatment, but who work with women of childbearing age, on how to identify high-risk women who are chemically dependent (Indiana State Department of Health, 2013).

▶ CLINICAL MANIFESTATIONS

The clinical manifestations of prenatal substance use are listed in the Clinical Manifestations and Therapies feature.

▶ COLLABORATION

Care of the pregnant woman who is a substance abuser is most effective when the woman agrees to try to quit abusing and seeks both prenatal and addiction treatment early in her pregnancy.

Clinical Manifestations and Therapies **Prenatal Substance Exposure**

ETIOLOGY	CLINICAL MANIFESTATIONS	CLINICAL THERAPIES
Cocaine abuse	■ Placental abruption ■ Fetal demise ■ Cardiovascular effects: increased heart rate, vasoconstriction, hypertension, myocardial infarction, arrhythmias, cardiomyopathy ■ CNS effects: euphoria, increased energy, excitement, loss of appetite, feeling of increased physical and mental strength, dilated pupils, nausea, vomiting, headache, vertigo, emotional instability, muscle jerks, hallucinations, cocaine psychosis ■ Nasal and sinus diseases if cocaine is snorted	Substance withdrawal using: ■ Behavioral therapy ■ Recovery environment ■ Group supportive therapy ■ Detoxification.
Alcohol abuse	■ Increased risk of miscarriage and stillbirth ■ Low-birth-weight infant ■ Increased risk of learning, speech, attention span, and language disorders in the child born to a mother who abuses alcohol ■ Fetal alcohol syndrome	Substance withdrawal using: ■ Behavioral therapy ■ Recovery environment ■ Group supportive therapy ■ Detoxification ■ Medication therapy, which generally is not recommended during pregnancy.
Nicotine abuse	■ Miscarriage ■ Placental abruption ■ Premature rupture of membranes ■ Premature birth ■ Low-birth-weight infants ■ Increased risk that child born to a smoker will smoke later in life ■ Premature aging of placenta ■ Arterial spasm, including arteries to placenta ■ Polycythemia in the fetus, leading to possible fetal demise	Substance withdrawal using: ■ Behavioral therapy ■ Recovery environment ■ Group supportive therapy ■ Medication therapy in the form of nicotine replacement with gradual weaning of support.
Narcotic abuse (opioids)	■ Fetal narcotic abstinence syndrome ■ Increased risk of premature birth, low-birth-weight infant, newborn respiratory distress, newborn hypoglycemia, and fetal death ■ Respiratory depression in pregnant woman, possibly leading to hypoxia or death ■ Increased risk for infection secondary to use of dirty injection equipment	Substance withdrawal using: ■ Behavioral therapy ■ Recovery environment ■ Group supportive therapy ■ Detoxification ■ Medication therapy—choice of methadone or buprenorphine.

With the mother's permission, nurses, physicians, and therapists can share information to collaborate in supporting the mother during all phases of treatment.

 NURSING PROCESS

The nurse plays an important role in caring for the pregnant woman with a substance abuse problem. Compared to any other healthcare provider, nurses spend more time with the client; as a result, they are more likely to notice the often subtle signs of substance abuse. It is important for the nurse to follow the nursing process, using its cyclical nature for ongoing assessment and care.

Assessment

The substance user is difficult to identify prenatally. Because many drugs are illegal, women may be reluctant to volunteer information about their drug use. The nurse who is familiar with the woman may recognize subtle signs of drug use, including mood swings and appetite changes, and withdrawal symptoms such as depression, irritability, nausea, lack of motivation, and psychomotor changes. As the number of women of childbearing age using

Complementary and Alternative Therapy
Yoga for Pregnant Women

Yoga classes for women who are pregnant are available in most communities. Yoga can help reduce anxiety and stress, which can decrease a substance abuser's need to use in order to relieve anxiety. Pregnant mothers who want to try yoga should take a class specifically designed for pregnant women from a yoga practitioner who has been trained to work with pregnant women, because some poses are contraindicated during pregnancy.

substances increases, healthcare providers must be alert to early signs of use. It is often difficult for a nurse or physician to face the fact that a client is using an illegal substance, but ongoing alertness and an open, nonjudgmental approach are important for early detection. Care must be taken to ask open-ended questions in a nonjudgmental manner. For example, "How much alcohol do you drink per day?" is more helpful than "You don't drink alcohol, do you?" which leads the pregnant woman to believe that it would be inappropriate to admit to alcohol consumption.

Urine screening is valuable, but because cocaine is metabolized rapidly, the drug screen is negative within 24–48 hours after cocaine use. Thus, many expectant mothers who use cocaine probably are not identified.

SAFETY ALERT
Keep in mind that almost 1 out of 10 women in the United States, regardless of socioeconomic status or ethnic background, is currently abusing a substance. If you consider that possibility with every woman, you will ask the important questions about drug use and be alert for signs of substance abuse.

Because of the prevalence of substance abuse in society today, nurses and other care providers should screen all pregnant women for substance abuse during the health history. Several simple screening tools are available. In addition, the nurse needs to be alert for clues in the woman's history or appearance that suggest substance abuse (**Box 22–7 ●**).

If abuse is suspected, the nurse needs to ask direct questions, beginning with less threatening questions about use of tobacco, caffeine, and over-the-counter medications. The nurse can then progress to questions about alcohol consumption and finally to questions focusing on past and current use of illicit drugs. The nurse who uses a matter-of-fact and nonjudgmental approach is more likely to elicit honest responses.

Nursing assessment of the woman with a known substance abuse problem focuses on the woman's general health status, with specific attention paid to nutritional status, susceptibility to infections, and evaluation of all body systems. The nurse also assesses the woman's understanding of the impact of substance abuse on herself and her pregnancy.

Diagnosis
Nursing diagnoses that may apply to a woman at risk because of substance abuse include the following:

■ *Imbalanced Nutrition: Less Than Body Requirements* related to inadequate food intake secondary to substance abuse

Box 22–7   Possible Signs of Substance Abuse
HISTORY
■ History of vague or unusual medical complaints
■ Family history of alcoholism or other addiction
■ History of childhood physical, sexual, or emotional abuse
■ History of cirrhosis, pancreatitis, hepatitis, gastritis, sexually transmitted infections, or unusual infections such as cellulitis or endocarditis
■ History of high-risk sexual behavior
■ Psychiatric history of treatment and/or hospitalization

PHYSICAL SIGNS
■ Dilated or constricted pupils
■ Inflamed nasal mucosa
■ Evidence of needle "track marks" or abscesses
■ Poor nutritional status
■ Slurred speech or staggering gait
■ Odor of alcohol on breath

BEHAVIORAL SIGNS
■ Memory lapses, mood swings, hallucinations
■ Pattern of frequently missed appointments
■ Frequent accidents, falls
■ Signs of depression, agitation, euphoria
■ Suicidal gestures

■ *Risk for Infection* related to use of inadequately cleaned syringes and needles secondary to IV drug use
■ *Risk for Ineffective Health Maintenance* related to a lack of information about the impact of substance abuse on the fetus.

(NANDA-I © 2012)

Planning
Prevention of substance abuse during pregnancy is the ideal nursing goal and is best accomplished through education. Unfortunately, many women who abuse substances do not receive regular health care and may not seek care until they are far along in pregnancy. Other goals for client care may include the following:

■ The client will immediately reduce number of cigarettes smoked to ____ and develop a plan to quit smoking within 2 weeks.
■ The client will attend counseling sessions and/or drug treatment program within 48 hours.
■ The client will explain effects of substance being abused on fetal health.

Implementation
All women need to be counseled about the effects of alcohol in pregnancy. If heavy consumption is involved, the nurse can refer the pregnant woman to an alcoholism treatment program immediately. Counselors in these programs need to be made aware of a woman's pregnancy before drug therapy is suggested because certain drugs may be harmful to the developing fetus. For example, the drug disulfiram (Antabuse), often used in conjunction with alcohol treatment, is suspected to be a teratogenic agent. If the woman's behavior indicates possible substance abuse problems, the nurse can provide ongoing support and counseling and refer the woman to appropriate professionals.

The nurse's role in providing prenatal care for the woman who abuses substances focuses on ongoing assessment and client teaching. The nurse can provide information about the relationship between substance abuse and existing health problems and the implications for the woman's unborn child. By establishing a relationship of trust and support, the nurse may gain the woman's cooperation. The knowledgeable nurse can discuss possible strategies to help the woman quit (addiction treatment programs, 12-step programs, individual counseling) and suggest a referral for more in-depth assessment by a specialist. Relapse rates are high, even for motivated women, but the nurse's continued support and encouragement are important factors in helping women stop abusing substances.

One clinical study of pregnant substances abusers showed differences in their abstinence patterns. Discontinuation rates were lower for tobacco (22%), and higher for alcohol (65%) and marijuana (77%). Those who became abstinent experienced increased self-worth and decreased depression and anxiety compared to those who continued their addictions (Massey et al., 2011).

Preparation for labor and birth should be part of prenatal planning. Fear, tension, or discomfort may be relieved through nonnarcotic psychological support and careful explanation of the labor process. If pain medication is necessary, it should not be withheld; the notion that it will contribute to further addiction is mistaken. Preferred methods of pain relief include the use of psychoprophylaxis and regional blocks, such as epidurals or local anesthetics such as pudendal block and local infiltration. Immediate intensive care should be available for the newborn, who is often depressed, small for gestational age (SGA), and premature.

Evaluation

The ongoing and cyclical nature of the nursing process is especially evident in the prenatal setting. Throughout the course of pregnancy, however, certain criteria can be used to determine the quality of care provided. In essence, nursing care has been effective when the following occur:

- The woman avoids substances and situations that pose a risk to her well-being or that of her child.
- The woman seeks regular prenatal care.
- The woman describes the impact of her substance abuse on herself and her unborn child.
- The woman gives birth to a healthy infant.
- The woman agrees to accept a referral to social services (or another appropriate community agency) for follow-up care after discharge.

NURSING CARE PLAN   A Client Abusing Substances While Pregnant

ASSESSMENT	DIAGNOSIS	PLANNING
Kathy Sanderson is a 27-year-old woman who is visiting her gynecologist. She reports a positive home pregnancy test and has come to the physician's office for confirmation and prenatal care if the provider confirms pregnancy. Ms. Sanderson is in a long-term committed relationship and works full-time as a grammar school teacher. She denies use of alcohol, illegal substances, or any medications. The admitting nurse assesses her and notes dilated pupils, mildly increased temperature, increased heart rate and blood pressure, and extreme talkativeness with rapid speech. Ms. Sanderson has rhinorrhea but denies having a cold, saying she thinks it might be allergies. The nurse suspects possible cocaine use and shares assessment data with the provider, who orders a urine toxicology screen. The provider explains the need for a urine specimen and seeks consent, which the client provides. The results indicate that cocaine, cannabis (marijuana), and alcohol metabolites are present in the urine. When the results are shared with Ms. Sanderson, she begins to cry and admits she drinks occasionally, uses cocaine several times a week, and attended a party last night where marijuana was smoked but denies using it herself. She says that she was afraid to tell the nurse about her drug use because she would be fired from her job if her principal found out. Physical examination indicates the following: Height: 172 cm (5'8") Weight: 57 kg (125 lb) Temperature: 37.2°C (99°F) Pulse rate: 102 bpm Respirations: 22/min Blood pressure: 142/90 mmHg Urine toxicology positive for cannabis, cocaine, and alcohol Hemoglobin: 10.8 Hematocrit: 33.8%	■ *Knowledge Deficit* related to impact of cocaine and alcohol on the growing fetus and her own health status (NANDA-I © 2012)	■ The client will exhibit substance abuse control as evidenced by extensively describing the following: • Own risk for substance misuse • Adverse health effects of substance use • Signs of dependence during substance withdrawal • Benefits of eliminating substance use. ■ The client will exhibit knowledge of pregnancy evidenced by extensive description of the following: • Importance of prenatal care • Warning signs of pregnancy complications • Major fetal development milestones.

NURSING CARE PLAN (continued)

IMPLEMENTATION

- Establish a therapeutic relationship with Ms. Sanderson.
- Encourage Ms. Sanderson to take control of her own behavior.
- Assist Ms. Sanderson in identifying use of denial as a substitute for confronting the problem.
- Discuss with Ms. Sanderson the impact of substance abuse on her pregnancy and general health.
- Identify constructive goals with Ms. Sanderson to provide alternatives to the use of substances to reduce stress.

- Determine whether codependent or abusive relationships exist within the family.
- Determine Ms. Sanderson's learning needs.
- Appraise Ms. Sanderson's educational level.
- Select appropriate teaching methods and strategies.

EVALUATION

The goals related to Ms. Sanderson's knowledge deficit were met. At the prenatal visit, Ms. Sanderson admitted she had a cocaine addiction and agreed to begin rehabilitation therapy immediately. Through counseling, she was able to face her denial and recognize the people in her life who contributed to the problem, as well as those who could help her maintain her resolution to quit using cocaine. After completing an inpatient recovery program, she began attending a 12-step program for ongoing support. She received ongoing prenatal care through the rehabilitation and recovery phase and delivered a healthy, normal baby free of cocaine addiction at 39 weeks' gestation. She continues to attend group support sessions and has not relapsed since the baby was born.

CRITICAL THINKING

1. If the nurse had not noted the subtle assessment findings pointing to cocaine use, how might Ms. Sanderson's outcome have differed?
2. Could the provider have tested Ms. Sanderson's urine for toxicology if Ms. Sanderson had denied permission for the test? Why or why not?
3. While the nurse is working with her, Ms. Sanderson becomes very angry and says, "You don't understand. You've never had to go through this." How might the nurse respond?
4. If Ms. Sanderson had decided not to attend drug rehabilitation and delivered the baby while using cocaine, what follow-up care might the nurse have recommended for this new family?
5. Does the nurse have a responsibility to report Ms. Sanderson's drug use to the school system where she works? Explain your answer.

REVIEW Prenatal Substance Exposure

RELATE Link the Concepts and Exemplars

Linking the exemplar of prenatal substance exposure with the concept of development:

1. Explain why the goal of substance use and pregnancy is focused primarily on stopping substance abuse before the woman becomes pregnant.

2. What developmental complications could develop from substance abuse if the woman detoxifies from the substance immediately after the first prenatal visit?

Linking the exemplar of prenatal substance exposure with the concept of perfusion:

3. What substances reduce perfusion to the neonate?

4. What long-term effects are they likely to have on the growing fetus?

READY Go to Companion Skills Manual

REFER Go to Pearson Nursing Student Resources
nursing.pearsonhighered.com

- Additional review materials

REFLECT Case Study

Jessica Riley is an 18-year-old single mother of a 1-year-old son, Ryan. She lives in a small one-bedroom apartment with her boyfriend Casey, who is not Ryan's father. She has had no

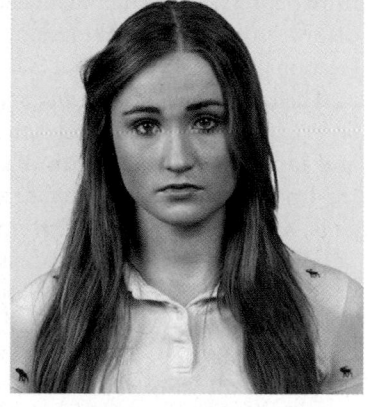

contact with Ryan's father since before Ryan was born. Jessica works full time as a waitress at a restaurant and struggles financially. She is very grateful for Casey's income because she doesn't know how she would make it financially without him. Jessica dropped out of community college when she learned she was pregnant again. She goes to the community clinic for prenatal care. She likes seeing the nurse midwife because she makes Jessica feel comfortable. At the 24-week visit, Jessica tells the midwife that she tried to stop smoking but hasn't been successful. She tells the midwife that she has stopped drinking alcohol, although she still drinks an occasional beer when Casey insists on having someone to drink with. At her 28-week visit, she reports a problem with constipation. The nurse midwife asks what types of fluids she consumes, and Jessica says that she drinks mostly Coke. The midwife suggests that Jessica decrease the number of soft drinks she consumes and increase her fluid and fiber intake. During the visit, Jessica learns from the ultrasound that the baby is a girl. It never dawns on Jessica to tell the midwife that Casey is smoking marijuana because she doesn't know that it has any impact on her or the baby.

1. What impact will Casey's marijuana use have on Jessica and the fetus?

2. Why would the nurse midwife tell Jessica to reduce her intake of soft drinks?

3. What effect will smoking cigarettes and an occasional beer (1–2 per week) have on the fetus?

4. If you were the nurse caring for Jessica, how would you help her make healthier choices to improve the outcome of her pregnancy?

EXEMPLAR 22.4 Substance Abuse

EXEMPLAR KEY TERMS
Amphetamine, *1563*
Caffeine, *1562*
Cannabis sativa, *1563*
Central nervous system (CNS) depressants, *1563*
Hallucinogens, *1564*
Inhalants, *1564*
Kindling, *1561*
Opiates, *1564*
Psychostimulants, *1563*
Substance abuse, *1560*
Substance dependence, *1560*

EXEMPLAR LEARNING OUTCOMES
After reading about this exemplar, you will be able to:

1. Describe the pathophysiology, etiology, clinical manifestations, and direct and indirect causes of substance abuse.

2. Identify risk factors associated with substance abuse.

3. Illustrate the nursing process in providing culturally competent care across the life span for individuals with a substance abuse disorder.

4. Formulate priority nursing diagnoses appropriate for individuals with a substance abuse disorder.

5. Summarize therapies used by interdisciplinary teams in the collaborative care of individuals with a substance abuse disorder.

6. Plan evidence-based care for individuals with a substance abuse disorder and their families in collaboration with other members of the healthcare team.

7. Evaluate expected outcomes for individuals with a substance abuse disorder.

▶ OVERVIEW

Substance abuse refers to the use of any chemical in a fashion inconsistent with medical or culturally defined social norms despite physical, psychological, or social adverse effects. Anxiety and depressive disorders frequently occur with substance abuse. More than 90% of people who commit suicide suffer from depression or other mental disorders, or a substance abuse disorder (often in combination with other mental disorders) (National Institute of Mental Health, 2010).

The current *Diagnostic and Statistical Manual of Mental Disorders* (DSM-5) includes substance abuse in "substance-related and addictive disorders" with 10 separate classes of drugs, ranging from alcohol, caffeine, and tobacco to cannabis, hallucinogens, opioids, sedatives, and stimulants. The DSM-5 notes that "all drugs that are taken in excess have in common direct activation of the brain reward system . . ." (American Psychiatric Association, 2013, p. 481).

Substance dependence occurs when an individual can no longer control use of a substance, continues to use despite adverse effects, and experiences withdrawal symptoms without continued use of the substance. Individuals who are dependent on drugs experience tolerance, requiring increasing quantities of the substance to meet the same level of need. They may spend a great deal of time obtaining drugs and limit their usual social, occupational, or recreational activities because of the substance use. As addiction continues, the need for the drug becomes so powerful that even addicts explicitly wanting to abstain find themselves "powerless to resist drugs, despite knowing that drug-taking may be a harmful course of action" (Kermati & Gutkin, 2013, p. 00). This exemplar focuses on substance dependence, which is the more severe form of the substance-related disorders.

Substance withdrawal symptoms are physiological, behavioral, cognitive, and affective symptoms that occur after reduction or discontinuance of a drug that has been used heavily over a long period of time. When experiencing withdrawal, most individuals find themselves craving the drug, which they know would relieve the withdrawal symptoms. Withdrawal symptoms are specific for each drug. Withdrawal is an uncomfortable state lasting several days and, depending on the amount of drugs consumed, may put the client in medical danger. Tolerance is a cumulative state in which a particular dose of the chemical elicits a smaller response than before. With increased tolerance, the individual needs higher and higher doses to obtain the desired effect. When an individual is physically addicted to the drug and stops taking it, withdrawal symptoms can occur within hours.

Chemical dependence is a complex, chronic progressive disease that can be fatal if left untreated. While it is true that a disease is not defined as a deficiency of willpower, chemical dependence is composed of several biochemical processes that are subject to voluntary control. In addition, there are psychological, sociological, and spiritual aspects to chemical dependence.

A number of types of psychoactive substances are associated with chemical dependence. The days of the so-called pure drug addict or alcoholic are gone. Most people who are chemically dependent are engaged in polysubstance abuse. They may use amphetamines or cocaine to get high and alcohol, diazepam (Valium), or marijuana to come down off the high. Some addicts use sedatives to sleep and amphetamines to wake up. Whatever the pattern, clients must be treated for all secondary, as well as primary, addictions.

While alcohol and nicotine are often abused, they are covered in separate exemplars in this concept. For the purpose of this exemplar, the term *substance abuse* refers specifically to drugs, both legal and illegal, that lead to addiction and dependence.

▶ PATHOPHYSIOLOGY AND ETIOLOGY

The pathophysiology of substance abuse was discussed earlier in the module. In summary, it is a complex, multifactorial process that involves a combination of biological, genetic, psychological, and sociocultural factors. In addition to these factors, specific factors associated with substance dependency may affect the process of recovery. For example, the craving that an individual has for a particular substance may be heightened by a phenomenon known as the kindling effect. **Kindling** refers to long-term changes in brain neurotransmission that occur after repeated detoxifications (Breese, Sinha, & Heilig, 2011). Recurrent detoxifications increase neuron sensitivity and are thought to intensify obsessive thoughts or cravings for a substance. Eventually, the brain responds spontaneously in a dysfunctional manner even when the substance is no longer being used (Stuart, 2008). This phenomenon may explain why subsequent episodes of withdrawal from a substance tend to get progressively worse.

Epidemiology

In 2011, an estimated 20.6 million people ages 12 or older were classified with substance dependence or abuse. This figure represents 8.0% of the American people ages 12 or older (SAMHSA, 2012a). Each year millions of people who have never tried illicit drugs begin to do so. In 2011, the largest group, 2.6 million people, "tried" marijuana followed by 1.9 million who tried nonmedical use of pain relievers (1.9 million), nonmedical use of tranquilizers (1.2 million), Ecstasy (0.9 million), and cocaine and stimulants (0.7 million) (SAMHSA, 2012a). The average age of first use varies. Among people ages 12 to 49, the average age at first use was 16.4 years for inhalants, 17.5 years for marijuana, 19.6 years for Ecstasy, 20.1 years for cocaine, 21.8 years for pain relievers, 22.1 years for heroin, 22.2 years for stimulants, and 24.6 years for tranquilizers (SAMHSA, 2012a).

Substance use disorders in the United States cost over $600 billion a year, including the costs of treatment, related health problems, absenteeism, lost productivity, drug-related crime and incarceration, and education and prevention. This includes $235 billion for alcohol, and $193 billion each for illicit drugs and for tobacco (NIDA, 2011a). The relapse rates for drug addiction are 40%–60%, comparable to relapse rates of other chronic illnesses, such as diabetes, hypertension, and asthma (NIDA, 2008).

Results of the *2011 National Survey on Drug Use and Health* showed that over 22 million Americans, about 9% of the population ages 12 or older, were currently using illicit drugs (SAMHSA, 2012a). The greatest rate of increase was seen in those ages 50 to 59 years old, whose use of illicit drugs zoomed to over 6% from under 3% in 2002. This reflects the baby boomer population's lifetime rate of illicit drug use being higher than that of older people of previous generations.

Illicit use of prescription drugs is on the rise, especially among adolescents who mistakenly believe that these drugs are safer than illegal drugs. Generally, the four categories of prescription-type drugs (pain relievers, tranquilizers, stimulants, and sedatives) include numerous medications that currently are or have been available by prescription. They also include drugs within these groupings that originally were prescription medications but currently may be manufactured and distributed illegally, such as methamphetamine, which is included under stimulants (SAMHSA, 2012a).

Risk Factors

Risk factors for substance abuse include being male; loneliness, depression, and/or low self-esteem; family history of addiction; peer pressure; presence of mental illness; lack of family involvement; and using highly addictive drugs such as cocaine and heroin (Mayo Clinic, 2011).

Impaired Nurses

In the 1970s, research on impaired nursing practice began to appear, and in 1982, the American Nurses Association (ANA) passed a resolution entitled "Action on Alcohol and Drug Misuse and Psychological Dysfunctions Among Nurses." The hope was to shift the focus from punishment to rehabilitation. In 2002, the ANA adopted an updated resolution entitled "The Profession's Response to the Problems of Addictions and Psychiatric Disorders in Nursing," calling attention again to impaired nursing practice, stressing the need for peer assistance programs (Heise, 2003). The ANA currently joins with the International Nurses Society on Addictions to promote a treatment-over-discipline approach.

Healthcare providers are as susceptible as anyone else to developing substance abuse. By the very nature of their roles, dentists, pharmacists, physicians, and nurses are in frequent contact with drugs and are at high risk for substance abuse problems. As a rule, nurses experience many pressures in the workplace and have easy access to drugs. Thomas and Siela (2011) estimated that 10%–15% of all nurses may be impaired or in recovery from alcohol or drug addiction. They also reported that the two best predictors of successful recovery from addiction are the length of treatment and the willingness of the nurse. Nurses who remained in treatment for at least a year are twice as likely to be drug free.

Substance abuse and dependence can lead to impaired professional practice; therefore, nurses must act responsibly when coworkers display signs of substance abuse. The American Nurses Association Code of Ethics for Nurses provides a framework for client safety. Four suggestions for implementing its philosophy are:

- Do not ignore poor performance.
- Do not lighten or change the nurses' client assignment.
- Do not accept excuses.
- Do not allow yourself to be manipulated or fear confronting a nurse if client safety is in jeopardy (Thomas & Siela, 2011).

If nurses are showing signs of a substance abuse problem, to help them, their colleagues can find information about impaired nurse programs through state boards of nursing. Warning signs of impaired nurses in the workplace are listed in **Table 22–6** ●.

TABLE 22–6   Warning Signs of Impaired Nurses in the Workplace

AT-RISK SITUATIONS	OBSERVABLE WARNING SIGNS
Easy access to prescription drugs	Inaccurate narcotic counts or drugs frequently missing Client complaints of ineffective pain control, denial of having received pain meds Excessive "wasting" of drugs Likelihood of volunteering to give medications to clients Frequent trips to the bathroom
Role strain	Frequent tardiness or absenteeism, especially before and after scheduled days off Haphazard, shoddy charting Judgment errors in client care Unorganized, erratic behavior; unkempt appearance
Depression	Irritability, unable to focus or concentrate Abrupt mood swings Isolating self, taking long breaks Apathetic, depressed, lethargic Unexplained absences from assigned unit
Signs of alcohol or drug use	Smell of alcohol on breath Excessive use of perfumes, mouthwash, or mints Slurred speech, flushed face, reddened eyes, unsteady gait Long sleeves worn in hot weather to cover up arms
Signs of withdrawal	Tremors, restlessness, sweating Watery eyes, runny nose, stomachaches

When nurses have an addiction, shame and guilt are magnified. They are not expected to have their own problems, certainly not an addiction that could lead them to take drugs from clients or be less than 100% in control when they are at work.

Nurses now have access to peer assistance and statewide programs to seek treatment and to maintain or reinstate their licenses. **Box 22–8** ● lists resources for impaired nurses.

▶ CLINICAL MANIFESTATIONS

Clinical manifestations, and their severity, are dependent on amount, frequency, and specific combination of substances used. Combining two CNS depressants, for example, will produce far more significant manifestations than the use of only one CNS depressant. Some symptoms can be alarming or even fatal. For example, long-term crack use can result in sensory hallucinations, and even the first use of cocaine can result in death for people with never diagnosed cardiac disorders. Specific manifestations are linked to specific substances in the following sections.

Box 22–8   Resources for Impaired Nurses

Most state nurses' associations have peer assistance programs. Resources vary by state, but generally are accessible through each state association's Web site. Many state boards of nursing offer programs designed to guide nurses to sobriety, rather than instituting immediate disciplinary consequences. Again, this information typically is available on the specific board of nursing's Web site. Additionally, larger agencies may offer programs for employees, including support groups. Regardless, nurses who feel they are developing a substance abuse problem are ethically required to seek help in order to prevent mistakes in the workplace. The ANA Web site (www.NursingWorld.org) includes the ANA Code of Ethics and an Impaired Nurse Resource Center.

Caffeine

Caffeine is a stimulant that increases the heart rate and acts as a diuretic. Although commonly consumed daily in soft drinks, coffee, tea, chocolate, and some pain relievers, an excessive amount of caffeine can cause negative physiological effects, especially cardiac-related risks. Approximately 300 mg/day is safe for most people, but over 600 mg is considered excessive and is not recommended (Kneisl & Trigoboff, 2013, p. 314). Individuals with a history of cardiac disease should be advised to cut down or eliminate caffeine intake altogether. Caffeine, if consumed in large quantities, also can cause higher total cholesterol levels and insomnia.

Many people in today's society recognize the adverse effects of too much caffeine in their system and voluntarily cut down by drinking decaffeinated beverages. A caffeine-addicted person who abruptly withdraws from caffeine will most likely experience headaches and irritability. However, even with evidence of withdrawal symptoms, some clinicians do not consider caffeine as addicting, because it does not have a major action on the mesolimbic dopamine system (McNeece & DiNitto, 2012, p. 50).

Regardless of the label, a rising number of adolescents are developing symptoms of caffeine dependence by consuming sizable quantities of caffeinated energy drinks. The caffeine content can be an "alarming" 505 mg per can or bottle (Reissig, Strain, & Griffiths, 2009). Researchers predict an increase in caffeine intoxication and problems with caffeine dependence and withdrawal. Genetic factors may also play a role in these clinical manifestations. Other studies suggest that caffeine in combination with alcohol may increase accidental injuries. As important, several studies raise the issue of energy drinks serving as a gateway to other forms of drug dependence (Reissig et al., 2009).

Cannabis

Cannabis sativa is the source of marijuana. The greatest psychoactive substances are in the flowering tops of the cannabis plant. Marijuana (also known as grass, weed, pot, dope, joint, and reefer) and hashish are the most common derivatives. The psychoactive component of marijuana is an oily chemical known as delta-9-tetrahydrocannabinol (THC). THC activates specific cannabinoid receptors in the brain. Evidence suggests that marijuana may act like opioids and cocaine in producing a pleasurable sensation, probably by causing release of endogenous opioids and then dopamine (Kneisl & Trigoboff, 2013).

The physiological effects of cannabis are dose related and can cause an increase in heart rate and bronchodilation in short-term use. Chronic long-term use can lead to airway constriction and inflammation, and increased incidence of acute and chronic bronchitis (World Health Organization, 2013). The reproductive system also is affected by marijuana use; it causes decreased spermatogenesis and testosterone levels in males and suppresses follicle-stimulating, luteinizing, and prolactin hormones in females, making breastfeeding impossible for new mothers. Birth defects also may be associated with cannabis use. Marijuana crosses the placental barrier and is spread to fetal tissues.

Euphoria and relaxation are the pleasurable effects most associated with marijuana use. Other subjective effects of marijuana include sedation and hallucinations. With increased use, marijuana can result in amotivational behaviors such as apathy, dullness, poor grooming, reduced interest in achievement, and disinterest. Memory impairment is common, due to the alteration of how information is processed in the hippocampus. At extremely high doses, tolerance and physical dependence result (NIDA, 2010c).

The *2011 National Survey on Drug Use and Health* found marijuana continues to be the most common illicit drug used (SAMHSA, 2012a). In 2011, over 18 million people in the United States had used marijuana in the past month, up from the 14.5 million using it in 2007.

Central Nervous System Depressants

Central nervous system (CNS) depressants, including barbiturates, benzodiazepines, paraldehyde, meprobamate, and chloral hydrate, also are subject to abuse. Cross-dependence exists among all CNS depressants, and cross-tolerance can develop to alcohol and general anesthetics. Chronic users of barbiturates require progressively higher doses to achieve subjective effects as tolerance develops, but they develop little tolerance to respiratory depression. The depressant effects related to barbiturates are dose dependent and range from mild sedation to sleep to coma to death. With larger doses over time and a combination of alcohol and barbiturates, the risk of death increases greatly.

The risk of accidental overdose and death resulting from barbiturates has resulted in decreased use, yet barbiturates are still clinically useful in treating seizure disorders and alcohol withdrawal. Benzodiazepines have replaced barbiturates as the drugs of choice for anxiety-related disorders. Benzodiazepines alone are safer than barbiturates because an overdose of oral benzodiazepines rarely results in death. However, when taken together, CNS depressants (for example, alcohol and benzodiazepines) can result in death.

Psychostimulants

Psychostimulants such as cocaine and amphetamines have a high potential for abuse. Euphoria is the main subjective effect associated with cocaine and amphetamines, leading to addiction. Powdered cocaine has been "snorted" (inhaled through the nostrils) for thousands of years, but a more dangerous method used today is called freebasing. Cocaine base (free-based cocaine, or "crack") is heat stable and is usually "cooked" in a baking soda solution and smoked (freebasing). Cocaine hydrochloride is diluted or cut before sale, and the pure form ("rocks") is administered intranasally (snorted) or injected intravenously. "Skin popping" is a subcutaneous method that many substance abusers are using to administer drugs, perhaps leading to the formation of abscesses under the skin.

The duration of euphoria achieved by cocaine depends on the route of administration. Regardless, the pleasurable effects do not last long, and its highly addictive properties can easily lead to overdose. A mild overdose of cocaine produces agitation, dizziness, tremor, and blurred vision. A severe overdose produces anxiety, hyperpyrexia, convulsions, ventricular dysrhythmias, severe hypertension, and hemorrhagic stroke with possible angina or myocardial infarction.

The use of cocaine during pregnancy is especially problematic because the drug crosses the placenta and enters the fetal bloodstream. Spontaneous abortion, premature delivery, IUGR, congenital abnormalities, and fetal addiction can result.

Long-term intranasal use of cocaine can cause atrophy of the nasal mucosa, necrosis and perforation of the nasal septum, and lung damage. Crack cocaine injection requires serious attention because this new drug use is associated with increased rates of high-risk behaviors (NIDA, 2010a).

Amphetamine is a powerful stimulant that poses a severe health risk to society due to its devastating physical and neurological consequences, including amphetamine-induced mental disorders. Methamphetamine is a highly addictive form of amphetamine whose use is widespread due to the fact that its manufacturing process can be carried out by individuals without special knowledge or expertise in chemistry. Methamphetamine is often taken in combination with other drugs such as cocaine and marijuana. Smoking or injection provides the greatest euphoria, although it may also be inhaled or ingested. Chronic use or abuse can result in paranoia, hallucinations, and compulsions. Some users experience delusions that insects are crawling over them, resulting in obsessive scratching. Psychosis characterized by violent behavior may also result (Partnership at Drugfree.org, 2013).

Amphetamines cause arousal and an elevation of mood with a sense of increased strength, mental capacity, self-confidence, and a decreased need for food and sleep. Tolerance to mood elevation, appetite suppression, and cardiovascular effects develops with amphetamines; however, dependence is more psychological than physical.

Withdrawal from amphetamines produces dysphoria and craving with fatigue, prolonged sleep, excessive eating, and depression. Methamphetamine addiction can be successfully treated. Programs using a combination of individual and group therapy designed to promote behavioral changes as well as incentive-based programs have been cited as effective. Although there is currently no proven pharmacologic therapy, research in that area continues (NIDA, 2011b).

Opiates

Opiates such as morphine, meperidine, codeine, hydrocodone, and oxycodone are narcotic analgesics. Some common brand names include Vicodin, Percocet, OxyContin, and Darvon. Narcotic analgesics are a type of pain reliever derived from natural or synthetic opiates. A small percentage of individuals are originally exposed to opiates in the context of prescription pain management; however, most people use opiates under social or illicit circumstances.

The problem of abuse of and addiction to prescribed narcotics resurfaced as a major issue for the United States in the early 2000s and has worsened at a dramatic rate. Americans, only 4.6% of the world's population, consume 80% of the global opiate supply, and 99% of the global hydrocodone supply. Americans use two thirds of the world's illegal drugs (Manchikanti et al., 2010).

This increase in opiate abuse seems to reflect, in part, changes in medication prescribing practices, changes in drug formulations, and fairly easy access via the Internet. Other factors include an increased awareness of the right to pain relief and aggressive marketing by the pharmaceutical industry (Manchikanti et al., 2012). Although the use of narcotic analgesics for acute pain management looks benign, long-term use has been associated with significant rates of abuse or addiction. Three problematic physiological effects have been pointed out: hyperalgesia, hypogonadism, and sexual dysfunction (Manchikanti et al., 2010).

According to data collected by the Drug Abuse Warning Network (DAWN), drug abuse–related ED visits involving narcotic analgesics increased 153% in the nation from 2004 to 2011, with 420,040 ED visits in 2011 (SAMHSA, 2013). The greatest increases during this period occurred for oxycodone (512%), methadone (176%), hydrocodone (159%), and morphine (116%).

Opiates are responsible for more deaths than fatalities from both suicide and motor vehicle crashes combined (Manchikanti et al., 2012).

Heroin is an opiate that has been abused for many centuries and is usually administered intravenously. It induces a "rush" or "kick" that lasts less than a minute, followed by a sense of euphoria lasting several hours. Tolerance develops to the euphoria, respiratory depression, and nausea, but not to constipation and miosis. Physical dependence occurs with long-term use of opiates. Initial withdrawal symptoms such as drug craving, lacrimation (tear production), rhinorrhea, yawning, and diaphoresis usually take 10 days to run their course. The second phase of opiate withdrawal lasts for months with insomnia, irritability, fatigue, and potential GI hyperactivity and premature ejaculation as problems.

Methadone is a synthetic opiate used to treat chronic pain and addiction to other opiates. Methadone does not hinder one's ability to function productively, as other narcotics do, and it is a viable support for withdrawal (Stuart, 2008).

Hallucinogens

Hallucinogens are also called *psychedelics* and include PCP, 3,4-MDMA, D-lysergic acid diethylamide (LSD), mescaline, dimethyltryptamine (DMT), and psilocin. Psychedelics bring on the same types of thoughts, perceptions, and feelings that occur in dreams. PCP (also called *angel dust*) was developed in the 1950s as an anesthetic similar to ketamine. Due to its severe side effects, its development for human use was discontinued. The most common route of administration is smoking tobacco, marijuana, or herbal cigarettes laced with PCP powder or the liquid form of PCP. In the clinical setting, clients experiencing PCP intoxication are often violent and difficult to control physically. A chemical restraint is frequently needed to protect other clients and staff from an agitated PCP user. Haloperidol (Haldol) has been evaluated as an effective medical intervention, without causing harm to the client (MacNeal et al., 2012).

As mentioned earlier, MDMA, commonly known as Ecstasy, was very popular in the 1980s as a recreational "club drug" associated with dance clubs and "raves" and has reappeared in recent years as a date or rape drug. According to the 2011 *National Survey on Drug Use and Health* data, approximately 922,000 people ages 12 and older used Ecstasy for the first time in 2011 (SAMHSA, 2012a). Parties where other drugs such as marijuana and alcohol are present may lead to easier access or availability of Ecstasy, thereby increasing the chances for first-time Ecstasy use. Females were more likely than males to report using multiple club drugs. Staying in school and getting married were associated with decreased odds of club drug use. On the other hand, criminal behaviors and recent alcohol abuse or dependence increased use of club drugs.

LSD was first used to simulate psychosis. It affects serotonin receptors at multiple sites in the brain and spinal cord. LSD is usually taken orally but can be injected or smoked, as in tobacco- or marijuana-laced cigarettes. The individual's response to a trip, the experience of being high on LSD, cannot be predicted. Psychological effects (e.g., seeing bursts of radiant colors and seeing objects that appear to breathe) and flashbacks are common. Serotonin imbalance is thought to affect impulse control and may be responsible for uninhibited sexual responses in women who have been given the drug without their knowledge. Other hallucinogens are similar to LSD but have a different potency and course of action. Because physical dependence to hallucinogens does not appear to occur, withdrawal symptoms are not present.

Inhalants

Inhalants are categorized into three types: anesthetics, volatile nitrites, and organic solvents. Nitrous oxide (laughing gas) and ether are the most abused anesthetics. Amyl nitrite, butyl nitrite, and isobutyl nitrite are volatile nitrites used especially by homosexual males to induce venodilation and anal sphincter relaxation. Amyl nitrite is manufactured for medical use, but butyl and isobutyl nitrites are sold for recreational use. Other names for butyl and isobutyl nitrites are *climax, rush,* and *locker room.* Street names for amyl nitrite are *poppers* and *snappers.* Brain damage or sudden death can occur the first, tenth, or hundredth time an individual uses an inhalant, resulting in "sudden sniffing death." This danger makes the use of inhalants more hazardous than some other substances.

Another danger is the wide assortment of organic solvents that are available to and inhaled by young children. Organic solvents are ingested by three different methods: bagging, huffing, and sniffing. *Bagging* involves pouring the solvent in a plastic bag and inhaling the vapor. *Huffing* refers to pouring the solvent on a rag and inhaling. *Sniffing* refers to inhaling the solvent directly from the container. Common organic solvents are toluene, gasoline, lighter fluid, paint thinner, nail polish remover, benzene, acetone, chloroform, and model airplane glue. The effects from inhaling organic solvents are similar to those of alcohol. Prolonged use can lead to multiple toxicities. There are no antidotes for these inhalants; therefore, management of overdose is supportive.

Inhalant users have higher rates of some mental health issues than nonusers of inhalants: major depression, suicidal ideation and attempts, anxiety disorders, and other substance use disorders. Some researchers believe that inhalant use might be related to an overall antisocial mind-set, rather than the chemicals causing subsequent drug use and negative psychosocial outcomes (Howard et al., 2010a, 2010b). This viewpoint is given substantiation by the finding that the first use of inhalants peaks at about 14 years of age, earlier than first use of cannabis or tobacco. A higher family income was protective against first use; on the other hand, parental drug use was a risk factor for first use (Nonnemaker et al., 2011).

▶ COLLABORATION

Effective treatment of substance abuse and dependence results from the efforts of an interdisciplinary team specializing in the treatment of psychiatric and substance abuse disorders. Therapies may include detoxification, aversion therapy to maintain abstinence, group and individual psychotherapy, psychotropic medications, cognitive-behavioral strategies, family counseling, and self-help groups. Clients who are substance abusers can be treated in either an inpatient or outpatient setting (**Figure 22–4** ●). A substance overdose is a life-threatening condition that requires emergency hospitalization to stabilize the client medically before any of the interventions mentioned are implemented. Several diagnostic tests can provide valuable information about the client's physical condition and set the course for treatment.

Diagnostic Tests

The body fluids most often tested for drug content are blood and urine, although saliva, perspiration, and even hair may be tested. More invasive procedures such as serum drug levels are useful in the ED and other hospital settings to treat drug overdoses or complications. Urine drug screening (UDS), which is noninvasive, is the preferred method for detecting substances in the body. Companies often require a UDS of prospective employees before hiring them. In addition, professional and college athletes are now required to submit to random drug testing. Results of UDS tests are also used in the court system to determine drug use in relation to criminal activity. The length of time that drugs can be found in blood and urine varies according to dosage and metabolic properties of the drug. All traces of the drug may disappear within 24 hours or may still be detectable 30 days later. THC, the psychoactive substance found in marijuana, is stored in fatty tissues (especially the brain and reproductive system) and can be detected in the body for up to 6 weeks (Kneisl & Trigoboff, 2013).

Pharmacologic Therapy

Common drugs used in the treatment of substance abuse and withdrawal are presented in **Table 22–7** ●.

Emergency Care for Overdose

The care of a client who has overdosed on any substance is a serious medical emergency. Respiratory depression may require mechanical ventilation. The client may become severely sedated and difficult to arouse. Every effort must be made to keep the client awake; however, stupor and coma often result. A seizure is another serious complication that requires emergency treatment. If the overdose was intentional, the client must be monitored constantly for further signs of suicidal ideation. An actively suicidal client must never be left alone. Signs of overdose and withdrawal from major substances are summarized in **Table 22–8** ● along with recommended treatments.

■ NURSING PROCESS

Nurses may interact with clients experiencing substance abuse or substance dependence in a variety of settings. The most common setting is an alcohol and drug abuse treatment program where clients are hospitalized for 20–30 days for detoxification and inpatient therapy. These clients may be voluntarily admitted or ordered by the court to undergo treatment. Clients with substance abuse or dependence have impaired senses and risk-taking behaviors that lead to injuries from falls and accidents requiring medical attention. Therefore, hospital emergency departments as well as medical and surgical units are places where nurses frequently encounter these clients. Occupational nurses and community health nurses also interact with

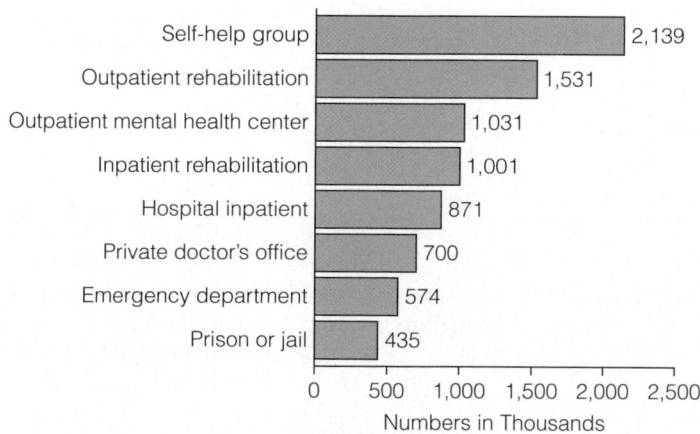

Figure 22–4 ● Locations where substance abuse treatment was received among individuals ages 12 or older in 2011.

TABLE 22-7 Drugs Used in the Treatment of Substance Abuse/Withdrawal

DRUG	DOSE	PURPOSE
Benzodiazepines		
1. Chlordiazepoxide (Librium)	15–100 mg	Diminishes anxiety and has anticonvulsant qualities to provide safe withdrawal. May be ordered q4h or PRN to manage adverse effects from withdrawal; then dose is tapered to zero.
2. Diazepam (Valium)	4–40 mg	
3. Oxazepam (Serax)	30–120 mg	
4. Lorazepam (Ativan)	2–6 mg	
Vitamins		
1. Thiamine (vitamin B$_1$)	100 mg/day	Prevents Wernicke encephalopathy
2. Folic acid	1 mg/day	Corrects vitamin deficiency caused by heavy, long-term alcohol abuse.
3. Multivitamins	1 tab/cap daily	
Anticonvulsants		
1. Phenobarbital	30–320 mg	Controls seizures and acts as a sedative.
2. Magnesium sulfate	1 g q6h	Reduces postwithdrawal seizures.
Abstinence Medications		
1. Disulfiram (Antabuse)	250 mg/day	Prevents breakdown of alcohol.
2. Naltrexone (ReVia)	50 mg/day	Diminishes cravings for alcohol and opioids.
3. Acamprosate (Campral)	666 mg BID	Decreases alcohol cravings.
4. Methadone	40 mg/day	Blocks craving for heroin.
Antidepressants		
1. Fluoxetine (Prozac)	20–80 mg/day	Enhances and stabilizes mood and diminishes anxiety.
2. Sertraline (Zoloft)	50–200 mg/day	

TABLE 22-8 Signs and Treatment of Overdose and Withdrawal

DRUG	OVERDOSE		WITHDRAWAL	
	SIGNS	TREATMENT	SIGNS	TREATMENT
CNS Depressants				
Alcohol Barbiturates Benzodiazepines	Cardiovascular or respiratory depression or arrest (mostly with barbiturates) Coma Shock Convulsions Death	*If awake:* Keep awake. Induce vomiting. Use activated charcoal to absorb drug. VS q 15 minutes. *Coma:* Clear airway, intubate IV fluids. Perform gastric lavage. Take seizure precautions. Administer hemodialysis or peritoneal dialysis if ordered. Assess VS as ordered. Assess for shock and cardiac arrest.	Nausea and vomiting Tachycardia Diaphoresis Anxiety or agitation Tremors Marked insomnia Grand mal seizures Delirium (after 5–15 years of heavy use)	Carefully titrated detoxification with similar drug *Note:* Abrupt withdrawal can lead to death.
Stimulants				
Cocaine/crack Amphetamines	Respiratory distress Ataxia Hyperpyrexia Convulsions Coma Stroke Myocardial infarction Death	Antipsychotics Management for: 1. Hyperpyrexia 2. Convulsions 3. Respiratory distress 4. Cardiovascular shock 5. Acidic urine (ammonium chloride for amphetamine).	Fatigue Depression Agitation Apathy Anxiety Sleepiness Disorientation Lethargy Craving	Antidepressants (desipramine) Dopamine agonist Bromocriptine
Opiates				
Heroin Meperidine Morphine Methadone	Pupil dilation due to anoxia Respiratory depression arrest Coma Shock Convulsions Death	Narcotic antagonist (Narcan) quickly reverses CNS depression	Yawning, insomnia Irritability Rhinorrhea Panic Diaphoresis Cramps Nausea and vomiting Muscle aches Chills and fever Lacrimation Diarrhea	Methadone tapering Clonidine-naltrexone detoxification Buprenorphine substitution

TABLE 22–8   Signs and Treatment of Overdose and Withdrawal (*continued*)

| DRUG | OVERDOSE | | WITHDRAWAL | |
	SIGNS	TREATMENT	SIGNS	TREATMENT
Hallucinogens				
LSD	Psychosis Brain damage Death	Ensure low stimuli with minimal light, sound, activity. Have one person "talk down client," reassure. Speak slowly and clearly. Administer diazepam or chloral hydrate for anxiety as ordered.	No pattern of withdrawal	
PCP	Possible hypertensive crisis Respiratory arrest Hyperthermia Seizures	Acidify urine to help excrete drug (cranberry juice, ascorbic acid); in acute stage: ammonium chloride. Minimize stimuli. Do *not* attempt to talk down; speak slowly in low voice. Administer diazepam or Haldol as ordered.		
Inhalants				
Volatile solvents such as butane, paint thinner, airplane glue, and nail polish remover	Intoxication Excitation Drowsiness Disinhibition Staggering Light-headedness Agitation Side effects: 1. Damage to nervous system 2. Death	Support affected systems	No pattern of withdrawal	
Nitrites	Enhanced sexual pleasure	Neurological symptoms may respond to vitamin B_{12} and folate.		
Anesthetics such as nitrous oxide	Giggling, laughter Euphoria	Chronic users may experience poly-neuropathy and myelopathy.		

substance-abusing clients in employee assistance programs and community health departments. Urgent care centers, pain clinics, and ambulatory care centers are other settings in which clients with substance abuse disorders frequently appear for minor health problems associated with chronic disorders related to substance abuse or dependence.

Nursing care of the client with substance abuse or dependence is challenging and requires a nonjudgmental atmosphere promoting trust and respect. Nurses should provide adults with information on healthy coping mechanisms and relaxation and stress reduction techniques to decrease the risks of substance abuse. Nurses have a responsibility to educate their clients about the physiological effects of substances on the body. Nurses must encourage and support periods of abstinence while assisting clients to make major changes in lifestyles, habits, relationships, and coping methods. See the Lifespan Considerations feature on page 1568 for a discussion of older clients with substance abuse problems.

Health promotion efforts are aimed at preventing drug use among children and adolescents and reducing the risks among adults. Adolescence is the most common phase for the first experience with drugs (Stuart, 2008); therefore, teenagers are a vulnerable population, often succumbing to peer pressure. Healthy lifestyles, parental support, stress management, good nutrition,

and information about ways to steer clear of peer pressure are important topics for the nurse to provide in school programs.

Assessment

If you have a stereotypical picture of what an addict "looks like," beware! Many high-functioning substance abusers do not fit the stereotypical picture of a drug or alcohol abuser. They are your friends and neighbors, functioning in many responsible roles. They may not drink or use drugs every day and they may still avoid the serious consequences that befall most addicts and their families. High-functioning addicts can spend years, even decades, in denial. The high-functioning substance abuser's denial may be compounded by family and friends who fail to recognize or confront the problem.

A comprehensive approach to the assessment of all clients for substance use is essential to ensure adequate and appropriate intervention. Therapeutic communication techniques should be used to establish trust prior to the assessment process.

It is important for the nurse to assess the client for a history of substance use and medical and psychiatric disorders as well as for the presence of psychosocial concerns. Open-ended questions that elicit more than a simple yes or no answer are more effective in eliciting truthful information and may help deter-

Box 22-9 Examples of Open-Ended Questions for Assessment of Substance Abuse

- On average, how many days per week do you use drugs?
- On a typical day when you use drugs, how much do you use?
- What is the greatest number of drugs you have used at any one time during the past month?
- What drug(s) did you take before coming to the hospital or clinic?
- How long have you been using the substances?
- How often and how much do you usually use?
- What problems has substance use caused for you and your family, friends, finances, and health?

mine the direction of future counseling. Examples of open-ended questions are provided in **Box 22-9** ●.

History of Past Substance Use

A thorough history of the client's past substance use is important in order to ascertain the possibility of tolerance, physical dependence, or withdrawal syndrome. The following questions are helpful in eliciting a pattern of substance use behavior:

- How many substances has the client used simultaneously in the past?
- How often, how much, and when did the client first use the substance(s)?
- Is there a history of blackouts, delirium, or seizures?
- Is there a history of withdrawal syndrome, overdoses, and complications from previous substance use?
- Has the client ever been treated in a drug abuse clinic?

- Has the client ever been arrested for driving under the influence or charged with any criminal offense while using drugs?
- Is there a family history of drug use?

Medical and Psychiatric History

The client's medical history is another important area for assessment and should include the existence of any concomitant physical or mental condition (e.g., HIV, hepatitis, cirrhosis, esophageal varices, pancreatitis, gastritis, Wernicke-Korsakoff syndrome, depression, schizophrenia, anxiety, or personality disorder). The nurse should ask about prescribed and over-the-counter medications as well as any allergies or sensitivity to drugs. A brief overview of the client's current mental status is also significant.

- Is there a history of abuse (physical or sexual) or family violence?
- How often does the client experience feelings of sadness or depression?
- What does the client do to relieve feelings of sadness or depression?
- Has the client ever tried to commit suicide?
- Is the client currently having suicidal or homicidal ideation?

Psychosocial Issues

Information about the client's level of stress and other psychosocial concerns can help in the assessment of substance use problems.

- Has the client's substance use affected his or her ability to hold a job?
- Has the client's substance use affected relationships with spouse, family, friends, or coworkers?

Lifespan Considerations Substance Abuse in the Older Adult

Older Adults

- Substance abuse in older adults is likely to increase as baby boomers reach retirement age. The number of adults 50 years and older with a substance use disorder is estimated to double from 2.8 million in 2006 to 5.7 million in 2020 (Wu & Blazer, 2011).

- People of any age can have substance abuse problems, but the consequences in older adults may be more critical. Falls and accidents can rob older adults of their independence, and substance abuse increases the risk of falls by affecting alertness, judgment, coordination, and reaction time.

- Older adults (especially older women) are more likely than younger people to use prescription or over-the-counter medicines, which can be harmful when mixed with alcohol and/or illicit drugs. Alcohol and drug abuse also can make certain medical problems hard to diagnose, for example, by dulling a pain sensation that might warn of a heart attack.

- Substance abuse and dependence are less likely to be recognized in older adults. A substance abuse problem in an older adult can be difficult to detect because many of the symptoms of abuse (e.g., insomnia, depression, loss of memory, anxiety, musculoskeletal pain) may be confused

with conditions commonly seen in older clients. This results in treating the symptoms of abuse rather than diagnosing and treating the abuse itself.

- Older adults who are alcoholics are at greater risk for numerous physical problems and premature death. Chronic alcohol abuse is associated with tissue damage to several organs. Alcohol interacts negatively with the natural aging process to increase risks for hypertension, alcoholic liver disease, breast cancer in menopausal women, dementia, and depression (Caputo et al., 2012).

- Because depression and alcohol abuse are the most frequently found disorders in completed suicides, nurses should routinely screen older adults for substance abuse and mental disorders.

- Older adults can have several potentially protective factors preventing illicit and nonmedical drug use: being married, never using alcohol or tobacco, and regularly attending religious services (Wu & Blazer, 2011).

- Prevention of drinking relapse in older alcoholics can be more successful than in younger clients. One study found that more than 20% of treated older adults with alcohol dependency remained abstinent after 4 years (Caputo et al., 2012).

- How does the client usually cope with stress?
- Does the client have a support system that helps in time of need?
- How does the client spend his or her leisure time?

Screening Tools

Screening tools such as the Brief Drug Abuse Screening Test (B-DAST or DAST) (Skinner, 1982) may help the nurse determine the degree of severity of substance abuse or dependence. Screening tools provide a nonjudgmental, brief, and easy method to ascertain patterns of substance abuse behaviors. The B-DAST is a yes/no self-administered 20-item questionnaire that is useful in identifying people who may be addicted to drugs other than alcohol. A positive response to one or more questions suggests significant drug abuse problems and warrants further evaluation. Because people do not always answer self-report tools truthfully, all clients who screen positive for drug addiction should be evaluated according to other diagnostic criteria.

Nurses working with clients who experience opiate withdrawal find two scales useful for assessing symptoms: First, the *Objective Opiate Withdrawal Scale (OOWS)* has the nurse rate 13 common, physically observable signs of opiate withdrawal as being either absent or present. Second, the *Subjective Opiate Withdrawal Scale (SOWS)* asks the client to rate 16 symptoms on a scale of 0 (not at all) to 4 (extremely). In either case, the summed total score can be used to assess the intensity of opiate withdrawal and determine the extent of a client's physical dependence on opioids. Higher scores mean a more intense withdrawal and more physical dependence (Handelsman et al., 1987). The two scales have also proven useful in clinical research studies in the 25 years since their creation. One example used the SOWS to measure withdrawal symptoms of clients with chronic low back pain taking extended-release hydromorphone (Jamison et al., 2013).

Diagnosis

Nursing diagnoses for clients with substance abuse problems are highly individualized depending on the substance abused, the length of time the client has abused the chemical, and the sources of support available to the client. Common diagnoses used in the care of these clients include the following:

- *Risk for Injury*
- *Risk for Violence*
- *Ineffective Denial*
- *Ineffective Coping*
- *Imbalanced Nutrition: Less Than Body Requirements*
- *Chronic or Situational Low Self-Esteem*
- *Deficient Knowledge*
- *Disturbed Sensory Perceptions*
- *Disturbed Thought Processes.*

(NANDA-I © 2012)

Planning

When planning care for a client who is abusing substances, it is important to keep goals and expectations reasonable. Substance abuse recovery takes many months and often requires several attempts before abstinence is obtained and maintained. As a result, setting both short- and long-term goals for the client is often most effective.

Short-term goals may include the following:

- The client will admit having a substance abuse problem and having lost control of her life as a result.
- The client will seek help to stop using the substance.
- The client will suffer no complications as a result of drug withdrawal symptoms.
- The client will enter a drug rehabilitation program to change the behavior.

Long-term goals may include the following:

- The client will explore the impact of the substance addiction on family, job, and friends.
- The client will describe and recognize her denial in avoiding the problems related to substance abuse.
- The client will change her thinking and behavior as a result of understanding the negative consequences of substance abuse.
- The client will regularly attend a support group to maintain sobriety from substance use.
- The client will remain free of substance and maintain sobriety.

Implementation

Implications for nursing care in acute and home care settings are combined in this discussion.

Promote Safety

- Assess the client's level of disorientation to determine specific risks to the safety of the client, family members, and others.
- Obtain a drug history as well as urine and blood samples for laboratory analysis of substance content. A client may not admit to using drugs at all or may admit to using only one drug recreationally, when in truth, the client is using one or more drugs regularly. Urine and blood samples provide accurate, objective information.
- Place the client in a quiet private room to decrease excessive stimuli and related agitation, but do not leave the client alone if excessive hyperactivity or suicidal ideation is present.
- If the client is disoriented, frequently orient the client to reality and the environment, ensuring that potentially harmful objects are stored outside the client's access. The client may harm self or others if disoriented and confused.
- Monitor vital signs every 15 minutes until stable. If treatment is dependent on blood or urine levels of a specific drug, reevaluate as instructed by the treating physician.

Promote Adherence to Treatment

- Be genuine, honest, and respectful of the client. Keep all promises and convey an attitude of acceptance of the client. The development of a nonjudgmental, therapeutic nurse–client relationship is essential for gaining the client's trust.

- Identify maladaptive behaviors or situations that have occurred in the client's life and discuss how the use of substances may have been a contributing factor. The first step in combating denial is for the client to recognize the relationship between substance use and personal problems.

- Do not accept the use of defense mechanisms such as rationalization or projection as the client attempts to blame others or make excuses for her behavior. Use confrontation with caring to avoid placing the client on the defensive. Confrontation interferes with the client's ability to use denial.

- Encourage client participation in therapeutic group activities such as NA meetings. Peer feedback is often more accepted than feedback from authority figures.

Promote Healthy Coping Skills

- Set limits on manipulative behavior and maintain consistency in responses. Addicted clients are often unable to set limits and must begin to accept responsibility without being manipulative.

- Encourage the client to verbalize feelings, fears, or anxieties. Use attentive listening and validate the client's feelings with observations or statements that acknowledge the feelings. Addicts are inexperienced at verbalizing and sharing feelings and anxieties.

- Explore methods of dealing with stressful situations other than resorting to substance use. Provide encouragement for changing to a healthier lifestyle. Teach healthy coping mechanisms (e.g., physical exercise, progressive muscle relaxation, deep breathing exercises, meditation, and imagery) that will help the client adapt to stress without resorting to drug use.

Promote Adequate Nutrition

- Administer vitamins and dietary supplements as ordered by the physician.

- Monitor lab work (e.g., total albumin, complete blood count, urinalysis, electrolytes, and liver enzymes) and report significant changes to the physician. Objective laboratory tests provide necessary information to determine the extent of malnourishment.

- Collaborate with a dietitian to determine the number of calories needed to provide adequate nutrition and a realistic weight. Document intake, output, and calorie count. Weigh the client daily if condition warrants. Weight loss or gain impacts development of the care plan.

- Teach the physical effects of malnutrition on body systems. Provide information about adequate nutrition using the federal MyPlate program. The client may have inadequate knowledge of proper nutritional habits.

Promote Healthy Self-Esteem

- Spend time with the client and convey an attitude of acceptance. Encourage the client to accept responsibility for his or her behaviors and feelings. An attitude of acceptance enhances self-worth.

- Encourage the client to focus on strengths and accomplishments rather than weaknesses and failures. Minimize attention to negative ruminations.

- Encourage participation in therapeutic group activities. Offer recognition and positive feedback for actual achievements. Success and recognition increase self-esteem.

- Teach assertiveness techniques and effective communication techniques such as the use of "I feel" rather than "You make me feel" statements. Previous patterns of communication may have been aggressive and accusatory, causing barriers to interpersonal relationships.

Provide Client Education

- Assess the client's level of knowledge and readiness to learn the effects of drugs and alcohol on the body. Baseline assessment is required to develop appropriate teaching material.

- Develop a teaching plan that includes measurable objectives. Include short-term goals so that the client sees some level of success at an early stage. Include significant others if possible. Lifestyle changes often affect all family members.

- Begin with simple concepts and progress to more complex issues. Use interactive teaching strategies and written materials appropriate to the client's educational level. Include information on physiological effects of substances, the propensity for physical and psychological dependence, and risks to the fetus if the client is pregnant. Active participation and handouts enhance retention of important concepts.

Promote Client Safety During Withdrawal

- Observe the client for withdrawal symptoms. Monitor vital signs. Provide adequate nutrition and hydration. These actions provide supportive physical care during detoxification.

Client Teaching Substance Abuse

Teach the client and family the following:

- The negative effects of substance abuse, including physical and psychological complications of substance abuse
- The signs of relapse and the importance of after-care programs and self-help groups to prevent relapse
- Information about specific medications that help reduce cravings and maintain abstinence, including the potential side effects, possible drug interactions, and any special precautions to be taken (e.g., avoiding over-the-counter medications such as cough syrup that may contain alcohol)
- Ways to manage stress, including techniques such as progressive muscle relaxation, abdominal breathing techniques, imagery, meditation, and effective coping skills.

In addition, suggest the following resources:

- AA, NA, and other self-help groups
- Employee assistance programs
- Individual, group, and family counseling
- Community rehabilitation programs
- National Alliance for the Mentally Ill (NAMI).

- Assess the client's level of orientation frequently. Orient and reassure the client of safety in the presence of hallucinations, delusions, or illusions.

- Explain all interventions before approaching the client. Avoid loud noises and talk softly to the client. Decrease external stimuli by dimming lights. Excessive stimuli increase agitation.

- Administer medications according to the detoxification schedule. Benzodiazepines may help minimize the discomfort of withdrawal symptoms.

- Provide positive reinforcement when thinking and behavior are appropriate or when the client recognizes that delusions are not based in reality. Drugs and alcohol can interfere with the client's perception of reality.

- Use simple step-by-step instructions and face-to-face interaction when communicating with the client. The client may be confused or disoriented.

- Express reasonable doubt if the client relays suspicious or paranoid beliefs. Reinforce accurate perception of people or situations. It is important to communicate that you do not share the false beliefs as reality.

- Do not argue with the client experiencing delusions or hallucinations. Convey acceptance that the client believes a situation to be true, but that you do not see or hear what is not there. Arguing with the client or denying the belief serves no useful purpose because it does not eliminate the delusions.

- Talk to the client about real events and real people. Respond to feelings and reassure the client that she is safe from harm. Discussions that focus on the delusions may aggravate the condition. Verbalization of feelings in a nonthreatening environment may help the client develop insight.

The community provides many options for treating substance abuse, including a mixture of individual, group, and family therapy. Medical detoxification can occur in hospitals, psychiatric units, special substance abuse units, methadone clinics, and outpatient settings. Less restrictive environments include residential rehabilitation programs, halfway houses, and partial hospitalization programs. These programs provide structured environments for the recovering substance abuser while the client maintains a viable presence in the community. In addition, clients can obtain vocational counseling, become involved in self-help groups such as AA or AN, and receive drug and health education.

Evaluation

The client is evaluated based on the ability to meet goals designed during the planning phase of nursing care. Potential positive outcomes may include the following:

- The client suffers no complications from withdrawing from substance.

- The client admits a problem with substance abuse and seeks help.

- The client enters a substance abuse program.

- The client can describe choices made that contributed to substance abuse.

- The client attends daily support group meetings after leaving rehabilitation facility.

- The client remains substance free for (insert time period—days, weeks, months—depending on progress and time sober).

NURSING CARE PLAN — A Client With Substance Abuse

ASSESSMENT	DIAGNOSES	PLANNING
Donna Smith is brought to the ED by her husband. She is agitated and can't stand still. Her husband tells the nurse that she has been getting high on crack cocaine on a regular basis. When she didn't come home last night, he called their cell phone company to activate her GPS and found her outside a motel on the highway. He took her home, where she began shouting, yelling, and throwing things and talking about the "men in the trees" who are after her. The nurse conducting the assessment determines that they have two children, ages 11 and 15, living at home.	■ *Risk for Injury* ■ *Altered Tissue Perfusion* ■ *Interrupted Family Processes* ■ *Ineffective Coping* ■ *Disturbed Sensory Perceptions* ■ *Disturbed Thought Processes* (NANDA-I © 2012)	Goals of care include the following: ■ Experience no adverse cardiac event. ■ Orient to time and place. ■ ECG will return to normal sinus rhythm. ■ Neurological assessment will return to pre-substance use baseline. ■ Agree to psychosocial intervention to assist in substance avoidance.
The nurse collects the following data during assessment: Temperature 99.4°F axillary; pulse 114 bpm; respirations 20/min; BP 168/92 mmHg Pupils constricted and equally responsive to light		
Client is muttering to herself in mostly unintelligible sentences, with phrases such as "men in trees," "gonna get me," and "don't worry" understood among gibberish words. Client says she hears voices and points out things that are not there—apparently having both visual and auditory hallucinations.		
Peripheral pulses are 3+ and bounding, sinus tachycardia noted on ECG with frequent premature ventricular contractions, hyperreactive reflexes.		
Client is admitted to monitored unit (telemetry) for observation until cardiac and neurological systems are stable.		

(continued on next page)

NURSING CARE PLAN *(continued)*

IMPLEMENTATION

- Monitor cardiorespiratory function.
- Assess orientation and maintain safety while hallucinating.
- Maintain low stimulation environment until effects of drug subside.
- Maintain hydration to promote excretion of drug from system.
- Obtain complete history of substance use when client's cognitive function returns.

- Administer sedatives and antiarrhythmics as required per orders
- Refer Mr. Smith to a support program for spouses and children.
- Refer to substance abuse program to assist in abstinence once drugs have been cleared from system if client is willing to participate.

EVALUATION

Evaluation of client response may be based on the following expected outcomes:
- The client experiences no cardiac event as the result of cocaine use.
- The client's cognition returns to prior baseline.
- The client admits to having a problem and agrees to seek treatment.

CRITICAL THINKING

1. While the client is experiencing both auditory and visual hallucinations, how will the nurse respond if the client insists there is something in the room that is not seen by the nurse?
2. What actions will the nurse implement to maintain the client's safety?
3. After detoxification the client regains normal cognitive function and informs the nurse she is leaving the facility because she wants to "get high again." What is the nurse's legal obligation to this client?

REVIEW Substance Abuse

RELATE Link the Concepts and Exemplars

Linking the exemplar of substance abuse with the concept of safety:

1. The nurse had surgery a few days ago and is taking a narcotic analgesic to control pain. Is it safe for the nurse to work assigned shifts while taking this medication? Why or why not?

2. You suspect that a coworker whom you admire for his experience and knowledge may be using an illegal drug. What is your best action to maintain client safety? How would you handle this issue?

Linking the exemplar of substance abuse with the concept of violence:

3. How does the abuse of substances affect the risk for violence committed by the client?

4. When working in a substance abuse treatment facility, how can you, as the nurse, encourage spouses at risk for acts of domestic violence by your clients seek support for their own health?

READY Go to Companion Skills Manual

REFER Go to Pearson Nursing Student Resources
nursing.pearsonhighered.com

- Additional review materials

REFLECT Case Study

Casey Holmes is a physically fit 23-year-old male who had a troubled youth. His parents divorced when he was very young, and he

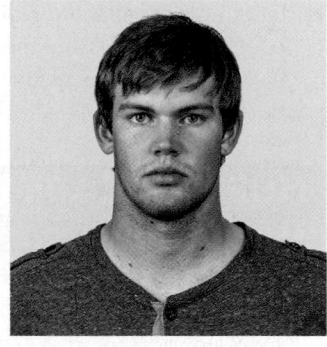

bounced back and forth between parents—both of whom remarried. Growing up, he often saw his father hit his stepmother when angry. As an adolescent, Mr. Holmes became involved with a gang and was arrested a few times for petty crimes, such as shoplifting and vandalism. He never finished high school and moved out on his own at the age of 18. Since that time, he has held a number of odd jobs and has made an effort to stay out of trouble.

Mr. Holmes lives with his pregnant girlfriend Jessica Riley and her son Ryan. He does not particularly like Ryan and thinks Jessica spoils him. He is very proud of the fact that Jessica is pregnant with his baby. He is controlling of Jessica and does not want anybody else looking at her. On most days after work and into the evening, Mr. Holmes drinks beer and smokes dope with his buddies. He is irritated that Jessica does not party with him as much as she did when they first met. Mr. Holmes also uses other drugs when he can afford to buy them.

1. What are the priority nursing diagnoses for Mr. Holmes?

2. What are the implications of his substance abuse on the family?

3. Mr. Holmes accompanies Jessica to the clinic for one of her prenatal visits. The nurse is aware of Mr. Holmes's drug use, which Jessica admitted on a prior visit. What should the nurse say to Mr. Holmes during this visit regarding the impact of his behavior on Jessica and the baby?

■ REFERENCES

Albrecht, S., Kelly-Thomas, K., Osborne, J. W., & Ogbager, S. (2011). The SUCCESS program for smoking cessation for pregnant women. *Journal of Obstetric, Gynecologic, and Neonatal Nursing, 40*(5), 520–531. doi:10.1111/j.1552-6909.2011.01280.x.

American Congress of Obstetricians and Gynecologists (ACOG). (2010). Committee opinion number 462: Moderate caffeine consumption during pregnancy. *Obstetrics and Gynecology, 116,* 467–468.

American Lung Association. (2013). *Smoking.* Retrieved from http://www.lung.org/stop-smoking/about-smoking/health-effects/smoking.html.

American Psychiatric Association. (2013). *Diagnostic and statistical manual of mental disorders* (5th ed.). Washington, DC: Author.

Ballinger, B., & Yalom, I. D. (1995). *The theory and practice of group psychotherapy* (4th ed.). New York, NY: Basic Books.

Behnke, M., & Smith, V. C. (2013). Prenatal substance abuse: Short- and long-term effects on the exposed fetus. *Pediatrics, 131*(3), e1009–e1024. doi:10.1542/peds.2012-3931.

Bernstein, P. M. (2013). *Trauma: Healing the hidden epidemic.* Petaluma, CA: Bernstein Institute for Integrative Psychotherapy and Trauma Treatment.

Bosch, O. G., Wagner, M., Jessen, F., Kühn, K. U., Joe, A., Seifritz, E., et al. (2013). Verbal memory deficits are correlated with prefrontal hypometabolism in (18)FDG PET of recreational MDMA users. *PLoS One, 8*(4). doi:10.1371/journal.pone.0061234.

Breese, G. R., Sinha, R., & Heilig, M. (2011). Chronic alcohol neuroadaptation and stress contribute to susceptibility for alcohol craving and relapse. *Pharmacology and Therapeutics, 129*(2), 149–171. doi:10.1016/j.pharmthera.2010.09.007.

Burns, M. J. (2013). *Delirium tremens (DTs): Prognosis.* Retrieved from emedicine.medscape.com/article/166032.

Caputo, F., Vignoli, T., Leggio, L., Addolorato, G., Zoli, G., & Bernardi, M. (2012). Alcohol use disorders in the elderly: A brief overview from epidemiology to treatment options. *Experimental Gerontology, 47*(6), 411–416. doi:10.1016/j.exger.2012.03.019.

Centers for Disease Control and Prevention (CDC). (2012). *Adolescent and school health.* Retrieved from http://www.cdc.gov/healthyyouth/alcoholdrug.

Centers for Disease Control and Prevention (CDC). (2013a). *Celebrate moms who protect children's health.* Retrieved from http://www.cdc.gov/Features/SmokeFreeMoms.

Centers for Disease Control and Prevention (CDC). (2013b). *Smoking and tobacco use.* Retrieved from http://www.cdc.gov/tobacco.

Centers for Disease Control and Prevention (CDC). (2013c). *Smoking and tobacco use. Fast facts.* Retrieved from http://www.cdc.gov/tobacco/data_statistics/fact_sheets/fast_facts.

Centers for Disease Control and Prevention (CDC). (2013d). *Tobacco use and pregnancy.* Retrieved from http://www.cdc.gov/reproductivehealth/TobaccoUsePregnancy/index.htm.

Chassin, L., Lee, M. R., Cho, Y. I., Wang, F. L., Agrawal, A., Sher, K. J., & Lynskey, M. T. (2012). Testing multiple levels of influence in the intergenerational transmission of alcohol disorders from a developmental perspective: The example of alcohol use promoting peers and μ-opioid receptor M1 variation. *Development and Psychopathology, 24*(3), 953–967. doi:10.1017/S0954579412000478.

Cosgrove, K. P. (2010). Imaging receptor changes in human drug abusers. *Current Topics in Behavioral Neurosciences, 3,* 199–217. doi:10.1007/7854_2009_24.

Czermak, C., Lehofer, M., Wagner, E. M., Prietl, B., Lemonis, L., Rohrhofer, A., et al. (2004). Reduced dopamine D$_4$ receptor mRNA expression in lymphocytes of long-term abstinent alcohol and heroin addicts. *Addiction, 99*(2), 251–257.

Ehlers, C. L., & Gizer, I. R. (2013). Evidence for a genetic component for substance dependence in Native Americans. *American Journal of Psychiatry, 170*(2), 154–164. doi:10.1176/appi.ajp.2012.12010113.

Ewing, J. A. (1984). Detecting alcoholism: The CAGE questionnaire. *Journal of the American Medical Association, 252*(14), 1905–1907.

Fontaine, K. L. (2010). *Complementary and alternative therapies for nursing practice* (3rd ed.). Upper Saddle River, NJ: Pearson-Prentice Hall.

Foroud, T., & Phillips, T. J. (2012). *Assessing the genetic risk for alcohol use disorders.* Retrieved from National Institute on Alcohol Abuse and Alcoholism Web site: http://alcoholism.about.com/gi/dynamic/offsite.htm?site=http://www.niaaa.nih.gov.

Green, K. E., & Feinstein, B. A. (2012). Substance use in lesbian, fay, and bisexual populations: An update on empirical research and implications for treatment. *Psychology of Addictive Behaviors, 26*(2), 265–278. doi:10.1037/a0025424.

Haber, J. R., Koenig, L. B., & Jacob, T. (2011). Alcoholism, personality, and religion/spirituality: An integrative review. *Current Drug Abuse Reviews, 4*(4), 250–260.

Handelsman, L., Cochrane, K. J., Aronson, M. J., Ness, R., Rubinstein, K. J., & Kanof, P. D. (1987). Two new rating scales for opiate withdrawal. *American Journal of Drug and Alcohol Abuse, 13*(3), 293–308.

Heise, B. (2003). The historical context of addiction in the nursing profession: 1850–1982. *Journal of Addictions Nursing, 14,* 117–124.

Howard, M. O., Perron, B. E., Sacco, P., Ilgen, M., Vaughn, M. G., Garland, E., & Freedenthal, S. (2010). Suicide ideation and attempts among inhalant users: Results from the National Epidemiologic Survey on Alcohol and Related Conditions. *Suicide & Life-Threatening Behavior, 40*(3), 276–286. doi:10.1521/suli.2010.40.3.276.

Howard, M. O., Perron, B. E., Vaughn, M. G., Bender, K. A., & Garland, E. (2010). Inhalant use, inhalant-use disorders, and antisocial behavior: Findings from the National Epidemiologic Survey on Alcohol and Related Conditions (NESARC). *Journal of Studies on Alcohol and Drugs, 71*(2), 201–209.

Indiana State Department of Health. (2013). *Prenatal substance use prevention program.* Retrieved from http://www.state.in.us/isdh/22243.htm.

Jamison, R. N., Edwards, R. R., Liu, X., Ross, E. L., Michna, E., Warnick, M., & Wasan, A. D. (2013). Relationship of negative affect and outcome of an opioid therapy trial among low back pain patients. *Pain Practices, 13*(3), 173–181. doi:10.1111/j.1533-2500.2012.00575.x.

Jansson, L. M., & Velez, M. (2012, April). Neonatal abstinence syndrome. *Current Opinion in Pediatrics, 24*(2), 252–258. doi:10.1097/MOP.0b013e32834fdc3a.

Jellinek, E. (1946). *Phases in the drinking history of alcoholics.* New Haven, CT: Hillhouse Press.

Johnston, L. D., O'Malley, P. M., Bachman, J. G., & Schulenberg, J. E. (2013). *Monitoring the future. National results on drug use: 2012 overview. Key findings on adolescent drug use.* Ann Arbor, MI: Ann Arbor Institute for Social Research, University of Michigan.

Jones, H. E., Finnegan, L. P., & Kaltenbach, K. (2012). Methadone and buprenorphine for the management of opioid dependence in pregnancy. *Drugs, 72*(6), 747–757.

Kash, T. L. (2012). The role of biogenic amine signaling in the bed nucleus of the stria terminals in alcohol abuse.

Alcohol, 46(4), 303–308. doi:10.1016/j.alcohol.2011.12.004.

Keegan, J., Parva, M., Finnegan, M., Gerson, A., & Belden, M. (2010, April). Addiction in pregnancy. *Journal of Addictive Diseases, 29*(2), 175–191. doi:10.1080/10550881003684723.

Keramati, M., & Gutkin, B. (2013). Imbalanced decision hierarchy in addicts emerging from drug-hijacked dopamine spiraling circuit. *PLoS One, 8*(4), e61489. doi:10.1371/journal.pone.0061489.

Kneisl, C. R., & Trigoboff, E. (2013). *Contemporary psychiatric–mental health nursing* (3rd ed.). Upper Saddle River, NJ: Pearson-Prentice Hall.

Knopik, V. S., Maccani, M. A., Francazio, S., & McGeary, J. E. (2012). The epigenetics of maternal cigarette smoking during pregnancy and effects on child development. *Development and Psychopathology, 24*(4). 1377–1390. doi:10.1017/S0954579412000776.

Kraft, A. M. (1966). The therapeutic community. In S. Arieti (Ed.), *American handbook of psychiatry* (Vol. 2). New York, NY: Basic Books.

Ling, P. M., Neilands, T. B., & Glantz, S. A. (2009). Young adult smoking behavior: A national survey. *American Journal of Preventive Medicine, 36*(5), 389–394. doi:10.1016/j.amepre.2009.01.028.

Liska, K. (2008). *Drugs and the human body* (8th ed.). Upper Saddle River, NJ: Prentice Hall.

MacNeal, J. J., Cone, D. C., Sinha, V., & Tomassoni, A. J. (2012). Use of haloperidol in PCP-intoxicated individuals. *Clinical Toxicology, 50*(9), 851–853. doi:10.3109/15563650.2012.722222.

Manasco, A., Chang, S., Larriviere, J., Hamm, L. L., & Glass, M. (2012). Alcohol withdrawal. *Southern Medical Journal, 105*(11), 607–612. doi:10.1097/SMJ.0b013e31826efb2d.

Manchikanti, L., Fellows, B., Ailinani, H., & Pampati, V. (2010). Therapeutic use, abuse, and nonmedical use of opioids: A ten-year perspective. *Pain Physician, 13*(5), 401–435.

Manchikanti, L., Helm, S., Fellows, B., Janata, J. W., Pampati, V., Grider, J. S., & Boswell, M. V. (2012). Opioid epidemic in the United States. *Pain Physician, 15*(3 Suppl.), ES9–ES38.

Massey, S. H., Lieberman, D. Z., Reiss, D., Leve, L. D., Shaw, D. S., & Neiderhiser, J. M. (2011). Association of clinical characteristics and cessation of tobacco, alcohol, and illicit drug use during pregnancy. *American Journal on Addictions, 20*(2), 143–150. doi:10.1111/j.1521-0391.2010.00110.x.

Mayo Clinic. (2011). *Drug addiction: Risk factors.* Retrieved from http://www.mayoclinic.com/health/drug-addiction/DS00183/DSECTION=risk-factors.

McNeece, C. A., & DiNitto, D. M. (2012). *Chemical dependency: A systems approach* (4th ed.). Upper Saddle River, NJ: Pearson.

Morgan, S., Koren, G., & Bozzo, P. (2013). Is caffeine consumption safe during pregnancy? *Canadian Family Physician, 59*(4), 361–362.

Morse, R. M., & Flavin, D. K. (1992). The definition of alcoholism. The Joint Committee of the National Council on Alcoholism and Drug Dependence and the American Society of Addiction Medicine to Study the Definition and Criteria for the Diagnosis of Alcoholism. *Journal of the American Medical Association, 268*(8), 1012–1014.

National Child Traumatic Stress Network. (2008). *Making the connection: Trauma and substance abuse.* Retrieved from http://www.nctsn.org/sites/default/files/assets/pdfs/SAToolkit_1.pdf.

National Council on Alcoholism and Drug Abuse. (2009). Children's role identification in the dysfunctional family. Retrieved from http://www.ncada-stl.org/factsheets/childrens_role.pdf.

National Institute on Aging. (2012). *Alcohol use in older adults*. Retrieved from http://www.nia.nih.gov/health/publication/alcohol-use-older-people.

National Institute on Alcohol Abuse and Alcoholism. (2013). NIAAA recognizes alcohol awareness month (News release). Retrieved from http://www.niaaa.nih.gov/news-events/alcohol-awareness-month-2013.

National Institute on Drug Abuse (NIDA). (2008). *Addiction science: From molecules to managed care*. Retrieved from http://www.drugabuse.gov/publications/addiction-science/relapse/relapse-rates-drug-addiction-are-similar-to-those-other-well-characterized-chronic-ill.

National Institute on Drug Abuse (NIDA). (2010a). *Cocaine abuse and addiction*. Retrieved from http://www.drugabuse.gov/publications/research-reports/cocaine-abuse-addiction.

National Institute on Drug Abuse (NIDA). (2010b). *Drugs, brains, and behavior: The science of addiction*. Retrieved from http://www.drugabuse.gov/publications/science-addiction.

National Institute on Drug Abuse (NIDA). (2010c). *Marijuana abuse: How does marijuana use affect your brain and body?* Retrieved from http://www.drugabuse.gov/publications/marijuana-abuse/how-does-marijuana-use-affect-your-brain-body.

National Institute on Drug Abuse (NIDA). (2010d). *What is drugged driving?* Retrieved from http://www.drugabuse.gov/publications/drugfacts/drugged-driving.

National Institute on Drug Abuse (NIDA). (2011a). *The science of drug abuse and addiction. DrugFacts: Understanding drug abuse and addiction*. Retrieved from http://www.drugabuse.gov/publications/drugfacts/understanding-drug-abuse-addiction.

National Institute on Drug Abuse (NIDA). (2011b). *Topics-in-brief: Methamphetamine addiction: Progress, but need to remain vigilant*. Retrieved from http://www.drugabuse.gov/publications/topics-in-brief/methamphetamine-addiction-progress-need-to-remain-vigilant.

National Institute on Drug Abuse (NIDA). (2012a). *Principles of drug addiction treatment: A research-based guide* (Publication No. 12-4180, 3rd ed.). Bethesda, MD: National Institutes of Health.

National Institute on Drug Abuse (NIDA). (2012b). *The science of drug abuse and addiction. DrugFacts: Nationwide trends*. Retrieved from http://www.drugabuse.gov/publications/drugfacts/nationwide-trends.

National Institute on Drug Abuse (NIDA). (2013a). *DrugFacts: Cocaine*. Retrieved from http://www.drugabuse.gov/publications/drugfacts/cocaine.

National Institute on Drug Abuse (NIDA). (2013b). *DrugFacts: Heroin*. Retrieved from http://www.drugabuse.gov/publications/drugfacts/heroin.

National Institute on Drug Abuse (NIDA). (2013c). *The science of drug abuse and addiction. Trends and statistics*. Retrieved from http://www.drugabuse.gov/related-topics/trends-statistics.

National Institute of Mental Health. (2010). *Suicide in the U.S.: Statistics and prevention* (No. 06-4594). Retrieved from http://www.nimh.nih.gov/health/publications/suicide-in-the-us-statistics-and-prevention/index.shtml.

Nellissery, M., Feinn, R. S., Covault, J., Gelernter, J., Anton, R. F., Pettinati, H., et al. (2003). Alleles of a functional serotonin transporter promoter polymorphism are associated with major depression in alcoholics. *Alcoholism: Clinical and Experimental Research, 27*(9), 1402–1408.

Niebyl, J. R., & Simpson, J. L. (2012). Drugs and environmental agents in pregnancy and lactation: Embryology, teratology, epidemiology. In Chapter 8 of S. G. Gabbe, J. R. Niebyl, H. L. Galan, E. R. M. Jauniaux, M. B. Landon, J. L. Simpson, & D. A. Driscoll (Eds.), *Obstetrics: Normal and problem pregnancies* (6th ed.). Philadelphia, PA: Saunders.

Nonnemaker, J. M., Crankshaw, E. C., Shive, D. R., Hussin, A. H., & Farrelly, M. C. (2011). Inhalant use initiation among U.S. adolescents: Evidence from the National Survey of Parents and Youth using discrete-time survival analysis. *Addictive Behaviors, 36*(8), 878–881. doi:10.1016/j.addbeh.2011.03.009.

Oesterle, S., Hawkins, J. D., & Hill, K. G. (2011). Men's and women's pathways to adulthood and associated substance misuse. *Journal of Studies on Alcohol and Drugs, 72*(5), 763–773.

Partnership at Drugfree.org (2013). *Methamphetamine*. Retrieved from http://www.drugfree.org/drug-guide/methamphetamine.

Peplau, H. (1952). *Interpersonal relations in nursing*. New York, NY: Putman.

Pettinati, H. M., & Dundon, W. D. (2011). Comorbid depression and alcohol dependence: New approaches to dual therapy challenges and progress. *Psychiatric Times, 28*(6).

Pettinati, H. M., O'Brien, C. P., & Dundon, W. D. (2013). Current status of co-occurring mood and substance use disorders: A new therapeutic target. *American Journal of Psychiatry, 170*(1), 23–30. doi:10.1176/appi.ajp.2012.12010112.

Pokorny, A. D., Miller, B. A., & Kaplan, H. B. (1972). The brief MAST: A shortened version of the Michigan Alcohol Screening Test. *American Journal of Psychiatry, 129*, 342–345.

Rappaport, D., Chuu, A., Hullett, C., Nematollahi, S., Teeple, M., Bhuyan, N., et al. (2013). Assessment of alcohol withdrawal in Native American patients utilizing the Clinical Institute Withdrawal Assessment of Alcohol Revised Scale. *Journal of Addiction Medicine, 7*(3), 196–199.

Reissig, C. J., Strain, E. C., & Griffiths, R. R. (2009, January 1). Caffeinated energy drinks—a growing problem. *Drug and Alcohol Dependence, 99*(1–3), 1–10. doi:10.1016.

Serec, M., Svab, I., Kolšek, M., Svab, V., Moesgen, D., & Klein, M. (2012). Health-related lifestyle, physical and mental health in children of alcoholic parents. *Drug and Alcohol Review, 31*(7), 861–870. doi:10.1111/j.1465-3362.2012.00424.x.

Singer, J. (2012). *Beating alcohol addiction in midlife*. Retrieved from http://www.nextavenue.org/article/2012-09/beating-alcohol-addiction-midlife.

Skinner, H. A. (1982). *Drug abuse screening test (DAST)* (p. 363). Langford Lance, UK: Elsevier Science.

Stern, S., & Morr, L. (2013). Portrayals of teen smoking, drinking, and drug use in recent popular movies. *Journal of Health Communication, 18*(2), 179–191. doi:10.1080/10810730.2012.688251.

Stuart, G. W. (2008). *Principles and practice of psychiatric nursing* (9th ed.). St. Louis, MO: Mosby.

Substance Abuse and Mental Health Services Administration (SAMHSA). (2011). *Drug abuse warning network, 2009: National estimates of drug-related emergency department visits* (HHS Publication No. SMA 11-4659, DAWN Series D-35). Rockville, MD: Author.

Substance Abuse and Mental Health Services Administration (SAMHSA). (2012a). *Results from the 2011 National Survey on Drug Use and Health: Summary of national findings* (NSDUH Series H-44, HHS Publication No. SMA 12-4713). Rockville, MD: Author.

Substance Abuse and Mental Health Services Administration (SAMHSA). (2012b). Substance use and mental disorders affect all individuals. In *2012 recovery month toolkit*. Rockville, MD: Author.

Substance Abuse and Mental Health Services Administration (SAMHSA). (2013). *The DAWN report: Highlights of the 2011 drug abuse warning network (DAWN) findings on drug-related emergency department visits*. Retrieved from http://www.samhsa.gov/data/2k13/DAWN127/sr127-DAWN-highlights.htm.

Sullivan, J. T., Sykora, K., Schneiderman, J., Naranjo, C. A., & Sellers, E. M. (1989). Assessment of alcohol withdrawal: The revised Clinical Institute Withdrawal Assessment for Alcohol Scale (CIWA-Ar). *British Journal of Addictions, 84*, 1353–1357.

Surgeon General. (2012). *Preventing tobacco use among youth and young adults: A report of the Surgeon General*. Retrieved from http://www.surgeongeneral.gov/library/reports/preventing-youth-tobacco-use.

Sussman, S., Black, D.S., & Rohrbach, L. A. (2010). A concise history of school-based smoking prevention research: A pendulum effect case study. *Journal of Drug Education, 40*(3), 217–226.

Sussman, S., Levy, D., Lich, K. H., Cené, C. W., Kim, M. M., Rohrbach, L. A., & Chaloupka, F. J. (2013). Comparing effects of tobacco use prevention modalities: need for complex system models. doi:10.1186/1617-9625-11-2. Retrieved from http://www.ncbi.nlm.nih.gov/pmc/articles/PMC3567972.

Thomas, C. M., & Siela, D. (2011). The impaired nurse: Would you know what to do if you suspected substance abuse? *American Nurse Today, 6*(8). Retrieved from http://www.medscape.com/viewarticle/748598_7.

Thompson, V. B., Koprich, J. B., Chen, E. Y., Kordower, J. H., Terpstra, B. T., & Lipton, J. W. (2012). Prenatal exposure to MDMA alters noradrenergic neurodevelopment in the rat. *Neurotoxicology and Teratology, 34*(1), 206–213.

Uscher, J. (2012). Alcohol and pregnancy: Is "a little bit" safe? Retrieved from http://webmd.com/baby/features/drinking-alcohol-during-pregnancy.

Varcarolis, E. M., & Halter, M. J. (2009). *Foundations of psychiatric mental health nursing: A clinical approach* (6th ed.). Philadelphia, PA: Saunders.

Wisner, K. L., Sit, D. K. Y., Altemus, M., Bogen, D. L., Famy, C. S., Pearlstein, T. B., et al. (2012). Mental health and behavioral disorders in pregnancy. In Chapter 52 of S. G. Gabbe, J. R. Niebyl, H. L. Galan, E. R. M. Jauniaux, M. B. Landon, J. L. Simpson, & D. A. Driscoll (Eds.), *Obstetrics: Normal and problem pregnancies* (6th ed.). Philadelphia, PA: Saunders.

World Health Organization (WHO). (2013). *Management of substance abuse: Cannabis*. Retrieved from http://www.who.int/substance_abuse/facts/cannabis/en.

Wu, L. T., & Blazer, D. G. (2011). Illicit and nonmedical drug use among older adults: A review. *Journal of Aging and Health, 23*(3), 481–504. doi:10.1177/0898264310386224.

Zhang, K., & Wang, X. (2013, May). Maternal smoking and increased risk of sudden infant death syndrome: A meta-analysis. *Legal Medicine (Tokyo, Japan), 15*(3), 115–321.

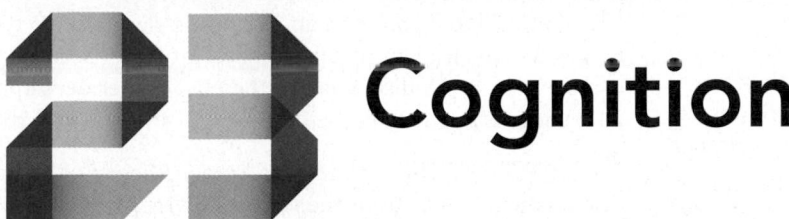

23 Cognition

MODULE AT-A-GLANCE

The Concept of Cognition, 1575

Exemplar 23.1
  Alzheimer Disease, 1594

Exemplar 23.2
  Confusion, 1605

Exemplar 23.3
  Schizophrenia, 1610

◪ THE CONCEPT OF COGNITION

Cognition is the complex set of mental activities through which individuals acquire, process, store, retrieve, and apply information. Many different processes are part of cognition, including awareness, remembering, reasoning, decision making, and understanding and using language.

Cognition is a function of the nervous system, so physical changes that affect this system often result in cognitive disturbances. Depending on their cause, these disturbances may be major or minor, chronic or acute, permanent or reversible. Even small disruptions in cognition can dramatically affect a client's quality of life, as well as the quality of life of others. For this reason, it is important that nurses understand why cognitive alterations occur, how these alterations can be prevented, and what they can do to help affected individuals. **‹‹**

Concept Learning Outcomes

After reading this concept, you will be able to:

1. Summarize the physiology of the neurological system in relationship to cognition.
2. Examine the relationship between cognition and other concepts/systems.
3. Identify commonly occurring alterations in cognition and their related therapies.
4. Differentiate common assessment procedures used to examine cognitive function across the life span.
5. Describe diagnostic and laboratory tests to determine the individual's cognitive status.
6. Explain management of alterations in cognition and prevention of cognitive dysfunction.
7. Demonstrate the nursing process in providing culturally competent and caring interventions across the life span for individuals with common alterations in cognition.
8. Compare and contrast common independent and collaborative interventions for clients with alterations in cognitive function.

Concept Key Terms

Adaptive behaviors, *1581*
Akathisia, *1584*
Anomia, *1584*
Aphasia, *1584*
Ataxia, *1584*
Carphologia, *1584*
Cerebrum, *1576*
Cognition, *1575*
Delusions, *1578*
Dementia, *1584*
Developmental
  disability, *1581*
Down syndrome, *1581*
Dysphagia, *1584*
Echolalia, *1584*
Fetal alcohol syndrome
  (FAS), *1581*

Fragile X syndrome, *1581*
Hallucinations, *1578*
Hemispheres, *1576*
Hippocampus, *1576*
Illusions, *1578*
Intellectual disability, *1581*
Intellectual
  functioning, *1581*
Learning disabilities, *1578*
Limbic system, *1576*
Lobes, *1576*
Mental retardation, *1581*
Neurons, *1576*
Neurotransmitters, *1576*
Psychosis, *1578*
Schemes, *1576*
Trisomy 21, *1581*

▶ NORMAL COGNITION

Normal cognition is the result of several factors. First, an individual's nervous system must be anatomically and physiologically sound. Second, the individual must have progressed through one or more stages of cognitive development typical of individuals in his age group.

Physiology Review

Cognition is primarily the brain's responsibility—and within the brain, most cognitive tasks occur in the cerebrum. The **cerebrum** is the largest, uppermost region of the brain. A deep fold divides this structure into two halves, or **hemispheres**, each of which consists of four **lobes**. Specific lobes are specialized for different functions. For example, the frontal lobe controls speech, learning, and intellect; the parietal lobe controls conscious awareness of sensory stimuli; the occipital lobe interprets visual stimuli; and the temporal lobe interprets auditory and olfactory stimuli.

Beyond the cerebral lobes, other parts of the brain are also involved in cognition. Notably, the **limbic system** is a set of structures located deep inside the brain, just below the cerebrum. One important component of the limbic system is the **hippocampus**, a small, curved body that plays a role in memory formation. (For more details on the regions of the brain, refer to the module on Intracranial Regulation.)

Like the rest of the nervous system, the brain consists of specialized cells called **neurons**, which carry and process information. Information travels along the length of individual neurons in the form of electrical impulses, and it moves between neurons by way of chemical messengers called **neurotransmitters**. Research suggests that abnormalities in neurotransmitter function are involved in many cognitive disorders. Research has also proven that even slight alterations in the brain's structure and chemical environment can produce a variety of cognitive disturbances—as described later in this concept.

Theories of Cognitive Development

It's obvious that newborns think differently than adults. But how, exactly, do human cognitive patterns change between birth and maturity? Researchers have proposed several theories of cognitive development in an attempt to describe the typical process by which an individual's mental processes become more complex. In-depth discussion of these and other developmental theories is provided in the module on Development.

PIAGET'S THEORY The best-known theory of cognitive development comes from the work of Swiss psychologist Jean Piaget (1896–1980). Piaget claimed that cognitive development is an orderly, sequential process in which children form adaptive cognitive structures—called **schemes**—in response to environmental stimuli. According to Piaget, as children learn more about the world by physically interacting with it, they actively revise their schemes to better fit with the reality they observe. Over time, as their brains mature and they are exposed to additional stimuli, children become capable of building more complex schemes—and as they do so, they move from one stage of development to the next. In fact, Piaget proposed that all children pass through four universal stages of cognitive development, as described in **Table 23–1 ●**: sensorimotor, preoperational, concrete operational, and formal operational (Piaget, 1966, 1972; Shaffer & Kipp, 2010).

VYGOTSKY'S THEORY Piaget's theory provides the framework for much of our understanding of cognitive development, but a few notable theories expand and refute Piaget's work. One important challenge comes from the work of Soviet psychologist Lev Vygotsky (1896–1934). Vygotsky's sociocultural theory of development proposed that children learn through their culture and through social interactions with other people. Whereas Piaget viewed children as independent learners, Vygotsky saw cognitive development as a socially mediated activity in which children build knowledge through cooperative dialogue with adults. He rejected Piaget's idea that all children progress through the same stages of development, proposing instead that individuals develop different skills depending on the values and teaching methods of their native culture. From Vygotsky's point of view, Piaget's theory ignores the impact of culture and language on learning (Shaffer & Kipp, 2010; Vygotsky, 1962).

TABLE 23–1 Piaget's Stages of Cognitive Development		
STAGE AND AGE RANGE	DESCRIPTION	DEVELOPMENTS
Sensorimotor Birth to 2 years	Infants use motor and sensory capabilities to explore the physical environment. Learning is largely trial and error.	Children develop a sense of "self" and "other" and come to understand object permanence. Behavioral schemes begin to produce images or mental schemes.
Preoperational 2–7 years	Young children use symbols (images and language) to explore their environment. Thought is egocentric, and children cannot adopt the perspectives of others.	Children participate in imaginative play and begin to recognize that others don't see the world the same way they do.
Concrete operational 7–11 years	Older children acquire cognitive operations, or mental activities that are an important part of rational thought. Logical reasoning is possible but limited to concrete (observable) problems.	Children are no longer fooled by appearances. They understand the basic properties of and relations among objects and events, and they are proficient at inferring motives.
Formal operational 11 years and beyond	Adolescents' cognitive operations are organized in a way that permits them to think about thinking. Thought is now systematic and abstract.	Logical thinking is no longer limited to the concrete or observable. Children engage in systematic, deductive reasoning and ponder hypothetical issues.

INFORMATION-PROCESSING THEORY Another influential theory of cognitive development is the information-processing perspective, which emerged in the second half of the 20th century. Information-processing theory views the mind as a continuously evolving computational system that takes in information, operates on it, and converts it to answers. According to this theory, physical changes associated with brain maturation are the most important determinant of cognitive ability, although culture and environment also affect development because they provide information to the brain. The information-processing perspective differs substantially from Vygotsky's theory in that it turns away from culture as the main factor in cognitive development and looks at the brain's inner workings. The difference between information-processing theory and Piaget's theory is even more radical, as the former theory rejects the notion of stages, instead proposing a continuous process of development from birth to adulthood (Shaffer & Kipp, 2010).

APPLICATION TO NURSING Though psychologists continue to debate their merits, Piaget's theory, Vygotsky's theory, and information-processing theory are all valuable in nursing practice. Piaget's theory provides an overview of childhood cognitive development, an important concept for the pediatric nurse. Vygotsky's theory acknowledges the role of cultural differences in learning—something all nurses should keep in mind when interacting with clients from different socioeconomic and ethnic backgrounds. Lastly, the information-processing perspective provides a scheme for understanding cognitive growth as a fluid process, a useful concept to keep in mind when dealing with clients of all ages.

A working knowledge of cognitive theory is perhaps most important in pediatric nursing. To design appropriate activities, develop effective teaching plans, and better prepare children for procedures, nurses must understand their young clients' thought processes and cognitive capabilities. For example, nurses might opt to explain healthcare measures to toddlers through the use of stories, pictures, or manipulative toys. In comparison, adolescents are likely in the formal operational stage and able to engage in higher-level reasoning. They also value the input of their peers. Thus the nurse might describe the possible consequences of a procedure to a teenage client so that she can make a rational decision about whether to undergo the procedure. The nurse might also suggest the teen participate in a support group with other adolescents who are sharing similar experiences or offer visitation time with the teenager's friends.

Of course, not all individuals develop cognitive skills according to the time frame described by Piaget—and some individuals may not acquire certain higher-level skills at any point in their lives. As Vygotsky's theory and information-processing theory emphasize, the normal range of cognitive development is broad and variable. Therefore nurses should attempt to gauge adult clients' abilities to process new information and engage in rational thought, then plan their teaching strategies as appropriate.

Genetic Considerations and Nonmodifiable Risk Factors

Under normal conditions, individuals' cognitive skills become increasingly complex as they advances from childhood to adulthood. In some cases, these skills appear to decline with advancing age—but this decline is not as dramatic as widely believed, nor does it affect all individuals. Although genetic factors may be involved in age-related cognitive changes, researchers are challenged when trying to distinguish between genetic effects and environmental influences on cognition—not only in older adults, but across the entire life span (Deary et al., 2012; Lee et al., 2010).

As individuals move from early and middle adulthood into late adulthood, their brains change in specific ways. In most individuals, a slow, steady decrease in brain mass is accompanied by decreased cerebral blood flow and increased levels of cerebrospinal fluid (Deary et al., 2009). These changes are a normal part of aging, and their cognitive effects appear to be minor. In fact, multiple studies have shown that normal, healthy aging does not dramatically change an individual's cognition or mental health. Although some cognitive skills decline slightly, others stay the same or improve with age. The American Psychological Association (2013b) reports the following findings:

- As individuals age, their information-processing speed decreases, as does their ability to split attention between tasks. Most individuals find it harder to maintain attention, filter out irrelevant details, and rapidly switch attention between auditory inputs.
- Generally, older adults' short-term memory changes very little. However, their long-term memory shows more noticeable declines.
- The ability to use and understand word combinations remains stable with age. In some cases, vocabulary improves. Still, many older adults have increased difficulty finding and rapidly listing words.
- The ability to engage in visuospatial tasks (such as drawing and constructing) decreases. Many individuals also undergo a slight decline in their mental flexibility and ability to engage in abstract thought.
- Most older adults continue to acquire practical information until the end of their lives.

The timing and degree of cognitive change vary by individual. For instance, some individuals might notice a decline in their recall abilities around age 65, others might notice this change around age 80, and others may not notice any decrease at all. This variability seems to be linked to several factors, including genetics, presence of diseases or disorders (especially cardiovascular disease), inflammation, dietary intake, activity level, and overall lifestyle. In general, the healthier individuals are, the less likely they are to experience significant cognitive decline. Interestingly, individuals who have higher educational levels and/or come from higher social classes also tend to experience less decline—probably because they often have safer home and work environments and better access to care (Deary et al., 2009).

Most age-related cognitive changes are relatively minor, as are their associated limitations. Many older adults adopt strategies to cope with those declines that do occur. Some of these actions have the added benefit of helping prevent further cognitive deterioration. Common coping strategies include the following:

- Participating in daily activities that call on a variety of cognitive skills (e.g., reading, playing cards, completing puzzles)
- Keeping lists and calendars, and writing reminder notes to oneself

- Using mnemonic strategies such as word associations and interactive imagery, especially when learning new information
- Avoiding distractions and making an effort to focus attention on the task at hand
- Establishing routines for important daily tasks and not rushing through them
- Always putting objects in the same place when done using them
- Engaging in regular physical activity, which can help preserve brain function
- Staying social and seeking support from family and friends
- Refusing to accept common stereotypes about aging
- Remaining positive about the future, and keeping a sense of humor about any cognitive lapses that do occur (American Psychological Association, 2013a, 2013b)

Above all, older adults should remember that significant cognitive declines are *not* inevitable and *not* a normal part of the aging process. When such changes are severe enough to affect an individual's quality of life, they usually are a sign of illness or impairment. Common physical causes of cognitive dysfunction include circulatory problems, medication or alcohol use, sensory impairment, infection, dehydration, nutritional deficiency, thyroid imbalance, and Alzheimer disease (discussed in detail later in this concept). Similarly, many psychological conditions manifest as confusion or memory loss in older adults—especially depression and severe anxiety (APA, 2013a). Depending on their cause, some declines in cognition may be reversible, while others might stay the same or even worsen. By promptly assessing older clients who show signs of cognitive deterioration, nurses may be able to help reverse or slow further decline.

SAFETY ALERT

Changes in cognition require immediate attention. Cognitive disturbances put clients at increased risk of injury, so rapid institution of safety measures is critical. Also, prompt assessment of a client's cognitive impairment may allow the medical team to more quickly identify and treat the root cause.

▶ ALTERATIONS TO COGNITION

Normal cognition is contingent on normal brain function—and an individual's brain will not work correctly unless precise chemical conditions are in place. Disruption of nearly any phys-iological system may cause cognitive impairment. See the Concepts Related to Cognition feature for examples. In these cases, resolution of the underlying problem often restores normal cognition. Other times, cognitive impairment is the primary or defining characteristic of a given condition. Prominent examples of such conditions include learning disabilities, intellectual disability, and dementia. Cognitive dysfunction, including that associated with dementia and schizophrenia, may be accompanied by psychosis. **Psychosis** is an abnormal mental state that alters an individual's thoughts, feelings, perceptions, and/or behaviors. Psychosis may be characterized by a number of features, including delusions, hallucinations, and illusions. **Delusions** are rigid, false beliefs, for example, believing that members of a hospital care team are actually government spies assigned to gather secret information about a client. **Hallucinations** are imagined sensory experiences, for example, hearing voices or seeing people, animals, or things that are not present in reality. **Illusions** are distorted perceptions of actual sights, sounds, and other stimuli, for example, interpreting a shadow on the wall as being an angel or an alarming infusion pump as being the sound of a telephone ringing.

Learning Disabilities

Learning disabilities are a group of disorders that impair an individual's ability to receive and process information, causing reduced functioning in verbal, linguistic, reasoning, and academic skills. These disorders first become evident in childhood, although they may not be diagnosed until a child is old enough to read and write. Individuals with learning disabilities are of at least average intelligence but face challenges to knowledge acquisition that can last a lifetime (National Center for Learning Disabilities, 2013).

ALTERATIONS AND MANIFESTATIONS   The principal sign of a learning disability is an unaccountable gap between an individual's expected level of academic performance and his actual achievement. All learning disabilities can range in severity from mild to profound, and affected individuals are frequently diagnosed with more than one of these conditions.

As mentioned, learning disabilities can impact an individual's reasoning, spelling, writing, reading, speaking, listening, and mathematics abilities (National Center for Learning Disabilities, 2013). Common disabilities include dyslexia, dyscalculia, dysgraphia, and dyspraxia, all of which are described in **Table 23–2 ●**.

TABLE 23–2   Common Learning Disabilities

DISORDER	FUNCTION AFFECTED	CLINICAL MANIFESTATIONS	EXAMPLES
Dyslexia	Language processing	Challenges with spelling, reading, and writing	Slow reading rate; confusing letters and their sounds; problems combining sounds into words
Dyscalculia	Mathematics skills	Challenges with computation and other mathematical tasks	Problems in learning to count; impaired mental math abilities
Dysgraphia	Written communication	Challenges with writing, spelling, and composition	Illegible writing; trouble organizing ideas before and during the composition process
Dyspraxia	Fine motor skills	Challenges with tasks that require manual dexterity and coordination	Problems with object manipulation and physical crafts (e.g., drawing, using scissors, tying shoes)

Source: Based on National Center for Learning Disabilities. (2013). *What are learning disabilities?* Retrieved from http://www.ncld.org/types-learning-disabilities/what-is-ld/what-are-learning-disabilities.

Concepts Related to **Cognition**

Even slight hypoxia can cause mild to moderate deficits in memory and judgment, because the brain's neurons aren't receiving enough oxygen to function properly. Further decreases in cerebral oxygen levels bring about more dramatic changes, such as confusion, speech deficits, and loss of consciousness. If cerebral hypoxia continues as few as 5 minutes, coma and brain death may result (Cleveland Clinic, 2010).

The presence of foreign substances such as alcohol and drugs can also wreak havoc on an individual's ability to think, speak, reason, and remember. Alcohol in particular has a wide range of damaging effects. Upon entering the bloodstream, alcohol travels to the brain, where it alters neuronal membranes and interferes with enzyme and neurotransmitter function. The net result is a decrease in cognitive function, ranging from slurred speech and forgetfulness up to blackout and even death (Mukherjee et al., 2008). Long-term alcohol abuse can also damage the brain in several ways. Excessive consumption may result in diminished red blood cell production and anemia, thus limiting the blood's ability to carry oxygen to the brain. Frequent use can also affect platelet function, which increases the risk of cerebral clotting and hypoxia (Ballard, 1997). In addition, long-term alcohol use causes irreversible liver damage. When the liver can no longer remove metabolic waste products from the blood, these substances accumulate in the brain and cause widespread cognitive impairment (Mayo Clinic, 2012a).

Of course, many other factors can disrupt an individual's cognition, including inflammation and altered fluid and electrolyte levels. Nurses should have a general understanding of these factors, their effects, and related nursing interventions.

CONCEPT	RELATIONSHIP TO COGNITION	NURSING IMPLICATIONS
Fluids and Electrolytes		
■ Fluid and electrolyte imbalance	Fluid and ion imbalances can result in abnormal intracranial pressure, disrupted O_2 transport, and/or poor neuronal function, all of which may lead to cognitive impairment.	■ Monitor vital signs, I&O, daily weight, ABGs, and serum ion levels. ■ *Anticipate:* IV fluids, dietary restrictions, pharmacotherapy
Inflammation		
	Inflammation involves changes in vascular permeability, which may lead to abnormal brain chemistry and cognitive impairment.	■ Monitor vital signs and white cell count. ■ Assess for pain, warmth, redness, and edema. ■ Watch for infection or injury that may be causing inflammation. ■ Encourage fluid intake. ■ Position client for comfort and elevate inflamed areas as appropriate. ■ *Anticipate:* Antipyretics, analgesics, cold packs, IV fluids
Oxygenation		
■ Acute respiratory distress syndrome ■ Asthma ■ Chronic obstructive pulmonary disease	Decreases in the amount of O_2 reaching the brain can result in cognitive impairment, coma, and death.	■ Monitor vital signs, ABGs, and airway clearance. ■ Watch for cyanosis and/or impaired perfusion. ■ Administer oxygen. ■ Position client for optimum blood flow. ■ *Anticipate:* Bronchodilators, corticosteroids, sputum testing, respiratory therapy, client education
Perfusion		
	Inadequate perfusion of brain tissue results in low O_2 levels and impaired cognitive function.	■ Monitor vital signs, ABGs, and cardiac sounds. ■ Assess perfusion, including pulses, nail beds, and skin color. ■ Administer oxygen. ■ Position client for optimum blood flow. ■ Watch for chest pain and signs of cardiac disruption. ■ *Anticipate:* Pharmacotherapy, IV fluids, stress/exercise tests, echocardiogram, possible cardiac catheterization and/or surgery

(continued on next page)

Concepts Related to **Cognition** (continued)

CONCEPT	RELATIONSHIP TO COGNITION	NURSING IMPLICATIONS
Addiction		
■ Alcohol abuse ■ Substance abuse	Drugs and alcohol interfere with normal neuronal functioning, blood flow, and/or waste removal, resulting in cognitive impairment.	■ Monitor vital signs. ■ Provide for client safety. ■ Watch for symptoms of withdrawal and provide supportive care as necessary. ■ *Anticipate:* Pharmacotherapy, substance abuse counseling, patient education
Legal Issues		
■ Advance directives	By preparing advance directives, clients with recurring or worsening cognitive alterations can ensure their care wishes are known should they become unable to speak for themselves.	■ Ask whether client has established an advance directive or is interested in doing so. ■ Document the advance directive and all conversations about it in the client's chart. ■ Advocate on the client's behalf by ensuring the advance directive is followed. ■ *Anticipate:* Patient education, referral to counseling resources

PREVALENCE   There are few reliable statistics about the prevalence of learning disabilities across all age groups, because self-report surveys are the only information source for the adult population. The most recent data set, collected in 2005, indicates that 1.8% of the U.S. population age 6 and older has learning disabilities. That adds up to 4.67 million individuals, many of whom are school-age children. In fact, just under 4% of American schoolchildren have been diagnosed with a learning disorder. Prevalence rates decline with age, ranging from 2.7% of adults under age 24 to 0.4% of adults age 85 and older (Cortiella, 2011).

Beyond age, the prevalence of learning disorders varies by gender, economic status, and ethnicity. Males are more likely to be diagnosed than females. Among school-age children, boys have a prevalence rate of 3.9%, while girls have a rate of 2.0%. This disparity is smaller, yet still present, in the adult population. Prevalence is also higher among poor families. Whereas 4.1% of families living below the poverty line report having a child with learning disabilities, only 2.7% of nonpoor families report the same. In terms of ethnicity, rates are similar among Whites, Blacks, and Latinos; lower among Asians; and higher among multiracial populations and members of smaller ethnic groups, such as Native Americans (Cortiella, 2011).

Despite these statistics, actual learning disability rates are probably more even across genders and age groups. Researchers believe that the higher rate among males is related to the fact that boys and their families are often more willing to admit to learning problems. Similarly, higher prevalence rates among children and young adults reflect enhanced diagnostic efforts over the past four decades, largely due to passage of federal laws that require educational assistance for children with special needs (Cortiella, 2011).

GENETIC CONSIDERATIONS AND NONMODIFIABLE RISK FACTORS   There is frequently no evident cause of learning disabilities, although they appear to involve differences in brain structure that affect an individual's ability to process information. Experts aren't sure how these differences arise, but genetics seems to be a major factor. For example, between 35% and 45% of individuals in a family with reading disabilities are likely to be affected (Horowitz, 2013). Though genetic factors cannot be counteracted, knowledge of a family history of learning disorders provides an opportunity for early diagnosis and treatment.

PREVENTION   Many learning disabilities are unavoidable, especially when they involve genetic factors. Still, women can take several steps to reduce the likelihood their children will be affected. Parents and nurses also can work together to identify affected children as early as possible through recognizing abnormalities in growth and development and promptly seeking treatment, thus increasing the chances of early intervention.

Although heritable traits are known to contribute to learning disabilities, modifiable risk factors also play a role. Some learning disabilities are congenital and result from maternal behaviors such as alcohol consumption, drug use, and smoking during pregnancy (Horowitz, 2013). Other conditions that can lead to learning disabilities include fetal oxygen deprivation, low birth weight, and premature or prolonged labor. Childhood experiences such as traumatic injury, nutritional deprivation, and toxin exposure are also thought to give rise to the neurological changes associated with learning disabilities (Cortiella, 2011).

Nurses play a central role in detecting learning disabilities, as the doctor's office is frequently a parent's first stop when she suspects a child has developmental problems. Whenever parents express concern about a child's development, academic performance, or behavior, the nurse should determine whether there is a family history of learning difficulties. The nurse should also review the child's health history for prematurity, low birth weight, head injury, seizures, and other chronic conditions. In addition, the nurse should be aware that absence of any of the following skills may indicate a learning disability:

■ Ability to speak in sentences by 2.5 years of age

■ Ability to use intelligible speech at least 50% of the time by age 3

- Ability to tie shoes, hop, use buttons and snaps, and cut with scissors by kindergarten
- Ability to pay attention to a short story by 3–5 years of age (Kelly & Aylward, 2005)

Whenever learning disability is suspected, the nurse should refer the family to the child's school or a different testing resource, such as a learning specialist. There, the child will undergo a battery of cognitive and developmental tests before a diagnosis is made. Although magnetic resonance imaging (MRI) of the brain is a promising method for uncovering diagnostic clues, this technology is not yet available in most communities.

In the event the child is diagnosed with a learning disability, the nurse should work with the family to plan for the child's needs. This includes creating a home setting that maximizes learning potential, promoting activities that build the child's self-esteem, and helping the family collaborate with the child's school to establish appropriate learning goals. Referral to government or community resources may also be appropriate. Early intervention is essential. With proper assistance, most children can learn to compensate for their learning disability and live successful, productive lives.

Intellectual Disability

Intellectual disability, previously known as **mental retardation**, involves significant limitations in intellectual functioning and adaptive behavior that begin prior to age 18.

- **Intellectual functioning** refers to general intelligence or mental capacity, including the abilities to learn, use logic, and solve problems. An IQ score of 70–75 or below is considered indicative of limited intellectual functioning.
- **Adaptive behaviors** involve three categories of everyday skills: conceptual skills (such as the abilities to read, use language, and tell time); social skills (such as the abilities to follow rules and appropriately interact with others); and practical skills (such as the abilities to engage in work and activities of daily living).

A low IQ score alone does not necessarily correlate with limitations in an individual's adaptive behaviors. Before diagnosing a child with intellectual disability, practitioners must also consider how the child functions within the contexts of his specific culture and community.

Intellectual disability is a form of developmental disability. A **developmental disability** is one of various chronic conditions first noticed during early childhood that involve physical and/or intellectual impairments (American Association on Intellectual and Developmental Disabilities, 2013). For more information on developmental disabilities, refer to the module on Development.

ALTERATIONS AND MANIFESTATIONS Intellectual disability can result from prenatal errors in central nervous system (CNS) development, external factors that damage the CNS, or pre- or postnatal changes in an individual's biological environment. Regardless of category, all causes of intellectual disability act by disrupting the normal form or function of the CNS. Sometimes, these changes produce only mental limitations. Other times, intellectual disability is one of a constellation of symptoms linked to a particular cause.

Of the various conditions associated with intellectual disability, three deserve special mention because of the range of physical and cognitive alterations they involve. **Down syndrome, fragile X syndrome**, and **fetal alcohol syndrome (FAS)** are all caused by problems during prenatal development, although the first two conditions involve genetic errors while the third involves alcohol consumption during pregnancy. All three conditions are present at birth and affect an individual for the rest of his life. See **Table 23–3** ● for a summary of physical traits associated with these conditions.

- ***Down syndrome*** occurs when an individual's cells contain a third full or partial copy of the 21st chromosome (National Down Syndrome Society, 2012b). Usually, a full copy of the extra chromosome is present, a situation known as **trisomy 21**. In either case, the excess genetic material leads to intellectual disability and physical impairments that can range from mild to severe.

  Individuals with Down syndrome are at increased risk of several problems not normally seen in childhood. Roughly 40% are born with congenital heart defects. Children with Down syndrome are also more likely to experience hearing loss, gastrointestinal blockages, celiac disease, cataracts, strabismus, thyroid disease, skeletal abnormalities, orthodontic problems, leukemia, and eventual dementia. With appropriate support, affected individuals can lead healthy lives and sometimes live and work independently. Average life expectancy for individuals with Down syndrome is about 55 years, although some individuals live 10 or even 20 years longer (Centers for Disease Control, 2011a; National Association for Down Syndrome, 2013).
- ***Fragile X syndrome*** arises from a single recessive abnormality on the X chromosome. Specifically, a mutation in the *FMR-1* gene causes a small section of DNA to be repeated 200 or more times, rather than the normal 5–40 times. This change renders the gene unable to make its associated protein, and absence of the protein leads to errors in brain development and function.

  A variety of signs and symptoms are associated with fragile X syndrome. The most notable is intellectual disability, typically accompanied by behavioral problems such as attention-deficit/hyperactivity disorder (ADHD). Affected children may also exhibit autistic behaviors; speech problems; anxiety and mood problems; delays in learning to sit, walk, and talk; and enhanced sensitivity to environmental stimuli. Most individuals with fragile X syndrome are in generally good health and have a normal life span. Still, between 5% and 15% of affected children experience seizures and require anticonvulsant medications.

  Interestingly, boys usually experience the effects of fragile X syndrome to a much greater degree than girls. Because females have two copies of the X chromosome, one X chromosome's *FMR-1* gene is able to produce enough protein to partially compensate for the amount normally produced by the other copy. Boys, however, have just one X chromosome, so no compensatory mechanism is available (March of Dimes, 2010).
- ***Fetal alcohol syndrome.*** Unlike Down syndrome and fragile X syndrome, fetal alcohol syndrome (FAS) is a completely preventable condition caused by maternal alcohol intake

TABLE 23–3 Physical Traits Associated With Three Causes of Intellectual Disability

DOWN SYNDROME (See Figure 23–1 ●)	FRAGILE X SYNDROME (See Figure 23–2 ●)	FETAL ALCOHOL SYNDROME (See Figure 23–3 ●)
Broad hands with a single traverse palmar crease	Crossed eyes	Small eyes
Congenital cataracts	Enlarged testicles	Abnormal joints and bones
Decreased muscle tone	Epicanthic eye folds	CNS abnormalities
Epicanthic eye folds	Excessively flexible joints	Flattened nasal bridge
Flattened nose	High palate Increased likelihood of middle ear infections	Growth deficits
Hearing impairment		Hearing impairment
Increased likelihood of diabetes, leukemia, and heart defects	Increased seizure risk	Lack of coordination
	Large ears	Small nose that turns up at the tip
Protruding tongue	Long head with protruding jaw	Small palpebral fissures
Short, stocky neck	Scoliosis	Smooth philtrum
Small ears located low on the head		Thin vermillion border
Small head		
Wide space between first two toes		

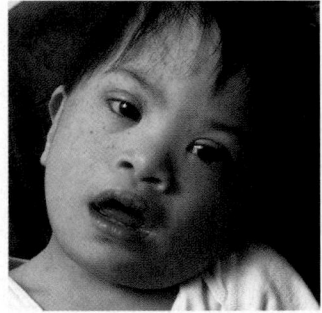

Figure 23–1 ● A child with Down syndrome.

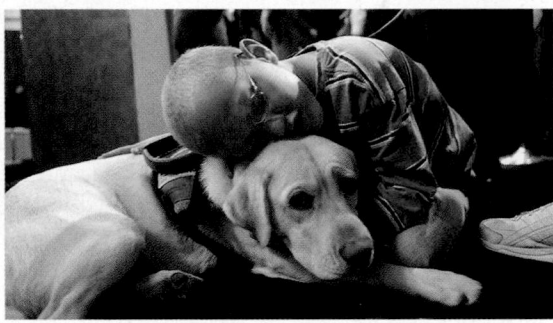

Figure 23–2 ● A child with fragile X syndrome.
Source: © ZUMA Press, Inc./Alamy.

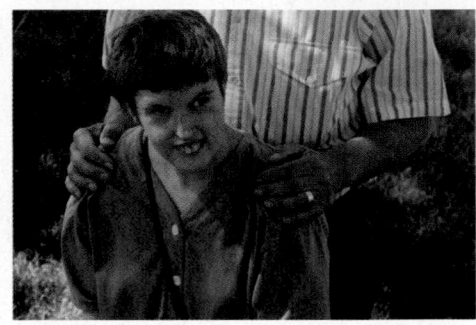

Figure 23–3 ● A child with fetal alcohol syndrome.
Source: © STUART WONG/KRT/Newscom.

during pregnancy. (See the Client Teaching feature.) FAS is the most severe of several fetal alcohol spectrum disorders (FASDs), all of which involve some degree of physical, intellectual, behavioral, and/or learning disability.

FAS and related disorders result from the presence of alcohol in a woman's bloodstream. Because alcohol crosses the placenta and the fetal liver cannot process it, the fetus has the same blood alcohol content as its mother, regardless of the type or amount of alcohol consumed (National Organization on Fetal Alcohol Syndrome, 2012b). Given the fetus's size and immaturity, even small amounts of alcohol can dramatically disrupt prenatal development, causing facial, skeletal, and organ abnormalities, along with a variety of other problems. However, for a diagnosis of FAS (as opposed to another fetal alcohol spectrum disorder), a child must exhibit all of the following conditions:

- Growth deficits
- Characteristic facial abnormalities, including a smooth philtrum (ridge between the nose and upper lip), thin vermillion border (line between the lips and surrounding skin), and small palpebral fissures (separations between the upper and lower eyelids)
- Central nervous system abnormalities (structural, neurological, and/or functional; National Organization on Fetal Alcohol Syndrome, 2012a)

These nervous system abnormalities almost always result in some degree of mental impairment, such as intellectual disability, learning disability, communication problems, poor memory, or limited attention span. Although the many effects of FAS last a lifetime, early treatment can help lessen some symptoms and improve an affected individual's quality of life (Centers for Disease Control, 2011b).

Client Teaching **Fetal Alcohol Syndrome**

In the United States, roughly 12% of women admit consuming at least one alcoholic drink during pregnancy, while about 2% report having five or more drinks at one time (Beck, 2012). These statistics indicate that all women need clear, timely messages about the damaging effects of alcohol on the fetus.

Client teaching must emphasize that the *only* way to prevent FAS is to abstain from all alcohol of all types for the entire duration of pregnancy. This message should be communicated to all female clients of childbearing age, including teenagers, so they understand how important it is to stop drinking immediately should they become pregnant. Nurses should also explain that the most dangerous time for fetal alcohol exposure may be early in pregnancy—often before a woman even knows she's expecting.

PREVALENCE   Intellectual disability is the most prevalent developmental disability in the United States today, with approximately 6.5 million Americans diagnosed with some degree of impairment. The condition is so common that it affects roughly 10% of all children who receive special education services in public schools (National Dissemination Center for Children with Disabilities, 2011).

Various causes of intellectual disability have different prevalence rates. Of the three conditions described earlier—Down syndrome, fragile X syndrome, and FAS—Down syndrome is most common, affecting 1 in every 691 babies born in the United States (National Down Syndrome Society, 2012a). Fragile X syndrome is significantly less common. Several studies indicate that the prevalence in males is approximately 1 in 3,600–4,000, while that in females is approximately 1 in 4,000–6,000 (National Fragile X Foundation, 2013). The prevalence of fetal alcohol syndrome is more difficult to determine, and estimates vary widely. However, studies conducted by the U.S. Centers for Disease Control and Prevention have found that FAS rates range from 0.2 to 1.5 cases for every 1,000 live births, depending on state and region (Centers for Disease Control, 2012).

GENETIC CONSIDERATIONS AND NONMODIFIABLE RISK FACTORS   Intellectual disability can be caused by any condition that inhibits brain development before birth, during birth, or in the childhood years. Of the known sources of intellectual disability, many are nonmodifiable in origin. Often, they involve inherited gene disorders or prenatal gene abnormalities, as is the case with Down syndrome and fragile X syndrome. Another common cause of intellectual disability is phenylketonuria (PKU), a single-gene disorder that renders individuals unable to process the amino acid phenylalanine. Without treatment, phenylalanine builds up in the blood and inflicts severe brain damage.

PREVENTION   Nurses can help reduce the risk of intellectual disability by instructing clients about several modifiable risk factors. Nurses also play a key role in screening for intellectual disability and related conditions, especially in pediatric clients.

FAS is the leading preventable cause of intellectual disability—and a mother can ensure her child doesn't develop FAS simply by abstaining from alcohol during pregnancy. Other modifiable risk factors include the following:

- Certain events and behaviors during pregnancy can lead to intellectual disability in infants. These include maternal drug use, smoking, malnutrition, exposure to environmental toxins, and illness.

- Prematurity and low birth weight forecast disability more reliably than any other conditions. Difficulties at delivery, such as oxygen deprivation or birth injury, may also cause problems in intellectual functioning.

- Diseases such as whooping cough, chickenpox, measles, and *Haemophilus influenzae* type B (Hib) can damage the brain in childhood. So can head injuries and near-drowning. Childhood exposure to lead, mercury, and other toxins can also cause irreparable damage to the nervous system.

- Children who live in poverty are at higher risk for malnutrition, childhood diseases, and exposure to environmental health hazards, as well as a lack of intellectual stimulation early in life. All of these factors have been linked to intellectual disability.

Over the last three decades, several advances have helped reduce the prevalence of intellectual disability. In the United States, rates have dropped thanks to public health measures that mandate newborn screening for PKU and require vaccinations for Hib, measles, encephalitis, and rubella. Comprehensive prenatal care, including testing for diseases and administering folic acid to expectant mothers, also reduces the risk of intellectual disability.

Various screenings look for the conditions that give rise to intellectual disability and for the disability itself. For example, all 50 states now require that newborns be tested for PKU and hyperthyroidism. The PKU screening consists of a blood test performed a day or two after birth, a mandatory measure that has significantly reduced the incidence of intellectual disabilities across the country (Mayo Clinic, 2011).

Genetic counseling is another screening process that provides information to individuals who may be at risk of passing on conditions that cause intellectual disability. Counseling should be considered if there is a family history of such conditions, if any of a couple's previous births resulted in a child with a genetic disorder, or if a mother has had two or more miscarriages. Genetic counseling should also be recommended if the mother is over age 35, if either partner is part of an ethnic group with a high incidence of certain genetic conditions, or if the partners are blood relatives (The Arc, 2011).

As previously mentioned, prematurity and low birth weight are major risk factors for intellectual disability. Therefore nurses should ensure infants who are born too early or too small receive frequent neurological and developmental screenings for at least the first 2 years of life. Premature infants generally achieve developmental milestones on a delayed schedule that corresponds with how early they were born. So an infant who is 6 weeks premature should be expected to display the same level of development as a child who is chronologically 6 weeks younger but was born at full term. Most premature children catch up to their peers developmentally sometime around their second birthday. If a child is not catching up by this time, further evaluation for possible intellectual disability may be necessary.

Diagnosis of intellectual disability is a complex issue that is not decided by any one test. The American Association on Intellectual and Developmental Disabilities stresses that when making a diagnosis, professionals must consider factors such as linguistic diversity, cultural differences in communication and behavior, and the community environment typical of an individual's culture. Still, formal IQ tests are a key part of measuring intellectual function. An IQ of roughly 70–75 is considered indicative of disability. Other tests that gauge conceptual, social, and practical skills are used to complement IQ tests in the diagnostic process (AAIDD, 2013).

When working with clients who have an intellectual disability, the nurse plays a key role in monitoring for signs of abuse. Children with intellectual disability are at greater risk of abuse than unaffected children, in part because of the emotional and financial stresses they place on their families, albeit unintentionally. Still, nurses should remember that some conditions cause injuries that resemble abuse. Nurses should also note that children with intellectual disability may have difficulty verbalizing what's happened to them. If, after careful assessment, a nurse suspects a child is the victim of abuse, the nurse should follow organizational protocols for reporting suspected abuse and ensure law enforcement is notified.

Dementia

Dementia is a progressive loss of cognitive function. It is not a specific disease, but rather a set of symptoms caused by various disorders that affect the brain. Dementia is sometimes confused with delirium, but it is critical to distinguish between the two. While delirium is an acute and reversible syndrome, dementia is the steady, irreversible loss of global brain function. (For discussion about delirium, see the exemplar on Confusion in this module.)

Dementia affects multiple cortical functions. In fact, doctors diagnose dementia only if two or more brain functions are significantly impaired. For individuals who suffer from dementia, this impairment interferes with normal activities and relationships. Affected individuals lose their ability to solve problems and maintain emotional control. They also experience personality changes and behavioral problems, such as agitation, delusions, and hallucinations. While memory loss is a common symptom, memory loss by itself is not indicative of dementia (National Institute of Neurological Disorders and Stroke, 2012).

ALTERATIONS AND MANIFESTATIONS All forms of dementia result from neuronal death and subsequent changes in brain structure. These changes are caused by a variety of conditions, including Alzheimer disease, vascular dementia, Lewy body dementia, frontotemporal dementia, Huntington disease, and Creutzfeldt-Jakob disease. For more information on the most common causes, see **Table 23–4** ●. Beyond these diseases, researchers have identified numerous other conditions that can cause dementia, including medication reactions; metabolic problems; nutritional deficiencies; infections; poisoning; brain tumors, anoxia, or hypoxia; and cardiovascular and pulmonary problems (National Institute of Neurological Disorders and Stroke, 2012). A heritable component clearly plays a part in some cases of dementia, but there is no known family history in many affected individuals.

A variety of conditions can mimic dementia, especially in older individuals. These include the following:

- *Age-related cognitive decline related to mild memory impairment and slower information processing.* With advancing age, the brain naturally loses some neurons, decreasing in volume in the process. These changes are normal and not symptomatic of dementia.
- *Mild cognitive impairment.* This condition may progress to dementia, but in its initial stages, it is not severe enough to be diagnosed as such.

- *Depression and other emotional problems.* Emotional disturbances may cause some individuals to become passive, forgetful, slow, or disoriented.
- *Delirium characterized by confusion, rapidly changing mental states, disorientation, and personality changes.* Delirium typically results from treatable physical or mental health problems. When these problems are addressed, affected individuals experience full recovery from their delirium.

More information about these conditions can be found elsewhere in the text, including **Table 23–5** ● and the exemplar on Confusion in this module.

Individuals with dementia may experience a variety of cognitive limitations, ranging from mild to severe. Some of these deficits affect an individual's bodily actions; examples include **akathisia** (restlessness), **carphologia** (involuntary, repeated lint picking), **ataxia** (lack of muscle coordination), and **dysphagia** (difficulty swallowing). Other conditions—such as **anomia** (difficulty naming people and things), **aphasia** (inability to express and understand language), and **echolalia** (involuntary repetition of sounds)—manifest in terms of cognition and social behavior.

SAFETY ALERT Individuals with dementia are at increased risk of malnutrition, dehydration, and noncompliance with their drug regimen, as they may forget to eat, drink, or take medication. They are also more likely to get lost or wander. For these and other reasons, daily supervision should be a key part of any dementia care plan.

PREVALENCE Dementia is not a natural part of aging, although it is substantially more common in older adults. Whereas fewer than 2% of individuals ages 65–69 have dementia, the condition affects approximately 5% of individuals ages 71–79; 24% of individuals ages 80–89; and 37% of individuals age 90 and older (Plassman et al., 2007). Alzheimer disease is the most common cause, followed by vascular dementia and dementia with Lewy bodies. In 2012, approximately 5.4 million Americans had Alzheimer disease (Alzheimer's Association, 2012).

GENETIC CONSIDERATIONS AND NONMODIFIABLE RISK FACTORS Although genetic factors contribute to some cases of dementia, the exact degree and mechanism of involvement vary by type of dementia. For example, researchers know that many cases of early-onset Alzheimer disease (which mani-

TABLE 23–4 Dementia: Common Etiologies

ETIOLOGY	CAUSE AND PRIMARY PATHOPHYSIOLOGY
Alzheimer disease	Form of dementia that causes problems with memory, thinking, and behavior. Although the cause is unknown, the disease clearly involves two types of brain abnormalities: amyloid plaques and neurofibrillary tangles. Alzheimer disease is progressive, worsening with time.
Vascular dementia	Involves brain damage from circulatory problems, mainly stroke. May also arise when blood vessels in the brain are damaged by chronic disorders like extreme hypotension. (*Note:* Vascular brain changes frequently coexist with other conditions, such as Alzheimer disease.)
Dementia with Lewy bodies (DLB)	A progressive dementia that results from abnormal deposits that accumulate in brain cells. Called *Lewy bodies*, these deposits kill the cells over time. The cause of DLB is usually unknown, although it sometimes seems to run in families.
Frontotemporal dementia (FTD)	A group of disorders caused by progressive cell degeneration in the frontal or temporal lobes. As nerve cells degenerate, brain tissue shrinks. Some affected individuals develop neurofibrillary tangles.

TABLE 23-5   Dementia and Delirium Compared

	DEMENTIA	DELIRIUM
PROGRESSION	Onset is slow and subtle. Condition consistently worsens over months or years, culminating in death.	Onset is usually sudden and severe. Condition is typically brief (hours to days) but may persist for months.
DEFINING CHARACTERISTIC	Irreversible and increasing loss of cognition and global brain function.	Temporary, reversible disturbance in consciousness and other brain functions.
MOTOR SIGNS	None until late in course of disease.	Restlessness; tremor; movement may be either slow or hyperactive.
EFFECTS ON SPEECH	Increased difficulty finding words in early stages of disorder. As condition progresses, communication skills deteriorate. Eventually, many individuals become uncommunicative.	Speech may suddenly become slurred, disorganized, or nonsensical.
EFFECTS ON MENTAL STATUS	Normal attention in early stages, with increasing levels of distraction as condition progresses.	Attention is fluctuating and often fleeting.
EFFECTS ON MEMORY	Memory gradually worsens over time. Recent memory is typically the first area to be affected.	Memory remains, although it may be limited by problems with attention.
PERCEPTUAL CHANGES	Individuals may experience paranoia and delusions as their cognitive skills decline.	Individuals often experience visual, auditory, and/or tactile hallucinations.
EFFECTS ON MOOD	Individuals may display lack of interest, anhedonia, and/or lack of inhibition.	Individuals may display fear, paranoia, anxiety, irritability, depression, and/or high levels of elation and excitement.
SYSTEMIC INVOLVEMENT	Primary etiology usually related to impaired brain function, with subsequent impact on other body systems.	Manifestations related to temporary, reversible brain impairment. Primary etiology often linked to exposure to toxins or systemic illness.

fests before age 65) are caused by three heritable gene mutations. If an individual carries one of these mutations, her children have a 50% chance of inheriting the disease. In contrast, late-onset Alzheimer disease exhibits a more complex pattern of inheritance. Scientists continue to identify genes that increase risk, but none of these genes directly cause the disease. Thus, while children of individuals with late-onset Alzheimer disease have an increased likelihood of illness, the condition is not inevitable.

Other forms of dementia also exhibit varying patterns of heritability. Frontotemporal dementia clearly runs in families, as about one third of affected individuals have two or more relatives with the disease. The role of genetics in vascular dementia and dementia with Lewy bodies is less obvious. Researchers have yet to identify any genes that directly cause either disorder, although they suspect some risk factors may be passed from generation to generation (Alzheimer's Society, 2013c).

Beyond genetics, other nonmodifiable risk factors for dementia include age, gender (with women slightly more likely to be affected), diabetes, Parkinson disease, multiple sclerosis, Down syndrome, kidney disease, HIV, and some learning disabilities (Alzheimer's Society, 2013a).

PREVENTION   Because the causes of dementia vary, a number of preventive actions can help reduce the risk of disease. Similarly, various screening methods may be appropriate depending on what form of dementia an individual has.

Several modifiable factors can increase an individual's risk of dementia, including:

■ Medical conditions that are preventable or remediable (e.g., cardiovascular disease)

■ Environmental, psychological, and interpersonal traits and behaviors (e.g., repeated head trauma)

■ Depression in older adults

To reduce risk, individuals should follow their treatment plans for medical conditions. Consuming fruits and vegetables is especially important, because they contain vitamins and antioxidants believed to help prevent dementia. Weight control and smoking cessation improve cardiovascular function, and limiting alcohol consumption reduces dementia risk. Use of personal protective equipment while cycling and participating in contact sports also reduces the likelihood of head trauma.

Engaging in regular social activity can help prevent depression, especially in older adults. Moreover, social activity itself decreases dementia risk, as does taking part in mental activities like reading, games, and puzzles (Alzheimer's Society, 2013a).

No specific screenings for dementia exist, in part because the condition has so many different causes. The most effective way to screen individuals is to simply observe them in their daily lives. Early signs of dementia include difficulty finding words, as well as regularly forgetting recent events and everyday information. As the disease progresses, many individuals undergo mood changes and are often agitated or scared about their symptoms. With time, more deficits start to emerge, but they appear so gradually that they are frequently overlooked or wrongly attributed to normal aging. Often, affected individuals deny having any cognitive problems whatsoever.

All older adults should be monitored for dementia, but some require closer screening. Individuals who have experienced stroke or head trauma should undergo regular cognitive assessment, as should individuals with a family history of Alzheimer disease. Individuals from families with early-onset Alzheimer disease may also opt for screenings that look for the three genes implicated in this condition.

CASE STUDY \\ PART 1

Victor Wallace is a 74-year-old Caucasian male who was diagnosed with moderate Alzheimer disease 2 years ago. Mr. Wallace lives with his 50-year-old daughter, Anne Marie, who is his primary caretaker. His wife of 52 years died of pancreatic cancer 18 months ago.

Mr. Wallace presents at his gerontologist's office at 9:30 on Thursday morning. Ms. Wallace requested the appointment because she is concerned about the changes she has seen in her father over the past month. As the nurse working with Mr. Wallace's gerontologist, you conduct an initial assessment and interview with Mr. Wallace and Ms. Wallace. Ms. Wallace reports that Mr. Wallace has exhibited increased confusion and anxiety at home and at the adult day care center he attends each day while she is at work. In the past, Mr. Wallace only had these problems in unfamiliar settings. He is also experiencing a decline in language, increasingly using the wrong words to describe common objects and relying on scanning speech to find words. However, Ms. Wallace's main concern is her father's refusal to carry out the basic ADLs he is still capable of performing. When you ask Mr. Wallace about the ADLs, he says, "There's no point in trying because I won't be able to do them much longer."

As you observe Mr. Wallace, you note that he seems agitated. He is sitting on the edge of his chair, tapping his foot and rapping his hands on his knees. When you ask him basic questions, he has a hard time coming up with answers. When he can't find the words he wants, he just repeats the phrase "That's how it is."

Mr. Wallace's vital signs and weight are normal, and his physical condition is good for a man his age. You administer the Cornell Scale for Depression in Dementia and his score is 17, indicating high probability of depression. The gerontologist maintains Mr. Wallace's current dose of 28 mg of memantine (Namenda) per day to slow the progression of his Alzheimer symptoms. She then adds sertraline (Zoloft), an SSRI, to treat his depression symptoms. Mr. Wallace is to start out taking 50 mg of sertraline per day, gradually working up to 150 mg per day over a 6-week period.

Clinical Reasoning Questions Level I

1. How do your observations of Mr. Wallace correlate with the changes Ms. Wallace reports?
2. What aspects of Mr. Wallace's presentation prompt you to test him for depression?
3. Why might Mr. Wallace's increased confusion in familiar settings be a concern for Ms. Wallace?

Clinical Reasoning Questions Level II

4. Why is it important to distinguish between Mr. Wallace's refusal to perform ADLs and an inability to do so?
5. Would speech therapy be an appropriate intervention for Mr. Wallace? Why or why not?
6. *Refer to the exemplar on Alzheimer disease in this module:* How would a change in Mr. Wallace's Alzheimer medication from an angiotensin-converting enzyme inhibitor like memantine to a cholinesterase inhibitor like donepezil affect the doctor's choice of SSRI for depression?

Alterations and Therapies **Cognition**

ALTERATION	DESCRIPTION/DEFINITION	MANIFESTATIONS	INTERVENTIONS AND TREATMENTS
Learning disabilities	Group of disorders that impair an individual's ability to receive and process information, causing reduced functioning in verbal, linguistic, reasoning, and academic skills	Dyslexia Dyscalculia Dysgraphia Dyspraxia	■ Special educational accommodations ■ Teach compensatory strategies that rely on an individual's other capabilities ■ Refer to learning specialists
Intellectual disability	Condition that involves significant limitations in intellectual functioning and adaptive behavior that begin before age 18	Down syndrome Fragile X syndrome Fetal alcohol syndrome Intellectual disability related to metabolic diseases (e.g., PKU)	■ Special educational accommodations ■ Refer to community resources ■ Provide a safe environment ■ Teach about dangers of alcohol consumption during pregnancy ■ Address potentially causative metabolic diseases
Dementia	Progressive, irreversible loss of global brain function	Alzheimer disease Vascular dementia Frontotemporal dementia Dementia with Lewy bodies	■ Pharmacological therapy (e.g., Aricept) ■ Refer to community resources ■ Provide a safe environment ■ Encourage healthy lifestyle choices

▶ ASSESSMENT

When it comes to cognition, many assessment methods are condition specific. For example, IQ tests are routinely administered to children with suspected intellectual disability, but not to individuals who display signs of dementia. Assessment methods appropriate for clients with cognitive impairment of any type and etiology are described below.

Nursing Assessment

A thorough physical assessment is critical for all clients, as it can help the nurse pinpoint the cause of the problem. The nurse should also assess the client's cognition by way of a mental status examination. A mental status exam involves a variety of actions meant to gauge a client's language abilities, orientation, memory, calculation ability, mood, perceptions, and thought processes, as described in the Assessment feature on pages 1588–1589. The nurse might opt to use one or more formal assessment tools, such as those listed in **Table 23–6** ●. Of these, the Mini-Mental State Exam (MMSE) is among the most common. Although the MMSE is frequently used to screen for Alzheimer disease, it is useful for all clients with cognitive disruption in that it provides a quick snapshot of their dysfunction.

With older adults, the nurse should also screen for depression. This is important because many symptoms of depression, including memory lapses, decreased motivation, and slowed speech and movement, are also symptoms of dementia. To better determine whether an individual suffers from depression, dementia, or both, the nurse can rely on specialized assessment tools like the Geriatric Depression Scale (GDS) and the Cornell Scale for Depression in Dementia. The full-length Patient Health Questionnaire (PHQ), which is another mental health screening tool, is designed to assess for several alterations in mental health, including depression and anxiety, as well as somatic symptoms and related disorders (American Psychological Association, n.d.). Specific components of the PHQ may be used to more selectively identify signs and symptoms of depression; for example, the PHQ-9 contains nine items and the PHQ-2 contains two items (American Psychological Association, n.d.). For more information on these assessments, see Table 23–6.

Nurses must always be conscious of clients' reactions when conducting a mental status exam. Many clients who are experiencing disturbed cognition are already anxious about their condition, and direct questioning may exacerbate their anxiety. Direct questioning may also increase confusion and abnormal behaviors in clients who are delusional or hallucinating. In such cases, indirect questioning may be more appropriate.

Lifespan and Cultural Considerations

Many factors can complicate assessment of clients who are experiencing cognitive alterations. For example, individuals with known intellectual disability may be unable to answer some questions simply because they lack the faculties to do so, not because they have any other underlying problem. Similarly, the nurse must consider a pediatric client's level of cognitive development before asking questions that involve calculation, judgment, or abstract thought. Even children with normal cognition will be unable to respond appropriately if they have not yet achieved the level of development necessary for these activities.

TABLE 23–6 Common Mental Status Assessments

ASSESSMENT NAME	DESCRIPTION
Confusion Assessment Method (CAM)	Interview-style exam that can be conducted in around 5 minutes Screens specifically for signs of delirium
Cornell Scale for Depression in Dementia	Nineteen-question tool that involves interviews with both clients and their caregivers Assesses for signs of depression in individuals known to have dementia
General Health Questionnaire	Written questionnaire, the most common version featuring 28 items Screens for individuals who have or are likely to develop problems with depression, anxiety, somatic symptoms, and/or social withdrawal
Geriatric Depression Scale (GDS)	Brief questionnaire (15 or 30 items) that asks clients how they've felt over the past 7 days Assesses for depression in older adults
Hamilton Rating Scale for Depression (HRSD)	Seventeen-question, 20-minute examination Assesses severity of depression in adult clients
Mini-Mental State Examination (MMSE)	Thirty-question interview-style exam that assesses a client's memory, language skills, attention level, and ability to engage in mental tasks Also known as the Folstein Mini-Mental State Examination
Short Portable Mental Status Questionnaire (SPMSQ)	Ten-item, clinician-administered questionnaire Assesses degree of organic brain deficit in elderly clients
Patient Health Questionnaire (PHQ)	Full-length 11-item tool that screens for depression and anxiety, somatic symptoms, and related disorders Abbreviated forms (PDQ-9 and PDQ-2) used to more selectively screen for depression

Sources: Data from Alexopoulous, G. S., Abrams, R. C., Young, R. C., & Shamoian, C. A. (1988). Cornell Scale for Depression in Dementia. Biological Psychiatry, 23(3), 271–284; Greenberg, S. A. (2012). The Geriatric Depression Scale (GDS). Try This: Best Practices in Nursing Care to Older Adults, 4, 1–2. Retrieved from http://consultgerirn.org/uploads/File/trythis/try_this_4.pdf; Hamilton, M. (1960). A rating scale for depression. Journal of Neurology, Neurosurgery, and Psychiatry, 23(1), 56–62. Retrieved from http://www.ncbi.nlm.nih.gov/pmc/articles/PMC495331/?page=1; Jackson, C. (2007). The General Health Questionnaire. Occupational Medicine, 57(1), 79; Pfeiffer, E. (1975). A short portable mental status questionnaire for the assessment of organic brain deficit in elderly patients. Journal of the American Geriatrics Society, 23(10), 433–441; Waszynski, C. M. (2012). The Confusion Assessment Method (CAM). Try This: Best Practices in Nursing Care to Older Adults, 13, 1–2. Retrieved from http://consultgerirn.org/uploads/File/trythis/try_this_13.pdf; American Psychological Association. (n.d.). Patient health questionnaire PHQ-9 and PHQ-2. Retrieved from http://www.apa.org/pi/about/publications/caregivers/practice-settings/assessment/tools/patient-health.aspx.

Mental Status Assessment

ASSESSMENT/METHOD	NORMAL FINDINGS	ABNORMAL FINDINGS	LIFESPAN OR DEVELOPMENTAL CONSIDERATIONS
Step 1: Prepare the Client			
Tell the client you will be performing a series of tests. Describe what equipment you'll use. Explain that the exam should be comfortable, and ask the client to inform you should difficulties arise. Provide an overview of the assessment activities and the order in which they'll occur.	■ Client pays attention and asks questions as appropriate. ■ Client may be nervous, but this shouldn't interfere in the assessment process.	■ Client displays high levels of confusion, anxiety, or agitation. ■ Client shows signs of delusions or hallucinations. ■ Client pays no attention to the information you provide. ■ Client is partially or fully uncommunicative.	■ A number of assessment tools are available, with some tailored to specific conditions and/or populations. (See Table 23–6.) ■ Direct questioning may not be appropriate for clients who are experiencing hallucinations, delusions, or extreme anxiety.
Step 2: Position and Observe the Client			
Take note of the client's general appearance, including hygiene, posture, body language, and expression. Observe the client's ability to follow your instructions.	■ Client follows directions. ■ Client's hygiene and overall appearance are acceptable. ■ Client's expressions and body language are appropriate to the situation.	■ Poor hygiene and/or inappropriate expressions and body language might be reflective of depression, schizophrenia, dementia, or another cognitive disorder.	■ In some cases, a client's appearance and hygiene may be negatively affected by socioeconomic factors rather than mental status.
Step 3: Assess the Client's Language Abilities			
Note the tone, rate, pronunciation, and volume of the client's speech throughout the course of the exam. Consider the client's vocabulary and whether he seems to understand what you are saying.	■ Client's tone, rate, pronunciation, and volume are appropriate. ■ Client speaks easily and naturally, without searching for words. ■ Client understands what you are saying and indicates this through verbal and physical reactions.	■ Problems with language could be a result of anxiety, dementia, depression, or aphasia.	■ Consider whether the client's hearing may be impaired, especially when working with older adults. ■ Don't assume all clients are native English speakers. Some clients may simply be unable to communicate well in English.
Step 4: Assess the Client's Level of Orientation			
Check whether the client knows the date and time. Ask if the client knows where she is and why. Gauge the client's level of consciousness.	■ Client knows the correct date and time, where she is, and why. ■ Client is fully conscious and alert.	■ Reduced or varying consciousness may be due to hypoglycemia, stroke, seizure, delirium, or organic brain disease.	■ Noticeable decreases in consciousness during the exam may necessitate immediate medical attention.
Step 5: Assess the Client's Memory			
See whether the client knows her name, birth date, and address. Ask the client for a brief summary of places lived and jobs held. Attempt to verify all responses.	■ Client can recall basic personal information and provide an accurate biography.	■ Inability to recall events from one's past may be suggestive of dementia, especially Alzheimer disease.	■ In Alzheimer disease, loss of short-term memory typically precedes loss of long-term memory.
Step 6: Assess the Client's Computational Ability			
Have the client answer several arithmetic problems. Start with basic facts and work toward more complicated questions.	■ Client can compute the correct values.	■ Inability to perform simple calculations may be suggestive of brain disease.	■ Clients' responses may be negatively affected by language barriers, anxiety, and/or limited experience or education in mathematics.

Mental Status Assessment (continued)

ASSESSMENT/METHOD	NORMAL FINDINGS	ABNORMAL FINDINGS	LIFESPAN OR DEVELOPMENTAL CONSIDERATIONS
Step 7: Assess the Client's Emotions and Mood			
Note the client's affect. Ask the client how he feels and whether this is typical. If not, ask about events that may have prompted the change.	■ Client's affect corresponds with the tone and content of his speech. ■ Client's emotions and mood are appropriate given past events and current situation.	■ Mismatch between the client's affect and speech may reflect neurological or psychological problems. ■ Absent, excessively subdued, or excessively animated expressions and responses may be indicative of psychological disorders.	
Step 8: Assess the Client's Perceptions and Thinking Abilities			
Note whether the client's statements are complete, rational, and pertinent, and whether she seems aware of reality. Then, ask the client to compare two different things or explain the meaning of a common phrase.	■ Client is aware of reality. ■ Client's statements are logical and complete. ■ Client correctly compares two objects and/or explains the meaning of a phrase.	■ Clients who are unaware of reality may be experiencing neurological disturbances or a mental disorder. ■ Illogical, incomplete statements suggest problems with concrete thought and may be indicative of a mental disorder. ■ Absent or strange comparisons and explanations are frequent symptoms of psychological disorders.	■ Clients' responses may be negatively affected by language barriers; unfamiliarity with the objects or phrase presented; and/or intellectual disability.
Step 9: Assess the Client's Decision-Making Ability			
Ask the client about a personal situation that requires good judgment. Determine whether the client's responses reflect consideration of viable options and logical decision making.	■ Client considers possible, probable, and appropriate options.	■ Client considers impossible, improbable, or inappropriate options. ■ Client's decision reflects absent or inadequate consideration of available options.	■ Consider whether the client's options and decisions make sense—not whether they reflect the choice you would make. ■ A number of neurological and psychological conditions, including schizophrenia and bipolar disorder, can impair decision-making ability.

The nurse must also remember that not all clients are English-language proficient, nor have they all had similar exposure to education or mainstream U.S. culture. In some cases, it may be necessary to omit assessment activities that require familiarity with mathematics, idioms, or culturally specific information. Use of an interpreter may also be required.

Physical limitations to communication are another area of concern. Some clients (especially older adults) may fail to respond to assessment questions or perhaps respond inappropriately due to hearing problems rather than impaired cognition. Other clients may be unable to speak clearly, if at all, making traditional interview-based assessment impossible.

Here, the nurse should explore use of assistive devices, such as hearing aids, pencil and paper, or erasable whiteboards. If assistive devices are not a viable solution, the nurse may need to rely on a client's caregivers for more information about the client's mental state.

Diagnostic Tests

Because cognitive disorders take a wide variety of forms, no single diagnostic test is appropriate for all clients. Furthermore, most cognitive disorders cannot be diagnosed using just one testing method. Instead, practitioners rely on multiple tests and gradually rule out unlikely conditions through differential diagnosis.

Assessment Interview **Cognition**

When conducting mental status examinations, the nurse may find it helpful to ask clients one or more of the following questions that assess:

Orientation

- What is your name?
- When and where were you born?
- What is today's date?
- What day of the week is it?
- Do you know where you are and why you're here?

Memory (Moving From Recent to Remote)

- When was your last meal? What did you eat?
- Who were the past two presidents?
- Where did you go to high school?

Cognitive Function

- Count by 5s from 0 to 100.
- Say the alphabet backward, beginning with Z.
- Please draw a five-sided star with a circle around it.

Thought Processes

- What are the similarities and differences between an airplane and a helicopter?
- What is meant by the phrase "Don't count your chickens before they're hatched?"
- Do you ever have trouble thinking clearly? If so, what sort of problems do you experience?

Judgment

- What would you do if you were on a sinking ship?
- If you won $10,000, how would you spend it?
- Do you find it easy or difficult to make decisions? Tell me about your usual decision-making process.

Perception

- Do you ever see objects or hear voices that other people do not?
- If you see objects, what are they? If you hear voices, what do they say? Do they make sense?
- Do you ever confuse or misinterpret sights, sounds, smells, tastes, or sensations of touch?

Still, some procedures are used relatively frequently in clients with suspected cognitive alterations. IQ tests, for example, are routinely administered to help distinguish between possible learning disabilities and intellectual disability. Individuals whose IQs are below 70 or 75 are considered to have limited intellectual functioning. For a diagnosis of intellectual disability, however, these clients must also display significant limitations in adaptive behaviors.

Brain imaging is another method used in the diagnosis of cognitive disorders. MRI and CT scanning can reveal structural or functional abnormalities, and they are valuable in identifying tumors, fluid buildup, and stroke damage. Despite their usefulness, the results of imaging studies are only suggestive (rather than conclusive) of dementia, schizophrenia, and a host of other conditions. In fact, the only way to confirm a diagnosis of dementia is to conduct a brain autopsy.

Genetic testing is an emerging field with many potential applications. Currently, just a handful of cognitive disorders can be diagnosed via genetic analysis—primarily, conditions like Down syndrome and fragile X syndrome, which involve large-scale chromosomal abnormalities. Genetic testing can also reveal whether an individual carries various genes associated with Alzheimer disease, but the presence of these genes only means that individuals are at increased risk, not that they will inevitably suffer from the disorder.

CASE STUDY \\ PART 2

In the winter after his visit to the gerontologist, Mr. Wallace begins experiencing increased agitation and wandering in the afternoons and evenings. One afternoon at the adult day care center, Mr. Wallace slips out the door undetected. By the time the day care providers realize he's gone, he has left the grounds and is wandering the neighborhood. The day care providers call Ms. Wallace and 911, and a search for Mr. Wallace commences. Ms. Wallace and two police officers find Mr. Wallace 2 miles from the day care center. He has no idea where he is or how he got there. He has taken a fall, and his face and hands are covered in scrapes.

The officers radio for an ambulance as Ms. Wallace attempts to talk to Mr. Wallace. He panics because he does not recognize his daughter, and he pushes her to the ground. He then throws punches at the officers when they prevent him from running away. The paramedics arrive and restrain Mr. Wallace. Once he is restrained, Ms. Wallace is able to calm him down. He is then transported to the emergency department, where you are the admitting nurse.

Mr. Wallace is calm upon his arrival at the hospital, and you are able to treat his injuries without incident. You attempt to speak with him, but he indicates he is tired and promptly falls asleep. You use this opportunity to interview Ms. Wallace. She states that aggression has become common during her father's increasingly frequent periods of confusion. Sometimes he doesn't recognize her; other times, he mistakes her for his sister. He is also increasingly unable to use basic objects—such as pencils, toothbrushes, and combs—and relies on Ms. Wallace for many basic ADLs. In addition, he occasionally experiences urinary and fecal incontinence. Ms. Wallace is shaken by the day's events and the situation in general, and she begins to cry.

When Mr. Wallace's gerontologist arrives in the ED, you inform her of these developments. She adds 20 mg of buspirone (BuSpar) three times daily (tid) to Mr. Wallace's treatment regimen to lessen his agitation and aggression. The doctor also tells Ms. Wallace that Mr. Wallace is starting to transition from moderate to severe Alzheimer disease, and she recommends that Ms. Wallace begin looking for a nursing home that specializes in the care of individuals with this condition.

Clinical Reasoning Questions Level I

1. What are the priorities for Mr. Wallace's care to decrease his risk of wandering and injury during his remaining time at home?

2. What independent interventions can you perform to address the caregiver role strain felt by Ms. Wallace?

3. What additional information or education do you anticipate Ms. Wallace will need in light of the doctor's recommendation?

Clinical Reasoning Questions Level II
Referring to the exemplar on Alzheimer disease in this module:

4. Which of Mr. Wallace's symptoms indicate he is transitioning from moderate to severe AD?

5. What steps can Ms. Wallace take at home to lessen the incidence and severity of Mr. Wallace's sundowning episodes?

6. Why is it important for Ms. Wallace to find an institutional care situation for Mr. Wallace now rather than waiting until he reaches a more severe stage of AD?

▶ INTERVENTIONS AND THERAPIES

A variety of interventions and therapies may be appropriate for individuals with cognitive impairment, yet some general principles and practices apply.

Independent

Perhaps the most important nursing intervention is to create a safe environment. Depending on the client's diagnosis, this may include limiting access to medications and other potentially harmful substances, taking steps to prevent the client from wandering, or minimizing fall and fire hazards. The nurse should attempt to orient the client to time and place, for example, by displaying a simple calendar or pictures that depict what the weather is like. Limiting environmental stimuli can also be useful, as many clients are easily overwhelmed by an abundance of sights and sounds.

Education is another critical nursing task. The nurse should help clients and their families understand their diagnosis, along with the causes and course of their disorder. If environmental modifications are needed to ensure the client's safety, the nurse should explain them to caregivers and perhaps even make a home visit.

Equally important, the nurse must attempt to preserve the client's dignity to the greatest degree possible. Because individuals with cognitive alterations may not have the same comprehension, social, or communication skills as individuals with normal cognition, they are at greater risk of being ignored, exploited, or mistreated. Nurses must remain vigilant for any signs of possible harm or neglect—physical, emotional, financial, or otherwise. Nurses should also remember the principle of dignity in their own dealings with these clients, never forgetting that they have the same innate worth and deserve as much respect as any other individual.

Collaborative

When caring for clients with cognitive alterations, collaboration often means referring clients and their families to community resources. Nurses may also collaborate with others to ensure clients are following their prescribed course of drug therapy.

Community-Based Care **Legal Protections for Clients With Cognitive Dysfunction**

Individuals with cognitive alterations and their families should be informed of several key laws that may affect them. For example:

- The Americans with Disabilities Act of 1990 ensures individuals with disabilities have equal access to government services, employment, and public accommodations.

- The Education for All Handicapped Children Act of 1975 requires that children with any type of disability have access to free public education. An amendment to this act in 1986 provides federal funding to states that offer early intervention services.

- The Developmental Disabilities and Bill of Rights Act of 2000 provides federal funding to state, public, and nonprofit agencies that provide community-based training activities and education to individuals with developmental disabilities. The law also created the U.S. Administration on Developmental Disabilities to oversee these efforts.

COMMUNITY RESOURCES Because cognitive dysfunction can have such severe, wide-ranging effects, clients frequently need support from a variety of community resources. It is the nurse's responsibility to be aware of such resources and refer clients to them as appropriate. The nurse should also be prepared to collaborate with different resource providers to ensure that all parties are working in concert to help clients and their families achieve the best quality of life possible.

Government resources are one source of assistance for many clients and their families. Depending on an individual's age and diagnosis, she may be eligible for Medicare, Medicaid, or Social Security disability benefits. Federal law also requires that all individuals with physical and/or mental disabilities receive certain legal protections, and it mandates that children with disabilities be provided access to special education at no cost to parents. At the state level, early intervention services are offered to parents of children with certain disabilities. In addition, many state and local governments have programs that provide free or low-cost transportation, assistive devices, and in-home care services to disabled individuals of all ages.

Nongovernmental advocacy groups are another resource for many clients with cognitive alterations. Organizations such as the Alzheimer's Association, American Association on Intellectual and Developmental Disabilities, and National Alliance on Mental Illness offer education and sponsor ongoing research. These organizations also provide referrals to many different types of services, including counselors, legal services, day care centers, support groups, and respite services for caregivers. The assistance these groups provide to family members is invaluable, since caring for individuals with cognitive alterations can be a physically and mentally exhausting task.

PHARMACOLOGIC THERAPY Because nurses play a key role in medication administration, education, and compliance, they must be familiar with the different classes of drugs pre-

Medications **Cognitive Alterations**

CLASSIFICATION AND DRUG EXAMPLES	MECHANISM OF ACTION	NURSING CONSIDERATIONS
Anti-Alzheimer Medications ■ Acetylcholinesterase inhibitors ■ NMDA receptor antagonists *Drug examples:* ■ donepezil (Aricept) ■ rivastigmine (Exelon) ■ galantamine (Razadyne) ■ memantine (Namenda)	Acetylcholinesterase inhibitors reduce acetylcholine breakdown, whereas NMDA receptor antagonists limit the effects of glutamate. Both drugs slow an individual's rate of cognitive decline. *May also be used for:* —Vascular dementia —Parkinson-related dementia	■ Monitor for GI distress and bleeding. ■ Monitor cardiovascular status, as some drugs may cause hypotension or bradycardia. ■ Watch for headache and/or dizziness. ■ Monitor I&O, as some medications may cause urinary retention.
Antipsychotics *Drug examples:* ■ haloperidol (Haldol)	Blocks dopamine receptors in the brain, leading to a decrease in symptoms of psychosis (including delusions and hallucinations) that may accompany dementia. *May also be used for:* —Schizophrenia and other psychotic disorders —Tourette syndrome	■ Monitor for extrapyramidal side effects, including tardive dyskinesia. ■ Monitor for neuroleptic malignant syndrome, especially in clients who have hypertension or are taking lithium. ■ Watch for rapid mood shifts and exacerbation of seizure activity.
Atypical Antipsychotics *Drug examples:* ■ risperidone (Risperdal) ■ olanzapine (Zyprexa)	Limits dopamine's ability to bind with receptors in the brain, thereby decreasing symptoms of psychosis. *May also be used for:* —Schizophrenia and other psychotic disorders —Bipolar disorder	■ Monitor for seizure activity. ■ Monitor cardiovascular status, watching for palpitations and changes in blood pressure. ■ Monitor for possible dyspnea. ■ Watch for signs of tardive dyskinesia and neuroleptic malignant syndrome. ■ Regularly assess serum glucose; closely monitor clients with diabetes for loss of glycemic control. ■ Monitor for excessive weight gain. ■ Regularly assess serum lipids and monitor for hyperlipidemia.
Anxiolytics *Drug examples:* ■ buspirone (BuSpar)	Inhibits serotonin reuptake and activates dopamine receptors in the brain, leading to a decrease in symptoms of anxiety. *May also be used for:* —Anxiety	■ Monitor for dystonia, restlessness, and involuntary movements. ■ Watch for swollen ankles, decreased output, and other signs of fluid retention. ■ Monitor for nausea, vomiting, itchiness, and jaundice. ■ Encourage clients to discuss alcohol and OTC drug use with prescriber.
Selective Serotonin Reuptake Inhibitors (SSRIs) *Drug examples:* ■ sertraline (Zoloft) ■ citalopram (Celexa) ■ fluoxetine (Prozac)	Inhibits reuptake of serotonin in the central nervous system, leading to a decrease in symptoms of depression. *May also be used for:* —Depression —Anxiety —Obsessive-compulsive disorder —Posttraumatic stress disorder —Social anxiety disorder	■ Monitor for worsening of symptoms or suicidal ideation. ■ Watch for dizziness or drowsiness. ■ Monitor older adults for adverse effects, including fluid and sodium imbalances. ■ Educate clients on importance of alcohol avoidance.
Cerebral Stimulants *Drug examples:* ■ methylphenidate (Ritalin) ■ amphetamine sulfate (Adderall)	Exerts a stimulant effect on the cerebral cortex, leading to increased alertness and decreased symptoms of ADHD.	■ Monitor for insomnia, decreased appetite, increased heart rate, and hypertension. ■ Monitor clients with diabetes for loss of glycemic control. ■ Watch for signs of abuse and/or dependence. ■ Educate clients on high potential for abuse.

scribed to individuals with cognitive alterations. Unfortunately, there are few such medications available. Most conditions that cause cognitive alterations involve irreversible changes in the brain that cannot be remedied by pharmacologic therapy. Those drugs that do exist are primarily aimed at slowing further brain changes—specifically, those associated with Alzheimer disease.

Currently, there are two main classes of drugs used in the treatment of Alzheimer disease: acetylcholinesterase inhibitors and NMDA (N-methyl-D-aspartate) receptor antagonists. Both types of medication alter the function of neurotransmitters in the brain, although they target different chemicals (acetylcholine and glutamate, respectively) and act on them in different ways. While neither class of drug can stop or reverse Alzheimer disease, they slow cognitive decline in many clients. Both acetylcholinesterase inhibitors and NMDA receptor antagonists have relatively mild side effects, including nausea, diarrhea, headaches, and tiredness (Alzheimer's Society, 2013b). For more information on these drugs and other potential pharmaceutical treatments for Alzheimer disease, please refer to the exemplar on Alzheimer Disease in this module.

Several other categories of drugs are commonly administered to clients with cognitive disorders, although they are aimed at reducing symptoms rather than slowing or reversing the disorders themselves. For example, atypical antipsychotics like risperidone (Risperdal) and olanzapine (Zyprexa) may be given to clients who are experiencing agitation in relation to delusions, dementia, or hallucinations. These drugs are generally preferred over traditional antipsychotics like haloperidol (Haldol) because of the lower risk of side effects. Similarly, various medications may be prescribed to clients who suffer from anxiety and depression in relation to their condition. Frequently used drugs include certain anxiolytics, such as buspirone (BuSpar), and SSRI antidepressants including sertraline (Zoloft), citalopram (Celexa), and fluoxetine (Prozac). It is also common for children with FAS or fragile X syndrome to receive stimulants that control symptoms of ADHD, such as methylphenidate (Ritalin) and amphetamine sulfate (Adderall).

SAFETY ALERT
Nurses must assess clients with cognitive alterations to determine their ability to self-administer medication. Many clients will require caregiver administration of pharmaceuticals. Missed doses may result in a return or exacerbation of symptoms and increase the client's risk for injury.

REVIEW The Concept of Cognition

RELATE Link the Concepts

Linking the concept of cognition with the concept of perfusion:

1. Describe how alterations in perfusion can affect a client's risk of specific types of dementia.
2. What measures might you implement when caring for a client with impaired perfusion to limit the risk of dementia?

Linking the concept of cognition with the concept of development:

3. What considerations should a nurse apply when designing developmentally appropriate activities for an 8-year-old with Down syndrome?
4. What treatment measures used for clients with ADHD might also be useful for clients with fragile X syndrome? Why?

Linking the concept of cognition with the concept of family:

5. How might a family's normal processes and interactions be affected when one member is diagnosed with a cognitive disorder?
6. What actions can nurses take to support family members of clients with cognitive alterations?

READY Go to Companion Skills Manual

REFER Go to Pearson Student Nursing Resources
nursing.pearsonhighered.com

- Additional review material

REFLECT Case Study \\ Part 3

After his wandering episode, Mr. Wallace's condition rapidly declines. His communication skills are almost completely gone; he speaks infrequently and uses only two- or three-word sentences. He no longer recognizes Ms. Wallace, cannot perform ADLs, and is indifferent to food. His tendency toward wandering and aggression has disappeared. In fact, he rarely leaves his room. For his safety and to allow for provision of the care he needs, Mr. Wallace is admitted to an extended care facility that specializes in treating clients with Alzheimer disease.

You are the nurse assigned to care for Mr. Wallace. As part of his daily assessment, you obtain his vital signs, which include temperature 99.8°F oral; pulse 92 bpm; respirations 32/min; and blood pressure 108/74 mmHg. Auscultation of Mr. Wallace's lungs reveals faint bibasilar crackles. On reviewing his chart, you note that he has experienced a 5% weight loss since the previous month. You notify the attending physician about Mr. Wallace's vital signs, breath sounds, and weight loss. The physician orders a chest x-ray and complete blood count (CBC).

Clinical Reasoning Questions Level I

1. What is the significance of Mr. Wallace's vital signs and breath sounds?
2. What effect might Mr. Wallace's weight loss have on his cognitive condition?
3. What important pieces of information might be gleaned from tracking Mr. Wallace's food intake and weight?

Clinical Reasoning Questions Level II

4. What is the priority nursing diagnosis for Mr. Wallace at this time?
5. What independent interventions can you perform to optimize Mr. Wallace's respiratory status? What positive effects might these have on other aspects of his health?
6. *Refer to the exemplar on Alzheimer disease in this module:* Would Mr. Wallace's condition improve with the addition of a cholinesterase inhibitor to his treatment regimen? Why or why not?

EXEMPLAR 23.1   Alzheimer Disease

EXEMPLAR KEY TERMS

Alzheimer disease (AD), *1594*
Amyloid plaques, *1595*
Familial AD (FAD), *1594*
Galanin, *1594*
Neurofibrillary tangles, *1595*
Sporadic AD, *1594*
Sundowning, *1597*

EXEMPLAR LEARNING OUTCOMES

After reading about this exemplar, you will be able to:

1. Describe the pathophysiology, etiology, clinical manifestations, and direct and indirect causes of Alzheimer disease.

2. Identify risk factors and prevention methods associated with Alzheimer disease.

3. Illustrate the nursing process in providing culturally sensitive care across the life span for individuals with Alzheimer disease.

4. Formulate priority nursing diagnoses appropriate for an individual with Alzheimer disease.

5. Summarize therapies used by interdisciplinary teams in the collaborative care of an individual with Alzheimer disease.

6. Plan evidence-based care for an individual with Alzheimer disease and his or her family in collaboration with other members of the healthcare team.

7. Evaluate expected outcomes for an individual with Alzheimer disease.

▶ OVERVIEW

Dementia is a progressive, irreversible loss of cognitive function that may be caused by several conditions and disorders. Of these causes, **Alzheimer disease (AD)** is by far most common, accounting for 60%–80% of all dementia cases in individuals age 65 and older (Alzheimer's Association, 2013g). Over 5 million Americans suffer from AD, and this number is predicted to reach 7 million by 2025 and 14 million by 2050. AD is the sixth leading cause of death in the United States and resulted in $203 billion in direct healthcare costs in 2013. This number does not include the estimated $216 billion in unpaid care provided by friends and family of individuals with AD (Alzheimer's Association, 2013c).

Although AD usually manifests after age 65, some individuals experience symptoms as early as their 30s. Most individuals with AD survive between 4 and 8 years after diagnosis; those who are diagnosed at younger ages may live up to two decades. Clients typically spend more time in the most severe stage of AD than in any other stage. Eventually, they die from complications of the disease. One frequently fatal complication is aspiration pneumonia caused by AD-related swallowing difficulties (Alzheimer's Association, 2012).

AD takes a harsh toll on the family and friends of those who have the disease. Because AD gradually renders individuals incapable of all activities of daily living, caregivers face an ever-increasing set of responsibilities. The physical burden of these duties, coupled with emotional strain of having a loved one with a terminal condition, leaves many caregivers exhausted. Nurses must therefore consider both client and caregiver needs when working with individuals with AD.

▶ PATHOPHYSIOLOGY AND ETIOLOGY

There are two basic types of AD: familial and sporadic. **Familial AD (FAD)** has a strong inherited component and is also called *early-onset AD* because it usually manifests before age 65. **Sporadic AD** shows no clear pattern of inheritance, although genetic factors may be involved. Because it typically develops after age 65, sporadic AD is sometimes referred to as *late-onset AD*, and it is more common than its early-onset counterpart, accounting for 90% or more of all cases (Lladó & Sánchez-Valle, 2011). FAD and sporadic AD both involve the same set of pathophysiological changes. Why these changes occur and how to prevent them remain active areas of research, although some answers have begun to emerge.

Individuals who suffer from AD show a pattern of degenerative changes related to neuronal death throughout the brain. The cells die in a characteristic order, beginning with neurons in the limbic system, including the hippocampus. Damage to this region results in emotional problems and loss of recent memory. From there, the destruction spreads up and out toward the cerebral surface. Eventually, neuronal death in the cerebral lobes produces a range of symptoms, including loss of remote memory, as outlined in **Table 23–7** ●.

As AD progresses and more neurons die, two characteristic abnormalities develop in the brains of affected individuals. The first is thick protein clots called *neurofibrillary tangles*, and the second is insoluble deposits known as *amyloid plaques*. Researchers continue to investigate whether these abnormalities are a cause or a result of AD, as described in the section on etiology.

Beyond plaques and tangles, researchers have noted several other brain irregularities associated with AD. One such finding is elevated levels of the neuropeptide **galanin**, which is released by neurons as they are injured. The exact role of galanin in AD remains unclear. Some studies suggest it exerts a protective effect, increasing acetylcholine release by the remaining neurons and slowing cognitive decline. Other studies suggest that an overabundance of galanin contributes to AD symptoms by reducing memory and learning capacity (Counts, Perez, & Mufson, 2008; Turkington & Mitchell, 2010).

Some other abnormal findings associated with AD are a bit less mysterious. For example, CT scans of the brains of AD sufferers show reduced blood flow, enlarged ventricles, and gross cerebral atrophy, all of which are consequences of widespread neuronal death (Cleveland Clinic, 2011). Decreased numbers of neurons also result in low levels of several neurotransmitters, including acetylcholine, which is thought to have a negative effect on cognition.

TABLE 23–7 Cerebral Effects of AD

REGION	SYMPTOMS OF DAMAGE
Limbic system (including hippocampus)	Loss of memory (recent before remote); fluctuating emotions; depression; difficulty learning new things
Frontal lobe	Problems with intentional movement; difficulty planning; emotional lability; loss of walking, talking, and swallowing ability
Occipital lobe	Loss of reading comprehension; hallucinations
Parietal lobe	Difficulty recognizing places, people, and objects; hallucinations; seizures; unsteady movement; expressive aphasia; agraphia; agnosia
Temporal lobe	Impaired memory; difficulty learning new things; receptive aphasia

Etiology

Researchers are not sure why most cases of AD arise, although a variety of genetic and environmental factors appear to be involved. Moreover, the exact biochemical origins of AD remain unknown, even in clients who clearly have an inherited form of the disease. Researchers have thus proposed several theories that seek to explain the disease process, including the cholinergic, amyloid, and tau hypotheses.

CHOLINERGIC HYPOTHESIS The cholinergic hypothesis emerged in the early 1980s after nearly 20 years of investigation into the role of neurotransmitters. Researchers noted that lowered levels of acetylcholine (a cholinergic neurotransmitter) appeared to produce memory deficits. Autopsies also revealed that brains of individuals with AD had markers characteristic of decreased acetylcholine function. These findings suggested that AD was caused by below-normal production of acetylcholine in the brain. Although the cholinergic hypothesis was widely accepted at the time of its proposal, it has lost much of its support in recent years, primarily because drugs that boost acetylcholine function have had only modest therapeutic results (Contestabile, 2011).

AMYLOID HYPOTHESIS Today, the amyloid and tau hypotheses are considered more likely explanations of the biochemistry of AD. The amyloid hypothesis states that AD arises when the brain cannot properly process a substance called *amyloid precursor protein (APP)*. Incorrect processing leads to the presence of short, sticky fragments of APP known as *beta-amyloid*. Eventually, the fragments clump together, forming insoluble deposits called **amyloid plaques**. These plaques damage the surrounding neurons, killing them and provoking an inflammatory response that may result in further brain damage (Khan, 2013).

TAU HYPOTHESIS The tau hypothesis focuses on a protein known as *tau*. Normally, tau holds together the microtubules responsible for intracellular transport within the axons of neurons. With AD, however, individuals have abnormal tau proteins that join and twist, forming **neurofibrillary tangles** instead of the microtubule network necessary for cellular survival.

OTHER HYPOTHESES Beyond these three theories, several other mechanisms of AD have been proposed. Some researchers theorize that AD arises due to excessive myelin breakdown. (Myelin is the fatty substance that sheathes the axons of neurons and speeds message transmission.) Other scientists propose that oxidative stress—or buildup of by-products from oxidative metabolic reactions—plays a role in AD onset (Bartzokis, 2004; Praticò, 2008). Although these hypotheses are intriguing, they, too, have yet to garner definitive experimental support.

Risk Factors

For the majority of individuals with AD, it's impossible to trace their disease to any one source. However, a variety of factors appear to increase the risk of developing AD. Age is among the most prominent risk factors. Statistics show that as individuals age, their likelihood of suffering from AD increases dramatically. In fact, whereas only 13% of all individuals age 65 and older have the disease, approximately 45% of individuals age 85 and older are affected. Still, it is important to note that AD and other forms of dementia are not a normal part of the aging process.

Family history and gender also increase the odds of AD. As mentioned, a small number of AD cases are directly traceable to certain inherited genes. However, most cases are believed to involve gene variants that increase an individual's risk but do not directly cause the disease. This theory is supported by the fact that individuals with one or more first-degree relatives with AD are at higher risk of developing the disease. Being female also appears to increase an individual's risk, although this may be partially because women tend to live longer than men.

Not all AD risk factors have to do with age or inherited characteristics. Individuals who experience moderate head injury are twice as likely to develop AD, and individuals who experience severe head trauma have roughly 4.5 times the normal risk. AD is also more likely to affect individuals who have frequent yet comparatively mild head injury, such as football players and boxers. The connection between head trauma and AD remains unclear, although it may involve increased levels of amyloid protein and/or various inflammatory processes (Alzheimer's Association, 2012). In fact, emerging research suggests that inflammation is a major contributor to many brain changes associated with AD (Heneka et al., 2013). Research has also implicated cardiovascular disease as a risk factor, most likely because it impedes the transport of oxygen and nutrients to brain tissue (Alzheimer's Association, 2012).

It is important to note that some factors previously linked to AD are no longer considered problematic. Exposure to aluminum, aspartame, dental fillings, and flu vaccine have all been ruled out as potential contributors (Alzheimer's Association, 2013d).

Prevention

There is no way to prevent AD, but certain actions appear to limit an individual's risk. One important step is weight control, as long-term studies have shown that obesity doubles an individual's risk of AD. Eating a diet that is low in cholesterol and saturated fat reduces the likelihood of obesity. It also helps prevent cardiovascular disease, high blood pressure, and high cholesterol, all of which increase the likelihood of AD. Regular exercise is another behavior that combats obesity, promotes good circulation and cardiovascular health, and therefore protects against AD.

In addition to avoiding saturated fats and cholesterol, individuals should seek to consume certain protective foods. Vitamin E, omega-3 fatty acids, and antioxidants appear to protect the brain against AD, and they also reduce cardiovascular disease risk. Vitamin C, vitamin B12, and folate may also exert a protective effect (Alzheimer's Association, 2013a).

Use of drugs and alcohol can both limit and increase a person's chances of AD, depending on the substance and amount consumed. Cigarette smoking was previously thought to protect against AD, but recent research suggests the opposite is true (Goldacre, 2010; Moreno-Gonzalez et al., 2012). Drinking moderate amounts of green tea and red wine seems to interrupt formation of amyloid plaques. However, black tea and other types of alcohol do not have this effect (Rushworth, Griffiths, Watt, & Hooper, 2013). Similarly, long-term use of nonsteroidal anti-inflammatory drugs (NSAIDs) like naproxen may help prevent AD if taken before the disease process begins, though not all evidence supports this conclusion (Breitner et al., 2011).

Finally, individuals who stay mentally and socially active have a significantly reduced risk of AD. One study found that older adults who engaged in frequent social activity cut their rate of cognitive decline by 70% (James et al., 2011). Research also suggests that greater levels of cognitive activity in early and middle adulthood can slow or perhaps even stop beta-amyloid deposition in the brain (Landau et al., 2012). Examples of beneficial activities include word puzzles, games, and reading.

▶ CLINICAL MANIFESTATIONS

The initial symptoms of AD emerge gradually and may be almost unnoticeable. The first manifestation is usually subtle memory loss that becomes increasingly apparent as time passes. Other early signs include difficulty finding words and performing familiar tasks; impaired judgment and abstract thinking; disorientation to time and place; and frequently misplacing things. These alterations go beyond the changes sometimes seen with normal aging, as described in The Concept on Cognition. Changes in mood or personality are also common. Early in the course of AD, many individuals exhibit decreased initiative, odd behavior, and signs of depression. As the disease progresses, the continued deterioration in clients' cognition is accompanied by physical decline. At some point, affected individuals lose the ability to perform everyday tasks and must rely wholly on their caregivers.

Because many manifestations of AD are similar to those of other conditions, it is important to rule out other disease processes before concluding a client has AD (Franzen & Getz,

2010). One useful tool for remembering conditions that mimic AD is the **DEMENTIA** mnemonic:

Drug or alcohol use
Emotional disorders
Metabolic or endocrine disorders
Eye and ear dysfunctions
Nutritional deficiencies
Tumors, trauma, or toxins
Infections
Atherosclerotic effects on the heart and brain

Individuals with AD progress through several stages of the disease. In general, clients with FAD move from the initial to the later stages of the disease faster than clients with sporadic AD. However, individuals' rate of progression is affected by a variety of factors, including their overall health and the type of care they receive following diagnosis.

In the past, AD was described in terms of three stages: stage 1 (early), stage 2 (moderate), and stage 3 (severe). Recently, many practitioners have abandoned this system in favor of the seven-stage model proposed by Dr. Barry Reisberg (Reisberg & Franssen, 1999). **Table 23–8** ● outlines each of Reisberg's stages and the related symptoms.

▶ COLLABORATION

To provide the best care possible, nurses must be familiar with a range of collaborative interventions related to AD. These include diagnostic tests, medications, and nonpharmacologic and alternative therapies.

Diagnostic Tests

There is no definitive way to diagnose AD other than performing a brain autopsy. Thus practitioners rely on differential diagnosis, ruling out potential causes of a client's symptoms until AD remains the most likely explanation. In doing so, they use multiple techniques, including blood tests for drugs, alcohol, toxins, and metabolic or endocrine imbalances, as well as screenings for infection, nutritional deficiencies, eye and ear problems, and emotional disorders. MRI, CT, and other brain-imaging studies may be conducted to look for tumors, impaired blood flow, fluid accumulation, or stroke damage. In some cases, genetic testing may be useful, and in all cases, clients should be asked about their family history of AD. Of course, ongoing interviews are critical, as they allow practitioners to track changes in a client's mental and physical status. For more information on many of these procedures, refer to the Diagnostic Tests section on page 1589.

Pharmacologic Therapy

There is currently no cure for AD. Thus the main goal of drug therapy is to slow a client's decline to the greatest degree possible. Several categories of medication are used for this purpose, with limited success. Some clients also receive other drugs aimed at controlling related symptoms such as anxiety, depression, and psychosis.

As discussed in the Pharmacologic Therapy section on pages 1591–1593, two classes of medication are prescribed specifically to slow AD progression: acetylcholinesterase inhibitors and

TABLE 23–8 The Seven Stages of AD

STAGE	DESCRIPTION
Stage 1: No impairment	Individuals have no symptoms of memory problems or any other cognitive impairment.
Stage 2: Normal aged forgetfulness	Individuals experience mild cognitive decline that may be related to either normal aging or AD. They may have trouble recalling names, remembering where they placed an object, or finding the correct word for something. However, these symptoms are not noticed by others.
Stage 3: Mild cognitive impairment	Memory lapses and decreased concentration become apparent to others. Affected individuals commonly experience the following: ■ Decreased job performance ■ Trouble carrying out tasks in social or work settings ■ Noticeable problems remembering names and finding words ■ Inability to recall recently learned information ■ Frequently losing important objects ■ Increasing difficulty planning or organizing events

Stage 4: Mild or early-stage AD	At this stage, symptoms of impairment are obvious and allow for a considerably accurate diagnosis of AD. Cognitively, individuals may have trouble recalling recent events, personal history, and/or the day, week, or month. They may also find it hard to perform complicated mental activities, such as counting backward by 7s.
	    Functionally, individuals begin to have difficulty performing complex ADLs, such as shopping, preparing meals for others, and managing finances. However, they may be able to continue living independently.
	    Emotionally, individuals may become moody or exhibit flat affect. They also tend to withdraw from social situations and challenging mental activity.

Stage 5: Moderate AD	In stage 5, individuals lose the ability to live independently. They may be unable to choose appropriate clothing or prepare food, and they are vulnerable to strangers who may want to take advantage of them. Individuals' cognitive skills continue to decline. Clients may forget their address or phone number. They often have trouble recalling information from recent memory, such as major news events. Remote memory also begins to fail, with individuals commonly forgetting where or when they went to school. Disorientation is common, as is an inability to perform less complex mental activities, such as counting backward by 2s.

Stage 6: Moderately severe AD	In this stage, individuals become unable to perform even basic activities of daily living. They first need help dressing and bathing, then performing other hygiene-related activities such as brushing their teeth. Eventually, they lose the ability to use the toilet independently because they forget to do things like wipe and flush. At some point, they become incontinent.
	    Cognitive declines are steep in stage 6. Individuals can remember their name but few other personal details. They recognize faces but forget the names or confuse the identity of close family members. They also lose awareness of their surroundings, along with the ability to perform simple mental tasks like counting backward by 1s. By the end of this stage, individuals are largely unable to speak.
	    Emotionally, most clients undergo major personality changes, often becoming fearful and suspicious. Delusions and compulsive, repetitive behaviors are common. Individuals may experience **sundowning**, or increased agitation, disorientation, and tendency to wander at night. Angry and/or violent outbursts may occur.

Stage 7: Severe AD	During stage 7, individuals completely lose the ability to respond to their surroundings and function without continuous assistance. They need help eating, toileting, and ambulating. Gradually, they lose the ability to speak, then walk. Next, the abilities to sit unaided, smile, and hold up the head disappear. Toward the end of stage 7, individuals become physically rigid and develop abnormal reflexes. Even the ability to swallow is impaired. Clients frequently die from aspiration pneumonia or infected pressure ulcers.

Sources: Based on Reisberg, B., & Franssen, E. H. (1999). Clinical stages of Alzheimer's disease. In M. J. deLeon (Ed.), *An Atlas of Alzheimer's Disease* (pp. 11–20). Pearl River, NY: Parthenon; Alzheimer's Association. (2013f). *Seven stages of Alzheimer's.* Retrieved from http://www.alz.org/alzheimers_disease_stages_of_alzheimers.asp; Mayo Clinic. (2012e). *Alzheimer's disease.* Retrieved from http://www.mayoclinic.com/health/alzheimers-stages/AZ00041.

NMDA receptor antagonists. Acetylcholinesterase inhibitors have been standard treatment for the past decade. They work by reducing acetylcholine breakdown. Because individuals with Alzheimer disease are gradually losing neurons that communicate by using this substance, the presence of extra acetylcholine increases communication among the remaining neurons. This appears to temporarily stabilize symptoms related to language, memory, and reasoning for an average of 6–12 months.

Commonly prescribed acetylcholinesterase inhibitors include donepezil (Aricept), rivastigmine (Exelon), and galantamine (Razadyne). Rivastigmine and galantamine are approved for early to moderate stages of AD, while donepezil is approved for all stages. Although these drugs all act similarly, not all individu-

als respond to them in the same way, if at all. In fact, about half of individuals who take these drugs see no delay in symptom progression. Acetylcholinesterase inhibitors generally produce few side effects. Those that do occur are usually mild and may include decreased appetite, nausea, diarrhea, headaches, and dizziness (Alzheimer's Association, 2013e; Alzheimer's Society, 2013b).

NMDA receptor antagonists differ from acetylcholinesterase inhibitors in several ways. Instead of boosting acetylcholine levels, they block the effects of glutamate. Large amounts of this neurotransmitter are released when neurons are damaged by AD, and it appears they contribute to further brain deterioration. Thus NMDA receptor antagonists do not remedy existing damage, but they do slow the rate at which new damage occurs. Also unlike acetylcholinesterase inhibitors, NMDA receptor antagonists generally are not prescribed until an individual is in the moderate to severe stages of AD. In some cases, they may be given in conjunction with acetylcholinesterase inhibitors.

Currently, memantine (Namenda) is the only NMDA receptor antagonist approved by the U.S. Food and Drug Administration (FDA). Its side effects are less common and usually less severe than those associated with donepezil, rivastigmine, and galantamine. They include dizziness, constipation, confusion, headache, fatigue, and increased blood pressure (Alzheimer's Association, 2013e; Alzheimer's Society, 2013b).

Researchers continue to investigate other medications that may have a protective effect against AD. Some studies suggest that several classes of antihypertensive drugs—including angiotensin-converting enzyme (ACE) inhibitors, angiotensin receptor blockers (ARBs), and calcium channel blockers—may be useful, although the results of these studies are far from conclusive (Poon, 2008; Li et al., 2010; Sink et al., 2009).

Because there are so few drugs aimed at AD, practitioners often rely on other medications to address clients' symptoms, such as atypical antipsychotics (to treat delusions or hallucinations), anxiolytics (to treat anxiety), and SSRI antidepressants (to treat depression). For more details on these drugs, please refer to the Medications feature on page 1592.

Nonpharmacologic Therapy

Clients with AD can benefit from a range of nonpharmacologic interventions. Individuals who are starting to experience language deficits may be able to slow this decline by working with a speech therapist. Similarly, physical therapy can help individuals improve their muscle tone, maintain coordination, and maintain their range of motion. Occupational therapy may be appropriate, especially for clients in the earlier stages of the disease, because it can help them maintain the ability to perform many activities of daily living. Clients and their caregivers may also benefit from referral to community organizations. Government agencies and social workers may be able to assist with such things as receiving disability benefits, obtaining assistive devices, and securing transportation. AD advocacy groups such as the Alzheimer's Association can link families with a range of other community-based resources, including adult day care centers, caregiver respite services, long-term care facilities, legal assistance, and support groups.

Complementary and Alternative Therapy

In the quest to prevent or slow AD, individuals have turned to a variety of alternative therapies. Many involve dietary supplements, including those described in **Table 23–9** ●. As shown in

TABLE 23–9 Common Supplements Taken by Clients With AD

SUPPLEMENT(S)	PROPOSED MECHANISM OF ACTION	EFFECTIVENESS	WARNINGS
Antioxidants ■ vitamin C ■ vitamin E ■ coenzyme Q10 ■ carotenoids (beta-carotene, lycopene, etc.)	Antioxidants are purported to prevent neuronal damage caused by by-products from oxidative metabolic reactions.	Several studies suggest that antioxidants may have protective value against oxidative damage. However, no clear connection between antioxidants and reduced AD risk has been established.	High doses can increase the risk of stroke and certain cancers. Some antioxidants may interact with anticoagulant, anticholesterol, and anticancer medications.
resveratrol	Resveratrol is a naturally occurring chemical in red grapes. It is also available as a dietary supplement. Proponents claim resveratrol counteracts AD by preventing or reducing neuronal changes.	Animal studies suggest resveratrol reduces beta-amyloid deposits in the brain. Researchers are currently examining the substance's effectiveness in human subjects, but clear results aren't yet available.	Supplemental forms of resveratrol are not regulated by the FDA, so their safety remains unclear.
gingko biloba	Gingko biloba is a plant extract believed to act as an antioxidant, fight inflammation, protect cell membranes, and balance neurotransmitter function. Each of these effects may help prevent or delay AD.	A major, multioffice study conducted by the National Institutes of Health found that gingko biloba offered no more benefits than a placebo in combating AD.	Supplemental forms of gingko biloba are not regulated by the FDA, so their safety remains unclear.
omega-3 fatty acids	Research suggests omega-3 fatty acids may stave off AD by promoting cardiovascular health, combating inflammation, and protecting neuronal membranes.	Current evidence is mixed. Some studies show individuals who take omega-3s perform better on memory tests, while others show that omega-3s are no more effective than a placebo.	Omega-3 supplements are not regulated to the same degree as food, so clients should be encouraged to seek dietary sources of these supplements.

Sources: Data from Alzheimer's Association. (2013b). *Alternative treatments.* Retrieved from http://www.alz.org/alzheimers_disease_alternative_treatments.asp; Alzheimer's Association. (2013e). *Medications for memory loss.* Retrieved from http://www.alz.org/alzheimers_disease_standard_prescriptions.asp; National Institute on Aging. (2012). *Preventing Alzheimer's disease: What do we know?* Retrieved from http://www.nia.nih.gov/alzheimers/publication/preventing-alzheimers-disease/search-alzheimers-prevention-strategies; Galasko, D. R., Peskind, E., Clark, C. M., Quinn, J. F., Ringman, J. M., Jicha, G. A., ... Aisen, P. (2012). Antioxidants for Alzheimer disease: A randomized clinical trial with cerebrospinal fluid biomarker measures. *Archives of Neurology, 69*(7), 836–841; National Center for Alternative and Complementary Medicine. (2012). *Antioxidants and health: An introduction.* Retrieved from http://nccam.nih.gov/health/antioxidants/introduction.htm#safety; National Center for Alternative and Complementary Medicine. (2013). *Resveratrol.* Retrieved from http://nccam.nih.gov/health/resveratrol?nav=gsa.

the table, the usefulness of these substances is unclear. Some supplements clearly offer no benefit, while others have not yet been proven to be either helpful or ineffective. Individuals who take supplements should be made aware of the latest research on their usefulness. The nurse should also inform clients that even seemingly harmless supplements may ultimately be dangerous because their safety and likelihood of producing negative reactions aren't always monitored by the FDA. Clients should always consult with their physician before starting any supplement regimen (Alzheimer's Association, 2013b).

Beyond supplements, several alternative therapeutic processes may be useful in managing AD. Music therapy can help fight depression and anxiety in clients with mild to moderate AD, as well as reduce problematic behavior in clients in the moderate to late stages of the disease. Studies have also found that music therapy temporarily boosts cognitive function (Wollen, 2010). Therapeutic touch has proven effective in reducing restlessness, agitation, and aggression (Hawranik, Johnston, & Deatrich, 2008; Woods, Beck, & Sinha, 2009), and aromatherapy appears to bring about improvements in orientation and may improve cognitive

Clinical Manifestations and Therapies **Alzheimer Disease**

ETIOLOGY	CLINICAL MANIFESTATIONS	CLINICAL THERAPIES
Mild cognitive impairment	■ Reduced concentration and memory lapses noticeable by others ■ Difficulty learning and remembering new things ■ Problems functioning in work or social settings ■ Frequently losing or misplacing important objects ■ Difficulties with planning and organization	■ Use of cuing devices such as to-do lists, calendars, written schedules, and verbal reminders ■ Deliberate establishment of and adherence to daily routines ■ Counseling regarding possible retirement or withdrawal from the more challenging aspects of one's job
Mild AD (early stages)	■ Difficulty recalling recent events, personal history, or the current date ■ Trouble performing complicated mental calculations ■ Difficulty finding words ■ Problems performing complex ADLs, including shopping, preparing meals for others, and managing finances ■ Withdrawal from social situations and challenging mental activity ■ Increased moodiness, flat affect, or signs of depression and/or anxiety	■ Continued use of cuing devices and established routines ■ Assistance with complex ADLs (may permit client to continue living independently) ■ Administration of anti-AD acetylcholinesterase inhibitors, including rivastigmine (Exelon), galantamine (Razadyne), and donepezil (Aricept) ■ Administration of SSRIs and/or anxiolytics to address mood-related symptoms ■ Occupational therapy ■ Consultation with a dietitian or nutritionist ■ Referral to community resources, support groups, and/or counseling services
Moderate AD (middle stages)	■ Inability to carry out less complex ADLs, such as preparing meals for oneself and choosing appropriate clothing ■ Loss of ability to live independently ■ Difficulty recalling one's address or phone number ■ Increased problems finding words and communicating clearly ■ Inability to recall information from recent memory ■ Increasing difficulty remembering details from remote memory ■ Disorientation to time and place ■ Increased tendency to become lost ■ Inability to perform less complex mental calculations	■ Assistance with a wider range of ADLs ■ Continuation of earlier behavioral and pharmacologic therapies ■ Addition of anti-AD NMDA receptor antagonists, including memantine (Namenda) ■ Occupational, physical, and/or speech therapy ■ Institution of safety measures to help prevent injuries, wandering, and accidents

(continued on next page)

Clinical Manifestations and Therapies **Alzheimer Disease** (continued)

ETIOLOGY	CLINICAL MANIFESTATIONS	CLINICAL THERAPIES
Severe AD (late stages)	■ Gradual inability to perform any ADLs, including bathing and toileting ■ Eventual urinary and fecal incontinence ■ Inability to identify family and caregivers ■ Extreme confusion and lack of awareness of one's surroundings ■ Gradual loss of remote memory and ability to speak ■ Inability to perform simple mental calculations ■ Dramatic personality changes, including extreme suspiciousness and fearfulness ■ Sundowning, delusions, compulsions, agitation, and violent outbursts ■ Gradual loss of ability to walk, sit unaided, and hold one's head up ■ Development of abnormal reflexes ■ Physical rigidity ■ Loss of swallowing ability	■ Assistance with all ADLs ■ Continuation of earlier behavioral and pharmacologic therapies ■ Addition of atypical antipsychotics, as appropriate ■ Round-the-clock care and/or admittance to a skilled nursing facility ■ Frequent repositioning ■ Liquid nutrition or feeding tubes as appropriate ■ Respite care for family members and other caregivers

function (Jimbo et al., 2009). Researchers continue to investigate other alternative therapies, including interactions with therapy pets, which appear to have a calming effect on clients (Fisher Center for Alzheimer's Research Foundation, 2007).

 NURSING PROCESS

The nurse's primary goal in working with individuals with AD is to provide a safe, supportive environment that meets their changing abilities and needs. The nurse must also take steps to support clients' family members as they cope with the emotional and physical demands of caring for a loved one with AD.

Assessment

Like all client assessments, a nurse's assessment of individuals with AD consists of two main elements: a health history and a complete physical examination. During the history portion of the assessment, the nurse should take care to ask about factors associated with an increased likelihood of AD, including:

- Family history of AD and other dementias
- Personal history of stroke, cardiovascular disease, brain injury, or brain infection
- Changes in behavior, cognition, memory, and/or communication ability
- Alterations in mood
- Disrupted sleep patterns
- Difficulty performing activities of daily living
- Drug and alcohol use
- Possible exposure to environmental toxins

Next, during the physical assessment, the nurse should evaluate the client's height, weight, vital signs, and overall physical condition. Throughout the exam, the nurse should remain alert for

possible signs of abuse, neglect, depression, malnutrition, elimination difficulties, and alterations in skin and tooth integrity, as AD increases the risk for all of these. The nurse should also inquire about any medications and supplements the client is taking, both to check for possible interactions and to assess whether any of these substances increase the client's risk for injury. Some blood pressure medications, for example, may contribute to an increased likelihood of dizziness, disorientation, and falls.

For clients with AD, a thorough mental status examination is critical. Nurses can choose from a variety of assessment instruments, as described in the Assessment section on pages 1586–1591. Of these tools, the Mini-Mental State Exam (MMSE) is particularly useful as it quickly evaluates multiple areas of functioning and is appropriate for clients of all ages.

Following the health history, physical exam, and mental status exam, several steps may be appropriate. For an individual suspected of having but not yet diagnosed with AD, laboratory testing and imaging studies may help rule out other health problems. When working with a client who has already been diagnosed with AD, the nurse should note any significant changes in the client's symptoms since the last assessment. The nurse must also investigate the client's living situation, including caregiver ability and availability. Lastly, caregivers themselves should be assessed for signs of emotional and/or physical distress, as they are increasingly likely to experience burnout as the client's condition deteriorates.

Diagnosis

Appropriate nursing diagnoses for clients with AD vary by stage of the disease. Some common diagnoses for individuals in the earlier stages of AD are as follows:

- *Risk for Injury*
- *Imbalanced Nutrition: Less Than Body Requirements*
- *Impaired Memory*

- *Chronic Confusion*
- *Ineffective Denial*
- *Anxiety*
- *Hopelessness*

(NANDA-I © 2012)

As the disease progresses, additional nursing diagnoses may also be applicable. Note that some of these diagnoses, especially those related to anxiety and role strain, can also be applied to caregivers and should be addressed by the nurse. Examples of nursing diagnoses that may be appropriate for inclusion in the nursing plan of care for the client with AD include the following:

- *Risk for Aspiration*
- *Self-Care Deficit (Bathing, Dressing, Feeding, and/or Toileting)*
- *Impaired Social Interaction*
- *Impaired Verbal Communication*
- *Functional Urinary Incontinence*
- *Impaired Physical Mobility*
- *Wandering*
- *Impaired Swallowing*
- *Risk for Compromised Human Dignity*
- *Risk for Caregiver Role Strain*

(NANDA-I © 2012)

Planning

The planning portion of the nursing process involves identifying desired client outcomes and formulating steps for achieving them. Appropriate goals and actions will vary depending on a client's physical and mental status and current living situation, and they may include the following:

- Client will utilize lists, calendars, and other memory aids as needed.
- Client will perform instrumental activities of daily living with caregiver assistance.
- Client will remain free from injury.
- Client will exhibit reduced anxiety, agitation, and restlessness.
- Client will take all medications as prescribed.

The nurse should also consider caregiver and family needs during the planning process. Some suggested outcomes are as follows:

- Caregiver will utilize respite care resources as necessary.
- Caregiver will learn effective strategies for coping with the stresses of supporting a loved one with AD.
- Caregiver will obtain the sleep and nutrition necessary to preserve personal health.

Implementation

Providing care to clients with AD becomes increasingly challenging as their condition worsens. Further complicating care is the fact that clients in the moderate to late stages of the disease no longer have the cognitive capacity necessary to consent to care. For this reason, clients should be encouraged to make their wishes known before they lose the ability to do so. Nurses should emphasize the importance of advance directives and planning for long-term institutional care.

Implementation involves more than simply encouraging clients to plan for their future. The nurse must also engage in interventions aimed at maintaining clients' physical and cognitive functioning to the greatest degree possible. Most interventions fall into several broad categories, as described in the following sections.

Promote Effective Coping Strategies

Clients and caregivers require assistance coping with the memory loss that accompanies early-stage AD. Cuing devices that remind clients of important people, events, and actions may be helpful. The nurse might encourage individuals with AD to keep a detailed appointment calendar, write to-do lists, post notes around their home, or have a friend or family member remind them of upcoming events. Electronic devices, such as alarm clocks and cellular phones, can be programmed to deliver reminders at designated times. Less complex assistive tools, such as date-labeled medication boxes and lists of loved ones' contact information, may also be useful. Because stress aggravates memory loss, nurses should encourage clients to engage in relaxation-promoting activities such as meditation, exercise, and therapeutic touch. Referral to a psychologist or support group can also help clients cope with emotional turmoil related to memory loss.

Similarly, a number of interventions can greatly assist clients who are coping with chronic confusion. One easy action is to label frequently used objects and locations, like keys, doors, and drawers. Another is to minimize environmental stimuli, including loud noises, flashing lights, and rapid movements. Large, easy-to-read clocks and calendars can help orient confused individuals to time and date, as can frequent verbal references to what season or day it is. A variety of interpersonal actions are also useful in limiting confusion. For instance, continuity in which nurses care for which clients can help put affected individuals at ease, as can adherence to the communication tips outlined in **Box 23–1** ●.

Prevent Injury

Because of the many physical and mental challenges associated with AD, affected individuals are at particularly high risk of harm from falls. Thus nurses should take steps to minimize clients' likelihood of falling, such as clearing the environment of tripping hazards (e.g., electrical cords and throw rugs); making sure clients have sturdy, well-fitting shoes; and applying skid-

---

Box 23–1   The Client With AD: Recommended Communication Strategies

- Begin every interaction by introducing yourself and stating the client's name.
- Face the client when speaking, and maintain an open, relaxed posture.
- Talk calmly, slowly, and at moderate to low volume.
- Use simple vocabulary and brief, straightforward sentences.
- Ask only one question at a time. Use questions that require yes or no answers, and provide sufficient response time.
- Repeat questions, explanations, and instructions as required.
- Do not question the client's interpretation of reality, as this may lead to agitation and noncompliance.
- If the client seems anxious or upset, adjust your approach in an attempt to reduce these emotions.

proof tape to stairs and slick surfaces. Use of night-lights, brighter daytime lighting, or glow-in-the-dark floor tape may be appropriate in hard-to-navigate areas. The nurse should also check whether clients' medications increase their risk of balance problems, as well as work with physical therapists to ensure clients engage in exercises that support strength and mobility.

A number of other injury-prevention measures have nothing to do with falls. For example, nurses should ensure that potential hazards, such as knives, guns, medications, matches, lighters, and toxic chemicals, are inaccessible to individuals with moderate to late-stage AD. In some cases, it may be necessary to disconnect or place childproofing devices on a client's stove or oven. Doors should have a double-lock mechanism or alarm to prevent clients from accessing forbidden areas or wandering away, and areas such as balconies and porches should be modified for increased safety. Fenced yards with locked gates are another good wandering deterrent.

Finally, for everyone's safety, individuals with AD must not be allowed to drive. Unfortunately, many clients refuse to willingly surrender their car keys, and they become angry when their family raises the topic. In such cases, the nurse can take several steps to assist family members in limiting their loved one's access to automobiles. For example, the nurse can reinforce the dangers of driving in conversations with the client or can offer the client a self-assessment tool for gauging his ability to drive. The nurse can also work with the physician to contact the local bureau of motor vehicles, asking that the client's driving ability be reevaluated or his license revoked for medical reasons.

SAFETY ALERT
Individuals with AD are at increased risk of burns. Nurses can help prevent burn injuries by teaching clients and their families about protective strategies, including locking away caustic chemicals; limiting access to lighters, matches, and cigarettes; using microwaves rather than stoves for cooking; and setting water heaters at a cooler temperature.

Promote Balance Between Rest and Activity
In the later stages of AD, restless behavior is common in the afternoons and evenings due to sundowning. Overstimulation can also lead clients to become agitated. Examples of nursing interventions that may prevent fatigue and agitation include the following:

- Watch clients for early signs of restless, tiredness, or anxiety. When clients seem agitated or fatigued, take action quickly. Consider moving them to a quiet place where they can rest and calm themselves.
- Prevent fatigue by giving clients adequate time to rest throughout the day. Consistent scheduling of daily activities also helps clients feel more familiar with their surroundings and therefore less anxious.
- Set aside "quiet time" in the late afternoon and early evening. Low lighting and calming activities like listening to music can help decrease the likelihood of sundowning.
- If clients cannot achieve relief of their anxiety or agitation, look for possible physical causes, such as electrolyte imbalance, infection, or fever; then take action as appropriate.

Promote Psychosocial Wellness
Clients with AD often suffer from heightened anxiety and restlessness, both before and after major cognitive and physical declines become apparent. Sudden life changes can exacerbate this problem and lead to further deterioration. For example, events such as hospitalization, moving, or a change in caregivers may precipitate confusion and declines in cognitive and physical health. To help minimize the risk of such declines, all foreseeable life transitions should be well planned and carried out in a way that minimizes client anxiety.

Hopelessness and depression are also common among clients with AD and their caregivers, and these emotions may wax and wane as the disease progresses. A variety of nursing interventions can help manage feelings of hopelessness and thereby increase clients' and families' quality of life. For instance, the nurse should provide realistic information about the disease at a level appropriate to the client's and/or family's level of understanding. All parties should feel free to express their feelings in a judgment-free environment that promotes mutual respect. The nurse should also foster open discussion and further questions, as clear communication based in fact (rather than myth) is central to good decision making. Similarly, clients should be encouraged to make as many of their own health decisions as possible, both to increase their autonomy and reduce the burden on family members. Lastly, the nurse should encourage clients and families to seek counseling and/or spiritual guidance if they so desire.

Facilitate Stress Management for Caregivers
Caregivers of individuals with AD experience a wide range of stressors that can lead to feelings of fatigue and isolation. Often, a client's spouse is the primary caregiver, and this individual is also struggling with fear of the future and eventual loss of a mate. Other times, the burden of care falls on the client's children, who may already be overwhelmed by families of their own. In either case, caregivers may turn to the nurse for support. When this happens, the nurse should refer them

Community-Based Care Resources for Caregivers of Individuals With AD

There are a range of community resources available to individuals who are caring for loved ones with AD, including:

- In-home care services
- Adult day centers and other respite care providers
- Residential facilities
- Local support group meetings
- Caregiver training workshops

Stay Current: For more information on these and other resources, nurses should refer clients and their families to organizations such as the local affiliate of the Alzheimer's Association. Additional details are also available via the Alzheimer's Association's Web site at **http://www.alz.org/care/overview.asp**.

Focus on Diversity and Culture Attitudes Toward Caring for Aging Family Members

Members of different cultural groups may have differing views of their role in caring for loved ones with AD. For example, individuals from traditional Hispanic or Asian cultures may feel the duty to provide their loved ones with all necessary care until the end of life. Nurses must be sensitive to cultural preferences and keep them in mind when planning and making recommendations, especially referrals to community resources.

to various community resources as appropriate. The nurse should also validate the caregivers' emotions, telling them that what they're feeling is normal and not a sign of weakness or being a bad person. This is especially important when caregivers express feelings of guilt for wanting a "break" from their caregiving duties. In such situations, referrals to respite care agencies can be useful in promoting and preserving caregivers' mental, physical, and emotional health.

Evaluation

Ongoing evaluation is a critical element of the nursing process for individuals with AD, as their condition is continually worsening. Nurses must assess these clients on a frequent basis, regularly adjusting diagnoses, goals, and interventions to achieve optimal outcomes. Although there is no cure for AD, nurses can and should help clients live out their days with as much autonomy, comfort, and dignity as possible.

Evaluation of the nursing care plan depends on client-specific nursing diagnoses and goals. Some examples of potential achieved outcomes include the following:

- The client remains free from injury.
- The client's nutritional intake meets his nutritional and metabolic needs.
- The client maintains and follows her medication regimen.
- The client effectively uses memory aids, such as lists and calendars.
- The caregiver utilizes available community resources, such as respite care services.

NURSING CARE PLAN A Client With Alzheimer Disease

Sixty-one-year-old Loretta Gordon arrives at her general practitioner's office complaining of memory problems and depression that began about a month ago. Ms. Gordon is currently taking sertraline for her depression. She is afraid her medication is causing her current complaints, so she came to see the doctor.

ASSESSMENT	DIAGNOSES	PLANNING
Gretchen Burchett, RN, obtains a client history and conducts a physical examination of Ms. Gordon. Nurse Burchett notes that Ms. Gordon retired 2 years ago after 35 years as an elementary school music teacher. Shortly after retirement, Ms. Gordon began to experience depression and was prescribed sertraline; until recently, her symptoms were well controlled by the medication. Ms. Gordon receives a "comfortable pension" from the school and lives alone in a small house. She has never been married and has no children, but she maintains a close relationship with her brother, who is 15 years younger. Her primary social outlet is a group of women friends she's known since college, though she says she hasn't been attending their weekly get-togethers because she "has a hard time following the conversation." Ms. Gordon is an avid piano player but admits to recent frustration over her inability to follow sheet music. Ms. Gordon is clean and well groomed, and her weight is healthy for someone her age and height. She struggles to find the right words when answering Nurse Burchett's questions. Nurse Burchett also notes a family history of AD and that Ms. Gordon sustained a serious head injury in a car accident 8 years ago. Ms. Gordon's vital signs include temperature 99.2°F oral; pulse 67 bpm; respirations 18/min; and blood pressure 116/72 mmHg. Suspecting mild or early-stage AD, Nurse Burchett administers the MMSE. Ms. Gordon scores 23, indicating mild cognitive impairment. The physician orders blood tests to check for metabolic and endocrine problems and an MRI to assess for impaired blood flow and fluid accumulation in the brain. All of Ms. Gordon's test results are negative, and a diagnosis of probable mild or early-stage FAD is made. The physician prescribes donepezil, 5 mg orally, increasing to 10 mg after 6 weeks. He also increases her sertraline from 150 mg orally to 175 mg and instructs her to return in 6 months.	- *Risk for Injury* related to impaired cognitive function - *Impaired Memory* related to diminished neurological function - *Chronic Confusion* related to deterioration of cognitive function - *Impaired Verbal Communication* related to intellectual changes - *Anxiety* related to awareness of physiological and cognitive changes (NANDA-I © 2012)	Goals for Ms. Gordon's care include: - The client will remain free from injury. - The client will verbalize an understanding of her disease and its stages. - The client will utilize lists, calendars, and other memory aids as needed. - The client will participate in speech and language therapy. - The client will exhibit decreased signs and symptoms of anxiety and depression. - The client will take all medications as prescribed. - The client will remain in the home environment as long as possible.

(continued on next page)

NURSING CARE PLAN (continued)

IMPLEMENTATION

- Teach about AD, and provide informational materials and recommendations for community resources.
- Collaborate with the primary care provider about potential home visits to regularly assess the client's functional capabilities and identify any safety concerns.
- Emphasize the use of calendars and electronic devices to record appointments and alert to important activities, such as medication administration.
- Instruct about the prescribed medications, potential side effects, and dietary changes that can minimize negative side effects.

- Refer to a speech therapist.
- Stress the importance of relaxation techniques and therapies—such as music therapy—to decrease anxiety and promote relaxation.
- Promote activities that encourage social, emotional, and cognitive well-being.
- Encourage collaborating with family members to plan for care during more advanced stages of AD.

EVALUATION

Nurse Burchett refers Ms. Gordon to a speech therapist, and therapy sessions are scheduled for twice weekly. During therapy, Ms. Gordon engages in a series of exercises designed to slow her decline in communication skills. She has also mastered the electronic calendar and alarm on her cell phone, programming reminders for even basic daily functions. She enjoys an hour of music in the evenings, although she listens to recordings rather than playing her piano. After 6 months of pharmacologic treatment and speech therapy, Ms. Gordon's cognitive condition is stable and she once again scores 23 on her MMSE.

Ms. Gordon continues to display symptoms of depression, primarily stemming from the realization that there is no cure for her condition. She attends a local AD support group, which helps her verbalize and cope with her anxiety. With the help of her brother, who has invited Ms. Gordon to move into his home, she has created a long-term care plan.

CRITICAL THINKING

1. Ms. Gordon is fortunate that her brother is willing to be involved in her care. How would you adapt the care plan if Ms. Gordon had no family or her family was unwilling to be involved?
2. Ms. Gordon finds comfort in a support group for AD clients. Identify resources in your area that provide these kinds of services to AD clients and caregivers.
3. Develop a care plan for the nursing diagnoses of Self-Care Deficit related to cognitive decline and physical limitations.

◤ REVIEW Alzheimer Disease

RELATE Link the Concepts and Exemplars

Linking the exemplar of Alzheimer disease with the concept of tissue integrity:

1. Why might clients with AD be at a heightened risk of impaired tissue integrity? What types of impairments would you most expect to see, and during which stages of AD would they most likely occur?
2. When caring for the client with AD, what nursing interventions are appropriate when seeking to limit the risk of impaired tissue integrity?

Linking the exemplar of Alzheimer disease with the concept of spirituality:

3. How might a client's spirituality be affected by a diagnosis of AD? How might a client's diagnosis of AD affect her family and loved ones?
4. What nursing interventions might be appropriate for clients and families who are experiencing spiritual distress related to the cognitive and physical alterations associated with AD?

Linking the exemplar of Alzheimer disease with the concept of legal issues:

5. Why are issues of informed consent often problematic for individuals with AD?

6. What actions might nurses recommend to prevent such issues from arising?

READY Go to Companion Skills Manual

REFER Go to Pearson Student Nursing Resources
nursing.pearsonhighered.com

- Additional review material

REFLECT Case Study

Robert Moser, a 75-year-old Caucasian male, is brought to the emergency department by State Trooper Kelly just before midnight. Law enforcement had received reports of a car driving erratically along the highway and pulled Mr. Moser over. Trooper Kelly tells you that when he stopped Mr. Moser, Mr. Moser was able to get out his wallet but unable to tell Trooper Kelly his name. Mr. Moser stated he was trying to find the hospital where his wife is located, but he could not name the hospital or say where it is. Trooper Kelly pulled up the list of contacts in Mr. Moser's cell phone. When Mr. Moser confirmed one of the contacts was his son, Trooper Kelly contacted the son and asked him to meet them at the hospital. The son, who informs Trooper Kelly that Mr. Moser recently was diagnosed with Alzheimer disease, lives out of town and will arrive in about an hour. Mr. Moser is polite and compliant, but he keeps asking "Is this a hospital?" over and over again. As you begin your assessment, Mr. Moser has difficulty finding the words he needs to respond.

1. What additional assessment information do you need?

2. Identify three other conditions that may produce symptoms that mimic dementia.

3. How will you go about the assessment since Mr. Moser is unable to participate fully?

4. What are Mr. Moser's priorities for care at this time?

5. What stage of Alzheimer disease is Mr. Moser likely experiencing?

EXEMPLAR 23.2 **Confusion**

EXEMPLAR KEY TERMS

Ageism, *1607*
Confusion, *1605*
Confusion Assessment Method (CAM), *1607*
Delirium, *1605*
Sundowning, *1606*

EXEMPLAR LEARNING OUTCOMES

After reading about this exemplar, you will be able to:

1. Describe the pathophysiology, etiology, clinical manifestations, and direct and indirect causes of confusion.

2. Identify risk factors and prevention methods associated with confusion.

3. Illustrate the nursing process in providing culturally sensitive care across the life span for individuals with confusion.

4. Formulate priority nursing diagnoses appropriate for an individual with confusion.

5. Summarize therapies used by interdisciplinary teams in the collaborative care of an individual with confusion.

6. Plan evidence-based care for an individual with confusion and his or her family in collaboration with other members of the healthcare team.

7. Evaluate expected outcomes for an individual with confusion.

▶ OVERVIEW

Confusion is a condition in which individuals have increased difficulty thinking clearly, making judgments, or focusing attention. In most cases, confusion is a symptom of another health alteration, rather than a stand-alone diagnosis. Common causes of confusion include hypoxia, inadequate perfusion, medications, and a number of diseases. Depending on causative agent, the onset of confusion may be sudden or gradual. Confusion may be a one-time occurrence, a recurrent alteration, or an ever-present state of mind.

Confusion is closely related to **delirium**, which is an acute cognitive disorder that affects an individual's functional independence. The primary distinction is that confusion often presents more slowly and subtly and may be chronic, whereas delirium is severe and sudden. In the past, health professionals frequently used the terms *acute confusion* and *delirium* interchangeably. Similarly, the term *chronic confusion* was often used to describe what is now commonly referred to as *dementia* (Steis & Fick, 2012). Regardless of terminology, nurses should understand the differences between acute confusion (delirium) and chronic confusion (dementia), as timely assessment and diagnosis may allow for better control and perhaps even reversal of a client's cognitive impairment. (For additional information on distinguishing between delirium and dementia, refer to Table 23–5 on page 1585.)

▶ PATHOPHYSIOLOGY AND ETIOLOGY

Usually, individuals with acute confusion are aware of their symptoms and will seek help. In many cases, once the underlying cause is identified and treated, the confusion will resolve. Even so, clients who experience confusion should be closely monitored for signs of delirium. When left unchecked, delirium can contribute to increased mortality, hospital costs, and long-term cognitive and functional impairment (Tullmann, Fletcher, & Foreman, 2012). The pathophysiology of both confusion and delirium varies, depending on the causative condition.

Etiology

Delirium affects individuals of all ages, although it is commonly (and mistakenly) conceptualized as something seen only in older adults. A wide variety of conditions can result in delirium, including infections, metabolic imbalances, trauma, nutritional deficiencies, central nervous system disease, hypoxia, hypothermia, hyperthermia, circulatory problems, low blood glucose, toxin exposure, sleep deprivation, and drug and alcohol use and withdrawal (Gower, Gatewood, & Kang, 2012).

Delirium occurs in 10%–24% of the general hospital population (Whitlock, Vannucci, & Avidan, 2011), 15%–53% of postsurgical clients, and 70%–87% of clients in the intensive care unit. Among hospitalized individuals over age 65, approximately 14%–56% experience delirium, as do 22%–89% of older clients with documented dementia (Fong, Tulebaev, & Inouye, 2009; Flanagan & Fick, 2010). Statistics range widely for several reasons, including the fact that delirium is undetected or misdiagnosed by medical professionals in up to two thirds of all cases (Trzepacz & Meagher, 2008).

Risk Factors and Prevention

Although anyone can develop delirium, certain traits increase the likelihood of this condition. Age is a major risk factor. Older adults (men in particular) are at higher risk due to normal age-related cognitive decline. Age-related vision and hearing loss can contribute to delirium by impairing individuals' ability to accurately and effectively interpret their surroundings. Older clients are also more likely to experience many of the underlying physical causes of delirium, such as central nervous system and circulatory disease. Among younger individuals, children are more prone to delirium than are adolescents and younger adults. Again, physiology is a primary factor, as children's bodies are less equipped to cope with insults such as fever, infection, and toxin exposure.

Other characteristics linked to elevated delirium risk include dementia, diabetes, undertreated pain, onset of a new illness, or exacerbation of a chronic illness. Hospitalization is a prominent risk factor, in part due to environmental factors such as unfamiliar surroundings and increased potential for sleep deprivation, stress, and sensory overload. Individuals with depression and other emotional disorders are at increased susceptibility as well, especially when faced with the added strain of illness, loss, or a change in environment. In addition to infection and inadequate nutrition, alcohol and drug use are also risk factors. This includes use of prescriptions, most notably analgesics, hypnotics/sedatives, antihistamines, anxiolytics, antidepressants, anti-Parkinson drugs, anticonvulsants, antispasmodics, and asthma medications (Mayo Clinic, 2012b).

Methods of preventing delirium vary depending on an individual's risk factors. For example, preventive measures vary greatly when caring for a pediatric postsurgical client versus an adult client whose medications produce anxiolytic and analgesic effects. Still, nearly all at-risk clients can benefit from routine screenings for delirium. Certain standardized protocols may also be helpful. Many hospitals, for example, require that older clients receive a geriatric consultation, are closely monitored for dehydration and nutritional imbalances, and are provided with environmental modifications that foster orientation, facilitate sleep, and maximize mobility (Tullman et al., 2012).

▶ CLINICAL MANIFESTATIONS

Typical manifestations of confusion include reduced awareness, impaired thinking skills, and/or changes in behavior. See **Table 23–10** ● for an overview of common symptoms from each of these categories. The intensity of manifestations varies, with some clients having only subtle symptoms and others experiencing acute loss of most or all cognitive function.

Delirium is characterized by fluctuation of symptoms. An individual may be largely unresponsive at one point in the day but hypervigilant just a few hours later, with a period of normal behavior in between. Likewise, the individual's psychomotor activity may be hyperactive, hypoactive, or a mixture of both at various times throughout the day. Confusion that intensifies in the evening or at bedtime is referred to as **sundowning**. Sundowning is not a disorder in and of itself; rather, it is a feature of dementia that affects some individuals.

Lifespan and Cultural Considerations

As described earlier, children and older adults are at greater risk for delirium; however, a number of factors can complicate diagnosis among these clients. In children, delirium is often mistaken as uncooperative or willful behavior rather than a medical emergency. Similarly, in older clients, delirium may be confused with normal forgetfulness or dementia. Careful, ongoing assessment is key to recognizing the abrupt onset and fluctuation of symptoms characteristic of delirium.

Culture may also affect the diagnosis process. When working with clients from Hispanic, Asian, African American, and other cultural groups, the nurse must remember that these cultures may promote different conceptions of time, place, and person in comparison to Anglo-American culture. Thus what the nurse might perceive as a lack of orientation to time might be perfectly normal, acceptable behavior to a client and his family. Cultural beliefs may also impact the interpretation of manifestations such as hallucinations and incoherent speech. Clients

TABLE 23–10 Manifestations of Confusion

CATEGORY	COMMON SIGNS AND SYMPTOMS
Reduced awareness	■ Difficulty shifting attention from one topic to another ■ Limited or absent span of attention ■ High distractibility ■ Difficulty keeping track of what has been said ■ Inability to answer questions or engage in conversation ■ Little activity or response to the environment
Impaired thinking skills	■ Impaired memory (especially recent memory) ■ Disorganized thought ■ Disorientation to place, time, date, and/or person ■ Rambling, incoherent, illogical, or absent speech ■ Poor word-finding ability ■ Difficulty reading, writing, or understanding speech ■ Hallucinations and/or illusions
Changes in behavior	■ Agitation, irritability, restlessness, or combative behavior ■ Altered sleep patterns ■ Mood swings and extreme emotions ■ Fear, anxiety, and/or depression ■ Withdrawal

Sources: Based on Mayo Clinic. (2012e). *Alzheimer's disease.* Retrieved from http://www.mayoclinic.com/health/alzheimers-stages/AZ00041; Tullman, D. F., Fletcher, K., & Foreman, M. D. (2011). Delirium: Prevention, early recognition, and treatment. In M. Boltz, E. Capezuti, T. T. Fulmer, D. Zwicker, & A. O'Meara (Eds.), *Evidence-based geriatric nursing protocols for best practice* (4th ed.). New York, NY: Springer; Osborn, K. S., Wraa, C. E., Watson, A., & Holleran, R. S. (2013). *Medical-surgical nursing: Preparation for practice* (2nd ed.). Upper Saddle River, NJ: Pearson.

and their families may view these experiences as spiritual or religious events rather than signs of illness. In such cases, the nurse must be careful not to discount or disparage the client's cultural preferences and beliefs. Promotion of trust and acceptance is necessary for building an effective nurse–client relationship.

▶ COLLABORATION

Nurses must be familiar with a range of collaborative interventions related to confusion. These include diagnostic tests, surgeries, medications, and nonpharmacologic therapies. Psychosocial considerations are directed toward both clients and their family members.

Focus on Diversity and Culture
Cultural Literacy and Cognitive Assessment

When assessing an individual's cognitive skills and orientation, remember that not all clients will have the same level of general knowledge or cultural literacy. While a question like "Who is the president?" may seem simple, the answer may not be obvious to a newly immigrated U.S. resident or an individual who is not exposed to mainstream news and culture. For these clients, incorrect responses to questions like these are not necessarily indicative of cognitive impairment.

Diagnostic Tests

Medical professionals use any number of diagnostic procedures to determine the underlying source of a client's delirium. The first steps usually include conducting a physical exam and obtaining a detailed medical history. Cognitive testing, such as the Confusion Assessment Method (CAM) test (described later in this exemplar), can also be useful for determining whether a client is suffering from reversible confusion or another form of impairment.

Based on assessment data, the primary care provider will choose appropriate diagnostic procedures. Examples of tests that may be appropriate for identifying underlying causes of confusion include the following:

- Detailed neurological examination
- Drug and alcohol screening
- Laboratory testing of blood and urine for signs of metabolic, nutritional, and other imbalances
- Tests for the presence of infection
- Screening for depression and other psychological conditions

Surgery

In some cases, confusion may be reversible through surgical treatment of the underlying cause. For instance, surgical removal of a brain tumor or insertion of a shunt to relieve hydrocephalus may lead to alleviation of delirium associated with these conditions. However, there is no single surgical procedure that can effectively resolve delirium.

Pharmacologic Therapy

No one drug or class of drugs is appropriate for all clients with delirium, but some medications may effectively treat the causative condition. For example, antipsychotics may be appropriate for clients with delirium related to an underlying psychotic disorder, and SSRIs and other antidepressants can help minimize confusion in some individuals with mood disorders. In other cases, discontinuation of medications may be the best course of action, especially for individuals who are experiencing drug-related delirium.

Nonpharmacologic Therapy

Numerous nonpharmacologic interventions may benefit individuals with confusion, depending on their pathology. These interventions fall into three categories: physical, environmental, and cognitive.

- *Physical interventions* target anatomical or biological factors that may be contributing to delirium. Common physical interventions that promote enhanced cognition include oxygen administration, IV delivery of fluids and/or electrolytes, and provision of appropriate nutrition.
- *Environmental interventions* involve enhancing clients' level of comfort within their surroundings, as this helps minimize the likelihood of confusion. Often, these interventions focus on preventing under- or overstimulation, maintaining safety, and promoting consistency. (See the Nursing Process section).

- *Cognitive interventions* involve orienting clients to person, place, and time, as well as providing reassurance that they are safe and that their delirium will be resolved. (Again, see the Nursing Process section below.)

SAFETY ALERT

In some situations, use of restraints may be necessary to protect clients and staff members from physical harm. Due to legal and ethical concerns, restraints should be employed only when no other appropriate therapeutic interventions are effective. For more information on the use of restraints, see the module on Safety.

NURSING PROCESS

One of the nurse's primary duties in caring for a client with acute confusion is to promote resolution of whatever condition is causing the client's cognitive impairment. The nurse must also take steps to keep the client safe, promote better cognitive functioning, and minimize the likelihood of further episodes of confusion.

Assessment

Nursing assessment for the client with delirium typically involves three main elements: a health history, a physical examination, and a mental status examination. The history is critical to identifying potential causes of the client's confusion and highlighting areas that require further assessment. For the client with delirium, basic components of the health history include the following:

- Age
- History of other disease processes
- Recent history of infection and/or fever
- Vision and/or hearing impairments
- Alcohol and drug use (including medications)
- Possible toxin exposure (e.g., in the workplace)
- Dietary patterns
- Untreated or undertreated pain
- History of depression or other mood disorders
- Recent life changes that may be contributing to cognitive and/or emotional upset

Next, during the physical assessment, the nurse should evaluate the client's height, weight, vital signs, and overall condition. For any areas of concern identified during the health history, a focused assessment is indicated. For example, for a client who reports that he is hard of hearing, the nurse should attempt to determine the degree of impairment and explore the possibility that this impairment may be contributing to the client's confusion.

To differentiate between delirium and dementia, the **Confusion Assessment Method (CAM)** may be used. This instrument, which consists of two parts, accounts and controls for **ageism**, which is a form of stereotyping that may lead healthcare providers to recognize lethargy and cognitive impairment as inevitable consequences of aging. The first portion of the CAM screens for overall cognitive impairment, while the second screens specifically for traits associated with reversible confusion. Although the CAM is highly effective in identifying delirium, it does not

Clinical Manifestations and Therapies **Confusion**

ETIOLOGY	CLINICAL MANIFESTATIONS	CLINICAL THERAPIES
Variable etiologies; may include the following: ■ Infection ■ Metabolic imbalance ■ Trauma ■ Nutritional deficiency ■ Central nervous system disease ■ Hypoxia ■ Hypothermia ■ Hyperthermia ■ Acute circulatory alteration ■ Hypoglycemia (decreased serum glucose) ■ Toxin exposure ■ Sleep deprivation ■ Drug and alcohol use or withdrawal	■ Reduced awareness, as evidenced by: • Limited span of attention • Difficulty focusing or logically shifting from one topic to another • Inability to answer questions or engage in conversation • Limited response to the environment ■ Impaired thinking skills, as evidenced by: • Impaired memory • Disorganized thought • Disorientation to place, time, date, and/or person • Impaired speaking, reading, and comprehension ability ■ Behavioral changes, such as: • Hyperactivity, hypoactivity, or a combination thereof • Hallucinations • Agitation and/or restlessness • Fear, anxiety, and/or depression • Altered sleep patterns • Mood swings • Withdrawal ■ Acute onset and fluctuation of symptoms ■ Appearance of symptoms at specific times of day (e.g., sundowning)	■ Physical interventions aimed at correcting biological causes of delirium: • Supplemental oxygen • IV fluids and/or electrolytes • Supplemental nutrition ■ Environmental interventions: • Preventing under- or over-stimulation • Instituting safety measures • Promoting consistency ■ Cognitive interventions: • Orienting client toward place, time, date, and/or person • Providing reassurance that delirium is temporary ■ Pharmacologic therapies aimed at the underlying cause of delirium (as appropriate) ■ Surgical treatment of the underlying cause of delirium (as appropriate)

measure the severity of a client's delirium, so the nurse must rely on other instruments for this purpose (Waszynski, 2012).

Stay Current: *A current version of the CAM can be accessed online at* **http://consultgerirn.org/uploads/File/trythis/try_this_13.pdf.**

In addition to screening for dementia, the nurse may also choose to screen the client for depression, because this condition is often linked to confusion in older adults. For discussion of testing instruments designed for this purpose, refer to the Nursing Assessment section in the Concept of Cognition.

Because delirium has a fluctuating course, ongoing assessment is important. The nurse should reassess clients with delirium at least once every 8 hours. Some clients, such as those with delirium related to poor oxygenation, may require more frequent assessment.

Diagnosis

Appropriate nursing diagnoses for clients with delirium vary, depending on the cause and severity of their condition. Still, some diagnoses are likely to apply to many, if not most, clients with acute confusion. These include:

- *Risk for Injury*
- *Self-Care Deficit (Bathing, Dressing, Feeding, and/or Toileting)*
- *Disturbed Sleep Pattern*
- *Acute Confusion*
- *Impaired Memory*
- *Impaired Verbal Communication*
- *Impaired Social Interaction*
- *Risk for Compromised Human Dignity*

(NANDA-I © 2012)

Planning

The planning portion of the nursing process involves identifying desired outcomes and choosing evidence-based interventions that facilitate their achievement. Again, goals and interventions will vary depending on the cause and severity of a client's delirium. Appropriate outcomes may include the following:

- Client will remain free from injury.
- Client will be oriented to time, place, date, and person.
- Client will return to baseline cognitive status (i.e., status prior to onset of confusion).
- Client will demonstrate the ability to communicate in a clear and logical manner.
- Client will obtain adequate sleep and rest.
- Client will exhibit reduced anxiety, agitation, and restlessness.
- Client will be able to perform activities of daily living.

Implementation

Typically, nursing interventions for the client with confusion revolve around provision of a safe, therapeutic environment that prevents further cognitive impairment and promotes resolution of the condition causing the client's delirium. The following measures may be useful for most clients:

- Maintaining appropriate levels of noise and lighting in an attempt to prevent under- or overstimulation
- Preventing access to potential hazards (e.g., knives, guns, medications, lighters, and chemicals)
- Locking doors and taking other precautions to prevent wandering
- Promoting consistency by assigning the same caregivers (if possible) and scheduling activities at the same time each day
- Providing an environment that allows for adequate sleep
- Ensuring access to assistive devices, including glasses and hearing aids
- Providing adequate pain management
- Keeping familiar items in the client's environment without allowing the environment to become disorganized or cluttered
- Using calendars, clocks, and signs to help orient the client to time, date, and place
- Encouraging loved ones to visit the client (unless this contributes to hyperactivity)

The nurse can also employ various communication strategies to limit confusion. The nurse should always wear a name tag and introduce himself during client interactions. The nurse should then verbally orient the client to date, time, and place. When talking with the client, the nurse should speak clearly and allow time for response. All explanations of treatments or procedures should be brief and as easy to understand as possible. The nurse should reinforce reality by helping clients interpret confusing or unfamiliar stimuli. Any misconceptions of events or situations should be gently corrected but not directly disputed as this can cause agitation and increased confusion. The nurse should also reassure clients that their delirium is temporary and that they aren't "going crazy."

> **SAFETY ALERT**
> Never directly dispute a client who is delusional or misinterpreting reality. Doing so can cause the client to become agitated, leading to further confusion and the threat of physical aggression.

Teaching is especially important when clients have an ongoing health issue that predisposes them to delirium. For example, if clients are taking medications that increase their risk of confusion, they and their loved ones should be informed of common symptoms of delirium and what to do when these symptoms arise. Similarly, clients with diabetes should be taught about signs of confusion related to abnormal blood glucose. In addition, family members and caregivers should be assisted with developing an action plan for assisting the client during hyperglycemic or hypoglycemic episodes.

Evaluation

Ongoing evaluation is critical for all clients with confusion, as it allows nurses to monitor their condition and adjust the nursing plan of care as needed. Some examples of potential achieved outcomes include the following:

- Client sustains no injuries.
- Client is oriented to time, place, date, and person.
- Client demonstrates an absence of confusion.
- Client communicates clearly and transitions logically between topics.
- Client is able to perform activities of daily living.

◢ REVIEW **Confusion**

RELATE Link the Concepts and Exemplars

Linking the exemplar of confusion with the concept of infection:

1. How might confusion increase the client's risk for infection?
2. Why are clients with infection at a heightened risk for delirium? What types of infections do you think would most increase a client's likelihood of delirium?

Linking the exemplar of confusion with the concept of stress and coping:

3. Why are clients more likely to experience confusion during periods of increased stress? What sorts of events are likely to be most stressful and thus result in confusion?
4. For the confused client, what nursing interventions could be implemented to help reduce stress and promote effective coping?

Linking the exemplar of confusion with the concept of safety:

5. How might caring for clients with confusion put a nurse's safety in jeopardy?
6. What interventions could a nurse implement to protect her own safety when caring for a client with delirium? What legal or ethical issues are associated with these measures?

READY Go to Companion Skills Manual

REFER Go to Pearson Student Nursing Resources
nursing.pearsonhighered.com

- Additional review material

REFLECT Case Study

Clifford Allen is a 64-year-old male who has been married to his wife, Pam, for 40 years. Their only child, 24-year-old Gary, has Down syndrome and lives with them. Mr. Allen is a middle manager for a small manufacturing company where he has worked for the last 20 years.

Overall, Mr. Allen is in good health, although he has recently been undergoing conservative treatment for benign prostate hypertrophy. He has a history of depression, including a brief episode during college for which he did not seek treatment. Mr. Allen had another episode shortly after his son was born, and at the encouragement of his wife, he sought treatment, which consisted of counseling and antidepressant medications. He quit taking the medications after 6 months and decided he would just learn to deal with depression on his own. Although he has had several mild episodes of depression since that time,

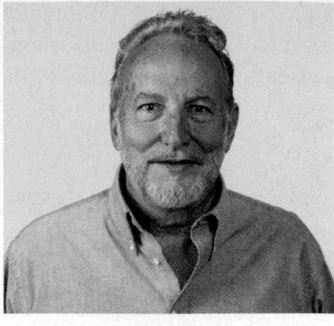 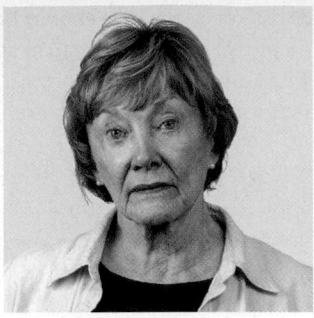

Mr. Allen has been unwilling to seek treatment because he fears the social stigma of being labeled medically depressed and is concerned his employer will discover it through his use of his medical benefits. It is Mr. Allen's opinion that his employer would perceive depression as a sign of weakness. Overall, Mr. Allen has done well without the medications.

Mr. Allen has been thinking about retiring in the next few years. He and his wife have always planned to do some traveling, but mostly he looks forward to escaping his busy, stressful work environment. Mr. Allen and his son are involved in church activities; they also enjoy a walk each evening after supper. Mr. Allen belongs to a bowling league and is at the bowling alley a couple of evenings a week.

Mr. Allen is admitted to the acute care hospital for a transurethral resection of the prostate (TURP). He has been very anxious about the procedure because of the risk of impotence. The surgery goes smoothly, and he experiences no complications. In the immediate postoperative period, Mr. Allen has a three-way Foley catheter inserted, with continuous bladder irrigation. He experiences pain and occasional bladder spasms because of blood clots. The day after surgery, the nurse enters Mr. Allen's room, and he asks why the hospital bed was brought to his room and calls the nurse by his wife's name. The nurse assesses Mr. Allen and determines he is confused.

1. What factors may increase the risk of confusion in this client?

2. What interventions would the nurse initiate for Mr. Allen if he were to continue to display confusion?

3. What nursing diagnosis would be appropriate for Mr. Allen if he were to continue to display confusion?

4. What assessment tools would the nurse use to assess Mr. Allen if he were to continue to display confusion?

EXEMPLAR 23.3 Schizophrenia

EXEMPLAR KEY TERMS
Alogia, *1614*
Anhedonia, *1614*
Assertive community treatment (ACT), *1619*
Avolition, *1614*
Bidirectional influence, *1613*
Brief psychotic disorder, *1615*
Catatonia, *1614*
Clang, *1613*
Communication deviance, *1612*
Concrete thinking, *1614*
Delusions, *1611*
Disorganized behavior, *1614*
Disorganized thinking, *1613*
Double-bind theory, *1612*
Dystonia, *1618*
Electroconvulsive therapy (ECT), *1620*
Extrapyramidal side effects, *1617*
Flat affect, *1614*
Hallucinations, *1611*
Illusions, *1611*
Loose association, *1613*
Movement disorders, *1614*
Negative symptoms, *1613*
Neologisms, *1613*
Neuroleptic malignant syndrome, *1617*
Paranoia, *1611*
Perseveration, *1613*
Positive symptoms, *1613*

Psychosis, *1611*
Schizoaffective disorder, *1615*
Schizophrenia, *1610*
Schizophreniform disorder, *1615*
Sensory overload, *1613*
Tardive dyskinesia, *1618*
Thought blocking, *1613*
Thought disorders, *1613*
Transcranial magnetic stimulation (TMS), *1620*

EXEMPLAR LEARNING OUTCOMES
After reading about this exemplar, you will be able to:

1. Describe the pathophysiology, etiology, clinical manifestations, and direct and indirect causes of schizophrenia.

2. Identify risk factors and prevention methods associated with schizophrenia.

3. Illustrate the nursing process in providing culturally sensitive care across the life span for individuals with schizophrenia.

4. Formulate priority nursing diagnoses appropriate for an individual with schizophrenia.

5. Summarize therapies used by interdisciplinary teams in the collaborative care of an individual with schizophrenia.

6. Plan evidence-based care for an individual with schizophrenia and his or her family in collaboration with other members of the healthcare team.

7. Evaluate expected outcomes for an individual with schizophrenia.

▶ OVERVIEW

Schizophrenia is the most common psychotic disorder. Manifestations of schizophrenia include various features associated with psychosis, such as disorganized thinking (which makes clear thought and decisions difficult), sensory and perceptual disturbances (which complicate interpretation of reality), and abnormal and disruptive behavior (which causes difficulty with social interaction). Affected individuals often have a normal childhood. Then, following subtle changes associated with puberty, more severe signs and symptoms manifest in the late teen and early adult years. These symptoms are often devastating, damaging individuals' relationships and preventing them from becoming productive members of society.

Like many forms of severe mental illness, schizophrenia is associated with **psychosis**, an abnormal mental state characterized by a number of features, including **delusions**, or false beliefs without basis in reality; **hallucinations**, or sensory experiences of things that aren't present; and **illusions**, or distorted perceptions of actual sights, sounds, and other stimuli. Individuals who are suffering from psychosis have disorganized behavior and difficulty with interpersonal interaction, and many experience **paranoia**, or a belief that others are "out to get them," either by following them or intending to harm them. These features make it difficult for affected individuals to determine what is real as they interact with the world around them.

Psychosis is classified as either acute or chronic. Whereas acute psychotic episodes occur over a period as short as hours or days, chronic psychoses can evolve over months or years. Both acute and chronic psychoses sometimes originate from a definable cause, like brain damage, medication overdose, severe depression, substance dependence, or genetic factors. For most clients, however, the cause of their psychosis cannot be determined.

Although schizophrenia is a single diagnosis, it is one of several disorders included in the 2013 *Diagnostic Statistical Manual of Mental Disorders*, 5th ed. (DSM-5) within the category of "schizophrenia spectrum and other psychotic disorders." Manifestations of schizophrenia range in severity, and this disorder has symptoms and etiologies that may overlap with other disorders. Medical diagnoses sometimes associated with schizophrenia include schizoid personality disorder, schizotypal personality disorder, paranoid personality disorder, schizoaffective disorder, schizophreniform disorder, delusional disorder, and brief psychotic disorder.

▶ PATHOPHYSIOLOGY AND ETIOLOGY

Research clearly shows evidence of abnormal brain development in individuals with schizophrenia. The primary problem appears to be abnormal development and migration of neurons in the brain, either during early development or as a result of progressive neuronal degeneration. The end result is miscommunication between portions of the brain, or "faulty wiring."

Neurons in the cerebral cortex of affected individuals also seem to function incorrectly. However, it is unclear whether these neurons are abnormal from the start or whether they form normally but then fail to flourish.

While brain abnormalities associated with schizophrenia may be identifiable during early development, the fact that symptoms often fail to manifest until the late teens or later suggests that other developmental factors are also important. One reason for this delay could be that myelination of neurons in the brain does not occur until late adolescence, and formation of myelin sheaths may have some sort of triggering effect. Another factor could be changes in cortical actions that typically occur between ages 16 and 22. Specifically, schizophrenia may somehow relate to improper reorganization of the left prefrontal and temporal regions.

Beyond these factors, pathophysiological mechanisms associated with schizophrenia may include abnormalities in neurotransmitter levels and/or function. Research continues to look at the role of neurotransmitters, including dopamine, serotonin, norepinephrine, glutamate, and gamma-aminobutyric acid (GABA). Glutamate in particular may be connected to the cognitive symptoms of schizophrenia. Glutamate is required for the degradation of dopamine and several other neurotransmitters that influence prefrontal information processing. Glutamate receptors also help control the migration of neurons during brain development, which means they may be involved in the abnormalities mentioned earlier. Similarly, increased dopamine activity has been associated with paranoid symptoms of schizophrenia, and high levels of norepinephrine have been linked with positive symptoms of psychosis. (Positive symptoms are described in depth later in the exemplar.) Still, no single neurotransmitter or set of neurotransmitters is definitively responsible for schizophrenia. Some researchers argue that the disorder may not involve abnormal neurotransmitter levels at all, but rather too many neurotransmitter receptors or perhaps receptors that are too sensitive. There may also be some chemical factor at work that scientists have yet to discover.

In addition to abnormal neurotransmitter levels, certain central nervous system irregularities have been noted in brain-imaging studies of individuals with schizophrenia. Some parts of the brain appear enlarged, including the ventricles and sulci (Elkis et al., 1995). Other areas show decreased volume and/or activity, as described in **Table 23–11** ●. Many individuals with schizophrenia also have defects in the corpus

TABLE 23–11 Typical CNS Abnormalities Observed in Individuals with Schizophrenia

	INCREASED SIZE	DECREASED VOLUME	DECREASED BLOOD FLOW	DECREASED BLOOD GLUCOSE	DECREASED O$_2$ USE	DECREASED ACTIVITY	DECREASED NICOTINIC RECEPTORS
Ventricles	X						
Sulci	X						
Temporal lobes		X	X				
Hippocampus		X					X
Prefrontal cortex		X				X	
Thalamus		X					
Basal ganglia			X	X	X		
Frontal lobes			X	X	X		

callosum, which negatively affect communication between the cerebral hemispheres.

One notable finding associated with schizophrenia is reduced blood flow to the thalamus, which can interfere with the brain's filter, turning the normal flow of sensory information into an overload. Another interesting abnormality is a decreased number of nicotinic receptors in the hippocampus, which makes it harder for affected individuals to form new memories and interpret sensory stimuli. Many individuals with schizophrenia may unknowingly compensate for this deficiency by smoking. In fact, between 70% and 85% of diagnosed individuals regularly smoke, as compared with roughly 22.5% of Americans without schizophrenia (National Institute of Mental Health, 2009).

Etiology

The exact causes of schizophrenia are not completely understood. Genetics, while not entirely predictive, seems to be one important factor, as individuals with a parent, brother, or sister with the disease have a 10 times higher risk of schizophrenia than the general population.

Schizophrenia affects about 1% of the population, both in the United States and worldwide, with men and women diagnosed at equal rates (National Institute of Mental Health, 2009). Among individuals with schizophrenia, the onset and progression can vary widely. In most cases, the disorder emerges during or soon after adolescence, although about 23% of individuals are older than age 40 when their symptoms first manifest (Raiji, Ismail, & Mulsant, 2009). Age also appears to affect the type and intensity of symptoms. For example, aging is sometimes associated with a reduction in hallucinations and delusions in individuals who experience early-onset schizophrenia, while individuals with a later onset often have paranoia and fewer negative symptoms (Simon, 2012). Such findings have led some scientists to suggest that late-onset schizophrenia may even represent a distinct disorder (Vahia et al., 2010; Howard et al., 2000).

> ### SAFETY ALERT
> Schizophrenia does not make individuals more violent, but it does greatly increase their suicide risk. For this reason, nurses should closely monitor all clients with schizophrenia for possible warning signs of suicide.

Risk Factors

Multiple factors appear to influence the development of schizophrenia. Some researchers believe that, even when schizophrenia is present, the disorder may not fully manifest until an individual is exposed to certain environmental or social factors. Research studies have examined genetic, biological, environmental, and social factors both jointly and separately.

BIOLOGICAL FACTORS Genetic factors significantly impact the risk for developing schizophrenia. Although some gene targets have been identified, no single gene or set of genes has been implicated as a marker for the disorder. Recent studies identified multiple genes that appear to contribute to schizophrenia by causing errors in either neurochemical function or growth and development of the central nervous system (Ota et al., 2013;

Jackson et al., 2013; Umeda-Yano et al., 2013; Hoerder-Suabedissen et al., 2013). Certain genetic defects, while not directly leading to schizophrenia, may render individuals susceptible to symptom onset in the presence of certain environmental factors, such as toxins or other stressors (Niwa et al., 2013). Still other studies have focused exclusively on the role of external events like birth complications, in utero viral exposure, and poor prenatal care (Giovanoli et al., 2013; Sutterland et al., 2013; Zugno et al., 2013; Hamlyn et al., 2013).

At present, the most compelling evidence for the role of genetics is that individuals are multiple times more likely to develop schizophrenia when one of their family members is affected. For instance, whereas members of the general population have a 1% risk of schizophrenia, individuals with an affected third-degree relative such as a cousin have a risk of 2%, and individuals with an affected second-degree relative such as an aunt, uncle, half sibling, or grandparent have a risk of 2%–6%. An individual who has an affected first-degree relative such as a parent or sibling has a risk of schizophrenia that jumps to as much as 46% (Gaebel, 2011; Gottesman, 1991; Lichtenstein et al., 2009; Gottesman et al., 2010; Cardno & Gottesman, 2000). Genetics, however, is not the only determinant of individual risk; 60% of individuals with schizophrenia have no close afflicted relatives (Simon, 2012; Gaebel, 2011).

One intriguing biological risk factor for schizophrenia is advanced paternal age. A large Swedish study showed that children with fathers in their 40s and 50s had double and triple the risk, respectively, of developing schizophrenia as compared to children with fathers under age 25. This increase is believed to be due to cumulative mutations in the fathers' sperm, but the exact reason remains unknown (Sipos et al., 2004; Smith et al., 2012).

SOCIAL-ENVIRONMENTAL FACTORS Although genetic factors can predispose an individual toward developing schizophrenia, it often takes a further social-environmental trigger for symptoms to emerge. Researchers have identified **communication deviance** as one such trigger. Communication deviance refers to communication patterns that are distracting and confusing to listeners who are trying to share a common focus or meaning with a speaker (Davey, 2011). For example, a parent's response to a child's question may be completely off-topic and therefore confusing to the child. Studies have shown that parental communication deviance was predictive for psychotic disorders in genetically at-risk children, whereas children with a low genetic risk showed no such association (Tienari et al., 2004; Asarnow et al., 1988). A similar concept known as **double-bind theory** posits that schizophrenia symptoms are partially an expression of contradictory family interactions (Bateson et al., 1956). Essentially, the individual is placed in a "no-win" situation by one or more family members, which results in manifestation of psychotic symptoms. For example, a parent who abuses a young child and yet assures the child that he is loved places the child in a double bind. For the dependent child, there is no option for escaping the abuse and, due to yet-undeveloped communication skills, the child is unable to identify and question the incongruence between the abusive parent's words and actions. As a result, the child is left to try and reconcile the contradictory verbal and nonverbal messages. Moreover, the child may equate love, which is desirable, with the undesirable act of physical abuse.

Beyond communication deviance and double-bind theory, family interactions also may yield other detrimental effects. For example, high levels of familial expressed emotion, such as hostility, overinvolvement, and criticism, correlate to worse negative symptoms in recent-onset cases of schizophrenia. In addition, relapse rates for individuals with schizophrenia are much greater in high-expressed-emotion homes (Subotnik et al., 2012; Pharoah et al., 2010; Hogarty et al., 1986). **Bidirectional influence** can also pose a problem for both individuals with schizophrenia and their families. Bidirectional influence refers to the fact that while an individual's family can negatively affect her emotional health (especially if the individual has schizophrenia), the individual can also negatively affect the emotional health of her family members, thus contributing to a downward emotional and behavioral spiral. Even without negative family situations, stress can elevate the risk of schizophrenia, especially for genetically predisposed individuals. Increased levels of daily stress and/or stressful life events may trigger schizophrenia onset, exacerbation of symptoms, and even relapse (Tessner, Mittal, & Walker, 2011).

Additional environmental factors that may play a role include virus exposure, malnutrition, and other problems in utero. For example, complications during birth and various psychosocial factors are considered likely contributors (National Institute of Mental Health, 2009).

Prevention

Among individuals who are predisposed to developing schizophrenia, the majority will not develop symptoms unless exposed to one or more of the environmental stressors discussed. Certain protective measures, such as reducing stress, getting adequate sleep, and avoiding illegal drug use, can lower the likelihood of schizophrenia (Mayo Clinic, 2012d). Community-based programs that involve education and social support also have beneficial outcomes (Primm et al., 2010), as do family-based programs that emphasize communication, crisis management, caregiver care, advocacy, and utilization of community services (National Alliance on Mental Illness, 2013b). In general, the more protective factors an individual has, the lower his chance of developing schizophrenia.

▶ CLINICAL MANIFESTATIONS

The major manifestations of schizophrenia are generally described as either **positive symptoms** or **negative symptoms**, depending on whether they involve the presence of unusual behaviors or the absence of typical behaviors, respectively. Both types of symptoms can greatly impact a person's affect, perception, cognitive function, and relationships with others. Some common examples of positive and negative symptoms are listed in **Table 23–12** ●.

Positive symptoms are additional psychotic behaviors not commonly observed in adults, often causing them to lose touch with reality. One example is hallucinations, which are extrasensory experiences that occur without an external stimulus. Hallucinations can involve any of the five senses—sight, sound, taste, touch, or smell—but individuals with schizophrenia most often have auditory hallucinations, with 60%–80% of

TABLE 23–12 Positive and Negative Symptoms of Schizophrenia

POSITIVE SYMPTOMS	NEGATIVE SYMPTOMS
Hallucinations	Anhedonia
Delusions	Memory impairment
Thought disorders:	Flat affect
■ Disorganized thinking	Lack of focus
■ Sensory overload	Avolition
■ Thought blocking	Alogia
■ Neologisms	Neglect of personal hygiene
■ Loose associations	Social withdrawal
■ Clang	Poor problem solving
■ Perseveration	Concrete thinking
Disorganized behavior:	
■ Bizarre behavior	
■ Overreactive affect	
■ Inappropriate affect	
■ Poor impulse control	
Movement disorders:	
■ Additional body movements	
■ Catatonia	

affected individuals experiencing this symptom. Auditory hallucinations generally take the form of voices and may initially be misinterpreted as self-talk. These voices may provide a commentary on daily life, carry on conversations, warn of danger, or provide commands that the individual feels compelled to obey. Although less common, visual hallucinations are experienced by 24%–72% of affected individuals (Amad et al., 2013). This type of hallucination involves seeing things that aren't really there.

Delusions, or beliefs that have no basis in reality, are another positive symptom of schizophrenia. These fixed, false beliefs will persist, despite ample evidence to the contrary. Delusions can assume various themes, the most common of which are described in **Table 23–13** ●.

Beyond hallucinations and delusions, **thought disorders** are another category of positive symptoms of schizophrenia. These disorders involve abnormal or unusual ways of thinking. Affected individuals often have a difficult time organizing their thoughts, which becomes apparent in their speech patterns. These disorders take a variety of forms, including the following:

■ *Disorganized thinking*. The individual has trouble logically connecting thoughts, leading to a garbled way of speaking.

■ *Sensory overload*. The brain's natural filtering mechanism is impaired, which results in an abundance of sensory information that cannot be correctly processed.

■ *Thought blocking*. The individual stops speaking in mid-sentence as if the thought disappeared from her head.

■ *Neologisms*. The individual uses meaningless words that only have meaning to her.

■ *Loose association*. The individual rapidly switches from one topic to another, with no apparent connection between them.

■ *Clang*. The individual repeatedly uses rhyming words without apparent meaning.

■ *Perseveration*. The individual uses the same words or phrases over and over.

TABLE 23–13   Common Categories of Delusions

TYPE	EXAMPLE
Delusions of control	"My neighbor is manipulating all of my thoughts and actions through use of a special remote control device."
Erotomanic delusions	"Every woman on the planet wants to go out with me. I'm so busy turning them down that I barely have time for all my dates with Angelina Jolie."
Delusions of grandeur	"I am Abraham Lincoln. The country needs me at this critical time of division, and they will be calling on me any day now."
Delusions of persecution	"The letter carrier is really a covert government agent. He's watching me through my vents and monitoring my communications. He'll do whatever he can to get to me."
Delusions of reference	"That billboard is giving me orders for a secret mission. It's telling me to watch the employees in the grocery store for antigovernment activity, then report back with my observations."
Religious delusions	"An angel contacted me through the crucifix in my bedroom. He told me I'm a new prophet and must spread God's word in the streets to save people from eternal damnation."
Delusions of sin and guilt	"Everything I do is wrong, and everyone despises me because of it. My family hates me, my friends hate me, and even God hates me."
Somatic delusions	"Green worms are slowly eating my body from the inside out. Pretty soon, all of my organs are going to stop working."
Delusions involving thought broadcasting	"I know that you know what I'm thinking right now. You can hear all my thoughts. In fact, everyone can."
Delusions involving thought insertion	"My thoughts are not my own. The CIA is inserting thoughts and ideas into my head."
Delusions involving thought withdrawal	"I can't remember what I was going to tell you. Someone keeps stealing the thoughts from my head before I share them with you."

Although the biological mechanism of thought disorders is currently unknown, there is evidence that genetic components may be involved (Levy et al., 2010).

A further class of positive symptoms involves **disorganized behavior**, or an inability to start or finish goal-oriented activities that interferes with an individual's ability to lead a normal life. Disorganized behavior can manifest in a number of ways, including bizarre or purposeless actions, problems with impulse control, overreactive affect (in which an individual's reaction is suitable but out of proportion to the circumstances), and inappropriate affect (in which an individual's emotional response is incongruent with the situation). **Movement disorders** are yet another type of positive symptom. These disorders take two general forms. The first involves additional body movements, which may appear agitated, repetitive, and purposeless. The second involves **catatonia**, or unresponsiveness to the environment or others. Here, the affected individual may adopt bizarre postures and/or resist attempts at repositioning. Possible causes of catatonia include cerebral folate deficiency or dysfunction of the medial motor system, which involves self-initiated movements. Although catatonia may be present with schizophrenia, it is also associated with conditions such as major depression and bipolar disorder (Fink, Shorter, & Taylor, 2010; Scheuerecker et al., 2009; Ho et al., 2010).

Compared with the aforementioned symptoms, the negative symptoms of schizophrenia are sometimes more difficult to notice, because they involve an absence of normal behavior and emotions and may be confused with other conditions, such as depression. Common negative symptoms include the following:

- **Flat affect**. The affected individual shows minimal facial expression and movement, sometimes speaking in a monotone voice.

- **Alogia**. The individual experiences impoverished thinking, resulting in nominal speech patterns, even during forced interaction.

- **Avolition**. Due to a lack of motivation, the individual is progressively unable to function in daily life, at home, work, or in social interactions.

- **Anhedonia**. The individual is unable to feel pleasure and loses interest in life, which can result in decreased social interaction and withdrawal.

- *Neglect of personal hygiene.* The individual forgets to bathe or change and wash his clothes, which serves to further his social isolation.

- **Concrete thinking**. The individual has a tendency to focus primarily on facts and details, coupled with an inability to think abstractly.

- *Memory impairment.* The individual couples incorrect recall of facts and events with a certainty that this recalled information is correct, leading to impaired decision-making ability.

- *Poor problem solving.* Impairments in the individual's cognitive skills lead to faulty reasoning, which affects everyday functioning and social relationships.

- *Lack of focus.* The individual displays high distractibility and reduced concentration due to obstructed information processing and response mechanisms.

Physiologically, negative symptoms have been correlated with CNS white matter abnormalities and changes in dopamine function, as well as late prenatal immune activation (Laruelle et al., 1996; White et al., 2011; Bitanihirwe et al., 2010).

In addition to age of onset, the rate of onset seems to make a difference in the overall course of the disease. In acute cases of schizophrenia, symptoms can quickly manifest and disappear.

In chronic cases, where symptoms appear over months or years, individuals may eventually achieve a steady state with respect to the disease or experience a gradual decline in cognition as the disease progresses. Gender is another influencing factor. Although the prevalence of schizophrenia is the same for both sexes, women generally have later onset, often in their 20s and 30s (Cleveland Clinic, 2009b). In addition, women tend to respond better to pharmaceutical treatment, have fewer negative symptoms, experience fewer relapses of shorter duration, and have a more favorable course of illness (Abel et al., 2010).

The physical and psychological toll of schizophrenia is evident in the life expectancy of affected individuals, which is about 25 years shorter than that of the general population. One major reason for this difference in life expectancy is that between 10% and 30% of individuals with schizophrenia commit suicide. Among affected individuals who do not commit suicide, the leading causes of death are similar to those for all Americans—heart disease, pulmonary disease, diabetes, and other conditions—but they occur at two to three times the rate seen in the general population. This higher rate is partially due to the fact that individuals with schizophrenia often have greater difficulty accessing and paying for healthcare services because of functional impairments related to their symptoms. For the same reasons, affected individuals are also more vulnerable to higher rates of homelessness, victimization, unemployment, poverty, poor nutrition, substance abuse, unsafe sexual behavior, incarceration, social isolation, and disease exposure in group home/shelter settings (Parks et al., 2006; Gay et al., 2008).

Subtypes, Specifiers, and Dimensions

In the past, the American Psychiatric Association (APA) advocated a system in which schizophrenia was divided into different subtypes depending on clients' symptoms and pattern of onset. However, in the most recent version of the *Diagnostic and Statistical Manual of Mental Disorders* (DSM-5), published in May 2013, the APA did away with this system due to its low reliability and poor validity. Specifically, many individuals with schizophrenia had fluctuating symptoms that did not place them squarely or permanently in any one subtype. Moreover, none of the subtypes were found to exhibit a distinctive course or response to treatment.

The APA now advocates that mental health practitioners describe schizophrenia in terms of specifiers rather than subtypes. For example, individuals who exhibit symptoms of catatonia would now be said to have "schizophrenia with catatonia" rather than "schizophrenia of the catatonic subtype." The DSM-5 also includes a dimensional approach to rating the core symptoms of schizophrenia on a scale ranging from 0 to 4, based on an individual's behaviors over the past month. This new approach better reflects the wide variety of symptom types and severities observed in affected individuals.

Related Disorders

To further complicate the diagnostic process, there are a number of related psychotic disorders that share many symptoms with schizophrenia. These include the following:

- *Schizoaffective disorder*. As with schizophrenia, clients with schizoaffective disorder experience hallucinations, delusions, disorganized thought, and disorganized behavior, although they also suffer from at least one manic episode or period of major depression. In order for diagnosis to be made, an affected individual's psychotic symptoms must persist for 2 weeks or more in the absence of depression or mania. Moreover, individuals must experience depressive or manic episodes at least 50% of the time throughout the entire course of their illness. Schizoaffective disorder affects approximately 1% of the population but is often misdiagnosed (Duckworth & Freedman, 2012c).

- *Brief psychotic disorder*. This disorder is characterized by a brief episode of typically positive psychotic behavior, such as hallucinations, delusions, thought disorders, and disorganized behavior. The episode lasts between 1 day and 1 month.

- *Schizophreniform disorder*. Schizophreniform disorder presents similarly to schizophrenia. However, symptoms last from 1 to 6 months, whereas a 6-month duration is required for a diagnosis of schizophrenia. In addition, affected individuals may not have as much difficulty functioning in daily life as do individuals with schizophrenia.

To avoid misdiagnosis and provide appropriate treatment, practitioners must understand the major signs and symptoms of these disorders and how they differ from those associated with schizophrenia.

Comorbid Disorders

Many clients also experience a comorbid, nonpsychotic psychological disorder at some point during the course of their schizophrenia. One common comorbid disorder is addiction, with at least 47% of individuals with schizophrenia demonstrating a diagnosis of substance abuse in their life (Buckley et al., 2009). Alcohol abuse is prevalent among this population: Clients are approximately 9–13 times more likely to abuse alcohol than members of the general population (Volkow, 2009). As previously discussed, smoking is more prevalent among individuals with schizophrenia. Illicit drug use is problematic as well. Not only is drug use higher among individuals with schizophrenia, but it also correlates with a younger age of onset, more positive symptoms, higher relapse rates, a greater risk of violence and suicide, additional legal complications, and more pharmaceutical side effects (Buckley et al., 2009).

Various psychiatric disorders, including panic disorder, posttraumatic stress disorder (PTSD), and generalized anxiety disorder, are also comorbid with schizophrenia. For example, approximately 15%–25% of individuals with schizophrenia exhibit panic attacks and panic disorder, respectively, compared with a lifetime prevalence in the general U.S. population of 2%–5%. Individuals with comorbid panic disorders are more likely to experience positive symptoms of psychosis, suicidal ideation, and vulnerability to substance abuse (Buckley et al., 2009).

Similarly, mood disorders are present in many clients with schizophrenia. Depression is seen in a majority of afflicted individuals, although exact percentages are difficult to determine because of factors such as medication side effects, negative symptoms, and comorbid substance abuse. Among those with schizophrenia, depression is related to increased risk of psychotic relapse, as well as heightened suicide risk (Buckley et al., 2009; Simon, 2012). Comorbid obsessive-compulsive disorder

(OCD) and obsessive-compulsive symptoms (OCS) also commonly accompany schizophrenia. In fact, OCD was observed in approximately 23% of individuals with schizophrenia, while comorbid OCS was noted in roughly 25%. Lifetime prevalence rates for both conditions among the general U.S. population are only 2%. OCD and OCS have been linked to earlier onset of psychotic symptoms, more severe neuropsychological impairment, more severe paranoia, and more psychotic symptoms (Buckley et al., 2009; Duckworth & Freedman, 2012b).

Individuals with schizophrenia also experience high rates of comorbid medical illness. Type 2 diabetes is not uncommon: In one study, individuals with schizophrenia had type 2 diabetes about twice as often as members of a control population (11.3% vs. 6.3%), with over 10% greater mortality (Schoepf et al., 2012). This risk does not appear to have a strong genetic correlation (Lin & Shuldiner, 2010). Although some of the added risk is believed to result from avolition and poor self-care, antipsychotic medications have been found to play a significant role. Drugs such as olanzapine, clozapine, and various other first- and second-generation antipsychotics tend to produce weight gain, higher blood cholesterol, and higher blood glucose levels, all of which boost an individual's likelihood of type 2 diabetes (Rummel-Kluge et al., 2010).

Lifespan and Cultural Considerations

Although most clients first notice symptoms of schizophrenia at some point between late adolescence and early adulthood, about 4% of sufferers experience earlier onset, with some cases reported in children as young as age 3. In general, among men, psychotic features associated with schizophrenia most commonly surface during the early to mid 20s. For women, schizophrenia-related psychotic symptoms tend to emerge during the mid 20s (American Psychiatric Association, 2013).

Early-onset schizophrenia (EOS) appears to affect males and females with approximately equal frequency (Vyas, Kumra, & Puri, 2010; Vyas, Patel, & Puri, 2011). EOS also tends to display a more chronic onset, with a majority of parents describing their child's behavior as unusual and marked by symptoms of shyness, hesitancy, withdrawal, and cognitive dysfunction. Individuals with EOS generally show greater childhood maladjustment than individuals with adult-onset schizophrenia (AOS). In addition, various developmental delays are common among these clients. Numerous studies show evidence of motor impairment and poor coordination in up to 60% of clients with EOS, as well as speech and language impairment rates of around 50%. Lower IQ scores have also been noted (Kinros, Reichenberg, & Frangou, 2010).

EOS differs from AOS in several other ways. At onset, one of the most common EOS symptoms is hallucinations, observed in around 80% of cases; unlike AOS hallucinations, these are more child-themed, involving toys, monsters, and animals. Delusions, however, are less prominent in EOS than AOS. In addition, EOS is associated with a more chronic course of disease; neurodevelopmental abnormalities; more hospitalizations; worse symptoms; and greater educational, occupational, and social development maladjustment, with earlier onset correlating with even worse symptoms and disease outcomes (Vyas, Kumra, & Puri, 2010; Amminger et al., 2011).

Focus on Diversity and Culture
Schizophrenia

Cultural practices and beliefs can affect an individual's interpretation of various symptoms of schizophrenia. For example, in some cultures, it may be normal or even desirable for someone to hear voices or see visions as part of a religious experience. Thus individuals from these cultures may not view hallucinations as indicative of a mental disorder. The nurse should report the client's delusions/hallucinations in the context they were described as having occurred to the healthcare provider for further evaluation and medical diagnosis, if indicated.

▶ COLLABORATION

To provide the best care possible, nurses must be familiar with a range of collaborative interventions related to schizophrenia. These include various diagnostic tests, medications, and non-pharmacologic and alternative therapies.

Diagnostic Tests

There is no single definitive test for schizophrenia. Instead, physicians, psychiatrists, and psychologists diagnose this disorder based upon symptoms exhibited by the client. See **Box 23–2** ● for specific diagnostic criteria for schizophrenia.

Early diagnosis of schizophrenia can be difficult, as an individual's initial symptoms may be no more than social withdrawal, poor school performance, or irritability. Furthermore, many other conditions, including depression, bipolar disorder, drug abuse, brain tumors, and medication reactions, share symptoms with schizophrenia, so they must be ruled out through psychological evaluation, blood tests, and imaging studies. Diagnosis is also complicated by the fact that most individuals with schizophrenia do not believe they have the disease (National Institute of Mental Health, 2009; Simon, 2012; Mayo Clinic, 2012d).

Although primarily employed for research, imaging studies can be used to look for neurological changes typical of schizophrenia, such as enlarged ventricles, reduced gray matter volume, and so on. These studies are also useful in ruling out brain tumors. Common brain-imaging techniques include magnetic resonance imaging (MRI), positron emission tomography (PET), and single photon emission computed tomography (SPECT) (**Figure 23–4** ●).

Pharmacologic Therapy

Because there is no surgery that can treat schizophrenia, pharmacologic therapy is often the first line of intervention. The principal objective of pharmacologic treatment is to decrease the positive symptoms of the disorder (e.g., hallucinations and delusions) with the lowest possible dosage. For clients who have been hospitalized, another major goal is to facilitate their discharge and return them to as normal a life as possible.

Of the one third of Americans with schizophrenia who receive treatment, about half will show improvement over time. However, even individuals who are undergoing drug therapy have an increased risk of mortality. Psychotropic medications

Box 23–2 DSM-5 Diagnostic Criteria for Schizophrenia

A. Two (or more) of the following, each present for a significant portion of time during a 1-month period (or less if successfully treated). At least one of these must be (1), (2), or (3):

1. Delusions.
2. Hallucinations.
3. Disorganized speech (e.g., frequent derailment or incoherence).
4. Grossly disorganized or catatonic behavior.
5. Negative symptoms (i.e., diminished emotional expression or avolition).

B. For a significant portion of the time since the onset of the disturbance, level of functioning in one or more major areas, such as work, interpersonal relations, or self-care, is markedly below the level achieved prior to the onset (or when the onset is in childhood or adolescence, there is failure to achieve expected level of interpersonal, academic, or occupational functioning).

C. Continuous signs of the disturbance persist for at least 6 months. This 6-month period must include at least 1 month of symptoms (or less if successfully treated) that meet Criterion A (i.e., active-phase symptoms) and may include periods of prodromal or residual symptoms. During these prodromal or residual periods, the signs of the disturbance may be manifested by only negative symptoms or by two more symptoms listed in Criterion A present in an attenuated form (e.g., odd beliefs, unusual perceptual experiences).

D. Schizoaffective disorder and depressive or bipolar disorder with psychotic features have been ruled out because either 1) no major depressive or manic episodes have occurred concurrently with the active-phase symptoms, or 2) if mood episodes have occurred during active-phase symptoms, they have been present for a minority of the total duration of the active and residual periods of the illness.

E. The disturbance is not attributable to the physiological effects of a substance (e.g., a drug of abuse, a medication) or another medical condition.

F. If there is a history of autism spectrum disorder or a communication disorder of childhood onset, the additional diagnosis of schizophrenia is made only if prominent delusions or hallucinations, in addition to the other required symptoms of schizophrenia, are also present for at least 1 month (or less if successfully treated).

Source: American Psychiatric Association. (2013). *Diagnostic and statistical manual of mental disorders* (5th ed.). Washington, DC: Author, pp. 99–100.

can mask illnesses and exacerbate existing medical symptoms. They can also cause side effects such as reduced sensitivity to pain, weight gain, metabolic syndrome, high cholesterol, and diabetes. Furthermore, multiple medications are sometimes required for treatment, which increases the likelihood of side effects, makes it harder for clients to adhere to the treatment regimen, and elevates the risk of sudden death (Parks et al., 2006; Gay et al., 2008). Still, for many individuals, early diagnosis and treatment can improve overall outcomes and reduce the duration of symptoms.

With the advent of conventional or typical antipsychotic medications in the 1950s, drugs such as chlorpromazine (Thorazine) and haloperidol (Haldol) became the treatment of choice for positive symptoms of schizophrenia. These medications generally work by blocking dopamine receptors (National Alliance on Mental Illness, 2013b). Although these drugs have beneficial effects for many clients, they often produce devastating side effects, such as hypotension; sudden cardiac death; **neuroleptic malignant syndrome**, a sometimes fatal condition characterized by fever and rigidity; and increased prolactin levels, which can lead to infertility, impotence, and higher risk of osteoporosis and breast cancer. Also, roughly 70% of clients who take conventional antipsychotics experience **extrapyramidal side effects**, which affect the functioning of various nerves and muscles that

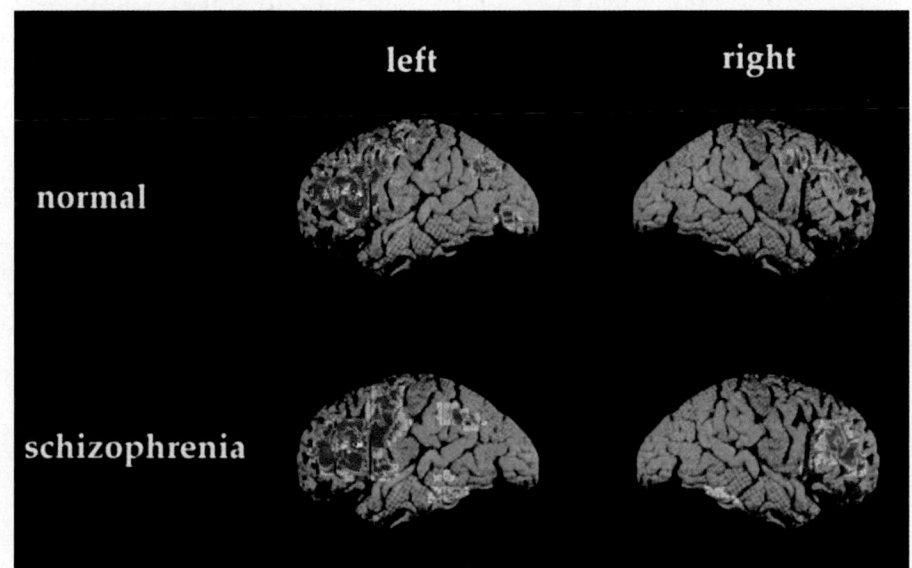

Figure 23–4 ● These PET scans show the difference between the brains of a normal client and a client with schizophrenia during a verbal fluency task, i.e., the clients were asked to speak words. The red and yellow areas were activated when the subjects spoke the words. In the normal subject (top row), the brain shows much activity in the prefrontal and motor areas, and less activity in the parietal area on the left side. In the subject with schizophrenia (bottom row), there is also activity in the middle temporal gyrus (lower center of brain), which is not seen in the normal subject.

Source: Wellcome Department of Cognitive Neurology/Science Source.

control coordination and movement. Extrapyramidal side effects often bear a resemblance to symptoms of Parkinson disease and include **tardive dyskinesia** (repetitive, involuntary body movements of varying severity that may not cease after medication cessation), acute **dystonia** (unusual muscle spasms in the neck, jaw, trunk, or eyes), agitation, slow speech, retarded movement, and tremor. These side effects can sometimes be counteracted by ceasing conventional antipsychotic therapy and/or administering anticholinergics, which function by raising dopamine levels. Benzodiazepines may also be effective (Simon, 2012).

Beginning in 1989, a generation of drugs known as atypical antipsychotics was introduced. These drugs, which now include clozapine (Clozaril), risperidone (Risperdal), and olanzapine (Zyprexa), generally function by affecting dopamine and other neurotransmitters. Their main benefit over conventional antipsychotics is a reduction in extrapyramidal side effects, but other advantages include improved mental functioning, control of both positive and negative symptoms, and reduced depression, hostility, and suicide risk. Still, atypical antipsychotics have their own side effects, including diabetes, weight gain, elevated cholesterol, seizures, hypotension, neutropenia (a major

drop in white blood cell count), cataracts, increased prolactin levels, and heart problems (Simon, 2012).

More recently, a new class of drugs called *dopamine system stabilizers* were approved for use in the United States. One example is aripiprazole (Abilify). Like atypical antipsychotics, these medications reduce positive and negative symptoms of schizophrenia, but with lower instance of weight gain, diabetes, sexual dysfunction, and extrapyramidal effects (Kirino, 2012). Common side effects of dopamine system stabilizers include nausea, vomiting, headache, dizziness, anxiety, restlessness, and insomnia (Otsuka America Pharmaceutical, 2013).

Unfortunately, even with these newer-generation pharmaceuticals, adherence to a medication regimen is a challenge for many individuals with schizophrenia. Some clients stop taking their medication because it stops working. In fact, studies estimate that 20%–30% of individuals with schizophrenia become resistant to antipsychotics (Repo-Tiihonen et al., 2012). Other clients stop taking medication when they start feeling better or because they cannot tolerate the side effects. For these individuals, drug discontinuation results in relapse or worsening of symptoms within 2 years or less (Simon, 2012).

Medications **Schizophrenia**

CLASSIFICATION AND DRUG EXAMPLES	MECHANISM OF ACTION	NURSING CONSIDERATIONS
Conventional/Typical Antipsychotics *Drug examples:* - chlorpromazine (Thorazine) - haloperidol (Haldol) - perphenazine - fluphenazine	Block postsynaptic dopamine receptors in the brain, thus reducing symptoms of schizophrenia. *May also be used for:* —Bipolar disorder —Psychoses that accompany dementia —Tourette syndrome —Severe behavior problems in children —Severe nausea and vomiting	- Monitor for extrapyramidal side effects, including tardive dyskinesia. - Monitor for neuroleptic malignant syndrome, especially in clients who have hypertension or are taking lithium. - Watch for rapid mood shifts and exacerbation of seizure activity. - Monitor clients with diabetes (and those who are prediabetic) for reduced glucose control. - Teach clients about dangers of abrupt drug discontinuation. - Note that anticholinergics and/or benzodiazepines may be administered in an attempt to counteract side effects.
Atypical Antipsychotics *Drug examples:* - clozapine (Clozaril) - risperidone (Risperdal) - olanzapine (Zyprexa)	Limit dopamine's ability to bind with receptors in the brain, thereby decreasing symptoms of schizophrenia. *May also be used for:* —Bipolar disorder —Psychoses that accompany dementia	- Monitor for seizure activity. - Regularly test for agranulocytosis (clozapine only) and neutropenia. - Monitor cardiovascular status, watching especially for palpitations and changes in blood pressure. - Monitor respiratory status for possible dyspnea. - Watch for signs of tardive dyskinesia and neuroleptic malignant syndrome. - Monitor clients with diabetes (and those who are prediabetic) for reduced glucose control. - Emphasize importance of taking medication as ordered.
Dopamine System Stabilizers *Drug examples:* - aripiprazole (Abilify)	Enhances dopamine and serotonin activity in regions of the brain where these substances are deficient, yet inhibits serotonin activity in areas where there is an abundance of this neurotransmitter. *May also be used for:* —Bipolar disorder —Major depressive disorder —Irritability associated with autism —Restless leg syndrome	- Monitor for increased or worsening depression or thoughts of suicide, especially in children and adolescents. - Monitor cardiovascular status, watching especially for changes in blood pressure. - Watch for signs of tardive dyskinesia and neuroleptic malignant syndrome. - Monitor clients with diabetes (and those who are prediabetic) for reduced glucose control.

Nonpharmacologic Therapy

Although pharmaceuticals can be of great help in treating schizophrenia, affected individuals usually have better results when drug therapy is combined with nonpharmacologic therapy. Therapies employed in the treatment of schizophrenia include psychiatric/psychosocial rehabilitation, group therapy, assertive community treatment, hospitalization, and electroconvulsive therapy.

PSYCHIATRIC/PSYCHOSOCIAL REHABILITATION

Individuals with schizophrenia typically have the same goals and dreams as healthy individuals, and most believe that better access to housing, jobs, and transportation would improve their likelihood of achieving these goals (Gay et al., 2008). However, due to the debilitating symptoms of their disorder, many clients have problems with even basic self-care, work, communication, and social situations. For these clients, psychiatric or psychosocial rehabilitation can increase their likelihood of success in relationships, work, and daily living, which in turn helps them comply with their medication regimens and reduces the number of relapses and hospitalizations.

Psychiatric or psychosocial rehabilitation involves a number of parties, including physicians, nurses, mental health therapists, family, and friends. Therapists educate clients about the disorder, including its causes, symptoms, medications, and common complications, empowering them to take an active role in disease management and make educated decisions about their care and treatment. For example, during rehabilitation, the therapist might teach a client about coping skills and how to respond to early signs of relapse. Rehabilitation frequently also includes treatment for substance abuse, as this is a common problem for individuals with schizophrenia. In addition, many clients greatly benefit from cognitive-behavioral therapy, especially when their symptoms persist despite antipsychotic administration. This type of therapy teaches individuals how to examine the reality of their perceptions, how to ignore the voices, and how to motivate themselves, which can reduce the symptom severity and chances of relapse (Cleveland Clinic, 2009a).

Rehabilitation frequently also includes job and social training, as these skills are often underdeveloped in individuals with schizophrenia. Such training may include help with vocational counseling, money management skills, using public transportation, and social and on-the-job communication skills. Successful employment can greatly improve overall therapeutic outcomes for clients with schizophrenia. For example, studies have found that after 1 year of paid work, 40% of individuals reported improvement in all symptoms of schizophrenia and 50% reported improvement in positive symptoms, whereas unpaid workers with schizophrenia did more poorly by comparison (Simon, 2012).

The nurse is an important member of the rehabilitation team and must be both sympathetic and empathetic. The nurse not only helps ensure the client is adhering to the prescribed treatment regimen but also educates the client with regard to various vocational and social situations. In addition, it is the nurse's responsibility to help the client find support services in the community. These and other important nursing interventions are described in greater detail in the Nursing Process portion of the exemplar.

GROUP THERAPY

One of the most beneficial nonpharmacologic interventions for many clients with schizophrenia is participation in group therapy. Self-help groups provide ongoing support and encouragement for affected individuals. These groups let clients know they are not alone in their illness, and they also provide an opportunity for social engagement that might not otherwise be available.

Family therapy and education are also included under the umbrella of group therapy. Family therapy is often an important part of the rehabilitation process, as loved ones frequently play an active role in helping clients continue their treatment and function in the community. During therapy, family members learn about schizophrenia, including common symptoms, problems, therapeutic medications, and signs of relapse. In addition, they are educated about coping skills, outpatient and other support services, and their loved one's specific treatment program. Family therapy is especially important for families that are overly emotional, critical, or hostile, since this behavior may lead to anxiety, withdrawal, depression, and relapse in the individual with schizophrenia (Simon, 2012; Cleveland Clinic, 2009a).

ASSERTIVE COMMUNITY TREATMENT

Assertive community treatment (ACT) can be an especially effective therapeutic regimen for individuals with schizophrenia who are disabled by their symptoms. Often, these clients aren't capable of locating the many services they need in their community, much less keep up with all of their appointments and treatment plans. ACT is therefore a service delivery model that provides clients with individually tailored services right in their own community, rather than acting simply as a case management program. It is a proactive process that attempts to prevent further crises, ensures compliance with the medication regimen, and assists the client with daily functioning. The usefulness of ACT has been validated by research, which shows that treatment of this nature decreases clients' hospitalization time and severity of symptoms while improving their stability and quality of life (Cleveland Clinic, 2009a). See the Community-Based Care feature for more information on ACT.

HOSPITALIZATION

Most clients with schizophrenia are able to succeed in outpatient settings, especially when treatment involves therapy or ACT services. For some clients, however, hospitalization is necessary. Often, an individual's first hospital

---

Community-Based Care Assertive Community Treatment (ACT)

ACT programs provide clients with schizophrenia with a wide range of interventions right in their own home or another community setting. For example, trained professionals might visit clients to assist them with taking their prescriptions as directed or to provide individualized cognitive-behavioral therapy. Other services often provided through ACT programs include substance abuse treatment, mobile crisis intervention, occupational therapy and job placement, family counseling, assistance with activities of daily living, educational planning, and help accessing legal services, financial services, transportation, and safe and affordable housing (National Alliance on Mental Illness, 2013a).

stay comes with his initial psychotic episode. During this admission, the client undergoes a variety of physical and psychological tests. Medications are administered to bring symptoms under control, at which point the client is discharged, usually with referrals to outpatient treatment services. Further hospitalizations may also be necessary under certain circumstances. The primary reason for subsequent hospital stays is a relapse of symptoms. Clients may also be hospitalized if they threaten or are violent toward others, or if they are at serious risk of suicide. In these latter two cases, admission may be involuntary.

ELECTROCONVULSIVE THERAPY **Electroconvulsive therapy (ECT)** is a process by which electric currents are passed through an individual's brain to trigger a brief seizure and thereby reduce symptoms of psychosis. Originally developed in 1938, ECT now has a negative reputation due to past instances of unsafe usage, many of which produced side effects including memory loss and broken bones. Today, however, ECT treatment is delivered in a safer and more controlled manner (National Institute of Mental Health, 2013).

Modern-day ECT typically is employed in situations where pharmaceutical and psychological interventions are unsuccessful. Common symptoms addressed with ECT include severe depression, depression with psychosis, severe suicidal thoughts and behaviors, and treatment-resistant symptoms of mania, all of which can also be symptoms of schizophrenia. ECT often works more quickly than pharmaceutical treatment, which can sometimes take 2–3 months to be effective, but it is not without its risks. Acute side effects include headaches, confusion, and muscle pains. Between 25% and 67% of clients also experience chronic memory effects, such as problems with new memory formation, which can last a few days or weeks or sometimes much longer (Duckworth & Freedman, 2012a).

Complementary and Alternative Therapy

Some individuals with schizophrenia become frustrated with the lack of progress in the course of their disease or with the significant side effects of traditional treatments. These reasons, along with cultural beliefs and other lifestyle preferences, lead some clients to try a number of alternative therapeutic measures for schizophrenia, with varying degrees of success.

One somewhat promising alternative therapy is **transcranial magnetic stimulation (TMS)**. This method involves applying an electromagnetic stimulus to the scalp to affect brain activity in the cerebral cortex. Because the cerebral cortex is thought to be involved with auditory hallucinations, TMS may be effective in treating both the length and regularity of these hallucinations. An initial review demonstrated that TMS may indeed help control auditory hallucinations, but further research about the effectiveness of this method is still needed (Simon, 2012).

Whereas antipsychotic medications often have debilitating side effects, another alternative therapy, use of omega-3 fatty acid supplements, can produce positive results without significant adverse effects. Some scientists believe that a malfunction in fatty acid metabolism may be involved in schizophrenia. This may explain why one study found that individuals with subthreshold psychosis symptoms who were at high risk of an initial psychotic episode saw a significant decrease in their progression to full-blown psychotic disorder after taking omega-3 fatty acids. Moreover, these individuals also experienced improved cognitive functioning and a reduction in positive, negative, and general symptoms as compared with members of a placebo group (Amminger et al., 2010). A similar study of women with psychotic-like symptoms found a lower symptom rate in those who consumed omega-3 and omega-6 fatty acids (Hedelin et al., 2010). However, other studies have shown no measurable benefits of omega-3 fatty acid intake, so further research remains to be done.

Aromatherapy, in which various plant oils are inhaled or applied to the skin, is another potential complementary treatment. The effects of aromatherapy are believed to stem from stimulation of the olfactory receptors in the nose. These receptors relay the message to the limbic system, which is the part of the central nervous system that controls emotions (Bauer, 2011). Some studies have shown that aromatherapy can reduce stress (Kim et al., 2011), anxiety levels (Y. L. Lee et al., 2011), and symptoms of dementia, and it can also improve cognitive function, quality of life, and independent living ability (Fung, Tsang, & Chung, 2012). However, not all studies have shown conclusive effects (M. S. Lee et al., 2012), and further research is warranted. Also, there can be side effects of aromatherapy, including allergic reactions, skin irritation, and sun sensitivity (Bauer, 2011).

◼ NURSING PROCESS

Primarily, nursing goals for clients with schizophrenia include promoting symptom control and facilitating effective coping to help the client achieve optimal mental, physical, and social functioning. Ideally, the client will avoid further episodes of psychosis and be able to function successfully in the community to the greatest degree possible.

Assessment

Nursing assessment of a client with schizophrenia typically involves three main elements: a health history, a physical examination, and a mental status examination. The health history can reveal risk factors for schizophrenia, as well as help identify early signs of psychosis in clients who have not yet been diagnosed. For the client with known or suspected schizophrenia, elements of the health history should include the following:

- Age
- Family history of schizophrenia and other psychotic disorders
- Recent changes in behavior, cognition, memory, and/or communication ability
- Alterations in mood
- Disrupted sleep patterns
- Difficulty performing activities of daily living
- Drug and alcohol use
- Paternal age
- Possible birth complications, in utero viral exposure, and/or poor prenatal care
- Poor family communication patterns, especially during childhood
- History of commonly comorbid disorders (e.g., addiction, anxiety disorders, mood disorders)
- Presence or emergence of major life stressors

Clinical Manifestations and Therapies **Schizophrenia**

ETIOLOGY	CLINICAL MANIFESTATIONS	CLINICAL THERAPIES
Positive symptoms of psychosis	■ Hallucinations ■ Delusions ■ Thought disorders ■ Disorganized behavior ■ Movement disorders	■ Administration of conventional antipsychotics, atypical antipsychotics, and/or dopamine system stabilizers ■ Psychiatric/psychosocial rehabilitation, including education about symptom management and signs of relapse ■ Cognitive-behavioral therapy ■ Assertive community treatment ■ Group and/or family therapy ■ Hospitalization (for first psychotic episode and later episodes as necessary) ■ Electroconvulsive therapy ■ Transcranial magnetic stimulation ■ Omega-3 fatty acids ■ Aromatherapy
Negative symptoms of psychosis	■ Anhedonia ■ Impaired memory ■ Flat affect ■ Avolition and lack of focus ■ Poverty of speech ■ Poor personal hygiene ■ Poor problem solving	■ Administration of atypical antipsychotics and/or dopamine system stabilizers ■ Psychiatric/psychosocial rehabilitation, including education about symptom management and signs of relapse ■ Cognitive-behavioral therapy ■ Assertive community treatment ■ Group and/or family therapy ■ Hospitalization (for first psychotic episode and later episodes as necessary) ■ Electroconvulsive therapy ■ Omega-3 fatty acids ■ Aromatherapy
Impaired social functioning	■ Withdrawal ■ Isolation ■ Difficulty maintaining relationships	■ Psychiatric/psychosocial rehabilitation, including practice interacting in social situations ■ Group and/or family therapy ■ Assertive community treatment
Impaired occupational functioning	■ Lack of job skills ■ Inability to adhere to work schedule ■ Difficulty interacting with others in the workplace	■ Psychiatric/psychosocial rehabilitation, including practice interacting in workplace situations ■ Occupational therapy ■ Job training and placement ■ Group and/or family therapy ■ Assertive community treatment
Inability to live independently	■ Poor coping skills ■ Inability to carry out activities of daily living (bathing, dressing, money management, etc.)	■ Psychiatric/psychosocial rehabilitation, including practice and assistance with performing activities of daily living ■ Occupational therapy ■ Group and/or family therapy ■ Assertive community treatment (with a focus on maintaining compliance with prescribed drug regimen)

For the client diagnosed with schizophrenia, the nurse should also ask about possible risk factors for exacerbations or signs of relapse, such as:

- Poor compliance with the prescribed treatment regimen (especially pharmacologic therapy)
- Possible development of resistance to antipsychotic medications
- Presence of mild to full-blown symptoms of psychosis
- Recent life events that may increase the likelihood of relapse

Next, during the physical assessment, the nurse should evaluate the client's height, weight, vital signs, and overall physical condition. Throughout the physical exam, the nurse should remain alert for possible signs of malnutrition, drug/alcohol abuse, poor self-care, depression, and elevated anxiety, as schizophrenia increases the risk for all of these. The nurse should specifically inquire about any medications and supplements the client is taking, not only to monitor drug compliance, but also to check for possible interactions and adverse effects. In addition, the physical examination is a good time to look for common side effects of antipsychotic therapy, such as tardive dyskinesia and acute dystonia.

Finally, individuals with known or suspected schizophrenia should receive a thorough mental status examination. Nurses can choose from a variety of assessment instruments, as described in the Mental Assessment feature on pages 1588–1589. Regardless of which tool is used, the nurse should closely monitor for possible manifestations of schizophrenia throughout the mental status exam, including communication difficulties, delusions, movement disorders, and sensory and perceptual abnormalities. The nurse should also keep the client's cultural and religious background in mind, as this can affect an individual's description and interpretation of symptoms like auditory and visual hallucinations.

Following the health history, physical exam, and mental status examination, several steps may be appropriate. For an individual suspected of having but not yet diagnosed with schizophrenia, referral to a psychologist, psychiatrist, or other physician may be warranted. Laboratory testing and imaging studies may also be necessary to rule out other potential health problems. When working with a client who has already been diagnosed with schizophrenia, the nurse should note any significant changes in the client's signs, symptoms, and behaviors since the last assessment. In addition, the nurse should investigate the client's living situation and compliance with the prescribed treatment regimen.

Diagnosis

Appropriate nursing diagnoses for clients with schizophrenia vary depending on an individual's symptoms and level of functioning. Still, some diagnoses are likely to apply to many, if not most, clients. Some examples of such diagnoses include:

- *Risk for Injury*
- *Imbalanced Nutrition: Less Than Body Requirements*
- *Risk for Imbalanced Nutrition: More Than Body Requirements*
- *Ineffective Health Maintenance*
- *Self-Care Deficit (Bathing and/or Dressing)*
- *Acute Confusion*
- *Impaired Memory*
- *Impaired Verbal Communication*

- *Impaired Social Interaction*
- *Ineffective Coping*
- *Noncompliance*

(NANDA-I © 2012)

Other diagnoses may be appropriate for clients who are experiencing acute or severe psychosis and are unable to function outside the healthcare setting. Examples include the following:

- *Risk for Suicide*
- *Risk for Self-Directed Violence*
- *Risk for Other-Directed Violence*
- *Self-Neglect*
- *Stress Overload*
- *Dysfunctional Family Processes*
- *Disabled Family Coping*
- *Adult Failure to Thrive*
- *Social Isolation*

(NANDA-I © 2012)

Planning

The planning portion of the nursing process involves identifying desired client outcomes and formulating steps for achieving those outcomes. For clients with schizophrenia, appropriate nursing outcomes typically fall into one of three broad categories: symptom reduction, improved quality of life, and helping clients achieve life goals. Examples of specific outcomes in each category are provided in **Box 23–3** ●.

Implementation

Implementation involves evidence-based nursing interventions that facilitate the client's achievement of identified goals of care. Although appropriate interventions will vary, the following principles apply to most clients diagnosed with schizophrenia.

Box 23–3   Sample Nursing Outcomes for Clients With Schizophrenia

OUTCOMES RELATED TO SYMPTOM REDUCTION:

- Client will no longer experience hallucinations and delusions.
- Client will experience a reduction in disordered thought.
- Client will demonstrate appropriate affect.
- Client will experience fewer negative symptoms of schizophrenia.
- Client will take all medications as prescribed.

OUTCOMES RELATED TO QUALITY OF LIFE:

- Client will demonstrate appropriate self-care and personal hygiene.
- Client will obtain adequate sleep.
- Client will refrain from use of alcohol and/or illicit drugs.
- Client will demonstrate improved coping skills.
- Client will make a concerted effort to interact with others and avoid social isolation.

OUTCOMES RELATED TO ACHIEVING LIFE GOALS:

- Client will cultivate appropriate occupational skills.
- Client will find a job and maintain gainful employment.
- Client will retain responsibility for personal finances.
- Client will live independently in the community.

Prevent Injury

The nurse's first priority of care should be to provide a safe environment for clients with schizophrenia and prevent them from engaging in violence toward self or others. When hallucinating or interpreting others' actions and statements from the standpoint of delusions, the client may believe herself to be in danger, regardless of whether there is a factual basis for her fear. Under such circumstances, both the client and perceived aggressors may be at risk for injury.

Nursing interventions directed toward promoting safety and preventing injury may include administering antipsychotic medications as ordered, ensuring that the client's surroundings are free of potentially harmful objects, minimizing environmental stimuli, appropriately using physical restraints if necessary, and referring the client for hospitalization.

Provide Symptomatic Treatment

The nurse's second priority should be promoting control of the client's current symptoms and minimizing the likelihood that additional symptoms will arise. Applicable nursing interventions may include orienting the client to person and place; avoiding overwhelming or overstimulating the client; remaining calm and consistent when speaking with the client; and always informing the client before touching him. When the client appears to be experiencing hallucinations or delusions, the nurse should explain that she is not experiencing or thinking these things, yet she understands that they are real for the client. In some cases, the nurse may opt to explore the content of the client's delusions or hallucinations in an attempt to learn more about his state of mind. Of course, the nurse must also ensure that clients understand and are able to follow all parts of their treatment regimen. Many times, clients will require referral to various community agencies that can assist with such things as finding support groups, remembering to take their medications, and obtaining transportation to and from doctors' appointments and therapy sessions.

Educate Clients and Significant Others

Teaching and encouragement are another vital area of intervention for both clients with schizophrenia and their families. Inform clients and their loved ones about the symptoms and course of the disease, available therapeutic options and how they work, possible medication side effects, and potential signs of relapse. The nurse should also explore clients' and families' current communication and coping skills and encourage the development of new and potentially more effective strategies. Clients themselves should be encouraged to adopt healthier behaviors, such as discontinuing use of nicotine and alcohol, obtaining adequate sleep, and eating a balanced diet. Social skills training is often appropriate, as is encouraging clients to participate in activities that minimize their likelihood of social isolation and withdrawal. In addition, many individuals derive great benefit from training (or perhaps retraining) in how to perform various occupational skills and activities of daily living. To keep clients on the path toward fuller functioning and possibly even independent living, the nurse should be sure to provide frequent positive reinforcement for desired actions and behaviors.

Demonstrate Client Advocacy

The nurse must take steps to advocate on behalf of clients with schizophrenia. Here, the nurse should ensure that all interventions and therapies are actually in a client's best interests and not merely intended to ease the burden on the client's family and caregivers. The nurse should also make sure clients understand their legal rights to the greatest degree possible. Because individuals with schizophrenia are often unable to understand or independently exercise these rights during periods of acute psychosis, they should be encouraged to develop advance directives and similar documents explaining their wishes at times when their schizophrenia is well controlled.

Evaluation

Ongoing evaluation is critical for clients with schizophrenia, as it allows nurses to monitor their condition and adjust any client-specific diagnoses, goals, and interventions as necessary. Some general examples of potential achieved outcomes for clients with schizophrenia include the following:

- The client maintains and follows the medication regimen.
- The client demonstrates utilization of available community resources.
- The client communicates clearly and transitions logically between topics.
- The client reports an absence of hallucinations and/or delusions.
- The client is able to perform activities of daily living.
- The client refrains from use of nicotine, alcohol, and illicit drugs.
- The client engages in paid work in a structured setting.

Client Teaching **Family Communication**

Poor family communication skills may contribute to the development of schizophrenia—as well as to symptom relapse in affected individuals. By teaching families more effective communication skills, nurses not only help minimize the likelihood of relapse, but they also provide family members with the tools they need to more effectively deal with the stress of having a loved one with schizophrenia.

One useful method for teaching improved communication skills is for the nurse to describe a nonthreatening event, then guide the family through new ways of talking about that event. Throughout this process, the nurse should be sure to model the following skills:

- Using "I" language to express positive feelings (e.g., "I am happy when you decide to sit down for dinner with us")
- Engaging in active listening (e.g., asking questions and nodding in agreement when another person speaks)
- Making positive, specific requests for change that are linked to emotions (e.g., "I would really like it if you could play a game with us tonight")
- Expressing negative feelings with "I" rather than "you" language (e.g., saying "I'm worried that you may not be getting enough sleep" instead of "You never get enough sleep at night")

After teaching these skills, the nurse should have family members schedule a time for practice. It's also important for the nurse to emphasize that the more often family members use these skills, the more natural they will become.

NURSING CARE PLAN   A Client With Schizophrenia

Lauren Hildebrand, age 22, is brought to a private mental health center by her father, Peter, who is concerned about recent changes in her behavior. He reports that she is demonstrating increasing difficulty expressing her thoughts and that she often stops talking midsentence, as though she's forgotten what she was saying. He also states that Ms. Hildebrand dropped out of her graduate program in engineering 4 months ago because she suddenly was unable to maintain her grades. Mr. Hildebrand believes these problems are tied to cocaine use.

ASSESSMENT

Angel Sanchez, the RN at the health center, obtains a patient history and physical examination of Ms. Hildebrand. Mr. Sanchez notes that Ms. Hildebrand was adopted as an infant and little is known about her birth mother beyond the fact that she was homeless at the time Ms. Hildebrand was born. Until 10 months ago, Ms. Hildebrand was an A student at the local university and was awarded a position as a graduate assistant in the engineering department. Shortly after beginning her assistantship, she began having problems expressing herself. At first, she simply seemed distracted, rapidly switching from one topic to another in conversation; this eventually segued into problems logically connecting thoughts and completing sentences. Within 6 months, Ms. Hildebrand was no longer able to maintain her grades and job responsibilities and was forced to drop out of the graduate program. Around this time, her friends became aware of her drug problem. Out of concern, they contacted her parents.

Ms. Hildebrand's clothes are relatively new and fashionable, but they are rumpled and smell strongly of body odor. It appears that Ms. Hildebrand hasn't bathed or combed her hair in several days. Her affect is flat. Mr. Sanchez detects redness in and around Ms. Hildebrand's nostrils and notices that she frequently rubs her nose, both of which suggest insufflation of cocaine. Ms. Hildebrand admits that she uses but states that she hasn't used in 3 days. She has difficulty answering Mr. Sanchez's other questions; her speech is garbled and relies heavily on rhyming words that do not make sense when strung together. Ms. Hildebrand is very thin, and the shape of her arm, hand, and clavicle bones stands out clearly under her skin. Her vital signs include T 100.1°F oral, P 95 bpm; R 22/min; and BP 131/88 mmHg.

Based on his mental status assessment of Ms. Hildebrand, Mr. Sanchez suspects schizophrenia. The psychiatrist orders an MRI to rule out abnormalities such as brain tumors. Aside from slightly enlarged ventricles, Ms. Hildebrand's MRI does not reveal any unusual findings. After speaking with Ms. Hildebrand's father, the psychiatrist interviews Ms. Hildebrand, after which he diagnoses her with probable acute schizophrenia. Based on her mental state and substance abuse, the psychiatrist recommends Ms. Hildebrand complete a 28-day inpatient stay at the mental health center, where she will receive treatment for her psychiatric condition and substance abuse. He also prescribes olanzapine, 5 mg/day for 1 week, to be followed by 2.5 mg/day increases each week until Miss Hildebrand exhibits improvement, not to exceed 20 mg/day.

DIAGNOSES

- *Risk for Injury* related to disorganized thinking patterns and substance abuse
- *Impaired Social Interaction* related to altered cognitive function
- *Impaired Verbal Communication* related to perceptual and cognitive impairment
- *Ineffective Health Maintenance* related to perceptual and cognitive impairment
- *Self-Care Deficit* (Bathing/hygiene) related to cognitive impairment and substance abuse
- *Imbalanced Nutrition: Less Than Body Requirements* related to cognitive impairment and substance abuse

(NANDA-I © 2012)

PLANNING

Goals for Ms. Hildebrand's care include:

- The client will remain free from injury.
- The client will demonstrate clear communication patterns.
- The client will verbalize logical thought processes.
- The client will exercise appropriate self-care and hygiene measures, including bathing or showering daily and completing oral hygiene care twice daily.
- The client will discontinue cocaine use.
- The client will gain 1 to 2 lbs of weight per week.
- The client will engage in appropriate rehabilitation and group therapy activities while hospitalized and after release.

IMPLEMENTATION

- Monitor the client for indicators that suggest the potential for injury to self or others.
- Ensure the client receives care that promotes physical and psychological safety.
- Administer all medications as ordered.
- Counsel client about cocaine dependence and monitor for signs and symptoms of withdrawal.
- Assist the client with establishing a pattern of self-care that includes adequate nutritional intake and hygiene.

- Teach client and family members how to cope with schizophrenia and how to respond to signs of relapse.
- Encourage the client to attend and engage in group therapy sessions.
- Prepare the client for release and assertive community treatment at the end of the inpatient rehabilitation period.

NURSING CARE PLAN   (continued)

EVALUATION

Mr. Sanchez works closely with Ms. Hildebrand during her stay at the mental health center. While at the center, Ms. Hildebrand receives education about her disorder, its causes and symptoms, and complications commonly associated with it. She also receives substance abuse counseling, cognitive-behavioral therapy, and vocational counseling to prepare her to find a job after she is released. Her medication is gradually increased over the course of her stay until she reaches an effective dose of 12.5 mg/day. By the end of her inpatient stay, Ms. Hildebrand is able to demonstrate appropriate self-care skills related to hygiene, nutrition, and medication administration. She can also clearly and logically describe the symptoms of her condition and verbalize strategies for coping with them. She is scheduled to return to the center twice each week for group therapy and has an appointment to meet with an ACT provider.

CRITICAL THINKING

1. Based on the little we know of Ms. Hildebrand's birth mother, can we draw any conclusions about either Ms. Hildebrand's genetic predisposition to schizophrenia or environmental factors prior to her birth that may have predisposed her to this disorder? Why is it reasonable to draw these conclusions?
2. Research ACT in your geographical area. What types of services are offered, and which of these services would you recommend to Ms. Hildebrand if she were your client? Why would you recommend them?
3. Develop a care plan for the nursing diagnosis Risk for Self-Directed Violence related to disruptions in cognitive processes.

REVIEW Schizophrenia

RELATE Link the Concepts and Exemplars

Linking the exemplar of schizophrenia with the concept of immunity:

1. Why might clients with schizophrenia be at a heightened risk of HIV infection and AIDS?
2. What measures might you implement when caring for a client with schizophrenia to limit the risk of HIV exposure?

Linking the exemplar of schizophrenia with the concept of addiction:

3. Why are clients with schizophrenia more likely to abuse nicotine, alcohol, and illicit drugs? Be sure to explore physical, social, and psychological factors in your response.
4. What special challenges might arise when addressing addiction behaviors in clients with schizophrenia (as opposed to other clients)? Why? How might the nurse attempt to overcome these challenges?

Linking the exemplar of schizophrenia with the concept of managing care:

5. Why are care coordination and case management especially important for clients with schizophrenia?
6. What sort of professionals might be involved in the overall plan of care for a client with schizophrenia? How could the nurse promote better collaboration and communication among these providers?

READY Go to Companion Skills Manual

REFER Go to Pearson Student Nursing Resources
nursing.pearsonhighered.com

•Additional review material

REFLECT Case Study

Dwight Gibson, a 46-year-old male, is brought to the emergency department by his landlord, Ms. Alder. Ms. Alder is concerned about Mr. Gibson's current mental state. She reports that his behavior has always been eccentric for the 5 years she's known him. For example, he perpetually seems worried that someone is "out to get him" and has installed extra locks on his doors and windows.

Lately, however, Ms. Alder has felt that Mr. Gibson's behavior is progressing from merely unusual to severely disturbed. Ms. Alder explains that she lives in the apartment below Mr. Gibson's, and several times over the past month, she's heard him yelling. When Ms. Alder goes to check on him, he tells her he's arguing with the "voices," yet there's never anyone else in the apartment with him. Ms. Alder also mentions that Mr. Gibson seems to be letting garbage accumulate in his apartment, as it smells quite bad. Upon observation, Mr. Gibson's hair is dirty, and his clothes are stained and torn. As the nurse conducting Mr. Gibson's initial assessment, you introduce yourself to him and ask how he is feeling. He replies that he is feeling fine. Next, you ask Mr. Gibson if you may check his blood pressure. He appears agitated and states, "They told you to do that, didn't they? They're trying to steal my spirit. They're afraid my spirit will tell me the truth. I will not let you do that."

1. What additional assessment information do you need?
2. How should you respond to Mr. Gibson's refusal to allow you to assess his blood pressure?
3. What are Mr. Gibson's priorities of care at this time?
4. Should Mr. Gibson be determined to be suffering from schizophrenia, what nursing diagnoses would be appropriate for inclusion in his plan of care?

■ REFERENCES

Abel, K. M., Drake, R., & Goldstein, J. M. (2010). Sex differences in schizophrenia. *International Review of Psychiatry, 22*(5), 417–428.

Alexopoulous, G. S., Abrams, R. C., Young, R. C., & Shamoian, C. A. (1988). Cornell Scale for Depression in Dementia. *Biological Psychiatry, 23*(3), 271–284.

Alzheimer's Association. (2012). *2012 Alzheimer's Disease Facts and Figures.* Retrieved from http://www.alz.org/downloads/facts_figures_2012.pdf.

Alzheimer's Association. (2013a). *Adopt a brain-healthy diet.* Retrieved from http://www.alz.org/we_can_help_adopt_a_brain_healthy_diet.asp.

Alzheimer's Association. (2013b). *Alternative treatments.* Retrieved from http://www.alz.org/alzheimers_disease_alternative_treatments.asp.

Alzheimer's Association. (2013c). *Alzheimer's facts and figures.* Retrieved from http://www.alz.org/alzheimers_disease_facts_and_figures.asp.

Alzheimer's Association. (2013d). *Alzheimer's myths.* Retrieved from http://www.alz.org/alzheimers_disease_myths_about_alzheimers.asp.

Alzheimer's Association. (2013e). *Medications for memory loss.* Retrieved from http://www.alz.org/alzheimers_disease_standard_prescriptions.asp.

Alzheimer's Association. (2013f). *Seven stages of Alzheimer's.* Retrieved from http://www.alz.org/alzheimers_disease_stages_of_alzheimers.asp.

Alzheimer's Association. (2013g). *Types of dementia.* Retrieved from http://www.alz.org/dementia/types-of-dementia.asp.

Alzheimer's Society. (2013a). *Am I at risk of developing dementia?* Retrieved from http://www.alzheimers.org.uk/site/scripts/documents_info.php?documentID=102.

Alzheimer's Society. (2013b.) *Drug treatments for Alzheimer's disease.* Retrieved from http://www.alzheimers.org.uk/site/scripts/documents_info.php?documentID=147.

Alzheimer's Society. (2013c). *Genetics of dementia.* Retrieved from https://www.alzheimers.org.uk/factsheet/405.

Amad, A., Cachia, A., Gorwood, P., Pins, D., Delmaire, C., Rolland, B., . . . Jardri, R. (2013). The multimodal connectivity of the hippocampal complex in auditory and visual hallucinations. *Molecular Psychiatry* (January 15 e-Publication).

American Association on Intellectual and Developmental Disabilities. (2013). *FAQ on intellectual disability.* Retrieved from http://www.aaidd.org/content_104.cfm.

American Psychiatric Association. (2013). *Diagnostic and Statistical Manual of Mental Disorders* (5th ed.). Washington, DC: Author.

American Psychological Association. (n.d.). *Patient health questionnaire PHQ-9 and PHQ-2.* Accessed from http://www.apa.org/pi/about/publications/caregivers/practice-settings/assessment/tools/patient-health.aspx.

American Psychological Association. (2013a). *Memory and aging.* Retrieved from http://www.apa.org/pi/aging/memory-and-aging.pdf.

American Psychological Association. (2013b). *What practitioners should know about working with older adults.* Retrieved from http://www.apa.org/pi/aging/resources/guides/practitioners-should-know.aspx#.

Amminger, G. P., Henry, L. P., Harrigan, S. M., Harris, M. G., Alvarez-Jimenez, M., Herrman, H., . . . McGorry, P. D. (2011). Outcome in early-onset schizophrenia revisited: Findings from the Early Psychosis Prevention and Intervention Centre long-term follow-up study. *Schizophrenia Research, 131*(1), 112–119.

Amminger, G., Schäfer, M., Papageorgiou, K., Klier, C. M., Cotton, A. M., Mackinnon, A., . . . Berger, G. E. (2010). Long-chain ω-3 fatty acids for indicated prevention of psychotic disorders: A randomized, placebo-controlled trial. *Archives of General Psychiatry, 67*(2), 146–154.

The Arc. (2011). *Resources.* Retrieved from http://www.thearc.org/page.aspx?pid=2453.

Asarnow, J. R., Goldstein, M. J., & Ben-Meir, S. (1988). Parental communication deviance in childhood onset schizophrenia spectrum and depressive disorders. *Journal of Child Psychology and Psychiatry, 29*(6), 825–838.

Ballard, H. S. (1997). The hematological complications of alcoholism. *Alcohol Heath and Research World, 21*(1), 42–52. Available online at http://pubs.niaaa.nih.gov/publications/arh21-1/42.pdf.

Bartzokis, G. (2004). Age-related myelin breakdown: A developmental model of cognitive decline and Alzheimer's disease. *Neurobiology of Aging, 25*(1), 5–18.

Bateson, G., Jackson, J., Haley, J., & Weakland, J. (1956). Toward a theory of schizophrenia. *Behavioral Science, 1*(4), 251–264.

Bauer, B. (2011). *What are the benefits of aromatherapy?* Retrieved from http://www.mayoclinic.com/health/aromatherapy/AN02140.

Beck, M. (2012). Stricter thinking on alcohol use during pregnancy. *Wall Street Journal,* January 24. Retrieved from http://online.wsj.com/article/SB10001424052970203718504577178850309081474.html.

Bitanihirwe, B. K., Peleg-Raibstein, D., Mouttet, F., Feldon, J., & Meyer, U. (2010). Late prenatal immune activation in mice leads to behavioral and neurochemical abnormalities relevant to the negative symptoms of schizophrenia. *Neuropsychopharmacology, 35*(12), 2462–2478.

Breitner, J. C., Baker, L. D., Montine, T. J., Meinert, C. L., Lyketsos, C. G., Ashe, K. H., . . Tariot, P. N. (2011). Extended results of the Alzheimer's disease anti-inflammatory prevention trial. *Alzheimer's and Dementia, 7*(4), 402–11.

Buckley, P. F., Miller, B. J., Lehrer, D. S., & Castle, D. J. (2009). Psychiatric comorbidities and schizophrenia. *Schizophrenia Bulletin, 35*(2), 383–402.

Cardno, A., & Gottesman, I. (2000). Twin studies of schizophrenia: From bow-and-arrow concordances to star wars mx and functional genomics. *American Journal of Medical Genetics, 97*(1), 12–17.

Centers for Disease Control and Prevention. (2011a). *Facts about Down syndrome.* Retrieved from http://www.cdc.gov/ncbddd/birthdefects/DownSyndrome.html.

Centers for Disease Control and Prevention. (2011b). *Facts about FASDs.* Retrieved from www.cdc.gov/NCBDDD/fasd/facts.html.

Centers for Disease Control and Prevention. (2012). *Fetal alcohol spectrum disorders (FASDs): Data and statistics.* Retrieved from http://www.cdc.gov/ncbddd/fasd/data.html.

Cleveland Clinic. (2009a). *Schizophrenia.* Retrieved from http://my.clevelandclinic.org/disorders/Schizophrenia/hic_Schizophrenia_2.aspx.

Cleveland Clinic. (2009b). *Schizophrenia overview.* Retrieved from http://my.clevelandclinic.org/disorders/schizophrenia/hic_schizophrenia.aspx Cleveland Clinic. (2010). *Cerebral hypoxia.* http://my.clevelandclinic.org/disorders/cerebral_hypoxia/hic_Cerebral_Hypoxia.aspx.

Cleveland Clinic. (2011). *Alzheimer's disease: Overview of diagnostic tests.* Retrieved from http://my.clevelandclinic.org/disorders/alzheimers_disease/hic_alzheimers_disease_overview_of_diagnostic_tests.aspx.

Contestabile, A. (2011). The history of the cholinergic hypothesis. *Behavioural Brain Research, 221*(2), 334–40.

Cortiella, C. (2011). *The state of learning disabilities.* New York, NY: National Center for Learning Disabilities. Retrieved from http://www.ncld.org/images/stories/OnCapitolHill/PolicyRelatedPublications/stateofld/2011_state_of_ld_final.pdf.

Counts, S. E., Perez, S. E., & Mufson, E. J. (2008). Galanin in Alzheimer's disease: Neuroinhibitory or neuroprotective? *Cellular and Molecular Life Sciences, 65*(12), 1842–1853.

Crow, T. J. (1980). Molecular pathology of schizophrenia: More than one disease process? *British Medical Journal, 280*(6207), 66.

Davey, G. (Ed.). (2011). *Applied psychology.* West Sussex, UK: Wiley.

Deary, I. J., Corley, J., Gow, A. J., Harris, S. E., Houlihan, L. M., Marioni, R. E., . . . Starr, J. M. (2009). Age-associated cognitive decline. *British Medical Bulletin, 92*(1), 135–152.

Deary, I. J., Yang, J., Davies, G., Harris, S. E., Tenesa, A., Liewald, D., . . . Visscher, P. M. (2012). Genetic contributions to stability and change in intelligence from childhood to old age. *Nature, 482,* 212–215.

Duckworth, K., & Freedman, J. (2012a). *Electroconvulsive therapy.* Retrieved from http://www.nami.org/Content/NavigationMenu/Inform_Yourself/About_Mental_Illness/About_Treatments_and_Supports/Electroconvulsive_Therapy_%28ECT%29.htm.

Duckworth, K., & Freedman, J. (2012b). *Obsessive-compulsive disorder.* Retrieved from http://www.nami.org/Template.cfm?Section=By_Illness&Template=/ContentManagement/ContentDisplay.cfm&ContentID=142546.

Duckworth, K., & Freedman, J. (2012c). *Schizoaffective disorder.* Retrieved from http://www.nami.org/Template.cfm?Section=By_Illness&Template=/ContentManagement/ContentDisplay.cfm&ContentID=23043.

Elkis, H., Friedman, L., Wise, A., & Meltzer, H. Y. (1995). Meta-analyses of studies of ventricular enlargement and cortical sulcal prominence in mood disorders: Comparisons with controls or patients with schizophrenia. *Archives of General Psychiatry, 52,* 735–746.

Fink, M., Shorter, E., & Taylor, M. A. (2010). Catatonia is not schizophrenia: Kraepelin's error and the need to recognize catatonia as an independent syndrome in medical nomenclature. *Schizophrenia Bulletin, 36*(2), 314–320.

Fisher Center for Alzheimer's Research Foundation. (2007). *Therapy pets proving soothing to people with Alzheimer's.* Retrieved from http://www.alzinfo.org/02/articles/caregiving-13.

Flanagan, N. M., & Fick, D. M. (2010). Delirium superimposed on dementia: Assessment and intervention. *Journal of Gerontological Nursing, 36*(11), 19–23.

Fong, T. G., Tulebaev, S. R., & Inouye, S. K. (2009.) Delirium in elderly adults: Diagnosis, prevention and treatment. *Nature Reviews Neurology, 5*(4), 210–220.

Franzen, M., & Getz, G. (2010). *Screening for brain impairment.* New York, NY: Springer.

Fung, J. K. K., Tsang, H. W., & Chung, R. C. (2012). A systematic review of the use of aromatherapy in treatment of behavioral problems in dementia. *Geriatrics and Gerontology International, 12*(3), 372–382.

Gaebel, W. (Ed.). (2011). *Schizophrenia: Current science and clinical practice.* Hoboken, NJ: Wiley-Blackwell.

Galasko, D. R., Peskind, E., Clark, C. M., Quinn, J. F., Ringman, J. M., Jicha, G. A., . . Aisen, P. (2012). Antioxidants for Alzheimer disease: A randomized clinical trial with cerebrospinal fluid biomarker measures. *Archives of Neurology, 69*(7), 836–841.

Gay, K., Duckworth, K., Aron, L., Carolla, B., & Lehman, C. (2008). *Schizophrenia: Public attitudes, personal needs.* Retrieved from http://www.nami.org/Content/NavigationMenu/NAMILand/COMMschizophreniareport.pdf.

Giovanoli, S., Engler, H., Engler, A., Richetto, J., Voget, M., Willi, R., . . . Meyer, U. (2013). Stress in puberty unmasks latent neuropathological consequences of prenatal immune activation in mice. *Science, 339*(6123), 1095–1099.

Goldacre, B. (2010). Smoking prevents Alzheimer's? It depends who you ask. *Guardian,* March 5. Retrieved from http://www.guardian.co.uk/science/2010/mar/05/smoking-alzheimers-goldacre-bad-science.

Gottesman, I. I. (1991). *Schizophrenia genesis: The origins of madness.* New York, NY: Freeman.

Gottesman, I. I., Laursen, T. M., Bertelsen, A., & Mortensen, P. B. (2010). Severe mental disorders in offspring with two psychiatrically ill parents. *Archives of General Psychiatry, 67*(3), 252–257.

Gower, L. E. J., Gatewood, M. O., & Kang, C. S. (2012). Emergency department management of delirium in the elderly. *Western Journal of Emergency Medicine, 13*(2), 194–201.

Greenberg, S. A. (2012). The Geriatric Depression Scale (GDS). *Try This: Best Practices in Nursing Care to Older Adults 4*, 1–2. Retrieved from http://consultgerirn.org/uploads/File/trythis/try_this_4.pdf.

Hamilton, M. (1960). A rating scale for depression. *Journal of Neurology, Neurosurgery, and Psychiatry, 23*(1), 56–62. Retrieved from http://www.ncbi.nlm.nih.gov/pmc/articles/PMC495331/?page=1.

Hamlyn, J., Duhig, M., McGrath, J., & Scott, J. (2012). Modifiable risk factors for schizophrenia and autism: Shared risk factors impacting on brain development. *Neurobiology of Disease, 53*, 3–9.

Hawranik, P., Johnston, P., & Deatrich, J. (2008). Therapeutic touch and agitation in individuals with Alzheimer's disease. *Western Journal of Nursing Research, 30*(4), 417–434.

Hedelin, M., Löf, M., Olsson, M., Lewander, T., Nilsson, B., Hultman, C. M., & Weiderpass, E. (2010). Dietary intake of fish, omega-3, omega-6 polyunsaturated fatty acids and vitamin D and the prevalence of psychotic-like symptoms in a cohort of 33,000 women from the general population. *BMC Psychiatry, 10*(1), 38.

Heneka, M. T., Kummer, M. P., Stutz, A., Delekate, A., Schwartz, S., Vieira-Saecker, A.,. . . Golenbock, D. T. (2013). NLRP3 is activated in Alzheimer's disease and contributes to pathology in APP/PS1 mice. *Nature, 493*, 674–678.

Ho, A., Michelson, D., Aaen, G., & Ashwal, S. (2010). Cerebral folate deficiency presenting as adolescent catatonic schizophrenia: A case report. *Journal of Child Neurology, 25*(7), 898–900.

Hoerder-Suabedissen, A., Oeschger, F. M., Krishnan, M. L., Belgard, T. G., Wang, W. Z., Lee, S.,. . . Molnár, Z. (2013). Expression profiling of mouse subplate reveals a dynamic gene network and disease association with autism and schizophrenia. *Proceedings of the National Academy of Sciences, 110*(9), 3555–3560.

Hogarty, G., Anderson, C., Reiss, D., Kornblith, S. J., Greenwald, D. P., Javna, C. D., & Madonia, M. J. (1986). Family psychoeducation, social skills training, and maintenance chemotherapy in the aftercare treatment of schizophrenia: One-year effects of a controlled study on relapse and expressed emotion. *Archives of General Psychiatry, 43*(7), 633–642.

Horowitz, S. H. (2013). *The neurobiology of learning disorders.* Retrieved from http://www.ncld.org/types-learning-disabilities/what-is-ld/neurobiology-learning-disabilities.

Howard, R., Rabins, P., Seeman, M., & Jeste, D. (2000). Late-onset schizophrenia and very-late-onset schizophrenia-like psychosis: An international consensus. *American Journal of Psychiatry, 157*(2), 172–178.

Jackson, C. (2007). The General Health Questionnaire. *Occupational Medicine, 57*(1), 79.

Jackson, K., Fanous, A., Chen, J., Kendler, K., & Chen, X. (2013). Variants in the 15q25 gene cluster are associated with risk for schizophrenia and bipolar disorder. *Psychiatric Genetics, 23*(1), 20–28.

James, B. D., Wilson, R. S., Barnes, L. L, & Bennett, D. A. (2011). Late-life social activity and cognitive decline in old age. *Journal of the International Neuropsychological Society, 17*(6), 998–1005.

Jimbo, D., Kimura, Y., Taniguchi, M., Inoue, M., & Urakami, K. (2009). Effect of aromatherapy on patients with Alzheimer's disease. *Psychogeriatrics, 9*(4), 173–179.

Kelly, D. P., & Aylward, G. P. (2005). Identifying school performance problems in the pediatric office. *Pediatric Annals, 34*, 288–298.

Khan, A. (2013). The amyloid hypothesis and potential treatments for Alzheimer's disease. Retrieved from http://www.alzheimers.org.uk/site/scripts/documents_info.php?documentID=383&pageNumber=6.

Kim, S., Kim, H. J., Yeo, J. S., Hong, S. J., Lee, J. M., & Jeon, Y. (2011). The effect of lavender oil on stress, bispectral index values, and needle insertion pain in volunteers. *Journal of Alternative and Complementary Medicine, 17*(9), 823–826.

Kinros, J., Reichenberg, A., & Frangou, S. (2010). The neurodevelopmental theory of schizophrenia: Evidence from studies of early onset cases. *Israel Journal of Psychiatry and Related Sciences, 47*(2), 110.

Kirino, E. (2012). Efficacy and safety of aripiprazole in child and adolescent patients. *European Child and Adolescent Psychiatry, 21*(7), 361–368.

Landau, S. M., Marks, S. M., Mormino, E. C., Rabinovici, G. D., Oh, H., O'Neil, J. P.,. . . Jaqust, W. G. (2012). Association of lifetime cognitive engagement and low β-amyloid deposition. *Archives of Neurology, 69*(5), 623–629.

Laruelle, M., Abi-Dargham, A., Van Dyck, C. H., Gil, R., D'Souza, C. D., Erdos, J.,. . . & Innis, R. B. (1996). Single photon emission computerized tomography imaging of amphetamine-induced dopamine release in drug-free schizophrenic subjects. *Proceedings of the National Academy of Sciences, 93*(17), 9235–9240.

Lee, M. S., Choi, J., Posadzki, P., & Ernst, E. (2012). Aromatherapy for health care: An overview of systematic reviews. *Maturitas, 71*(3), 257–260.

Lee, M. S., Shin, B. C., Ronan, P., & Ernst, E. (2009). Acupuncture for schizophrenia: A systematic review and meta-analysis. *International Journal of Clinical Practice, 63*(11), 1622–1633.

Lee, T., Henry, J. D., Trollor, J. N., & Sachdev, P. S. (2010). Genetic influences on cognitive functions in the elderly: A selective review of twin studies. *Brain Research Reviews, 64*(1), 1–13.

Lee, Y. L., Wu, Y., Tsang, H. W., Leung, A. Y., & Cheung, W. M. (2011). A systematic review on the anxiolytic effects of aromatherapy in people with anxiety symptoms. *Journal of Alternative and Complementary Medicine, 17*(2), 101–108.

Levy, D. L., Coleman, M. J., Sung, H., Ji, F., Matthysse, S., Mendell, N. R., & Titone, D. (2010). The genetic basis of thought disorder and language and communication disturbances in schizophrenia. *Journal of Neurolinguistics, 23*(3), 176–192.

Li, N. C., Lee, A., Whitmer, R. A., Kivipelto, M., Lawler, E., Kazis, L. E., & Wolozin, B. (2010). Use of angiotensin receptor blockers and risk of dementia in a predominantly male population: Prospective cohort analysis. *British Medical Journal, 340*, b5465.

Lichtenstein, P., Yip, B., Bjork, C., Pawitan, Y., Cannon, T. D., Sullivan, P. F., & Hultman, C. M. (2009). Common genetic determinants of schizophrenia and bipolar disorder in Swedish families: A population-based study. *Lancet, 373*(9659), 234–239.

Lin, P. I., & Shuldiner, A. R. (2010). Rethinking the genetic basis for comorbidity of schizophrenia and type 2 diabetes. *Schizophrenia Research, 123*(2–3), 234–243.

Lladó, A., & Sánchez-Valle, R. (2011). Focusing on atypical symptoms for improved diagnosis of early-onset Alzheimer's disease. *Future Neurology, 6*(5), 575–578.

March of Dimes. (2010.) *Birth defects: Fragile X syndrome.* Retrieved from http://www.marchofdimes.com/baby/birthdefects_fragilex.html.

Mayo Clinic. (2011). *Phenyketonuria (PKU): Tests and diagnosis.* Retrieved from http://www.mayoclinic.com/health/phenylketonuria/DS00514/DSECTION=tests-and-diagnosis.

Mayo Clinic. (2012a). *Alcoholic hepatitis: Complications.* Retrieved from http://www.mayoclinic.com/health/alcoholic-hepatitis/DS00785/DSECTION=complications.

Mayo Clinic. (2012b). *Delirium: Causes.* Retrieved from http://www.mayoclinic.com/health/delirium/DS01064/DSECTION=causes.

Mayo Clinic. (2012c). *Delirium: Symptoms.* Retrieved from http://www.mayoclinic.com/health/delirium/DS01064/DSECTION=symptoms.

Mayo Clinic. (2012d). *Schizophrenia. Prevention.* Retrieved from http://www.mayoclinic.com/health/schizophrenia/DS00196/SECTION=prevention.

Mayo Clinic. (2012e). *Alzheimer's disease.* Retrieved from http://www.mayoclinic.com/health/alzheimers-stages/AZ00041.

Moreno-Gonzalez, I., Estrada, L. D., Sanchez-Mejias, E., & Soto, C. (2012). Smoking exacerbates amyloid pathology in a mouse model of Alzheimer's disease. *Nature Communications, 4*, 1495.

Mukherjee, S., Das, S. K., Vaidyanathan, K., & Vasudevan, D. M. (2008). Consequences of alcohol consumption on neurotransmitters: An overview. *Current Neurovascular Research, 5*, 266–272.

National Alliance on Mental Illness. (2013a). *Assertive community treatment.* Retrieved from http://www.nami.org/Template.cfm?Section=About_Treatments_and_Supports&template=/ContentManagement/ContentDisplay.cfm&ContentID=8075.

National Alliance on Mental Illness. (2013b). *Schizophrenia: Treatment, services and support.* Retrieved from http://www.nami.org/Template.cfm?Section=Schizophrenia9&Template=/ContentManagement/ContentDisplay.cfm&ContentID=118061.

National Association for Down Syndrome. (2013). *Facts about Down syndrome.* Retrieved from http://www.nads.org/pages_new/facts.html.

National Center for Alternative and Complementary Medicine. (2012). *Antioxidants and health: An introduction.* Retrieved from http://nccam.nih.gov/health/antioxidants/introduction.htm#safety.

National Center for Alternative and Complementary Medicine. (2013). *Resveratrol.* Retrieved from http://nccam.nih.gov/health/resveratrol?nav=gsa.

National Center for Learning Disabilities. (2013). *What are learning disabilities?* Retrieved from http://www.ncld.org/types-learning-disabilities/what-is-ld/what-are-learning-disabilities.

National Dissemination Center for Children with Disabilities. (2011). *Intellectual disabilities: NICHCY fact sheet #8.* Retrieved from http://nichcy.org/disability/specific/intellectual#def.

National Down Syndrome Society. (2012a). *CDC study on prevalence of Down syndrome.* Retrieved from http://www.ndss.org/About-NDSS/Media-Kit/Position-Papers/CDC-Study-on-Prevalence-of-Down-Syndrome-/.

National Down Syndrome Society. (2012b). *What is Down syndrome?* Retrieved from http://www.ndss.org/Down-Syndrome/What-Is-Down-Syndrome/.

National Fragile X Foundation. (2013). *Prevalence.* Retrieved from http://www.fragilex.org/fragile-x-associated-disorders/prevalence/.

National Institute of Mental Health. (2009). *Schizophrenia.* Retrieved from http://www.nimh.nih.gov/health/publications/schizophrenia/schizophrenia-booket-2009.pdf.

National Institute of Mental Health. (2013). *Brain stimulation techniques.* Retrieved from http://www.nimh.nih.gov/health/topics/brain-stimulation-therapies/brain-stimulation-therapies.shtml.

National Institute of Neurological Disorders and Stroke. (2012). *NINDS dementia information page.* Retrieved from http://www.ninds.nih.gov/disorders/dementias/dementia.htm.

National Institute on Aging. (2012). *Preventing Alzheimer's disease: What do we know?* Retrieved from http://www.nia.nih.gov/alzheimers/publication/preventing-alzheimers-disease/search-alzheimers-prevention-strategies.

National Organization on Fetal Alcohol Syndrome. (2012a). *FAQs.* Retrieved from http://www.nofas.org/faqs.

National Organization on Fetal Alcohol Syndrome. (2012b). *FASD.* Retrieved from http://www.nofas.org/about-fasd.

Niwa, M., Jaaro-Peled, H., Tankou, S., Seshadri, S., Hikida, T., Matsumoto, Y., . . . Sawa, A. (2013). Adolescent stress-induced epigenetic control of dopaminergic neurons via glucocorticoids. *Science, 339*(6117), 335–339.

Osborn K. S., Wraa, C. E., Watson, A., & Holleran, R. S. (2013). *Medical-surgical nursing: Preparation for practice* (2nd ed.). Upper Saddle River, NJ: Pearson.

Ota, V., Gadelha, A., Assunção, I., Santoro, M., Christofolini, D., Bellucco, F., . . . Jackowski, A. (2013). *ZDHHC8* gene may play a role in cortical volumes of patients with schizophrenia. *Schizophrenia Research, 145*(1–3), 33–35.

Otsuka America Pharmaceutical. (2013). *Abilify.* Retrieved from http://www.abilify.com/Index.aspx.

Parks, J., Svendsen, D., Singer, P., Foti, M., & Mauer, B. (2006). *Morbidity and mortality in people with serious mental illness.* Retrieved from http://www.dsamh.utah.gov/docs/mortality-morbidity_nasmhpd.pdf.

Pfeiffer, E. (1975). A short portable mental status questionnaire for the assessment of organic brain deficit in elderly patients. *Journal of the American Geriatrics Society, 23*(10), 433–441.

Pharoah, F., Mari, J., Rathbone, J., & Wong, W. (2010). Family intervention for schizophrenia. *Cochrane Database of Systematic Reviews, 11.*

Piaget, J. (1966). *Origins of intelligence in children.* New York, NY: Norton.

Piaget, J. (1972). *The child's conception of the world.* Totowa, NJ: Littlefield, Adams.

Plassman, B. L., Langa, K. M., Fisher, G. G., Heeringa, S. G., Weir, D. R., Ofstedal, M. B., . . . Wallace, R. B. (2007). Prevalence of dementia in the United States: The aging, demographics, and memory study. *Neuroepidemiology, 29*(1–2), 125–132.

Poon, I. O. (2008). Effects of antihypertensive drug treatment on the risk of dementia and cognitive impairment. *Pharmacotherapy, 28*(3), 366–375.

Praticò, D. (2008). Oxidative stress hypothesis in Alzheimer's disease: A reappraisal. *Trends in Pharmacological Sciences, 29*(12), 609–615.

Primm, A., Vasquez, M., Mays, R., Sammons-Posey, D., McKnight-Eily, L., Presley-Cantrell, L., . . . Perry, G. S. (2010). The role of public health in addressing racial and ethnic disparities in mental health and mental illness. *Preventing Chronic Disease, 7*(1), A20.

Raiji, T. K., Ismail, Z., & Mulsant, B. H. (2009). Age at onset and cognition in schizophrenia: Meta-analysis. *British Journal of Psychiatry, 195,* 286–293.

Reisberg, B., & Franssen, E. H. (1999). Clinical stages of Alzheimer's disease. In M. J. deLeon (Ed.), *An Atlas of Alzheimer's Disease* (pp. 11–20). Pearl River, NY: Parthenon.

Repo-Tiihonen, E., Hallikainen, T., Kivistö, P., & Tiihonen, J. (2012). Antipsychotic polypharmacy in clozapine resistant schizophrenia: A randomized controlled trial of tapering antipsychotic co-treatment. *Mental Illness, 4*(1), e1.

Rummel-Kluge, C., Komossa, K., Schwarz, S., Hunger, H., Schmid, F., Lobos, C. A., . . . Leucht, S. (2010). Head-to-head comparisons of metabolic side effects of second generation antipsychotics in the treatment of schizophrenia: A systematic review and meta-analysis. *Schizophrenia Research, 123*(2–3), 225.

Rushworth, J. V., Griffiths, H. H., Watt, N. T., & Hooper, N. M. (2013). Prion protein-mediated toxicity of amyloid-β oligomers requires lipid rafts and the transmembrane LRP1. *Journal of Biological Chemistry,* February 5. Retrieved from http://www.jbc.org/content/early/2013/02/05/jbc.M112.400358.full.pdf+html.

Scheuerecker, J., Ufer, S., Käpernick, M., Wiesmann, M., Brückmann, H., Kraft, E., . . . & Meisenzahl, E. M. (2009). Cerebral network deficits in post-acute catatonic schizophrenic patients measured by fMRI. *Journal of Psychiatric Research, 43*(6), 607–614.

Schoepf, D., Potluri, R., Uppal, H., Natalwala, A., Narendran, P., & Heun, R. (2012). Type-2 diabetes mellitus in schizophrenia: Increased prevalence and major risk factor of excess mortality in a naturalistic 7-year follow-up. *European Psychiatry, 27*(1), 33–42.

Shaffer, D. R., & Kipp, K. (2010). *Developmental psychology: Childhood and adolescence* (8th ed.). Belmont, CA: Wadsworth, Cengage Learning.

Simon, H. (2012). *Schizophrenia: Risk factors.* Retrieved from http://health.nytimes.com/health/guides/disease/schizophrenia/risk-factors.html.

Sink, K. M., Leng, X., Williamson, J., Kritchevsky, S. B., Yaffe, K., Kuller, L., . . . Goff, D. C., Jr. (2009). Angiotensin-converting enzyme inhibitors and cognitive decline in older adults with hypertension: Results from the Cardiovascular Health Study. *Archives of Internal Medicine, 169*(13), 1195–1202.

Sipos, A., Rasmussen, F., Harrison, G., Tynelius, P., Lewis, G., Leon, D. A., & Gunnell, D. (2004). Paternal age and schizophrenia: A population based cohort study. *British Medical Journal, 329*(7474), 1070.

Smith, R., Reichenberg, A., Kember, R., Buxbaum, J., Schalkwyk, L., Fernandes, C., & Mill, J. (2012). Advanced paternal age is associated with altered DNA methylation at brain-expressed imprinted loci in inbred mice: Implications for neuropsychiatric disease. *Molecular Psychiatry* (June 26 e-publication).

Steis, M. R., & Fick, D. M. (2012). Delirium superimposed on dementia: Accuracy of nursing documentation. *Journal of Gerontological Nursing, 38*(1), 32–42.

Subotnik, K. L., Schell, A. M., Chilingar, M. S., Dawson, M. E., Ventura, J., Kelly, K. A., . . . Nuechterlein, K. H. (2012). The interaction of electrodermal activity and expressed emotion in predicting symptoms in recent-onset schizophrenia. *Psychophysiology, 49*(8), 1035–1038.

Sutterland, A., Dieleman, J., Storosum, J., Voordouw, B., Kroon, J., Veldhuis, J., . . . Sturkenboom, M. (2013). Annual incidence rate of schizophrenia and schizophrenia spectrum disorders in a longitudinal population-based cohort study. *Social Psychiatry and Psychiatric Epidemiology* (January e-publication), 1–9.

Tessner, K. D., Mittal, V., & Walker, E. F. (2011). Longitudinal study of stressful life events and daily stressors among adolescents at high risk for psychotic disorders. *Schizophrenia Bulletin, 37*(2), 432–441.

Tienari, P., Wynne, L. C., Sorri, A., Lahti, I., Läksy, K., Moring, J., . . . Wahlberg, K. (2004). Genotype-environment interaction in schizophrenia-spectrum disorder: Long-term follow-up study of Finnish adoptees. *British Journal of Psychiatry, 184,* 216–222.

Trzepacz, P. T., & Meagher, D. J. (2008). Neuropsychiatric aspects of delirium. In S. C. Yudofsky & R. E. Hales (Eds.), *The American Psychiatric Publishing textbook of neuropsychiatry and behavioral neurosciences.* Arlington, VA: American Psychiatric.

Tullman, D. F., Fletcher, K., & Foreman, M. D. (2012). Delirium: Prevention, early recognition, and treatment. In M. Boltz, E. Capezuti, T. T. Fulmer, D. Zwicker, & A. O'Meara (Eds.), *Evidence-based geriatric nursing protocols for best practice* (4th ed.). New York, NY: Springer. Retrieved from http://consultgerirn.org/topics/delirium/want_to_know_more.

Turkington, C., & Mitchell, D. (2010). *The encyclopedia of Alzheimer's disease.* New York, NY: Infobase.

Umeda-Yano, S., Hashimoto, R., Yamamori, H., Okada, T., Yasuda, Y., Ohi, K., . . . Takeda, M. (2013). The regulation of gene expression involved in TGF-β signaling by ZNF804A, a risk gene for schizophrenia. *Schizophrenia Research, 146*(1–3), 273–278.

Vahia, I. V., Palmer, B. W., Depp, C., Fellows, I., Golshan, S., Kraemer, H. C., & Jeste, D. V. (2010). Is late-onset schizophrenia a subtype of schizophrenia? *Acta Psychiatrica Scandinavica, 122*(5), 414–426.

Volkow, N. D. (2009). Substance use disorders in schizophrenia: Clinical implications of comorbidity. *Schizophrenia Bulletin, 35*(3), 469–472.

Vyas, N. S., Kumra, S., & Puri, B. K. (2010). What insights can we gain from studying early-onset schizophrenia? The neurodevelopmental pathway and beyond. *Expert Review of Neurotherapeutics, 10*(8), 1243.

Vyas, N. S., Patel, N. H., & Puri, B. K. (2011). Neurobiology and phenotypic expression in early onset schizophrenia. *Early Intervention in Psychiatry, 5*(1), 3–14.

Vygotsky, L. (1962). *Thought and language.* Cambridge, MA: MIT Press.

Waszynski, C. M. (2012). The Confusion Assessment Method (CAM). *Try This: Best Practices in Nursing Care to Older Adults, 13,* 1–2. Retrieved from http://consultgerirn.org/uploads/File/trythis/try_this_13.pdf.

White, T., Magnotta, V. A., Bockholt, H. J., Williams, S., Wallace, S., Ehrlich, S., . . . Lim, K. O. (2011). Global white matter abnormalities in schizophrenia: A multisite diffusion tensor imaging study. *Schizophrenia Bulletin, 37*(1), 222-232.

Whitlock, E. L., Vannucci, A., & Avidan, M. S. (2011). Postoperative delirium. *Minerva Anestesiologica, 77*(4), 448–456.

Wollen, K. A. (2010). Alzheimer's disease: The pros and cons of pharmaceutical, nutritional, botanical, and stimulatory therapies, with a discussion of treatment strategies from the perspective of patients and practitioners. *Alternative Medicine Review, 15*(3), 223–244.

Woods, D. L., Beck, C., & Sinha, K. (2009). The effect of therapeutic touch on behavioral symptoms and cortisol in persons with dementia. *Forschende Komplementärmedizin, 6*(3), 181–189.

Zugno, A., Fraga, D., De Luca, R., Ghedim, F., Deroza, P., Cipriano, A., . . . Quevedo, J. (2013). Chronic exposure to cigarette smoke during gestation results in altered cholinesterase enzyme activity and behavioral deficits in adult rat offspring: Potential relevance to schizophrenia. *Journal of Psychiatric Research, 47*(6), 740–746.

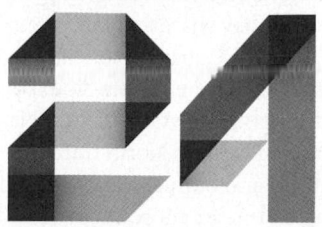 **Culture and Diversity**

MODULE AT-A-GLANCE

The Concept of Culture and Diversity, 1629

☑ THE CONCEPT OF CULTURE AND DIVERSITY

Culture refers to the patterns of behavior and thinking that people living in social groups learn, develop, and share. The term **diversity** refers to the array of differences among individuals, groups, and communities. Today's nurses must be able to work with diverse populations of clients—clients of varying socioeconomic, cultural, and spiritual backgrounds and clients with varying values and belief systems. To be able to provide culturally aware nursing, nurses must examine their own cultural values and beliefs. **<<**

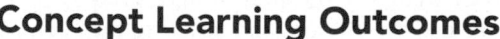

Concept Learning Outcomes

1. Describe how belief systems impact the provision of health care.
2. Describe how cultural values and beliefs are learned or transmitted.
3. Discuss how cultural and religious preferences may impact an individual's lifestyle and healthcare choices.
4. Compare and contrast the diverse needs of vulnerable populations.
5. Distinguish variations of social behaviors found in diverse groups.
6. Identify disparities in the provision of or access to health care among cultural groups and vulnerable populations.
7. Examine personal beliefs, prejudgment, and areas for professional development related to cultural differences and vulnerable populations.
8. Plan care for clients that reflects inclusion of a client's cultural values and beliefs.

Concept Key Terms

Acculturation, *1634*
Ageism, *1637*
Alternative therapies, *1643*
Assimilation, *1634*
Bias, *1635*
Classism *1635*
Complementary therapies, *1643*
Cultural competence, *1640*
Cultural groups, *1633*
Cultural humility, *1630*
Cultural values, *1632*
Culture, *1629*
Discrimination, *1630*
Diversity, *1629*
Enculturation, *1633*
Ethnic groups, *1630*
Healthcare disparity, *1638*
Heterosexism, *1636*

Homophobia, *1636*
Intersex, *1634*
Minority, *1630*
Multiculturalism, *1630*
Prejudice, *1641*
Race, *1635*
Racism, *1635*
Religion, *1638*
Sexism, *1635*
Sexual orientation, *1636*
Social justice, *1634*
Stereotyping, *1634*
Subculture, *1638*
Transgender, *1634*
Transsexual, *1634*
Vulnerable populations, *1637*
Worldview, *1632*

▶ CULTURAL DIVERSITY

Any discussion of culture and diversity must be informed by the terms and language that are part of that discussion. **Discrimination**, or the restriction of justice, rights, and privileges of individuals or subcultural groups, may occur when dominant groups reinforce their rules and regulations in a way that limits opportunities for others. A dominant group may be one that is dominant by reason of its numbers or as a result of having influence, power, money, and position to remain dominant while reinforcing rules and norms that benefit its own interests. The term **minority** usually refers to an individual or group of individuals who are outside the dominant group. Examples of subculture or minority groups may be people associated with religious sects, rural residency, special interests, music, philosophy, or even ethnicity.

Multiculturalism is defined as many subcultures coexisting within a given society in which no one culture dominates. In a multicultural society, human differences are accepted and respected. Classrooms in an academic setting may be considered multicultural whereby all students are socialized to succeed and all learning styles are valued and understood.

In the United States, one driver of multiculturalism has been immigration. People from nearly every country in the world have come to the United States in search of a new way of life. Each year, approximately 1 million individuals obtain legal permanent resident status in the United States. Of these, the majority (some 75%) come from other North American countries or from Asia (U.S. Department of Homeland Security, 2011).

Many individuals coming to America have sought freedom from an oppressive government. Others coming to our country have sought religious freedom, and still others freedom from poverty (**Figure 24–1** ●). Each family or group of immigrants brings its own culture, adding to what has been described as, to use a metaphor, the "melting pot." The image of a melting pot implies the assimilation of multiple ethnic groups and their cultural practices into a single national identity with national allegiance and values. Typically, families and groups from the same country will relocate to a specific area or neighborhood, which helps them to maintain their native language, traditions, and ways of worship. These **ethnic**

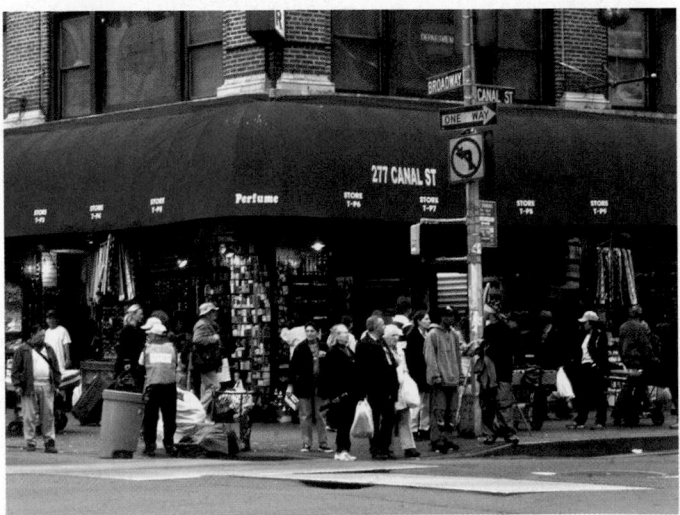

Figure 24–1 ● A crowded street in New York City where 36% of the city's population is foreign born.

Source: Tim Knox © Dorling Kindersley.

groups have common characteristics, including nationality, language, values, and customs, and they share a cultural heritage. Examples of ethnic groups are the large Cuban American population living in and around Miami, Florida; the Lakota Sioux, one of three major ethnic groups that make up the Great Sioux Nation; and the Hmong populations living in western North Carolina.

In addition to different cultural and ethnic groups, individuals in the United States belong to one or more races. The U.S. Census Bureau (2011) identifies the following races:

- White
- Black or African American
- American Indian or Alaska Native
- Asian
- Native Hawaiian or Other Pacific Islander

Individuals of Hispanic, Latino, or Spanish origin may be of any race.

Cultural, ethnic, racial, and other differences make nursing care both a privilege and a challenge. Nurses who are able to develop cultural competence and practice evidence-based care that is relevant to all of their clients will gain confidence in their abilities and greater personal benefit from their work with individual clients. A culturally competent practice begins with gaining a greater understanding of the differing values and beliefs of others (**Box 24–1** ●) and recognizing how these differing values and beliefs affect clients in all aspects of providing care (see the Concepts Related to Culture and Diversity feature).

▶ VALUES AND BELIEFS

Culture includes a society's values, beliefs, assumptions, principles, myths, legends, and norms. People living within a culture typically share many of the prevailing society's values and beliefs. People use these values and beliefs to help them define meaning, identify acceptable behaviors, choose emotional reactions, and determine appropriate actions in given situations. Values and belief systems are part of a culture, as are family relationships and roles. To understand client behaviors in more depth, a nurse must identify which cultures are prevalent demographically in a given area, learn more about those cultures by reading or attending a class about them, and apply that knowledge and experiences when providing client care.

Box 24–1 **Nurse's Self-Awareness**

Professional nurses must possess self-awareness. Self-awareness is critical to developing sensitivity to differences while supporting a sense of cultural humility rather than superiority over others. **Cultural humility** occurs when a healthcare provider recognizes that her personal cultural values are not superior over the cultural values of others, thus preventing the provider from taking an authoritative stance or engaging in abuse of power (Dayer-Berenson, 2011).

As a nursing student, you may find your personal values to be in conflict with professional values. For example, you may like to sleep in late in the day or may be frequently tardy for social or professional appointments, but these behaviors are in opposition to the professional time-oriented expectations found in U.S. healthcare systems. To be successful as a nurse, you must be on time for appointments and possess good time management skills. Your values and beliefs about timeliness and professional behavior impact how others perceive you. They also impact how you perceive others, including how you perceive clients and their families.

Concepts Related to **Culture and Diversity**

Differences among clients that are attributable to culture, ethnicity, race, gender, sexuality, and vulnerability impact the nursing care of clients in a variety of ways. Within the concept of communication, it is important to understand that clients use language differently, speak different languages, and recognize nonverbal cues differently. Therapeutic communication, interpreters, shared languages, and awareness of nonverbal cues can help nurses communicate more effectively with clients from diverse backgrounds.

Within healthcare systems, the resources available to the different types of clients depend on a variety of factors, especially whether or not the clients have health insurance and access to resources such as transportation. Clients who live in poverty or are homeless may need referrals to additional resources. Nurses must advocate for services such as interpreters or mental health resources for their clients who do not have the influence to ask for such changes on their own.

The professional behavior of nurses must be built on a moral and ethical code. Nursing as a discipline has a culture of its own. Nurses must understand collegial and regional differences to effectively work collaboratively with interdisciplinary teams. Self-awareness, emotional intelligence, and lifelong learning should be characteristics of a nurse's professional behavior.

Another concept related to culture and diversity is sexuality. Gender roles and the timing and type of sexual relationships vary among groups of people. Heterosexual and homosexual variations may also be culturally embedded.

Another concept related to culture and diversity is spirituality. Although spirituality may be defined more broadly than religion, cultural variations exist around religious and church doctrines such as Hinduism, Judaism, Christianity, and Muslim practices. Religious practices commonly influence eating or fasting patterns, types of worship, and family roles and responsibilities.

CONCEPT	RELATIONSHIP TO CULTURE AND DIVERSITY	NURSING IMPLICATIONS
Communication		
	Listening, clarification, reflection, and all therapeutic communication techniques are important when communicating with people different from you. Verbal/nonverbal differences	■ Use therapeutic communication skills. Identify translation and interpreter resources in your organization. ■ Common language
Healthcare Systems		
	Availability of health care for vulnerable populations may be difficult. Availability of resources	■ Unequal distribution of facilities and resources ■ Recognize cultural and group differences among healthcare providers. Seek to advocate for vulnerable populations. ■ Refer clients in need of additional resources to social services and nonprofit service agencies.
Comfort		
■ Pain	The verbalization of pain and preferred comfort measures may differ across cultural groups and gender roles.	■ Client's reaction to pain may range from stoicism to hysterics. Nurses must assess and accept a variety of client responses to pain and provide a myriad of interventions that include opioids, nonopioids, adjunct therapy, and complementary and alternative methods for reducing pain and increasing comfort.
Professional Behaviors		
	Recognize personal values and professional values.	■ Self-awareness of cultural competence
Sexuality		
	Sexual orientation, homophobia, heterosexism	■ Assist in advocating for LGBT healthcare needs and access. ■ Recognize same sex partners as family and client support.

(continued on next page)

Concepts Related to **Culture and Diversity** (continued)

CONCEPT	RELATIONSHIP TO CULTURE AND DIVERSITY	NURSING IMPLICATIONS
Spirituality		
	Recognize religious beliefs related to dietary regimen or times of fasting.	■ Show respect for religious differences, leaders, and practice. ■ Recognize that your personal spiritual and religious beliefs will not be universally shared with your clients. ■ Be nonjudgmental of differences. ■ Support client religious practices.

Values reflect an underlying system of beliefs. **Cultural values** describe preferred ways of behaving or thinking that are sustained over time and used to govern a cultural group's actions and decisions. When people live together in a society, cultural values often determine the rules people live by each and every day. These rules may be variously stated, but they basically address similar values. Examples of some rules in Western (which usually refers to North America and parts of Europe) culture may include the following:

■ Don't steal from others.

■ Respect other people's property.

■ Don't hurt others.

■ Don't cheat on spouse or significant other.

■ Share your food and clothing with those who are in need.

■ Speak truthfully based on what you see.

■ Respect your elders for their wisdom and experience.

■ Respect God or a higher power.

■ Respect nature and your environment.

Cultural characteristics include observable behaviors as well as the unseen values that influence those behaviors. Cultural practices have meanings that give the group its worldview and that reflects the social organization of the culture as a whole. The organization of a culture or society includes the following elements:

■ *A physical element.* The geographic area in which a society is located

■ *An infrastructure element.* The framework of the systems and processes that keep a society functioning

■ *A behavioral element.* The way people in a society act and react to each other

■ *A cultural element.* All the values, beliefs, assumptions, and norms that comprise a code of conduct for acceptable behaviors within a society.

Each culture has its own worldview or understanding of the world. A **worldview** refers to how the people in a culture perceive ideas and attitudes about the world, other people, and life in general. A culture's worldview supports its overall *belief system*, which is developed to explain the mysteries of the universe and of life that each society tries to understand:

■ What is the meaning of life?

■ How do individuals know their purpose in life?

■ What is reality?

■ How much can be known about values and beliefs?

■ Is there a God or power beyond me?

■ How was the universe created?

■ What happens after death?

■ How do we care for the sick?

A cultural belief system influences an individual's decisions and actions in society regarding everything from preparing food and caring for the sick to rituals of death and burial. Scientific and medical advancements may or may not impact a culture's belief systems. Belief systems differ in every culture. The beliefs of a society are passed from generation to generation by word of mouth and by rituals, such as reading certain stories or books on holidays (**Figure 24–2 ●**). In many cases, cultural practices are rooted in the individual's religious faith or practices (see the module on Spirituality). Children learn the belief system of their culture from parents and other family members who teach them any number of values and beliefs, including those about

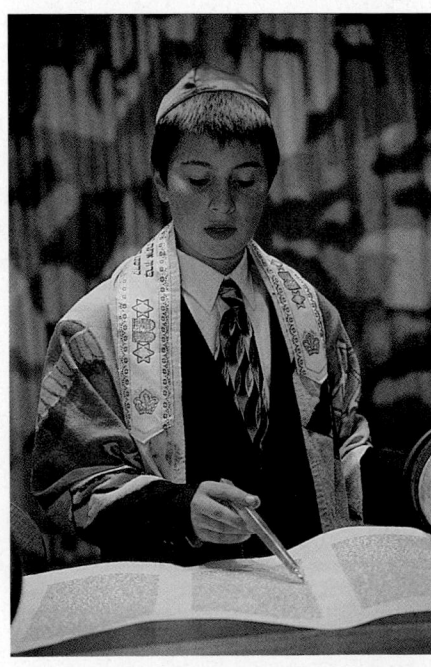

Figure 24–2 ● Cultures try to understand and give meaning to life through spiritual beliefs, social values, and acceptable behaviors.

The Concept of Culture and Diversity

"right or wrong." Differing opinions may originate from religious beliefs or social conditions. People make decisions about "right or wrong," and as things change, people adapt and the culture evolves.

Belief systems are based on people's experiences and exposures to differences found in our world. As people's knowledge and understanding grow, their belief systems expand. Knowing why we believe what we believe builds self-awareness and understanding of differences in our own beliefs compared with the beliefs of others.

Culturally based beliefs and traditions can affect the course and outcome of disease and illness. Healthcare providers and clients bring their respective cultural backgrounds and expectations to each interaction. These differences can impact both the expectations and practices of the client and the provision of services by nurses and other healthcare professionals. Some of these many differences are listed in **Table 24–1 ●**.

Cultural differences can present barriers to necessary care. Some areas in which barriers can arise include the following:

- The importance, or lack of importance, for family members in managing illness and disease
- Lack of trust in the healthcare system and providers
- The belief that illnesses are not linked to scientific pathophysiology
- Refusing to believe the mind–body connection
- Fear or denial of death or life after death
- Cultural assumptions about disease and illness that may influence the presentation of symptoms or the response to treatments
- Failure of clients to see a pattern of repeated illness as a chronic condition rather than their symptoms as unrelated occurrences
- Cultural beliefs that discussing prognosis and risks with clients can influence outcomes or be dangerous.

TABLE 24–1 Examples of Differences in Core Beliefs

AMERICAN OR WESTERN CULTURES	NON-WESTERN CULTURES
Health is viewed by many as the absence of disease.	Health is a state of harmony that encompasses the mind, body, and spirit.
Use of specialty practitioners (e.g., pediatricians, obstetricians)	Preference for respected healers from the culture of origin (e.g., herbalists, midwives, curandos)
Recognition that food affects biophysical processes, functions	Belief that food can restore imbalances
Independence, individualism, freedom are valued.	Interdependence with family, community, and group acceptance are valued.
Use of first names promotes familiarity, trust.	Use of first names is a sign of disrespect.

Source: Based on U.S. Department of Health and Human Services, Office of Minority Health (2004, March). *Physician toolkit and curriculum: Resources to implement cross-cultural clinical practice guidelines for Medicaid practitioners.* Retrieved from http://minorityhealth.hhs.gov/assets/pdf/checked/1/toolkit.pdf.

Although cultural beliefs and behaviors change over the years as a cultural group adapts to new ideas and conditions, some individuals may retain traditional behaviors and thinking and continue to follow the beliefs and practices as always. Tension can arise when different health belief systems conflict with each other. The result may be anxiety, anger, or fear. The healthcare provider's cultural competence may reduce this discomfort by showing a nonjudgmental attitude of respect. A nurse must also recognize the common defense mechanisms such as anger, avoidance, denial, intellectualization, or projection that may be used when an individual feels threatened (Berman & Snyder, 2012). See the module on Stress and Coping for information about defense mechanisms.

Professional nurses work with and care for people who have differing values and beliefs. It is important for nurses to understand how their own cultural beliefs and practices inform who they are as nurses, in part to strengthen their own value systems but also to ensure they are sufficiently self-aware to prevent projecting their own beliefs and values onto their clients.

Cultural Transmission

A society is a group of people who share a common culture, rules of behavior, and basic social organization. Culture is transmitted, or learned and shared, by people living together in a society. Cultural characteristics, such as customs, beliefs, values, language, and socialization patterns, are passed from generation to generation. **Cultural groups** can be categorized around racial, ethnic, religious, or socially common practice patterns. These groups often have common cultural characteristics such as language, customs, beliefs, and values. See **Box 24–2 ●**.

Culture is transmitted from one generation to the next through language, material objects, rituals, customs, institutions, and art. Through the use of a common language, people learn how to live by the rules governing the society and how to earn money or trade goods or services to meet basic needs, such as food and shelter. Culture can influence everything the members of a society think and do.

Enculturation, or cultural transmission, is exemplified by a process children use to learn cultural characteristics from adults. These characteristics are often normalized, meaning that certain

Box 24–2   Cultural Characteristics

- History of origin
- Holiday customs
- Styles of dress
- General worldview
- Religious beliefs and practices
- Food preferences and eating patterns
- Values
- Roles and patterns of relationships
- Leadership structure
- Health and illness beliefs and behaviors
- Social systems
- Concept of time
- Concept of personal space
- Gestures and facial expressions
- Concept of self
- Common language

Box 24–3 How Cultural Behaviors are Learned

Cultural behaviors are learned by:

- Observing others' actions
- Hearing instructions on what behaviors are right or wrong
- Imitating others doing a behavior
- Getting reinforcement (either positive or negative) for enacting a behaviors
- Internalizing behaviors
- Spontaneously doing the behaviors without thinking about it

characteristics are used to define acceptable rules and procedures of behaviors. People biologically inherit physical traits and behavioral instincts, but they socially inherit cultural characteristics. An individual learns culture from other people in a society. Enculturation occurs in families until the children are ready to leave and establish their own values, beliefs, and practices through exposure to other cultural or societal practices through work, marriage, or higher education. However, enculturation may continue among family members who live close to each other, celebrate religious holidays together, or otherwise work to maintain the culture within their family and limit their exposure to cultural differences. The great variety of cultural characteristics provides a broader perspective of cultural differences and respect.

People in a society have cultural characteristics that are embedded in art, music, food, religion, and traditions. Because culture is adaptive, these characteristics may be modified over the years as people use culture to adjust to changes in the world around them. See **Box 24–3** on how cultural behaviors are learned.

Different societies can come together and share or exchange cultures as well. People may evolve from one cultural group to another. **Assimilation** is the process of adapting to and integrating characteristics of the dominant culture as one's own. People typically benefit by exchanging ideas, natural resources, and goods. **Acculturation** is the process of not only adapting to another culture but also accepting the majority group's culture as one's own. Because culture is complex, members of a cultural group may engage in many behaviors and habits unconsciously, making them difficult to explain to others. Sometimes assimilation and acculturation are implicit and covert, whereas other times assimilation can be overt and coercive.

As individuals go through the process of acculturation, they may choose to discard some practices from their culture of origin in exchange for practices of the dominant culture. Therefore, nurses need to ask appropriate questions to assess individual cultural practices rather than make assumptions. For example, some clients of Chinese background may be practicing Buddhists who prefer traditional Chinese practices such as herbs and acupuncture; others may belong to a different faith and completely embrace Western medicine; while still others may blend practices in ways that make sense to them. Careful assessment of the individual client is necessary to avoid making assumptions and stereotyping.

Diversity

Cultural differences are not the only hallmarks of diversity. Gender, race, class, sexual orientation, and age are just a few of the differences among individuals living in the United States. In many instances, these factors carry important implications for nursing. For example, African American women are at greater risk for heart disease than any other single population, older adults are at greater risk for injury due to falls, and children are at greater risk for accidental injury. Nurses must be prepared to work with the each individual who walks in the door, regardless of that individual's own personal background.

The concept of **social justice** is a framework to explore the complexities surrounding the variety of factors that impact diverse and vulnerable populations (Clingerman, 2011). Using a lens of social justice enables individuals and organizations to follow a code of ethics that promotes equitable distribution of resources and seeks equitable rights for all individuals, thus providing advocacy for people who lack access to resources. Culturally competent nurses should respect and advocate for human dignity. Stereotyping, prejudice, and discrimination can threaten the delivery of healthcare services and adversely affect client outcomes. Nurses need to understand and recognize these attitudes in themselves and others in order to reduce their effects on the clients they serve. In summary, to overcome barriers to multiculturalism, a nurse must have a deep understanding of vulnerable clients who are impacted by racism, sexism, classism, and heterosexism.

GENDER Traditionally gender has been dichotomized into two groups: men and women. However, it is known that some people do not fit neatly into these categories of gender. For example, physical genitalia may be blended as male and female. **Intersex** is a general term used for a variety of conditions in which an individual is born with a reproductive or sexual anatomy that does not seem to fit the typical definitions of female or male (Intersex Society of North America [ISNA], n.d.a). People who identify as **transgender** are born with typical male or female anatomies but feel as though they have been born into the "wrong body" (ISNA, n.d.b). For example, an individual who identifies as transgender may have typical female anatomy but feel like a male. Those who seek to change genders by taking hormones or electing to have gender reassignment surgeries are called **transsexual**. New information and public awareness about gender spectrum or transgender people are helping to illuminate specific healthcare needs (Brill & Pepper, 2008).

Differences between men and women go beyond anatomy and physiology and cultural or social definitions. Compared to women, men typically are less verbal and more action oriented and have stronger skills in logic, mathematics, and coordination; women tend to be more skilled in languages, perceiving and responding to others' needs, and the arts. However, these are general tendencies and taking them at face value may lead to **stereotyping**. Stereotyping is an overgeneralization of group characteristics that reinforces societal biases and distorts individual characteristics (Grandbois & Sanders, 2012). Even within genders, individual diversity is expected; for example, some women may be highly coordinated, mathematically skilled, and disinterested in the arts. No conclusion about an individual can ever be drawn based on a simple term such as *woman* or *man*.

The genders also differ in access to and control over resources and decision-making power in the family and community. The extent of these differences is often cultural. Gender roles, often in interaction with socioeconomic circumstances, influence exposure to health risks, access to health information and services, health outcomes, and the social and economic consequences of ill health. This can be demonstrated by viewing the differences in mortality and morbidity between men and women of different cultures as well as their involvement in health prevention and health promotion programs. Therefore, nurses must recognize the root causes of gender inequities when designing a nursing plan of care. To obtain positive outcomes, health promotion and disease prevention and treatment need to address gender differences. For example, millions of women are injured as the result of spousal or significant other abuse, but the magnitude and health consequences of domestic violence against women have often been neglected in both research and policy.

Generally, there seems to be an assumption that interventions will be just as effective for men as for women. Many health promotion programs may be gender-blind and are based on research that neither accounted for nor controlled for the gender of the study participants. Until the last decade, many medications were tested only on White men, with no consideration that women or people of other ethnicities respond differently. Only in the mid-1990s did pharmaceutical companies begin to look at pharmacokinetic differences between males and females. Understanding the differences in responses between genders has led to research on how drugs affect women as well as those from different races and cultural backgrounds. As a result, scientists are finding that some drugs are more effective for women while others are more effective for men. In addition to the way in which men and women respond to health promotion, they also display different needs with regard to their response to the same diagnosis. For example, the traditional symptom of crushing chest pain as a primary indicator of myocardial infarction has been found to be primarily a male response. Women with myocardial infarction are more likely to experience extreme fatigue that extends to pain in the jaw, back, or shoulder if not treated early in the symptomatology. Biological differences such as genetics, hormones, and metabolic influences combine to play a part in shaping different symptoms as well as morbidity and mortality rates (Casper et al., n.d.; Schuiling & Likis, 2013).

By improving their understanding of how gender differences impact client health, nurses can develop a plan of care that meets the specific and unique healthcare needs of each client. It is important that nurses not allow their own gender bias or preconceived beliefs to affect their ability to assess and plan appropriate care for the individual client. Health-promoting interventions aimed at inclusion in a safe and supportive environment promote a trusting nurse–client relationship. Nurses should promote an environment in which clients can access essential services that address the differences between men and women in an equitable manner. When planning care, nurses who take into consideration the biological differences and social vulnerability of men and women are more likely to see positive outcomes for their clients.

Bias can be defined as favoring a group or individual over another. Gender bias results in **sexism,** and occurs when male values, beliefs, or activities are preferred over female. Sexism may be overt or covert. Institutional bias related to gender results in sexist practices within an organization. Nurses need an awareness of cultural variations of gender as they will be caring for diverse client needs.

RACE   The concept of race is very complex. Historically, **race** has often been defined by physical attributes linked to continents of origin, for example, Asia, Europe, Africa, and the Americas. The variations of skin color and hair texture have traditionally been used as markers of race. The dialogue about race and genetics is ongoing (Social Science Research Council, n.d.). However, the 2010 U.S. census data were collected by racial designation.

Stay Current: *To learn more about the U.S. census racial categories, search the U.S. Census Bureau's Web site:* **www.census.gov/prod/cen2010/briefs/c2010br-02.pdf**.

The oppression of a group of people based on perceived race is known as **racism.** Although racism is often perceived as overt acts of hostility, racism can also be insidious policies, procedures, traditions, and rules that benefit one group of people over another. For example, not providing translation services or not offering expensive diagnostic or treatment modalities to minority groups contributes to unequal treatment and injustice.

CLASS   Socioeconomic variations contribute to a society stratification based on money and access to resources. **Classism** is the oppression of groups of people based on their socioeconomic status. The lack of access to resources is apparent in some of the people at the lowest economic level such as the homeless, those living in poverty, or undocumented immigrants.

Homelessness   Among the most vulnerable clients are those who are homeless. Homeless clients presents unique and complex challenges because they often live in dangerous, unsanitary conditions; have diets that are severely lacking in nutrients; and have very few resources for coping with illness. They must find shelter and food every day and cannot predict what the next day will bring. People who are homeless have difficulty obtaining, keeping, and storing medications. A high incidence of substance abuse and mental illness limits their ability to provide self-care still further. An important nursing intervention in addition to providing care to those who are homeless is to identify resources to help these clients.

Stay Current: *To explore the details of homelessness, go to the Web site* **www.endhomelessness.org/pages/snapshot_of_homelessness**. *Find the region you will be practicing in to determine the demographics and to increase your knowledge base about the reasons for homelessness.*

Poverty   Although people who are homeless can be considered impoverished, many families with adequate shelter live in poverty. Children and those living in female-headed households are at greatest risk of living in poverty (U.S. Department of Health and Human Services [USDHHS], 2012):

- U.S. Census Bureau data indicate that the overall poverty rate in 2011 was 15.0%—statistically unchanged from 15.1% in 2010. This represents 46.2 million people living in poverty in 2011.

- Median household income was $50,054 in 2011, which is a statistically significant decrease of 1.5% from 2010.

- Just over 16 million children (people under age 18) were living in poverty in 2011, not significantly changed from 2010. The child poverty rate was 21.9%; again, not significantly changed from the 2010 rate of 22.0%.

- For African American children, the poverty rate was 37.4% for 2011. The rate for Hispanic children was 34.1%. For non-Hispanic, White children, the rate was 12.5%.

- Children living in female-headed families with no spouse present had a poverty rate of 47.6%, over four times the rate of children in married-couple families (10.9%).

- The 2011 poverty rate for people ages 65 and over was 8.7%, statistically unchanged from 2010.

- In 2011, 6.6% of all people, or 20.4 million people, lived in deep poverty (had incomes of less than one half the poverty threshold, or $11,511 for a family of four).

- The overall poverty rate of 15.0% in 2011 did not change significantly from 2010. In contrast, the poverty rate had risen significantly in 7 of the prior 10 years from a recent low of 11.3% in 2000.

- These figures reflect cash income only and do not reflect in-kind public supports, tax credits, most expansions funded by the American Recovery and Reinvestment Act (ARRA), and temporary reductions in the payroll tax.

Undocumented Immigrants Undocumented immigrants often do not seek health care until their condition becomes critical. This behavior results from a complex combination of factors. Many are uninsured, do not speak English, and have not yet learned the culture of their new homeland. Many believe that accessing health care will result in legal consequences, up to and including deportation. For some, the differences between the U.S. healthcare system and the medical practices and beliefs of their culture of origin create an additional barrier. These factors combine to create fear in the undocumented immigrant client who needs medical attention.

Special healthcare concerns related to this population include lack of preventive care, inadequate immunization status, and lack of past medical records. Because they enter the country without border screening, risks of diseases such as tuberculosis and HIV are much higher. Many receive their health information from television, the Internet, or family members, which can lead to misinformation and improper treatment.

States and regional politics vary across the country with regard to whether or not government or healthcare facilities are required to ask for proof of citizenship when providing care. Further, some states require reporting nondocumented people, which also impedes their willingness to seek care. You need to familiarize yourself with the laws within your state of nursing practice. When providing care to clients who may be or are known to be undocumented immigrants, the nurse has the ethical and moral imperative to deliver the same high-quality care delivered to any client. Use of an interpreter will improve the quality of communication if the client does not speak English or does not speak English well enough to understand the information presented. Thorough screening, nursing history, and assessment contribute to determining both current condition as well as risks, preventive care needs, and understanding of self-care upon discharge. Because access to health care for this pop-ulation is unpredictable, nurses should maximize each opportunity to care for and teach self-care to these clients.

SEXUAL ORIENTATION **Sexual orientation** is a continuum ranging from those who have a strong preference for a partner of the same sex to those who strongly prefer someone of the opposite sex. *Homosexual* individuals prefer a partner of the same sex, with the term *lesbian* used to describe women who prefer to develop intimate relationships with other women. The term *gay* may refer to homosexual women or men, but is more commonly used to describe men who are homosexual. *Heterosexual* individuals prefer to develop an intimate relationship with a partner of the opposite sex. *Bisexual* individuals are physically attracted to both males and females. The most common biases related to sexual orientation are **homophobia** (fear, hatred, or mistrust of gays and lesbians often expressed in overt displays of discrimination) or **heterosexism** (view of heterosexuality as the only correct sexual orientation). Often bias toward homosexual individuals is displayed in subtle and invisible ways that create obstacles to achieving full equality for the homosexual client (Irwin, 2007). Current state laws against gay marriage are examples of laws that were created based on heterosexism. Laws differ by state on the legality of same-sex marriage, civil unions, and the rights of the homosexual partner to make healthcare decisions when the client is unable to make independent decisions. Nurses should know the laws of the states in which they practice.

Social determinants affecting the health of lesbian, gay, bisexual, and transgender (LGBT) individuals largely relate to oppression and discrimination. Examples include:

- Legal discrimination in access to health insurance, employment, housing, marriage, adoption, and retirement benefits

- Lack of laws protecting against bullying in schools

- Lack of social programs targeted to and/or appropriate for LGBT youth, adults, and older adults

- Shortage of healthcare providers who are knowledgeable about and culturally competent in providing LGBT health.

In addition, nurses must advocate for a physical environment that contributes to healthy LGBT individuals, including:

- Safe schools, neighborhoods, and housing

- Access to recreational facilities and activities

- Availability of safe meeting places

- Access to health services.

The Institute of Medicine (IOM) (2011) of the National Academies has published a book addressing LGBT health issues throughout the life span and found an ongoing need for healthcare professionals to improve culturally competent health care and to eliminate health care disparities.

DISABILITY STATUS Many clients have physical or cognitive disabilities. During the past 30 years, various terms have been used to describe people with intellectual disabilities. *Mental deficiency*, *mental retardation*, *mental handicap*, *developmental disability*, and *learning disability* are examples. Clients with an intellectual disability and their families experience poorer health care compared with the general population. Living with an intellectual disability is often challenged by coexisting complex and chronic conditions and can lead to economic hardship and family conflict. Both intellectual and physical disability can impair the individual client's ability to participate in health promotion and to provide self-care. The American Association of People with Disabilities (2012) is the nation's largest disability rights organization. It is an important advocacy, resource, and referral organization for individuals with disabilities and their families, friends, and advocates. Nurses working with clients with disabilities must develop trusting relationships so they can successfully assist clients with disabilities and their families and caregivers and enable them to find resources.

AGE Children and older adults are considered vulnerable populations. Both older adults and children often depend on others for nutrition, health care, transportation, and personal safety. Many older adults live on limited incomes. In 2011, one half of all older adults living in the United States had annual incomes of less than $20,000, with one half of older adult *households* earning less than $33,200 per year from all income sources (Pension Rights Center, n.d.). **Ageism** is defined as discrimination against older adults. U.S. culture places an emphasis on youth, beauty, and productivity, which minimizes respect and access to opportunities for older adults. The increasing use of the Internet and technology as a primary means of sharing and retrieving information also has implications. Older adults are less likely to be fluent in the latest technologies (Zickuhr & Maden, 2012).

▶ DISPARITIES AND DIFFERENCES

In many ways the United States is a nation that celebrates culture and diversity. From Greek festivals to soul food to Tex-Mex, from gay pride parades to Chinese New Year, there is plenty in our diverse heritage and society to celebrate. Unfortunately, these differences also give rise to disparities of opportunity, and these include disparities that relate to health care. In 2002, the Institute of Medicine released a report on disparities in the United States regarding the types and quality of health services that racial and ethnic minorities receive. This historical report explored factors that may contribute to inequities in care, and recommended policies and practices to eliminate these inequities. More than 10 years later, despite much progress, inequities still exist and researchers are attempting to identify and prevent the causes of disparities (**Figure 24–3 ●**). Nurses should be alert to practices in their work environment that impact the quality of care offered to individuals of any ethnic group. Healthcare practices should be accessible and culturally relevant, and client preferences should be at the core of decision making. Nurses should work collaboratively to ensure quality care and provision of best practice methods to all clients.

The recommendations for reducing these disparities in health care include increasing awareness of them among the public, healthcare providers, insurance companies, and policy makers. In addition, more minority healthcare providers are needed in underserved communities, and more interpreters are needed in clinics and hospitals to improve the quality of care. IOM reports suggest educating healthcare professionals to increase their cultural competence with different populations and inform them of how discrimination and racism affect the provision of health care. Including information about health-

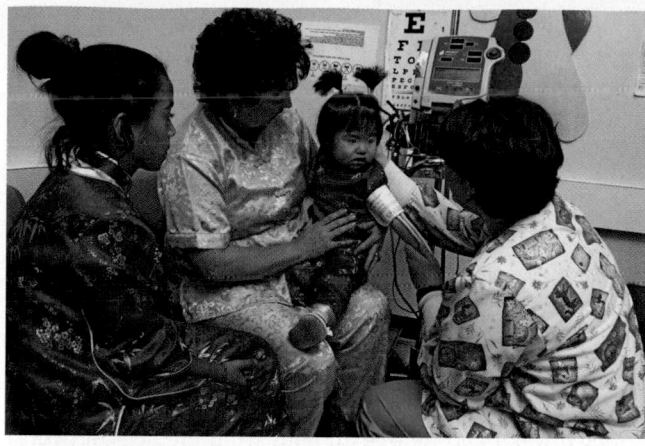

Figure 24–3 ● Although much has been done to improve the quality of health services received by American cultural and ethnic minorities, these services are still in need of continued reform.

care disparities in the curriculum is one way to educate nurses early in their careers (IOM, 2002, 2011).

Stay Current: *To see recent statistics and demographics specific to disease processes and ethnic variations, you are encouraged to explore* **www.ahrq.gov/research/findings/nhqrdr/nhqr11/index.html**.

Vulnerable Populations

The concept of multiculturalism assumes that all cultural groups are equally valued and respected by others. Unfortunately, this is rarely the case. Historically, the United States has had norms, values, and even laws based on stratification of gender, race, and class divisions. The term **vulnerable population** refers to groups of people in our culture who are at greater risk for diseases and reduced life span due to lack resources and exposure to more risk factors. People may be made vulnerable by financial circumstances, place of residence, education, age, functional or developmental status, inability to communicate effectively, presence of chronic or terminal illness or disability, personal characteristics, sexual preferences, immigration status, or oppression (Clingerman, 2011). *Oppression*, or the systematic limitation of access to resources, may be covert or subtle and typically is linked to laws, education, or even healthcare norms and regional access to services and transportation. All vulnerable populations are less able than others to safeguard their needs and interests adequately. In conceptual terms, the most vulnerable are those households with the fewest choices and the greatest number of disabling factors.

Clients from vulnerable populations are more likely to develop health problems because they have the greatest number of risk factors and the fewest options for managing those risks. These individuals often have limited access to health care and are more dependent on others for helping them meet their healthcare needs. Those from vulnerable populations are likely to be older, living in poverty, homeless, in abusive relationships, mentally ill, chronically ill, or children. It is not uncommon for vulnerable individuals to belong to more than one of these groups. They face multiple challenges, statistically poorer outcomes and shorter life spans, and higher mortality and morbidity rates due to cumulative or combinations of risk factors. They may be from any culture, ethnicity, age, or gender, although they are more likely to be women than men. Nurses face many challenges when caring for individuals who are vulnerable. Their physical, social, and emotional needs are complex and many have multiple chronic conditions that can complicate care still further. Assessing the client from a vulnerable population requires the nurse to investigate all systems, determine stressors and coping mechanisms, and help the client identify potential resources.

The welfare of vulnerable populations depends on the nation's willingness to provide the necessary programs to promote health and well-being. Other issues impacting the provision of health care to vulnerable populations include accessibility and transportation. Impoverished children living in very rural communities, for example, may not have access to fluoridated water and may be an hour from the nearest dentist who accepts Medicaid.

A primary focus of health care, as outlined by *Healthy People 2020*, is to reduce the disparity of access to health care among groups. **Healthcare disparity** is defined as a difference in a "measurement of access to or quality of health care services between an individual or group possessing a defined characteristic when other variables have been controlled, such as individual health choices, disease courses, and other variations from the normative measure" (Fink, 2009, p. 355). Some examples of vulnerable group affiliations are highlighted in this module.

Social Differences

People learn the social behaviors practiced in their cultures and communities. These behaviors differ from culture to culture, from community to community. They may also be practiced by members of subcultures who decide to maintain traditional cultural practices, while others from the same culture living nearby choose to adapt to the dominant culture (**Figure 24–4 ●**). The terms **subculture** and *minority* are sometimes used to label groups characterized by specific norms, beliefs, and values that coexist or even oppose those of the dominant culture. Some common social behavioral variations among people of different cultures involve communication, environmental control, hygiene, space, time, and social organization. These ethnic differences exist within smaller cultural groups within a larger society. Within the United States, social differences are evolving as individuals from different cultural groups relocate for college or work and interact with people from other cultures, and as the numbers of individuals of different cultural groups change over time. For example, from 2000 to 2010, U.S. Census records indicate that Asian and Hispanic/Latino populations increased by 43% each (Humes, Jones, & Ramirez, 2010).

COMMUNICATION Cultural groups may speak a unique language or a variation of another language. The meaning of words can differ among various groups of people, and misunderstandings may result from lack of common communication. Languages vary in terms of references to time, gender, roles, or common concepts and definitions. Translation of concepts from one language to another may miss contextual embedded meanings and lead to misunderstandings. Misinterpretation of nonverbal communication also may lead to

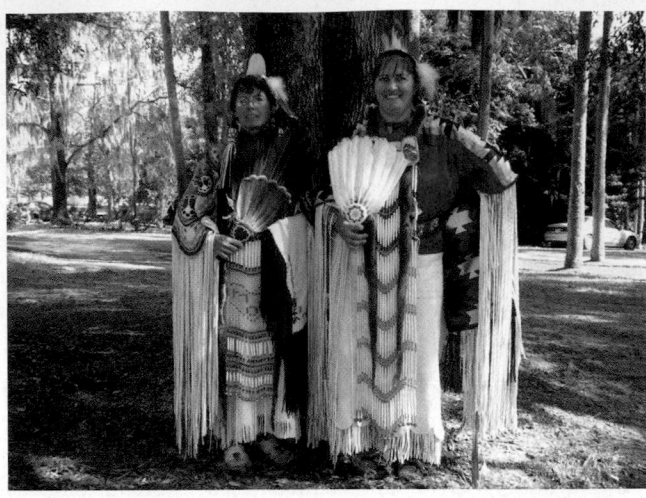

Figure 24–4 ● Subcultures can maintain heritage and identity through dress, foods eaten, and cultural festivities.
Source: © namwar69/Fotolia.

problems. Direct eye contact may show disrespect in some cultures and be a sign of interest and active listening in others. An example of a nonverbal communication difference is when up-and-down head nodding does not reflect agreement, but may instead be an attempt to acknowledge respect for authority.

ENVIRONMENTAL CONTROL An individual's relationship to nature varies among cultures. Different health practices, values, and experiences with illness can be associated with an external or internal locus of control. An internally focused individual recognizes how she can personally influence her health by appropriate diet, exercise, and wellness practices. In contrast, an externally focused perspective may reflect a fatalistic attitude, suggesting that health and illness are influenced solely by outside sources (Dayer-Berenson, 2011). Therefore, these individuals and groups would most likely not be as engaged in preventive measures. Also, environmental control may also influence whether an individual values herbs and natural remedies in contrast to standardized medical protocols.

RELIGIOUS VARIATIONS Many religions are practiced, including Protestant Christianity, Catholicism, Judaism, Hinduism, Islam, and Buddhism. **Religion** refers to a set of doctrines accepted by a group of people who gather together regularly to worship that offer a means to relate to God or a higher power, nature, and their spiritual being. Religion plays a greater role in some communities than in others. One town may sponsor a living nativity at Christmas, while the next may ban religious spectacles on government property altogether. See the module on Spirituality for more information.

SPACE Culture defines an individual's perception of personal space. Comfort may result from honoring the boundaries of personal space, whereas anxiety can result when these boundaries are not followed. Practices regarding proximity to others, body movements, and touch differ among groups. Variations of intimate zones and social public distance occur among

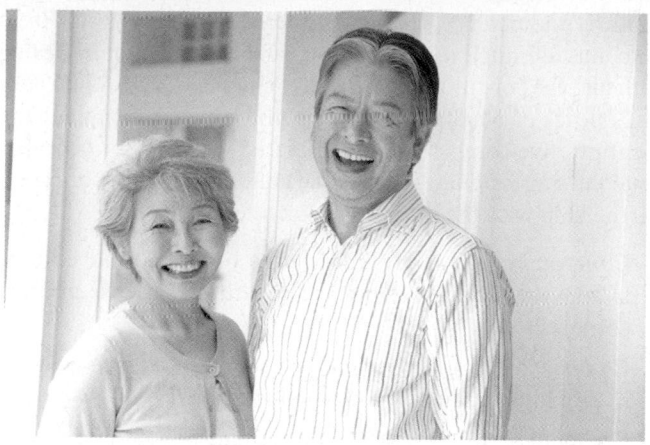

Figure 24–5 ● People from different cultures vary biologically. This couple of Japanese descent is likely to have higher blood glucose levels than the general population.
Source: © paylessimages/Fotolia.

cultural groups, and a healthcare provider needs to be aware that what he perceives as "normal" may be anxiety producing for others (Dayer-Berenson, 2011).

TIME   The concepts of time, duration of time, and points in time vary among cultures. Past-oriented cultures, for example, value tradition. Individuals from cultures that closely follow tradition may not be receptive to new procedures or treatments. Present-oriented cultures focus on the here and now, and individuals from these cultures may not be receptive to preventive healthcare measures. Some cultural groups have no understanding of linear time, and individuals from these cultures may miss appointments or be late. Healthcare providers are very regulated by clock hours influencing wake, sleep, work, and mealtimes. Not all cultural groups are regulated by clock hours.

BIOLOGICAL VARIATIONS   People differ genetically and physiologically. These biological variations among individuals, families, and groups produce differences in susceptibility and response to various diseases among people of different cultures and all walks of life (**Figure 24–5 ●**). The field of ethnopharmacology addresses variations in pharmacodynamics and pharmacokinetics among cultural groups. Nurses must be aware of these differences because they are responsible for monitoring clients' responses to the drugs they give. In addition, some enzyme deficiencies occur more commonly in some cultural groups. For example, lactose deficiency (the inability to absorb milk by-products) or other malabsorption disorders are seen with increased incidence in Asian and African cultural groups.

SUSCEPTIBILITY TO DISEASE   Certain ethnic groups or races may tend toward developing specific diseases. African Americans, for example, have a higher incidence of hypertension and sickle cell disease. Cardiovascular disease is the number-one killer of American women, and African American women are at greater risk from this disease compared to women

TABLE 24–2   Additional Cultural and Social Differences

CATEGORY	IMPLICATIONS
Hygiene	Cleanliness practices can vary among cultural groups. Whether or not body odor is disguised, ignored, or enhanced can vary by culture, as can hairstyles and grooming practices.
Nutrition	Food preferences can be an indicator of or cause of disease. Cooking techniques vary and may increase risk for disease in susceptible populations. Social patterns around eating and food choices also have implications for health promotion and direct nursing care.
Skeletal and growth and development differences	Skeletal variations occur across racial and cultural lines. For example, small-framed White women of European descent are at greater risk for osteoporosis. Pubertal developmental changes occur at different times.
Social organization	Across cultures and communities, the roles of older adults and the respect given them vary. Differences among who is the recognized head of household and gender roles also exist. Work and recreational patterns and norms vary. The role of adult children and caretaking expectations also vary among groups.

from any other ethnic group. Sometimes, however, an individual's susceptibility to disease is not so obvious but may be discerned as a nurse takes a health history, including the health of any parents, grandparents, and siblings.

SKIN COLOR   Historically, skin color has been associated with racial definitions. However, labeling of people based on their skin color should be avoided. Healthcare providers need to explore ethnic variations and not make assumptions based on skin color. As a nurse, when doing skin assessment it is important to know that darker skin tones require closer inspection and enhanced lighting to observe changes (e.g., when assessing for changes in oxygenation). Skin color changes such as erythema and cyanosis are subtle, and palpation and lighting will need to be used for skin assessment. In addition, skin color does impact some prevalence statistics since African Americans and Native Americans have lower incidences of skin cancer due to higher levels of melanin.

Additional cultural and social differences are outlined in **Table 24–2 ●**.

CASE STUDY \\ A

Susan Moore is a 16-year-old who comes to a local family practice clinic for a first-time appointment complaining of painful, irregular, and heavy menstrual periods. Her mother comes with her to the clinic visit. Susan's assessment is notable for her lack of participation in regular medical care. Her parents homeschool Susan and her sisters, and her mother tells you that they hardly ever see a physician. Following a thorough nursing assessment and physical examination, the family nurse practitioner diagnoses Susan with endometriosis and recommends hormonal contraceptives. Susan's mother is adamant that Susan not take any medication, saying they believe in using only "natural" therapies and do not use prescription drugs. Susan begins to cry, complaining of how much pain she is in constantly, and she pleads with her mother to let her try the medication.

Critical Thinking Questions

1. What are the priorities for care for Susan based on the information presented here?
2. How can you show cultural sensitivity to Susan and her mother and promote evidence-based care?
3. Using therapeutic communication, what could you say or do to affect Susan's mother's decision regarding her daughter's treatment?

▶ DEVELOPING CULTURAL COMPETENCE

Cultural competence is the ability to apply the knowledge and skills needed to provide high-quality, evidence-based care to clients of diverse backgrounds and beliefs to overcome barriers and access resources promoting health and wellness. Cultural competence has some basic characteristics:

1. Valuing diversity
2. Capacity for cultural self-assessment
3. Awareness of the different dynamics present when cultures interact
4. Knowledge about different cultures
5. Adaptability in providing nursing care that reflects an understanding of cultural diversity.

Cultural competence can be considered a process as well as an outcome, although no one person can be competent in dealing with all types of cultural variations. The American Association of Colleges of Nursing (2008) has published a document that identifies five competencies considered essential for baccalaureate nursing graduates to provide culturally competent care in partnership with the interprofessional team:

- *Competency 1.* Apply knowledge of social and cultural factors that affect nursing and health care across multiple contexts.
- *Competency 2.* Use relevant data sources and best evidence in providing culturally competent care.
- *Competency 3.* Promote achievement of safe and quality outcomes of care for diverse populations.
- *Competency 4.* Advocate for social justice, including commitment to the health of vulnerable populations and the elimination of health disparities.
- *Competency 5.* Participate in continuous cultural competence development.

Because the concept of culture is very complex, scholars have identified models of cultural competence to facilitate the continuous process of cultural competence. The purpose of using a model is to help communicate and enhance the understanding of a complex concept. A theoretical model may provide a nurse or student with a deeper understanding of how concepts are related. Many models have been published. Some focus on the process of becoming culturally competent, such as the ASKED model by Campinha-Bacote (2007) and the LEARN model from the American Medical Student Association (2007).

The LEARN model (American Association of Medical Colleges, 2005; Berlin & Fowkes, 1983) can be used as a tool for

---

Focus on Diversity and Culture **How Culturally Competent Are You?**

To help you identify areas where you can improve when providing nursing care to culturally different people, answer the following questions by checking "Yes" or "No":

____ Yes ____ No I accept values of others even when different from my own.

____ Yes ____ No I accept beliefs of others even when different from my own.

____ Yes ____ No I accept that the male and female roles may vary among different cultures.

____ Yes ____ No I accept that religious practices may influence how a client responds to illness, health problems, and death.

____ Yes ____ No I accept that alternative medicine practices may influence a client's response to illness and health problems.

____ Yes ____ No I accept cultural diversity in my clients.

____ Yes ____ No I attend educational programs to enhance my knowledge and skills in providing care to diverse cultural groups.

____ Yes ____ No I understand that clients who are unable to speak English may be very proficient in their own languages.

____ Yes ____ No I try to have written materials in the client's language available when possible.

____ Yes ____ No I use interpreters when available to improve communication.

If you have more No responses than Yes responses, you may not be as culturally competent as you could be. The purpose of this self-assessment is to increase your awareness of areas where you can improve your cultural competence.

developing cultural competency. Below is a modification of the **LEARN** model that can help nurses include cultural behaviors in a client's health care:

Listen to the client's perception of the problem.

Explain your perception of the problem and of the treatments ordered by the physician.

Acknowledge and discuss the differences and similarities between these two perceptions.

Review the ordered treatments while remembering the client's cultural parameters.

Negotiate agreement. Assist the client in understanding the medical treatments ordered by the physician, and have the client help to make decisions about those treatments as appropriate (e.g., choosing cultural foods that are permitted on an ordered diet).

CASE STUDY \\ B

An Arab couple has come to a local clinic because the wife, who is 6 months pregnant, is not feeling well. The husband speaks English fluently, but the wife's proficiency in English is more limited. Both are dressed in American-style clothes. During the assessment, the registered nurse, Clea Smith, determines that the couple has a 9-month-old and a 2-year-old at home. Ms. Smith also learns that the husband is the head of the household, making most of the major decisions for the family, and that the wife has sole responsibility for the family's care and daily living needs. The wife presents with exhaustion and elevated blood pressure. After obtaining a urine specimen, the physician diagnoses toxemia and orders the wife to be on strict bed rest and to return in 2 weeks. While the husband conveys concern for his wife's health, he is reluctant to have her treatment disrupt the household routine.

Critical Thinking Questions

1. What are the priorities of care for the wife?
2. What additional information would you like to collect about this family?
3. Using either the ASKED or LEARN model, describe how the nurse working with this family could understand and address this situation and the physician's recommendations with both the husband and wife.

In addition to the ASKED and LEARN models, nursing scholars have identified models that illuminate a variety of areas for nurses to explore to deepen their understanding of cultural competence.

Purnell's (2012) model of cultural competence identifies how individuals, families, communities, and the global society all possess 12 domains of culture:

1. Overview, inhabited localities, and topography
2. Communication
3. Family roles and organization
4. Workforce issues
5. Biocultural ecology
6. High-risk behaviors

7. Nutrition
8. Pregnancy and childbearing practices
9. Death rituals
10. Spirituality
11. Healthcare practices
12. Healthcare practitioners.

No one becomes culturally aware or culturally competent overnight. As healthcare providers, it is imperative that we recognize common prejudices. **Prejudices** are prejudgments about cultural groups or vulnerable populations that are unfavorable or false because they have been formed without the background knowledge and context upon which to form an accurate opinion. There is a process by which nursing students (and other individuals) learn cultural confidence, with learning taking place in a fairly predictable sequence:

1. Students begin by developing cultural awareness of how culture shapes beliefs, values, and norms.
2. Students develop cultural knowledge about the differences, similarities, and inequalities in experience and practice among various societies.
3. Students develop cultural understanding of problems and issues facing societies and cultures when values, beliefs, and behaviors are compromised by another culture.
4. Students develop cultural sensitivity to the cultural beliefs, values, and behaviors of their clients. This reflects an awareness of their own cultural beliefs, values, and behaviors that may influence their nursing practice.
5. Students and nurses develop cultural competence and provide care that respects the cultural values, beliefs, and behaviors of their clients.
6. Nurses practice lifelong learning through ongoing education and exposure to cultural groups.

Standards of Competence

Maintaining cultural competence is an ongoing process. Nurses continually assess, modify, and evaluate the care provided to culturally diverse clients. In 2011, Douglas et al. addressed current

Evidence-Based Practice A Model of Ethical Multiculturalism

The Harper model is an evidenced-based model of ethical multiculturalism (**Figure 24–6 ●**) developed and presented at the 34th Annual Transcultural Nursing Society Conference (Harper, 2006). This model includes key attributes of cultural competence and the relationship to a continuum of ethical philosophies. Dr. Harper has said, "Cultural competence occurs on a continuum. Even when you believe you are competent, you can always learn more!" (Harper, 2006).

Critical Thinking Questions

1. How do beneficence and nonmaleficence relate to the concept of cultural competence?
2. Where on Harper's continuum do you think most nurses are? Most student nurses? What would help you become more culturally competent?

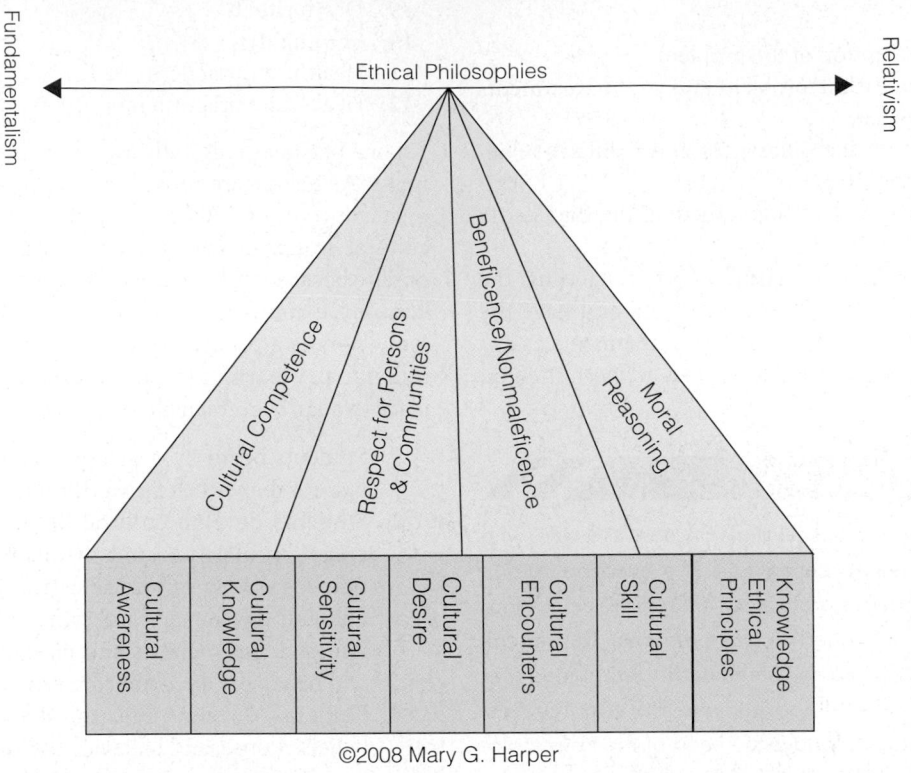

Revised Model of Ethical Multiculturalism
Balance = Protection, Preservation, Dignity, Value

©2008 Mary G. Harper

Figure 24–6 ● This model shows how components of cultural competence are obtained through ethical influences, knowledge, and experience with culture.

Source: Mary Harper, University of Central Florida. Reprinted with permission.

standards for culturally competent nursing care. Their 12 standards are:

1. Social justice
2. Critical reflection
3. Knowledge of cultures
4. Culturally competent practice
5. Cultural competence in healthcare systems and organizations
6. Client advocacy and empowerment
7. Multicultural workforce
8. Education and training in culturally competent care
9. Cross-cultural communication
10. Cross-cultural leadership
11. Policy development
12. Evidence-based practice and research.

Institutions such as hospitals also need to develop and implement cultural competence to address the cultural and language needs of an increasingly multicultural client population. Purnell and colleagues (2011) developed a guide to assessing a culturally competent organization and suggested the following areas be addressed:

■ *Administration and governance.* Some areas for an organization to consider being culturally competent is congruence with a mission statement and implementation of policies and procedure. All administrators must walk the talk and promote organizational practices that promote cultural competence. Organizations should initiate a continuous monitoring process for assessment and evaluation of cultural and language needs. These practices may be hiring protocols, having an ethics or cultural committee to resolve conflicts, having a cafeteria with diverse food choices, and instituting effective communication policies. In addition, monies must be allocated to provide resources and training throughout the organization. Handouts and marketing plans should reflect diverse groups in their narrative, illustrations, and relevant terminology (Byrne et al., 2003).

■ *Orientation and education.* The orientation or professional development for *all* employees should address concepts of cultural competency. An organization should have a philosophy of respect for all of its employees and have resources for multicultural and multilingual employees and community partners.

■ *Language.* The United States is a country of many cultures, and healthcare professionals need to have a basic understanding of how language impacts healthcare delivery systems. Clients with limited proficiency in English often run into barriers when they try to enter the healthcare system. They may delay making an appointment because of difficulties communicating over the telephone, for example, and during this delay, the health problem may become more severe, requiring more expensive treatment. If the client does make an appointment, there may be misunderstandings about the scheduled date, time, or location. Nurses need to know that translation services and interpreter access are federal mandates. Note, too, that translation services involve written communication and interpreters refer to oral communication.

- **Staff competencies.** The last area for organizational cultural competency is providing opportunities for all staff to learn about a variety of cultural groups and become educated as culturally competent providers. Being competent is both an individual and organizational moral imperative for which the organization should provide resources and opportunities for education and multicultural experiences.

Using an Interpreter

Many clients do not speak English, and many who do speak some English are of limited proficiency. Any facility receiving federal funding from the U.S. Department of Health and Human Services is required to communicate effectively with clients or risk the loss of that funding. Having bilingual nurses available is one strategy to address the language barrier. Another strategy is providing access to language banks through electronic or telephone systems that nurses can dial for interpreter services. Unless a client brings an interpreter with her, however, an interpreter may not have any previous knowledge of the client. Nurses can ask a client or family with limited English proficiency if the family works with any area service organizations that provide interpreters. These organizations attempt to provide competent interpreters who build relationships with families over time.

Guidelines for using an interpreter include the following:

- When possible, use an interpreter to translate and provide meaning behind the words.
- To protect client confidentiality and to guard against the possibility of the interpreter misunderstanding medical information, avoid using a family member as an interpreter.
- If possible, use an interpreter of the same gender as the client.
- Address your questions to the client, not the interpreter, but maintain eye contact with both the client and the interpreter.
- Avoid using metaphors, medical jargon, similes, and idiomatic phrases.
- Observe the client's nonverbal communication.
- Plan what to say, and avoid rephrasing or hesitating.
- Use short questions and comments. Ask one question at a time.
- Speak slowly and distinctly, but not loudly.
- Provide written materials in the client's language as available.

Stay Current: Explore this Web site to learn about best practices for using interpreters in health care: **http://minorityhealth. hhs.gov/templates/browse.aspx?lvl=2&lvlID=15**.

CASE STUDY \\ C

Henry Lee is approximately 55 years old. Born in China, he has been living in the United States for the last 10 years, working as a professor at a local university. Following surgery for a broken arm, he refuses pain medication, explaining that his discomfort is bearable and he can survive without medication.

When you next check on him, you find him restless and uncomfortable. You have a standing order to administer medication as needed, and again offer to administer medication. Mr. Lee again refuses, saying that your other responsibilities are more important than his discomfort and he does not want to impose.

Critical Thinking Questions

1. What do you think is behind Mr. Lee's refusal to accept medication?
2. What can you do or say to change Mr. Lee's perception of the situation?
3. What additional information might influence your nursing care?

▶ PROVIDING CULTURALLY COMPETENT NURSING CARE

The provision of culturally competent care begins with incorporating culture into the initial nursing assessment. Areas for assessment include use of herbal supplements and alternative therapies, such as acupuncture; cultural practices related to food preparation or practices at specific times of day or during the week; health beliefs; and preferences for care, such as whether or not women prefer to be examined by a female nurse.

When clients speak languages other than English or are not proficient in English, minimal assessment information from clients can be obtained with the following questions:

- What language do you speak? Do you speak any English?
- How long have you lived here?
- Describe the illness or problem that brings you here today.
- What do you think caused your problem?
- When did it start?
- Why do you think it started when it did?
- What does your sickness do to you?
- How severe is your sickness?
- What do you fear about your sickness?
- What kind of treatment do you think you need?
- Are there any religious practices we need to know about?
- Who is your family?
- Who makes decisions most of the time?
- Who can you go to for help when you need it?

Assessment of cultural influences and practices is imperative because differences in cultural behaviors, beliefs, and values may result in barriers to clients achieving positive outcomes. Cultural misunderstandings or miscommunications also may result from different perceptions of health and of the illness diagnosed.

Nursing assessment of the client's values and beliefs includes assessing for the use of complementary and alternative therapies. The term **complementary therapies** refers to any of a diverse array of practices, therapies, and supplements that are not considered part of conventional or traditional medicine that are used *in addition to* conventional treatments. **Alternative therapies** is a term used to describe use of these diverse therapies *instead of* conventional therapies (see the Complementary and Alternative Therapies feature). Assessing the client for use of these therapies is important to determine client preferences for care and if there are any therapies the client is currently using that are contraindicated.

Once the assessment is complete, nurses can begin to form diagnoses appropriate to the individual or family seeking care. Examples of NANDA nursing diagnoses that may be appropriate for clients of different cultures include:

- *Powerlessness*
- *Spiritual Distress*
- *Risk for Impaired Religiosity*
- *Disturbed Thought Processes*
- *Fear*
- *Decisional Conflict*
- *Noncompliance*
- *Anxiety*
- *Ineffective Health Maintenance*
- *Ineffective Coping*
- *Impaired Social Interaction.*

(NANDA-I © 2012)

Planning care in collaboration with the client increases the likelihood that the client will follow the care plan. At times it can be challenging to incorporate a client's cultural preferences and practices into the care plan, especially in the hospital setting. For example, practicing Muslims observe prayer rituals at five specific times each day. By providing time and space for

> ## Complementary and Alternative Therapy
> ### Overview of CAM
>
> The National Center for Complementary and Alternative Medicine reports that approximately 38% of Americans use complementary and alternative medicine (CAM). Types and examples of CAM include:
>
> - *Natural products.* Dietary supplements
> - *Mind and body medicine.* Meditation, yoga, acupuncture
> - *Manipulative and body-based practices.* Spinal manipulation, massage therapy
> - *Other CAM.* Movement therapies, energy therapies, whole medical systems such as traditional Chinese medicine, homeopathy.
>
> **Stay Current:** For more information on complementary and alternative therapies, go to the NCCAM Web site: **http://nccam.nih.gov**.

these clients to practice their faith, nurses promote therapeutic client relationships and help instill client confidence in the healthcare system.

Evaluating how successfully the client is able to follow the treatment regimen while observing cultural practices and rituals is essential to determining client outcomes but also provides a way for nurses to evaluate whether or not they provided culturally competent care that promoted improved client outcomes.

REVIEW The Concept of Culture and Diversity

RELATE Link the Concepts

Linking the concept of culture and diversity with the concept of development:

1. How might a pediatric client's development be impacted if his or her mother is homeless?

2. How might an adolescent's development be impacted by the realization that he or she is homosexual?

You are a nurse working in a children's rehabilitation center. A 6-year-old girl who is recovering from a car crash comes to your center for an extended stay. She speaks a little English. Her family has recently moved here from China, and her parents speak very little English. Although they are grateful for the help they are receiving, they are very stressed about their daughter's situation.

Linking the concept of culture and diversity with the concept of communication:

3. How might the nurse assess this family's values and beliefs in light of the family's inability to speak English?

4. How might involvement of an interpreter to facilitate communication impact the client and her family's values and beliefs? How can you overcome this problem?

Linking the concept of culture and diversity with the concept of advocacy:

5. How can you advocate for this client's values and beliefs while she is institutionalized?

6. The client's family wishes to pray at the child's bedside using candles, which are not allowed because of the risk for fire related to oxygen use. How can you advocate for this family while maintaining safety?

REFER Go to Pearson Nursing Student Resources
nursing.pearsonhighered.com

- Additional review materials
- Additional case study

REFLECT Case Study

Mrs. Rivera, a 79-year-old woman of Mexican heritage, is admitted to a long-term care facility. Neither she nor her immediate family members speak, write, read, or understand English. She has been a lifelong member of an orthodox Catholic Church and will not allow staff to help her undress. She tells a translator she is very modest and does not want the nursing staff to examine her under her clothing. When asked about advance directives, living wills, or medical power of attorney, both the client and the family inform the staff, "That is none of your business."

1. What client teaching will the nurse provide through the use of a medical interpreter?

2. How can the nurse advocate for Mrs. Rivera's diversity requirements while maintaining facility policy and meeting the client's healthcare needs?

3. What nursing diagnoses and interventions would be appropriate for Mrs. Rivera's plan of care?

■ REFERENCES

American Association of Colleges of Nursing. (2008). *Cultural competency in baccalaureate nursing education.* Retrieved from http://www.aacn.nche.edu/leading-initiatives/education-resources/competency.pdf.

American Association of People with Disabilities (2012). *AAPD mission.* Retrieved from http://www.aapd.com/what-powers-us/aapd-mission.html.

Association of American Medical Colleges. (2005). *Cultural competence education.* Retrieved from https://www.aamc.org/download/54338/dataf.

Berlin, E. A., & Fowkes, W. C. (1983). A teaching framework for cross-cultural health care. *Western Journal of Medicine, 139,* 934–938.

Berman, A., & Snyder, S. (2012). *Fundamentals of nursing: Concepts, process and practice.* Upper Saddle River, NJ: Pearson Education.

Brill, S., & Pepper, R. (2008). *The transgender child: A handbook for families and professionals.* Berkeley, CA: Cleis Press.

Byrne, M., Weddle, C., Davis, E., & McGinnis, P. (2003). The Byrne guide for inclusionary cultural content. *Journal of Nursing Education, 42*(6), 277–281.

Campinha-Bacote, J. (2007). *The journey continues: The process of cultural competence in the delivery of healthcare services.* Cincinnati, OH: Transcultural C.A.R.E. Associates.

Casper, M., Barnett, E., Halverson, J., Elmes, G., Braham, V., Majeed, Z., et al. (2000). *Women and heart disease: An atlas of racial and ethnic disparities in mortality* (2nd ed.). Morgantown, WV: Office for Social Environment and Health Research, West Virginia University.

Clingerman, E. (2011). Social justice: A framework for culturally competent care. *Journal of Transcultural Nursing, 22*(4), 334–341. doi:10.1177/1043659611414185.

Dayer-Berenson, L. (2011). *Cultural competencies for nurses: Impact on health and illness.* Sudbury, MA: Jones & Bartlett.

Douglas, M. K., Pierce, J. U., Rosenkoetter, M., Pacquiao, D., Callister, L. C., Hattar-Pollara, M., et al. (2011). Standards of practice for culturally competent nursing care: 2011 update. *Journal of Transcultural Nursing, 22*(4), 317–333. doi:10.1177/1043659611412965.

Fink, A. (2009). Toward a new definition of health disparity: A concept analysis. *Journal of Transcultural Nursing, 20*(4), 349–357. doi:101177/1043659609340802.

Grandbois, D., & Sanders, G. (2012). Resilience and stereotyping: The experiences of Native American elders. *Journal of Transcultural Nursing, 23*(4), 389–396. doi:10.1177/1043659612451614.

Harper, M. G. (2006). Ethical multiculturalism: An evolutionary concept analysis. *Advances in Nursing Science, 29*(2), 110–124.

Humes, K., Jones, N., & Ramirez, R. (2010). *Overview of race and Hispanic origin: 2010.* Washington, D.C.: U.S. Census Bureau.

Institute of Medicine (IOM). (2002). *Unequal treatment: Confronting racial and ethnic disparities in health care.* Washington, DC: National Academy of Sciences.

Institute of Medicine (IOM). (2011). *The health of lesbian, gay, bisexual, and transgender people: Building a foundation for better understanding.* Washington, DC: National Academy of Sciences.

Intersex Society of North America (ISNA). (n.d.a). *What is intersex?* Retrieved from http://www.isna.org/faq/what_is_intersex.

Intersex Society of North America (ISNA). (n.d.b). *What's the difference between being transgender or transsexual and having an intersex condition?* Retrieved from http://www.isna.org/faq/transgender.

Irwin, L. (2007). Homophobia and heterosexism: Implications for nursing and nursing practice. *Australian Journal of Advanced Nursing, 25*(1), 70–76.

Pension Rights Center. (n.d.). *Income of today's older adults.* Retrieved from http://www.pensionrights.org/publications/statistic/income-today%E2%80%99s-older-adults.

Purnell, L. (2012). *Transcultural health care: A culturally competent approach* (4th ed.). Philadelphia, PA: F. A. Davis.

Purnell, L., Davidhizar, R, Giger, J, Strickland, O, Fishman, D., & Allison, D. (2011). A guide to developing a culturally competent organization. *Journal of Transcultural Nursing, 22*(1), 7–14. doi:10.1177/1043659610387147.

Schuiling, K. D., & Likis, F. E. (2013). *Women's gynecologic health* (2nd ed.). Sudbury, MA: Jones & Bartlett.

Social Science Research Council. (n.d.). *Is race "real"?* Retrieved from http://raceandgenomics.ssrc.org.

U.S. Census Bureau. (2011). *Overview of race and Hispanic origin 2010.* Retrieved from http://www.census.gov/prod/cen2010/briefs/c2010br-02.pdf.

U.S. Department of Health & Human Services (USDHHS). (2012). *Information on poverty and income statistics: A summary of 2012 current population survey data.* Retrieved from http://aspe.hhs.gov/hsp/12/povertyandincomeest/ib.shtml.

U.S. Department of Health and Human Services, Office of Minority Health (2004, March). *Physician toolkit and curriculum: Resources to implement cross-cultural clinical practice guidelines for Medicaid practitioners.* Retrieved from http://minorityhealth.hhs.gov/assets/pdf/checked/1/toolkit.pdf.

U.S. Department of Homeland Security. (2011). *2010 yearbook of immigration statistics.* Retrieved from http://www.dhs.gov/xlibrary/assets/statistics/yearbook/2010/ois_yb_2010.pdf.

Zickuhr, K., & Maden, M. (2012). *Pew Internet and American life project: Older adults and internet use.* Retrieved from http://www.pewinternet.org/Reports/2012/Older-adults-and-internet-use.aspx.

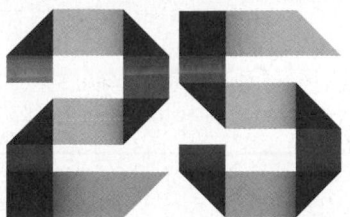 **Development**

MODULE AT-A-GLANCE

The Concept of Development, 1647

Exemplar 25.1
Attention-Deficit/Hyperactivity Disorder, 1680

Exemplar 25.2
Autism Spectrum Disorder, 1688

Exemplar 25.3
Cerebral Palsy, 1695

Exemplar 25.4
Failure to Thrive, 1701

◩ THE CONCEPT OF DEVELOPMENT

The terms *growth* and *development* both refer to dynamic processes. Often used interchangeably, these terms have different meanings. **Growth** refers to physical change and increase in size. Indicators of growth include height, weight, bone size, and dentition. The pattern of physiological growth is similar for all people. However, growth rates vary during different stages of growth and development. The growth rate is rapid during the prenatal, neonatal, infancy, and adolescent stages and slows during childhood. Physical growth is minimal during adulthood.

    Development is an increase in the complexity of function and skill progression, the capacity and skill of an individual to adapt to the environment. Development is the behavioral aspect of growth (e.g., an individual develops the ability to walk, to talk, and to run). **<<**

Concept Learning Outcomes

After reading about this concept, you will be able to:

1. Summarize the physiological and psychological factors that impact development.
2. Examine the relationship between development and other concepts/systems.
3. Identify commonly occurring alterations in development and their related therapies.
4. Differentiate common assessment procedures used to examine developmental health across the life span.
5. Describe diagnostic and laboratory tests to determine the individual's developmental status.
6. Explain promotion of developmental health and prevention of developmental alterations.
7. Demonstrate the nursing process in providing culturally competent and caring interventions across the life span for individuals with common alterations in development.
8. Compare and contrast common independent and collaborative interventions for clients with alterations in development.

Concept Key Terms

Accommodation, *1653*
Adaptation, *1653*
Adaptation phase, *1655*
Adaptive mechanisms, *1649*
Adjustment phase, *1655*
Animism, *1665*
Assimilation, *1653*
Associative play, *1665*
Autosomal chromosomes, *1659*
Centration, *1665*
Cephalocaudal, *1648*
Cognitive development, *1653*
Conservation, *1665*
Cooperative play, *1667*
Defense mechanism, *1649*
Development, *1647*

Developmental stage, *1648*
Developmental task, *1652*
Dramatic play, *1665*
Ecological theory, *1656*
Ego, *1649*
Egocentrism, *1665*
Expressive jargon, *1664*
Expressive speech, *1662*
Fixation, *1650*
Growth, *1647*
Id, *1649*
Libido, *1650*
Magical thinking, *1665*
Moral, *1657*
Moral behavior, *1657*
Moral development, *1657*
Morality, *1657*

(continued on next page)

Nature, *1655*

Nurture, *1656*

Object permanence, *1665*

Parallel play, *1663*

Personality, *1649*

Protective factors, *1654*

Proximodistal, *1648*

Puberty, *1668*

Receptive
speech, *1662*

Resilience, *1654*

Risk factors, *1655*

Self-efficacy, *1654*

Sex chromosomes, *1659*

Solitary play, *1661*

Superego, *1649*

Temperament, *1658*

Transductive
reasoning, *1665*

Unconscious mind, *1649*

▶ NORMAL DEVELOPMENT

Growth and development are independent, yet interrelated processes. For example, an infant's muscles, bones, and nervous system must grow to a certain point before the infant is able to sit up or walk. Growth generally takes place during the first 20 years of life; development takes place throughout the life span. Principles of growth and development include:

- Growth and development are continuous, orderly, sequential processes influenced by maturational, environmental, and genetic factors.

- All humans follow the same pattern of growth and development.

- The sequence of each stage is predictable, although the time of onset, the length of the stage, and the effects of each stage vary with each individual.

- Each **developmental stage** (level of achievement) has its own characteristics. For example, Piaget suggested that in the sensorimotor stage (birth to 2 years) children learn to coordinate simple motor tasks.

- Growth and development occur in a **cephalocaudal** direction, that is, starting at the head and moving toward the trunk, legs, and feet (**Figure 25–1 ●**). This pattern is

particularly obvious at birth, when the head of the infant is disproportionally large.

- Growth and development occur in a **proximodistal** direction, that is, from the center of the body outward (see Figure 25–1). For example, infants can roll over before they can grasp an object with the thumb and second finger.

- Development proceeds from simple to complex, or from single acts to integrated acts. To accomplish the integrated act of drinking and swallowing from a cup, for example, the child must first learn a series of single acts: eye–hand coordination; grasping; hand–mouth coordination; controlled tipping of the cup; and then mouth, lip, and tongue movements to drink and swallow.

- Development becomes increasingly differentiated. Differentiated development begins with a generalized response and progresses to a specific skilled response. For example, an infant's initial response to a stimulus involves the total body, but a 5-year-old child can respond more specifically with laughter or fear.

- Certain stages of growth and development are more critical than others. It is known, for example, that the first 10–12 weeks after conception are critical. The incidence of congenital anomalies as a result of exposure to certain viruses, chemicals, or drugs is greater during this stage than during others.

- The pace of growth and development is uneven. It is known that growth is greater during infancy than during childhood. Asynchronous development is demonstrated by rapid growth of the head during infancy and the extremities at puberty.

- The rate of growth and development is highly individual; however, the sequence of growth and development is predictable. Stages of growth usually correspond to certain developmental changes (**Table 25–1 ●**).

Theories of Growth and Development

Theories help to explain one or more aspects of an individual's growth and development. Typically, theorists examine only one aspect of development, such as the cognitive, moral, or physical aspect. The area chosen for examination usually reflects the researcher's academic discipline and personal interest. The theorists may also limit the population that is studied to a particular part of the life span, such as infancy, childhood, or adulthood.

Although such theories can be useful, they have limitations. First, while a given theory may explain one aspect of the growth and development process, an individual does not develop in fragmented sections but rather as a whole human being. Thus, application of several theories may be necessary to gain insight about an individual's growth and development.

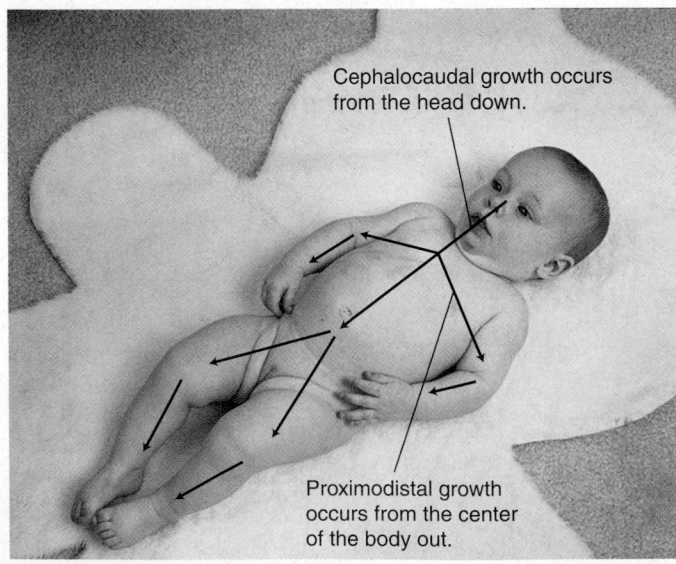

Cephalocaudal growth occurs from the head down.

Proximodistal growth occurs from the center of the body out.

Figure 25–1 ● In normal cephalocaudal growth, the child gains control of the head and neck before the trunk and limbs. In normal proximodistal growth, the child controls arm movements before hand movements. For example, the child reaches for objects before being able to grasp them. Children gain control of their hands before their fingers; that is, they can hold things with the entire hand before they can pick something up with just their fingers.

TABLE 25–1 Stages of Growth and Development

STAGE	AGE	SIGNIFICANT CHARACTERISTICS	NURSING IMPLICATIONS
Neonatal	Birth–28 days	Behavior is largely reflexive and develops to more purposeful behavior.	Assist parents to identify and meet unmet needs.
Infancy	1 month–1 year	Physical growth is rapid.	Control the infant's environment so that physical and psychological needs are met.
Toddlerhood	1–3 years	Motor development permits increased physical autonomy. Psychosocial skills increase.	Safety and risk-taking strategies must be balanced to permit growth.
Preschool	3–6 years	The preschooler's world is expanding. New experiences and the preschooler's social role are tried during play. Physical growth is slower.	Provide opportunities for play and social activity.
School age	6–12 years	This stage includes the preadolescent period (10–12 years). Peer group increasingly influences behavior. Physical growth is slower.	Allow time and energy for the school-age child to pursue hobbies and school activities. Recognize and support child's achievement.
Adolescence	12–18 years	Self-concept changes with biological development. Values are tested. Physical growth accelerates. Stress increases.	Assist adolescents to develop coping behaviors. Help adolescents develop strategies for resolving conflicts.
Young adulthood	18–40 years	A personal lifestyle develops. Individual establishes a relationship with a significant other and a commitment to something.	Accept adult's chosen lifestyle and assist with necessary adjustments relating to health. Recognize the individual's commitments. Support change as necessary for health.
Middle adulthood	40–65 years	Lifestyle changes due to other changes; for example, children leave home, occupational goals change.	Assist clients to plan for anticipated changes in life, to recognize the risk factors related to health, and to focus on strengths rather than weaknesses.
Older Adulthood Young-old	65–74 years	Adaptation to retirement and changing physical abilities is often necessary. Chronic illness may develop.	Assist clients to keep mentally, physically, and socially active and to maintain peer group interactions.
Middle-old	75–84 years	Adaptation to decline in speed of movement, reaction time, and increasing dependence on others may be necessary.	Assist clients to cope with loss (e.g., hearing, sensory abilities, eyesight, death of loved one). Provide necessary safety measures.
Old-old	85 years and older	Increasing physical problems may develop.	Assist clients with self-care as required, and with maintaining as much independence as possible.

Another limitation of some theories is the suggestion that certain tasks are performed at a specific age. In most cases, the child or adult does accomplish the task at the time specified by the guidelines. In other cases, however, the nurse may find that an individual does not accomplish the task or meet the milestone at the exact time the theory suggests. Such individual differences are not easily defined or categorized by a single theory.

Growth and development are commonly thought of as having five major components: psychosocial, cognitive, moral, spiritual, and biophysical. Researchers have advanced several theories about the various stages and aspects of growth and development, particularly with regard to infant and child development. A discussion of some of the major theories follows.

PSYCHOSOCIAL THEORIES Psychosocial development refers to the development of personality. **Personality** can be considered an outward expression of the inner (intrapersonal) self. It encompasses an individual's temperament, feelings, character traits, independence, self-esteem, self-concept, behavior, ability to interact with others, and ability to adapt to life changes.

Freud (1856–1939) Sigmund Freud introduced a number of concepts about psychosocial development that are still used today. The **unconscious mind** is the part of an individual's mental life of which she is unaware. This concept of the unconscious is one of Freud's major contributions to the field of psychiatry. The **id** resides in the unconscious and, operating on the pleasure principle, seeks immediate pleasure and gratification. The **ego**, the realistic part of the individual, balances the gratification demands of the id with the limitations of social and physical circumstances. The ego uses defense mechanisms to fulfill the needs of the id in a socially acceptable manner. **Defense mechanisms**, or **adaptive mechanisms** as they are more commonly called today, are the result of conflicts between the id's impulses and the anxiety created by the conflicts due to social and environmental restrictions. The third aspect of the personality, according to Freud, is the superego. The **superego** contains the conscience and the ego ideal. The conscience consists of society's "do not's," which usually result from parental and cultural expectations. The ego ideal comprises the standards of perfection toward which the individual strives. Freud also proposed that the underlying

TABLE 25–2 Freud's Five Stages of Development

STAGE	AGE	CHARACTERISTICS	IMPLICATIONS
Oral	Birth–1½ years	Mouth is the center of pleasure (major source of gratification and exploration). Security is primary need. Major conflict: weaning.	Feeding produces pleasure and a sense of comfort and safety. Feeding should be pleasurable and provided when required.
Anal	1½–3 years	Anus and bladder are the sources of pleasure (sensual satisfaction, self-control). Major conflict: toilet training.	Controlling and expelling feces provide pleasure and sense of control. Toilet training should be a pleasurable experience.
Phallic	4–6 years	The child's genitals are the center of pleasure. Masturbation offers pleasure. Other activities can include fantasy, experimentation with peers, and questioning of adults about sexual topics. Major conflict: the Oedipus or Electra complex, which resolves when the child identifies with parent of same sex. (The Oedipus complex refers to the male child's attraction to his mother and hostile attitudes toward his father. The Electra complex refers to the female child's attraction to her father and hostile attitudes toward her mother.)	The child identifies with the parent of the opposite sex and later takes on a love relationship outside the family. Encourage identity.
Latency	6 years–puberty	Energy is directed toward physical and intellectual activities. Sexual impulses tend to be repressed. Relationships between peers of the same sex develop.	Encourage child with physical and intellectual pursuits. Encourage sports and other activities with same-sex peers.
Genital	Puberty and after	Energy is directed toward full sexual maturity and function and development of skills needed to cope with the environment.	Encourage separation from parents, achievement of independence, and decision making.

motivation to human development is a dynamic, psychic energy, which he called **libido**. According to Freud's theory of psychosexual development, the personality develops in five overlapping stages from birth to adulthood. The libido changes its location of emphasis within the body from one stage to another. Therefore, a particular body area has special significance to a client at a particular stage. The first three stages (oral, anal, and phallic) are called *pregenital stages*. The culminating stage is the *genital stage*. **Table 25–2** ● indicates characteristics for each stage.

Freudian theory asserts that the individual must meet the needs of each developmental stage to move successfully to the next. For example, during the oral stage, nurses can assist an infant's development by making feeding a pleasurable experience. This provides comfort and security for the infant. Freud also emphasized the importance of infant–parent interaction. Therefore, the nurse, as a caregiver, should provide a warm, caring atmosphere for an infant and assist parents to do so when the infant returns to their care.

Unsuccessful progression through a given stage can result in fixation. **Fixation** is immobilization or the inability of the personality to proceed to the next stage because of anxiety. For example, making toilet training a positive experience during the anal stage enhances the child's feeling of self-control. If, however, the toilet training was a negative experience, the resulting conflict or stress can delay or prolong the child's progression through that stage or cause the child to regress to a previous stage. Ideally, an individual progresses through each stage with balance between the id, ego, and superego.

Erikson (1902–1994) Erik H. Erikson (1963, 1968) adapted and expanded Freud's theory of development to include the entire life span, believing that people continue to develop throughout life. He described eight stages of development (**Table 25–3** ●).

Erikson's theory proposes that life is a sequence of developmental stages or levels of achievement. Each stage signals a task that must be accomplished. The resolution of the task can be complete, partial, or unsuccessful. Erikson believed that the more successful an individual is at each developmental stage, the healthier the personality of the individual will be. Failure to complete any developmental stage interferes with the individual's ability to progress to the next level. These developmental stages can be viewed as a series of crises. Successful resolution of these crises supports healthy ego development. Failure to resolve the crises damages the ego.

Erikson's eight stages reflect both positive and negative aspects of the critical life periods. The resolution of the conflicts at each stage enables the individual to function effectively in society. Each phase has its own developmental task, and the individual must find a balance between, for example, trust and mistrust (stage 1) or integrity and despair (stage 8). See **Figures 25–2** ● and **25–3** ●.

When using Erikson's developmental framework, nurses should be aware of indicators of positive and negative resolution of each developmental stage. According to Erikson, the environment is highly influential to development. Nurses can enhance a client's development by being aware of the individual's developmental stage and assisting with the development of coping skills related to stressors experienced at that specific level. Nurses can

TABLE 25–3   Erikson's Eight Stages of Development

STAGE	AGE	PRIMARY TASK	OUTCOMES OF SUCCESSFUL TASK ACCOMPLISHMENT	OUTCOMES OF FAILED TASK ACCOMPLISHMENT
Infancy	Birth to 18 months	Trust versus mistrust	Development of basic trust and sense of security	Lack of trust, sense of fear
Early childhood	18 months to 3 years	Autonomy versus shame and doubt	Basic awareness of independence; sense of autonomy and self-control	Self-doubt, sense of helplessness, heightened dependence on caregivers
Late childhood	3 to 5 years	Initiative versus guilt	Emergence of basic sense of self-guidance and self-discipline	Impaired self-initiative, insecurity regarding leadership ability
School age	6 to 12 years	Industry versus inferiority	Confidence in ability to attain goals, initial formation of identity apart from nuclear family, successful peer group integration	Sense of incompetence, low self-esteem, difficulty integrating into peer groups
Adolescence	12 to 20 years	Identity versus role confusion	Formation of strong sense of identity as an individual and as a member of society, identification of personal and occupational goals	Role confusion, social alienation, potential substance abuse, potential development of antisocial personality disorder
Young adulthood	18 to 25 years	Intimacy versus isolation	Development of healthy romantic relationships without compromising personal identity	Avoidance of intimacy, fear of commitment, isolation
Adulthood	25 to 65 years	Generativity versus stagnation	Productivity and creativity, desire to care for and guide offspring (or, if childfree, to guide the next generation)	Self-preoccupation, primary attainment of pleasure through self-indulgence, stagnation
Maturity	65 years to death	Integrity versus despair	Sense of peace concerning life experiences, life choices framed within a meaningful context, development of wisdom	Life experiences framed by bitterness and/or regret; may progress to hopelessness and depression

Source: Based on Erikson, E. (1963). *Childhood and society.* New York, NY: W.W. Norton; Weber, J. R., & Kelley, J. H. (2010). *Health assessment in nursing* (4th ed.). Philadelphia: Lippincott Williams & Wilkins; Watts, J., Cockcroft, K., & Duncan, N. (Eds.). (2010). *Developmental psychology* (2nd ed.). Cape Town, South Africa: UCT Press.

strengthen a client's positive resolution of a developmental task by providing the individual with appropriate opportunities and encouragement. For example, a 10-year-old child (industry versus inferiority) can be encouraged to be creative, to finish schoolwork, and to learn how to accomplish these tasks within the limitations imposed by health status. An older adult can be encouraged to maintain generativity (care for and connection with others) to avoid a sense of stagnation, or a feeling of disconnectedness that increases self-absorption and loneliness.

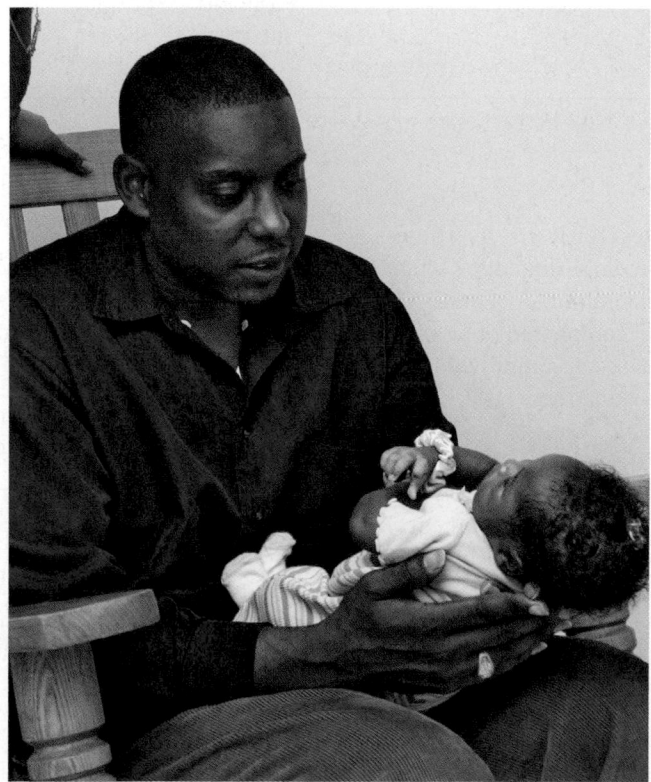

Figure 25–2 ● Note that the parent's and infant's faces are in the same plane. This *en face* position enables both to examine the other's face and establish eye contact, fostering attachment between parent and child.

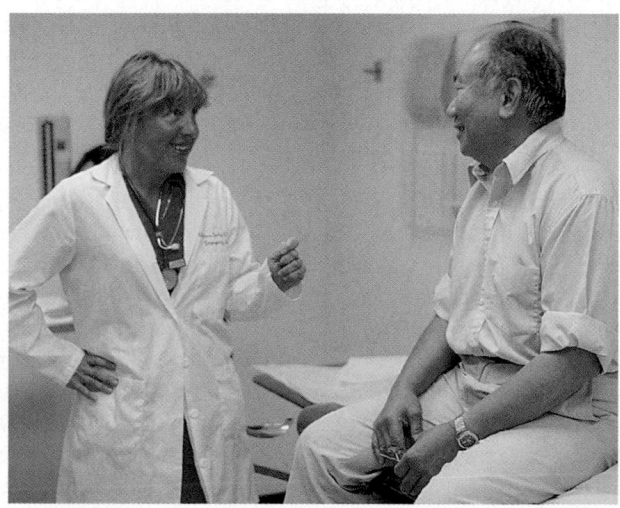

Figure 25–3 ● Regular assessments can help older adults maintain their health and independence, contributing to achievement of integrity versus despair.

TABLE 25–4 Age Periods and Developmental Tasks

Infancy and Early Childhood
1. Learning to walk
2. Learning to take solid foods
3. Learning to talk
4. Learning to control the elimination of body wastes
5. Learning sex differences and sexual modesty
6. Achieving psychological stability
7. Forming simple concepts of social and physical reality
8. Learning to relate emotionally to parents, siblings, and other people
9. Learning to distinguish right from wrong and developing a conscience

Middle Childhood
1. Learning physical skills necessary for ordinary games
2. Building wholesome attitudes toward oneself as a growing organism
3. Learning to get along with age-mates
4. Learning an appropriate masculine or feminine social role
5. Developing fundamental skills in reading, writing, and calculating
6. Developing concepts necessary for everyday living
7. Developing conscience, morality, and a scale of values
8. Achieving personal independence
9. Developing attitudes toward social groups and institutions

Adolescence
1. Achieving new and more mature relations with age-mates of both sexes
2. Achieving a masculine or feminine social role
3. Accepting one's physique and using the body effectively
4. Achieving emotional independence from parents and other adults
5. Achieving assurance of economic independence
6. Selecting and preparing for an occupation

7. Preparing for marriage and family life
8. Developing intellectual skills and concepts necessary for civic competence
9. Desiring and achieving socially responsible behavior
10. Acquiring a set of values and an ethical system as a guide to behavior

Early Adulthood
1. Selecting a mate
2. Learning to live with a partner
3. Starting a family
4. Rearing children
5. Managing a home
6. Getting started in an occupation
7. Taking on civic responsibility
8. Finding a congenial social group

Middle Age
1. Achieving adult civic and social responsibility
2. Establishing and maintaining an economic standard of living
3. Assisting teenage children to become responsible and happy adults
4. Developing adult leisure-time activities
5. Relating oneself to one's spouse as a person
6. Accepting and adjusting to the physiological changes of middle age
7. Adjusting to aging parents

Later Maturity
1. Adjusting to decreasing physical strength and health
2. Adjusting to retirement and reduced income
3. Adjusting to death of a spouse
4. Establishing an explicit affiliation with one's age group
5. Meeting social and civil obligations
6. Establishing satisfactory physical living arrangements

Source: Havighurst, R. J. (1972). *Developmental tasks and education* (3rd ed.). New York, NY: David McKay Company, Inc.

Erikson emphasized that people must change and adapt their behavior to maintain control over their lives. In his view, no stage in personality development can be bypassed, and people can become fixated at one stage or regress to a previous stage under anxious or stressful conditions. For example, a middle-aged woman who has never satisfactorily resolved the identity versus role confusion task might regress to an earlier stage when stressed by an illness with which she cannot cope.

Havighurst (1900–1991) Robert Havighurst believed that learning is basic to life, and people continue to learn throughout life. He described growth and development as occurring in six stages, each associated with 6–10 tasks to be learned (**Table 25–4 ●**).

Havighurst (1972) promoted the concept of developmental tasks in the 1950s. A **developmental task** is "a task which arises at or about a certain period in the life of an individual, successful achievement of which leads to his happiness and to success with later tasks, while failure leads to unhappiness in the individual, disapproval by society, and difficulty with later tasks" (p. 2).

Havighurst's developmental tasks provide a framework that the nurse can use to evaluate an individual's general accomplishments. However, some nurses find that the broad catego-

ries limit its usefulness as a tool in assessing specific accomplishments, particularly those of infancy and childhood. In addition, in a multicultural society, the definition of successful completion of tasks may vary with values and belief systems (e.g., not all individuals may wish to marry or bear children), making these tasks less relevant for some.

Peck (1919–2002) Theories and models about adult development are relatively recent compared with theories of infant and child development. Research into adult development has been stimulated by a number of factors, including increased longevity and healthier old age. In the past, development was viewed as complete by the time of physical maturity, and aging was considered a decline following maturity. The emphasis was on the negative rather than positive aspects of aging. However, Robert Peck (1968) believes that, although physical capabilities and functions decrease with old age, mental and social capacities tend to increase in the latter part of life.

Peck (1968) proposes three developmental tasks during old age, in contrast to Erikson's one (integrity versus despair):

1. ***Ego differentiation versus work-role preoccupation.*** An adult's identity and feelings of worth are highly dependent

on that individual's work role. On retirement, people may experience feelings of worthlessness unless they derive their sense of identity from a sufficient number of roles that one such role can replace the work role or occupation as a source of self-esteem. For example, a man who likes to garden or golf can obtain ego rewards from those activities, replacing rewards formerly obtained from his occupation.

2. *Body transcendence versus body preoccupation.* This task calls for the individual to adjust to decreasing physical capacities and at the same time maintain feelings of well-being. Preoccupation with declining body functions reduces happiness and satisfaction with life.

3. *Ego transcendence versus ego preoccupation.* Ego transcendence is the acceptance without fear of one's death as inevitable. This acceptance includes being actively involved in one's own future beyond death. Ego preoccupation, by contrast, results in holding onto life and a preoccupation with self-gratification.

Gould (1935–)

Roger Gould is another theorist who has studied adult development. He believes that transformation is a central theme during adulthood: "Adults continue to change over the period of time considered to be adulthood and developmental phases may be found during the adult span of life" (Gould, 1972, p. 33). According to Gould, in his 20s the individual assumes new roles, in the 30s role confusion often occurs, in the 40s the individual becomes aware of time limitations in relation to accomplishing life's goals, and in the 50s the acceptance of each stage as a natural progression of life marks the path to adult maturity.

- **Stage 1 (ages 16–18).** Individuals consider themselves part of the family rather than individuals; they begin to want to separate from their parents.

- **Stage 2 (ages 18–22).** Although individuals have established autonomy, they feel it is in jeopardy; they feel they could be pulled back into their families.

- **Stage 3 (ages 22–28).** Individuals feel established as adults and autonomous from their families. They see themselves as well defined but still feel the need to prove themselves to their parents. They see this as the time for growing and building for the future.

- **Stage 4 (ages 28–34).** Marriage and careers are well established. Individuals question what life is all about and wish to be accepted as they are, no longer finding it necessary to prove themselves.

- **Stage 5 (ages 34–43).** This is a period of self-reflection. Individuals question long-held values as well as life itself. They see time as finite, with little time left to shape the lives of adolescent children.

- **Stage 6 (ages 43–50).** Personalities are seen as set. Time is accepted as finite. Individuals are interested in social activities with friends and spouse and desire both sympathy and affection from spouse.

- **Stage 7 (ages 50–60).** This is a period of transformation, with a realization of mortality and a concern for health. There is an increase in warmth and a decrease in negativism. The spouse is seen as a valuable companion (Gould, 1972, pp. 525–527).

Continuity Theory

This theory advances the idea that successful aging involves maintaining or continuing previous values, habits, preferences, family ties, and all other linkages that have formed the basic underlying structure of adult life. Older age is not viewed as a time that should trigger major life readjustment, but rather as just a time to continue being the same individual (Havighurst, Neugarten, & Tobin, 1963). According to this theory, the pace of activities may be slowed. The older adult may drop activities pursued in earlier life that did not bring satisfaction and genuine happiness. For some, relief from constant time pressures and deadlines is one of the benefits of old age.

PIAGET'S THEORY OF COGNITIVE DEVELOPMENT

Cognitive development refers to the manner in which people learn to think, reason, and use language. It involves a person's intelligence, perceptual ability, and ability to process information. Cognitive development represents a progression of mental abilities from illogical to logical thinking, from simple to complex problem solving, and from understanding concrete ideas to understanding abstract concepts.

The most widely known cognitive theorist is Jean Piaget. His theory of cognitive development has contributed to other theories, such as Kohlberg's moral development and Fowler's development of faith theories, both discussed in this module.

According to Piaget (1966), cognitive development is an orderly, sequential process in which a variety of new experiences (stimuli) must exist before intellectual abilities can develop. Piaget divides cognitive development into five major phases: the sensorimotor phase, the preconceptual phase, the intuitive thought phase, the concrete operations phase, and the formal operations phase. A detailed discussion of these phases, and how the nurse can incorporate his or her knowledge of them into nursing plans and interventions, can be found in the Cognition module.

An individual develops through each of these phases; each phase has its own unique characteristics (**Table 25–5 ●**). In each phase, the individual uses three primary abilities: assimilation, accommodation, and adaptation. **Assimilation** is the process through which humans encounter and react to new situations by using mechanisms they already possess. In this way, people acquire knowledge and skills as well as insights into the world around them. **Accommodation** is a process of change whereby cognitive processes mature sufficiently to allow the individual to solve problems that were unsolvable before. This adjustment is possible chiefly because new knowledge has been assimilated. **Adaptation**, or coping behavior, is the ability to handle the demands made by the environment.

Nurses can use Piaget's theory of cognitive development when developing teaching strategies. For example, a nurse can expect a toddler to be egocentric and literal; therefore, explanations to the toddler should focus on the needs of the toddler rather than on the needs of others. A 13-year-old can be expected to use rational thinking and to reason; therefore, when explaining the need for a medication, a nurse can outline the consequences of taking and not taking the medication, enabling the adolescent to make a rational decision. Nurses must remember, however, that the range of normal cognitive development is broad, despite the ages arbitrarily associated with each level. When teaching adults, nurses may become aware that some adults are more comfortable

TABLE 25–5 Piaget's Phases of Cognitive Development

PHASES AND STAGES	AGE	SIGNIFICANT BEHAVIOR
Sensorimotor phase	Birth–2 years	
Stage 1: Use of reflexes	Birth–1 month	Uses reflexes: sucking, rooting, grasping.
Stage 2: Primary circular reaction	1–4 months	Infant responds reflexively. Objects are extension of self.
Stage 3: Secondary circular reaction	4–8 months	Awareness of environment grows. Changes in the environment are actively made as infant recognizes cause and effect.
Stage 4: Coordination of secondary schemata	8–12 months	Intentional behavior occurs. Object permanence begins.
Stage 5: Tertiary circular reaction	12–18 months	Toddlers discover new goals and ways to attain goals. Rituals are important.
Stage 6: Mental combinations	18–24 months	Language gives toddlers a new tool to use.
Preoperational phase	2–7 years	Young children think by using words as symbols. Everything is significant and relates to "me." They explore the environment. Language development is rapid. Words are associated with objects.
		As children get older, egocentric thinking diminishes. They think of one idea at a time. Words express thoughts.
Concrete operational phase	7–11 years	Children solve concrete problems, begin to understand relationships such as size, understand right and left, and recognize various viewpoints.
Formal operational phase	11–15 years	Children use rational thinking. Reasoning is deductive and futuristic.

Source: Data from Piaget, J. (1966). The origin of intelligence. Copyright © 1966 International Universities Press, Inc.

with concrete thought and are slower to acquire and apply new information than are other adults.

BEHAVIORISM Behaviorist theory states that learning takes place when an individual's reaction to a stimulus is either positively or negatively reinforced. The more rapid, consistent, and positive the reinforcement, the more likely a behavior is to be learned and retained.

B. F. Skinner believed that organisms learn as they respond to or "operate on" their environment. His research led to the concept of *operant conditioning*, in which he maintained that rewarded or reinforced behavior will be repeated; behavior that is punished will be suppressed. Most of his work was with laboratory animals.

SOCIAL LEARNING THEORY Albert Bandura (1925–), a contemporary psychologist, believes that children learn attitudes, beliefs, customs, and values through their social contacts with adults and other children. Children imitate (or model) the behavior they see; if the behavior is positively reinforced, they tend to repeat it. However, Bandura also believes that people can consciously choose how to act, such as deciding to handle problems by talking rather than using violence. The external environment (the behavior of others) and the child's internal processes are both key elements in the behaviors the child manifests (Bandura, 1986, 1997a).

Bandura believes that an important determinant of behavior is **self-efficacy**, or the expectation that someone can produce a desired outcome. For example, if adolescents believe they can avoid use of drugs or alcohol, they are more likely to do so. A child who has confidence in his or her ability to exercise regularly or lose weight has a greater chance of success with these behavior changes. Parents who have confidence in their ability

to care adequately for their infants are more likely to do so (Bandura, 1997b).

TEMPERAMENT THEORY Chess and Thomas (1995, 1996) recognize the innate qualities of personality that each individual brings to the events of daily life. They view the child as an individual who both influences and is influenced by the environment. However, Chess and Thomas focus on one specific aspect of development: the wide spectrum of behaviors possible in children and how they respond to daily events. Infants generally display clusters of responses, which Chess and Thomas have classified into three major personality types (**Box 25–1 ●**). Although most children do not demonstrate all behaviors described for a particular type, they usually show a grouping indicative of one personality type (Chess & Thomas, 1995, 1996).

Longitudinal research has demonstrated that personality characteristics displayed during infancy are often consistent with those seen later in life. The ability to predict future characteristics is not possible, however, because of the complex and dynamic interaction of personality traits and environmental reactions.

RESILIENCY THEORY Why do some children have such different behavioral outcomes from others coming from similar backgrounds? A theory that examines the individual's characteristics as well as the interaction of those characteristics with the environment is the resiliency model. **Resilience** is the ability to function with healthy responses, even when experiencing significant stress and adversity (Masten et al., 2009). In this model, the individual or family members experience a crisis that provides a source of stress, and the family interprets or deals with the crisis based on resources available. Families and individuals have **protective factors** that provide strength and

Evidence-Based Practice Self-Efficacy

Problem

Nurses often provide information for parents and children that will encourage them to adopt healthy lifestyles. Providing information, however, may not be enough. Many of us know about healthy behaviors, but do not consistently apply them. The concept of self-efficacy helps to explain why some people take on healthy behaviors, whereas others do not. People who are convinced they can make a positive change are more likely to do so. A number of research projects test and apply self-efficacy in teaching about health. Two examples follow.

Evidence

A federally funded study sought to measure the effectiveness of a preventive parent training program among low-income families with small children. The weekly sessions involved viewing a videotape and discussing positive and negative parenting skills observed. The researchers compared characteristics of the parents who chose to attend the sessions, including a measure of parental self-efficacy, or belief that they could manage a range of tasks and situations in caring for their young children. Parents with lower self-efficacy scores were significantly more likely to enroll in and attend the parenting training sessions (Gross et al., 2009).

Mothers who have a greater degree of self-efficacy about their ability to breastfeed are significantly more likely to begin and to continue breastfeeding. A Breastfeeding Self-Efficacy Scale has been developed to identify both risk and protective factors that influence the self-efficacy of new mothers. Educational level, support from other women, quality of postpartum care, maternal anxiety, and plans made for feeding method all influence the breastfeeding self-efficacy scores of women. Additionally, the instrument is effective when used among diverse ethnic populations (Gregory et al., 2008).

Implications

In addition to providing information about health behaviors, nurses need to integrate methods to increase self-efficacy in teaching projects with families. Assessments should be designed to identify self-efficacy of parents and children around health topics of interest. Interventions can then be planned to enhance the self-efficacy of family members.

Critical Thinking Application

Nurses can apply the concept of self-efficacy in teaching children and families.

1. Plan a teaching project for school-age children to foster healthy eating. Include expected outcomes for the children and interventions.

2. Could your outcome be improved if you focus not just on getting the content across, but also on increasing the belief and confidence that the children will be able to integrate the new behaviors into their lives?

3. What activities could your teaching plan include that would be likely to improve the self-efficacy of these school-age children?

Box 25–1   Patterns of Temperament— Chess and Thomas

- **"Easy" child.** The "easy" child is generally moderately active; shows regularity in patterns of eating, sleeping, and elimination; and is usually positive in mood and when subjected to new stimuli. The easy child adapts to new situations and is able to accept rules and work well with others. About 40% of children in the New York Longitudinal Study displayed this personality type.

- **"Difficult" child.** The "difficult" child displays irregular schedules for eating, sleeping, and elimination; adapts slowly to new situations and persons; and displays a predominantly negative mood. Intense reactions to the environment are common. The New York Longitudinal Study found that approximately 10% of children display this personality type.

- **"Slow-to-warm-up" child.** The "slow-to-warm-up" child has reactions of mild intensity and is slow to adapt to new situations. The child displays initial withdrawal followed by gradual, quiet, and slow interactions with the environment. About 15% of children in the New York Longitudinal Study displayed this personality type.

The remaining 35% of children studied showed some characteristics of each personality type.

Source: Data from Chess S. & Thomas, A. (1996) *Temperament: Theory and Practice*, Philadelphia: Brunner/Mazel Publishers.

---

assistance in dealing with crises and **risk factors** that promote or contribute to their challenges. Protective and risk factors can be identified in children, in their families, and in their communities. A typical crisis for a young child might be a transfer to a new childcare provider. Protective factors for a child transferring to a new provider could involve past positive experiences with new people and an "easy" temperament. An additional protective factor might be the level of understanding the new childcare provider has about the adaptation needs of young children to new experiences. Risk factors for a child experiencing this type of transition might include repeated moves to new care providers, limited close relationships with adults, and a "slow-to-warm-up" temperament.

Once confronted by a crisis, the child and family first experience the **adjustment phase**. This phase is characterized by disorganization and unsuccessful attempts at meeting the crisis. In the **adaptation phase**, the child and family meet the challenge and use resources to deal with the crisis (Walsh, 2011). Adaptation may lead to increasing resilience, as the child and family learn about new resources and inner strengths and develop the ability to deal more effectively with future crises.

ECOLOGICAL THEORY   The relative importance in human development of heredity versus environment—or nature versus nurture—is controversial among theorists. **Nature** refers to the genetic or hereditary capability of an individual. **Nurture** refers to the effects of the environment on a person's performance. Contemporary developmental theories increasingly recognize the interaction of nature and nurture in determining the child's development.

The ecological theory of development was formulated by Urie Bronfenbrenner to explain the child's unique relationship in all of life's settings, from close to remote (Bronfenbrenner, 1986, 2005; Bronfenbrenner et al., 1996). **Ecological theory** emphasizes the presence of mutual interactions between the child and these various settings. Neither nature nor nurture is considered more important. Bronfenbrenner believes each child brings a unique set of genes—and specific attributes such as age, gender, health, and other characteristics—to his or her interactions with the environment. The child then interacts in many settings at different levels or systems (**Figure 25–4 ●**). The five systems of ecological theory are the microsystem, mesosystem, exosystem, macrosystem, and chronosystem.

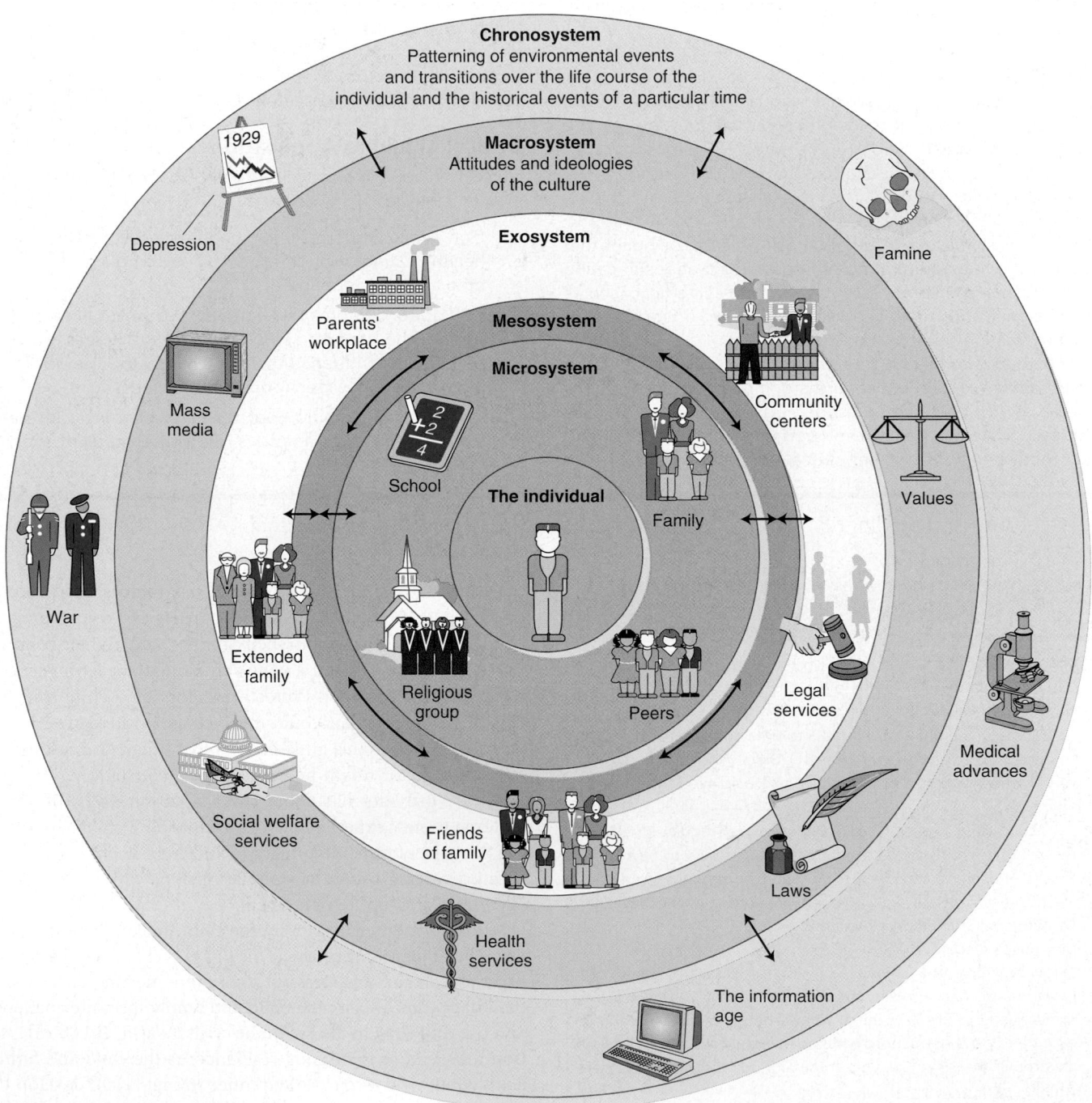

Figure 25–4 ● Bronfenbrenner's ecological theory of development views the individual as interacting within five levels or systems.
Source: Redrawn from Santrock, J. W. (2005). *Life span development.* Madison, WI: Brown & Benchmark. Based on Bronfenbrenner's (1979, 1986) works in Contexts of child rearing: Problems and prospects. *American Psychologist, 34,* 844–850; Ecology of the family as a context for human development: Research perspectives. *Developmental Psychology, 22,* 723–742.

Microsystem   This level is defined as the daily, consistent, close relationships such as home, child care, school, friends, and neighbors. For the child with a chronic illness requiring regular care, the healthcare providers may even be part of the microsystem. In the ecological model, the child influences each of these settings in addition to being influenced by them, with reciprocal interactions.

Mesosystem   This level includes relationships of microsystems with one another. For example, two microsystems for most children are the home and the school. The relationships between these microsystems are shown by parents' involvement in their children's school. This involvement, in turn, influences the effects of both the home and school settings on the children.

Exosystem   This level of ecological theory is composed of those settings that influence the child even though the child is not in close daily contact with the system. Examples are the parents' jobs and the governing board of the local school district. Although the child may not go to the parents' workplaces, he or she can be influenced by policies related to health care, sick leave, inflexible work hours, overtime, travel, or even the mood of the boss (through its impact on the parent). The child's needs may influence a parent to give up a certain job or to work harder to obtain money for the child's education. Likewise, when a local school board votes to ban certain books or to finance a field trip, the child is influenced by these decisions; the child, in turn, can help establish an atmosphere that will guide future school board decisions.

Macrosystem   This level includes the beliefs, values, and behaviors expressed in the child's environment. Culture is a powerful influence on the macrosystem, as is the political system. For instance, a democratic system creates different beliefs, values, and even eating practices from those of an anarchic system.

Chronosystem   This final level brings the perspective of time to the previous settings. The time period during which the child grows up influences views of health and illness. For example, the experiences of children with influenza in the 19th versus the 20th century were quite different.

MORAL THEORIES   Moral development is a complex process that is not fully understood. It involves learning what a person should and should not do, but it is more than merely the imprinting of parents' rules and virtues or values on children. The term **moral** means "relating to right and wrong." The terms *morality, moral behavior,* and *moral development* need to be distinguished from each other. **Morality** refers to the requirements necessary for people to live together in society, **moral behavior** is the way an individual perceives and responds to those requirements, and **moral development** is the pattern of change in moral behavior with age.

Kohlberg (1927–1987)   Lawrence Kohlberg's theory specifically addresses moral development in children and adults (Kohlberg, 1981, 1984). Kohlberg was not concerned with the morality of an individual's decision; rather, he focused on the reasons an individual makes a decision. According to Kohlberg, moral development progresses through three levels and six stages. Levels and stages are not always linked to a certain developmental stage, because some people progress to a higher level of moral development than others.

At Kohlberg's first level, called the *premoral* or *preconventional level,* children are responsive to cultural rules and labels of good and bad, right and wrong. However, children interpret these in terms of the consequences of their actions—punishment or reward. At the second level, the *conventional level,* the individual is concerned about maintaining the expectations of the family, group, or nation, and sees this as right. The emphasis at this level is on conformity and loyalty to an individual's own expectations as well as society's. Level III is called the *postconventional, autonomous,* or *principled level.* At this level, people make an effort to define valid values and principles without regard to outside authority or to the expectations of others (**Table 25–6 ●**).

Gilligan (1936–)   After more than 10 years of research with female subjects, Carol Gilligan (1982) reported that women often consider the dilemmas Kohlberg used in his research to be irrelevant. Women scored consistently lower on Kohlberg's scale of moral development despite the fact that they approached moral dilemmas with considerable sophistication. Gilligan believed that most frameworks for research in moral development do not include the concepts of caring and responsibility.

Gilligan proposed that moral development proceeds through three levels and two transitions, with each level representing a more complex understanding of the relationship of self and others and each transition resulting in a crucial reevaluation of the conflict between selfish and responsibility (Campbell, 2010; Murray & Zentner, 2001, p. 251):

- *Level 1: Caring for oneself.* At this level of development, the individual is concerned only with caring for the self. The individual feels isolated, alone, and unconnected to others. There is no concern or conflict with the needs of others because the self is the most important. The focus of this stage is survival. The transition out of this stage occurs when the individual begins to view this approach as selfish and moves toward responsibility. The individual begins to realize a need for relationships and connections with other people.

- *Level 2: Caring for others.* At this level, the individual recognizes the selfishness of earlier behavior and begins to understand the need for caring relationships with others. The individual now approaches relationships with a focus on not hurting others. This approach causes the individual to be more responsive and submissive to others' needs, often to the exclusion of meeting his own needs. A transition from goodness to truth occurs when the individual recognizes that the lack of balance between caring for himself and caring for others in this approach can cause difficulties with relationships. The individual makes decisions on personal intentions and consequences of actions rather than on how he thinks others will react (Campbell, 2010; Murray & Zentner, 2001, p. 253).

- *Level 3: Caring for self and others.* During this last stage, an individual sees the need for a balance between caring for others and caring for the self. Care remains the focus on which decisions are based. However, the individual recognizes the interconnections between the self and others and realizes that if her own needs are not met, other people may also suffer.

Gilligan (1982) proposes that because women often see morality in the integrity of relationships and caring, the moral problems they encounter are different from those of men. Men

TABLE 25–6 Kohlberg's Stages of Moral Development

LEVEL	STAGE	AVERAGE AGE
I. Preconventional Individual is responsive to cultural rules of good and bad, right or wrong. Externally established rules determine right or wrong actions. Individual reasons in terms of punishment, reward, or exchange of favors. Egocentric focus	1. Punishment and obedient orientation Fear of punishment, not respect for authority, is the reason for decisions, behavior, and conformity. 2. Instrumental relativist orientation Conformity is based on egocentricity and narcissistic needs. There is no feeling of justice, loyalty, or gratitude. "I'll do something if I get something for it or because it pleases you."	Toddler to 7 years Preschooler through school age
II. Conventional Individual is concerned with maintaining expectations and rules of the family, group, nation, or society. A sense of guilt has developed and affects behavior. The individual values conformity, loyalty, and active maintenance of social order and control. Conformity means good behavior or what pleases or helps another and is approved. Societal focus	3. Interpersonal concordance orientation Decisions and behavior are based on concerns about others' reactions; the individual wants others' approval or a reward. An empathic response, based on understanding of how another individual feels, is a determinant for decisions and behavior. ("I can put myself in your shoes.") 4. Law-and-order orientation The individual wants established rules from authorities, and the reason for decisions and behavior is that social and sexual rules and traditions demand the response. ("I'll do something because it's the law and my duty.")	School age through adulthood (Most American women are in this stage.) Adolescence and adulthood (Most men are in this stage.)
III. Postconventional The individual lives autonomously and defines moral values and principles that are distinct from personal identification with group values. He or she lives according to principles that are universally agreed on and that the individual considers appropriate for life. Universal focus	5. Social contract legalistic orientation The social rules are not the sole basis for decisions and behavior because the individual believes a higher moral principle applies, such as equality, justice, or due process. 6. Universal ethical principle orientation Decisions and behaviors are based on internalized rules, on conscience rather than social laws, and on self-chosen ethical and abstract principles that are universal, comprehensive, and consistent.	Middle-aged or older adult (Only 20% or fewer of Americans achieve this stage.) Middle-aged or older adult (Few people attain or maintain this stage. Examples of this stage are seen in times of crisis or extreme situations.)

Source: Murray, R. B., Zentner, J. P., & Yakimo, R. (2009). Health promotion strategies through the life span (pp. 32–33). Upper Saddle River, NJ: Pearson Prentice Hall. Adapted with permission.

tend to consider what is right to be what is just, whereas for women what is right is taking responsibility for others as a self-chosen decision (p. 140). The ethic of justice, or fairness, is based on the idea of equality: Everyone should receive the same treatment. This is the development path usually followed by men and widely accepted by moral theorists. By contrast, the ethic of care is based on the premise of nonviolence: No one should be harmed. This is the path typically followed by women but given little attention in the literature of moral theory.

In discussing the development of maturity, Gilligan (1982) stated that both viewpoints blend "in the realization that just as inequality adversely affects both perspectives in an unequal relationship, so too violence is destructive for everyone involved" (p. 174). The blending of these two perspectives could give rise to a new view of human development and a better understanding of human relations.

SPIRITUAL THEORIES The spiritual component of growth and development refers to individuals' understanding of their relationship with the universe and their perceptions about the direction and meaning of life.

Fowler (1940–) James Fowler describes the development of faith as a force that gives meaning to a person's life. He uses the

term *faith* as a form of knowing, a way of being in relation to "an ultimate environment." To Fowler, "faith is a relational phenomenon; it is an active 'mode-of-being-in-relation' to another or others in which we invest commitment, belief, love, risk and hope" (Fowler & Keen, 1985, p. 18). Fowler is influenced by the work of Piaget, Kohlberg, and Erikson. Fowler believes that the development of faith is an interactive process between the individual and his or her environment (Fowler, Streib, & Keller, 2004).

Westerhoff (1933–) John Westerhoff describes faith as a way of being and behaving that evolves from an experienced faith, guided by parents and others during a person's infancy and childhood, to an owned faith that is internalized in adulthood and serves as a directive for personal action (**Table 25–7 ●**). For the client who is ill, faith—whether in a higher authority (e.g., God, Allah, Jehovah), in the client's own self, in the healthcare team, or in a combination of all—provides strength and trust.

Genetic Considerations

The genetic inheritance of an individual is established at conception. It remains unchanged throughout life and determines physical characteristics (e.g., eye color); gender; and, to some extent, **temperament**, that combination of biological and

TABLE 25–7 Westerhoff's Four Stages of Faith

STAGE	AGE	BEHAVIOR
Experienced faith	Infancy/early adolescence	Experiences faith through interaction with others who are living a particular faith tradition.
Affiliative faith	Late adolescence	Actively participates in activities that characterize a particular faith tradition; experiences awe and wonderment; feels a sense of belonging.
Searching faith	Young adulthood	Through a process of questioning and doubting own faith, acquires a cognitive as well as an affective faith.
Owned faith	Middle adulthood/old age	Puts faith into personal and social action and is willing to stand up for what the individual believes, even against the nurturing community.

Source: Westerhoff, J. (1976). *Will our children have faith?* New York, NY: Seabury Press. Reprinted with permission from the author.

physical characteristics that is specific to each individual and influences personality and behavior. Each child inherits 23 chromosomes from the mother's egg and 23 from the father's sperm, resulting in a unique individual with 46 chromosomes. Two of these are **sex chromosomes**, which determine the child's gender; the rest, called **autosomal chromosomes**, govern all remaining characteristics. Every chromosome carries many genes that determine physical characteristics, intellectual potential, personality type, and other traits. Children are born with the potential for certain features; however, their interaction with the environment influences how and to what extent particular traits are manifested. For example, a child may have the potential for a high level of intellectual performance, but if he or she lives in an environment without access to supports such as education and proper nutrition, that potential may never be reached.

▶ GROWTH AND DEVELOPMENT THROUGH THE LIFE SPAN

Individuals constantly change and evolve throughout their lives. While some changes are subtle and highly individualized, others are apparent and represent milestones common to all human beings at or near a specific phase of growth and development.

Infants (Birth to 1 Year)

Immense changes occur during the child's first year of life. The child emerges totally dependent on others, his actions primarily reflexive in nature. By the end of his first year, the infant can walk and communicate. Never again in life is development so swift.

PHYSICAL GROWTH AND DEVELOPMENT The infant's birth weight usually doubles by about 5 months and triples by the end of the first year. Height increases by approximately 1 foot during this year. Teeth begin to erupt at about 6 months, and by the end of the first year, the infant has six to eight deciduous teeth. Physical growth is closely associated with type and quality of feeding.

Body organs and systems, although not fully mature at 1 year of age, function differently than they did at birth. Kidney and liver maturation helps the 1-year-old excrete drugs or other toxic substances more readily than in the first weeks of life. The changing body proportions mirror changes in developing internal organs (**Figure 25–5 ●**). Maturation of the nervous system is demonstrated by increased control over body movements, enabling the infant to sit, stand, and walk. Sensory function also increases as the infant begins to discriminate visual images, sounds, and tastes (**Table 25–8 ●**).

COGNITIVE DEVELOPMENT The brain continues to increase in complexity during the first year of life. Most of the

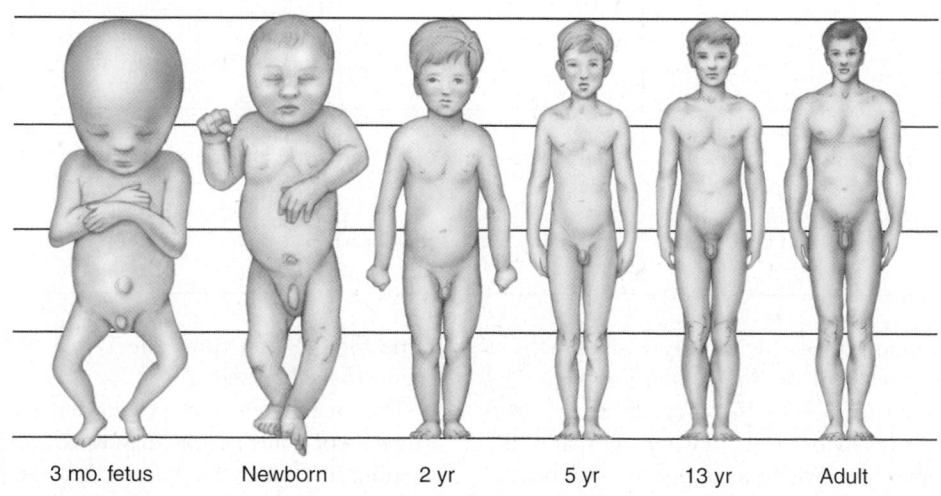

3 mo. fetus   Newborn   2 yr   5 yr   13 yr   Adult

Figure 25–5 ● Body proportions at various ages.

TABLE 25-8 Growth and Development Milestones During Infancy

AGE	PHYSICAL GROWTH	FINE MOTOR ABILITY	GROSS MOTOR ABILITY	SENSORY ABILITY
Birth–1 month	Gains 140–200 g (5–7 oz)/week. Grows 1.5 cm (1/2 in.) in first month. Head circumference increases 1.5 cm (1/2 in.)/month.	Holds hand in fist. Draws arms and legs to body when crying.	Inborn reflexes such as startle and rooting are predominant activity. May lift head briefly if prone. Alerts to high-pitched voices. Comforts with touch.	Prefers to look at faces and black-and-white geometric designs. Follows objects in line of vision.
2–4 months	Gains 140–200 g (5–7 oz)/week. Grows 1.5 cm (1/2 in.)/month. Head circumference increases 1.5 cm (1/2 in.)/month. Posterior fontanel closes. Eats 120 mL/kg/24 hr (2 oz/lb/24 hr).	Holds rattle when placed in hand. Looks at and plays with own fingers. Brings hands to midline.	Moro reflex fading in strength. Can turn from side to back and then return. Head lag when pulled to sitting position decreases; sits with head held in midline with some bobbing. When prone, holds head and supports weight on forearms.	Follows objects 180 degrees. Turns head to look for voices and sounds.
4–6 months	Gains 140–200 g (5–7 oz)/week. Doubles birth weight in 5–6 months. Grows 1.5 cm (1/2 in.)/month. Head circumference increases 1.5 cm (1/2 in.)/month. Teeth may begin erupting by 6 months. Eats 100 mL/kg/24 hr (1 1/2 oz/lb/24 hr).	Grasps rattles and other objects at will; drops them to pick up another offered object. Mouths objects. Holds feet and pulls to mouth. Holds bottle. Grasps with whole hand (palmar grasp). Manipulates objects.	Holds head steady when sitting. Has no head lag when pulled to sitting. Turns from abdomen to back by 4 months and then back to abdomen by 6 months. When held standing supports much of own weight.	Examines complex visual images. Watches the course of a falling object. Responds readily to sounds.
6–8 months	Gains 85–140 g (3–5 oz)/week. Grows 1 cm (3/8 in.)/month. Growth rate slower than first 6 months.	Bangs objects held in hands. Transfers objects from one hand to the other. Pincer grasp begins at times.	Most inborn reflexes extinguished. Sits alone steadily without support by 8 months. Likes to bounce on legs when held in standing position.	Recognizes own name and responds by looking and smiling. Enjoys small and complex objects at play.
8–10 months	Gains 85–140 g (3–5 oz)/week. Grows 1 cm (3/8 in.)/month.	Picks up small objects. Uses pincer grasp well.	Crawls or pulls whole body along floor by arms. Creeps by using hands and knees to keep trunk off floor. Pulls self to standing and sitting by 10 months. Recovers balance when sitting.	Understands words such as "no" and "cracker." May say one word in addition to "mama" and "dada." Recognizes sound without difficulty.
10–12 months	Gains 85–140 g (3–5 oz)/week. Grows 1 cm (3/8 in.)/month. Head circumference equals chest circumference. Triples birth weight by 1 year.	May hold crayon or pencil and make mark on paper. Places objects into containers through holes.	Stands alone. Walks holding onto furniture. Sits down from standing.	Plays peek-a-boo and patty cake.

growth involves maturation of cells, with only a small increase in cell number. This growth of the brain is accompanied by development of its functions, something easily understood when one compares the behavior of the newborn to that of the 1-year-old. The newborn's eyes widen in response to sound; the 1-year-old turns to the sound and recognizes its significance. The 2-month-old cries and coos; the 1-year-old says a few words and understands many more. The 6-week-old grasps a rattle for the first time; the 1-year-old reaches for toys and begins to feed herself.

The infant's behaviors provide clues about thought processes. Piaget's work outlines the infant's actions in a set of rapidly progressing changes in the first year of life. The infant receives stimulation through sight, sound, and feeling, which the maturing brain interprets. This input from the environment interacts with internal cognitive abilities to enhance cognitive functioning.

PSYCHOSOCIAL DEVELOPMENT The infant relies on interactions with primary care providers to meet needs and then begins to establish a sense of trust in other adults and in children. As trust develops, the infant becomes comfortable in interactions with a widening array of people.

Play Play for an 8-month-old infant might include grasping blocks and banging them on the floor. When a parent walks by, the infant laughs and waves hands and feet wildly (**Figure 25–6 ●**). The infant plays primarily alone with toys (**solitary play**) but enjoys the presence of adults or other children. Physical capabilities enable the infant to move toward and reach for objects of interest.

Cognitive ability is reflected in manipulation of the blocks to create different sounds. Social interaction enhances play. The presence of a parent or other individual increases interest in surroundings and teaches the infant different ways to play.

The play of infants begins in a reflexive manner. When infants move extremities or grasp objects, they experience the foundations of play. They gain pleasure from the feel and sound of these activities, and gradually perform them purposefully. For example, when a parent places a rattle in the hand of a 6-week-old infant, the infant grasps it reflexively. As the hands move randomly, the rattle makes an enjoyable sound. The infant learns to move the rattle to create the sound and then finally to grasp the toy at will to play with it.

The next phase of infant play focuses on manipulative behavior. The infant examines toys closely, looking at them, touching them, and placing them in his or her mouth. The infant learns a great deal about texture, qualities of objects, and all aspects of the surroundings. At the same time, interaction with others becomes an important part of play. The social nature of play is obvious as the infant plays with other children and adults.

Toward the end of the first year, the infant's ability to move in space enlarges the sphere of play. Once infants crawl or walk,

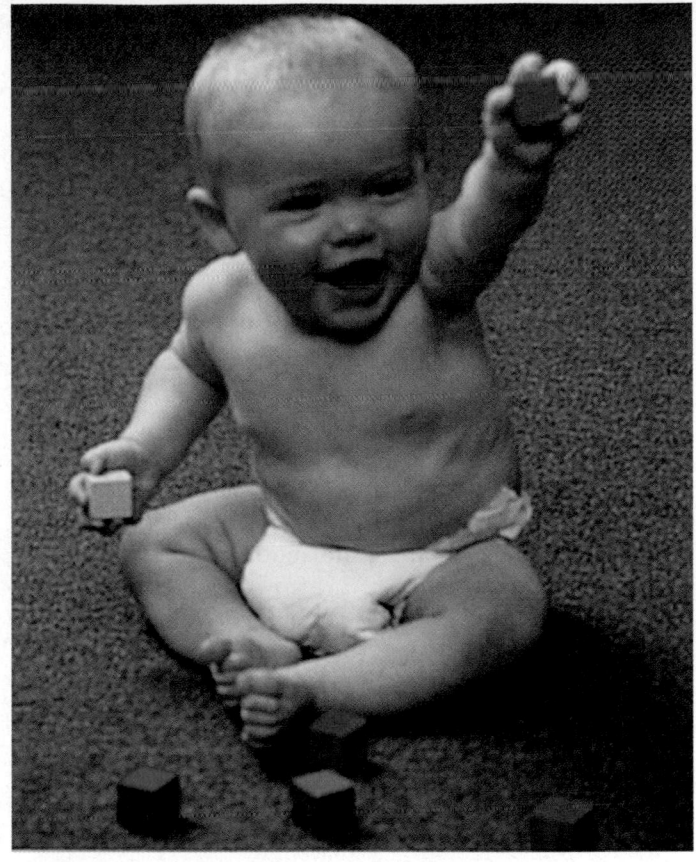

Figure 25–6 ● Garrett shows us that an 8-month-old child can play with blocks, demonstrating physical, cognitive, and social capabilities.

they can get to new places, find new toys, discover forgotten objects, or seek out other people for interaction. Play is a reflection of every aspect of development, as well as a method for enhancing learning and maturation (**Table 25–9 ●**).

TABLE 25–9 Psychosocial Development During Infancy

AGE	PLAY AND TOYS	COMMUNICATION
Birth–3 months	■ Prefers visual stimuli of mobiles, black-and-white patterns, mirrors. ■ Responds to auditory stimuli such as music boxes, tape players, soft voices. ■ Responds to rocking and cuddling. ■ Moves legs and arms while adult sings and talks. ■ Likes varying stimuli—different rooms, sounds, visual images.	■ Coos. ■ Babbles. ■ Cries.
3–6 months	■ Prefers noise-making objects that are easily grasped like rattles. ■ Enjoys stuffed animals and soft toys with contrasting colors.	■ Vocalizes during play and with familiar people. ■ Laughs. ■ Cries less. ■ Squeals and makes pleasure sounds. ■ Babbles multisyllabically (mamamamama).
6–9 months	■ Likes teething toys. ■ Increasingly desires social interaction with adults and other children. ■ Favors soft toys that can be manipulated and mouthed.	■ Increases vowel and consonant sounds. ■ Links syllables together. ■ Uses speechlike rhythm when vocalizing with others.
9–12 months	■ Enjoys large blocks, toys that pop apart and go back together, nesting cups and other objects. ■ Laughs at surprise toys like a jack-in-the-box. ■ Plays interactive games like peek-a-boo. ■ Uses push-and-pull toys.	■ Understands "no" and other simple commands. ■ Says "dada" and "mama" to identify parents. ■ Learns one or two other words. ■ Receptive speech surpasses expressive speech.

Personality and Temperament Personality and temperament vary widely among infants. For example, one infant will awaken frequently in the night, while another will sleep soundly for 8–10 hours. One infant may smile and react positively to interactions, while another withdraws around unfamiliar people and frequently frowns and cries. Such differences in responses to the environment are believed to be inborn characteristics of temperament. Infants are born with a tendency to react in certain ways to noise and to interact differently with people. They may display varying degrees of regularity in activities of eating and sleeping, and manifest a capacity for concentrating on tasks for different amounts of time.

The nursing assessment identifies personality characteristics of the infant that the nurse can share with the parents. With this information, the parents can appreciate more fully the uniqueness of their infant and design experiences to meet the infant's needs. Parents can learn to modify the environment to promote adaptation. For example, an infant who does not adapt easily to new situations may cry, withdraw, or develop another way of coping when adjusting to new people or places. Parents might be advised to use one or two babysitters rather than engaging new sitters frequently. If the infant is easily distracted when eating, parents can feed the infant in a quiet setting to encourage a focus on eating. Although the infant's temperament is unchanged, the ability to fit with the environment is enhanced.

Communication Communication skills are evident even at a few weeks of age. Infants communicate and engage in two-way interaction; they express comfort by soft sounds, cuddling, and eye contact. The infant displays discomfort by thrashing the extremities, arching the back, and crying vigorously. From these rudimentary skills, communication ability continues to develop until the infant speaks several words at the end of the first year of life (see Table 25–9). Nonverbal methods continue to be a primary method of communication between parent and child.

Nurses assess communication to identify possible abnormalities or developmental delays. Language ability may be assessed with the Denver II developmental test or other specialized language screening tools. Normal infants and toddlers understand (**receptive speech**) more words than they can speak (**expressive speech**). Abnormalities may be caused by a hearing deficit, developmental delay, or lack of verbal stimulation from caretakers. Further assessment may be required to pinpoint the cause of the abnormality.

Nursing interventions focus on providing a stimulating and comforting environment. Parents are encouraged to speak to infants and teach words. Hospital nurses should include the infant's known words when providing care, and provide nonverbal support by hugging and holding. Nurses planning interventions should consider the family's cultural patterns for communications and development.

Toddlers (1 to 3 Years)

Toddlerhood is sometimes called the first adolescence. The child from 1–3 years of age, who months before was merely an infant, is now displaying independence and negativism. Pride in newfound accomplishments emerges during this time.

PHYSICAL GROWTH AND DEVELOPMENT The rate of growth slows during the second year of life. The child requires limited food intake during this time, a change that may cause concern to the parent. The nurse reassures parents with these concerns that this is a normal occurrence in their child's development. By age 2 years, the birth weight has usually quadrupled and the child is about one half of the adult height. Body proportions begin to change, with longer legs and a smaller head in proportion to body size than during infancy. The toddler has a pot-bellied appearance and stands with feet apart to provide a wide base of support. By approximately 33 months, eruption of the 20 deciduous teeth is complete.

Gross motor activity develops rapidly (**Table 25–10** ●) as the toddler progresses from walking to running, kicking, and riding a tricycle. As physical maturation occurs, the toddler develops the ability to control elimination patterns.

TABLE 25–10 Growth and Development Milestones During Toddlerhood

AGE	PHYSICAL GROWTH	FINE MOTOR ABILITY	GROSS MOTOR ABILITY	SENSORY ABILITY
1–2 years	▪ Gains 227 g (8 oz) or more per month. ▪ Grows 9–12 cm (3.5–5 in.) during this year. ▪ Anterior fontanel closes.	▪ By end of second year, builds a tower of four blocks. ▪ Scribbles on paper. ▪ Can undress self. ▪ Throws a ball.	▪ Runs. ▪ Walks up and down stairs. ▪ Likes push- and pull-toys.	Visual acuity 20/50
2–3 years	▪ Gains 1.4–2.3 kg (3–5 lb)/year. ▪ Grows 5–6.5 cm (2–2.5 in.)/year.	▪ Draws a circle and other rudimentary forms. ▪ Learns to pour. ▪ Is learning to dress self.	▪ Jumps. ▪ Kicks ball. ▪ Throws ball overhand.	

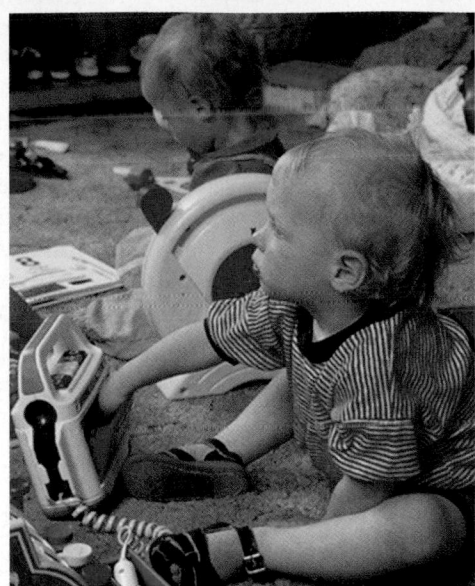
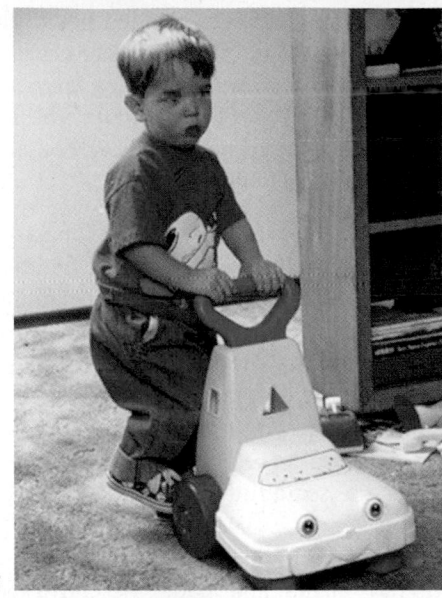

A   B

Figure 25–7 ● *A,* Two children are displaying typical parallel play, since they enjoy playing near other children, but are not engaging in social interactions with each other. Which cognitive and motor skills are these children developing? *B,* Imitative play such as pushing and pulling a vacuum allows this toddler to develop gross and fine motor skills.

COGNITIVE DEVELOPMENT   During the toddler years, the child moves from the sensorimotor to the preoperational stage of development. The early use of language awakens in the 1-year-old the ability to think about objects or people when they are absent. Object permanence is well developed.

At about 2 years of age, the increasing use of words as symbols enables the toddler to use preoperational thought. Rudimentary problem solving, creative thought, and an understanding of cause-and-effect relationships are now possible.

PSYCHOSOCIAL DEVELOPMENT   The toddler is soundly rooted in a trusting relationship and feels more comfortable asserting autonomy and separating from primary care providers. It is important for toddlers to begin asserting their autonomy within the context of safe places and relationships that promote their interaction with both adults and other children.

Play   Patterns of play emerge and change between infancy and toddlerhood. The toddler's motor skills enable him to bang pegs into a pounding board with a hammer. The social nature of toddler play is also visible. Toddlers find the company of other children pleasurable, even though socially interactive play may not occur. Toddlers tend to play with similar objects side by side, occasionally trading toys and words (**Figure 25–7 ●**). This is called **parallel play**. Playing with other children assists toddlers to develop social skills. Toddlers engage in play activities they have seen at home, such as pounding with a hammer and talking on the phone. This imitative behavior helps them to learn new actions and skills.

Physical skills are manifested in play as toddlers push and pull objects, climb in and out and up and down, run, ride a Big Wheel, turn the pages of books, and scribble with a pen. Both gross motor and fine motor abilities are enhanced during this age period.

Cognitive understanding enables the toddler to manipulate objects and learn about their qualities. Stacking blocks and placing rings on a building tower teach spatial relationships and other lessons that provide a foundation for future learning. Various kinds of play objects should be provided for the toddler to meet play needs. These play needs can easily be met whether the child is hospitalized or at home (**Table 25–11 ●**).

Personality and Temperament   The toddler retains most of the temperamental characteristics identified during infancy, but may demonstrate some changes. The normal developmental progression of toddlerhood plays a part in responses. For

TABLE 25–11 Psychosocial Development During Toddlerhood		
AGE	**PLAY AND TOYS**	**COMMUNICATION**
1–3 years	■ Refines fine motor skills by use of cloth books, large pencil and paper, wooden puzzles. ■ Facilitates imitative behavior by playing kitchen, grocery shopping, toy telephone. ■ Learns gross motor activities by riding Big Wheel tricycle, playing with a soft ball and bat, molding water and sand, tossing ball or bean bag. ■ Cognitive skills develop through exposure to educational television shows, music, stories, and books.	■ Increasingly enjoys talking. ■ Vocabulary grows exponentially, especially when spoken and read to. ■ Needs to release stress by pounding board, frequent gross motor activities, and occasional temper tantrums. ■ Likes contact with other children and learns interpersonal skills.

example, the infant who previously responded positively to stimuli, such as a new babysitter, may appear more negative in toddlerhood. The increasing independence characteristic of this age is shown by the toddler's use of the word *no*. The parent and child constantly adapt their responses to each other and learn anew how to communicate with each other.

Communication Because the individual's capacity for development of language skills is greatest during the toddler period, adults should communicate frequently with children in this age group. This communication is critical not only to the toddler's ability to communicate simple wants and needs, but also to cognitive and language development, which affects the toddler's future literacy. Toddlers also begin to learn the subtleties of language, as they begin to imitate words and speech intonations, as well as the social interactions and nonverbal gestures that they observe.

At the beginning of toddlerhood, the child may use four to six words in addition to "mama" and "dada." Receptive speech (the ability to understand words) far outpaces expressive speech. By the end of toddlerhood, however, the 3-year-old has a vocabulary of almost 1,000 words and uses short sentences.

Communication occurs in many ways, some of which are nonverbal. Toddler communication includes pointing, pulling an adult over to a room or object, and speaking in **expressive jargon** (using unintelligible words with normal speech intonations as if truly communicating in words). Other communication methods include crying, pounding or stamping feet, displaying a temper tantrum, or other means that illustrate dismay. These powerful communication methods can upset parents, who often need suggestions for handling them. Adults can best assist the toddler by verbalizing the feelings shown by the toddler, by saying things like "You must be very upset that you cannot have that candy. When you stop crying you can come out of your room." Verbalizing the child's feeling and then ignoring further negative behavior ensures that the parent is not unintentionally reinforcing the inappropriate behavior. While the toddler's search for autonomy and independence creates a need for such behavior, an upset toddler may respond well to holding, rocking, and stroking.

Parents and nurses can promote a toddler's communication by speaking frequently, naming objects, giving single-step directions, explaining procedures in simple terms, expressing feelings that the toddler seems to be displaying, and encouraging speech. The toddler from a bilingual home is at an optimal age to learn two languages. If the parents do not speak English, the toddler will benefit from a child care experience that will expose her to English in addition to her native language.

The nurse who understands the communication skills of toddlers is able to assess expressive and receptive language and communicate effectively, thereby promoting positive healthcare experiences for these children. Parents often need suggestions for ways to communicate with the young child.

Preschool Children (3 to 6 Years)

The preschool years are a time of new initiative and independence. Most children are in a child care center or school for part of the day, and they learn a great deal from this social contact. Language skills are well developed, and the child is able to understand and speak clearly. Endless projects characterize the world of busy preschoolers. They may work with play dough to form animals, then cut out and paste paper, then draw and color.

PHYSICAL GROWTH AND DEVELOPMENT Preschoolers grow slowly and steadily, with most growth taking place in long bones of the arms and legs. The short, chubby toddler gradually gives way to a slender, long-legged preschooler (**Table 25–12 ●**).

Physical skills continue to develop. The preschooler runs with ease, holds a bat, and throws balls of various types. Writing ability increases, and the preschooler enjoys drawing and learning.

The preschool period is a good time to encourage good dental habits. Children can begin to brush their own teeth with parental supervision and help in reaching all tooth surfaces. Parents should floss children's teeth, give fluoride as ordered if the water supply is not fluoridated, and schedule the first dental visit so the child can become accustomed to the routine of periodic dental care.

COGNITIVE DEVELOPMENT The preschooler exhibits characteristics of preoperational thought. Symbols or words are used to represent objects and people, enabling the young child to think about them. This is a milestone in intellectual development; however, the preschooler still has some limitations in thought (**Table 25–13 ●**).

It is important to understand the preschooler's thought processes in order to plan appropriate teaching for health care and development of health habits.

PSYCHOSOCIAL DEVELOPMENT The preschooler is more independent in establishing relationships with others.

TABLE 25–12 Growth and Development Milestones During the Preschool Years			
PHYSICAL GROWTH	FINE MOTOR ABILITY	GROSS MOTOR ABILITY	SENSORY ABILITY
Gains 1.5–2.5 kg (3–5 lb)/year. Grows 4–6 cm (1 1/2–2 1/2 in.)/year.	Uses scissors. Draws circle, square, cross. Draws at least a six-part person. Enjoys art projects such as pasting, stringing beads, using clay. Learns to tie shoes at end of preschool years. Buttons clothes. Brushes teeth. Eats three meals, with snacks. Uses spoon, fork, and knife.	Throws a ball overhand. Climbs well. Rides tricycle.	Visual acuity continues to improve. Can focus on and learn letters and numbers.

TABLE 25–13   Characteristics of Thought Identified by Piaget

CHARACTERISTIC	DEFINITION	DEVELOPMENT STAGE	NURSING IMPLICATIONS
Object permanence	Ability to understand that when something is out of sight it still exists	Sensorimotor period, especially in coordination of secondary schemes substage from 8–12 months	Before development of object permanence, babies will not look for toys or other objects out of sight; as the concept is developing they are concerned when a parent leaves, since they are not certain the parent will return.
Egocentrism	Ability to see things only from one's own point of view	Preoperational thought	Peers or others who have gone through an experience will not impress the preschooler; teaching should focus on what an experience will be like for the child himself.
Transductive reasoning	Connecting two events in a cause-and-effect relationship simply because they occur together in time	Preoperational thought	Ask the child what she thinks caused an occurrence; ask how the two events are connected; correct misconceptions to lessen child's guilt.
Centration	Focusing only on one particular aspect of a situation	Preoperational thought	Listen to the child's comments and deal with concerns in order to be able to present new concepts to the child.
Animism	Giving lifelike qualities to nonliving things	Preoperational thought	Ask preschool children to describe how a machine works, or how the trees move. Provide opportunities to learn about machines that may move and make noises (intravenous pumps, magnetic resonance imaging) to decrease fears.
Magical thinking	Believing that events occur because of one's thoughts or actions	Preoperational thought	Ask young children how they became ill, or what caused a parent's or sibling's illness. Correct misconceptions when the child blames self for causing problems by wishing someone ill or having bad behavior.
Conservation	Knowing that matter is not changed when its form is altered	Concrete operational thought	Before conservation of thought is reached, the child may think that gender can be changed when hair is cut, the leg under a cast is broken in separate pieces. Ask perceptions and clarify misconceptions.

The child interacts closely with children and adults and is able to plan and carry out activities.

Play   Play for the preschooler takes on a new dimension as the preschooler begins to interact with others. One child cuts out colored paper while his friend glues it on paper in a design. This new type of interaction is called **associative play**.

In addition to this social dimension, other aspects of play also differ. The preschooler enjoys large motor activities such as swinging, riding a tricycle, and throwing a ball (**Figure 25–8 ●**). Preschoolers demonstrate increasing manual dexterity as they create more complex drawings and manipulations of blocks and modeling. As these changes are observed, playtime should evolve to accommodate appropriate activities. Preschool programs and child-life departments in hospitals help meet this important need.

Materials provided for play can be simple but should guide activities in which the child engages. Because fine motor activities are popular, paper, pens, scissors, glue, and a variety of other such objects should be available. The child can use them to create important images such as pictures of people, hospital beds, or friends. A collection of dolls, furniture, and clothing can be manipulated to represent parents and children, nurses and physicians, teachers, or other significant people. Because fantasy life is so powerful at this age, the preschooler readily uses props to engage in **dramatic play** (the living out of the drama of human life).

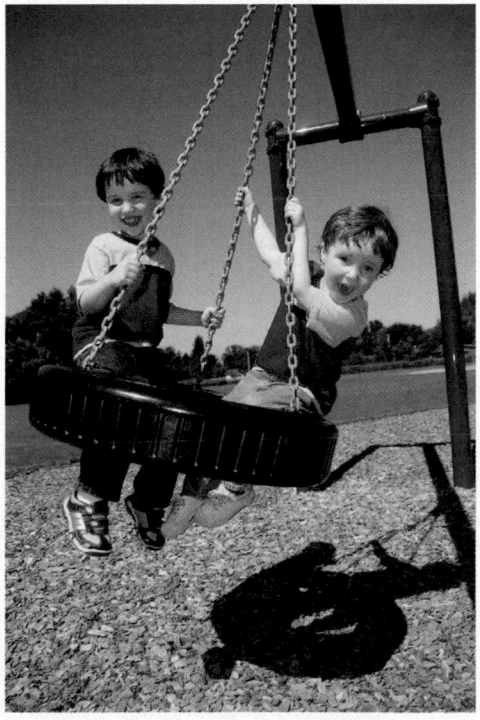

Figure 25–8 ● Preschoolers have well-developed large motor skills and enjoy activities such as swinging.
Source: Rossario/Shutterstock

TABLE 25–14 *Psychosocial Development During Preschool Years*

AGE	PLAY AND TOYS	COMMUNICATION
3–6 years	Associative play is facilitated by simple games, puzzles, nursery rhymes, songs. Dramatic play is fostered by dolls and doll clothes, play houses and hospitals, dress-up clothes, puppets. Stress is relieved by pens, paper, glue, scissors. Cognitive growth is fostered by educational television shows, music, stories and books.	Develops and uses all parts of speech, occasionally incorrectly. Communicates with a widening array of people. Play with other children is a favorite activity. Health professionals can: ■ Verbalize and explain procedures to children. ■ Use drawings and stories to explain care. ■ Use accurate names for bodily functions. ■ Allow the child to talk, ask questions, and make choices.

The nurse can use playtime to assess the preschooler's developmental level, knowledge about health care, and emotions related to healthcare experiences. Observations about objects chosen for play, content of dramatic play, and pictures drawn can provide important assessment data. The nurse can also use play periods to teach the child about healthcare procedures and offer an outlet for expressing emotions (**Table 25–14** ●).

Personality and Temperament   Characteristics of personality observed in infancy tend to persist over time. The preschooler may need assistance as these characteristics are expressed in the new situations of preschool or nursery school. An excessively active child, for example, will need gentle, consistent handling to adjust to the structure of a classroom. Encourage parents to visit preschool programs to choose the one that would best foster growth in their child. Some preschoolers enjoy the structured learning of a program that focuses on cognitive skills, while others are happier and more open to learning in a small group that provides much time for free play. Nurses can help parents to identify their child's personality or temperament characteristics and to find the best environment for growth.

Communication   Language skills blossom during the preschool years. The vocabulary grows to over 2,000 words, and children speak in complete sentences of several words and use all parts of speech. They practice these newfound language skills by endlessly talking and asking questions.

The sophisticated speech of preschoolers mirrors the development occurring in their minds and helps them to learn about the world around them. However, this speech can be quite deceptive. Although preschoolers use many words, their grasp of meaning is usually literal and may not match that of adults. These literal interpretations have important implications for healthcare providers. For example, the preschooler who is told she will be "put to sleep" for surgery may think of a pet recently euthanized; the child who is told that a dye will be injected for a diagnostic test may think he is going to die; mention of "a little stick" in the arm can cause images of tree branches rather than of a simple immunization.

Concrete visual aids such as pictures of a child undergoing the same procedure or a book to read together enhance teaching by meeting the child's developmental needs. Handling medical equipment such as intravenous bags and stethoscopes increases interest and helps the child to focus. Teaching may have to be done in several short sessions rather than one long session.

Some general approaches include the following:

■ Allow time for the child to integrate explanations.
■ Verbalize frequently to the child.
■ Use drawings and stories to explain care.
■ Use accurate names for bodily functions.
■ Allow choices.

The preschooler's social growth and increased communication skills make these years the perfect time to introduce concepts related to problem solving and conflict resolution. Puzzles and manipulative toys help foster early problem-solving skills. Children in this age group can learn to calm themselves by learning how to take deep breaths and count to 3 or 5 when they are upset. Many preschool programs employ special curricula that help teachers and parents assist children in developing essential conflict resolution skills. Using language to resolve conflict is a protective factor that decreases the likelihood of children choosing inappropriate or violent behavior to try to get what they want or bring a distressing interaction to a close.

School-Age Children (6 to 12 Years)

School-age children demonstrate common characteristics of their age group. They are in a stage of industry in which it is important to the child to perform useful work. Meaningful activities take on great importance and are usually carried out in the company of peers. A sense of achievement in these activities is important to developing self-esteem and to preventing a sense of inferiority or poor self-worth.

PHYSICAL GROWTH AND DEVELOPMENT   School age is the last period in which girls and boys are close in size and body proportions. As the long bones continue to grow, leg length increases (see Figure 25–5). Fat gives way to muscle, and the child appears leaner. Jaw proportions change as the first deciduous tooth is lost at 6 years and permanent teeth begin to erupt. Body organs and the immune system mature, resulting in fewer illnesses among school-age children. Medications are less likely to cause serious side effects, because they can be metabolized more easily. The urinary system can adjust to changes in fluid status. Physical skills are also refined as children begin to play sports, and fine motor skills are well developed through school activities (**Table 25–15** ●).

Although it is commonly believed that the start of adolescence (age 12 years) heralds a growth spurt, the rapid increases

TABLE 25–15   Growth and Development Milestones During the School-Age Years

PHYSICAL GROWTH	FINE MOTOR ABILITY	GROSS MOTOR ABILITY	SENSORY ABILITY
Gains 1.4–2.2 kg (3–5 lb)/ year.	Plays card and board games.	Roller skates or ice skates.	Is able to concentrate for longer periods.
Grows 4–6 cm (1 1/2–2 1/2 in.)/year.	Enjoys craft projects.	Jumps rope. Rides two-wheeler.	Can read.

in size commonly occur during school age. Girls may begin a growth spurt as early as 9 or 10 years of age and boys a year or so later (**Figure 25–9** ●). Nutritional needs increase dramatically with this spurt.

The loss of the first deciduous teeth and the eruption of permanent teeth usually occur at about age 6 years, or at the beginning of the school-age period. Of the 32 permanent teeth, 22–26 erupt by age 12 years and the remaining molars follow during the teenage years. See the module on Health, Wellness, and Illness for a discussion of oral care for school-age children.

COGNITIVE DEVELOPMENT   The child enters the stage of concrete operational thought at about age 7 years. This stage enables school-age children to consider alternative solutions and solve problems. However, school-age children continue to rely on concrete experiences and materials to form their thought content.

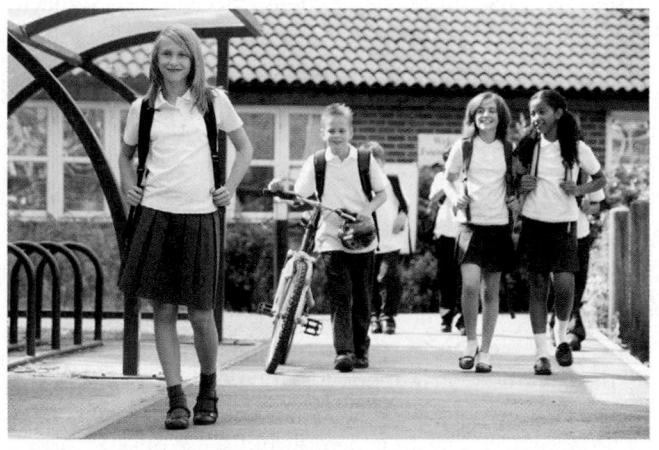

Figure 25–9 ● Because girls have a growth spurt earlier than boys, girls often are taller than boys of the same age.
Source: © Monkey Business/Fotolia

During the school-age years, the child learns the concept of conservation (that matter is not changed when its form is altered). At earlier ages, a child believes that when water is poured from a short, wide glass into a tall, thin glass, there is more water in the taller glass. The school-age child recognizes that, although it may look like the taller glass holds more water, the quantity is the same. The concept of conservation is helpful when the nurse explains medical treatments. The school-age child understands that an incision will heal, that a cast will be removed, and that an arm will look the same as before once the intravenous infusion is removed.

PSYCHOSOCIAL DEVELOPMENT   The school-age child has many friends and cooperatively interacts with others to accomplish tasks. The child develops a sense of accomplishment from activities and relationships.

Play   Play for the school-age child is enhanced by increasing fine and gross motor skills. By 6 years of age, children have acquired the physical ability to hold the bat properly and may occasionally hit the ball. School-age children also understand that everyone has a role—the pitcher, the catcher, the batter, the outfielders. They cooperate with one another to form a team, are eager to learn the rules of the game, and want to ensure that these rules are followed exactly (**Table 25–16** ●).

The characteristics of play exhibited by the school-age child include cooperation with others and the ability to play a part in order to contribute to a unified whole. This type of play is called **cooperative play**. The concrete nature of cognitive thought leads to a reliance on rules to provide structure and security. Children have an increasing desire to spend much of their playtime with friends, which demonstrates the social component of play. Play is an extremely important method of learning and living for the school-age child. Active physical play has decreased in recent years as television viewing and playing of computer games have increased, leading to poor nutritional status and high rates of overweight among children.

TABLE 25–16   Psychosocial Development During the School-Age Years

AGE	ACTIVITIES	COMMUNICATION
6–12 years	Gross motor development is fostered by ball sports, skating, dance lessons, water and snow skiing/boarding, biking. A sense of industry is fostered by playing a musical instrument, gathering collections, starting hobbies, playing board and video games. Cognitive growth is facilitated by reading, crafts, word puzzles, schoolwork.	Use of language is mature. Is able to converse and discuss topics for increasing lengths of time. Spends many hours at school and with friends in sports or other activities. Health professionals can: ■ Assess child's knowledge before teaching. ■ Allow the child to select rewards following procedures. ■ Teach techniques such as counting or visualization to manage difficult situations. ■ Include both parent and child in healthcare decisions.

Complementary and Alternative Therapy Music and Art Therapy

Most children are accustomed to listening to music via earphones or earbuds. They should be encouraged to bring their favorite music to the hospital as a means of stress reduction. It may also reduce the need for sedation during diagnostic tests or uncomfortable procedures (Kulkarni et al., 2012). Musical instruments and artistic tools such as paints and brushes, markers, and clay are frequently used in hospital and other care settings to help children express fears and anxieties about their illnesses. Just as important, these tools can assist children in sharing their desires and dreams for health and wellness.

When a child is hospitalized, the separation from playmates can lead to feelings of sadness and purposelessness. School-age children often feel better when placed in multibed units with other children. Normal, rewarding parts of play should be integrated into care. Friends should be encouraged to visit or call a hospitalized child. Discharge planning for the child who has had a cast or brace applied should address the activities in which the child can participate and those the child must avoid. Nurses should reinforce the importance of playing games with friends to both parents and children.

Personality and Temperament Characteristics seen in earlier years tend to endure in the school years. The child classified as "difficult" at an earlier age may now have trouble in the classroom. Nurses may advise parents to provide a quiet setting for homework and to reward the child for concentration. For example, after completing homework, the child may be allowed to have "screen time" (play a video game, watch television, or play on the computer or tablet). Creative efforts and alternative methods of learning should be valued. Encourage parents to see their children as individuals who may not all learn in the same way. The "slow-to-warm-up" child may need encouragement to try new activities and to share experiences with others, whereas the "easy" child will readily adapt to new schools, people, and experiences.

Communication During the school-age years, children should learn how to use language correctly, including correcting any lingering pronunciation or grammatical errors, and learning the pragmatic (social) uses of language. Vocabulary increases, and the child learns about parts of speech in school. School-age children enjoy writing and, while in the hospital, can be encouraged to keep a journal of their experiences as a method of dealing with anxiety. The literal translation of words characteristic of preschoolers is uncommon among school-age children.

Some communication strategies helpful with the school-age child include:

- Provide concrete examples of pictures or materials to accompany verbal descriptions.
- Assess knowledge before planning the instruction.
- Allow child to select rewards following procedures.
- Teach techniques such as counting or visualization to manage difficult situations.
- Include child in discussions and history with parent.

Sexuality Awareness of gender differences and sexuality becomes more pronounced during the school years. Although children become aware of sexual differences between genders during preschool years, they deal much more consciously with sexuality during the school-age years. As children mature physically, they need information about their bodily changes so that they can develop a healthy self-image and an understanding of the relationships between their bodies and sexuality. Children become interested in sexual issues and are often exposed to erroneous information on television shows, in magazines, or from friends and siblings. Schools and families need to use opportunities to teach school-age children factual information about sex and to foster healthy concepts of self and others. It is advisable to ask occasional questions about sexual issues to learn how much the child knows and to provide correct information when answers demonstrate confusion.

Both friends and the media are common sources of erroneous ideas. Appropriate and inappropriate touch should be discussed, with lists of trusted people who can be approached (teachers, clergy, school counselors, family members, neighbors) to discuss any episodes with which the child feels uncomfortable. Because even these trusted people can be implicated in inappropriate episodes, the nurse should encourage the child to go to more than one person, an important approach if the child is uncomfortable about a relationship with any individual.

Adolescents (12 to 18 Years)

Adolescence is a time of passage signaling the end of childhood and the beginning of adulthood. Although adolescents differ in behaviors and accomplishments, they are all in a period of identity formation. If a healthy identity and sense of self-worth are not developed during this period, role confusion and purposeless struggling will ensue. The adolescents in your care will represent various degrees of identity formation, and each will offer unique challenges.

PHYSICAL GROWTH AND DEVELOPMENT The physical changes ending in **puberty**, or sexual maturity, begin near the end of the school-age period. The prepubescent period is marked by a growth spurt at an average age of 10 years for girls and 13 years for boys, although there is considerable variation among children. The increase in height and weight is generally remarkable and is completed in 2–3 years (**Table 25–17** ●). The growth spurt in girls is accompanied by an increase in breast size and growth of pubic hair. Menstruation occurs last and signals achievement of puberty. In boys, the growth spurt is accompanied by growth in size of the penis and testes and by growth of pubic hair. Deepening of the voice and growth of facial hair occur later, at the time of puberty.

TABLE 25–17 Growth and Development Milestones During Adolescence

PHYSICAL GROWTH	FINE MOTOR ABILITY	GROSS MOTOR ABILITY	SENSORY ABILITY
Variation in age of growth spurt During growth spurt, girls gain 7–25 kg (15–55 lb) and grow 2.5–20 cm (2–8 in.); boys gain approximately 7–29.5 kg (15–65 lb) and grow 11–30 cm (4 1/2–12 in.).	Skills are well developed.	New sports activities are attempted and muscle development continues. Some lack of coordination is common during growth spurt.	Sensory ability is fully developed.

During adolescence children grow stronger and more muscular and establish characteristic male and female patterns of fat distribution. The apocrine and eccrine glands mature, leading to increased sweating and a distinct odor to perspiration. All body organs are now fully mature, enabling the adolescent to take adult doses of medications.

The adolescent must adapt to a rapidly changing body for several years. These physical changes and hormonal variations offer challenges to identity formation.

COGNITIVE DEVELOPMENT   Adolescence marks the beginning of Piaget's last stage of cognitive development, the stage of formal operational thought. The adolescent no longer depends on concrete experiences as the basis of thought but develops the ability to reason abstractly. Such concepts as justice, truth, beauty, and power can be understood. The adolescent revels in this newfound ability and spends a great deal of time thinking, reading, and talking about abstract concepts.

The ability to think and act independently leads many adolescents to rebel against parental authority. Through these actions, adolescents seek to establish their own identity and values. While this behavior is normal for adolescents, it can create a number of difficulties at home and school as adolescents try to balance their need to express themselves against the expectations of parents, teachers, and other authority figures.

PSYCHOSOCIAL DEVELOPMENT   The adolescent is mature in relationships with others. The key aspect that teens work on during relationships and activities is establishing a meaningful identity.

Activities   Activities represent a central focus for the adolescent. Maturity leads to new activities. Adolescents may drive, ride buses, or bike independently. They are less dependent on parents for transportation and spend more time with friends. Activities include participation in sports and extracurricular school activities, as well as "hanging out" and attending movies or concerts with friends. Activities also drive psychosocial development, as the peer group becomes the focus of activities, regardless of the teen's interests. Peers are important in establishing identity and providing meaning. Although same-sex interactions dominate, boy–girl relationships are more common than at earlier stages. Adolescents thus participate in and learn from social interactions fundamental to adult relationships. They also begin to develop abstract thought and analysis through conversations at home and at school.

Personality and Temperament   Characteristics of temperament manifested during childhood usually remain stable in the teenage years. For instance, the adolescent who was a calm, scheduled infant and child often demonstrates initiative to regulate study times and other routines. Similarly, the adolescent who was an easily stimulated infant may now have a messy room, a harried schedule with assignments always completed late, and an interest in many activities. It is also common for an adolescent who was an easy child to become more difficult because of the psychological changes of adolescence and the need to assert independence.

As during the child's earlier ages, the nurse's role may be to inform parents of different personality types and to help them support the teen's uniqueness while providing necessary structure and feedback. Nurses can help parents understand their teen's personality type and work with the adolescent to meet expectations of teachers and others in authority.

Communication   All parts of speech are used and understood by the adolescent. Colloquialisms and slang are commonly used with the peer group. The adolescent often studies a foreign language in school, having the ability to understand and analyze grammar and sentence structure.

The adolescent increasingly leaves the home base and establishes close ties with peers. These relationships become the basis for identity formation. A period of stress or crisis generally occurs before a strong identity can emerge. The adolescent may try out new roles by learning a new sport or other skills, experimenting with drugs or alcohol, wearing different styles of clothing, or trying other activities. It is important to provide positive role models and a variety of experiences to help the adolescent make wise choices.

The adolescent also has a need to leave the past, to be different, and to change from former patterns to establish a self-identity. Rules that are repeated constantly and dogmatically will probably be broken in the adolescent's quest for self-awareness. This poses difficulties when the adolescent has a health problem that requires ongoing care, such as diabetes or a heart problem. Introducing the adolescent to other teens who manage the same problem appropriately usually is more successful in getting the adolescent to comply with a care plan than telling the adolescent what to do.

Teens need privacy during client interviews or interventions. Even if a parent is present for part of a health history or examination, the adolescent should be given the opportunity to relay information to or ask questions of the healthcare provider alone. The adolescent should be given a choice of whether to have a parent present during an examination or while care is provided. Most information shared by an adolescent is confidential. Some states mandate disclosure of certain information to parents such as an adolescent's desire for an abortion. In these cases, the adolescent should be informed of what information will be disclosed to the parent.

In the hospital setting, nurses and care staff should allow adolescents the freedom of choice whenever possible, including preferences for evening or morning bathing, the type of clothes to wear while hospitalized, timing of treatments, and visitation guidelines. Use of contracts with adolescents may increase adherence with healthcare recommendations. Firmness, gentleness, choices, and respect must be balanced during care of adolescent clients.

Some specific communication strategies that help with the adolescent:

- Provide written and verbal explanations.
- Direct history and explanations to teen alone; then include parent.
- Allow for safe exploration of topics by suggesting that the teen is similar to other teens. ("Many teens with diabetes have questions about. . . . How about you?")
- Arrange meetings for discussions with other teens.

Sexuality Sexuality is influenced by physical maturation and increased hormonal secretion, which are integral to the adolescent's development of physiological sexual maturity. Psychosocially, this complex process involves growing interactions with members of the opposite sex, an interplay of the forces of society and family, and identity formation. The early adolescent progresses from attending dances and other social events with members of the opposite sex to the late adolescent who is mature sexually and may have regular sexual encounters. About 47% of all high school students in the United States have had intercourse and 34% are currently sexually active (i.e., have had sex in the past 3 months). Fewer than 40% of adolescents used a condom at their last sexual encounter, putting this age group at high risk of acquiring sexually transmitted infections (STIs) (Centers for Disease Control and Prevention [CDC], 2012h).

Teenagers need information about their bodies and emerging sexuality. Many school districts now provide some teaching on STIs and HIV. Health histories include questions on sexual activity, STIs, and birth control use and understanding. Most hospitals routinely perform pregnancy screening on adolescent girls before elective procedures.

Adolescents will benefit from clear information about sexuality, an opportunity to develop relationships with adolescents in various settings, an open atmosphere at home and school where problems and issues can be discussed, and previous experience in problem solving and decision making. Alternatives and support for their decisions should be available.

Some adolescents identify as lesbian, gay, bisexual, or transgendered (LGBT). These teens are at particular risk of being stigmatized and harassed by other youth or adults. They are more likely to suffer problems such as isolation, rejection by significant others, violence, suicide, and sexual risk-taking (Moran, 2011; Rew et al., 2005). Nurses are instrumental in helping these youths by providing information for them and their parents, integrating LGBT content into sexual education curricula, and providing referrals for health and social care when needed. Nurses must examine their own beliefs and communication styles to provide culturally competent care. They can promote trust and acceptance among youth and in the general school community (Saha, Beach, & Cooper, 2008). Additionally, the nurse who encounters a sexually active teenager should remember that she may be the very first healthcare provider with whom the teenager discusses his or her sexuality. The nurse who refrains from asserting her own beliefs and who emphasizes open communication and active listening will strengthen the teen's confidence in the healthcare system and increase the likelihood that the teen will seek help from a healthcare professional in the future.

Adults

The adult years commonly are divided into three stages: young adulthood (ages 18–40), middle adulthood (ages 40–65), and older adulthood (over age 65). Although developmental markers are not as clearly delineated in the adult as in the infant or child, specific changes in intellectual, psychosocial, and spiritual development, as well as in physical structures and functions, do occur with aging (see Tables 25–3, 25–4, 25–6, and Multisystem Effects of Aging on page 1672). Applying a variety of developmental theories is important to the holistic care of the adult client as nurses perform assessments, implement care, and teach.

YOUNG ADULTS From ages 18–25, the healthy young adult is at the peak of physical development. All body systems are functioning at maximum efficiency. During the 30s, some normal physiological changes begin. A comparison of physical status for young adults during their 20s and 30s is shown in **Table 25–18** •.

Many individualized psychosocial stressors may affect the young adult. Choices must be made about education, occupa-

TABLE 25–18 Physical Status and Changes in the Young Adult Years

ASSESSMENT	STATUS DURING THE 20s	STATUS DURING THE 30s
Skin	Smooth, even temperature	Beginning of wrinkles
Hair	Slightly oily, shiny Beginning of balding	Beginning of graying Balding
Vision	Snellen 20/20	Some loss of visual acuity and accommodation
Musculoskeletal	Strong, coordinated	Some loss of strength and muscle mass
Cardiovascular	Maximum cardiac output 60–90 beats/min Mean BP: 120/80	Slight decline in cardiac output 60–90 beats/min Mean BP: 120/80
Respiratory	Rate: 12–20 Full vital capacity	Rate: 12–20 Decline in vital capacity

TABLE 25–19   Physical Changes in the Middle Adult Years

ASSESSMENT	CHANGES
Skin	Decreased turgor, moisture, and subcutaneous fat result in wrinkles. Fat is deposited in the abdominal and hip areas.
Hair	Loss of melanin in hair shaft causes graying. Hairline recedes in men.
Sensory	Visual acuity for near vision decreases (presbyopia) during the 40s. Auditory acuity for high-frequency sounds decreases (presbycusis); more common in men. Sense of taste diminishes.
Musculoskeletal	Skeletal muscle mass decreases by about age 60. Thinning of intervertebral discs results in loss of height (about 2.5 cm [1 in.]). Postmenopausal women may have loss of calcium and develop osteoporosis.
Cardiovascular	Blood vessels lose elasticity. Systolic blood pressure may increase.
Respiratory	Loss of vital capacity (about 1 L from age 20–60) occurs.
Gastrointestinal	Large intestine gradually loses muscle tone; constipation may result. Gastric secretions are decreased.
Genitourinary	Hormonal changes occur: menopause, women (↓ estrogen); andropause, men (↓ testosterone).
Endocrine	Gradual decrease in glucose tolerance occurs.

tion, relationships, independence, and lifestyle. The young adult without adequate education or job skills may face unemployment, poverty, homelessness, and limited access to health care.

Physical assessment of the young adult includes height and weight, blood pressure, and vision. During the health history, the nurse should ask specific questions about substance use, sexual activity and concerns, exercise, eating habits, menstrual history and patterns, coping mechanisms, any familial chronic illnesses, and family changes.

MIDDLE ADULTS   The middle adult, ages 40–65, has physical status and function similar to that of the young adult. However, many changes take place between ages 40 and 65. **Table 25–19** ● lists the physical changes that normally occur in the middle years.

Physical assessment of the middle adult includes all body systems, including blood pressure, vision, and hearing. Monitoring for risks and onset of cancer symptoms is essential. During the health history, the nurse should ask specific questions about food intake and exercise habits, substance use, sexual concerns, changes in the reproductive system, coping mechanisms, and family history of chronic illnesses.

OLDER ADULTS   The older adult period begins at age 65, but it can be further divided into three periods: the young-old (65–74 years), the middle-old (75–84 years), and the old-old (age 85 years and older). With increasing age, a number of normal physiological changes occur, as listed in **Table 25–20** ●.

The older adult population is increasing more rapidly than any other age group. In the past century, the number of adults in the United States living to age 65 or older increased from 3.1 million in 1900 to an estimated 42.5 million in 2012. The average life expectancy in the United States is 76 years for men and 81 years for women (*CIA World Factbook*, 2013). One in five, or about 70 million, people will be classified as older adults by the year 2030, more than twice the number in 2000 (Vincent & Velkof, 2010).

The increasing number of older adults has important implications for nursing. Clients needing health care in all settings will be older, requiring nursing interventions and teaching specifically designed to meet needs that differ from those of young and middle adults.

▶ ALTERATIONS FROM NORMAL

Developmental disabilities are a cluster of conditions that occur as the result of impairment in physical function, language development, behavioral patterns, or learning ability (CDC, 2012f). To recognize developmental delays or deviations from normal patterns, the nurse must be knowledgeable about normal developmental milestones. While this module focuses on impairments that affect pediatric development, it is important to remember that development continues throughout the life span and alterations may occur at any point. Any noted alteration should be investigated further. Management of developmental delays varies and may require use of a multidisciplinary team, depending on the nature of the alterations and the individual's needs. In addition, nurses assess each client's individual developmental level and incorporate that into the plan of care. This is especially important when considering client teaching and planning for the client's care needs following discharge. See the Concepts Related to Development feature for an overview of how clients' development can impact other concepts and systems.

Alterations and Manifestations

Certain alterations in development have a single manifestation; however, the alteration may stem from one of many different etiologies. For example, congenital anomalies, infantile glaucoma, and retinopathy of prematurity can all lead to visual impairment in neonates. In other cases, a single defect may manifest in an array of signs and symptoms. For example, fragile X syndrome (FXS) is a genetic disorder in which the absence

Multisystem Effects of Aging

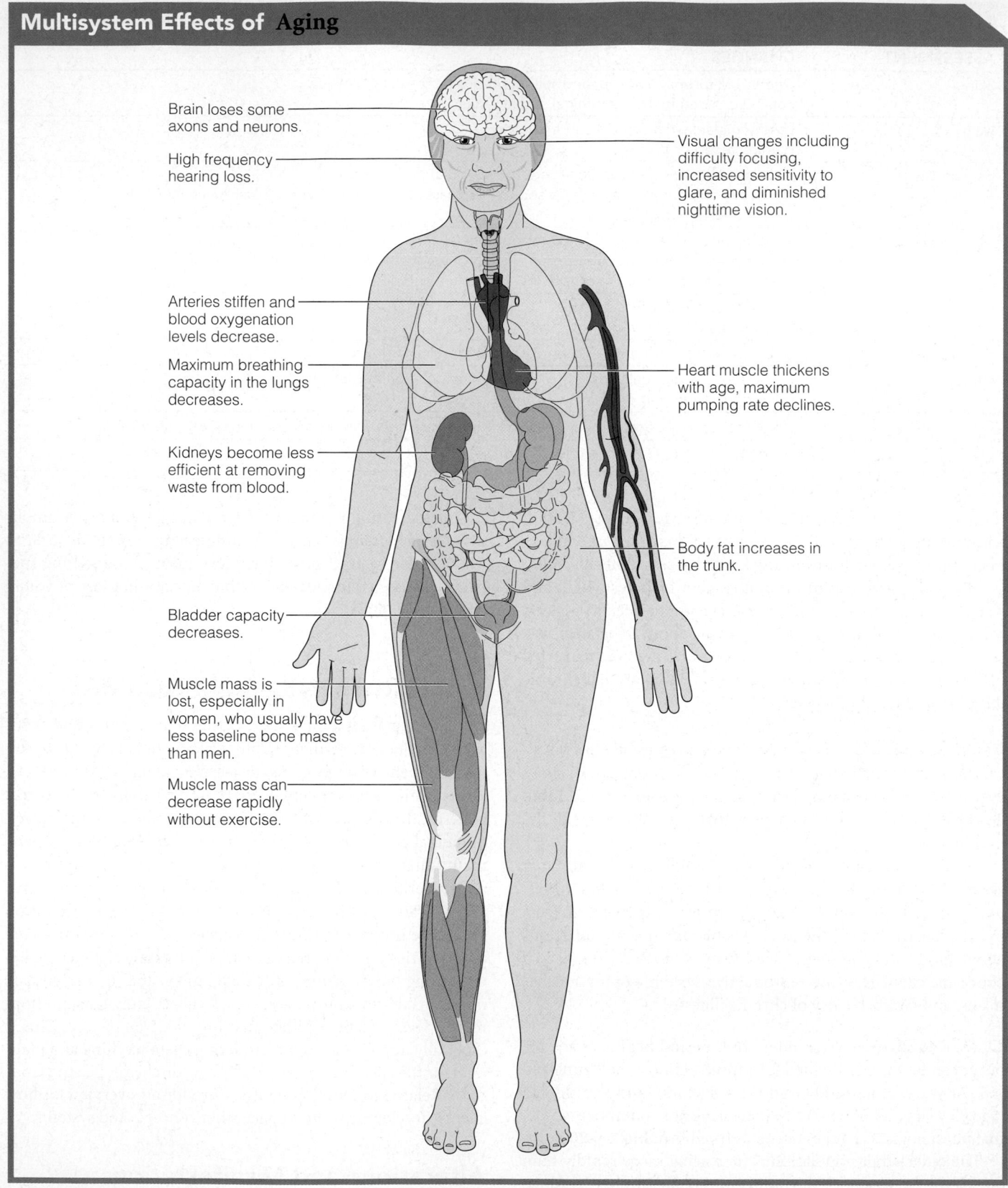

Brain loses some axons and neurons.

High frequency hearing loss.

Visual changes including difficulty focusing, increased sensitivity to glare, and diminished nighttime vision.

Arteries stiffen and blood oxygenation levels decrease.

Maximum breathing capacity in the lungs decreases.

Heart muscle thickens with age, maximum pumping rate declines.

Kidneys become less efficient at removing waste from blood.

Body fat increases in the trunk.

Bladder capacity decreases.

Muscle mass is lost, especially in women, who usually have less baseline bone mass than men.

Muscle mass can decrease rapidly without exercise.

of one protein impairs brain development and may yield multiple effects, including impairments related to language, learning, and social interaction (CDC, 2012g).

The exemplars in this module explore four developmental impairments commonly seen in pediatric clients: attention-deficit/hyperactivity disorder (ADHD), autism spectrum disorder

(ASD), cerebral palsy (CP), and failure to thrive (FTT). (For an overview of manifestations associated with these disorders, see the Alterations and Therapies feature.)

🌐 **Stay Current:** *For discussion of additional pediatric developmental disorders, visit the CDC's information center at* **www.cdc.gov/ncbddd/developmentaldisabilities/index.html**.

TABLE 25–20   Physical Changes in the Older Adult Years

ASSESSMENT	CHANGES
Skin	Decreased turgor and sebaceous gland activity result in dry, wrinkled skin. Melanocytes cluster, causing "age spots" or "liver spots."
Hair and nails	Scalp, axillary, and pubic hair thins; nose and ear hair thickens. Women may develop facial hair. Nails grow more slowly; may become thick and brittle.
Sensory	Visual field narrows, and depth perception is distorted. Pupils are smaller, reducing night vision. Lenses yellow and become opaque, resulting in distortion of green, blue, and violet tones and increased sensitivity to glare. Production of tears decreases. Sense of smell decreases. Age-related hearing loss progresses, involving middle- and low-frequency sounds. Threshold for pain and touch increases. Alterations in proprioception (sense of physical position) may occur.
Musculoskeletal	Loss of overall mass, strength, and movement of muscles occurs; tremors may occur. Loss of bone structure and deterioration of cartilage in joints result in increased risk of fractures and limitation of range of motion.
Cardiovascular	Systolic blood pressure rises. Cardiac output decreases. Peripheral resistance increases, and capillary walls thicken.
Respiratory	Loss of vital capacity continues as the lungs become less elastic and more rigid. Anteroposterior chest diameter increases; kyphosis occurs. Although blood carbon dioxide levels remain relatively constant, blood oxygen levels decrease by 10%–15%.
Gastrointestinal	Production of saliva decreases, and declining number of taste buds reduces the number of accurate receptors for salt and sweet. Gag reflex is decreased, and stomach motility and emptying are reduced. Both large and small intestines undergo some atrophy, with decreased peristalsis. The liver decreases in weight and storage capacity; incidence of gallstones increases; pancreatic enzymes decrease.

Genitourinary	Kidneys lose mass, and the glomerular filtration rate is reduced (by nearly 50% from young adulthood to old age).
	Bladder capacity decreases, and the micturition reflex is delayed. Urinary retention is more common.
	Women may have stress incontinence; men may have an enlarged prostate gland.
	Reproductive changes in men occur:
	    Testosterone decreases.
	    Sperm count decreases.
	    Testes become smaller.
	    Length of time to achieve an erection increases; erection is less full.
	Reproductive changes in women occur:
	    Estrogen levels decrease.
	    Breast tissue decreases.
	    Vagina, uterus, ovaries, and urethra atrophy.
	    Vaginal lubrication decreases.
	    Vaginal secretions become alkaline.

Endocrine	Pituitary gland loses weight and vascularity. Thyroid gland becomes more fibrous, and plasma T_3 decreases. Pancreas releases insulin more slowly; increased blood glucose levels are common. Adrenal glands produce less cortisol.

Prevalence

According to the CDC (2012e), approximately 1 in 6 children in the United States is impaired by one or more developmental disabilities or by other forms of developmental delays. Based on parental reporting, an estimated 9.5% of children between the ages of 4 and 17 were diagnosed with ADHD in 2007. Compared to girls, boys are more than twice as likely to be diagnosed with ADHD (CDC, 2011a).

In 2008, approximately 1 in 88 children was diagnosed with ASD. In comparison, in 2000, an estimated 1 in 150 children was diagnosed with this disorder (CDC, 2012a), while the

prevalence of CP varies between states, the prevalence of this disorder among 8-year-old children is estimated to be 1 in 303 (CDC, 2012c). Among children in the United States, FTT is diagnosed in approximately 3%–5% of children assessed in hospital settings. In primary care settings, FTT is seen in approximately 5%–10% of children (Cole & Lanham, 2011).

Genetic Considerations and Nonmodifiable Risk Factors

In some cases, developmental delays are inevitable due to genetic abnormalities. Because chromosomes and genes carry

Concepts Related to **Development**

The relationship between stress and development is complex. How children respond to stress depends, in large part, on their developmental level. For example, young infants will cry or turn their heads from noxious stimulation and try to sooth themselves by engaging in activities such as thumb sucking. Adolescents, on the other hand, have a more highly developed cognitive ability to cope with stressful situations and can employ strategies such as humor. This is also a time when harmful coping mechanisms to stress can develop (Folkman, S., 2010).

Nurses incorporate knowledge of development in their roles as client educators. For example, the use of dolls to explain medical procedures and body parts related to illness can be useful for preschool children (U.S. National Library of Medicine, 2012a, 2012d, 2012e). When teaching adult clients, it is important to assess their literacy skills in order to provide effective and appropriate teaching (Rudd, 2010). Clients will also have different learning styles: visual, auditory, read/write, or kinesthetic (VARK) (Neider, Borges, & Pearson, 2011). Client teaching should ideally be conducted in the preferred learning method whenever possible. Nurses working with older adults experiencing dementia or memory loss understand that these conditions impair the client's ability to learn (Merrill & Small, 2011). Loss of sensory function can occur at any part of the life cycle and also can impact learning ability.

Developmental status has legal implications. A child's psychosocial development may be adversely effected by adoption, divorce, and custody disputes (Potter, 2010). Divorced adults no longer have a spouse to rely on for support and may rely more heavily on their children or social services to fill that gap (Brown & Lin, 2012). Developmental status of a client should also be considered when obtaining informed consent and discussing end-of-life decisions such as do-not-resuscitate (DNR) orders. Lastly, abuse has many forms and can occur at any point during the life cycle. Any occurrence of abuse can affect a client's ability to meet developmental milestones. Individuals with developmental disabilities are at greater risk for abuse and neglect.

CONCEPT	RELATIONSHIP TO DEVELOPMENT	NURSING IMPLICATIONS
Stress and Coping		
■ Stressors and the coping process ■ Manifestations of stress ■ Assessment of stress	Stress can yield either positive or negative developmental effects. Coping mechanisms will vary based on developmental stage as well as on the individual.	■ Assess the client's developmental level to determine signs of stress the client may exhibit. ■ Consider the client's level of development in employing coping mechanisms to help the client through an illness or procedure.
Teaching and Learning		
■ Learning theories ■ Factors facilitating learning ■ Factors inhibiting learning ■ Client/consumer education	Ability to learn will vary based on client's developmental level. Clients will have different learning styles.	■ The developmental level of the client should be considered when planning teaching. ■ Teaching of minors and clients with sensory perception alterations should always include the parent, guardian, or other responsible adult. ■ Whenever possible, utilize the client's preferred method of learning.
Legal Issues		
■ Strategies to prevent incidents of professional negligence ■ Selected laws that affect nursing practice ■ Advance directives ■ HIPAA ■ Mandatory reporting	The client's developmental level should be considered when signing legal documents pertaining to health care. Many social issues can affect a client's development.	■ Nurses should be alert for signs of abuse or neglect across the life span and report it to the appropriate agency. ■ A victim of abuse or neglect at any age may need assistance meeting developmental milestones.

Alterations and Therapies **Development**

ALTERATION	DESCRIPTION	MANIFESTATIONS	INTERVENTIONS AND THERAPIES
Attention-deficit/ hyperactivity disorder (ADHD)	Pervasive pattern of inattention and hyperactivity combined with impulsivity that interferes with daily functioning in more than one setting (e.g., home, school, and work)	Manifestations of inattention may include making careless mistakes during completion of homework assignments, routinely losing items needed to complete activities or tasks, and avoiding (or disliking) activities that require mental focus. Manifestations of hyperactivity and impulsivity include excessive fidgeting or an apparent inability to sit still, excessive talking and/or verbal outbursts, and habitual interruption of others during conversation.	▪ Pharmacologic stimulants ▪ Behavioral therapy ▪ Modification of teaching styles to meet the individual's needs in the educational setting
Autism spectrum disorder (ASD)	Disorder characterized by chronic impaired social interaction and communication, particularly as this skill pertains to balanced "give and take" aspects of social interaction and communication. Also includes repetitive and limited behaviors, interests, or activities. Manifestations of this disorder impair the individual's routine daily living.	Manifestations of social communication impairment may include preferring not to play with others, avoiding eye contact, inappropriate or emotionless facial expressions, inability to be comforted by others during periods of distress, and difficulty comprehending one's own emotions or the emotions of others. Repetitive, restrictive patterns of interests, behaviors, or activities may include repetition of phrases or words (echolalia), repeated flapping of the hands or spinning of the body, and obsessive organization of toys or other items. Extreme irritability may lead to temper tantrums, self-harm, and outward aggression. Deficits manifest in early childhood but may not become fully pronounced until later years.	Pharmacologic treatments, including antipsychotics, antidepressants, and stimulants ▪ Occupational therapy ▪ Sensory integration therapy (desensitization of the individual to certain sounds, sights, and smells to minimize the distress associated with the stimuli) ▪ Facilitated communication ▪ Dietary and nutritional therapies
Cerebral palsy (CP)	Condition of impaired muscle control due to damage to the developing brain or abnormal brain development	Inadequate balance and coordination (ataxia); uncontrolled movements (dyskinesia); muscle stiffness (spasticity)	▪ Pharmacologic treatments including antispasmodics, anticholinergics (to reduce excessive salivation and uncontrolled physical movements), anticonvulsants (if a coexisting seizure disorder is present) ▪ Orthopedic surgery ▪ Orthotic devices ▪ Occupational therapy ▪ Physical therapy ▪ Speech therapy

(continued on next page)

Alterations and Therapies **Development** (continued)

ALTERATION	DESCRIPTION	MANIFESTATIONS	INTERVENTIONS AND THERAPIES
Failure to thrive (FTT)	Inability to meet or maintain developmental milestones related to physical growth due to undernutrition	Baseline criteria for diagnosis include weight for age that falls below the fifth percentile on numerous occasions or weight loss that crosses two major percentile lines on a growth chart.	▪ Hospitalization if outpatient treatment is unsuccessful, if abuse or neglect is suspected, or if severe caregiver psychosocial dysfunction is suspected ▪ Home nursing visits to facilitate client treatment and caregiver education ▪ Dietary and nutritional education for caregiver

Source: Based on American Psychiatric Association (APA). (2013). *Diagnostic and statistical manual of mental disorders* (5th ed.). Arlington, VA: Author; APA. (n.d.b). *DSM-5 video series: Changes to autism spectrum disorder.* Retrieved from http://www.psychiatry.org/practice/dsm/dsm5/dsm-5-video-series-changes-to-autism-spectrum-disorder; Centers for Disease Control and Prevention (CDC). (2010). *Autism spectrum disorders—Signs and symptoms.* Retrieved from http://www.cdc.gov/ncbddd/autism/signs.html; CDC. (2012a). *Autism spectrum disorders (ASDs)—Data & statistics.* Retrieved from http://www.cdc.gov/ncbddd/autism/data.html; CDC. (2012b). *Autism spectrum disorders (ASDs)—Treatment.* Retrieved from http://www.cdc.gov/ncbddd/autism/treatment.html#types; CDC. (2012d). *Cerebral palsy (CP)—Facts about cerebral palsy.* Retrieved from http://www.cdc.gov/ncbddd/cp/facts.html; CDC. (2012e). *Developmental disabilities.* Retrieved from http://www.cdc.gov/ncbddd/developmentaldisabilities/index.html; Cole, S. Z., & Lanham, J. S. (2011). Failure to thrive: An update. *American Family Physician, 83*(7), 829–834; National Alliance on Mental Illness (NAMI). (2010). *Mental illnesses—Attention-deficit/hyperactivity disorder.* Retrieved from http://www.nami.org/Template.cfm?Section=By_Illness&Template=/TaggedPage/TaggedPageDisplay.cfm&TPLID=54&ContentID=23047.

messages that encode for certain characteristics, they also can carry diseases. Although some genetic mutations are incompatible with life and result in fetal death, live births can occur with others.

Chromosomal disorders may be caused by an array of factors, such as radiation exposure, parental age, or parental disease states; however, sometimes their causes cannot be determined. For example, there is an increased incidence of autism spectrum disorder (ASD) among children with parents or siblings who have ASD (CDC, 2012e). Some children inherit genes that lead to diseases such as cystic fibrosis; others may have a mutation that manifests in the disease. A family history of these diseases is usually present, but because genes sometimes mutate, an initial incidence of a genetic disorder may appear with no identifiable history.

Premature birth, multiple gestation, and low birth weight are also linked to an increased risk for several types of developmental disorders (CDC, 2012e). In all cases, early identification and referral to appropriate resources can help a client to achieve his highest level of developmental functioning possible based on the abnormality.

CASE STUDY \\ PART 1

Ms. Lacy Galleret, 30 years old, arrives at the nurse practitioner's office with her 5-month-old daughter, Annabelle. Ms. Galleret reports that for the past week, Annabelle has had a runny nose and also has been sneezing on occasion. Annabelle was born slightly premature (at 35 weeks of age) and has no other health history.

Annabelle has been afebrile with no vomiting, diarrhea, or any other apparent signs or symptoms of illness. Ms. Galleret reports that her daughter's urine output is good and that she has a good

appetite. On examination, Annabelle is active and in no acute distress, and her skin is pink, warm, and dry. Her mucous membranes are pink and moist. Her lungs are clear to auscultation bilaterally. Annabelle's vital signs, which are within normal limits, include the following: temperature 97.8°F tympanic; pulse 112 bpm; and respirations 28/min. (BP is deferred.) Her weight is 15 pounds (6.8 kg). When asked if Annabelle seems to have any other indicators of potential problems or unusual changes, Ms. Galleret replies, "No, I don't think so. I'm probably just making a big deal out of nothing. Annabelle is our only child, and my husband says I worry too much."

The nurse practitioner diagnoses Annabelle with a viral cold and instructs her mother to encourage fluid intake and to return immediately if Annabelle develops a fever, or if she begins vomiting or has diarrhea. She also tells Ms. Galleret to encourage fluid intake and to contact the clinic if Annabelle's urine output decreases. Ms. Galleret verbalizes understanding of her daughter's discharge instructions and agrees to notify the clinic if Annabelle does not show signs of improvement within the next few days.

One week later, during a follow-up call to Ms. Galleret, she reports that Annabelle's runny nose and sneezing have resolved and that she is healthy.

Clinical Reasoning Questions Level I

1. Identify three developmental milestones Annabelle should have achieved by 5 months of age. Describe methods of assessing Annabelle for achievement of these milestones.

2. Using Erikson's theory of developmental stages, what is Annabelle's current developmental task? What is Annabelle's mother's developmental task?

Clinical Reasoning Questions Level II

4. Identify two nursing diagnoses that are appropriate for inclusion in the plan of care for Annabelle.

5. Identify two nursing diagnoses that are appropriate for inclusion in the plan of care for Ms. Galleret (Annabelle's mother).

6. Is Annabelle's weight within normal limits for her age? Based on her weight and age, in which percentile does Annabelle fall? (See the CDC's growth chart at www.cdc.gov/growthcharts/data/set1/chart02.pdf.)

▶ PREVENTION

Prevention of some developmental delays can be achieved by educating the pregnant client about proper nutrition and avoidance of harmful substances during pregnancy. After birth, the focus shifts to helping parents achieve healthy parent–child interactions. Nurses should stress the importance of safety throughout the life span. An injury that causes brain damage or loss of sensory perception can have a major impact on a client's ability to meet developmental milestones.

Modifiable Risk Factors

While genetic risk factors usually are not modifiable, a number of risk factors can be avoided. During the prenatal period, avoiding fetal exposure to harmful substances, including chemicals and infection, is essential to healthy development. Cultural influences also impact development. After birth, factors such as family dynamics, nutrition, and environment play significant roles in an individual's development.

PRENATAL CONSIDERATIONS   The mother's nutrition and general state of health play a part in pregnancy outcome. Poor nutrition can lead to low-birth-weight infants and infants with compromised neurological performance, slow development, or impaired immune status with resultant high disease rates. Low maternal stores of iron can result in anemia in the infant (Kleinman, 2009). Maternal smoking is associated with low-birth-weight infants. Ingestion of alcoholic beverages, including beer and wine, during pregnancy may lead to fetal alcohol syndrome or fetal alcohol effects. Substance abuse by the mother may result in neonatal addiction, convulsions, hyperirritability, poor social responsiveness, and other neurological disturbances of the infant, as well as changes in neurobehavioral and cognitive function of children (Minnes, Lang, & Singer, 2011).

Even prescription or nonprescription drugs may adversely affect the fetus. Differences in physiology related to gastric emptying, renal clearance, drug distribution, and other factors contribute to variations in pharmacokinetics during pregnancy. Drugs can cause teratogenesis (abnormal development of the fetus) or mutagenesis (permanent changes in the fetus's genetic material) (Minnes et al., 2011). Certain drugs can cause bleeding, stained teeth, impaired hearing, or other defects in the infant. The U.S. Food and Drug Administration (FDA) has established risk categories for drugs in pregnancy.

Some maternal illnesses are harmful to the developing fetus. One example is rubella (German measles), which is rarely a serious disease for adults but can cause deafness, vision defects, heart defects, and mental retardation in the fetus if it is acquired by a pregnant woman. A fetus can also acquire diseases such as AIDS and HIV infection or hepatitis B from the mother.

Chronic maternal distress or depression can affect the fetus. Excess stress hormones such as cortisol pass through the placenta, and can result in lower birth weight and size (Bolten et al., 2011).

The best outcomes for infants occur when mothers eat well; exercise regularly; seek early prenatal care; refrain from use of drugs, alcohol, tobacco, and excessive caffeine; and follow general principles of good health.

ENVIRONMENTAL FACTORS   An environmental factor that is extremely important in the development of children is the profile of family characteristics. The family is an important component in every child's life and plays an essential role in fostering the development of youth. Parenting is a significant concept in families. The effects of parenting interact with a child's individual characteristics to influence risk and protective factors, personality characteristics, and developmental outcomes. See the module on Family for more information.

Adequate nutrition is an essential component of growth and development. For example, poorly nourished children are more likely to get infections than are well-nourished children. In addition, poorly nourished children may not attain their full height potential. Inadequate nutrition during pregnancy and the first few years of life may also impact brain development. See the module on Nutrition for more information.

Other environmental factors that can influence growth and development are the living conditions of the child (e.g., homelessness), socioeconomic status (e.g., poverty versus financial stability), climate, and community (e.g., providing developmental support versus exposing the child to hazards). Illness or injury can affect growth and development. Being hospitalized is stressful for a child and can affect the child's coping mechanisms. Prolonged or chronic illness may affect normal developmental processes, including psychosocial development.

Screenings

Well-child visits are perhaps the most effective initial method of screening for developmental disorders. Through regularly assessing the child at set intervals, the healthcare provider is able to identify the child's degree of achievement of milestones related to growth and development. Developmental assessments are performed in the clinical setting, as well as in home, school, and community settings. Because development is multifaceted, screenings for specific developmental disorders are tailored to particular conditions.

⚙ *Stay Current: For more information on specific developmental screenings, visit the CDC's child development and screening information center at* **www.cdc.gov/ncbddd/childdevelopment/freematerials.html***.*

▶ ASSESSMENT

In nursing, developmental theories can be useful in guiding assessment, explaining behavior, and providing a direction for nursing interventions. An understanding of a child's intellectual ability helps a nurse to anticipate and explain certain reactions, responses, and needs. Nurses can then encourage client behavior that is appropriate for that particular developmental stage.

Theories are also useful in planning nursing interventions. For example, choosing the appropriate toy for a 3-year-old boy requires some knowledge of the physical and cognitive development of the child, as well as a sensitivity to individual preferences.

In adult care, knowledge about the physical, cognitive, and psychological aspects of the aging process is a fundamental aspect of administering sensitive nursing care. For example, nurses can use their familiarity with the theories of development to help clients understand and anticipate the psychosocial changes that take place after retirement or the physical limitations that come with aging.

Nursing Assessment

Nurses use information about developmental milestones to assess children, to identify those with delays, and to plan interventions that will foster development. To do so requires a comprehensive understanding of expected physical growth and development, cognitive abilities, and psychosocial characteristics (Papalia, Olds, & Feldman, 2009). Potential risks—such as prematurity, international adoption, and presence of health problems—necessitate a more frequent and in-depth assessment of observed milestones. Nurses compare the expected findings with assessment results, make referrals for further evaluation when appropriate, and use the results to plan nursing interventions.

Lifespan and Cultural Considerations

Culture influences development in numerous ways, including through traditional practices and genetic variations among some ethnic groups. The traditional customs of the many cultural groups represented in North America influence the development of children in these groups. Nutritional practices of various ethnic groups may influence the rate of growth for infants. In addition, development may be influenced by childrearing practices. For example, the Native American practice of carrying infants on boards often delays walking compared to the norm measured in some developmental tests. Children who are carried by straddling the mother's hips or back for extended periods have a low incidence of developmental hip dysplasia since this keeps their hips in an abducted position. It is important for nurses to take cultural practices into account when performing developmental screening; some tests may not be culturally sensitive and can inaccurately label a child as delayed when the pattern of development is simply different in the group, perhaps due to family's childrearing practices. In these cases there is no lasting delay in any milestone, but variation in acquiring skills may occur.

All cultural groups have rules regarding patterns of social interaction. Schedules of language acquisition are determined by the number of languages spoken and the amount of speech in the home. The particular social roles men and women assume in the culture affect school activities and ultimately career choices. Attitudes toward touching and other methods of encouraging developmental skills vary among cultures.

Genetic traits common in certain ethnic or cultural groups may predispose children to being at the upper or lower ranges

of growth and may influence other physical characteristics. Genetic variations also make certain groups more prone to develop certain diseases.

Diagnostic Tests

Laboratory diagnostic tests generally are not used to determine developmental status. Observational tools, questionnaires, and screening tests are some of the tools that are most helpful in determining developmental status. These are discussed in detail in each of the exemplars that follow.

CASE STUDY \\ PART 2

When Annabelle Galleret is 9 months old, her mother brings her to the clinic for her wellness exam. Ms. Galleret reports that her daughter has had no health issues since her cold a few months ago. However, Ms. Galleret reports that Annabelle "feels stiff sometimes" when she holds her. Additionally, she states her daughter "seems like she keeps her left fist clenched a lot."

Ms. Galleret denies noticing any other unusual behaviors by Annabelle. In reviewing Ms. Galleret's personal health history, you discover that she has a seizure disorder. In addition, she and her husband underwent fertility treatment prior to conceiving Annabelle. When you begin to ask more questions about her seizure disorder, Ms. Galleret says, "You don't think Annabelle has a seizure disorder, do you? My daughter feels stiff in general, not just for short periods of time. She doesn't look like she's having a seizure."

Clinical Reasoning Questions Level I
1. How should the nurse practitioner respond to Ms. Galleret's question about Annabelle potentially having a seizure disorder?
2. In addition to her premature delivery at 35 weeks, what other factor may increase Annabelle's risk for cerebral palsy?

Clinical Reasoning Questions Level II
3. *Refer to the exemplar on Cerebral Palsy within this module.* Describe the components of a developmental assessment for the pediatric client suspected of having cerebral palsy.
4. Based on Annabelle's age, what additional motor activities should be assessed during her examination by the nurse practitioner? If Annabelle does have CP, what findings would she most likely demonstrate?
5. At this time, what are the priorities for care for Annabelle?

▶ INTERVENTIONS AND THERAPIES

Often, clients with impaired development will demonstrate alterations in more than one area of function. For that reason, the treatment approach is varied. Many of the interventions relevant to care of the client with a developmental disorder will require collaboration on the part of the healthcare team.

Independent

As with all client care, safety is the highest priority. All children with impaired mobility are at an exceptionally high risk for injury. For ambulatory children, the nurse should ensure that the child is assisted with activities as needed and that properly fitted orthotic devices are being effectively used. Additionally, range-of-motion (ROM) exercises should be implemented in order to promote flexibility and reduce contracture formation. Families and caregivers should be instructed about injury prevention within the home, including keeping walkways free from loose rugs, electrical cords, or any other obstacles.

Impulsivity and impaired decision-making ability also increase the child's risk for injury (Merrill et al., 2009). In addition to carefully monitoring clients who face these challenges, the nurse should teach families and caregivers about creating a safe home environment, including restricting access to potentially hazardous materials.

Clients affected by developmental impairment, as well as their caregivers and family members, face challenges that extend into the physical and psychosocial realm. For those individuals who require lifelong treatment of a severe condition, financial stress is a serious concern. The nurse caring for these individuals and their families should offer to facilitate connections with support groups and community resources, including agencies that offer assistance through financial aid or services.

Collaborative

In addition to the team providing primary care to the client and client's family, integral care team members may include physical therapists, occupational therapists, speech and language pathologists, psychologists, psychiatrists, and social workers. For pediatric clients diagnosed with FTT, nutritionists play an integral role in teaching caregivers about the client's dietary requirements.

PHARMACOLOGIC THERAPY Pharmacologic therapies are available for use in some instances for both ASD and CP. They are widely used in the treatment of ADHD. Although pharmacologic therapies specific to each condition are discussed in their respective exemplars and can be very helpful to children, it is important to understand that children benefit from interdisciplinary care that is planned according to each child's individual need.

REVIEW The Concept of Development

RELATE Link the Concepts

Linking the concept of development with the concept of infection:

1. Explain the impact of infection on prenatal development.

2. When caring for pregnant clients, how might the nurse promote infection prevention for both mother and fetus?

Linking the concept of development with the concept of family:

3. Explain the interrelationship between an individual's successful achievement of developmental milestones and the developmental health of the individual's family unit.

4. Describe specific aspects of family function that may be impacted when one family member is diagnosed with a developmental disorder.

Linking the concept of development with the concept of ethics:

5. You are caring for an 8-month-old infant who appears to be undernourished. Along the infant's arms and back, you note what appear to be bruises. The child's mother reports that she recently lost her job and can barely afford to pay her rent or other bills. As a nurse, what is the primary issue and what actions are required of you?

6. Identify potential ethical concerns that may arise as a result of utilizing prenatal testing (e.g., amniocentesis and chorionic villus sampling) to diagnose developmental disorders in utero.

READY Go to Companion Skills Manual

REFER Go to Pearson Student Nursing Resources
nursing.pearsonhighered.com

- Additional review materials

REFLECT Case Study \ \ Part 3

Following Annabelle's 9-month wellness examination, the nurse practitioner referred Ms. Galleret and Annabelle to Dr. Barens, who is a pediatric neurologist. After completing a developmental assessment, Dr. Barens was unable to conclusively diagnose Annabelle with CP; however, he was also unable to rule out the possibility that she had the disorder. Ms. Galleret is instructed to bring her daughter back for a follow-up visit with Dr. Barens when she reaches 12 months of age or sooner, if her condition appears to be worsening.

One month prior to Annabelle's follow-up visit with Dr. Barens, Annabelle's mother calls to schedule another appointment with the nurse practitioner. For this visit, both Mr. and Ms. Galleret are present with Annabelle. Ms. Galleret reports that Annabelle has been coughing a lot lately, both when she is eating and when she is simply resting quietly. According to Ms. Galleret, Annabelle has been afebrile and demonstrates no other signs or symptoms of illness; however, she is afraid her daughter will choke while she is asleep. Annabelle's vital signs are within normal limits and she appears to be in no acute distress. She is resting quietly in her mother's arms with her head against her mother's shoulder.

When the nurse practitioner asks for more information about Annabelle's current problem, Ms. Galleret suddenly begins to cry, and states, "I read that making extra saliva is a sign of CP. I don't know what we're going to do if our little girl has that disease. I feel like my heart is breaking into a million pieces!" Mr. Galleret puts his arm around his wife's shoulder in an attempt to console her, but he looks as though he is also near tears.

Clinical Reasoning Questions Level I

1. What concerns do you have about Annabelle?

2. What is an appropriate therapeutic response to make to her mother's expression of sadness?

Clinical Reasoning Questions Level II

3. *Refer to the exemplar on Cerebral Palsy within this module.* What is the link between excess saliva production and cerebral palsy?

4. What are the priorities for care for Annabelle at this time?

5. Identify two nursing interventions that may facilitate Mr. and Ms. Galleret's ability to cope with their current challenges.

EXEMPLAR 25.1 **Attention-Deficit/Hyperactivity Disorder**

EXEMPLAR KEY TERMS
Attention deficit disorder (ADD), *1680*
Attention-deficit/hyperactivity disorder (ADHD), *1680*

EXEMPLAR LEARNING OUTCOMES
After reading about this exemplar, you will be able to:

1. Describe the pathophysiology, etiology, clinical manifestations, and direct and indirect causes of attention-deficit/hyperactivity disorder (ADHD).
2. Identify risk factors and prevention methods associated with ADHD.
3. Illustrate the nursing process in providing culturally competent care across the life span for individuals with ADHD.
4. Formulate priority nursing diagnoses appropriate for an individual with ADHD.
5. Summarize therapies used by interdisciplinary teams in the collaborative care of an individual with ADHD.
6. Plan evidence-based care for an individual with ADHD and his or her family in collaboration with other members of the healthcare team.
7. Evaluate expected outcomes for an individual with ADHD.

▶ OVERVIEW

At one time, **attention-deficit/hyperactivity disorder (ADHD)** was considered a childhood condition, outgrown in adolescence and of little consequence for adults. Research indicates, however, that the disorder persists into adulthood in 30%–70% of individuals. Classic characteristics exhibited by an individual with ADHD include difficulty completing tasks that require focused concentration, as well as hyperactivity, hyperkinesis (excessive movement), and impulsivity (American Psychiatric Association [APA], n.d.a). Hyperactivity and impulsivity may improve as the child nears adulthood, with inattentiveness appearing as the most persistent characteristic. The adolescent may have difficulty due to the increasing cognitive demands of school (Kent et al., 2011). Physical hyperactivity often changes to verbal hyperactivity in adults (Gibbons et al., 2011). ADHD is a known risk factor among adults for antisocial behavior, substance abuse, involvement in serious accidents, academic underachievement, and low occupational success. In adults, inattention is more persistent than hyperactivity or impulsivity.

Roughly one third of adults with ADHD are not diagnosed until after 18 years of age. Approximately 41% of adults with ADHD go on to have a child with the disorder, suggesting a genetic component to the disease (Takeda et al., 2010).

The term **attention deficit disorder (ADD)** is sometimes used to describe individuals who experience the inattentiveness and difficulty concentrating related to ADHD, but who are without the associated hyperactivity that accompanies ADHD. However, the American Psychiatric Association officially recognizes only ADHD, the manifestations of which are described using specifiers (APA, 2013).

▶ PATHOPHYSIOLOGY AND ETIOLOGY

The pathophysiology of ADHD is unclear, but some brain characteristics provide clues. Some children may have a deficit in the catecholamines dopamine and norepinephrine, which lowers the threshold for stimuli input. The disorder is marked by a delay in brain maturation in the areas of self-regulation. Increased input from stimuli and decreased self-regulation cause the hallmark inability to inhibit stimuli and motor activity. Some children exhibit additional problems such as aggressive behaviors, learning disabilities, and motor disorders.

Etiology

Although a variety of physical and neurological disorders are associated with ADHD, children with identifiable causes represent a small proportion of this population. ADHD may result from several different mechanisms involving interaction of genetic, biologic, and environmental risk factors. Examples of known associations include exposure to high levels of lead in childhood and prenatal exposure to alcohol or tobacco smoke. Other prenatal factors associated with a higher incidence of ADHD include preterm labor, impaired placenta functioning, and impaired oxygenation. Seizures and serious head injury are other potential associations.

Risk Factors

Genetic factors are implicated in the development of ADHD. Although ADHD occurs more commonly within families (25% have a first-degree relative with the disorder), a single gene has not been located and a specific mechanism of genetic transmission is not known. It is believed that a genetic predisposition interacts with the child's environment, so that both factors contribute to the appearance of the condition. Family stress, poverty, and poor nutrition may be contributing factors in some cases. Daily television exposure at ages 1–3 years is associated with attentional problems at 7 years (Swing et al., 2010).

Prevention

At this time, there is no known way to prevent the development of ADHD. Clients should avoid smoking, drugs, and alcohol during pregnancy to help prevent behaviors that are similar to ADHD. Learning good parenting skills and having consistent behavior rules, as well as teaching attention skills through reading and puzzles rather than television, can help children with or without ADHD (Swing et al., 2010).

▶ CLINICAL MANIFESTATIONS

Children with ADHD have problems related to decreased attention span, impulsiveness, and/or increased motor activity (**Figure 25–10 ●**). Symptoms can range from mild to severe. The child has difficulty completing tasks, fidgets constantly, is frequently loud, and interrupts others. Sleep disturbances are common. Because of these behaviors, the child often has difficulty

Clinical Manifestations and Therapies ADHD

ETIOLOGY	CLINICAL MANIFESTATIONS	CLINICAL THERAPIES
ADHD may have a genetic basis; however, there is no clearly established cause for this disorder.	■ Symptoms of ADHD fall into three groups: Hyperactivity Impulsive behavior Lack of attention	■ Make environmental modifications. ■ Reduce environmental stimuli. ■ Encourage planned seating in classrooms, group settings. ■ Promote consistent limit setting. ■ Behavioral therapy: Reward appropriate behavior. Apply timely, appropriate consequences for inappropriate behavior. Teach strategies to improve focus, coping. ■ Medications: *See Medications feature.*

developing and maintaining social relationships and may be shunned or teased by other children. This only increases the anxiety of the already compromised child, whose behavior is set on a downward-spiraling course (Hong et al., 2012).

Typically, girls with ADHD show less aggression and impulsiveness than boys, but far more anxiety, mood swings, social withdrawal, rejection, and cognitive and language problems. Girls tend to be older at the time of diagnosis.

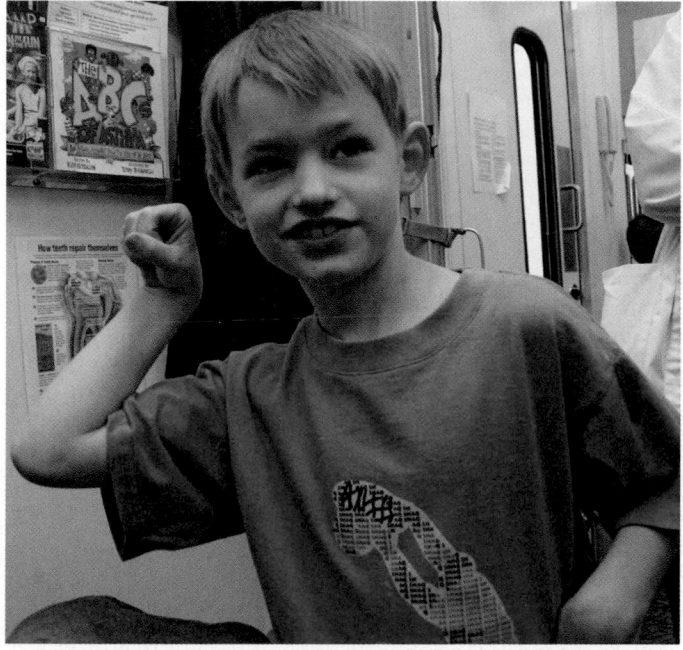

Figure 25–10 ● This child with ADHD was challenged by a visit to a healthcare facility for dental care. He found it difficult to remain in the chair for the examination, and once it was over, he rapidly ran from one piece of equipment to another in the facility. He asked what things were for but did not wait for answers. His engaging personality emerged as he posed briefly for a picture. Such behaviors can be exhausting for parents to manage and may create safety hazards in the healthcare setting.

▶ COLLABORATION

The successful diagnosis and treatment of the child or adult with ADHD requires a collaborative effort that may involve any combination of the following: parents, nurses, and physicians; teachers and school personnel or coworkers; and mental health specialists and speech and language therapists.

Diagnostic Tests

Diagnosis begins with a careful history of the child, including family history, birth history, growth and developmental milestones, behaviors such as sleep and eating patterns, progression and patterns in school, social and environmental conditions, and reports from parents and teachers. A physical examination should be performed to rule out neurological diseases and other health problems. The mental health specialist then tests the child and administers questionnaires to the parent and teacher. It is important to identify other conditions that may mimic ADHD or exist in conjunction with the disorders. These conditions may include depression, anxiety, learning disorder, conduct disorder, or oppositional defiant disorder (Gupta & Kar, 2010).

Specific diagnostic criteria must be applied to all children with the potential diagnosis of ADHD (see **Box 25–2 ●**). Behaviors at home and school or at day care must be evaluated because abnormal patterns in two settings are needed for diagnosis. A variety of tests are available for the trained professional to use in establishing the diagnosis (**Table 25–21 ●**).

Based on the findings, desired outcomes are established for the child's performance and management of the disorder. Treatment is established to meet the desired behavioral outcomes and includes a combination of approaches, such as environmental changes, behavior therapy, and pharmacotherapy (U.S. National Library of Medicine, 2012b). Treatment is expected to be long term.

Children are usually brought for evaluation when behaviors escalate to the point of interfering with the daily functioning of teachers or parents. When children have learning disabilities or anxiety disorders, the problem is commonly misdiagnosed as

Box 25–2 DSM-5 Diagnostic Criteria for Attention-Deficit/Hyperactivity Disorder

A. A persistent pattern of inattention and/or hyperactivity-impulsivity that interferes with functioning or development, as characterized by (1) and/or (2):

1. *Inattention:* Six (or more) of the following symptoms have persisted for at least 6 months to a degree that is inconsistent with developmental level and that negatively impacts directly on social and academic/occupational activities (*Note:* The symptoms are not solely a manifestation of oppositional behavior, defiance, hostility, or failure to understand tasks or instructions. For older adolescents and adults (age 17 and older), at least five symptoms are required.):

   a. Often fails to give close attention to details or makes careless mistakes in schoolwork, at work, or during other activities (e.g., overlooks and misses details, work is inaccurate).

   b. Often has difficulty sustaining attention in tasks or play activities (e.g., has difficulty remaining focused during lectures, conversations, or lengthy reading).

   c. Often does not seem to listen when spoken to directly (e.g., mind seems elsewhere, even in the absence of any obvious distraction).

   d. Often does not follow through on instructions and fails to finish schoolwork, chores, or duties in the workplace (e.g., starts tasks but quickly loses focus and is easily sidetracked).

   e. Often has difficulty organizing tasks and activities (e.g., difficulty managing sequential tasks; difficulty keeping materials and belongings in order; messy, disorganized work; has poor time management; fails to meet deadlines).

   f. Often avoids, dislikes, or is reluctant to engage in tasks that require sustained mental effort (e.g., schoolwork or homework; for older adolescents and adults, preparing reports, completing forms, reviewing lengthy papers).

   g. Often loses things necessary for tasks or activities (e.g., school materials, pencils, books, tools, wallets, keys, paperwork, eyeglasses, mobile telephones).

   h. Is often easily distracted by extraneous stimuli (for older adolescents and adults, may include unrelated thoughts).

   i. Is often forgetful in daily activities (e.g., doing chores, running errands; for older adolescents and adults, returning calls, paying bills, keeping appointments).

2. *Hyperactivity and impulsivity:* Six (or more) of the following symptoms have persisted for at least 6 months to a degree that is inconsistent with developmental level and that negatively impacts directly on social and academic/occupational activities (*Note:* The symptoms are not solely a manifestation of oppositional behavior, defiance, hostility, or failure to understand tasks or instructions. For older adolescents and adults (age 17 and older), at least five symptoms are required.):

   a. Often fidgets with or taps hands and feet or squirms in seat.

   b. Often leaves seat in situations when remaining seated is expected (e.g., leaves his or her place in the classroom, in the office or other workplace, or in other situations that require remaining in place).

   c. Often runs about or climbs in situations where it is inappropriate. (*Note:* In adolescents or adults, may be limited to feeling restless.)

   d. Often unable to play or engage in leisure activities quietly.

   e. Is often "on the go," acting as if "driven by a motor" (e.g., is unable to be or uncomfortable being still for extended time, as in restaurants, meetings; may be experienced by others being restless or difficult to keep up with).

   f. Often talks excessively.

   g. Often blurts out an answer before a question has been completed (e.g., completes other people's sentences; cannot wait for turn in conversation).

   h. Often has difficulty waiting his or her turn (e.g., while waiting in line).

   i. Often interrupts or intrudes on others (e.g., butts into conversations, games, or activities; may start using other people's things without asking or receiving permission; for adolescents and adults, may intrude into or take over what others are doing).

B. Several inattentive or hyperactive-impulsive symptoms were present prior to age 12 years.

C. Several inattentive or hyperactive/impulsive symptoms are present in two or more settings (e.g., at home, school, or work; with friends or relatives; in other activities).

D. There is clear evidence that symptoms interfere with, or reduce the quality of, social, academic, or occupational functioning.

E. The symptoms do not occur exclusively during the course of schizophrenia or another psychotic disorder and are not better explained by another mental disorder (e.g., mood disorder, anxiety disorder, dissociative disorder, personality disorder, substance intoxication or withdrawal).

Source: American Psychiatric Association. (2013). *Diagnostic and statistical manual of mental disorders* (5th ed.). Arlington, VA: Author.

ADHD without further evaluation of the child's symptoms. Obtaining an accurate diagnosis by a pediatric mental health specialist is vital (U.S. National Library of Medicine, 2012b). Careful management of ADHD in childhood may lead to better social functioning later in life.

Pharmacologic Therapy

Children with moderate to severe ADHD are treated with pharmacotherapy (see the Medications feature). The psychostimulant methylphenidate (Ritalin, Concerta) is most often prescribed. Paradoxically, in clients with ADHD, this medication helps to improve focus and attention, as opposed to yielding increased hyperactivity. A skin patch that releases medication over a 9-hour period is now available, facilitating ease of administration (Liberatore & McBarron, 2010). Usually, a favorable response (a decrease in impulsive behaviors and an increase in the ability to sit still and attend to an activity for at least 15 minutes) is seen in the first 10 days of treatment and frequently with the first few doses. Other medications that may be used include dextroamphetamine (Dexedrine or Adderall), dexmethylphenidate, and atomoxetine (Wolraich et al., 2011). All of these medications are Schedule II drugs, which means that a monthly prescription must be obtained from a healthcare practitioner. Side effects include headaches, insomnia, tachycardia, and anorexia. A child's growth pattern should be carefully monitored while taking these medications. A "drug holiday," during which the child does not take the medication

TABLE 25–21 Screening Tests for ADHD

TEST	SOURCE
Vanderbilt Parent and Teacher Scales	www.brightfutures.org/mentalhealth/pdf/professionals/bridges/adhd.pdf
Conners' Parent and Teacher Rating Scales—Revised—Long Form	http://www.mhs.com/product.aspx?gr=cli&id=overview&prod=conners3
Swanson, Nolan, and Pelham Questionnaire II Teacher and Parent Rating Scale (SNAP-IV)	www.ourgirlwednesday.com/downloads/snap-iv-instructions.pdf
Disruptive Behavior Disorder Scale	http://vinst.umdnj.edu/VAID/TestReport.asp?Code=DBRSF
ADHD Rating Scale	www.fmpe.org/en/documents/appendix/Appendix%201%20-%20ADHD%20Rating%20Scale.pdf
Revised Behavior Problem Checklist	http://vinst.umdnj.edu/VAID/TestReport.asp?Code=RBPC
Child Behavior Checklist	http://vinst.umdnj.edu/VAID/TestReport.asp?Code=CBCA

during weekends or over school breaks, can be considered and discussed with the prescribing provider.

Currently, one nonpsychostimulant medication has been approved for treatment of ADHD. Atomoxetine (Strattera) was originally developed as a drug to treat depression, but studies did not support this use. It was found to be beneficial in treating symptoms of ADHD. One major side effect that clients and their parents should be aware of is the increased risk of suicidal ideation. It can also cause nausea and hepatic dysfunction. Liver function should be monitored while taking this medication. It should be used with caution in clients with heart disease or a family history of heart disease especially with long-QT syndrome or arrhythmias (RX List, 2012).

SAFETY ALERT
Many medications used to treat ADHD are central nervous system stimulants. As such, they have a potential for abuse, especially among teens and young adults who take them as an appetite suppressant or in order to stay awake.

Nonpharmacologic Therapy
Although medications are an important part of the treatment plan for the client with ADHD, nonpharmacologic therapies are also integral components of care. Environmental modification and behavioral therapy can greatly improve outcomes for the client with ADHD and enhance their daily quality of life.

Medications **ADHD**

CLASSIFICATION AND DRUG EXAMPLES	MECHANISMS OF ACTION	NURSING CONSIDERATIONS
Psychostimulants *Drug examples:* ■ amphetamine-dextroamphetamine (Adderall) ■ dexmethylphenidate (Focalin) ■ methylphenidate (Ritalin, Concerta)	The mechanisms of action for stimulants in the treatment of ADHD is poorly understood. It is thought to block the reuptake of dopamine and norepinephrine. *May also be used for:* ■ Narcolepsy	■ Teach clients and parents about side effects such as headaches, insomnia, and anorexia. ■ Monitor client's growth while on this medication. ■ Ask about a "drug holiday" on weekends and school breaks. ■ *Potential for abuse:* Some children will sell the drug at school.
Nonstimulants *Drug example:* ■ atomoxetine (Strattera)	The mechanism of action of nonstimulants in the treatment of ADHD is poorly understood. Atomoxetine is a selective norepinephrine reuptake inhibitor.	■ Has less abuse potential since nonstimulant. ■ Teach parents to be alert for serious side effects including psychosis and suicidal tendencies. ■ Monitor hepatic function while on this medication. ■ Use with caution in clients with heart disease.
Psychostimulant Skin Patch *Drug example:* ■ methylphenidate (Daytrana)	The mechanisms of action for stimulants in the treatment of ADHD is poorly understood. It is thought to block the reuptake of dopamine and norepinephrine.	■ Teach clients to alternate patch placement between left and right hips. ■ Watch for skin irritations. ■ Teach client to remove patch after 9 hr. ■ Same side effect profile as oral medications.

Source: Data from Liberatore, D., & McBarron, J. (2010). *US FDA approves first skin patch for ADHD.* Retrieved from http://www.dukeandthedoctor.com/2010/01/us-fda-approves-first-skin-patch-for-adhd; RX List. (2012). *Strattera.* Retrieved from http://www.rxlist.com/strattera-drug.htm; Wilson, B. A., Shannon, M. T., & Shields, K. M. (2013). *Nurse's drug guide.* Upper Saddle River, NJ: Pearson Education; Wolraich, M., Brown, L., & Brown, R. T. (2011). Subcommittee on Attention-Deficit/Hyperactivity Disorder; Steering Committee on Quality Improvement and Management. ADHD: Clinical practice guideline for the diagnosis, evaluation, and treatment of attention-deficit/hyperactivity disorder in children and adolescents. *Pediatrics, 128,* 1007–1022.

Complementary and Alternative Therapy ADHD

Common alternative and complementary therapies used in treatment of the client with ADHD include elimination of dietary components such as highly processed foods, sugar, aspartame, or yeast. Other therapies include use of supplements such as iron, magnesium, zinc, and vitamin B_6. Herbs such as Pycnogenol, melatonin, *Echinacea*, St. John's wort, and ginkgo biloba are sometimes used, as are visual and auditory training. Parents do not typically tell healthcare providers about the use of herbs; 70%–75% of parents have not discussed their use during healthcare visits. Reviews of scientific literature find no systematic proof that Pycnogenol, hypericum, or ginkgo biloba is effective in treating the symptoms of ADHD. Treatment of ADHD with vitamin supplements has not been scientifically proven effective unless there is evidence of specific nutrient deficiencies. Controlled studies of elimination diets (especially the Feingold diet) in the treatment of ADHD have more often disproved their efficacy than supported it (National Resource Center on AD/HD, 2008).

ENVIRONMENTAL MODIFICATION Children with ADHD often benefit from environmental changes. Decreasing stimulation by turning off the television, keeping the environment quiet, and maintaining an orderly and clutter-free desk or study area may help the child to stay focused on the task at hand. Another relatively simple change is appropriate classroom placement, preferably in a small class with a teacher who can provide close supervision and a structured daily routine. Consistent limits and expectations should be set for the child. Children living in chaotic homes and communities may function better if the environment can be simplified. When aggressive behaviors occur, therapeutic approaches such as play and group therapy may be useful.

BEHAVIORAL THERAPY Behavioral therapy involves rewarding the child for desired behaviors and applying consequences for undesirable behaviors. Children may be rewarded by praise or earn points toward a movie or another desired outing for staying seated during meals or quietly listening in a classroom. Cues are established so that a child can subtly be reminded when impulsive or hyperactive behaviors are escalating. Behavioral therapy is most effective when all adults who are in close contact with the child, such as parents and teachers, are involved in and supportive of the program.

■ NURSING PROCESS

Especially when caring for pediatric clients, parents and caregivers are integral to each phase of the nursing process. In particular, because collection of assessment data depends largely on client interviews, the nurse should establish effective communication patterns with the parents and caregivers

Assessment

The nurse often encounters the family who is concerned about the child's behavior before a diagnosis has been made. Ask about family and birth history and have the parents describe the child's behaviors. Perform developmental testing and look specifically for attention span and physical activity. Refer the family to their pediatric healthcare home for further assessment, then to a mental healthcare specialist who is experienced in diagnosing ADHD.

The nurse may encounter the child with ADHD in the hospital when parents bring the child for treatment of an injury (e.g., fracture) or another problem. Explore in detail the parents' report of the child's attention span. Usually within a few minutes in an unstructured setting or waiting area, the child with ADHD becomes restless and searches for distraction. Gather information about the child's activity level and impulsiveness. Find out how the family manages at home and what treatments are being applied.

Diagnosis

Examples of nursing diagnoses that may be appropriate for a child with ADHD include the following:

- *Risk for Injury*
- *Impaired Verbal Communication*
- *Impaired Social Interaction*
- *Chronic Low Self-Esteem*
- *Risk for Caregiver Role Strain.*

(NANDA-I © 2012)

Planning

Prevention can focus on discouraging regular television exposure for young children ages 1–3 years and encouraging daily vigorous physical activity for all children.

The nursing care of the hospitalized child with ADHD focuses on administering medications, managing the child's environment, implementing behavioral management plans, providing emotional support to the child and family, promoting self-esteem, and ensuring ongoing care. Care in the community includes using the same components along with guiding parents to appropriate resources when needed.

Implementation

Children with ADHD present a number of challenges to their parents and teachers. The nurse may need to provide client teaching to both parents and teachers regarding medications and their side effects, the importance of decreasing stimuli and minimizing distractions, and the need for consistency and patience with behavior management plans. Some trial and error may be necessary before the child's treatment team (including parents and teachers) finds the combination of therapies that is most effective for the child.

Administer Pharmacologic Treatments

Stimulant and nonstimulant medications increase the child's attention span and decrease distractibility. Interventions related to pharmacologic treatment include the following:

- Teach parents to be alert for the common side effects of these medications, including anorexia, insomnia, and tachycardia.
- Administer medication early in the day to help alleviate insomnia. Anorexia can be managed by giving medication at mealtimes.
- Perform careful periodic monitoring of weight, height, and blood pressure.
- Instruct families about the abuse potential of stimulant drugs; they should be locked up and administered only as directed.

Minimize Environmental Distractions

Children with ADHD benefit from fewer environmental distractions:

- Keep potentially harmful equipment out of reach.
- Limit and monitor "screen" time.
- Provide a quiet, clutter-free area for study time.
- Use shades to darken the room during naps or at bedtime and minimize noise.
- Teach parents to minimize distractions at home during periods when the child needs to concentrate (e.g., when doing schoolwork) (**Figure 25–11 ●**).
- When the child is hospitalized, minimizing environmental distractions may mean placement in a room with only one other child.

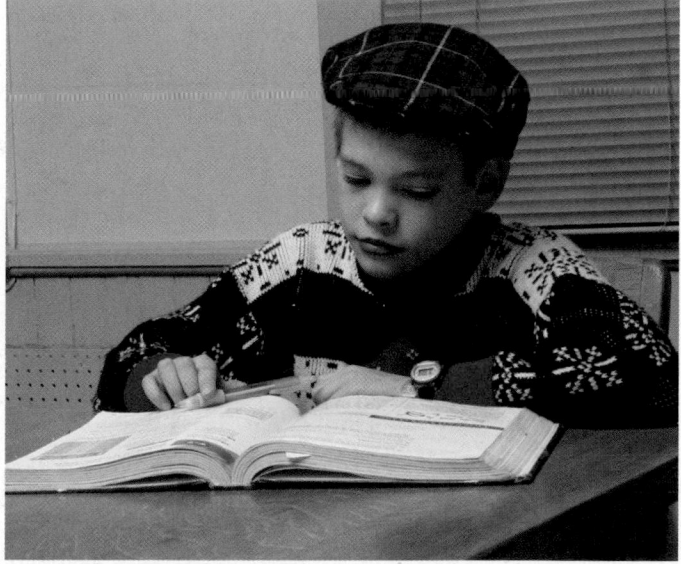

Figure 25–11 ● Managing the environment to provide quiet places with minimal distractions is often necessary for the child with ADHD. This boy reads and does homework in a room with few pictures, no music, and only the book with homework on the table. He also is assisted by structure, such as a scheduled time for homework, with short breaks to walk around every 10–15 minutes.

Implement Behavioral Management Plans

Behavior modification programs can help reduce specific impulsive behaviors. An example is setting up a reward program for the child who has taken medication as ordered or completed a homework assignment. Depending on the child's age, the rewards may be daily as well as weekly or monthly. For example, one completed homework assignment might be rewarded with 30 minutes of basketball or a bike ride, and assignments completed for a week might be rewarded with participation in an activity of the child's choice on the weekend.

If punishment is necessary, the behavior should be corrected while simultaneously supporting the child as an individual. Punishment is generally withdrawal of a privilege and should follow the offense quickly, as the child may not otherwise connect the punishment with the behavior.

Provide Emotional Support

Children with ADHD offer a special challenge to parents, teachers, and healthcare providers.

Family support is essential. Educate both the parents and the child about the importance of appropriate expectations and consequences of behaviors. Teach skills that will help as the child grows older: making lists of tasks to accomplish; following routines for eating, sleeping, recreation, and schoolwork; minimizing stimuli in the environment when completing work; and asking teachers and friends to identify when behavior is inappropriate.

When the child is hospitalized for another condition, the time may provide a brief respite from constant care by the parent. The activity, impulsivity, and general high energy of children with ADHD can fatigue parents. When the child is hospitalized, parents may want to spend a few hours each day at home or at a nearby residence for families. Ask them how they manage at home and offer ideas for respite care.

Promote Self-Esteem

Children with ADHD are easily frustrated, in part by their own behaviors and in part by the reactions of others. This frustration easily leads to loss of self-esteem. Nurses help children with ADHD understand the disorder at a developmentally appropriate level, and also facilitate a trusting relationship with healthcare providers. Children with ADHD who build healthy relationships with healthcare providers are more likely to seek help as they grow into adulthood. Interventions to promote self-esteem may include (U.S. National Library of Medicine, 2012b):

- Assist the child with social skills through the use of role playing, small group play, and modeling.
- Promote the child's self-esteem by emphasizing the positive aspects of behavior and treating instances of negative behavior as learning opportunities.
- Help the child to develop ego strengths (the conscious ability to screen outside stimuli and to control internal demands), which will result in better impulse control and thus increase the child's self-esteem over time.
- Encourage skills at which the child excels and consider the use of support groups for children in school.
- Praise the hospitalized child for lying still for a procedure, taking a medication on time, or helping a staff member carry toys around to other children.

Box 25–3 Optimizing the Educational Experience for the Child With ADHD

Parents can work with teachers to provide a school environment that fosters attention and learning. Some ideas that may be helpful include the following:

- Have the child sit near the front of the class, preferably away from doors or windows.
- Plan a reminder (for the child) that is apparent to the teacher and student but not to other children when the child needs to concentrate on attention. This might be an object placed on the student's desk or a light hand placed on the shoulder or arm.
- Go over assignments and tests with the child in person to explain areas that are understood and those that need attention. Give instructions verbally and in written form and repeat them more than once.
- Provide opportunities to take notes and make lists of assignments and mark off when accomplished. Have a planned time to go through the child's backpack daily to find notices and to ensure that homework is completed and in a uniform location.

- Use computers, note-taking partners, or recording devices for making lists and taking notes.
- If the child has well-developed fine or gross motor skills, integrate motor movement into learning situations whenever possible. Allow the child to run occasional errands to provide additional opportunities for movement.
- Provide quiet places with minimal distraction for examinations. Offer additional time.
- Allow time for organizing clothing, desk, and other areas.
- Find the child's areas of excellence and allow for performance in these ways. Some children are talented in dance; others, in art or extemporaneous speech.
- Never call the child names, make fun of behavior or performance, or call the child "hyperactive" in front of other children, teachers, or parents.
- Incorporate social and behavioral skills into the child's learning plan.

Source: Based on Call-Schmidt, T., & Maharaj, G. (2004). Using nonpharmacological treatments in conjunction with stimulant medications for children with ADHD. *Journal of Pediatric Health Care, 18,* 255–259; National Alliance on Mental Illness (NAMI). (n.d.). ADHD and school: Helping your child succeed in the classroom. Retrieved from http://www.nami.org/Template.cfm?Section=ADHD&Template=/ContentManagement/ContentDisplay.cfm&ContentID=106379; Stein, M. A., & Barren, M. (2003). Welcome progress in the diagnosis and treatment of ADHD in adolescence. *Contemporary Pediatrics, 20*(8), 83–107.

Educate Families

Parents need support to understand the diagnosis and to learn how to manage the child. Explain what the diagnosis is and what is known about attention deficit disorders. Provide written materials, Internet sites, and an opportunity to ask questions.

Emphasize the importance of a stable environment at home as well as at school. At home, the child may have difficulty staying on task. Parents need to consider the child's age and developmental appropriateness of tasks, give clear and simple instructions, and provide frequent reminders to ensure completion. Routines in the evening can promote good sleep patterns.

The nurse can serve as a liaison to teachers and school personnel or as the case manager for the child. See **Box 25–3** ● for suggestions on how parents and teachers can work together to optimize the child's educational experience. An individualized education plan (IEP) may be needed, with clear expected outcomes stated for the child's behaviors. IEPs or periods of instruction free from the distractions of the entire class may enable the child to improve school performance. Parents may have difficulty understanding the need for these approaches because the child often tests at above-average intelligence.

Reinforce the importance of providing a structured environment free from unnecessary external stimuli. Make sure that parents understand behavioral approaches that will help the child, the administration of prescribed medications, and the importance of returning for healthcare visits to monitor for side effects. Medication should be safely locked away at home to keep it away from other children and to prevent illegal use of the controlled substance.

Parents may have heard about ADHD in the media and may have questions about its cause and management. Providing information about complementary and alternative treatments is a nursing role. The National Institutes of Health sponsors the National Center for Complementary and Alternative Medicine (NCCAM), which is a reliable source for parents and professionals.

As the child grows older, provide explanations about the disorder and information about techniques that will assist in dealing with problems. Emphasize the importance of doing homework or other tasks requiring concentration in a quiet environment without background noise from a television or radio. Encourage children with ADHD to keep assignment notebooks and use checklists to help them accomplish specific tasks.

Evaluation

Expected outcomes of nursing care for the child with ADHD include the following:

- The parents and child demonstrate understanding of the disorder.
- The family accurately and safely manages medication administration.
- The child demonstrates an increase in attentiveness and a decrease in hyperactivity, impulsivity, and sleep disturbance.
- The child displays formation of a positive self-image.
- The child manifests formation of healthy social interactions with peers and family.
- The child achieves educational performance to maximum potential.

Focus on Diversity and Culture
Mental Health and Stigma

Many families who have a child with ADHD are embarrassed and feel shame because of the diagnosis, especially in certain cultures (e.g., some Asian groups) and in very structured and highly achieving families. When taking histories from family members, be sensitive to the stigma some may feel. In a private setting, ask about the family's feelings regarding a mental health disorder. Is there someone in the family with whom they can talk about the diagnosis? Provide information in a nonjudgmental manner and, if appropriate, provide support from other families with similar experiences.

NURSING CARE PLAN A Client With Attention-Deficit/Hyperactivity Disorder

ASSESSMENT

Melanie Taylor, 8 years old, visits her pediatrician's office for a routine checkup. Her mother, Mrs. Taylor, reports Melanie is not doing well in school and she is a difficult child to raise. Upon further questioning Mrs. Taylor reports her daughter is forgetful, has trouble focusing, and often does not respond to her name being called. She has to repeatedly ask her to perform her chores, get ready for bed, or do her homework. Melanie does not sleep well at night, and most nights she crawls into her parents' bed. One night Mrs. Taylor awoke to find Melanie watching TV at 2 a.m. in the family room. Melanie's teacher has suggested she be evaluated for possible ADHD.

The nurse interviews Melanie who says she doesn't like school because "it's too hard" and the teacher "always tells me to sit still."

Upon reviewing Melanie's medical history the nurse finds the client's growth and development have been normal to date. Mrs. Taylor's pregnancy and delivery were unremarkable.

The physical examination is normal although the nurse notes Melanie often requires repetition of instructions such as "Touch your finger to your nose" before she complies. Both Melanie and her mother appear tired and yawn several times during the nurse's time with them.

The provider speaks with Melanie and Mrs. Taylor suggesting the signs and symptoms are highly suspicious of ADHD and provides a referral for the family to meet with a psychologist specializing in the care of clients with this disorder.

The nurse provides Ms. Taylor with a Conners' Parent Rating Scale to complete and gives her a copy of the Teacher Rating Scale to give to Melanie's teacher for completion before seeing the counselor, who will evaluate the results.

DIAGNOSES

- *Risk for Situational Low Self-Esteem*
- *Disturbed Sleep Pattern*
- *Risk for Caregiver Role Strain*
- *Fatigue*

(NANDA-I © 2012)

PLANNING

- The client (Melanie) will sleep through the night, remaining in her own bed.
- The client will participate in a therapeutic regimen as recommended by the physician.
- The client's parents and teachers will participate in the therapeutic regimen.
- The client will increase her ability to remain on task by 5-minute intervals over a period of 6–8 weeks, until she can remain on task for a minimum of 20 minutes at a time.
- The client will keep track of her belongings.
- The client will respond when spoken to the first time.

IMPLEMENTATION

- Explain diagnosis in terms Melanie can understand and help Melanie understand she is not "abnormal" but "unique" in how her brain works.
- Help Mrs. Taylor set rules related to sleep that will promote Melanie's sleep hygiene.
- Assist client to understand how her potential diagnosis of ADHD impacts her thinking as well as how treatment can help her perform better in school.
- Determine if Melanie or Mrs. Taylor have questions related to ADHD.

- Suggest strategies for helping Melanie improve her concentration and memory.
- Teach positive behavioral skills through role play, role modeling, and discussion.
- Convey confidence in client's and mother's ability to handle situation.
- Encourage increased responsibility for self, as appropriate.
- Encourage Melanie to accept new challenges.
- Monitor Melanie's statements of self-worth and frequency of self-negating verbalizations.

EVALUATION

Mrs. Taylor and Melanie return at the end of 3 months. Mrs. Taylor reports that Melanie is doing better at paying attention both at home and at school, and that she is able to maintain attention for 20 minutes "most of the time." Both of them are sleeping better. Melanie is able to answer the nurse's questions readily and describes things that she does to keep track of her belongings and try to stay on task. Melanie voices pride in her improvement at school.

CRITICAL THINKING

1. *Mrs. Taylor asks the nurse, privately out of range of Melanie's hearing, if the diagnosis resulted from something she did as a parent or while pregnant. How would you respond?*
2. *Melanie tells the nurse, "I'm so stupid compared to the other kids in my class. I guess ADHD means I'm brain damaged." How would you respond?*
3. *Is it possible to adequately treat ADHD without the use of medications? Explain your answer.*

REVIEW Attention-Deficit/Hyperactivity Disorder

RELATE Link the Concepts and Exemplars

Linking the exemplar of attention-deficit/hyperactivity disorder with the concept of family:

1. How can the nurse support the family of a child with ADHD?
2. What if the family is a single parent? A grandparent?

Linking the exemplar of attention-deficit/hyperactivity disorder with the concept of safety:

3. What interventions are important for the nurse to initiate to maintain the safety of a client with ADHD?
4. When caring for an adolescent with ADHD how would you teach automobile safety?

REFER Go to Pearson Nursing Student Resources nursing.pearsonhighered.com

- Additional review materials

REFLECT Case Study

Jason is an active, healthy 11-year-old boy. He is currently in fifth grade at the public elementary school near his home. He lives with his mother Evelyn and his 14-year-old sister Jenna. He has not had much contact with his father. Jason's home life has been somewhat stressful the past year or so because of ongoing fights between his mother and oldest sister Jessica; the conflict resulted in Jessica moving out of the house. Jason gets along well with his mother, but he has typical sibling conflicts with Jenna.

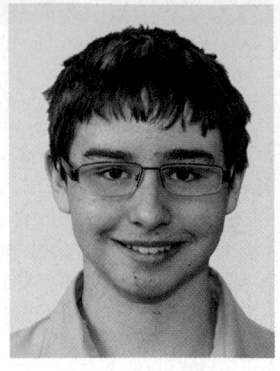

Jason has had problems in school for the past 3 years. Teachers report that he has difficulty staying on task and won't follow directions. Although he made some progress last year with his fourth-grade teacher, his grades have been consistently poor. His mother tries to help him with homework after school or in the evening; these sessions frequently turn into battlegrounds. It takes Jason hours to complete fairly simple assignments, resulting in a great deal of frustration for both Jason and his mother. The fact that he frequently comes home from school with headaches further aggravates the situation.

In addition to problems with academics, Jason has problems with social interactions. His teachers find him to be disruptive in the classroom. During the past year, he has often been sent to the principal's office for misbehaving. He has few friends and is a frequent target of teasing at school. Most of his time at home is spent playing video and computer games and watching TV.

1. What are the priorities of nursing care for Jason?
2. What outcomes would be appropriate for this client?
3. What independent nursing interventions would you initiate for this client?

EXEMPLAR 25.2 Autism Spectrum Disorder

EXEMPLAR KEY TERMS

Autism spectrum disorder (ASD), *1688*
Echolalia, *1689*
Stereotypy, *1689*

EXEMPLAR LEARNING OUTCOMES

After reading about this exemplar, you will be able to:

1. Describe the pathophysiology, etiology, clinical manifestations, and direct and indirect causes of autism spectrum disorder (ASD).
2. Identify risk factors and prevention methods associated with ASD.
3. Illustrate the nursing process in providing culturally competent care across the life span for individuals with ASD.
4. Formulate priority nursing diagnoses appropriate for an individual with ASD.
5. Summarize therapies used by interdisciplinary teams in the collaborative care of an individual with ASD.
6. Plan evidence-based care for an individual with ASD and his or her family in collaboration with other members of the healthcare team.
7. Evaluate expected outcomes for an individual with ASD.

▶ OVERVIEW

The client with **autism spectrum disorder (ASD)** characteristically demonstrates impaired communication and social interaction patterns, and the presence of repetitive, restrictive, and stereotyped behaviors. Manifestations of ASD range across a spectrum from mild to severe.

Children and adults with ASD often suffer from impairments of language, cognition, and social skills that make them seem different from others.

🔅 *Stay Current: Keep abreast of statistics, research, and treatment at* **www.autismspeaks.org**.

▶ PATHOPHYSIOLOGY AND ETIOLOGY

Although the etiology of ASD is unknown, it is believed to be associated with a complex interplay between genetic, immunologic, and environmental factors. Current research is investigating the role of environmental exposure to certain drugs during pregnancy; the role of neurotransmitters such as dopamine and serotonin, which are abnormal in some children with ASDs; and other factors (CDC, 2010). As discussed in the module on Immunity, no link has been found between mercury-containing vaccinations and autism spectrum disorders (U.S. National Library of Medicine, 2012c).

Risk Factors

Without a specific etiology, determining risk for autism is difficult. However, some factors appear to be linked. A maternal age of 40 or older and a paternal age of 50 and above increase the risk that a child will be born with autism. Maternal smoking or the use of alcohol, valproic acid, or misoprostol during pregnancy also increases rates of autism (Duchan & Patel, 2012).

Children with genetic abnormalities such as tuberous sclerosis, fragile X syndrome, Down syndrome, congenital rubella syndrome, and neurofibromatosis have an increased occurrence of autism. Boys have a higher rate of ASD than girls. Premature or low birth weight babies carry a higher risk (Duchan & Patel, 2012).

Prevention

Although there is no way to prevent autism, some factors can be modified to reduce the risk of occurrence, maternal health being the most important. Women who are pregnant should be counseled to avoid use of tobacco products and exposure to secondhand smoke; refrain from drinking alcohol or using illegal substances; and disclose the pregnancy to any healthcare provider, including their pharmacist, when they learn they are pregnant.

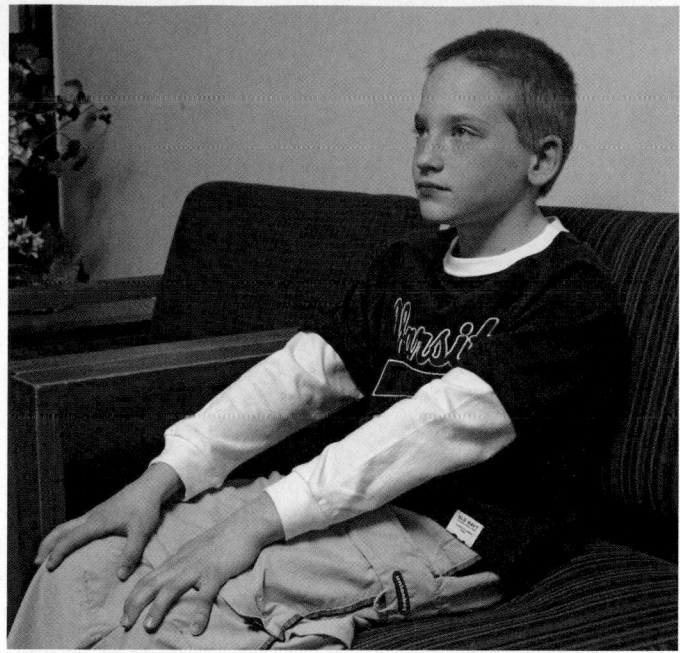

Figure 25–12 ● This child with autism sits stiffly in the chair and engages in rhythmic rocking behavior. He has a disengaged appearance and does not readily interact with other children or adults who are in his environment.

▶ CLINICAL MANIFESTATIONS

The essential features typically become apparent by the time a child is 3 years of age. They reflect impairments in the following:

- Social interactions
- Communication
- Ability to adapt to new situations
- Attention span and ability to organize responses to situations (Roeyers, Desoete, & Dereu, 2011)

Social interactions are always complex and involve perceptions of the other individual as well as social behaviors. The client with ASD does not learn the common characteristics of these social interchanges. As a result, these individuals may be unable to converse normally, may fail to initiate conversations, and may fail to understand or observe nonverbal behavior.

Children with ASD manifest disturbances in the rate or sequence of development, with onset of abnormal functioning in at least one of the following areas prior to age 3: social interaction, language used in social interactions, and imaginative play.

A primary finding is impairment in social interactions, particularly as this pertains to relating to others or responding to social and emotional cues. In addition, **stereotypy**, or rigid and obsessive behavior, may be observed. Characteristically, these repetitive behaviors in affected children include head banging, twirling in circles, biting themselves, and flapping their hands or arms (**Figure 25–12 ●**). Frequently, a child's behavior is self-stimulating or self-destructive. Responses to sensory stimuli are frequently abnormal and include an extreme aversion to touch, loud noises, and bright lights. Emotional lability (rapid, significant mood changes) is common.

Communication difficulties or delays in speech and language are common and are often the first symptoms that lead to diagnosis. Absence of babbling and other communication by 1 year of age, absence of two-word phrases by 2 years, and deterioration of previous language skills are characteristic of autism. Language acquisition, including verbal and nonverbal communication patterns, such as eye contact, will vary based on the severity of the disorder. Some children and adults with ASD can participate fully in conversations, but may show characteristic behaviors such as marked lack of eye contact and lack of emotional reciprocity. They may or may not understand humor and other subtleties of language.

For children with ASD, speech patterns are likely to show certain abnormalities, such as the following:

- Using *you* in place of *I*
- Engaging in **echolalia** (a compulsive parroting of a word or phrase just spoken by another)
- Repeating questions rather than answering them
- Being fascinated with rhythmic, repetitive songs and verses.

Behaviors of children with autism spectrum disorders show several differences from other children's behaviors. Children with ASD may have a great difficulty dealing with new situations and typically show agitation and withdrawal when routines are changed. Children with ASD do not commonly explore objects, but have stereotyped behaviors. They may line up objects, play with the same objects over and over, and have certain rituals that must be performed. They often become upset if these normal routines are disrupted. Rituals may involve eating only certain types or colors of foods or eating in specific patterns.

Clients with ASD may manifest disturbances in the rate or sequence of development. Pediatric clients may be cognitively

Lifespan Considerations Adults With ASD

Childhood ASD persists into adulthood. Children who receive timely intervention and whose parents and treatment teams collaborate to find the best treatment for them as individuals have the greatest chance of becoming successfully functioning adults. Adults with ASD continue to struggle with communication skills, especially understanding nonverbal communication, and socialization. These clients are most successful when they seek employment opportunities and activities that play to their strengths.

Many communities provide job training and supervised work programs for adults with ASD. Many adults with less severe ASD are active community members, becoming fully employed and living independently. Others need more support and may choose to continue to live with their parents or to reside in a group living environment that provides additional support. A number of government programs exist to assist these individuals with financial support. Information on

these programs is available from the Social Security Administration (National Institute of Mental Health, 2009).

Unfortunately, research on adults with ASD is lacking, especially for the geriatric population. Few clinics exist that specifically treat adults with ASD, making it challenging for these adults to get the best level of care. Many adults with ASD who cannot function independently or whose families can no longer provide care for them end up being financially subsidized by the state. With the steady rise in the number of children diagnosed with this disorder comes a resulting increase in the number of adults with the disorder. The financial impact on state governments is significant and is likely to increase steadily for many years. This is all the more reason why children with ASD need to be identified early, so that they may have access to treatments and therapies that give them the best chance to become fully functioning adults.

impaired, but they can demonstrate a wide range of intellectual ability and functioning. Cognitive impairment may be manifested early in life by slow developmental progression, particularly in social skills. Some children with ASD are of at least average intelligence, and some are highly gifted. Some children with autism spectrum disorder are impaired in particular areas of development, while others are above normal. About 25% have macrocephaly, with reduced head size at birth, followed by excessive growth at 1–2 months and 6–14 months (Freitag et al., 2009). However, most children with ASD have a normal appearance. The clinical manifestations and therapies for ASD are outlined in the following feature.

▶ COLLABORATION

A number of agencies and resources are available to support the child with autism spectrum disorder. Many communities have an interdisciplinary task force or team that meets regularly to review services available in their area for children with special

needs, including ASD. By law, public schools are charged with the responsibility of facilitating and providing services for children with ASD and other disabilities. Nurses frequently serve on multidisciplinary teams to ensure that medical and mental health needs of these clients are included in supportive plans. Team members for a client with ASD may include parents, nurses, physicians, teachers, mental health professionals, occupational therapists, and physical therapists.

Diagnostic Tests

Diagnosis is based on the presence of specific criteria, as described in the American Psychiatric Association's *Diagnostic and Statistical Manual of Mental Disorders*, fifth edition (DSM-5) (see **Box 25–4** ●). **Table 25–22** ● lists several screening tests that are useful in identifying characteristics that are congruent with ASD. Additional testing is done to rule out other causes of the child's behavior. Tests may include neuroimaging (computed tomography [CT] scan or MRI), lead screening, DNA analysis, and electroencephalography.

Clinical Manifestations and Therapies Autism Spectrum Disorder

ETIOLOGY	CLINICAL MANIFESTATIONS	CLINICAL THERAPIES
Autism spectrum disorder (ASD)	■ Impaired social, communicative, and behavioral development is usually noted in the first year of life.	■ Early intervention is key to maximal performance. ■ Interventions focus on improving behaviors and communication skills, providing physical and occupational therapy, structuring play interactions with other children, and educating parents about the child's needs.
	■ Impaired social interactions with normal language development for age; pitch, tone, and other speech characteristics may be abnormal. Verbal skills involving spelling and vocabulary are high, with concept formation, language flexibility, and comprehension low.	■ Social interactions and speech and language therapy for pragmatics are the focus of therapy.
	■ Severe social impairment without meeting DSM criteria for other types of ASD.	■ Behavioral therapy focuses on building social and language skills.

Box 25–4 DSM-5 Diagnostic Criteria for Autism Spectrum Disorder

A. Persistent deficits in social communication and social interaction across multiple contexts, as manifested by the following, currently or by history (examples are illustrative, not exhaustive; see text):

1. Deficits in social-emotional reciprocity, ranging, for example, from abnormal social approach and failure of normal back-and-forth conversation; to reduced sharing of interests, emotions, or affect; to failure to initiate or respond to social interactions.
2. Deficits in nonverbal communicative behaviors used for social interaction, ranging, for example, from poorly integrated verbal and nonverbal communication; to abnormalities in eye contact and body language or deficits in understanding and use of gestures; to a total lack of facial expressions and nonverbal communication.
3. Deficits in developing, maintaining, and understanding relationships, ranging, for example, from difficulties adjusting behavior to suit various social contexts; to difficulties in sharing imaginative play or making friends; to absence of interest in peers.

B. Restricted, repetitive patterns of behavior, interests, or activities, as manifested by at least two of the following, currently or by history (examples are illustrative, not exhaustive; see text):

1. Stereotyped or repetitive motor movements, use of objects, or speech (e.g., simple motor stereotypies, lining up toys or flipping objects, echolalia, idiosyncratic phrases).
2. Insistence on sameness, inflexible adherence to routines, or ritualized patterns of verbal or nonverbal behavior (e.g., extreme distress at small changes, difficulties with transitions, rigid thinking patterns, greeting rituals, need to take same route or eat same food every day).

3. Highly restricted, fixated interests that are abnormal in intensity or focus (e.g., strong attachment to or preoccupation with unusual objects, excessively circumscribed or perseverative interests).
4. Hyper- or hyporeactivity to sensory input or unusual interest in sensory aspects of the environment (e.g., apparent indifference to pain/temperature, adverse response to specific sounds or textures, excessive smelling or touching of objects, visual fascination with lights or movement.

C. Symptoms must be present in the early developmental period (but may not become fully manifested until social demands exceed limited capacities, or may be masked by learned strategies in later life).

D. Symptoms cause clinically significant impairment in social, occupational, or other important areas of current functioning.

E. These disturbances are not better explained by intellectual disability (intellectual developmental disorder) or global developmental delay. Intellectual disability and autism spectrum disorder frequently co-occur; to make comorbid diagnosis of autism spectrum disorder and intellectual disability, social communication should be below that expected for general developmental level.

Note: Individuals with a well-established DSM-IV diagnosis of autistic disorder, Asperger's disorder, or pervasive developmental disorder should be given the diagnosis of autism spectrum disorder. Individuals who have marked deficits in social communication, but whose symptoms do not otherwise meet criteria for autism spectrum disorder, should be evaluated for social (pragmatic) communication disorder.

Source: American Psychiatric Association. (2013). *Diagnostic and statistical manual of mental disorders* (5th ed.). Arlington, VA: Author.

Pharmacologic Therapy

For some clients, medications are used to manage manifestations and associated symptoms. Medications used in the care of clients with ASD may include stimulants, selective serotonin reuptake inhibitors (SSRIs), and mood stabilizers.

The overall prognosis for children with ASD to become functioning members of society is guarded. The extent to which adequate adjustment is achieved varies greatly. Successful adjustment is more likely for children with higher IQs, adequate speech, and access to specialized programs.

Nonpharmacologic Therapy

Early intervention assists in maximizing the child's potential by improving developmental skills, decreasing severity of symptoms,

TABLE 25–22 Screening Tests for Autism Spectrum Disorders

TEST	SOURCE
Clinical Practice Guidelines—Early Intervention Program of the New York State Department of Health	www.health.ny.gov/community/infants_children/early_intervention/disorders/autism/
Checklist for Autism in Toddlers (CHAT) or Modified Checklist for Autism in Toddlers (MCHAT)	www.aheadwithautism.com/chat_screening.html www.firstsigns.org/downloads/m-chat.PDF
Autism Diagnostic Interview—Revised	Kim, S. H., & Lord, C. (2012). New Autism Diagnostic Interview–Revised algorithms for toddlers and young preschoolers from 12 to 47 months of age. *Journal of Autism and Developmental Disorders, 42*(1), 82–93. http://portal.wpspublish.com/portal/page?_pageid=53,70436&_dad=portal&_schema=PORTAL
Communication and Symbolic Behavior Scales Developmental Profile (CSBS DP)	www.brookespublishing.com/store/books/wetherby-csbsdp/checklist.htm
Screening Tool for Autism in Two-Year-Olds	http://kc.vanderbilt.edu/triad/training/page.aspx?id=821
Autism Diagnostic Observation Schedule—Generic (ADOS-G)	www.ehow.com/how_2095042_use-adosg.html
Childhood Autism Rating Scale (CARS)	http://oreilly.com/medical/autism/news/diag_tools.html
Developmental Checklist–Early Screen (DBC-ES)	www.med.monash.edu.au/spppm/research/devpsych/download/dbc-info-package.pdf

Hispanics are diagnosed with autism far less frequently than are members of non-Hispanic groups (Palmer et al., 2010). This is more likely the result of lack of access to services and lack of Spanish-speaking professionals in the United States than to any biomedical or genetic factor. As with any other culture, early intervention is critical to identifying and providing appropriate therapies and supports to the Hispanic child with autism. Nurses working with Hispanic families who do not have insurance should refer them to the local health department or department of social services to see whether their children qualify for Medicaid or the Children's Health Insurance Plan. Nurses working in hospitals or health departments should ask whether families have a medical home and help them find one if they do not. Clinics offering developmental screenings to children should have at least one staff member trained to administer a valid, reliable screening tool that has been developed specifically for use with Spanish-speaking children and is not simply a tool that has been translated into Spanish.

and establishing helpful support for parents (Boyd et al., 2010; Peters-Scheffer et al., 2011; Warren et al., 2011). Children are taught how to focus and apply learning. Treatment focuses on behavior management to reward appropriate behaviors, foster positive or adaptive coping skills, and facilitate effective communication. The goals of treatment are to reduce rigidity or stereotypy (repetitive, obsessive, machinelike movements) and other maladaptive behaviors.

Complementary and Alternative Therapy

Some parents who have a child with autism choose to use complementary and alternative medicine (CAM), such as touch therapy or a gluten-free diet, in an attempt to help the child. It is important to note that CAM therapies have not been adequately evaluated; therefore, there is an insufficient research base to support or refute them individually or as a whole.

One approach includes dietary therapy with vitamin A, vitamin C, vitamin B_6, magnesium, and omega-3 fatty acids. The use of gluten-free or casein-free diets has gained popularity in recent years. Parents have tried drug therapies that include secretin, a pancreatic gastrointestinal peptide, and Pepcid or other antacids. Some parents believe that detoxification by limiting certain dietary intake or using Epsom salt baths can be helpful (Whiteley et al., 2012).

Nurses can help parents evaluate studies on complementary care and encourage parents to initiate only one treatment at a time; the effectiveness of any one treatment cannot be measured properly if it is initiated in conjunction with other therapies. At each healthcare interaction, the nurse working with a client with ASD should ask about therapies being used and discuss safeguards to avoid any undesired side effects.

NURSING PROCESS

Throughout application of the nursing process, the client's parents or caregivers will be integral team members. Because much of the assessment data is collected by way of interview, the nurse should prioritize the establishment of effective, open communication patterns with the client's primary caregivers and family members.

Assessment

The nurse may encounter the child with ASD when parents seek care for a suspected hearing impairment, speech difficulty, or developmental delay. Early and frequent developmental screening of all children can help in referral for thorough assessment and identification of cases. Parents may report abnormal interaction such as lack of eye contact, disinterest in cuddling, minimal facial responsiveness, and failure to talk. Be alert to observations by the parents that the baby or young child does not look at them or provide other developmental or behavioral cues (Wallace & Rogers, 2010). Initial assessment focuses on language development, response to others, and hearing acuity. Become familiar with the following "red flags" of the American Academy of Neurology and Child Neurology Society that require immediate evaluation (Pickles et al., 2009):

- No babbling or communication gestures by 12 months
- No single word by 16 months
- No spontaneous two words by 24 months
- Loss of language or social skills previously achieved.

Ask about birth history, including possible neonatal exposure to drugs or alcohol. Carefully evaluate the child for history of developmental milestones and refer for abnormalities. Perform developmental screening that considers several areas of development, including motor activity, social skills, and language, or refer the family to a professional or community resource that provides such screenings. Recall that the child may have normal performance in one area such as motor skills, but delayed development in another area such as language skills. Likewise, language may be normal for age, but social interactions delayed. Include questions about adaptive skills such as toilet training and feeding patterns. Inquire about school performance because

Complementary and Alternative Therapy The GFCF Diet

Many parents of children with ASD choose to implement a gluten-free, casein-free (GFCF) diet. This has gained sufficient popularity that there are entire Web sites and programs devoted to this diet. Essentially, the GFCF diet eliminates the proteins gluten and casein from the client's diet. Gluten is normally found in wheat, barley, and rye. Casein is found in dairy products, including milk, cheese, and eggs. Nurses working with clients considering the GFCF diet should encourage them to consult with a nutritionist or registered dietitian who can help them make sure that they plan GFCF meals that will meet their child's nutritional needs.

some areas may be normal while others are delayed. Observe the child in play situations and evaluate the use of creative and exploratory play versus more repetitive patterns. Perform hearing and vision screening if possible to rule out sensory problems.

When a child with a diagnosis of autistic disorder is hospitalized for a concurrent problem, obtain a history from the parents regarding the child's routines, rituals, and likes and dislikes, as well as ways to promote interaction and cooperation. Autistic children may carry a special toy or object that they play with during times of stress. Ask parents about these objects and their use.

Ask about the child's behaviors and observe them on admission. Obtain a history of acute and chronic illnesses and injuries. Ask about eating patterns and food restrictions. Inquire about CAM in a nonjudgmental and supportive manner.

Diagnosis

Nursing diagnoses must be tailored to fit the individual needs of the child. Nursing diagnoses that may be appropriate for inclusion in the plan of care for pediatric clients with ASD include the following:

- *Risk for Injury*
- *Impaired Verbal Communication*
- *Impaired Social Interaction related to developmental disability*
- *Risk for Caregiver Role Strain related to the chronic demands of child's condition*
- *Compromised Family Coping.*

(NANDA-I © 2012)

Planning

Nursing care focuses on preventing injury, stabilizing environmental stimuli, providing supportive care, enhancing communication, giving the parents anticipatory guidance, and providing emotional support. Appropriate outcomes for a child with ASD may include the following:

- The child will remain free of injury.
- The child will acquire communication strategies that enable communication with others.
- The child will be able to perform self-care to maximum potential.
- The child will demonstrate consistent developmental progress.
- The child will participate in small group activities with family members or peers.
- The child's symptoms will be managed successfully.

Implementation

Working with children with autism spectrum disorder and their families requires patience, sensitivity, and understanding. While some parents may be aggressive about seeking information and resources, others may be too overwhelmed and exhausted from caring for their child to do this. For these parents, the nurse may be the most important, most accessible, and most caring resource available to them. Nurses must take the time to provide client teaching and support and affirm parents' efforts to help their children.

Prevent Injury

Monitor autistic children at all times, including bath time and bedtime. Close supervision ensures that the child does not obtain any harmful objects or engage in dangerous behaviors. For the child who engages in head banging or other abusive behaviors, bicycle helmets and hand mitts can be the least restrictive method for providing safety. They enable the child to participate in activities and engage in a social environment to the degree possible.

Provide Anticipatory Guidance

Many children with autism spectrum disorders will require lifelong supervision and support, especially if the disorder is accompanied by mental retardation. Some children may grow up to lead independent lives, although they will have social limitations with impaired interpersonal relationships. Encourage parents to promote the child's development through behavior modification and specialized educational programs. The overall goal is to provide the child with the guidance, education, and support necessary for optimal functioning.

Stabilize Environmental Stimuli

Children with ASD interpret and respond to the environment differently than other individuals. Sounds that are not distressing to the average individual may be interpreted by autistic children as louder, more frightening, and overwhelming. They may respond to different sounds or environments by withdrawing, crying, or using ritualistic behaviors such as arm-flapping, which may or may not be self-injurious.

The child needs to be oriented to new settings such as a classroom or hospital room and may adjust best to a small classroom or a hospital room with only one other child. Encourage parents to bring the child's favorite objects from home. To avoid distressing the client, minimize relocation of objects within the environment.

Provide Supportive Care

Developing a trusting relationship with the autistic child is often difficult. Adjust communication techniques and teach to the child's developmental level. Ask parents about the child's usual home routines and maintain these routines as much as possible when the child is out of the home.

Because self-care abilities are often limited, the child may need assistance to meet basic needs. When possible, schedule daily care and routine procedures at consistent times to maintain predictability. Identify rituals for nap time and bedtime and maintain them to promote rest and sleep. Integrate patterns that facilitate intake of nutritious foods at mealtimes. School programs and individualized education plan (IEPs) can help the child learn self-care skills. Parents are integral parts of the treatment team when the child's learning goals are established in early intervention or school programs. If the child is hospitalized, encourage parents to remain with the child and to participate in daily care planning.

All clients with ASD need emotional support. Children who are developing successfully may face new challenges with the onset of the emotional and hormonal changes of adolescence. As social circles develop in middle and high school, the adolescent with autism may become more painfully aware of being different from other teenagers (Kenworthy et al., 2010.) The nurse may see this when a parent brings in a child after a scuffle at school or for help with increasing self-destructive behaviors as the child struggles to deal with the many changes. The nurse can provide crucial information about the physical changes adolescents experience and help the parent modify the plan of care to include opportunities for building new skills the child needs to navigate this difficult time.

Enhance Communication

Because children with autism have impaired communication skills, nursing care focuses on utilizing and improving communication with the child. Speech is used when possible; short, direct sentences are usually best (Maher, 2012). If the child responds well to visual cues, then pictures, computers, and other visual aids may form an important part of interaction. Some children are able to learn and communicate through sign language.

Children with autism spectrum disorders benefit greatly from speech and language therapy. Encourage parents of these children to maintain close contact with speech therapists. Use of consistent communication techniques at home and at school provides further stability for the child and increases opportunities for successful communication.

Facilitate Community-Based Care

Families of autistic children need a great deal of support to cope with the challenges of caring for the autistic child. They experience the challenges of families who have a child with a chronic disorder. Participating in parent support groups and learning how to reframe the condition to view its positive aspects are helpful strategies (Hall & Graff, 2011). Many communities offer training programs for parents, in addition to support groups. Help parents identify resources for child care, such as special toddler programs and preschools.

The child may need specialized transportation services or other social supports. The school-age child will need an individualized education plan (IEP). The parent or primary caretaker often has difficulty obtaining respite care and may need assistance to find suitable resources. Siblings of the autistic child may need help explaining the disorder to their friends or teachers. The nurse can be instrumental in assisting these siblings in understanding and explaining autism. Family support programs are available in some states to provide assistance to parents.

Genetic counseling should be offered to the family. Information on immunizations is necessary because parents may have heard about a potential connection between immunization and the disorder. They should be encouraged to have the child immunized on the recommended schedule. Parents may have questions about where to find information on complementary and alternative therapies.

Local support groups for parents of autistic children are available in most areas. Families can also be referred to the Autism Society of America for information.

Evaluation

At each healthcare interaction, the nurse discusses the child's progress with the parents, including any injuries that have occurred since the previous visit and the steps being taken to prevent recurrence. The nurse asks parents what type of environments the child is in during the day, paying particular attention to the frequency of transitions and changes in caregivers. For example, a child with ASD who attends school or an early intervention program at a preschool will do well having the same caregiver drop off the child in the morning and pick up the child at the end of the school day.

For children who are enrolled in early intervention programs or who have IEPs at school, the nurse should participate as part of the treatment team when possible. If this is not possible, the nurse should ask the parent how the child's treatment is progressing and continue to encourage open communication between the parents and the treatment team. For children who are taking medication to treat a comorbid disorder such as depression or ADHD, the nurse should, with parent permission, provide the necessary information to the treatment team so that the team is aware of potential side effects.

◢ REVIEW Autism Spectrum Disorder

RELATE Link the Concepts and Exemplars

Linking the exemplar of autism spectrum disorder with the concept of family:

1. How can the nurse support the family of a child with ASD?
2. How might other children in the family be impacted by a sibling with ASD?

Linking the exemplar of autism spectrum disorder with the concept of safety:

3. What interventions are important for the nurse to initiate to maintain the safety of a client with autism?
4. What would be important at school?

REFER Go to Pearson Nursing Student Resources
nursing.pearsonhighered.com

- Additional review materials

REFLECT Case Study

Chad, age 4, was recently diagnosed with autism spectrum disorder. Chad's mother keeps ruminating about her pregnancy, wondering what she did that "caused" Chad's illness. Chad recently became angry and reacted by banging his head against the wall. His parents told the nurse they do not believe that the doctor made the right diagnosis.

1. Based on the case study, what are the priorities of nursing care for Chad?
2. Based on the statement made by Chad's parents, what are his parents experiencing?
3. How might the nurse locate resources to help Chad's parents learn more about having a child with autism? What resources might the nurse find?

EXEMPLAR 25.3   **Cerebral Palsy**

EXEMPLAR KEY TERM
Cerebral palsy (CP), 1695

EXEMPLAR LEARNING OUTCOMES
After reading about this exemplar, you will be able to:

1. Describe the pathophysiology, etiology, clinical manifestations, and direct and indirect causes of cerebral palsy (CP).
2. Identify risk factors and prevention methods associated with CP.
3. Illustrate the nursing process in providing culturally competent care across the life span for individuals with CP.

4. Formulate priority nursing diagnoses appropriate for an individual with CP.
5. Summarize therapies used by interdisciplinary teams in the collaborative care of an individual with CP.
6. Plan evidence-based care for an individual with CP and his or her family in collaboration with other members of the healthcare team.
7. Evaluate expected outcomes for an individual with CP.

▶ OVERVIEW

Cerebral palsy (CP) is a group of chronic conditions affecting body movement, coordination, and posture that results from a nonprogressive abnormality of the immature brain. CP often is the result of some type of insult to the developing brain of the fetus, neonate, or infant that occurs in the later stages of pregnancy, during birth, or within the first 2 years after birth. The impact of the disease can range from mild to profound mobility issues; CP may or may not include mental retardation.

Cerebral palsy occurs in an estimated 1 per 308 births (Kirby et al., 2011). Four types of motor dysfunction are seen with CP—spastic, dyskinetic, ataxic, and mixed—and are related to the location of brain insult. Children with severe impairment of mobility, epilepsy, and intellectual disability are at greater risk of compromising lung infections and have a greater risk of dying during childhood (Fitzgerald, Follett, & Van Asperen, 2009).

▶ PATHOPHYSIOLOGY AND ETIOLOGY

The exact insult leading to CP may not be identifiable if it occurs during the prenatal period. After delivery, the cause of the insult is more likely to be identified. Insults may include any combination of hypoxic-ischemic encephalopathy, vascular, metabolic, infectious, toxic, teratogenic, traumatic, or genetic events. The insult alters muscle tone, muscle stretch reflexes, postural reactions, and primitive reflexes; it may also result in seizures, mental retardation, and/or hearing problems. The outcome depends on the area of the brain affected, the severity of the event, the duration of the insult, and the child's age at the time of the event.

The exact pathogenesis is multifactorial and not clearly understood. It is believed that damage is done to the motor areas of the brain, impairing the body's ability to control movement and adjust posture appropriately. CP is neither contagious nor inherited, and it is not progressive. It cannot be cured, but it can be managed.

CP often is identified when children fail to meet expected developmental milestones and diagnostic testing is ordered to pinpoint the reason for the delay. Symptoms and manifestations vary from person to person depending on the exact neurological impact of the event.

Etiology

Most CP cases are believed to be caused by congenital, hypoxic, ischemic, or infectious intrauterine insults to the central nervous system (CNS) (Pakula, Van Naarden Braun, & Yeargin-Allsopp, 2009). The risk for CP is increased when intrauterine infection (chorioamnionitis) is documented (Shatrov et al., 2010). Injury to the immature periventricular white matter in fetuses and premature infants is thought to be the most common cause of CP (Rutherford et al., 2010). At one time, hypoxia was considered the primary culprit for CP, but studies revealed that premature birth is responsible for most cases. Birth defects and adverse labor events also are significant contributors to CP (Sukhov et al., 2012).

The rate of CP increases with decreasing gestational age. Infants born before 27 weeks' gestational age are diagnosed with CP at a much higher rate than are those with a higher gestational age (McElrath et al., 2009). Birth asphyxia is believed to account for a significant number of CP cases, but still far fewer than previously believed. No reduction of incidence of CP has been noted since the use of electronic fetal heart rate monitoring was implemented (Grimes & Peipert, 2010). In young children, CNS infection and head trauma are the major sources of acquired brain injury and subsequent motor dysfunction.

Risk Factors

Increased risk for CP is found in mothers older than 40 or younger than 20 years of age, fathers who are 20 years of age or younger, and mothers or fathers with African American ethnicity. The risk is highest in first-born children and in children born subsequent to the fourth child. Prematurity, multiple births, low birth weight, blood type incompatibility, neonatal sepsis, and hyperbilirubinemia place the infant at higher risk for development of CP. Multiple risk factors at the same time can further increase the odds of developing CP.

Certain maternal medical problems, such as seizure disorders and thyroid conditions, may slightly increase a child's risk for CP. Children conceived by way of assisted reproductive technology (ART) and through infertility treatments are also at a greater risk for this disorder. Maternal viral infection during pregnancy (e.g., cytomegalovirus, rubella, and chicken pox) is also associated with an increased incidence of CP (CDC, 2011b).

Prevention

Because maternal infection is associated with the development of pediatric CP, infection prevention, including maintaining

TABLE 25–23 Clinical Characteristics of Cerebral Palsy

CLINICAL CHARACTERISTICS	DEFINITIONS
Hypotonia	Floppiness, increased range of motion of joints, diminished reflex response
Hypertonia	Tense, tight muscles
Rigidity Spasticity	Uncoordinated, awkward, stiff movements; scissoring or crossing of the legs; exaggerated reflex reactions
Athetosis	Constant involuntary writhing motions that are more severe distally
Ataxia	Poor muscle control during voluntary movement, poor balance
Hemiplegia	Involvement of one side of the body, with the upper extremities being more dysfunctional than the lower extremities
Diplegia	Involvement of all extremities, but the lower extremities are more affected than the upper, usually spastic
Quadriplegia	Involvement of all extremities with the arms in flexion and legs in extension

good hand hygiene, is a primary goal. Keeping current with vaccinations is also a means by which a pregnant client can reduce the risk for having a baby born with CP. Injury prevention, including properly securing infants during motor vehicle travel and taking measures to prevent falls, serves to protect the child from brain trauma. Additionally, women at risk for preterm labor should discuss methods of risk reduction with their healthcare provider. Some research suggests magnesium sulfate may reduce the risk of CP among surviving infants who are born preterm (CDC, 2011b).

▶ CLINICAL MANIFESTATIONS

Cerebral palsy is characterized by abnormal muscle tone and lack of coordination, with spasticity found in the majority of cases. Children have a variety of symptoms depending on their age. See **Table 25–23** ● for symptoms by type of central nervous system injury. Symptoms vary depending on the area of the brain involved and the degree of insult.

Children with CP usually are delayed in meeting developmental milestones. For example, at 6 months of age, they may have persistent back arching, show little spontaneous movement, and be unable to sit up. They frequently have other problems, including visual defects such as strabismus (abnormal alignment of the eyes or "crossed eyes"), nystagmus (involuntary rapid eye movement), or refractory errors; hearing loss; language delay; speech impediment; or seizures. Feeding may be difficult because of oral motor involvement. Approximately 40% of children with CP also have some form of intellectual disability (Kirby et al., 2011).

▶ COLLABORATION

Care of the client with CP requires a collaborative care team of nurses, physical therapists, occupational therapists, physicians, orthotics, speech therapists, dietitians, and social services. Cerebral palsy is a lifelong condition that requires special consideration, particularly in the growing child who quickly outgrows orthotic devices and must meet changing developmental needs.

Stay Current: For more information on CP, visit the National Institutes of Health at **www.nlm.nih.gov/medlineplus/cerebralpalsy.html**.

Diagnostic Tests

Diagnosis is usually based on clinical findings. CP is difficult to diagnose in the early months of life, because it must be distinguished from other neurological conditions and signs may be subtle. Suspicious findings include an infant who is small for his or her age or has a history of prematurity; low birth weight; low Apgar score (0–3 at 5 minutes); or the occurrence of an inflammatory, traumatic, or anoxic event (Ahlin et al., 2013). However, the majority of children who develop CP have normal Apgar scores at birth. Ultrasonography can be used to detect fetal and neonatal abnormalities of the brain, such as intraventricular hemorrhage. Neuromotor tests are used to evaluate the presence of normal movement patterns and absence of primitive reflexes and abnormal tone. Once CP is suspected, CT scans, MRI, and positron emission tomography may be performed.

Surgery

Surgical interventions may be required to improve function by balancing muscle power and stabilizing uncontrollable joints. The Achilles tendon may be lengthened to increase range of motion in the ankle, which allows the heel to touch the floor and thus improves ambulation. The hamstrings may be released to correct knee flexion contractures. Other procedures may be performed to improve hip adduction or correct the foot's natural position. A dorsal rhizotomy may be performed for spastic diplegia to cut the afferent fibers that contribute to spasticity; however, some muscle weakness may result from the procedure and there is evidence that it does not prevent contractures or improve functioning in the long term (Tedroff et al., 2011).

Pharmacologic Therapy

Medications are given to control seizures, to control spasms (skeletal muscle relaxants, baclofen, and benzodiazepines), and

Clinical Manifestations and Therapies **Cerebral Palsy**

ETIOLOGY	CLINICAL MANIFESTATIONS	CLINICAL THERAPIES
Spastic	■ Persistent hypertonia, rigidity	■ Physical therapy ■ Muscle relaxants ■ Braces, splints, and orthotics
Cerebral cortex or pyramidal tract injury	■ Exaggerated deep tendon reflexes	■ In addition to therapies used for spastic CP, surgery may be required to loosen contractures or to repair curvature of the spine.
Most common form of CP, comprising 80% of cases (CDC, 2012d)	■ Persistent primitive reflexes ■ Leads to contractures and abnormal curvature of the spine	
Dyskinetic	■ Impairment of voluntary muscle control accompanied by appearance of involuntary movements (e.g., tics, chorea)	
Extrapyramidal, basal ganglia injury	■ Bizarre twisting movements ■ Tremors, difficulty with fine and purposeful motor movements ■ Exaggerated posturing ■ Rigid muscle tone when awake and normal or decreased muscle tone when asleep ■ Inconsistent muscle tone that may change hour to hour or day to day	
Ataxic cerebellar (extrapyramidal) injury	■ Abnormalities of voluntary movement involving balance and position of the trunk and limbs ■ Difficulty controlling hand and arm movements when reaching ■ Increased or decreased muscle tone ■ Hypotonia in infancy ■ Muscle instability and wide-based, unsteady gait	■ Canes, crutches, walkers, and other orthotics may be needed to promote mobility.
Mixed injuries to multiple areas	■ No dominant motor pattern ■ Unique compensatory movements and posture to maintain control over specific neuromotor deficits ■ Combination of characteristics from other types	

to minimize gastrointestinal side effects (cimetidine or ranitidine). Baclofen is administered by intrathecal pump to decrease muscle tone and vasospasms when oral administration is ineffective or causes side effects (Tasseel-Ponche et al., 2011). See **Figure 25–13 ●**. Botulinum toxin injection into specific muscles is a relatively new therapy used to help control spasticity (Hoare et al., 2010).

Nonpharmacologic Therapy

Clinical therapy focuses on helping the child develop to a maximum level of independence. Referrals are made for physical, occupational, and speech therapy, as well as special education to improve motor function and ability. Braces and splints, serial casting, and positioning devices (prone wedges, standers, and side-lyers) are used to promote range of motion, skeletal alignment, stability, and control of involuntary move-

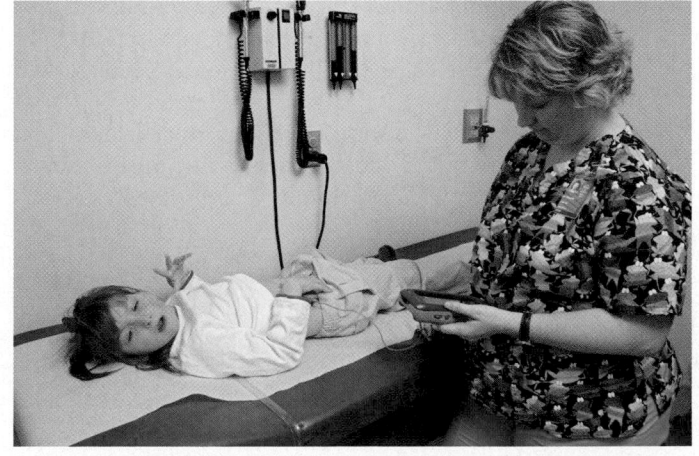

Figure 25–13 ● This child is having a baclofen pump filled.

ments. They are also used to prevent contractures. Physical therapy and occupational therapy promote optimal independent functioning.

EARLY INTERVENTION PROGRAMS   The prognosis for infants and children with CP depends on the level of physical involvement and on the presence of intellectual, visual, or hearing deficits. Early intervention programs can significantly improve performance. Many children with hemiplegia or ataxia show some improvement with maturation and are able to ambulate. Others need assistance with mobility and activities of daily living. They are usually cared for in their homes, although some receive care in long-term care facilities.

 NURSING PROCESS

Nursing care focuses on early intervention, prevention of complications, and support of children and families to help them cope with the diagnosis of CP.

Assessment

Be alert for children whose histories indicate an increased risk for CP. It is not uncommon for children who are delayed in meeting developmental milestones or have neuromuscular abnormalities at 1 year of age to show gradual improvement in function. Studies have shown that of the risk factors, assessment of general movements has a high predictive validity of CP among infants less than a year old (Bouwstra et al., 2010; Einspieler et al., 2012).

Assess all children at each healthcare visit for developmental delays. Note any orthopedic, visual, auditory, or intellectual deficits. Assess for newborn reflexes, which may persist beyond the normal age in a child with CP. Identify infants who appear to have abnormal muscle tone or abnormal posture (child has an arched back, child becomes stiff when moving against gravity, child's neck or extremities have increased or decreased resistance to passive movement). A child with asymmetric or abnormal crawling using two or three extremities indicates a motor problem. Hand dominance before the preschool years is another sign of a motor problem. Record dietary intake as well as height and weight percentiles for children suspected to have or to be diagnosed with the condition.

Evaluate all infants who show symptoms of developmental delays, feeding difficulties caused by poor sucking, or abnormalities of muscle tone. Two simple screening assessments are helpful:

- Place a clean diaper on the 6- to 12-month-old infant's face. The infant without special needs will use two hands to remove it, but the infant with CP will use one hand or will not remove the cloth at all.
- Turn the infant's head to one side. A persistent asymmetric tonic neck reflex (beyond 6 months of age) indicates a pathological condition. Suspect CP in any infant who has persistent primitive reflexes.

Diagnosis

Nursing diagnoses appropriate for inclusion in the care of the child with CP vary depending on the type of CP, the particular child's symptoms and age, and the family situation. Examples of nursing diagnoses relevant to caring for the client with CP may include the following:

- *Risk for Injury*
- *Impaired Mobility*
- *Risk for Constipation*
- *Impaired Tissue Integrity*
- *Impaired Verbal Communication*
- *Impaired Home Maintenance*
- *Chronic Pain*
- *Delayed Growth and Development*
- *Caregiver Role Strain.*

(NANDA-I © 2012)

Planning

Because the condition can range from mild to severe and may involve numerous manifestations, care planning must be highly individualized on the basis of the specific needs of each individual. It may include the following goals:

- The client will remain free from injury.
- The client will demonstrate appropriate growth and development.
- The client will maintain an appropriate diet to meet nutritional needs.
- The client and family will monitor bony prominences to avoid altered skin integrity.

Implementation

Interventions need to be adapted to the particular child and family. Nursing care focuses on providing adequate nutrition, maintaining skin integrity, promoting physical mobility, promoting safety, promoting growth and development, teaching parents how to care for the child, and providing emotional support. See the Community-Based Care feature for more information on supporting client's with CP.

Prevent Injury

Clients with CP have varying degrees of mobility. The nurse should ensure that the client receives the degree of assistance required for safe ambulation, and that orthotic and assistive devices are properly used. Maintaining a safe environment includes eliminating all potential obstacles from walkways and providing adequate lighting. Assess caregivers and family members for awareness of safety precautions and provide teaching as needed.

Safety belts should be used for children in strollers and wheelchairs. An adaptive car safety seat may be needed to transport the child safely. A child with chronic seizures should wear a helmet to protect against further injury.

Community-Based Care The Community's Role in Supporting Individuals With CP

Children with CP need continuous support in the community. A case manager, such as the parent or a nurse, is often needed to coordinate care. Parents may need financial assistance to provide for the child's needs and to obtain appliances such as braces, wheelchairs, or adaptive utensils. As they grow, children need new adaptive devices, ongoing developmental assessment and care planning, and sometimes surgery. Although the brain lesion does not change, it manifests differently as the child grows. For example, once the child begins to walk, the extensor tone may cause tightening of the Achilles cord. Braces may decrease deformities, but surgery may be needed eventually.

Early intervention programs can help parents meet their child's special needs, by providing physical, occupational, and speech therapy. Early education programs also help meet the child's educational needs. The child often needs an individualized education plan (IEP) or an individualized family service plan (for children younger than 3 years of age) to maximize learning potential. The nurse can be instrumental in helping parents meet the needs of the child with CP in preschools, schools, offices, clinics, and other settings. In addition, the nurse makes referrals, as appropriate, to support groups and organizations such as the United Cerebral Palsy Association and Shriners Hospitals.

An individualized transition plan developed during adolescence assists the family and adolescent with CP to develop plans for adult living. Vocational training options can be explored. The young adult (18–21 years) may be able to move into a group home or live independently if desired.

Provide Adequate Nutrition

Children with CP require high-calorie diets or supplements to the diet because of feeding difficulties associated with spasticity. Many children have difficulty chewing and swallowing. Give the child small amounts of soft foods at a time. Utensils with large, padded handles may be easier for the child to use.

Maintain Skin Integrity

Take special care to protect the bony prominences from skin breakdown. Monitor the skin under splints and braces for redness. If the skin is red, the braces or splints should be removed and not replaced until the redness is gone.

Proper body alignment should be maintained at all times. Support the child with pillows, towels, and bolsters whether the child is in bed or in a chair. Support the head and body of a floppy infant. A child with spasticity may have scissored, extended legs, and a child with athetoid movements may be difficult to carry and transport.

Promote Physical Mobility

Range-of-motion exercises are essential to maintain joint flexibility and to prevent contractures. Consult with the child's physical therapist and help with recommended exercises. Teach parents to position the child to foster flexion rather than extension so that the child can more easily interact with the environment (for example, by bringing objects closer to the face). Consider the use of therapeutic massage or relaxation training to manage pain associated with spasticity and stretching exercises (Glew et al., 2010).

Adaptive and assistive technology may be needed to promote mobility and communication. Assistive technology is any item, equipment, or product customized for use to promote the functional capabilities and independence of an individual with disabilities. Examples include computers, adaptive utensils, and customized wheelchairs. Refer parents to the appropriate resources for help obtaining adaptive devices. Encourage parents to bring in the child's adaptive appliances (braces, positioning devices) for use during hospitalization.

Promote Growth and Development

Remember that many children with CP have physical disabilities but not necessarily intellectual disabilities. Use terminology appropriate for the child's developmental level. Help the child develop a positive self-image to ensure emotional health and social growth. Adaptive devices may be available to help the child with CP to communicate more independently. Children with a hearing impairment may need a referral to learn American Sign Language or other communication methods. Provide audio and visual activities for the child who is quadriplegic.

Foster Parental Knowledge

Teach parents about the disorder and arrange sessions to teach them about all of the child's special needs. Teach administration, desired effects, and side effects of medications prescribed for seizures. Make sure parents are aware of the need for dental care for children taking anticonvulsants and other medications, because they can impact oral health.

Parents also may need suggestions for amending parenting strategies to promote the child's autonomy and abilities.

Provide Emotional Support

Parents require emotional support to help them cope with the diagnosis. Listen to the parents' concerns and encourage them to express their feelings and ask questions. Explain what they can expect from future treatment. Refer parents to individual and family counseling if appropriate. Work with other healthcare professionals to help families adjust to this chronic disease.

Evaluation

Clients are evaluated based on their ability to meet goals identified in the plan of care, which may include the following:

- Client's growth is appropriate for age.
- Client meets developmental milestones appropriate for age.
- Client's nutritional status is adequate for age and energy needs.

NURSING CARE PLAN A Client With Cerebral Palsy

ASSESSMENT

Justine McBride is a 2-year-old African American child. Her mother was 41 when she delivered Justine, and Justine's father was 45. Justine is the seventh child in the family. Her mother works as a chemistry teacher at the local high school, and her father is an accountant for a large firm. Justine's mother became concerned that Justine was not walking when she turned 14 months old; all of her other children were walking by 12 months of age. Diagnostic tests were performed, and Justine was diagnosed with spastic CP.

Examination of Justine demonstrates scissoring of the legs when prone, stiff movements of arms and legs, hyperreflexia, and muscular rigidity.

DIAGNOSES

- *Impaired Physical Mobility* related to decreased muscle strength and control
- *Imbalanced Nutrition: Less Than Body Requirements* related to difficulty in chewing and swallowing and high metabolic needs
- *Ineffective Therapeutic Regimen Management: Family* related to excessive demands made on family with child's complex care needs

(NANDA-I © 2012)

PLANNING

Goals for Justine's care include the following:
- Justine will reach maximum physical mobility and all developmental milestones.
- Justine will receive adequate visual sensory/perceptual input to maximize developmental outcome.
- Justine will exhibit normal growth patterns for height, weight, and other physical parameters.
- Justine's family will successfully support all of its members.
- Justine will participate in activities to maximize development.

IMPLEMENTATION

Recreation Therapy: *Purposeful use of recreation to promote relaxation and enhancement of social skills.*
- Refer the family to an early intervention program. Encourage contact with other children. If Justine is hospitalized, place her in a room with other children whenever possible.
- Investigate recreational programs for children with disabilities and share information with the parents.

Family Mobilization: *Utilization of family strengths to influence Justine's health in a positive direction.*
- Allow chances for parents to verbalize the impact of CP on the family. Refer to other parents and support groups.
- Explore community services for rehabilitation, respite care, child care, and other needs and refer family as appropriate.
- During home and office visits, review Justine's achievements and praise the family for care provided.
- Teach the family skills needed to manage Justine's care (e.g., medication administration, muscle stretching, physical rehabilitation, seizure management).
- Teach case management techniques.
- Assess needs of siblings; involve them in Justine's care as appropriate. Review with parents the needs of all children in the family.

Nutrition Management: *Assistance with or provision of a balanced dietary intake of foods and fluids.*
- Monitor height and weight and plot on a growth grid. Perform hydration status assessment.

- Teach the family techniques to promote caloric and nutrient intake.
- Position Justine upright for feedings.
- Place foods far back in the mouth to overcome tongue thrust.
- Use soft and blended foods.
- Allow extra time for chewing and swallowing.
- Obtain adaptive handles for utensils and encourage self-feeding skills.
- Apply manual jaw control technique if it helps the child to control jaw movement.
- Perform frequent respiratory assessment. Teach the family to avoid aspiration pneumonia.

Exercise Therapy, Joint Mobility: *Use of active and passive body movement to maintain or restore joint flexibility.*
- Perform development assessment and record age of achievement of milestones (e.g., reaching for objects, sitting).
- Plan activities to use gross and fine motor skills (e.g., holding a crayon or eating utensils, reaching for toys and rolling over).
- Allow time for the child to complete activities.
- Perform range-of-motion exercises every 4 hours for the child who is unable to move body parts. Position the child to promote tendon stretching (e.g., foot plantar flexion instead of dorsiflexion, legs extended instead of flexed at knees and hips).
- Arrange for and encourage parents to keep appointments with physical or rehabilitation therapist and other members of the collaborative team.

EVALUATION

The client's progress in meeting the goals of care is based on the following expected outcomes:
- Justine reaches maximum physical mobility and all developmental milestones.
- Justine shows normal growth patterns for height, weight, and other physical parameters.
- Justine demonstrates appropriate growth and developmental progress. The family successfully supports all of its members.
- Justine engages in activities to maximize development.

CRITICAL THINKING

1. What support groups or professional organizations exist in your area that could help Justine's family cope with this diagnosis?
2. Why is involvement of the older siblings important?
3. How would you assess Justine's cognitive ability? Is cognition always impacted by CP?

REVIEW Cerebral Palsy

REVIEW Link the Concepts and Exemplars

Linking the exemplar of cerebral palsy with the concept of comfort:

1. How might you help to promote comfort in a child with CP who is required to wear braces and orthotics to bed at night?

2. If spasticity of muscles causes pain, what nonpharmacologic strategies might you recommend?

Linking the exemplar of cerebral palsy to the concept of cognition:

3. While caring for a child diagnosed with CP who also has mild cognitive impairment, how would you help the child become increasingly autonomous in performing range-of-motion exercises?

4. How might you encourage this child's parents to promote autonomy?

READY Go to Companion Skills Manual

REFER Go to Pearson Nursing Student Resources
nursing.pearsonhighered.com

- Additional review materials

REFLECT Case Study

Frangelica Gonzalez, 12 years old, was born with CP. She began working with physical therapists when she was less than 1 year old and has worn braces on her legs and used crutches to allow her greater mobility for as long as she can remember. Her mother and father have always told her she can overcome any challenge and do anything other children do if she tries hard enough. As a result of her parent's encouragement and support, Frangelica is a member of the school swim team, plays jazz piano, and has a large circle of friends. She has a younger brother who is 9 years old, an older brother who is 15 years old, and an identical twin sister who is healthy and does not have CP.

Lately her parents have noticed that Frangelica is moody, often seeming depressed, and her twin sister told their mother that Frangelica is "tired of being different." Frangelica has been waking in the morning offering various physical complaints as reasons why she can't go to school that day, ranging from a stomachache to a sore foot.

1. Why might Frangelica suddenly be feeling different and trying to find reasons not to go to school?

2. What strategies might you recommend to Frangelica's parents to help her cope with the developmental changes she is experiencing?

3. What strategies might you recommend to Frangelica to explore and cope with her feelings?

EXEMPLAR 25.4 Failure to Thrive

EXEMPLAR KEY TERMS
Failure to thrive (FTT), *1701*
Geriatric failure to thrive (GFTT), *1701*

EXEMPLAR LEARNING OUTCOMES
After reading about this exemplar, you will be able to:

1. Describe the pathophysiology, etiology, clinical manifestations, and direct and indirect causes of failure to thrive (FTT).

2. Identify risk factors and prevention methods associated with FTT.

3. Illustrate the nursing process in providing culturally competent care across the life span for individuals with FTT.

4. Formulate priority nursing diagnoses appropriate for an individual with FTT.

5. Summarize therapies used by interdisciplinary teams in the collaborative care of an individual with FTT.

6. Plan evidence-based care for an individual with FTT and his or her family in collaboration with other members of the healthcare team.

7. Evaluate expected outcomes for an individual with FTT.

▶ OVERVIEW

Failure to thrive (FTT) most commonly describes a syndrome in which an infant falls below the fifth percentile for weight and height on a standard growth chart or is falling in percentiles on a growth chart. This disorder accounts for 1%–5% of pediatric hospitalizations in children under 1 year of age, and many more children are managed in community settings. From 5% to 10% of low-birth-weight infants are affected (Cole & Lanham, 2011).

Geriatric failure to thrive (GFTT) is a similar disorder seen in older adults.

✳ Visit **nursing.pearsonhigher.com** *for a minimodule on geriatric failure to thrive (GFTT).*

▶ PATHOPHYSIOLOGY AND ETIOLOGY

FTT may stem from inadequate caloric intake, inadequate caloric absorption, or excessive caloric expenditure. In all cases, undernutrition results. Biological and psychosocial factors may also influence the development of FTT.

Etiology

The cause of FTT can be organic, as in congenital AIDS, inborn errors of metabolism, neurological disease, and esophageal reflux. However, most cases of FTT are nonorganic in origin. FTT resulting from nonorganic causes is called *feeding disorder of infancy or early childhood.*

Risk Factors

Infants who are deprived of mothering, especially those 3–15 months of age, will not learn to form significant relationships or to trust others. Touch, cuddling, and visual and auditory stimulation are all critical for the infant. Through these mechanisms, the baby comes to know self and the environment. Infants who fail to establish a loving, responsive relationship with a caregiver often fail to develop normally.

Infants and children whose parents or caretakers suffer from depression, substance abuse, mental retardation, or psychosis, or who have a history of abuse are at risk for FTT. Their parents may be socially and emotionally isolated or may lack knowledge of infant nutritional and nurturing needs. A multifactorial and reciprocal interaction pattern may exist whereby the parent does not offer enough food or is not responsive to the infant's hunger cues and, as a result, the infant is irritable, not soothed, and does not give clear cues about hunger.

Prevention

Research suggests that educating caregivers regarding an infant's dietary and nutritional needs may help guard against development of FTT in children. Likewise, home nursing visits significantly impacted caregivers' delivery of adequate nutrition to children within the home (Cole & Lanham, 2011).

▶ CLINICAL MANIFESTATIONS

The characteristics of this feeding disorder are persistent failure to eat adequately with no weight gain or with weight loss in a child under 6 years of age. While FTT may be caused by a physical disorder, in 80% of cases, no definitive underlying physical disorder is identified (Cole & Lanham, 2011). Infants with feeding disorders refuse food, may have erratic sleep patterns, are irritable and difficult to soothe, fall well under expected growth patterns, and are often developmentally delayed (**Figure 25–14 ●**).

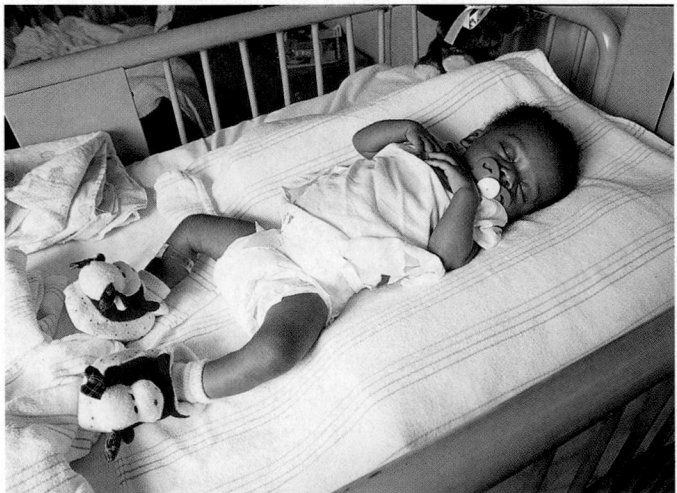

Figure 25–14 ● Infants with failure to thrive may not look severely malnourished, but they fall well below the expected weight and height norms for their age and population. This infant, who appears to be about 4 months old, is actually 8 months old. He has been hospitalized for examination of his failure to thrive and treatment of an eating disorder.

Infants with inorganic FTT show delayed development without any physical cause. They are often malnourished and fail to gain weight and grow normally. Behavior may be apathetic, withdrawn, demonstrate poor eye contact, and the child may lack anticipated stranger danger.

▶ COLLABORATION

A thorough history and physical examination are needed to rule out any chronic physical illness. The infant or child may be hospitalized so that healthcare providers can establish a routine for feeding and sleeping. The goals of treatment are to provide adequate caloric and nutritional intake, promote normal growth and development, and assist parents in developing feeding routines and responding to the infant's cues of physical and psychological hunger.

Stay Current: *For a description of a collaborative healthcare team addressing FTT, visit the Web site of the Kennedy Krieger Institute's Feeding Disorder Clinic at* **www.kennedykrieger.org/patient-care/patient-care-programs/outpatient-programs/feeding-disorders-clinic**.

Diagnostic Tests

Diagnosis of FTT occurs primarily through assessment. Because of the relative ineffectiveness of laboratory diagnostics to identify this condition, routine laboratory testing is not recommended (Cole & Lanham, 2011).

Surgery

Surgical management of the client with FTT will vary based on the physiological impairment. For example, possible surgical interventions may include cleft palate repair or alleviation of a bowel obstruction.

Pharmacologic Therapy

No medications are indicated for primary treatment of FTT. Rather, the approach to treatment includes identifying the cause, resolving any barriers to obtaining and absorbing adequate caloric intake, and providing nutritional supplementation to treat deficiencies.

Nonpharmacologic Therapy

Developmentally appropriate education for caregivers regarding nutrition and home care visits are believed to reduce to incidence of FTT among children. For clients who choose to breastfeed, the nurse should assess the client's knowledge and efficacy, and provide or facilitate the provision of additional teaching as needed.

■ NURSING PROCESS

Nursing care is directed toward improving the child's nutritional intake with the end result of increasing the growth and health of the child. This may be accomplished through parent teaching; observation of child–parent interactions, especially during feeding times; and careful recording of height and weight on growth charts.

Focus on Diversity and Culture
Growth Measurement

Each child should maintain a height and weight growth pattern similar to the population standard. It may be normal for children of Asian descent to be below the fifth percentile on growth charts and not have an eating disorder. American children tend to be larger, and growth charts are based on American averages. Suspect an eating disorder when the infant or child falls one standard deviation below the curve and fails to gain weight or loses weight over several months.

Assessment

Assessment of the child is essential for establishing the best intervention plan. Take accurate measurement of weight, height, BMI, and percentiles each time a child interacts with a healthcare provider to develop an important record of growth patterns over time. See the Focus on Diversity and Culture feature for more information on measuring growth. This helps to identify the child with an eating disorder. The child's activity level, developmental milestones, and interaction patterns also provide important information. When feeding the child, observe how the child indicates hunger or satiety, the ability of the child to be soothed, and general interaction patterns such as eye contact, touch, and cuddliness.

Ask parents about stressors in their lives that may prevent or interfere with appropriate interaction with the child. Questions about the pregnancy and delivery can elicit information about early disturbances in the child–parent relationship. Ask whether there are other children in the family and whether they have experienced feeding problems. It is important for the nurse to observe the child's and parents' behaviors when the parents feed the child; cues given by each individual and interactional modes such as rocking, singing, talking, and body postures are important.

Diagnosis

Nursing diagnoses pertinent for the young child with failure to thrive may include the following:

- *Imbalanced Nutrition*
- *Delayed Growth and Development*
- *Risk for Impaired Parenting*
- *Fatigue.*

(NANDA-I © 2012)

Planning

The goals of nursing care for the child with failure to thrive may include the following:

- Child will attain adequate growth and normal development.
- The parent–child relationship will improve.
- Parental understanding of the child's nutritional requirements will improve.
- Complications associated with poor nutrition will be prevented.

Implementation

Nursing care centers on performing a thorough history and physical assessment, observing parent–child interactions during feeding times, and providing necessary teaching to enable parents to respond appropriately to their child's needs. The child may be hospitalized initially so that staff members can establish feeding and sleeping patterns and evaluate the child's physical growth. Accurate weights, nutritional assessments, and developmental evaluation should be done to see if the child begins to grow more normally. Additional diagnostic tests may be given to rule out organic causes of the poor growth.

Once a diagnosis of nonorganic FTT is confirmed, parents become involved in feeding the child. Observations of feeding and continued careful physical assessments are needed. Teach parents to record carefully the child's intake at each meal or feeding. Teach parents how to understand and respond to the child's cues of hunger and satiety. Teach them to hold, rock, and touch the infant during feeding and to establish eye contact with infants and older children.

Upon discharge, refer parents to an early childhood intervention agency that can continue monitoring the home situation. Agency staff can observe feeding during a home visit and evaluate stresses and behavior patterns among family members. Frequent growth measurement and development must be ensured so that the child is adequately nourished. Parents may need referral to community resources to help them manage stressful situations and to enhance their parenting skills.

Evaluation

The child's outcomes are largely evaluated based on the following:

- Growth and development of the child improve.
- The parent–child relationship improves.
- The parent voices a specific action plan to improve and maintain appropriate growth of child.
- The child experiences no long-term complications as a result of FTT.

REVIEW Failure to Thrive

RELATE Link the Concepts and Exemplars

Linking the exemplar of failure to thrive with the concept of acid–base balance:

1. How might excessive protein metabolism as the result of inadequate sources of energy supply from dietary intake impact the client's acid–base balance?

2. How might altered glucose metabolism as a result of inadequate caloric intake impact the client's acid–base balance?

Linking the exemplar of failure to thrive with the concept of elimination:

3. How might inadequate caloric and nutrient intake impact elimination?

4. If caloric and nutrient intake is increased suddenly, how might the client's elimination habits be impacted?

READY Go to Companion Skills Manual

REFER Go to Pearson Nursing Student Resources
nursing.pearsonhighered.com

- Additional review materials
- **Minimodule:** Geriatric Failure to Thrive

REFLECT Case Study

Hilary is born 8 weeks prematurely at 32 weeks' gestation to a single adolescent mother. Hilary remains in the neonatal intensive care unit for 10 weeks until she is stable enough to be discharged. Her mother tries to visit at least once a week and is sometimes able to visit more often depending on whether someone can give her a ride to and from the hospital.

Hilary returns in 6 weeks following discharge and is found to have gained only 2 ounces, increasing her weight from 2.32 kg (5 lb 2 oz) to 2.38 kg (5 lb 4 oz). The provider schedules a follow-up visit for 2 weeks later, and the nurse explains Hilary's nutritional requirements. When Hilary returns, she has lost 1 ounce in weight.

1. Does Hilary qualify as having FTT? Explain your answer.
2. Do you suspect an organic or inorganic cause of her failure to gain weight?
3. Develop a nursing plan of care for Hilary.

■ REFERENCES

Ahlin, K., Himmelmann, K., Hagberg, G., Kacerovsky, M., Cobo, T., Wennerholm, U. B., & Jacobsson, B. (2013). Non-infectious risk factors for different types of cerebral palsy in term-born babies: A population-based, case–control study. *International Journal of Obstetrics & Gynaecology, 120*(6), 724–731.

American Psychiatric Association (APA). (n.d.a). *Children: Children's mental health—Attention-deficit/hyperactivity disorder (ADHD).* Retrieved from http://www.psychiatry.org/mental-health/people/children.

American Psychiatric Association (APA). (n.d.b). *DSM-5 video series: Changes to autism spectrum disorder.* Retrieved from http://www.psychiatry.org/practice/dsm/dsm5/dsm-5-video-series-changes-to-autism-spectrum-disorder.

American Psychiatric Association (APA). (2013). *Diagnostic and statistical manual of mental disorders* (5th ed.). Arlington, VA: Author.

Bandura, A. (1986). *Social foundations of thought and actions: A social cognitive theory.* Englewood Cliffs, NJ: Prentice Hall.

Bandura, A. (1997a). *Self-efficacy: The exercise of control.* New York, NY: W. H. Freeman.

Bandura, A. (1997b). *Self-efficacy in changing societies.* New York, NY: Cambridge University Press.

Bolten, M. I., Wurmser, H., Buske-Kirschbaum, A., Papoušek, M., Pirke, K. M., & Hellhammer, D. (2011). Cortisol levels in pregnancy as a psychobiological predictor for birth weight. *Archives of Women's Mental Health, 14*(1), 33–41.

Bouwstra, H., Dijk-Stigter, G. R., Grooten, H. M., Janssen-Plas, F. E., Koopmans, A. J., Mulder, C. D., et al. (2010). Predictive value of definitely abnormal general movements in the general population. *Developmental Medicine & Child Neurology, 52*(5), 456–461.

Boyd, B. A., Odom, S. L., Humphreys, B. P., & Sam, A. M. (2010). Infants and toddlers with autism spectrum disorder: Early identification and early intervention. *Journal of Early Intervention, 32*(2), 75–98.

Bronfenbrenner, U. (1986). Ecology of the family as a context for human development: Research perspectives. *Developmental Psychology, 22,* 723–742.

Bronfenbrenner, U. (Ed.). (2005). *Making human beings human: Bioecological perspectives on human development.* Thousand Oaks, CA: Sage.

Bronfenbrenner, U., McClelland, P. D., Ceci, S. J., Moen, P., & Wethington, E. (1996). *The state of Americans.* New York, NY: Free Press.

Brown, S., & Lin, I. (2012). The gray divorce revolution: Rising divorce among middle-aged and older adults, 1990–2010. *Journal of Gerontology, 67*(6), 731–741.

Call-Schmidt, T., & Maharaj, G. (2004). Using nonpharmacological treatments in conjunction with stimulant medications for children with ADHD. *Journal of Pediatric Health Care, 18,* 255–259.

Campbell, T. (2010). Ethics of care. In R. H. Corrigan & M. E. Farrell (Eds.), *Ethics: A university guide* (pp. 79–107). Gloucester, UK: Progressive Frontiers Press.

Centers for Disease Control and Prevention (CDC). (2010). *Autism spectrum disorders—Signs and symptoms.* Retrieved from http://www.cdc.gov/ncbddd/autism/signs.html.

Centers for Disease Control and Prevention (CDC). (2011a). *Attention-deficit/hyperactivity disorder—Data and statistics.* Retrieved from http://www.cdc.gov/ncbddd/adhd/data.html.

Centers for disease Control and Prevention (CDC). (2011b). *Cerebral palsy (CP)—Causes and risk factors of cerebral palsy.* Retrieved from http://www.cdc.gov/ncbddd/cp/causes.html.

Centers for Disease Control and Prevention (CDC). (2012a). *Autism spectrum disorders (ASDs)—Data & statistics.* Retrieved from http://www.cdc.gov/ncbddd/autism/data.html.

Centers for Disease Control and Prevention (CDC). (2012b). *Autism spectrum disorders (ASDs)—Treatment.* Retrieved from http://www.cdc.gov/ncbddd/autism/treatment.html#types.

Centers for Disease Control and Prevention (CDC). (2012c). *Cerebral palsy (CP)—Data & statistics for cerebral palsy.* Retrieved from http://www.cdc.gov/ncbddd/cp/data.html.

Centers for Disease Control and Prevention (CDC). (2012d). *Cerebral palsy (CP)—Facts about cerebral palsy.* Retrieved from http://www.cdc.gov/ncbddd/cp/facts.html.

Centers for Disease Control and Prevention (CDC). (2012e). *Developmental disabilities.* Retrieved from http://www.cdc.gov/ncbddd/developmentaldisabilities/index.html.

Centers for Disease Control and Prevention (CDC). (2012f). *Developmental disabilities—Facts about developmental disabilities.* Retrieved from http://www.cdc.gov/ncbddd/developmentaldisabilities/facts.html.

Centers for Disease Control and Prevention (CDC). (2012g). *Fragile x syndrome (FXS)—Facts about fragile x syndrome.* Retrieved from http://www.cdc.gov/ncbddd/fxs/facts.html.

Centers for Disease Control and Prevention (CDC). (2012h). Youth risk behavior surveillance—United States, 2011. *Morbidity and Mortality Weekly Report, 61,* SS-4.

Chess, S., & Thomas, A. (1995). *Temperament in clinical practice.* New York, NY: Guilford Press.

Chess, S., & Thomas, A. (1996). *Temperament: Theory and practice.* Philadelphia, PA: Brunner/Mazel Publishers.

CIA World Factbook. (2013). *United States: People and society.* Retrieved from https://www.cia.gov/library/publications/the-world-factbook/geos/us.html.

Cole, S. Z., & Lanham, J. S. (2011). Failure to thrive: An update. *American Family Physician, 83*(7), 829–834.

Duchan, E., & Patel, D. (2012). Epidemiology of autism spectrum disorders. *Pediatric Clinics of North America, 59*(1), 27–43.

Einspieler, C., Marschik, P. B., Bos, A. F., Ferrari, F., Cioni, G., & Prechtl, H. F. (2012). Early markers for cerebral palsy: Insights from the assessment of general movements. *Future Neurology, 7*(6), 709–717.

Erikson, E. (1963). *Childhood and society.* New York, NY: W. W. Norton.

Erikson, E. (1968). *Identity: Youth and crisis.* New York, NY: W. W. Norton.

Fitzgerald, D. A., Follett, J., & Van Asperen, P. P. (2009). Assessing and managing lung disease and sleep disordered breathing in children with cerebral palsy. *Paediatric Respiratory Reviews, 10*(1), 18–24.

Folkman, S. (Ed.). (2010). *The Oxford handbook of stress, health, and coping.* New York, NY: Oxford University Press.

Fowler, J., & Keen, S. (1985). *Life maps: Conversations in the journey of faith.* Waco, TX: Word Books.

Fowler, J. W., Streib, H., & Keller, B. (2004). *Manual for faith development research* (3rd ed.). Bielefeld, Germany: Research Center for Biographical Studies in Contemporary Religion; Atlanta, GA: Center for Research in Faith and Moral Development, Emory University.

Freitag, C. M., Luders, E., Hulst, H. E., Narr, K. L., Thompson, P. M., Toga, A. W., et al. (2009). Total brain volume and corpus callosum size in medication-naive adolescents and young adults with autism spectrum disorder. *Biological Psychiatry, 66*(4), 316.

Gibbins, C., Toplak, M. E., Flora, D. B., Weiss, M. D., & Tannock, R. (2011). Evidence for a general factor model of ADHD in adults. *Journal of Attention Disorders, 16*(8), 635–644.

Gilligan, C. (1982). *In a different voice: Psychological theory and women's development.* Cambridge, MA: Harvard University Press.

Glew, G. M., Fan, M. Y., Hagland, S., Bjornson, K., Beider, S., & McLaughlin, J. F. (2010). Survey of the use of massage for children with cerebral palsy. *International Journal of Therapeutic Massage & Bodywork, 3*(4), 10.

Gould, R. L. (1972). The phases of adult life: A study in developmental psychology. *American Journal of Psychiatry, 129,* 33–43.

Gregory, A., Penrose, K., Morrison, C., Dennis, C. L., & MacArthur, C. (2008). Psychometric properties of the Breastfeeding Self-Efficacy Scale-Short Form in an ethnically diverse UK sample. *Public Health Nursing, 25*(3), 278–284.

Grimes, D. A., & Peipert, J. F. (2010). Electronic fetal monitoring as a public health screening program: The arithmetic of failure. *Obstetrics & Gynecology, 116*(6), 1397.

Gross, D., Garvey, C., Julion, W., Fogg, L., Tucker, S., & Mokros, H. (2009). Efficacy of the Chicago Parent Program with low-income African American and Latino parents of young children. *Prevention Science, 10*(1), 54–65.

Gupta, R., & Kar, B. R. (2010). Specific cognitive deficits in ADHD: A diagnostic concern in differential diagnosis. *Journal of Child and Family Studies, 19*(6), 778–786.

Hall, H. R., & Graff, J. C. (2011). The relationships among adaptive behaviors of children with autism, family support, parenting stress, and coping. *Issues in Comprehensive Pediatric Nursing, 34*(1), 4–25.

Havighurst, R. J. (1972). *Developmental tasks and education* (3rd ed.). Boston, MA: Allyn & Bacon.

Havighurst, R., Neugarten, B., & Tobin, S. (1963). Disengagement, personality, and life satisfaction. In P. Hansen (Ed.), *Age with a future* (pp. 319–324.) Copenhagen, Holland: Munksgaard.

Hoare, B. J., Wallen, M. A., Imms, C., Villanueva, E., Rawicki, H. B., & Carey, L. (2010). Botulinum toxin A as an adjunct to treatment in the management of the upper limb in children with spastic cerebral palsy (UPDATE). *Cochrane Database of Systematic Reviews*, Issue 1. Art. No.: CD003469. doi:10.1002/14651858. CD003469.pub4.

Hong, J. S., Espelage, D. L., Grogan-Kaylor, A., & Allen-Meares, P. (2012). Identifying potential mediators and moderators of the association between child maltreatment and bullying perpetration and victimization in school. *Educational Psychology Review, 24*(2), 167–186.

Jung, C. (1960). *Psychology and religion.* New York, New York, NY: Pantheon Books.

Kent, K. M., Pelham, W. E., Molina, B. S., Sibley, M. H., Waschbusch, D. A., Yu, J., et al. (2011). The academic experience of male high school students with ADHD. *Journal of Abnormal Child Psychology, 39*(3), 451–462.

Kenworthy, L., Case, L., Harms, M. B., Martin, A., & Wallace, G. L. (2010). Adaptive behavior ratings correlate with symptomatology and IQ among individuals with high-functioning autism spectrum disorders. *Journal of Autism and Developmental Disorders, 40*(4), 416–423.

Kim, S. H., & Lord, C. (2012). New autism diagnostic interview-revised algorithms for toddlers and young preschoolers from 12 to 47 months of age. *Journal of Autism and Developmental Disorders, 42*(1), 82–93.

Kirby, R. S., Wingate, M. S., Van Naarden Braun, K., Doernberg, N. S., Arneson, C. L., Benedict, R. E., et al. (2011). Prevalence and functioning of children with cerebral palsy in four areas of the United States in 2006: A report from the Autism and Developmental Disabilities Monitoring Network. *Research in Developmental Disabilities, 32*(2), 462–469.

Kleinman, R. E. (Ed.). (2009). *Pediatric nutrition handbook* (6th ed.). Elk Grove Village, IL: American Academy of Pediatrics.

Kohlberg, L. (1981). *Essays on moral development: Vol. 1. The philosophy of moral development.* San Francisco, CA: Harper & Row.

Kohlberg, L. (1984). *Essays on moral development: Vol. 2. The psychology of moral development.* San Francisco, CA: Harper & Row.

Kulkarni, S., Johnson, P., Kettles, S., & Kasthuri, R. (2012). Music during interventional radiological procedures, effects on sedation, pain and anxiety: A randomised controlled trial. *British Institute of Radiology, 85*(1016), 1059–1063.

Liberatore, D., & McBarron, J. (2010). *US FDA approves first skin patch for ADHD.* Retrieved from http://www. dukeandthedoctor.com/2010/01/us-fda-approves-first-skin-patch-for-adhd.

Maher, E. M. (2012). Promoting social responsiveness within a developmental relationship-based approach with primary caregivers and young children with autism. *Neuropsychiatrie de l'Enfance et de l'Adolescence, 60*(5), S133–S134.

Masten, A. S., Cutuli, J. J., Herbers, J. E., & Reed, M. G. (2009). Resilience in development. In *Oxford handbook of positive psychology* (pp. 117–132). New York, NY: Oxford University Press.

McElrath, T. F., Allred, E. N., Boggess, K. A., Kuban, K., O'Shea, T. M., & Paneth, N. (2009). Maternal antenatal complications and the risk of neonatal cerebral white matter damage and later cerebral palsy in children born at an extremely low gestational age. *American Journal of Epidemiology, 170*(7), 819–828.

Merrill, D., & Small, G. (2011). Prevention in psychiatry: Effects of healthy lifestyle on cognition. *Psychiatric Clinics of North America, 34*(1), 249–261.

Merrill, R. M., Lyon, J. L., Baker, R. K., & Gren, L. H. (2009). Attention deficit hyperactivity disorder and increased risk of injury. *Advances in Medical Sciences, 54*(1), 20–26.

Minnes, S., Lang, A., & Singer, L. (2011). Prenatal tobacco, marijuana, stimulant, and opiate exposure: Outcomes and practice implications. *Addiction Science & Clinical Practice, 6*(1), 57.

Moran, M. (2011). Data sound alarm on gay teens' heightened suicide risk. *Psychiatric News, 46*(9), 9–28.

Murray, R. B., & Zentner, J. P. (2001). *Health promotion strategies through the life span* (7th ed.). Upper Saddle River, NJ: Prentice Hall.

National Alliance on Mental Illness (NAMI). (n.d.). ADHD and school: Helping your child succeed in the classroom. Retrieved from http://www.nami.org/Template. cfm?Section=ADHD&Template=/ContentManagement/ContentDisplay.cfm&ContentID=106379.

National Alliance on Mental Illness (NAMI). (2010). *Mental illnesses—Attention-deficit/hyperactivity disorder.* Retrieved from http://www.nami.org/Template. cfm?Section=By_Illness&Template=/TaggedPage/ TaggedPageDisplay.cfm&TPLID=54&ContentID=23047.

National Institute of Mental Health. (2009). *Adults with autism spectrum disorder.* Retrieved from http://www. nimh.nih.gov/health/publications/autism/adults-with-an-autism-spectrum-disorder.shtml.

National Resource Center on AD/HD. (2008). *Diagnosis & treatment: Complementary and alternative treatments.* Retrieved from http://www.help4adhd.org/en/treatment/complementary/WWK6.

Neider, G., Borges, N., & Pearson, J. (2011). Medical student use of online lectures: Exam performance, learning styles, achievement motivation and gender. *Medical Science Educator, 21*(3), 222–228.

Pakula, A. T., Van Naarden Braun, K., & Yeargin-Allsopp, M. (2009). Cerebral palsy: classification and epidemiology. *Physical Medicine and Rehabilitation Clinics of North America, 20*(3), 425.

Palmer, R. F., Walker, T., Mandell, D., Bayles, B., & Miller, C. S. (2010). Explaining low rates of autism among Hispanic schoolchildren in Texas. *American Journal of Public Health.* Retrieved from http://www.ncbi.nlm.nih.gov/ pmc/articles/PMC2804636.

Papalia, D. E., Olds, S. W., & Feldman, R. D. (2009). *Human development* (11th ed.). Boston, MA: McGraw-Hill.

Peck, R. (1968). Psychological developments in the second half of life. In B. L. Neugarten (Ed.), *Middle age and aging.* Chicago, IL: University of Chicago Press.

Peters-Scheffer, N., Didden, R., Korzilius, H., & Sturmey, P. (2011). A meta-analytic study on the effectiveness of comprehensive ABA-based early intervention programs for children with autism spectrum disorders. *Research in Autism Spectrum Disorders, 5*(1), 60–69.

Piaget, J. (1966). *Origins of intelligence in children.* New York, NY: W. W. Norton.

Pickles, A., Simonoff, E., Conti-Ramsden, G., Falcaro, M., Simkin, Z., Charman, T., et al. (2009). Loss of language in early development of autism and specific language impairment. *Journal of Child Psychology and Psychiatry, 50*(7), 843–852.

Potter, D. (2010). Psychological well-being and relationship between divorce and children's academic achievement. *Journal of Marriage and Family, 72*(4), 933–946.

Rew, L., Whittaker, T. A., Taylor-Seehafer, M. A., & Smith, L. R. (2005). Sexual health risks and protective resources in gay, lesbian, bisexual, and heterosexual homeless youth. *Journal for Specialists in Pediatric Nursing, 10*(1), 11–19.

Roeyers, H., Desoete, A., & Dereu, M. (2011). Early signs of autism spectrum disorders in infants and toddlers (dissertation). Faculty of Psychology and Educational Sciences, Ghent University, Belgium.

Rudd, R. (2010). Improving Americans' health literacy. *New England Journal of Medicine, 363*(24), 2283–2285.

Rutherford, M. A., Supramaniam, V., Ederies, A., Chew, A., Bassi, L., Groppo, M., et al. (2010). Magnetic resonance imaging of white matter diseases of prematurity. *Neuroradiology, 52*(6), 505–521.

RX List. (2012). *Strattera.* Retrieved from http://www.rxlist. com/strattera-drug.htm.

Saha, S., Beach, M. C., & Cooper, L. A. (2008). Patient centeredness, cultural competence and healthcare quality. *Journal of the National Medical Association, 100*(11), 1275.

Shatrov, J. G., Birch, S. C., Lam, L. T., Quinlivan, J. A., McIntyre, S., & Mendz, G. L. (2010). Chorioamnionitis and cerebral palsy: A meta-analysis. *Obstetrics & Gynecology, 116*(2, Part 1), 387–392.

Stein, M. A., & Barren, M. (2003). Welcome progress in the diagnosis and treatment of ADHD in adolescence. *Contemporary Pediatrics, 20*(8), 83–107.

Sukhov, A., Wu, Y., Xing, G., Smith, L. H., & Gilbert, W. M. (2012). Risk factors associated with cerebral palsy in preterm infants. *Journal of Maternal–Fetal and Neonatal Medicine, 25*(1), 53–57.

Swing, E. L., Gentile, D. A., Anderson, C. A., & Walsh, D. A. (2010). Television and video game exposure and the development of attention problems. *Pediatrics, 126*(2), 214–221.

Takeda, T., Stotesbery, K., Power, T., Ambrosini, P., Berrettini, W., Hakonarson, H., et al. (2010). Parental ADHD status and its association with proband ADHD subtype and severity. *Journal of Pediatrics, 157*(6), 995–1000.

Tasseel-Ponche, S., Ferrapie, A. L., Chenet, A., Menei, P., Gambart, G., Ménégalli Bogeli, D., et al. (2011). Intrathecal baclofen in cerebral palsy. A retrospective study of 25 wheelchair-assisted adults. *Annals of Physical and Rehabilitation Medicine, 54*(1), 16.

Tedroff, K., Löwing, K., Jacobson, D. N., & Åström, E. (2011). Does loss of spasticity matter? A 10-year follow-up after selective dorsal rhizotomy in cerebral palsy. *Developmental Medicine & Child Neurology, 53*(8), 724–729.

U.S. National Library of Medicine. (2012a). *Adolescent test or procedure preparation.* Retrieved from http://www. nlm.nih.gov/medlineplus/ency/article/002054.htm.

U.S. National Library of Medicine. (2012b). Attention deficit hyperactivity disorder . Retrieved from http://www. ncbi.nlm.nih.gov/pubmedhealth/PMH0002518.

U.S. National Library of Medicine. (2012c). *Autism.* Retrieved from http://www.ncbi.nlm.nih.gov/pubmedhealth/PMH0002494.

U.S. National Library of Medicine. (2012d). *Preschooler test or procedure preparation.* Retrieved from http://www. nlm.nih.gov/medlineplus/ency/article/002057.htm.

U.S. National Library of Medicine. (2012e). *School age test or procedure preparation.* Retrieved from http://www. nlm.nih.gov/medlineplus/ency/article/002058.htm.

Vincent, G. K., & Velkof, V. A. (2010). *The next four decades: The older population in the United States 2010 to 2050.* Retrieved from U.S. Census Bureau Web site: http://www.census.gov/prod/2010pubs/p25-1138.pdf.

Wallace, K. S., & Rogers, S. J. (2010). Intervening in infancy: implications for autism spectrum disorders. *Journal of Child Psychology and Psychiatry, 51*(12), 1300–1320.

Walsh, F. (2011). Family resilience: A collaborative approach in response to stressful life challenges. In S. M. Southwick, B. T. Litz, D. Charney, & M. J. Friedman

(Eds.), *Resilience and mental health: Challenges across the lifespan* (pp. 149–161). Cambridge, UK: Cambridge University Press.

Warren, Z., McPheeters, M. L., Sathe, N., Foss-Feig, J. H., Glasser, A., & Veenstra-VanderWeele, J. (2011). A systematic review of early intensive intervention for autism spectrum disorders. *Pediatrics, 127*(5), e1303–e1311.

Westerhoff, J. (1976). *Will our children have faith?* New York, NY: Seabury Press.

Whiteley, P., Shattock, P., Knivsberg, A. M., Seim, A., Reichelt, K. L., Todd, L., et al. (2012). Gluten- and casein-free dietary intervention for autism spectrum conditions. *Frontiers in Human Neuroscience, 6,* 1–8.

Wilson, B. A., Shannon, M. T., & Shields, K. M. (2013). *Nurse's drug guide.* Upper Saddle River, NJ: Pearson Education.

Wolraich, M., Brown, L., & Brown, R. T. (2011). Subcommittee on Attention-Deficit/Hyperactivity Disorder; Steering Committee on Quality Improvement and Management. ADHD: Clinical practice guideline for the diagnosis, evaluation, and treatment of attention-deficit/hyperactivity disorder in children and adolescents. *Pediatrics, 128,* 1007–1022.

Zhu, P., Tao, F., Hao, J., Sun, Y., & Jiang, X. (2010). Prenatal life events stress: Implications for preterm birth and infant birthweight. *American Journal of Obstetrics and Gynecology, 203*(1), e1–e8.

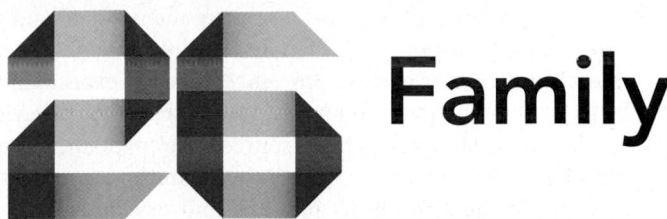 # Family

MODULE AT-A-GLANCE

The Concept of Family, 1707

Exemplar 26.1
Family Health Promotion, 1724

Exemplar 26.2
Family Response to Health Alterations, 1730

◪ THE CONCEPT OF FAMILY

For most individuals, family serves as a primary developmental influence. Numerous family structures exist, from single-parent families to families headed by two mothers or two fathers. Regardless of structural variations, every family is subject to the challenges of life, including economic hardship, illness, and stress. This concept will explore the role of the family in terms of development, childrearing, health promotion, and response to alterations in health status. In addition, the nurse's role in caring for the family unit will be examined. **<<**

Concept Learning Outcomes

After reading about this concept, you will be able to:

1. Summarize the makeup of the family structure.
2. Examine the relationship between family and other concepts/systems.
3. Identify commonly occurring alterations in family and their related therapies.
4. Differentiate common assessment procedures used to examine family health across the life span.
5. Explain management of family health and prevention of stress.
6. Demonstrate the nursing process in providing culturally competent and caring interventions across the life span for individual members of a family.
7. Compare and contrast common independent and collaborative interventions for clients with alterations in family health.

Concept Key Terms

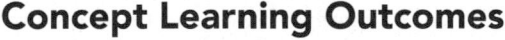

Adolescent family, *1710*
Binuclear family, *1711*
Blended family, *1710*
Boundaries, *1714*
Childless family, *1710*
Discipline, *1717*
Ecomap, *1720*
Emotional availability, *1716*
Extended family, *1709*
Extended-kin network family, *1710*
Family, *1708*
Family-centered care, *1708*
Family-centered nursing, *1708*
Family cohesion, *1715*
Family communication, *1716*

Family coping mechanisms, *1715*
Family development, *1712*
Family flexibility, *1716*
Foster family, *1710*
Genogram, *1720*
Intragenerational family, *1711*
Joint custody, *1711*
Limit setting, *1717*
Nuclear family, *1709*
Parenting, *1708*
Punishment, *1717*
Resiliency, *1715*
Single-parent family, *1710*
Stepfamily, *1710*
Two-career family, *1710*

▶ NORMAL PRESENTATION

The family is a basic unit of society. It consists of those individuals, male or female, youth or adult, legally or not legally related, genetically or not genetically related, whom the others consider to be their significant persons. The U.S. Census Bureau (2012b) defines a **family** as two or more individuals who are joined together by marriage, blood, or adoption, and are residing in the same household. More broadly, families are generally characterized by bonds of emotional closeness, sharing, and support. Family members can also include "honorary relatives" of the family, whether or not they are related by blood, marriage, or adoption, or even living in the same household. The family as defined by its members is likely to be dynamic with membership changing over time. In today's world it is even more likely that extended family members will live in different cities, states, or even countries. So, there is no *typical* family.

Within families, members are guided by a common set of values that binds them together. These family values are greatly influenced by external factors including cultural background, social norms, education, environmental influences, and socioeconomic status, as well as beliefs held by peers, coworkers, political and community leaders, and other individuals outside the family unit. Because of the influence of these external factors, a family's values may change considerably over the years.

A family is generally understood to be a safe haven for its members as they learn group values, norms, and acceptable behaviors. However, child abuse and neglect are significant problems and can occur within any family configuration.

In a healthy, functional family unit, roles include the following:

- Caring, nurturing, and educating children; teaching children how to get along in the world

- Maintaining the continuity of society by transmitting the family's knowledge, customs, traditions, values, and beliefs to children

- Receiving and giving love

- Preparing children to become productive members of society

- Meeting the needs of its members, including protection and economic support

- Serving as a buffer between family members and environmental and societal demands while advocating or addressing the interests and needs of the individual family members.

Individual family members take on certain social and gender roles and hold a designated status within the family based on the values and beliefs that bind the family together. These values and beliefs may evolve from the family's religious or cultural values and practices, social norms, education, and other influences to which parents were exposed during their childhood, adolescence, and early adult years. Parental roles, including childrearing practices and beliefs, are usually learned through a socialization process that occurs during childhood and adolescence.

Parents have important roles that involve childrearing and the long-term care of children until they reach adulthood. The role of **parenting** is a leadership role in the family; parents guide children as they learn the family's acceptable behaviors, beliefs, morals, and rituals and become socially responsible members of the community. Depending on their other roles in society, parents work to nurture and rear children, helping them meet role expectations. Parents must also meet the needs of and provide economic support for the family. Children also learn specific roles through a socialization process. Parents set expectations of behavior with discipline and modeling of appropriate behavior.

Ideally, the family is a child's source of strength and support, the major constant in the child's life. Families are intimately involved in their children's physical and psychological well-being, and they play a vital role in the health promotion and health maintenance of their children. By respecting the family's role, strengths, and experiences with the healthcare system, nurses have an opportunity to develop an effective partnership with the child and family as they make healthcare decisions that promote the child's health. This partnership between nurses and families is known as **family-centered care**. Nursing that considers the health of the family as a unit in addition to the health of individual family members is called **family-centered nursing**.

Viewing the Family Holistically

Although each family is unique, all families have certain structural and functional features in common. Family structure (family roles and relationships) and family function (interactions among family members and with the community) provide the following:

- *Interdependence.* The behaviors and level of development of individual family members constantly influence and are influenced by the behaviors and level of development of all other members of the family.

- *Maintaining boundaries.* The family creates boundaries that guide its members, providing a distinct and unique family culture. This culture, in turn, provides values.

- *Adapting to change.* The family changes as new members are added, current members leave, and the development of each member progresses.

- *Performing family tasks.* Essential tasks maintain the stability and continuity of the family. These tasks include physical maintenance of the home and the people in the home, the production and socialization of family members, and the maintenance of the psychological well-being of members.

In addition to providing an environment conducive to physical growth and health, the family creates an atmosphere that influences the cognitive and the psychosocial growth of its members. Children and adults in healthy, functional families receive support, understanding, and encouragement as they progress through predictable developmental stages, as they move in or out of the family unit, and as they establish new family units. In families where members are physically and emotionally nurtured, individuals are encouraged to achieve their potential in the family unit. As individual needs are met, family members are able to reach out to others in the family, the community, and the larger society.

Families from different cultures are an integral part of North America's rich heritage. Each family has values and beliefs that are unique to its culture of origin and shape the family's structure, methods of interaction, healthcare practices, and coping mechanisms. These factors interact to influence the health of families. Families of a particular culture may cluster

Evidence-Based Practice Parental Presence During Procedures

Problem

Few hospitals have formal policies regarding parental or family presence during procedures. Many parents wish to be present during their child's care, and find that it helps the child's anxiety if a parent or family member is present during procedures.

Evidence

Increasingly, parents are permitted to be present during medical procedures performed on their children. Historically, resistance to parental presence was based on the fear that parents would delay or interfere with the procedure, distract or increase the anxiety of the health professionals performing the procedure, or experience heightened anxiety of their own. Studies have investigated parental presence in various situations involving medical procedures such as anesthesia induction, intravenous starts, and resuscitation. In most cases, parents are less anxious if they are able to be present when their child has a procedure, and the ability of health professionals to perform procedures is not affected (Ahmann & Dokken, 2009; Bowden & Greenberg, 2009; Pye, Kane, & Jones, 2010).

Hospitals that do allow parent or family presence during procedures such as resuscitation will often provide support staff to explain the actions being taken by healthcare professionals. This support may be in the form of a nurse, a social worker, or a chaplain, and has shown to be helpful overall. In fact, 97.5% of family members interviewed about being present during a child or family member's resuscitation reported that they did not regret the decision and that they felt they had the right to be present (Doolin et al., 2011).

Implications

Understanding the potential effectiveness of parental and family involvement with procedures is beneficial to nurses. Parents and nurses should collaborate when working with children who may be anxious about being in a hospital or about the procedure in general. Parental involvement also facilitates better communication between parents and healthcare professionals.

Critical Thinking Application

Consider how parents could be helpful during procedures performed on children. Describe two procedures in which parental involvement and collaboration could make the situation less anxiety inducing for the child. How could nurses work to further collaboration efforts with parents when working with pediatric clients?

---

to form mutual support systems and to preserve their heritage; however, this practice may isolate them from the larger society (**Figure 26–1 ●**).

Diversity in Family Structures and Roles

Families consist of individuals (structure) and their responsibilities within the family (roles). Governmental data are grouped by types of *households*: married couples with children, married couples without children, other family households (single-parent families), men living alone, women living alone, and other nonfamily households. Some families live in houses, some in apartments; some live in urban areas, some in rural towns, and some are homeless.

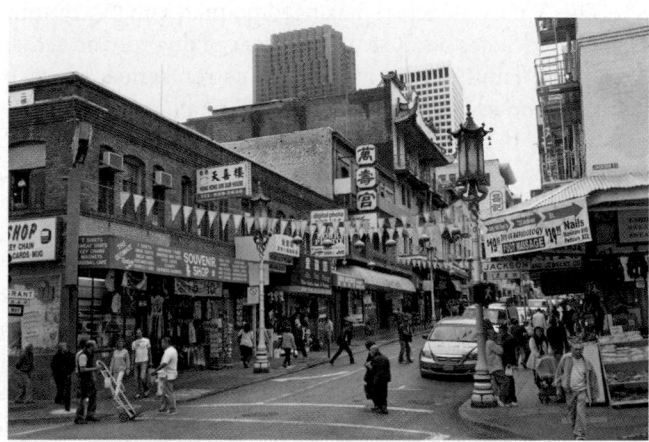

Figure 26–1 ● An example of cultural clustering can be seen in San Francisco's Chinatown.
Source: © Peter Horree/Alamy

The family protects the physical health of its members by providing adequate nutrition and healthcare services. Family nutritional and lifestyle practices directly affect the developing health attitudes and lifestyle practices of the children. In most cases, the family's economic resources are secured by adult members.

When considering families from the standpoint of the tasks associated with functioning as a unit, many families are similar. However, family units in the United States are diverse in terms of structure and with regard to which family member assumes a given role.

NUCLEAR FAMILY   A family structure of two parents and their offspring is known as the **nuclear family**. The nuclear family consists of a husband, a wife, and their shared biological children. In 2011, the U.S. Census Bureau (2012a) reported 24.7 million fathers in married-couple families, 176,000 of whom were stay-at-home fathers (caring for 332,000 children).

EXTENDED FAMILY   The relatives of nuclear families, such as grandparents or aunts and uncles, compose the **extended family**. In some families, members of the extended family live with the family (**Figure 26–2 ●**). Although members of the extended family may live in different areas, they may be a source of emotional or financial support for the family. An extended family may share household and childrearing responsibilities with parents, siblings, or other relatives. According to the U.S. Census Bureau (2011b), as of 2009, 7.8 million children lived in an extended family with at least one grandparent. Grandparents may raise children because the parents are unable to care for them. Grandparents endure emotional, physical, and financial stresses when taking on the childrearing role of one or more grandchildren.

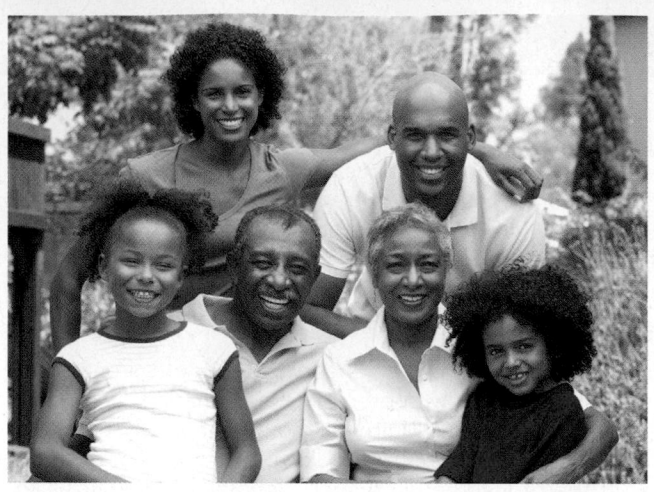

Figure 26–2 ● Three generations of a family enjoying a day in the park.
Source: © Monkey Business/Fotolia

EXTENDED-KIN NETWORK FAMILY Another example of an extended family is the **extended-kin network family**. This is a specific form of an extended family in which two nuclear families of primary or unmarried kin live in proximity to each other. The family shares a social support network, chores, goods, and services. This type of family model is common in the Latino community. Multigenerational arrangements of this sort are more common in non-U.S. cultures and working-class families.

TWO-CAREER FAMILY In **two-career families** (or dual-career families), both partners are employed by choice or by necessity. They may or may not have children. Two-career families have steadily increased since the 1960s because of increased career opportunities for women, a desire to increase the family's standard of living, and economic necessity. The U.S. Bureau of Labor Statistics (2012) reported that the percentage of married dual-career families rose to 58.5% in 2011. Two-career families have to address issues related to child care, household chores, and spending time together, with finding good-quality, affordable child care being one of the greatest stressors.

SINGLE-PARENT FAMILY As of 2010, there were 11.7 million **single-parent families** in the United States. Of those, 9.8 million were headed by single mothers, while 1.8 million were headed by single fathers. The number of single-parent families has increased steadily during the past decade (U.S. Census Bureau, 2010, 2012d).

There are many reasons for single parenthood, including death of a spouse, separation, divorce, birth of a child to an unmarried woman (whether or not the pregnancy was planned), or adoption of a child by a single man or woman. The stresses of single parenthood are many: child care concerns, financial concerns, role overload and fatigue from managing daily tasks, and social isolation. Single-parent families may face difficulties because the sole parent may need assistance with childrearing issues, lack social and emotional support, or have financial issues. Single-parent families experience higher rates of poverty, which has important implications for the children. In 2010, poverty was highest among single-parent families headed by women, with 31.6% living in poverty. In addition, 15.8% of single-parent families headed by men were

living at or below the poverty line (National Poverty Center, 2010). Single mothers are at risk for poverty due to lack of child support and unequal pay for work performed. Additional risk factors may include work skill deficiencies and cutbacks in social welfare programs, such as childcare subsidy programs. Nurses working with single parents assess their strengths and needs in providing care to the child, such as afterschool and backup child care arrangements that enable the parent to fulfill work commitments. Nurses also determine if the family has access to all resources available to support growth and development, such as school breakfast and lunch programs that provide nutritional support.

ADOLESCENT FAMILY The birth rate among teenagers peaked in 1991 and has decreased progressively since then to 34.2 births per 1,000 women ages 15–19 in 2010. This is the lowest birth rate for teenagers reported in more than 70 years. Rates are highest among Hispanic females, followed by Black females, and then White females (Martin et al., 2012). The parents in **adolescent families** are often developmentally, physically, emotionally, and financially ill prepared to undertake the responsibility of parenthood. Adolescent pregnancies frequently interrupt or stop formal education. Children born to adolescents are often at greater risk for health and social problems.

FOSTER FAMILY Children who can no longer live with their birth parents may require placement with a family that has agreed to include them temporarily. The legal agreement between the **foster family** and the court to care for the child includes the expectations of the foster parents and the financial compensation they will receive. A family (with or without its own children) may house more than one foster child at a time or different children over many years. Hopefully, at some time the fostered child can return to the birth parent(s) or be legally and permanently adopted by other parents.

CHILDLESS FAMILY **Childless families** (also known as child-free families) are a growing trend. In some cases a family is childless by choice; in other cases, a family is childless because of issues related to infertility or other medical conditions that present risks to the woman or fetus should the woman become pregnant.

STEPFAMILY A **stepfamily** consists of a biological parent with children and a new spouse who may or may not have children. This family structure has become increasingly common in the United States because of high rates of divorce and remarriage. These families also are known as remarried, reconstituted, or **blended families**. In 2009, 16% of all children, or 11.7 million, lived in blended families; at least 8 million of these children were living with a half sibling (U.S. Census Bureau, 2011b).

Stepfamily models have both strengths and challenges. Stepfamilies may have fewer financial issues and may offer a child a new support person and role model. Remarriage also provides a new opportunity for a successful relationship for the parents; however, the relationship between stepparents and stepchildren can be strained. Stresses occur as blended families get acquainted with each other, learn to respect differences, and establish new patterns of behavior. These stresses can include discipline issues, adjustment problems, role ambiguity, strain with the other biological parent, and communication issues. When blended families with children form after the divorce or death of a parent, adjustment can be particularly challenged by the normal processes of grief and loss. An important nursing consideration is to direct families to resources that may help reduce the potential conflicts associated with different parenting styles, discipline, and manipulative behaviors of children that can develop within a blended family.

BINUCLEAR FAMILY   A **binuclear family** is a postdivorce family in which the biological children are members of two nuclear households, both that of the father and that of the mother. The children alternate between the two homes. This is also called coparenting and involves joint custody. In **joint custody**, both parents have equal responsibility and legal rights, regardless of where the children live. The binuclear family model enables both parents to be involved. It is a model for effective communication. It enables both biological parents to be involved in a child's upbringing and provides additional support and role models in the form of extended family members. Special nursing considerations in this family type involve ensuring that health promotion guidance and education for care of the child with an acute or chronic condition are communicated effectively to both biological parents.

INTRAGENERATIONAL FAMILY   In some cultures, and as people live longer, more than two generations may live together in an **intragenerational family**. Children may continue to live with their parents even after having their own children, or the grandparents may move in with their grown children's families after some years of living apart. In other situations, a generation is skipped or missing; that is, grandparents live with and care for their grandchildren, but the children's parents are not a part of this family. Many life events and choices can result in this type of family structure.

HETEROSEXUAL COHABITING FAMILY   Cohabiting (or communal) families consist of unrelated individuals or families who live under one roof. This may include never-married individuals as well as divorced or widowed persons. According to the 2011 U.S. Census, approximately 1.9 million children under 18 years of age live with a parent and unmarried partner (U.S. Census Bureau, 2011a). Biological children may result from the relationship, or in some cases children of one parent are present and help form a blended cohabitating family.

An important nursing consideration for children who live in informal cohabiting families is that the nonbiological parent has no legal authority to seek emergency medical care for the child. However, in the case of a true emergency that could result in loss of life or diminished functioning, health professionals are obligated to provide care and obtain consent as soon as possible afterward. The nonbiological parent also may not have any knowledge of the child's medical history.

GAY AND LESBIAN FAMILIES   Gay and lesbian families include those in which two or more people who share a same-sex orientation live together (with or without children), and those in which a gay or lesbian single parent rears a child (**Figure 26–3 ●**). Children in these families may be from a previous heterosexual union, or be born to or adopted by one or both member(s) of the same-sex couple. For example, a biological child may be born to one of the partners through artificial insemination or through a surrogate mother. Lesbian and gay couples function much like heterosexual couples, and children who are adopted or born into the family are highly valued. Children raised in gay and lesbian

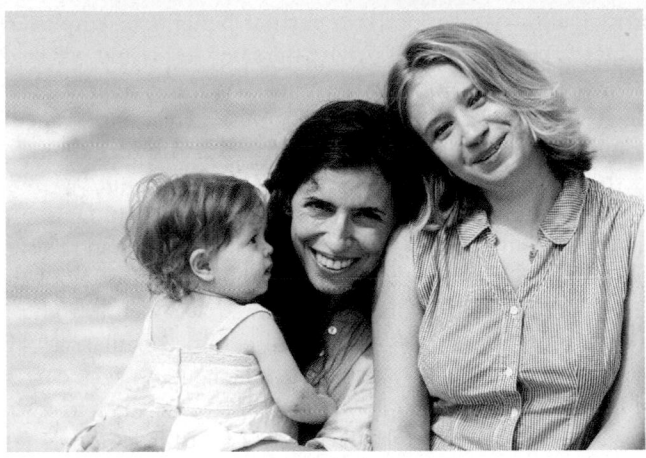

Figure 26–3 ● A lesbian couple and their daughter.
Source: © dubova/Fotolia

families may face unique issues when interacting with peers and when revealing their parents' sexual orientation.

Homosexual adults form gay and lesbian families based on the same goals of caring and commitment seen in heterosexual relationships. In addition, the structure of gay and lesbian families is as diverse as that of heterosexual families—including stepfamilies and single-parent families. Children raised in these family units develop sex role orientations and behaviors similar to those of children in the general population. These children have been found to have the same advantages and expectations for health, adjustment, and development as children born into heterosexual families. Lesbian and gay parents are believed to be as effective as heterosexual couples in providing a supportive and healthy environment for their children (Weber, 2010).

SAFETY ALERT
When obtaining consent to provide health care and medical treatments to children and adolescents, the healthcare provider should identify the biological or adoptive parent or confirm a caregiver's possession of legal documentation proving the right to make medical decisions on the child's behalf.

Children in these families typically have only one biological or adoptive legal parent. In many states, the other partner is the coparent and has no legal parental status. Various states have now taken legislative action to ensure the security of children whose parents are gay or lesbian by guaranteeing access to the second parent of joint adoption rights.

Coparent adoption provides for either parent to give consent for health care and make other important decisions on behalf of the child. It also has implications for child custody and financial support in the event the parents separate or a death occurs, ensuring the child's right to a continuing relationship with and financial support from both parents. Nursing considerations for individuals in gay and lesbian families emphasize respect for the relationship between partners and recognition of the nurturing capacity in these families.

Legal issues for same-sex couples are significant and constantly changing. Many, but by no means all, companies and municipalities offer domestic partner benefits to employees. Domestic partner policies extend the same rights and privileges to the partner of a nonmarried employee of the same or opposite gender as would be offered to spouses. Health insurance is an example of a benefit that often is offered under domestic partner policies. California Family Code Section 297–297.5 defines domestic partners as "two adults who have chosen to share one another's lives in an intimate and committed relationship of mutual caring" (State of California Franchise Tax Board, 2013). Numerous state and federal laws have been introduced in the United States to allow or prohibit same-sex marriages or civil unions. The nurse may find it challenging to keep current on how such legislation affects healthcare issues such as insurance coverage and the right to consent for health care.

Stay Current: *To view the up-to-date legislative policies on adoption by state, visit this Web site:* **www.childwelfare.gov/ systemwide/laws_policies/state**.

SINGLE ADULTS LIVING ALONE Individuals who live by themselves represent a significant portion of today's society. Of younger adults 18–34 years of age, about 16% live alone, with more males living alone than females. However, among adults 65 years and older, about 22% of men live alone, whereas about 47% of women live alone (U.S. Census Bureau, 2012c). Singles include young self-supporting adults who have recently left the nuclear family as well as older adults living alone. Young adults typically move in and out of living situations and may have membership in family, nonfamily household, and living alone categories at different times. Older adults may find themselves single through divorce, separation, or the death of a spouse, but generally remain living alone for the remainder of their lives.

Developmental Stages

Family development refers to the dynamics or changes that a family experiences over time, including changes in relationships, communication patterns, roles, and interactions (**Box 26–1 ●**). Although each family is unique, the members go through a set of fairly predictable changes. For example, Duvall (1977) developed an eight-stage family life cycle that describes the developmental process each family encounters. This model is based on the nuclear family (**Table 26–1 ●**). The oldest child serves as a marker for the family's developmental stages except in the last two stages, when children are no longer present. Couples with

---

Box 26–1 The "Sandwich Generation"

Adults who care for their own children and one or more of their own parents belong to a group that has come to be known as the "sandwich generation." This group of adults faces an incredible amount of stress trying to meet the diverse needs of young children and adolescents as well as aging parents. One of the chief sources of stress for these families is financial insecurity. A family with limited financial resources may face taking the aging parent into their own home or placing an aging parent who is no longer independent into a senior care facility that is below standard. If a family has very young children, taking an aging parent with dementia into the home can present either real or perceived hazards to the young children, increasing the stress level of the entire family. In addition, a member of the sandwich generation often faces additional stress addressing an older parent's needs while still trying to get children off to school and to extracurricular activities and maintain a full-time job. End-of-life issues can be a great source of stress and conflict for these families.

A nurse who is assessing an adult who cares for both her own children and her aging parents may diagnose any one of several conditions including, but not limited to, the following:

Ineffective Self-Health Management
- Disturbed Sleep Pattern
- Risk for Situational Low Self-Esteem
- Interrupted Family Processes
- Compromised Family Coping.

(NANDA-I © 2012)

CRITICAL THINKING APPLICATION

In small groups, discuss what assessment questions would be appropriate when working with a client who is a member of the "sandwich generation." Discuss what caring interventions might be appropriate and what outcomes could be developed in collaboration with the client.

STAGE	CHARACTERISTICS
Stage I	Beginning family, newly married couples*
Stage II	Childbearing family (oldest child is an infant through 30 months of age)
Stage III	Families with preschool children (oldest child is between 2.5 and 6 years of age)
Stage IV	Families with schoolchildren (oldest child is between 6 and 13 years of age)
Stage V	Families with teenagers (oldest child is between 13 and 20 years of age)
Stage VI	Families launching young adults (all children leave home)
Stage VII	Middle-aged parents (empty nest through retirement)
Stage VIII	Family in retirement and old age (retirement to death of both spouses)

TABLE 26–1 Eight-Stage Family Life Cycle

*Keep in mind that this was the norm at the time the model was developed, but today families form through many different types of relationships.
Source: Adapted from Duvall, E. M. (1977). *Marriage and family development* (5th ed.). Philadelphia, PA: Lippincott; Duvall, E. M., & Miller, B. C. (1985). *Marriage and family development* (6th ed.). New York, NY: Harper Row; Friedman, M. M., Bowden, V. R., & Jones, E. G. (2003). *Family nursing: Research, theory, and practice* (5th ed.). Upper Saddle River, NJ: Prentice Hall; Gedaly-Duff, V., Nielsen, A., Heims, M. L., & Pate, M. D. (2010). Family child health nursing. In J. R. Kaakinen, V. Gedaly-Duff, D. P. Coehlo, & S. M. H. Hanson, *Family health care nursing: Theory, practice, and research* (4th ed., pp. 332–378). Philadelphia, PA: F. A. Davis..

more than one child may find themselves in overlapping stages, with developmental advances occurring simultaneously. Other family development models have been developed to address the stages and developmental tasks facing the unattached young adult, the gay and lesbian family, those who divorce, and those who remarry.

▶ FACTORS THAT SHAPE FAMILY DEVELOPMENT

Choosing to become a parent is a major life change for adults. Beginning when they first learn they are expecting a child (whether through pregnancy or adoption), parents experience stresses and challenges along with feelings of pride and excitement. Mothers and fathers adjust their lifestyles to give priority to parenting. Babies and very young children are dependent for total care 24 hours a day, and this often results in sleep deprivation, irritability, less personal time, and less time for the couple's relationship. In addition, the family with a new baby often experiences a change in financial status.

Several factors influence how well the parents adjust to their new role. Social support provided to the mother, especially by the father, is important for the mother's adjustment. Marital happiness during pregnancy is an important factor for the adjustment of both parents. Infants with significant health conditions or those with difficult temperaments can cause parents extra stress and affect their adjustment to the parenting role.

With the birth of the first child, mothers and fathers both have challenges related to renegotiating their employment to accommodate family and child care time (Box 26–2 ●). Fathers are sometimes additionally challenged to develop closeness with the infant and learn how to care for the infant, especially when they may not have had role models or any previous child care experience. Most parents find that caring for infants and children takes more time than anticipated.

As you study the factors that shape family development, consider also how the concept of Family relates to other concepts, as discussed in the Concepts Related to Family feature.

Box 26–2   Family and Medical Leave Act

Eligible parents of newborns and adopted children are entitled to 12 weeks of unpaid leave during any 12-month period, as initially authorized by the federal Family and Medical Leave Act of 1993. Vacation or sick leave may be used to pay for time away from work, depending on the employer's leave policies. This act also applies if a child, spouse, or parent of the employee develops a serious health condition. The employee is entitled to return to the previous position or an equivalent position with all the same pay, benefits, and other conditions. The act carries some additional conditions and requirements, including that employees are only eligible if they have worked for a covered employer for 1,250 hours over the previous 12 months.

💧 **Stay Current:** More information on the Family and Medical Leave Act can be found at **www.dol.gov/whd/fmla**.

Source: Based on the Family and Medical Leave, Public Law 103-3, February 5, 1999. 5 U.S.C. 6381–6387; 5 CFR part 630, subpart L. Retrieved from http://www.opm.gov/pca/leave/HTMS/fmlafac2.asp.

Parent–Child Interaction

The qualities of family relationships and behaviors are important aspects of family strengths and functioning. Positive family relationships are characterized by parent–child warmth and supportiveness. Warm parent–child relationships can buffer children from stress and promote positive cognitive and social outcomes. Parents who are warm and place high demands on their children for appropriate behavior have children who tend to be content, self-reliant, self-controlled, and open to learning in school.

Mothers and fathers both contribute to the psychological, emotional, and social health and development of their children. Both parents provide affection, nurturing, and comfort. They teach children life skills and healthy lifestyles. Both mothers and fathers promote the social competence, academic achievement, and problem-solving abilities of their children.

Family Size

The size of the family influences the amount of attention parents are able to give individual children. In small families parents often have more time to give attention to the children, encourage achievement, meet family expectations, and support involvement in community activities. Children in larger families are encouraged to be cooperative to support family functioning. The children usually receive less personal attention from the parents and often turn to others in the family for needed support. Family finances may be more limited. Children may adopt a specialized family role to gain recognition, such as the "responsible one," "the clown," or "the black sheep."

Sibling Relationships

Siblings are a child's first peers and often have a lifelong relationship. Siblings, especially those of the same gender or who are close in age, tend to have a close relationship because they often share many common experiences through childhood and adolescence. In general, the parents have greater influence than siblings on children who are more widely spaced in age. However, an older sibling may be a very strong role model for younger siblings.

Sibling rivalry between children exists at times in all families. Within the family children learn to share, compete, and compromise with siblings. Some siblings take on roles such as protector, problem solver, friend, and supporter for dealing with issues in the family and in the environment. Some siblings learn to work well together to maintain privacy or to form a coalition for negotiating with the parents. An older sibling helps reinforce rules and roles in the family by prompting and inhibiting certain patterns of behavior in the younger siblings. However, one sibling may test the waters by breaking a previously implicit rule to determine what rule flexibility is allowed in the family.

Studies indicate that birth order contributes to personality differences among genetically related children who are raised in the same house. Research findings collected during the past 15 years and involving evaluation of various cultures suggest a correlation between an individual's birth order and personality. Firstborn children have been identified as having a tendency to assume a surrogate parent role, while the youngest child will

Concepts Related to Family

A family is a dynamic collection of relationships that strengthen and/or dwindle over time. Familial relationships and dynamics are influenced by a number of factors, and the actions of one family member can affect the family unit as a whole. For example, when an individual suffers from addiction to illegal substances or alcohol, his addictive behaviors are likely to affect close family members in a number of ways. Life-threatening health conditions can result in anticipatory grieving, loss of financial security, and caregiver burden, increasing the stresses with which families cope on a daily basis. Alternatively, the birth of a child can result in the strengthening or weakening of bonds and relationships within the family. Family members may be drawn closer through shared interests in the welfare of the child. Conversely, the addition of a new family member can add financial and emotional stressors that strain familial relationships.

CONCEPT	RELATIONSHIP TO FAMILY	NURSING IMPLICATIONS
Addiction		
■ Alcohol abuse ■ Substance abuse	Substance and/or alcohol abuse can affect individual family members as well as the family unit as a whole. Potential stressors may be psychosocial, physiological, financial, or spiritual in nature.	■ Be alert to the signs of addiction. ■ Propose interventions appropriate to addiction behavior. ■ Evaluate the individual's potential for being a danger to herself or others. ■ Recommend community resources to family members to help them process and cope with resultant complications.
Grief and Loss		
■ Loss of a loved one	May result in alterations in family dynamics, particularly if the deceased individual was in a position of family leadership or was the primary source of financial support. Grief reactions can also affect how family members relate to one another.	■ Be alert to the signs of intense grief reactions, such as lasting depression, anger, or denial. ■ Consider the nature of the loss and its possible ramifications. ■ Offer appropriate support and referral, such as therapy or grief counseling.
Reproduction		
■ Antepartum care ■ Postpartum care	Addition of a family member may strengthen familial bonds through shared interests in the child's welfare or may instead strain relationships in terms of increased physical, emotional, and financial demands.	■ Teach about prenatal care and maternal health. ■ Encourage all family members to engage in educational activities. ■ Assess the involved individuals' responses to pregnancy and sensitively address potentially harmful issues, such as ineffective communication patterns. ■ Be alert to signs of postpartum depression. ■ Advise parents of potential jealousies and complications with toddlers and new infants.

generally work to develop talents and skills not possessed by the other siblings in order to stand out in the family as deserving of recognition. Outside influences and experiences also impact an individual's overall personality, but it is believed that the basis of these traits is affected by birth order (Badger & Reddy, 2009).

Boundaries

Boundaries are the invisible lines that define the amount and kind of contact allowable among members of a family and between the family and outside systems. Boundaries determine the patterns of how, when, and to whom family members relate. Boundaries define the divisions among the spousal, parental, and sibling subsystems.

- *Clear boundaries.* Firm yet flexible; family members are supported and nurtured but also allowed a certain degree of autonomy.

- *Rigid boundaries.* Family members are isolated from one another and there is little room for negotiation and individual development.

■ *Diffuse boundaries.* Everyone is into everyone else's business; there is little distinction between family members and there is too much negotiation, resulting in a loss of autonomy

In the modern Western nuclear family, competent families have clear hierarchical boundaries between generations in terms of power, authority, and responsibility. Competent adult leadership provides an emotional climate that considers everyone's needs and provides a sense of security. Members spend time apart, as well as time together. Mutual respect is also a boundary issue. Competent families respect and value the individual's opinions and feelings. The family system tolerates individual differences and honors different opinions.

Boundaries are a social construction and, as such, are culturally determined. What appears to be a boundary violation in one culture may be acceptable in another culture. For example, how family members respect privacy in regard to toileting, bathing, changing clothes, and sleeping arrangements varies by culture. Multigenerational boundaries in terms of power and authority vary from culture to culture.

Family Cohesion

Family cohesion is defined as the emotional bonding between family members. The four levels of cohesion are (**Figure 26–4** ●):

1. Disengaged (very low)
2. Separated (low to moderate)
3. Connected (moderate to high)
4. Enmeshed (very high).

In Western, developed societies, the central ranges of cohesion (separated and connected) are believed to contribute to optimal family competency. The extremes (disengaged or enmeshed) are seen as less adaptive. Disengaged families seem almost like a group of strangers who happen to be living together. A disengaged family does not experience much loyalty or close-

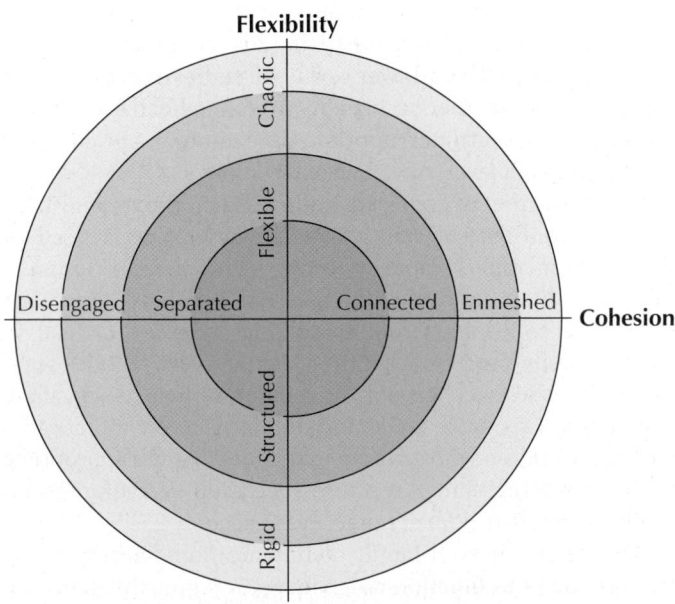

Figure 26–4 ● Levels of family cohesion.

Box 26–3   Characteristics of Family Cohesion

DISENGAGED
■ Little closeness
■ Little loyalty
■ High independence.

SEPARATED
■ Low–moderate closeness
■ Some loyalty
■ Interdependent with more independence than dependence.

CONNECTED
■ Moderate–high closeness
■ High loyalty
■ Interdependent with more dependence than independence.

ENMESHED
■ Very high closeness
■ Very high loyalty
■ High dependency.

---

ness. Members of enmeshed families cannot develop a separate identity, and each person must yield autonomy to belong to the family. Uniqueness is experienced as distance, and individuality is viewed as alienation and disloyalty (Olson, 1996). See **Box 26–3** ● for characteristics of family cohesion.

Resiliency

More important than the form or type of family are the family's relational resources and adaptive abilities. The most distinctive trait of competent families is the ability to manage stress productively. Simply put, adaptive families evolve and shift with changing situations. This is often referred to as **resiliency**. F. Walsh (2011) explains that resilience enables individuals to overcome adversity, and then heal from the experience, thus allowing themselves to move on to a more fulfilling life. Life crises and developmental transitions can stimulate family growth and transformation. Resilient families make it through crises such as disability and death with a renewed sense of confidence and purpose.

Family Coping Mechanisms

Family coping mechanisms are the behaviors families use to deal with stress or changes imposed from either within or without the family. Coping mechanisms can be viewed as an active method of problem solving developed to meet life's challenges. The coping mechanisms families and family members develop reflect their individual resourcefulness. Families may use coping patterns rather consistently over time or may change their coping strategies when new demands are made on the family. The success of a family largely depends on how well it copes with the stresses it experiences.

Nurses working with families realize the importance of assessing coping mechanisms as a way of determining how families relate to stress. The resources available to the family also are important. Internal resources, such as knowledge, skills, effective communication patterns, and a sense of mutuality and purpose within the family, assist in the problem-solving process. In addition, external support systems promote coping and adaptation. These external systems may be extended family, friends, religious affiliations, healthcare professionals, or social service agencies. The development of social support systems is particularly valuable today because many families, due to stress, mobility, or poverty, are isolated from the resources that would traditionally have helped them cope with stress.

Emotional Availability

Families that cope well encourage their members to express a wide variety of feelings. The emotional climate is one of intimacy and predictability. In other families, the emotional climate may be angry, cold, or distant and unpredictable. **Emotional availability** is another way to describe the quality of parent–child interactions. Areas for assessment include parental sensitivity, structuring, nonintrusiveness, and nonhostility. Parental sensitivity is assessed by how parents pick up on children's emotional signals and how appropriately parents express their own emotions. Parental structuring refers to the ability of parents to support learning and exploration without overwhelming the child's autonomy. Parental nonintrusiveness refers to the parents' availability to the child without being interfering, overprotective, or overwhelming. Nonhostility refers to ways of interacting with the child that are patient and pleasant. When angry, parents express their anger in an appropriately controlled manner (Biringen, 2000).

Inability to express anger appropriately often carries consequences for the family. Family violence is one potential consequence. Family violence includes abuse between intimate partners, child abuse, and elder abuse, and it may include physical, mental, and verbal abuse as well as neglect. Nurses should be alert to the symptoms of family violence and take appropriate measures to report it and obtain resources for the family. See the module on Violence for more information on this topic.

Family Flexibility

Family flexibility includes the amount of change in a family's leadership, role relationships, and relationship rules, but it also refers to the family's ability to respond to stress. There are four levels of flexibility (see Figure 26–4):

1. Rigid (very low)
2. Structured (low to moderate)
3. Flexible (moderate to high)
4. Chaotic (very high).

As with the levels of family cohesion, it is believed that the central ranges (structured and flexible) are more conducive to family adaptation, with the extremes (rigid and chaotic) being less competent (Olson, 1996). See **Box 26–4** ● for characteristics of family flexibility.

Rules determine appropriate roles and relationship patterns within the family. Rules express the family's values, forming a boundary around each family that screens outside information for compatibility with its value system. If the message is not congruent with the family's values, statements such as "That is not the way we do things in this family" or "I don't care what Marc is allowed to do. In this family, we . . ." will be voiced.

Box 26–4   Characteristics of Family Flexibility

CHAOTIC
- Lack of leadership
- Dramatic role shifts
- Erratic discipline
- Too much change.

FLEXIBLE
- Shared leadership
- Democratic discipline
- Role-sharing change
- Change when necessary.

STRUCTURED
- Leadership sometimes shared
- Somewhat democratic discipline
- Roles stable
- Change when demanded.

RIGID
- Authoritarian leadership
- Strict discipline
- Roles seldom change
- Too little change.

Family Communication Patterns

Family communication is measured by focusing on the listening and speaking skills, self-disclosure, and tracking abilities of the family as a group. In high-functioning families each person does the following:

- *Listens.* Is empathetic and attentive.
- *Speaks.* Speaks for oneself and does not speak for others.
- *Self-discloses.* Shares personal feelings about oneself and others in the family.
- *Tracks.* Stays on the topic at hand.

Family members who communicate well are better able to adapt and cope. Family members who find communication difficult may experience lower levels of expressiveness, vague requests to one another, an inability to comprehend each other's messages, frequent interruption of one another, speaking for others, and high levels of verbalized hostility.

Another aspect of family communication is the strategy used to resolve conflict. The ability to resolve differences is based on the family members' capacity to talk about areas of disagreement and their mutual willingness to negotiate and reach acceptable solutions. Problem-solving skills are critical to smooth family functioning. Without these skills, families seem to use strategies such as confrontation or avoidance, which are ineffective in reducing stress and do not resolve conflict satisfactorily. Children who grow up in families that use appropriate problem-solving skills are more successful at avoiding and resolving conflicts both at home and in school.

The effectiveness of family communication determines the family's ability to function as a cooperative, growth-producing unit. Messages are constantly being communicated among family members, both verbally and nonverbally. The information transmitted influences how members work together, fulfill their assigned roles in the family, incorporate family values, and develop skills to function in society. Intrafamily communication plays a significant role in the development of self-esteem, which is necessary for the growth of personality.

Parenting Styles

Parents have responsibility for providing children stability through nurturance, safety, and structure in a family that undergoes frequent changes over time. The child needs to have physical and emotional space to grow and develop. Parents also provide their children with the values, beliefs, rituals, and behaviors learned and transmitted across family generations.

To be successful, parents should implement reasonable, consistent **limit setting** (established rules or guidelines for behavior) on children's autonomy while the children are still learning values and self-control. At the same time, parents need to foster their children's curiosity, initiative, and sense of competence. Parents use different styles to parent their children. Parental warmth and control are two major factors that are important in children's development. Parental warmth refers to the amount of affection and approval displayed. Parental control refers to how restrictive the parents are regarding rules. See **Table 26–2** ● for the characteristics associated with parental warmth and control.

Diana Baumrind (1971), an important contemporary child developmentalist, proposed classifications of parenting styles that are still well accepted today. She identified three main types of parenting styles—(*authoritarian, authoritative,* and *permissive*)—and described the influences each style has on children. One additional parenting style, called *indifferent,* exists in some families. Although families generally tend to use one style, they may vary their style for certain situations.

AUTHORITARIAN PARENTS   Authoritarian parents tend to be punitive and adhere to rigid rules, or to be more dictatorial. Parents who use this style might say, "Because I'm your parent, that's why," "A rule is a rule," or "Just do what I say." This style sets firm limits, and those limits or rules are not negotiable or open to any discussion. Parents expect family beliefs and principles to be accepted without question. Children have no opportunity to participate in the family decision-making process. Children with authoritarian parents do not develop the skills to examine why a certain behavior is desirable or how their actions might influence others.

AUTHORITATIVE PARENTS   Authoritative parents use firm control to set limits, but they establish an atmosphere with open discussion or are more democratic than authoritarian parents. Limits for behavior are clear, consistent, and reasonable, but the children are encouraged to talk about why certain behaviors occurred and how the situations might be handled differently another time. Parents set and stick to established routines, so children have clear expectations of appropriate behavior. Authoritative parents provide explanations about inappropriate behaviors at a child's level of understanding. Children are allowed to express their opinions and objections, and some flexibility is permitted when appropriate. However, parents make it clear that they are the ultimate authority for decisions. Children with authoritative parents develop a sense of social responsibility because they converse about their responsibilities and approaches.

PERMISSIVE PARENTS   Permissive parents show a great deal of warmth, but set few controls or restraints on the children's behavior. Parents are so intent on showing unconditional love that they fail to perform some important parenting functions. Children are allowed to regulate their own behavior. Discipline is inconsistent, and parents may threaten punishment but not follow through. Both extremes result in excessive permissiveness, and the children do not learn socially acceptable limits of behavior. Because the parents do not impose any controls on the children, the children end up controlling the parents.

INDIFFERENT PARENTS   Indifferent parents do not display much interest in their children or in their roles as parents. They do not demonstrate affection or approval of the children, and they do not set limits or controls on the children. This may occur because they do not care, or because their lives are so stressed that they have no time or energy left for the children.

Discipline and Limit Setting

Discipline is a method for teaching children the rules for how to behave in society and what is expected in different circumstances. **Punishment** is the action taken to enforce the rules when the

TABLE 26–2 Characteristics of Significant Parenting Attributes		
PARENTING ATTRIBUTE	PARENTAL WARMTH	PARENTAL CONTROL
High level	■ Warm, nurturing ■ Expressing affection and smiling at children frequently ■ Limiting criticism, punishment ■ Expressing approval of child	■ Restrictive control of behavior ■ Surveying and enforcing compliance with rules ■ Encouraging children to fulfill their responsibilities ■ Sometimes limiting freedom of expression
Low level	■ Cool, hostile ■ Quick to criticize or punish ■ Ignoring children ■ Rarely expressing affection or approval ■ Sometimes rejecting children	■ Permissive, minimally controlling ■ Making fewer demands ■ Making fewer restrictions on behavior or expression of emotion ■ Permitting freedom in exploring environment

---

Client Teaching Guidelines for Promoting Acceptable Behavior in Children

The nurse can assist parents in handling their child's misbehavior by helping them to:

- Set realistic expectations and directions for behavior based on the child's age and understanding; consistently enforce the expected directions and behaviors.
- Focus on promoting appropriate and desirable behaviors in the child.
- Model or suggest appropriate behavior.
- Review expected behavior for special situations, such as a family party, going to the movies, or other social event.
- Help the child distinguish between inside and outside voices and behaviors.
- Praise or reward the child using appropriate behaviors.
- Tell the child about his or her inappropriate behavior as soon as it begins, and offer guidelines for changing behavior or provide a distraction.

- When reprimanding the child, focus on the behavior rather than stating that the child is bad. Explain how the behavior is inappropriate, how it makes you, as the parent, and any other person involved feel. Avoid ridicule or accusation that can take the form of shame or criticism, because these actions can affect the child's self-esteem if repeated often enough.
- Be alert for situations when the child could misbehave, such as when tired or overexcited. Use a distraction to control or calm the child.
- Help children gain self-control with friendly reminders (e.g., count to 3, as soon as the clothes are on the doll, as soon as you finish the game) regarding the timing for transition to the next event of the day, such as bedtime, putting the toys away, or washing hands before dinner.
- Discuss reasons and social rules for expected behaviors when the child is old enough to understand.

---

child misbehaves. Parenting styles play an important role in the type of discipline and punishment parents use with children. When clear limits are set and consistently maintained, as with authoritative parenting, punishment may be needed less often. Limit setting and firm control of those limits are important discipline methods that allow children to learn to what extent they can safely and independently operate within the environment. Firm limits also help children feel secure; they are reassured by consistency and the sense of protection the limits are perceived to provide. Punishment helps children learn that misbehavior has consequences, and may affect other individuals. This helps children develop a sense of responsibility for their behavior.

Genetic Considerations and Nonmodifiable Risk Factors

Familial relationships can be complicated by the presence or development of certain genetic disorders or irregularities. Many childhood behavioral disorders are believed to have at least some basis in genetics; these include anxiety disorders, attention-deficit/hyperactivity disorder, bipolar disorder, conduct disorders, and learning disorders. Behavioral management issues alone may strain familial relationships. Additionally, the diagnosis and treatment of some of these conditions may be further complicated by societal stigmas attached to the disorder. Side effects of prescription medications used in the treatment of these individuals may lead to alterations in family dynamics, as well. For example, the primary medications used to treat bipolar disorder in children are associated with side effects that include exhaustion and restlessness (National Institute of Mental Health, 2013).

CASE STUDY \\ PART 1

Maria Rodriguez, age 30, and her wife Daniella Marshall, age 32, were recently married and decided to start a family. Following donor insemination, Mrs. Rodriguez became pregnant. The couple arrives at the obstetrician's office for Mrs. Rodriguez's routine health

exam. You are familiar with the couple and have provided care to them in the past. Today, you are assigned to care for Mrs. Rodriguez, who is now at 7 months' gestation. After talking to the couple for a few minutes, you notice that Mrs. Rodriguez is more reserved than usual and seems a bit depressed. When you ask how things are coming along with planning for the new arrival, both women are silent. Finally, Mrs. Marshall explains that they are struggling to cope with reactions from other participants of the birthing classes they have been attending, and it is making them both more stressed. Mrs. Rodriguez then tells you that she no longer wishes to attend the birthing classes, even though Mrs. Marshall wishes to complete the course.

Clinical Reasoning Questions Level I

1. What additional information would be useful in assessing the challenges faced by Mrs. Rodriguez and Mrs. Marshall?
2. Which characteristics of communication would best promote open discussion between you and this couple?
3. What are some societal challenges that same-sex couples face?

Clinical Reasoning Questions Level II

4. Describe two nursing diagnoses that may be applicable in the care of Mrs. Rodriguez and Mrs. Marshall.
5. What are some of the dangers of stress at this stage in Mrs. Rodriguez's pregnancy?
6. Explain some of the benefits of birthing classes in terms of both safe delivery of the child and family planning.

▶ PREVENTION

Education is a key to preventing many alterations in family function. Nurses should emphasize that help and resources are available to assist with challenges and to guide families in learning healthy coping strategies. Not all familial complications and hardships can be prevented; however, trauma, abuse, and neglect

Alterations and Therapies **Family**

ALTERATION	DESCRIPTION	MANIFESTATIONS	INTERVENTIONS AND THERAPIES
Abuse	Physical, emotional, or sexual abuse directed toward another individual	■ Withdrawn emotions and a decrease in communication and/or socialization with family and friends ■ Behavioral changes, such as anger, depression, acting out in school or at home, and changes in appetite or sleep patterns ■ Bruises, broken bones, concussion, and other physical markers ■ Fear of a specific person or situation (e.g., family events, arguments, school dances)	■ As mandated reporters, nurses are required to report child abuse to law enforcement. Reports to supervisors that are not submitted to law enforcement can result in prosecution of both the nurse and the supervisor. Follow hospital policy while ensuring that all incidents are properly reported (Lazoritz, Rossiter, & Whiteaker, 2010). ■ Treat physical injuries (e.g., broken bones, cuts, concussions) and emphasize the importance of follow-up care. ■ Offer resources for emotional manifestations, for example, counseling or therapy. ■ Provide proficient, nonjudgmental client care.
Divorce	The separation of a couple from a marital bond with or without children	■ Anxiety ■ Depression ■ Stress and resulting manifestations such as restlessness, weight loss, headaches, and sleeplessness ■ Behavioral modifications in children (e.g., acting out in school, withdrawal, anger, confusion, nightmares)	■ Provide information about counseling, therapy, and support groups. ■ Advise about healthy coping mechanisms for stress; for example, exercise, new hobbies, and writing. ■ Educate about the importance of health maintenance and nutrition even during times of high stress and anxiety.
Death of family member	The loss of a spouse, child, parent, or other family member	■ Grief as evidenced by sadness, anger, denial, and pain associated with the loss ■ Depression manifested in a lack of enjoyment in normal activities, intense feelings of sadness, and changes in appetite ■ Sleeplessness ■ Weight loss or weight gain ■ Anxiety	■ Provide information about therapy and support groups. ■ Teach about healthy coping strategies. ■ Assess for signs of complicated or traumatic grief. ■ Facilitate referrals to grief counselors and other professional resources.

can be prevented or stopped if recognized early enough. Although identifying abuse is not always possible, certain warning signs and risk factors can be considered predictive. Frequent outbursts of uncontrolled or improperly expressed anger can be a warning sign. Poverty is also associated with potentially traumatic experiences (Collins et al., 2011). Interventions sensitively aimed at addressing a family's specific needs can improve the family's circumstances and promote healthy family dynamics.

Modifiable Risk Factors

Risk factors for family dysfunction may not always be evident. At times, the risk factors are masked by the absence of obvious problems. Stress, for example, can lead to many problems within a family, as the effects of unmanaged and unresolved stress can impact normal family functioning. Parental coping methods can also determine how their children will learn to

Family Assessment Guide

The family assessment provides important information about family structure, including which individuals are responsible for making healthcare decisions for specific family members. The following data may be useful in informing planning and care:

Family Structure

■ Which adults spend the most time with the children? What is the nature of sibling relationships?

■ Who has legal custody, that is, who is able to make healthcare decisions for the child?

■ For older adults or those living with serious illness, has a family member been legally designated as having a healthcare power of attorney?

Family Roles/Functions/Resources

■ Who provides for the child or family financially? Does the child/client/family have health insurance?

■ Who else helps the parent(s) care for the children? What other support systems does the family have in place?

Physical Health Status

■ What is the health status of each member of the family? How do family members perceive their own health?

■ What preventive practices does the family use (e.g., status of immunizations, oral hygiene practices, regularity of vision examinations)?

■ To what extent do family members receive routine health care?

Family Interactions and Values

■ How do family members express feelings? Communicate with each other?

■ What cultural and religious practices does the family observe? What relationship do these practices have to family health and well-being?

■ What are the family's health values? How much emphasis is put on exercise, diet, and preventive health care?

---

handle stress, since children often model the actions of their parents (American Psychological Association [APA], 2013). Stress in families results from numerous situations, including financial worry, job loss, marriage difficulties, and personal stress. The response to stressors can be exacerbated by a real or perceived sense of powerlessness over circumstances, such as poverty, unemployment, or abuse.

One debilitating and self-sustaining form of strain is sometimes referred to as "poverty-related stress." Economic strain impacts individual well-being and physical health. Poverty-related stress can have a detrimental effect on the family unit by straining the parental relationship, which ultimately leads to an increase in the stress level of any children in the family (Wadsworth & Rienks, 2012). Nurses can help alleviate some of this stress by facilitating connections with community resources that can help families meet their food, safety, and job-related needs (Collins et al., 2011).

▶ ASSESSMENT

The purpose of family assessment is to determine the level of family functioning, clarify family interaction patterns, identify family strengths and weaknesses, and describe the health status of the family and its individual members. Also important are family living patterns, including communication, childrearing, coping strategies, and health practices. Family assessment gives an overview of the family process and helps the nurse identify areas that need further investigation.

Nursing Assessment

Nurses carry out a detailed assessment in targeted areas as they become more acquainted with the family and begin to understand family needs and strengths more fully. An understanding of a family's structure helps provide insight into the family's support system and needs. In planning interventions, nurses need to focus not only on problems, but also on family strengths and resources as part of the nursing care plan (see the Family Assessment Guide feature).

To obtain an accurate and concise family assessment, the nurse needs to establish a trusting relationship with the parent(s) and the family. Data are best collected in a comfortable, private environment, free from interruptions.

HEALTH HISTORY Assessment begins with a complete health history. The nurse focuses first on the family unit and then on the individuals in that family. Taking a health history is one of the most effective ways to identify existing or potential health problems. Using a genogram will aid the nurse in visualizing familial relationships and patterns of chronic conditions occurring within the family unit. **Genograms** consist of visual representations of gender showing lines of birth descent through the generations (**Figure 26–5 ●**). The history is followed by physical assessment of family members. If further evaluation is indicated, a referral is made to the appropriate healthcare professional.

INTERPERSONAL INTERACTIONS How a family interacts within the community can provide useful information, especially when trying to determine how to support families who are having difficulty coping. **Ecomaps** are an assessment tool that can help nurses visualize how the family unit interacts with the external community environment, including schools, religious commitments, occupational duties, and recreational pursuits (**Figure 26–6 ●**). Developing an ecomap can help the nurse and family members see where family members are spending energy and identify possible sources of support during times of crisis. As part of the assessment, the nurse observes intrafamily communication patterns closely, paying special attention to who does the talking for the family, which members are silent, how disagreements are handled,

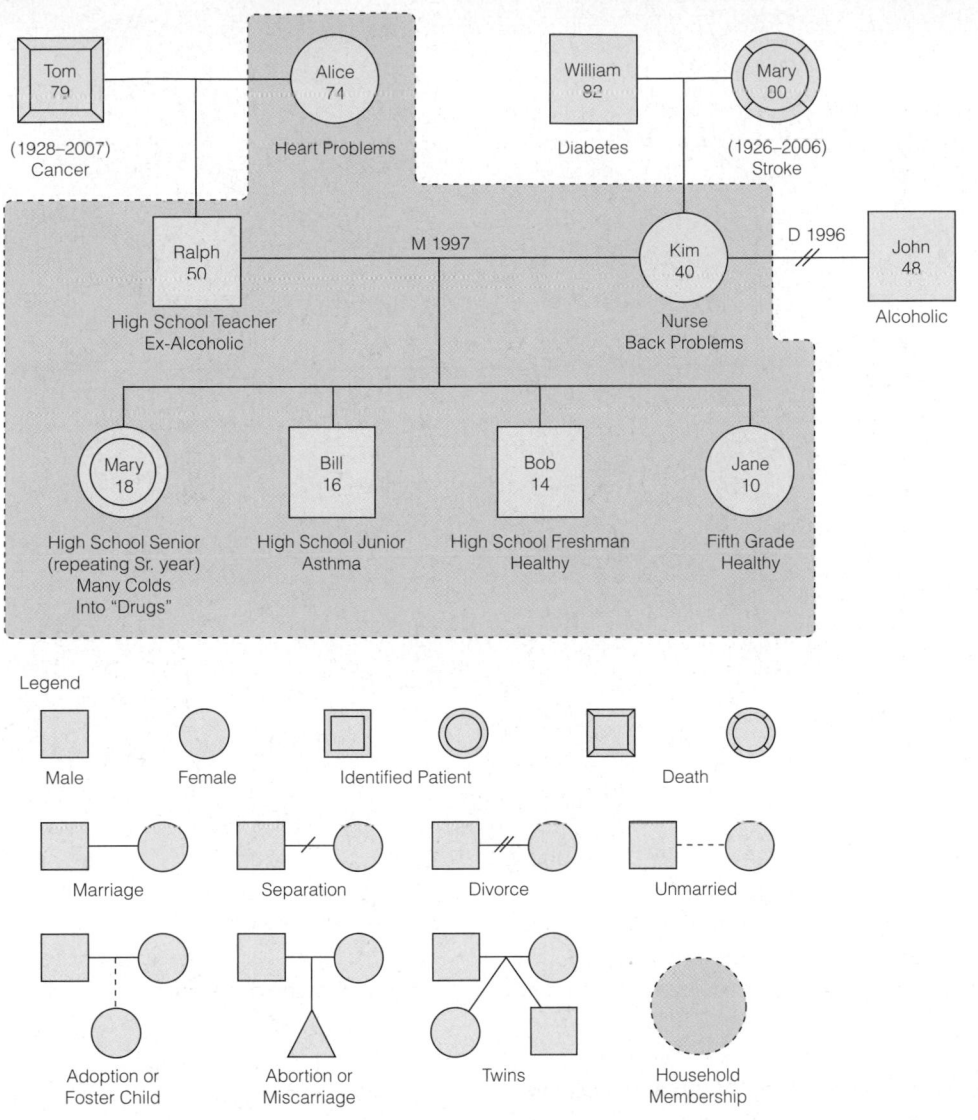

Legend

Male · Female · Identified Patient · Death

Marriage · Separation · Divorce · Unmarried

Adoption or Foster Child · Abortion or Miscarriage · Twins · Household Membership

Figure 26–5 ● Example of a family genogram with accompanying legend (symbols used in genograms).

and how well the members listen to one another and encourage the participation of others. Nonverbal communication is important because it gives valuable clues about what people are feeling.

LIFESPAN AND CULTURAL CONSIDERATIONS Family assessment requires consideration of the ages of all family members, as well as the cultural practices of the family. The age of the child or children will influence the family dynamic; for example, tasks associated with raising a toddler are vastly different from those pertinent to raising a teenager. Family activities and interaction will also vary depending on the age of the child. When raising a toddler, a majority of the parents' focus will likely be on meeting the child's developmental and social needs, whereas a teenager will generally work to meet these needs on his own, and the parental roles incorporate guiding the teenager in making life choices.

Cultural practices may influence the child's diet, behavior, and even sleep patterns. Some cultural and religious traditions may involve vegetarianism, while others may involve periods of fasting. The manner in which a child is expected to behave in public and at home can be impacted by culture, as can the

child's degree of respect for older adults. Culture can also affect the behavior of the entire family unit depending on matriarchal or patriarchal views. For example, in a matriarchal structure, the mother may be expected to take responsibility for making family healthcare decisions, to the near-exclusion of the father and children. Although it is neither realistic nor necessary for the nurse to be an expert as to each culture's beliefs, through open and nonjudgmental communication, the nurse can ascertain a great deal about the family's cultural influences.

PARENTING STYLES Nurses assess parenting styles by asking families how they handle situations that require limit setting. As previously described, an authoritative style is preferred because of its positive outcomes for child behavior and learning. The nurse in all settings is often in a position to discuss parenting styles and to offer suggestions for managing certain types of child behaviors that are frustrating to the family. Keep in mind that children are all different, and parents often must vary their parenting styles for different children in the family. For example, the child's temperament is often tied to her behavioral style. One child may need very clear limits, with discus-

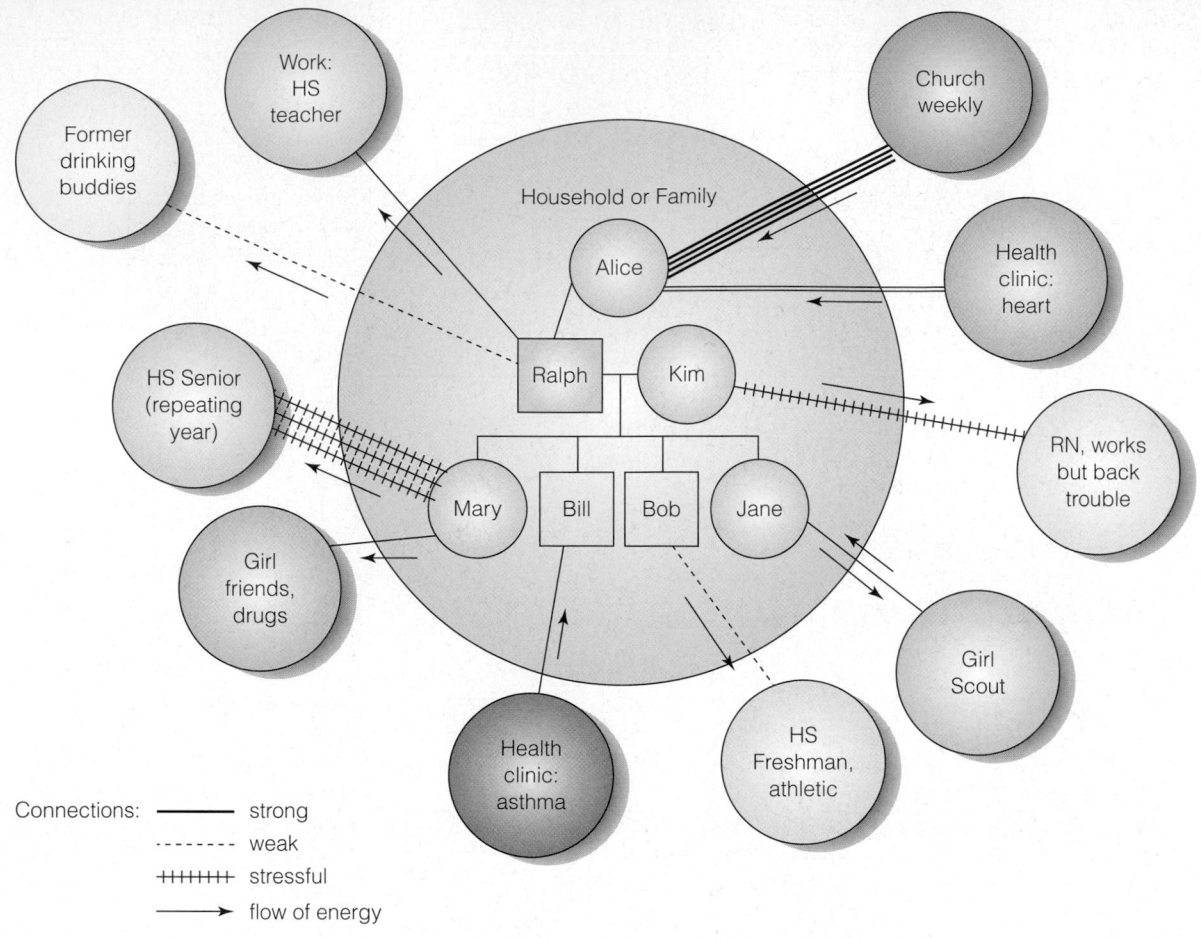

Figure 26–6 ● Example of a family ecomap. Many more components may be added to the map.

sion and reinforcement, whereas a sibling may immediately respond to the parents' limit setting without a need for discussion of the situation.

CASE STUDY \\ PART 2

After expressing concern for Mrs. Rodriguez and Mrs. Marshall, you begin to explore their birthing class experiences in greater detail. Mrs. Rodriguez explains that many of the other couples in the class are rude to her and her wife, and that the woman conducting the class is cold to them as well. The couple continues to tell you about similarly negative reactions they have experienced while searching for a birthing center. During the discussion, you notice that Mrs. Rodriguez becomes increasingly upset. When Mrs. Marshall asks for a few moments alone with Mrs. Rodriguez, you step out of the room. Upon your return, Mrs. Rodriguez apologizes for "losing control of my emotions." You assure her that she is welcome to express her emotions and that you are committed to providing her with the best possible care, including recommending some potential alternatives to her current birthing classes. You continue your physical assessment of Mrs. Rodriguez. Her vital signs are T 98.8°F oral, P 86 bpm, R 24/min, and BP 168/90 mmHg. Mrs. Rodriguez denies any physical complaints or unusual changes in her condition. You leave the room to talk with the physician. The

physician comes in to examine Mrs. Rodriguez and notes that everything appears to be fine but expresses concern about Mrs. Rodriguez's elevated blood pressure.

Clinical Reasoning Questions Level I
1. Presuming that Mrs. Rodriguez has no other health issues and no pregnancy-related complications, why might her blood pressure be elevated?
2. Identify three nursing actions described in this scenario that reflect respect and nonjudgmental care of this couple.

Clinical Reasoning Questions Level II
3. Describe two nursing interventions appropriate for inclusion in the care of this couple.
4. What steps might you take to assist Mrs. Rodriguez with identifying alternative providers of birthing classes?
5. What are some concerns associated with hypertension during the third trimester of pregnancy?

▶ INTERVENTIONS AND THERAPIES

Variations among families are shaped by multiple factors, including life experiences, current and past challenges, coping abilities, cultural diversity, individual personalities, and the age of the family members. Nurses can employ different interventions—

both independently and collaboratively—to assist families with navigating through challenges or difficult circumstances, as well as to promote the optimal use of each individual's strengths.

Independent

Client education is an essential component of family-centered care. Through tactful, nonjudgmental communication, the nurse can identify areas of knowledge deficiency. Effective communication also requires the nurse to demonstrate cultural competence and an awareness of each client's current health beliefs.

PROVIDING CULTURALLY COMPETENT CARE Proficient nursing care requires cultural awareness. As previously noted, the nurse is not expected to become an expert about every culture. Rather, the nurse should strive to become knowledgeable about the cultures predominantly served in his clinical setting and seek additional information when caring for clients whose cultural beliefs are unfamiliar to him. Nurses should also acknowledge the numerous variations of family structures, while avoiding making assumptions and judgments.

FACILITATING THE TRANSITION TO PARENTHOOD Nurses can help parents through this important transition by listening to the challenges the parents describe during the infant's first health visits. Encourage fathers as well as mothers to attend and participate in health promotion visits with the healthcare provider. Answer questions and offer ideas to address described problems that the parents may be too tired to solve on their own. Help parents recognize that their frustrations and feelings regarding the challenges of infant care are normal.

Encourage both parents to become active in caring for the infant and to gain comfort in that care. Help both parents find activities that they enjoy with regard to infant care that will encourage interaction and bonding with the infant.

EXPLORING HEALTH BELIEFS AND PROVIDING EDU-CATION Health beliefs may reflect a lack of information or misinformation about health or disease. They may also include folklore and practices from different cultures. Because of the many advances in medicine and health care during the past few decades, clients may have outdated information about health, illness, treatment, and prevention. The nurse is frequently in a position to give information or correct misconceptions. This function is an important component of the nursing care plan.

Collaborative

When working with families, nurses will often need to collaborate with other healthcare professionals. In some cases, collaboration may include working with experts who specialize in social work, psychology, or mental health care. For families in need of counseling, financial assistance may be available. Generally, community-funded organizations offer free or discounted services. When making these recommendations, nurses should be aware of some stigmas surrounding therapy and counseling, and work to assure families of the potential benefits of these modes of care. For new or expectant parents, referral to parenting classes may be valuable. Families facing economic challenges should be made aware of community resources, including wellness clinics and food banks.

REVIEW The Concept of Family

RELATE Link the Concepts

Linking the concept of family with the concept of culture:

1. Explain how culture influences the family unit. What are three values or beliefs that could impact how a family functions?

2. What impact does stereotyping have on family? Describe at least two negative effects stereotyping can have on the family unit.

Linking the concept of family with the concept of self:

3. What are two measures that could be implemented for a teenager you suspect is suffering from anorexia nervosa?

4. While you are providing care to a family of four (two parents, two children), the parents ask for advice on helping their daughter, who they believe has become bulimic. What suggestions do you provide the parents? Explain your answers.

READY Go to Companion Skills Manual

REFER Go to Pearson Student Nursing Resources
nursing.pearsonhighered.com

- Additional review materials

REFLECT Case Study \\ Part 3

The physician requests that Mrs. Rodriguez remain at the office so that her blood pressure can be reassessed. While Mrs. Rodriguez is relaxing, you check with some of the staff and learn that a newly hired certified nurse midwife (CNM) offers a birthing class

once per week. The CNM reports that two of her clients are a lesbian couple and that they are warmly welcomed by the other clients. You also consult with two of the physicians and compile a list of three birthing centers in the area that they prefer.

Upon return to Mrs. Rodriguez's room, you reassess her blood pressure, which is now 122/82 mmHg. You provide the couple with the information you have gathered about the birthing class and the three birthing centers. Both Mrs. Rodriguez and her wife express gratitude for your compassion and efforts to assist them. Mrs. Rodriquez is scheduled to return for a follow-up appointment in 2 weeks. She reports that she has a blood pressure monitor at home and tells you she'll check her blood pressure at least once daily. Mrs. Rodriguez agrees to contact the clinic if her blood pressure is elevated or if she has any unusual changes.

Clinical Reasoning Questions Level I

1. Do you think Mrs. Rodriguez and Mrs. Marshall are wellness oriented? Explain your answer.

2. What recommendations would you provide to help Mrs. Rodriguez keep her stress level down during her pregnancy?

Clinical Reasoning Questions Level II

3. What are some of the negative effects of stress on families?

4. According to the laws of your state, when the couple in this case study has their child, who will have parental rights?

5. If Mrs. Rodriguez's blood pressure had not decreased, what interventions could have been proposed?

EXEMPLAR 26.1 Family Health Promotion

EXEMPLAR KEY TERMS
Community-based care, 1724
Health promotion, 1724

EXEMPLAR LEARNING OUTCOMES
After reading about this exemplar, you will be able to:

1. Describe the purpose and general goals of family health promotion.
2. Identify risk factors and prevention methods associated with impaired family health processes.
3. Illustrate the nursing process in application of culturally competent family health promotion strategies across the life span.
4. Formulate priority nursing diagnoses appropriate for family health promotion.
5. Summarize therapies used by interdisciplinary teams in the collaborative promotion of family health.
6. Plan evidence-based health promotion strategies for families in collaboration with other members of the healthcare team.
7. Evaluate expected outcomes related to family health promotion.

▶ OVERVIEW

The World Health Organization (2013) defines **health promotion** as a process enabling individuals to assert control over, and subsequently improve, their health. Ideally, this process leads to physical, mental, and social well-being. Health promotion also involves **community-based care**, which focuses on the political, social, institutional, and physical environments of this client. Using a community-based approach, healthcare professionals view the environment as a contributing force to an individual's overall well-being. An understanding of health promotion is essential to holistic nursing care.

Health promotion within the family unit can be challenging. In some cases, family members will respond positively to nursing suggestions and interventions; in other cases, clients may feel they are unable to change their lifestyle either due to socioeconomic conditions, stress, or other factors. Individuals also may interpret health promotion as an attempt to control their behaviors. Nurses should approach families on a case-by-case basis, recognizing that each family unit will need different forms of care and different nursing approaches.

Wellness Promotion

Actual and potential levels of wellness vary among clients, families, and communities. In addition to outward manifestations, wellness is also considered to be a state of mind. Rather than reflecting a set goal with well-defined limits, achievement of optimal wellness is an ongoing goal without limitations (Strout, 2012). The National Wellness Institute (NWI) (2013) defines wellness as "an active process through which people become aware of, and make choices toward, a more successful existence." In accordance with this definition, the NWI explains that wellness is ever evolving and includes mental and spiritual well-being, as well as lifestyle and environmental factors.

Dr. Bill Hettler (1976), cofounder of the NWI, proposed six dimensions of wellness: occupational, physical, social, intellectual, spiritual, and emotional wellness. These dimensions are all interconnected, contributing to an individual's overall well-being.

⚙ **Stay Current:** *For an in-depth discussion of the six dimensions of wellness, visit* **www.nationalwellness.org/?page=Six_Dimensions**.

When working with families, nurses should consider wellness from not only an individual perspective, but also in terms of the family unit. Family wellness promotion emphasizes addressing each individual family member's contribution to the health and well-being of the family. If one family member is experiencing difficulties, the entire family unit will be affected. For example, any number of occupational or environmental problems could alter the individual's physical and emotional wellness. A physical ailment—such as a broken leg or lead poisoning—can be treated, but if occupational (e.g., physically demanding and personally unsatisfying hard labor) and environmental (e.g., house with lead-based paint in a dangerous neighborhood) aspects are not addressed, the wellness of the individual and the family remain at risk. To complete a full wellness assessment for a family, nurses need to look at all contributing factors. Similarly, nurses need to focus on healthy members of the family, too, in order to promote higher levels of wellness.

Family wellness and health promotion strategies involve empowering clients to make beneficial changes in their lives (Strout, 2012). Some common health promotion strategies include encouraging tobacco cessation, increased exercise, healthy eating habits, and use of stress reduction techniques. Each individual will have different needs and circumstances, requiring nurses to modify health promotion suggestions. For example, consider a stay-at-home mother of three who is seeking stress relief. For this client, the nurse might suggest a community activity that promotes exercise (for stress relief) and a chance to connect with others in the community (for social wellness). Clients may decline to follow the nurse's suggestion; however, the nurse's role is to offer health- and wellness-promoting options without judgment and then allow the client to decide.

Empowering clients requires nurses to help clients set goals for their own personal wellness and the wellness of their families. The choice of goals is dependent on the family's needs, both as individual members and as a unit. One family may set the goal of participating in a family game night once a week to promote emotional, social, and intellectual wellness, whereas another family could set the goal of going hiking or biking every 2 weeks as a family to promote physical and even spiritual wellness. Nurses can help families set goals by working to understand the needs and wants of the family (Strout, 2012).

Family Developmental Stages and Tasks

The family, like the individual, has developmental stages and tasks. Each stage brings change, requiring adaptation; each new stage also brings family-related risk factors for alterations in health and wellness. The nurse must consider the client's needs both at specific developmental stages and within a family with specific developmental tasks. Family developmental stages and developmental tasks are described next; related risk factors and health problems for each stage are listed in Table 26–3 ●.

COUPLE Two people living together (with or without being married) are in a period of establishing themselves as a couple. The developmental tasks of the couple include adjusting to living together as a couple, establishing a mutually satisfying relationship, relating to kin, and deciding whether to have children (in those of childbearing age).

TABLE 26–3 Wellness Promotion for the Family at Risk for Health Alterations

DEVELOPMENTAL STAGE AND ASSOCIATED RISK FACTORS	POTENTIAL HEALTH CONSEQUENCES	WELLNESS PROMOTION STRATEGIES
Couple, or family with infants and preschoolers ■ Lack of knowledge about family planning, contraception, and sexual and marital roles ■ Inadequate prenatal care ■ Altered nutrition: inadequate nutrition, overweight, underweight ■ Smoking, alcohol/drug abuse ■ Lack of knowledge about child health and safety ■ Low socioeconomic status ■ First pregnancy before age 16 or after age 35	■ Premature pregnancy ■ Low-birth-weight infant ■ Birth defects ■ Injury to infant or child ■ Accidents	■ Promote prenatal care if applicable. ■ Provide education related to contraception and sexually transmitted infection (STI) prevention. ■ Facilitate nutritional assessment and counseling. ■ Offer referrals to appropriate resources for smoking cessation programs and alcohol/drug abuse counseling. ■ Educate about basic child health and safety protocols. ■ Identify resources for financial assistance and facilitate appropriate referrals.
Family with school-age children ■ Unsafe home environment ■ Working parents with inappropriate or inadequate resources for child care ■ Low socioeconomic status ■ Child abuse or neglect ■ Multiple, closely spaced children ■ Repeated infections, accidents, and hospitalizations ■ Unrecognized and unattended health problems ■ Poor or inappropriate nutrition ■ Toxic substances in the home	■ Behavior problems ■ Speech and vision problems ■ Learning disabilities ■ Communicable diseases ■ Physical abuse ■ Developmental delay ■ Obesity, underweight	■ Educate about preventive healthcare measures. ■ Provide information about community assistance and healthcare programs. ■ Educate about contraception. ■ Provide information about adequate nutrition.
Family with adolescents and young adults ■ Family values of aggressiveness and competition ■ Lifestyle and behaviors that lead to chronic illness (substance abuse, inadequate diet) ■ Lack of problem-solving skills ■ Conflicts between parent and children	■ Violent death and injury ■ Alcohol/drug abuse ■ Unwanted pregnancy ■ Suicide ■ STIs ■ Domestic abuse	■ Promote healthy problem-solving skills. ■ Educate about healthy anger and emotion management techniques. ■ Provide information about healthcare resources. ■ Teach about contraception. ■ Facilitate learning about substance and alcohol abuse prevention.
Family with middle adults ■ High-cholesterol diet ■ Obesity ■ Hypertension ■ Smoking, alcohol abuse ■ Physical inactivity ■ Personality patterns related to stress ■ Exposure to environment: sunlight, radiation, asbestos, or water or air pollution ■ Depression ■ Age	■ Cardiovascular disease (coronary artery disease, cerebrovascular disease) ■ Cancer ■ Accidents ■ Suicide ■ Mental illness	■ Educate about nutrition and exercise. ■ Provide information about mental health counseling and facilitate referrals. ■ Educate about healthcare options.
Family with older adults ■ Depression ■ Drug interactions ■ Chronic illness ■ Death of spouse ■ Reduced income ■ Poor nutrition ■ Lack of exercise ■ Past environmental exposure to toxins and adverse lifestyle choices	■ Impaired vision and hearing ■ Hypertension ■ Acute illness ■ Chronic illness ■ Infectious diseases (influenza, pneumonia) ■ Injuries from burns and falls ■ Depression ■ Alcohol abuse	■ Educate about nutrition and exercise. ■ Provide information about community-based programs for health care. ■ Facilitate mental health counseling.

FAMILY WITH INFANTS AND PRESCHOOLERS The family with infants or preschoolers must adjust to having and supporting the needs of more than two members, with at least one being completely dependent on the other members. Other developmental tasks of the family at this stage are developing an attachment between parents and children, adjusting to the economic costs of having more members, coping with energy depletion and lack of privacy, and carrying out activities that enhance growth and development of the children.

FAMILY WITH SCHOOL-AGE CHILDREN The family with school-age children has the developmental tasks of adjusting to the expanded world of children in school and encouraging educational achievement. A further task is promoting joint decision making between children and parents.

FAMILY WITH ADOLESCENTS AND YOUNG ADULTS The developmental tasks of the family with adolescents and young adults focus on transition. While providing a supportive home base and maintaining open communications, parents must balance freedom with responsibility and release adult children as they seek independence.

FAMILY WITH MIDDLE ADULTS The family with middle adults (in which the parents are middle aged and children are no longer at home) has the developmental tasks of maintaining ties with older and younger generations and planning for retirement. If the family consists of just the middle-aged couple, they have the developmental task of reestablishing the relationship and (if necessary) acquiring the role of grandparents.

FAMILY WITH OLDER ADULTS The older adult family has the developmental tasks of adjusting to retirement, adjusting to aging, and coping with the loss of a spouse. If a spouse dies, further tasks include adjusting to living alone or closing the family home.

Risk Factors

Individuals born into families with a history of certain diseases, such as diabetes or cardiovascular disease, are at greater risk of developing these conditions. A detailed family health history that includes genetically transmitted disorders, lifestyle, and environmental information is essential to the identification of persons and families at risk. These data are used not only to monitor the health of individual family members, but also to recommend modifications in health and lifestyle practices that potentially reduce the risk, minimize the consequences, or postpone the development of genetically related conditions as well as other factors affecting wellness.

Some family units or family members may be at risk of developing a disease by reason of gender or race. Men, for example, are at greater risk of having cardiovascular disease at an earlier age than women, and women are at greater risk of developing osteoporosis, particularly after menopause. Although it is sometimes difficult to separate genetic factors from cultural factors, certain risk factors seem to be related to race. Sickle cell disease, for example, is a hereditary disease that is more prevalent among those whose ancestral origins include Africa, South or Central America, the Caribbean, Saudi Arabia, India, and certain Mediterranean regions (National Heart, Lung, and Blood Institute, 2012a). As another example, Tay-Sachs is a neurodegenerative disease that occurs primarily in descendants of eastern European Jews (Centers for Disease Control and Prevention [CDC], 2011).

Poverty is a major problem that affects not only the family but also the community and society. Poverty is a real concern among the rising number of single-parent families. As the number of these families increases, poverty will affect a larger number of growing children. When ill, the poor are likely to put off seeking services until the illness reaches an advanced state and requires longer or more complex treatment.

Prevention

Many diseases are preventable, the effects of some diseases can be minimized, or the onset of disease can be delayed through lifestyle modifications. Lifestyle diseases include certain cancers, cardiovascular disease, adult-onset diabetes, and tooth decay. The incidence of lung cancer, for example, would be greatly reduced if individuals stopped smoking. Good nutrition, dental hygiene, and use of fluoride—in the water supply, in toothpaste, as a topical application, or as a supplement—have been shown to reduce dental decay or caries, one of America's most prevalent health problems.

The five leading chronic diseases in Americans include heart disease, cancer, stroke, diabetes, and arthritis. Among Americans, 50% of annual deaths are linked to heart disease, stroke, or cancer (CDC, 2012). Nursing health promotion measures can be powerful tools in disease prevention. For examples, nurses can educate clients about the relationship between nutrition and regular exercise and the subsequent reduced risk for developing heart disease, type 2 diabetes, and certain forms of cancer.

Modification of environmental, lifestyle, and occupational variables can help reduce the risk of stroke, arthritis, and some forms of cancer. For example, smoking cessation, avoiding occupational exposure to known carcinogens or excessive stress, and avoiding excessive alcohol consumption are all disease prevention strategies. Today, health professionals have the knowledge to prevent or minimize the effects of some of the main causes of disease, disability, and death. The challenge is to disseminate information about prevention and to motivate families to make lifestyle changes before the onset of illness.

Lifespan and Cultural Considerations

Families with members at both ends of the age continuum are at risk of developing health problems. Families entering childbearing and childrearing phases experience many changes in roles, responsibilities, and expectations. The many, often conflicting, demands on the family cause stress and fatigue, either or both of which may impede growth of individual family members and the functioning of the group as a unit. Adolescent mothers, because of their developmental level and lack of knowledge about parenthood, are more likely to develop health problems, as are single-parent families because of role overload experienced by the head of the household. Many older adults feel a lack of purpose and decreased self-esteem. These feelings can reduce their motivation to engage in health-promoting behaviors, such as exercise or community and family involvement.

▶ COLLABORATION

Wellness promotion is an essential aspect of family health and focuses on increasing healthy behaviors and optimizing lifestyle choices. Educating clients and facilitating appropriate referrals (e.g., to nutritionists, educational programs, and community service providers) will not only improve the family's quality of life, but also reduce the risk of illness. Depending on the needs of the client, nurses may collaborate with a variety of healthcare providers and professionals, including physicians, counselors, social workers, and mental health specialists.

■ NURSING PROCESS

Nursing care for families requires caring for each individual as well as for the family unit as a whole. Wellness promotion emphasizes identifying and capitalizing on individual and group strengths, while also minimizing the risks associated with alterations in health.

Assessment

In the context of wellness promotion, nursing assessment includes identifying and optimizing current positive behaviors and lifestyle choices, as well as recognizing the family's needs for disease prevention. In addition to client interviews and observation of family processes, several tools are available for completing a multifaceted family assessment that takes into consideration a number of factors, including physiological, psychosocial, spiritual, and environmental components.

Family Ecomap

An ecomap illustrates the family's relationships and interactions with the social networks in the community, enabling the nurse and other healthcare providers to visualize the family's social network. By having family members participate in preparing the ecomap, the nurse can obtain information about how the family perceives or receives social support, as well as the strength of family relationships with significant other individuals and organizations. The ecomap provides an opportunity to identify the community resources the family uses and to highlight any potential community resources that may help promote the family's health. See **Figure 26–7 ●** for a sample ecomap.

Family APGAR

The Family APGAR is a quick, five-item questionnaire that may be used as an initial screening tool for family assessment. The five family concepts measured are family adaptability, partnership, growth, affection, and resolve (**Table 26–4 ●**). This five-item questionnaire can be administered quickly to family members over 10 years of age. Ask all family members to complete a separate copy of the questionnaire to gain a picture of the family's perspective on family functioning. Be concerned if the majority of responses fall in the "hardly ever" category or if

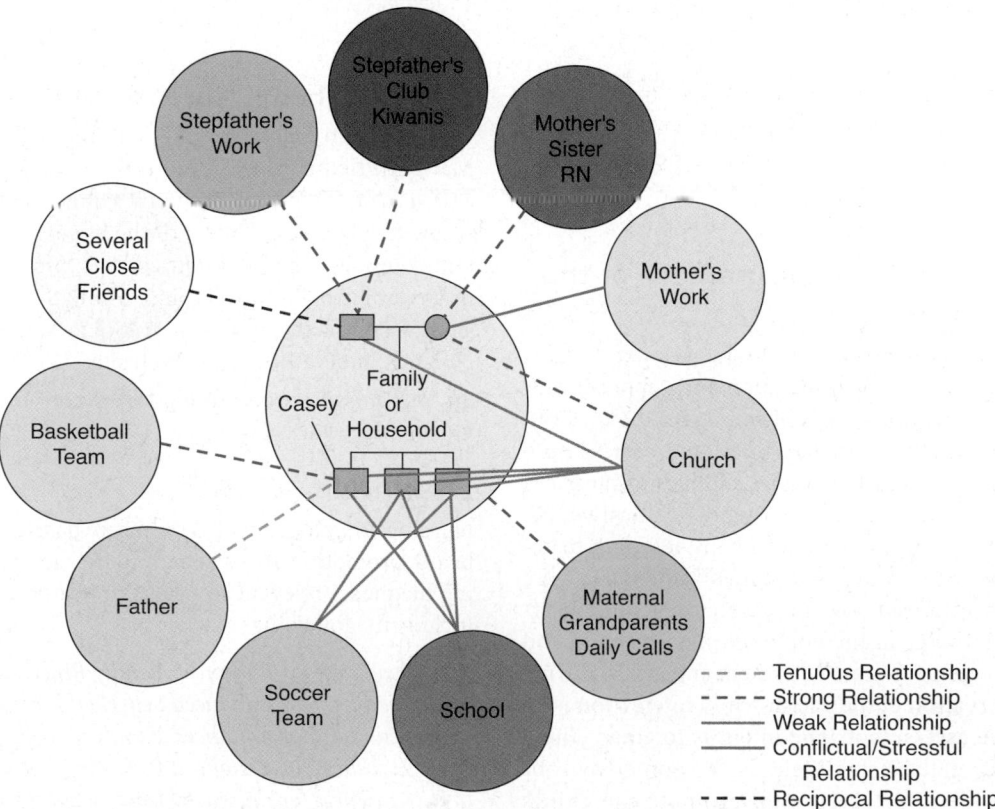

Figure 26–7 ● An ecomap illustrates one family's relationships and interactions with groups and individuals in the immediate external environment.

TABLE 26–4 The Family APGAR Questionnaire

Directions: The following questions have been designed to help us better understand you and your family. You should feel free to ask questions about any item in the questionnaire. The space for comments should be used when you wish to give additional information or if you wish to discuss how the question is applied to your family. Please try to answer all questions. Family is defined as the individual(s) with whom you usually live. If you live alone, your "family" consists of persons with whom you now have the strongest emotional ties.*
For each question, check only one box.

	ALMOST ALWAYS 2	SOME OF THE TIME 1	HARDLY EVER 0
I am satisfied that I can turn to my family for help when something is troubling me. Comments: _____			
I am satisfied with the way my family talks over things with me and shares problems with me. Comments: _____			
I am satisfied that my family accepts and supports my wishes to take on new activities or directions. Comments: _____			
I am satisfied with the way my family expresses affection and responds to my emotions, such as anger, sorrow, and love. Comments: _____			
I am satisfied with the way my family and I share time together. Comments: _____			

**Note:* Depending on which member of the family is being interviewed, the interviewer may substitute for the word *family* either *spouse, significant other, parents,* or *children.* Responses are scored 2, 1, 0 and totaled. The total score ranges from 0 to 10. The larger the score, the greater amount of satisfaction that family member has with family functioning.

Source: Adapted from Smilkstein, G. (1978). The family APGAR: A proposal for a family function test and its use by physicians. *Journal of Family Practice, 6,* 1231–1239.

responses vary a lot among family members. This may indicate a family that needs much more support to cope with the demands of daily life and provide insight into health maintenance and health promotion needs.

Home Observation for Measurement of the Environment (HOME)

The HOME Inventory is an assessment tool developed to measure the quality and quantity of stimulation and support available in the home environment (Caldwell & Bradley, 1984). Four age-specific scales are available (birth to 3 years, 3 to 6 years, 6 to 10 years, and 10 to 15 years). Examples of subscales within each age-specific scale are parental responsiveness, acceptance of child, the physical environment, learning materials, variety in experience, and parental involvement. Data are collected during an informal, low-stress interview and observation over 45–90 minutes in the home setting. The child and his or her primary caregiver must be present and awake during the interview. Observation of the parent–child interaction is an essential part of the assessment. The intent is to allow family members to act normally. Assessment of the home environment will help to identify factors that promote the child's growth and development. Nursing interventions that could result from the HOME assessment include recommending items that can be used in the home for toys and suggesting strategies for interacting with the child to promote learning.

Friedman Family Assessment Tool

The Friedman Family Assessment Tool (FFAM), developed by Marilyn Friedman, was designed to assist nurses with family assessment. This tool provides a method for examining the whole family in the context of the larger community where the family resides. The interview collects information about a family's relationships, functioning, strengths, and problems. The short form for this assessment tool is available at the Pearson Nursing Student Resources Web site.

❈ *Visit* **nursing.pearsonhighered.com** *to see the Friedman Family Assessment Tool.*

Diagnosis

Nursing diagnoses will be chosen based on which areas of health promotion are of benefit to the family. Examples of nursing diagnoses relevant to health promotion for the family unit include the following:

- *Readiness for Enhanced Family Processes*
- *Readiness for Enhanced Self-Health Management*
- *Readiness for Enhanced Family Coping*
- *Readiness for Enhanced Parenting*
- *Readiness for Enhanced Immunization Status*
- *Readiness for Enhanced Knowledge*
- *Readiness for Enhanced Communication*
- *Readiness for Enhanced Decision Making.*

(NANDA-I © 2012)

Planning

Families need support to increase their resources and coping behaviors so they can successfully manage the multiple stressors, strains, and challenges of daily living.

The nurse working with a family to develop a care plan identifies potential resources in the community that match the child's and the family's needs for support. The nurse will collaborate with the family to discuss those resources and to select the ones that are acceptable to the family, to increase the likelihood that the family will follow through with the plan. In some cases it may be necessary to collaborate with a multidisciplinary team, including social workers, to help the family obtain assistance to overcome, for example, transportation or financial problems or any others that interfere with the child's health care. The nurse should make sure the family has a care coordinator, especially when a family member initially seems unable to assume the case management role. The nurse may also assist the family in obtaining resources by such actions as role rehearsal, providing instructions and support when making an initial call, or connecting with another family support person who can help with resource linkage. The nurse will refer families with moderate or severe dysfunction to community resources for social support and counseling as appropriate.

Outcomes are determined based on the needs of the family and may include any of the following:

- Children will achieve developmental milestones in social, self-regulatory behavior or cognitive, language, or gross or fine motor skills.
- Family will display or describe actions to manage stressors that tax family resources.
- Family will meet the needs of its members during developmental transitions.
- Family members will demonstrate actions to improve the overall health and social competence of the family unit.

Implementation

Establishing a therapeutic relationship with the family is an important intervention in and of itself. This relationship should be characterized by empathy and trust, as well as the development of mutually identified goals for the family's needs. To help families develop resiliency, the nurse should focus on family competence and strengths, and acknowledge and validate their emotions. The nurse provides information in a clear, timely, and sensitive manner. Questions are asked to help direct the family's thinking rather than providing them with all of the answers. The nurse works with families by teaching them to identify solutions until they are able to problem solve independently. The family's ethnic and religious background needs to be considered in developing intervention recommendations.

Evaluation

Evaluation is based on the family's progress toward goals and outcomes mutually determined by the family and nurse. Although evaluation depends on the nursing diagnoses and identified outcomes specific to a given family, the following indicators are general examples of achieved outcomes:

- Parents report enhanced understanding and achievement of parental tasks.
- Family members demonstrate more frequent engagement in activities that involve the entire family unit.
- Each family member is up to date with all vaccinations.
- Individual family members report a decrease in or cessation of behaviors associated with adverse health conditions and disease, such as smoking, excessive drinking, and maintaining a sedentary lifestyle.
- Family members' behaviors collectively demonstrate cohesion, strength, and emotional bonding.
- The family demonstrates the capacity to successfully adapt and function competently after adversity or crisis.

NURSING CARE PLAN — A Single-Parent Family With Childcare Issues

ASSESSMENT	DIAGNOSES	PLANNING
Ms. Wilson, a newly divorced single mother, brings her 3-year-old son in for routine immunizations. After he has received his immunizations, while waiting the required 20 minutes before leaving, Ms. Wilson reveals that she recently lost her job because her company was bought by another. She says that she has found a new job, and that the salary is much higher, but the only available shift is from midnight to 7:00 a.m. She asks if there are any certified childcare providers who provide services during nighttime hours. She notes that her parents have offered to keep her son while she is at work, but she is worried about burdening her parents and being viewed as incapable of taking care of her child independently.	■ *Readiness for Enhanced Immunization Status* ■ *Readiness for Enhanced Parenting* ■ *Readiness for Enhanced Knowledge* ■ *Readiness for Enhanced Decision Making* (NANDA-I © 2012)	■ Ms. Wilson will be able to state the risks related to leaving a child home alone. ■ Ms. Wilson will learn of other resources available to help her care for her child in a safe environment. ■ Ms. Wilson will discuss available choices she has without risking her child's safety.

IMPLEMENTATION

- Explore client's reluctance to accept her parents' offer to assist her.
- Assist with identifying additional sources of support, including support groups and classes geared toward meeting the needs of single parents.
- Reinforce and support the client's concern for her child's well-being, including his physiological and psychosocial wellness.
- Provide referrals to social services to help meet financial needs.
- Encourage and support client's desire to be financially self-sufficient.
- Assess client's knowledge of pediatric vaccination schedules and provide appropriate teaching, including in written form.

(continued on next page)

NURSING CARE PLAN *(continued)*

EVALUATION

Ms. Wilson agrees to explore the option of accepting her parents' offer to care for her child while she is at work. She also agrees to attend classes designed to educate and assist individuals with overcoming challenges that accompany single parenting.

CRITICAL THINKING

1. Is the nursing diagnosis of Readiness for Enhanced Parenting *appropriate? Why or why not?*
2. In what ways might Ms. Wilson's recent divorce have affected her family's level of wellness?
3. How might Ms. Wilson's fear of appearing dependent negatively impact her level of personal and family wellness?

REVIEW Family Health Promotion

RELATE Link the Concepts and Exemplars

Linking the exemplar of family health promotion with the concept of culture:

1. How does the nurse incorporate the family's cultural beliefs into health promotion teaching?
2. How might the family's cultural beliefs impact their health behaviors?

Linking the exemplar of family health promotion with the concept of advocacy:

3. How can the nurse advocate for families from vulnerable populations in the community?
4. What responsibilities does the nurse have to advocate for families?

REFER Go to Pearson Nursing Student Resources
nursing.pearsonhighered.com

- Additional review materials
- The Friedman Family Assessment Tool

REFLECT Case Study

The home health nurse has been visiting a 90-year-old woman and her younger sister who live alone in a large farmhouse. The women have been active in caring for each other and their residence. During one of the home visits, they confide that the farm is too much for them, but they admit that they do not want to tell their families because they are afraid that they will be put into a nursing home.

1. What community resources are available to assist the sisters to live independently?
2. How should the family be involved in the decision making?
3. What signs can alert the nurse that the sisters are unable to care for themselves?
4. Should the nurse contact the family without the sisters' knowledge? Why or why not?

EXEMPLAR 26.2 Family Response to Health Alterations

EXEMPLAR KEY TERMS
Family burden, *1731*
Family recovery, *1732*
Family support, *1732*
Friend support, *1732*
Objective family burden, *1731*
Professional support, *1732*
Spiritual support, *1732*
Stigma, *1732*
Subjective family burden, *1732*

EXEMPLAR LEARNING OUTCOMES
After reading about this exemplar, you will be able to:

1. Describe the factors that influence a family's response to health alterations.

2. Identify risk factors and prevention methods associated with a family's response to health alterations.
3. Illustrate the nursing process in providing culturally competent care across the life span to families responding to health alterations.
4. Formulate priority nursing diagnoses appropriate for a family's response to health alterations.
5. Summarize therapies used by interdisciplinary teams in the collaborative care of a family responding to health alterations.
6. Plan evidence-based care for a family responding to health alterations in collaboration with other members of the healthcare team.
7. Evaluate expected outcomes for a family responding to health alterations.

▶ OVERVIEW

Although some clients are totally alone in the world, most have one or more people who are significant in their lives. These significant others may be related or bonded to the client by birth, adoption, marriage, or friendship. Although not always meeting traditional definitions, people (or even pets) significant to the client are the client's family. The nurse includes the family as an integral component of care in all healthcare settings.

▶ THE IMPACT OF ILLNESS ON THE FAMILY SYSTEM

Illness of a family member is a crisis that affects the entire family system. The family is disrupted as members abandon their usual activities and focus their energy on restoring family equilibrium. Roles and responsibilities of the ill family member are delegated to other family members, or those functions remain undone for the duration of the illness. Family members experi-

Box 26–5 Factors Determining the Impact of Illness on the Family

- The nature of the illness, which can range from minor to life threatening
- The duration of the illness
- The residual effects of the illness, ranging from none to permanent disability
- The meaning of the illness to the family and its significance to family systems
- The financial impact of the illness, which is influenced by factors such as insurance and ability of the ill family member to return to work
- The effect of the illness on future family functioning (for instance, previous patterns may be restored or new patterns may be established).

ence anxiety about the sick individual and the resolution of the illness. This anxiety is compounded by additional responsibilities that leave less time or motivation to complete the normal tasks of daily living. See **Box 26–5** ● for some factors that determine the impact of illness on the family unit.

The family's ability to deal with the stress of illness depends on the members' coping skills. Families with good communication skills are better able to discuss how they feel about the illness and how it affects family functioning. They can plan for the future and are flexible in adapting these plans as the situation changes. An established social support network provides strength, encouragement, and services to the family during the illness. During health crises, families must realize that turning to others for support is a sign of strength rather than weakness. Nurses can be part of the support system for families, or they can identify other sources of support in the community.

During a crisis, families are often drawn together by a common purpose. In this time of closeness, family members have the opportunity to reaffirm personal and family values and their commitment to one another. Indeed, illness may provide a unique opportunity for family growth.

Nurses committed to family-centered care involve both the client and the client's family in the nursing process. Through their interaction with families, nurses can give support and information, although the client needs to give permission regarding what information can be shared with family members. Nurses make sure that not only the client but also each family member understands the disease, its management, and the effect of these two factors on family functioning.

Chronic Illness and the Family

The client with a chronic illness may be hospitalized when he or she experiences acute exacerbations, but the care of the client is primarily and usually provided at home. Chronic illness in a family member is a major stressor that may cause changes in family structure and function, as well as in how family developmental tasks are performed.

Many different factors affect family responses to chronic illness; family responses in turn affect the client's response to and perception of the illness. Factors influencing response to chronic illness include personal, social, and economic resources; the nature and course of the disease; and demands of the illness

as perceived by family members. Clients with chronic illness, and their families, may be at risk for depression. Nursing considerations for a client with a chronic illness include being alert to symptoms of depression, both in the client and in his or her close family members.

Severe Mental Illness and the Family

Family members of individuals with mental illness often share in the many losses that accompany the illness. Families are the major source of support and rehabilitation for their loved ones. In the United States, care for individuals with mental illness has become as much family based as community based. Caring for a family member with a mental illness can result in overwhelming emotional and economic stress on the family system, particularly if caregiver strain becomes a contributing factor. Symptoms associated with severe mental illness can significantly impair daily functioning, requiring a great deal of time and energy from family members who live with or care for the individual. Thus, it is common for the individual with severe mental illness to become a large focus within the family dynamic, causing other members of the family to feel neglected or even ignored. In some situations this can cause a strain on the family unit as a whole (Mental Health America, 2013).

FAMILY BURDEN Families have important needs of their own in response to their loved one's mental illness. Severe and persistent mental illness often puts the family under catastrophic levels of stress. As families respond to the grief and trauma, they need empathy and support from healthcare professionals.

Family burden is the overall level of distress experienced as a result of the mental illness. The **objective family burden** is related to the actual, identifiable family problems associated with the individual's mental illness. One burden the family must manage relates to *symptomatic behaviors*. The deficit behaviors of the individual with a mental illness—such as lack of motivation, difficulty in completing tasks, isolation from others, inability to manage money, poor grooming and personal care, and poor eating and sleeping behavior—can be of great concern to families. Intrusive or acting-out behaviors—such as lack of consideration for others, excessive arguing, conflicts with neighbors and friends, damaging material possessions, inappropriate sexual behavior, suicide attempts, substance abuse, and violent outbursts—are very disturbing to family members. These behaviors may be more episodic than the deficit behaviors but may have more severe immediate consequences. This family burden may lead to loss of independence and increased responsibility as families try to cope with day-to-day living. This burden includes disruption in household functioning, restriction of social activities, and financial hardship due to medical bills and the cost of their loved one's economic burden.

Another objective burden related to family problems is caregiving. Families may find that community services are not always available and not always satisfactory. Inadequate funding results in lack of treatment programs and lack of services for families themselves. Families also find themselves negotiating with the legal and criminal justice system. With few long-term psychiatric facilities available, many people who would have previously been cared for in state hospitals now find themselves in jails and prisons. Often, the "crimes" with which they are charged are misdemeanors resulting from their symptoms of mental illness, such as disorderly conduct, trespassing, and drunkenness.

A third objective burden that families must cope with is the burden of **stigma**, which is a collection of negative attitudes and beliefs that lead people to fear, reject, avoid, and discriminate against people with mental illness. In response to stigma, individuals with mental disorders internalize these attitudes and become ashamed of themselves and their illness. They continue to be ostracized from mainstream society. Families may become isolated as they avoid others who misunderstand the illness. When a family member has cancer or heart disease, others respond with kindness. When a family member has a mental disorder, the response is often avoidance because there is a perception of unpredictability and danger. Thus, stigma severely limits support from extended family and friends. As they and their loved one face multiple discriminations, families may feel isolated and shameful, may lose self-esteem, and may run the risk of self-stigmatization (Mayo Clinic, 2011; Mental Health America, 2013).

The **subjective family burden** is defined as the psychological distress of the family members in relation to the objective burden. They often experience frustration, anxiety, depression, hopelessness, and helplessness. Families also experience intense feelings of grief and loss. They must mourn for the person they knew before the onset of the illness and the potential loss of hopes, dreams, and expectations. They live with a sense of chronic sorrow for those loved ones who experience periods of remission and relapse. There is also a sense of empathetic pain as they watch their family member become a victim of the illness. Living with and caring for an individual with mental illness can have a tremendous impact on the family. Some families cope fairly well, whereas others are easily exhausted and give up (Corrigan et al., 2009). See **Box 26–6** ● for descriptions of the language of family pain.

FAMILY RECOVERY   Family response to the mental illness of a family member can vary depending on what stage the family (or members of a family) is in. Family response, formally known as "**family recovery**" to mental illness within the family, has three pronounced stages. A nurse may adjust his or her approach toward caring interventions for a family depending on the family's stage of recovery.

Box 26–6   The Language of Family Pain

Catastrophe. Watching as your loved one slips away. This is like a horror movie in which the hero/heroine (loved one) is utterly transformed by some unseen, monstrous force.

Torture. The agony of watching a loved one experience relentless pain and suffering without being able to make it stop. The absolute panic when he or she refuses your assistance, rejects your help, resists your protection at the time when it is most needed.

Anguish. The pain of having loved ones turn on those who are trying to help them, attack them angrily, or blame them for their difficulties.

Horror/fear. A dread that the ill person will do something terrible to him- or herself or others.

Nightmare. Rejection, labeling, and ostracism by the mental health system when we are trying to help.

Source: Reprinted with permission from NAMI (2013). *NAMI Provider Education program.* Arlington, VA: National Alliance for the Mentally Ill.

Stage 1 of family recovery involves discovery and denial. Family members are often the first to notice that another member is exhibiting unusual behavior. The family's initial response may range from minimizing ("It's not so serious") to denial ("It's just a phase"). This response is a temporary, rather than maladaptive, reaction to avoid a painful reality.

Stage 2 of family recovery involves recognition and acceptance. As it becomes more evident that a significant problem exists, families begin to search for reasons and solutions by gathering available information. Families start to develop their own image of the disease process and expectations of mental health professionals.

Stage 3 of family recovery involves coping and competence. This includes the day-to-day efforts necessary to cope with all the changes in the family. When people become persistently and severely mentally ill, they may have difficulty carrying out their family roles and responsibilities. In this case, other family members must assume those roles and come to terms with an altered family lifestyle. Family members develop cognitive, emotional, and behavioral coping strategies for living with their loved one who is experiencing a mental disorder. As they take stock of the challenges, constraints, and resources, they are better able to make the most of their options.

Coping strategies protect the affected family member and maintain the stability of family functioning. These strategies include expressing affection, suggesting alternatives, reducing conflict, seeking social support, and trying to make the best of the family members' experiences by focusing on the positive parts of the relationship with the ill family member.

Individuals seek out four main types of support when working through trying situations: professional support, friend support, family support, and spiritual support. **Professional support** may come from any one or a number of professionals in the community who exhibit a nonblaming and respectful attitude toward families, and who provide information on how to respond to symptoms and help in locating community resources, such as housing or vocational training. **Friend support** comes from non–family members, such as close friends and coworkers. Friend support is most valued when the concern is genuine and stigma is minimized. **Family support** often comes in the form of tangible assistance, such as respite care for family members and physical presence in times of crisis. Many families find emotional strength from their religious faith. They find **spiritual support** as they search for meaning through relationships and feeling connected with others. Supportive relationships build and sustain courage, helping families make the best of their difficult lives.

When families learn to cope effectively, the intense focus on the ill family member lightens as other members, moving through the adjustment process, begin to focus on caring for themselves and reconnecting with others outside the family. The family adapts to its changed circumstances and continues to function successfully.

The final stage of family recovery is personal and political advocacy. This stage involves working with the mental health system to obtain treatment. Family members want to be seen as partners in treatment and do not want to be excluded from discussions and treatment recommendations. Ideally, professionals, clients, and families all work together in joint problem solving. At times, the issue of client confidentiality is raised. Family members generally respect confidentiality but do need information about treatments, medications, resources, and ways to cope with certain behaviors.

Some families go on to educate the public about mental illness and lobby for improved public policy and legislation, often through the National Alliance on Mental Illness (NAMI), an organization composed of clients, families, and professionals. NAMI actively lobbies for improved legislation and improved healthcare benefits at local, state, and federal levels.

Pediatric Illness and the Family

Collaborating with families in providing health care is essential to promoting the best outcome when caring for children. Families have important knowledge to share about their child, their child's health condition, and how their child responds to various actions and events. They also need access to information that will make it possible for them to fully participate in planning and decision making.

Family-centered care is a philosophy of health care in which a mutually beneficial partnership develops between families, the nurse, and other health professionals as appropriate. In this way the priorities and needs of the family are addressed when the family seeks health care for the child. Each party respects the knowledge, skills, and experience that the other brings to the healthcare encounter (Table 26–5 ●). This contrasts family-focused care, in which health professionals provide care from the position of an expert. In family-focused care, the expert health professional directs care, tells the family what to do, and intervenes for the child and family as a unit.

TABLE 26–5 Elements of Family-Centered Care and Recommendations for Nursing Practice

ELEMENTS	NURSING PRACTICE RECOMMENDATIONS
Family at the center: ■ Incorporate into policy and practice the recognition that the family is the constant in a child's life, while the service systems and support personnel within those systems fluctuate, and that the illness or injury of a child affects all members of the family system.	■ Establish a therapeutic relationship with the family. ■ Perform a comprehensive family assessment in collaboration with the family, identifying both strengths and needs. ■ Use the family assessment when working with the family to plan, implement, and evaluate care, considering the impact of the child's illness or injury on the entire family, with special attention to the siblings. ■ Provide siblings with information about their sibling's illness/injury at an appropriate developmental level and answer questions honestly. ■ Promote sibling visitation in hospital settings and participation in home care activities. ■ Identify extended family members who should receive information and be included in the educational process.
Family–professional collaboration: ■ Facilitate family professional collaboration at all levels of hospital, home, and community care for the following: ■ Care of an individual child ■ Program development, implementation, evaluation, and evolution ■ Policy formation.	■ Develop provider–family relationships that are guided by the goals and expectations of both the family and the provider. ■ Ensure that parents are integral and critical collaborators in the decision-making process about their child's care. Involve children and adolescents in the decision-making process as appropriate for their cognitive and emotional development. ■ Assure parents 24-hour access to their child and facilitate their participation in the child's care. ■ Provide parents with the option to stay with their child during procedures and tests, and provide ways for parents to support the child during the procedure. ■ Provide comfort and hygiene facilities for families who spend long hours at the facility or travel great distances. ■ Promote the family's development of expertise in the special care of their child, fostering family independence and empowerment. ■ Incorporate parents and children into the quality assessment/improvement process. ■ Integrate family members into institutional and community advisory groups and involve them in policy development.
Family–professional communication: ■ Exchange complete and unbiased information between families and professionals in a supportive manner at all times.	■ Provide information about the child's problem, prognosis, and needs in a manner that respects the child and family as individuals and promotes two-way dialogue. ■ Encourage the family to share information about the child and the illness/injury so that care planning and decisions are made in the most informed and collaborative manner.
Cultural diversity of families: ■ Incorporate into policy and practice the recognition and honoring of cultural diversity, strengths, and individuality within and across all families, including ethnic, racial, gender, spiritual, social, economic, educational, and geographic diversity.	■ Practice family-centered care in a culturally competent manner with respect and sensitivity for the wide range of families with diverse values and beliefs. ■ Seek to understand the family's beliefs and practices related to race, culture, gender, and ethnicity when developing relationships and collaborating in the child's health care. ■ Seek to understand and respect the family's religious/spiritual beliefs and practices and integrate these into the child's care, as the family desires. ■ Assist the family to address care issues related to socioeconomic status, insurance status, geography, and access to health care. ■ Integrate training programs on diversity, cultural understanding, and culturally competent care into staff development programs.

(continued on next page)

TABLE 26–5 Elements of Family-Centered Care and Recommendations for Nursing Practice (*continued*)

ELEMENTS	NURSING PRACTICE RECOMMENDATIONS
Coping differences and support: ■ Recognize and respect different methods of coping. Implement comprehensive policies and programs that provide families with the developmental, educational, emotional, spiritual, environmental, and financial support needed to meet their diverse needs.	■ Assess the strengths and weaknesses of the family's coping strategies and its resiliency factors and characteristics. Identify maladaptive coping mechanisms and assist the family to augment its coping efforts. ■ Assess and support the family's needs and desires for support and assist the family in accessing and accepting assistance from support networks as needed or desired.
Family-centered peer support: ■ Encourage and facilitate family-to-family support and networking.	■ Educate parents about parent-to-parent and family support resources and assist them to access such resources in the institution and community. ■ Provide access to psychoeducational groups that might be useful to parents, siblings, or ill/injured children.
Specialized service and support systems: ■ Ensure that hospital, home, and community service and support systems for children needing specialized health and developmental care and their families are flexible, accessible, and comprehensive in responding to diverse family-identified needs.	■ Provide collaborative, flexible, accessible, comprehensive, and coordinated services to children and their families. ■ Provide comprehensive case management/care coordination for children and families with ongoing care needs. ■ Along with families, take an active role in advocating for the needs of ill and injured children.
Holistic perspective of family-centered care: ■ Appreciate families as families and children as children, recognizing that they possess a wider range of strengths, concerns, emotions, and aspirations beyond their need for specialized health and developmental services and support.	■ Encourage attention to the normal developmental needs and developmental tasks of the entire family unit and individual family members. ■ Encourage and facilitate the development of individual and family identities beyond a focus on illness or injury. ■ Facilitate "normalization" as valued and desired by the family.

Source: Reprinted with permission from NAMI (2013). *NAMI Provider Education program.* Arlington, VA: National Alliance for the Mentally Ill.

Parents often need to assess their strengths in managing their ongoing family and caregiving responsibilities before planning how to add more caregiving responsibilities to their routine. Individuals who become family caregivers are at risk for considerable strain and stress, especially if they are unable to balance their own needs with those of the child. Nurses should be aware of the possibility of caregiver strain (APA, 2013). The nurse and parents should also collaborate in developing the plan for the child's care, so as not to conflict with the family's cultural and ethnic illness-related behaviors, experiences, and beliefs. The child's opinions should also be integrated in the strategies for care. In almost all cases, the child leaves the healthcare setting and the family assumes responsibility for providing needed care in the home. The family caregivers must not feel alienated from a healthcare system they need for continuing assistance. See **Box 26–7** ● for guidelines for effective collaboration.

Family involvement is also valuable in the development of policies and guidelines for family-centered care in all types of healthcare settings. A family's experiences while receiving care may reveal valuable insights, perspectives, and realities that could lead to improved quality of care and satisfaction with care. Feedback could be provided on such issues as how comfortable they felt in the setting, their understanding of information provided to them, and the attitudes they sensed from health professionals. Parents who have been supported in developing leadership skills can be empowered to serve on advisory boards or councils representing the family and community perspectives (Warren, 2012).

Box 26–7 Guidelines for Effective Parent–Provider Collaboration

Parents have a role in developing an effective collaborative relationship with nurses and other health professionals. Parents often become experts in their child's health condition, and learn to advocate for their child. They also must learn to communicate effectively with the health professionals caring for their child, and in the process develop a trusting relationship.

Tips for parents for improved communication are as follows:

■ Keep a journal that includes your observations about your child's behavior, eating habits, illness, temperature, or anything else that might be helpful to the healthcare providers caring for your child.

■ Keep a copy of your child's medical records, including test and procedure results.

■ Write out questions and do not hesitate to ask for clarification if you do not understand an answer provided.

■ Be realistic about what you can expect from your child's nurses and doctors. They may not have all of the answers to your questions right away, but if you give them time they will answer your questions. Try to let your healthcare providers know you appreciate their time and efforts on behalf of your child (Dowshen, 2013).

Communication tips for nurses include the following:

■ Provide information and honestly discuss issues of concern to both the family and healthcare providers.

■ Engage in creative problem solving and identify options for needed care that conform to the family's values and functioning.

■ Demonstrate respect for the family's choices and methods for providing needed care.

■ Continue to collaborate with the child and family and be willing to continue problem solving as new issues arise.

When working to establish a family-centered relationship with families of various ethnic groups, consider the possibility that an extended family may need to be consulted. For example, Native Americans may consult tribal elders (considered part of the extended family) before agreeing to health care for their child. In some Hispanic cultures, major decisions for the child's health care are made with input from grandparents and other extended family members. The nurse should strive to learn more about the strengths of the family network to better assist the family in planning the child's care at home (K. Walsh, 2011).

Some healthcare facilities are developing family resource centers to provide consumer information and support. In most cases, the resource center is a consumer-oriented health library with staffing, but peer support services may be coordinated through the center as well (Institute for Family Centered Care, 2011). Families can be supported in accessing useful information that helps them become informed decision makers about their child's care. Resources can often be provided in the preferred language and at an appropriate reading level.

When providing care to children, be aware that the family is central to all healthcare interventions with parents and child as the partners in care. It is important to consider how a healthcare setting's written policies, procedures, and literature for families refer to families and what attitudes these materials convey. Words like *policies*, *allowed*, and *not permitted* imply that hospital personnel have authority over families in matters concerning their children. Words like *guidelines*, *working together*, and *welcome* communicate an openness and appreciation for families in the care of their children.

Risk Factors

The physical or mental illness of one family member places the entire family unit at risk for alterations in function. Among families, coping with illness may lead to family disputes, financial difficulties, and caregiver strain, as well as a number of other challenges. Financial challenges associated with illness are multifactorial; however, two common sources include medical bills and a member of the family leaving employment to help take care of another family member. Illness alone adds a considerable amount of stress to each family member's life—financial strains further compound the stress (Wadsworth & Rienks, 2012). High stress levels, especially among family caregivers, have been linked to health problems and an increased risk for premature mortality. Similarly, for the caregiver, impaired or inadequate coping function may lead to unhealthy choices, such as using tobacco and/or alcohol to manage stress levels (APA, 2013).

Prevention

Families who are made aware of the challenges associated with illness early in the process may benefit from having additional time to consider and plan for some of the upcoming circum-

stances. Successful coping with caregiver and family challenges comes as a result of accepting the illness, whether it is temporary or chronic, and then working to keep the family unit healthy. Talking about the illness as a family can be extremely beneficial, as can family counseling. Family support for one another is essential to get through this difficult time (Mental Health America, 2013). Nurses can help families by advising them of the challenges they will face and connecting them with the appropriate supportive resources, including counselors and sources of financial assistance as indicated.

▶ CLINICAL MANIFESTATIONS

Each family's reaction to a particular illness will vary based on their previous experiences, personal opinions, and cultural influences. Nurses must be alert to manifestations that signal the family is having difficulty coping with managing the illness and be able to respond appropriately to help family members improve their coping skills and access helpful resources (see the Clinical Manifestations and Therapies feature). Primary caregivers may benefit from education about techniques to relieve stress, participation in support groups, and respite care.

▶ COLLABORATION

Interventions vary based on the identified risks and actual or potential alterations in health. Nurses may collaborate with various healthcare professionals during the course of caring for the client and family, including social workers, grief counselors, psychiatrists, physicians, pediatricians, surgeons, and pharmacists. Nurses also need to understand the importance of collaborating with parents. Nurses working with pediatric clients may collaborate with the school nurse, homebound teacher, guidance counselors, and other professionals. Collaboration with parents is key, because they often are the experts not only on their child but also on their child's illness, making them an extremely valuable member of the healthcare team.

▶ NURSING PROCESS

Nurses assess both the family and the client when one family member is experiencing health problems. Families should be assessed for coping abilities, as well as possible complications that can arise from stress as a result of the family member's illness. Data from assessment of the client and family will determine priorities for care.

Assessment

Assessment of the family facing challenges related to illness leads to the identification of family strengths and weaknesses. When indicated, the nurse also assesses the family's readiness and ability to provide continued care and supervision at home. Key components to consider when performing any family assessment and developing a client's plan of care include the following:

- Cohesiveness and communication patterns within the family
- Family interactions that support self-care
- Number of friends and relatives available

Clinical Manifestations and Therapies **Family Stressors**

ETIOLOGY (PRIMARY STRESSOR)	CLINICAL MANIFESTATIONS	CLINICAL THERAPIES
Chronic illness in the family	■ Increased stress resulting in weight loss or gain, headaches, and anxiety ■ Lifestyle changes (e.g., job loss and financial difficulties) ■ Depression as evidenced by fatigue, lack of enjoyment, loss of interest in regular activities ■ Decreased participation in social activities; withdrawal ■ Unhealthy coping mechanisms (e.g., smoking, alcohol use, substance use)	■ Teach about healthy forms of stress management. ■ Provide resources for family counseling. ■ Educate about healthy eating habits to reduce risk for further illness and increase nutrition. ■ Discuss the benefits of exercise for stress relief and health.
Mental illness in the family	■ Confusion over changes occurring within the family unit ■ Stress related to helping the family member suffering from mental illness (possibly financial stress) ■ Anxiety ■ Depression ■ Feelings of loss related to changes in family member's behavior ■ Fear over the changes that are occurring ■ Changes in social activities, often resulting in decreased socialization	■ Educate about the benefits of counseling for the family to help with the changes that are occurring. ■ Advise about healthy stress management techniques. ■ Provide resources for support groups involving other families in similar circumstances. ■ Educate about the realities of the mental illness to dispel any misinformation and/or stigmas.
Illness of a child	■ Fear of death of the child ■ Anxiety, stress, depression in accordance with the child's illness and its effect on the parents and family ■ Decreased job performance, job loss and financial difficulties resulting from taking the child to doctor appointments or spending time in the hospital ■ Confusion and anger resulting from a lack of control over the child's illness and health	■ Promote awareness of available counseling services. ■ Emphasize the importance of healthy eating habits and exercise. ■ Advise the primary caregivers to take time for themselves to avoid burnout. ■ Teach about healthy coping mechanisms and stress management. ■ Answer any questions the parents may have about their child's illness.

■ Family values and beliefs about health and illness
■ Cultural and spiritual beliefs
■ Developmental level of the client and family.

Nursing assessment requires obtaining a complete family history, including genetic influences that may impact health. A family genogram (see Figure 26–5) may be helpful in collecting information, as detailed health histories should incorporate data regarding the client's parents, siblings, grandparents, and even great-grandparents if information is available. If aunts, uncles, or cousins have had any health concerns, these should be noted as well. When assessing a family's history of mental illness, nurses should be aware that many individuals—especially from older generations—might not have volunteered knowledge about their mental illness. As such, the client may not know that a grandparent was diagnosed with a mental illness. Clients who were adopted and have no information about their birth parents will have no genetic health history to report, but information can be gathered about their health and environmental conditions during childhood, such as exposure to secondhand smoke, dietary patterns, or childhood illnesses.

Nurses must also focus attention on the family, both as the context for the individual and as the unit of care. It is important to assess and involve families because they are in a position to be affected by and to influence the course of a client's illness. Clients, families, and nurses collaborate to identify the family's strengths, resources, and social support and try to identify problems that might cause stress for any of the family members. Factors in assessing clients and their families include family communication, conflict resolution, boundaries, cohesion, flexibility, emotional availability, leadership patterns, and overall family functionality.

Diagnosis

Data gathered during a family assessment may lead to the following nursing diagnoses:

- *Interrupted Family Processes*
- *Readiness for Enhanced Family Coping*
- *Disabled Family Coping*
- *Impaired Parenting*
- *Impaired Home Maintenance*
- *Caregiver Role Strain.*

(NANDA-I © 2012)

Planning

Being sensitive to cultural differences is important in assessment and planning care. The nurse should determine who makes most of the decisions in the family, especially healthcare decisions, so he knows whom to obtain information from and whom to instruct. The extended family unit is found in many cultures, and different health beliefs and health practices may exist within the family. Building a trusting relationship with these families by talking with them about their beliefs and practices is the first step toward planning more effective care.

Nursing care includes assisting the family with planning realistic goals/outcomes and strategies that enhance family functioning, such as improving communication skills, identifying and utilizing support systems, and developing and rehearsing parenting skills. Anticipatory guidance may assist well-functioning families in preparing for predictable developmental transitions that occur in the life of families.

To help families reintegrate the client into the home following hospitalization or rehabilitation, nurses use data gathered during family assessment to identify family resources and deficits. By formulating mutually acceptable goals for reintegration, nurses help families cope with the realities of the illness and the changes it may have brought about. Such changes may include new roles and functions of family members or the need to provide continued medical care to the client. Working together, nurses and families can create environments that restore or reorganize family functioning during illness and throughout the recovery process.

Implementation

While teaching is a core nursing intervention, it is important to remember that standardized teaching plans may not be effective for clients with chronic illness and their families. These clients and their families should be encouraged to choose appropriate literature and to find self-help or support groups so they can interact with others who have the same illness.

For families who will be providing care in the home setting, extensive teaching may be required. When the plan of care includes medication administration and equipment use, family members and caregivers may feel overwhelmed by the technical aspects of the client's care. As much as possible, teaching sessions should be organized and divided into segmented presentations to avoid overloading the family and caregivers with information. After carefully planned instruction and practice, families are given an opportunity to demonstrate their ability to provide care under the supportive guidance of the nurse. When the care indicated is beyond the capability of the family, nurses work with families to identify available resources that are socially and financially acceptable.

Evaluation

In evaluating the efficacy of the family nursing care plan, the nurse identifies the degree to which the family members have achieved the identified outcomes relevant to each nursing diagnosis. During evaluation, the nurse also examines all aspects of the nursing care plan to determine the effectiveness of nursing interventions, as well as to evaluate the continued relevance of original nursing diagnoses. Based on evaluation, the nursing care plan is modified to meet the family's current needs.

While the process of evaluation varies depending on the components of the family-specific nursing care plan, examples of criteria that may reflect successful achievement of identified outcomes include the following:

- Family members demonstrate the ability to identify realistic personal and family goals.
- Family members identify and demonstrate healthy coping strategies.
- Caregiver(s) demonstrate safe and effective implementation of care to their family member.
- Family members demonstrate support of the primary caregiver(s).

REVIEW Family Response to Health Alterations

RELATE Link the Concepts and Exemplars

Mrs. Ann Bell, an 82-year-old widow, was diagnosed with Alzheimer disease several years ago. She lives with her daughter and son-in-law and their two children, ages 16 and 10 years. Mrs. Bell has begun wandering, especially at night, and has started small fires when she attempts to cook and forgets about the pot on the stove. Mrs. Bell's daughter, Laura, accompanies her mother to her physician's appointment today and relates that the stress of caring for her mother, in addition to her other obligations to her husband and children, is becoming increasingly difficult.

Linking the exemplar of family response to health alterations with the concept of grief and loss:

1. How can the nurse help the family members to cope with the loss they feel related to Mrs. Bell's cognitive degeneration?

2. What strategies might help Mrs. Bell's grandchildren identify their feelings of grief and loss and work as a family to deal with these feelings?

Linking the exemplar of family response to health alterations with the concept of stress and coping:

3. What strategies can you suggest to help this family deal with the stress of Mrs. Bell's cognitive degeneration?

4. What referrals can you make to reduce Mrs. Bell's daughter's caregiver role strain?

REFER Go to Pearson Nursing Student Resources **nursing.pearsonhighered.com**

• Additional review materials

REFLECT Case Study

Casey, a 16-year-old, is recuperating from injuries sustained in a motor vehicle crash in which he was the passenger. He was not wearing a seat belt and experienced a brain injury after striking the windshield. His cognitive and motor functions are impaired. After a 7-day acute care hospital stay, he was moved to an inpatient rehabilitation hospital, where he has been for the past 5 days. He is much more responsive to stimuli and to family members 12 days after his injury. Physical therapy is provided twice a day to promote range of motion and muscle tone and to prevent contractures. Plans are being made to discharge him home with outpatient rehabilitation care within the next 5 days. A case manager will be assigned to coordinate his healthcare services.

Casey lives with his mother, two half-brothers (10 and 6 years old), and stepfather. Both his mother and stepfather are employed full time and are trying to determine how to manage care for Casey once he returns home. Casey's father has not been actively involved in his life since his parents divorced 12 years ago. Casey's grandparents reside in the same town and may provide the family some support.

1. What family supports will Casey need as he continues his rehabilitation for the brain injury?

2. What family assessment information is needed to effectively plan nursing care for this adolescent and his family?

3. Identify two strengths and coping strategies that will help Casey's family members adapt to his disability.

Casey's family is coping with his initial survival of a serious brain injury, and facing a long rehabilitation process. The family is just now recognizing that life as they have known it is changing. Casey is totally dependent for care, including bathing, toileting, feeding, and mobilizing. While he is expected to regain self-care abilities, the impact of the injury on his cognitive ability and future functioning is unknown.

Casey's extended family has provided support for the family during the past 12 days, but the level of support in the future weeks will decrease because of other family obligations. Casey's mother has already initiated a leave of absence from work so she can care for him when he returns home; however, this will mean the family has reduced income during that time period. Casey's younger brothers have been able to visit him, and they are very anxious because Casey cannot talk with them. They have been trying to avoid bothering their mother and father during this time, but they are wondering when life will be more normal and they can again participate in their usual afterschool activities.

4. What information about the family's strengths, needs, and resilience can be identified from the case study scenario?

5. What additional information would be helpful to know about family strengths and needs prior to developing a nursing care plan?

6. Based on your assessment of the family and challenges facing them, what is the priority nursing diagnosis for Casey and his family at this time? Why do you believe it is the priority?

7. Describe the use of family-centered care principles in planning Casey's nursing care in collaboration with the family.

8. What potential parenting issues could this family anticipate for Casey and his brothers?

■ REFERENCES

Ahmann, E., & Dokken, D. (2009). Parental presence in pediatric trauma resuscitation: One hospital's experience. *Pediatric Nursing, 35*(6), 376–380.

American Psychological Association (APA). (2013). *Risks for family caregivers.* Retrieved from http://www.apa.org/pi/about/publications/caregivers/faq/risks.aspx.

Badger, J., & Reddy, P. (2009). The effects of birth order on personality traits and feelings of academic sibling rivalry. *Psychology Teaching Review, 15*(1), 45–54. Retrieved from http://www.eric.ed.gov/PDFS/EJ860620.pdf.

Baumrind, D. (1971). Current patterns of parental authority. *Developmental Psychology, 4*, 1–103.

Biringen, Z. (2000). Emotional availability: Conceptualization and research findings. *American Journal of Orthopsychiatry, 70*(1), 104–114.

Bowden, V. R., & Greenberg, C. S. (2009). Should family members be present when their child is being resuscitated? *Pediatric Nursing, 35*(4), 254–256.

Burland, J. (1999). *NAMI provided education program.* Arlington, VA: National Alliance for the Mentally Ill.

Caldwell, B. M., & Bradley, R. H. (1984). *The home observation for measurement of the environment.* Little Rock, AR: University of Arkansas.

Centers for Disease Control and Prevention (CDC). (2011). *Sickle cell disease.* Retrieved from http://www.cdc.gov/ncbddd/sicklecell/data.html.

Centers for Disease Control and Prevention (CDC). (2012). Chronic disease prevention and health promotion.

Retrieved from http://www.cdc.gov/chronicdisease/overview/index.htm.

Collins, K. S., Strieder, F. H., DePanfilis, D., Tabor, M., Clarkson-Freeman, P. A., Linde, L., & Greenberg, P. (2011). Trauma adapted family connections: Reducing developmental and complex trauma symptomology to prevent child abuse and neglect. *Child Welfare, 90*(6), 29–47.

Corrigan, P. W., Mueser, K. T., Bond, G. R., Drake, R. E., & Solomon, P. (2009). *Principles and practice of psychiatric rehabilitation: An empirical approach.* New York, NY: Guilford Press.

Doolin, C. T., Quinn, L. D., Bryant, L. G., Lyons, A. A., & Kleinpell, R. M. (2011). Family presence during cardiopulmonary resuscitation: Using evidence-based knowledge to guide the advanced practice nurse in developing formal policy and practice guidelines. *Journal of the Academy of Nurse Practitioners, 23*, 8–14.

Dowshen, S. (2013). *How to talk to your child's doctor.* Retrieved from http://kidshealth.org/parent/general/sick/talk_doctor.html#.

Duvall, E. M. (1977). *Marriage and family development* (5th ed.). New York, NY: Harper & Row.

Family and Medical Leave Act, Public Law 103-3, February 5, 1999. 5 U.S.C. 6381–6387; 5 CFR part 630, subpart L. Retrieved from http://www.opm.gov/pca/leave/HTMS/fmlafac2.asp.

Friedman, M. M. (1998). *Family nursing: Research, theory, and practice* (4th ed., p. 113). Upper Saddle River, NJ: Pearson Education.

Hettler, B. (1976). *The six dimensions of wellness model.* Retrieved from http://c.ymcdn.com/sites/www.nationalwellness.org/resource/resmgr/docs/sixdimensions-factsheet.pdf.

Institute for Family Centered Care. (2011). *Patient and family resource centers.* Retrieved http://www.ipfcc.org/advance/topics/pafam-resource.html.

Lazoritz, S., Rossiter, K., & Whiteaker, D. (2010). What every nurse needs to know about the clinical aspects of child abuse. *American Nurse Today, 5*(7). Retrieved from http://www.americannursetoday.com/article.aspx?id=6902&fid=6846.

Martin, J. A., Hamilton, B. E., Ventura, S. J., Osterman, M. J. K., Wilson, E. C., & Matthews, T. J. (2012). Births: Final data from 2010. *National Vital Statistics Reports, 61*(1), 1–71. Retrieved from http://www.cdc.gov/nchs/data/nvsr/nvsr61/nvsr61_01.pdf#table06.

Mayo Clinic. (2011). *Mental illness.* Retrieved from http://www.mayoclinic.com/health/mental-health/MH00076.

Mental Health America. (2013). *Mental illness and the family: Recognizing warning signs and how to cope.* Retrieved from http://www.nmha.org/go/information/get-info/mi-and-the-family/recognizing-warning-signs-and-how-to-cope.

National Heart, Lung, and Blood Institute. (2012). *Explore sickle cell anemia*. Retrieved from http://www.nhlbi.nih.gov/health/health-topics/topics/sca.

National Institute of Mental Health. (2013). *Bipolar disorder in children and teens: A parent's guide*. Retrieved from http://www.nimh.nih.gov/health/publications/bipolar-disorder-in-children-and-teens-a-parents-guide/what-treatments-are-available-for-children-and-teens-with-bipolar-disorder.shtml.

National Poverty Center. (2010). *Poverty in the United States*. Retrieved from http://www.npc.umich.edu/poverty

National Wellness Institute. (2013). *The six dimensions of wellness*. Retrieved from http://www.nationalwellness.org/?page=Six_Dimensions.

Olson, D. H. (1996). Clinical assessment and treatment interventions using the family circumplex model. In F. W. Kaslow (Ed.), *Handbook of relational diagnosis and dysfunctional family patterns* (pp. 59–77). New York, NY: John Wiley & Sons.

Pye, S., Kane, J., & Jones, A. (2010). Parental presence during pediatric resuscitation: The use of simulation training for cardiac intensive care nurses. *Journal for Specialists in Pediatric Nursing, 15*(2), 172–175. doi:10.1111/j.1744-6155.2010.00236.x.

Smilkstein, G. (1978). The family APGAR: A proposal for a family function test and its use by physicians. *Journal of Family Practice, 6,* 1231–1239.

State of California Franchise Tax Board. (2013). *Domestic partners*. Retrieved from https://www.ftb.ca.gov/individuals/faq/dompart.shtml.

Strout, K. (2012). Wellness promotion and the institute of medicine's future of nursing report: Are nurses ready? *Holistic Nursing Practice, 26*(3), 129–136.

U.S. Bureau of Labor Statistics. (2012). *Employment characteristics of families—2012*. Retrieved from http://www.bls.gov/news.release/pdf/famee.pdf.

U.S. Census Bureau. (2010). *America's family and living arrangements: 2010*. Retrieved from http://www.census.gov/population/www/socdemo/hh-fam/cps2010.html.

U.S. Census Bureau. (2011a). *America's family and living arrangements: 2011*. Retrieved from http://www.census.gov/population/www/socdemo/hh-fam/cps2011.html.

U.S. Census Bureau. (2011b). *Living arrangements of children: 2009*. Retrieved from http://www.census.gov/prod/2011pubs/p70-126.pdf.

U.S. Census Bureau. (2012a). *America's family and living arrangements: 2012*. Retrieved from http://www.census.gov/hhes/families/data/cps2012.html.

U.S. Census Bureau. (2012b). *Definition: Family*. Retrieved from http://www.census.gov/cps/about/cpsdef.html.

U.S. Census Bureau. (2012c). *Persons living alone by sex and age: 1990–2010*. Retrieved from http://www.census.gov/compendia/statab/2012/tables/12s0072.pdf.

U.S. Census Bureau. (2012d). *Single-parent households: 1980–2009*. Retrieved from http://www.census.gov/compendia/statab/2012/tables/12s1337.pdf.

Wadsworth, E., & Rienks, S. L. (2012). *Stress as a mechanism for poverty's ill effects on children: Making a case for family strengthening interventions that counteract poverty-related stress*. Retrieved from http://www.apa.org/pi/families/resources/newsletter/2012/07/stress-mechanism.aspx.

Walsh, F. (2011). *Strengthening family resilience* (2nd ed.). New York, NY: Guilford Press.

Walsh, K. (2011). *Grief and loss: Theories and skills for the helping professions* (2nd ed.). Upper Saddle River, NJ: Pearson.

Warren, N. (2012). Involving patient and family advisors in the patient and family-centered care model. *Medsurg Nursing, 21*(4), 233–239.

Weber, S. (2010). Nursing care of families with parents who are lesbian, gay, bisexual, or transgendered. *Journal of Child and Adolescent Psychiatric Nursing, 23*(1), 11–16. doi:10.1111/j.1744-6171.2009.00211.x.

World Health Organization. (2013). *Health promotion*. Retrieved from http://www.who.int/topics/health_promotion/en.

27 Grief and Loss

MODULE AT-A-GLANCE

The Concept of Grief and Loss, 1741

Exemplar 27.1
  Children's Response to Loss, 1751

Exemplar 27.2
  Death and Dying, 1757

Exemplar 27.3
  Older Adult's Response to Loss, 1763

Exemplar 27.4
  Perinatal Loss, 1767

◢ THE CONCEPT OF GRIEF AND LOSS

Loss and grief are inherent in the human experience. Even so, reactions to loss and manifestations of grief vary widely. Each individual's methods of processing and coping with grief are influenced by numerous variables, including personality, age, culture, the nature of the loss, and the availability of a functional support system. In addition to the loss of a loved one, numerous other sources of loss can also prompt grief reactions; for example, loss of a friend or relationship, loss of mobility, loss of independence, loss of a limb, and loss of hair from illness. By understanding the emotional and physical aspects associated with grief, nurses are better prepared to care for clients who have experienced loss, as well as to support these clients during the grieving process. ≪

Concept Learning Outcomes

After reading about this concept, you will be able to:

1. Summarize the physiology of grief and loss.

2. Examine the relationship between grief and other concepts/systems.

3. Identify commonly occurring alterations in grief or loss and their related therapies.

4. Differentiate common assessment procedures used to examine grief responses across the life span.

5. Explain management of mental health and prevention of complicated grief reactions.

6. Demonstrate the nursing process in providing culturally competent and caring interventions across the life span for individuals with common alterations in grief or loss.

7. Compare and contrast common independent and collaborative interventions for clients with alterations in grief or loss.

Concept Key Terms

Actual loss, *1742*
Anticipatory grief, *1742*
Anticipatory loss, *1742*
Bereavement, *1742*
Complicated grief, *1743*
Disenfranchised grief, *1742*

Grief, *1742*
Hospice, *1750*
Loss, *1742*
Mourning, *1742*
Perceived loss, *1742*

▶ NORMAL PRESENTATION OF GRIEF AND LOSS

Grief is the combination of various psychological, biological, and behavioral responses to a loss. Psychological responses may include anger, denial, and depression. Biological responses to grief include sleep disturbances, decreased appetite, and weight loss. Behavioral responses include personality changes and decreased socialization. Bereavement and mourning can also accompany grief. **Bereavement** is the response to having lost another through death. **Mourning** involves the processing and resolution of grief, generally through cultural and/or spiritual beliefs and practices. Grief can be triggered by any number of situations or occurrences, from the loss of a loved one or acquaintance to being diagnosed with a terminal illness. Grief can also result from the end of a significant relationship with a partner or a close friend or relation. In most cases, grief is a normal, healthy reaction to loss, as it helps the individual to process the situation. Grief should not be avoided, as avoidance often prolongs and intensifies the experience. For some individuals, the grieving process may also be prolonged by failure to mourn the loss according to an individual's cultural or spiritual practices.

The Process of Grieving

The process of grieving is different for all who experience a loss. There is no correct way to grieve, nor is there a timetable for how long the grieving process should last. Manifestations associated with grief are highly individualized and depend on numerous factors including the nature of the loss, the circumstances surrounding the loss, the developmental age and personality of the individual grieving, and the individual's history of grief and/or depression, among many other factors. Intense feelings of grief over the loss of a loved one are generally believed to lessen over a few months, and to resolve—or at least partly resolve—within 1–2 years (Walsh, 2012). This timetable does not apply in every case, and if the grief becomes complicated in any way—for example, when a loss is especially sudden or traumatic—resolution and acceptance take longer. Different types of grief should also be considered, as these often coincide with the type of loss experienced.

TYPES AND SOURCES OF LOSS **Loss** occurs when something or someone of value is rendered inaccessible or drastically changed. Examples of loss include the death of a loved one or friend; the death of a pet; divorce; the end of a job or career; and severe illness or injury resulting in long-term physiological change, such as the loss of a limb (**Figure 27–1 ●**). Everyone experiences various types of loss over the course of a lifetime. The three main types of loss are **actual loss**, loss that is identified and recognized by others, such as the loss of a spouse; **anticipatory loss**, which occurs when an individual knows a loss is coming, such as the impending death of a friend or family member from a fatal illness; and **perceived loss**, which is felt by an individual but cannot be verified as a loss from outside, for example, loss of control or loss of self-esteem.

The source of the loss may impact the range of an individual's emotional responses. For example, individuals who have lost a limb due to amputation lose an aspect of themselves. They may experience disturbance of body image, depression, loss of inde-

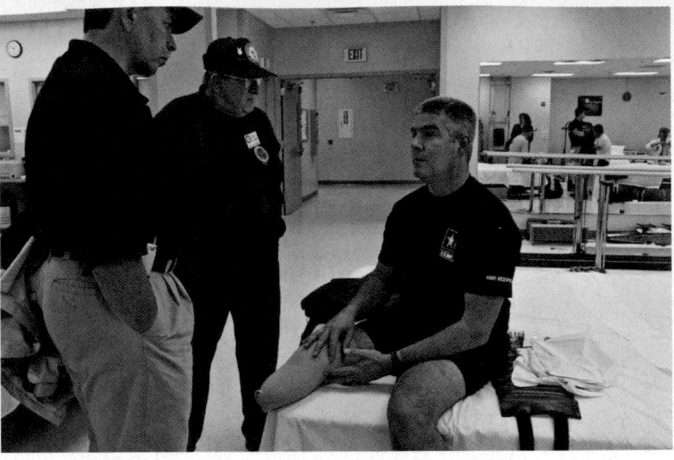

Figure 27–1 ● Loss of an aspect of self is common in those serving in the military, as loss of an appendage or a functional ability is one of the hazards of serving in combat.
Source: David S. Holloway/Getty Images.

pendence, and frustration as they learn to live without use of the limb. Loss of an aspect of self can be very similar to loss of a loved one, in that the individual must learn to function despite the loss. Loss of independence itself is a serious loss, and it may occur with the loss of mobility due to injury or with debilitating illnesses such as dementia or multiple sclerosis.

Since September 11, 2001, families in the United States have experienced increased losses related to the wars in Iraq and Afghanistan. The deployment of military personnel carries a number of consequences that may result in grief responses. Long-term absence of a deployed parent creates additional responsibility for the parent remaining at home and a sense of loss for the entire family, as well as fear for the safety of the deployed family member. In cases where both parents are deployed, children may be relocated away from their childhood home and support systems to live with other relatives. Personnel returning with traumatic injuries may have difficulty rejoining the family unit. Finally, death of a family member overseas brings great loss to a family.

TYPES OF GRIEF Grief presents itself in many different forms ranging from anticipatory grief to complicated grief. Similar to anticipatory loss, **anticipatory grief** is grief that is experienced before the event occurs. This can occur in anticipation of the death of a loved one, or in response to the diagnosis of an individual's own terminal illness. For example, a man's wife has a terminal illness and is expected to live only another three months. He may experience anticipatory grief in advance of his wife's death, grieving for her while she is still alive. Not all individuals experience anticipatory grief. Despite the many debates on the subject, no conclusive studies have proven whether anticipatory grief actually lessens the grieving process after a loved one has died.

Disenfranchised grief occurs when individuals cannot acknowledge their loss to others, typically when the loss is not one that is socially recognized (sometimes referred to as an *ambiguous loss*). Disenfranchised grief may result from the loss of a partner in a socially unrecognized relationship, the loss of a child due to abortion, the loss of someone from suicide or a drug overdose, or even the loss of a pet. When a loss is considered socially unacceptable, the individual grieving the loss may experience not only intense grief but also feelings of isolation. Unable to participate in culturally appropriate expressions of mourning, the bereaved may find it very difficult to resolve their feelings and responses to the loss.

Individuals who are unable to process their grief to a point of resolution may experience **complicated grief**. Complicated grief is generally not diagnosed until 6 months after a loss. If at this time the grief has not diminished and has become debilitating, making daily activities difficult or impossible, the grief may be deemed complicated. Some have proposed renaming this type of grief and calling it *prolonged grief disorder* (*PGD*). The two terms are sometimes used interchangeably (Robinaugh et al., 2012).

Theories Related to Grieving

Different theories have been proposed to explain the grieving process. Typically these theories identify different stages of grief. Grief theorists include Elizabeth Kübler-Ross, George Engel, and Catherine Sanders.

KÜBLER-ROSS AND THE FIVE STAGES OF GRIEF One of the first grief theorists, Elizabeth Kübler-Ross (1969) proposed five stages of grief: denial, anger, bargaining, depression, and acceptance. A psychiatrist, Kübler-Ross based her theory on work she did with dying clients, so some criticism holds that these stages cannot, therefore, be ascribed to those mourning the loss of another. Other critics contend that the stages of grief do not always occur sequentially, as Kübler-Ross described them; stages can overlap or occur individually (Buglas, 2010, p. 45).

Denial, the first stage of grieving identified by Kübler-Ross, may serve to soften the initial blow of the loss. A small amount of denial early in the grieving process is healthy, as it allows the individuals who have undergone a loss to retreat into themselves so as to eventually accept the loss more fully. Nurses working with clients in denial should not force their clients to accept the loss; neither should they reinforce the denial. Denial generally occurs for only a short time, as most individuals eventually begin to accept the loss in their own way, so nurses should be understanding and supportive.

Anger is one of the most difficult stages for all those involved. During this stage, bereaved individuals direct their anger toward anyone who is around them, sometimes without even the slightest apology. Clients who are angry in their grief over a significant loss may direct their anger at staff, nurses, and doctors. This behavior should not be taken personally, as it usually has nothing to do with the actions of the nurse, doctor, or staff member.

The third stage is bargaining. Those who are in this phase of grieving try to make a bargain, generally with God or a higher power, or even with a doctor, for more time. Kübler-Ross found through interviews with clients that this stage sometimes results from the individual's guilt over something from the past. A nurse can help during this stage by listening sympathetically to the client's expression of fears and guilt.

Depression follows the bargaining stage. Depression, a profound sense of deep and penetrating loss felt during the grieving period, is part of the normal work of loss. Nurses support clients during this phase by encouraging and allowing them to express their sadness and sometimes simply by sitting with them silently as they work through these emotions on their own.

After depression, the final stage of the grieving process is acceptance. During acceptance the client is free from anger and depression; this is not a happy stage, but one almost lacking in emotions. Generally, during this time, a terminally ill client's family needs more support and comfort than the client, who often experiences a decreased desire for visits from family and loved ones. At this point, the dying individual has fully accepted the loss and gone through the various stages of grieving in order to arrive at acceptance.

ENGEL AND SANDERS Other theories about the grieving process describe similar experiences with grief, but focus on the individual grieving for the loss of another as opposed to individuals grieving the loss of their own lives. George Engel's (1964) theory describes six stages of grief: shock, disbelief, awareness, restitution, idealization, and outcome. Shock and awareness are very similar to Kübler-Ross's stages of denial and anger, while restitution, idealization, and outcome deal primarily with the acceptance and understanding of the loss.

The work of Catherine Sanders (1988) focuses on the five distinct phases of grief: shock, awareness, conservation, healing, and renewal. The phases of shock and awareness resemble Kübler-Ross's stages of denial and anger, during which the client is still working to come to terms with the loss. In the conservation/withdrawal phase, the individual begins to feel depressed and weakened from the loss, needing time to work through the emotions. Healing and renewal are the final stages, during which the emotions associated with grief begin to abate, and the individual is left with a feeling of acceptance.

Lifespan Considerations

Children and adults experience grief differently, and manifestations of grief vary across the life span (**Figure 27–2 ●**). Children do not generally show or express their emotions regarding loss as openly as adults. Because young children may not express their grief in a way that is expected by an adult, they are sometimes believed to be too young to fully recognize the loss. However, this is not always the case. The child may be grieving

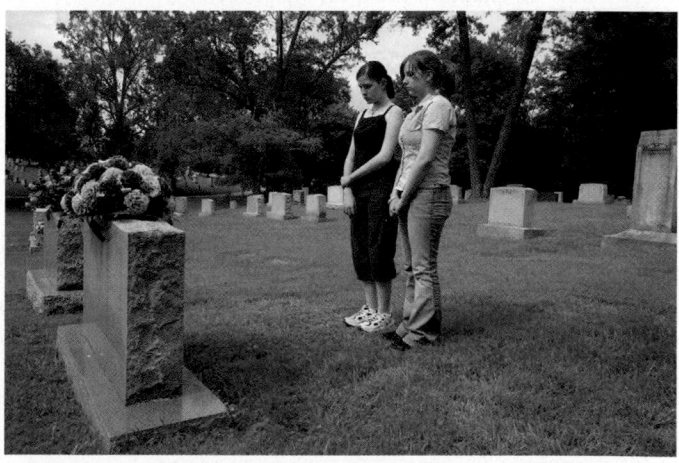

Figure 27–2 ● Children experience grief differently depending on their developmental age.
Source: © EditorialByDarrellYoung/Alamy.

in her own way and sometimes expresses this grief after the loss through art, imaginary games, playing, or behavioral changes. Behavioral changes, such as decreased socialization, irritability, and confusion, may occur more frequently among adolescents than in very young children (Walsh, 2012). Losses experienced by children that may result in grieving include any of the following: loss of parent, grandparent, or sibling; loss of a pet; loss of a relationship with a parent due to divorce; loss of a childhood friend or mentor; and loss of support systems if the family relocates to another city or country.

Adults from early to middle adulthood experience a range of losses that are not as common in childhood, such as the death of a parent or a close friend. Other losses typical of adulthood include the loss of a significant other through death or divorce. Unfortunately, it is not uncommon for adults to experience the death of their own sibling or child. Because of developmental factors, including life experiences and learned coping skills, adults process grief differently from children. Adults can understand cognitively the permanence of the loss and can recognize and rely on coping mechanisms such as mourning rituals and distractions (e.g., work, exercise). However, in contrast to the grief work for children, the grief work of adults may be complicated by the various responsibilities of adulthood. When adults experience a loss—whether a death or a symbolic loss such as a divorce—they still have day-to-day responsibilities such as work, caring for children, and providing emotional support for other family members. These responsibilities may influence adults' grieving processes in various and significant ways.

In addition to the effects of personality and age, experience with previous losses can also impact how an individual handles grief. While older adults grieve in much the same way as others, their grief may sometimes seem more intense, as the loss they are experiencing now can trigger memories of the other significant losses in their lives (Walsh, 2012, p. 58). In the same respect, younger and middle-age adults, or even adolescents who have encountered a multitude of losses, may respond to grief much differently from those who have not experienced as much loss. This reaction may be more intense or less intense. No set formula for grieving exists, but certain factors, such as age, personality, and an individual's previous experiences with loss, do have an effect on the grieving process.

Sociological Considerations

When considering the process of grieving, it is important to take into account the nature of the individual's loss as well as the support system. The nature of the loss and the individual's current health and financial status affect the amount and type of support needed. A loss that impacts daily functioning, such as the death of an income-earning spouse or of a primary caregiver, results in a variety of consequences. Individuals experiencing this type of loss typically require greater support than those who experience the loss of, say, a distant relative or casual acquaintance. Similarly, individuals who experience ambiguous losses—such as perinatal loss, the death of a pet, or the death of an ex-spouse—require a wholly different form of support. In general, individuals seek support from those who were close to the deceased or from those who have experienced similar losses. Researchers have found that among participants in a study of the importance of social support during bereavement,

the majority of respondents said it was helpful to talk to others who had undergone similar experiences, or who could truly understand the feelings of the individual grieving. In the same study, many participants reported that whether or not they took advantage of professional support such as therapy, they were comforted by knowing it was available to them if needed (Benkel, Wijk, & Molander, 2009, pp. 144–145).

▶ ALTERATIONS FROM NORMAL

Normal grief reactions are difficult to define, as all individuals grieve differently, but in general it is normal to experience sadness, anxiety, guilt, anger, confusion, sleep disturbances, and loss of appetite, among other reactions. The amount of time these emotions last varies. Alterations from normal grief arise from the circumstances surrounding the loss, and/or the individual's own personal response to grief. These alterations can cause a prolonged grief response, or, in extreme cases, an inability to process the grief in a healthy manner.

Grief and loss can impact individual functioning in a variety of areas, among them the individual's comfort, ability to cope with stress, and possible resultant addiction. See Concepts Related to Grief and Loss for more information on integrating these concepts.

Alterations and Manifestations

Because each individual grieves differently depending on the nature of the loss, "normal" grief cannot be defined. Typically, however, the intense feelings of grief begin to dissipate over the first 3–6 months following the loss, resurfacing on holidays, birthdays, and other important reminders of the loss. When grief becomes complicated, the intense emotions begin to impact the individual's ability to carry out daily activities. Similarly, these forms of grief may begin to affect the individual's health through loss of appetite, extreme depression, and sleeplessness. It is important for nurses to know the signs of different forms of grief reactions. Disenfranchised grief, described earlier, may result in a prolonged grief reaction, in part due to the individual's inability to mourn the loss in a socially acceptable way. Consider, for example, the case of a mother who gives up her child for adoption. Others do not know why she has made this decision, and individuals may assume that she did not want the child. Others are also likely to refrain from offering support or from asking questions, unsure how to treat the mother who is giving up her child. As a result, the birth mother may feel that society has told her she has no right to grieve the loss of this infant because she decided to give it up for adoption. Her grief may then become disenfranchised because she cannot acknowledge her loss to others. It is critical that nurses provide both physical care and psychosocial support to clients experiencing disenfranchised grief. When a mother has released her child for adoption, the nurse might mention the subject of the adoption, letting the client know she is free to talk if she chooses. Often, the nurse's willingness to listen without offering advice helps the client greatly by allowing her a safe, nonjudgmental place to grieve. The nurse could also offer the birth mother an opportunity to hold the infant and say good-bye, thus allowing a sense of closure (Aloi, 2009, p. 30).

Concepts Related to Grief and Loss

Grief is an important consideration when working with end-of-life clients. Not only are these clients learning how to come to terms with the loss of their own lives, but their families experience a variety of hardships during this time, from the financial burden of caring for the dying to anticipatory grieving. Nurses need to understand the grieving process in order to help end-of-life clients and their families work through grief. When working with grieving clients, it is equally important to obtain a full history in order to determine if those clients have a history of anxiety or depression, as these conditions can compli-

cate or elongate the grieving process. Clients who have experienced a traumatic loss, such as a perinatal loss or a death due to violence, or who have witnessed a death are at risk for developing posttraumatic stress disorder and should be made aware of the signs. Similarly, clients who have a history of posttraumatic stress disorder have a higher risk of developing a complicated grief reaction later in life. When grief becomes overwhelming, some individuals turn to alcohol or other substances to numb their emotions. Masking the impact of a loss only serves to prolong the grieving process.

CONCEPT	RELATIONSHIP TO GRIEF AND LOSS	NURSING IMPLICATIONS
Comfort		
■ End-of-life care	Palliative care can help further the grieving process for both clients and their families, providing both physical and psychological comfort.	■ Help dying clients to grieve for their own loss of life. ■ Assist family members in understanding the signs of grief and acceptance of death. ■ Provide referral to such assistance as hospice, support groups, and spiritual resources.
Stress and Coping		
■ Posttraumatic stress disorder	Existing anxiety disorders and posttraumatic stress disorder can prolong or intensify the effects of grief.	■ Look for signs of posttraumatic stress disorder in clients who have experienced traumatic losses. ■ Obtain an extensive history from clients experiencing any grief reactions. ■ Encourage clients who are already in treatment to continue their treatment plan and to communicate their loss to their provider.
Addiction		
■ Alcohol abuse ■ Substance abuse	Alcohol and substance abuse can mask the emotions associated with grief and cause a longer and sometimes more intensified grief reaction.	■ Look for signs of alcohol or substance use as an unhealthy coping mechanism for grief. ■ Teach the client about healthy coping mechanisms. ■ Maintain a nonjudgmental attitude.

COMPLICATED GRIEF For the individual suffering from complicated grief, the grieving process does not progress. Instead, an overwhelming sense of grief persists and sometimes worsens over a period of months. The individual may experience profound emotions associated with memories of the deceased, along with an inability to accept the reality of the loss. Auditory and visual hallucinations are not uncommon for those suffering this form of prolonged grief. In addition to these symptoms, bereaved individuals may become distrustful or uncaring toward others, forcing themselves into a form of self-imposed isolation. Complicated grief arises in approximately 6%–25% of the bereaved who still feel intense, disruptive grief for a prolonged period of many months, or even years, while typically grief begins to lessen in intensity within 3–6 months. In the first 6 months after a loss, an indi-

vidual is expected to experience some of the same symptoms seen in individuals with complicated grief, such as extreme distress and an inability to function normally in day-to-day activities. However, if after 6 months these symptoms have not lessened and individual functioning is significantly impaired or the individual is at an increased risk for suicide, then complicated grief may be diagnosed. The earliest this diagnosis can be made is 6 months; however, many still debate about how much time must elapse before this diagnosis can be made (Robinaugh et al., 2012).

Treatment of complicated grief is often in the form of psychotherapy targeting specific symptoms related to the disorder. Physician Katherine Shear (2005) developed Complicated Grief Treatment (CGT), a form of psychotherapy administered over 16 sessions in accordance with a published manual that describes this treatment. According to Shear, healing from a loss is composed of a loss-oriented process and a restoration-oriented process. During the first process, the individual accepts the loss; during the restoration process, the individual begins to move on to a life without the deceased (Robinaugh et al., 2012, p. 32). CGT has been shown to be helpful to clients on its own, but some have used it in combination with antidepressants. While recent studies have shown that antidepressants may be helpful to those with depression related to grief, they do not appear to be as effective for clients with complicated grief. However, combining the use of antidepressants with CGT has proved to be quite effective in helping clients to work through their grief.

Factors That Affect the Grieving Process

As previously stated, any number of factors can affect the grieving process; however, the age and gender of the client and the client's use of or experience with substances carry particular considerations for nurses and other healthcare providers.

AGE Children who experience loss at an early age are at greater risk of an intense grieving period, especially children who lose a parent or primary caregiver. This risk increases further when the remaining parent or caregiver fails to recognize the child's grief and assumes that the child is too young to be affected by the loss. If children do not receive support and explanation after a substantial loss, they may view the loss as a betrayal, giving rise to feelings of guilt and anger. This reaction may result in the development of trust issues later in life (Walsh, 2012, p. 33). Children's grief responses can also be more complicated if the individual lost was physically or mentally abusive, or both. In such cases, especially young children may find it difficult to process the loss because, while there is a considerable amount of sadness, there might also be some relief that the abuse is over. The guilt that comes with relief at the death of a loved one is difficult to handle at any age, but particularly for a young child, especially if the child is unable to express these feelings.

Adults' reactions to grief and loss can become abnormal if the loss cannot be, or is not, acknowledged by others, or if extreme grief responses do not lessen after a substantial amount of time. The complicated or disenfranchised grief responses in adults have more to do with personality, circumstance, support systems, and other factors. By middle adulthood, loss and grief begin to be expected and accepted as a normal occurrence. While losses are certainly not easy, they typically are processed in a healthy manner. Older adults may be at greater risk for a complicated grief reaction because their support system may have become limited as a result of past losses, including the death of close family members and friends and even children and grandchildren (Walsh, 2012, p. 72). For example, an older adult who has already lost her husband may be more likely to experience complicated grief if her child dies, as she finds herself without her partner to help her mourn the loss of their child. Further, these accumulated substantial losses may result in complicated grieving. Having a past history of numerous losses may make the grieving process harder for older adults, as a new loss may serve as a reminder of past losses.

Symbolic losses are also more prevalent among older adults; for example, older adults are more at risk than other age groups of losing their independence, their memory, and their mobility, as well as other significant assets. Symbolic losses may occur as a consequence of the death of a spouse or caregiver. For example, a husband with limited mobility may rely on his wife for transportation, cooking, and assistance with daily living. If she dies, man faces a number of losses in addition to mourning her death.

GENDER Gender often is a factor in grief when society or culture influences how individuals perceive the grieving process. From the Western perspective, it is considered acceptable for women to show emotion in response to loss, but men are not expected to grieve openly. This is not necessarily true for other cultures (Walsh, 2012, p. 82). Due to this cultural stigma, men may be at greater risk for disenfranchised grief. Grief reactions in general, though, cannot truly be understood or analyzed based on the individual's gender alone. Other factors, such as age, personality, culture, and the nature of the loss, must also be taken into account when in the assessment of grief reactions.

SUBSTANCE AND ALCOHOL ABUSE Periods of grief and loss are very vulnerable times. Grief can have devastating effects that, if not acknowledged and dealt with, can result in various forms of self-medicating. Nurses encourage healthy coping mechanisms such as seeking counsel from support systems, seeking comfort from religious practices, going to support groups, and doing therapeutic writing. Unhealthy coping mechanisms can complicate grief resulting in alcohol or drug use as a way to numb the pain of loss. This type of unhealthy coping is often employed in the early stages of grief, if at all, and may result in a prolonging of the grieving process. Because substance use only masks the pain and delays the work of grief, addiction may result quickly.

The signs of substance or alcohol abuse are not always easy to spot, especially in a client who is going through a period of heightened grief. Some drugs used over a long period, or used in excess, can present in physical ways such as weight loss and a general physical deterioration. In situations where the nurse suspects alcohol or substance abuse, the nurse remains nonjudgmental and uses a therapeutic approach to ask how the client has been handling the grief and adjusting to the loss. If clients admit to depending on alcohol or substances, the nurse can provide support and referral for the dependency and can also provide client teaching related to healthy coping responses.

ASKING FOR HELP Depending on an individual's paradigm, as well as the views of society or an individual's culture, grief may carry a stigma. Some cultural beliefs can also affect the grieving process, such as the belief that men should not openly grieve for a loss. Neglecting to grieve or being unable to seek comfort and strength from support systems can lead to feelings of isolation. Nurses encourage clients to ask for help if they feel that the effects of loss are becoming overwhelming. Nurses also provide information about support systems and services available in the community. A strong support system can positively impact the grieving process.

Alterations and Therapies **Grief**

ALTERATION	DESCRIPTION / DEFINITION	MANIFESTATIONS	INTERVENTIONS AND THERAPIES
Disenfranchised grief	The result of being unable to acknowledge a loss to others, generally because the grief is not socially recognized	▪ Hiding grief from others as opposed to allowing support from friends and family ▪ Not seeking support after a loss due to feelings of shame, guilt, or lack of recognition of the loss ▪ Intensified emotions associated with grief as opposed to those found in a normal grief reaction ▪ More pronounced feelings of anger and depression due to resentment over the unacknowledged loss	▪ Refer the client to support groups that acknowledge the loss and feelings of grief. ▪ Recognize and support the client's right to grieve the loss. ▪ Facilitate the client's spiritual and cultural needs.
Complicated grief	Prolonged or intensified grief causing an individual to be unable to proceed with the grieving process	▪ Intense grieving for 6 months or more with little to no indication of grief resolution ▪ Inability to proceed with daily activities after the loss ▪ Visual and/or auditory hallucinations of the individual who has died ▪ Growing distrust of friends and family members, making the individual seem cold or uncaring ▪ Avoidance of places associated with memories of the deceased ▪ Intense feelings of depression, at times accompanied by suicidal thoughts or tendencies	▪ Psychotherapy ▪ Monitoring for suicidal behaviors ▪ Assessment for signs of alcohol and/or substance abuse ▪ Appropriate referrals when signs of suicidal ideation and drug/alcohol abuse are present

CASE STUDY \\ PART 1

Josie Duncan is a 32-year-old African American woman whose 7-year-old daughter, Tasha, died 3 months ago after fighting leukemia. Mrs. Duncan took a week off from work after her daughter died and then returned to her job. She visits her primary care physician's office complaining of difficulty falling asleep over the past 2 weeks. After checking her vital signs, weight, and temperature, you notice that Mrs. Duncan has lost 15 pounds since her last visit 6 months ago. Her blood pressure and temperature are both normal. You observe that she looks exhausted and has deep circles under her eyes; the clothes she is wearing are at least a size too large. She also seems to be very distracted.

Clinical Reasoning Questions Level I

1. Why might Mrs. Duncan be having trouble sleeping?
2. What are some factors that influence an individual's grief response?
3. What additional questions would you want to ask Mrs. Duncan? Why?

Clinical Reasoning Questions Level II

4. Is Mrs. Duncan at risk for a complicated grief reaction? Explain your answer.
5. Do you think the doctor will prescribe medication for Mrs. Duncan's sleeplessness? What other interventions could be performed?

▶ ASSESSMENT

Assessment related to grief and loss should include exploration of the client's current grief, as well as interviewing the client regarding any past significant losses. Obtaining a complete history of any medical conditions is also necessary. A mental health assessment and information about current coping abilities should also be attained. A complete nursing assessment also includes identifying the client's cultural and spiritual needs.

Nursing Assessment

Assessment of the client who has experienced a loss includes assessing the many factors that contribute to an individual's grief reaction, such as the client's age, coping mechanisms, support system, history of previous losses, history of depression, culture, and personality. When conducting an assessment, it is also important to be attentive to the client's needs and to maintain a nonjudgmental attitude. If the nurse discovers the client has an extensive history of loss, the nurse should ascertain how the client dealt with these losses and whether the client has achieved resolution or acceptance of those losses. Through a sensitive and thorough assessment, the nurse promotes openness and creates an environment in which the client can feel safe in discussing emotions.

Assessment Interview Grief and Loss

Current Loss
- When did the loss occur?
- What was the nature of the loss?
- Are you having trouble carrying on with your normal activities?
- Have you experienced any trouble sleeping or eating?
- Have you talked to anyone about the loss? (For example, a spouse, friends, family, or counselor.)
- Are you taking any medications and/or antidepressants?

History of Loss and Grief Reactions
- Have you experienced similar losses in the past?
- Did your grief manifest in similar ways to your grief for this loss?
- Are you experiencing any unresolved grief?

Lifestyle
- Do you have an active support system?
- Do you drink on a regular basis?
- What types of coping mechanisms have you employed to work through your grief?

Spiritual and Cultural Considerations

Accurate assessment of the grieving process requires awareness of an individual's cultural influences. While it would be unreasonable to expect nurses and other medical professionals to know the practices and beliefs of every culture, in many cases valuable information can be gleaned during a simple client interview. Understanding the client's culture may also give meaning to his reaction toward professionals who offer assistance, particularly as certain cultural or religious practices view seeking help as unfavorable. The nurse should avoid the tendency to view individual behaviors and cultural practices through a "Western" lens, which leads to deeming the traditions and practices of others as odd because they do not fit into the nurse's own expectations and experiences. In most settings, client populations offer a diversity of cultural backgrounds. Respect for the practices of others is essential to building trust, establishing a relationship, and, ultimately, to providing effective client care.

Awareness of the client's cultural beliefs and values can prevent miscommunication and conflict. For example, some

Grief and Loss Assessment

ASSESSMENT/METHOD	NORMAL FINDINGS	ABNORMAL FINDINGS	LIFESPAN OR DEVELOPMENTAL CONSIDERATIONS
Loss Assessment			
Ask about previous losses. Discover the different types of losses, as well as their frequency.	Experiencing a number of losses is normal at almost any age. In the first few months after the loss, sadness, sleep disturbance, loneliness, and intermittent periods of decreased motivation or activity are to be expected.	■ Inability or unwillingness to process the loss ■ Denial of the loss for a prolonged time ■ Inability or unwillingness to discuss the loss ■ Accumulation of losses with little to no resolution ■ Grief that interferes with daily functioning and lasts 6 months or longer should trigger additional assessment.	■ Children are likely to process losses differently from adults; it should not be assumed that they do not understand loss because of their age. ■ Older adults are likely to develop numerous losses over their lifetime, and these can begin to pile up.
Grief Assessment			
Assess client's current and past grief reaction. Determine the nature of the loss causing the grief.	Grief is intense over the first 2–6 months after the loss and then begins to lessen. Resolution/acceptance generally occurs within 1–2 years after the loss.	■ *Complicated Grieving* ■ *Grief* related to traumatic loss ■ *Grief* related to disenfranchised loss ■ Post-Trauma Syndrome	■ Children and older adults are at a high risk for complicated grief. ■ Older adults are at high risk for depression. Loss of a spouse or caregiver may impact independence and requires additional assessment and referral.

cultures see death as a beginning rather than an end and choose to celebrate the individual's life on earth and the movement to the next life. Misinterpretation of cultural belief may lead clinicians to try to promote coping mechanisms that may not have meaning to the individual client. It is important to understand that clients view death and grief from their own perspective.

Mourning practices vary widely among cultures and religions. Some mourn openly and in public, while others mourn at home for a set period before moving back into society. In the Jewish faith, for example, followers practice the tradition of shivah, a 7-day mourning period during which the closest family members—such as parents, siblings, and spouse—stay together to mourn their loss and receive visitors. Other cultures may emphasize the need to continue with normal activities, such as school or work, during the mourning period, in place of taking time away to mourn privately.

Similarly, cultural and religious practices are important to a client who is dying. If a client has specific spiritual or religious requests, such as seeing a priest or a rabbi or having ceremonial traditions performed by an elder of the religion, these requests should be facilitated whenever possible. Some requests have greater impact on nursing and clinical staff than others. For example, it would be imprudent to have a male nurse responsible for the end-of-life care of a female client who is a Muslim or who practices Orthodox Judaism, as in these religions men are generally not permitted to touch women (Spector, 2013, p. 155).

CASE STUDY \\ PART 2

Mrs. Duncan tells you that she has been working a lot since her daughter died because she needs something to occupy her mind. For the last year of Tasha's life, Mrs. Duncan spent all of her free time taking Tasha to doctor appointments and treatments; now that Tasha is gone, Mrs. Duncan does not know what to do with her spare time. She reports that her appetite decreased before her daughter died, and she has not really had any desire to eat since then. Lately Mrs. Duncan has not wanted to see any of her friends because they act differently around her; they also have children, and Mrs. Duncan admits she does not want to be around children right now. She reports her sleeplessness started 2 weeks ago, shortly after the Christmas holiday. She and her husband tried to celebrate, but they felt it was not the same without their daughter. Mrs. Duncan admitted that she does not think her husband understands how upset she is over their loss.

Clinical Reasoning Questions Level I

1. Why was Mrs. Duncan's appetite poor before her daughter died?

2. What are two nursing diagnoses that apply to Mrs. Duncan?

Clinical Reasoning Questions Level II

3. Based on what you know about grief and loss, why do you think Mrs. Duncan began to experience sleep disturbances after Christmas?

4. How would you characterize Mrs. Duncan's support system? Is it strong, moderate, or weak? Explain your answer.

5. Do you think Mrs. Duncan is working through the grieving process, avoiding grief, or both? Justify your answer using data from the case study.

▶ INTERVENTIONS AND THERAPIES

Nurses can employ various interventions to help clients with their grief. While certain general principles apply to many clients across the cultural spectrum, the plan of care must be tailored and individualized to meet each client's needs. Some situations require collaboration with other professionals, such as social workers, chaplains, and hospice.

Independent

When an individual is grieving, it is sometimes hard to know what to say or do, and nurses may find themselves reluctant to pose questions that clients may see as an invasion of their privacy. It is important to know that there are many ways to offer a client support and a forum to discuss any difficulties (**Figure 27–3** ●). Open-ended questions, such as asking how the client has been doing since the loss or what challenges the client is facing, may be effective for engaging the client in discussion. Once the client begins to speak, the nurse should use active listening techniques to show full engagement in the interaction. Body language also conveys the nurse's engagement in the conversation. A nurse's body language should be open and attentive, and when possible, both individuals should be positioned so they are at eye level with one another. (See the exemplar on Therapeutic Communication in the Communication module for a discussion of active listening techniques.)

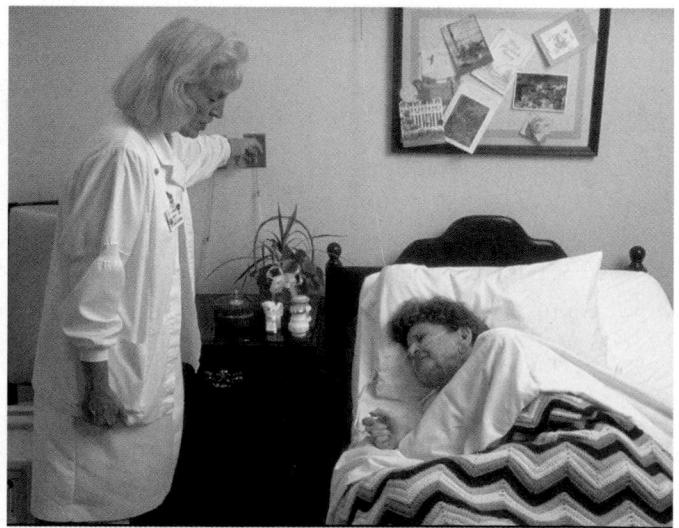

Figure 27–3 ● Providing compassionate and holistic end-of-life care allows the nurse to apply a wide range of skills.

Medications **Antidepressants**

CLASSIFICATION AND DRUG EXAMPLES	MECHANISM OF ACTION	NURSING CONSIDERATIONS
Antidepressants ■ Selective serotonin reuptake inhibitors (SSRIs) ■ Serotonin and norepinephrine reuptake inhibitors (SNRIs) ■ Tricyclic and tetracyclic antidepressants ■ Monoamine oxidase inhibitors (MAOIs) *Drug examples:* Escitalopram, fluoxetine, sertraline, duloxetine, doxepin, phenelzine	May be used to treat the symptoms of moderate or severe depression as the result of grief or loss. *May also be used for:* —Treatment of complicated grief in conjunction with psychotherapy	■ Monitor for signs of suicidal thoughts. ■ Teach clients about risks associated with specific antidepressants. ■ Monitor for signs of allergic reaction. ■ Monitor for signs of drug interactions.

Collaborative

Collaboration may include facilitating meetings between the hospital chaplain and the client or the family, or requesting a referral to a social worker who can provide expert guidance about coping with loss or assist with linking clients with additional resources (**Figure 27–4 ●**). Group therapy, bereavement groups, and grief therapists can all be resources for clients who have experienced a loss. **Hospice** is an organization that provides end-of-life care for clients either in their homes or in a hospital setting. Area hospice programs also provide an array of other services, depending on the community resources available. (See the exemplar on Death and Dying in this module for more information on hospice and palliative care.)

If pharmacologic interventions are appropriate, antidepressant medications may be prescribed. Although impaired sleep patterns may be associated with grieving, medications to promote sleep usually are not indicated for these clients. In addition to the addictive potential of certain pharmacologic sleeping aids, these medications may be used to mask the client's grief response, which can prolong the process. If these medications are prescribed, the client should be carefully monitored for signs and symptoms that they are being used to blunt the emotional impact of grieving.

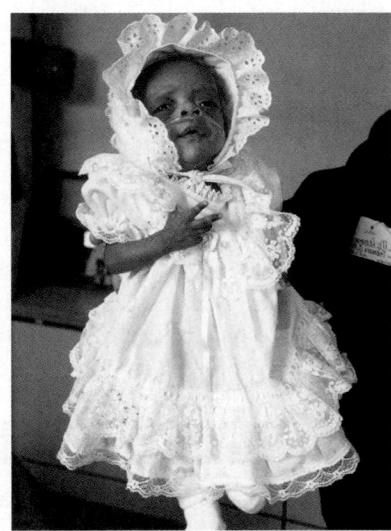

Figure 27–4 ● Religious rituals such as baptism and the blessing of an ill infant may provide great comfort to the family. When the infant is stable, a traditional baptism may be performed in the home or church with family and friends present. When the infant has a life-threatening illness, baptism may be performed in the hospital by a chaplain or health professional.

REVIEW The Concept of Grief and Loss

RELATE Link the Concepts

Linking the concept of grief and loss with the concept of addiction:

1. Describe appropriate interventions for a 30-year-old woman who has begun abusing alcohol to bury her grief.

2. What preventive measures could be taken in the case of a 60-year-old recovered alcoholic whose wife has recently died? How would you work with the client to help prevent him from using alcohol to deal with his grief?

Linking the concept of grief and loss with the concept of violence:

3. You are caring for a 25-year-old woman who has suffered a perinatal loss as the result of domestic abuse. Describe at least four factors that put this client at a high risk for a complicated grief reaction.

4. An 8-year-old boy has been physically abused by his father until 2 months ago, when the father died suddenly. What nursing interventions would be appropriate for this boy's grief? How could his history of abuse make the grief more difficult?

READY Go to Companion Skills Manual

REFER Go to Pearson Student Nursing Resources
nursing.pearsonhighered.com

• Additional review materials

REFLECT Case Study \\ Part 3

Before the doctor talks with Mrs. Duncan, you discuss her complaints of sleeplessness and weight loss with him. You also inform him of Mrs. Duncan's difficulties since her daughter has died. After the doctor talks to Mrs. Duncan, he recommends that she consider talking with a grief counselor about the loss of her daughter. He also recommends that she try to eat more, and that she begin exercising at least three times a week—even if she only goes for a 10-minute walk. Mrs. Duncan and the doctor agree that she should try a combination of counseling, a healthy diet, and exercise before they consider the possibility of pharmacotherapy. Mrs. Duncan schedules a follow up appointment for next month.

Clinical Reasoning Questions Level I

1. Why do you think the doctor recommended exercise?
2. What are some of the benefits of grief counseling?

Clinical Reasoning Questions Level II

3. Do you think Mrs. Duncan's grief reaction is normal after the loss of a child? Explain your answer.
4. Why did the doctor not prescribe pharmaceutical sleep aids immediately? What are some risk factors associated with taking controlled substances while grieving?
5. Do you think Mrs. Duncan has demonstrated healthy coping mechanisms for dealing with her grief?

EXEMPLAR 27.1   Children's Response to Loss

EXEMPLAR KEY TERMS
Childhood traumatic grief, *1753*
Death anxiety, *1751*

EXEMPLAR LEARNING OUTCOMES
After reading about this exemplar, you will be able to:

1. Describe the grief responses, clinical manifestations, and direct and indirect causes of childhood loss and grief.
2. Identify risk factors and prevention methods associated with childhood grief and loss.
3. Illustrate the nursing process in providing culturally sensitive care across the life span for individuals dealing with childhood grief.
4. Formulate priority nursing diagnoses appropriate for an individual working through childhood grief.
5. Summarize therapies used by interdisciplinary teams in the collaborative care of an individual working through childhood grief.
6. Plan evidence-based care for an individual experiencing childhood grief and his or her family in collaboration with other members of the healthcare team.
7. Evaluate expected outcomes for an individual experiencing childhood grief.

▶ OVERVIEW

During childhood, all losses contribute to the formation of the child's pattern of response to loss and grief. Losses during the formative years may include loss of a pet, loss of a grandparent, loss of a parent, loss of a home due to moving or foster care, loss of a friend who moves away or transfers to another school, and loss of a sense of security. A child's reaction to these losses generally depends on the relationship to the individual or object that has been lost. From infancy to late teens, individuals depend on others such as parents, grandparents, or caregivers for security, love, and shelter, so the loss of a provider and caregiver may be accompanied by a sense of losing emotional and physical security.

▶ CHILDREN'S GRIEF RESPONSE

Children's grief responses vary depending on a number of factors, most notably the child's developmental stage and the significance of the loss. When caring for a grieving child, it is important to remember that cognitive development greatly influences grief response. While young children have the capacity to understand loss to some degree, their grief is displayed in ways that differ from grief reactions seen in other age groups. Children also experience **death anxiety**, which manifests as feelings of fear and/or apprehension connected with death.

Developmental Stage

Children grieve differently at different stages of development. Quite a few similarities exist as well. Grief responses in children across the developmental stages are often behavioral: The child acts out emotionally or physically in one way or another.

Worden and Silverman (1996) proposed four tasks that help children adapt to loss:

1. Accept the loss and its permanence.
2. Experience the emotions associated with grief, such as anger, fear, sadness, guilt, and loneliness.
3. Adjust to daily life without the individual who has been lost.
4. Come to see the relationship with the deceased as one based on memories in place of continuing experience.

During the first task, the child must come to understand the loss. In the case of a death, the child must understand that the one who has been lost will not return. Many childhood movies, television shows, and books involve storylines where an important individual dies but is then magically brought back to life. While a child may intellectually understand this is not possible, the desire for the return of the individual who has been lost may be so great that it is easier for the child to believe that the individual will come back in some way. Although the child should not be forced to accept the death, nurses and other caregivers can explain and reinforce the reality that the beloved individual is not returning. During the second task, children experience emotions similarly to those of adults as they grieve loss. Nurses support children in this task by encouraging emotional expression and by helping parents to understand that these expressions are normal and appropriate. It also is helpful for adults to recognize that emotions can be triggered long after the loss by holidays, birthdays, or other special events. The third and fourth tasks of this model take time to process and accept (Howarth, 2011, pp. 23–24). Adults can help children in these tasks by listening, by helping children adjust to changes in routines, and by encouraging activities that promote new memories.

AGES 2–4 Children from ages 2–4 cannot yet fully comprehend or express the ideas associated with loss. At this stage, they also see death as temporary or even reversible, believing that the individual or pet who has been lost will come home again. Reaction to grief at this age can also result in changes to sleeping and eating habits, as well as regression in the area of toilet training. Other habits also may change in reaction to loss; for example, the child may lose interest in normal activities or may crave more attention and affection. This type of behavior often manifests as the child becoming clingy or screaming when not being held. When dealing with loss at this age, it is best for caregivers to respond to the child's changes from grief by trying to maintain as normal a routine as possible. Similarly, providing extra reassurance and attention can also be helpful. It is easy to believe that children at such a young age do not understand the concept of loss or death, but they most certainly do notice and understand when change occurs. Therefore it is important for parents to provide honest answers to questions about grief when they are asked.

AGES 5–7 During the developmental stage after toddlerhood, death is still seen as reversible. It is also common during this age span for children to think of death as another place; according to this thinking, the loved one is still alive but has moved to a place the child cannot reach. Other common thought processes at this age revolve around feelings of guilt or blame. In the case of the death of a loved one, a child may fear having caused the death, especially as a result of negative thoughts about the individual or engaging in some type of misbehavior just before the death. Feelings of responsibility such as these are referred to as *magical thinking,* and are quite normal in this stage of development. Children at this age may or may not verbalize these feelings, so parents or caregivers are advised to discuss the loss honestly and help the child realize the loss is not the child's fault. A child experiencing grief at this age may also act as though nothing has changed—this is a common reaction for children at this stage and is not by itself cause for alarm.

Grief responses for children ages 5–7 may include changes in eating and sleeping patterns, as well as an increase in nightmares. It is also quite normal for the child to be concerned that other important individuals may die as well. Some children express these fears verbally, while others express them through artwork or even writing. These expressions vary based on the individual, but the child should be encouraged to participate in these types of activities, especially if the activity appears to be therapeutic for the child. Parents and caregivers can help children with reassurances about their safety and well-being, and also by inviting children to talk about their grief or ask any questions. It is best for adults to answer questions simply and honestly, providing the child with further explanations when needed.

AGES 8–11 As children advance in age, their understanding of loss and, in particular, death also increases. From around age 8 to age 11, children begin to understand that death means the individual is gone and will not be coming back. During this developmental stage, children become more curious about death and what happens after people (or pets) die. As in the previous developmental stage, children in this age group also tend to believe their thoughts or misbehaviors could be the cause of a loved one's death. It is common for a child to feel that the death of a loved one is a form of punishment for some mis-

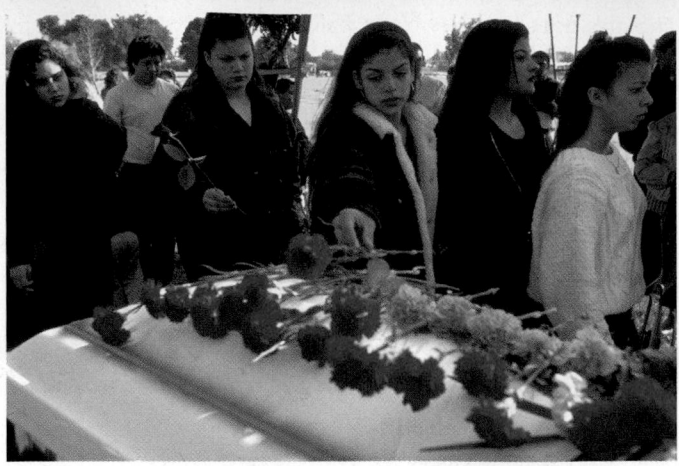

Figure 27–5 ● Hispanic teenagers lay red carnations on the casket of the victim of a drive-by shooting.
Source: A. Ramey/PhotoEdit Inc.

behavior. Grief responses at this stage are typically behavioral and may involve becoming more aggressive, acting out in school or misbehaving at home, or the child may respond by becoming more withdrawn and engaging in solitary activities.

AGES 12–18 By the time children reach adolescence, they are more capable of understanding the abstract idea of death. During this time, children stop believing their thoughts or behaviors can result in the death of others. Adolescent grief responses are very similar to those of most adults, and they may display a wide range of emotions, including depression, denial, and anger. It is very common for individuals in this age group to direct grief-related anger toward their parents. Adolescents should be encouraged, but not forced, to voice their feelings about the loss. Sometimes individuals in this age group feel more comfortable talking to peers or those outside the family (**Figure 27–5** ●).

Significance of the Loss

The significance of a loss impacts the child's grief experience. For many children, their first encounter with loss is the death of a pet; regardless of the type of pet (fish or dog, cat or hamster), the loss carries meaning for the child. Some parents hide the death of the pet, saying that the cat or dog has gone to live somewhere else, or that the lizard escaped in the middle of the night, but the child still feels the loss. With the death of a pet, the child may react with an abbreviated grief response and, depending on age, ask a number of questions. For more significant losses, though, such as the death of a parent, grandparent, sibling, or friend, a child's grief response is likely to be much more developed.

DEATH OF A PARENT Approximately 2.5 million children in the United States lose a parent before the age of 18 (Howarth, 2011, p. 21). In many ways the death of a parent, especially for a young child, is one of the most devastating losses the child will experience. The death of a parent is not only the loss of an important person, for many children the death results in the loss of an entire way of life. Children depend on their parents or caregivers for almost everything, from their home, meals, and security to their sense of love and belonging. When a parent dies, children sense that all of those things are threatened. Children are very habit oriented, so a parent's death brings chaos and confusion to their daily routine. The death of one parent also puts numerous different stresses on the other parent, and the child may not receive as much attention or discipline as before. Depending on the developmental stage of the child, the death of one parent could also introduce profound fear that the other parent will die soon as well. This sense of impending loss can stimulate a great deal of anxiety for the child. How the surviving parent or guardian handles the adjustment period after the death has a large impact on how the child copes with the loss. Many children are said to adjust to a parent's death after about a year, but a large percentage still experience changes in behavior, such as social withdrawal and problems with schoolwork, well beyond the first year.

DEATH OF A GRANDPARENT The death of a grandparent generally is one of the first significant losses children experience. How a child handles the death depends on the child's relationship with that grandparent. For example, if the child has met her grandfather only once because he lives in another state and does not visit often, the impact of the loss will be far less than if the grandparent has lived with and helped raise the child. In this case, the impact of the grandparent's death is similar to that of a parent dying. Children who realize the significance of the grandparent's relationship to their own parent may become concerned about the possibility of losing their parents.

DEATH OF A SIBLING In many ways, the loss of a sibling can be as traumatic as losing a parent or primary caregiver. Siblings often spend much of their childhood together, and they share experiences and relationships with loved ones. For siblings who share a bedroom, the connection is intensified. At a minimum, the death of a sibling generates questions about mortality; related concerns may lead to fear and worry. If unaddressed, fear and worry may cause behavioral problems, developmental regression, and a heightened fear of anything the child believes may be harmful. Depending on the developmental stage of the child, feelings of guilt and confusion may also be associated with the death of a sibling. Children from ages 5 to 11 often indulge in a certain amount of magical thinking, believing that their negative thoughts or wishes could be the cause of another's death. This type of thinking is particularly difficult in connection with siblings, as most siblings fight from time to time, so if a child's sister dies, he may believe that his mean thoughts toward her were the cause of her death.

DEATH OF A FRIEND Similar to the death of a sibling, the loss of a friend causes difficulties for children because it is the death of someone their own age. When a parent or grandparent dies, children often fear for the surviving adults; however, when another child dies, children fear for themselves and their friends. This fear can affect the child's sense of security in the world. If a child becomes friends with a schoolmate who is terminally ill, parents can work to prepare the child for the loss. If the death occurs suddenly, however, there is no time to prepare, and parents and caregivers should work to assure children of their safety.

OTHER LOSSES Like adults, children experience losses other than death that can trigger a grief response. Parental divorce alone can be a significant loss, but it is further complicated if the divorce results in the child's separation from the noncustodial parent by a great distance. Similarly, deployment of a parent serving in the military or other parental absence creates a loss for the child and other family members. Moving can result in loss of school friends, teachers, and other support systems. Long-term or severe acute or chronic illness or injury may result in lifestyle modifications, loss of a limb or body part, or loss of independence. Children experiencing these losses need as much support as, and sometimes more support than, children who experience the death of a loved one.

Complications

Children can experience complications in the grief process as the result of circumstances surrounding the loss, or the significance of the loss. When children experience a significant or traumatic loss, they need a very strong support system to help them work through their feelings of grief, which are most likely difficult for them to understand. If this support is not received either because the child does not show any obvious signs of grief, or because a support system is not present, then the child is at an increased risk for developing a grief reaction that has been complicated in some way.

COMPLICATED GRIEF REACTIONS Loss of an abuser can lead to development of a complicated grief reaction. In such circumstances, feelings of grief are mixed with a sense of relief at knowing the abuse has ended. Regardless of age, coping with mixed emotions related to the death of an abuser presents serious challenges. For children, who lack the cognitive ability to fully understand death, the impact is even more complex. Furthermore, if the abuse has been hidden, the child's experience can be even more confusing. The child who is grappling with mixed emotions observes the others involved mourning the loss. With no confidantes, the child has no one with whom to discuss the conflicted feelings. This need to hide emotions related to grief due to feelings of guilt or shame can result in a complicated grief reaction.

CHILDHOOD TRAUMATIC GRIEF **Childhood traumatic grief** is a grief reaction to the traumatic death of an individual who is important in a child's life. Examples are a child's witnessing a loved one's death in a motor vehicle accident, fire, suicide, or act of violence. Or the child may find it traumatic to see a beloved individual's body after death . According to the National Child Traumatic Stress Network's seminal report in 2004, children who experience traumatic grief are often prevented from moving through grief as they normally would have. All thoughts of the individual who died are now mixed up with the trauma of having seen the death or the circumstances around that death. It even becomes difficult for the child to think of the loved one in the context of any happy memories. This type of grief reaction results in both trauma and grief symptoms for the child. Not all children who are involved in a traumatic death experience develop traumatic grief, and if they do, it may not present immediately; in fact, the symptoms sometimes do not surface for 1–2 years after the death (Goodman et al., 2004).

▶ CLINICAL MANIFESTATIONS

When children encounter death, they often do not grasp the idea entirely. As a result, their minds often work to protect them from the overwhelming feelings caused by grief. In some cases, children may not even react to loss outwardly. There is nothing wrong with this reaction: Their minds may act to protect them from experiencing emotions for which they have no point of reference. When children do react, though, their reactions often revolve around behavioral changes, which may include emotional and behavioral regression.

Behavioral Response to Grief

Behavioral responses to grief vary depending on developmental age, temperament, and other factors discussed in this exemplar. Behavioral changes following loss may be immediate or may occur over an extended period of time. A child's behavior change often presents in one of two ways: withdrawal or acting out. Some children are more withdrawn at home but act out more frequently at school. The responses depend on the child. For children who withdraw, they will be quieter than usual, may seem shy around others, and their primary method of play may be in activities they can do alone, such as drawing, reading, or simply engaging in solitary play. In rare cases, a school-age child may revert to total silence, refusing to speak to anyone. If this behavior goes on for an extended period, a doctor or therapist should be consulted.

Some children may respond to grief with anger and aggression. Anger typically is directed toward the individual who has passed away or at the loss itself but often is taken out on family, friends, or teachers. Other responses may involve trouble eating and sleeping, or an overall feeling of anxiety. Adolescents who are grieving may turn to alcohol, tobacco, or drugs as a method of coping with the loss.

Watching a child's behavior change drastically after an individual dies can be terrifying for a parent or guardian. Nurses work to assure parents that the changes they are seeing in their children are a normal response to the loss and that each individual grieves differently. Nurses and other clinicians encourage parents to allow children to express their grief, either verbally or artistically, and provide parents with information about warning signs of unhealthy coping. For example, preoccupation with thoughts of death, engaging in dangerous activities, and drug or alcohol use are considered unhealthy coping mechanisms.

Cultural Considerations

How children handle their grief at the loss of a loved one is greatly influenced by the cultural or spiritual practices of the child's immediate family. For example, children may be raised to believe that someone who dies goes on to an afterlife. Other cultural traditions teach children that an individual's soul is reincarnated in a new body after death. Some practices teach children that no existence of any sort continues after death, and that death is simply the end of life. Nurses take the cultural and spiritual traditions of clients into consideration, especially when speaking to children about grief. For example, if a child's father has told her that the individual who has died will now be reincarnated in a new existence, and another individual who is not familiar with the family's culture tells the child that this individual is now in heaven, the child will most likely be very confused. The nurse who is unaware of a family's beliefs should avoid inadvertently imposing his own belief system on the child. Similarly, if the family has decided not to offer any explanation of an afterlife or lack thereof to the child, that is the parents' decision, and the nurse should not use spiritual beliefs to help the child work through her grief.

▶ COLLABORATION

In most cases, childhood grief progresses naturally and in a healthy manner with the help of supportive family members and friends. Young children's minds are equipped to protect them from experiencing the full range of grief all at once and for prolonged periods. This is one of the many reasons children grieve differently from adults. When faced with a challenge that is beyond their emotional capacity, young children have defense mechanisms that allow them to compartmentalize the event. As a result, the child can focus on play or daily activities, as opposed to being overwhelmed. Young children experience intense grief for short periods before their mind moves on to another focus (National Cancer Institute, 2013). In some cases, however, parents or guardians need to work with medical professionals to help their child process grief.

Pharmacologic Therapy

In most cases involving a child who is having difficulty working through grief, nonpharmacologic options such as therapy or group counseling are effective; these options should be used before medication is considered. Pharmacologic therapies can keep children from developing their own coping and healing mechanisms and may therefore cause problems later in life. In addition, many medications used as pharmacotherapy for extended grief responses are difficult to stop; most must be tapered slowly. Parents or guardians should be informed of all the side effects of these medications so that they can make an informed decision. If cognitive-behavioral therapy and other nonpharmacologic interventions are given a significant trial and still prove ineffective, and if the child is at an increased risk for hurting himself or others, low doses of antidepressants may be suggested. At this time, fluoxetine (Prozac) is the only antidepressant approved for the treatment of childhood depression. For adolescents 12 or older, the FDA has also approved the use of escitalopram (Lexapro). In 2004, the FDA revealed findings from clinical trials indicating that children taking antidepressants are at a higher risk for suicidal thoughts or behaviors. When the prescription of antidepressants is being considered for children, the increased risk for suicidal behaviors should be discussed with parents. If the child is prescribed antidepressants, regular follow up appointments should be scheduled for at least the first 12 weeks after beginning the medication. Antidepressants can also be used in combination with nonpharmicologic options to help the child work through her grief and eventually move on to acceptance (Mayo Clinic, 2010a; U.S. Food and Drug Administration, 2005).

Nonpharmacologic Therapy

Individual sessions with a therapist or participation in a bereavement group can help children work through a difficult loss.

Clinical Manifestations and Therapies **Childhood Grief**

ETIOLOGY	CLINICAL MANIFESTATIONS	CLINICAL THERAPIES
Normal grief	■ Feelings of depression, sadness, or anger associated with the loss ■ Behavioral regression, such as wetting the bed or baby talk ■ Confusion and restlessness ■ Preoccupation with, and an attempt to understand, death as a concept	■ Explain death in an honest, age-appropriate manner. ■ Provide reassurance. ■ Promote discussion of the child's feelings and thoughts about the loss.
Childhood traumatic grief	■ Abnormal or nonexistent progression through the grieving process ■ Conflicted feelings of grief due to trauma ■ Withdrawal from normal activities and socialization ■ Change in regular behavior	■ Grief counseling ■ Bereavement groups
Complicated grief	■ Prolonged and intensified grief ■ Drastic changes to normal ■ behavior ■ Nightmares and/or sleeplessness ■ Decrease in appetite	■ Complicated grief treatment ■ Psychotherapy

Children's bereavement groups often include activities involving drawing, writing, or other forms of arts and crafts. During these activities, the child may be encouraged to draw expressions depicting how he feels about the loss. He may also be given the option of creating a scrapbook or a memory box about the individual who has died (Walsh, 2012, p. 113). Older children and adolescents may be encouraged to practice forms of writing therapy, which can involve keeping a journal about their feelings. Other activities in writing therapy include writing a letter to the deceased. In these writings, individuals are encouraged to be entirely honest without any fear of judgment from others or from themselves. The main idea behind this form of therapy is that in writing about intense feelings of grief, pain, or trauma, the feelings will eventually begin to subside. Many individuals are not comfortable talking about these emotions or thoughts and find it easier to express their emotions openly in writing. Therapeutic writing can also be suggested for terminally ill children as a way to express their fears and uncertainties.

NURSING PROCESS

Nursing care of the pediatric or adolescent client and his family who are experiencing loss will change depending on whether the child is grieving a loss is terminally ill and grieving his own life. The nursing process connected with childhood grief begins with an assessment of the child's overall state. For the pediatric or adolescent client who is dying, primary considerations should be given to the client's comfort and psychological well-being. The psychological health of the immediate family should also be addressed. The nurse should acknowledge and encourage the client's feelings about the illness while providing options for resolution of those feelings. Depending on the developmental stage of the child, different reactions should be expected. Parents should be made aware of these reactions.

Assessment

The nurse assesses the child's and the parents' history of previous losses, coping skills, psychosocial supports, and cultural and spiritual practices and preferences. In the case of a pediatric or adolescent child experiencing grief from a recent loss, the overall health and reactions of the child should be assessed. Some families have difficulty talking about death, and the nurse needs to assess the ability of family members to support the child's grief responses. Additional parent education and referral may be necessary to help parents support their child as she grieves the loss.

Diagnosis

A child anticipating his own death or the death of a loved one can experience varying complications and changes in health. Many of these complications can come due to a fear of death, or even a fear of the change the death of a loved one will bring. Death can be quite difficult for children to fully understand. Some potential nursing diagnoses are:

- *Grieving* related to anticipation of a pending death
- *Ineffective Coping*
- *Fear*
- *Death Anxiety*
- *Spiritual Distress*

(NANDA-I © 2012)

Planning

When creating goals for a child's care involving grief, it is important to consider the child's developmental stage. Children who are 5 years old will have a different grief reaction than those who are 13 years old. Some goals for a child experiencing grief are the following:

- Child will demonstrate healthy and age-appropriate coping mechanisms.
- Child will express fears concerning death.

Implementation

Nursing interventions for childhood grief include providing emotional support for both the client and family as appropriate.

For a child who is dying, comfort measures are essential. Some comfort measures are:

- Provide pain medication as needed to keep the client comfortable.
- Involve parents by suggesting measures to help the child, including massages, warm or cool blankets as needed, singing, and reading.
- Allow parents to stay with the child as much as possible.
- Offer resources for any spiritual or cultural traditions requested by the child or family.

Some emotional support measures are:

- Encourage the child and family to ask any questions they may have.
- Educate the parents about the signs of impending death.
- Provide information about the normal coping mechanisms generally displayed during the developmental stage of the child.

- Assist in helping the parents find meaning in the child's death; this has been shown to help facilitate acceptance.

For more information, see the exemplar on End-of-Life Care in the module on Comfort, particularly the section on End-of-Life Care for Children.

For a child who is grieving the loss of a loved one or friend, appropriate nursing interventions include the following:

- Encourage the child to honestly express any feelings about the loss.
- Assure the child that it is normal to feel angry, sad, and even confused when someone dies.
- Educate the child and parents about some healthy outlets for childhood grief, such as drawing, painting, or writing to the deceased.
- Provide the parents with information about explaining death in an honest and age-appropriate manner.

Evaluation

In evaluating a child's response to death, it is imperative to remember that children often do not acknowledge their own emotions and fears related to death. Children should be encouraged to discuss any emotions they may be experiencing. Some desired outcomes are as follows:

- The client expresses fears related to death or the dying process.
- The client acknowledges grief felt at the loss of a loved one.

NURSING CARE PLAN   Loss of a Parent by a Pediatric Client

Johnny Ferris, age 8, is brought in to his regular doctor's office by his father. Since Johnny's mother died 8 months ago, Johnny has been very withdrawn and quiet. In the last 2 weeks, he has stopped eating regularly, and his sleeping habits have been irregular.

ASSESSMENT	DIAGNOSES	PLANNING
Mr. Ferris tells Johnny's regular nurse, an RN named Fatima Forez, that Johnny has been acting very strangely since his mother died. He has stopped playing with his regular friends or with anyone else. Johnny has also been very quiet, only speaking to others if he is required to. The school has reported that Johnny's grades have been declining. About a month ago, Johnny explained to his father that his mother had been physically abusing him in the year before her sudden death. At first, Mr. Ferris thought Johnny was experiencing normal grief reactions, but 2 weeks ago he stopped eating almost entirely, and he has been sleeping only a few hours a night. Ms. Forez checks Johnny's vitals and discovers that his blood pressure and temperature are both normal. When she checks Johnny's weight, Ms. Forez notices that he has lost 7 pounds since his last visit 2 months ago. When Ms. Forez asks Johnny why he has been having trouble eating and sleeping, he refuses to answer the question and looks down at the floor instead. After discussing Johnny's case with his regular pediatrician, Ms. Forez recommends that Johnny start seeing a grief counselor once a week for help working through a probable complicated grief reaction.	- *Complicated Grieving* related to psychosocial conflicts associated with coping with the loss of an abusive parent - *Imbalanced Nutrition: Less than Body Requirements* related to loss of appetite secondary to grief and feelings of guilt - *Disturbed Sleep Pattern* related to unexpressed emotions - *Ineffective Coping* related to complicated grief reaction (NANDA-I © 2012)	Goals for Johnny's care include: - The client will keep weekly appointments with grief counselor. - The client will eat at least one full meal per day and eat whenever he feels hungry. - The client will regain a relatively normal sleep schedule.

IMPLEMENTATION

- Teach about complicated grief reactions.
- Emphasize the importance of eating to maintain and increase weight.

- Explain the benefits of grief counseling.

NURSING CARE PLAN *(continued)*

EVALUATION

Johnny begins going to grief counseling every week. His therapist works with Johnny to develop healthy coping mechanisms to work through his emotions and grief. Johnny starts to get his appetite back, and his sleeping habits begin to improve. After 2 months of grief counseling, Johnny goes to his follow up appointment; his weight and disposition have returned to normal.

CRITICAL THINKING

1. If Johnny had not improved after 2 months with a grief counselor, how would you change the nursing care plan?
2. How would this nursing care plan have been different had Johnny's grief not been complicated by an abusive parent?

◣ REVIEW Children's Response to Loss

RELATE Link the Concepts and Exemplars

Linking the exemplar children's response to loss with the concept of immunity:

1. How does the stress of losing a loved one impact the functioning of the immune system? For pediatric clients, what age-specific implications should be considered?

2. What strategies could you implement to promote optimal immune function for the pediatric client who is experiencing grief and loss?

Linking the exemplar children's response to loss with the concept of development:

3. While assessing a 4-year-old whose mother died 2 years ago, you find the child has some small delays in developmental milestones. Why might this have happened?

4. What interventions can you initiate to help this child meet future developmental milestones?

READY Go to Companion Skills Manual

REFER Go to Pearson Student Nursing Resources
nursing.pearsonhighered.com

- Additional review materials

REFLECT Case Study

Jason Riley is an active, healthy 11-year-old boy. He is currently in the fifth grade at the public grade school near his home. He lives with his mother, Evelyn, and his 14-year-old sister Jenna. He has never had much contact with his father. Jason's home life has been somewhat stressful this last year because of fighting between his mom and oldest sister Jessica, who moved out and lives in her own apartment with her new baby. Jason gets along well with his mom and oldest sister but has typical sibling conflicts with his sister Jenna.

This year, Jason is not doing well in school, academically or socially. He tells his sister that he gets teased a lot because he doesn't have a father. His mother has been told by the teachers that he is disruptive in class. Jason and his mom are in the clinic for a well-child check today.

1. Based on Jason's developmental level, what loss might he be grieving?

2. How is Jason's grief impacting his daily life?

3. As the nurse, how might you guide both Jason and his mother to help Jason discuss and cope with his feelings of loss more constructively?

◣ EXEMPLAR 27.2 Death and Dying

EXEMPLAR LEARNING OUTCOMES

After reading about this exemplar, you will be able to:

1. Describe the pathophysiology, etiology, clinical manifestations, and direct and indirect causes of death.

2. Identify the physiological changes associated with death.

3. Illustrate the nursing process in providing culturally sensitive care across the life span for individuals who are dying.

4. Formulate priority nursing diagnoses appropriate for an individual who is dying.

5. Summarize therapies used by interdisciplinary teams in the collaborative care of an individual who is dying.

6. Plan evidence-based care for an individual who is dying and his or her family in collaboration with other members of the healthcare team.

7. Evaluate expected outcomes for an individual who is dying.

▶ OVERVIEW

Death, the process of dying, and the client's response to and perception of that process are highly individualized. The client with terminal lung cancer dies differently from the client killed instantly in a motor vehicle crash. The former has time to consider death and perhaps even to fear it or accept it; the latter is relieved of any of these feelings and considerations. Similarly, responses of family members to death—whether imminent or sudden, expected or unexpected—vary greatly. To support the range of clients and their families (and their various responses), the nurse needs a solid understanding of the physiological process of death and dying. Before understanding these processes and working with the dying client, however, nurses must examine their own thoughts and fears about death.

▶ PATHOPHYSIOLOGY AND ETIOLOGY

Various signs and symptoms of death can present themselves up to 3 months before a client's death. Some of these are changes in attitude, while others involve physiological changes such as decreasing blood pressure and abnormal breathing. If clients have accepted the illness they are suffering from, they may be more willing to acknowledge the signs of death. Family members of clients are sometimes not as willing to accept these signs. It is the nurse's responsibility to keep the client informed about his condition and about any changes he can expect. Similarly, keeping the family informed (with the client's permission) about expected changes in the client can also be beneficial. For example, individuals who have accepted the terminal nature of their illness often become withdrawn for a time. If the nurse is able to alert the family to this potential common response or explain it when it occurs, it may make this period of withdrawal easier for both the client and family.

Etiology

Death may be the result of an accident, injury, violent act, suicide, or illness. The actions leading to an individual's death often determine how the client, family members, and care team react. For example, clients dying as a result of a progressive illness will have more time to accept the situation, as will the family, and the care team will design a care plan accordingly. When death comes suddenly, there is little or no time to prepare, even though the realization of the death may be immediate and profound. Regardless of the catalyst, the ultimate medical cause of death is the cessation of all vital organ functions, primarily the heart, brain, and respiratory functions. If the individual is on life support, then death is defined as the absence of brain waves for 24 hours or more (Berman & Snyder, 2011, p. 1108).

▶ CLINICAL MANIFESTATIONS

Signs of impending death may be physiological or psychological. Nurses caring for clients who are dying will work to address not only clients' physical needs, but also their emotional needs, such as grief and anxiety. The family's needs should also be addressed, as this will make the process easier for both the client and family.

Anticipatory Grief

Anticipatory grief can affect both the client who is dying and the client's family. This type of grief is experienced in advance of an individual's death. When anticipatory grief is experienced by clients who are dying, this grief is not only directed at their own death, but also at the loss of everything they love that will soon be gone. Anticipatory grieving can be a catalyst for saying good-bye to loved ones and resolving any unfinished affairs. However, it can also result in the clients' distancing themselves from friends and family members in an effort to decrease the pain of loss (Walsh, 2012, p. 92). Clients' family members may also experience anticipatory grieving, which in some cases could help to lessen the intensity of grief after the clients' death. Not all individuals who know of a loved one's death will experience anticipatory grieving, but it is common. If possible, nurses can try to encourage clients and family members to be honest with one another about how they are feeling.

Helping the Client Cope With Death

Clients who are working to accept the reality of their own death often experience a wide range of emotions, from anger and fear to denial and sadness. At times, some of these emotions can be directed at the nurse, even though the client is likely angry as a result of grief and not anything the nurse has done. Nurses should be aware of the possibility of such emotional reactions and try not to take them personally. It is during this time, when clients are beginning to cope with the fact of impending death, that nurses can be of considerable assistance. Nurses have the benefit of not only knowing about the illness or condition the clients are suffering from, but also about the grieving process and the process of dying. In providing clients with information about the types of symptoms and changes they will experience both physically and emotionally, nurses help to prepare the clients for these coming changes. Death in itself is often seen as terrifying and mysterious, but by warning clients about what is to be expected, nurses help to demystify the experience. Aiding clients and their families in understanding the dying process also helps to reinforce positive coping mechanisms that move away from denial and toward acceptance.

Lifespan and Cultural Considerations

The nurse who provides end-of-life care generally interacts with the client more often than almost any other healthcare provider. During this particularly stressful time for both the client and the family, it is imperative that the relationship between the nurse and the client be built on respect and mutual goals. Nurses should refrain from judging the cultural preferences of clients and should work to help them die in the way they choose. A lot of control has already been taken away from the dying client, but she can still choose what cultural traditions she would like observed, and who should be with her when she dies. If these needs can be facilitated in any way by the nurse, then they should be. For example, some cultures perform last rites ceremonies involving incense, scented candles, and possibly even chanting. These rituals could be disruptive to other individuals if performed in the client's room, but the nurse could find another area where these traditions could take place.

Pain management often plays a large role in end-of-life care. However, some cultures view pain as an important part of life and consider pain at the end of life an act of purification. This belief may cause difficulty for the nurse, who sees that the client is suffering from intense pain, but the client's wishes should be honored (Guido, 2010, p. 148). Culture, and for that matter an individual's personality, may also contribute to how a client expresses his needs. Some clients may feel less inclined to tell the nurse if they are uncomfortable or concerned in any way because they do not want to bother the nurse. This can make it very difficult to provide adequate care for the client, as the nurse may not know the individual is in pain. Nurses should encourage open lines of communication with clients, so that their needs do not go unmet. When working with children who are dying, nurses should reassure them that it is important to report any pain they may be feeling. See the exemplar on Acute and Chronic Pain in the module on Comfort for information on assessing pain in children.

Physiological Changes in the Dying Client

A number of physiological changes occur when an individual's body begins to stop functioning. Some of these changes can be of great concern to the client and/or the client's family, so the nurse should make them aware of such alterations. Nurses should inform clients and their families about the normal progression of physiological symptoms, depending on the client's illness; this will help them prepare for what to expect in the coming days or weeks.

DYSPNEA Dyspnea occurs when the client has trouble breathing normally. This can be caused by a number of factors, including chemotherapy, heart failure, abdominal ascites, and infection. The treatment will depend on the client's desires for medical interventions during end-of-life care. Oxygen via nasal cannula can be used to lessen the symptoms of breathlessness. If the client permits pharmacologic interventions, opioids can be administered, as well as benzodiazepines for any underlying anxiety. Of the opioids, morphine is the most commonly administered medication for clients receiving end-of-life care. Nonpharmacologic nursing interventions may include positioning the client with the upper body elevated to a level of improved comfort, as well as teaching the client relaxation techniques to reduce anxiety.

HYPOTENSION Low blood pressure, or hypotension, occurs as a client's body begins to near death. This is often accompanied by cool skin and an irregular pulse rate. Hypotension can lead to blurry vision, as well as confusion and dizziness; however, etiologies other than low blood pressure may also be the source of these symptoms.

ANOREXIA, NAUSEA, AND DEHYDRATION Anorexia involves a client's loss of appetite and desire to eat. This may be a symptom of the client's illness, but it is also a common occurrence in clients at the end of life. Loss of appetite often will be of less concern to clients than to their families. Nurses should explain that anorexia is normal at this stage in the individual's illness. Clients may consider trying to eat their favorite meals, which should be prepared with strong spices, as these will help the meal to be more appealing to the client. Alcoholic beverages, which are normally high in calories, can also help to improve a client's appetite, provided alcohol is not contraindicated with any of the client's medications.

Nausea is also very common at the end of life. Nausea may result from a variety of causes, including medications, constipation, anxiety, or overwhelming odors. Nonpharmacologic interventions include drinking ginger ale, eating crackers, and practicing relaxation techniques. If the client allows pharmacologic interventions, an antiemetic may be prescribed to reduce nausea.

Dehydration is rarely a cause for distress in clients at this stage. Often the client will complain of a dry mouth, for which nurses should assess and provide care every 2 hours. Intravenous fluids are not recommended, as they will generally make the client more uncomfortable. Small sips of water should be offered.

Most families are unfamiliar with the signs of dying and may take some of them as a sign that the client is "giving up." Families should be reassured that symptoms such as loss of appetite and nausea are a normal part of the dying process.

ALTERED LEVELS OF CONSCIOUSNESS Clients at the end of life may experience confusion as the result of infection, electrolyte abnormalities, medications, illness progression, and pain, as well as from many other causes. During periods of altered consciousness, the client may begin rambling or acting contrary to normal behaviors; concentration is also poor during these periods. If the client's actions become uncontrollable or put the client at risk, sedation may be necessary. In cases such as this, haloperidol or chlorpromazine generally is used. Clients in their last hours who are suffering from altered levels of consciousness can also be treated with morphine. It is helpful for these clients to be surrounded with familiar family and staff, as changes will only cause more confusion.

PAIN Pain and pain management are primary concerns for the client in need of end-of-life care. If a client is dying from a terminal illness or an untreatable injury or condition, the client will also likely be suffering from pain. At this stage in the client's care, pain medication should be administered as needed, as there is no longer a concern about long-term effects or addiction. Nurses conduct a thorough pain assessment to ensure appropriate interventions. (See the exemplar on Acute and Chronic Pain in the concept of Comfort). Morphine or other opioids are the most common pain medications used, but coanalgesic drugs and nerve blocks may also be considered. To be effective, pain management should be reassessed at least twice a day, with modifications in treatment and dosage being made as needed.

PSYCHOSOCIAL NEEDS As clients approach death, nurses should encourage the client and family to say good-bye and make any final arrangements in accordance with the client's final wishes. This stage can be very difficult for the client's family, so nurses should explain that it benefits the client to have as much resolution as possible before dying. Any final cultural or religious practices should also be arranged in accordance with the client's requests (see the Focus on Diversity and Culture feature).

When a client dies, nurses may be present with both the client and family members. In nursing homes and memory care centers, for example, it is not uncommon for nurses and other staff members who have cared for the client to be in the room

Focus on Diversity and Culture Culture and the Dying Client

■ Cultural and religious beliefs and traditions are often of paramount importance for end-of-life clients and their families. Nurses should work to facilitate requests to every extent possible. For example, some cultures (in particular, those who practice the Islamic faith) observe a ritual of cleansing the body immediately after death. Others may call for a priest or spiritual leader to say prayers with the client who is dying and family members.

■ If a nurse is uncomfortable with the cultural practices and traditions of the client, then another nurse, possibly with a similar cultural background, should be asked to work with that client.

■ For clients who do not speak English, nurses should seek the assistance of a qualified interpreter to ensure that they

understand the client's and family's needs, and that the client and family understand the care being provided. In some instances, the interpreter may be able to help facilitate cultural and religious practices.

■ The parents' decision to tell a child who is terminally ill of impending death may also be based on cultural practices; some cultures consider it imperative that the dying, especially the very young and the very old, not be told of their illnesses (Walsh, 2012).

■ Expressions of grief also may be culturally influenced. Some cultures see it as a sign of weakness to grieve or cry openly. Nurses must refrain from assuming that loved ones are not grieving simply because they do not show grief to others.

with the client and family as the client dies. This can provide great comfort to the family, especially when nurses have taken the time to build a therapeutic relationship with both the client and family.

Once the client has died, family members may desire to spend time alone with the deceased. It is important that this be allowed. In particular, nurses encourage parents of children and adolescents to hold their child and take as much time as they need to say good-bye. Families should also be allowed time and space to observe cultural and spiritual practices.

DETERMINATION OF DEATH   The following signs and symptoms indicate that death has occurred:

■ Flat encephalogram

■ No pulse or respiratory activity

■ No response to external stimuli

■ No reflexes

■ No muscle movement

▶ THE NURSE'S RESPONSE TO DEATH AND DYING

All nurses will encounter death of a client at some point in their practice, although nurses in care settings such as oncology, hospice, the emergency department, and intensive care units will experience client deaths with some frequency. All nurses, but especially those who work with terminally ill clients, should assess their own needs to grieve and process a loss. If these needs are not addressed, the nurse is more likely to experience burnout (Guido, 2010, p. 162).

Nurses not accustomed to working with dying clients should also assess their own feelings regarding death. Nurses who are not comfortable with the topic of dying may not be prepared when confronted by a client who is dying and in need of support. When this happens, nurses may cope by encouraging the client or family member to talk about something else. While this may seem more conducive to the client's happiness, it can be detrimental to the client's overall well-

Clinical Manifestations and Therapies Death and Dying

ETIOLOGY	CLINICAL MANIFESTATIONS	CLINICAL THERAPIES
Dyspnea	■ Difficulty breathing ■ Breathlessness ■ Wheezing	■ Oxygen by nasal cannula ■ Morphine ■ Elevated bed position ■ Anxiety reduction
Nausea	■ Feeling nauseated ■ Loss of appetite ■ Sometimes vomiting	■ Ginger or ginger ale ■ Crackers ■ Anxiety reduction ■ Antiemetics
Confusion	■ Restlessness ■ Rambling ■ Poor concentration ■ Acting contrary to normal behavior	■ Haloperidol ■ Chlorpromazine

being. Similarly, the nurse who is uncomfortable with the topic of death may try to avoid the topic by providing the client with false hope, saying things such as "You are going to be fine; don't worry." This type of false reassurance is not beneficial to either the client or the family (Berman & Snyder, 2011, p. 1108). Nurses need to honestly assess their own feelings about death and handle them properly so as not to impose these feelings on the client. For example, a nurse who is obviously anxious about and fearful of death can make a client more fearful of death.

Coping With the Loss of a Client

Nurses are not immune to the effects of grief over the death of a client. When working with a client who has a terminal illness, or a client who has been fatally injured, it is easy for a nurse to form a bond with this individual. These bonds can result not only in normal feelings of grief, such as sorrow, but also in feelings of guilt, as nurses sometimes wonder if they could have done more to help their clients. In such cases, it is important that nurses acknowledge and process their feelings of guilt rather than ignore them. Similarly, nurses should seek support for any grief they may feel at the loss of a client (**Figure 27–6** ●). Resources for support may include coworkers, professional therapists or social workers, and grief counseling resources offered through employers. It is important that nurses make time to seek and find the support they need to process their own grief in a healthy manner. In acknowledging and process-

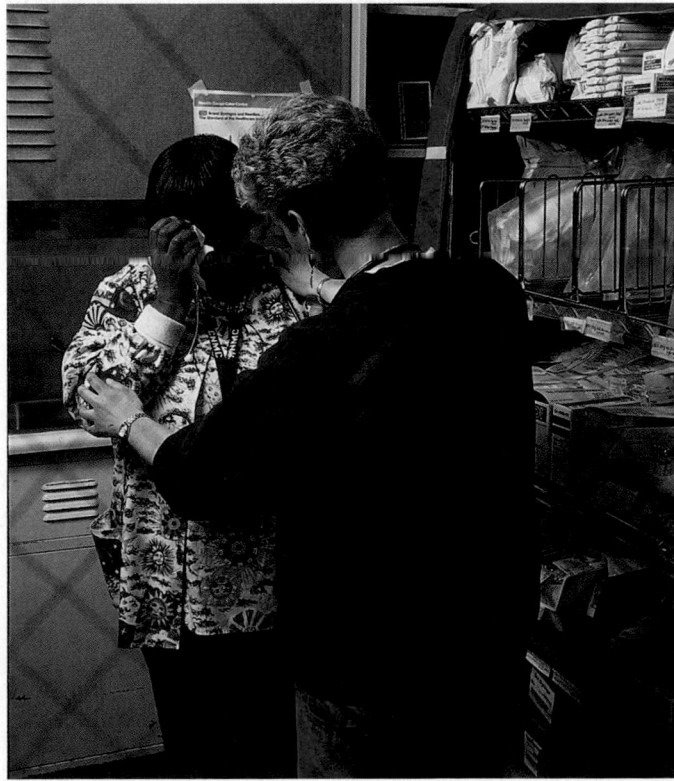

Figure 27–6 ● Nurses need to express their own grief in a supportive environment after a child's death. Sharing with colleagues the sadness and grief or futility of resuscitation efforts often helps nurses provide supportive care to the next family who needs it.

ing their grief over a client's death, nurses will be better able to help future clients and their families through the processes of death and grief.

▶ COLLABORATION

End-of-life clients often will benefit from working with social workers as their illness progresses. Social workers can help both the client and the family to plan for the coming days, weeks, or months of the client's life, as well as helping them to prepare for what will happen after the client dies. Nurses and social workers can collaborate to develop the plan of care for the client that will be most beneficial, and that reflects the desires of the client. For clients who belong to a specific religion, collaboration with the client's faith leader or the hospital chaplain also may provide comfort to the client and family.

Pharmacologic Therapy

Pharmacologic therapy for end-of-life clients is generally in the form of pain management, as well as any medications needed to treat symptoms that may arise either from the pain medicines or from underlying conditions. Some clients will refuse any medications or treatments other than pain management as they do not wish to prolong their life, while others will accept medications for any symptoms that may arise during their care. Pain management is a vital part of end-of-life care and can be administered to most clients without sedating them. As stated earlier, opioids, morphine in particular, are the preferred pharmacotherapy for pain at the end of life. Effective management of pain will require scheduled doses as well as rescue doses for any breakthrough pain. Clients who have had chronic pain for many years are harder to treat for pain management, but it is possible. Treatment for these clients should be strategically planned and continuously reassessed (Guido, 2010).

Nonpharmacologic Therapy

Various other therapies can be used in combination with pain management and other pharmacologic interventions. Most of these therapies involve comfort and anxiety reduction measures:

- Massage and touch in general can help the client to relax and also help relieve any muscle spasms.
- Heat therapy helps with relaxation and muscle cramps and spasms.
- Acupuncture can be used for multiple types of pain relief.
- Mouth and oral care, including cleaning and moistening the lips, mouth, and tongue, increases comfort.
- Meditation and breathing techniques can be employed for anxiety reduction.

Clients may not always verbalize discomfort or pain. For that reason, observation for physical cues and interviewing the client are keys to assessment for discomfort. (For further discussion of pain assessment, see the concept of Comfort.) Sometimes something as simple as helping the client to sit up in bed and readjusting her pillows can go a long way toward the client's overall comfort.

NURSING PROCESS

Caring for dying clients requires nurses to consider the needs not only of the client, but also of the client's family. Some clients come to an acceptance of their death, while others may be less accepting and more anxious. Either of these reactions can be difficult for the family; nurses can help by explaining the dying and grieving process to both the client and the family.

Assessment

Nurses assess client comfort and anxiety levels regularly. Pain assessments should be performed at least twice a day, if not more often, depending on the client's pain levels. If the client reports that pain is not subsiding, nurse should consult the physician about raising the dosage or changing the medication regimen. In addition to pain management and physical comfort, nurses assess the client's social and spiritual needs. The client may request to be surrounded by comforting objects, have the window open, listen to a particular type of music, or have access to a religious text; the nurse facilitates these requests to the greatest extent possible.

As the client approaches death, the nurse assesses vital signs often, watching for hypotension, abnormal pulse rates, and a cooling of the skin and body temperature. The nurse makes the family aware of any changes as they occur.

Diagnosis

Diagnoses involving the end-of-life client and that individual's family vary depending on multiple factors, including personality, culture, and the circumstances surrounding the client's illness or condition. For additional examples of nursing diagnoses relevant to physiological needs associated with the dying process, see the module on Comfort. Within the realm of psychosocial concerns for the client who requires end-of-life care, some potential nursing diagnoses are:

- *Fear*
- *Death Anxiety*
- *Grieving* related to impending death

(NANDA-I © 2012)

Planning

The nurse, healthcare team, client, and family members or caregivers as designated by the client collaborate to develop the plan of care. The nurse facilitates the client's wishes to the greatest extent possible, in order to increase comfort and reduce anxiety about the dying process. When working with family members, it is important for the nurse to help the family consider the best interests of the client. Appropriate outcomes may include the following:

- The client will maintain dignity throughout the dying process.
- The client will remain free of pain throughout the dying process.
- The client will participate in the decision-making process as long as competent to do so.
- The family will receive the emotional support needed throughout the dying process.

Implementation

The nurse working with the dying client and the family is responsible for communicating changes in client health status and providing a wide array of caring interventions at a time when the client and family are most in need of support and consideration.

All terminally ill clients reach a point when they can no longer care for themselves. Nurses are responsible for implementing caring interventions to prevent impairments in skin integrity, prevent and alleviate pain, and maintain client hygiene. Nursing care for the comatose client or the client with a very low level of consciousness or cognition includes:

- Using artificial tears if the client does not blink
- Keeping lights at a low level
- Keeping the client's skin clean and dry
- Covering the client only with a light blanket
- Using adult incontinence pads or pants for incontinence
- Turning the client every 2 hours and maintaining joint positions

The nurse can assist the client in addressing fears by ensuring comfort and support. Often the nurse is present for the client and family and can communicate compassion through caring acts such as adjusting the client's position in bed or gently massaging the client's hands with lotion. Nurses also can help alleviate fears by providing family members the opportunity to observe religious and spiritual rituals with the client. Offering to call the family's minister or spiritual leader, providing space and time, and scheduling nursing interventions around specific prayer times can provide a great deal of comfort to clients and families during this time. Additional supportive interventions may include the following:

- Refer clients and families to social services and other agencies that provide financial support.
- Provide bedside activities and distractions to decrease boredom and to limit obsessing about death. Schools, churches, and civic organizations are excellent sources of volunteers who read to clients; play cards or board games with clients; or sit, pray, or simply listen to music with clients.
- Encourage clients who are able to form support groups to discuss fears and ways to alleviate them.
- Ensure that clients who are still competent have the opportunity to visit with their lawyer or financial representative so that they can make the necessary arrangements regarding wills and advanced directives.

Evaluation

Outcomes for the dying client are centered on physiological comfort and emotional support. A client should never have to fear dying in pain. Some desired outcomes are as follows:

- The client expresses fears related to death or the dying process.
- The client informs the nurse about increases in pain.
- The client is made comfortable.
- The client's family remains informed of any changes in the client's condition.

REVIEW Death and Dying

RELATE Link the Concepts and Exemplars

Linking the exemplar of death and dying with the concept of culture and diversity:

1. When caring for a client who just died, how can you support the family's request to hold a ceremony and prepare the body according to its customs?

2. What priority interventions will you implement for the family visiting the bedside of the client who is dying from lung cancer if the family members are from South America and speak no English?

Linking the exemplar of death and dying with the concept of comfort:

3. What appropriate response will you make to a family member who states that he or she cannot stand to watch his or her father gasp for air and asks you to do something to make him more comfortable?

4. What are your priorities of care for the client dying at home and his or her family?

READY Go to Companion Skills Manual

REFER Go to Pearson Nursing Student Resources
nursing.pearsonhighered.com

- Additional review materials

REFLECT Case Study

Julianna Converse, a 38-year-old, has been diagnosed with metastatic breast cancer. She had a radical mastectomy of the left breast 1 month ago. Diagnostic tests indicate metastasis to the brain and bone. She is currently being treated with chemotherapy and radiation. Julianna and her husband, Frank, have three children: Paul, age 17; Mary, age 12; and Johnny, age 8. Julianna recently quit her job as a buyer for a major clothing chain due to her treatments and extreme fatigue. Julianna has been told her chance for survival is very slim, and she has accepted her likely death. She is trying to put her affairs in order while she has the energy to do the things that are important to her. She has contacted friends and family to help her plan for the future care of her children. Julianna is in the clinic today for chemotherapy and appears depressed and sad. Her chest is excoriated from the radiation treatments, her hair is brittle and falling out, and she has very little energy.

1. How can you assess your assumption of depression and sadness?

2. What nursing diagnoses are appropriate for Julianna? Which take priority at this time?

3. Describe a conversation you might have with Julianna using therapeutic communication to help her express her feelings?

4. What resources could you recommend to Julianna to help her plan for her family's future?

EXEMPLAR 27.3   Older Adult's Response to Loss

EXEMPLAR KEY TERM
Ageism, *1763*

EXEMPLAR LEARNING OUTCOMES
After reading about this exemplar, you will be able to:

1. Describe the pathophysiology, etiology, clinical manifestations, and direct and indirect causes of loss and grief in the older adult.

2. Identify risk factors and prevention methods associated with loss or grief in the older adult.

3. Illustrate the nursing process in providing culturally competent care across the life span for older adults experiencing loss or grief.

4. Formulate priority nursing diagnoses appropriate for an older adult experiencing loss or grief.

5. Summarize therapies used by interdisciplinary teams in the collaborative care of an older adult experiencing grief.

6. Plan evidence-based care for an older adult experiencing grief and his or her family in collaboration with other members of the healthcare team.

7. Evaluate expected outcomes for an older adult experiencing loss or grief.

▶ OVERVIEW

Older adults' responses to grief and loss can be intricate because of inherent factors unique to this age demographic. Older adults are defined as anyone 65 years of age or older. At this point in life, the older adult has more than likely accumulated a number of losses, both symbolic and actual. This accumulation may compound any new grief felt by the individual: A new loss may bring up grief from one or more previous losses.

▶ PATHOPHYSIOLOGY AND ETIOLOGY

Grief and loss as experienced by older adults can be more complicated than at other ages. A single death may trigger multiple losses. For example, a woman in the early stages of Alzheimer

disease may be able to live in her home while her husband is in good health. When he dies and she moves in with one of her children, her loss of independence may accelerate. Older adults will lose friends and acquaintances in their age group, and as that happens they begin to anticipate their own death as well as the death of their partners (Walsh, 2012).

Etiology

Losses associated with aging are varied and may include loss of independence, loss of mobility, loss of health, and loss of memory. Unfortunately, these create a misperception among some younger adults that with age inevitably comes frailty and deterioration of mental function. Misperceptions such as this are considered a form of **ageism**, which involves forming stereotypes about older adults. Nurses must guard against such misperceptions. Many older adults live active, healthy, fulfilling lives.

Factors Affecting the Grieving Process

Older adults are at greater risk of depression following significant real or symbolic losses. Depression in older adults is rarely the result of only one factor. Among the most common causes of depression in this population are the death of a loved one, loss of independence, illness, and isolation and loneliness. Untreated depression can worsen and is very serious. It can lead to the prolonging of other illnesses, and even to suicide. As of 2009, suicide in older adults had started to decline and finally dipped below the rate of suicide in individuals from ages 25 to 64. From 1987 to the early 2000s, the rate of suicide in older adults had surpassed the rate of every other age demographic. Among older adults, the highest percentage of individuals who committed suicide were Caucasian males. Various studies over the years have shown that approximately 75% of older adults who committed suicide had seen a doctor within a month of their death. These adults were very likely suffering from depression at the time of their appointment (American Association of Suicidology, 2009; National Institute of Mental Health, 2010; Centers for Disease Control and Prevention, 2012). Grief is a powerful emotion, particularly when coupled with other losses. Older adults should be assessed for signs of serious depression, especially after the loss of a spouse or other loved one.

> **SAFETY ALERT**
> Suicide in older adults is commonly the result of untreated depression. In the past, the chronic underdiagnosis of minor depression in older adults led to high suicide rates—particularly in males. Nurses should assess for signs of depression, even if it appears minor, and then assess for increased risk of suicide.

▶ CLINICAL MANIFESTATIONS

Manifestations of grief in older adults may be more profound than those observed in younger clients. Accumulating losses in combination with existing health conditions and medication side effects may contribute to a complicated grief reaction. As a result, grief in older adults that may present as a response to the loss of a single person, object, or freedom may actually be a reaction to numerous losses that have accumulated over time. How older adults handle loss depends on the circumstances of the loss, as well as the overall health of the individual—both physically and mentally.

Older Clients' Response to Grief

Grief initially presents in older adults much as it presents in younger adults; anger, sadness, longing, disbelief, and depression may be present. The duration and intensity of these emotions vary from client to client. Older adults may seem to experience the emotional aspects of grief more acutely than younger adults; for example, older adults may show pronounced and overwhelming feelings of anger or sadness in response to a death. It also is common for older adults—particularly those living alone—to respond to intense grief by neglecting their own needs. Eating habits, personal hygiene, and health maintenance may fluctuate during periods of bereavement. Nurses need to be particularly observant of these changes in regular nutrition, hygiene, and health, as they indicate that clients are not taking care of themselves and may need additional support.

CLIENT'S HISTORY In working with older adults who are experiencing grief, it is important to inquire about other recent losses, as well as any present health concerns such as dementia, Alzheimer disease, or a history of depression or suicide attempts. If a client has recently experienced a number of losses, a common experience for older adults, the accumulation of these losses can be overwhelming. When assessing the span of loss in older adults, it is important to consider all losses. For example, the loss of mobility, the loss of independence, and even the loss of a beloved pet can all contribute to feelings of overwhelming grief.

For clients with dementia or Alzheimer disease, the death of a loved one is very complicated. The affected client may have been told about the individual's death and been emotional, but may then have forgotten that this individual has died. Even in the early stages of Alzheimer disease, newly learned information is often forgotten quickly (Alzheimer's Association, 2013). A client's loss of memory of a loved one's death can be hard on the nurse and/or the client's caretaker, as the individual may ask to see the loved one who has died. Similarly, the client may become very upset because the deceased has not come to visit. If the client were to be reminded daily of the loss, then he would experience fresh grief for the individual who had died. With the progression of Alzheimer disease, the grieving process becomes virtually impossible as it constantly requires time to accept and process the loss.

COMPLICATED GRIEF Complicated grief in older adults manifests in feelings of unrelenting preoccupation and yearning resulting from the loss, experienced over an increased duration of time (at least 6 months or more). Memories, even those that are happy, illicit strong emotions, which may be coupled with an avoidance of familiar places or individuals who trigger thoughts of the deceased or regret of the loss. Clients may also manifest trust issues, suspecting once close friends and family members of judging their pain or not understanding their emotions. Because of these feelings of judgment or betrayal, the clients may appear distant and even uncaring. This may be especially true of older adults who have experienced a loss of independence or mobility. Nurses need to be observant of the progression of grief in older adults. If symptoms intensify or affect the client's overall health, appropriate assessments and interventions need to be made. Signs of intense depression should also be monitored, as complicated grief and depression are often comorbid disorders (Robinaugh et al., 2012).

Lifespan and Cultural Considerations

It is a common misconception that all older adults are frail, have dementia, or cannot handle upsetting news as well as others. However, these generalizations are simply not true for every older adult. An individual does not become frail or weak simply because she has reached 65 years of age. When assessing grief in older adults, it is important to take into consideration the many difficulties that can occur later in life, but it is equally important to assess each client individually rather than to automatically apply generalizations about the aging.

Many older adults find deep meaning in their religious or spiritual beliefs and practices, possibly because these individuals were raised during a time when religious practices were more widespread than they are currently. A client may turn to religion

- Depression is prevalent among older adults, especially those with decreased support systems.
- Depression can present itself in older adults in combination with other illness, such as diabetes, heart disease, and cancer.
- The risk factors for both dementia and Alzheimer disease increase with age.
- One in every eight older American adults has Alzheimer disease (Alzheimer's Association, 2012).

in times of grief or loss. If the client is in a nursing home, hospital, hospice, or an extended care facility and is working through grief, nurses should inquire if the client would like to participate in any specific form of religious practice. Nurses should assist clients in meeting these needs when possible.

► COLLABORATION

Older adults experiencing significant losses may require support in a variety of areas. Nurses must assess their need for support carefully. Clients might find it helpful to talk to others who have had similar losses, or they might want to speak individually with a professional therapist. Some clients may need referral to a social worker to learn more about means of financial support, including financial assistance with groceries or housing. Some clients may require pharmacologic therapy.

Pharmacologic Therapy

Two conditions involving grief may require pharmacologic therapies: depression and complicated grief. Treatment of depression begins with assessment to determine the underlying cause of the depression. Most of the time depression can be treated quite

Focus on Diversity and Culture
Loss Among Older Adults

Nurses practice culturally sensitive care by assessing clients' cultural and spiritual beliefs and practices and incorporating them into the care plan appropriately. This aspect of nursing is particularly important in work with older adults experiencing loss.

- Those who uphold traditional Asian cultural beliefs have a great respect for older adults and are expected to take care of their parents if they need assistance in later life.
- Muslims are instructed by the Qur'an to honor, respect, and care for their parents as they age. It would be considered dishonorable for an older Muslim adult to be placed in a retirement or nursing home if a child or grandchild is still available to see to the client's care.
- Native American traditions consider the elders of the tribe the keepers of wisdom and knowledge. Older adults are cared for by all members of the tribe. Death is not something to be feared, as the soul is considered immortal.

effectively through nonpharmacologic therapies, but in cases where they proves ineffective, antidepressants may be used. Antidepressants should be used with caution in older adults, as various other medications have adverse reactions with some forms of antidepressants. Similarly, some conditions that are particularly prevalent in older adults—such as diabetes, dementia, and heart problems—can be made worse by antidepressants (Wiese, 2011).

Treatment of complicated grief sometimes involves antidepressants, generally in the form of serotonin reuptake inhibitors (SSRIs). Some of the common SSRIs used are escitalopram, paroxetine, and nortriptyline. These are used in combination with Complicated Grief Treatment, as they have not proved effective when used alone to treat complicated grief (Robinaugh et al., 2012). Both escitalopram and nortriptyline are mildly contraindicated for use in older adults and are to be used with caution; similarly, paroxetine may cause negative side effects in clients with heart disease (Wilson, Shannon, & Shields, 2013). Older adults who are prescribed antidepressants for grief should be monitored closely for any side effects or complications.

Nonpharmacologic Therapy

Treatment of grief in older adults can be successful without medications. Group therapies can be quite effective, as they can be a means of support that the individual may be lacking, as well as a place where the client can discuss any concerns in a judgment-free setting. This type of therapy can also be particularly helpful as it introduces the client to other individuals who have experienced the same loss, and who may be having similar grief responses. For some clients, depending on their personality and preferences, group therapy may not be a good option, but individual therapy may be helpful. Complicated grief is generally treated with a form of psychotherapy called Complicated Grief Treatment, which treats the symptoms of complicated grief while helping the client to move through the grieving process (Shear, 2005). The goal of the treatment is acceptance of the loss, as well as natural healing. Support groups have also proved effective in the treatment of complicated grief in older adults.

🜚 **Stay Current:** For more information on Complicated Grief Treatment, visit The Center for Complicated Grief at **http://www. complicatedgrief.org/about/profile/katherine-shear-m.d/**

◼ NURSING PROCESS

Nursing care for older adults who are working through loss and grief requires a certain amount of sensitivity and understanding. Older adults may be reluctant to admit difficulty coping with grief, in part due to ageism and the stigma attached to conditions such as depression and dementia and mental health treatment. It is important for nurses to remember that, because of a client's history with previous losses, a current loss that does not seem significant to the nurse may be very significant to the client. Careful, holistic assessment is necessary for nurses to gain an accurate picture of the client's care needs.

Assessment

Nurses working with older adults who have experienced a loss and are subsequently grieving should complete a full assessment of the client's history—both physical and mental health—as well as an assessment of the client's coping mechanisms. Older adults, especially older adult males, are at a particularly high risk for both depression and suicide, so the nurse should assess for signs of depression. The client's support system should also be evaluated. If the client has been grieving for 6 months or more and the grief has not lessened, or has significantly increased, then the nurse should assess for signs of a complicated grief reaction. Collaboration with social workers can be quite helpful when working with clients who are grieving.

The nurse should provide the client with any assistance involving spiritual or cultural needs. If the client would like to attend religious services or talk to a pastor, rabbi, or other spiritual leader, then the nurse should help to facilitate these needs. Similarly, the nurse should try to help the client who mentions finding comfort in religious or spiritual texts, but not having access to them.

Diagnosis

An older adult's response to loss and grief varies based on the nature of the loss. Nurses should take into consideration the client's past history before making any diagnoses. Various diagnoses can be made in connection with an older adult's responses to grief and loss:

- *Self-Neglect*
- *Disturbed Sleep Pattern*
- *Grieving*
- *Complicated Grieving*
- *Risk for Situational Low Self-Esteem*

(NANDA-I © 2012)

Planning

The nurse should collaborate with the client to develop the plan of care that works best for the client's grief response, personality, and history. Potential outcomes include:

- The client will participate in group therapy or one-on-one therapy, depending preference.
- The client will use healthy coping mechanisms.

- The client will discuss any instances of depression or suicidal thoughts with the nurse or another healthcare provider.
- The client will move on to acceptance of the loss.

Implementation

Implementation of the client's care depends on a number of factors, including the nature of the loss, the client's health, the client's use of coping mechanisms, and the client's personality. Interventions helpful in working with older adults who are grieving include:

- Teach the client about the grieving process and its general progression.
- Discuss the benefits of different forms of therapy, as well as the differences between modes of therapy such as group therapy, psychotherapy, and one-on-one therapy.
- Inform the client about the warning signs of intense depression and/or suicidal thoughts.
- Teach the client about healthy coping mechanisms as opposed to unhealthy coping mechanisms.
- Provide a judgment-free area for the client to discuss experiences and fears about grief.
- Encourage the client to share emotions and fears with close family members or friends.
- Provide referral to resources that can assist the client to maintain as much independence as possible.

Evaluation

The grieving process takes time, and the amount of time is different for each individual. When working with older adults, it is important to set realistic goals for movement through grieving toward acceptance. Some outcomes may include the following:

- The client employs healthy coping mechanisms.
- The client asks for help and support when needed.
- The client begins to accept the loss as evidenced by a return to normal activities and a decrease (or cessation) of the emotions associated with grief.

NURSING CARE PLAN   A Client With a Normal Grief Reaction

Mary O'Connor, age 72, comes in for an appointment at her general practitioner's office. She has recently been restless and depressed.

ASSESSMENT	DIAGNOSES	PLANNING
Khalid Riza is Mrs. O'Connor's regular RN. Mr. Riza checks Mrs. O'Connor's temperature and vitals. Her temperature is 98.8° F, her blood pressure is 137/82 mmHg, and her pulse is 85 bpm. Mrs. O'Connor explains that she has been very restless over the past 2 months since her husband died, and in the last month she has been unable to sleep. She has been thinking about her husband constantly and sometimes wakes up forgetting he is gone. Once she remembers his death, she is so upset that she finds it difficult to fall back asleep. Mr. Riza asks about Mrs. O'Connor's children and grandchildren and finds that they have not been around very much since Mr. O'Connor died. Mrs. O'Connor lives alone and is able to take care of herself quite efficiently. She has never shown signs of dementia or Alzheimer disease. She exercises regularly, maintains a healthy diet, and has no history of depression. After talking with the physician, Mr. Riza suggests that Mrs. O'Connor consider attending a group therapy meeting with other older adults who have recently lost their spouses. He explains that this is a very common practice and that it may help Mrs. O'Connor with both her anxiety and her sleep troubles.	■ *Grieving* related to death of a spouse ■ *Disturbed Sleep Pattern* related to grief and anxiety ■ *Ineffective Coping* related to death of a spouse ■ *Ineffective Role Performance* related to alteration in familial and societal role secondary to death of a spouse (NANDA-I © 2012)	Goals for Mrs. O'Connor's care: ■ The client will go to group therapy once a week. ■ The client will learn about the normal progression of grief. ■ The client will demonstrate healthy coping mechanisms. ■ The client's sleep patterns will return to normal.

NURSING CARE PLAN (continued)

IMPLEMENTATION

- Teach about the effectiveness of group therapy.
- Discuss the grief cycle and the stages of grief.
- Emphasize the warning signs of depression and suicide.

EVALUATION

Mr. Riza finds a group therapy session close to Mrs. O'Connor's house. Mrs. O'Connor begins attending group therapy; after a few sessions, she feels comfortable enough to discuss the loss of her husband. She finds that many of the other members of the group have had grief reactions similar to her own. Mrs. O'Connor stays in group therapy for 8 weeks and develops not only a support system, but also healthy coping mechanisms for her grief. By the end of the 2 months, her sleep patterns have returned to normal.

CRITICAL THINKING

1. If Mrs. O'Connor's husband had died 9 months prior to this appointment, how would the nursing care plan have changed? What diagnosis could have been added?
2. How would the plan of care change if Mrs. O'Connor had a history of depression? Of suicide attempts?

REVIEW Older Adult's Response to Loss

RELATE Link the Concepts and Exemplars

Linking the exemplar of older adult's response to loss with the concept of mood and affect:

1. Describe the types of losses older adults experience and why those losses put them at risk for depression.
2. How will you assist the elderly man who has had to give up his home and move to an assisted living facility to adjust to this change? What other losses do you anticipate this client may experience?

Linking the exemplar of older adult's response to loss with the concept of mobility:

3. What are your goals for the older adult client who has lost the use of his or her legs?
4. Create a plan of care for an older adult client who lives alone and is wheelchair bound.

READY Go to Companion Skills Manual

REFER Go to Pearson Nursing Student Resources
nursing.pearsonhighered.com

- Additional review materials

REFLECT Case Study

Peter Murphy is an 86-year-old man who has arthritis that is particularly advanced in his lower extremities due to injuries he sustained playing pro football. He has also been diagnosed with congestive heart failure and peripheral vascular disease. His lower extremities are becoming increasingly weak, and he has fallen several times. His primary provider is strongly encouraging him to use a wheelchair for safety.

Mr. Murphy's wife died 3 years ago, and he now lives in their second-floor apartment by himself. With help from neighbors, he manages to care for himself and his small dog. His neighbor, Mary, does his laundry for him once a week and takes him to the local senior center every morning with her husband. Mr. Murphy gets his breakfast and lunch at the center and returns home around 4 p.m. He is extremely upset by the idea of being confined to a wheelchair because he feels his independence is being threatened. Mary's car is not big enough to take him and a scooter or wheelchair to the senior center, where he finds his primary source of support and friendship. He is at the clinic today for follow-up care, and his primary provider is encouraging him to decide about the type of wheelchair he would like to use.

1. What assessment data would help you determine Mr. Murphy's risk for depression or, possibly, suicide?
2. How can you help Mr. Murphy cope with his grief over the need to rely on a wheelchair?
3. What are your priority nursing diagnoses and goals of care for Mr. Murphy?

EXEMPLAR 27.4 Perinatal Loss

EXEMPLAR KEY TERMS
Blighted ovum, *1768*
Disseminated intravascular
 coagulation (DIC), *1768*
Fetal demise, *1768*
Intrauterine fetal death (IUFD), *1768*
Miscarriage, *1768*
Perinatal loss, *1768*
Placental abruption, *1768*
Rh disease, *1768*

Spontaneous abortion, *1768*
Stillbirth, *1768*

EXEMPLAR LEARNING OUTCOMES
After reading about this exemplar, you will be able to:

1. Describe the pathophysiology, etiology, clinical manifestations, and direct and indirect causes of perinatal loss.
2. Identify risk factors and prevention methods associated with perinatal loss.

3. Illustrate the nursing process in providing culturally competent care across the life span for individuals experiencing perinatal loss.

4. Formulate priority nursing diagnoses appropriate for an individual experiencing perinatal loss.

5. Summarize therapies used by interdisciplinary teams in the collaborative care of an individual experiencing perinatal loss.

6. Plan evidence-based care for an individual experiencing perinatal loss and her family in collaboration with other members of the healthcare team.

7. Evaluate expected outcomes for an individual experiencing perinatal loss.

▶ OVERVIEW

Perinatal loss is the death of an infant or fetus at any time from the point of conception to 28 days after birth. Perinatal loss is a traumatic event for the infant's parents as well as other family members. In the past, some have proposed that perinatal loss results in less intense grief because the parents and family have not had time to form a close bond with the infant; this theory has since been proven incorrect. In fact, the grief associated with the loss of a child can be more intense than most other losses (Kersting & Wagner, 2012).

▶ PATHOPHYSIOLOGY AND ETIOLOGY

Perinatal loss can be difficult for the mother both physically and emotionally. If the fetus is lost during the first 20 weeks of gestation, it is referred to as a **miscarriage** or a **spontaneous abortion**. This is a significant loss for the mother and should not be discounted for any reason. Loss of the infant after 20 weeks' gestation is known as **intrauterine fetal death (IUFD)**, but is more commonly referred to as **fetal demise** or **stillbirth**. It is typical to assume that a stillbirth will produce a more difficult grief reaction for mothers; however, a study researching both miscarriages and stillbirths found that the grief responses in the mothers were essentially the same (Sutan et al., 2010). The grief experienced by fathers after the loss of a child through either miscarriage or a stillbirth often presents differently from the grief of mothers. The father of the child is likely to be quite upset, but he may not show his grief as openly. This response varies, of course, depending on the individual.

Etiology

The loss of a fetus while it is in the womb results from a variety of circumstances that can occur between conception and birth. These include biological conditions such as infection, an abnormality in the fetus, problems with the placenta, or accidents involving the umbilical cord. Environmental conditions also can contribute to, or cause, perinatal loss; for example, domestic abuse, motor vehicle crashes, or other accidents, such as a fall.

MISCARRIAGE One of the most common causes of miscarriage is **blighted ovum**, which occurs when the egg has been fertilized and both the membrane and placenta have formed, but the embryo has not formed. This condition sometimes results from chromosomal abnormalities in the fetus. Health conditions in the mother can also contribute to miscarriage; in particular, infections, hormonal problems, unmanaged diabetes, and thyroid disease. Miscarriages generally occur during the first trimester of pregnancy; although second trimester losses are less common, they can occur (Mayo Clinic, 2010b).

STILLBIRTH It may be impossible to know the reason for a stillbirth, even in the later stages of pregnancy. Some known factors that may contribute to and/or cause fetal demise include birth defects or chromosomal disorders, placental abruption, infections, slow fetal growth, and umbilical cord problems. **Placental abruption** occurs when the placenta detaches from the uterine wall before delivery. This condition does not always result in fetal demise, but the fetus's survival depends on the stage of development and prompt medical treatment ("Placenta Abruptio," 2012). Umbilical cord abnormalities are relatively unusual, but if a knot in the cord occurs it could cause oxygen deprivation in the fetus. Another rare cause of fetal demise is **Rh disease**, where the mother is Rh negative and the child is Rh positive. If this condition arises, the mother's body sees the Rh-positive cells in the fetus as foreign and produces antibodies to fight off the Rh-positive cells. Rh disease results in the death of the fetus only in extreme causes.

Risk Factors

Risk factors for perinatal loss include age, health conditions, and previous instances of perinatal loss. Increased age at the time of conception, particularly for women 40 or older, can increase the risk for complications during pregnancy. A woman's medical history also factors into the risk for complications. Generally having one past experience with a miscarriage or spontaneous abortion does not impact future pregnancies—depending on the cause—but past instances of multiple complications put a woman at higher risk. Similarly, contributing factors involving a weak cervix or other health conditions such as diabetes or thyroid disease can lead to miscarriage or fetal demise (Mayo Clinic, 2010c). The use of drugs, alcohol, or tobacco increases the risk for pregnancy complications, as does exposure to harmful chemicals.

When fetal demise transpires and the mother does not go into labor naturally, labor is induced, or a cesarean section is performed. In cases of elongated retention of the fetus, a condition known as **disseminated intravascular coagulation (DIC)** may occur. DIC is a disorder where the proteins controlling clotting of the blood become abnormally active, causing excessive clotting. In addition to DIC, both infection and sepsis can set in if the dead fetus remains in the woman's womb for an extended period.

Prevention

In the majority of cases it is not possible to prevent perinatal loss. As mentioned in the previous sections, many cases are circumstantial and/or biological and cannot often be detected until the miscarriage or fetal demise has occurred. The best prevention for parents is knowledge of factors that can compromise the mother's health. Women who are pregnant should avoid drugs, chemicals, tobacco, alcohol, and infectious diseases, as they may cause perinatal loss or other health complications for the fetus. Proper maternal care is also important, as some pregnancy complications can be caught early and treated before any harm is done to the fetus or mother.

▶ CLINICAL MANIFESTATIONS

The manifestations of perinatal loss involve both physical and emotional changes. The physical changes are either changes to the mother's body, including spotting, severe back pain, and cramping, or changes in fetal movement or heart rate. These manifestations indicate that something has occurred that could lead to fatal complications. After a perinatal loss, the parents and family of the infant experience various, and often intense, forms of grief.

Changes in Fetal Activity

Some warning signs of pregnancy complications can be detected through fetal movement or fetal heartbeat. Mothers can generally first detect fetal movement between 18 and 20 weeks' gestation. From this point onward, fetal movement becomes more regular and predictable, with the mother detecting the greatest movement while sitting or lying down. A significant decrease in or stopping of fetal movement before labor may be a sign of complications, such as the fetus's receiving too little oxygen. Mothers should be observant of fetal movements, but not overly anxious. An infant that does not move for an hour may be sleeping. Similarly, during the last trimester of pregnancy, the infant may not move as much as in earlier weeks. When a significant decrease in fetal movement is detected, the clinician checks the fetal heart rate. If the heart rate is abnormal or cannot be detected, an ultrasound is done to check for complications. If complications are found and the infant is still alive, early delivery or a cesarean section may be performed.

Grief

The loss of an infant during any stage of pregnancy can be an extremely traumatic event for both parents, and intense feelings of grief are to be expected. The intensity and duration of this grief depend on the individual, but it should not be assumed that this form of grief resolves quickly simply because the parents have not yet established a direct relationship with their baby. Studies have shown very little difference between the intensity of grief felt when a close family member dies and the grief felt after a perinatal death (Kersting & Wagner, 2012).

Grief in cases of perinatal loss may be intensified by the circumstances involving the loss. Many factors impact the parents' ability to resolve their emotions, including how the loss occurred, how the parents learned about the loss, and if the loss could have been prevented. Perinatal loss may also have a stigma attached to it, as some believe that it is unnecessary to mourn the loss of a child whom the parents have never come to know or raise. Beliefs such as these may hinder the parents' grieving process. These emotions can be further complicated for the mother if she feels guilt associated with the loss, and/or if postpartum depression becomes a factor.

DISENFRANCHISED GRIEF The loss of an infant before, or immediately following, birth result in disenfranchised grief. Perinatal loss is often not a socially recognized loss, particularly if that loss occurred in the early stages of pregnancy. Early miscarriages are generally not discussed except between the parents and healthcare professionals; in such a case, the grief is unacknowledged socially. Losses that occur in the early stages of pregnancy can be more difficult to grieve, as no funeral services or other formal mourning traditions are practiced (Kersting & Wagner, 2012). The result may be that the parents feel they have no right to mourn or feel grief over the loss of their child. Disenfranchised or complicated grief can also occur if the pregnancy had to be terminated for health reasons. Many parents in this situation choose to tell friends and family that the loss of the child was due to miscarriage or fetal demise.

POSTPARTUM DEPRESSION Postpartum depression is a form of depression that occurs in the first few weeks after a child has been born. Many do not realize that postpartum depression can also occur in women who have suffered perinatal loss; in fact, two of the major risk factors for developing postpartum depression are experiencing complications during the pregnancy and suffering a perinatal loss. The exact cause of postpartum depression is unknown, but the symptoms are similar to those of other forms of depression and may include anxiety, difficulty concentrating, lack of enjoyment, feelings of inadequacy, sleeplessness, decreased appetite, and suicidal thoughts ("Postpartum Depression," 2012). Experiencing these symptoms while trying to mourn the loss of a child can make both the grief and the depression worse. Women who are experiencing these emotions should be encouraged to discuss their thoughts, and should be monitored closely for a worsening of symptoms.

SAFETY ALERT
Mothers who have lost a child and develop postpartum depression should be closely monitored for signs of serious depression and/or suicidal thoughts. Signs of depression include loss of interest in once-enjoyable activities, alterations in appetite, fatigue, and unexplainable crying spells. Suicidal thoughts may be evidenced by intense periods of depression accompanied by statements such as "everyone would be better off without me," or "I wish I was dead/had died instead." Individuals contemplating suicide may also begin to give away items once valued, explaining that the items are not needed anymore.

Lifespan and Cultural Considerations

Parents who have lost a child may desire to speak with a religious or spiritual leader. Nurses can call for the hospital chaplain to meet with the parents or facilitate the presence of a chaplain from the same spiritual background as the client. If the infant is born alive but not expected to live long, the parents may want the child to be baptized or to receive a form of last rites as soon as possible, depending on their beliefs. Nurses facilitate the family's participation in these rituals.

Religious or spiritual beliefs may affect how the parents mourn the loss of a child. Clients of the Catholic faith may worry that their child was a stillborn and therefore unable to be

Following a late-stage perinatal loss, many hospitals recommend that nurses offer to create a kit for the parents containing keepsakes, such as a lock of hair, hand- and footprints, and a picture of the infant. While these kits may be comforting to some parents, they can be distressing to others—especially if any part of the kit's creation clashes with their cultural beliefs. For example, members of the traditional Amish culture would very likely decline any photographs of their child, as photographs are evidence of overabundant pride. As a component of culturally competent care, nurses need to explore the parent's cultural preferences before creating memory kits for them.

baptized, and this may cause considerable anxiety. Those of the Jewish faith are not allowed to mourn for a child who has been alive less than 30 days, and so parents of these children are unable to hold any traditional services. Some traditions, such as Islam, believe the child is instantly admitted into heaven. Others, such as Buddhism and Hinduism, believe the child's soul will be reincarnated. Nurses should be respectful of clients' beliefs and offer to meet any needs that arise.

▶ COLLABORATION

After a perinatal loss, tests can be performed on both the mother and the fetus to determine the cause of the fetal demise. Some parents refuse this testing for personal or religious reasons, and that decision must be honored. Parents who have lost a child may also need additional support in the coming months; many support groups and bereavement counselors can be recommended.

Diagnostic Tests

A series of tests are available to determine potential cause of fetal demise, but often it is impossible to determine the exact

cause. After delivery, with the parents' consent, the fetus will undergo blood tests and placental tests, x-rays and MRIs, as well as chromosomal studies. These tests are done to determine a possible cause of the pregnancy complications and generally include an autopsy. Mothers also undergo a series of blood tests. These tests check to see if the mother has diabetes or thyroid disease, or if she has contracted any infectious disease that could have affected the fetus. A Betke-Kleihauer test may also be performed to check the mother's Rh antibodies to determine if Rh disease was a contributing factor. These tests can help the parents to know of possible similar problems with future pregnancies.

Pharmacologic Therapy

Depending on the circumstances surrounding the fetal demise, medications may be administered to treat the mother for any infections or complications. If a placental abruption has occurred, the mother may need IV fluids, as well as a blood transfusion if the blood loss is substantial ("Placenta Abruptio," 2012). In cases where the fetal demise goes untreated and the dead fetus is retained, resulting disseminated intravascular coagulation may result requires treatment for the clotting, possible plasma transfusions, and treatment for sepsis, depending on how long the fetus has been retained ("Disseminated Intravascular Coagulation," 2012). The mother may also need antibiotics if the blood work indicates the presence of infection.

The mother is at risk for developing postpartum depression within the first 4 weeks after a perinatal loss. If this depression becomes overwhelming, especially in combination with the grief, two pharmacologic therapies may be recommended: antidepressants and hormone therapy. Antidepressants have been shown to be effective in the treatment of postpartum depression and can be used in combination with other forms of therapy and counseling. Hormone therapy, in the form of estrogen replacement, may help to dispel some of the symptoms of postpartum depression, but research on this treatment is unsubstantial. Women should be made aware of the risks

Clinical Manifestations and Therapies **Perinatal Loss**

ETIOLOGY	CLINICAL MANIFESTATIONS	CLINICAL THERAPIES
Miscarriage	■ Spotting ■ Cramping ■ Lower back pain	■ Antibiotics if a resultant infection occurs
Placental abruption	■ Back pain ■ Uterine contractions ■ Vaginal bleeding ■ Abdominal pain	■ IV fluids ■ Blood transfusion ■ Delivery of the fetus ■ Antibiotics if infection occurs
Disseminated intravascular coagulation as a result of a retained fetus.	■ Bleeding ■ Blood clots ■ Drop in blood pressure	■ Delivery of the fetus ■ Treatment of clotting ■ Plasma transfusions, if needed ■ Antibiotics if sepsis occurs

and benefits of all treatments so they may make an informed decision.

Nonpharmacologic Therapy

The grief resulting from perinatal loss can be intense and even overwhelming. Mothers may feel unnecessary guilt, believing that they, or their bodies, failed in some way and led to the infant's death. Intense grief and even feelings of guilt are entirely normal after the death of an infant and may last for a few weeks or possibly a few months. These emotions generally lessen on their own, but if they do not, or if the parents require further support, different forms of therapy can be helpful. Group therapy in cases of perinatal loss may be useful, or it may be more painful, depending on the clients. Some clients may find it therapeutic and reassuring to talk to other parents who have lost an infant, while others may see it as disorienting and painful to share others' experiences of such a traumatic event. In these cases, individual grief counseling is preferable.

Lifestyle changes may also assist mothers experiencing postpartum depression and grief. In place of isolation, mothers should seek out a strong support system after the loss; sharing their feelings about the loss as well as any trauma experienced has been proven to help prevent or alleviate any posttraumatic stress disorder (Sutan et al., 2010). Physical activity and proper nutrition can also help to lessen the effects of depression.

◼ NURSING PROCESS

Appropriate nursing care after a perinatal loss is extremely important, as it can help parents through a difficult and traumatic experience. Nurses remain patient and kind, informing the parents of all the different steps and procedures that will be taken during the birth of the stillborn infant. Parents play an active role in developing the plan of care after a perinatal loss.

Assessment

Perinatal loss can occur at any point in a pregnancy for a multitude of different reasons. Mothers who are suspected of having suffered a perinatal loss should be evaluated immediately. A fetal heart monitor can be used to check the heart rate of the fetus. If a heartbeat cannot be found, an ultrasound should be done to determine if fetal demise has occurred. The safety of mother and fetus takes priority; if the assessment determines the infant is in distress, immediate action is necessary.

Following confirmation of fetal demise, the parents are informed. Institutional policies vary with regard to when parents are notified of fetal demise. In some cases, the parents are not informed until after the delivery. It is important to adhere to institutional policies and procedures.

The nurse begins assessing the parents' needs and resources as well as planning for needs that will arise during delivery. The nurse assesses the parents' spiritual needs by asking if they would like to speak to the hospital chaplain or if they would like the presence of another spiritual leader. Nurses also collaborate with social workers or grief counselors to provide further assistance to the parents after the birth.

Diagnosis

Diagnoses depend on the cause of the perinatal loss in addition to any further complications. Potential diagnoses include:

- *Grieving*
- *Risk for Complicated or Disenfranchised Grieving*
- *Risk for Spiritual Distress*
- *Risk for Infection* related to a retained fetus
- *Risk for Bleeding* related to placental abruption

(NANDA-I © 2012)

Planning

In working with clients who have experienced a perinatal loss, it is imperative for the nurse to work with both parents to develop an appropriate plan of care. Clients' needs vary in this situation and should be honored and facilitated when possible. The mother's comfort and safety during and following delivery should be a top priority. Some possible goals are:

- Parents will ask any questions regarding the loss, the delivery, or any other aspects of care.
- The client will choose how she wishes to deliver the fetus, as well as the atmosphere of the delivery room.
- The client's health and safety will be monitored and preserved during and after labor.
- Parents will have access to resources and support systems to help them cope with the loss.
- Parents will express grief over the loss of the fetus.
- Parents will avoid taking undue or unreasonable responsibility for fetal loss.

Implementation

When parents are admitted with a possible perinatal loss, they should be put in a private room as far away from the other mothers as possible. If it is determined that perinatal loss has occurred, the privacy provided is likely to benefit both parents. Once tests are performed and perinatal loss is confirmed, parents are informed of the test results and encouraged to ask any questions they may have. Nurses should allow parents time to process their grief before asking about the mother's birthing preferences. When the parents have indicated that they are ready to discuss the birthing process, the nurse should explain what will happen in the delivery of a stillborn infant; the parents should also be informed about the methods of inducing labor, if induction is to occur. The mother's birthing preferences determine how the birth takes place. Nurses consult her regarding how the room should be lit, who she would like in the birthing room with her, if she would like relaxing music playing, and what position she would prefer to give birth in. The mother's comfort and understanding are an important priority for a nurse during the birthing process.

Before the child is born, the nurse should establish when and if the parents would like to see the infant. Parents should be gently encouraged to see the infant for their own sense of acceptance. If the parents wish to see the infant, the nurse should prepare them for how the child may look. For example, if the child is not fully developed, if the child is slightly blue or yellow from complications, or if the child is deformed in any way, the parents should be told before viewing the infant. It is important for nurses to respect parents' wishes if they would like time alone with the infant. The nurse also consults the parents to determine if they would like to take home keepsakes of the child, such as a picture, a lock of hair, or foot- or handprints.

After the birth has taken place and the parents have seen the infant, the nurse should again ask if they have any questions. The nurse assures both parents that any questions they may have are normal, even if the parents feel their questions are odd or morbid in some way. The nurse provides time and space for the parents to express their feelings, being careful to address feelings of guilt by explaining that most cases of perinatal loss cannot be prevented. Nurses provide information on discharge regarding the need to report any signs of infection, such as fever, chills, or dizziness. Nurses also make referrals for grief counseling and other sources of support the parents may require.

Evaluation

Parents should be encouraged to ask any questions they have during this difficult experience. Nurses should work with the parents to ensure that their needs are being met. Some potential outcomes of the nursing process are as follows:

- Parents ask questions regarding the birthing process.
- Parents make their preferences for the birthing process known.
- Parents express grief over the loss of their child.
- Parents are given resources to help with their grief.
- Parents develop healthy coping mechanisms for working through the grieving process.

NURSING CARE PLAN   A Client With a Perinatal Loss

Gina Worton, age 30, and her husband arrive at the birthing center. Ms. Worton reports that her infant's movements were irregular this morning when she woke, and that in the 4 hours since she woke up, the infant's movements have been decreasing. Ms. Worton is 36 weeks into her pregnancy and so far has had no complications.

ASSESSMENT

On admission Grant Schmidt, the RN at the birthing center, obtains a history from Mrs. Worton. She reports that she has been seeing her obstetrician frequently throughout the pregnancy and everything has been going well. She does not smoke, drink, or take illicit drugs; her past tests for gestational diabetes and thyroid disease have been negative; and she has not experienced any accidents or trauma during the pregnancy. An electronic fetal heart monitor is used to check the fetal heartbeat. When none is found, an ultrasound is performed. The ultrasound reveals that the Wortons' child has died in the womb. Mr. and Mrs. Worton are informed of the death and advised to take some time to process their loss before delivery is induced. Mrs. Worton is moved to a private room in the birthing center away from the other mothers. During delivery, the room is kept quiet; Mr. and Mrs. Worton are both quite upset and Mrs. Worton is weeping. Mr. Schmidt tells the Wortons what they should expect during the delivery and offers to call the hospital chaplain. The Wortons decline.

After the child is born, Mrs. Worton asks to see her. Mr. Schmidt inspects the baby and then explains that the child will appear slightly blue when they see her. He explains that the cause is a knot in the umbilical cord. Once the Wortons have been prepared to see the child, Mr. Schmidt brings in the infant and hands her to the mother. He then leaves the room to give the Wortons time to grieve. Mr. Schmidt stays close to the Wortons' room in case they would like the infant removed suddenly. After an hour alone with their daughter, the Wortons give the infant to Mr. Schmidt. Mrs. Worton shows no signs of resultant complications, and they are prepared for discharge 3 hours later.

DIAGNOSES

- *Ineffective Coping* related to traumatic pregnancy experience
- *Disabled Family Coping* related to perinatal loss
- *Interrupted Family Processes* related to psychosocial trauma for each family member secondary to perinatal loss
- *Complicated Grieving* related to perinatal loss.

(NANDA-I © 2012)

PLANNING

Proposed goals for Ms. Worton's care include:

- The client will follow up with her obstetrician.
- The client will report any dizziness, fever, or heavy bleeding immediately.
- The client will repeat an understanding of the signs of postpartum depression.
- The client will maintain healthy coping mechanisms for her grief.

IMPLEMENTATION

- Teach about perinatal loss and normal grief.
- Teach about postpartum depression.
- Emphasize the need to report any symptoms of infection.

- Instruct about resources for grief as a result of perinatal loss.
- Provide referrals to appropriate professionals and, if desired by the client, to support groups.

EVALUATION

Mrs. Worton conveys that she understands how the loss happened and agrees to see her obstetrician for a follow up appointment. She watches for any signs of infection but does not develop one. Mrs. Worton develops healthy coping mechanisms for her grief and shares her emotions with close friends and family members.

CRITICAL THINKING

1. How would the nursing care plan have changed if the client had developed DIC?
2. As a nurse, what support could you offer to parents who have experienced a perinatal loss?
3. What resources could be recommended to the client?

REVIEW Perinatal Loss

RELATE Link the Concepts and Exemplars

Linking the exemplar of perinatal loss with the concept of family:

1. What impact does perinatal loss have on the entire family, including father, siblings of the fetus, and grandparents?

2. How can the family members be helped to both support the mother and cope with their own feelings of loss?

Linking the exemplar of perinatal loss with the concept of reproduction:

3. What implications does a perinatal loss have for future pregnancies?

4. How might the needs of this mother differ if she had experienced other perinatal losses and was currently childless?

READY Go to Companion Skills Manual

REFER Go to Pearson Nursing Student Resources
nursing.pearsonhighered.com

- Additional review materials

REFLECT Case Study

Betty Jane Walker, 29 years old, is 30 weeks pregnant. She lives with her husband, Rick, and their three children ages 6, 5, and 3. She and Rick describe their marriage as average. He has a history of alcohol abuse but is currently functioning well and owns his own business in the city, commuting via train. Betty is a stay-at-home mom who enjoys reading and playing the piano when she can find the time. Betty is an excellent cook, likes to play bridge, and enjoys golf. She rarely gets time to pursue her hobbies but does find time to read a few evenings a week. Rick ignores the children for the most part, working all day and burying himself in the newspaper and TV at night. Betty learned last week that the fetus has died, and the provider recommended waiting for the normal labor process to begin. Betty visits her provider today because she isn't feeling well.

1. What is the priority nursing diagnosis for Betty?

2. How can you assess Betty's current coping related to the perinatal loss?

3. Betty asks you how to tell her other children about the loss of the baby. What counseling will you provide?

4. How will you respond if Betty tells you that, in some ways, she is somewhat relieved by the loss of the fetus?

■ REFERENCES

Aloi, J. A. (2009). Nursing the disenfranchised: Women who have relinquished an infant for adoption. *Journal of Psychiatric and Mental Health Nursing, 16,* 27–32.

Alzheimer's Association. (2012). *2012 Alzheimer's disease facts and figures.* Retrieved from http://www.alz.org/downloads/facts_figures_2012.pdf.

Alzheimer's Association. (2013). *Symptoms of Alzheimer's.* Retrieved from http://www.alz.org/alzheimers_disease_what_is_alzheimers.asp#symptoms.

American Association of Suicidology. (2009). *Elderly suicide fact sheet.* Retrieved from http://www.suicidology.org/c/document_library/get_file?folderId=232&name=DLFE-242.pdf.

Benkel, I., Wijk, H., & Molander, V. (2009). Family and friends provide most social support for the bereaved. *Palliative Medicine, 23,* 141–149.

Berman, A. J., & Snyder, S. (2011). *Kozier & Erb's fundamentals of nursing: Concepts, process, and practice* (9th ed.). Upper Saddle River, NJ: Pearson.

Buglas, E. (2010). Grief and bereavement theories. *Nursing Standard, 24*(41), 44–47.

Centers for Disease Control and Prevention. (2012). *National suicide statistics at a glance.* Retrieved from http://www.cdc.gov/violenceprevention/suicide/statistics/trends02.html.

Disseminated intravascular coagulation. (2012). In *A.D.A.M Medical Encyclopedia.* Retrieved from http://www.nlm.nih.gov/medlineplus/ency/article/000573.htm.

Engel, G. L. (1964). Grief and grieving. *American Journal of Nursing, 64,* 93–98.

Goodman, R. F., Cohen, J., Epstein, C., Kliethermes, M., Layne, C., Macy, R., & Ward-Wimmer, D. (2004). *Childhood traumatic grief educational materials for parents.* Retrieved from http://rems.ed.gov/docs/SAMHSA_ChildhoodTraumaticGriefForParents.pdf.

Guido, G. W. (2010). *Nursing care at the end of life.* Upper Saddle River, NJ: Pearson.

Howarth, R. A. (2011). Promoting the adjustment of parentally bereaved children. *Journal of Mental Health Counseling, 33*(1), 21–32.

Kersting, A., & Wagner, B. (2012). Complicated grief after perinatal loss. *Dialogues in Clinical Neuroscience, 14*(2), 187–194. Available at http://www.ncbi.nlm.nih.gov/pmc/articles/PMC3384447/.

Kübler-Ross, E. (1969). *On death and dying.* New York, NY: Macmillan.

Mayo Clinic. (2010a). *Antidepressants for children. Explore the pros and cons.* Retrieved from http://www.mayoclinic.com/health/antidepressants/MH00059.

Mayo Clinic. (2010b). *Miscarriage: Causes.* Retrieved from http://www.mayoclinic.com/health/miscarriage/DS01105/DSECTION=causes.

Mayo Clinic. (2010c). *Miscarriage: Risk factors.* Retrieved from http://www.mayoclinic.com/health/pregnancy-loss-miscarriage/DS01105/DSECTION=risk-factors.

National Cancer Institute. (2013). *Children and grief.* Retrieved from http://www.cancer.gov/cancertopics/pdq/supportivecare/bereavement/Patient/page1/AllPages#6.

National Institute of Mental Health. (2010). *Older adults: Depression and suicide facts.* Retrieved from http://www.nimh.nih.gov/health/publications/older-adults-depression-and-suicide-facts-fact-sheet/index.shtml.

Placenta abruptio. (2012). In *A.D.A.M Medical Encyclopedia.* Retrieved from http://www.ncbi.nlm.nih.gov/pubmedhealth/PMH0001903/.

Postpartum depression. (2012). In *A.D.A.M Medical Encyclopedia.* Retrieved from http://www.ncbi.nlm.nih.gov/pubmedhealth/PMH0004481/.

Robinaugh, D. J., Marques, L., Bui, E., & Simon, N. M. (2012). Recognizing and treating complicated grief: Timing and severity of symptoms can help identify this distinct syndrome. *Current Psychiatry, 11*(8), 30–34.

Sanders, C. M. (1998). *Grief: The mourning after: Dealing with adult bereavement* (2nd ed.). New York, NY: Wiley.

Shear, K., Frank, E., Houck, P. R., & Reynolds, C. F. (2005). Treatment of complicated grief: A randomized controlled trial. *Journal of the American Medical Association, 293*(21), 2601–2608. Retrieved from http://jama.jamanetwork.com/article.aspx?articleid=200995.

Spector, R. E. (2013). *Cultural diversity in health and illness* (8th ed.). Upper Saddle River, NJ: Pearson.

Sutan, R., Amin, R. M., Ariffin, K. B., Teng, T. Z., Kamal, M. F., & Rusli, R. Z. (2010). Psychosocial impact of mothers with perinatal loss and its contributing factors: An insight. *Journal of Zhejiang University Science B, 11*(3), 209–217. Doi: 10.1631/jzus.B0900245.

U.S. Food and Drug Administration. (2005). *Medication guide: About using antidepressants in children and teenagers.* Retrieved from http://www.fda.gov/downloads/drugs/drugsafety/informationbydrugclass/UCM161646.pdf.

Walsh, K. (2012). *Grief and loss: Theories and skills for the helping professions* (2nd ed.). Upper Saddle River, NJ: Pearson.

Wiese, B. S. (2011). Geriatric depression: The use of antidepressants in the elderly. *BC Medical Journal, 53*(7), 341–347. Available at http://www.bcmj.org/articles/geriatric-depression-use-antidepressants-elderly.

Wilson, B. A., Shannon, M. T., & Shields, K. M. (2013). *Pearson nurse's drug guide.* Upper Saddle River, NJ: Pearson.

Worden, J. W., & Silverman, P. R. (1996). Parental death and the adjustment of school-age children. *Omega: Journal of Death and Dying, 29,* 219–230.

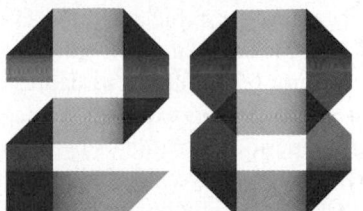 # Mood and Affect

MODULE AT-A-GLANCE

The Concept of Mood and Affect, 1775

Exemplar 28.1
Depression, 1798

Exemplar 28.2
Adjustment Disorder With Depressed Mood, 1805

Exemplar 28.3
Bipolar Disorders, 1808

Exemplar 28.4
Postpartum Depression, 1816

◪ THE CONCEPT OF MOOD AND AFFECT

Emotions are feeling responses to a wide variety of stimuli. Positive emotions such as joy stimulate the individual to remain in the situation, whereas negative emotions such as fear stimulate the individual to avoid or withdraw from the situation. **Mood** is an individual's internal, subjective, sustained emotional state (like climate). Only the individual is capable of describing his or her mood. Nurses and other clinicians must be careful not to assume they know the client's mood based solely on their observations. **Affect** is the immediate emotional expression of mood that people communicate verbally and nonverbally. It can be externally observed and is a more changeable emotional state (like the weather). Words commonly used to describe emotional states include *happiness, pleasure, frustration, anger,* or *sadness.* Nonverbal cues to emotions include facial expressions such as smiling, frowning, and looking blank; motor activities such as clenching hands into fists and pacing; and physiological responses such as sweating profusely and experiencing increased heart rate or respirations. Although an individual may choose not to communicate verbally to others, it is difficult to prevent nonverbal expression of feelings. **≪**

Concept Learning Outcomes

After reading about this concept, you will be able to:

1. Summarize the structure and physiological processes of the neurological system related to mood and affect.

2. Examine the relationship between mood and affect and other concepts/systems.

3. Identify commonly occurring alterations in mood and affect and their related therapies.

4. Differentiate common assessment procedures used to examine mood and affect across the life span.

5. Describe diagnostic and laboratory tests used to determine causes of alterations in an individual's mood and affect.

6. Explain prevention of and management strategies for alterations in mood and affect.

7. Demonstrate the nursing process in providing culturally competent and caring interventions across the life span for individuals with common alterations of mood and affect.

8. Compare and contrast common independent and collaborative interventions for clients with alterations of mood and affect.

Concept Key Terms

Adjustment disorder with depressed mood, *1778*
Affect, *1775*
Aggressive behavior, *1789*
Anhedonia, *1776*
Anxious distress, *1776*
Assertive behavior, *1789*
Biological rhythms, *1780*
Bipolar disorder, *1779*
Depressive disorder with peripartum onset, *1779*
Double depression, *1778*
Dysthymic disorder, *1778*
Electroconvulsive therapy (ECT), *1795*
Emotions, *1775*
Hypomania, *1776*
Major depressive disorder (MDD), *1778*
Mania, *1776*
Monoamine oxidase inhibitors (MAOIs), *1792*

Mood, *1775*
Mood stabilizers, *1793*
Passive behavior, *1789*
Persistent depressive disorder, *1778*
Postpartum blues, *1779*
Postpartum depression, *1779*
Postpartum psychosis, *1779*
Seasonal affective disorder (SAD), *1780*
Selective serotonin reuptake inhibitors (SSRIs), *1791*
Serotonin syndrome, *1790*
Somatization, *1787*
Tricyclic antidepressants (TCAs), *1790*
Unipolar depression, *1778*

▶ NORMAL MOOD AND AFFECT

Healthcare professionals describe affect in terms of appropriateness, range, stability, intensity, and congruence (**Table 28–1** ●). The normal range of mood generally is stable and appropriate to the situation. Emotions, mood, and affect become dysfunctional when they occur in inappropriate situations, when the response is out of proportion to the stimulus, or when they shift dramatically or rapidly out of proportion to external events.

Genetic and Lifespan Considerations

The study of genetic influences on normal mood is in its infancy. A study of middle-age male twins indicated that mood intensity and lability (shift from normal mood to anger or depression or between depression and anxiety) indicated a strong genetic influence for all. In addition, environmental influences (apart from shared experiences) also had a strong influence on the ability to self-regulate mood intensity and shifts (Coccaro et al., 2012). There are no lifespan considerations in normal mood and affect; however, there are in alterations of mood and affect, which are addressed in the following section.

▶ ALTERATIONS TO MOOD AND AFFECT

When alterations in mood and affect become significant enough to impair functioning, they may rise to the level of a mood disorder as defined by the American Psychiatric Association (APA). Mood disorders are best understood as syndromes with a core cluster of symptoms. Mood disorders are categorized into several subtypes, each with different patterns and symptoms. Individuals with depressive disorders exhibit depressed mood characterized by feelings of sadness, discouragement, and hope-

lessness. Other core symptoms include **anhedonia**, a loss of interest or inability to engage in pleasurable activities; fatigue and sleep disturbance; and somatic complaints. In children and adolescents, irritability is a common symptom of depression. Individuals with bipolar disorders typically experience a depressive episode alternating with a period of mania or hypomania. **Mania** is an abnormal, persistent expansive, elevated mood that lasts a week or more and that significantly impairs functioning (usually) to the extent of requiring hospitalization. **Hypomania** is a similar impairment of mood that lasts less than a week; its symptoms, although significant, do not rise to the level of requiring hospitalization (APA, 2013). Because of the degree to which mood disorders can impact daily functioning, they can impact individuals across a wide variety of systems and situations (see Concepts Related to Mood and Affect).

Anxious distress is associated with depressive and bipolar disorders with sufficient frequency that the *Diagnostic and Statistical Manual of Mental Disorders,* 5th ed. (DSM-5), includes it as a specifier clinicians may add to a diagnosis of depression or bipolar disorder. **Anxious distress** is a combination of symptoms often associated with anxiety, including restlessness, impaired concentration due to worry, fear of something awful happening, and fear of losing control. Clients experiencing anxious distress in combination with a depressive or bipolar disorder typically are harder to treat and are at greater risk for suicide (APA, 2013).

The National Institute of Mental Health (NIMH) (n.d.a) reports that mood disorders affect nearly 10% of adults, with 45% of cases classified as severe. Mood disorders impact individuals of every race and age. Treatment is critical: Without it, approximately one in six individuals with serious depression will commit suicide (NIMH, 2003). Mood disorders also carry economic costs. For example, depression is associated with lower rates of productivity, increased absenteeism, and increased rates of short-term disability (NAMI, n.d.). Nurses should take note that clients

TABLE 28–1 Descriptors of Affect

AFFECT	DEFINITION	BEHAVIORAL EXAMPLE
Appropriate	Affect is congruent with the immediate situation.	Juan cries when learning of the death of his father.
Inappropriate	Affect is not related to the immediate situation.	When Sue's husband tells her about his terrible pain, Sue laughs out loud.
Full range	Shows range of emotional response appropriate to the situation or conversation.	During an assessment interview, Tessa laughs at a joke, and appears sad when speaking of her mother's illness.
Stable	Affect is resistant to sudden changes when there is no provocation in the environment.	During a party, Dan smiles and laughs at the appropriate social interchanges.
Labile	Affect shifts suddenly in a way that cannot be understood in the context of the situation.	During a friendly game of checkers, Dorothy, who was laughing, suddenly knocks the board off the table in anger. She then laughs and wants to continue the game.
Elevated	Affect is one of extreme elation not necessarily related to the immediate situation.	Sean runs around the dayroom, laughing, singing, and telling other patients how wonderful everything is.
Depressed	Affect is one of despondency not necessarily related to the immediate situation.	Leo sits slumped in a chair with a sad facial expression, teary eyes, and minimal body movement.
Overreactive	Affect is appropriate to the situation but out of proportion to the immediate situation.	Karen screams and curses when her child spills a glass of milk.
Blunted	Response to the immediate situation is dulled.	When Tom learns of his full-tuition scholarship, he responds with only a small smile.
Flat	There are no visible cues to the person's emotions.	When Juanita is told about her best friend's death, she says "Oh" and does not give any indication of an emotional response.

Concepts Related to **Mood and Affect**

Mood disorders are characterized by disturbances in nutrition and sleep as well as in emotions and psychological functioning. A major priority in the care of individuals with any alteration in mood or affect is to maintain physiological health and functioning. Therefore, the goal of overall health, wellness, and illness is of utmost importance. Individuals with depression typically experience difficulty falling asleep or staying asleep or experience early morning awakening. During a manic state the individual may not sleep for several days. Individuals with mood disturbances may neglect their physical health and personal hygiene.

Nutrition may be affected in mood disorders. Individuals with depressive disorders may experience decreased appetite and subsequent weight loss. Those with bipolar disorders may go without eating for long periods. The increased psychomotor activity associated with the manic states may increase caloric requirements. It is essential for nurses to monitor nutritional status and be knowledgeable regarding this concept.

Violence is another important concept related to mood and affect because alterations in mood and affect can result in violence toward self in the form of suicide. Hopelessness and intense psychological suffering may lead clients who are depressed to believe killing themselves is the only way to escape the intolerable. Suicide prevention is the most important goal of nursing care for individuals with mood disorders. Many people develop depression following interpersonal violence such as assault; rape trauma; physical, sexual, or emotional abuse or neglect; or family violence. Therefore, an understanding of the concept of violence will assist the nurse in providing individualized care for a depressed person who has survived violence.

Prolonged and overwhelming stress can result in depression. Anxiety disorders such as generalized anxiety disorder, obsessive compulsive disorder, and posttraumatic stress disorder (PTSD) and symptoms associated with anxiety such as agoraphobia and panic attacks often occur along with depression. Figure 28–1, presented later in this module, shows the relationship between life events and depression.

The rate of comorbidity between mood disorders and substance use disorders is high. Results of the National Epidemiologic Survey on Alcohol and Related Conditions showed that of those surveyed with current alcohol dependence, 20.5% also had an independent major depressive disorder. Individuals who reported alcohol dependence were 3.7 times more likely to have major depression than those who were not dependent on alcohol. Of those with current alcohol abuse or dependence who were seeking treatment, 40.7% also had at least one current independent mood disorder (Pettinati & Dundan, 2011). Bipolar disorders are associated with some of the highest rates of alcohol and substance abuse (Petrakis, Rosenheck, & Desai, 2011). There is a clear link between addiction and mood disorders. In some people the depressive disorder develops as a result of the substance abuse. In others, it is thought that the substance use disorder grows out of attempts to self-medicate to relieve symptoms of the mood disorder. Although research is limited, the integrated approach (treating both disorders simultaneously) was superior to other methods in terms of drug and alcohol outcomes in five randomized clinical trials (Hesse, 2009).

CONCEPT	RELATIONSHIP TO MOOD AND AFFECT	NURSING IMPLICATIONS
Health, Wellness, and Illness		
■ Sleep–rest patterns ■ Physical fitness and exercise	Depression = ↓ sleep/nutrition/wellness → physical illness → sick role = ↑ depression	■ Promote adequate rest and sleep. ■ Encourage self-care in personal hygiene. ■ Assess for signs of physical illness. ■ Promote routine health maintenance, screening, healthy lifestyle, preventive care.
Violence		
■ Abuse ■ Assault and homicide ■ Suicide	Mood disorders = ↑ suicide risk Experiencing violence → depression	■ Assess for suicide risk. ■ Assess for history of violence. ■ Provide safe environment. ■ Educate regarding community resources. ■ Anticipate need to develop a behavioral contract with the client.

(continued on next page)

Concepts Related to **Mood and Affect** (continued)

CONCEPT	RELATIONSHIP TO MOOD AND AFFECT	NURSING IMPLICATIONS
Stress and Coping		
■ Anxiety disorders ■ Crisis ■ PTSD	↑ Stress → depression or triggers mania Ineffective coping → depression and/or anxiety Exposure to trauma → depression and/or posttraumatic stress disorder	■ Assist client in developing effective coping mechanisms. ■ Assess for exposure to traumatic event. ■ Assess for symptoms of anxiety. ■ Assist client in identifying triggers for anxiety symptoms. ■ Teach stress reduction techniques.
Addiction		
■ Alcohol abuse ■ Substance abuse	Addiction → depression Mood disorders → addiction Mood disorders + addiction = ↑ severity of both	■ Assess for substance use. ■ Provide concurrent treatment for mood disorders and substance abuse. ■ Refer to community resources. ■ Assess and educate family regarding codependency issues. ■ Anticipate client denial of substance use.
Nutrition		
	Mood disorder → ↓ or ↑ in appetite and weight Manic state → increased caloric requirements	■ Monitor appetite and weight. ■ Provide nutritious snacks. ■ Educate clients on importance of eating balanced diet even when not hungry. ■ Provide nutritional supplements as needed.

with mood disorders are found in the community and in all types of clinical settings. This has a wide impact for nursing: Mood disorders can affect a client's communication skills, family relationships, and ability or motivation to adhere to a treatment plan.

Alterations and Manifestations

Alterations in mood and affect may be seen at any point across the life span. Brief periods of sadness, irritability, and excitement are common as individuals encounter hardship, challenge, and joy. At times these periods extend beyond just a few days or weeks depending on the nature of the stressor or situation and the individual's own ability to respond. When altered mood and affect begin to interfere with daily activities, individuals may need professional assistance to help them return to functioning and return to a normal mood state.

DEPRESSION What most Americans think of as *depression* is **major depressive disorder (MDD)**, also called **unipolar depression**. MDD is diagnosed when the client experiences either depressed mood or loss of interest most of the day, almost every day, for at least 2 weeks. The depression or anhedonia must be accompanied by at least four core symptoms, which may include any of the following (APA, 2013):

■ Sleep disturbances

■ Fatigue

■ Feelings of worthlessness or guilt

■ Restlessness, psychomotor agitation

■ Suicidal ideation or attempt.

Another depressive disorder, **persistent depressive disorder** (or **dysthymic disorder**), is also commonly referred to as *depression*, but it is different from MDD. Persistent depressive disorder is a chronic disorder in which periods of depressed mood are interspersed with normal mood. With this disorder, people experience a depressed mood for most of the day more days than not for at least 2 years. Symptoms in dysthymic disorder tend to be less severe than those in MDD, and the individual experiences fewer physiological symptoms (i.e., disturbed sleep, altered appetite, and weight loss or gain). Individuals with dysthymic disorder also may also experience one or more episodes of MDD. Sometimes this is referred to as **double depression**, but it is important to note that this is not a bona fide diagnosis.

ADJUSTMENT DISORDER WITH DEPRESSED MOOD Individuals often experience dramatic life changes because of losses due to death, relocation, loss of autonomy, illness, and financial stress. One or a combination of life changes or stressors may contribute to the development of **adjustment disorder with depressed mood**, sometimes referred to as situational depression. The essential feature of adjustment disorder with depressed mood is a maladaptive reaction to an identifiable psychosocial stressor or stressors that occurs within 3 months after the onset of the stressor and has persisted for no longer than 6 months (APA, 2013). Symptoms of adjustment disorder with depressed mood are similar to those of the other depressive disorders but to a lesser degree, although a higher level of anxiety may be present. Newer work has reconceptualized adjustment disorders as primarily stress response syndromes in which the level of distress is out of proportion to the actual stressor. The main feature is impairment in functioning in school, work, relationships, or other areas of daily life in response to an identifiable stressor (Friedman et al., 2011).

BIPOLAR DISORDERS   Bipolar-related disorders include bipolar I, bipolar II, cyclothymic disorder, and other related disorders. The medical diagnosis of **bipolar disorder** is given when an individual's mood alternates between the extremes of depression and mania or hypomania, interspersed with periods of normal mood. *Bipolar I disorder* is characterized by the occurrence of one or more manic episodes and one or more depressive episodes. *Bipolar II disorder* is characterized by one or more hypomanic episodes (less severe) and one or more depressive episodes. Paris (2009) reports that there may be additional subtypes of bipolar disorder such as *bipolar III* disorder, in which hypomanic episodes occur only after taking antidepressant medication, and *bipolar IV*, an ultra-rapid-cycling disorder. As yet, however, no conclusive evidence has been found to support these proposed diagnoses. A relationship exists between unipolar depression and bipolar disorder. Paris (2009) states that "when unipolar depression has an early onset, a recurrent course, atypical symptomatology, or irritability and hostility, it may go on to present with manic or hypomanic episodes or be associated with family histories of bipolarity" (p. 209). He goes on to cite 42 studies that support his statement.

Bipolar disorders may be further classified as follows (APA, 2013):

- *With mixed features.* The individual experiences symptoms of depression (e.g., depressed mood, loss of interest in pleasurable activities, and suicidal ideation or attempt) during episodes of mania or hypomania; or the individual experiences manic symptoms during the depressive episode.

- *With rapid cycling.* Four or more episodes of illness (mania, hypomania, or depressive) within a 12-month period, with at least 2 months between each episode OR with alternating episodes (e.g., a period of mania followed by a depressive episode). Rapid cycling occurs in 13%–24% of people with a bipolar disorder in Western countries. People with rapid cycling are more likely to be female, have an earlier age of onset, and be more resistant to treatment (Lee et al., 2010).

POSTPARTUM MOOD DISORDERS   It is not uncommon for women to experience depressive symptoms during and shortly after pregnancy. During pregnancy, levels of estrogens, glucocorticoids, and amino acids increase by as much as 200 times, only to drop sharply within 24 hours after delivery. This results in a hypoactive hypothalamic–pituitary axis that may last for months. Symptoms can be described along a continuum from postpartum blues to postpartum depression to the rare form, postpartum psychosis. **Postpartum blues** begin within the first 10 days postpartum and last a few days to 2 weeks with

symptoms disappearing spontaneously. The woman's mood may be unstable, accompanied by sadness, weepiness, irritability, anxiety, and fatigue. As many as 70% of new mothers may experience these symptoms, which are thought to be caused by hormonal fluctuations (Office of Women's Health [OFW], 2009). Any symptoms lasting longer than 2 weeks qualify as postpartum depression.

Depressive disorder with peripartum onset, typically called **postpartum depression**, refers to moderate to severe depression experienced either during pregnancy or up to a year after giving birth; in up to 50% of cases, the depression begin during the pregnancy (APA, 2013). Most often it occurs within the first 3 months after delivery (Zieve & Merrill, 2012). It affects both men and women. *Both* parents are at highest risk for depression in the first year after the birth of their child. Parents with a prior history of depression, of younger age, and from deprived areas are most vulnerable to depression. Men and women with a history of any type of depression are more vulnerable to postpartum depression (Beyond the "baby blues," 2011; Davé et al., 2012). According to the *Harvard Medical Letter* (Beyond the "baby blues," 2011), "10% of women who have never been depressed develop postpartum depression, compared with 25% of those who have been depressed. And at least 50% of women who recover from one episode of postpartum depression experience a relapse of symptoms after another delivery" (p. 2). Women who give birth to multiple children and/or to preterm children also are at higher risk for postpartum depression.

Symptoms of postpartum depression include insomnia, loss of energy, inability to concentrate, anxiety, mood swings, periods of crying, and feelings of despair as the individual ruminates over perceived inadequacies as a parent. If depression goes untreated, it may affect the individual's ability to parent and to cope with stressful situations. Contributing factors are hormonal changes, family history of depression, feelings of being overwhelmed by parenting tasks, changes in family dynamics, and inadequate support.

One to 2 women in 1,000 with no history of a mood disorder experiences a **postpartum psychosis**—a medical emergency that usually requires hospitalization (Beyond the "baby blues," 2011). The incidence of relapse for women who have a diagnosed bipolar disorder is 25%–40% during postpartum, or 260 women per 1,000 deliveries. The symptoms usually occur between the first 2–6 weeks after delivery but may occur as early as 48 hours postpartum. Symptoms develop rapidly and include insomnia, mood lability, delusions, hallucinations, agitation, and bizarre feelings or behavior. An inordinate concern with the baby's health, guilt about lack of love, and delusions about the infant being dead or defective also may be present. The mother may deny having given birth or hear voices that command her to hurt the baby. In extreme cases, the mother may even kill the child and/or herself.

Theories of Depression

Mood disorders are currently considered to be caused by an interaction of individual genetic, biological, environmental, and psychosocial factors. Depressive disorders are considered spectrum disorders, occurring along a continuum of mild to severe. Most cases fall somewhere between these two extremes.

Alterations and Therapies **Mood and Affect**

ALTERATION	DESCRIPTION	THERAPIES
Depression (including major depressive disorder and persistent depressive disorder)	Depressed mood that varies from mild to severe with severe phases lasting longer than 6 weeks. Symptoms include: ■ Feelings of sadness, hopelessness, powerlessness, apathy, or guilt ■ Changes in sleep and/or appetite ■ Anhedonia (lack of pleasure in normally pleasing activities) ■ Inability to concentrate. ■ Psychomotor retardation or agitation.	■ Antidepressant medications: SSRIs, SNRIs, Bupropion, TCAs, MAOIs ■ Antidepressants may be combined with low-dose antipsychotic medication in resistant cases. ■ Electroconvulsive therapy ■ Cognitive-behavioral therapy (CBT) ■ Transcranial magnetic stimulation (TMS) ■ Vagus nerve stimulation (VNS)
Bipolar disorders	Extreme alterations in mood with intermittent periods of normal mood (mood swings)	■ Mood stabilizing medication ■ Psychotherapy ■ Hospitalization or partial hospitalization during severe episodes
Depressive disorder with peripartum onset (postpartum depression)	Severe depression appearing during pregnancy or within the first year following birth of a child. Symptoms include: ■ Insomnia ■ Fatigue ■ Crying ■ Feelings of despair ■ Anxiety ■ Mood swings.	■ Combination of antidepressants and psychosocial interventions is most effective.
Adjustment disorder with depressed mood (situational depression)	■ Hyperreaction to an identifiable, life-altering (but not life-threatening) stressor that occurs within 3 months after the onset of the stressor and persists for no more than 6 months; symptoms are similar to but less severe than those of major depressive disorder.	■ Psychotherapy alone may be sufficient to relieve symptoms and return client to premorbid level of functioning.

In understanding clients with mood disorders, the nurse must look at how factors interacted in the individual's past and how the individual interacts in present circumstances. An individual may have a genetic predisposition to abnormalities in neurotransmission. The abnormalities may occur only when certain psychological mechanisms are present, and these mechanisms may operate only when particular social interactions occur. Many factors in the individual and the environment increase or decrease the risk of mood disorders. Different forms of the illness may have different risk factors. In some forms, predisposition may have a stronger role, and in other forms, stressors may play more of a role. Mood disorders likely represent a common final pathway of multiple underlying factors, with most individuals with mood disorders possessing multiple risk factors. By applying genetic, neurobiological, intrapersonal, learning, cognitive, social, and gender bias theories, the nurse can approach the client from a holistic perspective.

BIOLOGICAL RHYTHMS Another hypothesis involves biological rhythms. **Biological rhythms** are regular fluctuations of a variety of physiological factors over a period of time. In some individuals, internal desynchronization may result in depression. The tendency toward internal desynchronization is probably inherited, but stresses, lifestyle, and normal aging also influence it. It is unclear, however, whether changes in circadian rhythms cause mood disturbances or whether changes in mood alter circadian rhythms. (See the module on Health, Wellness, and Illness for a more detailed discussion of circadian rhythms.)

Some forms of mood disorders are related to the time of year and the amount of available sunlight. In **seasonal affective disorder (SAD)**, the individual typically experiences depression during fall and winter, returning to normal mood in spring and summer, although rarely a version of SAD may be seen in which the individual experiences depression in the spring and summer (Mayo Clinic, 2012b). For those with fall/winter SAD, the depressive state appears to be directly related to the amount of natural sunlight because symptoms disappear when the person is exposed to more sunlight. Light has an inhibiting effect on the production of melatonin, a hormone that affects mood, sensations of fatigue, and sleepiness. The majority of SAD sufferers are women with a family history of mood disorders. Unlike major depression, in which symptoms for children and adults differ, children and adults with SAD exhibit similar symptoms: fatigue, decreased activity, irritability, sadness, crying, worrying, and decreased concentration. A symptom seen more frequently in SAD compared to the other mood disorders is increased appetite, carbohydrate craving, and weight gain.

INTRAPERSONAL FACTORS   Intrapersonal theory focuses on the theme of loss, either real or symbolic. The loss may be of another person, a relationship, an object, self-esteem, or security. When grief concerning the loss is unrecognized or unresolved, depression may result. A normal feeling accompanying all loss is anger, a compensatory response to feelings of powerlessness. Individuals who have been taught that it is inappropriate to experience and express anger learn to repress it. The result is that anger is turned inward and against the self. Some theorists believe that the repressed anger and aggression against the self are the cause of depressive episodes. Other theorists believe that the cause of depression is an inability to achieve desired goals, the loss of those goals, and a feeling of lack of control in life.

Individuals who are unusually sensitive to loss or abandonment issues are said to have dependent traits. Those who are unusually sensitive to failure to achieve their goals are said to have self-critical traits. Both of these cognitive-personality features increase the likelihood that environmental stressors will lead to depression.

LEARNING THEORY   Learning theory states that individuals learn to be depressed in response to an external locus of control, in which they perceive themselves lacking control over their life experiences. Individuals with depression typically experience little success in achieving gratification and little positive reinforcement for their attempts to cope with negative incidents. These repeated failures teach them that what they do has no effect on the final outcome. The more stressful their life events, the more their sense of helplessness is reinforced. When these individuals reach the point of believing they have no control, they no longer have the will or energy to cope with life, and a depressive state results.

COGNITIVE THEORY   Cognitive thought processes influence the way individuals with mood disorders experience themselves and others. Those who are depressed focus on negative messages in the environment and ignore positive experiences. These negative thought processes, or schemas, contribute to a view of the self as incompetent, unworthy, and unlikable. All present experiences are viewed as negative, and the individual sees no hope for the future. In the manic phase, individuals focus on positive messages in the environment and ignore negative experiences. These positive schemas contribute to manic clients' grandiose view of themselves. Everything that occurs is seen as positive, and the future holds no limits. When individuals get caught up in this process, a number of cognitive distortions may occur.

SOCIOCULTURAL FACTORS   Another sociocultural factor that may contribute to depression is the occurrence of stressful life events. Some events cause expansion of the family system: marriage, births, adoptions, and other people moving into the home. Other events cause a reduction of the family system: children leaving, marital separations, divorce, and death. Some life events involve a threat, as in job difficulties,

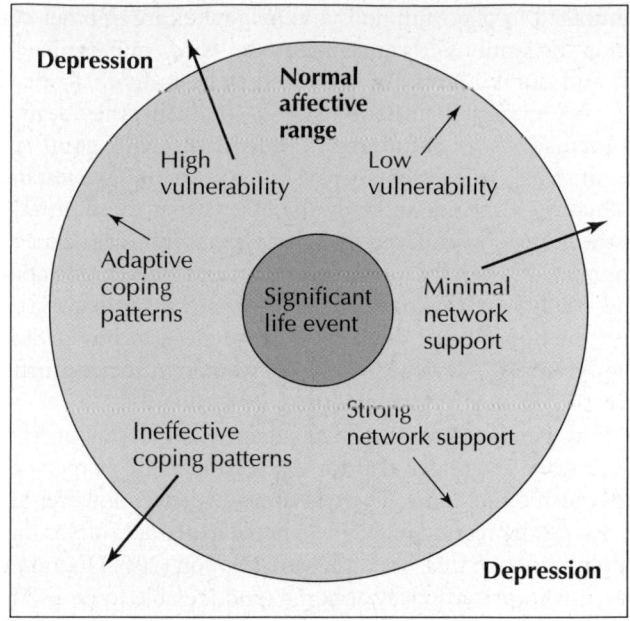

Figure 28–1 ● The relationship between life events and depression.

encounters with law enforcement, and illness. Other events can be emotionally exhausting, such as celebrating holidays, changing residences, and arguing with family and friends. Many individuals who experience stressful events do not become depressed. However, for those who are vulnerable to depression, stressors may play a significant role in the exacerbation and course of the disorder.

A number of factors influence the degree of stress that accompanies significant life events. **Figure 28–1 ●** illustrates the relationship between life events and depression. The presence of a social support network can decrease the impact that an event may have on an individual. Individuals who have developed adaptive coping patterns such as problem solving, direct communication, and use of resources are more likely to maintain their normal mood. Those who feel out of control, are unable to problem solve, and ignore available resources are more apt to feel depressed. Thus, an individual's perception and interpretation of significant events may contribute to depression.

Childhood sexual abuse is a significant risk factor for depression during both childhood and adulthood. Although the depressive episodes do not seem to be more severe, the onset is often earlier and the survivors are more likely to self-mutilate and attempt suicide (Lu et al., 2008).

GENDER BIAS THEORY   Throughout the world, women experience more depression than do men. Certainly, there are cross-cultural similarities in the way women are socialized and in the inferior status they experience in many societies. Psychosocial stressors, including multiple work and family responsibilities, poverty, sexual and physical abuse, gender discrimination, lack of social supports, and traumatic life experiences, may contribute to women's increased vulnerability to depression. In the United States and Canada, African American women are at higher risk for depression than Caucasian women. Gender socialization differences may be a factor in the higher rate of depression in women. It starts early, when many girls are encouraged to play with dolls and help take care of other children in the family. Girls are taught to be "nice," nonargumentative, and docile. Boys are socialized to be individualistic, to speak up, to raise their hand in class. Gradually, they begin to see themselves as autonomous individuals with good self-esteem. Many disciplines—psychology, sociology, nursing, psychiatry—continue to study the effects that these differing messages have on children and adolescents, and how expectations related to gender roles impact men and women into adulthood. Many have theorized that popular messages to girls (e.g., "Don't be bossy") that differ from those given to boys ("Stand up for yourself") devalue the roles of women in society, further increasing women's vulnerability to depression.

Many gender theorists have suggested that stay-at-home mothers are at greater risk for depression than women who work outside the home. There is some evidence, however, that the risk for depression in women related to gender roles is more complicated than this. Usdansky and Gordon (2011) found that women who prefer to stay at home (and are able to do so) and women who work in high-quality jobs are at lower risk for depression than women who want to work but are not employed, and they are also at lower risk for depression than women who are employed in low-paying jobs that provide little opportunity for individual success.

Gender bias theory can also be applied to the situation in which some older adults find themselves. In a society that places a premium on youth, older people feel useless, unimportant, incapable, and at times even repulsive. Role changes and losses may threaten their self-esteem. With aging, physiological changes may lead to a self-perception of being unfit, which then extends to further thoughts of being ineffectual and inferior. All of these changes may contribute to despair about one's life and a sense of hopelessness about the limited future. Considering these effects, it is not surprising to find a higher rate of depression among older people. See **Table 28–2** ● for an overview of the etiologies of mood disorders, with specific relevance to women and older adults.

Prevalence

Mood disorders include both depressive and bipolar disorders. Approximately 9.5% of U.S. adults (over 20 million) reported current depression (Kessler et al., 2005).

In the following discussion, *lifetime prevalence* indicates the number of people diagnosed with a depressive disorder at anytime during their lifetime. *Twelve-month prevalence* indicates the number of people with the disorder in a given year.

MAJOR DEPRESSIVE DISORDER   According to data from the National Co-morbidity Study (Kessler et al., 2005), the lifetime prevalence rates for U.S. adults with major depressive disorder are:

- All ages: 16.6%
- Ages 18–29: 15.4%
- Ages 30–44: 19.8%
- Ages 45–59: 18.8%
- Ages 60 and older: 10.6%
- Females: 20.2%
- Males: 13.2%.

The Substance Abuse and Mental Health Services Administration (SAMHSA) collects data on the national prevalence of depression each year through the National Survey on Drug Use and Health (NSDUH). Their most recent data are for 2008 (SAMHSA, 2008) and show the 12-month prevalence of depression among adults in the United States as 6.4%, with 8.1% of females reporting a major depressive episode female and 4.6% of males (NIMH, n.d.c). According to the Centers for Disease Control and Prevention (CDC) (2013), those with the highest prevalence of depression include:

- Individuals ages 45–64
- Women
- Blacks, Hispanics, non-Hispanic persons of other races or multiple races

TABLE 28–2   Causative Theories of Mood Disorders

THEORY	MAIN POINTS	RELEVANCE TO WOMEN AND OLDER ADULTS
Neurobiological	Impaired neurotransmission; limbic dysfunction	The central nervous system of women and older people have higher levels of monoamine oxidase (MAO).
Biological rhythms	Internal desynchronization of circadian rhythms	
Sunlight	A decrease in production of melatonin with decreased exposure to sunlight	Older adults may avoid going outdoors during the winter months.
Intrapersonal	Loss of person, object, self-esteem; hostility turned against the self; unachieved goals	Older adults suffer multiple losses.
Learning	Lack of control over experiences; learned helplessness; difficulty in adaptation	Expectation of women's dependency may reinforce helplessness; older adults may have increased stress with decreased resources, which may contribute to feelings of powerlessness.
Cognitive	Negative view of self, the present, and the future; focus on negative messages; cognitive errors	May apply regardless of age or gender.
Feminist	Internalization of cultural norms of behavior; rigid gender role and age expectations	Women's identity may be limited to the role of homemaker; employment positions are less prestigious; women may hold two full-time jobs. Older adults may suffer from the American cultural value placed on youth and endure many role changes and losses.

- Individuals with less than a high school education
- Individuals unable to work or who are unemployed
- Individuals without health insurance coverage
- Residents of southern states (Oklahoma, Louisiana, Mississippi, Alabama, Tennessee, West Virginia) and Puerto Rico.

DYSTHYMIA   The prevalence rates for dysthymia are as follows (NCS, n.d.):

- All ages: 2.5%
- Ages 18–29: 1.8%
- Ages 30–44: 2.8%
- Ages 45–59: 2.8%
- Ages 60 and older: 1.3%
- Females: 3.1%
- Males: 1.8%.

BIPOLAR DISORDERS   Approximately 5.7 million U.S. adults (2.6% of the population) reported a current bipolar disorder, with over 82% of these cases described as severe (Kessler et al., 2005). Men and women have equal rates of bipolar I disorder. Substance abuse and divorce rates among those with bipolar disorders are almost twice those of the general population.

POSTPARTUM DEPRESSION   In a national CDC survey, 8%–19% of women reported having frequent postpartum depressive symptoms (Ko et al., 2012). Interestingly, 4% of fathers reported depression in the year following the birth of a child (Davé et al., 2012), but the true prevalence of paternal postpartum depression is unknown.

Genetic Considerations and Nonmodifiable Risk Factors

Increasingly, genetics and neurobiology have been found to play a role in the development of mood disorders. Note, however, that all individuals operate within the contexts of their environments. Genetics and neurobiology inform nursing care and treatment for individuals with mood disorders, but nurses and clinicians must not overlook other determinants when providing care.

GENETICS   Some evidence suggests that people who experience mood disorders have a genetic predisposition to them. It is not yet clear what is inherited: neurobiological vulnerability, cognitive vulnerability, or social vulnerability. The rate of recurrent unipolar depression in the general population is 8%. Children of depressed parents (top-down sampling as shown in **Figure 28–2 ●**) have twice the risk, or about 16%, of experienc-

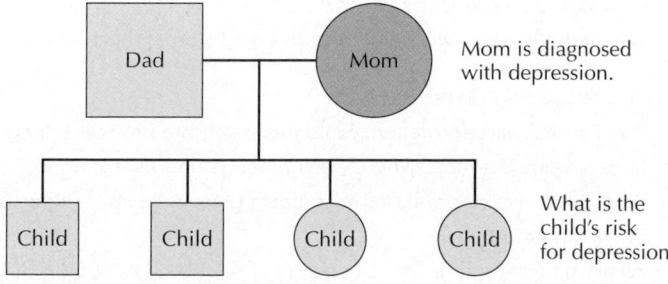

Figure 28–2 ● Top-down sampling.

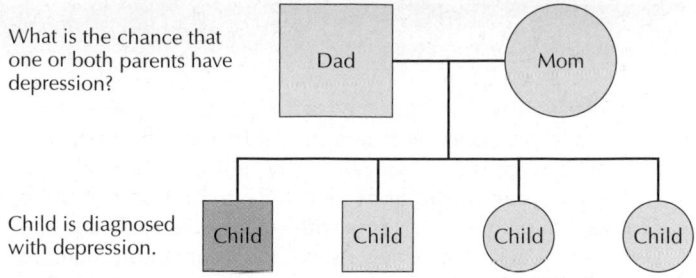

Figure 28–3 ● Bottom-up sampling.

ing depression over a lifetime. If both parents have depression, the risk rises to 75%. First-degree relatives of depressed children (bottom-up sampling as depicted in **Figure 28–3 ●**) also have twice the risk of depression. Studies of the incidence in twins show that in 60% of monozygotic twins, both twins developed a unipolar depression, compared with only 12% of dizygotic twins (Faraone et al., 2004).

Bipolar disorders have the greatest inheritability; about 85% of the risk appears to be inherited. Early onset of the disorder may be the result of a particularly strong genetic effect. Studies of the incidence in twins demonstrate that in 50%–80% of monozygotic twins, both twins developed bipolar disorders, compared with only 17%–24% of dizygotic twins (Badner, 2003; Fisfalen et al., 2005).

Studies suggest that rather than a single dominant gene, a complex mode of inheritance exists. The individual mix of these multiple genes likely determines differences such as age of onset, symptoms, severity, and course of the mood disorders. Evidence also suggests that environmental factors, such as maternal care in early childhood, may play a role in expression of genetic predisposition to mood disorders (Lau & Eley, 2010).

NEUROBIOLOGY   The *prefrontal cortex* has been the subject of increasing research on mood disorders. Studies of individuals with depression have shown lower-than-normal activity, low glucose metabolism, and decreased blood flow in the anterior cingulate cortex. These abnormalities may be associated with abnormal processing of emotion. Neuroimaging findings in bipolar disorders include ventricular enlargement and smaller volumes in the posterior hippocampus, left amygdala, and temporal lobe. The amygdala plays a role in keeping social and emotional behavior within bounds, both of which are impaired in manic episodes (Caetano et al., 2006; Frazier et al., 2005; Neumeister, Charney, & Drevets, 2005).

The *neurotransmission hypothesis* is specifically concerned with the levels of serotonin (5-HT), dopamine (DA), norepinephrine (NE), and acetylcholine (ACh) in the central nervous system (CNS). It is believed that there is a functional deficiency of these neurotransmitters during a depressive episode and a functional excess during a manic episode (Meyer et al., 2003).

Most likely there are different combinations of problems with the neurotransmitter systems. Both DA and the balance between DA and ACh are responsible for difficulties with motivation. ACh is implicated in the sleep disturbances of both bipolar and unipolar disorders. NE is important in motor arousal, movement, energy, concentration, and motivation. The principal neurotransmitter for mood states is 5-HT, which is associated with anxiety and aggression, especially self-destructive

Lifespan Considerations Prevalence of Mood and Affect Disorders Across the Life Span

Children

Prevalence of mood disorders in children is difficult to determine, and prevalence reports vary between 5% and 11%. This may, in part, result from reluctance on the part of some clinicians to diagnose children with serious mental illness and also from a lack of qualified providers in some communities (NAMI, 2008). Certainly some children experience depression, although onset of clinical depression typically occurs sometime between puberty and young adulthood. Onset of bipolar disorders typically does not begin until late adolescence or when individuals are in their 20s (APA, 2013).

Adolescents

The lifetime prevalence of depressive disorders (MDD and persistent depressive disorder) among 13–18 years old in a large U.S. national sample was 11.2%. Of those, 3.3% had a "severe" depressive disorder. Broken down further, lifetime prevalence was 15% for females and 7.5% for males; 7.4% for 13- to 14-year-olds, 12.2% for 15- to 16-year-olds, and 15.4% for 17- to 18-year-olds (Merekangas et al., 2010).

Older Adults

Depression affects nearly 5 million of the 31 million Americans ages 65 and older. Thirteen percent of people ages 80 and older have clinically significant symptoms of depression. The prevalence of MDD in community-dwelling older adults is 8%–16%. In hospitalized older adult medical surgical clients, 10%–12% had MDD, and an additional 23% had significant depressive symptoms (Blazer, 2009).

---

behavior. A newly found protein named p11 appears to regulate how brain cells respond to 5-HT by increasing the number of receptors. Compared to people who are not depressed, people who are depressed have lower levels of p11. In addition, endogenous opioids are necessary to moderate sad moods. The interactions between these different neurotransmitters explain how clinical features tend to vary among individuals (Svenningsson et al., 2006).

One way this imbalance may occur is through the action of the enzyme *monoamine oxidase (MAO)*, which is responsible for deactivating neurotransmitters after they have been released from the receptor sites. If there is an excess of MAO, neurotransmitter levels will be low, resulting in decreased impulse transmission. If there is insufficient MAO to deactivate the neurotransmitters, they will accumulate at the synapse and increase the transmission of impulses.

This hypothesis may be one explanation for the higher incidence of depression in women and older adults. Throughout life, women and older adults have consistently higher levels of MAO than do men and younger people. The result may be a functional decrease in the necessary neurotransmitters.

Another part of the hypothesis concerns the *sensitivity of the receptors* to the neurotransmitters. During depression, the receptors may be subsensitive, so fewer impulses are transmitted. During the manic state, receptors may be supersensitive, resulting in an increase in the transmission of impulses.

Continuing research into the relationship between stress and mood disorders indicates that the limbic system of the brain is the major site of stress adaptation. With stress, neurotransmitter production in the limbic system increases. When the stress becomes chronic or recurrent, the body can no longer adapt as efficiently, and a shortage of neurotransmitters results. During manic episodes, the feedback mechanism in the limbic system appears to be defective. Even after the stressful event has been resolved, the limbic system continues to produce excessive neurotransmitters; the increased transmission of impulses continues. Different areas of the limbic system play a major role in the regulation of emotions such as fear, rage, excitement, and euphoria. The signs and symptoms of limbic dysfunction correlate to the characteristics seen in the mood disorders.

CASE STUDY \\ PART 1

Jason is a 22-year-old college student. He has missed several classes and did not turn in a major paper. When contacted by his professor, Jason admits to feeling so depressed that he has not been able to concentrate on his course work, and has not left his apartment for several days. His professor expresses concern and suggests Jason go to the campus health center, which takes walk-ins. Jason agrees to go to the campus health center as a condition of getting an extension on the paper. Once there, he tells the nurse he has no appetite and complains of difficulty falling asleep. Jason says he feels guilty for not getting his assignments done and is not doing well in any of his classes. He states he doesn't know what is wrong with him, he just can't seem to get motivated and he doesn't know why. He looked forward to going to college and was excited to be accepted and move away from home for the first time. Jason did very well last semester, and in the beginning of this semester. He was active in several clubs and was thinking of running for the student senate and joining the track team, but recently things just seemed to fall apart. Although Jason has many acquaintances through his classes and activities, he has no close friends in the area. During the intake interview, the nurse observes that Jason sits hunched forward in his chair with his eyes downcast. He becomes tearful at times and never smiles.

Clinical Reasoning Questions Level I

1. What is the most important issue the nurse should assess?
2. How would you describe Jason's affect?
3. What are the physical health priorities for Jason at this time?

Clinical Reasoning Questions Level II

4. What additional information would the healthcare providers need to determine the most likely cause of Jason's depressed mood?
5. What are the considerations in contacting Jason's family regarding his situation?
6. What sociocultural factors or stressors might be contributing to Jason's distress?

▶ PREVENTION

There is no definitive way to prevent depression, due to causative and contributing genetic and biological factors that cannot be modified. Some strategies can be useful, however, for modifying stressors and environmental factors that can contribute to depressive illnesses. Teaching and promoting the use of healthy coping strategies and building social support may help increase resilience to stress and loss, and therefore prevent depression associated with loss or life events. Proper diet, exercise, and rest are important in maintaining physical and mental well-being. Abstaining from illegal drugs and using alcohol only in moderation can prevent substance use disorders that are associated with depression and can complicate treatment. Teaching people of all ages to recognize the symptoms of depression and to seek treatment promptly if they occur can lead to early detection and treatment. Awareness of individual risk factors such as family history, low self-esteem, and common comorbid conditions can be helpful. Regular visits to the healthcare provider and treatment compliance can help prevent recurrence.

Prevention Programs

Prevention programs may be useful for children and adolescents. A meta-analysis included 46 studies involving 32 depression prevention programs targeting children between the ages of 10 and 19 years. Larger effects were seen in programs for high-risk individuals than for universal trials. It was thought that higher level of distress or symptoms may have led to increased motivation in high-risk participants. Shorter programs had greater effects than longer ones. Program content was not related to effect size. Programs that included homework assignments had greater effects than those that did not, presumably because it allowed participants to apply acquired knowledge and skills in the real world. Prevention programs delivered by professional interventionists had greater effects than those delivered by teachers (Stice et al., 2009).

Screenings

No diagnostic tests are available to screen for mood disorders, however several self-report scales exist that can assist in screening for depression (see the Assessment section that follows). Clients scoring in the range indicating depression or mood disorder should be referred to a mental health professional for a thorough diagnostic evaluation. Two screening instruments—the Reynolds Child Depression scale and the PHQ-2—can be used in a variety of settings to screen individuals to determine if referral is necessary.

The Reynolds Child Depression scale was designed for school or class screenings of depression in children ages 7–13 years. It contains 30 items and takes about 10–15 minutes to complete. It must be purchased and comes with normative data and a short form (Reynolds, 1989). An adolescent version is also available (Reynolds, 1987).

There is evidence that asking two simple questions (PHQ-2) related to feelings of sadness and anhedonia can accurately screen for depression in adults (Kroenke, Spitzer, & Williams, 2003), adolescents (Borner et al., 2010), and postpartum women (Gjerdingen et al., 2009). This is a quick and easy method that can be done in any setting. Depending on the setting, a longer, more comprehensive screening tool may be administered following a positive response to the PHQ-2. In any case, the client must be referred for psychiatric evaluation.

▶ ASSESSMENT

The first and most important aspect in conducting an assessment is to establish a therapeutic relationship based on mutual trust. The nurse should ask open-ended questions and allow adequate time for client response. It is important that the nurse remain nonjudgmental and validate the client's feelings. It may be necessary to reduce the client's anxiety. The nurse should communicate with brief, clear statements, verify the client's understanding, and clarify areas that may not be understood. Refer to the exemplar on Therapeutic Communication in the module on Communication for additional information.

Assessment of clients with mood disorders may need to be done in segments of 15–20 minutes each. Individuals who are severely depressed may not have the energy to talk for longer periods, and those who are in a manic phase may be unable to concentrate and sit still for longer periods. Clients who are depressed may require more time to answer questions due to psychomotor retardation or difficulty concentrating; the nurse may need to repeat questions. If family members are present, the nurse should discourage them from answering questions for the client who is responding slowly.

Clients in a manic phase of bipolar disorder with flight of ideas must be refocused frequently on the topic at hand. Their elevated mood may interfere with their ability to give accurate information.

Individuals with mood disorders display a variety of characteristics involving changes in behavior, affect, cognition, and physiology. Somewhat similar changes occur for people experiencing grief.

The nurse conducting an assessment of the client who is suspected of having a mood disorder must remember that these disorders affect individuals in a variety of ways. The nurse should be aware that individuals with mood disorders may display changes in a number of characteristics, including behavioral, cognitive, and physiological. **Table 28–3** ● lists some of the most common characteristics of mood disorders.

Self-Report Scales

Nurses may use self-reporting scales as part of the assessment process.

ADULTS   The Beck Depression Inventory is a self-rating scale that is used to screen for depression. The client can complete the questionnaire in about 10 minutes. If necessary, the nurse can verbally read the questions to clients who are unable to complete the questionnaire independently.

The Center for Epidemiological Studies Depression Scale–Revised (CESD-R) is a 20-item self-rating scale that asks people to rate how often during the past week they experienced symptoms associated with depression. A score of 16 or above indicates depression. This scale is useful for a wide age range of populations including older adults (Lewinsohn et al., 1997). It was originally developed for use in epidemiological studies (Radloff, 1977), but is now widely used as a screening tool as well as a research measure.

TABLE 28–3   Characteristics of Mood Disorders

CHARACTERISTIC	DEPRESSED STATE	MANIC STATE
Behavioral		
Desire to participate in activities	Decreased to absent	Interested in all activities; increase in high-risk behaviors
Interaction with others	Limited; client withdraws	Talkative, gregarious
Affiliation needs	Increased dependency	Independent, self-sufficient
Affective		
Mood	Despair, desolation	Unstable: euphoric and irritable
Guilt	High level	Unable to experience guilt
Crying spells	Frequent crying to inability to cry	May have brief episodes
Gratification	Loss of interest in pleasurable activities	Constantly seeking fun and excitement
Emotional attachments	Indifference to others	Forms intense attachments rapidly
Cognitive		
Self-evaluation	Focuses on failures; sees self as incompetent; catastrophizes and personalizes	Grandiose beliefs about self
Expectations	Believes present and future are hopeless; overgeneralizes one experience or fact	Inordinate positive expectations; unable to see potential negative outcomes
Self-criticism	Harshly critical of self; is a perfectionist; anticipates disapproval from others	Approves of own behavior; irate if criticized by others
Concentration	Decreased	Decreased
Decision-making ability	Decreased ability or inability to make decisions	Difficulty due to distractibility and impulsiveness
Flow of thought	Decreased rate and number of thoughts	Flight of ideas; cannot be interrupted
Body image	Believes self to be unattractive or ugly	Believes self unusually beautiful
Delusions	Somatic delusions	Delusions of grandeur
Hallucinations	Occur in 15%–25% of cases	Occur in 15%–25% of cases
Sociocultural		
Sexual desire	Loss of desire	Increase in activity and partners
Physiological		
Appetite	Increased or decreased in mild and moderate depression; decreased in severe depression	Difficulty eating due to inability to sit still
Amount of sleep	Increased or decreased in mild and moderate depression; decreased in severe depression	Sleeps only 1 or 2 hours a night
Activity level	Impaired motor activity; loss of energy	Hyperactivity; high energy
Bowel activity	Constipation	Constipation
Physical appearance	Unkempt; poor hygiene	Bright clothing; frequently changes clothing

💠 *Stay Current:* Visit **http://cesd-r.com** *to see or take the CESD-R.*

The Mood Disorders Questionnaire (MDQ) was developed to screen for bipolar disorder in adults in primary care (Hirschfeld et al., 2000). It contains 13 questions plus items that assess symptom clusters and functional impairment. A version is available for use with adolescents (Wagner et al., 2006). Use of the MDQ was recently called into question because some were using it as a diagnostic proxy or case finding test instead of as a screening tool. Zimmerman (2012) pointed out that most people referred for evaluation through MDQ screening will not be diagnosed with bipolar disorder. However, due to most clinicians' unfamiliarity with the disorder and the underdiagnosis of bipolar disorder, a screening tool such as the MDQ is still useful for determining when to make a referral. There is no substitute for the clinical diagnostic interview by a mental health professional to diagnose bipolar disorder.

💠 *Stay Current:* Visit **www.integration.samhsa.gov/ images/res/MDQ.pdf** *to see or take the MDQ.*

CHILDREN   The Center for Epidemiological Studies–Depression Scale for Children (CES-DC) is a 20-item self-rating scale developed for use in children that is similar to the CESD-R. A score of 15 or above indicates depression (Weissman et al., 1980). Another widely used screening tool is the Children's Depression Inventory 2 (CDI-2). It consists of 28 items, each containing three statements that screen for depression in children and adolescents ages 7–17 years and can be used in a variety of settings. There is also a 10-item version. This scale must be purchased. The kit comes with normative data and parent and teacher report forms. Children who score in the depressed range on any screening tool must be referred to a mental health clinician who specializes in the diagnosis and treatment of children and/or adolescents.

🔖 *Stay Current: Visit* **www.brightfutures.org/mentalhealth/pdf/professionals/bridges/ces_dc.pdf** *to see the CES-DC.*

There is a version of the MDQ specifically designed to screen adolescents for bipolar disorder (Wagner et al., 2006). Prompt referral for diagnostic evaluation by a specialist in adolescent mental health is warranted for those who screen positive.

OLDER ADULTS   The Geriatric Depression Scale (GDS) can be used to assess depression in older adults. Older adults may complete the scale themselves or have a healthcare provider read it to them and score their answers. Older adults scoring above 10 on the GDS should be referred for further assessment. The GDS may be used with older adults with cognitive impairment as well as those with alterations in physical health. The Cornell Depression Scale (CDS) can be used to screen for depression in older adults with severe cognitive impairments (mini-mental health status examination below 15). The CDS relies on observations of behaviors and functional measures instead of client responses. Clients who score 12 or above on the CDS should be referred for further assessment. The MDQ has been used to screen for bipolar disorder in a wide range of adults, however age of onset for bipolar disorder is usually in adolescence or young adulthood.

POSTPARTUM DEPRESSION   The Edinburgh Postnatal Depression Scale is the most widely used screening tool for postpartum depression in large populations of women. The tool has been validated, computerized, and used in telephone screening. Mothers who score above 12 are likely to be suffering from postpartum depression. Another tool is Beck's (2002) Postpartum Depression Predictors Inventory–Revised (PDPI-R). This tool also is a practical and simple screening checklist for use during routine care with all postpartum women to identify those who might be experiencing postpartum depression, ensuring that early management can be initiated. See the exemplar on Postpartum Depression later in this module for more information.

Lifespan and Cultural Considerations

Older, single White males have one of the highest rates of suicide in the United States (American Association of Suicidology, 2013). This is of particular concern because many older adults who complete suicide were seen by their primary care provider sometime during the month before their suicide (Cornwell, 2009). Older adults face a number of life changes that may increase their risk for depressive disorders or that may increase the risk for relapse in adults who have successfully managed a depressive disorder over time. Life changes such as retirement or disability related to the onset of illness or injury may precipitate changes in mood. In all clinical settings, nurses working with older adults need to assess for risk for and symptoms of depression and suicidal ideation.

Appropriate expressions of mood are largely culturally determined. For example, situations in which people are expected to experience sadness, anger, loneliness, frustration, joy, or happiness are defined by the culture. Culture also determines how people are to behave when experiencing a variety of feelings.

For example, cultural expectations of grieving individuals may be self-control and a "stiff upper lip" or may be loud mourning and ripping of clothing. Extreme pleasure may be expressed with a nod and a smile or may be expressed with loud laughter and exuberant behavior.

The Western interpretation of feelings is that emotions are intrapersonal. In contrast individuals from cultures that do not normally focus on or discuss mood states (e.g., Middle Eastern, African, Hispanic, and Chinese cultures) may report somatic (bodily) complaints at a higher rate than individuals from Western cultures (Culture and depression, 2008). The process by which psychological distress is experienced and communicated in the form of somatic symptoms is called **somatization**.

Emotions of suffering and depression have dramatically different meaning and forms of expression in different cultures. Many Americans view suffering as unexpected or unacceptable and perceive depression as something to overcome through personal striving. Latin American cultures associate suffering with a deep sense of tragedy. Shi'ite Muslims view suffering within a religious context of martyrdom, while Buddhist cultures view suffering as a positive feature of life. Throughout the entire world, most cases of depression are experienced and expressed in bodily terms such as fatigue, headaches, heart distress, and dizziness. When nurses assess clients from cultures different from their own, they must understand the impact of culture on both the expression of depression as well as culture-related risks for depression. Immigrants are at higher risk for depression as they cope with multiple stressors such as long-distance family relationships, unemployment or underemployment, discrimination, language problems, and a new environment. Immigrant children are at risk for depression as they are often expected to interpret the concerns of adult family members to outside authority figures such as physicians, nurses, teachers, and government officials (Aroian & Norris, 2002; Smith, 2011).

Rather than seeking professional help, African Americans and Latinos often look to their family and faith communities for help. There is a strong fear of hospitalization and involuntary commitment, both of which are more likely for African Americans and Latinos than for Caucasians. A survey of Medicare beneficiaries (2001–2005) indicated that African Americans are diagnosed with depression at a rate of 4.2% versus 6.4% for Caucasians. The survey also found greater distrust of the medical community among African Americans, communication challenges, and financial considerations. For example, White clients receiving Medicare services are far more likely to participate in a supplemental insurance program (Nauert, 2011).

Although nurses need to take cultural factors into account during assessment (e.g., ensuring careful assessment that includes access to financial resources and attitudes toward the healthcare community), nurses must take care not to stereotype clients during the assessment process. When nurses engage in stereotyping they risk failing to assess for important indicators and are likely to increase barriers to trust and understanding when they should be building the therapeutic alliance and gaining client trust.

Diagnostic Tests

Although no diagnostic tests exist for mood disorders, a thorough workup is necessary to rule out any underlying medical

TABLE 28–4   Differences Between Depression and Grief

TRAIT	DEPRESSION	GRIEF
Trigger	Specific trigger not necessary, but may be present.	Trigger is usually loss or multiple losses.
Active/passive	Passive behavior tends to keep client "stuck" in sadness.	Actively feel their emotional pain and emptiness.
Emotions	Generalized feeling of helplessness, hopelessness.	Experience a range of emotions that are usually intense.
Ability to laugh	Likely to be humorless and incapable of being happy or even temporarily cheered up; likely to resist support.	Sometimes will be able to laugh and enjoy humor; more likely to accept support.
Activities	Lacks interest in previously enjoyed activities.	Can be persuaded to participate in activities, especially as they begin to heal.
Self-esteem	Low self-esteem, low self-confidence; feels like a failure.	Self-esteem usually remains intact; does not feel like a failure unless it relates directly to the loss.
Feeling of failure	May dwell on past failures, catastrophize feelings.	Any self-blame or guilt relates directly to the loss; feelings resolve as they progress toward healing.

condition that could mimic or cause symptoms of mood disorders, or to detect comorbid medical illness that could contribute to symptoms and functional abnormalities. Diagnostic and laboratory tests may include:

- Thyroid function tests since thyroid disorders may mimic depression or hypomania
- Electrolyte panel, urinalysis, toxicology to rule out substance abuse
- Liver function tests since antidepressant medications are metabolized in the liver
- Other tests based on the client's individual symptoms and history.

A pregnancy test may be ordered in females of reproductive age since antidepressants may affect fetal development.

Differentiating Depression From Grief

In some clients, depression and grief may present similarly on initial assessment. Nurses must distinguish whether a client who exhibits sadness and anhedonia is depressed or grieving (Table 28–4 ●). Although this may appear to be easy, it can be difficult when working with new clients with whom the nurse has not yet developed a therapeutic relationship. Careful assessment includes determining if the feelings described by the client were triggered by a loss or losses (such as the death of a family member).

CASE STUDY \\ PART 2

Following a clinical interview and administration of the Beck Depression Inventory, the healthcare provider at the campus health center diagnosed Jason with major depressive disorder and prescribed extended-release venlafaxine (Effexor XR). One month later, Jason comes to the health center for his follow-up appointment. The nurse notes his behavior is nearly the opposite of what she observed at the initial visit. He describes his current mood as "fabulous." He states he is only sleeping about 2 hours a night but that "It's OK," that he feels great and is getting so much done in the extra hours of wakefulness. Jason also reports a heightened sexual desire and urges and attributes this to his decreased need for sleep. Jason tells the nurse that he completed his required paper and that

it is so good, he is turning it into a book about the secret to the meaning of life, although he has not yet received a grade. He is running for student senate, tried out for the track team, and volunteered at the campus tutoring center. The increased participation in activities has resulted in making new friends with whom he goes drinking 2–3 nights a week. Jason is considering taking five accelerated courses during the summer.

During the interview, Jason's speech is loud, rapid, and pressured. He is restless, unable to sit still for more than 5 minutes. He offers to give the nurse his autograph because he is convinced his intended book will win a Pulitzer Prize. Jason denies side effects of the medication, and considers it a miracle drug because he feels better than he ever has in his entire life. When questioned about thoughts of suicide, he denies them stating "A person as special as I am needs to be cloned, not killed!"

Clinical Reasoning Questions Level I
1. What else should the nurse assess?
2. How would you describe Jason's affect during this visit?
3. What are the priority health and safety considerations for Jason?

Clinical Reasoning Questions Level II
4. What could be responsible for Jason's remarkable change in mood, affect, and behavior?
5. What are the priority topics to address in Jason's healthcare teaching plan during this visit?
6. How would you rate Jason's risk for suicide?

▶ INTERVENTIONS AND THERAPIES

Independent

Nurses are in the singular position to provide a number of caring interventions for depressed clients and their families. The most important of these are preventing client suicide and promoting client and family safety.

PREVENTING SUICIDE AND PROMOTING SAFETY There are few times when *always* and *never* are applicable. Client safety, however, *always* takes priority over other nursing care concerns. Clients experiencing severe depression are at a high risk for suicide and violent behaviors.

Box 28–1   Preventing Inpatient Suicide and Promoting Safety

Check the policy and procedures of the individual inpatient treatment facility and implement those guidelines as well.

- Evaluate the level of suicide intent regularly and institute the appropriate level of staff supervision following unit protocol.
- Let suicidal clients know that the environment is safe for them. Remove sharp objects, razors, breakable glass items, mirrors, matches, and straps or belts and explain why these objects are being removed. Monitor the use of scissors, razors, and other potential weapons.
- Clients at risk for suicide should not be left alone. In acute care hospitals or residential settings, one-to-one observation must be instituted until a psychiatrist or qualified physician determines the client is no longer at risk. Family members cannot substitute for staff in performing one-to-one observation. In psychiatric inpatient settings, checking the client every 15 minutes is acceptable.

Documentation of client behavior and one-to-one observation and 15 minute checks are required.

- Avoid establishing a predictable pattern of observation during the day and especially at night.
- Be particularly alert during change of shifts and on holidays or other times when staffing is limited and during times of distraction, such as mealtimes and visiting hours.
- Examine items brought by visitors and monitor for safety. Many units have policies regarding what can and cannot be brought into the unit. Most prohibit food of any kind from outside of the facility.
- Encourage clients to seek a staff member when experiencing suicidal thoughts or impulses. Discussing these thoughts and impulses may be sufficient to diminish them and prevent a crisis from occurring. Avoid discussing suicidal ruminations in repetitious detail, as this may reinforce maladaptive behavior.

When the risk for self-directed violence is high, immediate intervention is necessary. The risk of suicide increases as clients in the severest stage of depression begin to improve; it is then that clients have sufficient energy and cognitive ability to plan and successfully implement a suicide plan. When a client expresses suicidal ideation, confidentiality does **not** apply. It is the nurse's duty to report suicidal thoughts or actions to the treatment team, or take necessary steps to have the client transported via ambulance or police to a community crisis screening center, hospital emergency department, or other appropriate facility according to state guidelines. See **Box 28–1** for guidelines to help prevent inpatient suicide and promote safety. The module on Violence contains detailed information on suicide along with a nursing care plan for a suicidal client.

Encourage clients to discuss all of their feelings. Clients need to know that all feelings are valid and that it benefits them to express their emotions—particularly anger and hopelessness—rather than act them out through maladaptive behaviors. Having the feeling is always acceptable. Acting on the feeling, however, may be problematic. More important is what an individual decides to do about the feeling. Nurses should assist in the transition from hospital to home by helping clients identify people in their usual environments to whom they can express feelings candidly without being judged.

Use a calm, reassuring approach and teach calming measures such as time-outs and controlled breathing. Provide safe physical outlets for expression of anger or increasing tension.

Partner with clients to identify community resources to which they can turn if suicidal thoughts recur outside the treatment setting. Most communities provide hotlines that are staffed around the clock with trained volunteers or professionals who are available to discuss feelings before they reach crisis proportions. With client's permission, discuss with the client's family the risks for injury in the home (e.g., the presence of firearms) and to understand how the family plays a role in the client's illness.

TEACHING ASSERTIVE BEHAVIOR   Nurses working with clients can model, encourage, and teach assertive behavior. Assertiveness is a learned behavior. Everyone has assertiveness potential, but not everyone is born knowing how to be assertive. Children learn patterns of communicating from the adults around them. People can unlearn poor communication patterns that do not work and learn new ones, which is the idea behind assertiveness training. The goal is to help individuals express themselves without fear of disapproval from others. Being assertive does not guarantee that others will agree, but it does provide an individual the satisfaction of offering a personal opinion without ignoring the opinions of others.

Aggressive behavior is directed toward getting what one wants without considering the feelings of others. Aggressive communicators want to get their own way at any cost. They want others to "back off," and they use intimidation to convey this message. An example of aggressive behavior is insisting on going to a certain movie even though you know your companion does not enjoy that type of movie. The outcome of aggressive behavior is that although you may get what you want in the short run, others feel discredited and tend to avoid you.

Passive behavior consists of avoiding conflict at any cost, even at the expense of one's own happiness. An example of passive behavior is agreeing to go to a movie you do not want to see because your friend pressures you to go. Passive communicators hold their feelings in and allow anger to build up. Anger can explode suddenly or can be expressed in passive–aggressive behavior. An example of passive–aggressive behavior is taking a long time to get ready to go out while your friend is waiting because you are angry at him for insisting on seeing a movie you do not want to see. The outcome is that the passive person gives up control and is left with resentment, which usually emerges in other ways that damage relationships.

Assertive behavior consists of expressing one's wishes and opinions, or taking care of oneself, but not at the expense of others. An example of assertive communication is saying, "I really don't care for violent movies. Let's look at the movie listings and see if there is something playing that we can both enjoy." The outcome of assertive behavior is self-confidence and self-esteem. Helpful references include the following books, which can be obtained through a local library or bookseller: *The Assertiveness Handbook (Overcoming Common Problems),* by Mary Hartley, 2007; *Peace at Any Price: How to Overcome the Please Disease,* by Deborah Day Poor, 2005; and *Civilized Assertiveness for Women: Communication with Backbone . . . Not Bite,* by Judith Selee McClure, 2007.

MINIMIZING MALADAPTIVE DEPENDENCE   Hopeless clients have a tendency to form dependent relationships. Nurses must work from the first contact with these clients to minimize the likelihood that maladaptive dependence occurs in the nurse–client relationship. Strategies to minimize maladaptive dependence include the following:

- Emphasize the short-term nature of the relationship.
- Recognize that a client who singles out one staff member exclusively and refuses to relate to others is developing dependence.
- Avoid giving dependent clients the hope that the nurse–client relationship can continue after therapy has ended.
- Refuse (kindly but firmly) requests for your address or telephone number.
- Remind clients that social contact will not be allowed.

If you find yourself wanting to continue relationships with certain clients, discuss these feelings with your instructor (if you are a student), your supervisor, or a respected professional peer (if you are a practicing nurse). It is essential that you separate your professional life from your social life.

Collaborative

Collaborative interventions for clients with mood disorders include pharmacotherapy, cognitive-behavioral therapy and other psychotherapies, and complementary therapies. Often the use of therapies in combination leads to greater success. Nurses help clients determine what combination of therapies may be most helpful for them, encourage adherence to the treatment plan, and suggest alternatives if a sufficient trial of a treatment or therapy (typically at least 6 weeks) proves ineffective.

PHARMACOLOGIC THERAPY FOR DEPRESSION   A number of medications are available for the treatment of mood disorders. Often they achieve greatest effect when used in combination with psychotherapy.

Drugs used to treat depression are categorized as antidepressants. Antidepressants treat major depression by enhancing mood. Antidepressants are also sometimes prescribed to treat anxiety disorders. Recent studies link depression and anxiety to similar neurotransmitter dysfunction, and both seem to respond to treatment with antidepressant medications. Antidepressants are also beneficial in treating psychological and physical signs of pain, especially in clients without MDD (e.g., when mood problems are associated with debilitating conditions such as fibromyalgia or muscle spasticity).

SAFETY ALERT

The Food and Drug Administration (FDA) requires a "black box warning" to be included at the beginning of the drug package inserts and drug information sheets of **all** antidepressants. They warn of the increased risk for suicidal thoughts and behaviors associated with taking antidepressant medications. The nurse must be aware of this and educate clients and families to monitor for this and provide 24-hour emergency center contact numbers for use if this occurs. Those ages 24 or younger are especially at risk.

Depression is associated with dysfunction of neurotransmitters in certain regions of the brain. Although medication does not completely restore normal chemical balance, it may help reduce depressive symptoms while the client develops effective means of coping.

It is thought that antidepressants exert their effect through their action on certain neurotransmitters in the brain, including norepinephrine, dopamine, and serotonin. The two basic mechanisms of action are blocking the enzymatic breakdown of norepinephrine and slowing the reuptake of serotonin. The four primary classes of antidepressant drugs are tricyclic antidepressants (TCAs), selective serotonin reuptake inhibitors (SSRIs), monoamine oxidase inhibitors (MAOIs), and atypical antidepressants, which include the serotonin–norepinephrine reuptake inhibitors (SNRIs). Nurses working with clients taking antidepressants must be alert to the symptoms of **serotonin syndrome**, which can occur in individuals taking two or more medications that increase serotonin levels. In addition to antidepressants, over-the-counter (OTC) agents such as dextromethorphan, pseudoephedrine, and St. John's wort can increase serotonin levels. Symptoms of serotonin syndrome include hypertension or hypotension, agitation, shivering, changes in mental status, symptoms of gastrointestinal distress, restlessness, tremor, muscle rigidity, unreactive pupils, and tachypnea. Typically supportive measures and discontinuing the medications involved will resolve the client's symptoms.

Tricyclic Antidepressants   Named for their three-ring chemical structure, **tricyclic antidepressants (TCAs)** were the mainstay of depression pharmacotherapy from the early 1960s until the 1980s. They are still used today, although less frequently.

TCAs act by inhibiting the reuptake of both norepinephrine and serotonin into presynaptic nerve terminals. TCAs are used mainly for major depression. TCAs have some unpleasant and serious side effects. The most common side effect is orthostatic hypotension, which is due to alpha$_1$ blockade on blood vessels. The most serious adverse effect occurs when TCAs accumulate in cardiac tissue. Although rare, cardiac dysrhythmias can occur.

Sedation is a frequently reported complaint at the initiation of therapy, though clients may become tolerant to this effect after several weeks of treatment. Most TCAs have long half-lives, which increases the risk of side effects for clients with delayed excretion. Anticholinergic effects such as dry mouth, constipation, urinary retention, excessive perspiration, blurred vision, and tachycardia are common. These effects are less severe if the drug is gradually increased to the therapeutic dose over 2–3 weeks. Significant drug interactions can occur with CNS depressants, sympathomimetics, anticholinergics, and MAOIs. For clients over the age of 40, an electrocardiogram may be ordered prior to initiation of treatment to detect preexisting arrhythmias. Since the advent of newer antidepressants that have fewer side effects, TCAs are less frequently used as first-line drugs in the treatment of depression and/or anxiety.

- *Nursing considerations.* The role of the nurse in TCA therapy involves careful monitoring of a client's condition and providing education as it relates to the prescribed drug treatment. The therapeutic effects of TCAs may take 2–6 weeks to occur. Monitor the client closely for suicidal ideation and behaviors throughout treatment. As clients begin to recover from both psychological and physical depression (psychological depression slows all body processes), their energy levels rise.

Assessing previous health history is essential. Tricyclic antidepressants are contraindicated in clients in the acute recovery phase of an MI, with heart block, or with a history of dysrhythmias because of the effects of TCAs on cardiac tissue. Because TCAs lower the seizure threshold, carefully monitor clients with epilepsy. Clients with urinary retention, narrow-angle glaucoma, or prostatic hypertrophy may not be good candidates for TCAs because of anticholinergic side effects. Anticholinergic effects, coupled with the weight gain effect of TCAs, may lead to noncompliance. Tricyclics must be given with extreme caution to clients with asthma, cardiovascular disorders, gastrointestinal disorders, alcoholism, and other psychiatric disorders including schizophrenia and bipolar disorders. Most TCAs are pregnancy category C or D, so they are used during pregnancy or lactation only when medically necessary.

■ **Drug interactions.** Significant drug interactions may occur with TCAs. Less commonly used than other opioids, a single dose of meperidine (Demerol) can cause seizures, delirium, hyperpyrexia, circulatory collapse, coma, and death in clients taking MAOIs. Oral contraceptives may decrease the effectiveness of TCAs. TCAs affect the effectiveness of clonidine (Catapres) and guanethidine (Ismelin). Use with St. John's wort may cause serotonin syndrome. The nurse should observe clients for the effects of drugs that enhance the effects of TCAs, such as antidysrhythmics, antihistamines, antihypertensives, and CNS depressants. Clients who take cimetidine and atropine also should be monitored. Some drugs increase the rate of TCA metabolism and excretion from the body. These include cimetidine (Tagamet), carbamazepine (Tegretol), phenytoin (Dilantin), and rifampin (Rifadin). Cigarette smoking also diminishes the effect of TCAs.

■ **Client education.** Client education as it relates to TCAs should include the aforementioned risk of increased suicidal thoughts and behaviors, goals of therapy, the reasons for obtaining baseline data such as vital signs and the existence of underlying cardiac and renal disorders, and possible drug side effects. Include the following points when teaching clients about TCAs:
  ● It may take several weeks or more to achieve the full therapeutic effect of the drug.
  ● Keep all scheduled follow-up appointments with your healthcare provider.
  ● Understand that sweating, along with anticholinergic side effects such as dry mouth, constipation, blurred vision, and increased heart rate, may occur.
  ● If decreased urination or difficulty urinating occurs, call healthcare provider immediately.
  ● Take the medication exactly as prescribed and report side effects if they occur.
  ● Do not take other prescription drugs, OTC medications, or herbal remedies without notifying your healthcare provider.
  ● Avoid using alcohol and other CNS depressants.
  ● Change positions slowly to avoid dizziness.
  ● Do not drive or engage in hazardous activities until the drug's sedative effect is known.
  ● Take the drug at bedtime if sedation occurs.

  ● Immediately discuss with your healthcare provider an intention or desire to become pregnant.
  ● Do not discontinue abruptly; these drugs must be withdrawn over several weeks due to risk of arrhythmias.

Selective Serotonin Reuptake Inhibitors   Drugs that slow the reuptake of serotonin into presynaptic nerve terminals are called **selective serotonin reuptake inhibitors (SSRIs)**. Their mechanism of action is to increase the availability of serotonin in the synaptic cleft for post-synaptic receptors. They are considered first-line therapy in the treatment of depressive disorders due to their favorable side effect profiles.

Serotonin is a natural neurotransmitter in the CNS, found in high concentrations in certain neurons in the hypothalamus, limbic system, medulla, and spinal cord. Serotonin is important to several body activities, including the cycling between NREM and REM sleep, pain perception, and emotional states. Lack of adequate serotonin in the CNS can lead to depression. Serotonin is metabolized to a less active substance by the enzyme monoamine oxidase (MAO). Serotonin is also known by its chemical name, 5-hydroxytryptamine (5-HT).

Whereas the TCAs inhibit reuptake of both norepinephrine and serotonin, the SSRIs selectively target serotonin. Increased levels of serotonin in the synaptic gap induce complex neurotransmitter changes in presynaptic and postsynaptic neurons in the brain. Presynaptic receptors become less sensitive, and postsynaptic receptors become more sensitive.

■ **Nursing care.** Although the SSRIs are safer than other antidepressants, serious adverse effects can still occur. Obtain baseline liver function tests because SSRIs are metabolized in the liver, and hepatic disease can result in higher serum levels. Obtain a baseline body weight to monitor weight gain.

■ **Client education.** In terms of SSRIs, client education should include the goals of therapy, the reasons for obtaining baseline data such as vital signs and the existence of underlying disorders or concurrent medication use, and possible drug side effects. Include the following points when teaching clients about SSRIs:
  ● Know that SSRIs may take up to 5 weeks to reach their maximum therapeutic effectiveness.
  ● Do not take any prescription drugs, OTC drugs, or herbal products without notifying your healthcare provider.
  ● Keep all follow-up appointments with your healthcare provider.
  ● Report side effects, including nausea, vomiting, diarrhea, sexual dysfunction, and fatigue.
  ● Sexual side effects include decreased desire and difficulty or inability to achieve orgasm or ejaculation.
  ● Do not drive or engage in hazardous activities until the drug's sedative effect is known.
  ● Do not stop taking the drug suddenly after long-term use because withdrawal symptoms can occur. Although these symptoms are not life threatening, they are uncomfortable.
  ● Take most SSRIs in the morning with food to avoid gastrointestinal upset and insomnia. If the client complains of feeling sedated or tired, the SSRI may be taken in the evening. Take mirtazapine (Remeron) at bedtime because it usually causes excessive drowsiness, especially at lower doses.
  ● Exercise and monitor caloric intake to avoid weight gain.

The role of the nurse in SSRI therapy involves careful monitoring of a client's condition and providing education as it relates to the prescribed drug treatment. Assess the client's needs for antidepressant therapy by noting the intensity and duration of symptoms and identifying factors that led to depression, such as life events and health changes. Obtain a careful drug history, including the use of CNS depressants, alcohol, and other antidepressants, especially MAOI therapy, and use of OTC medications and supplements, especially St. John's wort and gingko biloba because these may interact with SSRIs. Assess for hypersensitivity to SSRIs. Assess for suicidal ideation. Because these drugs have a high incidence of sexual side effects, obtain a history of any disorders of sexual function. Note any history of eating disorders; some SSRIs may cause weight gain, which may contribute to noncompliance in clients with distortions and concerns about body image.

Monoamine Oxidase Inhibitors The group of drugs called **monoamine oxidase inhibitors (MAOIs)** inhibit monoamine oxidase, the enzyme that terminates the actions of neurotransmitters such as dopamine, norepinephrine, epinephrine, and serotonin. Because of their low safety margin, these drugs are reserved for clients who have not responded to TCAs or SSRIs.

The MAOIs were the first drugs approved to treat depression, introduced in the 1950s. They are as effective as TCAs and SSRIs in treating depression. However, because of drug–drug and food–drug interactions, hepatotoxicity, and the development of safer antidepressants, MAOIs are now reserved for clients who are not responsive to other antidepressant classes.

- *Adverse effects.* Common side effects of the MAOIs include orthostatic hypotension, headache, insomnia, and diarrhea. A primary concern is that these agents interact with a large number of foods and other medications—sometimes with serious effects. A hypertensive crisis can occur when an MAOI is used concurrently with other antidepressants or sympathomimetic drugs. Combining an MAOI with an SSRI can produce serotonin syndrome. If MAOIs are given with antihypertensives, the client can experience excessive hypotension. MAOIs also potentiate the hypoglycemic effects of insulin and oral antidiabetic drugs. Hyperpyrexia is known to occur in clients taking MAOIs with meperidine (Demerol), dextromethorphan (commonly found in cough and cold remedies), and TCAs. Ginseng, ephedra, ma huang, and St. John's wort can cause hypertensive crisis when taken with MAOIs.

A hypertensive crisis also can result from an interaction between MAOIs and foods containing tyramine, a form of the amino acid tyrosine. Tyramine is formed by the breakdown of certain proteins as food ages. Tyramine is usually degraded by MAO in the intestines. If a client is taking MAOIs, however, tyramine enters the bloodstream in high amounts and displaces norepinephrine in presynaptic nerve terminals. The result is a sudden release of norepinephrine, causing acute hypertension. Symptoms usually occur within minutes of ingesting the food and include occipital headache, stiff neck, flushing, palpitations, diaphoresis, and nausea. Myocardial infarctions (MIs) and cerebrovascular accidents (CVAs), although rare, are possible consequences as well. Calcium channel blockers may be given as an antidote. Because of their serious side effects when taken with

food and drugs, the use of MAOIs is limited to clients with symptoms that are resistant to the more typical antidepressants and who are likely to comply with the restrictions regarding foods and drugs. In general, the older the protein-containing food, the higher the tyramine content. The fresher the food, the less likely problem will occur. Examples of tyramine-containing foods to avoid are any aged, fermented, or spoiled foods; aged cheeses such as cheddar; sour cream; aged or cured meats such as salami, sausage, and bologna; yeast supplements such as Brewer's yeast, Marmite yeast extract, Vegemite supplement (baked goods prepared with yeast are acceptable); sauerkraut; fermented soybean products (soy sauce, miso); broad (fava) bean pods, bean curd; beer, and red and white wine, especially chianti; anchovies, pickled or salted fish or meats; caviar, meat, fish or shrimp paste; avocados; bananas; overripe or canned figs; protein extracts; and chocolate. Caffeine intake should be severely limited. Keep in mind that this is not a comprehensive list. Clients should be referred to a dietitian or nutritionist. A pharmacist should also be consulted. Food restrictions should be continued for a minimum of 2 weeks following discontinuation of MAOIs.

- *Nursing care.* The role of the nurse in MAOI therapy involves careful monitoring of a client's condition and providing education, including education related to foods containing tyramine. Assess cardiovascular status because these agents may affect blood pressure. Phenelzine (Nardil) is contraindicated in cardiovascular disease, heart failure, stroke, hepatic or renal dysfunction, and paranoid schizophrenia. Obtain a CBC because MAOIs can inhibit platelet function. Assess for the possibility of pregnancy because these agents are pregnancy category C and enter breast milk. Use MAOIs with caution in clients with epilepsy because they may lower the seizure threshold.

Take a careful drug history; common drugs that may interact with an MAOI include other MAOIs, insulin, caffeine-containing products, other antidepressants, buspirone (BuSpar), meperidine (Demerol), and possibly opioids and methyldopa (Aldomet). There must be at least a 14-day interval between the use of MAOIs and these other drugs.

Some clients may not achieve the full therapeutic benefits of an MAOI for 4–8 weeks. Because depression continues during this time, clients may discontinue the drug if they believe it is not helping them. Symptoms of sleep disorder or anxiety are treated with short-term antianxiety agents and sleep aids until the therapeutic effects of the medication are achieved.

Because of the serious side effects that are possible with MAOIs, client education is vital. The client's ability to comprehend restrictions and be compliant with them may be impaired when the client is in a severely depressed state.

- *Client education* as it relates to MAOIs should include the goals of therapy, the reasons for obtaining baseline data such as vital signs and the existence of underlying disorders, and possible drug side effects. Include the following points when teaching clients and their caregivers about MAOIs:
  - Strictly observe dietary restrictions for foods containing tyramine. Make sure the client has a readily available list of such foods.

- Do not take any prescription, OTC drugs, or herbal products without notifying your healthcare provider.
- Avoid caffeine and chocolate.
- Wear a medic alert bracelet identifying the MAOI medication.
- It may take several weeks or more to obtain the full therapeutic effect of the drug.
- Keep all follow-up appointments with your healthcare provider.
- Do not drive or engage in hazardous activities until the drug's sedative effect is known; it may be taken at bedtime if sedation occurs.
- Observe for and report signs of impending stroke or MI.

Atypical Antidepressants The atypical antidepressants do not fit into the three major drug classes. Duloxetine (Cymbalta) and venlafaxine (Effexor), examples of atypical antidepressants, are serotonin–norepinephrine reuptake inhibitors (SNRIs). They inhibit the reabsorption of serotonin and norepinephrine and elevate mood by increasing the levels of serotonin, norepinephrine, and dopamine in the CNS. Venlafaxine (Effexor) is available in an intermediate-release form that requires two or three doses a day and an extended-release form taken just once a day. The next generation of venlafaxine is desvenlafaxine (Pristiq), available in once-daily dosing that does not require titration to achieve an effective dosage.

Bupropion (Wellbutrin) not only inhibits the reuptake of serotonin, but may also affect the activity of norepinephrine and dopamine. It should be used with caution in clients with seizure disorders because it lowers the seizure threshold. It is prescribed under the brand name Zyban for smoking cessation. Mirtazapine (Remeron) is an SNRI. In lower doses it is highly sedating and should be taken at bedtime. It is associated with increased appetite and weight gain. Duloxetine (Cymbalta) is another SNRI used for depression that is also approved for relieving neuropathic pain.

PHARMACOLOGIC THERAPY FOR BIPOLAR DISORDERS

Drugs used to treat bipolar disorders are called **mood stabilizers** because they have the ability to moderate extreme shifts in emotions between mania and depression. Some anticonvulsive drugs are used for mood stabilization in bipolar clients. Medications commonly prescribed for the treatment of bipolar disorders include lithium carbonate (Eskalith); atypical antipsychotics, such as aripiprazole (Abilify) and olanzapine (Zyprexa); and anticonvulsants such as carbamazepine (Tegretol) and valproic acid (Depakote). Side effects and adverse effects of these drugs are many and vary. Generally speaking, however, nursing considerations for clients receiving pharmacologic therapy for bipolar disorders include the following (Wilson, Shannon, & Shields, 2014):

- Monitor drug levels (especially lithium), blood glucose levels, and electrolyte panels periodically. (Note that older adults require more frequent monitoring for drug toxicity.)
- Monitor for and report increased signs of suicidality and suicidal ideation. (Children and adolescents may need more frequent monitoring.)
- Monitor for and report changes in cardiovascular status, particularly orthostatic hypotension. (Older adults require more frequent monitoring.)
- Monitor for and report signs of extrapyramidal symptoms or neuroleptic malignant syndrome.
- Monitor neurological and neuromuscular status in older adults.

> **SAFETY ALERT**
> Clients with bipolar disorders who are in the depressive phase and prescribed only an antidepressant are at high risk for switching to a manic episode. For that reason, mood stabilizers are always prescribed at the same time. A study funded by the National Institutes of Health found that adding an antidepressant medication to a mood stabilizer was not more effective than the mood stabilizer alone (Sachs et al., 2007).

Lithium Therapy The role of the nurse in lithium therapy involves carefully monitoring a client's condition and providing education as it relates to prescribed drug treatment. Because lithium is a salt, clients with a history of cardiovascular and kidney disease should not take it. Clients frequently experience dehydration and sodium depletion; therefore, clients on a low-salt diet should not be prescribed lithium. Assess for and identify signs and symptoms of lithium toxicity, which include diarrhea, lethargy, slurred speech, muscle weakness, ataxia, seizures, edema, hypotension, and circulatory collapse. Serum lithium levels should be ordered every 1–3 days when therapy is initiated and periodically thereafter. They should be drawn at least 8 hours after the last dose. This is essential because lithium is nephrotoxic, and hemodialysis may be necessary if overdose occurs (Adams, Holland, & Urban, 2014).

- **Client education.** As it relates to lithium therapy, client education should include the goals of therapy; the reasons for obtaining baseline data such as vital signs and the existence of cardiac, renal, thyroid, or seizure disorders; and possible drug side effects. Include the following points when teaching clients about lithium:
  - Take medication as ordered because compliance is the key to successful treatment.
  - Keep all scheduled laboratory visits to monitor lithium levels.
  - Do not change diet or decrease fluid intake because any changes in diet and fluid status can affect therapeutic drug levels.
  - Avoid alcohol use.
  - Do not take other prescription medications, OTC drugs, or herbal products without notifying your healthcare provider.

Further information about pharmacologic therapies for bipolar disorders is provided in Exemplar 28.3.

NONPHARMACOLOGIC THERAPY

A number of nonpharmacologic therapies are available to those clients experiencing depression. Psychotherapy is used most frequently, often in combination with pharmacologic therapy. Electroconvulsive therapy is typically reserved for clients who are difficult to treat, while alternative therapies are often tried by clients in addition to more traditional therapies.

Both medication and psychotherapy alone are effective in treating depression, however, the combination of both medication

Lifespan Considerations Pharmacologic Therapy for Mood Disorders

Children and Adolescents

Initially, many parents choose to try psychotherapy alone to treat depressive disorders in their children. However, if this proves unsuccessful, medication is indicated. Currently, fluoxetine (Prozac) is the only antidepressant that is FDA approved for use in children. However, many healthcare providers prescribe other SSRIs for children with depression. For example, sertraline (Zoloft) is approved for use in treating obsessive-compulsive disorder in children but not depression. This is considered "off-label" use. Most prescribers will start children on a lower dose of antidepressant than is normally prescribed for adults and titrate up to a dose that is effective in symptom relief. Note that the FDA does **not** recommend paroxetine (Paxil) to treat depression in children and adolescents (NIMH, 2013a).

After a comprehensive review of published and unpublished controlled clinical trials of antidepressants in children and adolescents, the FDA issued a public warning in October 2004 regarding increased risk of suicidal thoughts or behavior in children and adolescents treated with SSRI antidepressant medications. In 2006, the warning was extended to age 25 years (NIMH, 2013a). More recent results of a comprehensive review of pediatric trials conducted between 1988 and 2006 suggested that the benefits of antidepressant medications outweigh the risks to children and adolescents with major depression and anxiety disorders (Bridge et al., 2007).

Older Adults

Care must be taken in treating depression in older adults, but it must be treated. A thorough evaluation is necessary to rule out medical causes of depressive symptoms before medication is prescribed. As with most medications in older adults, the cardinal rule is "start low and go slow." Older adults may respond to a lower antidepressant dose, but it is important to treat to remission. The majority of antidepressant medications are metabolized in the liver, so care must be taken in older adults with liver disease. Lithium is contraindicated in liver or kidney disease and should be used cautiously in thyroid disease. TCAs must be used with care and are not considered first line due to risk of arrhythmias. ECGs should be evaluated prior to initiation of TCA treatment. With most antidepressants, sedation may occur and clients should be educated to report excessive daytime sleepiness. If sedation occurs, the medication can be taken at bedtime.

Due to risk of orthostasis, clients should be educated to sit before standing and stand before walking to reduce fall risk. A study concluded that the "increased risk of falling with an antidepressant is about the same as the excess risk found in clients with untreated depression" (Darowski, Chambers, & Chambers, 2009). The client and family should be educated on fall-risk reduction strategies. A thorough medication history and periodic medication reconciliation should be conducted due to the risk of medication interactions and polypharmacy. Of special note is that the SSRIs may interact with some anticoagulants.

Atypical antipsychotics, often used to treat bipolar disorder, all have an FDA "black box" warning that they may increase mortality in elderly clients with dementia-related psychosis. Older adults treated with these medications for bipolar disorder should be monitored carefully.

Pregnancy

To date, no psychotropic medication has been approved by the FDA for use during pregnancy. However, abrupt discontinuation of maintenance medications including antipsychotics, antidepressants, and mood stabilizers has been associated with a high, early relapse risk. Abrupt discontinuation of these medications to minimize potential birth defects can place a woman and her fetus at risk due to impulsive or self-injurious behavior, substance abuse, or inattention to prenatal care. Untreated mood disorders during pregnancy have been associated with premature delivery, low birth weight, and lower Apgar scores in infants.

TCAs and SSRIs have not generally been associated with a high risk of major birth defects. Lamotrigine (Lamictal) appears to be safer than the other anticonvulsants. If lithium is continued during pregnancy, serum lithium levels must be monitored frequently to prevent toxicity. Lithium doses should be decreased at the onset of labor to avoid maternal toxicity at delivery. Divalproex (Depakote) should be switched to another mood stabilizer before conception because of the higher-than-average risk for neural tube defects. Carbamazepine (Tegretol) is contraindicated in pregnancy.

---

and psychotherapy is most effective. Therefore, psychotherapy is almost always recommended.

One of the most successful forms of psychotherapy is cognitive-behavioral therapy. However, a number of different forms of psychotherapy can be considered. The best approach to psychotherapy is chosen based on the cause and symptoms of the depressive condition as well as the client's needs and personality.

Cognitive-Behavioral Therapy Cognitive-behavioral therapy (CBT) focuses on skill training and problem solving to help clients reorient patterns of negative thinking and negative behaviors. The clinician or therapist works with clients to identify the most troubling problems in their lives and erroneous thought patterns or behaviors that may reinforce or exacerbate them. The therapist then helps clients problem solve by asking questions that help clients reflect and reconsider troubling situations. Examples of questions include:

- What happens? What do you *think* when this happens? What do you *feel*? What do you *do*?

- When does this happen? Where? With whom? What are the consequences?

- Why do you think this happens to you?

- What would need to happen for you to feel differently? What might you do to change the situation?

Cognitive-behavioral therapists utilize various techniques. One is *cognitive modification* of negative thought patterns. Every individual has automatic thought patterns, some of which are helpful and some of which are negative. An example is that of a teenage daughter who is 1 hour late for her curfew and has not called. The mother's automatic thought might be one of the following:

- "She must have been in an accident and can't call."
- "She cares so little for me that she can't call even though she knows how much I worry."
- "She is just trying to push my buttons."
- "She is usually very responsible, so I am sure she will be home soon and will be able to tell me what happened."

Cognitive-behavioral therapists help clients identify these patterns of irrational thinking and find ways to replace them with more logical and fact-based patterns of thinking. For example, a mother suffering depression may constantly choose to believe the worst in a number of given scenarios involving her children. In CBT, the therapist may help the mother view her children as they really are and begin to reorient her expectations. For example, the mother of a teen may change her thinking from "Something must have happened to Sarah!" to recognizing more likely scenarios: "Sarah is late for curfew, but she was at the football game with some friends. They probably went to get something to eat afterward and she's forgotten to call."

A technique promoted in cognitive-behavioral therapy that may specifically help clients with depression is mindfulness training. Most often people go through daily routines with little awareness or attention. People read while they eat, exercise while watching television, or cook while talking to their children, and the nuances of these experiences are lost. This situation might be called living mindlessly by ignoring present moments. *Mindfulness* is the art of conscious living by focusing one's full attention on the activity at hand. While it may be simple to practice mindfulness, it is not necessarily easy. Habitual unawareness is persistent, and mindfulness requires effort and discipline. Cognitive-behavioral therapists believe that the way for people to start changing their minds is not to force the change, but to watch it. Through the process of mindfulness, people can learn to identify destructive thought patterns, simply label them, and watch them pass by whenever they come to mind. As people learn how their brains "tell stories," they can begin to change their negative thought patterns.

Electroconvulsive Therapy   **Electroconvulsive therapy (ECT)** is a treatment procedure that passes an electric current through the brain to induce a seizure. It has been used clinically since the 1930s. It is usually given 2–3 times a week until a course of 12 treatments is completed. A systematic review of ECT (Allan & Ebmeier, 2011) cited the following findings from studies completed within the past 10 years:

- ECT is effective in treating depression, with responses of over 80%.
- Response is even higher in clients who have depression with psychotic features.
- Response is relatively rapid (greater than 60% within 3 weeks).
- ECT is associated with improved mood, functional status, anxiety, and quality of life.
- It is effective in treating depression in all ages.
- Older adult clients, even those with cognitive impairment, tolerate and respond well to ECT.

- It does not cause a switch to mania when used to treat bipolar depression, and may also be used in clients with bipolar disorder with mixed features.
- It is especially useful for severely depressed clients who are resistant to other treatments, those who are severely suicidal, and those with severe psychomotor retardation.

A review of ECT in pregnancy demonstrated its effectiveness in treating depression, with low rates of fetal and maternal complications (Anderson & Reti, 2009). Risks and benefits of ECT must be weighed carefully on an individual case basis before deciding to treat a pregnant woman with ECT.

The procedure is done under anesthesia. A thorough medical examination is required prior to the procedure to clear the client for anesthesia. Muscle relaxants are usually administered. The client is ventilated during the procedure. EEG and ECG, oxygen saturation via pulse oximetry, and vital signs are monitored during the procedure, which only takes a few minutes. Mild confusion following the procedure (a postictal state) is typical. Vital signs must be monitored frequently for several hours after the procedure. During a course of ECT, a transient short-term memory loss (anterograde amnesia) is expected. This is distressing to some clients, and they need to be reassured that memory is usually restored. In rare cases, however, retrograde amnesia occurs and may be permanent. There are the usual risks associated with anesthesia. It is essential that all the potential risks and benefits of ECT be explained to and understood by the client. A written, informed consent form must be signed by the client before the procedure. Clients have the right to refuse treatments at any time during the course of therapy. Nursing considerations for clients receiving ECT are outlined in **Box 28–2** ●.

Transcranial Magnetic Stimulation   Repetitive transcranial magnetic stimulation (rTMS) is an FDA-approved treatment for depression that involves the use of a magnetic field that passes through the skull, causing cells in the cerebral cortex to fire. Repetitive transcranial magnetic stimulation in depression is the most studied clinical application in psychiatry. The target area is the left prefrontal cortex, which is the brain area thought to be disrupted in depression. Targeting the opposite lobe, the right prefrontal cortex, has therapeutic effects in manic episodes. This therapy has a rapid onset of action of 1–2 weeks, which is faster than most psychotropic medications. Electroconvulsive therapy and rTMS have the same effectiveness in depression without psychosis, while depression with psychosis is best treated with ECT.

COMPLEMENTARY AND ALTERNATIVE THERAPY   In community surveys, depression, fatigue, insomnia, and anxiety are among the most commonly reported reasons for the use of alternative therapies. The following are some alternative therapies used for mood disorders. Note that these types of therapies should be used as complementary, rather than alternative, therapies in clients experiencing significant disruption in functioning related to mood disorders. Further, clients taking pharmacologic therapy should be encouraged to consult their prescribing provider before trying herbs or dietary supplements.

Exercise   Numerous studies have been conducted on the effect of exercise on depression. Short periods of vigorous

---

Box 28–2 Nursing Considerations for Clients Receiving Electroconvulsive Therapy

- Prepare the client by explaining the procedure and answering all questions as completely as possible.
- If part of responsibility, have client sign a separate consent for treatment because ECT requires the administration of anesthesia. Although informing clients and obtaining consent forms is legally a medical responsibility, in practice, it is often shared by nurses.
- Client should have nothing by mouth for at least 4 hours before treatment.
- Just prior to treatment, request that the client empty the bladder and remove contact lenses, jewelry, hairpins, and dentures.
- Monitor vital signs and oxygenation.
- The anesthetic preparation usually consists of the following:
  a. Generally, an atropine-like medication such as glycopyrrolate (Robinul) is given to decrease secretions and block cardiac vagal reflexes during the seizure.
  b. A short-acting anesthetic such as methohexital sodium (Brevital) is administered intravenously.
  c. Following induction, a skeletal muscle relaxant such as succinylcholine chloride (Anectine) is administered to prevent injuries during the seizure.
  d. The client must be artificially ventilated until the muscle relaxant is fully metabolized, usually in 2–3 minutes. Oxygen is administered with a rubber bite block in place. If necessary, oxygen may be administered by positive pressure.
- An electric current is passed through the brain by means of unilateral or bilateral electrodes placed on the temples. This causes a generalized (or tonic–clonic) seizure, the effects of which are masked by the muscle relaxant. Often the only observable signs of seizure are a fluttering of the eyelids and carpopedal spasms.
- Clients are recovered in the lateral recumbent position to facilitate drainage and to prevent aspiration. Upon awakening, they will be confused and somewhat disoriented. After they are fully recovered and have been reoriented by the nurse, they may eat. Memory loss may be short term or permanent.

---

aerobic exercise or longer periods of nonaerobic exercise for at least several weeks is most helpful in mild to moderate depression. Exercise raises levels of endorphins, which enhance an individual's feelings of well-being. Exercise also increases levels of DA, 5-HT, and NE, which are related to feelings of reward, motivation, and attention.

Yoga has been found to improve wellness and prevent disorders such as depression. The gentle nature of the exercises allows its use in almost any condition. People who practice yoga on a regular basis report improved life satisfaction, alertness, enthusiasm, and mental and physical energy, all of which are the opposite of the symptoms of depression (Kabat-Zinn, 2003). It is thought that both yoga and qigong have the common effect of increasing self-control of movement and cognition. This sense of control "allows individuals to manage their mental health more efficiently in the sense that negative mental states and thoughts, emotions, moods could be recognized and controlled when they occur" (Posadzki, Parekh, & Glass, 2010, p. 84).

St. John's Wort   St. John's wort (*Hypericum perforatum*) is the most widely publicized alternative treatment for mild to moderate depression, but studies conducted by the National Center for Complementary and Alternative Medicine (NCCAM) and the National Institute of Mental Health question its benefits (NCCAM, 2012). The side effects of St. John's wort in higher doses are similar to those of SSRIs. The dosage is 300–600 mg/day of 0.3% hypericin, the active component in St. John's wort. It should *not* be combined with prescription antidepressants. It also may interfere with the action of anticonvulsants. There are insufficient data to recommend this herb for children. St. John's wort has been found to reduce the effectiveness of birth control pills, HIV treatment medications, and the asthma medication theophylline (NCCAM, 2012; Wilson et al., 2014). If taken with SSRIs, TCAs, or some atypical antidepressants, serotonin syndrome may result.

SAMe   A nutritional supplement called SAMe (pronounced "sammy") has been used by more than 1 million people in Europe, primarily for depression and arthritis. SAMe (S-adenosylmethionine), a compound made by every cell in the body, helps produce DA, 5-HT, and NE. Numerous trials have found SAMe to be effective in treating depression, postpartum depression, and postmenopausal depression. It may, however, worsen bipolar depression. Its rapid onset (10–12 days), few side effects (no weight gain or sexual dysfunction), and ability to boost antioxidants give it many advantages in the treatment of depression. The dose is 800–1,600 mg/day and is best taken 30 minutes before meals. It has been successfully used as augmentation of all categories of antidepressants without adverse effects, and there is no evidence that it interacts with other medications. Side effects are generally mild and temporary (headaches, loose bowels, anxiety, and insomnia). Like TCAs, SAMe should be used with caution in people who have a history of cardiac arrhythmia. Infants normally have a three to four times naturally higher level of SAMe than do adults. Given this knowledge, the amount of SAMe passing to infants through breast milk may be inconsequential (Goren et al., 2004).

Vitamin B   Vitamin B is necessary for the production of DA, 5-HT, and NE, as well as for the natural synthesis of SAMe. One study found that individuals with a significant vitamin B deficiency were at twice the risk of depression than those who had normal levels. Depression itself could cause low levels through decreased appetite and resulting decreased food intake. In addition, many of the TCAs deplete the body of vitamin B (Hvas et al., 2004).

Tyrosine   Tyrosine, an amino acid, is the precursor for DA and NE and, as such, acts as a mood elevator. Supplemental tyrosine has been used in depression, stress reduction, anxiety, and chronic fatigue. People taking MAOIs should not take any supplements containing tyrosine, as it may lead to a hypertensive crisis. Tyrosine combined with vitamin B_6 and vitamin C will provide better absorption.

Melatonin   Insomnia is a frequent complaint among people suffering from depression. Melatonin, a hormone secreted by the pineal gland, plays a critical role in the regulation of the day–night cycle. Studies have shown that melatonin is effective in inducing sleep and has no notable side effects. Slow-release melatonin combined with standard antidepressant treatment often improves the sleep pattern in depressed individuals.

Omega-3 Fatty Acids   A number of studies have been done on the effects of omega-3 fatty acids from concentrated fish oils on mood disorders. Omega-3 fatty acids are thought to act on cells in a manner similar to that of lithium. Like the other mood stabilizers, these fatty acids block calcium channels and help regulate 5-HT. Omega-3 appears to be an antidepressant, an antimanic, and a mood stabilizer. Research shows significantly low levels of omega-3 fatty acids in depression, and the lower the levels, the more severe the depression. The recommended dose is 5 grams per day, which is usually seven or eight capsules. The maximum dose is 15 grams daily. Taking the capsules at night with orange juice cuts down on the fishy aftertaste (Basch & Ulbricht, 2005).

Acupuncture   Acupuncture is helpful in relieving feelings of depression and anxiety, most likely related to the rise in endorphin levels as a result of the treatment. Adding electrostimulation to acupuncture needles usually increases the effectiveness of the treatment. After only a single session, many people report a sense of well-being. Two rigorous studies found acupuncture to be as effective as TCAs. It is unclear how helpful acupuncture is for bipolar disorders. Client response appears to be quite variable at the present time (Larzelere & Wiseman, 2002).

Animal-Assisted Therapy   Companionship with animals is associated with people experiencing less depression and loneliness. Animals provide meaningful and substantial comfort for many individuals. Studies show that older women (who are at higher risk for depression) who live alone tend to be in better emotional health when they live with an animal. They were less lonely, more optimistic, and more interested in the future than women who lived alone without a pet (Hart, 2000).

Music Therapy   Clients may benefit from enrolling in art or music therapy, which is now widely available in a number of clinical settings. Based on the idea that creativity can assist healing, art and music therapy have been found to reduce anxiety and stress (American Cancer Institute, 2008).

Care of the client experiencing depression requires an individualized plan of care that is revised based on the client's response. Different treatment options may need to be tried before the one that works best for the client is found. Careful assessment of the client's mental status, screening for suicidal ideation, and ongoing evaluation to determine client response to treatment is a primary focus of nursing care. It is also important to reassure the client that depression is often successfully treated because hope can help the client focus on the future.

◢ REVIEW   **The Concept of Mood and Affect**

RELATE Link the Concepts

Linking the concept of mood and affect with the concept of development:

1. Explain how failure to master the developmental tasks of older adulthood could contribute to the development of depression (refer to developmental theories).

2. How can resiliency theory be applied to the development or prevention of depression?

Linking the concept of mood and affect with the concept of family:

3. How can the burden of having a family member with a severe mental illness such as bipolar disorder affect the family system?

4. How does the stage that the family is in affect family recovery from a mood disorder?

Linking the concept of mood and affect with the concept of self:

5. How would you assess self-esteem in a client suspected of having a mood disorder?

6. What are some strategies that can be used to enhance the low self-esteem often experienced by clients with mood disorders?

READY Go to Companion Skills Manual

REFER Go to Pearson Nursing Student Resources
nursing.pearsonhighered.com

- Additional review materials

REFLECT Case Study \\ Part 3

Reread Parts 1 and 2 of the case study. Jason was admitted to the short-term acute care psychiatric unit of the local hospital. He was diagnosed with bipolar I disorder and started on aripiprazole (Abilify). Jason reports feeling as if he has to keep moving all the time, and he has mild dystonic symptoms involving muscle twitches in his hands. He is currently taking 20 mg of aripiprazole daily. He is attending individual and group therapy sessions. He is sleeping and eating more normally; his speech is no longer rapid and pressured. Jason no longer believes he has special talents. He says he now feels stupid about his previous behavior and ashamed that he ended up being hospitalized. He states, "I can't face anyone I know now that they know I am crazy. I don't want to live the rest of my life like this. What's the point?"

Clinical Reasoning Questions Level I

1. What symptoms should be reported to the physician and therapist?

2. Based on the information provided, what does the nurse need to assess immediately?

3. What is the probable cause of Jason's feelings of restlessness and muscle twitches? What additional treatments might be indicated to address them?

Clinical Reasoning Questions Level II

4. What do Jason's statements indicate and how should the nurse respond?

5. What is the priority nursing diagnosis for Jason at this time?

6. Why do you think Jason was not prescribed an antidepressant?

EXEMPLAR 28.1 **Depression**

EXEMPLAR KEY TERMS
Anergy, *1799*
Anhedonia, *1799*
Depression, *1798*
Dysthymic disorder, *1800*
Hypersomnia, *1799*
Insomnia, *1799*
Major depressive disorder (MDD), *1798*
Major depressive episode, *1798*
Persistent depressive disorder, *1800*
Psychomotor retardation, *1799*
Seasonal affective disorder (SAD), *1800*

EXEMPLAR LEARNING OUTCOMES
After reading about this exemplar, you will be able to:

1. Describe the pathophysiology, psychopathology, and clinical manifestations of depressive disorders.

2. Identify risk factors associated with depression.
3. Illustrate the nursing process in providing culturally competent care across the life span for individuals with depression.
4. Formulate priority nursing diagnoses appropriate for an individual with depression.
5. Summarize therapies used by interdisciplinary teams in the collaborative care of an individual with depression.
6. Plan evidence-based care for an individual with depression and his or her family in collaboration with other members of the healthcare team.
7. Evaluate expected outcomes for an individual with depression.

▶ OVERVIEW

Depression is a disorder characterized by a sad or despondent mood or loss of interest in usual activities. Many symptoms are associated with depression, including lack of energy; sleep disturbances; anxious distress; abnormal eating patterns; psychomotor retardation or agitation; and/or feelings of despair, guilt, and hopelessness. Depression is one of the most common mental health disorders and encompasses a variety of physical, emotional, cognitive, and social considerations. The National Alliance on Mental Illness (NAMI) (2013) reports that some 25 million Americans will suffer a depressive episode in a given year but only half will receive treatment.

The majority of clients suffering from depression are not found in psychiatric hospitals, but in mainstream everyday settings. Proper diagnosis and treatment require collaboration among healthcare providers. Because clients with depression are present in multiple settings and in all areas of practice, every nurse should be proficient in the assessment and nursing care of clients with this disorder.

Risk factors for depression include the following:

- History of child abuse or neglect, spousal abuse, loss of a close family member or intimate friend, other significant loss

- Dysfunctional family relationships, with or without the presence of substance abuse

- Personal or family history of mental illness or substance abuse.

Prevention

As discussed at the beginning of this module, there is no definitive way to prevent depression, due to causative and contributing genetic and biological factors that cannot be modified. However, some strategies are useful in modifying stressors that can contribute to depressive illnesses. These include:

- Exercise
- Proper diet and rest
- Avoiding alcohol and illicit drugs.

In addition, it is helpful to provide client education related to recognizing the symptoms of depression and the need to seek treatment promptly, because early detection and treatment result in better client outcomes. If the nursing assessment yields risk factors for depression, including a history of child abuse or trauma, further assessment is needed. If assessment for depression is negative, provide client teaching regarding depression risks, symptoms, and strategies for promoting mental health.

▶ CLINICAL MANIFESTATIONS

Some of the clinical manifestations of depression seem fairly obvious: feelings of sadness and despair and sleep disturbances, for example. Others may not be as obvious, such as anger and physical complaints. Manifestations of depression also can differ according to culture. It is important for nurses involved with all levels of depression to know and recognize the symptoms.

Major Depressive Disorder

A **major depressive episode** is characterized by a change in several aspects of an individual's emotional state and functioning consistently over a period of 14 days or longer. The most important factor is the client's mood, which the client may not describe in terms of "depression." Instead, the client may describe feelings of sadness, discouragement, or hopelessness. Or the client may complain of having no feelings at all or of feeling blah. Some clients may report vague somatic (physical) complaints such as aches and pains; other clients may report increased anger, frustration, and irritability, with uncharacteristic outbursts over minor matters. It is not difficult to imagine that someone who looks and feels sad or empty is depressed. A diagnosis of depression is more likely to be missed when an individual simply seems anxious or irritable.

Major depressive disorder (MDD) may consist of a single episode or may exhibit as recurrent major depression at various points in life. The description of the diagnostic criteria for single-episode and recurrent major depression is found in **Box 28–3** ●. Key facts about MDD are listed in **Box 28–4** ●.

Box 28–3 DSM-5 Diagnostic Criteria for Major Depressive Disorder

A. Five (or more) of the following symptoms have been present during the same 2-week period and represent a change from previous functioning; at least one of the symptoms is either (1) depressed mood or (2) loss of interest or pleasure.

1. Depressed mood most of the day, nearly every day, as indicated by either subjective report (e.g., feels sad, empty, hopeless) or observation made by others (e.g., appears tearful). (**Note:** In children and adolescents, can be irritable mood.)

2. Markedly diminished interest or pleasure in all, or almost all, activities most of the day, nearly every day (as indicated by either subjective account or observation).

3. Significant weight loss when not dieting or weight gain (e.g., a change of more than 5% of body weight in a month), or decrease or increase in appetite nearly every day. (**Note:** In children, consider failure to make expected weight gain.)

4. Insomnia or hypersomnia nearly every day.

5. Psychomotor agitation or retardation nearly every day (observable by others, not merely subjective feelings of restlessness or being slowed down).

6. Fatigue or loss of energy nearly every day.

7. Feelings of worthlessness or excessive or inappropriate guilt (which may be delusional) nearly every day (not merely self-reproach or guilt about being sick).

8. Diminished ability to think or concentrate, or indecisiveness, nearly every day (either by subjective account or as observed by others).

9. Recurrent thoughts of death (not just fear of dying), recurrent suicidal ideation without a specific plan, or a suicide attempt or a specific plan for committing suicide.

B. The symptoms cause clinically significant distress or impairment in social, occupational, or other important areas of functioning.

C. The episode is not attributable to the direct physiological effects of a substance (e.g., a drug of abuse, a medication) or a general medical condition (e.g., hypothyroidism).

D. The occurrence of the major depressive episode is not better explained by schizoaffective disorder, schizophrenia, schizophreniform disorder, delusional disorder, or other specified an unspecified schizophrenia spectrum and other psychotic disorders.

E. There has never been a manic episode or a hypomanic episode.

Note: Do not include symptoms that are clearly attributed to another medical condition.
Source: Reprinted with permission from American Psychiatric Association. (2013). *Diagnostic and statistical manual of mental disorders* (5th ed.). Washington, DC: American Psychiatric Publishing.

SAFETY ALERT

Healthcare providers often use language that is unfamiliar to clients and their families. To help clients and families understand the symptoms of a major depressive episode, nurses should discuss symptoms and characteristics using terms clients and families are more likely to understand. For example, rather than using the phrase "psychomotor retardation," nurses can inquire if the client is experiencing difficulty or slowness in speaking or in performing tasks.

Individuals with a history of a manic or hypomanic episode are considered to have a bipolar disorder and are not classified under the categories of depressive disorders.

Box 28–4 Key Facts About Major Depressive Disorder

■ The average age of onset of MDD is the mid-twenties, although the disorder can begin at any age and seems to be occurring in younger people.

■ Women are two to three times as likely to develop depression as men.

■ First-degree biological relatives (parents or siblings) of people with MDD are two to four times as likely to develop depression as are members of the general population (APA, 2013).

■ Symptoms of MDD usually develop over a period of time. The person may experience anxiety and mild depression for several days, weeks, or months before the onset of a full major depressive episode.

■ If untreated, major depression lasts 6 or more months. In some individuals, depressive symptoms persist for longer periods ranging from months to years. This is considered a partial remission and thought to be predictive of later depressive episodes and the development of chronic depression.

Individuals experiencing MDD often no longer enjoy activities that previously brought pleasure, such as hobbies, sports, and sex. This is a condition known as **anhedonia**. Changes in appetite, usually experienced as a reduction or loss of interest in food, are often seen, although increased appetite and cravings are also reported.

Sleep disturbances, particularly **insomnia** (inability to fall or stay asleep or, in some individuals, early morning awakening), are common in depressed individuals. Two types of insomnia are most often experienced by people having a major depressive episode. *Middle insomnia* refers to waking up during the night and having difficulty falling asleep again. *Terminal insomnia* refers to waking at the end of the night and being unable to return to sleep. Depressed clients also may report **hypersomnia**, in which the individual sleeps for prolonged periods at night as well as during the day but still wakes up tired or fatigued. These sleep disturbances are discussed at length in the module on Comfort.

Fatigue and decreased energy, which are characteristic symptoms of depression, may be referred to as **anergy** or *anergia*. Anergic individuals report being tired upon awakening regardless of how long they have slept. Even the smallest task seems insurmountable, and routine activities require substantial effort and take longer to accomplish. Decreased energy may be manifested in **psychomotor retardation**, in which thinking and body movements are noticeably slowed and speech is slowed or absent. Psychomotor agitation also may occur, in which the individual cannot sit still; paces; wrings the hands; and picks at the fingernails, skin, clothing, bedclothes, or other objects.

Other common symptoms in individuals with moderate to severe depression include guilt or a sense of worthlessness, self-blame, impaired concentration and decision-making ability (even about trivial things), and suicidal ideation. The characteristics of a major depressive episode are illustrated in **Figure 28–4 ●**.

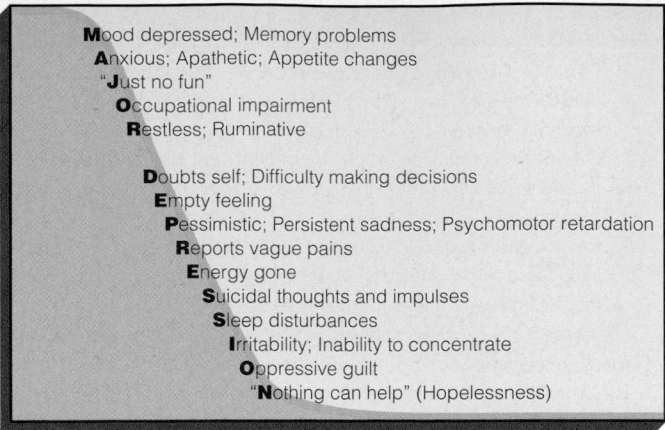

Mood depressed; Memory problems
Anxious; Apathetic; Appetite changes
"**J**ust no fun"
Occupational impairment
Restless; Ruminative

Doubts self; Difficulty making decisions
Empty feeling
Pessimistic; Persistent sadness; Psychomotor retardation
Reports vague pains
Energy gone
Suicidal thoughts and impulses
Sleep disturbances
Irritability; Inability to concentrate
Oppressive guilt
"**N**othing can help" (Hopelessness)

Figure 28–4 ● Characteristics of major depression.

Persistent Depressive Disorder

The term **persistent depressive disorder**, also known as **dysthymic disorder**, describes chronic depression for the majority of most days for at least 2 years (1 year for children and adolescents). Throughout those 2 years, no more than 2 months can be described as symptom free. The symptoms of dysthymic disorder, while distressing, tend to be less severe than those in MDD, with fewer physiological symptoms, but the degree of impact to individual functioning can be as great or greater than that of MDD. Individuals with persistent depressive disorder are at higher risk for developing other mental health disorders than those with MDD (APA, 2013).

Persistent depressive disorder often occurs in childhood, adolescence, or early adulthood and tends to be chronic. While both females and males are equally affected as children, there are two to three times as many adult females as males with dysthymic disorder. Factors that contribute to poorer long-term outcomes include the presence of a comorbid anxiety or conduct disorder, greater symptom severity, and greater impairment in functioning (APA, 2013).

Seasonal Affective Disorder

Seasonal affective disorder (SAD) is not an official DSM diagnosis, but rather a specifier of MDD "with seasonal pattern." Natural light is frequently taken for granted, and most people may be unaware of how it influences the human experience. As early as the days of Hippocrates, observers of human behavior noticed that some people suffer mood changes as the seasons change.

The relationships between light, biological rhythms, and mood have been the subject of robust and thorough scientific study. This research focuses on the use of light in the treatment of SAD, usually during winter months. Natural light may help modulate daily rhythms that influence sleep and activity patterns, neuroendocrine functions, and brain chemical systems.

Many antidepressants are typically used to treat the depressive features of SAD, but only one is currently indicated for this diagnosis by the FDA. Bupropion extended-release (Wellbutrin ER) may prevent major depressive episodes in people with SAD. Treatment for SAD has entered areas well beyond therapy and medication. Researchers are exploring the application of different forms of light to the skin and eyes at different times of the day, and the results indicate a reduction of fatigue and depression as well as improved alertness (Joseph, 2006). The exact relationship among SAD and light, biological rhythms, and events at the cellular level has not yet been determined.

*Stay Current: Information on SAD and the clinical application of light therapy is available through the Society for Light Treatment and Biological Rhythms (**www.sltbr.org**),the National Institutes of Health (**www.ncbi.nlm.nih.gov/pubmed-health/PMH0002499/**), and the National Alliance on Mental Illness (**www.nami.org/Template.cfm?Section=By_Illness&Template=/ContentManagement/ContentDisplay.cfm&ContentID=23051**).*

Clinical Manifestations and Therapies **Depressive Disorders**

ETIOLOGY	CLINICAL MANIFESTATIONS	CLINICAL THERAPIES
Major depressive disorder	Symptoms must last 14 days or longer and may include: ■ Feelings of sadness and hopelessness ■ Somatic complaints such as pain, stomachaches ■ Anxiety, anger, irritability ■ Loss of interest in pleasurable activities ■ Sleep disturbances	■ Pharmacologic therapies include: • Selective serotonin reuptake inhibitors (SSRIs) • Tricyclic antidepressants (TCAs) • Atypical antidepressants • Electroconvulsive therapy (most often used for those who are resistant to treatment with medications) ■ Cognitive-behavioral therapy
Persistent depressive disorder (dysthymic disorder)	Symptoms are not as severe as those of major depressive disorder, but last beyond 2 years with period of relief lasting less than 2 months.	■ Pharmacologic therapies are the same as for MDD. ■ Electroconvulsive therapy (most often used for those who are resistant to treatment with medications) ■ Cognitive-behavioral therapy
Seasonal affective disorder	Depressive symptoms occur in relation to the seasons; usually during the winter months, when days are shorter.	■ Bupropion extended-release ■ Light therapy ■ Cognitive-behavioral therapy

Lifespan Considerations Symptoms of Depression

Symptoms of depression can vary among age groups, although sadness and anhedonia are common at all ages. Differences include the following:

Children and Adolescents

■ Toddlers can show regressive behaviors in toileting and other activities.

■ Preschoolers have less symbolic and other play activities and demonstrate self-destructive play themes. They may whine and show irritability, disinterest, and lack of confidence.

■ School-age children may show a decrease in academic performance, increased or decreased physical activity, somatic complaints, and loss of friends. The older school-age child may talk of running away or show signs of boredom and low self-esteem.

■ The adolescent can have a wide array of symptoms (e.g., decreased social contact, poor school performance, lack of involvement in typical activities, poor self-care, difficulty with parents and teachers, or a focus on violence).

Older Adults

Depression is common among older adults, but it is important to note that it is not a normal part of aging. Manifestations of depression in older adults may include memory problems, social withdrawal, sleep disturbances, loss of appetite, and irritability. Some individuals may experience delusions or hallucinations. Depression in older adults can complicate treatment of other conditions because impairment of functioning due to depression may impair the individual's ability or motivation to participate in treatment. Other medical conditions can complicate treatment of depression if nurses and clinicians dismiss symptoms as related to another medical condition (or side effects of treatment) without doing a full assessment for depression.

▶ COLLABORATION

The healthcare team for a client with a depressive disorder will normally include nurses, the client's treating physician, a psychiatrist or psychologist (or a psychiatrist working with a licensed mental health therapist), and family members. The nurse's role as a member of the healthcare team is detailed in the Nursing Process section.

Diagnostic Tests

Although there is no diagnostic test to determine depression, clinicians typically perform a complete medical history and thorough physical exam to rule out the possibility of an underlying medical condition causing the client's depressive symptoms. If no physical illness is found, diagnosis will be determined by a licensed mental health provider. Existing medical illnesses, such as diabetes, may inform selection of medication therapy if determined appropriate.

Pharmacologic Therapy

Antidepressant medications are often prescribed for clients with depression. Because individuals experience depletion of different neurotransmitters, different individuals respond differently to various antidepressants. A period of trial and error may be necessary to determine which medication is most effective for the client. See the Interventions and Therapies section of this module for a more detailed discussion of these medications.

Psychotherapy

Psychotherapy often is used in combination with medications to treat major depression. Some of the psychosocial problems associated with depression (ability to relate to others, motivation, problem-solving ability) cannot be resolved with medications. Psychotherapy promotes effective coping skills and positive, helpful patterns of thinking and behavior. Clients with mild depression may benefit from therapy alone. Cognitive-behavioral therapy is the most effective type of psychotherapy for depression.

Other Therapies

As discussed earlier in this module, electroconvulsive therapy and complementary therapies may be appropriate for the client diagnosed with depression. The nurses role includes assessing for safety, assessing for potential contraindications, encouraging client communication with all healthcare providers (e.g., primary care provider and mental health provider or therapist), and providing client teaching related to types of therapies and the importance of adhering to the treatment plan.

■ NURSING PROCESS

Priorities of nursing care are focused on safety and meeting functional needs until the client's condition improves. Risk of suicide must always be a consideration when caring for clients who are depressed. Clients with depression may not meet their daily hygiene, sleep, nutrition, or other needs and the nurse can initiate strategies to help them until they are able to function autonomously.

Assessment

Assess for the signs and symptoms of depression discussed throughout the Concept section, being sure to assess for history of manic or hypomanic episodes or behavior. Clients with depressive disorders may articulate any of the following clinical manifestations:

■ Feelings of sadness

■ Fatigue

■ Lack of interest in relationships and activities that previously brought pleasure

■ Impaired concentration

■ Feelings of worthlessness or guilt

Box 28–5 Physical Complaints and Depression

Frequently, individuals will feel aches and pains more acutely when they are depressed. The natural reaction to pain is to seek help from a primary medical healthcare provider. One out of every six clients going to a medical office is depressed. Out of *those* clients, only one in six is actually diagnosed and treated for depression. It is important for individuals who are suffering from depression to talk to their healthcare providers about other experiences and symptoms during their lifetime.

People seldom self-diagnose depression. They are more likely to assume that not enjoying their usual activities, experiencing changes in eating or sleeping habits, and feeling bad in one way or another are caused by a medical problem. Determining the real cause of distress will help to ensure effective responses to treatment.

- Anxious distress
- Sleep disturbances or excessive sleep
- Changes in appetite and/or weight
- Withdrawal/social isolation.

Clients will often describe how long it takes them to complete activities that they formerly accomplished easily, such as preparing a simple meal. Tearfulness and emotional outbursts also may be a part of their description of the problem. Clients may or may not mention a loss or disappointment that they relate to the feelings.

Somatic concerns are often the presenting complaint. Depressed clients may complain of abdominal pains, headaches, and vague body aches. A problem with sexual functioning or lack of desire also may be a presenting complaint. Constipation is a common result of the general slowing of metabolism due to inactivity. Clients from some cultures are more likely to express symptoms of depression through complaints about body function and discomfort. See **Box 28–5** • for information on how depression evidenced by somatic concerns can be detected in other settings.

Suicide Assessment

Assess all clients for suicide risk by using direct questioning. Ask whether the client has thoughts of self-harm (*suicidal ideation*), how often these thoughts occur, and whether or not the person would act on these thoughts (intent). Inquire whether or not the client has a plan regarding carrying out suicide (*plan/method*). If a plan exists it is important to assess lethality or the plan: degree of effort required, specificity of plan, accessibility of means to carry out the plan. A history of prior suicide attempts or family history of suicide should be elicited and, if present, signals increased risk. Note that asking about suicide will not "plant the idea" in the client's mind. Rather, it is often a relief for the client to be able to openly discuss these feelings and thoughts. See the exemplar on Suicide in the module on Violence. If a client is considered at risk for suicide, he or she must not be left alone, the environment assessed for safety, and suicide precautions initiated per agency policy. The client should be assessed by a psychiatrist or qualified suicide screener to determine whether hospitalization and/or a higher level of care or transfer to a psychiatric facility is indicated.

Assess for Comorbidities

Assess for the presence of medical illnesses. This is important not only to rule out the possibility of an underlying medical condition causing the client's symptoms of depression, but also because some illnesses may trigger depression. These include autoimmune, oncological, metabolic, and endocrine disorders. Chronic illnesses, such as asthma and diabetes, are associated with increased risk of depression. A diagnosis of a chronic or life-threatening illness may also trigger a depressive episode.

Alcohol, which is a CNS depressant, and certain legal and illegal drugs can cause or complicate depression. Through matter-of-fact questioning, obtain a complete list of all substances and medications the client uses. A few prescription medications have depression as a side effect, and they should not be overlooked in the complete assessment. Birth control pills, sedatives, reserpine, glucocorticoids, and anabolic steroids have all been associated with the development of depression.

Assessment of Children

Careful and thorough assessment of a child suspected of having depression is necessary to rule out physical illness that can be linked to depressive symptoms. Other tests, such as hearing and vision tests, may be indicated as well. It is essential to question parents, caregivers, or guardians regarding their observations of the child's behavior and recent changes or precipitating factors. Diagnostic evaluation must be performed by a child psychiatrist, psychiatric nurse practitioner, or other mental health professional experienced in the diagnosis and treatment of children and adolescents. A variety of scales and techniques are used; however, very little guidance is available relating to evaluation of children under 6 years of age. See the Concept section of this module for commonly used screening tools. Thorough assessment for both physical and mental health disorders is necessary because comorbidities (appearance with other disorders) are common. Examples of these include a history of bullying or substance abuse.

Assessment of Older Adults

Due to the increased risk older adults have for medical illness, careful assessment of the older adult is critical. Polypharmacy issues may make prescribing for older adults a challenge, and older adults taking psychotropic medications often require more frequent monitoring and laboratory tests (e.g., blood glucose levels). The Geriatric Depression Scale can be useful in screening older adults for depression and determining the need for further evaluation (Sheikh, et al., 1991).

Diagnosis

A number of nursing diagnoses may be appropriate for clients with depression, including the following:

- *Risk for Self-Directed Violence*
- *Situational Low Self-Esteem or Chronic Low Self-Esteem*
- *Hopelessness*
- *Social Isolation*
- *Ineffective Health Maintenance.*

(NANDA-I © 2012)

Planning

Together with the client, the nurse will design a plan of care that may include any of the following objectives:

- The client will remain free of injury.
- The client will refrain from attempts to injure self or others.
- The client will participate in recreational activities.
- The client will articulate taking steps to feeling better, such as engaging in recreational activities or exercise *before* beginning to feel better.
- The client will comply with the treatment regimen.

Implementation

When implementing interventions designed to help clients with depression, keep two general principles in mind:

1. It is impossible to make clients with depression feel better by being cheerful. In fact, an overly cheerful attitude tends to make them feel even worse because it trivializes or minimizes the impact of their feelings. Try to adopt a more emotionally neutral attitude while maintaining confidence that they will feel better.
2. Recognize that working with clients with depression may eventually lower your own mood and make you feel "down" yourself. This is called *emotional contagion*. The nurse should be aware of personal feelings and, if necessary, ask to be assigned to a different type of client for a time.

Improve Self-Esteem

While low self-esteem is a chronic problem, the nurse can take a number of actions to reduce negative thinking, thereby promoting improved self-esteem:

- Provide distraction from self-absorption by involving the client in recreational activities and pleasant pastimes. Simple conversation with a staff member or another client helps interrupt the pattern of negative thoughts. Use care to select activities that are not too complex for the client's current level of functioning. Experiences of success, not more failures, are needed. Increase the complexity of activities as the client progresses.
- Dispel the notion that clients often have that *when* they feel better, they will want to engage in activities. Explain that they must begin doing things *in order* to feel better. Being active promotes a more balanced feeling state. Acknowledge that it takes self-discipline and energy to do something when one doesn't really feel like it.
- Recognize accomplishment, but do not use flattery or excessive praise. Give positive, matter-of-fact reinforcement, such as "I notice that you combed your hair," rather than overly enthusiastic compliments such as "What a great hairstyle!" Appropriate recognition increases the likelihood that the client will continue the positive behavior, while insincerity can be perceived as ridicule or infantilizing.
- Be accepting of clients' negative feelings, but set limits on the amount of time spent discussing accounts of past failures. Be alert for opportunities to interrupt negative conversational patterns with more neutral ones.
- Teach assertiveness techniques, such as the ability to say "no" to protect one's rights while respecting the rights of others.

Clients with low self-esteem often allow others to take advantage of them. Defining passive, aggressive, and assertive behavior and giving examples of each also are helpful when teaching assertiveness. Practice these techniques with the client, providing feedback on how it feels to the recipient of assertive communication or an assertive action.

Instill Hope

It is equally important to help clients identify the aspects of their lives that are not within their control. Being able to accept what *cannot* be changed is just as essential as developing the ability to bring about positive change. This skill is particularly helpful in reorienting clients from feelings of hopelessness to a more hopeful aspect. Other interventions to help clients combat hopelessness include the following:

- Help clients identify their personal strengths. It may be useful to write these down. Recognize that it often takes time for clients to realize that they have any strengths. Recognizing strengths helps a client design an activity or engagement plan that the client is more likely to enjoy and find successful.
- Engage clients in setting goals for themselves. Direct clients to focus on small goals at first. For example, instead of "going to yoga twice a week," the initial goal might be to go to the yoga center and get a list of class times and teachers or sit in on a class.
- Help clients weigh and choose alternatives. Taking responsibility even for small choices such as when or where to eat helps the client regain self-esteem.
- Explore problem-solving models with the client, including practicing problem solving. "When you found out the toaster was broken, you threw it against the wall. You said all that did was put a dent in the wall and make a mess for you to clean up. What might you do differently next time that might be more helpful?"
- Help clients to identify resources such as family, community, or friends who can provide support and encouragement in overcoming problems they identify.

Planning for discharge should begin with the first client contact and is particularly important with hopeless, dependent clients. Help these clients and their families and significant others identify resources in the community they can use to build support systems. Support groups, therapy groups, and social groups can help clients separate from caregivers more readily when the time comes to end therapy.

Evaluation

Client progress is evaluated based on the ability to meet the expected outcomes. These should be modified based on each client's unique situation.

- The client meets daily functional needs appropriately such as eating three meals a day, bathing regularly, or sleeping 8 hours per night.
- The client does not demonstrate suicidal behavior or express suicidal ideation.
- The client describes hopefulness for the future.
- The client is able to resume normal activity patterns such as returning to work or school.

NURSING CARE PLAN A Client With Depression

ASSESSMENT

You are the hospice nurse assigned to Pam Allen, who is dying of cancer. During your assessment of her husband, Clifford Allen, he discloses the following:

- He was diagnosed with depression years ago but is not currently receiving treatment.
- Years ago his brother committed suicide.
- He feels helpless about Pam's situation. He says that he has been a terrible husband and father.
- He is not currently receiving any treatment for depression.
- He has two or three alcoholic drinks every night after Pam goes to bed.
- He is not sure how he is going to cope with caring for their son, Gary, who has Down syndrome, after Pam is gone.

DIAGNOSES

- *Powerlessness*
- *Anticipatory Grieving*
- *Situational Low Self-Esteem*
- *Risk for Caregiver Role Strain*
- *Ineffective Health Maintenance*
- *Anxiety*

(NANDA-I © 2012)

PLANNING

The next day the hospice nurse talks further with Mr. Allen. Together they create a plan of care that will help Mr. Allen:

- Investigate resources for helping him care for Gary.
- Develop a plan of exercise and recreation.
- Stop drinking.
- Begin treatment for depression as recommended by a mental health professional.

IMPLEMENTATION

- Provide teaching to Mr. Allen about the need to begin treatment for depression again in order to prevent deterioration in mood and affect.
- Refer Mr. Allen to a mental health professional for diagnosis and treatment.
- Encourage Mr. Allen to explore his feelings regarding his wife's terminal condition and what his life will be like after her death.
- Encourage Mr. Allen to talk with his wife about her wishes regarding her death and funeral care in order to take a more active role in meeting her needs.

- Support Mr. Allen's need to grieve for his wife and help him to recognize that sadness is a normal part of the process.
- Encourage Mr. Allen to see that maintaining his own health is an important contribution to both Pam and Gary's care.
- Refer Mr. Allen to agencies serving clients with disabilities to determine what assistance may be available to help him care for Gary.
- Help Mr. Allen develop a plan of exercise and recreation.
- Support Mr. Allen's need to obtain assistance in caring for Pam and Gary to reduce caregiver role strain.

EVALUATION

Mr. Allen demonstrates improvement by meeting the following expected outcomes:
- He begins seeing a mental health professional to treat depression.
- He is taking medications as prescribed.
- He finds a day care program that specializes in treating adults with Down syndrome.
- He discusses his wife's terminal condition with her, her desires for end of life care, and her postmortem wishes.
- He learns that his medical insurance will pay for someone to come to the home to provide for Pam's care 4 hours a day and initiates these visits immediately.

CRITICAL THINKING

1. What expected outcome would you anticipate for Mr. Allen if he fails to obtain treatment for depression?
2. What community programs might you suggest to Mr. Allen to help him care for Gary and Pam?
3. What follow-up care can the hospice nurse provide Mr. Allen when making daily visits to Pam?

REVIEW Depression

RELATE Link the Concepts and Exemplars

Linking the exemplar of depression with the concept of addiction:

1. Why might dependence on alcohol promote depression?
2. What impact might dependence on nicotine have on mood and affect?

Linking the exemplar of depression with the concept of elimination:

3. What aspects of depression increase the risk for constipation?
4. How might alterations in elimination put an older client at risk for depression?

READY Go to Companion Skills Manual

REFER Go to Pearson Nursing Student Resources
nursing.pearsonhighered.com

- Additional review materials

REFLECT Case Study

Melvin Thomas is a 14-year-old African American male whose mother brings him to their family physician's office because this is the third day in a row that Melvin "hasn't felt well." Melvin has been getting in trouble at school for arguing with teachers, and he has missed a lot of school, complaining of stomachaches. Melvin's mother says that he rarely sees his dad but that her second husband tries to spend time with Melvin when he can. When they do spend time together, they go shooting at the gun range or play video games. Melvin's expression at the physician's office is sullen, and he keeps his arms crossed in front of him. He answers the nurse by giving one-syllable responses or by nodding or shaking his head.

1. What assessment findings would make you suspect Melvin is depressed?
2. What priority teaching would you want to provide Melvin's mother if the diagnosis of depression is confirmed?
3. What impact is depression having on Melvin's ability to meet developmental milestones?

EXEMPLAR 28.2   Adjustment Disorder With Depressed Mood

EXEMPLAR KEY TERMS

Adjustment disorder with depressed mood, *1805*
Resilience, *1805*
Situational depression, *1805*

EXEMPLAR LEARNING OUTCOMES

After reading about this exemplar, you will be able to:

1. Describe the features, clinical manifestations, and direct and indirect causes of adjustment disorder with depressed mood.
2. Identify risk factors associated with adjustment disorder with depressed mood.

3. Illustrate the nursing process in providing culturally competent care across the life span for individuals with adjustment disorder with depressed mood.
4. Formulate priority nursing diagnoses appropriate for an individual with adjustment disorder with depressed mood.
5. Summarize therapies used by interdisciplinary teams in the collaborative care of an individual with adjustment order with depressed mood.
6. Plan evidence-based care for an individual with adjustment disorder with depressed mood and his or her family in collaboration with other members of the healthcare team.
7. Evaluate expected outcomes for an individual with adjustment disorder with depressed mood.

▶ OVERVIEW

Adjustment disorder with depressed mood represents a change in mood and affect following a stressor, such as the end of a relationship, or multiple stressors; it may also be called **situational depression.** Symptoms generally begin 3 months after the event and typically last no more than 6 months. Adjustment disorder with depressed mood is differentiated from an appropriate change in mood following a sad or stressful event in that the distress experienced by the client is out of proportion to the event and results in significant impairment in functioning (APA, 2013).

Risk Factors

Any life-altering event can create risk for the occurrence of adjustment disorder with depressed mood. This risk is further increased by a preexisting mental health issue, ineffective or unhealthy coping mechanisms, or lack of a support network. Clients with these preexisting conditions may find that adjustment disorder with depressed mood has exacerbated their condition. For example, in an attempt to diminish feelings of depression, a client who has remained sober after a history of alcohol abuse may resume drinking as a coping mechanism following a stressful event.

Older adults are at high risk for adjustment disorder with depressed mood, especially when they experience two or more stressors in proximity. Loss of independence, be it cognitive, physical, or otherwise, often results in adjustment disorder with depressed mood in the older adult. Even those older adults who "see the glass as half full" are challenged by these types of stressors. The loss of driving privileges (due to physical or cognitive changes) is a huge loss to older adults, often putting a great deal of strain on family members who must accommodate the older adult who can no longer drive, as well provide support as the individual learns to cope with this loss of independence.

Resilience Factors

The capacity to respond successfully to stressors is called **resilience.** Resilience is the ability not only to survive and bounce

back from difficult and traumatic experiences, but also to continue to grow and develop emotionally and psychologically. The notion of resilience encompasses the biological and psychological characteristics intrinsic to an individual, such as personality style and quality of interpersonal relationships, that confer protection against the development of psychopathology (Bhui & Dinos, 2011). Resilience probably explains why not all individuals who experience stress or social isolation develop mental health problems as adults (Cacioppo, Reis, & Zautra, 2011). Researchers and clinicians alike have been surprised by the prevalence of the capacity for resilience, and clinicians are beginning to focus on uncovering and energizing pathways to resilience in their clients.

Individuals without a history of mental illness can succumb to adjustment disorder with depressed mood following a stressful event. Resilience factors can make a great deal of difference in preventing the adjustment disorder with depressed mood from becoming a depressive disorder. Nurses working with clients experiencing adjustment disorder with depressed mood should help them identify their resilience factors and use those factors as supportive mechanisms during this critical time. Resilience factors may include a close-knit family, close friends, a good job with benefits, membership in a volunteer organization, or any other number of factors.

▶ CLINICAL MANIFESTATIONS

The symptoms of adjustment disorder with depressed mood are similar to those of the other depressive disorders and include sleep disturbances, feelings of hopelessness and sadness, loss of self-esteem, irritability, difficulty concentrating, and anhedonia. Behaviors that may occur include ignoring financial responsibilities; arguing and fighting; performing poorly at work or school; and behaving recklessly, such as driving while intoxicated or vandalizing others' property.

Clinical Manifestations and Therapies Adjustment Disorder With Depressed Mood

ETIOLOGY	CLINICAL MANIFESTATIONS	CLINICAL THERAPIES
Sleep disturbances	■ Insomnia, hypersomnia	■ Improved sleep hygiene ■ Short-term sedative
Feelings of sadness, despair Loss of self-esteem Irritability	■ Crying ■ Avoiding pleasurable activities ■ Avoiding family and friends	■ Cognitive-behavioral therapy alone may be sufficient to help the individual return to normal. ■ Alternative therapies such as massage therapy or acupuncture may provide relief. ■ Antidepressant therapy
Behavioral changes	■ Ignoring financial responsibilities ■ Performing poorly at work and school ■ Fighting, behaving recklessly	■ Cognitive behavior therapy ■ Family therapy ■ Antidepressant therapy

▶ COLLABORATION

Cognitive-behavioral therapy often is sufficient to help clients put things in perspective and return to a normal state. If a client exhibits behavioral changes that are affecting the family, such as ignoring financial responsibilities, direct intervention by a key family member may be helpful. Family therapy also may be helpful depending on how close or involved the family is as a whole.

The nurse's responsibilities as part of a collaborative team are discussed in detail in the Nursing Process section.

Pharmacologic Therapy

An antidepressant or antianxiety medication may be prescribed for the client with adjustment disorder with depressed mood. Some of these medications require several weeks to take full effect, and clients suffering from adjustment disorder with depressed mood are at a high risk for self-medicating with alcohol or other drugs. Client teaching regarding appropriate use of prescribed medications as well as the need to refrain from self-medicating is critical.

Exercise

Extensive evidence indicates that exercise is effective in reducing symptoms of depression. However, an extensive search of the research literature revealed no studies specifically investigating the role of exercise in adjustment disorder with depressed mood or situational depression. Gill, Womack, and Safranen (2010) summarized the results of a 2009 Cochrane systematic review of exercise and depression. It clearly showed that exercise is beneficial in reducing depressive symptoms. Further analysis showed that resistance exercise, or resistance exercise combined with aerobic exercise, was more effective than aerobic exercise alone, and that exercising three times a week or more was more effective than exercising only once a week. In the United States, exercise is not recognized as a first-line treatment for depression. However, in the United Kingdom, the National Institute for Health and Clinical Excellence recommends structured, supervised exercise programs, three times a week (45- to 60-minute sessions) for 10 to 14 weeks to treat mild depression, and exercise program referrals are available for clients consulting physicians for a complaint

of depression. There is some evidence that physical exercise is as effective as CBT or medication in reducing depression, but further research is needed (aan het Rot, Collins, & Fitterling, 2009; Gill et al., 2010). Mindful exercise practices, such as yoga, qigong, and tai chi, that combine cognitive meditation with physical movement were found to significantly improve symptoms of depression in five out of six studies in a systematic review (Tsang, Chan, & Cheung, 2008). Based on the evidence, physical exercise should be recommended to clients who are diagnosed with adjustment disorder with depressed mood.

NURSING PROCESS

Priorities of care for clients with adjustment disorder with depressed mood focus on maintaining clients' safety, encouraging them to work through their feelings of sadness, and helping them identify strengths that will help them overcome their feelings of hopelessness and fear.

Assessment

Assessment of the client with adjustment disorder with depressed mood includes a nursing history to determine the precipitating stressor and symptoms the client is experiencing. The nurse also assesses the client's risk factors for depression, as well as the presence of resilience factors. If the precipitating stressor was a physical assault or accident, such as a motor vehicle crash, a physical examination may be necessary to confirm healing of any injuries. Depression scales or inventories may be used, such as the Beck Depression Inventory.

Diagnosis

The following nursing diagnoses may be appropriate for the client with adjustment disorder with depressed mood:

- *Helplessness*
- *Disturbed Sleep Pattern*
- *Disrupted Family Processes*
- *Situational Low Self-Esteem*
- *Ineffective Coping.*

(NANDA-I © 2012)

Planning

Appropriate goals for clients with adjustment disorder with depressed mood may include the following:

- The client will obtain adequate sleep and rest.
- The client will refrain from reckless or irresponsible behaviors.
- The client will return to normal daily routines.
- The client will remain free of injury.

Implementation

When initiating interventions, it is important to prioritize care to meet the client's most immediate needs first. Involving the client, when possible, in planning priorities can promote independence and a feeling of control.

Promote Hope

Nursing interventions to help clients return to a hopeful attitude include exploring their previous achievements, encouraging them to identify their strengths and abilities, and facilitating the evaluation of their behavior. Help clients to identify ways in which they have control of their lives. Help them learn to identify situations in which they can become more autonomous, especially through vocational, social, and community activities.

Many people with mood disorders believe they have lost control over their lives, rights, and responsibilities and have lost the ability and right to effectively advocate for themselves. Nursing activities designed to help clients advocate for themselves provide them with hope and self-esteem. The nurse may assist clients in the following ways:

- Encourage them to believe in themselves.
- Inform them of their rights.
- Help them clarify what they need and want by setting clear goals.
- Provide accurate information, preferably in writing.
- Help them strategize by using the problem-solving process.
- Identify and facilitate resources such as friends, family, self-help groups, and advocacy organizations.
- Encourage identification of the best person(s) to assist with this problem.

- Foster effective communication so clients can get their message across; use suggestions such as these: Be brief, stick to the point, do not get diverted, and state the concern and how things should be changed.
- Promote firmness and persistence so clients can get what they need for themselves.

Support Family Function

Mood disorders affect not only the client, but also family and friends. Nurses must provide care to the family as well as to the client with situational depression. During acute episodes, clients may be dependent and needy or may need firm direction and limit setting. Help caregivers acknowledge clients' dependency and assume appropriate responsibility. Provide information about clients' condition in accordance with client preferences, remembering the importance of confidentiality. Provide the family with a list of community resources and encourage them to participate in support groups.

In some cases, the stressor that causes the client's adjustment disorder with depressed mood also directly disrupts family processes. For example, a mother who is injured in a motor vehicle crash and confined to bed rest for more than a few days requires someone to step in and assume her normal roles until she is able to perform them again. In cases like this in which family processes and patterns are disrupted, the nurse can support the family by providing referrals to outside resources and by helping the father or another adult family member develop a plan to "cover the bases" until the mother returns to health.

Families who have experienced a loss or stressor that disrupts family processes are at increased risk for family conflict. Nurses working with these families should encourage them to resolve disagreements in a healthy manner and not allow the situation to overrun their family strengths. Box 22–4 in the module on Addiction outlines eight steps to resolving family disagreements.

Evaluation

Expected outcomes for a client in crisis may include:

- The client clarifies what is needed and has set clear goals.
- The client has used a problem-solving process.
- The client understands and uses resources for support.

NURSING CARE PLAN — A Client With Adjustment Disorder With Depressed Mood

ASSESSMENT	DIAGNOSES	PLANNING
Kara Garner is a 70-year-old African American widow who was recently admitted to a rehabilitation facility following a stroke with mild right-side hemiplegia. She is right-handed. She does not feed herself and has little appetite. Mrs. Garner is alert and oriented to person and place. She cooperates with having her activities of daily living (ADL) done for her, but she does not try to help. Her affect appears sad. She refuses to attend activities, preferring to stay in her room alone. The nurse working with Mrs. Garner thinks she might be depressed, and the attending physician agrees to order a psychiatric consult. The psychiatric nurse practitioner diagnoses Ms. Garner with adjustment disorder with depressed mood, explaining she does not meet full criteria for MDD. She tells the nurse that Mrs. Garner misses her family, but is afraid she will not be able to care for herself and does not want to become a burden to them. The nurse practitioner will provide psychotherapy but does not think that Mrs. Garner requires antidepressant medication at this time. She recommends working on assisting Mrs. Garner to regain independence and increase socialization.	Three priority nursing diagnoses were identified for this client: - *Powerlessness* - *Self-Care Deficit* in bathing/hygiene, dressing/grooming, feeding, and toileting - *Impaired Social Interaction* (NANDA-I © 2012)	The goals for Mrs. Garner's plan of care are as follows: - The client will identify two areas in which she feels some control. - The client will assist with all her ADLs, and feed herself independently within 2 weeks. - The client will demonstrate increased social interaction as evidenced by attending at least four activities in the next week.

(continued on next page)

NURSING CARE PLAN (continued)

IMPLEMENTATION

- Gradually offer Mrs. Garner simple choices regarding dressing, bathing, prioritizing care needs, and activities. This will help her begin to assist in her own care and eventually regain control.
- Encourage self-care by helping Mrs. Garner use her left hand to feed and bathe herself.
- Encourage social contact by promoting involvement in activities and introducing Mrs. Garner to other clients with similar interests.

- Identify local community stroke support groups and encourage Mrs. Garner to participate in one.
- Provide positive reinforcement for Mrs. Garner as she assumes increasing responsibility for her own care and begins to socialize with others.
- Discuss Mrs. Garner's care with her primary provider to provide ongoing assessment of depression and risk for suicide.

EVALUATION

Within 2 weeks Mrs. Garner begins to assist in bathing herself and learns to eat with her left hand by choosing foods that are easy to stab and bring to her mouth. The psychiatric nurse practitioner discusses attending a stroke support group and she agrees to participate. She develops a few friendships with other clients and appears less sad. She expresses hopefulness that she will continue to regain function and is looking forward to going home to her family.

CRITICAL THINKING

1. Why did the nurse suspect Mrs. Garner was depressed?
2. What factors promoted Mrs. Garner's depressed mood?
3. When a client such as Mrs. Garner experiences adjustment disorder with depressed mood how can the depression best be resolved? Explain your answer.

REVIEW Adjustment Disorder With Depressed Mood

RELATE Link the Concepts and Exemplars

Linking the exemplar of adjustment disorder with depressed mood with the concept of family:

1. How might the client with adjustment disorder with depressed mood be at risk for impaired parenting?
2. What normal but stressful events in a family's life might be likely to be met with an out-of-proportion, depressive response by one or more family members?

Linking the exemplar of adjustment disorder with depressed mood with the concept of nutrition:

3. How might adjustment disorder with depressed mood impact a client's nutritional status?
4. What client teaching should the nurse provide to the client with adjustment disorder with depressed mood regarding nutrition?

READY Go to Companion Skills Manual

REFER Go to Pearson Nursing Student Resources
nursing.pearsonhighered.com

- Additional review materials

REFLECT Case Study

Jill Adkins is an 18-year-old, African American woman in her second semester at a major university, where she is on a prestigious academic scholarship. Just before midterms, she gets a call from her aunt, who informs Ms. Adkins that her mother, who has diabetes, has taken a turn for the worse and requires a kidney transplant. Ms. Adkins phones her mother, who tells her to study hard and take her midterms. Ms. Adkins tries to study, but she keeps thinking about her mother. She has trouble sleeping, and her roommate has to encourage her to eat. The weekend after midterms, Ms. Adkins's uncle comes to take her home to see her mother, who looks very ill and is very weak but is in good spirits. Ms. Adkins's mother convinces her to return to school, where Ms. Adkins learns that she did poorly on her midterms. Ms. Adkins feels poorly over the next couple of days. She decides to go to the student health center at the urging of her roommate.

1. What are the priority nursing considerations for Ms. Adkins? What nursing diagnoses are appropriate?
2. What risk factors does Ms. Adkins have for adjustment disorder with depressed mood? What resilience factors does she have?
3. If you were the nurse at the student health center, what would your plan of care for Ms. Adkins include?

EXEMPLAR 28.3 Bipolar Disorders

EXEMPLAR KEY TERMS

Bipolar disorders, *1809*
Cyclothymic disorder, *1811*
Flight of ideas, *1809*
Hypomania, *1809*
Mania, *1809*

EXEMPLAR LEARNING OUTCOMES

After reading about this exemplar, you will be able to:

1. Describe the pathophysiology, psychopathology, and clinical manifestations of bipolar disorders.
2. Identify risk factors associated with bipolar disorders.

3. Illustrate the nursing process in providing culturally competent care across the life span for individuals with bipolar disorders.

4. Formulate priority nursing diagnoses appropriate for an individual with bipolar disorder.

5. Summarize therapies used by interdisciplinary teams in the collaborative care of an individual with bipolar disorder.

6. Plan evidence-based care for an individual with bipolar disorder and his or her family in collaboration with other members of the healthcare team.

7. Evaluate expected outcomes for an individual with bipolar disorder.

▶ OVERVIEW

The **bipolar disorders** are a group of mood disorders that include manic hypomanic, and depressive episodes. Cyclothymic disorder, a related disorder, is characterized by alternating periods of hypomanic and depressive symptoms that are not significant enough to meet the criteria for hypomania or depression. Although less than 2% of the population is diagnosed with bipolar disorders, these types of disorders can have a tremendous impact on those closest to the person with the disorder (APA, 2013, p. 136).

▶ PATHOPHYSIOLOGY AND ETIOLOGY

No definitive cause or specific pathophysiology has been identified for bipolar spectrum disorders. Rather, they are thought to arise from a complex combination of genetic, physiological, environmental and psychosocial factors. Immunological abnormalities may contribute to the pathophysiology of mania and bipolar disorder. Mitochondrial dysfunction and oxidative stress also may be involved in bipolar disorder (Andreazza et al., 2010). Children of parents with bipolar disorders have a 4%–15% risk of having a bipolar disorder. Stressful life events (especially suicide of a family member); sleep cycle disruptions; family or caregivers with high expressed emotion; and an emotionally overinvolved, hostile and critical communication pattern are factors associated with heritability. Bipolar disorders, schizophrenia, and major depressive disorders share biological susceptibility and inheritance patterns. Several genes and loci that may be associated with bipolar disorders, including glycogen synthase kinase-3β have been discovered (Price & Marzani-Nissen, 2012).

Bipolar I disorder consists of one or more manic or mixed episodes, and the course of illness is usually accompanied by major depressive episodes. *Bipolar II disorder* consists of one or more major depressive episodes accompanied by at least one hypomanic episode.

Bipolar disorders tend to be recurrent and have the unusual tendency to increase in frequency as the individual ages. Many clients return to normal functioning during remission periods, but approximately 30% of those with bipolar disorder will exhibit functional impairment at work. Of clients with bipolar II disorder, at least 15% will continue to experience dysfunction between episodes, and up to 20% will not experience any recovery between alternating episodes of hypomania and depression (APA, 2013).

Bipolar disorders typically appear between the ages of 15 and 30. Risk factors include a family history of bipolar disorders, drug abuse, periods of very high stress, and a major life-altering event. Women and men are at equal risk of having bipolar disorders, although women are more likely to experience rapid cycling and depressive symptoms and are at greater risk for comorbid alcohol abuse than men (APA, 2013).

▶ CLINICAL MANIFESTATIONS

The manifestations experienced by the individual define the type of bipolar disorder. Nurses must recognize these manifestations, understand how clients respond during various stages, and provide client and family teaching regarding symptoms and treatments. See **Box 28–6** ● for the diagnostic criteria for bipolar I disorder.

Mania and Hypomania

Mania is characterized by an abnormal and persistently elevated, expansive, or irritable mood and increased energy (or activity) present for most of the time, nearly every day, or a week or more and accompanied by specific symptoms as articulated in the DSM-5 (see Box 28–6). **Flight of ideas** (rapidly changing, fragmented thoughts), pressured speech patterns, and increasing goal-directed activities are common during manic episodes. Psychotic symptoms such as delusions or hallucinations may be a feature of severe mania.

Hypomania is a less extreme form of mania that is not severe enough to markedly impair functioning or require hospitalization. Individuals experiencing hypomania feel wonderful, "on top of the world," and do not recognize changes in themselves. Those who know them well, however, are aware of the changes in mood and behavior. There are no psychotic features in hypomania.

The onset of manic episodes usually occurs in the early twenties but may begin at any age. It often follows a severe disappointment, embarrassment, or other psychic stressor. The mood of clients experiencing a manic episode is euphoric, or "high." Their behavior is excessive and out of bounds. During mania, individuals typically exhibit overly enthusiastic involvement in projects of an interpersonal, political, religious, or occupational nature. When someone or something gets in the way or appears to put a snag in their way, they become irritable. Moods alternate between euphoria and irritability. Increased sexual behaviors are common, including flirting, making sexual overtures, having inappropriate sexual relationships, and feeling compelled to seduce and be seduced. Women may dress in an uncharacteristically flashy or seductive manner and wear garish makeup. Grandiosity can reach delusional proportions. Clients with mania rarely believe they are sick, even when they are in financial or legal trouble, and may vehemently protest the need for treatment. The characteristics of a manic episode are illustrated in **Figure 28–5** ●.

Depressive Episodes

A diagnosis of bipolar disorder does not always mean that manic or hypomanic behaviors will be manifested in the current episode of illness. Bipolar I and bipolar II disorder are characterized by periods of mania/hypomania alternating with depressive episodes. Mood stabilizers are the drug of choice, so it is important when assessing clients who present with depression to determine

Box 28–6   DSM-5 Diagnostic Criteria for Bipolar I Disorder

For a diagnosis of bipolar I disorder, it is necessary to meet the following criteria for a manic episode. The manic episode may have been preceded by and may be followed by hypomanic or major depressive episodes.

MANIC EPISODE

A. A distinct period of abnormally and persistently elevated, expansive, or irritable mood, and abnormally and persistently increased goal-directed activity or energy, lasting at least 1 week and present for most of the day, nearly every day (or any duration if hospitalization is necessary).

B. During the period of mood disturbance and increased energy or activity, three (or more) of the following symptoms (four if the mood is only irritable) are present to a significant degree and represent a noticeable change from usual behavior:
   1. Inflated self-esteem or grandiosity.
   2. Decreased need for sleep (e.g., feels rested after only 3 hours of sleep).
   3. More talkative than usual or pressure to keep talking.
   4. Flight of ideas or subjective experience that thoughts are racing.
   5. Distractibility (i.e., attention too easily drawn to unimportant or irrelevant external stimuli), as reported or observed.
   6. Increase in goal-directed activity (either socially, at work or school, or sexually) or psychomotor agitation (i.e., purposeless non-goal-directed activity).
   7. Excessive involvement in pleasurable activities that have a high potential for painful consequences (e.g., engaging in unrestrained buying sprees, sexual indiscretions, or foolish business investments).

C. The mood disturbance is sufficiently severe to cause marked impairment in social occupational functioning or to necessitate hospitalization to prevent harm to self or others, or there are psychotic features.

D. The episode is not attributable to the physiological effects of a substance (e.g., a drug of abuse, a medication, other treatment) or to another medical condition.

HYPOMANIC EPISODE

A. A distinct period of abnormally and persistently elevated, expansive, or irritable mood and abnormally and persistently increased activity or energy, lasting at least 4 consecutive days and present most of the day, nearly every day.

B. During the period of mood disturbance and increased energy and activity, three (or more) of the following symptoms (four if the mood is only irritable) have persisted, represent a noticeable change from usual behavior, and have been present to a significant degree:
   1. Inflated self-esteem or grandiosity.
   2. Decreased need for sleep (e.g., feels rested after only 3 hours of sleep).
   3. More talkative than usual or pressure to keep talking.
   4. Flight of ideas or subjective experience that thoughts are racing.
   5. Distractibility (i.e., attention too easily drawn to unimportant or irrelevant external stimuli), as reported or observed.
   6. Increase in goal-directed activity (either socially, at work or school, or sexually) or psychomotor agitation.

7. Excessive involvement in pleasurable activities that have a high potential for painful consequences (e.g., engaging in unrestrained buying sprees, sexual indiscretions, or foolish business investments).

C. The episode is associated with an unequivocal change in functioning that is uncharacteristic of the individual when not symptomatic.

D. The disturbance in mood and the change in functioning are observable by others.

E. The episode is not severe enough to cause marked impairment in social or occupational functioning or to necessitate hospitalization. If there are psychotic features, the episode is, by definition, manic.

F. The episode is not attributable to physiological effects of a substance (e.g., a drug of abuse, a medication, or other treatment).

MAJOR DEPRESSIVE EPISODE

A. Five (or more) of the following symptoms have been present during the same 2-week period and represent a change from previous functioning; at least one of the symptoms is either (1) depressed mood or (2) loss of interest or pleasure.
   1. Depressed mood most of the day, nearly every day, as indicated by either subjective report (e.g., feels sad, empty, or hopeless) or observation made by others (e.g., appears tearful). (**Note:** In children and adolescents, can be irritable mood.)
   2. Markedly diminished interest or pleasure in all, or almost all, activities most of the day, nearly every day (as indicated by either subjective account or observation).
   3. Significant weight loss when not dieting or weight gain (e.g., a change of more than 5% of body weight in a month), or decrease or increase in appetite nearly every day. (**Note:** In children, consider failure to make expected weight gain.)
   4. Insomnia or hypersomnia nearly every day.
   5. Psychomotor agitation or retardation nearly every day (observable by others; not merely subjective feelings of restlessness or being slowed down).
   6. Fatigue or loss of energy nearly every day.
   7. Feelings of worthlessness or excessive or inappropriate guilt (which may be delusional) nearly every day (not merely self-reproach or guilt about being sick).
   8. Diminished ability to think or concentrate, or indecisiveness, nearly every day (either by subjective account or as observed by others).
   9. Recurrent thoughts of death (not just fear of dying), recurrent suicidal ideation without a specific plan, or a suicide attempt or a specific plan for committing suicide.

B. The symptoms cause clinically significant distress or impairment in social, occupational, or other important areas of functioning.

C. The episode is not attributable to the physiological effects of a substance or another medical condition.

BIPOLAR I DISORDER

A. Criteria have been met for at least one manic episode (Criteria A–D under "Manic Episode" above).

B. The occurrence of the manic and major depressive episode(s) is not better explained by schizoaffective disorder, schizophrenia, schizophreniform disorder, delusional disorder, or other specified or unspecified schizophrenia spectrum and other psychotic disorder.

Source: Reprinted with permission from American Psychiatric Association. (2013). *Diagnostic and statistical manual of mental disorders* (5th ed.). Washington, DC: American Psychiatric Publishing.

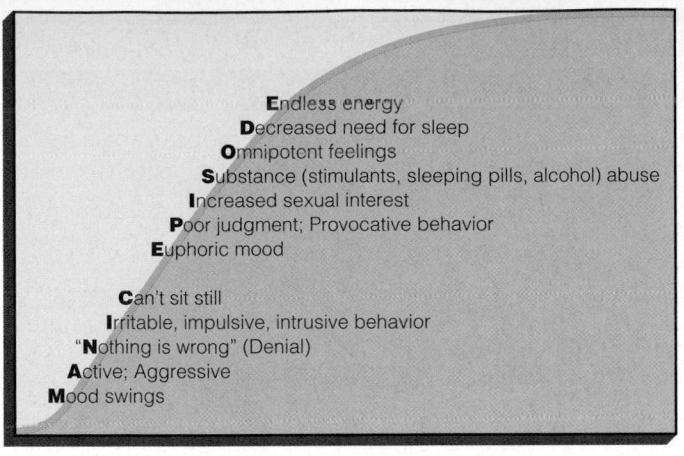

Endless energy
Decreased need for sleep
Omnipotent feelings
Substance (stimulants, sleeping pills, alcohol) abuse
Increased sexual interest
Poor judgment; Provocative behavior
Euphoric mood

Can't sit still
Irritable, impulsive, intrusive behavior
"**N**othing is wrong" (Denial)
Active; Aggressive
Mood swings

Figure 28–5 ● Characteristics of a manic episode.

if the client has ever had a manic or hypomanic episode. Antidepressant medications should be used with care, at low doses, and only during the severe depressive episode to reduce the chance of switching to a manic state.

Many clients with bipolar disorders are not correctly diagnosed in a timely manner. This can mean that an individual loses years to an illness that could have been successfully managed if it had been correctly diagnosed and treated.

Mixed Features

The DSM-5 recognizes certain specifiers for bipolar and related disorders. These include a specifier *with mixed features*, which recognizes that depressive episodes may occur and be accompanied by symptoms of mania or hypomania; and manic or hypomanic episodes may occur and be accompanied by symptoms characteristic of depressive episodes (APA, 2013).

Rapid Cycling

Individuals with either bipolar I or bipolar II disorder may exhibit rapid cycling—four mood episodes occurring within

a year with periods of partial or full remission of 2 months or more *or* with immediate alternate periods of mania/hypomania and depression. Individuals can experience episodes more than once a week and even more than once a day (NIMH, n.d.b).

Cyclothymic Disorder

When clients have suffered at least 2 years from "chronic, fluctuating mood disturbance involving numerous periods of hypomanic symptoms and numerous periods of depressive symptoms," they are diagnosed with **cyclothymic disorder** (APA, 2013). They must be free of severe symptoms that qualify for the diagnosis of manic disorder or MDD. These individuals are often considered to be moody, unpredictable, or temperamental, and they may go on to develop an overlay of symptoms that are of major depressive or manic intensity. **Figure 28–6 ●** compares mood in MDD, bipolar disorders, dysthymia, and cyclothymia.

Cyclothymic disorder begins early, usually in adolescence or early adulthood. Although not common, with a lifetime risk of only 0.4%–1.0% of the general population, cyclothymic disorder is thought to predispose individuals to other mood disorders. The incidence is approximately equal between males and females (APA, 2013).

Lifespan Considerations

Children with bipolar disorders present with mood changes (such as being overly silly or joyful when that is unusual for the child) and behavioral changes (such as sleeping little but not feeling tired, and talking a lot and having racing thoughts). Lifetime prevalence of bipolar disorders in adolescents is 0%–3% (NIMH, 2013b).

The rate of attempted suicide in those with bipolar disorders is high, as is co-occurrence with other disorders such as ADHD, anxiety, and substance abuse, all of which complicate diagnosis (NIMH, 2013c).

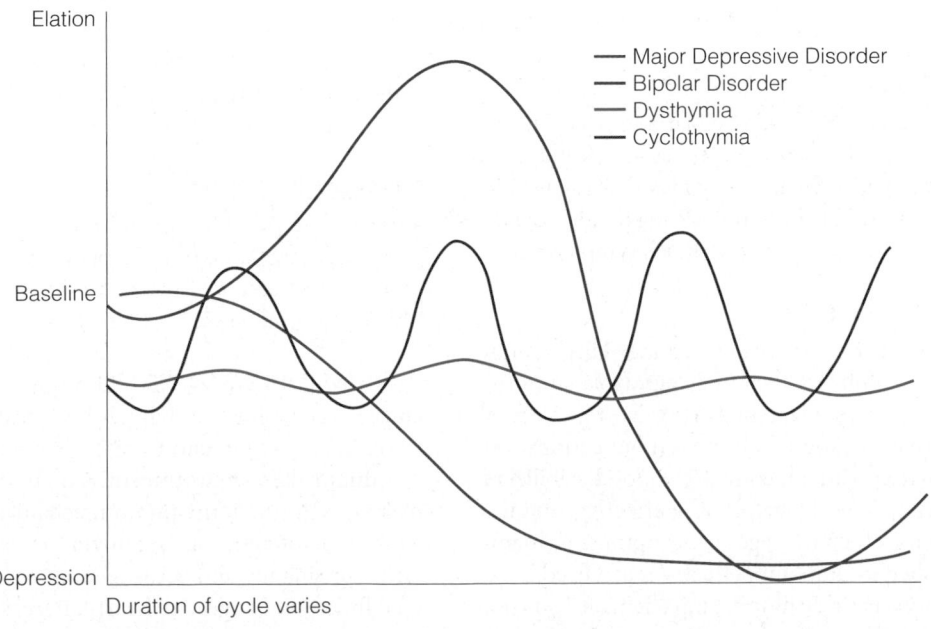

Figure 28–6 ● Comparison of affect (mood) in major depressive disorder, bipolar disorder, dysthymia, and cyclothymia.

Clinical Manifestations and Therapies Bipolar Disorders

ETIOLOGY	CLINICAL MANIFESTATIONS	CLINICAL THERAPIES
Mania/manic episode	Characterized by elevated, expansive, or irritable mood and increased activity or energy that significantly impairs social or occupational functioning and is accompanied by at least three of the following: ■ Increased self-esteem ■ Decreased need for sleep ■ Pressure of speech ■ Flight of ideas ■ Distractibility ■ Increased involvement in goal-directed activities ■ Psychomotor agitation ■ Excessive involvement in pleasurable activities that carry a high risk of painful consequences	■ Administer mood stabilizers such as lithium. ■ Remove or limit environmental stimuli. ■ Set limits; teach limit setting. ■ Orient to self, place, and time.
Hypomania	■ Less extreme than mania; individuals describe themselves as feeling "wonderful" and do not recognize changes in their behavior, although friends and family can observe changes.	■ Administer mood stabilizers such as lithium. ■ Remove or limit environmental stimuli. ■ Set limits or teach limit setting.
Depressed episode	■ Symptoms of depression	■ Administer antidepressant with mood stabilizer.

▶ COLLABORATION

Care of the client with a bipolar disorder requires a multidisciplinary effort that includes the nurse, the client, the primary care provider, a mental health specialist, a nurse case manager, and possibly a pharmacist as the team works to find a successful therapeutic regimen. The nurse should take special care to encourage the client to track feelings, behaviors, and side effects, especially during the first few weeks of trying a new medication.

Diagnostic Tests

There is no diagnostic test to determine bipolar and related disorders. Diagnosis is made based on clinical manifestations and client history. A physical examination, which may include drug testing, assists in ruling out the possibility of an underlying medical condition or substance abuse as the source of the client's symptoms.

Pharmacologic Therapy

Hyperactive and agitated behavior usually responds fairly rapidly to antipsychotic mood stabilizers such as aripiprazole (Abilify), risperidone (Risperdal), and olanzapine (Zyprexa). The atypical antipsychotics, effective as mood-stabilizing medications, are often given in conjunction with anticonvulsive mood stabilizers. Because lithium takes 1–3 weeks before it is effective, atypical antipsychotics are used to help manage the symptoms of mania for individuals prescribed lithium until efficacy is achieved.

Nursing interventions include monitoring clients for adverse side effects of antipsychotic medications. These include extrapyramidal effects such as Parkinson-like symptoms (e.g., rigidity, tremor, or "pill rolling" movements of the fingers); dystonia,

which is abnormal tonic contractions of the muscles (muscle spasms); and akathisia (subjective need to move, "jumping out of my skin"). Extrapyramidal symptoms should be reported and are usually treated by administration of an anticholinergic medication such as benztropine (Cogentin), diphenhydramine (Benadryl), or trihexyphenidyl (Artane). Acute dystonic reactions may be severe and require immediate medical intervention. These side effects can be distressing to the client. The nurse must reassure the client and explain what is occurring.

Several psychopharmacologic agents have proven effective in the long-term treatment of mania. One effective and widely used agent is lithium carbonate.

SAFETY ALERT

For clients with bipolar disorder, the orally disintegrating form of olanzapine may be prescribed to reduce instances of "med cheeking," where clients hide the tablet until in their mouth or cheek until they can dispose of it.

LITHIUM CARBONATE   Lithium carbonate is a potentially dangerous alkali metal that has been used in the treatment and prevention of acute manic episodes since the 1960s.

Lithium alters neurotransmission in the CNS. It is thought to interfere with the ionic pump mechanism in brain cells, but its exact mode of action is unknown. Its use is not recommended during pregnancy and breastfeeding or in clients with impaired renal function, congestive heart failure, sodium-restricted diets, organic brain disease, and impaired CNS functioning.

Administered orally, the onset of action ranges from 1 to 3 weeks. The dosage is gradually increased until the recommended therapeutic blood level of 0.8–1.2 mEq/L is achieved. Once the desired effect is achieved, the dosage is adjusted downward to the maintenance blood level of 0.6–1.2 mEq/L. There are cultural considerations to the therapeutic blood level: People of Asian descent may have toxic reactions at dosages as low as 0.6 mEq/L. Monitor therapeutic effect as well as side effects.

Toxic symptoms begin appearing at blood levels above 1.5 mEq/L. Because there is such a narrow margin of safety, serum concentrations must be closely monitored until stabilized.

ANTICONVULSANTS Common agents used in mania therapy are the anticonvulsants valproic acid (Depakote, Depakene), lamotrigine (Lamictal), and carbamazepine (Tegretol). These medications cannot be discontinued abruptly.

ATYPICAL ANTIPSYCHOTICS The atypical antipsychotics aripiprazole (Abilify), olanzapine (Zyprexa), quetiapine (Seroquel), and risperidone (Risperdal) are approved for bipolar mania and are becoming first-line treatments for bipolar mania. Olanzapine and aripiprazole come in an injectable form for use in acute agitation. These agents, especially the injectable forms, work quickly to calm the client.

 NURSING PROCESS

Because the nursing care of clients experiencing depressive symptoms is the same whether the diagnosis is MDD, dysthymic disorder, or depressed episode bipolar disorder, this section focuses on hypomania and mania, which constitute the other half of the bipolar continuum of behaviors.

Assessment

The onset of a hypomanic or manic episode may be gradual or dramatic. Affect is euphoric or elated but can change quickly to irritability or hostility if the individual is confronted with limits or is otherwise frustrated. The signs and symptoms range in severity from mild (in hypomania) to extreme (in a frank manic episode).

Clients who have mania are not usually able to cooperate fully in the assessment process. In many cases, nurses find it necessary to rely on their own assessment skills and secondary sources such as family members to obtain essential assessment data. Family members often can provide detailed information about the onset and progression of symptoms, as well as information about any previous episodes. Manic behaviors may include:

- Changes in the client's thought processes, evidenced by statements such as "I feel like my thoughts are racing."
- Inflated self-esteem, sometimes to the extent of having delusions of grandeur. Delusions of persecution also may be a feature.
- Clients ignoring fatigue, hunger, and even hygiene, being too involved in activity to focus on physiological sensations.
- Distractibility. The client experiencing a manic episode often suffers from an inability to concentrate and is easily distracted by the slightest stimulus in the environment.
- Hallucinations.
- A surprising sense of well-being. Individuals who are hypomanic and those early in manic episodes feel wonderful and do not understand why people are upset with their behavior.

Clients who are experiencing their first mania are most likely to be young people in their twenties, although adolescents are

sometimes affected. The hallmark of mania is constant motor activity. During a manic episode, clients may not stop to eat. They do not rest, have disordered sleep patterns, and may go for days without sleep. Bruises and other injuries sometimes result from the constant activity. Other indicators include the following:

- Rapid, loud, pressured speech
- Flight of ideas
- Poor judgment and impulsivity as reported by family members, such as shopping sprees, drug use, or sexual activity that is out of character with the client's usual behavior
- Unusual appearance (e.g., dressing inappropriately and using garish makeup or being disheveled and unkempt).

Impairment in occupational functioning may result in being laid off from work, being placed on a leave of absence, or being fired because the behavior is disruptive in the workplace. People who have mania cause interpersonal chaos by behaving manipulatively, testing limits, and playing one person against another. If their attempts at manipulation fail, they become irritable or hostile, and such behavior further alienates others.

Diagnosis

Several nursing diagnoses are common in the care of clients who have mania. These include the following:

- *Risk for Injury*
- *Disturbed Thought Processes*
- *Impaired Social Interaction*
- *Self-Care Deficit*
- *Sleep Deprivation*
- *Risk for Suicide.*

(NANDA-I © 2012)

Planning

Outcomes for mood disorders include the expectation of a return to normal functioning. While these will vary by client, appropriate outcomes for a client with bipolar disorder include the following:

- The client will remain free of injury.
- The client will remain oriented.
- The client will be able to focus on a specific stimulus for more than 10 minutes at a time.
- The client will be able to choose between two or more alternatives.
- The client will use appropriate behaviors in a variety of social settings.
- The client will maintain self-care.
- The client will no longer experience sleep disturbances.

Implementation

With clients who are manic, maintain a calm, relaxed, but firm and matter-of-fact demeanor, particularly when communicating limits. The nurse's behavior serves as a model and can be reassuring to out-of-control clients. As with all clients, building a trusting relationship is important (**Box 28-7** •).

Box 28-7   Potential Reactions of Nurses Working With Clients Who Have Mania

Working with clients who have mania will challenge your maturity, self-control, and professionalism. When you work with clients who have mania, you may experience some of the following feelings. Think about and discuss with your classmates and instructor how you might handle each of these reactions in order to maintain a positive nurse–client relationship.

- I feel annoyed by the client's demanding behavior.
- I feel outsmarted and outmaneuvered. I question whether my judgments and actions are appropriate.
- I develop rescue fantasies in response to a client's flattery and think I am the only one who understands this client.
- I become defensive and angry when colleagues point out a client's manipulative behavior.
- I feel anxious and insecure when a client turns on me, saying, "I'm not progressing because you're cold and mean."
- I have difficulty being objective about clients who have manic symptoms.
- I disagree emphatically with colleagues about how to handle a client's manipulative behavior. The client sits back and watches nurses fight with each other.
- I become angry and unsure of my judgment when a client consistently exceeds established limits.
- I withdraw and avoid clients who have mania so I do not feel embarrassed or experience self-doubt.

Promote Client Safety

Taking steps to ensure the safety of clients and others in the environment is a priority.

- Provide a safe environment by reducing environmental stimuli. For inpatient clients, this means providing a simply furnished private room that has had all unnecessary items removed. It should be in a quiet location to reduce noise stimulation. Low lighting also can be calming to the hyperactive client. Some hospitals have "quiet units." From there, clients can be transferred to milieu units when they are better able to deal with the distractions of community living.
- Remove or prohibit smoking materials. These are particularly hazardous in the hands of agitated clients. They may burn themselves or leave burning cigarettes lying around when they become distracted by other stimuli. While not an issue in most institutions, allow the client who is experiencing mania to smoke only under supervision.
- Monitor activities. Scheduling a program of appropriate activity interspersed with rest periods helps provide an outlet for tension while protecting clients from exhaustion. Appropriate activities include walking, exercising, or dancing with the supervision of an activity therapist and supervised vacuuming or sweeping chores. Avoid highly competitive activities that bring out hostility and overtly aggressive behaviors.
- Set and enforce limits on unsafe or socially inappropriate behavior when clients are unable to control their impulses. Matter-of-fact intervention rather than angry scolding is the most effective approach. Clients may respond to verbal reminders, or you can use their distractibility to redirect them into safer and more appropriate activities. Remember to reward appropriate behavior with positive reinforcement

such as "I enjoyed our walk today because you were able to walk with me rather than running ahead."

Promote Reality-Based Thinking

Present reality by spending time with clients. Identify yourself, the time and day, the location, and other orienting information as needed. Engage clients in reality-based, somewhat concrete activities (e.g., discussing a current event).

Consistency is reassuring to clients with altered thought processes. Establish consistency by following a schedule to help clients understand what is expected of them. Consistency also is enhanced by assigning the same caregivers to work with the same clients whenever possible.

When dealing with delusional or hallucinating clients, the nurse should communicate acceptance of their need for false beliefs while clearly stating that he or she does not share their perceptions. A statement such as "I understand that you believe you are the owner of this facility, but I see it differently" conveys acceptance without supporting delusional thinking.

It is not therapeutic to argue or try to reason with delusional clients. Arguing with a client often serves to harden the belief system and can impair the development of trust. Instead, use statements such as "I find that hard to believe" or "That is extremely unusual" to instill reasonable doubt as a therapeutic intervention.

When clients communicate perceptions of altered reality, reflect their statements back to them for validation. For example, asking "Are you saying that your husband is trying to poison you with monosodium glutamate?" can help a client understand how her perceptions sound to others. You will recognize that clients are becoming less delusional when they make statements such as "I know this sounds bizarre, but. . . ." Remember to give positive reinforcement when clients begin to focus on reality.

Enhance Socialization

Nursing activities are designed to facilitate the client's ability to interact with others by identifying needed behavior changes and assigning tasks that will improve the client's interactions with others. This may require mediating between the client and others when the client exhibits negative behavior. Nursing actions should encourage and demonstrate honesty and respect for others' rights.

Manipulation, a maladaptive behavior of clients who are manic, significantly impairs social interactions. This may take a simple form, such as borrowing money from others rather than using their own, or it may be highly complex, such as pitting staff members against one another by giving them false information about each other.

Manipulation meets a need for the client. It serves the purpose of increasing the client's sense of control and interpersonal power. (The mania can be frightening as it spins out of control.) Nursing interventions, such as setting limits, promote client security and often enable clients to curb their manipulative behavior or give it up entirely. Nurses should be aware of their own need for control and provide opportunities for clients to be in control when appropriate. Forming a therapeutic alliance with the client, discovering his or her expectations, and providing opportunities for interpersonal interactions have been linked with positive long-term outcomes for people with bipolar disorders (Gaudiano & Miller, 2006).

Set Limits

Out-of-control, manipulative behavior requires setting limits. All staff members must agree on the established limits and enforce them consistently. Violations of limits must have established consequences, also agreed on by all staff members. Clients must know what behaviors are expected and what consequences will result if they exceed the limits. Inconsistent application of consequences will result in a failure to decrease manipulative behavior.

Nurses should expect clients to give charming explanations of why they exceeded this or that limit, but should not be disarmed by these explanations. They are another form of manipulative behavior. Matter-of-fact limit enforcement and the consistent application of consequences are essential in promoting adaptive behaviors.

Promote Improved Self-Care

Well-being is compromised when clients do not receive sufficient nourishment and fluids for extended periods of time, particularly during periods of hyperactivity. Monitoring intake and output is an important nursing activity. The hyperactive client who is unable to sit down and eat is most likely to consume frequent small snacks that can be eaten on the go. For the inpatient client, work with a dietitian to ensure that high-calorie finger foods and nutritious liquids are available on the nursing unit until the client is able to attend regular meals. For outpatient clients or those preparing for discharge, collaborate with the client and dietitian to determine client preferences and create a list of easily prepared foods that the client finds palatable and can make or eat on the go.

A minimal level of personal hygiene is needed to ensure health, self-esteem, and healthy social interactions. Assist hyperactive clients who are unwilling or unable to bathe, brush their teeth, shave, wash their hair, change clothes, or use the toilet. Autonomy is desirable, so allow clients to do as much for themselves as possible with verbal encouragement. Reinforce any attempts at self-care with recognition; for example, "I see you shaved today, Mr. Adams."

Incontinence of urine or feces is occasionally seen in severely regressed clients during mania. This can be very disturbing to other clients and staff and insults the dignity of the client who is experiencing incontinence. Nursing activities include establishing a schedule of frequent, regular toileting. Accompany the client to the bathroom every hour or half hour until "accidents" no longer occur.

A more common elimination problem is constipation. Hyperactive clients suppress the urge to defecate and may become severely constipated. The anticholinergic effect of some medications also may exacerbate constipation. Frequent fluid intake and a high-fiber diet can reduce constipation.

Enhance Rest and Sleep

Clients in the manic phase of bipolar disorder appear deceptively energetic when they may actually be nearing the point of exhaustion. Design nursing activities to facilitate regular sleep–wake cycles. Monitor clients closely for signs of fatigue and make provisions for rest periods. Promote nighttime sleeping by limiting extended daytime naps.

Sleep may promote the rapid resolution of first episodes of mania. Prior to bedtime, decrease light and noise and encourage quiet activities and pre-sleep routines such as listening to soothing music. A warm bath and snack or a backrub may aid relaxation. Administer medications that do not suppress REM sleep, such as zolpidem tartrate (Ambien), as prescribed.

If clients experience extended nighttime wakefulness, avoid engaging them in long conversations or otherwise stimulating them or giving extra attention at night. Firmly encourage clients to stay in their darkened room with the expectation that they will fall asleep. If they will not stay in their room, assign a monotonous, repetitive task such as folding towels or sorting papers to encourage drowsiness.

When clients are able to sleep, avoid waking them for nonessential care or activities. Allow for sleep cycles of at least 90 minutes.

Evaluation

Specific client behaviors indicate that nursing interventions have been successful. Evaluation and outcome criteria answer the question "How do we know that the client's condition has improved?"

NURSING CARE PLAN   A Client With Bipolar Disorder

ASSESSMENT	DIAGNOSES	PLANNING
Mr. Grey, a 52-year-old engineer, is brought to the emergency psychiatric clinic by two adult sons at 2 a.m. Their mother called them to come help with their father, who has not slept in 3 days. When they arrived at their parents' home, they found their father working on a large landscaping project in the backyard that involved stonework, a waterfall, a fish pond, and extensive plantings of trees, shrubs, and flowers. According to the sons, Mr. Grey has had three prior episodes of manic behavior, beginning when he was in the army many years ago. He was stabilized on lithium carbonate for years but stopped taking it about a year ago because he felt so good. The current episode began about 1 week ago, after he was passed over for a promotion at work. He then took a leave of absence from his job to create what he called "the world's first home-based theme park." Any attempt by his wife to talk him out of the project has been met with anger and renewed resolve. Mr. Grey angrily tells the admitting nurse, "I don't know why these boys brought me here! I need to get back to work! I'm going to get millions for this franchise."	■ *Disturbed Thought Processes* ■ *Sleep Deprivation* ■ *Caregiver Role Strain* ■ *Interrupted Family Processes* ■ *Ineffective Therapeutic Regimen Management* (NANDA-I © 2012)	Goals for care include: ■ The client will comply with instructions for taking medications as ordered. ■ The client will sleep through the night. ■ The client will be oriented to time and place. ■ Family members will return to normal activities. ■ Family members will support medication administration.

(continued on next page)

NURSING CARE PLAN (continued)

IMPLEMENTATION

- With Mr. Grey and family members, develop a plan of activity that will help Mr. Grey disperse energy at appropriate times.
- Help family members set and enforce limits. For example, "From 8 p.m. until 6 a.m., Mr. Grey will remain indoors, engaged in sleep-promoting activities or sleeping."

- Refer Mr. Grey and his family to a therapist who can help them learn how to orient Mr. Grey to reality when his mind begins to stray.
- Help Mr. Grey and his wife learn how to promote sleep by decreasing environmental stimuli in the bedroom and engaging in good sleep hygiene.

EVALUATION

Expected outcomes to evaluate the client's care include:
- The client maintains therapeutic drug levels indicating compliance with medication regimen.
- The client and family report Mr. Grey obtains 6–8 hours of sleep per night.
- The client demonstrates orientation to time and place.
- The family reports a return to normal daily routine.
- The client regularly attends counseling sessions.

CRITICAL THINKING

1. What client teaching can the nurse provide to reduce the risk of medication noncompliance once Mr. Grey feels well and is no longer symptomatic?
2. What teaching will the nurse provide the family to help them cope with the client's diagnosis?
3. How can the nurse assist the client to meet his nutritional needs during manic phases of the illness?

REVIEW Bipolar Disorders

RELATE Link the Concepts and Exemplars

Linking the exemplar of bipolar disorders with the concept of family:

1. How might bipolar disorder affect parenting styles?
2. How might different family processes affect a child's treatment for bipolar disorder?

Linking the exemplar of bipolar disorders with the concept of nutrition:

3. How might bipolar disorder affect a client's nutritional status?

Linking the exemplar of bipolar disorders with the concept of health, wellness, and illness:

4. What consumer education resources are available to clients with bipolar disorders and their families to help them maintain their health during periods of relapse?

READY Go to Companion Skills Manual

REFER Go to Pearson Nursing Student Resources
nursing.pearsonhighered.com

- Additional review materials

REFLECT Case Study

Brittany Mathews, who is 21 years old and attending college, has been diagnosed with bipolar I disorder and is in the manic phase. Since admission 2 days ago, she has been averaging 2 hours of sleep a night. The rest of the night she spends pacing the hallways and talking to staff. She is in constant motion and brags about how much energy she has. Her clothing consists of startling bright miniskirts, low-cut sweaters, and high heels. Every few hours she changes clothes and reapplies her makeup to match.

1. What strategies might the nurse implement to maintain Ms. Mathews's safety at this time?
2. What risks to health does Ms. Mathews face during the manic phase of her illness and how can the nurse reduce these risks?

EXEMPLAR 28.4 Postpartum Depression

EXEMPLAR KEY TERMS
Acquaintance phase, *1819*
Engrossment, *1819*
Major depressive disorder with peripartum onset, *1817*
Maternal role attainment (MRA), *1817*
Phase of mutual regulation, *1819*
Postpartum blues, *1817*
Postpartum depression, *1817*
Postpartum psychosis, *1821*
Puerperium, *1817*

EXEMPLAR LEARNING OUTCOMES
After reading about this exemplar, you will be able to:

1. Describe the pathophysiology, etiology, clinical manifestations, and direct and indirect causes of postpartum depression.
2. Identify risk factors associated with postpartum depression.
3. Illustrate the nursing process in providing culturally competent care across the life span for women with postpartum depression.
4. Formulate priority nursing diagnoses appropriate for a woman with postpartum depression.

5. Summarize therapies used by interdisciplinary teams in the collaborative care of a woman with postpartum depression.
6. Plan evidence-based care for an individual with postpartum depression and her family in collaboration with other members of the healthcare team.

7. Evaluate expected outcomes for an individual with postpartum depression.

▶ OVERVIEW

The postpartum period is a time of readjustment and adaptation for the entire family, but especially for the mother. The woman experiences a variety of responses as she adjusts to a new family member, postpartum discomforts, changes in her body image, and the reality that she is no longer pregnant. The **puerperium** is that time immediately following childbirth when physiological changes that occurred during pregnancy begin to return to normal. **Postpartum blues**, commonly known as "baby blues," are a common occurrence after childbirth. Symptoms include mood swings; feeling sad, anxious, or overwhelmed; crying spells often for no reason; decreased appetite; and problems sleeping. These symptoms are not severe and do not require treatment. They usually resolve within a few days or a week (OWH, 2009). **Postpartum depression,** a depressive disorder associated with pregnancy, is now recognized to begin *during* pregnancy approximately 50% of the time, and is called **major depressive disorder with peripartum onset** in the DSM-5. Women who experience a depressive episode during pregnancy typically experience severe anxiety, and panic attacks are not uncommon. Mood and anxiety during pregnancy and postpartum blues are both associated with greater risk for postpartum depression (APA, 2013). This exemplar discusses the psychological struggles that women face after giving birth and how nurses can support them during this critical time.

▶ NORMAL PRESENTATION

Pregnancy is a time of great joy for many mothers, but it can also be a time of great anxiety. First-time mothers need to discuss their preconceptions about birth and obtain information to ensure a healthy pregnancy. The first day or two after birth, the mother may seem passive about the event and may seem more concerned with her own needs. Food and sleep are priority needs, and she begins to process the event. By the second or third day, the new mother is ready to resume control of her mothering and of her body and life and general. At this stage, however, she may experience anxiety and requires assurance that she is doing well as a mother. Difficulties with feedings may be a particular source of anxiety.

Maternal Role Attainment

Maternal role attainment (MRA) is the process by which a woman learns mothering behaviors and becomes comfortable with her identity as a mother. Formation of a maternal identity occurs with each child a woman bears. As the mother grows to know this child and forms a relationship, the mother's maternal identity gradually and systematically evolves and she "binds in" to the infant (Rubin, 1984).

Maternal role attainment often occurs in four stages (Mercer, 1995):

1. *The anticipatory stage* occurs during pregnancy. The woman looks to role models, especially her own mother, for examples of how to mother.
2. *The formal stage* begins when the child is born. The woman is still influenced by the guidance of others and tries to act as she believes others expect her to act.
3. *The informal stage* begins when the mother starts making her own choices about mothering. The woman begins to develop her own style of mothering and finds ways of functioning that work well for her.
4. *The personal stage* is the final stage of maternal role attainment. When the woman reaches this stage, she is comfortable with the notion of herself as "mother."

In most cases, MRA occurs within 3–10 months after birth. Social support, the woman's age and personality traits, the marital relationship, the presence of underlying anxiety or depression, the woman's previous child care experiences, the temperament of her infant, and the family's socioeconomic status all influence the woman's success in attaining the maternal role.

The postpartum woman faces a number of challenges as she adjusts to her new role (Mercer, 1995):

- For many women, finding time for themselves is one of the greatest challenges of motherhood. It is often difficult for the new mother to find time to read a book, talk to her partner, or even eat a meal without interruption.

- Women also report feelings of incompetence because they have not mastered all aspects of the mothering role. Many times mothers find themselves unsure of what to do in a given situation.

- The next greatest challenge involves fatigue resulting from sleep deprivation. The demands of nighttime care are tremendously draining, especially when the woman has other children.

- Another challenge for the new mother involves the feeling of responsibility that having a child brings. A woman experiences a sense of lost freedom, an awareness that she will never again be quite as carefree as she was before becoming a mother.

- Finding time for older children following the birth of a new baby also presents challenges. Many women feel guilty because the new baby takes up so much of their time. Sibling rivalry or ill feelings about the baby from other children can put additional stress on the mother.

- Mothers sometimes cite the infant's behavior as a challenge, especially when the child is about 8 months old. The baby develops stranger anxiety, begins crawling and getting into things, and may be fussy from teething. In addition, the baby's tendency to put things in his or her mouth requires constant vigilance by the parent.

Focus on Diversity and Culture Middle Eastern Initial Postpartum Experience

In many countries in the Middle East that follow a patriarchal system, the new mother and her infant stay with the husband's family following the birth of the infant. Frequent visits from the woman's family are discouraged and may even be viewed as burdensome by the husband's family. Typically, only women visit the new mother during the postpartum period. For the birth of the first baby, the wife's parents are expected to purchase all of the baby's supplies and clothing.

In some cultures, the father may have little involvement in newborn care. In the Muslim culture, for example, emphasis on childrearing and infant care is on the mother and extended female family members. Nurses need to be aware of cultural differences when evaluating a father's interaction with his newborn.

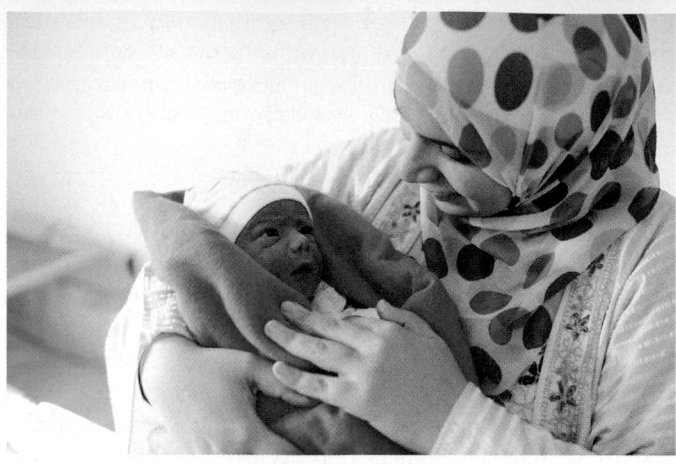

Figure 28–7 ● New mother *en face* with her infant.
Source: ZouZou/Shutterstock.

In 2004, Mercer proposed replacing the term *maternal role attainment* (MRA) with the term *becoming a mother* (BAM). She stated that BAM "more accurately encompasses the dynamic transformation and evolution of a woman's persona than does MRA, and the term MRA should be discontinued."

Nurses caring for families in the postpartum stage need to be aware of the long-term adjustments and stresses that the family faces as its members adjust to new and different roles. Nurses can help by providing anticipatory guidance about the realities of being a parent and by giving the postpartum family parenting literature for reference at home. Ongoing parenting groups give parents an opportunity to discuss problems and become comfortable in new roles.

Development of Family Attachment

A mother's first interaction with her infant is influenced by many factors, including her involvement with her family of origin, her relationships, the stability of her home environment, the communication patterns she has developed, and the degree of nurturing she received as a child. These factors shaped the person she has become. The following personal characteristics are also important:

- *Level of trust.* What level of trust has this mother developed in response to her life experiences? What is her philosophy of childrearing? Will she be able to treat her infant as a unique individual with changing needs that should be met as much as possible?
- *Level of self-esteem.* How much does she value herself as a woman and a mother? Is she generally able to cope with the adjustments of life?
- *Capacity for enjoying herself.* Is the mother able to find pleasure in everyday activities and human relationships?
- *Adequacy of knowledge about childbearing and childrearing.* What beliefs about the course of pregnancy, the capabilities of newborns, previous experiences with infants or children, and the nature of her emotions may influence her behavior at first contact with her infant and later?
- *Prevailing mood or usual feeling tone.* Is the woman predominantly content, angry, depressed, or anxious? Is she sensitive to her own feelings and those of others? Will she be able to accept her own needs and to obtain support in meeting them?

- *Reactions to the present pregnancy.* Was the pregnancy planned? Did it go smoothly? Were there ongoing life events that enhanced her pregnancy or depleted her reserves of energy? How have other life roles changed because of her pregnancy and motherhood?

By the time of birth, each mother has developed some kind of emotional orientation to the baby based on these factors.

Initial Maternal Attachment Behavior

After labor and birth, a new mother demonstrates a fairly regular pattern of maternal behaviors as she continues to familiarize herself with her newborn. In a progression of touching activities, the mother proceeds from fingertip exploration of the newborn's extremities toward palmar contact with larger body areas and finally to enfolding the infant with the whole hand and arm. The time she takes to accomplish these steps varies from minutes to days. The mother increases the proportion of time spent in the *en face* position—she arranges herself or the newborn so that she has direct face-to-face and eye-to-eye contact (**Figure 28–7 ●**). There is an intense interest in having the infant's eyes open. When the infant's eyes are open, the mother characteristically greets the newborn and talks to the baby in high-pitched tones.

In most instances, the mother relies heavily on her senses of sight, touch, and hearing in getting to know what her baby is really like. She also tends to respond verbally to any sounds emitted by the newborn, such as cries, coughs, sneezes, and grunts. The sense of smell may be involved as well.

SAFETY ALERT
Newborns are sometimes taken from their parents immediately after birth and placed in a special care or intensive care nursery. This separation can interfere with the normal attachment process. If this occurs, take the parents to the nursery as soon as possible to interact with their infant and allow them to hold and care for their infant as much as possible. If the infant is in an incubator and cannot be held, encourage the parents to stroke the infant's hand, foot, or cheek. Provide reassurance that this will not hurt the infant and is actually beneficial.

While interacting with her newborn, the mother may be experiencing shock, disbelief, or denial. She may state, "I can't believe she's finally here" or "I feel like he is a stranger." On the other hand, feelings of connectedness between the newborn and the rest of the family can be expressed in positive or negative terms: "She's got your cute nose, Daddy" or "Oh, no! He looks just like Matthew, and he was an impossible baby." A mother's facial expressions or the frequency and content of her questions may demonstrate concerns about the infant's general condition or normality, especially if her pregnancy was complicated or if a previous baby was not healthy.

During the first few days after her child's birth, the new mother applies herself to the task of getting to know her baby. This is termed the **acquaintance phase**. If the infant gives clear behavioral cues about needs, the infant's responses to mothering will be predictable, which will make the mother feel effective and competent. Other behaviors that make an infant more attractive to caretakers are smiling, grasping a finger, nursing eagerly, and being easy to console.

During this time, the newborn also is becoming acquainted. Within a few days after birth, infants show signs of recognizing recurrent situations and responding to changes in routine. To the extent that their mother is their world, it can be said that they are actively acquainting themselves with her.

During the **phase of mutual regulation**, mother and infant seek to determine the degree of control each will exert in their relationship. In this phase of adjustment, a balance is sought between the needs of the mother and the needs of the infant. The most important consideration is that each should obtain a good measure of enjoyment from the interaction. During this phase, negative maternal feelings are likely to surface or intensify. Because "everyone knows that mothers love their babies," these negative feelings often go unexpressed and are allowed to build up. If they are expressed, the response of friends, relatives, or healthcare personnel is often to deny the feelings to the mother: "You don't mean that." Some negative feelings are normal in the first few days after birth, and the nurse should be supportive when the mother vocalizes these feelings.

When mother and infant primarily enjoy each other's company, reciprocity has been achieved. Reciprocity is an interactional cycle that occurs simultaneously between mother and infant. It involves mutual cuing behaviors, expectancy, rhythmicity, and synchrony. The mother develops a new relationship with an individual who has a unique character and evokes a response entirely different from the fantasy response of pregnancy. When reciprocity is synchronous, the interaction between mother and infant is mutually gratifying and is sought and initiated by both.

FATHER–INFANT INTERACTIONS In Western cultures, commitment to family-centered maternity care has fostered interest in understanding the feelings and experiences of the new father. Evidence suggests that the father has a strong attraction to his newborn and that the feelings he experiences are similar to the mother's feelings of attachment. The father's characteristic sense of absorption, preoccupation, and interest in the infant demonstrated during early contact is termed **engrossment**. Differences in involvement still exist among fathers in Western culture and may be influenced by factors other than

culture (e.g., previous experience with paternal role or exposure to male/father role models).

SIBLINGS AND OTHERS Infants are capable of maintaining a number of strong attachments without loss of quality. These attachments may include siblings, grandparents, aunts, and uncles. The social setting and personality of the individual seem to be significant factors in the development of multiple attachments. Birth centers are especially geared toward the family's inclusion in the birth process. In the hospital setting, the advent of open visiting hours and rooming-in permits siblings and others to participate in the attachment process.

Cultural Influences in the Postpartum Period

Whereas Western culture places primary emphasis on the events of birth, many other cultures place greater emphasis on the postpartum period. For women who are not from the dominant American culture, the new mother's culture and personal values influence her beliefs about her postpartum care. Her expectations about food, fluids, rest, hygiene, medications and relief measures, support, and counsel—as well as other aspects of her life—are influenced by the beliefs and values of her family and cultural group. Sometimes a new mother's preferences differ from the expectations of the certified nurse-midwife, physician, or nurse. Nurses must assess each mother's preferences let the mother exercise her choices whenever possible, and provide support for those choices.

Although describing particular practices of different cultural groups involves some generalization, it is helpful for nurses to understand some of the possible differences in beliefs and practices. Women of European heritage may expect to eat a full meal and have large amounts of iced fluids after the birth, in the belief that the food restores energy and the fluids help replace fluid lost during labor. They may want to ambulate shortly after the birth, shower, wash their hair, and put on a fresh gown. They may expect a short stay in the hospital and may or may not be interested in educational classes. Women of the Islamic faith may have specific modesty requirements: The woman must be completely covered, with only her feet and hands exposed, and no man, other than the husband or a family member, may be alone with her (Al-Oballi Kridli, 2002; Lauderdale, 2008).

In many cultures, the extended family plays an essential role during the puerperium. The grandmother is often the primary helper to the mother and newborn. She brings wisdom and experience, allowing the new mother time to rest and giving her ready access to someone who can help with problems and concerns as they arise. It is important to ensure that all family members have access to the mother and newborn, with the prior permission of the mother. Visiting hours may be waived to allow family members or authority figures access to the mother and newborn. These practices show respect and foster a blending of old and new behaviors to meet the goals of all concerned (Purnell & Paulanka, 2012). African American mothers model their mothering skills after their older female relatives. In addition, these same older female relatives usually provide needed child care (Purnell & Paulanka, 2012). People of Jewish faith observe a Sabbath from sundown Friday to sundown Saturday. During this time, Orthodox Jews do not perform any manual labor. Further, they may not request that anyone perform labor on their behalf. For the postpartum woman who is an Orthodox Jew, this includes turning the lights on and off, pressing the call bell, or raising/lowering the head of the bed (Gebers, 2003). Nurses may need to assess client comfort more frequently and intervene to assist clients of the Jewish faith. Jewish clients also may request a Kosher diet.

Postpartum Blues

As stated previously, the postpartum blues represent the transient period of depression that occurs in as many as 50%–75% of women during the first few days following labor (Beck, 2008b, 2008c). Postpartum blues may be manifested by mood swings, anger, weepiness, anorexia, difficulty sleeping, and a feeling of letdown. This mood change frequently occurs while the woman is still hospitalized, but it may occur at home as well. Changing hormone levels are a factor; psychological adjustments, an unsupportive environment, and insecurity also have been identified as potential causes. In addition, fatigue, discomfort, and overstimulation may play a role. The postpartum blues usually resolve naturally within 10–14 days, but if symptoms persist or worsen, the woman may need evaluation for postpartum depression. Ideally, a depression assessment should be completed each trimester to update a pregnant woman's risk status (Beck, 2002). If an assessment was not done previously, the nurse assesses the woman for predisposing factors during labor and the postpartum stay. Several depression scales are available for assessing postpartum depression. The routine use of a screening tool such as the Edinburgh Postnatal Depression Scale or Postpartum Depression Predictors Inventory–Revised significantly increases the diagnosis (Beck, 2008a).

A key feature of postpartum blues is episodic tearfulness, often without an identifiable cause. Often when the woman is asked why she is crying, she responds that she does not know. Cunningham et al. (2010) speculate that several factors contribute to the blues:

- Emotional letdown that follows labor and childbirth
- Physical discomfort typical in the early postpartum period
- Fatigue
- Anxiety about caring for the newborn after discharge
- Depression during pregnancy or previous depression unrelated to pregnancy
- Severe PMS (premenstrual syndrome).

Validating the existence of this phenomenon, labeling it as a real but normal adjustment reaction, and providing reassurance can offer a measure of relief. Assistance with self-care and infant care, rest, good nutrition, information, and family support aids recovery. The partner should be encouraged to watch for and report signs that the new mother is not returning to a normal mood, but is slipping into a deeper depression.

IMPORTANCE OF SOCIAL SUPPORT   The psychological outcomes of the postpartum period are far more positive when the parents have access to a support network. Women and their partners may find that family relationships become increasingly important, but the increased family interaction itself can be a source of stress. New parents also may have increasing contact with other parents of small children but find that contact with coworkers declines. Of great concern are women and their partners who have no family or friends with whom to form a social network. Isolation at a time when the woman feels an increased need for support can result in tremendous stress and is often a contributing factor in situations of postpartum depression, child neglect, or abuse. New mother support groups are helpful for women who lack a social support system.

Postpartum doulas can be of great help during this critical time. Doulas are professionals trained to help the new mother after the birth of the baby. As a "mother helper," postpartum doula services are tailored to help the new mother feel as rested as possible and well nourished and to place her household in good order so that she can focus her energy on her new baby.

▶ POSTPARTUM MOOD DISORDERS

Postpartum Depression

Postpartum depression, or major depressive disorder with peripartum onset, is major depression that occurs during or in the first 4 weeks following birth. It has an overall prevalence rate of 3% to 6% in women during pregnancy or in the first 4 weeks following delivery (APA, 2013, p. 186). Postpartum depression may or may not be accompanied by psychotic symptoms.

Many of the symptoms of this major depression are indistinguishable from serious depression at other times in life: sadness, frequent crying, insomnia or excessive sleeping, appetite change, difficulty concentrating or making decisions, feelings of worthlessness, obsessive thoughts of inadequacy as an individual and parent, lack of interest in activities that are usually associated with pleasure (including sexual relations), and lack of concern about personal appearance. Persistent anxiety further contributes to the woman's feeling of being out of control. Irritability and hostility toward others, including the newborn, may be evident. Women participating in Beck's qualitative research on postpartum depression described a sense of living their daily life in a sort of fog, from which they believed they would never emerge. Once they improved, they often grieved over the time lost with their newborns while in this "fog." The duration of symptoms varies but as many as half continue to be symptomatic at 6 months or longer. Delayed treatment of major depression is associated with longer duration (Doucet et al., 2009).

RISK FACTORS   Risk factors for postpartum depression include the following:

- Primiparity (first pregnancy)
- Ambivalence about maintaining the pregnancy
- History of postpartum depression or bipolar illness
- Lack of social support
- Lack of a stable and supportive relationship with parents or partner
- The woman's lack of a supportive relationship with her parents, especially her father, as a child
- The woman's dissatisfaction with herself, including body image problems and eating disorders.

Focus on Diversity and Culture Postpartum Depression

Postpartum depression is a universal phenomenon, not restricted to specific cultures. It is seen in both industrialized and nonindustrialized countries (O'Mahoney & Donnelly, 2010).

The gender of an infant may influence the development of postpartum depression. In Sweden, births of boys were associated with recall of postpartum sadness in all ethnicities except those from the Middle East (Lagerberg & Magnusson, 2012; Sylven et al., 2011). Female gender of offspring is "nonpreferred" in Asia (Klainin & Arthur, 2009). Countries such as India, China, and Turkey show a traditional gender preference for male children (Dey & Chaudhuri, 2009). Male offspring are preferred in countries where gender equity is

low (Mills & Begall, 2010). Pakistani women who had already given birth to three female children had a higher mean depression score if the fourth child was female than if it was male (Gul et al., 2011).

An alarming cultural consideration in the United States is the disparity of health care for postpartum depression in low-income women. A study of over 29,000 New Jersey Medicaid recipients found that Black and Latina women were significantly less likely than White women to initiate treatment for postpartum depression. Among those who did, Black and Latina women were less likely than White women to receive follow-up care, continue care, or refill antidepressant prescriptions (Kozhimannil et al., 2011).

Women with postpartum depression are at risk for suicide, most prominently as they enter or exit the deeply depressed state. In a deep depression, the woman is unlikely to be able to plan and carry out suicide. For that reason, signs of improvement in depression should be celebrated with some caution. Whereas the woman with postpartum psychosis may attempt suicide because of illogical thought processes, the woman with major depression attempts suicide because her suffering is so great that dying seems a more favorable option than continuing to live in such pain. She also may attempt suicide to save her newborn from some perceived or real threat—including the possibility that she herself might harm the baby. The risk of suicide is greater in women who have attempted suicide previously, have a specific plan, and can access the means or weapon identified in the plan. The more specific the plan, the greater the probability of an attempt.

GENETIC CONSIDERATIONS   There is increasing support for the gene and environment interaction theory of depression and postpartum depression. Variants in genes that code enzymes affecting serotonin, dopamine, and noradrenalin (neurotransmitters affecting mood) were associated with development of depression in the peripartum period (Doornbos et al., 2009). Several studies implicated a serotonin-related transporter genotype to postpartum depression (Binder et al., 2010; Shapiro, Frasier, & Séguin, 2012). Other studies implicated MAO-related genes in postpartum depression (Corwin et al., 2010). More research is needed to definitively identify the role of specific genes in postpartum depression.

Postpartum Psychosis

Postpartum psychosis (postpartum mood episodes with psychotic features) occurs in 1 in every 500 to 1,000 deliveries (APA, 2013, p. 187). The risk is increased in first deliveries, in women with prior postpartum depression, and in those with a history of depressive or bipolar disorder. Although relatively rare, postpartum psychosis gains considerable national attention when an incident of infanticide occurs. Symptoms include agitation, hyperactivity, insomnia, mood lability, confusion, irrationality, difficulty remembering or concentrating, poor

judgment, delusions, and hallucinations that tend to be related to the infant. With appropriate treatment, 95% of women experience improvement of symptoms within 2–3 months. Recurrence in subsequent pregnancies may be as high as 20%–30%.

Postpartum psychosis is considered an emergency because of the risk of suicide and/or infanticide (Mayo Clinic, 2012a). The psychotic woman may experience delusions or hallucinations that support her perceptions that the infant should not be allowed to live. Illogical thinking or evidence of bonding difficulties may serve as cues to infanticide and suicide risk; however, this assessment is often challenging because of the lucidity seen in some psychotic clients.

▶ COLLABORATION

Women with a history of postpartum psychosis or depression or other risk factors should be referred to a mental health professional for counseling and biweekly visits between the second and sixth week postpartum for evaluation. Medication, individual or group psychotherapy, and practical assistance with child care and other demands of daily life are common treatment measures for both disorders; however, specific therapies may vary. Treatment of postpartum depression is not unlike treatment of any other significant depression: psychotherapy and antidepressant medications, usually selective serotonin reuptake inhibitors. The nurse's responsibilities as part of the healthcare team are discussed in detail in the Nursing Process section.

Diagnostic Tests

The routine use of a screening tool in a matter-of-fact approach significantly improves the diagnosis. The Edinburgh Postnatal Depression Scale (**Box 28–8** ●) and the Postpartum Depression Predictors Inventory (PDPI) (**Box 28–9** ●) are appropriate tools for use in assessing clients for postpartum depression.

Pharmacologic Therapy

The use of antidepressant medications in breastfeeding women is a controversial issue. A recent systematic review

Clinical Manifestations and Therapies **Postpartum Depression**

ETIOLOGY	CLINICAL MANIFESTATIONS	CLINICAL THERAPIES
Postpartum depression	■ Severe depression that occurs within the first year of giving birth, with increased incidence at about the fourth week postpartum, just before menses resumes, and upon weaning	■ Sertraline (Zoloft) or paroxetine (Paxil) ■ Support groups ■ Assistance with care of the newborn, taking care to promote self-confidence in mothering ■ Mental health counseling ■ Assistance with building self-esteem and self-confidence in mothering skills
Postpartum psychosis	■ Agitation ■ Hyperactivity ■ Insomnia ■ Mood lability ■ Confusion ■ Irrationality ■ Difficulty remembering or concentrating ■ Delusions and hallucinations that tend to be related to the infant	■ Lithium or antipsychotics ■ Should be supervised at all times when caring for infant or other children. ■ Support groups ■ Short-term institutionalization may be required.

Box 28–8   Edinburgh Postnatal Depression Scale

In the past 7 days:

1. I have been able to laugh and see the funny side of things.
   As much as I always could
   Not quite so much now
   Definitely not so much now
   Not at all

2. I have looked forward with enjoyment of things.
   As much as I ever did
   Rather less than I used to
   Definitely less than I used to
   Hardly at all

*3. I have blamed myself unnecessarily when things went wrong.
   Yes, most of the time
   Yes, some of the time
   Not very often
   No, never

4. I have been anxious or worried for no good reason.
   No, not at all
   Hardly ever
   Yes, sometimes
   Yes, very often

*5. I have felt scared or panicky for no very good reason.
   Yes, quite a lot
   Yes, sometimes
   No, not much
   No, not at all

*6. Things have been getting on top of me.
   Yes, most of the time I haven't been able to cope at all
   Yes, sometimes I haven't been coping as well as usual
   No, I have been coping quite well
   No, I have been coping as well as ever

*7. I have been so unhappy that I have had difficulty sleeping.
   Yes, most of the time
   Yes, sometimes
   Not very often
   No, not at all

*8. I have felt sad or miserable.
   Yes, most of the time
   Yes, quite often
   Not very often
   No, not at all

*9. I have been so unhappy that I have been crying.
   Yes, most of the time
   Yes, quite often
   Only occasionally
   No, never

*10. The thought of harming myself has occurred to me.
   Yes, quite often
   Sometimes
   Hardly ever
   Never

Note: Response categories are scored 0, 1, 2, and 3 according to increased severity of the symptoms. Items marked with an asterisk are reverse-scored (3, 2, 1, 0). The total score is calculated by adding together the scores for each of the 10 items. A score above the threshold of 12 to 13 out of 30 indicates with 86% sensitivity that the woman is suffering from postpartum depression.

Source: Cox, J. L., Holden, J. M., & Sagovsky, R. (1987). Detection of postnatal depression: Development of the 10-item Edinburgh Postnatal Depression Scale. *British Journal of Psychiatry, 150,* 782–786. Users may reproduce the scale without further permission provided they respect copyright by quoting the names of the authors, the title, and the source of the paper in all reproduced copies.

Box 28–9 Postpartum Depression Predictors Inventory–Revised

DURING PREGNANCY

Marital status	Check One
1. Single	○
2. Married/cohabitating	○
3. Separated	○
4. Divorced	○
5. Widowed	○
6. Partnered	○
Socioeconomic status	○
Low	○
Middle	○
High	○

Self-esteem	Yes	No
Do you feel good about yourself as a person?	○	○
Do you feel worthwhile?	○	○
Do you feel you have a number of good qualities as a person?	○	○
Prenatal depression	○	○

1. Have you felt depressed during your pregnancy?
   If yes, when and how long have you been feeling this way?
   If yes, how mild or severe would you consider your depression?

Prenatal anxiety		
Have you been feeling anxious during your pregnancy?	○	○

If yes, how long have you been feeling this way?

Unplanned/unwanted pregnancy		
Was the pregnancy planned?	○	○
Is the pregnancy unwanted?	○	○

History of previous depression		
1. Before this pregnancy, have you ever been depressed?	○	○
If yes, when did you experience this depression?	○	○
If yes, have you been under a physician's care for this past depression?	○	○
If yes, did the physician prescribe any medication for your depression?	○	○

Social support		
1. Do you feel you receive adequate emotional support from your partner?	○	○
2. Do you feel you receive adequate instrumental support from your partner (e.g., help with household chores or baby-sitting)?	○	○
3. Do you feel you can rely on your partner when you need help?	○	○
4. Do you feel you can confide in your partner? (repeat same questions for family and again for friends)	○	○

Marital satisfaction		
1. Are you satisfied with your marriage (or living arrangement)?	○	○
2. Are you currently experiencing any marital problems?	○	○
3. Are things going well between you and your partner?	○	○

Life stress	Yes	No
1. Are you currently experiencing any stressful events in your life such as:	○	○
Financial problems	○	○
Marital problems	○	○
Death in the family	○	○
Serious illness in the family	○	○
Moving	○	○
Unemployment	○	○
Job change	○	○

(continued on next page)

AFTER DELIVERY, ADD THE FOLLOWING ITEMS

Childcare stress

	Yes	No
1. Is your infant experiencing any health problems?	○	○
2. Are you having problems with your baby feeding?	○	○
3. Are you having problems with your baby sleeping?	○	○

Infant temperament

	Yes	No
1. Would you consider your baby irritable or fussy?	○	○
2. Does your baby cry a lot?	○	○
3. Is your baby difficult to console or soothe?	○	○

Maternity blues

	Yes	No
1. Did you experience a brief period of tearfulness and mood swings during the 1st week after delivery?	○	○

concluded "(1) knowledge of pharmacokinetic characteristics are scarcely useful to assess safety and (2) the majority of antidepressants are not usually contraindicated: (a) Selective serotonin reuptake inhibitors and nortriptyline have a better safety profile during lactation, (b) fluoxetine must be used carefully, (c) the tricyclic doxepin and the atypical nefazodone should better be avoided, and (d) lithium, usually considered as contraindicated, has been recently rehabilitated" (Davanzo et al., 2011, p. 89). Recommendations are that a combination of antidepressants and psychosocial interventions be used regardless of whether or not the woman is breastfeeding. Many of the drugs used in treating postpartum psychiatric conditions may be contraindicated in breastfeeding women. Fluoxetine (e.g., Prozac and Sarafem) is not recommended for lactating women because of its long half-life (Beck, 2008). Some of the antidepressant drugs have been linked to an increase in congenital defects, so birth control also should be emphasized. The woman and her partner should be reminded that antidepressants may take several weeks to have an effect. Providers may prefer to start antidepressants before the birth of the baby (usually at 36 weeks' gestation) so that a therapeutic blood level is achieved before the birth of the baby.

Support Groups

Support groups have proven to be successful adjuncts to such treatment. In a support group of postpartum women and their partners, a couple may feel consolation that they are not alone in their experience. Moreover, the group provides a forum for exchanging information about postpartum depression, learning stress reduction measures, and experiencing renewed self-esteem and support. The most effective support groups provide for safe child care to facilitate attendance. If a support group is not available locally, the woman and her family may be encouraged to contact Depression After Delivery (DAD), now a national Web-based support network that provides education and volunteers, or Postpartum Support International.

Other Therapy

Treatment of postpartum psychosis is directed at the specific type of psychotic symptoms displayed and may include lithium, antipsychotics, or electroconvulsive therapy in combination with psychotherapy, removal of the infant, and social support. It is important for the nurse to realize that many of the drugs used in treating postpartum psychiatric conditions are contraindicated in breastfeeding women. The risks and benefits of treatment options must be considered and discussed with the client and family.

■ NURSING PROCESS

The priority of nursing care for the client with postpartum depression is to maintain safety of both client and family. Nurses may hesitate to assess clients for risk of harm to themselves or others for fear of introducing an idea that had not occurred to the client. Not only is this not the case, but questioning the client's thoughts of harming self or others can actually contribute to saving lives and should be a component of care for any client experiencing depression.

Assessment

Because depression may occur during pregnancy, assessment of risk factors for depression and psychosis should be made early in the pregnancy. Questions designed to detect problems can be included as part of the routine prenatal history interview or questionnaire. Women with a personal or family history of psychiatric disease, particularly postpartum depression or psychosis, need prenatal instructions on the signs and symptoms of depression and may need additional emotional support. Ideally, a depression assessment should be completed each trimester to update a pregnant woman's risk status (Beck, 2002). If one was not done previously, the nurse assesses the woman for predisposing factors during labor and the postpartum stay.

No matter what approach the nurse uses to assess for postpartum depression, enabling the woman to voice her feelings of maternal role transition and how she is adjusting in this vulnerable time is of inestimable value (Beck, 2008). Listening to her story provides a critical emic (insider's) view of her circumstances as opposed to an etic (outsider's) view.

In providing daily care, the nurse observes the woman for objective signs of depression—anxiety, irritability, poor concentration, forgetfulness, sleep difficulties, appetite change, fatigue, and tearfulness—and listens for statements indicating feelings of failure and self-accusation. Severity and duration of symptoms should be noted. Behavior and verbalizations that are bizarre or seem to indicate a potential for violence against herself or others, including the infant, are reported as soon as possible for further evaluation.

The nurse needs to be aware that many normal physiological changes of the puerperium are similar to symptoms of depression (lack of sexual interest, appetite change, fatigue). It is essential that observations be as specific and as objective as possible and that they be carefully documented. Beck and Indman (2005) found that anxiety was a prominent feature of illness for some women and suggested that women be assessed for their level of anxiety, particularly regarding infant care. Because of the strong association of interrupted sleep and postpartum depression and the finding that severe fatigue was an excellent predictor of postpartum depression (Corwin et al., 2005), assessing fatigue level at 2 weeks postpartum by telephone may be helpful in predicting depression risk early. Restorative sleep improves a woman's ability to cope and make decisions, thereby producing a sense of better self-control.

A central challenge for nursing is identifying women at risk of suicide. Asking the client directly if she has thoughts of self-harm is best. If the client responds "yes," the client must be screened by a qualified mental health professional as soon as possible; she is not left alone until this has been accomplished. Family members of the depressed woman also should be alert to signals that she may be intent on self-harm; they must be advised that threats are to be taken seriously. Contact information for community mental health and crisis resources should be given to both the client and family, along with the National Suicide Hotline toll-free number. Family members should be told to be especially vigilant for suicide when the woman seems to be feeling better.

Diagnosis

Possible nursing diagnoses that may apply to a woman with a postpartum psychiatric disorder include the following:

- *Ineffective Coping*
- *Risk for Impaired Parenting*
- *Risk for Violence, Self-Directed*
- *Risk for Violence, Other-Directed*

(NANDA-I © 2012)

Planning

Appropriate goals for the woman experiencing postpartum depression may include the following:

- The client and family will remain free of injury.
- Family members and support persons will provide appropriate care for the newborn.

- The client will articulate feelings and concerns.
- The client will adhere to the plan of care.
- The client will integrate the newborn into the family (with assistance as appropriate).

Implementation

Nurses working in antepartum settings (including the pediatrician's office) or teaching childbirth classes play indispensable roles in helping prospective parents appreciate the lifestyle changes and role demands associated with parenthood. Offering realistic information and anticipatory guidance and debunking myths about the perfect mother or perfect newborn may help prevent postpartum depression. Social support teaching guides are available for nurses to use in helping postpartum women explore their needs for postpartum support.

- Alert the mother, spouse, and other family members to the possibility of postpartum blues in the early days after birth and reassure them of the short-term nature of the condition.
- Describe symptoms of postpartum depression and encourage the mother to call her healthcare provider if symptoms become severe, if they fail to subside quickly, or if at any time she feels she is unable to function.
- Encourage the mother to plan how she will manage at home and provide concrete suggestions on how to cope in her adjustment to motherhood.

In all postpartum women, the presence of three symptoms of depression on 1 day or one symptom for 3 days may signal serious depression and requires immediate referral to a mental health professional. Make an immediate referral if rejection of the infant or threatened or actual aggression against the infant has occurred. In such cases, the newborn is never left unattended with the mother. Depression does appear to interfere with optimal mothering; there is less interaction between mother and child, an increased incidence of mood and cognitive development problems, and more visits to the physician in children whose mothers experience depression (Beck, 2002).

A diagnosis of postpartum depression or other psychiatric disorder poses major problems for the family, especially the father. The symptoms of these disorders are difficult to witness and may be harder to understand than physical problems such as hemorrhage and infection. The father may feel hurt by his partner's hostility; worry that she is becoming insane; or be baffled by her mood swings and lack of concern about herself, the newborn, or household responsibilities. He may be troubled by their lack of intimacy or deteriorating communication. Certainly, he has cause for concern about how the newborn and any other children are being affected. Very real practical matters—running the household; managing the children, including the totally dependent newborn; and caring for the mother—may be added to his usual routines and work responsibilities. It is not surprising that even in the most supportive families, relationships may suffer in response to these circumstances. It is often the father or another close family member who, in desperation, makes contact with the healthcare agency. This is especially difficult when the mother is reluctant to

Evidence-Based Practice   Prevention of, Identification of, and Interventions for Postpartum Depression

Problem

How can the risk of postpartum depression be identified early in a pregnancy? What is the most effective way to prevent postpartum depression? When it occurs, how can it be treated?

Evidence

Postpartum depression is a serious condition that occurs in the first 12 weeks after birth; approximately 13% of new mothers will experience it. Untreated, the condition may have consequences for mothers, infants, and their families. It often goes undetected, as symptoms may be hidden or misinterpreted. A team of advanced practice nurses developed recommendations for AWHONN, the professional association for nurses practicing in women's and neonatal health (McQueen et al., 2008). Their recommendations focused on identification and prevention of depression and were based on a systematic review of research and expert opinion. Other evidence included a meta-analysis of studies focused on effective treatment of postnatal depression (Bledsoe & Grote, 2006). This type of integrative review provides the strongest evidence for practice. Further evidence comes from Sit and Wisner (2009) in their paper on identifying postpartum depression.

The strongest evidence supported individualized, flexible postpartum care that focused on the identification of risk for depression and/or signs of depression early in the pregnancy. Routine screening for depression should be part of the prenatal and postnatal assessment. A rating on the Edinburgh Postnatal Depression Scale of ≥13 was determined to be an acceptable cut-point for identifying women at risk for major depression (Sit & Wisner, 2009). The best outcomes are achieved when early preventive strategies accompany depression screening. When depression symptoms appear, supportive weekly interactions and ongoing assessment focused on mental health needs should be part of the routine postnatal treatment plan. Peer support (via technology or group) can help mediate depressive symptoms and encourage problem solving. Standard instruments should be used to identify mothers who are at risk for depression so that they can be referred to their primary care physician or a specialist in mental health for treatment.

Although various methods were shown to be effective in treating postnatal depression, no one therapy emerged as a definitive treatment.

Implications

Nurses are in a particularly good position to screen mothers for depression during the prenatal period and for at least 12 weeks after birth. You should use a standard instrument for screening at each encounter, and increased risk of depression should be cause for referral to a medical provider. Early detection and prevention will produce better outcomes for the mother, baby, and family. Diverse treatments—both pharmaceutical and counseling based—have been shown to be effective in mediating the symptoms of depression. The treatment program should be matched to the specific client characteristics and needs.

Critical Thinking Application

1. Why do you think providing early prevention strategies with early screening for depression improves client outcomes?

2. What advantages might "supportive weekly interactions" offer?

3. Why does postpartum care need to be individualized and flexible?

Community-Based Care   Primary Prevention Strategies for Postpartum Depression

Nurses can encourage new mothers and parents to participate in a number of strategies to help prevent postpartum depression. Suggestions include the following:

- Celebrate childbirth but appreciate that it is a life-changing transition that can be stressful—at times it can seem overwhelming. Share your feelings with your partner and/or others.

- Consider keeping a journal in which you write down feelings. It not only is emotionally cathartic, but also provides a great memory book.

- Appreciate that you do not have to know everything to be a good parent—it is okay to seek advice during this transition.

- Connect to others who are parents—use them as a support and information network.

- Set a daily schedule and follow it even if you do not feel like it. Structuring activity helps counteract the inertia that comes with feeling sad or unsettled.

- Prioritize daily tasks. Decide what must be done and what can wait. Try to get one major thing done every day.

- Remember that you do not have to entertain or care for everyone who drops by. Doing something for someone else, however, often tends to make you feel better.

- If someone volunteers to lend a hand with tasks or baby care, accept the person's help. While your volunteer is in action, do something pleasurable or get some rest.

- Maintain outside interests. Plan some time every day—even if it is just 15 minutes—to do something exclusively for you that is pleasurable.

- Eat a healthful diet. Limit alcohol. Quit smoking. Get some exercise. (All of these can positively affect the immune system.)

- Get as much sleep as possible. Rest whenever you can, such as when the baby is napping. If you have other young children, bring them onto your bed to read or play quietly while you lie down.

- If things get overwhelming and you feel yourself slipping into depression, reach out to someone for help.

- Attend a postpartum support group if one is available. Also consider an international program such as Postpartum Support International, which provides an emergency contact phone number at 1-800-944-4PPD as well as a Web site at http://postpartum.net.

admit she is suffering emotional difficulty or is too ill to recognize her own needs.

Information, emotional support, and assistance in providing or obtaining care for the infant may be needed. The nurse can assist family members by identifying community resources, making referrals to public health nursing services and social services, and providing a list of telephone numbers as well as emergency services that the mother may need. Postpartum follow-up is especially important, as are visits from a psychiatric home health nurse.

Evaluation

Expected outcomes of nursing care include the following:

- The client's signs of depression are identified and she receives prompt intervention.
- The newborn is effectively cared for by the father or other support persons until the mother is able to provide care.
- The mother and newborn remain safe.
- The newborn is successfully integrated into the family unit.

NURSING CARE PLAN   A Client With Postpartum Depression

ASSESSMENT

Salma al-Hussein, a 30-year-old woman who was born in Jordan but has lived in the United States for nearly 20 years, is brought to her primary care provider's office by her mother. Ms. al-Hussein gave birth to her third child nearly 6 weeks ago. Her mother is worried because her daughter is showing almost no interest in the baby and very little interest in her older children. Ms. al-Hussein's mother and sister have been providing most of the care for the children. At first, Ms. al-Hussein is slow to answer the nurse's questions and keeps her eyes on the floor during the assessment. Ms. al-Hussein's mother says that her daughter is not normally like this, that she is usually full of life and outgoing and polite with others, even those she does not know well. With the encouragement of her mother, Ms. al-Hussein becomes more cooperative. The nurse uses the Edinburgh Postnatal Depression Scale; Ms. al-Hussein scores 14 out of 30.

DIAGNOSES

- *Impaired Parenting*
- *Risk for Powerlessness*
- *Impaired Social Interaction*
- *Ineffective Coping*

(NANDA-I © 2012)

PLANNING

- The client will commit to safety.
- The client will express her feelings.
- The client will agree to participate in mental health counseling.
- The family will continue to provide care for the children and support Ms. al-Hussein as she begins the treatment process.

IMPLEMENTATION

- Refer to mental health professional.
- Attempt to persuade Ms. al-Hussein to commit to safety for both herself and the children.
- Teach family to supervise mother's interaction with the infant and other children at all times to promote safety.
- Explain impact of postpartum depression to the family and help them cope with the impact on the family.
- Identify community resources for assisting with treatment.

- Encourage family to continue providing care for the infant and other children.
- Help Ms. al-Hussein to recognize the signs of depression and accept the diagnosis of postpartum depression.
- Explain to both Ms. al-Hussein and her family members that postpartum depression is not uncommon and can be successfully treated but risk for reoccurrence is high if she has other children.

EVALUATION

Ms. al-Hussein's care is evaluated based on the following expected outcomes:
- The client begins treatment with a mental health counselor and is taking her prescribed medications regularly.
- Family members continue to provide supervision and care of the children until Salma's condition improves.
- The client commits to safety for herself and her children.

CRITICAL THINKING

1. How would you persuade Ms. al-Hussein to commit to safety for herself and her children?
2. What specific questions would you ask to determine if Ms. al-Hussein is thinking about harming herself or her children?
3. If Ms. al-Hussein admitted having fantasies of harming her children, how could you advocate for the family?

◣ REVIEW Postpartum Depression

RELATE Link the Concepts and Exemplars

Linking the exemplar of postpartum depression with the concept of development:

1. How might a mother's postpartum depression impact the development of her 3-year-old daughter?
2. What is your priority developmental concern for the newborn when the mother has severe postpartum depression?

Linking the exemplar of postpartum depression with the concept of comfort:

3. What are your concerns for the mother who has postpartum depression regarding sleep and rest?
4. How will fatigue impact postpartum depression and the care of the newborn?

READY Go to Companion Skills Manual

REFER Go to Pearson Nursing Student Resources
nursing.pearsonhighered.com

- Additional review materials

REFLECT Case Study

Jessica Riley is a single 17-year-old new mother of a 1-month-old infant son named Ryan whose father ended his relationship with Jessica when she was 4 months pregnant. Jessica's relationship with her mother has been strained for the past few years and worsened when she became pregnant. Because she was constantly fighting with her mother, Jessica moved to a small apartment when she was 6 months pregnant. Jessica's father left the family when Jessica was 7 years old. She recently completed her GED and is now trying to go to school part time for an associate's degree in cosmetology. She also works nearly full time as a waitress, but because she is supporting herself and her baby, she struggles financially.

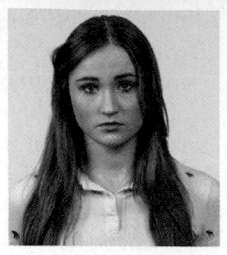

1. What information in Jessica's history puts her at risk for postpartum depression?
2. How would you assess Jessica for potential postpartum depression?
3. What interventions can you implement to reduce Jessica's risk of postpartum depression?

■ REFERENCES

aan het Rot, M., Collins, K.,& Fitterling, H. (2009). Physical exercise and depression *Mount Sinai Journal of Medicine, 76*(2), 204–214.

Adams, M., Holland, N., & Urban, C. (2014). *Pharmacology for nurses: A pathophysiologic approach.* Upper Saddle River, NJ: Pearson Education.

Al-Oballi Kridli, S. (2002). Health beliefs and practices among Arab women. *American Journal of Maternal Child Nursing, 27*(3), 178–182.

Allan, C. L., & Ebmeier, K. P. (2011). The use of ECT and MST in treating depression. *International Review of Psychiatry, 23*(5), 400–412.

American Association of Suicidology. (2013). *Suicide in the USA based on 2010 data.* Retrieved from http://www.suicidology.org.

American Cancer Society. (2008). *Art therapy.* Retrieved from http://www.cancer.org/treatment/treatmentsand-sideeffects/complementaryandalternativemedicine/mindbodyandspirit/art-therapy.

American Psychiatric Association. (2013). *Diagnostic and statistical manual of mental disorders* (5th ed.). Washington, DC: American Psychiatric Publishing.

Anderson, E. L., & Reti, I. M. (2009). ECT in pregnancy: A review of the literature from 1941 to 2007. *Psychosomatic Medicine, 71*, 235–242.

Andreazza, A. C., Shao, L., Wang, J. F., & Young, L. T. (2010). Mitochondrial complex I activity and oxidative damage to mitochondrial proteins in the prefrontal cortex of patients with bipolar disorder. *Archives of General Psychiatry, 67*(4), 360–368.

Aroian, K. J., & Norris, A. (2002). Assessing risk for depression among immigrants at two-year follow-up. *Archives of Psychiatric Nursing, 16*(6), 245–253.

Badner, J. A. (2003). The genetics of bipolar disorder. In B. Geller & M. P. Delbello (Eds.), *Bipolar disorder in childhood and early adolescence* (pp. 247–254). New York, NY: Guilford Press.

Basch, E. M., & Ulbricht, C. E. (2005). *Natural standard: Herb & supplement handbook.* St. Louis, MO: Elsevier Mosby.

Beck, A. T., Ward, C. H., Mendelson, M., Mock, J., & Erbaugh, J. (1961). Inventory for measuring depression. *Archives of General Psychiatry, 4*, 561–571.

Beck, C. T. (2002). Revision of the Postpartum Depression Predictors Inventory. *Journal of Obstetric, Gynecologic, and Neonatal Nursing, 31*(4), 394–402.

Beck, C. T. (2008a). *Postpartum mood and anxiety disorders: Case studies, research, and nursing care* (2nd ed.). Washington, DC: Association of Women's Health, Obstetric and Neonatal Nurses.

Beck, C. T. (2008b). State of the science on postpartum depression: What nurse researchers have contributed—Part 1. *American Journal of Maternal Child Nursing, 33*(2), 121–126.

Beck, C. T. (2008c). State of the science on postpartum depression: What nurse researchers have contributed—Part 2. *American Journal of Maternal Child Nursing, 33*(3), 151–156.

Beck, C. T., & Indman, P. (2005). The many faces of depression. *Journal of Obstetric, Gynecologic, and Neonatal Nursing, 34*(5), 569–576.

Beyond the "baby blues": Postpartum depression is common and treatable. (2011). *Harvard Medical Letter, 28*(3), 1–3.

Bhui, K., & Dinos, S. (2011). Preventive psychiatry: A paradigm to improve population mental health and well-being. *British Journal of Psychiatry, 198*, 417–419.

Binder, E. B., Jeffrey Newport, D., Zach, E. B., Smith, A. K., Deveau, T. C., Altshuler L., … Cubells, J. F. (2010). A serotonin transporter gene polymorphism predicts peripartum depressive symptoms in an at-risk psychiatric cohort. *Journal of Psychiatric Research, 44*(10), 640–646.

Blazer, D. G. (2009). Depression in late life: Review and commentary. *FOCUS, 7*(1), 118–136.

Bledsoe, S., & Grote, N. (2006). Treating depression during pregnancy and the postpartum: A preliminary meta-analysis. *Research on Social Work Practice, 16*, 109–120.

Borner, I., Braunstein, J., St. Victor, R., & Pollack, J. (2010). Evaluation of a 2-question screening tool for detecting depression in adolescents in primary care. *Clinical Pediatrics, 49*(10), 947–953.

Bridge, J., Iyengar, S., Salary, C., Barbe, R., Birmaher, B., Pincus, H., … Brent, D. (2007). Clinical response and risk for reported suicidal ideation and suicide attempts in pediatric antidepressant treatment: A meta-analysis of randomized controlled trials. *Journal of the American Medical Association, 297*, 1683–1696.

Caicoppo, J. T., Reis, H. T., & Zautra, A. J. (2011). Social resilience: The value of social fitness with an application to the military. *American Psychologist, 66*(1), 43–51.

Caetano, S. C., Kaur, S., Brambilla, P., Nicoletti, M., Hatch, J. P., Sassi, R. B., … Soares, J. C. (2006). Smaller cingulated volumes in unipolar depressed patients. *Biological Psychiatry, 59*(8), 702–706.

Centers for Disease Control and Prevention (CDC). (2013). *An estimated 1 in 10 U.S. adults report depression.* Retrieved from http://www.cdc.gov/features/dsdepression.

Coccaro, E., Ong, A., Seroczynski, A., & Bergeman, C. (2012). Affective intensity and lability: Heritability in adult male twins. *Journal of Affective Disorders, 136*(3), 1011–1106.

Cornwell, Y. (2009) Suicide prevention in later life: A glass half full, or half empty? *American Journal of Psychiatry, 166*(8), 845–849.

Corwin, E. J., Brownstead, J., Barton, N., Heckard, S., & Merin, K. (2005). The impact of fatigue on the development of postpartum depression. *Journal of Obstetric, Gynecologic, and Neonatal Nursing, 34* (5), 577–586.

Corwin, E., Kohen, R., Jarrett, M., & Stafford, B. (2010). The heritability of postpartum depression. *Biological Research for Nursing, 12*(1), 73–83.

Culture and depression. (2008). *Science Daily.* Retrieved from http://www.sciencedaily.com/releases/2008/07/080715071401.htm.

Cunningham, F. G., Leveno, K. J., Bloom, S. L., Hauth, J. C., Gilstrap, L. C., & Wenstrom, K. D. (2010). *Williams obstetrics* (23rd ed.). New York, NY: McGraw-Hill.

Darowski, A., Chambers, S., & Chambers, D. (2009). Antidepressants and falls in the elderly. *Drugs and Aging, 26*(5), 381–394.

Davanzo, R., Copertino, M., De Cunto, A., Minen, F., & Amaddeo, A. (2011). Antidepressant medications and breastfeeding: A review of the literature. *Breastfeeding Medicine, 6*(2), 89–98.

Davé, S., Petersen, I., Sherr, L., & Nazareth, I. (2012). Incidence of maternal and paternal depression in primary care: A cohort study using a primary care database. *Archives of Pediatrics & Adolescent Medicine, 164*(11), 1038–1044.

Dey, I., & Chaudhuri, R. (2009). Gender preference and its implications on reproductive behavior of mothers in a rural area of West Bengal. *Indian Journal of Community Medicine, 34*, 65–67.

Doornbos, B., Dijck-Brouwer, D., Kema, I., Tanke, M., van Goor, S., Muskiet, F., & Korf, J. (2009). The development of peripartum depressive symptoms is associated with gene polymorphisms of MAOA, 5-HTT and COMT. *Progress in Neuro-Psychopharmacology & Biological Psychiatry, 33*(7), 1250–1254.

Doucet, S., Dennis, C. L., Letourneau, N., & Blackmore, E. R. (2009). Differentiation and clinical implications of postpartum depression and postpartum psychosis. *Journal of Obstetric, Gynecologic, and Neonatal Nursing, 38*(3), 269–279.

Faraone, S. V., Glatt, S. J., Su, J., & Tsuang, M. T. (2004). Three potential susceptibility loci shown by a genome-wide scan for regions influencing the age at onset of mania. *American Journal of Psychiatry, 161*(4), 625–630.

Fisfalen, M. E., Schulze, T. G., DePaulo, J. R., DeGroot, L. J., Badner, J. A., & McMahon, F. J. (2005). Familial variation in episode frequency in bipolar affective disorder. *American Journal of Psychiatry, 162*(7), 1266–1272.

Frazier, J. A., Chiu, S., Breeze, J. L., Makris, N., Lange, N., Kennedy, D. N., … Biederman, J. (2005). Structural brain magnetic resonance imaging of limbic and thalamic volumes in pediatric bipolar disorder. *American Journal of Psychiatry, 162*(7), 1256–1265.

Friedman, M., Resick, P., Bryant, R., Strain, J., Horowitz, M., & Spiegel, D. (2011). Classification of trauma and stressor-related disorders in DSM-V. *Depression and Anxiety, 28*(9), 737–749.

Gaudiano, B. A., & Miller, I. W. (2006). Patients' expectancies, the alliance in pharmacotherapy, and treatment outcomes in bipolar disorder. *Journal of Consulting and Clinical Psychology, 74*(4), 671–676.

Gebers, L. (2003). Care of the Orthodox Jewish patient. *Advance for Nurses.* Retrieved from http://nursing.advanceweb.com/Article/Care-of-the-Orthodox-Jewish-Patient.aspx.

Gill, A., Womack, R., & Safranen, E. (2010). Does exercise alleviate symptoms of depression? *Journal of Family Practice, 59*(9), 530–531.

Gjerdingen, D., Crow, S., McGovern, P., Miner, M., & Center B. (2009). Postpartum depression screening at well-child visits: Validity of a 2-question screen and the PHQ-9. *Annals of Family Medicine, 7*(1), 63–70.

Goren, J. L., Stoll, A. L., Damico, K. E., Sarmiento, I. A., & Cohen, B. M. (2004). Bioavailability and lack of toxicity of s-adenosyl-l-methionine (SAMe) in humans. *Pharmacotherapy, 24*(11), 1501–1507.

Gul, M., Bajwa, S., Niaz, S., Haroon, M., Liaqat, S., Ahmad, M., . . . Late, H. (2011). Postnatal depression and its comparison with the gender of newborn in fourth pregnancy. *International Journal of Culture and Mental Health.* doi:10.1080/17542863.2011.602543.

Hart, L. A. (2000). Psychosocial benefits of animal companionship. In A. H. Fine (Ed.), *Handbook on animal-assisted therapy* (pp. 59–78). San Diego, CA: Academic Press.

Hesse, M. (2009). Integrated psychological treatment for substance use and co-morbid anxiety or depression vs. treatment for substance use alone. A systematic review of the published literature. *BMC Psychiatry, 9*, 6.

Hirschfeld, R., Williams, B., Spitzer, R., Calabrese, R., Flynn, L., Keck, P., . . . Zajecka, J., (2000). Development and validation of a screening instrument for bipolar spectrum disorder: The Mood Disorder Questionnaire. *American Journal of Psychiatry, 157*(11), 1873–1875.

Hvas, A. M., Juul, S., Bech, P., & Nexo, E. (2004). Vitamin B$_6$ level is associated with symptoms of depression. *Psychotherapy and Psychosomatics, 73*(6), 340–343.

Joseph, A. (2006). *The impact of light on outcomes in healthcare settings.* Concord California Center for Health Design, Issue Paper #2.

Kabat-Zinn, J. (2003). Mindful yoga movement & meditation. *Yoga International, 70*, 86–93.

Kessler, R., Chiu, W., Demler, O., & Walters, E. (2005). Prevalence, severity, and comorbidity of twelve-month DSM-IV disorders in the National Comorbidity Survey Replication (NCS-R). *Archives of General Psychiatry, 62*(6), 617–627.

Klainin, P., & Arthur, D. (2009). Postpartum depression in Asian cultures: A literature review. *International Journal of Nursing Studies, 46*, 1355–1373.

Ko, J., Farr, S., Dietz, P., & Robbins, C. (2012). Depression and treatment among U.S. pregnant and nonpregnant women of reproductive age, 2005–2009. *Journal of Women's Health, 21*(8), 830–836.

Kozhimannil, K. B., Trinacty, C. M., Busch, A. B., Huskamp, H. A., & Adams, A. S. (2011). Racial and ethnic disparities in postpartum depression care among low-income women. *Psychiatric Services, 62*(6), 619–625.

Kroenke, K., Spitzer, R., & Williams, J. (2003). The Patient Health Questionnaire-2: Validity of a two-item depression screener. *Medical Care, 41*(11), 1284–1292.

Lagerberg, D., & Magnusson, M. (2012). Infant gender and postpartum sadness in the light of region of birth and some other factors: A contribution to the knowledge of postpartum depression. *Archives of Women's Mental Health, 15*, 121–130.

Larzelere, M. M., & Wiseman, P. (2002). Anxiety, depression, and insomnia. *Primary Care, 29*(2), 339–360.

Lau, J. Y. F., & Eley, T. C. (2010). The genetics of mood disorders. *Annual Review of Clinical Psychology, 6*, 313–337. doi:10.1146/annurev.clinpsy.121208.131308.

Lauderdale, J. (2008). Transcultural perspectives in child bearing. In M. M. Andrews & J. S. Boyle (Eds.), *Transcultural concepts in nursing care* (5th ed.). Philadelphia, PA: Lippincott Williams & Wilkins.

Lee, S., Tsang, A., Kessler, R., Jin, R., Sampson, N., Andrade, L., . . . Petukhova, M. (2010). Rapid-cycling bipolar disorder: Cross-national community study. *British Journal of Psychiatry,196*, 217–225.

Lewinsohn, P. M., Seeley, J. R., Roberts, R. E., & Allen, N. B. (1997). Center for Epidemiological Studies-Depression Scale (CES-D) as a screening instrument for depression among community-residing older adults. *Psychology and Aging, 12*, 277–287.

Lu, W., Mueser, K. T., Rosenberg, S., & Jankowsi, M. K. (2008). Correlates of adverse childhood experiences among adults with severe mood disorders. *Psychiatric Services, 59*(9), 1018–1026. doi:10.1176/appi.ps.59.9.1018.

Mayo Clinic. (2012a). *Postpartum depression.* Retrieved from http://www.mayoclinic.com/health/postpartum-depression/DS00546/DSECTION=symptoms.

Mayo Clinic. (2012b). *Seasonal affective disorder.* Retrieved from http://www.mayoclinic.com/health/seasonal-affective-disorder/DS00195.

McQueen, K., Montgomery, P., Lappan-Gracon, S., Evans, M., & Hunter, J. (2008). Evidence-based recommendations for depressive symptoms in postpartum women. *Journal of Obstetric, Gynecologic, and Neonatal Nursing, 37*, 127–136.

Mercer, R. T. (1995). *Becoming a mother.* New York, NY: Springer.

Mercer, R. T. (2004). Becoming a mother versus maternal role attainment. *Journal of Nursing Scholarship, 36*(3), 226–232.

Merikangas, K., He, J., Burstein, M., Swanson, S., Avenevoli, S., Cui, L., . . . Swendsen, J. (2010). Lifetime prevalence of mental disorders in U.S. adolescents: Results from the National Comorbidity Study-Adolescent Supplement (NCS-A). *Journal of the American Academy of Child & Adolescent Psychiatry, 49*(10), 980–989.

Meyer, J. H., McMain, S., Kennedy, S. H., Brown, G. M., DaSilva, J. N., Wilson, A. A., . . . Links, J. (2003). Dysfunctional attitudes and 5-HT2 receptors during depression and self-harm. *American Journal of Psychiatry, 160*(1), 90–99.

Mills, M., & Begall, K. (2010). Preferences for the sex-composition of children in Europe: A multilevel examination of its effect on progression to a third child. *Population Studies 64*, 77–95.

National Alliance on Mental Illness (NAMI). (2008). *Getting an accurate diagnosis for your child: 10 steps for families.* Retrieved from http://www.nami.org/Template.cfm?Section=Child_and_Teen_Support&template=/ContentManagement/ContentDisplay.cfm&ContentID=63784.

National Alliance on Mental Illness (NAMI). (2013). *Major depression fact sheet.* Retrieved from http://www.nami.org/factsheets/depression_factsheet.pdf.

National Alliance on Mental Illness (NAMI). (n.d.). *The impact and cost of mental illness: The case of depression.* Retrieved from http://www.nami.org/Template.cfm?Section=Policymakers_Toolkit&Template=/ContentManagement/ContentDisplay.cfm&ContentID=19043.

National Center for Complementary and Alternative Medicine. (2012). *St. John's wort.* Retrieved from http://nccam.nih.gov/health/stjohnswort/ataglance.htm.

National Institute of Mental Health (NIMH). (2003). *Breaking ground, breaking through: The strategic plan for mood disorders research of the National Institute of Mental Health.* Retrieved from http://www.nimh.nih.gov/about/strategic-planning-reports/breaking-ground-breaking-through-the-strategic-plan-for-mood-disorders-research.pdf.

National Institute of Mental Health (NIMH). (2013a). *Antidepressant medication for use in children and adolescents: Information for parents and caregivers.* Retrieved from http://www.nimh.nih.gov/health/topics/child-and-adolescent-mental-health/antidepressant-medications-for-children-and-adolescents-information-for-parents-and-caregivers.shtml.

National Institute of Mental Health (NIMH). (2013b). *Bipolar disorder among children.* Retrieved from http://www.nimh.nih.gov/statistics/1BIPOLAR_CHILD.shtml.

National Institute of Mental Health (NIMH). (2013c). *Bipolar disorder in children and teens: A parent's guide.* Retrieved from http://www.nimh.nih.gov/health/publications/bipolar-disorder-in-children-and-teens-a-parents-guide/index.shtml.

National Institute of Mental Health (NIMH). (n.d.a). *Any mood disorder in adults.* Retrieved from http://www.nimh.nih.gov/statistics/1ANYMOODDIS_ADULT.shtml.

National Institute of Mental Health (NIMH). (n.d.b). *Bipolar disorder.* Retrieved from http://www.nimh.nih.gov/health/publications/bipolar-disorder/nimh-bipolar-adults.pdf.

National Institute of Mental Health (NIMH). (n.d.c). *National Comorbidity Survey: Table 1. Lifetime prevalence of DSM-IV/WMH-CIDI disorders by sex and cohort.* Retrieved from http://www.hcp.med.harvard.edu/ncs/ftpdir/NCS-R_Lifetime_Prevalence_Estimates.pdf.

Nauert, R. (2011). *Ethnic disparities persist in depression diagnosis, treatment.* Retrieved from http://psychcentral.com/news/2011/12/22/ethnic-disparities-persist-in-depression-diagnosis-treatment/32902.html.

Neumeister, A., Charney, D. S., & Drevets, W. C. (2005). Depression and the hippocampus. *American Journal of Psychiatry, 162*(6), 1057.

Office of Women's Health (OWH), U.S. Department of Health and Human Services. (2009). *Depression during and after pregnancy fact sheet.* Retrieved from http://www.womenshealth.gov/publications/our-publications/fact-sheet/depression-pregnancy.cfm.

O'Mahony, J., & Donnelly, T. T. (2010). Immigrant and refugee women's post-partum depression help-seeking experiences and access to care: A review and analysis of the literature. *Journal of Psychiatric and Mental Health Nursing, 17*, 917–928.

Paris, J. (2009). Bipolar spectrum: A critical perspective. *Harvard Review of Psychiatry, 17*(3), 206–209.

Petrakis, I., Rosenheck, R., & Desai, R. (2011). Substance use comorbidity among veterans with posttraumatic stress disorder and other psychiatric illness. *American Journal on Addictions, 20*, 185–189.

Pettinati, H., & Dundan, W. (2011). Comorbid depression and alcohol dependence: New approaches to dual therapy challenges and progress. *Psychiatric Times 28*(6), 1–8. Retrieved from http://www.nlm.nih.gov/medlineplus/ency/article/007215.htmetriev.

Posadzki, P., Parekh, S., & Glass, P. (2010). Yoga and qigong in the psychological prevention of mental health disorders: A conceptual synthesis. *Chinese Journal of Integrated Medicine, 16*(1), 80–86.

Price, A. L., & Marzani-Nissen, G. R. (2012). Bipolar disorder: A review. *American Family Physician, 85*(5), 483–493. Retrieved from http://www.aafp.org/afp/2012/0301/p483.html.

Purnell, L. D., & Paulanka, B. J. (2012). *Transcultural health care: A culturally competent approach* (4th ed.). Philadelphia, PA: F. A. Davis.

Radloff, L. S. (1977). The CES-D scale: A self report depression scale for research in the general population. *Applied Psychological Measurements, 1*, 385–401.

Reynolds, W. M. (1987). *Reynolds Adolescent Depression Scale: Professional manual.* Lutz, FL: Psychological Assessment Resources.

Reynolds, W. M. (1989). *Reynolds Child Depression Scale: Professional manual.* Odessa, FL: Psychological Assessment Resources.

Rubin, R. (1984). *Maternal identity and the maternal experience.* New York, NY: Springer.

Sachs, G., Nierenberg, A., Calabrese, J., Marangell, L., Wisniewski, S., Gyulai, L., . . . Thase, M. (2007). Effectiveness of adjunctive antidepressant treatment for bipolar depression. *New England Journal of Medicine, 356*(17), 1711–1722.

Shapiro, G., Fraser W., & Séguin J. (2012). Emerging risk factors for postpartum depression: serotonin transporter genotype and omega-3 fatty acid status. *Canadian Journal of Psychiatry, 57*(11), 704–712.

Sheikh, J. I., Yesavage, J. A., Brooks, J. O., III, Friedman, L. F., Gratzinger, P., Hill, R. D., . . . Crook, T. (1991). Proposed factor structure of the Geriatric Depression Scale. *International Psychogeriatrics, 3,* 23–28.

Sit, D. K., & Wisner, K. L. (2009). The identification of postpartum depression. *Clinical Obstetrics and Gynecology, 52*(3), 456–468. Retrieved from http://www.ncbi.nlm.nih.gov/pmc/articles/PMC2736559.

Smith, M. (2011). Immigration increases risk for depression. *Medpage Today.* Retrieved from http://www.medpagetoday.com/Psychiatry/Depression/25708.

Stice, E., Shaw, H., Bohon, C., Marti, C. N., & Rohde, P. (2009). A meta-analytic review of depression prevention programs for children and adolescents: Factors that predict magnitude of intervention effects. *Journal of Consulting Clinical Psychology, 77*(3), 486–503.

Substance Abuse and Mental Health Services Administration (SAMSHA). (2008). *Results from the 2007 National Survey on Drug Use and Health: National findings* (NSDUH Series H-34, DHHS Publication No. SMA 08-4343). Rockville, MD: Author.

Svenningsson, P., Chergui, K., Rachleff, I., Flajolet, M., Zhang, X., Yacoubi, M. E., . . . Greengard, P. (2006). Alterations in 5-HT1B receptor function by p11 in depression-like states. *Science, 6*(5757), 77–80.

Tsang, H. W., Chan, E. P., & Cheung, W. M. (2008). Effects of mindful and non-mindful exercises on people with depression: A systematic review. *British Journal of Clinical Psychology, 47,* 303–322.

Usdansky, M. L., & Gordon, R. A. (2011). *Working mothers, stay-at-home mothers, and depression risk.* Retrieved from http://www.contemporaryfamilies.org/children-parenting/working-mothers-stay-at-home-mothers-and-depression-risk.html.

Wagner, K., Hirschfeld, R., Emslie, G., Findling, R., Gracious, B., & Reed, M. (2006). Validation of the Mood Disorder Questionnaire for bipolar disorders in adolescents. *Journal of Clinical Psychiatry, 67*(5), 827–830.

Weissman, M. M., Orvaschel, H., & Padian, N. (1980). Children's symptoms and social functioning self-report scales: Comparison of mothers' and children's reports. *Journal of Nervous Mental Disorders, 168*(12), 736–740.

Wilson, B., Shannon, M., & Shields, K. (Eds.). (2014). *Pearson nurse's drug guide.* New York, NY: Pearson Education.

Zieve, D., & Merrill, D. (2012). Postpartum depression. *Medline Plus.* Retrieved from http://www.nlm.nih.gov/medlineplus/ency/article/007215.htm.

Zimmerman, M. (2012). Misuse of the Mood Disorders Questionnaire as a case-finding measure and a critique of the concept of using a screening scale for bipolar disorder in psychiatric practice. *Bipolar Disorders, 14,* 127–134.

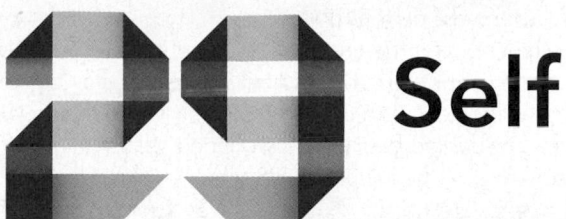 **Self**

MODULE AT-A-GLANCE

The Concept of Self, 1831

Exemplar 29.1
Feeding and Eating Disorders, 1843

Exemplar 29.2
Personality Disorders, 1852

◢ THE CONCEPT OF SELF

By nature, the nurse's role centers on recognizing and meeting the needs of others. In order to identify and meet clients' needs, the nurse must use physiological and cognitive resources, such as time, energy, and knowledge. However, before being able to use these resources, the nurse must first possess them.

At the simplest level, caring for clients requires the nurse to be physically present in the care setting. Physical presence in the workplace requires adhering to a work schedule and honoring a commitment to an employer and to clients. However, the energy needed to maintain employment and to care for others requires that the nurse obtain adequate nutrition and rest. Likewise, the knowledge needed to apply the nursing process first requires education and training in the field of nursing.

On a deeper level, to assess and care for clients from a holistic perspective and to establish therapeutic relationships, the nurse must draw from psychosocial resources that include caring, empathy, and compassion. (See the module on Caring Interventions for a discussion of caring.) As with time, energy, and knowledge,

(continued on next page)

Concept Learning Outcomes

After reading about this concept, you will be able to:

1. Summarize the psychosocial processes related to self-concept.
2. Examine the relationship between self-concept and other concepts/systems.
3. Identify commonly occurring alterations in self-concept and their related therapies.
4. Differentiate common assessment procedures used to examine self-concept across the life span.
5. Describe diagnostic and laboratory tests to explore the individual's self-concept.
6. Explain management of psychosocial wellness and prevention of alterations in self-concept.
7. Demonstrate the nursing process in providing culturally competent and caring interventions across the life span for individuals with common alterations in self-concept.
8. Compare and contrast common independent and collaborative interventions for clients with alterations in self-concept.

Concept Key Terms

Anorexia nervosa (AN), *1838*
Body image, *1833*
Bulimia nervosa (BN), *1838*
Erik Erikson, *1836*
Feeding and eating disorders, *1836*
Global evaluative dimension of the self, *1834*
Global self-esteem, *1834*
Ideal body image, *1833*
Ideal self, *1832*
Introspection, *1834*
Personal identity, *1832*
Personality disorder (PD), *1838*
Prader-Willi Syndrome (PWS), *1836*

Psychoanalytic theory, *1835*
Public self, *1833*
Purging, *1838*
Real self, *1832*
Role, *1833*
Role ambiguity, *1834*
Role conflicts, *1834*
Role development, *1833*
Role mastery, *1834*
Role performance, *1833*
Role strain, *1834*
Self-awareness, *1834*
Self-concept, *1832*
Self-esteem, *1834*
Specific self-esteem, *1834*

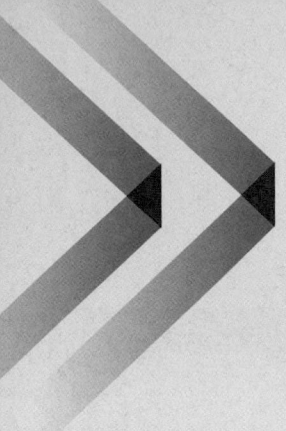

in order to share these resources with others, the nurse must first possess them. However, unlike physical and cognitive resources, attainment of these psychosocial resources is far more personal in nature.

Nurses recognize that caring for others is not one dimensional in nature; that is, caring for a client extends beyond the treatment of injury or illness. For example, treatment of a pediatric client who has sustained a forehead laceration incorporates far more than ensuring physiological stability and providing wound care. Along with these priority concerns, other facets of nursing care include addressing the wounded child's pain, anxiety, and fear as well, and recognizing and addressing the concerns of the injured child's family or loved ones. In this light, just as clients are not one-dimensional beings, neither are nurses. In turn, as the client's needs extend beyond the physiological domain, so do the needs of the nurse.

To promote health and wellness in others, nurses must first recognize and understand their own thoughts, emotions, perceptions, abilities, and limitations. Recognition of one's own needs requires an understanding of the concept of self. In application to nursing care, accurate assessment of a client's degree of psychosocial health requires that the nurse be capable of recognizing signs and symptoms of impairments and alterations. Additionally, the nurse must be able to identify evidence-based interventions that are effective in the promotion of psychosocial well-being.

Both personally and professionally, wellness promotion requires the nurse to understand and apply principles related to the concept of self, which is an individual's overall self-image and self-perception. Included within the self are all personal traits, characteristics, beliefs, and behaviors. This module will explore the concept of self, as well as its various components. **<<**

▶ NORMAL PRESENTATION

Physiological alterations often produce visible findings or manifestations that can be discerned through laboratory and diagnostic tests. In many cases, identification of abnormal physiological findings is further simplified through the use of established algorithms or parameters that guide the nurse in recognizing whether or not assessment findings are normal. For example, the nurse is taught that, in a symptomatic adult client, a heart rate of less than 60 bpm (bradycardia) usually is considered to be too slow, while a heart rate greater than 100 bpm (tachycardia) is considered to be abnormally fast. Likewise, the nurse can use institutional guidelines to determine whether or not a client's measured hemoglobin level is within normal limits.

In comparison to identifying discrete abnormalities within the physiological realm, identification of abnormal psychosocial function requires a different approach. Rather than following objective algorithms and guidelines, normal parameters within the psychosocial realm often range along a continuum. Moreover, to identify what is normal or abnormal, the nurse must assess the degree to which the psychosocial concern is affecting the client. *Normal* is more easily defined within the physiological realm, while *healthy* is the term that more readily applies to the psychosocial realm.

Development of self is a dynamic process that is influenced by interpersonal interactions throughout an individual's lifetime. Numerous theorists, including famed psychologists Erik Erikson and Jean Piaget, proposed theories to describe the processes of human growth and development, including specific stages and tasks associated with each phase of life. From a broad standpoint, principles of growth and development apply to mastery of numerous tasks, as well as to achievement of milestones related to physiological, cognitive, psychosocial, spiritual, and moral development. For many developmental tasks throughout the life span, successful task completion is rooted in interpersonal interaction.

While this module will offer an overview of the development of self, the primary focus will include exploring and describing the impact of self on client health, as well as its importance to nursing care. (For in-depth discussion of theories related to psychosocial development, see the module on Development.)

Three major components of self include self-concept, self-esteem, and self-awareness (Osborn et al., 2013). This module will explore the concept of self from the standpoint of each of these components.

Self-Concept

Self-concept, which is integral to psychosocial development, is the personal perception of self that forms in response to interactions with others and the environment throughout the course of an individual's lifetime. Self-concept affects an individual mentally, physically, and spiritually. A negative self-concept can lead to struggles with adapting to change and building interpersonal relationships. In addition, a negative self-concept can increase an individual's susceptibility to physical and psychological illnesses. Within the psychosocial domain, effective nursing care includes assessing clients' self-concept, as well as assisting them with the development of a healthy, positive self-perception (Berman & Snyder, 2012). Because each individual's self-concept impacts the nature and efficacy of her interpersonal interactions, including nurse–client relationships, the nurse is responsible for exploring and optimizing her own self-concept. In nursing, components of self-concept are often considered to include personal identity, body image, role performance, self-esteem, and self-awareness, each of which will be discussed.

PERSONAL IDENTITY **Personal identity** can be evaluated from the standpoint of three aspects of self: the ideal self, the real self, and the public self. The **ideal self** reflects qualities an individual believes she should possess, as well as those she aspires to develop. The **real self** represents the perceived true self (Ciccarelli & White, 2013). The real self may include observations about self or self-perceived qualities that the individual hides from others or does not readily share. For example, the real self may house perceptions such as "I am greedy," or "I am judgmental." The **public self** is formed on the basis of how the individual wishes to be perceived by others. For example, in the workplace, an individual's public self may lead to behaviors that inspire others to deem him as being friendly, competent, and team-oriented. While the ideal self reflects "who I should be and who I want to be," the real self represents "who I really am." The public self reflects "who I believe others think I am."

When considering the real self, characteristics that make up personal identity include objective descriptors, such as name, age, gender, marital status, and occupation. In addition, personal identity can include an individual's cultural background and ethnic origin. Values, beliefs, and self-expectations also shape personal identity. When an individual chooses values that she believes to be important and acts in accordance with those values, her sense of personal identity is strengthened (Eby & Brown, 2009). This has direct impact on nursing care, as congruence of the nurse's behavior with her personal character and values impacts the extent to which clients and coworkers find her to be trustworthy (Starr, 2008).

BODY IMAGE   **Body image** is an individual's mental picture of his physical self. How an individual perceives the appearance and size of his body and his emotional reaction to those perceptions are components of body image. However, the impact of an individual's body image extends far beyond these two components. Elements of body image include those within the perceptual, cognitive, behavioral, affective, and subjective satisfaction dimensions (**Table 29-1** ●; Ginis, Bassett-Gunter, & Conlin, 2012). Body image takes into account prosthetic devices, including hairpieces and artificial limbs, as well as assistive devices, such as wheelchairs, walkers, eyeglasses, and hearing

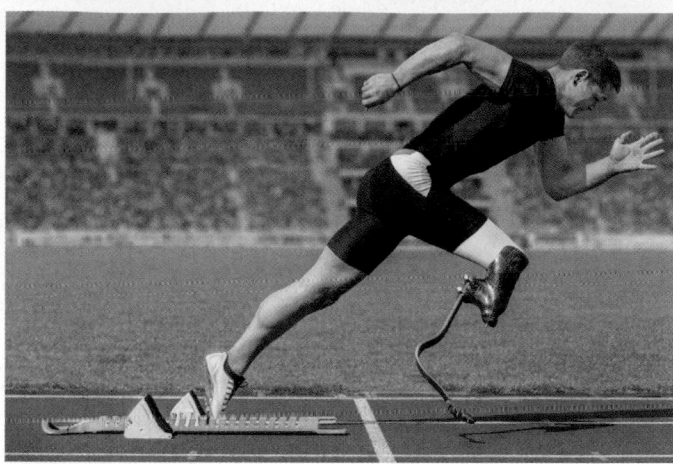

Figure 29–1 ● Body image is the sum of a person's conscious and unconscious attitudes about his or her body. How do you think the runner pictured here views his body image?
Source: © mezzotint_fotolia/Fotolia.

aids (**Figure 29–1** ●). The individual's perception of his need to use assistive devices is also part of body image.

Culture and society significantly impact body image, including the **ideal body image**, which is a mental representation of what an individual believes his body should look like. In particular, visual media—such as movies and magazine images—are viewed by some as promoting an unrealistic ideal body image. For example, in the United States, the modeling and advertising industries often feature women who are extremely thin, which is a topic that has sparked cultural debate with regard to the effects of this practice on the development of ideal body image among young females. Typically, the more congruent an individual's perceived body image is with her ideal body image, the greater her level of satisfaction with her body image will be.

ROLE PERFORMANCE   A nursing student is also a son or daughter, perhaps a brother or sister, and may be a father or mother as well. Each of these positions or roles—student, offspring, sibling, and parent—is associated with certain behavioral expectations. A **role** encompasses a grouping of behavioral expectations associated with a specified societal or organizational position. Role expectations may be defined by numerous entities, including society, culture, religion, tribal leadership, an employer, or any organization of which the individual is a member. The demonstration of behaviors or actions associated with a given role is called **role performance**.

Teaching and modeling the behaviors needed to successfully assume a role are part of **role development**, which is essential for effective role performance. Role development also includes socialization of the individual who is preparing to assume a given role. For example, a graduate nurse who accepts a position in a medical-surgical hospital unit will most often complete an orientation program, which includes exposure of the newly employed nurse to basic aspects related to working in that clinical setting, such as institutional protocols and guidelines, equipment management, charting requirements, introduction to nursing colleagues and administrative leaders, and familiarization with routine practices. After orientation, the nurse (usually) will be assigned a preceptor who models expected nursing behaviors and assists the nurse with continued role development.

TABLE 29–1	Elements of Body Image
ELEMENT	DESCRIPTION
Perceptual	Mental image of the body; includes one's perception of physical appearance and how one perceives her body when viewing herself in a mirror.
Cognitive	Includes beliefs and attitudes about one's body, as well as the degree to which body image is valued and the individual's level of investment in physical appearance.
Behavioral	Encompasses behavioral manifestations that may reveal cues about an individual's feelings and perceptions about her body; for example, indicators may include wearing revealing clothing and engaging in activities that require physical exposure (e.g., wearing a swimsuit to the swimming pool).
Affective	Represents feelings about one's body, in terms of both appearance and function. May be negative (e.g., shame or embarrassment) or positive (e.g., pride or satisfaction).
Subjective satisfaction	Reflects an individual's degree of satisfaction with his body, both as a whole and in terms of individual parts or regions.

Ineffective role development can lead to **role ambiguity**, which occurs when an individual lacks clarity regarding the expectations, behaviors, or demands associated with fulfilling a given role. Individuals who feel incapable of fulfilling a role may experience **role strain**. In some cases, role strain may be the result of sexual stereotyping. For example, a female firefighter who is told or given the impression by male colleagues that she is physically incapable of handling the rigorous demands associated with a male-dominated occupation may experience role strain. Both role ambiguity and role strain can negatively impact self-concept.

When role-related expectations clash or are incongruent, **role conflicts** may occur. If needs for recognition, accomplishment, and independence are not met, the role conflict can produce embarrassment, increased stress, and decreased self-esteem (Berman & Snyder, 2012). Conflicts may transpire between one or more individuals (interpersonal) or within one individual (intrapersonal), as well as between groups and organizations. Forms of role conflict include the following:

- *Interpersonal conflict.* Occurs when individuals hold varying or conflicting expectations about tasks and behaviors associated with a specific role; for example, a husband and wife may have conflicting expectations about who is responsible for completing household chores and preparing meals.

- *Interrole conflict.* Occurs when roles create competing demands; for example, for an individual who is balancing college enrollment with parenting, the demands associated with being a student may impinge on the demands related to raising a child.

- *Person–role conflict.* Occurs when role expectations are in opposition to the values and beliefs of the one who fills the role; for example, despite the Western healthcare practice of promoting truth telling and autonomy, in some instances, a family may ask that their family member not be informed that he has been diagnosed with a terminal illness (Coolen, 2012).

Role mastery occurs when an individual's behaviors within a role meet or exceed predetermined expectations. The inability to achieve role mastery can lead to stress, internal conflict, and impaired self-esteem (Berman & Snyder, 2012).

Self-Esteem

Self-esteem, which is separate from self-concept, is an individual's opinion of himself. In essence, self-esteem describes the degree to which an individual approves of, values, or likes himself (Blascovich & Tomaka, 1991).

While self-concept reflects how an individual perceives himself, self-esteem, which is the evaluative component of self-concept (Berk, 2010), describes the individual's judgments and opinions about those perceived characteristics. Positive or high self-esteem is associated with greater levels of achievement, increased financial prosperity, and decreased incidence of depression (Orth et al., 2009; Orth, Trzesniewski, & Robins, 2010).

Researchers have proposed two categories of self-esteem: global and specific. **Global self-esteem**, or the **global evaluative dimension of the self**, is the degree to which an individual likes herself overall, as a whole being. **Specific self-esteem**, however, reflects an individual's positive regard for certain aspects of herself (Gentile et al., 2009), such as physical appearance, athletic ability, parenting skills, or academic achievement.

Specific self-esteem influences global self-esteem (Berman & Snyder, 2012). For example, if an individual who highly values athletic ability possesses exceptional athletic skills, that individual's athletic performance will impact his global self-esteem. However, if that same individual assigns little value to academic achievement, his global self-esteem will be minimally influenced by failing a college course.

In their landmark study, DeHart, Pelham, and Tennen (2006) identified early parent–child interactions as significantly influencing the development of self-esteem. Young adult children who reported exposure to greater levels of parental nurturing also reported higher self-esteem, while parental overprotectiveness was linked to lower self-esteem (DeHart et al., 2006). Additionally, both behavioral and neural studies (using MRI scanning) have identified a link between an individual's perceived experience of rejection and the expression of a sense of low self-esteem (Eisenberger et al., 2011; Leary, 2006).

In studies of individuals between the ages of 14 and 30, high risk-taking behaviors, low sense of mastery, and poor health status effectively predicted lower levels of self-esteem (Erol & Orth, 2011). In addition, in older adults, self-esteem was higher among individuals who had completed more education (Orth et al., 2010).

Despite a heightened interest among researchers regarding the topic of self-esteem, to a great degree the question as to how self-esteem develops—including which factors influence its development—remains a mystery. Along these lines, conflict also exists as to the relationship between self-esteem and psychological disorders in terms of causation. Specifically, researchers have questioned whether poor self-esteem leads to psychopathology or vice versa (Zeigler-Hill, 2011).

Self-Awareness

Formation of a reality-based perception of the real self requires **self-awareness**. Development of self-awareness begins in infancy, as infants learn to distinguish themselves from other individuals and objects in their environment. With the ability to differentiate his own voice and body from the voices and bodies of others, the infant's self-awareness increases (Berk, 2010). Self-awareness development is an ongoing process that requires intense examination of one's personal perspectives, beliefs, and values. Moreover, self-awareness includes identifying relationships that connect actions to self. By establishing connections between past experiences and current actions or choices, the individual who is self-aware gains insight into the meaning of his behaviors. As opposed to viewing life experiences as being isolated events, many of which are perhaps inexplicable, development of self-awareness requires that actions and behaviors are viewed within the context of the individual's deep-seated values and beliefs (Eckroth-Bucher, 2010). Essentially, the individual who is self-aware understands why he does what he does, and his behaviors and actions can be linked to his core beliefs and values.

The process of developing self-awareness requires **introspection**, which is personal exploration and evaluation of one's own thoughts, emotions, behaviors, and values. Introspection also incorporates both verbal and nonverbal feedback from others (Eckroth-Bucher, 2010). While the process of introspection is intimate and personal in nature, the outcome of this process is greatly influenced by a number of external factors. In many ways, an individual's view of himself is significantly shaped by how others perceive him.

Psychosocial Development

The topic of self is both complex and vast, and even just the definition of self is subject to much debate. To one extreme, including within certain philosophical and religious realms, some theorists and leaders have argued that the self does not exist. To yet another extreme, some theorists and researchers have argued that the self is not only real, but that the unknown self—or unconscious—serves as a driving force behind an individual's actions.

NO-SELF THEORY   The absence of self has been proposed by philosophers and is a principle ascribed to by certain religions. For example, Buddhism, which is based upon the teachings of Siddhartha Gautama (563–483 B.C.), teaches that no phenomenon, experience, or thing is permanent. In addition, existence is neither inherent nor eternal. Physical death is followed by rebirth (Taylor, 2012). However, as opposed to reincarnation—which is not a teaching inherent to orthodox Buddhism—this rebirth refers to transmigration of an existence that possesses neither self nor soul (Faure, 2009).

Also in keeping with the absence of self, Scottish philosopher David Hume (1711–1776) is widely known as having proposed the "no-self theory," which asserts that a human being exists only within the context of experience, that is, when she is actively perceiving a stimulus. Thus, when unable to perceive stimuli—including when asleep—Hume questioned whether or not an individual existed (Wright, 2009).

SELF THEORY   Numerous behavioral theorists and scientists have proposed theories to describe the development of personality as a component of self. Among the most famous developmental theories are those originated by Sigmund Freud and Erik Erikson. While Freud's theory is grounded in psychosexual elements and the human response to impulses, Erikson's theory incorporates social, cultural, and interpersonal components (Kneisl & Trigoboff, 2013).

Freud's Psychosexual Theory of Development
Psychoanalytic theory is a framework for personality development that emphasizes the presence of unconscious impulses and their influence on behaviors and the formation of self. The conscious and unconscious selves were most famously described by renowned neurologist, psychiatrist, and founder of psychoanalysis, Sigmund Freud (1856–1939).

In his 1923 text *The Ego and the Id*, Freud introduced *the structural model of the mind*, in which he described the human personality as comprising three primary elements: the id, the ego, and the superego (Freud, 1923/1962). According to Freud, each of these three components of personality has a specific role and associated functions, some of which are in opposition to one another (see **Table 29–2 ●**). In accordance with Freudian theory, the id, which is motivated by the desire for pleasure, is in conflict with the perfectionistic superego, which serves as the conscience. The ego, which is based in reality, serves as a mediator between the id and superego. When the superego and ego join forces to oppose the id, guilt may result (Kneisl & Trigoboff, 2013). According to Freud, human motivation is primarily driven by instinct and sexual desire (Hatala, 2010), and personality is formed during childhood by way of successfully achieving tasks related to five psychosexual stages. (For additional discussion of Freudian theory, see the module on Development.)

Erikson's Psychosocial Theory of Development
The theory of psychosocial development originated by German-born

TABLE 29 2   Freud's Psychoanalytic Theory: Elements of Personality

THE ID	THE SUPEREGO	THE EGO
■ Motivated by the desire for pleasure ■ Seeks to avoid pain ■ Represents an entirely unconscious component of the personality ■ Animalistic in nature ■ Encompasses sexual desires (including those deemed to be socially unacceptable) ■ Can be aggressive ■ Seeks instant gratification ■ Unbound by social rules ■ Dictates "what I want"	■ Motivated by the desire to adhere to social norms and rules ■ Functions in opposition to the id ■ Serves as the social conscience ■ Contains the "ego ideal," which is an image of perfection an individual strives to attain ■ Primarily unconscious, but also contains aspects that are conscious (i.e., known to the individual) ■ Reflects societal norms, as well as standards imparted by parents, teachers, and other significant authority figures ■ Developed during early childhood ■ Guides the individual in recognizing and demonstrating socially acceptable behavior. Responsible for self-judgment ■ Imparts guilt and shame ■ Dictates "what I should want"	■ Motivated by reality ■ Not concerned with social norms or rules ■ Functions as the decision maker of the personality ■ Recognizes the consequences of behaviors and weighs the impact of potential outcomes ■ Primarily conscious, but also contains aspects that are unconscious (i.e., hidden from the individual) ■ Serves as a mediator between the id and superego ■ Attempts to fulfill the id's desires in ways that are socially acceptable ■ Determines how to get what the id wants, but through use of methods and tactics that are both rational and socially acceptable

Sources: Based on Freud, S. (1962). *The ego and the id.* New York: W. W. Norton; Kneisl, C. R., & Trigoboff, E. (2013). *Contemporary psychiatric-mental health nursing.* Upper Saddle River, NJ: Pearson Education; Osborn, K. S., Wraa, C. E., Watson, A., & Holleran, R. S. (2013). *Medical-surgical nursing: Preparation for practice* (2nd ed.). Upper Saddle River, NJ: Pearson.

psychologist and psychoanalyst **Erik Erikson** (1902–1994) is still widely taught today. Erikson's theory, which comprises eight stages, describes age-related tasks faced by an individual throughout the life span. Achievement of each task is associated with mastery of a developmental stage, while failure to achieve the task is associated with failure to achieve a developmental milestone. In addition to addressing psychosocial aspects of the self and personality, Erikson's theory also includes biological, social, cultural, and interpersonal elements of development. (For discussion of Erikson's developmental theory, see Table 3 in the module on Development.)

Genetic and Lifespan Considerations

Researchers Erol and Orth (2011) studied levels of self-esteem in males and females between the ages of 14 and 30. Overall findings suggested self-esteem increases during adolescence and, to a lesser degree, into young adulthood. Regardless of age, participants who were extraverted, emotionally stable, and conscientious reported higher self-esteem than did those participants who were deemed introverted, emotionally unstable, and less conscientious. In addition, among all ages studied, low risk-taking behaviors, high sense of mastery, and better health status reliably predicted higher levels of self-esteem.

In 2010, Orth, Trzesniewski, and Robins published findings of a study designed to evaluate the development of self-esteem between young adulthood and old age. Participants ranged in age from 25 to 104 years old. Study findings included an apparent increase in self-esteem during young and middle adulthood, with self-esteem levels ultimately peaking around 60 years of age. After age 60, self-esteem declined. Higher self-esteem was reported by participants who had completed more education. Overall, results suggested that the declining self-esteem reported by older adults was primarily caused by changes in physical health and socioeconomic status (Orth et al., 2010).

▶ ALTERATIONS FROM NORMAL

Alterations in self may stem from a variety of factors, including issues pertaining to the primary components of self-concept, self-esteem, and self-awareness. Within the component of self-concept, some researchers suggest conflicts related to body image may lead to the development of feeding and eating disorders. Alterations in one or more components of self may manifest through the development of personality disorders.

Although aspects of self may be difficult to measure in the absence of an extreme response such as a feeding and eating disorder, they are essential to everyday nursing practice. How individuals view themselves has implications for how they wish to be cared for, their ability to care for themselves, and the extent to which they are likely to participate in a plan of care. Examples of how the concept of self interacts with other concepts and systems can be found in Concepts Related to Self.

Alterations and Manifestations

FEEDING AND EATING DISORDERS **Feeding and eating disorders** are marked by chronic disturbances in eating or eating-related practices with resultant impairment in food con-

sumption or absorption to the extent that daily functioning is impaired and physical and psychological health are significantly impaired (American Psychiatric Association, 2013). Individuals who have feeding and eating disorders suffer deeply both emotionally and physically. These disorders cause low self-esteem, self-hatred, fear, and hopelessness and put the individual at risk for a variety of physiological problems. Those with feeding and eating disorders often also have other mental disorders such as anxiety disorder (see the module on Stress and Coping), substance abuse (see module on Addiction), and depression (see module on Mood and Affect) (Grilo et al., 2009). Feeding and eating disorders can be fatal. Nurses should not underestimate the significance of these disorders.

The most common feeding and eating disorders include anorexia nervosa, bulimia nervosa, and binge-eating disorder, each of which is discussed in detail in the exemplar on Feeding and Eating Disorders within this module. The characteristic features of these three disorders are presented in **Table 29–3** ●. Other disorders that may impact body image include nocturnal sleep-related eating disorder and Prader-Willi syndrome. Additional disorders often clustered with the more prevalent feeding and eating disorders include pica, rumination disorder, and avoidant/restrictive food intake disorder.

Nocturnal sleep-related eating disorder (NSRED) is characterized by an initial period of insomnia, followed by an episode of sleepwalking or semiconsciousness, during which time the affected individual consumes unusual foods or nonfood items. Primary manifestations associated with NSRED include obesity and difficulty losing weight. For these clients, interventions include referral to a nutritionist and evaluation of mood and stress. In recent trials, sertraline (Zoloft®) has been shown useful in the treatment of clients with NSRED (Sim et al., 2010).

Pica refers to a continuing pattern of behavior in which the individual consumes nonnutritive, nonfood substances (e.g., chalk, paper, soap, dirt, metal, string, hair). Pica is more commonly reported in children, although it may appear in adults with intellectual disability or mental disorders. Pica may manifest in pregnancy related to cravings for nonfood substances (American Psychiatric Association, 2013).

Rumination disorder describes the repeated regurgitation of food outside the presence of a medical condition (e.g., pyloric stenosis, gastroesophageal reflux). Onset may occur at any age, but if rumination begins in the first year of life, it may result in medical emergency if it does not resolve spontaneously or if treatment is not initiated (American Psychiatric Association, 2013).

Avoidant/restrictive food intake disorder is characterized as a disturbance in eating patterns manifested by failure to meet nutritional needs. Significant weight loss, nutritional deficiency, and dependency on enteral feeding or nutritional supplements may be observed along with impairment of psychosocial functioning. This disorder is seen more commonly in children and may result in impaired family functioning due to increased stress related to meals and around functions including meals (American Psychiatric Association, 2013).

Prader-Willi Syndrome (PWS) is a chromosomal disorder, the characteristic features of which include mental retardation, poor muscle tone, and an incessant desire to eat (Mayo Clinic, 2011). Obesity occurs as a result of indiscriminate and

Concepts Related to **Self**

An individual's self-concept and self-esteem may be affected by alterations in other systems. For example, an individual who is challenged by alterations in mobility may experience difficulty with accomplishing even simple tasks associated with daily living. Loss of independence and autonomy may negatively impact self-concept or self-esteem. Similarly, a positive self-concept and high self-esteem may help motivate the individual to move beyond the impairment and learn to adapt and function independently.

As discussed earlier, family plays a role in the development of healthy self-esteem. Overprotective parenting has been associated with lower self-esteem (DeHart et al., 2005). Authoritative parenting, interfamilial violence, and the loss of a close family member may also impact an individual's self-esteem.

Decreased self-esteem has been associated with an increased risk for depression. Alterations in mood and affect influence an individual's level of resilience when coping with life's challenges. Clients with personality disorders who have difficulty adhering to treatment regimens may experience negative consequences, including shame and stigmatization, as a result of their behaviors. These perceptions can lead to further impairment of self-esteem.

Nurses have an ethical responsibility to engage in self-care, as outlined by the American Nurses Association (ANA). In particular, Provision 5 of the ANA Code of Ethics for Nurses requires the nurse to provide the same level of self-care as that which is provided to others, including with regard to character, integrity, and self-respect (ANA, 2001). Effectively caring for others requires first recognizing and adequately fulfilling one's own personal needs, including those within the physiological, psychosocial, and spiritual realms.

CONCEPT	RELATIONSHIP TO SELF	NURSING IMPLICATIONS
Mobility		
■ Back problems ■ Fractures ■ Multiple sclerosis ■ Osteoarthritis ■ Parkinson disease ■ Spinal cord injury	Mobility → independence in daily living →↑ self-esteem. Impairment of mobility → increased dependence on others → may ↓ self-esteem and negatively impact self-concept. High self-esteem and positive self-concept → greater resilience → increased likelihood for adaptation and achievement of optimal independence despite impairment.	■ Assess self-concept and self-esteem in the client with alterations in mobility. ■ Collaborate with other healthcare providers, including physical therapists and occupational therapists, to assist the client with achieving maximum independence and autonomy. ■ Encourage the client to focus on strengths and abilities, as opposed to limitations.
Family		
■ Factors that shape family development ■ Nurturing parenting style ■ Overprotective parenting style	↑ parental nurturing → ↑ self-esteem. ↑ parental overprotectiveness → ↓ self-esteem.	■ Interview the client regarding his perception of his familial style of parenting. ■ Assess client's level of self-esteem.
Mood and Affect		
■ Depression	↓ self-esteem linked to ↑ risk for depression.	■ Assess clients who exhibit low self-esteem for presence of signs and symptoms of depression. ■ In the clinical setting, report signs and symptoms of depression to the client's primary care provider. ■ Facilitate referrals to mental health professionals for clients at risk for depression.
Ethics		
■ Nursing codes of ethics ■ Ethical issues in nursing practice	Nurses are required to administer self-care that is at the same level as that which is provided to others.	■ Perform self-assessment and strive for self-awareness both personally and professionally. ■ Identify and meet personal needs in order to promote optimal physical, psychosocial, and spiritual self-wellness.

TABLE 29–3 Characteristic Manifestations of Common Feeding and Eating Disorders

EATING DISORDER	CHARACTERISTICS
Anorexia nervosa (AN)	■ Obsessive focus on weight and body size ■ Abnormally low body weight (usually 85% or less of the normal/expected weight) ■ Extreme fear of weight gain ■ May include **purging** behaviors (e.g., vomiting, diuretic use, laxative abuse) ■ Average age of onset 19 years
Bulimia nervosa (BN)	■ Obsessive focus on weight and body size ■ Classified by presence or absence of purging behaviors ■ Purging type: includes episodes of binge eating followed by purging through self-induced vomiting or use of diuretics or laxatives ■ Nonpurging type: includes episodes of binge eating followed by fasting, intense and frequent exercise, or restrictive dieting ■ Average age of onset 20 years
Binge-eating disorder (BED)	■ Episodic compulsive consumption of excessive amounts of food within a 2-hour time period ■ Overeating typically conducted in private/secrecy ■ Not associated with purging behaviors ■ Average age of onset 25 years

Sources: Based on Sim, L. A., McAlpine, D. E., Grothe, K. B., Himes, S. M., Cockerill, R. G., & Clark, M. M. (2010). Identification and treatment of eating disorders in the primary care setting. *Mayo Clinic Proceedings, 85*(8), 746–751; Osborn, K. S., Wraa, C. E., Watson, A., & Holleran, R. S. (2013). *Medical-surgical nursing: Preparation for practice* (2nd ed.). Upper Saddle River, NJ: Pearson; National Institute of Mental Health. (n.d.). Statistics—Serious mental illness (SMI). Retrieved from http://www.nimh.nih.gov/statistics/index.shtml; PubMed Health. (2012a). *Anorexia nervosa.* Retrieved from http://www.ncbi.nlm.nih.gov/pubmedhealth/PMH0001401/.

excessive food consumption (Osborn et al., 2013). Because individuals with PWS have a constant sense of hunger and desire to eat, treatment includes ensuring good nutritional habits and providing the client with the proper amount of food intake. Due to hormonal deficiencies, these clients exhibit impaired physical growth and hypogonadism (underdevelopment of the sex organs). Treatment for clients with PWS may include hormonal therapies, as well as mental health services to address comorbid conditions. Speech, physical, and occupational therapy may also be of benefit to these clients (Mayo Clinic, 2011).

PERSONALITY DISORDERS A **personality disorder (PD)** manifests as a pervasive pattern of behaviors, personal perceptions, and internal experiences that are significantly incongruent with an individual's cultural expectations. This persistent pattern of behaviors, perceptions, and experiences is relatively inflexible and causes distress or functional impairment (**Figure 29–2 ●**). Manifestations of the PD frequently lead to disruption of the individual's personal, social, and professional interactions. Typically, the onset of PDs is during adolescence or early adulthood (American Psychiatric Association, 2013). At present, the American Psychiatric Association recognizes the following 10 forms of PD, each of which is discussed in the exemplar on Personality Disorders in this module (American Psychiatric Association, 2013):

■ Antisocial Personality Disorder (ASPD)

■ Avoidant Personality Disorder (APD)

■ Borderline Personality Disorder (BPD)

■ Dependent Personality Disorder (DPD)

■ Histrionic Personality Disorder (HPD)

■ Narcissistic Personality Disorder (NPD)

■ Obsessive-Compulsive Personality Disorder (OCPD)

■ Paranoid Personality Disorder (PPD)

■ Schizoid Personality Disorder

■ Schizotypal Personality Disorder.

See the Alterations and Therapies feature for a summary of the manifestations and therapies for feeding and eating disorders and personality disorders.

Prevalence

Although feeding and eating disorders can impact individuals at any age, from the standpoint of clients who are officially diagnosed with an eating disorder, these conditions are reportedly

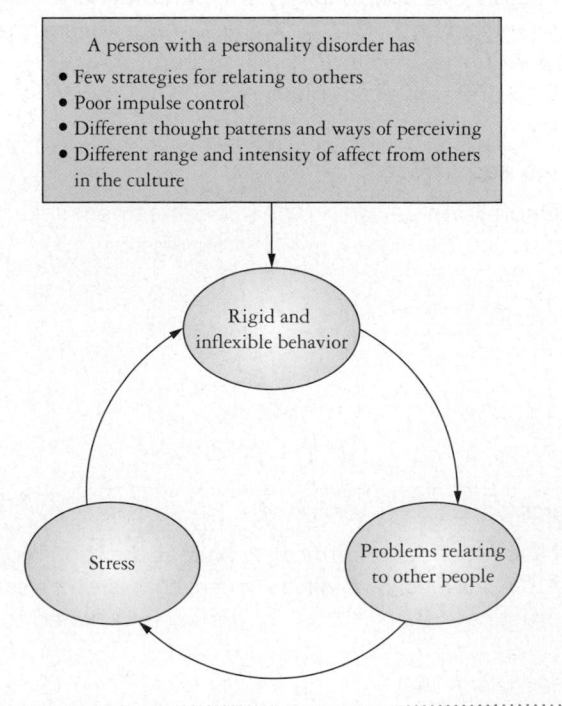

A person with a personality disorder has

● Few strategies for relating to others
● Poor impulse control
● Different thought patterns and ways of perceiving
● Different range and intensity of affect from others in the culture

Rigid and inflexible behavior

Stress

Problems relating to other people

Figure 29–2 ● Vicious cycle of personality disorders.

Alterations and Therapies Feeding and Eating Disorders and Personality Disorders

ALTERATION	DESCRIPTION	MANIFESTATIONS	INTERVENTIONS AND TREATMENTS
Feeding and eating disorders ■ Body image distortion	Impaired perception of body size and/or shape; e.g., a thin individual believing herself to be obese when she is excessively thin	■ Refusal to eat ■ Verbalized self-perception of obesity ■ Verbalized negative perception of body image	■ Cognitive behavioral therapy (CBT) ■ Pharmacologic therapy for management of comorbid disorders or to treat acute symptoms of depression or anxiety
Feeding and eating disorders ■ Absence or loss of appetite	Extreme restriction or prohibition of oral intake through self-imposed starvation	■ Absence of appetite ■ Emaciation ■ Potential nutritional deficiencies, dehydration, and electrolyte imbalances ■ Potential death	■ Cognitive behavioral therapy (CBT) ■ In extreme cases, forced nutritional supplementation and hydration (e.g., through nasogastric feeding tube)
Feeding and eating disorders ■ Binge eating	Unrestrained consumption of excessive amounts of food within a 2-hour time period; eating continues even after sensing satiation	■ Weight exceeds recommended guidelines ■ If obesity is present, may have secondary physiological alterations	■ Cognitive behavioral therapy (CBT) ■ Nutritional counseling and weight management programs
Feeding and eating disorders ■ Purging	Self-induced expulsion of food and/or products of digestion through use of forced vomiting, laxatives, enemas, and/or diuretics	■ Dental caries (cavities) and damage to tooth enamel due to caustic effects of stomach acid if frequent vomiting is occurring ■ Potential nutritional deficiencies, dehydration, and electrolyte imbalances; in particular, decreased serum potassium and serum chloride due to frequent vomiting can lead to metabolic alkalosis ■ Relatively stable weight patterns ■ Relatively normal weight and body mass index (BMI)	■ Cognitive behavioral therapy (CBT) ■ Nutritional counseling, including encouragement to eat foods that provide replacement of electrolytes lost through vomiting (e.g., bananas, nuts, and dried cereals, and potatoes for potassium replacement)
Personality disorders ■ Absence or reduction of insight as to effects of behaviors ■ Externalized stress response ■ Failure to accept consequences of behaviors ■ May include egocentricity, grandiosity, or perfectionism	■ Pervasive pattern of behaviors, personal perceptions, and internal experiences that are significantly incongruent with an individual's cultural expectations ■ Behaviors, perceptions, and experiences are relatively inflexible and cause distress or functional impairment	■ Impaired function and disruption within personal, social, and professional realms ■ Impulsivity with disregard for consequences of actions ■ Outbursts of emotion, including anger and frustration ■ Attempts to control external environment, including other individuals ■ Potential self-directed violence ■ Potential suicidal ideations and suicide attempts ■ Potential other-directed violence ■ Potential psychosis	■ Cognitive behavioral therapy (CBT) ■ Dialectical behavioral therapy (DBT) ■ Schema-focused therapy (SFT) ■ Family-focused therapy ■ Expressive therapy ■ Pharmacologic treatment with antidepressants (e.g., selective serotonin reuptake inhibitors [SSRIs], such as fluoxetine) for management of obsessive-compulsive, aggressive, and self-destructive behaviors ■ Antipsychotics for cognitive-perceptual symptoms ■ Pharmacologic mood stabilizers for control of impulsive behavior and anger

Sources: Based on Sim, L. A., McAlpine, D. E., Grothe, K. B., Himes, S. M., Cockerill, R. G., & Clark, M. M. (2010). Identification and treatment of eating disorders in the primary care setting. *Mayo Clinic Proceedings, 85*(8), 746–751; Wilson, B. A., Shannon, M. T., & Shields, K. M. (2013). *Pearson nurse's drug guide.* Upper Saddle River, NJ: Pearson; Eby, L., & Brown, N. J. (2009). *Mental health nursing care* (2nd ed.). Upper Saddle River, NJ: Pearson Education.

more common among adolescents and young adults. In the United States, among adolescents and teens between the ages of 13 and 17, an estimated 2.7% have an eating disorder. Bulimia nervosa is most prevalent among Hispanic adolescents, while anorexia nervosa is most prevalent among non-Hispanic White adolescents (Swanson et al., 2011). Bulimia nervosa (BN) is more common than is anorexia nervosa (AN) (Sim et al., 2010).

Among individuals 18 years and older, the overall prevalence of personality disorders in the United States is estimated at 9.1% (Lenzenweger et al., 2007). Prevalence associated with specific PDs is discussed in the exemplar on Personality Disorders in this module.

Genetic Considerations and Nonmodifiable Risk Factors

Compared to boys, girls are more than twice as likely to develop an eating disorder (Swanson et al., 2011). Gender prevalence varies with regard to specific personality disorders.

Research suggests obsessive-compulsive personality disorder may have a genetic component, as may certain personality characteristics that can promote the development of PDs, such as pervasive anxiety, fear, and aggression. Being a victim of childhood trauma or sexual abuse or trauma may promote the development of borderline personality disorder. Verbal abuse during childhood may be linked to adult development of borderline, narcissistic, paranoid, and obsessive-compulsive personality disorders (American Psychological Association, n.d.).

CASE STUDY \\ PART 1

Jocelyn LeMandre, a 28-year-old female, is transported to the emergency department (ED) by a friend. Although Ms. LeMandre is alert, oriented, and denies any complaints, her friend reports that Ms. LeMandre "passed out during an aerobics class" and also notes Ms. LeMandre has been complaining of being light-headed for the past few weeks. Ms. LeMandre reports she is finishing her doctoral degree in chemistry and currently teaches university courses.

When questioned about her symptoms, Ms. LeMandre admits to "feeling a little light-headed" but also notes that she hasn't been drinking enough fluids lately. She reports that she exercises daily for 2 hours prior to teaching her first course and occasionally exercises for another hour before going to bed. When asked about her dietary habits, Ms. LeMandre quietly replies, "I eat almost anything I want to eat. I might as well—I'm still going to be fat," and then looks away. When asked, Ms. LeMandre reports her height and weight as 5'7" tall and 154 pounds. By observation, Ms. LeMandre's weight is relatively proportionate to her height. Upon assessment, Ms. LeMandre's vital signs, which are within normal limits, include temperature 97.8°F oral; pulse 89 bpm; respirations 20/min; and BP 92/52 mmHg.

Clinical Reasoning Questions Level I
1. Considering the report provided by Ms. LeMandre's friend and Ms. LeMandre's statements, what may be the cause of her light-headedness?

2. Based on Ms. LeMandre's educational background, occupation, and exercise regimen, what aspects of her personality are apparent?

Clinical Reasoning Questions Level II
3. At this time, what nursing diagnoses may be appropriate for inclusion in Ms. LeMandre's plan of care?
4. Based on the available information, what additional assessment data might you expect the primary healthcare provider to order for Ms. LeMandre?

▶ PREVENTION

Because of the numerous variables believed to influence the development of feeding and eating disorders and personality disorders, prevention depends upon the individual. Ideally, prevention includes recognition of alterations in self (including those that manifest as negative self-concept or poor low-esteem) and promotion of self-wellness prior to development of disorders. With regard to wellness promotion, which is a core function of nursing, the nurse can play a vital role in recognizing manifestations associated with alterations in self and assisting clients with identification of strategies to promote a healthy self-concept.

Screenings

Identification of manifestations associated with personality disorders and medical diagnosis of such is guided by the fifth edition of the American Psychiatric Association's *Diagnostic and Statistical Manual of Mental Disorders* (DSM-5). Screening for eating disorders may include administration of the SCOFF questionnaire (Morgan, Reid, & Lacy, 1999). The **SCOFF** questionnaire was developed in England and has been found to reliably identify core elements of early-stage anorexia nervosa and bulimia nervosa (Sim et al., 2010).

S: Do you make yourself **S**ick because you feel uncomfortably full?
C: Do you worry you have lost **C**ontrol over how much you eat?
O: Have you recently lost more than **O**ne stone (14 pounds) in a 3-month period?
F: Do you believe yourself to be **F**at when others say you are too thin?
F: Would you say that **F**ood dominates your life?

One point for every "yes"; a score of ≥2 indicates a likely case of anorexia nervosa or bulimia.

▶ ASSESSMENT

Assessment of the client with suspected impairments related to self requires that priority consideration be given to establishing and maintaining a safe environment. In particular, because certain personality disorders may be associated with impulsive or aggressive behavior, the nurse should ensure that neither the client, the nurse, nor anyone else in the area is at risk for physical injury throughout the client's care. The second priority is the establishment of a therapeutic relationship, which requires the nurse to build trust and apply principles of therapeutic communication.

Nursing Assessment

After establishing trust, the nursing assessment begins with tactfully interviewing the client regarding components related to self-concept, self-esteem, and self-awareness. The simplest means by which to begin a psychosocial assessment is to ask the client his name, followed by asking about marital status and inquiring about ethnic and cultural origins (Kneisl & Trigoboff, 2013). While it is important to complete a thorough assessment, the nurse should avoid asking personal questions that are unlikely to substantially add to the assessment data. For examples of basic components of a psychosocial assessment, see **Table 29–4** ●.

Diagnostic Tests

In the diagnosis and treatment of clients with alterations in self, particularly those who are diagnosed with feeding and eating disorders and personality disorders, there are no specific laboratory diagnostics that can be used to conclusively confirm a diagnosis. Most often, for these clients, laboratory and diagnostic tests are initially used to rule out physiological causes that might be the source of associated signs and symptoms.

For clients diagnosed with feeding and eating disorders, laboratory and diagnostic testing may be used to assess for additional impairments that have occurred as a result of the primary disorder. For example, in the care of a client with anorexia nervosa who is severely dehydrated and malnourished, laboratory studies may include a complete blood count (CBC) and electrolyte studies, as well as tests to assess kidney function, such as blood urea nitrogen (BUN) and creatinine, and liver function tests. Other diagnostic exams may include electrocardiogram, thyroid screening, and urinalysis.

CASE STUDY \\ PART 2

After assessing Ms. LeMandre, the ED physician orders a complete blood count (CBC) and serum electrolytes, as well as administration of intravenous fluids for treatment of acute dehydration. When you return to insert Ms. LeMandre's IV catheter, she asks if she can first use the restroom. You respond that she is welcome to use the restroom; however, because of her recent loss of consciousness and history of light-headedness, policy dictates that she must be transferred to the restroom by wheelchair. Ms. LeMandre replies, "That's ridiculous. I'm perfectly capable of walking to the restroom!" Against your wishes, Ms. LeMandre quickly rises from the ED gurney and proceeds to ambulate to the restroom with you following at her side. She staunchly refuses to allow you to assist her. As you wait outside the restroom door, you hear water running, followed by retching sounds. When you knock on the door and ask if she is okay, Ms. LeMandre replies, "I'm fine—I'll be out shortly."

Less than a minute later, Ms. LeMandre emerges with what appears to be a small amount of emesis on the front of her hospital gown. When you ask if she vomited, she replies, "I just ate too much before I worked out this morning. Sometimes, when I eat too much, I get an upset stomach."

Ms. LeMandre denies any further complaints and, at your insistence, she agrees to allow you to return her to her ED room via

TABLE 29–4   Sample Psychosocial Assessment Criteria

DIMENSION	SAMPLE ASSESSMENT CRITERIA
Personal identity	Name Age Gender Marital status Occupation Cultural background, practices Ethnic origin Religious or spiritual affiliation, practices Self-perception: "How do you describe yourself?" Perceived image viewed by others: "How do others describe you?" Values: "In your life, what is most important to you?"
Physical history	Current physical illness History of physical illness Level of energy Disabilities
Communication skills and behaviors	Emotional tone Ability to follow conversation Verbal expression of emotion Verbal and nonverbal cues
Role performance	Current roles Presence of role conflicts, or recent changes (e.g., retirement, death of spouse) Level of congruence between current developmental life stage and role performance Past behaviors used in management of role conflict
Body image	*Perceptual:* "What do you think when you look at your body in a mirror?" *Cognitive:* "How important is physical appearance to you?" *Behavioral:* "Are you comfortable in clothing that exposes more of your body, such as a swimsuit?" *Affective:* "In one or two words, how do you feel about your body?" *Subjective satisfaction:* "Overall, how satisfied are you with your body? Which is your favorite body part or region? Which is your least favorite body part or region?"
Self-esteem	(Global) "How satisfied are you with yourself?" (Global) "Overall, do you feel you're the person you should be?" (Specific) "What do you like most about yourself?" (Specific) "What do you like least about yourself?"

Sources: Based on Kneisl, C. R., & Trigoboff, E. (2013). *Contemporary psychiatric-mental health nursing.* Upper Saddle River, NJ: Pearson Education; Berman, A., & Snyder, S. J. (2012). *Kozier and Erb's fundamentals of nursing: Concepts, process, and practice.* Upper Saddle River, NJ: Pearson Education; Eby, L., & Brown, N. J. (2009). *Mental health nursing care* (2nd ed.). Upper Saddle River, NJ: Pearson Education; Ginis, K. A. M., Bassett-Gunter, R. L., & Conlin, C. (2012). Body image and exercise. In E. O. Acevedo (Ed.), *The Oxford handbook of exercise psychology* (pp. 55–75). New York, NY: Oxford University Press.

wheelchair. You insert her IV catheter without incident and begin infusion of 500 mL of lactated Ringer solution, as ordered. Per Ms. LeMandre's request, you provide her with magazines to read while she awaits her lab draw and further assessment.

Clinical Reasoning Questions Level I

1. How does Ms. LeMandre's initial refusal to allow you to assist her to the restroom coincide with other aspects of her personality?

2. Does Ms. LeMandre's vomiting episode seem congruent with her explanation? How might Ms. LeMandre's vomiting contribute to her light-headedness?

Clinical Reasoning Questions Level II

3. Based on all available data, including nursing observations, what nursing diagnoses may be appropriate for inclusion in Ms. LeMandre's plan of care?

4. What actions should the nurse take next? What information should be reported to the primary care physician?

▶ INTERVENTIONS AND THERAPIES

In the promotion of psychosocial wellness, nurses have the unique opportunity to build trusting relationships with clients and to create a safe environment in which the client can openly discuss both positive and negative aspects of himself as a holistic being. Through assessment of a client's psychosocial wellness, the nurse can assist clients with identifying areas of strength and weakness, which enhances the client's level of self-awareness.

For the client diagnosed with an eating disorder or personality disorder, treatment centers on counseling and therapy, and most often entails collaboration with a psychiatrist, psychologist, psychiatric advanced practice nurse, and/or other mental health professionals. In some cases, for management of symptoms associated with comorbid disorders, such as anxiety or depression, therapies may include pharmacologic intervention.

Independent

Establishment of trust and application of therapeutic communication techniques require the nurse to exercise authenticity. The principle of authenticity includes remaining committed to promoting the client's health and well-being (Myrick, Yonge, & Billa, 2010). In particular, for clients with alterations in self, trust and respect are keys to both assessment and treatment. When caring for these clients, building a therapeutic relationship can be especially challenging. Clients with personality disorders may already be impacted by the stigma and shame often associated with mental illness, and they may have limited social support systems. For clients with feeding and eating disorders, many of whom maintain their condition and behaviors in secrecy, speaking openly about their self-perceptions and eating patterns may be especially difficult. Likewise, recovery rates are poor and dropout rates are high among clients who receive inpatient treatment for feeding and eating disorders (K. M. Wright, 2010).

For clients who are challenged by feeding and eating disorders, promotion of adequate nutrition is a difficult but critical intervention. In addition to being affected by the psychopathology underlying these conditions, these clients often have an exceptionally strong need for self-determination and control (K. M. Wright, 2010). Moreover, in most cases, the physiological consequences of inadequate nutrition are not enough to convince these clients to change their behaviors. When offering nutritional counseling, the nurse should keep in mind that these clients may perceive any encouragement to eat and drink as being an attempt to control them. In the clinical setting, nutritional programs for clients with feeding and eating disorders are medically directed. (For discussion of basic nutritional guidelines, see the module on Nutrition.)

Collaborative

For many clients with feeding and eating disorders or personality disorders, counseling and therapy are the mainstays of treatment. In particular, cognitive behavioral therapy (CBT), which emphasizes focusing on immediate problems and developing solutions through activities such as repatterning the client's thinking or developing healthy coping behaviors to replace maladaptive ones, has been deemed promising in the treatment of the clients with feeding and eating disorders (National Institute of Mental Health, 2012). Other forms of therapy include dialectical behavioral therapy (DBT) and schema-focused therapy (SFT); these are discussed in the exemplar on Personality Disorders in this module.

In the treatment of anxiety and depression, which often co-occur with feeding and eating disorders, antidepressants and anxiolytics (antianxiety medications) may be prescribed. Pharmacologic treatment of personality disorders varies, depending upon the nature and symptomatology of the disorder, as well as the presence of comorbid conditions. For example, antipsychotic medications may be indicated in the care of clients who are experiencing delusions, hallucinations, or other manifestations associated with psychosis.

◤ REVIEW The Concept of Self

RELATE Link the Concepts

Linking the concept of self with the concept of fluids and electrolytes:

1. Explain how alterations in self may affect fluid and electrolyte balance. Which personality disorders might lead the client to be most vulnerable to alterations in fluid and electrolyte balance?

2. Describe at least three independent and collaborative nursing interventions that are appropriate for implementation in the plan of care for a client with an alteration in fluid and electrolyte balance due to an eating disorder. Include discussion of diagnostic testing that may be useful for evaluating fluid and electrolyte balance in these clients.

Linking the concept of self with the concept of ethics:

3. Describe ethical considerations related to the nurse's self-care. How might a nurse's self-concept affect the ethical aspects of his behavior, both personally and professionally?

4. Describe ethical considerations that impact the care of a client who is known or believed to be at risk for self-injury.

5. In the course of caring for a client with an eating disorder who refuses to eat, what ethical considerations might the nurse face?

READY Go to Companion Skills Manual

REFER Go to Pearson Student Nursing Resources **nursing.pearsonhighered.com**

- Additional review material

REFLECT Case Study \\ Part 3

You report Ms. LeMandre's vomiting episode to the primary care physician. Shortly thereafter, Ms. LeMandre's CBC and serum electrolyte findings are available; all findings are within normal limits, although both her potassium level (3.7 mEq/L) and chloride level (99 mmol/L) are on the low end of the normal range. The physician diagnoses Ms. LeMandre with dehydration. However, in light of her laboratory results, rigorous exercise regimen, statements about her eating patterns, expressed body image, and vomiting episode, the physician is concerned that Ms. LeMandre's signs and symptoms may be manifestations of an eating disorder. He asks you to accompany him while he speaks with Ms. LeMandre. After speaking with her for several minutes about her dietary patterns and what she now describes as "occasionally getting sick when my stomach is too full," the physician asks Ms. LeMandre if he may ask her a few questions about her overall physical health and her views about food. Reluctantly, Ms. LeMandre agrees.

The physician proceeds to administer the SCOFF Questionnaire. Ms. LeMandre responds "yes" to two of the questions contained in the questionnaire: "Do you make yourself sick because you feel uncomfortably full?" and "Do you worry you have lost control over how much you eat?" Subsequently, the ED physician requests that Ms. LeMandre speak with the on-call psychiatrist. Once again, Ms. LeMandre reluctantly agrees. Following the consultation, the psychiatrist diagnoses Ms. LeMandre with bulimia nervosa and schedules her for a follow-up appointment in 3 days for further evaluation and treatment.

Clinical Reasoning Questions Level I

1. What is the SCOFF Questionnaire? What criteria suggest the potential presence of anorexia nervosa or bulimia nervosa?

2. If Ms. LeMandre does have an eating disorder, why do you think her weight is within normal limits?

3. How does anorexia nervosa differ from bulimia nervosa?

Clinical Reasoning Questions Level II

4. Based on all available data, including nursing observations, what nursing diagnoses may be appropriate for inclusion in Ms. LeMandre's plan of care?

5. What is the most likely cause of Ms. LeMandre's near-hypokalemia (low serum potassium) and near-hypochloremia (low serum chloride)? In light of these deficiencies, what dietary recommendations might be appropriate for her?

6. What long-term risks are associated with feeding and eating disorders? How might Ms. LeMandre's personality traits affect her willingness to follow treatment protocols?

EXEMPLAR 29.1 **Feeding and Eating Disorders**

EXEMPLAR KEY TERMS

Anorexia nervosa (AN), *1845*
Binge eating, *1846*
Binge-eating disorder (BED), *1848*
Bulimia nervosa (BN), *1846*
Metabolism, *1843*
Nutrients, *1843*
Purging, *1846*

EXEMPLAR LEARNING OUTCOMES

After reading about this exemplar, you will be able to:

1. Describe the pathophysiology, etiology, clinical manifestations, and direct and indirect causes of feeding and eating disorders.

2. Identify risk factors and prevention methods associated with feeding and eating disorders.

3. Illustrate the nursing process in providing culturally competent care across the life span for individuals with feeding and eating disorders.

4. Formulate priority nursing diagnoses appropriate for an individual with an eating disorder.

5. Summarize therapies used by interdisciplinary teams in the collaborative care of an individual with an eating disorder.

6. Plan evidence-based care for an individual with an eating disorder and his or her family in collaboration with other members of the healthcare team.

7. Evaluate expected outcomes for an individual with an eating disorder.

▶ OVERVIEW

Food is essential to life. The body requires an adequate supply of **nutrients** to meet energy requirements such as thermoregulation, cellular regulation, and metabolism. Feeding and eating disorders are complex conditions that stem from myriad social, cultural, and psychological causes, and that culminate in the disruption of the body's nutrient supply. These disorders can cause either under- or overnutrition, both of which have negative physiological effects. In the absence of a food source to use for energy, the body digests body fat and muscles. When it has excess food in proportion to energy use,

weight gain and obesity result. Feeding and eating disorders result from complex mental processes but produce biochemical and physiological interruptions of the metabolism that endanger the whole body. **Metabolism** is the complex process by which the body breaks down and converts food and fluids into energy sources.

For many individuals, the act of eating is associated with home, family, and comfort. It is thought of in relation to health, security, and pleasure to the degree that throughout the world, food takes on a heightened significance. Normal eating patterns are disrupted for a variety of reasons. For some individuals, cultural and social expectations of thinness take on extreme importance, resulting in self-starvation and depression. In addition, stress can produce unhealthy eating patterns, leading to both inadequate and excessive food consumption.

Feeding and eating disorders include pica, rumination disorder, avoidant/restrictive food intake disorder, anorexia nervosa, bulimia nervosa, and binge-eating disorder. The three disorders discussed in this exemplar are anorexia nervosa, bulimia nervosa, and binge-eating disorder. Anorexia nervosa (AN) is a condition characterized by an extreme aversion to gaining weight, as well as the physiological and mental consequences of this form of perfectionism. Bulimia nervosa (BN) is characterized by a cycle of binging and purging. Binge-eating disorder (BED) is characterized by the consumption of large amounts of food and a feeling of loss of control during binges. These three conditions create biological, physiological, and social imbalances that ravage an individual's health and self-concept. For individuals with feeding and eating disorders, the irregular supply of the nutrients necessary for physical health is compounded by psychological states such as depression, isolation, and self-destructive tendencies.

▶ PATHOPHYSIOLOGY AND ETIOLOGY

Feeding and eating disorders are not defined by body weight and external appearance, but rather by the psychological states that give rise to inadequate nutrition. There are many causes for feeding and eating disorders that are outcomes of biological, psychological, and social processes. At present, researchers believe that an individual's family, social context, and culture provide triggers, but that hormones, brain chemicals, and genetics cause individuals to push themselves to starvation or obesity.

Etiology

Although many studies have been performed and published on the causes of feeding and eating disorders, there is no medical consensus on the etiology of these conditions. Biological theories, cognitive-behavioral theories, and psychoanalytic theory are all relevant to the development of these alterations. An understanding of these theories allows the nurse to take a holistic approach when caring for clients with feeding and eating disorders.

It seems clear that biology—including genetic and neurological factors—plays a part in the origination of feeding and eating disorders. Research shows that relatives of clients with feeding and eating disorders are 5–10 times more likely to develop a disorder. Studies of twins have demonstrated that feeding and eating disorders occur for both twins at a rate of 55%–60%, indicating that a genetic predisposition may play into the development of these conditions. Neurological factors include neurotransmitter dysregulation. The neurotransmitter in question is 5-HT, or serotonin, which is synthesized partially of carbohydrates. A low level of 5-HT typically reduces an individual's satiety and increases the consumption of nutrients; a high level of the neurotransmitter increases satiety and decreases food intake. A current theory of binge eating holds that repeated binge episodes may result from a deficiency in

serotonin, and that the tendency of individuals with bulimia to binge carbohydrate-rich foods is a manifestation of the body's attempt to replenish serotonin. However, 5-HT is not the only neurotransmitter involved in feeding and eating disorders. Norepinephrine and neuropeptide Y increase food consumption, while dopamine inhibits eating. In addition, endogenous opioids, such as endorphins, increase food intake and elevate mood. Individuals who are significantly underweight typically have significantly lower endorphin levels than individuals of normal weight. The fact that endorphin levels return to normal when weight returns to normal outlines the complex relationship between biology, nutrition, and psychology in feeding and eating disorders (Kneisl & Trigoboff, 2013).

Cognitive-behavioral theories see feeding and eating disorders as learned patterns of behavior based on irrational thought and beliefs. These theories look at the affected individual's cognition and behavior to stimuli, whether physiological, psychological, or social, and attempt to help the client with the disorder by changing the maladaptive behavior and replacing it with a healthier response. An essential element of cognitive-behavioral theory is that the individual's thought patterns give rise to destructive behavioral patterns, and that irrational thoughts are at the heart of the network of problems that leads to feeding and eating disorders (Murphy et al., 2010; Kneisl & Trigoboff, 2013).

The psychoanalytic theory of feeding and eating disorders takes into account the importance of eating to psychological growth and development. Psychoanalytic theory considers feeding and eating disorders to be signs of unconscious conflicts in an individual's mind, without reference to biological or cultural factors. The psychoanalytic theory views individuals with anorexia as fearing sexual maturity, for instance, and frequently relies on explanations that do not take into account the real-world forces that play on the minds of individuals who are susceptible to feeding and eating disorders. There is little empirical evidence for the effectiveness of psychoanalysis in the treatment of feeding and eating disorders, and the capacity of psychoanalytic theory to explain the origination of feeding and eating disorders is questioned by researchers in favor of other explanations (Kneisl & Trigoboff, 2013).

Risk Factors

Because the origination of feeding and eating disorders is so complex, the risk factors for feeding and eating disorders are closely related to their etiologies. Biology, sociocultural factors, and family systems all contribute to the psychological conditions that prime an individual for an eating disorder.

Increasingly, research is pointing to genetic factors as a major risk factor for feeding and eating disorders. Contemporary genetic research works with the behavioral, neurobiological, and temperamental variables that are core features of disorders. Behavioral conditions that may be related to genetics are perfectionism, orderliness, low tolerance for unfamiliar situations, low self-esteem, and high anxiety. The genetic underpinnings of these conditions can cause individuals to develop an eating disorder even when their culture does not commonly induce feeding and eating disorders (Kneisl & Trigoboff, 2013).

Sociocultural risk factors are elements of an individual's social and cultural context that exert the pressure that initiates an eating disorder. In the American culture, portrayals of men's and women's bodies in the media and a pervasive cultural understanding of a trim body as the "ideal" lead to the unrealistic expectation that everyone should have a low weight. In addition to glamorizing an unrealistically trim body shape, the cultural obsession with thinness leads to a bias against those who are overweight. These social factors diminish the self-esteem of those who believe they do not fit the "ideal" body shape and enhance self-worth for those who are deemed attractive. Females are hardest hit by the cultural emphasis on thin bodies: Magazines targeted at adolescent girls present dieting as a sensible solution to the crises of adolescents and contain 90% more articles promoting weight control than magazines targeted at teenage males. For many young women, self-esteem becomes centered on concerns about weight.

In recent years, the American ideal of male attractiveness has also shifted toward the unhealthy. Men and boys are confronted every day with images of male beauty that center on muscle-bound figures defined by their strength. The use of anabolic steroids is common among men with feeding and eating disorders, because in addition to seeking thinness they also seek improved muscle tone (National Association of Men With Eating Disorders, 2011). Because of the pressure that the media, social, and cultural expectations exert, feeding and eating disorders like anorexia and bulimia can be considered culture-reactive syndromes in the United States and the rest of the Western world. Negative body image, degraded self-worth, and body dissatisfaction create the stress that leads to feeding and eating disorders (Kneisl & Trigoboff, 2013).

Family systems theories do not necessarily hold that harmful family patterns cause feeding and eating disorders, but rather that the family enables maladaptive behaviors. Some individuals with feeding and eating disorders are survivors of childhood and adolescent abuse—including sexual abuse—much of which occurs in immediate and extended family systems. In addition to abuse, many families of eating disorder clients have impaired conflict resolution skills. Another factor that enables the development of feeding and eating disorders is a family-wide emphasis on achievement and performance, with ambition for the family's success being one of the principal goals of the parents. Body shape frequently is related to success in these families, and an emphasis on fitness combined with a desire for control may become obsessive. In addition to the family system impacting the development of an eating disorder, the appearance of a disorder can disrupt the fragile order of a family unit. After the diagnosis or appearance of a disorder such as anorexia, certain families become enmeshed: The boundaries between members become weak, interactions intensify, members become more dependent, and autonomy decreases. Each family member becomes less stable and more involved with the other members' private concerns. In this situation, the parents become overprotective, and food can take on extreme importance. A family's system of interpersonal relations influences the development of an eating disorder, and the presence of an eating disorder impacts the way a family conducts itself in a harmful cycle (Kneisl & Trigoboff, 2013).

Prevention

Prevention is a systematic attempt to change the circumstances that facilitate feeding and eating disorders. Prevention can involve reducing negative risk factors such as body dissatisfaction, depression, and basing self-esteem on appearance. Prevention also involves increasing protective factors such as basing self-esteem on factors other than appearance, and replacing unhealthy dieting with an appreciation for the body's natural functionality. A culturewide emphasis on prevention is essential for the global reduction of the suffering associated with feeding and eating disorders (National Eating Disorders Association, 2013).

Healthcare providers should target two types of audiences when implementing eating disorder prevention. Universal prevention, the first type, should be aimed at the general public, even at those individuals that show no signs of feeding and eating disorders. This type of prevention aims to promote healthy development and understanding of the many complex issues that cause disorders, as a way of spreading the information that can cut disorders off before they begin. Targeted prevention, the second type of prevention, educates individuals who are beginning to show symptoms of feeding and eating disorders. These individuals may have high levels of body dissatisfaction. The goal of targeted prevention is to provide enough information to stop an eating disorder from developing (National Eating Disorders Association, 2013).

After years of studying feeding and eating disorders and disordered-eating prevention programs, experts believe that carefully developed programs can alter the populace's knowledge, attitudes, and behaviors. Both universal and targeted programs have had success preventing disorders, though targeted programs seem to be more effective. When targeted programs use cognitive dissonance methods—that is, methods that ask individuals to question media portrayals of ideal body weight—outcomes are particularly encouraging for adolescent and young adult women. Additionally, research shows that programs designed to prevent both obesity and feeding and eating disorders can be combined into single programs that promote healthy eating habits. Despite the encouraging evidence that prevention programs work, much more research is required to determine how best to discourage the development of feeding and eating disorders in children, males, and all ethnic groups (National Eating Disorders Association, 2013).

▶ CLINICAL MANIFESTATIONS

Clinical manifestations of the different feeding and eating disorders vary, but similarities include body image disturbance, anxiety, and ineffective coping skills. Commonly occurring feeding and eating disorders include anorexia nervosa, bulimia nervosa, and binge-eating disorder.

Anorexia Nervosa

Anorexia nervosa (AN) is a potentially deadly eating disorder that compels individuals to lose more weight than is healthy for their age and height. Clients with anorexia have an intense phobia of gaining weight, even when they show the symptoms of being dangerously underweight. Individuals with anorexia engage in dieting and exercising to the point of dangerous malnutrition to avoid gaining weight (PubMed Health, 2012a). The DSM-5 diagnostic criteria for anorexia nervosa are summarized in **Box 29–1** ●.

Anorexia nervosa typically begins during the teen years, and it is more commonly diagnosed in females. In particular, AN is

---

Box 29–1 DSM-5 Diagnostic Criteria for Anorexia Nervosa

A. Restriction of energy intake relative to requirements, leading to a significantly low body weight in the context of age, sex, developmental trajectory, and physical health. *Significantly low weight* is defined as a weight that is less than minimally normal or, for children and adolescents, less than that minimally expected.

B. Intense fear of gaining weight or becoming fat, or persistent behavior that interferes with weight gain, even though at a significantly low weight.

C. Disturbance in the way in which one's body weight or shape is experienced, undue influence of body weight or shape on self-evaluation, or persistent lack of recognition of the seriousness of the current low body weight.

Specify whether:

Restricting type: During the last 3 months, the individual has not engaged in recurrent episodes of binge eating or purging behavior (i.e., self-induced vomiting or the misuse of laxatives, diuretics, or enemas). This subtype describes presentations in which weight loss is accomplished primarily through dieting, fasting, and/or excessive exercise.

Binge-eating/purging type: During the last 3 months, the individual has engaged in recurrent episodes of binge eating or purging behavior (i.e., self-induced vomiting or the misuse of laxatives, diuretics, or enemas).

Specify if:

In partial remission: After full criteria for anorexia nervosa were previously met, Criterion A (low body weight) has not been met for a sustained period, but either Criterion B (intense fear of gaining weight or becoming fat or behavior that interferes with weight gain) or Criterion C (disturbances in self-perception of weight and shape) is still met.

In full remission: After full criteria for anorexia nervosa were previously met, none of the criteria have been met for a sustained period of time.

Specify current severity:

The minimum level of severity is based, for adults, on current body mass index (BMI) (see below) or, for children and adolescents, on BMI percentile. The ranges below are derived from World Health Organization categories for thinness in adults; for children and adolescents, corresponding BMI percentiles should be used. The level of severity may be increased to reflect clinical symptoms, the degree of functional disability, and the need for supervision.

Mild: BMI ≥ 17 kg/m^2
Moderate: BMI 16–16.99 kg/m^2
Severe: BMI 15–15.99 kg/m^2
Extreme: BMI <15 kg/m^2

Source: American Psychiatric Association. (2013). *Diagnostic and statistical manual of mental disorders* (5th ed.). Arlington, VA: Author.

---

more prevalent among White females with a history of high academic achievement. See the Evidence-Based Practice feature for a discussion of how those with feeding and eating disorders are affected by the Internet. These women frequently have goal-oriented families or personalities, and they develop rigid "rules" that they use to control weight. These rituals can be simple, such as cutting food into tiny pieces, or elaborate, such as preparing lavish dinners for friends or family without consuming any food themselves. Criteria for diagnosis of AN include possessing an intense fear of weight gain, refusal to maintain a healthy weight, and perceiving a distorted body image. In previous years, amenorrhea (absence of menstruation for 3 or more months) was also a diagnostic criterion for AN; however, this is no longer the case. In order to maintain low body weight, individuals with anorexia severely limit food consumption and offset consumption with excessive exercise. Other behaviors include self-induced vomiting; refusing to eat in the presence of others; using diuretics, laxatives, and diet pills; and cutting food into small pieces as a way of pretending to eat (PubMed Health, 2012a).

As an individual loses body weight and becomes malnourished, hair and nails become brittle, skin becomes dry and yellow, and a fine layer of hair called *lanugo* appears on previously hairless parts of the body. Individuals with anorexia may constantly feel cold, as the body loses its ability to retain heat. The starvation resulting from anorexia can cause damage to vital organs like the brain, kidneys, and heart. Pulse rate and blood pressure drop, and irregular heart rhythms can cause heart failure. Loss of nutrients can lead to brittle bones and even changes in the brain, which in turn lead to impaired thinking. In the worst cases of anorexia, clients can starve themselves to death. The condition has the highest mortality rate of any mental illness, due to the complications of malnutrition and the high rate of suicide in the population (National Alliance on Mental Illness, 2013a).

Bulimia Nervosa

Bulimia nervosa (BN) is a condition in which individuals binge on food or have episodes of overeating in which they feel a loss of control. After periods of binging, the individuals use methods such as vomiting or laxative abuse to prevent weight gain. Binging may also be followed by periods of extreme exercise. Many individuals who have bulimia also have anorexia nervosa. Individuals with bulimia are obsessed with their body appearance and engage in the destructive pattern of binging and purging to control weight (PubMed Health, 2012b).

For diagnosis of bulimia nervosa, the individual must demonstrate binge eating in association with unhealthy compensatory behaviors (e.g., purging or excessive exercise) at least once per week over a 3-month period (American Psychiatric Association, 2013). **Binge eating** is the rapid consumption of an uncommonly large amount of food in a short amount of time, for example, over a 2-hour time period (American Psychiatric Association, 2013). Individuals who binge-eat feel out of control during the episode, and although eating binges may involve any kind of food, they usually consist of junk foods, fast foods, and high-calorie foods. Binging may be pleasant initially, but the individual who is binging quickly becomes distressed. A binge usually ends only when abdominal pain becomes powerful, when the individual is interrupted, or when the individual runs out of food. After the binge, the individual with bulimia feels guilt and engages in purging activities to rid the body of excess calories (National Alliance on Mental Illness, 2013b).

Purging behaviors are frequently dangerous and include a wide variety of activities that are meant to remove all food from the body. Those with bulimia use self-induced vomiting, enemas, or diuretics to remove food from the body. Restrictive dieting and extreme exercising also are common. For many with bulimia, purging becomes a purification ritual and a

Evidence-Based Practice Feeding and Eating Disorders and the Internet

Problem

For a client coping with an eating disorder, the Internet can be perilous territory. Not only does the Internet offer Web sites dedicated to encouraging and celebrating feeding and eating disorders, but some research suggests that sites provide erroneous diagnostic criteria that can be detrimental to clients and their families. Especially for adolescent clients who spend hours every day engaged with media, information on the Internet can both prompt and exacerbate disordered eating behaviors.

Evidence

Adolescents today have unprecedented access to new media: Recent research revealed that 93% of youth ages 12–17 are online, and 71% have a cell phone. Of young Internet users, 65% use social networking sites, and 28% use the Web to access health information (Strasburger et al., 2010).

Digital media have become an important source of the social pressure, cultural expectations, and health misinformation that contribute to the development of feeding and eating disorders in adolescents. Neuroscientists worry about the effect of new communication technology on the teenage brain, particularly because sites such as the *more than 100* proanorexia Web sites not only encourage feeding and eating disorders but also offer specific advice on anorexic and bulimic techniques (Strasburger et al., 2010). These pro-eating-disorder Web sites offer advice on binging, purging, and extreme forms of weight control, and they provide interactive resources such as message boards. Research indicates that the sites are alarmingly easy to access and understand: One study found that half of the sites were written at less than a high school reading level. The sites frequently feature glorified images of malnourished models, celebrities, and regular individuals, and they feature "thinspiration"—original poetry or artwork designed to provide inspiration for extreme weight control. Pro-eating-disorder Web sites are readily accessible communities with dynamic, user-distributed content (Borzekowski et al., 2010).

In addition to sites that provide information that explicitly promotes feeding and eating disorders, Web sites that purport to provide medical information can spread damaging information to individuals of all ages. Research shows that the quality of medical content related to the diagnosis and treatment of feeding and eating disorders is relatively low. Few sites fully describe the criteria for diagnosis, complications, and treatment options of any eating disorder, and some provide a good deal of erroneous information. Some sites use inaccurate "diagnostic" terms—"bulimerexia," for example—as well as multiple "optimal" treatment options for each of the feeding and eating disorders. Inaccurate information is particularly dangerous for adolescents with disordered eating, and it may interfere with the family's decision to seek medical treatment (Smith et al., 2011).

Implications

The fact that almost all adolescents have easy access to the Internet and its variety of viewpoints brings with it a new set of problems for the nurse. The Web offers an interactive way for impressionable adolescents and young adults to engage with unhealthy cultural expectations of thinness. Additionally, the myriad viewpoints expressed online include pathological Web sites that support the damaging behaviors associated with anorexia and bulimia. Even sites that purport to present medical information and treatment options for eating disorders often contain flawed and medically inadequate information.

Critical Thinking Application

Consider a consultation with an adolescent female client who has been exhibiting the behaviors associated with anorexia nervosa for the past 3 years. This client has also been taking part in proanorexia message boards online for the past 2 years. She knows that anorexia is unhealthy but embraces the damage she deals her body by fasting and exercising, partly because she learned most of what she knows about the condition from Web sites full of incorrect "information." Identify a communication strategy that will enable you to correct her misconceptions about anorexia nervosa while attempting to communicate the grim reality of her disorder.

---

means of regaining self-control in addition to a mechanism for emptying the body of nutrients (National Alliance on Mental Illness, 2013b).

Bulimia nervosa is frequently underdiagnosed because many of those who have the condition are either overweight or of normal weight. The typical age of onset is late adolescence or early adulthood. The disorder mainly affects females, though at least 1 in 10 individuals with the condition is male. BN is more common than anorexia, and it occurs in approximately 3% of the population. Additionally, BN is often comorbid with other psychiatric disorders, such as mood disorders, anxiety disorders, substance abuse, and disorders of self-injurious behavior (National Alliance on Mental Illness, 2013b).

The principal indicator of bulimia nervosa is an incessant obsession with food and body weight. Other important indicators are physical signs of binging and purging. These include the trash produced by the large quantity of food required for binging, and the products—enemas and laxatives—used in purging. Individuals affected by BN may also experience menstrual irregularity and depressed mood, in addition to the unexplained stomach pain and sore throat that binging and purging produce. The signs of self-induced vomiting—unexplained damage to teeth, scarring on the backs of fingers, and swollen cheeks due to the damage to parotid glands—often indicate to doctors and dentists that there is a problem.

Behaviors associated with BN can lead to severe physiological damage, even if the individual's weight remains normal. Binging and purging cause unhealthy nutritional patterns, and self-induced vomiting can cause serious injury to the digestive tract. Tooth decay, esophageal and stomach injury, and acid reflux are all common in individuals with the condition.

Purging behaviors can lead to dehydration and changes in the body's electrolytes. Because stomach acid contains potassium and chloride, electrolyte disturbances associated with purging include low potassium (hypokalemia) and low chloride (hypochloremia). Frequent vomiting, diuretic use, or laxative abuse may cause hypokalemia; in each case, metabolic alkalosis may result (Roerig et al., 2010). Bloating and slowed peristalsis (movement of gastric contents through the intestines) also may accompany BN (Sim et al., 2010). Complications stemming from electrolyte disturbances, severe dehydration, and undernutrition associated with BN may include cardiac arrhythmias, heart failure, and possibly even death (National Alliance on Mental Illness, 2013b).

Binge-Eating Disorder

Persons with **binge-eating disorder (BED)** experience periods of rapid food consumption, episodes during which they are unable to stop eating. Individuals with the disorder may continue to eat until long after they are full, and they may experience embarrassment about their behavior. For some individuals with BED, binging can produce a sense a relief or fulfillment that gives way as the episode progresses into feelings of disgust, guilt, worthlessness, and depression (National Alliance on Mental Illness, 2013c).

There is no specific test that can diagnose someone with binge-eating disorder. Rather, a diagnosis is made by a mental health practitioner based on an assessment that includes a formal history and collateral information. Any client diagnosed with the condition should have a full physical exam performed in order to screen for complications of the illness. These complications include obesity, high cholesterol, type 2 diabetes, and heart disease. In cases of extreme weight gain, complications can include arthritis, obstructive sleep apnea, and other weight-related conditions (National Alliance on Mental Illness, 2013c).

Lifespan and Cultural Considerations

Feeding and eating disorders are often thought of as conditions limited to affecting adolescent and teen populations, but anorexia, bulimia, and binge-eating disorder frequently affect older adults as well. Recent research has found that eating disorder symptoms are common in older adults. In a study of women age 50 and older, 62% of respondents said their weight or shape negatively impacts their life, and 64% think about their weight at least once a day. Fully 13.3% of women 50 and older exhibited eating disorder symptoms. Binging and purging are both prevalent among women in their early 50s, but in women older than 75 as well. Participants in research reported using unhealthy methods to lose weight and maintain thinness, including diet pills, excessive exercise, diuretics, laxatives, and vomiting. Feeding and eating disorders are detrimental to the health of individuals of all ages, but they can be particularly damaging to the bodies of older adults. The damaging effects of bulimia and anorexia exacerbate preexisting osteoporosis, cardiovascular problems, and gastroesophageal reflux disease (Gagne et al., 2012).

▶ COLLABORATION

Feeding and eating disorders are diagnosed through a combination of laboratory tests to detect the effects of irregular nutrition and consultation with a medical professional. Once a disorder is diagnosed, the reestablishment of adequate nutrition, the cessation of binge–purge behaviors, and the reduction of excessive

Clinical Manifestations and Therapies **Feeding and Eating Disorders**

ETIOLOGY	CLINICAL MANIFESTATIONS	CLINICAL THERAPIES
Anorexia nervosa	■ Obsession over body shape and food ■ Extreme perfectionism ■ Rigidity, overcontrol, obsessive rituals ■ Significant weight loss ■ Body disturbances ■ Strenuous exercises ■ Reductions in heart rate, blood pressure, metabolic rate, and in production of estrogen or testosterone ■ Extreme sensitivity to cold ■ Feelings of depression	■ Antidepressants ■ Cognitive-behavioral therapy ■ Group therapy ■ Family therapy
Bulimia nervosa	■ Cycle of binging and purging food ■ Body image disturbances ■ Abuse of laxatives, enemas, and diuretics ■ Extreme exercise to compensate for binging ■ Hoarding food ■ Secretive behaviors	■ Antidepressants ■ Cognitive-behavioral therapy ■ Family therapy
Binge-eating disorder	■ Binging once a week for at least 3 months ■ Absence of purging ■ Sense of loss of control ■ Allowing eating and weight to interfere with personal relationships ■ Sense of embarrassment, disgust after overeating	■ Antidepressants ■ Cognitive-behavioral therapy

exercise are the essential points of treating feeding and eating disorders. These goals are accomplished through a combination of pharmacologic and nonpharmacologic therapies, including psychotherapy. Treatment plans are tailored to individual needs but include counseling, medication, and even hospitalization in extreme cases (National Institute of Mental Health, 2012).

Diagnostic Tests

Laboratory tests can reveal the physiological hallmarks of feeding and eating disorders. Screening for anorexia may include tests for albumin, total protein, electrolyte levels, a complete blood count (CBC), and a bone density test to check for signs of osteoporosis. Other diagnostic exams include an electrocardiogram; kidney, thyroid, and liver function tests; and urinalysis. These exams determine whether there is a severe deficiency of any nutrients or any wasting of the body as a result of malnutrition (PubMed Health, 2012a).

Diagnostic tests for bulimia nervosa consider many more visible symptoms of disease than do the tests for anorexia because of the physical damage induced by purging. The dentist is often the first medical professional to identify signs of bulimia, including cavities and gum infections. The enamel of teeth may be worn or pitted because of exposure to the acid in vomit. Loss of stomach acid can lead to metabolic alkalosis. A physical exam may discover broken blood vessels in the eyes (from the stress of vomiting), a dry mouth, pouchlike cheeks, rashes and pimples, and cuts and calluses on the finger joints. Laboratory tests might show an electrolyte imbalance or dehydration from purging (PubMed Health, 2012b).

In order to diagnose a binge-eating disorder, a physician typically conducts a physical exam, followed by blood and urine tests. A psychological evaluation is necessary to complete the evaluation, including a discussion of the client's eating habits. Following diagnosis, the other tests should be performed to check for the common health implications of BED, including heart problems and gallbladder disease (Mayo Clinic, 2012a). Some clients require hospitalization to treat problems caused by severe malnutrition. An inpatient stay at a hospital can also be used to ensure that the clients are eating if they are severely underweight and to establish new eating patterns in a supportive environment (National Institute of Mental Health, 2012).

Pharmacologic Therapy

There is presently no surgical treatment indicated for any of the feeding and eating disorders. Treating anorexia nervosa involves restoring the client to a healthy weight, treating underlying psychological issues, and eliminating behaviors that might lead to malnutrition and relapse. Research suggests that antidepressants, antipsychotics, or mood stabilizers may be modestly effective in treating clients with anorexia. Medications can treat some of the psychological states that undergird the eating disorder, but it is not yet clear whether medications are effective in preventing relapse. No medication has yet been shown to be effective in assisting weight gain.

The antidepressant fluoxetine (Prozac) is the only medication approved by the U.S. Food and Drug Administration for treating bulimia. This and other antidepressants may help individuals for whom depression and anxiety are at the root of bulimic behavior. Fluoxetine appears to lessen binging and purging behaviors, reduce the likelihood of relapse, and improve attitudes toward eating.

The pharmacologic options for treating binge-eating disorder are similar to the treatments for bulimia nervosa. Antidepressants, particularly fluoxetine, have been found to reduce binge-eating episodes and help ease depression (National Institute of Mental Health, 2012).

Nonpharmacologic Therapy

Though pharmacologic treatments play a role in the treatment of feeding and eating disorders, therapies that do not make use of medication have proven to be more consistently effective. In the treatment of anorexia nervosa, individual, group, and family-based psychotherapy can address the psychological reasons for the illness. A therapy called the *Maudsley approach* has been shown to be particularly effective in the treatment of adolescents with anorexia. In the Maudsley approach, the parents of the affected adolescent take responsibility for feeding the child. Research shows that for clients with anorexia, a combined approach of medical attention and psychotherapy produces more complete recoveries than psychotherapy alone. There is no cure-all approach for anorexia nervosa, but evidence points to the fact that individualized treatment programs frequently achieve success, and that specialized treatment may help reduce the risk of death.

The nonpharmacologic treatment of bulimia nervosa frequently involves a combination of options and depends on the need of the individual client. The most effective psychotherapy for clients with bulimia is cognitive behavioral therapy (CBT), which helps individuals focus on their present problems and how to solve them. CBT may be individualized or group-based, and it is effective in changing binge-and-purge behaviors and attitudes to eating.

Nonpharmacologic treatment options for binge-eating disorder are very similar to the options for bulimia nervosa. Psychotherapy, especially cognitive-behavioral therapy that is individualized, has shown to be effective in many cases (National Institute of Mental Health, 2012).

A common format for the treatment of severe feeding and eating disorders is inpatient therapy. An inpatient stay provides a structured and contained environment in which clients have access to clinical support at all times. The close proximity of medical help reduces the chance of relapse while improving the chances of recovery. Inpatient programs are now frequently affiliated with daytime programs so that clients can move to the correct level of care. The majority of inpatient programs only treat clients with anorexia, bulimia, and binge-eating disorder so that the symptoms can be isolated and treated as effectively as possible (Academy for Eating Disorders, 2013).

Complementary and Alternative Therapy

For individuals with feeding and eating disorders, a variety of alternative and complementary medical techniques can help improve recovery outcomes. However, those with feeding and eating disorders sometimes use alternative medical techniques to achieve the unhealthy goals of disordered eating. The numerous herbal dietary supplements that are used as appetite suppressants or as weight loss aids are sometimes abused by clients with feeding and eating disorders. Herbal supplements can be dangerous when they interact with other products, such as laxatives and diuretics, which are frequently used by those with feeding and eating disorders. Health professionals have not determined conclusively that any complementary or alternative therapies are helpful for individuals with anorexia, bulimia, or BED, but some research indicates that some therapies may help reduce anxiety. Chamomile tea, acupuncture, massage, yoga, and biofeedback, among other treatments, have been shown to improve mood and reduce the stress associated with feeding and eating disorders (Mayo Clinic, 2012b).

◼ NURSING PROCESS

When assessing the client with a known or suspected eating disorder, the nurse should keep in mind that denial is often inherent to these conditions. As such, the nurse should recognize that deceit and manipulation on the part of the client are characteristics of the disorder and not necessarily consciously chosen behaviors on the part of the client.

Assessment data serves as the basis for application of the nursing process. For the client with an eating disorder, assessment combines a thorough review of both physiological and psychosocial function as well as careful observations for the physiological manifestations associated with feeding and eating disorders. In consideration of significant weight gain or loss, the nurse should not automatically assume the client has an eating disorder. Numerous physiological conditions can lead to muscle wasting and weight loss, including cancer, hyperthyroidism, and impaired gastrointestinal function. Likewise, weight gain may occur due to a variety of causes, including endocrine disorders and medication side effects. Before the primary care provider establishes the diagnosis of an eating disorder, other causes for weight alteration must be ruled out (Fontaine, 2009; Kneisl & Trigoboff, 2013).

Focused assessment of the client's nutritional status incorporates data obtained through the client interview, physiological assessment findings, and review of laboratory and diagnostic test results. Assessment of nutritional status includes height, weight, BMI, mid-arm circumference (MAC), and waist-to-hip ratio. It also includes assessment of the skin, the oral mucosa and tongue, the shape of the abdomen, and the nature and presence of bowel sounds. Assess the teeth and gums for any irregularities.

On physical assessment, clients with anorexia nervosa will appear emaciated. Their skin may be dry and covered by a fine layer of hair called *lanugo*, and they also may appear jaundiced (yellow-orange in color). As a result of malnourishment, hair and nails will appear to be brittle. Undernutrition may impair the function of any body system, including the brain, musculoskeletal system, kidneys, and heart. In particular, cardiovascular manifestations may include bradycardia, hypotension, and cardiac dysrhythmias. Because the potential effects of undernutrition are numerous, for these clients a complete physical assessment is warranted.

Assessment of clients with known or suspected bulimia nervosa usually includes completion of a physical exam by the primary healthcare provider, followed by psychological evaluation

and laboratory diagnostics. Clients with bulimia nervosa typically maintain a body weight that meets or exceeds normal weight limits. For these clients, focused assessment of the oral cavity can be very revealing. If purging behaviors include vomiting, clients' teeth may demonstrate pitting and enamel erosion, as well as an increased incidence of dental caries. Clients who purge by vomiting may also exhibit ruptured blood vessels in the eyes, as well as a hoarse voice due to throat irritation. General appearance may include pouchlike cheeks, skin lesions, and cuts and calluses on the finger joints. Laboratory tests might reveal electrolyte imbalances or dehydration due to purging (PubMed Health, 2012b). In particular, clients with bulimia nervosa are susceptible to metabolic acidosis. If dehydrated, they may demonstrate a variety of manifestations, including hypotension, dry mouth, poor skin turgor, complaints of light-headedness or dizziness, general weakness, decreased urine production, and concentrated urine.

Diagnosis

Nursing diagnoses that may be appropriate for inclusion in the plan of care for the client with an eating disorder may include the following:

- *Risk for Injury* related to orthostatic hypotension, fluid volume deficiency, and electrolyte imbalances
- *Deficient Fluid Volume*
- *Imbalanced Nutrition: Less Than Body Requirements*
- *Impaired Oral Mucous Membrane*
- *Disturbed Body Image*
- *Ineffective Coping*
- *Chronic Low Self-Esteem*
- *Anxiety*

(NANDA-I © 2012)

Planning

Client goals are measurable, client-specific outcomes that allow for evaluation of the efficacy of nursing interventions. Goals of care should be realistic and tailored to the client. Ultimately, the primary long-term goals of care for the client with an eating disorder include restoring nutritional status and fluid and electrolyte balance, maintenance of body weight within an acceptable range, and development of a healthy body image. Because these clients face significant psychosocial barriers, including body image distortion and rigid behavioral patterns, intensive psychological care is often necessary for achieving long-term outcomes. Examples of short-term client goals that may be applicable to the nursing plan of care for the client with an eating disorder include the following:

- The client will remain free from injury.
- The client will demonstrate manifestations of fluid volume balance, including adequate urine production, vital signs that range within normal limits, and absence of symptoms such as light-headedness or dizziness.
- The client's laboratory testing will demonstrate electrolyte levels that are within normal limits.
- The client will not engage in purging behaviors.
- The client will actively participate in individual and/or group therapy.

Implementation

Care of the client who is diagnosed with an eating disorder is highly complex. Priorities of care include protecting the client from physiological effects of the eating disorder. However, the ultimate goal is identification and treatment of the cause of the alterations, which is the eating disorder itself. For these clients, the primary intervention involves intensive therapy provided by a mental health professional who is specially trained in the treatment of clients with feeding and eating disorders. While recognizing the complexity of the origin and treatment of feeding and eating disorders, the nurse can promote wellness through preventing client injury and encouraging healthy client behaviors and thought patterns.

Prevent Injury

With all clients, injury prevention and safety promotion are priorities of nursing care. By nature, clients with feeding and eating disorders are at constant or near-constant risk for injury due to undernutrition and its consequences. The effects of purging behaviors also keep the client at risk for injury. For these clients, eating patterns and behaviors such as purging and excessive exercise are compulsive in nature, meaning that they are outside the clients' realm of control. Behavioral contracts that outline prohibited actions and their consequences may prove effective in the care of clients who are at risk for injurious behaviors. However, especially early in the course of treatment of clients with feeding and eating disorders, behavioral contracts may have adverse effects, particularly as asking clients to promise to control compulsive behaviors is unrealistic. For these clients, many of whom are already struggling with shame, the inability to adhere to the contract could serve to heighten the sense of shame and further diminish self-esteem. For clients in the clinical setting, constant monitoring and supervision may be necessary to ensure adequate nutritional intake and prevent purging behaviors.

In extreme cases, intake of nutrients and fluids may be medically ordered and administered to clients whose lives are at risk. For all clients, such issues raise ethical concerns and require the nurse to be aware of legal considerations related to forced care. Among experts in the field of feeding and eating disorders, the practice of forcing client interventions to prevent injury (including death) is the subject of intense debate (Fox & Goss, 2012).

Promote a Therapeutic Relationship

Many clients with feeding and eating disorders have maintained secrecy with regard to their nutritional habits and purging behaviors. Treatment requires clients to be open about their behaviors, as well as to discuss sensitive topics and issues that may be psychologically painful. Transitioning from secrecy to openness is a major challenge that requires great courage on the part of the client, as well as establishment of trust between the client and the healthcare provider. With these clients, respect, consistency, and patience are keys to establishing trust, which is part of the foundation of a therapeutic relationship.

Evaluation

Evaluation is a dynamic, ongoing feature of the nursing process that includes identifying the degree to which clients have achieved the goals and outcomes established in conjunction with each nursing diagnosis. While goals and outcomes for the client with an eating disorder will vary based upon client individuality and the client's nursing diagnoses, examples of potential outcomes relevant to the care of these clients may include the following:

- The client remains free from injury.
- The client's vital signs remain within normal limits.
- The client's serum electrolytes remain within normal limits.
- The client demonstrates production of non-concentrated urine.
- The client denies light-headedness or dizziness.
- The client does not demonstrate purging behaviors.
- The client actively participates in individual and/or group therapy.

◢ REVIEW **Feeding and Eating Disorders**

RELATE Link the Concepts and Exemplars

Linking the exemplar on feeding and eating disorders with the concept of teaching and learning:

1. In the context of caring for a client diagnosed with an eating disorder, describe the barriers the nurse faces with regard to teaching about nutrition.

2. The nurse is caring for a 17-year-old female client who is diagnosed with anorexia nervosa. The client's father states, "Once she starts eating regularly, she'll get better. She's just being stubborn." To effectively teach the father about the basis of anorexia nervosa, how should the nurse respond?

Linking the exemplar on feeding and eating disorders with the concept of acid–base balance:

3. How does purging by way of self-induced vomiting most often affect the individual's acid–base balance? How does purging through laxative abuse most often affect acid–base balance?

4. What potential cardiac complications may arise as a result of acid–base imbalances associated with feeding and eating disorders?

READY Go to Companion Skills Manual

REFER Go to Pearson Student Nursing Resources
nursing.pearsonhighered.com

- Additional review materials

REFLECT Case Study

Anisha Robinson is an 18-year-old college student who received a full scholarship for gymnastics. At 5'2" and 101 pounds, Ms. Robinson is tiny, but she frequently complains about being overweight. When she is not practicing with the gymnastics team, she spends much of her time studying. Although her grades are outstanding, she worries that she will not be admitted into pharmacy school. Sometimes she is so wound up at night that she can't sleep. In order not to keep her roommate up, she'll go out and run 2–3 miles in the middle of the night. Her friends worry about her because they don't know how she can keep her strength up when she eats so little, despite the fact that she'll exercise for an hour or more after every meal. Her roommate becomes worried when they return from Thanksgiving break and she hears the gymnastics coach complaining that Ms. Robinson has gained 3 pounds over the holiday. Ms. Robinson tearfully resolves to eat less and work out more.

1. What are the priority nursing diagnoses for Ms. Robinson?
2. What nursing interventions may be appropriate for inclusion in Ms. Robinson's nursing plan of care?
3. What assessment findings may indicate that Ms. Robinson's health is deteriorating?

EXEMPLAR 29.2 Personality Disorders

EXEMPLAR KEY TERMS
Antagonism, 1854
Antisocial personality disorder (ASPD), 1855
Avoidant personality disorder (APD), 1855
Borderline personality disorder (BPD), 1855
Dependent personality disorder (DPD), 1857
Depersonalization, 1860
Derealization, 1860
Detachment, 1855
Disinhibition, 1855
Ego-syntonic, 1853
Histrionic personality disorder (HPD), 1858
Impulsiveness, 1852
Manipulation, 1852
Narcissism, 1852
Narcissistic personality disorder (NPD), 1859
Negative affectivity, 1855
Obsessive-compulsive personality disorder (OCPD), 1859
Paranoid personality disorder (PPD), 1859
Personality, 1852
Personality disorder (PD), 1852
Personality traits, 1852
Psychoticism, 1855
Schizoid personality disorder, 1859

Schizotypal personality disorder, 1860
Splitting, 1857

EXEMPLAR LEARNING OUTCOMES
After reading about this exemplar, you will be able to:

1. Describe the pathophysiology, etiology, clinical manifestations, and direct and indirect causes of personality disorders.
2. Identify risk factors and prevention methods associated with personality disorders.
3. Illustrate the nursing process in providing culturally competent care across the life span for individuals with personality disorders.
4. Formulate priority nursing diagnoses appropriate for an individual with a personality disorder.
5. Summarize therapies used by interdisciplinary teams in the collaborative care of an individual with a personality disorder.
6. Plan evidence-based care for an individual with a personality disorder and his or her family in collaboration with other members of the healthcare team.
7. Evaluate expected outcomes for an individual with a personality disorder.

▶ OVERVIEW

The American Psychological Association (2013) defines **personality** as enduring characteristic patterns of thinking, feeling, and behavior that make an individual unique. These patterns begin to take shape in childhood and are set by early adulthood. Character and temperament constitute two important aspects of a person's personality. *Character* refers to moral and ethical value judgments, whereas *temperament* refers to innate characteristics, such as nervousness or sensitivity.

The elements that comprise an individual's personality are called **personality traits**. They number in the hundreds, and examples include affability, impulsiveness, and honesty. In the field of psychology, however, special emphasis has been placed on the five-factor model: neuroticism, extraversion, openness, agreeableness, and conscientiousness (Butcher, Mineka, & Hooley, 2013). Psychologists generally use these traits to describe an individual's personality, as they are considered to be universal; however, recent research raises questions as to their universality in non-Western preindustrialized societies (Gurven, von Rueden, & Massenkoff, 2013).

An individual's personality determines how that individual interacts with others. When established personality patterns result in repeated conflicts with others and impair the individual's ability to function in society, that individual is said to suffer

from a **personality disorder (PD)**. PDs affect all aspects of an individual's life and are marked by overly rigid and maladaptive behaviors that make it difficult for the individual to adapt to social demands and change. PDs are independent of mental disorders and substance abuse and are generally consistent over time and across varying situations.

▶ PATHOPHYSIOLOGY AND ETIOLOGY

PDs typically manifest themselves during adolescence and continue throughout the life span, although in some cases symptoms diminish with age. Symptoms include interpersonal difficulties, identity problems that result in a weak sense of self, a lack of intimate relationships, and clumsy social skills that hinder cooperation. Individuals with PDs exhibit behaviors that may include **manipulation** (controlling and taking advantage of others); **narcissism** (believing oneself superior and worthy of special treatment); and **impulsiveness** (acting without regard to potential consequences; Kneisl & Trigoboff, 2013).

The nature of these dysfunctions is not fully understood. The American Psychiatric Association has described several PDs, but because clinical definitions lack precision, there is often overlap. Consequently, individuals suffering from a PD are usually diagnosed with more than one. That said, all individuals with PDs demonstrate three common behaviors. First, they manage stress by attempting to change the environment rather than themselves; second, they fail to assume responsibility for the consequences of their actions; and lastly, they illustrate a lack of understanding as to how their behavior affects others. In effect, individuals with PDs are **ego-syntonic**, meaning that they behave according to the beliefs, desires, and values that concur with their disorder; in other words, they see themselves and their behavior as normal and view the problems that arise with others as external to themselves, often believing they are being victimized (Fontaine, 2009; Kneisl & Trigoboff, 2013).

PDs are also characterized by deficits in the areas of cognition, affect, interpersonal relationships, and impulse control; individuals with PDs manifest problems and difficulties in at least two of these areas of functioning (Kneisl & Trigoboff, 2013). In addition to this impairment, developing healthy coping strategies proves to be a challenge as individuals with PDs are typically inflexible. This lack of adaptability feeds into a continual negative cycle in which the same behaviors are consistently exhibited, sabotaging opportunities to gain new skills, and ultimately leading to social isolation (Eby & Brown, 2009).

Etiology

Much about PDs remains unknown, and studies on PDs are hampered by several factors. For example, the lack of diagnostic uniformity makes it difficult for researchers to define samples and replicate previous studies. Another problem is that most individuals suffering from PDs do not come to the attention of mental health professionals. Many individuals with PDs fail to recognize themselves as abnormal and see no need to seek out treatment (inpatient or outpatient). Consequently, mental health professionals only come in contact with individuals who are pushed to enter the mental health system by family members or are referred by the courts (Fontaine, 2009; Kneisl & Trigoboff, 2013).

In part because of the lack of engagement of these individuals with the healthcare system, the causes and origins of PDs are not entirely understood. It is known that, unlike posttraumatic stress disorder or major depression, PDs are not caused by a single stressful episode. Instead, the inflexible personality and behavioral patterns that characterize these disorders appear to develop gradually, often with origins in childhood (Butcher et al., 2013). PDs do not appear to be the result of any one cause. Instead, they seem to be the result of an interaction between biological and environmental factors.

GENETICS There does appear to be a genetic causal relationship with certain PDs. According to the Mayo Clinic (2013a), a family history of schizotypal PD and/or schizophrenia increases the likelihood of an individual developing schizotypal PD. Similarly, Gunderson et al. (2011) interviewed individuals in a psychiatric hospital as well as their families and concluded that a family history of borderline PD was an important factor in the development of this type of PD. A study on fraternal and identical twins with antisocial personality disorder (ASPD) found genetic factors to be a greater influence than environmental factors (Kendler, Aggen, & Patrick, 2012). The American Psychiatric Association (2013) reports on increasing

evidence of the link among specific genes, obsessive-compulsive personality disorder (OCPD), and the personality traits of aggressiveness, anxiety, and fear.

NEUROBIOLOGY Research points to several neurobiological factors as contributors to the development of PDs. For example, Terburg, Morgan, and van Honk (2009) found that high levels of testosterone combined with low levels of cortisol are associated with the aggressive behaviors typically exhibited by those with ASPD. Neuroimaging studies of individuals with borderline personality disorder (BPD) revealed activity variations in the areas of the brain that control emotions and impulses (Dell'Orso et al., 2010). Another neuroimaging study found that trait anxiety might cause emotional interference and disrupt cognitive processing in individuals with BPDs (Holtmann et al., 2013). Stanley and Siever (2010) suggest that "altered neuropeptide function" (p. 36) may contribute to BPD.

INTRAPERSONAL FACTORS Individuals with different PDs interact with others in a variety of ways. They may project their feelings onto those around them, demonstrate problems in developing genuine intimate relationships, lack a sense of guilt, or behave childishly, depending on their personality dysfunction (Kneisl & Trigoboff, 2013).

Various studies point to childhood trauma as playing a key role in the development of these personality patterns. Early parent–child interactions can significantly affect a person's developing sense of self, and as a result, a child's perception of reality may become distorted if parents are insensitive to the child's needs. Individuals with a family background of criminality and parental separation, or a childhood marked by continually changing caregivers or care institutions, show a higher propensity for PDs (Gibbon, Ferriter, & Duggan, 2009). The American Psychiatric Association (2013) also reports that individuals diagnosed with BPDs have a higher incidence of childhood sexual trauma. Additionally, a longitudinal study of almost 800 mothers and their children showed that the incidence of borderline, narcissistic, obsessive-compulsive, and paranoid PDs increased threefold in children who were verbally abused by their mothers, independent of other factors such as sexual or physical abuse, the temperament of the child, and any coexisting psychiatric disorders (Johnson et al., 2001). Lastly, although mood and anxiety disorders are distinct from PDs, overlapping features among the three types of disorders exist, which makes the correlation between childhood verbal abuse by a parent and the later development of mood and anxiety disorders noteworthy (Tomoda et al., 2011).

SOCIOCULTURAL FACTORS The influence of social and cultural factors in personality disorders is not fully understood, yet it is known that they contribute to personal development. For example, when certain groups are discriminated against in a society, it is difficult for the members of that group to develop a healthy self-image. In traditional cultures, such as those found in Japan, there is societal pressure to conform and adhere to group norms. In the United States, on the other hand, emphasis is placed on the personal versus the communal, leading to the prevalence of a me-first mentality. Thus individuals from different parts of the world have a greater propensity for certain kinds of PDs according to their sociocultural backdrop.

There is evidence that histrionic disorders are less common in Asian cultures, where individuals tend to be more reserved, than in Hispanic cultures, where individuals tend to be more expressive. In the United States, African Americans and Caucasians are less prone to develop BPDs than Hispanics, but they differ with respect to schizotypal PD, with African Americans showing a greater propensity than Caucasians for developing such a disorder (Butcher et al., 2013).

FAMILY THEORY   Individuals with PDs often report dysfunctional families, but this may be the result of projecting blame on their parents. Similarly, children with certain personality traits, such as an impulsive temperament, may be treated badly by parents and peers or rejected socially, leading to the development of a PD. For instance, ASPD may be associated with emotional deprivation, similar to the link between BPD and family enmeshment and abandonment issues (Kneisl & Trigoboff, 2013). There is strong evidence linking BPD and various forms of childhood abuse, including emotional, physical, and sexual. For example, more than 70% of individuals with BPD report being emotionally abused as children. The likelihood of BPD developing as a result of some sort of childhood abuse seems to hold across cultures, although it appears that the varying types of abuse contribute differently to the development of this disorder in different cultures (Huang et al., 2012).

Risk Factors

As discussed in the concept section of this module, both genetic and environmental factors are believed to influence the development of a PD. According to the Mayo Clinic (2013a), notable risk factors include genetics, such as having relatives diagnosed with a PD or another mental illness; family life, such as an unstable home life or parental loss via death or divorce; childhood abuse, such as verbal, physical, and sexual abuse or neglect; diagnosis of other disorders, such as childhood conduct disorder; and low socioeconomic status. That said, diagnosing PDs in children can prove to be challenging because the behavioral and thinking patterns that may indicate such a disorder could actually be the consequence of a developmental phase or the experimentation that often occurs during adolescence.

Prevention

PDs can be prevented if the developing patterns of behavior, feeling, and thought are identified before they become set. This generally requires intervention during childhood and early adolescence (Evans, 2009). Consequently, prevention programs have been created to address both developmental and environmental risk factors, and to break the cycle of repeating problematic patterns by providing interventions at school and in the home. Screening programs have been implemented in schools and primary care settings to help detect risk factors and identify patterns that indicate a PD may be forming. Instruments for use with children have been specifically created for this purpose (Evans, 2009).

In terms of interventions, there are several programs in the United States focused on imparting parenting skills to address aggressive and antisocial behaviors. The Nurse-Family Partnership Program is one of them. Under this program, registered nurses visit at-risk families with newborn children starting at the prenatal period and lasting through the child's second birthday. The nurses impart parenting skills and work with family members to change poor habits, such as smoking and unhealthy eating choices. Another is the Incredible Years Program, which uses video recordings of scenarios with parents to promote positive parent–child interactions. The program also includes a classroom management component for teachers and uses puppets to teach children social skills. A third program, New Beginnings, is designed to help children in the case of divorce by strengthening parenting skills; the program has reduced problem behaviors in children and improved parenting warmth and discipline. The parenting interventions included in these and other programs have demonstrated a positive correlation between sociable behavior and a child's self-esteem (Evans, 2009).

A positive role model can also help a child avoid developing a PD. Evans (2009) also cites the Big Brothers Big Sisters Program, a community-based program that matches adult volunteers with children ages 6–18 from single-parent homes. Children participating in the program tend to have higher grades in school, improved parental relationships, and less aggressive behavior than nonparticipating children in similar circumstances. Regardless of the type of intervention, the earlier preventive measures start, the more likely they are to be effective. Interventions should be used in tandem with other efforts to counter the many influences that may lead a child to develop a PD.

▶ CLINICAL MANIFESTATIONS

Published by the American Psychiatric Association, the *Diagnostic and Statistical Manual of Mental Disorders*, most commonly referred to as the DSM, provides the classification system and diagnostic criteria for mental health disorders. The current version of the DSM is the fifth edition, and thus is written "DSM-5." With regard to PDs, the DSM-5 specifies that individuals with PDs must exhibit dysfunctional behavior toward self and others, and they must also maintain persistent, rigid thoughts and beliefs that are incongruent with sociocultural norms (American Psychiatric Association, 2013). Using a categorical approach, each of the 10 PDs is viewed as being a clinically distinct syndrome. However, the American Psychiatric Association also outlines criteria that are characteristic of a PD in general. The DSM-5 diagnostic criteria for a general personality disorder are summarized in **Box 29–2** ●.

As an alternative to the categorical approach, clinicians may opt to apply the dimensional perspective for diagnosis of a PD (American Psychiatric Association, 2013). For application of the dimensional model, the DSM-5 outlines five domains of personality characteristics and specific traits (also referred to as *trait facets*) associated with each domain. This approach is based upon the premise that PDs result from dysfunctional variations of personality traits from one or more of five primary domains: antagonism, detachment, disinhibition, negative affectivity, and/or psychoticism (American Psychiatric Association, 2013). When a trait domain is associated with a specific PD, that does not necessarily mean that all of the traits within that domain must apply to the PD.

The first trait domain is **antagonism**, which is composed of manipulativeness (common use of deception for selfish

Box 29–2 DSM-5 Diagnostic Criteria for General Personality Disorder

A. An enduring pattern of inner experience and behavior that deviates markedly from the expectations of the individual's culture. This pattern is manifested in two (or more) of the following areas:
   1. Cognition (i.e., ways of perceiving and interpreting self, other people, and events).
   2. Affectivity (i.e., the range, intensity, lability, and appropriateness of emotional response).
   3. Interpersonal functioning.
   4. Impulse control.

B. The enduring pattern is inflexible and pervasive across a broad range of personal and social situations.

C. The enduring pattern leads to clinically significant distress or impairment in social, occupational, or other important areas of functioning.

D. The pattern is stable and of long duration and its onset can be traced back at least to adolescence or early adulthood.

E. The enduring pattern is not better explained as a manifestation or consequence of another mental disorder.

F. The enduring pattern is not attributable to the physiological effects of a substance (e.g., a drug of abuse, a medication) or another medical condition (e.g., head trauma).

Source: American Psychiatric Association. (2013). *Diagnostic and statistical manual of mental disorders* (5th ed.). Arlington, VA: Author.

purposes); deceitfulness (lying); callousness (no interest in other individuals' suffering or misfortune, aggression, and no sense of guilt for negative actions committed against others); hostility (common presence of anger and vindictive behavior); grandiosity (feelings of superiority over others); and attention seeking (behaviors that aim to attract the attention of others). A second trait domain is **detachment**, which is broken down into withdrawal (evasion of social interaction); intimacy avoidance (eschewal of sexual and authentic relationships); anhedonia (apathetic reaction to pleasant activities); and restricted affectivity (little to no demonstration of emotions). Another trait domain is **disinhibition**, noted for the presence of irresponsibility (uninterested in following through with obligations); impulsivity (lack of self-control); and risk taking (participation in dangerous activities while ignoring the potential consequences). Fourth is **negative affectivity**, which refers to anxiousness (the extreme sensations of worry and/or panic); emotional lability (common mood swings not necessarily related to a specific situation); separation insecurity (intense fear of abandonment); depressivity (consistently sad and pessimistic feelings and outlook); perseveration (repetitive behavior that does not produce desired results); and suspiciousness (lack of trust in others that involves feeling mistreated or bullied). The last trait domain is **psychoticism**, composed of eccentricity (abnormal or inappropriate conduct); cognitive and perceptual dysregulation (unconventional way of thinking, communicating, and perceiving); and unusual beliefs and experiences (perception of reality is seen as peculiar).

Stay Current: *For additional detail regarding each trait domain and trait facet, visit the Web site for the American Psychiatric Association at* **www.psych.org**.

The DSM-5 lists 10 PDs. The PDs are categorized into three clusters: Cluster A includes those PDs that may be characterized by odd or eccentric behaviors; Cluster B includes the PDs characterized by dramatic, erratic, or emotional behaviors; and Cluster C includes those PDs typified by avoidant, dependent, or obsessive-compulsive behaviors (American Psychiatric Association, 2013). The currently recognized PDs are presented in alphabetical order. For an overview of the primary PDs, see **Table 29–5** ●.

Antisocial Personality Disorder

One of the first named PDs was **antisocial personality disorder (ASPD)**, which is distinguished by the individual's propensity to manipulate or violate others' rights with a disregard for their feelings and/or the consequences (U.S. National Library of Medicine, 2012). As reported by the NIMH (2013a), risk factors include having a caregiver who has ASPD or alcoholism and being a victim of child abuse. An estimated 1.0% of the U.S. population has ASPD with approximately twice as many men having the disorder than women (Eby & Brown, 2009). Due to the lack of remorse and inclination for risk-taking behavior associated with ASPD, it's not surprising that a high incidence of individuals with ASPD is found in prison and substance abuse treatment centers.

To confirm diagnosis of ASPD, an individual must illustrate dysfunction as illustrated by egocentric behaviors, including pleasure-seeking and unlawful behaviors. In addition, impairments must exist in interpersonal functioning either via a lack of empathy and remorse for wrongdoings or the inability to form and maintain intimate relationships, which often includes deceptive or coercive behaviors. Two trait domains are associated with ASPD: antagonism and disinhibition. In addition to the other general criteria for PDs, an individual with ASPD must be at least 18 years of age (American Psychiatric Association, 2012).

Avoidant Personality Disorder

Avoidant personality disorder (APD) is characterized by extreme shyness and fear of rejection. Despite the desire to connect and bond with others, their insecurities and concern for other individuals' perception of them prevent individuals with this disorder from forming relationships of substance. Approximately 1.0% of individuals in the United States have APD (National U.S. Library of Medicine, 2012).

Low self-esteem, poor social skills, extreme sensitivity to criticism, and unrealistic expectations related to goal achievement and interacting in groups are characteristics of individuals with APD. They also typically experience a pronounced distrust of individuals' interest in relationship building. Detachment and negative affectivity are the two trait domains associated with APD, with negative affectivity being characterized by anxiety (American Psychiatric Association, 2013).

Borderline Personality Disorder

In 1938, psychoanalyst Adolf Stern established the label of **borderline personality disorder (BPD)**, as he believed the symptoms of BPD sat on the dividing line or "border" between psychosis and neurosis. Currently, many mental healthcare professionals don't agree with Stern's assessment and argue that *borderline* is misleading and can reinforce already existing

TABLE 29–5 Personality Disorders and Associated Characteristics

BEHAVIORAL TRAITS	AFFECTIVE TRAITS	COGNITIVE TRAITS	SOCIAL TRAITS
Antisocial Personality Disorder			
■ Impulsive; difficulty in delaying gratification ■ Dishonest ■ Irresponsible ■ Risk taking ■ Criminal behavior	■ Has no problems with self-expression yet remains detached in interactions ■ Lack of guilt and remorse for committing harmful acts ■ Callous ■ Easily agitated ■ Hostile ■ Failure to empathize	■ Egocentric ■ Grandiose ■ Despite lack of long-term planning, exhibits confidence in future success	■ Cannot form intimate relationships ■ Exploits others as form of interaction ■ Exhibits controlling and abusive behaviors ■ Aggressive
Avoidant Personality Disorder			
■ Intense discomfort in social situations ■ Avoids social contact unless feels will be fully accepted	■ Timid ■ Fearful of rejection ■ Intense worry and anxiety especially with regard to forming relationships	■ Hypersensitive to others' opinions of self ■ Acceptance of others' negative evaluations	■ Wants to have intimate relationships but an extreme fear of being embarrassed, judged, or rejected by others often prevents it ■ Possesses very few close relationships that aren't familial
Borderline Personality Disorder			
■ Impulsive ■ Dangerous risk taking ■ Can self-mutilate and have suicidal tendencies ■ Unpredictable	■ Intense anxiety ■ Difficulty empathizing and feeling guilt ■ Psychotic episodes are common ■ Reactive moods ■ Difficulty in controlling anger ■ Consistently low mood; rarely experiences satisfaction or happiness	■ Unstable perception of self, ranging from grandiosity to self-loathing	■ Highly unstable relationships ■ Manipulative ■ Intense fear of abandonment ■ Mistrust ■ Behavior swings from all-encompassing interest in another individual to complete withdrawal
Dependent Personality Disorder			
■ Passive by nature ■ Seeks out others who are dominant and who will control the relationship	■ Strives to appear friendly and helpful ■ Will subordinate personal desires and needs and instead prioritize the desires and needs of others	■ Insecure with personal decision making ■ Pervasive sense of inferiority	■ Intense fear of rejection ■ Separation from the dominant other may produce extreme anxiety and depression
Histrionic Personality Disorder			
■ Flamboyant ■ Dramatic ■ Seeks to be the center of attention	■ Appears inconsiderate and incapable of empathy ■ Pervasive craving for excitement	■ Egocentric ■ Tends to prefer creative and artistic endeavors as opposed to academic achievement	■ May use sexual behaviors to manipulate others ■ May engage in high-risk sexual behaviors
Narcissistic Personality Disorder			
■ Very competitive in search of power, fame, and love ■ Arrogant ■ Manipulates others to achieve own ends	■ Difficulty in expressing emotions ■ Empathy is a challenge ■ Anxiety and fear in relation to failure	■ Grandiosity ■ Believes is better than others ■ Spends much time fantasizing about being powerful, famous, loved, and beautiful	■ Balanced reciprocal relationships are rare ■ Seeks out relationships as a way to boost own self-esteem
Obsessive-Compulsive Personality Disorder			
■ Perfectionist ■ Inflexible ■ Hardworking ■ High achiever ■ Compulsive; engages in repetitive or ritualistic checking	■ Difficulty in expressing emotions ■ Empathy is a challenge ■ Anxiety and fear in relation to failure	■ Extreme fear of making mistakes; may procrastinate or avoid tasks due to fear of failure	■ Tends to be controlling in relationships, which limits intimacy

TABLE 29–5 Personality Disorders and Associated Characteristics (*continued*)

BEHAVIORAL TRAITS	AFFECTIVE TRAITS	COGNITIVE TRAITS	SOCIAL TRAITS
Paranoid Personality Disorder			
■ Suspicious and mistrusting of others ■ Rigid, fixed worldview	■ Inflexible about beliefs, perceptions, and suspicions ■ Argumentative	■ Generally intelligent and highly capable of arguing in support of personal beliefs	■ Extreme jealousy may impair intimate relationships with significant others ■ Tends to believe every action by others is driven by malevolent intent or ulterior motive
Schizoid Personality Disorder			
■ Loners; tend to prefer solitary activities ■ Uninterested in socialization	■ Generally appear apathetic ■ Flat (emotionless) affect	■ Generally indifferent to situations and circumstances ■ May appear to be cognitively impaired	■ Uninterested in intimate relationships ■ Prefers social isolation and avoids roles that require socialization
Schizotypal Personality Disorder			
■ Bizarre behaviors, appearance, and speech ■ Prefers solitary activities ■ Frequent lack of eye contact	■ Indifferent ■ Nonreactive or inappropriate in emotional situations	■ Extreme suspicion of others ■ Paranoid fears of persecution ■ Odd or distorted thoughts	■ Excessive anxiety in social situations ■ Fears intimate relationships ■ Alienation ■ Lacks the desire to form close relationships ■ Introverted

Sources: Eby, L., & Brown, N. J. (2009). *Mental health nursing care* (2nd ed.). Upper Saddle River, NJ: Pearson Education; Fontaine, K. L. (2009). *Mental health nursing.* Upper Saddle River, NJ: Prentice Hall; Oltmanns, T. F., & Emery, R. E. (2012). *Abnormal psychology.* Upper Saddle River, NJ: Pearson Education; U.S. National Library of Medicine. (2012). *Diseases and conditions.* Retrieved from http://www.ncbi.nlm.nih.gov/pubmedhealth/s/diseases_and_conditions/a; Kneisl, C. R., & Trigoboff, E. (2013). *Contemporary psychiatric-mental health nursing.* Upper Saddle River, NJ: Pearson Education.

negative perceptions of individuals with BPD (Centre for Addiction and Mental Health, 2009). For more information about the stigma attached to BPD, see the Evidence-Based Practice feature.

Impulsivity, unstable emotions, and depression are key symptoms of BPD; self-harm is also common (see **Figure 29–3 ●**), with suicide occurring in up to 9% of those with this disorder (National Institute of Mental Health, 2013d). **Splitting**, the inclination to perceive people or situations as one extreme or the other (e.g., all good or all bad) is also commonly found among individuals with BPD; this feature contributes to their frequent extreme shifts in mood (Oltmanns & Emery, 2012). Gender plays a significant role in that 75% of diagnosed cases are women (American Psychiatric Association, 2013). Approximately 20% of psychiatric inpatients have BPD and 2% of the general population is affected. Risk factors include childhood abuse and abandonment and a strong genetic link: Individuals are five times more likely to be diagnosed with BPD if a first-degree relative also has the disorder. Antisocial personality disorder, mood disorders, and substance abuse disorders are also much more probable in families where individuals are affected with BPD (American Psychiatric Association, 2013).

SAFETY ALERT
Borderline personality disorder is often associated with self-mutilation, which can include cutting or carving into the skin (see Figure 29–3), burning, pulling out hair, and head banging. Nurses must be extremely cognizant of the signs of self-injury and demonstrate sensitivity when conducting an assessment. Clients often hide their injuries by wearing long sleeves or pants, even in warmer weather (Mayo Clinic, 2013b; National Institute of Mental Health, 2013d).

Low self-esteem, intense self-criticism, and disassociation are associated with BPD. Interpersonal functioning is marked by the tendency to take offense easily or an intense fear of abandonment, which creates conflict-ridden and unstable relationships. The dysfunctional personality traits in BPD fall within the trait domains of negative affectivity (including emotional lability), disinhibition, and antagonism (American Psychiatric Association, 2012). The DSM-5 diagnostic criteria for borderline personality disorder are summarized in **Box 29–3 ●**.

Dependent Personality Disorder

Central features of **dependent personality disorder (DPD)** include a pervasive need to be cared for, difficulty with decision making, separation anxiety, and impaired self-confidence.

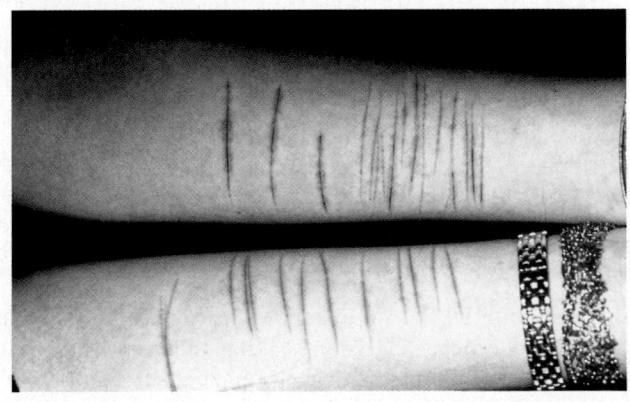

Figure 29–3 ● Some individuals with borderline personality disorder engage in self-mutilating behavior such as cutting.
Source: Dr. P. Marazzi/Science Photo Library/Science Source.

Evidence-Based Practice   Overcoming the Stigma Attached to Borderline Personality Disorder

Problem

On December 4, 2012, personality disorders were the topic of the day on National Public Radio's *Talk of the Nation* (2012). Early in the broadcast, a psychiatric technician at an inpatient hospital called in to share her observations about the stigma attached to clients with BPD. "If the diagnosis was major depressive disorder or an anxiety disorder or even a psychotic disorder ... the stigma didn't seem to be as strong," she said. Later in the program, a nurse in Green Bay, Wisconsin, sent in an email confessing to having a bias against clients with BPD. She described them as "manipulative, demanding, and unpleasant." Further, she reported that despite the conscious efforts of mental health professionals to overcome their negative feelings, she suspected BPD clients were receiving inferior care because they are unlikeable.

Evidence

The stigma attached to BPD is widely acknowledged in the research literature. McGrath and Dowling (2012) discuss several characteristics of BPD that are challenging to nurses, including unstable and intense interpersonal relationships, manipulative behavior, and threats of harming others and themselves, with the latter being reported as the most disturbing. Nurses interacting with clients with BPD report feelings of helplessness, being used and underappreciated, anger, betrayal, and frustration. For their part, clients with BPD report feeling stigmatized and believing that mental health professionals view their acts of self-harm as a form of attention-seeking manipulation. In their study, McGrath and Dowling interviewed 17 nurses who worked with BPD clients at a community mental health clinic in Ireland and surveyed them using the Staff-Patient Interaction Response Scale (SPIRS); they found the words *challenging* and *difficult* repeated often in nurse descriptions of working with BPD clients, many expressing frustration with their clients' attention-seeking behaviors and lack of personal responsibility for their actions. What's more, nurses reported limiting their interactions with clients with BPD as much as possible, as well as providing minimal care and often at the end of the day in order to avoid exploring the client's current needs or concerns in any great detail.

Bodner, Cohen-Fridel, and Iancu (2011) surveyed nurses, psychiatrists, and psychologists working in public psychiatric institutions on their attitudes toward clients with BPD and found that although there were some differences in specific attitudes among the varying professions (e.g., nurses scored lower overall on empathy compared to psychiatrists and psychologists), all groups agreed that the suicidal aspects of BPD were the primary cause of the negative feelings toward such clients. Additionally, Liebman and Burnette (2013) explored countertransference reactions to BPD in 560 clinicians via an online survey and found them to be markedly more negative than with any other disorder, which concurs with previous research.

Implications

Liebman and Burnette (2013) suspect that the high burnout rate among mental health professionals working with BPD may be a consequence of that disorder type's uncommonly high incidence of negative countertransference reactions. They propose a possible solution to the matter: They found that mental health professionals with a postgraduate degree or special BPD training had more positive reactions. Therefore training and education combined with experience seemed to make clinicians more aware of their negative feelings and thus more capable of managing countertransference.

Similarly, based on their findings, McGrath and Dowling (2012) recommend improved nurse training and education aimed at fostering a holistic view of BPD in order to better understand its causes and resulting behaviors. They cite CBT for nurses and BPD workshops as possible models.

In this same vein, Bodner et al. (2011) suggest that the mapping of the varying emotional and cognitive attitudes toward BPD expressed by the different members of the mental health team can be used to specialize staff education and training in the management of BPD clients. Liebman and Burnette (2013) also call for specially tailored training designed according to the education, training, professional discipline, and experience of clinicians; they also suggest that supervised hands-on experiences with clients with BPD can help novice professionals develop competency early on.

Critical Thinking Application

In their study, McGrath and Dowling (2012) asked nurses to react to several scenarios in which clients with BPD say things such as "You're the only one who listens to me" and "I don't want to go to group. It's a waste of time." Mental health professionals sometimes do not know how to react to clients with BPD, often either ignoring comments such as these or replying with platitudes or policy statements in an effort to protect themselves from being manipulated. Many times, the prevailing notion is that clients with BPD have greater control over their behaviors than others, and therefore their transgressions are not as easily forgiven.

1. What steps might an individual nurse take to overcome negative feelings against clients with BPD?
2. How might a nurse help other colleagues do the same?
3. What steps might an institution take?

Individuals with DPD tend to seek out partners with dominant traits who will dictate decision making and choices. Viewing themselves as "dumb" or "inadequate," individuals with DPD will acquiesce to the wants and needs of others, often in an attempt to build or maintain a relationship. At times, these individuals will agree to perform undesirable tasks with the goal of receiving praise or acceptance from others (Kneisl & Trigoboff, 2013).

Histrionic Personality Disorder

Characteristically, individuals with **histrionic personality disorder (HPD)** are self-centered (egocentric) and dramatic. In an attempt to garner attention, they may behave erratically, even going to extremes that appear "silly." Behind the attention-seeking behaviors is a strong sense of inadequacy and

Box 29–3   DSM-5 Diagnostic Criteria for Borderline Personality Disorder

A pervasive pattern of instability of interpersonal relationships, self-image, and affects, and marked impulsivity, beginning by early adulthood and present in a variety of contexts, as indicated by five (or more) of the following:

1. Frantic efforts to avoid real or imagined abandonment. (*Note:* Do not include suicidal or self-mutilating behavior covered in Criterion 5.)
2. A pattern of unstable and intense interpersonal relationships characterized by alternating between extremes of idealization and devaluation.
3. Identity disturbance: markedly and persistently unstable self-image or sense of self.
4. Impulsivity in at least two areas that are potentially self-damaging (e.g., spending, sex, substance abuse, reckless driving, binge eating). (*Note:* Do not include suicidal or self-mutilating behavior covered in Criterion 5.)
5. Recurrent suicidal behavior, gestures, or threats, or self-mutilating behavior.
6. Affective instability due to a marked reactivity of mood (e.g., intense episodic dysphoria, irritability, or anxiety usually lasting a few hours and only rarely more than a few days).
7. Chronic feelings of emptiness.
8. Inappropriate, intense anger or difficulty controlling anger (e.g., frequent displays of temper, constant anger, recurrent physical fights).
9. Transient, stress-related paranoid ideation or severe dissociative symptoms.

Source: American Psychiatric Association. (2013). *Diagnostic and statistical manual of mental disorders* (5th ed.). Arlington, VA: Author.

helplessness. In many cases, the individual with HPD's motivation for behaviors is rooted in a search for excitement and activity. For these clients, an apparent insincerity and inability to establish emotional commitment cause problems in the context of interpersonal relationships. The simultaneous need for love and reassurance experienced by the individual with HPD is counterbalanced by failure to demonstrate empathy and lack of consideration for significant others (Kneisl & Trigoboff, 2013).

Clients with HPD may demonstrate highly sexualized behaviors, appearing provocative and seductive. Seduction and sexuality serve as methods of manipulating others. For some clients with HPD, acting out may include impulsive sexual encounters and promiscuity, which lead to an increased risk for contracting and transmitting sexually transmitted infections (STIs). Additionally, when needs for attention and affection are unfulfilled, the client with HPD may act out through demonstration of suicidal behaviors (Kneisl & Trigoboff, 2013).

Narcissistic Personality Disorder

At the heart of **narcissistic personality disorder (NPD)** is a sense of grandiosity, an inability to empathize with others, and attention-seeking behaviors. Eby and Brown (2009) note that substance-abuse disorders, feeding and eating disorders, and depression are commonly found in conjunction with NPD. More men than women are diagnosed, and it is estimated that less than 1% of the general population suffers from the disorder.

Narcissistic personality disorder is characterized by extreme reliance on other individuals' perceptions and/or an inflated sense of self, or by approval seeking and either an extremely low or high set of personal standards. A failure to identify with others and their emotions or a hypersensitivity to others creates difficulty in developing meaningful relationships. NPD aligns with the trait domain of antagonism, specifically the trait facets of grandiosity and attention seeking (American Psychiatric Association, 2012).

Obsessive-Compulsive Personality Disorder

Obsessive-compulsive personality disorder (OCPD) is characterized by significant impairments in social functioning and relationships and an all-consuming desire to achieve perfection in all tasks. It is important to note that OCPD is not the same as obsessive-compulsive disorder (OCD), which is an anxiety disorder. (See the module on Stress and Coping.) Although they share similar traits, key differences exist. The International OCD Foundation (2012) specifies that individuals with OCPD do not see anything dysfunctional about their way of thinking or acting, whereas those with OCD recognize that their thoughts are disruptive and not normal, making them more likely to seek treatment. Additionally, individuals with OCPD can demonstrate great productivity on the job, but their symptoms place strain on their interpersonal relationships; OCD generally causes disruptions in all areas. Men are twice as likely to suffer from OCPD as women, and approximately 1 in 100 individuals in the United States are believed to have this disorder.

Impaired personality functioning associated with the self involves an identity primarily based on the individual's career or efficiency, or problems with task completion due to extremely inflexible personal standards and values. Additional manifestations identified include a lack of empathy, or viewing relationships as less important than accomplishments and work (American Psychiatric Association, 2013). Abnormal personality traits for OCPD fall within two trait domains: compulsivity, notable by rigid perfectionism, and negative affectivity, characterized by perseveration (American Psychiatric Association, 2012).

Paranoid Personality Disorder

Individuals with **paranoid personality disorder (PPD)** tend to demonstrate an inability to trust others. Actions and intentions of others are perceived as having an underlying theme of malevolence. From the suspicious, mistrusting vantage point of the individual with PPD, others are viewed as being deceptive and disloyal. The pathological jealousy sometimes associated with PPD can damage relationships with significant others. Tending toward being prejudicial and judgmental, individuals with PPD often maintain rigid, inflexible worldviews and will reject logic or proof that contradicts their beliefs. Hypervigilance combined with certainty that others' actions are prompted by hidden motives can lead to isolation for the client with PPD (Kneisl & Trigoboff, 2013).

Schizoid Personality Disorder

Central features of **schizoid personality disorder** include a seeming aloofness, a tendency to prefer solitary activities, absence of humor, and uninterested in forming relationships, including those of a romantic nature. Generally disengaged and uninterested in social interaction, individuals with schizoid personality disorder may appear to be cognitively impaired. Functional abilities and levels of adjustment vary among these clients; some are able to live independently and maintain marginal to adequate function within society, while others are institutionalized (Kneisl & Trigoboff, 2013).

Schizotypal Personality Disorder

Schizotypal personality disorder is distinguishable by extreme social anxiety and eccentric behavior. Commonly, **depersonalization** occurs, in which the individual feels apart from his body or an overall strangeness related to the physical self. Individuals with schizotypal personality disorder can also experience **derealization**, or feeling disconnected from their own body (Kneisl & Trigoboff, 2013). Schizotypal personality disorder and schizophrenia share similar criteria but they are two different disorders, with schizophrenia being more severe. (For discussion of schizophrenia, see the module on Cognition.) For some individuals, symptoms of schizotypal personality disorder progress to a point where a diagnosis of schizophrenia is applied. Schizophrenia is commonly seen in families where another member is diagnosed with schizotypal personality disorder (Eby & Brown, 2009).

Individuals with this disorder experience difficulty in establishing boundaries between self and other individuals and frequently possess aims that are unrealistic or unclear. They frequently misunderstand other individuals' motives and actions, exhibit a lack of understanding of how their own behavior affects others, and experience challenges in establishing intimate relationships primarily due to anxiety and a lack of trust. The DSM-5 outlines three trait domains in schizotypal PD. The first is psychoticism, which is distinguished by eccentricity, cognitive and perceptual dysregulation, and unusual beliefs and experiences. The second trait domain is detachment, characterized by restricted affectivity and withdrawal, and the final trait domain is negative affectivity, which is defined by the trait facet of suspiciousness (American Psychiatric Association, 2012).

Stay Current: *In addition to the American Psychiatric Association's Web site, additional information about PDs can be found at* **www.MayoClinic.com** *and the National Institute for Mental Health at* **www.nimh.nih.gov.**

Lifespan and Cultural Considerations

The DSM-5, as well as previous versions of the DSM, has stated that the abnormal personality traits and impairments in functioning outlined for each PD should remain more-or-less consistent over time (American Psychiatric Association, 2012). However, as Ferguson (2010) outlines, "Debate continues about whether personality, both normal and disordered, can change significantly or is mainly stable across the life span" (p. 659). One faction maintains the historical perspective on personality development is correct: While personality often changes and fluctuates throughout childhood and adolescence, it remains fairly stable after the approximate age of 30 (Costa & McCrae, 2006). In contrast, other researchers argue that "personality continues to change, albeit more slowly, well into adulthood,

and that the maladaptive manifestations of personality disorder are much less stable than previously believed" (Clark, 2009, p. 27). Adding some clarity to this issue is Ferguson's research (2010), which examined 47 studies and the impact of measurement error on the final results. After analyzing the studies and accounting for such errors, Ferguson concluded that personality is quite changeable throughout adolescence "yet quickly becomes stable by early adulthood. Personality remains generally stable throughout adulthood, particularly after the late 20s, and remains stable throughout later adulthood" (p. 663).

As environmental influences play a part in the development of personality, nurses and other healthcare professionals must take care not to deem a personality trait or behavior maladaptive or dysfunctional without first considering the influence of culture. Fontaine (2009) offers a few examples: Individuals who are new to the United States may present as paranoid or overly suspicious of others when in fact their behavior could simply be a result of their unfamiliarity with American customs; some cultures condition girls and women to avoid social situations; and individuals from Latin cultures are generally much more expressive and exuberant than those from Britain. Cultural competence and being aware of one's own biases is crucial in providing quality care for clients. For additional examples, see the Focus on Diversity and Culture feature.

► COLLABORATION

The treatment of personality disorders requires a collaborative effort that includes the client, the multidisciplinary team responsible for the client's care, and the client's family. The multidisciplinary team working with the client may include a primary medical care provider; a psychiatrist or psychologist; a licensed mental health professional; an advanced practice nurse who specializes in psychiatric mental health care; the registered nurse; and other professionals. The registered nurse can fill several important functions, including providing education and follow up related to the therapeutic regimen, and instilling hope in the client and family that achieving a more normal level of functioning is possible.

Treating personality disorders is a considerable challenge and can generate frustration and try the patience of healthcare workers. All those involved, including nurses, ought to understand that an individual's personality developed over that individual's lifetime, reflecting learned experiences, and is therefore unlikely to change drastically. The aim instead should be realistic, short-term outcomes. Eventually, clients should be encouraged to seek long-term therapy, which is considered the most effective in the treatment of personality disorders; long-term therapy demands time, dedication, and buy-in from the client (Eby & Brown, 2009). Nurses should also be especially cognizant of establishing and maintaining boundaries with clients. Friendship should not be encouraged, but rather caring professional treatment should be the priority (Eby & Brown, 2009; Fontaine 2009).

Diagnostic Tests

There isn't any one test mental health professionals use to diagnose PDs. Instead, PDs are typically diagnosed through an interview with the client that covers issues such as symptoms,

Focus on Diversity and Culture Mental Health and Religious Beliefs

When caring for clients with personality disorders, nurses should be aware that some clients may interpret their condition in the context of deeply held religious and spiritual beliefs. More specifically, the symptoms of delusions and hallucinations may be viewed not as mental health issues, but rather as demonic possession or the work of evil spirits. Tajima-Pozo et al. (2011) report on the case of a young woman in Spain who suffered from kinesthetic hallucinations and was diagnosed with paranoid schizophrenia; the client also had high scores for NPD and histrionic personality disorder. She was convinced that half of her symptoms were attributed to an evil presence dwelling within her body, subsequently submitting to several exorcisms at the hands of Catholic priests. This is one example of many as the influence of spirituality and religion in mental health care extends to several of the world's diverse faiths, from Christianity to Buddhism to Islam (Mohr, 2011).

In both the distant and recent past, the medical community viewed religious and spiritual influences as more likely to be harmful than helpful in client care. As a consequence, individuals with personality disorders who maintained a strong spiritual or religious practice often chose not to enter the mental health system, either out of shame or fear of how their beliefs would be perceived, or from their conviction that only religious and spiritual healing could help them (Pargament & Lomax, 2013).

Today, the role of religion is viewed much differently. Partly due to a greater awareness of the need for cultural competence in mental health care, professional caregivers are more willing to integrate religious and spiritual elements into treatment (Pargament & Lomax, 2013). For example, CBT has been adapted for use with Christian clients who suffer from depression and anxiety and feeding and eating disorders by applying its approaches in a religious context that includes biblical imagery and teachings. In Saudi Arabia, clients with schizophrenia who presented with auditory hallucinations were treated with CBT that included Muslim accommodations. And Buddhist principles have been incorporated into treatments such as dialectical behavior therapy (DBT) and Windhorse therapy, which seeks to create an environment tailored to the client's mental health needs (Mohr, 2011). Studies on populations as diverse as Malaysian Muslims with anxiety disorder, Australian clients with depression and schizophrenia, and Jewish clients with anxiety are providing evidence that integrating the client's spiritual and religious beliefs into treatment programs improves the effectiveness of traditional approaches to mental health (Pargament & Lomax, 2013).

family history, and thoughts of violence, suicide, or self-injury. A physical exam and laboratory tests also help rule out other factors that could be the cause of abnormal behavior, such as drug and alcohol abuse (National Institute of Mental Health, 2013; Mayo Clinic, 2013b).

Although mental health professionals refer to the specific diagnostic criteria for each PD found in the most recent version of the DSM, identifying the specific PD a client is suffering from can be complicated due to the frequent overlap of symptoms across disorders. The subjectivity of the client's descriptions and the care provider's interpretation of those descriptions also pose a challenge (Mayo Clinic, 2013a). In this respect, there are a number of psychological tests that can help mental health professionals arrive at a more definitive diagnosis, including personality inventories in a true/false or yes/no format, such as the Personality Diagnostic Questionnaire commonly used to identify NPD, and open-ended projective tests, such as the Thematic Apperception Test frequently used to identify personality traits (D'Agostino et al., 2012; Hopwood et al., 2012).

The presence of a PD does not necessarily require hospitalization (Fontaine, 2009). However, if the disorder becomes so pronounced that an individual is unable to provide self-care or is in imminent jeopardy of causing harm to self or others, then the individual should be hospitalized. Different inpatient options exist, such as day hospitalization or residential treatment (Mayo Clinic, 2013b).

Pharmacologic Therapy

Individuals with personality disorders often are prescribed medications to control their symptoms. Obsessive-compulsive, aggressive, and self-destructive behaviors may be held in check with the use of selective serotonin reuptake inhibitors (SSRIs), such as Prozac. Symptoms associated with avoidant and border-line disorders may be minimized with antidepressants, just as acute psychosis may be ameliorated with antipsychotic drugs. Medications, however, should be used to complement a comprehensive treatment plan that includes therapy (ideally long-term) that incorporates various approaches (Fontaine, 2009; Eby & Brown, 2009).

Psychotherapy

Long-term psychotherapy is the most highly recommended treatment for individuals with PDs. There are various different types of psychotherapy, some more suitable to certain types of PDs than others. Medical professionals usually draw from and combine elements of the different types of psychotherapy to meet a particular client's needs (National Institute of Mental Health, 2013c). All of the therapies described here are generally available as both outpatient and inpatient services.

COGNITIVE-BEHAVIORAL THERAPY Cognitive-behavioral therapy (CBT) combines cognitive aspects to change thoughts and beliefs with behavioral aspects to alter problematic action patterns. It focuses on skill training and problem solving. Typically, the therapist serves as a guide to assist the client in recognizing harmful ways of thinking and erroneous beliefs and works with the individual to purge them by analyzing and reinterpreting both past and current experiences, thus helping the client adopt positive behaviors and interactions with others. This type of therapy can address the symptoms of depression by encouraging the client to change negative thought patterns and also help them identify behaviors that exacerbate depression so that they can be avoided. It can also assist clients with anxiety disorders and those who experience anxiety as a symptom of a personality disorder by providing them a supportive setting in which they can confront their fears. Exposure therapy is a type of CBT in which clients are repeatedly exposed to the source of their anxiety within the safety of a treatment setting. It aims to reduce symptoms by offering clients the chance to develop concrete coping strategies in conjunction with the therapist. CBT can also help individuals with mood disorders recognize when their mood is about to shift, thus giving them the foresight to apply coping strategies to deal with it (American Psychiatric Association, 2013; National Institute of Mental Health, 2013c).

DIALECTICAL BEHAVIORAL THERAPY   A combination of cognitive and behavior therapy, dialectical behavioral therapy (DBT) originally was developed to treat individuals with suicidal thoughts. *Dialectical* refers to striking a balance between two extremes; the therapist displays understanding and validates the client's behaviors and feelings while at the same time imposing limits and making the client responsible for changing unhealthy patterns. It has proven effective in treating borderline personality disorder, showing lower dropout rates than other therapies and lowering the frequency of suicide attempts. Through DBT, clients learn to accept things as they are and apply techniques to control strong emotions that might otherwise overwhelm them. Mindfulness is one such technique, where clients learn to become aware of and explore emotions without reacting to them. This type of therapy usually relies on individual sessions to teach new skills and strategies, and then group sessions to apply them. Traditional and cognitive approaches are also used in conjunction with DBT to help clients foster better relationships with others (American Psychiatric Association, 2013; National Institute of Mental Health, 2013c; Oltmanns & Emery, 2012).

SCHEMA-FOCUSED THERAPY   Schema-focused therapy (SFT) combines aspects of CBT with other forms of psychotherapy to change a client's self-perception. This is often applied to personality disorders, where the individual typically has a poor self-image. SFT aims to help clients view themselves differently so they can create new and more effective ways of interacting with their environment and others (National Institute of Mental Health, 2013c). Research has shown that SFT is an extremely effective treatment option for individuals with BPD, sometimes leading to recovery (Farrell, Shaw, & Webber, 2009).

GROUP THERAPY   Group therapy is also important to the treatment of certain PDs. For example, it can be helpful in strengthening empathic skills for individuals with ASPD in that it allows for feedback about the perceptions of the other group members (Eby & Brown, 2009). Another example of group therapy is the Systems Training for Emotional Predictability and Problem Solving (STEPPS), consisting of 20 two-hour sessions led by a social worker. According to the National Institute of Mental Health (2013c), the STEPPS program, when combined with other approaches, such as pharmacologic treatments and psychotherapy, has alleviated depression and improved the quality of life of individuals with borderline personality disorder.

FAMILY-FOCUSED THERAPY   It is often useful for the family members of clients with PD to participate in family-focused therapy (FFT) so as to cope with the stress of living with a loved one with a personality disorder and avoid behaviors that might worsen the client's condition. FFT educates family members about their loved one's disorder, giving them the necessary knowledge to improve interactions and play an active role in supporting the client. For example, the client's family can develop a course of action in case warning signs of a relapse appear. Additionally, family therapy programs like Family Connections address the needs and concerns of the client's family members. DBT family therapy helps family members understand and support relatives with PD by teaching them skills and strategies and having them participate in the client's treatment sessions (National Institute of Mental Health, 2013c).

ADDITIONAL THERAPIES   Other therapies used to treat PDs include expressive therapy, which relies on creative arts such as music or writing to reduce symptoms of depression, and animal therapy, which brings the client in contact with animals such as dogs or horses to help them work through behavioral and emotional issues. Additionally, psychodynamic therapy can provide greater self-awareness by exploring how subconscious motivations and feelings can drive behaviors. This type of therapy is usually used in combination with others, such as CBT. Psychoeducation is also commonly used in raising awareness about the individual's specific disorder, treatment approaches, and coping strategies. Social skills training also can prove effective with PDs like schizotypal and avoidant (National Institute of Mental Health, 2013c; Mayo Clinic, 2013b).

Complementary and Alternative Therapy

Although there isn't a specific form of complementary or alternative therapy that is recommended for clients with PDs, CAM therapies may provide some relief from certain symptoms, such as anxiety and depression. For instance, yoga, meditation, breathing exercises, and chamomile tea can help individual with anxiety to relax, while vitamin B12 and omega-3 fatty acids can ease depression (Fontaine, 2009). Studies indicate that omega-3 fatty acids may also serve to prevent psychosis from fully emerging in young individuals who show signs of developing such a disorder (Amminger et al., 2010).

◼ NURSING PROCESS

Just as the care of clients with personality disorders will be specific to each client and the manifestations of the disorder, certain features of the nursing assessment will vary as well. Nurses working with clients with personality disorders should remember that some of the symptoms (e.g., labile affect and impairments in social skills) make it difficult to develop the nurse–client relationship, especially when the client denies the presence of symptoms or problems.

Assessment

Assessment data serves as the basis for application of the nursing process. However, assessment of the client with a personality disorder may be complicated by a number of factors, including the following characteristics often associated with PDs:

- Lack of insight/self-awareness
- Denial of the existence of a disorder or manifestations of a disorder

Clinical Manifestations and Therapies **Personality Disorders**

ETIOLOGY	CLINICAL MANIFESTATIONS	CLINICAL THERAPIES
Antisocial	■ Impulsive ■ Lack of remorse ■ Failure to empathize ■ Easily agitated, aggressive, and controlling	■ Group therapy ■ Anger management therapy ■ Psychodynamic therapy ■ Psychoeducation ■ Pharmacologic therapy (antidepressants, mood stabilizers, antianxiety medications, antipsychotics)
Avoidant	■ Extreme discomfort socially ■ Hypersensitive ■ Intense anxiety related to social contact ■ Easily internalizes negative comments by others	■ Social skills training ■ Cognitive-behavioral therapy ■ Group therapy ■ Pharmacologic therapy (antidepressants, antianxiety medications) ■ Alternative therapy
Borderline	■ Extreme risk-taking ■ Impulsive ■ Self-injury, suicidal ■ Intense anxiety ■ Consistently low mood ■ Unstable relationships due to intense mistrust of others	■ Schema-focused therapy ■ Dialectical behavior therapy ■ Cognitive-behavioral therapy ■ Pharmacologic therapy (antidepressants, antianxiety medications, antipsychotics, mood stabilizers) ■ Group therapy (e.g., STEPPS) ■ Alternative therapy
Dependent	■ Pervasive need to be under control by a dominant other ■ Insecure about making decisions ■ Chronic sense of inadequacy	■ Psychotherapy ■ Pharmacologic treatment of symptoms with antidepressants or anxiolytics; caution to monitor for dependence on medications
Histrionic	■ Flamboyant, highly seductive in behavior and/or appearance ■ May be sexually manipulative ■ Demands to be center of attention ■ Constantly seeks excitement and activity	■ Psychotherapy may be effective ■ Group therapy not recommended due to attention-seeking behaviors
Narcissistic	■ Grandiosity ■ Rage ■ Depression, anxiety ■ Manipulative ■ Lack of empathy	■ Cognitive-behavioral therapy ■ Family-focused therapy ■ Pharmacologic therapy (antidepressants, antianxiety medications)
Obsessive-compulsive	■ Inflexible, controlling ■ Anxiety ■ Difficulty with empathy ■ Perfectionist	■ Cognitive-behavioral therapy ■ Pharmacologic therapy (SSRIs) ■ Alternative therapy
Paranoid	■ Unable to trust others ■ Rigid, fixed worldview that often is conspiratorial in nature ■ Believes others' actions are based on ulterior motives	■ Psychotherapy ■ If accepted by the client, pharmacologic therapy may include antidepressants, anxiolytics, and antipsychotic medications
Schizoid	■ Prefers solitude, uninterested in interpersonal relationships ■ Generally unable to perceive or express strong emotions	■ Cognitive-behavioral therapy ■ Group therapy with others who are also learning interpersonal skills ■ Pharmacologic treatment may include antidepressant and antipsychotic medications

(continued on next page)

Clinical Manifestations and Therapies Personality Disorders (continued)

ETIOLOGY	CLINICAL MANIFESTATIONS	CLINICAL THERAPIES
Schizotypal	■ Odd mannerisms and speech patterns ■ Cold demeanor, inappropriate responses ■ Lack of affect ■ Distorted thoughts ■ Intense anxiety in social situations ■ Paranoid fears of persecution	■ Cognitive-behavioral therapy ■ Family-focused therapy ■ Pharmacologic therapy (antidepressants, antianxiety medications, antipsychotics) ■ Alternative therapy

Sources: Eby, L., & Brown, N. J. (2009). *Mental health nursing care* (2nd ed.). Upper Saddle River, NJ: Pearson Education; Fontaine, K. L. (2009). *Mental health nursing.* Upper Saddle River, NJ: Prentice Hall; Gunderson, J. G., & Choi-Kain, L. W. (2012). *Personality disorders.* Retrieved from http://www.merckmanuals.com/home/mental_health_disorders/personality_disorders/personality_disorders.html; International OCD Foundation. (2012). *Obsessive-compulsive personality disorder (OCPD).* Retrieved from http://www.ocfoundation.org/materials.aspx; Mayo Clinic. (2013a). *Personality disorders: Risk factors.* Retrieved from http://www.mayoclinic.com/health/personality-disorders/DS00562/DSECTION=risk-factors; Oltmanns, T. F., & Emery, R. E. (2012). *Abnormal psychology.* Upper Saddle River, NJ: Pearson Education; U.S. National Library of Medicine. (2012). *Diseases and conditions.* Retrieved from http://www.ncbi.nlm.nih.gov/pubmedhealth/s/diseases_and_conditions/a.

■ Lack of trust

■ Ineffective communication skills and/or communication abilities.

Within the realm of psychosocial assessment, the primary goals of assessment include identification of behaviors, beliefs, or thought patterns that disrupt the client's social, professional, and personal life. When the client lacks insight about the existence or effects of a PD, pertinent information may be gleaned from reports by family members or others who are closely associated with the client. However, because maintenance of client confidentiality is essential, the nurse must avoid overstepping the client's personal and legal boundaries during data collection.

Data collection should include assessing work history; history of behavior problems, including violence directed at self or others; history of suicidal ideation; methods of resolving conflicts; alcohol and drug use; and nature of relationships with family members, coworkers, and friends. Ask questions that encourage the client to describe aspects of self:

■ When was the last time you were upset? What upset you? How did you handle it?

■ How do others describe you?

■ How would you describe yourself?

■ What do you like about yourself? What would you like to change?

■ How do you usually relate to others?

Assess for signs of self-directed violence, such as cutting (see Figure 29–3); assess for evidence of alcohol or drug use.

Diagnosis

Selection of nursing diagnoses depends on client-specific needs and strengths, as well as functional capability. For example, high-functioning clients who have insight as to the nature and effects of their PD may be well suited for client teaching, while clients who demonstrate significant functional impairment and lack of insight may not benefit from teaching. General examples of nursing diagnoses that may be appropriate for

inclusion in the plan of care for the client with a PD may include the following:

■ *Risk for Injury*
■ *Risk for Self-Directed Violence*
■ *Risk for Other-Directed Violence*
■ *Self-Mutilation*
■ *Ineffective Coping*
■ *Anxiety*
■ *Social Isolation*
■ *Impaired Social Interaction*
■ *Ineffective Role Performance*
■ *Disturbed Personal Identity*
■ *Interrupted Family Processes*

(NANDA-I © 2012)

Planning

Client goals are measurable, client-specific outcomes that allow for evaluation of the efficacy of nursing interventions. Goals of care should be realistic and tailored to the client. Examples of client goals that may be applicable to the nursing plan of care for the client with a PD include the following:

■ The client will remain free from injury.
■ The client will refrain from violent behaviors.
■ The client will report a reduction in anxiety.
■ The client will verbalize emotions to staff.
■ The client will adhere to established rules and guidelines.
■ The client will actively participate in one-on-one and/or group therapy sessions.

Implementation

As with assessment and planning, implementation of the nursing plan of care will vary based on the manifestations and effects of the client's PD. In general, nursing interventions for clients diagnosed with a PD will include preventing injury and maintaining physical safety of the client, as well as protecting the safety of individuals with whom the client interacts. In addition, promotion of comfort—both physical and psychosocial—is a priority of care. Psychosocial aspects of comfort promotion include building a therapeutic relationship with the client and effectively managing conflicts. In a respectful, professional manner, the nurse establishes clear boundaries and limits for the client. For clients who are amenable to socialization, the nurse identifies client-specific interventions that will afford the client the opportunity to learn and practice social skills.

Promote Safety

With all clients, priorities of care include injury prevention and safety promotion. For clients with PDs, some of whom are prone to self-destructive and impulsive behavior, the emphasis on injury prevention is heightened. Behavioral contracts that outline prohibited actions and the consequences of those actions may be used to establish clear guidelines and expectations with regard to any form of behavior, including that related to injuring self or others. Basic precautions include ensuring that the client's environment is free from items that may be used in the process of harming self or others, as well as ensuring that clients are not left unsupervised or unmonitored. As opposed to trying to independently manage strong emotions, clients should be encouraged to seek assistance from members of the healthcare team when they need to process their feelings, including when they perceive that their stress levels are rising.

Promote the Therapeutic Relationship

The ineffective social skills and impaired perceptions that often accompany PDs can create unique challenges in the establishment of a therapeutic nurse–client relationship. Moreover, for clients who struggle with trust issues, unplanned admission to a hospital or treatment center can exacerbate their anxiety and sense of mistrust. Consistency with client care—including demonstration of respect for the client at all times—is one of the first steps to building trust.

Establish Boundaries

Boundaries are limits that define what is acceptable to an individual in every facet of life, including the physical, mental, emotional, sexual, relational, spiritual, and professional realms. A breach of boundaries occurs when those limitations are ignored or exceeded. In many ways, definition of boundaries occurs during childhood, beginning in infancy, through experiencing how others treat us. Breach of boundaries during childhood, such as when a child is the victim of sexual abuse, may render the affected individual unable to form or enforce healthy boundaries later in life. Culture, as well as other factors, also influences boundaries. Intact boundaries clarify the delineation between self and others and promote a sense of well-being. Failure to establish and maintain healthy boundaries can lead to a number of alterations in psychosocial well-being, including depression, anxiety, identity confusion, and excessive dependency (Cloud, 1996).

In the context of the nurse–client relationship, establishing and maintaining healthy boundaries establishes a sense of safety and predictability for the client. As the result of past experiences, including a history of abuse and a sense of shame that may accompany the stigmatization often associated with mental illness, the client with a PD may have unhealthy, unclear, or nonexistent boundaries. The nurse can help the client to understand and set healthy boundaries through interventions such as teaching, as well as through role playing with the client. In helping the client establish healthy boundaries, the nurse can use role play to simulate situations in which the client is faced with potential boundary violations, assess the client's coping skills, and teach the client about healthy responses to attempted boundary violation (Fontaine, 2009).

Because manipulation, which often includes a breach of boundaries, is inherently linked to many PDs, nurses and other members of the healthcare team should be alert to behaviors that suggest exploitation of others, including other clients. Particularly for clients who exhibit splitting behaviors, healthcare providers must work as a team in order to prevent conflict between nurses and clients, as well as among themselves.

Regardless of the client's behaviors, the nurse is responsible for maintaining healthy professional boundaries. Provision 2 of the American Nurses Association's (ANA) Code of Ethics (2001) requires the nurse to establish and maintain boundaries, and to effectively set limits with clients. Establishing professional boundaries includes choosing which of the nurse's personal information is appropriate for sharing with the client. Especially because of the intimate nature of the nurse–client relationship, the client also may ask personal questions, for example, whether or not the nurse is married or has children. Sharing some degree of background information in an appropriate, professional manner can strengthen the nurse–client relationship; however, the oversharing of personal information is detrimental and nontherapeutic. Through sharing details of personal problems and struggles with the client, the nurse can create an unnecessary—and unethical—burden for the client, who is the one seeking care. Boundary violations occur when meeting the nurse's needs takes precedence over meeting the client's needs (Gutheil & Brodsky, 2011; Holder & Schenthal, 2007). For further illustration of maintaining professional boundaries in nursing, see **Table 29–6** .

Evaluation

Evaluation is a dynamic, ongoing feature of the nursing process that includes identifying the degree to which clients have achieved the goals and outcomes established in relationship to each nursing diagnosis. While goals and outcomes for the client with a PD will vary based upon client individuality and the nursing diagnoses included in the nursing plan of care, examples of achieved outcomes relevant to the evaluation of client care may include the following:

- The client remains free from injury.
- The client does not demonstrate violent behaviors toward self or others.
- The client verbalizes understanding of the concept of boundaries.
- The client verbalizes understanding of the principles of respecting boundaries related to self and others.
- The client actively participates in individual and/or group therapy.

TABLE 29–6   Maintaining Professional Boundaries in Nursing

BOUNDARIES MAINTAINED	BOUNDARIES BREACHED
Keeping one's personal life private and focusing on the client's needs	Sharing details of personal life, issues, and/or problems with a client
Sharing limited details about basic background information when asked, such as marital status, number of children, educational background, and professional nursing background	Discussing the state of one's marriage (e.g., marital separation or currently in the process of divorce); sharing about one's children's behavioral problems or medical challenges; discussing personal, emotional, or legal problems or setbacks
Maintaining all client-related information as confidential, and discussing only relevant aspects of the client's condition and care with the necessary healthcare team members in the workplace	Revealing client-related information to anyone who is not involved in planning or administering care to the client
Limiting discussion of clients and their care to within the clinical setting	Discussing clients and their care in the hospital cafeteria, hallways, or other nonclinical areas; sharing any client-related information through any format, including via social media
Interacting with the client only during scheduled duty hours for professional intents and purposes	Visiting the client during off-duty hours, in or away from the clinical setting; communicating with the client by any means for purposes other than those directly related to the client's plan of health care
Demonstrating respect for one's institution or organization, work policies, and other members of the healthcare team, and declining to discuss workplace-related conflicts or criticisms	Venting to the client about issues or concerns regarding one's employer, work policies, or other members of the healthcare team
Facilitating referrals for clients with financial needs to appropriate organizations or assisting the client in connecting with official agencies who can provide assistance	Giving clients personal items or financial assistance
Identification and referral to appropriate healthcare team members for resolution of the client's personal conflicts	Choosing to side with a client during conflict between clients and their spouses, family members, or significant others

Sources: Based on Remshardt, M. A. (2012). Do you know your professional boundaries? *Nursing Made Incredibly Easy, 10*(1), 5–6; Holder, K. V., & Schenthal, S. J. (2007). Watch your step: Nursing and professional boundaries. *Nursing Management, 38*(2), 24–29; Gutheil, T. G., & Brodsky, A. (2011). *Preventing boundary violations in clinical practice.* New York, NY: Guilford Press.

NURSING CARE PLAN   A Client With Borderline Personality Disorder

Kathryn Vannosa is an 18-year-old Hispanic female client who is transported to the emergency department (ED) by law enforcement. Officer Rick Natami, the attending police officer, reports that Ms. Vannosa broke a window with her fist while arguing with her boyfriend. Subsequently, Ms. Vannosa told her boyfriend she was going to kill herself. At that point, Ms. Vannosa's boyfriend called 911. In addition to law enforcement, emergency medical personnel also responded to the call. Officer Natami reports Ms. Vannosa was combative at the scene and would not allow the paramedics to assess her injuries, nor would she permit them to transport her to the ED by ambulance. As a result, because of her injuries and her threat to commit suicide, Officer Natami handcuffed and transported Ms. Vannosa in his squad car for physical and psychiatric evaluation.

Upon arrival to the ED, Ms. Vannosa is cursing at Officer Natami, as well as anyone with whom she makes eye contact, including her attending nurse. When the ED physician asks if he can assess Ms. Vannosa's injuries, she replies, "Yeah, if you tell the cop to take these handcuffs off me and make him leave! You're cool, but he's a total jerk!" The ED physician tells Ms. Vannosa he will ask the police officer to remove the handcuffs and stand outside the examination room, but only if she agrees to remain calm and noncombative. Ms. Vannosa agrees, and the officer removes her handcuffs and steps outside the room. Because Ms. Vannosa has previously been treated at the facility, her electronic medical record (EMR) is accessible. Based on her EMR, her past medical history includes borderline personality disorder and previous treatment for self-inflicted superficial leg lacerations. Before the ED physician evaluates Ms. Vannosa's lacerations, he quietly asks the nurse to order a psychiatric consultation for the client.

ASSESSMENT	DIAGNOSES	PLANNING
Following closure of her lacerations, Ms. Vannosa agrees to allow the nurse to assess her vital signs and auscultate her heart and lungs. Vital signs include temperature 97.3°F oral, pulse 90 bpm, respirations 20/min, and BP 133/71 mmHg. Ms. Vannosa's heart tones are normal; however, the nurse hears faint, bibasilar wheezes in her lungs. When the nurse asks if Ms. Vannosa has had any recent respiratory problems, she replies, "I have no idea. I don't have health insurance and nobody cares anyway. I'm just a piece of garbage." Ms. Vannosa begins to cry and states, "I don't know why I get so mad. I'm such an idiot! My boyfriend should dump me, just like everybody else does." The nurse verbally reassures Ms. Vannosa that she is safe and will receive the best possible care. Ms. Vannosa replies, "I'm sorry I called you names earlier—you're the nicest nurse I've ever met. The nurses on the psych floor are mean. They're only going to make me take a bunch of pills. I wish I could stay here, with you."	■ *Risk for Injury* ■ *Risk for Self-Directed Violence* ■ *Risk for Other-Directed Violence* ■ *Impaired Skin Integrity* ■ *Ineffective Coping* (NANDA-I © 2012)	■ The client will sustain no further physical injury. ■ The client will not injure others. ■ The client's wound will be closed and protected from further injury or contamination. ■ The client will express her emotions to members of the healthcare team in a nondestructive manner.

NURSING CARE PLAN *(continued)*

IMPLEMENTATION

- Maintain or delegate a team member to maintain constant observation of the client to assess for and prevent injurious behavior.
- Outline behavioral guidelines for the client, including the requirement that she cannot injure herself or attempt to injure others.
- Follow institutional guidelines for the application of physical restraints as needed.

- Seek to establish rapport with the client through demonstrating respect and establishing therapeutic communication patterns.
- Encourage the client to verbalize her emotions and use active listening techniques.
- Educate the client about dressing changes and basic principles of wound care.

EVALUATION

Following evaluation by the on-call psychiatrist, Ms. Vannosa was admitted to the psychiatric unit and hospitalized for 3 days. During her stay, she was argumentative with several of the staff nurses and client care technicians, but she appeared to favor one of the nurses, Jim. When Jim was on duty, she first insisted that he be assigned to care for her but later refused to allow him to be her nurse, stating, "He's a jerk, just like my boyfriend." In meetings with the clinical psychologist, Ms. Vannosa reported a history of physical abuse during childhood, including sexual abuse by an uncle, as well as several physically abusive dating relationships. When asked about abuse in her current relationship, Ms. Vannosa denied any abuse and reported that her boyfriend was "the only person who ever cared" about her. The psychologist referred Ms. Vannosa to a counselor who specialized in dialectical behavior therapy (DBT), but Ms. Vannosa declined and stated, "I don't want to keep talking about stuff that happened when I was a kid. I just need to stop getting so mad at my boyfriend." She sustained no further injury during her hospitalization and was not physically abusive toward staff. Upon discharge, Ms. Vannosa agreed to return to the ED in 7 days for suture removal.

CRITICAL THINKING

1. What other nursing interventions might be appropriate for inclusion in the plan of care for Ms. Vannosa?
2. Describe two instances in which Ms. Vannosa demonstrated splitting. How should the nurse address clients who demonstrate splitting behaviors?
3. Why did the psychologist recommend dialectical behavior therapy (DBT) for Ms. Vannosa? How is DBT believed to be beneficial to clients diagnosed with BPD?

REVIEW **Personality Disorders**

RELATE Link the Concepts and Exemplars

Linking the exemplar on personality disorders with the concept of stress and coping:

1. In relationship to personality disorders (PDs), describe three behaviors that reflect impaired coping.

2. How does manipulation, which is a behavior associated with several PDs, affect the nurse's morale and stress level? Explain how the nurse can effectively cope with manipulation in the course of a therapeutic relationship.

Linking the exemplar on personality disorders with the concept of safety:

3. Which PDs are associated with a high risk for injury? How does impulsiveness increase the risk for injury?

4. A client who is diagnosed with schizotypal personality disorder tells her nurse she hears voices that are ordering her to cut her wrists. How should the nurse respond? To protect the client from injury, what actions should the nurse take?

READY Go to Companion Skills Manual

REFER Go to Pearson Student Nursing Resources
nursing.pearsonhighered.com

- Additional review materials

REFLECT Case Study

Steffan Richter, a 32-year-old male, recently was diagnosed with avoidant personality disorder. The psychiatrist who made the diagnosis recommended that Mr. Richter begin psychotherapy, but Mr. Richter declined after learning that group therapy may be indicated at some point during treatment. To Mr. Richter, psychotherapy would be almost unbearable, but talking about his issues in a group setting would be impossible.

Since graduating from college 10 years ago, Mr. Richter has worked as a mailroom clerk. Having earned a bachelor's degree in accounting, Mr. Richter is qualified to apply for other, higher paying positions within the company. However, he chooses to maintain his current position, as his present job responsibilities greatly limit his need to interact with other individuals. Several years earlier, he was offered a supervisory position; however, he declined the offer. The promotion would have increased his salary significantly, but the job responsibilities included a great deal of interaction with the mailroom team and administrators.

During lunchtime, the mailroom shuts down operations so all employees can eat their meals together in the staff lounge. Because he finds the lunchtime social interaction in the staff lounge to be forced, unpleasant, and overwhelming, Mr. Richter remains in the quiet mailroom and reads a book during his break. Company policy restricts employees from eating in any areas other than the staff lounge, and employees are forbidden to leave the building during their work shift. As such, Mr. Richter never eats lunch during the week.

Because Mr. Richter is extremely shy and quiet, several of his coworkers refer to him as "the invisible man." He is also very underweight and some of his coworkers tease him about his size. Although he finds his nickname and the teasing to be cruel and humiliating, Mr. Richter does not share his feelings; instead, he resolves to stay as far away as possible from the group. Several of his coworkers have invited him to join the group for social activities outside of work; however, he declines their invitations, as he knows his coworkers will only further demean and embarrass him. To avoid being humiliated or rejected, Mr. Richter does not build friendships at or away from his workplace.

1. How are the effects of avoidant personality disorder impacting Mr. Richter's occupational and professional advancement?

2. In what ways does avoidant personality disorder impact Mr. Richter socially, both in and out of his workplace?

3. How does avoidant personality disorder affect Mr. Richter's nutritional habits?

REFERENCES

Academy for Eating Disorders. (2013). *Treatment.* Retrieved from http://www.aedweb.org/Treatment/1533.htm.

American Nurses Association. (2001). *Code of ethics for nurses with interpretive statements.* Silver Spring, MD: Author. Retrieved from, www.nursingworld.org/MainMenuCategories/EthicsStandards/CodeofEthicsforNurses/Code-of-Ethics.pdf.

American Psychiatric Association. (2012). *DSM-IV and DSM-5 criteria for the personality disorders.* Retrieved from http://www.dsm5.org/Documents/Diagnostic%20Criteria%20for%20Personality%20Disorder%20%28Comparison%20of%20DSM-IV%20DSM-5%20old%20DSM-5%20new.pdf.

American Psychiatric Association. (2013). *Diagnostic and statistical manual of mental disorders* (5th ed.). Arlington, VA: Author.

American Psychological Association. (n.d.). *What causes personality disorders?* Retrieved from http://www.apa.org/topics/personality/disorders-causes.aspx.

American Psychological Association. (2013). *Psychology topics: Personality.* Retrieved from http://www.apa.org/topics/personality/index.aspx.

Amminger, G. P., Schäfer, M. R., Papageorgiou, K., Klier, C. M., Cotton, S. M., Harrigan, S. M., … Berger, G. E. (2010). Long-chain omega-3 fatty acids for indicated prevention of psychotic disorders: A randomized, placebo-controlled trial. *Archives of General Psychiatry, 67*(2), 146–154.

Berk, L. E. (2010). *Development through the lifespan* (5th ed.). Boston, MA: Pearson Education.

Berman, A., & Snyder, S. J. (2012). *Kozier and Erb's fundamentals of nursing: Concepts, process, and practice* (9th ed.). Upper Saddle River, NJ: Pearson Education.

Blascovich, J., & Tomaka, J. (1991). Measures of self-esteem. In J. P. Robinson, P. R. Shaver, & L. S. Wrightsman (Eds.), *Measures of personality and social psychological attitudes* (Vol. 1, pp. 115–160). New York, NY: Academic. Press.

Bodner, E., Cohen-Fridel, S., & Iancu, I. (2011). Staff attitudes toward patients with borderline personality disorder. *Comprehensive Psychiatry, 52*(5). Retrieved from http://www.sciencedirect.com/science/article/pii/S0010440X10001719.

Borzekowski, D. L. G., Schenk, S., Wilson, J. L., & Peebles, R. (2010). e-Ana and e-Mia: A content analysis of pro-eating disorder Web sites. *American Journal of Public Health, 100,* 1526–1534.

Butcher, J. N., Mineka, S., & Hooley, J. M. (2013). *Abnormal psychology* (15th ed.). Upper Saddle River, NJ: Pearson.

Centre for Addiction and Mental Health. (2009). *Borderline personality disorder.* Retrieved from http://www.camh.ca/en/hospital/health_information/a_z_mental_health_and_addiction_information/borderline_personality_disorder_an_information_guide_for_families/Pages/default.aspx.

Ciccarelli, S. K., & White, J. N. (2013). *Psychology: An exploration* (3rd ed.) (Chap. 13). Upper Saddle River, NJ: Pearson.

Clark, L. A. (2009). Stability and change in personality disorder. *Current Directions in Psychological Science, 18*(1), 27–31. doi:10.1111/j.1467-8721.2009.01600.x.

Cloud, H. (1996). *Changes that heal: How to understand your past to ensure a healthier future.* Grand Rapids, MI: Zondervan.

Coolen, P. R. (2012). *Cultural relevance in end-of-life care.* Retrieved from http://ethnomed.org/clinical/end-of-life/cultural-relevance-in-end-of-life-care.

Costa, P. T., & McCrae, R. R. (2006). Age changes in personality and their origins: Comment on Roberts, Walton, and Viechtbauer, 2006. *Psychological Bulletin, 32*(1), 26–28.

D'Agostino, A., Manni, R., Limosani, I., Terzaghi, M., Cavallotti, S., & Scarone, S. (2012). Challenging the myth of REM sleep behavior disorder: No evidence of heightened aggressiveness in dreams. *Sleep Medicine, 13*(6), 714–719.

DeHart, T., Pelham, B. W., & Tennen, H. (2006). What lies beneath: Parenting style and implicit self-esteem. *Journal of Experimental Social Psychology, 42*(1), 1–17.

Dell'Osso, B., Berlin, H. A., Serati, M., & Altamura, A. C. (2010). Neuropsychobiological aspects, comorbidity patterns and dimensional models in borderline personality disorder. *Neuropsychobiology, 61*(4), 169–179.

Eby, L., & Brown, N. J. (2009). *Mental health nursing care* (2nd ed.). Upper Saddle River, NJ: Pearson Education.

Eckroth-Bucher, M. (2010). Self-awareness. A review and analysis of a basic nursing concept. *Advances in Nursing Science, 33*(4), 297–309.

Eisenberger, N. I., Inagaki, T. K., Muscatell, K. A., Haltrom, K. E. B., & Leary, M. R. (2011). The neural sociometer: Brain mechanisms underlying state self-esteem. *Journal of Cognitive Neuroscience, 23*(11), 3448–3455.

Erol, R. Y., & Orth, U. (2011). Self-esteem development from age 14 to 30 years: A longitudinal study. *Journal of Personality and Social Psychology, 101*(3), 607–619.

Evans, M. E. (2009). Prevention of mental, emotional, and behavioral disorders in youth: The Institute of Medicine report and implications for nursing. *Journal of Child and Adolescent Psychiatric Nursing, 22*(3), 154–159.

Farrell, J. M., Shaw, I. A., & Webber, M. A. (2009). A schema-focused approach to group psychotherapy for outpatients with borderline personality disorder: A randomized controlled trial. *Journal of Behavior Therapy and Experimental Psychiatry, 40*(2), 317–328.

Faure, B. (2009). *Unmasking Buddhism.* West Sussex, UK: Wiley.

Ferguson, C. J. (2010). A meta-analysis of normal and disordered personality across the life span. *Journal of Personality and Social Psychology, 98*(4), 659–667. doi: 10.1037/a0018770.

Fontaine, K. L. (2009). *Mental health nursing.* Upper Saddle River, NJ: Prentice Hall.

Fox, J. R. E., & Goss, K. (2012). *Eating and its disorders.* Sussex, UK: Wiley.

Freud, S. (1962). *The ego and the id.* New York, NY: W.W. Norton.

Gagne, D. A., Von Holle, A., Brownley, K. A., Runfola, C. D., Hofmeier, S., Branch, K. E., & Bulik, C. M. (2012). Eating disorder symptoms and weight and shape concerns in a large Web-based convenience sample of women ages 50 and above: Results of the gender and body image (GABI) study. *International Journal of Eating Disorders, 45,* 832–844.

Gentile, B., Grabe, S., Dolan-Pascoe, B., Twenge, J. M., Wells, B. E., & Maitino, A. (2009).

Gender differences in domain-specific self-esteem: A meta-analysis. *Review of General Psychology, 13*(1), 34–45.

Gibbon, S., Ferriter, M., & Duggan, C. (2009). A comparison of the family and childhood backgrounds of hospitalised offenders with schizophrenia or personality disorder. *Criminal Behaviour and Mental Health, 19*(3), 207–218.

Ginis, K. A. M., Bassett-Gunter, R. L., & Conlin, C. (2012). Body image and exercise. In E. O. Acevedo (Ed.), *The Oxford handbook of exercise psychology* (pp. 55–75). New York, NY: Oxford University Press.

Grilo, C. M., White, M. A., & Masheb, R. M. (2009). DSM-IV psychiatric disorder comorbidity and its correlates in binge eating disorder. *International Journal of Eating Disorders, 42*(3), 228–234.

Gunderson, J. G., & Choi-Kain, L. W. (2012). *Personality disorders.* Retrieved from http://www.merckmanuals.com/home/mental_health_disorders/personality_disorders/personality_disorders.html.

Gunderson, J. G., Zanarini, M. C., Choi-Kain, L. W., Mitchell, K. S., Jang, K. L., & Hudson, J. I. (2011). Family study of borderline personality disorder and its sectors of psychopathology. *Archives of General Psychiatry, 68*(7), 753–762.

Gurven, M., von Rueden, C., & Massenkoff, M. (2013). How universal is the Big Five? Testing the five-factor model of personality variation among forager–farmers in the Bolivian Amazon. *Journal of Personality and Social Psychology, 104*(2), 354–370.

Gutheil, T. G., & Brodsky, A. (2011). *Preventing boundary violations in clinical practice.* New York, NY: Guilford Press.

Hatala, A. R. (2010). Frankl and Freud: Friend? or foe? Towards cultural and?developmental?perspectives of theoretical ideologies. *Psychology and Society, 3*(1), 1–25?.

Holder, K. V., & Schenthal, S. J. (2007). Watch your step: Nursing and professional boundaries. *Nursing Management, 38*(2), 24–29.

Holtmann, J., Herbort, M. C., Wüstenberg, T., Soch, J., Richter, S., Walter, H., Roepke, S., & Schott, B. H. (2013). Trait anxiety modulates fronto-limbic processing of emotional interference in borderline personality disorder. *Frontiers in Human Neuroscience, 7*(54). doi: 10.3389.

Hopwood, C. J., Donnellan, M. B., Ackerman, R. A., Thomas, K. M., Morey, L. C., & Skodol, A. E. (2012). The validity of the Personality Diagnostic Questionnaire–4 Narcissistic Personality Disorder Scale for assessing pathological grandiosity. *Journal of Personality Assessment.* DOI:10.1080/00223891.2012.732637.

Huang, J., Yang, Y., Wu, J., Napolitano, L. A., Xi, Y., & Cui, Y. (2012). Childhood abuse in Chinese patients with borderline personality disorder. *Journal of Personality Disorders, 26*(2), 238–254.

International OCD Foundation. (2012). *Obsessive-compulsive personality disorder (OCPD).* Retrieved from http://www.ocfoundation.org/materials.aspx.

Johnson, J. G., Cohen, P., Smailes, E. M., Skodol, A. E., Brown, J., & Oldham, J. M. (2001). Childhood verbal abuse and risk for personality disorders during adolescence and early adulthood. *Comprehensive Psychiatry, 42*(1), 16–23.

Kendler, K. S., Aggen, S. H., & Patrick, C. J. (2012). A multivariate twin study of the DSM-IV criteria for antisocial personality disorder. *Biological Psychiatry, 71*(3), 247–253.

Kneisl, C. R., & Trigoboff, E. (2013). *Contemporary psychiatric-mental health nursing* (3rd ed.). Upper Saddle River, NJ: Pearson Education.

Leary, M. (2006). Motivational and emotional aspects of the self. *Annual Review of Psychology, 58,* 317–344.

Lenzenweger, M. F., Lane, M. C., Loranger, A. W., & Kessler, R. C. (2007). DSM-IV personality disorders in the National Comorbidity Survey Replication. *Biological Psychiatry, 62*(6), 553–564.

Liebman, R. E., & Burnette, M. (2013). It's not you, it's me: An examination of clinician- and client-level influences on countertransference toward borderline personality disorder. *American Journal of Orthopsychiatry, 83*(1), 115–125. DOI: 10.1111.

Mayo Clinic. (2011). *Prader-Willi syndrome.* Retrieved from http://www.mayoclinic.com/health/prader-willi-syndrome/DS00922.

Mayo Clinic. (2012a). *Binge eating disorder: Tests and diagnosis.* Retrieved from http://www.mayoclinic.com/health/binge-eating-disorder/DS00608/DSECTION=tests-and-diagnosis.

Mayo Clinic. (2012b). *Eating disorders: Alternative medicine.* Retrieved from http://www.mayoclinic.com/health/binge-eating-disorder/DS00608/DSECTION=tests-and-diagnosis.

Mayo Clinic. (2013a). *Personality disorders: Risk factors.* Retrieved from http://www.mayoclinic.com/health/personality-disorders/DS00562/DSECTION=risk-factors.

Mayo Clinic. (2013b). *Self injury/cutting: Symptoms.* Retrieved from http://www.mayoclinic.com/health/self-injury/DS00775/DSECTION=symptoms.

McGrath, B., & Dowling, M. (2012). Exploring registered psychiatric nurses' responses towards service users with a diagnosis of borderline personality disorder. *Nursing Research and Practice, 2012.* Retrieved from http://www.hindawi.com/journals/nrp/2012/601918.

Mohr, S. (2011). Integration of spirituality and religion in the care of patients with severe mental disorders. *Religions, 2*(4), 549–565. doi:10.3390/rel2040549.

Morgan, J. F., Reid, F., & Lacey, J. H. (1999). The SCOFF questionnaire: Assessment of a new screening tool for eating disorders. *BMJ, 319,* 1467–1468.

Murphy, R., Straebler, S., Cooper, Z., & Fairburn, C. G. (2010). Cognitive behavioral therapy for eating disorders. *Psychiatric Clinics of North America, 33*(3), 611–627.

Myrick, F., Yonge, O., & Billa, D. (2010). Preceptorship and practical wisdom: A process of engaging in authentic nursing practice. *Nurse Education in Practice, 10*(2), 82–87.

National Alliance on Mental Illness. (2013a). *Anorexia nervosa.* Retrieved from http://www.nami.org/Template.cfm?Section=By_Illness&template=/ContentManagement/ContentDisplay.cfm&ContentID=7409.

National Alliance on Mental Illness. (2013b). *Bulimia nervosa.* Retrieved from http://www.nami.org/Content/ContentGroups/Helpline1/Bulimia.htm.

National Alliance on Mental Illness. (2013c). *Binge eating disorder.* Retrieved from http://www.nami.org/Content/ContentGroups/Helpline1/Binge_Eating_Disorder.htm.

National Association of Men with Eating Disorders. (2011). Anabolic steroid use among males with eating disorders. Retrieved from http://www.namedinc.org/newsdetails.asp?id=55.

National Collaborating Centre for Mental Health. (2009). *Borderline personality disorder: Treatment and management.* National Clinical Practice Guideline, Number 78. The British Psychological Society and the Royal College of Psychiatrists, London.

National Eating Disorders Association. (2013). *Eating disorder prevention.* Retrieved from http://www.nationaleatingdisorders.org/eating-disorder-prevention.

National Institute of Mental Health. (n.d.) Statistics—Serious mental illness (SMI). Retrieved from http://www.nimh.nih.gov/statistics/index.shtml.

National Institute of Mental Health. (2012). *How are eating disorders treated?* Retrieved from http://www.nimh.nih.gov/health/publications/eating-disorders/how-are-eating-disorders-treated.shtml.

National Institute of Mental Health. (2013a). *The numbers count: Mental disorder in America.* Retrieved from http://www.nimh.nih.gov/health/publications/the-numbers-count-mental-disorders-in-america/index.shtml.

National Institute of Mental Health. (2013b). *Borderline personality disorder.* Retrieved from http://www.nimh.nih.gov/health/publications/borderline-personality-disorder/borderline_personality_disorder_508.pdf.

National Institute of Mental Health. (2013c). *Psychotherapies.* Retrieved from http://www.nimh.nih.gov/health/topics/psychotherapies/index.shtml.

National Institute of Mental Health. (2013d). *Borderline personality disorder: What are the symptoms of borderline personality disorder?* Retrieved from http://www.nimh.nih.gov/health/publications/borderline-personality-disorder/what-are-the-symptoms-of-borderline-personality-disorder.shtml.

National Public Radio. (2012). *Talk of the Nation: The challenge of treating personality disorders.* Retrieved from http://www.npr.org/2012/12/04/166503627/the-challenges-posed-by-personality-disorders.

Oltmanns, T. F., & Emery, R. E. (2012). *Abnormal psychology.* Upper Saddle River, NJ: Pearson Education.

Orth, U., Robins, R. W., Trzesniewski, K. H., Maes, J., & Schmitt, M. (2009). Low self-esteem is a risk factor for depressive symptoms from young adulthood to old age. *Journal of Abnormal Psychology, 118,* 472–478.

Orth, U., Trzesniewski, K. H., & Robins, R. W. (2010). Self-esteem development from young adulthood to old age: A cohort-sequential longitudinal study. *Journal of Personality and Social Psychology, 98*(4), 645–658.

Osborn K. S., Wraa, C. E., Watson, A., & Holleran, R. S. (2013). *Medical-surgical nursing: Preparation for practice* (2nd ed.). Upper Saddle River, NJ: Pearson.

Pargament, K. I., & Lomax, J. W. (2013). Understanding and addressing religion among people with mental illness. *World Psychiatry, 12*(1), 26–32.

Paris, J. (2010). Estimating the prevalence of personality disorders. *Journal of Personality Disorders, 24*(4), 405–411.

PubMed Health. (2012a). *Anorexia nervosa.* Retrieved from http://www.ncbi.nlm.nih.gov/pubmedhealth/PMH0001401/.

PubMed Health. (2012b). *Bulimia.* Retrieved from http://www.ncbi.nlm.nih.gov/pubmedhealth/PMH0001381/.

Remshardt, M. A. (2012). Do you know your professional boundaries? *Nursing Made Incredibly Easy, 10*(1), 5–6.

Roerig, J. L., Steffen, K. J., Mitchell, J. E., & Zunker, C. (2010). Laxative abuse. *Drugs, 70*(12), 1487–1503.

Sim, L. A., McAlpine, D. E., Grothe, K. B., Himes, S. M., Cockerill, R. G., & Clark, M. M. (2010). Identification and treatment of eating disorders in the primary care setting. *Mayo Clinic Proceedings, 85*(8), 746–751.

Smith, A. T., Kelly-Weeder, S., Engel, J., McGowan, K. A., Anderson, B., & Wolfe, B. E. (2011). Quality of eating disorders Web sites: What adolescents and their families need to know. *Journal of Child and Adolescent Psychiatric Nursing, 24,* 33–37.

Stanley, B., & Siever, L. J. (2010). The interpersonal dimension of borderline personality disorder: Toward a neuropeptide model. *American Journal of Psychiatry, 167*(1), 24–39.

Starr, S. S. (2008). Authenticity: A concept analysis. *Nursing Forum, 43*(2), 55–61.

Strasburger, V. C., Jordan, A. B., & Donnerstein, E. (2010). Health effects of media on children and adolescents. *Pediatrics, 125,* 756–767.

Swanson, S. A., Crow, S. J., LeGrange, D., Swendsen, J., & Merikangas, K. R. (2011). Prevalence and correlates of eating disorders in adolescents: Results from the national comorbidity survey replication adolescent supplement. *Archives of General Psychiatry, 68*(7), 714–723.

Tajima-Pozo, K., Zambrano-Enriquez, D., de Anta, L., Moron, M. D., Carrasco, J. L., Lopez-Ibor, J. J., & Diaz-Marsá, M. (2011). Practicing exorcism in schizophrenia. *BMJ Case Reports,* doi:10.1136/bcr.10.2009.2350. Retrieved from http://www.ncbi.nlm.nih.gov/pmc/articles/PMC3062860/.

Taylor, E. J. (2012). *Religion: A clinical guide for nurses.* New York, NY: Springer.

Terburg, D., Morgan, B., & van Honk, J. (2009). The testosterone–cortisol ratio: A hormonal marker for proneness to social aggression. *International Journal of Law and Psychiatry, 32*(4), 216–223.

Tomoda, A., Sheu, Y., Rabi, K., Suzuki, H., Navalta, C. P., Polcari, A., & Teicher, M. H. (2011). Exposure to parental verbal abuse is associated with increased gray matter volume in superior temporal gyrus. *NeuroImage, 54*(1), S280–S286.

U.S. National Library of Medicine. (2012). *Diseases and conditions.* Retrieved from http://www.ncbi.nlm.nih.gov/pubmedhealth/s/diseases_and_conditions/a/.

Wilson, B. A., Shannon, M. T., & Shields, K. M. (2013). *Pearson nurse's drug guide.* Upper Saddle River, NJ: Pearson.

Wright, J. P. (2009). *Hume's 'a treatise of human nature': An introduction (Cambridge introductions to key philosophical texts).* Cambridge, UK: Cambridge University Press.

Wright, K. M. (2010). Therapeutic relationship: Developing a new understanding for nurses and care workers within an eating disorder unit. *International Journal of Mental Health Nursing, 19,* 154–161.

Zeigler-Hill, V. (2011). The connections between self-esteem and psychopathology. Journal of Contemporary Psychotherapy, 41, 157–164.

30 Spirituality

MODULE AT-A-GLANCE

The Concept of Spirituality, 1871

Exemplar 30.1
Morality, 1878

Exemplar 30.2
Religion, 1883

Exemplar 30.3
Spiritual Distress, 1890

◢ THE CONCEPT OF SPIRITUALITY

Spirituality, faith, and religion are separate entities, yet the words are often used interchangeably. The word *spiritual* derives from the Latin word *spirare*, which means "to blow" or "to breathe," and has come to connote that which gives life or essence to being human. A nursing concept analysis concluded with the following definition for **spirituality**: "that most human of experiences that seeks to transcend self and find meaning and purpose through connection with others, nature, and/or a Supreme Being, which may or may not involve religious structures of traditions" (Buck, 2006, p. 288). Spirituality generally involves a belief in a relationship with some higher power, creative force, divine being, or infinite source of energy. For example, an individual may believe in God, Allah, the Great Spirit, or a Higher Power. Spirituality includes the following aspects (Martsolf & Mickley, 1998):

- Meaning (having purpose, making sense of life)
- Value (having cherished beliefs and standards)
- Transcendence (appreciating a dimension that is beyond the self)
- Connecting (relating to others, nature, Ultimate Other)
- Becoming (involves reflection, allowing life to unfold, and knowing who one is).

(continued on next page)

Concept Learning Outcomes

After reading about this concept, you will be able to:

1. Define the concept of spirituality.
2. Identify characteristics of spiritual health.
3. Examine the relationship between spirituality and other concepts.
4. Identify commonly occurring alterations in spirituality and their related therapies.
5. Differentiate common assessment procedures used to examine spirituality across the life span.
6. Explain management of spiritual health and prevention of spiritual illness.
7. Demonstrate the nursing process in providing culturally competent and caring interventions across the life span for individuals with common alterations in spirituality.
8. Compare and contrast common independent and collaborative interventions for clients with alterations in spirituality.

Concept Key Terms

Agnostic, *1873*
Atheist, *1873*
Faith, *1873*
Hope, *1873*
Kosher, *1876*
Monotheism, *1873*
Polytheism, *1873*

Religion, *1873*
Spiritual distress, *1873*
Spiritual health, *1872*
Spiritual well-being, *1872*
Spirituality, *1871*
Transcendence, *1874*

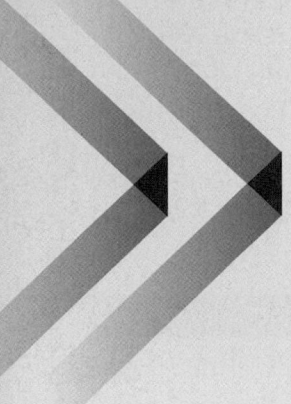

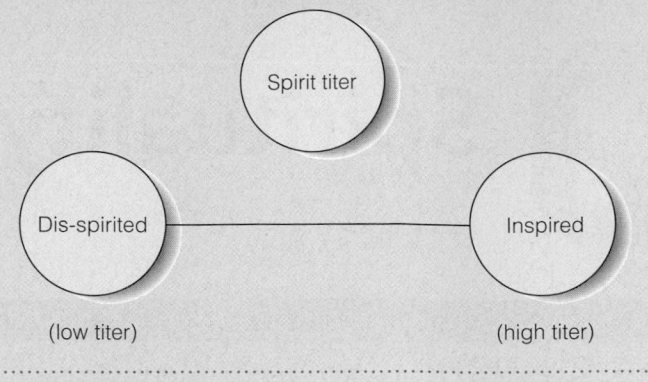

Figure 30–1 ● Spirit titer.

Words or concepts that are reflective of spirituality, such as *faith*, *courage*, *cheer*, and *hope*, may be used in ordinary speech when discussing spirituality.

Spirituality can be described by measuring it, so to speak, on a "spirit titer" (Jourard, 1971). One's spirit titer is influenced by numerous factors, such as life experiences, coping skills, social supports, and individual belief systems. Individuals experience multiple changes and losses over their life span, and if their spirit titer is low, they may become dispirited or depressed. If they have a high spirit titer, they will lean toward being inspired and becoming an inspiration to others in spite of hardships they experience (**Figure 30–1 ●**). Nurses need to direct their goals and planning to assist clients in attaining and maintaining a high spirit titer.

A recent study (Giske & Cone, 2012) was conducted to determine undergraduate nursing students' perspectives on spiritual care and how they learn to assess and provide spiritual care to clients. The researchers found that nurses need a wide range of competences to fulfill the nursing focus on holistic client care and that nursing education should prepare students to recognize and act on spiritual cues. This learning is best accomplished when a trusting relationship is built with the client and respectful and sensitive communication is used to assist students to discover what is important to their clients.**<<**

▶ COMPONENTS OF SPIRITUALITY

Spirituality incorporates a number of components including spiritual needs, spiritual health and well-being, spiritual distress, and core aspects of spirituality such as religion, faith, and hope. Having a solid understanding of spirituality itself, how spirituality influences a client's decision making, and how spirituality can be affected by illness is crucial for nurses.

Spiritual Needs

Just as everybody has a spiritual dimension, all clients have needs that reflect their spirituality. These needs are often accentuated by an illness or other health crisis. Clients who have well-defined spiritual beliefs may find that their beliefs are challenged by their health situation or may hold to their beliefs more firmly and appreciatively. Clients who have no defined beliefs may suddenly come face to face with challenging questions such as "Why me?" and others related to the meaning and purpose of life. Nurses need to be sensitive to indications of the client's spiritual needs and respond appropriately. Examples of spiritual needs are listed in **Box 30–1 ●**.

Spiritual Health and Well-Being

Spiritual health, or **spiritual well-being**, is manifested by a feeling of being "generally alive, purposeful, and fulfilled" (Ellison, 1983, p. 332). According to Pilch (1998), spiritual wellness is "a way of living, a lifestyle that views and lives life as purposeful and

---

Box 30–1   Examples of Spiritual Needs

NEEDS RELATED TO THE SELF
- Need for meaning and purpose
- Need to express creativity
- Need for hope
- Need to transcend life challenges
- Need for personal dignity
- Need for gratitude
- Need for vision
- Need to prepare for and accept death.

NEEDS RELATED TO OTHERS
- Need to forgive others
- Need to cope with loss of loved ones.

NEEDS RELATED TO THE ULTIMATE OTHER
- Need to be certain there is a God or Ultimate Power in the universe
- Need to believe that God is loving and personally present
- Need to worship.

NEEDS AMONG AND WITHIN GROUPS
- Need to contribute or improve one's community
- Need to be respected and valued
- Need to know what and when to give and take.

Note: From Taylor, E. J. (2002). *Spiritual care: Nursing theory, research, and practice.* Upper Saddle River, NJ: Prentice Hall. Reprinted by permission of Pearson Education, Inc., Upper Saddle River, New Jersey.

pleasurable, that seeks out life-sustaining and life-enriching options to be chosen freely at every opportunity, and that sinks its roots deeply into spiritual values and/or specific religious beliefs" (p. 31). Spiritual health, as defined by the Nursing Outcomes Classification project (Moorhead, Johnson, & Maas, 2004) is the "connectedness with self, others, higher power, all life, nature and the universe that transcends and empowers the self" (p. 519). Indicators of spiritual health include, but are not limited to, faith and hope; meaning and purpose in life; ability to love, forgive, pray, and worship; participation in spiritual rites; expression through music, art, or writing; and connectedness with others.

Individuals nurture or enhance their spirituality in many ways. Some focus on development of the inner self; others focus on the expression of their spiritual energy with others or the outer world. Relating to one's inner self or soul may be achieved by conducting an inner dialogue with a higher power or with oneself through prayer or meditation, by analyzing dreams, by communing with nature, or by experiencing the inspiration of art (e.g., drama, music, dance). The expression of an individual's spiritual energy to others is manifested in loving relationships with and service to others, joy and laughter, participation in religious services and associated fellowship gatherings and activities, and expression of compassion, empathy, forgiveness, and hope. In a retrospective study focusing on spiritual care by nurses, a positive correlation between spiritual care perceptions (or the way nurses attend to their own spirituality) and spiritual care practice among nurses was shown to exist (Chan, 2010). The greater the nurse's spiritual care perceptions, the more frequently spiritual care was included in that nurse's practice.

Another study reviewing the nursing practice and its relation to spiritual care shows there are many commonalities between good nursing and spiritual care. These commonalities can be found in both personal and professional attributes of the nurse. Personal attributes of the nurse are described in similar terms in research on spiritual care and good nursing. Professional attributes common to good nursing and spiritual care are the nurse–client relationship, assessment skills, and communication skills (Biro, 2012).

Spiritual Distress

Spiritual distress refers to a challenge to one's spiritual well-being or to the belief system that provides strength, hope, and meaning to life. Some factors that may be associated with or contribute to an individual's spiritual distress include physiological problems, treatment-related concerns, and situational concerns. Physiological problems include having a medical diagnosis of a terminal or debilitating disease, experiencing pain, experiencing the loss of a body part or function, or experiencing a miscarriage or stillbirth. Treatment-related factors include a recommendation for blood transfusions, abortion, surgery, dietary restrictions, amputation of a body part, or isolation. Situational factors include the death or illness of a significant other, inability to practice one's spiritual rituals, or feelings of embarrassment when practicing them (Carpenito-Moyet, 2012).

Core Aspects of Spirituality

Because spirituality is a reflection of an inner experience that is expressed individually, it includes as many representations as

there are human beings. Core aspects of spirituality include religion, faith, hope, transcendence, and forgiveness.

RELIGION   Religion is an organized system of beliefs and practices. It offers a way of spiritual expression that provides guidance for believers in responding to life's questions and challenges. According to Vardey (1996, p. xv), organized religions offer the following:

- A sense of community bound by common beliefs
- The collective study of scripture (the Torah, Bible, Koran, or others)
- The performance of ritual
- The use of disciplines and practices, commandments, and sacraments
- Ways of taking care of the individual's spirit (such as fasting, prayer, and meditation).

Many traditional religious practices and rituals are related to such life events as birth, transition from childhood to adulthood, marriage, illness, and death. Religious rules of conduct, typically influenced concurrently by culture, may also apply to matters of daily life such as dress, food, social interaction, menstruation, and sexual relationships.

Religious development of an individual refers to the acceptance of specific beliefs, values, rules of conduct, and rituals. Religious development may or may not parallel spiritual development. For example, an individual may follow certain religious practices and yet not internalize the symbolic meaning behind the practices. Often religious development strengthens and enhances spirituality by providing a system of belief that can suggest areas of growth to the believer. For example, the daily prayers of the Muslims bring the believers into direct relationship with the profound questions of life several times per day.

An **agnostic** is an individual who doubts the existence of God or a supreme being or who believes that the existence of God has not been proved. An **atheist** is an individual who does not believe in any god. **Monotheism** is the belief in the existence of one god, while **polytheism** is the belief in more than one god.

FAITH   **Faith** is belief in or commitment to something or someone. Fowler (1981) described faith as being present in both religious and nonreligious individuals. Faith gives life meaning, providing the individual with strength in times of difficulty. For the client who is ill, faith—whether in a higher authority (e.g., God, Allah, Jehovah), in oneself, in the healthcare team, or in a combination of all of these—provides strength and hope. The term *faith* may be used in a way that is interchangeable with the term *religion*. For example, the term *faith-based organization* is often used to refer to an organization or agency that is affiliated with a particular religion or religious faith.

HOPE   **Hope** is a concept that incorporates spirituality. Stephenson (1991) suggested this definition: "a process of anticipation that involves the interaction of thinking, acting, feeling, and relating, and is directed toward a future fulfillment that is personally meaningful" (p. 1459). In the absence of hope, the client gives up, losing spirit. In the client who has lost hope, illness is likely to progress more rapidly.

Lifespan Considerations Spiritual Development

Children

The development of spirituality in children parallels their cognitive and psychosocial development. As children mature, they are increasingly capable of understanding spiritual matters, stating spiritual beliefs, and incorporating spirituality into their lives.

A developing spirituality includes the following:

- A sense of wholeness, having internal resources and identity
- Being attached to others, and being a part of a greater, even transcendent, world
- Having a sense of meaning and purpose in one's life
- Being able to express hope, even in the face of fear, uncertainty, and serious illness (Howden, 1992).

Nurses should help ill or injured children and their parents identify and express these qualities. Helping in this way can be done by actively listening, by offering opportunities to practice religious rituals, and by providing materials for nonverbal expression (e.g., painting, play, music).

Older Adults

Many older adults frequently use and highly value religious coping strategies such as prayer. Evidence shows spiritual well-being to be directly correlated with mental health and less medical illness among older adults (Koenig, 2002). Addressing the spiritual issues of this population is significant to their nursing care. Older adults may be especially concerned about living a purposeful life, about maintaining loving relationships to avoid social isolation, and about preparing for a good death. Nursing care for older adults that attends to such spiritual issues includes the following:

- Supporting meaning-making activities (e.g., conducting a life review or reminiscence therapy; allowing the client to weave together the strands of lived life; encouraging the client to become dedicated to some social, political, religious, or artistic cause; supporting the client to leave a legacy or do an altruistic deed). Such activities provide older adults with a sense of purpose for their life and assist them to make sense of the life that they have lived.
- Allowing open discussions about suffering and dying, encouraging client disclosure by asking open-ended questions, and providing responses that are respectful and compassionate. Do not avoid discomforting topics and questions that older adults raise by imposing positivity, giving pat answers, or otherwise minimizing or avoiding their spiritual pain.
- As appropriate, supporting older adults to reframe the "losses" of aging as "liberations." For example, older adults possess great wisdom and are in a season of life that promotes spiritual growth.

Clients with dementia present special circumstances for spiritual caregiving. Nurses can help those with early stages of dementia to focus on the positives, the "haves" rather than the losses. Allowing older adults with dementia to tell their stories helps them to maintain some identity (amidst a disease that threatens the very sense of self) and gives the nurse a window into their world. Clients with dementia can also worship and express their hope and creativity through various art forms (e.g., movement, painting, music). These clients are often able to experience the compassion of others when they feel their caring touch or hear their soothing voice.

TRANSCENDENCE The term **transcendence** is often used interchangeably with self-transcendence, which Coward (1990) defined as "the capacity to reach out beyond oneself, to extend oneself beyond personal concerns and to take on broader life perspectives, activities, and purposes" (p. 162). Transcendence is also thought to involve an individual's recognition that there is something other or greater than the self and a seeking and valuing of that greater other, whether it is an ultimate being, force, or value.

FORGIVENESS The concept of forgiveness is receiving increased attention among healthcare professionals. For many clients, illness or disability brings a sense of shame or guilt. The health problem is interpreted as a punishment for past sins (e.g., "Having sex before I got married is why I have breast cancer"). Clients facing imminent death may seek forgiveness from others as well as from God. Mickley and Cowles's (2001) research suggested that nurses can play a pivotal role in assisting clients to understand the process of forgiveness and to persevere through it.

Spiritual Development

Just as individuals develop physically, cognitively, and morally, they also develop spiritually. Several theologians have identified specific linear stages through which individuals may progress while maturing spiritually. Westerhoff (1976), for example, described faith as a way of behaving that evolves from a faith guided by parents and others during infancy and childhood to an owned faith that is internalized in adulthood and serves as a

directive for action. See also the Lifespan Considerations feature above.

Integrating the Concepts

Spirituality is integrated with many other concepts, some of which are outlined in the Concepts Related to Spirituality feature on page 1875.

CASE STUDY \\ PART 1

Tom Denton, a young adult male, is brought into the emergency department with a GI bleed. He is vomiting blood, hypotensive, pale, and diaphoretic, and his pulse is weak and thready. He is alert enough to hear Sharon Hynes, the ED physician, order a type and cross for four units of blood. Mr. Denton interrupts and states that he does not want the blood transfusion because of personal beliefs. Dr. Hynes orders volume-expanding agents to be used instead. Mr. Denton's wife Melissa arrives not long before he loses consciousness, and they discuss the use of the volume expanders versus blood transfusions. She agrees with his decision and tells him she loves him. He tells her he loves her also.

Critical Thinking Questions

1. What are the primary concerns for Mr. and Mrs. Denton?
2. How are the staff and others likely to react to the couple's decision? Why?
3. How do the principles of autonomy affect this scenario?

Concepts Related to **Spirituality**

CONCEPT	RELATIONSHIP TO SPIRITUALITY	NURSING IMPLICATIONS
Culture and Diversity		
■ Values and beliefs ■ Disparities and differences	Culture and diversity often influence the spirituality of an individual particularly in terms of religion and morality.	■ Be aware of cultural influences and protect the rights of clients related to their spirituality.
Health, Wellness, and Illness		
■ Health promotion ■ Variables influencing health	Health beliefs are often influenced by spirituality.	■ Assess the influence of spirituality on health beliefs and behaviors.
Sexuality		
■ Family planning	Sexuality and practices related to sexuality such as family planning/birth control may be influenced by spirituality.	■ Assess the influence of spirituality on sexuality and associated practices.
Ethics		
■ Strategies to enhance ethical decisions and practice ■ Ethical dilemmas ■ Patient rights	Choices associated with ethics often stem from spirituality or morality.	■ Be aware of possible influences based on spirituality of client.
Legal Issues		
■ Advance directives	Advance directive choices and choices associated with autonomy and self-determination may be influenced by spirituality.	■ Be aware of legal aspects of spirituality of clients.

▶ ASSESSMENT

Data about a client's spiritual beliefs are obtained from the client's general history (religious preferences or orientation); through a nursing history; and by clinical observations of the client's behavior, verbalizations, mood, and interactions with others. Nurses should never assume that a client follows all of the practices of the client's stated religion.

Nursing Assessment

The Joint Commission (2008) mandates that each client admitted to an institution's care be assessed for spiritual beliefs and practices. Several experts (Cole, Benore, & Pargament, 2004; Koenig, 2002; Massey, Fitchett, & Roberts, 2004; Taylor, 2002) recommend a two-tiered approach to spiritual assessment. All clients can be asked a general question or two (e.g., "What spiritual beliefs or practices are important to you now while you live with illness?" "How would you like your healthcare team to support you spiritually?"). Only clients who manifest some type of unhealthful spiritual need or are at risk for spiritual distress need be subjected to a more thorough spiritual assessment. Even this assessment can be streamlined to hone in on the particular spiritual concern present.

Although the nurse will continually be assessing, the initial spiritual assessment is best taken at the end of the assessment process or following the psychosocial assessment, after the nurse has developed a relationship with the client and/or the client's support person. A nurse who has demonstrated sensitivity and personal warmth, earning some rapport, will be more successful during a spiritual assessment.

Remembering an acronym such as **FICA** can also help the nurse to ask appropriate questions:

> **Faith or beliefs:** For example, "What spiritual beliefs are most important to you?"
>
> **Implications or influence:** For example, "How is your faith affecting the way you cope now?"
>
> **Community:** For example, "Is there a group of like-minded believers with whom you regularly meet?"
>
> **Address:** For example, "How would you like your healthcare team to support you spiritually?" (Dameron, 2005; Massey et al., 2004).

Assessment Interview **Spirituality**

- Are any particular religious practices important to you? If so, could you please tell me about them?
- How will being sick interfere with your religious practices?
- How is your faith helpful to you? In what ways is it important to you right now?
- In what ways can I support your spirit? For example, would you like me to read your prayer book to you?
- Would you like a visit from your spiritual counselor or the hospital chaplain?
- What are your hopes and your sources of strength right now? What comforts you during hard times?

Cues to spiritual and religious preferences, strengths, concerns, or distress may be revealed by one or more of the following (Taylor, 2002):

- *Environment.* Does the client have a Bible, Torah, Koran, other prayer book, devotional literature, religious medals, rosary, cross, Star of David, or religious get-well cards in the room? Does a church send altar flowers or Sunday bulletins?

- *Behavior.* Does the client appear to pray before meals or at other times or read religious literature? Does the client have nightmares and sleep disturbances or express anger at religious representatives or at a deity?

- *Verbalization.* Does the client mention God or a higher power, prayer, faith, a church, a synagogue, a temple, a spiritual or religious leader, or religious topics? Does the client ask about a visit from the clergy? Does the client express fear of death, concern with the meaning of life, inner conflict about religious beliefs, concern about a relationship with a deity, questions about the meaning of existence or the meaning of suffering, or questions about the moral or ethical implications of therapy?

- *Affect and attitude.* Does the client appear lonely, depressed, angry, anxious, agitated, apathetic, or preoccupied?

- *Interpersonal relationships.* Who visits? How does the client respond to visitors? Does a minister or other spiritual mentor come? How does the client relate to other clients and nursing personnel?

To provide holistic care, it is important for the nurse to understand the spiritual needs and beliefs of the client. Understanding and support of a client's spiritual beliefs and practices builds trust in the nurse–client relationship, makes the client feel more comfortable in strange environments, and individualizes the nursing plan of care to meet each individual's unique needs. Specific considerations and appropriate interventions are detailed in the exemplars that follow.

CASE STUDY \\ PART 2

Mr. Denton has slipped into a coma. Mrs. Denton is crying and begging her husband not to leave her. The staff members continue to treat the client with the volume expanders, but there is no significant improvement. Dr. Hynes speaks to Mrs. Denton and asks whether she has changed her mind.

Critical Thinking Questions

1. Does Dr. Hynes have the right to ask Mrs. Denton this question? Why or why not?
2. Who could be called to help Mrs. Denton during this time?
3. How should the nurse assess the needs of Mr. and Mrs. Denton at this time?

▶ SPIRITUAL PRACTICES AFFECTING NURSING CARE

Clients frequently identify religious practices such as prayer as important strategies for coping with illness (Carson & Koenig, 2008; Taylor, 2007b). The most common practices affecting the nursing care of clients include practices associated with diet, nutrition, healing, dress, birth, and death.

Nurses should avoid unethically imposing personal spiritual beliefs on clients, whose circumstances inherently leave them vulnerable. Observing guidelines for ethical conduct in spiritual caregiving is essential. The following guidelines for nurses were offered by Winslow and Wehtje-Winslow (2007):

- First seek a basic understanding of clients' spiritual needs, resources, and preferences (i.e., assess).
- Follow the client's expressed wishes regarding spiritual care.
- Do not prescribe or urge clients to adopt certain spiritual beliefs or practices, and do not pressure them to relinquish any of their beliefs or practices.
- Strive to understand personal spirituality and how it influences caregiving.
- Provide spiritual care in a way that is consonant with personal beliefs.

Although some clients are eager for nurses' overt offers of "spiritual care," others may be uncertain or opposed to such offers (Taylor, 2007a). Clients often confuse religiosity with spirituality; this may contribute to their uncertainty about receiving spiritual care from nurses. Observing and using the client's language for spirituality (e.g., "being at peace" or "faith") and exhibiting large measures of sensitivity and respect will help nurses to converse therapeutically with clients to provide spiritual care.

Before sharing personal beliefs or practices, a nurse must consider questions such as the following:

- For what purpose am I sharing my beliefs or practices? By doing so, am I meeting my needs or my client's?
- Is my spiritual care reflecting a spiritual assessment?
- Am I preying on a vulnerable client?
- Am I offering my beliefs or practices in a manner that allows my client to comfortably refuse?
- Does my spiritual care hurt or contribute to a therapeutic relationship with the client?

Beliefs Affecting Diet and Nutrition

Many religions have proscriptions regarding diet. There may be rules about which foods and beverages are allowed and which are prohibited. For example, Orthodox Jews are not to eat shellfish or pork, and Muslims are not to drink alcoholic beverages or eat pork. Members of the Church of Jesus Christ of Latter-Day Saints (Mormons) are not to drink coffee, tea, or alcoholic beverages and may abstain from caffeine. Older Catholics may choose not to eat meat on Fridays because it was proscribed in years past, and abstinence from meat is still required on some days during Lent. Buddhists and Hindus are generally vegetarian, not wanting to take life to support life. Religious law may also dictate how food is prepared; for example, many Jewish individuals require **kosher** food, which is food prepared according to Jewish law.

Some solemn religious observances are marked by fasting, which is the abstinence from food for a specified period of time. Fasting in some religions may also require restricting beverages; others allow drinking of water or other sustaining beverages on fast days. Examples of religions that observe fasting include Islam, Judaism, and Catholicism. During the month of Ramadan, devout Muslims eat no food and avoid beverages during daylight hours; the fast is broken after sunset. Members of Jewish synagogues fast on Yom Kippur, and devout Catholics may fast on the Lenten holy days of Ash Wednesday and Good Friday. Most religions lift the fasting requirements for seriously ill believers for whom fasting may be a detriment to health (e.g., clients with diabetes). Some religions may exempt nursing mothers or menstruating women from fasting requirements.

Healthcare providers should prescribe diet plans with an awareness of the client's dietary and fasting beliefs.

Beliefs Related to Healing

Clients may have religious beliefs that attribute illness to a spiritual disruption. Healing for such clients may appear to be unrelated to current treatment practices. The nurse needs to assess the client's beliefs and, if possible, include some aspects of healing that are part of the client's belief system in the planning of care.

Beliefs Related to Dress

Many religions have laws or traditions that dictate dress. For example, Orthodox and Conservative Jewish men believe that it is important to have their heads covered at all times and therefore wear yarmulkes. Orthodox Jewish women cover their hair with a wig or scarf as a sign of respect to God. Many Muslim women also cover their hair in accordance with their particular ethnic or national background. Mormons may wear temple undergarments in compliance with religious law.

Some religions require women to dress in a conservative manner, which may include wearing sleeves and modestly cut tops, and skirts that cover the knees. Some religions, such as Islam, may require that the body (torso, arms, and legs) be covered. Hindu women accustomed to wearing saris prefer to cover all of the body except arms and feet (**Figure 30–2 ●**). Hospital gowns may make women who wish to comply with religious dress codes uneasy and uncomfortable. Clients may be especially disconcerted when undergoing diagnostic tests or treatments, such as mammography, that require body parts to be bared.

Beliefs Related to Birth

For all religions, the birth of a child is an important event giving cause for celebration. Many religions have specific ritual ceremonies that consecrate the new child to God. When a Muslim child is born, "someone recites the call to prayer in the infant's ear." On the seventh day after birth, the child is named, and a tuft of hair is shaved from the head (Denny, 1993, p. 682).

In the Christian faith, baptism and christening ceremonies may take place after the birth of a child to confirm that the "infant [was] born into a Christian family as part of the organism of the church" (Frankiel, 1993, p. 556). Christian parents of seriously ill newborns may want baptism performed by the nurse or primary care provider if a chaplain or clergy person is not present.

In the Jewish religion, the ritual circumcision conducted on male children on the eighth day after birth is an expression of the religious bond between the prophet Abraham, his descendants, and their God. Following the ritual circumcision by the trained person, called a *mohel*, the child is named. Girls are named in the synagogue on the Sabbath after the birth (Fishbane, 1993).

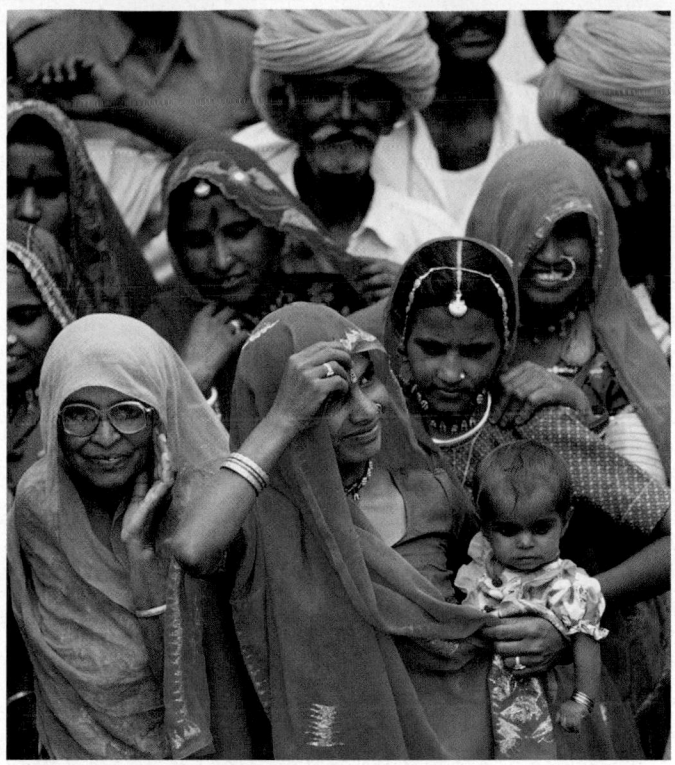

Figure 30–2 ● Hindu women dressed in saris.
Source: Charlie Westerman/Stone/Getty Images.

When nurses are aware of the religious needs of families and their infants, they can assist families in fulfilling their religious obligations. This is especially important when the newborn infant is seriously ill or in danger of dying, because some individuals believe that if religious obligations are not fulfilled the infant will not be accepted into the community of the faithful after death.

Beliefs Related to Death

Spiritual and religious beliefs play a significant role in the believer's approach to death just as they do in other major life events. Many believe that the individual who dies transcends this life for a better place or state of being.

Some religions have special rituals surrounding dying and death that must be observed by the faithful. Observance of these rituals provides comfort to the dying individual and his or her loved ones. Some rituals are carried out while the individual is still alive, and can include special prayers, singing or chants, and reading of sacred scriptures. Roman Catholic priests perform the sacrament of Anointing of the Sick (previously referred to as the Last Rites or Extreme Unction) when clients are very ill or near death. Muslims who are dying want their body or head turned toward Mecca (Denny, 1993).

Jews have a tradition of burial within 24 hours following death, except on the Sabbath, and they sit Shiva (gather to pay respects), draping any mirrors in black to ensure that guests are focused on memory of the deceased rather than on themselves. Tibetan Buddhists read the *Tibetan Book of the Dead* within 7 days of the death to release the soul of the deceased from the Bardos, or netherworlds. Hindus cremate the body within 24 hours to release the soul from any earthly attachment.

Griffith (1996) suggested that during a terminal illness the client and family should be queried about observances or rituals that follow death. Some religions require that the body of the deceased be touched only by members of that individual's faith. In both the Muslim (Denny, 1993) and Jewish (Fishbane, 1993) religions, believers may require that a ritual bath be given after death by a family member or by a ritual burial society. Religious symbols or objects should be treated with respect and kept with the body (Griffith, 1996). The nurse can support family members of the deceased by providing an environment conducive to the performance of their traditional death rituals.

REVIEW The Concept of Spirituality

RELATE Link the Concepts

Linking the concept of spirituality with the concept of development:

1. How might a nurse address the spiritual needs of an 8-year-old child who has leukemia?

2. How might a nurse address the spiritual needs of a teenager with cystic fibrosis?

Linking the concept of spirituality with the concept of culture and diversity:

3. What could a nurse say to a Muslim client who wants to fast during the day because it is the month of Ramadan, even though his physician has ordered a clear liquid diet?

4. How could you help a female Muslim client who is disturbed by wearing a hospital gown that exposes her arms and legs?

REFER Go to Pearson Nursing Student Resources nursing.pearsonhighered.com

- Additional review materials

REFLECT Case Study \\ Part 3

Mr. Denton's minister arrives, and Mrs. Denton and the minister discuss the situation. They agree that the situation has been handled according to Mr. Denton's beliefs. Mr. Denton dies, and Mrs. Denton states, "He died as he believed; God's will has been done." Members of the ED staff are overheard saying things like "He was too young to die" and "If only they had allowed the blood transfusion."

Clinical Reasoning Questions Level I

1. What should the nurse do to help Mrs. Denton at this time?

2. What resources are available to help Mrs. Denton?

3. What should the staff members do to help deal with their own feelings?

Clinical Reasoning Questions Level II

4. If the client in the case study had been 10 years old and the parents had made the decision to treat with volume expanders only, with the same results, what would have been the staff's responsibility?

5. What ethical and legal issues would be involved in the decision-making process in this situation?

6. How would you assess the needs of the young client and his family?

EXEMPLAR 30.1 Morality

EXEMPLAR KEY TERMS
Accountability, *1880*
Autonomy, *1880*
Beneficence, *1880*
Bioethics, *1878*
Consequence-based (teleological) theories, *1879*
Ethics, *1878*
Fidelity, *1880*
Justice, *1880*
Moral development, *1879*
Moral rules, *1879*
Morality, *1879*
Nonmaleficence, *1880*
Nursing ethics, *1878*
Principles-based (deontological) theories, *1879*
Relationship-based (caring) theories, *1879*
Responsibility, *1880*

Utilitarianism, *1879*
Utility, *1879*
Veracity, *1880*

EXEMPLAR LEARNING OUTCOMES
After reading about this exemplar, you will be able to:

1. Define the concept of morality as it relates to nursing and health care.

2. Identify factors associated with conflicts in, or alterations of, morality.

3. Describe theories, frameworks, and principles of moral development.

4. Describe nursing interventions to support clients experiencing moral dilemmas or distress.

5. Identify desired outcomes for clients experiencing moral dilemmas or distress.

▶ OVERVIEW

The term **ethics** has several meanings in common use. It refers to (a) a method of inquiry that helps individuals to understand the morality of human behavior (i.e., it is the study of morality), (b) the practices or beliefs of a certain group (e.g., medical ethics, nursing ethics), and (c) the expected standards of moral behavior of a particular group as described in the group's formal code of ethics. The term **bioethics** describes the application of ethics to issues of human life or health (e.g., to decisions about abortion or euthanasia). The term **nursing ethics** refers to the application of ethics to issues that occur in nursing practice. The American Nurses Association's revised *Scope and Standards of Practice* (2010b) holds nurses accountable for their ethical conduct. Nurses are repeatedly named as among the most ethical of professionals in various surveys (Gallup Poll, 2012).

Morality (or morals) is similar to ethics, and many individuals use the terms interchangeably. **Morality** usually refers to private, personal standards of what is right and wrong in conduct, character, and attitude. Sometimes the first clue to the moral nature of a situation is an aroused conscience or an awareness of feelings such as guilt, hope, or shame. Another indicator is the tendency to respond to the situation with words such as *ought, should, right, wrong, good,* and *bad*. Moral issues are concerned with important social values and norms; they are not about trivial things.

Nurses must be able to distinguish between morality and law. Laws reflect the moral values of a society, and they offer guidance in determining what is moral. However, an action can be legal but not moral. For example, an order for full resuscitation of a dying client is legal, but one could still question whether the act is moral. Conversely, an action can be moral but illegal. For example, if a child stops breathing at home, it is moral but not legal to exceed the speed limit when driving to the hospital. Legal aspects of nursing practice are covered in the module on Legal Issues.

Nurses should also distinguish between morality and religion as they relate to health practices, although the two concepts are related. For example, according to some religious beliefs, women should undergo procedures such as female circumcision that may cause physical mutilation. Other religions or groups may consider this practice to be an ethical violation of the human right to self-determination and an action that discriminates against women. Other common instances of differences in moral perspectives on health involving religious beliefs include blood transfusions, abortion, sterilization, and contraceptive and safer sex counseling.

Moral Development

Ethical decisions require individuals to think and reason. Reasoning is a cognitive function and is, therefore, developmental. **Moral development** is the process of learning to tell the difference between right and wrong and of learning what ought and ought not to be done. This process is complex, beginning in childhood and continuing throughout life.

Theories of moral development attempt to answer questions such as these: How does an individual become moral? What factors influence the way an individual behaves in a situation involving a question of morals? Two well-known theorists of moral development are Lawrence Kohlberg (1981, 1984) and Carol Gilligan (1982). Kohlberg's theory emphasizes rights and formal reasoning; Gilligan's theory emphasizes care and responsibility, although it points out that individuals use the concepts of both theorists in their moral reasoning. For a full discussion of these two theories, see the module on Development.

Moral Frameworks

Moral theories provide different frameworks through which nurses can view and clarify client care situations. Nurses can use moral theories in developing explanations for their ethical decisions and actions and in discussing problem situations with others. Three types of moral theories are widely used, and they can be differentiated by their emphasis on (a) consequences, (b) principles and duties, or (c) relationships.

Consequence-based (teleological) theories look to the outcomes (consequences) of an action in judging whether that action is right or wrong. **Utilitarianism**, one form of consequentialist theory, views a good act as one that brings the most good and the least harm for the greatest number of people and is called the principle of **utility**. This approach is often used in making decisions about the funding and delivery of health care. Teleological theories focus on issues of fairness.

Principles-based (deontological) theories involve logical and formal processes and emphasize individual rights, duties, and obligations. The morality of an action is determined not by its consequences, but by whether it is done according to an impartial, objective principle. For example, following the rule "Do not lie," a nurse might believe he or she should tell the truth to a dying client, even though the physician has given instruction not to do so. There are many deontological theories; each justifies the rules of acceptable behavior differently.

Relationship-based (caring) theories stress courage, generosity, commitment, and the need to nurture and maintain relationships. Unlike the two preceding types of theories, which frame problems in terms of justice (fairness) and formal reasoning, caring theories judge actions according to a perspective of caring and responsibility. Principles-based theories stress individual rights, but caring theories promote the common good or the welfare of the group.

A moral framework guides moral decisions, but it does not determine the outcome. Imagine a situation in which a frail older client has made it clear that he does not want further surgery but the family and surgeon insist. Three nurses have each decided that they will not help with preparations for surgery and that they will work through proper channels to try to prevent it. Using consequence-based reasoning, Nurse A thinks, "Surgery will cause him more suffering; he probably will not survive it anyway, and the family may even feel guilty later." Using principles-based reasoning, Nurse B thinks, "This violates the principle of autonomy. This man has a right to decide what happens to his body." Using caring-based reasoning, Nurse C thinks, "My relationship to this client commits me to protecting him and meeting his needs, and I feel such compassion for him. I must try to help the family understand that he needs their support." Each of these different perspectives is based on the nurse's moral framework.

Moral Principles

Moral principles are statements about broad, general, philosophical concepts such as autonomy and justice. They provide the foundation for **moral rules**, which are specific prescriptions for actions. For example, the rule "People should not lie" is based on the moral principle of respect for individuals (autonomy). Principles are useful in ethical discussions because even if individuals disagree about which action is right in a situation, they may be able to agree on the principles that apply. Such an agreement can serve as the basis for a solution that is acceptable to all parties. For example, most individuals would agree to the principle that nurses are obligated to respect their clients, even if they disagree as to whether the nurse should deceive a particular client about his or her prognosis.

Autonomy refers to the right to make one's own decisions. Nurses who follow this principle recognize that each client is unique, has the right to be who or what he or she is, and has the right to choose personal goals. Individuals have "inward autonomy" if they have the ability to make choices; they have "outward autonomy" if their choices are not limited or imposed by others.

Honoring the principle of autonomy means that the nurse respects a client's right to make decisions even when those choices seem to the nurse not to be in the client's best interest. It also means treating others with consideration. In a healthcare setting, this principle is violated, for example, when a nurse disregards clients' subjective accounts of their symptoms (e.g., pain). Finally, respect for autonomy means that no individual should be treated as an impersonal source of knowledge or training. This principle comes into play, for example, in the requirement that clients provide informed consent before tests, procedures, or involvement as a research participant can be carried out.

Nonmaleficence is the duty to "do no harm." Although this would seem to be a simple principle to follow, in reality it is complex. Doing harm can mean intentionally causing harm, placing someone at risk of harm, and unintentionally causing harm. In nursing, intentional harm is never acceptable. However, placing an individual at risk of harm has many facets. A client may be at risk of harm as a known consequence of a nursing intervention that is intended to be helpful. For example, a client may react adversely to a medication. Unintentional harm occurs when the risk could not have been anticipated. For example, while catching a client who is falling, a nurse might grip the client tightly enough to cause bruises to the client's arm. Caregivers do not always agree on the degree of risk that is morally permissible in order to attempt the beneficial result.

Beneficence means "doing good." Nurses are obligated to do good, that is, to implement actions that benefit clients and their support individuals. However, doing good can also pose a risk of doing harm. For example, a nurse may advise a client about a strenuous exercise program to improve general health, but the nurse should not recommend such a program if the client is at risk of a heart attack.

Justice is often referred to as *fairness*. Nurses often face decisions in which a sense of justice should prevail. For example, a nurse making home visits finds one client tearful and depressed and knows that she could help by staying for 30 more minutes to talk. However, that would take time from her next client, who has diabetes and needs a great deal of teaching and observation. The nurse will need to weigh the facts carefully in order to divide her time justly among her clients.

Fidelity means to be faithful to agreements and promises. By virtue of their standing as professional caregivers, nurses have responsibilities to clients, employers, government, and society, as well as to themselves. Nurses often make promises such as "I'll be right back with your pain medication" or "I'll

find out for you." Clients take such promises seriously, and so should nurses.

Veracity refers to telling the truth. Although this seems straightforward, in practice choices are not always clear. Should a nurse tell the truth when it is known that it will cause harm? Does a nurse tell a lie when it is known that the lie will relieve anxiety and fear? Lying to sick or dying individuals is rarely justified. The loss of trust in the nurse and the anxiety caused by not knowing the truth, for example, usually outweigh any benefits derived from lying.

Nurses must also have professional accountability and responsibility. According to the *Code of Ethics for Nurses* (ANA, 2010a), **accountability** means "answerable to oneself and others for one's own actions," while **responsibility** refers to "the specific accountability or liability associated with the performance of duties of a particular role." Thus, the ethical nurse is able to explain the rationale behind every action and recognizes the standards to which he or she will be held.

▶ MORALITY AND THE PRACTICE OF NURSING

The *Stanford Encyclopedia of Philosophy* states that morality can be used to "normatively refer to a code of conduct that, given specified conditions, would be put forward by all rational persons." Given that nurses are seen as among the most ethical of professionals, it is difficult to accept that there are nurses who abuse their clients and nurses who witness abuse or are cognizant of it and say nothing. Unfortunately, such unethical or immoral behavior does occur. Although only a very few individuals in the nursing profession exhibit this behavior, all nurses must be able to identify, discourage, and report it. Every nurse must understand that to know about the abuse of a client by a nurse or other healthcare professional and not report it is a violation of the *Code of Ethics for Nurses*; condoning or ignoring abuse is a violation of the nurse–client relationship.

The idea of a nurse willfully harming a client or allowing a client to be harmed is almost unthinkable, yet it happens. In a series of articles in the fall of 2008, *Nursing Standard* explored the reasons why some nurses abuse, and sometimes kill, clients in their care (Wright, 2008). In a survey conducted by *Nursing Standard* and *Nursing Elder People*, 58% of 848 nurses surveyed said they would not report abuse of an older client or other client in their care for fear of "misinterpreting" the situation. Some respondents also cited fear of becoming a target of the abuser as a reason for not making a report (Doughty, 2007).

Another "unthinkable" situation is described in a 2007 report of the American Red Cross, which found that nurses, physicians, and other healthcare professionals at Guantanamo Bay, a U.S. detention camp in Cuba, witnessed and condoned the torture of prisoners. Some detainees even reported that healthcare professionals had, at times, given interrogators instructions "to continue, to adjust, or to stop particular methods" of interrogation (Shane, 2009).

To rise above questionable and unethical practices, nurses must have a thorough understanding of their own morality and what constitutes right and wrong for them as individuals. They must also have a thorough understanding of their professional code of ethics and be able to identify when the ethics of another professional or another agency are contrary to the *Code of Ethics for Nurses.*

 NURSING PROCESS

Just as the nurse will encounter clients of various cultural and religious backgrounds, the nurse will encounter clients at various stages of moral development, clients with questionable or confusing morals, and even clients who are immoral. Nursing ethics and professional codes of conduct require nurses to deliver high-quality, professional care to all clients, regardless of client morality. Doing so can sometimes challenge even the most professional, experienced nurse. Examples of these challenges include the following scenarios:

1. A client with HIV is transferred to the critical care unit (CCU) of a hospital from the prison infirmary. In addition to having HIV, the client is paraplegic with no ability to move his legs. He is serving a life sentence in prison for repeated child molestation and rape.
2. A young woman comes to the local free health clinic with her boyfriend to get a pregnancy test. The test is positive. The boyfriend immediately starts talking to her about how she'll have to get an abortion.
3. An older woman is brought to the emergency department by a friend who came to visit and found her lying in her own feces. She is weak and dehydrated. The friend says that the older woman lives with her son and his wife.

To care for clients such as these, nurses must have an awareness of their own ethics, a thorough understanding of the requirements they must follow under the professional code of ethics, and an understanding of the reporting requirements in their own state and the procedures they must follow in their place of employment. The nurse's own personal beliefs, morality, and bias will influence how he or she manages each situation. Every nurse should remember his or her moral duty to provide the best possible care, no matter what the client's morality or immorality may be. A nurse must never allow personal feelings about a client to affect care.

Assessment

As with any client, the assessment of the client who is immoral or who is exposed to immorality leading to abuse or mistreatment includes a nursing history and physical examination. Clients who are immoral may not be able to participate in a trusting nurse–client relationship and may not respond to attempts at therapeutic communication. The nurse attempting to interview these clients should maintain a calm, nonjudgmental manner and should ask open-ended questions in a matter-of-fact tone.

Diagnosis

Nursing diagnoses for an individual with moral dilemmas or distress or a client with a family member or significant other with questionable morals will vary. Diagnoses in the scenarios mentioned earlier may include the following:

- The prisoner transferred to the CCU will have a number of diagnoses appropriate to his medical condition. In addition, the following nursing diagnoses may be appropriate:
  a. *Risk-Prone Health Behavior*
  b. *Moral Distress*
  c. *Noncompliance*
  d. *Social Isolation.*

  (NANDA-I © 2012)

- The young woman who has just found out she is pregnant may be diagnosed with the following:
  a. *Risk for Situational Low Self-Esteem*
  b. *Impaired Individual Resilience.*

  (NANDA-I © 2012)

- The older woman who was brought to the emergency department by a friend may be diagnosed with the following:
  a. *Interrupted Family Process*
  b. *Powerlessness*
  c. *Chronic Low Self-Esteem*
  d. *Social Isolation*
  e. *Post-Trauma Syndrome.*

  (NANDA-I © 2012)

Planning

Individuals with moral dilemmas or distress may exhibit difficulty in participating in the planning process; in fact, they may even show disdain for it. The nurse may try to obtain cooperation by capitalizing on needs the client presents during the assessment. "I remember that you said you didn't want to be in pain any more. We need to run these tests to find out what is causing your pain, so that we can treat it." "I know you don't like the food here, but remember we discussed that to feel better, you have to get appropriate nutrition." While outcomes for these clients will vary widely, a few appropriate outcomes include the following:

- The client will participate appropriately as able in the therapeutic regimen.
- The client will refrain from causing disruptions that affect other clients and staff.
- The client will be appropriately supervised during caring interventions, diagnostic procedures, and other activities. For example, a security staff member or member of law enforcement will be present during caring interventions for a client with a history of assault.

Implementation

Caring for individuals with moral dilemmas or distress can be challenging, unpleasant, and time consuming. Interventions that may be appropriate in working with these clients may include any of the following:

- Following procedures that ensure the safety of staff working with the client. For example, the nurse working with a client who is potentially dangerous should stay between the client and the door and should notify security to be present as necessary.

- Adding precautions or procedures as necessary to ensure safety of other clients and staff. This may include restraining the client, providing additional staff for interventions and procedures, and transporting the client for procedures when hallways and other areas have the fewest people around.
- Encouraging clients to make informed decisions without pressure from others. In the earlier example of the young woman who learned she was pregnant, her boyfriend was attempting to influence her decision. While clients are free to seek advice from whomever they wish, the nurse must ensure that the client makes a treatment decision free from coercion.
- Refer clients to spiritual leaders or mental health professionals as necessary to help the clients in the decision-making process.

Evaluation

Treatment decisions that challenge individual morality and ethics, such as abortion and organ transplantation, are often the decisions that leave clients and family members second guessing the decisions after they are made. Evaluation of the client who is faced with making a decision that poses a challenge to the client's morality or evaluation of the client who is without morality is based on the question "Is the client comfortable that the best possible decision was made?" Nurses working with clients in these situations should support autonomy; provide a listening, nonjudgmental ear; and continue to support the client's decision following the conclusion of treatment.

NURSING CARE PLAN — A Client Presenting Morality Issues

ASSESSMENT

Michael Dunham is a 50-year-old male with paraplegia, who also has HIV. He has a history of IV drug use and having sexual relations with female sex workers. He is admitted to the critical care unit of the local hospital from the prison infirmary, where he has been for more than a month. He is on oxygen by cannula. He is restrained to his bed. Almost every time members of the nursing staff work with him, he tries to spit on them in an effort to "give" them his disease. Upon arrival, the prison transport unit informs the head nurse that Mr. Dunham is serving a life sentence for molesting children and that he used his disability to trick preteen girls into coming close enough for him to handcuff them to his wheelchair so they could not escape his sexual abuse. Before releasing them, he would threaten to kill their parents if the girls told anyone what happened.

Upon physical examination, the nurses working with this client find the following:

- Temperature 37.9°C oral (100.2°F), P 104 bpm, R 32/min, BP 102/60 mmHg
- Oxygen saturation 84%; breath sounds reveal coarse crackles in the left lower base
- Mild cyanosis of nail beds and mucous membranes
- Use of accessory muscles to breathe with intercostal and suprasternal retractions
- Flaccid paralysis of lower extremities since he was 8 years old
- ECG shows 2–3 premature ventricular contractions per minute
- HIV positive with CD4 T-cell count of 64, CBC showed WBC of 9.8, elevated lymphocyte and low segs
- Chest x-ray shows characteristic appearance of *Pneumocystis jiroveci.*

DIAGNOSES

- *Moral Distress*
- *Impaired Social Interaction*
- *Social Isolation*
- *Impaired Gas Exchange*
- *Risk-Prone Health Behavior*

(NANDA-I © 2012)

PLANNING

- The client will participate appropriately as able in the therapeutic regimen.
- The client will refrain from causing disruptions that affect other clients and staff.
- The client will be appropriately supervised during caring interventions, diagnostic procedures, and other activities.
- Nursing staff will take appropriate precautions to prevent spread of HIV.

IMPLEMENTATION

- A correctional officer or member of the hospital security staff will be present during any intervention in which removing the restraints is necessary.
- Nurses will provide care in groups of two or more.
- The client will be offered counseling and a referral to the hospital chaplain.

- The nurses caring for the client will share their concerns with their supervisor or mentor.
- The client will be consulted and asked to give permission for all treatments and therapies.
- Additional interventions will be used as warranted for medical condition and ordered by the attending physician.

EVALUATION

Mr. Dunham's condition continued to deteriorate, and he was placed on the mechanical ventilator. As it became increasingly difficult to meet his oxygenation needs, he was given paralytics. He ultimately died of cardiorespiratory failure.

CRITICAL THINKING

1. *Does a nurse who is assigned to care for this client have the option of requesting a different assignment based on the nurse's feelings of revulsion, disgust, or anger at the client's past history and behavior? Why or why not?*
2. *What interventions would be the most difficult for you to provide this client? Explain your answer.*
3. *How would your moral beliefs regarding this client's history and behavior affect your nursing care of this client? Is it appropriate to reduce the quality of care you provide as a result? Explain your answer.*

REVIEW Morality

RELATE Link the Concepts and Exemplars

A mother brings her 13-year-old daughter to her gynecologist's office for the daughter's first pelvic examination. The daughter is autistic and has a spoken vocabulary of less than 500 words. The mother tells the nurse she wants to talk to the physician about getting her daughter's tubes tied "or some other" procedure that will keep her daughter from getting pregnant if anyone molests her.

Linking the exemplar of morality with the concept of ethics:

1. How would you respond to this mother's request?
2. What ethical responsibilities do you have to the daughter in this situation?

Linking the exemplar of morality with the concept of comfort:

3. What moral or ethical issues are involved in clients' advance directives and do-not-resuscitate orders?
4. What are your feelings about the morality of do-not-resuscitate orders? How would you keep these feelings from influencing your discussions with a client about do-not-resuscitate orders? Would your feelings change if the client were a child or adolescent?

READY Go to Companion Skills Manual

REFER Go to Pearson Nursing Student Resources
nursing.pearsonhighered.com

- Additional review materials

REFLECT Case Study

The nurse on the day shift at an inpatient rehabilitation center makes her morning rounds. She finds a young female client awake in her bed, crying. The woman has bruises on her wrists and forearms that were not there when the nurse last saw the client the previous afternoon. When the nurse asks the client what happened, she responds only by shaking her head, and she pulls away when the nurse reaches out to comfort her. The nurse checks the visitor logs and confirms the client had no visitors the night before.

1. What are the priorities of care for the client at this moment?
2. What steps should the nurse take to try to determine what happened to this client?
3. How should the nurse document her findings, and with whom should the nurse share them?
4. Does the nurse have an obligation to report these findings? If so, to whom must she report them?

EXEMPLAR 30.2 Religion

EXEMPLAR KEY TERMS
Denomination, *1885*
Holy day, *1884*
Meditation, *1885*
Prayer, *1884*

EXEMPLAR LEARNING OUTCOMES
After reading about this exemplar, you will be able to:

1. Define the concept of religion as it relates to nursing and health care.
2. Identify components of different religious practices.
3. Describe how religious practices may impact nursing care.
4. Describe culturally competent nursing interventions to support religious needs of clients.
5. Identify desired outcomes for clients and their families at risk for impaired religiosity.

▶ OVERVIEW

Religion is an organized, communal approach to human spirituality. In its simplest terms, a religion provides its members with the constructs of beliefs, moral values, and spiritual practices that guide its members' expressions of their spirituality. While religion is typically practiced in a community setting, such as a church, synagogue, or mosque, most religious individuals also practice their religion outside of this setting in various ways, and individuals who are separated from their religious community will often continue their observations of holy days and rituals in private.

Religions have more differences than they have similarities, but all religions share some characteristics. These include the following:

- *Belief in a god or higher power.* Some religions, including Hinduism and Buddhism, worship multiple gods.
- *Belief that the god or higher power has influence over humanity.*
- *Forms of communication.* Members believe they communicate with the higher power, usually in the form of prayer or rituals.

- *Community.* Religions are typically practiced in a communal setting, such as a church, synagogue, or mosque.
- *Rituals to honor the god or gods.* Some religions use rituals to incorporate the community into the religious faith. Baptism is an example of a ritual that brings the newly baptized into the Christian faith.
- *Ethical or moral codes.* Probably the single best-known example of a religious moral code is the Ten Commandments.

Beyond these shared characteristics, religions have various similarities and differences, including how they approach medicine and certain aspects of health care. The very brief descriptions included later in this exemplar are mere snapshots intended to raise the nurse's awareness of some important areas of health care that an individual's religion can affect. Nurses should ask appropriate questions to determine whether a client practices a particular religion and to learn how the client's religion affects the client's healthcare decision-making processes. Nurses should elicit information about religious holy days, sacred writings and symbols, and times and needs regarding prayer and meditation.

Holy Days

A **holy day** is a day set aside for special religious observance; all the world religions observe certain holy days. For example, Christians observe Easter and Christmas, Jews observe Yom Kippur and Passover, Buddhists observe the birthday of the Buddha, Muslims observe the month-long holy period of Ramadan, and Hindus observe Mahashivratri, a celebration of Lord Shiva. Many religions require fasting, extended prayer, and reflection or ritual observances on sacred (or high holy) days. Believers who are seriously ill are often exempted from such requirements.

The concept of the Sabbath is common to Christianity and Judaism, in response to the biblical commandment "Remember the Sabbath day to keep it holy." Most Christians observe the Sabbath on Sunday, whereas Jews and sabbatarian Christians (e.g., Seventh-Day Adventists) observe Saturday as their Sabbath. Clients who are devout in their religious practices may want to avoid any special treatments or other intrusions on their day of rest and reflection.

Muslims follow the practice of praying five times a day (**Figure 30–3 ●**). The Muslim client may need assistance to maintain this commitment. In addition, Muslims traditionally gather on Friday at noon to worship and learn about their faith. Both Hindus and Buddhists practice meditation, and the nurse can help by creating a quiet time for them to meditate.

Solemn religious observances throughout the year may be referred to as *high holy days* and may include fasting, reflection, and prayer. Examples of such holy days are Rosh Hashanah and Yom Kippur (Jewish), Good Friday (Christian), and Ramadan (Islam). Many hospitals and health organizations facilitate ritual observances for clients and staff on holy days. Because many religions follow calendars other than the Gregorian calendar, a multifaith calendar can be used to identify the holy days of the various religious groups (Griffith, 1996).

Sacred Writings

Each religion has sacred and authoritative scriptures that provide guidance for its adherents' beliefs and behaviors. In addition,

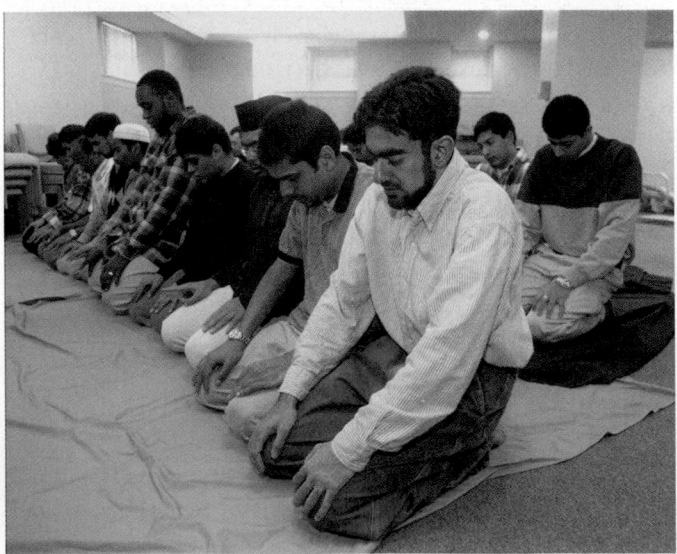

Figure 30–3 ● Muslim students at Johns Hopkins University at their weekly prayer meeting.
Source: AP Photo/John Gillis.

sacred writings frequently tell instructive stories of the religion's leaders, kings, and heroes. In most religions, these scriptures are thought to be the word of the Supreme Being as written down by prophets or other human representatives. Christians rely on the Bible, Jews on the Torah and Talmud, and Muslims on the Koran; Hindus have several holy texts, or Vedas; and Buddhists value the teachings of the Tripitakas. Scriptures generally set forth religious law in the form of admonitions and rules for living (e.g., the Ten Commandments). This religious law may be interpreted in various ways by subgroups of a religion's adherents and may affect a client's willingness to accept treatment suggestions. For example, blood transfusions are in conflict with the religious admonitions of Jehovah's Witnesses.

Individuals often gain strength and hope from reading religious writings when they are ill or in crisis. Examples of scriptural stories that may give comfort to clients are Job's suffering, in both the Jewish and Christian scriptures, and Jesus's healing of individuals who were physically or mentally ill, in the New Testament.

Sacred Symbols

Sacred symbols include jewelry, medals, amulets, icons, totems, or body ornamentation (e.g., tattoos) that carry religious or spiritual significance. They may be worn to pronounce one's faith, to remind the practitioner of the faith, to provide spiritual protection, or to be a source of comfort or strength. Individuals may wear religious medals at all times, and they may wish to wear them when they are undergoing diagnostic studies, medical treatment, or surgery. Individuals who are Roman Catholic may carry a rosary for prayer; an individual who is Muslim may carry a mala, or string of prayer beads (**Figure 30–4 ●**).

Individuals may have religious icons or statues in their home, car, or place of work as a personal reminder of their faith or as part of a personal place of worship or meditation. Hospitalized clients or long-term care residents may wish to have their spiritual icons or statues with them as a source of comfort.

Prayer and Meditation

Prayer is a spiritual practice; for many, it is also a religious practice. An encyclopedia of religion defines **prayer** simply as "human communication with divine and spiritual entities" (Gill, 1987, p. 489). Some argue that because prayer requires a belief in a divine or spiritual entity, not all individuals pray, while others consider prayer a universal phenomenon that does not require such belief. Ulanov and Ulanov (1983), for example, proposed that everyone prays: "People pray whether or not they call it prayer. We pray every time we ask for help, understanding, or strength, in or out of religion . . . who and what we are speak out of us. . . . To pray is to listen to and hear this self who is speaking" (p. 1). Prayer is intention plus love, often communicated with "the Absolute," according to Dossey (1999); that is, prayer is a loving wish or thought for oneself or another and not an invocation of positive or negative forms of magic.

Prayer experiences vary. Poloma and Gallup (1991) categorized them as follows:

- ■ *Ritual* (e.g., the Lord's Prayer, memorized prayers that can be repeated)
- ■ *Petitionary* (e.g., "God, cure me!" or intercessory prayers when one is requesting something of the divine)

Meditation is the act of focusing one's thoughts or engaging in self-reflection or contemplation. Some individuals believe that, through deep meditation, one can influence or control physical and psychological functioning and the course of illness.

Religion and Medical Care

There are many broad forms, or categories, of religions. Within each category are any number of **denominations**, groups of members that adhere to the same practices and beliefs. Even within a specific denomination, such as the Baptist faith, there may be further sects or denominations within the larger group. For example, the Southern Baptist Church has a number of different groups, including traditionalists, fundamentalists, and revivalists (Wax, 2008). Because of the great number of different groups that may be affiliated with a particular religion, nurses must be careful not to make assumptions about a client's beliefs and practices based on what religion the client professes. The client may belong to a group that practices the religion somewhat differently or may have belonged to the religion as a child and has since modified his or her practices to suit evolving beliefs. In addition to the following information, see **Box 30–2** ● for health-related information about specific religions.

JUDAISM   Typically, Jewish individuals participate actively in their medical care and seek treatment from modern Western doctors. Some Jews keep to the traditional kosher diet. This is a complex dietary code laid out in the Torah, the first five books of the Old Testament. Some of its rules are not eating meat and dairy foods together and not eating meat from animals that do not both chew their cud and have cleft feet; this includes pork.

Traditionally Jews will use all medical care necessary to extend life. Because there are prescribed Jewish rituals for individuals who are near death and for the time of and after death, Jewish families will often request the presence of a rabbi, a Jewish spiritual leader, when they know a loved one is near death. Jewish burial customs require the dead to be buried as soon as possible, preferably within 24 hours.

ISLAM   Islam is the second largest religion in the world, and those who practice Islam are called Muslims. Most Muslims live outside Arab countries. Because many Muslims view events in their lives as a direct result of God's will, they may view illness or death as the will of God and therefore believe that healing can take place only through God's will. Cleanliness and modesty are of great importance; ideally, the Muslim client should have a nurse of the same gender. Practicing Muslims follow dietary codes similar to those of Judaism, particularly regarding pork and pork-based products. During the holy period of Ramadan, Muslims fast. If a client wishes to fast and doing so may endanger his or her health, a nurse or physician may want to consult a Muslim elder, or imam, to speak with the client, because some exceptions to the fasting laws are allowed. Muslims pray five times a day, so nurses working with Muslim clients, especially those in a hospital or institutional setting, should take their prayer times into consideration.

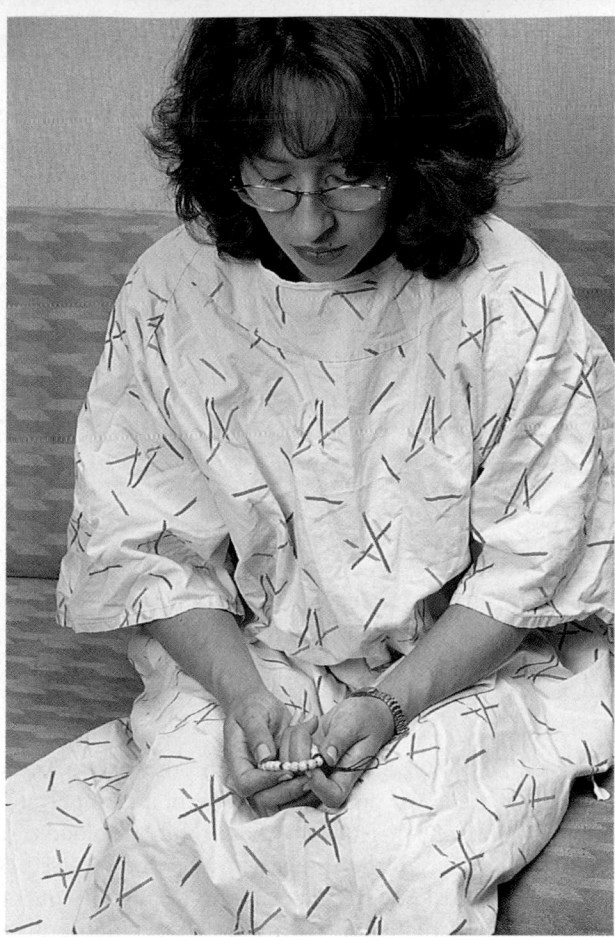

Figure 30–4 ● Clients may bring objects to the hospital to use in prayer or other religious rituals. Caregivers should respect such objects, because they usually have great significance for clients.

- *Colloquial* (i.e., conversational prayers)
- *Meditational* (e.g., moments of silence focused on nothing, a meaningful phrase, or a certain aspect of the divine).

Although meditational and colloquial prayer experiences have been found to be associated with spiritual well-being and good quality of life in healthy adults, ritual and petitionary prayer experiences may be most comforting and appropriate for those who are ill.

Some religions have prescribed prayers that are printed in a prayer book, such as the Anglican/Episcopal *Book of Common Prayer* or the Catholic missal. Some religious prayers are attributed to the source of faith; for example, the Lord's Prayer for Christians is attributed to Jesus, and the first sutra for Muslims is attributed to Mohammed.

Some religions require daily prayers or dictate specific times for prayer and worship: the five daily prayers, or Salat, of the Muslims (performed while facing east toward Mecca at dawn, noon, midafternoon, sunset, and evening), the daily Kaddish of the Jews, or the seven canonical prayers of the Roman Catholics. Individuals who are ill may want to continue or increase their prayer practices (Moschella et al., 1997). They may need uninterrupted quiet time during which they have their prayer books, rosaries, malas, or other icons available to them.

Box 30–2 Health-Related Information About Specific Religions

A SAMPLER

Amish, Mennonites. Likely will not have insurance coverage; rely on religious community for support.

Anglicans, Episcopalians, Roman Catholics. Appreciate receiving Eucharist (Holy Communion), a ritual of ingesting bread and wine (or grape juice) led by clergy or lay leaders to commemorate the death of Jesus. Lenten season (Ash Wednesday to Easter) may involve some degree of abstention from food.

Buddhists. May be vegetarian. Facilitate meditation (may desire incense, visual focal point, use breathing or chanting, etc.).

Christian Scientists. Typically oppose Western medical interventions, relying instead on lay and professional Christian Science practitioners.

Hindus. Most eat no beef; many are vegetarian. Cleanliness highly valued. Many food preferences (e.g., foods fresh or cooked in oil).

Jehovah's Witnesses. Abstain from most blood products; need to discuss alternative treatments such as blood conservation strategies, autologous techniques, hematopoietic agents, nonblood volume expanders, and so on; contact local Jehovah's Witness hospital liaison committee.

Jews. Some observe kosher diet to varying degrees (e.g., avoid pork and shellfish, do not mix dairy and meat). Sabbath observance varies

(e.g., Orthodox Jews avoid traveling in vehicles, writing, turning on electric appliances and lights).

Latter-Day Saints (LDS or Mormons). Avoid alcohol, coffee, tea, and smoking. May avoid caffeine. Prefer to wear temple undergarments. Arrange for priesthood blessing if requested.

Muslims. Respect modesty, avoid nakedness. Provide same-gender nurse if possible. Support prayers five times daily (may need to assist with ritual washing and positioning beforehand). Allow for family and imam (religious leader) to follow Islamic guidelines for burial when client dies. Eat no pork. Children, pregnant, older adults, and sick exempt from daytime fast during month of Ramadan.

Roman Catholics. Sacrament of the Anointing of the Sick appropriate for the ill. Be aware that some clients may think that an offer of this sacrament means they are dying; in fact, it may be administered to anyone who is seriously ill or about to undergo a major operation.

Seventh-Day Adventists. Avoid unnecessary treatments on Saturday (Sabbath). Sabbath begins at Friday sundown and ends at Saturday sundown. Adventists prefer restful, spirit-nurturing, family activities on Sabbaths. Likely to be vegetarian and abstain from caffeinated beverages. Do not smoke or drink alcohol.

ROMAN CATHOLICISM Roman Catholics generally participate in Western medicine. Catholics typically have a great respect for life, so a Catholic's religious beliefs will most likely inform decisions about childbearing and end-of-life care. This is not always true, however. Many Roman Catholics use birth control despite religious laws against it. Roman Catholics have a great deal of respect for the rituals of the sacrament of Anointing of the Sick. Nurses working with a very sick or dying member of the Roman Catholic faith will want to make sure that the family has the opportunity to call for a priest to administer this sacrament.

PROTESTANT CHRISTIANITY The umbrella of Protestant Christianity covers many religions. Episcopalians, Methodists, Southern Baptists, African Methodist Episcopalians, and Lutherans are just a few of them. Protestants generally embrace Western medicine, although they may differ in their views about birth control and end-of-life care.

HINDUISM Hinduism is a religion practiced by individuals from India and other parts of Asia. Typically, Hindus embrace Western medicine, but they will also employ alternative therapies from their culture such as yoga and various homeopathic remedies. Hindus generally do not eat meat and may prefer not to use medications that are derived from animals. Hindus generally believe that they have more than one life, and as a result may choose not to participate in organ donation. As with many other religions, Hinduism had ceremonial rites that are practiced at the time of dying and immediately after death.

BUDDHISM Practicing Buddhists generally prefer Eastern medicine, believing that most illnesses can be cured through the mind and the use of herbs. Many Buddhists also use acupuncture. This does not mean that Buddhists will refuse Western medicine. In fact, Buddhists see giving blood as a great gift. However, a Buddhist client or client of Asian origin may use traditional therapies in addition to those prescribed by a physician or nurse practitioner.

JEHOVAH'S WITNESSES Although Jehovah's Witnesses are not one of the larger populations of faith, it is important to note that traditionally their religion has prohibited blood transfusions, to the extent of shunning members who received certain types of transfusions. This can have important consequences for care in emergency and labor and delivery departments. Organ donation and organ transplants, however, are seen as personal decisions.

▶ ALTERATIONS

Any number of situations can threaten an individual's or community's ability to express or practice religion. Many countries do not guarantee their citizens the kind of freedom of religion that is guaranteed in the United States. In some countries, certain religious faiths are prohibited. For example, according to the U.S. Department of State (2011), Saudi Arabia's basic law establishes the country as a sovereign Arab Islamic state. Neither the government nor society in general accepts the concept of separation of church and state. Within the United States, active, passionate discussions take place about the separation of church and state, with many Christians feeling that the Christian religion should be practiced in public schools, on public property, and at public events, despite knowing that the United States has no official religion and guarantees freedom of religion for all individuals.

■ NURSING PROCESS

Determining the client's religious practices during the admissions process is important. If the client denies a formal religious affiliation, the nurse must determine whether the client holds to any practices the client may not identify as religious that are spiritual in nature and would affect the delivery of care. Meditating at regular intervals is one example of such a practice.

Assessment

As discussed in the Concept section of this module, assessment of the client's religious faith, practices, and spirituality occurs as part of the nursing history. Certainly the nurse should assess the religious and spiritual needs of any client who will be receiving care in an institution for more than a few hours. The longer the client's hospitalization or institutionalization, the more important this assessment becomes. In addition, any client with an illness or injury that may result in a threat to life should be assessed for religious practices and spiritual needs. Nurses should inquire about religious practices related to all of the following:

- Diet and nutrition, including types of foods prohibited and any required meals or mealtimes
- Prayers observed, including any requirements regarding the times that prayers must be observed
- Use of sacred objects or texts during prayers
- Prohibitions regarding medical procedures (if any)
- Other medical-related requirements or prohibitions.

Diagnosis

Any number of medical situations can threaten an individual's ability to practice his or her religion. NANDA International has three nursing diagnoses that reflect client religious issues (NANDA-I © 2012): *Impaired Religiosity, Risk for Impaired Religiosity,* and *Readiness for Enhanced Religiosity* (Carpenito-Moyet, 2012).

The religious client and family may practice a number of observations of their faith at home, and these may be an essential part of each day in the life of the family. *Interrupted Family Processes* and *Readiness for Enhanced Family Coping* may also be appropriate diagnoses if these normal daily practices are disturbed by hospitalization. Because the individual's sense of self may be closely tied to his or her religious practices, *Risk for Compromised Human Dignity* and *Risk for Powerlessness* may also be appropriate diagnoses.

Impaired religiosity is the impaired ability to exercise reliance on religious beliefs and/or participate in rituals of a particular faith tradition. Illness or injury that disrupts religious practice can impair the client's religiosity and result in emotional distress. An example of impaired religiosity might be the situation of the Roman Catholic client who attends daily Mass but is on enforced bed rest or requires an extended hospitalization, or the Muslim client who says evening prayers daily at the local mosque and is in the same situation.

In certain situations a medical condition may require a decision that is in conflict with a client's or family's religious practice. For example, a pregnant client who believes that life begins at conception discovers at 20–22 weeks' gestation learns that she will not be able to carry the fetus to term and attempting to do so will most likely result in her death. How will she decide what to do? If she had been trying for years to get pregnant without success, how would that influence her decision? How would her decision be affected if she had two small children at home? In such a situation in which a medical condition presents a complication that is at odds with a client's faith, the nursing diagnosis of *Risk for Impaired Religiosity* may be appropriate.

The relationship between the individual and his or her religion and religious practices is complex. Sometimes events that might threaten one individual's faith strengthen the faith of another. *Readiness for enhanced religiosity* is defined as the ability to increase reliance on religious beliefs and/or participate in rituals of a particular faith tradition. *Spiritual distress* is discussed in detail in the exemplar that follows.

Planning

When planning care, the nurse attempts to preserve the client's and family's ability to observe their religious practices to every extent possible. This may include the following outcomes of care:

- The client will be able to participate in religious observances if he or she desires.
- The client will be able to participate in prayer at prescribed times without interruption.
- The client will receive meals in keeping with religious dietary restrictions or requirements.
- The client will have access to religious resources, including ministers, prayer partners, sacred texts, and sacred objects.

Implementation

Providing care related to the client's religious needs must be done with great tact and sensitivity. The nurse's own religious beliefs may influence the approach to implementing care, but the nurse should never preach or proselytize his or her own beliefs and practices; rather, the nurse should focus on supporting the needs of the client.

Support Religious Practices

During the assessment of the client, the nurse obtains specific information about the client's religious preference and practices. Nurses need to consider specific religious practices that will affect nursing care, such as the client's beliefs about birth, death, dress, diet, prayer, sacred symbols, sacred writings, and holy days. See **Box 30–3** ● for ways in which the nurse can help clients to continue their usual spiritual practices.

Assist Clients with Prayer

Prayer involves a sense of love and connection, as well as a reaching out. It has many health benefits and healing properties (Dossey, 1996). It offers a means for someone to talk to a greater power, a mechanism for expressing care, and a sense of serenity and connection with something greater.

Clients may choose to participate in private prayer or may want group prayer with family, friends, or clergy. In such situations the nurse's major responsibility is to ensure a quiet environment and privacy. Nursing care may need to be adjusted to accommodate periods for prayer.

Illness can interfere with some clients' ability to pray (Taylor, 2003). Feelings such as anxiety, fear, guilt, grief, despair, and isolation can produce barriers to relationships in general and to the relationship the individual has with the Divine. In these instances, the client may ask the nurse to pray with him or her. Praying with clients should be done only when there is mutual agreement between the clients and those praying with them. Nurses who are unaccustomed to praying aloud or in public may find it helpful to have a formal prayer or a scriptural passage readily available. Because prayer can evoke deep feelings,

Box 30–3   Supporting Religious Practices

- Create a trusting relationship with the client so that any religious concerns or practices can be openly discussed and addressed.
- If unsure of the client's religious needs, ask how nurses can assist in having these needs met. Avoid relying on personal assumptions when caring for clients.
- Do not discuss personal spiritual beliefs with a client unless the client requests it. Be sure to assess whether such self-disclosure contributes to a therapeutic nurse–client relationship.
- Inform clients and family caregivers about spiritual support available at your institution (e.g., chapel or meditation room, chaplain services).
- Allow time and privacy for, and provide comfort measures prior to, private worship, prayer, meditation, reading, or other spiritual activities.
- Respect and ensure safety of the client's religious articles (e.g., icons, amulets, clothing, jewelry).
- If desired by the client, facilitate clergy or spiritual care specialist visitation. Collaborate with the chaplain (if available).
- Prepare the client's environment for spiritual rituals or clergy visitations as needed (e.g., have a chair near the bedside for clergy, create private space).
- Make arrangements with the dietitian so that dietary needs can be met. If the institution cannot accommodate the client's needs, ask the family to bring food. (Most religions have some recommendations about diet, such as espousing vegetarianism, rejecting alcohol.)
- Acquaint yourself with the religions, spiritual practices, and cultures of the area in which you are working.
- Remember the difference between facilitating/supporting a client's religious practice and participating in it yourself.
- Ask another nurse to assist you if a particular religious practice makes you uncomfortable.
- All spiritual interventions must be done within agency guidelines.

the nurse needs to spend time with the client following a prayer to enable the client to express these feelings.

Clients' preferences for prayer reflect their personalities. That is, introverts may prefer being alone to pray, and their prayers will reflect their capacity for introspection. In contrast, extroverts' prayers may revolve around their relationships with others and be expressed in creative, verbal ways. Similarly, a prayer of a feeling-type client may be emotion filled, whereas the prayer of a thinking-type client may be based on ideas and logic. The nurse should structure prayer interventions accordingly (**Box 30–4 ●**).

Evaluation

Expected outcomes of nursing care with regard to the client's religious needs include the following:

- The client has been provided the opportunity to practice religious rituals, including prayers.
- The nursing and dietary staff made appropriate considerations regarding dietary restrictions.
- The client successfully maintained connection with his or her religious practices and community of faith.

Box 30–4   Praying With Clients

- When a client asks the nurse to pray, talk to the client to determine prayer preferences before starting. Clients may prefer praying silently, while others may want the nurse to lead the prayer or the nurse to listen to the client's prayer.
- Assess how the client approaches the addressee of prayer. For example, a Baptist may pray to Jesus, whereas a Jew would pray directly to God, or Yahweh. Use universal terms such as "Higher Power" or "Creator" until you know your client's preference.
- Before praying, assess what the client would like you to pray. Listen carefully. The answer may provide greater insight into the client's fears and concerns.
- Personalize the prayer. Present your client's name and personal concerns to the Divine.
- Prayer can be used to summarize a conversation. This lets the client know you have heard what was said. It may also help the client to view circumstances more objectively.
- Prayer may be the springboard to further discussion or catharsis. Stay with the client after a prayer until there has been time for conversation.
- Follow a prayer with nonverbal communication (e.g., eye contact or touch) to conclude the session.
- Be mindful of one difference between magic and prayer. Magic invokes a greater power for personal gain. Prayer allows the greater power to do the greater good ("Thy will be done").
- Praying with a client may not involve verbalization. You may feel it will be more comfortable or appropriate if you remain quiet and fully present, praying silently.
- Facilitate the client's prayer practices. Schedule time when the client will be undisturbed, palliate distressing symptoms that interfere with praying, help with articles that accompany prayers (e.g., rosaries, prayer garments, books of prayers), and so on.
- In times of distress, a client or loved one may not be able to construct a prayer spontaneously. You may want to teach a centering prayer that is very brief (e.g., "Lord, have mercy/healing"). Nurses can discuss with care recipients what prayer would benefit them most and encourage them to use it while alone. These prayers may be more beneficial when they are framed in a positive sense. To illustrate, "Jesus loves me" or "The Lord has mercy."
- Encourage clients to think (privately or with you) about what prayer means to them. Offer questions such as these: Why do you pray? What do you expect from your praying? Are these expectations appropriate? How content are you with your prayer experiences? Is there a yearning for something more in your prayer experience?

Sources: Based on Taylor, E. J. (1998). Caring for the spirit. In C. C. Burke (Ed.), *Psychosocial dimensions of oncology nursing care* (pp. 55–75). Pittsburgh, PA: Oncology Nursing Press; Hubbartt, B., Corey, D., and Kautz, D.D. (n.d.). Nurse, please pray with me. Retrieved from http://rnjournal.com/journal-of-nursing/nurse-please-pray-with-me; Thieman, L. (2012). Nursing care: should you pray for your patients? Retrieved from http://www.nursetogether.com/nursing-care-should-you-pray-for-your-patients

NURSING CARE PLAN A Client at Risk for Impaired Religiosity

ASSESSMENT

Mohammed Al-Hussein is a 45-year-old husband and father of four who was badly hurt in a motor vehicle crash. Upon admission to the rehabilitation center, where he is expected to stay for several weeks, he informs the nurse that he is Muslim and a strict follower of prayer rituals and dietary restrictions. Dr. Al-Hussein and his wife are both science professors at the nearby university. His wife teaches an early class and has to leave for work before the school bus arrives. His oldest child, a daughter, is 16, and Dr. Al-Hussein says that she has been helping her mother with the younger children since the accident, almost a week ago. He admits that he is concerned that the extra burden on his daughter may affect her schoolwork but says that she does not complain. He says he can deal with the pain and discomfort but that he misses the company of his wife and children greatly. Currently confined to a wheelchair because of a hip fracture, Dr. Al-Hussein has orders for daily physical and occupational therapy.

DIAGNOSES

- Risk for Impaired Religiosity
- Impaired Physical Mobility
- Impaired Transfer Ability
- Risk for Caregiver Role Strain
- Interrupted Family Processes

(NANDA-I © 2012)

PLANNING

Together with Dr. Al-Hussein and his wife, the nurse develops a plan of care that includes the following:

- The client will observe all five prayer times daily.
- The client's diet will follow Islamic restrictions.
- The client will talk with the imam at his mosque about the possibilities of additional help around the house while the client is in rehab.
- The entire family will visit regularly to pray together and to talk about what is happening at home and school while the client is in the rehabilitation center.

IMPLEMENTATION

- Talk with the occupational and physical therapists about scheduling therapy sessions around the client's prayer schedule.
- Talk with the supervisor about moving the client's bed to face east so that even though he cannot kneel, he can pray in the appropriate direction.

- Facilitate the client contacting his imam.
- Notify the registered dietitian of the client's needs for dietary considerations and follow-up with the client after the first meal.

EVALUATION

Evaluation of Mr. Al-Hussein's plan of care should include checking with him to make sure that his meals meet his requirements and that staff members are not interrupting him during prayer times. The nurse should also follow up with his wife to make sure that no additional considerations need to be made for the family.

CRITICAL THINKING

1. What are the prescribed times for daily Islamic prayers? Which times might be most difficult for nursing staff to accommodate? Why?
2. What other interventions can the nurse make to support Mr. Al-Hussein as he tries to maintain his religious observations while in the rehab unit?
3. Where can the nurse go for more information about the Islamic faith?

REVIEW Religion

RELATE Link the Concepts and Exemplars

Linking the exemplar of religion with the concept of stress and coping:

1. How might the client's inability to perform customary religious rituals during times of illness result in anxiety?

2. How does helping the client meet his or her religious needs, thus reducing anxiety, help the client to recover more quickly?

Linking the exemplar of religion with the concept of development:

3. How do an individual's religious beliefs change as the client ages?

4. In assisting the client to meet his or her needs related to religion, how might the nurse's interventions differ based on the developmental stage of the client?

READY Go to Companion Skills Manual

REFER Go to Pearson Nursing Student Resources
nursing.pearsonhighered.com

- Additional review materials

REFLECT Case Study

Olivia Rossi is an 80-year-old woman who attends Catholic Mass at her church every day. She enjoys shopping at the Italian market that is within walking distance of her home. A couple of years ago she was diagnosed with Parkinson disease. At first she did well, thanks to medication and therapy, but in the past few months her symptoms have become worse, and she is afraid to continue to live on her own. After going to visit several assisted living centers, she and her adult children chose one that is very nice, with a very well-qualified staff, but is a 15-minute drive from the nearest Catholic church. After a few weeks, the nurse working on Mrs. Rossi's floor notices that Mrs. Rossi has become depressed. The nurse approaches Mrs. Rossi and begins to talk with her about the changes she's experienced since moving to the center. Mrs. Rossi expresses her sadness at not being able to attend Mass and says that she misses her church community.

1. What are the priority nursing diagnoses for Mrs. Rossi?

2. What caring interventions could the nurse implement to help Mrs. Rossi?

3. What are the possible outcomes if Mrs. Rossi does not receive any nursing interventions?

EXEMPLAR 30.3 Spiritual Distress

EXEMPLAR KEY TERM
Presencing, 1891

EXEMPLAR LEARNING OUTCOMES
After reading about this exemplar, you will be able to:

1. Define the concept of spiritual distress as it relates to nursing and health care.

2. Identify components of spiritual health and well-being.

3. Describe nursing interventions to support clients with spiritual distress.

4. Identify desired outcomes for clients with spiritual distress.

▶ OVERVIEW

When working with clients and their families, assessing for spiritual health is essential. Faith, a firm connection with others, and a belief in the future and in a higher power can be a strongly sustaining influence for critically or chronically ill clients and their families. In diagnosing spiritual health, the nurse may find that spiritual problems provide the diagnostic label or that spiritual distress is the etiology of the problem.

Carpenito-Moyet (2012) offers the following as defining characteristics of spiritual distress:

■ Expresses lack of hope, meaning and purpose in life, forgiveness of self

■ Expresses being abandoned by or having anger toward God

■ Refuses interaction with friends, family

■ Undergoes sudden changes in spiritual practices

■ Requests to see a religious leader

■ Lacks interest in nature, reading spiritual literature.

No list could be complete, however, considering the complexity and variability of individuals and their spiritual dimensions.

▶ SPIRITUAL OR RELIGIOUS DISTRESS AS THE ETIOLOGY

Spiritual distress may affect other areas of functioning and indicate other diagnoses. In these instances, spiritual distress becomes the etiology. Examples of nursing diagnoses related to spiritual distress include the following:

■ *Fear* related to apprehension about the soul's future after death and unpreparedness for death

■ *Chronic* or *Situational Low Self-Esteem* related to failure to live within the precepts of one's faith

■ *Disturbed Sleep Pattern* related to spiritual distress

■ *Ineffective Coping* related to feelings of abandonment by God and loss of religious faith

■ *Decisional Conflict* related to conflict between treatment plan and religious beliefs.

(NANDA-I © 2012)

■ NURSING PROCESS

Clients in spiritual distress require the nurse's thoughtful interventions. Although the nurse may not be able to provide the spiritual guidance clients require, the nurse can help clients explore their feelings and work through their distress and help them talk with an individual who can provide the necessary spiritual guidance such as a religious leader, spiritual guide, or elder in their community. Sensitivity and tact are important skills for the nurse to employ.

Assessment

As part of the assessment of the client, the nurse should ask questions to determine the client's spiritual beliefs and practices and how they affect or are affected by the client's health condition. Asking open-ended questions such as "How did you feel when the doctor told you about the risks associated with the surgery?" serve to build the nurse–client relationship as well as eliciting information the nurse will need to formulate the plan of care. Client statements such as "Why is God doing this to me?" "I don't care anymore," and "I wish I were dead" indicate that the client is in spiritual distress. A recent quality improvement project related screening for spiritual distress to client satisfaction with and trust in their overall care for clients on an inpatient oncology unit (Blanchard, 2012). The findings concluded that nurses are interested in the spiritual well-being of their clients and assess for spiritual distress. The nurses who were more likely to utilize referrals to chaplains after a brief spiritual screening protocol improved the client outcomes and reduced the harmful effects of spiritual distress as reported by the clients themselves.

Diagnosis

Carpenito-Moyet (2012) recognizes three diagnoses related to spirituality:

■ *Spiritual Distress* is "impaired ability to experience and integrate meaning and purpose in life through an individual's connectedness with self, others, art, music, literature, nature, or a power greater than oneself."

■ *Readiness for Enhanced Spiritual Well-Being* recognizes that spiritual well-being is the "ability to experience and integrate meaning and purpose in life through an individual's connectedness with self, others, art, music, literature, nature, or a power greater than oneself." This wellness diagnosis describing spiritual health acknowledges that some individuals respond to adversity with an increased sensitivity to spirituality or spiritual maturation.

- *Risk for Spiritual Distress* is defined by NANDA as being "at risk for an impaired ability to experience and integrate meaning and purpose in life through an individual's connectedness with self, other individuals, art, music, literature, nature, and/ or a power greater than oneself." This diagnosis may be appropriate for a client who currently shows no indication of this disruption of spirit yet may if a nurse fails to intervene.

(NANDA-I © 2012)

Planning

In the planning phase, the nurse identifies interventions to help the client achieve the overall goal of maintaining or restoring spiritual well-being so that the client may realize spiritual strength, serenity, and satisfaction. Outcomes of care may include the following:

- The client will fulfill religious obligations.
- The client will draw on and use inner resources more effectively to meet the present situation.
- The client will maintain or establish a dynamic, personal relationship with a supreme being in the face of unpleasant circumstances.
- The client will find meaning in existence and the present situation.
- The client will feel a sense of hope.
- The client will have access to spiritual resources as needed.

Implementation

Numerous nursing actions are available to help clients meet their spiritual needs (Cole et al., 2004; Mauk & Schmidt, 2004; Taylor, 2002). Spiritual care may include any of the following diverse actions:

- Recognize and validate the inner resources of an individual, such as coping methods, humor, motivation, self-determination, positive attitude, and optimism.
- Assist the client to leave a legacy by storytelling and/or recording life stories for family and friends, and encouraging creative expression through art, music, and writing. (This keeps the imagination alive and serves to regenerate the body, mind, and spirit.)
- Foster ways for clients to keep in touch with nature and maintain a sense of wonder, which are forms of spiritual care.
- Recognize that the seasons, the emergence of flowers in spring, the phases of the moon, the migrations of birds, and the unchanging stars provide examples of orderliness in the universe, even in the midst of chaos and loss.

A client with a good measure of spiritual health will find hope, meaning, purpose, and value in existence. Although nursing therapeutics that enhance spiritual health are diverse, some of the most common and most desired include (a) providing presence, (b) supporting religious practices, (c) assisting clients with prayer, and (d) referring clients for spiritual counseling (Taylor & Mamier, 2005).

Provide Presence

Presencing is defined as being present, being there, or just being with a client. This term identifies one of the competencies incorporated by expert nurses (Zerwekh, 1997). Pettigrew (1990) identified four distinguishing features of presencing:

1. Giving of self in the present moment
2. Being available with all of the self
3. Listening, with full awareness of the privilege of doing so
4. Being there in a way that is meaningful to another individual.

Fredriksson (1999) noted that presencing is a "gift of self" given by the nurse who maintains an attitude of attentiveness toward the client. Thus, nurses who listen attentively to clients yet fail to give of self (i.e., inwardly "make room") diminish their effectiveness.

Presencing exists on many levels. Osterman and Schwartz-Barcott (1996) identified four ways of being present for clients:

1. Presence (when a nurse is physically present but not focused on the client)
2. Partial presence (when a nurse is physically present and attending to some task on the client's behalf but not relating to the client on any but the most superficial level)
3. Full presence (when a nurse is mentally, emotionally, and physically present; intentionally focusing on the client)
4. Transcendent presence (when a nurse is physically, mentally, emotionally, and spiritually present for a client; involves a transpersonal and transforming experience).

Presencing is often the best and sometimes the only intervention to support a client who suffers under circumstances that medical interventions cannot address. When a client is helpless, powerless, and vulnerable, a nurse's presencing can be most beneficial. Rather than worrying about saying or doing "the right thing," nurses should focus on being fully present (Taylor, 2002).

Refer Clients for Spiritual Counseling

In some cases spiritual care is best referred to other members of the healthcare team. Referrals can be made for hospitalized clients and their families through the hospital chaplain's office if one is available. Nurses in home and community health settings can identify spiritual resources by checking directories of community service agencies, telephone directories, or religious directories that describe available spiritual counselors and the services provided through the religious community. Many religious counselors will provide assistance to members of their faith who are not members of their specific religious community. For example, a priest may attend a client in the hospital or at home even though the individual is not a member of the priest's parish.

When the nurse's spiritual beliefs conflict with the client's, the nurse must remember his or her role is as a healthcare provider and not a spiritual counselor. If the conflict is minor, the nurse may be able to support the client's beliefs and help the client to resolve issues of concern. However, if the conflict is great and the nurse cannot support the client in an objective manner, the nurse should find a spiritual counselor who shares the client's beliefs. The client's permission is needed before seeking an outside counselor in order to protect the client's right to confidentiality.

Referrals may be necessary when the nurse makes a diagnosis of spiritual distress. In this situation, the nurse and religious counselor can work together to meet the client's needs. One situation the nurse may encounter is client refusal of necessary medical intervention because of religious tenets. In this case, the nurse encourages the client, primary care provider, and spiritual adviser to discuss the conflict and consider alternative methods of therapy. The nurse's major roles are to provide information the client needs to make an informed decision and to support the client's decision.

Evaluation

Using the measurable desired outcomes developed during the planning stage, the nurse collects data needed to judge whether client goals and outcomes have been achieved. Appropriate outcomes for the client who needs to maintain or be restored to spiritual health include the following:

- The client participates in religious observance, such as observing prayer times.
- The client articulates a sense of hopefulness about the future.
- The client articulates faith in a higher power.
- The client articulates how to access spiritual resources.
- The client finds meaning and existence in the present situation.

NURSING CARE PLAN A Client With Spiritual Distress

ASSESSMENT	DIAGNOSIS	PLANNING
Mrs. Sally Horton is a 60-year-old hospitalized homemaker who is recovering from a right radical mastectomy. Her primary care provider told her yesterday that due to metastases of the cancer, her prognosis is poor. This morning her nurse finds her tearful, stating that she slept poorly and has no appetite. She asks the nurse, "Why has God done this to me? Perhaps it's because I have sinned in my life. I've not gone to church or spoken to a minister in several years. Is there a chapel in the hospital where I could go and pray? I'm terribly afraid of dying and what awaits me." **Physical Examination** Height: 165.1 cm (5'5')	■ *Spiritual Distress* related to feelings of guilt and alienation from God as evidenced by questioning why "God has done this"; inquiries about praying in a chapel; insomnia; no appetite (NANDA-I © 2012)	■ The client will interact with a spiritual leader from her faith. ■ The client will observe a spiritual practice that provides her comfort. ■ The client will connect with others to share thoughts, feelings, beliefs.

IMPLEMENTATION

- Create an accepting, nonjudgmental atmosphere.
- Be open to Mrs. Horton's feelings about illness and death.
- Assist her to express and relieve anger in appropriate ways.
- Encourage the use of spiritual resources, if desired by the client.

- Encourage her to list values that guide behavior in times of tragedy.
- Encourage verbalization of feelings, perceptions, and fears. Allow time for grieving.

EVALUATION

Mrs. Horton has been visited on several occasions by her minister. She reads scripture each day and has found consolation in reading the book of Psalms. She states, "God is merciful and will help me bear my suffering."

CRITICAL THINKING

1. What spiritual resources might you recommend for this client?
2. If Mrs. Horton's spiritual leader supports the concept that disease is a result of sins committed throughout life, how could you help this client?
3. If your religious beliefs would help this client obtain spiritual well-being, what actions could you take to help this client?

◢ REVIEW Spiritual Distress

RELATE Link the Concepts and Exemplars

Linking the exemplar of spiritual distress with the concept of oxygenation:

1. Describe the risk for spiritual distress faced by the parents of a child who has just died from sudden infant death syndrome.
2. What caring interventions would you offer to the child's parents?

Linking the exemplar of spiritual distress with the concept of development:

3. What signals or words might indicate that an 8-year-old child from a Protestant Christian family is in spiritual distress? What caring interventions would be appropriate for a child this age?
4. How might a teenager communicate spiritual distress? What interventions would be appropriate for a teenager that would not be appropriate for a younger child?

READY Go to Companion Skills Manual

REFER Go to Pearson Nursing Student Resources
nursing.pearsonhighered.com

- Additional review materials

REFLECT Case Study

Terry Mears is a 32-year-old male who received several pints of blood following an automobile crash 10 years ago. Five years ago he was diagnosed with AIDS, and he is now in the hospital with pneumonia and severe diarrhea. He is very ill and very discouraged. While you are caring for Mr. Mears, he comments, "I might as well die right now because I'm not going to get well. My folks were Methodist, but I guess I'm being punished because I'm not very religious."

1. Mr. Mears stated that he was "not very religious." Does that mean that he is not spiritual? Explain.
2. What data suggest that Mr. Mears may be experiencing spiritual distress?
3. How might illness affect one's spiritual beliefs? Religious beliefs?
4. How might a spiritual assessment be of benefit to both you and Mr. Mears?

■ REFERENCES

American Nurses Association. (2010a). *ANA nursing code of ethics.* Retrieved from http://www.nursingworld.org/Mobile/Code-of-Ethics.

American Nurses Association (ANA). (2010b). *Scope and standards of practice* (2nd ed.). Silver Spring, MD: American Nurses Association.

Biro, A. L. (2012). Creating conditions for good nursing by attending to the spiritual. *Journal of Nursing Management, 20*(8), 1002–1011.

Blanchard, J. (2012). Screening for spiritual distress in the oncology inpatient: a quality improvement pilot project between nurses and chaplains. *Journal of Nursing Management, 20*(8), 1076–1084.

Buck, H. G. (2006). Spirituality: Concept analysis and model development. *Holistic Nursing Practice, 20,* 288–292.

Carpenito-Moyet, L. J. (2012). *Nursing diagnosis: Application to clinical practice* (14th ed.). Philadelphia, PA: Lippincott.

Carson, V. B., & Koenig, H. G. (Eds.). (2008). *Spiritual dimensions of nursing practice.* West Conshohocken, PA: Templeton Foundation.

Chan, M. F. (2010). Factors affecting nursing staff in practising spiritual care. *Journal of Clinical Nursing, 19*(15/16), 2128–2136.

Cole, B., Benore, E., & Pargament, K. I. (2004). Spirituality and coping with trauma. In S. Sorajjakool & H. Lamberton (Eds.), *Spirituality, health, and wholeness* (pp. 49–76). New York, NY: Haworth Press.

Coward, D. D. (1990). The lived experience of self-transcendence in women with advanced breast cancer. *Nursing Science Quarterly, 3*(4), 162–160.

Dameron, C. M. (2005). Spiritual assessment made easy. . . with acronyms! *Journal of Christian Nursing, 22*(1), 14–16.

Denny, F. M. (1993). Islam and the Muslim community. In H. Byron Earhart (Ed.), *Religious traditions of the world* (pp. 603–713). New York, NY: HarperSanFrancisco.

Dossey, L. (1996). *Prayer is good medicine. How to reap the benefits of prayer.* New York, NY: HarperCollins.

Dossey, L. (1999). Healing and the nonlocal mind: Interview by Bonnie Horrigan. *Alternative Therapies in Health and Medicine, 5*(6), 85–93.

Doughty, S. (2007). Six in ten nurses would turn "blind eye" to the abuse of the elderly. *The Daily Mail Online.* Retrieved from http://www.dailymail.co.uk/health/article-478352/Six-10-nurses-turn-blind-eye-abuse-elderly.html.

Ellison, C. W. (1983, April). Spiritual well-being: Conceptualization and measurement. *Journal of Psychology and Theology, 11,* 330–340.

Fishbane, M. (1993). Judaism: Revelation and traditions. In H. Byron Earhart (Ed.), *Religious traditions of the world* (pp. 373–484). New York, NY: HarperSanFrancisco.

Fowler, J. W. (1981). *Stages of faith: The psychology of human development and the quest for meaning.* San Francisco, CA: Harper & Row.

Frankiel, S. S. (1993). Christianity: A way of salvation. In H. Byron Earhart (Ed.), *Religious traditions of the world* (pp. 484–601). New York, NY: HarperSanFrancisco.

Fredriksson, L. (1999). Modes of relating in a caring conversation: A research synthesis on presence, touch, and listening. *Journal of Advanced Nursing, 30,* 1167–1176.

Gallup Poll. (2012). *Honesty/ethics in professions.* Retrieved from http://www.gallup.com/poll/1654/honesty-ethics-professions.aspx.

Gill, S. D. (1987). Prayer. In M. Eliade (Ed.), *The encyclopedia of religion* (pp. 489–492). New York, NY: Macmillan.

Gilligan, C. (1982). *In a different voice: Psychological theory and women's development.* Cambridge, MA: Harvard University Press.

Giske, T., & Cone, P.H. (2012 July). Opening up to learning spiritual care of patients: a grounded theory study of nursing students. *Journal of Clinical Nursing, 21*(13–14), 2006–2015. doi:10.1111/j.1365-2702.2011.04054.x. Epub 2012 May 8.

Griffith, J. K. (1996). *The religious aspects of nursing care.* Vancouver, BC: Author.

Howden, J. W. (1992). *Development and psychometric characteristics of the Spirituality Assessment Scale* (unpublished doctoral dissertation). Texas Woman's University, Denton, TX.

Joint Commission. (2008). *Provision of care, treatment, and services: Spiritual assessment.* Retrieved from http://www.jointcommission.org/mobile/standards_information/jcfaqdetails.aspx?StandardsFAQId=290&StandardsFAQChapterId=29.

Jourard, S. (1971). *The transparent self.* London, UK: Van Nostrand.

Koenig, H. G. (2002). *Spirituality in patient care: Why, how, when, and what.* Radnor, PA: Templeton Press.

Kohlberg, L. (1981). *Essays on moral development: The philosophy of moral development* (Vol. 1). San Francisco, CA: Harper & Row.

Kohlberg, L. (1984). *Essays on moral development: The philosophy of moral development* (Vol. 2). San Francisco, CA: Harper & Row.

Martsolf, D. S., & Mickley, J. R. (1998). The concept of spirituality in nursing theories: Differing world-views and extent of focus. *Journal of Advanced Nursing, 27,* 294–303.

Massey, K., Fitchett, G., & Roberts, P. A. (2004). In K. L. Mauk & N. K. Schmidt (Eds.), *Spiritual care in nursing practice. Assessment and diagnosis in spiritual care* (pp. 209–242). Philadelphia, PA: Lippincott Williams & Wilkins.

Mauk, K. L., & Schmidt, N. K. (2004). *Spiritual care in nursing practice.* Philadelphia, PA: Lippincott Williams & Wilkins.

Mickley, J. R., & Cowles, K. (2001). Ameliorating the tension: Use of forgiveness for healing. *Oncology Nursing Forum, 28,* 31–38.

Moorhead, S., Johnson, M., & Maas, M. (2004). *Iowa intervention project: Nursing outcome classification.* St. Louis, MO: Mosby.

Moschella, V. D., Pressman, K. R., Pressman, P., & Weissman, D. E. (1997). The problem of theodicy and religious responses to cancer. *Journal of Religion & Health, 36*(1), 17–20.

Osterman, P., & Schwartz-Barcott, D. (1996). Presence: Four ways of being there. *Nursing Forum, 31*(2), 23–30.

Pettigrew, J. (1990). Intensive nursing care: The ministry of presence. *Critical Care Nursing Clinics of North America, 2,* 503–508.

Pilch, J. J. (1998, May/June). Wellness spirituality. *Health Values, 12,* 28–31.

Poloma, M. M., & Gallup, G. H., Jr. (1991). *Varieties of prayer: A survey report.* Philadelphia, PA: Trinity Press International.

Shane, S. (2009). Report outlines medical workers' role in torture. *New York Times.* Retrieved from http://www.nytimes.com/2009/04/07/world/07detain.html.

Stephenson, C. (1991). The concept of hope revisited for nursing. *Journal of Advances in Nursing, 16,* 1456–1461.

Taylor, E. J. (1998). Caring for the spirit. In C. C. Burke (Ed.), *Psychosocial dimensions of oncology nursing care.* Pittsburgh, PA: Oncology Nursing Press.

Taylor, E. J. (2002). *Spiritual care: Nursing theory, research, and practice.* Upper Saddle River, NJ: Prentice Hall.

Taylor, E. J. (2003). Nurses caring for the spirit: Patients with cancer and family caregiver expectations. *Oncology Nursing Forum, 30,* 585–594.

Taylor, E. J. (2007a). Client perspectives about nurse requisites for spiritual caregiving. *Applied Nursing Research, 20*(1), 44–48.

Taylor, E. J. (2007b). Spiritual pain. *Advance for Nurses, 9*(21), 15–16.

Taylor, E. J., & Mamier, I. (2005). Spiritual care nursing: What cancer patients and family caregivers want. *Journal of Advanced Nursing, 49*(3), 260–267.

Ulanov, A., & Ulanov, B. (1983). *Primary speech: A psychology of prayer.* Atlanta, GA: John Knox Press (classic).

U.S. Department of State. (2011). *Saudi Arabia.* Retrieved from http://www.state.gov/j/drl/rls/irf/2011/nea/192905.htm.

Vardey, L. (1996). *God in all worlds.* Toronto, Canada: Vintage Canada.

Wax, T. (2008). Seven types of Southern Baptists. Retrieved from http://trevinwax.com/2008/06/10/7-types-of-southern-baptists.

Westerhoff, J. (1976). *Will our children have faith?* New York, NY: Seabury Press.

Winslow, G. R., & Wehtje-Winslow, B. J. (2007). Ethical boundaries of spiritual care. *Medical Journal of Australia, 186*(10 Suppl.), S63–S66.

Wright, S. (2008). When nurses do. *Nursing Standard, 23*(6), 18–20.

Zerwekh, J. V. (1997). The practice of presencing. *Seminars in Oncology Nursing, 13,* 260–262.

31 Stress and Coping

MODULE AT-A-GLANCE

The Concept of Stress and Coping, 1895

Exemplar 31.1
Anxiety Disorders, 1917

Exemplar 31.2
Crisis, 1927

Exemplar 31.3
Obsessive-Compulsive Disorder, 1934

Exemplar 31.4
Phobias, 1939

Exemplar 31.5
Posttraumatic Stress Disorder, 1945

◢ THE CONCEPT OF STRESS AND COPING

Although everyone experiences stress, what triggers stress in one individual may not cause stress in another. These triggers are known as stressors. A **stressor** is an external influence that threatens to disrupt the equilibrium that is needed to maintain homeostasis. **Homeostasis** describes the body's ability to maintain a stable, balanced internal environment despite the constant challenges posed by external influences (Cannon, 1929). When healthy and functioning properly, the body adapts to these external influences, or stressors, and promotes maintenance or restoration of homeostasis. Homeostasis is demonstrated by the body's ability to maintain fluid and electrolyte balance, oxygenation, and thermoregulation (the control of heat production and heat loss to maintain a steady body temperature). In particular, physiological maintenance of the body's delicate acid–base balance provides a classic example of homeostasis in action (Cannon, 1932).

Stressors may be physical, mental, or emotional in nature; they also may be positive or negative, depending on several variables, including the individual's perception of the experience. However, by definition, all stressors share one commonality: They have the capacity to cause stress. **«**

Concept Learning Outcomes

After reading about this concept, you will be able to:

1. Summarize the physiological response to stress and the psychodynamics of coping.

2. Examine the relationship between stress and coping and other concepts/systems.

3. Identify commonly occurring alterations in coping and their related therapies.

4. Differentiate common assessment procedures used to examine stress levels and coping mechanisms across the life span.

5. Explain management of stress to facilitate healthy coping and prevent stress-related illness.

6. Demonstrate the nursing process in providing culturally competent and caring interventions across the life span for individuals with common alterations in coping.

7. Compare and contrast common independent and collaborative interventions for clients with alterations in coping.

Concept Key Terms

Adaptation, *1900*

Allostasis, *1896*

Allostatic load, *1896*

Anger, *1904*

Anxiety, *1904*

Approach coping, *1899*

Avoidance coping, *1899*

Biogenic stressors, *1897*

Burnout, *1907*

Cognitive appraisal, *1898*

Cognitive structuring, *1904*

Cognitive-behavioral therapy (CBT), *1914*

Coping, *1896*

Countershock phase, *1901*

Depression, *1904*

Diseases of adaptation, *1901*

Distress, *1896*

Ego defense mechanisms, *1904*

Emotion-focused coping, *1899*

Eustress, *1896*

External environmental stressors, *1898*

Fantasizing, *1904*

Fear, *1902*

General adaptation syndrome (GAS), *1900*

Hassles, *1898*

Hildegard Peplau, *1902*

(continued on next page)

Homeostasis, *1895*

Internal environment, *1898*

Local adaptation syndrome (LAS), *1900*

Maslow's hierarchy of needs, *1899*

Meaning-focused coping, *1899*

Nursing transactional model, *1902*

Primary appraisal, *1902*

Problem solving, *1904*

Problem-focused coping, *1899*

Psychosocial stressors, *1897*

Reappraisal, *1902*

Response-based stress model, *1900*

Secondary appraisal, *1902*

Self control, *1904*

Shock phase, *1901*

Stage of exhaustion, *1901*

Stage of resistance, *1901*

Stimulus-based stress model, *1900*

Stress, *1896*

Stress mediators, *1896*

Stress response, *1896*

Stressor, *1895*

Suppression, *1904*

▶ STRESS AND HOMEOSTASIS

The term *stress* has appeared in the literature since approximately the 14th century, at which time it was applied in reference to hardship, adversity, or some form of affliction (Lumsden, 1981). However, the present-day understanding of the concept of stress initially was made famous through the research and publications of Dr. Hans Selye (1907–1982). Selye was an endocrinologist and a pioneer in the study of stress and the stress response. Selye (1956) defined **stress** as the body's general, nonspecific response to the demands placed on it by a stressor. Selye further asserted that not all stress is bad; in some cases, stress can help an individual to achieve desired goals or exceed self-imposed limitations (Cherry, 1978; Selye, 1956, 1976). Good stress, which Selye called **eustress**, is associated with accomplishment and victory. The opposite of eustress is **distress**, which is stress that is associated with inadequacy, insecurity, and loss. In sum, eustress may be considered the stress of winning, while distress may be viewed as the stress of losing (Cherry, 1978; Selye, 1956).

In further refining Canon's conceptualization of homeostasis from a more holistic standpoint, Sterling and Eyer (1988) originated the term **allostasis**, which refers to the necessary changes that must occur to achieve the characteristic stability of homeostasis. Current literature defines allostasis as encompassing all of the body's responses to a challenge or demand for change (McEwen & Gianaros, 2010). In essence, homeostasis is the goal, while allostasis is the means to reach that goal. The process of allostasis includes the psychosocial and physiological changes that occur in response to stress, many of which are triggered by activation of the sympathetic nervous system. In addition to other functions, the sympathetic nervous system triggers the body's "fight-or-flight" response, which is necessary for survival. Activation of the sympathetic nervous system causes release of hormones such as epinephrine, which increases the heart rate and blood pressure to assist in the delivery of oxygen to tissues and organs. Epinephrine also causes bronchial dilation, which allows for increased oxygen uptake. This increase in oxygen uptake and delivery is intended to meet the increased metabolic demands associated with facing a stressor (fight) or escaping the stressor (flight).

Formally referred to as the **stress response**, physiological changes triggered by stress include activation of the neural, neuroendocrine, and endocrine systems, as well as activation of target organs (Everly & Lating, 2013). The two primary stress mediators are glucocorticoids (such as cortisol) and catecholamines (such as epinephrine). These hormonal **stress mediators** are intended to promote adaptation through mechanisms such as triggering a necessary increase in heart rate and blood pressure when faced with physical danger.

Under ideal conditions, the stress response permits the body to compensate for the impact of stressors and to either maintain or regain homeostasis, which is necessary for an organism's survival. However, repeated activation of the stress response takes a toll on the individual. The physical cost of adaptation to physiological or psychosocial stressors is referred to as the **allostatic load**. In addition to hormonal changes, the allostatic load also includes behavioral responses to stress, not all of which may be favorable; for example, smoking, drinking alcohol, and poor dietary habits. Chronic, prolonged overexposure to stress mediators, as well as inefficiency of the stress response and unhealthy behavioral responses to stress, can lead to illness (McEwen, 1998).

How an individual responds to stress varies and depends both on the individual and the stressor. **Coping** is a dynamic process through which an individual applies cognitive and behavioral measures to handle internal and external demands that are perceived by the individual as exceeding his available resources (Lazarus & Folkman, 1984). Individuals cope by integrating environmental and cognitive measures to mitigate or diminish the stress response (Everly & Lating, 2013). For example, a nursing student who is studying for final exams might cope with stress through application of environmental measures, such taking a walk or enjoying a mocha with friends at a favorite coffee shop. Cognitively, the nursing student might alter her appraisal of the upcoming examination, choosing not to see it as an insurmountable barrier, but rather as a challenge for which she can prepare and successfully master.

When an individual is unable to adapt to stress in a sufficient way to maintain homeostasis, functional impairment may occur. For example, feelings of worry and panic accompanied by elevated heart rate may make it difficult for a student to concentrate on studying for an exam or for a professional to concentrate at work. A young child may become irritable and not be able to sit in the circle during morning carpet time and may strike out at a classmate.

A husband and father returning from military deployment may experience nightmares and flashbacks associated with a traumatic event from his deployment. He may turn to behaviors that prevent sleep and avoid activities that he associates with the event. Individuals who experience impairment of functioning related to stress and coping may develop one of several disorders of anxiety, stress, or trauma. This module provides a discussion of stress and coping as well as a more detailed picture of specific related disorders including anxiety disorders, crisis, obsessive-compulsive disorder, phobias, and posttraumatic stress disorder.

▶ STRESSORS AND THE COPING PROCESS

When clients present to clinics, emergency departments, or mental health centers with distress, nurses assist in the assessment of the source of the stress and help the client cope with the stressor. To be able to respond appropriately, nurses must have a working knowledge of types of stressors; how human beings respond to, or cope, with stress; and theoretical models of stress and coping that provide insight into stress and coping and how nurses can support clients during types of stress.

Not everyone will agree as to what constitutes a stressor. For example, one individual may view bungee jumping as a terrifying, life-threatening event that should be avoided, while another individual may consider this activity to be an exhilarating form of stress release. In this case, identification of a stressor depends on the individual's personal perception of the event or circumstance. However, certain stressors naturally evoke the physiological stress response in all individuals, without regard to personal perception.

Types of Stressors

Stressors may be categorized using a variety of methods. From a broad standpoint, stressors often are categorized as being either biogenic or psychosocial (Girdano, Dusek, & Everly, 2009).

Biogenic stressors directly trigger the stress response without any necessary cognitive process on the part of the individual; that is, the individual does not need to recognize the experience or circumstance as being stressful. Common examples of biogenic stressors include caffeine and nicotine, as well as extreme temperatures (Girdano et al., 2009). **Psychosocial stressors**, which are environmental events, may be either real or imagined. Rather than directly triggering the stress response, psychosocial stressors can facilitate its activation, depending on how the individual views the stressor (*cognitive appraisal,* discussed later in this module) (Girdano et al., 2009). For example, an individual who interprets the sound of distant thunder as gunshots may respond differently than an individual who perceives the same sound as signaling an approaching rainstorm.

Just as the severity (or perceived severity) of a stressor impacts the magnitude of the stress response, so does the length of time to which the individual is exposed to the stressor. This is true regardless of whether the stressor is biogenic or psychosocial in

nature—both can be equally powerful. In fact, anticipation of a stressor can produce the same physiological response that occurs when faced with the stressor in reality (Romero, Dickens, & Cyr, 2009). For example, anticipating or imagining a potential physical attack can evoke the release of the same stress hormones that would be released when an individual is engaged in an actual physical fight.

From the standpoint of duration of exposure, stressors may be classified into four categories:

1. Acute and time limited
2. Sequential events following an initial stressor
3. Chronic intermittent
4. Chronic permanent.

See **Table 31–1** ● for examples of each classification.

To understand the reciprocal and dynamic relationship between the individual and the environment, the discussion of stressors must be broadened to include sources of stress and types of stressors. The degree of a stressor's impact ranges from the benign (nonthreatening) hassles of daily living to traumatic events within an individual, family, and society. Examples of traumatic events include rape, life-threatening illness or injury, and natural disasters such as Hurricane Sandy in 2012. **Box 31–1** ● lists some common stressors.

DEVELOPMENTAL STRESSORS Developmental stressors include the challenges faced by each individual when progressing through the life span. For example, the transition from childhood to adolescence involves numerous challenges, including navigating relationships with peers and completing performance-related tasks, such as academic assignments that require public speaking. Researchers who studied the impact of adolescent challenges in relationship to the stress response have identified several physiological patterns. For example, among adolescents, research suggests that peer rejection stimulates an increase in systolic blood pressure and in the production of saliva α-amylase (sAA), which is an enzyme that is reflective of sympathetic nervous system activation. Additionally, stressors related to performance-based challenges were associated with increased cortisol production and increased diastolic blood pressure (Stroud et al., 2009). (For discussion of

TABLE 31–1 Classifications and Examples of Stressors

CLASSIFICATION OF STRESSORS	EXAMPLES
1. Acute and time limited	Roller-coaster ride
	Nursing licensure exam
2. Sequential events following an initial stressor	Losing a job and subsequently filing for bankruptcy
3. Chronic intermittent	Strained relationship with in-laws
	Shared caretaking for an elderly parent
4. Chronic permanent	Paralysis
	Disability (e.g., blindness, deafness)

Box 31–1 Types of Stressors

DEVELOPMENTAL STRESSORS

Starting school
Playing and working with peers
Puberty
Education
Changes
Marriage
Birth of children
Aging

DAILY HASSLES

Roles of living
Caring for children
Pets
Work responsibility
Paying bills
Traffic
Neighbors

ENVIRONMENTAL STRESSORS

Major cataclysmic changes affecting a large number of people (natural disasters, war, floods, hurricanes)
Major changes affecting one or a few people (divorce, bereavement)

INTERNAL STRESSORS

Cognition (thoughts)
Spirituality
Emotions

TABLE 31–2 Factors Affecting an Individual's Stress Response

INDIVIDUAL FACTORS	ENVIRONMENTAL FACTORS
Genetic predisposition	Family support and connectedness
Past experience coping with stressors	Community support
Ability to meet own basic human needs	Financial resources
Cultural beliefs and customs	Community resources
Holistic health and well-being	Access to health care and education
Personal worldview and appraisal	Family appraisal
Coping mechanisms and history of coping successes	Social support

developmental tasks throughout the life span, see the module on Development.)

INTERNAL STRESSORS The **internal environment** includes the physical, spiritual, cognitive, emotional, and psychological well-being of an individual and depends on the satisfaction of these basic human needs. According to Lazarus and Folkman (1984), the drive to fulfill human needs internally sparks the stimulus to produce the energy to seek gratification. This individual day-to-day tension is commonly referred to in stress and coping research as daily **hassles**. The holistic health and balance of individuals experiencing stressors affect their ability to cope with daily hassles. Examples of daily hassles include making it through a day of work or school or having to care for a small child after a poor night's sleep. Physical, emotional, and spiritual health affects whether or not the individual views a hassle as a minor inconvenience or a major strain. Alterations of health in any of these areas may overwhelm an individual's ability to cope with a specific stimulus or event, no matter how mild.

Dossey and Keegan (2009) address the spiritual dimension of the human condition as part of the individual's internal environment. The authors define *spirituality* as the essence of who we are and how we relate to the world. They incorporate elements of spirituality that include individual values, our place or fit in the world, and a sense of peace. Recent research has identified interconnectedness with the self, individuals, and the world around us as important components of spirituality. (See the module on Spirituality.)

ENVIRONMENTAL STRESSORS **External environmental stressors** include triggers outside of the individual that demand change or disrupt homeostasis. Positive stressors, such

as graduation from college, generally produce eustress. Negative stressors, such as the inability to find employment, tend to cause distress. Stressors also may be simultaneously positive and negative, as with the combination of pending college graduation and imminent lack of employment. An event is a stressor if it creates a change in the individual or the individual's circumstances. **Table 31–2** ● outlines specific individual and environmental factors that affect an individual's response to a stressor.

The Coping Process

As described earlier individual responses to stress include physiological, psychological, and behavioral responses. Coping is the process by which individuals can control or modify their responses. Successful coping allows individuals to maintain or return to homeostasis within a reasonable amount of time. Individuals who are unable to cope successfully may experience a range of symptoms requiring intervention from nurses and other healthcare professionals.

COGNITIVE APPRAISAL **Cognitive appraisal** is a key factor in the client's ability to cope with stressors. As the individual experiences exposure to a stressor, he appraises the stressor; that is, the individual mentally sorts, assesses, categorizes, evaluates, and frames the significance of an event or stressor with respect to his own well-being. The *primary appraisal* is the "first impression," occurring immediately on exposure to a stressor. Based on the transactional model, there are three ways in which an individual categorizes a stimulus or demand: (1) irrelevant, (2) benign-positive, or (3) stressful. Irrelevant stressors are appraised as having no meaningful effect on the individual or his circumstance, and are disregarded. Benign-positive stressors are demands for change that are perceived as preserving or enhancing well-being, such as taking a driver's education class. Stressors or stimuli categorized as stressful include those viewed as harmful, threatening, or disturbing, such as the death of a family member or a threat to life or safety.

During the secondary appraisal, the individual attempts to predict the impact, intensity, and duration of the coping behavior necessary to respond to the stressor. At this time the individual selects a coping response.

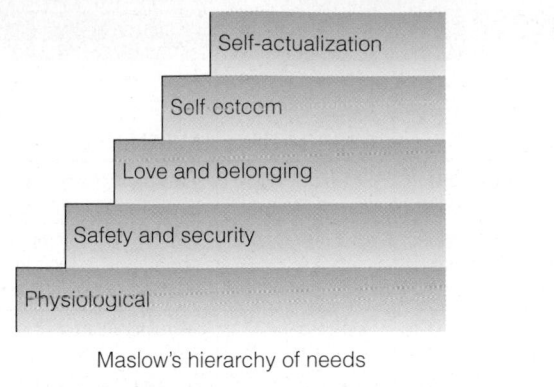

Figure 31–1 ● Maslow's hierarchy of needs.

In some cases, the intensity of an individual's stress response may appear to be incongruent with the stressor. For example, for some individuals, the loss of a family pet may be devastating and can elicit an extreme stress response, whereas other individuals may demonstrate a response that is mild in intensity when faced with a similar loss. Likewise, some students may view earning a grade of C on an examination as being successful, because it is a passing grade; for others, earning anything less than an A is distressing. Keeping in mind that each individual is unique, **Maslow's hierarchy of needs** offers a model that is useful for understanding the significance of stressors within the context of human needs.

MASLOW'S HIERARCHY OF NEEDS

When Abraham Maslow introduced his hierarchy of needs in 1943, he proposed the existence of levels of human needs that could be organized into five categories: physiological, safety, love and belonging, self-esteem, and self-actualization (**Figure 31–1 ●**). Physiological needs represent the first and most important requirements, with each subsequent category of needs presented in order of importance. Although Maslow later expanded his model to include three additional categories of needs (cognitive, aesthetic, and self-transcendence), the five-stage model is widely used and can be used to assist nurses and other professionals in identifying and prioritizing client needs and interventions (Koltko-Rivera, 2006; Maslow, 1968, 1987). According to Maslow, unmet lower order needs will dominate the individual and prohibit higher-order needs from emerging. For example, for an individual who is experiencing extreme hunger or starvation, the quest for food becomes life's focus. As each category of needs is met, the individual's focus shifts to meeting higher-order needs. As such, once hunger is satiated, the need for safety and protection emerges and becomes the individual's primary goal. The satisfaction of both physiological and safety needs allows for the emergence of needs related to love and belonging. This process continues as the individual is able to meet each stage of needs (Maslow, 1987).

It is important to note that individual traits and variations lead to flexibility with regard to the sequencing of Maslow's hierarchy of needs. As a result, the prioritization of needs may vary, depending on the individual (Maslow, 1987). As an example, for an individual who demonstrates an extremely powerful drive to achieve professional success, esteem needs (e.g., respect from others, empowerment, competence) may supersede needs related to love and belonging. Likewise, mental illness may lead to the exclusion of certain categories of needs (Maslow, 1987). For example, antisocial personality disorder is characterized by a lack of concern for the safety needs of self or others.

EFFECTIVE COPING   Effective coping is a learned process, not an inherent personality trait. It includes all efforts mobilized by the individual to manage stressors. Coping involves constant change by the individual and includes spiritual, emotional, cognitive, and behavioral efforts to manage the demand. A stressor is appraised in terms of its effects or alterations on the physical, emotional, and spiritual conditions of the individual and/or on the individual's unmet needs or drives. Lazarus and Folkman's (1984) transactional model describes *coping* as a means to manage or alter the problem causing the distress. The appraisal process allows the individual to inform the coping response by incorporating the person's own spiritual, cognitive, affective, and inherent vulnerability. In essence, every person responds to a stressor according to his or her unique worldview and condition.

Two forms of coping are (1) **problem-focused coping**, which is aimed at managing or altering the stressor, event, or circumstance, and (2) **emotion-focused coping**, which is directed at regulating the emotional response to the distress. Emotion-focused coping is used most when the stressor is perceived to be beyond the individual's control. In problem-focused coping, generally the perception is that the stressor can be changed (Lazarus & Folkman, 1984). Additional subcategories of coping include **avoidance coping** (using both behaviors and cognitive processes to avoid the stressor) and **approach coping** (confronting and trying to change the stressor by taking direct action). Finally, there is also **meaning-focused coping**, which involves revaluation to reduce the appraisal of a threat (Carver & Connor-Smith, 2010).

It is crucial for nurses to understand that any form of coping is an individual process influenced by the number of stressors; their source, type, intensity, and duration; and the individual's support, experience, and vulnerability. Nurses need to be aware of their own coping styles and maintain a nonjudgmental attitude about the coping mechanisms of individuals experiencing stressors. **Table 31–3 ●** depicts the various forms and examples of coping with stressors.

Healthcare professionals and researchers have clearly established the strong and complex relationship among stress, coping, and physical and psychological illness (Juster, McEwen, & Lupien, 2010). Lazarus and Folkman (1984) note that it is the reaction to the demand, not the stimulus itself, that causes stress. The nursing transactional model allows the nurse to consider individual client preferences, resources, culture, and environment in the assessment of the client's abilities to respond to stress and to assist the client in returning to homeostasis.

REAPPRAISAL AND ADAPTATION   Following attempts to cope with the stressor, the individual engages in a reappraisal process. During this time, the individual evaluates what coping mechanisms were successful and what were not and, ideally, begins another attempt to respond to the stressor and return to homeostasis. In terms of its effects on the body, stress is not viewed as "good" or "bad," but merely according

TABLE 31–3 Examples of Types of Coping

TYPES	EMOTION-FOCUSED COPING (DEFENSIVE)	PROBLEM-FOCUSED COPING	AVOIDANCE	APPROACH	MEANING
Cognitive	Minimizing the event: "Oh it's not that bad!"	Information gathering: "What are my odds of surviving?"	Denial of a situation or limiting information about stressful situations: "This is a bad dream!"	Confronting the situation	Identifying positive changes associated with stressful events; for example, personal illness that leads to increased family bonding
Behavioral	Performing physical activity to avoid thinking about a stressful situation	Adhering to a healthcare plan	Refusing to get a mammogram when a history of breast cancer runs in the family	Seeking means to exercise control	Attempting to fit into the environment: "I'll make the best of the situation."
Affective	Hoping for a miracle	Keeping feelings from interfering	Dealing with feelings later	Using feelings to motivate change	Seeking control of environment; regulating the emotional response to stress

to how much, what kinds, and under what conditions is it harmful or helpful (Lazarus & Folkman, 1984). **Adaptation** incorporates all the processes, including physiological and psychological, employed by an organism in response to stress in an attempt to survive and thrive (Smith & Lazarus, 1990). Adaptation and the development of health alterations are influenced by personal variables, with cognitive appraisal of the stressor, genetic predisposition to illness, and behavioral responses to stress being among the most significant factors (Juster et al., 2010).

Theoretical Models of Stress and Coping

A number of theories and models exist to explain the phenomenon of stress. In this section we discuss stimulus-based and response-based stress models briefly, before presenting the transactional model in more detail.

STIMULUS-BASED STRESS MODELS **Stimulus-based stress models** view "stress" as being synonymous with "stressor." These models define stress as being a life event that requires change or adaptation on the part of the individual who is experiencing the life event. Exposure to such life events leads to physiological and psychological "wear and tear," and can increase the individual's susceptibility to illness (Holmes & Rahe, 1967; Lyon, 2012). In their classic work, Holmes and Rahe (1967) proposed the Social Readjustment Rating Scale (SRRS), which quantified the impact of 43 significant life events—with none of the events classified as being either positive or negative—by assigning a numerical value to each individual experience. Examples of life events included marriage, divorce, change of residence, and loss of a job. Variations of the SRRS questionnaire are still in use today. In 1997, a 77-item version of the SRRS was created (Miller & Rahe, 1997). In 2002, a shortened version was designed (Rahe & Tolles, 2002).

When considering the validity of the SRRS and similar scales, note that perception of a life event will vary among individuals, particularly with regard to cognitive appraisal of the event as being a stressor. Likewise, the impact of significant events must be considered from the standpoint of the individual's simultaneous exposure to routine stressors. According to Lazarus and Folkman (1984), in comparison to experiencing significant life events, exposure to life's daily hassles was more likely to lead to stress-related alterations.

RESPONSE-BASED STRESS MODELS In **response-based stress models**, stress is considered to be a response to a stressor. According to Selye (1956, 1976), stress is "the nonspecific response of the body to any kind of demand made upon it" (1976, p. 1). Selye's (1976) model described the stress response as a three-stage chain of events called the **general adaptation syndrome (GAS)** or *stress response*. Selye used the term *stressor* to distinguish between the stimulus and the response. Within the context of GAS, stressors are any stimuli that evoke the stress response. Selye (1974) also proposed that not every instance of disruption of homeostasis qualifies as an occurrence of stress. For example, a close-flying insect that stimulates an individual to blink excessively may disturb the body's equilibrium, but this event does not necessarily trigger the GAS.

Within the framework of the GAS, in response to genuine stress, physiological changes occur. These changes include hormonal production and release, as well as alterations in organs and structures. For example, prolonged exposure to stress may lead to significant enlargement of the adrenal glands and pronounced shrinkage (atrophy) of the lymphatic structures, including the lymph nodes, thymus, and spleen. Additionally, within the gastrointestinal tract, ulcers may develop.

Although the stress response may be global (or generalized) in nature, the stress response can also manifest itself locally. A local stress response, during which one organ or body system reacts to stress, may produce **local adaptation syndrome (LAS)**. For example, local inflammation in response to a scrape or minor laceration is an example of LAS. However, according to Selye (1976), both GAS and LAS produce a three-stage response: alarm reaction, resistance, and exhaustion (see **Figure 31–2** ●).

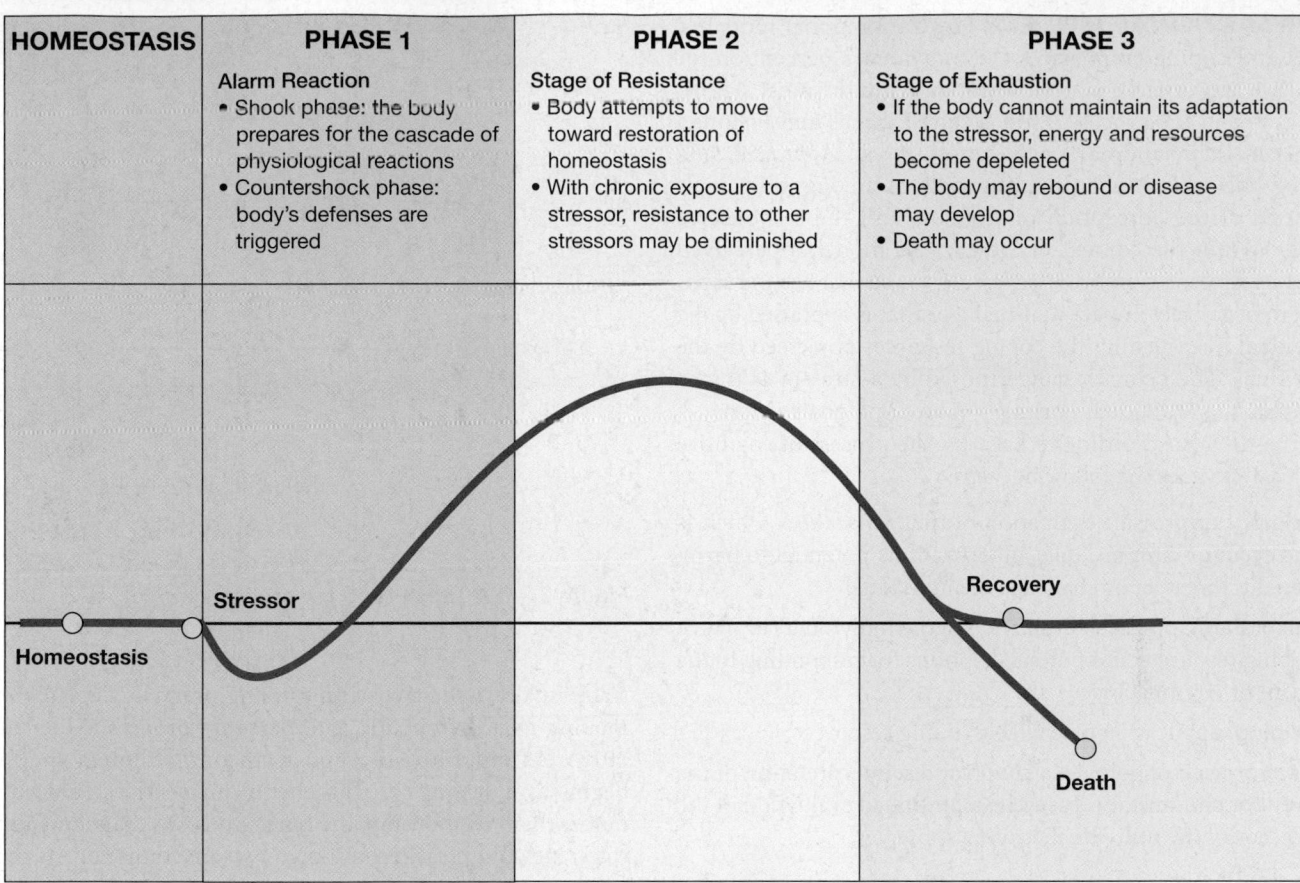

HOMEOSTASIS	PHASE 1	PHASE 2	PHASE 3
	Alarm Reaction	**Stage of Resistance**	**Stage of Exhaustion**
	• Shock phase: the body prepares for the cascade of physiological reactions • Countershock phase: body's defenses are triggered	• Body attempts to move toward restoration of homeostasis • With chronic exposure to a stressor, resistance to other stressors may be diminished	• If the body cannot maintain its adaptation to the stressor, energy and resources become depleted • The body may rebound or disease may develop • Death may occur

Figure 31–2 ● The three stages of adaptation to stress: the alarm reaction, the stage of resistance, and the stage of exhaustion.

Alarm Reaction   The body's initial response is the two-part alarm reaction, which begins with the **shock phase**. During the shock phase, as the body prepares for the cascade of physiological reactions to the stressor, the sympathetic nervous system is suppressed and the individual may experience manifestations such as hypotension, decreased body temperature, and decreased muscle tone. During the second part of the alarm reaction, which is referred to as the **countershock phase**, sympathetic nervous system stimulation triggers the body's defenses, which in turn stimulates the hypothalamus. The hypothalamus releases corticotrophin-releasing hormone (CRH), which stimulates the anterior pituitary gland to release adrenocorticotropic hormone (ACTH). This sympathetic stimulation results in secretion of epinephrine and norepinephrine. Significant body responses to epinephrine include increased myocardial activity, bronchial dilation, and increased fat mobilization. This adrenal hormonal activity prepares the individual for *fight or flight*. This primary response is short lived, lasting from 1 minute to 24 hours.

Stage of Resistance   During the second stage of the GAS, which is the **stage of resistance**, the body attempts to move toward restoration of homeostasis while continuing to respond to the stressor. With chronic exposure to a stressor, although the body may maintain resistance to the primary stressor, resistance to other stressors may be diminished. For example, an individual who is going through the divorce process may become emotionally and psychologically stable, giving an outward appearance of effectively coping with the emotional impact of the divorce. However, the prolonged physiological stress response—which includes increased production of catecholamines (such as epinephrine and norepinephrine), glucose, and cortisol—may lead to increased susceptibility to physical illness, including peptic ulcers and hypertension. Selye (1946) called stress-related illnesses **diseases of adaptation**.

Stage of Exhaustion   During the third stage, the **stage of exhaustion**, if the body cannot maintain its adaptation to the stressor, the stressor overwhelms the individual's ability to cope or mount a continued defense, resulting in the depletion of energy and resources. The body may rebound from the stressor after a period of rest or disease may develop. Death also may ensue. The end of this stage depends largely on the adaptive energy resources of the individual, the severity of the stressor, and the external adaptive resources that are provided. An example of this can be seen in the client who lives with chronic pain. The client may be able to tolerate the pain during the day, but at night finds the pain far more stressful because her energy resources are diminished to the point that the pain is intolerable.

TRANSACTIONAL MODEL   The transactional model of stress and coping emphasizes the individual's perception, or cognitive appraisal, of a given threat as being the most significant factor in the process. Proposed by Lazarus and Folkman (1984) in their landmark publication, *Stress, Appraisal, and Coping,* this model incorporates variations among individuals in terms of the perception of stressors and the response to stress. Within the context of the Lazarus model, a perceived threat or stressor is an event or circumstance that has the capability to negatively impact well-being or that is appraised by the individual as exceeding the coping resources possessed by the individual. The primary danger posed by a stressor is that it threatens the individual's primary values and goals (Monat & Lazarus, 1991). According to Lazarus, the process of cognitive appraisal includes the following steps:

- **Primary appraisal:** evaluation of the *transaction*, which is the event or circumstance, in terms of its potential to harm, benefit, threaten, or challenge the individual
- **Secondary appraisal:** evaluation of the individual's available coping resources and potential options for responding to the event or circumstance
- **Coping:** application of available coping resources
- **Reappraisal:** ongoing evaluation and reinterpretation of the event or circumstance, as well as continued evaluation of the efficacy of the individual's coping strategies.

Culturally competent nursing care requires recognizing that cultural influences, as well as characteristics that are unique to the individual (including personality and temperament), impact both cognitive appraisal and coping styles.

The nursing transactional model is an adaptation of Lazarus and Folkman's work. The **nursing transactional model** is defined as the relationship between the nurse, the client, and the environment in which they interact (**Figure 31–3** ●). This interaction or relationship is dynamic—with each transaction the individual and the stressor engage to form a new transaction with a particular meaning. This model has numerous implications for the profession of nursing and care of the individual experiencing stress. The emphasis is on the relationship among stress, the client, the nurse, and both the internal and external environment.

In considering the complexity of a client's response to stress, the nurse must consider the client as an individual person as well as a member of a family, community, culture, and environment. The astute nurse collects important information from each context to build a foundation for understanding, assessing, intervening, and mediating the harmful effects of stress on the individual client and his or her family, community, and society.

The nursing transactional model emphasizes communication and the development of an interpersonal relationship with the client with the intent of decreasing the client's anxiety and increasing or improving the client's coping resources. This perspective and approach is largely based on the work of nursing theorist **Hildegard Peplau,** who is widely considered to be the mother of psychiatric nursing. In 1952, as the first nurse to publish a nursing theory since Florence Nightingale (Pokorny, 2010), Peplau published her classic textbook, *Interpersonal Relations in Nursing.* As opposed to the task-oriented focus

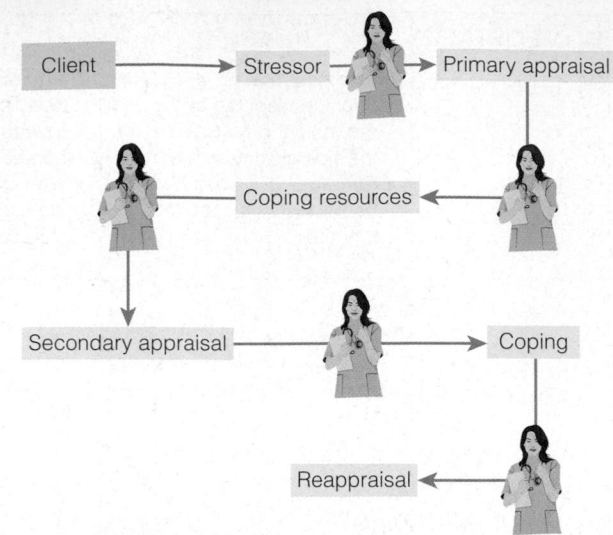

Figure 31–3 ● The nursing transactional model.

traditionally associated with nursing practice, Peplau viewed nursing as a therapeutic interpersonal process (Elder et al., 2013). As described in Peplau's theory, although the nurse begins as a stranger to the client, during the course of the nurse–client relationship, the nurse proceeds to assume several roles, including teacher, resource person, counselor, surrogate, and leader (Peplau, 1952).

▶ MANIFESTATIONS OF STRESS

Just as each individual is unique in terms of cognitive appraisal and coping methods, individuals also may vary in terms of the internal and external manifestations of stress. In addition to the physiological domain, stress also may yield manifestations in various other domains, including psychological and cognitive.

Physiological Indicators

Physiological manifestations of stress primarily result from stimulation of the sympathetic and neuroendocrine systems. (See **Table 31–4** ● for an overview of physiological indicators of the stress response.) As previously discussed, cognitive appraisal is crucial to activation of the stress response; that is, the individual's perception of the potential stressor is the key to triggering the physiological manifestations of stress. Prolonged exposure to perceived stressors and chronic activation of the stress response can lead to disease and may even be fatal. The relationship between this mind–body connection is illustrated in the Multisystem Effects of Stress feature on page 1903.

Psychological Indicators

Individual manifestations of stress within the psychological domain may include fear, anxiety, anger, depression, and a variety of other responses.

Fear is a sense of apprehension triggered by a perceived threat to safety or well-being, including a painful stimuli or dangerous event. Fear may be aroused by memories of an actual past experience,

Multisystemic Effects of Stress

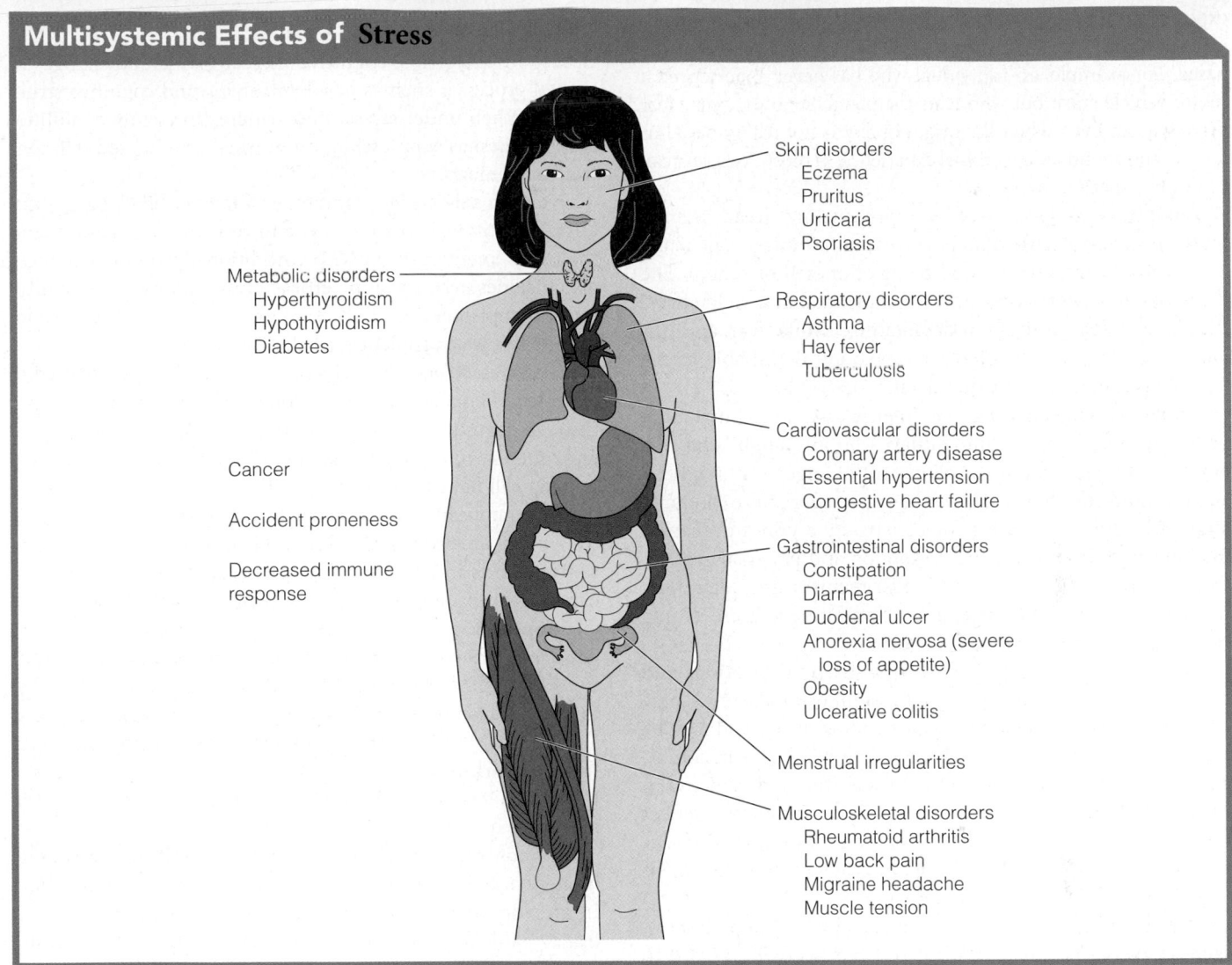

Metabolic disorders
  Hyperthyroidism
  Hypothyroidism
  Diabetes

Cancer

Accident proneness

Decreased immune
response

Skin disorders
  Eczema
  Pruritus
  Urticaria
  Psoriasis

Respiratory disorders
  Asthma
  Hay fever
  Tuberculosis

Cardiovascular disorders
  Coronary artery disease
  Essential hypertension
  Congestive heart failure

Gastrointestinal disorders
  Constipation
  Diarrhea
  Duodenal ulcer
  Anorexia nervosa (severe
    loss of appetite)
  Obesity
  Ulcerative colitis

Menstrual irregularities

Musculoskeletal disorders
  Rheumatoid arthritis
  Low back pain
  Migraine headache
  Muscle tension

TABLE 31–4   Overview of Physiological Manifestations of the Stress Response

BODY SYSTEM	RESPONSE
Respiratory	■ Increased ventilatory rate and depth of respirations
	■ Dilation of bronchioles to facilitate increased oxygenation
Cardiac	■ Increased heart rate and cardiac output to promote transport of oxygen and nutrients throughout the body
Integumentary	■ Increased sweat production (diaphoresis) to offset increased body temperature secondary to increased metabolism
	■ Skin pallor secondary to vasoconstrictive effects of norepinephrine
Gastrointestinal	■ Inhibition of the parasympathetic nervous system leads to decreased motility of gastric and intestinal contents (peristalsis) through the gastrointestinal tract, which may cause constipation and excess flatus (intestinal gas)
	■ Dry mouth due to decreased salivation secondary to inhibition of the parasympathetic nervous system
Urinary	■ Increased sodium and water retention due mineralocorticoid release, which leads to decreased urine output and increased blood volume
Ophthalmic	■ Pupillary dilation to allow entrance of more light and enhanced visual perception
Neurological	■ Enhanced awareness and alertness in response to severe threats
Musculoskeletal	■ Increased muscular tension in preparation for defense (fight) or rapid mobility (flight)
Endocrine	■ Increased release of glucocorticoids and increased gluconeogenesis, which leads to increased serum glucose (blood sugar)

exposure to a present threat, or anticipated exposure to an event or circumstance. Events that trigger fear may or may not be reality based. For example, an individual who has never experienced a motor vehicle crash but who fears the possibility of one may fear driving a car. Even when the origin of fear is not reality based or founded on an individual's actual experience, in most cases, fear can be tied to a specific source.

Anxiety is characterized by apprehension, dread, mental uneasiness, and a sense of helplessness in response to an actual or perceived threat to the well-being of oneself or others. The degree of anxiety experienced by an individual may yield effects that range from minimal to debilitating. Unlike fear, an individual's anxiety may not have an apparent identifiable cause. Anxiety is discussed in greater detail in Exemplar 31.1.

Anger is a subjective sense of intense displeasure, irritation, or animosity. For those individuals who are taught that this emotion is unacceptable, development of anger may trigger a sense of guilt or shame. However, processing and expressing anger through application of constructive communication methods may lead to conflict resolution and personal growth. Constructive communication of anger requires clear identification of the source of the anger and a commitment to preventing escalation of anger during discussions.

Escalation of anger may lead to destructive emotions and behaviors, including hostility, aggression, or violence. Generally, hostility is characterized by open antagonism, and may be expressed through both verbal and nonverbal means in combination with behaviors ranging from insensitive to destructive in nature. Aggression describes unprovoked actions that reflect hostility, attempts to cause injury, or a desire to cause destruction. Violence is the application of physical force with the intent to abuse or injure one or more individuals.

Depression is a persistent feeling of emptiness, hopelessness, sadness, or despair. A loss of interest (apathy) with regard to activities, including those related to daily living, often accompanies this emotional state. Manifestations of depression include behavioral, emotional, and physical signs and symptoms (see **Table 31–5** for examples of manifestations of depression). Depression may occur as a normal response to loss, such as when grieving the death of a loved one, following termination of employment, or following divorce. Chronic, recurrent, or extended periods of depression signal the need for evaluation and potential treatment (see the module on Mood and Affect).

Cognitive Indicators

In response to stress, cognitive indicators include changes in mental processes such as problem solving and cognitive structuring. When under stress, impairments in cognitive abilities may manifest as suppression, diminished or impaired self-control, and fantasizing.

Problem solving incorporates evaluating a challenging situation, identifying potential steps to resolve the situation, and then implementing those steps. Additionally, problem solving also includes evaluating the efficacy of solutions, and identifying and implementing alternative approaches as needed to adequately resolve a problem or challenge.

Cognitive structuring refers to the mental processes used to interpret and make sense of environmental stimuli. For example, through cognitive structuring, a nurse working in the hospital environment interprets the sound associated with an activated nursing call light to mean that a client needs assistance. More complex application of cognitive structuring includes drawing from previous experiences with problem solving and the associated outcomes and then, through general application of those past experiences, forming a plan for resolving a present challenge.

Suppression, which is a defense mechanism, is the active, conscious process of denying unacceptable thoughts or emotions (Kneisl & Trigoboff, 2013). Suppression can be healthy; for example, an individual may suppress anger related to a disagreement with his significant other in order to effectively perform his work-related duties and demonstrate a positive attitude toward his coworkers. However, suppression may also lead to avoidance of facing problems or challenges.

Self-control is the ability to restrain oneself from acting on impulse or to behave in such a manner as to delay gratification. In an extreme example, exercising self-control may prevent fear or panic from overriding logic when faced with a stressful situation. However, attempts at exercising self-control—or a desire to appear to have self-control—can lead to ignoring or denying emotions and neglecting to ask for needed assistance.

Fantasizing or *daydreaming*, is imagining the fulfillment of desires or wishes, or mentally picturing the resolution of a situation in a manner that is more favorable than the resolution that occurred in reality. Fantasizing can be healthy and may even lead to identifying solutions to problems. However, excessive use of fantasy as a form of coping or in an attempt to avoid facing challenges can delay problem resolution.

Ego Defense Mechanisms

Frequently referred to as *defense mechanisms*, **ego defense mechanisms** were proposed and defined by Sigmund Freud (1946) as being unconscious psychological processes developed for the purpose of defending the personality (or self). Individuals use defense mechanisms to balance the tensions that emerge during times of stress and to protect themselves from anxiety and its adverse effects. See **Table 31–6** for a description of the primary defense mechanisms, as well as examples of their functional purpose and effects, which may be positive or negative.

Defense mechanisms are essential to psychological survival. Just as the fight-or-flight response supports individual physical survival, defense mechanisms protect our psychological state. Nurses must not only identify the defense mechanisms used by

TABLE 31–5	Manifestations of Depression
DOMAIN	**MANIFESTATIONS**
Behavioral	Difficulty concentrating, withdrawal from socialization, impaired decision-making ability, diminished libido (sexual desire), crying, disturbed sleep patterns, inability to complete activities of daily living (including personal hygiene)
Emotional	Sadness, despair, loss of interest (apathy) in normal activities, emptiness, hopelessness, irritability, sense of powerlessness
Physical	Weight loss, loss of appetite (anorexia), constipation; various somatic complaints, including dizziness, headache, generalized pain, and fatigue

TABLE 31–6 Ego Defense Mechanisms

DEFENSE MECHANISM	EXAMPLE(S)	USE/PURPOSE
Compensation: covering up weaknesses by emphasizing a more desirable trait or by over-achievement in a more comfortable area	A high school student too small to play football becomes the star long-distance runner for the track team.	Allows an individual to overcome weakness and achieve success
Denial: attempting to screen or ignore unacceptable realities by refusing to acknowledge them	A woman, though told her father has metastatic cancer, continues to plan a family reunion 18 months in advance.	Temporarily isolates an individual from the full impact of a traumatic situation
Displacement: transferring or discharging emotional reactions from one object or person to another object or person	A husband and wife are fighting, and the husband becomes so angry he hits a door instead of his wife. A student gets a C on a paper she worked hard on and goes home and yells at her family.	Allows for feelings to be expressed through or to less dangerous objects or people
Identification: attempting to manage anxiety by imitating the behavior of someone feared or respected	A student nurse imitates the nurturing behavior she observes one of her instructors using with clients.	Helps an individual avoid self-devaluation
Intellectualization: evading the emotional response that normally would accompany an uncomfortable or painful incident by using rational explanations that remove from the incident any personal significance and feelings	The pain over a parent's sudden death is reduced by saying, "He wouldn't have wanted to live disabled."	Protects an individual from pain and traumatic events
Introjection: a form of identification that allows for the acceptance of others' norms and values into oneself, even when contrary to one's previous assumptions	A 7-year-old tells his little sister, "Don't talk to strangers." He has introjected this value from the instructions of parents and teachers.	Helps an individual avoid social retaliation and punishment; particularly important for the child's development of superego
Minimization: not acknowledging the significance of one's behavior	An individual says, "Don't believe everything my wife tells you. I wasn't so drunk I couldn't drive."	Allows an individual to decrease responsibility for his or her own behavior
Projection: blaming others or the environment for unacceptable desires, thoughts, shortcomings, and mistakes	A mother is told her child must repeat a grade in school, and she blames this on the teacher's poor instruction. A husband forgets to pay a bill and blames his wife for not giving it to him earlier.	Allows an individual to deny the existence of shortcomings and mistakes; protects self-image
Rationalization: justifying certain behaviors by faulty logic and ascription of motives that are socially acceptable but did not in fact inspire the behavior	A mother spanks her toddler too hard and says it was all right because he couldn't feel it through the diapers anyway.	Helps an individual cope with the inability to meet goals or certain standards
Reaction formation: a mechanism that causes people to act exactly opposite to the way they feel	An executive resents his bosses for calling in a consulting firm to make recommendations for change in his department, but verbalizes complete support of the idea and is exceedingly polite and cooperative.	Aids in reinforcing repression by allowing feelings to be acted out in a more acceptable way
Regression: resorting to an earlier, more comfortable level of functioning that is characteristically less demanding and responsible	An adult throws a temper tantrum when he does not get his own way. A critically ill client allows the nurse to bathe and feed him.	Allows an individual to return to a point in development when nurturing and dependency were needed and accepted with comfort
Repression: an unconscious mechanism by which threatening thoughts, feelings, and desires are kept from becoming conscious; the repressed material is denied entry into consciousness	A teenager, seeing his best friend killed in a car crash, becomes amnesic about the circumstances surrounding the accident.	Protects an individual from a traumatic experience until he or she has the resources to cope
Sublimation: displacing energy associated with more primitive sexual or aggressive drives into socially acceptable activities	An individual with excessive, primitive sexual drives invests psychic energy into a well-defined religious value system.	Protects an individual from behaving in irrational, impulsive ways
Substitution: replacing a highly valued, unacceptable, or unavailable object with a less valuable, acceptable, or available object	A woman wants to marry a man exactly like her dead father and settles for someone who looks a little bit like him.	Helps an individual achieve goals and minimizes frustration and disappointment
Undoing: performing an action or using words designed to cancel some disapproved thoughts, impulses, or acts in which the person relieves guilt by making reparation	A father spanks his child and the next evening brings home a present for him. A teacher writes an examination that is far too easy, then constructs a grading curve that makes it difficult to earn a high grade.	Allows an individual to appease guilty feelings and atone for mistakes

Concepts Related to **Stress and Coping**

The physiological and psychological effects of stress have numerous implications for both the client and the nurse. For example, stress-related activation of the sympathetic nervous system triggers the release of catecholamines and glucocorticoids, prompting considerations related to perfusion, metabolism, and oxygenation. In the clinical setting, acute stress-related events, including impending surgery, can be stressful for clients. For all individuals, including the nurse, chronic exposure to stress may increase susceptibility to a variety of illnesses and lead to negative consequences.

CONCEPT	RELATIONSHIP TO STRESS AND COPING	NURSING IMPLICATIONS
Perfusion		
■ Factors affecting the pulse ■ Factors affecting blood pressure ■ Normal changes of aging ■ Assessment interview: perfusion	Stress response → release of catecholamines epinephrine and norepinephrine → ↑ blood pressure and ↑ heart rate	■ Assess clients for hypertension and tachycardia. ■ Be aware that prolonged exposure to stress can lead to long-term hypertension and secondary complications, including cardiovascular disease, cerebrovascular accident (CVA or stroke), and renal damage. ■ Educate clients about stress management techniques, including regular physical exercise. ■ Facilitate referrals to counselors as ordered.
Metabolism		
■ Diabetes ■ Diabetes in children	Stress response → release of glucocorticoids and ↑ gluconeogenesis → increased serum glucose (blood sugar) → ↑ risk for hyperglycemia and poor glucose control in clients with diabetes	■ Assess all clients with diabetes for exposure to acute and chronic stress. ■ Educate clients with diabetes about the effects of stress on serum glucose level. ■ Counsel clients experiencing acute or chronic stress about methods of stress reduction, including regular physical exercise and the importance of eating properly.
Caring Interventions		
■ Caring for the caregiver: self-care in nursing	Unmanaged nursing-related stress → ↑ risk for burnout → ↑ risk for emotional and physiological alterations and ↑ risk for adverse effects on client care and ↓ client satisfaction	■ Recognize and acknowledge manifestations of stress. ■ Identify healthy coping mechanisms, including ensuring adequate time away from the workplace and incorporation of recreational activities into personal life. ■ Seek out support and assistance when needed.
Oxygenation		
■ Asthma	Stress → ↑ release of epinephrine → bronchial dilation → increased oxygen uptake Stress → release of epinephrine → ↑ heart rate and ↑ blood pressure → increased tissue and organ perfusion	■ Be aware of the unseen impact of chronic stress, including complications related to hypertension and cardiovascular disease. ■ Assess and monitor changes in vital signs; report abnormalities to the client's primary healthcare provider. ■ Encourage the client to regularly engage in activities that are enjoyable and relaxing. ■ Educate the client about available relaxation techniques (such as meditation and massage) and provide information about techniques that are of interest to him.

Concepts Related to **Stress and Coping** (continued)

CONCEPT	RELATIONSHIP TO STRESS AND COPING	NURSING IMPLICATIONS
Perioperative Care		
■ Preparing the client ■ Psychosocial assessment ■ Lifespan considerations: preparing the pediatric client	Anticipation of surgery and anesthesia → stress → ↑ release of stress hormones, including catecholamines and glucocorticoids → potential for ↑ heart rate, ↑ blood pressure, and ↑ serum glucose preoperatively	■ Assess vital signs preoperatively; recognize the potential for stress-related increases in heart rate and blood pressure. ■ Interview the client regarding her level of anxiety and encourage open expression of concerns and emotions. ■ Encourage questions from the client and family members. ■ Administer preoperative anxiolytic medications as ordered; prior to anxiolytic administration, ensure that the surgeon and anesthesia provider have performed their preprocedure evaluations and that the client has signed all necessary consents for care prior to administration of anxiolytic medications.

clients, but also how they themselves use defense mechanisms to gain insight into their own defensive coping patterns. It is important to remember that defenses protect the individual and the ego. Providing a safe and nonjudgmental environment helps clients to let go of protective defenses and begin to cope with reality.

Integrating the Concepts

Stress and coping are intricately linked to physiological function. As previously discussed, the stress response triggers activation of the sympathetic nervous system, which in turn prompts the release of numerous neurotransmitters and hormones, with the primary stress mediators being catecholamines and glucocorticoids. Among numerous potential effects, chronic exposure to stress can increase susceptibility to a variety of illnesses, including cardiovascular disease and complications for clients with preexisting diabetes (American Diabetes Association, n.d.).

The effects of stress impact not only healthcare clients, but also their caregivers, including nursing professionals. Left unmanaged, what initially manifests as stress can translate into something far more serious. Due to occupation-specific demands, including irregular work schedules and increased workloads due to staffing shortages, nurses are at particularly high risk for **burnout**. In addition to adverse emotional and physical effects on the nurse, burnout also is associated with reduced quality of care and decreased client satisfaction with nursing care (McHugh et al., 2011).

See Concepts Related to Stress and Coping for more information on the relationship between stress and coping and other concepts.

▶ ALTERATIONS FROM NORMAL COPING RESPONSES

When an individual experiences stress so disabling that functioning is adversely affected, the individual is highly susceptible to the development of a disorder of anxiety, stress, or trauma. Until 2013,

these disorders were categorized as anxiety disorders in the American Psychiatric Association's *Diagnostic and Statistical Manual of Mental Disorders*, Fourth Edition, Text Revision (DSM-IV). With the 2013 publication of the DSM-5, the American Psychiatric Association (APA) recognizes three different classifications of disorders recognized as impairments in stress and coping:

■ *Anxiety disorders*, which include separation anxiety disorder, selective mutism, specific phobia, social anxiety disorder (social phobia), panic disorder, agoraphobia, generalized anxiety disorder, substance/medication-induced anxiety disorder, anxiety disorder due to another medical condition, other specified anxiety disorder, and unspecified anxiety disorder.

■ *Obsessive-compulsive and related disorders*, which include obsessive-compulsive disorder, body dysmorphic disorder, hoarding disorder, trichotillomania (hair-pulling disorder), excoriation (skin-picking disorder), substance/medication-induced obsessive-compulsive and related disorder, obsessive-compulsive and related disorder due to another medical condition, other specified and obsessive-compulsive and related disorder, and unspecified obsessive-compulsive and related disorder. Of these, obsessive-compulsive disorder is discussed in detail in Exemplar 31.3.

■ *Trauma- and stressor-related disorders*, which include reactive attachment disorder, disinhibited social engagement disorder, posttraumatic stress disorder, acute stress disorder, adjustment disorders, and other specified trauma- and stressor-related disorder. Posttraumatic stress disorder is discussed in Exemplar 31.5 along with a brief overview of acute stress disorder.

Children and Anxiety

In the early stages of development, some degree of anxiety is normal, particularly when children are separated from their parents or caregivers. Likewise, stranger anxiety is most pronounced dur-

Alterations and Therapies **Stress and Coping**

ALTERATION	DESCRIPTION	MANIFESTATIONS	INTERVENTIONS AND THERAPIES
Generalized anxiety disorder	Excessive worry about a number of everyday problems for at least 6 months, with anxiety that is more intense than the situation warrants	■ Anticipation of disaster and preoccupation with health issues, money, familial problems, or challenges at work ■ Difficulty relaxing, tendency to startle easily, trouble concentrating and falling asleep ■ Various somatic complaints, which may include fatigue, headache, muscle tension and aches, digestive issues, irritability, shortness of breath or dyspnea, and hot flashes	■ Psychotherapy, including cognitive-behavior therapy (CBT) ■ Pharmacologic treatments, which may include antidepressants (e.g., SSRIs), anxiolytic medications (e.g., benzodiazepines), beta-blockers, and antipsychotic medications ■ Relaxation techniques, such as massage and guided imagery ■ Mental health counseling
Phobias	An intense, persistent, irrational fear of something dreaded; may be an object, situation, or activity that elicits panic and automatic avoidance of or repelling urge to stay away	■ Fear and anxiety in response to exposure (or, in some cases, imagined exposure) to the phobia-related object, situation or activity	■ Pharmacologic treatments, which may include short-term use of benzodiazepines, or administration of SSRIs or tricyclic antidepressants ■ CBT ■ Desensitization and implosion therapy for specific phobias ■ Dietary changes, including alcohol and caffeine restrictions
Panic disorder	A sudden attack of terror that can produce a sense of unreality, impending doom, or a fear of losing control	■ Somatic manifestations may include pounding heart, rapid heart rate (tachycardia), rapid respirations (tachypnea), weakness, sweatiness, light-headedness, or dizziness	■ Reduced environmental stimuli or placement in a quiet, nonstimulating environmental setting ■ CBT ■ Pharmacologic treatments, which may include antidepressants (e.g., SSRIs or tricyclic antidepressants), anxiolytic medications (e.g., benzodiazepines), beta-blockers, and antipsychotic medications ■ Relaxation techniques, such as massage and guided imagery ■ Mental health counseling
Posttraumatic stress disorder (PTSD)	A trauma- and stressor-related disorder that can evolve after exposure to a traumatic or overwhelming event in which an individual's physical health was endangered (e.g., violent personal assaults, natural or human-caused disasters, accidents, military combat, dismemberment, incest and child abuse, traumatic childbirth, or invasive medical procedures)	■ May include flashbacks, nightmares, and recurrent, intrusive memories of the adverse event(s); hypervigilance or the appearance of "being on edge"; avoidance of stimuli associated with the traumatic event; dissociative symptoms may be present.	■ CBT ■ Exposure-based CBT (application of principles of CBT combined with reexposure to the stressful event, including through use of imagination, verbal discussion, or written exercises) (Benedek et al., 2009)

Alterations and Therapies Stress and Coping (continued)

ALTERATION	DESCRIPTION	MANIFESTATIONS	INTERVENTIONS AND THERAPIES
	characterized by exaggerated stress responses to the event Signs and symptoms endure for more than 1 month (APA, 2013). Onset of symptoms usually occurs within 3 months following exposure to the trauma; however, symptoms may present immediately following exposure to the traumatic event or may manifest months or years after the traumatic exposure (APA, 2013).	■ May include intense physiological reactions when exposed to cues that are similar to or representative of some part of the traumatic experience.	■ Eye movement desensitization and reprocessing (EMDR) ■ Exposure therapy, which may include simulated or "virtual" exposure to the associated stimuli (Mayo Clinic, 2011a) ■ Pharmacologic treatments, which may include antipsychotic agents, antidepressants (e.g., SSRIs), anxiolytic medications (e.g., benzodiazepines) ■ Relaxation techniques, such as massage and guided imagery ■ Mental health counseling
Acute stress disorder	Like PTSD, acute stress disorder is a trauma- and stressor-related disorder that can evolve after exposure to a traumatic or overwhelming event in which an individual's physical health was endangered (e.g., violent personal assaults, natural or human-caused disasters, accidents, military combat, dismemberment, incest and child abuse, traumatic childbirth, or invasive medical procedures) characterized by exaggerated stress responses to the event. Unlike PTSD, the individual with acute stress disorder experiences signs and symptoms that endure for 3 days to 1 month following exposure to traumatic event (APA, 2013). ■ May progress to PTSD if symptoms persist for longer than 1 month (APA, 2013). ■ Onset of symptoms usually occurs immediately following exposure to the traumatic event (APA, 2013).	■ May include flashbacks, nightmares, and recurrent, intrusive memories of the adverse event(s); hypervigilance or the appearance of "being on edge"; avoidance of stimuli associated with the traumatic event. ■ May include intense physiological reactions when exposed to cues that are similar to or representative of some part of the traumatic experience. ■ Manifestations may include some form of dissociation; for example, viewing oneself from the perspective of another individual or, being unable to recall certain events related to the traumatic event (APA, 2013).	■ CBT ■ Exposure-based CBT (application of principles of CBT combined with reexposure to the stressful event, including through use of imagination, verbal discussion, or written exercises) (Benedek et al., 2009) ■ EMDR ■ Pharmacologic treatments, which may include antipsychotic agents, beta-blockers, antidepressants (e.g., SSRIs), and anxiolytic medications (e.g., benzodiazepines) (Benedek et al., 2009) ■ Relaxation techniques, such as massage and guided imagery ■ Mental health counseling
Obsessive-compulsive disorder (OCD)	Characterized by obsessive thoughts and compulsive repetitive behaviors formed in response to the obsessive thoughts to lower the level of anxiety experienced	Signs and symptoms vary, depending on the theme of the specific obsessions and compulsions (see Exemplar 31.3). For example, OCD that features a theme of excessive cleanliness may include a fixation on the need to clean oneself and/or the environment (and fear of contamination), along with repetitive behaviors related to cleaning.	■ CBT ■ Antidepressants

ing the first 2 years of life. As a result of normal cognitive development, usually around the toddler stage, children become more adept at distinguishing between dangerous and nondangerous situations, and fears begin to abate. Along with this developing sense of discernment, toddlers also begin to learn how to cope with fear (Berk, 2012). In children, anxiety disorders are the result of anxiety and fear that persist beyond the expected age of resolution and endure for 6 months or longer (APA, 2013).

Prevalence

According to the Anxiety and Depression Association of America (ADAA) (n.d.a), anxiety disorders are the most common mental health disorders in the United States. Among adults over the age of 18 years, the prevalence of anxiety disorders is approximately 18%, which equates to affecting nearly 40 million individuals (ADAA, n.d.a). Generalized anxiety disorder (GAD) affects 6.8 million adults in the United States, and twice as many women as men. The disorder can develop at any time in the life cycle, though people are at the highest risk for the condition in early adulthood, between childhood and middle age (National Institute of Mental Health [NIMH], 2009). Additional U.S. prevalence rates for disorders that are discussed in this module's exemplars include the following (ADAA, n.d.a):

- Obsessive-compulsive disorder (OCD) affects approximately 2.2 million individuals or an estimated 1.0% of the population.

- Phobias affect an estimated 19 million individuals, which is approximately 8.7% of the population.

- Posttraumatic stress disorder (PTSD) affects approximately 7.7 million individuals or an estimated 3.5% of the population.

Genetic Considerations and Nonmodifiable Risk Factors

In the development of disorders related to anxiety, stress, and trauma, gender is a significant risk factor. Overall, anxiety disorders are more common or reported more in women, at least twice as frequently as in men. However, when considering specific disorders, gender-based variations do occur (ADAA, n.d.a). For example, men are twice as likely to develop a phobia, whereas OCD is equally common among men and women.

Brain chemistry and genetic factors influence the potential for developing anxiety disorders, as do certain life experiences. For example, although PTSD is more common among women, a history of childhood sexual abuse greatly increases the susceptibility to developing this disorder, regardless of gender. Victims of rape are also at high risk for developing PTSD; among rape victims, an estimated 65% of men and 45.9% of women develop this disorder (ADAA, n.d.a).

CASE STUDY \\ PART 1

Kevin DeLarno is a 23-year-old student who is completing his second year of graduate school in the study of anatomy and physiology. He presents to the university student health services center

with complaints of frequent headaches, including a current headache that he describes as "a throbbing in the front of my head." He rates his pain as 7 on a scale of 0 to 10, with 10 being the worst imaginable pain. During his client interview, he denies any past medical history or any additional complaints, including trauma, visual disturbances, dizziness, weakness, or neurological changes. According to Mr. DeLarno, his headaches are "interfering with my study schedule. I have exams every week and I can't concentrate on studying. If I don't get these headaches under control, I'm going to end up failing at least one class this semester." He reports that he drinks "about a pot of coffee a day" and occasionally smokes a cigar when he is socializing with his friends.

Upon arrival, Mr. DeLarno's vital signs include temperature 97.9°F oral; pulse 92 bpm; respirations 18/min; and BP 153/82 mmHg. Auscultation of his heart and lungs reveals no abnormal findings. Mr. DeLarno insists he is "fine, except for these stupid headaches. I'm sure it's just stress. I need something to help me get them under control so I can get my work done." During his assessment interview, the nurse asks if Mr. DeLarno has made any recent changes to his daily routine or health habits. He replies, "There aren't any recent changes, but soon, there will be. I'm getting married in three months and my fiancé and I will be moving off campus. We're in the process of buying a house." Mr. DeLarno further states that he is "excited about getting married," but feels the wedding planning has gotten out of hand, as he and his fiancé have already exceeded their wedding budget. When asked what activities he engages in for enjoyment and recreation, he replies, "I don't have time for anything except classes and studying. I used to work out and play racquetball three times a week, but I don't have the time for that right now."

Clinical Reasoning Questions Level I

1. Based on Mr. DeLarno's statements, what are his current potential sources of stress?

2. In addition to his complaints of recurrent headaches, which assessment data might reflect manifestations of the stress response?

3. Describe the effects of coffee and nicotine intake, including how these effects are similar to those evoked by the stress response.

Clinical Reasoning Questions Level II

4. Do positive stressors and negative stressors differ in terms of physiological effects? Explain your answer.

5. Presuming Mr. DeLarno's headaches are stress related, what nursing diagnoses would be appropriate for inclusion in his nursing plan of care?

6. What nursing interventions could be implemented to promote stress reduction for Mr. DeLarno?

▶ PREVENTION

Factors that influence the development of anxiety disorders include personality-related characteristics; for example, shy children are at an increased risk (University of and Medical Center [UMM], 2009). Traumatic events, including a history of spousal or childhood abuse and being bullied, also increase the risk of impairment. Social factors, especially limited or absent socialization and living in a threatening environment, increase an individual's susceptibility to developing an anxiety disorder. Even hypersensitivity of the amygdala—which is the brain's "worry center"—is believed to be a potential factor that may increase the likelihood for development of an anxiety-related disorder (UMM, 2009).

Family wellness promotion is essential to enhancing physiological and psychosocial outcomes for clients of all ages. The link between the development of mental illness and childhood abuse and neglect serves to emphasize this point. Research suggests childhood abuse is associated with an increased risk for physical and psychological disorders, including depression and anxiety. These increased risks remain in effect decades after the abuse occurs (Springer et al., 2007). Even when overt abuse and neglect are not factors, family dynamics and parenting styles can pose serious threats to a child's psychosocial well-being. For example, even when adequate child care is provided, frequent changes in caregivers may predispose a child to the development of separation anxiety disorder or reactive attachment disorder (APA, 2013; Mayo Clinic, 2011b). (See the modules on Family and Violence for further discussion.)

Many of the causative factors associated with development of a disorder of anxiety, stress, or trauma are outside the realm of the individual's control and therefore are not modifiable. As a result, prevention of exacerbation of these disorders and control of their manifestations is most often the focus. Although not always possible, complete healing is the ultimate goal; however, from a nursing standpoint, optimization of wellness is both realistic and achievable.

Screenings

Screening tests are available for use in the identification of many disorders of anxiety, stress, and trauma, including generalized anxiety disorder, obsessive-compulsive disorder, posttraumatic stress disorder, and specific phobias.

Stay Current: *To view a sample of these screening tools, visit the Anxiety and Depression Association of America's online library at* **www.adaa.org/living-with-anxiety/ask-and-learn/screenings**.

▶ ASSESSMENT

Appraisal is to the transactional model of stress and coping what assessment is to the nursing process. Just as the nurse assesses and prioritizes client health concerns, individuals evaluate (appraise) and prioritize stressors. During the assessment, the nurse will help clients identify stressors that trigger unhealthy coping responses as well as the potential effects of those responses.

Many clients with anxiety or trauma responses will present complaining of physical symptoms. In the case study example, Mr. DeLarno's presenting complaint is a headache, which he then attributes to "just stress." Some clients, however, will be unable to articulate anxiety or trauma, either due to lack of awareness or understanding of the source of their symptoms, or due to a reluctance to disclose what they consider to be very personal information. Through developing the therapeutic nurse–client relationship, the nurse may be able to encourage reluctant clients to disclose necessary information or come to an awareness that stress and anxiety are impacting the client's physical health.

Nursing Assessment

During the nursing assessment, the nurse acknowledges and affirms the client's concerns. **Box 31–2** ● describes application of the nursing transactional model with regard to specific communication strategies that may be appropriate for use during assessment of the client with anxiety.

Box 31–2 Application of the Nursing Transactional Model to Assessment of the Client With Anxiety

In the nursing transactional model, the nurse is part of the anxious client's environment and can influence changes in the client with both verbal and nonverbal cues. From the very first interaction with the client, the nurse's demeanor conveys a great deal of information to the client about how the client can expect to be treated. Initial nursing actions that inspire client confidence and that may help calm anxious clients include the following:

- Make eye contact, focusing on the person.
- Take a nonthreatening stance.
- Validate the client's feelings: "I know you are very uncomfortable; we will do everything we can to help you feel better."
- Determine and address the client's immediate concerns: "What can I do right away to help you?"
- Remember to address the client by name. Some clients find terms of endearment such as "Honey" or "Sweetie" impersonal or demeaning. Using the client's first name may be seen as patronizing if the client is expected to use the nurse's last name. On the other hand, some clients respond positively to the informality of first name use. Ask clients how they would prefer to be addressed and never use the first name of anyone over age 18 without permission.

Mrs. Arlene Betts is a 35-year-old woman who has come to her primary care physician's office with a number of complaints. The receptionist informs the nurse that Mrs. Betts is obviously anxious and is rambling a lot. As the nurse walks into the examination room, Mrs. Betts immediately begins talking about a number of issues. Wide-eyed, she complains of tingling in her arms, lack of sleep, and feeling like her heart is racing. She bombards the nurse with so many issues that he becomes confused. Sitting down, the nurse asks Mrs. Betts, "Tell me, which of those issues are you most concerned about?" Sitting down conveys that the nurse has time for Mrs. Betts. Asking her to prioritize her concerns helps the nurse prioritize them as well.

Mrs. Betts replies, "I am having a heart attack and no one believes me." The nurse responds, "We know you're uncomfortable right now, and you must be worried. We're definitely going to check out your cardiac status. It will take a little time. What can I do to make you feel more comfortable right now?" By providing assurance and information, the nurse both empowers Mrs. Betts and assists her in making a secondary appraisal, deciding which concern is the next most important. This secondary appraisal is an important tool in helping Mrs. Betts learn the steps needed to lower her anxiety level. It also helps the nurse learn more about Mrs. Betts within a very short period of time.

Box 31–3 Stress Assessment Checklist

BEHAVIORAL

Always doing too much
Argumentativeness
Grinds teeth during sleep
Increase in compulsive behaviors (eating, drinking, nail biting, sexual activity, smoking)
Looks at watch or clock often
Loud voice
Pacing
Talks too fast
Vigilance
Withdrawal
Work on multiple projects simultaneously

COGNITIVE

Ambivalence
Difficulty concentrating or listening
Fear of the unknown
Forgetfulness
Lack of creativity
Lack of initiative
Lack of a sense of humor
Memory lapses/loss
Short attention span
Trouble thinking
Wanting to run away
Worrying

EMOTIONAL

Agitation/anger
Anxiety and feeling pressured
Crying

Defensiveness
Easily annoyed
Fear
Feeling overwhelmed
Feeling powerless
Hostility
Irritability
Isolation
Jumpiness and nervousness
Sadness
Suspiciousness

PHYSICAL

Constipation
Diaphoresis
Diarrhea
Difficulty falling asleep
Dry mouth
Fatigue
Gastrointestinal upsets or butterflies
Headaches
Increase in blood sugar levels
Increase in respiration rate
Insomnia
Muscular stiffness and tension
Pallor
Racing or pounding heart
Restlessness
Shakiness
Sweaty palms
Urinary frequency

The client interview should include collection of data related to the client's current and past illnesses, specific physical complaints, general health history, client-perceived stressors or stressful incidents, manifestations of stress, and past and present coping strategies. In addition to an assessment interview, the nurse may use a simple checklist while talking with and observing the client to note indications of stress. Box 31–3 provides a checklist for use in identifying symptoms of stress. As mentioned earlier, stress and stressors are a part of everyday life. The first step in mediating the effect of the stressor is conscious awareness of the manifestations of stress. Review the symptom checklist to increase your awareness of and assess your own stress reactions and behaviors.

The checklist in **Box 31–3** ● is not meant to be all encompassing; it is, however, intended to provide points of reference to improve your conscious awareness of your own stress reactions and those of individuals with whom you interact. The experience of stress is an individual process; therefore, experiences that you have had or those of other individuals you know may not be listed in Box 31–3.

Physical assessment should include observation of the client for verbal, motor, cognitive, or other physical manifestations of stress. Remember, however, that stress-related manifestations may not be apparent when cognitive coping is effective.

Lifespan and Cultural Considerations

Psychosocial assessment of the pediatric client should be age and developmentally specific (see the module on Development) and should take into consideration that children may exhibit manifestations of disorders in ways that vary significantly from those demonstrated by adult clients. For example, in children with PTSD who are under 6 years of age, reexperiencing the trauma may take the form of playing in such a way as to overtly or indirectly recreate the traumatic event (APA, 2013). Very young children with PTSD may demonstrate reexperiencing the traumatic event by drawing pictures that symbolize the event (APA, 2013).

For older adults, recognizing alterations due to disorders related to anxiety, stress, or trauma can be complicated by preexisting physical illness or cognitive changes. Fear of stigmatization is also a significant consideration. Because many older adults were raised during a time when mental illness carried a heavy stigma, they may be especially resistant to reporting any symptoms of mental disorders (ADAA, n.d.b).

When working with clients from different cultures, nurses must take care not to inadvertently attribute a normal, healthy cultural response as inappropriate or maladaptive. Cultural expressions of distress vary. A thorough assessment of stressors, the individual client's responses, and the client's efforts to seek help or reduce distress will help distinguish each client's individual stress responses. The Cultural Formulation Interview (CFI) outlined in the DSM-5 may be used to assist healthcare providers in interviewing clients as part of a comprehensive mental health assessment. The CFI is a series of 16 questions designed to assess clients in four areas (APA, 2013):

- Cultural definition of the problem
- Cultural perceptions of cause and support
- Cultural factors affecting coping and past help-seeking behaviors
- Cultural factors affecting current help-seeking behaviors.

Diagnostic Tests

For identification of disorders of anxiety, stress, or trauma, diagnostic criteria are collected primarily through client interviews and reports of subjective symptoms. Medical testing is conducted to rule out other causes of particular manifestations; for example, a rapid heart rate or heart palpitations indicate either the presence of cardiovascular dysfunction or anxiety. To that effect, numerous medical conditions may produce signs and symptoms that are similar to those associated with anxiety; for example, hyperthyroidism and hypoglycemia may cause tachycardia and nervousness. Likewise, certain medical conditions may produce genuine anxiety, including disorders that cause dyspnea (e.g., asthma) or pain. Likewise, clients with disorders related to stress and coping may present with somatic (physical) complaints and may not initially articulate any anxiety or trauma. Although clients may present to primary care providers with complaints that appear to be related to exposure to stress or due to impaired coping mechanisms, diagnosis of associated psychiatric disorders requires evaluation by a trained mental health professional, such as a psychiatrist or advanced practice psychiatric nurse.

CASE STUDY \\ PART 2

Mr. DeLarno is awaiting evaluation by the university healthcare clinic's nurse practitioner. He agrees to dimming of his room lights while he waits. After resting quietly for 10 minutes, he falls asleep. When the nurse awakens Mr. DeLarno to reassess him, he states, "I'm surprised I fell asleep. Usually, I can't fall asleep no matter how hard I try to relax. I'm only sleeping a few hours each night." He reports his headache "feels quite a bit better, but I know it's going to come back with a vengeance as soon as I start studying again." He rates his pain as 3 on a scale of 0 to 10, with 10 being the worst imaginable pain. His blood pressure has decreased to 128/72 mmHg and his pulse is now 78 bpm.

Upon arriving to assess Mr. DeLarno, the nurse practitioner introduces herself and asks the client to describe his current complaints, as well as any similar problems he has experienced in the past. Mr. DeLarno states, "My headache is better, but I need something to help me control it when I'm studying. I think alprazolam would help—I have a friend who takes that when he gets stressed." The nurse practitioner responds by noting that she would like to further assess Mr. DeLarno, as well as ask him a few questions

before making any treatment recommendations. Mr. DeLarno replies, "The nurse I saw earlier already listened to my heart and lungs, and she already asked me a bunch of questions. Headaches are my only problem—I don't need any additional workup. I can't stay here all day. Are you able to help me or not?"

Clinical Reasoning Questions Level I

1. Explain the most likely reasons for Mr. DeLarno's decreased headache and decrease in blood pressure and heart rate.
2. What is the significance of Mr. DeLarno's reported sleep habits?

Clinical Reasoning Questions Level II

3. In the event that Mr. DeLarno's complaints are related to anxiety, is a prescription for alprazolam a preferable first approach to treatment? Why or why not?
4. How should the nurse practitioner respond to Mr. DeLarno's seeming frustration with the need for additional assessment?

▶ INTERVENTIONS AND THERAPIES

Nursing care of clients with alterations in stress and coping includes independent interventions such as the use of therapeutic communication and offering education regarding nonpharmacologic relaxation techniques. Collaborative interventions for these clients include administration of prescribed pharmacologic therapies and facilitation of counseling, psychotherapy, and other therapies as ordered.

Independent

Independent nursing interventions include encouraging the client to maintain or achieve optimal health, as well as assisting the client with identifying strategies that will help him meet his goals. Because physical and psychosocial wellness are intricately connected, many wellness-related nursing interventions focus on physical health. However, certain primary aspects of wellness promotion are more administrative in nature, such as time management. For an overview of examples of nursing interventions that pertain to wellness promotion for the client with alterations related to stress and coping, see **Table 31–7** ●.

Additional independent nursing interventions include utilizing therapeutic communication and implementing cognitive-behavioral interventions, such as teaching relaxation techniques, as well as encouraging client and family participation in support groups. Validating the client's feelings is essential to building self-esteem and fostering healthy coping. Reinforcing positive coping efforts, offering hope and reassurance to the individual about her ability to cope, and helping her to identify successes in life provide a sense of personal power and hope. Spiritual distress occurs when an individual loses hope of ever resolving or coping more adaptively. The chronic nature of anxiety disorders can be devastating and can erode an individual's sense of power and self-worth.

In the care of clients diagnosed with mental illness, one of the nurse's most crucial roles concerns client advocacy. Covert discrimination against individuals with mental illness still exists today in society and the healthcare system. According to the National Coalition for the Homeless, in 2009, an estimated

TABLE 31–7 Wellness Promotion for Clients With Stress-Related Disorders

NURSING INTERVENTION	RATIONALE
Physical Exercise	
■ Promote regular physical exercise. ■ Educate the client about the benefits of physical exercise.	■ Regular physical exercise offers physiological benefits, including improved cardiac and pulmonary function, enhanced muscle tone and joint mobility, and weight control. ■ Psychological benefits include tension relief, stress reduction, enhanced sense of well-being, and promotion of relaxation following activity.
Sleep/Rest Patterns	
■ Promote balance between sleep/rest and activity. ■ Teach relaxation techniques to promote relaxation and sleep.	■ Adequate sleep and rest are essential to survival. ■ Sleep allows for physical healing, restoration, and removal of free radicals, which are believed to be associated with illness and disease. ■ Adequate sleep enhances cognitive function.
Nutrition	
■ Provide education related to balanced nutrition. ■ Facilitate referrals to dietary professionals and nutritionists.	■ Inadequate nutrition reduces physical resistance to illness and increases susceptibility to disease and illness. ■ Excessive intake of caffeine and use of nicotine may interfere with sleep/rest patterns.
Time Management	
■ Promote balance between fulfilling personal responsibilities (e.g., related to work, family, school) and time for rest, socialization, and extracurricular activities. ■ Assist with identifying potential schedule modifications to allow for more effective time management. ■ Encourage implementation of personal boundaries.	■ Effective time management is associated with an increased sense of control and decreased sense of stress. ■ Identification of the client's roles and demands allows for identification of potential stressors. ■ Boundaries aid in determining the appropriateness of requests/demands made by others and allow the individual to identify which requests/demands can be fulfilled while still maintaining her or his wellness.

20%–25% of homeless individuals suffered from mental illness. Even when provided with housing, these individuals were unlikely to remain off the streets unless they received access to continued healthcare treatment and services.

Stay Current: To learn more about advocating for individuals with mental illnesses, visit NAMI's Web site, **www.nami.org**. NAMI is the nation's largest organization for individuals suffering from mental illness and their families. NAMI has affiliates in every state and in more than 1,100 local communities across the country.

Every individual and nurse who cares enough about the plight of individuals living with mental illnesses has the ability to impact public policy. Organizations such as NAMI provide a platform for individuals to work collaboratively. Turning our conscience to the side as we pass homeless individuals with mental illness on the street does not make them disappear.

The Internet offers a wealth of information on issues that affect individuals living with mental illnesses in our global society. Ethical nursing practice involves developing expertise in accessing relevant current data and resources for the individual, hospital, and community.

SAFETY ALERT
Legal requirements to maintain client confidentiality do not apply in the event of a client's threat to harm himself or others. Immediately report any threats to injure self or others to the client's primary care provider.

Collaborative

A number of collaborative interventions may be appropriate for the client who is having difficulty coping with stressors. In addition to being well informed about various interventions and treatment options, such as psychotherapy, nurses should be able to recognize and manage their own responses to stress.

PSYCHOTHERAPY Psychotherapy is a preferred method of treating anxiety and other psychiatric disorders. Psychotherapy involves talking with a mental health professional, such as a psychiatrist, mental health nurse, advanced practice psychiatric nurse, psychologist, social worker, or counselor, to explore the nature and symptom management of the disorder (NIMH, 2009). The severity of symptoms may warrant hospitalization in a safe therapeutic *milieu*, or social setting, for the individual. Such an intervention provides needed protection from environmental stressors and the additional support of group therapy. The impact of overwhelming and disabling anxiety can create vulnerability to depression, suicidal thoughts, or self-harm.

COGNITIVE-BEHAVIORAL THERAPY (CBT) **Cognitive-behavioral therapy (CBT)** combines cognitive techniques and behavior modification to change detrimental beliefs and thought patterns. The goals of CBT include enhancing problem-solving and coping skills. Usually, the therapist guides the client in identifying detrimental or distorted thought patterns, and assists her with restructuring these thoughts and beliefs. Through analysis and reinterpretation of past and current experiences, the client is able to learn and apply new skills that promote healthy behaviors and positive interpersonal interactions. In caring for a client with an anxiety disorder, CBT provides a supportive environment in which the client can safely confront her fears (APA, 2013; NIMH, 2013b).

Box 31–4   Additional Cognitive-Behavioral Therapeutic Techniques

The following techniques are also commonly used as a part of CBT:

- *A comprehensive assessment interview* is the first step in developing a contract with the goal of behavioral change. The purpose of the interview is to develop a complete picture of the client's stress responses (e.g., negative thought patterns, feelings of worry or fear, or maladaptive behaviors such as repeated hand washing), so that strategies for changing these responses may be targeted. The interview process identifies problematic behavior and divides it into four areas:
  - The behavioral area, which asks what the client is doing
  - The cognitive component, which asks what the client is thinking
  - The affective component, which asks what the client is feeling
  - The physiological component, which probes the physical reality of the situation.
- *Thought stopping* is a technique that is used to help the client change her thinking processes. Many individuals who suffer with anxiety have difficulty with repetitive, maladaptive thinking, and thought stopping is used to halt destructive thoughts before they get out of control. In this technique, the client learns to stop destructive thoughts by visualizing a specific image, sensation, or circumstance. The thought-stopping agent can be the image of a traffic stop sign, the sound of the word *stop*, the tactile sensation of leaning against a closed door, or the visualization of pushing one's negative thoughts out the back door. Successful thought stopping should be implemented whenever maladaptive thoughts occur, so that over time, the client learns to stop such thoughts reflexively.
- *A behavioral contract* outlines the behavioral changes that the client and the mental health professional agree should take place. When negotiating a behavioral contract, a mental health provider engages the client and family as colleagues, avoids jargon, and ensures the client and family are comfortable with the contract. Possible problems with behavioral contracts include a lack of understanding, a lack of commitment, a lack of adequate follow-up, and the lack of a defined plan of care. Continuing assessment, regular evaluation, and trouble-shooting meetings can determine whether adjustments to the contract are necessary. Contracts can be adjusted in many ways, from changes in the prioritization of objectives to the appropriate revision of goals.

Source: Based on Kneisl, C. R., & Trigoboff, E. (2013). *Contemporary psychiatric–mental health nursing* (3rd ed.). Upper Saddle River, NJ: Pearson Education.

Exposure-based CBT combines the techniques used in CBT with exposure of the client to a controlled version of the situation that triggers the anxiety. By inducing mild anxiety under the supervision of a mental health expert, exposure-based CBT can help an individual with panic disorder learn that his panic attacks are not heart attacks, for example (NIMH, 2009). Additional cognitive-behavioral techniques are listed in **Box 31–4** •.

PHARMACOLOGIC THERAPY   The therapeutic goal of psychopharmacology is to manage symptoms and alleviate distress. Generally speaking, pharmacologic therapies are most successful when used in combination with psychotherapy. Many clients require medication for only short periods of time. Some treatment-resistant clients, however, may require longer courses of medication. With proper treatment, many people with anxiety disorders can lead normal, fulfilling lives (NIMH, 2009).

Medications used in the treatment of anxiety disorders include benzodiazepines. These medications may be used for short-term treatment during an acute phase of an anxiety disorder. Clients experiencing anxiety secondary to short-term medical therapies, such as mechanical ventilation, also may find benzodiazepines helpful. They may be effective in quickly lowering the severity of a client's anxiety, but they are generally not recommended for use beyond a few weeks because of their addictive properties. Additionally, some research suggests long-term use of benzodiazepines may cause permanent cognitive dysfunction, including in the areas of information processing and verbal learning (Stewart, 2005). Despite current guidelines that recommend the use of benzodiazepines primarily during the acute phase of treatment for anxiety, in reality, these medications sometimes are prescribed for long-term use (Cloos, 2010). Clients should consult with their prescribing provider about the potential side effects of long-term benzodiazepine use.

For long-term management of certain anxiety disorders, prescribers may consider an antidepressant. Selective serotonin reuptake inhibitors (SSRIs) are helpful in the treatment of phobias, symptoms of OCD, and panic symptoms. Fluoxetine (Prozac), paroxetine (Paxil), and sertraline (Zoloft) are examples of SSRIs that may be used in the treatment of clients with disorders of anxiety, stress, and trauma. Tricyclic antidepressants, such as imipramine (Tofranil) or amitriptyline (Elavil), may be used. These are contraindicated in clients with a history of heart dysfunction or heart attack (Adams, Holland, & Urban, 2014).

Monoamine oxidase inhibitors (MAOIs) such as phenelzine (Nardil), atypical antidepressants such as serotonin–norepinephrine reuptake inhibitors (SNRIs), and antipsychotic agents may be prescribed for the treatment of these disorders. Beta-blockers may be used to block the effects of sympathetic nervous system stimulation and reduce manifestations of anxiety. See the Medications feature.

Herbal supplements, including valerian, kava, and passion flower, are used by some individuals in the treatment of anxiety. However, these medications have not been conclusively proven to be effective and may cause various side effects (Mayo Clinic, 2012a). The nurse should caution the client to consult with his primary healthcare provider before adding herbal supplements to his medication regimen.

SAFETY ALERT

The antihistamine diphenhydramine (Benadryl) is not suitable for use in the long-term treatment of anxiety-related disorders. Although diphenhydramine does produce sedation, research suggests that this drug's sedative effects are not effective for achieving anxiolysis (reduction of anxiety) (Baas et al., 2009). Moreover, cessation of diphenhydramine after long-term use can cause withdrawal symptoms. Clients with anxiety-related signs and symptoms should seek professional evaluation and guidance.

Medications **Disorders of Anxiety, Stress, or Trauma**

CLASSIFICATION AND DRUG EXAMPLES	MECHANISMS OF ACTION	NURSING CONSIDERATIONS
Antidepressants *Drug examples:* - SSRIs, such as fluoxetine (Prozac), paroxetine (Paxil), and sertraline (Zoloft) - tricyclic antidepressants, such as imipramine (Tofranil)	SSRIs inhibit reuptake of the neurotransmitter serotonin in the brain, resulting in circulation of increased levels of serotonin. Although primarily used for treatment of depression, certain SSRIs are also effective in the treatment of clients with anxiety, OCD, and panic disorder. Tricyclic antidepressants block presynaptic neuronal reuptake of serotonin and norepinephrine, resulting in increased circulating levels of these neurotransmitters. Tricyclic antidepressants may be used in the treatment of clients with panic disorders.	- Monitor for development of suicidal ideation or worsening of symptoms - Assess for adverse effects, including dizziness or drowsiness. - Counsel clients to avoid alcohol in combination with SSRIs or tricyclic antidepressants. - Periodically obtain complete blood count (CBC) with differential, serum electrolyte panel, and liver and kidney function studies.
Antipsychotics *Drug examples:* - risperidone (Risperdal) - olanzapine (Zyprexa)	Interfere with action of serotonin and dopamine in the brain; as a result, for some clients, they promote reduction of compulsive behaviors and decreased agitation. In conjunction with other therapies, may be used in the treatment of clients with OCD or panic disorders.	- Monitor for neuroleptic malignant syndrome and tardive dyskinesia, and immediately report signs and symptoms of these conditions. - Assess for side effects including drowsiness, excess sedation, somnolence, or increased agitation. - Monitor CBC, kidney and liver function studies, serum electrolytes, and serum glucose level.
Anxiolytics *Drug example:* - buspirone (BuSpar)	Act as a dopamine agonist in the brain and also inhibit serotonin reuptake (leading to increased circulating serotonin), producing antianxiety effect. Used to treat GAD.	- Assess for side effects including nausea, headaches, and dizziness. - Monitor for dystonia, motor restlessness, and involuntary repetitive muscle movements (primarily facial or in the cervical neck region). - Advise client this medication requires daily administration for at least 2 weeks to produce antianxiety effect.
Benzodiazepines *Drug examples:* - alprazolam (Xanax) - clonazepam (Klonopin) - diazepam (Valium) - lorazepam (Ativan) - temazepam (Restoril)	Potentiate the effect of the naturally occurring inhibitory neurotransmitter gamma-aminobutyric acid (GABA), leading to promotion of relaxation and a decrease in the subjective experience of anxiety.	- Not recommended for long-term use due to habit-forming properties. - Monitor client for excess sedation and dizziness. - Use cautiously in clients with impaired hepatic function and monitor liver function studies for these clients. - Counsel client to avoid alcohol in combination medications in this classification.
Beta-Blockers *Drug example:* - propranolol (Inderal)	Selectively block cardiac and bronchial beta receptors, compete with epinephrine and norepinephrine, and reduce effects of sympathetic nervous system stimulation, such as increased heart rate, increased cardiac contractility, and increased blood pressure. Unlabeled uses include management of anxiety states and prevention of acute panic states (such as those related to public speaking).	- Assess blood pressure and heart rate prior to administration. Withhold medication if systolic blood pressure <90 mmHg or apical pulse rate <60 bpm, or if blood pressure and apical pulse rate do not meet parameters defined by the prescribing provider. - Monitor for adverse effects, including bradycardia, confusion, fatigue, and drowsiness.

◢ REVIEW **The Concept of Stress and Coping**

RELATE Link the Concepts

Linking the concept of stress and coping with the concept of communication:

1. Describe the application of therapeutic communication in the nursing care of clients with disorders related to stress and coping.
2. Particularly during the care of clients with disorders related to stress and coping, why is giving advice contraindicated?

What specific communication strategies are recommended for these clients?

Linking the concept of stress and coping with the concept of ethics:

3. What is client confidentiality and how does this principle pertain to clients who seek treatment for alterations related to stress and coping? Under what circumstances is the requirement to maintain client confidentiality not applicable?

4. While in the hospital cafeteria, a nurse overhears a nursing colleague discussing a client's recent hospital admission for treatment related to an unusual phobia. Although the nursing colleague does not specify the client's name, she includes a detailed discussion of the client's complaints. How should this situation be addressed?

READY Go to Companion Skills Manual

REFER Go to Pearson Student Nursing Resources
nursing.pearsonhighered.com

- Additional review materials

REFLECT Case Study \\ Part 3

Following Mr. DeLarno's assertion that he cannot "stay here all day" and his prompting for rapid treatment, the nurse practitioner replies, "I can imagine that your headaches are interfering with every aspect of your life, Mr. DeLarno. In particular, it must be miserable to try to study while you have a pounding headache, much less to take an exam. I want to help you find the best solution, which means I'll need some more information from you." She further explains to Mr. DeLarno that additional assessment is needed to accurately identify the cause of his headaches, as well as to choose the appropriate treatment approach. Initially, Mr. DeLarno is disappointed about not receiving a prescription for alprazolam, which he again suggests will fully resolve his headaches. However, after talking with the nurse practitioner, he agrees with the plan for further assessment.

The nurse practitioner performs a focused neurological assessment, including assessing Mr. DeLarno's pupillary response to light and his extremity strength. She also interviews him as to the presence of any alterations in sensory perception, including numbness, tingling, or other unusual sensations. With the exception of his headache and sleep disturbances, which Mr. DeLarno reports began about 8 months earlier, his assessment findings reveal no abnormalities.

Based on assessment findings, the nurse practitioner suspects Mr. DeLarno may have developed generalized anxiety disorder (GAD). For further evaluation and treatment, she refers him to the student wellness center, the staff of which includes a psychiatrist and other mental health specialists. She further instructs Mr. DeLarno to avoid caffeine and nicotine, and to contact the clinic if his headaches worsen, or if he experiences any alterations in sensory perception. Additionally, she offers to refer Mr. DeLarno to a local massage therapist who offers one free massage to students referred by the university student health services center. The client agrees to follow up with the student wellness center and pleasantly accepts the referral for massage, stating, "I'm calling the massage therapist as soon as I walk out of here."

Clinical Reasoning Questions Level I

1. Which of the nurse practitioner's statements represent validation of the client's complaints? Explain how validation can serve to diffuse a tense verbal interaction with a client.

2. How could the staff nurse support and facilitate the interventions prescribed by the nurse practitioner?

Clinical Reasoning Questions Level II

3. Identify three nursing diagnoses that are appropriate for inclusion in Mr. DeLarno's nursing plan of care.

4. What additional recommendations could be offered by the staff nurse to promote healthy sleep/rest patterns for this client?

EXEMPLAR 31.1 **Anxiety Disorders**

EXEMPLAR KEY TERMS

Anxiety, *1917*
Free-floating anxiety, *1918*
Generalized anxiety disorder (GAD), *1920*
Panic disorder, *1921*
Vulnerability, *1918*

EXEMPLAR LEARNING OUTCOMES

After reading about this exemplar, you will be able to:

1. Describe the pathophysiology, etiology, clinical manifestations, and direct and indirect causes of anxiety disorders.

2. Identify risk factors and prevention methods associated with anxiety disorders.

3. Illustrate the nursing process in providing culturally competent care across the life span for individuals with anxiety disorders.

4. Formulate priority nursing diagnoses appropriate for an individual with an anxiety disorder.

5. Summarize therapies used by interdisciplinary teams in the collaborative care of an individual with an anxiety disorder.

6. Plan evidence-based care for an individual with an anxiety disorder and his or her family in collaboration with other members of the healthcare team.

7. Evaluate expected outcomes for an individual with an anxiety disorder.

▶ OVERVIEW

Anxiety is a stress response characterized by feelings of mental uneasiness, apprehension, dread, foreboding, and a feeling of helplessness related to an impending or actual threat to oneself or significant relationships. Generally anxiety helps an individual cope; it is a reaction to a stressor and is part of daily living. Anxious energy is a productive force for most people, and the experience of anxiety is influenced by an individual's genetic makeup as well as emotional, developmental, physical, cognitive, sociocultural, and spiritual factors.

Anxiety disorders may occur when normal feelings of anxiety get out of control and begin to impair individual functioning.

Anxiety disorders are mental illnesses that cause people to feel extremely uneasy, distressed, or frightened during everyday situations. Left untreated, anxiety disorders can damage personal relationships and the ability to work. Anxiety disorders impair daily activity and can lead to low self-esteem, drug abuse, and social isolation. Anxiety disorders are the most common mental illnesses in the United States, typically afflicting around 20% of the population. Effective treatments exist for anxiety disorders, but many people do not seek treatment because they do not realize how severe their symptoms are, or because family, friends, and even physicians have difficulty recognizing the symptoms (NAMI, 2012).

The ability to differentiate healthy and expected stress responses from those that are harmful is an essential psychosocial competency for all nurses. Every individual experiences anxiety at times. The individual's anxiety is no longer healthy when the anxiety level reaches the point at which it prevents the individual from returning to homeostasis through healthy coping and adaptation.

▶ PATHOPHYSIOLOGY AND ETIOLOGY

Research suggests that people are more likely to suffer from anxiety disorders if their parents have anxiety disorders. However, it is not clear whether biological or environmental factors play a greater role in the development of these conditions. Research suggests traumatic brain injury may increase an individual's susceptibility for development of an anxiety disorder. In any case, scientists have found that certain areas of the brain, including the amygdala, function differently in people with anxiety disorders (NAMI, 2012).

The appearance of an anxiety disorder in an individual of any age requires attention by both healthcare professionals and caregivers. Family and friends may be the first to notice anxiety symptoms. Healthcare professionals recognize that many medical problems—including hormonal and neurological conditions—might cause symptoms of anxiety. The primary symptom of anxiety disorders is what psychiatrists sometimes refer to as **free-floating anxiety**. This is characterized by excessive worry about everyday events, worry that is hard to control and the focus of which may shift from moment to moment. Free-floating anxiety is anxiety that is not connected to a specific stimulus (Kneisl & Trigoboff, 2013). Examples of anxiety disorders are listed in the concept section earlier in this module; this exemplar discusses three of them: generalized anxiety disorder, separation anxiety, and panic disorder.

Etiology

Across the range of anxiety disorders, there are some important similarities in the basic causes of the anxious response. Biological causes seem to play a significant role in the development of anxiety disorders. Abnormal function of structures in the limbic system and certain parts of the cortex seem to be involved. The neurotransmitters most closely involved with the anxiety response are gamma aminobutyric acid (GABA), norepinephrine, and serotonin. Genetic contributions to each of the common disorders play a role as well, with at least part of the genetic vulnerability being nonspecific, or common across the disorders. Psychosocial and behavioral causal factors include the classical conditioning of fear and a perception of lack of control over one's environment, an attitude that begins in childhood (Butcher, Mineka, & Hooley, 2013).

Vulnerability refers to the individual's susceptibility to react to a specific stressor. Individual vulnerability stems from biological and environmental sources, both of which have

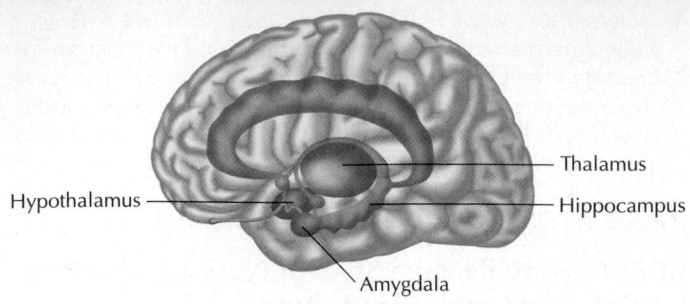

Figure 31–4 ● The limbic system. Just above the inner core, yet surrounded by the cerebral cortex, the limbic system plays a role in motivation, emotion, and memory. The system is composed of many structures, including the thalamus, amygdala, hippocampus, and hypothalamus.

been the subjects of etiological research. Current explanations of the origin of anxiety disorders include neurobiological, neurochemical, psychosocial, behavioral, genetic, and humanistic theories.

NEUROBIOLOGICAL THEORIES   Several areas of the brain orchestrate the experience of anxiety and the expression of the symptoms (**Figure 31–4 ●**). The amygdala is known as the "emotional brain" and is the focus of much research related to feelings of anxiety, fear, and anger, which are elicited in this area. The hippocampus stores memory related to fear. The locus coeruleus stimulates arousal, and contains almost half of all the neurons that use norepinephrine as a neurotransmitter. Stimulating an animal's locus coeruleus produces anxious behaviors. Heart rate and respirations are regulated by the brainstem, and the hypothalamus activates the entire response. The frontal cortex assists with appraisal of a threat and is the center of cognitive processes. The thalamus integrates all sensory stimuli, and the basal ganglia are responsible for the tremors associated with anxiety (Dubuc, 2013). Individual differences in the structure of the brain or injury to the brain will also alter the anxiety response.

NEUROCHEMICAL THEORIES   Communication within the brain occurs between neurons through the transmission of electrical stimuli (**Figures 31–5 ●** and **31–6 ●**). To transmit a signal, a neuron releases chemicals called neurotransmitters. These chemicals deliver messages by binding to the receptors on the surface of another neuron, causing the neuron to fire and transmit the electrical impulse. Once the message is delivered, the neurotransmitter is taken back to a vesicle in the presynaptic cell (NIMH, 2013a). Any disruption in these transporters, binding sites, or cell structure can cause an alteration in cell functioning, leading to misfiring.

Structural anatomical differences, dysregulation of neurotransmitters, sensitivity of neuronal receptor sites, and the balance of neurotransmitters in the synaptic cleft all have an effect on the anxiety reaction. The brain's benzodiazepine (BZD) receptor system enhances the activity of GABA, an inhibitory neurotransmitter that "shuts down" or slows excitability in the cell. It is present in the locus coeruleus, where norepinephrine is produced. Norepinephrine is an excitatory

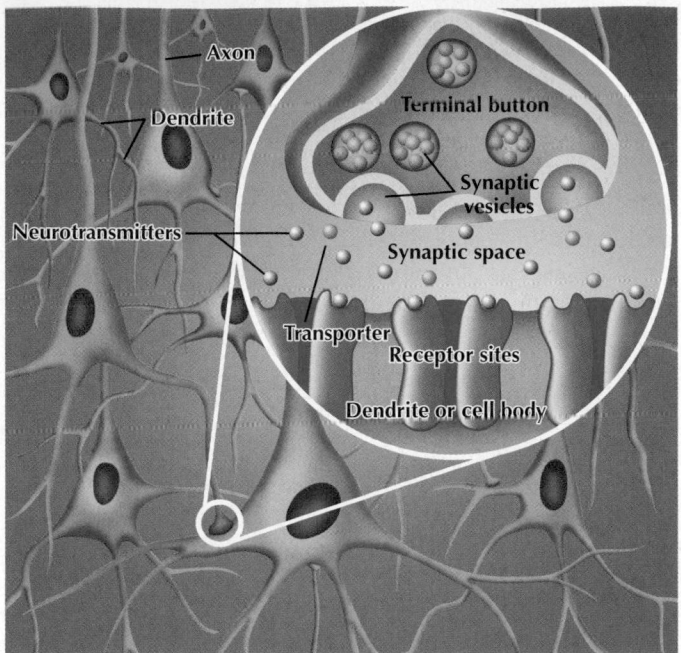

Figure 31–5 ● Neurotransmission: How neurons communicate.

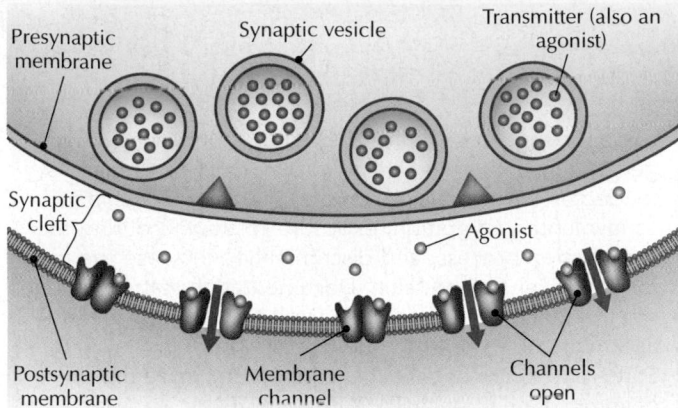

(**A**) Strong agonist activates receptors without transmission.

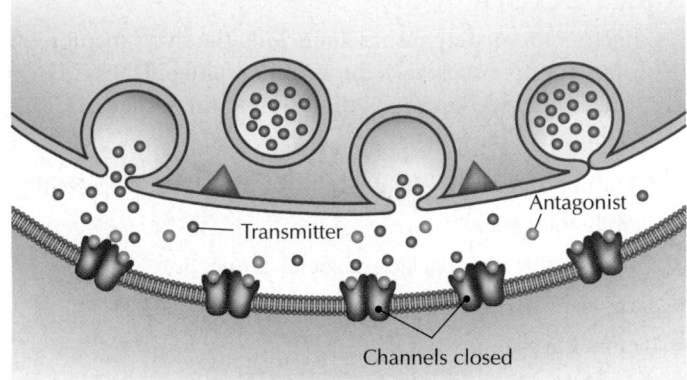

(**B**) Antagonist blocks receptors. Agonist cannot act.

Figure 31–6 ● Ligands: Agonists and antagonists. Agonists and antagonists bind to the same binding site as transmitters. A, An agonist has potency, so it activates the cell biologically, while B, antagonists bind and have no potency. An antagonist produces its effect by blocking the binding site, preventing a transmitter from binding and producing its biological effect.

neurotransmitter that signals arousal and hyperarousal. Researchers believe that an imbalance in the regulation of these two neurotransmitters produces anxiety disorders: When GABA is decreased and norepinephrine is increased, anxiety results (Kneisl & Trigoboff, 2013). Serotonin is also implicated in the pathology of anxiety. It is thought to produce a feeling of well-being and is believed to be correlated with a decrease in anxiety (Butcher et al., 2013).

PSYCHOSOCIAL THEORIES Psychoanalytic theory views anxiety as a sign of internal conflict resulting from the threatened emergence of repressed emotions into consciousness. According to the theory, an individual fears expressing forbidden emotions, and so becomes anxious. Neo-Freudian analytical views of anxiety believe that the state can be traced back to birth trauma, whereas interpersonal theorists stress the importance of the transmission of the mother's anxiety to the child (Kneisl & Trigoboff, 2013). Psychosocial theorists actively debate the origin of anxiety, but these debates typically have little to do with clinical practice.

BEHAVIORAL THEORIES Behaviorists believe that the faulty thinking and behavior are learned dysfunctional responses to stressors. They believe individuals can unlearn unhealthy behaviors by engaging in behavior modification, a treatment approach that teaches clients new ways to behave in response to stress. Behavior modification therapies use conditioning techniques—positive and negative reinforcements—in order to produce systematic desensitization, a process in which the client builds up tolerance to anxiety through gradual exposure to a series of anxiety-provoking stimuli. Behavioral therapists tend to avoid mediation because they believe that it may interfere with the client's ability to shape his or her own responses (Kneisl & Trigoboff, 2013).

GENETIC THEORIES Research suggests that genetic predisposition may play a part in the development of anxiety disorders. According to twin studies, panic disorder and OCD feature a genetic factor, with first-degree relatives of people with panic disorder being four to seven times more likely to develop the condition. One quarter of people with generalized anxiety disorder have a family history of the problem (Kneisl & Trigoboff, 2013). Genetic predisposition can produce the biological conditions necessary for an anxiety disorder to develop, priming an individual for anxious behavior.

HUMANISTIC THEORIES A humanistic, holistic explanation of anxiety disorder etiology is essential to a useful understanding of the ways in which these conditions come about. Biological, psychological, behavioral, and genetic causes do not exist in isolation—they interact with one another to produce the complex of symptoms we call anxiety disorders. The humanistic perspective has generated a nuanced approach to client care that integrates psychotherapeutic interventions, steps to develop social support systems, techniques to reduce external stress, and psychopharmacologic therapy.

Focus on Diversity and Culture Anxiety Disorders in Immigrant Populations

Evidence suggests that the migration experiences of first-generation immigrant Latino youth contribute to their risk for depression and anxiety. Unique migration stressors such as involuntary migration, exposure to trauma during the immigration process, and discrimination increase the risk for anxiety and depression. Documentation status plays a significant role in the adaptation and acculturation process, and migration supports, such as time spent in the United States and family and teacher support, minimize the stress of immigration (Potochnick & Perreira, 2010).

Risk Factors

Risk factors for anxiety disorders include the dysregulation of neurotransmitters such as serotonin, norepinephrine, GABA, and a neuropeptide known as cholecystokinin. Other risk factors include the following:

- Childhood adversity, including witnessing traumatic events
- Family incidence
- Social factors, such as lack of social connection
- Serious or chronic illness
- Traumatic events
- Personality factors such as shyness and worrying
- Multiple stressors, such as chronic illness concurrent with loss of employment (UMM, 2009).

CHILDREN Childhood anxiety disorders are reported more frequently in girls than in boys. Symptoms are more prevalent in girls and minority children from low socioeconomic backgrounds. All children from disadvantaged socioeconomic backgrounds are more vulnerable to emotional illness than their more advantaged peers. Familial predisposition is also a contributing vulnerability factor. Studies suggest that, in general, 3%–5% of children and adolescents have an anxiety disorder of some kind. Children with anxiety disorders run the risk of developing other anxiety disorders, depression, and substance abuse (UMM, 2009).

OLDER ADULTS Older adults with cognitive impairments or one or more chronic physical impairments are at increased risk for developing anxiety. Significant emotional loss, such as the death of a spouse, also increases the older adult's risk for anxiety. In older adults, manifestations of anxiety may overlap with medical illness, resulting in older adults presenting first to their primary care provider. Although the prevalence rates of anxiety disorders in older adults are lower than in the general population, this may be due as much to the lack of appropriate diagnosis rather than to an actual lower rate of anxiety in older adults. Risk factors for anxiety disorders in older adults include lower education levels, presence of multiple chronic illnesses, and being unmarried (Bassil, Ghandour, & Grossberg, 2011).

Prevention

Prevention of anxiety disorders is dependent on an individual's knowledge of her own growing anxiety. Individuals at risk for anxiety disorders should seek medical help early, because these conditions become harder to treat as they progress. Keeping track of patterns of worrying can also help stop anxiety before it grows out of control. Mental health professionals advise that individuals at risk for anxiety disorders keep journals to catalog stressors and sources of relief and to manage priorities. Finally, individuals with multiple risk factors should avoid unhealthy substance use, including the abuse of alcohol, illegal drugs, and even nicotine and caffeine. These drugs can stimulate anxiety, and for people who are addicted, quitting can worsen anxiety (Mayo Clinic, 2012b).

▶ CLINICAL MANIFESTATIONS

Anxiety disorders are clustered around a range of physiological, psychological, behavioral, and cognitive manifestations. Though each of the disorders is distinct (generalized anxiety disorder is completely distinct from acute stress disorder, and so on), the symptoms of all the disorders cluster around excessive, irrational fear and dread (NIMH, 2009). Worry is a major component of each of the anxiety disorders. Individuals in anxiety states experience the emotion as both a subjective condition and as a range of physical symptoms resulting from muscular tension and autonomic nervous system activity. Chronic anxiety can lead to bodily discomforts and disabilities, including constipation, diarrhea, epigastric distress, and heartburn, as well as musculoskeletal aches and pains. Anxiety can come either suddenly or gradually, and it may be expressed as either relatively mild bodily symptoms or as an incapacitating outbreak of acute anxiety (Kneisl & Trigoboff, 2013). See **Table 31–8** ● for an overview of three prominent anxiety disorders; each is discussed in more detail in the following sections.

Generalized Anxiety Disorder

People with **generalized anxiety disorder (GAD)** go through their days filled with intense tension and worry, even if no external stressors are present. They anticipate disaster and are preoccupied with health issues, money, familial problems, or challenges at work. GAD is diagnosed when an individual becomes excessively anxious about everyday problems for at least 6 months. People with the condition cannot rid themselves of their anxious state, even though they can usually recognize that their anxiety is more intense than the situation requires. People with GAD have difficulty relaxing, startle easily, and have trouble concentrating and falling asleep. Somatic symptoms of GAD include fatigue, headache, muscle tension and aches, digestive issues, irritability, feeling out of breath, and hot flashes. Adults with mild GAD can function in social situations and hold down jobs, but those with severe forms of the condition have great difficulty carrying out daily tasks. GAD affects 6.8 million adults in the United States, and twice as many women as men. The disorder can develop at any time in the life cycle, though people are at the highest risk for the condition in early adulthood, between childhood and middle age (NIMH, 2009).

GAD can also appear in children with all the same symptoms as in adults. Children with GAD feel significantly distressed and, as with adults, the principal sign of GAD is intense worry over a long period of time. GAD is common among children and adolescents and is treated mostly with psychotherapy,

TABLE 31–8 Summary of Criteria for Anxiety Disorders

The following are summaries of the criteria for the anxiety disorders discussed in this exemplar. Refer to the DSM-5 for the complete diagnostic criteria.

DISORDER	SUMMARY
Generalized anxiety disorder	■ Characterized by intense tension and worry, even in the absence of external stressors. ■ May demonstrate anticipation of disaster and/or preoccupation with health issues, money, familial problems, or work-related challenges. ■ Affected individuals usually recognize that their anxiety is disproportionate to the circumstances. ■ Manifestations include difficulty relaxing, pronounced startling, trouble concentrating, and difficulty falling asleep. ■ Somatic symptoms include fatigue, headache, muscle tension and aches, digestive issues, irritability, feeling out of breath, and hot flashes. ■ Diagnostic criteria include excessive anxiety about everyday problems for at least 6 months.
Separation anxiety disorder	■ Developmentally inappropriate and excessive anxiety about separation from home and people to whom the person is attached. ■ Evidence for this condition includes recurrent distress when separated from home and family, persistent and excessive worry about harm befalling major attachment figures, persistent refusal to leave attachment figures, persistent fear of being alone, persistent reluctance to go to sleep away from a major attachment figure, and complaints of physical symptoms. ■ Duration of symptoms of at least 4 weeks. ■ Onset before age 18 years. ■ Clinically significant distress or impairment in important areas of functioning. ■ Disturbance does not occur exclusively during the course of other disorders.
Panic disorder	■ Recurrent unexpected panic attacks, when at least one of the attacks has been followed by 1 month of persistent concern about having more attacks, worry about the implications of the attack, or a significant change in behavior related to the attacks. ■ The attacks are not due to the physiological effects of a substance. ■ The attacks are not better accounted for by another mental disorder.

Sources: Based on BehaveNet. (2013a). *Panic disorder without agoraphobia.* Retrieved from http://behavenet.com/panic-disorder-without-agoraphobia; BehaveNet. (2013b). *Separation anxiety disorder.* Retrieved from http://behavenet.com/separation-anxiety-disorder; National Institute of Mental Health. (2009). *Anxiety disorders.* Retrieved from http://www.nimh.nih.gov/health/publications/anxiety-disorders/anxiety_disorders_en_ln.pdf; and American Psychiatric Association. (2013). *Diagnostic and statistical manual of mental disorders* (5th ed.). Arlington, VA: Author.

the goal of which is to build up health and constructive responses to anxiety (Boston Children's Hospital, 2012). The DSM-5 criteria for GAD are outlined in **Box 31–5** ●.

Separation Anxiety Disorder

An individual experiences separation anxiety disorder (SAD) when she has excessive worry about being apart from people to whom she is most attached. The condition is most common in children, for whom symptoms include a refusal to sleep alone, repeated nightmares with a theme of separation, excessive worry about family members, and a refusal to go to school. Other symptoms may include a reluctance to be alone, frequent physical complaints, muscle aches, excessive worry, and an excessive "clinginess" even when at home. Children with the condition fear being lost from their family or fear something bad happening to a loved one. Symptoms of fear must last for at least 4 weeks to be considered SAD. The disorder is distinct from stranger anxiety, which is normal for children between 7 and 11 years old. Symptoms of SAD are more severe than the normal separation anxiety that most children experience between the ages of 18 months and 3 years. In children, SAD occurs equally in males and females, and the first indications of the condition often occur between the ages of 7 and 9. Approximately 4% of younger children have the condition, and the estimate for adolescents is slightly lower (Children's Hospital of Pittsburgh, 2013).

The adult form of the condition, adult separation anxiety disorder (ASAD), is newly recognized by the mental healthcare community. ASAD can have its first onset in adulthood, although in a portion of cases, it represents the persistence or recurrence of childhood SAD. Clinical studies have shown that ASAD is associated with high levels of disability, as well as a likelihood of poor outcomes when clients are treated using cognitive-behavioral therapy (Manicavasagar et al., 2010).

Panic Disorder

Panic disorder is characterized by sudden attacks of terror, sometimes accompanied by a pounding heart, sweating, fainting, or dizziness. In a panic attack, an individual with panic disorder will feel flushed or chilled, his hands will tingle or become numb, and he may experience nausea, chest pain, and a sense of breathlessness, in addition to a sense of unreality, a fear of impending death, and a terror of losing control. A fear of one's own unexplained symptoms is itself a symptom of panic disorder. People in the grip of a panic attack sometimes believe they are dying or losing their minds; between episodes, they may worry intensely about the next panic attack (APA, 2013; NIMH, 2009). Attacks can occur at any time of day, and even during sleep. An attack usually lasts only around 10 minutes, but some symptoms may last much longer. The disorder affects around 6 million people in the United States, and is twice as common in women as men (NIMH, 2009).

People who have full-fledged panic disorder can become incapacitated by their condition and should seek treatment before they start to avoid situations where attacks have

Box 31–5 DSM-5 Diagnostic Criteria for Generalized Anxiety Disorder

A. Excessive anxiety and worry (apprehensive expectation), occurring more days than not for at least 6 months, about a number of events or activities (such as work or school performance).

B. The individual finds it difficult to control the worry.

C. The anxiety and worry are associated with three (or more) of the following six symptoms (with at least some symptoms having been present for more days than not for the past 6 months):

   Note: Only one item is required in children.

   ■ Restlessness or feeling keyed up or on edge.
   ■ Being easily fatigued.
   ■ Difficulty concentrating or mind going blank.
   ■ Irritability.
   ■ Muscle tension.
   ■ Sleep disturbance (difficulty falling or staying asleep, or restlessness, unsatisfying sleep).

D. The anxiety, worry, or physical symptoms cause clinically significant distress or impairment in social, occupational, or other important area of functioning.

E. The disturbance is not attributable to the physiological effects of a substance (e.g., a drug of abuse, a medication) or another medical condition (e.g., hyperthyroidism).

F. The disturbance is not better explained by another medical disorder (e.g., anxiety or worry about having panic attacks in panic disorder, negative evaluation in social anxiety disorder [social phobia], contamination or other obsessions in obsessive-compulsive disorder, separation from attachment figures in separation anxiety disorder, reminders of traumatic events in posttraumatic stress disorder, gaining weight in anorexia nervosa, physical complaints in somatic symptom disorder, perceived appearance flaws in body dysmorphic disorder, having a serious illness in illness anxiety disorder, or the content of delusional beliefs in schizophrenia or delusional disorder).

Source: American Psychiatric Association. (2013). *Diagnostic and statistical manual of mental disorders* (5th ed.). Arlington, VA: Author.

---

occurred. In severe cases, people who have panic attacks avoid normal activities. One third of people who have panic disorder become housebound and are able to confront a feared situation only when accompanied by a loved one or trusted friend. If the client seeks treatment early, however, and the illness is correctly diagnosed, the disorder can usually be cleared up, because panic disorder is one of the most treatable anxiety disorders (NIMH, 2009).

Levels of Anxiety

Levels of anxiety range from mild to panic. The client's level of anxiety greatly impacts nursing care. For clients experiencing panic or severe anxiety, safety is a priority. Because the individual will be unable to take in any new information during these stages, interventions focus on reducing the anxiety level prior to providing any new information. Immediate interventions include reducing exposure to stimuli and providing comfort measures to assist in reducing symptom severity. Distractions and relaxation techniques may be helpful. Once the client's anxiety level decreases, additional interventions to reduce anxiety, such as beginning a course of medication and starting psychotherapy, may be introduced. Clients who experience mild anxiety may benefit from nonpharmacologic interventions, such as yoga, deep breathing, and journaling.

▶ COLLABORATION

The treatment of anxiety disorders is more apt to occur in the home and community than in the hospital, with the exception of panic disorder. Considering the level of distress that accompanies anxiety disorders, it is not difficult to understand the vulnerability of individuals with anxiety and the correlating increased incidence of substance abuse and/or depression. This combination is a threat to treatment success and positive outcomes for the individual. Because the individual is part of a family and a larger community, nurses need to support positive outcomes for individuals by involving both the individual and his or her family in the treatment process. Such treatment is multimodal and involves the assessment of age, education, health and health practices, spirituality, and culturally specific needs (NIMH, 2013b).

Lifespan Considerations Separation Anxiety Disorder

Infants and Toddlers

■ From 8–14 months, children often become frightened when they meet new people or visit unknown places.

■ When infants are separated from their parents, they feel unsafe. This is called separation anxiety, and is a normal developmental phase.

■ Normal separation anxiety usually ends when the child is around 2 years old (MedlinePlus, 2010).

Children and Adolescents

■ A child's feeling of anxiety when separated from loved ones is diagnosed as SAD when symptoms are powerful enough to interfere with daily life and last for at least 4 weeks.

■ Children with the condition have an overwhelming fear of being lost from their family or that something bad will happen to a loved one.

■ In children, SAD occurs equally in males and females, and the first indications of the condition usually occur between the ages of 7 and 9.

■ Approximately 4% of younger children have the condition, and the estimate for adolescents is slightly lower (Children's Hospital of Pittsburgh, 2013).

Adults

■ Adult separation anxiety disorder (ASAD) usually has its first onset in adulthood, although it can represent the persistence or recurrence of childhood SAD.

■ ASAD is associated with high levels of disability, and may interfere with committed relationships, work, and interactions with family and friends (Manicavasagar et al., 2010).

Clinical Manifestations and Therapies **Anxiety Disorders**

LEVEL OF SEVERITY OF ANXIETY	CLINICAL MANIFESTATIONS	CLINICAL THERAPIES
Mild	■ Increase in sensory perception and arousal ■ Increase in alertness ■ Sleeplessness ■ Increase in motivation ■ Restlessness and irritability	■ Mild anxiety typically is resolved by an individual's coping mechanisms. Mild anxiety may be helpful to the client to accentuate focus and concentration. ■ Clients who are distressed by mild anxiety may benefit from ■ Improved sleep hygiene ■ Relaxation techniques ■ Behavior therapy ■ Massage ■ Aromatherapy.
Moderate	■ Narrowing of perceptual field and attention span (a process called "selective inattention") ■ Reduction in alertness and awareness of surroundings ■ Feeling of discomfort and irritability with others ■ Self-absorption ■ Increased restlessness ■ Increase in respirations, heart rate, and muscle tension ■ Increase in perspiration ■ Rapid speech, louder tone, and higher pitch	■ Cognitive and behavior therapy to identify triggers and learn improved coping techniques ■ Relaxation techniques ■ Complementary and alternative therapies such as yoga, acupuncture, massage ■ Low-dose antianxiety medications if symptoms do not improve with other therapies or if the medications exacerbate chronic conditions
Severe	■ Perceptual field greatly reduced ■ Difficulty following directions ■ Feelings of dread, horror ■ Need to relieve anxiety ■ Headache ■ Dizziness ■ Nausea, trembling, insomnia ■ Palpitations, tachycardia, hyperventilating, diarrhea	■ Cognitive and behavior therapy to learn to identify triggers and to learn better coping techniques ■ Antianxiety medications (may include benzodiazepines) ■ Relaxation techniques ■ Complementary therapies such as yoga, acupuncture, massage ■ Hospitalization may be required initially to manage severe anxiety until improved coping mechanisms are developed
Panic	■ Inability to focus ■ Perception distorted ■ Terror ■ Feelings of doom ■ Bizarre behavior ■ Dilated pupils ■ Trembling, sleeplessness, palpitations, pallor, diaphoresis, muscular incoordination ■ Immobility or hyperactivity, incoherence	Immediate, structured intervention required. Immediate therapies include the following: ■ Placing client in a quiet, less stimulating environment ■ Use of repetitive or physical task to diffuse energy ■ Administration of antianxiety medications Long-term therapies include the following: ■ Cognitive and behavioral therapy ■ Pharmacologic therapy ■ Relaxation techniques ■ Improved sleep hygiene ■ CAM therapies such as massage, acupuncture, yoga, hydrotherapy ■ Nutrition consultation ■ Mental health counseling (Kneisl & Trigoboff, 2013)

Evidence-Based Practice Anxiety Disorders, Oxidative Stress, and Illness

Problem

Oxidative stress (OS) is a loss of balance in oxidation–reduction reactions. OS is characterized by the reduced ability of the body's antioxidant defense system to efficiently eliminate the excess of reactive oxygen species (ROS) production, making oxygen toxic and bringing about detrimental effects at the cellular level. Research has observed a close relationship between anxiety and oxidative stress in humans.

Evidence

Recent findings indicate that oxidative metabolism is a plausible pathway for the regulation of anxiety. This hypothesis has gained favor due to the intrinsic oxidative vulnerability of the brain, a lipid-rich organ that uses large quantities of oxygen. Conditions in the brain are favorable to the production of free-radical chain reactions that cause membrane fluidity and damage to membrane proteins. Oxidation of neuronal membrane lipids and proteins and oxidation of other sensitive brain components can alter overall brain activity, giving rise to a variety of neurological diseases, including anxiety disorders (Bouayed, 2011).

Using experiments on mice, researchers have found that elevated anxiety levels in mice are accompanied by markedly boosted levels of ROS in neuronal and glial cells within the cerebellum and hippocampus, as well as in neurons of the cerebral cortex and in blood monocytes, granulocytes, and lymphocytes. These findings show a clear link between oxidative stress and trait anxiety, but the results do not necessarily show a causal relationship (Bouayed et al., 2009). Another study shows a relationship between the renin–angiotensin system, its active peptide angiotensin II (AngII), oxidative stress, and anxiety. In clients with high blood pressure, a certain gene was associated with both high plasma AngII and oxidase-generated ROS. The collective results of this study indicate that angiotensin II is involved with the oxidative stress associated with anxiety disorders (Liu et al., 2012).

Implications

Accumulating evidence indicates that oxidative stress is linked to the development of anxiety in humans. Antioxidants play a crucial role in maintaining redox homeostasis by maintaining the level of ROS necessary for optimal physiological functioning. Diet is the principal source of antioxidants. Research suggests that a relative deficiency of dietary antioxidants may increase an individual's vulnerability to the destructive effects of oxidative stress. Vitamin E, vitamin C, carotenoids, zinc, selenium, and polyphenols constitute the principal dietary antioxidants in food. These nutrients may benefit health for reasons other than their antioxidant properties, but there is evidence that antioxidants can also exhibit a cognitive-enhancing effect, psychostimulant activity, and even antidepressant and antianxiety properties (Bouayed, 2011).

Critical Thinking Application

Consider the oxidative stress-based explanation of the etiology of anxiety. How do you think this mechanism relates to an individual's environment and upbringing? Do you think oxidative stress is triggered by an individual's lifestyle, or might a state of oxidative stress impact the way an individual handles stressors in his or her environment? Is this physiological theory relevant to clinical practice? With this theory in mind, would you recommend dietary or lifestyle changes?

Diagnostic Tests

If symptoms of an anxiety disorder are present, the provider begins an evaluation by performing a complete medical history and physical exam. Currently no laboratory tests are available to diagnose any of the anxiety disorders, but various diagnostic tests may be used to rule out physical illness as the cause of the symptoms. If no physical illness is found, the client may be referred to a mental health professional trained to diagnose and treat mental illnesses. These specialists use specially designed interview and assessment tools to evaluate an individual for an anxiety disorder. The mental health professional bases the diagnosis on the client's subjective report of the duration and intensity of symptoms, including any interference with daily functioning. The client's own observation of her affect and behavior may be considered in determining whether symptoms and degree of dysfunction indicate a specific disorder. The diagnosis is typically made according to the standard reference manual on the subject, the *Diagnostic and Statistical Manual of Mental Disorders* (DSM-5), published by the American Psychiatric Association (Cleveland Clinic, 2012).

Pharmacologic Therapy

Medication does not cure anxiety disorders, but it can control the associated signs and symptoms while the client enters psychotherapy. Medication may be prescribed by a psychiatrist or advanced practice psychiatric/mental health nurse, or by a primary care provider (e.g., physician, nurse practitioner). The medications usually used for anxiety disorders are antidepressants, antianxiety drugs, and beta-blockers, though antipsychotics are sometimes used as well. See the Medications feature in this module's concept section for more information.

Antidepressants were developed to treat depression, but the drugs are also effective for anxiety disorders. These medications begin to alter brain chemistry after the first dose, but their full effect requires a few weeks because a series of neurobiological changes must take place before the mediations achieve efficacy. Selective serotonin reuptake inhibitors (SSRIs) alter the levels of the neurotransmitter serotonin in the brain. SSRIs are commonly prescribed for anxiety disorders. SSRIs are generally started at low doses and then increased as their effectiveness becomes apparent. SSRIs have fewer side effects than previous generations of antidepressants, but they sometimes generate nausea, jitters, and occasionally sexual dysfunction.

The most commonly used antianxiety drugs are benzodiazepines. These drugs have few side effects other than drowsiness, but higher and higher doses may be necessary over a long period of time, so benzodiazepines are typically prescribed for a short time. Because they take only hours to reach efficacy, they often are prescribed for clients experiencing severe or panic levels of anxiety. Clients with panic disorder can typically take benzodiazepines for up to a year without harm. Examples of benzodiazepines used in the treatment of anxiety include alprazolam

(Xanax), diazepam (Valium), lorazepam (Ativan), and chlordiazepoxide (Librium) (Adams et al., 2014).

Some clients experience withdrawal symptoms if they stop taking benzodiazepines abruptly, and anxiety can return immediately after cessation. These potential problems have led some physicians to shy away from using these drugs. Buspirone, an azapirone, is a newer antianxiety medication used to treat GAD. Possible side effects include nausea, headaches, and dizziness. Unlike benzodiazepines, buspirone must be taken consistently for at least 2 weeks to achieve an antianxiety effect.

Beta-blockers, such as propranolol, which is used to treat heart conditions, can prevent the physical abnormalities (such as blushing and hyperventilation) that accompany certain anxiety disorders, particularly social phobia. When a feared situation can be predicted, the physician may prescribe a beta-blocker to keep the physical symptoms of the anxiety under control (NIMH, 2009).

At times, antipsychotic medications—drugs typically reserved for conditions such as bipolar disorder and schizophrenia—are used to treat anxiety disorders. Typical antipsychotics, the first drugs of this type, include haloperidol, chlorpromazine, and loxapine. These drugs have been shown to produce a significant reduction in neurotic anxiety. Atypical antipsychotics, a later generation of antipsychotics, provide potential benefits for clients with generalized anxiety disorder. Extended-release quetiapine has been shown to prevent relapse anxiety in clients with GAD, but more studies need to be performed to examine the risks and benefits of using antipsychotic medications for anxiety disorders (Jewell, 2010).

Nonpharmacologic Therapy

Nonpharmacologic therapy provides the most effective treatment for anxiety disorders. Complementary and alternative health practices can be used in conjunction with pharmaceutical therapy to bring relief to clients with anxiety disorders, but the most effective nonpharmacologic therapy is psychotherapy, including cognitive-behavioral therapy. Psychotherapy involves talking with a mental health professional, such as a psychiatrist, psychologist, social worker, or counselor, to uncover what caused an anxiety disorder and to determine how to work through its symptoms. The most effective treatment strategy for most people with anxiety disorders is a combination of cognitive-behavioral therapy and medication (NIMH, 2009).

COGNITIVE-BEHAVIORAL THERAPY
Cognitive-behavioral therapy (CBT) is a useful nonpharmacologic intervention for treating anxiety disorders. The cognitive aspect of this treatment helps the client change the thought patterns that support his fears, and the behavioral aspect helps the client change the way he reacts to anxiety-provoking situations. This intervention has been proven to reduce the symptoms of all types of anxiety disorders. For additional discussion of CBT, refer to the concept section of this module.

COMPLEMENTARY AND ALTERNATIVE THERAPY
Though conventional medical therapies are consistently shown to ease the symptoms of anxiety disorders, alternate and complementary therapies have been shown to ease the symptoms of anxiety as well. These alternative therapies include herbal preparations, massage and touch, and yoga and meditation.

Herbal Preparations Overall, herbal preparations show little promise as potential therapies for the symptoms of anxiety. However, a few different plant species seem to have moderate effects on anxiety disorders. Kava is a native plant of the islands of the South Pacific, a member of the pepper family. Scientific studies provide evidence that kava may be beneficial for anxiety management, but the U.S. Food and Drug Administration (FDA) has warned that kava supplements have been linked to a risk of severe liver damage. In addition, kava has been associated with cases of dystonia, drowsiness, and scaly, yellowed skin. It is also suspected to interact with drugs used to treat Parkinson disease.

Lavender is currently used as a traditional remedy for anxiety, among other psychological conditions. It is most commonly used for aromatherapy, in which the essential oil from the flowers is inhaled. Dried lavender flowers can be used to make teas or liquid extracts that can be taken orally. Small studies on lavender show mixed results, and topical use of diluted lavender and the use of the oil for aromatherapy is considered safe for adults. However, the undiluted oil irritates skin, is poisonous by mouth, and may cause drowsiness (National Center for Complementary and Alternative Medicine [NCCAM], 2013).

Chamomile is a traditional remedy in widespread use, and a recent study has found that the plant has modest benefits for some people with mild to moderate GAD. The plant has been shown to compare favorably with placebo in the reduction of anxiety, and it is well tolerated by clients. However, there are reports of allergic reactions in people who have eaten chamomile products, especially individuals who are allergic to plants in the daisy family, including ragweed, chrysanthemums, marigolds, and daisies (NCCAM, 2009a).

Massage and Therapeutic Touch Scientific research on massage and touch therapy is limited, but evidence suggests that massage may benefit some clients. A single session of massage therapy can reduce state anxiety (a reaction to a particular situation), blood pressure, and heart rate, and multiple sessions can reduce "trait anxiety" (an individual's predisposition to anxiety), depression, and pain. It is not currently known how massage therapy has these effects on the body. *Gate control theory*, for instance, suggests that massage may provide stimulation to block pain signals sent to the brain. Other theories suggest that massage may stimulate the release of chemicals such as serotonin or endorphins or cause mechanical changes in the body.

Relaxation Techniques, Yoga, and Meditation In addition to being a state of mind, relaxation physically changes the way the body functions, in the process relieving stress. When the body relaxes, breathing slows, blood pressure and oxygen consumption decrease, and well-being increases. Being able to produce the relaxation response using relaxation techniques may counteract the long-term stress that can lead to anxiety disorders. Relaxation techniques often combine breathing and focused attention to calm the mind and body, and usually only require brief instruction from a practitioner before they can be done without assistance. Common relaxation techniques include autogenic training, biofeedback, deep breathing, guided imagery, progressive relation, and self-hypnosis.

Yoga, a tradition linked to Indian spiritual practice, can also be used to produce a relaxation response. Yoga is currently widely used as a complementary health practice and for exercise purposes. Many people who practice yoga do so to maintain well-being, improve fitness, and relieve stress, in addition to addressing specific health conditions such as back pain, arthritis, and anxiety (NCCAM, 2013).

Evidence also suggests that religious or secular meditation can be used to combat the effects of anxiety. In particular, a recent study found that transcendental meditation (TM) helped participants decrease psychological distress and increase coping ability. The college students who practiced TM in the study were more likely to handle academic, financial, and social pressures without developing significant anxiety (NCCAM, 2009b).

▓ NURSING PROCESS

Nursing interventions are focused on reducing the severity of the symptoms of anxiety. Specific interventions include establishing a rapport, communicating therapeutically, supporting and enhancing coping skills, assessing and identifying maladaptive coping, fostering mental health, maintaining a therapeutic milieu, minimizing the deleterious effects of anxiety, and promoting the health of the individual. The generalist nurse provides case management, home health care, psychoeducation, and medication administration.

Assessment

Assessment of clients with anxiety includes interviewing the client with regard to his current and previous illnesses, medication (and supplement) regimen, and past and present stressors. In addition, the nurse should tactfully interview the client about current and previous methods of coping, including the use of alcohol and drugs, particularly because certain coping methods may actually compound the individual's sense of anxiety and may predispose the client to developing an illness or other health alteration. Physical assessment should include a general assessment, as well as a focused assessment of any body systems that are relevant to the client's current complaints.

Diagnosis

Selection of nursing diagnoses should be client specific and depends on numerous factors, including the degree to which anxiety is impacting the client's daily life and social interaction. Examples of nursing diagnoses that may be appropriate for inclusion in the plan of care for the client with GAD may include the following:

- *Anxiety*
- *Ineffective Coping*
- *Disturbed Sleep Pattern*
- *Impaired Social Interaction*
- *Risk for Ineffective Self-Health Management*
(NANDA-I © 2012)

Planning

The nursing plan of care, designed in collaboration with the client, may include the following goals:

- The client will report a decrease in level of and frequency of anxiety.
- The client will articulate successful coping mechanisms.

- The client will report increasing use of successful coping mechanisms.
- The client will participate in psychotherapy or group counseling activities as outlined by the primary care provider.

Implementation

Nursing interventions for individuals experiencing mild anxiety focus on appraisal. To gain understanding about the individual, the nurse acquires information about how the person appraises and prioritizes stressors. To facilitate the adaptive coping process, the nurse critically evaluates thoughts that may be increasing the person's anxiety.

Clients experiencing mild anxiety are often able to learn information and acquire new behaviors easily. The nurse is able to provide valuable information to these clients, teaching them ways to manage stress and modify thinking processes and behaviors.

Both mild and moderate anxiety need appropriate intervention to prevent the client from progressing to severe anxiety and panic. Due to the increase in physical autonomic responses described earlier, appropriate caring interventions for an individual with moderate anxiety include both cognitive reframing and physical exertion to expend the client's excess energy due to excessive catecholamines. Walking briskly, running, or working out large muscle groups assists the individual to manage his or her own physical body.

Severe anxiety and panic require immediate intervention. The safety of the individual is at risk due to the narrowing of perception and inability to process information and think rationally. It is imperative to isolate the severely anxious or panicked client to prevent the client's distress from impacting, disturbing, or threatening others. Provide the individual with a safe, quiet, protective environment; do not leave the person unattended; and administer medications or other interventions as ordered by the healthcare provider. Benzodiazepines typically are used to treat severe anxiety and panic.

The mind–body connection has been well documented through scientific research. As such, promotion of psychosocial wellness incorporates principles related to physical health. For clients with stress-related disorders, wellness promotion and education should include applicable interventions related to physical exercise, sleep/rest patterns, nutrition, and time management (refer back to Table 31–7 for an overview of the basic principles related to these considerations). Depending on the client's current level of wellness and specific needs, the relevant nursing interventions will vary.

Evaluation

Evaluation of the client experiencing anxiety is based on the symptoms with which she presented and her strengths and weaknesses. Suggested expected outcomes may include:

- The client's anxiety has diminished as reflected by vital signs returning to baseline and client's report of anxiety level.
- The client demonstrates new or improved coping measures to reduce anxiety.
- The client self-moderates the anxiety response when stressors occur.

REVIEW Anxiety Disorders

RELATE Link the Concepts and Exemplars

Linking the exemplar of anxiety disorders with the concept of perfusion:

1. What impact does anxiety have on perfusion?
2. What medications normally prescribed for anxiety would be contraindicated for an individual with a history of heart disease?

Linking the exemplar of anxiety disorders with the concept of acid–base balance:

3. How might anxiety impact acid–base balance?
4. What nursing interventions might the nurse recommend for the client with anxiety that is altering acid–base balance?

READY Go to Companion Skills Manual

REFER Go to Pearson Nursing Student Resources
nursing.pearsonhighered.com

- *Additional review materials*

REFLECT Case Study

Heather O'Malley is a 34-year-old woman who is newly separated from her husband. She has been a stay-at-home mother of children ages 7, 5, and 4, along with a 3-month-old infant. Her days are very busy caring for her young children, and she wonders how she will manage on her own, especially because she will need to find a job in order to provide for the financial needs of the household now that her husband has moved out. Although he is paying court-ordered child support, it is not enough to meet the living expenses of Ms. O'Malley and all four children. Her attempts to work with a lawyer to get additional money in the form of alimony are on hold because she does not have money to pay the lawyer.

Ms. O'Malley worked as a nurse before quitting when the oldest child was born. She looks into taking a refresher course so she can return to nursing and learns that several hospitals provide the course free of charge if she agrees to work for them after successful completion. She applies to one of these hospitals and is called for an interview. Ms. O'Malley wakes up early on the morning of the interview, feeds the older children and sends them to school, then takes the youngest child to the house of a neighbor who has agreed to babysit. She returns home to dress for her interview, thinking about how she will find good child care if she takes a full-time job and trying to figure out what salary she will need to meet her financial obligations if they are to stay in their home. As she is starting the car, Ms. O'Malley suddenly finds she can't catch her breath, she feels light-headed and dizzy, and she has acute chest pressure. She sits in the car concentrating on her breathing until the feeling subsides and then returns to the house to cancel her interview. She reschedules twice and each time the same physical symptoms begin before she can get to the interview. When she calls to reschedule a third time the hospital declines to set up another interview.

1. What stressors are impacting Ms. O'Malley at this time?
2. If Heather came to the clinic and you were admitting her to the office, what assessment questions would you ask to explore her methods of coping?
3. Describe three nursing diagnoses that may be appropriate for inclusion in Ms. O'Malley's nursing plan of care.
4. For each nursing diagnosis, list at least two relevant nursing interventions.

EXEMPLAR 31.2   Crisis

EXEMPLAR KEY TERMS
Anticipatory guidance, *1930*
Crisis, *1927*
Crisis counseling, *1930*
Crisis intervention, *1930*
Crisis intervention centers, *1931*
Maturational crisis, *1928*
Resilience, *1928*
Scaling, *1932*
Situational crisis, *1928*

EXEMPLAR LEARNING OUTCOMES
After reading about this exemplar, you will be able to:

1. Describe the physiology, etiology, clinical manifestations, and direct and indirect causes of a crisis response.

2. Identify risk factors and prevention methods associated with crisis.
3. Illustrate the nursing process in providing culturally competent care across the life span for individuals in crisis.
4. Formulate priority nursing diagnoses appropriate for an individual in crisis.
5. Summarize therapies used by interdisciplinary teams in the collaborative care of an individual in crisis.
6. Plan evidence-based care for an individual in crisis and his or her family in collaboration with other members of the healthcare team.
7. Evaluate expected outcomes for an individual in crisis.

▶ OVERVIEW

By necessity, life and the human condition include the experience of crisis. A **crisis** occurs when an event or circumstance overwhelms an individual's inherent ability to resolve, manage, or process the event. A crisis refers to any acute incident that can evolve from a situation or event and that overwhelms an individual's normal coping process. Such an event may be a developmental, biological, psychosocial, environmental, or spiritual stressor. Crises occur when the typical or normal means an individual utilizes to cope with stressful situations no longer reduces the anxiety or resolves the situation, producing an acute state of disequilibrium and turmoil. Adaptation and successful resolution of a crisis may involve a number of adjustments and may result in a change in the individual's coping process. A crisis also affords the individual an opportunity to grow and change as a result of successful adaptation to the crisis.

▶ PATHOPHYSIOLOGY AND ETIOLOGY

A crisis is, by definition, an acute situation and is precipitated by an event that creates disequilibrium. Crises occur in the lives of all individuals. The characteristics of a crisis are listed in **Box 31–6** ●. The experience of crisis is an individual event. What is a crisis for one person may not constitute a crisis for someone else.

All crises provide opportunities for growth or deterioration (Townsend, 2009). There typically are three possible resolutions to a crisis. Generally, an individual will either (1) adapt to the crisis and return to the previous level of functioning, (2) utilize the opportunity to improve as an individual and cope with life more effectively, or (3) deteriorate to a lower level of functioning.

The contributions of Caplan (1964) to the prevention of mental illness have long provided the groundwork on which to build what we know today as *crisis theory*. Individuals interact constantly with the environment; internally, they struggle to meet Maslow's hierarchy of needs (see Figure 31–1). These needs, which include physical, psychological, social, and spiritual needs, are different as an individual progresses through the life span. The individual's ability to fulfill needs, maintain homeostasis, regulate affect, mobilize resources, and maintain reality testing impacts whether or not the individual is able to achieve adaptation. The individual's perception of the crisis, resources, support, and ego strength all impact his or her capacity to return to prior levels of functioning after crisis. The intensity of the stressor and crisis can induce a range of symptoms from severe emotional pain and anxiety to the loss of reality testing.

Types of crises include both situational and maturational crises. A **situational crisis** involves an unexpected stressor or circumstance that occurs in the course of daily living (**Figure 31–7** ●). Individuals experience acute stressors from the external environ-

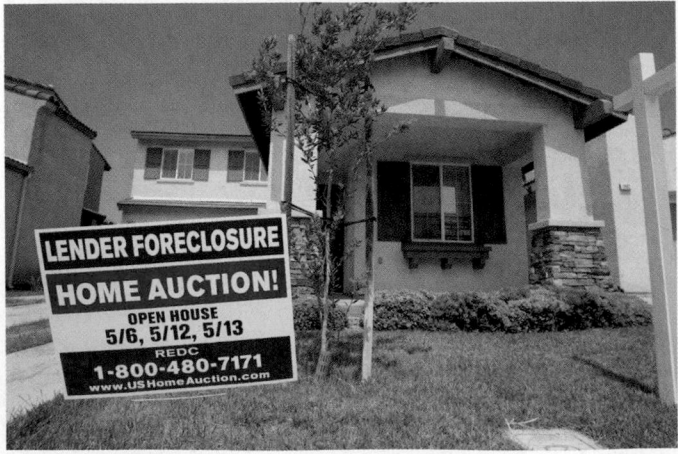

Figure 31–7 ● Economic turmoil in the United States starting in 2008 created crises for many families as they lost jobs and homes.
Source: REUTERS/Mark Avery.

ment, such as tornadoes or earthquakes; the internal environment, such as critical illness or disfigurement; and relational or interpersonal sources, such as the death of a loved one or a lost relationship. **Maturational crisis** occurs normally as individuals progress through the life cycle. Everyone experiences predictable stages of human growth and development as outlined by Erikson (1968). During each stage, the individual is subject to unique stressors. A failure at any one stage compromises the next stage of development.

Holistically, achievement of the milestones of growth and development requires a tremendous amount of energy. Unexpected life events may alter the person's ability to adapt successfully to either a maturational or situational crisis. This increases an individual's vulnerability, often requiring supportive interventions from healthcare providers.

Resilience

Resilience describes the personal patterns, behaviors, or processes that promote an individual's recovery from or adaptation to adversity (Reich, Zautra, & Hall, 2010). Resilience appears to buffer the effects of a crisis or adverse situation (Girdano et al., 2009). Rather than being a static characteristic or personality trait, resilience is dynamic in nature. That is, an individual may demonstrate varying degrees of resilience when exposed to the same or similar stressors throughout the life span. An individual also may tend to be more or less resilient when faced with certain stressors or situations than with others (Reich et al., 2010).

Among the factors that influence an individual's resilience, optimism and perceived self-efficacy appear to be primary determinants (Girdano et al., 2009). Optimism refers to a sense of confidence and hope with regard to positive or favorable resolution of a situation or set of circumstances. Perceived self-efficacy refers to an individual's beliefs concerning his ability to identify and perform the actions needed for accomplishment of goals, and to influence events that impact his life (Bandura, 1994; Girdano et al., 2009).

Psychologist Dr. Albert Bandura, whose contributions to the field of psychology include his famous *social learning theory*, conducted in-depth research in the area of self-efficacy. According to Bandura (1994), an individual's perception of self-efficacy is significantly shaped by the following influences:

- *Mastery experiences:* Personal experiences with conquering obstacles through tenacious efforts and perseverance; a pattern of easy achievement of success may lead an individual to expect victory and to be discouraged by failure.

- *Vicarious experiences:* In the context of observing other individuals who one believes to be similar to himself, the apparent ability or inability of those individuals to accomplish goals and achieve success.

- *Social persuasion:* The extent to which an individual is verbally persuaded by others to believe he is capable of achieving success and to accomplish given tasks.

- *Somatic and emotional states:* Incorporates self-judgments regarding an individual's stress response and physical abilities, as well as mood state. Individuals may be self-critical of their stress response or sense of tension when faced with stressors; in turn, these same individuals may perceive their physical response to stress as rendering them susceptible to failure. In comparison to a negative mood, a positive mood is associated with greater perceived self-efficacy (Bandura, 1994).

Resilience, along with factors such as cognitive appraisal and coping style (as discussed in the concept section of this module), affect both the physical and psychological manifestations of an individual's response to crisis.

▶ CLINICAL MANIFESTATIONS

Individuals in crisis need immediate assistance and support. The Clinical Manifestations and Therapies feature outlines the common clinical symptoms and manifestations of individuals in crisis.

The impact of a crisis may elicit intense emotions. To facilitate adaptive coping, it is essential that nurses support individuals in expressing their feelings and listen attentively. Nurses encourage individuals to vent and emote and facilitate this process. The goal in crisis is to stabilize the reactions of the individual, thereby initiating the process of adaptation by reducing the disruption created by the crisis. The nurse is an active participant in the intervention process. The generalist nurse serves as communicator, facilitator, and resource expert for the individual.

Lifespan and Cultural Considerations

The response to trauma varies throughout the life span, as well as among cultures. In general, very young children are unable to identify specific emotions; likewise, they lack the ability to cope with crisis and trauma. For young children, changes in behavior may signify a crisis response. Parents are expert sources of information with regard to identifying behavioral changes in their children. For pediatric clients, the nurse collaborates with the client's parents to establish a baseline (i.e., normal behavior) and to identify behavioral changes. Children of all ages who are able to express themselves verbally should be encouraged to express their feelings and thoughts.

Depending on their beliefs and family values, older clients may be resistant to expressing what they perceive as negative emotions. Some older adults perceive sadness, grief, and fear to be private matters that are not appropriate for discussion. Still, for clients of all ages, the nurse should seek to establish a therapeutic relationship that is built on trust and that represents a safe place in which clients can verbalize feelings and emotions.

Cultural factors may also present barriers to expression of emotions. In certain cultures, expressions of pain, sorrow, or fear are viewed as signs of weakness. The nurse should be aware of the client's cultural background and, while maintaining respect for the client's privacy, gently offer the client the opportunity to express himself.

▶ COLLABORATION

Caring for clients during times of crisis may include facilitating counseling referrals, connecting clients and families with community agencies, and implementing crisis interventions. For some clients, an extended or severe response to crisis may warrant pharmacologic intervention.

Diagnostic Tests

The client interview and physical assessment provide the most valuable data for use in planning client care. In addition, tools are available for use in evaluating the impact of a crisis event. For example, the Horowitz Impact of Event Scale (IES), which originally was developed in 1979 and revised in 1997, allows for measurement of an individual's stress response following traumatic or impactful life experiences (Horowitz, Wilner, & Alverez, 1979; Weiss & Marmer, 1997). Some researchers found the IES-R to be especially useful in helping to identify signs and symptoms associated with posttraumatic stress disorder (PTSD).

⚙ *Stay Current:* To view the IES-R, visit **http://consultgerirn. org.**

Clinical Manifestations and Therapies **Crisis**

ETIOLOGY	CLINICAL MANIFESTATIONS	CLINICAL THERAPIES
▪ Physical trauma (including rape, assault, and exposure to violence)	▪ Difficulty problem solving	▪ Counseling
▪ Emotional trauma (including psychological and verbal abuse)	▪ Disorganized thought processes with difficulty processing information	▪ Crisis intervention
▪ Exposure to violence, including in the school or workplace settings	▪ Disorientation	▪ Inpatient hospitalization and intensive counseling
▪ Illness and health-related alterations	▪ Vulnerability	▪ Couple, family, and/or group therapy
▪ Significant loss (including death of a loved one or significant other)	▪ Increased tension and helplessness	▪ Pharmacologic treatment for specific stress-related manifestations, if indicated (e.g., short-term administration of benzodiazepines for treatment of anxiety) or as indicated based on client-specific needs (e.g., prophylactic antibiotics)
▪ Exposure to natural and environmental disasters	▪ Fearfulness and sense of being overwhelmed	
▪ Exposure to acts of terrorism	▪ Intense emotional reactions	
▪ Financial stressors	▪ Increased sensory input and bombardment	
▪ Legal stressors (including divorce, child custody disputes, and identity theft)	▪ Hypervigilance	
	▪ Intense physical reactions depicted in the fight-or-flight response	
	▪ By definition, event usually is time limited and resolves within 6 weeks	

Pharmacologic Therapy

Pharmacologic therapies may be prescribed to address immediate medical needs, which vary widely depending on the nature of the crisis. Immediate needs that may require pharmacologic treatment include:

- Pain following injury (e.g., associated with a motor vehicle crash)
- Threat of infection following injury or exposure to a bacterial infection (e.g., prophylactic treatment for tuberculosis following a lengthy stay in a hurricane shelter)
- Sleep disturbance
- Anxiety or depression.

For additional discussion about medications used in the treatment of clients with manifestations such as anxiety and depression, see the Medications feature in the concept section of this module.

Nonpharmacologic Therapy

Nursing care of clients in crisis includes establishing a therapeutic relationship; ensuring client safety from the first moment of contact; mobilizing support through the significant other, family, relatives, friends, church support groups, and healthcare institutions; and collaborating with mental health professionals. Directive suggestion may be helpful, such as gently advising the mother of a critically sick child to go home and sleep while assuring her that she will be called immediately if her child's condition changes. Offering time, attention, and direction is most critical during a crisis. An arrangement for a follow-up care appointment suggests concern for the individual's well-being. The opportunities to offer care in crisis are endless and may involve only a moment of time.

THERAPEUTIC COMMUNICATION   Communicating with individuals in crisis requires frequent, brief, simple, and often directive communication. Biologically speaking, the brain of the individual in crisis is in the process of being bombarded with electrochemical reactions. Concentration and the ability to remember and retain information can be impaired. The nurse must continually reassess what the individual has heard or interpreted. In applying the transactional model, it is important to remember primary appraisal. What does the individual believe is happening? How can the nurse add resources and information to the reappraisal process to facilitate adaptive coping? Continual observation of patterns of communication within the family and/or group is essential. Due to the hyperarousal that occurs during the crisis, the nurse must be cognizant of nonverbal communication, tone, inflection, and mannerisms while communicating. For more information see the exemplar on Therapeutic Communication in the module on Communication.

Communication may also be a powerful tool in the prevention of the development of a crisis. **Anticipatory guidance** incorporates recognition of the potential for a crisis and assisting the client with identifying potential methods for averting the crisis. Examples of anticipatory guidance include counseling pregnant women about prenatal nutrition recommendations and facilitating connections between respite care organizations and caregivers of clients with chronic illness. For more information on anticipatory guidance, see the exemplar on Client/Consumer Education in the module on Teaching and Learning.

In times of crisis, the nurse may be the one responsible for communicating bad news regarding injury or death of loved ones.

Box 31–7   Communicating Painful Information

One of the uncomfortable roles of the nurse is to communicate painful information to individuals. This task can be unnerving. A few simple guidelines convey a professional attitude of concern and care for those receiving dire news:

1. Greet the individuals with warmth, a kind smile, and an introduction.
2. Inform them that you are there and will assist during this difficult time.
3. Provide privacy, tissues, a drink, and a place to sit down to discuss the information.
4. Inquire about what they know, answer questions, and provide support.
5. Apprise them of the current circumstances in terms that they can understand.
6. Respond to their feelings and offer support.
7. Ask what they need from you and what has helped in the past to cope with difficult situations.
8. Incorporate cultural and religious practices of the individual in crisis to provide comfort.
9. Inform them you will facilitate communication and provide direction about the best means of accessing information.
10. Focus on the immediate reaction and needs of the individuals in crisis.
11. Write down specific contact numbers and instructions.
12. Inform them and check back with them as needed to see how they are doing.

As in all care settings, the nurse uses therapeutic communication strategies to impart this information and to provide support to family or friends as they process the information (**Box 31–7 ●**).

CRISIS COUNSELING   **Crisis counseling** is focused on brief solutions, focused interventions, and supportive care. During the course of a crisis, nurses should consider each individual's physical vulnerability and degree of emotional stability, with special emphasis on determining the client's risk for self-harm or potential for harming others. While prioritizing the safety of the client and others, the nurse should assess the client's perception of and response to the crisis, while also ensuring that the client's basic needs are met. The alarm reaction, anxiety, and fear may prevent the person from resting, sleeping, or eating. Important members of the healthcare team during a crisis may include the hospital chaplain or family minister, a grief counselor, a social worker, a child and family therapist, and a teacher. See **Box 31–8 ●** for an overview of the components of crisis counseling.

CRISIS INTERVENTION   A **crisis intervention** is an emergent approach to care that is intended to assist clients with recognizing a crisis situation and identifying and implementing an immediate, short-term solution. For the client, the ultimate goal of crisis intervention is restoration to a level of functioning that is at or above the level of the precrisis state. This approach often incorporates the client's family members and loved ones, as well as those individuals who are significant to the client in terms of providing social support. Depending on the circumstances, a crisis intervention also may include professionals from a variety of specialties, such as school guidance counselors, law enforcement or probation officers, rescue workers, and clergy members. Successful completion of a crisis intervention depends on the client's needs; for example, some crisis interventions may culminate in the client's receiving outpatient counseling or guidance, while others may require immediate hospital admission or transfer to a facility that provides treatment for clients with substance abuse disorders.

Box 31–8 ABCs of Crisis Counseling

ACHIEVE RAPPORT

In the first stage of crisis counseling, the nurse or therapist works to achieve rapport with the client by using therapeutic communication; in particular, attentive and reflective listening. Helping victims/clients clarify feelings and perceptions of the event first will help them vent initial emotions, lower their anxiety levels, and create an environment that will support building of the therapeutic relationship and development of a plan of care.

- Introduce yourself, your role.
- Ensure the client's immediate safety (physical and emotional).
- Be respectful. Ask the client's name, preferred way of being addressed.
- Use calm, consistent verbal and nonverbal communication.
- Use open-ended questions and clarifying questions.
- Assess immediate needs. For example, does the client take medication or need medical treatment?
- Identify the victim's feelings, reactions, and perceptions of the event.

BOIL DOWN THE PROBLEM (IDENTIFY, VALIDATE, AND INTERVENE)

At this stage, the nurse or therapist helps the client to identify the problem, providing validation and intervention. Communication with the client at this stage focuses on identifying the problem, assessing how the client is thinking and feeling about the problem, and the client's functional ability since the crisis event.

- Ask the client to describe what happened.
- Encourage the client to talk about the present.
- Assess for ongoing safety concerns (e.g., suicide, abuse, self-harm, substance abuse, physical or psychological illness).
- Ask what is the most pressing problem (one at a time).
- Identify how the client thinks and feels about the crisis.
- Ask whether the client has ever experienced a similar situation or crisis in the past. Assess what coping mechanisms were

successful or helpful. Look for opportunities to help the client regain control.

In some situations, clients may not have a previous experience and coping mechanisms that they can articulate. Giving clients small choices, such as asking what they would like to drink or if they would like to make a phone call, can help build their confidence.

Assessment and intervention will vary greatly depending on the client and the crisis. The safety assessment of a client with asthma following a natural disaster will be very different than the safety assessment of a client who is being abused by her partner.

COPE WITH THE PROBLEM (RESOLUTION AND REFERRAL)

At this stage, the nurse or therapist determines what is necessary to help the client cope with the problem. Maslow's hierarchy of needs is a good framework to use when prioritizing care for clients in crisis, focusing on basic needs of shelter, food, water, and physiological safety. For clients who are victims of violence, physiological and emotional safety needs will be very closely related. Consider both short- and long-term needs for resolution and referral.

- What does the client want to happen? Are the client's expectations realistic?
- What will help the client meet the most important need or address the most pressing problem?
- Help the client formulate an action plan and steps for follow-up. For example, following a natural disaster, help the client identify sources of shelter, food, and water.
- Support the client's need for validation, hope for the future. Use hopeful terms of a "new normal" or a "new reality."
- Arrange for follow-up with the client.
- Refer the client to resources that will help the client develop coping skills and manage the aftermath of the crisis.

Sources: Based on ABCD tip card developed by the Association of Traumatic Stress Specialists, *"Recognizing Standards of Excellence in Response, Treatment & Service,"* P.O. Box 2747, Georgetown, TX, 78627, 512-868-3677, 512-868-3678 fax, www.atss.info; Grice, R. (2010). *ABC model crisis counseling.* Retrieved from http://www.livinghealthy360.com/index.php/abc-model-crisis-counseling-16607; Mental Health Academy. (2012). *Crisis counseling: The ABC model.* Retrieved from http://www.mentalhealthacademy.net/video_details.php?catid=15.

Crisis intervention centers provide telephone consultation for clients in crisis. Some organizations also offer consultation by way of e-mail and online chatting. In most cases, call-in crisis intervention centers, also known as crisis hotlines, are staffed by trained volunteers who follow protocols to assist the client and who have professional consultation available to them, such as mental health counselors and psychologists. These 24-hour services allow callers to remain anonymous. For individuals who use crisis hotline services, primary goals include preventing the caller from inflicting harm directed at herself or others, giving the individual an opportunity to share her emotions and conflicts, and encouraging follow-up care with a local mental health professional if needed.

A step-by-step intervention is outlined in **Box 31–9** ●. A crisis connection provides a lifeline for the client in crisis and allows the nurse to determine immediate needs.

TEMPORARY RELOCATION Clients in crisis—in particular, those who are homeless and those who are subject to abuse—may require assistance with meeting one of the most basic needs: finding shelter. Nurses should be aware of community organizations and representatives who can assist clients with finding emergency living arrangements.

ALTERNATIVE THERAPY As discussed in the concept section of this module, the mind–body connection has been established through research. Elicitation of the stress response by way of cognitive appraisal of a stressor is a classic example of this connection. Building on this relationship, a holistic approach to nursing care acknowledges a connection between not only the mind and body, but also the spirit.

In the United States, results of a 2002 study revealed that prayer for self and prayer for others (intercessory prayer) are the two most common forms of alternative therapies implemented by adults when faced with illness (Barnes et al., 2004). Concerning the effects of prayer on healing and wellness, research is hindered

Box 31–9 Crisis Connection

1. Make contact and connect with the individual.
2. Assess immediate safety needs.
3. Determine thought processes.
4. Scan for physical distress.
5. Listen intently, supporting emotional reactions.
6. Explore perceptions of the crisis.
7. Identify coping strengths.
8. Develop a support plan and a follow-up plan.

by obvious limitations, including that the measurement of psychosocial wellness is largely subjective and, as such, is difficult to measure quantitatively. Moreover, the inclusion of treatments that are in addition to prayer, such as pharmacologic interventions, complicate the study of the effects of prayer alone. What is clear is that, among clients, prayer is a widely used approach in the quest for healing. For nurses, the implications of this finding include assessing and respecting the spiritual beliefs of each individual client, including those who are atheists.

■ NURSING PROCESS

The primary focus of a crisis intervention is to ensure the client's safety, as well as the safety of others. Once safety is established, the ideal goals include guiding the client to acknowledgment of the crisis state and assisting the client with identification of a resolution.

Assessment

The nurse systematically assesses the client in crisis, beginning with making contact and connecting with the client. The first part of the assessment is focused on the individual client and should include assessing the safety of the self or others (explore suicidal and homicidal intent, feelings of hopelessness or threat to self or others, and/or potential for violence). If necessary, to ensure the client's safety, emergent admission to a hospital or treatment center may be necessary. Ideally, assessment also includes interviewing the client's family or significant others.

Individual Assessment

During the assessment process, the nurse must also determine the client's thought processes, orientation, and ability to process information. Assessment of the client's physical condition includes any physical complaints and determining if the client is able to fulfill basic needs such as eating, rest, sleeping, and self-care. Due to the intensity of the fight-or-flight reaction, vulnerable individuals may be at risk for physical illness during a crisis.

Psychosocial assessment includes data collection about the client's perception of the precipitating event, impact of the crisis, and his ability to cope with the crisis. The nurse should also interview the client regarding his current and past coping methods, as well as his support system. Particularly for disaster survivors, the issue of survivor's guilt should be explored. For these clients, guilt may stem from the act of surviving while knowing others have died. Survivors may also harbor guilt as a result of the actions taken to allow for survival.

Scaling assessment questions involve asking the client to rate the severity of symptoms or problems. This allows the nurse to determine the perceptions of the client. For example, the nurse may ask, "Mr. Smith, on a scale of one to ten, with ten being absolutely intolerable, how would you score your distress right now?" Assessment information is prioritized on the basis of input from the individual. It is essential that the nurse be attuned to caring for individuals' basic needs in a crisis, such as eating, sleeping, resting, self-care, and physical stability.

It is important to remember that the expression of feelings and interpretations of an event are culturally influenced and must be considered within the context of the individual's life. Sociocultural factors greatly impact an individual's interpretation of a crisis or traumatic event, as well as her response to the

event. The client's interpretation of manifestations of the stress response, as well as her feelings about the appropriateness of seeking assistance, also are impacted by sociocultural factors. For example, among members of some cultures, persistent anxiety is considered to be a sign of weakness, as opposed to being a potential sign of a stress-related disorder. This belief is particularly prevalent among women in the Pacific Islander and Asian cultures; as a result, these women may not reach out for help until they enter a crisis stage (U.S. Department of Health and Human Services [USDHHS], Office on Women's Health, 2010).

Cultural competence extends beyond the identification of a client's cultural and ethnic background; it encompasses awareness of a client's health practices and beliefs and demonstrating respect for the client's preferences. However, the nurse also has a responsibility to identify health practices that may be detrimental to the client's well-being. Identification and evaluation of the client's culturally based health practices require sensitive, nonjudgmental exploration of the topic. For example, the client interview may include items such as "I want to try to understand how this experience may be affecting you. Will you please tell me more about how you feel?" and "How would you expect your family or close friends to react to a similar experience?"

Family Assessment

Traumatic experiences and crises also may impact the affected individual's interactions with family, friends, and significant others, particularly as they seek to help the client who is in distress. Likewise, those closest to the client may be well suited to offer insight as to her coping methods and the availability of social support. Inclusion of individuals who are most closely associated with the client may allow for more accurate assessment of the client's needs, as well as identification of potential stress-related concerns among those who are impacted by the client's crisis experience. The nurse should adhere to protocols regarding client confidentiality when incorporating others into the client's care.

Community Assessment

Nurses may be among the first civilians called on to offer assistance in the wake of a disaster. For the community faced with crisis, following triage and treatment of clients in need, the top priorities include assessment of living conditions and availability of basic resources, such as food, water, and shelter. Identification of the community's mental health and support resources, as well as the availability of financial and organizational resources (such as disaster assistance organizations), is also essential.

Diagnosis

Selection of nursing diagnoses depends on the client's crisis response and associated manifestations. Examples of nursing diagnoses that may be appropriate for inclusion in the nursing plan of care for a client in a state of crisis may include the following:

- *Risk for Self-Harm*
- *Risk for Injury*
- *Ineffective Self-Health Management*
- *Anxiety*
- *Ineffective Coping*
- *Social Isolation*

- *Impaired Social Interaction*
- *Post-Trauma Syndrome.*

(NANDA-I © 2012)

Planning

Planning involves the selection of realistic goals and identified outcomes that promote resolution of the selected nursing diagnoses. Examples of client goals and outcomes that may be relevant to the nursing care of a client in crisis may include the following:

- The client will remain free from injury or self-harm.
- The client will verbalize awareness of effective coping strategies.
- The client will identify and utilize his social support network.
- The client will request assistance from staff when necessary.
- The client will actively participate in counseling and group therapy activities as outlined by the primary care provider.
- The client will report a reduction in perceived anxiety.

Implementation

Establishment of trust and application of therapeutic communication techniques serve as the foundation for building a relationship with the client in crisis. Therapeutic communication incorporates verbal and nonverbal communication. Maintaining eye contact, nodding when appropriate, and avoiding distractions all signal genuine concern for the client. Paraphrasing and repeating the client's statements may also be useful for validating the nurse's understanding of the client and seeking clarification; for example, "I hear you saying that you feel like everything's a mess. Can you please share with me what that means to you?" or "I understand you feel anxious when you try to relax. Will you please tell me more about what happens when you try to rest?"

Although encouraging the expression of emotions is important, when appropriate, silence is also an effective communication tool. In addition to demonstrating respect for the client's privacy and willingness to share, periods of silence also allow the client to reflect on her thoughts and emotions in order to more effectively express them. The nurse should avoid minimizing the

---

Box 31–10 Some Do's and Don'ts of Crisis Communication

DO SAY:

- "These are normal reactions to an abnormal situation."
- "It is understandable that you feel this way."
- "It wasn't your fault; you did the best you could."
- "I am sorry that this happened."
- "Things will get better, and you will feel better, although they may never be the same again."

DON'T SAY:

- "It could have been worse."
- "You can always get another pet/car/house [or have another child, get married again, etc.]."
- "It's best if you just stay busy."
- "I know just how you feel."
- "You need to get on with your life."
- "If I were you, I would . . ."

Source: Adapted from USDHHS, Substance Abuse and Mental Health Services Administration. (2007). *Disaster counseling.* Retrieved from http://www.samhsa.gov.

---

client's feelings or offering false reassurances of hope. See **Box 31–10** ● for examples of statements that may be appropriate for inclusion during communication with clients in crisis, as well as for examples of statements that should be avoided.

Evaluation

Expected outcomes that may be appropriate for the client experiencing a crisis include:

- The client determines strengths and resources available to assist with crisis management.
- The client accurately perceives and describes events occurring as a result of crisis.
- The client creates a plan of action to cope with the crisis.
- The client verbalizes a feeling of control over managing the crisis.

NURSING CARE PLAN   A Client in Crisis

ASSESSMENT	DIAGNOSES	PLANNING
Deborah Smith is a 30-year-old African American woman who comes to the emergency department following a fall down the stairs outside her apartment. She breaks down in tears during the assessment. Not only is her ankle painful and swollen, but the father of her two small children has recently been arrested for nearly killing his girlfriend. She has no idea when he will be able to pay child support again, and she is afraid she will not be able to return to work at her job as a waitress if her ankle is sprained. The physical assessment reveals the following: ■ Vital signs include temperature 90.0°F oral; pulse 96 bpm; respirations 18/min; and BP 136/86 mmHg. ■ Hands are trembling, client is tearful and crying ■ Circular scars noted on both forearms the size of pencil erasers ■ Left ankle is edematous and painful to touch, unable to perform range of motion in ankle ■ Abrasions on the palm of the right hand, left elbow, and both knees.	Nursing diagnoses applicable to the plan of care for Ms. Smith include the following: ■ *Acute Pain* ■ *Anxiety* ■ *Risk for Caregiver Role Strain* ■ *Risk for Compromised Resilience.* (NANDA-I © 2012)	Nursing goals for Ms. Smith's care include: ■ Identify community resources that can provide assistance until Ms. Smith can return to work. ■ Identify Ms. Smith's strengths in terms of available resources and family support. ■ Manage pain to allow Ms. Smith to maintain comfort. ■ Teach client crutch walking and self-care for injured ankle.

(continued on next page)

NURSING CARE PLAN (continued)

IMPLEMENTATION

- Encourage Ms. Smith to express her feelings.
- Ask Ms. Smith whom she can look to for help. Are the children's grandparents supportive? Does she have a supportive spiritual community? Does her workplace have a sick leave policy? Are there resources within the community that can provide support and assistance?
- Provide referral to the hospital's department of social services to determine potential community resources.

- Encourage Ms. Smith to identify her strengths that can help her resolve her current crisis.
- Establish a follow-up plan for both Ms. Smith's physical as well as psychosocial needs.
- Provide teaching on care of ankle injury, symptoms to report to provider immediately, crutch walking, and wound care.

EVALUATION

Social services assisted Ms. Smith in obtaining unemployment insurance during her medical leave of absence and provided anticipatory guidance to help her retain her job until she was able to return. Ms. Smith developed a stronger relationship with her church community who assisted in picking up the children from school, delivered meals, and helped to perform tasks such as laundry that Ms. Smith could not perform with limited mobility.

CRITICAL THINKING

1. If you were the nurse caring for Ms. Smith and lived in the same community, would it be appropriate for you to offer to provide home care for her and the children when you had time available? Why or why not?
2. Is it appropriate for you, as the nurse caring for Ms. Smith, to solve problems for her? Explain your answer.
3. What functions can social service provide to help clients in crisis like Ms. Smith?

REVIEW Crisis

RELATE Link the Concepts and Exemplars

Linking the exemplar of crisis with the concept of addiction:

1. When a crisis results from addiction behavior, what is the nurse's priority intervention? Explain your answer.
2. When a client's spouse is demonstrating addiction behavior that has caused the client's crisis, what community referrals might you consider suggesting to help the client?

Linking the exemplar of crisis with the concept of culture and diversity:

3. Why might one series of events trigger a crisis for one client but not another?
4. How do coping strategies differ during times of crisis for clients from vulnerable populations versus those who are less vulnerable? How would your nursing interventions differ for each client?

READY Go to Companion Skills Manual

REFER Go to Pearson Nursing Student Resources
nursing.pearsonhighered.com

- Additional review materials

REFLECT Case Study

Carol Holland is a 51-year-old mother of three. She is a nurse educator and works full time at a community college. Her son Paul recently moved back to live with her to attend college full time. Along with Paul, Mrs. Holland lives with her husband Tom and their other son Mike. Her oldest and only daughter Angela lives in an apartment nearby. The Hollands receive a call in the wee hours of the morning. One of Mike's friends tells them that Mike has been in a terrible accident, and they need to come to the hospital immediately. Arriving at the trauma unit at 3:00 a.m., the Hollands and their son Paul enter the satellite unit. Mike is intubated and requires mechanical ventilation. Mrs. Holland scans Mike's motionless body for signs of independent life, but he is motionless. His face is so swollen that he is nearly unrecognizable to her. What appears to be a blue cable cord holds together a laceration that encompasses most of his head. His left arm is swollen three times its size, and is blue and seeping from lacerations. As Paul collapses in a nearby chair and begins weeping, the nurse quietly gathers vital information from Mrs. Holland. She directs Mike's family to the lounge where they will wait during a procedure to insert a ventricular shunt. The neurosurgeon is unsure Mike will survive the night.

1. What type of crisis is this family experiencing?
2. Given the information presented thus far, which nursing diagnoses might be applicable?
3. List possible psychosocial interventions.
4. List specific interventions for this family.
5. What basic needs might this family require throughout the night?

EXEMPLAR 31.3 Obsessive-Compulsive Disorder

EXEMPLAR KEY TERMS
Compulsion, 1935
Hoarding, 1936
Obsession, 1935
Obsessive-compulsive disorder (OCD), 1935

EXEMPLAR LEARNING OUTCOMES
After reading about this exemplar, you will be able to:

1. Describe the pathophysiology, etiology, clinical manifestations, and direct and indirect causes of obsessive-compulsive disorder (OCD).

2. Identify risk factors and prevention methods associated with OCD.

3. Illustrate the nursing process in providing culturally competent care across the life span for individuals with OCD.

4. Formulate priority nursing diagnoses appropriate for an individual with OCD.

5. Summarize therapies used by interdisciplinary teams in the collaborative care of an individual with OCD.

6. Plan evidence-based care for an individual with OCD and his or her family in collaboration with other members of the healthcare team.

7. Evaluate expected outcomes for an individual with OCD.

▶ OVERVIEW

Obsessive-compulsive disorder (OCD) is a disabling disorder characterized by obsessive thoughts and compulsive, repetitive behaviors that dominate an individual's life. An **obsession** is a recurrent, unwanted, and often distressing thought or image that leads to feelings of fear and anxiety. A **compulsion** is a repetitive behavior or mental activity (such as counting) used in response to the obsessive thoughts to help the individual lower his or her anxiety level (APA, 2013). To be diagnosed with OCD, the individual must experience distress and lose time (more than 1 hour a day) due to the consuming rituals and repetitive behaviors associated with the disorder (APA, 2013).

▶ PATHOPHYSIOLOGY AND ETIOLOGY

Conducting a review of recent research on OCD, Grados and Wilcox (2007) report that significant gains have been made in the past decade. A specific gene has not yet been isolated, but epidemiological studies with families and twins strongly support a genetic linkage. The neurobiology of OCD also suggests that the frontosubcortical regions are affected. Abnormal neuroimaging in the basal ganglia and the orbitofrontal cortex has been found in individuals with OCD. Biochemical studies implicate dysregulation of serotonin in the etiology of OCD (Townsend, 2009), and a recent study conducted by German scientists suggests that both environmental and genetic factors strongly influence the disorder (Walitza et al., 2008).

Studies conducted by the surgeon general (2008), as well as other researchers, suggest that the development of OCD in children may be linked to streptococcal infection (Swedo, Leckman, & Rose, 2012).

Lifespan Considerations
OCD in Childhood and Adolescence

Current research suggests that some children with OCD develop the condition after experiencing one type of streptococcal infection (Swedo et al., 2012). Initially referred to by the acronym PANDAS, which stands for pediatric autoimmune neuropsychiatric disorders associated with streptococcal infections, researchers have proposed revision of this condition to pediatric acute-onset neuropsychiatric syndrome (PANS). Its hallmark is a sudden and abrupt exacerbation of OCD symptoms after a strep infection. The cause of this form of OCD appears to be antibodies mistakenly attacking a region of the brain. The SSRIs appear effective in alleviating symptoms of OCD in children. Several randomized, controlled trials revealed SSRIs to be effective in treating children and adolescents with OCD. CBT has been used to treat OCD, but the evidence is not conclusive.

Diagnosis of OCD may be challenging for those who are untrained or uninformed about the disease. It is also made difficult by the variances that occur in the disorder, which are explained in detail in the Clinical Manifestations section. Contamination obsessions combined with washing and cleaning compulsions are probably the best-known variance of the disorder.

Etiology

Approximately 2.2 million Americans have OCD (NIMH, 2009). Obsessive-compulsive disorder typically begins in adolescence or early adulthood, although some cases do begin in childhood. It affects men and women equally, but men develop the disorder earlier. Among males, approximately 25% of those with OCD demonstrate onset before 10 years of age (APA, 2013). Without treatment, the rate of remission is estimated to be low. However, for individuals who experience childhood onset of OCD, approximately 40% may experience remission by the time they reach early adulthood (APA, 2013).

Risk Factors

Risk factors for OCD include having a first-degree relative with the disorder. A history of childhood sexual or physical abuse also increases the risk, as does exposure to other stressful or traumatic events during childhood (APA, 2013).

▶ CLINICAL MANIFESTATIONS

Obsessive-compulsive disorder is not to be confused with *obsessive-compulsive personality disorder*. The clinical manifestations of the personality disorder involve more of a preoccupation with perfection and are characterized by inflexibility.

The most frequently reported obsessions in OCD are repeated thoughts about contamination from shaking hands, repeated doubts with fear of having hurt someone or leaving a door unlocked, and a need to have things in a certain order. Aggressive impulses are often of a sexual nature or obscene. The obsessions are not rational or real-life problems. The client with OCD is, at some point, aware that the obsessions are not real (APA, 2013).

Compulsions are also part of OCD. Commonly reported repetitive behaviors include hand washing, ordering, checking, and counting. Common themes of the associated intrusive, repetitive thoughts include those which are considered by the individual to be forbidden or taboo; for example, religious or sexual obsessions and fears related to self-harm or injury of others (APA, 2013). For additional examples of commonly occurring obsessions and their related compulsions, see **Table 31–9** ●. Compulsive behavior does not produce a sense of pleasure for the client with OCD. Rather, the individual feels driven to perform the compulsion to reduce the anxiety produced by the obsession.

TABLE 31–9 Examples of Commonly Occurring Obsessions and Compulsions

OBSESSION	ASSOCIATED COMPULSIONS
Symmetry	■ Counting ■ Ensuring orderliness of items ■ Fixation on maintaining symmetrical positioning of items
Cleaning	■ Repetitive environmental cleaning ■ Avoiding contamination ■ Repetitive performance of decontamination practices
Forbidden or taboo thoughts	■ Acting out aggressive or sexual behavior toward self or others ■ Conducting religious behaviors or practices that are incongruent with the accepted norm for a particular religious group or community (e.g., repeated recitation of prayers to the extent that the activity interferes with daily life)
Injury	■ Extreme avoidance of activities or circumstances that may cause injury
Hoarding	■ Excessive collection and accumulation of objects ■ Extreme cluttering of the living environment ■ Lack of insight with regard to the embarrassment of family members or others whose living space is impacted by the appearance of the home environment ■ Often associated with reluctance or refusal by family members to allow outsiders to enter the home, leading to social isolation

Sources: Data from American Psychiatric Association (APA). (2013). *Diagnostic and statistical manual of mental disorders* (5th ed.). Arlington, VA: Author; Duckworth, J., & Freedman, J. L. (2012). *Obsessive-compulsive disorder.* Retrieved from http://www.nami.org/Template.cfm?Section=By_Illness&Template=/ContentManagement/ContentDisplay.cfm&ContentID=142546; and Fontaine, K. L. (2009). *Mental health nursing* (6th ed.). Upper Saddle River, NJ: Pearson.

▶ COLLABORATION

When caring for the client with OCD, the nurse may collaborate with a variety of healthcare team members, including primary care physicians, psychiatrists, psychologists, and counselors. Community and school agencies may also collaborate in the care of these individuals. Because the impact of OCD can range from mild to disabling, the client's needs will vary.

The most common therapy for OCD is pharmacologic, followed by psychotherapies. In particular, CBT has proven to be useful for clients with OCD. Using CBT, the affected individual is gradually exposed to the object of his or her obsession

Clinical Manifestations and Therapies **Obsessive-Compulsive Disorder**

ETIOLOGY	CLINICAL MANIFESTATIONS	CLINICAL THERAPIES
Aggressive, sexual, and religious obsessions with checking compulsions	■ Checks doors, locks, appliances, written work. ■ Confesses frequently (to anything). ■ Needs to ask others repeatedly for assurance.	Pharmacologic therapies include SSRIs: ■ fluoxetine (Prozac) ■ sertraline (Zoloft) ■ fluvoxamine (Luvox) ■ paroxetine (Paxil)
Symmetry obsessions with ordering, arranging, and repeating compulsions	■ Needs to have objects in fixed and symmetrical positions. ■ Repeats movements, such as going in and out of doorways, getting in and out of chairs, touching objects. ■ Counts or spells silently or aloud.	■ Antipsychotic medications such as risperidone (Risperdal) may be helpful for those who do not respond to SSRIs. ■ Cognitive behavior therapy may include *desensitization therapy* in which the person is carefully exposed over a period of time to an object that promotes fear. For example, the therapist and client may, at an appropriate time, agree that the client will touch the door knob. ■ Other therapies; for example, *deep brain stimulation* may be helpful to those who are treatment resistant.
Contamination obsessions with washing and cleaning compulsions	■ Repeatedly washes hands, showers, bathes, brushes teeth. ■ Cleans personal space frequently.	
Hoarding, saving, and collecting symptoms	■ Compulsively acquires items. ■ Has difficulty discarding items. ■ Lives with extreme clutter.	

Box 31–11 Guideline Summary for the Treatment of Individuals With Obsessive-Compulsive Disorder

PSYCHIATRIC MANAGEMENT

OCD is usually a chronic illness. Treatment is necessary when the symptoms interfere with functioning or cause significant distress. Therapeutic management consists of a variety of therapeutic interventions throughout the course of the illness.

PSYCHIATRIC ASSESSMENT

The psychiatrist will usually consider a medical evaluation and assessment of common comorbid conditions, such as depression, bipolar symptoms, other anxiety disorders, tics, impulse-control disorders, anorexia nervosa, bulimia nervosa, alcohol use, attention-deficit/hyperactivity disorder, and a history of panic attacks.

PHARMACOLOGIC TREATMENT

- Clomipramine, fluoxetine, fluvoxamine, paroxetine, and sertraline are approved by the FDA for treatment of OCD. The SSRIs have fewer side effects than clomipramine and are recommended for the first medication trial.
- Successful medication treatment should be continued for 1–2 years before gradually tapering and while observing for symptom exacerbation.

PSYCHOTHERAPY

CBT that relies primarily on behavioral techniques such as exposure and response prevention (ERP) is recommended because it has the best evidentiary support. Family therapy may reduce interfamily tensions due to the individual's OCD symptoms.

Sources: Adapted from the National Guideline Clearinghouse. (2007). *Practice guideline for the treatment of patients with obsessive-compulsive disorder.* Retrieved from http://www.guideline.gov/content.aspx?id=11078; and American Psychiatric Association. (2007). *Practice guideline for the treatment of patients with obsessive compulsive disorder* (p. 570). Arlington, VA: Author.

or fear and is taught healthy methods of coping with the associated anxiety (Mayo Clinic, 2010). The National Guideline Clearinghouse guidelines for treatment of OCD are summarized in **Box 31–11** ●.

Diagnostic Tests

No definitive laboratory findings have been identified for diagnosing OCD. Abnormal laboratory findings have been noted in groups of individuals with OCD in comparison to control groups.

Pharmacologic Therapy

For the client with OCD, SSRIs are often prescribed as part of the treatment regimen. Clomipramine, which is a tricyclic antidepressant (TCA), also may be administered (Mayo Clinic, 2010). While the SSRIs tend to have fewer side effects than do the TCAs, all medications carry risks and potential adverse effects. The nurse's role includes educating the client about the safe administration of medications, as well as the potential side effects.

Nonpharmacologic Therapy

Psychotherapy is an integral component of treatment for the client with OCD. In addition to focusing on the client, therapy and counseling sessions may include the client's family members or significant others. In particular, CBT, which involves restructuring thought patterns and behaviors, has been found to be effective for these clients (Mayo Clinic, 2010). For a discussion of CBT, refer to the concept section of this module.

◼ NURSING PROCESS

The primary nursing goals for the client with OCD are to ensure client safety and to alleviate anxiety and distress. Care must be taken not to prevent the performance of rituals that the client uses to reduce anxiety, but rather to promote new behavioral patterns and coping mechanisms to make the rituals unnecessary while maintaining the safety of the client.

Assessment

The nursing assessment interviews of clients with OCD share many similarities to those used with clients who have other anxiety disorders. A thorough physical examination may determine physical problems resulting from manifestations of OCD. For example, excessive hand washing or the use of irritating cleansing agents may result in loss of tissue integrity.

Diagnosis

Appropriate nursing diagnoses for OCD may vary depending on the nature of the obsessive thoughts and compulsive behaviors and the severity of the illness. The presence of comorbid or co-occurring disorders must also be taken into consideration. For example, a hoarder who has allergic asthma may be at risk for ineffective airway clearance and ineffective breathing pattern due to the presence of dust and debris in the house. Possible diagnoses for OCD clients include the following:

- *Anxiety*
- *Fear*
- *Ineffective Coping*
- *Stress Overload*
- *Disturbed Sleep Pattern*
- *Insomnia*
- *Fatigue*
- *Deficient Knowledge*
- *Risk for Caregiver Role Strain.*

(NANDA-I © 2012)

Planning

Planning in collaboration with the client should be prioritized according to what the client identifies as most important and may include the following goals:

- The client will identify triggers for obsessive-compulsive behaviors.
- The client will create a quiet, restful environment.
- The client will learn to identify strengths that can be used to reorder thinking in order to reduce obsessive-compulsive behaviors.

Assessment Interview Obsessive-Compulsive Disorder

Current and Past Medical History

- Does anyone in your family suffer from an anxiety disorder?
- Have you experienced intrusive or unwanted thoughts? Please describe the nature of the unwanted thoughts.
- Do you find yourself performing repetitive actions and behaviors to alleviate your anxiety? Please describe.
- Describe how these compulsions have interfered with your life.
- How old where you when you first experienced these obsessive-compulsive thoughts and behaviors? Age of diagnosis?
- Approximately how much time out of your day is interrupted by dealing with these obsessions and compulsions?
- On a scale of 0–10, please rate your current level of distress (0 = no distress, 10 = intolerable anxiety).
- What have you tried in the past to alleviate the anxiety? What do you think was successful?

- Describe any repetitive or ritualistic behaviors.
- Do you use counting when feeling anxious?
- Have you experienced depression? Have you considered suicide? If yes, please rate on a scale from 0 to 10 how likely you are to act on these thoughts or impulses (0 = not at all, 10 = I will kill myself).
- Do you drink or use illicit drugs to manage your anxiety? If so, please list name, frequency, and amount.

Activities of Daily Living

- Is your health at risk as a result of the obsessions and compulsions?
- Describe a typical day (sleep, eating, activities, employment).
- How has this disorder affected your relationships?
- How has this disorder affected your spirituality?
- How has this disorder affected you emotional well-being and mental health?

- The client will recognize that continued obsessive-compulsive behaviors are not an indication of treatment failure and that reductions in behavior signify positive progress.

Implementation

A supportive and nonjudgmental demeanor is essential when working with clients with OCD. Often the individual is aware that the compulsive behaviors are unreasonable and feels embarrassed. Compulsive behaviors are designed to lower the level of anxiety or defensively "undo" the obsessive thoughts. Interrupting an individual during a ritual or compulsive behavior creates more anxiety and frequently leads to redoing or repeating the behavior to reduce anxiety. Working with the client to fit the ritual into the routine of the hospital may be necessary until relief is experienced from the pharmacologic agents or CBT. Administration of medications to lower anxiety and reevaluation of the client's response to the medication are the responsibility of the nurse in collaboration with the healthcare provider and the client.

Evaluation

Client response to nursing care may be evaluated by using the following expected outcomes:

Client Teaching Adaptive Coping

Establishing a therapeutic relationship provides the nurse with an opportunity to promote healthy adaptive coping. Client teaching about the nature of obsessive thinking is critical to lowering the client's feelings of shame and anxiety. The nurse can help the client realize that fears of hurting or killing family members arise from the *disease*, not from any actual desire of the client to harm others. Nurses can help clients reframe how they think about their disease and help them reframe thought processes in order to reduce ritual performance, such as helping the client meditate versus performing a ritual and then recognizing that nothing bad happened as a result of the absence of the ritual. The nurse has an essential role in helping the client with OCD understand that he or she can decrease anxiety and gain control over the disease through pharmacologic and behavior therapies.

- The client reports a reduction in the performance of ritualistic compulsive behaviors.
- The client demonstrates adequate coping skills to control anxiety related to the absence of ritualistic compulsive behaviors.

REVIEW Obsessive-Compulsive Disorder

RELATE Link the Concepts and Exemplars

Linking the exemplar of obsessive-compulsive disorder with the concept of mood and affect:

1. How might mood be impacted in the client who is unable to control his ritualistic compulsive disorders?

2. Is assessment for suicidal ideation important when admitting a new client with OCD? Why or why not?

Linking the exemplar of obsessive-compulsive disorder with the concept of advocacy:

3. If a client's rituals involve an act that places her in danger, what actions can the nurse take to advocate for the client while not causing increased anxiety that can result from not being able to perform the ritual?

4. While working on a medical unit in a local hospital you admit an adult client for surgery. While collecting the admission

assessment you note what you suspect is ritualistic compulsive behavior. How can you best advocate for this client?

READY Go to Companion Skills Manual

REFER Go to Pearson Nursing Student Resources **nursing.pearsonhighered.com**

- Additional review materials

REFLECT Case Study

Karleen Lassiter, a married, 40-year-old mother of three children, is admitted to a hospital psychiatric unit with complaints of anxiety, inability to relax, and intrusive thoughts that she states are "horrific." When asked to describe her thoughts, she states, "I'm afraid I'm going to hell as punishment for what goes through my mind sometimes. It's really dark stuff." In conjunction with her intrusive thoughts, Ms. Lassiter recites the same prayer up to 50 times daily. Ms. Lassiter is trained as a respiratory therapist, but she has not practiced in the clinical setting for the past 5 years. In part, she reports that her departure from her position as a respiratory therapist was related to her need to complete her prayer rituals. Ms. Lassiter explains that her employment was terminated due to her being late for work on several occasions, because "I needed to finish praying before I could leave for work." She is aware that her behavior is irrational and that it is negatively impacting her life; however, she is unable to control or cease the behavior.

Ms. Lassiter's medical history includes panic attacks between the ages of 18 and 21, during college enrollment. She denies suicidal ideation; however, she states, "I don't think I can handle living like this. My husband and kids think I'm crazy, and they're right."

1. Based on the available assessment data, identify Ms. Lassiter's apparent obsessions and compulsions.

2. Describe appropriate communication strategies for encouraging Ms. Lassiter to further describe her intrusive thoughts.

3. Based on the client's statements, identify the priority nursing diagnosis for Ms. Lassiter.

EXEMPLAR 31.4 **Phobias**

EXEMPLAR KEY TERMS
Agoraphobia, *1940*
External locus of control, *1940*
Internal locus of control, *1940*
Locus of control, *1940*
Phobia, *1939*
Social anxiety disorder, *1941*
Specific phobia, *1940*

EXEMPLAR LEARNING OUTCOMES
After reading about this exemplar, you will be able to:

1. Describe the pathophysiology, etiology, clinical manifestations, and direct and indirect causes of phobias.

2. Identify risk factors and prevention methods associated with phobias.

3. Illustrate the nursing process in providing culturally competent care across the life span for individuals with phobias.

4. Formulate priority nursing diagnoses appropriate for an individual with a phobia.

5. Summarize therapies used by interdisciplinary teams in the collaborative care of an individual with a phobia.

6. Plan evidence-based care for an individual with a phobia and his or her family in collaboration with other members of the healthcare team.

7. Evaluate expected outcomes for an individual with a phobia.

▶ OVERVIEW

A **phobia** is defined as an intense, persistent, irrational fear of a simple thing or social situation that compels the individual to avoid the stressor that elicits the fear. The stressor can be anything; needles and syringes, airplanes, spiders, dogs, closed areas, performing, and social activities are a few examples. The individual with a phobic disorder will experience severe panic upon contact with the stressor. The intensity of the fear drives the individual to avoid the situation at all costs. Adults suffering from a phobic disorder are aware that the fear is irrational; children are not always able to make that distinction.

The maladaptive coping mechanism associated with phobias is the defensive mechanism known as displacement. The individual's unconscious, unresolved emotional issues are symbolically placed on the external object or situation. The individual moderates his or her anxiety by avoiding the object of fear. To be classified as a disorder, the phobia must be severe enough to interfere with the individual's daily functioning.

▶ PATHOPHYSIOLOGY AND ETIOLOGY

The complex neurochemical and neuroendocrine systems are the focus of recent research studies linking dysregulation of neurotransmitters to anxiety disorders such as phobias. According to Antai-Otang (2008), recent data suggest that the dysregulation of three major neurotransmitters, norepinephrine (NE), serotonin (5-HT), and gamma aminobutyric acid (GABA), is implicated in the origin of anxiety disorders.

Etiology

In the United States, an estimated 5%–10% of the population is affected by some type of phobia. Less conservative estimates suggest that up to 25% of the population may demonstrate some type of phobia (Sadock & Sadock, 2008). The causes of specific phobias have not yet been determined. Evidence suggests that the development of certain phobias may run in families (Sadock & Sadock, 2008). If the feared situation can be avoided, people with specific phobias often do not seek treatment. It is when daily functioning is jeopardized that individuals most often seek help.

Risk Factors

According to the Mayo Clinic (2009), risk factors for developing phobias include the following:

- *Age.* Social anxiety disorder (formerly known as social phobia) typically develops between the ages of 11 and 15 and almost never after the age of 25. Situational phobias generally develop by the mid-20s.
- *Gender.* Girls and women are twice as likely to develop phobias as men, although this figure may be slightly skewed because men are less likely to seek help for anxiety disorders.
- *Family.* Individuals are at higher risk of developing a phobia if an immediate family member has the phobia.

An additional factor predisposing individuals to anxiety and phobias is an external locus of control. Lazarus and Folkman (1984) describe **locus of control** as the extent to which an individual believes he has control over the events in his life. Individuals with an **internal locus of control** believe their actions, choices, and behaviors impact life events. Those with an **external locus of control** believe that powers outside of themselves, such as luck or fate, determine life events.

According to the APA (2013), factors that may predispose an individual to development of a phobia include the following:

- Traumatic events (e.g., animal attack, being trapped in an elevator)
- Witnessing others as they experience traumatic events
- Unexpected panic attacks while in a specific environment (e.g., experiencing a panic attack while traveling via airplane, which may lead to subsequent panic attacks in relationship to air travel)
- Exposure to extensive reports of traumatic events (e.g., media coverage of terrorist attacks, plane crashes, environmental disasters, or natural disasters).

▶ CLINICAL MANIFESTATIONS

Primary categories of phobias include specific phobias, agoraphobia, and social anxiety disorder (formerly known as *social phobia*).

Specific phobia refers to intense or extreme fear with regard to a particular object or situation. The object or situation that triggers the fear is referred to as the *phobic stimulus*. Both actual and anticipated exposure to the phobic stimulus may evoke a response, the intensity of which may vary from the sudden onset of fear to an incapacitating panic attack (APA, 2013). Examples of specific phobias are presented in **Table 31–10** ●.

Phobias adversely impact the affected individual's quality of social, occupational, and academic function and also interfere with activities of daily living. In many cases, adults with phobias recognize their fear as being disproportionate to the given

TABLE 31–10   Examples of Specific Phobias

SPECIFIC PHOBIA	ASSOCIATED FEAR
Acrophobia	Heights
Arachnophobia	Spiders
Aviophobia	Flying
Claustrophobia	Enclosed spaces
Hematophobia	Blood
Hydrophobia	Water
Nyctophobia	Darkness, nighttime

object or situation; however, they are prone to overestimating the degree of danger associated with the phobic stimulus. These clients usually practice *active avoidance* of the phobic stimulus, meaning that they minimize or avoid contact with it (APA, 2013).

Specific phobias frequently are comorbid with numerous other psychiatric alterations, including depressive disorders, anxiety disorders, bipolar disorders, and substance-related disorders.

Agoraphobia is characterized by anxiety associated with two or more of the following situations: being in enclosed spaces, being in open spaces, utilizing public transportation, being in a crowd or standing in a line of people, or being alone outside the home environment (APA, 2013). Anxiety related to the triggering circumstances is linked to a fear of the inability to escape or a fear that needed assistance may not be available in the event that panic-related symptoms develop. Alternatively, the client with agoraphobia may fear the development of other potentially embarrassing or debilitating manifestations. Most clients with agoraphobia also meet the criteria for diagnosis of other forms of mental illness (APA, 2013). **Figure 31–8** ● depicts a woman who is fearful of leaving her home environment.

As with most other behaviors, an individual's choice to remain inside the home environment is impacted by cultural influences. Additionally, in some cultures, remaining inside the

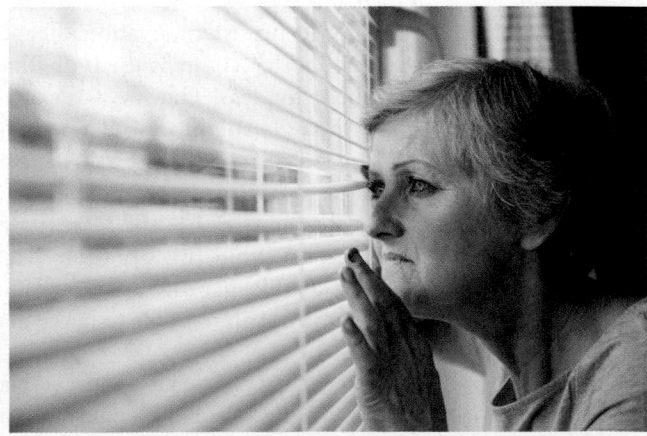

Figure 31–8 ● People with agoraphobia do not feel safe outside their own homes.

Source: Halfpoint/Shutterstock.

Clinical Manifestations and Therapies Phobias

TYPES OF PHOBIAS	CLINICAL MANIFESTATIONS	CLINICAL THERAPIES
Agoraphobia	■ Fear of places or situations where the individual feels unable to readily escape	The short-term use of antianxiety agents, such as the benzodiazepines, may be indicated in severe cases (should not be used more than 2–4 weeks). SSRIs may be used for longer periods. Tricyclic antidepressants are also recommended.
Social anxiety disorder (social phobia)	■ Fear of being criticized or ridiculed by others	Psychological therapies include:
Specific phobias	■ Unreasonable fear triggered by the presence of an object or dreaded situation (e.g., animals, insects, performing)	■ CBT ■ Supportive therapy ■ Desensitization and implosion therapy for specific phobias ■ Self-help groups and bibliotherapy (therapy that incorporates written forms of expression) based on CBT. ■ Discuss exercise and healthy nutrition. Phobic clients should decrease caffeine and nicotine intake. Assess alcohol intake.

Sources: Data from Mayo Clinic. (2009). *Phobias.* Retrieved from http://www.mayoclinic.com/health/phobias/DS00272; American Psychiatric Association. (2013). *Diagnostic and statistical manual of mental disorders* (5th ed.). Arlington, VA: Author; and Kneisl, C. R., & Trigoboff, E. (2013) *Contemporary psychiatric–mental health nursing* (3rd ed.). Upper Saddle River, NJ: Pearson Education.

home and limiting public social interaction may be a cultural expectation. Adherence to cultural expectations to remain inside one's home typically does not reflect agoraphobia.

Social anxiety disorder, formerly known as social phobia, is characterized by a pervasive, extreme fear of one or more social situations that may lead to scrutiny by others. Exposure to the particular situation (such as giving a speech, drinking or eating in the presence of others, or meeting strangers) usually triggers an immediate anxiety reaction. Although adolescents and adults usually recognize their fear as being excessive, pediatric clients do not always have this insight. Most clients with social anxiety disorder will avoid their phobic stimulus; however, some affected individuals will endure the experiences, despite an intense sense of anxiety or fear.

Typically, the anxiety, fear, or avoidant behaviors associated with social anxiety disorder persist for at least 6 months. Diagnosis of this disorder is made only if marked distress is present or if the individual's related anxiety, fear, or avoidance behaviors significantly interfere with her daily routine or occupational, academic, or social life. Affected individuals may also demonstrate inadequate attempts at assertiveness or excessively submissive behaviors. Less commonly, these clients may demonstrate excessive control of conversations (APA, 2013).

The physical symptoms associated with social anxiety disorder typically correlate with anxiety, and may include blushing, stammering speech, excessive sweating, and gastrointestinal distress. Some individuals may choose to self-medicate with drugs or alcohol prior to exposure to their phobic stimulus. Because of the limitations imposed by this disorder, establish-

ment and maintenance of friendships and interpersonal relationships may be extremely challenging.

▶ COLLABORATION

Short-term goals of care for clients with phobias include assisting the individual with learning strategies for successfully coping with the anxiety produced by the triggering object, event, or situation. Long-term goals include facilitating the collaborative care of these clients, which may include pharmacologic interventions and psychotherapy.

Pharmacologic Therapy

Pharmacologic therapy options for the phobic client include benzodiazepines, SSRIs, and some antipsychotics. Because of their addictive qualities, benzodiazepines should be used for only a short period of time. Benzodiazepines work rapidly to alleviate emotional distress and induce relaxation. The level of distress with phobias and panic is severe and readily alters the quality of life for the individual. A short course of benzodiazepines may sufficiently reduce anxiety to allow the client to begin participation in psychotherapy where the client can learn new ways of coping with anxieties. Clients who need pharmacologic support for a longer period of time may benefit from the use of SSRIs, which have fewer side effects than antipsychotics.

American culture has become a culture of immediate gratification. Pharmaceutical advertisements promoting chemicals for everything from headaches to anxiety, pain, and constipation are everywhere. The suggestion that human dis-

TABLE 31–11   Application of Cognitive-Behavioral Techniques in the Treatment of Clients With Phobias

TECHNIQUE	DESCRIPTION	EXAMPLE
Cognitive restructuring	Application of learned reframing/reinterpretation of anxiety- or fear-provoking stimuli to reduce the associated anxiety and fear.	A client who is terrified of thunder recognizes that thunder, in and of itself, poses no threat to life and that he is not at risk for harm as a result of the sound of thunder.
Systematic desensitization (exposure therapy)	Through exposure to situations that elicit increasing levels of anxiety, the client is desensitized to a given stimulus.	A client who is terrified of spiders is interviewed with regard to his fear. Next, the client is engaged in discussions about spiders until she is able to discuss them without extreme anxiety. The client is then exposed to photographs of spiders until she is able to complete the activity without extreme anxiety. Finally, the client is exposed to an actual spider, with the goal being that she may be so exposed without a sense of panic, fear, or anxiety.
Reciprocal inhibition	The phobic stimulus is combined with a stimulus that evokes a response that counteracts the undesired response.	The client who fears using public transportation uses biofeedback training to reduce his fear and anxiety while traveling on a public railway system.

comfort should be obliterated by chemicals and medication is epidemic and contributes to the addictive nature of contemporary society. Healthier coping mechanisms have taken a back seat to immediate gratification through chemistry. It is critical that the nurse working with a client with a phobia explain the importance of cognitive-behavioral therapy as a treatment for the client's phobia and that any medication used as treatment will be less effective if not used in combination with CBT.

Nonpharmacologic Therapy

Cognitive-behavioral therapy has demonstrated a high degree of success when used in the treatment of clients with anxiety disorders. (For discussion of CBT, see the concept section of this module.) **Table 31–11** • provides an overview

of CBT techniques that may be applicable to the care of clients with phobias.

NURSING PROCESS

The role of the professional nurse in caring for clients with phobic disorders is to provide comfort to the client and family and alleviate emotional distress. This supports adaptive coping while empowering the client by providing information, accessing resources, and communicating therapeutically.

Assessment

Accurate assessment of the client experiencing a phobic disorder is essential. Although the treatment regimen is similar for

---

Assessment Interview **Phobias**

Current and Past Medical History

- Do you have anxiety or avoid circumstances such as exposure to snakes or spiders?
- Do you avoid flying or are you afraid of heights?
- Do you avoid social situations where you might be evaluated by others such as eating or speaking in public?
- How often and in what circumstances do you leave home?
- Do you experience anxiety when anticipating or receiving criticism from others?
- Have you experienced feelings of irritability, guilt, depression, worthlessness, poor concentration, sleeplessness, suicidal intent?
- Have you sought treatment previously? What type of treatment have you tried? How helpful or effective was it?
- Do you have any history of substance abuse, alcohol abuse, or use of over-the-counter medication for anxiety? Do you use any herbs or supplements? Have you tried any alternative therapies, such as acupuncture or yoga?

- Whom can you rely on to understand and support you when you are distressed?
- Describe the qualities you like about yourself. What qualities do you dislike about yourself?
- Describe how family living patterns have changed around your fears.

Scaling Questions

- Ask the client to rank his or her anxiety on a scale of 0 (absence of symptoms) to 10 (completely disabling). Begin with current anxiety during the interview and progress to describe the "10," that is, the worst, experience of anxiety.
- Ask the client to rank how much the phobia interferes with daily routines or functioning.

Risk Factors

- Family history of anxiety disorders
- Family history of depression or substance abuse

the different types of phobias, it is important to obtain an accurate history from the individual about the attempts the individual has made to moderate his or her anxiety. Explore the possibility of comorbidity of depression and/or substance abuse, because the incidence for individuals suffering from anxiety disorders is high. Assess for any indication of suicidal ideation or past history of dangerous behavior.

Physical examination of the client should include assessment for symptoms related to substance abuse. Physical findings may be otherwise normal during the examination unless the client is currently experiencing anxiety related to the phobia.

Diagnosis

Examples of nursing diagnoses that may be appropriate for inclusion in the nursing plan of care for the client with a phobia may include the following:

- *Anxiety*
- *Fear*
- *Ineffective Health Maintenance*
- *Deficient Knowledge*
- *Ineffective Coping.*

(NANDA-I © 2012)

Planning

Based on the nursing diagnoses, client goals and identified outcomes are selected. Examples of goals that may reflect resolution of nursing diagnoses included in the nursing plan of care for the client with a phobia may include the following:

- The client will report a decrease in the frequency and severity of phobic episodes.
- The client will verbalize healthy ways of responding to fear.
- The client will demonstrate effective implementation of relaxation techniques.
- The client will participate in prescribed counseling and therapeutic treatments.

Implementation

Phobias with panic and severe anxiety must be treated immediately. As the level of an individual's anxiety increases, her judgment and ability to listen, remember, and learn is impaired. This is not the time to teach or present new information. The professional nurse does not argue with the individual regarding her perception of reality or reaction to the object of the phobia. Empathic nurses offer understanding, support, and direction to ensure safety. The nurse validates concerns and fears; offers a quiet, safe environment; and provides the following:

- **One-to-one supervision.** This helps alleviate the client's anxiety by providing assurance to the client that she is in no danger. One-to-one supervision should be provided until the antianxiety medications have begun to take affect and the nurse has assessed that the client can be safely left alone.

> ### Client Teaching Deep Breathing and Progressive Relaxation
>
> Essential teaching for individuals suffering from anxiety and phobias includes deep breathing and progressive relaxation techniques to lower anxiety responses. Avoidance of stimulants, caffeine, and nicotine is essential. Instructing individuals on the use of cognitive techniques can be helpful in lowering the individual's response to the threat. Strategies such as thought blocking, self-talk, and conversation with a support person all assist the individual to manage and empower more adaptive coping skills. Physical exercise that makes use of large muscle groups, such as walking, running, weight lifting, hiking, and various sport activities, can dissipate pent-up energy. Exercising also releases natural chemicals such as endorphins, improving mood and natural pain relief.

- **Structure and direction for the individual.** This includes informing the client about the next step in the treatment process (e.g., "We're waiting to the doctor to finish with another client; then he will see you"). It may include gentle reminders to the client such as "You're safe here. Let's practice deep breathing again."
- **Antianxiety agents as prescribed.**

Once the individual is stabilized, the nurse can effectively facilitate adaptive coping skills. The nurse encourages the client to vent feelings and describe his perception of the episode. As always, the nurse provides emotional support in a nonjudgmental manner. Specific interventions for the client experiencing phobia may include the following:

- Assist the individual to rethink or reframe the ability to manage his anxiety.
- Assist the client to reappraise the level of the threat as less damaging. The first opportunity to do this will likely occur after the antianxiety medication has begun to take effect and the client's immediate anxiety level has decreased.
- Teach the client relaxation techniques, such as deep breathing (see the Client Teaching feature).
- Assist the client to gain insight into his reactions.

Nurses working with the client over a period of time will have the opportunity to teach knowledge of defense mechanisms, to help the client work through unresolved issues and anxiety, and to help the client develop more adaptive coping mechanisms.

Evaluation

Evaluation of nursing care is largely based on the client's desire to overcome the phobia and willingness to follow the treatment regimen that requires confronting the phobia while controlling anxiety. When the client is able to encounter the phobia and not experience intolerable anxiety, he or she has met the goal of care. However, the ability to face the phobia and control the anxiety using improved coping strategies is an indication of a measure of success.

NURSING CARE PLAN A Client With Panic Disorder With Agoraphobia

ASSESSMENT

Mrs. Randolph is 43 years old, married, and the mother of four daughters in their late teens and early twenties. She is referred to the psychiatric outpatient clinic from the local emergency department following an acute panic attack with symptoms of racing heartbeat, sweating, feeling faint, and the belief that she was dying. She could not identify any events, thoughts, or feelings that precipitated the incident; it seemed to her to occur "out of the blue." She felt unable to cope with the severity of the symptoms of the attack: "I tried to talk myself out of it; to tell myself it would go away, but it only got worse." Mrs. Randolph reports she has had similar attacks lasting from 2 minutes to 2 hours in the past with no physical cause found by her family physician. Her daily routine has become restricted, and she will not leave the house without a family member. She is not comfortable alone in her home and can't sleep if any family member is still out. She is ashamed and angry about her growing disability and often tries to cover up her fears to friends and family. Recent life events include a hysterectomy 4 weeks ago and loss of employment resulting from hospitalization; the second anniversary of her father's sudden death is upcoming. She has no other history of mental health issues. She saw a therapist for her panic disorder when the attacks first started, "about the time I left home to marry" but did not follow up because she felt ashamed ("I've always been a strong and effective person!"), because the episodes were not so severe then, and because she found relief from the panic attacks after she had children. Her mother rarely left the house, never participating in social events unless they were in the home. She described her relationship with her husband as emotionally warm and supportive. She dreads seeing her daughters move from home.

Assessment findings:
- Is an attractive, carefully groomed woman who looks her stated age.
- Appears somewhat tense.
- Answers questions cooperatively, but at times with some hesitation, as if expecting criticism or judgment from the interviewer.
- Oriented to time, place, and person.
- Memory intact, good recall, no difficulty with calculations.
- Affect appears normal, with occasional evidence of anger in the form of irritability or sarcasm. Mood is within normal limits.
- Speech normal in flow and volume, pressured at times when she corrects an impression.
- Posture rigid at times, but she relaxes as she becomes more comfortable with the interview.

DIAGNOSES

- *Ineffective Role Performance* related to fear and anxiety level
- *Disturbed Thought Processes* related to high level of anxiety
- *Ineffective Coping* related to overwhelming fears

(NANDA-I © 2012)

PLANNING

Goals of care include:
- The client will describe specific changes in role function.
- The client will demonstrate appropriate decision making.
- The client will demonstrate effective coping as evidenced by employing behaviors to reduce stress and reporting fewer negative feelings.

IMPLEMENTATION

- Maintain a calm manner.
- Stay with the client.
- Use short, simple sentences.
- Direct client's attention to a repetitive or physical task.
- Administer pharmacologic agents as ordered.

- Teach relaxation exercises.
- Encourage client to identify previous coping skills.
- Help client identify coping resources (including social supports).
- Teach client relaxation techniques.
- Encourage client to verbalize feelings.

EVALUATION

Expected outcomes to evaluate the client's response to care include:
- The client demonstrates role performance as evidenced by the ability to meet role expectations, knowledge of role transition periods, and reported strategies for role changes.
- The client demonstrates ability to choose between two or more alternatives.
- The client uses actions to manage stressors that tax personal resources.

CRITICAL THINKING

1. What factors may be contributing to Mrs. Randolph's agoraphobia?
2. What interview questions would you like to ask Mrs. Randolph's family?
3. What strategies would you recommend to help Mrs. Randolph overcome her fear of leaving her house alone?

REVIEW **Phobias**

RELATE Link the Concepts and Exemplars

"My son Peter is scared to death to open his mouth! My friends come over to the house and he goes to his room or stands there like a fool and clams up. I tell him to say hello and he refuses. I think he does it to infuriate me."

Linking the exemplar of phobias with the concept of communication:

1. How could you respond therapeutically to this father's lack of empathy during the assessment process in an effort to educate the father about his son's phobia?

2. What strategies might you suggest to this father to improve communication between him and his son as well as reduce his son's anxiety related to talking with his father's friends?

Linking the exemplar of phobias with the concept of perfusion:

3. What impact on perfusion could be triggered by forcing someone to face a phobia prematurely?

4. What impact does acute anxiety have on perfusion?

READY Go to Companion Skills Manual

REFER Go to Pearson Nursing Student Resources
nursing.pearsonhighered.com

- Additional review materials

REFLECT Case Study

Returning to our discussion of Peter (introduced in the preceding Relate section), upon assessment the nurse collects the following data: Peter is an 8-year-old male who has a history of difficulty in school and refusal to go to school. Peter's mother recently caught Peter drinking pepper to induce vomiting in an attempt to feign illness in the hopes of staying home from school. Peter's mother is present during the initial nursing assessment. Peter barely responds during the assessment; he looks at the floor, shrugs his shoulders, and verbally responds in a barely audible voice "I don't know."

Objective data:

- Peter is having difficulty in school
- Poor attendance in school
- Peter is avoiding school
- Poor eye contact during the interview.

Subjective data:

- Peter responds "I don't know."

1. What further information would you want to collect about Peter from his mother?

2. What nursing diagnosis would be appropriate for Peter?

3. What do you suspect may be causing the described behaviors Peter is displaying?

EXEMPLAR 31.5 **Posttraumatic Stress Disorder**

EXEMPLAR KEY TERMS
Acute stress disorder, *1946*
Depersonalization, *1947*
Eye movement desensitization and reprocessing (EMDR), *1948*
Flashbacks, *1946*
Posttraumatic stress disorder (PTSD), *1945*

EXEMPLAR LEARNING OUTCOMES
After reading about this exemplar, you will be able to:

1. Describe the pathophysiology, etiology, clinical manifestations, and direct and indirect causes of posttraumatic stress disorder (PTSD).

2. Identify risk factors and prevention methods associated with PTSD.

3. Illustrate the nursing process in providing culturally competent care across the life span for individuals with PTSD.

4. Formulate priority nursing diagnoses appropriate for an individual with PTSD.

5. Summarize therapies used by interdisciplinary teams in the collaborative care of an individual with PTSD.

6. Plan evidence-based care for an individual with PTSD and his or her family in collaboration with other members of the healthcare team.

7. Evaluate expected outcomes for an individual with PTSD.

▶ OVERVIEW

Posttraumatic stress disorder (PTSD), once classified as an anxiety disorder, is one of a group of disorders now classified as trauma- and stressor-related disorders. This class of disorders also includes (APA, 2013):

- Reactive attachment disorder, which is a rare disorder seen in young children and associated with neglect; manifestations include an apparent aversion to engaging in interaction with adults

- Disinhibited social engagement disorder, which is most commonly diagnosed in young children and is associated with neglect; manifestations include an abnormal propensity for the child to interact with unfamiliar adults

- Acute stress disorder

- Adjustment disorders, which may be further characterized according to the client's manifestations (see the exemplar on

Adjustment Disorder With Depressed Mood in the module on Mood and Affect).

The APA (2013) characterizes PTSD as a disorder in which an individual who is exposed to a traumatic event develops, with regard to the traumatic event, intrusive symptoms, such as recurrent nightmares; patterns of persistent efforts to avoid stimuli associated with or reminiscent of the traumatic event; negative changes in cognition or mood; and marked changes in reactivity or arousal, such as hypervigilance or impaired concentration.

▶ PATHOPHYSIOLOGY AND ETIOLOGY

In the United States, recent events have brought discussion of PTSD to the forefront. For example, among those who experienced, witnessed, or attended to survivors of the World Trade Center attacks on September 11, 2001, some have spoken

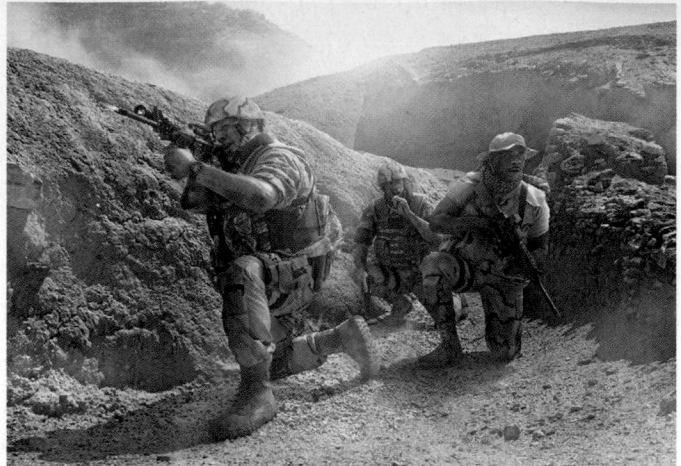

Figure 31–9 ● Many military personnel in or returning from the wars in Iraq and Afghanistan experience PTSD.
Source: Blend Images/Alamy.

publicly about their personal experiences with PTSD. Likewise, recent wars and conflicts, particularly those set in the Middle East, have resulted in a significant rise in the incidence of PTSD in military and civilian personnel deployed abroad (**Figure 31–9 ●**). Natural disasters, such as hurricanes and widespread fires, also provide sources of trauma as do the increasing incidences of mass shootings such as the 2012 shootings in a theater in Aurora, Colorado, and an elementary school in Newtown, Connecticut.

Traumatic events that may trigger PTSD include violent personal assaults, natural or human-caused disasters, motor vehicle crashes, military combat, being taken hostage or being tortured, imprisonment, dismemberment, incest, and child abuse. PTSD also can stem from sexual assault or from being subjected to sexual experiences during childhood (APA, 2013).

Even threats of violence or injury may prompt the development of PTSD. However, intentional infliction of harm or violence, such as torture or rape, is associated with a higher incidence of this disorder (APA, 2013).

PTSD may manifest through numerous signs and symptoms, including those related to fear-based reexperiencing of the event; alterations in emotional and behavioral states; dysphoric mood and negative cognitive states; and alterations in arousal and reactivity (APA, 2013). Some clients will experience manifestations that predominantly reflect one category of alterations, whereas others will experience a combination of manifestations (APA, 2013).

With regard to reexperiencing the traumatic event, the individual with PTSD may experience **flashbacks**, the recurrence of images, sounds, smells, or feelings from the traumatic event, which are often triggered by daily events, such as a car backfiring on the street or the smell of a perpetrator's cologne. In the affected individual's mind, flashbacks may be so lifelike that they appear to be happening in reality. Frequently, the individual experiences recurrent nightmares or intrusive memories related to the traumatic event.

Some individuals who experience trauma may experience acute stress during the immediate aftermath of the trauma. An acute stress or anxiety response sufficient to impair functioning

may result in acute stress disorder, discussed in **Box 31–12 ●**. Acute stress disorder shares several factors with PTSD, but is of a much shorter duration.

Etiology

Exposure to an overwhelming stressor can occur at any time or age in life. Childhood trauma, abuse, and molestation can create enduring effects and clinical symptoms that can last into adulthood. Additional factors that contribute to the development of PTSD are an individual history of a psychiatric disorder or a lack of emotional support or resources during the trauma. Among adults in the United States, the prevalence of PTSD is about 3.5 million (NIMH, n.d.), with women being more susceptible to its development (APA, 2013). Incidence among veterans is particularly high: One report documents that of military personnel who had been deployed in overseas combat presenting for treatment at Veterans Affairs healthcare centers, 21% were treated for PTSD. Incidence increases when traumatic brain injury (TBI) is present: 75% of combat personnel who experienced TBI had a concurrent diagnosis of PTSD (Congressional Budget Office, 2012).

Risk Factors

Individuals of any age and any cultural group may develop PTSD. In the United States, the incidence of this disorder is higher among military veterans, as well as law enforcement officers, firefighters, and emergency medical personnel (APA, 2013). Among the general population, risk factors for PTSD include the following:

- The severity of the event itself, including whether or not the individual was harmed or watched others be harmed or killed
- Little or no social or psychological support following the trauma
- Additional stressors immediately following the event, such as loss of a spouse or family member or loss of employment
- Presence of preexisting mental illness.

Clinical Manifestations and Therapies **Posttraumatic Stress Disorder**

PTSD	CLINICAL MANIFESTATIONS	CLINICAL THERAPIES
Anxiety disorder that evolves from exposure to actual trauma or threat of physical harm. Recovery varies from 1 month to several years. Comorbidity may include depression, substance abuse, or other anxiety disorders.	■ Persistent frightening thoughts and memories or flashbacks of the event: images, sounds, smells, or feelings ■ Emotional numbing ■ Sleep disorders ■ Hypervigilance and exaggerated startle response ■ Reexperiencing the event ■ Trouble with affection ■ Irritability, aggressiveness, or violence ■ Avoidance of trauma-related situations or general social contacts ■ Drug and alcohol abuse ■ Depression ■ Suicidal thoughts or violence	■ Holistic approach to treatment includes CBT ■ Eye movement desensitization and reprocessing ■ Supportive therapy ■ Group therapy ■ Pharmacologic therapy, including benzodiazepines, SSRIs, and antipsychotic agents. Prazosin, which is an antihypertensive medication that also inhibits the brain's response to norepinephrine, may be prescribed for treatment and prevention of nightmares (Mayo Clinic, 2011a).

▶ CLINICAL MANIFESTATIONS

Clients who experience flashbacks may lose touch with reality emotionally and may cognitively return to the traumatic incident as if it is happening all over again. Some may experience **depersonalization**, an emotional numbing and a loss of their sense of reality, feelings, and sense of self in relation to others. Clients who experience depersonalization may have difficulty in interpersonal relationships. They may have difficulty trusting or being affectionate. Things they formerly enjoyed may not provide pleasure for them anymore. Irritability, aggression, and even violence may be expressed when these would be out of character for the person before the incident.

Hyperarousal and hypervigilance are features associated with PTSD, rendering the affected individual in a near-constant state of "high alert." Dissociation, in which the individual blocks emotions related to the traumatic event, also may occur. The emotional numbness that can occur leads to impairment in establishing and maintaining social relationships. As with certain of the other anxiety disorders, depression also may accompany PTSD. Likewise, individuals with PTSD may abuse alcohol or other substances in an attempt to alleviate their symptoms.

Although manifestations of PTSD usually emerge within 3 months following exposure to the traumatic event, years may pass before the individual's signs and symptoms meet the criteria needed for an official diagnosis of PTSD (APA, 2013).

PTSD in Young Children

In pediatric clients with PTSD, manifestations of this disorder vary significantly from those demonstrated by adult clients. For example, children with PTSD who are under the age of 6 years may reexperience the trauma through playing in such a way as to overtly or indirectly recreate the traumatic event.

For very young children with PTSD, reexperiencing the traumatic event may take place through drawing pictures that symbolize the trauma. Children with PTSD may also behave recklessly or aggressively, or they may withdraw from interacting with others. Because of their undeveloped ability to express thoughts or identify emotions, expressions of PTSD in very young children often occur through changes in mood (APA, 2013).

▶ COLLABORATION

Caring for the client with PTSD requires the skillful ability to assess and facilitate the care of clients, families, and communities. As a client advocate, the nurse must effectively connect individuals with the resources they need to recover successfully from trauma. These resources may include financial resources, such as local departments of social services; medical resources, such as free clinics and mental health providers who treat uninsured clients on a sliding scale basis; and agencies that provide food and shelter.

Because of the all-encompassing impact of trauma on an individual's life, a holistic approach to treatment may be most effective, combining pharmacologic and alternative therapies, such as relaxation techniques, cognitive-behavioral therapy, eye movement desensitization and response therapy (discussed below), and support from a multiagency team of providers.

Pharmacologic Therapy

Depending on the severity and nature of a client's PTSD-related manifestations, pharmacologic therapy may include administration of benzodiazepines, antidepressants (in particular, SSRIs), and antipsychotic agents. Prazosin, which is an antihypertensive medication, has been shown effective in the reduction of nightmares associated with PTSD.

Nonpharmacologic Therapy

Eye movement desensitization and reprocessing (EMDR) is a form of psychotherapy that contains elements of a number of types of therapy, including cognitive-behavioral therapy and body-centered therapy. EMDR has been found effective in treating clients with PTSD. It is so named because one of the elements involves dual stimulation using eye movements, taps, or tones. *Dual stimulation* allows the client to reprocess or reappraise the trauma by focusing internally on the traumatic event or another stressor while simultaneously focusing on a different external stimulus (EMDR Institute, n.d.).

Preliminary research indicates that acupuncture may be effective in treating clients with PTSD. This research indicates the need for the client to participate in acupuncture on a regular basis for a period of 3 months or more (NCCAM, n.d.). Nurses working with clients who are interested in trying acupuncture as a treatment for PTSD should encourage the clients to add acupuncture as an adjunctive therapy and not to abandon cognitive-behavioral and more traditional therapies. Recommended treatments for sleep disturbances, which are common among clients with PTSD, include relaxation techniques such as guided imagery.

■ NURSING PROCESS

Clients with PTSD experiencing hyperarousal and vigilance may exhibit unpredictable, aggressive, or bizarre behavior. The nursing priorities for these clients are ensuring the safety of the client and others while quickly lowering client anxiety levels. The client with PTSD exhibiting extreme anxiety needs immediate pharmacologic intervention, a quiet and calm environment, and reassurance of his or her safety. Once anxiety levels are reduced, the client can be helped to learn a new process of appraisal and coping mechanisms.

Due to the complexity of trauma, families may also suffer from PTSD and require the nurse's assistance and support. Evaluation of the impact on the family must also be included in the assessment, evaluation, and decision-making process. Families play a key role in the support of the individual. In the case of national disasters, entire communities may be involved in the trauma.

Assessment

According to the National Guideline Clearinghouse (2010), recommendations for the assessment of clients with PTSD include assessing physical, psychological, social, and risk factors. The assessment tool utilized for anxiety and phobias is adapted to the individual who has experienced a traumatic event. Specific interview questions to ascertain the diagnosis of PTSD are aimed at the following clinical manifestations: reexperiencing or flashbacks, hyperarousal and vigilance, an exaggerated startle response, and sleep disturbances (see the Assessment Interview feature). In addition, the NGC (2010) suggests that identification of PTSD in children is improved when they are questioned directly about their experiences. Assessment of younger children involves questioning the child and/or the parents about significant changes in behavior and sleeping patterns. For children and vulnerable clients who are believed to be victims of abuse, the nurse should follow organizational protocols for reporting these situations (see the module on Violence).

Assessment Interview
Posttraumatic Stress Disorder

- How would you describe your mood?
- When do you feel most content? When do you feel least content?
- What are your favorite activities?
- What activities help you relax?
- How often do you socialize or participate in activities with others?
- Describe your sleep habits. Do you sleep soundly through the night? Do you feel rested when you awaken?
- Do you have friends or other individuals with whom you can be open and honest about your thoughts and emotions?
- How important is being able to share your thoughts and feelings?
- Are you currently working? If so, what type of work are you engaged in?

Because of the traumatization experienced by these clients, as well as the subsequent potential for emotional and physical isolation, establishment of trust can be especially challenging. For example, in the case of military veterans with PTSD, many of these individuals are resistant to openly sharing their thoughts and emotions even with their fellow veterans. During the assessment and throughout the care of all clients with PTSD, the nurse should be aware that direct questioning of the client with regard to traumatic experiences may inhibit establishment of a trusting relationship, and can even provoke frustration and anger in the client. The nursing assessment should include interview questions that allow for client assessment without pressuring the client to reveal information he is not ready or able to share. Through the inclusion of open-ended questions, the nurse affords the client the opportunity to express himself to the degree with which he is comfortable while demonstrating respect for the client's personal boundaries. (See the Assessment Interview feature).

Diagnosis

Evaluating assessment data for an individual with PTSD can be challenging. For some clients with PTSD, manifestations of the disorder can be compounded by substance abuse, depression, and insomnia. Appropriate diagnoses for the client with PTSD may include any of the following:

- *Risk for Self-Directed Violence*
- *Risk for Other-Directed Violence*
- *Post-Trauma Syndrome*
- *Anxiety*
- *Fear*
- *Ineffective Coping*
- *Compromised Family Coping*
- *Disturbed Sleep Patterns.*

(NANDA-I © 2012)

The nurse must explore the specific assessment questions directed at PTSD in order not to overlook the possibility of this diagnosis. It is important for the healthcare provider to involve the individual in the decision-making process and to facilitate the individual's preferences.

Planning

Planning includes identification of measurable, realistic client goals that are relevant to the selected nursing diagnoses. Examples of client goals that may be relevant to the care of the client with PTSD may include the following:

- The client will remain free from injury or harm.
- The client will report a decreased perception of anxiety.
- The client will report a reduction or cessation of nightmares.
- The client will discuss emotions related to traumatic experiences with at least one trusted mental health specialist or counseling professional.
- The client will verbalize awareness of nonpharmacologic stress reduction techniques.

Implementation

The presence of PTSD is not an inevitable outcome of a traumatic event. Some individuals may require only limited interventions. Clinically significant indicators are the severity of the event itself and the severity of the individual's initial response. For clients who develop this disorder, in addition to the interventions described previously, it is important to recognize the profound impact PTSD exerts on components related to multiple aspects of daily life, including within the social, interpersonal, and occupational domains. These clients may benefit

Client Teaching Typical Human Responses to Traumatic Events

Clients with PTSD should be given ample information about the typical human responses to traumatic events. Education about the process helps clients normalize the experience and gain information for reappraisal. Information and resources can lead to adaptive coping; conversely, a lack of resources may induce maladaptive coping. It is the responsibility of the nurse to provide information about the treatments available for PTSD to help the individual and family make informed choices.

from being connected with organizations and community resources that can facilitate long-term assistance, and that can also offer sensitive guidance as to the process for building trusting relationships with others.

Evaluation

The nurse evaluates the client's response to treatment using these suggested expected outcomes:

- The client utilizes self-calming techniques.
- The client experiences fewer cognitive distortions and fewer numinations or obsessions.
- The client decreases time spent ruminating over worries, verbalizing more accurate predictions of future events.

NURSING CARE PLAN A Client With Posttraumatic Stress Disorder

ASSESSMENT	DIAGNOSES	PLANNING
Sarah Green is a 44-year-old nurse whose 14-year-old son was killed in a motor vehicle crash (MVC) just over 6 months ago. At the time of the MVC, Ms. Green was driving her son to soccer practice when another vehicle crossed the interstate median and struck her vehicle. Her son died at the scene, and Ms. Green sustained serious injuries. Ms. Green also has a 17-year-old daughter and a 19-year-old son. At present, Ms. Green attends a support group for grieving parents, which she finds to be therapeutic. However, she has been having flashbacks about the night of the accident and can barely control herself when she knows one of her children is driving or riding in a car. Usually, when one of the children asks to borrow the car she just says "no" to avoid having to worry about them. Ms. Green knows she needs to see someone. She talks to a friend who is also a coworker, who recommends that she talk with an occupational health counselor at work. Ms. Green does not want anyone at work to know she is having trouble, but she agrees to see a mental health nurse that her friend recommends.	The mental health nurse develops the following nursing diagnoses: - *Post-Trauma Stress Syndrome* - *Anxiety* - *Fear* (NANDA-I © 2012)	Goals for Ms. Green's care include the following: - The client will utilize deep breathing to control escalating anxiety. - The client will express fears clearly. - The client will describe the symptoms associated with the various levels of anxiety. - The client will demonstrate breathing exercises to reduce anxiety.
At her initial appointment, Ms. Green freely shares her experiences with the flashbacks, which happen two or three times a week, usually at night. She says that when she knows her children are going anywhere, she can feel her heart racing, her breathing speeding up, and her palms getting sweaty. She tells the mental health nurse that she gets through these episodes by lying down and saying the Lord's Prayer out loud.		

(continued on next page)

NURSING CARE PLAN *(continued)*

IMPLEMENTATION

- Teach Ms. Green how to monitor her physiological level of arousal.
- Teach use of abdominal breathing at first sign of anxiety.
- Help client to express fears that interfere with her life.
- Encourage client to search for, confront, and relieve the source of the original anxiety.
- Teach distraction techniques that can control moderate levels of anxiety.

- Teach the use of positive imagery.
- Teach calming techniques such as muscle relaxation.
- Teach positive affirmations such as "I am calm and happy" or "I am very relaxed."
- Identify safe physical outlets for negative feelings such as exercise.

EVALUATION

- The client expresses feelings appropriately.
- The client spends less time thinking about the accident and instead turns thoughts to more positive memories.
- The client allows adolescent to borrow the car setting reasonable limits to reduce her anxiety.

CRITICAL THINKING

1. What impact does Ms. Green's PTSD have on her children's development?
2. How would you teach Ms. Green relaxation techniques?

REVIEW Posttraumatic Stress Disorder

RELATE Link the Concepts and Exemplars

Linking the exemplar of posttraumatic stress disorder with the concept of development:

Explore the incidence of childhood abuse, molestation, and incest in the Unites States.

1. What impact does childhood abuse, molestation, and incest have on the growth and development of a child?
2. Childhood abuse, molestation, and incest can negatively affect the physical, emotional, spiritual, and cognitive processes of individuals. What alterations in health are associated with abuse later in life?

Linking the exemplar of posttraumatic stress disorder with the concept of violence:

3. How might PTSD cause a previously nonviolent individual to become more violent in his or her interactions with others?
4. What anticipatory guidance can you provide the client with PTSD to reduce the risk of future violence?

READY Go to Companion Skills Manual

REFER Go to Pearson Nursing Student Resources
nursing.pearsonhighered.com

- Additional review materials

REFLECT Case Study

Melinda Burns lives in Manhattan. She is engaged to be married to a man she says she loves very much and although this should be the happiest time of her life, she is feeling very anxious and stressed.

She was 12 years old on September 11, 2001, when terrorists attacked the United States. She was in school when the planes hit the World Trade Center. They had to evacuate the school after the collapse of the buildings because the ash was so thick it made breathing difficult. Her father picked her up and they went to a hotel room in New Jersey because their apartment was also covered in ash and they weren't allowed to go home until several weeks later. Ms. Burns's grandmother stayed with her in the hotel room while her father tried to find her mother, who worked on the 92nd floor of the North Tower. Her Dad never found her mother and she never came home. Ms. Burns says the worst part is that her mother's body was never identified from the wreckage so she feels like she has no closure or confirmation that her mother is really dead. One of the New York fireman came to their home almost a year later to return a necklace that was found and the engraving helped them identify it as her mom's. Ms. Burns treasures the necklace even though it is badly damaged and burned.

Ms. Burns is seeking care because she is having trouble functioning normally. She reports severe anxiety whenever she hears a siren, has been waking from nightmares related to the World Trade Center several times a week, and she can't bring herself to watch any television programs or movies about the terrorist attack because they always make her cry. She has turned down a number of jobs because she can't bring herself to work on the upper levels of tall buildings. She says lately she has been having trouble concentrating, even when planning her wedding because she can't seem to think about anything other than the World Trade Center and what her mother's final minutes must have been like.

1. What nursing diagnosis is appropriate for Ms. Burns?
2. What collaborative actions can the healthcare team take to help Ms. Burns?
3. What independent nursing interventions would you initiate if Ms. Burns was your client?

■ REFERENCES

Adams, M. P., Holland, L., & Urban, C. (2014). *Pharmacology for nurses: A pathophysiologic approach* (4th ed.). Upper Saddle River, NJ: Prentice Hall.

American Diabetes Association. (n.d.). *Living with diabetes: Stress*. Retrieved from http://www.diabetes.org/living-with-diabetes/complications/stress.html.

American Psychiatric Association (APA). (2007). *Practice guideline for the treatment of patients with obsessive compulsive disorder* (p. 570). Arlington, VA: Author.

American Psychiatric Association (APA). (2013). *Diagnostic and statistical manual of mental disorders* (5th ed.). Arlington, VA: Author.

Antai-Otang, D. (2008). *Psychiatric nursing: Biological & behavioral concepts*. Clifton Park, NY: Delmar.

Anxiety and Depression Association of America (ADAA). (n.d.a). *Facts & statistics*. Retrieved from http://www.adaa.org/about-adaa/press-room/facts-statistics.

Anxiety and Depression Association of America (ADAA). (n.d.b). *Living and thriving with anxiety or depression means conquering your symptoms: Older adults— Symptoms*. Retrieved from http://www.adaa.org/living-with-anxiety/older-adults/symptoms.

Baas, J. M. P., Mol, N., Kenemans, J. L., Prinssen, E. P., Niklson, I., Xia-Chen, C., … & van Gerven J. (2009). Validating a human model for anxiety using startle potentiated by cue and context: The effects of alprazolam, pregabalin, and diphenhydramine. *Psychopharmacology (Berlin)*, 205(1), 73–84.

Bandura, A. (1994). Self-efficacy. In V. S. Ramachandran (Ed.), *Encyclopedia of human behavior* (Vol. 4, pp. 71–81). New York, NY: Academic Press.

Barnes, P., Powell-Griner, E., McFann, K., & Nahin, R. (2004). *Complementary and alternative medicine use among adults: United States, 2002* (CDC Advance Data Report #343). Hyattsville, MD: National Center for Health Statistics.

Bassil, N., Ghandour, A., & Grossberg, G. T. (2011). How anxiety presents differently in older adults. *Current Psychiatry 10*(3), 65–72. Retrieved from http://www.currentpsychiatry.com/pdf/1003/1003cp_article3.pdf.

BehaveNet. (2013a). *Panic disorder without agoraphobia*. Retrieved from http://behavenet.com/panic-disorder-without-agoraphobia.

BehaveNet. (2013b). *Separation anxiety disorder*. Retrieved from http://behavenet.com/separation-anxiety-disorder.

Benedek, D. M., Friedman, M. J., Zatzick, D., & Ursano, R. J. (2009). Guideline watch (March 2009): Practice guideline for the treatment of patients with acute stress disorder and posttraumatic stress disorder. *FOCUS: The Journal of Lifelong Learning in Psychiatry*, 7(2), 204–213.

Berk, L. (2012). *Child development* (9th ed.). Upper Saddle River, NJ: Prentice Hall.

Boston Children's Hospital. (2012). *Generalized anxiety disorder (GAD)*. Retrieved from http://www.childrenshospital.org/az/Site948/mainpageS948P0.html.

Bouayed, J. (2011). Relationship between oxidative stress and anxiety: Emerging role of antioxidants within therapeutic or preventive approaches. In Vladimir Kalinin (Ed.), *Anxiety disorders*. doi:10.5772/19214. Retrieved from http://www.intechopen.com/books/anxiety-disorders/relationship-between-oxidative-stress-and-anxiety-emerging-role-of-antioxidants-within-therapeutic-1.

Bouayed, J., Hassan Rammal, H., & Soulimani, R. (2009). Oxidative stress and anxiety: Relationship and cellular pathways. *Oxidative Medicine and Cellular Longevity*, 2(2), 63–67. Retrieved from http://www.ncbi.nlm.nih.gov/pmc/articles/PMC2763246.

Bryant, R. A., Friedman, M. J., Spiegel, D., Ursano, R. & Strain, J. (2011). A review of acute stress disorder in DSM-5. *FOCUS: The Journal of Lifelong Learning in Psychiatry*, 9(3), 335–350.

Butcher, J. N., Mineka, S., & Hooley, J. M. (2013). *Abnormal psychology* (15th ed.). Upper Saddle River, NJ: Pearson.

Cannon, W. B. (1929). Organization for physiological homeostasis. *Physiological Reviews*, 9(3), 399–431.

Cannon, W. B. (1932). *The wisdom of the body*. New York, NY: W. W. Norton.

Caplan, G. (1964). *Principles of preventive psychiatry*. New York, NY: Basic Books.

Carver, C. S., & Connor-Smith, J. (2010). Personality and coping. *Annual Review of Psychology*, 61, 679–704.

Cherry, L. (1978). On the real benefits of eustress: An interview with Hans Selye. *Psychology Today*, 11(10), 60–70.

Children's Hospital of Pittsburgh. (2013). *Separation anxiety disorder*. Retrieved from http://www.chp.edu/CHP/P02582.

Cleveland Clinic. (2012). *An overview of anxiety disorders*. Retrieved from http://my.clevelandclinic.org/disorders/anxiety_disorder/hic_an_overview_of_anxiety_disorders.aspx.

Cloos, J. M. (2010). Benzodiazepines and addiction: Myths and realities (Part 1). *Psychiatric Times*, 27(7), 6–29.

Congressional Budget Office. (2012). *The Veterans Health Administration's treatment of PTSD and traumatic brain injury among recent combat veterans*. Retrieved from http://www.cbo.gov/sites/default/files/cbofiles/attachments/02-09-PTSD.pdf.

Dossey, B. M., & Keegan, L. (Eds.). (2009). *Holistic nursing: A handbook for practice* (5th ed.). Sudbury, MA: Jones and Bartlett.

Dubuc, B. (2013). *Brain abnormalities associated with anxiety disorders*. Retrieved from http://thebrain.mcgill.ca/flash/i/i_08/i_08_cr/i_08_cr_anx/i_08_cr_anx.html.

Duckworth, J., & Freedman, J. L. (2012). *Obsessive-compulsive disorder*. Retrieved from http://www.nami.org/Template.cfm?Section=By_Illness&Template=/ContentManagement/ContentDisplay.cfm&ContentID=142546.

Elder, R., Evans, K., Nizette, D., & Trenoweth, S. (2013). *Psychiatric and mental health nursing* (3rd ed.). Sydney, Australia: Elsevier.

EMDR Institute. (n.d.). *What is EMDR?* Retrieved from http://www.emdr.com/general-information/what-is-emdr.html.

Erikson, E. H. (1968). *Identity: Youth and crisis*. New York, NY: Norton.

Everly, G. S., & Lating, J. M. (2013). *A clinical guide to the treatment of the human stress response* (3rd ed.). New York, NY: Springer.

Fontaine, K. L. (2009). *Mental health nursing* (6th ed.). Upper Saddle River, NJ: Pearson.

Freud, A. (1946). *The ego and mechanisms of defense*. New York, NY: International Universities Press.

Girdano, D. A., Dusek, D. E., & Everly, G. S. (2009). *Controlling stress and tension*. San Francisco, CA: Pearson Benjamin Cummings.

Grados, M. & Wilcox, H. C. (2007). Genetics of obsessive-compulsive disorder: A research update. *Expert Review of Neurotherapeutics*, 7(8), 967–980. Retrieved from http://www.ncbi.nlm.nih.gov/pubmed/18386211?ordinalpos=1&itool=EntrezSystem2.PEntrez.Pubmed.Pubmed_ResultsPanel.Pubmed_DefaultReportPanel.Pubmed_RVDocSum.

Holmes, T. H., & Rahe, R. H. (1967). The social readjustment rating scale. *Journal of Psychosomatic Research*, 11, 213–218.

Horowitz, M. J., Wilner, M., & Alverez, W. (1979). Impact of events scale: A measure of subjective stress. *Psychosomatic Medicine*, 41(3), 209–218.

Jewell, S. (2010). Antipsychotics for anxiety. *Livestrong.com*. Retrieved from http://www.livestrong.com/article/183286-antipsychotics-for-anxiety.

Juster, R. P., McEwen, B. S., & Lupien, S. J. (2010). Allostatic load biomarkers of chronic stress and impact on health and cognition. *Neuroscience and Biobehavioral Reviews*, 35(1), 2.

Kassin, S. (2001). *Psychology* (3rd ed.). Upper Saddle River, NJ: Prentice Hall.

Kneisl, C. R., & Trigoboff, E. (2013). *Contemporary psychiatric–mental health nursing* (3rd ed.). Upper Saddle River, NJ: Pearson.

Koltko-Rivera, M. E. (2006). Rediscovering the later version of Maslow's hierarchy of needs: Self-transcendence and opportunities for theory, research, and unification. *Review of General Psychology*, 10(4), 302–317.

Lazarus, R. S., & Folkman, S. (1984). *Stress, appraisal, and coping*. New York, NY: Springer.

Liu, F., Havens, J., Yu, Q., Wang, G., Davisson, R. L., Pickel, V. M., & Iadecola, C. (2012). The link between angiotensin II-mediated anxiety and mood disorders with NADPH oxidase-induced oxidative stress. *International Journal of Physiology, Pathophysiology and Pharmacology*, 4(1), 28–35. Retrieved from http://www.ncbi.nlm.nih.gov/pmc/articles/PMC3312460.

Lumsden, D. P. (1981). Is the concept of "stress" of any use, anymore? In *Contributions to primary prevention in mental health: Working papers*. Toronto, Canada: Toronto National Office of the Canadian Mental Health Association.

Lyon, B. L. (2012). Stress, coping, and health: A conceptual overview. In V. H. Rice (Ed.), *Handbook of stress, coping, and health: Implications for nursing research, theory, and practice* (2nd ed., pp. 1–20). Thousand Oaks, CA: Sage.

Manicavasagar, V., Marnane, C., Pini, S., Abelli, M., Rees, S., Eapen, V., & Silove, D., (2010). Adult separation anxiety disorder: A disorder comes of age. *Current Psychiatry Reports*, 12(4): 290–297.

Maslow, A. (1943). A theory of human motivation. *Psychological Review*, 50(4), 370–396.

Maslow, A. H. (1968). *Toward a psychology of being* (2nd ed.). New York, NY: Van Nostrand Reinhold.

Maslow, A. H. (1987). *Motivation and personality* (3rd ed.). New York, NY: Harper & Row.

Mayo Clinic. (2009). *Phobias*. Retrieved from http://www.mayoclinic.com/health/phobias/DS00272.

Mayo Clinic. (2010). *Obsessive-compulsive disorder (OCD)*. Retrieved from http://www.mayoclinic.com/health/obsessive-compulsive-disorder/DS00189.

Mayo Clinic. (2011a). *Post-traumatic stress disorder (PTSD)*. Retrieved from http://www.mayoclinic.com/health/post-traumatic-stress-disorder/DS00246.

Mayo Clinic. (2011b). *Reactive attachment disorder: Risk factors*. Retrieved from http://www.mayoclinic.com/health/reactive-attachment-disorder/DS00988/DSECTION=risk-factors.

Mayo Clinic. (2012a). *Anxiety*. Retrieved from http://www.mayoclinic.com/health/anxiety/DS01187/DSECTION=alternative-medicine.

Mayo Clinic. (2012b). *Anxiety: Prevention*. Retrieved from http://www.mayoclinic.com/health/anxiety/DS01187/DSECTION=prevention.

McEwen, B. S. (1998). Stress, adaptation, and disease: Allostasis and allostatic load. *Annals of the New York Academy of Sciences*, 840, 33–44.

McEwen, B. S., & Gianaros, P. J. (2010). Central role of the brain in stress and adaptation: Links to socioeconomic status, health, and disease. *Annals of the New York Academy of Sciences*, 1186, 190–222.

McHugh, M. D., Kutney-Lee, A., Cimiotti, J. P., Sloane, D. M., & Aiken, L. H. (2011). Nurses' widespread job dissatisfaction, burnout, and frustration with health benefits signal problems for patient care. *Health Affairs (Millwood)*, 30(2), 202–210.

MedlinePlus. (2010). *Separation anxiety.* Retrieved from http://www.nlm.nih.gov/medlineplus/ency/article/001542.htm.

Miller, M. A., & Rahe, R. H. (1997). Life changes scaling for the 1990s. *Journal of Psychosomatic Research, 43,* 279–292.

Monat, A., & Lazarus, R. S. (1991). *Stress and coping* (3rd ed.). New York, NY: Columbia University Press.

Morris, C. G., & Maisto, A. A. (2001). *Understanding psychology* (3rd ed.). Upper Saddle River, NJ: Prentice Hall.

National Alliance on Mental Illness (NAMI). (2012). *Mental illnesses: Anxiety disorders.* Retrieved from http://www.nami.org/Template.cfm?Section=By_Illness&Template=/ContentManagement/ContentDisplay.cfm&ContentID=142543.

National Center for Complementary and Alternative Medicine (NCCAM). (2009a). *Study shows chamomile capsules ease anxiety symptoms.* Retrieved from http://nccam.nih.gov/research/results/spotlight/040310.htm?nav=gsa.

National Center for Complementary and Alternative Medicine (NCCAM). (2009b). *Transcendental Meditation helps young adults cope with stress.* Retrieved from http://nccam.nih.gov/research/results/spotlight/051410.htm.

National Center for Complementary and Alternative Medicine (NCCAM). (2013). *Information for consumers about anxiety.* Retrieved from http://nccam.nih.gov/health/moreinfo/41/3888.

National Center for Complementary and Alternative Medicine (NCCAM). (n.d.). *Acupuncture may help symptoms of post-traumatic stress disorder.* Retrieved from http://nccam.nih.gov/research/results/spotlight/092107.htm.

National Coalition for the Homeless. (2009). *Mental illness and homelessness.* Retrieved from http://www.national-homeless.org/factsheets/Mental_Illness.pdf.

National Guideline Clearinghouse (NGC). (2007). *Guideline summary: Practice guideline for the treatment of patients with obsessive-compulsive disorder.* Retrieved from http://www.guideline.gov/content.aspx?id=11078.

National Guideline Clearinghouse. (2010). *Guideline summary: VA/DoD clinical practice guideline for management of post-traumatic stress.* Retrieved from http://www.guideline.gov/content.aspx?id=25628.

National Institute of Mental Health (NIMH). (2009). *Anxiety disorders.* Retrieved from http://www.nimh.nih.gov/health/publications/anxiety-disorders/anxiety_disorders_en_ln.pdf.

National Institute of Mental Health (NIMH). (2013a). *Brain basics.* Retrieved from http://www.nimh.nih.gov/health/educational-resources/brain-basics/brain-basics.shtml.

National Institute of Mental Health (NIMH). (2013b). *Psychotherapies.* Retrieved from http://www.nimh.nih.gov/health/topics/psychotherapies/index.shtml.

National Institute of Mental Health (NIMH). (n.d.). *Post-traumatic stress disorder among adults.* Retrieved from http://www.nimh.nih.gov/statistics/1ad_ptsd_adult.shtml.

Peplau, H. (1952). *Interpersonal relations in nursing.* New York, NY: Putnam.

Pokorny, M. E. (2010). *Nursing theorists of historical significance.* In A. M Tomey & M. Alligood (Eds.), *Nursing theorists and their work* (7th ed.). St. Louis, MO: Mosby/Elsevier.

Potochnick, S. R., & Perreira, K. M. (2010). Depression and anxiety among first-generation immigrant Latino youth: Key correlates and implications for future research. *Journal of Nervous and Mental Disease, 198*(7), 470–477.

Rahe, R., & Tolles, R. (2002). The brief stress and coping inventory: A useful stress management instrument. *International Journal of Stress Management, 9*(2), 61–70.

Reich, J. W., Zautra, A. J., & Hall, J. S. (2010). *Handbook of adult resilience.* New York, NY: Guilford Press.

Romero, L. M., Dickens, M. J., & Cyr, N. E. (2009). The reactive scope model—A new model integrating homeostasis, allostasis, and stress. *Hormones and Behavior, 55,* 375–389.

Sadock, B. J., & Sadock, V. A. (2008). *Kaplan & Sadock's concise textbook of clinical psychiatry* (3rd ed.). Philadelphia, PA: Lippincott Williams & Wilkins.

Selye, H. (1946). The general adaptation syndrome and the diseases of adaptation. *Journal of Clinical Endocrinology, 6*(1), 117–231.

Selye, H. (1956). *The stress of life.* New York, NY: McGraw-Hill.

Selye, H. (1974) *Stress without distress.* Philadelphia, PA: J. B. Lippincott.

Selye, H. (1976). *The stress of life* (revised ed.). New York, NY: McGraw-Hill.

Smith, C. A., & Lazarus, R. S. (1990). Emotion and adaptation. In L. A. Pervin (Ed.), *Handbook of personality: Theory and research* (pp. 609–637). New York, NY: Guilford.

Smock, T. K. (1999). *Physiological psychology: A neuroscience approach.* Upper Saddle River, NJ: Prentice Hall.

Springer, K. W., Sheridan, J., Kuo, D., & Carnes, M. (2007). Long-term physical and mental health consequences of childhood physical abuse: Results from a large population-based sample of men and women. *Child Abuse & Neglect, 31*(5), 517–530.

Sterling, P., & Eyer, J. (1988). Allostasis: A new paradigm to explain arousal pathology. In S. Fisher & J. Reason (Eds.), *Handbook of life stress, cognition and health* (pp. 629–649). New York, NY: John Wiley & Sons.

Stewart, S. A. (2005). The effects of benzodiazepines on cognition. *Journal of Clinical Psychiatry, 66*(Suppl. 2), 9–13.

Stroud, L. R., Foster, E., Papandonatos, G. D., Handwerger, K., Granger, D. A., Kivlighan, K. T., & Niaura, R. (2009). Stress response and the adolescent transition: Performance versus peer rejection stressors. *Development and Psychopathology, 21*(1), 47–68.

Swedo, S., Leckman, J. F., & Rose, N. R. (2012). From research subgroup to clinical syndrome: Modifying the PANDAS criteria to describe PANS (pediatric acute-onset neuropsychiatric syndrome). *Pediatrics & Therapeutics, 2*(2), 1–8.

Surgeon General. (2008). Evidence based mental health: A report of the surgeon general. *Children and Mental Health.* Retrieved from http://mentalhealth.samhsa.gov/features/surgeongeneralreport/chapter3/sec6.asp.

Swedo, S., Leckman, J. F., & Rose, N. R. (2012). From research subgroup to clinical syndrome: Modifying the PANDAS criteria to describe PANS (pediatric acute-onset neuropsychiatric syndrome). *Pediatrics & Therapeutics, 2*(2), 1–8.

Townsend, M. (2009). *Psychiatric mental health nursing: Concepts of care in evidence based practice* (6th ed.). Philadelphia, PA: F. A. Davis.

University of Maryland Medical Center (UMM). (2009). *Anxiety disorders—Risk factors.* Retrieved from http://www.umm.edu/patiented/articles/who_gets_anxiety_disorders_000028_3.htm.

U.S. Department of Health and Human Services (USDHHS), Office on Women's Health. (2010). *Minority women's health.* Retrieved from http://www.womenshealth.gov/minority-health.

U.S. Department of Health and Human Services (USDHHS), Substance Abuse and Mental Health Services Administration. (2007). *Disaster counseling.* Retrieved from http://www.samhsa.gov.

Walitza, S., Renner, T. J., Wewetzer, C., & Warnke, A. (2008). Klinik für Kinder- und Jugendpsychiatrie und Psychotherapie der Universität Würzburg [Genetic findings in obsessive-compulsive disorder in childhood and adolescence and in adulthood]. *Zeitschrift fur Kinder- und Jugendpsychiatrie und Psychotherapie, 36*(1), 45–52.

Weiss, D. S., & Marmer, C. R. (1997). The impact of event scale—Revised. In J. P. Wilson & T. M. Keane (Eds.), *Assessing psychological trauma and PTSD: A handbook for practitioners* (pp. 399–411). New York, NY: Guilford Press.

32 Violence

MODULE AT-A-GLANCE

The Concept of Violence, 1953

Exemplar 32.1
Abuse, 1964

Exemplar 32.2
Assault and Homicide, 1975

Exemplar 32.3
Rape and Rape-Trauma
Syndrome, 1983

Exemplar 32.4
Suicide, 1990

Exemplar 32.5
Unintentional Injury: Motor
Vehicle Crashes, 1998

◢ THE CONCEPT OF VIOLENCE

Violence is the use of excessive force against other individuals or oneself, often resulting in physical or psychological injuries or death. Despite the commonplace depiction of violence in the media, the incidence of violent crimes has been decreasing in the United States. As of 2011 the approximate number of violent crimes had decreased (by 3.8%) for the fifth consecutive year. In that same year, 1,203,567 violent crimes were reported to law enforcement officials.

According to the Federal Bureau of Investigation (FBI), a violent crime can involve one of four offenses: murder, rape, robbery, or aggravated assault. In the United States, the Southern region, which accounts for the largest population in the country, accounted for 41.3% of violent crimes, the West accounted for 22.9%, the Midwest 19.5%, and the Northeast made up the final 16.2%. Aggravated assaults constituted 62.4% of these crimes, robbery represented 29.4%, rape accounted for 6.9%, and murder comprised the final 1.2% (FBI, 2012a; 2012g).

Violence is not only limited to the violent crimes in the four major categories described above; it also represents all instances of abuse. Although violence in the United States may not be on the rise, it is certainly a cause for concern that impacts not only the law enforcement community, but also the healthcare community. Victims of violent acts may seek treatment at emergency departments, urgent care centers, or physician's offices. For injuries that are psychological in nature, affected individuals may seek treatment from counselors, therapists, or other mental health specialists. **<<**

Concept Learning Outcomes

After reading about this concept, you will be able to:

1. Summarize the physiology of aggression and violence.
2. Examine the relationship between violence and other concepts/systems.
3. Identify commonly occurring alterations in violent acts and their related therapies.
4. Differentiate common assessment procedures used to examine violent behavior across the life span.
5. Describe diagnostic and laboratory tests to determine if an individual has been the victim of violence.
6. Explain prevention efforts for violence.
7. Demonstrate the nursing process in providing culturally competent and caring interventions across the life span for individuals who have experienced violence.
8. Compare and contrast common independent and collaborative interventions for clients who have experienced violence.

Concept Key Terms

Blunt trauma, *1956*
Cycle of violence, *1955*
Interpersonal
   violence, *1954*
Minor trauma, *1956*
Multiple trauma, *1956*
Penetrating trauma, *1956*
Precipitating factors, *1954*

Predisposing factors, *1954*
Protective factors, *1954*
Risk factors, *1954*
Trauma, *1955*
Triage, *1963*
Violence, *1953*
Vulnerability
   factors, *1954*

► NORMAL PRESENTATION

Generally speaking, violence results from a combination of predisposing, precipitating, and protective factors in several areas. **Predisposing factors** are those that increase an individual's risk of violent victimization or perpetration of violence. Predisposing factors may be categorized as vulnerability factors or risk factors. In the context of violence, **vulnerability factors** increase an individual's risk of being a victim of violence; **risk factors** increase the potential that someone will perpetrate violence on others. **Precipitating factors** are those that give rise to a specific incident of violence. **Protective factors**, on the other hand, decrease the risk of violence perpetration and victimization. For example, connectedness to school has been found to be a protective factor for youth violence (Centers for Disease Control and Prevention [CDC], 2011b). Areas to be addressed in examining factors contributing to societal violence include biophysical, psychological, physical, environmental, sociocultural, behavioral, and healthcare system considerations.

Many factors influence violence, both in terms of factors that are likely to predispose an individual to becoming a victim of violence, and those that put an individual at risk for acting violently. Influencing factors do not cause violent behavior, nor do they wholly determine that an individual will be injured; rather, factors such as these can define trends and warning signs. For example, an individual may have a childhood history of being abused, reacting with anger, and experiencing academic failures from a young age. All of these elements are predisposing factors to violent behavior, but they are not determining factors (Office of Mental Health, 2012).

Predisposing Factors

Predisposing factors for violence include environmental, psychological, cultural, and behavioral variables. Geographical and environmental factors can deeply affect other aspects of an individual's life. Living in an impoverished community, especially one with a strong presence of gangs and drugs, puts an individual at increased risk for witnessing, experiencing, or even committing acts of violence (Collins et al., 2011; Office of Mental Health, 2012). These environmental situations can also become cyclical, with multiple generations feeling trapped in the same community with the same high levels of violence. Over time the stress and constant danger become traumatic, often feeding into more violence within the community, as well as within individual families.

Families themselves can be a predisposing factor to violence, especially if there is a history of abuse and neglect within the family, or if family members are involved in drug or alcohol abuse. Other influencing variables are individual or behavioral in nature, such as a preoccupation with danger or violence, a history of abusing or torturing animals, and a history of bullying (either as the victim or the perpetrator). Psychological factors should also be considered, including aggressive tendencies, uncontrolled anger, extreme emotional distress, emotional instability, and depression (CDC, 2011b; Office of Mental Health, 2012).

Protective Factors

In opposition to predisposing factors to violence are protective factors, which reduce the risk of violent behavior as well as being the target of violent actions. Many of these protective factors apply to adolescents. According to the CDC (2011b), some variables that decrease the risk associated with violence include:

- Determination and success in school
- Healthy and positive social relationships
- Parents who show interest in their child's experiences
- Involvement in the community
- Participation in family activities
- Participation in cultural or religious practices
- Strong emotional support from friends and family.

Note that regardless of an individual's predisposing or protective factors, anyone can become violent, and anyone can be a victim of violence.

► PHYSICAL VIOLENCE

Expressions of physical violence take different forms, including abuse and trauma. These behaviors can affect individuals of all ages, but some groups are considered to be at a greater risk for experiencing violence than others. Violence can affect the well-being of individuals, families, communities, cultures, and entire nations.

Alterations and Manifestations

Forms of abuse are extensive, and include child abuse, elder maltreatment, intimate partner abuse, sexual abuse, physical abuse, and emotional abuse. Reactions of clients who are impacted by these forms of abuse will vary depending on the individual circumstances (e.g., age, personality, and experiences of the individual who has been abused). Traumatic injuries may be intentional or unintentional.

ABUSE   As previously mentioned, violence takes many forms. When abuse occurs, it typically involves intentional harm or injury. Intimate partner abuse, child abuse, and elder maltreatment describe abusive situations that affect specific groups of people. Intimate partner abuse occurs when a partner or spouse inflicts harm that is physical, sexual, or psychological in nature. Child abuse involves any intentional mistreatment of a child under the age of 18 by someone in a custodial role (**Figure 32–1 ●**). Elder maltreatment represents the abuse and neglect of individuals 65 years of age and older. The perpetrator of elder maltreatment is typically the individual's trusted caregiver. Failure of the intended caregiver to provide care or protect an older person from harm also constitutes maltreatment (National Center on Elder Abuse, n.d.). As the older adult population in the United States grows, so does the occurrence of elder maltreatment, which is a form of abuse that often goes undetected.

Anyone can be a victim of sexual abuse, physical abuse, or emotional abuse. Sexual abuse involves any sexual contact that occurs without an individual's consent. Many who are sexually abused develop disorders, including depression, anxiety, posttraumatic stress disorder, trouble eating and sleeping, and attempted suicide (Mayo Clinic, 2010). **Interpersonal violence** is violence that occurs within relationships between family members, intimate partners, acquaintances, or strangers that does not

Concepts Related to **Violence**

Violence interrelates with various nursing practices, among them the concepts of communication, sexuality, and stress and coping. Communication is vital in all areas of nursing, especially when violence is a contributing factor. Clients who have been exposed to a violent situation are likely to be experiencing pain (both physical and emotional) and significant amounts of stress. Nurses need to employ therapeutic communication to help clients work through the stress and fear and ultimately accept that the situation they experienced cannot be reversed. If the client has suffered any form of sexual violence, he or she could also be experiencing fear regarding sexually transmitted infections, as well as the possibility of unwanted pregnancy.

CONCEPT	RELATIONSHIP TO VIOLENCE	NURSING IMPLICATIONS
Communication		
■ Therapeutic communication	Clear and therapeutic communication with clients after a violent experience can help to alleviate stress and facilitate acceptance.	■ Use therapeutic communication to facilitate healing and acceptance. ■ Encourage the client to ask questions. ■ Explain any procedures or tests suggested to the client. ■ Use appropriate nonverbal communication (body language) to encourage open communication.
Sexuality		
■ Sexually transmitted infections/disease ■ Responsible sexual behavior ■ Pregnancy	Sexual violence is a form of violence that can cause both psychological and physical trauma. Sexual violence can also result in diseases, infections, and unwanted pregnancy.	■ For victims of sexual assault, assessment may include use of a sexual assault evidence collection kit (also known as a rape kit), if permitted by the client. ■ Educate about options regarding the possibility of unwanted pregnancy (e.g., emergency contraception). ■ Educate about tests for sexually transmitted infections and diseases. ■ Facilitate referrals to resources such as support groups, therapy, and counseling.
Stress and Coping		
■ Anxiety ■ Crisis ■ PTSD	All forms of violence can cause stress, potentially leading to exacerbation of the injury and increased emotional strain.	■ Communicate with the client regarding needs to and wants, especially those in relation to stress relief (e.g., the presence of a family member or friend). ■ Answer questions regarding treatment and injuries calmly and honestly. ■ Employ comfort measures to decrease stress, such as warm blankets, relaxation techniques, and reassurance of safety.

aim to further the goals of a formal group or cause. Violence of this nature may include sexual assault, abusive relationships, or stalking (World Health Organization [WHO], 2013a).

It is not uncommon for more than one type of abuse to occur simultaneously. Violence may also occur with a patterned frequency, generally referred to as the **cycle of violence**. The cycle of violence consists of three phases. In the first phase, tension builds between individuals in a relationship as communication fails. An abusive or threatening incident occurs in the second phase. During this phase, the victim feels traumatized and the aggressor blames the victim for the incident. The third phase of the cycle is known as the honeymoon period, a time during which the aggressor may show love and affection and may also promise to change. During this phase, the victim may feel responsible for the abuse, consider reconciliation, and recant or minimize the incident.

Sometimes, the phrase *cycle of violence* refers to violence that occurs across multiple generations within a family. In this context, children witness or are subjected to patterned family violence committed by their parents. Physical damage and emotional damage incurred by children during these experiences cause them to perpetuate violence when they become adults.

TRAUMA **Trauma** is defined as injury to human tissues and organs resulting from the transfer of energy from an external environmental source, such as a motor vehicle, a fire, or a sharp object. In the past the term *trauma* has been associated with the word *accident*. Accident means that the injury occurred without intent, regardless of whether or not the injury could have been prevented (e.g., by wearing a seat belt). Rather than using the term *accident*, trauma professionals generally define trauma as

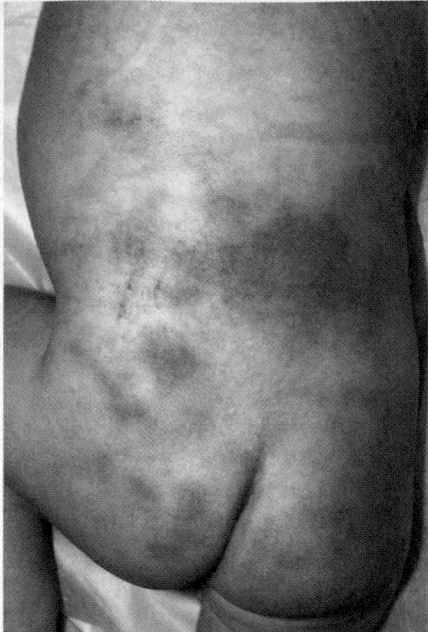

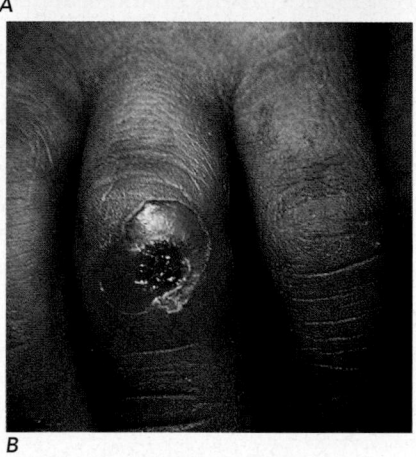

Figure 32–1 ● Examples of child abuse. *A,* Child who has been whipped. *B,* Child burned with a cigarette.

Source: Used with permission of the American Academy of Pediatrics, "Visual Diagnosis of Child Abuse Slide Kit". Copyright © AAP/Kempe (*A*) Biophoto Associates/Science Source. (*B*) NMSB/Custom Medical Stock Photo.

either *intentional* or *unintentional*. Intentional and unintentional trauma encompass a variety of injuries resulting from motor vehicle crashes, pedestrian injuries, gunshot wounds, falls, violence toward others, or self-inflicted violence. The injuries, disabilities, and deaths resulting from these incidents constitute a major healthcare challenge.

Trauma results from an abnormal exchange of energy between a host and a mechanism in a predisposing environment. The *host* is the person or group at risk of injury. Multiple factors influence the host's potential for injury: age, sex, race, economic status, preexisting illnesses, and use of substances such as street drugs and alcohol.

The *mechanism* is the source of the energy transmitted to the host. The energy exchanged can be mechanical, gravitational, thermal, electrical, physical, or chemical. Mechanical energy is the most common type of energy transferred to a host that results in trauma. The most common mechanical source of injury in all adult age groups is the motor vehicle. Guns are

another common mechanical source of injury. Trauma from gunshot wounds has steadily increased during the past 20 years and remains a major reason for emergency department and trauma center admissions, especially in large cities.

When describing a traumatic injury, *intention* is included as a component. Most gunshot and stab wounds are examples of intentional injuries. It is important to remember, however, that some gunshot wounds are unintentional, such as those that occur when children play with their parents' guns. Other common unintentional injuries result from motor vehicle crashes, falls, drownings, and fires. Although hunting accidents are rare in comparison to the number of people participating in the sport, hunting-related deaths and injuries have decreased with the implementation of mandatory "hunting safety" courses in some states.

The final component of trauma is the *environment.* For example, a road that has become slippery after a snowstorm is a physical environment that may contribute to an injury. Occupation is an important environmental factor to consider. Those in certain occupations face a high risk of trauma; examples include police officers, fire fighters, professional athletes, race car drivers, and taxi cab drivers. One's social environment also influences risk for injury.

Minor trauma causes injury to a single part or system of the body and is usually treated in a physician's office or in the hospital emergency department. A fracture of the clavicle, a small second-degree burn, and a laceration requiring sutures are examples of minor trauma. Major or **multiple trauma** involves serious single-system injury (such as the traumatic amputation of a leg) or multiple-system injuries. Multiple trauma is most often the result of a motor vehicle crash.

Trauma is further classified as either blunt or penetrating. **Blunt trauma** occurs when there is no communication between the damaged tissues and the outside environment; for example, a baseball batter being hit by a pitch. Blunt trauma is caused by various forces including *deceleration* (a decrease in the speed of a moving object), *acceleration* (an increase in the speed of a moving object), *shearing* (forces occurring across a plane, with structures slipping across each other), *compression*, and *crushing*. Blunt forces often cause multiple injuries that can affect the head, spinal cord, bones, thorax, and abdomen. Blunt trauma is frequently caused by motor vehicle crashes, falls, assaults, and sports activities.

Penetrating trauma occurs when a foreign object enters the body, causing damage to body structures. Structures commonly affected include the brain, lungs, heart, liver, spleen, intestines, and the vascular system. Examples of penetrating trauma are gunshot or stab wounds and impalement.

Other types of trauma include inhalation injuries from gases, smoke, or steam; burn or freezing injuries; and blast injuries from explosions. Blast injuries result from the temperature and velocity of air movement and the force of projectiles from the explosion. Blast injuries are more severe in water than in air because blast waves travel farther and faster in water. Trauma from blast injuries includes pulmonary edema and hemorrhage, damage to abdominal organs, burns, penetrating injuries, and ruptured tympanic membranes.

Prevalence

In the United States, violence is a widespread problem that affects people of all ages. Over 3 million child maltreatment cases are reported to state and local agencies each year, with over 740,000 youth hospitalized annually due to violence (CDC, 2012a). Data about elder maltreatment is harder to assess, largely because it is extremely underreported and often occurs at the hands of the person's intended caregiver. A study conducted in 2011 reported that 7.6%–10% of older adults had experienced abuse in the year prior to the study (National Center on Elder Abuse, n.d.).

Emergency departments handle 42 million trauma-related visits each year in the United States. Each year, roughly 2 million people are admitted to hospitals due to trauma. Violence accounts for about 10% of all traumatic brain injuries, including shaken baby syndrome, gunshot wounds, intimate partner violence (also called domestic violence), and child maltreatment (National Trauma Institute, 2012).

Genetic Considerations and Nonmodifiable Risk Factors

To better understand the causes and risk factors of the occurrence of violence, researchers have conducted studies about the influence that genetic predisposition, age, and gender have on people who commit violent acts. Each of these lenses explores the scope of violent behavior.

GENETIC PREDISPOSITIONS TOWARD VIOLENCE

Researchers continue to study whether a genetic predisposition toward violent behavior exists. They have found that while genetics may play a role in whether an individual becomes violent, environment is often a cofactor in its manifestation. Examples of environmental factors that may affect whether an individual becomes violent include prior abuse and exposure to violence. Researchers also believe there may be a link between expression of violence by genetically predisposed children and the parenting practices of their caregivers (Shannon, Mead, & Beauchaine, 2010).

Some studies have examined the X-linked gene *MAOA*, which is known to relate to an individual's propensity for developing violent behaviors. One such study found that external stimulation of neurotransmitters in the brain, namely, through spoken language, had different effects on how people process anger, how anger manifested as aggression, and how self-control was affected by stimulation.

Recent research has also examined how children believed to have a genetic predisposition toward violence are affected by maltreatment and whether or not they are apt to develop antisocial behavior or other disorders. In these studies, wherein children with similar environmental risk exposures were examined, the outcomes were varied. Some children became violent, others displayed signs of depression, and still others displayed no problematic behaviors (Shannon et al., 2010).

Genetic disorders that relate to social and mental health are often discussed in conjunction with studies that look at the genetic predisposition toward violence. Included in this discussion are bipolar disorder, paranoid schizophrenia, impulse control disorder, and depression. Mental health alone is not a predictor of future violent behavior. However, studies have shown that mental health disorders that go untreated can manifest in violent behaviors, especially when other risk factors— such as substance abuse, environmental stressors, and history of violence—are present (Elbogen & Johnson, 2009).

AGE   Patterns of violence evolve over an individual's lifetime, but are expressed at a particularly high rate during adolescence

and young adulthood. A nationwide 2010 study showed that 32.8% of youth in grades 9 through 12 reported having been in a physical fight during the year prior to the survey. A number of behaviors displayed in an individual's youth are considered warning signs for future violence. These include intense anger, frequent loss of temper or blow-ups, extreme irritability, extreme impulsiveness, and becoming easily frustrated. Environmental factors that increase risk of violence for youth include previous aggression, abuse, exposure to violence, use of drugs or alcohol, stressful socioeconomic factors at home, and brain damage from trauma (American Academy of Child and Adolescent Psychology, 2011).

GENDER   Gender has a strong influence on violence, according to statistics. Although people of any gender may become victims of violence, women are victims of intimate partner violence (IPV) and sexual violence more frequently than men are. In recent studies, women accounted for four out of every five victims of intimate partner violence. Though still prevalent in the United States, intimate partner violence has declined by over 60% for males and females in recent years. Severe physical violence at the hands of an intimate partner affected 24.3% of female intimate partner victims versus 13.8% of male victims (National Institute of Justice, 2010).

When it comes to intimate partner violence, several factors contribute to male aggression. Factors that relate to the family include having a criminal father figure, coming from a disrupted family, and having poor parental relationships. Individual risk predictors include impulsive behaviors and aggressiveness. Research has shown that these factors, when present in early childhood, can predict intimate partner violence in men. In addition, men who engaged in intimate partner violence often had struggles with employment, alcoholism, and using drugs (CDC, 2012b).

CASE STUDY \\ PART 1

A gunshot victim is en route to the emergency department (ED) by ambulance. You will be the client's admitting nurse. At present, you have minimal information about the client. The paramedics report that the bleeding is controlled and the client is alert. It is currently unclear how much blood loss has been sustained. Vital signs include temperature 97.0°F oral; pulse 92 bpm; respirations 22/min; and BP 105/75 mmHg. The ambulance ETA (estimated time of arrival) is 5 minutes.

Clinical Reasoning Questions Level I

1. How would severe blood loss affect the client's blood pressure?
2. What are the primary nursing considerations for this client?

Clinical Reasoning Questions Level II

3. Consider your perceptions of this client knowing only that this individual is a gunshot victim. What is your initial response?
4. How would your perceptions change if the client is a victim of intimate partner violence? A criminal assailant? Someone who was injured while protecting another individual from harm? Please explain your perceptions for each category.
5. Describe the symptoms of severe blood loss and shock. Describe the nursing interventions for a client who presents with severe blood loss.

Alterations and Therapies **Violence**

ALTERATION	DESCRIPTION	MANIFESTATIONS	INTERVENTIONS AND THERAPIES
Abuse	A pattern of behavior that dominates, controls, lowers self-esteem, or takes away freedom of choice. Can include elder abuse, child abuse, intimate partner abuse, and sexual abuse.	■ Bruises, broken bones, burns, and concussions, at times presenting with no explanation or improbable reasoning, such as "I fell down the stairs again" ■ Intense fear, manifesting primarily when discussing injuries or the abuser ■ Withdrawal from friends and family ■ Unexplained vaginal or anal bleeding or sores	■ Medical interventions for trauma ■ Legal interventions ■ Community response and resources ■ Behavioral therapy ■ Family therapy ■ Support groups
Assault/homicide	Injury from an act of violence where physical force is used with intent to harm, injure, or kill; in homicide, the injury is fatal.	■ Injuries such as knife wounds, gunshot wounds, bruises, broken bones, sprains, and/or dislocations ■ Death from injuries	■ Medical interventions for trauma ■ Legal intervention ■ Behavioral therapy ■ Support groups
Rape	The victim has physical and emotional responses to the act of rape.	■ Flashbacks of the rape days, months, or years after the event ■ Feelings of fear and anxiety ■ Depression ■ Sexual dysfunction ■ Shock ■ Eating and sleep disturbances ■ Feelings of guilt and self-blaming	■ Medical interventions for trauma ■ Support groups ■ Counseling ■ Medication ■ Legal intervention ■ Sexual assault evidence collection kit (rape kit) ■ Pregnancy interventions (e.g., emergency contraception) ■ Sexually transmitted infection and disease testing
Suicide	Suicide is the taking of one's own life.	■ Physical manifestations of suicide attempt could include wounds to wrists or throat, knife wounds, gunshot wounds, asphyxia, crushed trachea, or manifestations of pharmaceutical overdose. ■ Emotional manifestations may include pronouncements of wanting to die, severe depression, crying spells, anxiety, and emotional withdrawal.	■ Prevention ■ Medical interventions for injuries ■ Intervention if the attempt was not fatal; intervention may include pharmacotherapy and psychotherapy in combination. ■ Hospitalization may be necessary immediately following the attempt. ■ Support groups and other therapies for survivor, and/or surviving family members

▶ PREVENTION

Violence is preventable. Knowing the different warning signs of violent behavior as well as other forms of violence prevention can help promote safety. Individual violence prevention involves recognition of the warning signs of potentially violent behavior such as uncontrolled anger, threatening language, and aggression. Recognizing the indicators of violence can help individuals avoid potentially dangerous situations. Knowledge of protective measures is also imperative; some measures include not walking or running alone in deserted areas, asking for help when being abused, and reporting violent behaviors or crimes. Community-based prevention works to eliminate violence before it begins by changing the underlying roots of negative behavior in individual homes, schools, and within the community. Programs within communities focus on education regarding abuse, bullying, and neighborhood violence. Middle and high schools include a curriculum about dating violence, bullying, and overall safety. Adolescents have reported that this curriculum is both appropriate and helpful in responding to difficult or dangerous situations (Herrman, 2009). Many communities also have youth centers devoted to healthy recreational and educational activities in an effort to prevent youth violence.

Nurses help to prevent violence through educating clients about high-risk situations, such as spouses who have been abusive in the past, peer pressure in adolescent dating, and the dangers of date rape and violence. Assessing the signs of abuse and offering interventions can also help to prevent further violence. Nurses working at schools or other community settings can help to dispel myths about aggression and abuse, assuring clients that it is never acceptable for someone to control or injure them. Assessing for inadequate coping mechanisms, signs of inadequate anger management, or inappropriate behavior can help to identify potentially violent tendencies and implement behavior therapy before someone is victimized. Nurse must remain current with new, evidence-based practice initiatives to help protect individuals, clients, facilities, and the community from violence.

Modifiable Risk Factors

Abuse can be stopped, but many victims feel powerless against their abusers. By recognizing the signs of distress and injury that accompany abuse, nurses can help to prevent further attacks. Community and individual actions work to prevent trauma in the form of motor vehicle crashes and neighborhood violence. In working to prevent one act of violence, or one instance of abuse, and entire violent cycle could be ended.

ABUSE PREVENTION Nurses in all areas of practice (e.g., maternal/child health, school, community and occupational health, mental health, primary and acute care, and academic settings) need to take a proactive role to prevent family violence. Early screening of vulnerable individuals and efforts to promote a change in attitudes and beliefs about family violence are essential.

If they are to assist victims effectively, nurses must be aware of their own feelings about family violence. Nurses who are unclear about their own feelings about family violence may deny its existence, blame the victim in crisis, or minimize the effects of the violence. Individuals who have been abused often blame themselves. If this sense of blame is reinforced by healthcare providers, the victim will likely not seek assistance again if abused in the future. Factual, judgment free assessments of clients who have been subjected to violence are essential (Ford-Gilboe et al., 2011).

Nurses also can be instrumental as advocates for developing policies and programs and providing in-service training and education to healthcare professionals and the public. Comprehensive violence prevention programs require a variety of disciplines and organizations working together, such as state or provincial and local healthcare agencies, criminal justice agencies, and social service agencies.

TRAUMA PREVENTION Areas of health promotion and trauma prevention interventions for individuals and communities include the following:

- *Motor vehicle safety:* seat belts, air bags, helmets, driving under the influence of alcohol or drugs, reckless driving, visual or cognitive deficits in the older adult, cell phone use (dialing, talking, texting), driver fatigue
- *Relationships:* intimate partner violence, child abuse, elder abuse, or neglect
- *Communities:* gun control, gangs, condition of streets, neighborhood safety.

In providing information about trauma prevention to members of the community, the nurse serves as a healthcare educator, political activist, and safety advocate.

Many city and county governments have multidisciplinary child abuse and prevention teams or child fatality prevention teams. These teams meet monthly to review child abuse or child fatality cases to determine whether any recommendations need to be made at the state level. Typically, teams do not review cases until any legal actions have been taken and resolved. For example, a child fatality team will not review a child homicide until after the perpetrator has been to trial. All team members must sign confidentiality statements. Examples of recommendations that may result from the efforts of these multidisciplinary teams include recommendations regarding requirements for car seat or bicycle helmet use. Team members are usually mandated by law and frequently include community health nurses, school nurses, preschool directors and school principals, members of law enforcement, and representatives of the district attorney's office.

▶ ASSESSMENT

Assessment of a client who has been injured as the result of abuse or violent trauma will depend on the nature and extent of the injuries. The client may present with minor abrasions and bruises from abuse or with a gunshot wound to the abdomen from an attempted homicide. During the assessment phase it is imperative for nurses to consider the client's cultural and spiritual practices, because these can have bearing on further treatment and interventions.

Nursing Assessment

The priority when assessing any client always begins with the **ABC**s:

Airway
Breathing
Circulation.

Only when these priority needs have been met will the nurse go on to conduct a more complete physical survey. Abuse and trauma assessments are the most common assessments for violence, and cover a range of violent acts and their effects on clients. Nurses consider clients on a case-by-case basis; injuries from violence manifest differently depending on the client's overall disposition, experience, age, and history. Stereotypical mind-sets regarding abuse victims have no place in nursing; if a client presents with signs of abuse, that individual should be assessed for abuse regardless of his or her race, culture, gender, or socioeconomic status.

ABUSE ASSESSMENT   Often the nurse is the first person to discover that the client has been abused. Some victims may not disclose the abuse, may deny it despite obvious symptoms, or they may minimize its impact. However, it is the nurse's responsibility to be alert for symptoms of abuse. Because any client can be the victim of abuse, it is important for the nurse to not allow personal biases to impact who is assessed for these symptoms, but rather be alert for them in all client interactions. If the nurse acts on a bias that only certain types of individuals are abused, many abuse victims will not receive the care they need.

During the assessment interview, the nurse must ensure privacy. The victim must feel safe from the perpetrator. It may be difficult for the client to admit to the reality of family violence until a trusting nurse–client relationship evolves. The nurse should assure the client of a genuine desire to help the entire family system. The nurse should also approach this topic as if it were any other health risk with a professional and calm demeanor. In addition, the nurse can offer the option of answering questions about incidents of abuse with "sometimes" instead of "yes" or "no"; this may encourage the client to make a first step to acknowledge the abuse.

Victims of violence enter the healthcare system for a variety of conditions associated with abuse. For example, common physical complaints include chronic pelvic pain, headache, irritable bowel syndrome, arthritis, pelvic inflammatory disease, and neurological damage. Psychiatric illness (e.g., alcoholism) may also be the result of a history of sexual or physical abuse. Depression is also common. The assessment interview should include a detailed nursing history as well as a description of current symptoms.

Victims of physical abuse may suffer a variety of injuries. During a head-to-toe assessment, the nurse may observe for indications of abuse, such as the following:

- **Head:** bald patches on the scalp where hair has been pulled out; evidence of trauma from blows to the head, such as hematoma, facial bruises, facial fractures, bruised or swollen eyes, hemorrhages into the eyes; petechiae around the eyes from attempted strangulation
- **Skin:** swelling or tenderness, bruises, burns, or scars of past injuries on the skin, genitals, and rectal areas

- **Musculoskeletal system:** fractures or evidence of previous fractures, particularly of the face, arms/legs, and ribs; dislocated joints, especially in the shoulder when the victim is grabbed or pulled by the arm
- **Abdomen:** bruises, wounds, or intra-abdominal injuries, especially if the person is pregnant
- **Neurological system:** hyperactive reflexes due to neurological damage; paresthesias, numbness, or pain from old injuries.

If the nursing assessment reveals possible intimate partner violence, a team assessment needs to take place. The victim's medical condition and emotional state must be assessed. The severity and potential fatality of the situation must be considered, as well as the needs of dependent children and the legal ramifications.

TRAUMA ASSESSMENT   Violence results in traumatic injury that may involve multiple systems. Because of the serious consequences of trauma, it is important to identify the client's injuries and institute appropriate interventions immediately. When caring for the trauma victim, the nurse must always prioritize assessments with the **ABCDE**s as the highest priority concerns:

Airway maintenance with cervical spine protection
Breathing and ventilation
Circulation with hemorrhage control
Disability and neurological assessment
Exposure and environmental control.

Only after assessing the ABCDEs can the nurse go on to perform a detailed assessment of other systems or a focused assessment of the involved area of trauma.

Trauma usually occurs suddenly, leaving the client and family with little time to prepare for its consequences. Nurses provide a vital link in both the physical and psychosocial care of an injured client and family. In caring for the client who has experienced trauma, nurses must consider not only the initial physical injury, but also its long-term consequences, including rehabilitation and (in cases of accidents, abuse, or assault) prevention. Trauma may alter the client's previous way of life, potentially affecting independence, mobility, cognitive thinking, and appearance.

Death is a common result of serious traumatic injury, and may be immediate, early, or late. Immediate death happens at the scene from such injuries as a torn thoracic aorta or decapitation. Early death occurs within several hours of the injury from, for example, shock or delay in recognizing injuries. Late death generally occurs 1 or more days after the injury and results from multiple organ failure, sepsis, and blood loss.

Trauma may result in death or cause injury serious enough to alter both the client's and the family's lives. The suddenness and seriousness of the event are precipitating factors in the development of a psychological crisis. Nurses working with the client who has experienced trauma should assess the family for a variety of needs, including immediate social and spiritual support. For clients who will require long-term rehabilitation, nurses may provide referrals to family members for counseling or financial support services.

Most hospitals employ a variety of professionals who can provide support to families of trauma victims. Nurses may call on the hospital chaplain, foreign language interpreter, social worker, victim's advocate, or other professional to provide assistance to a client who is the victim of violence or trauma and/or the client's family.

Numerous factors help healthcare providers determine the seriousness of a client's injuries and the potential for survival when violence results in serious trauma. Scoring systems such as the Champion Revised Trauma Score system can be helpful. A rapid but comprehensive trauma assessment, completed on the scene, includes the following:

- *Airway and breathing assessments* to determine if the airway is patent, maintainable, or nonmaintainable, and if ventilations are impeded in any way, such as by rib fractures or a collapsed lung
- *Circulation assessment* to palpate peripheral and central pulses; to assess capillary refill, skin color, and temperature; and to identify any external sources of bleeding
- *Level of consciousness* and *pupillary function assessments*
- *Assessment for any obvious injuries.*

The Glasgow Coma Scale is another scoring system that is used to quantify the level of consciousness following traumatic brain injury. For more information on the Glasgow Coma Scale, see the module on Intracranial Regulation.

Lifespan and Cultural Considerations

No age group is immune to violence. However, some age groups (such as children and older adults) are less likely to report or admit to instances of violence. The abuse of older adults has become a growing problem in the United States. It is estimated that only 1 in every 14 cases of elder abuse is reported or recognized. Family members account for approximately 90% of abuse involving older adults (National Center on Elder Abuse, n.d.). Signs of abuse in older adults are often missed by healthcare professionals, which could be due to the misconception that this population is not at increased risk for violence. Nurses need to evaluate clients of all ages for signs of abuse, neglect, or violence.

Cultural and spiritual considerations in violence assessment are numerous, and will vary based on the incident (e.g., abuse vs. extensive trauma). Some considerations with regard to trauma injuries predominantly involve terms of treatment. Two primary spiritual beliefs to consider are those of Jehovah's Witnesses and Christian Scientists. Jehovah's Witnesses believe it is in defiance of their religious scripture to accept blood transfusions, even as a lifesaving procedure. Many hospitals are equipped to perform procedures without the use of blood transfusions, but in cases of extreme trauma the client may have already suffered dangerous levels of blood loss. Nurses and physicians should explain the dangers and potential outcomes (such as death, organ failure, or brain damage) of not accepting a needed blood transfusion, but ultimately the client's decision must be honored. Christian Scientists believe that healing is a matter of faith, and almost all medical interventions will be denied regardless of the risks and potential outcome.

Violence itself can also be an expected element of specific cultures; for example, gang culture and drug culture. Within gang culture violence is not only accepted, it is a value and a rite in the culture. Violence is at times an established form of initiation, and it is seen as an imperative for protecting the identity and social standing of the gang. Gang members also have a "code of behavior" with regard to injuries sustained from other members within the culture—including their gang and other gangs. It is often unacceptable for a member of this culture to report how an injury was received if it was related to gang activity. Similarly, due to fear of prosecution, some members of this culture will not seek immediate medical attention for injuries that result from gang violence (Howell & Moore, 2010). Nurses working with individuals from within this culture need to resign all negative preconceived notions and treat the client objectively.

Diagnostic Tests

The diagnostic tests ordered once the client reaches the hospital depend on the type of injury the client has sustained. Tests that may be ordered for victims of violence include the following:

- *Blood type and crossmatch* involves typing the client's blood for ABO antigens and Rh factor, screening the blood for antibodies, and crossmatching the client's serum and donor red blood cells.
- *Blood alcohol level* measures the amount of alcohol in a client's blood. Alcohol alters the client's level of consciousness and response to pain.
- *Urine drug screen* may also be ordered. Like alcohol, such drugs as cocaine alter the client's level of consciousness and overall response to the primary survey.
- *Pregnancy test* for any woman of childbearing age rules out the potential for pregnancy and fetal injury.
- *Focused assessment by sonography in trauma (FAST)* exam evaluates the unwelcome presence of blood in body cavities. Primary focus is on the peritoneum. It is also helpful in identification of blood in the pleura and pericardium.
- *Diagnostic peritoneal lavage* determines the presence of blood in the peritoneal cavity, which may indicate abdominal injury. This test is generally done in the emergency department. A local anesthetic (such as lidocaine) is injected subcutaneously, and a small incision is made in the lower abdomen. A catheter is placed into the peritoneal cavity, and any free blood is aspirated. If 10 mL of blood is found, the client is taken to the operating room for exploratory surgery. If no free blood is aspirated, 1 L of a warm isotonic solution (Ringer solution or normal saline) is rapidly infused into the peritoneal cavity and then allowed to drain by gravity. If the solution returns pink and is found to have a red blood cell count of 100,000 mm^3, a white blood cell count of >500, or bile, food, or feces, the test is considered positive and the client is taken to the operating room for exploratory surgery. This procedure has been used less since the inception of the FAST exam.
- *Computerized tomography (CT) scans* can reveal injuries to the brain, skull, spine, spinal cord, chest, and abdomen.
- *Magnetic resonance imaging (MRI) scans* can reveal injuries to the brain and spinal cord.

CASE STUDY \\ PART 2

The ambulance arrives at the ED and paramedics emerge with the client, Mark Alvarez, a 32-year-old Hispanic male police officer. Officer Alvarez was shot during a routine traffic stop, sustaining a bullet wound to his right shoulder. Upon arrival, the client is awake and alert. His clear speech suggests a patent airway. His respirations are regular and nonlabored. His skin is pink, warm, and dry. You obtain another set of vital signs, which include temperature 97.2°F oral; pulse 90 bpm; respirations 20/min; and BP 100/72 mmHg. Following thorough medical assessment by the ED physician, it is determined that Officer Alvarez is stable. He will require surgical intervention to explore and treat his shoulder injury. The ED physician orders laboratory diagnostics including complete blood count (CBC), serum electrolytes, and type and crossmatch for possible administration of blood products.

Following assessment and evaluation by the trauma surgeon, Officer Alvarez is scheduled for immediate surgical exploration of his right shoulder.

You remain with Officer Alvarez while he is waiting to be taken to surgery. The client seems slightly anxious. When you ask if he has any questions about his surgery, Officer Alvarez responds by asking if his wife has arrived yet. You report that she has not. Officer Alvarez seems disappointed to hear this; he asks you to make sure she is told he is going to surgery and you ensure him she will be informed as soon as she arrives. A nurse from the OR arrives to transport Officer Alvarez to surgery.

Clinical Reasoning Questions Level I

1. Explain two possible reasons for Officer Alvarez's decrease in blood pressure.
2. Why do you think Officer Alvarez seems more concerned about his wife's absence than his impending surgery?
3. How would the case have changed if Officer Alvarez's airway had not been patent?

Clinical Reasoning Questions Level II

4. Would Officer Alvarez's injury have been worse had he been shot in the left shoulder? Explain your answer.
5. Describe three long-term interventions for Officer Alvarez's care after surgery.
6. Describe two possible complications that could arise during the client's surgery.

▶ INTERVENTIONS AND THERAPIES

The nurse may be called on to care for the victim of violence, the perpetrator of violence, or both. Nurses must provide quality care to both the perpetrator and the victim. Personal biases, judgments, and retribution have no place in nursing care. Although caring for a victim of violence can arouse the nurse's sympathies, the nurse must maintain objectivity to optimize care.

Independent

Interventions for care will be both independent and collaborative, but the nurse may have first contact with the client during which time a number of independent interventions can be employed.

INTERVENTIONS FOR VICTIMS OF ABUSE   In cases of abuse the nurse may be the only professional to have contact with the client, so it is essential for the nurse to (a) determine the immediacy of danger, (b) convey that the person is not to blame and has the right to be safe, (c) explore options for help, and (d) provide information regarding available services. Nurses need to avoid a judgmental attitude and support the individual's choice about whether to leave the unsafe situation or return to the abusive relationship. Because severely battered women are at risk for homicide, the nurse needs to inform the client about associated risk factors and determine the immediacy of danger.

Nurses must familiarize themselves with agency protocols and resources available for victims of intimate partner violence. Most municipalities have crisis help lines and hotlines to provide assistance to victims of abuse. The nurse should also keep a record of telephone numbers for transition houses and rape crisis centers, alcohol and drug abuse information, support groups, religious organizations, and legal services. In addition, several national organizations offer toll-free contacts, such as the National Organization for Victim Assistance, the National Coalition Against Domestic Violence (in the United States), and the National Clearinghouse on Family Violence (in Canada).

The priority nursing consideration regarding the abused child is to ensure safety. Once the child's safety is ensured, developing a trusting relationship will allow the child to discuss his or her feelings and describe the abusive event. The child should not be required to repeat the story for multiple reports because each retelling carries the possibility of creating trauma for the child. All hospitals and agencies working with abused children have standard protocols that support the child and ensure adequate information needed by law enforcement is obtained without further victimizing the child through a repetitive or unfriendly process.

The nurse working with an abused child needs to say that he or she believes the child's story; the nurse also must reassure the child that he or she has done nothing wrong. The nurse should avoid making negative comments about the abuser and must follow established protocols for mandatory reporting, documentation, and use of available support services (e.g., the police department, social service agencies, and child welfare agency).

Short-term interventions for abused older adults include developing a positive relationship with both the victim and the abuser, exploring ways for the older person to maximize independence, and exploring the need for additional home care services or alternative living arrangements.

TRAUMA INTERVENTIONS   Victims of violence often present in the emergency department with life-threatening injuries including hypovolemia due to blood loss, organ damage, and multisystem complications. The client will often be in both physical and psychological shock. Medical care for the client in shock focuses on treating the underlying cause, increasing arterial oxygenation, and improving tissue perfusion. Depending on the cause and type of shock, interventions include emergency care measures, oxygen therapy, fluid replacement, and medication administration.

Care of the trauma client depends on a team approach. Providing trauma care with a team focus helps each team member know his or her role. Prompt delegation of tasks and responsibilities improves the client's chances for survival and decreases the morbidity that may result from traumatic injuries.

The nurse's role in trauma care begins with **triage**, the process of determining which client needs the most urgent medical intervention. Triage is based on the ABCDEs of trauma care. The nurse begins the triage process by performing a rapid general assessment including vital signs, level of consciousness, and a head-to-toe review looking for obvious physical alterations.

When caring for a client who experienced trauma, maintaining a patent airway and monitoring breathing and circulation are ongoing responsibilities. If the client has experienced blood loss, is in shock, or is in unstable condition, the initiation of an IV line is often a high priority because it allows for administration of medications, fluid, and blood products. Changes in the client's condition are often marked by subtle alterations, so the nurse's primary role is in performing ongoing assessments in order to correct problems before they become more acute.

Collaborative

The initial focus of care for the client with a traumatic injury is physiological stabilization. During this time, physical injuries are identified and treated. Pharmacologic treatment for these clients may include administering analgesics for pain; however, because certain analgesics may cause sedation, physical and neurological assessments are usually conducted prior to administering these medications. Depending on the severity of the client's injury, inotropic agents and vasopressors also may be indicated. (See the Medications feature.)

From the psychosocial standpoint, the best treatment for families experiencing violence generally involves a multidisciplinary approach with nurses, physicians, social workers, police, protective services personnel, and, often, lawyers. Most families are more open to accepting help during a time of crisis than at other times. They most likely will be willing to develop new behavior patterns for a short time following a crisis. If families are not helped during that time, they will most likely return to previous behavior patterns, including violence.

Nurses should know the laws associated with reporting abuse. In the United States and Canada, nurses are required to report any suspected child abuse. The courts and child protective agencies make decisions in the child's interest. They may allow a child to remain in the home but under court supervision; they may remove the child from the home; and, in instances of very severe abuse or repeated abuse despite intervention, they may terminate parental rights.

The nurse plays a critical role on a multidisciplinary team, working with families involved in abuse. The nurse is often the healthcare worker who spends the most time with clients and forms a trusting nurse–client relationship. As a result, the client may feel most comfortable when talking with the nurse and be more likely to relate details of the abusive situation. The nurse's role may include teaching, support, or role modeling behavior. For example, if a child is transferred to foster care, the nurse may provide client teaching to the foster family to provide for the child's healthcare needs. Violence may be prevented through anticipatory guidance, such as teaching the new mother normal developmental milestones and best ways of providing care for the infant to reduce frustration that can lead to violence. Read more about anticipatory guidance in the module on Teaching and Learning.

Adults and older adults experiencing violence need similar collaborative interventions, including physicians, social workers, counselors, and police and lawyers. Nurses facilitate referrals and honestly answer any questions asked by the client.

Medications **Trauma**

CLASSIFICATION AND DRUG EXAMPLES	MECHANISMS OF ACTION	NURSING CONSIDERATIONS
Inotropic drugs *Drug examples:* ■ dopamine (Dopastat, Intropin) ■ dobutamine (Dobutrex) ■ isoproterenol (Isuprel)	Inotropic drugs (drugs that increase myocardial contractility) may be given to increase cardiac output and improve tissue perfusion.	■ Administer only after fluid volume restoration. ■ Monitor for signs of extravasation; stop infusion immediately if extravasation occurs. ■ Watch for any side effects such as pain, irregular heartbeat, and rise in diastolic pressure.
Vasopressors *Drug examples:* ■ dopamine ■ epinephrine ■ norepinephrine ■ phenylephrine	Vasopressors may be administered in conjunction with fluid replacement to treat neurogenic, septic, or anaphylactic shock.	■ Monitor cardiovascular response to medications, including heart rate and rhythm, and blood pressure. ■ Use cautiously in children, volume-depleted clients (e.g., severely dehydrated or those who have sustained significant blood loss), and older adults. ■ Watch for signs of confusion and headache, which could be signs of water intoxication.
Opioids *Drug example:* ■ morphine	Opioids are used to treat pain. However, the effects of the pain medications may alter client responses to injury and mask potential injuries. For this reason, client assessment generally is performed prior to administration of opioids or other medications that may produce sedative effects.	■ Monitor for respiratory depression and administer reversal agent (naloxone) if needed. ■ Use cautiously in clients with head trauma.

RELATE Link the Concepts

Linking the concept of violence with the concept of cognition:

1. Describe how untreated schizophrenia could lead to instances of violence and/or violent behavior.

2. How would you assess and diagnose abuse in a client with advanced Alzheimer disease? What signs and symptoms would you look for in particular?

Linking the concept of violence with the concept of mood and affect:

3. You are caring for a client with severe depression who is at an increased risk for suicide. Explain three nursing interventions you could employ to prevent the client from attempting to commit suicide.

4. Could a woman suffering from postpartum depression be at increased risk for abusing her children or spouse? Explain your answer.

READY Go to Companion Skills Manual

REFER Go to Pearson Student Nursing Resources
nursing.pearsonhighered.com

- Additional review materials

REFLECT Case Study \\ Part 3

One month following his right shoulder injury and surgery, Officer Alvarez presents to the clinic for his post-op visit. His surgery was successful; the bullet was excised and damage to the surrounding tissues was minimal. Officer Alvarez has been attending physical therapy sessions, which he describes as "sort of helpful, but my shoulder swells a little bit after my therapy appointments." He reports that he is gaining range of motion in his right shoulder. On a scale of 1 to 10 (with 10 being extreme pain), Officer Alvarez rates his pain as 2.

When asked about his anticipated return to work, Officer Alvarez becomes very quiet. After a pause, he tells you he is expected to return to work in 3 days. He explains that he will be on light duty, which entails working in an administrative role inside the police department, until he has fully recovered. You notice that Officer Alvarez seems uncomfortable discussing his return to work, so you tactfully explore the topic. You begin by asking how he feels about returning to work. Officer Alvarez reports that he feels well physically; however, he has been having nightmares about the shooting. When you ask if he has discussed his nightmares or the actual shooting with anyone, he replies, "It's not something I really want to talk about. I have an appointment with the department shrink tomorrow, though. They're making me see her before I can go back to work." When you ask if he would like to speak with a counselor outside his department, Officer Alvarez replies, "I really don't want to talk about anything with anybody. I just want my shoulder to heal up."

Clinical Reasoning Questions Level I

1. What nursing interventions could you suggest to Officer Alvarez to promote comfort in his shoulder following therapy sessions?

2. What concerns might Officer Alvarez have with regard to his return to work, both in the psychosocial and physical realms?

Clinical Reasoning Questions Level II

3. Is Officer Alvarez at risk for developing posttraumatic stress disorder? Explain your answer.

4. In light of Officer Alvarez's statements, should the nurse proceed with exploring psychosocial considerations related to his injury? Why or why not?

EXEMPLAR 32.1 **Abuse**

EXEMPLAR KEY TERMS
Child abuse, *1965*
Elder abuse, *1965*
Intimate partner violence (IPV), *1966*
Sexual abuse, *1966*

EXEMPLAR LEARNING OUTCOMES
After reading about this exemplar, you will be able to:

1. Describe the pathophysiology, etiology, clinical manifestations, and direct and indirect causes of abuse.

2. Identify risk factors and prevention methods associated with abuse.

3. Illustrate the nursing process in providing culturally competent care across the life span for individuals who have been abused.

4. Formulate priority nursing diagnoses appropriate for an individual who has been abused.

5. Summarize therapies used by interdisciplinary teams in the collaborative care of an individual who has been abused.

6. Plan evidence-based care for an individual who has been abused and his or her family in collaboration with other members of the healthcare team.

7. Evaluate expected outcomes for an individual who has been abused.

▶ OVERVIEW

Abuse can happen to any individual of any age and from any demographic or sociocultural background. Abuse does not only happen to those with supposedly *weak* personalities; individuals with strong or dominant personalities can fall victim to abuse as well. Many generalizations and stereotypes exist in relation to abuse within families, but there have never been any accepted theories for predicting instances of family violence (Wallace & Roberson, 2011). Predisposing factors exist for all forms of abuse (e.g., child, intimate partner, sexual, and elder abuse); however,

even those factors do not always prove to be accurate. Abuse is a growing concern in the United States with many cases going unreported due to fear or threats from the abuser.

▶ PATHOPHYSIOLOGY AND ETIOLOGY

Abuse is often related to control; one individual attempts to control another individual and for this to happen a form of abuse must occur. The three main forms of abuse are physical, emotional, and sexual. All of these can work to break down an individual's self-confidence and self-worth. Some common elements of abuse are humiliation, intimidation, and physical injury (Benedictis, Jaffe, & Segal, 2012). Abuse sometimes start as emotional abuse—such as telling the victim he is not smart enough, or that no one will ever love him—but over time emotional abuse can escalate to physical abuse or even sexual abuse. Physical abuse is generally accompanied by emotional abuse. In cases of sexual abuse, especially childhood sexual abuse, victims will often be exposed to forms of psychological abuse whereby the perpetrator will use the child's need for love and approval against him in order to force the child to submit (American Psychological Association [APA], 2013). Ultimately cases of abuse involve both the use of control and manipulation.

Types of Abuse

The categorizing of abuse is often done in terms of the age of the victim or the form of abuse being perpetrated. Child abuse, elder abuse, sexual abuse, and intimate partner violence are the main categories discussed in this section. Each type of mistreatment presents differently within the life of the victim and has a common perpetrator; for example, child abuse is commonly committed by parents or caregivers. The physical and emotional manifestations of these types of abuse are presented in detail later in the exemplar.

CHILD ABUSE According to the Child Abuse Prevention and Treatment Act (CAPTA), **child abuse** and neglect are defined as "any recent act or failure to act on the part of a parent or caretaker which results in death, serious physical or emotional harm, sexual abuse or exploitation" or "an act or failure to act which presents an imminent risk of serious harm" (U.S. Department of Health & Human Services [USDHHS], 2010). In 2011, 676,569 children (ages newborn to 17) were reported to be victims of child abuse in the United States—this translates to 9.1 out of every 1,000 children. During the past 5 years, the rate of child abuse cases has been decreasing. From 2010 to 2011, 31 out of 51 states reported a marked decrease in cases of child mistreatment (USDHHS, 2012). However, many cases of child abuse still go unnoticed and unreported.

Approximately 47% of children who were abused in 2011 were 5 years old or younger, with 27% of these victims being 3 years of age or younger. Overall, the difference between boys and girls who were abused was almost negligible, with boys accounting for 48.6% and girls accounting for 51.1%. (The gender of some victims was not reported.) Child abuse is often defined as having three forms: neglect, physical abuse, or sexual abuse. Neglect accounts for the highest percentage of child mistreatment cases in the United States. Most often children are maltreated by their parents (81% in 2011), but other perpetrators are generally child care providers, relatives, or a partner or spouse of the child's parent (USDHHS, 2012).

Nurses working with potential victims need to be aware of different methods for helping victims to talk about their experiences. In a study conducted with a group of forensic nurses, the following five themes were highlighted as important when talking to potential victims: a child-friendly environment, building rapport and trust, active listening, believing the child, and the potential for false reports (Finn, 2011). The idea of a child-

friendly environment can be interpreted in various ways and does not necessarily relate directly to the design of the exam room. The nurses in this study reported that while having a room with calming and even fun pictures for the child was nice, it was not generally available or even necessary. Nurses can work to build the environment themselves by helping the child to feel safe. Children of abuse are often deprived of control, so it is important to shift control back to the child while helping her to feel empowered. Building trust is also imperative and will help the nurse to develop a rapport with the young client. Note that building trust with a child should never involve lying or making false promises; for instance, it is impossible to promise that the child's parent(s) will not get *in trouble* that is for Child Protective Services and the courts to decide. Nurses are also "mandatory reporters," meaning that if a child discloses information about abuse the nurse must report the situation; therefore, it would also be a false promise to say, or imply, that any information will be kept only between the nurse and the child. For more information, see the exemplar on Mandatory Reporting in the module on Legal Issues.

The use of age-appropriate language and communication helps the child feel comfortable speaking to the nurse. Active listening and observation must be employed at all times in order to fully engage the client. When starting the conversation, nurses need to begin with a discussion of safe topics, such as school, friends, favorite colors, or even books or television shows. From there, all questions concerning the potential abuse should be open ended as opposed to leading (Finn, 2011). It is not appropriate to ask "Did your mother break your arm?" (leading question); instead, it would be better to ask "How did you hurt your arm?" or "How did your arm break?"

One of the most important considerations for the nurse is believing the child no matter what is disclosed. Children who have been abused are often terrified and convinced that adults will not believe what has happened to them; if the nurse conveys disbelief, the child may shut down and refuse to tell about his experiences. False reports do occur—and nurses need to be mindful of this—but by using open-ended questions nurses cut down on the possibility of creating a false memory in the child's mind (Finn, 2011).

ELDER ABUSE **Elder abuse** is the intentional physical, emotional, or sexual mistreatment or neglect of an individual 65 years of age or older. Although other forms of abuse have been declining over recent years, elder abuse has been on the rise. It is believed that this upward trend is due to increased reporting of elder abuse as the problem receives more attention. Even so, recent studies estimate that only 1 in every 14 cases of elder abuse is actually reported. The reasons behind decreased reporting are numerous, but are believed to be the result of an unwillingness to report family members—who are the primary perpetrators of elder abuse. Other reasons for low reporting involve the physical or mental inability to report the abuse, as well as a heightened fear of retaliation from the abuser (National Center on Elder Abuse, n.d.).

The abuse of older adults—whether it is physical, emotional, or sexual—results in numerous consequences including decreased health, inability to heal from broken bones, and an increased risk for mortality. Studies have also shown that elder abuse that results in hospitalization for the victim often leads to the individual being discharged to a nursing home or long-term care facility, as opposed to returning home (Anetzberger, 2012). Nursing homes and other facilities are also not immune to mistreatment. A study conducted in 2009 reported that between nursing homes, assisted living facilities, and paid home care, residents of nursing homes reported the highest incidences of all forms of abuse, including neglect. The risk for being abused by a caretaker in a nursing home was the highest among all cases of caretaker abuse reported (Anetzberger, 2012). Nurses need to be vigilant in assessing for cases of maltreatment in older adults.

SEXUAL ABUSE **Sexual abuse**, also known as sexual violence, is defined by the CDC (2009b) as "any sexual act that is perpetrated against someone's will." Sexual abuse can include rape, attempted sexual acts, unwanted sexual contact, or even noncontact sexual abuse, which includes voyeurism and sexual harassment. All individuals can be at risk for sexual violence regardless of gender, age, education, IQ, or socioeconomic status. Sexual abuse is often perpetrated by an individual the victim knows such as an acquaintance, family member, teacher, authority figure, parent, sibling, or spouse. The majority of offenders involved in child sexual abuse are family members or are known to the child in some manner (APA, 2013).

INTIMATE PARTNER VIOLENCE **Intimate partner violence (IPV)** is the act of inflicting sexual, emotional, or physical harm on a current or previous partner or spouse. IPV can occur among any couple including same-sex couples, adolescent couples, and older adult couples. The four main forms include physical violence such as punching, kicking, or biting; sexual violence including forced sexual acts or physically violent sexual contact; threats of both physical and/or sexual violence; and emotional abuse such as humiliating the victim or controlling the victim by diminishing self-esteem. Stalking can also be a form of IPV and is defined as repeated harassment or threats often including action such as following the victim and/or vandalizing the person's property (CDC, 2010b).

Although IPV is commonly believed to be committed primarily by men, research does not support this perception. Family conflict studies suggest 50% of victims of IPV are men. Research indicates that men and women demonstrate similar motives for asserting control and inflicting harm when abusing their spouse (Hines & Douglas, 2010). Even so, societal views of IPV and misperceptions can influence the care and treatment of male victims. For example, a study of men who have sought help for instances of IPV described male victims who were ridiculed or arrested as they were assumed to have started the fight or been the aggressor. Even with proof of physical injuries, many men were denied help or ignored because it was considered inconceivable that a man could be abused by a woman (Douglas & Hines, 2011).

When conducting an assessment of a potential victim of IPV, nurses must remain nonjudgmental regardless of gender, sexual orientation, culture, or the socioeconomic status of the victim. Intimate partner violence can result in long-lasting physical and emotional complications, and if the victim feels helpless or as though she will not be believed, then the violence is likely to continue. Most cases of IPV begin as mild emotional or physical abuse, but they eventually escalate to more severe violence, and

can even end in death. Nurses can help to prevent this form of violence by being observant to the manifestations of IPV (discussed later in this section) and helping to empower the victim.

Stay Current: Jacquelyn C. Campbell, PhD, RN, FAAN, and Nancy Glass, PhD, MPH, RN, FAAN, have created an instrument that helps determine the level of risk an abused woman has of being killed by her intimate partner. Visit their Web site at **http://dangerassessment.org** to learn more about it.

Etiology

Many theories exist concerning the motivation for violent behavior and abuse within families. Some of those theories propose that individuals are genetically predisposed to violence, while other theories discuss the influences of society and family structure. No definite causes of family violence have ever been agreed on, but neurobiology, psychopathology theory, and social learning theory lead into one another to help highlight some contributing factors to abusive behavior.

NEUROBIOLOGY Genetics are believed to play a role in anger modulation and emotion control. Anger and its manifestations vary among individuals, with some having self-control and others expressing their anger by becoming abusers. Some studies have therefore suggested that genes can be linked to how the brain processes situations and emotions and then ultimately produces a reaction to anger. Gene studies show that individuals with low levels of the MAOA genotype (often associated with antisocial behavior and aggression) are more prone to become aggressive in high anxiety or emotional situations. Further research on the topic is needed to understand how genetics within families contribute to low levels of this gene. It is believed that individuals who have experienced abuse at an early age, while their nervous system was still developing, could be at higher risk for low levels of MAOA and thus more pronounced violent reactions (Alia-Klein et al., 2009).

PSYCHOPATHOLOGY THEORY The psychopathology theory suggests that some individuals who suffer from personality disorders and mental illnesses participate in family violence as a direct result of these illnesses. Although this is a popular theory, specific mental illnesses and personality disorders have never been indicated, and many with these illnesses are not violent. Some personality disorders and emotional illnesses when left untreated can result in violent tendencies (e.g., bipolar disorder, schizophrenia, paranoid personality disorder), but this does not always result in abuse or family violence (Wallace & Roberson, 2011).

SOCIAL LEARNING THEORY Social learning theory explains that individuals learn violent tendencies through association with others and a reinforcement of the abusive behavior. Children are especially susceptible to this form of learning because they model the behaviors of those around them. Children often model the behaviors of parents, siblings, other adults, or actions they see on television. Therefore, children have a high likelihood of adopting abusive tendencies perpetrated by their parents or siblings, thus furthering a cycle of abuse within the family. Environmental factors can also precipitate cases of abuse, with frustration and increased stress leading to unrestrained anger (Wallace & Roberson, 2011). Learned behaviors will not always result in physical abuse, the abuse may also be emotional or psychological in nature. For example, a child who grew up in a household where both parents were psychologically abusive towards her and each other, might then model that behavior and become psychologically abusive toward her own children. Social learning theory is not absolute, however, and many other factors can affect how an individual will behave later in life (such as environment and experience).

Risk Factors

Many risk factors exist in accordance with abuse, thereby helping to predict which populations are at a higher risk for victimization. Specific risk factors include age, gender, physiological development, cultural and socioeconomic factors, a spouse's history of substance abuse, and having firearms in the house. Abuse can happen to any individual regardless of how many personal risk factors they have, but it is helpful to understand the statistics and reasoning behind some areas of abuse.

AGE Some age groups, particularly younger children and older adults, are at increased risk for abuse due to abusers considering these age groups to be more helpless than others. Young children in particular are at the highest risk for an abuse injury with approximately 27% of all child abuse cases in 2011 occurring in children younger than 3 years old (USDHHS, 2012). In cases of elder abuse, it is virtually impossible to know the full extent of instances of abuse because many are not reported. However, it is known that as older adults age the risk for abuse increases. Abuse in older adults is commonly in the form of neglect, but can also be in terms of physical, emotional, or sexual abuse (Anetzberger, 2012; National Center on Elder Abuse, n.d.).

GENDER For some forms of abuse, gender can be a risk factor, whereas for other forms it does not play an active role. For example, in cases of child abuse there is virtually no difference between the number of female victims and the number of male victims (USDHHS, 2012). Intimate partner violence, however, does show a higher instance of women being abused (24.3% of the female population) than men (13.8% of the male population) (CDC, 2013a). Debates exist over reported numbers of IPV victims, with many claiming that the majority of male victims do not report being abused by their spouse. Some family conflict studies have even indicated that an equal percentage of men and women are victims of abuse from their spouse (Hines & Douglas, 2010). Trends in elder abuse, though, show a clear delineation of women being abused more often than men (National Center on Elder Abuse, n.d.).

PHYSIOLOGICAL DEVELOPMENT Physiological illnesses and disabilities may present one of the highest risk factors for all forms of abuse. Individuals with disabilities are more likely to be seen as easy targets for abuse, with perpetrators assuming that the victim will not, or cannot, report the crime. Some common reported disabilities associated with cases of abuse include intellectual disabilities, physical and learning disabilities, visual or hearing impairments, dementia, and Alzheimer disease (National Center on Elder Abuse, n.d.; USDHHS, 2012). Approximately 11% of all child abuse victims had a physical or emotional disability of some kind. A study of women with disabilities found that 67% had been subjected to physical abuse and 53% had been

sexually abused at some point in their lives. A similar study was conducted in men with disabilities and found that 55% had been physically abused at some time in their lives. It has also been discovered that intimate partner violence among individuals with disabilities is increasingly more prevalent and even disproportionate (National Center on Elder Abuse, n.d.).

CULTURAL FACTORS An individual's culture can also be a risk factor for abuse, with some cultures condoning acts that Western culture considers to be abusive. For example, some Asian cultures use shame as a method of teaching children respect, or for controlling individuals within the family unit. Shame in these instances could be considered a form of psychological abuse, as the individual being shamed may be verbally and continually confronted with his supposed shortcomings and mistakes—shaming could even go so far as to inform a member of the family that he is not good enough (or smart enough, or successful enough, etc.) to be considered a member of the family (Crosson-Tower, 2010). Physical abuse can also be a matter of cultural significance with some cultures employing and condoning punishments of a physical nature toward their children or spouses. Many cultures—including Hispanic Americans, traditional Asian cultures, and some Middle Eastern cultures—believe that children should be respectful and obedient to adults and should follow directions without questions. When children do not adhere to these standards, they may be physically disciplined through spanking or hitting. If these punishments become too forceful, the result can be mild to severe child abuse (Crosson-Tower, 2010).

Within cultures that are strictly patriarchal (or matriarchal) in nature, intimate partner violence may be more prevalent. In these situations one member of the relationship has more power than another, creating a potential for tension that could lead to violence. Instances of violence here could be either physical violence or psychological violence. Other cultures exist where the husband or male partner is strictly in control of the relationship and all members of the family, thus giving him the right to use punishments that he considers to be necessary. Problems can arise in situations such as this because if the woman or children within the family seek help from authorities or medical workers it is considered an act of defiance within the culture itself. The individual in this situation could essentially be shunned from their entire way of life for reporting instances of physical abuse (Montalvo-Liendo, 2009).

In rare, but increasingly more prevalent, instances some cultures may practice ritualistic forms of abuse. Many of these cultures acknowledge a belief and worship of Satan or another devil-like deity. Within the practices of these cultures, children (or new inductees) are continuously terrorized and tortured as a mode of control. Physical mutilation of the child or the child's pets is not uncommon; the pet may also be killed in front of the child as an example, likely causing extreme psychological damage. Ritualistic abuse can often be recognized by the presence of burns (often in a specific shape such as a pentagram or other symbol), tattoos, and/or brands. Injuries such as these when seen on children can be a strong indicator to nurses of the presence of abuse—whether ritual or otherwise. In cases of actual ritualistic abuse, victims are often told repeatedly that no one will ever believe them if report the abuse, making the victim less likely to seek help or admit to having been injured (Wallace & Roberson, 2011).

SOCIOECONOMIC FACTORS   Some researchers consider the culture of poverty to be the largest risk factor and predictor of child abuse and neglect. The stress and feelings of inevitability that come with poverty can lead to frustration, anger, and potentially physical and emotional abuse. Low socioeconomic neighborhoods have also been shown to be more prone to violent activities and to have a higher potential for gang and drug culture, thus feeding into a violent cycle that has been proven to infiltrate the family unit over generations (Collins et al., 2011). However, individuals from high socioeconomic backgrounds can also become the victims and perpetrators of abuse.

SUBSTANCE ABUSE   Substance or alcohol abuse is not necessarily a predictor of abusive behavior, but the excessive use of any mind-altering substances can make abusive situations much worse. For example, if an individual is already being extremely emotionally abusive the use of illegal substances or alcohol could push the perpetrator to physical or sexual abuse, or the emotional abuse could become intensified. Alcohol and other substances do not create an abusive situation; other factors also need to be considered such as the personality of the individual using the substances. However, substance and/or alcohol abuse is one of the leading risk factors for perpetrators of all forms of abuse.

FIREARMS IN THE HOME   It is controversial and virtually impossible to assign statistics for an increased risk for mortality in cases of abuse when a gun is present in the house because these statistics depend on too many reported variables such as the type of firearm (handgun, rifle, shotgun), the storage of the firearm (locked gun cabinet, nightstand drawer, secured gun room), and the location of the incident (city, urban, rural). However, according to the Pew Research Center (2013) and the FBI (2012b, 2012c, 2012d), the following 2011 statistics were reported regarding intimate partner homicide, firearm violence, and related factors:

- 36.5% of female victims (for whom the murderer was known) were killed by a husband or boyfriend.
- 42.9% of all murder victims (for whom the circumstance was known) were killed during arguments—including romantic arguments.
- 72.5% of weapons used during all murders were handguns.
- The murder rates and use of firearms were highest in metropolitan areas and lowest in rural areas.

Prevention

The prevention of abuse must come from various levels including individual, community, society, relationship, and parenting. In addition, the many factors that contribute to abusive relationships need to be addressed in order to stop abuse. Often, abuse is part of a familial or personal cycle that has been going on for years, and until the abuser acknowledges or realizes the cycle, it is likely to continue. Nurses can help prevent abuse by observing for the signs and symptoms of violence and then working to address the situation. When children are involved nurses must report the abuse, but in cases of intimate partner violence it is

ultimately the individual's choice to seek help in stopping the situation. In cases where the client does desire help to stop a violent and abusive situation, nurses can work to facilitate referrals to other healthcare providers, as well as police and lawyers.

> ### SAFETY ALERT
> Sudden unemployment or other forms of financial stress can greatly increase an individual's stress and thus, create a large risk factor for participating in abusive behavior toward another individual. Excessive stress can also lead to alcohol or substance use as a means of coping.

▶ CLINICAL MANIFESTATIONS

The signs of abuse can vary based on the population being abused, as well as the type of abuse. Intimate partner violence, for example, will often manifest with signs of intense fear and control, such as the victim not having access to cash and losing all contact with friends and family. The signs of physical and emotional abuse will also vary among populations with children reacting to psychological abuse differently than adults. In cases of sexual abuse, however, the signs are primarily consistent across age demographics. Nurses should be vigilant in assessing for signs of abuse in all clients.

Manifestations of Child Abuse

Many of the physical manifestations of child abuse are apparent, such as broken or fractured bones in different stages of healing, head injuries, excessive bruising, and burns or scars in specific shapes. More of these physical indicators are discussed in the Clinical Manifestations and Therapies table. Signs of long-term traumatic physical abuse can be evidenced by poor language, cognitive, and emotional development, primarily caused by the stress of abuse as an infant or young children. Advanced visual and motor impairment—such as blindness and spinal cord injuries—can also be indicators of physical abuse at a young age. Other indicators that a child is being abused can present in the form of behavioral changes. Some common changes include trouble sleeping, changes in eating habits, wetting the bed, avoiding specific situations or individuals (family gatherings, a once trusted friend or relative, etc.), and participation in high-risk behavior (drugs, alcohol, dangerous sports) (CDC, 2012a; Meadows, 2013).

Psychological manifestations of abuse can present in the form of childhood depression, anxiety disorders, eating disorders, and learning disorders. The child may also lose interest in academics and begin to perform poorly in school. Low self-esteem as well as a fear of adults and social situations can come as the result of chronic psychological torture. Children in these situations may also become noticeably uncomfortable around individuals who are angry or yelling for some reason; similarly, they may react drastically to simple mistakes—such as accidentally breaking something, or knocking something over—by apologizing profusely, becoming anxious, or crying (CDC, 2012a).

Manifestations of Elder Abuse

Elder abuse often manifests as neglect resulting in bedsores, untreated illnesses or injuries, soiled clothing or bed sheets, weight loss, and overall poor hygiene. The individual being abused could also show signs of depression or a withdrawal from normal activities. Bruises, contusions, or broken bones can be manifestations of elder abuse, but can also be easily explained away by a simple fall. Nurses should perform a complete assessment of the client if abuse is suspected, taking into consideration the client's physical and emotional well-being.

Manifestations of Sexual Abuse

Victims of sexual abuse may be withdrawn or combative, acting out in varied situations. Emotions such as guilt, anxiety, depression, suicidal thoughts, and fear are quite common. In children who have experienced sexual abuse, one of the most pronounced indicators is an early sexual knowledge and potentially early interest in sexual acts. Other children may regress instead, demonstrating behavioral difficulties, bed wetting, and insomnia (APA, 2013). Physical manifestations of sexual abuse at any age include injuries to genitals or anus, swollen genitals, bladder or kidney infections, sexually transmitted infections or diseases, unintended pregnancies, and pelvic inflammatory disease.

Manifestations of Intimate Partner Violence

Intimate partner violence presents with similar physical manifestations to other forms of violence, such as bruises, broken bones, knife wounds, head injuries, and headaches. Individuals experiencing this form of abuse may begin using alcohol and other substances to cope with and/or ignore the abuse. Depression, suicide attempts, fear, and an avoidance of social situations are not uncommon. Victims of IPV are often cut off from any form of support by their abuser; they are generally not encouraged to have relationships with family members or friends, and their freedoms are limited. It is interesting to note that victims of IPV and their children are at increased risk for violence when they are leaving the perpetrator.

Abusers will seek to control victims' finances and decision-making abilities in order to prevent them from leaving the relationship. Some perpetrators will even work to get their partner (or themselves) pregnant and then threaten to keep the child if the victim leaves. Individuals involved in IPV are likely to be intimidated by their abuser and reluctant to seek or accept help. Controlling abusers will likely accompany the victim to the hospital or treatment center for treatment of their injuries to ensure that the client does not ask for help, and depending on the type of abuse, to demonstrate repentance for the injuries (Benedictis et al., 2012; CDC, 2012b). In situations such as these, it may be very difficult or even impossible for the nurse to talk to the client alone. Nurses could try to schedule a follow-up appointment or express a willingness to help the client at a later date if the client wishes to come back alone.

Lifespan and Cultural Considerations

Cultural considerations in cases of abuse are twofold, with some acts or traditions presenting as signs of abuse (such as cupping or coin rubbing), and other cultures partaking in acts that Western culture considers abusive (hitting one's wife for disobedience, or hitting children with objects as a form of punishment). In cases of suspected abuse due to marks on the client's body, nurses must take cultural healing practices into consideration. The practices of cupping and coin rubbing—generally practiced by many Asian cultures, as well as individuals who participate in holistic healing—can both create marks on the body that could be misinterpreted as signs of abuse (**Figure 32–2 ●**) (Crosson-Tower, 2010). Cupping is the act of placing a glass cup on the skin, and then using heat to create suction; often this is performed to promote blood flow and overall healing. The result of the procedure can be circular red welts or even dark bruising, which are often found along the individual's back. Coin rubbing is used to treat a multitude of ailments from headaches and fevers to minor illnesses, but also leaves marks on the skin. In

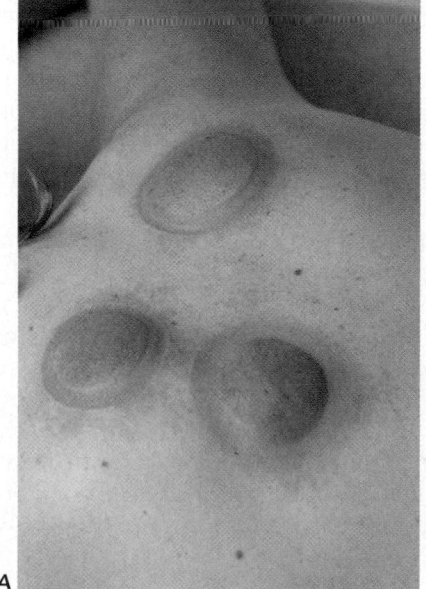
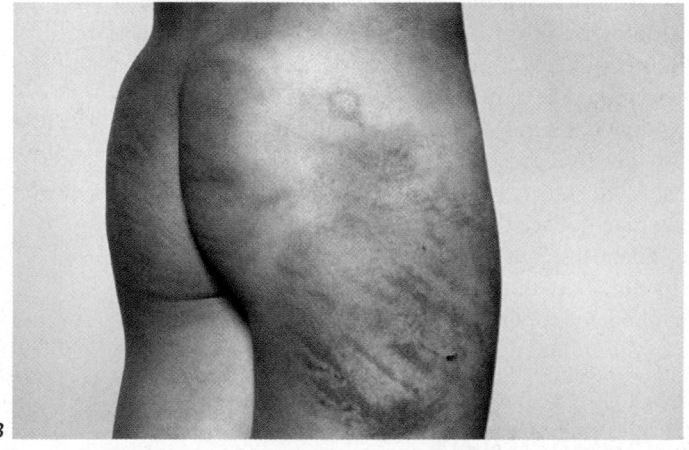

A   *B*

Figure 32–2 ● It is important to differentiate cultural practices such as *A*, cupping, and *B*, coining, from signs of child abuse.
Source: Used with permission of the American Academy of Pediatrics, "Visual Diagnosis of Child Abuse Slide Kit". Copyright © AAP/Kempe. (*A*) doc-stock/Alamy (*B*) Biophoto Associates/Science Source.

this treatment, warm oil is rubbed on the skin and then a coin is rubbed in a diagonal line until long marks appear. If these marks are seen without knowledge of their origin, they may look almost like marks from a whip. Neither of these treatments is abusive in nature, but are instead a form of healing.

Some cultural conceptions of punishment can be considered child abuse. Physical punishment of a child varies among cultures from spanking or hitting their hand, to burning the child, and even hitting the child with a cord to leave cuts (see the Focus on Culture and Diversity feature). Many of these practices may not seem acceptable from a Western perspective, but in some areas of Trinidad and Nigeria hitting a child with a cord is a common form of punishment. Similarly, it many cultures—particularly Chinese and Vietnamese—it is acceptable to discipline a child with the use of sticks. In America, until the early 1980s, it was considered fitting to hit a child by way of spanking or with a thin branch from a tree (commonly referred to as a switch) (Renteln, 2010). Burning a child, particularly with a shaped object, could be a tradition of punishment passed down within an individual family, whereby the mother was burned as a child so she deems it acceptable to do the same to her child. In cases of suspected culturally influenced abuse, nurses recognize that parents may not see the injuries to their child as inappropriate or even abusive, but rather as an unfortunate result of the child's behavior. It is not a nurse's place to judge; however, nurses are mandated reporters of child abuse, even if it is a cultural form of discipline.

▶ COLLABORATION

Usually, the best way to treat violent families is to use a multidisciplinary approach involving nurses, physicians, social workers, protective services personnel, law enforcement, and, often, lawyers. Most families are more open to accepting help during a time of crisis than at other times. They most likely will be willing to develop new behavior patterns for a short time following a crisis, but changing behaviors over time requires much difficult work and support. It is not uncommon for family members to return to previous, unhealthy behavior patterns, including those that condone or promote interpersonal violence.

Diagnostic Tests

Diagnostic tests cannot prove that an individual is being abused, but some tests, such as x-rays, MRIs, and CT scans, can show indicators of possible abuse. Most tests in abuse cases will be used to diagnose the full extent of the damage in order to properly treat the client. In cases of physical abuse, an ultrasound or a CT of the abdomen can check for abdominal or organ injuries, CT scans of the head will show hemorrhage or skull fractures, and an MRI of the spine will show any spinal injuries. For sexual abuse, swabs for DNA are needed to provide the abuser's identity, urine samples will show bladder or kidney infections, and sexually transmitted disease and infection testing should be conducted, as well as pregnancy testing for females. The range of testing to be conducted will depend on the type of abuse, injuries, and consent of the victim. For example, some individuals who have experienced sexual abuse may absolutely refuse to be tested for HIV due to the stigma that comes with the disease as well as the third-party disclosure laws in some states. Clients who have been victims of abuse may also refuse some testing, such as x-rays, so as to avoid healthcare professionals seeing the full extent of their past injuries.

Pharmacologic Therapy

Injuries associated with abuse will vary greatly depending on the situation and type of abuse. Therefore, the pharmacologic interventions will also change based on the type and severity of the injury. For injuries resulting from physical abuse such as broken bones and dislocations, pain medication, sedatives, and anti-inflammatories may be used while setting the injury and for resultant pain. Stabbings, gunshot wounds, or other penetrating injuries will require medications to prevent or heal infections from the injury. Tetanus boosters or vaccines will be needed for most deep penetrating wounds.

In cases of physical and emotional abuse, the client may suffer from posttraumatic stress disorder (PTSD) after the abuse, which could require medication in addition to therapy interventions. Selective serotonin reuptake inhibitors (SSRIs) are often used in conjunction with psychotherapy as a treatment for PTSD. The only two SSRIs approved by the U.S. Food and Drug Administration (FDA) for the treatment of PTSD are sertraline (Zoloft) and paroxetine (Paxil). Other medications may also be prescribed for insomnia or nightmares, such as mirtazapine (Remeron) and prazosin (Mayo Clinic, 2011).

Nonpharmacologic Therapy

The physical effects of abuse will often heal long before the emotional effects have even begun to fade; therefore, the nonpharmacologic therapies used with victims of abuse are numerous and important for the client. Therapy, counseling, and support groups are the most commonly prescribed forms of treatment in cases of abuse. The type of therapy will depend on the personality, needs, and desires of the client. For example, if an entire family unit has experienced abuse at the hands of a family member, then family therapy or group therapy will likely be appropriate. In cases of sexual abuse, group therapy may not be an option, especially if the individual if reluctant to talk about the experiences with others, a feeling that many victims of sexual abuse share.

DOMESTIC VIOLENCE SHELTERS   Today's domestic violence shelters offer a broad array of services. In addition to offering immediate shelter for women and their children, they also provide referrals to a number of agencies that provide services as well as group therapy for women and children, advocacy, and parent training. Many offer lists of attorneys and other professionals who make their services available at sliding scale fees. Nurses working with women and children should have available the contact information for the domestic violence shelters in their community.

PEDIATRIC CONSIDERATIONS   The nurse plays an important role in the multidisciplinary team providing treatment to the child who is the victim of abuse. The nurse should ensure that the team creates a safe and predictable environment in which the child feels supported at home, at school, and in whatever therapeutic environment the team chooses for the child.

As part of the team, the nurse should plan interventions that will encourage affective release in a supportive environment. Child victims must be able to experience a range of emotions. Play therapy helps these children play out traumatic themes, fears, and distorted beliefs. It is a nonthreatening way to process thoughts and feelings associated with the abuse, both symbolically and directly. Art therapy provides an opportunity to express feelings for which there are no words. Therapeutic stories present the traumatic issues of abuse, link victims' feelings and behavior, and describe new coping methods. Journal writing can help children cope with intrusive thoughts and feelings. They often choose to bring their journal into the one-on-one sessions with their therapist.

■ NURSING PROCESS

Care of an individual who has been abused will vary depending on the type of abuse and the age of the individual. A client's reaction to the abuse will also affect care, especially if fear, shame, and/or self-blaming are present. Nurses treat individuals on a client-by-client basis, assessing the need of a specific individual, rather than the needs of a supposedly *typical* abuse victim. Those who have experienced abuse may have similar injuries or mind-sets, but every client is different.

Assessment

The nurse's assessment in cases of abuse will be in order of the severity of the injuries. Airway function, head trauma, broken bones, internal injuries, knife wounds, and gunshot injuries will be assessed first, with cuts, bruises, and behavioral indications assessed after the client's safety is assured. A complete medical history will be performed to determine if the client has a history of injuries that could be the result of abuse. Nurses need to consider the client's emotional state; victims of abuse could be scared of their abuser, or of being blamed for the violence perpetrated against them. Similarly, some clients may be more nervous around male or female staff (depending on the gender of the abuser); if possible, adjustments should be made to the staff directly caring for that client. Some hospitals now assess victims of violence on locked units to minimize exposure of victims and hospital staff to perpetrators.

Diagnosis

Nursing diagnoses are dependent on the client's current physical and psychosocial status, including acute injuries. Clients who have experienced abuse could have a range of diagnoses depending on the mode of abuse. Diagnoses relevant to actual or suspected victims of child abuse, elder abuse, or interpersonal violence may include, but are not limited to, the following:

- *Risk for Trauma*
- *Risk for Self-Harm*
- *Powerlessness*
- *Post-Trauma Syndrome*
- *Risk for Sexual Dysfunction*
- *Social Isolation.*

(NANDA-I © 2012)

Planning

Goals for a client suffering from abuse will change according to the nursing diagnosis and the individual. The age of the client will also affect how an individual reacts to having been injured as the result of abuse. Examples of goals that may be appropriate for inclusion in the plan of care for the client who has experienced abuse are as follows:

- The client will be safe and free from harm.
- The client will ask for help in safely resolving the abusive situation.
- The client will honestly convey feelings of fear, helplessness, anger, or depression.
- The client will report any suicidal ideation.
- The client will acknowledge that she is not responsible for the abuse.
- The client will practice healthy coping mechanisms.

Implementation

The nurse's ability to implement care measures will in part depend on the client's willingness to accept help in leaving or reconciling the abusive situation. In most states, some forms of abuse, such as child and elder abuse, must be reported to the proper authorities. However, reporting other forms of abuse—including intimate partner violence and certain instances of sexual abuse—is often left to the discretion of the victim. Nurses need to understand the victim's fears and emotions in response to abuse in order to help the client in as complete a manner as possible.

Clinical Manifestations and Therapies Abuse

ETIOLOGY	CLINICAL MANIFESTATIONS	CLINICAL THERAPIES
Child abuse Physical, emotional, or sexual abuse of an individual less than 18 years of age	■ Bruises or welts in unusual places or in several stages of healing; distinctive shapes ■ Wary of physical contact with adults ■ Behavioral extremes of withdrawal or aggression ■ Burns (especially cigarette burns; immersion burns of hands, feet, or buttocks; rope burns; or distinctively shaped burns) ■ Apprehensive when other children cry ■ Fractures (multiple or in various stages of healing, inconsistent with explanations of injury) ■ Joint swelling or limited mobility ■ Long-bone deformities ■ Lacerations and abrasions to the mouth, lip, gums, eye, genitalia ■ Human bite marks ■ Signs of intracranial trauma ■ Deformed or displaced nasal septum ■ Bleeding or fluid drainage from the ears or ruptured eardrums ■ Broken, loose, or missing teeth ■ Difficulty in respirations, tenderness or crepitus over ribs ■ Abdominal pain or tenderness ■ Recurrent urinary tract infection ■ Emotional and/or behavioral problems	■ Treat physical injuries. ■ Give antibiotics for any infections. ■ Therapy may be behavioral, cognitive, group, or play therapy depending on developmental stage. ■ Reporting of the abuse is mandatory. ■ Ensure the safety and security of the child.
Elder abuse Emotional, physical, sexual, or financial abuse or neglect of an individual 65 years of age or older	■ Constant hunger or malnutrition ■ Listlessness ■ Poor hygiene ■ Social isolation ■ Inappropriate dress for the weather ■ Chronic fatigue ■ Unattended medical needs ■ Poor skin integrity or decubiti ■ Contractures ■ Urine burns/excoriation ■ Dehydration ■ Fecal impaction ■ Bruises and welts ■ Withdrawal ■ Burns ■ Confusion ■ Fractures ■ Fear or suspicion of caretaker, family members, healthcare providers ■ Sprains or dislocations ■ Lacerations or abrasions ■ Evidence of oversedation ■ Failure to meet financial obligations	■ Treat physical injuries. ■ Treat dehydration and malnutrition with increased fluids and food intake. ■ Treat psychological effects such as depression with medication or therapy. ■ Arrange for respite services. ■ Consider adult day care. ■ Refer to treatment or therapy for perpetrators. ■ Arrange transfer of legal authority.

Clinical Manifestations and Therapies Abuse (continued)

ETIOLOGY	CLINICAL MANIFESTATIONS	CLINICAL THERAPIES
Sexual abuse Can occur in any age demographic and is the performance of any sexual act against an individual's will.	■ Torn, stained, or bloody underwear ■ Pain or itching in genital areas ■ Bruises or bleeding from external genitalia, vagina, rectum ■ Poor peer relationships ■ Withdrawal ■ Sexually transmitted disease ■ Unwilling to participate in physical activities ■ Swollen or red cervix, vulva, or perineum ■ Wears long sleeves and several layers of clothing even in hot weather ■ Semen around the mouth or genitalia or on clothing ■ Pregnancy ■ Delinquency or running away ■ Inappropriate sexual behavior or mannerisms ■ Regressive behaviors	■ Treat physical injuries. ■ Test for sexually transmitted diseases and infections. ■ Administer pregnancy test. ■ Take DNA swabs for identification of the perpetrator. ■ Treat for depression and/or suicidal behavior. ■ Therapy may be behavioral, cognitive, group, or play therapy depending on developmental stage. ■ Consider behavioral therapy for perpetrators.
Intimate partner violence (IPV) Physical, emotional, or sexual abuse of an individual's spouse or partner	■ Chronic fatigue ■ Casual response to serious pain ■ Vague complaints, aches, and injury or excessively emotional response to a relatively minor injury ■ Frequent injuries ■ Recurrent sexually transmitted diseases ■ Frequent ambulatory or emergency department visits ■ Muscle tension ■ Nightmares ■ Facial lacerations ■ Depression ■ Injuries to chest, breasts, back, abdomen, or genitalia ■ Anorexia or other eating disorder ■ Bilateral injuries of arms or legs ■ Anxiety ■ Symmetric injuries ■ Drug or alcohol abuse ■ Obvious patterns of belt buckles, bite marks, fist or hand marks ■ Suicide attempts ■ Poor self-esteem ■ Burns of hands, feet, buttocks, or with distinctive patterns ■ Headaches ■ Gastrointestinal or stress ulcers	■ Treat physical injuries and physiological conditions. ■ Treat psychological effects such as depression with medication or therapy. ■ Suggest substance abuse counseling for perpetrator and victim, as needed.

Promote Safety

In cases of abuse, the client's safety is the primary concern. Due to mandatory reporting laws, nurses must report all suspected cases of child abuse. In some states it is also legally mandated for nurses to report the abuse or neglect of an older adult. Cases of intimate partner violence are often left to the victim to report, but some areas have laws concerning mandatory reporting of IPV. The use of specific weapons and the nature of the injuries are often a factor for mandatory reporting of IPV in states with those laws. Nurses must be aware of regulations within the state where they are practicing, and abide by those laws. When abuse is suspected, the nurse should follow institutional policies and guidelines for reporting. In the clinical setting, the nurse usually is required to notify a supervisor to begin the reporting process.

When mandatory reporting is not indicated, it is imperative for nurses to provide the client with information about resources for seeking help. Resources can be in the form of the client's friends and family members or community liaisons who can work to help the individual find a secure living environment. Other resources can be offered such as police, lawyers, and agencies that can provide ongoing assistance for the victim. Nurses encourage the client to accept help in seeking an abuse-free living situation, but the decision ultimately lies with the client. Some individuals will not be ready to seek help, and while the nurse may disagree with this decision, he must refrain from judgment and be respectful of the client's decision. All nurses can do in these situations is offer assistance and resources; this lets the victim know that help is available if it is needed in the future.

Establish a Therapeutic Relationship

Establishing appropriate modes of interaction with a client who has been abused, or who the nurse suspects has been abused, is vital. Adults who have experienced a form of abuse can be gently encouraged to seek assistance in promoting their own safety. If the client chooses not to seek assistance, then information should be provided in case assistance is ever needed. A large factor in establishing a therapeutic relationship is establishing trust. Were a healthcare worker to appear angry or disappointed in a client for not choosing to seek assistance in leaving an abusive situation, all forms of trust that had been established with that client would be shattered. Individuals who have experienced abuse are likely to have difficulty trusting anyone, particularly anyone who becomes annoyed or frustrated with them easily. Many cases of physical abuse also involve psychological abuse, which often belittles an individual's sense of self-worth and self-love sometimes to the point of feeling that it is impossible for them to do anything correctly. Nurses need to work to establish a trusting relationship with adults who have been abused, ensuring them that they are in a judgment-free and safe setting.

When nurses suspect child abuse, age-specific considerations must be employed. The child needs to feel safe and secure, particularly from the potential abuser. All early conclusions about the situation should be dismissed, because it is unwise to assume knowledge of a situation until all of the details are presented. Child abuse is a very serious situation and should never be taken lightly; however, nurses should be aware that cases of false reporting do exist. The majority of these cases are not malicious on the part of the child, but rather the result of a misunderstanding, or a leading question on the part of the healthcare professional. All forms of leading questions should be avoided when talking to children about abuse. It is appropriate to ask a child how she hit her head; it is inappropriate to ask a child if her mother slammed her head into a kitchen counter. Children in high-stress situations will sometimes work to tell an adult what they think that adult wants to hear. With this in mind, nurses should ask open-ended questions with no indication of the answer they expect to receive. It is imperative for nurses to follow organizational protocols with regard to suspected child abuse interviews.

Facilitate Communication

Accepting help after having experienced abuse for weeks, months, or years is sometimes exceptionally difficult for victims. Elements of fear of their abuser, lack of social support, decreased financial resources, and a sense of hopelessness all contribute to an apparent disinclination to accept assistance. Nurses need to understand these fears in order to better assist clients during this difficult situation. Many resources can be offered to help combat these individual reservations. For example, the client can be put in contact with local law enforcement agencies to file an order of protection against the abuser to ensure some degree of safety from retaliation. Connections can also be fostered with social workers, counselors, and community liaisons to find safe housing and assist with social and financial support. Nurses reassure clients that options and resources are available to help them move away from the abusive situation being experienced.

Promote Empowerment

Helping clients to achieve a sense of control within the situation is one of the first steps in helping them to accept assistance. All forms of abuse include an element of control on the part of the perpetrator, and generally result in taking control away from the victim. In working to help clients regain that sense of control, nurses can help empower them to leave the situation. Support groups and individual therapy are recommended in order to help the client talk about the abuse, and potentially connect with others who have experienced similar situations. Interventions here vary depending on the individual's age and circumstance, so referrals are made on a case-by-case basis.

Evaluation

All forms and cases of abuse are different depending on the age of the victim and the circumstances of the abuse; therefore, the outcomes in these cases will vary. It is important to set realistic goals for clients. Some desired outcomes include the following:

- The client remains free from injury or harm.
- The client seeks assistance when needed.
- The client demonstrates knowledge of the resources available to individuals in abusive situations.
- The client verbalizes awareness that she is not responsible for or deserving of abuse.
- The client openly communicates her fears with regard to the abusive situation.

◢ REVIEW Abuse

RELATE Link the Concepts and Exemplars

Linking the exemplar of abuse with the concept of development:

1. What protective factors would indicate a child probably has not experienced abuse? At age 3? At age 15?

2. What factors would put a child at risk for abuse?

Linking the exemplar of abuse with the concept of mood and affect:

3. What mood and affect would you anticipate a victim of abuse might display?

4. What nursing assessment regarding mood and affect would be a priority when admitting a client who was abused by a family member?

READY Go to Companion Skills Manual

REFER Go to Pearson Nursing Student Resources
nursing.pearsonhighered.com

- Additional review materials

REFLECT Case Study

Lucy Barnes, a 30-year-old woman who is 25 weeks pregnant, comes to the emergency department of Parkfield Community Hospital. She says she fell and hit her head at home and is having headaches. During the assessment the nurse notices multiple bruises in various stages of healing over her body and asks Lucy how she got them. Lucy says that she is just clumsy and falls a lot. While the nurse is assessing Lucy, another nurse enters the room to tell Lucy that her boyfriend is there to take her back home. At that point, Lucy becomes frightened and tells the nurse that her boyfriend has hit her many times before and had knocked her down today. She says he has threatened to kill her if she tells anyone and she does not want to leave with him.

1. Identify questions that the nurse could use in continuing her assessment and in documenting the discussion with Lucy.

2. What other people should be involved in Lucy's care in the emergency department?

3. Who should make the decision about where Lucy should go?

EXEMPLAR 32.2 Assault and Homicide

EXEMPLAR KEY TERMS
Aggravated assault, *1975*
Aggression, *1976*
Frustration, *1976*
Homicide, *1975*
Simple assault, *1975*

EXEMPLAR LEARNING OUTCOMES
After reading about this exemplar, you will be able to:

1. Describe the pathophysiology, etiology, clinical manifestations, and direct and indirect causes of assault and homicide.

2. Identify risk factors and prevention methods associated with assault and homicide.

3. Illustrate the nursing process in providing culturally competent care across the life span for individuals who have been assaulted.

4. Formulate priority nursing diagnoses appropriate for an individual who has been assaulted.

5. Summarize therapies used by interdisciplinary teams in the collaborative care of an individual who has been assaulted.

6. Plan evidence-based care for an individual who has been assaulted and his or her family in collaboration with other members of the healthcare team.

7. Evaluate expected outcomes for an individual who has been assaulted.

▶ OVERVIEW

Assault and homicide greatly impact the healthcare system, because the majority of victims of these crimes will eventually be treated by a healthcare provider within the community. According to the FBI (2012e, p. 50), **simple assault** is defined as "an unlawful physical attack by one person upon another where neither the offender displays a weapon, nor the victim suffers obvious severe or aggravated bodily injury involving apparent broken bones, loss of teeth, possible internal injury, severe laceration, or loss of consciousness." The legal definition of simple assault may vary among states. Additionally, simple assault is distinguished from the similar but more serious offense of aggravated assault. **Aggravated assault** is defined as "an unlawful attack by one person upon another for the purpose of inflicting severe or aggravated bodily injury. This type of assault usually is accompanied by the use of a weapon or by means likely to produce death or great bodily harm" (FBI, 2012e, pp. 49–50). **Homicide** is the killing of one individual by another; for legal purposes, this act is further specified by whether the act was intentional or the result of negligence (FBI, 2012e, p. 47).

Among violent crimes in the United States, assault is the most prevalent (62.4%), whereas homicide has the lowest prevalence (1.2%) (FBI, 2012g). In addition to caring for the victims of assault and homicide, nurses may also be responsible for caring for the perpetrators. All clients will receive the same quality of care regardless of the events that have led them to seek medical treatment. Nurses working in densely populated urban areas—particularly those with high crime rates—will be exposed to more clients who have been victim to these crimes than those in rural scarcely populated areas.

▶ PATHOPHYSIOLOGY AND ETIOLOGY

Whether an assault or homicide comes about through a robbery, an act of terror, a fight between strangers, a situation of domestic abuse, or a random act of cruelty, its origin can be traced to biological, situational, and cultural factors. The origins of violence in society must be understood through the lens of socioeconomic disparity and other demographic factors.

However, the pathophysiology of aggression and fear still plays a role, because these emotions lead to assault and homicide in the moment of the attack. Whether the assault consists of a verbal or a physical act, aggression and fear are the primary emotions at play.

Both the attacker and the victim in an incident of assault or homicide feel aggression during the encounter. Baron and Richardson (1994) offer the following widely accepted definition of **aggression**: "any form of behavior directed toward the goal of harming or injuring another living being who is motivated to avoid such treatment." A strong connection exists between feelings of aggression and stress. Stress itself activates two main physiological pathways: the sympatho-adrenomedullary (SAM) system and the hypothalamic-pituitary-adrenocortical axis. Frequently, a display of aggression is associated with the feeling of anger and an overall high emotional response. The other sort of aggression involved in assaults and homicides is instrumental aggression, which is executed in the absence of emotional arousal. This sort of aggression frequently takes place in individuals with antisocial disorders. A chronic physiological activation in response to stress can be one of the causes of the development of an aggressive personality. Stress can lead to a type of depression characterized by anxiety, anger, and aggressive outbursts, especially if early life experiences such as maltreatment or neglect are involved (Buchanan et al., 2012).

The principal feature of the fear felt by both participants in an assault or homicide is the stress-induced fight-or-flight response, which determines whether an organism will defend itself or flee in a situation of danger. The sympathetic division of the autonomic nervous system—which controls blood vessels, smooth muscles, and glands—mediates this response. An individual's reaction in a situation of extreme stress is a result of his or her physiological reaction. In this response, adrenaline flows through the body, the heart beats quickly, bronchial tubes in the lungs dilate, the liver releases glucose, and blood vessels dilate to permit oxygen-rich blood to go where it is needed. In addition, the pupils of the eyes dilate to make vision more acute, peristalsis in the gastrointestinal system is halted, the palms become sweaty, and the mouth becomes dry (Kneisl & Trigoboff, 2013).

The physical manifestations of an assault can include a variety of injuries: bruising, bleeding, lacerations, concussions, broken bones, and more. A homicide may feature any of these injuries, and the victim may seek medical attention before dying. Nurses are prepared to treat a variety of wounds and symptoms of pain, including shock.

Etiology

While some acts of violence are seemingly senseless, the majority have conscious or unconscious etiologies. In many cases, human biology and the socioeconomic imbalances within a culture form the basis for violence. Intense **frustration**, which occurs when an individual is prevented from reaching a desired goal, may trigger the violent aggressive tendencies that result in assault and homicide. Aggression itself can lead to assault, which is an act intended to frighten a victim. Aggression can also prompt aggravated assault, which is an act carried out with the intent to seriously hurt a victim,

and homicide, which is murder. Even seemingly minor factors, such as loud noise, excessive heat, or unpleasant odors can trigger frustration, aggression, and physical violence (Ciccarelli & White, 2013).

Frustration is the triggering mechanism for most forms of violent aggression, but biological and cultural characteristics can also cause assault and homicide. Research has proven that human aggression is partly genetic in origin. Twin studies show that if one identical twin has an aggressive temper, most likely, the same will be true of the other twin. Moreover, among identical twins, if one twin exhibits violent tendencies, the same is likely to be true of the other twin. Among fraternal twins, this correlation is not necessarily present.

Evidence suggests that a gene or a complex of genes renders some individuals vulnerable to exhibiting an aggressive response under the particular situational conditions. Other biological factors also have an impact on aggressive behavior. The amygdala and other structures of the limbic system have been shown to cause aggression when stimulated in humans and lab animals. Testosterone has been correlated with higher aggression levels in humans, which helps explain why many violent offenders are young males with muscular physiques. These individuals typically have high levels of testosterone and low levels of serotonin, the neurotransmitter commonly associated with satisfaction. Alcohol also causes the aggressive behavior that leads to assault and homicide. The drug reduces inhibitions by modifying the functioning of neurotransmitters, including a decrease in serotonin function (Ciccarelli & White, 2013).

While biology plays a significant role in aggression's etiology, family and society also play a major role in rates of assault and homicide. A child's formational years play a large part in determining his or her aggressive tendencies as an adult. Poor monitoring and supervision by parents and the use of harsh punishment for discipline are strong predictors of violence during adolescence and adulthood. Studies have also found that physical punishment by parents predicts, for boys, not only the child's probability of arrest for violence, but also the man's future harsh discipline of his own children and abuse of his spouse. Socioeconomic status also influences an individual's propensity for violence. In general, young males raised in socioeconomically challenged and impoverished urban neighborhoods are more likely to be involved in violent behaviors. The presence of gangs and drugs in a neighborhood only increases the likelihood that individuals will engage in aggressive behavior. The entanglement of youth gangs with drug dealing has increased the incidence of homicide among youths (World Health Organization, 2013c). While the situations that initiate assault and homicide frequently involve gang violence, robberies, intimate partner violence, and unregulated mental illness, the fundamental causes of aggression are biological and social in origin.

Risk Factors

For the individual, determinants of violent behavior include biological, psychological, and behavioral variables. These characteristics may become evident in childhood, and may be influenced by societal risks. The demographic risk factors for

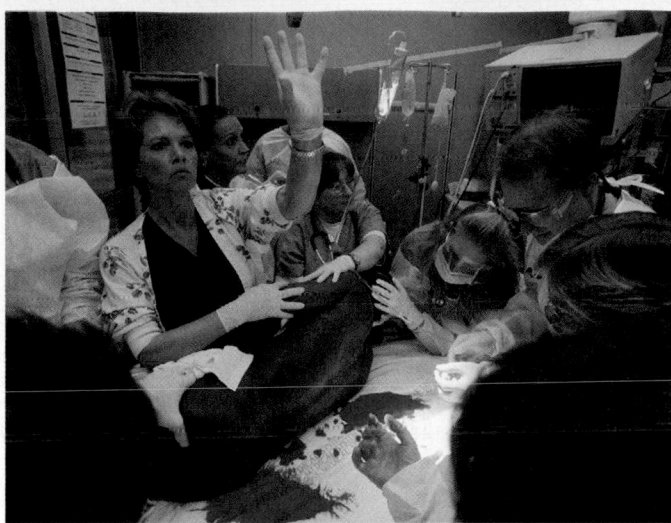

Figure 32–3 ● A nurse in the emergency department asks for a wipe to clean off blood from the victim of a stabbing.
Source: © Robert Tirey/Alamy

assault and homicide include youth, engagement with a subculture of violence, and low socioeconomic status. The demographics of both perpetrators and victims of violent crime are remarkably similar: In most cases, the assaulter and the person being attacked come from similar demographic circumstances (**Figure 32–3 ●**).

AGE Violence perpetrated by youths is one of the most visible forms of violence in society. In the United States and around the world, violence by youths flourishes in gangs, in schools, and in public areas. As with assault and homicide committed by individuals in any age demographic, the problem of youth violence cannot be viewed as isolated from other problem behaviors. Violent adolescents and young adults exhibit a range of problems, from truancy and dropping out of school to substance abuse, compulsive lying, reckless driving, and contraction of sexually transmitted diseases. The recklessness and instability of adolescence are partially responsible for high levels of youth violence, but there are close links between youth violence and experience in childhood. Witnessing violence in the family, being abused, and prolonged exposure to a community culture of violence can all condition children and adolescents to view violence as an acceptable means of solving problems (World Health Organization, 2013c). Adolescents and young adults may be the group likeliest to commit and be victimized by acts of assault and homicide, but other groups are at risk as well. For example, many ATM robbery victims are women, and many are alone at the time of the attack. Home invasion robbery usually victimizes people who are middle-aged and older, and frequently involves aggravated assault (Meadows, 2013).

CULTURE Both national culture and subculture affect an individual's predisposition to violence. Depictions of violence in the media and in video games are a major means through which modern mass culture endorses aggression as a normal method for resolving conflicts. Children's exposure to violent images in the media has increased significantly in the past few decades. The mass of evidence demonstrates that exposure to violence on television increases the chance of immediate aggres-

sive behavior and has an unknown effect in the longer term (World Health Organization, 2013c). Gang cultures are among the most visible subcultures that promote violence as a means of problem solving; they fail to provide nonviolent alternatives for conflict resolution. In addition to teaching the simple lesson that problems can be solved by assault and homicide, gangs foster violence by promising "easy money" for those willing to traffic drugs by whatever means necessary (World Health Organization, 2013c).

Within the United States, the cultural variation associated with geography plays a factor in the prevalence of assault and homicide. Urban centers, especially economically depressed areas, feature higher rates of violence than rural or suburban areas. Nationally, southern states have homicide rates that are significantly higher than those in other regions, although recently rates in the West have increased (Clinard & Meier, 2011).

SOCIOECONOMIC FACTORS Many studies have found that violent crime is heavily concentrated in the lower socioeconomic class. Several studies from the mid-20th century found that the vast majority of victims and offenders of homicides were from the lower class, and these findings hold true today. Living in poverty or an economically depressed area contributes significantly to the probability of an individual engaging in or becoming the victim of an assault or homicide. The specific circumstances of assault and homicide often vary by socioeconomic class. One study found dramatic differences among patterns in middle- and upper-class murders and lower-class homicides. In nearly three fourths of middle-class and upper-class murders, the offender killed principally for personal gain, and alcohol played no part in the crime. In contrast, the study found that alcohol was an element in almost two thirds of lower-class murders in Philadelphia (Clinard & Meier, 2011). Although the majority of assaults and homicides take place in the lower class, property owners of all socioeconomic classes are vulnerable to assault and homicide associated with robbery. Individuals involved in robberies frequently target people with particular demographic characteristics. Most victims of carjacking, for example, are lone females targeted by a lone male offender (Meadows, 2013).

OCCUPATION Workplace homicides are the fourth leading cause of job-related deaths. The workers at greatest risk are those who exchange money with the public, make deliveries, carry passengers in vehicles, work alone or in small groups during late night or early morning hours, or work in community settings in high-crime areas. Robbery is the primary motive of job-related homicide; together with disputes among coworkers and with customers or clients, they accounted for the most fatalities. For women, homicide is the leading cause of death in the workplace (Occupational Safety and Health Administration, 2011).

In the United States, healthcare professionals are at greater risk for violence than other service workers, and nurses are the healthcare professionals at greatest risk. The U.S. Occupational Safety and Health Administration published *Guidelines for Preventing Workplace Violence for Health Care & Social Service Workers* in 2002. These guidelines consist of four main components: (a) management commitment and employee involvement, (b) worksite analysis, (c) hazard prevention and control, and (d) safety and health training. The training for employees

Evidence-Based Practice Nurses Assaulted in the Workplace

Problem

Emergency department and psychiatric unit nurses experience high levels of assault at the hands of clients. This problem has not been decreasing in recent years, with some wondering if the problem is actually increasing. The physical assault of nurses by clients is overwhelmingly underreported.

Evidence

The National Advisory Council on Nurse Education and Practice (2007) has reported that "health care workers are more likely to be attacked than prison guards and police officers." A risk for assault from a client is present for all nurses, but emergency department and psychiatric unit nurses carry the highest levels of risk. In one study it was concluded that 72% of those working in emergency departments reported being assaulted during their career in the ED. Of those involved in the study, 42% stated they had been physically assaulted at work within the past 12 months (Taylor & Rew, 2010).

Another study documenting the nursing experiences with 2,726 clients highlighted some of the primary forms of assault experienced. Nurses reported violent clients kicking, biting, hitting, grabbing, punching, and throwing objects. As a result of these assaults nurses received abdominal injuries, falls, cuts to the skin, and contusions to both the sternum and coccyx. Among those clients who reacted aggressively, there were no overwhelmingly common diagnoses; instead, the physical and psychological ailments had a wide degree of variance (Ideker, Todicheeney-Mannes, & Kim, 2011).

Implications

High incidences of assault in the workplace lead to low job satisfaction, low retention rates, difficult recruitment, and detrimental effects to client care. Nurses who are continuously exposed to, or in fear of, physical assault from clients also report higher levels of stress and burnout (Anderson, Fitzgerald, & Luck, 2010).

Critical Thinking Application

Identify ways in which instances of violence in emergency departments and psychiatric units could be decreased. Consider how client care is affected by violent behavior. Describe some collaborative efforts that could be taken within the hospital setting to decrease cases of assault.

---

should include recognizing potential violence, defusing violence, and dealing with the aftermath of violence. Topics suggested for the training programs are as follows:

- The institution's workplace violence prevention policy
- Early recognition of escalating behavior
- Ways of defusing volatile situations, managing anger, and appropriately using medications.

▶ CLINICAL MANIFESTATIONS

Clinical manifestations of aggravated assault for the victim include injuries and wounds of varying severity, from minor surface injuries to severe injuries requiring prolonged medical attention. A common psychological outcome of surviving an aggravated assault is posttraumatic stress disorder (PTSD), a condition that is characterized by recurrent, subjective reexperiencing of the trauma.

If the perpetrator of homicide or assault belongs to a culture of violence or commits an assault or homicide in the course of a robbery of a stranger, he may show few signs of remorse after the crime (Meadows, 2013). However, violent personal crimes show a variety of different clinical manifestations. These crimes involve the accomplishment of a goal such as winning an argument, closing a dispute, or forcing sexual intercourse on an unwilling partner. The offenders in these cases typically do not pursue mastery of criminal skills or think of themselves as criminals. Murderers typically have very low rates of committing a second or third murder, because the crime often has to do with the execution of a specific goal. However, some offenders (including many with antisocial personality disorders) may go on to perform additional violent acts and to relish the reactions of others. In this way, the social reaction reinforces the offender's violence (Clinard & Meier, 2011).

Warning Signs

Most murders and violent assaults are violent responses to social interactions that involve differences in power. Therefore, the principal warning sign of assault or homicide is the social situation of the people involved, regardless of whether the situation is an incident as socioeconomically driven as a robbery or as private as a domestic dispute. Despite the prevalence of crime between strangers, more than half of all murderers know their victims as acquaintances. The offender and the victim may be friends, neighbors, work associates, gang members, or even client and healthcare practitioner. In an aggravated assault or homicide, the victim sometimes precipitates the attack. He may draw a weapon first, strike the first blow, or initiate the victimization in some other way. Most cases of violence develop from disputes that may seem trivial to outsiders, so even a minor dispute can be a warning sign for aggravated assault or homicide. Timing can also be a warning sign for assault or homicide, because conditions conducive to social interaction are typically conducive to homicide. Higher rates of homicide are present on weekends than during the workweek, and the homicide rate is generally higher during the summer than during the winter. These times encourage interaction and therefore violence, particularly in social spaces where alcohol is commonly consumed. Another significant warning sign for assault and homicide is a power differential between the perpetrator and the victim. Violence frequently results from an attempt by one person to establish a position of power over the other party. Acts of violence can flare up at times of upheaval between wives and husbands, business partners, parents and children, and siblings (Clinard & Meier, 2011).

A difference in power as a warning sign for assault or homicide is particularly relevant for the nurse working in the social space of a hospital or medical practice. Clients can become frustrated as they move through the healthcare system. A client who feels her power has been taken away may react violently toward a healthcare provider attempting to help. For this reason, the healthcare sector leads all other industries in assault, with 45% of all nonfatal assaults against healthcare workers resulting in lost workdays in the United States. From 2003 to 2009, eight registered nurses were fatally injured at work; all of them worked in private health practices. In 2009, registered nurses reported 2,050 nonfatal assaults. In the same, year, more than 50% of emergency department nurses experienced violence from a client. Twenty-five percent of emergency department nurses experienced 20 or more violent incidents in the past 3 years. In addition to violence between clients and nurses, there is a high incidence in the healthcare industry of lateral, or horizontal, violence, which consists of acts of abuse between healthcare workers. These acts can consist of verbal or physical assault, and have the damaging effect of diminishing the quality of the work environment and the quality of client care (American Nurses Association, 2013).

Lifespan and Cultural Considerations

Some cultures are more prone to assault and homicide than others due to circumstances and adherent belief systems. Gangs and those involved in the drug culture often participate in assault, and at times homicide, due to the nature of the culture itself. Religious and/or political extremists and hate groups are similarly known for their propensity for physically violent acts toward others. Groups such as the Ku Klux Klan, the Arm of the Lord, and Aryan Brotherhood will assault or even murder other individuals based on their religion, race, or sexual orientation. If members of these hate groups are injured during the act, they may react violently toward healthcare professionals from diverse backgrounds (Meadows, 2013).

Religious and political extremists who seek to injure or kill others as an act of homage to their belief system, or as an act of revenge against a political decision, pose a specific threat to all who encounter them. Individuals with these beliefs will attempt to assault or kill as many people as possible in order to fulfill their mission, and may also attempt to kill themselves after the

crimes have been committed. The level of violence within these particular groups has increased during the past decade (Meadows, 2013).

▶ COLLABORATION

A multidisciplinary approach is necessary when dealing with the violence of assault and homicide. Preventive activities at the community level involve school nurses and counselors, health department nurses, social workers, protective services personnel, police, and workplace programs. Professionals can identify those at risk for victimization and those at risk of committing violent acts and intervene by offering appropriate training, such as anger management or strategies for school safety.

Multidisciplinary approaches are also necessary when working with victims of homicide and assault and their families. Upon arriving at the hospital, a client with a serious gunshot wound, for example, will require care by the trauma team, which may include a trauma physician, a surgeon, several nurses, an infection specialist, a cardiologist, and a pulmonologist. An assault victim who has broken bones will require orthopedic care. The victim and family members may require counseling and spiritual guidance.

Diagnostic Tests

Due to the large number of potential injuries that could arise as the result of assault or attempted homicide, a number of diagnostic tests are performed depending on the nature of the injuries sustained. If internal bleeding is suspected, a CT, abdominal ultrasound, or MRI will be performed depending on the location of the original injury. For instances of potential broken or fractured bones as the result of an attack, an x-ray of the affected area(s) will be conducted. An MRI will also be performed if there is a risk for spinal cord injuries, injuries to the muscles, or abdominal injuries.

Pharmacologic Therapy

Individuals who have been injured in an assault will require different pharmacologic interventions in accordance with the type of injury presented. Pain medication are likely to be administered to clients suffering from intense pain. Opioids, particularly morphine, are generally used to control pain, but if the client has an allergy to morphine or another opioid, different medications are used. If a client has been shot, stabbed, or presents with lacerations to the skin, medications to treat possible infections are needed. Anti-inflammatories are used to reduce swelling and pain at the site of injury. Clients who have sustained deep lacerations, broken bones, or dislocations require local anesthesia in order to administer stitches or set the broken bone or dislocation.

Nonpharmacologic Therapy

One way in which many communities are providing a multidisciplinary approach is to offer violence prevention programs in schools, child care centers, churches, and other community programs where children and adults gather. A number of evidence-based curricula exist, which can be offered by nurses, teachers, social workers, or other professionals. Some of the most effective programs include a home teaching component

---

Focus on Diversity and Culture
Race and Homicide

- The homicide rate among African American individuals is considerably higher than among individuals of other races.
- Compared to other races, Caucasian individuals are significantly more likely to commit homicides involving multiple victims.
- Caucasian individuals are more likely to use poison as a means of homicide than any other weapon.
- The majority of familiar homicides (those committed by an acquaintance or family member) are interracial in nature.
- Stranger homicides typically are not interracial.
- Young adults (ages 18–24) have the highest homicide victimization rates of any age group across all races.
- Young adults (ages 18–24) have the highest homicide offense rates of any age group across all races (U.S. Department of Justice, 2011).

Clinical Manifestations and Therapies Assault

ETIOLOGY	CLINICAL MANIFESTATIONS	CLINICAL THERAPIES
Bone fractures resulting from physical attack	■ Inflammation, swelling, pain, and bruising. ■ In cases of a compound fracture, the skin around the broken bone will be punctured. X-rays will show a break in the bone.	■ Immobilization of the area to prevent further movement of the bone and allow for healing ■ Nonsurgical or surgical treatment of the fracture ■ Pain management ■ Physical therapy after healing
Gunshot wound	■ Shock, profuse bleeding, pain, and inflammation ■ Depending on the location of the injury, organ, bone, muscle, or nerve damage may be present.	■ Pain management ■ Surgery to remove bullet and/or repair damage ■ Medication to treat infection ■ Blood transfusion ■ Treatment for shock including treatment for potential hypothermia
Stabbing	■ Shock, bleeding, pain, and inflammation ■ Potential for organ, nerve, muscle, and bone damage depending on the location of the injury	■ Blood transfusion ■ Surgery to repair damage if needed ■ Pain management ■ Medication to treat infection ■ Treatment for shock ■ Stitches to close minor wounds
Internal bleeding as the result of blunt force trauma	■ Shock; dizziness; confusion; abdominal pain; chest pain ■ Blood in stool, urine, or vomit	■ Diagnostic tests to find the source of bleeding ■ Surgery to stop the bleeding and repair injury if necessary ■ Treatment for shock including treatment for hypothermia

that gets parents involved. Two such violence prevention programs are offered by the Committee for Children (www.cfchildren.org). *Second Step: A Violence Prevention Program* is designed to teach children of various ages how to solve problems and manage anger, and includes a home teaching component. *Steps to Respect: A Bullying Prevention Program* is designed to teach children why bullying is not appropriate, how it affects others, and how to manage their own anger.

SAFETY ALERT
Nurses are likely to treat both the perpetrators and victims of homicide. In situations where clients have the potential to become violent toward the healthcare professionals working to treat their injuries, nurses should take appropriate precautions. In the clinical setting, security personnel or police officers may be present when needed.

■ NURSING PROCESS

The nurse who is caring for a victim of assault needs to document all findings and care provided in specific detail. The likelihood of the medical record being entered into evidence at a legal proceeding against the person who committed the assault is high, and proper documentation can play a significant role in convicting the criminal. Wounds should be accurately and precisely described, the client's emotional state should be described as objectively as possible, and any specimens collected must follow the legal chain of custody procedure.

Assessment

The assessment of a client who has been involved in an assault should begin with an assessment of the airway, breathing, circulation, disability, and exposure (ABCDE). After these have been assessed and the client's immediate safety is ensured, nurses move on to the next immediate priority for the client. Prioritizing of injuries after the ABCDEs have been assessed depends on the injuries sustained by the client, as well as the client's emotional state. If the individual being treated is aggressive, violent, or poses a threat to the safety of the nurses or other staff, this will need to be one of the first conditions assessed. Nurses will request help from security and other staff as needed if the client begins to act in a violent manner. Physical injuries are then assessed by order of severity. For example, a gunshot or knife wound to the abdomen is assessed before a broken ankle.

Clients who are being treated in cases of assault, attempted homicide, or homicide will be assessed the same regardless of whether the nurse is treating the victim of the assault or the perpetrator. Both individuals have the potential to be angry or violent, and both clients are provided with the same quality of care.

Diagnosis

Individuals who have been assaulted can have a wide array of injuries all requiring different diagnoses. Injuries may yield effects ranging in severity from minimal to life threatening. Nursing diagnoses that are appropriate for inclusion in the plan of care for the client who is the victim of assault or attempted homicide may include:

- *Ineffective Airway Clearance*
- *Ineffective Breathing Pattern*
- *Ineffective Tissue Perfusion*
- *Risk for Infection*
- *Risk for Injury* related to secondary effects of trauma
- *Acute Pain*
- *Chronic Pain*
- *Impaired Physical Mobility*
- *Fear*
- *Ineffective Coping.*

(NANDA-I © 2012)

Planning

Goals for effective client care will be contingent on the type and severity of the injury sustained. Similarly, individuals who display violent or aggressive temperaments will have goals related to ineffective anger projection. Some goals for client care include:

- The client's airway will remain patent.
- The client will demonstrate effective breathing as evidenced by regular, nonlabored respirations; clear, equal breath sounds to auscultation; and oxygen saturation of at least 95%.
- The client's blood pressure and heart rate will remain within normal limits.
- The client will demonstrate no signs or symptoms of infection.
- The client's pain will be tolerable, with a client-reported rating of no greater than 3 on a 0–10 scale.
- The client will participate in all scheduled physical and occupational therapy activities.
- The client will seek to make the necessary changes to promote and enhance personal safety, including seeking help when needed.
- The client will verbalize emotions and concerns.

Implementation

Care of clients in cases of assault will be focused on infection control, health maintenance, and recovery. Injuries will be treated in order of severity, with some clients requiring emergency surgery to stop bleeding or repair organ damage. Nurses will work to keep clients stable, while preparing them for surgery, diagnostic testing, or other treatments to repair their injuries. Clients who have suffered physical trauma will be in pain and will generally be prescribed medication in order to control the pain. While some injuries sustained from assault will require basic interventions, other injuries will be more complex in nature.

For example, gunshot wounds require a specific and sometimes complex set of interventions. As a result, the entire trauma team is usually activated upon receiving notification by law enforcement or emergency services of the imminent arrival of the victim of a gunshot wound.

Possible injuries from gunshot wounds include, but are not limited to, the following:

- Eye injury, skull fracture, brain injury
- Pneumothorax, hemothorax, pulmonary contusion
- Organ and tissue damage, nerve and vascular damage.

Gunshot wounds may be classified in a variety of ways: by nature (e.g., contact or noncontact wound, entry or exit wound), size, or severity. Clinical priorities for the treatment of a gunshot wound are as following:

- Maintain airway and assist ventilation as necessary.
- Control hemorrhage.
- Prevent hypothermia.

Rapid, recurrent assessment of neurological status is also necessary, as is infection control. Bleeding can result in hypovolemia, leading to inadequate perfusion and oxygenation of tissues.

Family members of gunshot victims typically are very upset and often very angry. An experienced nurse should work closely with these families while the victim is being treated. Gunshot victims may themselves display dangerous behaviors. If law enforcement has not determined that the victim is free of weapons, such an assessment should be done before treatment is initiated. Violent or angry victims may need to be restrained during treatment for the protection of the trauma team. Law enforcement may assign officers to remain present during treatment.

Because the majority of gunshot wounds require an investigation by law enforcement, nurses working in emergency departments and trauma centers should be familiar with their agency's protocols for maintaining evidence required by law enforcement. Often, law enforcement does not want the victim's hands or the area around the victim's wounds cleansed. Clothes and personal items are often wanted as evidence (Taylor, 2009).

Evaluation

Evaluation of the client's response to care allows the nurse to gauge the efficacy of nursing interventions, discontinue nursing diagnoses that are no longer pertinent, and generate nursing diagnoses that reflect the client's current needs. For the client who is a victim of assault or attempted homicide, evaluation includes appraising the degree to which the client has achieved the identified outcomes of care and reassessing the client's physiological and psychosocial well-being.

NURSING CARE PLAN   A Client With Injuries From Assault

Kevin Rittrell, an 18-year-old White male, arrives in the emergency department accompanied by two police officers. Mr. Rittrell was apprehended by police while he was assaulting a clerk at a local grocery store. The client appears to have injured his right arm and has also experienced head trauma.

ASSESSMENT

Julia Miller, an RN, is informed by the police that Mr. Rittrell has been searched and cleared of all weapons. The client demonstrates no impairments related to airway, breathing, or circulation. Mr. Rittrell's vital signs include temperature 96.8°F tympanic; pulse 74 bpm; respirations 16/min; and BP 128/85 mmHg. Mr. Rittrell has remained silent throughout the examination process, looks very pale, and appears to be in pain whenever he moves his arm.

The client reports that he hit his head on a cement wall shortly after he hurt his arm. He denies loss of consciousness, neck pain, nausea, vomiting, visual changes, or any neurological problems. A dime-sized bruise is present on Mr. Rittrell's forehead; skin is intact and there is no apparent bleeding. While speaking with Mr. Rittrell, Mrs. Miller notes that his pupils appear to be dilated. Mr. Rittrell tells the nurse that the clerk at the grocery store was rude to him and accused him of stealing, after which point the client lost his temper and struck the clerk. He further states that he sustained his injuries during the physical altercation with the clerk in the grocery store.

Mr. Rittrell's right forearm is swollen, warm to the touch, and bruising has started to appear above his wrist. There is no obvious right arm bone deformity and the skin is intact. Mr. Rittrell has full range of motion of his right hand and his right radial pulse is strong. He says that his arm hurts a lot, especially when he attempts to move his fingers. Mr. Rittrell is sent for an x-ray of his arm, which reveals a fracture of the right distal radius. After intravenous administration of midazolam 1 mg for sedation and fentanyl 50 mcg for analgesia, the ED physician manually reduces Mr. Rittrell's right radial fracture and applies a splint to the injured arm. The ED physician refers Mr. Rittrell to a local orthopedic surgeon for follow-up in 1 week, but the client states, "I'm not going back to see anymore doctors." His discharge instructions include monitoring for changes in mobility or sensation in his injured arm, splint care, mobility restrictions, and instructions for self-administration of acetaminophen 500 mg every 6 hours as needed for pain for 1 week. He rates his right arm pain as "2" and refuses a prescription for pain medication. Mr. Rittrell is discharged in the custody of law enforcement.

DIAGNOSES

- *Acute Pain* related to right distal radius fracture
- *Risk for Other-Directed Violence*
- *Impaired Physical Mobility* related to right distal radius fracture
- *Risk for Ineffective Self-Health Management*
- *Risk for Noncompliance.*

(NANDA-I © 2012)

PLANNING

Goals for Mr. Rittrell's care include the following:

- The client will report pain is absent or tolerable as evidenced by a pain rating of 3 or less, using a pain scale of 0–10, where 0 equals no pain and 10 equals the worst possible pain.
- The client will report any changes in movement and sensation of his right arm.
- The client will regain full mobility in his right arm.
- The client will keep his splint clean, dry, and intact.
- The client will complete follow-up care as ordered.

IMPLEMENTATION

- Instruct the client about assessing and monitoring his injured extremity for changes in mobility and sensation and encourage the client to report any changes to the physician immediately.
- Instruct the client about splint care.
- Encourage the client to take acetaminophen as instructed.

- Encourage the client to seek follow-up orthopedic care as ordered by the physician.
- Encourage the client to seek counseling for personal growth and offer to facilitate referrals to community resources.

EVALUATION

Mr. Rittrell is taken into custody by the police and transferred to a county jail. He is released on bail 3 days after his incarceration. Mr. Rittrell visits the orthopedic physician as ordered and assessment reveals that his right arm is healing well. While he is at the orthopedic clinic, he asks about free counseling services that are available in the community. Mr. Rittrell is given educational brochures and contact information for local organizations that offer counseling and guidance at no cost.

CRITICAL THINKING

1. If the police had not informed the nurse that Mr. Rittrell had been checked for weapons, how should the nurse have proceeded?
2. How would the nursing care plan have changed if Mr. Rittrell had sustained a compound fracture of the right radius?
3. Identify at least three precautions nurses should take when working with a client who has been involved in a violent assault.

REVIEW Assault and Homicide

RELATE Link the Concepts and Exemplars

Linking the exemplar of assault and homicide with the concept of addiction:

1. You are caring for a client with addiction to alcohol who presents to the clinic for treatment of injuries incurred when he became aggressive while intoxicated. What teaching is appropriate for this client while he is under the influence of alcohol? What follow-up care will you recommend?

2. How will you intervene with the client who threatens to assault you in the ED and is known to be under the influence of cocaine?

Linking the exemplar of assault and homicide with the concept of family:

3. What nursing diagnoses might be appropriate for inclusion in the plan of care for family members of the victim of a hate crime, such as an individual who is assaulted because of his homosexuality?

4. What communication strategies might be appropriate when talking with an 8-year-old child whose mother was shot during a home robbery?

READY Go to Companion Skills Manual

REFER Go to Pearson Nursing Student Resources
nursing.pearsonhighered.com

- Additional review materials

REFLECT Case Study

Rose Clancy, age 14, is brought into her general practitioner's office after displaying aggressive behavior during the past month. Two weeks ago she was suspended from her high school for engaging in a physical altercation with another student, and 3 days ago she became angry with her mother and began throwing objects at her. Before this year Rose had never displayed aggressive or violent behavior and has always been a very successful student; however, recently her grades have been dropping considerably. During the past year Rose lost approximately 10 pounds and has started associating with a new group of friends her parents refer to as "troubled youths." Rose's parents are concerned about her change in behavior and have come into the office for advice. When Rose talks to the nurse she is polite, articulate, and kind, but when she addresses her parents she is considerably more aggressive.

1. Identify two primary nursing considerations for Rose's case.

2. What referrals could you provide Rose's parents to work through this aggressive behavior?

3. Name three potential nursing diagnoses for Rose's case. Explain each diagnosis.

EXEMPLAR 32.3 Rape and Rape-Trauma Syndrome

EXEMPLAR KEY TERMS
Acquaintance rape, *1984*
Marital rape, *1984*
Rape, *1983*
Rape-trauma syndrome (RTS), *1983*

EXEMPLAR LEARNING OUTCOMES
After reading about this exemplar, you will be able to:

1. Describe the pathophysiology, etiology, clinical manifestations, and direct and indirect causes of rape and rape-trauma syndrome.

2. Identify risk factors and prevention methods associated with rape.

3. Illustrate the nursing process in providing culturally competent care across the life span for individuals who have been raped.

4. Formulate priority nursing diagnoses appropriate for an individual who has been raped.

5. Summarize therapies used by interdisciplinary teams in the collaborative care of an individual who has been raped.

6. Plan evidence-based care for an individual who has been raped and his or her family in collaboration with other members of the healthcare team.

7. Evaluate expected outcomes for an individual who has been raped.

▶ OVERVIEW

Rape is one form of sexual violence. In the past this form of violence has had varying definitions, making it difficult to address what acts could actually be considered rape. However, in 2011 the 80-year-old federal definition of rape was officially updated by the FBI. According to this revised definition, **rape** is "penetration, no matter how slight, of the vagina or anus with any body part or object, or oral penetration by a sex organ of another person, without the consent of the victim" (FBI, 2012f). Individuals who have been raped will vary largely in their reactions to the incident. The variation in victim's reactions can be due to the individual's past history, personality, the circumstances of the event, if infection or pregnancy came as a result of the rape, and many other factors.

For decades, clinicians working with victims of rape have recognized **rape-trauma syndrome**, a series of psychological sequelae that many victims experience following rape in addition to physiological sequelae. Although symptoms and reactions vary widely, most victims of rape experience great emotional and physical impact. Many victims initially exhibit shock and disbelief, followed by fear, humiliation, shame, self-blame, and anger. Anxiety responses and mood swings are not uncommon. Physical symptoms generally exhibit in the area that was the focus of the sexual assault, and sleep disturbances following the rape are common. Some victims of rape may go on to experience symptoms so severe as to impact functioning to the extent that they may develop PTSD (American Psychiatric Association, 2013). (See also the exemplar on PTSD in the module on Stress and Coping.)

▶ PATHOPHYSIOLOGY AND ETIOLOGY

Individuals who experiences rape have their control taken from them in one way or another. Rape can occur under a number of circumstances, and can include physically violent elements (such as being threatened with a weapon or physically injured or tortured), as well as psychological elements (such as victims being told the rape was their own fault in some way). Regardless of the circumstances of the rape, after it is over the victim has lost something of herself. The extent of that loss will depend on the history and personality of the victim, as well as the circumstances of the incident. After being raped, victims will likely feel as though they have little to no control over what happens to them, and they may feel as though they have lost a part of themselves. Elements of fear, guilt, and anxiety will also often be present (CDC, 2009a).

Influencing Factors

Those who commit rape will often know the victim, either as a spouse, an ex-spouse, an acquaintance, a friend, or a relative. In a study conducted by the Bureau of Justice, 6 out of every 10 rape victims reported knowing their assailant (National Institute of Justice, 2010). Some factors influencing those who commit rape are environmental or social in nature, while others pertain to the individual's psychological well-being. It is imperative to remember that both men and women can commit rape.

INTRAPERSONAL AND INTERPERSONAL FACTORS

Multiple types of rapists exist, including those who know the victim and those who are strangers. Serial rapists are individuals who have committed sexual assault two or more times. To become a serial rapist, or even a first time offender, an individual needs to overcome the moral and ethical dilemma of taking away another individual's right to say no. Often this decision comes about through the use of drugs or alcohol; through powerful emotions such as anger, revenge, or a sense of entitlement; or through the use of self-delusion, convincing themselves that their victim actually wants to go through with the act despite protests. Depending on the rapist's own justifications, the act will either be physically violent with a result of profuse injuries to the victim, or emotionally violent where the perpetrator uses verbal coercion and only enough physical force to complete the rape. Some rapists may even apologize to their victims after the transgression as a way to absolve themselves of the crime, or they may blame the victim (Savino & Turvey, 2011).

No one form of rape is easier for the victim than another; however, different types of rapists cause varied reactions in their victims. For example, if the rapist was someone the individual knows on a personal level (e.g., a friend, relative, or spouse), the victim is likely to have serious trust issues as a result of the experience. Individuals who had a prior romantic relationship with the rapist are also prone to developing low self-esteem and higher levels of guilt, believing that their supposed poor judgment in character led to the event (DeAngelis, 2013).

SOCIOCULTURAL FACTORS   For an individual to commit rape, some sort of precipitating force needs to be present. This force could be emotional or substance based, as just discussed, or it could even be biological or environmental. Biological factors would include psychological disorders that cause impaired decision making, or deficient impulse control. Environmental factors that could influence an individual's decision to commit rape include growing up in a setting where physical, emotional, or sexual violence was common and perhaps even accepted. Similarly, being raised in a culture where women or men are seen as possessions rather than individuals could cause individuals to believe they have the right to take what they would like from others despite objections from the victim. Areas that have high crime rates and a seemingly increased tolerance for violence are also more prone to having a higher percentage of rape cases (CDC, 2009c).

Etiology

Approximately 83,046 cases of forcible rape were reported in 2011 in the United States, a number that has been decreasing steadily during the past 20 years (FBI, 2012e). A national survey of adults has shown that approximately 1 in 5 women and 1 in 71 men have reported being raped at some point in their lives. Of female victims, 42.2% were first raped before age 18, and 37.4% were first raped between ages 18 and 24. Of male victims, 27.8% reported being raped before the age of 11 (CDC, 2012c).

As discussed in previous sections, various forms of rape exist; two of the most common forms are marital rape and acquaintance rape. **Marital rape** occurs when one spouse forces the other to have sex against his or her will. Marital rape is considered a crime in all 50 states, and can occur in conjunction with both physical and emotional abuse. **Acquaintance rape** is a rather broad term used to describe a rape committed by an acquaintance or other familiar individual. The largest percentage of acquaintance rape cases occurs on college campuses, with many of them including factors such as the consumption of alcohol and illegal substances (on the part of both the perpetrator and the victim) (Meadows, 2013).

Acquaintance rape, regardless of where it takes place, can also involve the use of "date rape" drugs. The three most common date rape drugs are gamma hydroxybutyric acid (GHB), flunitrazepam (Rohypnol), and ketamine hydrochloride (ketamine). These three drugs are odorless and tasteless, and thus can be easily added to a victim's drink. After consuming the drugs the victim will feel mildly euphoric, sedated, and will often suffer from memory loss (Meadows, 2013).

The intense trauma associated with rape can lead to physical injuries, as well as intense emotional injuries. Individuals suffering from a traumatic experience will often display signs of shock and denial shortly after the experience.

Risk Factors

No specific individual risk factors exist for becoming a victim of rape. Individuals can be at a higher risk for rape if they are under the influence of drugs and/or alcohol, but these factors do not cause rape to occur. Similarly, being young could be considered to be a risk factor for rape, but only due to the fact that a large percentage of victims report having been raped before they were 18 years old.

The risk factors for committing a rape are also difficult to determine. While an individual may have all of the following risk factors, it does not necessarily mean that individual will one day become a rapist. Some of the risk factors for perpetration of rape are as follows:

- Alcohol and drug use
- Lacking inhibitions to suppress associations between sex and aggression
- Holding attitudes and beliefs supportive of sexual violence, including coercive sexual fantasies
- A pattern of behavior that is impulsive, antisocial, and hostile toward women
- Associating with sexually aggressive peers
- Having been sexually abused as a child
- Growing up in a family environment characterized by physical violence, little emotional support, and few economic resources (CDC, 2009c).

Prevention

The majority of preventive programs involving rape focus on stopping the perpetrator from committing the act. Programs such as these are often aimed at those who have committed sexual assault in the past, and work to help the individual accept responsibility for the crime. Preventive measures for victims include knowledge and awareness about situations that could foster those looking to commit rape, such as crowded bars, parties, raves, and fraternity or sorority parties on college campuses. Paying attention to surroundings and traveling in pairs or groups can also deter an individual looking to take a single unsuspecting victim. Self-defense classes and training aid in fighting off an individual attempting to commit sexual assault, and could give the victim a better chance of escaping (CDC, 2013c).

▶ CLINICAL MANIFESTATIONS

The clinical manifestations of rape vary depending on the genders of the assailant and the victim, the physical violence involved in the rape, and the type of rape. Common manifestations include oral, vaginal, or anal injuries and/or physical injuries with the presence of semen not belonging to the victim. Individuals who have been raped will also demonstrate psychological symptoms such as shock, denial, and confusion directly following the event.

Physical Injuries

Common physical injuries in rape victims include swelling, redness, and lacerations around the vagina and anus; injuries to the throat from forced oral sex or restraint; bruises; broken bones; and knife and gunshot wounds. Defensive and restraint injuries will present as wounds to the hands, arms, feet, and legs, often in the form of bruises, lacerations, and/or fractured and broken bones. If the victim was restrained (often with rope, handcuffs, or plastic zip ties), additional injuries will be found around the wrists, ankles, and possibly the neck. Internal injuries and bleeding could be present if the client was beaten before or after the rape, or raped with an object such as a bottle.

Long-term physical complications often present as pelvic pain, back pain, frequent headaches, gastrointestinal disorders, and potential pregnancy complications in women. Some of these long-term symptoms—such as headaches, gastrointestinal upset,

and even back pain—can be caused by a mix of intense stress and injuries from the rape (CDC, 2009a). Other long-term effects could be the result of sexually transmitted diseases or infections, such as gonorrhea, syphilis, chlamydia, hepatitis, or HIV.

Immediate Response

Initial responses to rape have already been briefly described in earlier sections and generally include feelings of shock, denial, and disbelief. Other early responses involve fear, anger, guilt, embarrassment, helplessness, loss of control, confusion, anxiety, and nervousness (CDC, 2009a; Meadows, 2013). The client who has recently experienced rape will be hesitant to trust others, and particularly resistant to those of the same gender as the attacker. Nurses understand this fear and work to reassure clients of their safety. If a woman has been raped by a male attacker, it may be necessary to have primarily female healthcare professionals working with this client. If a male staff member is needed, a female nurse should accompany him as reassurance to the client who will likely not want to be left alone with an unfamiliar male so soon after the incident.

An individual's first response after a rape is often to shower in an attempt to wash away the incident as well as what is left of the attacker's physical presence (such as the individual's smell, body fluids, etc.). If consulted, nurses will advise clients not to shower before being examined because this will remove potential evidence that could be collected and used to identify the attacker. Nurses recognize that this request is difficult for the client, and provide reassurance that a shower will be provided as soon as the examination is completed.

Some clients will present themselves as though nothing of consequence has happened, while acting relatively normal and unfazed by the situation. Nurses realize that this reaction is often an effect of shock and denial. Clients who react in this manner will be treated as sensitively as other clients who outwardly display their emotions. All procedures, tests, and examinations will be explained to the client in detail, and the client will be asked before any test or examination is performed. The individual who has been raped has already had control taken away by the attacker; nurses will work to empower the client's decision-making process.

Long-Term Response

After the initial shock of the incident subsides, clients will begin to accept that the rape has occurred. In the weeks following the incident, a variety of emotional responses will be present, and these responses will differ depending on the personality of the client. Common responses include anger, flashbacks of the incident, avoidance of previously enjoyed activities, avoidance of the setting where the rape occurred, insomnia, eating disturbances, sexual dysfunction, and depression (Meadows, 2013). Some individuals will cut all emotional ties to friends and family members, while others will seek the comfort of familiarity and respond very negatively to being alone. The emotional distress of the incident can trigger the use of unhealthy coping mechanisms such as drug and alcohol use, or abuse, and participating in high-risk sexual behavior (e.g., multiple partners, unprotected intercourse, and unhealthy partner choices). Pregnancy is also a concern for those who have been raped; more than 32,000 pregnancies occur each year as the result of forced sexual encounters (CDC, 2009a). How the client responds to the pregnancy depends on the emotional trauma associated with the incident, as well as the personality of the individual. It is highly probably that emotional difficulties will coincide with the progression of the pregnancy.

Depression and suicidal thoughts or actions are common after a rape has occurred. Nurses should be mindful of the warning signs of suicide, and employ appropriate interventions as needed (see the exemplar on Suicide later in this module). All individuals who have experienced forced sexual encounters are provided with resources for therapy, support groups, and/or counseling. Whether clients choose to utilize these resources is their decision, but it is the nurse's responsibility to provide clients with the means to seek help.

SAFETY ALERT

Individuals who have been raped are at a high risk for developing an eating disorder. The symptoms of this disorder could align with anorexia or bulimia, or the symptoms could be a crossover between the two. Eating disorders do not always develop out of an individual's desire to lose weight; often they come from an emotional disturbance. One of the main components of both anorexia and bulimia is control over what the individual is consuming, and over the nutrients that stay in the body or are forcefully discarded. In a rape situation the individual's control has been taken away, so an eating disorder may develop as a way to regain the control that has been lost (APA, 2011; CDC, 2009a).

Lifespan and Cultural Considerations

The cultural considerations in rape are numerous and often involve the culture's dominant definition of rape and what that act entails. Note that not all members of a culture will have the same beliefs about one particular topic, because their experiences and responses vary widely. In cultures that place an extreme importance on patriarchy and devalue the thoughts and rights of women, the forcible rape of a female will not be considered a matter of great importance. Because of these beliefs, women from radically patriarchal cultural backgrounds may not seek help or justice after an attack. Conversely, matriarchal cultures will view the rape of a woman as a paramount injustice, and the man will be ostracized and dishonored within the community or culture.

The idea of marital rape is not acknowledged in a number of countries and cultures around the world. If two individuals are married, then any sexual contact, regardless of whether it is desired or not, would be considered legal and warranted. Individuals from backgrounds with these beliefs (e.g., some Asian American and Mexican American cultures) would be hesitant to seek help if they were raped by their spouse; it could even be considered dishonorable to the victim's family to imply that a crime was committed.

Beliefs about rape in general vary widely even within similar belief systems and cultures. For example, numerous rape *myths* exist that blame the victim and exonerate the perpetrator. Beliefs such as these indicate that the individual who was raped deserved it either due to the nature of the clothes being worn, the setting of the rape (such as a party or rave), or the individual's consumption of alcohol or drugs. Other erroneous rape

Focus on Diversity and Culture
Rape Culture in Prisons and Jails

- In 2009 approximately 4.4% of all adult prison inmates and 3.1% of all jail inmates reported being raped by another inmate or a facility staff member.
- Females in prison or jail are more than twice as likely to be raped by another inmate than male prisoners.
- 19% of males in jail and 13% of males in prison were raped within the first 24 hours of admission (Beck & Harrison, 2010).
- 12% of individuals in juvenile facilities reported being raped by an inmate or staff member in 2009.
- Less than 1% of youths raped in juvenile facilities sought medical attention (U.S. Department of Justice, 2010).

myths imply that certain cultures or races are more sexually promiscuous than others and therefore welcome all forms of sexual contact, regardless of whether it is forced or permitted.

Individuals in the sex industry (e.g., prostitutes and escorts) can also be raped. Regardless of whether their job includes having sexual relations with others, if someone states an unwillingness to continue and the other person does not stop, then the act becomes defined as a rape. Nurses do not judge clients who claim to have been raped; they provide quality care to all individuals.

▶ COLLABORATION

A multidisciplinary team caring for clients who are victims of rape includes law enforcement personnel immediately after the rape, and nurses, physicians, and mental health professionals for ongoing treatment for emotional trauma. Sexual Assault Nurse Examiners (SANE) often participate in the assessment process. Many communities have victims' advocates who are available to guide rape victims through the process of prosecuting their attacker. These are sometimes volunteers trained by local health departments and district attorneys' offices. Some law enforcement agencies or district attorneys' offices employ trained staff to serve as victim's advocates, sometimes through grant funding made possible for the Violence Against Women Act and combinations of federal, state, and private funding.

Stay Current: *Visit the Web site of the International Association of Forensic Nurses (IAFN) at* **www.iafn.org** *to learn more about becoming a Sexual Assault Nursing Examiner.*

Diagnostic Tests

While not diagnostic in nature, specimens will likely be collected for the purpose of convicting the rapist, if caught. As a result, chain-of-custody laws must be followed and vary within jurisdictions. Specimens will include the following:

- Vaginal, oral, and anal swabs for DNA material
- Scrapings from under the client's fingernails for skin samples if the client scratched the rapist
- Combing of pubic hair for rapist's DNA
- Clothing worn by the victim (if the individual is brought directly to the ED following the rape).

Clinical Manifestations and Therapies Rape-Trauma Syndrome

ETIOLOGY	CLINICAL MANIFESTATIONS	CLINICAL THERAPIES
Acute phase of rape-trauma syndrome	Expressive styles vary: ■ Open expression of feelings—confusion, fear, crying, sobbing, pacing, hostility, inappropriate laughter ■ Controlled style—numbness, shock, disbelief, withdrawal ■ Compound reaction—reactivated symptoms of previous conditions, for example, psychotic behavior, depression, suicidal behavior, substance abuse ■ Somatic reactions—tension headache, fatigue, increased startle reaction, nausea, gagging ■ Outward appearance of adjustment with an attempt to restore equilibrium ■ Life activities are renewed, but superficially and mechanically ■ Periods of anxiety, fear, nightmares, depression, guilt, shame, vulnerability, helplessness, isolation, sexual dysfunctions	■ Counseling ■ Therapy ■ Follow-up care for emotional and physical trauma ■ Medication
Reorganization phase of rape-trauma syndrome	■ Anger at the assailant, at society, and at the judicial system ■ The need to talk to resolve feelings ■ The survivor seeks family and professional support.	■ Therapy ■ Support groups
Posttraumatic stress disorder (if unable to recover)	■ Anxiety ■ Flashbacks ■ Depression ■ Nightmares ■ Withdrawal	■ Therapy ■ Support groups ■ Antidepressants

In addition to the specimens collected for legal purposes, the victim is tested for sexually transmitted infections and potential pregnancy. Baseline testing is performed at the time of the initial examination and then follow-up HIV testing is done at 3, 6, and 12 months. Pregnancy testing related to the rape cannot be accurately performed until the woman has missed her first menstrual period.

Pharmacologic Therapy

Women who have been raped can be offered emergency contraception in order to prevent unwanted pregnancy. If the client is seen within 3 days of the attack, the contraceptive is more likely to be successful then if taken more than 3 days after intercourse has occurred. Some individuals will be opposed to using contraception; the nurse will explain the client's options and then be respectful of whatever decision is made.

Numerous sexually transmitted diseases and infections can be contracted during a rape—regardless of whether the attacker used a condom or not. The most common and treatable infections are listed below along with their prescribed pharmacologic treatment:

■ Syphilis, treated with penicillin
■ Chlamydia, treated with a dose of azithromycin or a week of doxycycline
■ Gonorrhea, treated with a combination of ceftriaxone and either azithromycin or doxycycline
■ Trichomoniasis, treated with metronidazole or tinidazole.

Nonpharmacologic Therapy

Support groups, therapy, and counseling are recommended to clients who have experienced a forced sexual encounter. Some clients will be more receptive to support groups where others who have had similar experiences come together to discuss the aftermath of the event and how they are working to heal from the experience. Other clients will prefer a more private setting and choose to work individually with a therapist to process their own personal experiences. While attending therapy clients will develop healthy coping mechanisms to process their emotions and work to release feelings of self-blame.

◼ NURSING PROCESS

Nursing care for a client who has been raped depends on a number of factors including the physical violence inflicted during the incident, the client's emotional state, and the client's willingness to allow an examination. Nurses know that this is an extremely difficult situation for the client, so they are both patient and understanding.

Assessment

When conducting a nursing assessment for a victim of rape, nurses first need to ensure the client's safety. If knife or gunshot wounds, organ damage, and/or severe head trauma are indicated, those injuries need to be assessed and treated first before any minor physical injuries or psychological injuries are assessed. Injuries to the vagina, anus, and throat are likely to be present, and should be assessed. The client may be in shock or outwardly emotionally distraught. Nurses should be aware that client's reactions to rape vary greatly in accordance with the situation and the personality of the client.

Once the physical safety of the client is assured, nurses work to comfort and empower the client, explaining their choices in examination and resources. Individuals who have been raped do not have to allow a rape kit, nor do they have to talk to a counselor; however, nurses should encourage both of these actions. If the client agrees to an examination and the collection of evidence, nurses will explain every step of the process and ask permission during the examination itself. While the client may be willing to allow evidence collection and DNA swabbing, she may not want any pictures taken of the injuries. Nurses need to remain understanding and supportive of the client's decisions. Disease, infection, and pregnancy testing and treatment are discussed with the client, and interventions planned accordingly.

The nurse assesses the clients' emotional needs, asking if the person would like a parent, friend, or rape advocate present during the examination. Resources for therapy and support groups are explained and provided for the client. Police involvement is also offered if the client chooses to file a statement about the incident.

Diagnosis

The client's diagnosis is contingent on the injuries and emotional state of the individual. Some potential nursing diagnoses include:

- *Risk for Infection*
- *Rape-Trauma Syndrome*
- *Fear*
- *Acute Pain*
- *Powerlessness*
- *Risk for Ineffective Coping*
- *Situational Low Self-Esteem*
- *Disturbed Self-Concept.*

(NANDA-I © 2012)

Planning

It is critical for the client who is the victim of rape to have control over the planning process. The client's input regarding both short-term and long-term goals is essential in order to prevent revictimization and to help the client regain control over self and environment. Appropriate short-term goals include the following:

- The client will receive treatment for physical injuries sustained during the rape.
- The client will participate in follow-up care for physical injuries.
- The client will follow a safety plan following release from medical care (e.g., stay with family or friends, change locks on doors, etc.).

It may be more than the client can manage to think beyond the first few days following the rape. The nurse can provide follow-up care to determine when the client is ready to engage in further planning. This follow-up care also allows the nurse to reassess how the client is meeting short-term goals. Appropriate long-term goals may include the following:

- The client will gain control over remembering—experiencing decreased flashbacks and nightmares.
- The client will work toward affect tolerance—ability to name feelings, feel them, and endure them without overwhelming arousal or numbing.
- The client will gain mastery over symptoms—anxiety, fear, depression, and sexual problems will decrease or become more tolerable.
- The client will reconnect—increasing his or her ability to trust and attach to others.
- The client will discover or attach some kind of meaning to the event, finding empowerment.

Implementation

Upon admission, individuals who have been raped are placed in a private room. All physical injuries are treated in order of severity. Nurses determine if the client has taken a shower or changed clothing. The nurse works with the client to relay the details of the incident, including whether a condom was used, as well as the type(s) of rape. Clients are assured of their safety and privacy, and nurses do not judge or make assumptions about the individual who has been raped or their decisions involving treatment and evaluation.

If the client chooses to have evidence collected, nurses explain every step of the process as it is being performed. Individuals are informed that they can ask to stop at any point in the process. DNA swabs and hair and skin samples are taken in an effort to identify the attacker. Tests for sexually transmitted diseases and infections are performed, and clients informed about appropriate treatments. Emergency contraception for cases of potential pregnancy is explained to the client and offered.

Nurses provide referrals to social workers, counselors, support groups, and law enforcement. If clients choose not to use these referrals, that is their decision, but nurses explain their options for seeking help. The need for continued HIV testing at regular intervals during the next year is discussed, and the client informed about potential outcomes.

Evaluation

Clients are encouraged to ask any questions they may have, either about the examination process or about future testing and resources. Nurses explore all options with the client as appropriate. Some potential outcomes are as follows:

- The client expresses emotions regarding the rape.
- The client is empowered to take control of the situation.
- The client discusses any fears or questions about the examination.
- The client employs healthy coping mechanisms.
- The client asks for, and accepts, help when needed.
- The client acknowledges that the rape was not his or her fault.

NURSING CARE PLAN

A Client Who Has Been Raped

Renee Meyers, age 23, comes into the emergency department after having been raped by her ex-boyfriend. She explains that the incident happened 4 hours ago, but she was hesitant to ask for help because she feels she holds some responsibility for the attack.

ASSESSMENT

Camilla Wright, an RN in the ED, escorts Ms. Meyers to a private examination room. Ms. Meyers is resistant to talk about the events, repeating multiple times that she feels that the attack was her own fault and that she cannot believe this could have happened. Nurse Wright is patient and tells the client to take her time in relaying the events as they occurred. The nurse also reassures the client that she is perfectly safe in the hospital and that no action will be taken without her permission.

After approximately 30 minutes, Ms. Meyers begins to discuss the details of the rape, reporting that her ex-boyfriend forced her to have sexual intercourse with him. When Ms. Meyers tried to resist, her attacker struck her repeatedly in the face with his fists. Nurse Wright notices slight discoloration near the client's right eye, and the left side of her face is moderately swollen. The client is visibly shaking, and she is fighting back tears. Ms. Meyers explains that the attacker did not use a condom, and says she is very worried about becoming pregnant.

Nurse Wright does not interrupt while Ms. Meyers is relaying the events, but when she is finished, she asks if the client has showered since the incident. Ms. Meyers reports that she has not showered. Nurse Wright then explains the process of collecting evidence and testing for sexually transmitted disease and infections, and asks Ms. Meyers if she is willing to consent to the examination and rape kit. At first Ms. Meyers is hesitant, but Nurse Wright does not try to pressure her into consent; instead, she asks the client if she would like some time alone to think it over.

Ms. Meyers takes some time alone and then informs Nurse Wright that she would like to have evidence collected. The client also requests to be tested for sexually transmitted diseases and infections.

DIAGNOSES

- *Risk for Infection*
- *Rape-Trauma Syndrome*
- *Fear* related to possible pregnancy
- *Acute Pain* related to physical trauma
- *Powerlessness*
- *Risk for Ineffective Coping.*

(NANDA-I © 2012)

PLANNING

Goals for Ms. Meyers' care include:

- The client will be tested and treated for any potential infections.
- The client will make an informed decision with regard to accepting or declining emergency contraceptive treatment.
- The client will report physical pain as absent or tolerable, as evidenced by client rating of pain as 3 or less on a scale of 0–10.
- The client will make an informed decision with regard to reporting the sexual assault to law enforcement officials.
- The client will make an informed decision with regard to evidence collection for potential future prosecution of the perpetrator.
- The client will openly express emotions and concerns to trusted confidantes.
- The client will seek follow-up counseling and psychosocial care.

IMPLEMENTATION

Nursing interventions for the client who is a victim of sexual assault vary based on the applicable nursing diagnoses, the client's personal preferences, and her willingness to report the crime to law enforcement. Examples of nursing interventions that may be appropriate for inclusion in these clients' care include the following:

Rape Trauma Treatment
- Refer to rape advocacy program.
- Administer medications to prevent sexually transmitted infections and pregnancy.

Client Teaching
- Support and educate about the physical examination and specimen collection process.
- Inform of HIV testing.
- Educate about legal procedures available to client.

Collect data to include the following:
- Events as client remembers them to have occurred
- Has client showered, bathed or douched since the rape
- Mental and physical state.

Collect specimens following chain of custody using a rape evidence kit:
- Pubic hair combing over a white paper sealed in an envelope and initialed by nurse
- Fingernail scrapings placed into an envelope that is sealed and initialed by nurse
- Clothing removed and placed in paper bag that is sealed and initialed by nurse
- Oral, rectal, and vaginal samples sealed and taken to laboratory for testing
- All specimens labeled with client's name, medical record number, date, time of collection, and nurse's initials
- Seal all specimens (except for those that go to the lab) in a large bag/folder and initial the seal and attach chain-of-custody form, which must be signed by the person who takes the bag for testing. Attach copy of chain-of-custody form on the client's medical record.

EVALUATION

Evaluation of the plan of care includes identifying the degree to which the client has achieved the identified outcomes associated with each nursing diagnosis. Examples of observed outcomes in which the client has demonstrated accomplishment of goals may include observation of the following actions:

- The client consents to collection of specimens and physical examination to promote conviction of rapist.
- The client talks with rape counselor.
- The client verbalizes understanding of the need for future HIV and pregnancy testing.

(continued on next page)

NURSING CARE PLAN (continued)

CRITICAL THINKING

1. *How should the nurse respond to Ms. Meyers if she refused to have specimens collected or a physical examination at this time?*
2. *Explain how the nurse should describe emergency contraceptives and their actions.*
3. *How might this client's emotional state change over the next 24–48 hours?*

REVIEW Rape and Rape-Trauma Syndrome

RELATE Link the Concepts and Exemplars

Linking the exemplar of rape and rape-trauma syndrome with the concept of stress and coping:

1. What teaching would you provide a client with rape-trauma syndrome about managing anxiety?
2. Describe the differences in communication strategy to assess for rape in a 12-year-old child versus a 30-year-old woman.

Linking the exemplar of rape and rape-trauma syndrome with the concept of self:

3. How will you plan to assist the victim of rape to regain her self-esteem?
4. When collecting specimens for use by law enforcement during the investigation of potential rape, what nursing interventions can be implemented to help the client maintain a positive self-concept?

READY Go to Companion Skills Manual

REFER Go to Pearson Nursing Student Resources
nursing.pearsonhighered.com

- Additional review materials

REFLECT Case Study

Damien Harris, a 31-year-old White male, transports himself to the ED after having been raped near a local bar. Mr. Harris has numerous bruises to his back, face, and ribs; he also has a shallow cut along his neck. He tells the nurse that a man approached him while he was outside a local bar having a cigarette; the man claimed to be having car trouble. Mr. Harris offered to help the stranger with his car, but once they were away from the bar the man began attacking him. The attacker put a knife to Mr. Harris's throat and threatened to kill him if he resisted. After the rape, the attacker struck Mr. Harris on the head and left him unconscious. Both his wallet and cell phone were taken by the attacker. Mr. Harris explains that his ribs hurt when he breathes and his head has begun throbbing since he regained consciousness. He has requested the use of a phone to call his wife.

1. What are the three primary nursing interventions for this client?
2. What resources can be offered to Mr. Harris?
3. Would the nursing care plan be any different if the client in this scenario were a female? Explain your answer.

EXEMPLAR 32.4 Suicide

EXEMPLAR KEY TERMS
Suicide, *1990*
Suicidal ideation, *1990*
Suicide attempt, *1990*

EXEMPLAR LEARNING OUTCOMES
After reading about this exemplar, you will be able to:

1. Describe the pathophysiology, etiology, clinical manifestations, and direct and indirect causes of suicide.
2. Identify risk factors and prevention methods associated with suicide.
3. Illustrate the nursing process in providing culturally competent care across the life span for individuals who have attempted suicide.
4. Formulate priority nursing diagnoses appropriate for an individual who has attempted suicide.
5. Summarize therapies used by interdisciplinary teams in the collaborative care of an individual who has attempted suicide.
6. Plan evidence-based care for an individual who has attempted suicide and his or her family in collaboration with other members of the healthcare team.
7. Evaluate expected outcomes for an individual who has attempted suicide.

▶ OVERVIEW

Suicide is the act of an individual inflicting self-harm resulting in death. When the individual's attempt was not fatal, but the intent to cause death was present, it is referred to as a **suicide attempt**. Cases of an individual constantly considering, planning, or thinking about suicide are considered **suicidal ideation**. In the United States suicide has become the 10th leading cause of death, even higher than homicide. In 2010, more than 38,000 individuals took their own lives, more than 1 million attempted

suicide, and more than 2 million adults considered suicide (CDC, 2012d).

▶ PATHOPHYSIOLOGY AND ETIOLOGY

One of the major changes that often accompanies individuals who commit suicide is depression. Approximately 67% of those who take their own lives were confirmed as being depressed at the time of the incident (American Association of Suicidology [AAS], 2012). Other changes that take place could be both biological and emotional in nature. An individual may express the desire to take his own life for an emotional reason (such as the end of a relationship, the death of a loved one, or the loss of a job), but that event could only be acting as a trigger to various biological factors (such as a genetic predisposition, a neurological disorder, or a neurotransmitter deficiency).

Influencing Factors

The majority of individuals who attempt or succeed at taking their own lives often cite a reason for wanting to die. However, suicide is generally influenced by a number of factors, not just one. In understanding the underlying causes of suicide, nurses can help to recognize potential warning signs for suicidal behavior, as well as identify individuals who are at greater risk.

GENETICS AND NEUROBIOLOGY Studies during the past 15 years have shown that suicidal tendencies have a genetic aspect in a number of cases. In fact, an individual's risk for suicide is five times higher if a biological relative has committed suicide in the past. Several neurobiological and genetic studies have also proposed that genes and situational stressors work together to create the conditions for suicidal behavior. The most commonly studied neurotransmitter proposed to be connected with suicide is serotonin, which is also believed to be linked to cases of major depression. Suicidal individuals have been found to have decreased levels of serotonin, which could cause increased impulsivity and suicidal behavior (Claydon et al., 2012).

INTERPERSONAL FACTORS Individuals contemplating suicide can be influenced by a number of interpersonal factors, such as a history of being abused, a history of being raped, loneliness, a recent separation from a significant other, and grief from the passing of a friend or loved one. Any significant emotional disturbance can cause an individual to become depressed, and if the depression becomes unmanageable, that can sometimes lead to suicidal thoughts and behaviors. Loss and grief can be profound influencing factors for suicidal behavior, especially if the individual lost (either by death or the end of a relationship) was of significant importance. Individuals who have lost a partner—especially those without other close family ties—should be monitored closely for warning signs of dangerous behavior.

Situations that take away an aspect of an individual's control over life should also be carefully monitored. For example, in cases of job loss, financial difficulties, or the loss of a house, the individual has experienced an extremely stressful event, and could feel that she has no way to make things better. Feelings of hopelessness such as these are at the root of many cases of suicide. The individual may come to believe that the easiest, and only, way to handle the loss of her job or finances is to kill herself.

COMORBID DISORDERS Approximately 90% of those who attempt or commit suicide have a comorbid disorder. Many of these disorders involve an element of depression, and it is estimated that 50% to 90% of individuals who succeed at taking their own lives were suffering from depression at the time, or were in the recovery phase of depression. The most common comorbid disorders for suicide are bipolar disorder, borderline personality disorders, conduct disorders, schizophrenia, and drug and alcohol dependence. All of these disorders have aspects of impaired impulse control, depression, and altered consciousness, thus making them the primary disorders associated with suicide attempts and completion (Butcher, Mineka, & Hooley, 2012).

Individuals with bipolar disorder are 15 to 20 times more likely to commit suicide than the general population. It is estimated that 25%–50% of those with the disorder will attempt suicide at some point in their lives. Risk percentages associated with this disorder decrease considerably when individuals are being actively treated. The most commonly studied treatment associated with decreased suicide risk was administration of lithium (Bipolar Foundation, 2013).

Numerous studies have shown that individuals with recurrent mood disorders have the highest risk of suicide. The general population has a 1.4% risk of committing suicide, whereas individuals with schizophrenia are shown to have a 10%–13% risk. Those with alcohol dependence carry a 3%–4% risk of suicide. Individuals with borderline personality disorder are often plagued with feelings of hopelessness and depression, making the prevalence of attempted and committed suicide quite high within that population. Similarly, conduct disorders and antisocial personality disorders are seen as predictors for suicidal behavior (Butcher et al., 2012).

SOCIAL FACTORS Society can also have an effect on suicide rates. Recessions, bullies, and/or dominant social beliefs can have an impact on individuals' mental health. Economic recessions can cause financial strain and job loss, which are both stressful events often cited as potential indicators of suicidal behavior. Bullies in schools or in the workplace are emotionally abusive toward their victims, harassing them to the point where the victims feel worthless or hopeless about life in general. Although many schools and community programs are working to eliminate bullying, it is still present across the country.

Etiology

Suicidal behavior comes from a feeling that death is the only option that will successfully solve the individual's current emotional strain. It is commonly said that suicide is a "cry for help," and while that may be true some of the time, suicide is a desire for a permanent solution to whatever catalyst has prompted the individual's behavior. Some who attempt suicide do so with the mind-set that they would like to die, but if they do not then at least others will realize how truly unhappy, or lonely, or desperate they feel. In cases such as these, a mild overdose on pharmaceuticals will often be used, or they will cause an injury that would be life threatening if no one found them in time. Individuals who have only death in mind will generally employ the use of a gun, hang themselves, or jump from a tall building because these methods are more likely to cause mortal injuries.

In cases where an individual has a comorbid disorder such as schizophrenia or bipolar disorder, the client may report having been instructed my voices in their mind to commit suicide. If these voices have been present for the majority of the individual's life, the individual may find it difficult hard to ignore such commands. However, if some part of the individual's mind still has the desire to survive, he might employ less drastic means of suicide in an effort to both satisfy the voices and get help in stopping them if he is able to survive the suicide attempt.

Box 32–1   Factors Contributing to High Suicidal Risk

- Euro-American
- Older adults, especially men, followed by adolescents and college students
- People who are isolated without support systems
- Individuals who are recently unemployed
- Recent loss of a significant relationship
- Separated, divorced, or widowed people
- Social isolation, including rural location
- Presence of a substance use disorder
- Presence of a mental disorder
- Feelings of failure and hopelessness
- Presence of a gun in the home
- Previous suicide attempts
- Positive family history of completed suicide

Risk Factors

Risk factors for suicide in the United States include depression or other mental disorders; a family history of abuse, violence, or suicide; substance abuse disorders; exposure to suicidal behavior; firearms in the home; or a previous suicide attempt (**Box 32–1 ●**).

Other risk factors include gender and age. Men in the United States are more likely to die from suicide, whereas women are twice as likely to attempt suicide. Suicide is currently the seventh leading cause of death in men (Butcher et al., 2012). From the late 1980s to the early 2000s, older adults were at the highest risk for committing suicide of any age group, and while their rates of completed suicide are still high, individuals in the age group of 25 to 64 are now more at risk for suicide than older adults. In 2006 the number of older adults completing suicide declined, while the number of adults ages 25 to 64 increased (CDC, 2013b).

Prevention

Prevention of suicide comes from knowing the warning signs and then employing effective responses and precautions. Individuals who are planning to commit suicide will display various warning signs, such as a preoccupation with death, talking about wanting their pain to end, talking about suicide, giving away once-prized possessions, and taking unnecessary risks. If nurses suspect an individual of being suicidal, it is important to discover if the client has made a plan for the act or set a specific date. Expressing genuine concern for the client's well-being is a good place for nurses to begin, as it is important to build a trusting rapport. It is also acceptable to ask if the client has formed a specific plan for suicide; a question such as this will in no way push the individual to harm himself, but could provide him with an outlet to discuss his concerns and fears.

Nurses who suspect a client to be at considerable risk for suicide will consider the client's safety as a main priority. If the nurse believes the client to be a danger to herself, then she will not be left alone at any point. All dangerous items (such as sharp tools, bags, wire coat hangers, and syringes) will be removed from the room where the client is staying. Nurses will contact the client's primary care physician, as well as a suicide prevention counselor or the psychiatric department of a hospital.

▶ CLINICAL MANIFESTATIONS

The clinical manifestations of suicidal ideation and behavior vary by age, but a few common factors underlie most suicidal behavior. Experts frequently cite impulsivity, aggression, pessimism, and an overall negative affect as personality traits associated with the condition. Though the specific events that lead to an individual's suicide attempt vary based on age, culture, individual psychology, and life history, suicide is often associated with negative events such as interpersonal crisis and financial catastrophe. The sense of a loss of meaning in life produces the painful, hopeless mental state conducive to suicide. Factors that predict suicidal behavior in the short term include major depression, psychic anxiety, delusions, and alcohol abuse. The fundamental clinical manifestation of suicidal ideation is the domination of the client's consciousness by an unrelenting stream of painful thoughts. The suicidal person feels that death is the only possible solution to escape a mental life of unrelenting stress, anxiety, and depression (Butcher et al., 2012).

Behavior

Behavioral cues provide a window into the mind of an individual who may be contemplating suicide. Though not all people who commit suicide behave abnormally beforehand, many people provide clues that an attempt is imminent. An individual contemplating suicide may mention feeling helpless in the face of stress, and may discuss life after death. He may also provide verbal cues such as "It won't matter for long" or "I can't take this much longer." Some behaviors may also demonstrate suicidal ideation, such as obtaining a weapon, withdrawing from relationships, and apathy toward school or work performance (Fontaine, 2009).

The American Association of Suicidology (2013) developed a mnemonic device for the short-term indications of suicidal intent with the phrase **IS PATH WARM**. The letters in the phrase indicate the following terms:

> **I**deation
> **S**ubstance abuse
>
> **P**urposelessness
> **A**nxiety
> **T**rapped
> **H**opelessness
>
> **W**ithdrawal
> **A**nger
> **R**ecklessness
> **M**ood Changes

All of these terms are indicators of possible suicidal behavior, and concern for the client's condition should increase if she exemplifies more than one of these behaviors. An individual at immediate risk for suicide will often display the warnings signs of acute risk. These include talking of wanting to hurt herself; looking for access to firearms, pills, or other means of suicide; and talking or writing about death. If these symptoms are observed, the individual should not be left alone and a mental health professional should be contacted (AAS, 2013).

Cognition

Children are at an increased risk for suicidal ideation if they have lost a parent or if they have been abused. However, psychopathology in childhood—including depression, antisocial behavior, and impulsivity—is a strong predictor of childhood suicide. Suicidal cognition in adolescents increases dramatically, most likely because of the collision of depression, anxiety, drug use, and conduct disorders in the teenage years. Exposure to the dramatic suicides of role-model celebrities also plays a role in the cognition of adolescents, who are highly susceptible to imitative behavior (Butcher et al., 2012).

Some individuals who attempt suicide will not be successful, either through a deliberate desire not to complete the act, or through healthcare professionals being involved soon after the attempt was made. After an unsuccessful suicide attempt, an easing of emotional stress typically takes place, especially if the attempt was expected to be lethal. This reduction is only temporary, and suicidal behavior will frequently recur. In the year after an attempt, repetition of suicidal behavior occurs in 15%–25% of cases, and there is an increased likelihood that the second or third attempt will be fatal. Long-term studies have shown that 7%–10% of individuals who seriously attempt suicide will eventually kill themselves, a risk of about five times greater than the average risk of 1.4% (Butcher et al., 2012).

Interpersonal Relationships

A common contributing factor to suicidal behavior is social stress or isolation. An individual may become suicidal when he becomes alienated from family and friends, or even when he has difficulty adapting to the demands of new social roles. Loss of a loved ones is a contributing factor related to suicide, as well as the loss of the ability to participate in once enjoyable activities. In general, women's motives for suicide tend to be related to painful or lost relationships or the death of a loved one, whereas men's tend to be linked to financial problems or a lost job (Fontaine, 2009).

The interpersonal motives for suicide vary by age group. Children most often attempt suicide in cases of physical or sexual abuse, an unstable family, humiliation in school, and the loss of a loved one. Adolescents may also attempt suicide because of a lack of meaningful relationships, sexual problems, and acute problems with parents. College students have additional risk factors, including anxiety about academics, new social situations and responsibilities, and anxiety about their place in the world. Adults over age 65 experience many changes that contribute to the risk for suicide, including loneliness and isolation, a loss of work deemed socially useful, and outliving good friends and loved ones (Fontaine, 2009).

Regardless of an individual's age, a stable social situation is essential to healthy mental functioning. The early 20th-century sociologist Emile Durkheim related the differences in suicide rates to differences in group cohesiveness, and concluded that the best deterrent to suicide is a sense of involvement and identity with other people. Durkheim's thesis is confirmed by the prevalence of suicide among people living in disorganized families and people experiencing social isolation (Butcher et al., 2012). The link between suicide and weak group organization is also corroborated by the relationship between unemployment and suicidal ideation: Unemployed individuals are cut off from both their sense of purpose and their social network.

Lifespan and Cultural Considerations

In the United States in 2009, individuals between the ages of 25 and 64 were the most likely to commit suicide, with a rate of 16.25 suicides per 100,000. Individuals over the age of 65 were the second likeliest to kill themselves, with a rate of 14.78 suicides per 100,000. Individuals from 10 to 24 years old were least likely to commit suicide, with a rate of 7.21 suicides per 100,000 in 2009 (CDC, 2013b).

Firearms, suffocation, and poison are by far the most common methods of suicide. A major concern in the treatment of suicide is the changing prevalence of suicide in different stages of development. In 2007, children ages 10 to 14 committed suicide at a rate of 0.9 per 100,000, adolescents ages 15 to 19 at a rate of 6.9 per 100,000, and young adults ages 20 to 24 killed themselves at a rate of 12.7 per 100,000 (National Institute of Mental Health [NIMH], 2010).

A similar trend of increasing suicide risk with increasing age is seen in older adults. Older White men are at the highest risk, with approximately 31.1 suicides per 100,000 each year. Men over age 85 are at the greatest risk of all age-gender groups, and though older adults attempt suicide less often than individuals in other groups, they have a higher rate of completion. One of the leading causes of suicide in the older population is depression, often undiagnosed, and the negative events that frequently come with long life: death of a loved one, illness, and isolation (AAS, 2009).

Also within the United States, the various ethnic groups exhibit substantial differences in suicide rates. For example, Whites and American Indian individuals have consistently higher rates of the condition than do African Americans, Hispanics, Asians, and Pacific Islanders (NIMH, 2010). Suicide rates also vary significantly among national cultures. The United States currently has a suicide rate of about 11 per 100,000, whereas countries like Greece, Spain, and the United Kingdom have rates of about 9 per 100,000. Hungary has a rate of about 40 per 100,000, the world's highest. Other European nations like Switzerland, Finland, Austria, Sweden, Denmark, and Germany have high rates due to a variety of cultural factors (Butcher et al., 2012).

Focus on Diversity and Culture
Suicide and LGBT Culture

- Lesbian, gay, bisexual, and transgender (LGBT) individuals are two times more likely to attempt suicide than heterosexual individuals.
- Gay and bisexual men are four times as likely to attempt suicide compared to heterosexual men.
- LGBT individuals are more likely to participate in suicide attempts and ideation compared to completed suicides.
- Increased risk for suicide in this population can be attributed to the presence of prejudice, stigmas, and discrimination.
- Adolescent LGBT individuals demonstrate a particularly high rate of suicide, attempted suicide, and suicidal ideation (APA, 2009).

Clinical Manifestations and Therapies **Suicide**

ETIOLOGY	CLINICAL MANIFESTATIONS	CLINICAL THERAPIES
Behavioral changes	■ Verbal cues indicating a desire to die or to "make it all stop" ■ Planning to commit suicide, including buying a gun, knife, or pills ■ Not participating in once-loved activities ■ Loss of interest in school or work ■ Participating in dangerous behavior such as drug use, driving too fast, not taking safety precautions	■ Treat underlying condition. ■ Behavioral therapy ■ Medication therapy ■ If a plan for suicide has been formed, make sure the person is not left alone. ■ Educate about therapy options.
Affect	■ Depression ■ Hopelessness ■ Loneliness ■ Anger ■ Anxiety	■ Treat underlying condition. ■ Behavioral therapy ■ Medication therapy ■ Express a sincere desire to help the individual.
Cognition	■ Rigid thinking ■ Fantasies about death or dying ■ Thought disorders ■ Preoccupation with death ■ Insomnia	■ Treat underlying condition. ■ Behavioral therapy ■ Medication therapy
Interpersonal relationships	■ Life stressors ■ Poor support systems ■ Social pressure ■ Feeling as though there is no one to ask for help ■ Feeling alienated from society ■ End of a relationship ■ Death of a close friend, spouse, or family member	■ Behavioral therapy ■ Medication therapy ■ Group therapy to recognize that other individuals are experiencing similar issues

Another cultural difference in the prevalence of suicide worldwide is gender disparity. Women are more likely to attempt suicide and men are more likely to complete suicide in the United States, but in India, Poland, and Finland, men are more likely to engage in nonfatal attempts. In China, India, and Papua New Guinea, women are more likely to complete suicide than men (Butcher et al., 2012).

Many religions are considered to be a protective factor for suicide. Faiths such as Catholicism and Islam strongly forbid suicide, and rates of suicide in nations that follow these religions are accordingly low. Many societies have strong cultural taboos against suicide in addition to formal declarations. However, some nations provide cultural exceptions to the rule outlawing suicide. Japanese culture is one of the few societies in which suicide has been approved as a socially acceptable solution to certain problems of disgrace or social cohesion. The suicidal zeal for a political and religious cause has found a new form in the suicide bombings of Muslim extremists in the Middle East. Across cultures, suicide can be a violent expression of inner turmoil, or an act motivated by national or religious fervor (Butcher et al., 2012).

▶ COLLABORATION

Suicidal attempts and tendencies, if caught early enough, can be addressed in a number of ways. The most common and effective method of treatment is to combine pharmaceutical interventions with talk or group therapy or counseling. For individuals who are also suffering from a comorbid disorder, the underlying disorder will also need to be treated in addition to the suicidal behavior because the two conditions may exacerbate each another. Nurses will work with the client, physicians, and therapists to create an effective plan of care.

Pharmacologic Therapy

The suicidal client should be assessed for the presence of comorbid disorders, especially major depressive disorder, bipolar disorder, and PTSD. Depending on the individual client's manifestations and the presence of comorbid disorders, pharmacologic therapy may be appropriate. The most likely choices of medications for the suicidal client will be antidepressants and mood stabilizers.

ANTIDEPRESSANTS The antidepressants most often used to treat depression (the underlying cause of the majority of suicide attempts) are fluoxetine (Prozac), citalopram (Celexa), sertraline (Zoloft), paroxetine (Paxil), and escitalopram (Lexapro). All five of these drugs are selective serotonin reuptake inhibitors (SSRIs), and are used to balance and stabilize the neurotransmitters in the brain that affect mood and emotional responses. Although all of these medications are used to treat depression, they also have the potential side effect of causing suicidal tendencies. According to the FDA, adolescents and young adults up to the age of 24 are at particular risk for suicidal thoughts and actions while taking antidepressants and should be monitored carefully. In addition, all adults taking antidepressants should be monitored for increased signs of depression or advanced suicidal thinking (NIMH, 2013). The use of antidepressants after a client has attempted or seriously considered suicide should be combined with other forms of nonpharmacologic therapy.

MOOD STABILIZERS AND ANTIPSYCHOTICS Drugs for bipolar disorder are called *mood stabilizers* because they have the ability to moderate extreme shifts in emotions between mania and depression. Some antiseizure drugs are also used for mood stabilization in bipolar clients. For more on drugs for bipolar disorder, see the exemplar on Bipolar Disorders in the module on Mood and Affect.

Medications used to treat schizophrenia are antipsychotics, and work to treat hallucinations and delusions. The treatment of these symptoms of the disease can help the suicidal client immensely by eliminating one of the underlying causes of the self-destructive thoughts. For more information about schizophrenia and the drugs used to treat the disorder, see the exemplar on Schizophrenia in the module on Cognition.

Nonpharmacologic Therapy

Therapeutic approaches to suicide prevention can be quite effective in many cases. The type of therapy employed will depend on both the client and the therapist, but the three most common forms of therapy used for suicidal clients are group therapy, individualized therapy, and family therapy. All three of these forms can be combined to further help the client work through her suicidal thoughts and behaviors. Family therapy will generally be used in tandem with either group or individualized therapy. The presence of the family can be very helpful in supporting the client, especially since most individuals who are truly contemplating suicide will work to isolate themselves from friends and family before the event. Family therapy can also help the client's family to understand what she is feeling and why she considered suicide, which can ultimately aid the family in taking an active role in supporting the client's recovery.

Cognitive behavior psychotherapy for suicide prevention (CBT-SP) is sometimes used with adolescents who display serious suicidal ideation or have recently attempted suicide. CBT-SP works to help the individual develop skills to prevent suicidal behavior in the future. The therapy works with the adolescent client to develop and employ healthy coping mechanisms and avoid all forms of self-harm (Stanley et al., 2009).

Clients who have attempted to take their own lives benefit from therapeutic interventions addressing healthy coping mechanisms. Writing therapy can be employed to help the client work through any suicidal thoughts or fantasies; similarly, a preoccupation with death and dying can be addressed through writing and keeping a journal. The journal will also serve to allow the client to see the progress that has been made from the start of therapy until its completion, with the goal of the writing changing tone from potentially hopeless at the start to more positive and hopeful at the end. Some therapists will also ask the client to sign a no-suicide contract, which says that the client will seek help before attempting suicide again.

■ NURSING PROCESS

Appropriate, nonjudgmental nursing care of the client who is suicidal is imperative. Clients who have experienced severe depression and considered or attempted suicide are emotional, and at times physically, vulnerable. Nurses will work to ensure the client's safety while helping to empower the client's need to refrain from self-harm. Every situation involving suicide is different, and nurses evaluate clients based on their individual cases and without any personal judgment or biases.

Assessment

Nurses working with clients who are considering suicide, or who have recently attempted suicide, should be direct but respectful when evaluating the client and asking questions. It is a common misconception that talking about suicide directly could cause the client to act in a suicidal manner, but this is not true. Individuals who are experiencing suicidal ideation respect direct acknowledgment of the situation as opposed to a restrained approach. For example, it is helpful to recognize the client's current state by talking about depression and asking directly "Are you considering suicide?" and "Do you currently have a plan for killing yourself?" Questions such as these will be much more effective than trying to avoid the reality of the situation by using phrases such as "hurting yourself" in place of suicide. Nurses recognize the severity and finality of the client's decision, and do not attempt to make light of the circumstances.

Nurses attain a full client and family history, focusing in particular on any mood disorders present in the client's family or with the client himself. It is also important to ascertain if the client has a history of suicide attempts or ideation, and if anyone in the client's family has ever committed suicide.

Discovering past instances of severe depression is necessary during the assessment process. Nurses can ask the client "Have you ever experienced severe, debilitating depression?" Or the question can be rephrased to discuss the most common symptoms of depression: "Have you ever felt hopeless, loss of interest in daily activities, or felt overwhelming guilt for long periods of time?"

During the assessment nurses determine the level of risk the client poses to himself. A low level of risk would be displays of mild depression and some curiosity about death. A high risk is represented by a client who talks about killing himself and has admitted to making a plan for suicide. Risk and protective factors are also assessed. Clients who are isolated from friends and family, and who show very little attachment to aspects of their lives have considerable risk factors for actually going through with the suicide. Individuals who have strong family connections, young children to take care of, and strong ties to religions that denounce suicide have strong protective factors against taking their own lives.

Diagnosis

The diagnoses for clients who demonstrate suicidal behavior, ideation, or have attempted suicide will change greatly depending on the assessment. Nurses recognize that each client is an individual case. Some nursing diagnoses for clients are as follows:

- *Risk for Suicide*
- *Risk for Self-Harm*
- *Risk for Vascular Trauma* secondary to wounds and lacerations
- *Hopelessness*
- *Powerlessness*
- *Disturbed Self-Esteem*
- *Disturbed Self-Concept.*

(NANDA-I © 2012)

Planning

Involving the client in the planning process can be beneficial depending on the individual's current emotional outlook. Empowering the client to take control of the goals of his care can be a small step in working toward those goals. Some potential goals are:

- The client will remain free from injury.
- The client will ask for help when needed.
- The client will discuss any extreme feelings of depression or hopelessness.
- The client will participate in regularly scheduled meetings with his therapist.
- The client will demonstrate healthy coping mechanisms.
- The client will begin to demonstrate a desire to live.

Implementation

The majority of suicidal individuals are also depressed. Nurses help clients by discussing the various symptoms of depression, including feelings of helplessness, worthlessness, and a lack of energy, while reassuring clients that it takes time for feelings associated with depression to dissipate. Similar discussions should be conducted with clients who have other comorbid disorders, especially bipolar disorder and schizophrenia. If any medications have been prescribed for clients with these disorders, nurses will explain how the medication works, its intended purpose, along with any potential side effects.

While clients are at increased risk to themselves due to suicidal ideation, nurses will ensure that they do not have access to any sharp objects, or other weapons or modes that could be used for suicidal purposes. Guests will be instructed as to what objects they cannot have while visiting the client, including knives, razor blades, and large quantities of pills. Nurses caring for suicidal clients will often ask them to sign a no-suicide contract, which says that the client will not attempt suicide while in the facility's or hospital's care, but will instead ask for help.

If a client is at an extremely high risk for suicide, nurses will ensure that the client is never left alone. A nurse, healthcare professional, or other healthcare worker will be with the client at all times until the risk for suicide decreases. Family will not be asked to perform this task for various reasons, the most paramount of which is a lack of training in how to handle the situation if the client does attempt suicide.

In situations where the nurse is caring for a client whom they suspect might be considering suicide, the nurse will alert the client's general healthcare practitioner as well as a mental health worker. Individuals who display suicidal warning signs will generally not ask for help in obvious ways, but will instead display signs associated with suicide, such as talking about wanting to die, giving away prized possessions, or saying that she will not be around much longer. These warning signs are the client's way of asking for help, and nurses should be able to recognize them and respond effectively.

Evaluation

The outcomes for clients demonstrating suicidal behavior can be varied. If the client is responsive to treatment, then the outcome has a chance of being favorable. However, if the client is truly determined to take his own life, then eventually the individual will succeed at achieving this goal. Nurses will sometimes feel responsibility or guilt for a client who has died while in their care, particularly if the client was suicidal. Although many interventions can be employed when a client demonstrates an unwillingness to live, none of these will prove successful if the individual does not have the desire to help himself. If a client dies while in a nurse's care and there is an emotional or guilt response, then the nurse should find someone to discuss her feelings with in regard to this event. Other nurses, physicians, therapists, or counselors are good sources of support for nurses who have lost a client.

Some potential outcomes for the client who is receiving treatment for suicidal ideation or attempted suicide include the following:

- The client remains free from injury.
- The client verbalizes emotions and concerns.
- The client participates in all scheduled meetings with therapists and counselors.
- The client demonstrates effective coping skills.
- The client seeks help when needed.

NURSING CARE PLAN   A Client Who Is Suicidal

Brandon Lewis, age 45, is admitted to the behavioral health unit after having threatened to attempt suicide. He was severely intoxicated at the time of his admission. Mr. Lewis is withdrawn and hesitant to speak to anyone who approaches him.

ASSESSMENT

Danielle Serrano, an RN in the psychiatric department, enters Mr. Lewis's room to obtain a health history and suicide risk assessment. Mr. Lewis does not readily respond to the nurse's questions, so Ms. Serrano waits and begins talking to the client about menial events such as the weather, a documentary she saw on television the evening before, and the lunch menu at the hospital for today. Eventually Ms. Serrano notices that Mr. Lewis seems to be more relaxed, so she asks him again if he would like to talk about what happened. When he does not reply, Ms. Serrano calmly explains that the client's daughter told the nurse she found him with a large knife and a bottle of painkillers, and then called 911. Mr. Lewis asks if his daughter is still at the hospital, and the nurse responds that she will be back this evening.

The client begins to explain that his wife left him 2 months ago, and then shortly after that he lost his job. Mr. Lewis has been drinking heavily for the past month. The night of his suicide attempt he wanted all of the pain to stop, so he tried to kill himself. Mr. Lewis's daughter walked in and got the knife away from him, then called for help. The client claims that he probably would not have tried to kill himself if he had not been intoxicated. Mr. Lewis has no previous history of suicide, depression, or any other comorbid disorders.

DIAGNOSIS

- *Risk for Suicide*
- *Risk for Self-Harm*
- *Hopelessness.*

(NANDA-I © 2012)

PLANNING

Identified outcomes for Mr. Lewis include:

- The client will remain free from injury.
- The client will discuss emotions and concerns.
- The client will ask for help.
- The client will demonstrate healthy coping mechanisms.
- The client will participate in treatment for alcohol dependence.

IMPLEMENTATION

- Assist Mr. Lewis to decrease or eliminate self-abusive behaviors.
- Facilitate development of a positive outlook for the future.
- Provide for safety, stabilization, recovery, and maintenance until Mr. Lewis's depression improves.
- Administer antidepressants as ordered.
- Teach visitors about restricted items (razors, scissors, etc.).
- Involve family, as client allows, in discharge planning.
- Initiate a multidisciplinary client care conference to develop a plan of care.

- Refer to mental healthcare provider.
- Initiate suicide precautions.
- Encourage Mr. Lewis to verbalize feelings.
- Contract with the client, as appropriate, for no self-harm for a specific period of time.
- Limit access to windows.
- Consider strategies to decrease isolation.

EVALUATION

Mr. Lewis agrees that he needs help to abstain from alcohol and agrees to be admitted to an alcohol rehabilitation facility. He says he probably would never have tried to harm himself if he had not been drinking, but agrees counseling is required and talks with a psychologist.

CRITICAL THINKING

1. *If you are the nurse caring for Mr. Lewis on the behavioral health unit, what actions will you take to keep the client safe?*
2. *Will you notify Mr. Lewis's wife of his admission? Explain your answer.*
3. *What strategies would you promote to Mr. Lewis to reduce hopelessness and have hope for the future?*

◢ REVIEW Suicide

RELATE Link the Concepts and Exemplars

Linking the exemplar of suicide with the concept of mood and affect:

1. Explain the relationship between depression and risk for suicide.
2. What questions will you ask the client you are admitting to the medical-surgical unit who admits to frequent bouts of depression to determine suicide risk?

Linking the exemplar of suicide with the concept of comfort:

3. Explain why the client with chronic pain should be assessed for risk of suicide.
4. How will you assess the client living with chronic pain for suicide risk?

READY Go to Companion Skills Manual

REFER Go to Pearson Nursing Student Resources
nursing.pearsonhighered.com
- Additional review materials

REFLECT Case Study

Jenny Vasquez, a 14-year-old female, presents to the emergency department after having consumed a box of diphenhydramine (Benadryl) tablets. Her left wrist has also been cut horizontally; the amount of blood loss is unknown. Upon ED arrival, Jenny is alert and angrily addressing emergency medical personnel and the ED staff. Two security guards are present in the examination room. When the ED physician asks if he can assess Jenny's wrist laceration, she attempts to slap him and threatens to "knock out" anyone who touches her. The ED physician orders application of physical restraints to Jenny's wrists and ankles for protection of herself and others.

Jenny's vital signs include temperature 96.2°F tympanic; pulse 118 bpm; and BP 152/96 mmHg. Respirations cannot be assessed due to Jenny's verbalization, but she does not appear to be in any acute respiratory distress. The ED physician quickly assesses Jenny's left wrist wound; there is no active bleeding and the wound is superficial with no deep tissue damage. A dressing is applied to the wound. Gastric lavage is performed immediately to remove the drugs from Jenny's stomach. Afterward, her wrist laceration is cleaned and sutured, and a sterile dressing is applied to the site.

Jenny is beginning to calm down and she pleads for removal of the physical restraints. The ED physician makes a verbal contract with Jenny; she agrees that she will not attempt to harm herself or others if the restraints are removed. After removal of the restraints, Jenny cries quietly. The security guards remain in the examination room.

Upon reassessment of Jenny, she speaks quietly and makes eye contact with the nurse. She explains that the teenagers at her school have been bullying her for the past year. Jenny is unsure about her sexual orientation, but was caught kissing another girl at the winter formal last year. Ever since then, she has been ostracized and teased constantly at school. The day of the suicide attempt she arrived at school to find that someone had spray painted slurs on her locker in red paint. Seeing no other way to stop the abuse, Jenny tried to kill herself.

1. Based on the information provided about Jenny's situation, do you believe she is at especially high risk for attempting suicide again? Please explain your answer.

2. Do you believe that Jenny was actually trying to kill herself, or was this incident more of a "cry for help"? Justify your answer with evidence from the case study.

3. Identify three nursing diagnoses that are appropriate for inclusion in Jenny's plan of care.

EXEMPLAR 32.5   Unintentional Injury: Motor Vehicle Crashes

EXEMPLAR KEY TERMS
Cervical collar (C-collar), *2003*
Dashboard knee, *2001*
Longboard spinal immobilization, *2003*
Motor vehicle crash (MVC), *1998*
Whiplash, *2001*

EXEMPLAR LEARNING OUTCOMES
After reading about this exemplar, you will be able to:

1. Describe the pathophysiology, etiology, clinical manifestations, and direct and indirect causes of motor vehicle crashes.

2. Identify risk factors and prevention methods associated with motor vehicle crashes.

3. Illustrate the nursing process in providing culturally competent care across the life span for individuals who have been involved in a motor vehicle crash.

4. Formulate priority nursing diagnoses appropriate for an individual who has been in a motor vehicle crash.

5. Summarize therapies used by interdisciplinary teams in the collaborative care of an individual who has been in a motor vehicle crash.

6. Plan evidence-based care for an individual who has been in a motor vehicle crash and his or her family in collaboration with other members of the healthcare team.

7. Evaluate expected outcomes for an individual who has been in a motor vehicle crash.

▶ OVERVIEW

Also referred to as a motor vehicle accident, a **motor vehicle crash (MVC)** is the unintentional collision of one or more motor vehicles with another vehicle or object. MVCs and the resultant injuries and deaths are a significant cause for concern in the United States (**Figure 32–4 ●**). Fatalities due to crashes have increased in recent years. In 2012 an estimated 34,080 individuals died as a result of motor vehicle crashes, which is a 5.3% increase from 2011. Injuries from accidents are far more prevalent, with 2,217,000 individuals injured in 2011. Accidents involving motor vehicles are currently the primary cause of death for individuals 11 to 27 years old.

Motorcyclist injuries and deaths have also increased, with 4,612 individuals involved in fatal crashes in 2010, representing a 2% increase from 2010. In 2011, 81,000 individuals were injured on a motorcycle. The number of injuries and deaths per year significantly impacts the healthcare industry, which provides medical treatment to these injured individuals (National Highway Traffic Safety Administration [NHTSA], 2013a).

▶ ETIOLOGY

Causes of motor vehicle crashes and injuries will vary based on location and the time of year (due to weather conditions such as snow, heavy rains, and high winds). The three main causes of fatal crashes in 2011 were alcohol-impaired driving, speeding, and lack of restraints. Some crashes involved all three factors, but the two most commonly combined were alcohol impairment and speeding. Among fatal crashes, 29% of motorcycle-related deaths and 24% of all fatal car crashes were influenced by alcohol. Individuals who represented the

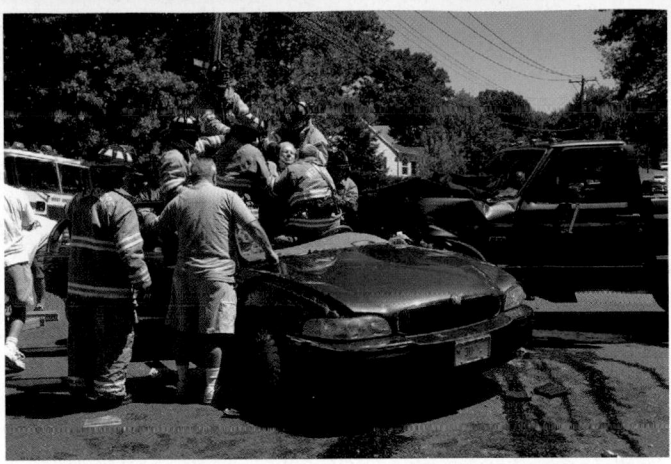

Figure 32–4 ● A man is extricated from a two-car crash by fire-fighters.

Source: © Enigma/Alamy.

largest percentage of alcohol-related MVC mortalities were those ages 21–24 (32%), those ages 25–34 (30%), and individuals ages 35–44 (24%). Speeding similarly contributed to a large percentage of mortalities on the road. In 2011, 35% of fatal motorcycle crashes and 22% of car crashes involved speeding (NHTSA, 2013b).

Hazardous driving conditions also result in fatalities and injuries. Approximately 24% of all motor vehicle crashes (1,511,000) are weather related. Every year an average of 7,130 individuals are killed and 629,000 are injured in weather-related accidents. Of these crashes, 75% are attributed to wet pavement, 15% occur during snow or sleet, 13% involve ice on the roadways, and 11% involve snowy or slushy pavement. Fog contributes to 3% of weather-related crashes. Hazardous weather conditions affect driver abilities, vehicle performance, and visibility, resulting in the potential for accidents (Federal Highway Administration, 2012).

Risk Factors

In the United States, the primary mode of travel is by motor vehicle, which means that a significant number of drivers are on the road at any time. Any individual driving in a motor vehicle is at risk for being injured in an accident. While some accidents are influenced by forces of nature, such as a deer or other forms of wildlife running across the road, or a sudden ice or rain storm, the primary cause of accidents is human error. Some of the main risk factors for motor vehicle incidents include age, speeding, distraction, aggressive driving, and impaired driving.

Both young drivers and older drivers are at particular risk for motor vehicle crashes. Beginning drivers ages 16–19 are still gaining experience with a variety of driving conditions and situations. They are also more likely to take risks while driving. Individuals in this age group are three times more likely to be involved in an accident than drivers ages 20 and older (CDC, 2012e). Older adult drivers (ages 65 and older) are at risk for incident not because of unsafe driving practices or inexperience, but rather due to preexisting health conditions, which can flare up while driving (such as heart or respiratory

problems), and decreases in sensory prevention (reduced eyesight and hearing).

Unsafe driving practices are a risk within every age group. Speeding and impaired driving in particular contribute to the vast majority of driving incidents. When a motor vehicle is moving too quickly, it is impossible to stop effectively if there is a sudden incident on the road—such as a car stopping suddenly, an animal walking across the road, a light changing to red, or a pedestrian unexpectedly crossing the street. Impaired driving limits the individual's ability to quickly react to a situation on the road, potentially leading to an accident due to delayed response time. Other driving traits that represent a risk for MVCs are driver distraction and aggressive driving. Distraction can result from talking on a cellphone or texting, dropping a beverage or food item while driving, or even having talking or crying children in the car. Aggressive driving leads to tailgating and partaking in other dangerous driving habits, which increase the risk for traffic accidents.

Prevention

Knowledge of the causes and at-risk groups directs prevention efforts. MVC-related injuries and deaths are preventable. Injury is the greatest health hazard for adolescents; therefore, injury prevention must be integrated into every health contact with youth.

Many teens learn to drive and have a license by 16 years of age. They often transport friends, get distracted by social interactions in the car, have little experience with actions to take if a car slides or has mechanical problems, may drink and drive, and are often tired when driving.

Several states have instituted graduated driver licensing to help decrease some risks. Graduated driver licensing is an approach used to decrease motor vehicle crashes among novice teen drivers. Common approaches are to increase the period required for a learner's permit, to decrease driving after dark, and to limit passengers in the car. Another method that has been suggested to improve safety records is to involve parents in practice driving times. Driving should always be presented as a privilege and a responsibility. Serious consequences such as losing the ability to drive for a time after any infraction can be suggested to parents. Because of the great risk of injury and death from car crashes, ask at each health visit if the teen drives or rides with other teens, what rules parents have established about driving, and whether the teen ever drinks and drives or rides with someone who does. Reinforce the need to wear a lap and shoulder belt at all times and to never drink and drive. Many common injuries are preventable by using protective gear and following safety guidelines.

Prevention efforts among older adults can be in the form of regular eye and hearing examinations, as well as considerations of the side effects of any medications being taken. For example, if a medication prescribed to an older client is known to cause drowsiness or vertigo, then the client should be advised of the dangers of driving while on this medication. If the client has a condition that could make driving a particular hazard, such as narcolepsy or severe epilepsy, then driving should be especially advised against. Various prevention efforts for all ages are listed in **Table 32–1 ●**.

TABLE 32-1 Strategies for Preventing Injuries Due to Motor Vehicle Crashes

AT-RISK GROUP OR BEHAVIOR	INJURY PREVENTION STRATEGY
Newborns/infants	■ Choose an infant-only seat or a convertible seat suitable for an infant. ■ Infant rides rear-facing until at least 1 year of age and more than 20 lb. ■ The safest place for all children to ride is in the backseat. Never place a rear-facing car safety seat in the front seat with an active passenger air bag. ■ Use a car safety seat every time the infant is in the car. ■ Read and follow the manufacturer's instructions for the car safety seat and the vehicle owner's manual for installation information. ■ Dress the infant in clothes that allow the straps to go between the legs. Never place blankets under the baby or under the belts. Buckle the baby into the seat, and place blankets over the baby. ■ To make sure the car safety seat is installed correctly and the baby is positioned correctly, go to a car seat inspection station. A certified child passenger safety (CPS) technician will assist you. Find a list of certified CPS technicians and safety seat inspection stations by state or zip code on the National Highway Traffic Safety Administration Web site: www.nhtsa.gov/cps/cpsfitting/index.cfm or 1–866-SEAT-CHECK.
Toddlers	■ Insist on safety seat use for all trips. Use approved safety seat only, such as forward-facing convertible seat. A toddler is not large enough to use car seat belts.
School-age	■ Verify that the child is belted in properly before starting car. Keep the child in a rear-facing seat until at least 1 year of age and 20 lb, but preferably longer, until achieving the highest weight or height recommended for the seat by the manufacturer. Forward-facing seats and booster seats are used in the backseat. These child restraint systems must be used until the child is 57 inches tall (or 8–12 years of age) and can safely use regular car safety belts. ■ For children over 40 lb (generally 4–8 years of age), use a belt-positioning, forward-facing booster seat located in the backseat. Always use both lap and shoulder belts. Make sure the lap belt fits low and tight across the lap/upper thigh area and the shoulder belt is snug across the chest and shoulder to avoid abdominal injuries. ■ Children 4'9" and taller can sit in a regular car seat restrained with lap and shoulder belt that are snug and correctly located across the lap and chest. The backseat is preferred for all children and should be the only location used for children 12 years and younger.
Adolescents	■ School-based education programs ■ Graduated driver's licensing programs ■ Enforce rules about safe driving. ■ Use seat belts for every trip. ■ Discourage drug and alcohol use.
Older adults	■ Regular vision exams ■ Driving ability screenings and community programs ■ Evaluate potential effects of medications.
Alcohol-related incidents	■ Enforce minimum drinking age laws. ■ Promote transportation alternatives, e.g., designated driver. ■ Conduct sobriety checkpoints. ■ Encourage treatment for alcohol abusers. ■ Conduct community-wide programs.
Speeding	■ Observe speed limits. ■ Enforce speed limits.
Motorcycle	■ Use helmet. ■ Observe speed limits.
Pedestrians and cyclists	■ Children: Teach young children never to go into the road. A safe, preferably enclosed, play yard is recommended. The child should be supervised at all times. Teach older children safe outside play, especially near streets. Teach biking safety rules and provide safe places for riding. Reinforce use of bike helmet. ■ Adults: Observe bike safety rules; wear helmet.

▶ CLINICAL MANIFESTATIONS

Motor vehicle crashes often result in a combination of physical and emotional injuries. Physical injuries can range from mild (minor scrapes and contusions) to severe (broken bones, head injuries, and even fatal injuries). When emotional injuries are present, they are often in the form of mild PTSD (especially if other passengers were severely or fatally injured) and/or a fear of future car accidents or of driving. Nurses will see a wide range of injuries as the result of motor vehicle crashes.

Common Injuries

Injuries are very common as the result of motor vehicle crashes, with some of the more prevalent injuries being whiplash, head and brain trauma, spinal cord injuries, facial injuries, internal organ damage, and a tearing of the posterior cruciate ligament in the knee. **Whiplash** results when a sudden impact to a motor vehicle causes an individual's head and neck to be forcibly contorted, resulting in injury to the spine. Spinal injuries are common in MVCs, and can result in partial or complete paralysis. When a motor vehicle is suddenly brought to rest from an advanced speed, the driver and passengers of the vehicle are often thrown forward or backward (depending on the type of crash), causing their bodies to strike forcibly into parts of the car. Facial and brain injuries often occur in this manner, as the individual's head hits the dashboard, steering wheel, or air bag. Tearing of the posterior cruciate ligament and other knee injuries result from the individual's knee slamming into the dashboard or back of a seat; this type of injury is colloquially referred to as "**dashboard knee**."

Although wearing a seat belt can save an individual's life, seat belts also can cause injuries during a crash. Common injuries from a seat belt are fractured ribs, fractured collar bone, internal injuries, and organ damage, as well as the potential for a punctured lung often resulting from broken ribs.

Cultural Considerations

Native American Indians and Alaska natives are at an especially high risk for motor vehicle crashes. Injuries from motor vehicle crashes are the leading cause of death for individuals within these cultures ages 1–44. Adults within this population are more than twice as likely to be involved in an accident as both Caucasians and African Americans. Some of the reasons for these high mortality rates include low seat belt use, low child safety seat use, and increased incidences of alcohol impairment while driving. Nurses should work to describe the lifesaving benefits of seat belt and child safety procedures to all individuals, particularly populations who are not required by law to use these restraints on their own property (CDC, 2010a).

Beliefs about medical interventions will need to be taken into account when caring for individuals who have been in

---

Focus on Diversity and Culture
Use of Safety Protection

Marked differences exist in behaviors that influence unintentional injuries. Males of all races are more likely to avoid seat belt use than females, with women being 10% more likely to use a seat belt than men. Individuals who live in urban and suburban areas are 10% more likely to wear safety belts than those who live in rural areas. Age also factors into seat belt use, with studies showing that adults from ages 18–34 are less likely to wear safety belts when compared to individuals 35 years of age or older (CDC, 2011a). How will you inquire about seat belt use in an open-ended manner during health promotion visits? Consider asking these questions: Where do you usually ride in the car? Who do you usually ride with? Does your car have seat belts? How often do you use them? Plan strategies that include all children and families, especially those at high risk of not using seat belts.

MVCs. Some individuals who are brought into the hospital after an MVC may refuse treatment—even lifesaving procedures—if it conflicts with their spiritual or cultural beliefs. This includes Christian Scientists (who do not allow most medical interventions) and Jehovah Witnesses (who cannot have blood transfusions). Other cultures also may refuse Western medical interventions, and although nurses should explain the potential medical consequences of not accepting treatment, they must ultimately be respectful of the client's decision.

▶ COLLABORATION

Collaborative care of the client who has sustained injury in a motor vehicle crash depends on a team approach. The team includes health personnel on site and the nurses, physicians, and surgeons at the hospital. Providing trauma care with a team focus helps each team member know his or her role. Prompt delegation of tasks and responsibilities improves the client's chances for survival and decreases the morbidity that may result from traumatic injuries.

Stay Current: *Many organizations such as the Society of Trauma Nurses and the American College of Surgeons offer courses in trauma care for nurses. For more information visit the Advanced Trauma Care for Nurses page at* **www.trauma-nurses.org/atcn-courses.html** *and the Advanced Trauma Life Support page at* **www.facs.org/trauma/atls/about.html**.

Prevention efforts require collaboration as well. Often local fire departments, law enforcement, and health departments will combine to offer awareness campaigns regarding issues related to motor vehicle crashes. Many communities offer programs that provide child car seats free of charge and provide training for parents on how to install and use child car seats correctly. Increasingly, states are mandating driver safety training for drivers who receive traffic citations for minor incidents in which no one was injured.

Diagnostic Tests

Because the injuries most commonly found with clients who have been in motor vehicle crashes vary widely, so do the diagnostic tests used to assess the severity of those injuries. Common diagnostic procedures performed include the use of MRIs, CTs, x-rays, and ultrasounds. These procedures can be used to determine the severity of head, neck, and back injuries and to identify the presence of internal bleeding, broken bones, or torn muscles. An electroencephalogram (EEG) can be used to diagnose changes in brain activity, which may indicate potential injuries that were sustained during the crash.

Surgery

The severity and life-threatening nature of some motor vehicle incidents will often lead to a client needing surgery to repair damage and/or stop internal bleeding. If internal organ damage is indicated—either due to organ rupture or a foreign object puncturing the abdominal cavity—emergency surgery will be needed to repair the damage or stabilize the client until a transplant can be performed.

Clinical Manifestations and Therapies **Motor Vehicle Crash Injuries**

ETIOLOGY	CLINICAL MANIFESTATIONS	CLINICAL THERAPIES
Mild head injury to brain, bruising, bleeding, and/or swelling	■ Headache ■ Sensitivity to light, blurred vision ■ Nausea, dizziness, balance problems ■ Changes in memory ■ Seizures and coma	■ CT, MRI, and/or EEG to determine the extent of the injury ■ Application of ice ■ Stitches for open wounds ■ Surgery if needed to stop bleeding or relieve pressure from swelling ■ Physical and/or speech therapy depending on the severity of the injury
Tearing or injury to the posterior cruciate ligament of the knee, commonly referred to as "dashboard knee"	■ Pain in the knee ranging from mild to moderate, swelling ■ More severe pain when bending the knee or walking up stairs ■ Instability in the knee	■ Pain relievers and anti-inflammatories, such as ibuprofen ■ Physical therapy to improve range of motion and function ■ Joint aspiration if swelling persists or impairs functioning ■ Surgery to repair the damage in severe cases
Whiplash	■ Neck stiffness and pain ■ Dizziness, blurred vision, headaches, ringing in the ears ■ Concentration and memory problems	■ Prescription pain relievers such as hydrocodone or oxycodone ■ Muscle relaxants to relieve muscle spasms ■ Lidocaine injections into the affected muscle to relieve pain and muscle spasms ■ Ice and heat therapy ■ Physical therapy ■ Immobilization collar to promote proper healing
Spinal cord injury, either incomplete or complete	■ Loss of sensation and movement below affected area ■ Pain if nerve damage is present ■ Breathing difficulty ■ Loss of bladder and bowel control ■ Numbness and tingling in extremities	■ Immobilization of the spine with a neck collar ■ Sedation to prevent further damage to the spine, if necessary ■ Methylprednisolone (Medrol) to decrease inflammation and nerve damage ■ Surgery if possible ■ Physical therapy and rehabilitation ■ Pain medications

Injuries involving severe head or spinal trauma may need surgery depending on the circumstances. Head injuries will not always need surgery; however, if an intracranial hemorrhage (ICH) is present and the bleeding does not stop on its own, surgery may be the only solution. Intracranial pressure (ICP) will be monitored when a head injury is present, and if the pressure rises to dangerous levels surgery will be performed to release some of the pressure. Spinal injuries are often irreversible once they have occurred, but in most cases surgery will be needed to remove bone fragments and stabilize the spine.

Pharmacologic Therapy

The majority of injuries sustained will be painful to clients and require some form of pain management. Less severe injuries involving sprains, minor cuts, and mild concussions do not require strong pain medicines, but rather a form of ibuprofen.

Deep cuts requiring sutures usually will be treated with lidocaine as a numbing agent before the suturing is conducted. In cases of more severe injuries, particularly those that require surgery, stronger pain medications—most often opioids—are administered. Sedation may be necessary if the client's reaction to the injuries or the pain puts her in danger of further injury. Nurses will follow proper sedation protocols, ensuring that the client is not oversedated.

Nonpharmacologic Therapy

Clients involved in MVCs will require empathy, understanding, and support from nurses. Because motor vehicle incidents are so common in the United States, nurses will be exposed to numerous clients who have sustained injuries in this manner, either recently or in the past. Although the injuries may seem common to nurses, clients may be terrified by the experience and the resultant injuries. Nurses will take the client's emotional state into consideration and respond effectively. Some individuals will be provided with a referral and resources for therapy and counseling due to emotional trauma resulting from the accident.

Physical therapy and rehabilitation are often required for severe injuries, including broken bones (especially compound fractures), spinal injuries, and some traumatic brain injuries. If the client falls into a coma or is put into a drug-induced coma, physical therapy and rehabilitation will be needed if muscle tone decreased significantly while the client was unconscious.

NURSING PROCESS

Nursing care of the client who has been injured begins with a primary assessment and the initiation of collaborative interventions for any life-threatening injuries. Nursing care is directed toward the client's specific responses to trauma.

Assessment

See the Concept of Violence section within this module for a complete assessment of the client experiencing trauma.

For the client who has sustained injury in a motor vehicle crash, primary consideration should be given to the airway: Assess if the airway is patent, maintainable, or nonmaintainable. Assess for manifestations of airway obstruction: stridor, tachypnea, bradypnea, cough, cyanosis, dyspnea, decreased or absent breath sounds, changes in oxygen levels, and changes in level of consciousness. Assessing the airway and initiating interventions are the first steps in managing the client with multiple injuries. A **cervical collar** (or **C-collar**), which stabilizes and maintains neutral alignment of the cervical spine, should be applied to clients with potential or suspected cervical spine injury. **Longboard spinal immobilization**, which provides support and immobilization of the entire spine below the level of the neck, should be instituted for clients with a potential or suspected spinal cord injury. Cervical and longboard spinal immobilization should be discontinued only by physician's order after determining that the client has not sustained a spinal injury. Although not always needed, this determination may require evaluation of the client's spine using CT scan.

Diagnosis

The trauma client has many complex and interrelated actual or potential alterations in health. The nursing care in this section focuses on client and family problems with respirations, infection, immobility, spirituality, and stress. Potential nursing diagnoses, which are numerous, may include the following:

- *Ineffective Airway Clearance*
- *Ineffective Breathing Pattern*
- *Risk for Decreased Cardiac Tissue Perfusion*
- *Risk for Impaired Peripheral Tissue Perfusion*
- *Risk for Deficient Fluid Volume*
- *Risk for Infection*
- *Impaired Physical Mobility*
- *Spiritual Distress*
- *Post-Trauma Syndrome.*

(NANDA-I © 2012)

Planning

Goals are based on individualized client needs, the type and amount of trauma sustained, and may include the following:

- The client's airway will remain patent.
- The client will demonstrate regular, nonlabored respirations and oxygen saturation levels of 95% or greater.
- The client's blood pressure will be maintained within normal limits.
- The client will not develop cardiac dysrhythmias.
- The client will demonstrate no signs or symptoms of infection.
- The client will demonstrate no motor or sensory deficits.
- The client will retain or regain mobility.

Implementation

As with any traumatic injury, nursing interventions begin with the ABCDEs. Only after ensuring an intact airway, appropriate breathing, and adequate circulation are other issues addressed.

Maintain Airway Patency and Ventilation

The client with multiple injuries is at great risk for developing airway obstruction and apnea. Facial injuries, loose teeth, blood, and vomitus increase the risk for aspiration and obstruction. Neurological injuries and cerebral edema alter the client's respiratory drive and ability to keep the airway clear.

- For clients who do not require tracheal intubation and controlled or assisted ventilation, administer supplemental oxygen as per hospital protocols, either by way of face mask or nasal cannula.
- Monitor oxygen saturation by applying a pulse oximeter. Adjust oxygen flow to maintain oxygen saturation from 95% to 100%. Decreased oxygen saturation readings despite a patent airway may indicate inadequate ventilation or ineffective

oxygen exchange at the tissue or cellular level. Pulse oximetry in clients who have been exposed to carbon monoxide (i.e., house fires) is unreliable since it cannot differentiate carboxy-hemoglobin from oxyhemoglobin.

■ Monitor level of consciousness. An early sign of an ineffective airway is change in the client's behavior. If the client becomes restless, anxious, combative, or unresponsive, the effectiveness of the airway needs to be immediately evaluated and appropriate interventions initiated.

Assess for Disability and Expose Obscured Areas

For a trauma assessment, disability and exposure are also assessed. Assessment for disability includes prompt recognition of neurological deficits through identifying decreased or altered level of consciousness, abnormal pupillary response to light, impaired or diminished mobility, and decreased or absent sensation.

Exposure requires removal of the client's clothing to allow for identification of injuries that may be obscured. Full assessment requires that the client be carefully rolled to one side for inspection of the back and the posterior aspect of the body. When rolling the client to one side, the trauma team will use a technique known as "logrolling," which allows for maintenance of neutral alignment of the spine. It is important to expose the client only as needed for assessment and treatment. To prevent hypothermia, warm blankets may be used to cover the client and the room temperature may be increased during periods for which exposure is required.

Promote Fluid Volume Balance

The plan of care for clients who sustain significant traumatic injuries, as well as for clients who may require administration of blood products, includes insertion of a large-bore IV catheter (at minimum, 18-gauge or larger in diameter). Both blood loss and the shifting of fluid from the intravascular space can lead to hypovolemia, which, if left untreated, may progress to cardiovascular shock. The nurse should administer IV fluid and blood products as per the physician's orders. Insertion of a Foley catheter may be required for continued assessment of urine production, which is an indirect reflection of the client's kidney function and fluid volume status.

Prevent Infection

Traumatic injuries are considered dirty wounds. Projectiles enter the body through dirty surfaces and clothing, carrying dirt and debris into the wound. Open fractures provide a portal for the entry of bacteria and dirt. Even with surgical intervention, the wounds often remain contaminated. Risk factors for wound infection include contamination, inadequate wound care, and the condition of the wound at the time of closure. Aseptic techniques used in applying and changing dressings reduce the entry of organisms:

■ Use careful hand hygiene practices. Hand hygiene remains the single most important factor in preventing the spread of infection.

■ Use strict standard precautions and aseptic technique when caring for wounds. Standard precautions are essential to protect the client and the nurse from infection. In addition, perform the following:
   a. Monitor wounds for odor, redness, heat, swelling, and copious or purulent drainage.
   b. Monitor hidden wounds, such as those under casts, by asking the client whether the pain has increased and observing for increased drainage and heat over the area of the wound.
   c. Ensure that cross-contamination between wounds does not occur. Collect drainage in ostomy bags if it is copious.

■ Take and record vital signs, including temperature, every 2–4 hours. Abnormal vital signs, particularly an elevated body temperature, indicate the presence of an infection.

■ Provide adequate fluids and nutrition. Adequate fluids, calories, and protein are essential to wound healing.

■ Assess for manifestations of gas gangrene: fever, pain, and swelling in traumatized tissues; drainage with a foul odor. Gas gangrene is usually caused by the organism *Clostridium perfringens*. This bacterium is found in the soil and can be introduced into the body during a traumatic injury. The organism grows in the tissues, causing necrosis; hydrogen and carbon dioxide are released, with resultant swelling of tissues. If the infection continues, tissues are progressively destroyed, and sepsis and death may result.

■ Assess status of tetanus immunization and administer tetanus toxoid or human toxin-antitoxin as prescribed.

■ Use strict aseptic technique when inserting catheters, suctioning, administering parenteral medications, or performing any other invasive procedure. Using aseptic technique during invasive procedures reduces the chances of infection.

Promote Mobility

The client with trauma injuries is often unable to change positions independently and is at risk for complications of the integumentary, cardiovascular, gastrointestinal, respiratory, musculoskeletal, and renal systems. Clients at greatest risk are those who have had multiple injuries, spinal cord injuries, peripheral nerve injuries, and traumatic amputations. Collaborate with the physical therapist and occupational therapist (if available) to determine the most effective types and schedule of exercises and assistive devices:

■ If active bleeding or edema is not present, provide active or passive exercises to affected and unaffected extremities at least once every 8 hours. Exercise improves muscle tone, maintains joint mobility, improves circulation, and prevents contractures.

■ Help the client turn, cough, and deep breathe, and use the incentive spirometer at least every 2 hours. Changing positions, coughing, deep breathing, and incentive spirometry reduce the risk of integumentary and respiratory complications.

■ If the client is unable to be moved and positioned, consider a specialty bed, such as the kinetic continuous rotation bed. The kinetic continuous rotation bed allows continuous turning of the client; the motion decreases pulmonary complications, venous stasis, postural hypotension, urinary stasis, muscle wasting, and bone demineralization.

■ Monitor the lower extremities each day for manifestations of deep venous thrombosis: heat, swelling, and pain. Measure and record the circumference of the thigh and calf each day. If antiembolic stockings or intermittent compression stockings are used, remove them for 1 hour during each shift and assess the skin. Venous stasis results when surrounding muscles are unable to contract and help move the blood through the veins. Thrombus (clot) formation in deep veins is a major risk for pulmonary embolism.

Offer Spiritual Comfort Measures

Trauma generally strikes without warning and carries potentially devastating consequences, including severe alterations in the lives of the victim and family, and death. The traumatic death of a loved one may be the most difficult event a family will ever experience. The decision to cease life support systems or to donate organs challenges the family's belief systems and psychological stability. Nursing care of the family (or client) experiencing spiritual distress includes the following:

■ Give the family information about the option to donate the client's organs. The decision to donate organs needs to be based on information about the client's condition, prognosis, and criteria by which brain death is determined. It is important to convey to family members that organ donation is only an option and that they should not feel they are obligated to consent or are doing something wrong if they do not consent.

■ Encourage the family members to ask questions and express their feelings about the traumatic event and/or organ donation. Allowing families to express their feelings may help prevent long-term consequences such as guilt.

■ Refer the family for follow-up care. Long-term follow-up is important for the family facing the sudden death of a loved one. Grieving is not an overnight process, and providing the family with resources that may be used in the future may help prevent future crises and dysfunction.

■ Provide the family of the dying or deceased client a place and time to pray or observe faith rituals together. Provide the family the opportunity to call for the family minister or spiritual leader. Praying or observing faith rituals helps the family begin a healthy process of grieving.

■ Be present for the family. The nurse's act of "presencing" provides a level of support and assures the family that they and their loved one are valued and respected. More information about presencing and providing spiritual support can be found in the module on Spirituality.

Promote Psychosocial Well-Being

Posttrauma syndrome is an intense, sustained emotional response to a disastrous event. It is characterized by emotions that range from anger to fear and by flashbacks or psychic numbing. In the initial stage, the client may be calm or may express feelings of anger, disbelief, terror, and shock. In the long-term phase, which begins anywhere from a few days to several months after the event, the client often experiences flashbacks and nightmares of the traumatic event. The client

may call on ineffective coping mechanisms, such as alcohol or drugs, and withdraw from relationships. Appropriate interventions may include the following:

■ Assess emotional responses while providing physical care. Observe for crying, sleep problems, suspiciousness, and fear during the initial phase of treatment. If the client is unconscious, encourage family members and friends to express their feelings. These assessments provide valuable information about the client's ability to cope with the trauma.

■ Be available if the client wishes to talk about the trauma, and encourage expression of feelings. The client may initially deny negative feelings; this denial is a coping mechanism in the initial phase of recovery.

■ Teach relaxation techniques, such as deep breathing, progressive muscle relaxation, or imagery. These techniques are often useful in coping when thoughts of the trauma recur.

■ Refer the client and family members for counseling, psychotherapy, or support groups as appropriate. Continued therapy may be necessary in assisting the client and family to resolve the acute and long-term effects of trauma.

Facilitate Community-Based Care

Address the following topics to prepare the client and family for home care:

■ The type of home environment to which the client will be returning, including any changes that will be required to let the client function in that environment

■ Medications, dressings, wound care, equipment, and supplies

■ Special diet, if needed

■ Rehabilitation plan and its effect on the client's family

■ Follow-up appointments with the physician or at the trauma clinic

■ Emotional changes that the client may undergo as a result of the trauma

■ Helpful resources:
   a. Home health care
   b. Community support groups
   c. National Institute of Neurological Disorders and Stroke.

Evaluation

The reaction and future care of each client to the trauma caused by a motor vehicle crash will vary. In some cases the client will be discharged the same day as the crash, whereas other clients will need treatment for a longer period of time. Some desired outcomes for clients include the following:

■ The client's airway remains free of obstruction.
■ The client's respiratory rate remains within normal limits.
■ The client's oxygen saturation is maintained at 95% or greater.
■ The client develops no cardiac dysrhythmias.
■ The client's blood pressure is maintained within normal limits.
■ The client demonstrates no signs or symptoms of infection.
■ The client demonstrates no neurovascular deficits.
■ The client retains mobility.
■ The client verbally expresses emotions and concerns.

NURSING CARE PLAN A Client With Multiple Injuries

Jane Souza is a 25-year-old married woman with two children who provides day care for preschool children in her home. As she is driving the interstate at 65 miles per hour, a car crosses the median and strikes her vehicle head-on. Ms. Souza, who is not wearing a seat belt, is thrown forward against the steering wheel. The front of her car is pushed up against her by the car that struck her, entrapping her lower extremities.

After extensive efforts to extricate her from the car, Ms. Souza is transported to the local trauma center. She is still conscious, is receiving high-flow oxygen by mask, and has one intravenous line in place. Her vital signs are a palpable systolic blood pressure of 80 mmHg, a pulse rate of 120 bpm, and a respiratory rate of 36/min. On arrival, she states that she is having difficulty breathing.

ASSESSMENT

- *Airway:* Maintainable with high-flow oxygen in place.
- *Breathing:* Respiratory rate of 36/min, multiple bruising and abrasions on right side of her chest, decreased breath sounds on the right side.
- *Circulation:* No palpable radial pulses; palpable brachial pulses. Monitor shows sinus tachycardia. No active external bleeding noted. Skin color pale, cool to the touch, and diaphoretic.
- *Neurological:* Moved her fingers when asked; complains of difficulty breathing; denies that she is hurt. Pupils 4 mm, equal, and react to light. Has a broken right arm and an open fracture of the left ankle; because of these injuries, extremity movement is limited.

Because of Ms. Souza's respiratory distress, she is intubated and ventilated with 100% oxygen. Another intravenous line is inserted and O-negative blood administered.

DIAGNOSES

- *Ineffective Breathing Pattern* related to multiple bruises and abrasions on the right side of the chest, and respiratory difficulty
- *Deficient Fluid Volume* related to acute internal blood loss (presumed because no active bleeding can be found)
- *Risk for Injury* related to trauma resuscitation

(NANDA-I © 2012)

PLANNING

Client goals are individualized, and may include the following:

- The client will maintain adequate oxygenation.
- The client will maintain adequate circulating blood volume.

IMPLEMENTATION

- Monitor airway and assist in any needed airway management.
- Explain all procedures.
- Monitor the effects of fluid and blood administration, including any changes in blood pressure and pulse.

- Prepare for transfer to the operating room for emergency surgery.
- Keep family informed about her condition.

EVALUATION

Ms. Souza is transferred to the operating room, where it is determined that she has a ruptured spleen and a serious pelvic fracture. Ms. Souza's treatment continues in the operating room.

CRITICAL THINKING

1. Is the nursing diagnosis of Deficient Fluid Volume *appropriate for Ms. Souza? Why or why not?*
2. *The assessment of a client who has experienced trauma is ABCDE. What is the rationale for this sequence?*
3. *Following surgery, Ms. Souza is moved to the surgical intensive care unit. She is very anxious and restless. What assessments would you make to identify the cause of her restlessness?*
4. *Infection is a common complication for the trauma client. Describe five risks for infection that are present from the time of injury to the time of hospital discharge.*

◢ REVIEW Unintentional Injury: Motor Vehicle Crashes

RELATE Link the Concepts and Exemplars

Linking the exemplar of unintentional injury with the concept of intracranial regulation:

1. What is the priority of care when your client who experienced a head injury in a car crash has a blood pressure of 90/60 mmHg and a heart rate of 51 bpm?
2. What nursing interventions would be appropriate for inclusion in the plan of care for the client who has a head injury from a car crash to prevent the rise of intracranial pressure?

Linking the exemplar of unintentional injury with the concept of perfusion:

3. Describe potential threats to a client's perfusion as a result of a motor vehicle crash. How would perfusion be impacted if

the client's mobility was altered due to traction or other immobilizing treatments?

4. How can you promote mobility for a client involved in a motor vehicle crash who has a casted left leg and right arm? How would this plan change if the client were an older adult with diminished mobility prior to the trauma?

READY Go to Companion Skills Manual

REFER Go to Pearson Nursing Student Resources
nursing.pearsonhighered.com

- Additional review materials

REFLECT Case Study

Lilia Hoffman, age 25, was the driver of a vehicle that was struck by another vehicle at an intersection. The driver of the car that hit her ran a red light. Ms. Hoffman was extracted from her car using the Jaws of Life and was moaning when initially removed, but did not respond to verbal commands. Her pupils were pinpoint and reactive to light. The paramedics at the scene provided initial emergent care. Her vital signs included temperature 96.2°F oral; pulse 110 bpm; respirations 12/min; and BP 90/50 mmHg. She had bleeding from facial and scalp lacerations as well as suspected rib fractures. Her lung sounds were clear and equal bilaterally, and her oxygen saturation was 97%. Ms. Hoffman 's airway was determined to be patent and oxygen was administered via face mask at 10 liters per minute.

The air bag in Ms. Hoffman's car deployed. It was unknown as to whether she sustained a head or neck injury. One of the paramedics immediately administered manual stabilization of Ms. Hoffman's cervical spine until a cervical collar (c-collar) was applied. In addition to c-spine immobilization, Ms. Hoffman was placed on a long spinal board to prepare for transport to the local emergency department. Circulatory status was assessed and an 18-gauge intravenous catheter was inserted in her left forearm, followed by intravenous administration of 0.9% normal saline at a rate of 150 mL/hr.

In the emergency department, Ms. Hoffman's vital signs were temperature 98°F oral; pulse 118 bpm; respirations 14/min; and BP 98/50 mmHg. An IV bolus of 250 mL of normal saline was administered and a Foley catheter inserted. Her airway remained patent and oxygen was continued.

1. What are three priority nursing diagnoses for Ms. Hoffman?
2. What laboratory and diagnostic tests should the nurse anticipate being ordered?
3. Under what circumstances can Ms. Hoffman's spinal precautions (cervical collar and longboard spinal immobilization) be discontinued?

■ REFERENCES

Alia-Klein, N., Goldstein, R. Z., Tomasi, D., Woicik, P. A., Moeller, S. J., Williams, B., … Volkow, N. D. (2009). Neural mechanisms of anger regulation as a function of genetic risk for violence. *Emotion, 9*(3), 385–396. doi:10.1037/a0015904.

American Academy of Child and Adolescent Psychology. (2011). *Understanding violent behavior in children and adolescents.* Retrieved from http://www.aacap.org/cs/root/facts_for_families/understanding_violent_behavior_in_children_and_adolescents.

American Association of Suicidology (AAS). (2009). *Elderly suicide fact sheet.* Retrieved from http://www.suicidology.org/c/document_library/get_file?folderId=232&name=DLFE-242.pdf.

American Association of Suicidology (AAS). (2012). *Some facts about suicide and depression.* Retrieved from http://www.suicidology.org/c/document_library/get_file?folderId=232&name=DLFE-246.pdf.

American Association of Suicidology (AAS). (2013). *Know the warning signs.* Retrieved from http://www.suicidology.org/stats-and-tools/suicide-warning-signs.

American Nurses Association. (2013). *Workplace violence.* Retrieved from http://nursingworld.org/workplace-violence.

American Psychiatric Association. (2013). *Diagnostic and statistical manual of mental disorders* (5th ed.). Arlington, VA: Author.

American Psychological Association (APA). (2009). *Diversity & suicidal behavior.* Retrieved from http://www.apa.org/divisions/div12/sections/section7/diversity_suic_factsheet.pdf.

American Psychological Association (APA). (2011). *Eating disorders.* Retrieved from http://www.apa.org/helpcenter/eating.aspx.

American Psychological Association (APA). (2013). *Understanding child sexual abuse: Education, prevention, and recovery.* Retrieved from http://www.apa.org/pubs/info/brochures/sex-abuse.aspx#.

Anderson, L., Fitzgerald, M., & Luck, L. (2010). An integrative literature review of interventions to reduce violence against ED nurses. *Journal of Clinical Nursing, 19*, 2520–2530.

Anetzberger, G. J. (2012). An update on the nature and scope of elder abuse. *Journal of the American Society on Aging, 36*(3), 12–20.

Beck, A. J., & Harrison, P. M. (2010). *Sexual victimization in prisons and jails reported by inmates, 2008–09.* Retrieved from http://bjs.gov/index.cfm?ty=pbdetail&iid=2202.

Baron, R. A., & Richardson, D. R. (1994). *Human aggression* (2nd ed.) New York, NY: Plenum.

Benedictis, T. D., Jaffe, J., & Segal, J. (2012). *Domestic violence and abuse: Types, signs, symptoms, causes, and effects.* Retrieved from American Academy of Experts in Traumatic Stress Wb site: http://www.aaets.org/article144.htm.

Bipolar Foundation. (2013). *Self-harm and suicide.* Retrieved from http://www.bipolar-foundation.org/bipolar-disorder/complications/self-harm-and-suicide.

Buchanan, T. W., Bagley, S. L., Standfield, R. B., & Preston, S. D. (2012). The emphatic, physiological resonance of stress. *Social Neuroscience, 7*(2), 191–201. doi:10.1080/17470919.2011.588723.

Butcher, J. N., Mineka, S., & Hooley, J. M. (2012). *Abnormal psychology* (15th ed.). Upper Saddle River, NJ: Pearson.

Centers for Disease Control and Prevention (CDC). (2009a). *Sexual violence: Consequences.* Retrieved from http://www.cdc.gov/violenceprevention/sexualviolence/consequences.html.

Centers for Disease Control and Prevention (CDC). (2009b). *Sexual violence: Definitions.* Retrieved from http://www.cdc.gov/violenceprevention/sexualviolence/definitions.html.

Centers for Disease Control and Prevention (CDC). (2009c). *Sexual violence: Risk and protective factors.* Retrieved from http://www.cdc.gov/violenceprevention/sexualviolence/riskprotectivefactors.html.

Centers for Disease Control and Prevention (CDC). (2010a). *Injuries among American Indians/Alaska natives (AI/AN): Fact sheet.* Retrieved from http://www.cdc.gov/Motorvehiclesafety/native/factsheet.html.

Centers for Disease Control and Prevention (CDC). (2010b). *Intimate partner violence: Definitions.* Retrieved from http://www.cdc.gov/violenceprevention/intimatepartnerviolence/definitions.html.

Centers for Disease Control and Prevention (CDC). (2011a). *Seat belts fact sheet.* Retrieved from http://www.cdc.gov/motorvehiclesafety/seatbelts/facts.html.

Centers for Disease Control and Prevention (CDC). (2011b). *Youth violence: Risk and protective factors.* Retrieved from http://www.cdc.gov/violenceprevention/youthviolence/riskprotectivefactors.html.

Centers for Disease Control and Prevention (CDC). (2012a). *Child maltreatment: Consequences.* Retrieved from http://www.cdc.gov/violenceprevention/childmaltreatment/consequences.html.

Centers for Disease Control and Prevention (CDC). (2012b). *Intimate partner violence: Consequences.* Retrieved from http://www.cdc.gov/violenceprevention/intimatepartnerviolence/consequences.html.

Centers for Disease Control and Prevention (CDC). (2012c). *Sexual violence.* Retrieved from http://www.cdc.gov/ViolencePrevention/pdf/SV-DataSheet-a.pdf.

Centers for Disease Control and Prevention (CDC). (2012d). *Suicide: Consequences.* Retrieved from http://www.cdc.gov/violenceprevention/suicide/consequences.html.

Centers for Disease Control and Prevention (CDC). (2012e). *Teen drivers: Fact sheet.* Retrieved from http://www.cdc.gov/motorvehiclesafety/teen_drivers/teen-drivers_factsheet.html.

Centers for Disease Control and Prevention (CDC). (2013a). *The national intimate partner and sexual violence survey.* Retrieved from http://www.cdc.gov/violenceprevention/nisvs.

Centers for Disease Control and Prevention (CDC). (2013b). *National suicide statistics at a glance.* Retrieved from http://www.cdc.gov/violenceprevention/suicide/statistics/trends02.html.

Centers for Disease Control and Prevention (CDC). (2013c). *Sexual violence: Prevention strategies.* Retrieved from http://www.cdc.gov/violenceprevention/sexualviolence/prevention.html.

Ciccarelli, S. K., & White, J. N. (2013). *Psychology: An exploration* (2nd ed.). Upper Saddle River, NJ: Pearson Education.

Clayden, R. C., Zaruk, A., Meyre, D., Thabane, L., & Samaan, Z. (2012). The association of attempted suicide with genetic variants in the SLC6A4 and TPH genes depends on the definition of suicidal behavior: A systematic review and meta-analysis. *Translational Psychiatry, 2.* doi:10.1038/tp.2012.96.

Clinard, M. B., & Meier, R. F. (2011). *Sociology of deviant behavior* (14th ed.). Belmont, CA: Wadsworth Cengage Learning.

Collins, K. S., Strieder, F. H., DePanfilis, D., Tabor, M., Clarkson-Freeman, P. A., Linde, L., & Greenberg, D. (2011). Trauma adapted family connections: Reducing developmental and complex trauma symptomology to prevent child abuse and neglect. *Child Welfare, 90*(6), 29–47.

Crosson-Tower, C. (2010). *Understanding child abuse and neglect* (8th ed.). Boston, MA: Pearson Education.

DeAngelis, T. (2013). *Rape takes global toll on women's lives, study finds.* Retrieved from http://www.apa.org/monitor/2013/01/rape.aspx.

Douglas, E. M., & Hines, D. A. (2011). The helpseeking experiences of men who sustain intimate partner violence: An overlooked population and implications for practice. *Journal of Family Violence, 26*(6), 473–485. doi:10.1007/s10896-011-9382-4.

Elbogen, E. B., & Johnson, S. C. (2009). The intricate link between violence and mental disorders: Results from the national epidemiologic society on alcohol and related conditions. *Archives of General Psychiatry, 66*(2), 152–161. doi:10.1001/archgenpsychiatry. 2008.537.

Federal Bureau of Investigation (FBI). (2012a). *Annual crime in the U.S. report released*. Retrieved from http://www.fbi.gov/news/stories/2012/october/annual-crime-in-the-u.s.-report-released.

Federal Bureau of Investigation (FBI). (2012b). *Crime in the United States 2011: Expanded homicide data Table 8*. Retrieved from http://www.fbi.gov/about-us/cjis/ucr/crime-in-the-u.s/2011/crime-in-the-u.s.-2011/tables/expanded-homicide-data-table-8.

Federal Bureau of Investigation (FBI). (2012c). *Crime in the United States 2011: Table 2*. Retrieved from http://www.fbi.gov/about-us/cjis/ucr/crime-in-the-u.s/2011/crime-in-the-u.s.-2011/tables/table-2.

Federal Bureau of Investigation (FBI). (2012d). *Expanded homicide data*. Retrieved from http://www.fbi.gov/about-us/cjis/ucr/crime-in-the-u.s/2011/crime-in-the-u.s.-2011/offenses-known-to-law-enforcement/expanded/expanded-homicide-data.

Federal Bureau of Investigation (FBI). (2012e). *Hate crimes data collection guidelines and training manual*. Washington, DC: Author.

Federal Bureau of Investigation (FBI). (2012f). *UCR program changes definition of rape*. Retrieved from http://www.fbi.gov/about-us/cjis/cjis-link/march-2012/ucr-program-changes-definition-of-rape.

Federal Bureau of Investigation (FBI). (2012g). *Violent crime*. Retrieved from http://www.fbi.gov/about-us/cjis/ucr/crime-in-the-u.s/2011/crime-in-the-u.s.-2011/violent-crime/violent-crime.

Federal Highway Administration. (2012). *How do weather events impact roads?* Retrieved from http://www.ops.fhwa.dot.gov/weather/q1_roadimpact.htm.

Finn, C. (2011). Forensic nurses' experience of receiving child abuse disclosures. *Journal for Specialists in Pediatric Nursing, 16*, 252–262. doi:10.1111/j.1744-6155.2011.00296.x.

Fontaine, K. L. (2009). *Mental health nursing* (6th ed.). New York, NY: Pearson Education.

Ford-Gilboe, M., Varcoe, C., Wuest, J., & Merrit-Gray, M. (2011). Intimate partner violence and nursing practice. In J. Humphreys & J. C. Campbell (Eds.), *Family violence and nursing practice* (2nd ed., pp. 115–154). New York, NY: Springer.

Herrman, J. W. (2009). There's a fine line…adolescent dating violence and prevention. *Pediatric Nursing, 35*(3), 164–170.

Hines, D. A., & Douglas, E. M. (2010). Intimate terrorism by women towards men: Does it exist? *Journal of Aggression, Conflict and Peace Research, 2*(3), 36–56. doi:10.5042/jacpr.2010.0335.

Howell J. C., & Moore, J. P. (2010). *History of street gangs in the United States*. Retrieved from http://www.national-gangcenter.gov/Content/Documents/History-of-Street-Gangs.pdf.

Ideker, K., Todicheeney-Mannes, D., & Kim, S.C. (2011). A confirmatory study of Violence Risk Assessment Tool (M55) and demographic predictors of patient violence. *Journal of Advanced Nursing, 67*(11), 2455–2462. doi:10.1111/j.1365-2648.2011.05667.x.

Kneisl, C. R., & Trigoboff, E. (2013). *Contemporary psychiatric-mental health nursing* (3rd ed.). New York, NY: Pearson Education.

Mayo Clinic. (2010). *Mayo clinic proceedings: Sexual abuse survivors have increased lifetime diagnoses of psychiatric disorders*. Retrieved from http://www.mayoclinic.org/news2010-rst/5858.html.

Mayo Clinic. (2011). *Post-traumatic stress disorder (PTSD)*. Retrieved from http://www.mayoclinic.com/health/post-traumatic-stress-disorder/DS00246/DSECTION=treatments-and-drugs.

Meadows. R. J. (2013). *Understanding violence and victimization* (6th ed.). Boston, MA: Pearson Education.

Montalvo-Liendo, N. (2009). Cross-cultural factors in disclosure of intimate partner violence: An integrated review. *Journal of Advanced Nursing, 65*(1), 20–34. doi:10.1111/j.1365-2648.2008.04850.x.

National Advisory Council on Nurse Education and Practice. (2007). *Violence against nurses: An assessment of causes and impacts of violence in nursing education and practice*. Retrieved from http://www.hrsa.gov/advisorycommittees/bhpradvisory/nacnep/Reports/fifthreport.pdf.

National Center on Elder Abuse. (n.d.). *Statistics/data*. Retrieved from http://www.ncea.aoa.gov/Library/Data/index.aspx.

National Highway Traffic Safety Administration (NHTSA). (2013a). *Just released: Research notes, crash stats, and reports*. Retrieved from http://www.nhtsa.gov/NCSA.

National Highway Traffic Safety Administration (NHTSA). (2013b). *Traffic safety facts: 2011 data*. Retrieved from http://www-nrd.nhtsa.dot.gov/Pubs/811753.pdf.

National Institute of Justice. (2010). *Victims and perpetrators*. Retrieved from http://www.nij.gov/topics/crime/rape-sexual-violence/victims-perpetrators.htm.

National Institute of Mental Health. (2010). *Suicide in the U.S.: Statistics and prevention*. Retrieved from http://www.nimh.nih.gov/health/publications/suicide-in-the-us-statistics-and-prevention/index.shtml#factors.

National Institute of Mental Health. (2013). *What medications are used to treat depression?* Retrieved from http://www.nimh.nih.gov/health/publications/mental-health-medications/what-medications-are-used-to-treat-depression.shtml.

National Trauma Institute. (2012). *Trauma statistics*. Retrieved from http://www.nationaltraumainstitute.org/home/trauma_statistics.html.

Occupational Safety and Health Administration. (2011). *Workplace violence*. Retrieved from http://www.osha.gov/SLTC/workplaceviolence.

Occupational Safety and Health Administration. (2002). *Guidelines for preventing workplace violence for health care & social service workers*. Retrieved from http://www.osha.gov/Publications/OSHA3148/osha3148.html.

Office of Mental Health. (2012). *Violence prevention: Risk factors*. Retrieved from http://www.omh.ny.gov/omh-web/sv/risk.htm.

Pew Research Center. (2013). *Why own a gun? Protection is now top reason*. Retrieved from http://www.people-press.org/2013/03/12/why-own-a-gun-protection-is-now-top-reason.

Renteln, A.D. (2010). Corporal punishment and the cultural defense. *Law and Contemporary Problems, 73*, 253–279.

Savino, J. O., & Turvey, B. E. (2011). Investigating serial rape. In J. O. Savino & B. E. Turvey (Eds.), *Rape investigation handbook* (431–435). Waltham, MA: Elsevier.

Shannon, K. E., Mead, H. K., & Beauchaine, T. P. (2010). Neurobiological adaptations to violence across development. *Developmental Psychopathology, 22*(1). doi:10.1017/S0954579409990228.

Stanley, B., Brown, G., Brent, D., Wells, K., Poling, K., Curry, J., … Hughes, J. (2009). Cognitive behavior therapy for suicide prevention (CBT-SP): Treatment model, feasibility and acceptability. *Journal of the American Academy of Child & Adolescent Psychiatry, 48*(10), 1005–1013. doi:10.1097/CHI.0b013e3181b5dbfe.

Taylor, I. (2009). Emergency care of patients with gunshot wounds. *Nursing Standard, 23*(40), 49–56.

Taylor, J. L., & Rew, L. (2011). A systematic review of the literature: Workplace violence in the emergency department. *Journal of Clinical Nursing, 20*(7–8), 1072–1085. Retrieved from http://www.ncbi.nlm.nih.gov/pubmed/20846214.

U.S. Department of Health and Human Services (USD-HHS). (2010). *Definitions of child abuse and neglect in federal law*. Retrieved from https://www.childwelfare.gov/can/defining/federal.cfm.

U.S. Department of Health and Human Services (USD-HHS). (2012). *Child maltreatment 2011*. Retrieved from http://www.acf.hhs.gov/sites/default/files/cb/cm11.pdf.

U.S. Department of Justice. (2010). *PREA data collection activities, 2010*. Retrieved from http://bjs.gov/content/pub/pdf/pdca10.pdf.

U.S. Department of Justice. (2011). *Homicide trends in the United States, 1980–2008: Annual rates for 2009 and 2010*. Retrieved from http://bjs.gov/content/pub/pdf/htus8008.pdf.

Wallace, H., & Roberson, C. (2011). *Family violence: Legal, medical, & social perspectives* (6th ed.). Boston, MA: Pearson Education.

World Health Organization. (2013a). *Definition and typology of violence*. Retrieved from http://www.who.int/violenceprevention/approach/definition/en.

World Health Organization. (2013b). *Elder abuse*. Retrieved from http://www.who.int/ageing/projects/elder_abuse/en.

World Health Organization. (2013c). *World report on violence and health*. Retrieved from http://www.who.int/violence_injury_prevention/violence/world_report/en/index.html.

Part III

Reproduction Module

Part III consists of the module on reproduction, which falls within the individual domain. This module presents the concept of reproduction, with exemplars designed to take the nursing student through the stages of pregnancy to caring for the newborn and the infant who is born prematurely. This module addresses care for infant, mother, and family, including biophysical and psychosocial needs.

Module 33   Reproduction   2011
    The Concept of Reproduction   2011
    Exemplar 33.1   Antepartum Care   2067
    Exemplar 33.2   Intrapartum Care   2112
    Exemplar 33.3   Postpartum Care   2170
    Exemplar 33.4   Newborn Care   2191
    Exemplar 33.5   Prematurity   2249

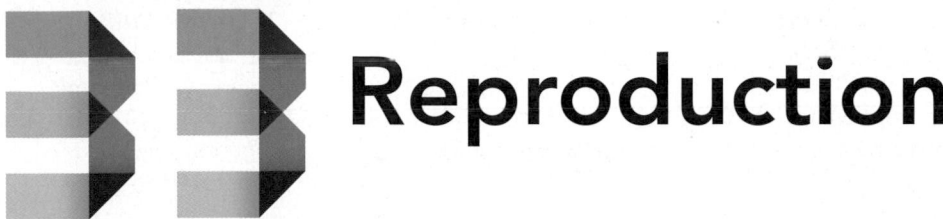

33 Reproduction

MODULE AT-A-GLANCE

The Concept of Reproduction, 2011

Exemplar 33.1
Antepartum Care, 2067

Exemplar 33.2
Intrapartum Care, 2112

Exemplar 33.3
Postpartum Care, 2170

Exemplar 33.4
Newborn Care, 2191

Exemplar 33.5
Prematurity, 2249

◢ THE CONCEPT OF REPRODUCTION

Understanding reproduction requires more than understanding sexual intercourse or the process by which the female and male sex cells unite. The nurse also must be familiar with the structures and functions that make childbearing possible and the phenomena that initiate it. The primary functions of both female and male reproductive systems are to produce sex cells and transport them to locations where their union can occur. The sex cells, called **gametes**, are produced by specialized organs called gonads. A series of ducts and glands in both the male and female reproductive system contributes to the production and transport of the gametes. ≪

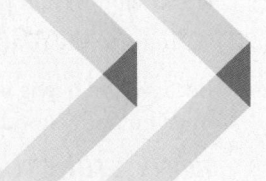

Concept Learning Outcomes

After reading about this concept, you will be able to.

1. Summarize the structure and physiology of the reproductive system related to childbearing.
2. Examine the relationship between reproduction and other concepts/systems.
3. Identify commonly occurring alterations in reproduction and their related therapies.
4. Differentiate common physical assessment procedures used to examine reproductive health across the life span.
5. Describe diagnostic and laboratory tests used to determine the individual's reproductive status.
6. Explain management of reproductive health and prevention of reproductive illness.
7. Demonstrate the nursing process in providing culturally competent and caring interventions across the life span for pregnant individuals and their families.
8. Compare and contrast common independent and collaborative interventions for clients with alterations in reproduction.

Concept Key Terms

Acrosomal reaction, *2021*
Amnion, *2023*
Amniotic fluid, *2023*
Aortocaval compression, *2031*
Ballottement, *2035*
Blastocyst, *2021*
Braxton Hicks contractions, *2025*
Capacitation, *2021*
Chadwick sign, *2030*
Chloasma, *2032*
Chorion, *2022*
Conjugate vera, *2014*
Corpus luteum, *2018*
Cotyledons, *2025*
Diagonal conjugate, *2013*
Diastasis recti, *2032*
Ductus arteriosus, *2028*
Ductus venosus, *2028*

Embryo, *2028*
Embryonic membranes, *2022*
False pelvis, *2013*
Female reproductive cycle, *2016*
Fertilization, *2020*
Fetus, *2028*
Foramen ovale, *2028*
Gametes, *2011*
Gametogenesis, *2020*
Gestational diabetes mellitus (GDM), *2045*
Goodell sign, *2030*
Graafian follicle, *2018*
Hegar sign, *2035*
McDonald sign, *2035*
Meiosis, *2019*
Melasma gravidarum, *2032*

(continued on next page)

Mitosis, *2019*
Morning sickness, *2035*
Morula, *2021*
Obstetric conjugate, *2013*
Oogenesis, *2020*
Ovulation, *2018*
Pelvic inlet, *2013*

Pelvic outlet, *2014*
Physiological anemia of
    pregnancy, *2031*
Placenta, *2023*
Postconception age, *2028*
Prenatal education, *2055*
Quickening, *2035*

Risk factors, *2052*
Spermatogenesis, *2020*
Striae, *2030*
Supine hypotensive
    syndrome, *2031*
Transverse diameter,
    2014

Trophoblast, *2021*
True pelvis, *2013*
Umbilical cord, *2023*
Vena caval syndrome,
    2031
Wharton jelly, *2023*
Zygote, *2020*

See also Box 33–1 on page *2051* for additional key terms.

▶ NORMAL PRESENTATION OF THE FEMALE REPRODUCTIVE SYSTEM

The female reproductive system is described in detail in the module on Sexuality. Two key components of the female reproductive system are discussed here in relation to their importance in conception and childbearing: the bony pelvis and the female reproductive cycle.

Bony Pelvis

The female bony pelvis has two unique functions:

- To support and protect the pelvic contents
- To form the relatively fixed axis of the birth passage.

Because the pelvis is so important to childbearing, its structure must be understood clearly.

BONY STRUCTURE   The pelvis is made up of four bones: two innominate bones, the sacrum, and the coccyx. The pelvis resembles a bowl or basin; its sides are the innominate bones, and its back is the sacrum and coccyx. Lined with fibrocartilage and held tightly together by ligaments, the four bones join at the symphysis pubis, the two sacroiliac joints, and the sacrococcygeal joints (**Figure 33–1 ●**).

The innominate bones, also known as the hip bones, are made up of three separate bones: the ilium, ischium, and pubis. These bones fuse to form a circular cavity, the acetabulum, which articulates with the femur.

The ilium is the broad, upper prominence of the hip. The iliac crest is the margin of the ilium. The ischial spines, the foremost projections nearest the groin, are the site of attachment for ligaments and muscles.

The ischium, the strongest bone, is under the ilium and below the acetabulum. The L-shaped ischium ends in a marked protuberance, the ischial tuberosity, on which the weight of a seated body rests. The ischial spines arise near the junction of the ilium and ischium and jut into the pelvic cavity. The shortest diameter of the pelvic cavity is between the ischial spines. The ischial spines serve as reference points during labor to evaluate the descent of the fetal head into the birth canal.

The pubis forms the slightly bowed front portion of the innominate bone. Extending medially from the acetabulum to the midpoint of the bony pelvis, each pubis meets the other to form a joint called the symphysis pubis. The triangular space

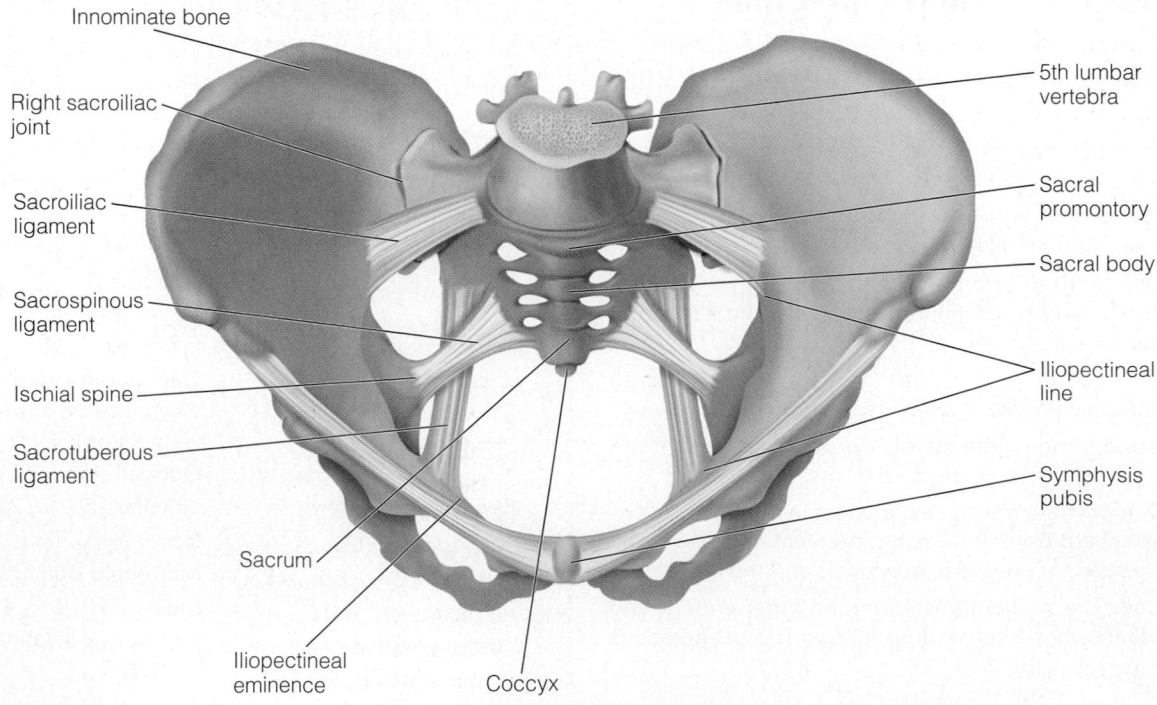

Labels: Innominate bone; Right sacroiliac joint; Sacroiliac ligament; Sacrospinous ligament; Ischial spine; Sacrotuberous ligament; Sacrum; Iliopectineal eminence; Coccyx; 5th lumbar vertebra; Sacral promontory; Sacral body; Iliopectineal line; Symphysis pubis

Figure 33–1 ● Pelvic bones with supporting ligaments.

Anterior

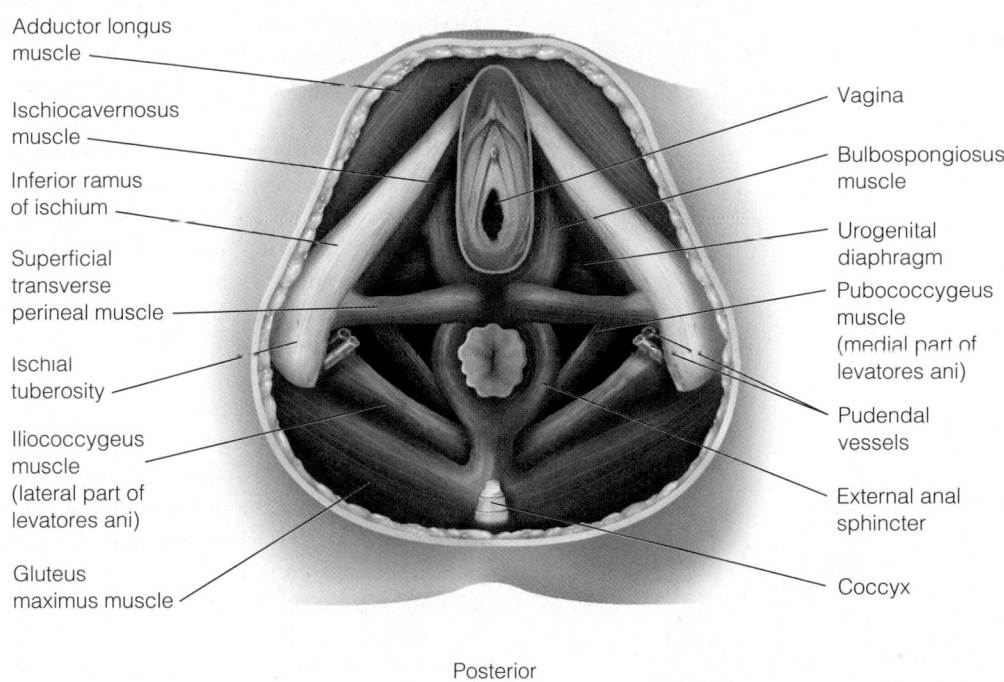

Adductor longus
muscle

Ischiocavernosus
muscle

Inferior ramus
of ischium

Superficial
transverse
perineal muscle

Ischial
tuberosity

Iliococcygeus
muscle
(lateral part of
levatores ani)

Gluteus
maximus muscle

Vagina

Bulbospongiosus
muscle

Urogenital
diaphragm

Pubococcygeus
muscle
(medial part of
levatores ani)

Pudendal
vessels

External anal
sphincter

Coccyx

Posterior

Figure 33–2 ● Muscles of the pelvic floor. (The puborectalis, pubovaginalis, and coccygeal muscles cannot be seen from this view.)

below this junction is known as the pubic arch. The fetal head passes under this arch during birth. The symphysis pubis is formed by heavy fibrocartilage and the superior and inferior pubic ligaments. The mobility of the inferior ligament increases during a first pregnancy and to a greater extent in subsequent pregnancies.

The sacroiliac joints also have a degree of mobility that increases near the end of pregnancy as the result of an upward gliding movement. The pelvic outlet may be increased by 1.5–2 cm in the squatting and sitting positions. These relaxations of the joints are induced by relaxin, one of the hormones of pregnancy.

The sacrum is a wedge-shaped bone formed by the fusion of five vertebrae. On the anterior upper portion of the sacrum is a projection into the pelvic cavity known as the sacral promontory. This projection is an obstetric guide in determining pelvic measurements.

The small triangular bone last on the vertebral column is the coccyx. It articulates with the sacrum at the sacrococcygeal joint. The coccyx usually moves backward during labor to provide more room for the fetus.

PELVIC FLOOR   The muscular pelvic floor of the bony pelvis is designed to overcome the force of gravity exerted on the pelvic organs. It acts as a supporting structure to the irregularly shaped pelvic outlet, providing stability and support for surrounding structures.

Deep fascia, the levator ani, and coccygeal muscles form the part of the pelvic floor known as the pelvic diaphragm. The components of the pelvic diaphragm function as a whole, yet they are able to move over one another. This feature provides an exceptional capacity for dilation during birth and return to pre-pregnancy condition following birth. Above the pelvic dia-

phragm is the pelvic cavity; below and behind it is the perineum. The sacrum is located posteriorly.

The levator ani muscle makes up the major portion of the pelvic diaphragm and consists of four muscles: the iliococcygeus, pubococcygeus, puborectalis, and pubovaginalis. The iliococcygeal muscle, a thin muscular sheet underlying the sacrospinous ligament, helps the levator ani support the pelvic organs. Muscles of the pelvic floor are shown in **Figure 33–2 ●**.

PELVIC DIVISION   The pelvic cavity is divided into the false pelvis and the true pelvis (**Figure 33–3A ●**). The false pelvis, the portion above the pelvic brim, or linea terminalis, supports the weight of the enlarged pregnant uterus and directs the presenting fetal part into the true pelvis below.

The **true pelvis** is the portion that lies below the linea terminalis (pelvic brim). The bony circumference of the true pelvis is made up of the sacrum, coccyx, and innominate bones and represents the bony limits of the birth canal. The relationship between the true pelvic cavity and the fetal head is of paramount importance: The size and shape of the true pelvis must be adequate for normal fetal passage during labor and at birth. The true pelvis consists of three parts: the inlet, the pelvic cavity, and the outlet (Figure 33–3B). Each part has distinct measurements that aid in evaluating the adequacy of the pelvis for childbirth.

The **pelvic inlet** is the upper border of the true pelvis and is typically rounded. Its size and shape are determined by assessing three anteroposterior diameters. The **diagonal conjugate** extends from the subpubic angle to the middle of the sacral promontory and is typically 12.5 to 13 cm in diameter. The diagonal conjugate can be measured manually during a pelvic examination. The **obstetric conjugate** extends from the middle of the sacral promontory to an area approximately 1 cm

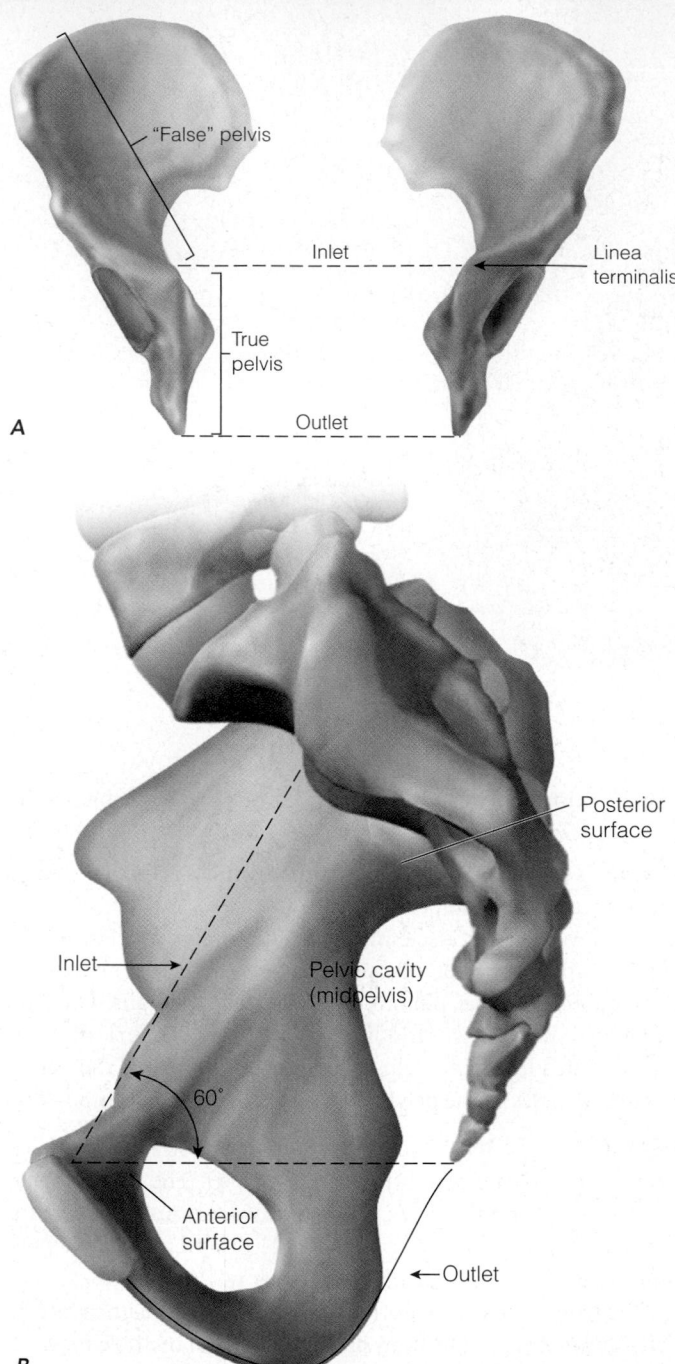

A

B

Figure 33–3 ● Female pelvis. *A*, False pelvis is a shallow cavity above the inlet; true pelvis is the deeper portion of the cavity below the inlet. *B*, True pelvis consists of inlet, cavity (midpelvis), and outlet.

below the pubic crest. Its length is estimated by subtracting 1.5 to 2 cm from the diagonal conjugate (**Figure 33–4 ●**). The fetus passes through the obstetric conjugate, whose diameter determines whether the fetus can move down into the birth canal for engagement to occur. The true (anatomic) conjugate, or **conjugate vera**, extends from the middle of the sacral promontory to the middle of the pubic crest (superior surface of the symphysis). One additional measurement, the transverse diameter, helps determine the shape of the inlet. The **transverse diameter** is the largest diameter of the inlet and is measured by using the linea terminalis as the point of reference.

The midpelvis or pelvic cavity (canal) is a curved canal with a longer posterior than anterior wall. A change in the lumbar curve can increase or decrease the tilt of the pelvis and influence the progress of labor because the fetus has to adjust itself to this curved path as well as to the different diameters of the true pelvis (see Figure 33–3*B*).

The **pelvic outlet** is at the lower border of the true pelvis. The size of the pelvic outlet can be determined by assessing the transverse diameter. The anteroposterior diameter of the pelvic outlet increases during birth as the presenting part pushes the coccyx posteriorly at the mobile sacrococcygeal joint. Decreased mobility, a large fetal head, and/or a forceful birth can cause the coccyx to break. As the fetus' head emerges, the long diameter of the head (occipital frontal) parallels the long diameter of the outlet (anteroposterior).

The transverse diameter (bi-ischial or intertuberous) extends from the inner surface of one ischial tuberosity to the other. It is the shortest diameter of the pelvic outlet and becomes even shorter when the woman has a narrowed pubic arch. The pubic arch is of great importance because the fetus must pass under it during birth. If it is narrow, the baby's head may be pushed backward toward the coccyx, making extension of the head difficult. This situation, known as outlet dystocia, may require the use of forceps or a cesarean birth. The shoulders of a large baby also may become wedged under the pubic arch, making birth more difficult.

PELVIC TYPES The Caldwell–Moloy classification of pelves is widely used to differentiate bony pelvic types (Caldwell & Moloy, 1933). The four basic types are gynecoid, android, anthropoid, and platypelloid (**Figure 33–5 ●**). However, variations in the female pelvis are so great that classic types are not usual. Each type has a characteristic shape, and each shape has implications for labor and birth. The types are described here, along with their implications for labor and birth.

Gynecoid Pelvis The most common female pelvis is the gynecoid type. The inlet is rounded with the anteroposterior diameter a little shorter than the transverse diameter. All of the inlet diameters are at least adequate for a vaginal birth. The posterior segment is broad, deep, and roomy, and the anterior segment is well rounded. The gynecoid midpelvis has nonprominent ischial spines; straight and parallel side walls; and a wide, deep sacral curve. The sacrum is short and slopes backward. All of the midpelvic diameters are at least adequate for a vaginal birth. The gynecoid pelvic outlet has a wide and round pubic arch; the inferior pubic rami are short and concave. The anteroposterior diameter is long; the transverse diameter, adequate. The overall capacity of the outlet is adequate for a vaginal birth. The bones are of medium structure and weight. Approximately 50% of female pelves are classified as gynecoid.

Android Pelvis The normal male pelvis is the android type; this type is occasionally seen in females. The inlet is heart shaped. The anteroposterior and transverse diameters are adequate for a vaginal birth, but the posterior sagittal diameter is too short, and the anterior sagittal diameter is long. The posterior segment is shallow because the sacral promontory is indented, resulting in a reduced capacity. The anterior segment is narrow, and the forepelvis is sharply angled. The android midpelvis has prominent ischial spines; convergent sidewalls; and a long, heavy sacrum inclining forward. All of the midpelvic

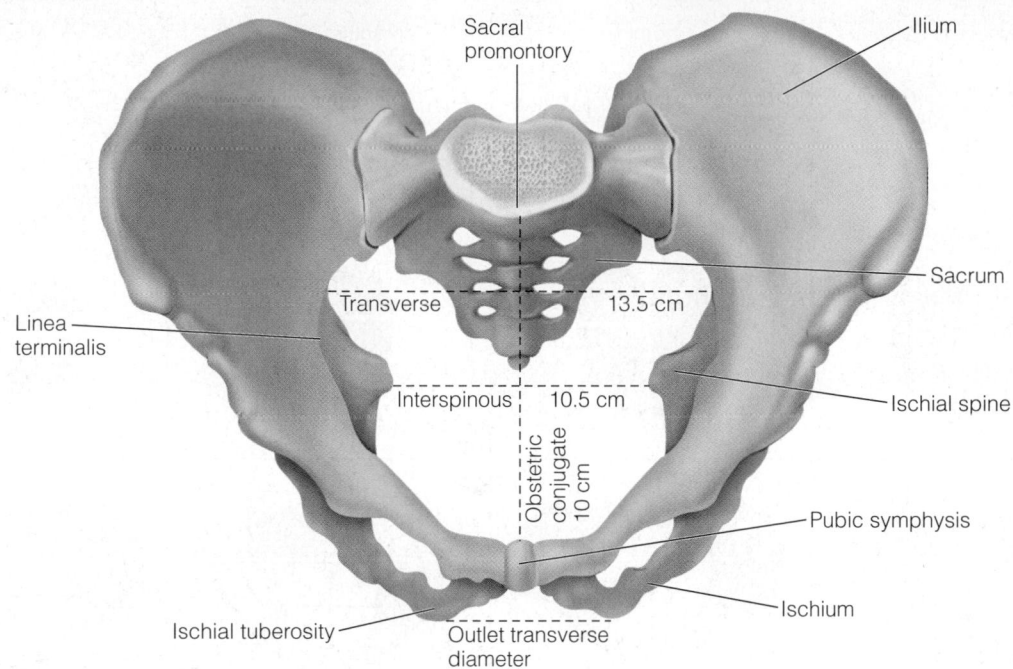

Sacral promontory
Ilium
Transverse
13.5 cm
Sacrum
Linea terminalis
Interspinous   10.5 cm
Ischial spine
Obstetric conjugate 10 cm
Pubic symphysis
Ischium
Ischial tuberosity
Outlet transverse diameter

Figure 33–4 ● Pelvic planes: coronal section and diameters of the bony pelvis.

diameters are reduced. The distance from the linea terminalis to the ischial tuberosities is long, yet the overall capacity of the midpelvis is reduced. The android outlet has a narrow, sharp, and deep pubic arch; the inferior pubic rami are straight and long. The anteroposterior diameter is short, and the transverse diameter is narrow. The capacity of the outlet is reduced. The bones are of medium to heavy structure and weight.

Approximately 20% of female pelves are classified as android. The structure of an android pelvis is not favorable for a vaginal birth. Descent of the fetus into the pelvis is slow. The fetal head usually engages in the transverse or occipital posterior diameter in asynclitism (oblique presentation) with extreme molding. Arrest of labor is frequent, requiring difficult forceps manipulation (rotation and extraction), and the deep, narrow pubic arch may lead to extensive perineal lacerations. Cesarean birth may be required.

Anthropoid Pelvis   The inlet of an anthropoid pelvis is oval, with a long anteroposterior diameter and an adequate but rather short transverse diameter. Both the posterior and anterior segments are deep; the posterior sagittal diameter is extremely long, as is the anterior sagittal diameter. The anthropoid midpelvis has variable ischial spines, straight side walls, and a narrow and long sacrum that inclines backward. The midpelvic diameters are at least adequate, making its capacity adequate for a vaginal birth. The anthropoid outlet has a normal or moderately narrow pubic arch; the interior pubic rami are long and narrow. The outlet capacity is adequate, and the bones are of medium weight and structure. Approximately 25% of female pelves are classified as anthropoid.

Platypelloid Pelvis   The platypelloid type refers to the flat female pelvis. The inlet is a distinctly transverse oval with a short anteroposterior and extremely short transverse diameter. The posterior sagittal and anterior sagittal diameters are short. Both the anterior and posterior segments are shallow. The platypelloid

midpelvis has variable ischial spines, parallel side walls, and a wide sacrum with a deep curve inward. Only the transverse diameter is adequate for a vaginal birth; thus the midpelvic capacity is reduced. The platypelloid outlet has an extremely wide pubic arch; the inferior pubic rami are straight and short. The transverse diameter is wide, but the anteroposterior diameter is short. The outlet capacity may be inadequate for a vaginal birth. The platypelloid bones are similar to those of a gynecoid pelvis. Only 5% of female pelves are classified as platypelloid.

Female Reproductive Cycle

The **female reproductive cycle** is composed of the ovarian cycle, during which ovulation occurs, and the uterine cycle, during which menstruation occurs. These two cycles take place simultaneously (**Figure 33–6 ●**).

EFFECTS OF FEMALE HORMONES   After menarche, a female undergoes a cyclic pattern of ovulation and menstruation, which is disrupted only by pregnancy, for a period of 30–40 years. This cycle is an orderly process under neurohormonal control. Each month multiple oocytes mature, with one rupturing from the ovary and entering the fallopian tube. The ovary, vagina, uterus, and fallopian tubes are major target organs for female hormones.

The ovaries produce mature gametes and secrete hormones (estrogens, progesterone, and testosterone). Estrogens cause the uterus to increase in size and weight due to increased glycogen, amino acids, electrolytes, and water. Blood supply is expanded as well. Under the influence of estrogens, myometrial contractility increases in both the uterus and fallopian tubes. Uterine sensitivity to oxytocin also increases. Estrogens inhibit follicle-stimulating hormone (FSH) production and stimulate luteinizing hormone (LH) production.

Estrogens have effects on many hormones and other carrier proteins. For example, they contribute to the increased amount

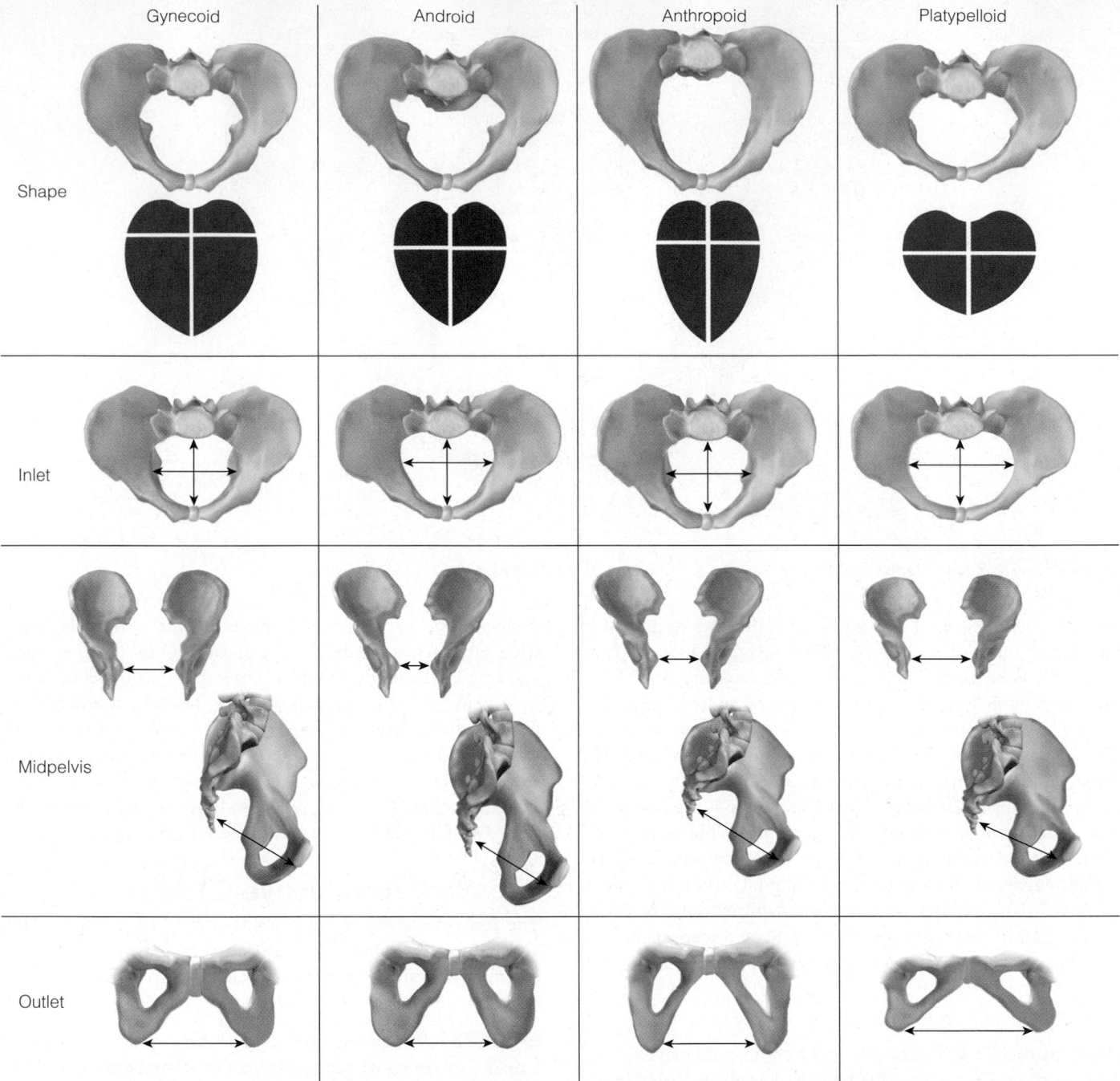

| Gynecoid | Android | Anthropoid | Platypelloid |

Figure 33–5 ● Comparison of Caldwell–Moloy pelvic types.

of protein-bound iodine in pregnant women and in women who use oral contraceptives containing estrogen. Estrogens also may increase libidinal feelings in humans. They decrease the excitability of the hypothalamus, which may cause an increase in sexual desire.

Progesterone   Progesterone is secreted by the corpus luteum and is found in greatest amounts during the secretory (luteal or progestational) phase of the menstrual cycle. Progesterone is often called the *hormone of pregnancy* because its effects on the uterus allow pregnancy to be maintained. Under the influence of progesterone, the vaginal epithelium proliferates and the cervix secretes thick, viscous mucus. Breast glandular tissue increases in size and complexity. Progesterone also prepares the breasts for lactation.

Prostaglandins   Prostaglandins (PGs), which are oxygenated fatty acids, are produced by the cells of the endometrium. They are classified as hormones. Prostaglandins have varied action in the body. The two primary types of PGs are group E and F. Generally, PGE relaxes smooth muscles and is a potent vasodilator; PGF is a potent vasoconstrictor and increases the contractility of muscles and arteries. Although the primary actions of PGE and PGF seem antagonistic, their basic regulatory functions in cells are achieved through an intricate pattern of reciprocal events.

Prostaglandin production increases during follicular maturation, is dependent on gonadotropins, and seems to be critical to follicular rupture (Cunningham et al., 2010). Extrusion of the ovum, resulting from follicular swelling and increased contractility of the smooth muscle in the theca externa layer of the mature follicle, is thought to be caused in part by $PGF_{2\alpha}$.

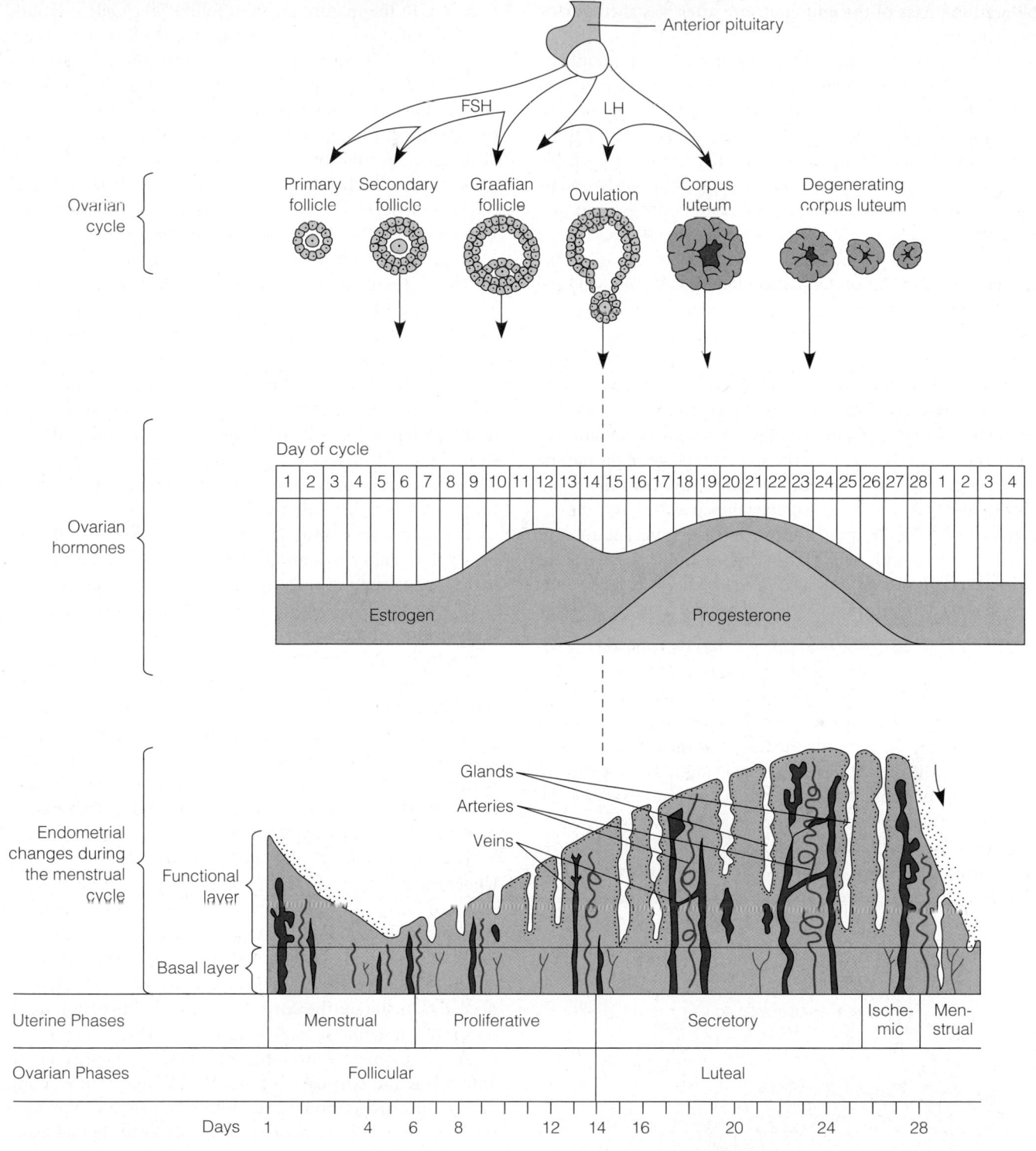

Figure 33–6 ● Female reproductive cycle: interrelationships of hormones with the four phases of the uterine cycle and the two phases of the ovarian cycle in an ideal 28-day cycle.

Significant amounts of PGs are found in and around the folli-cle at the time of ovulation.

NEUROHUMORAL BASIS OF THE FEMALE REPRODUCTIVE CYCLE
The female reproductive cycle is controlled by complex interactions between the nervous and endocrine systems and their target tissues. These interactions involve the hypothalamus, anterior pituitary, and ovaries.

The hypothalamus secretes *gonadotropin-releasing hormone* (GnRH) to the pituitary gland in response to signals received from the central nervous system (CNS). This releasing hormone is often called luteinizing hormone-releasing hormone (LHRH) and follicle-stimulating hormone-releasing hormone (FSHRH) (Blackburn, 2013).

In response to GnRH, the anterior pituitary secretes the gonadotropic hormones FSH and LH. FSH is primarily responsible for the maturation of the ovarian follicle. As the follicle matures, it secretes increasing amounts of estrogen, which enhance the development of the follicle (Cunningham et al., 2010). (This estrogen is also responsible for the re building or proliferation phase of the endometrium after it is shed during menstruation.)

Final maturation of the follicle cannot occur without the action of LH. The anterior pituitary's production of LH increases 6- to 10-fold as the follicle matures. The peak production of LH can precede ovulation by as much as 12 to 24 hours (Cunningham et al., 2010). The LH is also responsible for "luteinizing" the increase in production of progesterone by the granulosa cells of the follicle. As a result, estrogen production is reduced and progesterone secretion continues. Thus, estrogen levels fall a day before ovulation; tiny amounts of progesterone are in evidence. **Ovulation** takes place following the very rapid growth of the follicle, as the sustained high level of estrogen diminishes and progesterone secretion begins.

The ruptured follicle undergoes rapid change, complete luteinization occurs, and the mass of cells becomes the **corpus luteum**. The lutein cells secrete large amounts of progesterone with smaller amounts of estrogen. (Concurrently, the excessive amounts of progesterone are responsible for the secretory phase of the uterine cycle.) On day 7 or 8 following ovulation, the corpus luteum begins to involute. It loses its secretory function, severely diminishing the production of progesterone and estrogen. The anterior pituitary responds with increasingly large amounts of FSH; a few days later LH production begins. As a result, new follicles become responsive to another ovarian cycle and begin maturing.

OVARIAN CYCLE   The ovarian cycle has two phases: the *follicular phase* (days 1–14) and the *luteal phase* (days 15–28 in a 28-day cycle). **Figure 33–7 ●** depicts the changes the follicle undergoes during the ovarian cycle. In women whose menstrual cycles vary, usually only the length of the follicular phase varies because the luteal phase is of fixed length. During the follicular phase, the immature follicle matures as a result of FSH. Within the follicle, the oocyte grows.

A mature **graafian follicle** appears about the 14th day under dual control of FSH and LH. It is a large structure, measuring about 5 to 10 mm, which produces increasing amounts of

estrogen. In the mature graafian follicle, the cells surrounding the fluid-filled antral cavity are called granulosa cells. The mass of granulosa cells surrounding the oocyte and follicular fluid is called the cumulus oophorus. In the fully mature graafian follicle, the zona pellucida, a thick elastic capsule, develops around the oocyte. Just before ovulation, the mature oocyte completes its first meiotic division. As a result of this division, two cells are formed: a small cell, called a *polar body*, and a larger cell, called a secondary oocyte. The secondary oocyte matures into the ovum.

As the graafian follicle matures and enlarges, it comes close to the surface of the ovary. The ovary surface forms a blister-like protrusion 10-15 mm in diameter, and the follicle walls become thin. The secondary oocyte, polar body, and follicular fluid are pushed out. The ovum is discharged near the fimbria of the fallopian tube and pulled into the tube to begin its journey toward the uterus.

In some women, ovulation is accompanied by midcycle pain known as *mittelschmerz*. This pain may be caused by a thick tunica albuginea or by a local peritoneal reaction to the expulsion of the follicular contents. Vaginal discharge may increase during ovulation, and a small amount of blood (midcycle spotting) may be discharged as well.

The body temperature increases about 0.3–0.6°C (0.5–1.0°F) 24–48 hours after ovulation. It remains elevated until the day before menstruation begins. There may be an accompanying sharp drop in basal body temperature before the increase. These temperature changes are useful clinically to determine the approximate time ovulation occurs (Blackburn, 2013).

Generally, the ovum takes several minutes to travel through the ruptured follicle to the fallopian tube opening. The contractions of the tube's smooth muscle and its ciliary action propel the ovum through the tube. The ovum remains in the ampulla, where, if it is fertilized, cleavage can begin. The ovum is thought to be fertile for only 6–24 hours. It reaches the uterus 72–96 hours after its release from the ovary.

The luteal phase begins when the ovum leaves its follicle. Under the influence of LH, the corpus luteum develops from the ruptured follicle. Within 2 or 3 days, the corpus luteum becomes yellowish, spherical and increases in vascularity. If the ovum is fertilized and implants in the endometrium, the fertilized egg begins to secrete *human chorionic gonadotropin* (hCG), which is needed to maintain the corpus luteum. If fertilization does not occur, within about a week after ovulation, the corpus luteum begins to degenerate, eventually becoming a connective tissue scar called the corpus albicans. With degeneration comes a decrease in estrogen and progesterone. This allows for an increase in LH and FSH. These increases then trigger the hypothalamus.

MENSTRUAL CYCLE   *Menstruation* is cyclic uterine bleeding in response to cyclic hormonal changes. Menstruation occurs when the ovum is not fertilized and begins about 14 days after ovulation in an ideal 28-day cycle. The menstrual discharge, also referred to as the menses or menstrual flow, is composed of blood mixed with fluid, cervical and vaginal secretions, bacteria, mucus, leukocytes, and other cellular debris. The menstrual discharge is dark red and has a distinctive odor.

Menstrual parameters vary greatly among individuals. Generally, menstruation occurs every 29 days, but the cycle varies from 21 to 35 days. Some women have longer cycles, which can skew standard calculations of the estimated date of birth (EDB).

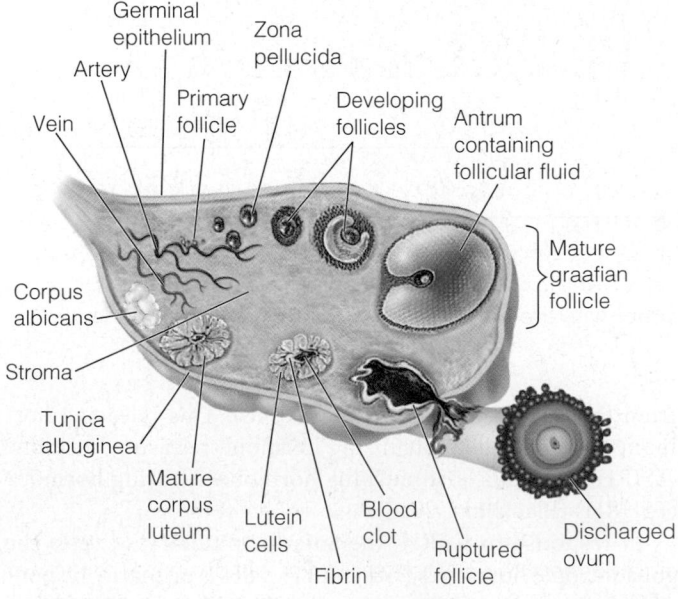

Figure 33–7 ● Various stages of development of the ovarian follicles.

Emotional and physical factors such as illness, excessive fatigue, stress or anxiety, and vigorous exercise programs can alter the cycle interval. Certain environmental factors such as temperature and altitude also may affect the cycle. The duration of menses is from 2 to 8 days, with the blood loss averaging 25–60 mL and the loss of iron averaging 0.5–1 mg daily.

The uterine (menstrual) cycle has four phases: menstrual, proliferative, secretory, and ischemic. Menstruation occurs during the *menstrual phase*. Some endometrial areas are shed, although others remain. Some of the remaining tips of the endometrial glands begin to regenerate. The endometrium is in a resting state following menstruation. Estrogen levels are low, and the endometrium is 1–2 mm deep. During this part of the cycle, the cervical mucosa is scanty, viscous, and opaque.

The *proliferative phase* begins when the endometrial glands enlarge, becoming twisted and longer in response to increasing amounts of estrogen. The blood vessels become prominent and dilated, and the endometrium increases in thickness six- to eightfold. This gradual process reaches its peak just before ovulation. The cervical mucosa becomes thin, clear, watery, and more alkaline, making the mucosa more favorable to spermatozoa. As ovulation nears, the cervical mucosa shows increased elasticity, called *spinnbarkeit*. At ovulation, the mucus will stretch more than 5 cm. The pH of the cervical mucosa increases from below 7.0 to 7.5 at the time of ovulation. On microscopic examination, the mucosa shows a characteristic ferning pattern (**Figure 33–8 ●**). This fern pattern is useful in assessing ovulation time.

The *secretory phase* follows ovulation. The endometrium, under estrogenic influence, undergoes slight cellular growth. Progesterone, however, causes such marked swelling and growth that the epithelium is warped into folds. The amount of tissue glycogen increases. The glandular epithelial cells begin to fill with cellular debris, become twisted, and dilate. The glands secrete small quantities of endometrial fluid in preparation for a fertilized ovum. The vascularity of the entire uterus increases greatly, providing a nourishing bed for implantation. If implantation occurs, the endometrium, under the influence of progesterone, continues to develop and becomes even.

If fertilization does not occur, the *ischemic phase* begins. The corpus luteum begins to degenerate, and as a result, both estrogen and progesterone levels fall. Areas of necrosis appear under the epithelial lining. Extensive vascular changes also occur. Small blood vessels rupture, and the spiral arteries constrict and retract, causing a deficiency of blood in the endometrium, which becomes pale. This ischemic phase is characterized by the escape of blood into the stromal cells of the uterus. The menstrual flow begins, thus beginning the menstrual cycle again. After menstruation, the basal layer remains so that the tips of the glands can regenerate the new functional endometrial layer. (For more about the female reproductive cycle, see the concept on Sexuality.)

▶ CONCEPTION AND FETAL DEVELOPMENT

Each human begins life as a single cell called a fertilized ovum, or zygote. This single cell reproduces itself and, in turn, each resulting cell reproduces itself in a continuing process. The new cells are similar to the cells from which they came. Cells are reproduced by mitosis or meiosis, two different but related processes.

Mitosis results in the production of diploid body (somatic) cells, which are exact copies of the original cell. Mitosis makes growth and development possible, and in mature individuals, it is the process by which the body's cells continue to divide and replace themselves. **Meiosis** is a process of cell division leading to the development of the eggs and sperm needed to produce a new organism. Unlike cells produced during mitosis, the cells produced during meiosis contain only half the genetic material or number of chromosomes (the haploid number).

Mitosis

During mitosis, the cell undergoes several changes, ending in cell division. As the last phase of cell division nears completion, a furrow develops in the cell cytoplasm, which divides it into two daughter cells, each with its own nucleus. Daughter cells have the same diploid number of chromosomes (46) and same genetic makeup as the cell from which they came. After a cell with 46 chromosomes goes through mitosis, the result is two identical cells, each with 46 chromosomes.

Meiosis

Meiosis is a special type of cell division by which diploid cells in the testes and ovaries give rise to gametes (sperm and ova) with the haploid number of chromosomes, which is 23.

Meiosis consists of two successive cell divisions. In the first division, the chromosomes replicate. Next, a pairing takes place between homologous chromosomes (Sadler, 2010). Instead of separating immediately, as in mitosis, the chromosomes become closely intertwined. At each point of contact, a physical exchange of genetic material takes place between the chromatids (the arms of the chromosomes). New combinations are provided by the newly formed chromosomes; these combinations account for the wide variation of traits in people (e.g., hair and eye color). The chromosome pairs then separate, and the members of the pair move to opposite sides of the cell. (In contrast, during mitosis, the chromatids of each chromosome separate and move to opposite poles.) The cell divides, forming two daughter cells, each with 23 double-structured chromosomes; thus it contains the same amount of deoxyribonucleic acid (DNA) as a normal somatic cell. In the second division, the

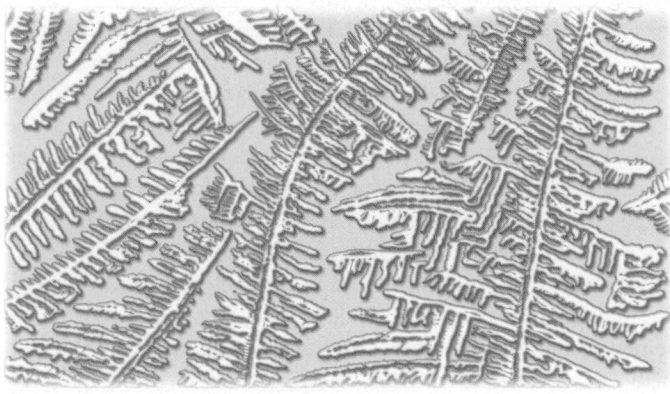

Figure 33–8 ● Ferning pattern.

chromatids of each chromosome separate and move to opposite poles of each of the daughter cells. Cell division occurs, resulting in the formation of four cells, each containing 23 single chromosomes (the haploid number of chromosomes). These daughter cells contain only half the DNA of a normal somatic cell (Sadler, 2010).

Mutations may occur during the second meiotic division if two of the chromatids do not move apart rapidly enough when the cell divides. The still-paired chromatids are carried into one of the daughter cells and eventually form an extra chromosome. This condition, autosomal nondisjunction (chromosomal mutation), is harmful to the offspring that may result should fertilization occur. Another type of chromosomal mutation can occur if chromosomes break during meiosis. If the broken segment is lost, the result is a shorter chromosome—a situation known as deletion. If the broken segment becomes attached to another chromosome, a harmful mutation called a translocation results.

Gametogenesis

Meiosis occurs during **gametogenesis**, the process by which germ cells, or gametes (*ovum* and *sperm*), are produced. These cells contain only half the genetic material of a typical body cell. The gametes must have a haploid number (23) of chromosomes so that when the female gamete (egg or ovum) and the male gamete (sperm or spermatozoon) unite to form the **zygote** (fertilized ovum), the normal human diploid number of chromosomes (46) is reestablished.

OOGENESIS   **Oogenesis** is the process that produces the female gamete, called an ovum (egg). The ovaries begin to develop early in the fetal life of the female. All of the ova that the female will produce in her lifetime are present at birth. The ovary gives rise to oogonial cells, which develop into oocytes. Meiosis begins in all oocytes before the female fetus is born, but stops before the first division is complete and remains in this arrested phase until puberty. During puberty, the mature primary oocyte proceeds (by oogenesis) through the first meiotic division in the graafian follicle of the ovary.

The first meiotic division produces two cells of unequal size with different amounts of cytoplasm but with the same number of chromosomes. These two cells are the secondary oocyte and the first polar body. Both the secondary oocyte and the first polar body contain 22 double-structured autosomal chromosomes and one double-structured sex chromosome (X).

At ovulation, a second meiotic division begins immediately and proceeds as the oocyte moves down the fallopian tube. Division is again not equal, and the secondary oocyte moves into the metaphase stage of cell division, where its meiotic division is arrested until and unless the oocyte is fertilized.

When the secondary oocyte completes the second meiotic division after fertilization, the result is a mature ovum with the haploid number of chromosomes and virtually all of the cytoplasm. In addition, the second polar body (also haploid) forms at this time. The first polar body now has also divided, producing two additional polar bodies. Thus, at the completion of meiosis, four haploid cells have been produced: the three polar bodies, which eventually disintegrate, and one ovum (Sadler, 2010).

SPERMATOGENESIS   During puberty, the germinal epithelium in the seminiferous tubules of the testes begins the process of **spermatogenesis**, which produces the male gamete (sperm). The diploid spermatogonium replicates before it enters the first meiotic division, during which it is called the primary spermatocyte. During this first meiotic division, the spermatogonium replicates and forms two haploid cells called secondary spermatocytes, each of which contains 22 double-structured autosomal chromosomes and either a double-structured X sex chromosome or a double-structured Y sex chromosome. During the second meiotic division, they divide to form four spermatids, each with the haploid number of chromosomes. The spermatids undergo a series of changes during which they lose most of their cytoplasm and become sperm (spermatozoa). The nucleus becomes compacted into the head of the sperm, which is covered by a cap called an acrosome that is, in turn, covered by a plasma membrane. A long tail is produced from one of the centrioles.

Fertilization

Fertilization is the process by which a sperm fuses with an ovum to form a new diploid cell, or zygote. The zygote begins life as a single cell with a complete set of genetic material, 23 chromosomes from the mother's ovum and 23 chromosomes from the father's sperm for a total of 46 chromosomes. The following events lead to fertilization.

PREPARATION FOR FERTILIZATION   The mature ovum and spermatozoa have only a brief time to unite. Ova are considered fertile for about 12–24 hours after ovulation. Sperm can survive in the female reproductive tract for 48–72 hours, but are believed to be healthy and highly fertile for only the first 24 hours.

The ovum's cell membrane is surrounded by two layers of tissue. The layer closest to the cell membrane is called the zona pellucida. It is a clear, noncellular layer whose thickness influences the fertilization rate. Surrounding the zona pellucida is a ring of elongated cells, called the corona radiata because they radiate from the ovum like the gaseous corona around the sun. These cells are held together by hyaluronic acid. The ovum has no inherent power of movement. During ovulation, high estrogen levels increase peristalsis in the fallopian tubes, which helps move the ovum through the tube toward the uterus. The high estrogen levels also cause a thinning of the cervical mucus, facilitating movement of the sperm through the cervix, into the uterus, and up the fallopian tube.

The process of fertilization takes place in the ampulla (outer third) of the fallopian tube. In a single ejaculation, the male deposits approximately 200–500 million spermatozoa into the vagina, of which only approximately one thousand sperm actually reach the ampulla (Sadler, 2010). Fructose in the semen, secreted by the seminal vesicles, is the energy source for the sperm. The spermatozoa propel themselves up the female tract by the flagellar movement of their tails. Transit time from the cervix into the fallopian tube can be as short as 5 minutes but usually takes an average of 2–7 hours after ejaculation (Sadler, 2010). Prostaglandins in the semen may increase uterine smooth muscle contractions, which help transport the sperm. The fallopian tubes have a dual ciliary action that facilitates movement of the ovum toward the uterus and movement of the sperm from the uterus toward the ovary.

The sperm must undergo two processes before fertilization can occur: capacitation and the acrosomal reaction. **Capacitation** is the removal of the plasma membrane overlying the spermatozoa's acrosomal area and the loss of seminal plasma proteins. If the glycoprotein coat is not removed, the sperm will not be able to fertilize the ovum (Sadler, 2010). Capacitation occurs in the female reproductive tract (aided by uterine enzymes) and is thought to take about 7 hours. Sperm that undergo capacitation take on three characteristics: (1) the ability to undergo the acrosomal reaction, (2) the ability to bind to the zona pellucida, and (3) the acquisition of hypermotility.

The **acrosomal reaction** follows capacitation, whereby the acrosomes of the sperm surrounding the ovum release their enzymes (hyaluronidase, a protease called acrosin, and trypsinlike substances) and thus break down the hyaluronic acid in the ovum's corona radiata (Sadler, 2010). Approximately a thousand acrosomes must rupture before enough hyaluronic acid is cleared for a single sperm to penetrate the ovum's zona pellucida successfully.

At the moment of penetration by a fertilizing sperm, the zona pellucida undergoes a reaction that prevents additional sperm from entering a single ovum. This is known as the block to polyspermy. This cellular change is mediated by release of materials from the cortical granules, organelles found just below the ovum's surface, and is called the cortical reaction.

THE MOMENT OF FERTILIZATION   After the sperm enters the ovum, a chemical signal prompts the secondary oocyte to complete the second meiotic division, forming the nucleus of the ovum and ejecting the second polar body. Then the nuclei of the ovum and sperm swell and approach each other. The true moment of fertilization occurs as the nuclei unite. Their individual nuclear membranes disappear, and their chromosomes pair up to produce the diploid zygote. Because each nucleus contains a haploid number of chromosomes (23), this union restores the diploid number (46). The zygote contains a new combination of genetic material that results in an individual different from either parent and from anyone else.

The sex of the zygote is determined at the moment of fertilization. The two chromosomes (the sex chromosomes) of the 23rd pair—either XX or XY—determine the sex of an individual. The X chromosome is larger and bears more genes than the Y chromosome. Females have two X chromosomes, and males have an X and a Y chromosome. Whereas the mature ovum produced by oogenesis can have only one type of sex chromosome—an X—spermatogenesis produces two sperm with an X chromosome and two sperm with a Y chromosome. When each gamete contributes an X chromosome, the resulting zygote is female. When the ovum contributes an X and the sperm contributes a Y chromosome, the resulting zygote is male. Certain traits are termed *sex-linked* because they are controlled by the genes on the X sex chromosome. Two examples of sex-linked traits are color blindness and hemophilia.

Preembryonic Development

The first 14 days of development, starting the day the ovum is fertilized (conception), make up the preembryonic stage, or the stage of the ovum. Development after fertilization can be divided into two phases: cellular multiplication and cellular differentiation. These phases are characterized by rapid cellular multiplication and differentiation and establishment of the primary germ layers and embryonic membranes. Synchronized development of the endometrium and the embryo is a prerequisite for implantation to succeed (Moore & Persaud, 2008). These phases and the process of implantation (nidation), which occurs between them, are discussed next.

CELLULAR MULTIPLICATION   Cellular multiplication begins as the zygote moves through the fallopian tube toward the cavity of the uterus. This transport takes 3 days or more and is accomplished mainly by a weak fluid current in the fallopian tube resulting from the beating action of the ciliated epithelium that lines the tube.

The zygote now enters a period of rapid mitotic divisions called cleavage, during which it divides into two cells, four cells, eight cells, and so on. These cells, called blastomeres, are so small that the developing cell mass is only slightly larger than the original zygote. The blastomeres are held together by the zona pellucida, which is under the corona radiata. The blastomeres eventually form a solid ball of 12–32 cells called the **morula**.

As the morula enters the uterus, two things happen: The intracellular fluid in the morula increases, and a central cavity forms within the cell mass. Inside this cavity is an inner solid mass of cells called the **blastocyst**. The outer layer of cells that surrounds the cavity and replaces the zona pellucida is the **trophoblast**. Eventually, the trophoblast develops into one of the two embryonic membranes, the *chorion*. The blastocyst develops into a double layer of cells called the embryonic disc, from which the *embryo* and the *amnion* (embryonic membrane) develop. The journey of the fertilized ovum to its destination in the uterus is illustrated in **Figure 33–9 ●**.

Early pregnancy factor (EPF), an immunosuppressant protein, is secreted by the trophoblastic cells. This factor appears in the maternal serum within 24–48 hours after fertilization and forms the basis of a pregnancy test during the first 10 days of development (Moore & Persaud, 2008).

IMPLANTATION (NIDATION)   While floating in the uterine cavity, the blastocyst is nourished by the uterine glands, which secrete a mixture of lipids, mucopolysaccharides, and glycogen. The trophoblast attaches to the surface of the endometrium for further nourishment. The most frequent site of attachment is the upper part of the posterior uterine wall. Between 7 and 10 days after fertilization, the zona pellucida disappears and the blastocyst implants itself by burrowing into the uterine lining and penetrating down toward the maternal capillaries until it is completely covered (Moore & Persaud, 2008). The lining of the uterus thickens below the implanted blastocyst, and the cells of the trophoblast grow down into the thickened lining, forming processes that will be called chorionic villi.

Under the influence of progesterone, the endometrium increases in thickness and vascularity in preparation for implantation and nutrition of the ovum. After implantation, the endometrium is called the decidua. The portion of the decidua that covers the blastocyst is called the decidua capsularis, the portion directly under the implanted blastocyst is the decidua basalis, and the portion that lines the rest of the uterine cavity is the decidua vera (parietalis). The maternal part of the placenta develops from the decidua basalis, which contains large numbers of blood vessels (magnified inset in Figure 33–9)

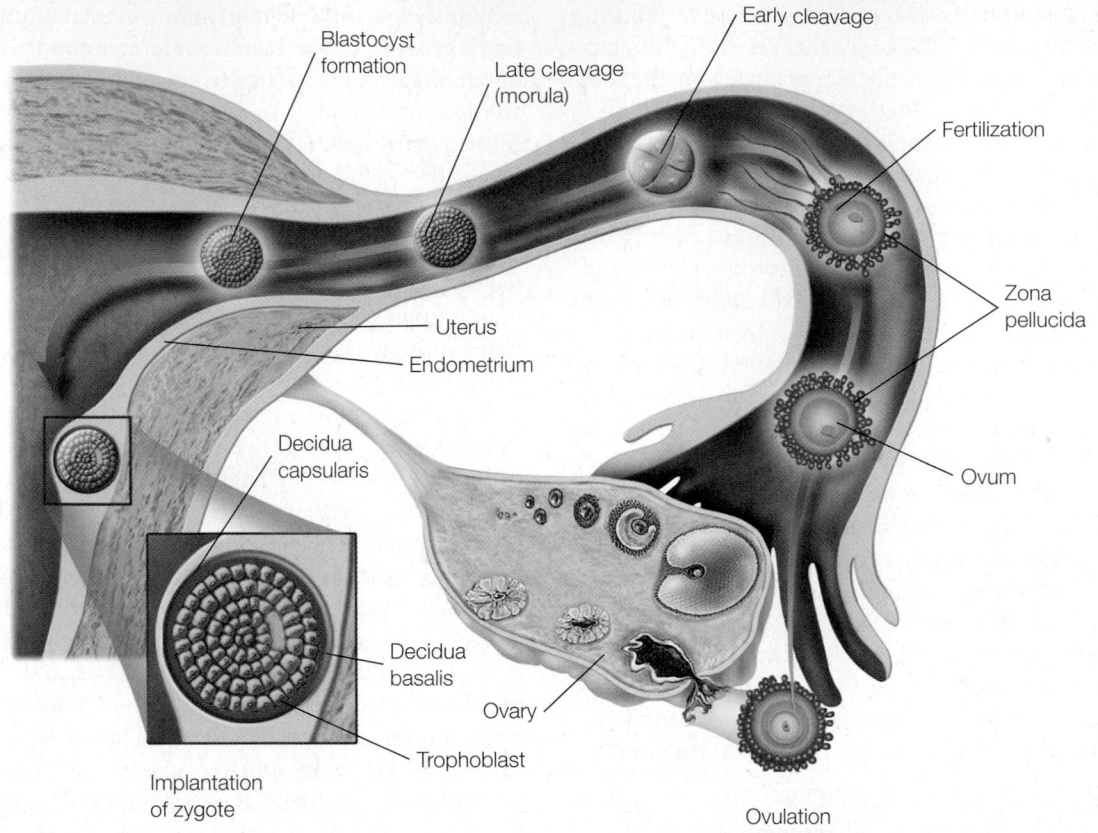

Figure 33–9 ● During ovulation, the ovum leaves the ovary and enters the fallopian tube. Fertilization generally occurs in the outer third of the fallopian tube. The figure depicts subsequent changes in the fertilized ovum from conception to implantation.

(Moore & Persaud, 2008). The chorionic villi (discussed shortly) in contact with the decidua basalis will form the fetal portion of the placenta.

CELLULAR DIFFERENTIATION

Primary Germ Layers About the 10th to 14th day after conception, the homogeneous mass of blastocyst cells differentiates into the primary germ layers. These three layers—the ectoderm, mesoderm, and endoderm—are formed at the same time as the embryonic membranes. All tissues, organs, and organ systems will develop from these primary germ cell layers.

Embryonic Membranes The **embryonic membranes** begin to form at the time of implantation (**Figure 33–10** ●). These membranes protect and support the embryo as it grows and develops inside the uterus. The first and outermost membrane to form is the **chorion**. This thick membrane develops from the trophoblast and has many fingerlike projections called chorionic villi on its surface. These chorionic villi can be used for early genetic testing of the embryo at 10–11 weeks' gestation by chorionic villi sampling (CVS). As the pregnancy progresses, the chorionic villi begin to degenerate, except for those just under the embryo, which grow and branch into depressions in the uterine wall, forming the fetal portion of the placenta. By the fourth month of pregnancy, the surface of the chorion is smooth except at the place of attachment to the uterine wall.

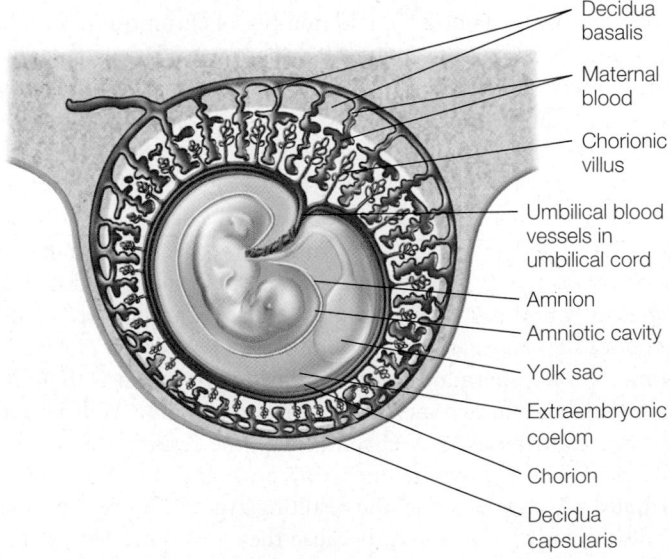

Figure 33–10 ● Early development of primary embryonic membranes. At 4½ weeks, the decidua capsularis (placental portion enclosing the embryo on the uterine surface) and decidua basalis (placental portion encompassing the elaborate chorionic villi and maternal endometrium) are well formed. The chorionic villi lie in blood-filled intervillous spaces within the endometrium. The amnion and yolk sac are well developed.

The second membrane to form, the amnion, originates from the ectoderm, a primary germ layer, during the early stages of embryonic development. The **amnion** is a thin protective membrane that contains amniotic fluid. The space between the membrane and the embryo is the amniotic cavity. This cavity surrounds the embryo and yolk sac, except where the developing embryo (germ-layer disc) attaches to the trophoblast via the umbilical cord. As the embryo grows, the amnion expands until it comes in contact with the chorion. These two slightly adherent membranes form the fluid-filled amniotic sac, which protects the floating embryo.

AMNIOTIC FLUID   The primary functions of **amniotic fluid** arc to:

- Act as a cushion to protect the embryo against mechanical injury.
- Help control the embryo's temperature (the embryo relies on the mother to release heat).
- Permit symmetrical external growth and development of the embryo.
- Prevent adherence of the embryo–fetus to the amnion (decreases chance of amniotic band syndrome) to allow freedom of movement so that the embryo–fetus can change position (flexion and extension), thus aiding in musculoskeletal development.
- Allow the umbilical cord to be relatively free of compression.
- Act as an extension of fetal extracellular space (hydropic infants have increased amniotic fluid).
- Act as a wedge during labor.
- Provide fluid for analysis to determine fetal health and maturity.

Amniotic fluid is slightly alkaline and contains albumin, urea, uric acid, creatinine, lecithin, sphingomyelin, bilirubin, fat, fructose, leukocytes, proteins, epithelial cells, enzymes, and fine hair called lanugo. The amount of amniotic fluid at 10 weeks is about 30 mL, and it increases to 350 mL at 20 weeks. After 28 weeks, the volume ranges from 700 to 1,000 mL. As the pregnancy continues, the fetus contributes to the volume of amniotic fluid by excreting urine. The fetus also swallows up to 262 mL/kg/day. About 400 mL of lung fluid flows out of the fetal lungs each day (Gilbert, 2007). Between 29-30 weeks, the amniotic fluid volume changes very little. After 39 weeks the amniotic fluid begins to dramatically decrease. Abnormal variations are oligohydramnios (less than 500 mL of amniotic fluid) and hydramnios (more than 2,000 mL or an amniotic fluid index greater than the 97.5 percentile for the corresponding gestational age). Hydramnios is also called *polyhydramnios.*

YOLK SAC   In humans, the yolk sac is small and it only functions in early embryonic life. It develops as a second cavity in the blastocyst on about day 8 or 9 after conception. It forms primitive red blood cells (RBCs) during the first 6 weeks of development, until the embryo's liver takes over the process. As the embryo develops, the yolk sac is incorporated into the umbilical cord, where it can be seen as a degenerated structure after birth.

UMBILICAL CORD   As the placenta develops, the **umbilical cord** is being formed from the mesoderm and is covered by the amnion. The body stalk, which attaches the embryo to the yolk sac, contains blood vessels that extend into the chorionic villi. The body stalk fuses with the embryonic portion of the placenta to provide a circulatory pathway from the chorionic villi to the embryo. As the body stalk elongates to become the umbilical cord, the vessels in the cord decrease to one large vein and two smaller arteries. About 1% of umbilical cords have only two vessels: an artery and a vein. This condition may be associated with congenital malformations primarily of the renal, gastrointestinal, and cardiovascular systems. A specialized connective tissue known as **Wharton jelly** surrounds the blood vessels in the umbilical cord. This tissue, in addition to the high blood volume pulsating through the vessels, prevents compression of the umbilical cord in utero. The umbilical cord has no sensory or motor innervation, so cutting the cord after birth is not painful. At term (38–42 weeks' gestation), the average cord is 2 cm (0.8 in.) across and about 55 cm (22 in.) long. The cord can attach itself to the placenta at various sites. Central insertion into the placenta is considered normal.

Umbilical cords appear twisted or spiraled, which is most likely caused by fetal movement. A true knot in the umbilical cord rarely occurs; if it does, the cord is longer than usual. More common are so-called false knots, caused by the folding of cord vessels. A nuchal cord is said to exist when the umbilical cord encircles the fetal neck.

Twins

Twins normally occur in approximately 1 in 80 pregnancies, and triplets occur in 1 in 8,000 pregnancies. Twins may be fraternal or identical (**Figure 33–11 ●**).

✳ Go to *nursing.pearsonhighered.com* for a MiniModule on twins.

Development and Functions of the Placenta

The **placenta** is the means of metabolic and nutrient exchange between the embryonic and maternal circulations. Placental development and circulation do not begin until the third week of embryonic development. The placenta develops at the site where the embryo attaches to the uterine wall. Expansion of the placenta continues until about 20 weeks, when it covers approximately one half of the internal surface of the uterus. After 20 weeks' gestation, the placenta becomes thicker but not wider. At 40 weeks' gestation, the placenta is about 15–20 cm (5.9–7.9 in.) in diameter and 2.5–3 cm (1–1.2 in.) in thickness. At that time, it weighs about 400–600 g (14–21 oz).

The placenta has two parts: the maternal and fetal portions. The maternal portion consists of the decidua basalis and its circulation. Its surface is red and fleshlike. The fetal portion consists of the chorionic villi and their circulation. The fetal surface of the placenta is covered by the amnion, which gives it a shiny gray appearance (**Figures 33–12 ●** and **33–13 ●**).

Development of the placenta begins with the chorionic villi. The trophoblastic cells of the chorionic villi form spaces in the tissue of the decidua basalis. These spaces fill with maternal

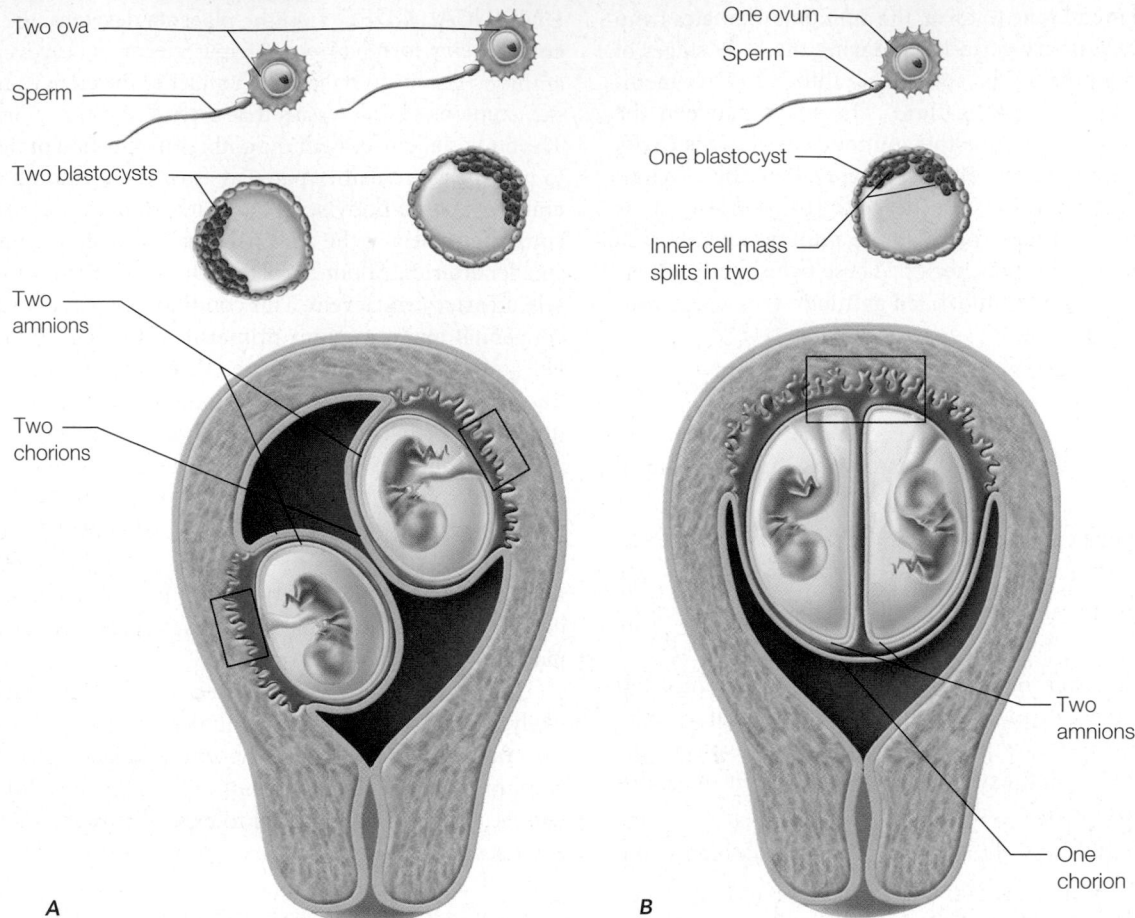

Two ova

Sperm

Two blastocysts

Two amnions

Two chorions

One ovum

Sperm

One blastocyst

Inner cell mass splits in two

Two amnions

One chorion

A

B

Figure 33–11 ● *A,* Dizygotic (fraternal) twins. (Note separate placentas.) *B,* Monozygotic (identical) twins.

blood, and the chorionic villi grow into them. As the chorionic villi differentiate, two trophoblastic layers appear: an outer layer, called the syncytium (consisting of syncytiotrophoblasts), and an inner layer, known as the cytotrophoblast. The cytotro-phoblast thins out and disappears around the fifth month, leaving only a single layer of syncytium covering the chorionic villi. The syncytium is in direct contact with the maternal blood in the intervillous spaces. It is the functional layer of the placenta, and it secretes the placental hormones of pregnancy.

A third inner layer of connective mesoderm develops in the chorionic villi, forming anchoring villi. These anchoring villi

Figure 33–12 ● Maternal side of placenta.
Courtesy of Marcia London.

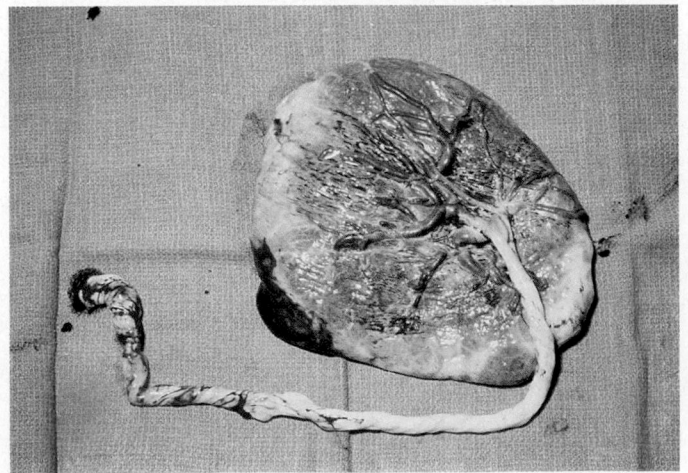

Figure 33–13 ● Fetal side of placenta.
Courtesy of Marcia London.

eventually form the septa (partitions) of the placenta. The septa divide the mature placenta into 15–20 segments called **cotyledons** (subdivisions of the placenta made up of anchoring villi and decidual tissue). In each cotyledon, the branching villi form a highly complex vascular system that allows compartmentalization of the uteroplacental circulation. The exchange of gases and nutrients takes place across these vascular systems.

Exchange of substances across the placenta is minimal during the first 3–5 months of development because the villous membrane is initially too thick, which limits its permeability. As the villous membrane thins, placental permeability increases until about the last month of pregnancy, when permeability begins to decrease as the placenta ages. In the fully developed placenta, fetal blood in the villi and maternal blood in the intervillous spaces are separated by three or four thin layers of tissue.

PLACENTAL CIRCULATION

After implantation of the blastocyst, the cells distinguish themselves into fetal cells and trophoblastic cells. The proliferating trophoblast successfully invades the decidua basalis of the endometrium, first opening the uterine capillaries and later opening the larger uterine vessels. The chorionic villi are an outgrowth of the blastocystic tissue. As these villi continue to grow and divide, the fetal vessels begin to form. The intervillous spaces in the decidua basalis develop as the endometrial spiral arteries are opened.

By the end of the fourth week, the placenta has begun to function as a means of metabolic exchange between embryo and mother. The completion of the maternal–placental–fetal circulation occurs about 17 days after conception, when the embryonic heart begins functioning (Moore & Persaud, 2008). By 14 weeks, the placenta is a discrete organ. It has grown in thickness as a result of growth in the length and size of the chorionic villi and accompanying expansion of the intervillous space.

In the fully developed placenta's umbilical cord, fetal blood flows through the two umbilical arteries to the capillaries of the villi, becomes oxygen enriched, and then flows back through the umbilical vein into the fetus (**Figure 33–14 ●**). Late in pregnancy a soft blowing sound (funic souffle) can be heard over the area of the umbilical cord. The sound is synchronous with the fetal heartbeat and fetal blood flow through the umbilical arteries.

Maternal blood, rich in oxygen and nutrients, moves from the arcuate artery to the radial artery to the uterine spiral arteries and then spurts into the intervillous spaces. These spurts are produced by the maternal blood pressure. The spurt of blood is directed toward the chorionic plate, and as the blood loses pressure, it becomes lateral (spreads out). Fresh blood enters continuously and exerts pressure on the contents of the intervillous spaces, pushing blood toward the exits in the basal plate. The blood then drains through the uterine and other pelvic veins. A uterine souffle, timed precisely with the mother's pulse, also is heard just above the mother's symphysis pubis during the last months of pregnancy. This souffle is caused by the augmented blood flow entering the dilated uterine arteries.

Braxton Hicks contractions are intermittent painless uterine contractions that may occur every 10–20 minutes; they occur more frequently near the end of pregnancy. These contractions are believed to facilitate placental circulation by enhancing the movement of blood from the center of the cotyledon through the intervillous space. Placental blood flow is enhanced when the woman is lying on her left side because venous return from the lower extremities is not compromised (Blackburn, 2013).

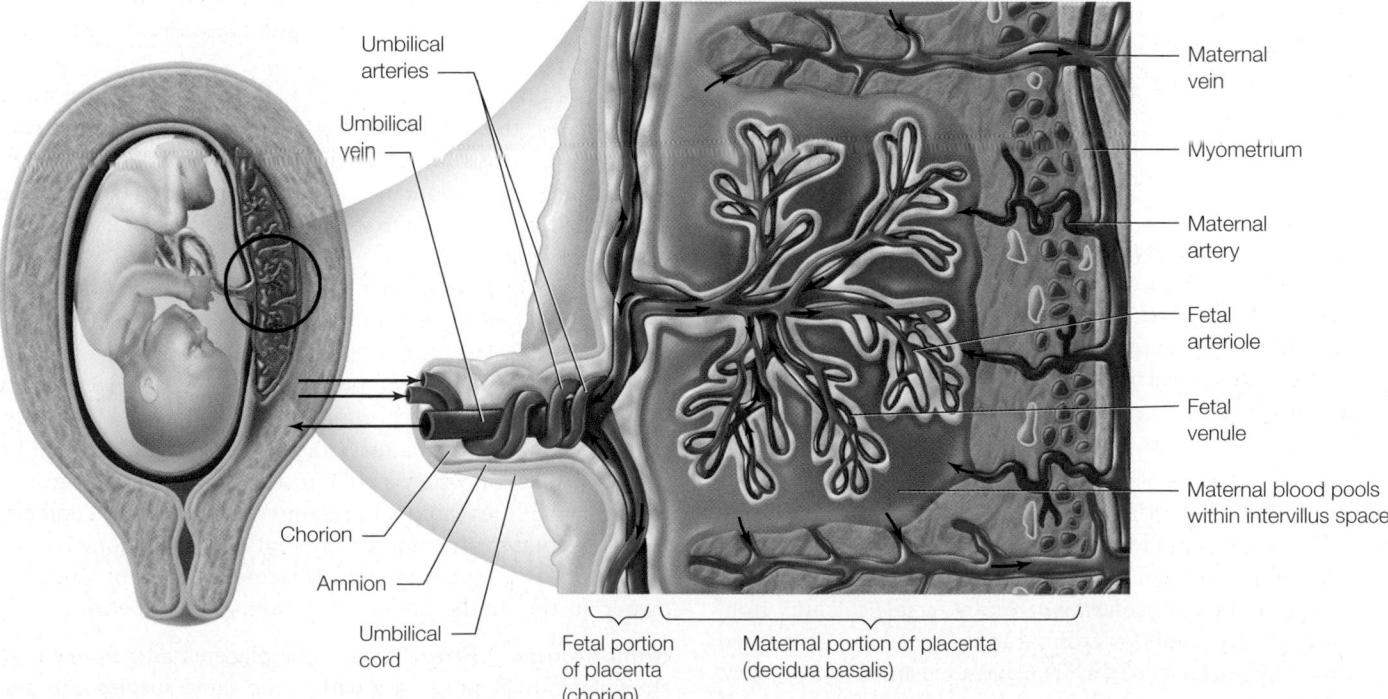

Figure 33–14 ● Vascular arrangement of the placenta. Arrows indicate the direction of blood flow. Maternal blood flows through the uterine arteries to the intervillous spaces of the placenta and returns through the uterine veins to maternal circulation. Fetal blood flows through the umbilical arteries into the villous capillaries of the placenta and returns through the umbilical vein to the fetal circulation.

PLACENTAL FUNCTIONS   Placental exchange functions occur only in those fetal vessels that are in intimate contact with the covering syncytial membrane. The syncytium villi have brush borders containing many microvilli, which greatly increase the exchange rate between maternal and fetal circulation (Sadler, 2010).

The placental functions, many of which begin soon after implantation, include fetal respiration, nutrition, and excretion. To carry out these functions, the placenta is involved in metabolic and transfer activities. In addition, it has endocrine functions and special immunological properties. (See the discussion later in this section.)

Metabolic Activities

The placenta continuously produces glycogen, cholesterol, and fatty acids for fetal use and hormone production. The placenta also produces numerous enzymes, such as sulfatase, which enhances excretion of fetal estrogen precursors, and insulinase, which increases the barrier to insulin. These enzymes are required for fetoplacental transfer. The placenta breaks down certain substances such as epinephrine and histamine (Blackburn, 2013). In addition, it stores glycogen and iron.

Transport Function

The placental membranes actively control the transfer of a wide range of substances by a variety of transport mechanisms.

- *Simple diffusion* moves substances from an area of higher concentration to an area of lower concentration. Substances that move across the placenta by simple diffusion include water, oxygen, carbon dioxide, electrolytes (sodium and chloride), anesthetic gases, and drugs. Insulin and steroid hormones originating from the adrenals, as well as thyroid hormones, also cross the placenta. However, this happens at a very slow rate. The rate of oxygen transfer across the placental membrane is greater than that allowed by simple diffusion, indicating that oxygen also is transferred by some type of facilitated diffusion transport. Unfortunately, many substances of abuse, such as cocaine and heroin, cross the placenta via simple diffusion.

- *Facilitated transport* involves a carrier system to move molecules from an area of greater concentration to an area of lower concentration. Molecules such as glucose, galactose, and some oxygen are transported by this method. Ordinarily, the glucose level in the fetal blood is approximately 20%–30% lower than the glucose level in the maternal blood because the fetus is metabolizing glucose rapidly. This, in turn, causes rapid transport of additional glucose from the maternal blood to the fetal blood.

- *Active transport* can work against a concentration gradient and allows molecules to move from areas of lower concentration to areas of higher concentration. Amino acids, calcium, iron, iodine, water-soluble vitamins, and glucose are transferred across the placenta this way. The measured amino acid content of fetal blood is greater than that of maternal blood, and calcium and inorganic phosphate occur in greater concentration in fetal blood than in maternal blood (Blackburn, 2013).

Other modes of transfer also exist. Pinocytosis is important for transferring large molecules such as albumin and gamma globulin. Materials are engulfed by amoeba-like cells, forming plasma droplets. Hydrostatic and osmotic pressures allow the bulk flow of water and some solutes. Also, fetal RBCs can pass into the maternal circulation through breaks in the capillaries and placental membrane, particularly during labor and birth. Certain cells (e.g., maternal leukocytes) and microorganisms such as viruses (e.g., HIV, which causes AIDS) and the bacterium *Treponema pallidum* (which causes syphilis) also can cross the placental membrane under their own power (Moore & Persaud, 2008). Some bacteria and protozoa infect the placenta by causing lesions and then entering the fetal blood system.

Reduction of the placental surface area, as with abruptio placentae (partial or complete premature separation of the placenta), lessens the area that is functional for exchange. Placental diffusion distance also affects exchange. In conditions such as diabetes and placental infection, edema of the villi increases the diffusion distance, thus increasing the distance the substance must be transferred.

Blood flow alteration changes the transfer rate of substances. Decreased blood flow in the intervillous space is seen in labor and with certain maternal diseases such as hypertension. Mild fetal hypoxia increases the umbilical blood flow, but severe hypoxia results in decreased blood flow.

As the maternal blood picks up fetal waste products and carbon dioxide, it drains back into the maternal circulation through the veins in the basal plate. Fetal blood is hypoxic in comparison to maternal blood; therefore, it attracts oxygen from the mother's blood. Affinity for oxygen increases as the fetal blood gives up its carbon dioxide, which also decreases its acidity.

Endocrine Functions

The placenta produces hormones that are vital to the survival of the fetus. These include hCG; human placental lactogen (hPL); and two steroid hormones, estrogen and progesterone.

The hormone hCG is similar to LH and prevents the normal involution of the corpus luteum at the end of the menstrual cycle. If the corpus luteum stops functioning before the 11th week of pregnancy, spontaneous abortion occurs. The hCG also causes the corpus luteum to secrete increased amounts of estrogen and progesterone.

After the 11th week, the placenta produces enough progesterone and estrogen to maintain pregnancy. In the male fetus, hCG also exerts an interstitial cell-stimulating effect on the testes, resulting in the production of testosterone. This small secretion of testosterone during embryonic development is the factor that causes male sex organs to grow. The hormone hCG may play a role in the trophoblast's immunological capabilities (ability to exempt the placenta and embryo from rejection by the mother's system). This hormone is used as a basis for pregnancy tests. (Placental hormones are discussed further in the Endocrine System section below.)

Immunological Properties

The placenta and embryo are transplants of living tissue within the same species and are, therefore, considered *homografts*. Unlike other homografts, the placenta and embryo appear exempt from immunological reaction by the host. Most recent data suggest that the placental hormones (progesterone and hCG) suppress cellular immunity during pregnancy. The chorionic villi may lack major histocompatibility (MHC) antigens and thus do not evoke rejection responses. They do, however, protect against antibody formation. Extravillous trophoblast (EVT) cells, which invade the uterine decidas, have human leukocyte antigen G (HLA-G), which is not readily recognized by sensitized T lymphocytes and natural killer cells (Cunningham et al., 2010).

Development of the Fetal Circulatory System

The circulatory system of the fetus has several unique features that, by maintaining the blood flow to the placenta, provide the

fetus with oxygen and nutrients while removing carbon dioxide and other waste products.

Most of the blood supply bypasses the fetal lungs because they do not carry out respiratory gas exchange. The placenta assumes the function of the fetal lungs by supplying oxygen and allowing the fetus to excrete carbon dioxide into the maternal bloodstream. **Figure 33–15** ● shows the fetal circulatory system. The blood from the placenta flows through the umbilical vein, which enters the abdominal wall of the fetus at the site that, after birth, is the umbilicus (belly button). As umbilical venous blood approaches the liver, a small portion of the blood enters the liver sinusoids, mixes with blood from the portal circulation, and then enters the inferior vena cava

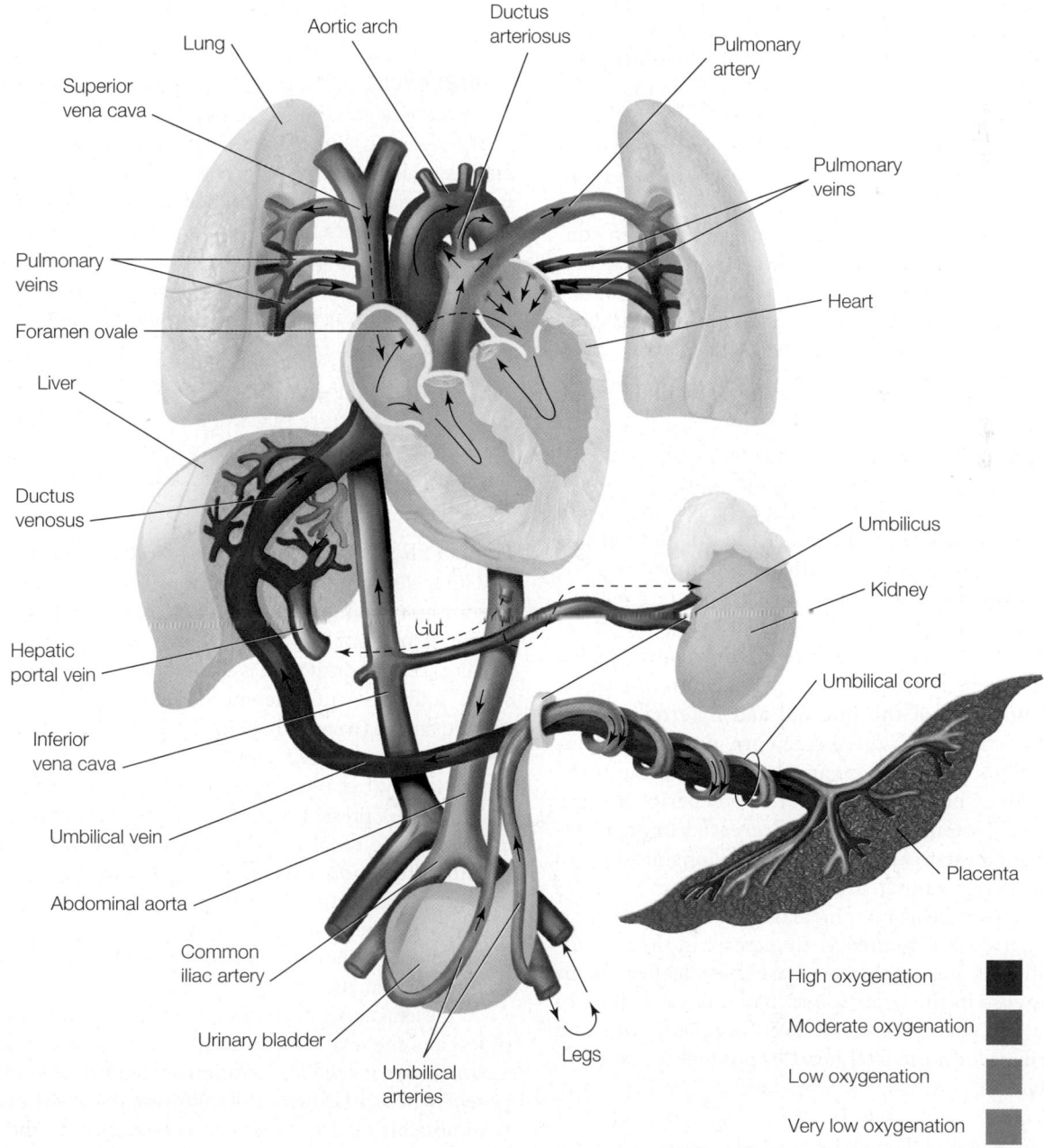

Figure 33–15 ● Fetal circulation. Blood leaves the placenta and enters the fetus through the umbilical vein. After circulating through the fetus, the blood returns to the placenta through the umbilical arteries. The ductus venosus, the foramen ovale, and the ductus arteriosus allow the blood to bypass the fetal liver and lungs.

via hepatic veins. Most of the umbilical vein's blood flows through the **ductus venosus** directly into the inferior vena cava, bypassing the liver. This blood then enters the right atrium; passes through the **foramen ovale** into the left atrium; and pours into the left ventricle, which pumps blood into the aorta. Some blood returning from the head and upper extremities by way of the superior vena cava is emptied into the right atrium and passes through the tricuspid valve into the right ventricle. This blood is pumped into the pulmonary artery, and a small amount passes to the lungs for nourishment only. The larger portion of blood passes from the pulmonary artery through the **ductus arteriosus** into the descending aorta, bypassing the lungs. Finally, blood returns to the placenta through the two umbilical arteries, and the process is repeated.

The fetus obtains oxygen via diffusion from the maternal circulation because of the gradient difference of PO_2 of 50 mmHg in maternal blood in the placenta to 30 mmHg PO_2 in the fetus. At term, the fetus receives oxygen from the mother's circulation at a rate of 20–30 mL/min (Sadler, 2010). Fetal hemoglobin facilitates obtaining oxygen from the maternal circulation because it carries as much as 20%–30% more oxygen than adult hemoglobin.

Fetal circulation delivers the highest available oxygen concentration to the head, neck, brain, and heart (coronary circulation) and a lesser amount of oxygenated blood to the abdominal organs and the lower body. This circulatory pattern leads to cephalocaudal (head-to-tail) development in the fetus.

FETAL HEART   The heart of the fetus, like that of the adult, is controlled by its own pacemaker. The sinoatrial (SA) node sets the rate and is supplied by the vagus nerve. Bridging the atrium and the ventricle is the atrioventricular (AV) node, also supplied by the vagus nerve. Baseline changes in the fetal heartbeat have been shown to be under the influence of this nerve. Atropine will block this effect. When the fetus is stressed, the sympathetic nervous system causes the release of norepinephrine, which increases the fetal heart rate. To counteract the increase in blood pressure, baroreceptors, which respond to the increase in pressure, are present in the vessel walls at the junction of the internal and external carotid arteries. When stimulated, these receptors, under the influence of the vagus and glossopharyngeal nerves, cause the heart rate to slow. Chemoreceptors in the fetal peripheral and central nervous systems respond to decreased oxygen tensions and to increased carbon dioxide tensions, leading to fetal tachycardia and an increase in blood pressure. The CNS also has control over heart rate. Increased activity of the fetus in a wakeful period is exhibited in an *increase* in the beat-to-beat variability of the fetal heart baseline. Sleep patterns involve a *decrease* in the beat-to-beat baseline variability. In cases of severe hypoxia, increased levels of epinephrine and norepinephrine act on the fetal heart to produce a faster and stronger rate.

Embryonic and Fetal Development

Pregnancy is calculated to last an average of 10 lunar months: 40 weeks, or 280 days. This period of 280 days is calculated from the onset of the last normal menstrual period to the time

of birth. Estimated date of birth, sometimes referred to as the estimated date of delivery (EDD), is usually calculated by this method. Most fetuses are born within 10–14 days of the calculated date of birth. The fertilization age (or **postconception age**) of the fetus is calculated to be *about* 2 weeks less, or 266 days (38 weeks), or 9.5 calendar months. The latter measurement is more accurate because it measures time from the fertilization of the ovum, or conception.

✳ Go to **nursing.pearsonhighered.com** for a chart on the basic events of organ development in the embryo and fetus.

In review, human development follows three stages. The preembryonic stage, as discussed earlier in this module, consists of the first 14 days of development after the ovum is fertilized. The embryonic stage covers the period from day 15 until approximately the end of the eighth week, and the fetal stage extends from the end of the eighth week until birth (**Figure 33–16 ●**).

EMBRYONIC STAGE   The stage of the **embryo** starts on day 15 (the beginning of the third week after conception) and continues until approximately the eighth week, or until the embryo reaches a crown-to-rump (C–R) length of 3 cm (1.2 in.). This length is usually reached about 56 days after fertilization (the end of the eighth gestational week). During the embryonic stage, tissues differentiate into essential organs and the main external features develop. The embryo is most vulnerable to *teratogens* during this period (**Figure 33–17 ●**).

FETAL STAGE   By the end of the eighth week, the embryo is sufficiently developed to be called a **fetus**. Every organ system and external structure that will be found in the full-term newborn is present. The remainder of gestation is devoted to refining structures and perfecting function. **Figure 33–18 ●** shows the fetus at 20 weeks' gestation.

FULL TERM   The fetus is considered full term at 38 weeks and up to 40 weeks after conception. The crown-to-heel (C–H) length varies from 48 to 52 cm (19 to 21 in.), with males usually longer than females. Males also usually weigh more than females. The weight at term is about 3,000–3,600 g (6 lb 10 oz–7 lb 15 oz) and varies in different ethnic groups. The skin is flesh colored and has a smooth, polished look. The only lanugo left is on the upper arms and shoulders. The hair on the head is no longer woolly, but is coarse and about 2.5 cm (1 in.) long. Vernix caseosa is present, with heavier deposits remaining in the creases and folds of the skin. The body and extremities are plump, with good skin turgor, and the fingernails extend beyond the fingertips. The chest is prominent but still a little smaller than the head, and mammary glands protrude in both sexes. In males, the testes are in the scrotum or are palpable in the inguinal canals.

As the fetus enlarges, amniotic fluid diminishes to about 500 mL or less and the fetal body mass fills the uterine cavity. The fetus assumes what is called its position of comfort, or lie. The head is generally pointed downward, following the shape of the uterus (and possibly because the head is heavier than the feet). The extremities, and often the head, are well flexed. After 5 months, patterns in feeding, sleeping, and activity become established; so at term, the fetus has its own body rhythms and individual style of response.

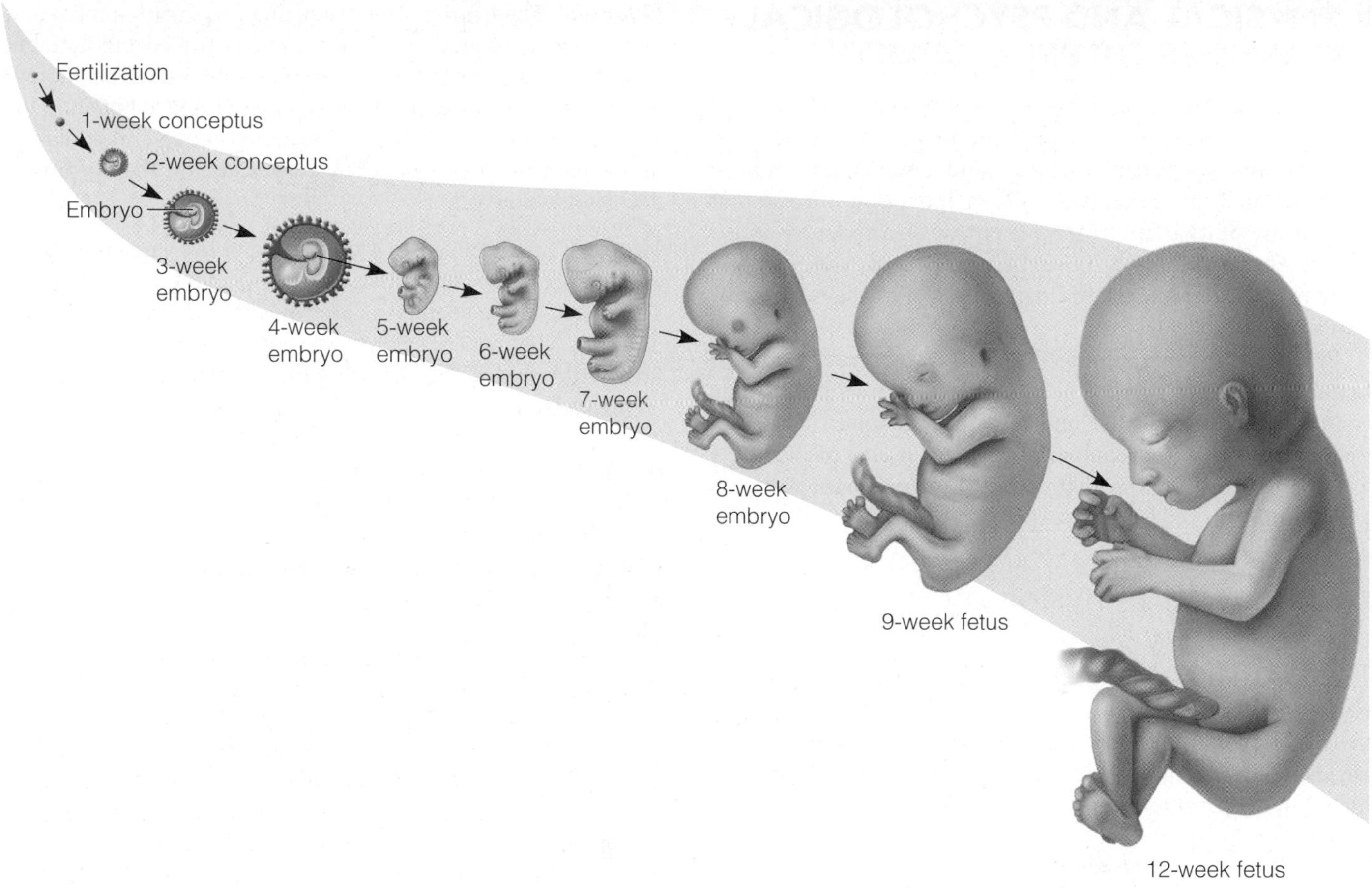

- Fertilization
- 1-week conceptus
  - 2-week conceptus
- Embryo
  - 3-week embryo
  - 4-week embryo
  - 5-week embryo
  - 6-week embryo
  - 7-week embryo
  - 8-week embryo
  - 9-week fetus
  - 12-week fetus

Figure 33–16 ● The actual size of a human conceptus from fertilization to the early fetal stage. The embryonic stage begins in the third week after fertilization; the fetal stage begins in the ninth week.

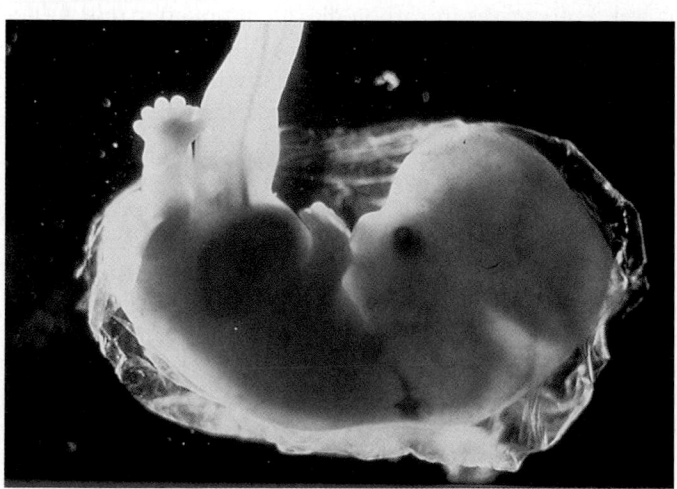

Figure 33–17 ● The embryo at 7 weeks. The head is rounded and nearly erect. The eyes have shifted forward and closer together, and the eyelids begin to form.
Source: Petit Format/Science Source.

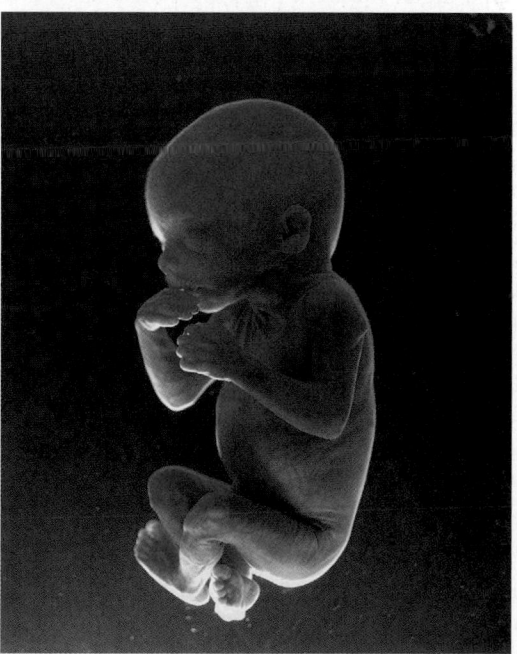

Figure 33–18 ● The fetus at 20 weeks. The fetus now weighs 435–465 g (15.2–16.3 oz) and measures about 19 cm (7.5 in.). Subcutaneous deposits of brown fat make the skin a little less transparent. "Woolly" hair covers the head, and nails have developed on the fingers and toes.
Source: Photo Researchers, Inc./Science Source.

► PHYSICAL AND PSYCHOLOGICAL CHANGES OF PREGNANCY

The growth of the developing fetus and the physical and psychological changes that occur in the pregnant mother continue to inspire feelings of awe and amazement, not to mention curiosity. First, it is nothing short of a miracle that the union of two microscopic entities—an ovum and a sperm—can produce a living being. Second, the woman's body must undergo extraordinary physical changes to maintain a pregnancy.

Pregnancy is divided into three trimesters, each approximately a 3-month period. Each trimester brings predictable changes for both mother and fetus. This section describes these physical and psychological changes. It also presents the various cultural factors that can affect a pregnant woman's well-being.

Anatomy and Physiology of Pregnancy

The changes that occur in the pregnant woman's body may result from hormonal influences, the growth of the fetus, and the mother's physiological adaptation to the pregnancy. Virtually every system must adapt to support the growing fetus and maintain the pregnant woman's body functions.

REPRODUCTIVE SYSTEM Some of the most dramatic changes of pregnancy occur in the reproductive organs.

Uterus The changes in the uterus during pregnancy are amazing. Before pregnancy, the uterus is a small, semisolid, pear-shaped organ measuring approximately 7.5 × 5 × 2.5 cm and weighing about 60 g (2 oz). At the end of pregnancy, it measures about 28 × 24 × 21 cm and weighs approximately 1,100 g (2.5 lb); its capacity also has increased from about 10 mL to 5,000 mL (5 L) or more (Cunningham et al., 2010).

The enlargement of the uterus is primarily caused by the enlargement (hypertrophy) of the preexisting myometrial cells as a result of the stimulating influence of estrogen and the distention caused by the growing fetus. Only a limited increase in cell number (hyperplasia) occurs. The fibrous tissue between the muscle bands increases markedly, which adds to the strength and elasticity of the muscle wall. The enlarging uterus, developing placenta, and growing fetus require additional blood flow to the uterus. By the end of pregnancy, one sixth of the total maternal blood volume is contained in the vascular system of the uterus.

Cervix Estrogen stimulates the glandular tissue of the cervix, which increases in cell number and becomes hyperactive. The endocervical glands secrete a thick, sticky mucus that accumulates and forms a mucous plug, which seals the endocervical canal and prevents the ascent of microorganisms into the uterus. This plug is expelled when cervical dilation begins. The hyperactivity of the glandular tissue also increases the normal physiological mucorrhea, at times resulting in profuse discharge. Increased cervical vascularity also causes both the softening of the cervix (**Goodell sign**) and its blue-purple discoloration (**Chadwick sign**).

Ovaries The ovaries stop producing ova during pregnancy. During early pregnancy hCG maintains the corpus luteum, which persists and produces hormones until 6-8 weeks of pregnancy. The corpus luteum secretes progesterone to maintain the endometrium until the placenta produces enough progesterone to maintain the pregnancy. The corpus luteum then begins to disintegrate slowly.

Vagina Estrogen causes a thickening of the vaginal mucosa, a loosening of the connective tissue, and an increase in vaginal secretions. These secretions are thick, white, and acidic (pH 3.5–6.0). The acid pH helps prevent bacterial infection but favors the growth of yeast organisms. Thus, the pregnant woman is more susceptible to *Candida* infection than usual.

The supportive connective tissue of the vagina loosens throughout pregnancy. By the end of pregnancy, the vagina and perineal body are sufficiently relaxed to permit passage of the infant. Because blood flow to the vagina is increased, the vagina may show the same blue-purple color (Chadwick sign) as the cervix.

BREASTS Estrogen and progesterone cause many changes in the breasts. They enlarge and become more nodular as the milk producing glands increase in size and number in preparation for lactation. Superficial veins become more prominent, the nipples become more erectile, and the areolas darken. Montgomery's follicles (sebaceous glands) enlarge, and **striae** (reddish stretch marks that slowly turn silver after childbirth) may develop.

Colostrum, an antibody-rich yellow secretion, may leak or be expressed from the breasts during the last trimester. Colostrum gradually converts to mature milk during the first few days after childbirth.

RESPIRATORY SYSTEM Many respiratory changes occur to meet the increased oxygen requirements of a pregnant woman. The volume of air breathed each minute increases 30%–40%. In addition, progesterone decreases airway resistance, permitting a 15%–20% increase in oxygen consumption as well as increases in carbon dioxide production and in the respiratory functional reserve.

As the uterus enlarges, it presses upward and elevates the diaphragm. The subcostal angle increases, so that the rib cage flares. The anteroposterior diameter increases, and the chest circumference expands by as much as 6 cm; as a result, there is no significant loss of intrathoracic volume. Breathing changes from abdominal to thoracic as pregnancy progresses, and descent of the diaphragm on inspiration becomes less possible. Some hyperventilation and difficulty in breathing may occur.

Nasal stuffiness and epistaxis (nosebleeds) also may occur because of estrogen-induced edema and vascular congestion of the nasal mucosa.

CARDIOVASCULAR SYSTEM During pregnancy, blood flow increases to organ systems with an increased workload. Thus, blood flow increases to the uterus, placenta, and breasts, whereas hepatic and cerebral flow remains unchanged. Cardiac output begins to increase early in pregnancy and peaks at 25–30 weeks' gestation at 30%–50% above prepregnant levels. It generally remains elevated in the third trimester.

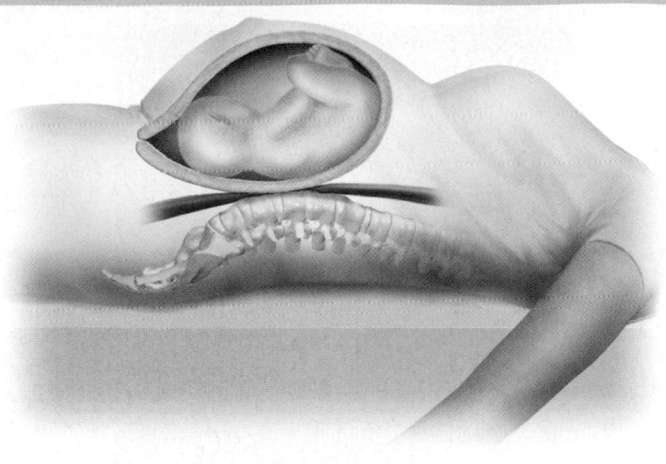

Figure 33–19 ● Vena caval syndrome. The gravid uterus compresses the vena cava when the woman is supine. This reduces the blood flow returning to the heart and may cause maternal hypotension.

The pulse may increase by as many as 10–15 bpm at term. The blood pressure decreases slightly, reaching its lowest point during the second trimester. It gradually increases to near prepregnant levels by the end of the third trimester.

The enlarging uterus puts pressure on pelvic and femoral vessels, interfering with returning blood flow and causing stasis of blood in the lower extremities. This condition may lead to dependent edema and varicosity of the veins in the legs, vulva, and rectum (hemorrhoids) in late pregnancy. This increased blood volume in the lower legs also may make the pregnant woman prone to postural hypotension.

When the pregnant woman lies supine, the enlarging uterus may press on the vena cava. This reduces blood flow to the right atrium; lowers blood pressure; and causes dizziness, pallor, and clamminess. Research indicates that the enlarging uterus also may press on the aorta and its collateral circulation (Cunningham et al., 2010). This condition is called **supine hypotensive syndrome**. It also may be referred to as **vena caval syndrome** or **aortocaval compression** (Figure 33–19 ●). It can be corrected by having the woman lie on her left side.

Blood volume progressively increases beginning in the first trimester, increases rapidly until about 30–34 weeks' gestation, and then plateaus until birth at about 40%–50% above nonpregnant levels. This increase occurs because of increases in both erythrocytes and plasma (Gordon, 2007).

The total erythrocyte (RBC) volume increases by about 25%. This increase in erythrocytes is necessary to transport the additional oxygen required during pregnancy. However, the increase in plasma volume during pregnancy averages about 50%. Because the plasma volume increase (50%) is greater than the erythrocyte increase (25%), the hematocrit, which measures the concentration of RBCs in the plasma, decreases slightly (Gordon, 2007). This decrease is referred to as the **physiological anemia of pregnancy** (pseudoanemia).

Iron is necessary for hemoglobin formation, and hemoglobin is the oxygen-carrying component of erythrocytes. Thus, the increase in erythrocyte levels results in the pregnant woman's increased need for iron. Even though the gastrointestinal absorption of iron is moderately increased during pregnancy, it is usually necessary to add supplemental iron to the diet to meet the expanded RBC and fetal needs. Women who are diagnosed with anemia prior to pregnancy may require more iron supplementation.

Leukocyte production increases slightly to an average of 8,500 mm³, with a range of 5,600–12,200 mm³. During labor and the early postpartum period, these levels may reach 20,000–30,000 mm³. Because of this normal increase in WBCs, the result should not be used clinically to diagnose the presence of infection (Gordon, 2007).

Both the fibrin and plasma fibrinogen levels increase during pregnancy. Although the blood-clotting time of a pregnant woman does not differ significantly from that of a nonpregnant woman, clotting factors VII, VIII, IX, and X increase; thus, pregnancy is a somewhat hypercoagulable state. These changes, coupled with venous stasis in late pregnancy, increase the pregnant woman's risk of developing venous thrombosis.

GASTROINTESTINAL SYSTEM Nausea and vomiting are common during the first trimester because of elevated hCG levels and changed carbohydrate metabolism. Gum tissue may soften and bleed easily. The secretion of saliva may increase and even become excessive (ptyalism).

Elevated progesterone levels cause smooth muscle relaxation, resulting in delayed gastric emptying and decreased peristalsis. As a result, the pregnant woman may complain of bloating and constipation. These symptoms are aggravated as the enlarging uterus displaces the stomach upward and the intestines are moved laterally and posteriorly. The cardiac sphincter also relaxes, and heartburn (pyrosis) may occur because of reflux of acidic secretions into the lower esophagus. Hemorrhoids frequently develop in late pregnancy from constipation and from pressure on vessels below the level of the uterus.

Only minor liver changes occur with pregnancy. Plasma albumin concentrations and serum cholinesterase activity decrease with normal pregnancy, as with certain liver diseases.

The emptying time of the gallbladder is prolonged during pregnancy as a result of smooth muscle relaxation from progesterone. This, coupled with the elevated levels of cholesterol in the bile, can predispose the woman to gallstone formation.

URINARY TRACT During the *first trimester*, the enlarging uterus is still a pelvic organ and presses against the bladder, producing urinary frequency. This symptom decreases during the *second trimester*, when the uterus becomes an abdominal organ and pressure against the bladder lessens. Frequency reappears during the *third trimester*, when the presenting part descends into the pelvis and again presses on the bladder, reducing bladder capacity, contributing to hyperemia, and irritating the bladder.

The ureters (especially the right ureter) elongate and dilate above the pelvic brim. The glomerular filtration rate (GFR) rises by as much as 50% beginning in the second trimester and remains elevated until birth. To compensate for this increase, renal tubular reabsorption also increases. However, glycosuria sometimes is seen during pregnancy because of the kidneys' inability to reabsorb all of the glucose filtered by the glomeruli. Glycosuria may be normal or may indicate gestational diabetes, so it always warrants further testing.

SKIN AND HAIR Changes in skin pigmentation commonly occur during pregnancy. Increased estrogen, progesterone, and α-melanocyte-stimulating hormone levels are thought to stimulate these changes. Pigmentation of the skin increases primarily in areas that are already hyperpigmented: the areola, the nipples, the vulva, the perianal area, and the linea alba. The linea alba refers to the midline of the abdomen from the pubic area to the umbilicus and above. During pregnancy, this area darkens and is referred to as the linea nigra (**Figure 33–20 ●**). Facial **chloasma**, or **melasma gravidarum** (also known as the "mask of pregnancy"), a darkening of the skin over the cheeks, nose, and forehead, may develop. Chloasma or melasma is more prominent in dark-haired women and is aggravated by exposure to the sun. The condition fades or becomes less prominent soon after childbirth, when the hormonal influence of pregnancy subsides.

The sweat and sebaceous glands are often hyperactive during pregnancy. Some women may notice heavy perspiration, night sweats, and the development of acne even if they have never experienced these symptoms before.

Striae may appear on the abdomen, thighs, buttocks, and breasts. They result from reduced connective tissue strength because of elevated adrenal steroid levels.

Vascular spider nevi—small, bright red elevations of the skin radiating from a central body—may develop on the chest, neck, face, arms, and legs. They may be caused by increased subcutaneous blood flow in response to elevated estrogen levels.

The rate of hair growth may decrease during pregnancy; the number of hair follicles in the resting or dormant phase also decreases. After birth, the number of hair follicles in the resting phase increases sharply and the woman may notice increased hair shedding for 1–4 months. Practically all hair is replaced within 6–12 months, however (Cunningham et al., 2010).

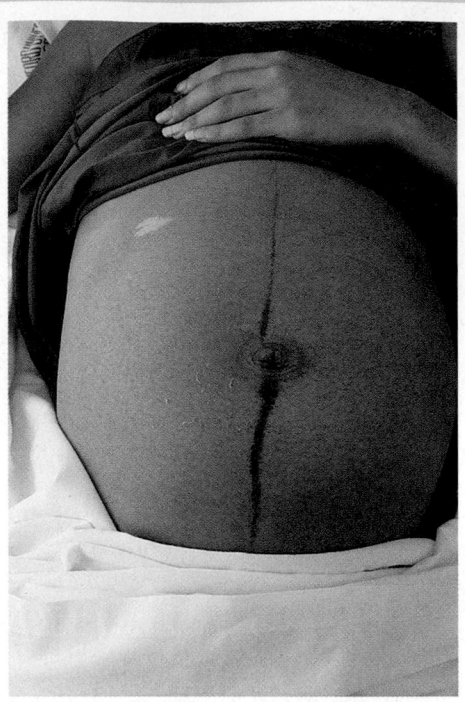

Figure 33–20 ● Linea nigra.

MUSCULOSKELETAL SYSTEM No demonstrable changes occur in the teeth of pregnant women. The dental caries that sometimes accompany pregnancy are probably caused by inadequate oral hygiene and dental care, especially if the woman has problems with bleeding gums or nausea and vomiting.

The joints of the pelvis relax somewhat because of hormonal influences. The result is often a waddling gait. As the pregnant woman's center of gravity gradually changes, the lumbodorsal spinal curve becomes accentuated and her posture changes (**Figure 33–21 ●**). This posture change compensates for the increased weight of the uterus anteriorly and frequently results in low backache.

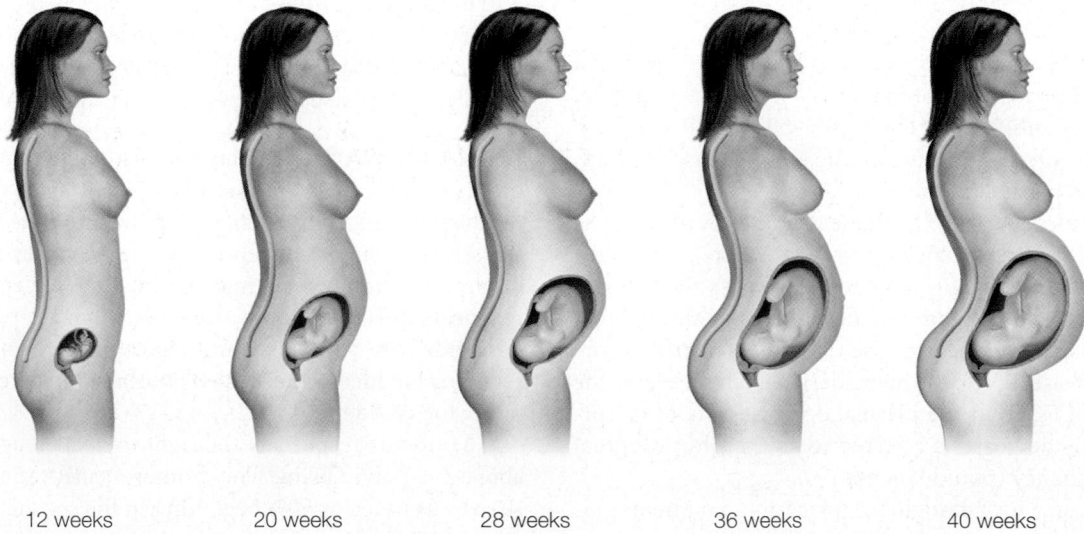

| 12 weeks | 20 weeks | 28 weeks | 36 weeks | 40 weeks |

Figure 33–21 ● Postural changes during pregnancy. Note the increasing lordosis of the lumbosacral spine and the increasing curvature of the thoracic area.

Pressure of the enlarging uterus on the abdominal muscles may cause the rectus abdominis muscle to separate, producing **diastasis recti**. If the separation is severe and muscle tone is not regained postpartum, subsequent pregnancies will not have adequate support and the woman's abdomen may appear pendulous.

EYES   Two changes generally occur in the eyes during pregnancy. First, intraocular pressure decreases, probably as a result of increased vitreous outflow. Second, a slight thickening of the cornea occurs, which is generally attributed to fluid retention. Although these changes are not readily perceived, some pregnant women experience difficulty wearing previously comfortable contact lenses (Cunningham et al., 2010). The change in the corneas generally disappears by 6 weeks postpartum.

CENTRAL NERVOUS SYSTEM   Pregnant women frequently describe decreased attention, concentration, and memory during and shortly after pregnancy, but few studies have explored this phenomenon. One study did compare a group of pregnant women and a control group, finding a decline in memory among the pregnant women that could not be attributed to depression, anxiety, sleep deprivation, or other physical changes of pregnancy. This memory loss disappeared soon after childbirth. Another study found that sleep problems are common in pregnancy. These include difficulty going to sleep, frequent awakenings, fewer hours of night sleep, and reduced sleep efficiency (Cunningham et al., 2010).

METABOLISM   Most metabolic functions accelerate during pregnancy to support the additional demands of the growing fetus and its support system. The expectant mother must meet her own tissue replacement needs, those of the fetus, and tissue changes preparatory for labor and lactation. No other event in life induces such profound metabolic changes.

Weight Gain   Growth of the uterus and its contents, growth of the breasts, and increases in intravascular fluids account for most of the weight gain in pregnancy. In addition, extra water, fat, and protein are stored, these are usually called *maternal reserves.*

Adequate nutrition and weight gain are important during pregnancy. The recommended total weight gain during pregnancy for a woman of normal weight before pregnancy is 11.5–16 kg (25–35 lb); for women who were overweight before becoming pregnant, the recommended gain is 6.8–11.5 kg (15–25 lb). Obese women are advised to limit weight gain to 5–9 kg (11–20 lb). Underweight women are advised to gain 12.7–18.1 kg (28–40 lb) (Institute of Medicine [IOM], 2009). Weight may decrease slightly during the first trimester because of nausea, vomiting, and food intolerances of early pregnancy. The lost weight is soon regained, and the IOM (2009) recommends a normal weight woman gain of 0.5–2 kg (1.1–4.4 lb) during the first trimester, followed by an average gain of about 0.45 kg (1 lb) per week during the last two trimesters.

Water Metabolism   Increased water retention is a basic chemical alteration of pregnancy. Several interrelated factors cause this phenomenon. The increased level of steroid sex hormones affects sodium and fluid retention. The lowered serum protein also influences the fluid balance, as do the increased intracapillary pressure and permeability. The extra water is needed for the products of conception—the fetus, placenta, and amniotic fluid—and the mother's increased blood volume, interstitial fluids, and enlarged organs.

Nutrient Metabolism   The fetus makes its greatest protein and fat demands during the second half of gestation, doubling in weight in the last 6–8 weeks. The increased protein retention that begins in early pregnancy is initially used for hyperplasia and hypertrophy of maternal tissues, such as the uterus and breasts. Protein must also be stored during pregnancy to maintain a constant level within the breast milk and to avoid depletion of maternal tissues.

Fats are more completely absorbed during pregnancy, resulting in a marked increase in the serum lipids, lipoproteins, and cholesterol and decreased elimination through the bowel. Fat deposits in the fetus increase from about 2% at midpregnancy to almost 12% at term. The excess nitrogen and lipidemia are considered to be a preparation for lactation. In addition, the woman's body switches from glucose metabolism to lipid metabolism once glucose from food intake has been used up. This leads to an increased tendency to develop ketosis between meals and overnight. The demand for carbohydrate increases, especially during the last two trimesters. Intermittent glycosuria is not uncommon during pregnancy. When it is not accompanied by a rise in blood sugar levels, glycosuria is secondary to the increased glomerular filtration rate. Fasting blood sugar levels tend to fall slightly, returning to more normal levels by the sixth postpartum month. The oral glucose tolerance test shows no change with pregnancy.

The possibility of diabetes must not be overlooked during pregnancy. Plasma levels of insulin increase during pregnancy (probably because of hormonal changes that cause increased tissue resistance) and rapid destruction of insulin takes place within the placenta. The woman's insulin production must increase during the second trimester, and any marginal pancreatic function quickly becomes apparent. The woman with diabetes often experiences increased exogenous insulin demands during pregnancy.

The demand for iron during pregnancy is accelerated, and the pregnant woman needs to guard against anemia. Iron is necessary for the increase in erythrocytes, hemoglobin, and blood volume, as well as for the increased tissue demands of both woman and fetus. Iron transfer takes place at the placenta in only one direction: toward the fetus. It has been demonstrated that approximately five sixths of the iron stored in the fetal liver is assimilated during the last trimester of pregnancy. This stored iron in the fetal liver compensates in the first 4 months of neonatal life for the normal inadequate amounts of iron available in breast milk and non-iron-fortified formulas.

The progressive absorption and retention of calcium during pregnancy have been noted. The maternal plasma concentration of bound calcium decreases as the levels of bindable plasma proteins fall. Approximately 30 g of calcium is retained in maternal bone for fetal deposition late in pregnancy.

ENDOCRINE SYSTEM

Thyroid   Pregnancy influences the thyroid gland's size and activity. Often a palpable change is noted, which represents an increase in vascularity and hyperplasia of glandular tissue. Total serum thyroxine (T_4) increases in early pregnancy, and thyroid-stimulating hormone (TSH) decreases. The elevated levels of total T_4 continue until several weeks postpartum, although the level of free serum T_4 returns to normal after the first trimester (Cunningham et al., 2010).

Increased thyroxine-binding capacity is evidenced by an increase in serum protein-bound iodine, probably due to the increased levels of circulating estrogens. The basal metabolic rate increases by as much as 20%–25% during pregnancy. The increased oxygen consumption is due primarily to fetal metabolic activity.

Parathyroid The concentration of the parathyroid hormone and the size of the parathyroid glands increase, paralleling the fetal calcium requirements. Parathyroid hormone concentration reaches its highest level of approximately twofold between 15 and 35 weeks of gestation, returning to a normal or even subnormal level before childbirth.

Pituitary Pregnancy is made possible by the hypothalamic stimulation of the anterior pituitary gland. The anterior pituitary produces *FSH*, which stimulates follicle growth in the ovary, and LH, which affects ovulation. Stimulation of the pituitary also prolongs the ovary's corpus luteal phase, which maintains the secretory endometrium in preparation for pregnancy. *Prolactin*, another anterior pituitary hormone, is responsible for initial lactation.

The posterior pituitary secretes *vasopressin* (antidiuretic hormone) and *oxytocin*. Vasopressin causes vasoconstriction, which results in increased blood pressure; it also helps regulate water balance. Oxytocin promotes uterine contractility and stimulates ejection of milk from the breasts (the let-down reflex) in the postpartum period.

Adrenals Little structural change occurs in the adrenal glands during a normal pregnancy. Estrogen-induced increases in the levels of circulating cortisol result primarily from lowered renal excretion. The circulating cortisol levels regulate carbohydrate and protein metabolism. A normal level resumes 1–6 weeks postpartum.

The adrenals secrete increased levels of aldosterone by the early part of the second trimester. The levels of secretion are even more elevated in the woman on a sodium-restricted diet. This increase in aldosterone in a normal pregnancy may be the body's protective response to the increased sodium excretion associated with progesterone (Cunningham et al., 2010).

Pancreas The islets of Langerhans are stressed to meet the increased demand for insulin during pregnancy, and a latent deficiency may become apparent during pregnancy, producing symptoms of gestational diabetes.

Hormones in Pregnancy Several hormones are required to maintain pregnancy. Most of these are produced initially by the corpus luteum; the placenta then assumes production.

- *Human chorionic gonadotropin:* The trophoblast secretes hCG in early pregnancy. This hormone stimulates progesterone and estrogen production by the corpus luteum to maintain the pregnancy until the placenta is developed sufficiently to assume that function.

- *Human placental lactogen:* Also called human chorionic somatomammotropin (hCS), hPL is produced by the syncytiotrophoblast. This hormone is an antagonist of insulin; it increases the amount of circulating free fatty acids for maternal metabolic needs and decreases maternal metabolism of glucose to favor fetal growth.

- *Estrogen:* Secreted originally by the corpus luteum, estrogen is produced primarily by the placenta as early as the seventh week of pregnancy. Estrogen stimulates uterine development to provide a suitable environment for the fetus. It also helps to develop the ductal system of the breasts in preparation for lactation.

- *Progesterone:* Progesterone, also produced initially by the corpus luteum and then by the placenta, plays the greatest role in maintaining pregnancy. It maintains the endometrium and also inhibits spontaneous uterine contractility, thus preventing early spontaneous abortion due to uterine activity. In addition, progesterone helps develop the ductal system of the breasts in preparation for lactation.

- *Relaxin:* Relaxin is detectable in the serum of a pregnant woman by the time of the first missed menstrual period. Relaxin inhibits uterine activity, diminishes the strength of uterine contractions, aids in the softening of the cervix, and has the long-term effect of remodeling collagen. Its primary source is the corpus luteum, but small amounts are believed to be produced by the placenta and uterine decidua throughout pregnancy.

Prostaglandins in Pregnancy Prostaglandins (PGs) are lipid substances that can arise from most body tissues but occur in high concentrations in the female reproductive tract and are present in the decidua during pregnancy. While their exact functions during pregnancy are still unknown, it has been proposed that PGs are responsible for maintaining reduced placental vascular resistance. Decreased PG levels may contribute to hypertension and preeclampsia. Prostaglandins are also believed to play a role in the complex biochemistry that initiates labor, although their specific functions are still being defined.

Signs of Pregnancy

Many of the changes women experience during pregnancy are used to diagnose the pregnancy itself. They are called the subjective, or presumptive, changes; the objective, or probable, changes; and the diagnostic, or positive, changes of pregnancy.

SUBJECTIVE (PRESUMPTIVE) CHANGES The subjective changes of pregnancy are the symptoms the woman experiences and reports. Because they can be caused by other conditions, they cannot be considered proof of pregnancy.

✳ *Go to* **nursing.pearsonhighered.com** *for a chart titled "Differential Diagnosis of Pregnancy—Subjective Changes."*

Amenorrhea, or the absence of menses, is the earliest symptom of pregnancy. The missing of more than one menstrual period, especially in a woman whose cycle is ordinarily regular, is an especially useful diagnostic clue. Excessive fatigue may be noted within a few weeks after the first missed menstrual period and may persist throughout the first trimester. Urinary frequency is experienced during the first trimester as the enlarging uterus presses on the bladder. This improves during the second trimester when the enlarging uterus escapes the pelvis, and then recurs in the third trimester when the growing fetus presses on the bladder.

Nausea and vomiting in pregnancy (NVP) occur frequently during the first trimester and may be the result of elevated hCG levels and changed carbohydrate metabolism. Because these symptoms often occur in the early part of the day, they are commonly referred to as **morning sickness**. In reality, the symptoms may occur at any time and can range from a mere distaste for food to severe vomiting. Research indicates that women who experience NVP often have a more favorable pregnancy outcome than those who do not (Gordon, 2007).

Changes in the breasts are frequently noted in early pregnancy. These changes include tenderness and tingling sensations, increased pigmentation of the areola and nipple, and changes in the Montgomery glands. The veins in the breasts also become more visible and form a bluish pattern beneath the skin.

Quickening, or the mother's perception of fetal movement, occurs about 18–20 weeks after the last menstrual period (LMP) in a woman pregnant for the first time, but may occur as early as 16 weeks in a woman who has been pregnant before. Quickening is a fluttering sensation in the abdomen that gradually increases in intensity and frequency.

OBJECTIVE (PROBABLE) CHANGES

An examiner can perceive the objective changes that occur in pregnancy. Because these changes also have other causes, they do not confirm pregnancy.

✳ Go to **nursing.highered.com** for a chart titled "Differential Diagnosis of Pregnancy—Objective Changes."

The only physical changes detectable during the first 3 months of pregnancy are caused by increased vascular congestion. These changes are noted on pelvic examination. As noted earlier, there is a softening of the cervix called the Goodell sign. The Chadwick sign is a bluish, purple, or deep red discoloration of the mucous membranes of the cervix, vagina, and vulva. (Some sources consider this a presumptive sign.) The **Hegar sign** is a softening of the isthmus of the uterus, the area between the cervix and the body of the uterus. The **McDonald sign** is an ease in flexing the body of the uterus against the cervix.

General enlargement and softening of the body of the uterus can be noted after the eighth week of pregnancy. The fundus of the uterus is palpable just above the symphysis pubis at about 10–12 weeks' gestation and at the level of the umbilicus at 20–22 weeks' gestation (**Figure 33–22 ●**).

Enlargement of the abdomen during the childbearing years is usually regarded as evidence of pregnancy, especially if it is continuous and accompanied by amenorrhea. Braxton Hicks contractions are palpable with abdominal palpation after week 28. As the woman approaches the end of pregnancy, these contractions may become uncomfortable.

Uterine souffle may be heard when the examiner auscultates the abdomen over the uterus. It is a soft blowing sound that occurs at the same rate as the maternal pulse. The funic souffle occurs at the same rate as the fetal heart rate (FHR).

The fetal outline may be identified by palpation in many pregnant women after 24 weeks' gestation. **Ballottement** is the passive fetal movement elicited when the examiner inserts two gloved fingers into the vagina and pushes against the cervix. This action pushes the fetal body up, and as it falls back, the examiner feels a rebound.

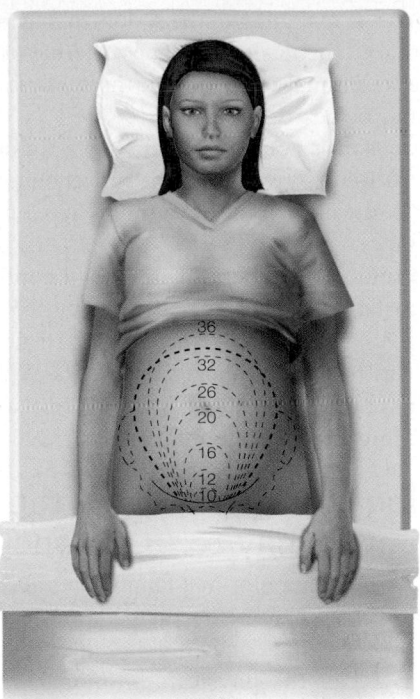

Figure 33–22 ● Approximate height of the fundus at various weeks of pregnancy.

Pregnancy tests are based on analysis of maternal blood or urine for the detection of hCG, the hormone secreted by the trophoblast. These tests are not considered positive signs of pregnancy because the similarity of hCG and the pituitary-secreted LH occasionally results in cross-reactions. In addition, certain conditions other than pregnancy can cause elevated levels of hCG.

Clinical Pregnancy Tests The most commonly used assay for pregnancy diagnosis is measuring the beta subunit of hCG in either urine or serum. Currently four main hCG tests are used: (1) radioimmunoassay, (2) immunoradiometric assay, (3) enzyme-linked immunosorbent assay (ELISA), and (4) fluoroimmunoassay. hCG is detectable in more than 97% of clients by day 11 after conception. False-negative or -positive results can also occur. In pregnancy, levels normally peak at 10–12 weeks' gestation and this initial rise is important in monitoring high-risk pregnancies where viability has not been documented. Failure to observe the expected rise may suggest an ectopic pregnancy or spontaneous abortion. An abnormally high level or accelerated rise can also prompt investigation into possible disorders such as molar pregnancy, multiple gestations, or chromosomal abnormalities. There is a decline in the hCG levels rapidly until 22 weeks' gestation when another gradual rise occurs (Cunningham et al., 2010).

DIAGNOSTIC (POSITIVE) CHANGES

The positive signs of pregnancy are completely objective, cannot be confused with a pathological state, and offer conclusive proof of pregnancy.

The fetal heartbeat can be detected with a fetoscope by approximately weeks 17–20 of pregnancy. With an electronic Doppler device, the fetal heartbeat can be detected as early as weeks 10–12. The fetal heart rate is between 110 and 160 bpm and must be counted and compared with the maternal pulse for differentiation. Auscultation of the abdomen may reveal sounds other than that of the fetal heart. The maternal pulse, emanating from the abdominal aorta, may be unusually loud, or a uterine souffle may be heard.

Fetal movement is actively palpable by a trained examiner after about 20 weeks' gestation. The movements vary from a faint flutter in the early months to more vigorous movements late in pregnancy.

Visualization of the fetus by ultrasound confirms a pregnancy. The gestational sac can be observed by 4–5 weeks' gestation (2–3 weeks after conception). Fetal parts and fetal heart movement can be seen as early as 8 weeks. A transvaginal, ultrasound has been used to detect a gestational sac as early as 10 days after implantation (Cunningham et al., 2010).

Psychological Response of the Expectant Family to Pregnancy

Pregnancy is a turning point in a family's life, accompanied by stress and anxiety, whether the pregnancy is desired or not. Especially when this is their first child, the expectant parents may be unaware of the physical, emotional, and cognitive changes of pregnancy and may anticipate no problems from such a normal event. Thus, they may be confused and distressed by new feelings and behaviors that are essentially normal.

For beginning families, pregnancy is the transition period from childlessness to parenthood. If the expectant woman is married or has a stable partner, she is no longer only a mate, but also must assume the role of mother. Her partner, whether male or female, will become a parent too. The anticipation of parenthood brings significant role changes for them. Career goals and mobility may be affected, and the couple's relationship takes on a different meaning to them and within the larger family and community. If the pregnancy results in the birth of a child, the couple enters a new, irreversible stage of their life together. With each subsequent pregnancy, routines and family dynamics are again altered, requiring readjustment and realignment.

In most pregnancies, finances are an important consideration. Today's society has many types of families, and pregnant women with or without stable partners recognize the financial impact of a child and may be concerned about financial issues. Decisions about financial matters need to be made at this time. Will both parents work outside the home during the pregnancy or after the child is born? If so, who will provide child care? Couples also may need to decide about the division of domestic tasks. Any differences of opinion must be discussed openly and resolved so that the family can meet the needs of its members.

If the pregnant woman has no stable partner, she must deal with the role changes, fears, and adjustments of pregnancy alone or seek support from family or friends. She also faces the reality of planning for the future as a single parent. Finances may be a major source of concern. Even if the pregnant woman plans to relinquish her infant, she still must deal with the adjustments of pregnancy. This can be especially difficult without a good support system.

DEVELOPMENTAL TASKS OF THE EXPECTANT COUPLE
Pregnancy can be viewed as a developmental stage with its own distinct developmental tasks. For a couple, it can be a time of support or conflict depending on the amount of adjustment each is willing to make to maintain the family's equilibrium.

During a first pregnancy, the couple plans together for the child's arrival, collecting information on how to be parents. At the same time, each member of the couple continues to participate in some separate activities with friends or family members. The availability of social support is an important factor in psychosocial well-being during pregnancy. The social network is often a major source of advice for the pregnant woman; however, both sound and unsound information may be conveyed.

During pregnancy, the expectant parents face significant changes and must deal with major psychosocial adjustments. Other family members, especially other children of the woman or couple and the grandparents-to-be, also must adjust to the pregnancy.

✳ Go to **nursing.pearsonhighered.com** to see a chart on *parental reactions to pregnancy.*

For some people, pregnancy is more than a developmental stage; it is a crisis. *Crisis* can be defined as "a disturbance or conflict in which the individual cannot maintain a state of equilibrium." Pregnancy can be considered a *maturational crisis*, because it is a common event in the normal growth and development of the family. During such a crisis, the individual or family is in disequilibrium. Egos weaken, usual defense mechanisms are not effective, unresolved issues from the past reappear, and relationships shift. This period of disequilibrium and disorganization is marked by unsuccessful attempts to solve the perceived problems. If the crisis is not resolved, it will result in maladaptive behaviors in one or more family members and possible disintegration of the family. Families that are able to resolve a maturational crisis will return successfully to normal functioning and can even strengthen the bonds in the family relationship.

THE MOTHER Pregnancy is a condition that alters body image and necessitates a reordering of social relationships and changes in the roles of family members. The way each woman meets the stresses of pregnancy is influenced by her emotional makeup, her sociological and cultural background, and her acceptance or rejection of the pregnancy. However, many women manifest similar psychologic and emotional responses during pregnancy, including ambivalence, acceptance, introversion, mood swings, and changes in body image.

A woman's attitude toward her pregnancy can be a significant factor in its outcome. Even if the pregnancy is planned, there is an element of surprise at first. Many women commonly experience feelings of ambivalence during early pregnancy. This ambivalence may be related to feelings that the timing is somehow wrong; worries about the need to modify existing relationships or career plans; fears about assuming a new role; unresolved emotional conflicts with the woman's own mother; and fears about pregnancy, labor, and birth. These feelings may be more pronounced if the pregnancy is unplanned or unwanted. Indirect expressions of ambivalence include complaints about considerable physical discomfort, prolonged or frequent depression, significant dissatisfaction with changing body shape, excessive mood swings, and difficulty in accepting the life changes resulting from the pregnancy.

Many pregnancies are unintended, but not all unintended pregnancies are unwanted. A pregnancy can be unintended and wanted at the same time. For some women, an unintended pregnancy has more psychological and social advantages than disadvantages. It provides purpose and direction to life and allows a woman to test the devotion and love of her partner and family. However, an unintended pregnancy can be a risk factor for depression. Women with an unintended pregnancy also may perceive life events as being more stressful than women with an intended pregnancy—another contributor to depression. Depression, in turn, can negatively impact a woman's health choices and behaviors (Messer et al., 2005).

Conflicts about adapting to pregnancy are no more pronounced for older pregnant women (ages 35 and over) than for younger ones. Moreover, older pregnant women tend to be less concerned about the normal physical changes of pregnancy and are confident about handling issues that arise during pregnancy and parenting. This difference may result because mature pregnant women have more experience with problem solving. However, mature pregnant women may have fewer pregnant peers and thus may have fewer people with whom to share concerns and expectations.

Pregnancy produces marked changes in a woman's body within a relatively short period of time. Pregnant women experience changes in body image because of physical alterations and may feel a loss of control over their bodies during pregnancy and later during childbirth. These perceptions are related to a certain extent to personality factors, social network responses, and attitudes toward pregnancy. Although changes in body image are normal, they can be very stressful for the woman. Explanation and discussion of the changes may help both the woman and her partner deal with the stress associated with this aspect of pregnancy.

Fantasies about the unborn child are common among pregnant women. The themes of the fantasies (baby's appearance, gender, traits, impact on parents, etc.) vary by trimester and differ among women who are pregnant for the first time and women who already have children.

First Trimester During the first trimester, feelings of disbelief and ambivalence are common. The woman's baby does not seem real, and she focuses on herself and her pregnancy. She may experience one or more of the early symptoms of pregnancy, such as breast tenderness or morning sickness, which are unsettling and at times unpleasant.

At this time, the expectant mother also begins to exhibit some characteristic behavioral changes. She may become increasingly introspective and passive. She may be emotionally labile, with characteristic mood swings from joy to despair. She may fantasize about a miscarriage and feel guilt because of these fantasies. She may worry that these thoughts will harm the baby in some way. Nursing responsibilities at this time include helping the mother to identify coping strategies and providing options and counseling for women experiencing a pregnancy that is both unintended and unwanted.

Second Trimester During the second trimester, quickening occurs around 20 weeks. This perception of fetal movement helps the woman think of her baby as a separate individual, and she generally becomes excited about the pregnancy even if she had not been looking forward to the pregnancy earlier. The woman becomes increasingly introspective as she evaluates her life, her plans, and her child's future. This introspection helps the woman prepare for her new mothering role. Emotional lability, which may be unsettling to her partner, persists. In some instances, the partner may react by withdrawing. This withdrawal is especially distressing to the woman because she needs increased love and affection. Once the couple understands that these behaviors are characteristic of pregnancy, it is easier for the couple to deal with them effectively, although to some extent they may be sources of stress throughout pregnancy. As pregnancy becomes more noticeable, the woman's body image changes. She may feel great pride, embarrassment, or concern. Generally, women feel best during the second trimester, which is a relatively tranquil time.

Third Trimester In the third trimester, the woman feels both pride about her pregnancy and anxiety about labor and birth. Physical discomforts increase, and the woman is eager for the pregnancy to end. She experiences increased fatigue, her body movements are more awkward, and her interest in sexual activity may decrease. During this time, the woman tends to be concerned about the health and safety of her unborn child and may worry that she will not cope well during childbirth. Toward the end of this period, the woman often experiences a surge of energy as she prepares for childbirth. Many women report bursts of energy, during which they vigorously clean and organize the home ("nesting").

Psychological Tasks of the Mother Rubin (1984) identified four major tasks that the pregnant woman undertakes to maintain her intactness and that of her family and at the same time to incorporate her new child into the family system. These tasks form the foundation for a mutually gratifying relationship with her infant:

1. **Ensuring safe passage through pregnancy, labor, and birth.** The pregnant woman feels concern for her unborn child and for herself. She looks for competent prenatal care to provide a sense of control. She may seek information from literature, observation of other pregnant women and new mothers, and discussion with others. She also attempts to ensure safe passage by engaging in self-care activities related to diet, exercise, alcohol consumption, and the like. In the third trimester, she becomes more aware of external threats in the environment—a toy on the stairs, the awkwardness of an escalator—that pose a threat to her well-being. She may worry if her partner is late or if she is home alone. Sleep becomes more difficult, and she longs for birth even though it, too, is frightening.

2. **Seeking acceptance of this child by others.** The birth of a child alters a woman's primary support group (her family) and her secondary affiliate groups. The woman slowly and subtly alters her network to meet the needs of her pregnancy. In this adjustment, the woman's partner is the most important figure. The partner's support and acceptance help form a maternal identity. If there are other children in the home, the mother also works to ensure their acceptance of the coming child. Acceptance of the anticipated change is sometimes stressful, and the woman may work to maintain special time with her partner or older children. The woman without a partner looks to others, such as a family member or friend, for this support.

3. ***Seeking commitment and acceptance of herself as mother to the infant (binding in).*** During the first trimester, the child remains a rather abstract concept. With quickening, however, the child begins to become a real individual and the mother begins to develop bonds of attachment. The mother experiences the movement of the child within her in an intimate, exclusive way, and out of this experience, bonds of love form. This binding-in process, characterized by its strong emotional component, motivates the pregnant woman to become competent in her role and provides satisfaction for her in the role of mother. This possessive love increases her maternal commitment to protect her fetus now and her child after he or she is born.

4. ***Learning to give of oneself on behalf of one's child.*** Childbirth involves many acts of giving. A man "gives" a child to a woman; she in turn "gives" a child to her partner. Life is given to an infant; a sibling is given to older children of the family. The woman begins to develop a capacity for self-denial and learns to delay immediate personal gratification to meet the needs of another. Baby showers and gifts are acts of giving that increase the mother's self-esteem and help her recognize the separateness and needs of the coming baby.

Accomplishment of these tasks helps the expectant woman develop her self-concept as a mother. The expectant woman who was well nurtured by her own mother may view her mother as a role model and emulate her; the woman who views her mother as a poor mother may worry that she will make similar mistakes. A woman's self-concept as a mother expands with experience and continues to grow through subsequent childbearing and childrearing. Occasionally, a woman fails to accept the mother role, instead playing the role of babysitter or older sister to her child.

THE FATHER Until fairly recently, the expectant father or partner was often viewed as a "bystander" or observer of the pregnancy. He was necessary for conception, for bill paying, and for providing male guidance as his child matured. This view has changed, and the father is now expected to be a nurturing, caring, involved parent as well as a provider. In response to societal pressures, the influence of the feminist movement, and the economic pressures that have resulted in more women being employed outside the home, shared parenting and shared breadwinning have become more common. Many men have actively sought to be more involved in the experience of childbirth and parenting.

Expectant fathers experience many of the same feelings and conflicts experienced by expectant mothers when the pregnancy has been confirmed. Initially, expectant fathers may feel pride in their virility, which pregnancy confirms, but also have ambivalent feelings. The extent of ambivalence depends on many factors, including the father's relationship with his partner, his previous experience with pregnancy, his age, his economic stability, and whether the pregnancy was planned. The expectant father must first deal with the reality of the pregnancy and then struggle to gain recognition as a parent from his partner, family, friends, coworkers, society—and from his baby as well. The expectant mother can help her partner be a participant and not merely a helpmate to her if she has a definite sense of the experience as *their* pregnancy and *their* infant and not *her* pregnancy and *her* infant.

Men whose partners are pregnant following a previous pregnancy loss may experience a variety of emotions attributable to the loss. These emotions might include an increased sense of risk, feelings of increased concern about the outcome of the current pregnancy, the recognition that something could go wrong again, and the sense that increased vigilance is essential. These fathers may call home more often to check on the mother's condition and the baby and may also feel an increased need to be involved more actively in the current pregnancy. They wish to be acknowledged as more than just a support person; they want their important role as family protector recognized (O'Leary & Thorwick, 2006).

In general, the expectant father faces psychological stress as he makes the transition from nonparent to parent or from parent of one to parent of two or more. Sources of stress include financial issues, unexpected events during pregnancy, concern that the baby will not be healthy and normal, worry about the pain the partner will experience in childbirth, and his role during labor and birth. Other sources of stress for expectant fathers include concern over the changing relationship with their partners, diminished sexual responsiveness in their partners or in themselves, changes in relationships with their families or male friends, and their ability to parent. Most men handle the transition to fatherhood well, and generally any anxieties they feel resolve over time. Fathers' feelings of anxiety often stem from inadequate preparation and can be addressed by recognizing paternal needs and including fathers more in prenatal education (Deave, Johnson, & Ingram, 2008).

The expectant father must establish a fatherhood role just as the expectant mother develops a motherhood role. The mother experiences biological changes of pregnancy that aid in the transition to motherhood. Fathers may feel left out because they are unable to experience what their partner is experiencing. The fathers who are most successful at developing a fatherhood role generally like children, are excited about the prospect of fatherhood, are eager to nurture a child, have confidence in their ability to be a parent, and share the experiences of pregnancy and childbirth with their partners (Lederman & Weis, 2009).

First Trimester After the initial excitement of announcing the pregnancy to friends and relatives and receiving their congratulations, an expectant father may begin to feel left out of the pregnancy. He is also often confused by his partner's mood changes and perhaps bewildered by his responses to her changing body. He may resent the attention given to the woman and the changes in their relationship as she experiences fatigue and a decreased interest in sex.

During this time, his child is a "potential baby." Fathers often picture interacting with a child of age 5 or 6 rather than a newborn. Even the pregnancy itself may seem unreal until the woman shows more physical signs.

Second Trimester The father's role in the pregnancy is still vague in the second trimester, but his involvement can be increased by his watching and feeling fetal movement. It is helpful if the father, as well as the mother, has the opportunity to hear the fetal heartbeat. That requires a visit to the nurse-midwife's or physician's office. Involvement of fathers in antepartum care is increasing and may even be an expectation of their partner. For many men, seeing the infant on ultrasound is an important experience in accepting the reality of the pregnancy.

Like expectant mothers, expectant fathers need to confront and resolve some of their own conflicts about the fathering they received. A father needs to sort out those behaviors in his own fathering that he wants to imitate and those he wishes to avoid. Research indicates that a father's beliefs about the fathering role are a strong predictor of his competence in parenting (Schoppe-Sullivan et al., 2008).

The anxiety experienced by the father-to-be is lessened if both parents agree on the support role the man is to assume during pregnancy and on his projected paternal role. For example, if both see his role as that of breadwinner, the man's stress is low. However, if the man views his role as that of breadwinner and the woman expects him to be actively involved in preparations and child care, his stress increases. An open and honest discussion about the expectations each parent has about their roles will help the father-to-be in his transition to fatherhood (Goodman, 2005).

The woman's appearance begins to alter at this time, and men react differently to the physical change. For some it decreases sexual interest; for others it may have the opposite effect. Both partners experience a multitude of emotions, and it continues to be important for them to communicate and accept each other's feelings and concerns. In situations in which the expectant mother's demands dominate the relationship, the expectant father's resentment may increase to the point that he is spending more time at work, involved in a hobby, or with his friends. The behavior is even more likely if the expectant father did not want the pregnancy or if the relationship was not a good one before the pregnancy.

Third Trimester

If the couple have communicated their concerns and feelings to one another and grown in their relationship, the third trimester is a special and rewarding time. A more clearly defined role evolves at this time for the expectant father, and it becomes more obvious how the couple can prepare together for the coming event. They may become involved in childbirth education classes and make concrete preparations for the arrival of the baby, such as shopping for a crib, car seat, and other equipment. If the expectant father has developed a detached attitude about the pregnancy before this time, however, it is unlikely that he will become a willing participant even though his role becomes more obvious.

Concerns and fears may recur. Many men are afraid of hurting the unborn baby during intercourse. The father may also begin to have anxiety and fantasies about what could happen to his partner and the unborn baby during labor and birth and feels a great sense of responsibility. The questions asked earlier in pregnancy emerge again. What kind of parents will he and his partner be? Will he really be able to help his partner in labor? Can they afford to have a baby?

The nurse needs to be prepared to meet the needs of lesbian or gay families as well. They face unique challenges in completing their developmental tasks. For example, they are frequently faced with discrimination and disapproval from mainstream society. In the past, many gay or lesbian families opt to keep their sexual orientation a secret. In most states, they do not have many of the benefits of marriage that heterosexual couples have, such as insurance benefits, rights to property custody issues, and family

> ### Focus on Diversity and Culture   Couvade
>
> Traditionally, the term *couvade* has referred to the male's observance of certain rituals and taboos to signify the transition to fatherhood. This observance affirms his psychosocial and biophysical relationship to the woman and child. Some taboos restrict his actions. For example, in some cultures, the man may be forbidden to eat certain foods or carry certain weapons before and immediately after the birth. More recently, the term has been used to describe the unintentional development of physical symptoms such as fatigue, increased appetite, difficulty sleeping, depression, headache, or backache by the partner of a pregnant woman. Men who demonstrate couvade syndrome tend to have a higher degree of paternal role preparation and be involved in more activities related to this preparation.

leave benefits associated with childbirth. Some states now recognize same-sex marriage and civil unions, which provide protection of rights for same-sex partners (Giger & Davidhizar, 2007).

SIBLINGS   The introduction of a new baby into the family often leads to sibling rivalry, which results from children's fear of change in the security of their relationships with their parents. Some of the behaviors demonstrating feelings of sibling rivalry may even be directed toward the mother during the pregnancy as she experiences more fatigue and less patience with her toddler, for example. Parents who recognize the situation early in pregnancy and make constructive responses can help minimize the problems of sibling rivalry.

Preparation of the young child for a new sibling should begin several weeks before the anticipated birth and is best designed according to the age and experience of the child. The mother may let the child feel the fetus moving in her uterus, explaining that this is "a special place where babies grow." The child can help the parents put the baby clothes in drawers or prepare the baby's room. Because they do not have a clear concept of time, young children should not be told too early about the pregnancy.

Consistency is important in dealing with young children. They need reassurance that certain people, special things, and familiar places will continue to exist after the new baby arrives. The crib is an important though transient object in a child's life. If it is to be given to the new baby, the parents should thoughtfully help the child adjust to this change. Any move from crib to bed or from one room to another should precede the baby's birth by several weeks or more. If the new baby is to share a room with one or more siblings, the parents must discuss this with them.

Some parents advocate cosleeping or bed sharing (one or both parents sleeping with their baby or young child), and so the crib is less of an issue. Cosleeping (infant sleeping in the same bed with the mother), which is common in many non-Western cultures, is on the increase in the United States. Opinion varies sharply about the advantages and risks of the practice. In 2005 the American Academy of Pediatrics (AAP) issued a policy statement recommending against cosleeping because of the increased risk of sudden infant death syndrome (SIDS). This policy statement was reaffirmed by the AAP in January 2009. The AAP stresses that the infant can be brought to the bed to be comforted or for breastfeeding but should be placed supine in a separate bed to sleep. Parents who choose to cosleep must make decisions about the sleeping arrangements of other siblings following the birth of the baby.

If the sibling is ready for toilet training, it is most effectively done several months before or after the baby's arrival. Parents should know that the older, toilet-trained child may regress to wetting or soiling because he or she sees the new baby getting attention for such behavior. The older, weaned child may want to drink from the breast or bottle again after the new baby comes. If the new mother anticipates these behaviors, they will be less frustrating during her early postpartum days.

During the pregnancy, older children should be introduced to a new baby for short periods to get an idea of what a new baby is like. This introduction dispels fantasies that the new arrival will be big enough to be a playmate. Pregnant women may also find it helpful to bring their children to a prenatal visit after they have been told about the expected baby. The children are encouraged to become involved in prenatal care and to ask any questions they may have. They are also given the opportunity to hear the fetal heartbeat, either with a stethoscope or with the Doppler device. This helps make the baby more real to them.

If siblings are school-age children, the pregnancy should be viewed as a family affair. Teaching about the pregnancy should be based on the child's level of understanding and interest. Over-eager parents may go into longer and more in-depth responses than the child is able to understand. Some children are more curious than others. Books at their level of understanding can be made available in the home. Involvement in family discussions, attendance at sibling preparation classes, encouragement to feel fetal movement, and an opportunity to listen to the fetal heart supplement the learning process and help make the school-age child feel part of the pregnancy. Sibling preparation classes assist in the transition process for both parents and children. After attending the classes, children often exhibit an increased ability to express their feelings and less anxiety.

Older children or adolescents may appear to have a sophisticated knowledge base, but it may be intermingled with many misconceptions. Thus, parents should make opportunities to discuss their concerns and should involve the children in preparation for the new baby.

Even after the birth, siblings need to feel that they are part of a family event. Changes in hospital regulations allowing siblings to be present at the birth or to visit their mother and the new baby facilitate this process. Participation in special programs for siblings may help in this process. On arrival at home, siblings can share in "showing off" the new baby.

Sibling preparation for the arrival of a new baby is essential, but other factors are equally important. These include the amount of parental attention focused on the new arrival, the amount of parental attention given the older child after the birth of the new arrival, and parental skill in dealing effectively with regressive or aggressive behavior.

GRANDPARENTS The first relatives told about a pregnancy are usually the grandparents. Often the expectant grandparents become increasingly supportive of the couple even if conflicts existed previously. But even sensitive grandparents may have difficulty knowing how deeply to become involved in the childrearing process.

Because grandparenting can occur over a wide expanse of years, people's response to this role varies considerably. Younger grandparents leading active lives may not demonstrate as much interest as the young couple would like. In other cases, expectant grandparents may freely give advice and gifts, sometimes to excess. For grandparents, conflict may be related to the expectant couple's need to feel in control of their lives or it may stem from events signaling changing roles in the grandparents' lives (e.g., retirement, financial concerns, menopause, or death of a friend). Some parents of expectant couples may already be grandparents with a developed style of grandparenting. This influences their response to the pregnancy.

Because childbearing and childrearing practices have changed, family cohesiveness is promoted by effective communication and frank discussion between young couples and interested grandparents about the changes and the reasons for those changes. Clarifying the role of the grandparents ensures a comfortable situation for all.

Classes for grandparents may provide information about changes in birth and parenting practices. These classes help familiarize grandparents with new parents' needs and may offer suggestions for ways in which the grandparents can support the childbearing couple.

Cultural Values and Pregnancy

A universal tendency exists to create ceremonial rituals or rites around important life events. Thus, rituals are often tied to pregnancy, childbirth, marriage, and death. The rituals and customs of a group are a reflection of the group's values. Therefore, the identification of cultural values is useful in predicting reactions to pregnancy. An understanding of male and female roles, family lifestyles, religious values, or the meaning of children in a culture may explain reactions of joy or shame.

Generalization about cultural characteristics or values is difficult because not every individual in a culture may display these characteristics. Just as variations are seen between cultures, variations are also seen within cultures. For example, because of their exposure to the American culture, a third-generation Chinese American family might have different values and beliefs from those of a Chinese family that has recently immigrated to America. For this reason, the nurse needs to supplement a general knowledge of cultural values and practices with a complete assessment of the individual's values and practices. The Focus on Diversity and Culture feature summarizes the key actions a nurse can take to become more culturally aware.

Cultural assessment is an important aspect of prenatal care. Increasingly, healthcare professionals know that they must address cultural needs during a prenatal assessment to provide culturally competent health care during pregnancy. The nurse needs to identify the prospective parents' main beliefs, values, and behaviors related to pregnancy and childbearing. This includes information about ethnic background, degree of affiliation with the ethnic group, patterns of decision making, religious preference, language, communication style, and common etiquette practices. The nurse also can explore the woman's (or family's) expectations of the healthcare system. Once this information has been gathered, the nurse can plan and provide care that is appropriate and responsive to family needs.

Focus on Diversity and Culture Providing Culturally Competent Care

Nurses who are interacting with expectant families from a different culture or ethnic group can provide more effective, culturally competent nursing care by

- Critically examining their own cultural beliefs
- Identifying personal biases, attitudes, stereotypes, and prejudices
- Making a conscious commitment to respect and study the values and beliefs of others
- Using sensitive, current language when describing others' cultures
- Learning the rituals, customs, and practices of the major cultural and ethnic groups with whom they have contact
- Including cultural assessment and assessment of the family's expectations of the healthcare system as a routine part of prenatal nursing care

- Incorporating the family's cultural and spiritual practices into prenatal care as much as possible
- Fostering an attitude of respect for and cooperation with alternative healers and caregivers when possible
- Providing for the services of an interpreter when language barriers exist
- Learning the language (or at least several key phrases) of at least one of the cultural groups with whom they interact
- Recognizing that ultimately it is the woman's right to make her own healthcare choices
- Evaluating whether the client's healthcare beliefs have any potential negative consequences for her health.

CASE STUDY \\ PART 1

Emma Halleck is a 22-year-old White female who presented at the antepartum clinic on June 15. She suspects that she is pregnant: A home pregnancy test was positive. Her last menstrual period began on April 10. She reports having urinary frequency, breast tenderness, fatigue, and occasional nausea and vomiting. She has begun to have some light-headedness and dizziness when she first gets up after sitting or sleeping.

Mrs. Halleck tells you she is married and states that this is her second pregnancy. She miscarried at 10 weeks approximately 6 months ago. She denies any history of drug or alcohol use, sexually transmitted infections (STIs), multiple partners, family violence, medical-surgical disorders, or mental illness. Mrs. Halleck is excited about the pregnancy, and she reports that her husband is too. She does express concern over carrying the pregnancy to term, although she feels relieved that she is beyond the time of her first pregnancy loss. This pregnancy was a planned pregnancy. Mrs. Halleck is a college graduate, employed as a teacher, and has group health insurance through the local public school system.

Exam

Weight 122 lb (prepregnant weight usually between 115 and 120 lb)

Height 5'4"

BP 110/60 mmHg, P 82 bpm, R 16/min

Hgb 12, Hct 33%, WBC 5,000

UA, blood glucose and protein all negative

Rubella titer—within normal limits

HIV, STIs—negative

Hepatitis antibody—negative

Immunoassay pregnancy test—positive

Mother: O Rh negative; father: O Rh positive.

On pelvic exam, the physician determines that Mrs. Halleck's uterus is enlarged and at the top of the symphysis pubis. The lower uterine segment is soft; the cervix is soft and bluish in color. There is an increase in vaginal and cervical secretions. The physician determines that Mrs. Halleck's pelvis is adequate for a normal vaginal birth. Vaginal ultrasound confirms pregnancy with fetal heart tones at 120 beats per minute.

Clinical Reasoning Questions Level I

1. Why is Mrs. Halleck experiencing urinary frequency?
2. Why is Mrs. Halleck having breast tenderness at this time?
3. Are light-headedness and dizziness normal? Why or why not? What nursing intervention should be taught to all pregnant women to avoid these symptoms?

Clinical Reasoning Questions Level II

4. Are the uterine changes assessed on examination considered normal? Why or why not?
5. How does the body maintain pregnancy during the first 12 weeks?
6. Which developmental stage of pregnancy is Mrs. Halleck in? How did you determine this?
7. How would you assess whether fetal attachment is occurring?

▶ ALTERATIONS IN REPRODUCTION THAT OCCUR DURING PREGNANCY

Pregnancy affects all body systems and many concepts. The Concepts Related to Reproduction table outlines some of the alterations to sexuality, safety, comfort, perfusion, nutrition, metabolism, and oxygenation that are related to pregnancy.

Adolescent Pregnancy

Adolescent pregnancy is a health and social issue with no single cause or cure. For the adolescent, pregnancy comes at a time when her physical development and the developmental tasks of adolescence are incomplete. She may not be prepared physically, psychologically, or economically for parenthood. Thus

Concepts Related to **Reproduction**

CONCEPT	RELATIONSHIP TO REPRODUCTION	NURSING IMPLICATIONS
Sexuality		
■ Family planning ■ Contraception ■ Sexually transmitted infections	Unprotected intercourse ↑ likelihood of pregnancy, ↑ risk for sexually transmitted infections.	■ Educate client regarding safer sex practices. ■ Assess risk factors. ■ Provide additional education related to risk factors.
Comfort		
■ Acute and chronic pain	Pregnancy discomforts Labor pain Postpartum pain	■ Pregnancy: provide comfort measures for common discomforts. ■ Labor: provide comfort measures for labor (relaxation, hot/cold, positioning, ambulating, birthing balls, hydrotherapy), medications for pain relief including IVP and epidurals. ■ Postpartum: Provide instruction on Kegel exercises, sitz baths.
Perfusion		
■ Perfusion assessment ■ Collaborative interventions and therapies ■ Congenital heart defects ■ Hypertensive disorders in pregnancy	↓ tissue perfusion creates oxygen deficit to organs.	■ Assess perfusion including pulses, nail beds, color, body position for comfort, orientation. ■ Be alert for tachycardia, then hypotension, cool clammy skin, altered LOC. ■ Administer oxygen. ■ Replace IV fluids. ■ Weigh pads. ■ Administer pharmacotherapy to contract uterus.
Nutrition		

■ Nutrition assessment
■ Nutritional status
■ Lifespan considerations: nutrition
	Prenatal nutrition is critical for a healthy fetus.
	Breastfeeding
		■ Educate client on need to increase calories and fluid intake and on safe food consumption during pregnancy.
		■ Provide health promotion strategies to enhance infant health:
		  • Easily digested foods
		  • Decreased allergies, risk for illness
		  • Promotion of self-regulation of feedings.

Metabolism		
■ Endocrine assessments ■ Diabetes	Diabetes, gestational diabetes ↑ risks to both mother and infant.	■ Assess for signs/symptoms of hypoglycemia and hyperglycemia. ■ Encourage 30 minutes of exercise after each meal. ■ Conduct fetal kick counts twice daily beginning at 28 weeks. ■ Teach blood glucose monitoring. ■ Refer to dietitian. ■ Encourage frequent prenatal visits. ■ Encourage verbalization of feelings related to diabetes diagnosis.
Oxygenation		
■ Oxygenation assessment ■ Asthma and pregnancy	Untreated or under-treated respiratory disease ↑ risk of inadequate oxygenation to fetus.	■ Educate client regarding need to adhere to therapeutic regimen for respiratory conditions such as asthma. ■ Refer clients who need specialized care who do not already have a provider (e.g., pulmonologist). ■ Assess respiratory status, client signs/symptoms at each healthcare interaction.

both she and her child are at high risk for a number of adverse outcomes. Compared with women of similar socioeconomic status who postpone childbearing, teen mothers are less likely to finish high school, less likely to go to college, more likely to be single, less likely to receive child support, and more likely to require public assistance. Babies of adolescent mothers are at an increased risk for preterm birth, low birth weight, and infant mortality. In addition, children of teen mothers are tend to score lower on assessments of knowledge, language development, and cognition. They are also more likely to grow up without a father. In addition, children of adolescent mothers are at an increased risk for abuse and neglect (National Campaign to Prevent Teen and Unplanned Pregnancy, 2010).

✳ To read more about adolescent pregnancy, see the Mini-Module at **nursing.pearsonhighered.com**.

Pregnancy Over Age 35

An increasing number of women are choosing to have their first baby after age 35. Many factors contribute to this trend, including the following:

- The availability of effective birth control methods
- The expanded roles and career options available to women
- The increased number of women obtaining advanced education, pursuing careers, and delaying parenthood until they are established professionally
- The increased incidence of later marriage and second marriage
- The high cost of living, which causes some young couples to delay childbearing until they are more secure financially
- The increased number of women in this older reproductive age group because of the baby boom between 1946 and 1964
- The increased availability of specialized fertilization procedures, which offers opportunities for women who had previously been considered infertile,

There are advantages to having a first baby after the age of 35. Single women or couples who delay childbearing until they are older tend to be well educated and financially secure. Usually their decision to have a baby was deliberately and thoughtfully made. Because of their life experiences, they are also more aware of the realities of having a child than younger women, and they recognize what it means to have a baby at their age. This delay in family allows for women to pursue advanced educational degrees and prepare financially for the impact children will have on their lives. Some women are ready to make a change in their lives, desiring to stay home with a new baby. Those who plan to continue working outside the home are typically able to afford good child care.

MEDICAL RISKS   In the United States and Canada during the past 30 years, the risk of death has declined dramatically for women of all ages as a result of advances in maternal health and obstetric practice. However, the risk for maternal death is significantly higher for women over age 35 and even higher for women ages 40 and older. These women also are more likely to have chronic medical conditions. Preexisting medical conditions, such as hypertension or diabetes, probably play a more

significant role than age in maternal well-being and the outcome of pregnancy. The incidence of low-birth-weight infants and preterm births is higher among women ages 35 and older (Delbaere et al., 2007). In addition, the rate of miscarriage is significantly higher in older women. Women over age 35 who become pregnant also have an increased risk for gestational diabetes mellitus, hypertension, placenta previa, difficult labor, and newborn complications (MOD, 2009). The cesarean birth rate is also higher in pregnant women over age 35. This practice may be related to increased concern by the woman and physician about the pregnancy outcome (MOD, 2009). However, these risks are much lower than previously believed for physically fit women without preexisting medical problems.

The risk of conceiving a child with Down syndrome does increase with age, especially over age 35. The American College of Obstetricians and Gynecologists (ACOG) (2007) recommends that all pregnant women, regardless of age, be screened for Down syndrome. Research has focused on the use of quadruple screening to detect Down syndrome and trisomy 18. First-trimester ultrasound assessment of the thickness of fetal nuchal folds (nuchal translucency, or NT) combined with serum screens of free beta-hCG and pregnancy-associated plasma protein A (PAPP-A) is increasing the detection of Down syndrome, trisomy 18, and trisomy 13. If the screening results are not in the normal range, follow-up testing using ultrasound and amniocentesis is often indicated (Cleveland Clinic, 2006).

Amniocentesis or non-invasive prenatal testing through cell free DNA are routinely offered to all women over age 35 to permit the early detection of several chromosomal abnormalities, including Down syndrome. Routine genetic testing has not been offered to couples when the only risk is advanced paternal age, because there is insufficient evidence to determine a specific paternal age at which to start genetic testing. Advanced paternal age is associated with adverse fetal and neonatal outcomes, including an increased risk for autism spectrum disorders.

SPECIAL CONCERNS OF THE EXPECTANT COUPLE OVER AGE 35   No matter what their age, most expectant couples have concerns regarding the well-being of the fetus and their ability to parent. The older couple has additional concerns related to their age, especially if they are over 40. Some couples are concerned about whether they will have enough energy to care for a new baby. Of greater concern is their ability to deal with the needs of the older child as they themselves age.

The financial concerns of an older couple are usually different from those of a younger couple. The older couple is generally more financially secure than the younger couple. However, when their "baby" is ready for college, the older couple may be near retirement and might not have the means to provide for their child.

While considering their financial future and future retirement, the older couple may be forced to face their own mortality. Certainly this is not uncommon in midlife, but instead of confronting this issue at 40–45 years of age or later, the older expectant couple may confront the issue several years earlier as they consider what will happen as their child grows.

The older couple facing pregnancy following a late or second marriage or after therapy for infertility may find themselves somewhat isolated socially. They may feel "different" because they are often the only couple in their peer group expecting their first baby. In fact, many of their peers are likely to be parents of adolescents or young adults and may be grandparents as well.

The response of older couples who already have children to learning that the woman is pregnant may vary greatly depending on whether the pregnancy was planned or unexpected. Other factors influencing their response include the attitudes of the couple's children, family, and friends to the pregnancy; the impact on their lifestyle; and the financial implications of having another child. Sometimes couples who had previously been married to other mates will choose to have a child together. The concept of blended family applies to situations in which "her" children, "his" children, and "their" children come together as a new family group.

The woman who has delayed pregnancy may be concerned about the limited amount of time that she has to bear children. When pregnancy does not occur as quickly as she hoped, the older woman may become increasingly anxious as time slips away on her "biological clock." When an older woman becomes pregnant but experiences a spontaneous abortion, her grief for the loss of her unborn child is exacerbated by her anxiety about her ability to conceive again in the time remaining to her.

Healthcare professionals may treat the older expectant couple differently than they would a younger couple. Older women may be offered more medical procedures, such as amniocentesis and ultrasound, than younger women. An older woman may be prevented from using a birthing room or birthing center even if she is healthy, because her age is considered to put her at risk.

Anemia During Pregnancy

Anemia indicates inadequate levels of hemoglobin (Hb) in the blood. Anemia is defined as hemoglobin less than 12 g/dL in nonpregnant women and less than 11 g/dL in pregnant women (ACOG, 2008a). Ethnicity, altitude, smoking, nutrition, and medications can affect the normal limits of hemoglobin. The lower limit of normal tends to be higher for women who smoke and those who live at higher altitudes because their bodies require a greater quantity of red blood cells to maintain their tissue oxygen levels. The common anemias of pregnancy are due either to insufficient hemoglobin production related to nutritional deficiency in iron or folic acid during pregnancy, or to hemoglobin destruction in inherited disorders, specifically sickle cell disease and thalassemia.

IRON DEFICIENCY ANEMIA   Iron deficiency anemia is the most common medical complication of pregnancy, primarily as a consequence of expansion of plasma volume without normal expansion of maternal hemoglobin mass (ACOG, 2008a). The greatest need for increased iron intake occurs in the second half of pregnancy. When the iron needs of pregnancy are not met, maternal hemoglobin falls below 11 g/dL. Serum ferritin levels, indicating iron stores, are below 12 mg/L.

The woman with iron deficiency anemia may be asymptomatic, but she is more susceptible to infection and has an increased chance of elevated blood pressure in pregnancy and postpartum hemorrhage. There is evidence of increased risk of low birth weight, prematurity, stillbirth, and neonatal death in infants of women with severe iron deficiency (maternal Hb less than 6 g/dL). The infant is not iron deficient at birth because of active transport of iron across the placenta, even when maternal iron stores are low. However, these babies do have lower iron stores and are at increased risk for developing iron deficiency during infancy.

The first goal of health care is to prevent iron deficiency anemia. To prevent anemia, the AAP and ACOG (2013) recommend that pregnant women supplement their diet with at least 30 mg of iron daily. This amount is contained in most prenatal vitamins. In addition, the woman should be encouraged to eat an iron-rich diet. If anemia is diagnosed, the dosage should be increased to 60–120 mg/day of iron. If the woman remains anemic after 1 month of therapy, further evaluation is indicated.

FOLIC ACID DEFICIENCY ANEMIA   Folate deficiency is the most common cause of megaloblastic anemia during pregnancy. Folic acid is needed for deoxyribonucleic acid (DNA) and ribonucleic acid (RNA) synthesis and cell duplication. In its absence, immature red blood cells fail to divide, become enlarged (megaloblastic), and are fewer in number. Even more significantly, an inadequate intake of folic acid has been associated with neural tube defects (NTDs) (spina bifida, anencephaly, meningomyelocele) in the fetus or newborn. With the tremendous cell multiplication that occurs in pregnancy, an adequate amount of folic acid is crucial. However, increased urinary excretion of folic acid and fetal uptake can rapidly result in folic acid deficiency.

Diagnosis of folic acid deficiency anemia may be difficult, and it is usually not detected until late in pregnancy or the early puerperium. This is because serum folate levels normally fall as pregnancy progresses. Even though folate levels are lower with deficiency, they will fluctuate with diet. Measurement of erythrocyte folate status is more reliable but indicates the folate status of several weeks previously. Women with true folic acid deficiency anemia often present with nausea, vomiting, and anorexia. Hemoglobin levels as low as 3–5 g/dL may be found. Typically the blood smear reveals that the newly formed erythrocytes are macrocytic.

Folic acid deficiency during pregnancy is prevented by a daily supplement of 0.4 mg of folate. Treatment of deficiency consists of 1-mg folic acid supplements. Because iron deficiency anemia almost always coexists with folic acid deficiency, the woman also needs iron supplements. The Food and Drug Administration (FDA) requires the addition of folic acid for all foods labeled "enriched." Even with this addition, the U.S. Public Health Service recommends that all women of childbearing age (15–45 years) consume 0.4 mg of folic acid daily. This recommendation is important because half of all U.S. pregnancies are unplanned and NTDs occur very early in pregnancy (3–4 weeks after conception), before most women realize they are pregnant (AAP & ACOG, 2013). Nurses can play a crucial role in helping young women become aware of this important recommendation.

Sickle Cell Disease

Sickle cell disease (SCD) is an autosomal recessive disorder in which the normal adult hemoglobin, hemoglobin A (HbA), is abnormally formed. This abnormal hemoglobin is called hemoglobin S (HbS). Approximately 1 in 12 African Americans has sickle cell trait and 1 in every 300 African American newborns has some form of sickle cell disease (ACOG, 2007). Diagnosis is confirmed by hemoglobin electrophoresis or a test to induce sickling in a blood sample. Prenatal diagnosis and newborn screening for sickle cell disease are important components of perinatal care (ACOG, 2007).

Women with sickle cell trait have a good prognosis for pregnancy if they have adequate nutrition and prenatal care. Maternal mortality due to sickle cell disease is rare. However, sickle cell crisis occurred in 47% of clients in one cohort study (Yu et al., 2009). Complications include anemia requiring blood transfusion, infections, and emergency cesarean births. Acute chest syndrome, congestive heart failure, or acute renal failure may also occur. Prematurity and intrauterine growth restriction (IUGR) are also associated with sickle cell disease. Fetal death is believed to be due to sickling attacks in the placenta.

Because the woman with sickle cell disease maintains her hemoglobin levels by intense erythropoiesis, additional folic acid supplements (4 mg/day) are required. Maternal infection should be treated promptly because dehydration and fever can trigger sickling and crisis. Vaso-occlusive crisis is best treated by a perinatal team in a medical center. Proper management requires close observation and evaluation of all symptoms. The term *sickle cell crisis* should be applied only after all other possible causes for the pain are excluded (Creary et al., 2007).

Diabetes During Pregnancy

Carbohydrate metabolism is affected early in pregnancy by a rise in serum levels of estrogen, progesterone, and other hormones. These hormones stimulate maternal insulin production and increase tissue response to insulin; therefore, anabolism (building up) of glycogen stores in the liver and other tissues occurs.

In the second half of pregnancy, the woman demonstrates prolonged hyperglycemia and hyperinsulinemia (increased secretion of insulin) following a meal. Although the mother is producing more insulin, placental secretion of hPL and prolactin (from the decidua), as well as elevated levels of cortisol (an adrenal hormone) and glycogen, causes increased maternal peripheral resistance to insulin. This resistance helps ensure that a sustained supply of glucose is available for the fetus. This glucose is transported across the placenta to the fetus, who uses it as a major source of fuel. Maternal amino acids are also actively transported by the placenta from the mother to her fetus. The fetus uses these amino acids for protein synthesis and as a source of energy. In addition to ensuring that glucose is available to the fetus, the increased maternal resistance to insulin means that the pregnant woman has a lower peripheral uptake of glucose to meet her own needs. This results in a catabolic (destructive) state during fasting periods (e.g., during the night and after meal absorption). Because increasing amounts of circulating maternal glucose are being diverted to the fetus, maternal fat is metabolized (lipolysis) during fasting periods much more readily than in a nonpregnant individual. This process is called *accelerated starvation*. Ketones may be present in the urine as a result of lipolysis.

The delicate system of checks and balances that exists between glucose production and glucose use is stressed by the growing fetus, who derives energy from glucose taken from the mother, and by maternal resistance to the insulin her body produces. This stress is referred to as the diabetogenic effect of pregnancy. Thus any preexisting disruption in carbohydrate metabolism is augmented by pregnancy, and any diabetic potential may precipitate gestational diabetes mellitus.

GESTATIONAL DIABETES MELLITUS   **Gestational diabetes mellitus (GDM)** is defined as a carbohydrate intolerance of variable severity with onset or first recognition during pregnancy. It results from (1) an unidentified preexisting disease, (2) the unmasking of a compensated metabolic abnormality by the added stress of pregnancy, or (3) is a direct consequence of the altered maternal metabolism stemming from changing hormonal levels. Diagnosis of GDM is important because even mild diabetes increases the risk of perinatal morbidity and mortality. Many women with GDM progress over time to overt type 2 diabetes mellitus.

INFLUENCE OF PREEXISTING AND GESTATIONAL DIABETES DURING PREGNANCY   Pregnancy can affect diabetes significantly. First, the physiological changes of pregnancy can drastically alter insulin requirements. Second, pregnancy may accelerate the progress of vascular disease secondary to diabetes.

The disease may be more difficult to control during pregnancy because insulin requirements are changeable. Insulin needs frequently decrease early in the first trimester. Levels of hPL, an insulin antagonist, are low; energy demands of the fetus are minimal; and the woman may be consuming less food because of nausea and vomiting. Nausea and vomiting may also cause dietary fluctuations, which can increase the risk of hypoglycemia or insulin shock. Insulin requirements usually begin to rise late in the first trimester as glucose use and glycogen storage by the woman and fetus increase. As a result of placental maturation and production of hPL and other hormones, insulin requirements may double or quadruple by the end of pregnancy.

Because her energy needs increase during labor, the woman with diabetes may require more insulin at that time to balance intravenous glucose. After delivery of the placenta, insulin requirements usually decrease abruptly with loss of hPL in the maternal circulation.

Other factors contribute to the difficulty in controlling the disease. As pregnancy progresses, the renal threshold for glucose decreases. There is an increased risk of ketoacidosis, which may occur at lower serum glucose levels in the pregnant woman with diabetes than in the nonpregnant woman with diabetes. The vascular disease that accompanies diabetes may progress during pregnancy. Hypertension may occur. Nephropathy may result from renal blood vessel impairment, and retinopathy may develop (from occlusion of the microscopic blood vessels of the eye).

INFLUENCE OF PREEXISTING AND GESTATIONAL DIABETES ON PREGNANCY OUTCOME   The pregnancy of a woman who has diabetes carries a higher risk of complications than a normal pregnancy, especially perinatal mortality and congenital anomalies. The risk has been reduced by the recent recognition of the importance of tight metabolic control (fasting, pre-meal, and bedtime blood glucose levels of 60-95 mg/dL; peak postprandial blood glucose levels of 100-129 mg/dL; and glycohemoglobin less than 6%). New techniques for monitoring blood glucose, delivering insulin, and monitoring the fetus have also reduced perinatal mortality (ACOG, 2005).

Maternal Risks   Maternal health problems in diabetic pregnancy have been greatly reduced by the team approach to preconception planning and early prenatal care and by the increased emphasis on maintaining tight control of blood glucose levels. The prognosis for the pregnant woman with gestational, type 1, or type 2 diabetes that has not resulted in significant vascular damage is positive. However, diabetic pregnancy still carries higher risks for complications than normal pregnancy.

Hydramnios, or an increase in the volume of amniotic fluid, occurs in 10%–20% of pregnant women with diabetes. It is thought to be a result of excessive fetal urination because of fetal hyperglycemia (Rinala, Dryfhout, & Lambers, 2009). *Preeclampsia–eclampsia* occurs more often in diabetic pregnancies, especially when diabetes-related vascular changes already exist.

Hyperglycemia due to insufficient amounts of insulin can lead to *ketoacidosis* as a result of the increase in ketone bodies (which are acidic) in the blood released when fatty acids are metabolized. Ketoacidosis usually develops slowly, but it may develop more rapidly in the pregnant woman because of the hyperketonemia associated with accelerated starvation in the fasting state. The tendency for higher postprandial glucose levels because of decreased gastric motility and the contrainsulin effects of hPL also predispose the woman to ketoacidosis. If the ketoacidosis is not treated, it can lead to coma and death of both mother and fetus.

Another risk to the pregnant woman with diabetes is a difficult labor (*dystocia*), caused by fetopelvic disproportion if fetal macrosomia (>4,000 g) exists. The pregnant woman with diabetes is also at increased risk for recurrent monilial vaginitis (yeast infection) and urinary tract infections because of increased glycosuria, which contributes to a favorable environment for bacterial growth. If untreated, asymptomatic bacteriuria can lead to pyelonephritis, a serious kidney infection.

Several studies have demonstrated that pregnancy worsens *retinopathy* in women with diabetes. Most investigators agree that during a diabetic pregnancy, good control of blood glucose levels and the use of laser photocoagulation (a treatment used to prevent retinal hemorrhage when the retina shows changes in the blood vessels) when indicated minimize the risk of the negative effects of pregnancy. Hence, women with preexisting diabetes should be referred to an ophthalmologist for evaluation during pregnancy (ACOG, 2005).

Fetal–Neonatal Risks   Many of the problems of the newborn result directly from high maternal plasma glucose levels. In the presence of severe maternal ketoacidosis, the risk of fetal death has ranged from 35% to a decrease more recently of 10% (ACOG, 2005). Fetal enzyme systems cease functioning in an acidic environment.

The incidence of *congenital anomalies* in diabetic pregnancies is 6%–12% and is the major cause of death for infants of mothers with diabetes. Research suggests that this increased incidence of congenital anomalies is related to multiple factors including high glucose levels in early pregnancy (Eriksson, 2009). The anomalies often involve the heart, CNS, and skeletal system. Septal defects, coarctation of the aorta, and transposition of the great vessels are the most common heart lesions seen. CNS anomalies include hydrocephalus, meningomyelocele, and anencephaly. One anomaly, *sacral agenesis*, appears only in infants of mothers with diabetes. In sacral agenesis, the sacrum and lumbar spine fail to develop and the lower extremities develop incompletely. To reduce the incidence of congenital anomalies, preconception counseling and strict diabetes control before conception and in the early weeks of pregnancy are indicated.

Characteristically, infants of mothers with diabetes are large for gestational age (LGA) as a result of high levels of fetal insulin production stimulated by the high levels of glucose crossing the placenta from the mother. Sustained fetal hyperinsulinism and hyperglycemia ultimately lead to *macrosomia*, and deposition of fat. If born vaginally, the macrosomic infant is at increased risk for birth trauma such as fractured clavicle or brachial plexus injuries due to shoulder dystocia. Shoulder dystocia occurs when, following birth of the head, the anterior shoulder of the macrosomic fetus does not emerge either spontaneously or with gentle traction (Cunningham et al., 2010). Macrosomia can be significantly reduced by tight maternal blood glucose control.

After birth, the umbilical cord is severed and, thus, the generous maternal blood glucose supply is eliminated. However, continued islet cell hyperactivity leads to excessive insulin levels and depleted blood glucose (hypoglycemia) within 2–4 hours after birth in the neonate. Infants of mothers with diabetes with vascular involvement (see the module on Metabolism) may demonstrate IUGR. This occurs because vascular changes in the mother decrease the efficiency of placental perfusion, and the fetus is not as well sustained in utero. *Respiratory distress syndrome* appears to result from inhibition, by high levels of fetal insulin, of some fetal enzymes necessary for surfactant production. Polycythemia in the newborn is due primarily to the diminished ability of glycosylated hemoglobin in the mother's blood to release oxygen. *Hyperbilirubinemia* is a result of the inability of immature liver enzymes to metabolize the increased bilirubin resulting from the polycythemia. Hypocalcemia, characterized by signs of irritability or even tetany, may occur. The cause of these low calcium levels in infants of mothers with diabetes is not known.

CLINICAL THERAPY   Gestational diabetes is more common than preexisting diabetes. It is estimated to occur in from 6% to 7% of pregnancies, depending on the population studied (ACOG, 2013). Therefore, screening for its detection is a standard part of prenatal care. If diabetes is suspected, further testing is undertaken for diagnosis.

All pregnant women should have their risk of diabetes assessed at the first prenatal visit. Women at high risk (prior history of GDM or birth of an LGA infant, marked obesity, diagnosis of polycystic ovarian syndrome, presence of glycos-uria, or a strong family history of type 2 diabetes mellitus [DM]) should be screened for diabetes as soon as possible. Various screening approaches may be used. Hb A_1c equal to or greater than 6.5% would be considered diagnostic as would a fasting plasma glucose level equal to or greater than 126 mg/dL (American Diabetes Association [ADA], 2010).

Two approaches to prenatal screening are currently available and performed at 24 to 28 weeks' gestation for all pregnant women not previously diagnosed with DM (ADA, 2014). In the two-step approach, the first step is to give the woman a non-fasting, 50-g, 1-hour oral glucose tolerance test (OGTT). The oral glucose load can be given at any time of the day with no requirement for fasting. One hour later plasma glucose is mea-sured. If plasma glucose levels are elevated (equal to or greater than 140 mg/dL, depending on the laboratory used), a 100-g, 3-hour glucose test is done. In the second step, a 100-g, 3-hour OGTT is administered. The woman eats an unrestricted diet, consuming at least 150 g of carbohydrates per day for at least 3 days before her scheduled test. She then ingests a 100-g oral glucose solution in the morning after an overnight fast. Plasma glucose is measured fasting and at 1, 2, and 3 hours. A diagnosis of GDM occurs if two or more of the following values are met or exceeded:

Fasting	95 mg/dL
1 hour	180 mg/dL
2 hours	155 mg/dL
3 hours	140 mg/dL

In the one-step approach the woman ingests a 75-g oral glu-cose solution in the morning after an overnight fast. Plasma glucose levels are determined fasting and at 1 and 2 hours. A diagnosed of GDM occurs if any one of the following values are equaled or exceeded:.

Fasting	92 mg/dL
1 hour	180 mg/dL
2 hours	153 mg/dL

Laboratory Assessment of Long-Term Glucose Control

Glycosylated hemoglobin (Hb A_1c) is a laboratory test that loosely reflects glucose control over the previous 4–8 weeks. It measures the percentage of glycohemoglobin in the blood. Gly-cohemoglobin is the hemoglobin to which a glucose molecule is attached. The test is not reliable for screening for gestational dia-betes and is not recommended at this time (Gandhia et al., 2008).

In women with known pregestational diabetes, however, abnormal Hb A_1c values correlate directly with the frequency of spontaneous abortion and fetal congenital anomalies. A value greater than 10% is associated with a fetal anomaly rate of 20%–25% (ACOG, 2005). Consequently, women with preexisting dia-betes who plan to become pregnant should work to achieve Hb A_1c levels at target levels (less than 6%) without significant hypoglycemia. Once the woman is pregnant, her Hb A_1c levels should be tested at the initial prenatal visit and every 2–3 months if target levels have been achieved (Kitzmiller et al., 2008).

Diet therapy and regular exercise form the cornerstone of intervention for GDM. Insulin therapy is indicated when

dietary management is unable to achieve a 1-hour postprandial blood glucose value of less than 130–140 mg/dL, a 2-hour post-prandial level of less than 120 mg/dL, or a fasting glucose of less than 95 mg/dL. In most instances, the overt diabetic manifesta-tion disappears postpartum, though subtle manifestations of impaired insulin secretory capacity may remain.

Oral hypoglycemics are used during pregnancy when needed, with Glyburide being the most common.

Evaluation of Fetal Status Information about the well-being, maturation, and size of the fetus is important for planning the course of the pregnancy and the timing of birth. Because pregnancies complicated by pre-existing diabetes are at increased risk of neural tube defects, a quadruple screen, which includes testing for maternal serum α-*fetoprotein (AFP)*, is offered at weeks 16–20 of gestation. Daily maternal evaluation of *fetal activity*, begun at about 28 weeks, is effective and simple to do. The woman is taught a particular method for counting fetal movements.

Nonstress testing (NST) may be started at about 28 weeks. If evidence of IUGR, preeclampsia, oligohydramnios, or poorly controlled blood glucose exists, testing may begin as early as 23 weeks and may be done more often. NSTs are increased to twice weekly at 32 weeks' gestation. If the NST is nonreactive, a fetal biophysical profile is performed. If the woman requires hospitalization (for example, to control glycemia or for compli-cations), NSTs may be done daily.

Ultrasound at 18 weeks confirms gestational age and diag-noses multiple pregnancy or congenital anomalies. It is repeated at 28 weeks to monitor fetal growth for IUGR or mac-rosomia. Some physicians order *fetal biophysical profiles* (ultra-sound evaluation of fetal well-being in which fetal breathing movements, fetal activity, reactivity, muscle tone, and amniotic fluid volume are assessed) as part of an ongoing evaluation of fetal status.

INTRAPARTUM MANAGEMENT OF PREEXISTING AND GESTATIONAL DIABETES MELLITUS
During the intrapartum period, medical therapy includes the following:

- *Timing of birth.* Most diabetic pregnancies go to term, with spontaneous labor, thereby decreasing the risk of respiratory distress in the newborn. Some clinicians do opt to induce labor in a woman at term to avoid problems related to decreased perfusion as the placenta ages. Cesarean birth may be indicated if evidence of nonreassuring fetal status exists. Birth before term may be indicated for women with diabetes who have vascular changes and worsening hyper-tension or if evidence of IUGR exists (ACOG, 2005). In pregnancies in which there is evidence of fetal macrosomia, fetal compromise, or elevated maternal Hb A_1c, amniocente-sis for fetal lung maturity may be indicated.

- *Labor management.* The degree of prenatal maintenance of normal maternal glucose levels (euglycemia) and the maintenance of maternal euglycemia during labor are important in preventing neonatal hypoglycemia. Maternal insulin requirements often decrease dramatically during labor. Consequently, maternal glucose levels are measured hourly to determine insulin need. The primary goal in controlling intrapartum maternal glucose levels is to prevent neonatal hypoglycemia (ACOG, 2005). During active labor, insulin may not be needed. Long-acting insulin should be reduced or stopped and regular insulin should be used to meet most or all of the woman's identified needs. Often two intravenous lines are used, one with a 5% dextrose solution and one with a saline solution. The saline solution is then available if a bolus is needed or for piggybacking insulin. Because insulin clings to the plastic intravenous bag and tubing, the intravenous tubing must be flushed with insulin before the prescribed amount is added to ensure that the woman receives the desired dose. During the second stage of labor and the immediate postpartum period, the woman may not need additional insulin. The intravenous insulin is discontinued with the completion of the third stage of labor.

POSTPARTUM MANAGEMENT OF PREEXISTING AND GESTATIONAL DIABETES MELLITUS

Maternal insulin requirements fall significantly postpartum because the levels of hPL, progesterone, and estrogen fall after placental separation, and their anti-insulin effect ceases, resulting in decreased blood glucose levels. The mother with diabetes may require no insulin for the first 24 hours or only one fourth to one half of her previous dose. Then, reestablishment of insulin needs based on blood glucose testing is necessary. Diet and exercise levels must also be re-established. Consequently, the woman with diabetes that is not controlled by diet alone may need insulin for a period of time (ACOG, 2005).

Women with GDM who did not require insulin during pregnancy generally do not need it during the postpartum period. Clinicians routinely discontinue insulin for women with GDM following childbirth and then monitor blood glucose levels. If elevated glucose levels develop, oral antihyperglycemic agents may be tried if the woman is not breastfeeding (ACOG, 2005). Antihyperglycemics are contraindicated during breastfeeding. The woman should be reassessed 6 weeks postpartum to determine whether her glucose levels are normal. If her levels are normal, she should be reassessed at a minimum of 3-year intervals (ACOG, 2009d).

Refer to the exemplar on Diabetes in the module on Metabolism for more information on diabetes.

Cardiac Disease During Pregnancy

Heart disease ranks fourth after hypertension, hemorrhage, and infection as a cause of maternal mortality. Currently, cardiac disease complicates about 1% of pregnancies. Although rheumatic heart disease used to dominate, at least half of all cases of heart disease currently encountered during pregnancy are caused by congenital heart defects (Curry, Swan, & Steer, 2009).

CONGENITAL HEART DEFECTS

Congenital heart defects have become a more common finding in pregnant women as improved surgical techniques enable females born with heart defects to live to childbearing age. The exact pathology depends on the specific defect. Congenital defects most often seen in pregnant women include tetralogy of Fallot, atrial septal defect, ventricular septal defect, patent ductus arteriosus, and coarctation of the aorta. When surgical repair can be accomplished with no remaining evidence of organic heart disease, pregnancy may be undertaken with confidence. In such cases, antibiotic prophylaxis is recommended to prevent subacute bacterial endocarditis at the time of birth. When congenital heart disease is associated with cyanosis, whether the defect was originally uncorrected or the correction failed to relieve the cyanosis, the woman should be counseled that the risk to both her and the fetus would be higher than in the general population. She also needs to know that there is an increased risk that the baby will inherit the disorder.

MARFAN SYNDROME

Marfan syndrome is an autosomal dominant disorder of connective tissue in which there may be serious cardiovascular involvement—usually dissection or rupture of the aorta. Because there may be a fivefold increase in morbidity during pregnancy, a pregnant woman with Marfan syndrome needs very careful cardiovascular assessment and counseling about her prognosis for pregnancy (Pacini et al., 2009). Because of its inheritance pattern, there is a 50% chance that the disease will be passed on to offspring.

PERIPARTUM CARDIOMYOPATHY

Peripartum cardiomyopathy is a dysfunction of the left ventricle that occurs in the last month of pregnancy or the first 5 months postpartum in a woman with no previous history of heart disease. This is a relatively rare but serious condition, which occurs in 1 in 3,000 to 4,000 live births. Early reports suggested a mortality rate of nearly 50%, but more recent studies indicate a 0%–5% rate in the United States (Ramaraj & Sorrell, 2009). The symptoms are related to CHF: dyspnea, orthopnea, chest pain, palpitations, weakness, and edema. The cause is unknown, although symptoms are often attributable to chronic hypertension, mitral stenosis, obesity, or viral myocarditis. The condition usually presents with anemia and infection; consequently, treatment focuses on underlying abnormalities. Digitalis, diuretics, vasodilators, anticoagulants, sodium restriction, and strict bed rest are often part of the treatment. Peripartum cardiomyopathy may resolve with bed rest as the heart gradually returns to its normal size. Subsequent pregnancy is strongly discouraged because the disease tends to recur during pregnancy.

MITRAL VALVE PROLAPSE

Mitral valve prolapse (MVP) is a usually asymptomatic condition commonly found in women of childbearing age. The condition is more common in women than in men and seems to be inherited. In MVP, the mitral valve leaflets tend to prolapse into the left atrium during ventricular systole because the chordae tendineae that support them are long and thin. As a result, some mitral regurgitation may occur. On auscultation a midsystolic click and a late systolic murmur are heard.

Women with MVP usually tolerate pregnancy well, and the prognosis is excellent. Most women require assurance that they can continue with normal activities. A few women experience symptoms such as palpitations, chest pain, and dyspnea, which are usually due to arrhythmias. They are often treated with propranolol hydrochloride. Limiting caffeine intake also helps decrease palpitations. Antibiotic prophylaxis is no longer recommended (Bonow et al., 2008).

CLINICAL THERAPY The primary goal of medical management of cardiac disease in a pregnant woman is early diagnosis and ongoing treatment. Auscultation of heart sounds along with a good history and physical are the first steps to diagnosis. Echocardiogram, chest x-ray, electrocardiogram, and sometimes cardiac catheterization may be necessary for establishing the type and severity of heart disease. The severity of heart disease can also be determined by the individual's ability to perform ordinary physical activity. The following classification of functional capacity for those with cardiac disease has been standardized by the Criteria Committee of the American Heart Association (2011):

- *Class I.* Individuals with cardiac disease but with no resulting limitation of physical activity and no symptoms of cardiac insufficiency. Ordinary physical activity causes no undue fatigue, dyspnea, or palpitations; anginal pain is not present.
- *Class II.* Individuals with cardiac disease that results in slight limitation of physical activity. They are comfortable at rest but ordinary physical activity causes fatigue, dyspnea, palpitation, or anginal pain.
- *Class III.* Individuals with cardiac disease that results in marked limitation of physical activity. They are comfortable at rest but less than ordinary physical activity results in fatigue, dyspnea, palpitation, or anginal pain.
- *Class IV.* Individuals with cardiac disease that results in the inability to carry on any physical activity without experiencing discomfort. Even at rest, they may experience symptoms of cardiac insufficiency or anginal pain; discomfort increases with any physical activity.

Women in classes I and II usually experience a normal pregnancy and have few complications. Those in classes III and IV are at risk for more severe complications, which may affect both maternal and fetal outcomes. Preconception counseling is important for women in classes III and IV to optimize maternal and fetal outcomes.

Because anemia increases the work of the heart, it should be diagnosed early and treated. Infection also increases the cardiac workload, so even minor infections should be treated thoroughly. To reduce the risk of pyelonephritis, monthly screening for asymptomatic bacteriuria is indicated, with antibiotic therapy as needed. As pregnancy progresses, it is important to minimize cardiac workload and promote tissue perfusion. Depending on the specific lesion, the woman's activity and weight gain may need to be limited (Bonow et al., 2008).

Drug Therapy Besides the iron and vitamin supplements prescribed during pregnancy, the pregnant woman with heart disease may need additional drug therapy to maintain health. Antibiotic prophylaxis is not indicated for uncomplicated vaginal or cesarean birth unless infection is suspected. If the woman develops coagulation problems, the anticoagulant heparin may be used. Heparin offers the greatest safety for the fetus because it does not cross the placenta. The thiazide diuretics and furosemide may be used to treat congestive heart failure if it develops. Digitalis glycosides and common antiarrhythmic drugs may be used to treat cardiac failure and arrhythmias. These agents do cross the placenta but have no reported teratogenic effect; however, they have not been adequately studied to establish their safety in pregnancy (Bonow et al., 2008).

Labor and Childbirth Spontaneous natural labor with adequate pain relief is usually recommended for clients in classes I and II. Special attention should be given to the prompt recognition and treatment of any signs of heart failure. Women in classes III and IV may need to be hospitalized before onset of labor for cardiovascular stabilization. They may also require invasive cardiac monitoring during labor.

Vaginal birth with low-dose regional analgesia (epidural) is recommended with the use of forceps or vacuum assistance if necessary to limit maternal pushing. The regional analgesia helps decrease maternal cardiac output and oxygen demand by reducing pain and related maternal anxiety (Burt & Durbridge, 2009). Cesarean birth is usually indicated only if fetal or maternal indications exist, not on the basis of heart disease alone.

Antepartum Period Nursing actions are designed to meet the physiological and psychosocial needs of the pregnant woman with heart disease. The woman and her family members should thoroughly understand her condition and its management and should recognize signs of potential complications. This will increase their understanding and decrease anxiety. When the nurse provides explanations, uses printed material, and offers frequent opportunities to ask questions and discuss concerns, the woman is better able to meet her own healthcare needs and seek assistance appropriately.

As part of health teaching, the nurse explains the purposes of the dietary and activity changes that are required. A diet is instituted that is high in iron, protein, and essential nutrients but low in sodium, with adequate calories to ensure normal weight gain. Such a diet best meets the nutrition needs of the client with cardiac disease. Excessive weight gain is avoided because it taxes the heart. To help preserve her cardiac reserves, the woman may need to restrict her activities. In addition, 8–10 hours of sleep and frequent daily rest periods are essential. The nurse can encourage the woman to rest in the side-lying position to promote optimal placental perfusion. Because upper respiratory infections may tax the heart and lead to decompensation, the woman must avoid contact with sources of infection and report symptoms of infection immediately.

During the first half of pregnancy, the woman is seen approximately every 2 weeks to assess cardiac status. During the second half of pregnancy, the woman is seen weekly. These assessments are especially important between weeks 28 and 30, when the blood volume reaches maximum amounts. If symptoms of cardiac decompensation occur, prompt medical intervention is indicated to correct the cardiac problem.

Intrapartum Period Labor and birth exert tremendous stress on the woman and her fetus. This stress could be fatal to the fetus of a woman with cardiac disease because the fetus may be receiving an inadequate oxygen and blood supply. Thus the intrapartum care of a woman with cardiac disease is aimed at reducing the amount of physical exertion and accompanying fatigue.

The nurse evaluates maternal vital signs frequently to determine the woman's response to labor. A pulse rate greater than 100 bpm or respirations greater than 24 per minute may indicate beginning cardiac decompensation, especially if accompanied by dyspnea, and require further evaluation. The nurse also auscultates the woman's lungs frequently for rales and carefully observes for other signs of developing decompensation. To ensure cardiac emptying and adequate oxygenation, the nurse encourages the laboring woman to assume either a semi-Fowler position with a lateral tilt or a side-lying position with her head and shoulders elevated. Oxygen by mask, diuretics to reduce fluid retention, sedatives and analgesics, prophylactic antibiotics, and digitalis may also be used as indicated by the woman's status.

Continuous electronic fetal monitoring is used to provide ongoing assessment of the fetus's response to labor. To prevent overexertion and the accompanying fatigue, the nurse encourages the woman to sleep and relax between contractions and provides her with emotional support and encouragement. During pushing, the nurse encourages the woman to use shorter, more moderate open glottis pushing, with complete relaxation between pushes. The nurse monitors vital signs closely during the second stage.

Postpartum Period The postpartum period is a significant time for the woman with cardiac disease. After birth, the intra-abdominal pressure and the venous pressure are reduced, the splanchnic vessels engorge, and blood flow to the heart increases. As extravascular fluid returns to the bloodstream for excretion, cardiac output and blood volume increase. This physiological adaptation places great strain on the heart and may lead to decompensation, especially in the first 48 hours postpartum.

So that the healthcare team can detect any possible problems, the woman may remain in the hospital longer than the low-risk woman postpartum. Her vital signs are monitored frequently, and she is assessed for signs of decompensation. She stays in the semi-Fowler or side-lying position, with her head and shoulders elevated, and begins a gradual, progressive activity program. Appropriate diet and stool softeners facilitate bowel movement without undue strain.

The postpartum nurse gives the woman opportunities to discuss her birth experience and helps her deal with any feelings or concerns that cause her distress. The nurse also encourages maternal–infant attachment by providing frequent opportunities for the mother to interact with her child.

Because there is no evidence that cardiac output is compromised during lactation, the only concern about breastfeeding for women with cardiovascular disease is related to medications that the mother may be taking. These must be evaluated for their ability to pass into the milk and for any effect of the drug on lactation. The nurse can assist the breastfeeding mother to a comfortable side-lying position with her head moderately elevated or to a semi-Fowler position. To conserve the mother's energy, the nurse should position the newborn at the breast and be available to burp the baby and reposition him or her at the other breast. The nurse can also encourage family members to provide the new mother with support and assistance as needed to help her avoid becoming fatigued.

In addition to providing the normal postpartum discharge teaching, the nurse stresses that follow-up for the new mother is imperative. Moreover, the nurse should ensure that the woman and her family understand the signs of possible problems resulting from her heart disease or from other postpartum complications. For women with heart disease, postpartum complications such as hemorrhage, thromboembolism, anemia, and infection pose a real threat and may even precipitate heart failure.

The nurse plans with the woman an activity schedule that is gradual, progressive, and appropriate to her needs and home environment. The nurse provides appropriate health teaching, including information about resumption of sexual activity and contraception. Visiting nurse or homemaker assistance referrals may be necessary, depending on the woman's status.

▶ ASSESSMENT

The nurse caring for a woman who is pregnant establishes an environment of comfort and open communication with each antepartum visit. The nurse conveys interest in the woman as an individual and discusses the woman's concerns and desires. Typically, the registered nurse may complete many areas of prenatal assessment. Advanced practice nurses such as certified nurse-midwives (CNMs) and certified women's health nurse practitioners have the education and skill to perform full and complete antepartum assessments. This section focuses on the initial prenatal assessment.

Nursing Assessment

The course of a pregnancy depends on a number of factors, including the woman's prepregnancy health, the presence of disease states, the woman's emotional status, and her past health care. A thorough history is useful in determining the status of a woman's prepregnancy health. Terms useful for recording the history of prenatal clients are listed in **Box 33–1** ●.

CLIENT PROFILE The history is essentially a screening tool that identifies factors that may place the mother or fetus at risk during the pregnancy. The following information is obtained for each pregnant woman at the first prenatal assessment:

1. *Current pregnancy*
   - First day of last normal menstrual period (Is she sure or unsure of the date? Do her cycles normally occur every 28 days, or do her cycles tend to be longer?)
   - Presence of cramping, bleeding, or spotting since LMP
   - Woman's opinion about the time when conception occurred and when infant is due
   - Woman's attitude toward pregnancy (Is this pregnancy planned? Wanted?)
   - Results of pregnancy tests, if completed
   - Any discomforts since LMP (e.g., nausea, vomiting, urinary frequency, fatigue, or breast tenderness)
2. *Past pregnancies*
   - Number of pregnancies
   - Number of abortions, spontaneous or therapeutic
   - Number of living children
   - History of previous pregnancies, length of pregnancy, length of labor and birth, type of birth (vaginal, forceps, or vacuum-assisted birth, or cesarean), type of anesthesia

Box 33–1   Definition of Terms

The following terms are used in recording the history of prenatal clients:

Abortion: Spontaneous loss or termination of pregnancy that occurs before the end of 20 weeks' gestation or the birth of a fetus–newborn who weighs less than 500 g (Cunningham et al., 2010)

Antepartum: Time between conception and the onset of labor; often used to describe the period during which a woman is pregnant; used interchangeably with *prenatal*

Gestation: The number of weeks since the first day of the last menstrual period

Gravida*: The number of pregnancies in the woman's lifetime, regardless of duration, including current pregnancy

Intrapartum: Time from the onset of true labor until the birth of the infant and placenta

Multigravida: A woman who is in her second or any subsequent pregnancy

Multipara: A woman who has had two or more births at more than 20 weeks' gestation

Nulligravida: A woman who has never been pregnant

Nullipara: A woman who has had no births at more than 20 weeks' gestation

Para*: Birth after 20 weeks' gestation regardless of whether the infant is born alive or dead

Postpartum: Time from birth until the woman's body returns to an essentially prepregnant condition

Postterm labor: Labor that occurs after 42 weeks' gestation

Prenatal: Time between conception and the onset of labor; antepartum

Preterm or **premature labor:** Labor that occurs after 20 weeks' gestation but before completion of 37 weeks' gestation

Primigravida: A woman who is pregnant for the first time

Primipara: A woman who has had one birth at more than 20 weeks' gestation, regardless of whether the infant was born alive or dead

Stillbirth: An infant born dead after 20 weeks' gestation

Term: The normal duration of pregnancy (38 to 42 weeks' gestation)

*The terms *gravida* and *para* are used in relation to pregnancies, not the number of fetuses. Thus, twins, triplets, etc., count as one pregnancy and one birth.

---

used (if any), woman's perception of the experience, and complications (antepartum, intrapartum, and postpartum)
- Neonatal status of previous children: Apgar scores, birth weights, general development, complications, and feeding patterns (breast milk or formula)
- Loss of a child (miscarriage, elective or medically indicated abortion, stillbirth, neonatal death, relinquishment, or death after the neonatal period) (What was the experience like for her? What coping skills helped? How did her partner, if involved, respond?)
- If Rh negative, was Rh immune globulin received during pregnancy and/or after birth/miscarriage/abortion to prevent sensitization?
- Prenatal education classes and resources (books)

3. *Gynecological history*
   - Date of last Pap smear; any history of abnormal Pap smear; any follow-up therapy completed
   - Previous infections: vaginal, cervical, tubal, sexually transmitted
   - Previous surgery (uterine/ovarian)
   - Age at menarche
   - Regularity, frequency, and duration of menstrual flow
   - History of dysmenorrhea
   - Sexual history
   - Contraceptive history (If birth control pills were used, did pregnancy occur immediately following cessation of pills? If not, how long after?)
   - Any issues related to infertility or fertility treatments

4. *Current medical history*
   - Weight
   - Blood type and Rh factor if known
   - General health, including nutrition (dietary practices such as vegetarianism) and regular exercise program (type, frequency, and duration)
   - Any medications currently being taken (including nonprescription, homeopathic, or herbal medications) or taken since the onset of pregnancy

- Previous or present use of alcohol, tobacco, or caffeine (Ask specifically about the amount of alcohol, cigarettes, and caffeine [specify coffee, tea, cola, and chocolate] consumed each day.)
- Illicit drug use or abuse (Ask about specific drugs such as cocaine, crack, methamphetamines, and marijuana.)
- Drug allergies and other allergies (Ask about latex allergies or sensitivities.)
- Potential teratogenic insults to this pregnancy, such as viral infections, medications, x-ray examinations, surgery, or cats in the home (possible source of toxoplasmosis)
- Presence of disease conditions such as diabetes, hypertension, cardiovascular disease, renal problems, or thyroid disorder
- Record of immunizations
- Presence of any abnormal symptoms

5. *Past medical history*
   - Childhood diseases
   - Past treatment for any disease condition
   - Surgical procedures
   - Presence of bleeding disorders or tendencies
   - Accidents requiring hospitalizations
   - Blood transfusions

6. *Family medical history*
   - Presence of diabetes, cardiovascular disease, cancer, hypertension, hematological disorders, tuberculosis, or preeclampsia–eclampsia
   - Occurrence of multiple births
   - History of congenital diseases or deformities
   - History of mental illness
   - Causes of death of deceased parents or siblings
   - Occurrence of cesarean births and cause if known

7. *Religious, spiritual, and cultural history*
   - Does the woman want to specify a religious preference on her chart? Does she have any spiritual beliefs or practices that might influence her health care or that of her child, such as prohibition against receiving

blood products, dietary considerations, or circumcision rites?
- What practices are important to maintaining her spiritual well-being?
- Might practices in her culture or that of her partner influence her care or that of her child?

8. *Occupational history*
   - Occupation
   - Physical demands (Does she stand all day, or are there opportunities to sit and elevate her legs? Any heavy lifting?)
   - Exposure to chemicals or other harmful substances
   - Opportunity for regular meals and breaks for nutritious snacks
   - Provision for maternity or family leave

9. *Partner's history*
   - Presence of genetic conditions or diseases in him or in his family history
   - Age
   - Significant health problems
   - Previous or current alcohol intake, drug use, or tobacco use
   - Blood type and Rh factor
   - Occupation
   - Educational level; methods by which he learns best
   - Attitude toward the pregnancy

10. *Personal information about the woman (social history)*
    - Age
    - Educational level; methods by which she learns best
    - Race or ethnic group (to identify need for prenatal genetic screening and racially or ethnically related risk factors)
    - Housing; stability of living conditions
    - Economic level
    - Acceptance of pregnancy, whether intended or unintended
    - Any history of emotional or physical deprivation or abuse of herself or children or any abuse in her current relationship (Ask specifically whether she has been hit, slapped, kicked, or hurt within the past year or since she has become pregnant. Ask whether she is afraid of her partner or anyone else. If yes, of whom is she afraid? *Note:* Ask these questions when the woman is alone.)
    - History of emotional problems
    - Support systems
    - Personal preferences about the birth (expectations of both the woman and her partner, presence of others, etc.)
    - Plans for care of child following birth
    - Feeding preference for the baby (breast milk or formula?)

OBTAINING DATA In many instances, a questionnaire is used to obtain information. The woman should complete the questionnaire in a quiet place with a minimum of distractions. The nurse can obtain further information in an interview, which allows the pregnant woman to clarify her responses to questions bland gives the nurse and client the opportunity to develop rapport.

The expectant father or partner can be encouraged to attend the prenatal examinations; he is often able to contribute to the history. The nurse should encourage partners to use the opportunity to ask questions or express concerns that are important to them.

PRENATAL HIGH-RISK SCREENING **Risk factors** are any findings that suggest that the pregnancy may have a negative outcome, for either the woman or her unborn child. Screening for risk factors is an important part of the prenatal assessment. Many risk factors can be identified during the initial assessment; others may be detected during subsequent prenatal visits. It is important to identify high-risk pregnancies early so that appropriate interventions can be started promptly. Not all risk factors threaten a pregnancy equally; thus, many agencies use a scoring sheet to determine the degree of risk. Information must be updated throughout the pregnancy as necessary. Any pregnancy may begin as low risk and change to high risk because of complications.

Physical Examination

The physical examination begins with assessment of vital signs; then the woman's body is examined. The pelvic examination is performed last. Before the examination, the woman should provide a clean urine specimen. When her bladder is empty, the woman is more comfortable during the pelvic examination and the examiner can palpate the pelvic organs more easily. After the woman has emptied her bladder, the nurse asks her to disrobe and gives her a gown and sheet or some other protective covering.

Increasing numbers of nurses (e.g., CNMs and other nurses in advanced practice) are prepared to perform complete physical examinations. The nurse who does not yet possess advanced assessment skills can assess the woman's vital signs, explain the procedures to allay apprehension, position her for examination, and assist the examiner as necessary. Each nurse is responsible for operating at the expected standard for his or her skill and knowledge base.

Thoroughness and a systematic procedure are the most important considerations when performing the physical portion of a prenatal examination. To promote completeness, the Prenatal Assessment, starting on page 2056, is organized in three columns that address the areas to be assessed (and normal findings), the variations or alterations that may be observed and their possible causes, and nursing responses to the data. The nurse should be aware that certain organs and systems are assessed concurrently with others during the physical portion of the examination.

A gestation calculator or wheel permits the caregiver to calculate the EDB even more quickly (**Figure 33–23 ●**).

If a woman with a history of menses every 28 days remembers her LMP and was not taking oral contraceptives before becoming pregnant, the Nägele rule may be a fairly accurate determiner of the EDB. However, *ovulation usually occurs 14 days before the onset of the next menses, not 14 days after the previous menses.* Consequently, if her cycle is irregular or more than 28 days long, the time of ovulation may be delayed. If she has been using oral contraceptives, ovulation may be delayed several weeks following her last menses. Then, too, a

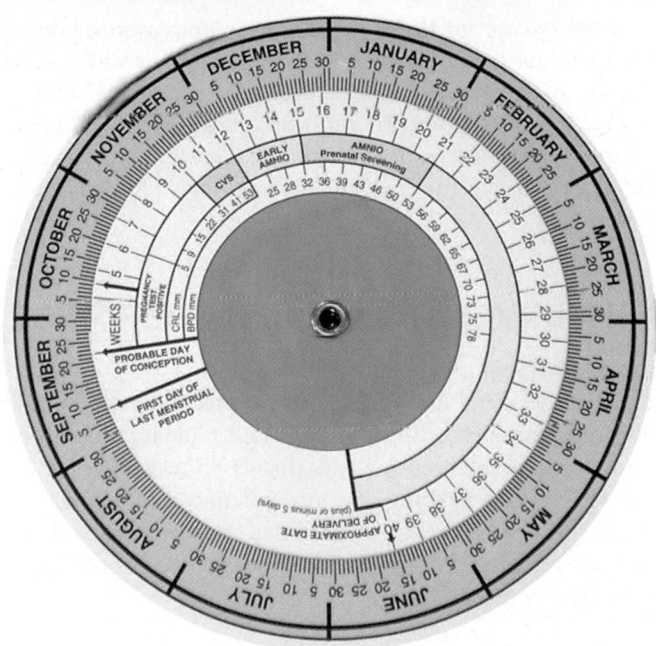

Figure 33–23 ● The EDB wheel can be used to calculate the due date. To use it, place the arrow labeled "1st day of last period" on the date of the woman's LMP. Then read the EDB at the arrow labeled 40. In this case, the LMP is September 8 and the EDB is June 17.

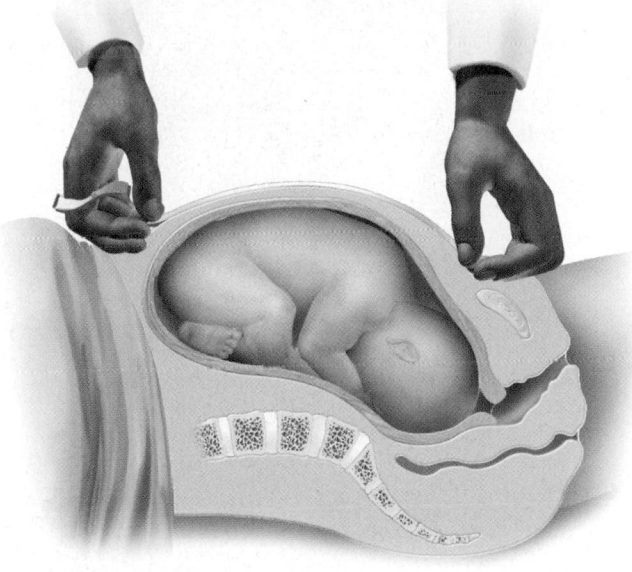

Figure 33–24 ● A cross-sectional view of fetal position when the McDonald method is used to assess the fundal height.

postpartum woman who is breastfeeding may resume ovulating but be amenorrheic for a time, making calculation impossible. Thus, the Nägele rule, although helpful, is not foolproof. The most accurate method of determining gestational age is using an EDB based on a fetal crown rump length measurement at 7-10 weeks gestation.

UTERINE ASSESSMENT

Physical Examination   When a woman is examined in the first 10–12 weeks of pregnancy and her uterine size is compatible with her menstrual history, uterine size may be the single most important clinical method for dating her pregnancy. In many cases, however, women do not seek prenatal care until well into their second trimester, when it becomes more difficult to evaluate specific uterine size. In women with obesity, it is difficult to determine uterine size early in a pregnancy because the uterus is more difficult to palpate.

Fundal Height   Fundal height may be used as an indicator of uterine size, although this method is less accurate late in pregnancy. A centimeter tape measure is used to measure the distance abdominally from the top of the symphysis pubis to the top of the uterine fundus (the McDonald method) (**Figure 33–24 ●**). Fundal height in centimeters correlates well with weeks of gestation after 20 weeks. The normal variation is gestational weeks plus or minus two centimeters. Thus, at 26 weeks gestation, fundal height is 24-28 centimeters depending on fetal position and maternal body habitus. The woman should have voided within 30 minutes of the exam and should lie in the same position each time. In the third trimester, variations in fetal weight decrease the accuracy of fundal height measurements. A lag in progression of mea-

surements of fundal height from month to month and from week to week may signal a fetus that is small for gestational age. A sudden increase in fundal height may indicate twins or hydramnios.

Small for gestational age is defined as a fetal weight estimated by ultrasound or a baby's actual birth weight that is less than the 10th percentile for gestational age. When no cause for this can be identified and the fetus or infant shows no evidence of compromise, it may be concluded that it is constitutionally small. When a fetus is small for gestational age in the setting of some pathology, this is called intrauterine growth restriction (IUGR). Causes include congenital anomalies, exposure to teratogens, maternal smoking and substance abuse, malnutrition, abnormal formation of the placenta, and decreased placental perfusion (King et al., 2015).

Leopold's Maneuvers   Leopold's maneuvers are a system of palpating the uterus externally, starting at the fundus and moving downward, to assess the baby's position and orientation. In the first maneuver, the examiner grips the fundus with both hands and identifies the fetal parts in the fundus. The second maneuver consists of palpating the sides of the uterus in to locate the fetal back and legs. The third maneuver consists of grasping the lower portion of the uterus to identify the fetal part that is lowest in the pelvis, called the presenting part. It should be the head in the third trimester. The fourth maneuver consists of identifying the position of the fetal brow or occiput to determine the degree of flexion or extension of the head (Gabbe,1996).

ASSESSMENT OF FETAL DEVELOPMENT

Quickening   Quickening may indicate that the fetus is nearing 20 weeks' gestation. However, quickening may be experienced between 16 and 22 weeks' gestation, so this method is not completely accurate.

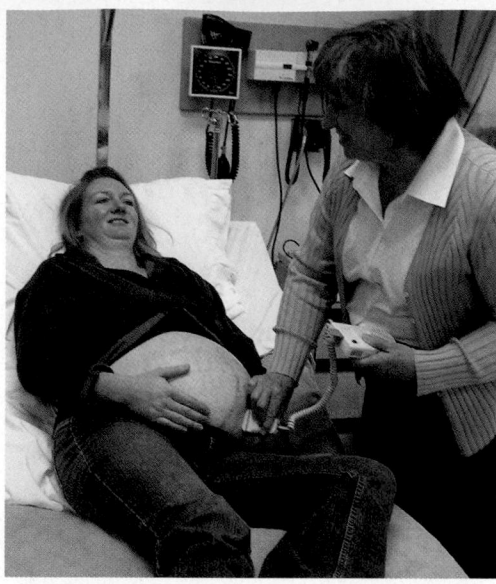

Figure 33–25 ● Listening to the fetal heartbeat with a Doppler device.

Fetal Heartbeat An ultrasonic Doppler device (**Figure 33–25** ●) is the primary tool for assessing fetal heartbeat. It can detect fetal heartbeat, on average, at 8–12 weeks' gestation. If such a device is not available, a fetoscope may be used, although in current practice, it is seldom necessary. The fetal heartbeat can be detected by fetoscope as early as week 16 and usually by 19 or 20 weeks' gestation.

Ultrasound In the first trimester, ultrasound scanning can detect a gestational sac as early as 5–6 weeks after the LMP, fetal heart activity by 6–7 weeks, and fetal breathing movement by 10–11 weeks of pregnancy. Crown-to-rump measurements can be made to assess fetal age until the fetal head can be visualized clearly. Biparietal diameter (BPD) can then be used. BPD measurements can be made by approximately 12–13 weeks and are most accurate between 20 and 30 weeks, when rapid growth in the BPD occurs.

ASSESSMENT OF PELVIC ADEQUACY (CLINICAL PELVIMETRY) The pelvis can be assessed vaginally by a process called *clinical pelvimetry*. It is performed by physicians or by advanced practice nurses such as CNMs or nurse practitioners. Some caregivers assess the pelvis as part of the initial physical examination. Others wait until later in the pregnancy, when hormonal effects are greatest and it is possible to make some determination of fetal size. Pelvic adequacy can, however, only be reliably determined by a trial of labor. Both radiographic and physical assessments of pelvic adequacy are poor predictors of the course of labor and birth.

Prenatal Tests

A number of tests may be used to detect hCG during pregnancy. In addition, a number of diagnostic and screening tests allow healthcare professionals (and the pregnant client) to monitor the safety of both mother and child. These tests are summarized in **Table 33–1** ●; some of them are discussed in greater detail in Exemplar 33.1.

Nursing care for the woman who is undergoing prenatal testing focuses on outcomes to ensure that she understands the reasons for the test, understands the test results, and has support during the test. In addition, other objectives include completing the tests without complication and ensuring that the safety of the mother and her unborn child has been maintained.

▶ INTERVENTIONS AND THERAPIES

Caring interventions for the pregnant woman are focused on teaching the client appropriate self-care techniques, especially with regard to protecting the fetus and relieving discomfort. Many of these interventions are discussed in Exemplars 33.1 and 33.2 on antepartum and intrapartum care, respectively. Those that are covered here are related to fetal safety and to some of the most common discomforts experienced by the pregnant woman.

Independent

It is important to recognize that pregnancy is usually a normal process that ends with the delivery of a healthy newborn. The nurse's role in these cases is health promotion and client teaching. However, alterations can result in injury to either the fetus or the client or both. The nurse assesses clients at each encounter in order to rapidly intervene, to minimize complications, and promote expected outcomes. Holistic, culturally appropriate care is important to make the experience as positive as possible for the client and her family.

PRENATAL EDUCATION **Prenatal education** programs provide important opportunities to share information about pregnancy and childbirth and to enhance the parents' decision-making skills. The content of each class is generally directed by the overall goals of the program. For example, in classes that aim to provide preconceptual information, preparations for becoming pregnant and optimizing the woman's health status are the major topics. Other classes may be directed toward childbirth choices available today, preparation of the mother and her partner for pregnancy and birth, preparation for a vaginal birth after a previous cesarean (VBAC) birth, and preparation for the birth by specific people such as grandparents or siblings. The nurse who knows the types of prenatal programs available in the community can direct expectant parents to programs that meet their special needs and learning goals.

From the expectant parents' point of view, class content is best presented in chronology with the pregnancy. It is important to begin the classes by finding out what each parent wants to learn and including a discussion of related choices. Classes for partners provide a forum for expectant fathers or partners to ask questions and interact with others who are in similar circumstances and have the same types of concerns (Premburg & Lundgren, 2006).

A family's culture may influence its beliefs about and practices surrounding many aspects of childbearing and childrearing. The accompanying Focus on Diversity and Culture feature describes some cultural beliefs and attitudes about pregnancy.

TABLE 33–1 Summary of Selected Antenatal Surveillance and Screening

GOAL	TEST	TIMING
To confirm intrauterine pregnancy and viability	Ultrasound: gestational sac volume	5 and 6 weeks after LMP by transvaginal ultrasound
To determine gestational age	Ultrasound: crown/rump length	6–10 weeks' gestation
	Ultrasound: BPD and fetal body measurement ratios	Greater than or equal to 14 weeks
To evaluate fetal growth	Ultrasound: BPD	Greater than or equal to 14 weeks
	Ultrasound: fetal body measurement ratios	Greater than or equal to 14 weeks
	Ultrasound: estimated fetal weight	About 23–42 weeks' gestation
To detect congenital anomalies and problems	Nuchal translucency testing	11–13 weeks' gestation
	Ultrasound	Greater than or equal to 18 weeks
	Chorionic villus sampling	10–14 weeks' gestation
	Amniocentesis	After 15 weeks' gestation
	First trimester integrated screen	10–13 weeks' gestation
	Cell free DNA	From 9 weeks onward
To determine placental location	Ultrasound	18–20 weeks initially. Repeated at 28–32 weeks for re-evaluation if needed
To assess fetal status	Biophysical profile	Approximately 23 weeks to birth
	Maternal assessment of fetal activity	Approximately 23 weeks to birth
	Nonstress test	Approximately 23 weeks to birth
To diagnose cardiac problems	Fetal echocardiography	Second and third trimesters
To assess fetal lung maturity with amniocentesis or vaginal pool sampled amniotic fluid	L/S ratio	32–39 weeks
	Phosphatidylglycerol	32–39 weeks
	Phosphatidylcholine	32–39 weeks
	Lamellar body counts	32–39 weeks
To determine fetal presentation	Ultrasound	At term or on admission for labor and birth

Prenatal education must include teaching the parents about teratogenic substances and the use of medications during pregnancy. Substances that adversely affect the normal growth and development of the fetus are called *teratogens*. Many substances are known or suspected teratogens, including, for example, certain medications, psychotropic drugs, and alcohol. The harmful effects of other teratogens, such as some pesticides and exposure to x-rays in the first trimester of pregnancy, also have been documented. It is essential that pregnant women receive information about recognized teratogens and environmental risks. An overview of the risks associated with medications and tobacco is provided here. For a more thorough discussion of the risks of substance abuse during pregnancy, see the exemplar on Prenatal Substance Exposure in the module on Addiction.

Medications The use of medications during pregnancy, including prescriptions, over-the-counter (OTC) drugs, and herbal remedies, is of great concern because maternal drug exposure is thought to account for at least 10% of birth defects (Black & Hill, 2003). Many pregnant women need medication for therapeutic purposes, such as the treatment of infections, allergies, or other pathological processes. In these situations, the problem can be complex. Known teratogenic agents are not prescribed and usually can be replaced with medications that are considered safe. Even when a woman is highly motivated to avoid taking any medications, she may have taken potentially teratogenic medications before her pregnancy was confirmed, especially if she has an irregular menstrual cycle.

The greatest potential for gross abnormalities in the fetus occurs during the first trimester of pregnancy, when fetal organs are first developing. The classic period of teratogenesis in a woman with a 28-day cycle extends from day 31 after the LMP (17 days after fertilization) to day 71 (54 days after fertilization) (Niebyl & Simpson, 2007). Many factors influence teratogenic effects, including the specific type of teratogen and the dose, the stage of embryonic development, and the genetic sensitivity of the mother and fetus. For example, the commonly prescribed acne medication isotretinoin (Accutane) is associated with a high incidence of spontaneous abortion and congenital malformations if taken early in pregnancy.

To provide information for caregivers and clients, the FDA has developed the following classification system for medications administered during pregnancy:

- *Category A:* Controlled studies in women have demonstrated no associated fetal risk. Few drugs fall into this category.
- *Category B:* Animal studies show no risk but there are no controlled studies in women, or animal studies indicate a risk but controlled human studies fail to demonstrate a risk. The penicillins fall into this category.

Prenatal Assessment

PHYSICAL ASSESSMENT/ NORMAL FINDINGS	ALTERATIONS AND POSSIBLE CAUSES*	NURSING RESPONSES TO DATA†
Vital Signs		
Blood pressure (BP): less than or equal to 140/90 mmHg	High BP (essential hypertension; renal disease; pregestational hypertension, apprehension or anxiety associated with pregnancy diagnosis, exam, or other crises; preeclampsia if initial assessment not done until after 20 weeks' gestation)	BP greater than 140/90 mmHg requires immediate consideration; establish woman's BP; refer to healthcare provider if necessary. Assess woman's knowledge about high BP; counsel on self-care and medical management.
Pulse: 60–90 bpm; rate may increase 10 bpm during pregnancy	Increased pulse rate (excitement or anxiety, cardiac disorders)	Count for 1 full minute; note irregularities.
Respirations: 12–22 breaths/min (or pulse rate divided by 4); pregnancy may induce a degree of hyperventilation; thoracic breathing predominant	Marked tachypnea or abnormal patterns	Assess for respiratory disease.
Temperature: 36.2°–37.6°C (97.0°–99.6°F)	Elevated temperature (infection)	Assess for infection process of disease state, or ruptured membranes, if temperature is elevated; refer to healthcare provider.
Body Mass Index (BMI)		
Between 18.5 and 24.9 based on pre-pregnant weight or weight on presentation to care if pre-pregnant weight is unknown	Less than 18.5 or greater than 30	Evaluate need for nutritional counseling; obtain information on eating habits, cooking practices, food regularly eaten, income limitations, need for food supplements, pica and other abnormal food habits. Note initial weight to establish baseline for weight gain throughout pregnancy.
Skin		
Color: consistent with racial background; pink nail beds	Pallor (anemia); bronze, yellow (hepatic disease; other causes of jaundice) Bluish, reddish, mottled; dusky appearance or pallor of palms and nail beds in dark-skinned women (anemia)	The following tests should be performed: complete blood count (CBC), bilirubin level, urinalysis, and blood urea nitrogen (BUN). If abnormal, refer to healthcare provider.
Condition: absence of edema (slight edema of lower extremities is normal during pregnancy)	Edema (possible preeclampsia); rashes, dermatitis (allergic response)	Counsel on relief measures for slight edema. Initiate preeclampsia assessment; refer to healthcare provider.
Lesions: absence of lesions	Ulceration (varicose veins, decreased circulation)	Further assess circulatory status; refer to healthcare provider if lesion is severe.
Spider nevi common in pregnancy	Petechiae, multiple bruises, ecchymosis (hemorrhagic disorders; abuse) Change in size or color (carcinoma)	Evaluate for bleeding or clotting disorder. Provide opportunities to discuss abuse if suspected. Refer to healthcare provider.
Pigmentation: pigmentation changes of pregnancy include linea nigra, striae gravidarum, melasma		Assure woman that these are normal manifestations of pregnancy and explain the physiological basis for the changes.
Café-au-lait spots	Six or more (Albright syndrome or neurofibromatosis)	Consult with healthcare provider.
	*Possible causes of alterations are identified in parentheses.	†This column provides guidelines for further assessment and initial nursing intervention.

Prenatal Assessment (continued)

PHYSICAL ASSESSMENT/ NORMAL FINDINGS	ALTERATIONS AND POSSIBLE CAUSES*	NURSING RESPONSES TO DATA†
Nose		
Character of mucosa: redder than oral mucosa; in pregnancy, nasal mucosa is edematous in response to increased estrogen, resulting in nasal stuffiness (rhinitis of pregnancy) and nosebleeds (epistaxis)	Olfactory loss (first cranial nerve deficit)	Counsel woman about possible relief measures for nasal stuffiness and nosebleeds; refer to healthcare provider for olfactory loss.
Mouth		
May note hypertrophy of gingival tissue because of estrogen	Edema, inflammation (infection); pale in color (anemia)	Assess hematocrit for anemia; counsel regarding dental hygiene habits. Refer to healthcare provider or dentist if necessary. Routine dental care is appropriate during pregnancy (no epinephrine, no nitrous anesthesia). Dental x-rays can be done during the second trimester if needed.
Neck		
Nodes: small, mobile, nontender nodes	Tender, hard, fixed, or prominent nodes (infection, carcinoma)	Examine for local infection; refer to healthcare provider.
Thyroid: small, smooth, lateral lobes palpable on either side of trachea; slight hyperplasia by third month of pregnancy	Enlargement or nodule tenderness (hyperthyroidism)	Listen over thyroid for bruits, which may indicate hyperthyroidism. Question woman about dietary habits (iodine intake). Ascertain history of thyroid problems; refer to healthcare provider.
Chest and Lungs		
Chest: symmetric, elliptic, smaller AP than transverse diameter	Increased AP diameter, funnel chest, pigeon chest (emphysema, asthma, chronic obstructive pulmonary disease [COPD])	Evaluate for emphysema, asthma, COPD.
Ribs: slope downward from nipple line	More horizontal (COPD) angular bumps (rachitic rosary) (vitamin C deficiency)	Evaluate for COPD. Evaluate for fractures. Consult healthcare provider. Consult nutritionist.
Inspection and palpation: no retraction or bulging of intercostal spaces (ICS) during inspiration or expiration; symmetric expansion	ICS retractions with inspirations, bulging with expiration; unequal expansion (respiratory disease)	Do thorough initial assessment. Refer to healthcare provider.
Tactile fremitus	Tachypnea, hyperpnea, Cheyne-Stokes respirations (respiratory disease)	Refer to healthcare provider.
Percussion: bilateral symmetry in tone	Flatness of percussion, which may be affected by chest wall thickness	Evaluate for pleural effusions, consolidations, or tumor.
Low-pitched resonance of moderate intensity	High diaphragm (atelectasis or paralysis), pleural effusion	Refer to healthcare provider.
Auscultation: upper lobes: bronchovesicular sounds above sternum and scapulas; equal expiratory and inspiratory phases	Abnormal if heard over any other area of chest	Refer to healthcare provider.
	*Possible causes of alterations are identified in parentheses.	†This column provides guidelines for further assessment and initial nursing intervention.

(continued on next page)

Prenatal Assessment (continued)

PHYSICAL ASSESSMENT/ NORMAL FINDINGS	ALTERATIONS AND POSSIBLE CAUSES*	NURSING RESPONSES TO DATA†
Remainder of chest: vesicular breath sounds heard; inspiratory phase longer (3:1)	Rales, rhonchi, wheezes; pleural friction rub; absence of breath sounds; bronchophony, egophony, whispered pectoriloquy	Refer to healthcare provider.
Breasts		
Supple: symmetric in size and contour; darker pigmentation of nipple and areola; may have supernumerary nipples. Axillary nodes unpalpable or pellet-sized	"Pigskin" or orange-peel appearance, nipple retractions, swelling, hardness (carcinoma); redness, heat, tenderness, cracked or fissured nipple (infection) Tenderness, enlargement, hard node (carcinoma); may be visible bump (infection)	Encourage monthly self-examination; instruct woman how to examine her breasts. Refer to healthcare provider if evidence of inflammation.
Pregnancy changes: 1. Size increase noted primarily in first 20 weeks. 2. Become nodular. 3. Tingling sensation may be felt during first and third trimester; woman may report feeling of heaviness. 4. Pigmentation of nipples and areolae darkens. 5. Superficial veins dilate and become more prominent. 6. Striae seen in multiparas. 7. Tubercles of Montgomery enlarge. 8. Colostrum may be present after 12th week. 9. Secondary areola appears at 20 weeks, characterized by series of washed-out spots surrounding primary areola. 10. Breasts less firm, old striae may be present in multiparas.		Discuss normalcy of changes and their meaning. Teach and/or institute appropriate relief measures. Encourage use of supportive, well-fitting brassiere.
Heart		
Normal rate, rhythm, and heart sounds	Enlargement, thrills, thrusts, gross irregularity or skipped beats, gallop rhythm or extra sounds (cardiac disease)	Complete an initial assessment. Explain normal pregnancy-induced changes. Refer to healthcare provider if indicated.
Pregnancy changes: 1. Palpitations may occur due to sympathetic nervous system disturbance. 2. Short systolic murmurs that increase in held expiration are normal due to increased volume.		
Abdomen		
Normal appearance, skin texture, and hair distribution; liver nonpalpable; abdomen nontender	Muscle guarding (anxiety, acute tenderness); tenderness, mass (ectopic pregnancy, inflammation, carcinoma)	Assure woman of normalcy of diastasis. Provide initial information about appropriate prenatal and postpartum exercises. Evaluate woman's anxiety level. Refer to healthcare provider if indicated.
	*Possible causes of alterations are identified in parentheses.	†This column provides guidelines for further assessment and initial nursing intervention.

Prenatal Assessment (continued)

PHYSICAL ASSESSMENT/ NORMAL FINDINGS	ALTERATIONS AND POSSIBLE CAUSES*	NURSING RESPONSES TO DATA†
Pregnancy changes: 1. Purple striae may be present (or silver striae on a multipara) as well as linea nigra. 2. Diastasis of the rectus muscles late in pregnancy. 3. Size: flat or rotund abdomen; progressive enlargement of uterus due to pregnancy. *10–12 weeks:* fundus slightly above symphysis pubis. *16 weeks:* fundus halfway between symphysis and umbilicus. *20–22 weeks:* fundus at umbilicus. *28 weeks:* fundus three finger breadths above umbilicus. *36 weeks:* fundus just below ensiform cartilage.	Size of uterus inconsistent with length of gestation (IUGR, multiple pregnancy, fetal demise, hydatidiform mole, polyhydramnios, inaccurate dating)	Reassess menstrual history regarding pregnancy dating. Use ultrasound to establish diagnosis.
4. Fetal heart rate: 110–160 bpm may be heard with Doppler at 10–12 weeks' gestation; may be heard with fetoscope at 17–20 weeks.	Failure to hear fetal heartbeat with Doppler (fetal demise, hydatidiform mole)	Refer to healthcare provider. Administer pregnancy tests. Use ultrasound to establish diagnosis.
5. Fetal movement palpable by a trained examiner after 18th week.	Failure to feel fetal movements after 20 weeks' gestation (fetal demise, hydatidiform mole)	Refer to healthcare provider for evaluation of fetal status.
6. Ballottement: during fourth to fifth month, fetus rises and then rebounds to original position when uterus is tapped sharply.	No ballottement (oligohydramnios)	Refer to healthcare provider for evaluation of fetal status.
Extremities		
Skin warm, pulses palpable, full range of motion; may be some edema of hands and ankles in late pregnancy; varicose veins may become more pronounced; palmar erythema may be present	Unpalpable or diminished pulses (arterial insufficiency); marked edema (preeclampsia)	Evaluate for other symptoms of heart disease; initiate follow-up if woman mentions that her rings feel tight. Discuss prevention and self-treatment measures for varicose veins; refer to healthcare provider if indicated.
Spine		
Normal spinal curves: concave cervical, convex thoracic, concave lumbar	Abnormal spinal curves; flatness, kyphosis, lordosis	Refer to healthcare provider for assessment of cephalopelvic disproportion.
In pregnancy, lumbar spinal curve may be accentuated	Backache	May have implications for administration of spinal anesthetics.
Shoulders and iliac crests should be even	Uneven shoulders and iliac crests (scoliosis)	Refer very young women to healthcare provider; discuss back-stretching exercise with older women.
Reflexes		
Normal and symmetric	Hyperactivity, clonus (preeclampsia)	Evaluate for other symptoms of preeclampsia.
	*Possible causes of alterations are identified in parentheses.	†This column provides guidelines for further assessment and initial nursing intervention.

(continued on next page)

Prenatal Assessment (continued)

PHYSICAL ASSESSMENT/ NORMAL FINDINGS	ALTERATIONS AND POSSIBLE CAUSES*	NURSING RESPONSES TO DATA†
Pelvic Area		
External female genitals: normally formed with female hair distribution; in multiparas, labia majora loose and pigmented; urinary and vaginal orifices visible and appropriately located	Lesions, hematomas, varicosities, inflammation of the Bartholin glands; clitoral hypertrophy	Explain pelvic examination procedure. Encourage woman to minimize her discomfort by relaxing her hips. Provide privacy.
Vagina: pink or dark pink, vaginal discharge odorless, nonirritating; in multiparas, vaginal folds smooth and flattened; may have episiotomy scar	Abnormal discharge associated with vaginal infections	Obtain vaginal smear. Provide understandable verbal and written instructions about treatment for woman and partner if indicated.
Cervix: pink color; os closed except in multiparas, in whom os admits fingertip	Eversion, reddish erosion, nabothian or retention cysts, cervical polyp; granular area that bleeds (carcinoma of cervix); lesions (herpes, human papilloma virus [HPV]); presence of string or plastic tip from cervix (intrauterine device [IUD] in uterus)	Provide woman with a hand mirror and identify genital structures for her; encourage her to view her cervix if she wishes. Refer to healthcare provider if indicated. Advise woman of potential serious risks of leaving an IUD in place during pregnancy; refer to healthcare provider for removal.
Pregnancy changes: *1–4 weeks' gestation:* enlargement in AP diameter *4–6 weeks' gestation:* softening of cervix (Goodell sign); softening of isthmus of uterus (Hegar sign); cervix takes on bluish coloring (Chadwick sign) *8–12 weeks' gestation:* vagina and cervix appear bluish violet in color (Chadwick sign) Uterus: pear-shaped, mobile; smooth surface	Absence of Goodell sign (inflammatory conditions, carcinoma) Fixed (pelvic inflammatory disease [PID]); nodular surface (fibromas)	Refer to healthcare provider. Refer to healthcare provider.
Ovaries: small, walnut-shaped, nontender (ovaries and fallopian tubes are located in adnexal areas)	Pain on movement of cervix (PID); enlarged or nodular ovaries (cyst, tumor, tubal pregnancy, corpus luteum of pregnancy)	Evaluate adnexal areas; refer to healthcare provider.
Pelvic Measurements		
Internal measurements: 1. Diagonal conjugate is at least 11.5 cm. 2. Obstetric conjugate is estimated by subtracting 1.5–2.0 cm from diagonal conjugate. 3. Inclination of sacrum. 4. Motility of coccyx; external intertubular diameter is greater than 8 cm.	Measurement below normal Disproportion of pubic arch Abnormal curvature of sacrum Fixed or malposition of coccyx	May be considered as a factor in protraction or arrest of labor.
Anus and Rectum		
No lumps, rashes, excoriation, tenderness; cervix may be felt through rectal wall	Hemorrhoids, rectal prolapse; nodular lesion (carcinoma)	Counsel about appropriate prevention and relief measures; refer to healthcare provider for further evaluation.
	*Possible causes of alterations are identified in parentheses.	†This column provides guidelines for further assessment and initial nursing intervention.

Prenatal Assessment (*continued*)

PHYSICAL ASSESSMENT/ NORMAL FINDINGS	ALTERATIONS AND POSSIBLE CAUSES*	NURSING RESPONSES TO DATA[†]
Laboratory Evaluation		
Hemoglobin: 12–16 g/dL; women residing in areas of high altitude may have higher levels of hemoglobin	Less than 11 g/dL (anemia)	*Note:* Wear nonlatex gloves when drawing blood. Hemoglobin less than 12 g/dL requires nutritional counseling; less than 11 g/dL requires iron supplementation.
ABO and Rh typing: normal distribution of blood types	Rh negative	If Rh negative, check for presence of anti Rh antibodies. Discuss the need for antibody titers during pregnancy, management during the intrapartum period, and possible need for Rh immune globulin. Determine the father's Rh status if possible.
CBC: Hematocrit: 38–47% physiological anemia (pseudoanemia) may occur	Marked anemia or blood dyscrasias	Perform CBC and Schilling differential cell count. Consider iron studies and hemoglobin electrophoresis.
RBCs: 4.2–5.4 million/microliter		
White blood cells (WBCs): 5,000–12,000/microliter	Presence of infection; may be elevated in pregnancy and with labor	Evaluate for other signs of infection.
Differential Neutrophils: 40%–60% Bands: up to 5% Eosinophils: 1%–3% Basophils: up to 1% Lymphocytes: 20%–40% Monocytes: 4%–8%		
Syphilis tests: serological tests for syphilis (STS), complement fixation test, Venereal Disease Research Laboratory (VDRL) test—nonreactive	Positive reaction STS—tests may have 25%–45% incidence of biological false-positive results; false results may occur in individuals who have acute viral or bacterial infections, hypersensitivity reactions, recent vaccinations, collagen disease, malaria, or tuberculosis	Positive results may be confirmed with the fluorescent treponemal antibody-absorption (FTA-ABS) test; all tests for syphilis give positive results in the secondary stage of the disease; antibiotic tests may cause negative test results.
First trimester integrated screen. Non invasive prenatal testing (NIPT)/ cell free DNA: Quad screen (Evaluates four factors—maternal serum alpha-fetoprotein (MSAFP), unconjugated estriol (UE), human chorionic gonadotropin (hCG), and inhibin-A: normal levels)	Abnormal fetal nasal bone an/or nuchal fold on ultrasound combined with abnormal lab values as in the quad screen Detection of abnormal fetal alleles in maternal serum Elevated MSAFP (neural tube defect, underestimated gestational age, multiple gestation). Lower than normal MSAFP (Down syndrome, trisomy 18). Higher than normal hCG and inhibin-A (Down syndrome). Lower than normal UE (Down syndrome)	Offered to all pregnant women at the gestational age appropriate for each test. If abnormal, further testing such as ultrasound or amniocentesis is offered.
	*Possible causes of alterations are identified in parentheses.	[†]This column provides guidelines for further assessment and initial nursing intervention.

(*continued on next page*)

Prenatal Assessment (continued)

PHYSICAL ASSESSMENT/ NORMAL FINDINGS	ALTERATIONS AND POSSIBLE CAUSES*	NURSING RESPONSES TO DATA†
Indirect Coombs Test: done on all pregnant women at the initial prenatal visit and repeated at 28 weeks for Rh negative women	Red blood cell (RBC) antibodies present (either Rhesus or non-Rhesus)	A number of RBC antigens may cause isoimmunization and fetal and newborn hemolytic disease. The most common of these is the D antigen, which may occur when an Rh negative mother carries an Rh positive fetus. This may be prevented through prenatal administration of Rh immune globulin (Rhogam).
Screening for Group B Streptococcus (GBS): Rectal and vaginal swabs obtained at 35–37 weeks' gestation for all pregnant women	Positive culture (maternal colonization)	Antibiotics administered during labor for infection prophylaxis in the neonate.
Glucose Tolerance Test: 50-g 1-hour glucose screen (done between 24 and 28 weeks' gestation)	Plasma glucose level greater than 130–140 mg/dL is considered abnormal, depending on provider preference. Be aware of your institution's guidelines.	Refer for a diagnostic 3-hour glucose tolerance test.
Urinalysis: normal color; specific gravity; pH 4.6–8.0	Abnormal color (porphyria, hemoglobinuria, bilirubinemia); alkaline urine (metabolic alkalemia, Proteus infection, old specimen)	Repeat urinalysis; refer to healthcare provider.
Urinalysis: negative for protein, RBCs, WBCs, casts	Positive findings (contaminated specimen, kidney disease)	Repeat urinalysis; refer to healthcare provider.
Urinalysis: glucose: negative (a small degree of glycosuria may occur in pregnancy)	Glycosuria (physiologic secondary to increased glomerular filtration of pregnancy, diabetes mellitus)	Assess blood glucose level; test urine for ketones.
Rubella titer: hemagglutination-inhibition (HAI) test—1:10 or above indicates woman is immune	HAI titer less than 1:10	Immunization will be given postpartum or within 6 weeks after childbirth. Instruct woman whose titers are less than 1:10 to avoid children who have rubella.
Hepatitis B screen for hepatitis B surface antigen (HbsAg): negative	Positive	If negative, consider referral for hepatitis B vaccine postpartum. If positive, refer to physician. Infants born to women who test positive are given hepatitis B immune globulin soon after birth, followed by first dose of hepatitis B vaccine.
HIV screen: offered to all women; encouraged for those at risk; negative	Positive	Refer to healthcare provider.
Illicit drug screen: offered to all women; negative	Positive	Refer to healthcare provider.
Hemoglobin screen for clients of African, Mediterranean, or south Asian descent: negative	Positive; test results would include a description of cells	Refer to healthcare provider.
Pap smear: negative	Test results that show atypical cells	Refer to healthcare provider. Discuss with the woman the meaning of the findings and the importance of follow-up.
Gonorrhea culture: negative	Positive	Refer for treatment.
	*Possible causes of alterations are identified in parentheses.	†This column provides guidelines for further assessment and initial nursing intervention.

Prenatal Assessment (*continued*)

CULTURAL ASSESSMENT[§]	VARIATIONS TO CONSIDER	NURSING RESPONSE TO DATA[§§]
Determine the woman's fluency in written and oral English.	Woman may be fluent in language other than English.	Work with a knowledgeable translator to provide information and answer questions.
Ask the woman how she prefers to be addressed.	Some women prefer informality; others prefer to use titles.	Address the woman according to her preference. Maintain formality in introducing oneself if that seems preferred.
Determine customs and practices regarding prenatal care:	Practices are influenced by individual preference, cultural expectations, or religious beliefs.	Honor a woman's practices and provide for specific preferences unless they are contraindicated for safety reasons.
■ Ask the woman if there are certain practices she expects to follow when she is pregnant.	Some women believe they should perform certain acts related to sleep, activity, or clothing.	Have information printed in the language of different cultural groups that live in the area.
■ Ask the woman if there are any activities she cannot do while she is pregnant.	Some women have restrictions or taboos they follow related to work, activity, sexual, environmental, or emotional factors.	Provide alternate activities if needed.
■ Ask the woman whether there are certain foods she is expected to eat or avoid while she is pregnant. Determine whether she has lactose intolerance.	Foods are an important cultural factor. Some women may have certain foods they must eat or avoid; many women have lactose intolerance and have difficulty consuming sufficient calcium.	Respect the woman's food preferences, help her plan an adequate prenatal diet within the framework of her preferences, and refer to a dietitian if necessary.
■ Ask the woman whether the gender of her caregiver is of concern.	Some women are comfortable only with a female caregiver.	Arrange for a female caregiver if it is the woman's preference.
■ Ask the woman about the degree of involvement in her pregnancy that she expects or wants from her support person, mother, and other significant people.	A woman may not want her partner involved in the pregnancy. The role may fall to the woman's mother or a female relative or friend.	Respect the woman's preferences about her partner's involvement; avoid imposing personal values or expectations.
■ Ask the woman about her sources of support and counseling during pregnancy.	Some women seek advice from a family member or traditional healer.	Respect and honor the woman's sources of support.
Psychological Status		
Excitement and/or apprehension, ambivalence	Marked anxiety (fear of pregnancy diagnosis, fear of medical facility)	Establish lines of communication. Active listening is useful. Establish trusting relationship. Encourage woman to take active part in her care.
	Apathy; display of anger with pregnancy diagnosis	Establish communication and begin counseling. Use active listening techniques.
Educational Needs		
May have questions about pregnancy or may need time to adjust to reality of pregnancy.		Establish educational, supporting environment that can be expanded throughout pregnancy.
Support System		
Can identify at least two or three individuals with whom she is emotionally intimate (partner, parent, sibling, friend).	Isolated (no telephone, unlisted number); cannot name a neighbor or friend whom she can call on in an emergency; does not perceive parents as part of her support system.	Institute support system through community groups. Help woman to develop trusting relationship with healthcare professionals.
[§]These are only a few suggestions. We do not mean to imply that this is a comprehensive cultural assessment; rather, it is a tool to encourage cultural competence.		[§§]This column provides guidelines for further assessment and initial nursing intervention.

Prenatal Assessment (*continued*)

CULTURAL ASSESSMENT[§]	VARIATIONS TO CONSIDER	NURSING RESPONSE TO DATA[§§]
Family Functioning		
Emotionally supportive Adequate communication Mutually satisfying Cohesiveness in times of trouble	Long-term problems or specific problems related to this pregnancy, potential stressors within the family, pessimistic attitudes, unilateral decision making, unrealistic expectations of this pregnancy or child	Help identify the problems and stressors, encourage communication, and discuss role changes and adaptations.
Economic Status		
Source of income is stable and sufficient to meet basic needs of daily living and medical needs.	Limited prenatal care; poor physical health; limited use of healthcare system; unstable economic status	Discuss available resources for health maintenance and the birth. Institute appropriate referral for meeting expanding family's needs (e.g., food stamps).
Stability of Living Conditions		
Adequate, stable housing for expanding family's needs	Crowded living conditions; questionable supportive environment for newborn	Refer to appropriate community agency. Work with family on self-help ways to improve situation.
[§]These are only a few suggestions. We do not mean to imply that this is a comprehensive cultural assessment; rather, it is a tool to encourage cultural competence.		[§§]This column provides guidelines for further assessment and initial nursing intervention.

- *Category C:* Either (1) no adequate animal or human studies are available or (2) animal studies show teratogenic effects but no controlled studies in women are available. Many drugs fall into this category, which, because of the lack of information, is a problematic one for caregivers. Epinephrine, beta-blockers, and zidovudine (a drug used to decrease perinatal transmission of HIV) fall into this category.

- *Category D:* Evidence of human fetal risk exists, but the benefits of the drug in certain situations are thought to outweigh the risks. Examples of drugs in this category include tetracycline, vincristine, lithium, and hydrochlorothiazide.

- *Category X:* The demonstrated fetal risks clearly outweigh any possible benefit. Examples of drugs in this category include isotretinoin (Accutane), the acne medication, which can cause multiple CNS, facial, and cardiovascular anomalies.

If a woman has taken a drug in category D or X, she should be informed of the risks associated with that drug and her alternatives. Similarly, a woman who has taken a drug in the safer categories can be reassured (Cunningham et al., 2010).

This system, although useful, has been criticized because the use of letters suggests a risk grading that is not necessarily accurate. More importantly, not all drugs in a category have the same risk level. The FDA is currently developing a new labeling system (Cunningham et al., 2010).

Although the first trimester is the critical period for teratogenesis, some medications are known to have a teratogenic effect when taken in the second and third trimesters. For example, tetracycline taken in late pregnancy is commonly associated with staining of teeth in children and has been shown to depress skeletal growth, especially in premature infants. Sulfonamides taken in the last few weeks of pregnancy are known to compete with bilirubin attachment of protein-binding sites, increasing the risk of jaundice in the newborn (Niebyl & Simpson, 2007).

Pregnant women need to avoid all medication—prescribed, homeopathic, or OTC—if possible. If no alternative exists, the woman should select a well-known medication rather than a newer drug whose potential teratogenic effects may not be known. When possible, the oral form of a drug should be used and it should be prescribed in the lowest possible therapeutic dose for the shortest time possible. Finally, the caregiver needs to consider the multiple components of the medication. Caution is the watchword for nurses caring for pregnant women who have been taking medications. It is essential that pregnant women check with their CNMs or physicians about any herbs or medications they were taking when pregnancy occurred and about any nonprescription drugs they are thinking of using. The advantage of using a particular medication must outweigh the risks. Any medication with possible teratogenic effects is best avoided.

Tobacco In the United States, smoking tobacco during pregnancy is one of the most significant, modifiable causes of poor pregnancy outcomes. Smoking during pregnancy has a strong association with low-birth-weight infants. In addition, mothers who smoke have an increased risk of preterm birth, premature rupture of the membranes, fetal demise, placentae previa, abruptio placentae, premature rupture of membranes, and preterm birth (Hartmann et al., 2007). Pregnant women who smoke tobacco and participate in other unhealthy behaviors, such as alcohol use, further increase their risk for low-birth-weight infants (Okah, Cai, & Hoff, 2005). Research also links maternal tobacco smoking, both during and after pregnancy, with an increased risk of SIDS. Maternal smoking exposes young children to other risks of secondhand smoke, including middle ear infections, acute and chronic respiratory tract illnesses, and behavioral and learning disabilities (Albrecht et al., 2004).

RELIEF OF THE COMMON DISCOMFORTS OF PREGNANCY The common discomforts of pregnancy result from physiological and anatomical changes and are fairly specific to

Focus on Diversity and Culture   Beliefs and Attitudes About Pregnancy

Children are generally valued all over the world, not only for the joy they bring, but also because they ensure continuation of the family and cultural values. This valuing of children may manifest itself in different ways, however. Families in the United States and many Western countries commonly have only one or two children out of a desire to provide the children with the best home and education the family can afford and so that the parents can spend as much free time with the children as possible. In contrast, in many cultures throughout the world, it is common to have as many children as possible.

In some cultures, a woman who gives birth achieves a higher status, especially when the child is male (Safadi, 2005). This is especially true in the traditional Chinese culture and in some Middle Eastern cultures (Do, 2005). Similarly, people of the Mormon faith view motherhood as the most important aspect of a woman's life, comparable with the male role of priesthood (Faust, 2005). In Mexican American society and among many other Latino groups, having children is evidence of the male's virility and is a sign of manliness or *machismo*, a desired trait.

Culture also may influence attitudes and beliefs about contraception. For example, Muslims from the Middle East may use birth control but do not believe in sterilization because it is a permanent method (Hammond, White, & Fetters, 2005). Other Muslims may not practice contraception because children are highly valued and it is believed that the traditional role of women is to bear children. In Chinese society, in contrast, where state policy limits the number of children a couple can have, contraception is common.

Health values and beliefs are also important in understanding reactions and behavior. Certain behaviors can be expected if a culture views pregnancy as a sickness, whereas other behaviors can be expected if the culture views pregnancy as a natural occurrence. For example, because Native Americans, African Americans, and Mexican Americans generally view pregnancy as a natural and desirable condition, prenatal care may not be a priority. In other cultures, pregnancy may be seen as a time of increased vulnerability. In Orthodox Judaism, for example, it is a man's responsibility to procreate, but it is a woman's right, not her obligation, to do so. This is because, according to Orthodox Jewish law, the health of the mother, both physically and mentally, is of primary concern and she should never be obliged to do something that threatens her life (Semenic, Callister, & Feldman, 2004).

Individuals of many cultures take certain protective precautions based on their beliefs. For example, many Southeast Asian women fear they will have a complicated labor and birth if they sit in a doorway or on a step. Thus, they tend to avoid areas near doors in waiting rooms and examining rooms. In the Mexican American culture, a common belief is that *mal aire*, or bad air, may enter the body and cause harm. Preventive measures such as keeping the windows closed or covering the head are used. Some Latinos place a raisin on the cord stump of newborns to prevent drafts from entering their bodies. A *taboo* is a behavior or thing to be avoided. Many cultures, including those in the United States, have taboos centered on the unborn baby and/or newborn that are meant to ensure that the baby will survive. For example, it is common among Muslims to avoid naming the baby until after birth; similarly, many Orthodox Jewish women wait to set up the nursery until after the baby is born.

In developing countries, mortality rates among infants and young children are extremely high; thus, certain traditions focus on protecting the baby from evil spirits. For example, many Muslim parents pin an amulet to the newborn's clothes as protection. This may be a palm, an eye, a blue stone, or a verse from the Quran. Following birth, it is common for a male family member to whisper prayers in the newborn baby's ear to declare faith and protect the baby (Cassar, 2006).

Some cultures subscribe to the *equilibrium model of health*, based on the concept of balance between light and dark, heat and cold. This model affects the treatment of pregnant women. Some Eastern philosophies focus on the notion of *yin* and *yang*. Yin represents the female (passive) principle—darkness, cold, wetness; yang is the masculine (active) principle—light, heat, and dryness. When the two are combined, they are all that can be. The hot–cold classification is seen in cultures in Latin America, the Near East, and Asia.

Some Mexican Americans consider illness to be an excess of either hot or cold. To restore health, imbalances are often corrected by the proper use of foods, medications, or herbs. These substances also are classified as hot or cold. For example, an illness attributed to an excess of cold is treated only with hot foods or medications. The classification of foods is not always consistent, but it conforms to a general structure of traditional knowledge. Certain foods, spices, herbs, and medications are perceived to cool or heat the body. These perceptions do not necessarily correspond to the actual temperature; some hot dishes are said to have a cooling quality.

Southeast Asians believe it is important to keep the woman "warm" after birth because blood, which is considered "hot," has been lost and the woman is at risk of becoming "cold." Therefore, they avoid cold drinks and foods following birth. In contrast, many women in India consider pregnancy a "hot" period and eat "cool" foods to balance the hot state (Holroyd, Twinn, & Yim, 2004).

The concepts of hot and cold are not as important in Native American or African American beliefs. Similarities exist in all of these groups, however, because of their emphasis on a balance in nature.

---

each of the three trimesters. Health professionals often refer to these discomforts as minor, but they are not minor to the pregnant woman. They can make her quite uncomfortable and, if they are unexpected, anxious.

✳ *Go to* **nursing.pearsonhighered.com** *for a chart that outlines the common discomforts of pregnancy, their possible causes, and the self-care measures that might relieve discomfort.*

Nausea and Vomiting   Nausea and vomiting are early, very common symptoms occurring in 70%–85% of pregnant women (ACOG, 2004). These symptoms appear sometime after the first missed menstrual period and usually cease by the fourth missed menstrual period. Some women develop an aversion to specific foods, many experience nausea upon arising in the morning, and others experience nausea throughout the day or in the evening.

The exact cause of nausea and vomiting in pregnancy (NVP) is unknown, but it is thought to be multifactorial. An elevated hCG level is believed to be a major factor, but changes in carbohydrate metabolism, fatigue, and emotional factors also may play a role. Research suggests that pregnant women should start taking a multivitamin before reaching 6 weeks' gestation to reduce the effects of NVP (ACOG, 2004).

Complementary and Alternative Therapy
Ginger for Morning Sickness

Women who experience NVP often try alternative approaches to relieve their symptoms because they are reluctant to take medication for fear of harming their fetus. Ginger, long used in traditional Chinese medicine for a variety of maladies ranging from gastrointestinal problems to headaches, is becoming an increasingly popular treatment for NVP, and its safety has been demonstrated in clinical trials (White, 2007). Ginger is available in a variety of forms, including the fresh root, capsules, tea, candy, cookies, crystals, inhaled powdered ginger, and sugared ginger (Lie, 2004). In the first trimester, the daily dosage should not exceed 2 g of dried ginger or 1 g of ginger syrup (Born & Barron, 2005).

In addition to the self-care measures identified in the chart at nursing.pearsonhighered.com, certain complementary therapies may be useful. For example, many women find that acupressure applied to pressure points in the wrists is helpful. Ginger also may relieve NVP (see the Alternative Therapy: Ginger for Morning Sickness box). Pyridoxine (vitamin B$_6$) or vitamin B$_6$ plus doxylamine (Unisom), an OTC antihistamine, is considered a first-line treatment. This is now available by prescription as a combined tablet under the brand name Diclegis. Antihistamine H$_1$-receptor blockers, phenothiazines, and antinausea medications such as Phenergan, Reglan, and Zofran are considered safe and effective for treating refractory cases. In severe cases, methylprednisolone, a steroid, may be used, but as a last resort because it poses a potential risk to the fetus (ACOG, 2004).

The nurse should advise a woman to contact her healthcare provider if she vomits more than once a day or shows signs of dehydration such as dry mouth and concentrated urine. In such cases, the physician/CNM might order an antiemetic such as promethazine (Phenergan).

Urinary Frequency Urinary frequency, a common discomfort of pregnancy, occurs early in pregnancy and again during the third trimester because of pressure of the enlarging uterus on the bladder. Although frequency is considered normal during the first and third trimesters, the woman is advised to report to her healthcare provider signs of bladder infection such as pain, burning with voiding, or blood in the urine. Fluid intake should never be decreased to prevent frequency. The woman needs to maintain an adequate fluid intake—at least 2,000 mL (eight to ten 8-oz glasses) per day. The nurse should also encourage her to empty her bladder frequently (about every 2 hours while awake).

Backache More than 50% of women experience backache during pregnancy (Johnson et al., 2007). Backache is due primarily to exaggeration of the lumbosacral curve that occurs as the uterus enlarges and becomes heavier. Maintaining good posture and using proper body mechanics throughout pregnancy can help prevent backache. The pregnant woman is advised to avoid bending over at the waist to pick up objects and should bend from the knees instead. She should place her feet 12–18 inches apart to maintain body balance. If the woman uses work surfaces that require her to bend, the nurse can advise her to adjust the height of the surfaces.

Collaborative

Members of the interdisciplinary team collaborate to coordinate quality, safe, and evidence-based care. Team members may include perinatologists, neonatologists, certified nurse-midwives, women's health practitioners, obstetricians, pediatricians, dietitians, social workers, mental health care providers, pharmacists, endocrinologists, cardiologists, and registered nurses.

PHARMACOLOGIC THERAPY A number of pharmacologic therapies may be safely used to protect the health and safety of the mother and fetus. A pregnant woman who lives with chronic illness or disease needs to discuss the treatment of her illness during her pregnancy with both her obstetrician and her treating physician. The nurse's responsibility is to elicit information about any preexisting illness when obtaining the client's health history. Particular consideration should be given to clients with existing respiratory or cardiac disease, diabetes mellitus, and HIV. Pregnant clients living with a chronic disease require additional teaching regarding management of their disease during pregnancy. Collaboration among all of the healthcare professionals working with these clients is essential to promoting client self-care and fetal well-being.

CASE STUDY \\ PART 2

When Mrs. Halleck returns to the clinic at 32 weeks' gestation, she says, "I feel like I need to pee all the time." Mrs. Halleck also states that she doesn't feel like exercising as much as she used to. She used to go to the gym three or four times a week, but now she only goes on the weekend, saying "I just don't feel like it. I keep getting these dull headaches, and all I seem to be able to do is sit on the sofa and eat and go to the bathroom." On examination, Mrs. Halleck has gained 12 pounds since her last appointment and her current weight is 150 lb. Her vital signs are T$_O$ 98.6°F, BP 139/90 mmHg, P 84 bpm, R 21/min. Otherwise her examination is normal. When the nurse asks Mrs. Halleck how her family has responded to her pregnancy, Mrs. Halleck replies, "Everyone's been great except my mother. She's only 45. She says she's too young to have a grandchild, and that I'm too young to have a baby." Mrs. Halleck looks away as she says this, adding, "I really wish I had her support."

Clinical Reasoning Questions Level I

1. How should the nurse respond to Mrs. Halleck's statements about her mother?
2. What interventions can the nurse recommend to help Mrs. Halleck with her nausea?
3. What interventions can the nurse recommend to Mrs. Halleck in response to her complaint about urinary frequency?

Clinical Reasoning Questions Level II

4. Which findings should concern the nurse caring for Mrs. Halleck?
5. *Referring to the exemplar on hypertensive disorders in pregnancy:* What other signs and symptoms of preeclampsia should the nurse assess in Mrs. Halleck?
6. *Referring to the exemplar on hypertensive disorders in pregnancy:* What clinical therapies would be appropriate for Mrs. Hallenbeck if the nurse observes edema in her extremities in addition to her high blood pressure?

REVIEW   The Concept of Reproduction

RELATE Link the Concepts

Linking the concept of reproduction with the concept of family:

1. Identify specific examples that demonstrate how the child-bearing family is meeting developmental tasks of pregnancy.

2. Discuss family adaptation to pregnancy.

3. Describe the impact of family stressors on pregnancy.

Linking the concept of reproduction with the concept of nutrition:

4. Develop health promotion strategies to promote optimal nutrition during pregnancy, postpartum, and throughout the first year of life.

5. Analyze the impact of nutritional deficits on birth outcomes.

6. Identify motivational strategies to improve nutritional status throughout the childbearing period.

Linking the concept of reproduction with the concept of perfusion:

7. Analyze fetal assessments to determine placental perfusion and fetal well-being.

8. Discuss the impact of poor perfusion on maternal–fetal outcomes.

9. Prioritize nursing care according to severity of postpartum hemorrhage.

READY Go to Companion Skills Manual

REFER Go to Pearson Nursing Student Resources
nursing.pearsonhighered.com

- Additional review materials
- MiniModule: Twins
- Chart 1: Organ Development in the Embryo and Fetus
- Chart 2: Differential Diagnosis of Pregnancy—Subjective Changes
- Chart 3: Differential Diagnosis of Pregnancy—Objective Changes
- Chart 4: Parental Reactions to Pregnancy
- MiniModule: Adolescent Pregnancy
- Chart 5: Self-Care Measures for Common Discomforts of Pregnancy
- Additional Case Study

REFLECT Case Study \\ Part 3

Mrs. Halleck is at the clinic for a weekly follow-up appointment. She reports that she has been taking her blood pressure at home, and her readings during the past 2 weeks have been consistently around 130/85 mmHg. On examination, her weight is 151 lb, T_O 98.5°F, BP 131/84 mmHg, P 85 bpm, R 20/min. Mrs. Halleck reports that she is very stressed about her blood pressure. She has already lost a baby and she is afraid she may lose this one. In addition, as a relatively young teacher, she does not have a lot of sick time built up and if she cannot return to work, she doesn't know how she and her husband will be able to pay their bills. "My parents won't help," she says, "my mother is still more worried about her image than she is about me." Mrs. Halleck begins to cry and states, "I cry all the time now. I can't sleep. My husband says he doesn't know what to do with me. I knew we should've waited before we tried to have another baby!"

Clinical Thinking Questions Level I

1. What is the priority for care for Mrs. Halleck at this time?

2. Based on the history of her pregnancy and the findings at this visit, what screenings do you anticipate the healthcare provider will order for Mrs. Halleck?

3. What do you think the nurse's responsibility to Mr. Halleck is at this time?

Clinical Thinking Questions Level II

4. What independent nursing interventions can the nurse implement to assist Mrs. Halleck at this time?

5. *Referring to the exemplar on postpartum depression:* What risk factors does Mrs. Halleck have for postpartum depression?

6. *Referring to the exemplar on postpartum depression:* What could the nurse do to assess Mrs. Halleck for possible depression with peripartum onset? The Edinburgh Postnatal Depression Scale and the Postpartum Depression Predictors Inventory may provide additional information to aid the nurse and the healthcare provider in determining if Mrs. Halleck needs further intervention at this time.

EXEMPLAR 33.1   Antepartum Care

EXEMPLAR KEY TERMS

Amniocentesis, *2088*
Contraction stress test (CST), *2088*
Dietary Reference Intakes (DRIs), *2091*
Estimated date of birth (EDB), *2107*
Fetal movement record, *2083*
Folic acid, *2096*
Kegel exercises, *2071*
Lactase deficiency, *2097*
Lacto-ovovegetarians, *2095*
Lactose intolerance, *2097*
Lactovegetarians, *2095*
Lecithin/sphingomyelin (L/S) ratio, *2090*
Nägele rule, *2107*
Nonstress test (NST), *2086*
Pelvic tilt, *2069*

Penta screen, *2090*
Pica, *2095*
Ptyalism, *2072*
Quadruple screen, *2090*
Surfactant, *2090*
Teratogens, *2074*
Ultrasound, *2083*
Vegans, *2095*

EXEMPLAR LEARNING OUTCOMES

After reading about this exemplar, you will be able to:

1. Summarize the care needs of the pregnant client and her family.

2. Examine the potential impact of risk factors on pregnancy.

3. Illustrate the nursing process in providing culturally competent care to the pregnant client and her family.

4. Formulate priority nursing diagnoses appropriate for the pregnant client.

5. Summarize therapies used by interdisciplinary teams in the collaborative care of the pregnant client.

6. Plan evidence-based care for a pregnant client and her family in collaboration with other members of the health-care team.

7. Evaluate expected outcomes for a pregnant client.

▶ OVERVIEW

From the moment a woman finds out she is pregnant, she faces a future marked by dramatic changes. Her appearance will alter. Her relationships will change. Even her psychological state will be affected. She will need to make adjustments in her daily life to cope with these changes. So, too, will her family. The roles and responsibilities of family members, for example, may alter as the woman's ability to perform certain activities changes. The family also must adapt psychologically to the expected arrival of a new member.

The expectant woman and her family will probably have many questions about the pregnancy and its impact on all of them, especially if this is a first pregnancy. Their daily activities and healthcare practices may affect the well-being of the unborn child. Addressing self-care and discomforts related to pregnancy, performing ongoing assessment to ensure fetal and maternal health and safety, and preparing for childbirth are the nursing priorities for the client experiencing a normal pregnancy.

▶ PROMOTING A HEALTHY PREGNANCY

The nurse can help promote maternal and fetal well-being by providing expectant couples with accurate, complete information about health behaviors and issues that can affect pregnancy and childbirth. Health behaviors, such as breast care, rest, sexual activity, and exercise, help protect both the fetus and the mother and decrease the discomfort of the mother during both pregnancy and labor (ACOG, 2011b). Issues that can affect pregnancy range from clothing to employment to travel. The nurse working with pregnant women needs to be able to provide client teaching in all of these areas.

Breast Care

Whether the pregnant woman plans to formula-feed or breast-feed her infant, support of the breasts is important to promote comfort and prevent back strain, particularly if the breasts become large and pendulous. The sensitivity of the breasts in pregnancy is frequently relieved by good support.

Wearing a well-fitting, supportive brassiere that has the following qualities is essential:

■ The straps are wide and do not stretch (elastic straps soon lose their tautness with the weight of the breasts and frequent washing).

■ The cup holds all breast tissue comfortably.

■ Tucks or other devices allow the brassiere to expand, thus accommodating the enlarging chest circumference.

■ The brassiere supports the nipple line approximately midway between the elbow and shoulder but is not pulled up in the back by the weight of the breasts.

Cleanliness of the breasts also is important, especially if they begin leaking colostrum, which may occur during the last

trimester (or earlier in women pregnant with multiples). If colostrum crusts on the nipples, it can be removed with warm water. The woman planning to breastfeed is advised not to use soap on her nipples because of its drying effect.

Some women have flat or inverted nipples. True nipple inversion, which is rare, is usually diagnosed during the initial prenatal assessment. Breast shells designed to correct inverted nipples are effective for some women, but others gain no benefit from them (**Figure 33–26 ●**).

Activity and Rest

Exercise during pregnancy helps maintain maternal fitness and muscle tone, leads to improved self-image, promotes regular bowel function, increases energy, improves sleep, relieves tension, helps control weight gain, and is associated with improved postpartum recovery. Regular aerobic exercise maintains or improves a pregnant woman's general fitness and body image (ACOG, 2011b). Normal participation in exercise can continue throughout an uncomplicated pregnancy and, in fact, is encouraged.

The client can check with her CNM or obstetrician about taking part in strenuous sports, such as skiing and horseback riding. In general, the skilled sportswoman is not discouraged from participating in these activities if her pregnancy is uncomplicated. However, pregnancy is not the appropriate time to learn a new sport.

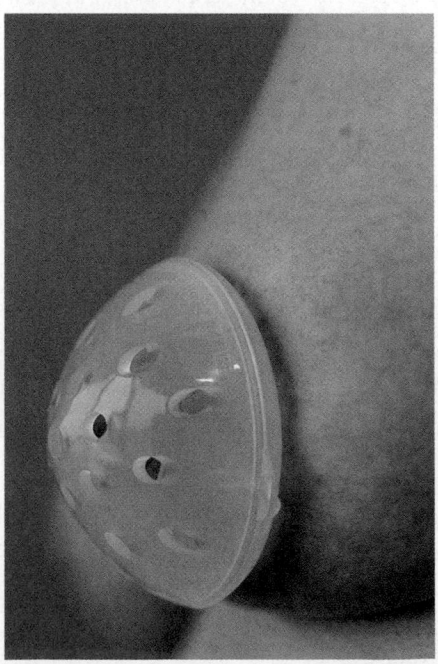

Figure 33–26 ● This breast shell is designed to increase the protractility of inverted nipples. Worn the last 3–4 weeks of pregnancy, it exerts gentle pulling pressure at the edge of the areola, gradually forcing the nipple through the center of the shield. It may be used after birth if necessary.

Certain conditions contraindicate exercise. These conditions include rupture of the membranes, preeclampsia–eclampsia, shortened cervix on transvaginal ultrasound or cerclage placement, persistent vaginal bleeding in the second and third trimesters, risk factors for preterm labor or a history of preterm labor in a prior or current pregnancy, placenta previa after 23 weeks of gestation, and chronic medical conditions that might be negatively impacted by vigorous exercise, such as significant heart disease (ACOG, 2002).

The following guidelines are helpful in counseling pregnant women about exercise:

- Even mild to moderate exercise is beneficial during pregnancy. Regular exercise—at least 30 minutes of moderate exercise daily or most days—is preferred (Penney, 2008).

- After the first trimester, women should avoid exercising in the supine position. In most pregnant women, the supine position is associated with decreased cardiac output. Because uterine blood flow is reduced during exercise as blood is shunted from the visceral organs to the muscles, the remaining cardiac output is further decreased. Similarly, women should avoid standing motionless for prolonged periods (ACOG, 2002; Penney, 2008).

- Because decreased oxygen is available for aerobic exercise during pregnancy, women should modify the intensity of their exercise based on their symptoms, should stop when they become fatigued, and should avoid exercising to the point of exhaustion. Non-weight-bearing exercises, such as swimming and cycling, are recommended because they decrease the risk of injury and provide fitness with comfort.

- As pregnancy progresses and the center of gravity changes, especially in the third trimester, women should avoid exercises in which the loss of balance could pose a risk to mother or fetus. Similarly, women should avoid any type of exercise that might result in even mild abdominal trauma.

- A normal pregnancy requires an additional 300 kcal/day of nutritional intake. Women who exercise regularly during pregnancy should be careful to ensure that they consume an adequate diet.

- To augment heat dissipation, especially during the first trimester, pregnant women should wear clothing that is comfortable and loose while exercising, ensure adequate hydration, and avoid the prolonged overheating associated with vigorous exercise in hot, humid weather because of the possible teratogenic effects of hyperthermia on the fetus (Cunningham et al., 2010). For the same reason, pregnant women are advised to avoid hot tubs and saunas.

- As a result of the cardiovascular changes of pregnancy, heart rate is not an accurate indicator in pregnant women for the intensity of exercise. If a pregnant woman is unable to maintain a conversation while exercising, then her exercise effort is too high (Field, 2012).

The nurse may suggest that the client wear a supportive bra and appropriate shoes when exercising. The nurse should advise the client to warm up and stretch to help prepare the joints for activity and, after exercising, to cool down with a period of mild activity to help restore circulation and avoid pooling of blood. A moderate, rhythmic exercise routine involving large muscle groups, such as swimming, cycling, or brisk walking, is best. Jogging or running is acceptable for women already conditioned to these activities as long as they avoid exercising at maximum effort and overheating.

During exercise, warning signs include pain of any kind, difficulty walking, dizziness, headache, muscle weakness, dyspnea before exertion, uterine contractions, vaginal bleeding, or fluid loss from the vagina (ACOG, 2002). The client should stop exercising if these symptoms occur and modify her exercise program. If the symptoms persist, the client should contact her healthcare provider.

Adequate rest in pregnancy is important for both physical and emotional health. Women need more sleep throughout pregnancy, particularly in the first and last trimesters when they tire easily. Without adequate rest, pregnant women have less resilience. Finding time to rest during the day may be difficult for women who work outside the home or have small children. The nurse can help the expectant mother examine her daily schedule to develop a realistic plan for short periods of rest and relaxation.

Sleeping becomes more difficult during the last trimester because of the enlarged abdomen, increased frequency of urination, and greater activity of the fetus. Finding a comfortable position becomes difficult for the pregnant woman. Progressive relaxation techniques similar to those taught in childbirth classes can help prepare the woman for sleep.

Exercises to Prepare for Childbirth

Certain exercises help strengthen muscle tone in preparation for birth and promote more rapid restoration of muscle tone after birth. Some physical changes of pregnancy can be minimized by faithfully practicing prescribed body-conditioning exercises. Many body-conditioning exercises for pregnancy are taught; a few of the more common ones are discussed here.

Handouts are a valuable tool for providing information, as are pictures. When combined, they are especially useful. Develop a handout that describes the correct way to perform prenatal exercises, and include drawings or photos. For exercises that may be new to a woman, such as the pelvic tilt, provide a handout for later reference, but also demonstrate the exercise and have the woman do a return demonstration.

The **pelvic tilt**, or pelvic rocking, is an exercise that helps prevent or reduce back strain as it strengthens abdominal muscles. To do the pelvic tilt in early pregnancy, the client lies on her back and puts her feet flat on the floor. This flexes the knees and helps prevent strain or discomfort. The client decreases the curvature in her back by pressing her spine toward the floor. With her back pressed to the floor, the client then tightens her abdominal muscles as she tightens and tucks in her buttocks. In the second and third trimesters of pregnancy, the client can also perform the pelvic tilt while on her hands and knees (**Figure 33–27 ●**), sitting in a chair, or standing with her back against a wall. The body alignment that results when the pelvic tilt is done correctly should be maintained as much as possible throughout the day.

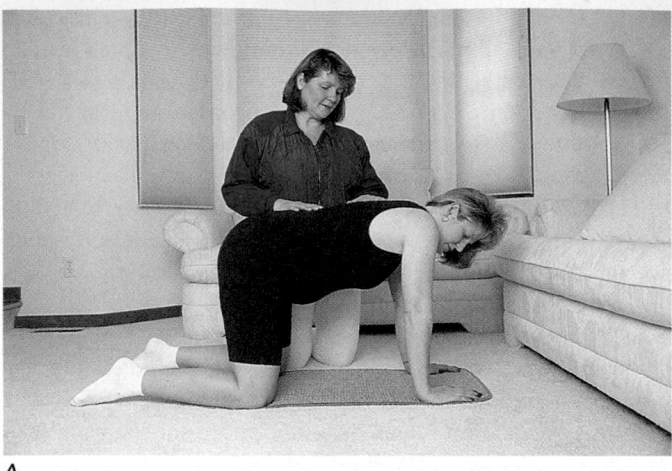

A

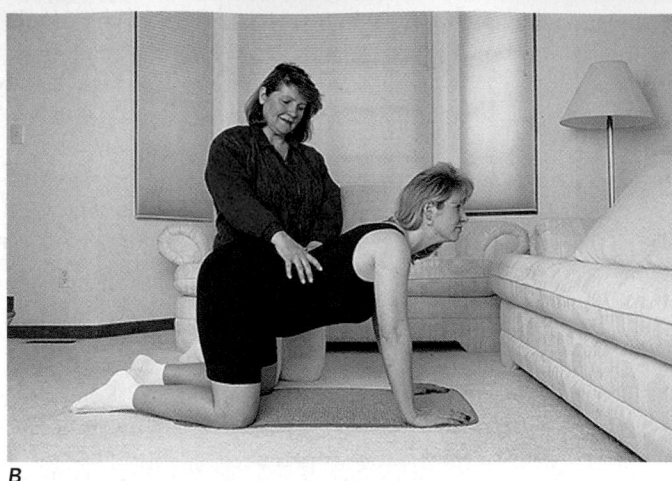

B

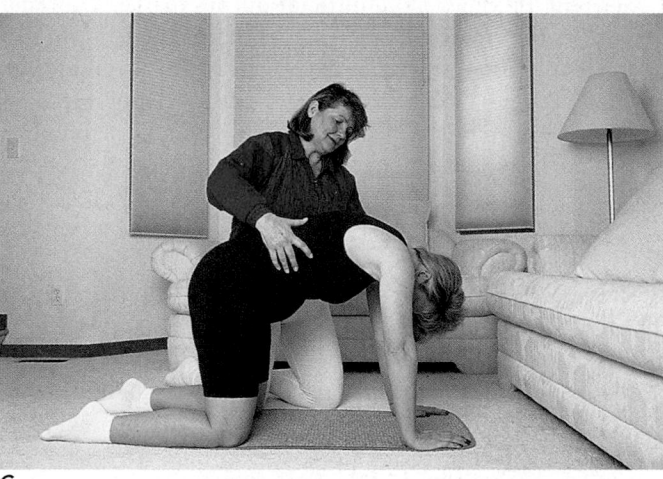

C

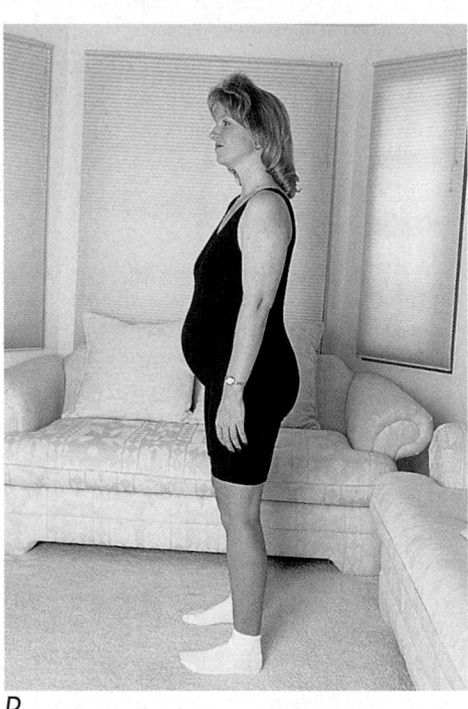

D

Figure 33–27 ● *A*, Starting position when the pelvic tilt is done on hands and knees. The back is flat and parallel to the floor, the hands are below the head, and the knees are directly below the buttocks. *B*, A prenatal yoga instructor offers pointers for proper positioning for the first part of the tilt: head up, neck long and separated from the shoulders, buttocks up, and pelvis thrust back, allowing the back to drop and release on an inhaled breath. *C*, The instructor helps the woman assume the correct position for the next part of the tilt. It is done on a long exhalation, allowing the pregnant woman to arch her back, drop her head loosely, push away from her hands, and draw in the muscles of her abdomen to strengthen them. Note that in this position, the pelvis and buttocks are tucked under, and the buttock muscles are tightened. *D*, Proper posture. The knees are slightly bent but not locked, and the pelvis and buttocks are tucked under, thereby lengthening the spine and helping support the weighty abdomen. With her chin tucked in, this woman's neck, shoulders, hips, knees, and feet are all in a straight line perpendicular to the floor. Her feet are parallel. This is also the starting position for doing the pelvic tilt while standing.

SAFETY ALERT
Doing the pelvic tilt on hands and knees may aggravate back strain. Teach women with a history of minor back problems to do the pelvic tilt only in the standing position.

ABDOMINAL EXERCISES   A basic exercise to increase abdominal muscle tone is tightening abdominal muscles with each breath. This exercise can be done in any position, but it is best learned during early pregnancy. The client lies supine with knees flexed and feet flat on the floor. The client expands her abdomen and slowly takes a deep breath. Exhaling slowly, she gradually pulls in her abdominal muscles until they are fully contracted. She relaxes for a few seconds and then repeats the exercise. The pregnant woman should avoid the supine position after the first trimester.

Partial sit-ups strengthen abdominal muscle tone and are best done according to individual comfort levels. In early pregnancy, partial sit-ups must be done with the knees flexed and the feet flat on the floor to avoid strain on the lower back. The client stretches

Complementary and Alternative Therapy   Yoga During Pregnancy

The following advice is important for women who practice yoga during pregnancy (Field, 2012):

- During pregnancy, some yoga poses or positions are contraindicated. Pregnant women should avoid poses that put pressure on the uterus as well as any extreme stretching positions.
- Because of the changed center of gravity that occurs as pregnancy progresses, pregnant women need to be especially careful to maintain balance when stretching.
- Pregnant women should avoid stomach-lying for any poses. After 20 weeks of gestation, they should lie on their left side rather than on their back for floor positions.

- In the last trimester, pregnant women may experience vena cava syndrome resulting in reduced blood flow back to the heart as the growing fetus puts pressure on the major vessels when lying flat on their backs.
- Pregnant women should immediately stop any pose that is uncomfortable.
- Warning signs that indicate the need to contact the physician or CNM immediately include dizziness, extreme shortness of breath, sudden swelling, contractions, leaking of fluid, and vaginal bleeding.

her arms toward her knees as she slowly pulls her head and shoulders off the floor to a comfortable level (if she has poor abdominal muscle tone, she may not be able to pull up very far). She then slowly returns to the starting position, takes a deep breath, and repeats the exercise while exhaling. To strengthen the oblique abdominal muscles, the client repeats the process but stretches the left arm to the side of her right knee, returns to the floor, takes a deep breath, and then, while exhaling, reaches with the right arm to the left knee. During the second and third trimesters, these exercises can be done on a large exercise ball. They can be done approximately five times in a sequence, and the sequence can be repeated at other times during the day as desired. It is important to do the exercises slowly to prevent muscle strain and overtiring.

PERINEAL EXERCISES   Perineal muscle tightening, also called **Kegel exercises**, strengthens the pubococcygeus muscle and increases its elasticity (**Figure 33–28 ●**). The woman can feel the specific muscle group to be exercised by stopping urination midstream. Doing Kegel exercises while urinating is discouraged because this practice has been associated with urinary stasis and urinary tract infection.

Childbirth educators sometimes use the following technique to teach Kegel exercises: Tell the woman to think of her perineal muscles as an elevator. When she relaxes, the elevator is on the

first floor. To do the exercises, she contracts, bringing the elevator to the second, third, and fourth floors. She keeps the elevator on the fourth floor for a few seconds and then gradually relaxes the area. If the exercise is properly done, the woman does not contract the muscles of the buttocks and thighs.

Kegel exercises can be done at almost any time. Some women use ordinary events—for instance, stopping at a red light—as a cue to remember to do the exercise. Others do Kegel exercises while waiting in a checkout line, talking on the telephone, or watching television.

INNER THIGH EXERCISES   The nurse can advise the pregnant woman to assume a seated position with the knees bent and the bottoms of the feet together. This "tailor sit" stretches the muscles of the inner thighs in preparation for labor and birth.

Sexual Activity

As a result of the physiological, anatomical, and emotional changes of pregnancy, couples usually have many questions and concerns about sexual activity during pregnancy. Often, these questions are about possible injury to the baby or the woman during intercourse and about changes in the desire each partner feels.

In the past, couples were often warned to avoid sexual intercourse during the last 6–8 weeks of pregnancy in order to prevent

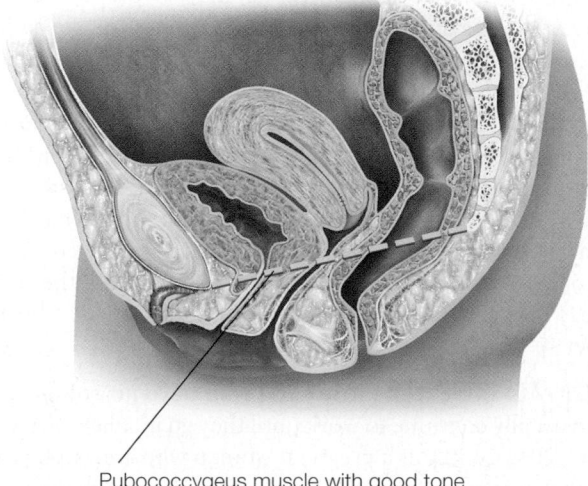

Pubococcygeus muscle with good tone

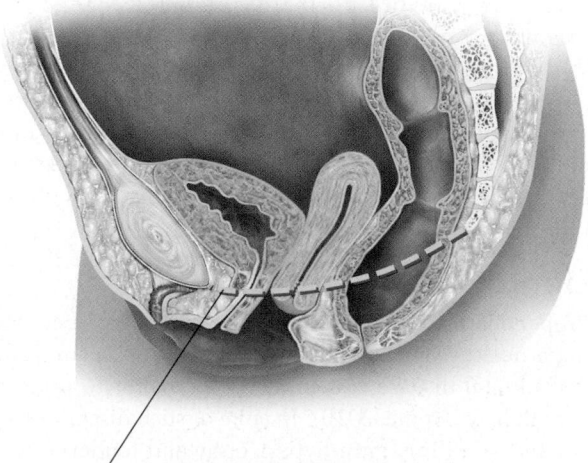

Pubococcygeus muscle with poor tone

Figure 33–28 ● Kegel exercises. The woman tightens the pubococcygeus muscle to improve support to the pelvic organs.

complications, such as infection or premature rupture of the membranes. However, these fears seem to be unfounded. In a healthy pregnancy, there is no medical reason to limit sexual activity. Intercourse is contraindicated for medical reasons, such as the bag of waters being ruptured or if the client has placenta previa (Katz, 2008).

The expectant mother may experience changes in sexual desire and response. Often, these changes are related to the various discomforts that occur throughout pregnancy. For instance, during the first trimester, fatigue or nausea and vomiting may decrease desire, and breast tenderness may make the woman less responsive to fondling of her breasts. During the second trimester, many of the discomforts have lessened, and with the vascular congestion of the pelvis, the woman may experience greater sexual satisfaction than she experienced before pregnancy.

During the third trimester, interest in coitus may again decrease as the woman becomes more uncomfortable and fatigued. In addition, shortness of breath, painful pelvic ligaments, urinary frequency, leg cramps, and decreased mobility may lessen sexual desire and activity. If they are not already doing so, the heterosexual couple should consider coital positions other than male superior, such as side by side, female superior, and vaginal rear entry.

Sexual activity does not have to include intercourse. Many of the nurturing and sexual needs of the pregnant woman can be satisfied by cuddling, kissing, and being held. The warm, sensual feelings that accompany these activities can be an end in themselves. Her partner, however, may choose to masturbate more frequently than before.

The sexual desires of partners of pregnant women are also affected by many factors in pregnancy. These factors include the previous relationship with the partner, acceptance of the pregnancy, attitudes toward the partner's change of appearance, and concern about hurting the expectant mother or baby. Some find it difficult to view their partners as sexually appealing while they are adjusting to the concept of their partners as mothers. Others find their partners' pregnancies arousing and experience feelings of increased happiness, intimacy, and closeness.

The expectant couple should be aware of their changing sexual desires, the normality of these changes, and the importance of communicating these changes to each other so that they can make nurturing adaptations. The nurse has an important role in helping the expectant couple adapt. The couple should feel free to express concerns about sexual activity and the nurse should be able to respond and give anticipatory guidance in a comfortable manner. See the Client Teaching feature.

Dental Care

Proper dental hygiene is important in pregnancy because ensuring a healthy oral environment is essential to overall health. Periodontal disease is a contributing factor to preterm labor (Babalola & Omole, 2010). In spite of such discomforts as nausea and vomiting, gum hypertrophy and tenderness, possible **ptyalism** (excessive, often bitter salivation), and heartburn, pregnant women need to maintain regular oral hygiene by brushing at least twice a day and flossing daily.

The nurse should encourage the pregnant woman to have a dental checkup early in her pregnancy. Dentistry should proceed as needed in pregnancy. Local anesthesia is fine, but epinephrine should not be used. The woman should inform her dentist of her pregnancy so that she is not exposed to teratogenic substances.

Other Self-Care Measures

A number of self-care measures not directly related to pregnancy are necessary to ensure the health of the mother and fetus. Some of these measures relate to immunizations, clothing, bathing, maternal employment, and travel.

IMMUNIZATIONS   All women of childbearing age need to be aware of the risks of receiving certain immunizations if pregnancy is possible. The influenza and Tdap vaccines are recommended for pregnant women (CDC, 2014b). Immunizations with attenuated live viruses, such as rubella vaccine, should not be given in pregnancy because of the teratogenic effect of the live viruses on the developing embryo. The most current recommendations on vaccines related to pregnancy should be obtained from the Centers for Disease Control and Prevention (CDC) Web site (www.cdc.gov).

CLOTHING   Traditionally, maternity clothes have been constructed with fuller lines to allow for the increase in abdominal size during pregnancy. However, maternity wear has changed in recent years and now also includes clothes that are more fitted, with little attempt to hide the pregnant abdomen. Maternity clothing can be expensive, and it is worn for a relatively short time. Women can economize by sharing clothes with friends, sewing their own garments, or buying used maternity clothes.

High-heeled shoes tend to aggravate back discomfort by increasing the curvature of the lower back. They are best avoided if the woman experiences backache or has problems with balance. Shoes should fit properly and feel comfortable.

BATHING   Because perspiration and mucoid vaginal discharge increase during pregnancy, hygiene is important. Practices related to cleansing the body are often influenced by cultural norms; thus, a pregnant woman may choose to cleanse only some portions of her body daily or may elect to take daily showers or tub baths. Caution is needed during tub baths because balance becomes a problem in late pregnancy. Rubber mats and hand grips are important safety devices. Vasodilation caused by warm water may make the woman feel faint when she attempts to get out of the tub, so she may require assistance, especially during the last trimester. During the first trimester, pregnant women should avoid hyperthermia associated with the use of a hot tub or Jacuzzi, because it may increase the risk for miscarriage or neural tube defects (Cunningham et al., 2010; Snijder et al., 2012).

EMPLOYMENT   Pregnant women who have no complications can usually continue to work until they go into labor (AAP & ACOG, 2013). Although pregnant women who are employed in jobs that require prolonged standing (>5 hours) do have a higher incidence of preterm birth, prolonged standing has no effect on fetal growth (Snijder et al., 2012).

Client Teaching Sexual Activity During Pregnancy

Discussion about various sexual activities requires that the nurse be comfortable with his or her sexuality and also tactful. A discussion of sexuality and sexual activity should stress the importance of open communication so that the couple feels comfortable expressing feelings, preferences, and concerns. The nurse can assist the couple regarding sexual activity during pregnancy with the following client teaching:

- Begin by explaining that the pregnant woman may experience changes in desire during the course of pregnancy. During the first trimester, discomforts such as nausea, fatigue, and breast tenderness may make intercourse less desirable for many pregnant women. Universal statements that give permission, such as "Many couples experience changes in sexual desire during pregnancy. What kind of changes have you experienced?" are often effective in starting discussion. Depending on the woman's (or couple's) level of knowledge and sophistication, part or all of this discussion may be necessary.

- In the second trimester, as symptoms decrease, desire may increase. In the third trimester, discomfort and fatigue may lead to decreased desire in the pregnant woman. If the partner is present, approach the partner in the same nonjudgmental way discussed previously. If not, ask the pregnant woman if she has noticed any changes in her partner or if her partner has expressed any concerns.

- Explain that partners of pregnant women may notice changes in their level of desire, too. Among other things, this change may be related to feelings about their partner's changing appearance, their belief about the acceptability of sexual activity with a pregnant woman, or concern about hurting the woman or fetus. Some partners find the changes of pregnancy erotic; others must adjust to the notion of their partners as mothers. Deal with any specific questions about the physical and psychological changes that the couple may have.

- Explain that the woman may notice that orgasms are much more intense during the last weeks of pregnancy and may be followed by cramping. Because of the pressure of the enlarging uterus on the vena cava, the pregnant woman

should not lie flat on her back for intercourse after about the fourth month. If the couple prefers that position, a pillow should be placed under the pregnant woman's right hip to displace the uterus. Alternative positions such as side by side, female superior, or vaginal rear entry may become necessary as her uterus enlarges.

- Stress that sexual activities both partners enjoy are generally acceptable. It is not advisable, however, for couples who favor anal sex to go from anal penetration to vaginal penetration because of the risk of introducing *Escherichia coli* into the vagina. The couple may be content with those approaches to meeting their sexual needs, or they may require assurance that such approaches are indeed "normal."

- Suggest that alternative methods of expressing intimacy and affection, such as cuddling, holding and stroking each other, and kissing may help maintain the couple's feelings of warmth and closeness. If the partner feels desire for further sexual release, the pregnant woman may help her partner masturbate to climax, or the partner may prefer to masturbate in private.

- Advise the pregnant woman who is interested in masturbation as a form of gratification that the orgasmic contractions may be especially intense during later pregnancy.

- Stress that sexual intercourse is contraindicated once the membranes have ruptured or if bleeding is present. Pregnant women with a history of preterm labor may be advised to avoid intercourse, because the oxytocin that is released with orgasm stimulates uterine contractions and may trigger preterm labor. Because oxytocin is also released with nipple stimulation, fondling the breasts may be contraindicated in those cases as well.

- Some couples are skilled at expressing their feelings about sexual activity. Others find it difficult and can benefit from specific suggestions. The nurse should provide opportunities for discussion throughout the talk. An explanation of the contraindications accompanied by their rationale provides specific guidelines that most couples find helpful. Specific handouts on sexual activity are helpful for couples and may address topics that were not discussed.

Fetotoxic hazards are always a concern to the expectant couple. The pregnant woman (or the woman contemplating pregnancy) who works in industry should contact her company physician or nurse about possible hazards in her work environment and do her own reading and research on environmental hazards as well. Similarly, a male partner can seek information about hazards in his workplace that might affect his sperm.

TRAVEL If medical or pregnancy complications are not present, there are no restrictions on travel. Pregnant women are advised to avoid travel if she has a history of bleeding or preeclampsia or if multiple births are anticipated. Availability of medical care at the destination is an important factor for the near-term woman who travels. It may be helpful to travel with a copy of the woman's medical record (Hezelgrave et al., 2011).

Travel by automobile can be especially fatiguing, aggravating many of the discomforts of pregnancy. The pregnant

woman needs frequent opportunities to get out of the car and walk. (A good pattern is to stop every 2 hours and walk around for approximately 10 minutes.) She should wear both lap and shoulder belts; the lap belt should fit snugly and be positioned under the abdomen and across the upper thighs. The shoulder strap should rest comfortably between the woman's breasts. Seat belts play an important role in preventing fetal and maternal morbidity and mortality with subsequent fetal death (ACOG, 2011a). Fetal death in car crashes is related to placental separation (abruptio placentae) as a result of uterine trauma. Use of the shoulder belt decreases the risk of traumatic flexion of the woman's body, thereby decreasing the risk of placental separation.

As pregnancy progresses, long-distance trips are best taken by plane or train. Currently, flying is considered to be safe up to 36 weeks of gestation in the absence of any complications (AAP & ACOG, 2013). Before flying, the woman should check with her airline to see if they have any travel restrictions. Prolonged air travel may lead to edema in the lower extremities and the development of venous thrombolytic events. To minimize complications, the traveler should consider wearing support stockings, maintain oral hydration, periodically move the lower extremities, change positions frequently, and move about the cabin at least every 2 hours when conditions are favorable (AAP & ACOG, 2013).

Complementary and Alternative Therapy

Many pregnant women elect to use complementary and alternative therapies, such as homeopathy, herbal medicine, acupressure and acupuncture, biofeedback, therapeutic touch, massage, and chiropractic, as part of a holistic approach to their healthcare regimens. The nurse should inquire about the use of complementary and alternative therapies as part of a routine antepartum assessment. The nurse working with pregnant women and childbearing families needs to develop a general understanding of the more commonly used therapies in order to be able to answer basic questions and provide resources as needed.

Pregnant women should understand that herbs are considered to be dietary supplements and are not regulated through the FDA as prescription or OTC drugs. Due to limited scientific evaluation of potential harmful effects on the fetus, herbal supplements should be avoided, particularly in the first trimester (Yankowitz, 2008).

Stay Current: Additional information about herbs, homeopathic remedies, and other alternative options may be accessed at the Web site for the National Center for Complementary and Alternative Medicine, **http://nccam.nih.gov**.

Teratogenic Substances

Substances that adversely affect the normal growth and development of the fetus are called **teratogens** (see the Concept section of this module and the exemplar on Prenatal Substance Exposure in the module on Addiction). The nurse who is caring for the pregnant client, or for the woman who is trying to become pregnant, should emphasize the need for that client to discuss the use of any and all medications with her obstetrician. Obstetricians and nurse-midwives are the most informed about the potential effects of medications on the fetus. The nurse should also instruct the client with a chronic condition, such as asthma or diabetes, to inform her treating physician if she is (or is trying to become) pregnant. The pregnant woman with a chronic condition should be encouraged to use a single pharmacy and to inform the pharmacy staff that she is pregnant. Discussing potential hazards in the work and home environments is important for preventing teratogenic effects on the fetus.

▶ RELIEF OF THE COMMON DISCOMFORTS OF PREGNANCY

The common discomforts of pregnancy result from physiological and anatomical changes and are fairly specific to each of the three trimesters (**Table 33–2** ●). Health professionals often refer to these discomforts as minor, but they are not minor to the pregnant woman. In fact, they can make her quite uncomfortable and, if they are unexpected, anxious.

SAFETY ALERT
At each prenatal visit, focus client teaching on changes or possible discomforts the pregnant woman might encounter during the coming month and the next trimester. If the pregnancy is progressing normally, spend a few minutes describing her baby at that particular stage of development.

TABLE 33–2 Self-Care Measures for Common Discomforts of Pregnancy

DISCOMFORT	INFLUENCING FACTORS	SELF-CARE MEASURES
First Trimester		
Nausea and vomiting	Increased levels of hCG Changes in carbohydrate metabolism Emotional factors Fatigue	Avoid odors or causative factors. Eat dry crackers or toast before arising in morning. Have small but frequent meals. Avoid greasy or highly seasoned foods. Take dry meals with fluids between meals. Drink carbonated beverages.
Urinary frequency	Pressure of uterus on bladder in both first and third trimesters	Void when urge is felt. Increase fluid intake during the day. Decrease fluid intake *only* in the evening to decrease nocturia.
Fatigue	Specific causative factors unknown May be aggravated by nocturia due to urinary frequency	Plan time for a nap or rest period daily. Go to bed early. Seek family support and assistance with responsibilities so that more time is available to rest.
Breast tenderness	Increased levels of estrogen and progesterone	Wear well-fitting, supportive bra.
Increased vaginal discharge	Hyperplasia of vaginal mucosa and increased production of mucus by the endocervical glands due to the increase in estrogen levels	Promote cleanliness by daily bathing. Avoid douching, nylon underpants, and pantyhose; cotton underpants are more absorbent.

TABLE 33–2 Self-Care Measures for Common Discomforts of Pregnancy (*continued*)

DISCOMFORT	INFLUENCING FACTORS	SELF-CARE MEASURES
Nasal stuffiness and nosebleed (epistaxis)	Elevated estrogen levels	May be unresponsive, but cool-air vaporizer may help; avoid use of nasal sprays and decongestants.
Ptyalism (excessive, often bitter salivation)	Specific causative factors unknown	Use astringent mouthwashes, chew gum, or suck hard candy.
Second and Third Trimesters		
Heartburn (pyrosis)	Increased production of progesterone, decreasing gastrointestinal motility and increasing relaxation of cardiac sphincter, displacement of stomach by enlarging uterus, thus regurgitation of acidic gastric contents into the esophagus	Eat small and more frequent meals. Use low-sodium antacids. Avoid overeating, fatty and fried foods, lying down after eating, and sodium bicarbonate.
Ankle edema	Prolonged standing or sitting Increased levels of sodium due to hormonal influences Circulatory congestion of lower extremities Increased capillary permeability Varicose veins	Practice frequent dorsiflexion of feet when prolonged sitting or standing is necessary. Elevate legs when sitting or resting. Avoid tight garters or restrictive bands around legs.
Varicose veins	Venous congestion in the lower veins that increases with pregnancy Hereditary factors (weakening of walls of veins, faulty valves) Increased age and weight gain	Elevate legs frequently. Wear supportive hose. Avoid crossing legs at the knees, standing for long periods, garters, and hosiery with constrictive bands.
Hemorrhoids	Constipation (see following discussion) Increased pressure from gravid uterus on hemorrhoidal veins	Avoid constipation. Apply ice packs, topical ointments, anesthetic agents, warm soaks, or sitz baths; gently reinsert into rectum as necessary.
Constipation	Increased levels of progesterone, which cause general bowel sluggishness Pressure of enlarging uterus on intestine Iron supplements Diet, lack of exercise, and decreased fluids	Increase fluid intake, fiber in the diet, and exercise. Develop regular bowel habits. Use stool softeners as recommended by healthcare provider.
Backache	Increased curvature of the lumbosacral vertebrae as the uterus enlarges Increased levels of hormones, which cause softening of cartilage in body joints	Use proper body mechanics. Practice the pelvic-tilt exercise.
	Fatigue Poor body mechanics	Avoid uncomfortable working heights, high-heeled shoes, lifting of heavy loads, and fatigue.
Leg cramps	Imbalance of calcium/phosphorus ratio Increased pressure of uterus on nerves Fatigue Poor circulation to lower extremities Pointing the toes	Practice dorsiflexion of feet to stretch affected muscle. Evaluate diet. Apply heat to affected muscles. Arise slowly from resting position.
Faintness	Postural hypotension Sudden change of position causing venous pooling in dependent veins Standing for long periods in warm area Anemia	Avoid prolonged standing in warm or stuffy environments. Evaluate hematocrit and hemoglobin.
Dyspnea	Decreased vital capacity from pressure of enlarging uterus on the diaphragm	Use proper posture when sitting and standing. Sleep propped up with pillows for relief if problem occurs at night.
Flatulence	Decreased gastrointestinal motility leading to delayed emptying time Pressure of growing uterus on large intestine Air swallowing	Avoid gas-forming foods. Chew food thoroughly. Get regular daily exercise. Maintain normal bowel habits.
Carpal tunnel syndrome	Compression of median nerve in carpal tunnel of wrist Aggravated by repetitive hand movements	Avoid aggravating hand movements. Use splint as prescribed. Elevate affected arm.

Sources: Davidson, M., London, M., & Ladewig, P. (2012). Olds' maternal-newborn nursing & womens' health across the lifespan (9th ed., Table 16-3, pp. 350–351). Upper Saddle River, NJ: Pearson Prentice Hall.

Focus on Diversity and Culture Self-Care Techniques During Pregnancy

BELIEF OR PRACTICE	NURSING CONSIDERATIONS
Home Remedies	
■ Pregnant women of Native American background may use herbal remedies. An example is the dandelion, which contains a milky juice in its stem believed to increase breast milk flow in mothers who choose to breastfeed (Spector, 2009). ■ Clients of Chinese descent may drink ginseng tea for faintness after childbirth or as a sedative when mixed with bamboo leaves. ■ Some individuals of African heritage may use self-medication for pregnancy discomforts—for example, laxatives to prevent or treat constipation (Spector, 2009).	Find out what medications and home remedies your client is using, and counsel your client regarding their overall effects. It is common for individuals to avoid telling healthcare workers about home remedies, because the client may feel the use of such remedies will be judged unfavorably. Phrase your questions in a sensitive, accepting way.
Nutrition	
■ Some women of Italian background may believe it is necessary to satisfy desires for certain foods in order to prevent congenital anomalies. Also, they may believe they must eat food that they smell, or else the fetus will move "inside," which will result in a miscarriage. ■ Some pregnant women of African descent may continue the tradition of eating clay, dirt, or starch, which they believe will benefit the mother and fetus (Spector, 2009).	Discuss the client's beliefs and practices in regard to nutrition during pregnancy. Obtain a diet history from the client. Discuss the importance of a well-balanced diet during pregnancy, with consideration of the client's cultural beliefs and practices. In some cases, you might want to suggest remedies that may be more effective—for example, eating high-fiber foods to reduce constipation. If the home remedy is not harmful, there is no reason to ask a client to discontinue this practice.
Alternative Healthcare Providers	
■ Some pregnant women of Mexican background may choose to seek out the care of a *partera* (midwife) for prenatal and intrapartum care. A *partera* speaks their language, shares a similar culture, and can care for pregnant women at home or in a birthing center instead of a hospital. ■ Some individuals in Hispanic-American communities may use a *curandero* (folk healer). A *curandero* frequently uses herbs, massage, and religious artifacts for treatment (Spector, 2009).	Discuss the variety of choices for healthcare providers available to the pregnant woman. Contrast the benefits and risks of different settings for prenatal care and birth. Provide reassurance that the goal of healthcare during pregnancy and birth is a healthy outcome for mother and baby, with respect for the specific cultural beliefs and practices of the client.
Exercise	
■ Some pregnant women of Italian descent may fear changing their body position in certain ways because they believe this may cause the fetus to develop abnormally (Spector, 2009). ■ Some individuals of European, African, and Mexican descent believe that reaching over the head during pregnancy can harm the baby.	Ask the client whether she is afraid of any activities because of the pregnancy. Assure her that reaching over her head will not harm the baby, and evaluate other activities for their effect on the pregnancy.
Spirituality	
■ Native Americans are aware of the mind–soul connection and may try to follow certain practices to have a healthy pregnancy and birth. These practices could include a focus on peace and positive thoughts as well as certain types of prayers and ceremonies. A traditional healer may assist them (Ogburn et al., 2012). ■ Some individuals of European background may tend to pay more attention to spirituality in their life to alleviate fears and ensure a safe birth.	Encourage the use of support systems and spiritual aids that provide comfort for the pregnant woman.

▶ ALTERATIONS

Even though pregnancy is a normal process, for some women it may become a life-threatening event because of potential or existing complications. These complications can result from factors such as age, parity, blood type, socioeconomic status, psychological health, or preexisting chronic illnesses. Effective prenatal care is directed toward identifying factors that increase a pregnant woman's risk and developing supportive therapies that promote optimal health of the mother and her fetus.

▶ ASSESSMENT OF FETAL WELL-BEING

A number of tests are used to obtain accurate and helpful data about the developing fetus. At times, just one test is done; in other circumstances, a combination of testing is necessary. Some of these assessment techniques pose risks to the fetus and, possibly, to the pregnant woman; the risk to both should be considered before deciding to perform the test. The healthcare provider must be certain that the advantages outweigh

Client Teaching Assessment of Fetal Well-Being

Before administration of any screening or diagnostic test, the nurse should use the following guide to ensure that the client knows the reason for performing the procedure:

1. Assess whether the woman knows the reason why the screening or diagnostic test is being recommended:
   - "Has your physician or nurse-midwife told you why this test is necessary?"
   - "Sometimes tests are done for many different reasons. Can you tell me why you are having this test?"
   - "What is your understanding about what the test will show?"
2. Provide an opportunity for questions:
   - "Do you have any questions about the test?"
   - "Is there anything that is not clear to you?"

3. Explain the test procedure, paying particular attention to any preparation the woman needs before the test:
   - "The test that has been ordered for you is designed to _____." (Add specific information about the particular test. Give the explanation in simple language.)
4. Validate the woman's understanding of the preparation:
   - "Tell me what you will have to do to get ready for this test."
5. Give permission for the woman to continue to ask questions if needed:
   - "I'll be with you during the test. If you have any questions at any time, please don't hesitate to ask."

Alterations and Therapies Pregnancy

ALTERATION	DESCRIPTION	THERAPY
Pregestational Factors		
Prenatal substance abuse	Use of tobacco, alcohol, or illegal substances, including cocaine, methamphetamines, narcotics, or abuse of prescription medications. Such use can be profoundly harmful to the fetus.	■ Nursing care is focused on motivating the client to abstain from substance use and on supporting the client through the withdrawal-and-recovery period. ■ For more information, see the exemplar on Prenatal Substance Exposure in the module on Addiction.
Diabetes mellitus	An endocrine disorder of carbohydrate metabolism resulting from inadequate production or use of insulin. The client may be diagnosed with diabetes before becoming pregnant or develop gestational diabetes during pregnancy.	■ Client teaching is important to promote self-care focused on stable glucose levels using a balance of diet, exercise, medications, and frequent monitoring. ■ For more information, see the exemplar on Diabetes in the module on Metabolism.
Anemia	Inadequate levels of hemoglobin in the blood, defined as levels of <11 g/dL during pregnancy (ACOG, 2008a) caused by either insufficient hemoglobin production related to nutritional deficiency in iron or folic acid or to hemoglobin destruction in inherited disorders, such as sickle cell disease.	■ Monitor clients for symptoms of anemia (fatigue, pallor, shortness of breath, and alterations in level of consciousness). ■ Promote good nutrition in order to meet the body's metabolic needs. For more information, see the exemplar on Anemia in the module on Cellular Regulation.
HIV/AIDS	Viral infection caused by the human immunodeficiency virus (HIV); called AIDS (acquired immunodeficiency syndrome) when symptoms of the disease appear.	■ Reassure the pregnant woman that risk of transmission to the fetus can be reduced by use of antiretroviral medication, that pregnancy is not believed to accelerate progression of the disease, and that most medications used to treat HIV can be safely taken during pregnancy. ■ Cesarean birth and abstaining from breastfeeding are recommended to reduce the risk of transmission to the baby. ■ For more information, see the exemplar on HIV and AIDS in the module on Immunity.

(continued on next page)

Alterations and Therapies **Pregnancy** (continued)

ALTERATION	DESCRIPTION	THERAPY
Heart disease	Pregnancy increases cardiac output, heart rate, and blood volume, which the normal heart can adapt to but which may put stress on the heart of a client with decreased cardiac reserve. Women in Class I or II usually experience a normal pregnancy; those in Class III or IV are at risk for more severe complications.	■ Assess the stress of pregnancy on functional capacity of the heart during all antepartum visits. This includes monitoring vital signs and comparing them with prepregnancy levels, activity level, and factors that increase strain on the heart, such as anemia, infection, anxiety, lack of a support system, and lifestyle demands (career, home life, and other children to care for). ■ For more information, see the module on Perfusion.
Asthma	An obstructive lung condition that can improve symptoms in some pregnant clients and worsen symptoms in others. Asthma has also been linked with higher rates of hyperemesis gravidarum, preeclampsia, uterine hemorrhage, and perinatal mortality.	■ Promote oxygenation to prevent hypoxia in both the client and the fetus. ■ Teach the client how to recognize signs of preterm labor, because premature birth is higher in clients with asthma. ■ The goal of therapy is to prevent maternal exacerbations, because even a mild exacerbation can cause severe hypoxia-related complications in the fetus. If an exacerbation occurs, inhaled albuterol is recommended. ■ For more information, see the exemplar on Asthma in the module on Oxygenation.
Epilepsy	Chronic disorder characterized by seizures. Many clients have uneventful pregnancies with excellent outcomes. Those with more frequent seizures before pregnancy may have exacerbations during pregnancy. Encourage clients to consult with their neurologists before and during pregnancy.	■ Teach the client to continue taking recommended antiseizure medication as well as supplementing with folic acid and vitamin K throughout the pregnancy to improve fetal outcome. ■ For more information, see the exemplar on Seizure Disorders in the module on Intracranial Regulation.
Hyperthyroidism	Enlarged, overactive thyroid gland. This can increase the risk for preeclampsia and postpartum hemorrhage in the mother and for abortion, intrauterine death, and stillbirth in the fetus if not well controlled. Even low doses of antithyroid drug in the mother may produce a mild fetal/neonatal hypothyroidism; higher dose may produce a goiter or mental deficiencies. Fetal loss is not increased in women who are euthyroid.	■ Nursing care is focused on early identification and treatment. ■ For more information, see the exemplar on Thyroid Disease in the module on Metabolism.
Hypothyroidism	Characterized by inadequate thyroid secretions (decreased thyroxine [T_4]: thyroxine-binding globulin [TBG] ratio), elevated thyroid-stimulating hormone (TSH), lowered basal metabolic rate, and enlarged thyroid gland (goiter). Long-term replacement therapy usually continues during pregnancy at the same dosage as before. If the mother is untreated, the rate of fetal loss is 50%, with a high risk for congenital goiter or true cretinism. Therefore, newborns are screened for T_4 level. Mild TSH elevations present little risk because TSH does not cross the placenta.	■ Nursing care is focused on early identification and treatment to prevent potential complications. ■ Teach the client the importance of taking a thyroid hormone supplement regularly to maintain stable levels. ■ For more information, see the exemplar on Thyroid Disease in the module on Metabolism.

Alterations and Therapies **Pregnancy** (continued)

ALTERATION	DESCRIPTION	THERAPY
Multiple sclerosis	Neurological disorder that destroys the myelin sheath of nerve fibers and affects primarily young women. Pregnancy is associated with remission and slightly increased relapse rates postpartum. Uterine contraction strength is not diminished, but labor may be almost painless because of diminished sensation.	■ Nursing care is focused on promoting rest and nutrition. ■ For more information, see the exemplar on Multiple Sclerosis in the module on Mobility.
Rheumatoid arthritis	Chronic inflammatory disease believed to have a genetic component. Remission of symptoms is common during the antepartum period, with relapse in the postpartum period. Heavy salicylate use may prolong gestation and lengthen labor. Salicylates may have possible teratogenic effects.	■ Monitor for anemia secondary to blood loss from salicylate therapy. ■ Encourage rest to relieve weight-bearing joints, but client needs to continue range-of-motion (ROM) exercises. ■ The client in remission may be advised to stop medications during pregnancy. ■ For more information, see the exemplar on Rheumatoid Arthritis in the module on Immunity.
Systemic lupus erythematosus (SLE)	Autoimmune collagen disease characterized by exacerbations and remissions. Women who conceive when the disease is in remission appear to have little risk for adverse outcomes. Those with active disease have less favorable outcomes, although pregnancy does not appear to alter the long-term prognosis (Nili et al., 2013). Incidences of spontaneous abortion, stillbirth, prematurity, and IUGR are increased. Infants born to women with SLE may have characteristic skin rash, which usually disappears by 12 months. Infants are at increased risk for complete congenital heart block, a condition that can be diagnosed prenatally. The prognosis for the fetus varies, but because the heart damage is permanent, a pacemaker may be necessary if the newborn is to survive (Branch, Silver, & Aagaard-Tillery, 2008).	■ Nursing care is focused on providing emotional support throughout the pregnancy and monitoring fetal well-being. Women with SLE have often experienced prenatal loss and may be very fearful about the outcome of pregnancy. ■ For more information, see the exemplar on Systemic Lupus Erythematosus in the module on Immunity.
Tuberculosis (TB)	An infection caused by *Mycobacterium tuberculosis*, which often affects the lungs. There has been a significant increase in diagnosis of TB, often associated with HIV infection, homeless shelters, and illicit drug users (Cunningham et al., 2010). Eighty percent of new cases are found in developing countries primarily in Africa and Asia. In the United States, the majority of cases occur in foreign-born people (Nhan-Chang & Jones, 2010). The relapse rate does not increase if TB is inactive because of prior treatment. Isoniazid crosses the placenta, but most studies show no teratogenic effects. Rifampin also crosses the placenta, and the possibility of harmful effects is still being studied.	■ When isoniazid is used during pregnancy, the woman should take supplemental pyridoxine (vitamin B_6). ■ Extra rest and limited contact with others are required until the disease becomes inactive. ■ If maternal TB is inactive, the mother may breastfeed and care for her infant. If TB is active, the newborn should not have direct contact with the mother until she is noninfectious. ■ For more information, see the exemplar on Tuberculosis in the module on Infection.

(continued on next page)

Alterations and Therapies **Pregnancy** (*continued*)

ALTERATION	DESCRIPTION	THERAPY
Gestational Onset		
Vaginal bleeding	Primarily the result of abortion (miscarriage) during the first and second trimesters. Bleeding can also result from complications, such as ectopic pregnancy or gestational trophoblastic disease. In the second half of pregnancy, bleeding is often caused by placenta previa and abruptio placentae.	<ul><li>Monitor blood pressure and pulse frequently.</li><li>Observe the woman for behaviors indicative of shock, such as pallor, clammy skin, perspiration, dyspnea, or restlessness.</li><li>Count and weigh pads to assess amount of bleeding over a given time period; save any tissue or clots expelled.</li><li>If at 12 weeks' gestation or beyond, assess fetal heart tones with a Doppler.</li><li>Prepare the woman for intravenous (IV) therapy. There may be standing orders to begin IV therapy on clients who are bleeding.</li><li>Prepare equipment for examination.</li><li>For more information, see the exemplar on Shock in the module on Perfusion and the exemplar on Menstrual Dysfunction in the module on Sexuality.</li></ul>
Spontaneous abortion (miscarriage)	Many pregnancies end in the first trimester by spontaneous abortion, often without the woman's awareness that she was even pregnant. Most miscarriages result from chromosomal abnormalities. Other causes include teratogens, faulty implantation because of an abnormal reproductive tract, weakened cervix, placental abnormalities, chronic maternal diseases, endocrine imbalances, and maternal infections.	<ul><li>Miscarriage during the first trimester can rarely be reversed, so nursing care is focused on providing emotional support and preventing complications.</li><li>Discourage use of hot tubs, because hyperthermia increases risk.</li></ul>
Ectopic pregnancy	Implantation of the fertilized ovum in a site other than the endometrial lining of the uterus. Ectopic pregnancy has many associated risk factors, including tubal damage caused by pelvic inflammatory disease, previous tubal surgery, congenital anomalies of the tube, endometriosis, previous ectopic pregnancy, presence of an intrauterine device, and in utero exposure to diethylstilbestrol.	<ul><li>Nursing care is focused on early identification, providing emotional support, and preventing complications secondary to blood loss.</li><li>Pain management is an important nursing intervention.</li><li>Assess hCG levels (often lower with ectopic pregnancy and do not increase normally).</li><li>Prepare the client for surgery.</li><li>Provide postoperative reassurance that pregnancy is still possible with one remaining fallopian tube.</li></ul>
Gestational trophoblastic disease (GTD)	Pathological proliferation of trophoblastic cells (the trophoblast is the outermost layer of embryonic cells). This includes hydatidiform mole, invasive mole (chorioadenoma destruens), and choriocarcinoma.	<ul><li>Teach the client about the need for regular screening for choriocarcinoma.</li><li>Assess all pregnant women for symptoms of GTD, including vaginal bleeding that is brown with greater uterine enlargement than expected for gestational age.</li><li>Follow quantitative hCG levels (discussed in greater detail in the Concept section of the module on Sexuality).</li></ul>

Alterations and Therapies **Pregnancy** (continued)

ALTERATION	DESCRIPTION	THERAPY
Hyperemesis gravidarum	Excessive vomiting during pregnancy that progresses to a point at which the woman not only vomits everything she swallows but also retches between meals. Increased hCG levels may play a role.	■ Assess hydration. ■ Administer IV fluids. ■ Assess nutritional status. ■ Total parenteral nutrition may be administered to prevent malnutrition. ■ Keep client away from food odors that may increase nausea and vomiting. ■ Maintain oral hygiene. ■ For more information on treating dehydration, see the exemplar on Fluid and Electrolyte Imbalance in the module on Fluids and Electrolytes.
Hypertensive disorders	Preeclampsia, eclampsia, chronic hypertension, and gestational hypertension.	■ Nursing care focuses on prevention and early detection. ■ For more information, see the exemplar on Hypertensive Disorders in Pregnancy in the module on Perfusion.
Alloimmunization	Destruction of fetal hemoglobin. When the mother is Rh negative and the fetus is Rh positive, alloimmunization may occur in second and successive pregnancies, whether the pregnancy was carried to term or not. Alloimmunization causes fetal anemia, resulting in marked fetal edema (hydrops fetalis). Congestive heart failure may result. Marked jaundice leading to neurological damage is also a risk.	■ Administer Rh immunoglobulin at 28 weeks of gestation if the pregnancy continues or immediately following a spontaneous miscarriage if the mother is Rh negative and the father is Rh positive. ■ Assess lab results for positive Coombs test, indicating sensitization, in which case Rh immunoglobulin is not administered.
ABO incompatibility	When a woman who has type O blood becomes pregnant with a type A, B, or AB fetus, an interaction occurs between the antibodies present in maternal serum and the antigen sites on the fetal red blood cells. ABO incompatibility does not normally cause the severity of hemolysis seen with Rh incompatibility.	■ Assess blood type during prenatal care, and document so that the infant can be followed after birth for potential hyperbilirubinemia if ABO incompatibility is likely.
Herpes simplex virus	Viral infection causing painful lesions in the genital area; may also occur on the cervix. This infection can profoundly affect the fetus. Primary infection has been associated with spontaneous abortion, low birth weight, and preterm birth. Transmission to the fetus usually occurs with membrane rupture and rarely via transplacental infection. If the fetus is infected, symptoms may include fever or hypothermia, jaundice, seizures, and poor feeding.	■ Prepare the mother for the need for cesarean birth if active lesions are present when she goes into labor.

(continued on next page)

Alterations and Therapies Pregnancy (continued)

ALTERATION	DESCRIPTION	THERAPY
Group B streptococcal (GBS) infection	Bacterial infection found in the lower gastrointestinal or urogenital tracts of 10%–30% of pregnant women (CDC, 2010). Women may transmit GBS infection to their fetus in utero or during childbirth. GBS is one of the major causes of early-onset neonatal infection. Newborns become infected by vertical transmission from the mother during birth or by horizontal transmission from colonized nursing personnel or colonized infants. GBS causes severe, invasive disease in infants.	▪ Nursing care is focused on detection and early intervention in order to resolve the infection before delivery.
Urinary tract infections	Dysuria, urgency, frequency; low-grade fever and hematuria. If not treated, infection may ascend and lead to acute pyelonephritis, which is associated with increased risk of premature birth and IUGR.	▪ Nursing care is focused on teaching the client the signs to report in order to allow quick intervention and to prevent potential complications. ▪ Oral sulfonamides taken in the last few weeks of pregnancy may lead to neonatal hyperbilirubinemia and kernicterus.
Vulvovaginal candidiasis	Fungal infection manifested by thick, white, curdy discharge as well as by severe itching, dysuria, and dyspareunia. If the infection is present at birth and the fetus is born vaginally, the fetus may contract thrush.	▪ Nursing care is focused on teaching the client the signs and symptoms of infection, preventive measures, and rapid recognition so that treatment can be initiated quickly.
Syphilis	Sexually transmitted infection manifested by chancre lasting ~4 weeks, then often asymptomatic until stage III. Syphilis can be passed transplacentally to the fetus. If untreated, one of the following can occur: second trimester abortion, stillborn infant at term, congenitally infected infant, or uninfected live infant.	▪ Screening for infections should be part of prenatal care in order to treat and eliminate the infection before delivery.

the potential risks and added expense. In addition, the diagnostic accuracy and applicability of these tests may vary. Although some tests are for screening purposes, meaning that they indicate the fetus *may* be at risk for a certain disorder or anomaly, others are diagnostic, meaning that they can diagnose the abnormality. Not all high-risk pregnancies require the same tests.

Selected conditions that indicate a pregnancy is at risk include the following:

- Maternal age less than 16 or more than 35 years
- Chronic maternal hypertension, preeclampsia, diabetes mellitus, or heart disease
- Presence of Rh isoimmunization (immune response to foreign antigen Rh-positive cells)
- Maternal history of fetal demise (stillbirth)
- Suspected IUGR
- Pregnancy prolonged past 42 weeks of gestation
- Multiple gestation

- Prior preterm birth
- Previous pregnancy losses before 20 weeks gestation or diagnosed cervical insufficiency.

Maternal Assessment of Fetal Activity

Clinicians now generally agree that vigorous fetal activity provides reassurance of fetal well-being and that a marked decrease in activity or cessation of movement may indicate possible fetal compromise (or even death), requiring immediate follow-up (Warrander & Heazell, 2011). Maternal assessment is typically used to monitor fetal well-being beginning at approximately 28 weeks of gestation. It provides a low-technology, inexpensive means to evaluate fetal well-being. A reduction of fetal movement has been associated with fetal hypoxia, fetal growth restriction, and fetal death (Warrander & Heazell, 2011).

Although there is no standard definition of how many movements should occur within a specified time, if there are fewer than 10 movements in a 3-hour period, or if the amount of movement is significantly less than normal, the client should

Sample Cardiff Count–to–Ten scoring card
Month: _____ Week of gestation at beginning of month: _____

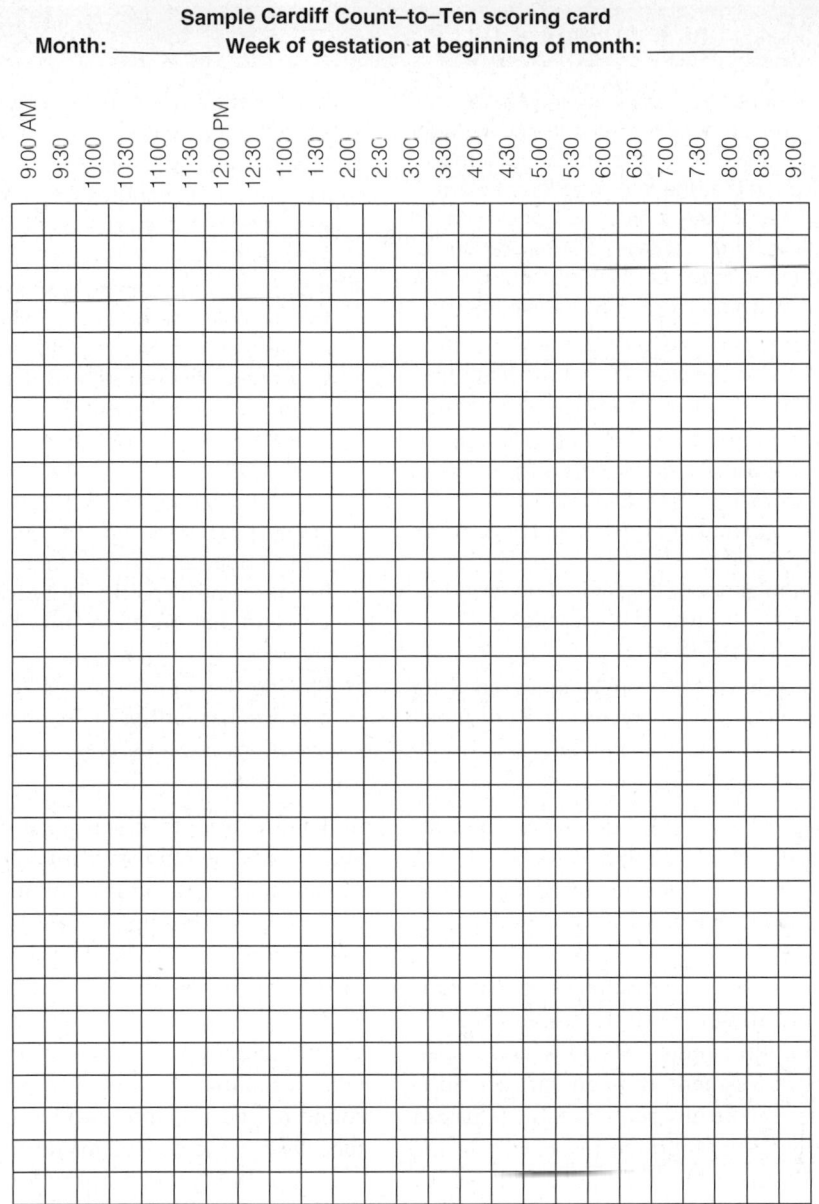

Figure 33–29 ● An adaptation of the Cardiff Count-to-Ten scoring card for assessment of fetal movement.

immediately notify her healthcare provider. A maternal perception of decreased movement occurring during a 24-hour period should cause concern and warrant antepartum fetal testing (Heazell et al., 2008).

Fetuses spend approximately 25% of their time making gross body movements. Fetal movements are directly related to the infant's sleep–wake cycle and vary from the maternal sleep–wake cycle (Blackburn, 2013; O'Neill & Thorp, 2012). Fetuses may react to maternal hypoglycemia by decreasing their activity level. In clients with a multiple gestation, daily fetal movements are significantly higher. After 38 weeks, fetuses spend 75% of their time in a quiet-sleep or active-sleep state. Other factors affecting fetal movement include sound, cigarette smoking, and drugs.

A variety of methods for tracking fetal activity have been developed. These methods focus on having the pregnant woman keep a fetal movement record, such as the Cardiff

Count-to-Ten method (**Figure 33–29 ●**). A **fetal movement record** is a noninvasive technique that enables the pregnant woman to monitor and record movements easily and without expense. See the Client Teaching feature.

The expectant mother's perception of fetal movements and her commitment to completing a fetal movement record may vary. When a client understands the purpose of the assessment, how to complete the form, whom to call with questions, and what to report—and has the opportunity for follow-up during each visit—she generally views completing the fetal movement record as an important activity. The nurse should be available to answer questions and clarify areas of concern.

Ultrasound

Valuable information about the fetus may be obtained from **ultrasound** testing, in which intermittent ultrasonic waves

Client Teaching   Maternal Assessment of Fetal Activity

- Explain that fetal movements are first felt around 18 weeks of gestation. From that time, the fetal movements get stronger and easier to detect. A slowing or stopping of fetal movement may be an indication that the fetus needs some attention and evaluation. The mother's perception of decreased fetal movement is sufficient in most cases. Formal tracking of fetal movement does not lead to improved outcomes in low risk pregnancies but may have value in high-risk situations.

- Describe the procedures, and demonstrate how to assess fetal movement. Sit beside the woman and show her how to place her hand on the fundus to feel fetal movement.

- Explain the procedure for the Cardiff Count-to-Ten method or the Daily Fetal Movement Record (DFMR). For both methods, advise the woman to do the following:
  a. Beginning at about 28 weeks of gestation, keep a daily record of fetal movement.
  b. Try to begin counting at about the same time each day, approximately 1 hour after a meal if possible.
  c. Lie quietly in a side-lying position.

- Using the Cardiff card, have the woman place an X for each fetal movement until she has recorded 10 of them.

- Movement varies considerably, but most women feel fetal movement at least 10 times in 3 hours (see Figure 33–29).

- Using the DFMR, have the woman count three times a day for 20–30 minutes each session. If fewer than three movements are felt in a session, have the woman count for 1 hour or more.

- Instruct the woman to contact her care provider in the following situations:
  a. If there are fewer than 10 movements in 3 hours.
  b. If overall the fetus's movements are slowing and it takes much longer each day to note 10 movements.
  c. If there are no movements in the morning.
  d. If there are fewer than three movements in 8 hours.

- Watch the woman fill out the record as examples are provided. Encourage her to complete the record each day and to bring it with her during each prenatal visit. Assure her that the record will be discussed at each prenatal visit and that questions may be addressed at that time if desired.

- Provide the woman with a name and phone number in case she has further questions.

(high-frequency sound waves) are transmitted by an alternating current to a transducer, which is applied to the client's abdomen. The ultrasonic waves are deflected by tissues within the client's abdomen, showing structures of varying densities (**Figures 33–30 ●** and **33–31 ●**).

Diagnostic ultrasound has several advantages. It is noninvasive, painless, and nonradiating to both the woman and the fetus. Serial studies (several ultrasound tests done over a span of time) may be done for assessment and comparison. Soft-tissue masses (e.g., tumors) can be differentiated, the fetus can be visualized, fetal growth can be followed (especially in the presence of multiple gestation), cervical length and impending cervical incompetence can be detected, and a number of other potential problems can be averted (Smith, Celik, et al., 2008; Verburg et al., 2008). In addition, the results are immediately available to the ultrasonographer or physician.

The use of four-dimensional ultrasound may eventually be able to generate future research regarding fetal well-being. Four-dimensional ultrasound combines the components of three-dimensional ultrasound with a fourth dimension, time, because it monitors live action. The technology produces images of photo-like quality, allowing healthcare providers to better visualize fetal structures and producing better guidance during invasive intrauterine procedures, such as amniocentesis and chorionic villus sampling. The use of three- and four-dimensional ultrasound has been helpful in identifying facial anomalies, neural tube defects, and skeletal malformations (Kurjak et al., 2007).

Although ultrasound is believed to serve as a useful tool in monitoring the fetus throughout pregnancy, it does have limitations. Ultrasound is limited by maternal body habits, fetal positioning, and technician or physician skill. Another limitation is that ultrasound cannot guarantee that a fetus does not

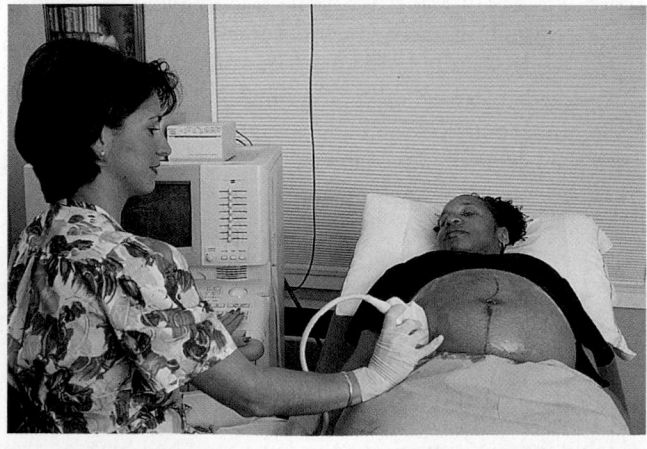

Figure 33–30 ● Ultrasound scanning permits visualization of the fetus in utero.

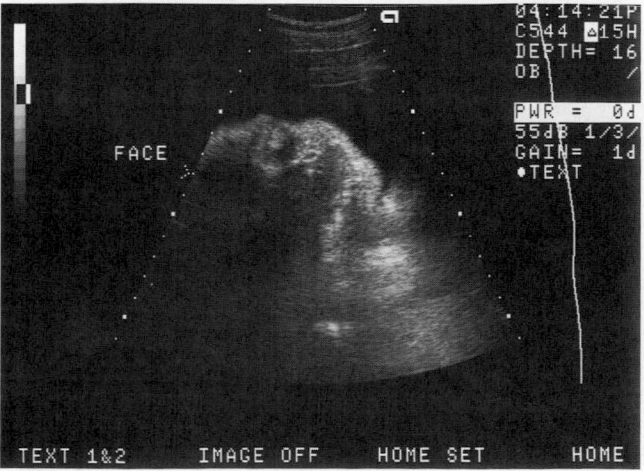

Figure 33–31 ● Ultrasound of fetal face.

have certain disorders or defects. Even though certain fetal problems can be diagnosed via the technology, sometimes abnormalities go unrecognized. A "normal" ultrasound is reassuring for the parents and the healthcare team, but it is important for parents to realize that a normal sonogram is not 100% reliable.

The two most common methods of ultrasound scanning are transabdominal and transvaginal.

TRANSABDOMINAL ULTRASOUND In the transabdominal approach, a transducer is moved across the client's abdomen. The client is often scanned with a full bladder, because when the bladder is full, the examiner can assess other structures, especially the vagina and cervix, in relation to the bladder. The ability to see the lower portion of the uterus and cervix is particularly important when vaginal bleeding is noted and placenta previa is the suspected cause. The client is directed to drink 1–1.5 quarts of water approximately 2 hours before the examination and to refrain from emptying her bladder. If the bladder is not sufficiently filled, she is asked to drink three to four 8-oz glasses of water and is rescanned 30–45 minutes later.

A water-based Mineral oil or a transmission gel is generously spread over the client's abdomen, and the sonographer slowly moves a transducer over the abdomen to obtain a picture of the uterine contents and surrounding structures. Ultrasound testing takes 20–30 minutes. The client may feel discomfort caused by pressure applied over a full bladder. In addition, if the client lies on her back during the test, she may develop shortness of breath. This may be relieved by elevating her upper body during the test.

TRANSVAGINAL ULTRASOUND The transvaginal approach uses a probe inserted into the vagina. Once inserted, the transvaginal probe is close to the structures being imaged; therefore, it produces a clearer, more defined image. The improved images obtained by transvaginal ultrasound have enabled sonographers to identify structures and fetal characteristics earlier in pregnancy (Kaur & Kaur, 2011). Internal visualization can also be used as a predictor for preterm birth in high-risk clients (Gilbert, 2011). Use of the ultrasound technique to detect shortened cervical length or funneling (a cone-shaped indentation in the cervical os) is helpful in predicting preterm labor, especially in clients who have a history of preterm birth (ACOG, 2009b).

After the procedure is fully explained to the client, she is prepared in the same manner as for a pelvic examination: in the lithotomy position, with appropriate drapes to provide privacy, and a female attendant in the room. It is important that her buttocks are at the end of the table so that, once inserted, the probe can be moved in various directions. A small, lightweight vaginal transducer is covered with a specially fitted sterile sheath, a condom, or one finger of a glove. Ultrasound gel is then applied to both the inside and outside of the covering, making insertion into the vagina easier and providing a medium for enhancing the ultrasound image. The transvaginal procedure can be accomplished with an empty bladder, and most women do not feel discomfort during the exam. The probe is smaller than a speculum, so insertion is usually completed with ease. The client may feel the movement of the probe during the exam as various structures are imaged. Some clients may want to insert the probe themselves to enhance their comfort, whereas others would feel embarrassed

even to be asked. The CNM, physician, or ultrasonographer offers the choice based on personal rapport with the client.

Ultrasound testing can be of benefit in the following ways:

- **Early identification of pregnancy.** Pregnancy may be detected as early as the fifth or sixth week after the last menstrual period by assessing the gestational sac and the presence of a fetal heart rate (FHR) after 6 weeks of gestation.

- **Observation of fetal heartbeat and fetal breathing movements.** Fetal breathing movements have been observed as early as 11 weeks of gestation.

- **Identification of more than one embryo or fetus.**

- **Comparison of the biparietal diameter of the fetal head, head circumference, abdominal circumference, and femur length to assess growth patterns.** These measurements help determine the gestational age of the fetus and identify IUGR.

- **Clinical estimations of birth weight.** This assessment helps identify macrosomia (infants >4,000 g at birth) and low-birth-weight infants (infants <2,500 g at birth). Macrosomia has been identified as a predictor of birth-related trauma and is a risk factor for both maternal and fetal morbidity (Bjorstadi et al., 2010) It is used only as a guideline in clinical decision making. Antenatal estimates of fetal weight are poor predictors of both actual fetal weight and outcomes in labor and birth.

- **Detection of fetal anomalies such as anencephaly and hydrocephalus.**

- **Examination of nuchal translucency in the first trimester to assess for Down syndrome and other fetal structural anomalies** (Sahota et al., 2012). Nuchal translucency describes an area in the back of the fetal neck that is measured via ultrasound during the first trimester of pregnancy. Nuchal translucency testing (NTT), also known as nuchal testing or nuchal fold testing, is performed at 11–13 weeks of gestation to screen for trisomies 13, 18, and 21 (Wright et al., 2008).

- **Examination of fetal cardiac structures (echocardiography).**

- **Length of fetal nasal bone.** The length of the fetal nasal bone during the NTT is used to indicate a risk factor for Down syndrome. Fetuses with a nonvisualized or shortened nasal bone are more likely to have trisomy 21 than are those with a normal-length nasal bone (Cusick et al., 2008).

- **Identification of amniotic fluid index (AFI).** Ultrasound can provide a rough measurement of the amount of amniotic fluid, which is an indicator of fetal well-being. The maternal abdomen is divided into quadrants using the umbilicus as the center point. The vertical diameter of the largest amniotic fluid pocket in each quadrant is measured. All measurements are totaled to obtain the AFI in centimeters. Women with an AFI of more than 24 cm are considered to have polyhydramnios, and women with an AFI of less than 5 cm at term are considered to have oligohydramnios. An AFI of between 5 and 24 cm is considered to be normal. After 39 weeks of gestation, the amniotic fluid volume begins to decline. Both polyhydramnios and oligohydramnios are associated with increased risk to the fetus, including nonreassuring fetal status, IUGR, meconium-stained amniotic fluid, and an increase in admissions to the neonatal intensive care unit (Magann et al., 2010).

- ■ *Location of the placenta.* The placenta is located before amniocentesis to avoid puncturing it during the procedure. Ultrasound is valuable in identifying and evaluating placenta previa (Cunningham et al., 2010).

- ■ *Placental grading.* As the fetus matures, the placenta calcifies. These changes can be detected by ultrasound and graded according to the degree of calcification. Placental grading can be used to identify internal placenta vasculature, in which abnormalities can be associated with preeclampsia and chronic hypertension. It can also identify disorders such as fetal growth abnormalities, triploidy, nonimmune hydrops, and infections (Moran et al., 2011).

- ■ *Detection of fetal death.* Inability to visualize the fetal heart beating and the separation of the bones in the fetal head are signs of fetal death.

- ■ *Determination of fetal position and presentation.*

- ■ *Accompanying procedures.* Ultrasound guidance is used in a variety of intrauterine procedures including amniocentesis and chorionic villus sampling.

Nonstress Test

The **nonstress test (NST)**, a widely used method of evaluating fetal status, may be used alone or as part of a more comprehensive diagnostic assessment called a biophysical profile. The NST is based on the knowledge that when the fetus has adequate oxygenation and an intact central nervous system, accelerations of the FHR occur with fetal movement. An NST requires an electronic fetal monitor to observe and record these FHR accelerations. A nonreactive NST is fairly consistent in identifying at-risk fetuses (Cunningham et al., 2010).

The advantages of the NST include the following:

- ■ It is quick to perform, permits easy interpretation, and is inexpensive.

- ■ It can be done in an office or clinic setting.
- ■ It is a noninvasive procedure.
- ■ There are no known side effects.

The disadvantages of the NST include the following:

- ■ It is sometimes difficult to obtain a suitable tracing.
- ■ The woman has to remain relatively still for at least 20 minutes.

PROCEDURE FOR NST The test can be done with the client in a reclining chair or in bed with the client in a left-tilted semi-Fowler or side-lying position. Research has shown that certain maternal positions can help produce more favorable results. Clients in left-tilted semi-Fowler, sitting, and left lateral positions are more likely to have a reactive tracing. Clients should not be placed in a supine position, because it decreases cardiac output and uterine perfusion, maternal back pain, and maternal shortness of breath (Cunningham et al., 2010). An electronic fetal monitor is used to obtain a tracing of the FHR and fetal movement. The nurse places the monitor under the client's clothing. Privacy should be provided. The examiner puts two elastic belts on the client's abdomen. One belt holds a device that detects uterine or fetal movement; the other belt holds a device that detects the FHR. As the NST is done, each fetal movement is documented so that associated or simultaneous FHR changes can be evaluated.

INTERPRETATION OF NST RESULTS An NST is indicated after 32 weeks at any time fetal well being needs to be established. It may be used between 26 and 32 weeks with modified criteria for interpretation. The results of the NST are interpreted as follows:

- ■ *Reactive test.* A reactive NST shows at least two accelerations of FHR with fetal movements of 15 bpm, lasting 15 seconds or more, over 20 minutes (**Figure 33–32** ●). This is the desired result.

- ■ *Nonreactive test.* In a nonreactive test, the reactive criteria are not met. For example, the accelerations do not meet the requirements of 15 bpm or do not last 15 seconds (**Figure 33–33** ●).

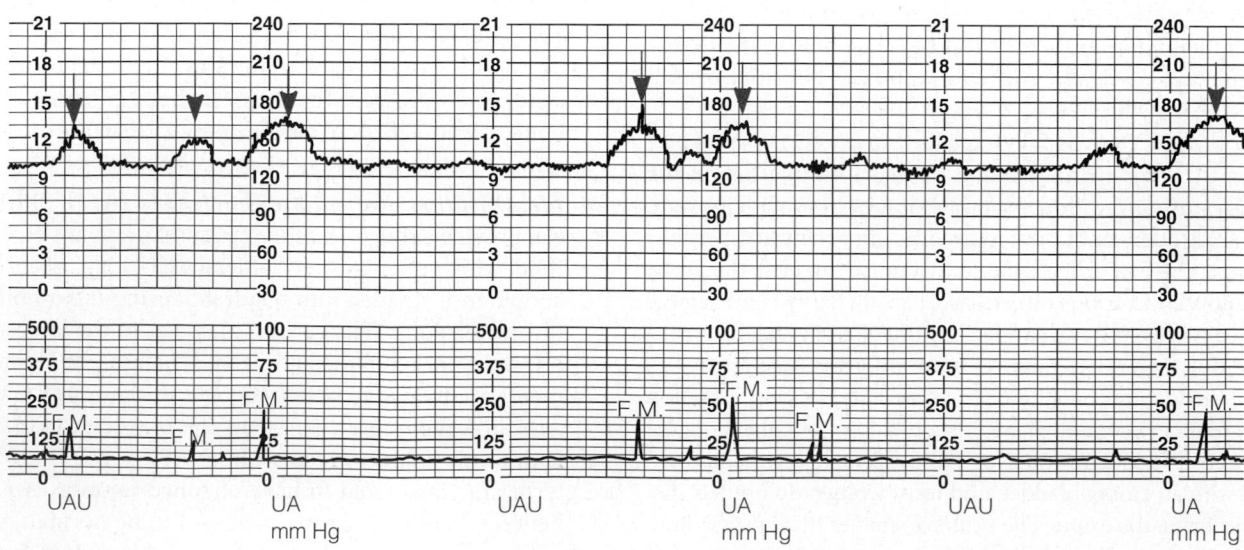

Figure 33–32 ● Example of a reactive nonstress test: accelerations of 15 bpm lasting 15 seconds with each fetal movement (FM). Top of strip shows fetal heart rate (FHR); bottom of strip shows uterine activity tracing. Note that FHR increases (above the baseline) at least 15 beats and remains at that rate for at least 15 seconds before returning to the former baseline.

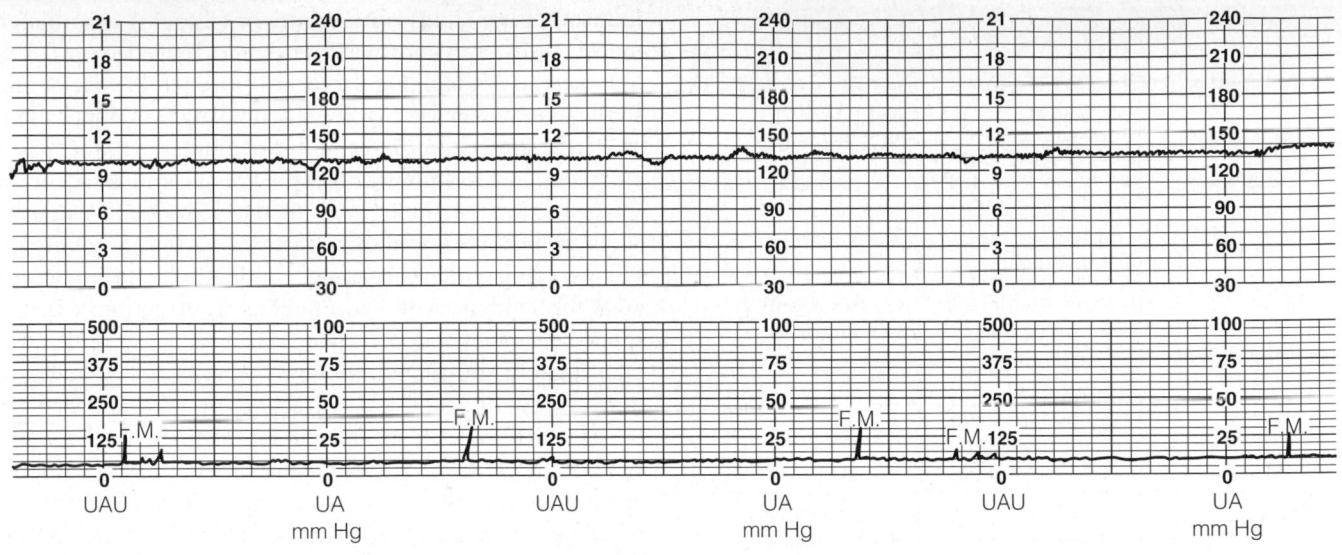

Figure 33–33 ● Example of a nonreactive nonstress test. There are no accelerations of the fetal heart rate (FHR) with fetal movement (FM). Baseline FHR is 130 bpm. The tracing of uterine activity is on the bottom of the strip.

■ *Unsatisfactory test.* An NST is unsatisfactory if the data cannot be interpreted or there was inadequate fetal activity.

It is important that anyone who performs the NST understand the significance of any decelerations of the FHR during testing. If decelerations are noted, the CNM or physician should be notified for further evaluation of fetal status.

Fetal Acoustic and Vibroacoustic Stimulation Tests

Acoustic (sound) and vibroacoustic (vibration and sound) stimulation of the fetus can be used as an adjunct to the NST. A handheld, battery-operated device is applied to the woman's abdomen over the area of the fetal head. This device generates a low-frequency vibration and a buzzing sound. These are intended to induce movement and associated accelerations of the FHR in fetuses with a nonreactive NST and in fetuses with decreased variability of the FHR during labor. The sound stimulus persists for 1 second; if no accelerations occur, it is then repeated at 1-minute intervals up to two times and then progresses to 2 seconds waiting 1 minute if no accelerations occur after the stimulus. Whether the fetus responds more to the vibration or to the sound is not known. Two FHR accelerations of 15 bpm, lasting 15 seconds, in a 10-minute period indicate a reactive test (Gilbert, 2011).

Advantages of the fetal acoustic stimulation test and the vibroacoustic stimulation test include the following:

■ Both are noninvasive techniques and are easy to perform.

■ Results are rapidly available.

■ Time for the NST is shortened.

Biophysical Profile

Use of the biophysical profile is indicated when there is risk of placental insufficiency or fetal compromise. The biophysical profile is a comprehensive assessment of five biophysical variables over a 30 minute period:

1. Fetal breathing movement
2. Fetal movements of body or limbs
3. Fetal tone (extension and flexion of extremities)
4. Amniotic fluid volume (visualized as pockets of fluid around the fetus)
5. FHR accelerations with activity (reactive NST).

The first four variables are assessed by ultrasound scanning; FHR reactivity is assessed with the NST. By combining these five assessments, the biophysical profile helps to identify the compromised fetus or to confirm the healthy fetus and also provides an assessment of placental functioning.

Specific criteria for normal and abnormal assessments are presented in **Table 33–3** ●. A score of 2 is assigned to each normal finding, and a score of 0 to each abnormal one, for a maximum score of 10. Scores of 8 and 10 are considered to be normal. Such scores have the least chance of being associated with a compromised fetus unless oligohydramnios is noted, in which case the infant's birth may be indicated (Thompson, Kuller, & Rhee, 2012).

Use of the biophysical profile may be indicated when there is risk of placental insufficiency or fetal compromise as in the following conditions:

■ IUGR

■ Maternal diabetes mellitus

■ Maternal heart disease

■ Maternal chronic hypertension

■ Maternal preeclampsia or eclampsia

■ Maternal sickle cell disease

■ Suspected fetal postmaturity (>42 weeks of gestation)

■ History of previous stillbirths

■ Rh sensitization

■ Abnormal estriol excretion

■ Hyperthyroidism

■ Renal disease

■ Nonreactive NST.

TABLE 33–3   Criteria for Biophysical Profile Scoring

COMPONENT	NORMAL (SCORE = 2)	ABNORMAL (SCORE = 0)
Fetal breathing movements	≥1 episode of rhythmic breathing lasting ≥30 seconds within 30 minutes	≤30 seconds of breathing in 30 minutes
Gross body movements	≥3 discrete body or limb movements in 30 minutes (episodes of active continuous movement considered as single movement)	≤2 movements in 30 minutes
Fetal tone	≥1 episode of extension of a fetal extremity with return to flexion or opening or closing of hand	No movements or extension/flexion
Amniotic fluid volume	Single vertical pocket >2 cm AFI >5 cm	Largest single vertical pocket ≤2 cm AFI <5 cm
Nonstress test	≥2 accelerations of ≥15 bpm for ≥15 seconds in 20–40 minutes	0 or 1 acceleration in 20–40 minutes

Contraction Stress Test

The **contraction stress test (CST)** is a means of evaluating the respiratory function (oxygen and carbon dioxide exchange) of the placenta. It enables the healthcare team to identify the fetus at risk for intrauterine asphyxia by observing the response of the FHR to the stress of uterine contractions (spontaneous or induced). During contractions, intrauterine pressure increases, and blood flow to the intervillous space of the placenta is momentarily reduced, thereby decreasing oxygen transport to the fetus. A healthy fetus usually tolerates this reduction well and maintains a steady heart rate. If the placental reserve is insufficient, however, then fetal hypoxia, depression of the myocardium, and a decrease in FHR occur.

In many areas, the CST has given way to the biophysical profile. It is still used, however, in areas where the availability of other technology is reduced (e.g., during night shifts) or limited (e.g., at small community hospitals or birthing centers). It may also be used as an adjunct to other forms of fetal assessment.

The CST is contraindicated in the client with third-trimester bleeding from placenta previa, marginal abruptio placentae or unexplained vaginal bleeding, previous cesarean section with classical incision (vertical incision in the fundus of the uterus), premature rupture of the membranes, incompetent cervix, cerclage in place (gathering stitch around cervix), anomalies of the maternal reproductive organs, history of preterm labor (if being done before term), or multiple gestation.

The critical component of the CST is the presence of uterine contractions. These contractions may occur spontaneously, which is unusual before the onset of labor, or they may be induced (stimulated) with oxytocin (Pitocin) administered intravenously (also known as an oxytocin challenge test). A natural method of obtaining oxytocin is through the use of breast stimulation (either via nipple self-stimulation or application of an electric breast pump); the posterior pituitary produces oxytocin in response to stimulation of the breasts or nipples.

An electronic fetal monitor is used to provide continuous data about the FHR and uterine contractions. After a 15-minute baseline recording of uterine activity and FHR, the tracing is evaluated for evidence of spontaneous contractions. If three spontaneous contractions of good quality and lasting 40–60 seconds occur in a 10-minute window, the results are evaluated, and the test is concluded. If no contractions occur, or if the contractions that do occur are insufficient for interpretation, then intravenous administration of oxytocin, breast self-stimulation, or application of an electric breast pump is done to produce contractions of good quality. The CST should be conducted only in a setting where tocolytic medications are available if a hyperstimulation pattern occurs or if labor is stimulated from the test.

The CST is classified as follows:

- ***Negative.*** A negative CST shows three contractions of good quality lasting 40 seconds or longer in a 10-minute period without evidence of late decelerations. This is the desired result and implies that the fetus can handle the hypoxic stress of uterine contractions.

- ***Positive.*** A positive CST shows repetitive, persistent, late decelerations with more than 50% of the contractions (**Figure 33–34 ●**). This is not a desired result. The hypoxic stress of the uterine contraction causes a slowing of the FHR. The pattern will not improve, and will most likely get worse with additional contractions.

- ***Equivocal.***
  a. An equivocal–suspicious test is one in which less than 50% of the contractions on the strip are late decelerations. Variability is usually good (Gilbert, 2011).
  b. An equivocal–hyperstimulation test is one in which uterine contraction frequency is every 2 minutes or in which contractions last greater than 90 seconds with a late deceleration. When this test result occurs, more information is needed.

- ***Unsatisfactory.*** In an unsatisfactory CST, the quality of the tracing is too poor to accurately interpret FHR with contractions or the frequency of three contractions lasting 40–60 seconds occurring in a 10-minute window of time cannot be obtained for the end point of the test.

A negative CST implies that the placenta is functioning normally, fetal oxygenation is adequate, and the fetus will probably be able to withstand the stress of labor. If labor does not occur in the ensuing week, further testing is done.

A positive CST with a nonreactive NST presents evidence that the fetus will not likely withstand the stress of labor. A positive CST may be able to identify a compromised fetus earlier than a nonreactive NST because of the stimulated interruption of intervillous blood flow (Cunningham et al., 2010). Although a negative CST is reliable in predicting fetal status, a positive result needs to be verified, such as with a biophysical profile.

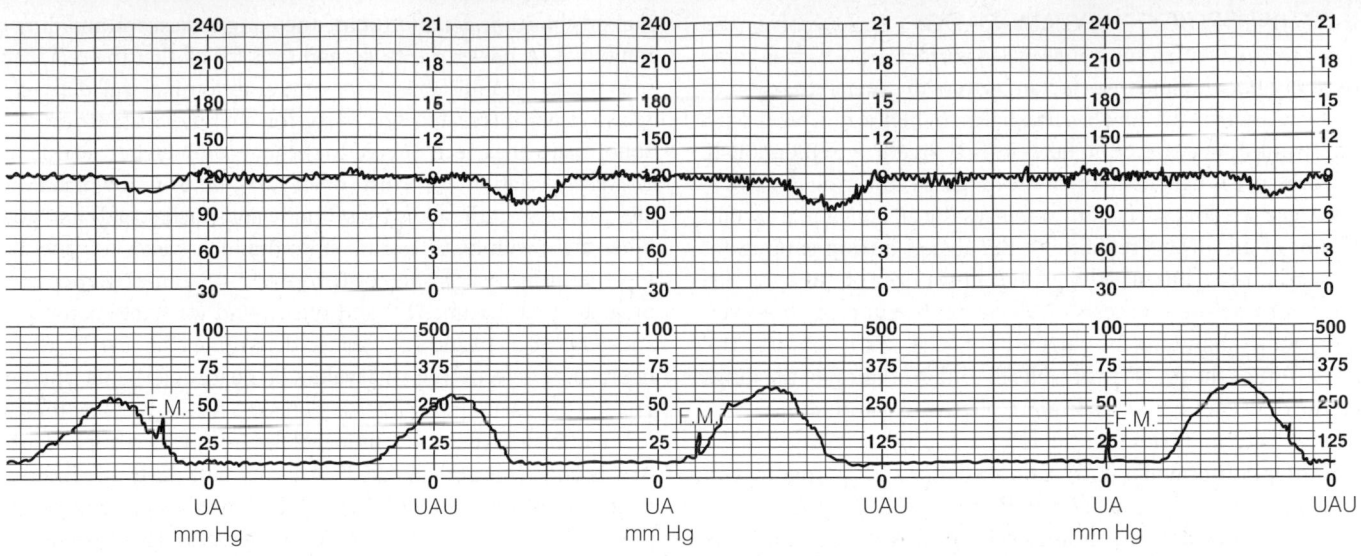

Figure 33–34 ● Example of a positive contraction stress test. Repetitive late decelerations occur with each contraction. Note that there are no accelerations of fetal heart rate (FHR) with three fetal movements (FM). The baseline FHR is 120 bpm. Uterine contractions (bottom half of strip) occurred four times in 12 minutes.

Amniotic Fluid Analysis

Amniocentesis is a procedure used to obtain amniotic fluid for genetic testing to determine fetal abnormalities or fetal lung maturity in the third trimester of pregnancy. During an amniocentesis, the physician scans the uterus using ultrasound to identify the fetal and placental positions and to identify adequate pockets of amniotic fluid. The skin is then cleaned with a Betadine solution. The use of a local anesthesia at the needle insertion site is optional. A 22-gauge needle is then inserted into the uterine cavity to withdraw amniotic fluid (**Figure 33–35** ●). After 15–20 mL of fluid have been removed, the needle is withdrawn, and the site is assessed for streaming (movement of fluid), which is an indication of bleeding. The FHR and maternal vital signs are then assessed. Rh immune globulin is given to all Rh-negative women. The analysis of amniotic fluid provides valuable information about fetal status. Amniocentesis is a fairly simple procedure, although complications do occur on rare occasions (<1% of cases).

A number of studies can be performed on amniotic fluid. These tests can provide information about genetic disorders, fetal health, and fetal lung maturity. Concentrations of certain substances in amniotic fluid provide information about the health status of the fetus. An amniocentesis is 99% accurate in diagnosing genetic abnormalities.

Because gestational age, birth weight, and the rate of development of organ systems do not necessarily correspond, amniotic fluid may also be analyzed to determine the maturity of the fetal lungs. Determination of fetal lung maturity is important when making clinical decisions regarding the timing of birth for women who may have complications, such as preeclampsia or diabetes.

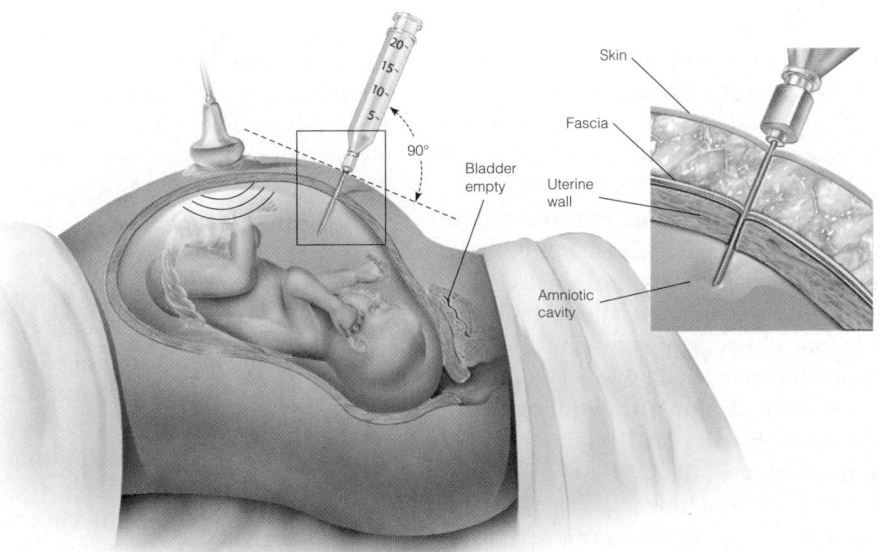

Figure 33–35 ● Amniocentesis. The woman is scanned by ultrasound to determine the placenta site and to locate a pocket of amniotic fluid. The needle is then inserted into the uterine cavity to withdraw amniotic fluid.

LECITHIN/SPHINGOMYELIN RATIO   The alveoli of the lungs are lined with a substance called **surfactant**, which is composed of phospholipids. Surfactant lowers the surface tension of the alveoli when the newborn exhales. When a newborn with mature pulmonary function takes its first breath, a tremendously high pressure is needed to open the lungs. By lowering the alveolar surface tension, surfactant stabilizes the alveoli, and a certain amount of air always remains in the alveoli during expiration. Thus, when the infant exhales, the lungs do not collapse. An infant born before synthesis of surfactant is complete, however, is unable to maintain lung stability. Each breath requires the same effort as the first. This results in underinflation of the lungs and the development of respiratory distress syndrome.

Fetal lung maturity can be ascertained by determining the **lecithin/sphingomyelin (L/S) ratio**. Lecithin and sphingomyelin are two components of surfactant. Early in pregnancy, the sphingomyelin concentration in amniotic fluid is greater than the concentration of lecithin, and so the L/S ratio is low (i.e., lecithin levels are low, and sphingomyelin levels are high). At approximately 32 weeks of gestation, sphingomyelin levels begin to fall, and the amount of lecithin begins to increase. By 35 weeks of gestation, an L/S ratio of 4:1 is usually achieved in the normal fetus. An L/S ratio of 2:1 indicates that the risk of respiratory distress syndrome is very low. Under certain conditions of stress, such as a physiological problem in the mother, placenta, and/or fetus (e.g., hypertension or placental insufficiency), the fetal lungs mature more rapidly (Torrance et al., 2008).

PHOSPHATIDYLGLYCEROL   Phosphatidylglycerol (PG) is another phospholipid in surfactant. PG is not present in the fetal lung fluid early in gestation. It appears when fetal lung maturity has been attained, at approximately 34 weeks of gestation. Because the presence of PG is associated with fetal lung maturity, when it is present, the risk of respiratory distress syndrome is low. Determination of PG is also useful in blood-contaminated specimens. Because PG is not present in blood or vaginal fluids, its presence is reliable in predicting fetal lung maturity.

Chorionic Villus Sampling

Chorionic villus sampling (CVS) involves obtaining a small sample of chorionic villi from the developing placenta.

The advantages of this procedure are early diagnosis and a short waiting time for results. Whereas amniocentesis is not done until at least 14 weeks of gestation, CVS is typically performed between 10 and 12 weeks of gestation. Previous studies that evaluated the use of CVS at 9 weeks of gestation found a possible association between limb-reduction birth defects and early CVS. Based on these findings, most practitioners do not recommend early CVS before 10 weeks of gestation (Cunningham et al., 2010). Risks of CVS include failure to obtain tissue, rupture of membranes, leakage of amniotic fluid, bleeding, intrauterine infection, maternal tissue contamination of the specimen, and Rh isoimmunization.

Because CVS testing is performed so early in the pregnancy, it cannot detect neural tube defects. Clients who desire screening for neural tube defects would need a quadruple screening or the AFP component of first trimester integrated screening at 15–20 weeks of gestation. The **quadruple screen** is a widely used test to screen for Down syndrome (trisomy 21), trisomy 18, and neural tube defects. The serum test assesses for appropriate levels of alpha-fetoprotein,

human chorionic gonadotropin, unconjugated estriol, and dimeric inhibin-A. A newer **penta screen** tests for all that the quadruple screen tests for and also tests for ventral abdominal wall defects. In recent years integrated screening for aneuploidy (chromosome abnormality) has been offered to pregnant women between 11 and 13 weeks gestation. It consists of an early ultrasound which evaluates markers on the fetus (nasal bone and nuchal fold) and combines these with hCG, estriol, and inhibin A values to generate a more accurate risk profile for trisomy 13, 18 and 21 earlier in the pregnancy. A serum AFP and ultrasound for fetal anatomy are added between 18 and 20 weeks to determine risk or presence of a neural tube defect. Abnormal values on quadruple, penta, and integrated screens are indicators of increased risk only. They must be followed by a diagnostic amniocentesis from which a fetal karyotype is done (Messerlian, 2013). Another new development in the diagnosis of fetal aneuploidy is non-invasive prenatal testing (NIPT), also called cell free DNA. This process detects fetal alleles in maternal serum and can provide accurate information on chromosomal abnormalities without the invasiveness and, albeit small, risk of amniocentesis from 9 weeks gestation onward (Wolfberg, 2015). Aneuploidy detection rates are similar for NIPT, CVS, and amniocentesis (King et al., 2015).

SAFETY ALERT
When explaining options for genetic testing to expectant parents, inform the mother that even if a CVS shows no chromosomal abnormality, it cannot screen for neural tube defects. Clients who have a normal CVS and an abnormal quadruple screen test are to be offered amniocentesis. Clients with risk factors for neural tube defects may want to consider amniocentesis instead of CVS because amniocentesis screens for both types of disorders.

The nurse assists the physician during the amniocentesis or CVS and supports the client undergoing the procedure. Although the physician has explained the procedure in advance so that the client can give informed consent, the client is likely to be apprehensive, both about the procedure itself and about the information it may reveal. She may become anxious during the procedure and need additional emotional support. The nurse can provide support by further clarifying the physician's instructions or explanations, by relieving the client's physical discomfort when possible, and by responding verbally and physically to the client's need for reassurance.

MATERNAL NUTRITION

A woman's nutritional status before and during pregnancy can significantly influence her health and that of her fetus. In most prenatal clinics and offices, nurses offer nutritional counseling directly or work closely with a nutritionist to provide nutritional assessment and teaching.

The following factors influence the pregnant woman's ability to achieve good prenatal nutrition:

- *General nutritional status before pregnancy.* Nutritional deficits, such as folic acid deficiency, present at the time of conception and during the early prenatal period may influence the outcome of the pregnancy.

- *Maternal age.* An expectant adolescent must meet her own growth needs in addition to the nutritional needs of pregnancy.
- *Maternal parity.* The mother's nutritional needs and the outcome of the pregnancy are influenced by the number of pregnancies she has had and by the interval between them.

Fetal growth occurs in three overlapping stages:

1. Growth by increase in cell number
2. Growth by increases in cell number and cell size
3. Growth by increase in cell size alone.

Nutritional problems that interfere with cell division may have permanent consequences. If the nutritional insult occurs when cells are mainly enlarging, the changes are usually reversible when normal nutrition resumes.

Growth of fetal and maternal tissues requires increased quantities of essential dietary components. These are listed in the federal government's **Dietary Reference Intakes (DRIs)** as specific allowances for pregnant and lactating women (**Table 33–4** ●). The DRIs are subdivided into the recommended dietary allowance (RDA) and adequate intake (AI). An RDA is the daily

TABLE 33–4 Dietary Reference Intakes (DRIs) for Nonpregnant, Pregnant, and Lactating Females, Vitamins and Elements

	AGE	VITAMIN A (MCG/DAY)	VITAMIN C (MG/DAY)	VITAMIN D (MCG/DAY)	VITAMIN E (MG/DAY)
Females	9–13 yr	600	45	15	11
	14–18 yr	700	65	15	15
	19–30 yr	700	75	15	15
	31–50 yr	700	75	15	15
	51–70 yr	700	75	15	15
	>70 yr	700	75	20	15
Pregnancy	14–18 yr	750	80	15	15
	19–30 yr	770	85	15	15
	31–50 yr	770	85	15	15
Lactation	14–18 yr	1200	115	15	19
	19–30 yr	1300	120	15	19
	31–50 yr	1300	120	15	19

	AGE	VITAMIN K (MCG/DAY)	THIAMINE (MG/DAY)	RIBOFLAVIN (MG/DAY)	NIACIN (MG/DAY)
Females	9–13 yr	60*	0.9	0.9	12
	14–18 yr	75*	1.0	1.0	14
	19–30 yr	90*	1.1	1.1	14
	31–50 yr	90*	1.1	1.1	14
	51–70 yr	90*	1.1	1.1	14
	>70 yr	90*	1.1	1.1	14
Pregnancy	14–18 yr	75*	1.4	1.4	18
	19–30 yr	90*	1.4	1.4	18
	31–50 yr	90*	1.4	1.4	18
Lactation	14–18 yr	75*	1.4	1.6	17
	19–30 yr	90*	1.4	1.6	17
	31–50 yr	90*	1.4	1.6	17

	AGE	VITAMIN B_6 (MG/DAY)	FOLATE[†] (MCG/DAY)	VITAMIN B_{12} (MCG/DAY)	CALCIUM (MG/DAY)
Females	9–13 yr	1.0	300	1.8	1300*
	14–18 yr	1.2	400	2.4	1300*
	19–30 yr	1.3	400	2.4	1000*
	31–50 yr	1.3	400	2.4	1000*
	51–70 yr	1.5	400	2.4	1200*
	>70 yr	1.5	400	2.4	1200*

(continued on next page)

TABLE 33–4 Dietary Reference Intakes (DRIs) for Nonpregnant, Pregnant, and Lactating Females, Vitamins and Elements (*continued*)

	AGE	VITAMIN B$_6$ (MG/DAY)	FOLATE[†] (MCG/DAY)	VITAMIN B$_{12}$ (MCG/DAY)	CALCIUM (MG/DAY)
Pregnancy	14–18 yr	1.9	600	2.6	1300*
	19–30 yr	1.9	600	2.6	1000*
	31–50 yr	1.9	600	2.6	1000*
Lactation	14–18 yr	2.0	500	2.8	1300*
	19–30 yr	2.0	500	2.8	1000*
	31–50 yr	2.0	500	2.8	1000*

	AGE	IODINE (MCG/DAY)	IRON (MG/DAY)	MAGNESIUM (MG/DAY)	PHOSPHORUS (MG/DAY)
Females	9–13 yr	120	8	240	1250
	14–18 yr	150	15	360	1250
	19–30 yr	150	18	310	700
	31–50 yr	150	18	320	700
	51–70 yr	150	8	320	700
	>70 yr	150	8	320	700
Pregnancy	≤18 yr	220	27	400	1250
	19–30 yr	220	27	350	700
	31–50 yr	220	27	360	700
Lactation	≤18 yr	290	10	360	1250
	19–30 yr	290	9	310	700
	31–50 yr	290	9	320	700

	AGE	SELENIUM (MCG/DAY)	ZINC (MG/DAY)
Females	9–13 yr	40	8
	14–18 yr	55	9
	19–30 yr	55	8
	31–50 yr	55	8
	51–70 yr	55	8
	>70 yr	55	12
Pregnancy	≤18 yr	60	11
	19–30 yr	60	11
	31–50 yr	60	13
Lactation	≤18 yr	70	12
	19–30 yr	70	12
	31–50 yr	70	12

*Values are adequate intakes rather than recommended dietary allowances (RDAs). All other values on the chart are RDAs.
[†]In view of evidence linking folate intake with neural tube defects in the fetus, it is recommended that all women capable of becoming pregnant consume 400 mcg from supplements or fortified foods in addition to intake of food folate from a varied diet.
Source: Based on Institute of Medicine. (2010). *Dietary reference intakes (DRIs): Recommended dietary allowances and adequate intakes, vitamins and elements.* Washington, DC: Food and Nutrition Board, Institute of Medicine, National Academies.

dietary intake that is considered to be sufficient to meet the nutritional requirements of nearly all individuals in a specific life stage and gender group. An AI is the value cited for a nutrient when the data are not sufficient to calculate an estimated average requirement. Most of the recommended nutrients can be obtained by eating a well-balanced diet each day. **Table 33–5** ● is a sample daily food plan for pregnancy and lactation.

▶ FACTORS INFLUENCING NUTRITION

It is important to consider the many factors that affect a client's nutrition. What environmental risks should the woman consider? What are her age, lifestyle, and culture? What food beliefs and habits does she have? What an individual eats is determined

TABLE 33–5   Daily Food Plan for Pregnancy and Lactation

FOOD GROUP	NUTRIENTS PROVIDED	FOOD SOURCE	RECOMMENDED DAILY AMOUNT DURING PREGNANCY	RECOMMENDED DAILY AMOUNT DURING LACTATION
Dairy products	Protein; riboflavin; vitamins A, D, and others; calcium; phosphorus; zinc; magnesium	Milk—whole, 2%, skim, dry, buttermilk	Four 8-oz cups (five for teenagers) used plain or with flavoring, in shakes, soups, puddings, custards, cocoa	Four 8-oz cups (five for teenagers); equivalent amount of cheese, yogurt, and so forth
		Cheeses—hard, semisoft, cottage	Calcium in 1 cup of milk equivalent to 1 1/2 cups of cottage cheese; 1 1/2 oz of hard or semisoft cheese; 1 cup of yogurt; 1 1/2 cups of ice cream (high in fat and sugar)	
		Yogurt—plain, low-fat		
		Soybean milk		
Meat and meat alternatives	Protein; iron; thiamine, niacin, and other vitamins; minerals	Beef, pork, veal, lamb, poultry, animal organ meats, fish, eggs; legumes; nuts, seeds, peanut butter, grains in proper vegetarian combination (vitamin B_{12} supplement needed)	Three servings (one serving = 2 oz), combination in amounts necessary for same nutrient equivalent (varies greatly)	Two servings
Grain products, whole grain or enriched	B vitamins; iron; whole grain also has zinc, magnesium, and other trace elements; provides fiber	Breads and bread products such as cornbread, muffins, waffles, hotcakes, biscuits, dumplings, cereals, pastas, and rice	6–11 servings daily: one serving = one slice bread, 3/4 cup or 1 oz of dry cereal; 1/2 cup of rice or pasta	Same as for pregnancy
Fruits and fruit juices	Vitamins A and C; minerals; raw fruits for roughage	Citrus fruits and juices, melons, berries, all other fruits and juices	Two to four servings (one serving for vitamin C): one serving = one medium fruit, 1/2–1 cup of fruit; 4 oz of orange or grapefruit juice	Same as for pregnancy
Vegetables and vegetable juices	Vitamins A and C; minerals; provides roughage	Leafy green vegetables; deep yellow or orange vegetables such as carrots, sweet potatoes, squash, tomatoes; green vegetables, such as peas, green beans, and broccoli; other vegetables, such as beets, cabbage, potatoes, corn, and lima beans	Three to five servings (one serving of dark green or deep yellow vegetable for vitamin A): one serving = 1/2 – 1 cup of vegetables; two tomatoes; one medium potato	Same as for pregnancy
Fats	Vitamins A and D; linoleic acid	Butter, cream cheese, fortified table spreads; cream, whipped cream, whipped toppings; avocado, mayonnaise, oil, nuts	As desired in moderation (high in calories): one serving = 1 tbsp butter or enriched margarine	Same as for pregnancy
Sugar and sweets		Sugar, brown sugar, honey, molasses, agave syrup	Occasionally, if desired	Same as for pregnancy
Desserts		Nutritious desserts such as fruits, puddings, custards, fruit whips, and crisps; other rich, sweet desserts and pastries	Occasionally, if desired	Same as for pregnancy
Beverages	Fluid	Coffee, decaffeinated beverages, tea, bouillon, carbonated drinks	As desired, in moderation	Same as for pregnancy
Miscellaneous		Iodized salt, herbs, spices, condiments	As desired	Same as for pregnancy

Note: The pregnant woman should eat regularly, three meals a day, with nutritious snacks of fruit, cheese, milk, or other foods between meals if desired. (More frequent but smaller meals are also recommended.) Between four and six 8-oz glasses of water, and a total of between eight and ten 8-oz cups of total fluid intake, should be consumed daily. Water is an essential nutrient.

by availability, economics, and symbolism. These factors and others influence the expectant mother's acceptance of the nurse's intervention.

Socioeconomic Influences

Socioeconomic level may be a determinant of nutritional status. Families living at the poverty level cannot afford the same foods that higher-income families can. Thus, pregnant women with low incomes are frequently at risk for poor nutrition. Because access to healthy proteins and fresh fruits and vegetables is critical for pregnant women and very young children, federal, state, and local programs exist to provide at-risk women and their children with nutritional support. The largest of these programs is the Special Supplemental Nutrition Program for Women, Infants and Children (WIC) program, a federal program administered at the state level. WIC provides food vouchers and nutrition education to low-income and at-risk pregnant and postpartum women and for at-risk infants and children up to 5 years old.

Stay Current: More information about this program can be found at the program Web site, **www.fns.usda.gov/wic**.

Cultural, Ethnic, and Religious Influences

Cultural, ethnic, and, occasionally, religious backgrounds determine an individual's experiences with food and influence that individual's food preferences and habits (**Figure 33–36 ●**). Individuals of different nationalities are accustomed to eating different foods because of the kinds of foodstuffs available in their countries of origin. The way food is prepared varies depending on the customs and traditions of the ethnic and cultural group. In addition, the laws of certain religions sanction particular foods, prohibit others, and direct the preparation and serving of meals. For an example, see the accompanying Focus on Diversity and Culture feature.

In each culture, certain foods have symbolic significance. Generally these symbolic foods are related to major life experiences such as birth and death. Although generalizations have been made about the food practices of ethnic and religious groups, there are many variations. The extent to which individ-

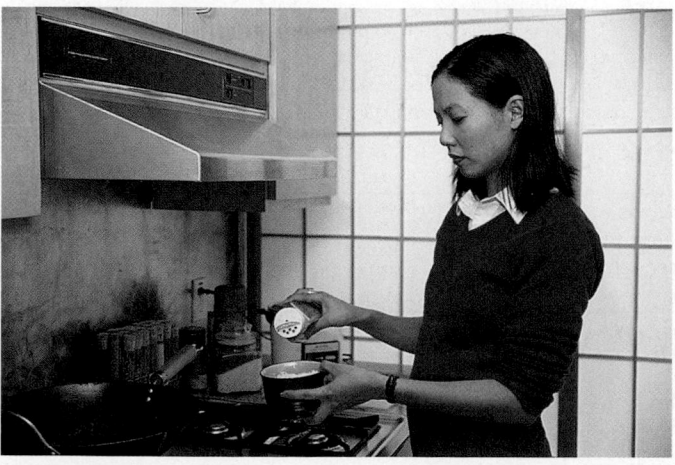

Figure 33–36 ● Cultural factors affect food preferences and habits.

uals continue to consume traditional ethnic foods and follow food-related ethnic customs is affected by the extent of their exposure to other cultures; by the availability, quality, and cost of traditional foods.

When working with pregnant women from any ethnic background, the nurse should understand the impact of the woman's cultural and spiritual beliefs on her eating habits and identify any beliefs she may have about food and pregnancy. Talking with the client can help the nurse determine the level of influence that traditional food customs exert. The nurse can then provide dietary advice that is meaningful to the client and her family.

Psychosocial Influences

The nurse should be aware of the various psychosocial factors that influence a woman's food choices. The sharing of food has long been a symbol of friendliness, warmth, and social acceptance in many cultures. Some foods and food practices are associated with status. Some foods are prepared "just for company"; others are served only on special occasions or holidays.

Knowledge about the basic components of a balanced diet is essential. Often, educational level is related to economic status, but even individuals on very limited incomes can prepare well-balanced meals if their knowledge of nutrition is adequate.

The expectant woman's attitudes and feelings about her pregnancy influence her nutritional status. For example, foods may be used as a substitute for expressing emotions, such as anger or frustration, or as a way of expressing feelings of joy. The client who is depressed or does not wish to be pregnant may manifest these feelings through loss of appetite or overindulgence in certain foods.

EATING DISORDERS Two serious eating disorders, anorexia nervosa and bulimia nervosa, develop most commonly in adolescent girls and young women. These conditions are described fully in the module on the Self.

Women with eating disorders who become pregnant are at risk for a variety of complications. The consequences of the restricting, bingeing, and purging behaviors characteristic of eating disorders can result in a lack of nutrients being available for the fetus. These clients are at increased risk for miscarriage, hyperemesis gravidarum, preeclampsia, and birth complications, whereas their infants have an increased incidence of preterm birth, low birth weight, low Apgar scores, and intrauterine death (Micali et al., 2012). Pregnant women with eating disorders are also at higher risk for cesarean birth and postpartum depression (Zerbe, 2007).

Pregnancy can be an especially difficult time for the client with an eating disorder, even if she has long desired a child. The consumption of additional food and the expectations that she will gain additional weight can result in feelings of fear, anxiety, depression, and guilt. Clients with eating disorders also have high rates of postpartum depression (Micali et al., 2012).

When a pregnant woman has an eating disorder, education and individualized meal plans can help the client increase her dietary intake while maintaining a sense of control. A multidisciplinary approach to treatment, involving medical, nursing, psychiatric, and dietetic practitioners, is indicated. Pregnant women with eating disorders need to be closely monitored and supported throughout their pregnancies.

PICA Pica is the craving for and persistent eating of nonnutritive substances not ordinarily considered to be edible or nutritionally valuable, such as soil, clay, and soap. Pica appears to occur worldwide but is underreported because women are often embarrassed to discuss it. In the United States, pica is more common among women who are economically disadvantaged, are of African American descent, live in rural areas, practiced pica before pregnancy, belong to a culture that encourages pica as important for fertility, and have family members who also practice pica (Ellis & Schnoes, 2012).

Iron deficiency anemia is the most common concern in pica. The connection of ice pica to iron deficiency is well known, but it is unclear if ingestion of large amounts of ice is a sign of iron deficiency or a contributing factor; however the pica often resolves with iron supplementation (King et al., 2015). The ingestion of laundry starch or certain types of clay may contribute to iron deficiency because they interfere with iron absorption. The ingestion of large quantities of clay could fill the intestine and cause fecal impaction, and the ingestion of starch may be associated with excessive weight gain. Lead poisoning, one of the most serious complications that can result from geophagia (eating soil or clay), may affect both the mother and her fetus. Geophagia may produce soil-borne parasitic infections, such as toxoplasmosis and toxocariasis. Gastrointestinal (GI) tract complications resulting from pica can be mechanical bowel problems, constipation, ulcerations, perforations, and intestinal obstructions. It also can result in impaired cognitive functioning, kidney damage, and encephalopathy. Consequently, blood lead levels should be determined in cases of diagnosed or suspected geophagia.

The nurse should be aware of pica and its implications for the client and fetus. Assessment for pica is an important part of a nutritional history. However, a client may be embarrassed about her cravings or reluctant to discuss them for fear of criticism. Using a nonjudgmental approach, the nurse can provide the client with information that is useful in decreasing or eliminating this practice.

VEGETARIANISM Vegetarianism is the dietary choice of many individuals for religious, health, or ethical reasons. There are several types of vegetarians. **Lacto-ovovegetarians** include milk, dairy products, and eggs in their diets. **Lactovegetarians** include dairy products but no eggs in their diets. **Vegans** will not eat any food from animal sources.

The expectant woman who is vegetarian must eat the proper combination of foods to obtain adequate nutrients. If her diet allows, the client can obtain ample and complete proteins from dairy products and eggs. Plant protein quality can be improved if it is consumed with these animal proteins.

If the client follows a vegan diet, careful planning is necessary to obtain complete proteins and sufficient calories. An adequate, pure vegan diet contains protein from unrefined grains (brown rice, whole wheat), legumes (beans, split peas, lentils), nuts in large quantities, and a variety of cooked and fresh vegetables and fruits. Adequate dietary protein can be obtained by consuming a varied diet with complementary amino acids, which together provide complete proteins. Complete proteins can be obtained by eating different types of plant-based proteins, such as beans and rice, peanut butter on whole-grain bread, and whole-grain cereal with soy milk, either in the same meal or over a day. Seeds may provide adequate protein in the vegetarian diet if the quantity is large enough. Obtaining sufficient calories to ensure adequate weight gain can be difficult, however, because vegan diets tend to be high in fiber and therefore filling. Figure 33–37 ● depicts a vegetarian food pyramid with suggestions for daily servings.

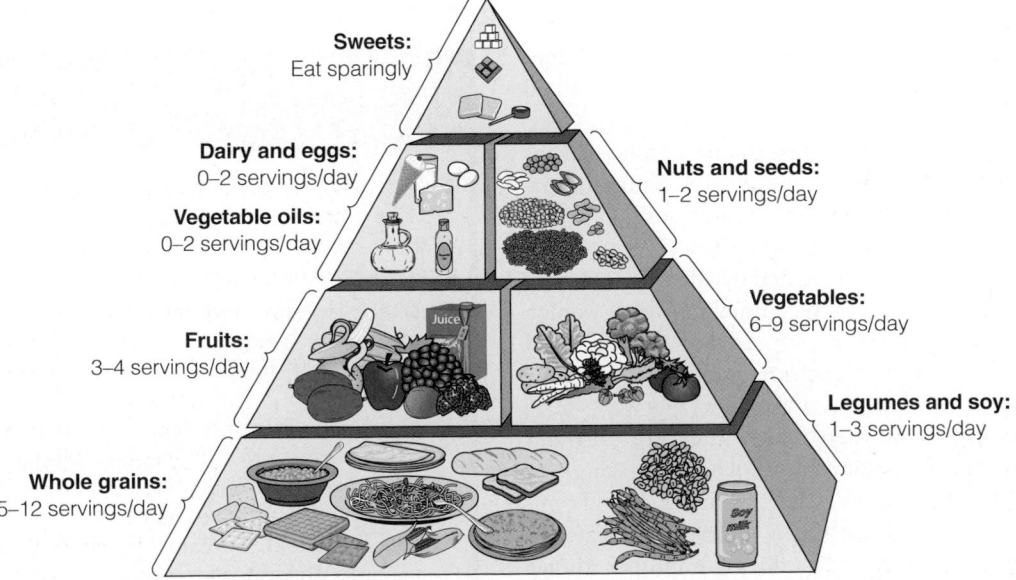

Figure 33–37 ● The vegetarian food pyramid.

TABLE 33–6 Vegetarian Food Groups

FOOD GROUP	MIXED DIET	LACTO-OVOVEGETARIAN	LACTOVEGETARIAN	VEGAN
Grain	Bread, cereal, rice, pasta	Bread, cereal, rice, pasta	Bread, cereal, rice, pasta	Bread, cereal, rice, pasta
Fruit	Fruit, fruit juices	Fruit, fruit juices	Fruit, fruit juices	Fruit, fruit juices
Vegetable	Vegetables, vegetable juices	Vegetables, vegetable juices	Vegetables, vegetable juices	Vegetables, vegetable juices
Dairy and dairy alternatives	Milk, yogurt, cheese	Milk, yogurt, cheese	Milk, yogurt, cheese	Fortified soy milk, rice milk, almond milk
Meat and meat alternatives	Meat, fish, poultry, eggs, legumes, tofu, nuts, nut butters	Eggs, legumes, tofu, nuts, nut butters	Legumes, tofu, nuts, nut butters	Legumes, tofu, nuts, nut butters

Both lacto-ovovegetarians and vegans should eat four servings of vitamin B_{12}–fortified foods (meat substitutes, tofu, cereals, soy milk, and nutritional yeast) daily. A daily supplement of vitamin B_{12} is also recommended during pregnancy and while breastfeeding (Penney & Miller, 2008).

The best sources of iron and zinc are animal products; consequently, vegan diets may also be low in these minerals. In addition, a high fiber intake may reduce mineral (calcium, iron, and zinc) bioavailability. Thus, pregnant women who are vegetarians should be advised to have approximately 1,200–1,500 mg/day of calcium, which is higher than the recommended levels for clients who are omnivores. Vitamin D supplements may be indicated for clients who do not have adequate exposure to sunlight (Penney & Miller, 2008).

To achieve optimum nutrition, the nurse should emphasize the use of foods that are nutrient dense and that provide a balanced diet. A vegetarian food group guide appears in **Table 33–6** ●.

Special Dietary Considerations

The pregnant client must carefully consider choices regarding foods and food additives. These include maintaining adequate levels of folic acid, use of artificial sweeteners, mercury levels in fish, and lactose intolerance.

FOLIC ACID   **Folic acid**, or folate, is required for normal growth, reproduction, and lactation and prevents the macrocytic, megaloblastic anemia of pregnancy. Megaloblastic anemia caused by folate deficiency is rarely found in the United States, but it does occur.

Even more significantly, an inadequate intake of folic acid has been associated with fetal neural tube defects (spina bifida, meningomyelocele). Although these defects are considered to be multifactorial, research indicates that 50%–70% of spina bifida and anencephaly cases could be prevented by adequate intake of folic acid (ACOG, 2011c). Experts recommend that all women of childbearing age (15–45 years) consume 400 mcg of folic acid daily because half of all U.S. pregnancies are unplanned and neural tube defects occur very early in pregnancy (3–4 weeks after conception), before most women realize they are pregnant (CDC, 2012). The best food sources of folate are fresh green leafy vegetables, liver, peanuts, and whole-grain breads and cereals. Folic acid can be made inactive by oxidation, ultraviolet light, and heating. It can easily be lost during improper storage and cooking. To prevent unnecessary loss, foods should be stored covered to protect them from light, cooked with only a small amount of water, and not overcooked.

USE OF ARTIFICIAL SWEETENERS   Sweeteners classified as Generally Recognized as Safe (GRAS) by the FDA are acceptable for use during pregnancy. As with other foods, moderation should be exercised when using artificial sweeteners, such as saccharin, which can cross the placenta and may remain in fetal tissues. Aspartame also appears to be safe if taken within FDA guidelines. Women affected by phenylketonuria should avoid aspartame because it contains phenylalanine. Splenda, or sucralose, is another artificial sweetener that is available to the public. The manufacturers of Splenda and Truvia (stevia) claim that they have no effects on fetal or neonatal development and are therefore safe for use by pregnant or lactating women.

MERCURY IN FISH   Seafood is an important source of omega-3 fatty acids, which are essential for neural development in the fetus. Research suggests that low maternal seafood consumption of omega-3 fatty acids is linked to suboptimal outcomes for verbal IQ, fine motor skills, communication, and social development in the child (Hibbeln, 2007).

Although the omega-3 in fish is beneficial, pregnant women need to be aware that fish can also contain mercury. Nearly all fish and shellfish contain traces of mercury. Although this is not a concern for most individuals, some fish and shellfish contain higher levels of mercury than others, and mercury can pose a threat to the developing nervous system of a fetus or young child. Mercury exposure also can have a negative effect on cognitive functioning,

---

Complementary and Alternative Therapy
Nutritional Content of Herbs

Several herbs are good sources of various vitamins and minerals. Like other "whole" foods, herbs contain all the necessary nutrients and enzymes to increase bioavailability versus isolated substances (e.g., in vitamin and mineral supplements):

- *Dandelion root and herb.* Contain high concentrations of vitamins A and C, beta-carotene, and potassium (National Center for Complementary and Alternative Medicine, 2012).
- *Oat straw.* Rich in calcium and magnesium, plus iron, manganese, and zinc (Natural Medicines Comprehensive Database, 2013a). Note that this is the same plant from which we derive oatmeal.
- *Raspberry leaf.* Contains vitamin A, B, C, and D plus the minerals phosphorous, potassium, and calcium and naturally chelated iron (Natural Medicines Comprehensive Database, 2013b).

resulting in deficiencies in language, attention, motor function, memory, and visual–spatial abilities (Womenshealth.gov, n.d.). Consequently, pregnant women need information about the importance of seafood in their diet, but also need to know that they should consume seafood that is low in mercury. The U.S. government has issued the following guidelines for women who are pregnant or may become pregnant, breastfeeding mothers, and young children (Agency for Toxic Substance and Disease Registry, 2013):

- Do not eat swordfish, shark, tilefish, or king mackerel, because these fish contain high levels of mercury.

- Eat up to 12 oz/week (two average meals) of a variety of shellfish and fish that are lower in mercury. Commonly eaten fish that are lower in mercury include canned light tuna, shrimp, salmon, catfish, and pollack. Albacore (white) tuna has more mercury than canned light tuna; therefore, only 6 oz/week of albacore tuna is recommended.

- Check local advisories about the mercury content of fish caught by family and friends. If no information is available, limit fish caught in local areas to 6 oz/week, and avoid consuming additional fish that week.

LACTASE DEFICIENCY (LACTOSE INTOLERANCE)

Some individuals have difficulty digesting milk and milk products. This condition, known as **lactase deficiency** or **lactose intolerance**, results from an inadequate amount of the enzyme lactase, which breaks down the milk sugar lactose into smaller, digestible substances.

Lactase deficiency is found in most adults of African, Mexican, Native American, Ashkenazi Jewish, and Asian descent and, indeed, in many other adults worldwide. Individuals who are not affected are mainly of northern European heritage. Symptoms include abdominal distention, discomfort, nausea, vomiting, loose stools, and cramps.

When counseling pregnant women who might be intolerant of milk and milk products, the nurse should be aware that even one glass of milk can produce symptoms. Milk in cooked form, such as custards, is sometimes tolerated, as are cultured or fermented dairy products, such as buttermilk, some cheeses, and yogurt. Lactase deficiency need not be a problem for pregnant women, because the enzyme is available over the counter in tablets or drops. Lactase-treated milk is also available commercially in most large grocery stores.

Foodborne Illnesses

Foodborne illnesses should be avoided by any individual, but especially by the pregnant client because they pose a threat to both fetus and mother. The nurse should provide client teaching about salmonella, listeriosis, and hepatitis E.

SALMONELLA Because of the risk for *Salmonella* contamination in raw eggs, advise pregnant women to avoid eating or tasting foods that may contain raw or lightly cooked eggs. These foods include cake batter; homemade eggnog; sauces made with raw eggs, such as Caesar salad dressing; and homemade ice cream (FDA, 2013).

LISTERIOSIS *Listeria monocytogenes* is another bacterium that poses a threat to an expectant mother and her fetus. *Listeria* is especially challenging because the organism can be found in refrigerated, ready-to-eat foods, such as unpasteurized milk and dairy products, meat, poultry, and seafood. To prevent listeriosis, advise pregnant women to do the following (FDA, 2013):

- Maintain the refrigerator at a temperature of 4°C (40°F) or below and the freezer at −18°C (0°F).

- Refrigerate or freeze prepared foods, leftovers, and perishables within 2 hours after eating or preparation.

- Do not eat hot dogs, deli meats, or luncheon meats unless they are reheated until steaming hot.

- Avoid soft cheeses, such as feta, brie, Camembert, blue-veined cheeses, queso fresco, or queso blanco (a soft cheese often used by Hispanic women in their cooking) unless the label clearly states that they are made with pasteurized milk.

- Do not eat refrigerated pates or meat spreads or foods that contain raw (unpasteurized) milk. Do not drink unpasteurized milk.

- Avoid eating refrigerated smoked seafood, such as salmon, trout, cod, tuna, or mackerel, unless it is in a cooked dish, such as a casserole. Canned or shelf-stable pates, meat spreads, and smoked seafood are considered safe.

HEPATITIS E Hepatitis E is a viral infection found most often in developing countries. This disease is spread through the feces of infected people or animals and is transmitted most often through unclean drinking water, but it can also be contracted by eating contaminated food. Hepatitis E is often more severe in pregnant women, especially during the third trimester, and may lead to maternal death (Bazaco, Albrecht, & Malek, 2008).

To prevent hepatitis E, pregnant women should wash their hands thoroughly after using the bathroom, changing diapers, or handling raw foods. When traveling to areas where the quality of the water is uncertain, they should avoid eating raw foods, unpeeled fruit, and uncooked fish. They should also avoid drinking tap water or using ice made with tap water. Rather, they should use bottled or boiled water for drinking, tooth brushing, and formula preparation (Bazaco et al., 2008).

▶ NUTRITIONAL CARE OF THE PREGNANT ADOLESCENT

Nutritional care of the pregnant adolescent is of particular concern to healthcare professionals. Many adolescents are nutritionally at risk because of a variety of complex and interrelated emotional, social, and economic factors. Important nutrition-related factors to assess in pregnant adolescents include low prepregnant weight, low weight gain during pregnancy, young age at menarche, smoking, excessive prepregnant weight, anemia, unhealthy lifestyle (drug or alcohol use), chronic disease, and history of an eating disorder.

Estimates regarding the nutritional needs of adolescents are generally determined by using the DRIs for nonpregnant teenagers (ages 11–14 or 15–18) and adding nutrient amounts recommended for all pregnant women (see Table 33–4). If the pregnant adolescent is physiologically mature (>4 years since menarche), her nutritional needs approach those reported for pregnant adults. However, adolescents who become pregnant less than 4 years after menarche are at risk because of their physiological and anatomical immaturity. These adolescents are more likely than older adolescents to still be growing, which can affect the fetus's development. Thus, young adolescents (ages 14 and younger) need to gain more weight than older adolescents (ages 18 and older) to produce babies of equal size.

In determining the optimal weight gain for the pregnant adolescent, the nurse adds the recommended weight gain for an adult pregnancy to that expected during the postmenarchal year in which the pregnancy occurs. If the teenager is underweight, additional weight gain is recommended to bring her to a normal weight for her height.

Specific Nutrient Concerns

Caloric needs of pregnant adolescents vary widely. Major factors in determining caloric needs include the physical activity level of the individual and whether her growth is complete. Figures as high as 50 kcal/kg have been suggested for young, pregnant adolescents who are very active physically. A satisfactory weight gain usually confirms an adequate caloric intake.

An inadequate iron intake is a major concern with the adolescent diet. Iron needs are high for the pregnant teen because of the requirement for iron by the enlarging maternal muscle mass and blood volume. Iron supplements—providing between 30 and 60 mg of elemental iron—are definitely indicated.

Calcium is another nutrient that demands special attention from pregnant adolescents. Inadequate intake of calcium is frequently a problem in this age group. Adequate calcium intake is necessary to support the normal growth and development of the fetus and the growth and maintenance of calcium stores in the adolescent. An extra serving of dairy products or other calcium-rich foods is usually suggested for teenagers. Calcium supplementation is indicated for teens who do not consume dairy products or other significant calcium sources in sufficient quantities.

Because folic acid plays a role in cell reproduction, it is also an important nutrient for pregnant teens. As previously indicated, a supplement is usually recommended for all pregnant clients, regardless of age.

Other nutrients and vitamins must be considered when evaluating the overall nutritional quality of the teenager's diet. Nutrients that have been found to be deficient in this age group include zinc and vitamins A, D, and B_6. Inclusion of a wide variety of foods—especially fresh and lightly processed foods—is helpful in obtaining adequate amounts of trace minerals, fiber, and vitamins.

Dietary Patterns

Healthy adolescents often have irregular eating patterns. Many skip breakfast, and most tend to be frequent snackers. Teens rarely follow the traditional three-meals-a-day pattern. Their day-to-day intake often varies drastically, and many eat food combinations that may seem bizarre to adults. Despite these practices, adolescents usually achieve a better nutritional balance than most adults would expect.

In assessing the diet of the pregnant adolescent, the nurse should consider the eating pattern over time, not simply a single day's intake. Once the pattern is identified, the nurse can direct counseling toward correcting deficiencies.

Counseling Issues

Counseling about nutrition and healthy eating practices is an important element of care for pregnant teenagers that nurses can provide effectively in a community setting. This counseling may be individualized, involve other teens, or provide a combination of both approaches. If an adolescent's family member does most of the meal preparation, it may be useful to include that individual in the discussion if the adolescent agrees. Involving the expectant father in counseling may also be beneficial. Clinics and schools often offer classes and focused activities designed to address this topic.

The pregnant teenager's understanding of nutrition will influence not only her well-being but also that of her child. However, teens tend to live in the present, and counseling that stresses long-term changes may be less effective than more concrete approaches. In many cases, group classes are effective, especially those that include other teens. In a group atmosphere, adolescents often work together to plan adequate meals including foods that are special favorites.

▶ MATERNAL WEIGHT GAIN

Maternal weight gain is an important factor in fetal growth and infant birth weight. The optimal weight gain depends on the woman's weight for height (body mass index) and her prepregnant nutritional state. An adequate weight gain indicates an adequate caloric intake. It does not, however, ensure that the woman has a sufficient nutrient intake. The pregnant woman must maintain the nutritional quality of her diet as her weight gain progresses.

The Institute of Medicine (2009) recommends weight gains in terms of optimum ranges. The IOM recommendations are shown in **Table 33–7** ●.

The pattern of weight gain is important. The ideal pattern for a normal-weight woman consists of a gain of 0.9–1.8 kg (2.0–4.0 lb) during the first trimester, followed by a gain of

TABLE 33–7 Institute of Medicine Weight Gain Recommendations for Pregnancy

PREPREGNANCY WEIGHT CATEGORY	BODY MASS INDEX*	RECOMMENDED RANGE OF TOTAL WEIGHT (LB)	RECOMMENDED RATES OF WEIGHT GAIN[†] IN THE SECOND AND THIRD TRIMESTERS (LB) (MEAN RANGE [LB/WK])
Underweight	<18.5	28–40	1 (1–1.3)
Normal weight	18.5–24.9	25–35	1 (0.8–1)
Overweight	25–29.9	15–25	0.6 (0.5–0.7)
Obese (includes all classes)	30+	11–20	0.5 (0.4–0.6)

*Body mass index is calculated as weight in kilograms divided by height in meters squared, or as weight in pounds multiplied by 703 divided by square of height in inches.
[†]Calculations assume a 1.1- to 4.4-lb weight gain in the first trimester.

Source: Based on Institute of Medicine. (2009). *Weight gain during pregnancy: Reexamining the guidelines.* Washington, DC: National Academies Press. ©2009 National Academy of Sciences. Retrieved from http://www.iom.edu/~/media/Files/Report%20Files/2009/Weight-Gain-During-Pregnancy-Reexamining-the-Guidelines/Report%20Brief%20-%20Weight%20Gain%20During%20Pregnancy.pdf.

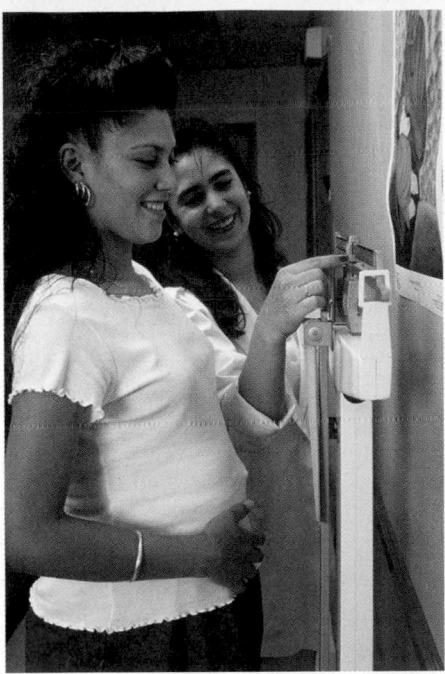

Figure 33–38 ● It is important to monitor a pregnant woman's weight over time.

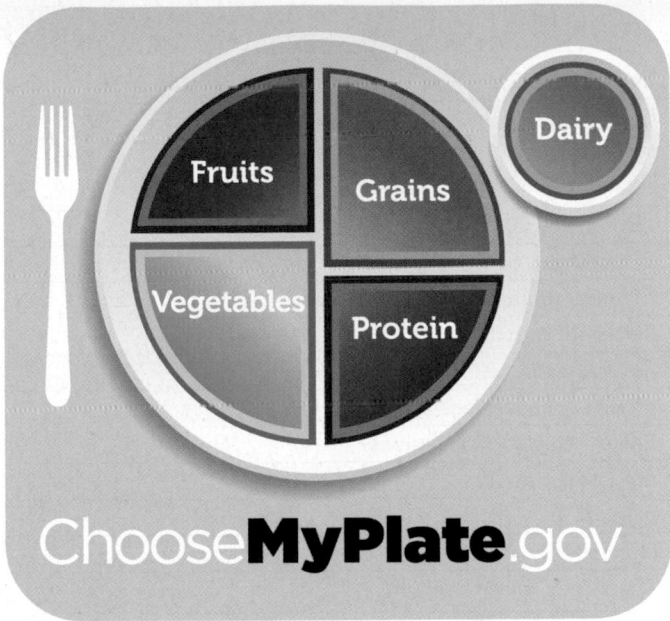

ChooseMyPlate.gov

Figure 33–39 ● ChooseMyPlate identifies the basic food groups and provides guidance about healthful eating. Grains, vegetables, and fruits are emphasized, with slightly less emphasis on dairy and protein. MyPlate is designed to remind Americans to eat healthfully.
Source: U.S. Department of Agriculture; U.S. Department of Health and Human Services.

approximately 0.3–0.5 kg (0.8–1 lb) per week during the second and third trimesters. The rate of weight gain in the second and third trimesters needs to be slightly higher for underweight women, and slightly lower (0.5–0.7 lb/week) for overweight women and 0.4–0.6 lb/week for women with obesity (IOM, 2009). A normal-weight woman who is expecting twins is advised to gain approximately 0.7 kg (1.5 lb) per week during the second and third trimesters of her pregnancy. Inadequate maternal weight gain has been associated with preterm birth and its associated problems for the newborn (IOM, 2009).

Obesity is becoming a major health problem in many developed countries, and more and more women are entering pregnancy already overweight or obese. Pregnant women who are obese are at an increased risk for medical and pregnancy-related complications, such as spontaneous abortion, gestational diabetes, preeclampsia, labor induction, and cesarean birth. They also have a higher incidence of fetal anomalies. They should be considered to be at high risk and counseled accordingly (ACOG, 2013a).

Maternal obesity also has implications for children. The children of mothers who are overweight and obese are predisposed to developing obesity and its related health concerns. In fact, the child of an overweight mother is three times more likely to be overweight by the age of 7 than is a child of a normal-weight mother (Reece, 2008).

Because of the association between maternal weight gain and pregnancy outcome, most healthcare providers pay close attention to weight gain during pregnancy (**Figure 33–38 ●**). Weight gain charts can be useful in monitoring the rate and pattern of weight gain over time.

Excessive weight gain during pregnancy also has long-term implications because weight gain during pregnancy is by far the most important predictor of the amount of weight that a woman will retain following childbirth (ACOG, 2013a). Counseling the pregnant woman to eat a variety of nutrients from each of the food groups places less emphasis on the amount of her weight gain and

more on the quality of her intake. It may also be helpful to encourage the woman to begin a simple exercise program such as walking.

The federal government's newly designed food choice program, ChooseMyPlate, offers users a colorful plan that emphasizes variety, proportionality, moderation, and physical activity. It is also designed to help guide individuals to make healthier choices (**Figure 33–39 ●**).

�“ *Stay Current: Go to **www.choosemyplate.gov/ pregnancy-breastfeeding.html** to see the USDA's nutrition recommendations for pregnant women and to **www.choosemyplate. gov/supertracker-tools/daily-food-plans/moms.html** to see how clients can get a "Daily Good Plan for Mom" using Choose-MyPlate's SuperTracker.*

SAFETY ALERT
Weight varies with time of day, amount of clothing, inaccurate scale adjustment, or weighing error. Do not overemphasize a single weight; rather, pay attention to the overall pattern of weight gain.

■ NURSING PROCESS

A written care plan or clinical pathway that incorporates the prenatal record, nursing diagnoses, and client goals is essential to ensure continuity of care. Prenatal care, especially for women with low-risk pregnancies, is community based, typically in a clinic or a private office. The healthcare community recognizes the value of providing a primary care nurse in these settings to coordinate holistic care for each childbearing family. The nurse in a clinic or health maintenance organization

TABLE 33–8   Danger Signs in Pregnancy

DANGER SIGN	POSSIBLE CAUSE
Sudden gush of fluid from vagina	Premature rupture of membranes
Vaginal bleeding	Abruptio placentae, placenta previa
	Lesions of cervix or vagina, "bloody show"
Abdominal pain	Premature labor, abruptio placentae
Temperature above 38.3°C (101°F) and chills	Infection
Dizziness, blurred vision, double vision, spots before eyes	Hypertension, preeclampsia
Persistent vomiting	Hyperemesis gravidarum
Severe headache	Hypertension, preeclampsia
Edema of hands, face, legs, and feet	Preeclampsia
Reflex irritability, convulsions	Preeclampsia, eclampsia
Epigastric pain	Preeclampsia, ischemia in major abdominal vessel
Oliguria	Renal impairment, decreased fluid intake, preeclampsia
Dysuria	Urinary tract infection
Absence of fetal movement	Maternal medication, obesity, fetal death

may be the only source of continuity for the woman, who may see a different physician or CNM at each visit.

Assessment

The nurse can complete many areas of prenatal assessment. Advanced practice nurses, such as CNMs and certified women's health nurse practitioners, have the education and skill to perform full and complete antepartum assessments. Areas of assessment may include the following:

- The woman's physical status
- The woman's understanding of pregnancy and the changes that accompany it
- The woman or family's attitudes about the pregnancy and expectations of the impact a baby will have on their lives
- Any health teaching needs
- The degree of support the woman has available to her
- The woman's knowledge of infant care.

Community-Based Care Delivering Prenatal Nursing Care in the Home

Home care can be of benefit to any pregnant woman, but it is especially effective in removing barriers for women who have difficulty accessing health care. These barriers may include lack of locally available healthcare facilities, problems with transportation to the facility, or schedule conflicts with available appointment times because of employment hours or family responsibilities. A prenatal home care visit or phone contact can also be useful for women who anticipate a short inpatient stay after childbirth. At the prenatal contact, the nurse explains the perinatal program and answers any questions the woman or her family have. Currently, home care is most often used for women with prenatal complications that can be managed without hospitalization if effective nursing assessment and care are provided in the home.

While gathering data, the nurse also has an opportunity to discuss important aspects of nutrition within the context of the family's needs and lifestyle. In addition, the nurse seeks information about psychological, cultural, and socioeconomic factors that may influence food intake.

At subsequent prenatal visits, the nurse continues to gather data about the course of the pregnancy to date and the woman's responses to it. The nurse also asks about the adjustment of the support person and of other children, if any, in the family. As the pregnancy progresses, the nurse inquires about the preparations the family has made for the new baby. The nurse asks specifically whether the woman has experienced any discomfort, especially the kinds of discomfort that are often seen at specific times during a pregnancy. The nurse also inquires about physical changes that relate directly to the pregnancy, such as fetal movement, and asks about the danger signs of pregnancy (Table 33–8 ●).

SAFETY ALERT
Pregnancy is a high-risk period for intimate partner abuse. It is important for the nurse to assess the client with suspicious or unexplained injuries for this possibility.

Other pertinent information includes any exposure to contagious illnesses, medical treatment and therapy prescribed for medical problems since the last visit, and any prescription or OTC medications or herbal supplements that were not prescribed as part of the woman's prenatal care.

During the antepartum period, it is essential for the nurse to begin assessing the readiness of the woman and her partner (if possible) to assume their responsibilities as parents successfully. The Assessment Interview feature identifies areas for assessment of parenting ability.

The accompanying Subsequent Prenatal Assessment feature provides a systematic approach to the regular physical examinations the pregnant woman should undergo for optimal antepartum care and also provides a model for evaluating both the pregnant woman and the expectant partner, if the partner is involved in the pregnancy.

Assessment Interview Prenatal Assessment of Parenting Ability

Perception of Complexities of Mothering

A. Desires baby for itself.

Positive:

1. The pregnancy is a planned or desired extension of a stable home life.

Negative:

1. Wants baby to meet own needs, such as someone to love her, someone to get her out of unhappy home, a way to repair faltering relationship.
2. The pregnancy is unwanted.
   - Was the pregnancy planned or a surprise?
   - How do you feel about being a mother?
   - Have you considered terminating the pregnancy or placing the baby for adoption?

B. Expresses consideration of the impact of mothering roles on other roles (relationship, career, school).

Positive:

1. Realistic expectations of how baby will affect job, career, school, and personal goals.
2. Interested in learning about child care.

Negative:

1. Lacks insight regarding the physical, emotional, and social demands of parenting.
2. Disinterested in learning about the needs of an infant.

C. Makes lifestyle changes for the baby's benefit.

Positive:

1. Gives up routines not good for baby (quits smoking, adjusts eating habits).
2. Initiates positive, proactive routines (childbirth classes, prenatal exercise classes, stress reduction).

Negative:

1. Rationalizes or denies behavior that places the baby at risk.
2. Expresses inability for or disinterest in proactive behavior.
   - What do you think it will be like to take care of a baby?
   - How do you think your life will be different after you have your baby?
   - How do you feel this baby will affect your job, career, school, and personal goals?
   - How will the baby affect your relationship with your significant other?
   - What can you do to help yourself and the baby be as healthy as possible?
   - What can you do to prepare for being a mother?

Attachment

A. Strong feelings regarding gender of baby.

Positive:

1. Verbalizes love and acceptance of either gender.

Negative:

1. Believes baby will be like negative aspects of self and partner.
2. Verbalizes belief that she will be unable to parent a child of a particular gender
3. Considers a particular gender as conferring more or less status on the family.
   - Why do you prefer a certain gender?
   - How will you feel and what will you do differently if your baby is a boy/girl?

B. Interested in data regarding fetus (e.g., growth and development, heart tones).

Positive:

1. Verbalizes positive thoughts about the baby.
2. Asks questions about the baby's development and status.

Negative:

1. Shows no interest in fetal growth and development, quickening, and fetal heart tones.
2. Expresses negative feelings about fetus.
3. Rejects counseling regarding nutrition, rest, hygiene.
   - Encourage interest in the fetus. Point out normal development.
   - Explore the mother's reasons for negative feelings and/or rejection of counseling.

C. Fantasizes about baby.

Positive:

1. Prepares for the addition of a baby to her household.
2. Speaks of the baby as her child and her other children's brother or sister.
3. Talks to the baby in utero.
4. Makes positive speculations about the baby's appearance and disposition.

Negative:

1. Bonding conditional depending on gender, age of baby, and/or labor and birth experience.
2. Woman considers only own needs when making plans for baby.
3. Exhibits no attachment behaviors.
4. Failure to prepare.
   - What did you think or feel when you first felt the baby move?
   - Have you started preparing for the baby?
   - What do you think your baby will look like?
   - How would you like your new baby to look?
   - Does this baby have a name?

Acceptance of Child by Significant Others

A. Acknowledges acceptance by significant others of the new responsibility.

Positive:

1. Acknowledges unconditional acceptance of pregnancy and baby by significant others.
2. Partner accepts new responsibility for child.
3. Shares experience of pregnancy with significant others.

Negative:

1. Significant others not supportively involved with pregnancy.
2. Conditional acceptance of pregnancy by significant others depending on gender, race, age of baby.
3. Decision making does not take in needs of fetus (e.g., food money spent on new car).
4. Partner and family with no/little responsibility for needs of pregnancy, woman/fetus.
   - How does your partner feel about this pregnancy?
   - How do your parents feel?
   - What do your friends think?
   - Does your partner have a preference regarding the baby's gender? If so, why?
   - How does your partner feel about being a parent?
   - What do you think your partner will be like as a parent?

(continued on next page)

Assessment Interview   Prenatal Assessment of Parenting Ability (continued)

- What do you think your partner will do to help you with child care?
- Have you and your partner talked about how the baby might change your lives?
- Who have you told about your pregnancy?
- Do you have family or friends who can help you take care of a new baby?

B. Concrete demonstration of acceptance of pregnancy/baby by significant others (e.g., baby shower, significant other involved in prenatal education).

Positive:

1. Baby shower.
2. Significant other attends prenatal class with client.
3. Commitment from the mother's community to help take care of the new baby (watch older children when she is in labor and immediately postpartum, meal planning, housework).
   - If partner attends clinic with client, note partner's degree of interest (e.g., listens to heart tones).
   - Significant other plans to be with client during labor and birth.
   - Partner is contributing financially.

Ensures Physical Well-Being

A. Concerns about having normal pregnancy, labor and birth, and baby.

Positive:

1. Preparing for labor and birth, attends prenatal classes, interested in labor and birth.
2. Aware of danger signs of pregnancy.
3. Seeks and uses appropriate health care (e.g., time of initial visit, keeps appointments, follows through on recommendations).

Negative:

1. Denies signs and symptoms that might suggest complications of pregnancy.
2. Verbalizes extreme fear of labor and birth—refuses to talk about labor and birth.
3. Misses appointments, fails to follow instructions, refuses to attend prenatal classes.
   - Encourage expression of fears so they can be addressed
   - Ask about reasons for missed appointments in order to assist with obtaining services (medical transportation, social working, home health nurse).

Note: When "Negative" is not listed in a section, the reader may assume that negative is the absence of positive responses.
Source: Modified and used with permission of the Minneapolis Health Department, Minneapolis, MN.

Subsequent Prenatal Assessment

PHYSICAL ASSESSMENT/ NORMAL FINDINGS	ALTERATIONS AND POSSIBLE CAUSES*	NURSING RESPONSES TO DATA†
Vital Signs		
Temperature: 36.2°–37.6°C (97°–99.6°F)	Elevated temperature (infection)	Evaluate for signs of infection. Refer to healthcare provider.
Pulse: 60–90 bpm Rate may increase 10 bpm during pregnancy	Increased pulse rate (anxiety, cardiac disorders)	Note irregularities. Assess for anxiety and stress.
Respiration: 12–22 breaths/min	Marked tachypnea or abnormal patterns (respiratory disease)	Refer to healthcare provider.
Blood pressure: less than 140/90 mmHg (falls in second trimester)	Greater than 140/90 mmHg	Assess for headache, edema, proteinuria, and hyperreflexia. Refer to healthcare provider.
		Schedule appointments more frequently.
Weight Gain		
First trimester: 1.6–2.3 kg (3.5–5 lb)	Inadequate weight gain (poor nutrition, nausea, small for gestational age)	Discuss appropriate weight gain.
Second trimester: 5.5–6.8 kg (12–15 lb)	Excessive weight gain (excessive caloric intake, edema, preeclampsia)	Provide nutritional counseling. Assess for presence of edema or anemia.
Third trimester: 5.5–6.8 kg (12–15 lb)		
	*Possible causes of alterations are identified in parentheses.	†This column provides guidelines for further assessment and initial nursing intervention.

Subsequent Prenatal Assessment (continued)

PHYSICAL ASSESSMENT/ NORMAL FINDINGS	ALTERATIONS AND POSSIBLE CAUSES*	NURSING RESPONSES TO DATA†
Edema		
Small amount of dependent edema, especially in last weeks of pregnancy	Edema in hands, face, legs, and feet (pre-eclampsia)	Identify any correlation between edema and activities, blood pressure, or proteinuria. Refer to healthcare provider if indicated.
Uterine Size		
See the Initial Prenatal Assessment feature in the Concept section for normal changes during pregnancy.	Unusually rapid growth (multiple gestation, hydatidiform mole, hydramnios, miscalculation of estimated date of birth)	Evaluate fetal status. Determine height of fundus. Use diagnostic ultrasound.
Fetal Heartbeat		
120–160 bpm Funic souffle	Absence of fetal heartbeat after 20 weeks of gestation (maternal obesity, fetal demise)	Evaluate fetal status.
Laboratory Evaluation		
Hemoglobin: 12–16 g/dL Pseudoanemia of pregnancy	Less than 11 g/dL (anemia)	Provide nutritional counseling. Hemoglobin check is repeated at 28–36 weeks of gestation. Consider a hemoglobin screen for women of Mediterranean, African, or south Asian descent.
Quad marker screen: blood test performed at 15–22 weeks of gestation. Evaluates four factors—maternal serum alpha-fetoprotein (MSAFP), unconjugated estriol (UE), human chorionic gonadotropin (hCG), and inhibin-A: normal levels	Elevated MSAFP (neural tube defect, underestimated gestational age, multiple gestation); lower-than-normal MSAFP (Down syndrome, trisomy 18); higher-than-normal hCG and inhibin-A (Down syndrome); lower-than-normal UE (Down syndrome)	Recommended for all pregnant women; especially indicated for women with any of the following risk factors: age 35 or over, family history of birth defects, previous child with a birth defect, insulin-dependent diabetes before pregnancy (Medline Plus, 2012). If quad screen abnormal, further testing such as ultrasound or amniocentesis may be indicated.
First trimester integrated screen	Provides the same information as the quad screen in a more accurate and timely fashion as information on trisomy 13, 18 and 21 is available between 11 and 13 weeks gestation and laboratory tests are combined with ultrasound of the fetal nasal bone and nuchal fold	
NIPT/ cell free DNA	Allows analysis of fetal alleles in maternal serum. Provides information on chromosomal anomalies.	
Repeat indirect Coombs test done on Rh-negative women: negative (done at 28 weeks of gestation)	Rh antibodies present (maternal sensitization has occurred)	If Rh negative and unsensitized, Rh immune globulin is given. If Rh antibodies are present, Rh immune globulin is not given; fetus is monitored closely for isoimmune hemolytic disease.
50-g, 1-hour glucose screen (done between 24 and 28 weeks of gestation)	Plasma glucose level greater than 140 mg/dL (GDM) *Note:* Some facilities use a level of greater than 130 mg/dL, which identifies 90% of women with GDM.	Discuss implications of gestational diabetes mellitus (GDM). Refer for a diagnostic 100-g oral glucose tolerance test.
Urinalysis: See the Initial Prenatal Assessment feature in the Concept section for normal findings.	See the Initial Prenatal Assessment feature in the Concept section for deviations.	Repeat urinalysis at 7 months of gestation. Repeat dipstick test at each visit.
	*Possible causes of alterations are identified in parentheses.	†This column provides guidelines for further assessment and initial nursing intervention.

(continued on next page)

Subsequent Prenatal Assessment (continued)

PHYSICAL ASSESSMENT/ NORMAL FINDINGS	ALTERATIONS AND POSSIBLE CAUSES*	NURSING RESPONSES TO DATA[†]
Protein: negative	Proteinuria, albuminuria (contamination by vaginal discharge, urinary tract infection, preeclampsia)	Obtain dipstick urine sample. Refer to healthcare provider if deviations are present.
Glucose: negative	Persistent glycosuria (diabetes mellitus)	Refer to healthcare provider.
Note: Glycosuria may be present because of physiological alterations in glomerular filtration rate and renal threshold.		
Screening for Group B streptococcus: rectal and vaginal swabs obtained at 35–37 weeks of gestation for all pregnant women.	Positive culture (maternal colonization)	Explain fetal/neonatal risks and the need for antibiotic prophylaxis in labor. Refer to healthcare provider for therapy.

CULTURAL ASSESSMENT[§]	VARIATIONS TO CONSIDER	NURSING RESPONSES TO DATA[†]
Determine the mother's (and family's) attitudes about the gender of the unborn child.	Some women have no preference about the gender of the child; others do. In many cultures, boys are especially valued as firstborn children.	Provide opportunities to discuss preferences and expectations; avoid a judgmental attitude to the response.
Ask about the woman's expectations of childbirth. Will she want someone with her for the birth? Whom does she choose? What is the role of her partner?	Some women want their partner present for labor and birth; others prefer a female relative or friend.	Provide information on birth options, but accept the woman's decision about who will attend.
	Some women expect to be separated from their partner once cervical dilation has occurred.	
Ask about preparations for the baby. Determine what is customary for the woman.	Some women may have a fully prepared nursery; others may not have a separate room for the baby.	Explore reasons for not preparing for the baby. Support the mother's preferences, and provide information about possible sources of assistance if the decision is related to a lack of resources.

Expectant Mother		
Psychological status	Increased stress and anxiety	Encourage woman to take an active part in her care.
First trimester: Incorporates idea of pregnancy; may feel ambivalent, especially if she must give up desired role; usually looks for signs of verification of pregnancy, such as increase in abdominal size or fetal movement.	Inability to establish communication; inability to accept pregnancy; inappropriate response or actions; denial of pregnancy; inability to cope	Establish lines of communication. Establish a trusting relationship. Counsel as necessary. Refer to appropriate professional as needed.
Second trimester: Baby becomes more real to woman as abdominal size increases and she feels movement; she begins to turn inward, becoming more introspective.		
Third trimester: Begins to think of the baby as a separate being; may feel restless, and may feel that the time of labor will never come; remains self-centered and concentrates on preparing place for baby.		
[§]These are only a few suggestions. We do not mean to imply that this is a comprehensive cultural assessment; rather, it is a tool to encourage cultural competence.		[†]This column provides guidelines for further assessment and initial nursing intervention.

Subsequent Prenatal Assessment (continued)

CULTURAL ASSESSMENT§	VARIATIONS TO CONSIDER	NURSING RESPONSES TO DATA†
Educational needs: Self-care measures and knowledge about the following: Health promotion 　Breast care 　Hygiene 　Rest 　Exercise 　Nutrition Relief measures for common discomforts of pregnancy Danger signs in pregnancy (see Table 33–8)	Inadequate information	Provide information and counseling.
Sexual activity: Woman knows how pregnancy affects sexual activity.	Lack of information about effects of pregnancy and/or alternative positions during sexual intercourse	Provide counseling.
Preparation for parenting: appropriate preparation	Lack of preparation (denial, failure to adjust to baby, unwanted child)	Counsel. If lack of preparation is caused by inadequacy of information, provide information.
Preparation for childbirth: Client is aware of the following: 1. Prepared childbirth techniques 2. Normal processes and changes during childbirth 3. Problems that may occur as a result of drug and alcohol use and of smoking	Continued abuse of drugs and alcohol; denial of possible effect on self and baby	If couple chooses a particular technique, refer to childbirth classes. Encourage prenatal class attendance. Educate woman during visits based on current physical status. Provide reading list for more specific information. Refer for thorough evaluation of substance abuse.
Woman has met other physician or nurse-midwife who may be attending her birth in the absence of primary caregiver	Introduction of new individual at birth may increase stress and anxiety for woman and partner.	Introduce woman to all members of group practice.
Impending labor: Client knows signs of impending labor. 1. Uterine contractions that increase in frequency, duration, and intensity 2. Bloody show 3. Expulsion of mucous plug 4. Rupture of membranes	Lack of information	Provide appropriate teaching, stressing importance of seeking appropriate medical assistance.
Expectant Partner		
Psychological status		
First trimester: May express excitement over confirmation of pregnancy; male partner may be pleased with evidence of his virility; concerns move toward providing for financial needs; energetic, may identify with some discomforts of pregnancy, and may even exhibit symptoms.	Increasing stress and anxiety; inability to establish communication; inability to accept pregnancy diagnosis; withdrawal of support; abandonment of the mother	Encourage expectant partner to come to prenatal visits. Establish line of communication. Establish trusting relationship.
§These are only a few suggestions. We do not mean to imply that this is a comprehensive cultural assessment; rather, it is a tool to encourage cultural competence.		†This column provides guidelines for further assessment and initial nursing intervention.

(continued on next page)

Subsequent Prenatal Assessment (continued)

CULTURAL ASSESSMENT§	VARIATIONS TO CONSIDER	NURSING RESPONSES TO DATA†
Second trimester: May feel more confident and be less concerned with financial matters; may have concerns about expectant mother's changing size and shape, her increasing introspection.		Counsel. Let expectant partner know that it is normal to experience these feelings.
Third trimester: May have feelings of rivalry with fetus, especially during sexual activity; may make changes in physical appearance and exhibit more interest in self; may become more energetic; fantasizes about child, but usually imagines older child; fears mutilation and death of woman and child.		Include expectant partner in pregnancy activities as the partner desires. Provide education, information, and support. Increasing numbers of expectant partners are demonstrating desire to be involved in many or all aspects of prenatal care, education, and preparation.
§These are only a few suggestions. We do not mean to imply that this is a comprehensive cultural assessment; rather, it is a tool to encourage cultural competence.		†This column provides guidelines for further assessment and initial nursing intervention.

SAFETY ALERT
When assessing blood pressure, have the pregnant woman sit up with her arm resting on a table so that her arm is at the level of her heart. Expect a decrease in her blood pressure from baseline during the second trimester because of normal physiological changes. If this decrease does not occur, evaluate further for signs of preeclampsia.

The woman's individual needs and the assessment of her risks should determine the frequency of subsequent visits. Generally, the recommended frequency of antepartum visits is as follows:

- Every 4 weeks for the first 28 weeks of gestation
- Every 2 weeks until 36 weeks of gestation
- After week 36, every week until childbirth.

During the subsequent antepartum assessments, most women demonstrate ongoing psychological adjustment to pregnancy. However, some women may exhibit signs of possible psychological problems, such as the following:

- Increasing anxiety
- Inability to establish communication
- Inappropriate responses or actions
- Denial of pregnancy
- Inability to cope with stress
- Intense preoccupation with the gender of the baby
- Failure to acknowledge quickening
- Failure to plan and prepare for the baby (e.g., living arrangements, clothing, and feeding methods)
- Indications of substance abuse.

If the woman's behavior indicates possible psychological problems, the nurse can provide ongoing support and counseling and also refer the woman to appropriate professionals.

Obstetric History

The nurse interviews the client regarding previous pregnancies, which affect the client's plan of care. A woman who has experienced previous miscarriages or complications of pregnancy may require increased monitoring and a greater level of support than a woman who has already had one or more successful pregnancies without complication.

The terms *gravida* and *para* are used in relation to pregnancies, not to the number of fetuses. Thus, twins, triplets, and other multiples count as one pregnancy and one birth. Miscarriages and fetal losses before viability at 24 weeks of gestation are called fetal demise. Those before 20 weeks are called abortions.

The following examples illustrate how these terms are applied in clinical situations:

1. Jean Sanchez has one child born at 38 weeks of gestation and is pregnant for the second time. At her initial prenatal visit, the nurse indicates her obstetric history as "gravida 2 para 1 ab 0." Jean Sanchez's present pregnancy terminates at 16 weeks of gestation. She is now "gravida 2 para 1 ab 1."
2. Tracy Hopkins is pregnant for the fourth time. At home, she has a child who was born at term. Her second pregnancy ended at 10 weeks of gestation. She then gave birth to twins at 35 weeks of gestation. One of the twins died soon after birth. At her antepartum assessment, the nurse records her obstetric history as "gravida 4 para 2 ab 1."

This approach is confusing, however, because it fails to identify the number of children that a woman might have. To provide more comprehensive data, a more detailed approach is used in some settings. Using the detailed system, *gravida* keeps the same meaning, but the meaning of *para* changes because the detailed system counts each infant born rather than the number of pregnancies carried to viability (Cunningham et al., 2010). For example, triplets count as one pregnancy but three babies.

A useful acronym for remembering the detailed system is **G TPAL**:

G: number of pregnancies (**G**ravida)
T: number of **T**erm infants born—that is, the number of infants born after 37 weeks of gestation
P: number of **P**reterm infants born—that is, the number of infants born after 20 weeks but before the completion of 37 weeks of gestation

Name	Gravida	Term	Preterm	Abortions	Living Children
Jean Sanchez	2	1	0	1	1
Tracy Hopkins	4	1	2	1	2

Figure 33–40 ● The **G TPAL** approach provides detailed information about a woman's pregnancy history.

A: number of pregnancies ending in either spontaneous or therapeutic Abortion
L: number of currently Living children

Using this approach, the nurse would have initially described Jean Sanchez (see the first example) as "gravida 2 para 1001." Following Jean's spontaneous abortion, she would be "gravida 2 para 1011." Tracy Hopkins would be described as "gravida 4 para 1212." **Figure 33–40 ●** illustrates this method.

> **SAFETY ALERT**
> In general, it is best to avoid an initial discussion of a woman's obstetric history in front of her partner. It is possible that the woman had a previous pregnancy she has not mentioned to her partner, and revealing this information could violate her right to privacy.

Determining Due Date

Families generally want to know the "due date," or the date around which childbirth will occur. Historically, the due date has been called the estimated date of confinement (EDC). However, the concept of *confinement* is rather negative, and many caregivers avoid it by referring to the due date as the estimated date of delivery. Even then, childbirth educators often stress that babies are not "delivered" like a package; they are born. In keeping with a view that emphasizes the normalcy of the process, this text refers to the due date as the **estimated date of birth (EDB)**.

To calculate the EDB, it is helpful to know the date of the woman's last menstrual period. However, some women have episodes of irregular bleeding or fail to keep track of menstrual cycles. Thus, other techniques also help determine how far along a woman is in her pregnancy—that is, at how many weeks of gestation she is. These techniques include evaluating uterine size, determining when quickening occurs, and auscultating FHR with a Doppler device or ultrasound and, later, with a fetoscope.

The most common method of determining the EDB is to use the **Nägele rule**. To use this method, one begins with the first day of the last menstrual period (LMP), subtracts 3 months, and adds 7 days. For example:

First day of LMP	November 21
Subtract 3 months	−3 months
	August 21
Add 7 days	+7 days
EDB	August 28

It is simpler to change the months to numeric terms:

November 21 becomes	11–21
Subtract 3 months	−3
	8–21
Add 7 days	+7
EDB	August 28

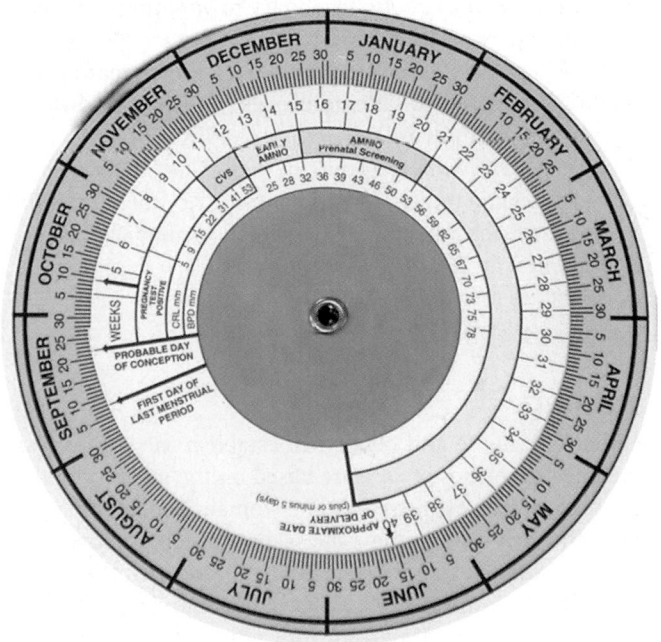

Figure 33–41 ● The EDB wheel can be used to calculate the due date. To use it, place the arrow labeled "1st day of last period" on the date of the woman's last menstrual period (LMP). Then read the EDB at the arrow labeled "40." In this case, the LMP is September 8 and the EDB is June 17.

A gestation calculator or wheel permits the caregiver to calculate the EDB even more quickly (**Figure 33–41 ●**).

If a woman with a history of menses every 28 days remembers her last menstrual period and was not taking oral contraceptives before becoming pregnant, the Nägele rule may be a fairly accurate determiner of the EDB. However, *ovulation usually occurs 14 days before the onset of the next menses, not 14 days after the previous menses*. Consequently, if the woman's cycle is irregular or is more than 28 days long, the time of ovulation may be delayed. If she has been using oral contraceptives, ovulation may be delayed for several weeks following her last menses. Then, too, a postpartum woman who is breastfeeding may resume ovulating but be amenorrheic for a time, making calculation impossible. Thus, the Nägele rule, although helpful, is not foolproof.

It is important to determine the EDB as accurately as possible, as the gestational age at which many prenatal screenings are done is extremely important. The most common reason for false positive results on aneuploidy and neural tube defect screening is inaccurate calculation of gestational age (Messerlain, 2013). It is also essential for evaluating fetal growth and deciding on the timing of intervention for postterm pregnancies. The most accurate estimation of gestational age is a 7-10 week crown rump length measurement consistent with LMP dating. If there is a discrepancy of more than 3 days between early ultrasound and LMP, the pregnancy is dated by the ultrasound (MacKenzie et al., 2015).

Diagnosis

Nursing diagnoses, of course, vary from pregnancy to pregnancy but may include the following:

- *Deficient Knowledge* related to self-care
- *Deficient Fluid Volume* secondary to vomiting/hyperemesis gravidarum
- *Decisional Conflict* related to unexpected pregnancy
- *Anxiety* related to change in role, deficient knowledge, reaction of family members, and so forth
- *Imbalanced Nutrition* (may be *Less Than Body Requirements* related to nausea and vomiting or *More Than Body Requirements* related to excessive caloric intake)
- *Readiness for Enhanced Parenting*
- *Readiness for Enhanced Family Processes.*

(NANDA-I © 2012)

Planning

Together, the nurse and client will establish the plan of care. Sometimes, priorities of care are based on the most immediate needs or concerns expressed by the woman. For example, during the first trimester, when she is experiencing nausea or is concerned about sexual intimacy with her partner, the woman likely will not want to hear about labor and birth. At other times, priorities may develop from findings during a prenatal examination. For example, a woman who is showing signs of preeclampsia may feel physically well and find it hard to accept the nurse's emphasis on the need for frequent rest periods.

Potential goals of nursing care during pregnancy may include the following:

- The client will increase her daily intake of calcium to the DRI level.
- The client will articulate the danger signs of pregnancy and when to call the physician's office or seek emergency care.
- The client will have the opportunity to express concerns and ask questions.
- The client will articulate methods of self-care.
- The client with a chronic condition will consult with her obstetrician and her treating physician during the pregnancy.

Implementation

When providing client care, the nurse should be sensitive to religious or spiritual, cultural, and socioeconomic factors that may influence a family's response to pregnancy as well as to the woman's expectations of the healthcare system. The nurse can avoid stereotyping clients simply by asking each woman about her expectations for the antepartum period. Although many women's responses may reflect what are thought to be traditional norms, other women may have decidedly different views or expectations that represent a blending of beliefs or cultures.

Promote Knowledge Related to Self-Care

The nurse may see a pregnant client only once every 4–6 weeks during the first several months of her pregnancy, during which time it is important to establish an environment of comfort and

open communication with each antepartum visit. The nurse conveys interest in the client as an individual and discusses the client's concerns and desires. The nurse can be extremely effective in working with the expectant family by answering questions; providing comprehensive information about pregnancy, prenatal healthcare activities, and community resources; and supporting the healthcare activities of the woman and her family.

Communities often have a wealth of services and educational opportunities available for pregnant women and their families, and the knowledgeable nurse can help expectant clients to assess and access these services. This approach supports the family's assumption of equal responsibility with healthcare providers in working toward their common goal of a positive birth experience.

Throughout the prenatal period, the nurse shares information with the family, both verbally and through written materials. This information is designed to help the family carry out self-care and wellness measures as needed and report changes that may indicate a health problem. The nurse also provides anticipatory guidance to help the family plan for changes that will occur after childbirth. The expectant woman and her partner and/or other family members are encouraged to identify and discuss issues that could be sources of postpartum stress. Issues to be addressed before the birth may include sharing of infant and household chores, help during the first few days after childbirth, options for baby-sitting to allow the mother (and couple) some free time, the mother's return to work after the baby's birth, and sibling rivalry. Families resolve these issues in different ways, but postpartum adjustment period tends to be easier for those who agree on the issues beforehand than for those who do not confront and resolve these issues.

Childbirth education classes are important in promoting adaptation to the event of childbirth for expectant couples. Classes for expectant parents over age 35 are now available in many communities.

Important topics for client teaching include the following:

- Self-care to promote positive outcomes (e.g., nutrition, activity, avoiding OTC medications, and delegating care of the litter box to other family members)
- Strategies to minimize the discomforts of pregnancy
- Childbirth preparation classes
- Danger signs to report to the provider
- Signs and symptoms of labor.

Evaluate Readiness for Enhanced Family Processes

The problems and concerns of the pregnant woman, the relief of her discomforts, and the maintenance of her physical, psychological, and spiritual health receive much attention during the antepartum period. However, her well-being is intertwined with the well-being of those to whom she is closest. Thus, the nurse also addresses the needs of the woman's family to help maintain the integrity of the family unit.

Periodic prenatal examinations offer the nurse an opportunity to assess the client's psychological needs and emotional status. If the woman's partner attends the antepartum visits, the nurse can also identify the partner's needs and concerns. The interchange between the nurse and the woman or her partner will be facilitated if it takes place in a friendly, trusting environment. The woman should have sufficient time to ask questions and air concerns. If the nurse provides the time and demonstrates genuine interest, the woman will be more at ease bringing up questions that she may believe are silly or has been afraid to verbalize. The nurse who has an accurate understanding of all the changes of pregnancy is most able to answer questions and provide information.

CARE OF THE PARTNER Although the pregnant client's partner is present in most cases, the partner's presence cannot be assumed. It is important to assess the client's support system to determine which significant individuals in her life will play a major role during her childbearing experience.

Anticipatory guidance of the expectant client's partner, if the partner is involved in the pregnancy, is a necessary part of any plan of care. The partner may need information about the anatomical, physiological, and emotional changes that occur during and after pregnancy, the couple's sexuality and sexual response, and the reactions that the partner is experiencing. The partner may wish to express feelings about breastfeeding versus formula feeding, the gender of the child, the partner's own ability to parent, and other topics.

If it is culturally acceptable to the couple and personally acceptable to the partner, the nurse may refer the couple to expectant parents' classes. These classes provide valuable information about pregnancy and childbirth using a variety of teaching strategies, such as discussion, films, demonstrations with educational models, and written handouts. Some classes even give the partner the opportunity to get a "feel" for pregnancy by wearing a pregnancy simulator. Such classes also offer the couple an opportunity to gain support from other couples.

The nurse assesses the partner's intended degree of participation during labor and birth and knowledge of what to expect. If the couple prefers that the partner's participation be minimal or restricted, the nurse must support the decision. With this type of consideration and collaboration, the partner is less apt to develop feelings of alienation, helplessness, and guilt during the pregnancy. As the couple's relationship is strengthened and the partner's self-esteem increases, the partner is better able to provide physical and emotional support to the client during labor and birth.

CARE OF SIBLINGS AND OTHER FAMILY MEMBERS The responses of siblings and other family members to the pregnancy are discussed in detail in the Concept section of this module. Briefly, these responses may include feelings of insecurity and even hostility. Thus, in the plan for prenatal care, the nurse incorporates a discussion about the negative feelings some children develop when anticipating the arrival of a sibling. Parents may be distressed to see an older child regress to "babyish" behavior or become aggressive toward the newborn. Parents who are unprepared for the older child's feelings of insecurity, anger, jealousy, and rejection may respond inappropriately in their confusion and surprise. The nurse emphasizes that open communication between parents and children (or acting out feelings with a doll if the child is too young to verbalize) helps children master their feelings. Children may feel less neglected and more secure if they know that their parents are willing to help with their anger and aggressiveness.

It is important not to make assumptions about a client's beliefs, because cultural norms vary greatly both within a culture and from generation to generation. The nurse should observe the client carefully and take the time to ask questions. Clients will benefit greatly from the nurse's increased awareness of their cultural beliefs and practices.

Nursing Care of Parents Over 35

In the United States and Canada the risk of death in childbirth has declined dramatically for women of all ages since 1950 because of advances in maternal health and obstetric practice. The risk of maternal death is significantly higher for women over age 35, however, and is even higher for women ages 40 and older. This is true regardless of a woman's parity, the time at which she begins prenatal care, and her level of education (Health Resources and Services Administration [HRSA], 2010).

The number of births in 2010 was 3% lower than in 2009. The general fertility rate also declined 3% in women ages 15–44. The teen birth rate fell 10%. The birth rate for women ages 40–44 continued to rise (HRSA, 2010). Women over age 35 and, even more, women over age 40 are more likely to have chronic medical conditions that can complicate a pregnancy. Preexisting medical conditions, such as hypertension or diabetes, probably play a more significant role than age in maternal well-being and the outcome of pregnancy. The incidence of low-birth-weight infants, very preterm births, and perinatal death is higher among women ages 35 and older (Kenny et al., 2013). In addition, the rate of miscarriage is significantly higher in older women. Women over age 35 who become pregnant also have an increased risk for gestational diabetes mellitus, hypertension, placenta previa, difficult labor, and newborn complications (Kenny et al., 2013; Lampinen et al., 2009).

The cesarean birth rate is also increased in pregnant women over age 35. This practice may be related to pregnancy complications as well as to increased concern by the woman and physician about the pregnancy outcome (Kenny et al., 2013; Lampinen et al., 2009).

The risk of conceiving a child with Down syndrome increases with maternal age, especially when the mother is over age 35. ACOG (2007) recommends that all pregnant women, regardless of age, be offered screening for Down syndrome.

No matter what their age, however, most expectant couples have concerns regarding the well-being of the fetus and their ability to parent. Expectant parents over age 35 often have additional concerns related to their age, especially the closer they are to age 40. Some couples are concerned about whether they will have enough energy to care for a new baby. Of greater concern is their ability to deal with the needs of the child as the parents age.

Older couples facing pregnancy following a late or second marriage or after therapy for infertility may find themselves somewhat isolated socially. They may feel different because they are often the only couple in their peer group expecting their first baby. In fact, many of their peers are likely to be parents of adolescents or young adults—or may even be grandparents.

The response of older couples who already have children to learning that the woman is pregnant may vary greatly depending on whether the pregnancy was planned or unexpected. Other factors influencing their response include their children's, family's, and friends' attitudes toward the pregnancy; the impact on their lifestyle; and the financial implications of having another child. Sometimes, couples who previously had other mates will choose to have a child together. The concept of blended family applies to situations in which each partner's children and the children they have together become a new family group.

Healthcare professionals may treat the older expectant couple differently than they would a younger couple. Older women may be offered more medical procedures, such as amniocentesis and ultrasound, than younger women. An older woman may be discouraged from using a birthing room or birthing center even if she is healthy, because her age is considered to put her at risk.

The increased risks that the pregnant woman over age 35 faces, combined with social, familial, and other healthcare concerns, place many of these clients and their families at risk for impaired family processes. In particular, women who are mothers of older children and who provide some level of care for their own older parents may find themselves at their wits' ends trying to find a way to juggle their many responsibilities. The arrival of a new baby in a blended family may cause jealousy among older siblings or strain relationships with in-laws or former partners. The nurse should engage in active listening with these clients and their partners, help them prioritize their concerns, and provide referrals to supportive resources as appropriate.

Often, because of their established routines, couples expecting their first child require assistance in understanding how to integrate a newborn into their daily routines. Secondary to increased risk to both the fetus and the pregnant woman, the family is often anxious and this anxiety can create stress in the household. Encourage the couple to express their fears and concerns and provide support and reassurance. Anxiety may be particularly high when they are waiting for diagnostic test results. Couples may report that they are fighting more than usual. The nurse should help these clients recognize that the role anxiety plays in disrupting their relationships is often an important step to improving the relationship.

If the couple has other children, especially if the siblings are in the teen or preteen age, they may find their older children are embarrassed by the pregnancy. Older siblings may also fear being asked to contribute to the newborn's care. It is important for the couple to take time to understand their older children's concerns and make it clear to the siblings that the newborn will be the responsibility of the parents, not the responsibility of the older children. Siblings should be welcomed to participate in newborn care but should not be placed in the position of taking on a majority of the responsibility. The nurse can provide a supportive role in this process by encouraging open family communication and trust.

Promote Balanced Nutrition

The nurse needs to assess the client's nutritional status in order to plan an optimal diet for her. From the woman's chart and by interviewing her, the nurse gathers information about the following:

- The woman's height and weight, as well as her weight gain during pregnancy
- Pertinent laboratory values, especially hemoglobin and hematocrit
- Clinical signs that have possible nutritional implications, such as constipation, anorexia, or heartburn
- Dietary history to evaluate the woman's views on nutrition as well as her specific nutrient intake.

Evidence-Based Practice Managing Excessive Weight Gain of Pregnancy

Problem

How can excessive weight gain in pregnancy be prevented? How can it be managed if it occurs?

Evidence

Excessive prenatal weight gain is a serious condition that affects not only a mother's physical and mental health but also the future health of her babies (Smith, Hulsey, & Goodnight, 2008). Up to 20% of women may retain excessive weight after pregnancy, increasing their vulnerability to a host of lifelong health problems (Walker, 2007). The American College of Obstetricians & Gynecologists cited research related to perinatal outcomes associated with obesity and excessive weight gain in pregnancy. The committee opinion focused on complications that occur at a higher rate, including an increase in spontaneous abortions and stillbirths, gestational diabetes, and an increase in cesarean deliveries. Fetal complications may include fetal macrosomia, prematurity, and congenital anomalies (ACOG, 2013c).

Implications

Women who are overweight before pregnancy, African American women, and women who have been treated for infertility were the most vulnerable to excessive gestational weight gain. Prenatal prevention activities were not as successful as postnatal interventions in managing long-term weight change. Interventions that began immediately after birth and lasted at least 10 weeks had the greatest success. Weight losses for women ranged from 4.8 to 7.8 kg (10.5 to 17.2 lb), with larger losses associated with longer interventions. Each successful program included the use of reduced-calorie diets, exercise, behavioral coaching, and motivational content.

Contrary to commonly held belief, breastfeeding was not shown to be protective against weight retention after pregnancy. Although exclusive breastfeeding for 6 months postpartum was associated with a small postpartum weight loss in one study, these effects were not seen if breastfeeding was not exclusive or was discontinued early. Postpartum interventions, although found to be efficacious, were tested almost exclusively with Caucasian women, so success with women of other ethnic backgrounds is not assured. Culturally competent interventions may need to be developed for women from specific ethnic communities. None of the studies mentioned postpartum depression and any impact it might have on weight outcomes.

Although you may be able to identify women at risk for excessive prenatal weight gain, it may be a difficult condition to prevent. Interventions to help mothers lose excess weight should begin immediately after birth and include low-calorie diets of 1,500 calories per day and an exercise component equal to walking 2 miles five times a week. Behavioral content delivered through group meetings and motivational content via telephone contact supplement the mother's physical efforts. Longer programs, lasting at least 10 weeks, are the most successful.

Critical Thinking Application

How might you approach a client who is gaining too much weight? How might you approach a new mother who has excess weight to lose?

The nurse can obtain a dietary history by asking the woman to complete a 24-hour diet recall, in which she lists everything she has eaten during the past 24 hours, including foods, fluids, and any supplements. At least 3 days of recall should be done to compensate for daily variations. Diet may also be evaluated using a food-frequency questionnaire. The questionnaire lists common categories of foods and asks the woman how frequently in a day (or a week) she consumes food from the list. Common categories include vegetables, fruits, milk or cheese, meat or poultry, fish, desserts or sweets, coffee or tea, and alcohol. This method may be less reliable than the 24-hour diet recall, however, because it requires an individual to be accurate about intake.

Most families can benefit from guidance about food purchasing and preparation. The nurse should suggest that the client plan food purchases thoughtfully by preparing general menus and a list before shopping. It is also helpful to advise the client to monitor sales, compare brands, and be cautious when purchasing "convenience" foods, which tend to be expensive. Other techniques for keeping food costs down without jeopardizing quality include buying food in season, using bulk foods when appropriate, using whole-grain or enriched products, buying lower-grade eggs (grading indicates color of the shell, delicacy of flavor, and so forth and has no relation to the egg's

nutritional value), and avoiding foods from specialty shops and foods in elaborate packaging. Specific recommendations for calcium include the following:

1. Plan with the woman how to add more milk or dairy products to the diet (specify amounts).
2. Encourage the use of other calcium sources, such as leafy greens and legumes.
3. Plan for the addition of powdered milk in cooking and baking.
4. If none of the preceding options is realistic or acceptable, consider the use of calcium supplements.

Identify Concerns and Promote Strengths

The nurse needs to discuss risks, identify concerns, and promote strengths. It is helpful in promoting a sense of well-being for the nurse to treat the pregnancy as normal unless specific health risks are identified. As the pregnancy continues, the nurse identifies and discusses concerns the woman may have related to her age or to specific health problems.

For couples who decide to have amniocentesis, the first few months of pregnancy are a difficult time. Amniocentesis is usually not done before 14 weeks of gestation, and the chromosomal

NURSING CARE PLAN The Pregnant Client

Martina de Herrara and her husband arrived in the United States from Puerto Rico 6 months ago. This is her first prenatal visit since her pregnancy was confirmed 2 days earlier. Mrs. de Herrara's first child is 3 years old and was born in Puerto Rico. Their families live in Puerto Rico, but Mrs. de Herrara's mother has come to visit and help her get settled in their new home. Mrs. de Herrara's husband speaks some English but is unable to attend the prenatal visit, so she has brought her mother to the prenatal clinic. Mrs. de Herrara's native language is Spanish. Both women speak very little English and seem uncomfortable as they wait for the provider. The nurse needs to complete a health history, collect some laboratory specimens, and get Mrs. de Herrara scheduled for her next appointment.

ASSESSMENT	DIAGNOSIS	PLANNING
Subjective: Shaking head side to side, no eye contact, anxious **Objective:** BP 128/82 mmHg, pulse 84 bpm, respirations 16/min, height 5'4", weight 140 lb, urine negative for protein and glucose	■ *Deficient Knowledge* about prenatal care related to barriers in communication and sociocultural factors. (NANDA-I © 2015)	■ The client will demonstrate understanding of health information received during prenatal visits.

IMPLEMENTATION

- Refer to posters with pictures to explain routine care and procedures during the prenatal exam.
- Use teaching models to demonstrate procedures.
- Provide brochures about prenatal care in the client's native language.

- Schedule an interpreter during prenatal visits.
- Refer the client to prenatal classes taught in her native language.
- Involve other members of the healthcare team to assist with prenatal care.

EVALUATION

- The client responds appropriately to the nurse by using an interpreter.
- The client demonstrates understanding by pointing to pictures and phrases on posters.
- The client uses hand gestures to demonstrate understanding.

CRITICAL THINKING

1. *Because of the loss of easily understandable tone and correlation with body language in this situation as the client speaks, how can the nurse assess the client's anxiety after providing client teaching?*
2. *Using an interpreter, how can the nurse determine the client's understanding of client teaching?*
3. *What questions would you ask to assess the client's cultural beliefs and needs related to her culture?*

studies take roughly 2 weeks to complete. The parents' fear that the fetus is at risk may delay the successful completion of the psychological tasks of early pregnancy. One of the advantages of NIPT is that it can be done early in pregnancy, thus reducing these kinds of difficulties.

The nurse can support couples who decide to have amniocentesis by providing information and answering questions about the procedure and by providing comfort and emotional support during the amniocentesis. If the results indicate that the fetus has Down syndrome or another genetic abnormality, the nurse can ensure that the couple has complete information about the condition, its range of possible manifestations, and its developmental implications.

Evaluation

Anticipated outcomes of nursing care include the following:

- The client and her partner are knowledgeable about the pregnancy and express confidence in their ability to make appropriate healthcare choices.
- The expectant client and her partner and their children, if any, are able to cope with the pregnancy and its implications for the future.
- The client receives effective health care throughout her pregnancy as well as during birth and the postpartum period.
- The client and her partner develop skills in child care and parenting.

REVIEW Antepartum Care

RELATE Link the Concepts and Exemplars

Linking the exemplar of antepartum care with the concept of fluids and electrolytes:

1. What recommendations would you make to reduce the risk of dehydration for the pregnant woman who reports vomiting one or two times per day?

2. What electrolyte levels would you want to monitor in the client with frequent morning sickness and vomiting?

Linking the exemplar of antepartum care with the concept of stress and coping:

3. You are caring for a client with four children who had a tubal ligation after delivery of her last baby. During this visit, the client finds she is pregnant. How can you help the client to cope with the discovery and reduce anxiety enough to allow decision making?

4. You are caring for a client who has been receiving infertility treatments for the past 2 years without success and has just learned she is pregnant. The client is very anxious about the possibility of miscarriage and fetal well-being. Design a plan of care to promote anxiety reduction.

READY Go to Companion Skills Manual

REFER Go to Pearson Nursing Student Resources
nursing.pearsonhighered.com

- Additional review materials

REFLECT Case Study

Jessica Riley is a single, 18-year-old mother with a 1-year-old son, Ryan. Jessica has had no contact with Ryan's father since before Ryan was born. Jessica and Ryan live in a small, one-bedroom apartment with Jessica's boyfriend, Casey. Jessica is now 6 months pregnant with Casey's child. Although Jessica works full

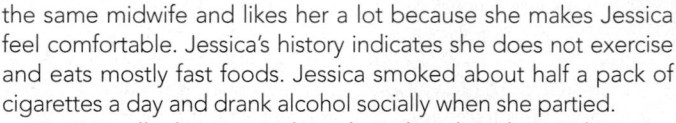

time at a restaurant, she has struggled financially. She is glad Casey contributes to paying the bills and is not sure how she could financially make it without him. Her mother, Evelyn, helps by watching Ryan in the evenings. Additionally, Jessica has government assistance in the form of WIC coupons and Medicaid. Ryan attends a government-assisted day care program.

Jessica goes to her 24-week prenatal visit. She continues to see the same midwife and likes her a lot because she makes Jessica feel comfortable. Jessica's history indicates she does not exercise and eats mostly fast foods. Jessica smoked about half a pack of cigarettes a day and drank alcohol socially when she partied.

Jessica tells the nurse who admits her that she tried to stop smoking but hasn't been able to. When asked about alcohol intake, Jessica tells the nurse she is no longer drinking. She shares with the nurse that Casey was giving her a hard time about not drinking, so she has been pretending to drink to keep him happy. While taking Jessica's blood pressure, the nurse notes bruises in the form of fingerprints on her upper arms. While helping Jessica prepare for the examination, the nurse also notes a bruise on her abdomen. When she asks Jessica how it happened, Jessica blushes, stutters, then looks down and mumbles, "I must have bumped into something."

1. Would you assess Jessica further to determine if she has been abused? If so, what specific questions would you ask?

2. What risk factors have you identified related to Jessica's fetus? What nursing strategies can you implement to reduce these risks?

3. What client teaching would you provide at this prenatal visit?

EXEMPLAR 33.2 Intrapartum Care

EXEMPLAR KEY TERMS

Accelerations, *2152*
Apgar score, *2135*
Artificial rupture of membranes, *2121*
Asynclitism, *2116*
Baseline fetal heart rate, *2149*
Baseline FHR variability, *2149*

Birthing room, *2113*
Bloody show, *2121*
Braxton Hicks contractions, *2121*
Cardinal movements, *2125*
Cervical ripening, *2128*
Cesarean birth, *2131*
Crowning, *2123*

Decelerations, 2152
Doula, 2164
Duration, 2118
Early deceleration, 2152
Effacement, 2119
Electronic fetal monitoring, 2148
Engagement, 2116
Episiotomy, 2131
Family-centered care, 2113
Fetal attitude, 2115
Fetal bradycardia, 2151
Fetal lie, 2115
Fetal position, 2116
Fetal presentation, 2115
Fetal tachycardia, 2151
Fontanelles, 2114
Forceps-assisted birth, 2130
Frequency, 2118
Hyperventilation, 2163
Intensity, 2118
Intrauterine pressure catheter, 2142
Labor induction, 2129
Late deceleration, 2152
Leopold maneuvers, 2142
Lightening, 2120
Malpresentations, 2115
Molding, 2114
Premature rupture of membranes (PROM), 2121
Presenting part, 2115
Preterm premature rupture of membranes (PPROM), 2121

Rupture of membranes, 2121
Spontaneous rupture of membranes (SROM), 2121
Station, 2116
Sutures, 2114
Synclitism, 2116
Vacuum extraction, 2130
Vaginal birth after cesarean (VBAC), 2135
Variable decelerations, 2152
Wandering baseline, 2149

EXEMPLAR LEARNING OUTCOMES

After reading about this exemplar, you will be able to:

1. Describe the physiology and clinical manifestations associated with normal labor and delivery.
2. Identify risk factors and prevention methods associated with normal labor and delivery.
3. Illustrate the nursing process in providing culturally competent care for a pregnant woman during labor and delivery.
4. Formulate priority nursing diagnoses appropriate for a pregnant woman during labor and delivery.
5. Summarize therapies used by interdisciplinary teams in the collaborative care of a pregnant woman during labor and delivery.
6. Plan evidence-based care for a pregnant woman during labor and delivery and her family members in collaboration with other members of the healthcare team.
7. Evaluate expected outcomes for a pregnant woman and her newborn during the intrapartum period.

▶ OVERVIEW

In the final weeks of pregnancy, both mother and baby begin to prepare for birth. The fetus develops and grows in readiness for life outside of the womb. At the same time, the expectant woman undergoes various physiological and psychological changes that prepare her for childbirth. During her prenatal visits, the mother is instructed to call her healthcare provider if any of the following occur:

- Rupture of membranes
- Regular, frequent uterine contractions (nulliparas, 5 minutes apart for 1 hour; multiparas, 6–8 minutes apart for 1 hour)
- Any vaginal bleeding
- Decreased fetal movement.

Increasingly, pregnant women and their families are seeking out family-centered care. **Family-centered care** is a model of care based on the philosophy that the physical, sociocultural, spiritual, and economic needs are combined and considered collectively when planning care for the childbearing family (Katz, 2012). To reflect the consumer demand for family-centered care, most birthing centers now have **birthing rooms**, single rooms where the woman and her partner or other family members will stay for the labor, birth, recovery, and possibly the postpartum period. These rooms may also be called labor, delivery, recovery, and postpartum (LDRP) rooms or single-room maternity care.

The atmosphere of a birthing room is more relaxed than that of a traditional hospital room, and families seem to feel more comfortable in birthing rooms. Another benefit is that the woman does not have to be transferred from one area to another for the actual birth. A birthing room setting not only helps the laboring woman create her own space to labor in, it also enhances the family's comfort and involvement. Birthing rooms usually have beds that can be adapted for birth by removing a small section near the foot. The decor is designed to produce a home-like atmosphere in which families can feel both safe and at ease.

This exemplar discusses in detail the normal progression of labor and culturally appropriate, family-centered care for the laboring mother, fetus, and close family members. A brief discussion of alterations that may occur in the intrapartum period is also provided.

▶ FACTORS IMPORTANT TO LABOR AN\D BIRTH

Five factors are important in the process of labor and birth (**Box 33–2 ●**):

1. The birth passage
2. The fetus
3. The relationship between the passage and the fetus
4. The physiological forces of labor
5. The psychosocial considerations.

The progress of labor is critically dependent on the complementary relationship among these five factors. Abnormalities affecting any one of these factors can alter the outcome of labor and jeopardize both the expectant woman and her baby.

Box 33–2   Critical Factors in Labor

1. BIRTH PASSAGE
   a. Size of the maternal pelvis (diameters of the pelvic inlet, mid-pelvis, and outlet)
   b. Type of maternal pelvis (gynecoid, android, anthropoid, platypelloid, or a combination)
   c. Ability of the cervix to dilate and efface, and ability of the vaginal canal and the external opening of the vagina (the introitus) to distend
2. FETUS
   a. Fetal head (size and presence of molding)
   b. Fetal attitude (flexion or extension of the fetal body and extremities)
   c. Fetal lie [the relationship of the fetal long axis (spine) to the maternal long axis]
   d. Fetal presentation (the body part of the fetus entering the pelvis in a single or multiple pregnancy)
3. RELATIONSHIP BETWEEN PASSAGE AND FETUS
   a. Engagement of the fetal presenting part
   b. Station (location of fetal presenting part in the maternal pelvis in relation to the ischial spine)
   c. Fetal position (relationship of the presenting part to one of the four quadrants of the maternal pelvis)
4. PHYSIOLOGICAL FORCES OF LABOR
   a. Frequency, duration, and intensity of uterine contractions
   b. Effectiveness of the maternal pushing effort
5. PSYCHOSOCIAL CONSIDERATIONS
   a. Mental and physical preparation for childbirth
   b. Sociocultural values and beliefs
   c. Previous childbirth experience
   d. Support from significant others
   e. Emotional status

The Birth Passage

The true pelvis, which forms the bony canal through which the fetus must pass, is divided into three sections:

1. The inlet
2. The pelvic cavity (midpelvis)
3. The outlet.

The Fetus

Several aspects of the fetal body and position are critical to the outcome of labor. Primary among these are the size and orientation of the fetal head.

FETAL HEAD   The head is the least compressible and largest part of the fetus. Once the fetal head has been born, the birth of the rest of the body is rarely delayed. The fetal skull (cranium) has three major parts:

1. The face
2. The base of the skull
3. The vault of the cranium (roof).

The bones of the face and cranial base are well fused and essentially fixed. The base of the cranium is composed of the two temporal bones, each with a sphenoid and ethmoid bone. The bones composing the vault are the two frontal bones, the two parietal bones, and the occipital bone (**Figure 33–42 ●**). These bones are not fused, allowing this portion of the head to adjust in shape as the presenting part passes through the narrow portions of the pelvis. The cranial bones overlap under

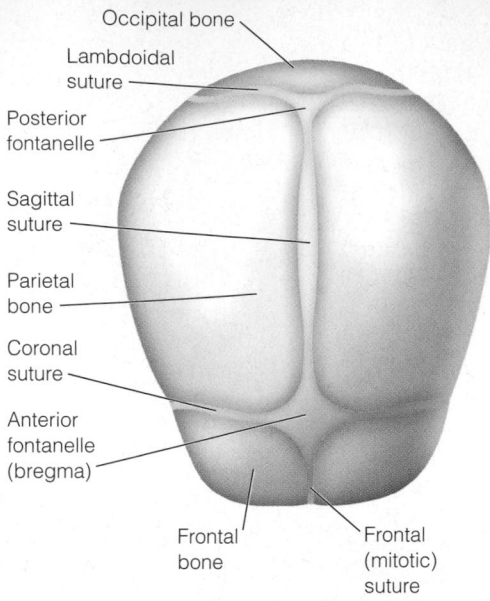

Figure 33–42 ● Superior view of the fetal skull.

pressure of the powers of labor and the resistance of the pelvis. This overlapping is called **molding**.

The **sutures** of the fetal skull are membranous spaces between the cranial bones. The intersections of these sutures are called **fontanelles**. Cranial sutures allow molding of the fetal head during birth and help the clinician to identify the position of the fetal head during vaginal examination. The important sutures of the cranial vault are as follows (see Figure 33–42):

- **Frontal (mitotic) suture.** Located between the two frontal bones, this becomes the anterior continuation of the sagittal suture.

- **Sagittal suture.** Located between the parietal bones, this divides the skull into left and right halves; it runs anteroposteriorly, connecting the two fontanelles.

- **Coronal suture.** Located between the frontal and parietal bones, this extends transversely left and right from the anterior fontanelle.

- **Lambdoidal suture.** Located between the two parietal bones and the occipital bone, this extends transversely left and right from the posterior fontanelle.

The anterior and posterior fontanelles (along with the sutures) are clinically useful in identifying the position of the fetal head in the pelvis and in assessing the neurological and hydration status of the newborn after birth. The anterior fontanelle is diamond shaped and measures approximately 2 by 3 cm. It permits growth of the brain by remaining unossified for as long as 18 months. The posterior fontanelle is much smaller and closes within 8–12 weeks after birth. It is shaped like a small triangle and marks the meeting point of the sagittal suture and the lambdoidal suture.

Following are several important landmarks of the fetal skull (**Figure 33–43 ●**):

- **Mentum.** This is the fetal chin.

- **Sinciput.** This anterior area is known as the brow.

- **Bregma.** This is a large diamond-shaped anterior fontanelle.

- **Vertex.** This is the area between the anterior and posterior fontanelles.

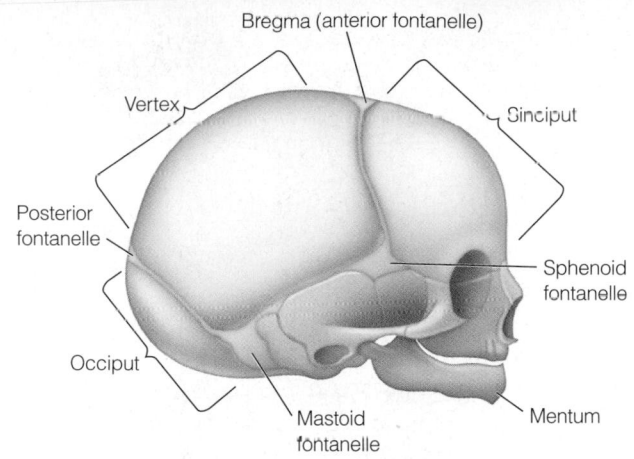

Figure 33–43 ● Lateral view of the fetal skull identifying the landmarks that have significance during birth.

- **Posterior fontanelle.** This is the intersection between posterior cranial sutures.
- **Occiput.** This is the area of the fetal skull occupied by the occipital bone, beneath the posterior fontanelle.

The diameters of the fetal skull vary considerably within its normal limits. Some diameters shorten and others lengthen as the head is molded during labor. Fetal head diameters are measured between the various landmarks on the skull. For example, the suboccipitobregmatic diameter is the distance from the undersurface of the occiput to the center of the bregma, or anterior fontanelle.

FETAL ATTITUDE **Fetal attitude** refers to the relation of the fetal parts to one another. The normal attitude of the fetus is one of moderate flexion of the head, flexion of the arms onto the chest, and flexion of the legs onto the abdomen.

FETAL LIE **Fetal lie** refers to the relationship of the cephalocaudal (spinal column) axis of the fetus to the cephalocaudal axis of the woman. The fetus may assume either a longitudinal (vertical) lie or a transverse lie. A longitudinal lie occurs when the cephalocaudal axis of the fetus is parallel to the woman's spine. A transverse lie occurs when the cephalocaudal axis of the fetus is at a right angle to the woman's spine.

FETAL PRESENTATION **Fetal presentation** is determined by fetal lie and by the body part of the fetus that enters the pelvic passage first. This portion of the fetus is referred to as the **presenting part**. Fetal presentation may be cephalic, breech, or shoulder. The most common presentation is cephalic. When this presentation occurs, labor and birth are likely to proceed normally. Breech and shoulder presentations are called **malpresentations** because they are associated with difficulties during labor. With a malpresentation, labor does not proceed as expected.

The fetal head presents itself to the passage in approximately 97% of term births. The cephalic presentation can be further classified according to the degree of flexion or extension of the fetal head (attitude) as follows:

- **Vertex presentation.** The fetal head is completely flexed onto the chest, and the smallest diameter of the fetal head (suboccipitobregmatic) presents to the maternal pelvis (**Figure 33–44A** ●). The occiput is the presenting part. Vertex is the most common type of presentation.
- **Military presentation.** The fetal head is neither flexed nor extended. The occipitofrontal diameter presents to the maternal pelvis (Figure 33–44B). The top of the head is the presenting part.
- **Brow presentation.** The fetal head is partially extended. The occipitomental diameter, the largest anteroposterior diameter, is presented to the maternal pelvis (Figure 33–44C). The sinciput is the presenting part (refer to Figure 33–43).
- **Face presentation.** The fetal head is hyperextended (complete extension). The submentobregmatic diameter presents to the maternal pelvis (Figure 33–44D). The face is the presenting part.

Breech presentations occur in 3% of all births (Cunningham et al., 2010). In all variations of the breech presentation, the

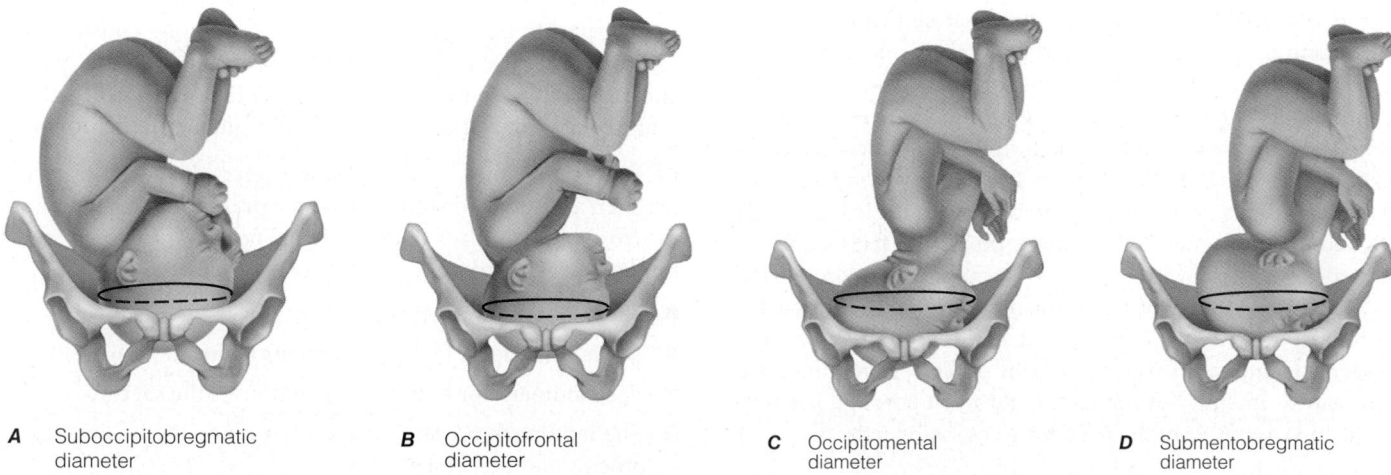

| **A** Suboccipitobregmatic diameter | **B** Occipitofrontal diameter | **C** Occipitomental diameter | **D** Submentobregmatic diameter |

Figure 33–44 ● Cephalic presentation. *A,* Vertex presentation. Complete flexion of the head allows the suboccipitobregmatic diameter to present to the pelvis. *B,* Military (median vertex) presentation with no flexion or extension. The occipitofrontal diameter presents to the pelvis. *C,* Brow presentation. The fetal head is in partial (halfway) extension. The occipitomental diameter, which is the largest diameter of the fetal head, presents to the pelvis. *D,* Face presentation. The fetal head is in complete extension, and the submentobregmatic diameter presents to the pelvis.

sacrum is the landmark to be noted. These presentations are classified according to the attitude of the fetus's hips and knees:

- In *complete breech*, the fetal knees and hips are both flexed, the thighs are on the abdomen, and the calves are on the posterior aspect of the thighs. The buttocks and feet of the fetus present to the maternal pelvis.
- In *frank breech*, the fetal hips are flexed, and the knees are extended. The buttocks of the fetus present to the maternal pelvis.
- In *footling breech*, the fetal hips and legs are extended, and the feet of the fetus present to the maternal pelvis. In a single footling breech, one foot presents; in a double footling breech, both feet present.

A shoulder presentation is also called a transverse lie. Most frequently, the shoulder is the presenting part, and the acromion process of the scapula is the landmark to be noted. However, the fetal arm, back, abdomen, or side may present in a transverse lie. The incidence of shoulder presentation is 0.1% of all births (Cunningham et al., 2010).

Relationship Between the Passage and the Fetus

When assessing the relationship of the maternal pelvis and the presenting part of the fetal body, the nurse considers engagement, station, and fetal position.

ENGAGEMENT   **Engagement** of the presenting part occurs when the largest diameter of the presenting part reaches or passes through the pelvic inlet. Whereas engagement confirms the adequacy of the pelvic inlet, it does not indicate whether the midpelvis and outlet are also adequate.

Engagement can be determined by vaginal examinations and Leopold maneuvers. In primigravidas, engagement occurs approximately 2 weeks before term. Multiparas, however, may experience engagement several weeks before the onset of labor or during the process of labor.

Another variable of engagement is the relationship of the fetal sagittal suture to the mother's symphysis pubis and sacrum. The terms *synclitism* and *asynclitism* describe this relationship. **Synclitism** occurs when the sagittal suture is midway between the symphysis pubis and the sacral promontory. Upon vaginal examination, the suture is felt to be midline between these two maternal landmarks and as though it is in alignment. **Asynclitism** occurs when the sagittal suture is directed toward either the symphysis pubis or the sacral promontory and is felt to be misaligned. Upon vaginal examination, the suture feels somewhat turned to one side within the pelvis, making it asymmetrical. Asynclitism can be either anterior or posterior. It is important to identify asynclitism, because it can lengthen the time of descent or interfere with the descent process. Sometimes, this can lead to inability of the fetal head to fit through the birth canal and can result in the need for a cesarean birth.

STATION   **Station** refers to the relationship of the presenting part to an imaginary line drawn between the ischial spines of the maternal pelvis. In a normal pelvis, the ischial spines mark the narrowest diameter through which the fetus must pass. As a landmark, the ischial spines have been designated as zero (0) station

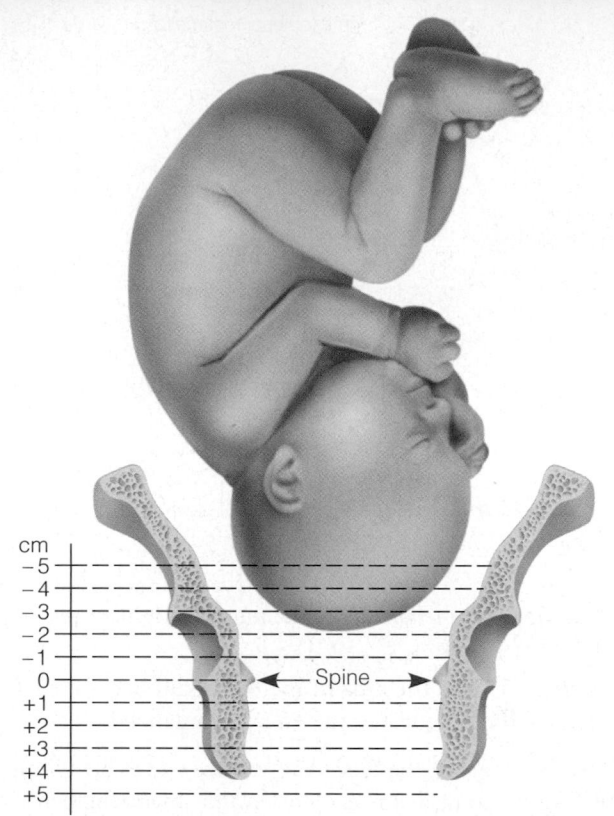

Figure 33–45 ● Measuring the station of the fetal head while it is descending. In this view, the station is –2/–3.

(**Figure 33–45 ●**). If the presenting part is higher than the ischial spines, a negative number is assigned, noting the number of centimeters above zero station. Engagement is represented when the fetal head reaches zero station. Positive numbers indicate that the presenting part has passed the ischial spines. Station –5 is at the pelvic inlet, and station +5 is at the outlet.

During labor, the presenting part should move progressively from the negative stations to the midpelvis at zero station and into the positive stations. If the presenting part can be seen at the woman's perineum, birth is imminent. Failure of the presenting part to descend in the presence of strong contractions may be caused by disproportion between the maternal pelvis and the fetal presenting part, malpresentation, asynclitism, or multiple fetuses. Station is assessed by vaginal examination.

FETAL POSITION   **Fetal position** refers to the relationship between a designated landmark on the presenting fetal part and the front, sides, or back of the maternal pelvis. The chosen landmarks differ according to presentation as follows:

- The landmark for vertex presentations is the occiput.
- The landmark for face presentations is the mentum.
- The landmark for breech presentations is the sacrum.
- The landmark for shoulder presentations is the acromion process on the scapula.

To determine position, the nurse notes which quadrant of the maternal pelvis the appropriate landmark is directed toward: left anterior, right anterior, left posterior, or right posterior. If the landmark is directed toward the side of the pelvis, fetal position is designated as transverse rather than anterior or posterior. In documentation, the following abbreviations are used:

- Right (R) or left (L) side of the maternal pelvis
- The landmark of the fetal presenting part: occiput (O), mentum (M), sacrum (S), or acromion process (A)
- Anterior (A), posterior (P), or transverse (T), depending on whether the landmark is in the front, back, or side of the pelvis.

These abbreviations help the healthcare team communicate the fetal position. For example, when the fetal occiput is directed toward the back and to the left of the birth passage, the abbreviation used is LOP (left-occiput-posterior). In the setting of a transverse lie, the fetal spine may be either superior or inferior. This is simply described as back up or back down, respectively (Strauss, 2013).

Assessment techniques to determine fetal position include inspection and palpation of the maternal abdomen and vaginal examination. The most common fetal presentation is occiput anterior. When this presentation occurs, labor and birth are likely to proceed normally. Presentations other than occiput anterior are more frequently associated with problems during labor; therefore, they are called malpresentations. Presentations and malpresentations are illustrated in **Figure 33–46 ●**.

Physiological Forces of Labor

Primary and secondary forces work together to achieve birth of the fetus, fetal membranes, and placenta. The primary force is uterine muscular contractions, which cause the changes of the first stage of labor: complete effacement and dilation of the cervix. The secondary force is the use of abdominal muscles to push during the second stage of labor, which also is known as bearing down.

CONTRACTIONS   In labor, uterine contractions are rhythmic but intermittent. Between contractions, there is a period of relaxation. This allows the uterine muscles to rest and provides respite for the laboring woman. It also restores uteroplacental circulation, which is important to fetal oxygenation and adequate circulation in the uterine blood vessels.

Each contraction has three phases:

1. *Increment:* the building up of the contraction (the longest phase)
2. *Acme:* the peak of the contraction
3. *Decrement:* the letting up of the contraction.

When describing uterine contractions during labor, healthcare providers use the terms *frequency, duration,* and *intensity* (**Figure 33–47 ●**). **Frequency** refers to the time between the beginning of one contraction and the beginning of the next contraction. **Duration** is measured from the beginning of a contraction to the completion of that same contraction. **Intensity** refers to the strength of the contraction during acme. In most instances, intensity can be estimated by an experienced examiner palpating the uterine fundus during a contraction, but it may be measured directly with an intrauterine catheter. When intensity is measured with an intrauterine catheter, the normal resting pressure in the uterus (between contractions) averages 10–12 mmHg. During acme, the intensity ranges from 25 to 40 mmHg in early labor, 50 to 70 mmHg in active labor, 80 to 100 mmHg during transition, and more than 100 mmHg while the woman is pushing in the second stage (Cunningham et al., 2010).

At the beginning of labor, the contractions are usually mild. As labor progresses, the duration, intensity, and frequency of the contractions increase. Because the contractions are involuntary, the laboring woman cannot control their duration, frequency, or intensity.

BEARING DOWN   After the cervix is completely dilated and the fetus has descended enough to stimulate a maternal urge to push, the maternal abdominal muscles contract as the woman pushes (Goer and Romano, 2012). This pushing action (also called bearing down) aids in expulsion of the fetus and placenta. If the cervix is not completely dilated, however, bearing down can cause cervical edema, which retards dilation, and may cause tearing and bruising of the cervix and maternal exhaustion.

Psychosocial Considerations

The final critical factor is the parents' psychosocial readiness, including their fears, anxieties, birth fantasies, excitement level, feelings of joy and anticipation, and level of social support. These psychosocial factors affect both parents. Both are making a transition into a new role, and both have expectations of themselves during the labor and birth experience and as caregivers for their child and their new family. Psychosocial factors that affect labor and birth include the couple's accomplishment of the tasks of pregnancy, usual coping mechanisms in response to stressful life events, support system, preparation for childbirth, and cultural influences. Even pregnant women and partners who attend childbirth preparation classes and have a solid support system can be concerned about what labor will be like. Many couples, even in the intense happiness and excitement of the event, may be concerned about whether they will be able to perform the way they expect, whether the pain will be more than the mother expects or can cope with, and whether the partner can provide helpful support. Although birth is usually a happy and joyful event, it is also a time of a physical and emotional stress. Whether that stress is positive or negative, it can affect a couple's responses to the labor itself.

A woman approaching her first labor faces a totally new experience, and the woman who has given birth before knows that this labor might be very different from her previous experience. Most women wonder whether they will live up to their expectations for themselves, whether they will experience a physical injury (e.g., lacerations, episiotomy, or cesarean incision), and whether significant others will be supportive. Many women are excited and happy that labor has occurred, however, even if they have concerns about the labor process itself.

Expectant women mentally prepare for labor through meaningful action and imaginary rehearsal. The actions frequently consist of "nesting behavior" (housecleaning, decorating the nursery) and a "psyching up" for the labor, which varies depending on the woman's self-confidence, self-esteem, and previous experiences with stress. Specific actions to prepare for labor may focus on becoming better informed and prepared. In addition, just as a woman tries on the maternal role during pregnancy, fantasizing about labor seems to help her understand and become better prepared for it. Fantasies about the excitement of the baby's birth and the sharing of the experience involve the woman in constructive preparation. Many pregnant women have dreams about their infant, labor, birth, and parenting.

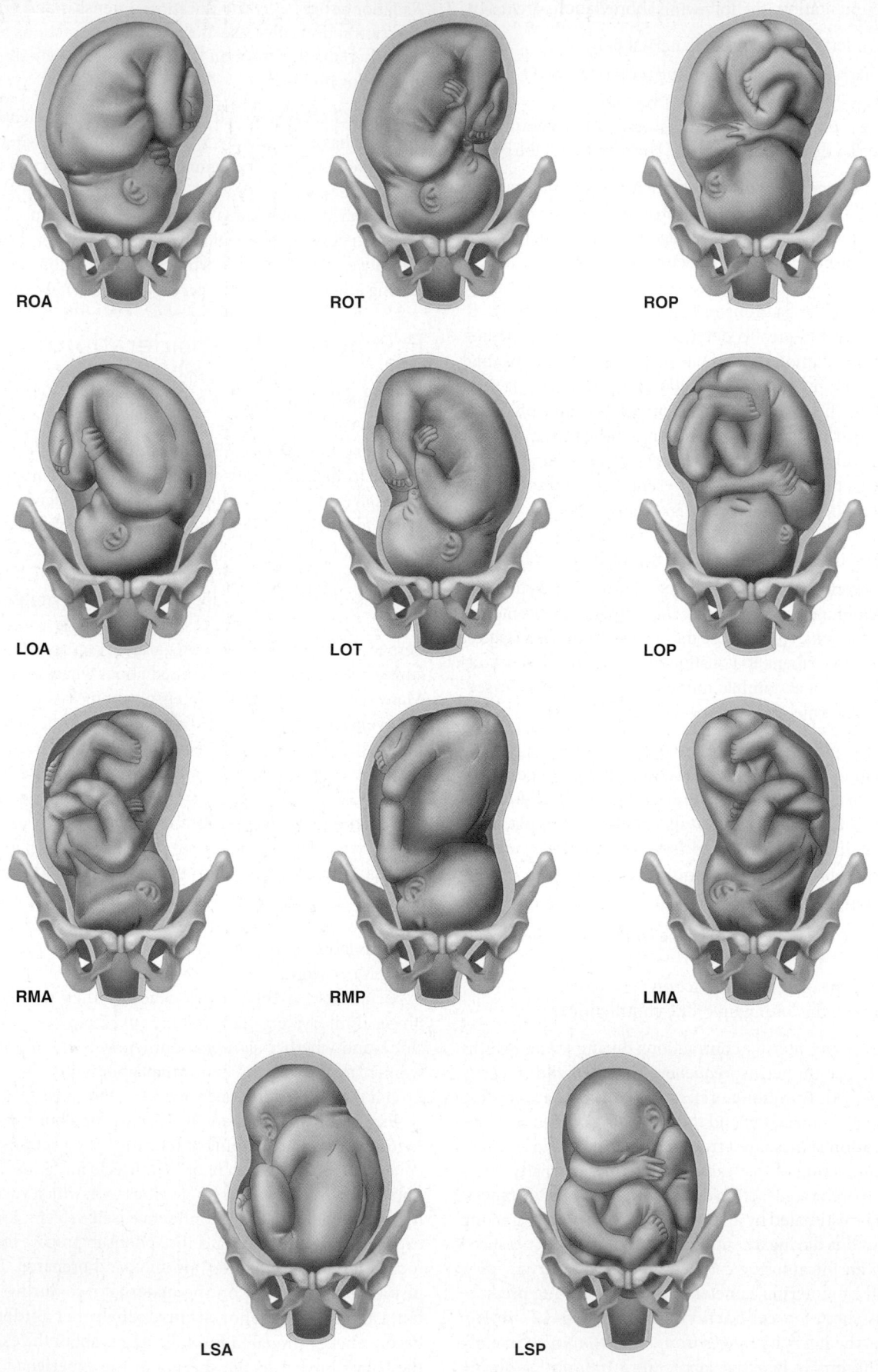

Figure 33–46 ● Presentations and malpresentations. Key: FIRST LETTER: R = right, L = left. SECOND LETTER: O = occiput, M = mentum, S = sacrum, A = acromion process. THIRD LETTER: A = anterior, P = posterior, T = transverse.

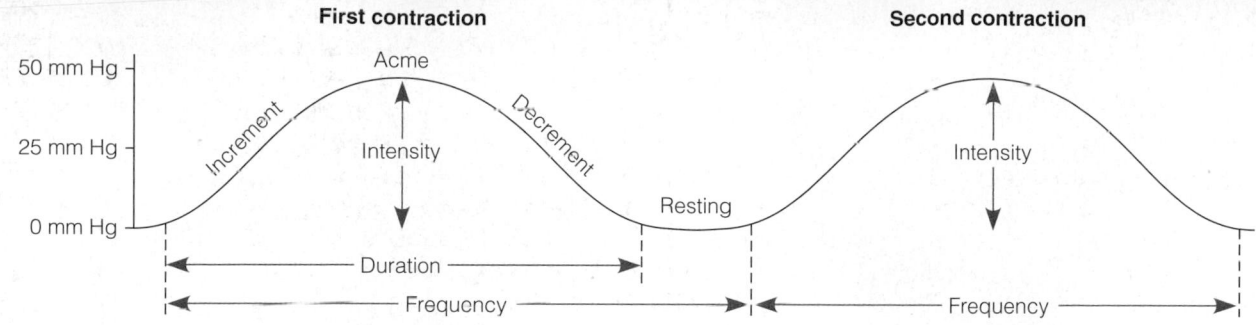

Figure 33–47 ● Characteristics of uterine contractions.

Some women may fear the pain of contractions, whereas others may welcome the opportunity to feel the birth process. Some women view the pain as threatening and associate it with a loss of control over their bodies and emotions. Others see the pain as a rite of passage into motherhood and a necessary means to an end. It is helpful for women to realize that she is safe and labor pain is not the same sign of danger as pain in other circumstances. Assurances from the nurse that labor is progressing normally can go a long way toward reducing anxiety (and thereby reducing pain) and providing positive reinforcement that the mother is doing a good job.

Empowerment and having control over one's body play a key role in determining whether the woman views her labor and birth positively. Women who viewed their birth experiences as being positive were also more likely to have a sense of well-being about themselves after the experience (Haines et al., 2013). Some women view the birth experience as a challenge in which they will have the opportunity to succeed and provide their baby with a joyful reception into the world.

The laboring woman's support system also influences the course of labor and birth. Some women prefer not to have a support person or family member with them during the birth process. For some, this process is a private moment that the woman may wish to reserve for herself. However, most women choose to have significant individuals (family members, partner, or friend) with them during labor and birth. This social support tends to have a positive effect. For some families, the birth event is a celebration in which they may want as many significant others present as possible. Some women may want to create a joyful, festive atmosphere that includes the grandparents, friends, and other children. A labor partner's presence at the bedside provides a means to enhance communication and to demonstrate feelings of love. Communication needs may include talking and the use of affectionate and reassuring words from the partner. Affection may also take the form of holding hands, hugging, touching, or gentle reassurance for the laboring woman.

How the woman views the birth experience in hindsight may affect her mothering behaviors. It appears that any activities by the expectant woman or by healthcare providers that enhance the birth experience benefit the mother–baby connection. Studies have shown that when some women are disappointed with their birth experience, they may have some initial difficulties and be at higher risk for postpartum mood disorders (Gurber et al., 2012). The partner's experience of the birth and opportunities for bonding may have important implications for parenting as well. Psychosocial factors associated with a positive birth experience are summarized in **Box 33–3** ●.

Box 33–3   Factors Associated With a Positive Birth Experience

- Motivation for the pregnancy
- Attendance at childbirth education classes
- A sense of competence or mastery
- Self-confidence and self-esteem
- Feelings of empowerment
- Positive relationship with mate
- Maintaining control during labor
- Support from partner or other individual during labor
- Not being left alone in labor
- Trust in the medical/nursing staff
- Having personal control of breathing patterns, comfort measures
- Choosing a physician/CNM who has a compatible philosophy of care
- Receiving clear information regarding procedures

▶ PHYSIOLOGY OF LABOR

In addition to considering the five critical factors affecting the progress of labor and birth, it is essential to explore the physiology of the normal birth experience.

Possible Causes of Labor Onset

The process of labor usually begins between 38 and 42 weeks of gestation, when the fetus is mature and ready for birth. Despite research, the exact cause of labor onset is not clearly understood. However, some important aspects have been identified: Progesterone relaxes smooth muscle tissue; estrogen stimulates uterine muscle contractions; and connective tissue loosens to permit the softening, thinning, and eventual opening of the cervix (Cunningham et al., 2010). Currently, researchers are focusing on the role of fetal membranes (chorion and amnion), the decidua, prostaglandin, corticotropin-releasing hormone, and progesterone withdrawal in relation to labor onset (Cunningham et al., 2010).

Myometrial Activity

In true labor, with each contraction the muscles of the upper uterine segment shorten and exert a longitudinal traction on the cervix, causing effacement. **Effacement** is thinning of the cervix as it is drawn upward into the uterine side walls. The cervix changes progressively from a long, thick structure to a structure that is tissue-paper thin (**Figure 33–48** ●). In primigravidas, effacement usually precedes dilation.

Contractions are stimulated by the hormone oxytocin. Oxytocin is a potent uterine stimulant and is frequently used as an agent

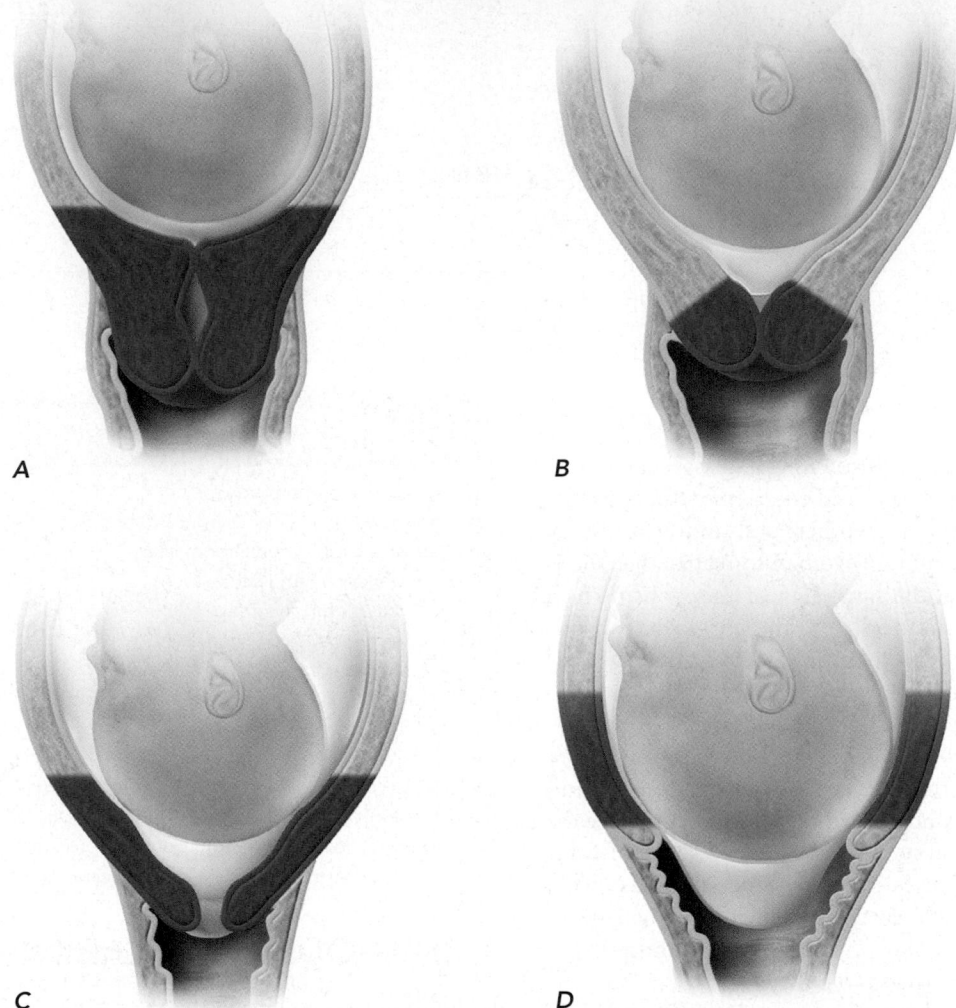

A

B

C

D

Figure 33–48 ● Effacement of the cervix in the primigravida. *A,* Beginning of labor. There is no cervical effacement or dilation. The fetal head is cushioned by amniotic fluid. *B,* Beginning cervical effacement. As the cervix begins to efface, more amniotic fluid collects below the fetal head. *C,* Cervix is about one-half (50%) effaced and slightly dilated. The increasing amount of amniotic fluid below the fetal head exerts hydrostatic pressure on the cervix. *D,* Complete effacement and dilation.

to induce or augment labor in term fetuses or when delivery is necessitated. Uterine sensitivity to oxytocin is increased during pregnancy (Blackburn, 2013). Oxytocin is produced in the hypothalamus and secreted into the bloodstream, but it is also produced in uterine tissues during late gestation, with concentrations increasing at the onset of labor. Oxytocin receptors are most likely formed in the gestational tissues, which when stimulated produce myometrial activity (Cunningham et al., 2010).

The uterus elongates with each contraction, decreasing the horizontal diameter. This elongation causes a straightening of the fetal body, pressing the upper portion against the fundus and thrusting the presenting part down toward the lower uterine segment and the cervix. The pressure exerted by the fetus is called the fetal axis pressure. As the uterus elongates, the longitudinal muscle fibers are pulled upward over the presenting part. This action and the hydrostatic pressure of the fetal membranes cause cervical dilation. The cervical os and cervical canal widen from less than 1 cm to approximately 10 cm, allowing birth of the fetus. When the cervix is completely dilated and retracted into the lower uterine segment, it can no longer be palpated. At

the same time, the round ligament pulls the fundus forward, aligning the fetus with the bony pelvis.

Musculature Changes in the Pelvic Floor

The levator ani muscle and fascia of the pelvic floor draw the rectum and vagina upward and forward with each contraction along the curve of the pelvic floor. As the fetal head descends to the pelvic floor, the pressure of the presenting part causes the perineal structure, which was once approximately 5 cm in thickness, to change to a structure less than 1 cm thick. A normal physiological anesthesia is produced as a result of the decreased blood supply to the area. The anus everts, exposing the interior rectal wall as the fetal head descends forward (Cunningham et al., 2010).

Premonitory Signs of Labor

Most primigravidas and many multiparas experience the following signs and symptoms of impending labor: lightening, Braxton Hicks contractions, cervical changes, bloody show, rupture of membranes, and a sudden burst of energy.

LIGHTENING **Lightening** describes the effects that occur when the fetus begins to settle into the pelvic inlet (engagement). With fetal descent, the uterus moves downward, and the fundus no longer presses on the diaphragm, so breathing is eased. However, with increased downward pressure of the presenting part, the woman may notice the following:

- Leg cramps or pains caused by pressure on the nerves that course through the obturator foramen in the pelvis
- Increased pelvic pressure
- Increased urinary frequency
- Increased venous stasis, leading to edema in the lower extremities
- Increased vaginal secretions resulting from congestion of the vaginal mucous membranes.

BRAXTON HICKS CONTRACTIONS Before the onset of labor, **Braxton Hicks contractions** (the irregular, intermittent contractions that have been occurring throughout the pregnancy) may become uncomfortable. The pain seems to be focused in the abdomen and groin but may feel like the "drawing" sensations experienced by some women with dysmenorrhea. Braxton Hicks contractions that are strong enough to disturb the mother without affecting cervical change or fetal descent are sometimes referred to as "false" labor. Pre-labor contractions may be exhausting. If the contractions are fairly regular, the woman has no way of knowing whether they are the beginning of active labor and she may come to the hospital or birthing center for a vaginal examination to determine whether cervical dilation is occurring. These pre-labor contractions may be exacerbated by inadequate fluid intake, a full bladder, sexual activity, or a urinary tract infection. An episode of regular contractions may resolve or continue, becoming active labor. It is important to remember that women with contractions that occur on a regular basis before 38 weeks of gestation should be assessed to determine whether they are experiencing preterm labor.

CERVICAL CHANGES Considerable change occurs in the cervix during the prenatal and intrapartum period. At the beginning of pregnancy, the cervix is rigid and firm, and it must soften so that it can stretch and dilate to allow passage of the fetus. This softening of the cervix is called ripening.

As term approaches, the action of enzymes, such as collagenase and elastase, breaks down the collagen fibers of the cervix. As the collagen fibers change, their ability to bind together decreases because of increasing amounts of hyaluronic acid, which loosely binds collagen fibrils, and decreasing amounts of dermatan sulfate, which tightly binds collagen fibrils. The water content of the cervix also increases. All these changes result in a weakening and softening of the cervix.

BLOODY SHOW During pregnancy, cervical secretions accumulate in the cervical canal to form a barrier called a mucous plug. With softening and effacement of the cervix, the mucous plug is often expelled, resulting in a small amount of blood loss from the exposed cervical capillaries. The resulting pink-tinged secretions are called **bloody show**. Bloody show is considered to be a sign that labor will begin within 24–48 hours. Vaginal examination that includes manipulation of the cervix may also result in a blood-tinged discharge, which is sometimes confused with bloody show.

RUPTURE OF MEMBRANES In approximately 12% of women, the amniotic membranes rupture before the onset of labor. After membranes rupture, 80% of women will experience spontaneous labor within 24 hours. Membrane rupture prior to the onset of labor is referred to as premature rupture of membranes (PROM) Many clinicians recommend induction of labor in the setting of term PROM to avoid intra-amniotic infection. There is, however, no quality evidence to support this practice and patients should be given the option of awaiting spontaneous labor (Goer and Romano, 2012).

At the beginning of labor, the amniotic membranes may bulge through the cervix in the shape of a cone. When the membranes rupture, the amniotic fluid may be expelled in large amounts. **Spontaneous rupture of membranes (SROM)** generally occurs at the height of an intense contraction with a gush of the fluid out of the vagina. If engagement has not occurred, the danger exists that a portion of the umbilical cord may be expelled with the fluid (prolapsed cord). In addition, because of these potential problems, the woman is advised to notify her certified nurse midwife (CNM) or physician and proceed to the hospital or birthing center. In some instances the fluid is expelled in small amounts and may be confused with episodes of urinary incontinence associated with urinary urgency, coughing, or sneezing. The discharge should be checked to ascertain its source and to determine further action. In some instances, the membranes are ruptured by the CNM or physician, using an instrument called an amniohook. This procedure is called *amniotomy* or **artificial rupture of membranes**.

When the membranes rupture and leakage of amniotic fluid from the vagina occurs before 37 weeks of gestation, the term **preterm premature rupture of membranes (PPROM)** is used. PPROM occurs in up to 25% of all cases of preterm labors, complicates more than 3% of pregnancies each year, and is associated with more than one third of preterm births (Goldenberg et al., 2008). Infection often precedes PPROM. When PPROM is suspected, strict sterile technique should be used in any vaginal examination.

SUDDEN BURST OF ENERGY Some women report a sudden burst of energy approximately 24–48 hours before labor. This often finds expression in nesting behaviors. The cause of this energy spurt is unknown. In prenatal teaching, warn prospective mothers not to overexert themselves during this energy burst in order to avoid being overtired when labor begins.

OTHER SIGNS Additional premonitory signs include the following:

- Weight loss of 1–3 lb resulting from fluid loss and electrolyte shifts produced by changes in estrogen and progesterone levels.
- Diarrhea, indigestion, or nausea and vomiting just before onset of labor. The cause of these signs is unknown.

Differences Between True and False Labor

The contractions of true labor produce progressive dilation and effacement of the cervix. They occur regularly and increase in frequency, duration, and intensity. The discomfort of true labor contractions usually starts in the back and radiates around to

TABLE 33–9 Comparison of True and False Labor

TRUE LABOR	FALSE LABOR
Contractions are at regular intervals.	Contractions are irregular.
Intervals between contractions gradually shorten.	Usually no change.
Contractions increase in duration and intensity.	Usually no change.
Discomfort begins in back and radiates around to abdomen.	Discomfort is usually in abdomen.
Intensity usually increases with change in activity.	Change of activity has no effect on contractions.
Cervical dilation and effacement are progressive.	No change.
Contractions do not decrease with rest or warm tub bath.	Rest and warm tub lessen contractions.

the abdomen. The pain is not relieved by ambulation; in fact, walking may intensify the pain.

The contractions of false labor do not produce progressive cervical effacement and dilation. Classically, they are irregular and do not increase in frequency, duration, and intensity. The contractions may be perceived as a hardening or "balling up" without discomfort, or discomfort may occur mainly in the lower abdomen and groin. The discomfort may be relieved by ambulation, changing positions, drinking a large amount of water, or taking a warm shower or tub bath (Cunningham et al., 2010).

The pregnant woman will find it helpful to know the characteristics of true labor contractions as well as the premonitory signs of ensuing labor. At times, however, the only way to differentiate accurately between true and false labor is to assess dilation. The woman must feel free to come in for accurate assessment of labor and should be counseled not to feel foolish if the labor is false. The nurse must reassure the woman that false labor is common and that it often cannot be distinguished from true labor except by vaginal examination. **Table 33–9** ● provides a comparison of true and false labor.

▶ STAGES OF LABOR AND BIRTH

To assist healthcare providers, common terms have been developed as benchmarks to subdivide the labor process into phases and stages of labor. It is important to note, however, that these represent theoretical separations in the process. A laboring woman will not usually experience distinct differences from one stage to another.

The first stage begins with the onset of true labor and ends when the cervix is completely dilated at 10 cm and the mother has the urge to push. The second stage begins with urge to push in the setting of complete dilation and ends with the birth of the newborn. The third stage begins with the birth of the newborn and ends with the delivery of the placenta.

Some clinicians identify a fourth stage. During this stage, which lasts 1–4 hours after delivery of the placenta, the uterus effectively contracts to control bleeding at the placental site (Cunningham et al., 2010).

First Stage

The first stage of labor is divided into the latent, active, and transition phases. Each phase of labor is characterized by physical and psychological changes and is summarized in **Table 33–10** ●.

LATENT PHASE The latent (or prodromal) phase starts with the beginning of regular contractions, which are usually mild. The client feels able to cope with the discomfort. She may

be relieved that labor has finally started and that the end of pregnancy has come. Although she may be anxious, she is able to recognize and express those feelings of anxiety. The client is often smiling and eager to talk about herself and answer questions. Excitement is high, and her partner or other support person is often equally elated.

Uterine contractions become established during the latent phase and increase in frequency, duration, and intensity. They may start as mild contractions lasting 30 seconds with a frequency of 10–30 minutes and progress to moderate ones lasting 30–40 seconds with a frequency of 5–7 minutes. As the cervix begins to dilate, it also effaces, although little or no fetal descent is evident. For a woman in her first labor (nullipara), the latent phase of the first stage of labor averages 8.6 hours but does not typically exceed 20 hours. The latent phase in multiparas averages 5.3 hours and does not typically exceed 14 hours. Such specific descriptions of the latent/ prodromal phase are guidelines and the actual experiences of women prior to the active phase vary widely. Timing and duration of contractions and time elapsed before the onset of the active phase do not, in themselves, require intervention or influence management. Maternal exhaustion may call for therapeutic rest or in hospital hydration (King et al., 2015).

At the beginning of labor, the amniotic membranes may bulge through the cervix in the shape of a cone. This spontaneous rupture of membranes generally occurs at the height of an intense contraction with a gush of fluid out of the vagina. In some instances, the membranes are ruptured by the physician or CNM using an instrument called an amniohook.

ACTIVE PHASE When the woman enters the early active phase, her anxiety and her sense of the need for energy and focus tend to increase as she senses the intensification of contractions and pain. She may begin to fear a loss of control or may feel the need to "really work and focus" on the contractions. Women will use a variety of coping mechanisms. Some women exhibit a sense of purpose and the need for regrouping, whereas others may feel a decreased ability to cope or a sense of helplessness. Women who have support persons and family available often experience greater satisfaction and have less anxiety compared to women without support.

During this phase, the cervix dilates from approximately 6–8 cm (1.6–2.8 in.). Fetal descent is progressive and the rate of cervical dilation most often increases. During the active phase, contractions become more frequent and longer in duration, and they increase in intensity. By the end of the active phase, contractions may have a frequency of 2–5 minutes, a duration of 40–60 seconds, and strong intensity.

TABLE 33–10 Characteristics of Labor

	FIRST STAGE			SECOND STAGE
	LATENT PHASE	ACTIVE PHASE	TRANSITION PHASE	
Nullipara	<20 hr in most cases	1.1–3.8 hr	1–3.2 hr	≤3 hr, may be longer than 3 hours with epidural anesthesia
Multipara	<14 hr in most cases	0.9–3.2 hr	0.6–2 hr	<1 hr, may be as much as 2 hours with epidural
Cervical dilation	0–6 cm	6–8 cm	8–10 cm	
Contractions Note: Contractions patterns may vary considerably. Patterns that do not fit the parameters outlined here are only classified as pathologic in the setting of protraction or arrest of labor.				
Frequency	Every 10–30 min	Every 2–5 min	Every 1.5–2.0 min	Every 1.5–2.0 min
Duration	30–40 sec	40–60 sec	60–90 sec	60–90 sec
Intensity	Begin as mild and progress to moderate; 25–40 mmHg by intrauterine pressure catheter (IUPC)	Begin as moderate and progress to strong; 50–70 mmHg by IUPC	Strong by palpation; 70–90 mmHg by IUPC	Strong by palpation; 70–100 mmHg by IUPC

TRANSITION PHASE The transition phase is the last part of the first stage of labor. When the client enters the transition phase, she may demonstrate an acute awareness of the need for her energy and attention to be completely focused to the task at hand. She may experience significant anxiety or feel out of control. She becomes acutely aware of the increasing force and intensity of the contractions. She may become restless, frequently changing position in an attempt to get comfortable.

By the time the client enters the transition phase, she is inner directed and often tired. She may not want to be left alone; at the same time, the support person may be feeling the need for a break. The nurse should reassure the woman that she will not be left alone. It is crucial that the nurse be available as relief support at this time and keep the client informed about where her labor support people are if they leave the room. Some women have the intuition that the end of labor is occurring and know that birth is near; an instinct to have support people remain often occurs.

During the transition phase, contractions have a frequency of approximately every 1.5–2 minutes, a duration of 60–90 seconds, and strong intensity. The transition phase does not usually last longer than 3 hours for nulliparas or longer than 2 hours for multiparas (Zhang et al., 2010). The total duration of the first stage may be increased by approximately 1 hour if epidural anesthesia is used.

As dilation approaches 10 cm, there may be increased rectal pressure and an uncontrollable desire to bear down, an increased amount of bloody show, and rupture of membranes (if it has not already occurred). With the peak of a contraction, the client may experience a sensation of pressure so great that she may fear that she will be "torn open" or "split apart." She may also fear that the sensations indicate that something is wrong. The nurse should inform the client that what she is feeling is normal in this stage of labor. Even with assurance, however, the client may increasingly doubt her ability to cope with

labor and may become apprehensive, irritable, and withdrawn. She may be terrified of being left alone, though she might not want anyone to talk to or touch her. However, with the next contraction, she may ask for verbal and physical support.

Other characteristics of this phase may include the following:

- Increasing bloody show
- Hyperventilation
- Generalized discomfort, including low backache, shaking and cramping in legs, and increased sensitivity to touch
- Increased need for partner's and/or nurse's presence and support
- Restlessness
- Increased apprehension and irritability
- An inner focusing on her contractions
- A sense of bewilderment, frustration, and anger at the contractions
- Requests for medication
- Hiccupping, belching, nausea, or vomiting
- Beads of perspiration on the upper lip or brow
- Increasing rectal pressure and feeling the urge to bear down.

The client in this phase is anxious to "get it over with." She may be amnesic and sleep between her now-frequent contractions. Her support persons may start to feel fatigue and may feel helpless, and they may want more participation from the nurse as their efforts to alleviate the woman's discomfort seem less effective.

Second Stage

The second stage of labor begins with complete cervical dilation and ends with birth of the infant. For primigravidas, the second stage should be completed within 3–4 hours after the cervix becomes fully dilated; for multiparas, the second stage is often less than 15 minutes long. Contractions continue with a frequency of about every 1.5–2 minute, a duration of 60–90 seconds, and strong intensity (Hanson, 2009). Descent of the fetal presenting part continues until it reaches the perineal floor.

As the fetal head descends, the woman usually has the urge to push because of pressure from the fetal head on the sacral and obturator nerves. As she pushes, intra-abdominal pressure is exerted from contraction of the maternal abdominal muscles. As the fetal head continues its descent, the perineum begins to bulge, flatten, and move anteriorly. Most women feel acute, increasingly severe pain and a burning sensation as the perineum distends. The amount of bloody show may increase.

The labia begin to part with each contraction, and between contractions, the fetal head appears to recede. With succeeding contractions and maternal pushing effort, the fetal head descends farther. **Crowning** when the head no longer recedes and remains visible at the vaginal introitus between contractions means that birth is imminent.

The woman may feel some relief that the transition phase of the first stage is over, the birth is near, and she can push. Some women feel a sense of purpose now that they can be actively involved. The client may be focused and should be encouraged to center all her energy into pushing. The nurse should encourage resting between contractions as well. The support person can offer

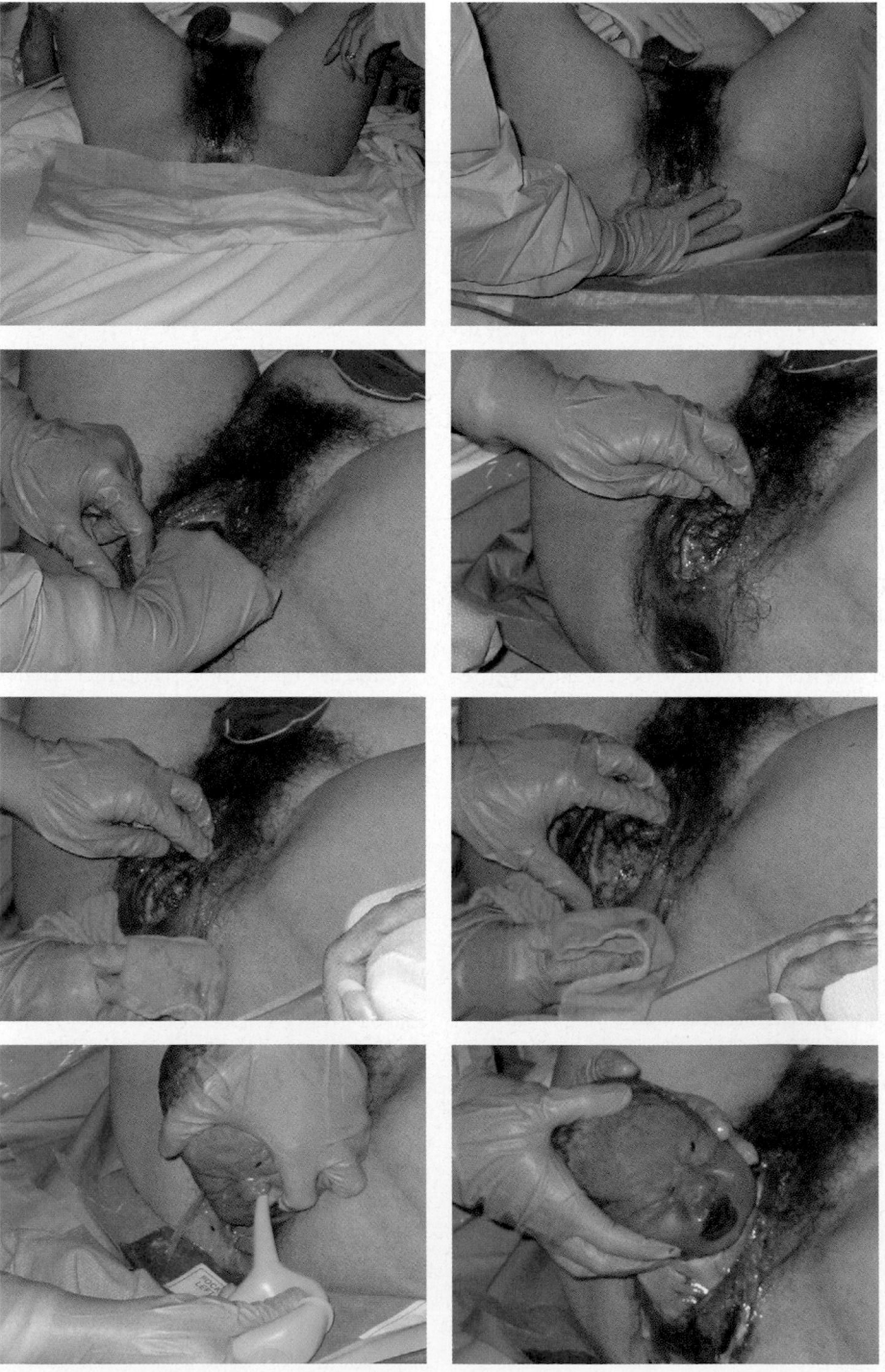

Figure 33–49 ● The birth sequence.

ice chips, fan the woman, who is often overheated and fatigued, offer verbal encouragement, and provide support to the legs.

For women without childbirth preparation, this stage can become frightening. The nurse should encourage the woman to work with her contractions and not fight them. A support person who has never seen a labor may also become disconcerted during this time. The nurse can assist the support person in performing activities and offering encouragement that assists the woman during the birth process. The woman may feel she has lost her ability to cope and may become embarrassed, or she may demonstrate extreme irritability toward the staff or her supporters as she attempts to regain control over her body. Some women feel a great sense of purpose and are unrelenting in their efforts to work with each and every contraction, and some women will be very forceful with and directive of staff and support persons. All of these reactions and emotions are common and should be supported as the woman works toward the birth.

SPONTANEOUS BIRTH (VERTEX PRESENTATION)
As the fetal head distends the vulva with each contraction, the perineum becomes extremely thin, and the anus stretches and protrudes. With time, the head extends under the symphysis pubis and is born. When the anterior shoulder meets the underside of the symphysis pubis, a gentle push by the mother aids in the birth of the shoulders. The body then follows (**Figure 33–49 ●**).

POSITIONAL CHANGES OF THE FETUS
For the fetus to pass through the birth canal, the fetal head and body must adjust to the passage by certain positional changes. These changes, called **cardinal movements** or mechanisms of labor, are described here in the order in which they occur (**Figure 33–50 ●**):

■ **Descent.** This occurs because of four forces: (1) pressure of the amniotic fluid, (2) direct pressure of the uterine fundus on the breech, (3) contraction of the abdominal muscles, and (4) extension and straightening of the fetal body. The head enters the inlet in the occiput transverse or oblique position because the pelvic inlet is widest from side to side. The sagittal suture is equidistant from the maternal symphysis pubis and the sacral promontory.

■ **Flexion.** This occurs as the fetal head descends and meets resistance from the soft tissues of the pelvis, the muscles of the pelvic floor, and the cervix. As a result of the resistance, the fetal chin flexes downward onto the chest.

■ **Internal rotation.** The fetal head must rotate to fit the diameter of the pelvic cavity, which is widest in the anteroposterior diameter. As the occiput of the fetal head meets resistance from the levator ani muscles and their fascia, the occiput rotates—usually from left to right—and the sagittal suture aligns in the anteroposterior pelvic diameter.

■ **Extension.** The resistance of the pelvic floor and the mechanical movement of the vulva opening anteriorly and forward assist with extension of the fetal head as it passes under the symphysis pubis. With this positional change, the occiput, and then the brow and face, emerge from the vagina.

■ **Restitution.** The shoulders of the fetus enter the pelvis inlet obliquely and remain oblique when the head rotates to the anteroposterior diameter through internal rotation. Because of this rotation, the neck becomes twisted. Once the head is born and is free of pelvic resistance, the neck untwists, turning the head to one side (restitution), and aligns with the position of the back in the birth canal.

■ **External rotation.** As the shoulders rotate to the anteroposterior position in the pelvis, the head turns farther to one side (external rotation).

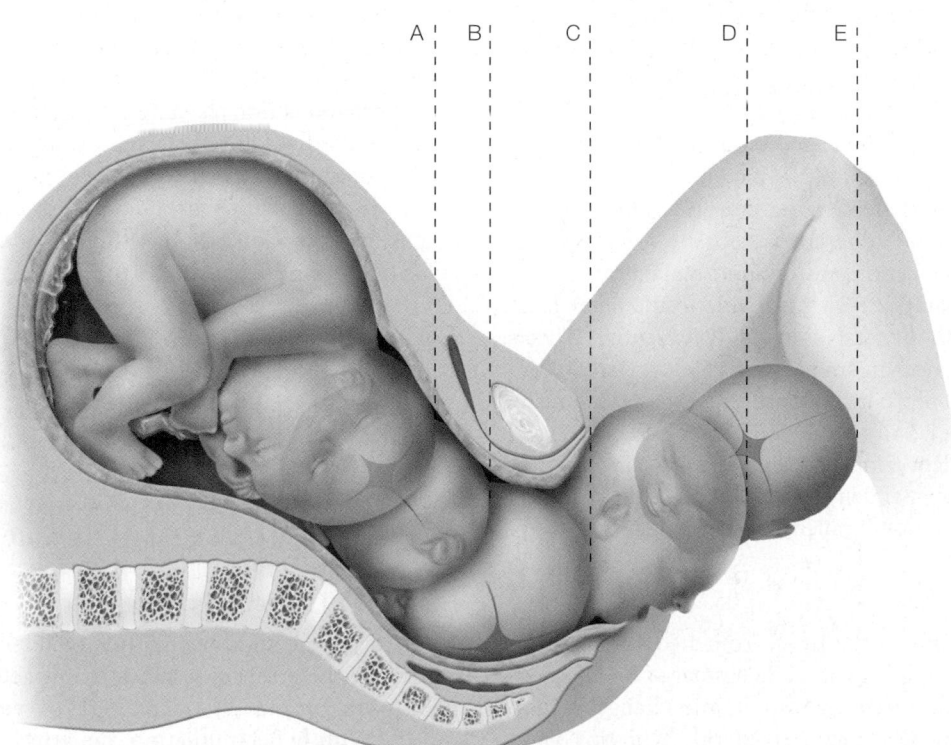

Figure 33–50 ● Mechanisms of labor. *A,* Descent. *B,* Flexion. *C,* Internal rotation. *D,* Extension. *E,* External rotation.

■ *Expulsion.* After the external rotation, and through the pushing efforts of the laboring woman, the anterior shoulder meets the undersurface of the symphysis pubis and slips under it. As lateral flexion of the shoulder and head occurs, the anterior shoulder is born before the posterior shoulder. The body follows quickly.

Third Stage

The third stage of labor is defined as the period of time from the birth of the infant until the completed delivery of the placenta. The third stage should be completed within 30 minutes of the birth of the infant. Intervention is required if separation of the placenta from the uterine wall has not occurred after 30 minutes.

PLACENTAL SEPARATION After the infant is born, the uterus contracts firmly, diminishing its capacity and the surface area of placental attachment. The placenta begins to separate because of this decrease in surface area. As this separation occurs, bleeding results in formation of a hematoma between the placental tissue and the remaining decidua. This hematoma accelerates the separation process. The membranes are the last to separate. They are peeled off the uterine wall as the placenta descends into the vagina.

Signs of placental separation are as follows:

■ A globular-shaped uterus

■ A rise of the fundus in the abdomen

■ A sudden gush or trickle of blood

■ Further protrusion of the umbilical cord out of the vagina.

PLACENTAL DELIVERY When the signs of placental separation appear, the woman may bear down to aid in placental expulsion. If this fails and the physician or CNM has ascertained that the fundus is firm, gentle traction may be applied to the cord while counter pressure is exerted on the lower uterine segment with the opposite hand to guard against uterine inversion. The direction of traction should follow the sacral and symphyseal curves and care should be taken to avoid allowing the placenta to fall into the collection pan in an uncontrolled fashion. This may snap off adherent membranes, leaving them in the uterus to cause infection and/or abnormal bleeding.

If the placenta separates from the inside to the outer margins, it is delivered with the fetal (shiny) side presenting. This is known as the Schultz mechanism of placental delivery or, more commonly, "shiny Schultz." If the placenta separates from the outer margins inward, it will roll up and present sideways, with the maternal surface delivering first. This is known as the Duncan mechanism of placental delivery and, because the placental surface is rough, is commonly called "dirty Duncan."

Fourth Stage

The fourth stage of labor is the time, from 1 to 4 hours after birth, during which physiological readjustment of the mother's body begins. With the birth, hemodynamic changes occur. Normal blood loss may be as much as 500 mL. With this blood loss and removal of the weight of the pregnant uterus from the surrounding vessels, blood is redistributed into venous beds.

This results in a moderate drop in both systolic and diastolic blood pressure, increased pulse pressure, and moderate tachycardia (Cunningham et al., 2010).

The uterus remains contracted in the midline of the abdomen. The fundus is usually midway between the symphysis pubis and umbilicus. Its contracted state constricts the vessels at the site of placental implantation. Immediately after birth of the placenta, the cervix remains open.

Nausea and vomiting usually cease. The woman may be thirsty and hungry. She may experience a shaking chill, which is thought to be associated with the ending of the physical exertion of labor. The bladder may be hypotonic because of trauma during the second stage and/or administration of anesthetics that decrease sensations. Hypotonic bladder can lead to urinary retention.

▶ MATERNAL SYSTEMIC RESPONSE TO LABOR

The labor and birth process affects nearly all maternal physiological systems.

Cardiovascular System

The mother's cardiovascular system is stressed both by the uterine contractions and by the pain, anxiety, and apprehension she experiences. During pregnancy, circulating blood volume increases by 50%. The increase in cardiac output peaks between the second and third trimester, although during labor there is a significant increase in cardiac output. With each contraction, 300–500 mL of blood volume are forced back into the maternal circulation, which results in an increase in cardiac output of as much as 10%–15% over the typical third-trimester levels (Cunningham et al., 2010). Further increases in cardiac output occur as the laboring woman experiences pain with uterine contractions and her anxiety and apprehension increase.

Maternal position also affects cardiac output. In the supine position, cardiac output decreases, heart rate increases, and stroke volume decreases. When the mother turns to a lateral (side-lying) position, cardiac output increases. Women with preexisting heart disease have higher rates of arrhythmias in labor (Cunningham et al., 2010).

Blood Pressure

As a result of increased cardiac output, blood pressure (both systolic and diastolic) rises during uterine contractions. In the first stage of labor, systolic pressure increases by 35 mmHg and diastolic pressure increases by approximately 25 mmHg. There may be further increases in the second stage during pushing (Blackburn, 2013; Cunningham et al., 2010).

Respiratory System

Oxygen demand and consumption increase at the onset of labor because of the presence of uterine contractions. As anxiety and pain from contractions increase, hyperventilation frequently occurs. With hyperventilation, the arterial partial pressure of carbon dioxide ($PaCO_2$) falls, and respiratory alkalosis results (Tomimatsu, Peña, & Longo, 2007).

By the end of the first stage of labor, most women develop a mild metabolic acidosis that is compensated for by respiratory alkalosis. As the woman pushes in the second stage of labor, her $PaCO_2$ levels may rise along with her blood lactate levels (because of muscular activity), leading to mild respiratory acidosis. By the time the baby is born (end of the second stage), the metabolic acidosis is uncompensated for by respiratory alkalosis (Blackburn, 2013).

The changes in acid–base status that occur in labor quickly reverse in the fourth stage because of changes in the woman's respiratory rate. Acid–base levels return to pregnancy levels by 24 hours after birth and to nonpregnant levels by a few weeks after birth (Blackburn, 2013).

Renal System

During labor, increases are seen in the maternal renin level, plasma renin activity, and angiotensinogen level. These elevations are thought to be important in the control of uteroplacental blood flow during birth and the early postpartum period (Blackburn, 2013).

Structurally, the base of the bladder is pushed forward and upward when engagement occurs. The pressure from the presenting part may impair blood and lymph drainage from the base of the bladder, leading to edema.

Gastrointestinal System

During labor, gastric motility and absorption of solid food are reduced. Gastric emptying time is prolonged, and gastric volume (amount of contents that remain in the stomach) remains increased, regardless of the time the last meal was taken (Blackburn, 2013). Some narcotics also delay gastric emptying time and add to the risk of aspiration if general anesthesia is used.

Immune System and Other Blood Values

The white blood cell (WBC) count increases to 25,000–30,000 cells/mm^3 during labor and the early postpartum period. The change in WBCs is mostly because of increased neutrophils resulting from a physiological response to stress. The increased WBC count makes it difficult to identify the presence of an infection.

Maternal blood glucose levels decrease during labor because glucose is used as an energy source during uterine contractions. The decreased blood glucose levels lead to a decrease in insulin requirements (Blackburn, 2013).

Pain

Pain during labor comes from a complexity of physical causes. Each mother experiences and copes with pain differently. Multiple factors affect a client's reaction to labor pain.

CAUSES OF PAIN DURING LABOR   The pain associated with the first stage of labor is unique in that it accompanies a normal physiological process. Even though perception of the pain of childbirth varies among women, a physiological basis exists for discomfort during labor. Pain during the first stage of labor arises from dilation of the cervix, which is the primary source of pain; stretching of the lower uterine segment; pressure on adjacent structures; and hypoxia of the uterine muscle cells during contraction (Blackburn, 2013). The areas of pain include the lower abdominal wall and the areas over the lower lumbar region and the upper sacrum.

During the second stage of labor, pain is caused by hypoxia of the contracting uterine muscle cells, distention of the vagina and perineum, and pressure on adjacent structures. Pain during the third stage of labor results from uterine contractions and cervical dilation as the placenta is expelled. This stage of labor is short, and afterward, anesthesia is needed primarily for episiotomy repair.

FACTORS AFFECTING RESPONSE TO PAIN   Many factors affect the individual's perception of and response to pain. For example, childbirth preparation classes may reduce the need for analgesia during labor. Preparing for labor and birth through reading, talking with others, or attending a childbirth preparation class frequently has positive effects for the laboring woman and her partner. The woman who knows what to expect and what techniques she may use to increase comfort tends to be less anxious during the labor. A tour of the birthing center and an opportunity to see and feel the environment also help reduce anxiety (especially with the first child), because during admission many new things are happening and they seem to occur all at once.

In addition, individuals tend to respond to painful stimuli in the way that is acceptable in their culture. In some cultures, it is natural for members to communicate pain, no matter how mild, whereas in other cultures, members stoically accept pain, either out of fear or because it is expected. Nurses need to be aware of cultural norms and demonstrate culturally competent care to women and their families in the intrapartum setting (Khademian & Vizeshfar, 2008).

Response to pain may also be influenced by fatigue and sleep deprivation. The fatigued client has less energy and ability to use such strategies as distraction or imagination to deal with pain. As a result, she may lose her ability to cope with labor and choose analgesics or other medications to relieve the discomfort.

A woman's previous experience with pain and anxiety also affects her ability to manage current and future pain. Women who have had experience with pain seem to be more sensitive to painful stimuli compared to those who have not. Unfamiliar surroundings and events may increase anxiety, as may separation from family and loved ones. Anticipation of discomfort and questions about whether the mother can cope with the contractions may increase anxiety as well.

Both attention and distraction influence the perception of pain. When the sensation of pain is the focus of attention, the perceived intensity is greater. A sensory stimulus, such as a back rub, can provide distraction and help refocus the woman's attention on the stimulus rather than the pain. Randomized controlled trials have shown that the continuous presence of a support person improves coping ability and maternal perception of her experience. Furthermore, consistent provision of social support and comfort measures shortens the duration of labor, use of analgesia and anesthesia, and reduces the rate of operative delivery (King et al., 2015).

▶ FETAL RESPONSE TO LABOR

When the fetus is healthy, the mechanical and hemodynamic changes of normal labor have no adverse effects.

Heart Rate

Fetal heart rate decelerations can occur with intracranial pressures of 40–55 mmHg as the head pushes against the cervix. The currently accepted explanation of this early deceleration is hypoxic depression of the central nervous system, which is under vagal control. The absence of these head-compression decelerations in some fetuses during labor is explained by the existence of a threshold that is reached more gradually in the presence of intact membranes and lack of maternal resistance. These decelerations are harmless in a normal fetus.

Acid–Base Status

Blood flow is decreased to the fetus at the peak of each contraction, leading to a slow decrease in pH status. During the second stage of labor, as uterine contractions become longer and stronger and the woman often holds her breath to push, the fetal pH decreases more rapidly. Although women are encouraged to maintain slow, evenly paced breathing, holding of the breath often occurs. As the base deficit increases, fetal oxygen saturation drops by approximately 10% (Blackburn, 2013).

Hemodynamic Changes

The adequate exchange of nutrients and gases in the fetal capillaries and intervillous spaces depends, in part, on the fetal blood pressure. Fetal blood pressure is a protective mechanism for the normal fetus in the anoxic periods caused by the contracting uterus during labor. The fetal and placental reserves are usually enough to ensure that the fetus comes through these anoxic periods unharmed (Blackburn, 2013).

Fetal Sensation

Beginning at approximately 37 or 38 weeks of gestation (full term), the fetus is able to experience sensations of light, sound, and touch. The full-term fetus is able to hear music and the maternal voice. Even in utero, the fetus is sensitive to light and will move away from a bright light source. Additionally, the full-term fetus is aware of pressure sensations during labor, such as the touch of the healthcare provider during a vaginal exam or the pressure on the head as a contraction occurs. Although the fetus may not be able to process this input, it is important to note that as the woman labors, the fetus also experiences the labor.

▶ ALTERATIONS DURING INTRAPARTUM CARE

Most births occur without the need for operative obstetric intervention. In some instances, however, procedures are necessary to maintain the safety of the woman and the fetus. The most common of these procedures are labor induction, episiotomy, cesarean birth, and vaginal birth following a previous cesarean birth.

Generally, women are aware of the possible need for an obstetric procedure during their labor and birth. However, some women expect to have a normal, physiologic experience and feel disappointed, angry, or even guilty when an unanticipated procedure becomes necessary. This conflict between expectation and the need for intervention presents a challenge to maternity nurses. The nurse provides information regarding any procedure to help the client and her partner or other support person understand what is proposed, the anticipated benefits and possible risks, and any alternatives.

Cervical Ripening

Induction of labor may be necessary or beneficial in certain clinical situations. When the cervix is unfavorable (usually defined as a Bishop score less than 6), the use of cervical ripening agents increases the likelihood of a successful induction of labor (see **Table 33–11** ●). Misoprostol (Cytotec) and formulations of prostaglandin E_2 (PGE_2) gel for **cervical ripening** (softening and effacing of the cervix) are drugs that may be used for the pregnant woman at or near term when there is a medical or obstetric indication for induction of labor. Mechanical methods designed to ripen the cervix employ the use of balloon catheters to encourage mechanical dilation.

USE OF MISOPROSTOL Misoprostol (Cytotec) is a synthetic PGE_1 analogue that can be used to soften and ripen the cervix and to induce labor. It is available as a tablet that is inserted into the vagina, or it can be taken orally or sublingually. The use of Cytotec for cervical ripening has fluctuated. Cytotec was widely used in the 1990s for cervical ripening and induction of labor until several reports showed an increase in the rates of uterine rupture. However, there is now a large body of research that supports its safety and efficacy when used appropriately (Phend, 2013). Cytotec is approved by the FDA for prevention of peptic ulcer disease and has had special labeling for indication of cervical ripening and induction of labor since 2002 (Phend, 2013).

Research has shown that the use of Cytotec for ripening the cervix and inducing labor is more effective than oxytocin or prostaglandin agents and is less costly. Women who receive Cytotec to induce labor typically deliver within 24 hours of administration. The use of Cytotec is also associated with lower cesarean birthrates. When compared with women who have been induced using prostaglandin agents or oxytocin, the adverse outcomes do not differ among the three methods (ACOG, 2009a). Most adverse maternal and fetal outcomes

TABLE 33–11	Bishop Scoring System				
			FACTOR		
SCORE	DILATION (CM)	POSITION OF CERVIX	EFFACEMENT (%)	STATION (FROM −3 TO +3)	CERVICAL CONSISTENCY
0	Closed	Posterior	0–30	−3	Firm
1	1–2	Midposition	40–50	−2	Medium
2	3–4	Anterior	60–70	−1, 0	Soft
3	5–6	—	80	+1, +2	—

Source: Bishop, E. H. (1964). Pelvic scoring for elective inductions. *Obstetrics & Gynecology, 24,* 266.

associated with misoprostol have been associated with the use of doses larger than the recommended 25 mcg. Intravaginal misoprostol has been found to be as efficacious or superior to dinoprostone gel (Cunningham et al., 2010). Guidelines for misoprostol induction include the following (ACOG, 2009a):

- The initial dosage should be 25 mcg.
- Recurrent administration should not exceed dosing intervals of more than 3–6 hours.
- Oxytocin should not be administered less than 4 hours after the last Cytotec dose.
- Cytotec should be administered only where the uterine activity and FHR can be monitored continuously for an initial observation period.

Contraindications for Cytotec include the following:

- Nonreassuring FHR tracing
- Frequent uterine contractions of moderate intensity.

USE OF PROSTAGLANDIN AGENTS   The two most commonly used types of prostaglandin gel are Prepidil and Cervidil. Prepidil gel contains 0.5 mg dinoprostone (a form of prostaglandin E_2 for intracervical application) and is placed intracervically. Cervidil is packaged in an intravaginal insert that resembles a 2-cm-square piece of cardboard. It is placed in the posterior vagina and is left in place to provide a slow release of 10 mg dinoprostone at a rate of 0.3 mg/hr over 12 hours (Cunningham et al., 2010).

The advantage of Cervidil is that it can be removed easily if an adverse reaction occurs (Beckmann et al., 2010). Both preparations have been demonstrated to cause cervical ripening, shorter labor, and lower requirements for oxytocin during labor induction. Vaginal birth is achieved within 24 hours for most women. The incidence of cesarean birth is reduced when prostaglandin agents are used before labor induction (Cunningham et al., 2010).

Risks of prostaglandin administration include uterine tachysystole (more than five contractions in 10 minutes), nonreassuring fetal status, higher incidence of postpartum hemorrhage, and uterine rupture that can occur even in the absence of a previous uterine incision (Creasy et al., 2008). Women with a previous uterine incision should not receive prostaglandin agents, because the risk of uterine rupture is greatly increased (ACOG, 2009a). Prostaglandin should be used with caution in women with compromised cardiovascular, hepatic, or renal function and in women with asthma or glaucoma (Creasy et al., 2008).

USE OF MECHANICAL METHODS   Balloon catheters are the safest and most common mechanical method of cervical ripening, though laminaria may still be used in some institutions. Advantages of mechanical agents for cervical ripening are similar efficacy when compared to hormonal agents, less costly, lower incidence of systemic side effects, and lower incidence of uterine tachysystole (Cunningham et al., 2010).

Balloon catheters have been used for cervical ripening for many years to promote mechanical dilation. A Foley catheter with a 25- to 80-mL balloon is passed through the undilated cervix and then inflated. The weighted balloon applies pressure on the internal os of the cervix and acts to ripen the cervix. This technique can be used alone or in conjunction with pharmacologic or additional mechanical methods. No evidence exists to show that any combination approach is superior to a balloon catheter alone (Wing, 2015).

One study examined cervical ripening after Foley catheter insertion and found that the mean change in the Bishop score was 3.56 after placement of a Foley bulb catheter. The average time from Foley bulb expulsion until birth was 8 hours and 27 minutes, which indicates that Foley bulb induction is a safe and effective means to induce cervical ripening (Marciniak et al., 2010). A systematic review of the evidence of mechanical methods of cervical ripening and induction found that in women with an unfavorable cervix, Foley catheter placement prior to induction with oxytocin significantly reduced the duration of labor and reduced the risk of a cesarean section (Fox et al., 2010).

NURSING CARE DURING CERVICAL RIPENING   Physicians, CNMs, and labor and delivery nurses who have had special education and training may administer agents for cervical ripening. Maternal vital signs are assessed for a baseline, and an electronic fetal monitor is applied for at least 20 minutes to obtain an external tracing of uterine activity, FHR pattern, and a reactive nonstress test (NST). If a nonreactive test is obtained, consultation with the physician or CNM is required. After the gel, intravaginal insert, or tablet has been inserted, the woman is instructed to remain lying down with a rolled blanket or hip wedge under her right hip to tip the uterus slightly to the left for the first 30–60 minutes to maintain the cervical ripening agent in place. Gel may leak from the endocervix. The nurse monitors the woman for uterine tachysystole and FHR abnormalities (changes in baseline rate, variability, and presence of decelerations) for 30 minutes to 2 hours if a prostaglandin gel agent is used (ACOG, 2009a). If tachysystole occurs, the woman is positioned on her left side and oxygen is administered if fetal stress is noted. The administration of a tocolytic agent (such as a subcutaneous injection of 0.25 mg terbutaline) should be considered if the uterine tachysystole pattern continues. The gel may be removed if severe nausea, vomiting, or tachysystole develops (Wilson, Shannon, & Shields, 2013). Treatment with antiemetics, antipyretics, and antidiarrheal agents usually is not indicated. Women who receive Cervidil or Cytotec tend to remain in the acute care setting so the contraction pattern and fetal status can be monitored continuously for an initial observation period (ACOG, 2009a).

Women undergoing induction via balloon catheters do not need continuous fetal monitoring. The nurse can perform intermittent monitoring along with the maternal vital signs. The nurse should also assess the location of the catheter to ensure that the catheter has not become displaced. This can be achieved by marking the catheter tubing at the introitus and noting whether movement has occurred. Vaginal examinations should not be performed.

Labor Induction

The ACOG defines **labor induction** as the stimulation of uterine contractions before the spontaneous onset of labor, with or without ruptured fetal membranes, for the purpose of accomplishing birth. Induction may be indicated in the presence of the following (ACOG, 2009a):

- Diabetes mellitus
- Renal disease

- Preeclampsia–eclampsia
- Chronic pulmonary disease
- Premature rupture of membranes
- Chorioamnionitis
- Postterm gestation greater than 42 weeks
- Mild abruptio placentae without evidence of nonreassuring fetal status
- Intrauterine fetal demise
- Intrauterine fetal growth restriction
- Isoimmunization
- Oligohydramnios
- Nonreassuring fetal status
- Nonreassuring antepartum testing.

Relative indications include chronic hypertension, systemic lupus erythematosus, gestational diabetes, coagulation disorders, cholestasis of pregnancy, polyhydramnios, fetal anomalies requiring specialized neonatal care, logistical factors (risk of rapid birth, distance from hospital, psychological factors, or advanced cervical dilation), previous stillbirth, and postterm gestation greater than 41 weeks (ACOG, 2009a).

All contraindications to spontaneous labor and vaginal birth are contraindications to the induction of labor. Maternal contraindications include, but are not limited to, the following (ACOG, 2009a):

- Client refusal
- Placenta previa or vasa previa
- Transverse fetal lie
- Previous classic uterine incision (or any vertical incision in the upper portion of the uterus)
- Active genital herpes infection
- Umbilical cord prolapse
- Absolute cephalopelvic disproportion.

Before induction is attempted, appropriate assessment must indicate that both the woman and the fetus are ready for the onset of labor. This includes evaluation of fetal maturity and cervical readiness. The gestational age of the fetus is best evaluated by accurate maternal menstrual dating and early ultrasound exams. Amniotic fluid studies provide valuable information regarding fetal lung maturity.

Forceps-Assisted Birth

Forceps are designed to assist the birth of a fetus by providing traction or by providing the means to rotate the fetal head to an occipitoanterior position. In medical literature and practice, **forceps-assisted birth** is also known as *instrumental delivery*, *operative delivery*, or *operative vaginal delivery*. There are many different types of forceps, each with special functions. The type of forceps used is determined by the physician assisting with the birth and the clinical situation.

INDICATIONS FOR USE OF FORCEPS Indications for the use of forceps include the presence of any condition that threatens the mother or fetus and that can be relieved by birth.

Conditions that put the woman at risk include heart disease, acute pulmonary edema or pulmonary compromise, certain neurological conditions, intrapartum infection, prolonged second stage, or exhaustion. Fetal conditions include premature placental separation, prolapsed umbilical cord, and nonreassuring fetal status. Forceps may be used electively when the fetal station is very low to shorten the second stage of labor and spare the woman's pushing effort (when exhaustion or heart disease is present) or when regional anesthesia or paralysis has affected the woman's motor innervation, and she cannot push effectively (Cunningham et al., 2010).

Risk factors for a forceps- or vacuum-assisted birth (discussion to follow) are as follows (Cunningham et al., 2010):

- Nulliparity
- Maternal age (35 and over)
- Maternal height of less than 150 cm (4 ft 11 in.)
- Pregnancy weight gain of more than 15 kg (33 lb)
- Postdate gestation (41 weeks or more)
- Epidural anesthesia
- Infant presentation other than occipitoanterior
- Presence of dystocia (labor dysfunction)
- Presence of a midline episiotomy
- Abnormal FHR tracing.

NEONATAL AND MATERNAL RISKS Some newborns may develop a small area of ecchymosis or edema, or both, along the sides of the face as a result of forceps application. Cephalohematoma (and subsequent hyperbilirubinemia) may occur as well as transient facial paralysis. Other reported complications include low Apgar scores, retinal hemorrhage, corneal abrasions, ocular trauma, other trauma (Erb palsy, fractured clavicle), elevated neonatal bilirubin levels, and prolonged infant hospital stay (Cunningham et al., 2010).

Maternal risks may include trauma such as lacerations of the birth canal, periurethral lacerations, and extensions of a median episiotomy into the anus, resulting in increased bleeding, bruising, hematomas, and pelvic floor injuries (Beckmann et al., 2010). Women who give birth with the assistance of forceps are more likely to have a third- or fourth-degree laceration and report more perineal pain and sexual problems in the postpartum period (Cunningham et al., 2010). In addition, an increase in postpartum infections, cervical lacerations, and prolonged hospital stays has been reported (Cunningham et al., 2010). Women who give birth with the assistance of forceps may also experience urinary and rectal incontinence, anal sphincter injury, and postpartum metritis (Cunningham et al., 2010).

Vacuum Extraction

Vacuum extraction is an obstetric procedure used by physicians and CNMs to assist the birth of a fetus by applying suction to the fetal head. The vacuum extractor accounts for 68% of all operative vaginal births. Its use has increased by 41% since 1990 and continues to rise (Cunningham et al., 2010). The vacuum extractor is composed of a soft suction cup attached to a suction bottle (pump) by tubing. The suction cup, which comes in various sizes, is placed against the occiput of the fetal head, avoiding the fontanels. Care must be taken to ensure that no cervical or vaginal tissue is trapped under the cup. The pump is used to create negative pressure (suction) of approximately 50–60 mmHg in a stepwise sequence or rapid application. An artificial caput ("chignon") is formed as the fetal scalp is pulled into the cup.

The longer the duration of suction, the more likely the newborn is to have a scalp injury. Although there are no data on the duration of use, ACOG advises a 30-minute time limit (Simpson & Creehan, 2013). Although there are no specifications on the number of attempts, failure to descend with multiple attempts is an indicator that a cesarean birth may be needed. In addition, if more than three "pop-offs" occur (the suction cup pops off the fetal head), the procedure should be discontinued. The most common indication for the use of the vacuum extractor is a prolonged second stage of labor or nonreassuring FHR pattern. Vacuum extraction is also used to relieve the woman of pushing effort, or when analgesia or fatigue interferes with her ability to push effectively, or in cases of nonreassuring fetal status when prompt birth is indicated. The vacuum extractor is preferred to forceps in cases of suspected cephalopelvic disproportion (CPD), when successful passage of the fetal head requires all potential space inside the vaginal canal. True CPD is an absolute contraindication to vacuum extraction. Other contraindications include nonvertex presentations, maternal or suspected fetal coagulation defects, known or suspected hydrocephalus, and fetal scalp trauma (Cunningham et al., 2010). Relative contraindications include suspected fetal macrosomia, high fetal station, face or breech presentation, gestation less than 34 weeks, incompletely dilated cervix, and previous fetal scalp blood sampling (Cunningham et al., 2010).

Neonatal complications include scalp lacerations, bruising, subgaleal hematomas, cephalohematomas, intracranial hemorrhages, subconjunctival hemorrhages, neonatal jaundice, fractured clavicle, Erb palsy, damage to the sixth and seventh cranial nerves, retinal hemorrhage, and fetal death. In addition, shoulder dystocia occurs more often (Cunningham et al., 2010). There appear to be more neonatal complications and injuries with use of a metal suction cup device than with soft cup devices. In the presence of a preterm gestation, risk of periventricular-intraventricular hemorrhage (PV-IVH) has been a concern, and some studies provide conflicting recommendations. Maternal complications include perineal trauma, edema, third- and fourth-degree lacerations, postpartum pain, and infection (Simpson & Creehan, 2013). Women who give birth with the aid of a vacuum extractor report more sexual difficulties in the postpartum period. Maternal genital tract and anal sphincter injuries occur less frequently with the vacuum extractor than with forceps.

Episiotomy

An **episiotomy** is a surgical incision of the perineal body to enlarge the outlet. The second most common procedure in maternal–child care, the episiotomy has long been thought to minimize the risk of lacerations of the perineum and overstretching of perineal tissues. However, episiotomy may actually increase the risk of fourth-degree perineal lacerations (Dudding, Vaizey, & Kamm, 2008). Research suggests, first, that rather than protecting the perineum from lacerations, the presence of an episiotomy makes it more likely that the woman will have anal sphincter tears and, second, that perineal lacerations heal more quickly than deep perineal tears (Frankman et al., 2009). In clinical practice, research has shown that the incidence of major perineal trauma (extension to or through the anal sphincter) is more likely to happen if a midline episiotomy is done (Frankman et al., 2009; Gural-Urganci et al., 2013). Women with previous episiotomies that resulted in a third- or fourth-degree extension were more likely to have a repeat occurrence when episiotomy was used initially compared to women who had a spontaneous laceration without the use of episiotomy (Frankman et al., 2009; Yogev et al., 2013). Additional complications associated with episiotomy are blood loss, infection, pain, and perineal discomfort that may continue for days or weeks past birth, including painful intercourse (Lyndon et al., 2012). Episiotomy is indicated for protection against injury to the anterior external genitalia, expediting delivery in the setting of non-reassuring fetal status, or enlarging the space in which to apply forceps or disimpact the fetal anterior shoulder. The American College of Obstetricians and Gynecologists discourages the use of episiotomy when it is not indicated. Rates have fallen from over 60% in 1979 to 12% in 2012 (Robinson, 2015).

Overall factors that place a woman at increased risk for episiotomy are primigravid status, large or macrosomic fetus, occipitoposterior position, use of forceps or vacuum extractor, and shoulder dystocia. Other factors that may be mitigated by nurses, physicians, and CNMs include the following:

- Use of lithotomy and other recumbent positions (causes excessive and uneven stretching of the perineum)
- Encouraging or requiring sustained breath holding during second-stage pushing (causes excessive and rapid perineal stretching, can adversely affect blood flow in mother and fetus, and requires woman to be responsive to caregiver directions rather than to her own urges to push spontaneously)
- Arbitrary time limit placed by the physician or CNM on the length of the second stage.

PREVENTIVE MEASURES   General tips to help reduce the incidence of lacerations and episiotomies include the following:

- Perineal massage during pregnancy for nulliparous women
- Natural pushing during labor and avoiding the lithotomy position or pulling back on legs, which tightens the perineum
- Side-lying position for pushing, which helps slow birth and diminish tears
- Warm or hot compresses on the perineum and firm counterpressure
- Encouraging a gradual expulsion of the infant at the time of birth by encouraging the mother to "push, take a breath, push, take a breath," thereby easing the infant out slowly
- Avoiding immediate pushing after epidural placement.

EPISIOTOMY PROCEDURE   The two types of episiotomy are midline and mediolateral, with midline being the most common in current use. Just before birth, when approximately 3–4 cm (1.2–1.6 in.) of the fetal head are visible during a contraction, the episiotomy is performed by using sharp scissors with rounded points (Kilpatrick & Garrison, 2007). The midline incision begins at the bottom center of the perineal body and extends

Evidence-Based Practice   Antenatal Perineal Massage for Reducing Perineal Trauma

Problem

What is the effectiveness of antenatal perineal massage on the incidence of perineal trauma at birth and its associated complications?

Evidence

Perineal trauma following birth can be associated with both short- and long-term complications. This type of trauma can result from surgical episiotomy as well as spontaneous tears. Rates of trauma are particularly high in primiparous women. Pain from perineal trauma can last up to 3 months, and this pain may impair a return to normal sexual function. Perineal massage during the antenatal period has been proposed as one method of enabling the perineum to expand more easily during birth. A systematic review published in the *Cochrane Database of Systematic Reviews* provided data comparing perineal trauma in 2,400 women who conducted antenatal perineal massage to women who did not (Beckman & Garrett, 2006; Beckman & Stock, 2013). This type of rigorous, unbiased review of multiple randomized, controlled trials represents the strongest evidence for practice.

Implications

Digital perineal massage performed by the woman herself or by her partner during the last 4–5 weeks of pregnancy reduced the number of needed episiotomies by approximately 15%. Perineal trauma—defined as an incidence of trauma requiring suturing—was also reduced when antenatal

perineal massage had been used. The benefit was greatest for women who were experiencing their first vaginal birth. When perineal trauma did occur, there was no difference in the extent of tearing in the group with perineal massage, so the advantage appears to be primarily in avoiding episiotomy. No differences were found in the incidence of instrument-assisted birth, resumption of sexual activity, or incontinence of urine or feces.

The number of women in these studies who were multiparous was small, so it cannot be definitively determined whether perineal massage is as effective when it is not the first vaginal birth. No testing of massage devices was included in these studies. No specific type of perineal massage was dictated, so a particular method cannot be recommended.

The nurse can suggest to primiparous women that perineal massage done by themselves or their partners will decrease the need for an episiotomy and may reduce the likelihood of perineal trauma with its associated, ongoing perineal pain. Perineal massage should be performed for at least the final 4–5 weeks of pregnancy to ensure the optimal therapeutic effect.

Critical Thinking Application

A prenatal client comes to you with this dilemma. In childbirth class, she was informed that perineal tear it less extensive and easier to heal than an episiotomy. Her physician disagreed and said that episiotomies heal better. How would you handle this situation?

---

straight down the midline to the fibers of the rectal sphincter. The mediolateral incision begins in the midline of the posterior fourchette and extends at a 45° angle downward to the right or left.

The episiotomy is usually performed with regional or local anesthesia but may be done without anesthesia in emergency situations. It is generally proposed that as crowning occurs, the distention of the tissues causes numbing. Repair of the episiotomy and any lacerations is completed either during the period between birth of the newborn and expulsion of the placenta or after expulsion of the placenta. Adequate anesthesia must be given for the repair.

Cesarean Birth

Cesarean birth (the birth of the infant through an abdominal and uterine incision) is one of the oldest known surgical procedures. Until the 20th century, cesarean procedures were used primarily to save the fetus of a dying woman. As the maternal and perinatal morbidity and mortality rates associated with cesarean birth steadily decreased throughout the 20th century, the proportion of cesarean births increased. Beginning in the early 1970s, the cesarean birth rate rose steadily for almost two decades. In 1989, however, in an effort to control healthcare costs, the number of cesarean births began to decline, but in 2009, the rate of cesarean births performed in the United States reached an all-time high of 32.9% (CDC, 2013). Since then, the rate has stabilized at 32.8% in both 2010 and 2011 (Martin et al., 2012).

Cesarean birth rates differ dramatically in other parts of the world. Worldwide, women living in urban areas are four times more likely to have a cesarean compared to women living in

rural areas (Bhutta et al., 2010). Countries with low cesarean birth rates (less than 17%) include the Netherlands, Finland, and Norway. The highest rates were found in Italy, Portugal, and the United States with rates greater than 30%. Overall, the incidence of cesarean birth has continued to increase worldwide (Declercq et al., 2011).

The increasing rate of cesarean births in the United States is linked to a rise in repeat cesarean births fueled by concerns about the risk of uterine rupture with a vaginal birth after a previous cesarean birth. There is also an increase in requests from women for cesarean births so that they can avoid the pain of labor and vaginal birth. Statements in some medical literature that vaginal births could result in pelvic floor damage during the birth process have led some women to consider cesarean births (Samarasekera et al., 2008). There is an emerging trend as well to "schedule" birth by cesarean section to meet specific needs of the parents, such as coordinating work projects, arranging for babysitting of older children, or allowing relatives who must travel from other geographic locations to be present for the birth itself.

Cesarean birth on request is associated with a reduction in maternal hemorrhage risk; however, it is also associated with increases in neonatal respiratory problems, longer hospitalizations, and increased complications in subsequent pregnancies, including placenta implantation problems and uterine rupture (ACOG, 2013b). Cesarean birth without medical indications should not be recommended for women desiring several children, for women less than 39 weeks of gestation, or when pregnancy dating is unknown or may be inaccurate. It should also not be motivated by the lack of anesthesia availability in an institution (ACOG, 2013b).

Many other factors have contributed to the rise in the cesarean birth rate and need to be considered in any discussion about decreasing the rate. These factors include an increased use of epidural anesthesia, maternal age over 35, failed labor inductions, decline in vaginal breech deliveries, decreases in operative vaginal deliveries, increased repeat cesarean rates, reduced vaginal birth after cesarean birth rates, increased physician scheduling of cesarean births for personal convenience, political pressure from malpractice insurance carriers who attempt to dictate practice standards, and fear of litigation (ACOG, 2013b).

INDICATIONS Commonly accepted indications for cesarean birth include complete placenta previa, breech presentation, transverse lie, placental abruption accompanied by non-reassuring fetal status, active genital herpes, umbilical cord prolapse, arrest of descent and/or arrest of dilation, nonreassuring fetal status, previous classical incision on the uterus (either previous cesarean birth or myomectomy), more than one previous cesarean birth, benign and malignant tumors that obstruct the birth canal, and cervical cerclage (Barber et al., 2011).

Certain maternal medical conditions are contraindications to a vaginal birth and warrant a cesarean birth (ACOG, 2010). These medical conditions include the following:

- Cardiac disorders
- Severe maternal respiratory disease
- Central nervous system disorders that increase intracranial pressure
- Mechanical vaginal obstruction, such as an ovarian mass or lower uterine segment fibroids

Other indications that are now commonly associated with cesarean birth, although in some circumstances may allow the child to be delivered vaginally, include breech presentation, previous cesarean birth, major congenital anomalies, and severe Rh isoimmunization

MATERNAL MORTALITY AND MORBIDITY Cesarean births have a higher maternal mortality rate than vaginal births. In the United States, women undergoing a cesarean birth have a twofold risk of most complications associated with delivery compared with women who give birth vaginally (Stranges, Wier, & Elixhauser, 2012). In England, emergency cesarean birth is associated with a ninefold risk of death when compared with vaginal delivery, and elective cesarean births have a threefold risk (Cunningham et al., 2010). Perinatal morbidity is also considerably higher in women who have had a cesarean. Common postoperative complications include infection, reactions to anesthesia agents, blood clots, and bleeding. Women who have had a cesarean birth are twice as likely to be rehospitalized within 60 days of birth when compared with women who have had a vaginal birth. Other sources of maternal morbidity that are directly associated with cesarean birth include ureteral injury, bladder laceration, and wound infection (Cunningham et al., 2010).

SKIN INCISIONS The skin incision for a cesarean birth is either transverse (Pfannenstiel) or vertical, and it is not indicative of the type of incision made into the uterus. Time factors,

client preference, previous vertical skin incision, or physician preference determines the type of skin incision.

The transverse incision is made across the lowest and narrowest part of the abdomen. Because the incision is made just below the pubic hairline, it is almost invisible after healing. The limitation of this type of skin incision is that it does not allow extension of the incision if needed. Because it usually requires more time to make and repair, this incision is used when time is not of the essence (e.g., with arrest of descent and/or arrest of dilation and stable fetal and maternal status).

The vertical incision is made between the navel and the symphysis pubis. This type of incision is quicker and, therefore, is preferred in cases of nonreassuring fetal status when rapid birth is indicated, with preterm or macrosomic infants, or when the woman is significantly obese (Cunningham et al., 2010).

UTERINE INCISIONS The two major locations of uterine incisions are in the lower uterine segment and in the upper segment of the uterine corpus. The type of uterine incision depends on the need for the cesarean. The choice of incision affects the woman's opportunity for a subsequent vaginal birth and her risks of a ruptured uterine scar with a subsequent pregnancy.

The lower uterine segment incision most commonly used is a transverse incision. The lower uterine segment incision is preferred for the following reasons (Cunningham et al., 2010):

- The lower segment is the thinnest portion of the uterus and involves less blood loss.
- It requires only moderate dissection of the bladder from the underlying myometrium.
- It is easier to repair, although repair takes longer.
- The site is less likely to rupture during subsequent pregnancies.
- There is a decreased chance for adherence of bowel or omentum to the incision line.

Disadvantages of this type of segment incision include the following:

- It takes longer to make a transverse incision.
- It is limited in size because of the presence of major vessels on either side of the uterus.
- It has a greater tendency to extend laterally into the uterine vessels.
- The incision may stretch and become a thin window, but it usually does not create problems clinically until subsequent labor ensues.

The lower uterine segment vertical incision is preferred for multiple gestation, abnormal presentation, placenta previa, nonreassuring fetal status, and preterm and macrosomic fetuses. Disadvantages of this type of incision include the following:

- The incision may extend downward into the cervix.
- More extensive dissection of the bladder is needed to keep the incision in the lower uterine segment; hemostasis and closure are more difficult.
- The vertical incision carries a higher risk of rupture with subsequent labor. Consequently, once a vertical incision is performed, future births need to be via cesarean.

One other incision, the classic incision, was the method of choice for many years but is used infrequently today. This vertical incision was made into the upper uterine segment. It resulted in greater blood loss and was more difficult to repair. Most important, it carried an increased risk of uterine rupture with subsequent pregnancy, labor, and birth, because the upper uterine segment is the most contractile portion of the uterus.

ANALGESIA AND ANESTHESIA   There is no perfect anesthesia for cesarean birth. Each has its advantages, disadvantages, possible risks, and side effects. Goals for the administration of analgesia and anesthesia include safety, comfort, and emotional satisfaction for the client.

PREPARATION FOR CESAREAN BIRTH   Because one of every four births is a cesarean, preparation for this possibility should be an integral part of all prenatal education. The nurse should encourage pregnant women and their partners to discuss the possibility of a cesarean birth, and their specific needs and desires under those circumstances, with their physician or CNM. Their preferences may include the following:

- Participating in the choice of anesthetic
- Partner or significant other being present during the procedures and/or birth
- Partner or significant other being present in the recovery or postpartum room
- Video recording and/or taking pictures of the birth
- Delayed instillation of eye drops to promote eye contact between parent and infant in the first hours after birth
- Physical contact or holding the infant while in the operating and/or recovery room (by the partner if the mother cannot hold the newborn)
- Breastfeeding in the recovery area within the first hour of birth.

Information that couples need about cesarean birth includes the following:

- What preparatory procedures to expect
- Description or viewing of the birthing room
- Types of anesthesia for birth and analgesia available postpartum
- Sensations that may be experienced
- Roles of significant others
- Interaction with newborn
- Immediate recovery phase
- Postpartum phase.

Preparing the woman and her family for cesarean birth involves more than the procedures of establishing an intravenous line, instilling a urinary indwelling catheter, and performing an abdominal prep. Good communication skills are essential in preparing the woman and her support person. The use of therapeutic touch and direct eye contact (if culturally acceptable and possible) assists the woman in maintaining a sense of control and lessens her anxiety.

If the cesarean birth is scheduled and not an emergency procedure, the nurse has ample time for preoperative teaching and to provide an opportunity for the woman and her support

person to express their concerns, ask questions, and develop a relationship with the nurse.

In preparation for surgery, the woman is given nothing by mouth. To reduce the likelihood of serious pulmonary damage if gastric contents are aspirated, antacids may be administered within 30 minutes of surgery. If epidural anesthesia is used, the nurse may assist with the procedure, monitor the woman's blood pressure and response, and continue electronic fetal monitoring. An abdominal and perineal prep is done, and an indwelling catheter is inserted to prevent bladder distention. An intravenous line is started with a large-bore needle to permit rapid administration of blood if that becomes necessary. Preoperative medication may be ordered. The pediatrician should be notified and preparation made to receive the new baby. The nurse ensures that the infant warmer is working and that resuscitation equipment is available.

The nurse assists in positioning the client on the operating table. Fetal heart rate is assessed before surgery and during preparation because fetal hypoxia can result from the mother lying in the supine position. The operating room table is adjusted so that it slants slightly to one side, or a hip wedge (folded blanket or towels) is placed under the right hip to tip the uterus slightly and reduce compression of blood vessels. The uterus should be displaced 15° from the midline. This helps relieve the pressure of the heavy uterus on the vena cava and lessens the incidence of vena cava compression and maternal supine hypotension. The suction should be in working order, and the urine collection bag should be positioned under the operating table to obtain proper drainage. Auscultation or electronic fetal monitoring of the fetal heart rate is continued until immediately before the procedure. If the fetus was monitored internally, a last-minute check is done to ensure that the fetal scalp electrode has been removed.

The nurse continues to provide reassurance and to describe the various procedures being performed (along with their rationale) to ease anxiety and give the woman a sense of control.

Women undergoing elective cesarean birth can be given information about the postoperative experience before their birth experience. Important components of client education that can be emphasized before birth include dealing with postoperative discomfort, splinting the incision to decrease pain, frequent deep breathing and coughing, and the importance of early ambulation. Clients who receive this information before the birth are more apt to remember it when the information is reviewed in the early postpartum period.

PREPARATION FOR REPEAT CESAREAN BIRTH   When a couple is anticipating a repeat cesarean birth, they have a general understanding of what will occur, which can help them make informed choices about their birth experience. Couples who have had previous negative experiences need an opportunity to describe what they felt. Encourage these couples to identify what they would like to be different and to list options that would make the experience more positive. Those who have already had positive experiences need reassurance that their needs and desires will be met in a similar manner. Provide all couples the opportunity to discuss any fears or anxieties. For women who previously labored and then had an unexpected cesarean birth, the experience may be perceived as negative. Emphasize the positive aspects of a repeat cesarean birth to all couples. These include participation in selecting the birth date, lack of fatigue related to labor, ability to prepare and make arrangements for other children, and the ability for other family members or friends to be present at the hospital during or immediately after birth if desired by the couple.

PREPARATION FOR EMERGENCY CESAREAN BIRTH

When the need for a cesarean birth emerges suddenly, the period preceding surgery must be used to its greatest advantage. It is imperative that the nurse use the most effective communication skills in supporting the couple. The nurse describes what the couple may anticipate during the next few hours and gives the woman information about (and the rationale for) any procedure before it begins. It is essential for the nurse to explain what is going to happen, why it is being done, and what sensations the woman may experience. This allows the woman to be informed and to consent to the procedure, which gives her a sense of control and reduces her feelings of helplessness.

SUPPORTING THE PARTNER

Every effort should be made to include the partner in the birth experience. When attending a cesarean birth, the partner wears protective coverings similar to those worn by others in the operating suite. A stool can be placed beside the woman's head so that the partner can sit nearby to provide physical touch, visual contact, and verbal reassurance.

To promote the participation of the partner who chooses not to be in the operating suite, the nurse can do the following:

- Allow the partner to be nearby, where the partner can hear the newborn's first cry.
- Encourage the partner to carry or accompany the infant to the nursery for the initial assessment.
- Involve the partner in postpartum care in the recovery room.

In some emergency circumstances, a support person may not be permitted in the operating room. Some facilities have policies that prohibit a support person from being in the operating room if the woman requires general anesthesia or if an emergency birth is being performed. In these situations, the support person should receive a thorough explanation of what is happening and why, be advised when the staff will return to provide information, know the expected length of time for the procedure, and be reassured that the mother is receiving the care she and the baby need. Because this exclusion is stressful for family members, staff need to provide information as soon as possible after providing emergency care to the mother.

IMMEDIATE POSTNATAL RECOVERY PERIOD

After birth, the nurse assesses the Apgar score and completes the same initial assessment and identification procedures used for vaginal births. The **Apgar score** is used to evaluate newborns at 1 minute and again at 5 minutes after birth. The total score is achieved by assessing five signs:

1. Heart rate
2. Respiratory effort
3. Muscle tone
4. Reflex irritability
5. Color.

Each of the signs is assigned a score of 0, 1, or 2. The highest possible score is 10. (Apgar scoring is described fully in Exemplar 33.4, Newborn Care.)

Infant identification bands must be placed on the infant and the mother (as well as on the support person, if present) before removing the infant from the operating room. The nurse should make every effort to assist the parents in bonding with their infant. If the mother is awake, one of her arms can be freed to enable her to touch and stroke the infant. The newborn may be placed on the mother's chest or held in an *en face* position. If physical contact is not possible, the nurse should provide a running narrative so that the mother knows what is happening with her baby. The nurse assists the anesthesiologist or nurse anesthetist with raising the mother's head so that she can see her infant immediately after birth. The parents can be encouraged to talk to the baby, and the partner can hold the baby until the family is taken to the recovery room.

The nurse caring for the postpartum woman assesses the mother's vital signs every 5 minutes until they are stable, then every 15 minutes for an hour, and then every 30 minutes until the woman is discharged to the postpartum unit. The nurse remains with the woman until she is stable.

The nurse evaluates the dressing and perineal pad every 15 minutes for at least an hour. Gently palpate the fundus to determine whether it is remaining firm; palpation may be performed by placing a hand to support the incision. Intravenous oxytocin is usually administered to promote the contractility of the uterine musculature. If the mother has been under general anesthesia, she should be positioned on her side to facilitate drainage of secretions, turned, and assisted with coughing and deep breathing every 2 hours for at least 24 hours. If she has received a spinal or epidural anesthetic, the level of anesthesia is checked every 15 minutes for the first 2 hours and then hourly until full sensation has returned. It is important for the nurse to monitor intake and output and to observe the urine for a bloody tinge, which could mean surgical trauma to the bladder. The physician prescribes medication to relieve the mother's pain and nausea, and that medication is administered as needed.

Bonding can be promoted by encouraging mother and baby skin-to-skin contact for the first hour uninterrupted and performing all assessments and procedures on the infant at the mother's bedside if both are stable.

Vaginal Birth After Cesarean

In the late 1980s there was an increasing trend to have a trial of labor after cesarean (TOLAC) and **vaginal birth after cesarean (VBAC)** in cases of nonrecurring indications for a cesarean (for example, twins, umbilical cord prolapse, placenta previa, nonreassuring fetal status). This trend was influenced by consumer demand and studies that support VBAC as a viable and safe alternative. VBAC rates peaked in the late 1990s and then the practice came under renewed scrutiny, causing rates to decline into the 2000s. This prompted the National Institutes of Health to review the matter and issue a statement on the safety of TOLAC. Consensus among providers is that all women who meet eligibility criteria should be offered TOLAC (King, 2015).

The American College of Obstetricians and Gynecologists (ACOG) guidelines state that the following aspects should be met when identifying candidates for a trial of labor (Cunningham et al., 2010):

- One previous cesarean birth and a low transverse uterine incision

- An adequate pelvis
- No other uterine scars or previous uterine rupture
- A physician who is able to do a cesarean needs to be available throughout active labor
- In-house anesthesia personnel are available for an emergency cesarean birth if warranted.

The absolute risks of VBAC are small. There is a 0.1%–0.7% risk of uterine rupture when women attempt a trial of labor after previously undergoing a cesarean birth (Algert et al., 2008). The significance is that, in the studies, there were no uterine ruptures in the group of women who had undergone an elective repeat cesarean birth. There is uncertainty about whether a trial of labor after cesarean (TOLAC) increases the risk of perinatal death compared to babies born by elective repeat cesarean section (ERCS). Some studies have found an increased perinatal death rate in babies in the TOLAC group compared to those in the ERCS group (Richter, Bergmann, & Dudenhausen, 2008). These findings, combined with nonmedical factors (rising malpractice premiums for providers, accessibility to an institution that provides VBAC services, provider attitudes), are primarily responsible for the decline of VBACs in the United States since the 1990s. Other risks associated with VBAC versus ERCS are listed in **Box 33–4** ●.

Success rates for VBAC have been encouraging. Women whose previous cesarean was performed because of nonrecurring indications have been reported to have an approximately 60%–80% chance of success with VBAC (Harper & Macones, 2008). Women whose previous cesarean was performed for breech presentation had the highest success rates for VBAC (91%). Women who had a previous cesarean birth for nonreassuring fetal status had an 84% success rate, whereas a woman diagnosed with previous dystocia had a 67% success rate. Women who were previously diagnosed with dystocia before 5-cm dilation had a 67% success rate, whereas women who had previously progressed to 6–9 cm had a 73% success rate. Women who had been labeled as having dystocia in the second stage had a 75% success rate (Cunningham et al., 2010).

The nursing care of a woman undergoing VBAC varies according to institutional protocols. Generally, if the woman is at low risk (has had one previous cesarean with a lower uterine segment incision), her blood count, type, and screen are obtained on admission; a heparin lock is inserted for intravenous access if needed; continuous electronic fetal monitoring (EFM) is used; and clear fluids may be taken. If the woman is at higher risk, NPO status should be maintained, and, in addition to the care listed, an intrauterine catheter may be inserted to monitor intrauterine pressures during labor.

Supportive and comfort measures are very important. The woman may be excited about this opportunity to experience labor and vaginal birth but apprehensive if she does not know what to expect from labor. The nurse provides information and encouragement for the laboring woman and her partner.

Intrapartum Risk Factors

A number of other alterations may occur during the intrapartum period. These include precipitous birth, abruptio placentae, placenta previa, premature rupture of membranes, preterm and postterm labor, hypertonic labor, hypotonic labor, fetal macrosomia, nonreassuring fetal status, prolapsed umbilical cord, amniotic fluid embolism, cephalopelvic disproportion, retained placenta, lacerations, placenta accreta, and perinatal loss. These alterations are described in the Alterations and Therapies feature. Perinatal loss is discussed in detail in the module on Grief and Loss.

✳ Go to **nursing.pearsonhighered.com** for a chart that describes intrapartum high-risk factors that increase the likelihood of labor complications.

■ NURSING PROCESS

Maternal–newborn nursing has kept pace with the changing philosophy of childbirth. Nurses who choose positions in a birthing area are presented with opportunities to interact with clients in a wide variety of situations, ranging from a family that wants maximum interaction to one that wants to be left alone as much as possible. In addition, despite the increasing focus on family-centered care, the nurse must always be ready to meet the needs and concerns of the single woman who is laboring alone. In every case, nurses strive to provide high-quality, individualized care.

The physiological and psychological events that occur during labor call for continual and rapid adaptations by the mother and fetus. Frequent and accurate assessments are crucial to the progress of these adaptations. In current nursing practice, the traditional assessment techniques of observation, palpation, and auscultation are augmented by the judicious use of technology, such as ultrasound and electronic monitoring. These tools may provide more detailed information for assessment; however, it is important for the nurse to remember that the technology only provides data. It is the nurse who truly monitors the mother and her baby.

Maternal Assessment

Assessment of the mother begins with a client history and screening for intrapartum risk factors. The nurse obtains a brief oral history when the client is admitted to the birthing area. Typically, the nurse assesses the maternal and fetal vital signs

---

Box 33–4 Complications Associated With VBAC

- Uterine rupture
- Scar dehiscence
- Hysterectomy
- Uterine infection
- Neonatal death
- Intrauterine fetal demise
- Stillbirth
- Transfusion
- Hypoxic ischemic encephalopathy

Alterations and Therapies **Intrapartum**

ALTERATION	DESCRIPTION	THERAPIES
Precipitous birth	Rapid progression of labor, with birth occurring within 3 hours or less.	<ul><li>The nurse's primary responsibility is to provide a physically and psychologically safe experience for the woman and her baby.</li><li>If birth is imminent, do not leave the mother alone, even for a minute.</li><li>Provide reassurance, and send auxiliary personnel to retrieve the emergency birth pack.</li></ul>
Abruptio placentae	Premature separation of a normally implanted placenta from the uterine wall; may be a catastrophic event depending on the severity of the resulting hemorrhage, which may be vaginal or may be unseen because it collects in the uterus or abdomen.	<ul><li>Monitor uterine resting tone, which is frequently increased with abruptio placentae.</li><li>Monitor abdominal girth measurements to determine internal blood collection.</li><li>Monitor vital signs, hemoglobin and hematocrit, and urine output.</li></ul>
Placenta previa	Implantation of the placenta in the lower uterine segment rather than the upper portion, resulting in placental separation with dilation of the cervix.	<ul><li>Teach all pregnant women the importance of reporting any bright-red vaginal bleeding, often scant at first.</li><li>Avoid vaginal examination if placenta previa is suspected.</li><li>Assess blood loss, pain, vital signs, fetal well-being, and uterine contractility.</li><li>Provide emotional support for the mother and family.</li></ul>
Premature rupture of membranes	Spontaneous rupture of the membranes before the onset of labor. Preterm PROM (PPROM) is the rupture of membranes occurring before 37 weeks of gestation associated with infection, previous history of PPROM, hydramnios, multiple pregnancy, urinary tract infection, amniocentesis, placenta previa, abruptio placentae, trauma, cervical insufficiency, bleeding during pregnancy, and maternal genital tract anomalies.	<ul><li>Assess for duration of rupture, appearance of amniotic fluid, and fetal well-being.</li><li>Monitor client for signs of infection, including WBC count and vital signs.</li><li>Assess for potential cord compression if witnessed rupture.</li><li>Educate the client and her partner regarding implications of PROM and all treatments.</li></ul>
Preterm labor	Labor that occurs between 20 and 36 completed weeks of pregnancy. Clients are admitted if at high risk for delivery in the setting of advanced cervical dilation, history of preterm delivery, or positive fetal fibronectin (fFN, a protein in the membranes found in vaginal secretions before 20 weeks and after 37 weeks. Detection of fFN on a vaginal swab between 24 and 34 weeks gestation increases suspicion of preterm labor) (King et al., 2015); if at low risk for imminent delivery, clients are sent home on pelvic rest and normal activity.	<ul><li>Administer IV magnesium sulfate for 12 hours maximum for fetal neuroprotection, and IM betamethasone. Monitor blood pressure every 10–15 minutes, serum magnesium levels, reflexes, respiratory rate, urinary output, and level of sedation, and be prepared to administer calcium if toxicity is suspected.</li><li>Provide emotional support to the woman who may be fearful of fetal well-being.</li><li>Teach client to recognize onset of labor, to perform home uterine activity monitoring, to evaluate contraction activity, and symptoms to report.</li></ul>
Postterm labor	A pregnancy that exceeds 42 weeks, occurring most frequently in primigravidas, women with history of postterm pregnancies, or fetal anencephaly.	<ul><li>Conduct ongoing assessment of fetal well-being.</li><li>Assess fluid for meconium following rupture of membranes.</li><li>Provide client education.</li><li>Provide emotional support, encouragement, and recognition of the woman's anxiety.</li></ul>

(continued on next page)

Alterations and Therapies **Intrapartum** (continued)

ALTERATION	DESCRIPTION	THERAPIES
Hypertonic labor	Ineffective uterine contractions of poor quality occurring in the latent phase of labor with increased resting tone of the myometrium and frequent contractions.	■ Provide comfort and support to the laboring woman and her partner. ■ Provide supportive measures such as change of position, quiet environment, back rubs, or guided imagery. ■ Consider therapeutic rest.
Hypotonic labor patterns	Usually developing in the active phase of labor, characterized by less than two to three contractions in a 10-minute period of low intensity causing minimal discomfort; often the result of overstretching of the uterus, bowel or bladder distention, arrest of descent, and fetal malposition.	■ Assess contractions, maternal vital signs, and FHR, watching for signs of infection or dehydration. ■ Promote maternal–fetal well-being. ■ Monitor for maternal exhaustion. ■ Assess for meconium if rupture of membranes. ■ Consider augmentation of labor.
Fetal malpresentation	Any presentation that is not right-occiput-anterior (ROA), occiput-anterior (OA), or left-occiput-anterior (LOA), which may prolong labor or require a cesarean section.	■ Assist with position change to promote fetal repositioning. ■ Promote rest if labor is prolonged. ■ Provide client education. ■ Prepare for surgery if cesarean section is required.
Fetal macrosomia	A newborn weight of >4,000 g at birth, often associated with excessive maternal weight gain, maternal obesity, uncontrolled maternal diabetes, grand multiparity, prolonged gestation, or those with a previous infant with macrosomia >4,000 g (ACOG, 2009d).	■ Identify women at risk, and assess FHR for nonreassuring fetal status. ■ Assess for labor dysfunction or lack of fetal descent. ■ Provide support, encouragement, and education. ■ Monitor for hemorrhage postpartum. ■ Assess newborn after delivery for cephalohematoma.
Nonreassuring fetal status	When the oxygen supply is insufficient to meet the physiological needs of the fetus, a nonreassuring fetal status may result, which may be transient or chronic; demonstrated by change in FHR, decreased fetal movement, meconium-stained amniotic fluid, or ominous FHR patterns.	■ Review prenatal history, and note any risk factors. ■ Assess fetal heart rate, and note characteristics of amniotic fluid with rupture. ■ Promote maternal positioning to maximize ureteroplacental fetal blood flow.
Prolapsed umbilical cord	The umbilical cord precedes the fetal presenting part, placing pressure on the cord and reducing or stopping blood flow to and from the fetus. Of greatest risk when rupture of membranes occurs before engagement of fetal presenting part.	■ Assess FHR, and observe for prolapse when membranes rupture for a full minute. If loop of cord is discovered, a gloved hand elevates the fetal presenting part to relieve pressure until the cesarean delivery can be accomplished. ■ Administer oxygen by face mask to increase fetal oxygenation. ■ If the presenting part is well applied to the cervix, then ambulation should be encouraged. If the presenting part is not well applied to the cervix, the woman is at an increased risk of cord prolapse and ambulation should be discouraged; however, the woman can sit with the head of the bed elevated or in a rocking chair to facilitate gravity.
Amniotic fluid embolism	In the presence of a small tear in the amnion or chorion high in the uterus, an area of separation in the placenta, or cervical tear, a small amount of amniotic fluid may leak into the chorionic plate and enter the maternal circulatory system as an amniotic fluid embolism. The more debris in the amniotic fluid (e.g., meconium), the greater the maternal danger.	■ Administer oxygen under positive pressure, and summon emergency assistance. ■ Establish intravenous access quickly. ■ Perform cardiopulmonary resuscitation if respiratory and cardiac arrest occur. ■ Call anesthesiologist immediately. ■ Provide support to the woman's partner and family members.

Alterations and Therapies **Intrapartum** (continued)

ALTERATION	DESCRIPTION	THERAPIES
Cephalopelvic disproportion (CPD)	Occurs when the fetal head is too large to pass through any part of the birth passage, which can result in prolonged labor, uterine rupture, necrosis of maternal soft tissues, cord prolapse, excessive molding of the fetal head, or damage to the fetal skull and central nervous system.	■ Assess adequacy of maternal pelvis for a vaginal birth, size of the fetus, and its presentation and position. ■ Suspect CPD when labor is prolonged, cervical dilation and effacement are slow, and engagement of the presenting part is delayed. ■ Provide support to the couple, and keep them informed of what is happening and about the procedures being performed. ■ Assess cervical dilation and fetal descent more frequently. ■ Monitor contractions and fetal well-being continuously. ■ Position to optimize pelvic diameters.
Retained placenta	Retention of the placenta beyond 30 minutes after birth, resulting in bleeding that may lead to shock.	■ Assess for excessive bleeding and uterine contraction after delivery. ■ Monitor maternal vital signs.
Lacerations	Tearing of the cervix or vagina, indicated by bright-red vaginal bleeding in the presence of a well-contracted uterus. The highest risk is in young or nulliparous women and during operative vaginal delivery (forceps or vacuum assisted).	■ Monitor for bright-red blood during labor. ■ Promote perineal massage prenatally. ■ If lacerations occur, manage pain and apply ice to the area after delivery to reduce edema. ■ Teach the mother to rinse the perineum after every elimination and use sitz baths to reduce discomfort.
Placenta accreta	The chorionic villi attach directly to the myometrium of the uterus in placenta accreta. Two other types of placental adherence are placenta increta, in which the myometrium is invaded, and placenta percreta, in which the myometrium is penetrated. The adherence itself may be total, partial, or focal, depending on the amount of placental involvement.	■ Assess for bleeding. ■ Monitor vital signs. ■ Prepare woman for surgical intervention and possible hysterectomy.
Shoulder dystocia	Impaction of the fetal anterior shoulder behind the maternal pubic bone after the birth of the head. Risk factors include macrosomia, history of shoulder dystocia, and rapid labor. However, most shoulder dystocias are not predictable. Pressure from the maternal bone on the fetal brachial plexus can result in paralysis of the arm. Failure to resolve the problem may lead to fetal hypoxia, encephalopathy, and death.	■ The provider will perform maneuvers to free the shoulder. ■ Call for assistance from the unit and nursery staff. ■ Maintain an orderly atmosphere and clear communication. ■ Emphasize the importance of helping the mother to co-operate with maneuvers and avoid pushing. ■ Monitor fetal status. ■ Monitor time from birth of the head to fetal expulsion. ■ Reposition the mother to maximize pelvic diameters. ■ Apply suprapubic pressure on provider request to assist in dislodging the shoulder.
Perinatal loss	Death of a fetus or infant from the time of conception through the end of the newborn period 28 days after delivery.	■ Covered in depth in the module on Grief and Loss and the exemplar on Perinatal Loss in that same module.

TABLE 33–12   Nursing Assessments in the First Stage

PHASE	MOTHER	FETUS
Latent	Blood pressure and respirations each hour if in normal range. Temperature every 4 hours unless over 37.5°C (99.6°F) or membranes ruptured, then every 2 hours. Uterine contractions every 30 minutes.	FHR every 60 minutes for low-risk women and every 30 minutes for high-risk women if normal characteristics are present (average variability, baseline in the 110–160 bpm range, without late or variable decelerations or assess the heart rate every 30 minutes if the provider orders intermittent auscultation in a low risk setting). Note fetal activity. If electronic fetal monitor is in place, assess for reactive nonstress test.
Active	Blood pressure, pulse, and respirations every hour if in normal range. Uterine contractions palpated every 15–30 minutes.	FHR every 30 minutes for low-risk women and every 15 minutes for high-risk women if normal characteristics are present.
Transition	Blood pressure, pulse, and respirations every hour. Contractions palpated every 15–30 minutes.	FHR every 15–30 minutes if normal characteristics are present.

immediately (Table 33–12 ●). If the vital signs are within normal limits, the interview continues. If a problem is identified, nursing care is then prioritized.

It is common for the healthcare provider to send the prenatal records to the labor and birthing unit before the client's due date. Review this information in a nonjudgmental manner to ensure changes have not occurred since the information was documented. During the initial interview, the nurse is building a trusting relationship. It is often helpful if the nurse sits down and appears unrushed, makes direct eye contact (if culturally appropriate), and begins the interview with a statement such as "I am going to be asking you some very personal and specific questions so that we can provide the best care for both you and your baby." This conveys a nonjudgmental approach, shows respect, and makes the expectant mother feel more at ease. Each agency has its own admission forms, but they usually include the following information:

- Woman's name and age
- Last menstrual period and estimated date of birth
- Attending physician or CNM
- Personal data: blood type; Rh factor; results of serology testing; prepregnant and present weight; allergies to medications, foods, or other substances; prescribed and OTC medications taken during the pregnancy; and history of drug and alcohol use and smoking during the pregnancy
- History of previous illness, such as tuberculosis, heart disease, diabetes, convulsive disorders, and thyroid disorders; asthma; sickle cell/Tay Sachs and other inherited disorders; or pregnancy-related complications (e.g., preterm labor, gestational diabetes, preeclampsia, or low platelets)
- Problems in the prenatal period, such as elevated blood pressure, bleeding problems, recurrent urinary tract infections, other infections, abnormal laboratory findings (e.g., abnormal glucose screen indicating gestational diabetes or low hemoglobin or hematocrit indicating anemia), or sexually transmitted infections
- Pregnancy data: gravida, para, abortions, and neonatal deaths
- Method chosen for infant feeding
- Type of childbirth education or infant care classes
- Previous infant care experience

- Woman's preferences regarding labor and birth, such as no episiotomy, no analgesics or anesthetics, or the presence or absence of the partner or others at the birth
- Pediatrician, family practice physician, or nurse practitioner
- Additional data: history of special tests, such as nonstress test, biophysical profile, or ultrasound; history of any preterm labor; onset of labor; amniotic fluid membrane status; and brief description of any previous labor and birth
- Onset of labor, status of amniotic membranes (intact, ruptured, time of rupture, color, and odor).

Because of the prevalence of domestic violence in our society (see the module on Violence), the nurse needs to consider the possibility that the pregnant woman may have experienced abuse at some point in her life. Many victims of domestic violence, sexual assault, or childhood abuse may be anxious about the labor process or may experience anxiety during labor. Therefore, it is essential to review the woman's prenatal record and any other available records for information that may indicate abuse or a history of victimization by violence.

Intrapartum High-Risk Screening

Screening for intrapartum high-risk factors is an integral part of assessing the woman in labor. As the history is obtained, the nurse notes the presence of any potential risk factors that may be considered high-risk conditions. For example, the woman who reports a physical symptom such as intermittent bleeding needs further assessment to rule out abruptio placentae or placenta previa before the admission process continues. It is important to determine the difference between vaginal bleeding and bloody show. In addition to identifying the presence of a high-risk condition, the nurse must recognize the implications of the condition for the laboring woman and her fetus. For example, if there is an abnormal fetal position, the nurse understands that the labor may be prolonged and that prolapse of the umbilical cord is more likely, thereby increasing the possibility of a cesarean birth.

Although physical conditions are frequently listed as the major factors that increase risk during the intrapartum period, socioeconomic and cultural variables, such as poverty, nutrition, the amount of prenatal care, crowded living conditions,

Box 33–5 Selected Intrapartum Risk Factors

- Intermittent bleeding
- Abnormal fetal presentation
- Poverty
- Poor nutrition
- Lack of prenatal care
- Mental illness
- Post-traumatic stress disorder (PTSD)
- Smoking
- Drug use
- Alcohol use

cultural beliefs regarding pregnancy, and communication patterns, may also precipitate a high-risk situation. Mental illness is a risk factor as well, because it can result in episodic prenatal care or the need to take psychotropic medications during the pregnancy (ACOG, 2008b). In addition, recent research indicates that women who suffer from posttraumatic stress disorder may be at increased risk for some pregnancy complications (Seng et al., 2009). Other risk factors include smoking, drug use, and consumption of alcohol during pregnancy. The nurse can quickly review the prenatal record for number of prenatal visits; weight gain during pregnancy; progression of fundal height; assistance, such as Medicaid and WIC participation; exposure to environmental agents; and history of traumatic life events, including abuse.

A partial list of intrapartum risk factors appears in **Box 33–5** ●. Keep these factors in mind during the assessment.

Intrapartum Physical and Psychosociocultural Assessment

A physical examination is part of the admission procedure and part of the ongoing care of the client. Although the intrapartum physical assessment is not as complete and thorough as the initial prenatal physical examination (see the Concept section of this module), it does involve assessment of some body systems and the actual labor process. The Intrapartum Assessment feature provides a framework the nurse can use when examining the laboring woman.

The physical assessment portion includes assessments performed immediately on admission as well as ongoing assessments. Nurses conduct ongoing assessments in all clinical situations. For example, when the woman is changing into her gown, the nurse can assess the skin for bruises, needle marks, burns, or other abnormalities. The nurse can also determine whether the woman appears to be undernourished or overnourished. When labor is progressing rapidly, however, the nurse may not have time for a complete assessment. In that case, the critical physical assessments include maternal vital signs, labor status, fetal status, and laboratory findings.

Assessment of psychosocial history is a critical component of intrapartum nursing assessment. More than 500,000 pregnancies annually are affected by some type of mental illness that is either present before or emerges with pregnancy (ACOG, 2008b). An estimated one third of all pregnant women are exposed to some type of psychotropic medication during their pregnancies. In addition, an estimated 17% of

pregnant women have diagnosed depression during pregnancy, and up to 70% report depressive symptoms while pregnant (ACOG, 2008b). Any mental illness can play a role in how the client copes with the labor and birth experience and should be assessed by the admitting nurse. Clients with identified disorders will need ongoing assessment during the labor and birth.

The nurse can begin gathering data about sociocultural factors as the woman enters the birthing area. The nurse observes the communication pattern between the woman and her support person and their responses to admission questions and initial teaching. If the woman and her support person do not speak English and translators are not available among the birthing unit staff, the course of labor and the nurse's ability to interact and provide support and education are affected. The couple must receive information in their primary language to make informed decisions. Communication may also be affected by cultural practices, such as beliefs about when to speak, who should ask questions, or whether it is acceptable to let others know about discomfort. People from certain cultures may want to experience birth naturally and may decline pain medications. In some cultures, the partner is not expected to be present in the birthing area. Nurses need to be culturally competent so that this is not interpreted as disinterest in the birth, the mother, or the infant (Spector, 2009).

Individualized nursing care can best be planned and implemented when nurses know and honor the values and beliefs of the laboring woman (Spector, 2009). To avoid stereotyping clients, the nurse always asks the woman and her family about individual beliefs and preferences. Nurses who feel uncertain about what to ask or to consider need to explore the varying cultural values and beliefs of the people residing in their community. While some communities have a prominent culture that may follow certain rituals, the nurse should still ask each client about her own individual beliefs and preferences.

The final section of the assessment guide addresses ideas, knowledge, fantasies, and fears about childbearing. The nurse should ask the client whether she has any special needs. However, because some women may not know what needs may arise, ongoing assessment is imperative. It is important for the nurse to pay specific attention to body language, eye contact, and other nonverbal cues that may indicate the woman is experiencing anxiety or other feelings. By assessing the client's cultural and psychosocial status, the nurse can better meet the woman's needs for information and support. The nurse can then assist the woman and her partner; in the absence of a partner, the nurse may become the support person.

Assessment of Contractions

Once contractions begin, the nurse must assess the nature of the contractions and any accompanying pain. When palpating a woman's uterus during a contraction, compare the consistency to your nose, chin, and forehead to determine the intensity. Many experienced nurses note that the feel during mild contractions is similar in consistency to the tip of the nose, moderate contractions feel more like the chin, and with strong contractions, the uterus feels firm, much like the forehead.

It is also important to assess the laboring woman's perception of pain. How does she describe the pain? What is her affect? Is this contraction more uncomfortable than the last one? Is the nurse's palpation of intensity congruent with the client's perception? (For instance, the nurse might evaluate a contraction as mild in intensity, whereas the laboring woman evaluates it as very strong.) A nurse's assessment is not complete unless the laboring woman's affect and response to the contractions are also noted and charted.

Electronic monitoring of uterine contractions provides continuous data. Electronic monitoring is routinely used in many birth settings for high-risk clients and those having oxytocin-induced labor. Electronic monitoring may be done externally, with a device that is placed against the maternal abdomen, or internally, with an intrauterine pressure catheter.

EXTERNAL ELECTRONIC MONITORING OF CONTRACTIONS

When monitoring contractions by external means, the portion of the monitoring equipment called a tocodynamometer, or "toco," is positioned against the fundus of the uterus and held in place with an elastic belt. The toco contains a flexible disk that responds to pressure. When the uterus contracts, the fundus tightens and the change in pressure against the toco is amplified and transmitted to the electronic fetal monitor. The monitor displays the uterine contraction as a pattern on graph paper.

External monitoring offers several advantages, including a continuous recording of the frequency and duration of uterine contractions, and it is noninvasive. However, it does not accurately record the intensity of the uterine contraction, and it is difficult to obtain an accurate fetal heart rate in some women, such as those who are very obese, those who have hydramnios, or those with a very active fetus. In addition, the client may be bothered by the belt if it requires frequent readjustment when she changes position. Electronic monitoring allows the nurse to continually monitor the fetus if concerns arise based on the fetal heart rate. It also enables the nurse and physician or CNM to observe the pattern of the FHR over a period of time by examining the electronic fetal monitoring strip.

INTERNAL ELECTRONIC MONITORING OF CONTRACTIONS

Internal intrauterine monitoring provides the same data as external monitoring, as well as accurate measurement of uterine contraction intensity (the strength of the contraction and the actual pressure within the uterus). After membranes have ruptured, the physician or CNM (or the nurse in some facilities) inserts the **intrauterine pressure catheter** into the uterine cavity and connects it by a cable to the electronic fetal monitor. It is important to first assess the fetal position and to review a past ultrasound to determine the location of the placenta, because the internal monitor should be placed away from the placenta. If an ultrasound has not been previously obtained, the physician or CNM may wish to do one on the unit or have the sonographer perform such an exam.

The pressure within the uterus in the resting state and during each contraction is measured by a small micropressure device located in the tip of the catheter. Internal electronic monitoring is used when it is imperative to have accurate intrauterine pressure readings to evaluate the stress on the uterus or to determine the adequacy of contractions. The advantage of the intrauterine pressure monitor is that it can directly measure the intensity of the contraction. It can be used when the external monitor may not be accurately assessing the contraction strength, such as in cases of maternal obesity. It can also be used when oxytocin is being administered to ensure that uterine contractions are adequate.

During internal electronic monitoring, the nurse should also evaluate the woman's labor status by palpating the intensity and resting tone of the uterine fundus during contractions. Technology is a useful tool if used as an adjunct to good assessment skills, but it is not a replacement for those skills.

Internal monitoring has both risks and benefits. It provides a more accurate fetal tracing and is more effective in monitoring the fetal status. Placement of an intrauterine pressure catheter, however, can cause vaginal bleeding. In rare cases, the scalp electrode can be placed on the fetal fontanelle or, if the fetus is in a face presentation, on an eye, thus causing fetal injury. Women with certain medical conditions, such as HIV infection, should not be monitored with internal monitoring, because it can increase the risk of viral transmission.

Cervical Assessment

Cervical dilation and effacement are evaluated directly by vaginal examination. The vaginal examination can provide information about the adequacy of the maternal pelvis, membrane status, characteristics of amniotic fluid, and fetal position and station.

Fetal Assessment

A complete intrapartum fetal assessment requires determination of the fetal position and presentation as well as evaluation of the fetal status.

Assessment of Fetal Position

Fetal position is determined in the following ways:

- Inspection of the woman's abdomen
- Palpation of the woman's abdomen
- Vaginal examination to determine the presenting part
- Ultrasound
- Auscultation of fetal heart rate.

INSPECTION Observe the woman's abdomen for size and shape. Assess the lie of the fetus by noting whether the uterus projects up and down (longitudinal lie) or left to right (transverse lie).

PALPATION: LEOPOLD MANEUVERS Leopold maneuvers are a systematic way to evaluate the maternal abdomen. Frequent practice increases the examiner's skill in determining fetal position by palpation. Leopold maneuvers may be difficult to perform on women who are obese or those who have excessive amniotic fluid (hydramnios). Before performing Leopold maneuvers, the nurse should have the woman empty her bladder and then lie on her back with her feet on the bed and her knees bent.

Intrapartum Assessment: First Stage of Labor

PHYSICAL ASSESSMENT/ NORMAL FINDINGS	ALTERATIONS AND POSSIBLE CAUSES*	NURSING RESPONSES TO DATA†
Vital Signs		
Blood pressure (BP): less than 140 systolic and 90 and greater than 90/50 diastolic	High blood pressure (essential hypertension, preeclampsia, renal disease, apprehension, anxiety, or pain) Low blood pressure (supine hypotension) Hemorrhage/hypovolemia Shock Drugs Side effect of epidural anesthesia	Evaluate history of preexisting disorders, and check for presence of other signs of preeclampsia. Do not assess during contractions; implement measures to decrease anxiety and reassess. Provide quiet environment. Have O_2 available Notify anesthesiologist.
Pulse: 60–90 bpm (normal, nonpregnant) Additional 10–20 bpm during pregnancy	Increased pulse rate (excitement or anxiety, cardiac disorders, early shock, drug use)	Evaluate cause, reassess to see if rate continues; report to physician/CNM.
Respirations: 16–24 breaths/min (or pulse rate divided by 4)	Marked tachypnea (respiratory disease), hyperventilation in transition phase Decreased respirations (narcotics)	Assess between contractions; if marked tachypnea continues, assess for signs of respiratory disease or respiratory distress.
	Hyperventilation (anxiety/pain)	Encourage slow breaths if woman is hyperventilating.
Pulse oximetry 95% or greater	Pulse oximetry less than 90%: hypoxia, hypotension, hemorrhage	Administer O_2; notify physician/CNM.
Temperature: 36.2°–37.6°C (97°–99.6°F)	Elevated temperature (infection, dehydration, prolonged rupture of membranes, epidural regional block)	Assess for other signs of infection or dehydration.
Weight		
25–35 lb greater than prepregnant weight	Weight gain greater than 35 lb (fluid retention, obesity, large infant, diabetes mellitus, preeclampsia) Weight gain less than 15 lb (small for gestational age, substance abuse, psychosocial problems)	Assess for signs of edema. Evaluate dietary patterns from prenatal record.
Lungs		
Normal breath sounds, clear and equal	Rales, rhonchi, friction rub (infection), pulmonary edema, asthma	Reassess; refer to physician/CNM.
Fundus		
At 40 weeks of gestation, located just below the xiphoid process	Uterine size not compatible with estimated date of birth (small for gestational age, large for gestational age, hydramnios, multiple pregnancy, placental/fetal anomalies, malpresentation)	Reevaluate history regarding pregnancy dating. Refer to physician/CNM for additional assessment.
Edema		
Slight amount of dependent edema	Pitting edema of face, hands, legs, abdomen, sacral area (preeclampsia)	Check deep tendon reflexes for hyperactivity; check for clonus; refer to physician/CNM.
Hydration		
Normal skin turgor, elastic	Poor skin turgor (dehydration)	Assess skin turgor; refer to physician/ CNM for deviations. Provide fluids per physician/CNM orders.
	*Possible causes of alterations are identified in parentheses.	†This column provides guidelines for further assessment and initial nursing intervention.

(continued on next page)

Intrapartum Assessment: First Stage of Labor (continued)

PHYSICAL ASSESSMENT/ NORMAL FINDINGS	ALTERATIONS AND POSSIBLE CAUSES*	NURSING RESPONSES TO DATA†
Perineum		
Tissues smooth, pink color	Varicose veins of vulva, herpes lesions/genital warts	Note on client record need for follow-up in postpartum period; reassess after birth, refer to physician/CNM.
Clear mucus; may be blood tinged with earthy or human odor	Profuse, purulent, foul-smelling drainage	Suspected gonorrhea or chorioamnionitis; report to physician/CNM; initiate care to newborn's eyes; notify neonatal nursing staff and pediatrician.
Presence of small amount of bloody show that gradually increases with further cervical dilation	Hemorrhage	Assess BP and pulse, pallor, diaphoresis, report any marked changes. Standard precautions.
Labor Status		
Uterine contractions: regular pattern	Failure to establish a regular pattern, prolonged latent phase Hypertonicity Hypotonicity Dehydration	Evaluate whether woman is in true labor. Ambulate if in early labor. Evaluate client status and contractile pattern. Obtain a 20-minute electronic fetal monitoring strip. Notify physician/CNM. Provide hydration.
Cervical dilation: progressive cervical dilation from size of fingertip to 10 cm (3.9 in.)	Rigidity of cervix (frequent cervical infections, scar tissue, failure of presenting part to descend)	Evaluate contractions, fetal engagement, position, and cervical dilation. Inform client of progress.
Cervical effacement: progressive thinning of cervix	Failure to efface (rigidity of cervix, failure of presenting part to engage); cervical edema (pushing effort by woman before cervix is fully dilated and effaced, trapped cervix)	Evaluate contractions, fetal engagement, and position. Notify physician/CNM if cervix is becoming edematous; work with woman to prevent pushing until cervix is completely dilated. Keep vaginal exams to a minimum.
Fetal descent: progressive descent of fetal presenting part from station −5 to + 4	Arrest of descent (abnormal fetal position or presentation, macrosomic fetus, inadequate pelvic measurements)	Evaluate fetal position, presentation, and size.
Membranes: may rupture before or during labor	Rupture of membranes more than 12–24 hours before onset of labor	Assess for ruptured membranes using Nitrazine test tape before doing vaginal exam. Follow standard precautions. Keep vaginal exams to a minimum to prevent infection. When membranes rupture in the birth setting, *immediately assess FHR* to detect changes associated with prolapse of umbilical cord (FHR slows).
Findings on Nitrazine test tape: Membranes probably intact: Yellow pH 5.0 Olive pH 5.5 Olive green pH 6.0	False-positive results may be obtained if large amount of bloody show is present, previous vaginal examination has been done using lubricant, or tape is touched by nurse's fingers	Assess fluid for consistency, amount, odor; assess FHR frequently. Assess fluid at regular intervals for presence of meconium staining. Follow standard precautions while assessing amniotic fluid.
Membranes probably ruptured: Blue-green pH 6.5 Blue-gray pH 7.0 Deep blue pH 7.5		Teach woman that amniotic fluid is continually produced (to allay fear of "dry birth"). Teach woman that she may feel amniotic fluid trickle or gush with contractions. Change pads often.
	*Possible causes of alterations are identified in parentheses.	†This column provides guidelines for further assessment and initial nursing intervention.

Intrapartum Assessment: First Stage of Labor (continued)

PHYSICAL ASSESSMENT/ NORMAL FINDINGS	ALTERATIONS AND POSSIBLE CAUSES*	NURSING RESPONSES TO DATA†
Amniotic fluid clear, with earthy or human odor, no foul-smelling odor	Greenish amniotic fluid (fetal stress) Bloody fluid (vasaprevia abruptio placentae) Strong or foul odor (amnionitis)	Assess FHR; do vaginal exam to evaluate for prolapsed cord; apply fetal monitor for continuous data; report to physician/CNM. Take woman's temperature and report to physician/CNM.

Fetal Status

FHR: 110–160 bpm	Less than 110 or greater than 160 bpm (nonreassuring fetal status); abnormal patterns on fetal monitor: decreased variability, late decelerations, variable decelerations, absence of accelerations with fetal movement	Initiate interventions based on particular FHR pattern.
Presentation: cephalic, 97%; breech, 3%	Face, brow, breech, or shoulder presentation	Report to physician/CNM; after presentation is confirmed as face, brow, breech, or shoulder, woman may be prepared for cesarean birth.
Position: left-occiput-anterior (LOA) most common	Persistent occipital-posterior (OP) position; transverse arrest	Carefully monitor maternal and fetal status. Reposition mother in side-lying or hands–knee position to promote rotation of fetal head.
Activity: fetal movement	Hyperactivity (may precede fetal hypoxia)	Carefully evaluate FHR; apply fetal monitor.
	Complete lack of movement (nonreassuring fetal status or fetal demise)	Carefully evaluate FHR; apply fetal monitor. Report to physician/CNM.
	*Possible causes of alterations are identified in parentheses.	†This column provides guidelines for further assessment and initial nursing intervention.

CULTURAL ASSESSMENT§	VARIATIONS TO CONSIDER	NURSING RESPONSES TO DATA§§
Cultural influences determine customs and practices regarding intrapartum care.	Individual preferences may vary.	
Ask the following questions:		
▪ Who would you like to remain with you during your labor and birth?	She may prefer only her partner or other support person to remain or may also want family and/or friends.	Provide support for her wishes by encouraging desired people to stay. Provide information to others (with the woman's permission) who are not in the room.
▪ What would you like to wear during labor?	She may be more comfortable in her own clothes.	Offer supportive materials, such as disposable pads, if needed to protect her clothing. Avoid subtle signals to the woman that she should not have chosen to remain in her own clothes. Have other clothing available if the woman desires. If her clothing becomes contaminated, it will be simple to place it in a plastic bag.
▪ What activity would you like during labor?	She may want to ambulate most of the time, stand in the shower, sit in the Jacuzzi, sit on a chair/stool/birthing ball, remain on the bed, and so forth.	Support the woman's wishes; provide encouragement and complete assessments in a manner so her activity and positional wishes are disturbed as little as possible.
§These are only a few suggestions. We do not mean to imply that this is a comprehensive cultural assessment; rather, it is a tool to encourage cultural competence.		§§This column provides guidelines for further assessment and initial nursing intervention.

(continued on next page)

Intrapartum Assessment: First Stage of Labor (continued)

CULTURAL ASSESSMENT[§]	VARIATIONS TO CONSIDER	NURSING RESPONSES TO DATA[§§]
■ What position would you like for the birth?	She may feel more comfortable in lithotomy position with stirrups and her upper body elevated, side-lying or sitting in a birthing bed, standing, or squatting, or on hands and knees.	Collect any supplies and equipment needed to support her in her chosen birthing position. Provide information to the support person regarding any changes that may be needed based on the chosen position.
■ Is there anything special you would like?	She may want the room darkened or to have curtains and windows open, music playing, her support person to cut the umbilical cord, to save a portion of the umbilical cord, to save the placenta, to videotape the birth, or other particular preferences.	Support requests, and communicate requests to any other nursing or medical personnel (so requests can continue to be supported and not questioned). If another nurse or physician does not honor the request, act as advocate for the woman by continuing to support her unless her desire is truly unsafe.
Ask the woman if she would like fluids, and ask what temperature she prefers.	She may prefer clear fluids other than water (tea, clear juice). She may prefer iced, room temperature, or warmed fluids.	Provide fluids as desired.
Observe the woman's response when privacy is difficult to maintain and her body is exposed.	Some women do not seem to mind being exposed during an exam or procedure; others feel acute discomfort.	Maintain privacy and respect the woman's sense of privacy. If the woman is unable to provide specific information, the nurse may draw from general information regarding cultural variation: Southeast Asian women may not want any family member in the room during exam or procedures. The woman's partner may not be involved with coaching activities during labor or birth. Muslim women may need to remain covered during the labor and birth and avoid exposure of any body part. The husband may need to be in the room but remain behind a curtain or screen so he does not view his wife at this time.
If the woman is to breastfeed, ask if she would like to feed her baby immediately after birth.	She may want to feed her baby right away or may want to wait a little while.	
[§]These are only a few suggestions. We do not mean to imply that this is a comprehensive cultural assessment; rather, it is a tool to encourage cultural competence.		[§§]This column provides guidelines for further assessment and initial nursing intervention.

PSYCHOSOCIAL ASSESSMENT	VARIATIONS TO CONSIDER	NURSING RESPONSES TO DATA[††]
Preparation for Childbirth		
Does the woman have some information regarding process of normal labor and birth?	Some women do not have any information regarding childbirth.	Add to present information base.
Does the woman have breathing and/or relaxation techniques to use during labor?	Some women do not have any method of relaxation or breathing to use, and some do not desire them.	Support breathing and relaxation techniques that the client is using; provide information if needed.
Have the woman and support person done extensive preparation for childbirth?	Some women have strong opinions regarding labor and birth preparation.	Support the woman's wishes to participate in her birth experience; support the woman's birth plan.
Response to Labor		
Latent phase: relaxed, excited, anxious for labor to be well established	May feel unable to cope with contractions because of fear, anxiety, or lack of information.	Provide support and encouragement, establish trusting relationship.
		[††]This column provides guidelines for further assessment and initial nursing intervention.

Intrapartum Assessment: First Stage of Labor (continued)

PSYCHOSOCIAL ASSESSMENT	VARIATIONS TO CONSIDER	NURSING RESPONSES TO DATA[††]
Active phase: becomes more intense, begins to tire	May remain quiet and without any sign of discomfort or anxiety, may insist that she is unable to continue with the birthing process.	Provide support and coaching if needed.
Transitional phase: feels tired, may feel unable to cope, needs frequent coaching to maintain breathing patterns		
Coping mechanisms: ability to cope with labor through use of support system, breathing, relaxation techniques, and comfort measures, including frequent position changes in labor, immersion in warm water, and massage	May feel marked anxiety and apprehension, may not have coping mechanisms that can be brought into this experience, or may be unable to use them at this time. Survivors of sexual abuse may demonstrate fear of intravenous lines or needles, may recoil when touched, may insist on a female caregiver, may be very sensitive to body fluids and cleanliness, and may be unable to labor lying down.	Support coping mechanisms if they are working for the woman; provide information and support if she exhibits anxiety or needs alternative to present coping methods. Encourage participation of partner or other individual if a supportive relationship seems apparent. Establish rapport and a trusting relationship. Provide information that is true and offer your presence.
Anxiety		
Some anxiety and apprehension is within normal limits.	May show anxiety through rapid breathing, nervous tremors, frowning, grimacing, clenching of teeth, thrashing movements, crying, increased pulse and blood pressure	Provide support, encouragement, and information. Teach relaxation techniques. Support controlled breathing efforts. May need to provide a paper bag to breathe into if woman says her lips are tingling. Note FHR.
Sounds During Labor		
	Some women are very quiet; others moan or make a variety of noises.	Provide a supportive environment. Encourage woman to do what feels right for her.
Support System		
Physical intimacy between mother and partner (or mother and support person/doula), caretaking activities, such as soothing conversation and touching	Some women would prefer no contact; others may show clinging behaviors.	Encourage caretaking activities that appear to comfort the woman; encourage support for the woman; if support is limited, the nurse may take a more active role.
Support person stays in proximity	Limited interaction may come from a desire for quiet.	Encourage support person to stay close (if this seems appropriate).
Relationship between mother and partner or support person: involved interaction	The support person may seem to be detached and maintain little support, attention, or conversation.	Support interactions; if interaction is limited, the nurse may provide more information and support. Ensure that the support person has short breaks, especially before transition.
		[††]This column provides guidelines for further assessment and initial nursing intervention.

VAGINAL EXAMINATION AND ULTRASOUND Other assessment techniques to determine fetal position and presentation include vaginal examination and the use of ultrasound to visualize the fetus. During the vaginal examination, the examiner can palpate the presenting part if the cervix is dilated. Information about the position of the fetus and the degree of flexion of its head (in cephalic presentations) can also be obtained. Visualization by ultrasound is used when the fetal position cannot be determined by abdominal palpation.

AUSCULTATION OF FETAL HEART RATE The handheld Doppler ultrasound is used to auscultate the FHR between, during, and immediately after uterine contractions. A fetoscope may also be used. Instead of listening haphazardly over the client's abdomen for the FHR, the nurse may choose to perform Leopold maneuvers first. Leopold maneuvers not only indicate the probable location of the FHR but also help determine the presence of multiple fetuses, fetal lie, and fetal presentation.

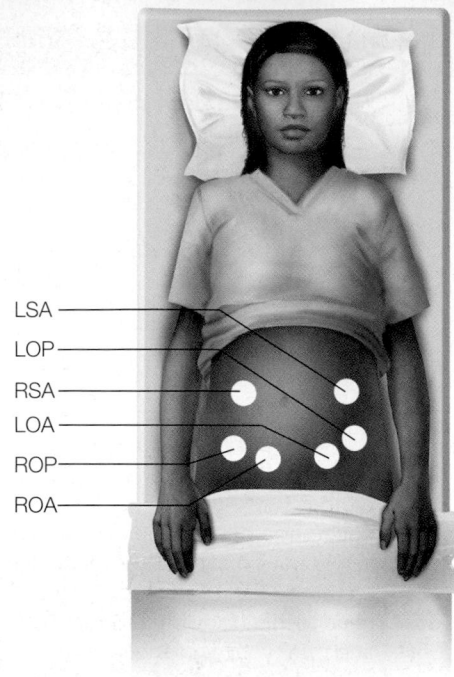

LSA
LOP
RSA
LOA
ROP
ROA

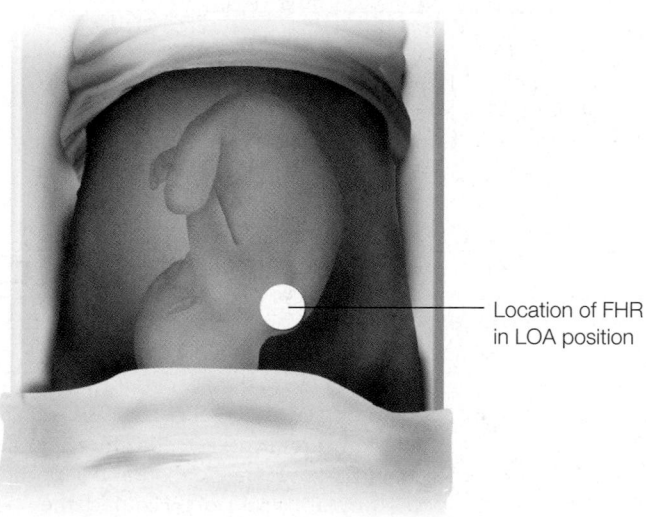

Location of FHR
in LOA position

Figure 33–51 ● Location of fetal heart rate in relation to the more commonly seen fetal positions. The FHR is heard more clearly over the fetal back.

The FHR is heard most clearly at the fetal back (**Figure 33–51 ●**). In a cephalic presentation, the FHR is best heard in the lower quadrants of the maternal abdomen. In a breech presentation, it is heard at or above the level of the maternal umbilicus. In a transverse lie, the FHR may be heard best just above or just below the umbilicus. As the presenting part descends and rotates through the pelvic structure during labor, the location of the FHR tends to descend and move toward the midline.

After the FHR is located, it is usually counted for 30 seconds, starting at the acme or immediately after a contraction, and multiplied by 2 in order to obtain the number of beats per minute. It is also appropriate to listen for a full minute, particularly after a change in status such as rupture of membranes (ACNM, 2010). If the FHR is irregular or has changed markedly from the last assessment, or if an audible deceleration is heard, the nurse listens for a full minute, through and immediately after a contraction. In these situations, continuous electronic fetal monitoring is warranted (Feinstein, Sprague, & Trepanier, 2008). It is important to note that intermittent auscultation has been found to be as effective as the electronic method for fetal surveillance.

Electronic Monitoring of Fetal Heart Rate

Electronic fetal monitoring produces a continuous tracing of the FHR, which allows many characteristics of the FHR to be visually assessed. A growing number of physicians and nurses, however, are beginning to question the widespread usage of this technology. Although fetuses who are monitored continuously have a reduction in seizures, there is no reduction in cerebral palsy, infant mortality, or adverse neonatal outcomes. Women who receive continuous fetal monitoring are more likely to undergo a cesarean birth or an instrument-assisted birth (Resnik, 2013).

INDICATIONS FOR ELECTRONIC MONITORING If one or more of the following factors are present, the FHR and contractions are monitored electronically:

- Previous history of a stillbirth at 38 or more weeks of gestation
- Presence of a complication of pregnancy (e.g., preeclampsia, placenta previa, abruptio placentae, multiple gestation, and prolonged or premature rupture of membranes)
- Induction of labor (labor that is begun as a result of some type of intervention [e.g., an intravenous infusion of oxytocin])
- Preterm labor
- Decreased fetal movement
- Nonreassuring fetal status
- Meconium staining of amniotic fluid (meconium has been released into the amniotic fluid by the fetus, which may indicate a problem)
- Trial of labor following a previous cesarean birth (ACOG, 2010)
- Maternal fever
- Placental problems.

METHODS OF ELECTRONIC MONITORING External monitoring of the fetus is usually accomplished by ultrasound. A transducer, which emits continuous sound waves, is placed on the maternal abdomen. When placed correctly, the sound waves bounce off the fetal heart and are picked up by the electronic monitor. The actual moment-by-moment FHR is displayed graphically on a screen (**Figure 33–52 ●**). In some instances, the monitor may track the maternal heart rate instead of the FHR. However, the nurse can avoid this error by comparing the maternal pulse to the FHR.

Recent advances in technology have led to the development of new ambulatory methods of external monitoring. Using a telemetry system, a small, battery-operated transducer transmits signals to a receiver connected to the monitor. This system, which is held in place with a shoulder strap, allows the client to ambulate, helping her to feel more comfortable and less confined

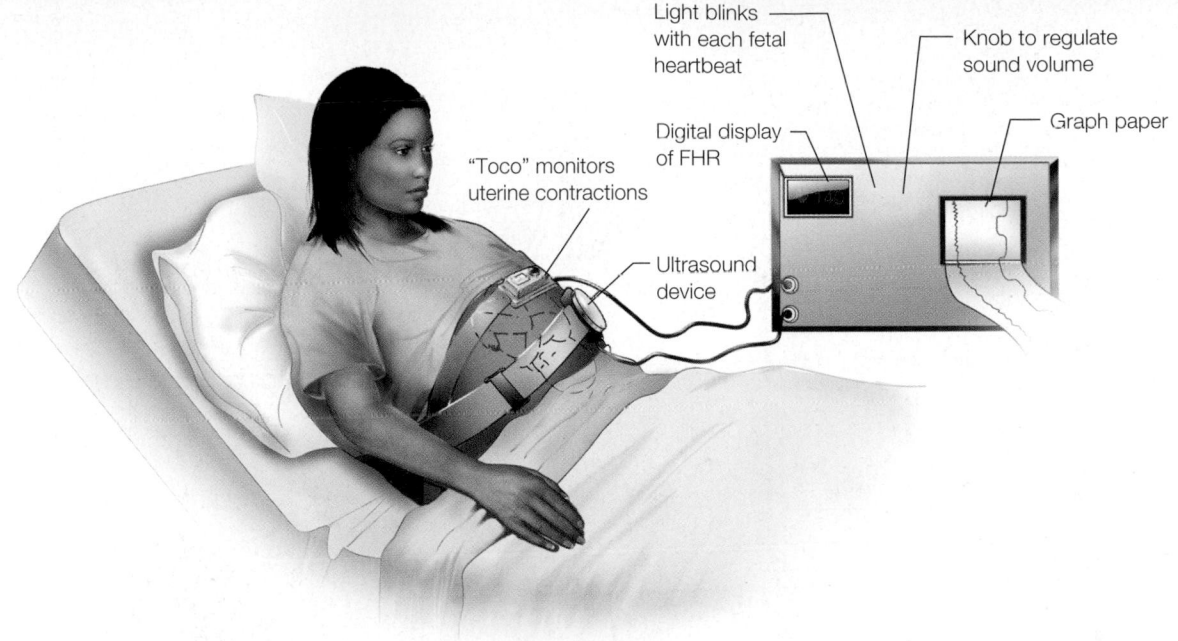

Figure 33–52 ● Electronic fetal monitoring by external technique. The ultrasound device, placed over the fetal back, transmits information on the fetal heart rate. Information from both the tocodynamometer and ultrasound device is transmitted to the electronic fetal monitor. The FHR is indicated in four ways: on the digital display, as a blinking light, by sound, and on special monitor paper. The uterine contractions are displayed on the graph paper.

during labor. Many of the newer models can also be worn in the tub and can be completely submerged in water, making a more natural birthing experience possible even for clients who require continuous monitoring for medical indications. In contrast, the system depicted in Figure 33–52 requires the laboring woman to remain close to the electrical power source for the monitor.

Internal monitoring requires an internal spiral electrode. Women who require internal monitoring are typically confined to bed and cannot ambulate. To place the spiral electrode on the fetal occiput, the amniotic membranes must be ruptured, the cervix must be dilated at least 2 cm (0.08 in.), the presenting part must be down against the cervix, and the presenting part must be known (i.e., the nurse must be able to detect the actual part of the fetus that is down against the cervix). If all these factors are present, the labor and birth nurse (if specialty training has been completed), the physician or CNM inserts a sterile internal spiral electrode into the vagina and places it against the fetal head. The spiral electrode is rotated clockwise until it is attached to the scalp. It is essential that the electrode not be placed over the eye or a fontanelle, so the fetal position must be determined before a scalp electrode is applied. Wires that extend from the spiral electrode are attached to a leg plate (placed on the woman's thigh) and then attached to the electronic fetal monitor. This method of monitoring the FHR provides more accurate continuous data than external monitoring because the signal is clearer and movement of the fetus or the woman does not interrupt it (**Figure 33–53 ●**).

Note that the metric system is used for measurement in labor and delivery. Dilation of the cervix is measured in centimeters, for example.

The FHR tracing at the top of **Figure 33–54 ●** was obtained by internal monitoring with a spiral electrode; the uterine contraction tracing at the bottom of the figure was obtained by external monitoring with a toco. Note that the FHR is variable (the tracing moves up and down instead of in a straight line). In Figure 33–54, each dark vertical line represents 1 minute; therefore, contractions are occurring about every 2.5–3 minutes. The FHR is evaluated by assessing an electronic monitor tracing for baseline rate, baseline variability, and periodic changes.

BASELINE FETAL HEART RATE
The **baseline fetal heart rate** refers to the average FHR rounded to increments of 5 bpm observed during a 10-minute period of monitoring. This excludes periodic or episodic changes, periods of marked variability, and segments of the baseline that differ by more than 25 bpm. The duration should be at least 2 minutes (Macones et al., 2008). Normal FHR (baseline rate) ranges from 110 to 160 bpm. There are two abnormal variations of the baseline rate—those above 160 bpm (tachycardia) and those below 110 bpm (bradycardia). Another change affecting the baseline is called **baseline FHR variability**, which is fluctuation in the FHR baseline of 2 cycles per minute or greater, with irregular amplitude and inconstant frequency (Cunningham et al., 2010).

A **wandering baseline** is a smooth, meandering, unsteady baseline in the normal range without variability (Cunningham et al., 2010). Possible causes for this pattern include congenital defects or metabolic acidosis. Immediate interventions are needed in order to enhance fetal oxygenation. Birth should be anticipated (Hamilton & Warrick, 2013).

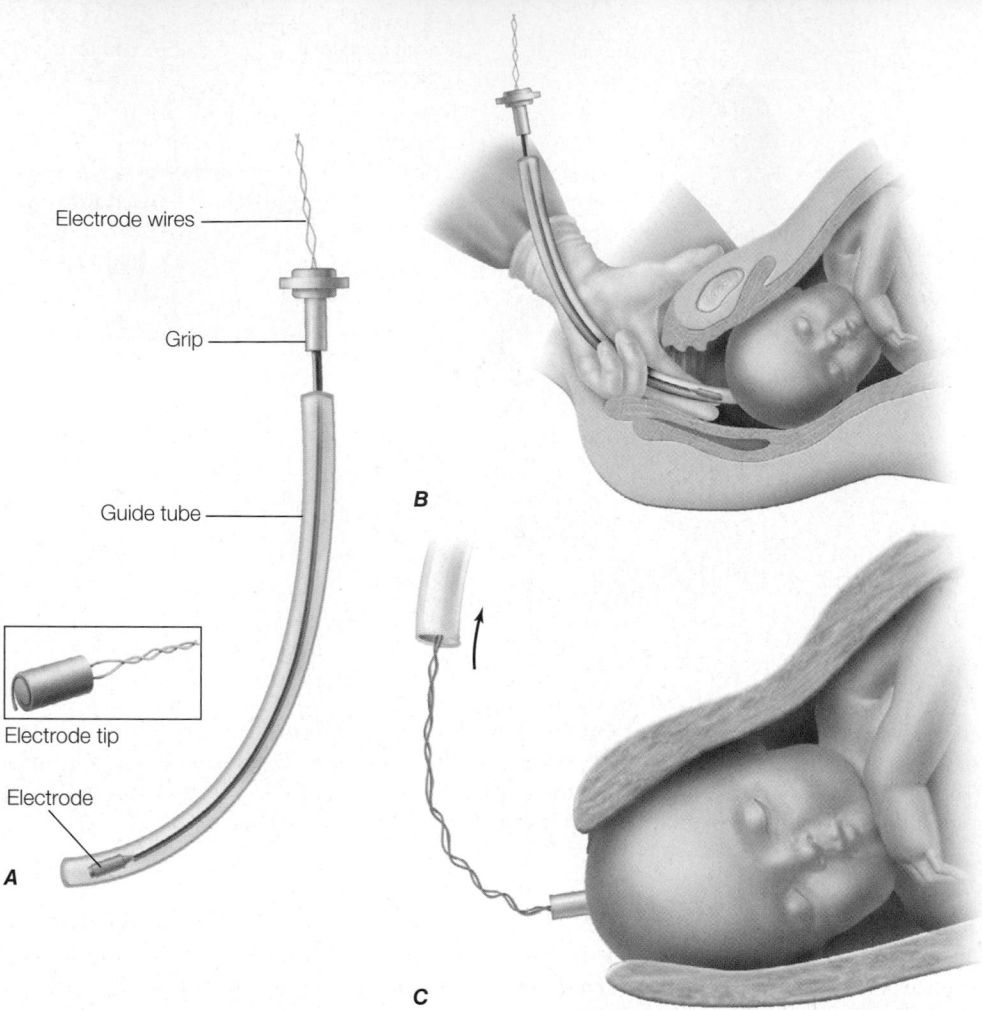

Electrode wires

Grip

Guide tube

Electrode tip

Electrode

A

B

C

Figure 33–53 ● Technique for internal, direct fetal monitoring. *A,* Spiral electrode. *B,* Attaching the spiral electrode to the scalp. *C,* Attached spiral electrode with the guide tube removed.

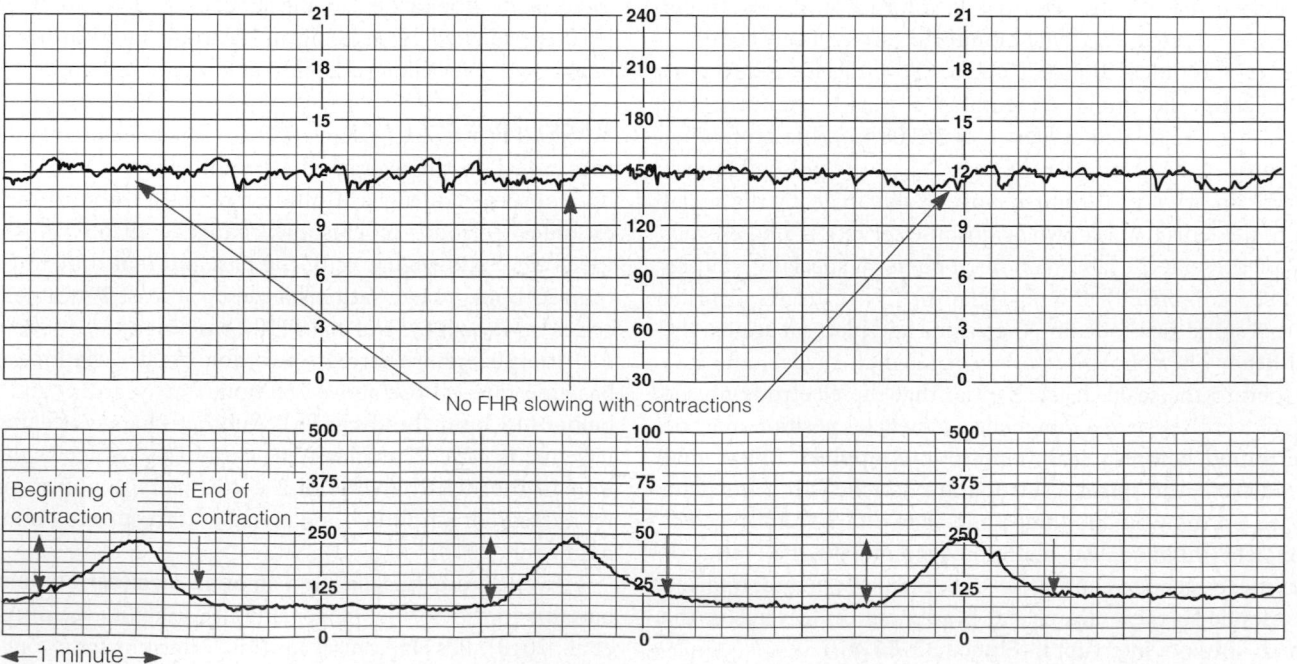

No FHR slowing with contractions

Beginning of contraction   End of contraction

←—1 minute—→

Figure 33–54 ● Normal fetal heart rate range is from 110 to 160 bpm. The FHR tracing in the upper portion of the graph indicates an FHR range of 140–155 bpm. The bottom portion depicts uterine contractions. Each dark vertical line marks 1 minute, and each small rectangle represents 10 seconds. The contraction frequency is about every 2.5 minutes, and the duration of the contractions is 50–60 seconds.

Fetal tachycardia is a sustained rate of 160 bpm or above. Marked tachycardia is 180 bpm or above. Causes of tachycardia include the following (Cunningham et al., 2010):

- Early fetal hypoxia, which leads to stimulation of the sympathetic system as the fetus compensates for reduced blood flow
- Maternal fever, which accelerates the metabolism of the fetus
- Maternal dehydration
- Beta sympathomimetic drugs, such as ritodrine, terbutaline, atropine, and isoxsuprine, which have a cardiac stimulant effect
- Amnionitis (fetal tachycardia may be the first sign of developing intrauterine infection)
- Maternal hyperthyroidism (thyroid-stimulating hormones may cross the placenta and stimulate FHR)
- Fetal anemia (the heart rate is increased as a compensatory mechanism to improve tissue perfusion)
- Tachydysrhythmias (fetal dysrhythmias occur in less than 1% of all pregnancies).

Tachycardia is considered to be an ominous sign if it is accompanied by late decelerations, severe variable decelerations, or decreased variability. If tachycardia is associated with maternal fever, treatment may consist of antipyretics and/or antibiotics.

Fetal bradycardia is a rate of less than 110 bpm during a 10-minute period or longer. Causes of fetal bradycardia include the following (Cunningham et al., 2010):

- Late (profound) fetal hypoxia (depression of myocardial activity)
- Maternal hypotension, which results in decreased blood flow to the fetus
- Prolonged umbilical cord compression (fetal baroreceptors are activated by cord compression, and this produces vagal stimulation, which results in decreased FHR)
- Fetal arrhythmia, which is associated with complete heart block in the fetus
- Uterine tachysystole
- Abruptio placentae
- Uterine rupture
- Vagal stimulation in the second stage (because this does not involve hypoxia, the fetus can recover)
- Congenital heart block
- Maternal hypothermia.

Bradycardia may be a benign or an ominous (preterminal) sign. If there is variability, the bradycardia is considered to be benign. Bradycardia accompanied by decreased variability and late decelerations is considered to be ominous and a sign of nonreassuring fetal status (Cunningham et al., 2010).

ARRHYTHMIAS AND DYSRHYTHMIAS Arrhythmias, a term often used interchangeably with dysrhythmias, are disturbances in the FHR pattern that are not associated with abnormal electrical impulse formation or conduction in the fetal cardiac tissue but are related to a structural abnormality or congenital heart disease (Tucker, Miller, & Miller, 2008). Fetal arrhythmias may be detected when listening to the FHR on a fetal monitor. It is important to rule out artifacts or electrical interference, which may occur. Most true arrhythmias are accompanied by baseline bradycardia, baseline tachycardia, or an abrupt baseline spiking. Ninety percent of fetal cardiac arrhythmias are benign. The most common serious arrhythmias are supraventricular tachycardia and complete heart block (Tucker et al., 2008).

VARIABILITY Baseline variability is a measure of the interplay (the push–pull effect) between the sympathetic and parasympathetic nervous systems. Baseline variability is fluctuations in the FHR of two cycles per minute or greater. **Figure 33–55** depicts the different ranges of variability. The amplitudes of the peaks and troughs in beats per minute are defined as follows (Macones et al., 2008):

- *Absent:* amplitude undetectable
- *Minimal:* amplitude detectable but less than 5 bpm
- *Moderate:* amplitude 6–25 bpm
- *Marked:* amplitude greater than 25 bpm.

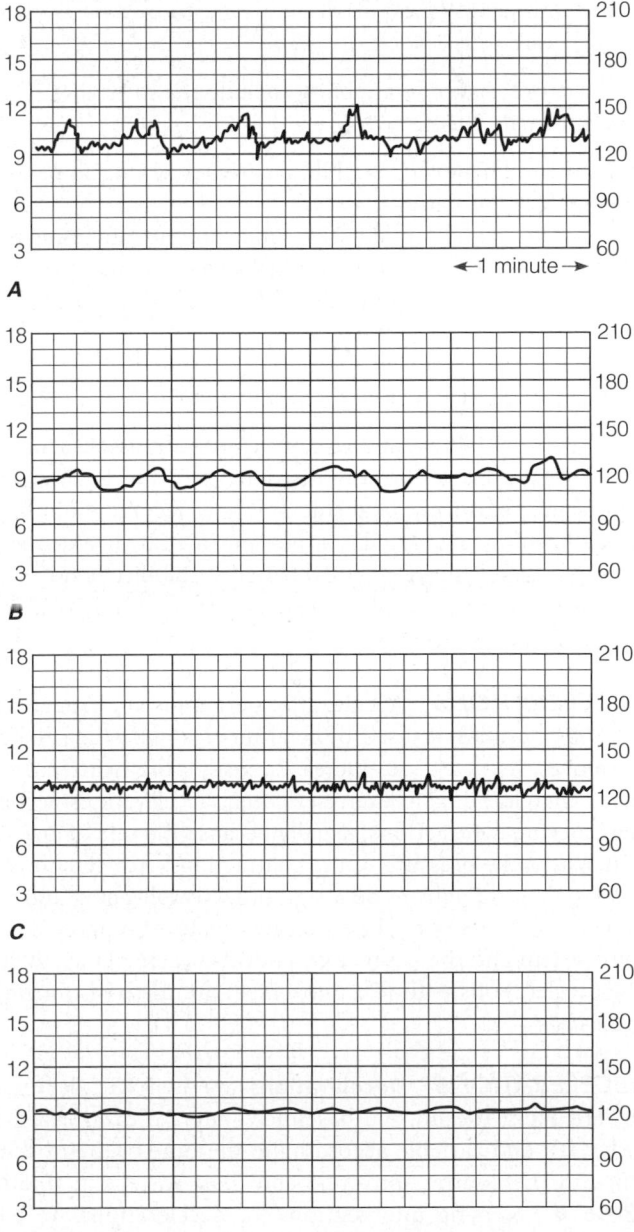

Figure 33–55 ● Variability. *A*, Marked variability. *B*, Moderate variability. *C*, Minimal variability. *D*, Absent variability.

Reduced variability is the best single predictor for determining fetal compromise (Cunningham et al., 2010). Fetal acidosis and subsequent hypoxia are highest in fetuses that have absent or minimal variability.

Causes of decreased variability include the following (Cunningham et al., 2010):

- Hypoxia and acidosis (decreased blood flow to the fetus)
- Administration of drugs such as meperidine hydrochloride (Demerol), diazepam (Valium), or hydroxyzine (Vistaril) that depress the fetal central nervous system
- Fetal sleep cycle (during fetal sleep, variability is decreased; fetal sleep cycles usually last for 20–40 minutes each hour)
- Fetus of less than 32 weeks of gestation (fetal neurological control of heart rate is immature)
- Fetal dysrhythmias
- Fetal anomalies affecting the heart, central nervous system, or autonomic nervous system
- Previous neurological insult
- Tachycardia.

Causes of marked variability include the following (Cunningham et al., 2010):

- Early mild hypoxia (variability increases as a result of compensatory mechanism)
- Fetal stimulation or activity (stimulation of autonomic nervous system because of abdominal palpation, maternal vaginal examination, application of spiral electrode on fetal head, or acoustic stimulation)
- Fetal breathing movements
- Advancing gestational age (greater than 30 weeks of gestation).

Absent variability that does not appear to be associated with a fetal sleep cycle or the administration of drugs is a warning sign of nonreassuring fetal status. It is especially ominous if absent or minimal variability is accompanied by late decelerations (explained shortly). If decreased variability is noted on monitoring, consider application of a spiral electrode to obtain more accurate information.

ACCELERATIONS Accelerations are transient increases in the FHR normally caused by fetal movement. When the fetus moves, its heart rate increases, just as the heart rates of adults increase during exercise. Often, accelerations accompany uterine contractions, usually because the fetus moves in response to the pressure of the contractions. Accelerations of this type are thought to be a sign of fetal well-being and adequate oxygen reserve. They indicate a mature autonomic nervous system and the absence of acidosis (Tucker et al., 2008). The accelerations with fetal movement are the basis for nonstress tests.

DECELERATIONS Decelerations are periodic decreases in FHR from the normal baseline. They are categorized as early, late, and variable according to the time of their occurrence in the contraction cycle and their waveform (**Figure 33–56 ●**). Nursing interventions for decelerations are outlined in **Table 33–13 ●**.

When the fetal head is compressed, cerebral blood flow is decreased, which leads to central vagal stimulation and results in **early deceleration**. The onset of early deceleration is associated with the onset of the uterine contraction. This type of deceleration is of uniform shape, is usually considered to be benign, and does not require intervention.

SAFETY ALERT
The presence of repetitive early decelerations may be a sign of advanced dilation or the beginning of the second stage of labor. If the monitoring strip shows reoccurring early decelerations, ask the laboring woman whether she is experiencing any pressure. Pressure that occurs only with the contractions typically indicates advanced dilation. Intense pressure that does not change or ease up when the contractions cease may indicate the beginning of the second stage. A vaginal examination may be performed to establish the amount of dilation.

Late deceleration is caused by uteroplacental insufficiency resulting from decreased blood flow and oxygen transfer to the fetus through the intervillous spaces during uterine contractions. The most common causes of late decelerations are maternal hypotension resulting from the administration of epidural anesthesia and uterine tachysystole associated with oxytocin infusion. Maternal hypertension, diabetes, collagen vascular disorders, and placenta abruption are also causative factors (Cunningham et al., 2010). The onset of the deceleration occurs after the onset of a uterine contraction and is of a uniform shape that tends to reflect associated uterine contractions. The late deceleration pattern is considered to be a nonreassuring sign and requires continuous assessment. If late decelerations continue and birth is not imminent, a cesarean birth may be indicated.

Variable decelerations occur if the umbilical cord becomes compressed, reducing blood flow between the placenta and fetus. The resulting increase in peripheral resistance in the fetal circulation causes fetal hypertension. Fetal hypertension stimulates the baroreceptors in the aortic arch and carotid sinuses, slowing the FHR. The onset of variable decelerations varies in timing with the onset of the contraction, and the decelerations are variable in shape. This pattern requires further assessment.

A sinusoidal pattern appears similar to a waveform. The characteristics of this pattern include absence of variability and the presence of a smooth, wave-like shape. The pattern resembles a perfect letter "S" lying on its side. These patterns can be pseudosinusoidal (benign) or true sinusoidal. The true pattern is associated with Rh alloimmunization, fetal anemia, severe fetal hypoxia, umbilical cord occlusion, twin-to-twin transfusion, or a chronic fetal bleed. Pseudosinusoidal patterns are usually temporary and commonly occur with the administration of medications such as meperidine (Demerol) or butorphanol tartrate (Stadol) (Cunningham et al., 2010).

Decelerations are also classified based on the rate in which the FHR leaves the baseline FHR:

- *Abrupt decelerations* occur in less than 30 seconds (Macones et al., 2008).
- *Variable decelerations* descend abruptly.

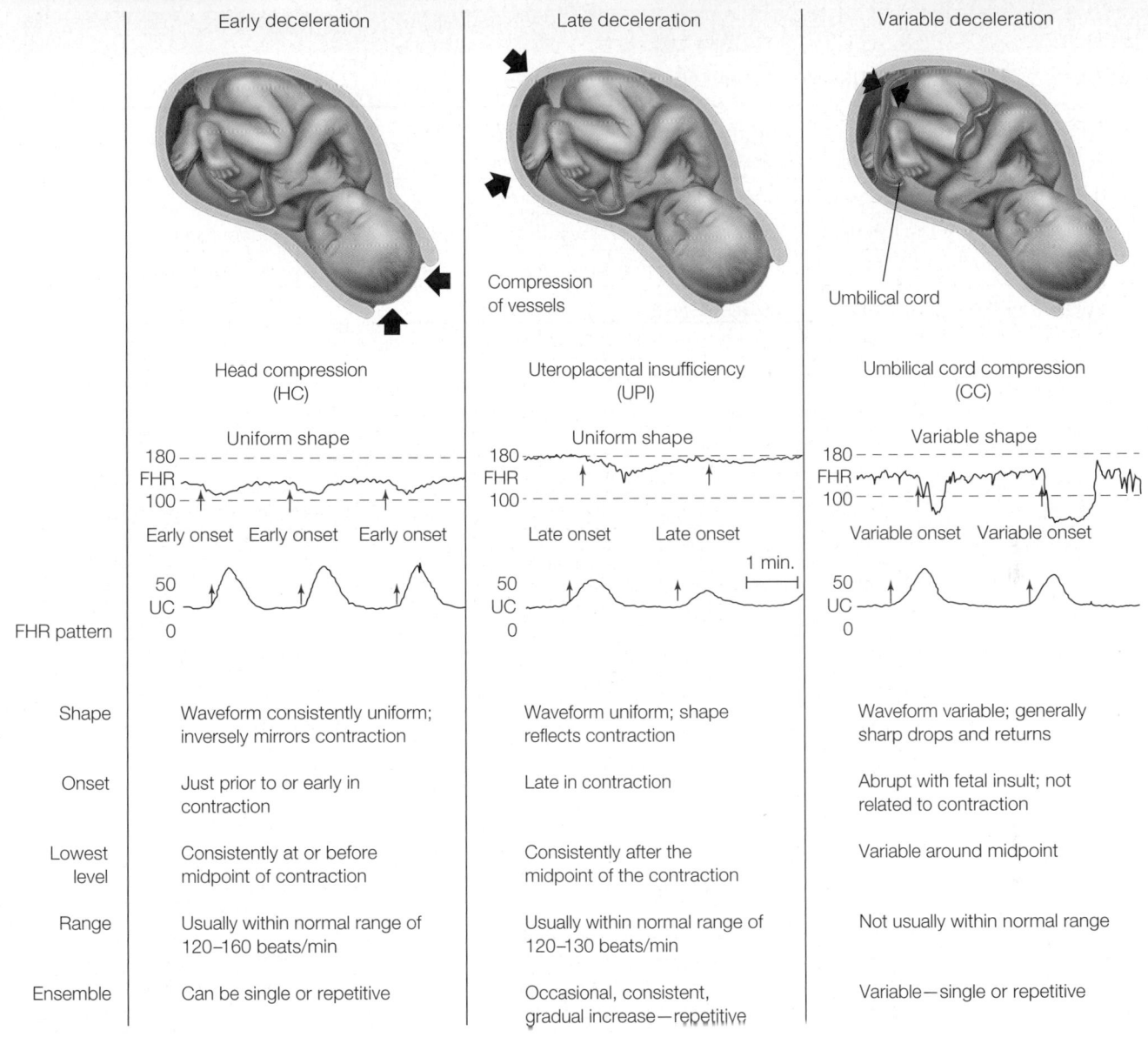

	Early deceleration	Late deceleration	Variable deceleration
	Head compression (HC)	Uteroplacental insufficiency (UPI)	Umbilical cord compression (CC)
Shape	Waveform consistently uniform; inversely mirrors contraction	Waveform uniform; shape reflects contraction	Waveform variable; generally sharp drops and returns
Onset	Just prior to or early in contraction	Late in contraction	Abrupt with fetal insult; not related to contraction
Lowest level	Consistently at or before midpoint of contraction	Consistently after the midpoint of the contraction	Variable around midpoint
Range	Usually within normal range of 120–160 beats/min	Usually within normal range of 120–130 beats/min	Not usually within normal range
Ensemble	Can be single or repetitive	Occasional, consistent, gradual increase—repetitive	Variable—single or repetitive

Figure 33–56 ● Types and characteristics of early, late, and variable decelerations.

- *Gradual decelerations* require 30 seconds or more to descend. Both early and late decelerations descend gradually.
- *Episodic decelerations* occur independently of the uterine contractions and are frequently the result of external stimulations, such as vaginal exams.
- *Periodic decelerations* refer to decelerations that occur with the contractions and are considered to be repetitive if they occur with 50% of the contractions
- *Prolonged decelerations* are those that leave the baseline for more than 2 minutes but less than 10 minutes.

EVALUATION OF FETAL HEART RATE TRACINGS

Evaluation of the electronic monitor tracing begins by looking at the uterine contraction pattern. To evaluate the contraction pattern, the nurse does the following:

1. Determine the uterine resting tone.
2. Assess the contractions: What is the frequency? What is the duration? What is the intensity?

The next step is to evaluate the FHR tracing as follows:

1. Determine the baseline: Is the baseline within the normal range? Is there evidence of tachycardia? Is there evidence of bradycardia?
2. Determine FHR variability: Is variability absent? Minimal? Moderate? Marked?
3. Determine whether a sinusoidal pattern is present.
4. Determine whether there are periodic changes: Are accelerations present? Do they meet the criteria for a reactive nonstress test? Are decelerations present? Are they uniform in shape? If so, determine whether they are early or late decelerations. Are they nonuniform in shape? If so, determine whether they are variable decelerations.

After evaluating the FHR tracing for the factors just listed, the nurse may further classify the tracing as reassuring (normal) or nonreassuring (worrisome). Reassuring patterns contain normal parameters and do not require additional treatment

TABLE 33–13   Guidelines for Management of Variable, Late, and Prolonged Deceleration Patterns

PATTERN	NURSING INTERVENTIONS
Variable decelerations	Report findings to physician/CNM and document in chart.
	Provide explanation to woman and partner.
Isolated or occasional, moderate	Change maternal position to one in which FHR pattern is most improved.
	Perform vaginal examination to assess for prolapsed cord or change in labor progress.
	Monitor FHR continuously to assess current status and for further changes in FHR pattern.
Variable decelerations, severe and uncorrectable	Administer oxygen by face mask at 7–10 L/min.
	Report findings to physician/CNM and document in chart.
	Provide explanation to woman and partner.
	Prepare for probable cesarean birth. Follow interventions previously listed.
	Prepare for vaginal birth unless baseline variability is decreasing or FHR is progressively rising, in which case cesarean, forceps, or vacuum birth is indicated.
	Maintain good hydration with intravenous (IV) fluids (normal saline or lactated Ringer solution).
Late decelerations	Administer oxygen by face mask at 7–10 L/min.
	Report findings to physician/CNM and document in chart.
	Provide explanation to woman and partner.
	Monitor for further FHR changes. Maintain maternal position on left side.
	Maintain good hydration with intravenous (IV) fluids (normal saline or lactated Ringer solution).
	Discontinue oxytocin if it is being administered and late decelerations persist despite other interventions.
	Monitor maternal blood pressure and pulse for signs of hypotension; possibly increase flow rate of IV fluids to treat hypotension.
	Follow orders of physician/CNM for treatment for hypotension if present.
	Increase IV fluids to maintain volume and hydration (normal saline or lactated Ringer solution).
	Assess labor progress (dilation and station).
Late decelerations with tachycardia or decreasing variability	Report findings to physician/CNM and document in chart.
	Maintain maternal position on left side.
	Administer oxygen by face mask at 7–10 L/min.
	Discontinue oxytocin if it is being administered.
	Assess maternal blood pressure and pulse.
	Increase IV fluids (normal saline or lactated Ringer solution).
	Assess labor progress (dilation and station).
	Prepare for immediate cesarean birth.
	Explain plan of treatment to woman and partner.
	Assist physician/CNM with fetal blood sampling (if ordered).
Prolonged decelerations	Perform vaginal examination to rule out prolapsed cord or to determine progress in labor status.
	Change maternal position as needed to try to alleviate decelerations.
	Discontinue oxytocin if it is being administered.
	Notify physician/CNM of findings/initial interventions and document in chart.
	Provide explanation to woman and partner.
	Increase IV fluids (normal saline or lactated Ringer solution).
	Administer tocolytic if hypertonus noted and if ordered by physician/CNM.
	Anticipate normal FHR recovery following deceleration if FHR previously normal.
	Anticipate intervention if FHR previously abnormal or deceleration lasts >3 minutes.

or intervention. Characteristics of reassuring FHR patterns include the following:

- Baseline rate is 110–160 bpm.
- Variability is present.
- Variability is at least two cycles per minute. Periodic patterns consist of accelerations with fetal movement, and early decelerations may be present.

Nonreassuring patterns may indicate that the fetus is becoming stressed and intervention is needed. Characteristics of nonreassuring patterns include the following:

- Severe variable decelerations (FHR drops below 70 bpm for longer than 30–45 seconds and is accompanied by rising baseline or decreasing variability or slow return to baseline.)
- Late decelerations of any magnitude
- Absence of variability
- Prolonged deceleration (a deceleration that lasts 60–90 seconds or more)
- Severe (marked) bradycardia (FHR baseline of 70 bpm or less).

Nonreassuring patterns may require continuous monitoring and more involved treatment and intervention (see Table 33–13).

After evaluating the FHR tracing for the factors listed, the nurse may categorize the tracing according to the Three-Tier Fetal Heart Rate Interpretation System shown in **Box 33–6**. The three-tier system for the categorization of FHR patterns is recommended by ACOG, Association of Women's Health, Obstetric, and Neonatal Nurses (AWHONN), and the National Institute of Child Health and Human Development (Macones et al., 2008). Categorization of the FHR tracing evaluates the fetus at that point in time; tracing patterns can and will change. A FHR tracing may move back and forth between categories

depending on the clinical situation and management strategies employed.

Category I FHR tracings are normal. They are strongly predictive of normal fetal acid–base status at the time of observation. The FHR tracings may be followed in a routine manner, and no specific action is required.

Category II FHR tracings are indeterminate. They are not predictive of abnormal fetal acid–base status, yet we do not have adequate evidence at present to classify these as Category I or Category III. Category II tracings require evaluation and continued surveillance and reevaluation, taking into account the entire associated clinical circumstances.

Category III FHR tracings are abnormal. They are predictive of abnormal fetal acid–base status at the time of observation. They require prompt evaluation. Depending on the clinical situation, efforts to expeditiously resolve the abnormal FHR pattern may include, but are not limited to, provision of maternal oxygen, change in maternal position, discontinuation of labor stimulation, and treatment of maternal hypotension.

It is important to provide information to the laboring woman regarding the FHR pattern and the interventions that will help her fetus. Sharing information with the laboring woman reassures her that a potential or actual problem has been identified and that she is an active participant in the interventions. Occasionally, a problem arises that requires immediate intervention. In that case, the nurse can say something like "It is important for you to turn on your side right now because the baby is having a little difficulty. I'll explain what is happening in just a few moments." This type of response lets the woman know that although an action needs to be accomplished rapidly, information will soon be provided. In the

---

Box 33–6 The Three-Tier Fetal Heart Rate Interpretation System

CATEGORY I

Category I FHR tracings include *all* of the following:

- Baseline rate: 110–160 bpm
- Baseline FHR variability: moderate
- Late or variable decelerations: absent
- Early decelerations: present or absent
- Accelerations: present or absent.

CATEGORY II

Category II FHR tracings include all FHR tracings not categorized as Category I or Category III. Category II tracings may represent an appreciable fraction of those encountered in clinical care. Examples of Category II FHR tracings include any of the following:

- Baseline rate
  - Bradycardia not accompanied by absent baseline variability
  - Tachycardia
- Baseline FHR variability
  - Minimal baseline variability
  - Absent baseline variability not accompanied by recurrent decelerations
  - Marked baseline variability

- Accelerations
  - Absence of induced accelerations after fetal stimulation
- Periodic or episodic decelerations
  - Recurrent variable decelerations accompanied by minimal or moderate baseline variability
  - Prolonged deceleration of 2 minutes or more but less than 10 minutes
  - Recurrent late decelerations with moderate baseline variability
  - Variable decelerations with other characteristics, such as slow return to baseline, "overshoots," or "shoulders."

CATEGORY III

Category III FHR tracings include:

- Absent baseline FHR variability and any of the following:
  - Recurrent late decelerations
  - Recurrent variable decelerations
  - Bradycardia
- Sinusoidal pattern.

Source: Macones, G. A., Hankins, G. D. V., Spong, C. Y., Hauth, J., & Moore, T. (2008). The 2008 National Institute of Child Health and Human Development Workshop report on electronic monitoring: Update on definitions, interpretation, and research guidelines. *The Journal of Obstetrics, Gynecology, and Neonatal Nursing, 37*(5), 510–515.

haste to act quickly, the nurse must not forget that it is the woman's body and her baby.

Labor and birth nurses must be skilled and competent in evaluating electronic FHR patterns and responding appropriately (see Table 33–13). Competence can be maintained through frequent in-services, formal courses, and continuing education programs.

RESPONSES TO ELECTRONIC MONITORING Responses to electronic fetal monitoring can be varied and complex. Many women have little knowledge of monitoring unless they have attended a prenatal class that dealt with this subject. Some women react to electronic monitoring positively, viewing it as a reassurance that "the baby is okay." They may also feel the monitor helps identify problems that develop in labor. Other women may have ambivalent or even negative feelings about the monitor. They may think the monitor is interfering with a natural process, and they do not want the intrusion. They may resent the time and attention that the monitor requires—time that could otherwise be spent providing nursing care. Some women may find that the equipment, wires, and sounds increase their anxiety. The discomfort of lying in one position and fear of injury to the baby are other objections.

Cord Blood Analysis at Birth

When significant abnormal FHR patterns have been noted, meconium-stained amniotic fluid is present, or the infant is depressed at birth, umbilical cord blood may be analyzed immediately following the birth to determine whether acidosis is present. The American Academy of Pediatrics (AAP) and ACOG (2013) recommend performing cord blood analyses when the Apgar score is below seven at 5 minutes of age (normal Apgar score is 7–10).

The cord is clamped before the infant takes the first breath. Using a third hemostat, the healthcare provider clamps a 20- to 25-cm (8- to 10-in.) portion of the umbilical cord. A small amount of blood (1.0 mL is required for a full panel) is aspirated with a syringe from one of the umbilical arteries or from an artery and a vein. If the cord blood will not be analyzed immediately, a heparinized syringe should be used. Normal fetal blood pH is above 7.25 (ACOG, 2012b). Lower levels indicate acidosis and hypoxia. Many healthcare providers order cord blood analysis to minimize medicolegal exposure.

Diagnosis

In the first stage of labor, appropriate nursing diagnoses may include the following:

- *Fear/Anxiety* related to discomfort of labor and unknown labor outcome
- *Acute Pain* related to uterine contractions, cervical dilation, and fetal descent
- *Readiness for Enhanced Childbearing Process* related to the normal labor process and comfort measures.

(NANDA-I © 2015)

In the second and third stages of labor, appropriate nursing diagnoses may include the following:

- *Acute Pain* related to uterine contractions, the birth process, and/or perineal trauma from birth
- *Readiness for Enhanced Childbearing Process* related to pushing methods to assist in the birth
- *Fear/Anxiety* related to the outcome of the birth process.

(NANDA-I © 2015)

In the fourth stage of labor, possible nursing diagnoses include the following:

- *Acute Pain* related to perineal trauma
- *Readiness for Enhanced Childbearing Process* related to the involution process and self-care needs
- *Readiness for Enhanced Family Processes* related to incorporation of the newborn into the family.

(NANDA-I © 2015)

Planning

When a plan of care is devised for the intrapartum period, the nurse can develop a general plan that encompasses the total process, from the beginning of labor through the fourth stage, or a plan can be developed for each stage of labor and birth. For instance, if the woman and her support person did not have the opportunity to attend childbirth education classes, a nursing goal is to provide desired information. To accomplish this goal, the nurse assesses the current level of the couple's understanding and then plans to provide brief explanations as labor progresses.

Implementation

The client in labor and her partner or support person tend to be concerned about arriving at the birth center in time for the birth. Sometimes, the labor is advanced and birth is imminent, but usually the woman is in early labor at admission. If time permits and the family is not familiar with what will occur during labor, the nurse can provide necessary information (see the Client Teaching feature).

Integrate Cultural Beliefs

Knowledge of values, customs, and practices of various cultures is as important during labor as it is in the prenatal period. Without this knowledge, a nurse is less likely to understand a family's behavior and may attempt to impose his or her personal values and beliefs on the woman and her family. As cultural sensitivity and competence increases, so does the likelihood of providing satisfying, high-quality care (Spector, 2017). In providing culturally appropriate care, it is important to familiarize yourself with cultural beliefs from various cultures. Be aware that examples regarding any culture or belief system need to be viewed as background information only. The understanding that individuals have unique cultural perspectives and may or may not identify to what may be considered their cultural roots or heritage is imperative. While it is important is to be familiar with different belief systems within cultural groups, healthcare providers should be cautioned to avoid making generalizations based on a client's perceived ethnicity, culture, or identity. As cultural understanding continues to emerge as an essential clinical skill, nurses will likely encounter more families with diverse cultural variations, including LGBTQ families (Ingraham, Wingo, Foster, & Roberts, 2017). Familiarizing yourself with the needs of diverse groups allows the nurse to deliver professional, respectful culturally sensitive care in a caring, professional manner. The nurse must always remain aware that an individual example of a birthing practice will never be pertinent to all women in a given group. Within every culture, each individual develops his or her set of beliefs, values, and behaviors. Culture is also discussed in the module on Culture and Diversity.

Client Teaching What to Expect During Labor

- Provide information on the basic assessment and care activities. Allow time for questions and discussion as the progress of labor permits. Describe aspects of the admission process, including the following:
  - Taking an abbreviated history
  - Physical assessment (maternal vital signs [VS], FHR, contraction status, status of membranes)
  - Assessment of uterine contractions (frequency, duration, intensity)
  - Orientation to surroundings
  - Introductions to other support staff
  - Determination of woman's and any support person's expectations of the nurse.
- Present aspects of ongoing physical care, such as when to expect assessment of maternal VS, FHR, and contractions.
- If the electronic fetal monitor is used, describe how it works and the information it provides. Demonstrate the fetal monitor. Orient the woman to the sights and sounds of the monitor. Explain what "normal" data will look like and what characteristics are being watched for.

- Note that assessments will increase as the labor progresses, especially during the transition phase (usually the time the woman would like to be left alone), to help keep the mother and baby safe by noting deviations from the normal course.
- Describe the vaginal examination and the information it elicits. Use a cervical dilation chart to illustrate the amount of dilation.
- Review comfort techniques that may be used in labor, and ascertain what the woman thinks will promote comfort. Focus on open discussion.
- Review the childbirth preparation the woman has learned so that you will be able to support her in their use. Ask the woman to demonstrate the techniques she has learned.
- Review comfort and support measures, such as positioning, back rub, effleurage, touch, distraction techniques, and ambulation.
- If the woman is in early labor, offer her a tour of the birthing area, and explain equipment and routines. Include the woman's partner.

MODESTY Modesty is an important consideration for most women regardless of culture. Many women are uncomfortable with the degree of exposure needed for certain procedures during the labor and birth process. Many women from a variety of backgrounds find it uncomfortable to be physically examined, so respecting the need for privacy with draping, inquiring the woman if she would like family members or her partner to leave the room, or other accommodations should be made whenever possible. Some women (including some Muslim women) may be uncomfortable when men are present and may feel more comfortable with women; others may be uncomfortable with exposure regardless of the gender of the healthcare providers. By explaining that examinations and assessments will need to be done, the nurse can explain that privacy will be given as much as possible. Questions that ascertain how the nurse can help the laboring woman feel more comfortable related to modesty can help empower the woman and her family to make informed choices and can allow personalization of goals to meet client preferences. It is more prudent to assume that embarrassment will occur with exposure and take measures to provide privacy than to assume that it will not matter to the woman if she is exposed.

While some Orthodox Jewish women may follow specific Jewish laws during the childbearing period, others may not adhere to certain traditional practices and beliefs. When a woman self-identifies with a cultural or religious preference, it is important to ask questions to gain a specific understanding of what that means to her and how she sees it impacting her care needs. For example, according to the law of *Tznuit*, women desire to maintain modesty in order to preserve dignity. For some women, this may be accomplished by providing a long sleeve gown that covers her elbows and knees, whereas other Orthodox Jewish women may voice no preferences. Additionally, it should not be assumed that a woman will wish to wear a hair covering, such as a wig or scarf, based on her stated religious preferences. While an understanding of cultural norms is imperative to provide a basis for a discussion on cultural needs and requests, making generalizations is inappropriate. It is important that the nurse balances

knowledge of cultural and religious beliefs with verbal or behavioral cues that support a woman's preferences. For example, offering to pull the curtain while an Orthodox Jewish woman changes into her client gown shows understanding that some women from this culture would prefer not to change in front of their husbands. For other women, it provides an opportunity for the woman to verbally decline, thus providing cues on her own belief and preferences (Neis, 2017).

EXPRESSION AND MEANING OF PAIN The manner in which a woman chooses to deal with the discomfort of labor varies widely. Some women seem to turn inward and remain very quiet during labor and birth, speaking only to ask others to leave the room or cease conversation. Others may be very vocal, with behaviors such as counting out loud, moaning, crying, or shouting. They may also turn from side to side or change positions frequently, often appearing restless. While some cultural influences impact the labor process, women react to labor based on a variety of factors, with culture being only a single variable; therefore, generalizations should not be used to anticipate a woman's responses. It is important to remember that a client's personal experiences, her own unique biopsychosocial factors, education level, family culture, partner opinions and expectations, and the woman's own perceptions of her preconceived labor responses will all play a part in how she experiences her labor and deals with the discomfort.

For some women from Asian cultures, it is important to act in ways that will not bring shame on the family. For some clients, this may manifest as laboring quietly and not expressing pain. While silence may be culturally more common in some Chinese societies, for example, it does not mean that all Chinese women will value or desire to labor quietly. It is important to explore each client's desires for her labor and to inquire how she would like to help manage her pain. Understanding how the woman wishes to control her labor is important and provides insight for the nurse to assist the woman with meeting her labor and birth expectations so a positive birth experience will occur. This is important because adverse birth events can increase postpartum mood disorders and

2158 Module 33 Reproduction

Focus on Diversity and Culture Childbirth Customs

Various cultures have different customs and beliefs surrounding childbearing and childbirth. Generalizations regarding cultural perspectives are discussed with examples designed to provide students with ways to integrate cultural customs into specific individualized labor and birth options for women.

Some Hmong women from Laos may prefer to stay active during labor. Some may prefer to squat during the second stage of labor. It is not unusual for the partner to be present and actively involved in providing comfort. Some laboring women may prefer only "hot" foods and warm water to drink (Spector, 2017). For some Hmong women, the family may request that the mother be given a soft-boiled egg to restore her energy as soon as birth occurs. The nurse may ask the woman about her own cultural beliefs and obtain specific requests for labor positioning, ambulation in labor, who she would like to provide labor support, preferred birth positions, temperature of oral fluids preferred, and advise her that a regular diet with her own food preferences can begin immediately following a vaginal birth.

Some Vietnamese women may show a strong sense of self-control throughout labor. They may prefer to walk during labor and to give birth in a squatting position. Like other Asian cultures, some may view labor as a "hot condition" and prefer cold beverages; however, during the postpartum period, which is viewed as a "cold" condition, she will prefer warm liquids (Kim, 2017). In some cultures, newborn praise can be perceived negatively, sometimes being referred to as is the "evil eye" which is associated with jealousy (Lloreda-Garcia, 2017).

It has been noted that in certain Latina subcultures women desire to have their partners present during labor and birth to provide support and reassure. As they labor, the women want their partners to show their love and to speak using affectionate words. Many Latina women also typically want their mothers present during the birth process (Attanasio, Hardeman, Kozhimannil, & Kjerulff, 2017). Again, knowledge of traditional cultural norms can provide the nurse with knowledge to effectively coordinate care for the woman and her family. The nurse may ask who the primary support person will be, others she may wish to have present during labor and birth, and preferences for medication to assist with pain. Cultural norms should guide, not dictate, the assessment process.

Some Muslim women may have their husband present whereas others may desire a female friend or relative with them during childbirth. Some fathers have a more passive, hands-off approach, speaking up only as an advocate as needed. Because modesty is of great concern for many Muslim women, care must be taken to cover the woman as much as possible (Spector, 2017). She may want to put her *khimar* (head covering) on before a male enters the room. For some Muslim families, it may be important for a female nurse, physician, or CNM to perform examinations when possible. Nurses should inquire about specific preferences if a male healthcare provider may be involved in a patient's care, such as a pediatrician or nurse. For women who express a preference for female care providers, it is important to discuss the possibility that a female provider may not always be present and that if a male is required, every effort to provide privacy and advanced notice will be given (Davidson, Ladewig, London, 2017). Some women may want their husbands to remain in the room in these circumstances. For some Muslim patients, traditions such as calling praise to Allah (*adhan*) into the newborn's right ear and cleaning the newborn may be requested. Familiarity with cultural norms is important as it shows a genuine respect for others personal and cultural beliefs (Spector, 2017).

Different religious practices are observed throughout the world. Some Orthodox Jewish women observe the law of *niddah*, which begins with the onset of regular uterine contractions or the appearance of bloody show or membrane rupture. Once this occurs, the *niddah* law mandates a physical separation of husband and wife (Neis, 2017). For couples who adhere to traditional beliefs, there is usually a lack of physical contact once this has occurred, although many fathers remain in the room or just outside the curtain around the bed. The nurse should inquire about specific observations so the best support and encouragement for the mother can be provided. If couples describe the preference for limited physical contact, it is important to remember that the nurse will need to assist the woman and serve as the primary caretaker. Sometimes, the laboring woman's mother or another female friend or relative may be present (Neis, 2017). During this time period, the father may read prayers, choose not to observe the birth, and wait to reenter the room until after the woman has completed the third stage of labor and has been assisted in resuming a comfortable position in bed.

can even create trauma which can have lasting psychological issues that persist for future pregnancies (DeGroot & Vik, 2017).

Another example is that while Japan may have a higher natural childbirth rate, it does not mean that all women of Japanese descent will desire a natural childbirth. While cultural background and heritage can be used to provide a basis for conversation and generate questions, the woman's own personal preferences and her personal goals and expectations are paramount in ensuring a positive birth experience.

Cultural norms can impact a woman's desire for who she would prefer to be present at her birth. For example, some Mexican women value support from female relatives and midwives throughout their pregnancy and childbirth experience; but the nurse should not assume that a woman accompanied by her mother and midwife does not also want her partner present at the birth. In order to integrate cultural beliefs and personal beliefs, the nurse should show cultural sensitivity and have knowledge of

cultural norms, yet show openness and acceptance to encourage the woman to describe her own needs and expectations.

Women demonstrate a wide variety of behaviors in response to pain, from silence to shouting. The nurse supports a woman's individual expression, as long as it is not harmful, in order to enhance the birthing experience for mother, baby, and family. Different cultures also have differing beliefs about the meaning and value of labor pain. Because childbearing is considered by ancient Chinese custom to be a woman's "career," some older adults may advise the pregnant woman not to fear childbirth. Other cultural assumptions, such as Latino culture, may view pain during labor as a symbol of love toward the baby—the more intense the pain, the more intense the love. As in all cultures, beliefs that were strongly held by one generation may change over time. External factors, such as immigration to other geographic areas, family influences, changes in cultural norms, and age can all impact cultural beliefs.

In the past, many Native American women viewed labor pain as natural and many used meditation, self-control, or indigenous plants or herbs, such as black cohosh, throughout their labor to aid them during birth (Spector, 2017). While some Native women may still adhere to these practices, others may no longer adhere to these beliefs and may want more modern approaches used to control pain. While some women may value pain as aiding in the birth of their baby and signaling that all is well, others may be irritable about the intensity of the pain and fear losing control. Labor and delivery nurses can provide culturally competent care by becoming acquainted with the beliefs and practices of the various subcultures while assessing each woman for her own unique preferences within a cultural context. In the birthing situation, the truly effective nurse supports the family's cultural practices as long as it is safe to do so. Do not assume, however, that a woman's preferences will always follow the norms of her ethnic or cultural group. Instead, the nurse assesses her individualized preferences and wishes.

Provide Nursing Care on Admission

The manner in which the maternity nurse greets the laboring woman and her partner influences the course of the woman's hospital stay. The arrival at the healthcare setting and the sometimes impersonal and technical aspects of admission can produce profound stress, fear, and anxiety. If women and their families are greeted in a brusque, harried manner, they are less likely to look to the nurse for support. A calm, pleasant manner indicates to the woman that she is important. It helps to instill in the couple a sense of confidence in the staff's ability to provide quality care during this critical time.

Following the initial greeting, the nurse escorts the client and support person to the birthing room and provides a quick yet thorough orientation to the facility, including the location of the restrooms, public phones, and nurse-call or emergency-call system. These simple steps can go a long way toward helping the couple feel more at ease. The nurse also explains the monitoring equipment or other unfamiliar technology. Every effort needs to be made to demystify the environment for the laboring woman and her support person. Some women prefer that their partner remain with them during the admission process, although others prefer to have the partner wait outside.

As the nurse helps the woman undress and get into a hospital gown, he or she can start to develop rapport and begin the assessment process. The experienced labor and birth nurse can obtain essential information about the woman and her pregnancy, initiate any immediate interventions needed, and establish individualized priorities and preferences within a few minutes after admission. Forming realistic objectives for laboring women is a major challenge for nurses, because each woman has different coping mechanisms and support systems.

Laboring women often face a number of unfamiliar procedures that may seem routine for healthcare providers. It is important to remember that all clients have the right to accept or reject care measures. The client's informed consent is needed before any procedure that involves touching her body. The admission process, therefore, includes signing an informed consent for treatment and providing information regarding advanced directives. Typically, an identification bracelet and an allergy band are attached to the expectant woman's wrist.

Laboring families have specific expectations of the labor and birth experience, of themselves, of the nurse, and of the physician or CNM. Sometimes, families have unrealistic expectations, which can increase anxiety, create stress, and end in disappointment if expectations are not met. The nurse should encourage all families to discuss their preferences and special requests. Some families may present to the birthing center with a birth plan. Reviewing the plan provides the nurse with the opportunity to explore the family's wishes. If requests cannot be met, explain the reasons thoroughly. All members of the healthcare team need to be informed of the family's requests.

Some families want the nurse present at all times, whereas others desire privacy and want to spend time alone. Couples may want a great deal of support if they have not attended childbirth education classes or if they are anxious. Others may want to enjoy the experience as a couple, with as few outside interruptions as possible. In this case, the nurse informs the couple of the nurse's availability and of the need to make intermittent assessments.

If indicated, the nurse assists the client into bed. A side-lying or semi-Fowler position rather than a supine position is most comfortable and prevents supine hypotensive syndrome (vena caval syndrome). After obtaining the essential information from the client and her records, the nurse begins the intrapartum assessment. Once the assessment is complete, the nurse can make effective nursing decisions about intrapartum care, including the following:

- Should ambulation, bed rest, or a combination of both be encouraged?
- Is more frequent or continuous electronic fetal monitoring needed?
- What preferences does the woman have for her labor and birth?
- Is a support person available?
- What special needs do this woman and her partner have?

The nurse auscultates the FHR. The nurse assesses the client's blood pressure, pulse, respirations, oral temperature, and level of pain or discomfort. The nurse also assesses contraction frequency, duration, and intensity (possibly while gathering other data). Before the vaginal examination, the nurse informs the client about the procedure and its purpose and obtains her consent; afterward, the nurse conveys the findings.

If signs of advanced labor are observed, a vaginal examination must be done immediately upon admission. If the woman shows signs of excessive bleeding or reports episodes of painless bleeding in the last trimester, refrain from performing a vaginal examination and notify the physician or CNM immediately.

Results of the FHR assessment, uterine contraction evaluation, and vaginal examination help determine whether the rest of the admission process can proceed at a leisurely pace or whether additional interventions are required. For example, an FHR of less than 110 bpm on auscultation indicates that a fetal monitor should be applied immediately to obtain additional data and that continuous fetal monitoring should be performed. The client's vital signs can be assessed once the monitor is in place.

SAFETY ALERT

If the fetal monitor is no longer recording the fetal heart tracing, check for adequate gel under the transducer and reposition it before assuming there is a problem with the fetus. Maternal and fetal movement are the most common causes of an inability to trace the FHR.

The admission process includes collecting a clean, voided, midstream urine specimen. The client with intact membranes may collect her specimen in the bathroom. Decisions regarding activity level are generally based on physical findings, clinician orders, the client's desires, agency policy, and safety concerns.

The nurse may test the woman's urine for the presence of protein, ketones, and glucose by using a dipstick before sending the sample to the laboratory. This procedure is especially important if edema or elevated blood pressure is noted on admission. Proteinuria of +1 or more may be a sign of impending preeclampsia. Glycosuria is frequently found in pregnant women because of the increased glomerular filtration rate in the proximal tubules and the inability of these tubules to increase reabsorption of glucose. It may also be associated with gestational diabetes, however, and should not be discounted. While the client is collecting the urine specimen, the nurse can gather the equipment for any preparation procedures ordered by the physician or CNM.

Laboratory tests are done during early admission. Hemoglobin and hematocrit values help determine the oxygen-carrying capacity of the circulatory system and the woman's ability to withstand blood loss at birth. Elevation of the hematocrit may indicate hemoconcentration of blood, which occurs with edema or dehydration. A low hemoglobin value, in the absence of other evidence of bleeding, suggests anemia. Blood may be typed and crossmatched if the woman is in a high-risk category. Platelets are evaluated as well, because low platelets can lead to bleeding problems. Low platelets are also a contraindication for epidural anesthesia. In addition, a type and screen is performed in case an obstetric emergency arises and the woman needs to get blood products. Additional serological testing may be performed as indicated. Offer HIV testing to all women who have not been previously screened (Office of AIDS Research Advisory Council, 2009).

Depending on how rapidly labor is progressing, the nurse notifies the healthcare provider before or after completing the admission procedures. The report includes the following information:

- Parity
- Cervical dilation and effacement
- Station
- Presenting part
- Status of the membranes
- Contraction pattern
- FHR
- Vital signs that are not in the normal range
- Any significant prenatal history
- The woman's birth preferences
- The woman's reaction to labor
- The woman's preferences for pain relief.

The nurse also enters an admission note into the computer or the charting system. The admission note should include the reason for admission, the date and time of the woman's arrival and notification of the physician or CNM, the condition of the woman and her baby, and labor and membrane status.

Provide Nursing Care During the First Stage of Labor

The nurse needs to evaluate physical parameters of the woman and her fetus. Maternal temperature is monitored every 2–4 hours unless the temperature is over 37.5°C (99.6°F), in which case it is taken every hour. When the amniotic membranes have ruptured, maternal temperature is assessed every 1–2 hours, depending on the policy of the institution. Blood pressure, pulse, respirations, and response to pain are monitored as indicated or according to unit policy. If the woman's blood pressure is greater than or equal to 140/90 mmHg or her pulse is more than 100 bpm, the nurse must notify the physician or CNM and reevaluate the blood pressure and pulse more frequently. Monitor the woman's pain level continually, because this can elevate the blood pressure and pulse, especially during contractions.

The nurse palpates uterine contractions for frequency, intensity, and duration every 30 minutes. The nurse also auscultates the FHR every 30 minutes in active labor for low-risk women and every 15 minutes for high-risk women as long as the FHR remains between 110 and 160 bpm and is reassuring (ACOG, 2009b). Auscultate the FHR throughout one contraction and for approximately 15 seconds after the contraction to ensure there are no decelerations. If the FHR baseline is not in the range of 110–160 bpm or if decelerations are heard, continuous electronic monitoring is recommended (see Table 33–13).

✳ Visit **nursing.pearsonhighered.com** to see a summary of labor progress, possible responses of the laboring woman, and support measures.

LATENT PHASE   The nurse offers foods and fluids as desired unless complications exist that may necessitate general anesthesia. Avoiding both liquids and solids during labor, which was once standard practice, is no longer necessary, because evidence-based practice research and new guidelines indicate that clear fluids can be consumed throughout labor and up to 2 hours before an elective cesarean birth. In a low risk setting, it is not necessary to restrict intake in any way.

Certain women with specific risk factors should be evaluated on a case-by-case basis to assess their specific risk factors and determine the most appropriate recommendation. Current guidelines suggest avoiding solids for 6–8 hours before a cesarean birth (ACOG, 2009c).

ACTIVE PHASE   During the active phase, the contractions have a frequency of 2–5 minutes, a duration of 40–60 seconds, and a moderate to strong intensity. As the contractions become more frequent and intense, a woman who has been ambulatory may choose to sit in a chair or lie down. Contractions need to be palpated every 30 minutes.

Vaginal exams may be performed to assess cervical dilation and effacement as well as fetal station and position. Vaginal examinations should be limited, however, because they introduce bacteria, which can lead to maternal infection. During the active phase, the cervix dilates from 6 to 8 cm, and vaginal discharge and bloody show increase; thus, the nurse needs to change the perineal pads more frequently.

The FHR is auscultated and evaluated every 30 minutes for low-risk women and every 15 minutes for high-risk women (ACOG, 2009b). Maternal blood pressure, pulse, and respirations are monitored during the FHR assessment or more frequently if indicated. The mother's level of pain and coping mechanisms are assessed continuously.

The woman is encouraged to void because a full bladder can interfere with fetal descent. If she is unable to void, catheterization or insertion of an indwelling Foley catheter may be necessary.

If the amniotic membranes have not ruptured previously, they may do so during this phase. When the membranes rupture, the nurse notes the amount, color, odor, and consistency of the amniotic fluid and the time of rupture and immediately auscultates the FHR. The fluid should be clear, with no odor. Nonreassuring fetal status may lead to intestinal and anal sphincter relaxation. This may result in the release of meconium into the amniotic fluid, which turns the fluid greenish brown. When the nurse notes meconium-stained fluid, an electronic monitor is applied to assess the FHR continuously. Current management of membrane rupture without labor varies. Providers may opt to deliver the fetus within 24–48 hours, or allow the pregnancy to continue while administering antibiotics to the mother, or allow the pregnancy to continue with no intervention other than monitoring unless the mother develops signs of infection. In this case, the Group B streptococcus status is evaluated, and intrapartum antibiotics are administered as indicated. Labor induction may be initiated on a case-by-case basis (CDC, 2010).

SAFETY ALERT

The highest-priority assessment following rupture of membranes is to check the fetal heart rate. As amniotic fluid is evacuated, the umbilical cord may become trapped between the fetal head and the maternal pelvis. The pressure on the umbilical cord slows or completely stops all blood flow to the fetus, which will be evidenced by a drop in FHR and ultimate fetal demise if not properly managed.

An additional potential issue during this phase is prolapse of the umbilical cord, which may occur when membranes rupture and the fetal presenting part is not well applied to the cervix. The concern is that the amniotic fluid coming through the cervix will propel the umbilical cord through the cervix (prolapsed cord). The FHR is auscultated because a drop in FHR might indicate an undetected prolapsed cord. Immediate intervention is necessary to remove pressure on a prolapsed umbilical cord.

✳ Visit **nursing.pearsonhighered.com** for a list of additional deviations from the normal labor process that require immediate intervention.

TRANSITION PHASE During transition, the contraction frequency may be every 1.5–2 minutes, duration is 60–90 seconds, and intensity is strong. Cervical dilation increases from 8 to 10 cm, effacement is complete (100%), and a heavy amount of bloody show is usually present. Contractions are palpated at least every 30 minutes. Sterile vaginal examinations may be done more frequently because this stage of labor usually is accompanied by rapid change. The FHR is auscultated every 30 minutes for low-risk women and every 15 minutes for high-risk women; maternal blood pressure, pulse, and respirations are monitored when the FHR is assessed or according to unit policy. Note that women may receive more frequent assessments based on individualized needs. The woman's pain level is monitored continuously.

Comfort measures become very important in this phase of labor, but continual assessment is required to ensure appropriate intervention. Women may also shake uncontrollably, feel nausea, or vomit during this stage. The woman may rapidly change

from wanting a back rub and other hands-on care to wanting to be left completely alone. The support person and the nurse need to follow the woman's cues and change interventions as needed. Because the woman is breathing more rapidly, the nurse can increase the woman's comfort by offering small spoons of ice chips to moisten her mouth or applying an emollient to dry lips. The nurse can encourage the woman to rest between contractions. If analgesics have been administered, a quiet environment enhances the quality of rest between contractions.

Some women have difficulty coping during this time and need help with their breathing. Either the support person or the nurse can breathe along with the woman during each contraction to help her maintain her pattern. A gentle reminder to "slow down your breathing" can help to prevent hyperventilation. It is helpful to encourage the woman and to assure her that she is doing a good job. The woman will begin to feel increased rectal pressure as the fetal presenting part moves down the birth canal. The nurse encourages the woman to refrain from pushing until the cervix is completely dilated. To help the woman avoid involuntary pushing during contractions, the nurse can encourage pant–blow breathing, suggesting that the woman "pant like a puppy" or "blow in short breaths as if you were blowing out a candle." This measure helps prevent cervical edema.

The end of the transition phase and the beginning of the second stage may be indicated by a change in the woman's voice or the sounds that she is making. As the fetus moves down and the woman feels increased pressure and a bearing-down sensation, her voice tends to deepen. If she moans during a contraction, it takes on a more guttural quality. Expert nurses recognize this sound as a sign of changes in the woman.

PROMOTION OF COMFORT The nurse identifies factors that may contribute to discomfort for the laboring woman. These factors include uncomfortable positions or infrequent position changes, diaphoresis, continual leaking of amniotic fluid, a full bladder, a dry mouth, anxiety, and fear. The nurse and client together plan interventions to minimize the effects of these factors.

Women in labor have many types of responses to pain. As the intensity of the contractions increases with the progress of labor, the woman becomes less aware of the environment and may have difficulty hearing and understanding verbal instructions. Some women may become irritable during this time. The pattern of coping with labor contractions varies from the use of highly structured breathing techniques to turning inward. As stated previously, the woman's responses to pain may have a cultural basis. Low moaning that begins deep in the throat, rocking or swaying, counting, facial grimacing, and using loud vocalizations are all effective means of dealing with the discomfort of labor and birth. Some women feel that making sounds helps them cope and do the work of labor, whereas others make loud sounds only as they lose their perception of control.

The most frequent physiological manifestations of pain are increased pulse and respiratory rates, dilated pupils, increased blood pressure, and muscle tension. During labor, these reactions are transitory because the pain is intermittent. Increased muscle tension is most significant because it may impede the labor process. Women in labor frequently tighten skeletal muscles voluntarily during a contraction and remain motionless. This method of dealing with the contractions may actually increase her discomfort, but the woman may believe it is the only acceptable way to cope with the pain.

A woman generally wants touching, massage, effleurage, and other forms of physical contact during the first part of labor, but when she moves into the transition phase, she may pull away. Alternatively, the woman may beseech her partner or the nurse to hold her hand or rub her back, or she may even reach out and grasp the support person. Some women are uncomfortable with being touched at all, regardless of the phase of labor; others do not welcome touch from a nonfamily member. It is important to validate the unique strengths and coping techniques of the individual and to meet each family on their own terms, always keeping in mind that this is *their* experience. Cultural influences can also affect how a woman will react to support and touch in labor. The nurse takes cues from the woman and makes adjustments in her care to meet the client's specific needs.

General Comfort   General comfort measures are of great importance during labor. By relieving minor discomforts, the nurse helps the woman optimize her coping abilities to deal with pain. The woman is encouraged to ambulate as long as there are no contraindications, such as vaginal bleeding or rupture of membranes before the fetus is engaged in the pelvis. Ambulation can increase comfort and aid in fetal descent. Even if the woman prefers not to walk around, upright positions, such as sitting in a rocker or leaning against a wall or bed, can enhance comfort. If the woman stays in bed, the nurse can encourage her to assume positions that she finds comfortable (Zwelling, 2010).

If the woman is more comfortable on her back, the nurse should elevate the head of the bed to relieve the pressure of the uterus on the vena cava. Pillows may be placed under each arm and under the knees to provide support. Because a pregnant woman is at increased risk for thrombophlebitis, it is important to avoid excessive pressure behind the knee and calf. The nurse needs to assess pressure points frequently. Frequent changes of position contribute to comfort and relaxation. The hands-and-knees posture may be used to relieve persistent back pain during labor (Simkin, 2010).

Wearing socks or slippers may alleviate cold feet, and adjusting the room's thermostat can offset excessive warmth. Attention to such details allows the woman to focus on the more

important issues of giving birth. The woman may be offered a warmed or cooled facial cloth, which is placed on her forehead or across or behind her neck. Providing a toothbrush and toothpaste for oral care can also increase comfort.

Diaphoresis and the constant leaking of amniotic fluid can dampen the woman's gown and bed linen. Offering fresh, smooth, dry bed linen promotes comfort. To avoid having to change the bottom sheet following rupture of the membranes, the nurse may replace absorbent underpads at frequent intervals (following standard precautions). To promote comfort and prevent infection, keep the perineal area as clean and dry as possible. A full bladder adds to discomfort during a contraction and may prolong labor by interfering with the descent of the fetus. The bladder should be kept as empty as possible. Even if the woman is voiding, urine may be retained because of the pressure from the fetal presenting part. The nurse can detect a full bladder by palpating directly over the symphysis pubis. Encourage the woman to empty her bladder every 1–2 hours. Some of the regional procedures for analgesia and anesthesia during labor contribute to the inability to void, and catheterization may be necessary.

The support person and any family members in attendance also need to be encouraged to maintain their own comfort. Because their attention is directed toward the laboring woman, they may forget their own needs. The nurse may have to encourage them to take breaks, to maintain food and fluid intake, and to rest. Many support persons and family members are reluctant to leave the woman unattended while they meet their own personal needs. Offer to stay with the woman during their absence. This provides reassurance to the support person or family member that the woman will be well cared for in his or her absence.

Handling Anxiety   The anxiety experienced by women beginning labor is related to a combination of factors inherent to the process. A moderate amount of anxiety about pain enhances the woman's ability to deal with it. However, an excessive degree of anxiety decreases her ability to cope with the pain. Women in the latent phase of labor who are experiencing increased levels of anxiety about their ability to cope and their own personal safety are much more likely to describe their pain as unbearable. Women at risk for greater anxiety during labor include those who are young, poor, and lacking in social support. Women with preexisting mental illness, such as depression and anxiety, are at a greater risk for developing posttraumatic stress disorder related to their labor and birth experience (Alcorn et al., 2010). Women with mental illness issues may need additional support to assist them with identifying effective coping mechanisms during the labor and birth process.

Ways to decrease anxiety not related to pain are to give information, which eases fear of the unknown; to establish rapport with the couple, which helps them preserve their personal integrity; and to express confidence in the couple's ability to work with the labor process. In addition to being a good listener, the nurse must demonstrate genuine concern for the laboring woman. Remaining with the woman as much as possible conveys a caring attitude and dispels fears of abandonment. Praise for breathing, relaxation, and pushing efforts not only encourages repetition of the behavior but also decreases anxiety about the ability to cope with labor.

Client Teaching   Providing truthful information about the nature of the discomfort that will occur during labor is important. Stressing the intermittent nature and maximum duration of the

Complementary and Alternative Therapy
Acupressure During Labor

Acupressure is an ancient Chinese medical treatment that involves using the fingers to press key pressure points on the surface of the skin. This pressure ultimately stimulates the immune system to promote healing by triggering the release of endorphins, reducing stress through muscle relaxation, and promoting circulation. The specific acupressure point used in laboring women is the San Yin-Jiao (SP-6) acupressure point. The SP-6 acupressure point is located on the medial side of the leg, in the calf region, approximately 3 cm (1.2 in.) superior to the prominence of the inner malleus. The use of acupressure in labor has been associated with shorter labors and lower subjective and objective pain scores. Women who receive acupressure typically use less pain medication than those who do not receive acupressure (Smith et al., 2011).

contractions can be helpful. The woman can cope with pain better when she knows that a period of relief will follow. Describing the type of discomfort and specific sensations that will occur as labor progresses helps the woman recognize these sensations when she does experience them as normal and expected.

Advise the client that although the strength and intensity of contractions are different for each woman, they may feel like a tightening sensation or a menstrual cramp initially. Over time, as the labor progresses, the contractions become more intense and more uncomfortable, with the uterus tightening and becoming very hard and with the pain radiating from the back around to the front. For some women, the pain takes their breath away, or they may feel anxiety and fear. As the contractions become more painful, they also occur closer together. The sensation of having to push occurs as the head progresses into the pelvis and feels like the woman has to have a bowel movement. Once the contraction goes away, this intense feeling of having to have a bowel movement usually lets up some.

Descriptions of sensations are best accompanied by information on specific comfort measures. As previously noted, some women experience the urge to push during the transition phase, when the cervix is not fully dilated and effaced. This sensation can be controlled by pant–blow breathing (it is difficult to pant or blow and bear down at the same time); the nurse should provide instructions about this technique before it is required.

Thorough orientation and explanation of surroundings, procedures, and equipment being used also decrease anxiety, thereby reducing pain. Attachment to an electronic monitor may produce fear because the woman may associate equipment of this type with people who are critically ill. It may also limit the woman's ability to move about and comfort herself with position changes and ambulation. If continuous electronic fetal monitoring is needed, the nurse can explain the beeps, clicks, and other strange noises and give a simplified explanation of the monitor strip. The nurse emphasizes that use of the fetal monitor provides a way to assess the well-being of the fetus during the course of labor. If available, a less intrusive telemetry monitor may be applied so that the woman has more freedom to move about. In addition, the nurse can show the woman and her partner or support person how the monitor can help them identify the beginnings of contractions. The nurse should encourage the woman to begin her breathing technique at the onset of each contraction; this may help lessen her perception of pain.

Labor and childbirth may be a critical time for the woman with a history of childhood physical, emotional, and/or sexual abuse or rape (Lukassi et al., 2010). To develop a competent plan of care, all laboring women should be evaluated on admission for a history of childhood abuse or rape. Depending on their cultural background, women may need specific examples of abuse to determine whether they have had these types of experiences, because some behaviors that are considered to be abusive in our society may be thought of as normal patterns of behavior in other cultures (Thombs et al., 2007). Women may or may not be able to address this issue with the nurse because sharing such personal information is difficult and may stir up painful memories. It is therefore especially important for the nurse to be alert for nonverbal cues, such as excessive unexplained anxiety, unrelenting pain, and/or intense fear during vaginal exams, and to be prepared to offer additional teaching to help offset the woman's anxiety.

> **SAFETY ALERT**
> If a woman is experiencing severe fear or anxiety about a vaginal examination, advise her to slowly count to 10 during the examination while continually wiggling her toes. This distraction may lessen her fear and anxiety. It also enables the woman to have a sense of control.

Supportive Relaxation Techniques   Tense muscles increase resistance to the descent of the fetus and contribute to maternal fatigue. This fatigue increases pain perception and decreases the woman's ability to cope with the pain. Comfort measures, massage, techniques for decreasing anxiety, and client teaching can contribute to relaxation. Adequate sleep and rest are also important. The laboring woman needs to be encouraged to use the period between contractions for rest and relaxation. A prolonged prodromal phase of labor (also known as false labor or Braxton Hicks contractions) may interfere with sleep. An aura of excitement naturally accompanies the onset of labor, making it difficult for the woman to sleep even though the contractions are mild and infrequent. The nurse may have to act as an advocate for the woman to limit the number of visitors, interruptions, and phone calls.

Distraction is another method of increasing relaxation and coping with discomfort. During early labor, conversation or activities such as watching television, light reading, or playing cards or other games can serve as distractions. One technique that is effective for relieving moderate pain is to have the woman concentrate on a pleasant experience she has had in the past. Other techniques include the use of a specific visual or mental focal point (e.g., a picture of a loved one), breathing techniques, counting or humming, or visualization.

Touch is another type of distraction. Although some women regard touching as an invasion of privacy or a threat to their independence, many want to touch and be touched during a painful experience. To determine whether the woman desires touch, the nurse can place a hand on the side of the bed within the woman's reach. The woman who needs touch will reach out for contact, and the nurse can follow through with this behavioral cue.

Specific touch techniques that are useful for relaxation include effleurage and massage. Mild to moderate abdominal discomfort during contractions may be relieved or lessened by effleurage. Back pain associated with labor may be relieved by firm pressure on the lower back or sacral area. To apply firm pressure, the nurse can place his or her hand or a rolled, warmed towel or blanket in the small of the woman's back or can instruct the woman's support person to do so.

In some instances, analgesics or regional anesthetic blocks may be used to enhance comfort and relaxation during labor. The nurse may also enhance the woman's relaxation by providing encouragement and support for her controlled breathing techniques.

Breathing Techniques   Breathing techniques may help the laboring woman. Used correctly, they raise the woman's pain threshold, permit relaxation, enhance her ability to cope with contractions, provide a sense of control, and allow the uterus to function more efficiently.

Various types of breathing techniques can be used in labor. Many women learn patterned-paced breathing during prenatal education classes. This type of controlled breathing often has three levels. The woman tends to begin with the first level and then proceed to the next when she feels the need. Regardless of the level of breathing used, a cleansing breath (involving only the chest) begins and ends each pattern. The cleansing breath consists of inhaling slowly through the nose until a sense of fullness in the lungs occurs and then exhaling slowly through pursed lips. The first pattern may also be called slow, deep breathing or slow-paced breathing. During the breathing movements, only the chest moves. The woman inhales slowly through her nose, moves her chest up and out during the inhalation, and exhales through pursed lips. The breathing rate is 6–9 breaths per minute.

The second pattern may be called shallow or modified-paced breathing. The woman begins with a cleansing breath. At the end of the cleansing breath, she pushes out a short breath. She then inhales and exhales through the mouth at a rate of about four breaths every 5 seconds. This pattern can be altered into a more rapid rate that does not exceed 2–2.5 breaths every second.

The third pattern, introduced earlier, is called pant–blow or patterned-paced breathing. It is similar to modified-paced breathing except that the breathing is punctuated every few breaths by a forceful exhalation through pursed lips. A pattern of 4 breaths may be used to begin. All breaths are kept equal and rhythmic. As the contraction becomes more intense, the woman may adjust the pattern as needed to 3:1, 2:1, and finally 1:1.

Abdominal breathing is another technique that can be effective in labor. In abdominal breathing, the woman moves the abdominal wall outward as she inhales and inward as she exhales. This method tends to lift the abdominal wall off the contracting uterus and thus helps to provide pain relief. The breathing is deep and rhythmic and typically relaxing. As transition approaches, the woman using abdominal breathing may feel the urge to breathe more rapidly. The pant–blow pattern discussed earlier can be suggested to slow the breathing and help the woman avoid the urge to bear down.

Hyperventilation is the result of an imbalance of oxygen and carbon dioxide (i.e., too much carbon dioxide is exhaled, and too much oxygen remains in the body). Hyperventilation may occur when a woman breathes very rapidly over a prolonged period. The signs and symptoms of hyperventilation are tingling or numbness in the tip of the nose, lips, fingers, or toes; dizziness; spots before the eyes; or spasms of the hands or feet (carpopedal spasms). If hyperventilation occurs, the nurse encourages the woman to slow her breathing rate and take shallow breaths. With instruction and encouragement, many women are able to change their breathing to correct the problem. Encouraging the woman to relax and counting out loud for her so that she can pace her breathing during contractions are also helpful actions. If the signs and symptoms continue or become more severe, the client is treated for hyperventilation as appropriate. The nurse remains with the woman to reassure her, because hyperventilation can increase anxiety levels.

ROLE OF THE DOULA   Throughout the first stage of labor, the nurse assesses and supports the interaction between the woman and her partner. In the absence of a partner, or when the partner desires a less active role, it is becoming more common for women to employ a paid caregiver who has experience in caring for laboring women. This caregiver, often called a **doula**, has typically received special training and may even be certified. The doula's role is to enhance the laboring woman's comfort and decrease her anxiety. A doula can be a valuable advocate for the laboring woman and her family as well as an asset to the labor nurse. For example, the doula

might support the woman by helping identify the beginning of each contraction and encouraging her as she breathes through it. A constant presence offering continued encouragement and support with each contraction throughout labor has immeasurable benefits.

Provide Nursing Care During the Second Stage of Labor

The second stage is reached when the cervix is completely dilated (10 cm [3.9 in.]). The uterine contractions continue as in the transition phase. Maternal pulse is assessed at the onset of the second stage. The blood pressure is assessed every 30 minutes, but assessment may be done more frequently if fetal decelerations or bradycardia occur. The FHR is assessed every 15 minutes in low-risk women and every 5 minutes in women with risk factors (Cunningham et al., 2010). Once the second stage is reached, the nurse remains with the woman continually and generally does not leave the room. Nursing care during the second stage focuses on providing care, promoting comfort, and assisting during the birth.

As the woman pushes during the second stage, she may make a variety of sounds. A low-pitched, grunting sound ("uhhh") usually indicates that the woman is working with the pushing. The nurse who feels comfortable with maternal sounds and stays sensitive to changes in the sounds may be able to detect if the woman is losing her ability to cope. For instance, if the woman feels afraid of the sensations produced by her pushing effort, her sound may change to a high-pitched cry or whimper.

It is not uncommon for the woman to be afraid to push. In these situations, the woman may talk or cry out during the contraction instead of actively pushing. During this time, the nurse provides support, reassurance, and clear directions for the woman to follow. Often, it is helpful to direct the woman to concentrate on a single voice, listen for suggestions, and let her body do the work. Many women find this type of interaction comforting because it allows them to focus on one individual.

When teaching the effective technique for pushing, instruct the woman to bear down and push into her bottom as if she is having a bowel movement. Watch the woman's perineum and rectum while she is pushing, and give verbal praise and encouragement when change in the perineum or rectum is seen, indicating she is successfully pushing.

During the second stage, the woman may feel intense rectal pressure. The instinctive response is to resist and to tighten muscles rather than bear down (push). A sensation of "splitting apart" or burning also occurs in the latter part of the second stage when the woman is pushing. The woman who expects these sensations and who understands that bearing down contributes to progress at this stage is more likely to do so.

When the urge to bear down becomes uncontrollable and pushing begins, the nurse can help by encouraging the client and by supporting her efforts. Most women push spontaneously and effectively in response to messages from their body. This more natural approach, which lets the mother wait to bear down until she feels an urge to push, may shorten the pushing phase, thereby reducing the incidence of physiological stress in the mother and acidosis in the newborn. This technique also decreases the incidence of instrument births and damage to maternal perineal tissue (Gennaro, Mayberry, & Kafulafula, 2007; Roberts, Gonzalez, & Sampselle, 2007). In some settings, however, sustained, forceful pushing may be useful. In that case, when the contraction begins, the nurse tells the woman to take a cleansing breath or two, then

Evidence-Based Practice Passive Descent Versus Active Pushing in Women With Epidural Anesthesia

Problem

Which method of pushing—passive descent or active pushing as soon as full cervical dilation is achieved—provides the most benefit for mothers with epidural anesthesia?

Epidural analgesia is a common method of pain management during active labor, but one of its side effects is a decrease in a woman's lower body sensations. This may inhibit the natural urge to push upon full cervical dilation. Women have traditionally been directed to push immediately once cervical dilation reaches 10 cm, whether they felt the urge to push or not. The chief concern leading to this practice was that an extended second stage of labor was deleterious for both mother and baby, leading to acidosis, maternal exhaustion, and neonatal morbidity.

The natural second stage of labor includes a period of time in which the fetus descends, which the literature refers to as "passive descent." Passive descent allows the woman to delay pushing until she feels the urge to push or until the head is visible.

Evidence

A group of obstetric and gynecologic nurse experts conducted a meta-analysis of studies comparing the effects and outcomes of immediate pushing versus passive descent in women with epidural anesthesia (Brancato, Church, & Stone, 2008). The results demonstrated that immediate pushing did not reduce the incidence of acidosis or shorten the second stage of labor. Indeed, prolonged active pushing was shown to increase the incidence of fetal and maternal acidosis, increase the risk of having an instrument-assisted birth, and decrease the chance a woman would have a spontaneous vaginal birth. Pushing time was lengthened with immediate pushing as compared to passive descent.

Furthermore, passive descent had additional benefits in that it allowed for further fetal descent and rotation, better situating the fetus in the woman's pelvis. It also caused further release of oxytocin that augmented the progress of labor.

Implications

These findings suggest that the duration of active pushing should be limited, not the duration of the second stage of labor.

Critical Thinking Application

1. How can the nurse help the mother recognize the urge to push at an effective time when epidural analgesia is in place?
2. How does a rest period during pushing influence perinatal outcomes?
3. What risk factors are associated with active pushing during the second stage of labor?
4. What are the evidence-based nursing interventions related to the second stage of labor?

---

to take a third large breath and hold it while pushing down with her abdominal muscles (called the Valsalva maneuver).

A nullipara is usually prepared for birth when perineal bulging is noted. A multipara usually progresses much more. As the birth approaches, the woman's partner or support person also prepares.

The nurse monitors the woman's blood pressure and the FHR between contractions, and the nurse assesses the contractions at least every 5 minutes until the birth. The nurse continually assesses the woman's level of pain or her ability to cope with the discomfort of labor. The nurse continues to assist the woman in her pushing efforts to keep both the woman and the support person informed of procedures and progress and to support them both throughout the birth.

PROMOTION OF COMFORT Most of the comfort measures that were used during the first stage remain appropriate during the second stage. Applying cool cloths to the face and forehead may help to cool the woman involved in the intense physical exertion of pushing. The woman may feel hot and want to remove some of her clothing or bed linens. Care still needs to be taken to provide privacy even though covers are removed. The nurse encourages the client to rest and relax all muscles during the periods between contractions. The nurse and support person can assist the woman into a pushing position with each contraction to further conserve energy. Between contractions, the woman should be assisted into a comfortable position. Sips of fluids or ice chips may be used to provide moisture and relieve dryness of the mouth. Positive reinforcement and encouragement should be continually provided.

ASSISTING DURING BIRTH In addition to assisting the woman and her partner, the nurse assists the healthcare provider in preparing for the birth. The provider dons a sterile gown and gloves and may place sterile drapes over the woman's abdomen and legs. An episiotomy may be performed just before the actual birth.

Shortly before the birth, the birthing room or delivery room is prepared with the equipment and materials that may be needed. These materials typically come in a prepackaged kit and contain the instruments and disposable drapes, gowns, and containers that will be used during the birth. The nurse ensures that all supplies and a pair of sterile gloves are placed on the instrument table. This table can be prepared before the birth and covered with a sterile drape. If the birth is to occur in a birthing room, family members do not need to change into other clothing; if the birth is to occur in a delivery room or surgery suite, they don a disposable scrub suit or scrubs provided by the facility. Thorough hand hygiene is required of the nurses and physician or CNM. Nurses who will be in direct contact with the mother at the time of birth need to wear protective clothing, such as an apron or gown with a splash apron, disposable gloves, and eye covering. The physician or CNM also needs to wear a plastic apron or a gown with a splash apron, eye covering, and sterile gloves.

If for any reason the laboring woman is to give birth in a location other than the birthing room (e.g., in the case of a forceps-assisted birth where a quick transition to cesarean delivery may

SAFETY ALERT

Some physicians and CNMs routinely use other equipment or supplies during the birth. Examples of such equipment include mineral oil, warm water, and clean washcloths for perineal massage. Gathering these supplies early can save time and enable the nurse to stay with the woman during pushing.

be necessary), she is moved on her bed or a cart shortly before birth. It is important that the woman move from one bed to another *between contractions*. During the contraction, the woman feels increased discomfort and may be involved in pushing efforts. Perineal bulging may be occurring, which adds to the discomfort and difficulty in moving. Take care to preserve her privacy during the transfer, and provide safety by raising the side rails. The bed itself should be placed in a locked position. The labor bed or transfer cart must be carefully braced against the delivery table to ensure the woman's safety during the transfer.

Even though the operating room setting is different from that of a birthing room, the family can still be together during the birth. It is important for nurses to provide encouragement for family members to participate, because the delivery room environment may be unfamiliar and seem intimidating. The family member may hesitate to continue providing support because of fear of interfering or being in the way. The nurse provides clear simple directions that help the support person participate throughout the birth process. The nurse can ensure the support person is sitting as close as possible to the woman. The nurse can also encourage hand holding and touching or stroking of the woman's face.

Maternal Birthing Positions The upright posture for birth was considered to be normal in most societies until modern times. Women variously selected squatting, kneeling, standing, and sitting positions for birth. During the mid-20th century, the recumbent position (lithotomy position) became common in North American hospitals because of the convenience it offered when applying new technology. In recent years, however, consumers and healthcare professionals have begun searching for alternative positions, refocusing on the comfort of the laboring woman rather than on the convenience of the physician or CNM.

✳ Visit **nursing.pearsonhighered.com** for a comparison of birthing positions.

Evidence-based practice research has shown that the squatting position results in fewer instrumental deliveries, fewer episiotomy extensions, and fewer perineal tears compared to the lithotomy position (Nasir, Korejo, & Noorani, 2007). An upright position, which has been found to be the most effective birthing position, is possible even for women who have epidural anesthesia (Gennaro et al., 2007).

The woman may be positioned for birth on a bed with use of leg supports in a squatting position, or perhaps on her hands and knees. If a birthing bed is used, the back is elevated 30°–60° to help the woman bear down. Stirrups, if needed and used, are padded to alleviate pressure. If the nurse is assisting the woman to place her legs in the stirrups, both the woman's legs should be lifted simultaneously to avoid strain on the abdominal, back, and perineal muscles. Stirrups are sometimes needed if the woman is unable to control her legs following epidural anesthesia, if forceps or a vacuum extractor is being used, or if a difficult birth is anticipated. The nurse should adjust the stirrups to fit the woman's legs. The feet are supported in the stirrup holders. The height and angle of the stirrups are adjusted so there is no pressure on the back of the knees or the calves, which might cause discomfort and postpartum vascular problems. Some practitioners may opt to leave the bed assembled and, instead, lower the foot of the bed into a lower position. Many times, women are more comfortable in this position. When stirrups are not used for the birth, the woman's legs may be placed in stirrups after the birth if a repair of the perineum is needed.

Cleansing the Perineum After the mother has been positioned for the birth, her vulvar and perineal area are cleansed to increase her comfort, to remove the bloody discharge that is present before the actual birth, and to prevent infection. Perineal cleansing methods range from use of warm, soapy water to aseptic technique depending on the agency protocol or on physician or CNM orders. Once the cleansing has been completed, the woman returns to the desired birthing position.

Supporting the Couple Both the woman's partner or support person and the nurse who has been with the woman during the labor continue to provide support during contractions. They encourage the woman to push with each contraction, and as the fetal head emerges, ask her to take shallow breaths or to pant to prevent pushing. The physician or CNM may instruct the woman to "push and breathe, push and breathe" in an effort to ease the fetal head out to prevent perineal trauma and tearing. While supporting the head, the physician or CNM assesses whether the umbilical cord is around the fetal neck and removes it if it is, then suctions the mouth and nose with a bulb syringe if there are any obvious obstructions to spontaneous breathing. The mouth is suctioned first to prevent reflex inhalation of mucus when the sensitive nares are touched with the bulb syringe tip. The woman is encouraged to push again as the rest of the newborn's body is born.

Provide Nursing Care During the Third Stage of Labor

Nursing care during the third stage of labor focuses on initial care of the newborn, enhancing attachment, assisting with delivery of the placenta, and providing care for the mother. Newborn care is discussed in Exemplar 33.4; this section discusses maternal care.

DELIVERY OF THE PLACENTA After birth, the physician or CNM prepares for the delivery of the placenta. The following signs suggest placental separation:

- The uterus rises upward in the abdomen.
- As the placenta moves downward, the umbilical cord lengthens.
- A sudden trickle or spurt of blood appears.
- The shape of the uterus changes from a disk to a globe.

While waiting for these signs, the nurse palpates the uterus to check for bogginess (soft or mushy feeling) and fullness caused by uterine relaxation and subsequent bleeding into the uterine cavity. After the placenta has separated, the woman may be asked to bear down to aid delivery of the placenta.

Oxytocics are frequently given at the time of the delivery of the placenta so that the uterus will contract and bleeding will be minimized. Oxytocin (Pitocin), 20 units, may be added to an intravenous infusion, or 10 units may be given intramuscularly. In the presence of hemorrhage caused by uterine atony, some physicians and CNMs may order up to 40 units of oxytocin in a liter of intravenous fluid; methylergonovine maleate (Methergine), 0.2 mg, administered intramuscularly; or carboprost tromethamine (Hemabate), 250 mcg/mL, administered intramuscularly. Cytotec has been commonly used when other pharmacologic interventions have failed. Cytotec is administered rectally in dosages of 800–1,000 mcg (Hofmeyr, Gülmezoglu, & Pileggi, 2013). In addition to administering the ordered medications, the nurse assesses and records maternal blood pressure before and after administration of oxytocics and assesses the amount of bleeding.

After delivery of the placenta, the physician or CNM inspects the placenta and membranes to make sure they are intact and that all cotyledons are present. If there is a defect or a part missing from the placenta, a manual uterine examination or uterine exploration is done. The nurse notes on the birth record the time of delivery of the placenta.

Provide Nursing Care During the Fourth Stage of Labor

The healthcare provider inspects the vagina, cervix, and perineum for lacerations and makes any necessary repairs. The episiotomy or laceration may be repaired now if it has not been done previously.

The nurse assesses the uterus for firmness by palpating the fundus. The normal position is at the midline and below the umbilicus. A displaced fundus may be caused by a full bladder or by blood collected in the uterus. The clots or blood accumulation in the uterus may be expelled by grasping the uterus transabdominally with one hand anteriorly and posteriorly and then squeezing. The nurse continues to palpate the uterine fundus at frequent intervals for at least 4 hours to ensure that it remains firmly contracted (**Figure 33–57 ●**), but it is not massaged unless it is soft (boggy). If the uterine fundus becomes soft (uterine atony) or appears to rise in the abdomen, the nurse massages it until firm; then, the nurse exerts firm pressure on the fundus in an attempt to express retained clots. During all aspects of fundal massage, the nurse uses one hand to provide support for the lower portion of the uterus and prevent damage to the round ligaments and uterine eversion. The uterus is very tender at this time; all palpation and massage should be performed as gently as possible.

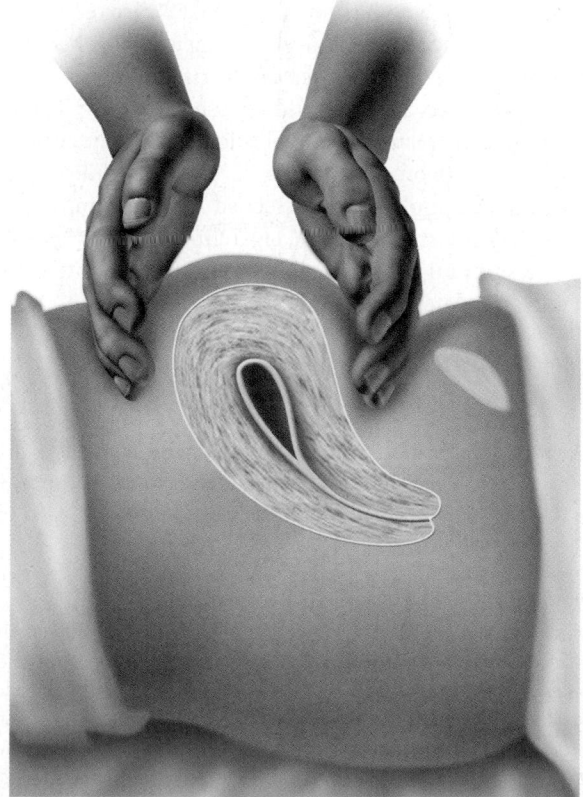

Figure 33–57 ● Suggested method of palpating the fundus of the uterus during the fourth stage. The left hand is placed just above the symphysis pubis, and gentle downward pressure is exerted. The right hand is cupped around the uterine fundus.

The nurse washes the woman's perineum with gauze squares and warmed solution and then dries the area well with a towel before placing the sanitary pad. Many times, an ice pack is also placed against the perineum to promote comfort and decrease swelling. If stirrups have been used, the woman's legs are removed from the stirrups at the same time to avoid muscle strain. The woman is encouraged to move her legs gently up and down in a bicycle motion. The woman remains in the same bed or is transferred to a recovery room bed, and the nurse helps her don a clean gown. Soiled linens are removed, and the woman is typically offered something to drink.

During the recovery period (1–4 hours) the nurse monitors the woman closely. The perineum is inspected for edema and hematoma formation, and frequent checking of vital signs for deviations from normal is required. The maternal blood pressure is monitored at 5- to 15-minute intervals to detect any changes. Blood pressure should return to the prelabor level because an increased volume of blood is returning to the maternal circulation from the uteroplacental shunt. Pulse rate should be slightly lower than it was during labor. Baroreceptors cause a vagal response, which slows the pulse. A rise in blood pressure may be a response to oxytocic drugs or may be caused by preeclampsia. Blood loss may be reflected by a lowered blood pressure and a rising pulse rate (**Table 33–14 ●**).

The nurse also monitors the woman's temperature. Frequently, women have tremors or uncontrollable shaking in the immediate postpartum period that may be caused by a difference in internal and external body temperatures (higher temperature inside the body than outside). Another theory is that the woman is reacting to the fetal cells that have entered the maternal circulation at the placental site. The nurse may place a heated blanket next to the woman's skin to alleviate the problem; this can be replaced as often as the mother desires.

The nurse assesses the mother's pain level. If the woman is experiencing any type of discomfort, pain medications can be administered as ordered. The nurse also assists with comfort measures, such as position changes, frequent ice pack changes, and administration of topical medications that are often ordered to reduce perineal edema and discomfort.

TABLE 33–14 Maternal Adaptations Following Birth	
CHARACTERISTIC	**NORMAL FINDING**
Blood pressure	Returns to prelabor level
Pulse	Slightly lower than in labor
Uterine fundus	In the midline at the umbilicus, or 1–2 fingerbreadths below the umbilicus
Lochia	Red (rubra), small to moderate amount (from spotting on pads to 1/4–1/2 of pad covered in 15 minutes); does not exceed saturation of one pad in first hour
Bladder	Nonpalpable
Perineum	Without hematomas or open lacerations. Mild to moderate bruising and/or edema is common.
Emotional state	Wide variation, including excited, exhilarated, smiling, crying, fatigued, verbal, quiet, pensive, and sleepy

The nurse inspects the bloody vaginal discharge for amount and charts it as minimal, moderate, or heavy and as with or without clots. This discharge (lochia rubra) should be bright red. A soaked perineal pad contains approximately 100 mL of blood. If the perineal pad becomes soaked in a 15-minute period or if blood pools under the buttocks, continuous observation is necessary. When the fundus is firm, a continuous trickle of blood may signal laceration of the vagina or cervix or an unligated vessel in the episiotomy.

If the fundus rises and displaces to the right, the nurse must be concerned about two factors:

1. As the uterus rises, the uterine contractions become less effective and increased bleeding may occur.
2. The most common cause of uterine displacement is bladder distention.

The nurse palpates the bladder to determine whether it is distended. The bladder fills rapidly with the extra fluid volume returned from the uteroplacental circulation (and with any fluid received intravenously during labor and birth). The postpartum woman may not realize that her bladder is full, because trauma to the bladder and urethra during childbirth and the use of regional anesthesia decrease bladder tone and the urge to void.

All measures should be taken to enable the mother to void. The nurse may place a warm towel across the lower abdomen or pour warm water over the perineum to relax the urinary sphincter and facilitate voiding. The woman may also try running warm water over her hand. If the woman is unable to void, catheterization is necessary.

SAFETY ALERT

In the immediate postbirth recovery period, report the following conditions to the physician or CNM:

- Hypotension
- Tachycardia
- Uterine atony
- Excessive bleeding
- Hematoma.

The woman and her partner or support person may be tired, hungry, and thirsty. Some agencies serve them a meal. Most women are very hungry after birth. The tired mother will probably drift off into a welcome sleep. The partner can also be encouraged to rest, because the supporting role is physically and mentally tiring. If the mother is not in a birthing room, she is usually transferred from the birthing unit to the postpartum or mother–baby area after 1 hour or more, depending on agency policy and whether the following criteria are met:

- Stable vital signs
- Stable bleeding
- Undistended bladder
- Firm fundus
- Sensations fully recovered from any anesthetic agent received during birth.

For some women, the childbirth experience has been extremely painful, filled with hours of feeling powerless or out of control. In this circumstance, the woman is at higher risk for developing posttraumatic stress disorder (Harris & Ayers, 2012).

Support the Adolescent During Birth

As with all women, each adolescent in labor is different. The nurse must assess what each teen brings to the experience as follows:

- Has the young woman received prenatal care?
- What are her attitudes and feelings about the pregnancy?
- Who will attend the birth, and what is each individual's relationship to the woman?
- What preparation has she had for the experience?
- What are her expectations and fears regarding labor and birth?
- How has her culture influenced her?
- What are her usual coping mechanisms?
- What are her plans for the newborn?

Any adolescent who has not had prenatal care requires close observation during labor. Fetal well-being is established by fetal monitoring. Adolescent women are at risk for pregnancy and labor complications and must be assessed carefully. The nurse must be especially alert for any physiological complications of labor. The young woman's prenatal record is carefully reviewed for risks, and the adolescent is screened for preeclampsia, cephalopelvic disproportion, anemia, cigarette smoking, alcohol and drugs ingested during pregnancy, sexually transmitted infections, and size–date discrepancies.

Lifespan Considerations Adolescents and Childbirth

- The very young adolescent (ages 14 and younger) has fewer coping mechanisms and less experience to draw on than her older counterparts. Because her cognitive development is incomplete, the younger adolescent may have fewer problem-solving capabilities. Her ego integrity may be more threatened by the experience of labor, and she may be more vulnerable to stress and discomfort. She may be more childlike and dependent than older teens. As a result, the very young adolescent needs someone to rely on at all times during labor. The nurse must be sure that instructions and explanations are simple and concrete. During the transition phase, this client may become withdrawn and unable to express her need to be nurtured. Touch, soothing encouragement, and measures to provide comfort help her maintain control and meet her needs for dependence. During the

second stage of labor, the young adolescent may feel as if she is losing control and may reach out to those around her. By remaining calm and giving directions, the nurse helps her cope with feelings of helplessness.

- The middle adolescent (ages 15–17 years) often attempts to remain calm and unflinching during labor. The experienced nurse realizes that a caring attitude will still help the young woman. Many older adolescents believe that they "know it all," but they may be no more prepared for childbirth than their younger counterparts. The nurse's reinforcement and nonjudgmental manner will help them save face. If the adolescent has not taken childbirth preparation classes, she may require preparation and explanations.

- The older teenager (ages 18–19 years) responds to the stresses of labor in a manner similar to that of the adult woman.

NURSING CARE PLAN | A Client Requiring Induction of Labor

Lakshmi Pandey is being admitted to labor and childbirth this morning for an induction. She is accompanied by her husband, Nitya. Mrs. Pandey is a primigravida at 42 weeks of gestation. She has been experiencing Braxton Hicks contractions during the past week, but a contraction pattern has not been established. Mrs. Pandey's membranes are intact, and her vital signs are within normal limits. Her cervix is soft and pliable, 80% effaced, and 3 cm, dilated. Fetal station is −1. The nurse places Mrs. Pandey on the external fetal monitor to obtain a baseline fetal heart rate pattern and evaluate uterine activity.

ASSESSMENT

Subjective: Braxton Hicks contractions, restlessness, backache, apprehension. Pain level reported as 5 out of 10.
Objective: Cervix is 3 cm dilated, 80% effaced; −1 station; amniotic membranes are intact. BP 120/84 mmHg, temperature 37.1°C (98.8°F), pulse 94 bpm, respirations 14/min, FHR 144 with average variability.

DIAGNOSES

- *Risk for Injury* related to tachy-systole of uterus caused by induction of labor
- *Anxiety*

(NANDA-I © 2015)

PLANNING

- The client will progress through the stages of labor without difficulty or complications.
- The client will have contractions every 2–3 minutes, with duration of 40–60 seconds, and moderate intensity.
- The client's labor will progress with cervical dilation, effacement, and fetal descent.
- The client's resting tone will return to baseline between contractions.
- The client's vital signs will remain within normal limits.

IMPLEMENTATION

- Obtain a baseline for maternal blood pressure, pulse, respirations, temperature, and pain level.
- Confirm medical, surgical, obstetric, and prenatal history; allergies and client identify.
- Place client on external fetal monitor for 20 minutes to obtain a baseline for FHR, variability and periodic changes (accelerations or decelerations).
- Insert intravenous line, and begin primary infusion with 1000 mL of electrolyte solution.
- Piggyback oxytocin solution into primary intravenous tubing, via pump, in the port closest to the intravenous insertion site.
- Monitor infusion pump and connections.
- Monitor and evaluate maternal blood pressure and pulse before each increase in the oxytocin infusion rate.

- Evaluate urine output.
- Evaluate and document FHR before each increase in the oxytocin infusion rate.
- Evaluate and document contraction pattern before each increase of the oxytocin infusion rate.
- Increase the oxytocin infusion dosage until adequate contractions are achieved or the maximum dose per agency protocol is reached.
- Evaluate contraction frequency, duration, and intensity before increasing the infusion rate. Discontinue the oxytocin infusion and infuse primary solution if signs of tachysystole of the uterus are detected.
- Initiate treatment measures to reverse the effects of the oxytocin infusion if fetal tachycardia or bradycardia occurs.

EVALUATION

- Contractions increased in frequency, duration, and intensity.
- Increase in cervical dilation, effacement, and intensity was achieved.
- Uterus remained soft between contractions.

CRITICAL THINKING

1. *Mrs. Pandey has been receiving an oxytocin infusion for the past 4 hours and is currently receiving 6 milliunits/min. Your assessment of Mrs. Pandey's contractions includes frequency every 3 minutes, lasting 60 seconds, with moderate intensity. FHR ranges from 140 to 155 bpm with average variability. Her cervix is now 6 cm (2.4 in.) dilated, 100% effaced, anterior, and the station is 0. Will you continue to monitor at the same infusion rate, increase the rate, or decrease the rate?*
2. *While monitoring a client with an oxytocin infusion, you assess that the client's contractions are now every 2 minutes and that the FHR has dropped to 100 bpm with a decrease in variability. Several late decelerations are also assessed. What is your initial nursing action?*

The support role of the nurse depends on the young woman's support system during labor. The adolescent may not be accompanied by someone who will stay with her during childbirth, or she may have her mother, the father of the baby, or a close friend as her labor partner. Regardless of whether the teen has a support person, the nurse needs to establish a trusting relationship with her. In this way, the nurse can help the teen understand what is happening to her. Establishing a nurturing rapport is essential. Some nurses may view adolescent pregnancy as a negative event; however, it is important to treat the young woman with respect. The adolescent who is given positive reinforcement will leave the experience with increased self-esteem despite the emotional problems that may accompany her situation.

If a support person accompanies the adolescent, that individual also needs the nurse's encouragement and support. The nurse must explain changes in the young woman's behavior and substantiate her wishes. The nursing staff needs to reinforce the adolescent's feelings that she is wanted and important.

The adolescent who has taken childbirth education classes is generally better prepared for labor compared to the adolescent who has not. However, the nurse must keep in mind that the younger the adolescent, the less she may be able to participate actively in the process, even if she has taken prenatal classes.

Adolescents, regardless of their age, need ongoing education throughout labor and in the early postpartum period. Provide clear explanations. Encourage these clients in particular to ask questions and seek information.

Even if the adolescent is planning to relinquish her newborn, she should be given the option of seeing and holding the infant. She may be reluctant to do this at first, but the grieving process is facilitated if the mother sees the infant. However, seeing or holding the newborn should be the young woman's choice.

Adolescents need individualized care for the issues that they face in the postpartum period. They may experience additional psychosocial issues unique to their age group and their developmental level. Adolescents are also at an increased risk for unintended subsequent pregnancies and abortions. Proper discharge teaching includes contraceptive options (Gavin et al., 2013).

Evaluation

Evaluation provides an opportunity to determine the effectiveness of nursing care. As a result of comprehensive nursing care during the intrapartum period, the following outcomes may be anticipated:

- The mother's physical and psychological well-being has been maintained and supported.
- The baby's physical and psychological well-being has been protected and supported.
- The mother and her family members have had input into the birth process and have participated as much as they desired.
- The mother and her baby have had a safe birth.

REVIEW Intrapartum Care

RELATE Link the Concepts and Exemplars

Linking the exemplar of intrapartum care with the concept of comfort:
You are caring for a mother in the transition stage of labor when she begins crying and says, "It hurts so much. I don't know if I can take this anymore." As you were admitting her, when contractions were less frequent and intense, the client told you it was very important to her that she deliver the baby without taking any pain medication and that she would feel like a failure if she gave in and took a narcotic.

1. Will you offer her a narcotic analgesic to reduce her discomfort? Explain your answer.
2. What nonpharmacologic strategies can you implement to help her manage her pain?

Linking the exemplar of intrapartum care with the concept of culture and diversity:

3. When admitting a client to the labor unit, what cultural assessment will you perform at this time?
4. The client tells you a cultural belief in her family is that a candle must be burning when the infant is born, because they believe the infant will move toward the light, thereby making labor easier and the baby will be born faster. How will you respond to this request?

READY Go to Companion Skills Manual

REFER Go to Pearson Nursing Student Resources
nursing.pearsonhighered.com

- Additional review materials
- Chart 6: Intrapartum High-Risk Factors
- Chart 7: Psychological Characteristics and Nursing Support During the First and Second Stages of Labor
- Chart 8: Deviations From Normal Labor Process Requiring Immediate Intervention
- Chart 9: Comparison of Birthing Positions

REFLECT Case Study

It's a busy night, and you admit two clients, one right after the other. The first client is a 24-year-old single woman in labor with her first pregnancy. Her contractions are 8 minutes apart, she is dilated 2 cm (0.8 in.), and is at the +3 station. She tells you the pain is almost more than she can stand during contractions and asks how soon the physician can start the epidural. The second client is 28 years old and in labor with her fourth child. Her contractions are also 8 minutes apart, and she is dilated to 2 cm (0.8 in.) and at the +2 station. She is laughing and joking with her partner between contractions and asks if it would be okay if they play cards while they wait for labor to progress.

1. What factors may be influencing the different responses of these women to the pain of labor?
2. How would your nursing care differ for these women?
3. Which client do you anticipate is likely to deliver first? Explain your answer.

EXEMPLAR 33.3 Postpartum Care

EXEMPLAR KEY TERMS
Afterpains, *2172*
Colostrum, *2174*
Diastasis recti
   abdominis, *2173*
Fundus, *2171*
Involution, *2171*
Lochia, *2172*

Lochia alba, *2172*
Lochia rubra, *2172*
Lochia serosa, *2172*
Mature milk, *2174*
Puerperium, *2171*
Subinvolution, *2172*
Transitional milk, *2174*
Uterine atony, *2172*

EXEMPLAR LEARNING OUTCOMES
After reading about this exemplar, you will be able to:

1. Describe the pathophysiology and clinical manifestations associated with the postpartum period.
2. Identify risk factors and prevention methods associated with the postpartum period.
3. Illustrate the nursing process in providing culturally competent care for postpartum clients.
4. Formulate priority nursing diagnoses appropriate for a postpartum client.
5. Summarize therapies used by disciplinary teams in the collaborative care of a postpartum client.
6. Plan evidence-based care for a postpartum client and her family in collaboration with other members of the healthcare team.
7. Evaluate expected outcomes for the postpartum client.

▶ OVERVIEW

During the **puerperium**, or postpartum period, the woman readjusts, both physically and psychologically, from pregnancy and birth. The period begins immediately after birth and continues for approximately 6 weeks, or until the body has returned to a near prepregnant state.

▶ PHYSICAL ADAPTATIONS

After delivery, the woman's body goes through many changes as it begins to return to a nonpregnant state.

Reproductive System

INVOLUTION The term **involution** describes the rapid reduction in size of the uterus and the return of the uterus to a nonpregnant state. Following separation of the placenta, the decidua of the uterus is irregular, jagged, and varied in thickness. The spongy layer of the decidua is cast off as lochia, and the basal layer of the decidua remains in the uterus to become differentiated into two layers. This occurs within the first 48–72 hours after birth. The outermost layer becomes necrotic and is sloughed off in the lochia. The layer closest to the myometrium contains the fundi of the uterine endometrial glands. These glands lay the foundation for the new endometrium. Except at the placenta site, this process is completed in approximately 3 weeks. Healing at the placenta site occurs gradually over 6 weeks, at which point the site is completely healed (Cunningham et al., 2010). Bleeding from the larger uterine vessels of the placenta site is controlled by compression of the contracted uterine muscle fibers. The clotted blood is gradually absorbed by the body. Some of these uterine vessels are eventually obliterated and replaced by new vessels with smaller lumens.

The placenta site heals by a process of exfoliation and growth of endometrial tissue. This occurs with upward endometrial growth in the decidua basalis under the placenta site, with simultaneous growth of endometrial tissue from the margins of the site. The infarcted superficial tissue then becomes necrotic and is sloughed off (Cunningham et al., 2010). Exfoliation is a very important aspect of involution; if healing of the placenta site leaves a fibrous scar, the area available for future implantation is limited, as is the number of possible pregnancies.

With the dramatic decrease in the levels of circulating estrogen and progesterone following placental separation, the uterine cells atrophy, and the hyperplasia of pregnancy begins to reverse. Proteolytic enzymes are released, and macrophages migrate to the uterus to promote autolysis (self-digestion), which breaks down and absorbs protein material in the uterine wall. Factors that enhance involution include an uncomplicated labor and birth, complete expulsion of the placenta and membranes, breastfeeding, manual removal of the placenta during a cesarean birth, and early ambulation.

✳ Go to **nursing.pearsonhighered.com** for a chart listing factors that slow uterine involution and a rationale for each factor.

The **fundus** (top portion of the uterus) is situated in the midline, and is palpable below the umbilicus (**Figure 33–58 ●**). Following expulsion of the placenta, the uterus contracts to the size of a large grapefruit. The uterine blood vessels are firmly compressed by the myometrium. Blood and clots that remain within the uterus and changes in support of the uterus by the ligaments cause the fundus of the uterus to rise to the level of the umbilicus within 6–12 hours after birth.

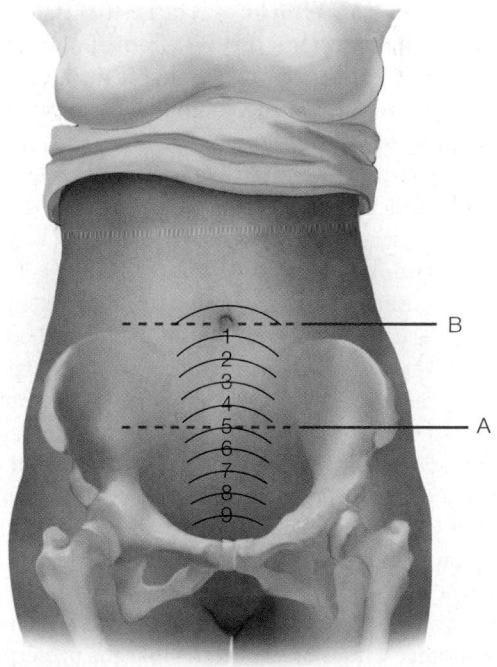

Figure 33–58 ● Involution of the uterus. *A,* Immediately after delivery of the placenta, the top of the fundus is in the midline and approximately halfway between the symphysis pubis and the umbilicus. Approximately 6–12 hours after birth, the fundus is at the level of the umbilicus. *B,* The height of the fundus then decreases about one fingerbreadth (~1 cm) each day.

A fundus that is above the umbilicus and is boggy (feels soft and spongy rather than firm and well contracted) is associated with excessive uterine bleeding. As blood collects and forms clots within the uterus, the fundus rises, interrupting firm contractions of the uterus and exacerbates **uterine atony** (relaxation of uterine muscle tone).

When the fundus is higher than expected on palpation and is not in the midline (usually deviated to the right), distention of the bladder should be suspected; the bladder should be emptied immediately and the uterus reassessed. If the woman is unable to void, in-and-out catheterization of the bladder may be required. In the immediate postpartum period, many women may not be aware of a full bladder. Because the uterine ligaments are still stretched, a full bladder can move the uterus. By the end of the puerperium, these ligaments regain their nonpregnant length and tension.

After birth, the top of the fundus remains at the level of the umbilicus for about half a day. On the first day postpartum, the top of the fundus is located about 1 cm (0.4 in.) below the umbilicus. The top of the fundus descends approximately one fingerbreadth (width of the index, second, or third finger), or 1 cm (0.4 in.), per day until it descends into the pelvis on about the 10th day.

If the mother is breastfeeding, the release of endogenous oxytocin from the posterior pituitary in response to suckling hastens involution of the uterus. Barring complications, such as infection or retained placental fragments, the uterus approaches its prepregnant size and location by 5–6 weeks. In women who had an oversized uterus during the pregnancy (because of hydramnios, birth of a large-for-gestational-age infant, or multiple gestation), the time frame for an immediate uterine involution process is lengthened. If intrauterine infection is present, foul-smelling lochia or vaginal discharge results. The infection irritates the uterine muscle, causing the fundus to descend much more slowly. When infection is suspected, other clinical signs, such as fever and tachycardia, and fundal tenderness must be assessed. Any slowing of descent is called **subinvolution**.

Afterpains (cramp-like pains caused by intermittent contractions of the uterus that occur after childbirth) are often more severe in multiparas than in primiparas. These afterpains may cause the mother severe discomfort for 2–3 days after birth. The administration of uterotonic agents (intravenous infusion with oxytocin or oral administration of methylergonovine maleate) stimulates uterine contraction and increases the discomfort of the afterpains. A warm water bottle placed against the lower abdomen may reduce this discomfort. In addition, the breastfeeding mother may find it helpful to take a mild analgesic agent approximately 1 hour before feeding her infant. The nurse can assure the mother who is breastfeeding that the prescribed analgesics are not harmful to the newborn and help improve the quality of the breastfeeding experience. If afterpains are interfering with the mother's rest, she may find it helpful to take an analgesic at bedtime.

LOCHIA   The uterus rids itself of the debris remaining after birth through a discharge called **lochia**, which is classified according to its appearance and contents. These classifications are lochia rubra, lochia serosa, and lochia alba.

Lochia rubra is dark red. It occurs for the first 2–3 days and contains epithelial cells, erythrocytes, leukocytes, shreds of decidua, and occasionally fetal meconium, lanugo, and vernix. Clotting is often the result of blood pooling in the upper portion of the vagina. A few small clots (no larger than a nickel) are common, particularly in the first few days after birth. However, lochia should not contain large (plum-size) clots; if it does, the cause should be investigated without delay.

Lochia serosa is a pinkish color. It follows from approximately day 3 until day 10. Lochia serosa is composed of serous exudate, shreds of degenerating decidua, erythrocytes, leukocytes, cervical mucus, and numerous microorganisms (Cunningham et al., 2010).

The red blood cell component decreases gradually, and a creamy or yellowish discharge persists for an additional week or two. This final discharge, termed **lochia alba** (from the Latin word for *white*), is composed primarily of leukocytes, decidual cells, epithelial cells, fat, cervical mucus, cholesterol crystals, and bacteria. Variation in the duration of lochia discharge is not uncommon; however, the trend should be toward a lighter amount of flow and a lighter color of discharge. When the lochia flow stops, the cervix is considered to be closed, and chances of infection ascending from the vagina to the uterus decrease.

Like menstrual discharge, lochia flow has a musty, stale odor that is not offensive. Microorganisms are always present in the vaginal lochia and contaminate the uterus with vaginal bacteria by the second day following birth. It is thought that infection does not develop because the organisms involved are relatively nonvirulent. Any foul smell to the lochia or used peripad suggests infection and the need for prompt additional assessment, such as white blood cell count and differential and assessment for uterine tenderness and fever.

The total average volume of lochia is approximately 225 mL, and the daily volume gradually decreases (Blackburn, 2013). Discharge is greater in the morning because of pooling in the vagina and uterus while the mother lies sleeping. The amount of lochia may also be increased by exertion or breastfeeding. Multiparous women usually have more lochia than first-time mothers. Women who undergo a cesarean birth typically have less lochia than women who give birth vaginally (Blackburn, 2013).

Evaluation of lochia is necessary not only to determine whether hemorrhage is present but also to assess uterine involution. The type, amount, and consistency of lochia determine the stage of healing of the placenta site; a progressive change from bright red at birth to dark red, then to pink, and then to white or clear discharge should be observed. Persistent discharge of lochia rubra or a return to lochia rubra may indicate subinvolution or late postpartum hemorrhage.

The nurse should exercise caution in evaluating bleeding immediately after birth. The continuous seepage of blood is more consistent with cervical or vaginal lacerations and may be effectively diagnosed when the bleeding is evaluated in conjunction with uterine consistency. Lacerations should be suspected if the uterus is firm and of expected size and if no clots can be expressed.

CERVICAL CHANGES   Following birth, the cervix is flabby, formless, and may appear bruised. The lateral aspects of the external os are sometimes lacerated during the birth process

(Cunningham et al., 2010). The external os is markedly irregular and closes slowly. It admits two fingers for a few days following birth, but by the end of the first week, it admits only a fingertip.

The first childbearing permanently changes the shape of the external os. The characteristic dimple-like os of the nullipara changes to the transverse slit (fish-mouth) os of the multipara. After significant cervical laceration or several lacerations, the cervix may appear lopsided. Because of the slight change in the size of the cervix, changes in maternal weight, muscle tone, and pelvic architecture, a diaphragm or cervical cap will need to be refitted if the woman uses one of these methods of contraception.

VAGINAL CHANGES   The vagina appears edematous and may be bruised following birth. The apparent bruising is caused by pelvic congestion and trauma and quickly disappears. Small, superficial lacerations may be evident, and the rugae are obliterated. The hymen, torn and jagged, heals irregularly, leaving small tags called carunculae myrtiformes.

The size of the vagina decreases, and rugae return within 3–4 weeks (Whitmer, 2011). This facilitates the gradual return to smaller, although not nulliparous, dimensions. By 6 weeks, the vagina of a woman who is not breastfeeding usually appears normal. The lactating woman is in a hypoestrogenic state because of ovarian suppression, and her vaginal mucosa may be pale and without rugae. The effects of the lowered estrogen level may lead to dyspareunia (painful intercourse), which may be reduced by the addition of a water-soluble personal lubricant.

Tone and contractility of the vaginal orifice may be improved by perineal tightening exercises, such as Kegel exercises. The woman may begin these soon after birth. The labia majora and labia minora are more flaccid in the woman who has borne a child than in the nullipara.

PERINEAL CHANGES   During the early postpartum period, the soft tissue in and around the perineum may appear edematous, with some bruising. If an episiotomy or a laceration is present, the edges should be approximated Initial healing of the episiotomy or laceration occurs in 2–3 weeks after the birth, although complete healing may take up to 4–6 months (Blackburn, 2013). Perineal discomfort may be present during this time.

OVULATION AND MENSTRUATION   The return of ovulation and menstruation varies for each postpartum woman. In mothers who are not breastfeeding, menstruation generally returns between 6 and 10 weeks after birth; 50% of the first cycles are anovulatory (Cunningham et al., 2010). The return of ovulation is directly associated with a rise in the serum progesterone level.

The return of ovulation and menstruation in breastfeeding mothers is usually prolonged. It is associated with the length of time the woman breastfeeds and whether formula supplements are used. If a mother breastfeeds for less than 1 month, the return of menstruation and ovulation is similar to that in the woman who is not breastfeeding. Women who exclusively breastfeed usually experience a delay in menstruation of at least 3 months. Suckling by the infant typically results in alterations in the gonadotropin-releasing hormone production, which is thought to be the cause of amenorrhea (Blackburn, 2013). Although exclusive breastfeeding helps to reduce the risk of pregnancy for the first 6 months after birth, it should be relied on only temporarily and if it meets the criteria for the lactational amenorrhea

method. Furthermore, because ovulation precedes menstruation and because women often supplement breastfeeding with bottles and pacifiers, breastfeeding is not considered to be a reliable means of contraception.

Abdomen

The uterine ligaments (notably the round and broad ligaments) are stretched and require the length of the puerperium to recover. Although the stretched abdominal wall appears loose and flabby, it responds to exercise within 2–3 months. However, the abdomen may fail to regain good tone and will remain flabby in the grand multipara, in the woman whose abdomen is overdistended, or in the woman with poor muscle tone before pregnancy. **Diastasis recti abdominis** (a separation of the abdominal muscle) may occur with pregnancy, especially in women with poor abdominal muscle tone. If diastasis occurs, part of the abdominal wall has no muscular support and is formed only by skin, subcutaneous fat, fascia, and peritoneum. This may be especially pronounced in women who have undergone a cesarean section, during which the rectus abdominis muscles are manually separated to access the uterine muscle. Improvement depends on the physical condition of the mother, the total number of pregnancies, pregnancy spacing, and the type and amount of physical exercise. Diastasis may result in a pendulous abdomen and increased maternal backache. Fortunately, diastasis responds well to exercise, and abdominal muscle tone can improve significantly.

The striae (stretch marks), which occur as a result of stretching and rupture of the elastic fibers of the skin, take on different colors based on the mother's skin color. The striae of light-skinned mothers are red to purple at the time of birth, then gradually fade to silver or white. The striae of mothers with darker skin, in contrast, are darker than the surrounding skin and remain darker. Striae gradually fade after a time, but they do remain visible.

Breasts and Lactogenesis

During pregnancy, increased levels of estrogen stimulate breast duct proliferation and development, and elevated progesterone levels promote the development of lobules and alveoli in preparation for lactation. Prolactin levels rise from approximately 10 mcg/mL before pregnancy to 200 mcg/mL at term. However, lactation is suppressed during pregnancy by elevated progesterone levels secreted by the placenta. Once the placenta is expelled at birth, progesterone levels fall, and the inhibition is removed, triggering milk production. This occurs whether the mother has breast stimulation or not. If breast stimulation is not occurring by the third or fourth day, however, prolactin levels begin to drop. By 2 weeks postpartum, if there is no stimulation, prolactin levels will be back to prepregnancy levels, and milk production will cease.

Initially, lactation is under endocrine control. The hormone prolactin is released from the anterior pituitary in response to breast stimulation from suckling or the use of a breast pump. Prolactin stimulates the milk-secreting cells in the alveoli to produce milk, then rapidly drops back to baseline. If more than approximately 3 hours elapse between stimulation, prolactin levels begin to drop below baseline. To reverse the overall decline in prolactin level, the mother can be encouraged to stimulate her breasts more frequently (e.g., every 1.5–2.0 hours). Mothers should be strongly encouraged to stimulate their breasts frequently if their infants are not effective feeders or if they are separated from their infants. Prolactin receptors are established during the first 2 weeks postpartum in response to frequency of breast stimulation (Human Milk Banking Association of North America, 2011). Inadequate development of prolactin receptors during this time is likely to negatively impact the mother's long-term milk volume.

The milk that flows from the breast at the start of a feeding or pumping session is called foremilk. The foremilk is watery milk that is high in protein and low in fat (1%–2%). This milk has trickled down from the alveoli between feedings to fill the lactiferous ducts, and it is low in fat because the fat globules made in the alveoli stick to each other and to the walls of the alveoli and do not trickle down. In addition to prolactin release, stretching of the nipple and compression of the areola signal the hypothalamus to trigger the posterior pituitary gland to release oxytocin. Oxytocin acts to cause the myoepithelial cells surrounding the alveoli in the breast tissue to contract, ejecting milk (including the fat globules present) into the ducts. This process is called the milk-ejection reflex but is better known in lay terms as the "let-down" reflex (response). The average initial let-down response occurs about 2 minutes after an infant begins to suckle, and between 4 and 10 let-down responses will occur during a feeding session. The milk that flows during "let-down" is called hindmilk. Hindmilk is rich in fat (which can exceed 10%) and, therefore, is high in calories. In a sample of expressed breast milk, the average total fat concentration is approximately 4% and the total caloric content is approximately 20 calories/oz.

By 6 months of breastfeeding, prolactin levels are only 5–10 mcg/mL (Riordan & Wambach, 2010), yet milk production continues. A whey protein called feedback inhibitor of lactation (FIL) has been identified as influencing milk production through a negative feedback loop. FIL is present in breast milk and functions to decrease milk production. The more milk that remains in the breast for a longer period of time, the more milk production is decreased. On the other hand, the more often the breasts are emptied, the lower the level of FIL and the faster milk is produced. This mechanism of regulating milk at the local level is called autocrine control. This process is key to understanding how a mother maintains or loses her milk supply (Riordan & Wambach, 2010). A number of factors can delay or impair lactogenesis. Maternal factors include the following (Riordan & Wambach, 2010):

- Cesarean birth
- Postpartum hemorrhage
- Type 1 diabetes
- Untreated hypothyroidism
- Obesity
- Polycystic ovary syndrome
- Retained placenta fragments
- Vitamin B_6 deficiency
- History of previous breast surgery
- Insufficient glandular breast tissue
- Significant stress.

Other factors that can interfere with breastfeeding include smoking, use of alcohol, and use of some prescription and OTC medications (e.g., antihistamines and combined birth control pills).

STAGES OF HUMAN MILK   During the establishment of lactation, there are three stages of human milk:

1. Colostrum
2. Transitional milk
3. Mature milk.

Colostrum is the initial milk that begins to be secreted during midpregnancy and that is immediately available to the baby at birth. It provides the infant with all the nutrition required until the mother's milk becomes more abundant in a few days. No routine supplementation of other fluids is necessary unless there is a medical indication. Colostrum is a thick, creamy, yellowish fluid with concentrated amounts of protein, fat-soluble vitamins, and minerals; it has lower amounts of fat and lactose compared with mature milk. It also contains antioxidants and high levels of lactoferrin and secretory IgA. It promotes the establishment of *Lactobacillus bifidus* flora in the digestive tract, which helps protect the infant from disease and illness. Colostrum also has a laxative effect on the infant, which helps the baby pass meconium stools, which in turn helps decrease hyperbilirubinemia.

After 30-72 hours, maternal milk production normally becomes noticeably more abundant. The milk "coming in" is called **transitional milk** and has qualities intermediate between those of colostrum and mature milk. It is still light yellow in color but is more copious than colostrum and contains more fat, lactose, water-soluble vitamins, and calories. By day 5, most mothers are producing approximately 500 mL/day.

Mature milk is white or slightly blue-tinged in color. It is present by 2 weeks postpartum and continues thereafter until lactation ceases. Mature milk contains approximately 13% solids (carbohydrates, proteins, and fats) and 87% water. Mature human milk's appearance, similar to that of skim cow's milk, may cause mothers to question whether their milk is "rich enough." The nurse should reassure the mother that this is the normal appearance of mature human milk and that mature milk provides the infant with all the necessary nutrients. Although gradual changes in composition do occur continuously over periods of weeks to accommodate the needs of the growing newborn, the composition of mature milk in general is fairly consistent with the exception of the fat content as noted previously. Milk production continues to increase slowly during the first month. By 6 months postpartum, a mother produces approximately 800 mL/day (Riordan & Wambach, 2010).

Gastrointestinal System

Following birth, the mother may be hungry and may enjoy a light meal. Frequently, she is quite thirsty and will drink large amounts of fluid. Drinking fluids helps replace those lost during labor, in the urine, and through perspiration.

The bowels tend to be sluggish following birth because of the lingering effects of progesterone, decreased abdominal muscle tone, and bowel evacuation associated with the labor and birth process. Women who have had an episiotomy or who have lacerations or hemorrhoids may tend to delay elimination because they fear increasing their pain or believe their stitches will be torn if they bear down. However, refusing or delaying the bowel movement may cause increased constipation and more pain when bowel elimination finally occurs.

There is no evidence in favor of restricting oral intake following a cesarean birth. While institutional policies may vary, evidence suggests that advancing the diet as desired restores the gastrointestinal system to a normal state more quickly than withholding solids and does not lead to an increased rate of complications (King et al., 2015). The woman may experience some initial discomfort from flatulence. This can be relieved by early ambulation and use of antiflatulence medications. Chamomile or peppermint tea may also be helpful in reducing discomfort from flatulence. It may take a few days for the bowel to regain its tone, especially if general anesthesia was used. The woman who has had a cesarean or a difficult birth may benefit from stool softeners.

Urinary System

The postpartum woman has increased bladder capacity, swelling and bruising of the tissue around the urethra, decreased sensitivity to fluid pressure, and decreased sensation of bladder filling. Consequently, she is at risk for overdistention, incomplete bladder emptying, and buildup of residual urine. Women who have had neuraxial anesthesia, such as an epidural or spinal, have inhibited neural functioning of the bladder and are more susceptible to bladder distention, difficulty voiding, and bladder infections. In addition, use of oxytocin to facilitate uterine contractions following expulsion of the placenta has an antidiuretic effect. Following cessation of the oxytocin, the woman will experience rapid bladder filling (Cunningham et al., 2010).

Urinary output increases during the early postpartum period (first 12–24 hours) because of postpartum diuresis. The kidneys must eliminate an estimated 2,000–3,000 mL of extracellular fluid with the normal pregnancy, which causes rapid filling of the bladder. Adequate bladder elimination is an immediate concern. Women with preeclampsia, chronic hypertension, and diabetes experience greater fluid retention than do other women, and postpartum diuresis is increased accordingly.

If urinary stasis exists, chances for urinary tract infection increase because of bacteriuria and the presence of dilated ureters and renal pelves, which persist for approximately 6 weeks after birth. A full bladder may also increase the tendency of the uterus to relax by displacing the uterus and interfering with its contractility, leading to hemorrhage. In the absence of infection, the dilated ureters and renal pelves return to prepregnant size by the end of the sixth week.

Vital Signs

With the exception of the first 24 hours after birth, the woman should be afebrile during the postpartum period. Epidural anesthesia for labor, which can interfere with heat dissipation, has a direct effect on maternal temperature but rarely results in overt fever (Shatken, Greenough, & McPherson, 2012). A maternal temperature of up to 38°C (100.4°F) may occur after childbirth as a result of the exertion and dehydration of labor. An increase in temperature to between 37.8°C and 39°C (100°–102.2°F) may also occur during the first 24 hours after the mother's milk comes in (Cunningham et al., 2010). However, in women not meeting these criteria, infection must be considered in the presence of an increased temperature.

Immediately following childbirth, many women experience a transient rise in both systolic and diastolic blood pressures, which spontaneously return to the prepregnancy baseline during the next few days (James, 2008). A decrease may indicate physiological readjustment to decreased intrapelvic pressure, or it may be related to uterine hemorrhage. Orthostatic hypotension, as indicated by feelings of faintness or dizziness immediately after standing up, can develop in the first 48 hours as a result of abdominal engorgement that may occur after birth. A low or decreasing blood pressure may reflect hypovolemia secondary to hemorrhage, but it is a late sign. Blood pressure elevations may result from excessive use of oxytocin or vasopressor medications. Because preeclampsia can persist into or occur first in the postpartum period, routine evaluation of blood pressure is needed. If a woman complains of headache, hypertension must be ruled out before analgesics are administered.

Puerperal bradycardia with rates of 50–70 bpm commonly occurs during the first 6–10 days of the postpartum period. This may be related to decreased cardiac effort, decreased blood volume following placental separation and contraction of the uterus, and increased stroke volume. A pulse rate of greater than 100 bpm may indicate hypovolemia, infection, fear, or pain and requires further assessment.

Frequently, the mother experiences intense tremors that resemble shivering from a chill immediately after birth. This shivering has been explained as

- a result of the sudden release of pressure on the pelvic nerves after birth,
- a response to a fetus-to-mother transfusion that occurred during placental separation,
- a reaction to maternal adrenaline production during labor and birth, or
- a reaction to epidural anesthesia.

If not followed by fever, this chill is of no clinical concern, but it is uncomfortable for the woman. The nurse can increase the woman's comfort by covering her with a warmed blanket and reassuring her that the shivering is a common, self-limiting situation. If the woman allows herself to go with the shaking, the shivering will last only a short time. Some women may find a warm beverage to be helpful. Later in the puerperium, chill and fever indicate infection and require further evaluation.

Blood Values

Blood values should return to the prepregnant state by the end of the postpartum period. Pregnancy-associated activation of coagulation factors may continue for variable amounts of time after birth. This condition, in conjunction with trauma, immobility, sepsis, obesity, African American ethnicity, diabetes, smoking, and advanced maternal age, predisposes the woman to development of thromboembolism (King et al., 2015). The incidence of thromboembolism is reduced by early ambulation.

Nonpathological leukocytosis often occurs during labor and in the immediate postpartum period, with white blood cell counts of 25,000–30,000 cells/mm^3 (Cunningham et al., 2010). These values typically return to normal levels by the end of the first postpartum week. Leukocytosis combined with the normal increase in erythrocyte sedimentation rate may obscure the diagnosis of acute infection at this time (Whitmer, 2011).

Hemoglobin and hematocrit levels may be difficult to interpret during the first 2 days after birth because of the changing blood volume. The loss of blood in the first 24 hours accounts for half the red blood cell volume gained during the course of the pregnancy. Blood loss averages 400 mL with a vaginal birth and nearly 1,000 mL with a cesarean birth (Rhode, 2011). Lochia constitutes less than 25% of this blood loss (James, 2008). As extracellular fluid is excreted, hemoconcentration occurs, with a concomitant rise in hematocrit. A drop in values indicates an abnormal blood loss. The following is a convenient rule to remember: A three to four percentage point drop in hematocrit equals a blood loss of 500 mL (Whitmer, 2011). After 3–4 days, mobilization of interstitial fluid leads to a slight increase in plasma volume. This hemodilution leads to a decrease in hemoglobin, hematocrit, and plasma protein by the end of the first postpartum week. Decreases in plasma volume reach nonpregnant levels by 4–6 weeks postpartum (Whitmer, 2011).

Platelet levels typically fall as a result of placental separation. They then begin to increase by the third to fourth day postpartum, gradually returning to normal by the sixth week postpartum. Fibrinolytic activity typically returns to normal during the hours following birth. The hemostatic system as a whole reaches its normal prepregnant status by 3–4 weeks postpartum; however, the diameter of deep veins can take up to 6 weeks to return to prepregnant levels (Blackburn, 2013). This explains the prolonged risk of thromboembolism in the first 6 weeks following birth.

Cardiovascular Changes

The mother's cardiovascular system undergoes dramatic changes during the birth that can result in cardiovascular instability because of an increase in cardiac output. The cardiac output typically stabilizes and returns to pregnancy levels within an hour following birth. Maternal hypervolemia acts to protect the mother from excessive blood loss. Cardiac output declines by 30% in the first 2 weeks and reaches normal levels by 6–12 weeks (Blackburn, 2013). For a more detailed description of cardiovascular changes that occur immediately following birth, consult a perinatal physiology text (Whitmer, 2011).

Diuresis in the first 2–5 days after birth assists in decreasing the extracellular fluid and results in a weight loss of 3 kg (6.6 lb) (James, 2008). Failure to have diuresis in the immediate postpartum period can lead to pulmonary edema and subsequent cardiac problems. This is seen more commonly in women with a history of preeclampsia or preexisting cardiac problems (Blackburn, 2013; James, 2008).

Neurological and Immunological Changes

Neurological problems and disorders can predispose women to higher rates of morbidity and mortality during pregnancy and the postpartum period. Headaches are the most common neurological symptoms encountered by postpartum women. Headaches may result from fluid shifts in the first week after birth, leakage of cerebrospinal fluid into the extradural space during spinal anesthesia, gestational hypertension, or stress (James, 2008). Migraine headaches may persist during pregnancy and

postpartum (Hoshiyama et al., 2012). It is more likely that a woman will have a seizure during labor or in the first 24 hours after birth than during pregnancy (Sibai, 2012). Women with epilepsy also have more feeding difficulties, irritability, and lethargy.

▶ PSYCHOLOGICAL ADAPTATIONS

The postpartum period is a time of readjustment and adaptation for the entire childbearing family but especially for the mother. The woman experiences a variety of responses as she adjusts to a new family member, postpartum discomforts, changes in her body image, and the reality that she is no longer pregnant. The psychological adaptations of the postpartum woman are discussed in detail in the exemplar on Postpartum Depression in the module on Mood and Affect.

The nurse plays a key role in assessing and assisting the mother–infant bond. As discussed in Exemplar 33.4, the nurse facilitates a number of activities that help strengthen maternal attachment, including feeding, bathing, and recognizing the infant's specific cues related to sleep and activity.

Ongoing assessment of the mother's psychological adaptation is critical because it allows the nurse to evaluate what client teaching needs to be provided. A detailed discussion of psychological assessment of the postpartum mother is included in the Nursing Process section of this exemplar.

▶ NUTRITION

An initial weight loss of approximately 4.5–5.4 kg (10–12 lb) occurs as a result of birth of the infant and expulsion of the placenta and amniotic fluid. Diuresis accounts for the loss of an additional 2.3 kg (5 lb) during the early puerperium. By the sixth to eighth week after birth, many women have returned to approximately their prepregnant weight if they had gained the average 11.4–13.6 kg (25–30 lb) during pregnancy. For others, a return to prepregnant weight may take longer. Women often express concern about the slow pace of their postpartum weight loss. Multiparas tend to be more positive than primiparas, probably because a multipara's previous experience has prepared her for the fact that the body does not immediately return to a prepregnant state.

Nutritional needs change following childbirth. Nutrient requirements vary depending on whether the mother decides to breastfeed. An assessment of postpartum nutritional status is necessary before giving nutritional guidance. Postpartum nutritional status is determined primarily by assessing the new mother's weight, hemoglobin and hematocrit levels, clinical signs, and dietary history.

Postpartum Nutritional Status

The amount of weight gained during pregnancy is a major determinant of weight loss after childbirth. Generally, women who gain excessive weight during pregnancy are more likely to sustain a weight gain 1 year following childbirth, putting them at increased risk of long-term overweight or obesity (Stuebe, 2009). The mother's weight should be considered in terms of ideal weight, prepregnancy weight, and weight gain during pregnancy. Women who desire information about weight reduction can be referred to a dietitian for individual counseling or to community-based educational programs. Educational programs need to address a variety of issues, such as the significance of the quality of food eaten rather than its quantity; the importance of regular physical activity in improving health, building lean muscle mass, and increasing metabolism; and the value of meal planning to ensure that healthy foods are readily available and to avoid pitfalls such as opting for fast foods, which are often high in fat (Stuebe, 2009).

Hemoglobin and erythrocyte levels should return to normal within 2–6 weeks after childbirth. Hematocrit levels gradually rise because of hemoconcentration as extracellular fluid is excreted. Iron supplements are generally continued for 2–3 months following childbirth to replenish stores depleted by pregnancy.

The nurse assesses clinical symptoms the new mother may be experiencing. Constipation is a common problem following birth. The nurse can encourage the woman to maintain a high fluid intake to keep the stool soft. Dietary sources of fiber, such as whole grains, fruits, and vegetables, are also helpful in preventing constipation.

The nurse obtains specific information on dietary intake and eating habits directly from the woman. Visiting the mother during mealtimes provides an opportunity for unobtrusive nutritional assessment. Which foods has the woman selected? Is her diet nutritionally sound? A comment focusing on a positive aspect of her meal selection may initiate a discussion of nutrition.

The nurse needs to inform the dietitian if a woman's cultural or religious beliefs require specific foods so that appropriate meals can be prepared for her. The nurse may also refer women with unusual eating habits or numerous questions about good nutrition. In addition, the nurse provides literature on nutrition so that the woman will have a source of appropriate information at home.

During the childbearing years, the risk for obesity becomes especially problematic for women. Consequently, it is critical to use the postpartum period to change behaviors and help promote effective weight management in women (Stuebe, 2009).

Nutritional Care of Formula-Feeding Mothers

After birth, the formula-feeding mother's dietary requirements return to prepregnancy levels. If the mother has a good understanding of nutritional principles, it is sufficient to advise her to reduce her daily caloric intake by approximately 300 kcal and to return to prepregnancy levels for other nutrients.

If the mother has a limited understanding of nutrition, now is the time to teach her the basic principles and importance of a well-balanced diet. Her eating habits and dietary practices will eventually be reflected in the diet of her child.

If the mother has gained excessive weight during pregnancy (or perhaps was overweight before pregnancy) and wishes to lose weight, the nurse should refer her to a dietitian. The dietitian can design weight-reduction diets to meet nutritional needs and food preferences. Weight loss goals of 0.45–0.9 kg (1–2 lb) per week are usually suggested.

In addition to meeting her own nutritional needs, the new mother is usually interested in learning how to provide for her infant's nutritional needs. A discussion of infant feeding that includes topics such as selecting infant formulas, formula preparation, and vitamin and mineral supplementation is appropriate and generally well received.

Nutritional Care of Breastfeeding Mothers

The nutritional needs of the mother are increased during breastfeeding. Table 33–4 in Exemplar 33.1 lists the Dietary Reference Intakes during breastfeeding for specific nutrients. Table 33–5 in Exemplar 33.1 provides a sample daily food plan for lactating women. It is especially important for the breastfeeding mother to consume sufficient calories because inadequate caloric intake can reduce milk volume. However, milk quality generally remains unaffected. The breastfeeding mother should increase her calories by approximately 200 kcal over her pregnancy requirement or 500 kcal over her prepregnancy requirement. This results in a total of approximately 2,500–2,700 kcal/day for most women.

Because protein is an important ingredient in breast milk, an adequate intake while breastfeeding is essential. An intake of 65 g/day during the first 6 months of breastfeeding, and of 62 g/day during the second 6 months, is recommended. As in pregnancy, it is important for the mother to consume adequate nonprotein calories to prevent the use of protein as an energy source.

Calcium is an important ingredient in milk production, and requirements during lactation remain the same as those during pregnancy—that is, an increase of 1,000 mg/day. If the intake of calcium from food sources is not adequate, calcium supplements are recommended.

Because iron is not a principal mineral component of milk, the needs of lactating women are not substantially different from those of nonpregnant women. As previously mentioned, however, supplementation for 2–3 months after childbirth is advised to replenish maternal stores depleted by pregnancy.

Liquids are especially important during lactation, because inadequate fluid intake may decrease milk volume. Fluid recommendations while breastfeeding are eight to ten 8-oz glasses daily, including water, juice, milk, and soups.

In addition to counseling nursing mothers on how to meet their increased nutrient needs during breastfeeding, it is important to discuss a few issues related to infant feeding. For example, many breastfeeding mothers are concerned about how specific foods they eat may affect their babies. Generally, the nursing mother need not avoid any foods except those to which she might be allergic. Occasionally, however, some nursing mothers find that certain foods may cause the infant to be colicky or to develop a skin rash. Onions, turnips, cabbage, chocolate, spices, and seasonings are common offenders. The best advice to give the nursing mother is to avoid those foods that she suspects cause distress in her infant. For the most part, however, she should be able to eat any nourishing food she wants without fear that her baby will be affected.

▶ ALTERATIONS

Alterations in health during the antepartum and intrapartum period cause increased risk during the postpartum period. **Table 33–15** ● lists risks associated with various conditions.

TABLE 33–15   Postpartum High-Risk Factors

Preeclampsia	↑ Blood pressure ↑ Central nervous system irritability ↑ Need for bed rest → ↑ risk thrombophlebitis ↑ Risk of seizures
Diabetes	Need for insulin regulation Episodes of hypoglycemia or hyperglycemia ↓ Healing
Cardiac disease	↑ Maternal exhaustion
Cesarean birth	↑ Recovery time ↑ Pain from incision ↑ Risk of infection ↑ Length of hospitalization
Overdistention of uterus (multiple gestation, hydramnios)	↑ Risk of hemorrhage ↑ Risk of thrombophlebitis ↑ Risk of anemia ↑ Risk of breastfeeding problems (cesarean section risk) ↑ Stretching of abdominal muscles ↑ Incidence and severity of afterpains
Abruptio placentae, placenta previa	Hemorrhage → anemia ↑ Uterine contractility after birth → ↑ infection risk
Precipitous labor (<3 hours)	↑ Risk of lacerations to birth canal → hemorrhage
Prolonged labor (>24 hours)	Exhaustion ↑ Risk of hemorrhage Nutritional and fluid depletion ↑ Bladder atony and/or trauma
Difficult birth	Exhaustion ↑ Risk of perineal lacerations ↑ Risk of hematomas ↑ Risk of hemorrhage → anemia
Extended period of time in stirrups at birth	↑ Risk of thrombophlebitis
Retained placenta	↑ Risk of hemorrhage ↑ Risk of infection

NURSING PROCESS

During the first several postpartum weeks, the woman must accomplish the following physical and developmental tasks:

- Restore physical condition.
- Develop competence in caring for and meeting the needs of her infant.
- Establish a relationship with her new child.
- Adapt to altered lifestyles and family structure resulting from the addition of a new member.

Assessment

Comprehensive care is based on a thorough assessment that identifies individual needs or potential problems. The nurse should remember the following principles in preparing for and completing the assessment of the postpartum woman:

- Use universal precautions including wearing gloves during this exam.

- Select a time that will provide the most accurate data. Palpating the fundus when the woman has a full bladder, for example, may give false information about the progress of involution. Ask the woman to void before assessment.
- Explain the purpose of regular assessment.
- Ensure that the woman is relaxed before starting. Perform the procedures as gently as possible to avoid unnecessary discomfort.
- Record and report the results as clearly as possible.
- Take appropriate precautions to prevent exposure to body fluids.

While performing the physical assessment, the nurse should also be teaching the woman. The assessment provides an excellent time to provide information about the body's postpartum physical and anatomical changes as well as the danger signs to report. Because the time that new mothers spend in the postpartum unit is limited, nurses need to use every available opportunity for client education about self-care. To assist nurses in recognizing these opportunities, examples of client teaching during the assessment are provided throughout the following discussion.

Psychological Assessment

Adequate assessment of the mother's psychological adjustment is an integral part of postpartum evaluation. This assessment focuses on the mother's general attitude, feelings of competence, available support systems, and caregiving skills. It also evaluates her fatigue level, sense of satisfaction, and ability to accomplish her developmental tasks.

Postpartum Psychological Adaptations

Soon after birth, during the taking-in period, the woman tends to be passive and somewhat dependent. The new mother follows suggestions, is hesitant about making decisions, and is still rather preoccupied with her needs (Rubin, 1984). She may spend time talking about her perceptions of her labor and birth. This helps her work through the process, sort out the reality from her fantasized experience, and clarify anything that she did not understand. Food and sleep are her major needs. The taking-hold phase is the second period of maternal adaptation, characterized by dependent and independent maternal behavior. If the woman is breastfeeding, she may worry about her technique or the quality of her milk. She may feel inadequate with her mothering abilities initially. She requires reassurance that she is doing well in her mothering abilities. The third period is the letting go where the mother reestablishes her relationships with other people. She adapts to parenthood through her role as a mother and she becomes more confident in her abilities to care for her newborn (Edelman & Mandle, 2010).

PSYCHOLOGICAL ASSESSMENT RISK FACTORS Some new mothers have little or no experience with newborns and may feel totally overwhelmed. They may show these feelings by asking questions and reading all available material or by becoming passive and quiet, because they simply cannot deal with their feelings of inadequacy. Unless a nurse questions the woman about her plans and previous experience in a supportive, nonjudgmental way, the nurse might conclude that

Postpartum Assessment: First 24 Hours After Birth

PHYSICAL ASSESSMENT/ NORMAL FINDINGS	ALTERATIONS AND POSSIBLE CAUSES*	NURSING RESPONSES TO DATA†
Vital Signs		
Blood pressure (BP): should remain consistent with baseline BP during pregnancy	High BP (preeclampsia, essential hypertension, renal disease, anxiety); drop in BP (may be normal; uterine hemorrhage)	Evaluate history of preexisting disorders and check for other signs of preeclampsia (edema, proteinuria). Assess for other signs of hemorrhage ($\uparrow$ pulse, cool clammy skin).
Pulse: 50–90 bpm	Tachycardia (difficult labor and birth, hemorrhage)	Evaluate for other signs of hemorrhage ($\downarrow$ BP; cool, clammy skin).
Respirations: 16–24 breaths/min	Marked tachypnea (respiratory disease)	Assess for other signs of respiratory disease.
Temperature: 36.6°–38°C (98°–100.4°F)	After first 24 hours, temperature of 38°C (100.4°F) or higher suggests infection	Assess for other signs of infection; notify physician/CNM.
Breasts		
General appearance: smooth, even pigmentation; changes of pregnancy still apparent; one may appear larger	Reddened area (mastitis)	Assess further for signs of infection.
Palpation: depending on postpartum day, may be soft, filling, full, or engorged	Palpable mass (caked breast, mastitis); engorgement (venous stasis); tenderness, heat, edema (engorgement, caked breast, mastitis)	Assess for other signs of infection: If blocked duct, consider heat, massage, and position change for breastfeeding. Assess for further signs. Report mastitis to physician/CNM.
Nipples: supple, pigmented, intact; become erect when stimulated	Fissures, cracks, soreness (problems with breastfeeding); not erectile with stimulation (inverted nipples)	Reassess technique; recommend appropriate interventions.
Lungs		
Sounds: clear to bases bilaterally	Diminished (fluid overload, asthma, pulmonary embolus, pulmonary edema)	Assess for other signs of respiratory distress.
Abdomen		
Musculature: abdomen may be soft, have a "doughy" texture; rectus muscle intact	Separation in musculature (diastasis recti abdominis)	Evaluate size of diastasis; teach appropriate exercises for decreasing the separation.
Fundus: firm, midline; following expected process of involution	Boggy (full bladder, uterine bleeding, retained products of conception)	Massage until firm. Assess bladder, and have woman void if needed. Attempt to express clots when firm. If bogginess remains or recurs, report to physician/CNM.
May be tender when palpated	Constant tenderness (infection)	Assess for evidence of endometritis.
Cesarean section incision dressing: dry and intact	Moderate to large amount of blood or serosanguineous drainage on dressing	Assess for hemorrhage. Reinforce dressing and notify physician/CNM.
Lochia		
Scant to moderate amount, earthy odor; no clots	Large amount, clots (hemorrhage) Foul-smelling lochia (infection)	Assess for firmness and express additional clots. Begin peripad count. Assess for other signs of infection; report to physician/CNM.
	*Possible causes of alterations are identified in parentheses.	†This column provides guidelines for further assessment and initial nursing actions.

(continued on next page)

Postpartum Assessment: First 24 Hours After Birth (continued)

PHYSICAL ASSESSMENT/ NORMAL FINDINGS	ALTERATIONS AND POSSIBLE CAUSES*	NURSING RESPONSES TO DATA†
Normal progression: first 1–3 days: rubra	Failure to progress normally or return to rubra from serosa (subinvolution)	Report to physician/CNM.
Following rubra: days 3–10: serosa (alba seldom seen in hospital)		
Perineum		
Slight edema and bruising in intact perineum	Marked fullness, bruising, increasing pain (vulvar hematoma)	Assess size. Apply ice glove or ice pack. Report to physician/CNM.
Episiotomy: no redness, edema, ecchymosis, or discharge; edges well approximated	Redness, edema, ecchymosis, discharge, or gaping stitches (infection)	Encourage sitz baths; review perineal care and appropriate wiping techniques.
Hemorrhoids: none present (if present, should be small and nontender)	Full, tender, inflamed hemorrhoids	Encourage sitz baths, side-lying position, Tucks pads, anesthetic ointments, manual replacement of hemorrhoids, stool softeners, and increased fluid intake.
Costovertebral Angle (CVA) Tenderness		
None	Present (kidney infection)	Assess for other symptoms of urinary tract infection (UTI); obtain clean-catch urine. Report to physician/CNM.
Lower Extremities		
No pain with palpation; negative Homans sign	Positive findings (thrombophlebitis)	Report to physician/CNM.
Elimination		
Urinary output: voiding in sufficient quantities at least every 4–6 hours; bladder not palpable	Inability to void (urinary retention); symptoms of urgency, frequency, dysuria (UTI)	Employ nursing interventions to promote voiding; if not successful, obtain order for catheterization.
		Report symptoms of UTI to physician/CNM.
Bowel elimination: should have normal bowel movement by second or third day after birth	Inability to pass feces (constipation caused by fear of pain from episiotomy, hemorrhoids, perineal trauma)	Encourage fluids, ambulation, roughage in diet, and sitz baths to promote healing of perineum; obtain order for stool softener.
	*Possible causes of alterations are identified in parentheses.	†This column provides guidelines for further assessment and initial nursing actions.

CULTURAL ASSESSMENT§	VARIATIONS TO CONSIDER	NURSING RESPONSES TO DATA§§
Determine customs and practices regarding postpartum care. Ask the mother whether she would like fluids, and ask what temperature she prefers.	Individual preference may include room temperature or warmed fluids rather than iced drinks.	Provide for specific request if possible. If woman is unable to provide specific information, the nurse may draw from general information regarding cultural variation.
Ask the mother what foods she would like.	Special foods or fluids to hasten healing after childbirth.	Mexican women may want food and fluids that restore hot–cold balance to the body.
		Women of European background may ask for iced fluids.
Ask the mother whether she would prefer to be alone during breastfeeding.	Some women may be hesitant to have someone with them when their breast is exposed.	Provide privacy as desired by the mother.
§These are only a few suggestions. We do not mean to imply this is a comprehensive cultural assessment; rather, it is a tool to encourage cultural competence.		§§This column provides guidelines for further assessment and initial nursing intervention.

Postpartum Assessment: First 24 Hours After Birth (continued)

PSYCHOSOCIAL ASSESSMENT/ NORMAL FINDINGS	VARIATIONS TO CONSIDER*	NURSING RESPONSES TO DATA†
Psychological Adaptation		
During first 24 hours: passive; preoccupied with own needs; may talk about her labor and birth experience; may be talkative, elated, or very quiet	Very quiet and passive; sleeps frequently (fatigue from long labor; feelings of disappointment about some aspect of the experience; may be following cultural expectation)	Provide opportunities for adequate rest, nutritious meals and snacks that are consistent with what the woman desires to eat and drink, and opportunities to discuss birth experience in nonjudgmental atmosphere if the woman desires to do so.
Usually by 12 hours: beginning to assume responsibility; some women eager to learn; easily feels overwhelmed	Excessive weepiness, mood swings, pronounced irritability (postpartum blues, feelings of inadequacy, culturally proscribed behavior)	Explain postpartum blues; provide supportive atmosphere. Determine support available for mother. Consider referral for evidence of profound depression.
Attachment		
En face position, holds baby close, cuddles and soothes, calls by name, identifies characteristics of family members in infant, may be awkward in providing care. Initially may express disappointment over gender or appearance of infant but within 1–2 days demonstrates attachment behaviors.	Continued expressions of disappointment with gender, appearance of infant; refusal to care for infant; derogatory comments; lack of bonding behaviors (difficulty in attachment, following expectations of cultural/ethnic group)	Provide reinforcement and support for infant caretaking behaviors; maintain nonjudgmental approach and gather more information if caretaking behaviors are not evident.
Client Education		
Has basic understanding of self-care activities and infant care needs; can identify signs of complications that should be reported.	Unable to demonstrate basic self-care and infant care activities (deficient knowledge; postpartum blues; following prescribed cultural behavior; may be cared for by grandmother or other family member)	Identify predominant learning style. Determine whether woman understands English, and provide interpreter if needed. Provide reinforcement of information through conversation and written material (remember that some women and their families may not be able to understand written materials because of language difficulties or inability to read). Provide information regarding infant care skills that are culturally consistent. Give woman an opportunity to express her feelings. Consider social service home referral for women who have no family or other support, are unable to take in information about self-care and infant care, and demonstrate no caretaking activities.
	*Possible causes of alterations are identified in parentheses.	†This column provides guidelines for further assessment and initial nursing actions.

the woman is disinterested, withdrawn, or depressed. Clues indicating adjustment difficulties include the following:

- Excessive continued fatigue
- Marked depression
- Excessive preoccupation with physical status or discomfort
- Evidence of low self-esteem
- Lack of support systems
- Marital problems
- Inability to care for or nurture the newborn
- Current family crises, such as illness or unemployment.

These characteristics frequently indicate a potential for maladaptive parenting, which may lead to child abuse or neglect (physical, emotional, or intellectual) and cannot be ignored. Referrals to public health nurses or other available community resources may provide greatly needed assistance and alleviate potentially dangerous situations.

Assessment of Early Attachment

A nurse in any postpartum setting can periodically observe and note progress toward attachment. Research shows that fathers experience attachment feelings similar to those experienced by mothers, and the assessment should include both parents when possible. This section, however, focuses primarily on the mother's attachment process.

The following questions can be addressed in the course of nurse–client interaction:

- Is the mother demonstrating attachment behaviors toward her newborn? To what extent does she seek face-to-face contact and eye contact? Has she progressed from fingertip touch, to palmar contact, to enfolding the infant close to her own body? Is attachment increasing or decreasing? If the mother does not exhibit increasing attachment, why not? Do the reasons lie primarily within her, the baby, or the environment?
- Is the mother inclined to nurture her infant by feeding every 2–3 hours?
- Is she progressing in her interactions with her infant?
- Does the mother act consistently? If not, is the source of unpredictability within her or her infant?
- Does she seek information and evaluate it objectively? Does she develop solutions based on adequate knowledge of valid data? Does she evaluate the effectiveness of her maternal care and adjust appropriately?
- Is the mother sensitive to the newborn's needs as they arise? How quickly does she interpret her infant's behavior and react to cues? Does she seem happy and satisfied with the infant's responses to her efforts? Is she pleased with feeding behaviors? How much of this ability and willingness to respond is related to the baby's nature and how much to her own?
- Does the woman state that she is pleased with her baby's appearance and gender? Is she reporting experiencing pleasure during interactions with her infant? What interferes with the enjoyment? Does she speak to the baby frequently and affectionately? Does she call him or her by name? Does she point out family traits or characteristics she sees in the newborn?
- Are there any cultural factors that might modify the mother's response? For instance, is it customary for the grandmother to assume most of the child care responsibilities while the mother recovers from childbirth?

When these questions have been addressed and the facts assembled, the nurse's intuition and knowledge should combine to answer three more questions:

1. Is there a problem in attachment?
2. If so, what is the problem?
3. What is its source?

The nurse can then devise a creative approach to the problem as it presents itself in the context of a unique, developing mother–infant relationship.

Diagnosis

Typical diagnoses related to the mother's needs may include any of the following:

- *Impaired Urinary Elimination*
- *Ineffective Breastfeeding*
- *Constipation*
- *Acute Pain*
- *Disturbed Sleep Pattern*.

(NANDA-I © 2015)

The postpartum family's needs, which should be identified during assessment, are also frequently used for developing nursing diagnoses. Examples of these diagnoses include the following:

- *Deficient Knowledge* related to information about infant care
- *Anxiety*
- *Readiness for Enhanced Family Coping*.

(NANDA-I © 2015)

Planning

Goals for care may include:

- The mother will demonstrate bonding with infant as evidenced by using the *en face* position.
- The mother will meet the infant's needs as they arise.

Implementation

Care of the mother during the postpartum period requires a great deal of client teaching in order to prepare her for discharge.

Promote Client Teaching

An important component of postpartum nursing care is client teaching, which must be individualized to the learning capability and readiness of the parents. Meeting the educational needs of the new mother and her family can be challenging. Each woman's educational needs will depend on her age, background, educational level, experience, and expectations. However, because the mother spends only a brief period of time in the postpartum area, it can be difficult for the nurse to identify and address individual instructional

Focus on Diversity and Culture
Postpartum Care

In many cultures, women and their families may embrace practices involving rest, seclusion, and dietary restraint, designed to assist the woman and her baby during the period of postpartum vulnerability. Chou (2017) notes a systematic review of over 50 studies that concludes that globally, most cultures identify a specified postpartum period, ranging 7 and 42 days, in which rest, specific dietary practices, and family support are common threads. In some cultures, including many Asian, African, and Latino cultures, there is also a period of seclusion which coincides with the period of lochial flow or postpartum bleeding. The nurse should not assume because a woman is of a certain ethnicity that she will automatically follow traditional cultural norms. The need to explore each woman's preferences for her postpartum needs and expectations is important to review prior to discharge. It should be noted that there are multifaceted variables that formulate a woman's personal beliefs and while cultural traditions will vary, the period of physiological recovery appears to coincide with the need for physical recovery in most cultures (Chou, 2017).

needs. Effective education provides the childbearing family with sufficient knowledge to meet many of its own health needs and to seek assistance if necessary.

The nurse first assesses the learning needs of the new mother through observation, sensitivity to nonverbal cues, and tactfully phrased questions. For example, "What plans have you made for handling things when you get home?" may elicit a response of several words and provide the opportunity for some information sharing and guidance. Some agencies also use checklists of common concerns for new mothers. The woman can check the concerns that are of interest to her.

Teaching during the postpartum period is a continuous process in which the nurse takes opportunities during interactions with the new parents to identify learning opportunities and offer teaching interventions. The nurse can also plan and implement teaching in a logical, nonthreatening way based on knowledge of and respect for the family's cultural values and beliefs. Unless the nurse believes a culturally related activity would be harmful, it can be supported and encouraged.

Nurses need to consider the mother's physical and psychosocial needs when conducting postpartum teaching. Initially, the woman may be exhausted from the birth experience, and her concentration may be impaired. Later, the new mother may be preoccupied with visitors and phone calls. Information should be delivered a little at a time and repeated to make sure that the parents understand what the nurse has discussed with them. Repetition is a valuable tool in the postpartum environment. In addition, many women are discharged during the first 48 hours after birth, making postpartum education difficult.

When the nurse is performing teaching sessions, the partner's schedule must also be considered. If the partner returns to work during the immediate postpartum period, teaching sessions in the late afternoon or early evening may be more convenient. In some cultures, such as the Hispanic culture, female relatives often assist the new mother and baby, so it is important to include any care providers in the teaching session.

Postpartum units use a variety of instructional methods, including handouts, formal classes, videotapes, and individual interaction. Printed materials are helpful for new mothers to consult if questions arise at home. Some facilities offer a hotline service in which new mothers can call with questions or concerns. As the cultural diversity in the United States continues to grow, the need for culturally competent information is imperative. Along with culturally diverse material, teaching aids should be presented in the woman's native language when possible. Written materials should be available, and translators or language lines should be utilized. Many clients are now accustomed to using the Internet and may prefer to use online support groups and access educational materials via the Internet. As technology expands, the nurse must remain current with the changing technology and the resources it creates. Evaluation of learning may also take several forms, such as return demonstrations, question-and-answer sessions, and even formal evaluation tools. Follow-up phone calls after discharge provide additional evaluative information and continue the helping process for the family.

Teaching content should include information on role changes and psychological adjustments as well as skills. Risk factors and signs of postpartum depression should be reviewed with every woman. Information is also essential for women with specialized educational needs, such as mothers who have had a cesarean birth, parents of twins, parents of an infant with congenital anomalies, parents with other young children, parents with a child who will require long-term hospitalization, and so on. More and more women with disabilities are now having children, and they may require additional support and education. Anticipatory guidance can help prepare parents for the many changes they will experience with a new family member.

Following discharge, various services are available in most communities to meet the needs of the postpartum family. These services range from educational, such as classes on nutrition, exercise, infant care, and parenting, to specific healthcare programs, such as well-baby checks, immunization clinics, family-planning services, new-mother support groups, and more. Some are offered by private caregivers, whereas others are the domain of city, county, state, or federal agencies. In all cases, the goal is to help ensure that all family members have the opportunity to meet healthcare needs, regardless of their resources.

Home health care is an important form of community-based nursing care offered to postpartum families. Home care visits and phone contacts help ensure that new parents have the necessary skills and resources to care for their infant.

Promote Comfort and Well-Being

The nurse can promote and restore maternal physical well-being by monitoring uterine status, vital signs, cardiovascular status, elimination patterns, nutritional needs, sleep and rest, and learning needs. Some women also require medication to relieve pain, treat anemia, provide immunity to rubella, and prevent development of antibodies in the nonsensitized Rh-negative woman. Most postpartum women need nursing interventions to promote their comfort and relieve stress.

❋ Go to **nursing.pearsonhighered.com** for a chart on essential information for common postpartum drugs.

It is important to ask the woman if she believes any special measures will be particularly effective and to offer her choices when possible. It is also important to remember that in some cultures or religions, such as Orthodox Judaism, women are prohibited from touching or changing their own perineal pads and will require the nurse or a family member to do so.

Many nursing interventions are available for the relief of perineal discomfort. Before selecting a method, the nurse needs to assess the perineum to determine the degree of edema and other problems. Application of ice to an episiotomy can promote comfort. The warmth of the water in the sitz bath provides comfort, decreases pain, and promotes circulation to the tissues, which promotes healing and reduces the incidence of infection. Gel pads, ice packs, and cool sitz baths have been found to be effective in reducing perineal edema and reducing the response of nerve endings that cause perineal discomfort (Petersen, 2011).

Client Teaching Perineal Care

Many women do not consider the episiotomy to be a surgical incision. Discussion helps them understand the importance of good wound care.

- Describe the process of wound healing. Discuss the risk of contamination of the episiotomy or laceration repair by bacteria from the anal area.
- Explain techniques that are used to keep the episiotomy clean and promote healing, such as
  a. a sitz bath, or
  b. use of a peri bottle following each voiding or defecation. Wash with soap and water at least once every 24 hours. Change peri pads at least four times per day.

- Demonstrate correct use of the peri bottle or sitz bath if necessary.
- Describe comfort measures:
  a. Ice pack, glove, or tea pad immediately following birth
  b. Sitz bath
  c. Judicious use of analgesics or topical anesthetics
  d. Tightening buttocks before sitting.
- Identify signs of suture line infection. Advise the woman to contact her caregiver if infection develops.
- Encourage discussion, and provide printed handouts. Some of this content may also be covered during a small postpartum class.

Some mothers experience hemorrhoidal pain after giving birth. Relief measures include the use of sitz baths, topical anesthetic ointments, rectal suppositories, or witch hazel pads applied directly to the anal area. The woman may be taught to digitally replace external hemorrhoids back into her rectum. Hand washing to prevent contamination to the vagina is essential. The woman may also find it helpful to maintain a side-lying position when possible and to avoid prolonged sitting. The mother is encouraged to maintain an adequate fluid intake, and stool softeners are administered to ensure greater comfort with bowel movements. Mothers should be advised to avoid straining with bowel movements, because this can increase the severity and discomfort associated with hemorrhoids. The hemorrhoids usually disappear a few weeks after birth if the woman did not have them before her pregnancy.

To reduce afterpains, the nurse can suggest that the woman lie prone, with a small pillow under her lower abdomen, and explain that the discomfort may feel intensified for approximately 5 minutes but then diminishes greatly, if not completely. The prone position applies pressure to the uterus and, therefore, stimulates contractions. When the uterus maintains a constant contraction, the afterpains cease. Additional nursing interventions include a sitz bath (for warmth), positioning, ambulation, or administration of an analgesic agent. For breastfeeding mothers, an analgesic administered 30 minutes to an hour before nursing helps promote comfort and enhances maternal–infant interaction.

Complementary and Alternative Therapy Lysine

Lysine, an essential amino acid, has been identified as a supplement that decreases the incidence of pain following an episiotomy. Lysine is available as a supplement. The recommended adult dosage is 12 mg/kg per day. It is also present in dietary sources, including meat, cheese, fish, eggs, soybeans, and nuts.

Discomfort may be caused by immobility. The woman who has been in stirrups or has pulled back on her legs for an extended period of time may experience muscular aches from such extreme positioning. It is not unusual for women to experience joint pains and muscular pain in both arms and legs, depending on the effort exerted during the second stage of labor. Early ambulation is encouraged to help reduce the incidence of complications, such as constipation and thrombophlebitis. It also helps promote a feeling of general well-being. The nurse provides information about ambulation and the importance of monitoring any signs of dizziness or weakness.

Enhance Attachment

The first few hours—and even minutes—after birth are an important period for the attachment of mother and infant.

If contact can occur during the first hour after birth, the newborn will be in the quiet state and able to interact with parents by looking at them. Newborns also turn their heads in response to a spoken voice. If possible and desired by the mother, the nurse may place the newborn on the woman's chest so that she can directly see her infant. This early interaction promotes attachment, early breastfeeding, and family interaction.

The first parent–newborn contact may be brief (a few minutes), and it may be followed by a more extended contact after the mother completes other uncomfortable procedures (expulsion of the placenta and suturing of the episiotomy or laceration). When the newborn is returned to the mother, the nurse can assist her to begin breastfeeding if the client so desires. The baby may seek out the mother's breast, and early contact between mother and infant can greatly affect breastfeeding success. Even if the newborn does not actively nurse, he or she can lick, taste, and smell the mother's skin. This activity by the newborn stimulates the maternal release of prolactin, which promotes the onset of lactation. These early interactions are associated with greater breastfeeding success.

Darkening the birthing room by turning out most of the lights causes newborns to open their eyes and gaze around. This in turn enhances eye-to-eye contact with the parents. (*Note:* If

Client Teaching Common Postpartum Concerns

Several postpartum occurrences cause special concern for mothers. The nurse will frequently be asked about the following events:

SOURCE OF CONCERN	EXPLANATION
Gush of blood that sometimes occurs when she first arises	Is a result of normal pooling of blood in the vagina when the woman lies down to rest or sleep. Gravity causes blood to flow out when she stands.
Passing clots	Blood pools at the top of the vagina and forms clots that are passed upon rising or sitting on the toilet.
Night sweats	Normal physiological occurrence that results as the body attempts to eliminate excess fluids that were present during pregnancy. May be aggravated by a plastic mattress pad.
Afterpains	More common in multiparas. Caused by contractions and relaxation of uterus. Increased by oxytocin and breastfeeding. Relieved with mild analgesics and time.
"Large stomach" after birth and failure to lose all weight gained during pregnancy	The baby, amniotic fluid, and placenta account for only a portion of the weight gained during pregnancy. The remainder takes approximately 6 weeks to lose. Abdomen also appears large because of decreased muscle tone. Postpartum exercises will help.

the healthcare provider needs a light source, the spotlight can be left on.) Treatment of the newborn's eyes with antibiotic eye ointment may also be delayed up to an hour after birth. Many parents who establish eye contact with the newborn are content to quietly gaze at their infant. Others may show more active involvement by touching or inspecting the newborn. Some mothers talk to their babies in a high-pitched voice, which seems to be soothing to newborns. Some couples verbally express amazement and pride when they see they have produced a beautiful, healthy baby. Their verbalization enhances feelings of accomplishment and ecstasy.

Encourage both parents to do whatever they feel most comfortable doing. Some parents prefer only limited contact with the newborn immediately after birth and, instead, desire private time together in a quiet environment. In spite of the current zeal for providing immediate attachment opportunities, nursing personnel need to be aware of parents' wishes. The desire to delay interaction with the newborn does not necessarily imply a decreased ability of the parents to bond with their newborn.

Discuss Suppression of Lactation

For the woman who chooses not to breastfeed, lactation may be suppressed by mechanical inhibition. Although signs of engorgement do not usually appear until the second or third day postpartum, engorgement is best prevented by beginning mechanical methods of lactation suppression as soon as possible after birth. Ideally, this involves having the woman begin wearing a supportive, well-fitting bra within 6 hours after birth. Some women may prefer a tight-fitting sports bra. The woman should wear the bra continuously until lactation is suppressed (usually ~5–7 days) and remove it only to shower. The bra provides support and eases the discomfort that can occur with tension on the breasts because of fullness. Ice packs should be applied over the axillary area of each breast for 20 minutes four times daily. This practice should begin soon

after birth. In addition, ice is useful in relieving discomfort if engorgement occurs.

The nurse should advise the mother to avoid any stimulation of her breasts by her baby, herself, breast pumps, or her sexual partner until the sensation of fullness has passed. Such stimulation increases milk production and delays the suppression process. Heat is avoided for the same reason; therefore, the mother is encouraged to let shower water flow over her back rather than her breasts.

Some mothers may inquire about suppression medications used in the past for nonnursing mothers. The nurse should inform these clients that because of concerns related to side effects, such medications are no longer used. Mechanical, rather than pharmacologic, methods are now employed.

Relieve Emotional Stress

The birth of a child, with the changes in role and the increased responsibilities it produces, is a time of emotional stress for the new mother. During the early postpartum period, the mother may be emotionally labile; mood swings and tearfulness are common. Initially the mother may repeatedly discuss her experiences of labor and birth. This allows the mother to integrate her experiences. If she believes that she did not cope well with labor, she may have feelings of inadequacy and may benefit from reassurance that she did well. Some women feel that they did not have any perception of time during the labor and birth and want to know how long it really lasted, or they may not remember the entire experience. In this case, it is helpful for the nurse to talk with the woman and provide the information that she is missing and desires.

During this time, the new mother must also adjust to the loss of her fantasized child and accept the child she actually has. This task may be more difficult if the child is not of the desired gender or if the infant has birth defects. Women who gave birth prematurely may experience guilt or have feelings of inadequacy. Immediately after the birth (the taking-in period), the mother is focused on bodily concerns and may not be fully ready to learn about personal and infant care. Following the initial dependent period, the mother becomes very concerned about her ability to be a successful parent (the taking-hold period). During this time, the mother requires reassurance that she is effective. She also tends to be receptive to teaching and demonstration designed to assist her in mothering successfully.

The depression, weepiness, and "let-down feeling" that characterize the postpartum blues are often a surprise for the new mother. She requires reassurance that these feelings are normal, an explanation of why they occur, and a supportive environment that permits her to cry without feeling guilty. The Edinburgh Postnatal Depression Scale (EPDS) is a widely used, validated screening tool that provides the nurse with clear information differentiating normal postpartum adjustment from postpartum depression. It consists of a ten item questionnaire in which each client response is given a score from 0-3. A total score greater than 12 is strongly associated with depression and indicates a need for intervention (Roy-Burne 2014).

Promote Rest

Energy is needed to make the psychological adjustments to a new infant and to assume new roles, so it is helpful for the new mother to know that fatigue may persist for several weeks or even months. Although most new mothers feel tired, if they have perceived the pregnancy and birth as a natural process, they tend to view themselves as healthy and well. Mothers who have other children may feel overwhelmed trying to meet the needs of the larger family.

Physical fatigue can affect other adjustments and functions of the new mother as well. For example, fatigue can reduce milk flow, thereby increasing problems with establishing breastfeeding. Persistent fatigue is especially common when mothers attempt to perform activities while the baby is napping instead of resting themselves. The nurse teaches women that failure to get adequate rest can lead to chronic fatigue and should be avoided. Fatigue can be a symptom of postpartum depression and should be discussed with the healthcare provider if symptoms continue or are accompanied by other signs of depression. Severe ongoing fatigue can also be a symptom of a thyroid disorder and should be evaluated by a healthcare provider (Gabbe, Niebyl, & Simpson, 2012).

Most mothers view the postpartum period as a time for recuperation. In many non-Western cultures, the 40 days following the birth are a time of recovery, when female relatives or friends assist the new mother in her daily activities (Eberhard, Garthus-Niegel, & Garthus-Niegel, 2010). In Mexico, during the first 7 days, nonhousehold members are not permitted to visit or enter the home. Mothers receive help with housework and eat special foods. It is recommended that they not be exposed to wind, and bathing is prohibited.

Specific groups of mothers at a higher risk for postpartum fatigue include the following:

- Mothers of multiples
- Mothers with infants who are still hospitalized and who engage in multiple trips to the hospital to visit their babies

- Mothers of infants with birth defects or special needs
- Mothers who lack social and familial support
- Mothers who return to work before the advised 6-week time period
- Mothers who have been on extended bed rest during the pregnancy.

Discuss Sexual Activity and Contraception

Typically, postpartum couples resume sexual intercourse once the episiotomy is healed and the lochial flow has stopped (James, 2008). Because this usually occurs by the end of the third week, before the 6-week follow-up, it is important that the woman and her partner have information about what to expect. The nurse may inform the couple that because the vaginal vault is "dry" (lacking estrogen), some form of water-soluble lubrication, such as K-Y jelly or Astroglide, may be necessary during intercourse. The female-superior and side-lying coital positions may be preferable, because they allow the woman to control the depth of penile penetration. Couples should be counseled that intercourse may be uncomfortable for the woman for some time and that patience is imperative.

Breastfeeding couples should be cautioned that during orgasm, milk may spurt from the nipples because of the release of oxytocin. Some couples find this spurt to be pleasurable or amusing, but others choose to have the woman wear a bra during sexual activity. Nursing the baby before lovemaking reduces the chance of milk release.

Other factors may inhibit satisfactory sexual experiences. For example, the baby's crying may be a distraction, the woman's changed body may seem unattractive to her or her partner, maternal sleep deprivation may reduce the woman's desire, or the woman's physiological response to sexual stimulation may be altered because of hormonal changes. By 3 months postpartum, many couples return to prepregnant levels of sexual interest and activity; however, this is highly variable. It is not abnormal for women, especially when breastfeeding, to experience decreased libido for several months. Decreased libido can be associated with hormonal changes, fatigue, stress, and lack of time because of family and work demands.

With anticipatory guidance during the prenatal and postpartum periods, the couple can be forewarned of potential temporary problems. Anticipatory guidance is enhanced if the couple can discuss their feelings and reactions as they experience them.

✳ *Go to* **nursing.pearsonhighered.com** *for more details on resuming sexual activity after childbirth.*

Information on contraception should be provided as part of discharge teaching if it is permissible within the healthcare agency. The nurse can also be an important resource for the woman and her partner during postpartum follow-up. Couples typically choose to use contraception to control the number of children they will have or to determine the spacing of future children. Some religious-based hospital facilities prohibit nurses and other healthcare providers from discussing contraception. If the nurse is discussing birth control, it is important to emphasize that in choosing a specific method, consistency of use is essential. The nurse needs to identify the advantages, disadvantages, risks, and contraindications of the various methods to help the couple, or the single mother, make an informed choice about the most practical and compatible method. Breastfeeding women are commonly concerned that a contraceptive method will interfere with their ability to breastfeed. Breastfeeding women should be given available options and choose the method that best fits their lifestyle, financial situation, and personal preference.

Promote Well-Being After Cesarean Birth

The mother who has a cesarean birth usually does extremely well postoperatively. Most women are ambulating by the day after the surgery. By the second postpartum day, the woman usually can shower, which seems to provide a mental as well as physical lift. Most women are discharged by the third day after birth.

The chances of pulmonary infection, however, are increased after a cesarean birth because of immobility after the use of narcotics and sedatives and because of the altered immune response in postoperative clients. Therefore, nurses should encourage the woman to cough and deep breathe every 2–4 hours while awake until she is ambulating frequently.

Nurses should also encourage leg exercises every 2 hours until the woman is ambulating. These exercises increase circulation, help prevent thrombophlebitis, and aid intestinal motility by tightening abdominal muscles.

Many of the complications that historically occurred after a cesarean birth were related to postpartum care practices in which mothers were encouraged to stay in bed for prolonged periods of time. Early ambulation, eating a low-roughage diet shortly after birth, and breastfeeding or infant feeding soon after birth all enhance the recovery of the mother and decrease complications in the postoperative period. Even though a cesarean birth is an operative procedure, most women giving birth are relatively healthy and, therefore, are less likely to experience postoperative complications when compared with other surgical clients.

The nurse monitors and manages the woman's pain experience during the postpartum period. Sources of pain include incisional pain, gas pain, referred shoulder pain, periodic uterine contractions (afterbirth pains), discomfort related to breastfeeding, and pain from voiding, defecation, or constipation. Nursing interventions are oriented toward preventing or alleviating pain or helping the woman cope with pain and include the following:

- Administer analgesics as needed, especially during the first 24–72 hours after childbirth. Use of analgesics relieves the woman's pain and enables her to be more mobile and active. Some facilities administer ibuprofen on a continuous basis in the early postpartum period to decrease swelling, reduce pain, and lower the need for, or frequency of, narcotic agents.
- Promote comfort through proper positioning, frequent changes of position, massage, back rubs, oral care, and reduction of noxious stimuli, such as noise and unpleasant odors.

- Encourage visits by significant others, including the newborn and older children. These visits distract the woman from the painful sensations and help reduce her fear and anxiety.
- Encourage the use of breathing, relaxation, guided imagery, and distraction (e.g., stimulation of cutaneous tissue) techniques taught in childbirth preparation class.

Epidural analgesia administered just after the cesarean birth is an effective method of pain relief for most women in the first 24 hours following birth. Other methods of pain relief that may be ordered by the physician include client-controlled analgesia and a continuous peripheral nerve block. A continuous epidural infusion is administered via an electric pump through an epidural catheter that is left in place following birth. The device has a button the woman can depress if additional pain relief is needed. Nursing assessments are hourly for women with a continuous epidural infusion in place and include vital signs, level of pain, amount of drug received, and amount of self-administration. The tubing is inspected to ensure connections are maintained, because movement by the woman in bed could disrupt the line. The epidural site should also be assessed to ensure the catheter has not been displaced.

Although the use of general anesthesia continues to decline, women who receive general anesthesia warrant additional assessments in the immediate postpartum period. Vital signs should be monitored continually until the woman has regained consciousness. Cardiopulmonary equipment should be in close range, with cardiac monitoring available as needed. The pulse oximeter should be used to determine the woman's oxygen status.

If a general anesthetic was used, abdominal distention may produce marked discomfort for the woman during the first few postpartum days. Measures to prevent or minimize abdominal distention include leg exercises, abdominal tightening, ambulation, avoiding carbonated or very hot or cold beverages, and avoiding the use of straws. Medical intervention for gas pain includes using rectal suppositories and enemas to stimulate passage of flatus and stool and encouraging the woman to lie on her left side. Lying on the left side allows the gas to pass from the descending colon to the sigmoid colon so that it can be expelled more readily.

Many physicians also order a nonsteroidal anti-inflammatory drug (NSAID) in addition to the previously mentioned agents once the woman is tolerating oral fluids well. NSAIDs assist with decreasing inflammation and do not have the negative side effects associated with many narcotics, such as sedation and constipation. NSAIDs are often given in combination with narcotic agents during the immediate postpartum period and often result in a decreased intake of narcotic agents.

Sometimes, women who have a cesarean birth have other discomforts that can be relieved with pharmacologic interventions. The nurse assesses the woman for other symptoms, such as nausea, itching (typically related to the morphine used in the epidural), and headache. If the woman is experiencing nausea, an antiemetic can be administered. Itching can also be relieved with pharmacologic interventions. NSAIDs are effective in managing headaches and other body aches.

The nurse can minimize discomfort and promote satisfaction as the mother assumes the activities of her new role. Instruction and assistance in assuming comfortable positions when holding or breastfeeding the infant will do much to increase the mother's sense of competence and comfort. The nurse should teach the woman to splint her incision when she ambulates to decrease pulling on the incision and the discomfort created by contraction of the abdominal muscles.

Other measures are aimed at needs that are unique to the woman who has had an operative birth. These measures include the following:

- Assess for the return of bowel sounds in all four quadrants every 4 hours, and assess the consistency of the abdomen. Women with a firm, distended abdomen may have difficulty passing flatus or stool.
- Assess the intravenous site, flow rate, and patency of the intravenous tubing.
- Monitor the condition of surgical dressings or the incision site using the REEDA scale (redness, edema, ecchymosis, discharge, and approximation of the suture line) along with skin temperature at and around the incision line.

Provide Postpartum Care of the Adolescent

The adolescent mother may have special postpartum needs, depending on her level of maturity and her support system. The nurse needs to assess maternal–infant interaction, roles of support people, plans for discharge, knowledge of childrearing, and plans for follow-up care. It is imperative that a community health service contact the adolescent shortly after discharge.

Contraception counseling is an important part of teaching the adolescent mother. The incidence of repeat pregnancies during adolescence is high. The younger the adolescent, the more likely she is to become pregnant again. Nurses should be aware of the state laws that govern their jurisdiction in order to determine if providing contraception without parental consent is allowed. In states where adolescents can obtain birth control without parental consent, it is often more comfortable for the adolescent to address these issues without others being present. Adolescents also may encounter obstacles when attempting to obtain contraceptives themselves. These may include embarrassment about discussing the topic; concerns about confidentiality, such as not wanting their parents to know or having to give permission; and lack of knowledge regarding available methods. Nurses can play a key role in overcoming these obstacles by providing teaching and referrals that address these barriers.

The nurse has many opportunities for teaching the adolescent about her newborn in the postpartum unit. Because the nurse is a role model, the manner in which nurses handle the newborn greatly influences young mothers. If the father is present, he should be included in as much of the teaching as possible. If the grandparents are going to take an active role in caring for the infant, they should also be included in teaching *if* this is desired by the new mother.

As with older parents, a newborn examination done at the bedside gives adolescents information about their baby's health and shows possible positions for handling the baby. The nurse can also use this time to provide information about newborn and infant behavior. Parents who have some idea of what to expect from their infant are less frustrated with the newborn's behavior.

The adolescent mother appreciates positive feedback about her newborn and her developing maternal responses. Praise and encouragement will increase her confidence and self-esteem. Young mothers with low self-esteem, family conflict, and few social supports are more likely to encounter postpartum depression (Lanzi, Bert, & Jacobs, 2009). Careful assessment of these factors should be made during the postpartum period so that appropriate referrals can be provided before discharge.

Group classes for adolescent mothers should include information about infant care skills, such as taking the baby's temperature, clearing the nose and mouth, monitoring growth and development, feeding the infant, providing well-baby care, and identifying danger signals in the ill newborn. These classes can also address unique needs of teen mothers, such as peer relationships, added responsibilities, and goal setting.

Ideally, teenage mothers should visit adolescent clinics for assessment of themselves and their newborn for several years after birth. In this way, the adolescent's enrollment in classes on parenting, need for vocational guidance, and school attendance can be supported and followed closely. Classes in the school system for young mothers are an excellent way of helping adolescents finish school and learn how to parent at the same time. Some public high schools have on-site child care centers to assist adolescent mothers and to provide an opportunity for them to learn important child development principles and child care tasks.

Provide Care for the Woman Who Relinquishes Her Infant

Women who choose to place their infants for adoption typically are single, White, never-married adolescents. It is much less common among Blacks and in Hispanic culture to consider adoption. The majority of women who relinquish their children have higher education and income levels, higher future educational or career goals, and mothers and fathers who favor adoption. Still others may feel that they are not emotionally ready for the responsibilities of parenthood, or their partner may strongly disapprove of the pregnancy. These and many other reasons may prompt the woman to relinquish her baby. The number of women who give their babies up voluntarily, however, is shrinking because of an increase in the acceptability of single motherhood and teenage parenting (Martin et al., 2009).

Increasingly, mothers are being forced to have their infants be placed in foster care because of illicit drug use, past history of abusing children, and incarceration. The number of infants placed for adoption because of these circumstances is unknown, but several factors must be met, including clear evidence that the parent is unfit and that severing the parental rights are in

NURSING CARE PLAN A Postpartum Client

Cathy McGhee delivered Callie, a healthy girl, 4 days ago. At the time of birth, Ms. McGhee was able to put the newborn to breast within the first hour. Callie was very alert at birth, latching on without difficulty. Ms. McGhee was able to breastfeed successfully during the remainder of her hospital stay. Today, Ms. McGhee has returned to the clinic complaining of pain and swelling in both breasts and a low-grade fever. She has also had trouble getting Callie to latch on.

ASSESSMENT

Subjective: Breast pain and tenderness, anxiety
Objective: Temperature 38°C (100.4°F). Breast tissue is firm, warm, and skin is shiny and taut. Swelling in axillary area and flattened nipples.

DIAGNOSIS

- *Acute Pain* related to increased breast fullness secondary to increased blood supply to breast tissue causing swelling of tissue around milk ducts

(NANDA-I © 2015)

PLANNING

- The client will remain free of breast fullness and pain.
- The client will experience decreased swelling of breast tissue.
- The client will exhibit no signs of breast tenderness or firmness.

IMPLEMENTATION

- Instruct client to breastfeed frequently.
- Instruct client to breastfeed at least 10–15 minutes on each breast per feeding.
- Assist client to pre-express milk onto nipple or baby's lips.
- Initiate pumping or manually express milk at the beginning of the feeding.

- Instruct client to pump, hand express, or massage to empty breast when feedings are missed.
- Administer analgesics before breastfeeding.
- Apply warm and/or cold compresses before breastfeeding.
- Apply fresh cabbage leaves to the breast between feedings.

EVALUATION

- No evidence of swelling found in breast tissue.
- Pain has decreased.
- Breast tissue is soft and without tenderness.

CRITICAL THINKING

1. The nurse preparing Ms. McGhee for discharge notices that Callie was breastfed 3 hours ago but for only 3–4 minutes on each breast. Ms. McGhee states that the baby is very sleepy and has slept most of the day. She says she will wait to breastfeed again until she is home and more comfortable, because her breasts hurt and are swollen. The nurse assesses the client's breasts, which are firm and tender, with some swelling under the arm. What should the nurse instruct the client to do before discharge? What can Ms. McGhee do to minimize the breast fullness and discomfort?
2. A postpartum nurse is teaching a breastfeeding class to new mothers. During the class, one client states she had a problem with engorgement after the birth of her first child and wants to know what she can do differently this time in order to avoid the problem again. What strategies can the nurse suggest to help prevent engorgement?

the best interest of the child (Child Welfare Information Gateway, 2013a). Many of these infants may be placed with relatives or in the foster care system.

In the 1990s, a number of infants were abandoned and left to die because the mothers did not want them and did not want others to know of their pregnancies. Starting in 1997, Infant Safe Haven Acts were passed that provided a means for a mother to place her baby up for adoption anonymously. The legislation was enacted to protect newborns from death caused by abandonment. Today, 47 states have legislation in place to ensure that relinquished babies are left with safe providers who can care for them and provide medical services. The relinquishing mother is protected from prosecution for neglect or abandonment under the law (Child Welfare Information Gateway, 2013b).

The mother who places her infant for adoption usually experiences intense ambivalence. Several factors contribute to this. First, there are social pressures against giving up one's child. Additionally, the woman has usually made considerable adjustments in her lifestyle to carry and give birth to this child, and she may be unaware of the growing bond between her and her child. Her attachment feelings may

peak upon seeing her baby. At the same time, she may not have told friends and relatives about the pregnancy and, therefore, may lack a support system to help her work through her feelings and support her decision making. After childbirth, the mother needs to complete a grieving process to work through her loss and its accompanying grief, loneliness, guilt, and other feelings. Mothers who relinquish their infants and have open adoptions experience less grief than those who have closed adoptions (Castle, 2012). When the relinquishing mother is admitted to the birthing unit, the nurse should be informed about the mother's decision to relinquish the baby. The nurse needs to respect any special requests for the birth and encourage the woman to express her emotions. After the birth, the mother should be allowed access to the baby; she is the one who will decide whether she wants to see the newborn. Seeing the newborn often aids in the grieving process and provides an opportunity for the birthmother to say goodbye. When the mother sees her baby, she may feel strong attachment and love. The nurse needs to assure the woman that these feelings do not mean that her decision to relinquish the child is wrong; relinquishment is often a painful act of love.

Postpartum nursing care also includes arranging ongoing care for the relinquishing mother. Some mothers may request an early discharge or a transfer to another medical unit. When possible, the nurse supports these requests.

Evaluation

Anticipated outcomes of comprehensive nursing care of the postpartum family include the following:

- The mother is reasonably comfortable and has learned pain relief measures.

- The mother is rested and understands how to add more activity during the next few days and weeks.
- The mother's physiological and psychological well-being have been supported.
- The mother verbalizes her understanding of self-care measures.
- The new parents demonstrate how to care for their baby.
- The new parents have had opportunities to form attachment with their baby.
- The new parents have information and access to community resources. This includes adoptive and relinquishing parents.

REVIEW Postpartum Care

RELATE Link the Concepts and Exemplars

Linking the exemplar of postpartum care with the concept of family:

1. What challenges would you anticipate for the new family following the delivery of twins or triplets?

2. How might you assess a family's ability to incorporate a newborn into the family unit?

Linking the exemplar of postpartum care with the concept of stress and coping:

3. What stressors must the mother of a newborn cope with after discharge?

4. How do these stressors impact the risk for child abuse? What nursing implementations and strategies can the nurse offer the new family to reduce this risk?

READY Go to Companion Skills Manual

READY Go to Pearson Nursing Student Resources
nursing.pearsonhighered.com

- Additional review materials
- Chart 10: Factors That Retard Uterine Involution
- Chart 11: Essential Information for Common Postpartum Drugs
- Chart 12: Resuming Sexual Activity After Childbirth

REFLECT Case Study

Jessica Riley is a single, 18-year-old mother with a 1-year-old son, Ryan. Jessica has had no contact with Ryan's father since before Ryan was born. Jessica and Ryan live in a small, one-bedroom apartment with Jessica's boyfriend, Casey. She is currently pregnant with Casey's baby.

Jessica took the evening off from work because she was feeling very tired. She fixes dinner for Casey before he has to go to work. While fixing dinner, Ryan is crying in the other room, and Jessica interrupts making dinner to attend to his needs.

When they all finally sit down to eat, Casey throws his plate against the wall and screams at her for making a "lousy dinner." He then proceeds to yank her out of her chair, hit her in the back, and knock her to the floor. She gets up crying, and he hits her in the abdomen and says, "You care more about these damn brats than me and what I want." She falls to the floor, and he kicks her in the abdomen. Jessica screams in pain. She somehow gets off the floor and makes it into the bedroom. The

neighbor in the next apartment hears the commotion and calls the police.

When the police arrive, they find Jessica on the bed doubled over and crying, Ryan in his crib crying, and Casey watching TV while smoking a joint. The police note that Jessica is pregnant and call for an ambulance. They ask her whether she was hit, and she tells them no. The police tell Jessica they are taking Casey in for

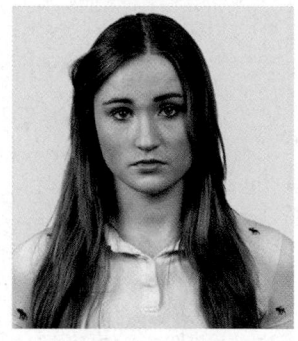

drug possession and further questioning. Jessica calls her mother and asks her to come get Ryan and then meet her at the hospital.

When the paramedics arrive, they start an intravenous line, place Jessica on oxygen, and transport her to the hospital. At the hospital, the OB triage nurse sends her directly to the labor and delivery unit. Jessica delivers a healthy female infant later in the evening. Because Jessica suffered a small abruption to the placenta, the midwife and physician suspect trauma from abuse.

In the immediate postpartum period, the midwife talks with Jessica privately. Jessica is told that she had a small abruption and that the placenta had an infarct. The midwife tells Jessica that in these situations, trauma is suspected. The midwife also shares with Jessica that sometimes women in abusive relationships get hit or kicked in the abdomen. Jessica cries and admits to the midwife that this is what happened, but she insists that Casey didn't mean to do it and is sure he will never do it again. She tells the midwife she will not press charges.

Social work is called for referral before Jessica goes home. The nurse midwife tells Jessica that a social work referral is required because of the risk of intimate partner violence and drug charges against Casey. Jessica worries about this, fearing that Casey will be angry. The social worker makes a visit the day after Jessica and the baby are discharged; Jessica is relieved that Casey is not home. Jessica tells the social worker everything is fine and that there are really no problems.

1. As the nurse caring for Jessica, what nursing diagnosis would be appropriate for the plan of care?

2. What risks to parental attachment do you anticipate for Jessica and her new daughter?

3. Create a teaching plan for Jessica before discharge.

EXEMPLAR 33.4 Newborn Care

EXEMPLAR KEY TERMS

Acrocyanosis, *2223*
Active acquired immunity, *2201*
Apgar score, *2210*
Babinski reflex (response), *2234*
Barlow maneuver, *2232*
Brazelton Neonatal Behavioral Assessment Scale, *2235*
Caput succedaneum, *2225*
Cephalohematoma, *2225*
Chemical conjunctivitis, *2226*
Circumcision, *2240*
Dubowitz tool, *2213*
Epstein pearls, *2227*
Erb-Duchenne paralysis (Erb palsy), *2231*
Erythema toxicum, *2223*
Forceps marks, *2224*
Gestational age assessment tools, *2213*
Grasping reflex, *2233*
Habituation, *2204*
Harlequin sign, *2223*
Jaundice, *2223*
Lanugo, *2212*
Meconium, *2200*
Milia, *2224*
Molding, *2225*
Mongolian spots, *2224*
Moro reflex, *2234*
Mottling, *2223*
Neonatal mortality risk, *2206*
Neonatal transition, *2191*
Neonatology, *2204*
Neutral thermal environment (NTE), *2196*
Nevus flammeus (port-wine stain), *2224*
Nevus vasculosus (strawberry mark), *224*
New Ballard Score, *2213*

Orientation, *2204*
Ortolani maneuver, *2232*
Passive acquired immunity, *2201*
Periodic breathing, *2194*
Physiological anemia of infancy, *2196*
Physiological jaundice, *2198*
Pseudomenstruation, *2201*
Rooting reflex, *2234*
Self-quieting ability, *2204*
Skin turgor, *2224*
Subconjunctival hemorrhages, *2227*
Sucking reflex, *2234*
Telangiectatic nevi (stork bites), *2224*
Thrush, *2227*
Tonic neck reflex, *2233*
Trunk incurvation (Galant reflex), *2234*
Vernix caseosa, *2224*

EXEMPLAR LEARNING OUTCOMES

After reading about this exemplar, you will be able to:

1. Describe the normal physiological adaptations of the newborn to extrauterine life.
2. Identify risk factors and prevention methods associated with the newborn period.
3. Illustrate the nursing process in providing culturally competent care for newborns and their families.
4. Formulate priority nursing diagnoses appropriate for a healthy newborn.
5. Summarize therapies used by interdisciplinary teams in the collaborative care of a newborn and his or her family.
6. Plan evidence-based care for a healthy newborn and his or her family in collaboration with other members of the healthcare team.
7. Evaluate expected outcomes for the newborn.

▶ OVERVIEW

The newborn (neonatal) period is the time from birth through the 28th day of life. During this period, the newborn adjusts from intrauterine to extrauterine life. The nurse needs to be knowledgeable about a newborn's normal physiological and behavioral adaptations and be able to recognize alterations.

▶ ADAPTATIONS TO EXTRAUTERINE LIFE

The first six hours of life, in which the newborn's body systems adapt to extrauterine life, is called the period of **neonatal transition**. The respiratory and cardiac systems undergo the most dramatic changes within the first minutes after birth.

Respiratory Adaptations

To begin life as a separate being, the newborn must immediately establish respiratory gas exchange in conjunction with marked circulatory changes. These radical and rapid changes are crucial to the maintenance of extrauterine life.

INITIATION OF RESPIRATION To maintain life, the lungs must function immediately after birth. Two changes are necessary for this to happen:

1. Pulmonary ventilation must be established through lung expansion.
2. A marked increase in the pulmonary circulation must occur.

The first breath of life—the gasp in response to mechanical and reabsorptive, chemical, thermal, and sensory changes associated with birth—initiates the serial opening of the alveoli. So begins the transition of the newborn from a fluid-filled environment to an air-breathing, independent, extrauterine life. **Figure 33–59 ●** summarizes the initiation of respiration.

During the latter half of gestation, the fetal lungs continuously produce fluid. This fluid expands the lungs almost completely, filling the air spaces. Some of the lung fluid moves up into the trachea and into the amniotic fluid; it is then swallowed by the fetus.

To prepare for birth, lung fluid production normally decreases and fetal breathing movement decreases 24–36 hours before the onset of true labor (Knuppel, 2007). However, approximately 80–100 mL of lung fluid remain in the respiratory passages of a normal term fetus at the time of birth. This fluid must be

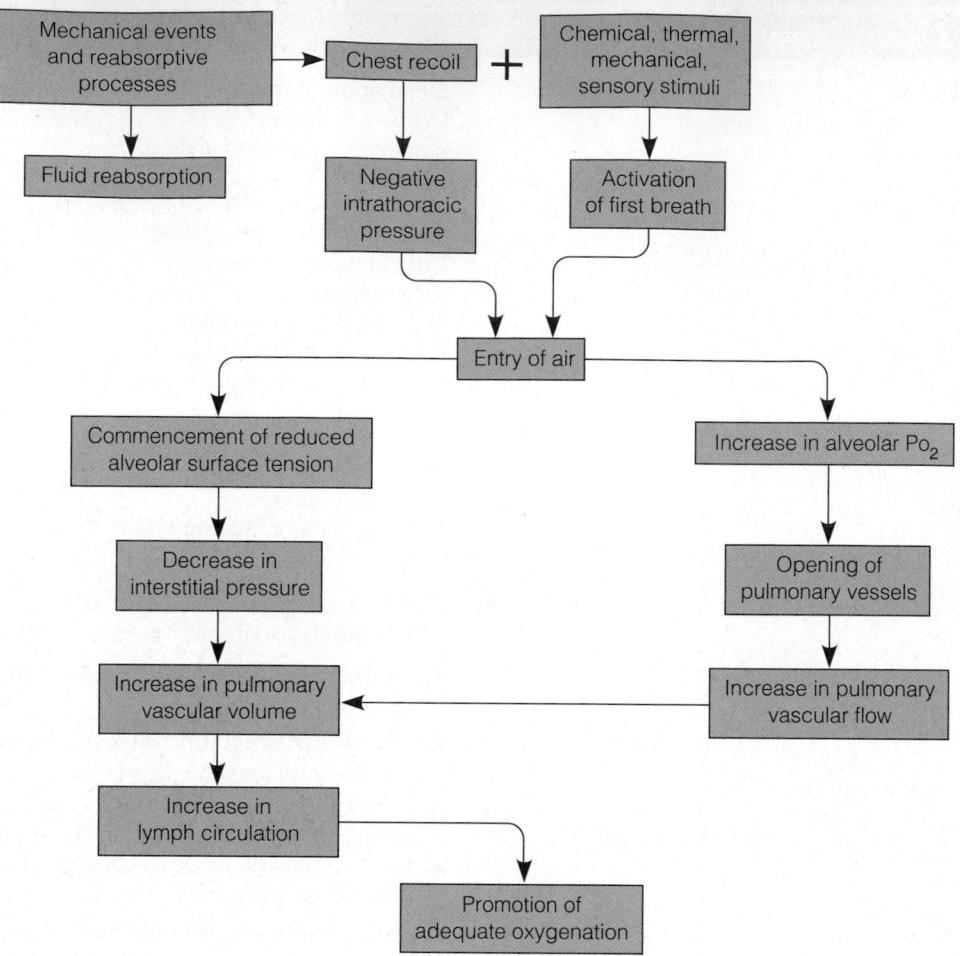

Figure 33–59 ● Initiation of respiration in the newborn.

removed from the lungs to permit adequate movement of air (Ramachandrappa & Jain, 2008).

During delivery, the fetal chest is compressed, increasing intrathoracic pressure and squeezing a small amount of the fluid out of the lungs. After the birth of the newborn's trunk, the chest wall recoils. This chest recoil creates a negative intrathoracic pressure, which is thought to produce a small, passive inspiration of air that replaces the fluid in the large airways that is squeezed out.

After this first inspiration, the newborn exhales, with crying, against a partially closed glottis, creating positive intrathoracic pressure. The high positive intrathoracic pressure distributes the inspired air throughout the alveoli and begins to establish functional residual capacity, which is the air left in the lungs at the end of a normal expiration. The higher intrathoracic pressure also increases absorption of fluid via the capillaries and lymphatic system. The negative intrathoracic pressure created when the diaphragm moves down with inspiration causes lung fluid to flow from the alveoli across the alveolar membranes into the pulmonary interstitial tissue.

At birth, the alveolar epithelium is temporarily more permeable. This permeability, combined with decreased cellular resistance at the onset of breathing, may facilitate passive liquid absorption. With each succeeding breath, the lungs continue to expand, stretching the alveolar walls and increasing the alveolar volume.

Protein molecules are too large to pass through capillary walls. The presence of more protein molecules in the pulmonary capillaries than in the interstitial tissue creates oncotic pressure. This pressure draws the interstitial fluid into the capillaries and lymphatic tissue to balance the concentration of protein. Lung expansion helps the remaining lung fluid move into the interstitial tissue. As pulmonary vascular resistance decreases, pulmonary blood flow increases, and more interstitial fluid is absorbed into the bloodstream. In the healthy term newborn, lung fluid moves rapidly into the interstitial tissue, but it may take several hours to move into the lymph and blood vessels. By 30 minutes of age most newborns have a normal functional residual capacity (FRC) with uniform lung expansion. Surfactant is essential for a normal FRC (Rosenberg, 2013).

Although the initial chest recoil assists in clearing the airways of accumulated fluid and permits further inspiration, most healthcare providers believe mucus and fluid should be suctioned from the newborn's mouth, nose, and throat. These providers use a bulb syringe to suction the mouth and nose as soon as the newborn's head and shoulders are delivered and again as the newborn adapts to extrauterine life and stabilizes.

Newborns may have problems clearing the fluid in the lungs and beginning respiration for a variety of reasons:

■ The lymphatic system may be underdeveloped, thus decreasing the rate at which the fluid is absorbed from the lungs.

■ Complications may occur before or during labor and birth that interfere with adequate lung expansion; thus, the decrease in pulmonary vascular resistance fails to occur, resulting in decreased pulmonary blood flow. These complications include the following:

a. Inadequate compression of the chest wall in very small newborns (small for gestational age or very low birth weight) because of immature muscular development

b. The absence of chest wall compression in a neonate born by cesarean birth, although this compression can be externally applied by skilled healthcare providers as they deliver the newborn from the uterus

c. Respiratory depression because of maternal analgesia or anesthesia agents

d. Aspiration of amniotic fluid, meconium, or blood.

Several chemical factors contribute to the onset of breathing. One of the most important is asphyxia of the fetus and newborn. The first breath is an inspiratory gasp, the result of central nervous system (CNS) reaction to sudden pressure, temperature change, and other external stimuli. This first breath is triggered by the slight elevation in partial pressure of carbon dioxide and decrease in pH and partial pressure of oxygen (PO_2), which are the natural result of a vaginal labor and birth. These changes, which are present in all newborns to some degree, stimulate the aortic and carotid chemoreceptors, initiating impulses that trigger the medulla's respiratory center. Although this brief period of asphyxia is a significant stimulator, prolonged asphyxia is abnormal and depresses respiration. Another chemical factor may result from clamping the umbilical cord, which may cause a drop in levels of a prostaglandin that inhibits respirations (Ramachandrappa & Jain, 2008). As a result, newborns can vigorously cry and be active before the cord is clamped or the placenta separates.

A significant decrease in environmental temperature after birth, from 37°C to between 21° and 23.9°C (98.6°F to 70°–75°F), results in sudden chilling of the moist newborn (Blackburn, 2013). The cold stimulates skin nerve endings, and the newborn responds with rhythmic respirations. Normal temperature changes that occur at birth are within acceptable physiological limits. Excessive cooling may result in profound respiratory depression and evidence of cold stress.

Upon birth the newborn experiences light, new sounds, and the full effects of gravity for the first time. As the fetus moves from the womb's familiar, comfortable, and quiet environment to one of sensory abundance, a number of physical and sensory influences help respiration begin. These stimuli include the following:

- The actual experience of birth, with its numerous tactile, auditory, and visual stimuli

- Joint movement, which results in enhanced proprioceptor stimulation to the respiratory center to sustain respirations

- Thorough drying of the newborn and placing the baby on the mother's chest and abdomen for skin-to-skin contact provides ample stimulation in a far more comforting way and also decreases heat loss.

FACTORS OPPOSING INITIATION OF RESPIRATION

Three major factors may inhibit the initiation of respiratory activity:

- The contracting force between alveoli (alveolar surface tension)

- Viscosity of lung fluid within the respiratory tract, which is influenced by surfactant levels

- The ease with which the lungs are able to fill with air (lung compliance).

Alveolar surface tension is the contracting force between the moist surfaces of the alveoli. This tension, which is necessary for healthy respiratory function, would nevertheless cause the small airways and alveoli to collapse between each inspiration were it not for the presence of surfactant. By reducing the attracting force between alveoli, surfactant prevents the alveoli from completely collapsing with each expiration and thus promotes lung expansion. Similarly, surfactant promotes lung compliance (the ability of the lung to fill with air easily). When surfactant decreases, compliance also decreases, and the pressure needed to expand the alveoli with air increases.

Resistive forces of the fluid-filled lung, combined with the small radii of the airways, necessitate pressures of 30–40 cm (11.8–15.7 in.) of water to open the lung initially (Niermeyer & Clarke, 2011).

The first breath usually establishes a functional residual capacity that is 30%–40% of the fully expanded lung volume. This functional residual capacity allows alveolar sacs to remain partially expanded on expiration, decreasing the need for continuous high pressures for each of the following breaths. Subsequent breaths require only 6–8 cm of water pressure to open alveoli during inspiration. Therefore, the first breath of life is usually the most difficult.

CARDIOPULMONARY PHYSIOLOGY As air enters the lungs, PO_2 rises in the alveoli, which stimulates the relaxation of the pulmonary arteries and triggers a decrease in pulmonary vascular resistance. As pulmonary vascular resistance decreases, the vascular flow in the lung increases rapidly and achieves 100% normal flow at 24 hours of life. This delivery of greater blood volume to the lungs contributes to the conversion from fetal circulation to newborn circulation.

After pulmonary circulation is established, blood is distributed throughout the lungs, although the alveoli may or may not be fully open. For adequate oxygenation to occur, the heart must deliver sufficient blood to functional, open alveoli. Shunting of blood is common in the early newborn period. Bidirectional blood flow, or right-to-left shunting through the ductus arteriosus, may divert a significant amount of blood away from the lungs, depending on the pressure changes of respiration, crying, and the cardiac cycle. This shunting in the newborn period is also responsible for the unstable transitional period in cardiopulmonary function.

OXYGEN TRANSPORT The transportation of oxygen to the peripheral tissues depends on the type of hemoglobin in the red blood cells (RBCs). In the fetus and newborn, a variety of hemoglobins exist, the most significant being fetal hemoglobin (HbF) and adult hemoglobin (HbA). Approximately 70%–90% of the hemoglobin in the fetus and newborn is of the fetal variety. The greatest difference between HbF and HbA relates to the transport of oxygen.

Because HbF has a greater affinity for oxygen than does HbA, the oxygen saturation in the newborn's blood is greater than that in the adult's, but the amount of oxygen available to the tissues is less. This situation is beneficial prenatally because the fetus must maintain adequate oxygen uptake in the presence of very low oxygen tension (umbilical venous PO_2 cannot exceed uterine venous PO_2). However, this high concentration of oxygen in the blood makes hypoxia in the newborn particularly difficult to recognize. Clinical manifestations of cyanosis do not appear until low blood levels of oxygen are present. In addition, alkalosis (increased pH) and hypothermia can result in less oxygen being available to the body tissues, whereas acidosis, hypercarbia, and hyperthermia can result in less oxygen being bound to hemoglobin and more oxygen being released to the body tissues.

MAINTAINING RESPIRATORY FUNCTION

The lung's ability to maintain oxygenation and ventilation (the exchange of oxygen and carbon dioxide) is influenced by such factors as lung compliance and airway resistance. Lung compliance is influenced by the elastic recoil of the lung tissue and anatomical differences in the newborn. The newborn has a relatively large heart and mediastinal structures that reduce available lung space. Also, the newborn chest is equipped with weak intercostal muscles and a rigid rib cage, with horizontal ribs and a high diaphragm, which restrict the space available for lung expansion. The large abdomen further encroaches on the high diaphragm to decrease lung space. Another factor that limits ventilation is airway resistance, which depends on the radii, length, and number of airways. Airway resistance is increased in the newborn compared with that in adults.

CHARACTERISTICS OF NEWBORN RESPIRATION

Initial respirations may be largely diaphragmatic, shallow, and irregular in depth and rhythm. The abdomen's movements are synchronous with the chest movements. When the breathing pattern is characterized by pauses lasting 5–15 seconds, **periodic breathing** is occurring. Periodic breathing is rarely associated with differences in skin color or heart rate changes, and it has no prognostic significance. Tactile or other sensory stimulation increases the inspired oxygen and converts periodic breathing patterns to normal breathing patterns during neonatal transition. With deep sleep, the pattern is reasonably regular. Periodic breathing occurs with rapid-eye-movement (REM) sleep, and grossly irregular breathing is evident with motor activity, sucking, and crying. Cessation of breathing lasting more than 20 seconds is defined as apnea and is abnormal in term newborns. Apnea may or may not be associated with changes in skin color or bradycardia (drop below 100 bpm). Apnea always needs to be further evaluated.

Newborns tend to be obligatory nose breathers: The nasal route is the primary route of air entry because of the high position of the epiglottis and the position of the soft palate (Blackburn, 2013). Although many term newborns can breathe orally, nasal obstructions can cause respiratory distress. Therefore, it is important to keep the nose and throat clear.

Immediately after birth, and for approximately the next 2 hours, respiratory rates of 60–70 breaths/minute are normal. Some cyanosis and acrocyanosis are normal for several hours; thereafter, the newborn's color improves steadily. If respirations drop below 30 or exceed 60 breaths/minute when the neonate is at rest, or if retractions, cyanosis, or nasal flaring and expiratory grunting occur, the healthcare provider should be notified. Any increased use of the intercostal muscles (retractions) may indicate respiratory distress, which should be reported immediately.

Cardiovascular Adaptations

During fetal life, blood with higher oxygen content is diverted to the heart and brain. Blood in the descending aorta is less oxygenated and supplies the kidney and intestinal tract before it is returned to the placenta. Limited amounts of blood, pumped from the right ventricle toward the lungs, enter the pulmonary vessels. In the fetus, increased pulmonary resistance forces most of this blood through the ductus arteriosus into the descending aorta.

✴ Go to **nursing.pearsonhighered.com** to see Chart 13: Fetal and Neonatal Circulation.

Marked changes occur in the cardiovascular system at birth. Expansion of the lungs with the first breath decreases pulmonary vascular resistance and increases pulmonary blood flow. Pressure in the left atrium increases as blood returns from the pulmonary veins. Pressure in the right atrium drops, and systematic vascular resistance increases as umbilical venous blood flow is halted when the cord is clamped. These physiological mechanisms mark the transition from fetal to neonatal circulation and show the interplay of cardiovascular and respiratory systems (**Figure 33–60 ●**).

Five major areas of change occur in cardiopulmonary adaptation:

1. *Increased aortic pressure and decreased venous pressure.* Clamping of the umbilical cord eliminates the placental vascular bed and reduces the intravascular space. Consequently, aortic (systemic) blood pressure increases. At the same time, blood return via the inferior vena cava decreases, resulting in a decreased right atrial pressure and a small decrease in pressure within the venous circulation.

2. *Increased systemic pressure and decreased pulmonary artery pressure.* With loss of the low-resistance placenta, systemic resistance pressure increases, resulting in greater systemic pressure. At the same time, lung expansion increases pulmonary blood flow, and the increased blood PO_2 associated with initiation of respirations dilates pulmonary blood vessels. The combination of vasodilation and increased pulmonary blood flow decreases pulmonary artery resistance. As the pulmonary vascular beds open, the systemic vascular pressure increases, enhancing perfusion of the other body systems.

3. *Closure of the foramen ovale.* Closure of the foramen ovale is a function of changing atrial pressures. In utero, pressure is greater in the right atrium, and the foramen ovale is open after birth. Decreased pulmonary resistance and increased pulmonary blood flow increase the pulmonary venous return into the left atrium, thereby increasing left atrial pressure slightly. The decreased pulmonary vascular resistance and the decreased umbilical venous return to the right atrium also decrease right atrial pressure. The pressure gradients across the atria are now reversed, with the left atrial pressure now greater, and the foramen ovale is functionally closed 1–2 hours after birth. However, a slight right-to-left shunting may occur in the early newborn period. Any increase in pulmonary resistance or right atrial pressure, such as occurs with crying, acidosis, or cold stress, may cause the foramen ovale to reopen, resulting in a temporary right-to-left shunt. Anatomical closure occurs within 30 months (Blackburn, 2013).

4. *Closure of the ductus arteriosus.* Initial elevation of the systemic vascular pressure above the pulmonary vascular pressure increases pulmonary blood flow by reversing the flow through the ductus arteriosus. Blood now flows from the aorta into the pulmonary artery. Furthermore, although the presence of oxygen causes the pulmonary arterioles to

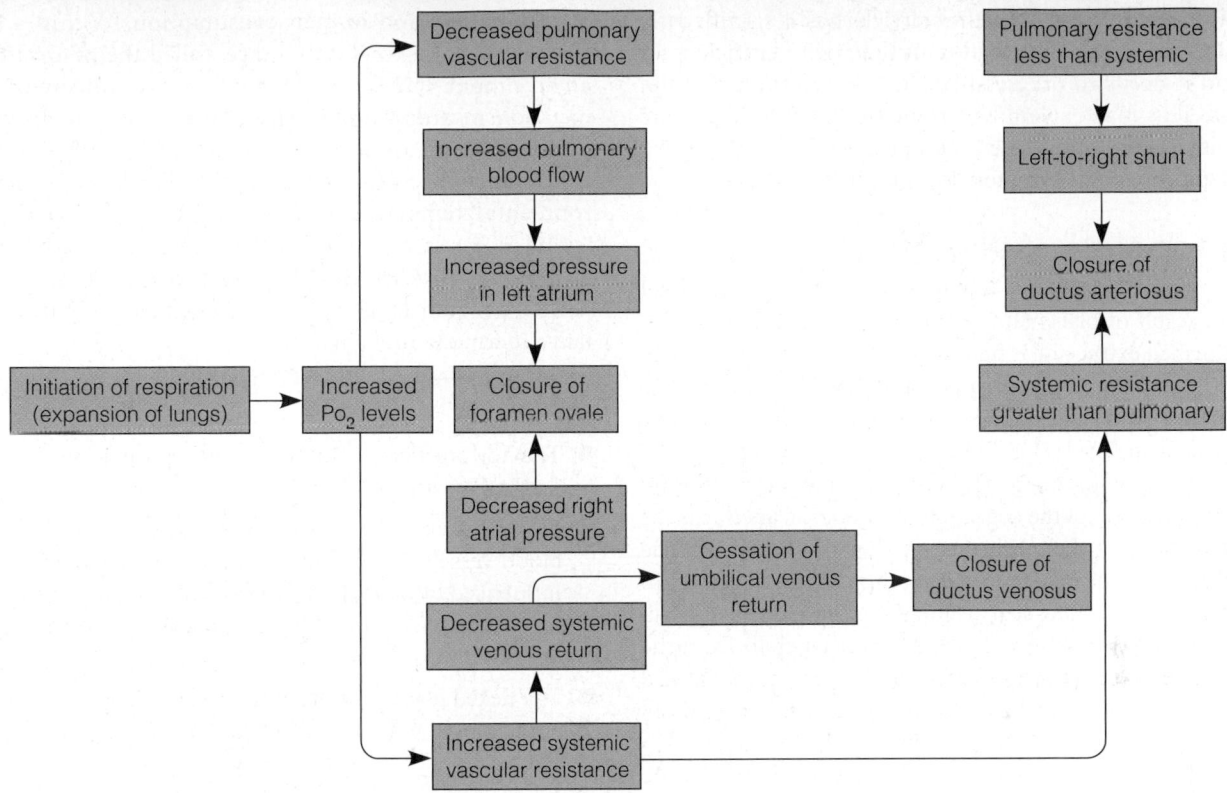

Figure 33–60 ● Transitional circulation: conversion from fetal to neonatal circulation.

dilate, an increase in blood PO_2 triggers the opposite response in the ductus arteriosus—that is, it constricts.

In utero, the placenta provides prostaglandin E_2, which causes ductus vasodilation. With the loss of the placenta and increased pulmonary blood flow, prostaglandin E_2 levels drop, leaving the active constriction by PO_2 unopposed. If the lungs fail to expand or if PO_2 levels drop, the ductus remains patent. Functional closure starts within 18 hours after birth, and fibrosis of the ductus occurs within 2–3 weeks after birth (Blackburn, 2013).

5. **Closure of the ductus venosus.** Although the mechanism initiating closure of the ductus venosus is not known, it appears to be related to mechanical pressure changes after severing of the cord, redistribution of blood, and cardiac output. Closure of the bypass forces perfusion of the liver. Fibrosis of the ductus venosus occurs within 2 months.

Assessment of the newborn's heart rate, blood pressure, heart sounds, and cardiac workload provides data for evaluating cardiac function. The newborn's blood pressure tends to be highest immediately after birth and then descends to its lowest level at about 3 hours of age. By days 4–6, the blood pressure rises and then plateaus at a level approximately the same as the initial level. Blood pressure is sensitive to the changes in blood volume that occur in the transition to newborn circulation. Peripheral perfusion pressure is a particularly sensitive indicator of the newborn's ability to compensate for alterations in blood volume before changes in blood pressure. Capillary refill should be less than 3 seconds when the skin is blanched.

Blood pressure values during the first 12 hours of life vary with the birth weight and gestational age. The average mean blood pressure is 31–61 mmHg in the full-term, resting newborn over 3 kg (6.6 lb) during the first 12 hours of life (AAP &

American Heart Association, 2011). Crying may cause an elevation in both the systolic and diastolic blood pressure; thus, accuracy is more likely in the quiet newborn. Currently two-point pulse oximetry (right hand and either foot) is recommended to screen for congenital heart disease. An SpO_2 of <95% needs to be referred to a cardiology clinic (Mahle et al., 2009).

Shortly after the first cry and the start of changes in cardiopulmonary circulation, the newborn heart rate can accelerate to 180 beats/min. The average resting heart rate in the first week of life is 110 to 160 beats/min in a healthy full-term newborn but may vary significantly during deep sleep or active awake states. In full-term newborns, the heart rate may drop to a low of 80 to 100 beats/min during deep sleep (Van Woudenberg et al., 2012).

Murmurs are produced by turbulent blood flow. Murmurs may be heard when blood flows across an abnormal valve or across a stenosed valve, when an atrial or ventricular septal defect is present, or when the flow across a normal valve is increased.

In newborns, 90% of all murmurs are transient *and not associated with anomalies.* These murmurs usually involve incomplete closure of the ductus arteriosus or foramen ovale. Soft murmurs may be heard as the pulmonary branch arteries increase their blood flow from 7% to 50% of the combined ventricular output during transition, causing a physiological peripheral pulmonary stenosis. Clicks may normally be heard at the lower left sternal border as the great vessels dilate to accommodate systolic blood flow in the first few hours of life. Murmurs are sometimes absent even in seriously malformed hearts.

Before birth, the right ventricle does approximately two thirds of the cardiac work, resulting in increased size and thickness of the right ventricle at birth. In the first 2 hours after birth, when the ductus arteriosus remains mostly patent, about one third of the left ventricular output is returned to the pulmonary circulation. As a result, the left ventricle has a significantly greater increase in volume load than the right ventricle after birth, and it needs to progressively increase in both size and thickness. This may explain why right-sided heart defects are better tolerated than left-sided ones and why left-sided heart defects rapidly become symptomatic after birth.

Hematopoietic Adaptations

In the first days of life, hematocrit may rise 1–2 g/dL above fetal levels as a result of placental transfusion, low oral fluid intake, and diminished extracellular fluid volume. By 1 week after birth, peripheral hemoglobin is comparable to fetal blood counts. The hemoglobin level declines progressively over the first 2 months of life (Blackburn, 2013). This initial decline in hemoglobin creates a phenomenon known as **physiological anemia of infancy**. A factor that influences the degree of physiological anemia is the nutritional status of the newborn. Supplies of vitamin E, folic acid, and iron may be inadequate given the amount of growth in the later part of the first year of life. Hemoglobin values fall, mainly from a decrease in red cell mass rather than from the dilutional effect of increasing plasma volume. The facts that red cell survival is lower in newborns than in adults and that red cell production is less also contribute to this anemia. Neonatal RBCs have a life span of 80–100 days, approximately two thirds the life span of adult RBCs. The normal RBC count in a term newborn is in the range of 5.1–5.3 million per milliliter during the first 24–48 hours of life (Bagwell, 2007).

Leukocytosis is a normal finding, because the stress of birth stimulates increased production of neutrophils during the first few days of life. Neutrophils then decrease to 35% of the total leukocyte count by 2 weeks of age. Lymphocytes play a role in antibody formation and eventually become the predominant type of leukocyte, and the total WBC count falls.

Blood volume is approximately 85 mL/kg for a term neonate (Bagwell, 2007). For example, a 3.6-kg (8-lb) newborn has a blood volume of 306 mL. Blood volume varies based on the amount of placental transfusion received during the delivery of the placenta as well as other factors, including the following:

- Delayed cord clamping and the normal shift of plasma to the extravascular spaces
- Gestational age
- Prenatal and/or perinatal hemorrhage
- Site of the blood sample.

SAFETY ALERT
Laboratory results may vary between capillary collection and venous collection. Greater variances can be expected if capillary collection was difficult or good blood flow was not obtained and the heel was squeezed excessively, which increases the risk of cellular damage within the specimen, increased serum levels, and micro blood clots.

Temperature Regulation

Newborns are homeothermic: They attempt to stabilize their internal (core) body temperatures within a narrow range in spite of significant temperature variations in their environment. Thermoregulation in the newborn is closely related to the rate of metabolism and oxygen consumption. Within a specific environmental temperature range, called the **neutral thermal environment (NTE)**, the rates of oxygen consumption and metabolism are minimal, and internal body temperature is maintained because of thermal balance (Brand & Boyd, 2010). For an unclothed term newborn, the NTE is an ambient environmental temperature range of 32°–34°C (89.6°–93.2°F) within 50% relative humidity. The limits for an adult are 26°–28°C (78.8°–82.4°F) (Brand & Boyd, 2010). Thus, the normal newborn requires higher environmental temperatures to maintain a thermoneutral environment.

Several newborn characteristics affect the establishment of thermal stability:

- The newborn has a thinner epidermis and less subcutaneous fat than an adult.
- Blood vessels in the newborn are closer to the skin than the blood vessels of an adult. Therefore, the circulating blood is influenced by changes in environmental temperature and, in turn, influences the hypothalamic temperature-regulating center.
- The flexed posture of the term newborn decreases the surface area exposed to the environment, thereby reducing heat loss.

Size and age may also affect the establishment of an NTE. For example, the small-for-gestational-age newborn has less adipose tissue and is hypoflexed and, therefore, requires higher environmental temperatures to achieve an NTE. Larger, well-insulated newborns may be able to cope with lower environmental temperatures. If the environmental temperature falls below the lower limits of the NTE, the newborn responds with increased oxygen consumption and metabolism, which results in greater heat production. As a result, prolonged exposure to the cold may result in depleted glycogen stores and acidosis. Oxygen consumption also increases if the environmental temperature is above the NTE.

A newborn is at a distinct disadvantage in maintaining a normal temperature. With a large body surface in relation to mass and a limited amount of insulating subcutaneous fat, the term newborn loses about four times the heat of an adult. The newborn's poor thermal stability is primarily because of excessive heat loss rather than impaired heat production. Because of the risk of hypothermia and possible cold stress, minimizing heat loss in the newborn after birth is essential. This topic is covered in more detail in the module on Thermoregulation.

Hepatic Adaptations

In the newborn, the liver is frequently palpable 2–3 cm (0.8–1.2 in.) below the right costal margin. It is relatively large and occupies approximately 40% of the abdominal cavity. The newborn liver plays a significant role in iron storage, carbohydrate metabolism, conjugation of bilirubin, and coagulation.

IRON STORAGE   As RBCs are destroyed after birth, the iron is stored in the liver until needed for new RBC production. Newborn iron stores are determined by total body hemoglobin content and length of gestation. The term newborn has approximately 270 mg of iron at birth, and approximately 140–170 mg of this amount is in the hemoglobin. If the mother's iron intake has been adequate, enough iron will be stored to last until the infant is about 5 months of age. After about 6 months of age, the

Evidence-Based Practice Thermoregulation and Heat Loss Prevention in Newborns

Problem

What is the best way to support thermoregulation in the newborn immediately after birth?

Evidence

Newborns have several risk factors for hypothermia after birth: a large surface-to-mass ratio, minimal subcutaneous tissue, and wet skin. The challenge of thermoregulation is increased if the infant is low birth weight, preterm, or sick. Cold stress can lead to harmful side effects or even death. Several systematic reviews of research on newborn thermoregulation have been published by professional groups interested in neonatal health: AWHONN, the American College of Nurse Midwives, and the American College of Pediatricians (Knobel & Holditch-Davis, 2007; Lyon, 2007; McCall et al., 2008; Mercer et al., 2007; Moore et al., 2012). These reviews have focused on healthy newborns as well as on newborns at risk. Multiple systematic reviews of multisite, randomized trials provide the strongest level of evidence for nursing practice.

Skin-to-skin contact of the newborn with its mother after birth is recommended as the mainstay of thermoregulation for most healthy newborns. When placed skin to skin, the baby gets heat directly from its mother via conduction. Skin-to-skin care is associated with both short- and long-term benefits, and it has been shown to be an effective method of thermoregulation for babies as small as 1,200 g. For smaller babies, or babies who are too ill to be placed on their mother's skin, resuscitation and other treatments may allow evaporative heat loss. Prewarming the delivery suite to 80°F and placing the infant in a plastic bag up to the neck during physiological stabilization prevents heat loss in high-risk babies. Heated mattresses are also effective in preventing hypothermia.

While plastic barriers have been shown to avoid hypothermia in high-risk newborns, no studies have demonstrated that these interventions reduce the long-term risk of death, brain injury, mean duration of oxygen therapy, or hospitalization. Some barrier methods (e.g., occlusive dressings) result in hyperthermia. Continuous monitoring of the newborn's body temperature should accompany any of the heat loss barrier methods.

Implications

Family-centered birth care provides the best environment for the newborn, including support of thermoregulation. You can avoid hypothermia in healthy newborns by drying the baby with a towel, placing the bare newborn in direct contact with the mother's bare skin, and placing a blanket over them both. Babies who are too small or too sick for skin-to-skin contact should be dried, placed on a heated mattress, and wrapped in plastic wrap up to the neck. A small cut can be made in the plastic for access to the umbilicus. In the case of plastic barriers, continuous monitoring of the baby's temperature is necessary to avoid overheating. Temperature can be continuously monitored using a temperature probe on the infant's skin connected to a monitoring device.

Critical Thinking Application

1. Discuss the evidence related to thermoregulation with skin-to-skin contact immediately after birth.
2. Identify nursing interventions that promote thermoregulation in the newborn.
3. Describe complications of cold stress in each physiological system in the newborn.

---

newborn requires foods containing iron or iron supplements to prevent anemia.

CARBOHYDRATE METABOLISM At term, the newborn's cord blood glucose level is 15 mg/dL lower than the maternal blood glucose level (Rosenberg, 2013). Newborn carbohydrate reserves are relatively low. One third of this reserve is in the form of liver glycogen. Newborn glycogen stores are twice those of the adult. The newborn enters an energy crunch at the time of birth, with the removal of the maternal glucose supply and the increased energy expenditure associated with the birth process and extrauterine life. The newborn consumes fuel sources at a faster rate because of the work of breathing, loss of heat when exposed to cold, activity, and activation of muscle tone. Glucose is the main source of energy in the first 4–6 hours after birth. During the first 2 hours of life, the serum blood glucose level declines, then rises, and finally reaches a steady state by 3 hours after birth (Rosenberg, 2013).

The nurse may assess the newborn's glucose level on admission if risk factors are present or per agency protocol. As stores of liver and muscle glycogen and blood glucose decrease, the newborn compensates by changing from a predominantly carbohydrate metabolism to fat metabolism. This allows the newborn to derive energy from fat and protein as well as from carbohydrates. The amount and availability of each of these "fuel substrates" depend on the ability of immature metabolic pathways, which lack specific enzymes or hormones, to function in the first few days of life.

CONJUGATION OF BILIRUBIN Conjugation of bilirubin is the conversion of yellow lipid-soluble pigment into water-soluble pigment. Unconjugated (indirect) bilirubin is a breakdown product derived from hemoglobin released primarily from destroyed RBCs. Unconjugated bilirubin is not in an excretable form and is a potential toxin. Total serum bilirubin is the sum of conjugated (direct) and unconjugated (indirect) bilirubin.

Fetal unconjugated bilirubin crosses the placenta to be excreted, so the fetus does not need to conjugate bilirubin. Total bilirubin at birth is usually less than 3 mg/dL unless an abnormal hemolytic process has been present in utero. After birth, the newborn's liver must begin to conjugate bilirubin. This produces a normal rise in serum bilirubin levels in the first few days of life.

The bilirubin formed after RBCs are destroyed is transported in the blood bound to albumin. The bilirubin is transferred into the hepatocytes and bound to intracellular proteins. These proteins determine the amount of bilirubin held in a liver cell for processing and, consequently, the amount of bilirubin uptake into the liver. Direct bilirubin is excreted into the tiny bile ducts, then into the common duct and duodenum. The conjugated (direct) bilirubin then progresses down the intestines, where bacteria transform it into urobilinogen (urine bilirubin) and stercobilinogen. Stercobilinogen is not reabsorbed; rather, it is excreted as a yellow-brown pigment in the stools.

Even after the bilirubin has been conjugated and bound, it can be changed back to unconjugated bilirubin via the enterohepatic circulation. In the intestines, beta-glucuronidase enzyme acts to split off (deconjugate) the bilirubin from glucuronic acid if it has not first been acted on by gut bacteria to produce urobilinogen. The free bilirubin is then reabsorbed through the intestinal wall and brought back to the liver via portal vein circulation. This recycling of the bilirubin and decreased ability to clear bilirubin from the system are prevalent in babies with very high beta-D-glucuronidase activity levels, those who are exclusively breastfed, and those with delayed bacterial colonization of the gut (e.g., because of the use of antibiotics). Very high beta-D-glucuronidase activity levels further increase the newborn's susceptibility to jaundice.

The newborn liver has relatively less glucuronyl transferase activity in the first few weeks of life than an adult liver. This reduction in hepatic activity, along with a relatively large bilirubin load, decreases the liver's ability to conjugate bilirubin and increases susceptibility to jaundice.

COAGULATION   The liver plays an important part in blood coagulation during fetal life, and it continues this function following birth. Coagulation factors II, VII, IX, and X (synthesized in the liver) are activated under the influence of vitamin K and, therefore, are considered to be vitamin K dependent. The absence of normal flora needed to synthesize vitamin K in the newborn gut results in low levels of vitamin K, which in turn results in a transient blood coagulation alteration between the second and fifth day of life. From a low point at approximately 2–3 days after birth, these coagulation factors rise slowly, but they do not approach adult levels until 9 months of age or later (Manco-Johnson, Rodden, & Hays, 2011). Other coagulation factors with low umbilical cord blood levels are factors XI, XII, and XIII. Fibrinogen and factors V and VII are near adult levels. Although newborn bleeding problems are rare, an injection of vitamin K (AquaMEPHYTON) is given prophylactically on the day of birth to combat potential clinical bleeding problems.

Platelet counts at birth are in the same range as for older children, but newborns may manifest mild transient difficulty in platelet aggregation functioning. This platelet problem is accentuated by phototherapy. Prenatal maternal therapy with phenytoin sodium (Dilantin) or phenobarbital also causes abnormal clotting studies and newborn bleeding in the first 24 hours after birth. Neonates born to mothers receiving warfarin (Coumadin) compounds may bleed because these agents cross the placenta and accentuate existing vitamin K–dependent factor deficiencies. Transient neonatal thrombocytopenia may occur in newborns born to mothers with severe hypertension or HELLP (**h**emolysis, **e**levated **l**iver enzymes, and **l**ow **p**latelet count) syndrome and in newborns born to mothers who have idiopathic isoimmune thrombocytopenic purpura.

PHYSIOLOGICAL JAUNDICE   **Physiological jaundice** (nonpathologic unconjugates hyperbilirubinemia) is caused by accelerated destruction of fetal RBCs, impaired conjugation of bilirubin, and increased bilirubin reabsorption from the intestinal tract. This condition does not have a pathological basis but is a normal biological response of the newborn.

McGrath and Hardy (2011) describe six factors—several of which can also be related to pathological events—whose interaction may give rise to physiological jaundice:

1. *Increased amounts of bilirubin delivered to the liver.* The increased blood volume because of delayed cord clamping combined with faster RBC destruction in the newborn leads to an increased bilirubin level in the blood. A proportionately larger amount of nonerythrocyte bilirubin forms in the newborn. Therefore, newborns have two to three times greater production or breakdown of bilirubin than adults. The use of forceps or vacuum extraction, which sometimes causes facial bruising or cephalohematoma (entrapped hemorrhage), can increase the amount of bilirubin to be handled by the liver.
2. *Defective hepatic uptake of bilirubin from the plasma.* If the newborn does not ingest adequate calories, the formation of hepatic binding proteins diminishes, resulting in higher bilirubin levels.
3. *Defective conjugation of bilirubin.* Decreased uridinediphosphoglucuronosyl activity, as in hypothyroidism or inadequate caloric intake, causes the intracellular binding proteins to remain saturated and results in greater unconjugated bilirubin levels in the blood. The fatty acids in breast milk are thought to compete with bilirubin for albumin-binding sites and, therefore, to impede bilirubin processing.
4. *Defective excretion of bilirubin.* A congenital infection may cause impaired excretion of conjugated bilirubin. Delay in introduction of bacterial flora and decreased intestinal motility can also delay excretion and increase enterohepatic circulation of bilirubin.
5. *Inadequate hepatic circulation.* Decreased oxygen supplies to the liver associated with neonatal hypoxia or congenital heart disease lead to a rise in the bilirubin level.
6. *Increased reabsorption of bilirubin from the intestine.* Reduced bowel motility, intestinal obstruction, or delayed passage of meconium increases the circulation of bilirubin in the enterohepatic pathway, thereby resulting in higher bilirubin values.

Approximately 50% of full-term newborns exhibit physiological jaundice on about the second or third day after birth. The characteristic yellow color results from increased levels of unconjugated (indirect) bilirubin, which are a normal product of RBC breakdown and reflect the body's temporary inability to eliminate bilirubin. Serum levels of bilirubin reach approximately 4–6 mg/dL before the yellow coloration of the skin and sclera appear. *The signs of physiological jaundice appear after the first 24 hours postnatally.* This time frame differentiates physiological jaundice from pathological jaundice, which is clinically seen at birth or within the first 24 hours of postnatal life. A major risk factor for developing severe hyperbilirubinemia in term neonates is a total serum or transcutaneous level in the high-risk zone on a bilirubin nomogram. The nomogram created by Bhutani, Johnson, and Sivieri (1999) and approved by the American Academy of Pediatrics (2004) is frequently used, as are bilirubin calculation tools available via the Internet.

Stay Current: *Visit* **www.bilitool.org** *to see a bilirubin calculation tool based on the nomogram by Bhutani et al. (1999).*

There is no consistent definition of neonatal hyperbilirubinemia; what is considered to be in that range varies with population characteristics and age (Blackburn, 2013). Peak bilirubin levels are reached between days 3 and 5 in the full-term newborn. These values are established for European and American White newborns. Chinese, Japanese, Korean, and Native American newborns have considerably higher bilirubin levels that are not as apparent and that persist for longer periods with no apparent ill effects (McGrath & Hardy, 2011).

The nursery or postpartum room environment, including lighting, may hinder early detection of the degree and type of jaundice. Pink walls and artificial lights mask the beginning of jaundice in newborns. Daylight assists the observer in early recognition by eliminating distortions caused by artificial light.

If jaundice is suspected, the nurse can quickly assess the newborn's coloring by pressing the skin, generally on the forehead or nose, with a finger. As blanching occurs, the nurse can observe the icterus (yellow coloring).

Several newborn care procedures will decrease the probability of high bilirubin levels:

- Maintain the newborn's skin temperature at 36.5°C (97.8°F) or above, because cold stress results in acidosis. Acidosis in turn decreases available serum albumin-binding sites, weakens albumin-binding powers, and causes elevated unconjugated bilirubin levels.

- Monitor stool for amount and characteristics. Bilirubin is eliminated in the feces; inadequate stooling may result in reabsorption and recycling of bilirubin. Encourage early breastfeeding, because the laxative effect of colostrum increases the excretion of meconium and transitional stool.

- Encourage early feedings to promote intestinal elimination and bacterial colonization and provide the caloric intake necessary for formation of hepatic binding proteins.

If jaundice becomes apparent, nursing care is directed toward keeping the newborn well hydrated and promoting intestinal elimination.

Physiological jaundice may be very upsetting to parents; they require emotional support and a thorough explanation of the condition. If the baby is placed under phototherapy, a few additional days of hospitalization may be required; this may also be disturbing to parents. The nurse can encourage parents to provide for the emotional needs of their newborn by continuing to feed, hold, and caress the baby. If the mother is discharged, the parents are encouraged to return for feedings and to telephone or visit when possible. In many instances, the mother, especially if she is breastfeeding, may elect to remain hospitalized with her newborn; the nurse should support this decision. If insurance limitations make this unrealistic, it may be possible to find an empty room for the discharged mother and her family to use while visiting the newborn. As an alternative to continued hospitalization, the newborn may be treated with home phototherapy.

BREASTFEEDING AND BREAST MILK JAUNDICE
Breastfeeding is implicated in prolonged jaundice in some newborns. Breastfeeding jaundice occurs during the first days of life in breastfed newborns. It appears to be related to inadequate fluid intake with some element of dehydration and not with any abnormality in milk composition (McGrath & Hardy, 2011).

Prevention of early breastfeeding jaundice includes encouraging frequent (every 2–3 hours) breastfeeding, avoiding supplementation if the newborn is not dehydrated, and accessing maternal lactation counseling. Breastfeeding jaundice is self-limiting; it peaks around day 3 as enteral intake increases, then resolves.

In breast milk jaundice, the bilirubin level begins to rise after the first week of life, when physiological jaundice is waning after the mother's milk has come in. The level peaks at 5–10 mg/dL at 2–3 weeks of age and then declines over the first several months of life (McGrath & Hardy, 2011).

In contrast to breastfeeding jaundice, breast milk jaundice is related to milk composition. Some women's breast milk contains several times the normal concentration of certain free fatty acids. These free fatty acids may compete with bilirubin for binding sites on albumin and inhibit the conjugation of bilirubin or increase lipase activity, which disrupts the RBC membrane. Increased lipase activity enhances absorption of bile across the gastrointestinal tract membrane, thereby increasing the enterohepatic circulation of bilirubin. Newborns with breastfeeding jaundice appear well, and at present, development of kernicterus (toxic levels of bilirubin in the brain) has not been documented. Temporary cessation of breastfeeding may be advised if bilirubin reaches presumed toxic levels of approximately 20 mg/dL or if the interruption is necessary to establish the cause of the hyperbilirubinemia. Most providers believe that breastfeeding may be resumed once other causes of jaundice have been ruled out and as long as serum bilirubin levels remain below 20 mg/dL. In cases of breast milk jaundice, the newborn's serum bilirubin levels begin to fall dramatically within 24–36 hours after breastfeeding is discontinued. With resumption of breastfeeding, the bilirubin concentration may have a slight rise of 2–3 mg/dL, with a subsequent decline. Breastfeeding mothers need encouragement and support in their desire to breastfeed their babies, assistance and instruction regarding pumping and expressing milk during the interrupted nursing period, and reassurance that nothing is wrong with their milk or mothering abilities (Academy of Breastfeeding Medicine Protocol Committee, 2010).

Gastrointestinal Adaptations
The term newborn has sufficient intestinal and pancreatic enzymes to digest most simple carbohydrates, proteins, and

Focus on Diversity and Culture
Interpreting Illness Through Cultural Beliefs

Cultural beliefs lead mothers to interpret illness within their cultural framework, especially when instructions are not given clearly or are not understood by the mother (D'Avanzo & Geissler, 2008). For example, some Latina women believe that showing strong maternal emotions during pregnancy and breastfeeding can be detrimental. They blame jaundice in their newborn on "bili" associated with anger. Careful explanations to the mothers about the diagnosis, prognosis, duration, and management options for jaundice and about the possibility for recurrence can minimize misunderstandings as well as negative or unrealistic maternal reactions.

fats. The carbohydrates requiring digestion in the newborn are usually disaccharides (lactose, maltose, and sucrose), which are split into monosaccharides (galactose, fructose, and glucose) by the enzymes of the intestinal mucosa. Lactose is the primary carbohydrate in the breastfeeding newborn and generally is easily digested and well absorbed. The only enzyme lacking in the newborn is pancreatic amylase, which remains relatively deficient during the first few months of life. Newborns have trouble digesting starches (changing more complex carbohydrates into maltose), so they should not be fed solid foods until after the first few months of life.

Although proteins require more digestion than carbohydrates, they are well digested and absorbed from the newborn intestine. The newborn digests and absorbs fats less efficiently because of the minimal activity of the pancreatic enzyme lipase. The newborn excretes approximately 10%–20% of the dietary fat intake, compared with 10% for the adult. The newborn absorbs the fat in breast milk more completely than the fat in cow's milk because breast milk consists of more medium-chain triglycerides and contains lipase.

By birth, the newborn has experienced swallowing, gastric emptying, and intestinal propulsion. In utero, fetal swallowing is accompanied by gastric emptying and peristalsis of the fetal intestinal tract. By the end of gestation, peristalsis becomes much more active in preparation for extrauterine life. Fetal peristalsis is also stimulated by anoxia, causing the expulsion of meconium into the amniotic fluid by more mature fetuses.

Air enters the stomach immediately after birth. The small intestine is filled with air within 2–12 hours, and the large bowel is filled within 24 hours. The salivary glands are immature at birth, and the newborn produces little saliva until about 3 months of age. The newborn's stomach has a capacity of approximately 50–60 mL. It empties intermittently, starting within a few minutes of the beginning of a feeding and ending 2–4 hours after a feeding. Bowel sounds are present within the first 30–60 minutes of birth; the newborn can successfully feed during this time. The newborn's gastric pH becomes less acidic about a week after birth and remains less acidic than that of adults for the next 2–3 months.

The cardiac sphincter is immature, as is neural control of the stomach. Therefore, some regurgitation may be noted in the newborn period. Regurgitation of the first few feedings during the first day or two of life can usually be lessened by avoiding overfeeding and by burping the newborn well both during and after the feeding.

When no other signs and symptoms are evident, vomiting is limited and ceases within the first few days of life. Continuous vomiting or regurgitation should be observed closely. If the newborn has swallowed bloody or purulent amniotic fluid, lavage of the stomach may be indicated in the term newborn to relieve the problem. Bilious vomiting is abnormal and must be evaluated thoroughly; it may represent a condition that warrants prompt surgical intervention.

Adequate digestion and absorption are essential for newborn growth and development. If optimal nutritional support is available, postnatal growth should parallel intrauterine growth; that is, after 30 weeks of gestation, the fetus gains 30 g per day and adds 1.2 cm (0.5 in.) to body length daily. To gain weight at the intrauterine rate, the term newborn requires 120 calories/kg per day. After birth, caloric intake is often insufficient for weight gain until the newborn is 5–10 days old. During this time, the term newborn may experience a weight loss of 5%–10%. Because insensible water loss and a shift of intracellular water to extracellular space account for the 5%–10% weight loss, failure to lose weight when caloric intake is inadequate may indicate fluid retention.

Term newborns usually pass **meconium** (their first stool) within 8–24 hours of life and almost always within 48 hours. Meconium is formed in utero from the amniotic fluid and its constituents, intestinal secretions, and shed mucosal cells. It is recognized by its thick, tarry-black or dark green appearance (**Figure 33–61A ●**). Transitional (thin brown to green) stools consisting of part meconium and part fecal material are passed for the next day or two (Figure 33–61B), and then the stools become entirely fecal (Figure 33–61C). Generally, the stools of a breastfed newborn are pale yellow (but may be pasty green); they are more liquid and more frequent than those of formula-fed newborns, whose stools are paler. Frequency of bowel movement varies but ranges from one every 2–3 days to as many as 10 daily. Mothers should be counseled that the newborn is not constipated as long as the bowel movement remains soft.

Urinary Tract Adaptations

Certain physiological features of the newborn's kidneys influence the newborn's ability to handle body fluids and excrete urine:

- The term newborn's kidneys have a full complement of functioning nephrons by 34–36 weeks of gestation.
- The glomerular filtration rate of the newborn's kidney is low in comparison with the adult rate. Because of this physiological decrease in kidney glomerular filtration, the newborn's kidney is unable to dispose of water rapidly when necessary.
- The juxtamedullary portion of the nephron has limited capacity to reabsorb HCO_3^+ and H^+ and to concentrate urine (reabsorb water back into the blood). The limitation of tubular reabsorption can lead to inappropriate loss of substances present in the glomerular filtrate, such as amino acids, bicarbonate, glucose, and sodium.

Full-term newborns are less able than adults to concentrate urine because their tubules are short and narrow. The limited tubular reabsorption of water and limited excretion of solutes (principally sodium, potassium, chloride, bicarbonate, urea, and phosphate) in growing newborns also reduce their ability to concentrate urine. Although feeding practices may affect the osmolarity of the urine, they have limited effect on the concentration of the urine. The ability to concentrate urine fully is attained by 3 months of age.

The newborn's difficulty concentrating urine makes the effect of excessive insensible water loss or restricted fluid intake unpredictable. The newborn kidney is also limited in its dilutional capabilities. Concentrating and dilutional limitations of renal function are important considerations in monitoring fluid therapy to prevent dehydration or overhydration.

Many newborns void immediately after birth; this voiding frequently goes unnoticed. A newborn who has not voided

(A) Day 1 and Day 2

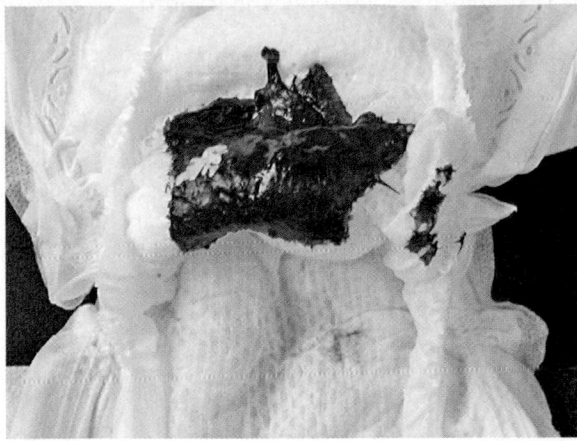

(B) Day 3 and Day 4

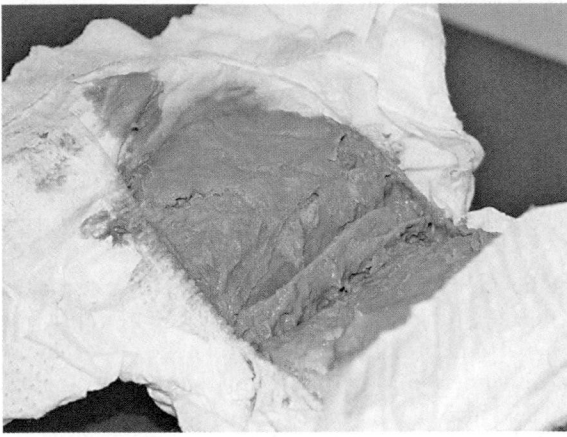

(C) Day 5

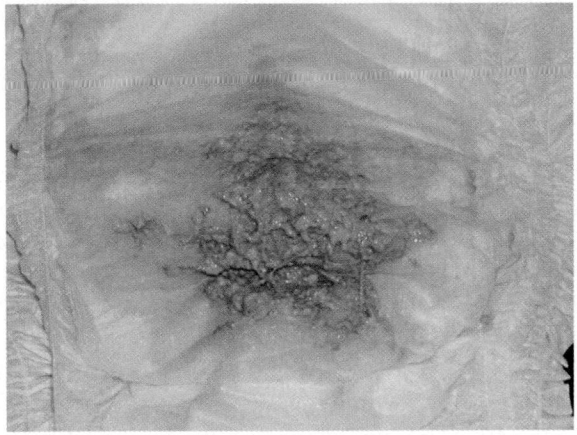

....

Figure 33–61 ● Examples of infant stools. *A,* Meconium. *B,* Transitional stools. *C,* Fecal stools.

Source: Courtesy of Brigitte Hall, RNC, MSN, IBCLC.

by 48 hours should be assessed for adequacy of fluid intake, bladder distention, restlessness, and symptoms of pain. The appropriate clinical personnel should be notified if indicated (Gabbe et al., 2012).

The initial bladder volume is 6–44 mL of urine. Unless edema is present, normal urinary output is often limited, and voidings are scanty until fluid intake increases. (The fluid of edema is eliminated by the kidneys, so newborns with edema have a much higher urinary output.) During the first 2 days after birth, the newborn voids 2–6 times daily, with a urine output of 15 mL/kg per day. The newborn subsequently voids 5–25 times every 24 hours, with a volume of 25 mL/kg per day.

Following the first voiding, the newborn's urine frequently appears cloudy (because of mucus content) and has a high specific gravity, which decreases as fluid intake increases. Occasionally, pink stains ("brick dust spots") appear on the diaper. These are caused by urates and are innocuous. Blood or whitish discharge may occasionally be observed on the diapers of female newborns; this **pseudomenstruation** is related to the withdrawal of maternal hormones. Males who are circumcised may have bloody spotting following the procedure. In the absence of apparent causes for bleeding, the healthcare provider should be notified. During the early neonatal period, normal urine is straw colored and almost odorless, although odor does occur when certain drugs are given, metabolic disorders exist, or infection is present. **Box 33–7** ● contains urinalysis values for the normal newborn.

Immunological Adaptations

The newborn's immune system is not fully activated until sometime after birth. Limitations in the newborn's inflammatory response result in failure to recognize, localize, and destroy invasive bacteria. As a result, the signs and symptoms of infection are often subtle and nonspecific in the newborn. The newborn also has a poor hypothalamic response to pyrogens; therefore, fever is not a reliable indicator of infection. In the neonatal period, hypothermia is a more reliable sign of infection.

Of the three major types of immunoglobulins that are primarily involved in immunity—IgG, IgA, and IgM—only IgG crosses the placenta. When the pregnant woman forms antibodies in response to illness or immunization, this process is called **active acquired immunity**. When IgG antibodies are transferred from the pregnant woman to the fetus in utero, **passive acquired immunity** results because the fetus does not produce the antibodies itself. IgG antibodies are very active against bacterial toxins.

Because the maternal IgG is transferred primarily during the third trimester, preterm newborns (especially those born before 34 weeks of gestation) may be more susceptible to infection than term newborns. In general, newborns have immunity to tetanus, diphtheria, smallpox, measles, mumps, poliomyelitis, and a variety of other bacterial and viral diseases. The period of resistance varies: Immunity against common viral infections, such as measles, may last 4–8 months; immunity to certain bacteria may disappear within 4–8 weeks.

Box 33–7   **Newborn Urinalysis Values**
■ Protein: <5–10 mg/dL
■ White blood cells: <2–3 cells/high-power field
■ Red blood cells: 0
■ Casts: 0
■ Bacteria: 0
■ Color: pale yellow.

The normal newborn can produce a protective immune response to vaccines, such as hepatitis B immunoglobulin vaccine, when given as early as a few hours after birth. It is customary to begin the majority of routine immunizations at 2 months of age so that the infant can develop active acquired immunity.

The IgM antibodies are produced in response to blood group antigens, gram-negative enteric organisms, and some viruses in the expectant mother. Because IgM does not normally cross the placenta, most or all of it is produced by the fetus beginning at 10–15 weeks of gestation. Elevated levels of IgM at birth may indicate placental leaks or, more commonly, antigenic stimulation in utero. Consequently, elevations of IgM suggest that the newborn was exposed to an intrauterine infection, such as syphilis or TORCH syndrome (**to**xoplasmosis, **ru**bella, **c**ytomegalovirus, **h**erpesvirus hominis type 2 infection). The lack of available maternal IgM in the newborn also accounts for the susceptibility to gram-negative enteric organisms, such as *Escherichia coli*.

The functions of IgA immunoglobulins are not fully understood. IgA appears to provide protection mainly on secreting surfaces, such as the respiratory tract, gastrointestinal tract, and eyes. Serum IgA does not cross the placenta and is not normally produced by the fetus in utero. Unlike the other immunoglobulins, IgA is not affected by gastric action. Colostrum (the forerunner of breast milk) is very high in the secretory form of IgA. Consequently, it may be of significance in providing some passive immunity to the neonate of a breastfeeding mother. Newborns begin to produce secretory IgA in their intestinal mucosa approximately 4 weeks after birth.

Neurological and Sensory–Perceptual Function

The newborn's brain is about one quarter the size of an adult's, and myelination of nerve fibers is incomplete. Unlike the cardiovascular and respiratory systems, which undergo tremendous changes at birth, the nervous system is minimally influenced by the actual birth process.

Because many biochemical and histological changes have yet to occur in the newborn's brain, the postnatal period is considered to be a time of risk with regard to development of the brain and nervous system. For neurological development—including development of intellect—to proceed, the brain and other nervous system structures must mature in an orderly, unhampered fashion.

INTRAUTERINE EXPERIENCE Newborns respond to and interact with the environment in a predictable pattern of behavior that is somewhat shaped by their intrauterine experience. This intrauterine experience is affected by intrinsic factors, such as maternal nutrition, and by external factors, such as the mother's physical environment. Depending on the newborn's intrauterine experience and individual temperament, neonatal behavioral responses to different stresses vary. Some newborns react quietly to stimulation, others become overreactive and tense, and still others exhibit a combination of the two.

Factors such as exposure to intense auditory stimuli in utero may eventually manifest in the behavior of the newborn. For example, the fetal heart rate initially increases when the pregnant woman is exposed to auditory stimuli, but repetition of the stimuli leads to decreased fetal heart rate. Thus, the newborn

who was exposed to intense noise during fetal life is significantly less reactive to loud sounds after birth.

CHARACTERISTICS OF NEWBORN NEUROLOGICAL FUNCTION Normal newborns are usually in a position of partially flexed extremities, with the legs near the abdomen. When awake, the newborn may exhibit purposeless, uncoordinated bilateral movements of the extremities. The organization and quality of the newborn's motor activity are influenced by a number of factors, including the following (Nugent, 2013):

- Intrauterine growth restriction
- Prenatal stress
- Environmental chemicals
- Obstetric medications
- Acute fetal distress
- Gestational and pregestational diabetes
- Intrauterine drug exposure
- Prematurity and low birth weight.

Eye movements are observable during the first few days of life. An alert newborn is able to fixate on faces and geometric objects or patterns, such as black-and-white stripes. A bright light shining in the newborn's eyes elicits the blinking reflex.

The cry of the newborn should be lusty and vigorous. High-pitched cries, weak cries, and no cries are causes for concern.

The newborn's body growth progresses in a cephalocaudal (head-to-toe), proximal–distal fashion. The newborn is somewhat hypertonic—that is, there is resistance to extending the elbow and knee joints. Muscle tone should be symmetric. Diminished muscle tone and flaccidity may indicate neurological dysfunction.

Specific symmetric deep tendon reflexes can be elicited in the newborn. The knee-jerk reflex is brisk; a normal ankle clonus may involve three to four beats. Plantar flexion is present. Other reflexes, including the Moro, grasping, Babinski, rooting, and sucking reflexes, are characteristic of neurological integrity. **Table 33–16 ●** provides a summary of stimulus for, and response for, the common newborn reflexes.

Performance of complex behavioral patterns reflects the newborn's neurological maturation and integration. Newborns who can bring a hand to their mouth may be demonstrating motor coordination as well as a self-quieting technique, thus increasing the complexity of the behavioral response. Newborns also possess complex, organized, defensive motor patterns, as exhibited by the ability to remove an obstruction, such as a cloth across the face.

PERIODS OF REACTIVITY The behavior of the newborn can be divided into two categories, the sleep state and the alert state (Brazelton, 1984; Gardner & Goldson, 2011). These postnatal behavioral states are similar to those that have been identified during pregnancy. Subcategories are identified under each major category.

Sleep States The sleep states are as follows:

- ***Deep or quiet sleep.*** Deep sleep is characterized by closed eyes with no eye movements; regular, even breathing; and jerky motions or startles at regular intervals. Behavioral

TABLE 33–16 Common Reflexes of the Newborn

REFLEX NAME	EVOKING STIMULUS	RESPONSE
Blinking reflex	Light flash	Eyelids close.
Pupillary reflex	Light flash	Pupil constricts.
Rooting reflex	Light touch of finger on cheek close to mouth	Head rotates toward stimulation; mouth opens and attempts to suck finger. Disappears by ~4 months of age.
Sucking reflex	Finger (or nipple) inserted into mouth	Rhythmic sucking occurs.
Moro reflex	Infant lying on back: slightly raised head suddenly released; infant held horizontally: lowered quickly 15 cm (~6 in.) and stopped abruptly	Arms are extended, head is thrown back, and fingers are spread wide; arms are then brought back to center convulsively with hands clenched; spine and lower extremities are extended. Disappears by ~6 months of age.
Startle reflex	Loud noise	Similar to Moro reflex flexion in arms; fists are clenched.
Grasping reflex	Finger placed in palm of hand	Newborn's fingers close around and grasp object.
Tonic neck reflex	Head turned to one side while infant lies on back	Arm and leg are extended on the side the infant faces. Opposite arm and leg are flexed.
Abdominal reflex	Tactile stimulation or tickling	Abdominal muscles contract.
Withdrawal reflex	Slight pinprick to the sole of the infant's foot	Leg flexes.
Stepping reflex	Infant supported in an upright position with feet lightly touching a flat surface	Rhythmic stepping (walking) movement. Disappears at ~4–8 weeks of age.
Babinski reflex	Gentle stroking on the sole of each foot	Fanning and extension of the toes (adults respond to this stimulation with flexion of toes).
Plantar, or toe-grasping, reflex	Pressure applied with the finger against the balls of the infant's feet	A plantar flexion of all toes. Disappears by the end of the first year of life.

Sources: Based on Ladewig, P. A. W., London, M. L., & Davidson, M. R. (2014). Table 25–2 in *Contemporary Maternal-Newborn Nursing Care*, 8th ed. Upper Saddle River, NJ: Pearson; MedlinePlus. (2011). Infant reflexes. Retrieved from http://www.nlm.nih.gov/medlineplus/ency/article/003292.htm; American Academy of Pediatrics. (2013). Newborn reflexes. Retrieved from http://www.healthychildren.org/English/ages-stages/baby/pages/Newborn-Reflexes.aspx.

responses to external stimuli are likely to be delayed. Startles are rapidly suppressed, and changes in state are not likely to occur. Heart rate may range from 100 to 120 bpm.

- **Active REM.** The baby has irregular respirations; eyes closed, with REM; irregular sucking motions; minimal activity; and irregular but smooth movement of the extremities. Environmental and internal stimuli may initiate a startle reaction and a change of state.

Newborn sleep cycles have been recognized and defined according to duration. The length of the sleep cycle depends on the age of the newborn. At term, REM active sleep and quiet sleep occur in intervals of 50–60 minutes (Gardner & Goldson, 2011). Approximately 45%–50% of the newborn's total sleep is active sleep, 35%–45% is quiet sleep, and 10% is transitional between these two periods. Growth hormone secretion depends on regular sleep patterns. Any disturbance of the sleep–wake cycle can result in irregular spikes of growth hormone. REM sleep stimulates the highest peaks of growth hormone and the growth of the neural system. Over a period of time, the newborn's sleep–wake patterns become diurnal (the newborn sleeps at night and stays awake during the day).

Alert States In the first 30–60 minutes after birth, many newborns display a quiet alert state. After a sleep phase that lasts from a few minutes to between 2 and 4 hours, a second alert state occurs. This second alert period lasts 4 to 6 hours in the normal newborn. The nurse should use these alert states to encourage bonding and breastfeeding.

The newborn's periods of alertness tend to be shorter during the first 2 days after birth; this allows the baby to recover from the birth process. Subsequent alert states are of choice or of necessity (Gardner & Goldson, 2011). Increasing choice of wakefulness by the newborn indicates a maturing capacity to achieve and maintain consciousness. Heat, cold, and hunger are but a few of the stimuli that can cause wakefulness by necessity. Once the disturbing stimuli have been removed, the baby tends to fall back asleep.

The following are subcategories of the alert state (Gardner & Goldson, 2011):

- **Drowsy or semidozing.** The behaviors common to the drowsy state are open or closed eyes; fluttering eyelids; semidozing appearance; and slow, regular movements of the extremities. Mild startles may be noted from time to time. Although the reaction to a sensory stimulus is delayed, a change of state often results.

- **Wide awake.** In the wide-awake state, the newborn is alert and follows and fixates on attractive objects, faces, or auditory stimuli. Motor activity is minimal, and the response to external stimuli is delayed.

- **Active awake.** In the active-awake state, the newborn's eyes are open, and motor activity is quite intense, with thrusting movements of the extremities. Environmental stimuli increase startles or motor activity, but individual reactions are difficult to distinguish because of the generally high activity level.

- **Crying.** Intense crying is accompanied by jerky motor movements. Crying serves several purposes for the newborn. It may be a distraction from disturbing stimuli, such as hunger and pain. Fussiness often allows the newborn to discharge energy and reorganize behavior. Most important, crying elicits an appropriate response of help from the parents.

BEHAVIORAL CAPACITIES OF THE NEWBORN Newborns have several behavioral capacities that assist them in adapting to extrauterine life. For example, **self-quieting ability** is the ability of newborns to use their own resources to quiet and comfort themselves. Their repertoire includes hand-to-mouth movements, sucking on a fist or tongue, and attending to external stimuli. Neurologically impaired newborns are unable to use self-quieting activities and require more frequent comforting from caregivers when stimulated. For example, drug-positive newborns often exhibit abnormal sleep and feeding patterns and irritability.

Habituation is the newborn's ability to process and respond to complex stimulation. For example, when a bright light is flashed into the newborn's eyes, the initial response is blinking, constriction of the pupil, and perhaps a slight startle reaction. However, with repeated stimulation the newborn's response repertoire gradually diminishes and disappears. The capacity to ignore repetitious, disturbing stimuli is a newborn defense mechanism that is readily apparent in the noisy, well-lit nursery.

SENSORY CAPACITIES OF THE NEWBORN Sensory capacities of the newborn include visual, auditory, olfactory, taste, and tactile capacities.

Visual Capacity **Orientation** is the newborn's ability to be alert to, follow, and fixate on appealing and attractive, complex visual stimuli. The newborn prefers the human face and eyes and The newborn is nearsighted and has best vision at a distance of 8 to 15 inches. As the face or object comes into the line of vision, the newborn responds with bright, wide eyes as well as still limbs and a fixed stare. This intense visual involvement may last several minutes. During this time, the newborn is able to follow the stimulus from side to side. The newborn uses this sensory capacity to become familiar with family, friends, and surroundings.

Auditory Capacity The newborn responds to auditory stimulation with a definite, organized behavioral repertoire. The stimulus used to assess auditory response should be selected to match the state of the newborn. A rattle is appropriate for light sleep, a voice for an awake state, and a clap for deep sleep. As the newborn hears the sound, the cardiac rate rises; a minimal startle reflex may be observed. If the sound is appealing, the newborn will become alert and search for the site of the auditory stimulus. Lack of auditory development is associated with an increased risk of sudden infant death syndrome. The AAP currently recommends that newborns receive hearing screening before discharge from the hospital (Russ et al., 2010); universal hearing screening before 1 month of age is a goal of *Healthy People 2020* (USDHHS, 2011).

Olfactory Capacity Newborns not only select their mother by smell, they apparently also can select other individuals by smell (Cheffer & Rannalli, 2011). Newborns are able to distinguish their mothers' breast pads from those of other mothers as early as 1 week after birth.

Taste and Sucking The newborn responds differently to varying tastes. Sugar, for example, increases sucking. Newborns fed with a rubber nipple versus the breast also show sucking pattern variations. When breastfeeding, the newborn sucks in bursts, with frequent regular pauses. The bottle-fed newborn, however, tends to suck at a regular rate, with infrequent pauses.

When awake and hungry, the newborn displays rapid searching motions in response to the rooting reflex. Once feeding begins, the newborn establishes a sucking pattern according to the method of feeding. Finger sucking is seen in utero as well as after birth. The newborn frequently uses nonnutritive sucking as a self-quieting activity, which assists in the development of self-regulation. For bottle-fed infants, there is no reason to discourage nonnutritive sucking with a pacifier. Pacifiers should be offered to breastfed infants only after breastfeeding is well established. If the pacifier is offered too soon, a phenomenon called "nipple confusion" may occur, in which the breastfed infant has difficulty learning to suck from the breast and will nurse less.

Tactile Capacity The newborn is very sensitive to being touched, cuddled, and held. Often, a mother's first response to an upset or crying newborn is touching or holding. Swaddling, placing a hand on the abdomen, or holding the arms to prevent a startle reflex are other methods of soothing the newborn. The quieted newborn is then able to attend to and interact with the environment. Touch is also used to rouse a drowsy newborn, making him or her more alert for feeding.

▶ ALTERATIONS

Neonatology is the field of medicine providing care for sick and premature neonates. Many levels of nursery care have evolved in response to increasing knowledge about at-risk newborns: special care, intensive care, and convalescent or transitional care. Along with the newborn's parents, the nurse is an important caregiver in all these settings. As a member of the multidisciplinary healthcare team, the nurse is a technically competent professional who contributes the high-touch, human care necessary in the high-tech, perinatal environment.

Various factors influence the outcome of at-risk neonates, including the following:

- Birth weight
- Gestational age
- Type and length of illness
- Environmental factors
- Maternal factors
- Maternal–newborn separation.

An at-risk newborn is one susceptible to illness (morbidity) or even death (mortality) because of dysmaturity, immaturity, physical disorders, or complications during or after birth. In most cases, the neonate is the product of a pregnancy involving one or more predictable risk factors, including the following:

- Low socioeconomic level of the mother
- Limited access to healthcare or no prenatal care
- Exposure to environmental dangers, such as toxic chemicals and illicit drugs
- Preexisting maternal conditions, such as heart disease, diabetes, hypertension, hyperthyroidism, and renal disease
- Maternal factors, such as age and parity
- Medical conditions related to pregnancy and their associated complications

■ Pregnancy complications, such as abruptio placentae, oligo-hydramnios, preterm labor, premature rupture of membranes, and preeclampsia.

Because these factors and the perinatal risks associated with them are known, the birth of at-risk newborns can often be anticipated. The pregnancy can be closely monitored, treatment can be started as necessary, and arrangements can be made for birth to occur at a facility with appropriate resources to care for both mother and baby.

Whether or not prenatal assessment indicates that the fetus is at risk, the course of labor and birth, as well as the newborn's ability to withstand the stress of labor, cannot be predicted. Thus, the nurse's use of electronic fetal heart monitoring or fetal heart auscultation by Doppler plays a significant role in detecting stress or distress in the fetus. Immediately after birth, the Apgar score may help identify the at-risk newborn, but it is not the only indicator of possible long-term outcome.

The newborn classification and neonatal mortality risk chart is another useful tool for identifying newborns at risk. Before this classification tool was developed, birth weight of less than 2,500 g was the sole criterion for determining prematurity. Healthcare providers then recognized that a newborn could weigh more than 2,500 g and still be premature. Conversely, an infant weighing less than 2,500 g might be functionally at term or beyond. As a result, birth weight and gestational age together

are now the criteria used to assess neonatal maturity, morbidity, and mortality risk.

According to the newborn classification and neonatal mortality risk chart, gestation (postmenstrual age) is divided as follows:

■ *Preterm:* less than 37 (completed) weeks

■ *Term:* 37–41 6/7 (completed) weeks

■ *Postterm:* greater than 42 weeks.

Late preterm is an emerging classification that refers to subgroups of infants between 34 and 37 weeks of gestation; however, it is not yet used consistently for a single age range (Cloherty, Eichenwald, & Stark, 2008).

As shown in **Figure 33–62** ●, large-for-gestational-age newborns are those who plot above the 90th percentile curve on an intrauterine growth chart. Appropriate-for-gestational-age newborns are those who plot between the 10th percentile and 90th percentile growth curves. Small-for-gestational-age newborns are those that plot below the 10th percentile growth curve. A newborn is assigned to a category depending on birth weight, length, occipitofrontal head circumference, and gestational age. For example, a newborn classified as Pr SGA is preterm and small for gestational age. The term newborn whose weight is appropriate for gestational age is classified F AGA. It is important to note that intrauterine growth charts are influenced by altitude and by the ethnicity of the newborn population used to

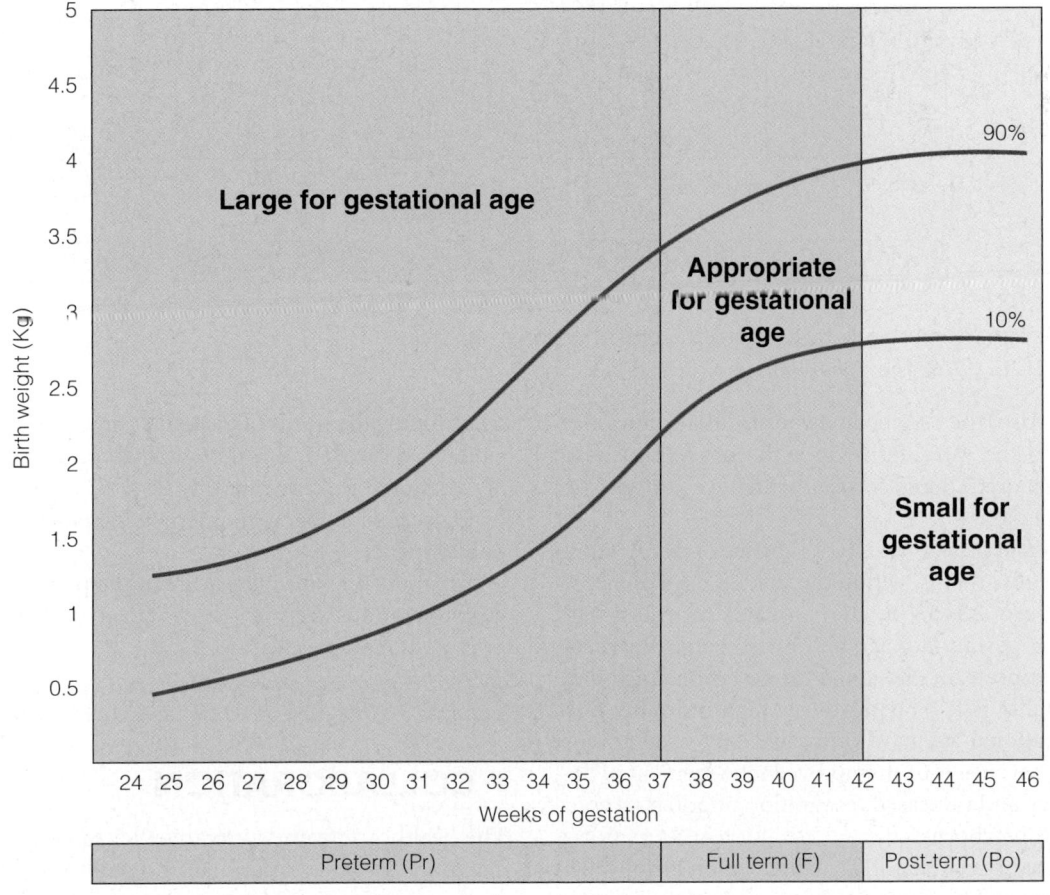

Figure 33–62 ● Intrauterine growth chart. Infants are classified according to weight as large for gestational age (LGA), appropriate for gestational age (AGA), or small for gestational age (SGA), and by gestation as preterm (Pr), term (F), or postterm (Po).

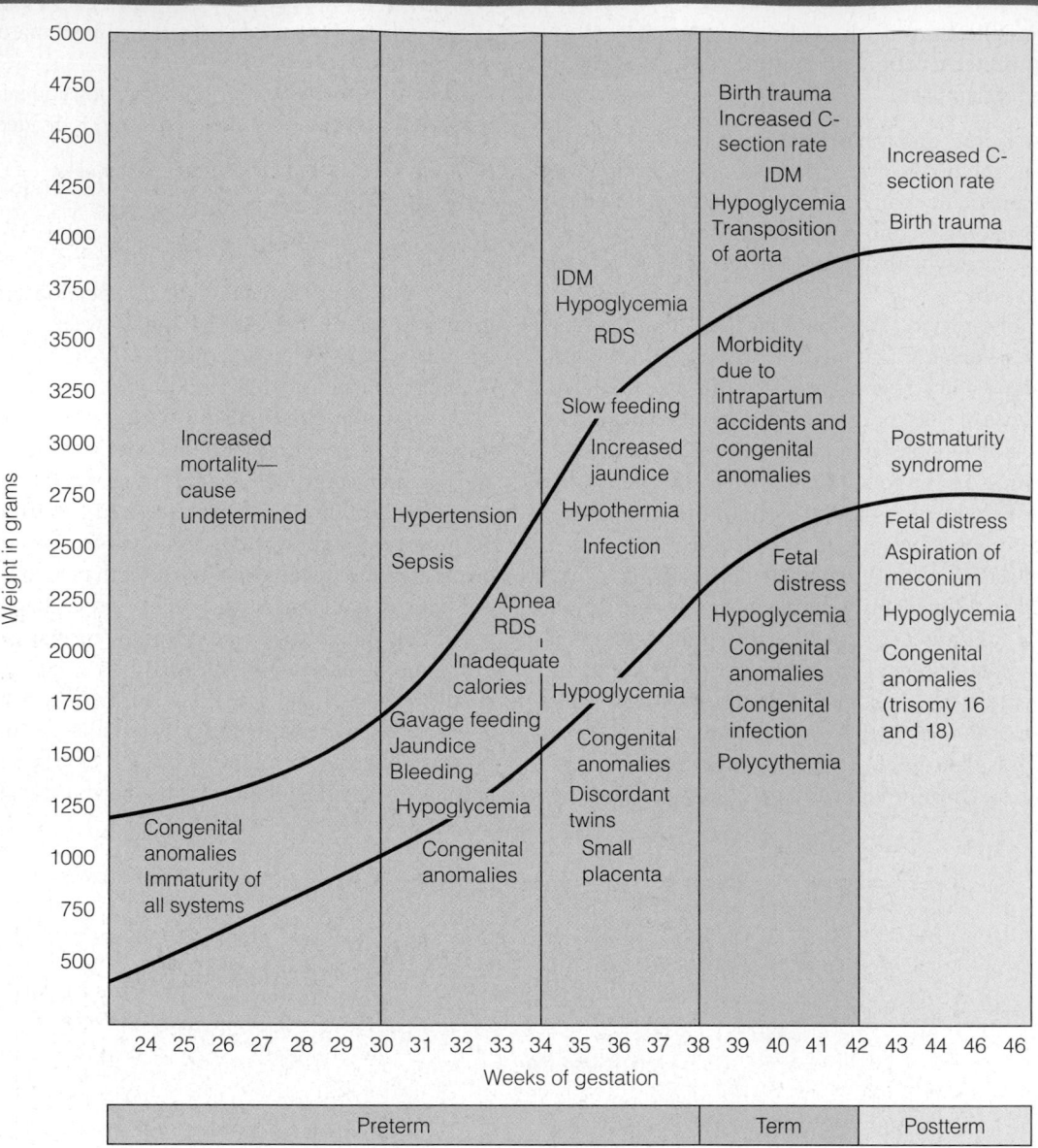

Figure 33–63 ● Neonatal morbidity by birth weight and gestational age.
Source: Lubchenco, L. O. (1976). *The high-risk infant* (p. 122). Philadelphia: Saunders.

create the chart. Also, the assigned newborn classification may vary according to the intrauterine growth curve chart used; therefore, the chart used should correlate with the characteristics of the client population.

Neonatal mortality risk is an infant's chance of death within the newborn period—that is, within the first 28 days of life. As indicated in **Figure 33–63 ●**, the neonatal mortality risk decreases as both gestational age and birth weight increase. Neonates who are preterm and small for gestational age have the highest mortality risk. The previously high mortality rates for large-for-gestational-age newborns have decreased at most perinatal centers because of both improved management of diabetes in pregnancy and increased recognition of potential complications of these newborns.

Neonatal morbidity can be anticipated based on birth weight and gestational age. In Figure 33–63, the newborn's birth weight is located on the vertical axis, and the gestational age in weeks is found along the horizontal axis. The area where the two meet on the graph identifies common problems. This tool assists in

determining the needs of particular newborns for special observation and care. For example, a newborn of 2,000 g at 40 weeks of gestation should be carefully assessed for evidence of distress, hypoglycemia, congenital anomalies, congenital infection, and polycythemia.

Exemplar 33.5 discusses care of the premature infant. Common alterations seen in the newborn are listed in the Alterations and Therapies feature.

✳ *Go to* **nursing.pearsonhighered.com** *to see Chart 14 on potential birth injuries and Chart 15 on congenital anomalies.*

▶ COLLABORATION

The healthcare team works together to care for the newborn. The nurse's role is described in detail in the Nursing Process section that follows. Needs of the newborn differ dramatically in the 4-hour period following birth versus later time periods. As a result, care is divided into initial care, subsequent care, and preparation for discharge.

Alterations and Therapies **Newborn Care**

ALTERATION	DESCRIPTION	THERAPIES
Growth		
Small for gestational age (SGA)	Less than the 10th percentile for birth weight; the newborn may be preterm, term, or postterm; often seen in women who smoke, have high blood pressure, or any condition that reduces blood flow to the fetus. Increased risk of perinatal asphyxia, perinatal mortality, polycythemia, and hypoglycemia.	■ Care is aimed at promoting growth. ■ Requires ongoing screening for potential complications related to SGA including polycythemia, cold stress, asphyxia, hypothermia, and hyperbilirubinemia. ■ Assess parents and family members because SGA may be an expected finding if short stature runs in the family.
Very small for gestational age (VSGA)	Less than the third percentile for birth weight; the newborn may be preterm, term, or postterm.	■ Promote weight gain. ■ Monitor blood sugar levels for hypoglycemia. ■ Promote smoking cessation or substance abstinence if that is a factor in the newborn's VSGA status.
Large for gestational age (LGA)	Newborn's weight is at or above the 90th percentile; often associated with maternal diabetes, genetic predisposition, multiparous women, erythroblastosis fetalis, Beckwith-Wiedemann syndrome, or transposition of the great vessels.	■ Accurate estimation of gestational age is important to determining LGA status. ■ Carefully assess for potential birth trauma, including effects of cephalopelvic disproportion and macrosomia, fractured clavicle, fractured femur as a result of shoulder dystocia. ■ Monitor for hypoglycemia, polycythemia, and hyperbilirubinemia.
Intrauterine growth restriction (IUGR)	Pregnancy circumstances of advanced gestation and limited fetal growth most commonly associated with lack of prenatal care, age extremes in the mother, low socioeconomic status, multiple gestation pregnancy, grand multiparity, and primiparity. Environmental factors such as excessive exercise, exposure to toxins, high altitudes, and maternal drug use have also been implicated.	■ Early identification is important to early intervention. ■ If IUGR is unexplained, an in utero infection must be ruled out. ■ Monitor newborn for hypoglycemia. ■ Provide client teaching to promote growth after discharge and participation in neonatal stimulation programs to promote neurological function.
Conditions Present at Birth		
Newborn of a mother with diabetes	Infants born to mothers with diabetes are often LGA, macrosomic, ruddy in color, and have excessive adipose tissue, decreased total body water, edema, cardiomegaly, and often trouble regulating blood sugar levels initially because of higher-than-normal insulin production in utero to cope with the mother's elevated blood sugar levels.	■ Assess blood sugar levels frequently. ■ Monitor for signs of hypoglycemia, including tremors, cyanosis, apnea, temperature instability, poor feeding, and hypotonia. ■ Seizures may occur in severe cases. ■ Assess lab results for hypocalcemia, hyperbilirubinemia, and polycythemia. ■ Initial assessment should observe for birth trauma due to large size.
Postterm newborn	Newborn born after 42 weeks of gestation; most often seen in those of Australian, Greek, and Italian heritage. Most are normal size but large because they continued to grow in utero and face higher risk for morbidity, with a 2–3 times higher mortality rate. Potential complications include hypoglycemia, meconium aspiration, polycythemia, congenital anomalies, seizures, and cold stress.	■ Many postterm neonates will adapt well to extrauterine life. ■ Monitor serum blood sugar. ■ Assess respiratory status, especially in the presence of possible meconium aspiration. ■ Maintain neutral thermal environment until newborn demonstrates temperature stability.

(continued on next page)

Alterations and Therapies **Newborn Care** (continued)

ALTERATION	DESCRIPTION	THERAPIES
Newborns with prenatal substance abuse exposure	Substance exposure may include tobacco, marijuana, prescription medications, narcotics, or any number of illegal substances.	■ Infants are at risk for IUGR, meconium aspiration, reduced birth weight, vomiting, seizures, or irritability depending on the substances the fetus was exposed to. ■ Sedate newborns to decrease irritability and tremors. ■ Provide IV fluid therapy for hydration. ■ Possibly advise against breastfeeding. ■ Care of infants with prenatal substance abuse is discussed in detail in the module on Addiction.
Newborns born to mothers with HIV/AIDS	HIV can be transmitted through the fetal circulation, but the mother who begins antiretroviral medications early in her pregnancy can reduce the risk to the newborn.	■ Advise client that taking most HIV medications during pregnancy is safe. ■ Neonate may be given prophylactic antiretroviral therapy to decrease risk of active infection. ■ Advise against breastfeeding. ■ This concept is discussed in detail in the exemplar on HIV and AIDS in the module on Immunity.
Congenital heart defects	Any number of abnormalities can impact the heart during fetal development, increasing the challenge for newborn adaptation to extrauterine life.	■ One third of neonates born with congenital heart defects develop life-threatening symptoms in the first few days of life. ■ Therapies range from palliative care to surgery. ■ This topic is discussed in more detail in the exemplar on Congenital Heart Defects in the module on Perfusion.
Phenylketonuria (PKU)	Amino acid disorders, in which phenylalanine found in dietary protein cannot be converted to tyrosine, result in accumulation of phenylalanine in the blood, which, in turn, results in damage to brain tissue that leads to progressive mental retardation.	■ Collect routine screening blood sample before discharge (24–48 hours after first enteral feeding). ■ Instruct parents that a second screening may be required if initial collection occurs before the initiation of enteral feedings. This follow-up screening often occurs between 7-14 days of life.
Maple syrup urine disease	Rapidly progressing and often fatal disease, when untreated, caused by enzymatic defect in the metabolism of the branched-chain amino acids leucine, isoleucine, and alloisoleucine.	■ Diagnosed by routine newborn screening and confirmed by plasma amino acid assay. ■ Instruct parents on importance of obtaining second screening exam, as noted for PKU.
Galactosemia	An inborn error of carbohydrate metabolism in which the body is unable to use the sugars galactose and lactose. Enzyme pathways in liver cells normally convert galactose and lactose to glucose. In galactosemia, one step in that conversion pathway is absent because of the lack of either the enzyme galactose 1-phosphate uridyl transferase or the enzyme galactokinase. High levels of unusable galactose circulate in the blood, resulting in cataracts, brain damage, and liver damage.	■ Instruct parents on importance of routine newborn screening for inborn errors of metabolism.
Homocystinuria	Disorder caused by a deficiency of the enzyme cystathionine beta-synthase, which causes an elevated excretion of homocystine and methionine.	■ Screening is done by a bacterial inhibition assay to detect increased blood methionine (Kaye & Committee on Genetics, 2006). ■ No symptoms are usually seen in the newborn period.

Alterations and Therapies **Newborn Care** (continued)

ALTERATION	DESCRIPTION	THERAPIES
Birth-Related Stressors		
Asphyxia	Asphyxia can occur for a number of reasons, including, but not limited to, abruptio placentae, prolapsed cord, maternal hypoxia or death, difficult or prolonged labor, meconium in the amniotic fluid, intrapartum bleeding, maternal infection, prematurity, multiple births, or narcotic use during labor.	■ Promote oxygenation, airway clearance, and breathing to reduce newborn hypoxia, which often includes resuscitation. ■ Monitor blood gas status. ■ Support parents and family. ■ Provide cardiorespiratory monitoring. ■ Newborn is usually taken to the neonatal intensive care unit.
Respiratory distress	May result from inadequate production of surfactant, prematurity, excessive airway secretions, narcotic administration to the mother during labor, meconium aspiration, or congenital anomalies, among other factors. Parenchymal damage results in hyaline membrane disease compounded by mechanical ventilation if required.	■ Continuous monitoring is conducted with a cardiorespiratory monitor. ■ Continuous oxygen saturation monitoring is provided. ■ Determine arterial blood gas levels frequently until stable. ■ May require assistance with respiration in the form of mechanical ventilation, CPAP, BiPaP, and/or oxygen administration. ■ Parents and family members require emotional support because it can be very frightening to see a small baby who is so sick and who requires mechanical ventilation.
Transient tachypnea of the newborn	Of particular risk to the LGA and late-preterm neonate because of inadequate clearing of the airways; the newborn will display increased work of breathing 1–6 hours after birth, with rapid respirations, grunting, nasal flaring, and/or mild respiratory and metabolic acidosis. Improvement is usually seen after 24–48 hours.	■ Monitor newborn's respiratory adaptation to extrauterine life, and report any signs of distress immediately to primary healthcare provider. ■ Administration of oxygen should be in conjunction with oxygen saturation monitoring to prevent complications related to oxygen toxicity. ■ Promote parental attachment because a newborn requiring oxygen may not be able to feed or spend as much time with parents until breathing improves.
Meconium aspiration syndrome (MAS)	Meconium is passed in-utero secondary to stress and/or hypoxia. This fluid may be aspirated into the tracheobronchial tree in utero or during the first few breaths taken by the newborn. Meconium causes chemical irritation and also forms small balls that become lodged in terminal airways, allowing some air to enter the alveoli but not allowing air to escape. As alveoli continue to expand, they eventually rupture. Complete respiratory collapse may be seen in severe cases.	■ Avoid positive end-expiratory pressure, which forces more air into the lungs and increases chance that alveoli might rupture. ■ Mechanical ventilation may be inadequate, and oscillating ventilators that administer 300–400 breaths/minute in small waves of air may be required. ■ Continuous cardiorespiratory and oxygen saturation monitoring is indicated. ■ Reduce oxygen demands by keeping the baby quiet; sedation may be required. ■ Hypoxic newborns should not be fed because oxygen is shunted from the gut; total parenteral nutrition may be administered to meet nutritional demands.

(continued on next page)

Alterations and Therapies **Newborn Care** (continued)

ALTERATION	DESCRIPTION	THERAPIES
Cold stress	Results from inadequate temperature regulation; can progress to respiratory distress.	■ Thermoregulation is discussed in the Nursing Process section that follows and in detail in the module on Thermoregulation.
Hypoglycemia	Abnormally low blood sugar (<40 mg/dL) can result from a number of conditions including a mother with diabetes, prematurity, or cold stress.	■ If possible, feed the baby to raise blood sugar levels. ■ If unable to feed, $D_{10}W$ may be administered intravenously. ■ Observe for signs of hypoglycemia, including jitteriness, crying, or in severe cases, seizures.
Polycythemia	Abnormally high hemoglobin levels; can result from placental transfusion caused by delayed cord clamping or cord stripping; fetal asphyxia, or twin-to-twin blood transfusion in utero.	■ Encourage fluids. ■ Monitor cardiorespiratory status for tachycardia or congestive heart failure, respiratory distress. ■ Assess jaundice caused by increased red blood cell breakdown. ■ May require patience with feeding because of feeding intolerance, poor feeding, and vomiting.

Initial Care of the Newborn

Immediately after birth, the provider places the newborn on the mother's abdomen or under the radiant-heated unit. Placing the newborn on the maternal abdomen promotes attachment and bonding and gives the mother the opportunity to immediately interact with her baby. Placing the baby on the mother's chest also promotes early breastfeeding opportunities. Even though the baby may not breastfeed immediately, placement on the mother's chest enables the baby to smell, touch, and lick the mother's nipples. The newborn is maintained in a modified Trendelenburg position, which aids drainage of mucus from the nasopharynx and trachea by gravity. The newborn is dried immediately, and wet blankets are removed. The nurse helps maintain infant warmth by placing warmed blankets over the newborn or by placing the newborn in skin-to-skin contact with the mother. If the newborn is under a radiant-heated unit, he or she is dried, placed on a dry blanket, and left uncovered under the radiant heat. Because radiant heat warms the outer surface of objects, a newborn wrapped in blankets will receive no benefit from radiant heat.

The newborn's nose and mouth are suctioned with a bulb syringe as needed. Most immediate care of the newborn can be accomplished while the newborn is in the parent's arms or under the radiant-heated unit. Many women request that their infant be left on their abdomen or chest while initial care is given. Unless a medical complication exists, the nurse should complete assessments in this position to promote parental attachment.

APGAR SCORING SYSTEM   The Apgar scoring system (**Table 33–17** ●) is used to evaluate the physical condition of the newborn at birth. The newborn is rated 1 minute after birth and again at 5 minutes and receives a total score (**Apgar score**) ranging from 0 to 10 based on the following assessments:

■ *Heart rate* is auscultated or palpated at the junction of the umbilical cord and skin. This is the most important assess-

ment. A newborn heart rate of less than 100 bpm indicates the need for immediate resuscitation.

■ *Respiratory effort* is the second most important Apgar assessment. Complete absence of respirations is termed apnea. A vigorous cry indicates adequate respirations.

■ *Muscle tone* is determined by evaluating the degree of flexion and resistance to straightening of the extremities. A normal newborn's elbows and hips are flexed, with the knees positioned up toward the abdomen.

■ *Reflex irritability* is evaluated by stroking the baby's back along the spine or by flicking the soles of the feet. A cry merits a full score of 2. A grimace is given 1 point, and no response is scored as 0.

■ *Skin color* is inspected for cyanosis and pallor. Generally, newborns have blue extremities with a pink body, which merits a score of 1. This condition is termed acrocyanosis and is present in 85% of normal newborns at 1 minute after birth. A completely pink newborn scores a 2, and a totally cyanotic, pale neonate

TABLE 33–17   The Apgar Scoring System

SIGN	SCORE		
	0	1	2
Heart rate	Absent	Slow—below 100 bpm	Above 100 bpm
Respiratory effort	Absent	Slow—irregular	Good crying
Muscle tone	Flaccid	Some flexion of extremities	Active motion
Reflex irritability	None	Grimace	Vigorous cry
Color	Pale blue	Body pink, blue extremities	Completely pink

Source: Apgar, V. (1966, August). The newborn (Apgar) scoring system, reflections and advice. *Pediatric Clinics of North America, 13,* 645.

scores a 0. Newborns with darker skin pigmentation will not be pink in color. Their skin color is assessed for pallor and acrocyanosis, and a score is selected on the basis of the assessment.

A score of 7–10 indicates a newborn in good condition who requires only nasopharyngeal suctioning and, perhaps, some oxygen near the face (called "blow-by" oxygen). If the Apgar score is less than 7 at 5 minutes, the scoring should be repeated every 5 minutes up to 20 minutes (ACOG, 2006), and resuscitative measures may need to be instituted. Apgar scores of less than 3 at 5 minutes may correlate with neonatal mortality (ACOG, 2006).

CLAMPING THE CORD   If the physician or CNM has not placed some type of cord clamp on the newborn's umbilical cord, the nurse must do so. Before applying the cord clamp, the nurse examines the cut end of the cord for the presence of two arteries and one vein. The umbilical vein is the largest vessel; the arteries are seen as smaller vessels. The number of vessels is recorded on the birth and newborn records. The cord is clamped approximately 1.3–2.5 cm (0.5–1 in.) from the abdomen to allow room between the abdomen and clamp as the cord dries. Abdominal skin must not be clamped, because this will cause necrosis of the tissue. The most common type of cord clamp is the plastic Hollister cord clamp (**Figure 33–64 ●**). The Hollister clamp is removed in the newborn nursery approximately 24 hours after the cord has dried.

Evidence-based practice suggests that delayed clamping may yield more benefits than immediate cord clamping (ACOG, 2012a). Delaying cord clamping for at least 30–60 seconds produces increased blood volume, reduced need from blood transfusions, decreased incidence of intracranial hemorrhage, and a lower frequency of iron deficiency anemia (ACOG, 2012a). One concern with delayed clamping is polycythemia, which is benign. Other concerns include delayed resuscitation of the newborn and interfering with cord blood banking collection (ACOG, 2012a).

BANKING CORD BLOOD   A growing number of parents are arranging for cord blood banking. Parents obtain a special container from the Cord Blood Registry, which they bring with them for the birth. Immediately after the newborn's umbilical cord is clamped and cut, the physician or CNM withdraws blood from the remaining umbilical cord by inserting a large-gauge needle into the umbilical vein. The needle allows the blood to be collected into the container. The nurse labels the specimen immediately and follows the directions required for storage and pickup. The collected cord blood can then be used to treat childhood cancers, rare genetic disorders, and cerebral palsy. There are both public and private cord blood banks. At private banks, the cord blood is stored for possible later use by the donor. Alternatively, cord blood may be donated to public banks for use by anyone in need, much like blood donations. Although cord blood can be donated at some hospital facilities, most hospitals do not have these services available. The main drawback of cord blood banking remains the cost.

NEWBORN IDENTIFICATION AND SECURITY   Identification bands typically come in a set of four, all preprinted with identical numbers. The nurse places two bands on the newborn—one on the wrist and one on the ankle. The newborn bands must fit snugly to prevent their loss. The nurse then gives the mother and partner each a band. The band number is documented in the maternal and newborn medical records. The bands allow access to the newborn care areas; they must not be removed until the newborn is discharged. In most facilities, as a security measure,

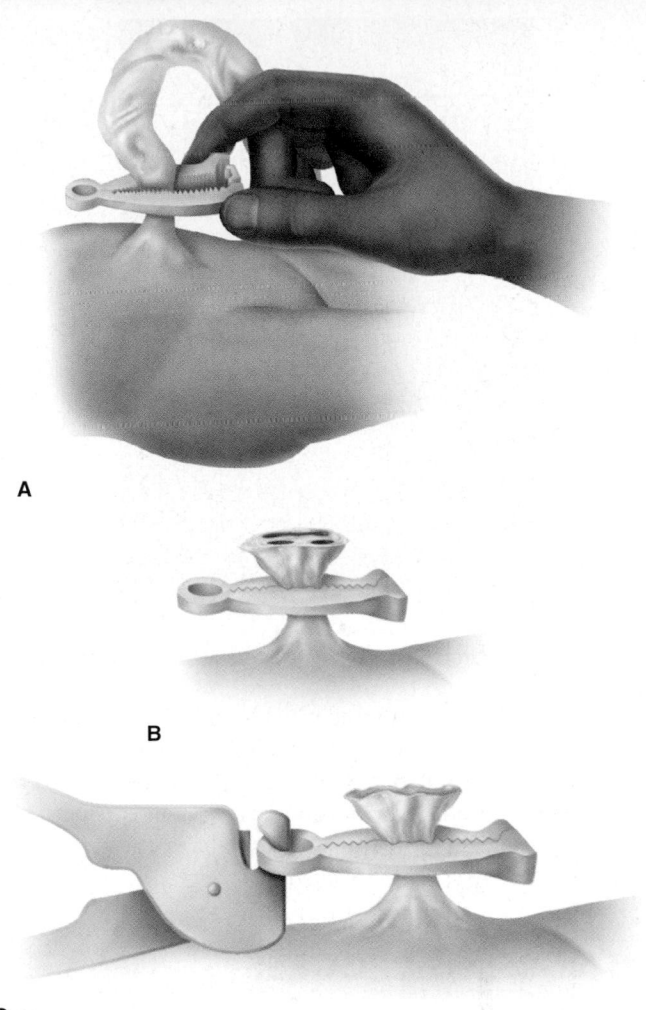

A

B

C

Figure 33–64 ● Hollister cord clamp. *A,* Clamp is positioned 1/2–1 in. from the abdomen and then secured. *B,* Cut cord. The one vein and two arteries can be seen. *C,* Plastic device for removing the clamp after the cord has dried. After the cord is cut, the nurse grasps the Hollister clamp on either side of the cut area and gently separates it.

only individuals with a band are given unlimited access to the newborn. Some facilities also include an umbilical clamp with a preprinted number identical to the number printed on the bands.

Although some institutions rely on an umbilical band system to ensure the safety of newborns, others attach an alarm to the band (**Figure 33–65 ●**). The alarm is triggered if the device is tampered with or if the newborn is removed from the parameters of the security field.

Additional hospital security measures are now commonplace in maternity settings. This includes mandating that all staff wear appropriate identification at all times. Parents are instructed that individuals without appropriate identification should not be allowed to remove their baby under any circumstances. The nurse also advises the parents to place their baby on the side of the bed away from the window and to have the baby returned to the nursery whenever the mother naps or showers and no other family member is present.

Although hospital infant abductions are rare, they are catastrophic for the family, hospital, and community. Many abductors pose as medical personnel to gain access to the mother and

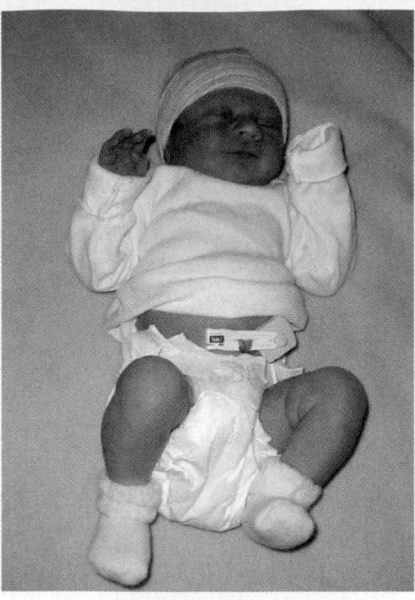

Figure 33–65 ● Umbilical alarm in place on a newborn infant.

baby. Women should be advised to ask all hospital personnel for proper identification. If the mother or family feels unsure of the individual, they should immediately use the call bell to alert the nurse and ask for other verification. If a woman is reluctant to allow a student nurse to transport her baby the staff nurse should be asked to assist the student.

◼ NURSING PROCESS

As with any client, the plan of care for the newborn is based on thorough and ongoing assessment. Thermoregulation and respiratory and cardiac function are the nurse's primary concerns. These and other interventions are discussed in this section.

Assessment

Unlike the adult, the newborn communicates needs primarily by behavior. Because nurses are the most consistent professional observers of the newborn, they can translate this behavior into information about the newborn's condition and respond with appropriate nursing interventions.

Assessment of the newborn is a continuous process designed to evaluate development and adjustments to extrauterine life. In the birth setting, the Apgar scoring procedure and careful observation form the basis of assessment and are correlated with information such as the following:

- Maternal prenatal care history
- Birthing history
- Maternal analgesia and anesthesia
- Complications of labor or birth
- Treatment instituted immediately after birth, in conjunction with determination of clinical gestational age
- Consideration of the classification of newborns by weight and gestational age and by neonatal mortality risk
- Physical examination of the newborn.

During the first 1–4 hours after birth, the nurse incorporates data from these sources with the assessment findings to formulate a plan for nursing intervention.

The various newborn assessments and the data obtained from them are valuable only to the degree to which they are shared with the parents. The parents must be included in the assessment process from the moment of their child's birth. The Apgar score and its meaning should be explained immediately to the family. As soon as possible, the parents should take part in the physical and behavioral assessments as well.

The nurse encourages the parents to identify the unique behavioral characteristics of their newborn and to learn nurturing activities. Attachment is promoted when parents have an opportunity to explore their newborn in private and identify individual physical and behavioral characteristics themselves. It is essential that the nurse provide supportive responses to parents' questions and observations throughout the assessment process. The newborn physical examination is the beginning of newborn health surveillance and health education for the newborn's family that will continue beyond discharge.

Timing of Newborn Assessments

During the first 24 hours of life, the newborn makes the critical transition from intrauterine to extrauterine life. The risk of mortality and morbidity is statistically high during this period. Assessment of the newborn is essential to ensure that the transition proceeds successfully.

There are three major time frames for assessments of newborns while they are in the birth facility:

1. The first assessment is done in the birthing area immediately after birth to determine the need for resuscitation or other interventions. The stable newborn can stay with the family after birth in order to initiate early attachment. The newborn with complications is usually taken to the nursery for further evaluation and intervention.
2. A second assessment is done by the nursery nurse as part of routine admission procedures. During this assessment, the nurse carries out a brief physical examination to estimate gestational age and evaluate the newborn's adaptation to extrauterine life. No later than 2 hours after birth, the admitting nursery nurse should evaluate the newborn's status and any problems that place the newborn at risk (AAP & ACOG, 2013).
3. Before discharge, a CNM, physician, or nurse practitioner will carry out a behavioral assessment and a complete physical examination to detect any emerging or potential problems. A general assessment is also done at this time.

Initial Physical Assessment

The nurse performs an abbreviated but systematic physical assessment in the birthing area to detect any abnormalities (Table 33–18 ●). First, the nurse notes the size of the newborn as well as the contour and size of the head in relationship to the rest of the body. The newborn's posture and movements indicate tone and neurological functioning.

The nurse inspects the skin for discoloration, presence of vernix caseosa and lanugo, and evidence of trauma and desquamation (peeling of skin). Vernix caseosa is a white, cheesy substance found normally on newborns. It is absorbed within 24 hours after birth. Vernix is abundant on preterm infants and absent on postterm newborns. **Lanugo** (fine hair) is seen on preterm newborns, especially on the shoulders, foreheads,

TABLE 33–18	Initial Newborn Evaluation
ASSESS	NORMAL FINDINGS
Respirations	30–60 breaths/min, irregular
	No retractions, no grunting
Apical pulse	110–160 bpm, somewhat irregular
Temperature	Skin temp above 36.5°C (97.8°F)
Skin color	Body pink with bluish extremities
Umbilical cord	Two arteries and one vein
Gestational age	Should be 38–42 weeks to remain with parents for an extended time
Sole creases	Sole creases that involve the heel

backs, and cheeks. Desquamation of the skin is seen in post-term newborns.

In general, expect a scant amount of vernix on upper back, axilla, and groin; lanugo only on upper back; ears with incurving of upper two thirds of pinnae and thin cartilage that springs back from folding; male genitals—testes palpated in upper or lower scrotum; female genitals—labia majora larger, clitoris nearly covered.

In the following situations, the newborn should generally be stabilized rather than remaining with parents in the birth area for an extended period of time:

- Apgar score of less than 8 at 1 minute and less than 9 at 5 minutes or baby requires resuscitation measures (other than "blow by" oxygen)
- Respirations below 30 or above 60 breaths/minute, with retractions and/or grunting
- Apical pulse below 110 or above 160 bpm, with marked irregularities
- Skin temperature below 36.5°C (97.8°F)
- Skin color pale blue or circumoral pallor
- Baby less than 38 weeks or more than 42 weeks of gestation
- SGA or LGA newborns
- Congenital anomalies involving open areas in the skin (meningomyelocele).

The nurse observes the nares for flaring and, as the newborn cries, inspects the palate for cleft palate. The nurse looks for mucus in the nose and mouth and removes it with a bulb syringe as needed. The nurse inspects the chest for respiratory rate and the presence of retractions. If retractions are present, the nurse assesses the newborn for grunting or stridor. A normal respiratory rate is 30–60 breaths/min. It is important to note that during the first few hours of life the newborn's respiratory rate may may be as high as 80 breaths/min. The nurse auscultates the lungs bilaterally for breath sounds. Absence of breath sounds on one side could indicate a pneumothorax. Because a small amount of fluid may remain in the lungs, rales may be heard immediately after birth; this fluid will be absorbed. Rhonchi indicate aspiration of oral secretions. If there is excessive mucus or respiratory distress, the nurse suctions the newborn with a mucous trap or wall suction. The nurse notes and records elimination of urine or meconium on the newborn record.

Establishing Gestational Age

The nurse must establish the newborn's gestational age in the first 4 hours after birth so that careful attention can be given to age-related problems. Once learned, the procedure can be done in a few minutes. Clinical gestational age assessment tools have two components:

1. External physical characteristics
2. Neurological or neuromuscular development.

Physical characteristics generally include sole creases, amount of breast tissue, amount of lanugo, cartilaginous development of the ear, and testicular descent and scrotal rugae or labial development. These objective clinical criteria are not influenced by labor and birth and do not change significantly within the first 12 hours after birth (Figure 33–66 ●).

Neurological examination facilitates assessment of functional or physiological maturation in addition to physical development. However, the newborn's nervous system is unstable during the first 24 hours of life. Therefore, neurological evaluation findings based on reflexes or assessments that are dependent on the higher brain centers may not be reliable. If the neurological findings drastically deviate from the gestational age derived by evaluation of external characteristics, a second assessment is done in 24 hours.

The neurological assessment components (excluding reflexes) can aid in assessing the gestational age of newborns of less than 34 weeks of gestation. Between 26 and 34 weeks, neurological changes are significant, whereas significant physical changes are less evident. One significant neuromuscular change is that muscle tone progresses from extensor tone to flexor tone in the extremities because the neurological system matures in a caudocephalad (tail-to-head) progression.

SAFETY ALERT
It is essential for the nurse to wear gloves when assessing the newborn in the early hours after birth and before the first bath until amniotic fluid, as well as vaginal and bloody secretions, on the skin are removed.

Ballard et al. (1991) developed the estimation of gestational age by maturity rating, a simplified version of the well-researched Dubowitz tool. The Ballard tool omits some of the neuromuscular tone assessments, such as head lag, ventral suspension (difficult to assess in very ill newborns or those on respirators), and leg recoil. In the Ballard tool, each physical and neuromuscular finding is given a value, and the total score is matched to a gestational age. The maximum score on the Ballard tool is 50, which corresponds to a gestational age of 44 weeks.

Postnatal gestational age assessment tools can overestimate preterm gestational age and underestimate postterm gestational age. The tools have been shown to lose accuracy when newborns of less than 28 weeks or more than 43 weeks of gestation are assessed. Ballard et al. (1991), in the New Ballard Score, added criteria for more accurate assessment of the gestational age of newborns between 20 and 28 weeks of gestation and less than 1,500 g. They suggest that the assessments should be made within 12 hours of birth to optimize accuracy, especially in infants with a gestational age of less than 26 weeks. Also, the Ballard assessment may be overstimulating to neonates of less than 27 weeks of gestation. Some maternal conditions, such as preeclampsia, diabetes, and maternal analgesia and anesthesia, may affect certain gestational assessment components and warrant further evaluation. Maternal diabetes, although it appears

Physical and Neuromuscular Characteristics of Gestational Age

Physical Characteristics

Skin. Assess for thickness, transparency, and texture. The preterm neonate's skin is thin and smooth and has visible blood vessels (see **Figure A ●**). The extremely preterm neonate has sticky, transparent skin. The term neonate has thick skin that may have a flaky texture, and the blood vessels are difficult to see.

A. Skin

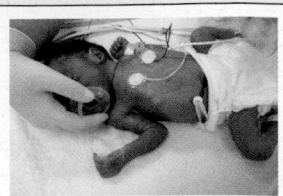

Lanugo. Assess for the quantity of lanugo, the fine soft hair covering the fetus during intrauterine development. This hair begins to appear at approximately 19–20 weeks' gestation and is most prominent at 27–28 weeks' gestation (see **Figure B ●**). It is mostly shed by 37 weeks' gestation. It first begins to thin over the lower back and then disappears last from the shoulders.

B. Lanugo

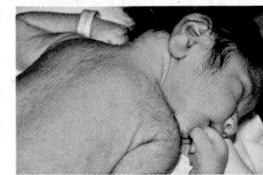

Source: Vanessa Howell RN, MSN.

Plantar surfaces. Assess the number of deep folds and creases over the sole of the foot. One to two creases appear at approximately 32 weeks' gestation (see **Figure C ●**). By 36 weeks' gestation, creases cover the anterior two thirds of the foot. At term, creases cover the entire foot (see **Figure D ●**). For extremely preterm neonates, measurement of the foot length from the tip of the great toe to the back of the heel is taken.

C. Plantar surface, 35 weeks' gestation

D. Plantar surface, term

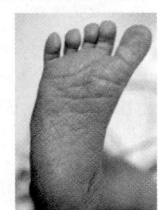

Breast. Assess the chest for visibility of the nipple and areola. Then assess the size of the breast bud when grasped between the thumb and forefinger. The extremely preterm neonate has no visible nipple and areola. The nipple and areola become more defined and raised by 34 weeks' gestation. A small breast bud appears by 36 weeks' gestation. At 38 weeks' gestation, the breast bud is 4 mm (see **Figure E ●**) and it grows to 5–10 mm in term infants (**Figure F ●**).

E. Breast bud, 38 weeks' gestation

F. Breast bud, term

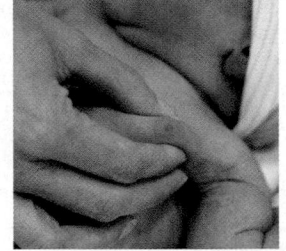
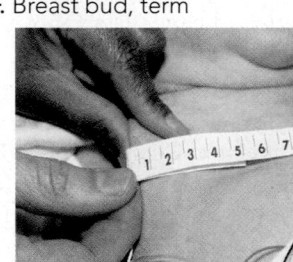

Eyes and ears. Assess the eye opening. In extremely preterm neonates, the eyelids are examined with gentle flexion to determine the amount of fusion. Eye opening begins at 22 weeks, and the lids are completely unfused by 28 weeks' gestation. Assess the formation of the ear cartilage and curving of the pinna. At earlier gestational ages the lack of cartilage allows the ear to fold easily and retain the fold. As gestational age increases, the resistance of the ear to folding increases and recoil is seen. In extremely preterm neonates the pinnae are flat. Incurving proceeds from the top down toward the lobes with advancing gestational age (see **Figures G ●** and **H ●**).

G. Ear at 36 weeks' gestation

H. Ear at term

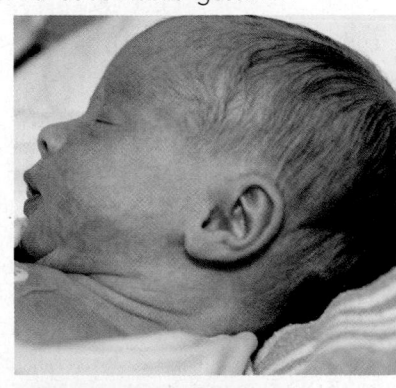

Male genitals. Assess whether the testicles are in the scrotum and for presence of rugae. The testicles are in the inguinal canal around 28 weeks' gestation and scrotal rugae are becoming visible (**Figure I ●**). By 36 weeks' gestation, the testicles are in the upper scrotum and rugae cover the anterior third of the scrotum. At term, rugae cover the scrotum (**Figure J ●**). At postterm, the testicles are pendulous.

I. Male genitals, preterm

J. Male genitals, term

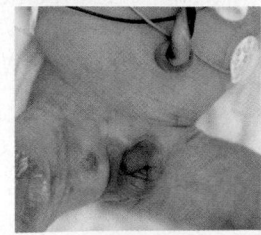
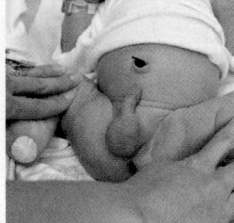

Figure 33–66 ● Physical and neuromuscular characteristics of gestational age.

Female genitals. Assess labial development. The clitoris is initially prominent and the labia minora are flat (**Figure K ●**). By 36 weeks' gestation, the labia majora are larger and the clitoris is nearly covered. At term, the labia majora are well developed and cover both the clitoris and labia minora (**Figure L ●**).

K. Female genitals, preterm

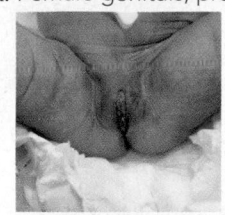

L. Female genitals, term

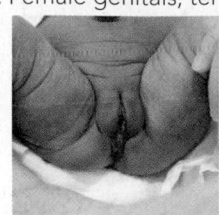

Neuromuscular Characteristics

Posture. Assess the position the supine neonate assumes at rest. The extremely preterm neonate will lie with arms and legs extended or in any position placed. With advancing gestational age, the neonate has more flexion in the arms and legs (**Figure M ●**). At term, the neonate lies with arms flexed to the chest, hands fisted, and legs flexed toward the abdomen (**Figure N ●**).

M. Resting posture, 31 weeks' gestation

N. Resting posture, term

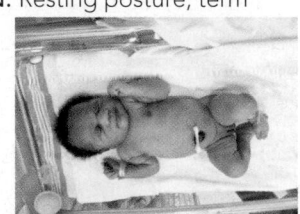

Square window sign. Assess the angle of the wrist when the palm is flexed toward the forearm. The extremely preterm neonate has no flexor tone and cannot achieve a 90-degree angle. The preterm neonate has poor flexion and is unable to flex the arm at the elbow more than 90 degrees. At 28–32 weeks' gestation, the angle is 90 degrees (see **Figure O ●**). The term neonate can achieve complete flexion against the forearm, at an angle of 30 degrees (**Figure P ●**).

O. Square window sign, 28–32 weeks' gestation

P. Square window sign, term

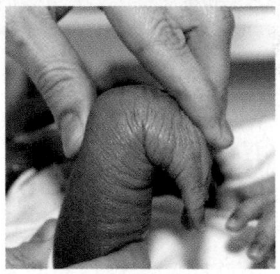

Arm recoil. Assess the amount of flexion by flexing the arms at the elbows for 5 seconds. Then extend the arms at the elbows (**Figure Q ●**). Release the arms to see the amount of recoil (**Figure R ●**). Very preterm neonates do not resist extension. They respond with weak and delayed flexion in a small arc. Term neonates resist extension and briskly return their arms to the flexed position.

Q. Extend arms at elbows

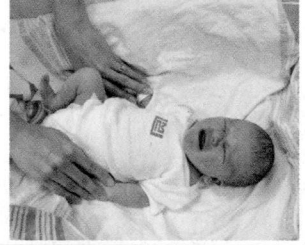

R. Release arms to see recoil

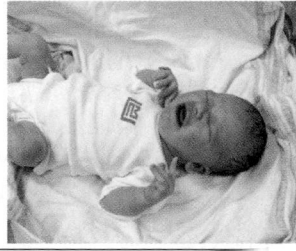

Popliteal angle. Assess the angle of the knee in the supine neonate. Holding the pelvis flat, flex and hold the thigh to the abdomen while extending the leg at the knee as (**Figure S ●**). Estimate the angle of the knee. The neonate with more advanced gestational age has greater flexion.

S. Popliteal angle

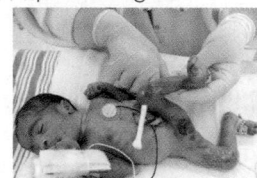

Scarf sign. Assess the neonate's resistance to pulling the arm across the chest toward the opposite shoulder. The neonate's elbow moves closer to the opposite shoulder with decreasing gestational age. Until approximately 30 weeks' gestation, the elbow moves past the midline with no resistance (**Figure T ●**). The term neonate's elbow will not cross the midline of the chest (**Figure U ●**).

T. Scarf sign, 30 weeks' gestation

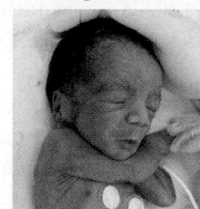

U. Scarf sign, term

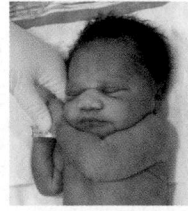

Heel-to-ear extension. Assess the amount of resistance to extension of the leg toward the ear without holding the knee or thigh in place (**Figure V ●**). The neonate's heel comes closer to the head with decreasing gestational age. Determine the distance between the heel and the head.

V. Heel-to-ear extension

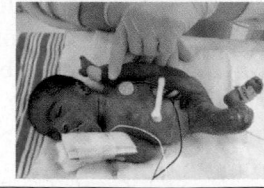

Figure 33–66 ● Physical and neuromuscular characteristics of gestational age. (*continued*)

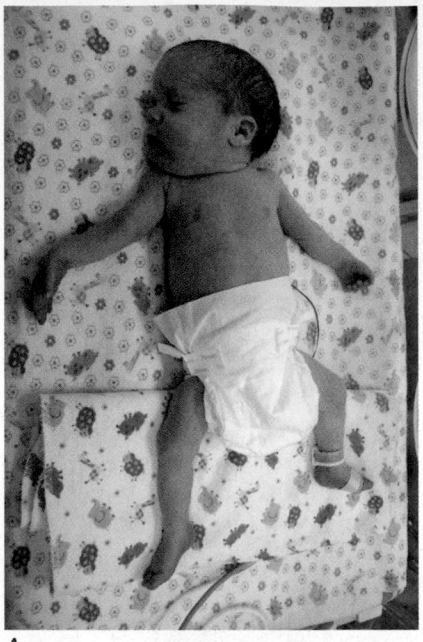 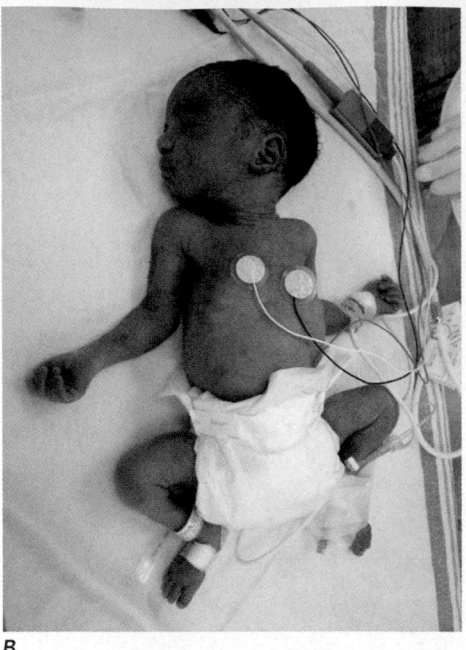 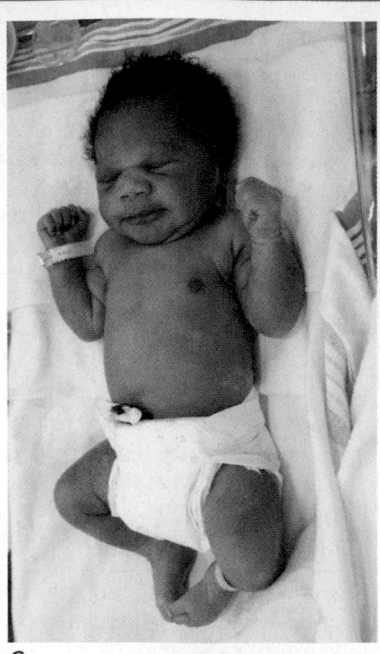

A   B   C

Figure 33–67 ● Resting posture. *A,* Newborn exhibits beginning of flexion of the thigh (score 1 or 2). The gestational age is approximately 31 weeks. Note the extension of the upper extremities. *B,* Newborn exhibits stronger flexion of the arms, hips, and thighs (score 3). The gestational age is approximately 35 weeks. *C,* The term newborn exhibits hypertonic flexion of all extremities (score 4).

to accelerate fetal physical growth, seems to retard maturation. Maternal hypertension states, which retard fetal physical growth, seem to speed maturation.

Newborns of women with preeclampsia have a poor correlation with the criteria involving active muscle tone and edema. Maternal analgesia and anesthesia may cause respiratory depression in the baby. Babies with respiratory distress syndrome tend to be flaccid and edematous and to assume a "frog-like" posture. These characteristics affect the scoring of the neuromuscular components of the assessment tool used.

ASSESSING PHYSICAL MATURITY CHARACTERISTICS

The nurse first evaluates observable characteristics without disturbing the baby. Selected physical characteristics common to the Dubowitz and Ballard gestational assessment tools are presented here in the order in which they might be most effectively evaluated:

1. *Resting posture,* although a neuromuscular component, should be assessed as the baby lies undisturbed on a flat surface (**Figure 33–67 ●**).
2. *Skin* in the preterm newborn appears thin and transparent, with veins prominent over the abdomen early in gestation. As the newborn approaches term, the skin appears opaque because of increased subcutaneous tissue. Disappearance of the protective vernix caseosa promotes skin desquamation; this is commonly seen in postmature neonates (neonates with a gestational age of more than 42 weeks) and those showing signs of placental insufficiency.
3. *Lanugo* decreases as gestational age increases. The amount of lanugo is greatest at 28–30 weeks and then disappears, first from the face and then from the trunk and extremities.

4. *Sole (plantar) creases* are reliable indicators of gestational age in the first 12 hours of life. Later, the skin of the foot begins drying, and superficial creases appear. Development of sole creases begins at the top (anterior) portion of the sole and, as gestation progresses, proceeds to the heel (**Figure 33–68 ●**). Peeling may also occur. Plantar creases vary with ethnicity; in newborns of African descent, sole creases may be less developed at term.
5. *Areola and breast bud tissue* should be inspected and gently palpated by applying the forefinger and middle finger to the breast area and then measuring the tissue between them in centimeters or millimeters (**Figure 33–69 ●**). At term gestation, the tissue measures between 0.5 and 1 cm (5 and 10 mm). During the assessment, the nurse should not grasp the nipple firmly, because skin and subcutaneous tissue will prevent accurate estimation of size. The nurse must do this procedure gently to avoid causing trauma to the breast tissue.

As gestation progresses, the breast tissue mass and areola enlarge. However, a large breast tissue mass can occur as a result of specific conditions other than advanced gestational age or the effects of maternal hormones on the baby. In the large-for-gestational-age neonate, the accelerated development of breast tissue in a mother with diabetes is a reflection of subcutaneous fat deposits. Small-for-gestational-age term or postterm newborns may have used subcutaneous fat, which would have been deposited as breast tissue, to survive in utero; as a result, their lack of breast tissue may indicate a gestational age of 34–35 weeks even though other factors indicate a term or postterm newborn.

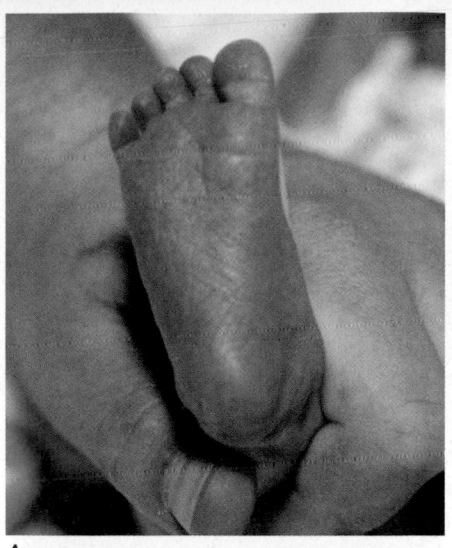
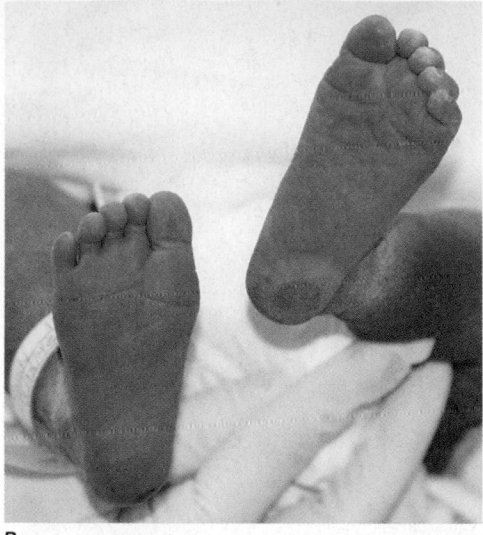
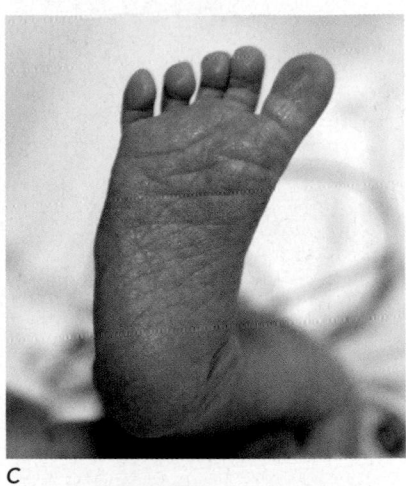

A   B   C

Figure 33–68 ● Sole creases. *A,* Newborn has a few sole creases on the anterior portion of the foot. Note the slick heel (score 2). The gestational age is approximately 35 weeks. *B,* Newborn has a deeper network of sole creases on the anterior two thirds of the sole. Note the slick heel (score 3). The gestational age is approximately 37 weeks. *C,* The term newborn has deep sole creases down to and including the heel as the skin loses fluid and dries after birth (score 4). Sole (plantar) creases can be seen even in preterm newborns.

6. ***Ear form and cartilage distribution*** develop with gestational age. The cartilage gives the ear its shape and substance (**Figure 33–70** ●). In a newborn of less than 34 weeks of gestation, the ear is relatively shapeless and flat. It has little cartilage, so the ear folds over on itself and remains folded. By approximately 36 weeks of gestation, some cartilage and incurving of the upper pinna are present, and the pinna springs back slowly when folded. (The nurse tests this response by holding the top and bottom of the pinna together with the forefinger and thumb and then releasing them or by folding the pinna of the ear forward against the side of the head, releasing it, and observing the response.) By term, the newborn's pinna is firm, stands away from the head, and springs back quickly from the folding.

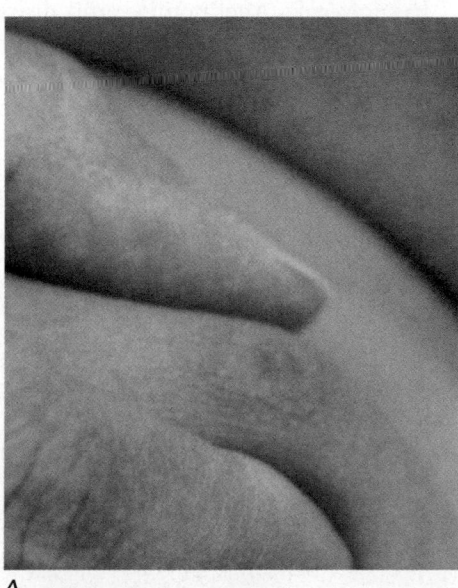
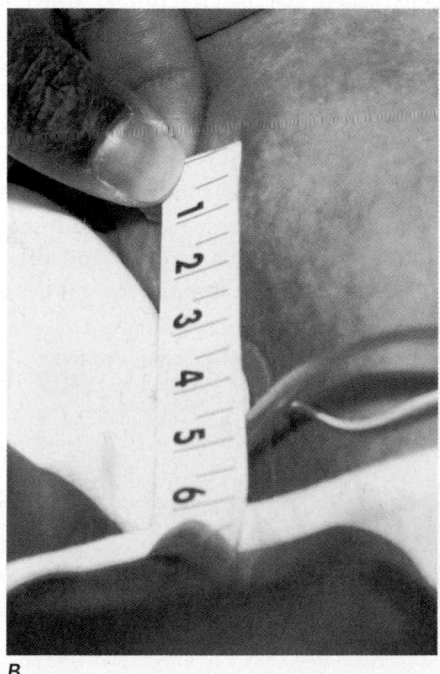

A   B

Figure 33–69 ● Breast tissue. *A,* Newborn has stippled areola, a visible raised area of 0.75 cm (0.3 in.) in diameter (score 3). The gestational age is 38 weeks.*B,* Gently compress the tissue between the middle and index fingers, and measure the tissue in centimeters or millimeters. Absence of or decreased breast tissue often indicates a premature or small-for-gestational-age newborn. *Source: C,* Vanessa Howell RN, MSN.

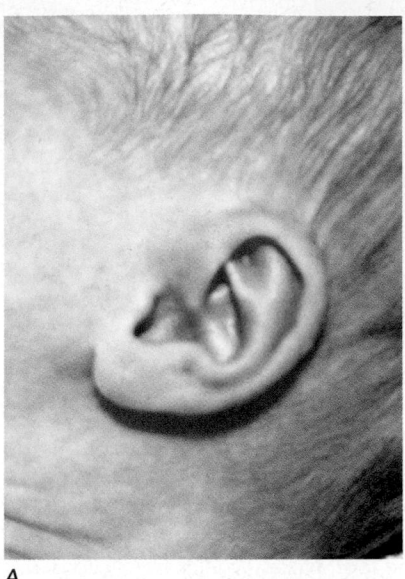 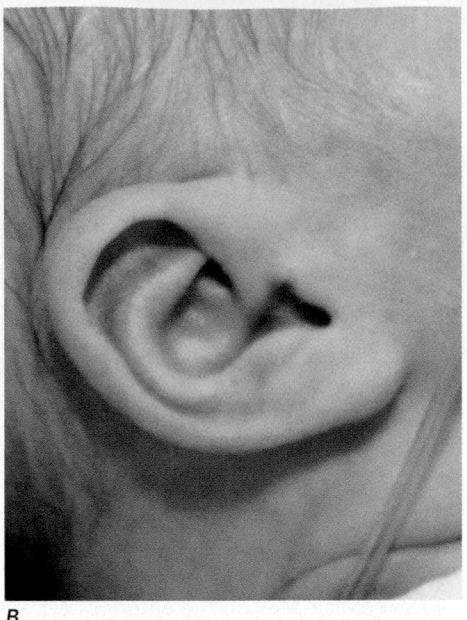 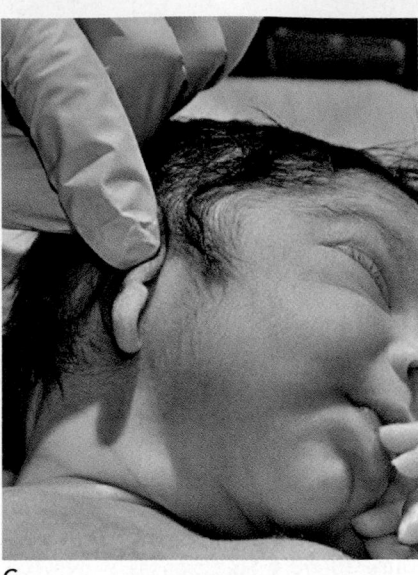

A   *B*   *C*

Figure 33–70 ● Ear form and cartilage. *A,* The ear of the newborn at approximately 36 weeks of gestation shows incurving of the upper two thirds of the pinna (score 2). *B,* Newborn at term shows well-defined incurving of the entire pinna (score 3). *C,* If the auricle stays in the position in which it is pressed or returns slowly to its original position, it usually means the gestational age is less than 38 weeks.

7. *Male genitals* are evaluated for size of the scrotal sac, presence of rugae (wrinkles and ridges in the scrotum), and descent of the testes (**Figure 33–71 ●**). Before 36 weeks of gestation, the scrotum has few rugae, and the testes are palpable in the inguinal canal. By 36–38 weeks, the testes are in the upper scrotum, and rugae have developed over the anterior portion of the scrotum. By term, the testes are generally in the lower scrotum, which is pendulous and covered with rugae.

8. *Female genital* appearance depends in part on subcutaneous fat deposition and, therefore, relates to fetal nutritional status (**Figure 33–72 ●**). The clitoris varies in size and, occasionally, is so swollen that it is difficult to identify the sex of the newborn. This swelling may be caused by adrenogenital syndrome, which causes the adrenals to secrete excessive amounts of androgen and other hormones. At 30–32 weeks of gestation, the clitoris is prominent, and the labia majora are small and widely separated. As gestational age increases, the labia majora increase in size. At 36–40 weeks, they nearly cover the clitoris. At 40 weeks and beyond, the labia majora cover the labia minora and clitoris.

Other physical characteristics assessed by some gestational age scoring tools include the following:

■ *Vernix* covers the preterm newborn. The postterm newborn has no vernix. After noting vernix distribution, the birthing area nurse (wearing gloves) dries the newborn to prevent evaporative heat loss, thus disturbing the vernix and potentially altering this gestational age criterion.

■ *Hair* of the preterm newborn has the consistency of matted wool or fur and lies in bunches rather than in the silky, single strands of the term newborn's hair.

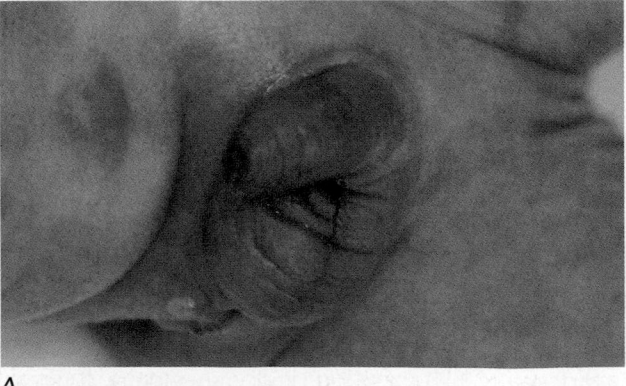 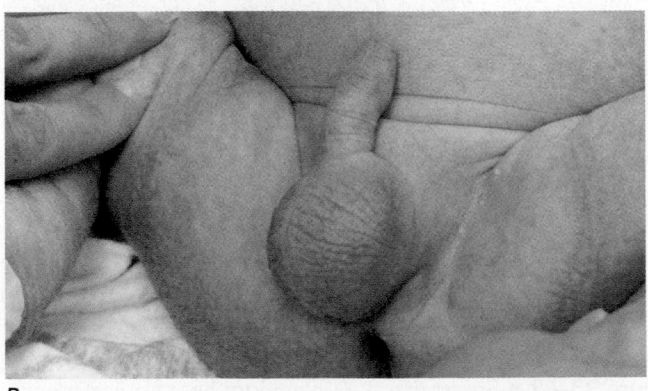

A   *B*

Figure 33–71 ● Male genitals. *A,* Preterm newborn's testes are not within the scrotum. The scrotal surface has few rugae (score 2). *B,* Term newborn's testes generally are fully descended. The entire surface of the scrotum is covered by rugae (score 3).

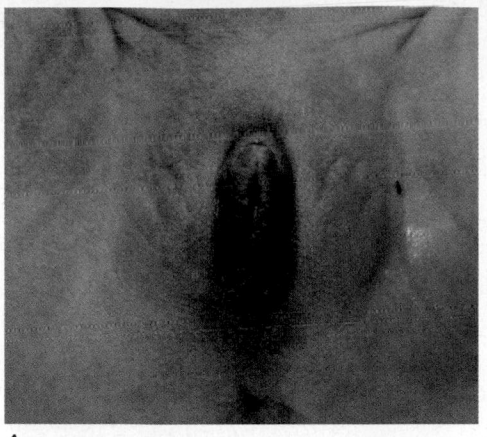
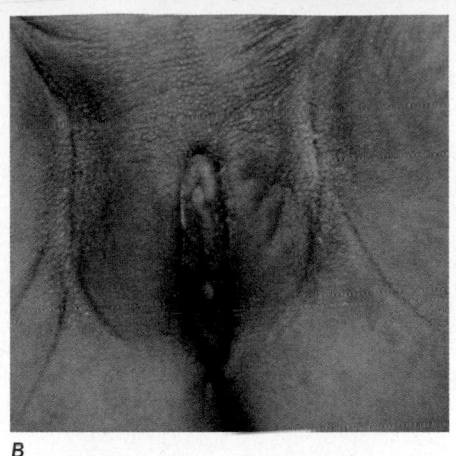
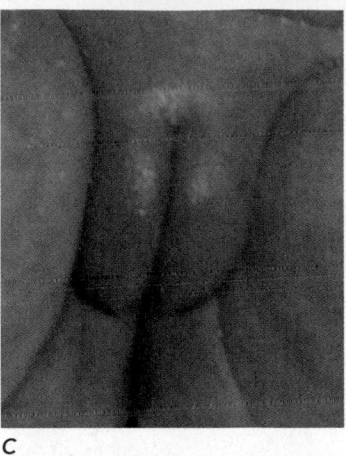

A   B   C

Figure 33–72 ● Female genitals. *A,* Newborn has a prominent clitoris. The labia majora are widely separated, and the labia minora, viewed laterally, would protrude beyond the labia majora (score 1). The gestational age is 30–36 weeks. *B,* The clitoris is still visible. The labia minora and labia majora are equally prominent (score 2). The gestational age is 36–40 weeks. *C,* The term newborn has developed large labia majora that cover both clitoris and labia minora (score 3).

- *Skull firmness* increases as the fetus matures. In a term newborn, the bones are hard, and the sutures are not easily displaced. The nurse should not attempt to displace the sutures forcibly.
- *Nails* appear and cover the nail bed at about 20 weeks of gestation. Nails extending beyond the fingertips may indicate a postterm newborn.

ASSESSING NEUROMUSCULAR MATURITY CHARACTERISTICS
The CNS of the fetus matures at a fairly constant rate. Tests have been designed to evaluate neurological status as manifested by development of neuromuscular tone. As noted earlier, neuromuscular tone in the fetus develops in a caudocephalad direction, from the lower to the upper extremities.

The neuromuscular evaluation of the newborn requires more manipulation and disturbances than the physical evaluation. The neuromuscular evaluation is best performed when the newborn has stabilized.

1. *The square window sign* is elicited by gently flexing the newborn's hand toward the ventral forearm until resistance is felt. The angle formed at the wrist is measured (**Figure 33–73 ●**).
2. *Recoil* is a test of flexion development. Because flexion first develops in the lower extremities, recoil is first tested in the legs. The nurse places the newborn on his or her back on a flat surface. With a hand on the newborn's knees, the nurse then places the baby's legs in flexion and extends them parallel to each other and flat on the surface. The response to this maneuver is recoil of the newborn's legs. According to gestational age, they may not move or may return slowly or quickly to the flexed position.

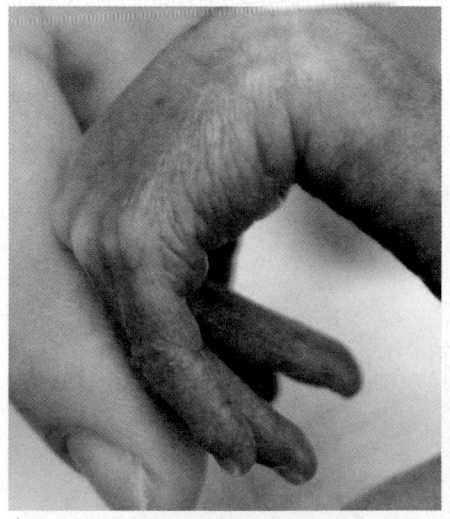
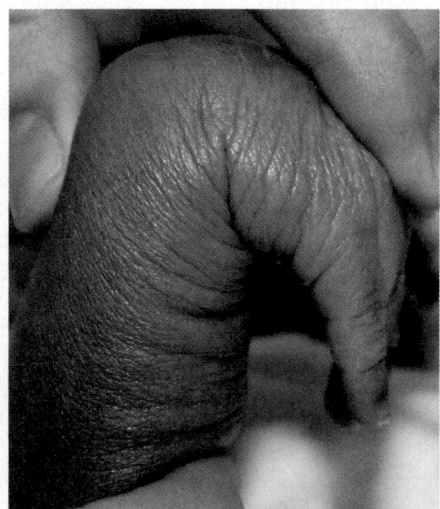
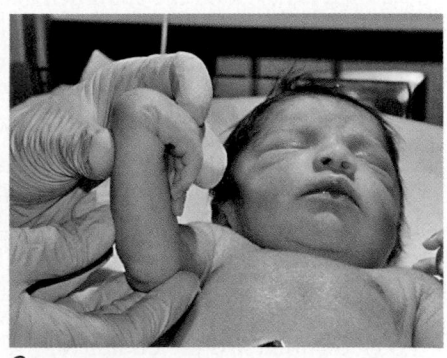

A   B   C

Figure 33–73 ● Square window sign. *A,* This angle is 90 degrees and suggests an immature newborn of 28–32 weeks of gestation (score 0). *B,* A 30- to 40-degree angle is commonly found from 38 to 40 weeks of gestation (score 2 to 3). *C,* A 0-degree-angle can occur from 40 to 42 weeks of gestation (score 4).
*Source: C,*Vanessa Howell RN, MSN.

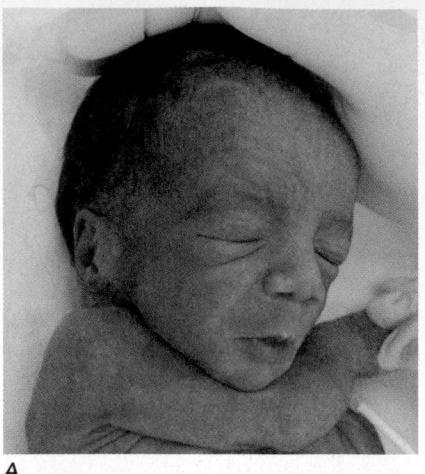
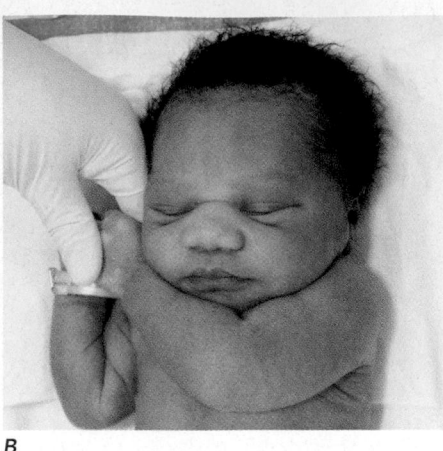
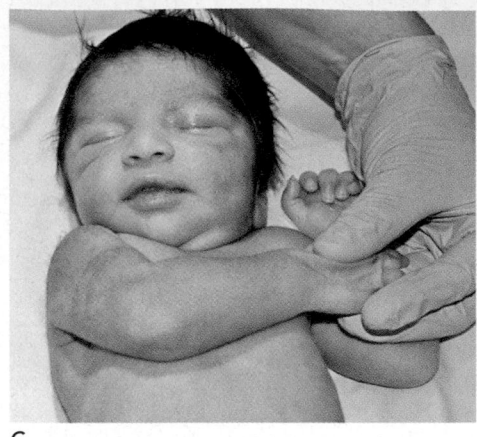

A   B   C

Figure 33–74 ● Scarf sign. *A,* No resistance is noted until after 30 weeks of gestation. The elbow moves readily past the midline (score 1). *B,* The elbow is at midline at 36–40 weeks of gestation (score 2). *C,* Beyond 40 weeks of gestation the elbow will not reach the midline (score 4).
Source: C, Vanessa Howell RN, MSN.

Preterm neonates have less muscle tone than term neonates, so preterm neonates have less recoil.

Arm recoil is tested by flexion at the elbow and extension of the arms at the newborn's side. While the baby is in the supine position, the nurse completely flexes both elbows, holds them in this position for 5 seconds, extends the arms at the baby's side, and releases them. On release, the elbows of a full-term newborn form an angle of less than 90 degrees and rapidly recoil back to a flexed position. The elbows of a preterm newborn have slower recoil time and form an angle of greater than 90 degrees. Arm recoil is also slower in healthy but fatigued newborns after birth; therefore, arm recoil is best elicited after the first hour postbirth, when the baby has had time to recover from the stress of the birth. The deep sleep state also decreases the arm recoil response. Assessment of arm recoil should be bilateral to rule out brachial palsy.

3. **The popliteal angle** (degree of knee flexion) is determined with the newborn flat on his or her back. The thigh is flexed on the abdomen and chest, and the nurse places the index finger of the other hand behind the newborn's ankle to extend the lower leg until resistance is met. The angle formed is then measured. Results vary from no resistance in the very immature newborn to an 80-degree angle in the term newborn.

4. **The scarf sign** is elicited by placing the newborn supine and drawing one of the newborn's arms across the chest toward the opposite shoulder until resistance is met. The location of the elbow is then noted in relation to the midline of the chest (**Figure 33–74** ●). A preterm neonate's elbow will cross the midline of the chest, whereas a full-term neonate's elbow will not cross midline.

5. **The heel-to-ear extension** is performed by placing the newborn in a supine position and then gently drawing the foot toward the ear on the same side until resistance is felt. The nurse should allow the knee to bend during the test. It is important to hold the buttocks down to keep from rolling the baby. Both the proximity of foot to ear and the degree of knee extension are assessed. A preterm, immature newborn's leg will remain straight, and the foot will go to the ear or beyond (**Figure 33–75** ●). With advancing gestational age, the newborn demonstrates increasing resistance to this maneuver. Maneuvers involving the lower extremities of newborns who had frank breech presentation should be delayed to allow for resolution of leg positioning.

6. **Ankle dorsiflexion** is determined by flexing the ankle on the shin. The nurse uses a thumb to push on the sole of the newborn's foot while the fingers support the back of the leg. Then, the angle formed by the foot and the interior leg is measured (**Figure 33–76** ●). This sign can be influenced by intrauterine position and congenital deformities.

7. **Head lag** (neck flexor) is measured by pulling the newborn to a sitting position and noting the degree of head lag. Total lag is common in newborns up to 34 weeks of

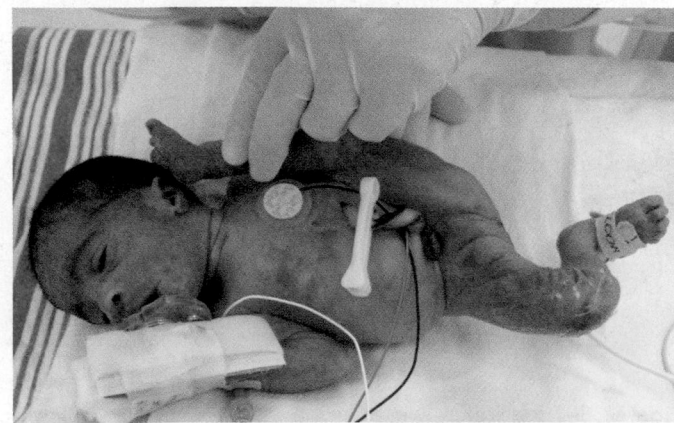

Figure 33–75 ● Heel to ear. No resistance. Leg fully extended (score 0).

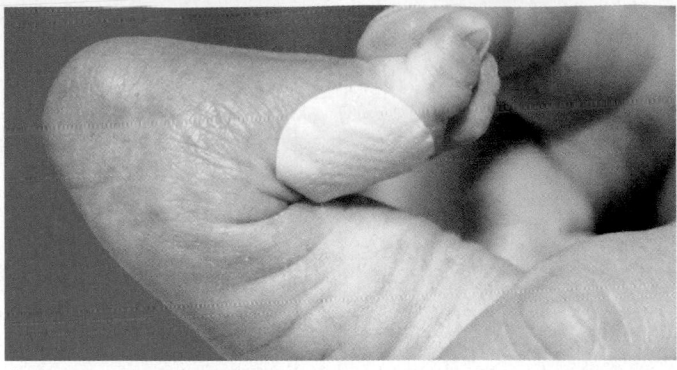
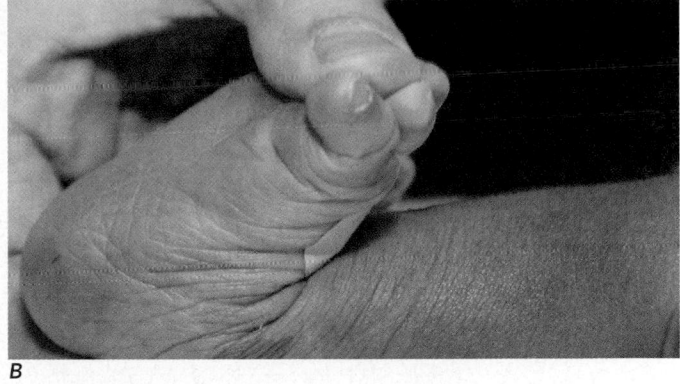

A   *B*

Figure 33–76 ● Ankle dorsiflexion. *A*, A 45-degree angle indicates 32–36 weeks of gestation. A 20-degree angle indicates 36–40 weeks of gestation (score 2 to 3). *B*, A 15- to 0-angle is common at 40 weeks or more of gestation (score 4).

gestation, whereas postterm newborns (>42 weeks) hold their heads in front of their body lines. Full-term newborns can support their heads momentarily.

8. *Ventral suspension* (horizontal position) is evaluated by holding the newborn prone on the nurse's hand. The position of the head and back and the degree of flexion in the arms and legs are noted. Some flexion of arms and legs indicates 36–38 weeks of gestation; fully flexed extremities, with the head and back even, are characteristic of a term newborn.

9. *Major reflexes*, such as sucking, rooting, grasping, Moro, tonic neck, Babinski, and others, are evaluated during the newborn exam.

A supplementary method for estimating gestational age (done by the physician or nurse practitioner) is to view the vascular network of the cornea with an ophthalmoscope. The nurse may need to delay administration of prophylactic eye ointment in preterm neonates until after this vascular eye exam has been done. The amount of vascularity present over the surface of the lens assists in identifying neonates with a gestational age of 27–34 weeks (Rosenberg, 2013).

When the gestational age determination and birth weight are considered together, the newborn can be identified as one whose growth is classified as follows (**Figure 33–77 ●**):

■ Below the 10th percentile, or small for gestational age
■ Between the 10th and 90th percentiles, or appropriate for gestational age
■ Above the 90th percentile, which is large for gestational age.

This determination enables the nurse to anticipate possible physiological problems. This information is used in conjunction with a complete physical examination to establish an appropriate plan of care for the individual newborn. For example, newborns who are small or large for gestational age are at risk for hypoglycemia and therefore often require frequent glucose monitoring and early feedings started soon after birth.

The nurse also plots the gestational age against the newborn's length, head circumference, and weight on an appropriate growth chart to determine if these measurements fall within the average range—the 10th–90th percentile for the corresponding gestational age. These correlations further document the level of maturity and appropriate category for the newborn. The

comparison of the newborn's weight–length ratio further facilitates identification of SGA newborns as having symmetric or asymmetric growth restriction. Measuring weight and height often aggravates newborns and may alter their vital signs. For better accuracy, take the newborn's vital signs before weighing and measuring the neonate.

Subsequent Physical Assessment

Once the initial assessment process is complete and gestational age has been established, the nurse carries out a thorough, systematic assessment of the newborn. Completing the physical assessment in the presence of the parents provides an opportunity to acquaint them with their unique newborn. The examination is performed in a systematic, head-to-toe manner, and all findings are recorded. When assessing the physical and neurological status of the newborn, the nurse should first consider general appearance and then proceed to specific areas.

GENERAL APPEARANCE The newborn's head is disproportionately large for its body. The neck looks short because the chin rests on the chest. Newborns have a prominent abdomen, sloping shoulders, narrow hips, and rounded chests. The center of the baby's body is the umbilicus rather than the symphysis pubis, as in the adult. The body appears long and the extremities short.

Newborns tend to stay in a flexed position similar to the one maintained in utero and will offer resistance when the extremities are straightened. This flexed position contributes to the short appearance of the extremities. The hands are tightly clenched. After a breech birth, the feet are usually dorsiflexed, and it may take several weeks for the newborn to assume the typical newborn posture.

WEIGHT AND MEASUREMENT The normal, full-term, newborn has an average birth weight of 3,405 g (7 lb, 8 oz). Newborns of African, Asian, or Mexican American descent may be somewhat smaller at term, whereas Native American newborns are often heavier at term (Teitler et al., 2007). Other factors that influence weight are age and size of the parents, health of the mother (smoking and malnutrition decrease birth weight), and the interval between pregnancies (short intervals, such as every year, result in lower birth weight). After the first week, and for the first 6 months, the baby's weight increases about 198 g (7 oz) weekly.

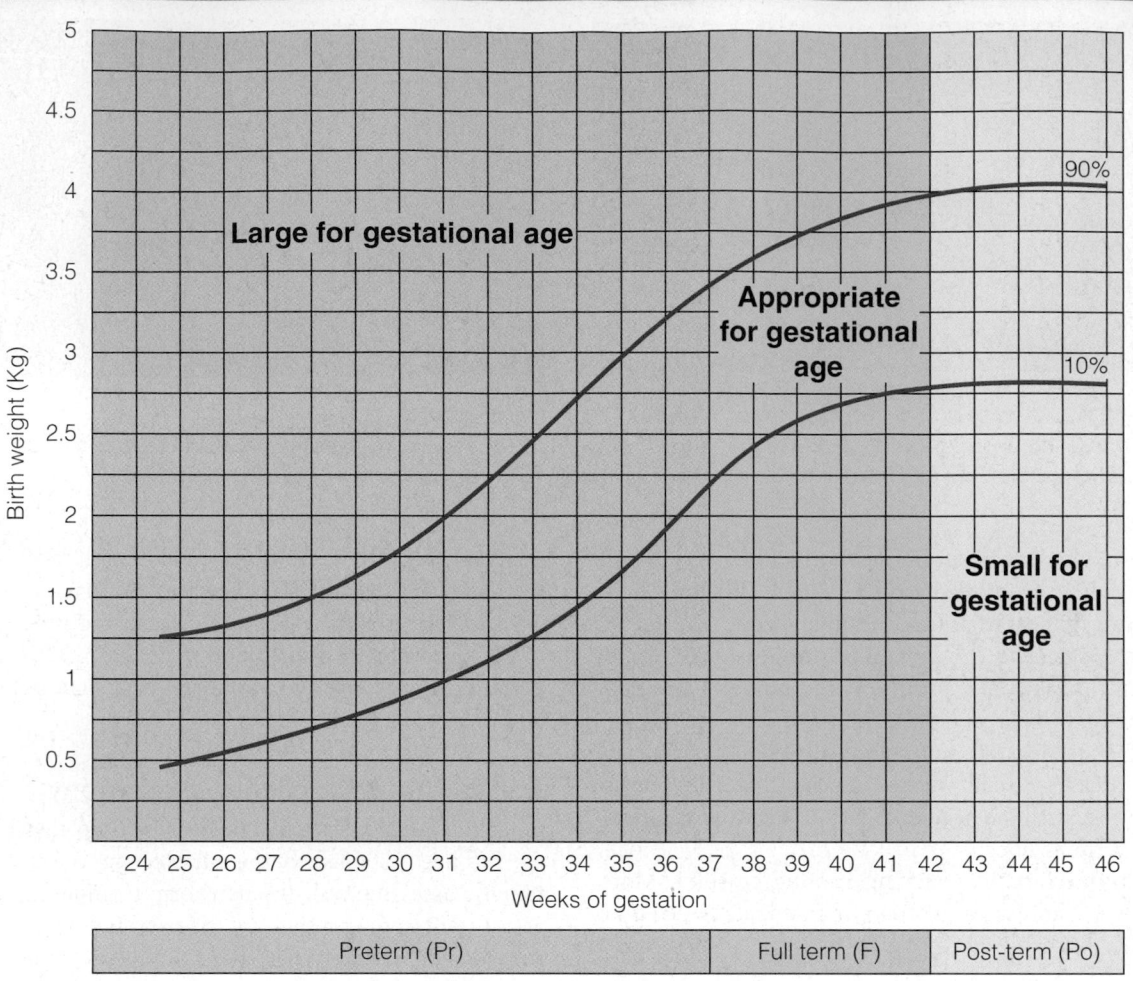

Figure 33–77 ● Classification of newborns by birth weight and gestational age. The nurse places the newborn's birth weight and gestational age on the graph and classifies the newborn as large for gestational age (LGA), appropriate for gestational age (AGA), or small for gestational age (SGA).

Approximately 70%–75% of the newborn's body weight is water. During the initial newborn period (the first 3–4 days), term newborns have a physiological weight loss of about 5%–10% because of fluid shifts. For the term newborn, weight loss that is greater than 10% indicates the need for clinical appraisal. Large babies also tend to lose more weight because of greater fluid loss in proportion to birth weight. Factors contributing to weight loss include insufficient fluid intake resulting from delayed breastfeeding or a slow adjustment to the formula, increased volume of meconium excreted, and urination. Weight loss may be marked in the presence of temperature elevation (because of associated dehydration) or consistent chilling (because of nonshivering thermogenesis).

The length of the average newborn is difficult to measure because the legs are flexed and tensed. To measure length, the nurse should place newborns flat on their backs with their legs extended as much as possible. The average length is 50 cm (20 in.), and the range is 46–56 cm (18–22 in.). The newborn will grow approximately 2.5 cm (1 in.) a month for the next 6 months. This is the period of most rapid growth.

At birth, the newborn's head is one third the size of an adult's head. The circumference (biparietal diameter) of the newborn's head is 32–37 cm (12.5–14.5 in.). For accurate measurement, the nurse places the tape over the most prominent part of the occiput and brings it just above the eyebrows. The circumference of the newborn's head is approximately 2 cm (0.8 in.) greater than the circumference of the newborn's chest at birth and will remain in this proportion for the next few months. It is best to take another head circumference on the second day if the newborn experienced significant head molding or developed a caput from the birth process.

The average circumference of the chest is 32 cm (12.5 in.) and ranges from 30 to 35 cm (12 to 14 in.). Chest measurements are taken with the tape measure placed at the lower edge of the scapulas and brought around anteriorly, directly over the nipple line. The abdominal circumference, or girth, may also be measured at this time by placing the tape around the newborn's abdomen at the level of the umbilicus, with the bottom edge of the tape at the top edge of the umbilicus.

TEMPERATURE   Initial assessment of the newborn's temperature is critical; if no heat conservation measures are started, skin temperature markedly decreases within 10 minutes after exposure to room air. The newborn's temperature should stabilize within 8–12 hours.

Temperature is monitored when the newborn is admitted to the nursery and at least every 30 minutes until the newborn's status has remained stable for 2 hours. Thereafter, the nurse should assess temperature at least once every 8 hours, or according to institutional policy (AAP & ACOG, 2013). For neonates who have been exposed to group B hemolytic streptococcus, more frequent temperature monitoring may be required.

Temperature can be assessed by the axillary skin method, a continuous skin probe, the rectal route, or a tympanic thermometer. Axillary temperatures are the preferred method and are considered to be a close estimation of the rectal temperature. Axillary temperature ranges from 36.5° to 37.0°C (97.7° to 98.6°F). Skin temperature is measured most accurately by means of a continuous skin probe, but this method generally is used only with small or sick newborns placed under radiant warmers or in isolettes. Normal skin temperature is 36°–36.5°C (96.8°–97.7°F). Rectal temperature is assumed to be the closest approximation to core temperature, but the accuracy of this method depends on the depth to which the thermometer is inserted. The rectal temperature is often measured during the initial newborn assessment to determine patency. This method is not recommended for routine use because of the risk of irritation to the rectal mucosa and increased chances of perforation (Blackburn, 2013). Normal rectal temperature is 36.6°–37.2°C (97.8°–99°F).

Temperature instability (a deviation of more than 1°C [2°F] from one reading to the next) or a subnormal temperature may indicate an infection. In contrast to an elevated temperature in older children, an increased temperature in a newborn may indicate a reaction to too many coverings, too hot a room, or dehydration. Dehydration, which tends to increase body temperature, occurs in newborns whose feedings have been delayed for any reason. Newborns may respond to overheating (temperature of >37.5°C [99.5°F]) by increased restlessness and, eventually, by perspiration after 35–40 minutes of exposure (Blackburn, 2013). The perspiration appears initially on the head and face and then on the chest.

SKIN CHARACTERISTICS Although the newborn's skin color varies with genetic background, all healthy newborns have a pink tinge to their skin. The ruddy hue results from increased RBC concentrations in the blood vessels and limited subcutaneous fat deposits.

Skin pigmentation is slight in the newborn period, so color changes may be seen even in darker-skinned babies. White newborns have a pinkish-red skin tone a few hours after birth, and African American newborns have a reddish-brown skin color. Hispanic and Asian newborns have an olive or yellow skin tone (Vargo, 2014). Skin pigmentation deepens over time; therefore, variations in skin color indicating illness are more difficult to evaluate in African American and Asian newborns (Vargo, 2014). A newborn who is cyanotic at rest and pink only with crying may have choanal atresia (congenital blockage of the passageway between the nose and pharynx). If crying increases

the cyanosis, heart or lung problems should be suspected. Very pale newborns may be anemic or have hypovolemia (low blood pressure) and should be evaluated for these problems.

Acrocyanosis (bluish discoloration of the hands and feet) may be present in the first 24–48 hours after birth. This condition is caused by poor peripheral circulation, which results in vasomotor instability and capillary stasis, especially when the baby is exposed to cold. Blue hands and nails are a poor indicator of decreased oxygenation in a newborn. If the central circulation is adequate, the blood supply should return quickly (2–3 seconds) to the extremity after the skin is blanched with a finger. The nurse should assess the face and mucous membranes for pinkness that reflects adequate oxygenation.

Mottling (lacy pattern of dilated blood vessels under the skin) occurs as a result of general circulation fluctuations. It may last several hours to several weeks, or it may come and go periodically. Mottling may be related to chilling or prolonged apnea, sepsis, or hypothyroidism.

Harlequin sign (clown) color change is occasionally noted: A deep red color develops over one side of the newborn's body while the other side remains pale, so the skin resembles a clown's suit. This color change results from a vasomotor disturbance in which blood vessels on one side dilate while the blood vessels on the other side constrict. It usually lasts from 1 to 20 minutes. Affected newborns may have single or multiple episodes, but they are transient and clinically insignificant. The nurse should document each occurrence.

Jaundice is yellow pigmentation of body tissues caused by the presence of bile pigments. It is first detectable on the face (where skin overlies cartilage) and the mucous membranes of the mouth, and it has a head-to-toe progression (Vargo, 2014). Jaundice regresses in the opposite direction (from toe to head). It is evaluated by blanching the tip of the nose, the forehead, the sternum, or the gum line. This procedure must be carried out in appropriate lighting. If jaundice is present, the area will appear yellowish immediately after blanching. Another area to assess for jaundice is the sclera. Evaluation and determination of the cause of jaundice must be initiated immediately to prevent possibly serious sequelae. The jaundice may be related to breastfeeding (extremely rare), hematomas, immature liver function, or bruises from forceps, or it may be caused by blood incompatibility, oxytocin (Pitocin) augmentation or induction, or a severe hemolytic process. Any jaundice noted before a newborn is 24 hours of age should be reported to the physician or neonatal nurse practitioner.

Erythema toxicum is an eruption of lesions in the area surrounding a hair follicle that are firm, vary in size from 1 to 3 mm, and consist of a white or pale yellow papule or pustule with an erythematous base. It is often called "newborn rash" or "flea bite" dermatitis. The rash may appear suddenly, usually over the trunk and diaper area, and is frequently widespread (**Figure 33–78 ●**). The lesions do not appear on the palms of the hands or the soles of the feet. The peak incidence is at 24–48 hours of life. The condition rarely presents at birth or after 5 days of life. The cause is unknown, and no treatment is necessary. Some healthcare providers believe it may be caused by irritation from clothing. The lesions disappear in a few hours or days. If a maculopapular rash

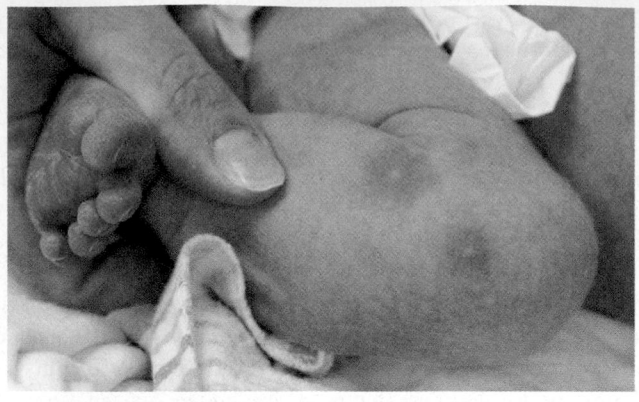

Figure 33–78 ● Erythema toxicum on leg.

appears, a smear of the aspirated papule will show numerous eosinophils on staining; no bacteria will be cultured.

Milia (exposed sebaceous glands) appear as raised white spots on the face, especially across the nose (**Figure 33–79** ●). No treatment is necessary, because they will clear spontaneously within the first month. Infants of African heritage have a similar condition called transient neonatal pustular melanosis (Silverman, 2012).

Skin turgor (the elasticity of the skin) is assessed to determine hydration status, the need to initiate early feedings, and the presence of any infectious processes. The usual place to assess skin turgor is over the abdomen, forearm, or thigh. Skin should be elastic and return rapidly to its original shape.

Vernix caseosa (a whitish, cheese-like substance) covers the fetus while in utero and lubricates the skin of the newborn. The skin of the term or postterm newborn has less vernix and is frequently dry; peeling is common, especially on the hands and feet.

Forceps marks may be present after a difficult forceps birth. The newborn may have reddened areas over the cheeks and jaws. It is important to reassure the parents that these marks will disappear, usually within 1 or 2 days. Transient facial paralysis resulting from the forceps pressure is a rare complication. Vacuum extractor suction marks on the vertex of the scalp are often seen when vacuum extractors are used to assist with the birth; these marks are benign and do not indicate underlying brain lesions.

BIRTHMARKS Birthmarks are frequently a cause of concern for parents. The mother may be especially anxious, fearing that she is to blame ("Is my baby 'marked' because of something I did?"). Feelings of guilt are common in the presence of misconceptions about the cause. Birthmarks should be identified and explained to the parents. By providing appropriate information about the cause and course of birthmarks, the nurse can relieve the fears and anxieties of the family. The nurse should note any bruises, abrasions, or birthmarks seen on admission to the nursery.

Telangiectatic nevi (stork bites) appear as pale pink or red spots and are frequently found on the eyelids, nose, lower occipital bone, and nape of the neck. These lesions are common in newborns with light complexions and are more noticeable during periods of crying. These areas have no clinical significance and usually fade by the second birthday.

Mongolian spots are macular areas of bluish-black or gray-blue pigmentation on the dorsal area and the buttocks (**Figure 33–80** ●). They are common in newborns of Asian, Hispanic, and African descent and in newborns of other dark-skin ethnicities. They gradually fade during the first or second year of life. They may be mistaken for bruises and should be documented in the newborn's chart.

Nevus flammeus (port-wine stain) is a capillary angioma directly below the epidermis. It is a nonelevated, sharply demarcated, red-to-purple area of dense capillaries. In newborns of African descent, it may appear as a purple-black stain. The size and shape vary, but it commonly appears on the face. It does not grow in size, does not fade with time, and as a rule, does not blanch. The birthmark may be concealed by using an opaque cosmetic cream. **Nevus vasculosus (strawberry mark)** is a capillary hemangioma. It consists of newly formed and enlarged capillaries in the dermal and subdermal layers. It is a raised, clearly delineated, dark red, rough-surfaced birthmark commonly found in the head region. Such marks usually grow (often rapidly) starting in the second or third week of life, and they may not reach their fullest size for 1–3 months (Tappero & Honeyfield, 2009). They begin to shrink and start to resolve spontaneously several weeks to months after they reach peak growth. A pale purple or gray spot on the surface of the hemangioma signals the start of resolution. The best cosmetic effect is achieved when the lesions are allowed to resolve spontaneously.

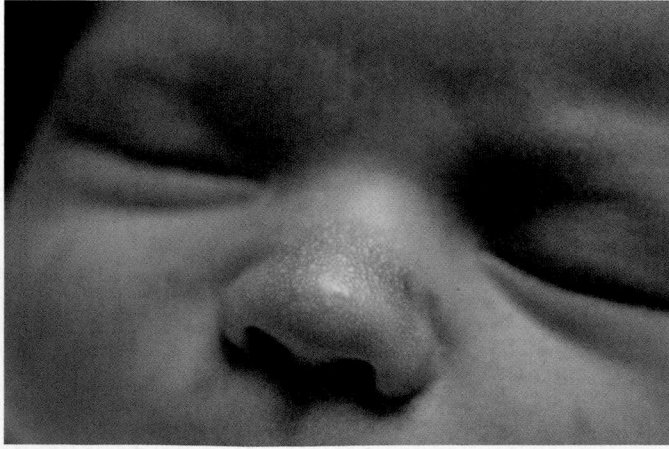

Figure 33–79 ● Facial milia.
Source: Jack Sullivan/Alamy.

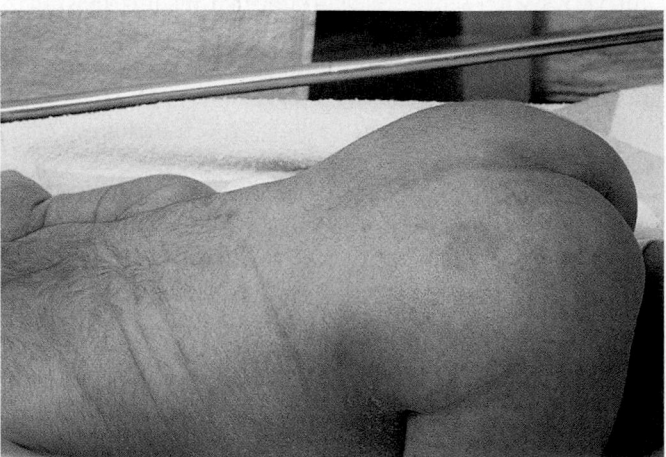

Figure 33–80 ● Mongolian spots.

HEAD The newborn's head is large (approximately one fourth of the body size), with soft, pliable skull bones. For most term neonates, the occipitofrontal circumference is 32–37 cm (12.6–14.6 in.).

The head may appear asymmetric in the newborn of a vertex birth. This asymmetry, called **molding**, is caused by overriding of the cranial bones during labor and birth. The degree of molding varies with the amount and length of pressure exerted on the head. Within a few days after birth, the overriding usually diminishes, and the suture lines become palpable. Because head measurements are affected by molding, a second measurement is indicated a few days after birth.

The heads of breech-born newborns and of those delivered by elective cesarean are characteristically round and well shaped because no pressure was exerted on them during birth. Any extreme differences in head size may indicate microcephaly (abnormally small head) or hydrocephalus (an abnormal buildup of fluid in the brain). Variations in the shape, size, or appearance of the head measurements may be caused by craniosynostosis (premature closure of the cranial sutures), which will need to be corrected through surgery to allow brain growth, and plagiocephaly (asymmetry caused by pressure on the fetal head during gestation) (Tappero & Honeyfield, 2009).

Two fontanelles ("soft spots") may be palpated on the newborn's head. Fontanelles, which are openings at the juncture of the cranial bones, can be measured with the fingers. Accurate measurement necessitates that the examiner's finger be measured in centimeters. The assessment should be carried out with the newborn in a sitting position and not crying. The diamond-shaped anterior fontanelle is approximately 3–4 cm (1.2–1.6 in.) long by 2–3 cm (0.8–1.2 in.) wide. It is located at the juncture of the frontal and parietal bones. The posterior fontanelle, smaller and triangular, is formed by the parietal bones and the occipital bone and is 0.5 by 1 cm. Because of molding, the fontanelles are smaller immediately after birth than they are several days later. The anterior fontanelle closes within 18 months, whereas the posterior fontanelle closes within 8–12 weeks.

The fontanelles are a useful indicator of the newborn's condition. The anterior fontanelle may swell when the newborn cries or passes a stool or may pulsate with the heartbeat, which is normal. A bulging fontanelle usually signifies increased intracranial pressure, and a depressed fontanelle indicates dehydration (Vargo, 2014).

The sutures between the cranial bones should be palpated for the amount of overlapping. In newborns whose growth has been restricted, the sutures may be wider than normal, and the fontanelles may also be larger because of impaired growth of the cranial bones. In addition to inspecting the newborn's head for degree of molding and size, the nurse should evaluate it for soft-tissue edema and bruising.

Cephalohematoma is a collection of blood resulting from ruptured blood vessels between the surface of a cranial bone (usually parietal) and the periosteal membrane (**Figure 33–81 ●**). The scalp in these areas feels loose and slightly edematous. These areas emerge as defined hematomas between the first and second days. Although external pressure may cause the mass to fluctuate, it does not increase in size when the newborn cries.

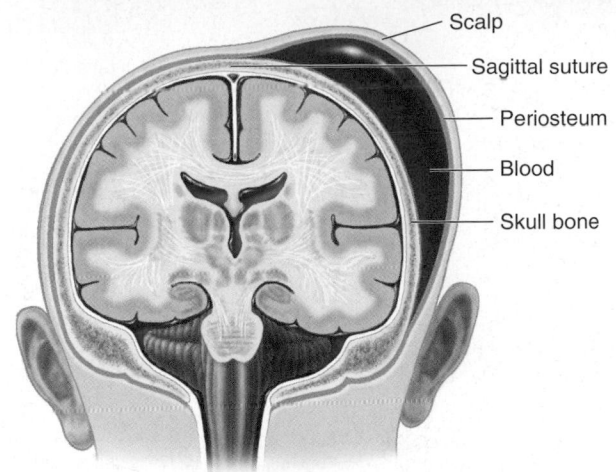

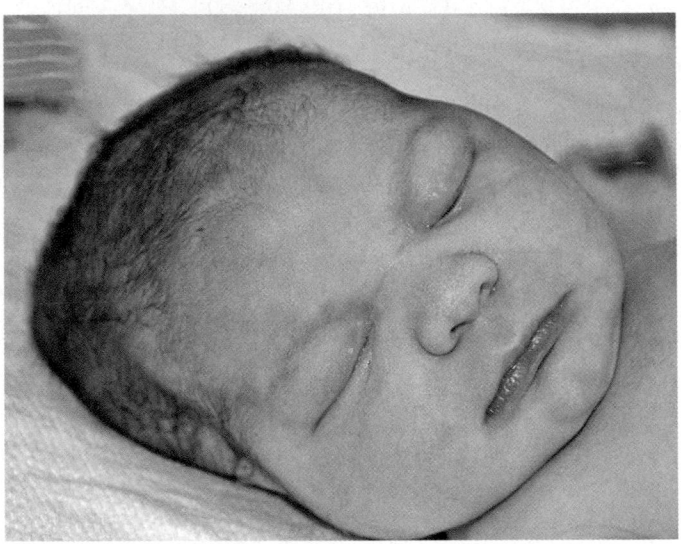

Figure 33–81 ● Cephalohematoma is a collection of blood between the surface of a cranial bone and the periosteal membrane. This is a cephalohematoma over the left parietal bone.
Source: Courtesy of Jo Engle, RN, MSN, NNP-BC, and Vanessa Howell RN, MSN.

Cephalohematomas may be unilateral or bilateral and do not cross suture lines. They are relatively common in vertex births and may disappear within 2 weeks to 3 months. They may be associated with physiological jaundice because extra RBCs are being destroyed within the cephalohematoma. A large cephalohematoma can lead to anemia and hypotension.

Caput succedaneum is a localized, easily identifiable, soft area of the scalp, generally resulting from a long and difficult labor or vacuum extraction. The sustained pressure of the presenting part against the cervix results in compression of local blood vessels, and venous return is slowed. This results in an increase of tissue fluids, edematous swelling, and occasional bleeding under the periosteum. The caput may vary from a small area to a severely elongated head. The fluid in the caput is reabsorbed within 12 hours to a few days after birth. Caputs resulting from vacuum extractors are sharply outlined, circular areas up to 2 cm (0.8 in.) thick. They disappear more slowly than naturally occurring edema. It is possible to distinguish

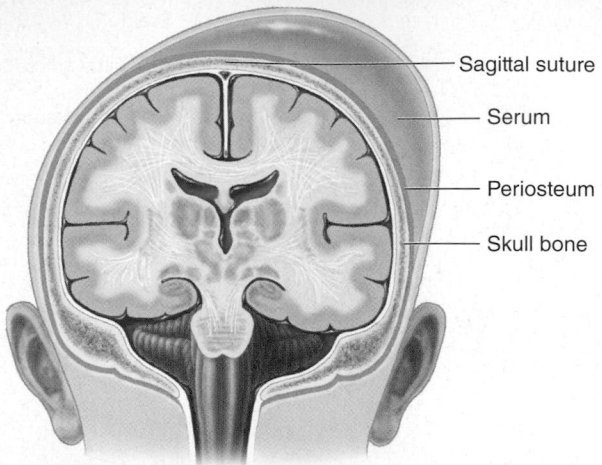

Sagittal suture

Serum

Periosteum

Skull bone

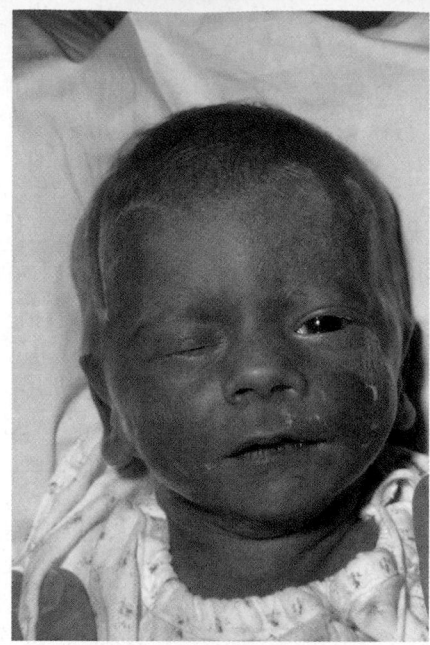

Figure 33–83 ● Facial paralysis. Paralysis of the right side of the face from injury to the right facial nerve.
Source: Wellcome Image Library/Custom Medical Stock Photo.

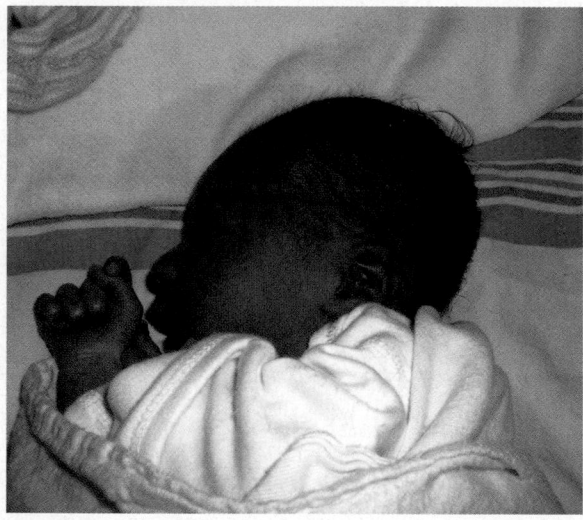

Figure 33–82 ● Caput succedaneum is a collection of fluid (serum) under the scalp.

between a cephalohematoma and a caput because the caput overrides suture lines (**Figure 33–82 ●**), whereas the cephalohematoma, because of its location, never crosses a suture line. Also, caput succedaneum is present at birth, whereas cephalohematoma generally is not.

✳ *Go to nursing.pearsonhighered.com to see Chart 16, which provides a comparison of cephalohematomas and caput succedaneums.*

Face The newborn's face is well designed to help the newborn suckle. Sucking (fat) pads are located in the cheeks, and a labial tubercle (sucking callus) is frequently found in the center of the upper lip. The chin is recessed, and the nose is flattened. The lips are sensitive to touch, and the sucking reflex is easily initiated.

Symmetry of the eyes, nose, and ears is evaluated. Symmetry of facial movement should be assessed to determine the presence of facial palsy.

Facial paralysis appears when the newborn cries: The affected side is immobile, and the palpebral (eyelid) fissure widens (**Figure 33–83 ●**). Paralysis may result from forceps-assisted

birth or pressure on the facial nerve caused by the maternal pelvis during birth. Facial paralysis usually disappears within a few days to 3 weeks, although in some cases it may be permanent.

EYES The eyes of the newborn range from a blue- or slate-gray color to a dark brown color. Scleral color tends to be bluish white in all newborns because of its relative thinness. A blue sclera is associated with osteogenesis imperfecta. The infant's eye color is usually established at approximately 3 months, although it may change any time up to 1 year.

The eyes should be checked for size, equality of pupil size, reaction of pupils to light, blink reflex to light, and edema and inflammation of the eyelids. The eyelids are usually edematous during the first few days of life because of the pressure associated with birth.

Erythromycin is frequently used prophylactically to reduce risk from bacteria to which the neonate may have been exposed during the birth process. Erythromycin is preferred over the once-popular silver nitrate because erythromycin does not usually cause chemical irritation of the eye. The instillation of silver nitrate drops in the newborn's eyes may cause edema, and **chemical conjunctivitis** (irritation of the conjunctiva by chemicals used to treat the eyes, resulting in a purulent greenish yellow discharge exudate) may appear a few hours after instillation but disappears in 1–2 days. Tetracycline is still used in some institutions (AAP & ACOG, 2013).

If infectious conjunctivitis exists, the newborn has the same purulent discharge exudate as in chemical conjunctivitis, but it is caused by gonococcus, *Chlamydia*, staphylococci, or a variety of gram-negative bacteria. It requires treatment with ophthalmic antibiotics. Onset is usually after the second day. Edema of the orbits or eyelids may persist

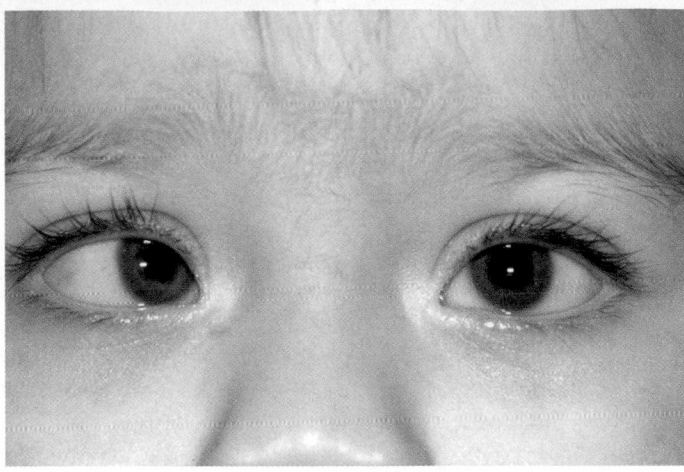

Figure 33–84 ● Transient strabismus may be present in the newborn because of poor neuromuscular control.
Source: Biophoto Associates/Science Source.

for several days until the newborn's kidneys can eliminate the fluid.

Small **subconjunctival hemorrhages** appear in approximately 10% of newborns and are commonly found on the sclera. These hemorrhages are caused by the changes in vascular tension or ocular pressure during birth. They will remain for a few weeks and are of no pathological significance. Parents need reassurance that the newborn is not bleeding from within the eye and that vision will not be impaired.

The newborn may demonstrate transient strabismus caused by poor neuromuscular control of eye muscles (**Figure 33–84 ●**). It gradually dissipates in 3–4 months. The "doll's-eye" phenomenon is also present for approximately 10 days after birth. As the newborn's head position is changed to the left and then to the right, the eyes move to the opposite direction. "Doll's eye" results from underdeveloped integration of head–eye coordination.

The nurse should observe the newborn's pupils for opacities or whiteness and for the absence of a normal red retinal reflex. Red retinal reflex is a red-orange flash of color observed when an ophthalmoscope light reflects off the retina. In a newborn with dark skin color, the retina may appear paler or more grayish. Absence of red reflex occurs with cataracts. Congenital cataracts should be suspected in newborns of mothers with a history of rubella, cytomegalic inclusion disease, or syphilis. Brushfield spots (black or white spots on the periphery of the iris) can be associated with Down syndrome (Vargo, 2014).

The cry of the newborn is commonly tearless because the lacrimal structures are immature at birth and are not usually fully functional until the second month of life. However, some babies produce tears during the newborn period.

Although poor oculomotor coordination and absence of accommodation limit visual abilities, newborns have peripheral vision, can fixate on objects near (20.3–38.1 cm [8–15 in.]) and in front of their face for short periods, can accommodate to large objects (7.6 cm [3 in.] tall × 7.6 cm [3 in.] wide), and can seek out high-contrast geometric shapes.

Newborns can perceive faces, shapes, and colors, and they begin to show visual preferences early. Newborns generally blink in response to bright lights, to a tap on the bridge of the nose (glabellar reflex), or to a light touch on the eyelids. Pupillary light reflex is also present. Examination of the eye is best accomplished by rocking the newborn from an upright position to the horizontal a few times or by other methods, such as diminishing overhead lights, which elicit an opened-eye response.

NOSE The newborn's nose is small and narrow. Babies are characteristically nose breathers for the first few months of life and generally remove obstructions by sneezing. Nasal patency is ensured if the newborn breathes easily with the mouth closed. If respiratory difficulty occurs, the nurse checks for choanal atresia (congenital blockage of the passageway between nose and pharynx). Historically, choanal atresia can be checked by attempting to gently pass a soft, #5 French catheter into both nostrils. Because of possible trauma with the catheter method, a cold, flat, metal object can instead be held under the nose to observe for fogging (Tappero & Honeyfield, 2009).

The newborn has the ability to smell after the nasal passages have been cleared of amniotic fluid and mucus. Newborns demonstrate this ability by the search for milk. Newborns turn their heads toward a milk source, whether bottle or breast. Newborns react to strong odors, such as alcohol, by turning their heads away or blinking.

MOUTH The lips of the newborn should be pink. A touch on the lips should produce sucking motions. Saliva is normally scant. The taste buds develop before birth, and the newborn can easily discriminate between sweet and bitter flavors.

The easiest way to examine the mouth completely is to stimulate the infant to cry by gently depressing the tongue, thereby causing the newborn to open the mouth fully. It is extremely important to examine the entire mouth to check for a cleft palate, which can be present even in the absence of a cleft lip. The examiner moves a gloved index finger along the hard and soft palate to feel for any openings. If the facility still provides gloves with powder, the glove powder should always be removed before examining the newborn's mouth.

Occasionally, an examination of the gums will reveal precocious teeth over the area where the lower central incisors will erupt. If they appear loose, they should be removed by the provider to prevent aspiration. Gray-white lesions (inclusion cysts) on the gums may be confused with teeth. On the hard palate and gum margins, **Epstein pearls** (small, glistening, white specks [keratin-containing cysts] that feel hard to the touch) are often present. They usually disappear in a few weeks and are of no significance. **Thrush** may appear as white patches that look like milk curds adhering to the mucous membranes, and bleeding may occur when patches are removed. Thrush is caused by *Candida albicans*, often acquired from an infected vaginal tract during birth, antibiotic use, or poor hand washing when the mother handles her newborn. Thrush is treated with an oral preparation of nystatin (Mycostatin).

A newborn who has ankyloglossia (tongue tied) has a ridge of frenulum tissue attached to the underside of the tongue at varying lengths from its base, causing a heart shape at the tip of the tongue. "Clipping the tongue," or cutting the ridge of tissue, is recommended only in severe cases. This ridge generally does not affect speech or eating, and cutting creates an entry for infection.

Transient nerve paralysis resulting from birth trauma may be manifested by asymmetric mouth movements when the newborn cries or by difficulty with sucking and feeding.

EARS The ears of the newborn are soft and pliable and should recoil readily when folded and released. In the normal newborn, the top of the ear (pinna) should be parallel to the outer and inner canthus of the eye. The ears should be inspected for shape, size, firmness of cartilage, and position. Low-set ears (**Figure 33–85 ●**) are characteristic of many syndromes. Although most often associated with Down syndrome, low-set ears may indicate other chromosomal abnormalities, intellectual disability, and internal organ abnormalities, especially bilateral renal agenesis. Preauricular skin tags may be present just in front of the ear. Visualization of the tympanic membrane typically is not done soon after birth because blood and vernix block the ear canal.

The first cry helps initiate hearing improvement as mucus from the middle ear is absorbed, the eustachian tube becomes aerated, and the tympanic membrane becomes visible. Newborns, especially when awake, should startle or respond to loud noise. Although this is not a completely accurate test, absence of this response requires further evaluation. This is one of the reasons why the AAP has endorsed universal newborn hearing screening before discharge from the birthing unit as the standard of care (Russ et al., 2010). If the birth occurs in the home or an alternative birthing center, referral for screening should be made within 1 month of birth. The current goal is to screen all babies by 1 month of age, confirm hearing loss with audiological examination by 3 months of age, and treat with comprehensive early intervention services before 6 months of age (AAP & ACOG, 2013). Families need to be educated about appropriate interpretation of screening test results and the appropriate steps for follow-up.

The newborn can discriminate the individual characteristics of the human voice and is especially sensitive to sound levels within the normal conversational range. The newborn in a noisy nursery may habituate to the sounds and not stir unless the sound is sudden or much louder than usual.

NECK A short neck, creased with skinfolds, is characteristic of the normal newborn. Because muscle tone is not well developed, the neck cannot support the full weight of the head, which rotates freely. The head lags considerably when the newborn is pulled from a supine to a sitting position, but the prone newborn is able to raise the head slightly. The neck is palpated for masses and the presence of lymph nodes and is also inspected for webbing. Adequacy of range of motion and neck muscle function is determined by fully extending the head in all directions. Injury to the sternocleidomastoid muscle (congenital torticollis) must be considered in the presence of neck rigidity.

The nurse evaluates the clavicles for evidence of fractures, which occasionally occur during difficult births or in newborns with broad shoulders. The normal clavicle is straight. If it is fractured, a lump and a grating sensation (crepitus) during movements may be palpated along the course of the side of the break. The nurse also elicits the Moro reflex to evaluate bilateral equal movement of the arms. If the clavicle is fractured, the response will be demonstrated only on the unaffected side.

CHEST The thorax is cylindrical and symmetric at birth, and the ribs are flexible. The general appearance of the chest should be assessed. A protrusion at the lower end of the sternum, called the xiphoid cartilage, is frequently seen. It is under the skin and will become less apparent after several weeks as adipose tissue accumulates.

Engorged breasts occur frequently in both male and female newborns. This condition, which occurs by the third day, is a result of maternal hormonal influences and may last up to 2 weeks (**Figure 33–86 ●**). A whitish secretion from the nipples may also be noted. The newborn's breast should not be massaged or squeezed, because this may cause a breast abscess. Extra nipples, or supernumerary nipples, are occasionally noted below and medial to the true nipples. These harmless pink or (in dark-skinned newborns) brown spots

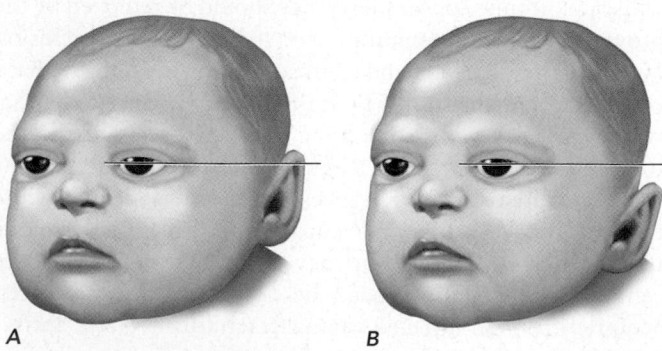

Figure 33–85 ● The position of the external ear may be assessed by drawing a line across the inner and outer canthus of the eye to the insertion of the ear. *A,* Normal position. *B,* True low-set position.

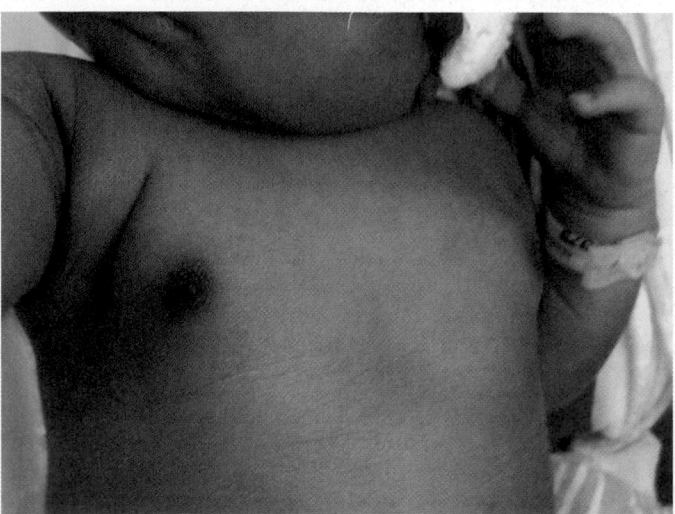

Figure 33–86 ● Breast hypertrophy.
Source: Michele Davidson.

vary in size and do not contain glandular tissue. Accessory nipples can be differentiated from a pigmented nevi (mole) by placing the fingertips alongside the accessory nipple and pulling the adjacent tissue laterally. The accessory nipple will appear dimpled. At puberty, the accessory nipple may darken.

CRY The newborn's cry should be strong, lusty, and of medium pitch. A high-pitched, shrill cry is abnormal and may indicate neurological disorders or hypoglycemia. Periods of crying usually vary in length after consoling measures are used. Babies' cries are an important method of communication and alert caregivers to changes in their condition and needs.

RESPIRATIONS Normal respiration for a term newborn is 30–60 breaths/minute and is predominantly diaphragmatic, with associated rising and falling of the abdomen during inspiration and expiration. The nurse notes any signs of respiratory distress, nasal flaring, intercostal or xiphoid retraction, expiratory grunt or sigh, seesaw respirations, or tachypnea (>60 breaths/minute). Hyperextension (chest appears high) or hypoextension (chest appears low) of the anteroposterior diameter of the chest should also be noted. The nurse auscultates both the anterior and posterior chest. Some breath sounds are heard best when the newborn is crying, but localizing and identifying breath sounds are difficult in the newborn. Upper airway noises and bowel sounds can be heard over the chest wall, making auscultation difficult. Because sounds may be transmitted from the unaffected lung to the affected lung, the absence of breath sounds may not be diagnosed. Air entry may be noisy in the first couple of hours until lung fluid resolves, especially after cesarean births. Brief periods of apnea (periodic breathing) occur, but no color or heart rate changes occur in healthy, term newborns. Sepsis should be suspected in term newborns experiencing apneic episodes.

HEART The nurse examines the heart for rate and rhythm, position of the apical impulse, and heart sound intensity. The pulse rate is variable and is influenced by physical activity, crying, state of wakefulness, and body temperature. The nurse auscultates the entire chest region (precordium) below the left axilla, and below the scapula. Auscultation for a full minute, preferably when the newborn is asleep, allows the nurse to obtain apical pulse rates.

A shift of heart tones in the mediastinal area to either side may indicate pneumothorax, dextrocardia (heart placement on the right side of the chest), or a diaphragmatic hernia. The nurse should auscultate heart sounds using both the bell and the diaphragm of the stethoscope. A slur or slushing sound (usually after the first sound) may indicate a murmur. Although 90% of all murmurs are transient and are considered to be normal, the nurse should document and report them. Many murmurs are secondary to closing of a patent ductus arteriosus or a patent foramen ovale, which should close 1–2 days after birth. A low-pitched, musical murmur just to the right of the apex of the heart is fairly common. Occasionally, significant murmurs are heard, such as the murmur of a patent ductus arteriosus, aortic or pulmonary stenosis, or small ventricular septal defect. Congenital cardiac defects are discussed in the module on Perfusion.

The nurse evaluates peripheral pulses (brachial, femoral, and pedal) to detect any lags or unusual characteristics. Brachial pulses are palpated bilaterally for equality and compared with the femoral pulses. Femoral pulses are palpated by applying gentle pressure with the middle finger over the femoral canal (**Figure 33–87 ●**). Decreased or absent femoral pulses may indicate coarctation of the aorta or hypovolemia and require additional evaluation. A wide difference in blood pressure between the upper and lower extremities also indicates coarctation of the aorta.

The measurement of blood pressure is best accomplished by using a noninvasive blood pressure device. If a blood pressure cuff is used, the newborn's extremities must be immobilized during the assessment, and the cuff should cover two thirds of the upper arm or upper leg. Movement, crying, and inappropriate cuff size can give inaccurate measurements of the blood pressure.

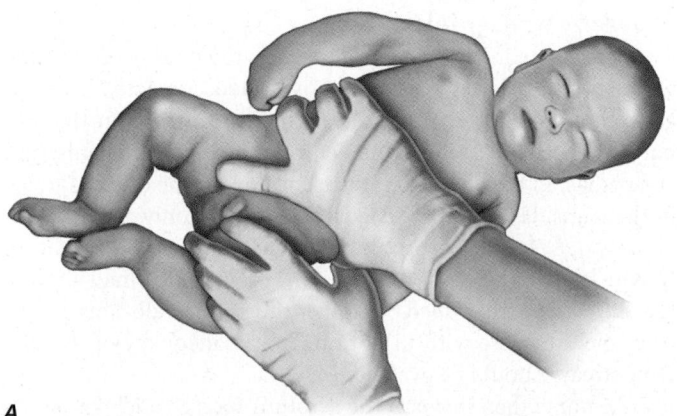 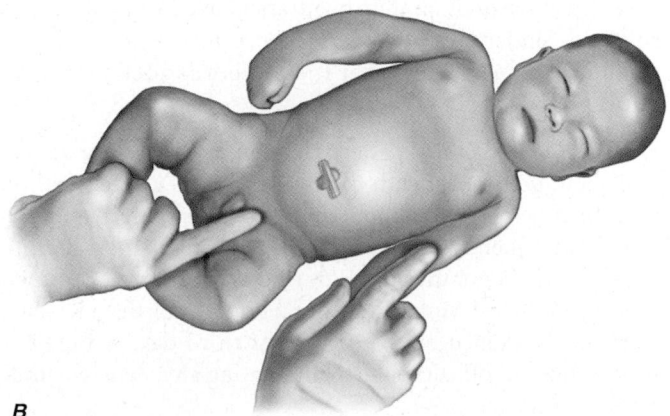

A *B*

Figure 33–87 ● *A,* Bilaterally palpate the femoral arteries for rate and intensity of the pulses. Press fingertip gently at the groin as shown. *B,* Compare the femoral pulses to the brachial pulses by palpating the pulses simultaneously for comparison of rate and intensity.

It is essential to measure blood pressure routinely for newborns who are in distress, premature, or suspected of having a cardiac anomaly (Tappero & Honeyfield, 2009). Neonates who have birth asphyxia and are on ventilators have significantly lower systolic and diastolic blood pressures compared with healthy neonates. If a cardiac anomaly is suspected, blood pressure is measured in all four extremities. At birth, systolic values usually range from 70 to 50 mmHg and diastolic values from 45 to 30 mmHg. By the 10th day of life, blood pressure rises to 90/50 mmHg.

ABDOMEN   The nurse can learn a great deal about the newborn's abdomen without disturbing the neonate. The abdomen should be cylindrical, protrude slightly, and move with respiration. A certain amount of laxness of the abdominal muscles is normal. A scaphoid (hollow-shaped) appearance suggests the absence of abdominal contents (often seen in diaphragmatic hernias). No cyanosis should be present, and few, if any, blood vessels should be apparent to the eye. There should be no gross distention or bulging. The more distended the abdomen, the tighter the skin becomes, with engorged vessels appearing. Distention is the first sign of many gastrointestinal abnormalities.

Before palpating the abdomen, the nurse should auscultate for the presence or absence of bowel sounds in all four quadrants. Bowel sounds may be present by 1 hour after birth. Palpation can cause a transient decrease in the intensity of bowel sounds.

The nurse palpates the abdomen systematically, assessing each of the four abdominal quadrants and moving in a clockwise direction until all four quadrants have been palpated for softness, tenderness, and the presence of masses. The nurse should place one hand under the newborn's back for support during palpation.

UMBILICAL CORD   The umbilical cord initially appears white and gelatinous, with the two umbilical arteries and one umbilical vein readily apparent. Because a single umbilical artery is frequently associated with congenital anomalies, the nurse should count the vessels during the newborn assessment. The cord begins drying within 1 or 2 hours of birth and is shriveled and blackened by the second or third day. Within 7–10 days, it sloughs off, although a granulating area may remain for a few days longer.

Cord bleeding is abnormal and may result because the cord was inadvertently pulled or the cord clamp was loosened. Foul-smelling drainage is also abnormal and is generally caused by infection, which requires immediate treatment to prevent septi-

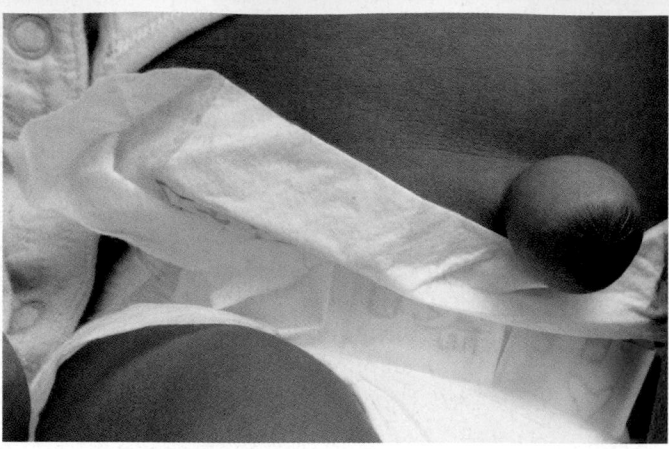

Figure 33–88 ● Umbilical hernia.

cemia. If the newborn has a patent urachus (abnormal connection between the umbilicus and bladder), moistness or draining urine may be apparent at the base of the cord. Another umbilical cord anomaly that can occur is umbilical cord hernia and associated patent omphalomesenteric duct (**Figure 33–88 ●**). Umbilical hernias are more common in infants of African American descent than in White infants (Tappero & Honeyfield, 2009).

Serous or serosanguineous drainage that continues after the cord falls off may indicate a granuloma. It appears as a small, red button deep in the umbilicus. Treatment involves cauterization by a healthcare provider with a topical silver nitrate stick (Tappero & Honeyfield, 2009).

GENITALS   For female neonates, the nurse examines the labia majora, labia minora, and clitoris and notes whether the size of each is appropriate for gestational age. A vaginal tag or hymenal tag is often evident and will usually disappear in a few weeks. During the first week of life, the female newborn may have a vaginal discharge composed of thick, whitish mucus. This discharge, which can become tinged with blood, is called pseudomenstruation and is caused by the withdrawal of maternal hormones. Smegma (a white, cheese-like substance) is often present between the labia. Removing it may traumatize tender tissue.

For male neonates, the nurse inspects the penis to determine whether the urinary orifice is positioned correctly. Possible alterations include hypospadias, which occurs when the urinary meatus is located on the ventral surface of the penis, and epispadias, in which the meatus is located on the dorsal surface of the glans. Hypospadias occurs most commonly among individuals of Western European descent. Phimosis is a condition in which the opening of the foreskin (prepuce) is small and the foreskin cannot be pulled back over the glans at all. This condition may interfere with urination, so the adequacy of the urinary stream should be evaluated.

The nurse then inspects the scrotum for size and symmetry. Scrotal color variations are especially prominent in African American, Indian, and Hispanic newborns (Vargo, 2014). Palpation allows the nurse to verify the presence of both testes and to rule out cryptorchidism (failure of testes to descend). The nurse palpates the testes separately between the thumb and forefinger, with the thumb and forefinger of the other hand placed together over the inguinal canal. Scrotal edema and discoloration are common in breech births. Hydrocele (a collection of fluid surrounding the testes in the scrotum) is common in newborns and should be identified. It usually resolves without intervention. The nurse should report the presence of a discolored or dusky scrotum and solid testis, because this may indicate testicular torsion.

ANUS   It is essential to inspect the anal area to verify that it is patent and has no fissure. Imperforate anus and rectal atresia may be ruled out by observation and through an initial rectal temperature. Digital examination, if necessary, is done by a physician or nurse practitioner. The nurse also notes the passage of the first meconium stool. Atresia of the gastrointestinal tract or meconium ileus with resultant obstruction must be considered if the newborn does not pass meconium in the first 24 hours of life.

EXTREMITIES   The nurse assesses the newborn's extremities for gross deformities, extra digits or webbing, clubfoot, and range of motion. Normal newborn extremities appear short, are generally flexible, and move symmetrically. Abnormalities should be noted so that the plan of care may be created.

Nails extend beyond the fingertips in term newborns. The nurse should count fingers and toes. Polydactyly is the presence of extra digits on either the hands or the feet. Syndactyly refers to fusion (webbing) of fingers or toes. The hands are inspected for normal palmar creases; a single palmar crease, called simian line (**Figure 33–89 ●**), is frequently present in children with Down syndrome.

Brachial palsy, paralysis of portions of the arm, results from trauma to the brachial plexus during a difficult birth. It occurs commonly when strong traction is exerted on the head of the newborn in an attempt to deliver a shoulder lodged behind the symphysis pubis in the presence of shoulder dystocia. Brachial palsy may also occur during a breech birth if an arm becomes trapped over the head and traction is exerted.

The portion of the arm affected is determined by the nerves damaged. **Erb-Duchenne paralysis (Erb palsy)** involves damage to the upper arm (fifth and sixth cervical nerves) and is the most common type. Injury to the eighth cervical and first thoracic nerve roots and the lower portion of the plexus produces the relatively rare lower arm injury. The whole-arm type results from damage to the entire plexus.

With Erb-Duchenne paralysis, the newborn's arm lies limply at the side. The elbow is held in extension, with the forearm pronated. The newborn is unable to elevate the arm, and the Moro reflex cannot be elicited on the affected side (**Figure 33–90 ●**). Lower arm injury causes paralysis of the hand and wrist; complete paralysis of the limb occurs with the whole-arm type.

The nurse carefully instructs the parents in the correct method of performing passive range-of-motion (ROM) exercises (to prevent muscle contractures and restore function) and arranges supervised practice sessions for the parents and referral to physical therapy follow-up within 2 weeks of discharge. In more severe cases, splinting of the arm is indicated until the edema decreases. The arm is held in a position of abduction and external rotation, with the elbow flexed 90 degrees; this is often called the "Statue of Liberty" position. The "Statue of Liberty" splint is commonly used, although similar results are obtained by attaching a strip of muslin to the head of the crib and tying the other end around the wrist, thereby holding the arm up.

Prognosis is related to the degree of nerve damage resulting from trauma and hemorrhage within the nerve sheath. With minimal trauma, complete recovery occurs within a few months. Moderate trauma may result in partial paralysis. With severe trauma, recovery is unlikely, and muscle wasting may develop.

The legs of the newborn should be of equal length, with symmetric skinfolds. However, they may assume a "fetal posture" secondary to position in utero, and it may take several days for the legs to relax into a normal position. To evaluate for hip dislocation or hip instability, the Ortolani and Barlow maneuvers are performed. The nurse (or, more commonly, the

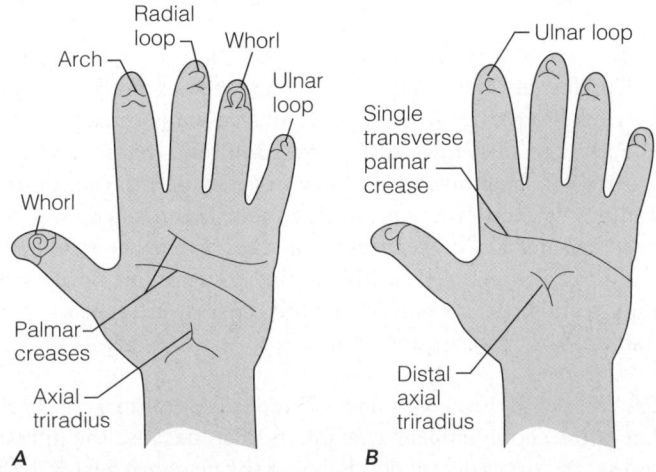

Figure 33–89 ● Dermatoglyphic patterns of the hands in *A*, a normal individual, and *B*, a child with Down syndrome. Note the single transverse palmar crease, distally placed axial triradius, and increased number of ulnar loops.

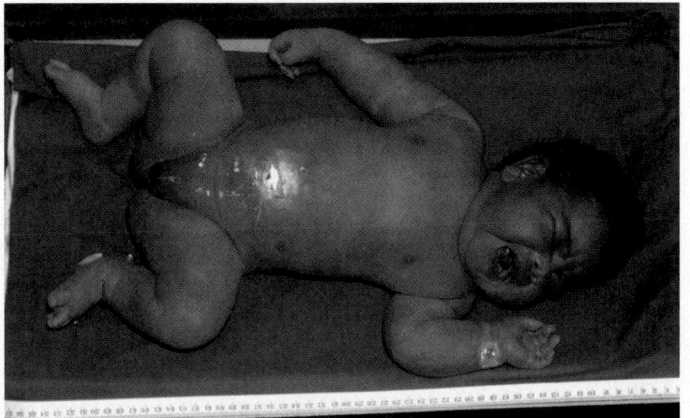

Figure 33–90 ● Right Erb palsy resulting from injury to the fifth and sixth cervical roots of the brachial plexus.

Source: Wellcome Image Library/Custom Medical Stock Photo.

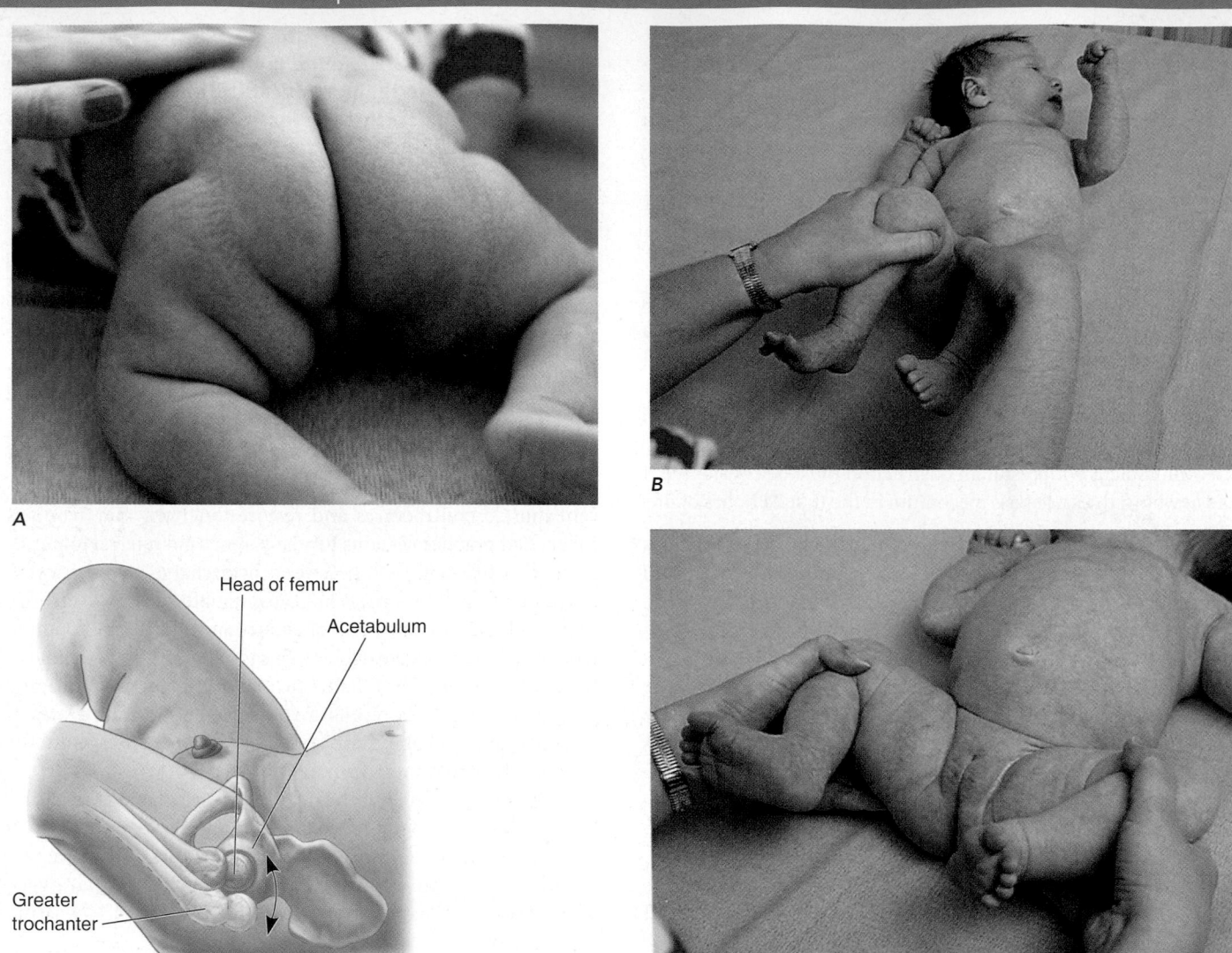

Figure 33–91 ● *A,* The asymmetry of gluteal and thigh fat folds seen in an infant with left developmental dysplasia of the hip. *B,* The Barlow (dislocation) maneuver. The baby's thigh is grasped and adducted (placed together) with gentle downward pressure. *C,* Dislocation is palpable as the femoral head slips out of the acetabulum. *D,* The Ortolani maneuver puts downward pressure on the hip and then inward rotation. If the hip is dislocated, this maneuver will force the femoral head back into the acetabular rim with a noticeable "clunk."

physician or nurse practitioner) performs the **Ortolani maneuver** to rule out the possibility of developmental dysplastic hip, also called congenital hip dysplasia (hip dislocatability). With the newborn relaxed, quiet, and on a firm surface, with hips and knees flexed at a 90-degree angle, the experienced nurse grasps the neonate's thigh with the middle finger over the greater trochanter and then lifts the thigh to bring the femoral head from its posterior position toward the acetabulum. With gentle abduction of the thigh, the femoral head is returned to the acetabulum. Simultaneously, the examiner feels a sense of reduction or a "clunk" as the femoral head returns. This reduction is palpable and may be heard. With the **Barlow maneuver,** the healthcare provider grasps and adducts the neonate's thigh and then applies gentle downward pressure. Dislocation is felt as the femoral head slips out of the acetabulum. The femoral head is then returned to the acetabulum using the Ortolani maneuver, confirming the diagnosis of an unstable or dislocatable hip (**Figure 33–91 ●**).

The feet are then examined for evidence of a talipes deformity (clubfoot). Intrauterine position frequently causes the feet to appear to turn inward (**Figure 33–92 ●**); this is termed a "positional" clubfoot. If the feet can easily be returned to the midline by manipulation, no treatment is indicated, and the nurse teaches ROM exercises to the family. Further evaluation is indicated when the foot will not turn to a midline position or align readily. This is considered the most severe type of "true clubfoot," or talipes equinovarus.

BACK   With the newborn prone, the nurse examines the back. The spine should appear straight and flat, because the lumbar and sacral curves do not develop until the newborn begins to sit. The base of the spine is examined for a dermal sinus. A nevus pilosus ("hairy nerve") is occasionally found at the base of the spine. This is significant because it is frequently associated with spina bifida. A pilonidal dimple should be examined to ascertain that there is no connection to the spinal canal.

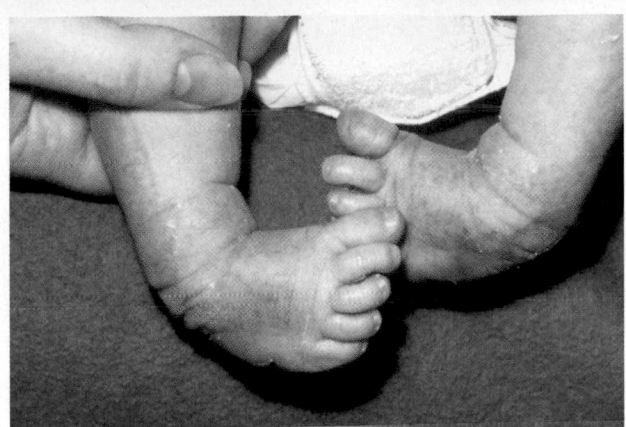

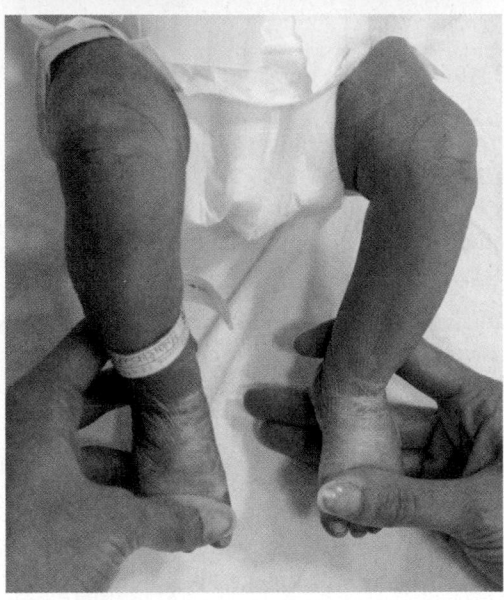

Figure 33–92 ● A, Unilateral talipes equinovarus (clubfoot). B, To determine the presence of clubfoot, the nurse moves the foot to the midline. Resistance indicates true clubfoot.

Source: A, Jim Stevenson/Science Source

Assessing Neurological Status

The nurse should begin the neurological examination with a period of observation, noting the general physical characteristics and behaviors of the newborn. Important behaviors to assess are the state of alertness, resting posture, cry, and quality of muscle tone and motor activity.

The usual position of the newborn is with partially flexed extremities, with the legs abducted to the abdomen. When awake, the newborn may exhibit purposeless, uncoordinated bilateral movements of the extremities. If these movements are absent, minimal, or obviously asymmetric, then neurological dysfunction should be suspected.

Eye movements are observable during the first few days of life. An alert newborn is able to fixate on faces and brightly colored objects. Shining a bright light in the newborn's eyes elicits the blinking response.

The nurse evaluates muscle tone by moving various parts of the body while the head of the newborn is in a neutral position. The newborn is somewhat hypertonic; that is, there should be resistance to extending the elbow and knee joints. Muscle tone

should be symmetric. Diminished muscle tone and flaccidity require further evaluation.

Tremors or jitteriness (tremor-like movements) in the term newborn must be evaluated to differentiate the tremors from convulsions. Tremors may also be related to hypoglycemia, hypocalcemia, or substance withdrawal. Environmental stimuli may initiate tremors. Jitteriness may be distinguished from tonic-clonic seizure activity because it usually can be stopped by the infant's sucking on the extremity or by the nurse holding or flexing the involved extremity. A fine jumping of the muscle is likely to be a CNS disorder and requires further evaluation. Newborn seizures may consist of no more than chewing or swallowing movements, deviations of the eyes, rigidity, or flaccidity because of CNS immaturity. In contrast to tremors, seizures are not usually initiated by stimuli, and they cannot be stopped by holding.

Specific deep tendon reflexes can be elicited in the newborn but have limited value unless they are obviously asymmetric. The knee jerk is typically brisk; a normal ankle clonus may involve three or four beats. Plantar flexion is present.

The newborn's immature CNS is characterized by a variety of reflexes. Because the newborn's movements are uncoordinated, methods of communication are limited, and control of bodily functions is restricted, the reflexes serve a variety of purposes. Some are protective (blink, gag, and sneeze), some aid in feeding (rooting and sucking) and may not be very active if the newborn has eaten recently, and some stimulate human interaction (grasping).

The following reflexes are the ones most commonly found in the normal newborn:

■ The **tonic neck reflex** (fencing position) is elicited when the newborn is supine and the head is turned to one side. In response, the extremities on the same side straighten, whereas on the opposite side, they flex (**Figure 33–93 ●**). This reflex may not be seen during the early newborn period, but once it appears, it persists until about the third month.

■ The palmar **grasping reflex** is elicited by stimulating the newborn's palm with a finger or object. The newborn grasps and holds the object or finger firmly enough to be lifted momentarily from the crib (**Figure 33–94 ●**).

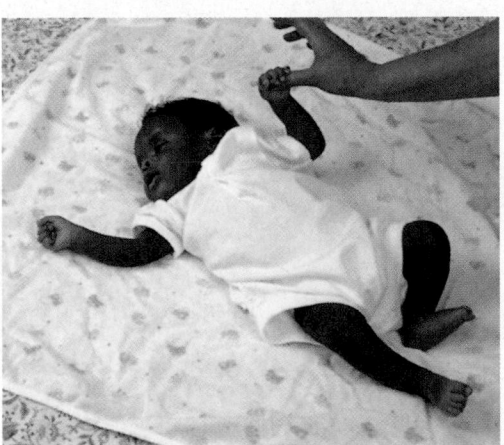

Figure 33–93 ● Tonic neck reflex.

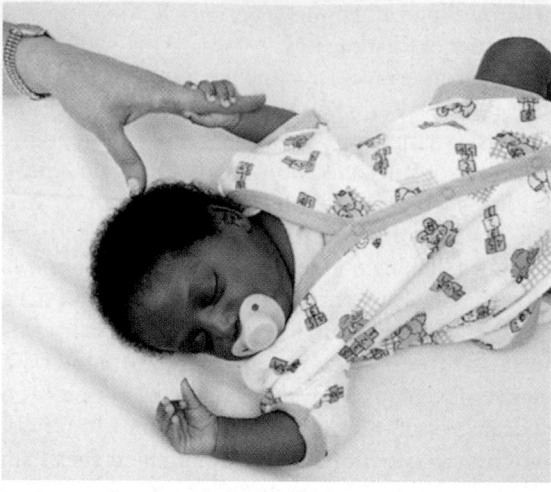

Figure 33–94 ● Palmar grasp.

- The **Moro reflex** is elicited when the newborn is startled by a loud noise or lifted slightly above the crib and then suddenly lowered. In response, the newborn straightens the arms and hands outward while the knees flex. Slowly, the arms return to the chest, as in an embrace. The fingers spread, forming a "C," and the newborn may cry (**Figure 33–95 ●**). This reflex may persist until approximately 6 months of age.
- The **rooting reflex** is elicited when the side of the newborn's mouth or cheek is touched. In response, the newborn turns toward that side and opens the lips to suck (if the newborn has not been fed recently) (**Figure 33–96 ●**).
- The **sucking reflex** is elicited when an object is placed in the newborn's mouth or anything touches the lips. Newborns suck even while sleeping; this is called nonnutritive sucking and can have a quieting effect on the baby.
- The **Babinski reflex (response)**, which is fanning and hyperextension of all toes and dorsiflexion of the big toe, occurs when the lateral aspect of the sole is stroked from the heel upward across the ball of the foot. In children older than 24 months, an abnormal response is extension or fanning of the

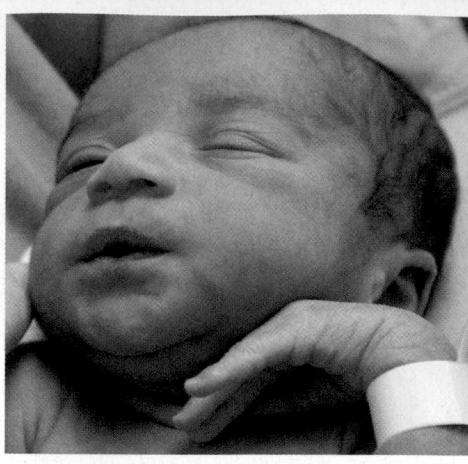

Figure 33–96 ● Rooting reflex.

toes; this Babinski response indicates upper motor neuron abnormalities (**Figure 33–97 ●**).
- **Trunk incurvation (Galant reflex)** is seen when the newborn is prone. Stroking the spine causes the pelvis to turn to the stimulated side.

In addition to these reflexes, newborns can blink, yawn, cough, sneeze, and draw back from pain (protective reflexes). They can even move a little on their own. When placed on their stomachs, they push up and try to crawl (prone crawl). When held upright with one foot touching a flat surface, the newborn puts one foot in front of the other and "walks" (stepping reflex) (**Figure 33–98 ●**). This reflex is more pronounced at birth and is lost after 4–8 weeks.

The nurse assesses CNS integration as follows:

1. The nurse inserts a gloved finger into the newborn's mouth to elicit a sucking reflex.
2. As soon as the newborn is sucking vigorously, the nurse assesses hearing and vision responses by noting changes in sucking in the presence of a light, a rattle, and a voice.
3. The newborn should respond to such stimuli with a brief cessation of sucking, followed by continuous sucking with repetitious stimulation.

This CNS integration exam demonstrates auditory and visual integrity as well as the ability to conduct complex behavioral interactions.

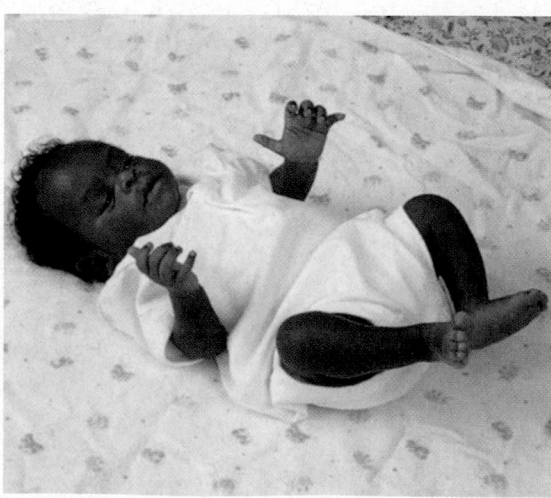

Figure 33–95 ● Moro reflex.

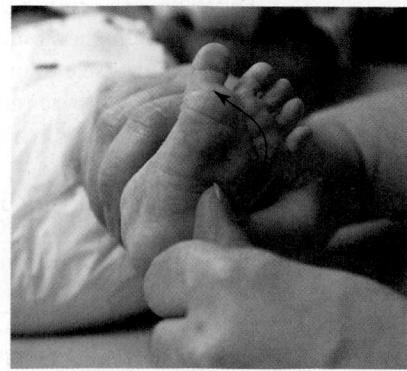

Figure 33–97 ● The Babinski reflex (response).

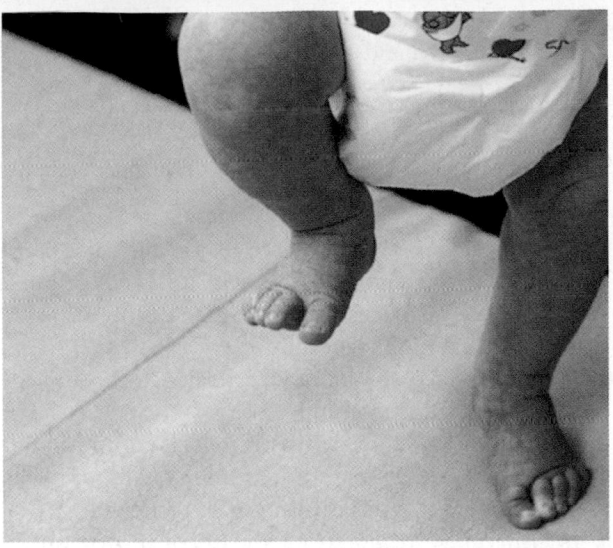

Figure 33–98 ● The stepping (walking) reflex disappears after approximately 4–8 weeks of age.

As healthcare providers carry out the newborn physical and neurological assessment, they are always on the alert to recognize possible alterations and possible injuries related to the birth process that require further investigation and intervention.

Assessing Newborn Behavior

The **Brazelton Neonatal Behavioral Assessment Scale** provides valuable guidelines for assessing the newborn's state changes, temperament, and individual behavioral patterns. It provides a way for the nurse, in conjunction with the parents (primary caregivers), to identify and understand the individual newborn's states and capabilities. Families learn which responses, interventions, or activities best meet the special needs of their newborn, and this understanding fosters positive attachment experiences.

The Brazelton assessment tool identifies the newborn's repertoire of behavioral responses to the environment and also documents the newborn's neurological adequacy and capabilities. The examination usually takes 20–30 minutes and involves approximately 30 tests. Some items are scored according to the newborn's response to specific stimuli. Others, such as consolability and alertness, are scored as a result of continuous behavioral observations throughout the assessment. (For a complete discussion of all test items and maneuvers, see Brazelton & Nugent, [1995].)

Because the first few days after birth are a period of behavioral disorganization, the complete assessment should be done on the third day after birth. The nurse should make every effort to elicit the best response. This may be accomplished by repeating tests at different times or by testing during situations that facilitate the best possible response, such as when the parents are holding, cuddling, rocking, and/or singing to their baby.

Assessment of the newborn should be carried out initially in a quiet, dimly lighted room, if possible. The nurse should first determine the newborn's state of consciousness, because scoring and introduction of the test items are correlated with the sleep or waking state. The newborn's state depends on physiological variables, such as the amount of time from the last feeding, positioning, environmental temperature, and health status; the presence of such external stimuli as noises and bright lights; and the sleep–wake cycle of the neonate. An important characteristic of the newborn period is the pattern of states, as well as the transitions from one state to another. The pattern of states is a predictor of the newborn's receptivity and ability to respond to stimuli in a cognitive manner. Babies learn best in a quiet, alert state and in an environment that is supportive and protective and that provides appropriate stimuli.

The nurse should observe the newborn's sleep–wake patterns, including the rapidity with which the newborn moves from one state to another, the newborn's ability to be consoled, and the newborn's ability to diminish the impact of disturbing stimuli. The following questions may provide the nurse with a framework for assessment:

- Does the newborn's response style and ability to adapt to stimuli indicate a need for parental interventions that will alert the newborn to the environment so that he or she can grow socially and cognitively?
- Are parental interventions necessary to lessen the outside stimuli, as in the case of the baby who responds to sensory input with intensity?
- Can the baby control the amount of sensory input that he or she must deal with?

The behaviors, and the sleep–wake states in which they are assessed, are categorized as follows:

- *Habituation.* The nurse assesses the newborn's ability to diminish or shut down innate responses to specific repeated stimuli, such as a rattle, bell, light, or pinprick to heel.
- *Orientation to inanimate and animate visual and auditory assessment stimuli.* The nurse observes how often and where the newborn attends to auditory and visual stimuli. Orientation to the environment is determined by an ability to respond to clues given by others and by a natural ability to fix on and follow a visual object both horizontally and vertically. This capacity and the parental appreciation of it are important for positive communication between infant and parents; the parents' visual (*en face*) and auditory (soft, continuous voice) presence stimulates their newborn to orient to them. Inability or a lack of response may indicate visual or auditory problems. It is important for parents to know that their newborn can turn to voices soon after birth or by 3 days of age and can become alert at different times with a varying degree of intensity in response to sounds.
- *Motor activity.* Several components are evaluated. Motor tone of the newborn is assessed in the most characteristic state of responsiveness. This summary assessment includes overall use of tone as the newborn responds to being handled—whether during spontaneous activity, prone placement, or horizontal holding—and overall assessment of body tone as the newborn reacts to all stimuli.

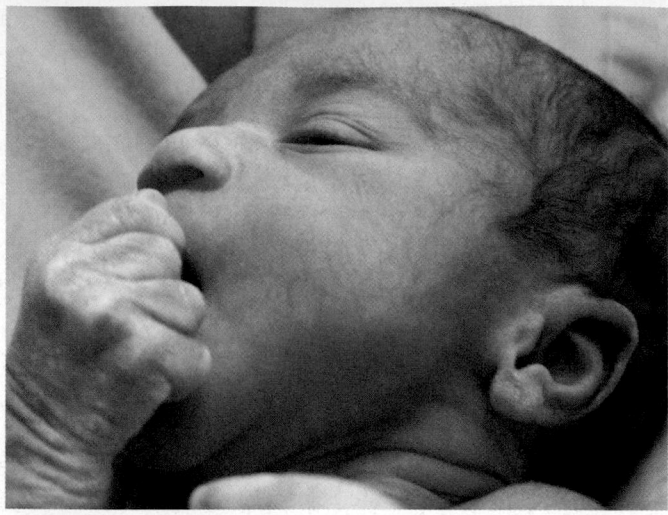

Figure 33–99 ● The newborn can bring hand to mouth as a self-soothing activity.

- **Variations.** Frequency of alert states, state changes, color changes (throughout all states as examination progresses), activity, and peaks of excitement are assessed.
- **Self-quieting activity.** This assessment is based on how often, how quickly, and how effectively newborns can use their resources to quiet and console themselves when upset or distressed. Considered in this assessment are such self-consolatory activities as putting a hand to mouth, sucking on a fist or the tongue, and attuning to an object or sound (**Figure 33–99** ●). The newborn's need for outside consolation must also be considered (e.g., seeing a face; being rocked, held, or dressed; using a pacifier; and being swaddled).
- **Cuddliness or social behaviors.** This area encompasses the newborn's need for, and response to, being held. These behaviors influence the couple's self-esteem and feelings of acceptance or rejection. Cuddling also appears to be an indicator of personality. Cuddlers appear to enjoy, accept, and seek physical contact; are easier to placate; sleep more; and form earlier and more intense attachments. Noncuddlers are active, restless, have accelerated motor development, and are intolerant of physical restraint. Smiling, even as a grimace reflex, greatly influences parent–newborn feedback. Parents identify this response as positive.

Once assessment has been completed, the nurse reviews the data and analyzes it to determine the newborn's specific needs.

Diagnosis

Nursing diagnoses of the newborn during the transition period are based on an analysis of the assessment findings. Physiological alterations of the newborn form the basis of many nursing diagnoses, as does the family members' incorporation of them in caring for the new baby. Nursing diagnoses that may apply to newborns include the following:

- *Airway Clearance, Ineffective* related to presence of mucus and retained lung fluid

- *Thermoregulation, Ineffective* related to evaporative, radiant, conductive, and convective heat losses
- *Pain, Acute* related to heelsticks for glucose or hematocrit tests or a vitamin K injection.

Examples of nursing diagnoses that may apply during daily care of the newborn include the following:

- *Breathing Pattern, Ineffective* related to periodic breathing
- *Nutrition, Imbalanced: Less Than Body Requirements* related to limited nutritional and fluid intake and increased caloric expenditure
- *Urinary Elimination, Impaired* related to meatal edema secondary to circumcision
- *Infection, Risk for* related to umbilical cord healing, circumcision site, immature immune system, or potential birth trauma (forceps or vacuum extraction birth)
- *Breastfeeding, Readiness for Enhanced* related to lack of information about breastfeeding
- *Parenting, Readiness for Enhanced* related to lack of information about basic baby care, male circumcision, and formula feeding
- *Family Processes, Interrupted* related to integration of newborn into family or demands of newborn care and feeding
- *Injury, Risk for* related to reabsorption of bilirubin and decreased defecation.

Nursing diagnoses that may apply to the newborn's family include the following:

- *Parenting, Readiness for Enhanced* related to appropriate behavioral expectations for the newborn
- *Family Processes: Readiness for Enhanced* related to integration of newborn into family unit or demands of newborn care and feeding.

(NANDA-I © 2015)

Planning

The broad goals of nursing care during this period are the following:

- The newborn will be healthy and well.
- The family unit will function well.

The nurse meets the first goal by providing comprehensive care to the newborn in the mother–baby unit. The nurse meets the second goal by teaching family members how to care for their new baby and by supporting their efforts so that they feel confident and competent. The nurse must be knowledgeable about family adjustments that need to be made as well as about the healthcare needs of the newborn. It is important for the family to return home with the positive feeling that they have the support, information, and skills to care for their newborn. Equally important is the need for each member of the family to begin a unique relationship with the newborn. The cultural and social expectations of individual families and communities affect the way in which normal newborn care is carried out.

Implementation

At the moment of birth, numerous physiological adaptations begin to take place in the newborn's body. Because of these dramatic changes, newborns require close observation to determine how smoothly they are making the transition to extrauterine life. Newborns also require specific care that enhances their chances of making this transition successfully. Immediately after birth, the baby is formally admitted to the healthcare facility by the nurse.

The nurse reviews the mother's prenatal record for information concerning possible risk factors for the newborn. These include infectious diseases screening results, drug or alcohol use by the mother, alterations to normal pregnancy and delivery, prolonged rupture of membranes, instrument or vacuum delivery, use of narcotic analgesia, presence of meconium, and any other data that may impact the newborn's ability to successfully transition to the extrauterine environment.

Care of the newborn is based on an analysis of assessment findings and the goals of the plan of care. This section covers some of the more common or essential interventions, both in the initial period immediately following birth and in the transition period that continues until the newborn and family are discharged.

Initial Care of the Newborn

The nurse responsible for the newborn first checks and confirms the newborn's identification with the mother's identification and then obtains and records all significant information.

MAINTENANCE OF A CLEAR AIRWAY For the neonate with any initial respiratory distress or excessive oral secretions, the nurse should position the newborn on the back (or the side if secretions are copious) and suction the airway using a bulb syringe. When possible, this procedure should be delayed for 10–15 minutes after birth to reduce the potential for severe vasovagal reflex apnea. Excessive secretions should be reported to the primary healthcare provider because they may indicate tracheoesophageal fistula.

MEASUREMENT OF VITAL SIGNS In the absence of any newborn distress, the nurse continues to admit the newborn by measuring vital signs. The vital signs for a healthy term newborn should be monitored at least every 30 minutes until the newborn's condition has remained stable for 2 hours (AAP & ACOG, 2013). The newborn's respirations may be irregular yet still be considered normal. Periodic breathing, lasting only 5–15 seconds with no color or heart rate changes, is considered to be normal. The normal pulse range is 110–160 bpm (a pulse anywhere from 100 to 205 bpm may be considered normal.), and the normal respiratory range is 30–60 breaths/minute. (during the first several hours after birth it is not uncommon for the newborn to have a respiratory rate as high as 80 breaths/min.)

PROMOTION OF THERMOREGULATION An NTE is best achieved by performing the newborn assessment and interventions with the newborn unclothed and under a radiant warmer. The radiant warmer's thermostat is controlled by the thermal skin sensor taped to the newborn's abdomen, upper thigh, or arm. The sensor indicates when the newborn's temperature exceeds or falls below the acceptable temperature range. The nurse should be aware that leaning over the newborn may block the radiant heat waves from reaching the neonate. In addition to placing the baby under a radiant warmer, it is common practice in some institutions to cover the newborn's head with a cap to prevent further evaporative heat loss (Blackburn, 2013).

When the newborn's temperature is normal and vital signs are stable (~2–4 hours after birth), the baby may be given a sponge bath. However, this admission bath may be postponed for some hours if the newborn's condition dictates or if the parents wish to give the first bath. In light of early discharge practices (12–48 hours), healthy term newborns can be bathed safely immediately after the admission assessment is completed. The baby is bathed while still under the radiant warmer. The newborn may be bathed in the parents' room and by the parents (Medves & O'Brien, 2004). Bathing the newborn offers an excellent opportunity for the nurse to teach and welcome parents' involvement in the care of their baby.

The nurse rechecks the baby's temperature after the bath and, if it is stable, dresses and places the newborn in an open crib at room temperature. If the baby's axillary temperature is below 36.5°C (97.7°F), the nurse returns the baby to the radiant warmer. The rewarming process should be gradual to prevent hyperthermia. Once the newborn is rewarmed, the nurse implements measures to prevent further neonatal heat loss, such as keeping the newborn dry, swaddled in one or two blankets with a hat on, and away from cool surfaces or instruments. Newborns are often "double-wrapped" in two or more blankets for temperature maintenance.

VITAMIN K DEFICIENCY A prophylactic injection of phytonadione (vitamin K) is recommended to prevent hemorrhage, which can occur because of low prothrombin levels in the first few days of life. The potential for hemorrhage is considered to result from the absence of intestinal bacterial flora, which influences the production of vitamin K in the newborn. Newborns should receive a single parenteral dose of 0.5–1 mg of phytonadione within 1 hour of birth; this dose may be delayed until after the first breastfeeding in the childbirth/birthing area (AAP & ACOG, 2013; Wilson et al., 2013). Current recommendations underscore the need for treatment in infants who are exclusively breastfed (Blackburn, 2013).

The phytonadione injection is given intramuscularly in the middle third of the vastus lateralis muscle, located in the lateral aspect of the thigh (**Figure 33–100 ●**). Before injecting, the nurse must thoroughly clean the newborn's skin site for the injection with a small alcohol swab. The nurse uses a 27-gauge, 0.5-in. needle for the injection. An alternative site is the rectus femoris muscle in the anterior aspect of the thigh. However, this site is near the sciatic nerve and femoral artery, so injections here should be done with caution (**Figure 33–101 ●**).

PREVENTION OF EYE INFECTION The nurse is responsible for giving the legally required prophylactic eye treatment for *Neisseria gonorrhoeae*, which may have infected the newborn of an infected mother during the birth process. A variety of topical agents appear to be equally effective. Ophthalmic ointments that are used include 0.5% erythromycin (Ilotycin Ophthalmic), 1% tetracycline, or per agency protocol (AAP & ACOG, 2013). All of these ointments are also

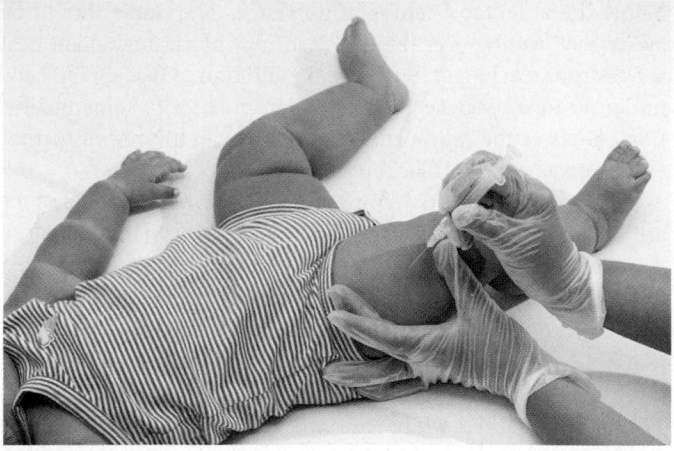

Figure 33–100 ● Procedure for vitamin K injection. Cleanse the area thoroughly with an alcohol swab and allow the skin to dry. Hold the tissue of the upper outer thigh (vastus lateralis muscle) taut, and quickly insert a 27-gauge, 0.5-in. needle at a 90-degree angle to the thigh. Aspirate, then slowly inject the solution to distribute the medication evenly and minimize the baby's discomfort. Remove the needle and gently massage the site with an alcohol swab.
Source: Marlon Lopez/Shutterstock.

effective against chlamydia, which has a higher incidence rate than gonorrhea.

Successful eye prophylaxis requires that the medication be instilled into the lower conjunctival sac of each eye (**Figure 33–102** ●). The nurse massages the eyelid gently to distribute the ointment. Instillation may be delayed up to 1 hour after birth to allow eye contact during parent–newborn bonding.

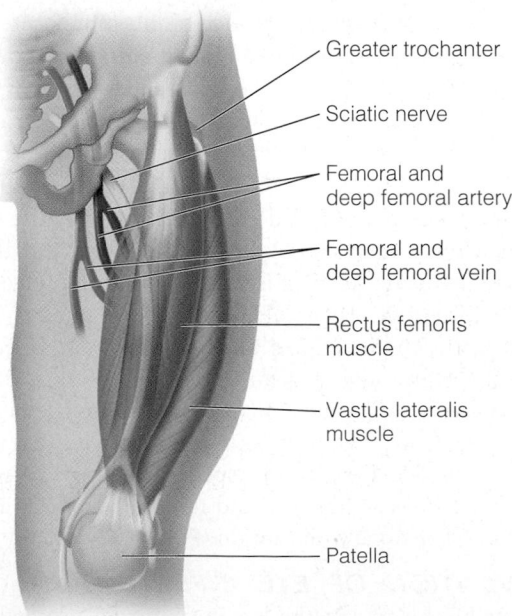

Figure 33–101 ● Injection sites. The middle third of the vastus lateralis muscle is the preferred site for intramuscular injection in the newborn. The middle third of the rectus femoris is an alternate site, but its proximity to major vessels and the sciatic nerve requires caution when using this site for an injection.

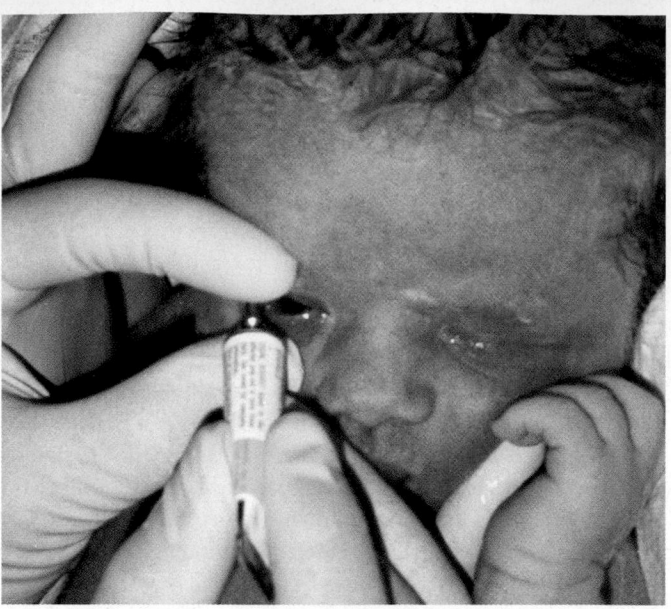

Figure 33–102 ● Ophthalmic ointment. Retract the lower eyelid outward to instill a 1-cm-(0.25-in.)-long strand of ointment from a single-dose tube along the lower conjunctival surface. *Make sure that the tip of the tube does not touch the eye.*

Eye prophylaxis medications can cause chemical conjunctivitis, which gives the newborn some discomfort and may interfere with the newborn's ability to focus on the parents' faces. The resulting edema, inflammation, and discharge may cause concern if the parents have not been informed that the side effects will clear in 24–48 hours and that this prophylactic eye treatment is necessary for the newborn's well-being.

EARLY ASSESSMENT OF NEONATAL DISTRESS   During the first 24 hours of life, the nurse is constantly alert for signs of distress. If the newborn is with the parents during this period, the nurse must take extra care to teach them how to maintain their newborn's temperature, recognize the hallmarks of newborn distress, and respond immediately to signs of respiratory problems. The parents learn to observe the newborn for changes in color or activity, grunting or "sighing" sounds with breathing, rapid breathing with chest retractions, or facial grimacing. Their interventions include nasal and oral suctioning with a bulb syringe, positioning, and vigorous fingertip stroking of the newborn's spine to stimulate respiratory activity if necessary. The nurse must be available immediately if the newborn develops distress.

INITIATION OF FIRST FEEDING   The timing of the first feeding varies depending on whether the newborn is to be breastfed or formula-fed and whether there were any complications during pregnancy or birth, such as maternal diabetes or intrauterine growth restriction. The nurse should encourage mothers who choose to breastfeed their newborns to put the baby to the breast during the newborn's first period of reactivity. This practice should be encouraged because successful, long-term breastfeeding during infancy appears to be related to beginning such feedings in the first few hours of life. Sleep–wake states affect feeding behavior and need to be considered when evaluating the newborn's sucking ability (Tedder, 2008).

Formula-fed newborns usually begin the first feedings by 5 hours of age, during the second period of reactivity when they awaken and appear hungry. Signs indicating newborn readiness for the first feeding are licking of the lips, placing a hand in or near the mouth, active bowel sounds, absence of abdominal distention, and a lusty cry that quiets with rooting and sucking behaviors when a stimulus is placed near the lips. Observing the earlier, more subtle cues that the baby is ready to nurse provides an opportunity to teach the parents to recognize these cues and respond before the baby is frustrated and crying.

FACILITATION OF PARENT–NEWBORN ATTACHMENT

To facilitate parent–newborn attachment, eye-to-eye contact between the parents and their newborn is extremely important during the early hours after birth, when the newborn is in the first period of reactivity. The newborn is alert during this time, the eyes are wide open, and the baby often makes direct eye contact with human faces within optimal range for visual acuity. It is theorized that this eye contact (*en face*) is an important foundation of establishing attachment in human relationships (Gurol & Polat, 2011). Parents who cannot be with their newborns in this first period because of maternal or neonatal distress may need reassurance that the bonding process can proceed normally as soon as both mother and baby are stable.

Another situation that can facilitate attachment is the interactive bath. While bathing their newborn for the first time, parents attend closely to their baby's behavior. In this way, the newborn becomes an active participant, and parents are drawn into an interaction with their baby. The nurse can interpret the newborn's behavior, model ways to respond to the behavior, and support parental strategies for doing so (Tedder, 2008).

Care of the Newborn Following Transition

Once a healthy newborn has demonstrated successful adaptation to extrauterine life, the neonate needs appropriate observations for the first 6–12 hours after birth and the remainder of his or her stay in the birthing facility.

MAINTENANCE OF CARDIOPULMONARY FUNCTION

The nurse assesses vital signs every 4–8 hours or more, depending on the newborn's status. The nurse places the newborn on the back (supine) for sleeping and keeps a bulb syringe within easy reach should the baby need oral–nasal suctioning. If the newborn has respiratory difficulty, the nurse clears the airway. Vigorous fingertip stroking of the baby's spine will frequently stimulate respiratory activity. A cardiorespiratory monitor may be used on newborns who are not being observed at all times and are at risk for decreased respiratory or cardiac function. Indicators of risk are pallor, cyanosis, ruddy color, apnea, and other signs of instability. Changes in skin color may indicate the need for closer assessment of temperature, cardiopulmonary status, hematocrit, glucose, and bilirubin levels.

MAINTENANCE OF A NEUTRAL THERMAL ENVIRONMENT

The nurse makes every effort to maintain the newborn's temperature within the normal range. The nurse must make certain the newborn is dried completely after the bath, dressed, and exposed to the air as little as possible and ensures that a head covering is used in maintaining body heat. The nurse monitors the ambient temperature of the room where the newborn is kept to prevent excessive cooling. Parents may be advised to dress the newborn in one more layer of clothing than is necessary for an adult to maintain thermal comfort. The use of layering allows flexibility as the newborn is moved from one area to another.

It is also important to avoid overheating the newborn. An overheated newborn will increase activity and respiratory rate in an attempt to cool the body. Both measures deplete caloric reserves, and the increased respiratory rate leads to increased insensible fluid loss (Blackburn, 2013).

PROMOTION OF ADEQUATE HYDRATION AND NUTRITION

The nurse records caloric and fluid intake and enhances adequate hydration by maintaining an NTE and offering early and frequent feedings. Early feedings promote gastric emptying and increase peristalsis, thereby decreasing the potential for hyperbilirubinemia by decreasing the amount of time fecal material is in contact with the enzyme beta-glucuronidase in the small intestine. This enzyme frees the bilirubin from the feces, allowing it to be reabsorbed into the vascular system.

The nurse records voiding and stooling patterns. The first voiding and the first passage of stool should occur within 24–48 hours. If they do not occur, the nurse continues the normal observation routine while assessing for abdominal distention, bowel sounds, hydration, fluid intake, and temperature stability.

The nurse weighs the newborn at the same time each day for accurate comparisons. The newborn must be kept warm during the weighing. A weight loss of up to 10% for term newborns is considered to be within normal limits during the first week of life. This weight loss is the result of limited intake, loss of excess extracellular fluid, and passage of meconium. Parents should be told about the expected weight loss, the reason for it, and the expectations for regaining the birth weight. Birth weight is usually regained by 2 weeks if feedings are adequate.

Excessive handling can cause an increase in the newborn's metabolic rate and caloric use and also cause fatigue. The nurse should be alert to the newborn's subtle cues of fatigue, including a decrease in muscle tension and activity in the extremities and neck as well as loss of eye contact, which may be manifested by fluttering or closure of the eyelids. The nurse quickly ceases stimulation when signs of fatigue appear. The nurse demonstrates to parents the need to be aware of newborn cues and to wait for periods of alertness for contact and stimulation.

The nurse also assesses the woman's comfort and latching-on techniques if breastfeeding. If the woman is not breastfeeding, the nurse assesses the mother's bottle-feeding techniques.

PROMOTION OF SKIN INTEGRITY

Newborn skin care, including bathing, is important for the health and appearance of the individual newborn and for infection control within the nursery. Ongoing skin care involves cleansing the buttock and perianal areas with fresh water and cotton or a mild soap and water during diaper changes. If commercial baby wipes are used, those without alcohol should be selected. Perfume-free and latex-free wipes are also available.

The nurse should assess the umbilical cord for signs of bleeding or infection. Removal of the cord clamp within 24–48 hours of birth reduces the chance of tension injury to the area. Keeping the umbilical stump clean and dry can reduce the chance for infection. Many types of routine cord care are practiced, including the use of triple dye, an antimicrobial agent (e.g., bacitracin), or application of 70% alcohol to the cord stump. These practices are largely based on tradition rather than current research findings. The skin absorption and toxicity of triple-dye agents in newborns have not been carefully studied. Studies have shown that alcohol used alone is not effective in preventing umbilical cord colonization and infection (omphalitis) (AAP & ACOG, 2013). Folding the diaper down to avoid covering the cord stump can prevent contamination of the area and promote drying. The nurse is responsible for cord care per agency policy. It is also the nurse's responsibility to instruct parents in caring for the cord and observing for signs and symptoms of infection after discharge, such as foul smell, redness and drainage, localized heat and tenderness, or bleeding.

PROMOTION OF SAFETY   Safety of the newborn is paramount. It is essential for the nurse and other caregivers to verify the identity of the newborn by comparing the numbers and names on the identification bracelets of the mother and newborn before giving a baby to a parent (AAP & ACOG, 2013). An additional form of identification band has a built-in sensor unit that sounds an alarm if the baby is transported beyond set birthing-unit boundaries. Individual birthing units should practice safety measures to prevent newborn abduction and provide information to parents regarding their role in this area and in general newborn safety measures.

The nurse should teach parents the following measures to prevent abduction and provide for safety:

- Parents should check that identification bands are in place as they care for their baby; if the bands are missing, parents should ask that they be replaced immediately.
- Parents should allow only individuals with proper birthing-unit picture identification to bring and/or remove the baby from the room. If parents do not know the staff person, they should call the nurse for assistance.
- Parents should report the presence of any suspicious individuals on the birthing unit.
- Parents should never leave their baby alone in their room. If they walk in the halls or take a shower, parents should have a family member watch the baby or should return the baby to the nursery.
- A parent who is feeling weak, faint, or unsteady should not lift the baby. Instead, the parent should call for assistance.
- Parents should always keep an eye and a hand on the baby when the newborn is out of the crib.
- Parents should ask visitors to leave if they have a cold, diarrhea, discharge from sores, or a contagious disease. Newborns need protection from infection even though they do possess some immunity.

PREVENTION OF COMPLICATIONS   Newborns are at continued risk for the complications of hemorrhage, late-onset cardiac symptoms, and infection. Pallor may be an early sign of hemorrhage and must be reported to the healthcare provider. The newborn with pallor is placed on a cardiorespiratory monitor to permit continuous assessment. Several newborn conditions put newborns at risk for hemorrhage. Cyanosis that is not relieved by oxygen administration requires emergency intervention, may indicate a congenital cardiac condition or shock, and requires ongoing assessment.

Infection in the nursery is best prevented by requiring that all personnel who have direct contact with newborns scrub for 2–3 minutes from the fingertips up to and including the elbows at the beginning of each shift. Each caregiver's hands must also be washed with soap and rubbed vigorously for 15 seconds before and after contact with every newborn and after touching any soiled surface, such as the floor or one's hair or face. Parents are instructed to practice appropriate hand hygiene before touching the baby. They are also instructed that anyone holding the baby should practice good hand hygiene, even after the family returns home. In some clinical settings family members are asked to wear gowns (preferably disposable) over their street clothes during their contact with newborns. These are good opportunities for the nurse to reinforce the efficacy of hand hygiene in preventing the spread of infection.

Jaundice in newborns is caused by the accumulation of the pigment bilirubin in the skin. Jaundice occurs in most newborns. Most jaundice is benign, but because of the potential toxicity of bilirubin, newborns must be monitored to identify those who might develop severe hyperbilirubinemia and, in rare cases, acute bilirubin encephalopathy or kernicterus (AAP & ACOG, 2013). Current recommendations include obtaining a total serum bilirubin level in any neonate who is visibly jaundiced in the first 24 hours of life and obtaining either a serum or transcutaneous bilirubin level before discharge. Nomograms for evaluating risk factors based on bilirubin levels and age of the neonate are available.

CIRCUMCISION   Circumcision is a surgical procedure in which the prepuce, an epithelial layer covering the penis, is separated from the glans penis and excised. This procedure permits exposure of the glans for easier cleaning. Controversy exists over the need to perform circumcisions.

Originally a religious rite practiced by Jews and Muslims, circumcision has gained widespread cultural acceptance in the United States but is much less common in Europe. Many parents choose circumcision because they want their male child to have a physical appearance similar to that of his father or the majority of other boys; some feel that it is expected by society. Another commonly cited reason for circumcising newborn males is to prevent the need for anesthesia, hospitalization, pain, and trauma if the procedure is needed later in life (AAP & ACOG, 2013). Failure to circumcise is a risk factor related to penile cancer in later life. During the prenatal period, the nurse ensures that parents have clear and current information regarding the risks and benefits of circumcision and supports their decision regarding the choice to circumcise.

As in the past, recommendations regarding circumcision have varied. The 1999 AAP policy statement was reaffirmed in 2005 and does not recommend *routine* circumcision, but it does acknowledge that medical indications for circumcision still exist (AAP & ACOG, 2013). The policy recommends that analgesia be used during circumcision to decrease procedural pain (AAP & ACOG, 2013); the dorsal penile nerve block and subcutaneous ring block are the most effective options (AAP & Canadian Paediatric Society [CPS], 2006). If a circumcision is to be performed, it should be done using the least painful method. Recent studies show that using oral sucrose for painful procedures can be effective in reducing pain for newborns and should be used with other nonpharmacologic measures to enhance its effectiveness (AAP & CPS, 2006).

Circumcision *should not be performed* if the newborn is premature or compromised, has a known bleeding problem, or is born with a genitourinary defect, such as hypospadias or epispadias, which may necessitate use of the foreskin in future surgical repairs.

The nurse plays an essential role in providing parents with current information regarding the medical, social, and psychological aspects of newborn circumcision. A well-informed nurse can allay parents' anxiety by sharing information and allowing them to express their concerns. In order for parents to make a truly informed decision, they must be knowledgeable about the potential risks and outcomes of circumcision. Hemorrhage, infection, difficulty in voiding, separation of the edges of the circumcision, discomfort, and restlessness are early potential problems. Later, there is a risk that the glans and urethral meatus may become irritated and inflamed from contact with the ammonia from urine. Ulcerations and progressive stenosis may develop. Adhesions, entrapment of the penis, and damage to the urethra are all potential complications of circumcision that could require surgical correction (AAP & ACOG, 2013).

The parents of a male newborn who will not be circumcised require information from the nurse about good hygienic practices. The nurse tells the parents that the foreskin and glans are two similar layers of cells that separate from each other. The separation process begins prenatally and is normally completed between 3 and 5 years of age. In the process of separation, sterile sloughed cells build up between the layers. This buildup looks similar to the smegma that is secreted after puberty, and it is harmless. Occasionally during the daily bath, the parent can gently test for retraction. If retraction has occurred, daily gentle washing of the glans with soap and water is sufficient to maintain adequate cleanliness. The parents should later teach the child to incorporate this practice into his daily self-care activities. Most uncircumcised males have no difficulty doing so.

If circumcision is desired, the procedure is performed when the newborn is well stabilized and has received his initial physical examination by a healthcare provider. The parents may also choose to have the circumcision done after discharge. However, parents need to be advised that if the baby is older than 1 month, the current practice is to hospitalize him for the procedure.

Before a circumcision, the nurse ensures that the physician has explained the procedure, determines whether the parents have any further questions about the procedure, and verifies that the circumcision permit is signed. As with any surgical procedure, the neonate's identification band should be checked to verify his identity before the procedure begins. The nurse gathers the equipment and prepares the newborn by removing the diaper and placing him on a padded circumcision board or some other type of restraint, but with only the legs restrained. These restraint measures, along with the application of warm blankets to the upper body, increase the newborn's comfort during the procedure. In Jewish circumcision ceremonies, the newborn is held by the father or godfather and is given wine before the procedure.

Various devices (Gomco clamp, Plastibell, and Mogen clamp) are used for circumcision (**Figures 33–103** ● and **33–104** ●), and all produce a small amount of bleeding. Therefore, the nurse should make special note of neonates with a family history of bleeding disorders or with mothers who took anticoagulants, including aspirin, prenatally. During the procedure, the nurse assesses the newborn's response. One important consideration is pain experienced by the newborn. A dorsal penile nerve block or ring block using 1% lidocaine without epinephrine or similar anesthetic significantly minimizes the pain and shifts in behavioral patterns, such as crying, irritability, and erratic sleep cycles, that are associated with circumcision. Other studies are investigating

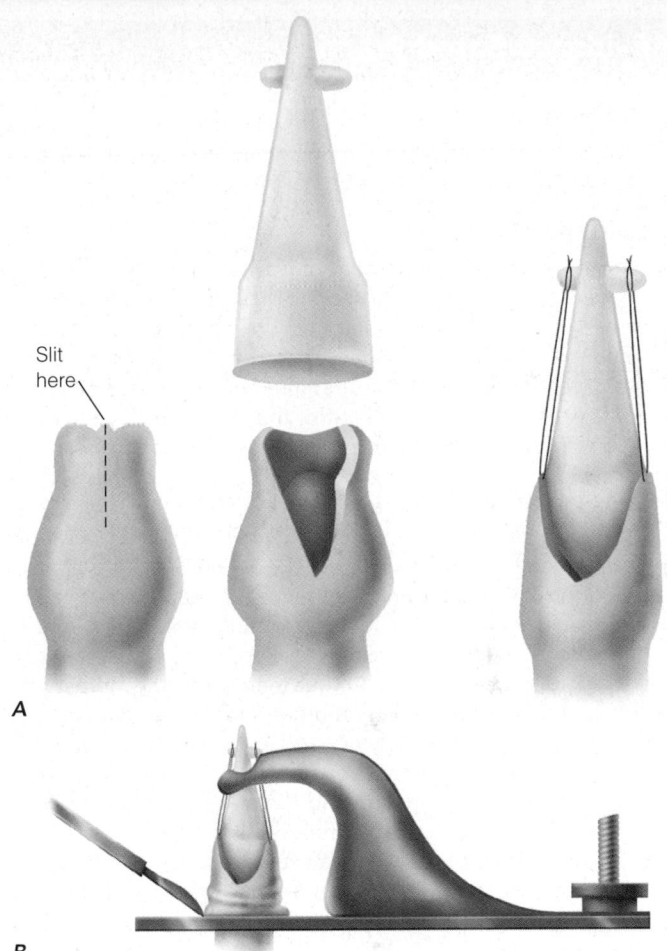

Slit here

A

B

Figure 33–103 ● Circumcision using a circumcision clamp. *A,* The prepuce is drawn over the cone and *B,* the clamp is applied. Pressure is maintained for 3–4 minutes, and then excess prepuce is cut away.

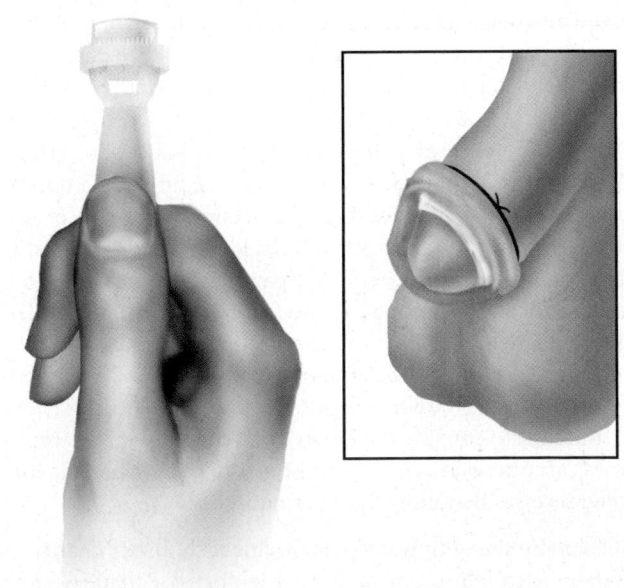

Figure 33–104 ● Circumcision using the Plastibell. The bell is fitted over the glans. A suture is tied around the bell's rim, and the excess prepuce is cut away. The plastic rim remains in place for 3–4 days until healing occurs. The bell may be allowed to fall off; it is removed if still in place after 8 days.

Evidence-Based Practice   Breastfeeding to Control Procedural Pain in Newborns

Problem

What nonpharmacologic methods can help reduce the pain associated with common neonatal procedures?

Evidence

Assessment and management of pain are important issues in neonatal care. Most newborns will experience a venipuncture or heel lance for blood sampling during their hospital stay. Although healthcare providers agree that newborns are capable of responding to painful stimuli, most providers do not administer medication to control the short-term pain associated with these common procedures. A Cochrane systematic review investigated the use of breastfeeding—specifically, the oral administration of breast milk—to control the pain associated with common procedures (Shah et al., 2012). Multiple systematic reviews with this quantity of randomized trials represent the strongest level of evidence for nursing practice.

Newborns who were feeding during heelsticks or venipuncture procedures demonstrated fewer physiological and behavioral signs of pain. Actual feeding at the breast was associated with a reduction in heart rate change, percentage time crying, duration of crying, and improvement in validated neonatal pain measures. Breastfeeding led to significantly lower increases in heart rate and decreased crying time compared to those who were swaddled. All groups that were fed during the procedure—whether it was breast milk from the mother or expressed breast milk—had better pain control

than babies who were swaddled, positioned, or given a pacifier without being held.

Implications

It does not appear that any of these measures completely eliminated the pain of routine procedures. Additionally, these studies were focused on healthy newborns undergoing minimally invasive, singular painful procedures. The effectiveness of either breast milk for repeated painful procedures was not studied. With regard to preterm or sick newborns, there is insufficient evidence to support the safety of breast milk or sucrose as a routine, repeated comfort measure. For preterm and sick full-term newborns who are subjected to repeated painful procedures during hospitalization, the ideal analgesic has not yet been identified.

Newborns undergoing single painful procedures, such as venipuncture or heelstick, should be breastfed by the mother during the procedure if at all possible. If not, the baby can be fed expressed breast milk with a syringe, a bottle, or by dipping a pacifier in the solution. Holding the baby while doing so achieves the best pain control.

Critical Thinking Application

1. What are the challenges with breastfeeding to control procedural pain in newborns?
2. How could we measure the influence of breastfeeding on newborn pain during procedures?

---

the use of topical anesthetic applied 60–90 minutes before prepuce removal, acetaminophen, and cryoanalgesia. Studies indicate that a combination of methods is most effective in reducing pain during circumcision (AAP & CPS, 2006).

Following the circumcision, the newborn should be held and comforted by a family member or the nurse. The nurse must be alert to any behavioral cues that these measures are overstimulating the newborn instead of comforting him. Such cues include turning away of the head, increased generalized body movement, skin color changes, hyperalertness, and hiccoughing.

Ideally, the circumcision should be assessed every 30 minutes for at least 2 hours following the procedure. It is important to observe for the first voiding after a circumcision in order to evaluate for urinary obstruction related to penile injury and/or edema. Petroleum ointment and gauze may be applied to the site immediately following the procedure to help prevent bleeding and can be used to protect the healing tissue afterward.

The nurse must also teach family members how to assess for unusual bleeding, how to respond if unusual bleeding is present, and how to care for the newly circumcised penis. Parents of babies circumcised with a method other than the Plastibell should receive the following information:

- Clean the site with warm water with each diaper change.
- Apply petroleum ointment for the next few diaper changes to help prevent further bleeding.
- If bleeding does occur, apply light pressure with a sterile gauze pad to stop the bleeding within a short time. If this is not effective, contact the physician immediately, or take the baby to the caregiver's office.

- The glans normally has granulation tissue (a yellowish film) on it during healing. Continued application of a petroleum ointment (or ointment suggested by the healthcare provider) can help protect the granulation tissue that forms as the glans heals.
- Report to the care provider any signs or symptoms of infection, such as increasing swelling, pus drainage, and cessation of urination.
- When diapering, ensure that the diaper is not loose enough to cause rubbing with movement and is not tight enough to cause pain.
- If the newborn's care provider recommends oral analgesics, follow instructions for proper measuring and administration.

If the Plastibell is used, parents should receive information about normal appearance and how to observe for infection. The parents are informed that the Plastibell should fall off within 8 days. If it remains on after 8 days, they should consult with their physician. No ointments or creams should be used while the bell remains, but application of petroleum ointment may protect granulation tissue afterward.

STRENGTHENING PARENT–NEWBORN ATTACHMENT   The nurse encourages parent–newborn attachment by involving all family members with the new member of the family. The nurse can discuss waking activities, such as talking with the baby while making eye contact, holding the baby in an upright position (sitting or standing), gently bending the baby back and forth while grasping under the knees and supporting the head and back with the other hand, or gently rubbing the baby's hands and feet. Quieting activities may include swaddling or bundling the baby to increase a sense of security; using slow, calming movements; and talking softly, singing, or humming to the baby (**Figure 33–105 ●**).

A Letter From Your Baby

Dear Parents:

I come to you a small, immature being with my own style and personality. I am yours for only a short time; enjoy me.

1. Please take time to find out who I am, how I differ from you, and how much I can bring you joy.

2. Please feed me when I am hungry. I never knew hunger in the womb, and clocks and time mean little to me.

3. Please hold, cuddle, kiss, touch, stroke, and croon to me. I was always held closely in the womb and was never alone before.

4. Please don't be disappointed when I am not the perfect baby that you expected, nor disappointed with yourselves that you are not the perfect parents.

5. Please don't expect too much from me as your newborn baby, or too much from yourself as a parent. Give us both six weeks as a birthday present—six weeks for me to grow, develop, mature, and become more stable and predictable, and six weeks for you to rest and relax and allow your body to get back to normal.

6. Please forgive me if I cry a lot. Bear with me and in a short time, as I mature, I will spend less and less time crying and more time socializing.

7. Please watch me carefully and I can tell you the things that soothe, console and please me. I am not a tyrant who was sent to make your life miserable, but the only way I can tell you that I am not happy is with my cry.

8. Please remember that I am resilient and can withstand the many natural mistakes you will make with me. As long as you make them with love, you cannot ruin me.

9. Please take care of yourself and eat a balanced diet, rest, and exercise so that when we are together, you have the health and strength to take care of me.

10. Please take care of your relationship with others. Relationships that are good for you, support both you and me.

Although I may have turned your life upside down, please realize that things will be back to normal before long.

Thank you,

Your Loving Child

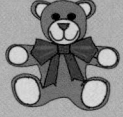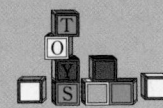

Figure 33–105 ● A letter from your baby.

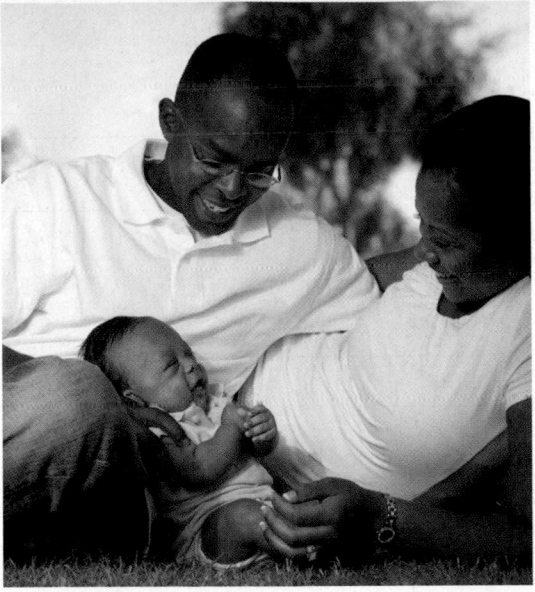

Figure 33–106 ● Parents must provide a nurturing environment to meet the emotional and physical needs of the infant. *Source:* aaron belford/Shutterstock

When fostering parent–newborn attachment, it is important to be sensitive to the cultural beliefs and values of the family. The nurse must also be aware of cultural variations in newborn care, such as naming the newborn, complimenting the baby, and using good luck charms.

Massage is a common child care practice in many parts of the world, especially Africa and Asia, that has recently gained attention in the United States. The nurse can teach parents to use massage as a method to facilitate the bonding process and to reduce the stress and pain associated with teething, constipation, inoculations, and colic. Massage not only induces relaxation for the baby, it also provides a calming and "feel-good" interaction for the parents that fosters the development of warm, positive relationships.

✳ Go to **nursing.pearsonhighered.com** to see Chart 17 on promoting attachment.

Prepare Family for Discharge

Although the adjustment to parenting is a normal process, going home presents a critical transition for the family. The parents become the primary caregivers for the newborn and must provide a nurturing environment in which the emotional and physical needs of the newborn can be met (**Figure 33–106 ●**). Nursing interventions focus on promoting health and preventing possible problems.

PARENT TEACHING Nearly every contact with the parents presents an opportunity for sharing information that can facilitate their sense of competence in newborn care. To meet the parents' need for information, the nurse who is responsible for the care of the mother and newborn should assume the primary responsibility for parent education. The nurse should teach the family all necessary caregiving methods before discharge. A checklist may be helpful to determine whether the teaching has been completed and to verify the parents' knowledge on leaving the birthing unit (**Figure 33–107 ●**). The nurse needs to review

PARENT TEACHING CHECKLIST	
Check off each item once parents understand your instructions	✓
General Baby Care	
Caring for skin	
Caring for cord	
Caring for circumcision and genital area	
What to do if baby is sick	
Using a thermometer	
Using a bulb syringe	
Burping baby	
Comforting baby	
Positioning baby	
Breastfeeding	
Waiting for milk to come in	
Understanding let-down reflex	
Positioning baby for feeding	
Getting baby to latch on	
When to breastfeed	
How long to breastfeed	
Removing baby from nipple	
Understanding supply and demand	
Supplementing	
Comfort measures for sore nipples	
Comfort measures for engorgement	
Using a breast pump	
Breastfeeding after returning to work	
Bottle-Feeding	
Choosing formula	
Mixing formula	
Feeding baby from a bottle	
Cleaning bottles	
Safety	
Placing baby to sleep on back	
Preventing shaken baby syndrome	
Using a car seat	
Managing pets	

Figure 33–107 ● A parent teaching checklist is completed by the time of discharge.

all areas for understanding by the mother and father, without rushing, and then take the time to resolve all of their queries. Any concerns of the parents or nurse are noted. Unless their care methods are harmful to the newborn, the parents' methods of giving care should be reinforced rather than contradicted.

Caring for newborns in the hospital setting means that the nurse will have contact with clients from a wide variety of racial, religious, and cultural backgrounds. The nurse needs to recognize and respect the many good ways of providing safe care and must be sensitive to the cultural beliefs and values of the family. Although it may not be possible to be conversant with all cultures, the nurse can demonstrate cultural sensitivity with both colleagues and clients as follows (Green-Hernandez et al., 2004):

■ Show respect for the inherent dignity of every human being, whatever the individual's age, gender, or religion.
■ Accept the rights of individuals to choose their care provider, participate in care, and refuse care.
■ Acknowledge personal biases, and prevent them from interfering with the delivery of quality care to individuals of other cultures.
■ Recognize cultural issues, and interact with clients from other cultures in culturally sensitive ways.
■ Incorporate the client's cultural preferences, health beliefs and behaviors, and traditional practices into the plan of care.
■ Develop appropriate educational materials that address the language and cultural beliefs of the client.
■ Access culturally appropriate resources to deliver care to clients from other cultures.
■ Assist clients to access high-quality care within a dominant culture.

Parents may be familiar with handling and caring for babies, or this may be their first time interacting with a newborn. If they are new parents, the sensitive nurse gently teaches them by example and provides instructions geared to their needs and previous knowledge about the various aspects of newborn care.

The length of stay in the birthing unit for mother and baby after birth is often 72 hours or less. The challenge for the nurse is to use every opportunity to teach, guide, and support individual parents, fostering their capabilities and confidence in caring for their newborn. Including mother–baby care and home care instruction on the night shift assists with education needs for early-discharge parents.

The nurse observes how parents interact with their newborn during feeding and caregiving activities. Even during a short stay, the nurse will have opportunities to provide information and observe whether the parents are comfortable with changing the diapers of, wrapping, handling, and feeding their newborn. Do both parents get involved in the newborn's care? Is the mother depending on someone else to help her at home? Does the mother give reasons (e.g., "I'm too tired," "My stitches hurt," or "I'll learn later") for not wanting to be involved in her baby's care? As the family provides care, the nurse can enhance parental confidence by giving them positive feedback. If the parents encounter problems, the nurse can express confidence in their abilities to master the new skills or information, suggest alternatives, and serve as a role model. All of these factors need to be considered when evaluating the educational needs of the parents.

Several methods may be used to teach families about newborn care. Daily newborn care videos and classes are nonthreatening ways

Focus on Diversity and Culture Examples of Cultural Beliefs and Practices Regarding Baby Care*

The culturally sensitive nurse knows that practices and beliefs vary among individuals of varying cultural groups. Assuming that a member of a particular cultural or ethnic group will perform certain rituals or hold certain beliefs could be a bias. Instead, the nurse should assess the client's desired practices and beliefs with open-ended questions. Then, the nurse can provide support for the client to practice these rituals.

Some variations from various cultures that the nurse might encounter include the following:

Umbilical Cord Care

After birth, some parents may desire to place abdominal binder or bellyband on the baby to protect against dirt, injury, and umbilical hernia.

Oils may be applied to the stump, or metal may be taped to the umbilicus to ward off evil spirits (D'Avanzo & Geissler, 2008).

Some families may expect a sterile cutting of the cord at birth. The parents will wait for the stump to air dry, and discard it after it falls off.

The stump may be cauterized with a candle flame, hot coal, or burning stick (World Health Organization [WHO], 1999).

In girls, the cord stump may be left long to prevent a small uterus and problems with childbirth (WHO, 1999).

Parent-Infant Contact

Some parents may pick up the baby as soon as it cries, or carry the baby at all times. Others may allow a baby to fuss or cry to teach the baby self-soothing skills.

Cradle boards, slings, or other infant carrying devices may be worn so that the infant can be with family even during work and feel secure (Andrews, 2008).

Some people may have specific rituals immediately after birth. There are some cultures where the father says a prayer in the newborn's right ear and cleans the infant after birth.

Feeding

Breastfeeding occurs across many cultures. The length of time a woman may breastfeed varies greatly. Some women choose to breastfeed for the first 1 to 2 years of life, while others breastfeed into toddlerhood. Weaning may occur after teeth are present, when the child is walking, or relative to other milestones.

Breastfeeding may be delayed because of a belief that colostrum is bad (D'Avanzo & Geissler, 2008).

Some women may avoid displaying "strong emotions" because they believe it can spoil milk (Lipson & Dibble, 2008).

Women may choose to breastfeed, formula feed, pump breastmilk and feed by bottle, or a combination of any of these options. The nurse should answer questions, provide education, and support the mother's decision.

Some women choose to provide a "comfort bottle" of formula in between feedings (Lipson & Dibble, 2008).

Women may have varying degrees of modesty around breastfeeding. Some may do so openly, while others will not breastfeed in public or in the presence of men. If the nurse is caring for a mother who will breastfeed or pump milk, the nurse should inquire about assisting with coverings or privacy.

Circumcision

Circumcision may be practiced as a religious ritual for the infant. Other cultures may practice circumcision as a rite of puberty (Lipson & Dibble, 2008; Ott, AlKhadhuri, & Al-Junaibi, 2003).

The nurse will also care for many infants who are not circumcised. As of 2016, an estimated 70% of males in the U.S. were circumcised and 30% were not (Morris et al,, 2016).

Health and Illness

There are a variety of practices to maintain health and avoid illness. The nurse should respect the desires of the client or family when able. Some practices the nurse many encounter include:

- Touching the face or head of an infant when admiring it to prevent the "evil eye."
- Avoiding cutting the baby's nails to avoid nearsightedness and, instead, putting mittens on the baby's hands to prevent scratching.
- Not allowing anyone to touch the baby's head without asking permission.
- Avoiding saying the baby's name before the formal naming ceremony to prevent harming the baby.
- Avoiding cutting a baby's hair or nails to prevent illness.

*Note: This information is meant only to provide examples of the behaviors that may be found within certain cultures. Not all members of a culture practice the behaviors described.

to convey general information. Individual instruction is helpful to answer specific questions or to clarify an item that may have been confusing in class. Currently, many birthing centers have 24-hour educational video channels or videos to be viewed in the mother's room on a variety of postpartum and newborn care issues.

One-to-one teaching while the nurse is in the mother's room is the most effective educational method. Both first-time and experienced postpartum parents rate individual teaching as the most effective method of instruction. Individual instruction is helpful both to answer specific questions and to clarify something that the parents may have found confusing in the educational video. With shorter stays, most teaching unfortunately tends to focus on newborn feeding and immediate physical care needs of the mothers, with limited anticipatory guidance provided in other areas.

✳ To address this deficit, go to **nursing.pearsonhighered. com** to see Chart 18, which provides a broad range of information important to share with new parents.

GENERAL INSTRUCTIONS FOR NEWBORN CARE

One of the first concerns of anyone who has not had the experience of picking up a baby is how to do it correctly. The newborn is easily picked up by sliding one hand under the neck and shoulders and the other hand under the buttocks or between the newborn's legs and then gently lifting upward. This technique provides security and support for the head, which the baby is unable to support until 3 or 4 months of age.

The nurse can be an excellent role model for families in the area of safety. Safety topics include proper positioning of the newborn on the back to sleep and correct use of the bulb syringe (discussed shortly). The baby should never be left alone anywhere but in the crib. The mother is reminded that while she and her newborn are together in the birthing unit, she should never leave her baby alone, both for security reasons and because newborns spit up frequently during the first day or two after birth.

Demonstrating a bath, cord care, and temperature assessment is the best way for the nurse to provide information on these topics to parents. Parents should be told to call their healthcare provider if redness, foul odor, bright-red bleeding, or greenish-yellow drainage occurs at the cord site or if the area remains unhealed 2–3 days after the cord stump has sloughed off. No single method of umbilical cord care (topical antimicrobials [triple dye, iodophor ointment, or hexachlorophene powder] or alcohol) has been proven to be superior in preventing colonization and disease (AAP & ACOG, 2013). The use of sterile water or air drying results in umbilical cords separating more quickly than those treated with alcohol (Fraser, 2013).

NASAL AND ORAL SUCTIONING

As mentioned, most newborns are obligatory nose breathers for the first months of life. They generally maintain air passage patency by coughing or sneezing. During the first few days of life, however, the newborn has increased mucus, and gentle suctioning with a bulb syringe may be indicated. The nurse can demonstrate the use of the bulb syringe in the mouth and nose and have the parents do a return demonstration. The parents should repeat this demonstration of suctioning and cleansing the bulb before discharge so that they feel confident in performing the procedure. Care should be taken to apply only gentle suction to prevent nasal bleeding.

To suction the newborn, the bulb syringe is compressed before the tip is placed in the nostril. The nurse or parent must take care not to occlude the passageway. The bulb is permitted to reexpand slowly by releasing the compression on the bulb. The bulb syringe is removed from the nostril, and drainage is then compressed out of the bulb and onto a tissue. The bulb syringe may also be used in the mouth if the newborn is spitting up and unable to handle the excess secretions. The bulb is compressed, the tip of the bulb syringe is placed approximately 2.5 cm (1 in.) to one side of the newborn's mouth, and compression is released. This draws up the excess secretions. The procedure is repeated on the other side of the mouth. The roof of the mouth and the back of the throat are avoided, because suction in these areas might stimulate the gag reflex. The bulb syringe should be washed in warm, soapy water and rinsed in warm water daily and as needed after use. Rinsing with a half-strength white vinegar solution followed by clear water may help to extend the useful life of the bulb syringe by inhibiting bacterial growth. A bulb syringe should always be kept near the newborn. New parents and nurses who are inexperienced with babies may fear that the baby will choke and are relieved to know how to take action if such an event occurs. They should be advised to turn the newborn's head to the side or hold the newborn with his or her head down as soon as there is any indication of gagging or vomiting and to use the bulb syringe as needed.

Some newborns may have transient edema of the nasal mucosa following suctioning of the airway after birth. The

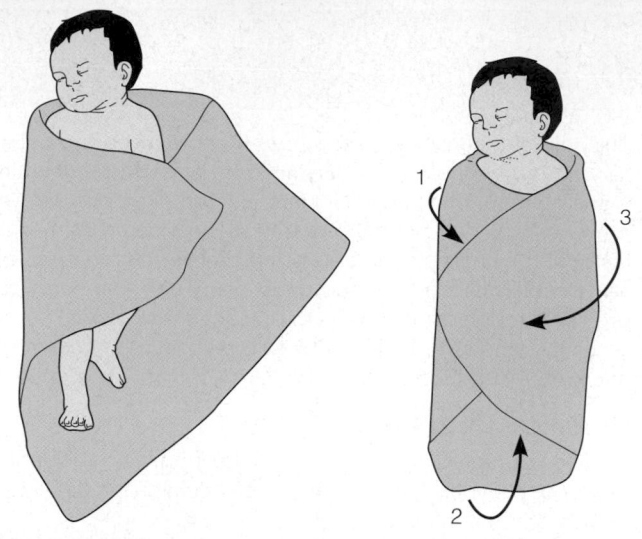

Figure 33–108 ● Steps in wrapping a baby.

nurse can demonstrate the use of normal saline to loosen secretions and instruct parents in the gentle and moderate use of the bulb syringe to avoid further irritation of the mucous membranes. If parents will be using humidifiers at home, they should be instructed to follow the manufacturer's cleaning instructions carefully so that molds, spores, and bacteria from a dirty humidifier do not enter the baby's environment.

SWADDLING THE NEWBORN

Swaddling (wrapping) helps the newborn maintain body temperature, provides a feeling of closeness and security, and may be effective in quieting a crying baby by having the newborn's hands near his or her mouth to allow sucking (Roach, 2004). A blanket is placed on the crib (or secure surface) in the shape of a diamond. The top corner of the blanket is folded down slightly, and the newborn's body is placed with the head at the upper edge of the blanket. The right corner of the blanket is wrapped around the newborn and tucked under the left side (not too tightly—the newborn needs a little room to move and to allow for hands to get to the mouth). The bottom corner is then pulled up to the chest, and the left corner is wrapped around the baby's right side (**Figure 33–108 ●**). The nurse can show this wrapping technique to new parents so that they will feel more skilled in handling their baby.

SLEEP AND ACTIVITY

The National Institute of Child Health and Human Development and the AAP recommend that healthy term newborns be placed on their backs to sleep. Parents are taught the importance of following "Safe to Sleep Guidelines" to reduce the incidence of sudden infant death syndrome (SIDS) (AAP, 2011). Though neonates may need to be placed on their sides initially because of copious or thick secretions, placing them on their backs in the newborn period serves to educate parents regarding safe sleep positioning. Studies indicate that parents position their babies in the same positions they observe in the hospital setting, so the nurse must demonstrate this behavior to reduce the risk of SIDS. If exceptions are warranted, these should be explained to families so that they do not misinterpret what they observe. The placement of babies in a prone position during wakeful play sessions ("tummy time") should be encouraged as well (AAP & ACOG, 2013).

Stay Current: *Visit the Safe to Sleep Web site at* **www.nichd.nih.gov/SIDS/Pages/sids.aspx** *to learn current recommendations for safe sleeping.*

Perhaps nothing is more individual to each baby than the sleep–activity cycle. It is important for the nurse to recognize the individual variations of each newborn and to assist parents as they develop sensitivity to their baby's communication signals and rhythms of activity and sleep.

CAR SAFETY CONSIDERATIONS   Half of the children killed or injured in automobile crashes could have been protected by the use of federally approved car seats. Newborns must go home from the birthing unit in a car seat adapted to fit them. Babies should never be placed in the front seat of a car equipped with a passenger-side airbag. The car seat should be positioned to face the rear of the car until the baby is 2 years old or until the child reaches the maximum height and weight for the seat (AAP, 2011a). The nurse need to ensure that all parents are knowledgeable about the proper installation and benefits of using a child safety seat. The nurse can encourage parents to have their safety seats checked by local groups trained specifically for that purpose. The Seat Check Initiative provides locations and information about child safety seats.

Stay Current: *Visit* **www.seatcheck.org** *to learn how to install car seats properly and about occupant protection laws in each state.*

NEWBORN SCREENING AND IMMUNIZATION PROGRAMS   Before the newborn and mother are discharged from the birthing unit, the nurse informs the parents about the newborn screening tests and tells them when to return to the birthing center or clinic if further tests are needed. Some of the disorders that can be identified from a few drops of blood obtained by a heelstick are cystic fibrosis, galactosemia, congenital adrenal hyperplasia, congenital hypothyroidism, maple syrup urine disease, phenylketonuria (PKU), sickle cell trait, biotinidase deficiency, and hemoglobinopathies.

Early discharge has affected both the timing of newborn metabolic screening tests and the acquisition of subsequent immunization. Early newborn discharge increases the risk for a delayed or even missed diagnosis of PKU and congenital hypothyroidism because of decreased sensitivity of screening before 24 hours of age. Newborns should be retested by 2 weeks of age if the first test was done before 24 hours of age. A second test for PKU is required in most states, usually between 1 week and 1 month of age, to minimize the chance of a positive child going undetected.

New technology is quickly increasing the number of metabolic and other disorders that can be detected in the newborn period. The Expanded Newborn Screening Program allows parents to have their babies screened for more than 20 disorders. Although controversy exists over the need for such comprehensive testing, it is recommended that states test for a core panel of 29 treatable congenital conditions and an additional 25 conditions that may be detected by screening (AAP, 2011b). While all states require screening for more than 50 congenital conditions, each state decides on the number and type of conditions (CDC, 2014).

Over 95% of newborns in the United States are screened for hearing loss prior to discharge. About 2% of screened newborns require follow-up (Russ et al., 2010).

Immunization programs against the hepatitis B virus during the newborn period and infancy are in place in many U.S. states, at least 20 countries, and high-incidence areas, such as American Samoa. Universal vaccination of infants is recommended. Babies should receive the first dose of hepatitis B vaccine during the period from birth to 2 months of age. The second dose should be administered at least 1 month after the first dose. The third dose should be administered at least 4 months after the first dose and at least 2 months after the second dose, but not before 6 months of age (AAP & ACOG, 2013). Parents need to be advised whether their birthing center provides newborn hepatitis vaccination so that an adequate follow-up program can be set in motion.

Stay Current: *Find up-to-date immunization schedules for infants in English and Spanish at the CDC Web site at* **www.cdc.gov/vaccines/schedules/easy-to-read/child.html**

COMMUNITY-BASED NURSING CARE   The nurse should discuss with parents ways to meet their newborn's needs, ensure safety, and appreciate the newborn's unique characteristics and behaviors. By assisting parents in establishing links with their community-based healthcare provider, the nurse can get the new family off to a good start. Parents also need to know the signs of illness, how to reach the pediatrician or after-hours clinic, and the importance of follow-up after discharge. Parents should also check with their healthcare provider for advice about OTC medications to be kept in the medicine cabinet.

The family should have the care provider's phone number, address, and any specific instructions. Having the birthing unit or nursery phone number is also reassuring to a newborn's family. They are encouraged to call with questions. Follow-up calls lend added support by providing another opportunity for parents to have their questions answered.

Some institutions have initiated postpartum and/or newborn follow-up home visits, especially for newborns discharged before 48 hours after birth. The follow-up home examination should be within 48 hours of discharge (AAP & ACOG, 2013) when the family is unable to visit their primary care physician within that time period. The home visit focuses on normal newborn care, assessment for hyperbilirubinemia (jaundice), extreme weight loss, feeding problems, and knowledge related to newborn care and feeding within the family unit.

Routine well-baby visits should be scheduled with the clinic, pediatric nurse practitioner, or physician. Regardless of the type of follow-up services available in the community, the nurse contributes to the newborn's health by stressing the importance of routine care and by helping families who have no follow-up plans to connect with local resources for care.

SAFETY ALERT
Infants with respiratory distress should not be fed orally because of an increased risk of aspiration.

NURSING CARE PLAN ⟩ A Small-for-Gestational-Age Newborn

Ellen, a term baby, was born 8 hours ago weighing 2,500 g at 40 weeks of gestation. Two hours after birth, Ellen's temperature was 37.1°C (98.8°F) under the radiant warmer. She was swaddled and placed in an open crib. One hour later, Ellen is returned to the radiant warmer with a falling temperature reading of 36.1°C (97°F). Acrocyanosis has also been detected. Glucose levels are 35 mg/dL. The nurse monitors the newborn for signs of hypothermia and hypoglycemia.

ASSESSMENT

Subjective: Alert and active.
Objective: 40 weeks of gestation; birth weight, 2,500 g; length, 48.3 cm (19 in.); head circumference, 30 cm (11.8 in.); chest circumference, 28 cm (11 in.); temperature, 36.1°C (97°F) axillary; pulse, 140 bpm; respirations, 45 breaths/minute; vigorous cry, alert, and wide-eyed; dry skin; thin, meconium-stained umbilical cord; glucose, 35 mg/dL; and tremors.

DIAGNOSES

- *Hypothermia* related to decrease in subcutaneous fat tissue and increased body surface exposure to environment
- *Nutrition, Imbalanced: Less Than Body Requirements* related to increased glucose consumption secondary to metabolic effects of hypothermia and poor hepatic glycogen stores
- *Injury, Risk for* related to hypoglycemia secondary to the metabolic effects of hypothermia and poor hepatic glycogen stores

(NANDA-I © 2015)

PLANNING

- The newborn will maintain stable body temperature within normal range of 36.5°–37.4°C (97.7°–99.4°F) in an open crib.
- The newborn will not exhibit signs of acrocyanosis, mottling, or lethargy.
- The newborn will maintain a glucose level above 40 mg/dL.
- The newborn's weight will remain stable.
- The newborn will not exhibit any unusual jitteriness or tremors.

IMPLEMENTATION

- Monitor axillary temperature every 4 hours and PRN.
- Monitor pulse and respirations every 4 hours and PRN.
- Assess skin color and temperature every 15–30 minutes in presence of color change.
- Place newborn under radiant warmer if temperature falls below 36.5°C (97.7°F).
- Place newborn in incubator if temperature is unstable.
- Initiate frequent feeding as tolerated (10 mL/kg is a general guideline for formula feeding).

- Initiate early feedings.
- Monitor glucose levels every 4 hours.
- Monitor for signs of hypoglycemia.
- Encourage on-demand feeding at least every 3–4 hours.
- Offer supplemental feedings or additional glucose.
- Maintain a neutral thermal environment.

EVALUATION

- The infant's temperature remains between 36.5° and 37.4°C (97.7° and 99.4°F) in an open crib.
- The skin is pink in color, with no signs of acrocyanosis or mottling.
- The glucose level remains above 45 mg/dL.
- The newborn's weight is stabilized.
- No signs of jitteriness or tremors are present.

CRITICAL THINKING

1. *What can the nurse do to prevent heat loss through convection when preparing the newborn for the open crib?*
2. *What measure can the nurse take to reduce heat loss through evaporation and conduction? How many calories can a SGA newborn lose through radiation?*
3. *Parents of an SGA newborn ask the nurse when they should expect their baby to catch up in weight to normal-growth newborns. What is the nurse's best response?*

Evaluation

When evaluating the nursing care provided during the period immediately after birth, the nurse may anticipate the following outcomes:

- The newborn's adaptation to extrauterine life is successful, as demonstrated by all vital signs being within acceptable parameters.
- The newborn's physiological and psychological integrity is supported.
- Positive interactions between parent and newborn are supported.

When evaluating the nursing care provided during the newborn period, the nurse may anticipate the following outcomes:

- The newborn's physiological and psychological integrity is supported by maintaining stable vital signs and interactions based on normal newborn behaviors.
- The newborn feeding pattern has been satisfactorily established.
- The parents express understanding of the bonding process and display attachment behaviors.

When evaluating the nursing care provided in preparation for discharge, the nurse may anticipate the following outcomes:

- The parents demonstrate safe techniques in caring for their newborn.
- Parents verbalize developmentally appropriate behavioral expectations of their newborn and knowledge of community-based newborn follow-up care.

REVIEW Newborn Care

RELATE Link the Concepts and Exemplars

Linking the exemplar of newborn care with the concept of stress and coping:

1. What stressors does a newborn place on the family?

2. What assessment findings might you anticipate in a family that is not coping appropriately with the stress brought on by caring for their newborn? What actions might the nurse take to improve coping strategies?

Linking the exemplar of newborn care with the concept of immunity:

3. What recommendations would you make to the parents during discharge teaching related to their newborn's immune system?

4. While planning for discharge from the hospital, the mother of a newborn asks you, "What vaccinations does my baby need first?" How would you respond to this question?

READY Go to Companion Skills Manual

REFER Go to Pearson Nursing Student Resources
nursing.pearsonhighered.com

- Additional review materials
- Chart 13: Fetal and Neonatal Circulation

- Chart 14: Potential Birth Injuries
- Chart 15: Congenital Anomalies: Identification and Care in the Newborn Period
- Chart 16: Comparison of Cephalohematoma and Caput Succedaneum
- Chart 17: Promoting Attachment
- Chart 18: What to Tell Parents About Infant Care

REFLECT Case Study

Maria and Carlos Ramirez are preparing to take their newborn daughter home. They have three other daughters at home, ages 7 years, 3 years, and 2 years. Mrs. Ramirez tells you that the middle child was very jealous when she brought the 2-year-old home from the hospital and is worried about how the children will respond to this new baby.

1. Mrs. Ramirez says she would like to breastfeed the baby, but wonders if that will increase the sibling rivalry among her other children. How would you respond to this concern?

2. What strategies might you recommend to Mrs. Ramirez to reduce sibling rivalry when introducing the new baby to the family?

3. Mr. Ramirez shares with you, while Mrs. Ramirez is out of the room, that he had really hoped this new baby would be a boy. What assessment questions might you ask of this father?

EXEMPLAR 33.5 Prematurity

EXEMPLAR KEY TERMS
Apnea of prematurity, *2254*
Minimal enteral nutrition, *2253*
Preterm newborn, *2249*

EXEMPLAR LEARNING OUTCOMES
After reading about this exemplar, you will be able to:

1. Describe the physiological differences in the premature neonate in comparison to the term neonate.

2. Identify risk factors associated with prematurity.

3. Illustrate the nursing process in providing culturally competent care for premature neonates and their families.

4. Formulate priority nursing diagnoses appropriate for the premature neonate.

5. Summarize therapies used by interdisciplinary teams in the collaborative care of a premature neonate.

6. Plan evidence-based care for a premature neonate and his or her family in collaboration with other members of the healthcare team.

7. Evaluate expected outcomes for a premature neonate.

▶ OVERVIEW

A **preterm newborn** is a baby born at less than 37 completed weeks of gestation (Gardner & Hernandez, 2011). The incidence of all preterm births in the United States is approximately 12% (Hamilton et al., 2013). With the help of modern technology, neonates are surviving at younger gestational ages, but not without significant morbidity. The rise in multiple birth rates has markedly influenced overall rates of low-birth-weight neonates. **Figure 33–109** ● shows a comparison of a premature neonate, a low-birth-weight neonate, and a full-term neonate.

▶ THE PRETERM NEWBORN

The major problem of the preterm newborn is the variable immaturity of all systems. The degree of immaturity depends on the length of gestation. The preterm newborn must traverse

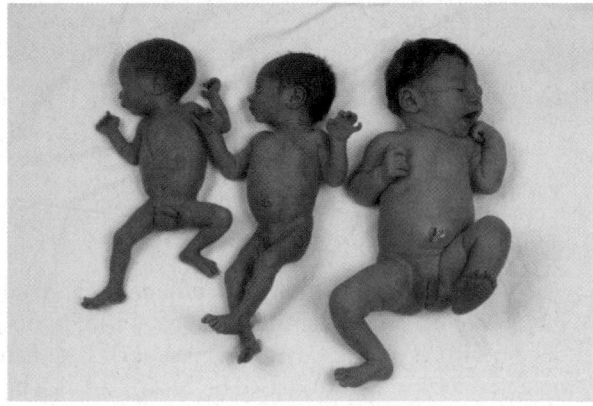

Figure 33–109 ● *From left to right:* A 4-week-old neonate who was born 9 weeks premature, a 2-week-old neonate who weighed 1,200 g at birth, and a full-term neonate, 2 days old, who weighed 3,730 g at birth.

the same complex, interconnected pathways from intrauterine to extrauterine life as the term newborn. Because of immaturity, however, the premature newborn is ill equipped to make this transition smoothly. Maintenance of the preterm newborn falls within narrow physiological parameters.

Respiratory and Cardiac Physiology

The preterm newborn is at risk for respiratory problems because the lungs are not fully mature and not fully ready to take over the process of oxygen and carbon dioxide exchange without assistance. Critical factors in the development of respiratory distress include the following:

- *The preterm neonate is unable to produce adequate amounts of surfactant.* Inadequate surfactant lessens compliance (ability of the lung to fill with air easily), thereby increasing the inspiratory pressure needed to expand the lungs with air. The collapsed (or atelectatic) alveoli will not facilitate an exchange of oxygen and carbon dioxide. As a result, the neonate becomes hypoxic, pulmonary blood flow is inefficient, and the preterm newborn's available energy is depleted.

- *The muscular coat of pulmonary blood vessels is incompletely developed.* As a result, the pulmonary arterioles do not constrict well in response to decreased oxygen levels. This lowered pulmonary vascular resistance leads to left-to-right shunting of blood through the ductus arteriosus, which increases the blood flow back into the lungs.

- *The ductus arteriosus of the preterm neonate, who is more susceptible to hypoxia, may respond to increasing oxygen and prostaglandin E levels by remaining open rather than by vasoconstriction, which is how the ductus responds in the term neonate.* A patent ductus increases the blood volume to the lungs, causing pulmonary congestion, increased respiratory effort, carbon dioxide retention, and bounding femoral pulses.

Thermoregulation

Heat loss is a major problem in premature newborns. Two factors limiting heat production are the availability of glycogen in the liver and the amount of brown fat available for heat production. Both of these limiting factors appear in the third trimester. In the cold-stressed baby, norepinephrine is released, which in turn stimulates the metabolism of brown fat for heat production. As a complicating factor, the hypoxic newborn cannot increase oxygen consumption in response to cold stress because of the already limited reserves; as a result, the hypoxic newborn becomes progressively colder. Preterm neonates have smaller muscle mass and diminished muscular activity, rendering them unable to shiver and further limiting heat production.

Five physiological and anatomical factors increase heat loss in the preterm neonate:

1. *The preterm baby has a higher ratio of body surface to body weight.* This means that the baby's ability to produce heat (based on body weight) is much less than the potential for losing heat (based on surface area). The loss of heat in a preterm neonate weighing 1,500 g is five times greater per unit of body weight than that of an adult.

2. *The preterm baby has very little subcutaneous fat, which is the human body's insulation.* Without adequate insu-

lation, heat is easily conducted from the core of the body (warmer temperature) to the surface of the body (cooler temperature). Heat is lost from the body as the blood vessels, which lie close to the skin surface in the preterm neonate, transport blood from the body core to the subcutaneous tissues.

3. *The preterm baby has thinner, more permeable skin than the term neonate.* This increased permeability contributes to a greater insensible water loss as well as to heat loss.

4. *The posture of the preterm baby influences heat loss.* Flexion of the extremities decreases the amount of surface area exposed to the environment. Extension increases the surface area exposed to the environment and thus increases heat loss. The gestational age of the neonate influences the amount of flexion, from completely hypotonic and extended at 28 weeks to strong flexion at 36 weeks.

5. *The premature baby has a decreased ability to vasoconstrict superficial blood vessels and conserve heat in the body core.* This lack of vasoconstriction allows heat to leave the premature neonate's body at a fast rate, thus leading to cold stress.

Thermoregulation is discussed more completely in the module on Thermoregulation. The essential point regarding thermoregulation of the premature neonate, however, is this: Gestational age is directly proportional to the ability to maintain thermoregulation; thus, the more preterm the newborn, the less able the neonate is to maintain heat balance.

The nurse can do much to prevent heat loss by providing a neutral thermal environment. This is one of the most important considerations in nursing management of the preterm neonate (see the Maintenance of a Neutral Thermal Environment section later in this exemplar). Cold stress, with its accompanying severe complications, can be prevented.

Gastrointestinal Physiology

The basic structure of the gastrointestinal (GI) tract is formed early in gestation. Maturation of the digestive and absorptive process is more variable, however, and occurs later in gestation. As a result of GI immaturity, the preterm newborn has the following ingestion, digestive, and absorption problems:

- A marked danger of aspiration and its associated complications because of the premature neonate's poorly developed gag reflex, incompetent esophageal cardiac sphincter, and poor sucking and swallowing reflexes. The ability to sucking, swallow, and breathing is not established until 32–34 weeks' gestation.

- Difficulty in meeting high caloric and fluid needs for growth because of small stomach capacity.

- Limited ability to convert certain essential amino acids to nonessential amino acids. Certain amino acids, such as histidine, taurine, and cysteine, are essential to the preterm neonate but not to the term neonate.

- Inability to handle the increased osmolarity of formula protein because of kidney immaturity. The preterm neonate requires a higher concentration of whey protein than of casein.

- Difficulty absorbing saturated fats because of decreased bile salts and pancreatic lipase. Severe illness of the newborn may also prevent intake of adequate nutrients.

- Initial difficulty with lactose digestion because processes may not be fully functional during the first few days of a preterm neonate's life. The preterm newborn can digest and absorb most simple sugars.

- Deficiency of calcium and phosphorus may exist because two thirds of these minerals are deposited in the last trimester. This can lead to rickets and significant bone demineralization.

- Increased basal metabolic rate and increased oxygen requirements caused by fatigue associated with sucking.

- Feeding intolerance and necrotizing enterocolitis (NEC) as a result of diminished blood flow and tissue perfusion to the intestinal tract because of prolonged hypoxia and hypoxemia at birth.

Renal Physiology

The kidneys of the premature neonate are immature compared with those of the full-term neonate, posing clinical problems in the management of fluid and electrolyte balance. Specific renal characteristics of the preterm neonate include the following:

- The glomerular filtration rate (GFR) is lower because of decreased renal blood flow. The GFR is directly related to lower gestational age, so the more preterm the newborn, the lower the GFR. The GFR is also decreased in the presence of diseases or conditions that decrease renal blood flow and perfusion, such as severe respiratory distress, hypotension, and asphyxia. Anuria and oliguria may also be observed.

- The preterm neonate's kidneys are limited in their ability to concentrate urine or to excrete excess amounts of fluid. This means that if excess fluid is administered, the neonate is at risk for fluid retention and overhydration. If too little fluid is administered, the neonate will become dehydrated because of the inability to retain adequate fluid.

- The kidneys of the preterm neonate begin excreting glucose (glycosuria) at a lower serum glucose level than those of the term infant. Glycosuria with hyperglycemia can lead to osmotic diuresis and polyuria.

- The buffering capacity of the kidney is reduced, predisposing the neonate to metabolic acidosis. Bicarbonate is excreted at a lower serum level, and acid is excreted more slowly. Therefore, after periods of hypoxia or insult, the preterm neonate's kidneys require a longer time to excrete the lactic acid that accumulates. Sodium bicarbonate is frequently required to treat metabolic acidosis in the premature neonate.

- The immaturity of the renal system affects the preterm neonate's ability to excrete drugs. Because excretion time is longer, many drugs are given over longer intervals (i.e., every 24 hours instead of every 12 hours). Urine output must be carefully monitored when the neonate is receiving nephrotoxic drugs, such as gentamicin and vancomycin. If urine output is poor, drugs can become toxic much more quickly in the neonate than in the adult.

Immunological Physiology

The preterm neonate is at much greater risk for infection than the term neonate. This increased susceptibility may be the result of an infection acquired in utero, which may have precipitated preterm labor and birth. However, all preterm neonates have immature specific and nonspecific immunity.

In utero, the fetus receives passive immunity against a variety of infections from maternal IgG immunoglobulins, which cross the placenta. Because most of this immunity is acquired in the last trimester of pregnancy, the premature neonate has few antibodies at birth, and these antibodies provide less protection and become depleted earlier than in a full-term neonate. The limited number of antibodies in the preterm neonate may be a contributing factor in the higher incidence of recurrent infection during the first year of life as well as in the immediate neonatal period.

The other immunoglobulin that is significant for the preterm neonate is secretory IgA, which does not cross the placenta but is found in breast milk at significant concentrations. The secretory IgA in breast milk provides immunity to the mucosal surfaces of the infant's GI tract, protecting the newborn from enteric infections such as those caused by *Escherichia coli* and *Shigella*.

Another altered defense against infection in the preterm neonate is the skin surface. In very small neonates, the skin is easily excoriated, and this factor, coupled with many invasive procedures, places the neonate at great risk for healthcare-associated infections. It is vital to use good hand hygiene in the care of these neonates in order to prevent unnecessary infection.

> ### SAFETY ALERT
> The sudden onset of apnea and bradycardia, coupled with metabolic acidosis in an otherwise healthy, growing premature neonate, may be suggestive of bacterial sepsis, especially if an invasive device, such as a central line or endotracheal tube, is in place.

Neurological Physiology

The general shape of the brain is formed during the first 6 weeks of gestation. Between the second and fourth months of gestation, the brain's total complement of neurons proliferates. These neurons migrate to specific sites throughout the central nervous system, and nerve impulse pathways organize. The final step in neurological development is the covering of these nerves with myelin, which begins in the second trimester of gestation and continues into adult life (Volpe, 2008).

The period of most rapid brain growth and development occurs during the third trimester of pregnancy; therefore, the closer to term an neonate is born, the better the neurological prognosis. A common interruption of neurological development in the preterm neonate is caused by intraventricular hemorrhage and intracranial hemorrhage. Hydrocephalus may develop as a consequence of an intraventricular hemorrhage caused by the obstruction at the cerebral aqueduct.

Reactivity and Behavioral States

The newborn neonate's response to extrauterine life is characterized by two periods of reactivity. The preterm neonate's periods of reactivity, however, are delayed. In the very ill neonate, these periods of reactivity may not be observed at all, because the neonate may be hypotonic and unreactive for several days after birth.

As the preterm newborn grows and the neonate's condition stabilizes, identifying behavioral states and traits unique to each neonate becomes increasingly possible. In general, stable preterm neonates do not demonstrate the same behavioral states as term neonates. Preterm neonates tend to be more disorganized in their sleep–wake cycles and are unable to attend as well to the human face and objects in the environment. Neurologically, their responses (sucking, muscle tone, and states of arousal) are weaker than those of full-term neonates.

By observing each neonate's patterns of behavior and responses, especially the sleep–wake states, the parents and nurse can plan nursing care around the times when the neonate is alert and best able to attend. In addition, the more knowledge parents have about the meaning of their newborn's responses and behaviors, the better prepared they will be to meet their newborn's needs and to form a positive attachment with their child. (See the Promote Developmentally Supportive Care section later in this exemplar.)

> **SAFETY ALERT**
> After observing an neonate's pattern of behavior and responses, especially the sleep–wake states, the nurse uses the time when the baby is alert and best able to attend to help parents learn about and provide newborn care.

Nutritional and Fluid Requirements

Beginning feedings as soon as possible is extremely valuable in maintaining normal metabolism and lowering the possibility of such complications as hypoglycemia, hyperbilirubinemia, and azotemia. However, the preterm neonate is at risk for complications that may develop because of immaturity of the digestive system. Advancement of feedings should occur only as the neonate demonstrates tolerance of enteral feedings. Clinical signs of feeding intolerance or illness dictate discontinuing or holding the advancement of feedings.

NUTRITIONAL REQUIREMENTS Oral (enteral) caloric intake necessary for growth in a healthy preterm newborn is 95–130 kcal/kg per day (Blackburn, 2013). In addition to these relatively high caloric needs, the preterm neonate requires more protein than the full-term neonate. To meet these needs, many institutions use breast milk or special preterm formulas.

Whether breast milk or formula is used, feeding regimens are established on the basis of the neonate's weight and estimated stomach capacity. Initial formula feedings are gradually increased as the neonate tolerates them. It may be necessary to supplement oral feedings with parenteral fluids to maintain adequate hydration and caloric intake until the baby is on full oral feedings. Preterm neonates who cannot tolerate any oral (enteral) feedings are given nutrition by total parenteral nutrition.

In addition to a higher calorie and protein formula, preterm neonates should receive supplemental multivitamins, including vitamins A, D, and E, as well as iron and trace minerals. A diet high in polyunsaturated fats, which preterm neonates tolerate best, increases the requirement for vitamin E. Preterm neonates who are fed iron-fortified formulas have higher red cell hemolysis and lower vitamin E concentrations and thus require additional vitamin E. Preterm formulas also need to contain medium-chain triglycerides and additional amino acids, such as cysteine, as well as calcium, phosphorus, and vitamin D supplements to increase mineralization of bones. Rickets and significant bone demineralization have

been documented in very-low-birth-weight neonates and otherwise healthy preterm neonates.

Nutritional intake is considered to be adequate when there is consistent weight gain of 20–30 g/day. Initially, no weight gain may be noted for several days, but total weight loss should not exceed 15% of the total birth weight or more than 1%–2% per day. Some institutions add the criteria of head circumference growth and increase in body length of 1 cm (0.4 in.) per week once the newborn is stable.

METHODS OF FEEDING The preterm infant is fed by various methods, depending on the neonate's gestational age, health and physical condition, and neurological status. The three most common oral feeding methods are bottle, breast, and gavage. In some cases, total parenteral nutrition is used.

Bottle Feeding Preterm neonates who have a coordinated and rhythmic suck–swallow–breathing pattern are usually between 32 and 34 weeks of postconceptual age and may be fed by bottle. Oral readiness to feed is best described by the following behaviors: remaining engaged in the feeding, organizing oral–motor functioning, coordinating the suck–swallow–breath skill, and maintaining physiological stability (Thomas, 2007).

Those premature neonates who root when their cheek is stroked and actively search for the nipple are neurodevelopmentally ready to initiate oral feeding. To avoid excessive expenditure of energy, a soft, yellow, single-hole nipple is generally used (milk flow is less rapid). The neonate is fed in a semisitting position and burped gently after each 0.5–1 oz. The feeding should take no longer than 30 minutes (nippling requires more energy than other methods). Premature neonates who are progressing from gavage feedings to bottle feeding should start with one session of bottle feeding a day and have the number of times per day a bottle is given slowly increase until the baby tolerates all feedings from a bottle.

In assessing the premature neonate's readiness for feeding, the nurse assesses the neonate's ability to suck. Sucking may be affected by age, asphyxia, sepsis, intraventricular hemorrhage, or other neurological insult. Before initiating nipple feeding, the nurse observes for signs of stress, such as tachypnea (>60 respirations/minute), respiratory distress, or hypothermia, which may increase the risk of aspiration. During the feeding, the nurse observes the neonate for signs of feeding difficulty (tachypnea, cyanosis, bradycardia, lethargy, or uncoordinated suck and swallow). Difficulty in bottle feeding is often associated with a milk bolus that is too large for the neonate's oral cavity, which can lead to aspiration. Demand feeding protocols, based on the neonate's hunger cues, should be considered for a growing premature neonate only when there is sufficient caloric intake to promote consistent weight gain (Kenner & Lott, 2007).

Breastfeeding Mothers who wish to breastfeed their preterm neonates are given the opportunity to put the baby to the breast as soon as the baby has demonstrated a coordinated suck and swallow reflex, is showing consistent weight gain, and can control body temperature outside of the incubator, regardless of weight. Preterm neonates tolerate breastfeeding with higher transcutaneous oxygen pressures and better maintenance of body temperature than during bottle feeding. Besides breast milk's many benefits for the neonate, breastfeeding allows the mother to contribute actively to the baby's well-being. The nurse should encourage mothers to breastfeed if they choose to do so. It is important for the nurse to be aware of both the advantages of breastfeeding and the possible disadvantages of breast milk as the sole source of food for the preterm neonate. Even if the neonate cannot be put to the breast, mothers can pump their breasts, and the breast milk can be given via gavage. Use of the double-pumping system produces higher levels of prolactin than are obtained using sequential pumping of the breasts.

By initiating skin-to-skin holding of premature neonates in the early intensive care phase, mothers can significantly increase milk volume, thereby overcoming lactation problems (Turnage-Carrier, 2010). The neonate is placed at the mother's breast. It has been suggested that the football hold is a convenient position for breastfeeding preterm babies. Feeding may take up to 45 minutes, and babies should be burped as they alternate breasts. The length of feeding time is monitored so that the preterm neonate does not burn too many calories.

The nurse should coordinate a flexible feeding schedule so that babies can nurse during alert times and be allowed to set their own pace. Feedings should be on demand, but a maximum number of hours between feedings should be set. A similar regimen should be used for the baby who is progressing from gavage feeding to breastfeeding. The mother begins with one feeding at the breast and then gradually increases the number of times during the day that the baby breastfeeds. When breastfeeding is not possible because the neonate is too small or too weak to suck at the breast, an option for the mother may be to express her breast milk into a cup. The milk touches the neonate's lips and is lapped by the protruding motions of the tongue.

> **SAFETY ALERT**
> For an otherwise healthy, growing premature neonate who is receiving total enteral intake and who has started to experience apnea and bradycardia, one differential diagnosis to think about is reflux rather than sepsis, although sepsis may need to be ruled out.

Gavage Feeding   The gavage feeding method is used with preterm neonates (<32–34 weeks of gestation) who lack or have a poorly coordinated suck-and-swallow reflex or who are ill and ventilator dependent. Gavage feeding may be used as an adjunct to nipple feeding if the neonate tires easily. It may also be used as an alternative if a neonate is losing weight because of the energy expenditure required for nippling.

Gavage feedings are administered by either the nasogastric or orogastric route and by intermittent bolus or continuous drip method. Bolus feedings may be preferred, because these are thought to be more like normal feedings than the continuous feeding method and may enhance the release of certain GI hormones necessary for development of gastrointestinal tissues (Kenner & Lott, 2007). Currently, no conclusive studies support one method over the other. In common practice, bolus feedings are usually initiated, but if intolerance occurs, then the feedings are changed to continuous.

Early initiation of **minimal enteral nutrition** via gavage is now advocated as a supplement to parenteral nutrition. Minimal enteral nutrition refers to small-volume feedings of formula or human milk (usually <24 mL/kg per day), which are designed to "prime" the premature neonate's intestinal tract, thereby stimulating many of its hormonal and enzymatic functions (AAP & ACOG, 2013; Kenner & Lott, 2007). Benefits of early feeding (as early as within the first 24–72 hours of life) include the following (Kenner & Lott, 2007):

- No increased incidence of NEC
- Fewer days on total parenteral nutrition, thereby decreasing the incidence of cholestatic jaundice
- Increased weight gain
- Increased muscle maturation of the GI function, which can lead to improved feeding tolerance
- Lower risk of osteopenia
- Possible decrease in the total number of hospital days in the neonatal intensive care unit (NICU).

> **SAFETY ALERT**
> Orogastric gavage catheter placement is preferable to nasogastric, because most neonates are obligatory nose breathers. If nasogastric is used, a #5 French catheter should be used to minimize airway obstruction.

Total Parenteral Nutrition   Total parenteral nutrition is used in situations that do not allow the neonate to be fed through the GI tract. This method provides complete nutrition to the neonate intravenously and uses hyperalimentation to provide calories, vitamins, minerals, protein, and glucose, and uses intra-lipids to provide essential fatty acids.

FLUID REQUIREMENTS   The calculation of fluid requirements must take into account the neonate's weight and postnatal age. Recommendations for fluid therapy in the preterm neonate are approximately 80–100 mL/kg per day for the first day, 100–120 mL/kg per day for the second day, and 120–150 mL/kg per day by the third day of life. These amounts may be increased up to 200 mL/kg per day if the neonate is very small, receiving phototherapy, or under a radiant warmer because of the increased insensible water losses. Fluid losses can be minimized through the use of heat shields and added humidification in the incubator. Daily weights (and, sometimes, twice-a-day weights) are the best indicator of fluid status in the preterm neonate. The expected weight loss during the first 3–5 days of life in a preterm neonate is 15%–20% of birth weight. Premature neonates who are being treated for complications such as respiratory distress syndrome or patent ductus arteriosus may be on diuretics that can influence their fluid requirements.

Long-Term Needs

The care of preterm neonates and their families does not stop on discharge from the nursery. Follow-up care is extremely important: Many developmental problems are not noted until an infant is older and begins to demonstrate motor delays or sensory disability.

Within the first year of life, low-birth-weight preterm infants face higher mortality rates than term infants. Causes of death include sudden infant death syndrome—which occurs about five times more frequently in the preterm baby—respiratory infections, and neurological defects. Morbidity is also much higher among preterm babies, those weighing less than 1,500 g being at the highest risk for long-term complications.

The most common long-term needs observed in preterm neonates include the following:

- *Retinopathy of prematurity (ROP).* Premature newborns are particularly susceptible to characteristic retinal changes, known as ROP, which can result in visual impairment. The premature newborn's retina does not have all of the blood vessels the term newborn's has. As the blood vessels fill in, they may grow abnormally with the development of fibrous tissue that can contract and scar, resulting in retinal detachment. The disease is now viewed as multifactorial in origin. Increased survival of very-low-birth-weight babies may be the most important factor in the increased incidence of ROP. The acute stages of ROP may be treated with laser photocoagulation and cryotherapy. Most acute changes with ROP regress spontaneously with no long-term visual impairment.

- *Bronchopulmonary dysplasia (BPD).* Long-term lung disease is a result of damage to the alveolar epithelium secondary to positive-pressure ventilator therapy and a high oxygen concentration. These babies have long-term dependence on oxygen therapy and an increased incidence of respiratory infection during their first few years of life.

- *Speech defects.* The most frequently observed speech defects involve delayed development of receptive and expressive ability that may persist into the school-age years.

- *Neurological defects.* The most common neurological defects include cerebral palsy (CP), hydrocephalus, seizure disorders, lower IQ, and learning disabilities. In the absence of major neurological defects, the socioeconomic climate and family support systems are extremely important influences on the child's eventual school performance. Families should be reminded that risk does not equal injury, injury does not equal damage, and description of damage does not allow a precise prediction about recovery or outcome.

- *Auditory defects.* Preterm babies have a 1%–4% incidence of moderate to profound hearing loss and should have a formal audiological exam before discharge and at 3–6 months (corrected age). Tests currently used to measure hearing functions of the newborn are the evoked otoacoustic emissions or the automated auditory brain response test. Any infant with repeated abnormal results should be referred to speech-and-language specialists.

When assessing the baby's abilities and disabilities, parents must understand that developmental progress must be evaluated on the basis of chronological age from the expected date of birth, not from the actual date of birth (corrected age). In addition, the parents need the consistent support of healthcare professionals in the long-term management of their child. Many new and ongoing concerns arise as the former premature neonate grows and develops; the goal is to promote the highest quality of life possible.

Many hospitals and NICUs provide referrals for parents of premature babies to local child health service coordination and early intervention service programs. Early intervention services for infants and toddlers are mandated under Part C of the Individuals with Disabilities in Education Act. Nurses working with these families, either in the NICU or hospital setting or in a pediatric setting, should be aware of their agency's referral process or know about services available in their area.

▶ ALTERATIONS

The goals of medical and nursing care are to meet the preterm neonate's growth and development needs and to anticipate and manage the complications associated with prematurity. The most common complications associated with prematurity are as follows:

1. *Apnea of prematurity.* **Apnea of prematurity** refers to cessation of breathing for 20 seconds or longer, or for less than 20 seconds when associated with cyanosis, pallor, and bradycardia. Apnea is a common problem in the preterm neonate less than 36 weeks' gestation, presenting between day 2 and day 7 of life. The etiology of apnea is multifactorial, but it is thought to be primarily a result of neuronal immaturity. This factor contributes to the preterm neonate's irregular breathing patterns. Other causes of apnea are obstructive apnea and gastroesophageal reflux. Obstructive apnea can occur when cessation of airflow is associated with blockage of the upper airway (resulting from a small airway diameter, increased pharyngeal secretions, or altered body alignment and positioning). Gastroesophageal reflux is defined as a movement of gastric contents into the lower esophagus caused by poor esophageal sphincter tone, in turn causing laryngospasm, which leads to bradycardia and apnea. Apnea of prematurity is then a diagnosis of exclusion.

2. *Patent ductus arteriosus (PDA).* The ductus arteriosus fails to close because of decreased pulmonary arteriole musculature and hypoxemia. Symptomatic PDA is often seen around the time when premature neonates are recovering from respiratory distress syndrome. PDA often prolongs the course of illness in a preterm newborn and leads to chronic pulmonary dysfunction.

> ### SAFETY ALERT
> A growing premature neonate who is showing clinical signs of worsening respiratory status (i.e., increased oxygen needs or increased ventilatory settings), acidosis, and hypotension may be exhibiting signs and symptoms of a PDA.

3. *Respiratory distress syndrome.* Respiratory distress results from inadequate surfactant production.

4. *Intraventricular hemorrhage.* Intraventricular hemorrhage is the most common type of intracranial hemorrhage in small preterm neonates, especially those weighing less than 1,500 g or of those less than 34 weeks of gestation. Up to 34 weeks, the preterm neonate's brain ventricles are lined by the germinal matrix, which is highly susceptible to hypoxic events, such as respiratory distress, birth trauma, and birth asphyxia. The germinal matrix is highly vascular, and these blood vessels rupture in the presence of hypoxia.

5. *Anemia of prematurity.* The preterm neonate is at risk for anemia because of the rapid rate of growth required, shorter red blood cell life, excessive blood sampling, decreased iron stores, and deficiency of vitamin E. The hemoglobin usually reaches its lowest level by 3–12 weeks and remains low for 3–6 months.

NURSING PROCESS

Subtle signs and symptoms can indicate a change in a neonate's condition that may require rapid interventions to prevent life-long complications. Nurses who want to care for premature neonates must obtain postgraduation specialized education offered by the hospital.

Assessment

The nurse needs to assess the physical characteristics and gestational age of the preterm newborn accurately. This allows the healthcare team to anticipate the special needs and problems of the baby.

Determining gestational age in preterm newborns requires knowledge and experience in administering gestational assessment tools. The tool used should be specific, reliable, and valid.

Physical characteristics vary greatly depending on gestational age, but the following characteristics are frequently present:

- *Color* is usually pink or ruddy but may show acrocyanosis. (Cyanosis, jaundice, and pallor are abnormal and should be noted.)
- *Skin* is reddened and translucent, blood vessels are readily apparent, and there is little subcutaneous fat.
- *Lanugo* is plentiful and widely distributed.
- *Head size* appears large in relation to the body.
- *Skull bones* are pliable; fontanelle is smooth and flat.
- *Ears* have minimal cartilage and are pliable, folded over.
- *Nails* are soft and short.
- *Testes* may not be descended and scrotum nonrugated.
- *Clitoris and labia minora* are prominent.
- *Resting position* is flaccid, frog-like.
- *Cry* is weak and feeble.
- *Reflexes* (sucking, swallowing, and gag) are poor.
- *Activity* consists of jerky, generalized movements. (Seizure activity is abnormal.)

Diagnosis

Nursing diagnoses that may apply to the preterm newborn include the following:

- *Gas Exchange, Impaired* related to immature pulmonary vasculature and inadequate surfactant production

- *Breathing Pattern, Ineffective* related to immature central nervous system
- *Tissue Perfusion: Cardiac, Risk for Decreased* related to hypotension related to decreased tissue perfusion secondary to PDA
- *Tissue Perfusion: Peripheral, Risk for Ineffective* related to anemia of prematurity
- *Nutrition, Imbalanced: Less than Body Requirements* related to weak suck-and-swallow reflexes and decreased ability to absorb nutrients
- *Thermoregulation, Ineffective* related to hypothermia secondary to decreased glycogen and brown fat stores
- *Fluid Volume: Deficient* related to high insensible water losses and inability of kidneys to concentrate urine
- *Coping: Family, Compromised* related to anger or guilt at having given birth to a premature baby.

(NANDA-I © 2015)

Planning

Important goals of nursing care for the premature neonate often include the following:

- The neonate's oxygenation and normal breathing patterns will be promoted.
- The neonate's weight gain and normal growth will be promoted.
- The neonate's developmental needs will be supported.
- The neonate's parents will be educated to provide care when discharged.
- The nurse will support the neonate's parents and suggest strategies to reduce parental anxiety.

Implementation

Priorities for care of the premature neonate are many. Maintenance of respiratory function, a neutral thermal environment, fluid and electrolyte status, and adequate nutrition are essential to giving the neonate the greatest chance for healthy growth and development. Prevention of infection and of fatigue during feeding is also important, as are promoting parent–infant attachment and developmentally supportive care and preparing for home care.

Maintain Respiratory Function

Premature newborns are at increased risk for respiratory obstruction because their bronchi and trachea are so narrow that mucus can obstruct the airway. The nurse must maintain patency through judicious suctioning, but only on an as-needed basis.

Positioning can also affect respiratory function. If the baby is in the supine position, the nurse should slightly elevate the head to maintain the airway, being careful to avoid hyperextension of the neck, which may cause the trachea to collapse. Also, because the newborn has weak neck muscles and cannot control head movement, place a small roll under the newborn's shoulders to maintain this head position. The prone position splints the chest wall and decreases the amount of respiratory effort used to move the chest wall, facilitating chest expansion and improving air entry and oxygenation. Weak or absent cough or gag reflexes increase the chance of aspiration in the premature newborn. The nurse should ensure that the newborn's position facilitates drainage of mucus or regurgitated formula.

The nurse monitors heart and respiratory rates with cardio-respiratory monitors and observes the newborn to identify alterations in cardiopulmonary status. Signs of respiratory distress include the following:

- Cyanosis (serious sign when generalized)
- Tachypnea (sustained respiratory rate >60 breaths/minute after first 4 hours of life)
- Retractions
- Expiratory grunting
- Nasal flaring
- Apneic episodes
- Presence of rales or rhonchi on auscultation
- Diminished air entry.

If respiratory distress occurs, the nurse administers oxygen per physician or nurse practitioner orders to relieve hypoxemia. If hypoxemia is not treated immediately, it may result in PDA or metabolic acidosis. If oxygen is administered to the newborn, the nurse monitors the oxygen concentration with a pulse oximeter and blood gas analysis. Periodic arterial blood gas sampling to monitor oxygen concentration in the baby's blood is essential because hyperoxemia may lead to ROP and other complications.

The nurse also needs to consider respiratory function before and during feedings. To prevent aspiration and increased energy expenditure and oxygen consumption, the nurse must ensure that the newborn's gag and suck reflexes are intact before starting oral feedings.

Maintain a Neutral Thermal Environment

Providing a neutral thermal environment minimizes the oxygen consumption required to maintain a normal core temperature; it also prevents cold stress and facilitates growth by decreasing the calories needed to maintain body temperature. The preterm newborn's small brown fat stores and immature central nervous system provide poor temperature control. A small premature neonate (>1,200 g) can lose 80 kcal/kg per day through radiation of body heat. To minimize heat loss and temperature instability for preterm and low-birth-weight newborns, the nurse should do the following:

- Monitor ambient temperature of the room where the newborn is kept.
- Allow kangaroo skin-to-skin contact between the parents and newborn to maintain warmth and foster security.
- Warm and humidify oxygen to minimize evaporative heat loss and decrease oxygen consumption.
- Place the baby in a double-walled incubator, or use a Plexiglas heat shield over small preterm neonates in single-walled incubators, to avoid radiative heat losses. Some institutions use radiant warmers and plastic wrap over the baby and pipe in humidity (swamping). Do not use Plexiglas shields on radiant warmer beds, however, because they block the infrared heat.
- Avoid placing the baby on cold surfaces, such as metal treatment tables and cold x-ray plates (conductive heat loss). Pad cold surfaces with diapers, and use radiant warmers during procedures. Place the preterm newborn on prewarmed mattresses, and warm hands before handling the baby to prevent heat transfer via conduction.

- Use warmed ambient humidity. Humidity can decrease insensible and transdermal water loss, especially in very-low-birth-weight newborns (Jones et al., 2011).
- Keep the newborn's skin dry (evaporative heat loss), and place a cap on the baby's head. The head makes up 25% of the total body size.
- Keep radiant warmers, incubators, and cribs away from windows or cold external walls (radiative heat loss) and out of drafts, which cause convection heat loss (conductive heat loss occurs when the newborn touches a cooler surface).
- Open incubator portholes and doors only when necessary, and use plastic sleeves on portholes to decrease convective heat loss.
- Use a skin probe to monitor the baby's skin temperature. Correlate ambient temperatures with the skin probe in the incubator using the servocontrol rather than the manual mode. The temperature should be 36°–37°C (96.8°–98.6°F). Temperature fluctuations indicate hypothermia or hyperthermia. Be careful not to place skin temperature probes over bony prominences; areas of brown fat; poorly vasoreactive areas, such as extremities; or excoriated areas.
- Warm formula or stored breast milk before feeding.
- Use a reflector patch over the skin temperature probe when using a radiant warmer bed so that the probe does not sense the higher infrared temperature as the baby's skin temperature and, therefore, decrease the heater output.

Once preterm newborns are medically stable, they can be clothed with a double-thickness cap, cotton shirt, and diaper and, if possible, swaddled in a blanket. The nurse begins the process of weaning to a crib when the premature newborn is medically stable, does not require assisted ventilation, weighs approximately 1,500–2,000 g (depending on facility policy), has had 5 days of consistent weight gain, and is taking oral feedings, and when apnea and bradycardia episodes have stabilized. The nurse should be familiar with the individual institution's protocol for weaning preterm babies to a crib.

Maintain Fluid and Electrolyte Status

The nurse maintains hydration by providing adequate fluid intake based on the newborn's weight, gestational age, chronological age, and volume of sensible and insensible water losses. Adequate fluid intake should compensate for increased insensible losses and the amount needed for renal excretion of metabolic products. Insensible water losses can be minimized by providing high ambient humidity, humidifying oxygen, using heat shields, covering the skin with plastic wrap, and placing the newborn in a double-walled incubator.

The nurse evaluates the hydration status of the baby by assessing and recording signs of dehydration. Signs of dehydration include the following:

- Sunken fontanelle
- Loss of weight
- Poor skin turgor (skin returns to position slowly when squeezed gently)
- Dry oral mucous membranes
- Decreased urine output
- Increased specific gravity (>1.013).

The nurse must also identify signs of overhydration by observing the newborn for edema or excessive weight gain and by comparing urine output with fluid intake.

The nurse weighs the preterm newborn at least once daily at the same time each day. *Weight change is one of the most sensitive indicators of fluid balance.* Weighing diapers is also important for accurate input and output measurement (1 mL = 1 g). A comparison of intake and output measurements over an 8- or 24-hour period provides important information about renal function and fluid balance. Assessment of patterns, and whether they show a net gain or loss over several days, is also essential to fluid management. In addition, the nurse monitors blood serum levels and pH to evaluate for electrolyte imbalances.

Accurate hourly intake calculations are needed when administering intravenous (IV) fluids. Because the preterm newborn is unable to excrete excess fluid, it is essential for the nurse to maintain the correct amount of IV fluid to prevent overload. Accuracy can be ensured by using neonatal or pediatric infusion pumps. To prevent electrolyte imbalance and dehydration, the nurse takes care to give the correct IV solutions as well as the correct volumes and concentrations of formulas. Urine-specific gravity and pH are obtained periodically. Urine osmolality provides an indication of hydration, although this factor must be correlated with other assessments (e.g., serum sodium). Hydration is considered to be adequate when the urine output is 1–3 mL/kg per hour.

Provide Adequate Nutrition and Prevent Fatigue During Feeding

The preterm newborn's feeding abilities and health status determine the feeding method. Both nipple and gavage methods are initially supplemented with IV therapy until oral intake is sufficient to support growth (110–130 kcal/kg per day). Early, small-volume enteral feedings, called minimal enteral nutrition via gavage, have proven to be beneficial for the very-low-birth-weight newborn (see Gavage Feeding earlier in this exemplar). GI priming with these small-volume feedings is not intended to contribute to the total nutritional intake but, rather, to enhance gut metabolism. Trophic feedings may also help encourage earlier advancement to full feedings, thereby decreasing the development of necrotizing enterocolitis and the complications of parenteral nutrition. Formula or breast milk (with or without fortifiers to increase caloric content) is incorporated into the feedings slowly. This is done to avoid overtaxing the digestive capacity of the preterm newborn. The nurse should carefully watch for any signs of feeding intolerance, including the following:

- Increasing gastric residuals
- Abdominal distention (measured routinely before feedings) with visible bowel loops
- Guaiac-positive stools (occult blood in stools)
- Lactose in stools (reducing substance in the stools)
- Vomiting
- Diarrhea
- Water-loss stools.

Before each feeding, the nurse measures abdominal girth and auscultates the abdomen to determine the presence and quality of bowel sounds. Such assessments permit early detection of abdominal distention, visible bowel loops, and decreased peristaltic activity, which may indicate necrotizing enterocolitis or paralytic ileus. The nurse also checks for residual formula in the stomach before feeding when the newborn is fed by gavage. This procedure also can be performed when the nipple-fed newborn presents with abdominal distention. The presence of increasing residual formula is an indication of intolerance to the type or amount of feeding or to the increase in amount of feeding.

Preterm newborns who are ill or who fatigue easily with nipple feedings are usually fed by gavage. The neonate is essentially passive with these methods, thus conserving energy and calories. As the baby matures, gavage feedings are replaced with nipple (breast or formula) feedings to assist in strengthening the sucking reflex and in meeting the newborn's oral and emotional needs. While their nutrition may come from gavage feedings, nonnutritive sucking is important to the preterm newborn's development and should be encouraged. Signs that indicate readiness for oral feedings include a strong gag reflex, presence of nonnutritive sucking, and rooting behavior. Both low-birth-weight and preterm newborns nipple-feed more effectively in a quiet state. The nurse establishes a gradual nipple-feeding program, such as one nipple feeding per day, then one nipple feeding per shift, and then a nipple feeding every other feeding. The nurse should weigh the baby daily, because a small weight loss often occurs when nipple feedings are started. After feedings, the nurse places the baby on the right side (with support to maintain this position) or on the abdomen. These positions facilitate gastric emptying and decrease the chance of aspiration if regurgitation occurs. Gastroesophageal reflux is not uncommon in preterm newborns. Long-term gavage feeding may create nipple aversion that will require developmental occupational therapy interventions.

The nurse involves the parents in feeding their preterm baby. This is essential to the development of attachment between parents and baby. In addition, it increases parental knowledge about the care of their baby and helps them cope with the situation.

Prevent Infection

The nurse is responsible for minimizing the preterm newborn's exposure to pathogenic organisms. An immature immune system as well as thin and permeable skin make the preterm newborn susceptible to infection. Invasive procedures, techniques such as umbilical catheterization and mechanical ventilation, and prolonged hospitalization also place the neonate at greater risk for infection.

The practice of strict hand hygiene and use of separate equipment for each neonate help minimize the preterm newborn's exposure to infectious agents. Most nurseries have adopted the Centers for Disease Control and Prevention standard precautions of isolating every baby and the Joint Commission requirement that staff members have short-trimmed nails and no artificial nails. Staff members are required to complete a

2- to 3-minute scrub using an antibacterial solution, which inhibits growth of gram-positive cocci and gram-negative rod organisms. Other specific nursing interventions include limiting visitors, requiring visitors to wash their hands, maintaining strict aseptic practices when changing IV tubing and solutions (IV solutions and tubing should be changed every 24 hours or per agency protocols), administering parenteral fluids, and assisting with sterile procedures. Incubators and radiant warmers should be changed weekly. The nurse prevents pressure-area breakdown by changing the baby's position regularly, doing ROM exercises, and using water-bed pillows or an air mattress. To avoid skin tears, a protective, transparent covering can be applied over vulnerable joints; however, this method is used sparingly (Blackburn, 2013). Chemical skin preps and tape may cause skin trauma and should be avoided as much as possible.

If infection (sepsis) occurs in the preterm newborn, the nurse may be the first to identify its subtle clinical signs, such as lethargy and increased episodes of apnea and bradycardia. The nurse informs the healthcare provider of the findings immediately and implements the treatment plan per clinician orders in the presence of infection.

Promote Attachment

In some cases, preterm newborns are separated from their parents for prolonged periods after illness or complications that are detected in the first few hours or days following birth. This interrupts the bonding process, necessitating intervention to ensure successful attachment.

Nurses need to take measures to promote positive parental feelings toward the preterm newborn. They can give photographs of the baby to parents to take home. Photographs also may be given to the mother if she is in a different hospital or, if in the same hospital, is too ill to come to the nursery and visit. By placing the newborn's first name on the incubator as soon as it is known, nurses help the parents feel that their baby is a unique and special individual. A number of other interventions promote the bonding process, including the following:

■ Give parents a weekly card with the baby's footprint, weight, and length.
■ Give parents the telephone number of the nursery or intensive care unit and the names of staff members so that they have access to information about their baby at any time of the day or night.
■ Encourage visits from siblings and grandparents.

Early involvement in the care of and decisions about their newborn provides the parents with realistic expectations for their baby. The individual personality characteristics of the newborn and the parents influence the bonding and contribute to the interactive process for the family. By observing each baby's patterns of behavior and responses, especially sleep–wake states, the nurse can teach parents the optimal times for interacting with their babies. The parents and nurse can plan nursing care around the times when the baby is alert and best able to attend.

Parents need education to develop caregiving skills and to understand the premature baby's behavioral characteristics. The more knowledge parents have about the meaning of their baby's responses, behaviors, and cues for interaction, the better they will be able to meet their newborn's needs and form a positive attach-

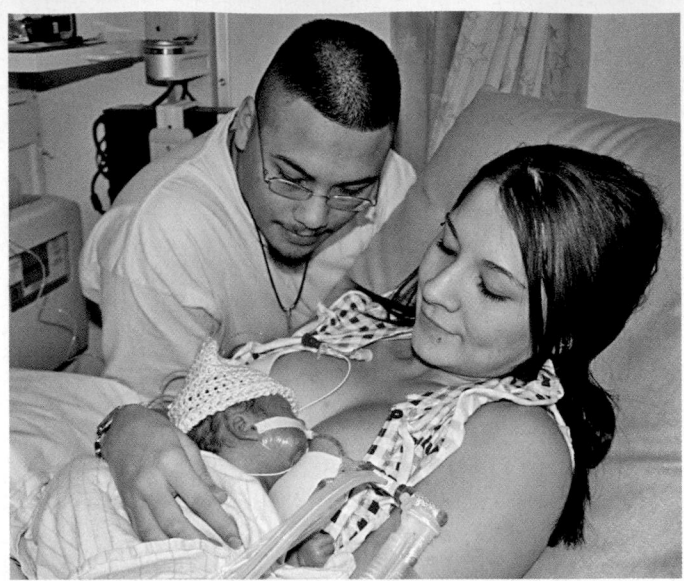

Figure 33–110 ● Kangaroo (skin-to-skin) care facilitates closeness and attachment between parents and their premature newborn.
Source: Carol Harrigan, RN, MSN, NNP-BC.

ment with their child. For parents who cannot stay with their preterm baby, the nurse should encourage their daily participation (if possible) as well as early and frequent visits. The nurse should provide opportunities for parents to touch, hold, talk to, and care for the baby. Skin-to-skin holding (kangaroo care) helps parents feel close to their small newborn (**Figure 33–110 ●**). Kangaroo care has been shown to improve sleep periods and parents' perception of their caregiving ability (Turnage-Carrier, 2010).

Some parents will progress easily to touching and cuddling their newborn; however, others will not. Parents need to know that their feelings are normal and that the progression of acquaintanceship can be slow. Rooming-in can provide another opportunity for the stable preterm newborn and family to get acquainted; it offers both privacy and readily available help.

Promote Developmentally Supportive Care

Prolonged separation and the NICU environment necessitate individualized baby sensory stimulation programs. The nurse plays a key role in determining the appropriate type and amount of visual, tactile, and auditory stimulation.

Some preterm newborns are not developmentally able to deal with more than one sensory input at a time. The Assessment of Preterm Infant Behavior (APIB) scale identifies individual preterm newborn behaviors according to five areas of development (Als et al., 1982). The preterm baby's behavioral reactions to stimulation are observed, and developmental interventions are then based on reducing detrimental environmental stimuli to the lowest possible level and providing appropriate opportunities for development (Turnage-Carrier, 2010).

Providing developmentally supportive, family-centered care improves the outcomes of the critically ill newborn. With this in mind, specially designed NICUs with the single-room care concept are being developed to minimize lighting and noise as well as to provide privacy for the parents of the convalescing newborn (Gibbins et al., 2008).

The NICU environment contains many detrimental stimuli that the nurse can help reduce. Simple actions that nurses can take include the following:

- If possible, replace alarms with lights to lower noise levels.
- Silence alarms quickly.
- Keep conversations away from newborns' bedsides.
- Use dimmer switches to shield newborns' eyes from bright lights.
- Place blankets over the top portion of each incubator.

Nursing care should also be planned to decrease the number of times the baby is disturbed. Signs (e.g., "Quiet Please") can be placed near the bedside to allow the baby some periods of uninterrupted sleep (Turnage-Carrier, 2010).

Some other suggested developmentally supportive interventions include the following:

- Facilitate handling by using containment measures when turning or moving the neonate or doing procedures such as suctioning. Use the hands to hold the neonate's arms and legs flexed close to the midline of the body. This helps stabilize the newborn's motor and physiological subsystems during stressful activities.
- Touch the preemie gently, and avoid sudden postural changes.
- Promote self-consoling and soothing activities, such as placing blanket rolls or approved manufactured devices next to the neonate's sides and against the feet to provide "nesting." Swaddle the preemie to maintain extremities in a flexed position while ensuring that the hands can reach the face. This permits the newborn to do hand-to-mouth activities, which can be consoling.
- Simulate the kinesthetic advantages of the intrauterine environment by using sheepskin and approved water beds. Water bed and pillow use has been reported to improve sleep and decrease motor activity as well as lead to more mature motor behavior, fewer state changes, and a decreased heart rate.
- Provide opportunities for nonnutritive sucking with a pacifier. This improves transcutaneous oxygen saturation; decreases body movements; improves sleep, especially after feedings; and increases weight gain.
- Provide objects for the preemie to grasp (e.g., a piece of blanket, oxygen tubing, or a finger) during caregiving. Grasping may comfort the baby.

The nurse teaches the parents how to read behavioral cues to help them move at their baby's own pace when providing stimulation. Parents are ideally equipped to meet the baby's need for stimulation. Stroking, rocking, cuddling, quiet singing, and talking to the baby can all be integral parts of the baby's care. Visual stimulation in the form of *en face* interaction with caregivers and mobiles is also important.

Kangaroo (skin-to-skin) care is becoming more prevalent in NICUs across the United States (see Figure 33–110). It was first practiced in Bogota, Colombia, in the early 1980s because of fear about the spread of infection by sharing incubators. Skin-to-skin care is defined as the practice of holding newborns skin-to-skin against their parents. The newborn is usually naked, except for a diaper, and is placed on his or her parent's bare chest. They are then both covered with a blanket. Benefits of skin-to-skin care as a developmental intervention include the following (Ludington, Morgan, & Abouelfettoh, 2008):

- Improved oxygenation, as evidenced by an increase in oxygen saturation levels
- Enhanced temperature regulation
- Decline in the episodes of apnea and bradycardia
- Increased periods of quiet sleep
- Stabilization of vital signs
- Positive interaction between parent and baby, which enhances attachment and bonding
- Increased growth parameters
- Early discharge.

Skin-to-skin care may be limited because of staff uneasiness when moving the neonate while attached to multiple IV lines, monitor leads, and a ventilator. The confines of the nursery may be another limiting factor.

Music therapy as a noninvasive auditory stimulus has been shown to be advantageous in full-term newborns but has not been well studied in the premature neonate (Loewy et al., 2012). The music used in NICUs primarily includes lullabies and soft acoustical pieces that are pleasant, soothing, and calming. Such music has been shown to affect newborn physiological responses, such as improving oxygenation and increasing weight gain. It also has behavioral effects, leading to enhanced parental bonding and increased intervals of nonnutritive sucking periods. Language development is also enhanced if the music is live and sung by the mother or another female, which is preferential to the newborn (Gardner & Goldson, 2011). However, the overall noise level in the NICU needs to be considered before including any extra auditory stimulation, including music therapy.

Massage and *gentle touch* have been practiced for many centuries. The types of stimulation include massage with stroking, gentle touch without stroking, and therapeutic touch or "hands-on" containment. Practitioners report such physiological benefits as stimulating blood and lymphatic flow, promoting weight gain in premature newborns, and regulating sleep patterns (Smith, 2012). Many emotional and behavioral benefits are also cited by practitioners. Classes are available to teach parents how to perform massage on their babies. Massage demonstrates compassion while increasing the parent's empathy and understanding of the baby. It helps parents learn to interpret their baby's behavioral cues, such as facial expression, various crying patterns, and other body language. At the same time, it helps newborns learn about their various body parts and boundaries and feel how those integrate into the whole. Therapeutic touch reduces motor activity and energy expenditure by the newborn and also promotes comfort.

Prepare for Home Care

Parents are often anxious when their premature newborn is transferred out of the NICU or is discharged home. Parents of preterm babies should receive the same postpartum teaching as any parent taking a new baby home. In preparing for discharge, the nurse encourages the parents to spend time caring directly for their baby. This familiarizes them with their baby's behavior patterns and helps them establish realistic expectations about the baby. Some hospitals have a special room near the nursery where parents can spend the night with their baby before discharge.

Discharge instruction includes breastfeeding and formula-feeding techniques, formula preparation, and vitamin administration. If the mother wishes to breastfeed, the nurse teaches her to pump her breasts to keep the milk flowing and provide milk even before discharge. The nurse gives information on bathing, diapering, hygiene, and normal elimination patterns and prepares the parents to expect changes in the color of the baby's stool, number of bowel movements, and timing of elimination when the baby is switched from formula-feeding to breastfeeding. This information can prevent unnecessary concern by the parents. The nurse also discusses normal growth and development patterns, reflexes, and activity for preterm newborns. In these discussions, the nurse should emphasize ways to promote bonding behaviors and deal with newborn crying. Caring for the preemie with complications, preventing infections, recognizing signs of a sick baby, and the need for continued medical follow-up are other key issues.

Families with preterm newborns usually do not need to be referred to community agencies, such as visiting nurse assistance. However, referral may be necessary if the preemie has severe congenital abnormalities, feeding problems, or complications with infections or respiratory problems, or if the parents seem unable to cope with an at-risk baby. Parents of preterm babies can benefit from meeting with others in a similar situation to share common experiences and concerns. Nurses should refer parents to support groups sponsored by the hospital or by others in the community and make connections for parents with early education intervention centers.

Preterm and low-birth-weight babies are at greater risk of increased morbidity from vaccine-preventable diseases (AAP & ACOG, 2013). The optimal timing to initiate hepatitis B therapy in preterm newborns weighing less than 2,000 g whose mothers are hepatitis B surface antigen negative has not been determined. Preterm newborns who weigh less than 2,000 g and are medically stable and thriving do show consistently high rates of seroconversion following the first dose of hepatitis B vaccine, even when the first dose is given as early as 1 month after birth (AAP & ACOG, 2013). The medically stable preterm baby and low-birth-weight newborns should receive full doses of diphtheria, tetanus, acellular pertussis, *Haemophilus influenzae* type b, poliovirus, and pneumococcal conjugate vaccines at a chronological age consistent with the schedule recommended for full-term infants (AAP & ACOG, 2013). The influenza vaccine should be administered at 6 months of age before the beginning of and during the influenza season. Palivizumab for respiratory syncytial virus (RSV) should be administered during the local RSV season and before hospital discharge to preterm newborns born at less than 35 weeks of gestation as well as to those with bronchopulmonary dysplasia or congenital heart disease (AAP & ACOG, 2013). Immunoprophylaxis should be continued on a monthly basis until the local RSV season ends.

Evaluation

Expected outcomes of nursing care include the following:

- The preterm newborn is free of respiratory distress and establishes effective respiratory function.
- The preterm newborn gains weight and shows no signs of fatigue or aspiration during feedings.
- The preterm newborn demonstrates a serial head circumference growth rate of 1 cm (0.4 in.) per week.
- The parents are able to verbalize their feelings of anger and guilt about the birth of a preterm baby and show attachment behavior, such as frequent visits and growing confidence in their participatory care activities.

NURSING CARE PLAN   A Premature Newborn

Baby Boy Johnson was born 12 weeks early at 28 weeks of gestation to Dennis and Alaina Johnson. He is their first child. The NICU nurse received the baby from the obstetrician after he was delivered vaginally. Apgar scoring was 5 at 1 minute, 5 at 5 minutes, and 4 at 10 minutes. He had a weak cry and was dusky and floppy, with an initial heart rate of greater than 100 bpm. During resuscitation, the nurse provided blow-by oxygen. When his oxygenation status not only failed to improve but dropped, indicating that resuscitation was not effective, the nurse practitioner inserted an oral endotracheal tube, and oxygen was administered by bagging. He was transported to the NICU in a warm isolette where he was admitted, placed on a ventilator, and had an umbilical artery catheter placed.

His parents come to see him when his mother is moved from the labor area to her room on the postpartum unit. Their first question to the nurse is "Is he okay?" Their next question is "When will he be able to come home?" The nurse encourages his parents to touch him and talk to him before they leave the nursery.

ASSESSMENT

- Vital signs 36°C (96.7°F) axillary; pulse 172 bpm; respiration 68/min; BP 42/24 mmHg
- Endotracheal tube taped in place to ventilator set to deliver 30 breaths/minute, with 4 mmHg of positive end-expiratory pressure
- Color pink with acrocyanosis
- Soft murmur audible in left midaxillary area
- Hypoactive bowel sounds in all quadrants
- Has not voided or stooled yet

DIAGNOSES

- *Airway Clearance, Ineffective* secondary to prematurity
- *Attachment, Risk for Impaired*
- *Body Temperature: Imbalanced, Risk for*
- *Gas Exchange, Impaired*

(NANDA-I © 2015)

PLANNING

- The newborn will maintain adequate gas exchange to meet tissue requirements.
- The newborn will maintain a clear airway to promote oxygenation.
- The parents will bond with the newborn and recognize the characteristics of their infant.
- The newborn will receive adequate nutrition and fluid to promote growth.

NURSING CARE PLAN — A Premature Newborn (continued)

IMPLEMENTATION

- Suction endotracheal tube as needed when secretions are heard in endotracheal tube.
- Monitor arterial blood gas studies to determine adequate gas exchange.
- Assist with surfactant administration as ordered to reduce alveolar collapse on expiration.
- Monitor daily weights.
- Monitor urine output and kidney function by testing urine for pH and specific gravity.
- Encourage parents to visit as often as possible, and point out the newborn's characteristics to help parents focus on the baby instead of the medical equipment.
- Assist parents to hold their baby, and offer the option of skin-to-skin (kangaroo) care to promote attachment.

- Monitor cardiorespiratory and oxygen saturation continuously. Change pulse oximeter location frequently (at least every 2 hours) to reduce the risk of altered skin integrity.
- Avoid use of tape to reduce altered skin integrity.
- Promote development by offering a pacifier for the newborn to suck on.
- Provide periods of reduced stimulation to promote rest and comfort.
- Maintain neonate in a neutral thermal environment, either on a radiant warmer or a heated isolette, until he is able to maintain a normal temperature independently.
- Monitor vital signs at a minimum of every 4 hours.

EVALUATION

After administration of surfactant, Baby Boy Johnson is extubated, placed on CPAP for 2 days, and then weaned to nasal cannula. Feedings are initiated via continuous gavage feedings. Once feedings are tolerated, he is changed to every-3-hour feedings. His murmur is diagnosed as a patent ductus arteriosus (PDA), and indomethacin is administered, which successfully closes the PDA. He begins to have occasional apneic episodes and is placed on caffeine every 12 hours.

Within 4 weeks, he is showing steady weight gain and is moved to the low-risk NICU. His parents begin participating more in providing care, such as bathing and feeding him, and he is discharged at 12 weeks of age.

CRITICAL THINKING

1. How would you respond to the parents when they ask when the baby is likely to come home?
2. How can you maintain the neonate's temperature while he is being held by his parents?
3. If the neonate weighs 900 g, what are his fluid and caloric needs per day?

REVIEW Prematurity

RELATE Link the Concepts and Exemplars

Linking the exemplar of prematurity to the concept of grief and loss:

1. What factors might induce feelings of loss for the parents of a premature newborn, even if the newborn is doing well?
2. What nursing interventions would you implement to help the parents who are feeling grief and loss over the birth of their premature newborn?

Linking the exemplar of prematurity with the concept of development:

3. What developmental needs does a premature newborn have?
4. What nursing care would you provide the premature newborn in order to promote development?

READY Go to Companion Skills Manual

REFER Go to Pearson Nursing Student Resources
nursing.pearsonhighered.com

- Additional review materials

REFLECT Case Study

Jessica Marshall, 15 years old, delivers a baby girl at 32 weeks of gestation. Jessica sees her baby briefly in the delivery room before the newborn is transported to the NICU. Jessica names the baby Shamika, after her best friend. On the way from the labor and delivery recovery room, the nurse brings Jessica to the nursery to see the baby, who is under an oxygen hood with an IV through her umbilicus and cardiac monitor leads on her chest. When Jessica sees her baby, she begins to cry and says, "She's so small and looks so sick. It's all my fault!" The nurse caring for Shamika points out the baby's beautiful curly hair, long fingers, and aquiline nose. Jessica stops crying and says, "Oh, you're right. Look how beautiful she is—and so perfect." Shamika's nurse takes Jessica to her new room, gives her some information about premature babies to read, and encourages her to come back to visit Shamika as soon as she feels up to it.

1. When assigned to care for Shamika, what nursing diagnoses would you consider to be the greatest priority regarding this family?
2. How would you help Jessica bond with her premature newborn?
3. What risks does this premature newborn face as the result of being born to an adolescent mother?

REFERENCES

Academy of Breastfeeding Medicine Protocol Committee. (2010). ABM clinical protocol No. 22: Guidelines for management of jaundice in the breastfeeding infant equal to or greater than 35 weeks' gestation. *Breastfeeding Medicine, 5*(2), 87–93.

Agency for Toxic Substance and Disease Registry (ATSDR). (2013). *Safeguarding communities from chemical exposure.* Retrieved from http://www.atsdr.cdc.gov/docs/apha-atsdr_book.pdf.

Albrecht, S. A., Maloni, J. A., Thomas, K. K., Jones, R., Halleran, J., & Osborne, J. (2004). Smoking cessation for pregnant women who smoke: Scientific basis for practice: AWHONN's SUCCESS Project. *Journal of Obstetric, Gynecologic, and Neonatal Nursing, 33*(3), 298–305.

Alcorn, K. L., O'Donovan, A., Patrick, J. L., Creedy, D., & Devilly, G. J. (2010). A prospective longitudinal study of the prevalence of PTSD resulting from childbirth events. *Psychological Medicine, 40*(11), 1849–1859.

Algert, C. S., Morris, J. M., Simpson, J. M., Ford, J. B., & Roberts, C. L. (2008). Labor before a primary cesarean delivery: reduced risk of uterine rupture in a subsequent trial of labor for vaginal birth after cesarean. *Obstetrics and Gynecology, 112*(5), 1061–1066. doi:10.1097/AOG.0b013e31818b42e3.

Als, H., Lester, B. M., Tronick, E., & Brazelton, T. B. (1982). Assessment of preterm infant behavior (APIB). In H. E. Fitzgerald, B. M. Lester, & M. W. Yogman (Eds.), *Theory and research in behavioral pediatrics* (Vol. 1). New York, NY: Plenum.

American Academy of Pediatrics (AAP). (2004). AAP Subcommittee on Hyperbilirubinemia. Clinical Practice Guideline: Management of hyperbilirubinemia in the newborn infant 35 or more weeks of gestation. *Pediatrics, 114,* 297.

American Academy of Pediatrics (AAP). (2011). Policy statement: SIDS and Other Sleep-Related Infant Deaths: Expansion of Recommendations for a Safe Infant Sleeping Environment. *Pediatrics,128*(5), 1030–1039.

American Academy of Pediatrics (AAP). (2011a). *AAP updates recommendation on car seats.* Retrieved from http://www.aap.org/en-us/about-the-aap/aap-press-room/Pages/AAP-Updates-Recommendation-on-Car-Seats.aspx.

American Academy of Pediatrics (AAP). (2011b). Newborn screening fact sheets. *Pediatrics, 118*(3), 934–963. Retrieved from http://pediatrics.aappublications.org/content/118/3/e934.full.

American Academy of Pediatrics (AAP) & American College of Obstetricians and Gynecologists (ACOG). (2013). *Guidelines for perinatal care* (7th ed.). Washington, DC: Author.

American Academy of Pediatrics (AAP) & American Heart Association. (2011). *Textbook of neonatal resuscitation* (6th ed.). Elk Grove Village, IL: Author.

American Academy of Pediatrics (AAP) & Canadian Paediatric Society (CPS). (2006). Prevention and management of pain in the neonate: An update. *Pediatrics, 118*(5), 2231–2241.

American College of Nurse Midwives. (2010). ACNM clinical bulletin #11. *Journal of Midwifery and Women's Health,* 55:397–492.

American College of Nurse-Midwives. (2011). Second stage of labor: pushing your baby out. Retrieved from http://onlinelibrary.wiley.com/doi/10.1111/j.1542-2011.2011.00145.x/full.

American College of Obstetricians and Gynecologists (ACOG). (2002). *Exercise during pregnancy and the postpartum period* (ACOG Technical Bulletin No. 267). Washington, DC: Author.

American College of Obstetricians and Gynecologists (ACOG). (2004). *Diagnosis and treatment of nausea and vomiting in pregnancy* (ACOG Practice Bulletin No. 52). Washington, DC: Author.

American College of Obstetricians and Gynecologists (ACOG). (2005). *Pregestational diabetes mellitus* (ACOG Practice Bulletin No. 60). Washington, DC: Author.

American College of Obstetricians & Gynecologists (ACOG). (2006). *Apgar score* (Committee Opinion No. 333). Washington, DC: Author.

American College of Obstetricians and Gynecologists (ACOG). (2007). *Hemoglobinopathies in pregnancy* (ACOG Practice Bulletin No. 78). Washington, DC: Author.

American College of Obstetricians and Gynecologists (ACOG). (2008a). *Anemia in pregnancy* (ACOG Practice Bulletin No. 95). Washington, DC: Author.

American College of Obstetricians and Gynecologists (ACOG). (2008b). *Use of psychiatric medications during pregnancy and lactation* (ACOG Practice Bulletin No. 92). Washington, DC: Author.

American College of Obstetricians and Gynecologists (ACOG). (2009a). *Induction of labor* (ACOG Practice Bulletin 107). Washington, DC: Author.

American College of Obstetricians and Gynecologists (ACOG). (2009b). *Intrapartum fetal heart rate monitoring: Nomenclature, interpretation, and general management principles* (ACOG Practice Bulletin 106). Washington, DC: Author.

American College of Obstetricians and Gynecologists. (2009c). *Oral intake during labor* (ACOG Committee Opinion No. 441). *Obstetrics & Gynecology, 114,* 714.

American College of Obstetricians and Gynecologists (ACOG). (2009d). *Postpartum screening for abnormal glucose tolerance in women who had gestational diabetes mellitus.* (ACOG Committee Opinion No. 435). Washington, DC: Author.

American College of Obstetricians and Gynecologists (ACOG). (2009e). *Ultrasonography in pregnancy* (ACOG Practice Bulletin No. 101). Washington, DC: Author.

American College of Obstetricians and Gynecologists (ACOG). (2010). *Vaginal birth after cesarean birth* (Technical Bulletin No. 115). Washington, DC: Author.

American College of Obstetricians and Gynecologists (ACOG). (2011a). *Car safety for you and your baby* (FAQ 18). Retrieved from http://www.acog.org/~/media/For%20Patients/faq018.pdf?dmc=1&ts=20130605T1627093666.

American College of Obstetricians and Gynecologists (ACOG). (2011b). *Exercise during pregnancy.* Retrieved from http://www.acog.org/~/media/For%20Patients/faq119.pdf?dmc=1&ts=20130605T1543597807.

American College of Obstetricians and Gynecologists (ACOG). (2011c). *Reduce birth defects with folic acid* (FAQ 146). Retrieved from http://www.acog.org/~/media/For%20Patients/faq146.pdf?dmc=1&ts=20130606T1419199364.

American College of Obstetricians & Gynecologists (ACOG). (2012a). *Timing of umbilical cord clamping after birth* (ACOG Committee Opinion No. 543). *Obstetrics and Gynecology, 120*(6), 1522–1526. doi:10.1097/01.AOG.0000423817.47165.48.

American College of Obstetricians and Gynecologists (ACOG). (2012b). *Umbilical cord blood gas and acid base analysis* (ACOG Committee Opinion No. 348). Washington, DC: Author.

American College of Obstetricians and Gynecologists (ACOG). (2013a). *Committee opinion: Obesity in pregnancy.* Retrieved from http://www.acog.org/~/media/Committee%20Opinions/Committee%20on%20Obstetric%20Practice/co549.pdf?dmc=1&ts=20130606T1559566932.

American College of Obstetricians and Gynecologists (ACOG). (2013b). *Non–medically indicated early-term deliveries* (Committee Opinion No. 561). Washington, DC: Author.

American College of Obstetricians and Gynecologists (ACOG). (2013c).*Obesity in pregnancy* (Committee Opinion No. 549). Washington, DC: Author.

American Diabetes Association (ADA). (2010). Diagnosis and classification of diabetes mellitus. *Diabetes Care, 33*(Suppl. 1), 62–69.

American Heart Association. (2011). *Classes of heart failure.* Retrieved from http://www.heart.org/HEARTORG/Conditions/HeartFailure/AboutHeartFailure/Classes-of-Heart-Failure_UCM_306328_Article.jsp.

Attanasio, L. B., Hardeman, R. R., Kozhimannil, K. B., & Kjerulff, K. H. (2017). Prenatal attitudes toward vaginal delivery and actual delivery mode: Variation by race/ethnicity and socioeconomic status. *Birth.* DOI: 10.1111/birt.12305

Andrews, M. M. (2008). Transcultural perspectives in the nursing care of children and adolescents. In M. M. Andrews & J. S. Boyle (Eds.), *Transcultural concepts in nursing care* (5th ed., pp. 116–145). Philadelphia, PA: Lippincott.

Apgar, V. (1966, August). The newborn (Apgar) scoring system, reflections and advice. *Pediatric Clinics of North America, 13,* 645.

August, P. (2015). Management of hypertension in pregnant and postpartum women. *UpToDate.* http://www.uptodate.com/contents/management-of-hypertension-in-pregnant-and-postpartum-women?source=machineLearning&search=hypertension+pregnancy&selectedTitle=1%7E150&sectionRank=1&anchor=H53704432#H198338096

Babalola, D. A., & Omole, F. (2010). Periodontal disease and pregnancy outcomes. *Journal of Pregnancy, 2010,* 293439. doi:10.1155/2010/293439.

Bagwell, G. A. (2007). Hematologic system. In C. Kenner & J. W. Lott (Eds.), *Comprehensive neonatal care: An interdisciplinary approach* (5th ed., pp. 221–253). St. Louis, MO: Saunders.

Ballard, J. L., Khoury, J. C., Wedig, K., Wang, L., Eilers-Walsmann, B. L., & Lipp, R. (1991). New Ballard Score, expanded to include extremely premature infants. *Journal of Pediatrics, 119*(3), 417–423.

Barber, E. L., Lundsberg, L. S., Belanger, K., Pettker, C. M., Funai, E. F., & Illuzzi, J. L. (2011). Indications contributing to the increasing cesarean delivery rate. *Obstetrics & Gynecology, 118*(1), 29–38.

Bazaco, M. C., Albrecht, S. A., & Malek, A. M. (2008). Preventing foodborne infection in pregnant women and infants. *Nursing for Women's Health, 12*(1), 46–54.

Beckman, M., & Garrett, A. (2006). Antenatal perineal massage for reducing perineal trauma. *Cochrane Database of Systematic Reviews,* Issue 1.

Beckman, M. M., & Stock, O. M. (2013). Antenatal message. *Cochrane Database of Systematic Reviews,* Issue 4.

Beckmann, C. R., Barzansky, B. M., Herbert, W. N., Douglas, W. N., Laube, W., & Ling, F. W. (2010). *Obstetrics & gynecology* (6th ed.). Philadelphia, PA: Lippincott Williams & Wilkins.

Bhutani, V. K., Johnson, L., & Sivieri, E. M. (1999). Predictive ability of a predischarge hour-specific serum bilirubin for subsequent significant hyperbilirubinemia in healthy term and near-term newborns. *Pediatrics, 103,* 6–14.

Bhutta, Z. A., Chopra, M., Axelson, H., Berman, P., Boerma, T., Bryce, J., . . . & Wardlow, T. (2010). Countdown to 2015 decade report (2000–10): Taking stock of maternal, newborn, and child survival. *Lancet, 375*(9730), 2032–2044. Retrieved from http://www.thelancet.com/journals/lancet/article/PIIS0140-6736(10)60678-2/abstract.

Bishop, E. H. (1964). Pelvic scoring for elective inductions. *Obstetrics & Gynecology, 24,* 266.

Bjorstadi, A. R., Irgens, H., Hanseni, I., Daltveiti, A. K., & Irgensi, L. M. (2010). Macrosomia: Mode of delivery and pregnancy outcome. *ACTA Obstetricia et Gynecologica, 89,* 664–669.

Black, R. A., & Hill, D. A. (2003). Over-the-counter medications in pregnancy. *American Family Physician, 67*(12), 2517–2524.

Blackburn, S. T. (2013). *Maternal, fetal, & neonatal physiology: A clinical perspective* (4th ed.). St. Louis, MO: Saunders.

Bonow, R. O., Carabello, B. A., Chatterjee, K., de Leon, A. C., Faxton, D. C., Freed, M. D., & Shanewise, J. S. (2008). Focused update incorporated into the ACC/AHA 2006 guidelines for the management of patients with valvular heart disease: A report of the American College of

Cardiology/American Heart Association Task Force on Practice Guidelines. *Circulation, 118*(15), e523.

Born, D., & Barron, M. L. (2005). Herb use in pregnancy. *American Journal of Maternal/Child Nursing, 30*(3), 201–206.

Brancato, R., Church, S., & Stone, P. (2008). A meta-analysis of passive descent versus immediate pushing in nulliparous women with epidural analgesia in the second stage of labor. *Journal of Obstetrical, Gynecological, and Neonatal Nursing, 37*(1), 4–12.

Branch, D. W., Silver, R. M., & Aagaard-Tillery, K. (2008). Immunologic disorders in pregnancy. In R. S. Gibbs, B. Y. Karlan, A. F. Haney, & I. E. Nygaard (Eds.), *Danforth's obstetrics and gynecology* (10th ed.). Philadelphia, PA: Wolters Kluwer/Lippincott Williams & Wilkins.

Brand, M. C., & Boyd, H. A. (2010). Thermoregulation. In M. T. Verklan & M. Walden (Eds.), *Core curriculum for neonatal intensive care nursing* (4th ed., pp. 110–119). St. Louis, MO: Saunders.

Bray, I., Gunnel, D., & Smith, G. D. (2006). Advanced paternal age: How old is too old? *Journal of Epidemiology and Community Health, 60,* 851–853.

Brazelton, T. B. (1984). *Neonatal behavioral assessment scale* (2nd ed.) London, England: Heinemann.

Brazelton, T. B., & Nugent, J. K. (1995). *The neonatal behavioral assessment scale* (3rd ed.). London, England: MacKeith.

Burt, C. C., & Durbridge, J. (2009). Management of cardiac disease of pregnancy. *Continuing Education in Anaesthesia Critical Care & Pain, 9*(2), 44–47.

Caldwell, W. E., & Moloy, H. C. (1933). Anatomical variations in the female pelvis and their effect on labor with a suggested classification [Historical article]. *American Journal of Obstetrics and Gynecology, 26,* 479–505.

Cassar, L. (2006). Cultural expectations of Muslims and Orthodox Jews in regard to pregnancy and the postpartum period: A study in comparison and contrast. *International Journal of Childbirth Education, 21*(2), 27–30.

Castle, P. (2012). Collaboration in open adoption: The birth mother's experience. *Australian Journal of Adoption, 6*(1), 1–9.

Centers for Disease Control and Prevention (CDC). (2010). *Prevention of perinatal group B streptococcal infection.* Retrieved from www.cdc.gov/mmwr/pdf/rr/rr5910.pdf.

Centers for Disease Control and Prevention (CDC). (2012). *Recommended dose of folic acid for pregnant women.* Retrieved from http://www.cdc.gov/ncbddd/folicacid/index.html.

Centers for Disease Control and Prevention (CDC). (2013). *Changes in cesarean delivery rates by gestational age: United States, 1996–2011.* Retrieved from http://www.cdc.gov/nchs/data/databriefs/db124.htm.

Centers for Disease Control and Prevention (CDC). (2014). *Newborn screening quality assurance program.* Retrieved from http://www.cdc.gov/labstandards/nsqap.html.

Centers for Disease Control and Prevention (CDC). (2014b). Guidelines for vaccinating pregnant women. Retrieved from http://www.cdc.gov/VACCINEs/pubs/preg-guide.htm

Cheffer, N. D., & Rannalli, D. A. (2011). Transition care of the newborn. In S. Mattson & J. E. Smith (Eds.), *Core curriculum for maternal–newborn nursing* (4th ed., pp. 345–361). St. Louis, MO: Saunders.

Child Welfare Information Gateway. (2013a). *Grounds for involuntary termination of parental rights.* Retrieved from http://www.childwelfare.gov/systemwide/laws_policies/statutes/groundtermin.cfm.

Child Welfare Information Gateway. (2013b). *Infant safe haven laws.* Retrieved from http://www.childwelfare.gov/systemwide/laws_policies/statutes/safehaven.cfm.

Chou, C. (2017). Traditional postpartum practices and rituals: A qualitative systematic review. Ci. Lee- Dennis, K. Fung, S. Grigoriadis, G. Erlick-Robinson, S. Romans & L. Ross. (Editors). *Embryo Project Encyclopedia.* Retrieved from https://embryo.asu.edu/

Cleveland Clinic. (2006). *Gestational diabetes. Hypoglycemia.* Retrieved from http://www.clevelandclinic.org/health/healthinfo/docs/2300/2354.asp?index=9012.

Cloherty, J. R., Eichenwald, E. C., & Stark, A. R. (2008). *Manual of neonatal care.* Philadelphia, PA: Lippincott Williams & Wilkins.

Creary, M., Williamson, D., & Kulkarni, R. A. (2007). Sickle cell disease: Current activities, public health implications, and future directions. *Women's Health, 16*(5), 575–582.

Creasy, R. K., Resnik, R., Iams, J. D., Lockwood, C. J., & Moore, T. R. (2008). *Creasy and Resnik's maternal fetal medicine* (6th ed.). Philadelphia, PA: Elsevier.

Cunningham, F. G., Leveno, K. J., Bloom, S. L., Hauth, J. C., Gilstrap, L. C., & Wenstrom, K. D. (2010). *Williams obstetrics* (23rd ed.). New York, NY: McGraw-Hill.

Curry, R., Swan, L., & Steer, P. J. (2009). Cardiac disease in pregnancy. *Current Opinion in Obstetrics and Gynecology, 21,* 508–513.

Cusick, W., Shevell, T., Duchan, L. S., Lupinacci, C. A., Terranova, J., & Crombleholme, W. R. (2008). Likelihood ratios for fetal trisomy 21 based on nasal bone length in the second trimester: How best to define hypoplasia? *Ultrasound in Obstetrics & Gynecology, 30*(3), 271–274.

D'Avanzo, C. E., & Geissler, E. M. (2008). *Pocket guide to cultural assessment* (4th ed.). St. Louis, MO: Mosby.

Davidson, M., London, M., & Ladewig, P. (2012). *Olds' maternal–newborn nursing & women's health across the lifespan* (9th ed.). Upper Saddle River, NJ: Pearson Prentice Hall.

Davidson, M.R., London, M.L., & Ladewig, P.L. (2017). *Old's maternal-newborn nursing & women's health.* (10th ed.). Boston: Pearson Education.

Deave, T., Johnson, D., & Ingram, J. (2008). Transition to parenthood: The needs of parents in pregnancy and early parenthood. *Pregnancy and Childbirth, 8,* 30–35.

Declercq, E., Young, R., Cabral, H., & Ecker, J. (2011). Is a rising cesarean delivery rate inevitable? Trends in the industrialized countries, 1987–2007. *Birth, 38*(2), 99–104.

DeGroot, J. M., & Vik, T. A. (2017). Disenfranchised grief following a traumatic birth. *Journal of Loss and Trauma, 22*(4), 346–356.

Delbaere, I., Verstraelen, H., Goetgeluk, S., Martens, G., DeBacker, G., & Temmerman, M. (2007). Pregnancy outcome in primiparas of advanced maternal age. *European Journal of Obstetrics, Gynecology, and Reproductive Biology, 135*(1), 41–46.

Do, H. (2005). Chinese culture. *Ethnomed.* Retrieved from http://ethnomed.org.

Dudding, T., Vaizey, C., & Kamm, M. (2008). Obstetrics anal sphincter injury: Incidence, risk factors, and management. *Annals of Surgery, 247*(2), 224–237.

Eberhard, M., Garthus-Niegel, S., & Garthus-Niegel, K. (2010). Postnatal care: A cross-cultural historical perspective. *Archives of Women's Mental Health, 13,* 459–466.

Edelman, C. K., & Mandle, C. L. (2010). *Health promotion throughout the life span.* St. Louis, MO: Mosby/Elsevier.

Ehrenkranz, R.A., Mercurio, M. (2015). Limit of Viability. *UpToDate.* http://www.uptodate.com/contents/limit-ofviability?source=machineLearning&search=fetal+viability&selectedTitle=1%7E150&sectionRank=1&anchor=H8144829#H8144829

Ellis, C. R., & Schnoes, C. J. (2012). Pica. *Medscape.* Retrieved from http://emedicine.medscape.com/article/914765-overview#a1.

Eriksson, U. J. (2009). Congenital anomalies in diabetic pregnancy. *Seminars in Fetal Neonatal Medicine, 14*(2), 85–93.

Faust, J. E. (2005). Instruments in the hands of God. *Liahona Archives.* Retrieved from www.lds.org.

Feinstein, N. F., Sprague, A., & Trepanier, M. J. (2008). *Fetal heart rate auscultation* (2nd ed.). Washington, DC: Association of Women's Health, Obstetric and Neonatal Nurses.

Field, T. (2012). Infant behavior and development. *Prenatal Exercise Research, 35*(3), 397–407.

Fleuriet, J. L. (2009). La Technologia y Las Monjitas: Constellation of authoritative knowledge at a religious brith center in south Texas. *Medical Anthropology Quarterly, 23*(3), 212–234.

Fox, N. S., Saltzman, D. H., Roman, A. S., Klauser, C. K., Moshier, E., & Rebarber, A. (2010). Intravaginal misoprostol versus Foley catheter for labour induction: A

meta-analysis. *British Journal of Obstetrics and Gynecology, 118*(6), 647–654.

Frankman, E. A., Wang, L., Bunker, C. H., & Lowder, J. L. (2009). Episiotomy in the United States: Has anything changed? *American Journal of Obstetrics & Gynecology, 200,* 573.

Fraser, D. (2013). Newborn adaptations to extrauterine life. In K. R. Simpson & P. A. Creehan, *Perinatal nursing* (4th ed.). Philadelphia, PA: Lippincott Williams & Wilkins.

Funai, E.F., Norwitz, E. (2014). Mechanism of normal labor and delivery. *UpToDate.* http://www.uptodate.com/contents/mechanism-ot-normal-labor-and-delivery?source=machineLearning&search=clinical+pelvimetry&selectedTitle=1%7E150&sectionRank=1&anchor=H3#H6

Gabbe, S.G., Niebyl, J.R, Simpson, J.P. (1996). Obstetrics: Normal & Problem Pregnancies, 3rd ed. Churchill Livingstone. New York.

Gabbe, S. G., Niebyl, J. R., & Simpson, J. L. (2012). *Obstetrics: Normal and problem pregnancies* (6th ed.). Philadelphia, PA: Churchill Livingstone.

Gandhia, R. A., Brown, J., Simmb, A., Pagea, R. C., & Idris, I. (2008). HbA1c during pregnancy: Its relationship to meal related glycaemia and neonatal birth weight in patients with diabetes. *European Journal of Obstetrics & Gynecology and Reproductive Biology, 138*(1), 45–48.

Gardner, S. L., & Goldson, E. (2011). The neonate and the environment: Impact on development. In S. L. Gardner, B. S. Carter, M. Enzman-Hines, & J. A. Hernandez (Eds.), *Merenstein & Gardner's handbook of neonatal intensive care* (7th ed., pp. 270–331). St. Louis, MO: Mosby.

Gardner, S. L., & Hernandez, J. A. (2011). Initial nursery care. In S. L. Gardner, B. S. Carter, M. Enzman-Hines, & J. A. Hernandez (Eds.), *Merenstein & Gardner's handbook of neonatal intensive care* (7th ed., pp. 78–112). St. Louis, MO: Mosby.

Gavin, L., Warner, L., O'Neil, M. E., Duong, L. M., Marshall, C., Hastings, P. A., . . . & Barfield, W. (2013). Vital signs: Repeat births among teens—United States, 2007–2010. *Morbidity and Mortality Weekly Report, 62*(13): 249–255. Retrieved from http://www.cdc.gov/mmwr/preview/mmwrhtml/mm6213a4.htm?s_cid=mm6213a4_w.

Gennaro, S., Mayberry, L. J., & Kafulafula, U. (2007). The evidence supporting nursing management of labor. *Journal of Obstetric, Gynecologic, & Neonatal Nursing, 36*(6), 598–604.

Gibbins, S., Hoath, S. P., Coughlin, M., Gibbins, A., & Franck, L. (2008). The universe of developmental care: A new conceptual model for application in a neonatal intensive care unit. *Advances in Neonatal Care, 8*(3), 141–147.

Giger, J. N., & Davidhizar, R. E. (2007). *Transcultural nursing: Assessment and interventions* (5th ed.). St. Louis, MO: Mosby.

Gilbert, E. (2011). *Manual of high risk pregnancy & delivery* (5th ed.). St. Louis, MO: Mosby-Elsevier.

Gilbert, W. M. (2007). Amniotic fluid disorders. In S. G. Gabbe, J. R. Niebyl, & J. L. Simpson (Eds.), *Obstetrics: Normal and problem pregnancies* (5th ed., pp. 834–845). Philadelphia, PA: Churchill Livingstone Elsevier.

Goer, H., Romano, A. (2012). Optimal Care in Childbirth: The Case for a Physiologic Approach. Classic Day: Seattle.

Goldenberg, R. L., Culhane, J. F., Iams, J. D., & Romero, R. (2008). Epidemiology and causes of preterm birth.*Lancet, 371*(9606), 75–84. doi:10.1016/S0140-6736(08)60074-4.

Goldstein.J., MacKenzie, A.P., Funai, E. F. (2015). Assessment of fetal lung maturity. UpToDate. http://www.uptodate.com/contents/assessment-of-fetal-lung-maturity?source=search_result&search=fetal+lung+maturity&selectedTitle=1%7E52

Goodman, J. H. (2005). Becoming an involved father of an infant. *Journal of Obstetric, Gynecologic, and Neonatal Nursing, 34*(2), 190–200.

Gordon, M. C. (2007). Maternal physiology. In S. G. Gabbe, J. R. Niebyl, & J. L. Simpson (Eds.), *Obstetrics: Normal and problem pregnancies* (5th ed.). New York, NY: Churchill-Livingstone.

Grant, G.J., (2014) Adverse effects of neuraxial analgesia and anesthesia for obstetrics. *UpToDate.* http://www.

uptodate.com/contents/adverse-effects-of-neuraxial-analgesia-and-anesthesia-for-obstetrics?source=related_link#H12559692

Green-Hernandez, G., Quinne, A., Falkenstern, S., Denman-Vitale, S., & Judge-Ellis, T. (2004, July/August). Making nursing care culturally competent. *Holistic Nursing Practice*, 215–218.

Gurber, S., Bielinski-Blattmann, D., Lemola, S., Jaussi, C., von Wyl, A., Surbek, D., & … Stadlmayr, W., (2012). Maternal mental health in the first 3 weeks postpartum: The impact of caregiver support and the subjective experience of childbirth–A longitudinal path model. *Journal of Psychosomatic Obstetrics and Gynaecology*, 33(4), 176–184.

Gurol, A., & Polat, S. (2011). The effects of baby massage on attachment between mothers and infants. *Asian Nursing Research*, 6, 35–41.

Gurol-Urganci, I., Cromwell, D., Edozien, L., Mahmood, T., Adams, E., Richmond, … & van der Meulen, J. (2013). Third- and fourth-degree perineal tears among primiparous women in England between 2000 and 2012: Time trends and risk factors. *British Journal of Obstetrics and Gynecology*, 120(12), 1534–1547. doi:10.1111/1471-0528.12363.

Haines, T. M., Hildingsson, I., Pallant, J. F., & Rubertsson, C. (2013). The role of women's attitudinal profiles in satisfaction with the quality of their antepartal and intrapartum care. *Journal of Obstetric, Gynecologic, and Neonatal Nursing*, 42(4), 428–441. Retrieved from http://www.ncbi.nlm.nih.gov/pubmed/23773005.

Hamilton, B. E., Martin, J. A., & Ventura, S. J. (2013). Births: Preliminary data for 2012. *National Vital Statistics Reports*, 62(3), 1–20. Retrieved from http://www.cdc.gov/nchs/data/nvsr/nvsr62/nvsr62_03.pdf.

Hamilton, E. F., & Warrick, P. A. (2013). New perspectives in electronic fetal surveillance. *Journal of Perinatal Medicine*, 41(1), 83–92.

Hammond, M. M., White, C. B., & Fetters, M. D. (2005). Opening cultural doors: Providing culturally sensitive healthcare to Arab American and American Muslim patients. *American Journal of Obstetrics & Gynecology*, 193(4), 1307–1311.

Hanson, L. (2009). Labor care challenges in spontaneous bearing down. *Journal of Perinatal-Neonatal Nursing*, 23(1), 31–39.

Harper, L. M., & Macones, G. A. (2008). Predicting success and reducing the risks when attempting vaginal birth after cesarean. *Obstetrical & Gynecological Survey*, 63(8), 538–545.

Harris, R., & Ayers, S. (2012). What makes labour and birth traumatic? A survey of intrapartum hot spots. *Psychology & Health*, 27(10), 1166–1177.

Hartmann, K. E., Wechter, M. E., Payne, P., Salisbury, K., Jackson, R. D., & Melvin, C. L. (2007). Best practice smoking cessation and resource needs of prenatal care providers. *Obstetrics & Gynecology*, 110(4), 765–770.

Health Resources and Services Administration (HRSA). (2010). *Women's health USA 2010: Maternal mortality*. Retrieved from http://mchb.hrsa.gov/whusa10/hstat/mh/pages/237mm.html.

Heazell, A. E., Green, M., Wright, C., Flenady, V., & Frøen, J. F. (2008). Midwives' and obstetricians' knowledge and management of women presenting with decreased fetal movements. *Acta Obstetricia et Gynecologica Scandinavica*, 87(3), 331–339.

Hezelgrave, N. L., Whitty, C. J., Shennan, A. H., & Chappell, L. C. (2011). Advising on travel during pregnancy. *British Medical Journal*, 28, 342. doi:10.1136/bmj.d2506.

Hibbeln, J. R. (2007). Maternal seafood consumption in pregnancy and neurodevelopment outcomes in childhood (ALSPAC Study): An observational cohort study. *Lancet*, 369(9561), 578–585.

Hofmeyr, G. J., Gülmezoglu, A. M., & Pileggi, C. (2013). Vaginal misoprostol for cervical ripening and induction of labour. *Cochrane Database of Systematic Reviews*, Issue 1. Art. No. CD000941.

Holroyd, E., Twinn, S., & Yim, I. W. (2004). Exploring Chinese women's cultural beliefs and behaviors regarding the practice of "doing the month." *Women's Health*, 40(3), 109–123.

Holtz, C., & Grisdale, S. (2008). Global health in reproduction and infants. In C. Holtz, *Global health care: Issues and policies* (1st ed., pp. 437–476). Boston, MA: Jones & Bartlett.

Hoshiyama, E., Muento, T., Histake, I., Watanabe, H., Noryuki, I., & Kolchi, H. (2012). Postpartum migraines: A long-term prospective study. *Internal Medicine*, 51(22), 3119–3123.

Human Milk Banking Association of North America. (2011). *Best practice for expressing, storing and handling human milk in hospitals, homes and child care settings*. Raleigh, NC: Author.

Ingraham, N., Wingo, E., Foster, D. G., & Roberts, S. (2017). Best practices for LGBTQ inclusion and exclusion in reproductive health research. *Contraception*, 96 (4), 299

Institute of Medicine (IOM). (2009). *Weight gain during pregnancy: Reexamining the guidelines* (rev. ed.). Retrieved from http://www.iom.edu/~/media/Files/Report%20Files/2009/Weight-Gain-During-Pregnancy-Reexamining-the-Guidelines/Report%20Brief%20-%20Weight%20Gain%20During%20Pregnancy.pdf.

Institute of Medicine (IOM). (2010). *Dietary reference intakes (DRIs): Recommended dietary allowances and adequate intakes, vitamins and elements*. Washington, DC: Food and Nutrition Board, Institute of Medicine, National Academies.

International Association of Diabetes and Pregnancy Study Groups (IADPSG), Consensus Panel. (2010). International Association of Diabetes and Pregnancy Study Groups recommendations on the diagnosis and classification of hyperglycemia in pregnancy. *Diabetes Care*, 33(3), 676–683.

James, D. C. (2008). Postpartum care. In K. R. Simpson & P. A. Creehan, *Perinatal nursing* (3rd ed., pp. 473–526). Philadelphia, PA: Lippincott Williams & Wilkins.

Johnson, T. R. B., Gregory, K. D., & Niebyl, J. R. (2007). Preconception and prenatal care: Part of the continuum. In S. G. Gabbe, J. R. Niebyl, & J. L. Simpson (Eds.), *Obstetrics: Normal and problem pregnancies* (5th ed.). New York, NY: Churchill-Livingstone.

Jones, J. E., Hayes, R. D., Starbuck, A. L., & Porcelli, P. J. (2011). Fluid and electrolyte management. In S. L. Gardner, B. S. Carter, M. I. Enzman-Hines, & J. A. Hernandez (Eds.), *Merenstein & Gardner's handbook of neonatal intensive care* (7th ed., pp. 333–352.). St. Louis, MO: Mosby.

Katz, B. (2012). New focus on family-centered maternity care. *International Journal of Childbirth Education*, 27(3), 99–102.

Katz, V. (2008). Prenatal care. In R. Gibbs, B. Karlan, A. Haney, & I. Nygaard (Eds.), *Danforth's obstetrics and gynecology* (10th ed., pp. 1–21). Philadelphia, PA: Lippincott, Williams & Wilkins.

Kaur, A., & Kaur, A. (2011). Trans-vaginal ultrasonography in first trimester pregnancy and its comparison with trans-abdominal ultrasonography. *Journal of Pharmacy and Bio-Allied Sciences*, 3(3), 329–338.

Kaye, C. I., & Committee on Genetics. (2006). Newborn screening facts sheets. *Pediatrics*, 118(3), 934–963.

Kenner, C., & Lott, J. W. (2007). *Comprehensive neonatal care: An interdisciplinary approach* (4th ed.). St. Louis, MO: Saunders/Elsevier.

Kenny, L. C., Lavender, T., McNamee, R., O'Neill, S. M., Mills, T., & Khashan, A. S. (2013). Advanced maternal age and adverse pregnancy outcome: Evidence from a large contemporary cohort. *PLOS ONE*, 8(2): e56583. doi:10.1371/journal.pone.0056583. Retrieved from http://www.plosone.org/article/info:doi/10.1371/journal.pone.0056583.

Khademian, Z., & Vizeshfar, F. (2008). Nursing students' perceptions of the importance of caring behaviors. *Journal of Advanced Nursing*, 61(4), 456–462.

Kilpatrick, S., & Garrison, E. (2007). Normal labor and delivery. In S. G. Gabbe, J. R. Niebyl, & J. L. Simpson (Eds.), *Obstetrics: Normal and problem pregnancies* (5th ed., pp. 303–321). Philadelphia, PA: Churchill Livingstone/Elsevier.

Kim, S. (2017). Sanhujori: Korea's traditional postnatal care culture. *International Journal of Childbirth Education*, 32(3).

King, T.K., Brucker, M.C., Kriebs, J.M., Fahey, J.O., Gegor, C.L., Varney, H. (2015). *Varney's Midwifery*. 5th Ed. Jones and Bartlett Learning: Burlington, MA.

Kitzmiller, J. L., Block, J. M., Brown, F. M., Catalano, P. M., Conway, D. L., Coustan, D. R., … & Kirkman, M. S. (2008). Managing preexisting diabetes for pregnancy: Summary of evidence and consensus recommendations for care. *Diabetes Care*, 31(5), 1060–1079.

Knobel, R., & Holditch-Davis, D. (2007). Thermoregulation and heat loss prevention after birth and during neonatal intensive-care unit stabilization of extremely low-birth-weight infants. *Journal of Gynecological, Obstetric, and Neonatal Nursing*, 36, 280–287.

Knuppel, R. A. (2007). Maternal–placental–fetal unit: Fetal and early neonatal physiology. In A. H. DeCherney, L. Nathan, T. M. Goodwin, & N. Laufer (Eds.), *Current obstetric & gynecologic diagnosis & treatment* (10th ed., pp. 159–186). New York, NY: Lang Medical Books/McGraw-Hill.

Krakow, D. (2008). Medical and surgical complications of pregnancy. In R. S. Gibbs, B. Y. Karlan, A. F. Haney, & I. E. Nygaard (Eds.), *Danforth's obstetrics and gynecology* (10th ed.). Philadelphia, PA: Wolters Kluwer/Lippincott Williams & Wilkins.

Kurjak, A., Miskovic, B., Andonotopo, W., Stanojevic, M., Azumendi, G., & Vrcic, H. (2007). How useful is 3D and 4D ultrasound in perinatal medicine? *Journal of Perinatal Medicine*, 35(1), 10–27.

Lampinen, R., Vehvilainen-Julkunen, K., & Kankkunen, P. (2009). A review of pregnancy in women over 35 years of age. *Open Nursing Journal*, 3, 33–38.

Landon, M. B., Catalano, P. M., & Gabbe, S. (2007). Diabetes mellitus complicating pregnancy. In S. G. Gabbe, J. R. Niebyl, & J. L. Simpson (Eds.), *Obstetrics: Normal and problem pregnancies*. Philadelphia, PA: Churchill Livingstone Elsevier.

Lanzi, R. G., Bert, S. C., & Jacobs, B. K. (2009). Depression among a sample of first-time adolescent and adult mothers. *Journal of Child and Adolescent Psychiatric Nursing*, 22, 194–202.

Lauderdale, J. (2008). Transcultural perspectives in childbearing. In M. M. Andrews & J. S. Boyle (Eds.), *Transcultural concepts in nursing care* (5th ed.). Philadelphia, PA: Lippincott Williams & Wilkins.

Lederman, R. P., & Weis, K. (2009). *Psychological adaptation to pregnancy* (3rd ed.). New York, NY: Springer.

Lie, D. (2004). Ginger helpful for nausea and vomiting of pregnancy. *Medscape CME*. Retrieved from www.medscape.com/viewarticle/466746_print.

Lipson, J. G., & Dibble, S. L. (2008). *Culture and clinical care* (7th ed.). San Francisco, CA: The Regents, University of California.

Loewy, J., Steward, K., Dassler, A., Telsey, A., & Homel, P. (2012). The effects of music therapy on vital signs, feedings, and sleep in premature infants. *Pediatrics*, 131, 902. doi:10.1542/peds.2012-1367.

Lloreda-Garcia, J. M. (2017). Religion, spirituality and folk medicine: Superstition in a neonatal unit. *Journal of Religion & Health*, 56: 2276. doi.org/10.1007/s10943-017-0408-y

Ludington, S., Morgan, K., & Abouelfettoh, A. (2008). A clinical guideline for implementation of kangaroo care with premature infants of 30 or more weeks post-menstrual age. *Advances in Neonatal Care*, 8(Suppl. 3): 3–23.

Lukassi, M., Vangen, S., Oian, P., Kumle, M., Ryding, E. L., & Schei, B. (2010). Childhood abuse and fear of childbirth—A population-based study. *Birth*, 37(4), 267–274.

Lundberg, P. C., & Thu, T. T. N. (2011). Vietnamese women's cultural beliefs and practices related to the postpartum period. *Midwifery*, 27, 731–736.

Lyndon, A., Lee, H. C., Gilbert, W. M., Gould, J. B., & Lee, K. A. (2012). Maternal morbidity during childbirth hospitalization in California. *Journal of Maternal–Fetal & Neonatal Medicine*, 12, 2529–2535.

Lyon, A. (2007). Temperature control in the neonate. *Paediatrics and Child Health, 18,* 155–160.

MacKenzie, A.P., Stevenson, C.D., Funai, E.F. (2015). Perinatal assessment of gestational age and estimated date of delivery. *UpToDate,* http://www.uptodate.com/contents/prenatal-assessment-of-gestational-age-and-estimated-date-of-delivery?source=machineLearning&search=biparietal+diameter&selectedTitle=1%7E18&sectionRank=1&anchor=H6#H6

Macones, G. A., Hankins, G. D. V., Spong, C. Y., Hauth, J., & Moore, T. (2008). The 2008 National Institute of Child Health and Human Development Workshop report on electronic monitoring: Update on definitions, interpretation, and research guidelines. *Journal of Obstetrics, Gynecology, and Neonatal Nursing, 37*(5), 510–515.

Magann, E. F., Doherty, D. A., Lutgendorf, M. A., Magann, M. I., Chauhan, S. P., & Morrison, J. C. (2010). Peripartum outcomes of high-risk pregnancies complicated by oligo- and polyhydramnios: A prospective longitudinal study. *Journal of Obstetrics and Gynaecology Research, 36*(2), 268–277.

Mahle, W. T., Newburger, J. W., Matheme, G. P., Smith, F. C., Hoke, T. R., Koppe, R., … & Grosse, S. D. (2009). Role of pulse oximetry in examining newborns for congenital heart disease. *Pediatrics, 124*(2), 823–836.

Manco-Johnson, M., Rodden, D., & Hays, T. (2011). Newborn hematology. In S. L. Gardner, B. S. Carter, M. Enzman-Hines, & J. A. Hernandez (Eds.), *Merenstein & Gardner's handbook of neonatal intensive care* (7th ed., pp. 503–530). St. Louis, MO: Mosby.

March of Dimes (MOD). (2009). *Pregnancy after 35.* Retrieved from http://www.marchofdimes.com/printableArticles/14332_1155.asp.

Marciniak, B., Leszczyn, ska-Gorzelak, B., Bartosiewicz, J., & Oleszczuk, J. (2010). [Effectiveness of intracervical catheter as a labor preinduction method]. *Ginekologia Polska, 81*(1), 31–36.

Marcones, G. (2015). Weight gain and loss in pregnancy. *UpToDate.* http://www.uptodate.com/contents/weight-gain-and-loss-in-pregnancy?source=see_link&sectionName=Overweight+and+obese+women&anchor=H20254135#H20254135

Martin, J. A., Hamilton, B. E., Sutton, P. D., Ventura, S. J., Menacker, F., Kimeyer, S., … & Mathews, T. J. (2009). Births: Final data for 2006. *National Vital Statistics Reports, 57*(7) .

Martin, J. A., Hamilton, B. E., Ventura, S. J., Osterman, M. J. K., Wilson, E. C., & Mathews, T. J. (2012). Births: Final data for 2010. *National Vital Statistics Reports, 61*(1). Retrieved from http://www.cdc.gov/nchs/data/nvsr/nvsr61/nvsr61_01.pdf.

Martin, J. A., Hamilton, B. E., Ventura, S. J., Osterman, M. J. K., Wilson, E. C., & Mathews, T. J. (2013). Births: Final data for 2011. *National Vital Statistic Reports, 62*(1). Retrieved from http://www.cdc.gov/nchs/data/nvsr/nvsr62/nvsr62_01.pdf.

McCall, E., Alderdice, F., Halliday, H., Jenkins, J., & Vohra, S. (2008). Interventions to prevent hypothermia at birth in preterm and/or low birthweight infants. *Cochrane Database of Systematic Reviews,* Issue 1.

McGrath, J. M., & Hardy, W. (2011). The infant at risk. In S. Mattson & J. E. Smith (Eds.), *Core curriculum for maternal–newborn nursing* (4th ed., pp. 362–414). St. Louis, MO: Saunders.

MedlinePlus. (2012). *Quadruple screen test.* Retrieved from http://www.nlm.nih.gov/medlineplus/ency/article/007311.htm.

Medves, J. M., & O'Brien, B. (2004). The effect of bather and location of first bath on maintaining thermal stability in newborns. *Journal of Obstetric, Gynecologic, and Neonatal Nursing, 33*(2), 175–182.

Mercer, J. S., Erickson-Owens, D. A., Graves, B., & Haley, M. (2007). Evidence-based practices for the fetal to newborn transition. *Journal of Midwifery and Women's Health, 52*(3), 262–272.

Messer, L. C., Dole, N., Kaufman, J. S., & Savitz, D. A. (2005). Pregnancy intendedness, maternal psychosocial factors and preterm birth. *Maternal and Child Health Journal, 9*(4), 403–412.

Messerlian, G.M., Farina, A., Palomaki, G.E. (2013). First trimester combined test and integrated test for screening for Down syndrome and trisomy 18. *UpToDate.* http://www.uptodate.com/contents/first-trimester-combined-test-and-integrated-tests-for-screening-for-down-syndrome-and-trisomy-18?source=machineLearning&search=aneuploidy+screening&selectedTitle=1%7E121&sectionRank=1&anchor=H2#H2

Micali, N., Stavola, B. D., Santos-Silva, I., Steenweg-de Graaff, J., Jansen, P. W., Jaddoe, V. W., … &Tiemeier, H. (2012). Perinatal outcomes and gestational weight gain in women with eating disorders: A population-based cohort study. *British Journal of Obstetrics and Gynecology, 119*(12), 1493–1502.

Moore, E. R., Anderson, G. C., Bergman, N., & Dowswell, T. (2012). Early skin to skin contact for mothers and their healthy newborn infants. *Cochrane Database Systematic Review.* Art. No.: CD0003519. doi:10.1002/14651858.CD003519.pub3.

Moore, K. L., & Persaud, T. V. N. (2008). *The developing human: Clinical oriented embryology* (8th ed.). Philadelphia, PA: Saunders.

Moran, M., Ryan, J., Higgins, M., Brennan, P. C., & McAuliffe, F. M. (2011). Poor agreement between operators on grading of the placenta. *Journal of Obstetrics and Gynecology, 31*(1), 24–28.

Mott, S. R., James, S. R., & Sperhac, A. M. (1990). *Nursing care of children and families: A holistic approach* (2nd ed.). Menlo Park, CA: Addison-Wesley Nursing.

Nasir, A., Korejo, R., & Noorani, K. J. (2007). Childbirth in squatting position. *Journal of Pakistanian Medical Association, 57*(1), 19–22.

National Campaign to Prevent Teen and Unplanned Pregnancy (NCPTUP). (2010). *Our mission: Goal.* Retrieved from http://www.thenationalcampaign.org/about-us/our-mission.aspx.

National Center for Complementary and Alternative Medicine. (2012). *Herbs at a glance: Dandelions.* Retrieved from http://nccam.nih.gov/health/dandelion.

Natural Medicines Comprehensive Database. (2013a). *Oat straw.* Retrieved from http://naturaldatabase.therapeuticresearch.com/nd/Search.aspx?cs=&s=ND&pt=9&Product=oat+straw&btnSearch.x=14&btnSearch.y=10.

Natural Medicines Comprehensive Database. (2013b). *Raspberry leaf.* Retrieved from http://naturaldatabase.therapeuticresearch.com/nd/Search.aspx?cs=&s=ND&pt=9&Product=raspberry+leaf&btnSearch.x=13&btnSearch.y=13.

Neis, R. (2017). The Reproduction of species: Humans, animals and species nonconformity in early Rabbinic science. *Jewish Studies Quarterly, 24*(4), 289–317.

Nhan-Chang, C., & Jones, T. B. (2010). Tuberculosis in pregnancy. *Clinical Obstetrics and Gynecology, 53*(2), 311–321.

Niebyl, J. R., & Simpson, J. L. (2007). Drugs and environmental agents in pregnancy and lactation: Embryology, teratology, epidemiology. In S. G. Gabbe, J. R. Niebyl, & J. L. Simpson (Eds.), *Obstetrics: Normal and problem pregnancies* (5th ed.). New York, NY: Churchill-Livingstone.

Niermeyer, S., & Clarke, S. (2011). Delivery room care. In S. L. Gardner, B. S. Carter, M. I. Enzman-Hines, & J. A. Hernandez (Eds.), *Merenstein & Gardner's handbook of neonatal intensive care* (7th ed., pp. 52–71). St. Louis, MO: Mosby.

Nili, F., McLeod, L., O'Connell, C., Sutton, E., & McMillan, D. (2013). Maternal and neonatal outcomes in pregnancies complicated by systemic lupus erythematosus: A population-based study. *Journal of Obstetrics and Gynaecology Canada, 35*(4), 323–328. Retrieved from http://www.ncbi.nlm.nih.gov/pubmed/23660039.

Noble, A., Rom, M., Newsome-Wicks, M., Englehardt, K., & Woloski-Wruble, A. (2009). Jewish laws, customs, and practice in labor, delivery, and postpartum care. *Journal of Transcultural Nursing, 20,* 323. doi:10.1177/1043659609334930.

Nugent, J. K. (2013). The competent newborn and the Neonatal Behavioral Assessment Scale: T. Berry Brazelton's legacy. *Journal of Child and Adolescent Psychiatric Nursing, 26,* 173–179.

Office of AIDS Research Advisory Council (OARAC), Panel on Treatment of HIV-Infected Pregnant Women and Prevention of Perinatal Transmission. (2009, April 29). *Recommendations for use of antiretroviral drugs in pregnant HIV-1-infected women for maternal health and interventions to reduce perinatal HIV transmission in the United States* (pp. 1–94). Retrieved from http://aidsinfo.nih.gov/ContentFiles/PerinatalGL.pdf.

Ogburn, J. A., Espey, E., Pierce-Bulger, M., Waxman, A., Allee, L., Haffner, W. II., & Howe, J. (2012). Midwives and obstetrician-gynecologists collaborating for Native American women's health. *Obstetrics & Gynecology Clinics of North America, 39*(3), 359–366. doi:10.1016/j.ogc.2012.05.004.

Okah, F. A., Cai, J., & Hoff, G. L. (2005). Term gestation low birth weight and health compromising behaviors during pregnancy. *Obstetrics and Gynecology, 105*(3), 543–550.

O'Leary, J., & Thorwick, C. (2006). Fathers' perspectives during pregnancy, postperinatal loss. *Journal of Obstetrics, Gynecology, &Neonatal Nursing, 35*(1), 78–86.

O'Neill, E., & Thorp, J. (2012). Antepartum evaluation of the fetus and fetal well-being. *Clinical Obstetrics and Gynecology, 55*(3), 722–730.

Ott, B., Al-Khadhuri, J., & Al-Junaibi, S. (2003). Preventing ethical dilemmas: Understanding Islamic health care practices. *Pediatrics, 29*(3), 227–230.

Pacini, L., Digne, F., Boumendil, A., Muti, C., Detaint, D., Boileau, C., & Jondeau, G. (2009). Maternal complication of pregnancy in Marfan syndrome. *International Journal of Cardiology, 136*(2), 156–161.

Penney, D. S. (2008). The effects of vigorous exercise during pregnancy. *Journal of Midwifery and Women's Health, 53*(2), 155–159.

Penney, D. S., & Miller, K. G. (2008). Nutritional counseling for vegetarians during pregnancy. *Journal of Midwifery & Women's Health, 53,* 37–44.

Petersen, M. R. (2011). Review of interventions to relieve postpartum pain from perineal trauma. *American Journal of Maternal Child Nursing, 36*(4), 240–245.

Phend, C. (2013). New form of misoprostol speeds up labor. *Medpage Today.* Retrieved from http://www.medpagetoday.com/MeetingCoverage/SMFM/37406.

Premburg, A., & Lundgren, I. (2006). Fathers' experiences of childbirth education. *Journal of Perinatal Education, 15*(2), 21–28.

Ramachandrappa, A., & Jain, L. (2008). Elective cesarean section: Its impact on neonatal respiratory outcome. *Clinics in Perinatology, 35,* 2.

Ramaraj, R., & Sorrell, V. L. (2009). Peripartum cardiomyopathy: Causes, diagnosis, and treatment. *Cleveland Clinic Journal of Medicine, 76*(5), 289–296.

Reece, E. A. (2008). Perspectives on obesity, pregnancy and birth outcomes in the United States: The scope of the problem. *American Journal of Obstetrics and Gynecology, 198*(1), 23–27.

Resnik, R. (2013). Electronic fetal monitoring: The debate goes on. *Obstetrics & Gynecology, 121*(5), 917–918.

Rhode, M. A. (2011). Postpartum complications. In S. Mattson & J. E. Smith (Eds.), *Core curriculum for maternal–newborn nursing* (4th ed., pp. 650–666). St. Louis, MO: Saunders/Elsevier.

Richter, R., Bergmann, R. L., & Dudenhausen, J. W. (2008). Previous cesarean or vaginal delivery: Which mode is a greatest risk of perinatal death at the second delivery? *European Journal of Obstetrics, Gynecology, and Reproductive Biology, 132*(1), 51–57.

Rinala, S. G., Dryfhout, V. L., & Lambers, D. S. (2009). Correlation of glucose concentrations in maternal serum and amniotic fluid in high-risk pregnancies. *American Journal of Obstetrics & Gynecology, 200*(5), e43–44.

Riordan, J., & Wambach, K. (2010). *Breastfeeding and human lactation* (4th ed.). Boston, MA: Jones & Bartlett.

Roach, J. A. (2004). Newborn stimulation: Preventing overstimulation is key for optimal growth and well-being. *AWHONN Lifelines, 7*(6), 531–535.

Roberts, J. M., Gonzalez, C. B., & Sampselle, C. (2007). Why do supportive birth attendants become directive of maternal bearing-down efforts in second-stage labor? *Journal of Nurse Midwifery & Women's Health, 52*(2), 134–141.

Robinson, J.N., (2015). Approach to episiotomy. *UpToDate.* http://www.uptodate.com/contents/approach-to-episiotomy?source=machineLearning&search=episiotomy&selectedTitle=1%7E52&sectionRank=1&anchor=H19#H19

Rosenberg, A. A. (2013). The neonate. In S. G. Gabbe, J. R. Niebyl, & J. L. Simpson (Eds.). *Obstetrics: Normal and problem pregnancies* (6th ed., pp. 523–565). Philadelphia, PA: Churchill Livingstone/Elsevier.

Roy-Burne, P.B. (2015). Postpartum blues and unipolar depression: Epidemiology, clinical features, assessment, and diagnosis. *UpToDate.* http://www.uptodate.com/contents/postpartum-blues-and-unipolar-depression-epidemiology-clinical-features-assessment-and-diagnosis?source=machineLearning&search=edinburgh+postnatal+depression+scale&selectedTitle=1%7E7&sectionRank=1&anchor=H6#H6

Rubin, R. (1984). *Maternal identity and the maternal experience.* New York, NY: Springer.

Russ, S. A., Hanna, D., DesGeorges, J., & Forsman, I. (2010). Improving follow-up to newborn hearing screening: A learning-collaborative experiences. *Pediatrics, 126*(Suppl. 1), 59–69. Retrieved from http://pediatrics.aappublications.org/content/126/Supplement_1/S59.full.

Russell, S. L., & Mayberry, L. J. (2008). Pregnancy and oral health. *American Journal of Maternal/Child Nursing, 33*(1), 32–37.

Sadler, T. W. (2006). *Langman's medical embryology* (10th ed.). Philadelphia, PA: Lippincott Williams & Wilkins.

Sadler, T. W. (2010). *Langman's medical embryology* (11th ed.). Philadelphia, PA: Lippincott Williams & Wilkins.

Safadi, R. (2005). Jordanian women: Perceptions and practices of first-time pregnancy. *International Journal of Nursing Practice, 11*(6), 269–276.

Sahota, D. S., Leung, W. C., To, W. K., Chan, W. P., Lau, T. K., & Leung, T. Y. (2012). Quality assurance of nuchal translucency for prenatal fetal Down syndrome screening. *Journal of Maternal–Fetal & Neonatal Medicine, 25*(7), 1039–1043. doi:10.3109/14767058.2011.614658.

Samarasekera, D. N., Bekhit, M. T., Wright, Y., Lowndes, R. H., Stanley, K. P., Preston, J. P., ... & Speakman, C. T. (2008, February 29). Long-term anal continence and quality of life following postpartum anal sphincter injury. *Colorectal Disease, 10*(8), 793–799. Retrieved from http://www.ncbi.nlm.nih.gov/pubmed/8266886.

Schoppe-Sullivan, S. J., Brown, G. L., Cannon, E. A., Mangelsdorf, S. C., & Sokolowski, M. S. (2008). Maternal gatekeeping, coparenting quality, and fathering behavior in families with infants, *Journal of Family Psychology, 22*(3), 389–398.

Semenic, S. E., Callister, L. C., & Feldman, P. (2004). Giving birth: The voices of Orthodox Jewish women living in Canada. *Journal of Obstetric, Gynecologic, and Neonatal Nursing, 33*(1), 80–87.

Seng, J. S., Kane Low, L. M., Sperlich, M., Ronis, D. L., & Liberzon, I. (2009). Prevalence, trauma history, and risk for posttraumatic stress disorder among nulliparous women in maternity care. *Obstetrics & Gynecology, 114*(4): 839–847. Retrieved from http://www.ncbi.nlm.nih.gov/pmc/articles/PMC3124073.

Shah, P. S., Herbozo, C., Aliwalas, L. L., & Shah, V. S. (2012). Breastfeeding or breast milk for procedural pain in neonates. *Cochrane Database of Systematic Reviews,* Issue 12. Art. No.: CD004950. doi:10.1002/14651858.CD004950.pub3.

Shatken, S., Greenough, K., & McPherson, C. (2012). Epidural fever and its implications for mothers and neonates: Taking the heat. *Journal of Midwifery and Women's Health, 57*(1): 82–85. doi:10.1111/j.1542-2011.00105.x.

Sibai, B. M. (2012). Etiology and management of postpartum hypertension-preeclampsia. *American Journal of Obstetrics and Gynecology,* doi:10.1016/j.ajog.2011.09.002.

Silverman, R. A. (2012). *Neonatal pustular melanosis.* Retrieved from http://emedicine.medscape.com/article/909753-overview.

Simkin, P. (2010). Fetal occiput posterior position: State of the science and a new perspective. *Birth, 37*(1), 61–70.

Simpson, K., & James, D. (2005). Effects of immediate versus delayed pushing during second-stage labor on fetal well-being: A randomized clinical trial. *Nursing Research, 54*(3), 149–157.

Simpson, K. R., & Creehan, P. A. (2013). *AWHONN's perinatal nursing* (4th ed.) Philadelphia, PA: Lippincott Williams & Wilkins.

Smith, C. A., Collins, C. T., Crowther, C. A., & Levett, K. M. (2011). Acupuncture or acupressure for pain management in labour. *Cochrane Database of Systematic Reviews,* Issue 7. Art. No.: CD009232.

Smith, G. C., Celik, E., To, M., Khouri, O., & Nicolaides, K. H. (2008). Cervical length at midpregnancy and the risk for primary cesarean delivery. *New England Journal of Medicine, 358*(13), 1346–1353.

Smith, J. R. (2012). Comforting touch in the very preterm hospitalized infant: An integrative review. *Advances in Neonatal Care, 12*(6), 349–365.

Smith, S. A., Hulsey, T., & Goodnight, W. (2008). Effects of obesity on pregnancy. *Journal of Obstetric, Gynecologic, and Neonatal Nursing, 37*(2), 176–184.

Snijder, C. A., Brand, T., Jaddoe, V., Hofman, A., Mackenbach, J. P., Steegers, E. P., & Burdorf, A. (2012). Physically demanding work, fetal growth and the risk of adverse birth outcomes: The Generation R study. *Occupational Environmental Medicine, 69*, 543–550.

Spector, R. E. (2009). *Cultural diversity in health and illness* (7th ed.). Upper Saddle River, NJ: Pearson/Prentice Hall.

Spector, R.E. (2017). *Cultural diversity in health & illness* (9th ed.). Boston: Pearson Education

Stranges, E., Wier, L. M., & Elixhauser, A. (2012). *Complicating conditions of vaginal deliveries and cesarean sections, 2009* (Healthcare Cost and Utilization Project Statistical Brief No. 131). Rockville, MD: Agency for Healthcare Research and Quality.

Stuebe, A. (2009). The risk of not breastfeeding for mother and infants. *Obstetrics and Gynecology, 2*(4), 222–231.

Tappero, E., & Honeyfield, M. E. (2009). *Physical assessment of the newborn: A comprehensive approach to the art of physical examination* (4th ed.). Santa Rosa, CA: NICU Ink Book Publisher.

Tedder, J. L. (2008). Give them the HUG: An innovative approach to helping parents understand the language of their newborn. *Journal of Perinatal Education, 17*(2), 14–20. doi:10.1624/105812408X29845.

Teitler, J. O., Reichman, N. E., Nepomnyaschy, L., & Martinson, M. (2007). A cross-national comparison of racial and ethnic disparities in low birth weight in the United States and England. *Pediatrics, 120*(5), e1182–e1189.

Thomas, J. A. (2007). Guidelines for bottle feeding for a premature baby. *Advances in Neonatal Care, 7*(6), 311–318.

Thombs, B. D., Bennett, W., Ziegelstein, R. C., Bernstein, D. P., Scher, C. D., & Forde, D. R. (2007). Cultural sensitivity in screening adults for a history of childhood abuse: Evidence from a community sample. *Journal of General Internal Medicine, 22*(3), 368–373.

Thompson, J. L., Kuller, J. A., & Rhee, E. H. (2012). Antenatal surveillance of fetal growth restriction. *Obstetrics and Gynecology Survey, 67*(9), 554–565.

Tomimatsu, T., Peña, J. P., & Longo, L. D. (2007). Fetal cerebral oxygenation: The role of maternal hyperoxia with supplemental CO_2 in sheep. *American Journal of Obstetrics and Gynecology, 196*(4), 359.

Torrance, H. L., Voorbij, H. A., Wijnberger, L. D., van Bel, F., & Visser, G. H. (2008). Lung maturation in small for gestational age fetuses from pregnancies complicated by placental insufficiency or maternal hypertension. *Early Human Development, 84*(7), 465–469.

Tucker, S. M., Miller, L. A., & Miller, A. (2008). *Mosby's pocket guide to fetal monitoring: A multidisciplinary approach.* St. Louis, MO: Mosby.

Turnage-Carrier, C. S. (2010). Development support. In M. T. Verklan & M. Walden (Eds.), *Core curriculum for neonatal intensive care nursing* (4th ed., pp. 208–232). St. Louis, MO: Saunders.

U.S. Department of Health and Human Services (USDHHS). (2011). *Healthy people 2020.* Retrieved from http://www.healthypeople.gov/2020/topicsobjectives2020/objectiveslist.aspx?topicid=26.

U.S. Food and Drug Administration (FDA). (2013). *Food safety for moms-to-be: At-a-glance.* Retrieved from http://www.fda.gov/Food/FoodborneIllnessContaminants/PeopleAtRisk/ucm081819.htm.

Vargo, L. (2014). Newborn physical assessment. In K. R. Simpson & P. A. Creehan (Eds.), *Perinatal nursing* (4th ed., pp. 597–625). Philadelphia, PA: Lippincott Williams & Wilkins.

Verburg, B. O., Steegers, E. A., De Ridder, M., Snijders, R. J., Smith, E., Hofman, A., ... Witteman, J. C. M. (2008). New charts for ultrasound dating of pregnancy and assessment of fetal growth: Longitudinal data from a population-based cohort study. *Ultrasound in Obstetrics & Gynecology, 31*(4), 388–396.

Volpe, J. J. (2008). *Neurology of the newborn* (5th ed.). Philadelphia, PA: Saunders.

Walker, L. O. (2007). Managing excessive weight gain during pregnancy and the postpartum period. *Journal of Obstetric, Gynecologic & Neonatal Nursing, 36*(5), 490–500.

Warrander, L., & Heazell, A. (2011). Identifying placental dysfunction in women with reduced fetal movements can be used to predict patients at increased risk of pregnancy complications. *Medical Hypotheses, 76*(1), 17–20.

Warren, J., & Silver, R. (2008). Genetics of pregnancy loss. *Clinical Obstetrics and Gynecology, 51*(1), 84–95.

Waskett, J. H. (2012). Global circumcision rates. *Circumcision Independent Reference and Commentary Service.* Retrieved from http://www.circs.org/index.php/Reviews/Rates/Global.

White, B. (2007). Ginger: An overview. *American Family Physician, 75*, 1689–1691.

Whitmer, T. (2011). Physical and psychologic change. In S. Mattson & J. E. Smith (Eds.). *Core curriculum for maternal–newborn nursing* (4th ed., pp. 301–314). St. Louis, MO: Saunders/Elsevier.

Wilson, B. A., Shannon, M. T., & Shields, K. M. (2013). *Pearson nurse's drug guide 2013.* Upper Saddle River, NJ: Pearson Education.

Womenshealth.gov. (n.d.). *Fish facts.* Retrieved from http://www.womenshealth.gov/publications/our-publications/fish-facts.pdf.

World Health Organization (WHO). (1999). *Care of the umbilical cord: A review of the evidence.* Retrieved from http://www.who.int/rht/documents/MSM98-4.

Wright, D., Kagan, K. O., Molina, F. S., Gazzoni, A., & Nicolaides, K. H. (2008). A mixture of nuchal translucency thickness in screening for chromosomal defects. *Ultrasound in Obstetrics and Gynecology, 31*(4), 376–383. doi:10.1002/uog.5299.

Yankowitz, J., (2008). Drugs in pregnancy. In R. S. Gibbs et al. (Eds.), *Danforth's obstetrics and gynecology* (10th ed.). Philadelphia, PA: Lippincott Williams & Wilkins.

Yogev, Y., Hiersch, L., Maresky, L., Wasserberg, N., Wiznitzer, A., & Melamde, N. (2013). Third and fourth degree perineal tears—The risk of recurrence in subsequent pregnancies. *Journal of Maternal–Fetal & Neonatal Medicine.* doi:10.3109/14767058.2013.806902. Retrieved from http://www.ncbi.nlm.nih.gov/pubmed/23682932.

Yu, C. K., Stasiowska, E., Stephens, A., Awogbade, M., & Davies, A. (2009). Outcome of pregnancy in sickle cell disease patients attending a combined obstetric and haematology clinic. *Journal of Obstetrics and Gynaecology, 29*(6), 512–516.

Zerbe, K. J. (2007). Eating disorders in the 21st century: Identification, management, and prevention in obstetrics and gynecology. *Best Practice & Research in Clinical Obstetrics and Gynaecology, 21*(2), 331–343.

Zwelling, E. (2010). Overcoming the challenges: Maternal movement and positioning to facilitate labor progress. *American Journal of Maternal/Child Nursing, 35*(2), 72–78.

Part IV
Nursing Domain

Part IV consists of modules that directly define and outline principles of nursing care, including assessment, clinical decision making, and communication. Each module presents a concept that directly relates to professional nursing and its impact on client health and well-being and selected principles or topics of that concept presented as exemplars. In the concept of clinical decision making, for example, the exemplars include the nursing process, the nursing plan of care, and prioritizing care. Each module addresses the impact of that concept and selected exemplars on the care of individuals across the life span, inclusive of cultural, gender, and developmental considerations.

Module 34   Assessment   2269
Module 35   Caring Interventions   2301
Module 36   Clinical Decision Making   2315
Module 37   Collaboration   2375
Module 38   Communication   2397
Module 39   Managing Care   2455
Module 40   Professional Behaviors   2479
Module 41   Teaching and Learning   2499

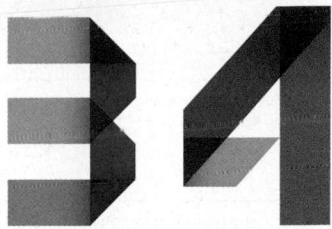

34 Assessment

MODULE AT-A-GLANCE

The Concept of Assessment, 2269

Exemplar 34.1
Holistic Health Assessment Across
the Life Span, 2285

⬛ THE CONCEPT OF ASSESSMENT

Health **assessment** may be defined as a systematic method of collecting data about a client for the purpose of determining the client's current and ongoing health status, predicting risks to health, and identifying health-promoting activities (D'Amico & Barbarito, 2012, p. 4). The focus of an assessment must include the problems presented by the client and the physical, social, cultural, environmental, and emotional factors that affect the overall well-being of the client in relation to the problems presented. Data gathered about the client's health status includes wellness behaviors, illness signs and symptoms, client strengths and weaknesses, and risk factors.

Knowledge of the natural and social sciences is a strong foundation for the nurse. Effective communication techniques and use of critical thinking skills are essential in helping the nurse to gather the detailed, complete, relevant data needed to formulate a plan of care to meet the needs of clients. Health assessment includes the interview and physical assessment, which must then be documented and interpreted. All future client care is directed by interpretation of findings from data collected throughout the assessment process.

Four different types of assessments are used: initial (or baseline) assessment, problem-focused (or system-specific) assessment, emergency assessment, and ongoing reassessment (see **Table 34–1** ●). **<<**

Concept Learning Outcomes

After reading about this concept, you will be able to:

1. Describe different types of assessments, indicating the proper use of each.

2. Relate the purposes of conducting a physical examination.

3. Propose actions required when preparing to conduct a physical examination.

4. Discriminate among positions appropriate for examination of different areas of the body.

5. Demonstrate use of each method of examination: inspection, palpation, percussion, and auscultation.

6. Discuss factors required to properly interpret findings from the nursing assessment.

7. Choose assessment tools as appropriate for clients' needs over their life spans.

Concept Key Terms

Assessment, 2269
Auscultation, 2280
Closed questions, 2274
Communication, 2284
Database, 2270
Directive interview, 2272
Dullness, 2280
Duration, 2281
Flatness, 2280
Holism, 2284
Hyperresonance, 2280
Inspection, 2278
Intensity, 2281
Interview, 2272
Leading question, 2275
Neutral question, 2275
Nondirective interview, 2272

Objective data, 2270
Open-ended questions, 2274
Palpation, 2278
Percussion, 2279
Pitch, 2280
Pleximeter, 2280
Plexor, 2280
Quality, 2281
Rapport, 2272
Resonance, 2280
Signs, 2270
Subjective data, 2270
Symptoms, 2270
Tympany, 2280
Validation, 2282

TABLE 34–1 Types of Assessment

TYPE	TIME PERFORMED	PURPOSE	EXAMPLE
Initial (or baseline) assessment	Performed within a specified time frame after admission to a healthcare agency (Refer to agency policy and procedure.)	To establish a complete baseline for problem identification, reference, and future comparison	Nursing admission assessment
Problem-focused (or system-specific) assessment	Ongoing process integrated with nursing care	To determine the status of a specific problem identified in an earlier assessment	Hourly assessment of client's fluid intake and urinary output in an intensive care unit (ICU)
			Assessment of client's ability to perform self-care while assisting a client to bathe
Emergency assessment	During any physiological or psychological crisis	To identify life-threatening problems	Rapid assessment of open airway, breathing status, and circulation during a cardiac arrest
		To identify new or overlooked problems	Assessment of suicidal tendencies or potential for violence
Ongoing reassessment	Minutes to months after initial assessment	To compare the client's current status to baseline data previously obtained	Reassessment of a client's functional health patterns in a home care or outpatient setting, or shift assessments at an acute care setting

▶ TYPES AND SOURCES OF DATA

Data collection is the process of gathering information about a client's health status. It must be both systematic and continuous to prevent the omission of significant data and to reflect a client's changing (in other words, not static) health status. Data can be constant or variable: Constant data is information that does not change over time such as race or blood type. Variable data can change quickly, frequently, or rarely and include data such as blood pressure, age, and level of pain.

A **database** contains all information about a client; it includes the nursing health history, physical assessment, primary care provider's history and physical examination, results of laboratory and diagnostic tests, and material contributed by other health personnel.

Client data should include past history as well as current problems. For example, a previous allergic reaction to penicillin is a vital piece of historical data. Past surgical procedures, folk healing practices that the client has used, and chronic diseases are also examples of historical data. Current data relate to present circumstances, such as pain, nausea, sleep patterns, and religious practices. To ensure accuracy, both the client and the nurse must participate actively in the data collection process. Data can be subjective or objective and may be constant or variable. Data can come from a primary or a secondary source.

Types of Data

Subjective data, also referred to as **symptoms** or covert data, are apparent only to the client affected and can be described or verified only by that client. Itching, pain, and feelings of worry are examples of subjective data. Subjective data include the client's sensations, feelings, values, beliefs, attitudes, and perception of personal health status and life situation.

Objective data, also referred to as **signs** or overt data, are detectable by an observer or can be measured or tested against an accepted standard. They can be seen, heard, felt, or smelled, and they are obtained by observation or physical examination. Examples of objective data include a discoloration of the skin and a blood pressure reading. During the physical examination, the nurse obtains objective data to validate subjective data and to complete the assessment phase of the nursing process.

Sources of Data

Sources of data are primary or secondary. The client is the primary source of data. Family members or other support people, other healthcare professionals, records and reports, laboratory and diagnostic analyses, and relevant literature are secondary or indirect sources. In fact, all sources other than the client are considered secondary sources. (Blood pressure measurements obtained by using an external cuff and manometer may be considered secondary or indirect data since they do not directly measure the pressure within the arteries.) All data from secondary sources should be validated if possible.

CLIENT The best source of data is usually the client, unless the client is too ill, young, or confused to communicate clearly. The client can provide subjective data that no one else can offer. Most often, primary data refer to statements made by the client but also include the objective data that the nurse can obtain directly from the client, such as gender. Some clients cannot or do not wish to provide accurate data. These include young children and clients who are confused, afraid, embarrassed, or distrustful, or who do not speak the nurse's language (D'Amico & Barbarito, 2012).

SUPPORT PEOPLE Family members, friends, and caregivers who know the client well often can supplement or verify information provided by the client. They might convey information about the client's response to illness, the stresses the client was experiencing before the illness, family attitudes on illness and health, and the client's home environment.

Support people are an especially important source of data for a client who is very young, unconscious, or confused. In some cases—a client who is physically or emotionally abused, for example—the individual giving information may wish to remain anonymous. Before eliciting data from support people, the nurse should ensure that the client, if mentally able, approves the gathering of such input. The nurse should also indicate on the nursing history that the data were obtained from a support person.

Information supplied by family members, significant others, or other healthcare professionals is considered subjective if it is not based on fact. If a client's daughter says, "Dad is very confused today," that is secondary subjective data because it is an interpretation of the client's behavior by the daughter. The nurse should attempt to verify the reported confusion by interviewing the client directly. However, if the daughter says, "Dad said he thought it was the year 1941 today," that may be considered secondary objective data since the daughter heard her father state this directly.

The presence or absence of support people in a client's life can itself be a significant assessment finding. A young child who is brought in for a clinic visit by foster parents will require a different combination of assessment tools than a child who is brought in by his or her own parent. Similarly, an older client who lives alone and is suspected of having dementia will require an assessment that differs somewhat from that of a healthy older client who lives an active life with his or her spouse.

CLIENT RECORDS   Client records include information documented by various healthcare professionals. Client records also contain data regarding the client's occupation, religion, and marital status. By reviewing such records before interviewing the client, the nurse can avoid asking questions for which answers have already been supplied. Repeated questioning can be stressful and annoying to clients and may cause concern about the lack of communication among health professionals. Types of client records include medical records, records of therapies, and laboratory records.

Medical records (e.g., medical history, physical examination, operative report, progress notes, and consultations done by primary care providers) provide information about a client's present and past health and illness patterns. These records also can provide the nurse with information about the client's coping behaviors, health practices, previous illnesses, and allergies.

Records of therapies provided by other health professionals, such as social workers, nutritionists, dietitians, or physical therapists, help the nurse obtain relevant data not expressed by the client. For example, a social agency's report on a client's living conditions or a home healthcare agency's report on a client's self-care abilities can inform the nurse's assessment of the client.

Laboratory records are another source of pertinent health information. For example, the determination of blood glucose level allows healthcare professionals to monitor the administration of oral hypoglycemic medications. Any laboratory data about a client must be compared to the agency or performing laboratory's norms for that particular test and for the client's age, gender, and other significant client data.

✳ *Go to **nursing.pearsonhighered.com** to see Appendix B for descriptions of diagnostic studies and their normal values.*

The nurse must always consider the information in client records in light of the present situation. For example, if the most recent medical record is 10 years old, the client's health practices and coping behaviors are likely to have changed. Older clients may have numerous previous records. These are very useful and contribute to a full understanding of the health history, especially if the client's memory is impaired.

HEALTHCARE PROFESSIONALS   Because assessment is an ongoing process, verbal reports from other healthcare professionals serve as potential sources of information about a client's health. Nurses, social workers, primary care providers, and physiotherapists, for example, may have information from either previous or current contact with the client. Sharing of information among professionals is especially important to ensure continuity of care when clients are transferred to and from home and healthcare agencies.

LITERATURE   Nursing and related literature, such as professional journals and reference texts, can provide additional information that can assist the nurse in developing or interpreting an assessment. The nurse may review literature to gather additional information on one or more of the following:

- Standards or norms against which to compare findings (e.g., height and weight tables, normal developmental tasks for an age group)
- Cultural and social health practices
- Spiritual beliefs
- Assessment data needed for specific client conditions
- Nursing interventions and evaluation criteria relevant to a client's health problems
- Medical diagnoses, treatment, and prognoses
- Current methodologies and research findings.

▶ COLLECTING DATA

The principal methods used to collect data are observing, interviewing, and examining. Observation occurs whenever the nurse is in contact with the client or support people. Interviewing is used mainly while the nurse is taking the nursing health history. Examining is the major method used in the physical health assessment.

In reality, the nurse uses all three methods simultaneously. For example, during the client interview the nurse observes, listens, asks questions, and mentally retains information to explore in the physical examination. These topics are covered further in the module on Communication.

Observing

Observation has two aspects: (a) noticing the data and (b) selecting, organizing, and interpreting the data (**Table 34–2 ●**). A nurse who observes that a client's face is flushed must relate that observation to findings such as body temperature, activity, environmental temperature, and blood pressure. The nurse often needs to focus on specific data so as not to be overwhelmed by a multitude of data. Observing, therefore, involves distinguishing data in a meaningful manner. For example, nurses caring for newborns learn to ignore the usual sounds of machines in the nursery but respond quickly to an infant's cry

TABLE 34–2 Using the Senses to Observe Client Data

SENSE	EXAMPLE OF CLIENT DATA
Vision	Overall appearance (e.g., body size, general weight, posture, grooming); signs of distress or discomfort; facial and body gestures; skin color and lesions; abnormalities of movement; nonverbal demeanor (e.g., signs of anger or anxiety); religious or cultural artifacts (e.g., books, icons, candles, beads)
Smell	Body or breath odors
Hearing	Lung and heart sounds; bowel sounds; ability to communicate; language spoken; ability to initiate conversation; ability to respond when spoken to; orientation to time, person, and place; thoughts and feelings about self, others, and health status
Touch	Skin temperature and moisture; muscle strength (e.g., hand grip); pulse rate, rhythm, and volume; palpatory lesions (e.g., lumps, masses, nodules)

or movement. Errors can occur in selecting, organizing, and interpreting data. For example, a nurse might not notice certain signs, either because they are unexpected or because they do not conform to preconceptions about a client's health.

The experienced nurse is often able to attend to an intervention (e.g., give a bed bath or monitor an intravenous infusion) and at the same time make important observations (e.g., note a change in respiratory status or skin color). The beginning student must learn to make observations and complete tasks simultaneously.

Interviewing

An **interview** is a planned communication or a conversation with a purpose. Interviews may be used to:

- Get or give information
- Identify problems of mutual concern
- Evaluate change
- Teach
- Provide support, counseling, or therapy.

One example of the interview is the nursing health history, which is a part of the nursing admission assessment. See **Box 34–1** ● for the components of a nursing health history.

Nurses use two approaches to interviewing: directive and nondirective. The **directive interview** is highly structured and elicits specific information. The nurse establishes the purpose of the interview and controls the interview—at least at the outset. The client responds to questions but may have limited opportunity to ask questions or discuss concerns. Nurses frequently use directive interviews to gather and to give information when time is limited (e.g., in an emergency situation).

During a **nondirective interview**, or rapport-building interview, the nurse allows the client to control the purpose, subject matter, and pacing. **Rapport** is an understanding between two or more people.

A combination of directive and nondirective approaches is usually appropriate during the information-gathering interview.

The nurse begins by determining areas of concern for the client. If, for example, a client expresses worry about surgery, the nurse pauses to explore the client's worry and to provide support. Simply noting the worry, without dealing with it, can leave the impression that the nurse does not care about the client's concerns or dismisses them as unimportant.

PLANNING THE INTERVIEW AND SETTING Before beginning an interview, the nurse reviews available information, for example, the operative report, information about the current illness, or literature about the client's health problem. The nurse also reviews the agency's data collection form to identify which data must be collected and which data are within the nurse's discretion to collect based on the specific client. If a form is not available, most nurses prepare an interview guide to help them remember areas of information and determine what questions to ask. The guide includes a list of topics and subtopics rather than a series of questions.

Both nurses and clients should be comfortable in order to encourage an effective interview by balancing several factors. Each interview is influenced by time, place, seating arrangement or distance, and language.

Time The nurse needs to plan interviews with clients when the client is physically comfortable and free of pain and when interruptions by friends, family, and other health professionals are minimal. The nurse should schedule interviews with clients in their homes at a time selected by the client.

Place A well-lighted, well-ventilated room that is relatively free of noise, movements, and distractions encourages communication. A place where others cannot overhear or see the client is essential.

Seating Arrangement The nurse who stands and looks down at a client who is in bed or in a chair risks intimidating the client. When a client is in bed, the nurse can sit at a 45-degree angle to the bed. This position is less formal than sitting behind a table or standing at the foot of the bed. During an initial admission interview, a client who is in bed may feel less confronted if an overbed table is placed between the client and the nurse. Sitting on a client's bed hems the client in and makes staring difficult to avoid. A seating arrangement with the nurse behind a desk and the client seated across creates a formal setting that suggests a business meeting between a superior and a subordinate. In contrast, a seating arrangement in which the parties sit on two chairs placed at right angles to a desk or table or a few feet apart, with no table between, creates a less formal atmosphere, and the nurse and client tend to feel on equal terms. In groups, a horseshoe or circular chair arrangement can avoid a superior or head-of-the-table position.

Distance The distance between the interviewer and interviewee should be neither too small nor too great, because people feel uncomfortable when talking to someone who is too close or too far away. Proxemics is the study of the use of space. As a species, humans are highly territorial, but we are rarely aware of it unless our space is somehow violated. Most people in Western cultures feel comfortable maintaining a distance of 2–3 feet during an interview. Some clients require more or less personal space, depending on their cultural and personal needs.

Box 34–1 Components of a Nursing Health History

BIOGRAPHICAL DATA

The client's name, address, age, sex, marital status, occupation, religious preference, healthcare financing, and usual source of medical care.

CHIEF COMPLAINT OR REASON FOR VISIT

The chief complaint is the answer given to the question "What is troubling you?" or "Can you tell me the reason you came to the hospital or clinic today?" It should be recorded in the client's own words.

HISTORY OF PRESENT ILLNESS

- When the symptoms started
- Whether the onset of symptoms was sudden or gradual
- How often the problem occurs
- Exact location of the distress
- Character of the complaint (e.g., intensity of pain or quality of sputum, emesis, or discharge)
- Activity in which the client was involved when the problem occurred
- Phenomena or symptoms associated with the chief complaint
- Factors that aggravate or alleviate the problem

PAST HISTORY

- *Childhood illnesses*, such as chickenpox, mumps, measles, rubella (German measles), rubeola (red measles), streptococcal infections, scarlet fever, rheumatic fever, and other significant illnesses
- *Childhood immunizations* and the date of the last tetanus shot
- *Allergies* to drugs, animals, insects, or other environmental agents; the type of reaction that occurs; and how the reaction is treated
- *Accidents and injuries:* how, when, and where the incident occurred, type of injury, treatment received, and any complications
- *Hospitalization for serious illnesses:* reasons for the hospitalization, dates, surgery performed, course of recovery, and any complications
- *Medications:* all currently used prescription and over-the-counter medications, such as aspirin, nasal spray, vitamins, or laxatives

FAMILY HISTORY OF ILLNESS

To ascertain risk factors for certain diseases, the ages of siblings, parents, and grandparents and their current state of health or, if they are deceased, the cause of death are obtained. Particular attention should be given to disorders such as heart disease, cancer, diabetes, hypertension, obesity, allergies, arthritis, tuberculosis, bleeding, alcoholism, and any mental health disorders.

LIFESTYLE

- *Personal habits:* the amount, frequency, and duration of use of tobacco, alcohol, coffee, cola, tea, and illicit or recreational drugs
- *Diet:* description of a typical diet on a normal day or any special diet, number of meals and snacks per day, who cooks and shops for food, ethnically distinct food patterns, and allergies
- *Sleep/rest patterns:* usual daily sleep–wake times, difficulties sleeping, and remedies used for difficulties

- *Activities of daily living (ADLs):* any difficulties experienced in the basic activities of eating, grooming, dressing, elimination, and locomotion
- *Instrumental ADLs (IADLs):* any difficulties experienced in food preparation, shopping, transportation, housekeeping, laundry, and ability to use the telephone, handle finances, and manage medications
- *Recreation/hobbies:* exercise activity and tolerance, hobbies and other interests, and vacations

SOCIAL DATA

- *Family relationships/friendships:* the client's support system in times of stress or need, what effect the client's illness has on the family, and whether any family problems are affecting the client
- *Ethnic affiliation:* health customs and beliefs; cultural practices that may affect health care and recovery
- *Educational history:* data about the client's highest level of education attained and any past difficulties with learning
- *Occupational history:* current employment status, the number of days missed from work because of illness, any history of accidents on the job, any occupational hazards with a potential for future disease or accident, the client's need to change jobs because of past illness, the employment status of spouses or partners and the way child care is handled, and the client's overall satisfaction with the work
- *Economic status:* information about how the client is paying for medical care (including what kind of medical and hospitalization coverage the client has) and whether the client's illness presents financial concerns
- *Home and neighborhood conditions:* home safety measures and adjustments in physical facilities that may be required to help the client manage a physical disability, activity intolerance, and ADLs; the availability of neighborhood and community services to meet the client's needs

PSYCHOLOGICAL DATA

- *Major stressors* experienced and the client's perception of them
- *Usual coping pattern* with a serious problem or a high level of stress
- *Communication style,* or the ability to verbalize appropriate emotion; nonverbal communication—such as eye movements, gestures, use of touch, and posture; interactions with support people; and the congruence of nonverbal behavior and verbal expression

PATTERNS OF HEALTH CARE

Patterns of health care are all healthcare resources the client is currently using and has used in the past. These include the primary care provider, specialists (e.g., ophthalmologist or gynecologist), dentist, folk practitioners (e.g., herbalist or *curandero*), health clinic, or health center; whether the client considers the care being provided adequate; and whether access to health care is a problem.

Language   Failure to communicate in a language the client can understand is a form of discrimination. The nurse must convert complicated medical terminology into common English usage. Interpreters or translators are needed if the client and the nurse do not speak the same language or dialect (a variation in a language spoken in a particular geographic region). Translating medical terminology is a specialized skill because not all individuals who are fluent in the conversational form of a language are familiar with anatomical or other health terms.

Interpreters, however, may make judgments about precise wording but also about subtle meanings that require additional explanation or clarification according to the specific language and ethnicity. Interpreters may also edit the original source to make the meaning clearer or more culturally appropriate.

If giving written documents to a client, the nurse must determine whether the client can read them, or if a translator is required. Live translation is preferred, since the client can then ask questions for clarification. Nurses must be cautious when asking family members, client visitors, or agency nonprofessional staff to assist with translation; issues of confidentiality or gender mismatch can interfere with effective communication. Services such as AT&T On Demand Interpreter, using Language Line Services, are available 24 hours a day in over 170 languages for a fee. Many large agencies have their own on-call translator services for the languages or dialects commonly spoken in their area.

SAFETY ALERT
Avoid asking family members to translate for the client. Family members may insert their own advice or alter information to reduce anxiety in the client.

Even among clients who speak English, there may be differences in understanding terminology. Clients from different parts of the country may have strong accents, and clients who are less well educated and teen clients may ascribe different meanings to words. For example, "cool" may imply something good to one client and something not warm to another. For some teens and young adults, the term "sick" means something very good. The nurse must always confirm accurate understandings.

TYPES OF INTERVIEW QUESTIONS   Questions are often classified as closed or open ended, and neutral or leading. **Closed questions**, used in the directive interview, are restrictive and generally require only "yes" or "no" or short factual answers giving specific information. Closed questions often begin with "when," "where," "who," "what," "do (did, does)," or "is (are, was)." Examples of closed questions are "What medication did you take?" "Are you having pain now? Show me where it is." "How old are you?" "When did you fall?" The highly stressed individual and the individual who has difficulty communicating will find closed questions easier to answer than open-ended questions.

Open-ended questions, associated with the nondirective interview, invite clients to discover and explore, elaborate, clarify, or illustrate their thoughts or feelings. An open-ended question specifies only the broad topic to be discussed, and invites answers longer than one or two words. Such questions give clients the freedom to divulge only the information that they are ready to disclose. The open-ended question is useful at the beginning of an interview or to change topics and to elicit attitudes.

Open-ended questions may begin with "what" or "how." Examples of open-ended questions are "How have you been feeling lately?" "What brought you to the hospital?" "How did you feel in that situation?" "Would you describe more about how you relate to your child?" "What would you like to talk about today?"

The type of question a nurse chooses depends on the needs of the client at the time. Nurses often find it necessary to use a combination of closed and open-ended questions throughout an interview to accomplish the goals of the interview and obtain needed information. See **Box 34–2** ● for advantages and disadvantages of open-ended and closed questions.

Box 34–2   Selected Advantages and Disadvantages of Open-Ended and Closed Questions

OPEN-ENDED QUESTIONS

Advantages	Disadvantages
They develop trust.	They take more time.
They let the client do the talking.	Clients may give only brief answers.
The nurse is able to listen and observe.	Valuable information may be withheld.
They are easy for the client to answer.	They can result in more information than necessary.
They reveal what the client thinks is important.	Responses may be difficult to document.
They may reveal the client's lack of knowledge.	The nurse requires skill in controlling an open-ended interview.
They can provide information the nurse may not ask for.	There may be language barriers if the nurse and client don't have the same first language.

CLOSED QUESTIONS

Advantages	Disadvantages
Questions and answers can be controlled more effectively.	They may provide too little information and require follow-up questions.
They require less effort from the client.	They may not reveal how the client feels.
They may be less threatening because they do not require explanations or justifications.	They do not allow the client to volunteer possibly valuable information.
They take less time.	They may inhibit communication and convey lack of interest by the nurse.
Information can be asked for sooner than it would be volunteered.	The nurse may dominate the interview with questions.
Responses are easily documented.	

Sources: Based on Stewart, C. J., & Cash, Jr., W. B. (2006). *Interviewing: Principles and practices* (11th ed.). New York, NY: McGraw-Hill; Richardson, J. V. (n.d.). *Open versus closed ended questions.* Retrieved from http://polaris.gseis.ucla.edu/jrichardson/dis220/openclosed.htm; McDonald, D. D., Shea, M., & Fedo, J. (2009). The effect of pain question phrasing on older adult pain information. *Journal of Pain and Symptom Management, 37*(6), 1050–1060.

A **neutral question** is a question the client can answer without direction or pressure from the nurse, is open ended, and is used in nondirective interviews. Examples are "How do you feel about that?" and "Why do you think you had the operation?" A **leading question**, by contrast, is usually closed, used in a directive interview, and thus directs the client's answer. Examples are "You're stressed about surgery tomorrow, aren't you?" "You will take your medicine, won't you?" The leading question gives the client less opportunity to decide whether the answer is true or not. Leading questions create problems if the client, in an effort to please the nurse, gives inaccurate responses. This can result in inaccurate data, which can negatively affect nursing care.

STAGES OF AN INTERVIEW   An interview has three major stages: the opening or introduction, the body or development, and the closing.

The Opening

The opening can be the most important part of an interview because it sets the tone for the remainder of the interview. What the nurse says, how the nurse says it, and the attitude the nurse projects to the client can make a huge difference in the client's attitude. The purposes of the opening are to establish rapport and orient the interviewee.

Establishing rapport is a process of creating goodwill and trust. It can begin with a greeting ("Good morning, Mr. Johnson") or a self-introduction ("Good morning. I'm Taylor James, a nursing student") accompanied by nonverbal gestures such as a smile, a handshake, and a friendly manner. The nurse must be careful not to overdo this stage; too much superficial talk can arouse anxiety and may appear insincere.

In orientation, the nurse explains the purpose and nature of the interview, for example, what information is needed, how long it will take, and what is expected of the client. The nurse tells the client how the information will be used and usually states that the client has the right not to provide information.

The following is an example of an interview introduction:

Step 1—Establish rapport:

Nurse: Hello, Ms. Goodwin, I'm Ms. Fellows. I'm a nursing student, and I'll be assisting with your care here today.
Client: Hi. Are you a student from the college?
Nurse: Yes, I'm in my final year. Are you familiar with the campus?
Client: Oh, yes! I'm an avid basketball fan. My nephew graduated in 2004, and I often attend basketball games with him.
Nurse: That's great! Sounds like fun.
Client: Yes, I enjoy it very much.

Step 2—Orientation

Nurse: May I sit down with you for about 10 minutes to talk about how I can help you while you're here?
Client: All right. What do you want to know?
Nurse: To help plan your care after your operation, I'd like to get some information about your usual daily activities and

what you expect here in the hospital. I'll take notes while we talk to get the important points and have them available to the other staff who will also look after you.
Client: OK. That's all right with me.
Nurse: If there is anything you don't want to talk about, please feel free to say so. Everything you tell me will be confidential and will be shared only with others who have the legal right to know it.
Client: Sure, that will be fine.

The Body

In the body of the interview, the client communicates what he or she thinks, feels, knows, and perceives in response to questions from the nurse. Effective development of the interview demands that the nurse use communication techniques that make both parties feel comfortable and serve the purpose of the interview. For communicating during an interview, follow these guidelines:

- Listen attentively, using all your senses, and speak slowly and clearly.
- Use language the client understands, and clarify points that are not understood.
- Plan questions to follow a logical sequence.
- Ask only one question at a time. Multiple questions limit the client to one choice and may confuse the client.
- Acknowledge the client's right to look at things the way they appear to him or her and not the way they appear to the nurse or someone else.
- Do not impose your own values on the client.
- Avoid using personal examples, such as saying, "If I were you. . . ."
- Nonverbally convey respect, concern, interest, and acceptance.
- Be aware of the client's and your own body language.
- Be conscious of the client's and your own voice inflection, tone, and affect.
- Sit down to talk with the client (be at an even level).
- Use and accept silence to help the client search for more thoughts or to organize them.
- Use eye contact and be calm, unhurried, and sympathetic.

The Closing

The nurse terminates the interview when the necessary information has been obtained. In some cases, however, a client terminates the interview. For example, the client may decide not to give any more information or may be unable to offer more information for some other reason—fatigue, for example. The closing is important for maintaining the rapport and trust and for facilitating future interactions. The following techniques are commonly used to close an interview:

1. *Offer to answer questions.* "Do you have any questions?" or "I would be glad to answer any questions you have." Be sure to allow time for the individual to answer, or the offer will be regarded as insincere.
2. *Conclude by saying* "Well, that's all I need to know for now" or "Well, those are all the questions I have for now."

Preceding a remark with the word "well" generally signals that the end of the interaction is near.

3. **Thank the client.** "Thank you for your time and help. The questions you have answered will be helpful in planning your nursing care." You may also shake the client's hand.

4. **Express concern for the client's welfare and future.** "Take care of yourself. I hope all goes well for you."

5. **Plan for the next meeting,** if there is to be one, or state what will happen next. Include the day, time, place, topic, and purpose: "Let's get together again here on the fifteenth at 9:00 a.m. to see how you are managing then." Or "Ms. Cho, I will be responsible for giving you care three mornings per week while you are here. I will be in to see you each Monday, Tuesday, and Wednesday between eight o'clock and noon. At those times, we can adjust your care as needed."

6. **Provide a summary to verify accuracy and agreement.** Summarizing serves several purposes, such as helping to terminate the interview, reassuring the client that the nurse has listened, checking the accuracy of the nurse's perceptions, clearing the way for new ideas, and helping the client to note progress and a forward direction: "Let's review what we have just covered in this interview." Summaries are particularly helpful for clients who are anxious or who have difficulty staying with the topic: "Well, it seems to me that you are especially worried about your hospitalization and chest pain because your father died of a heart attack five years ago. Is that correct? . . . I'll discuss this with you again tomorrow, and we'll decide what plans need to be made to help you."

CASE STUDY \\ A

Martha Whitman is a 59-year-old recently retired elementary school teacher, complaining of continued acute back pain. The findings from the physical assessment are all within normal limits. Ms. Whitman states that the pain started 2 weeks ago, and has been getting worse, with only temporary relief from aspirin. Before referring this client for diagnostic studies, the nurse asks about any activities or events associated with the onset of the pain. Ms. Whitman reveals that she had enthusiastically taken up a new hobby of quilting about 3 weeks ago. She has been sitting and working with an embroidery hoop almost every day for an hour or two. In addition, she proudly adds that her garden "has never looked better—not a weed in sight!"

Critical Thinking Questions

1. How does the additional interview information assist the nurse in interpretation of Ms. Whitman's back pain?

2. What recommendations could the nurse make to prevent further straining the muscles of Ms. Whitman's back?

3. What timetable should the nurse give Ms. Whitman to expect decreased symptoms? What is the plan if this target date is not met?

Examining

The physical examination or physical assessment is a systematic data collection method that uses observation (i.e., the senses of sight, hearing, smell, and touch) to detect health problems. To conduct the examination, the nurse uses techniques of inspection, auscultation, palpation, and percussion.

A physical examination can be any of three types: (a) an initial assessment (e.g., when a client is admitted to a healthcare agency), (b) a system-specific examination (e.g., the cardiovascular system), or (c) an examination of a body area (e.g., the lungs, when difficulty with breathing is observed).

Physical examinations typically reveal normal and abnormal findings. The nurse must analyze both types of findings and make critical decisions about their meaning and importance. For example, when the client is being admitted with a diagnosis of appendicitis, the presence of pain in the right lower quadrant would be a normal finding, while the absence of pain would be inconsistent with the diagnosis and might indicate that the appendix has ruptured.

When findings are different than anticipated, the nurse must make decisions about their importance and what to do with the information. If unsure about the significance of a finding or to whom it should be reported, the nurse should consult with a more experienced nurse regarding the best course of action to follow.

A complete physical examination starts at the head and proceeds in a systematic manner downward (head-to-toe assessment) or by systems (neurological system, respiratory system, etc.). Whichever approach is used, the nurse must adapt the examination according to the age of the individual, the severity of the illness, the preferences of the nurse, the environment for the examination, and the agency's policies and procedures. The order of a head-to-toe assessment is given in **Box 34–3 ●**. Regardless of the procedure used, the client's energy level and time constraints need to be considered. The physical assessment is conducted in a systematic and efficient manner with the fewest position changes for the client.

✳ Go to **nursing.pearsonhighered.com** for a table of normal vital signs across the life span.

Frequently, nurses assess a specific body area, instead of the entire body. These specific assessments are made in relation to client complaints, the nurse's observations, the client's presenting problem, available nursing interventions, and medical therapies. Examples of these situations and assessments are provided in **Table 34–3 ●**.

The purposes of a physical examination include the following:

- To obtain baseline data about the client's functional abilities

- To supplement, confirm, or refute data obtained in the nursing history

- To obtain data that will help establish nursing diagnoses and plans of care

- To evaluate the physiological outcomes of health care and thus the progress of a client in relation to health problems

- To make clinical judgments about a client's health status

- To identify areas for health promotion and disease prevention.

Box 34–3   Head-to-Toe Framework

GENERAL SURVEY

VITAL SIGNS

HEAD

- Hair, scalp, cranium, face
- Eyes and vision
- Ears and hearing
- Nose and sinuses
- Mouth and oropharynx
- Cranial nerves

NECK

- Muscles
- Lymph nodes
- Trachea
- Thyroid gland
- Carotid arteries
- Neck veins

UPPER EXTREMITIES

- Skin and nails
- Muscle strength and tone
- Joint range of motion
- Brachial and radial pulses
- Biceps tendon reflexes
- Tendon reflexes
- Sensation

CHEST AND BACK

- Skin
- Chest shape and size
- Lungs
- Heart
- Spinal column
- Breasts and axillae

ABDOMEN

- Skin
- Abdominal sounds
- Specific organs (e.g., liver, bladder)
- Femoral pulses

GENITALS

- Testicles
- Vagina
- Urethra

ANUS AND RECTUM

LOWER EXTREMITIES

- Skin and toenails
- Gait and balance
- Joint range of motion
- Popliteal, posterior tibial, and pedal pulses
- Tendon and plantar reflexes

Nurses use national guidelines and evidence-based practice while performing health assessments. For example, when screening for cancer, the nurse should keep in mind the American Cancer Society's guidelines (2013a) for early detection. These guidelines include methods for early identification of breast, colorectal, cervical, endometrial, lung, and prostate cancers.

TABLE 34–3   Nursing Assessments Addressing Selected Client Situations

SITUATION	PHYSICAL ASSESSMENT
Client complains of abdominal pain.	Inspect, auscultate, and palpate the abdomen; assess vital signs.
Client is admitted with a head injury.	Assess level of consciousness using the Glasgow Coma Scale (discussed in the module on Intracranial Regulation); assess pupils for reaction to light and accommodation; assess vital signs.
The nurse prepares to administer a cardiotonic drug to a client.	Assess apical pulse and compare with baseline data.
The client has just had a cast applied to the lower leg.	Assess peripheral perfusion of toes, capillary refill, pedal pulse if accessible, and vital signs.
The client's fluid intake is minimal.	Assess skin turgor, fluid intake and output, and vital signs.

Stay Current: Visit the American Cancer Society Web site at **www.cancer.org/healthy/findcancerearly/cancer-screeningguidelines/american-cancer-society-guidelines-for-the-early-detection-of-cancer** to see their guidelines for early detection of cancer.

PREPARING THE CLIENT   Most clients need an explanation of the physical examination process. Often clients are anxious about what the nurse will find. The nurse provides reassurance by explaining each step of the examination. The nurse should explain when and where the examination will take place, why it is important, and what will happen. The nurse should inform the client that all information gathered and documented during the assessment is kept confidential in accordance with the Health Insurance Portability and Accountability Act (HIPAA). Only healthcare providers who have a legitimate need to know the client's information will have access to it.

Health examinations are usually painless; however, it is important to determine in advance any positions contraindicated for a particular client. For example, clients having difficulty breathing may experience increased difficulty when lying in a supine position. The nurse assists the client as needed to undress and put on a gown. Clients should empty their bladders before the examination. Doing so helps them feel more relaxed and facilitates palpation of the abdomen and pubic area. If a urinalysis is required, the urine should be collected in a container for that purpose.

PREPARING THE ENVIRONMENT   It is important to prepare the environment before starting the assessment. The time for the physical assessment should be convenient to both the client and the nurse. The environment should be well lighted and the equipment organized for efficient use. A client who is physically relaxed will usually experience little discomfort. The room should be warm enough to be comfortable for the client.

Providing privacy is important. Most people are embarrassed if their bodies are exposed or if others can overhear or view them during the assessment. Culture, age, and gender of both the client and the nurse influence how comfortable the client will be and what special arrangements might be needed. For example, if the client and nurse are of different genders, the nurse should ask if it is acceptable to perform the physical examination or if a nurse of the same gender is preferred. Family and friends should not be present unless the client asks for someone.

POSITIONING   During the physical examination, the client may need to maintain several positions. The nurse must consider the client's ability to assume each position before asking him or her to do so. The client's physical condition, energy level, and age should also be taken into consideration. Some positions are embarrassing or uncomfortable and therefore should not be maintained for extended periods. By organizing the assessment so that several body areas can be assessed in one position, the nurse can minimize the number of position changes needed and maximize the client's comfort during the assessment (see **Table 34–4 ●**).

TABLE 34–4 Client Positions and Body Areas Assessed

POSITION	DESCRIPTION	AREAS ASSESSED	CAUTIONS
Dorsal recumbent	Back-lying position with knees flexed and hips externally rotated; small pillow under the head; soles of feet on the surface	Female genitals, rectum, and female reproductive tract	May be contraindicated for clients who have cardiopulmonary problems.
Supine (horizontal recumbent)	Back-lying position with legs extended; with or without pillow under the head	Head, neck, axillae, anterior thorax, lungs, breasts, heart, vital signs, abdomen, extremities, peripheral pulses	Tolerated poorly by clients with cardiovascular and respiratory problems.
Sitting	A seated position, back unsupported and legs hanging freely	Head, neck, posterior and anterior thorax, lungs, breasts, axillae, heart, vital signs, upper and lower extremities, reflexes	Older adults and weak clients may require support.
Lithotomy	Back-lying position with feet supported in stirrups; the hips should be in line with the edge of the table	Female genitals, rectum, and female reproductive tract	May be uncomfortable and tiring for older adults and embarrassing for most clients.
Sims	Side-lying position with lowermost arm behind the body, uppermost leg flexed at hip and knee, upper arm flexed at shoulder and elbow	Rectum, vagina	Difficult for older adults and people with limited joint movement.
Prone	Lies on abdomen with head turned to the side, with or without a small pillow	Posterior thorax, hip joint movement	Often not tolerated by older adults and people with cardiovascular and respiratory problems.

METHODS OF EXAMINING Four primary techniques are used in the physical examination: inspection, palpation, percussion, and auscultation. Each requires practice to develop expertise.

Inspection Inspection is visual examination or assessing by using the sense of sight. The process should be deliberate, purposeful, and systematic. The nurse inspects with the naked eye and with a lighted instrument such as an otoscope (used to view the ear). In addition to visual observations, olfactory (smell) and auditory (hearing) cues are noted. Nurses frequently use visual inspection to assess moisture, color, and texture of body surfaces, as well as shape, position, size, color, and symmetry of the body. Lighting must be sufficient for the nurse to see clearly; either natural or artificial light can be used. When using the auditory senses it is important to have a quiet environment. Observation can be combined with the other assessment techniques.

Palpation Palpation is the examination of the body using the sense of touch. The pads of the fingers are used because their concentration of nerve endings makes them highly sensitive to tactile discrimination. Palpation is used to determine the following characteristics:

- Texture (e.g., of the hair)
- Temperature (e.g., of a skin area)
- Vibration (e.g., of a joint)
- Position, size, consistency, and mobility of organs or masses
- Distention (e.g., of the urinary bladder)
- Pulsation
- The presence of pain upon touch or palpation.

There are two types of palpation: light and deep. *Light (superficial) palpation* should always precede *deep palpation*

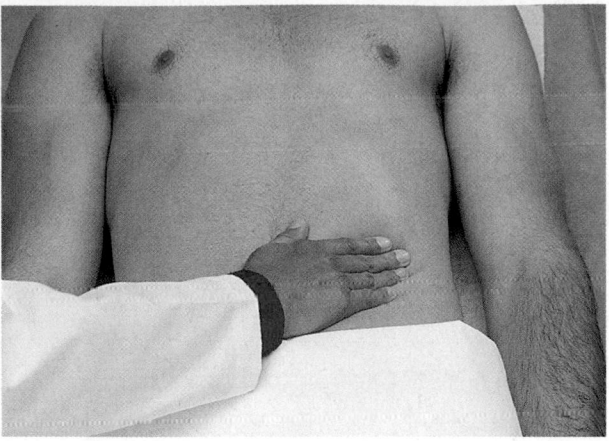

Figure 34–1 ● The position of the hand for light palpation.

because heavy pressure on the fingertips can dull the sense of touch. For light palpation, the nurse extends the dominant hand's fingers parallel to the skin surface and presses gently while moving the hand in a circle (see **Figure 34–1** ●). With light palpation, the skin is slightly depressed. If it is necessary to determine the details of a mass, the nurse presses lightly several times rather than holding the pressure. See **Table 34–5** ● for the characteristics of masses.

Deep palpation is done with one hand or with two hands (bimanually). In deep bimanual palpation, the nurse extends the dominant hand as for light palpation, then places the finger pads of the nondominant hand on the dorsal surface of the distal interphalangeal joints of the middle three fingers of the dominant hand (**Figure 34–2** ●). The top hand applies pressure while the lower hand remains relaxed to perceive the tactile sensations. For deep palpation using one hand, the finger pads of the dominant hand press over the area to be palpated. Often the other hand is used to support a mass or organ from below (**Figure 34–3** ●). Deep palpation is usually not done during a routine examination and requires significant practitioner skill. It is performed with extreme caution because pressure can damage internal organs. Deep palpation is usually not indicated in clients who have acute abdominal pain or pain that is not yet diagnosed.

To test skin temperature, the nurse should use the dorsal aspect (back) of the hand and fingers where the skin is thinnest. To test for vibration, the nurse should use the palmar

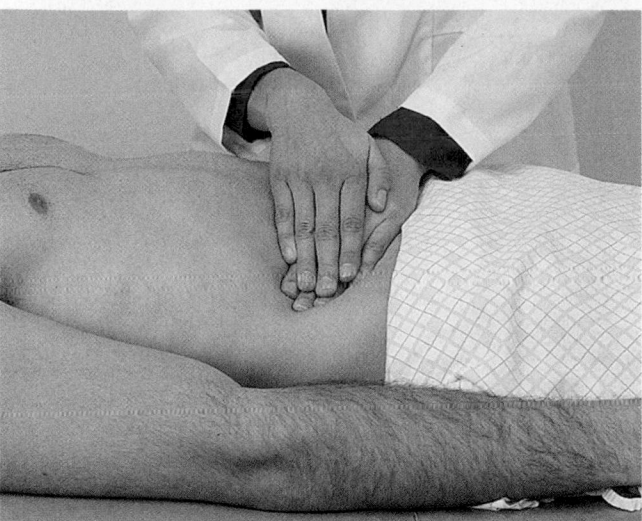

Figure 34–2 ● The position of the hands for deep bimanual palpation.

surface of the hand. General guidelines for palpation include the following:

- The nurse's hands should be clean and warm, and the fingernails should be short.
- Areas of tenderness should be palpated last.
- Deep palpation should be done after superficial palpation.

The effectiveness of palpation depends largely on the client's level of relaxation. The nurse can assist a client to relax by (a) gowning and/or draping the client appropriately, (b) positioning the client comfortably, and (c) ensuring that the nurse's own hands are warm before beginning. During palpation, the nurse should be sensitive to the client's verbal and nonverbal communication indicating discomfort.

Percussion   **Percussion** is the act of striking the body surface to elicit sounds that can be heard or vibrations that can be felt. There are two types of percussion: direct and indirect. In *direct*

TABLE 34–5   Characteristics of Masses

CHARACTERISTIC	DESCRIPTORS
Location	Site on the body, dorsal/ventral surface
Size	Length and width in centimeters
Shape	Oval, round, elongated, irregular
Consistency	Soft, firm, hard
Surface	Smooth, nodular
Mobility	Fixed, mobile
Pulsatility	Present or absent
Tenderness	Degree of tenderness to palpation

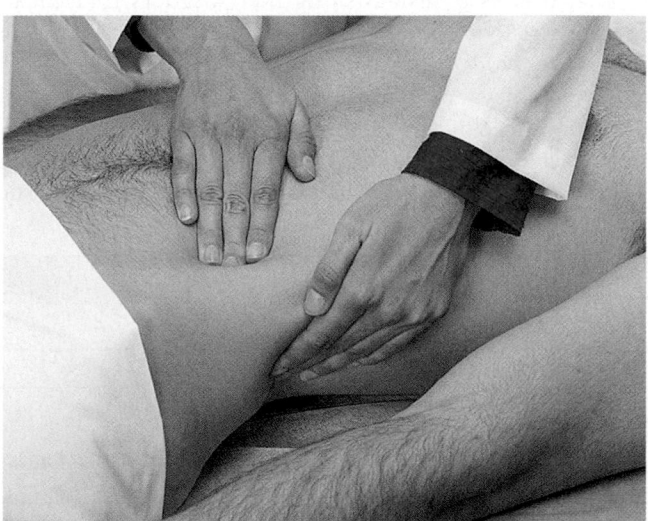

Figure 34–3 ● Deep palpation using the lower hand to support the body while the upper hand palpates the organ.

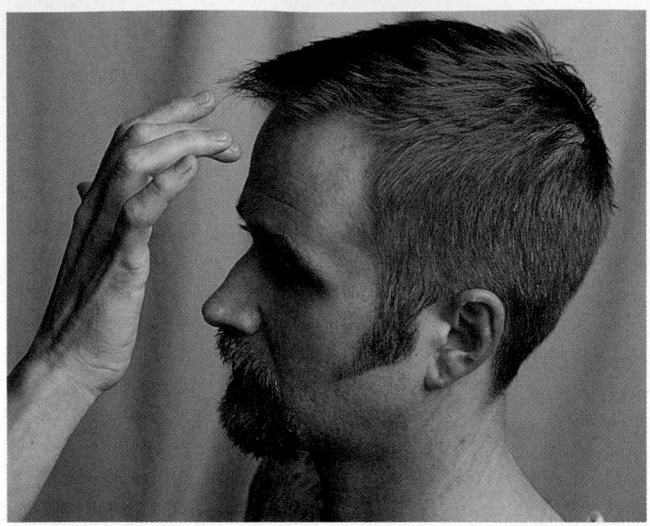

Figure 34–4 ● Direct percussion, in which one hand is used to strike the surface of the body.

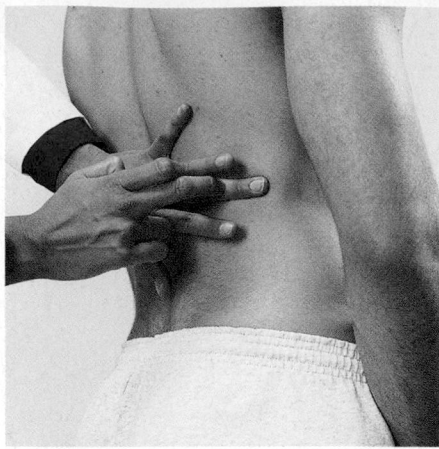

Figure 34–5 ● Indirect percussion, in which the finger of one hand taps the finger of the other hand.

percussion, the nurse strikes the area to be percussed directly with the pads of two, three, or four fingers or with the pad of the middle finger. The strikes are rapid, and the movement is from the wrist (see **Figure 34–4 ●**).

Indirect percussion refers to the striking of an object (e.g., a finger) held against the body area to be examined. In this technique, the middle finger of the nondominant hand, referred to as the **pleximeter**, is placed firmly on the client's skin. Only the distal phalanx and joint of this finger should be in contact with the skin. Using the tip of the flexed middle finger of the other hand, called the **plexor**, the nurse strikes the pleximeter, usually at the distal interphalangeal joint (see **Figure 34–5 ●**). Some nurses may find a point between the distal and proximal joints to be a more comfortable pleximeter point. The motion comes from the wrist; the forearm remains stationary. The angle between the plexor and the pleximeter should be 90 degrees, and the blows must be firm, rapid, and short to obtain a clear sound.

Percussion is used to determine the size and shape of internal organs by establishing their borders. It indicates whether tissue is fluid filled, air filled, or solid. Percussion elicits five types of sound: flatness, dullness, resonance, hyperresonance, and tympany. **Flatness** is an extremely dull sound produced by very dense tissue, such as muscle or bone. **Dullness** is a thudlike sound produced by dense tissue such as the liver, spleen, or heart. **Resonance** is a hollow sound, such

as that produced by lungs filled with air. **Hyperresonance** is not produced in the normal body. It is described as booming that can be heard over an emphysematous lung. **Tympany** is a musical or drumlike sound produced from an air-filled stomach. On a continuum, flatness reflects the most dense tissue (the least amount of air) and tympany the least dense tissue (the greatest amount of air). A percussion sound is described according to its intensity, pitch, duration, and quality (see **Table 34–6 ●**).

Auscultation   Auscultation is the process of listening to sounds produced within the body. Auscultation may be direct or indirect. An example of *direct auscultation* is the use of the unaided ear to listen to a respiratory wheeze or the grating of a moving joint. *Indirect auscultation* refers to the use of a stethoscope, which transmits the sounds to the nurse's ears. A stethoscope is used primarily to listen to sounds from within the body, such as bowel sounds or valve sounds of the heart and blood pressure.

The stethoscope tubing should be 30–35 cm (12–14 in.) long, with an internal diameter of about 0.3 cm (1/8 in.). The earpieces of the stethoscope should fit comfortably into the nurse's ears, facing forward. The amplifier of the stethoscope is placed firmly but lightly against the client's skin. If the client has excessive body hair, it may be necessary to dampen the hairs with a moist cloth so that they will lie flat against the skin and not interfere with clear sound transmission.

Auscultated sounds are described according to their pitch, intensity, duration, and quality. The **pitch** is the frequency of

TABLE 34–6   Percussion Sounds and Tones

SOUND	INTENSITY	PITCH	DURATION	QUALITY	EXAMPLE OF LOCATION
Flatness	Soft	High	Short	Extremely dull	Muscle, bone
Dullness	Medium	Medium	Moderate	Thudlike	Liver, heart
Resonance	Loud	Low	Long	Hollow	Normal lung
Hyperresonance	Very loud	Very low	Very long	Booming	Emphysematous lung
Tympany	Loud	High (distinguished mainly by musical timbre)	Moderate	Musical	Stomach filled with gas (air)

the vibrations (the number of vibrations per second). Low-pitched sounds, such as some heart sounds, have fewer vibrations per second than high-pitched sounds, such as bronchial sounds. The **intensity** (amplitude) refers to the loudness or softness of a sound. Some body sounds are loud, such as bronchial sounds heard from the trachea; others are soft, such as normal breath sounds heard in the lungs. The **duration** of a sound is its length (long or short). The **quality** of sound is a subjective description of a sound, for example, whistling, gurgling, or snapping.

EQUIPMENT The physical examination requires use of common healthcare tools such as the stethoscope, penlight, gloves, or water-soluble lubricant. The nurse determines what equipment will be required for the specific examination to be performed and collects the supplies in advance to avoid extending the time required of the client. The nurse should warm up cold equipment that will touch the client's skin. All equipment should be cleaned according to the recommendations for each instrument after each use. Table 34–7 ● describes some of the most commonly used tools.

TABLE 34–7   Tools Used for a Health Examination

SUPPLIES		PURPOSE
Flashlight or penlight		To assist viewing of the pharynx and cervix or to determine the reactions of the pupils of the eye
Nasal speculum		To permit visualization of the lower and middle turbinates; usually, a penlight is used for illumination
Ophthalmoscope		A lighted instrument to visualize the interior of the eye
Otoscope		A lighted instrument to visualize the eardrum and external auditory canal (a nasal speculum may be attached to the otoscope to inspect the nasal cavities)
Percussion (reflex) hammer		An instrument with a rubber head to test reflexes
Tuning fork		A two-pronged metal instrument used to test hearing acuity and vibratory sense
Vaginal speculum		To assess the cervix and the vagina
Cotton applicators		To obtain specimens
Gloves		To protect the nurse and the client
Lubricant		To ease insertion of instruments (e.g., vaginal speculum)
Tongue blades (depressors)		To depress the tongue during assessment of the mouth and pharynx

Clara and Roberto Galvez carry their screaming 7-year-old son Johnnie into the emergency department. They tell the triage nurse that Johnnie woke up before dawn, first complaining of his stomach hurting. He then vomited, and when touched, he felt very hot and sweaty. He now holds both hands tightly on his abdomen, and cannot be consoled.

The nurse conducts a physical examination that reveals the following: symmetrical abdomen, bowel sounds in all quadrants, tender to palpation in the lower quadrants, guarding. Johnnie has an oral temperature of 101.5°F, pulse of 122 bpm, and respiratory rate of 24/min.

Critical Thinking Questions

1. Classify the findings as objective or subjective data.
2. Prepare a narrative nursing note from the data.
3. What factors must be considered in conducting the comprehensive health assessment of Johnnie Galvez?
4. Prior to developing a nursing diagnosis, what must the nurse do?

▶ ORGANIZING DATA

The collected data must be documented at the time of collection or shortly thereafter. Complete coverage of documentation can be found in the exemplar on Documentation in the module on Communication.

As part of the documentation process, the nurse uses a written or digital format that organizes the assessment data systematically. This is often referred to as a nursing health history, nursing assessment, or nursing database form. Most schools of nursing and healthcare agencies have developed their own structured assessment format. Many of these are based on selected nursing models or frameworks. The format may be modified according to the client's physical status, such as one focused on musculoskeletal data for orthopedic clients.

Maslow's Hierarchy of Needs

Maslow's hierarchy of needs (see the module on Clinical Decision Making and the module on Stress and Coping for more information about Maslow's hierarchy) clusters data pertaining to the following:

- Physiological needs (survival needs)
- Safety and security needs
- Love and belonging needs
- Self-esteem needs
- Self-actualization needs.

Developmental Theories

Several physical, psychosocial, cognitive, and moral developmental theories may be used by the nurse in specific situations (see the module on Development). Examples include the following:

- Havighurst's age periods and developmental tasks
- Freud's five stages of development
- Erikson's eight stages of development

- Piaget's phases of cognitive development
- Kohlberg's stages of moral development.

Functional Health Patterns and Body Systems

Assessment data may also be organized by functional health patterns (see the exemplar on the Nursing Process in the module on Clinical Decision Making) or by body systems:

1. Immune system
2. Respiratory system
3. Cardiovascular system
4. Nervous system
5. Musculoskeletal system
6. Gastrointestinal system
7. Genitourinary system
8. Reproductive system.

Once data have been organized, they are validated.

▶ VALIDATING DATA

The information gathered during the assessment phase must be complete, factual, and accurate because the nursing diagnoses and interventions are based on this information. **Validation** is the act of double-checking or verifying data to confirm that they are accurate and factual. Validating data helps the nurse do the following:

- Ensure that assessment information is complete.
- Ensure that objective and related subjective data agree.
- Obtain additional information that may have been overlooked.
- Differentiate between cues and inferences.
- Avoid jumping to conclusions and focusing in the wrong direction to identify problems.

To collect data accurately, nurses need to be aware of their own biases, values, and beliefs and to separate fact from inference, interpretation, and assumption. For example, a nurse seeing a man holding his arm to his chest might assume that he is experiencing chest pain when in fact it is his hand that hurts.

Not all data require validation. For example, height, weight, birth date, and most laboratory studies that can be measured with an accurate scale can be accepted as factual. As a rule, the nurse validates data when discrepancies arise between data obtained in the nursing interview (subjective data) and the physical examination (objective data) or when the client's statements differ at different times in the assessment. Failure to validate can lead to an inaccurate or incomplete nursing assessment and could compromise client safety. Guidelines for validating data are shown in **Table 34–8** ●.

Once data have been collected, organized, and validated, they can be analyzed to determine priorities for client care.

▶ INTERPRETING DATA

Interpreting findings requires making determinations about all of the data collected in the health assessment process. The nurse must determine the following:

- Whether the findings fall within normal and expected ranges in relation to the client's age, gender, and race

TABLE 34–8 Validating Assessment Data

GUIDELINE	EXAMPLE
Compare subjective and objective data to verify the client's statements with observations made.	Client's perception of "feeling hot" needs to be compared with measurement of the body temperature.
Clarify any ambiguous or vague statements.	Client: "I've felt sick off and on for six weeks."
	Nurse: "Describe what your sickness is like. Tell me what you mean by 'off and on.'"
Be sure assessment data consist of cues and not inferences.	Observation: Dry skin and reduced tissue turgor.
	Inference: Dehydration.
	Action: Collect additional data that are needed to make the inference in the diagnosing phase. For example, determine the client's fluid intake, amount and appearance of urine, and blood pressure.
Double-check data that are extremely abnormal.	Observation: A resting pulse of 30 beats per minute or a blood pressure of 210/95 mmHg.
	Action: Repeat the measurement. Use another piece of equipment as needed to confirm abnormalities, or ask someone else to collect the same data.
Determine the presence of factors that may interfere with accurate measurement.	A crying infant will have an abnormal respiratory rate and will need quieting before accurate assessment can be made.
Use references (textbooks, journals, research reports) to explain phenomena.	A nurse considers tiny purple or bluish black swollen areas under the tongue of an older client to be abnormal until the nurse reads about physical changes of aging. Such varicosities are common.

■ The significance of the findings in relation to the client's health status and immediate and long-range health-related needs.

Interpretation of findings is influenced by a number of factors. These include the ability to obtain, recall, and apply knowledge; to communicate effectively; and to use a holistic approach.

Knowledge

Nurses obtain, recall, and apply knowledge from physical and social sciences, nursing theory, and all areas of research that affect current nursing practice. That knowledge includes human anatomy and physiology, growth and development across the life span, and characteristics specific to gender and race. Knowledge also reflects health-related and healthcare trends in groups and populations, such as the increased incidence of risk factors or actual illnesses in certain groups or populations. For example, in the United States one trend is the increased incidence of obesity in children and adults.

Nurses must be able to access and use reliable resources when interpreting findings. Resources include research; scientific literature; and charts, scales, and graphs to indicate ranges of norms and expectations about physical and psychological development. Examples of the latter include Denver Developmental scores, mental status examinations, weight, body mass index, and growth charts prepared by centers for health statistics (D'Amico & Barbarito, 2012, p. 9). Additionally, the nurse must be able to communicate effectively, to think critically, to recognize and act on client cues, to incorporate a holistic perspective, and to determine the significance of data in meeting immediate and long-term client needs. The nurse must be able to recognize situations that require immediate attention, initiate care, and seek appropriate assistance.

Expectations about interpretation of findings change as the nurse gains skills and experience in nursing practice and with advanced practice education. A nursing student is expected to recall and apply knowledge to discriminate between normal and abnormal findings and use resources to understand the findings in relation to wellness or illness for a particular client. For example, consider the findings from the assessment of Julie Connor, a 12-year-old girl: asymmetrical shoulders and elevated right scapula on inspection of the posterior thorax, and right lateral curvature of the thoracic spine on palpation of vertebrae. Normally, scapulae should be symmetrical and the vertebrae should be aligned. The findings are interpreted as a deviation from the normal. They do not, however, give sufficient information for the purposes of making nursing diagnoses. The nurse must collect more data to make diagnoses and design a plan of care for Julie.

The nurse gains confidence and ability to discriminate between normal and abnormal findings through experience and continuing education. With such experience, the nurse will learn to recognize patterns that predispose individuals to illness or are indicative of specific illnesses, and implement and evaluate appropriate nursing care.

CASE STUDY \\ C

James Long is a 46-year-old African American male: height 5'9", weight 220 lb, BP 156/94 mmHg. His mother died at age 62 from cerebrovascular accident (stroke), and his father died at age 42 from myocardial infarction (heart attack). Using knowledge of normal ranges of findings for vital signs, height, and weight, the nurse interprets Mr. Long's BP and weight results as abnormal findings: They indicate that he has high blood pressure and is obese. The nurse applies knowledge of trends associated with health problems to interpret the significance of the findings for this client. The nurse knows that hypertension occurs more frequently in African American males than in Caucasians. Hypertension, obesity, and a family history of coronary artery disease increase the risk of both acquiring hypertension and its associated complications. By combining knowledge of risk factors and complications with the findings themselves, the nurse working with Mr. Long can develop a plan of care. The nurse can collaborate with other healthcare professionals to address Mr. Long's need to reduce his weight and lower his blood pressure.

Critical Thinking Questions

1. What nursing diagnoses would be appropriate?
2. What client outcomes would you plan for Mr. Long?
3. What resources are available in your community to assist you with intervening or advocating for clients such as Mr. Long?

Communication

Effective communication is essential to the assessment process. **Communication** refers to the exchange of information, feelings, thoughts, and ideas. Verbal techniques, such as open-ended or closed questions, statements, clarification, and rephrasing, are just a few of the techniques used to gather information. The communication techniques must incorporate regard for the individual in relation to the purposes of the data collection, the client's age, and the client's level of anxiety. In addition, the nurse must use techniques that accommodate language differences or difficulties, cultural influences, cognitive ability, affect, demeanor, and special needs. Communication is discussed in greater detail in the module on Communication.

Holistic Approach

A holistic approach is an essential characteristic of nursing practice. **Holism** can best be defined as considering more than the physiological health status of a client. Holism includes all factors that affect the client's physical and emotional well-being. With a holistic approach, the nurse recognizes that developmental, psychological, emotional, family, cultural, and environmental factors affect immediate and long-term actual and potential health goals, problems, and plans.

Developmental Factors

The client's developmental level affects the health assessment. Sources of information may vary depending on the client's age and ability to communicate his or her symptoms. For clients with disabilities, findings must be interpreted according to the assessed developmental level, not the client's age. Parents or guardians are the primary sources for information about children and clients with disabilities or impairments that affect their ability to communicate. The developmental level of the client also influences the approach to assessment, including the words and terminology. For example, assessment of a pregnant adolescent would be different from assessment of a 38-year-old woman who is pregnant for the third time.

Psychological and Emotional Factors

Psychological and emotional factors affect physiological health and must be considered as predisposing or contributing factors when interpreting findings from a health assessment. One needs only to recall that anxiety triggers an autonomic response, resulting in increased pulse and blood pressure, to understand that relationship. Conversely, physical problems can affect emotional health. For example, childhood obesity can lead to problems with self-esteem and can affect socialization and development. Psychological problems such as anxiety and depression may interfere with the client's ability to fully participate in health assessment. Grieving may limit a client's ability to carry out required health practices or recognize health problems.

Family Factors

The nurse must consider family history of illness or health problems when conducting a health assessment and interpreting findings. Individuals with a family history of some illnesses are considered at high risk for contracting those diseases. For example, having a first-degree relative (mother, sister, or daughter) with breast cancer about doubles a woman's risk of developing breast cancer herself (American Cancer Society, 2013b). The nurse must recognize that family dynamics may influence one's approach to health care. In some families, health-related decisions are not made independently, but rather are made by the family leader or arrived at by group consensus. Circumstances within families can affect both physical and emotional health and must be considered as part of any health assessment. For example, children of people with alcoholism are not only at risk for alcoholism, but are also at risk for emotional issues not encountered by other children. Therefore, the nurse must view and interpret unexpected physical or emotional behaviors in relation to the alcoholic family situation.

Cultural Factors

The nurse must consider cultural factors when collecting data and interpreting findings. Culture affects language, expression, emotional and physical well-being, and health practices. Findings regarding physical and emotional health must be interpreted in relation to the cultural norms for the client. For example, many Asian cultures would not consider lack of eye contact during the interview as a lack of ability to interact, depression, or a problem with attention. The nurse must take care to provide clear explanations of abnormal findings, illnesses, and treatments because views of illness, causality, and treatment may be influenced by a client's culture. Refer to the module on Culture and Diversity for more information on cultural considerations.

Environmental Factors

Internal and external environmental factors affect health assessment and interpretation of findings. The nurse must always consider data in relation to norms and expectation for age, race, and gender and in relation to factors affecting the individual client.

Data from the comprehensive health assessment provide clues about the client's internal environment, including emotional state, response to medication and treatment, and physiological or anatomical alterations that influence findings and interpretations.

External environmental factors can also affect health, health assessment, and interpretation of findings. External factors may include any of the following:

- Inhaled toxins such as smoke, chemicals, and fumes
- Irritants that can be inhaled, ingested, or absorbed through the skin
- Noise, light, and motion
- Objects or substances encountered in the home, school, or workplace, such as animal dander or dust.

▶ NURSING PRACTICE

Nursing care always begins with assessment. The nurse should not develop a plan of care or initiate any intervention without first assessing the client. The nurse should gather and record carefully all information from the health history, focused interview, and physical assessment before beginning to interpret any of the data. The nurse must also document findings in the client's medical record as soon as possible.

Nursing care is based on a strong knowledge base and the application of critical thinking. The nurse's knowledge base is developed over time using information from the humanities and the biological, natural, and social sciences. Using evidence-based research data, standards of care, and the nursing process, the professional nurse provides competent care. Competent care includes promoting health and wellness, treating and caring for the ill, and caring for the dying individual while being supportive to family members. To perform these actions, the nurse works in a variety of settings including hospitals, clinics, nursing homes, clients' homes, schools, and workplaces.

Regardless of the setting, the role of the nurse is multifaceted. Each situation requires the nurse to use critical thinking and the nursing process. To provide care and utilize the nursing process, the nurse must develop strong assessment skills. The gathering of complete, accurate, and relevant data is required. While gathering the subjective and objective data from the client, the nurse must be attuned to the signs, symptoms, behaviors, and cues offered by the client. The collected data vary as the status of the client changes. The nurse functions as a teacher, caregiver, client advocate, and manager of client care.

◢ REVIEW The Concept of Assessment

RELATE Link the Concepts

Linking the concept of assessment with the concept of caring interventions:

1. You are assigned to care for a client who has been receiving tube feedings via a nasogastric tube that has been in place for several days. Prior to administering the first tube feeding of the shift, what assessments would you perform?

2. Would the assessment performed be an initial assessment or a problem-focused assessment? Explain your answer.

Linking the concept of assessment with the concept of clinical decision making:

3. You are assigned care of a 46-year-old man admitted for status asthmaticus. His condition has stabilized and discharge is planned for tomorrow. When you enter his room for the first time, you find that he is short of breath and he requests that you hand him his inhaler, which the physician ordered to be kept at the bedside for self-administration as needed. What will you do first?

4. What critical thinking would you apply to the above situation?

READY Go to Companion Skills Manual

REFER Go to Pearson Nursing Student Resources
nursing.pearsonhighered.com
- Additional review materials

REFLECT Case Study

To prepare for a follow-up visit, the nurse reads the health history of Mrs. Bernice Hall, a 39-year-old woman. From the regularity of her previous visits, it appears that Mrs. Hall has always taken good care of her physical and mental health. She bicycles to work and attends yoga classes semi-regularly. Her history recorded that she has dark, almost black, formed stools. The interviewer documented that Mrs. Hall stated that she has taken iron pills and eaten a lot of spinach and greens for years. She reported that her stools have always been consistently dark and formed.

1. What are the normal findings of stool color and consistency?

2. In Mrs. Hall's case, would her history indicate evidence of an abnormal finding?

3. What laboratory tests would be indicated to confirm that she is benefiting from taking iron medication?

◣ EXEMPLAR 34.1   Holistic Health Assessment Across the Life Span

EXEMPLAR KEY TERMS
Centration, *2292*
Hydrocephalus, *2290*
Overnutrition, *2290*
Undernutrition, *2290*

EXEMPLAR LEARNING OUTCOMES
After reading about this exemplar, you will be able to:

1. Correlate the role and impact of development on the nursing assessment, including the physical examination and interview for client history.

2. Differentiate how assessment of children varies from assessment of adults.

3. Propose differences in procedures when assessing a client in each stage of development.

4. Correlate specific health assessment needs with each stage of the life span.

5. Differentiate the needs of the older adult as related to the health assessment.

▶ OVERVIEW

Nursing assessment requires the ability to interpret how the complex interactions of heredity; environment; and physiological, cognitive, and psychological development affect an individual at a particular time. By developing an image of what is usual or expected of children and adults of various ages, the nurse has a basis for a comparison with the norm. This knowledge and an understanding of individual variations provide a foundation for assessment that helps individuals attain their maximum level of wellness.

▶ SPECIAL CONSIDERATIONS FOR ASSESSMENT OF CHILDREN

Children are not "little adults." Significant differences exist among infants, children, adolescents, and adults. These differences include variations in physiology, development, and cognition that must be incorporated into the nursing assessment. For instance, the head-to-toe approach to physical assessment is useful in many situations and with different types of clients, but it may not work with young children. Adults and adolescents will usually sit on an examination table, wear a paper gown, and follow the nurse's instructions. However, infants and toddlers often refuse to sit still or cooperate.

Furthermore, young children do not have the cognitive or verbal ability to describe symptoms or comply with complex instructions. The nurse must possess strong assessment skills to overcome the communication and situational challenges involved in pediatric physical assessment.

In assessing children, it may be helpful to conduct the nutrition history portion before the physical assessment in order to establish rapport and make the child more comfortable with the process. Rapport is essential, especially when assessing an adolescent. Infants and younger children need a caretaker present to assist with the assessment and to answer questions (**Figure 34–6 ●**). Adolescents may be more comfortable having privacy during an assessment. The nurse may discuss the assessment arrangement with the adolescent and caregiver separately to allow the adolescent to give an unpressured answer. A caregiver can be interviewed separately if appropriate.

The parameters of the physical assessment in children include anthropometric measurements and clinical observations appropriate for each child's age. Determination of developmental milestones provides critical information and is part of a complete assessment. Developmental milestones are covered in the module on Development.

Anthropometric measurements in children should be obtained using equipment appropriate for the pediatric population. Recumbent length and weight measurements are needed for infants and young children. An infant's or toddler's weight should be measured without the child wearing a diaper. Older children can have their height and weight measured while standing. Skinfold measurements should be done using calipers calibrated to 0.2 mm since small changes in measurement can cause changes in assessment classification. The World Health Organization (WHO) recommends weight for

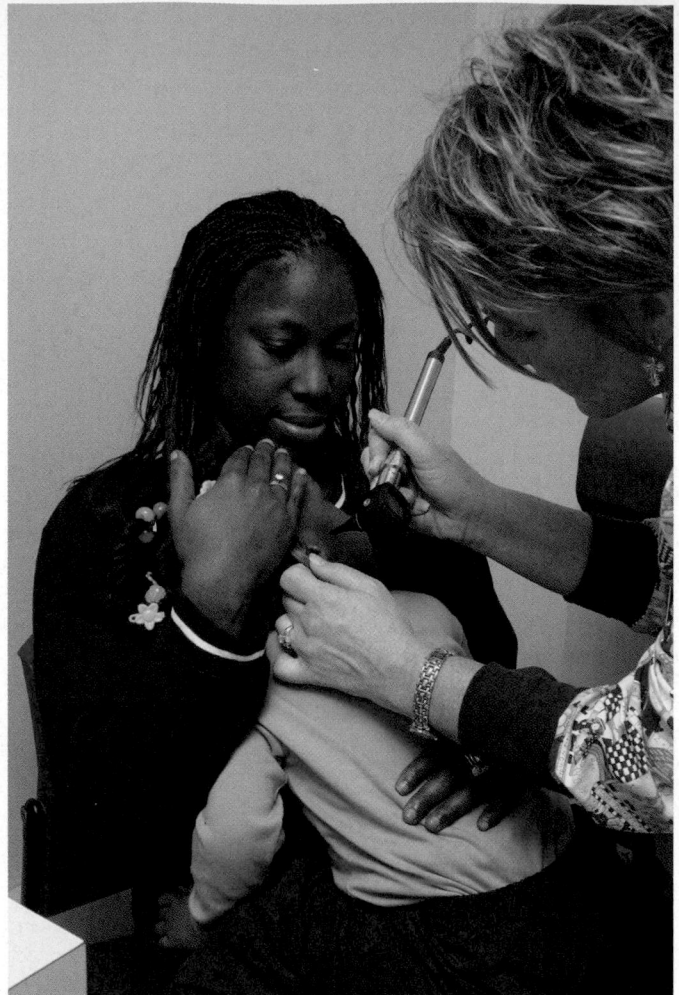

Figure 34–6 ● It is often helpful to have a young child sit on a parent's lap during an assessment.

height as the standard in measuring children since skinfold and circumference measurements are prone to errors that could result in misclassification of nutritional health. Head circumference is a measurement unique to the assessment of growth in children at or under 3 years of age. Beyond age 3, head circumference is not a valid tool for assessing growth and nutritional status.

Anthropometric measurements have age-specific references established by the Centers for Disease Control and Prevention and WHO. In children under 20 years of age, references are described using charts with age-specific percentiles for height, weight, body mass index (BMI), and, for children under 36 months, head circumference. Percentiles are used to assess growth rate and health. Percentile charts are derived from the distribution of data from population studies and are age- and gender-specific descriptions of anthropometric measurements. The charts may change as new data are incorporated. For example, breastfed infants normally grow at a slightly slower rate than do formula-fed babies, and newer infant growth charts are more representative of the population-matched prevalence of breastfed infants compared to charts published before 2000.

Infants, children, and adolescents can be compared to their age-matched peers to determine their individual percentile within the population. A best use of percentile charts is in monitoring individual growth over time. Normally, children will remain within a narrow percentile range for each measurement over the course of childhood. For example, a child assessed sequentially in the 25th percentile for height (length) for age may have a small frame and parents with small stature and may not be at risk for poor nutritional health. However, a child sequentially in the 50th percentile for height for age who drops to the 25th percentile may be at risk for undernutrition. A significant drop or increase in percentile category is cause for further investigation to assess for undernutrition or overnutrition. Overweight and obesity (overnutrition) in children is defined as a BMI for age greater than the 85th percentile and the 95th percentile, respectively. Undernutrition is defined as a BMI for age less than the 5th percentile. Separate growth references exist for children with some chronic diseases and for knee–height estimates of stature. See the module on Nutrition for more information on overnutrition and undernutrition.

Children are physically different from adults. Each concept in the individual domain (Modules 1–33) discusses lifespan differences that can be anticipated when conducting the physical examination.

The nurse should use a caring, supportive, yet firm approach with children. Whenever possible, play should be incorporated into the assessment process. It is helpful to allow children to touch and manipulate equipment. Adhesive bandages or empty syringes can be provided for play-acting with dolls. The nurse should encourage children to talk about their fears and concerns. Painful procedures should not be performed while a child is seated on a parent's lap. Children need to know they are safe from painful experiences when they are with their parents.

When a child is ill, parents suffer from increased stress that results from interrupted sleep, concern for the child's well-being, and frustration at the inability to understand what is hurting or bothering their child. Each of these factors may affect a parent's ability to recall information or to follow complex instructions. The nurse can help parents by providing them with written instructions as appropriate and encouraging clients and families to journal about their experiences or keep a notebook with information and details about the child's illness and treatment, including nutrition and activity levels. The nurse should consider parental stress levels when developing care plans.

The basic components of a health history are the same whether the nurse works with children or adults. However, a number of variations must be incorporated into a pediatric health history. It is essential for the nurse to determine the relationship between the child who seeks health care and the adult who presents with the child. State law determines which individuals can legally consent to medical treatment of a minor child. Federal privacy laws limit access to protected health information. One must never assume legal or family ties between children and the adults who accompany them.

Nannies, babysitters, friends, siblings, and stepparents often transport children to healthcare appointments. Asking directly about the relationships is the easiest way to ensure compliance with the legal and ethical concerns regarding the medical treatment of children.

Many children are nonverbal or have limited language ability; therefore, the nurse depends on parents and guardians for health history information. This can limit the specificity of the history information. However, it is important to ask preschoolers and older children about their chief complaint and symptoms even though the information they provide may not be as detailed as the information provided by their parents or guardians.

The nurse should determine prior to the health interview whether the parent is stressed or distracted. Many parents of ill children are sleep deprived because of their child's altered sleep patterns. Sleep deprivation can result in altered recall, limited ability to follow complex questions, and diminished ability to remember verbal instructions. The presence of other children can be distracting, especially if the children are loud, active, or irritable. The nurse can distract energetic or fussy children with books, crayons, or toys.

The nurse should listen carefully to the parent or primary caregiver and use open-ended questions to elicit health information. Parents know their children better than anyone else. They are able to detect subtle differences in their child's behavior. It is essential to pay special attention to the chief complaints that parents describe. A thorough physical assessment is then conducted based on the issues and concerns raised in the health history.

The nurse should call the child by his or her name and use words that the child understands. For example, most preadolescents are not familiar with the word *abdomen*, but most children have used the word *tummy* or *belly* from infancy. Instead of asking "Does your head hurt?" the nurse should ask the child to touch the head where it hurts. It is necessary to be patient. Children often pause between words or repeat phrases when they are excited or nervous.

The nurse should give children who are at least 10 years old the option of being examined without their parents or other accompanying adult present. The client is the child, not the parent. The nurse's legal and ethical responsibility is to the child first. The nurse must respect the confidentiality of the information provided by older children and be aware of state and federal laws regarding parental notification. The parent and the child should be told what the nurse can and cannot keep confidential. For example, statements such as "What you and I talk about will be between the two of us, unless you tell me that you are thinking about harming yourself or someone else, or if you tell me that someone is hurting you" help establish rapport and boundaries to the nurse–child and nurse–parent relationship. If a nurse is required to report health interview information to others (e.g., public health departments or child protective service agents), the nurse should always inform the child of the need to share the information with others prior to actually doing so. Failure to do so can jeopardize the rapport between nurse and child.

Focus on Diversity and Culture Considerations When Assessing Children

Most of the world's cultures value children. However, there is significant variation among cultures with respect to what constitutes acceptable child behavior and expectations for health or caregiving. The nurse must be aware of the cultural influences on children and families. For example, European cultures encourage independence at an early age whereas other groups, such as Asians, Hispanics, and Arab Americans, stress a strong commitment to family. Commonly, children from these cultural groups are taught to respect older family members and to place the needs of the family before their personal needs. Hispanics and Native Americans tend to be less strict with their children, especially with male children.

All of the dominant American cultures view mothers as the primary child caregivers. Overall, females are viewed as nurturers who are responsible for guiding and caring for children. Mothers commonly make the decisions regarding home care of child illness and complaints. However, many groups, including Arab Americans, have patriarchal hierarchies where the father must be consulted prior to the family making any professional healthcare decisions.

African American

- Newborns may have pustular melanosis, characterized by pustules that rupture, leaving 2- to 3-mm brown macules. These brown marks will disappear spontaneously within 3–4 months.
- Hair texture will become coarser with tighter curls over the first 6 months of life.
- Mongolian spots are commonly located over the lower back and buttocks; they will begin to fade by age 2 or 3.
- Infants should be tested for sickle cell disease at birth.
- Most infants are born with dark gray-brown eyes that will not change much as the baby gets older.
- Hypertension and insulin-resistant diabetes are more common in African American youths than in other ethnic groups.

Asian

- As a sign of respect, many Asian parents may be reluctant to disagree with or displease a healthcare provider.
- Direct eye contact may be viewed as impolite.
- Mongolian spots are common.
- Most infants have dark gray eye color at birth.
- Vietnamese families believe the head is sacred. The nurse should avoid touching the head of the mother and baby without first asking permission.
- Some Chinese individuals practice cupping, in which a heated cup is placed over the skin to draw out illness. Some Vietnamese individuals use coin rubbing, in which a coin is rubbed on the trunk. Neither practice should be considered abuse.
- Many Asian families use the concept of hot and cold illnesses. Certain illnesses are considered to be hot or cold, and treatments should counter the effect of the illness; in other words, hot illnesses should be treated with cold medicines and foods, whereas cold illnesses should be treated with hot medicines and foods.

Hispanic

- Most infants have dark gray-brown eye color at birth.
- Mongolian spots are common.
- Infants should be tested for sickle cell disease at birth.
- Many Mexican Americans consider it bad luck for an individual to touch a child's head.
- Many Hispanic families use the concept of hot and cold illnesses. Certain illnesses are considered to be hot or cold, and treatments should counter the effect of the illness; in other words, hot illnesses should be treated with cold medicines and foods, whereas cold illnesses should be treated with hot medicines and foods.
- Modesty may be important and should be respected.
- Some groups believe that complimenting a child without touching him or her can draw the "evil eye."
- Many individuals consider being overweight to be healthy, especially in women and young children.

Native American

- Many Native Americans have strong beliefs that children should be allowed to develop at their own rate. Parents may be reluctant to force a child to stop bottle or pacifier use or to start toilet training.
- Mongolian spots are common.
- Hypothyroidism is more common in Native Americans than in other ethnic groups (1 in 700). Newborn testing and vigilance for symptoms of hypothyroidism are recommended.
- It is taboo to purchase any clothing or items for the newborn prior to birth. This contrasts with customs in the Western culture.
- Hypertension and insulin-resistant diabetes are more common in Native American youths than in other ethnic groups.
- Direct eye contact may be avoided as a sign of respect.

Middle Eastern

- Direct eye contact may be viewed as impolite or improper, especially with members of the opposite gender.
- Physical examination by individuals of different gender is taboo after adolescence.
- Thalassemias are more common in children of Middle Eastern heritage than in children of European descent.
- Modesty may be important and should be respected.
- Females may defer to the male head of the family for healthcare decisions.

All Races and Cultures

- Babies within all races and cultures are born with lighter, pinker skin. The true color of the baby's skin will develop during the first year.
- All cultures and ethnic groups have folk beliefs that center around childbirth and childrearing. The nurse should assess for positive folk practices and incorporate them into nursing care.

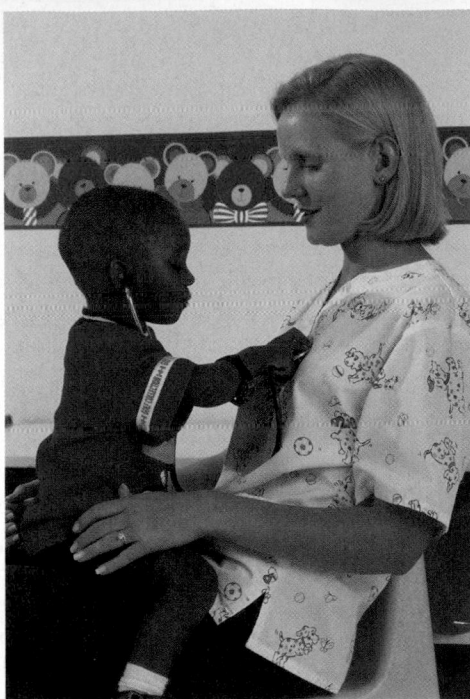

Figure 34–7 ● A nurse allows her client to play with her stethoscope before using it to assess his heart.
Source: Bill Lai/Getty Images.

There are many ways to make the examination tolerable. Allowing children to touch medical equipment is one technique (**Figure 34–7 ●**). For example, the nurse can ask a young child to put the otoscope's "hat" (i.e., speculum) on the light. Before examining the tympanic membrane, the nurse can ask toddlers and preschoolers if they have elephants or

Lifespan Considerations
Assessing the Pediatric Client

- Protect the modesty and privacy of children as you would for adults.
- Explain procedures and techniques in words that children can understand.
- Remember that young children are more comfortable and compliant when they sit on their parents' laps. However, this location still needs to be avoided when performing painful activities.
- Establish rapport with the parent and child before initiating any physical examination.
- Begin with the least threatening examinations; a flexible approach to assessment is essential.
- Perform painful or invasive procedures at the end of the assessment.
- Auscultate the thorax of the sleeping child.
- Allow children to touch equipment. Use games for examinations, such as asking children if they have elephants in their ears before examining the tympanic membrane.
- Use toys, for example, finger puppets, as distractions.
- Use standard precautions.

cartoon characters in their ear. Young children can be encouraged to take deep breaths by having them blow bubbles or blow out the light on the otoscope. Distracting children with toys is another way to make the assessment less frightening. Examples include finger puppets, small animals placed on the stethoscope, and whistles or small music boxes. Toys with small pieces should be kept out of the reach of infants, toddlers, and preschoolers.

▶ ASSESSMENT SPECIFIC TO STAGES OF THE LIFE SPAN

A comprehensive assessment includes information about physical, cognitive, and emotional growth and development including both subjective and objective data. When conducting health assessments, the nurse must be able to obtain accurate data and interpret findings in relation to expectations and predicted norms and ranges for clients at various stages of physical and emotional development. Knowledge of anatomical and physiological changes as well as theoretical information about cognitive, psychoanalytical, and psychosocial events and expectations at each stage of human development is invaluable for the nurse. Further information about growth and development can be found in the module on Development.

Physical growth and development change across the age span. Stages from infancy through adolescence are marked by spurts of rapid growth and development. Health assessment includes the use of clinical growth charts to compare individual client measurements of height and weight (and head circumference in infants) against expected normal values for age and gender. Additional indicators for normal growth and development throughout these stages include eating, sleeping, elimination, and activity patterns. Neurological and sensory functions are assessed by monitoring development of speech and language, muscular growth, strength and coordination, and tactile sensibility.

Puberty is a period of rapid physiological growth and development. Puberty occurs between the ages of 10 and 14 years in females and is marked by menarche, breast development, axillary and pubic hair growth, and a spurt in height. In males, puberty occurs between the ages of 12 and 16 years and is characterized by a spurt in height, development of the penis and testicles, and body hair growth (axillae, chest, facial), including pubic hair. Young adulthood is the stage marked by completed growth in physical and mental structures. Physical development continues to be assessed by comparing individual findings to clinical growth charts and by assessing eating, sleeping, and activity patterns.

Middle age, occurring between the ages of 45 and 60 years, is another period in which dramatic changes in physical development occur. Primary changes are related to hormonal changes in both men and women, resulting in menopause in women. During middle age, changes occur in all systems; these include decreases in basal metabolic rate, muscle size, nerve conduction, lung capacity, glomerular filtration, and cardiac output. The middle-aged client experiences increased adipose tissue deposit and skeletal changes leading to decreases in height, as well as changes in tactile sensibility, vision, and hearing. The physical changes continue into the stage of older adulthood. Middle-aged and older adults are at risk for obesity and associated health problems. Health assessment includes use of the BMI measurement to assess weight and risk for disease. Assessment also includes evaluation of the ability to carry out activities of daily living (ADLs) and regular testing of vision and hearing.

The leading causes of death throughout the life span are outlined in **Table 34–9** ●.

In addition to expectations about physical growth and development, there are expectations about cognitive, psychosocial, and emotional development across the age span. For example, attachment is an essential element in infant development. Attachment refers to the tie between the infant and caregivers that promotes physical and psychosocial well-being. Assessment of attachment includes observing caregivers for eye contact, apparent interest in the child, talking or cooing to the child, response to infant needs, and communication.

Children are expected to develop language and cognitive abilities that enable them to learn and become independent

over time. Young adults are expected to develop relationships with others and to become productive members of society. Maturity and aging lead individuals to contribute to the well-being of communities and their families and often to adapt to change and loss. Developmental milestones and crises occur in all stages of development and must be noted during assessment. A variety of instruments and scales can be used to identify developmental delays, behavioral patterns, and responses that indicate potential or actual problems with emotional, cognitive, and psychosocial development and adaptation in children and adults. **Table 34–10** ● includes a list and description of some of the instruments available to measure aspects of growth and development.

Assessment of Infants

Frequent assessments during the first year provide opportunities to monitor the infant's rate of growth and development as well as to compare the infant with the norm for age. Height, weight, and head circumference measurements are plotted on an appropriate growth chart at each assessment. The three measurements should fall within two standard deviations of each other. More importantly, each measurement should follow the expected rate of growth, following the same percentile throughout infancy.

Accurate assessment combining information obtained by history, physical assessment, and knowledgeable observation allows early identification of common problems that may easily be resolved with early intervention. Often basic parent education and support remedy problems that, if left untreated, could later result in significant health problems or disturbed parent–child interactions.

Overnutrition and undernutrition are identified by weight that crosses percentiles. In **overnutrition**, the rate of weight gain is accelerated; in **undernutrition** the rate of weight gain diminishes. Overnutrition may occur when caregivers do not learn to read infants' cues but instead assume that every cry signals hunger. Cultural beliefs that a plump baby is a healthy baby may also lead parents and other caregivers to overfeed infants.

Undernutrition may be caused by inadequate caloric intake. This may result from lack of knowledge of normal infant feeding, a lack of financial resources to obtain formula, or inappropriate mixing of formula. Some quiet or passive infants do not demand feedings, and parents or caregivers may misinterpret this passivity as lack of hunger.

Head growth that crosses percentiles requires evaluation, because it may indicate **hydrocephalus** (enlargement of the head caused by inadequate drainage of cerebrospinal fluid). Early diagnosis and intervention for rapid head growth prevent or diminish serious neurological effects.

Parents and caregivers generally enjoy relaying infants' new developmental milestones and can accurately describe infants' abilities. An infant who seems to be lagging behind on milestones may not be receiving appropriate stimulation. Assessment of caregivers' expectations and knowledge of infant development may reveal a knowledge deficit. Suggesting specific activities for caregivers to do with their infants may be the only intervention required. Infants who continue to lag

TABLE 34–9 Leading Causes of Death Throughout the Life Span

AGE RANGE	LEADING CAUSES OF DEATH AND NUMBER OF DEATHS IN 2010
Birth–age 10 years	■ Conditions originating in the perinatal period (short gestation, maternal pregnancy complications, placenta/cord/membranes): 6,791 ■ Congenital anomalies: 5,777 ■ Motor vehicle crashes and other unintentional injuries: 3,262 ■ Sudden infant death syndrome (SIDS): 2,063
Ages 11–24 years	■ Motor vehicle crashes and other unintentional injuries: 13,226 ■ Suicide: 4,867 ■ Homicide: 4,828 ■ Malignant neoplasms: 2,081 ■ Heart diseases: 1,145
Ages 25–64 years	■ Malignant neoplasms: 175,140 ■ Heart disease: 118,622 ■ Motor vehicle crashes and other unintentional injuries: 75,396 ■ Suicide: 27,489 ■ Diabetes: 19,682 ■ Homicide: 6,731 ■ Human immunodeficiency virus (HIV) infection: 5,762
Ages 65 and older	■ Heart disease: 477,338 ■ Malignant neoplasms (lung, colorectal, breast cancers): 396,670 ■ Chronic obstructive pulmonary disease: 118,031 ■ Cerebrovascular disease: 109,990 ■ Alzheimer disease: 82, 616 ■ Diabetes mellitus: 49,191 ■ Pneumonia and influenza: 42,846

Source: Centers for Disease Control and Prevention, *10 Leading Causes of Death by Age Group, United States—2010,* retrieved from http://www.cdc.gov/injury/wisqars/pdf/10LCID_All_Deaths_By_Age_Group_2010-a.pdf.

TABLE 34-10 Instruments to Assess Growth and Development

Ages & Stages Questionnaire (ASQ)	The ASQ is a parent questionnaire that covers developmental areas of communication, gross motor, fine motor, problem solving, and personal-social in children.
Battelle Developmental Inventory	This inventory tests developmental domains of cognition, motor, self-help, language, and social skills in children from birth through 8 years of age.
Brigance Screens	These screens assess speech-language, motor, readiness, and general knowledge at younger ages and also reading and math. Used from 21 to 90 months of age.
Child Development Inventory	Scales used to measure social, self-help, gross motor, fine motor, expressive language, language comprehension, letters, numbers, and general development in children from 15 months to 6 years of age.
Denver II	Screening test administered to well children between birth and 6 years of age. It is designed to test 20 simple tasks and items in four sectors: personal-social, fine motor adaptive, language, and gross motor.
Hassles and Uplifts Scale	Scale used to measure adult attitudes about daily situations defined as "hassles" and "uplifts." It focuses on evaluation of positive and negative events in daily life rather than on life events.
Life Experiences Survey	This self-administered questionnaire reviews life-changing events of a given year. Ratings are used to evaluate the level of stress an individual is experiencing.
McCarthy Scale of Children's Abilities	The McCarthy scale evaluates the general intelligence level of children ages 2½–8½ years. The scale identifies strengths and weaknesses in verbal, perceptual-performance, quantitative, memory, motor, and general cognitive skills.
Mini-Mental Status Examination (MMSE)	This brief, quantitative measure of cognitive status in adults can be used to screen for cognitive impairment, to estimate the severity of cognitive impairment at a given point in time, to follow the course of cognitive changes in an individual over time, and to document an individual's response to treatment. It is used frequently to track cognitive changes in clients with dementia.
Pediatric Symptom Checklist	Checklist of short statements used to identify conduct behaviors and behaviors associated with depression, anxiety, and adjustment in children ages 4–16 years. Item patterns determine the need for behavioral or mental health referrals.
Stanford-Binet Intelligence Scale: Fourth Edition	The Stanford-Binet test measures general intelligence. The areas of verbal reasoning, quantitative reasoning, abstract/visual reasoning, and short-term memory can be tested from ages 2 to 23 years.
Wechsler Preschool and Primary Scale of Intelligence—Revised (WPPSI-R)	The WPPSI-R is a standardized test of language and perception for children ages 4½–6 years.

significantly behind and are not achieving normal milestones require evaluation.

Healthy attachment is observed as a caregiver holds an infant close in a manner that encourages eye contact (the *en face* position). The caregiver looks at the infant, smiles, talks, and interacts with the infant. The infant responds by fixing on the caregiver's face, smiling, and cooing. The caregiver stays close to the infant, providing support and reassurance during examinations or procedures (**Figure 34–8 ●**).

Failure to engage the infant through eye contact, talking, or a smile limits available opportunities for the caregiver to receive positive feedback from the infant. The infant, in turn, finds efforts to engage the parent frustrating, resulting in decreased attempts to interact. A negative pattern is quickly established, requiring more extensive intervention the longer it persists.

Assessment of Toddlers

Although the rate of growth of toddlers decreases, it proceeds in an expected manner. Height and weight continue to follow a percentile, although slight variations are often seen. Assessing caloric intake by obtaining a 24-hour recall provides clues to inappropriate feeding patterns. Toddlers generally feed

themselves and begin to interact with the family at meals (**Figure 34–9 ●**). A favorite food one week may be refused the next, causing frustration and confusion in caregivers. Concern for the toddler's health may precipitate a power struggle as parents try to force the toddler to eat. Poor weight gain may result as the toddler exerts a newfound independence by refusing to eat. Excessive weight gain occurs when caregivers use food to quiet or bribe their toddlers. Discussing appropriate eating expectations and weight gain helps parents resolve eating problems.

Since cooperation of the young toddler is unlikely, a health history is often the best way to assess development. Older toddlers are more willing to play with developmental testing materials or explore the environment while in proximity to a caregiver, enabling direct observations of development. Because toddlers might not speak in a strange or threatening environment, language assessment can be difficult. Listening to the child talk in a playroom or waiting room increases the probability of assessing the toddler's language.

The toddler wanders a short distance from a caregiver to explore, returning periodically to "touch base." After receiving reassurance and encouragement, the child is ready for limits the duration of tantrums and keeps tantrums from becoming power struggles or attention-getting behavior.

Toddlers quickly turn to caregivers for comfort or when confronted with a stranger. Observing the adult–child interaction and listening to how the adult speaks to the child provide information about the quality of the relationship.

Continuous clinging of a toddler to a caregiver in a nonthreatening situation is unusual. Failure of the child to look to a caregiver for comfort and support may indicate that trust did not develop during infancy. Inappropriate caregiver expectations, such as expecting a toddler to sit quietly in a chair, may interfere with the normal progression of the toddler's development. Caregiver inattention to the child's activities and failure to set limits result in the child's inability to develop self-control.

Assessment of Preschoolers

Preschoolers are generally pleasant, cooperative, and talkative. They are often less anxious if their caretaker is in view but do not need to return to the caregiver for comfort except in threatening situations. Talking with preschoolers about favorite activities allows the nurse to assess language ability, cognitive ability, and development. The nurse evaluates the child's use of language to express thoughts, sentence structure, and vocabulary. It may be possible to identify **centration** (the ability to concentrate), magical thinking, and reality imitation as the child relays play activities. Lack of appropriate environmental stimulation may become evident, and the nurse may need to educate caregivers about age-appropriate activities for their children.

Preschoolers' slowed rate of growth is often of concern to caregivers. The nurse can allay anxiety by showing the preschooler's growth chart and discussing eating expectations.

A clinging, frightened preschooler in a nonthreatening situation may indicate a child who lacks a trusting relationship with his or her immediate caregivers. Lack of communication between caregiver and child limits the child's ability to learn appropriate social interaction and to practice language skills.

Children who do not exhibit appropriate achievement of developmental milestones should receive screenings and, if indicated, appropriate interventions. Periodic health assessments are necessary to ensure child well-being and to discuss child development with parents. Table 7–1: Health Screenings and Immunization Guidelines Across the Life Span in the module on Health, Wellness, and Illness provides a detailed listing of interventions recommended for newborns and infants, toddlers, and preschoolers. Depending on the results of the examination, additional screenings or referrals to agencies that conduct developmental screenings may be warranted.

Assessment of School-Age Children

The slow, steady growth and changing body proportions of school-age children make them appear thin and gangly. Assessing children's intake of nutrients and calories and reviewing their growth charts reassure parents that their children are not too thin. By educating parents to evaluate objectively their children's diets during the early school-age years, the nurse can help relieve family stress resulting from parents pushing children to eat and can help reinforce healthy eating habits that prevent obesity. Older school-age children have an increase in appetite as they

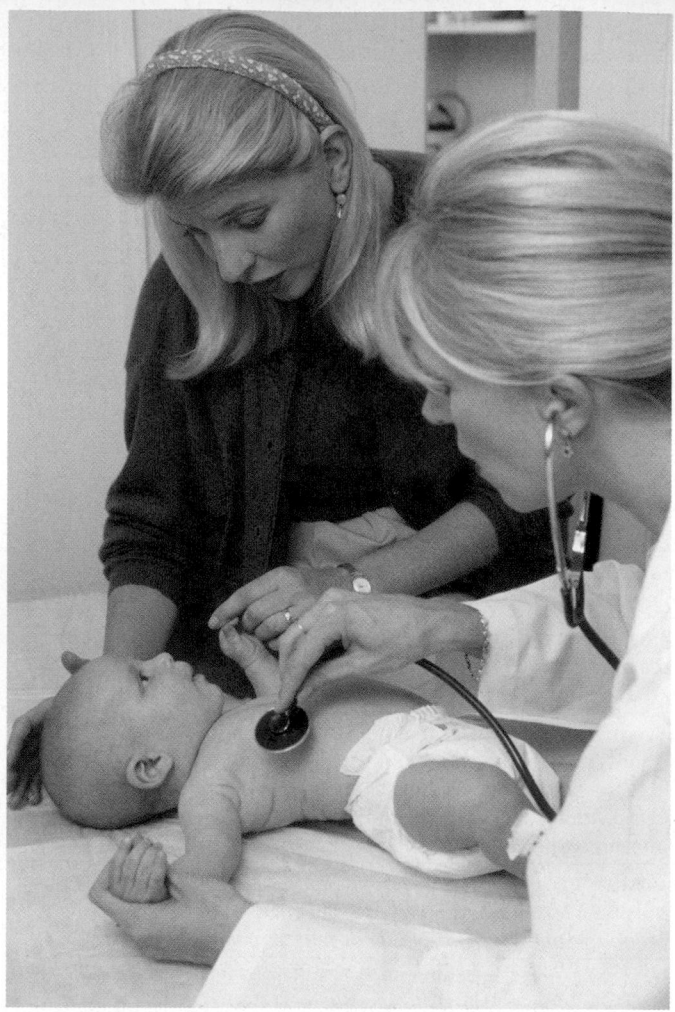

Figure 34–8 ● This mother interacts with her baby while the nurse performs an examination.
Source: MICHAEL KRASOWITZ/Getty Images

further exploration. Exploration provides learning opportunities but also places the toddler at risk for accidental injury or poisoning.

Toddlers have frequent tantrums, usually in response to unwanted limits or frustration. An attitude of calm understanding

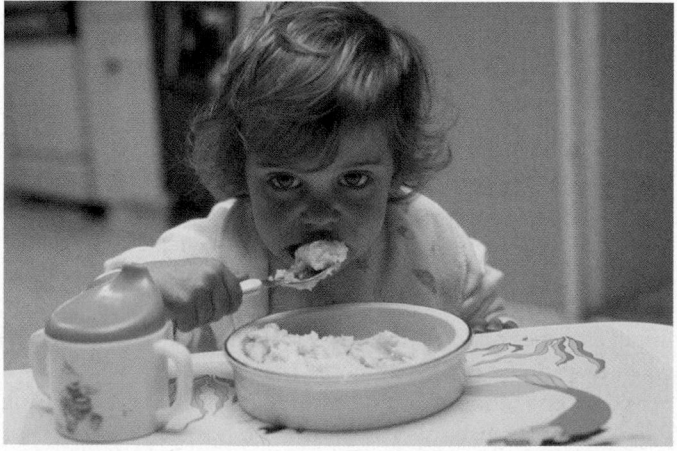

Figure 34–9 ● Toddlers can generally feed themselves.
Source: Felicia Martinez/PhotoEdit Inc.

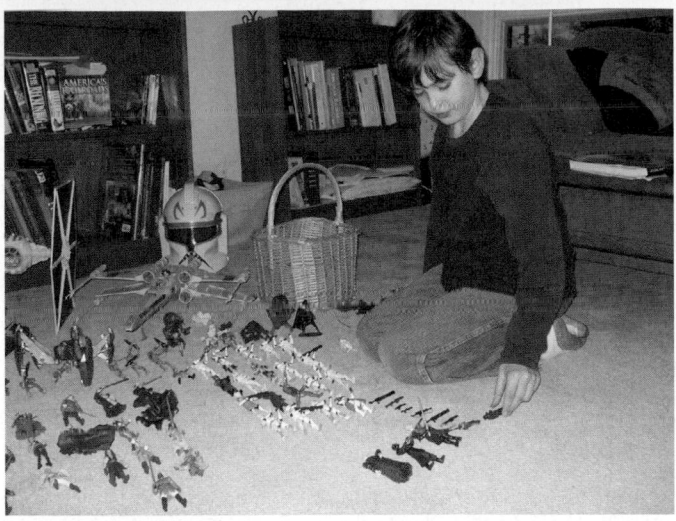

Figure 34–10 ● This school-age child enjoys sorting his collection of action figures.

enter the prepubertal growth spurt. During the growth spurt, height and weight increase and may normally cross percentiles.

School-age children are eager to talk about their hobbies, friends, school, and accomplishments. Increasing neurological maturity allows them to master activities requiring gross and fine motor control, such as sports, dancing, playing a musical instrument, artistic pursuits, or building things. School-age children enjoy showing off newly acquired skills, and families display pride in their children's accomplishments.

School-age children frequently sort and classify collections of rocks, sports cards, dolls, coins, stamps, or almost anything (Figure 34–10 ●). They are industrious in school, feeling pride in their accomplishments as they master difficult concepts and skills. Families provide positive feedback and encouragement to their children and speak of their children's successes with pride.

Adult family members and school-age children communicate openly, with adults setting appropriate and much-needed limits. Although peer relationships are becoming more important, the family remains the major influence during most of the school-age years. As children approach adolescence, the relationship with family may become strained as the children are drawn closer to peer groups and seek greater independence.

Children who lack hobbies or cannot think of any accomplishments may be environmentally deprived. Caregivers who are unable to think of anything positive to say about their children or who speak of them as a burden are likely to have a disturbed parent–child relationship. Children who lack encouragement and positive reinforcement at home for their achievements are at risk for gang recruitment. Gangs provide the "family" support children lack at home, increasing children's risk for violence, drug use, and illegal activity.

Problems in school may evolve at this time, and caregivers and children may have conflicts over grades and study time. The nurse can encourage the caregiver to help the child set a consistent place and time for homework. Caregivers should also be encouraged to communicate actively with the child's teacher. Teachers, adults, family members, and healthcare providers may identify learning disabilities at this time by careful observation.

Table 7–1: Health Screenings and Immunization Guidelines Across the Life Span in the module on Health, Wellness, and Illness provides a detailed listing of interventions recommended for school-age children.

Assessment of Adolescents

Parents and caregivers rarely express concern that their adolescents are not eating. The pubertal growth spurt requires adolescents to increase their caloric intake dramatically, causing parents concern that the adolescent eats constantly but never seems full. Despite this, adolescents (particularly women) are at risk for developing eating disorders. Information about eating disorders is included in the module on Self.

Adolescents often communicate better with peers and adults outside of the family than with family members. Assessing adolescents with their parents and then one-on-one affords a more complete picture of the adolescent–parent relationship and provides adolescents with an opportunity to express themselves and discuss concerns freely.

Most adolescents are able to hold an adult conversation and are often happy to discuss school, friends, activities, and plans for the future. They tend to be anxious about their bodies and the rapid changes that they are experiencing. Often adolescents are unsure if what is happening to them is normal, and they frequently express somatic complaints.

As adolescents become more independent, adult family members become anxious over their evolving lack of control. Parents may be uncomfortable with adolescents' sexuality, rebellious dress and hairstyles, and developing values that may differ from those of the parents. Communication between parents and adolescents is often challenging at this stage.

Severely restricting the activities and freedom of adolescents inhibits their ability to progress toward independence. Adolescents who lack social contacts and spend much time alone may be depressed and at high risk for suicide. Acting out and risk-taking behaviors place adolescents at risk for serious injury from accidents or drug or alcohol use. Alliance with gangs places adolescents at risk for violence and participation in illegal activities.

Table 7–1: Health Screenings and Immunization Guidelines Across the Life Span in the module on Health, Wellness, and Illness provides a detailed listing of interventions recommended for adolescents.

Assessment of Young Adults

Young adults tend to be busy, productive, and healthy. At their maximum physical potential, young adults actively pursue sports and physical fitness activities. They refine their creative talents and enjoy activities with peers.

Young adults form intimate partnerships with others in mature, cooperative relationships. Traditionally, such intimate relationships involved marriage. Increasingly, these relationships are formed and maintained without a formal marriage or between two people of the same sex. Developmentally, the important concept is the formation of the mature, intimate relationship.

People who want to have children in the 21st century have many more choices than their own parents and grandparents had: Surrogate motherhood, artificial insemination, in vitro fertilization, and other technological innovations make it possible for couples in a variety of situations to choose to become parents. Deciding not to have children and delaying having children are increasingly accepted, as are the decisions of single women to have children and single men to adopt children.

Young adults have chosen an occupation, established their values, and adopted a lifestyle. Career advancement, a quest for financial stability, and emotional investment characterize the young adult years.

The young adult without a steady job may lack direction and self-confidence. Marital discord may trigger feelings of failure and insecurity. Failing to achieve intimacy may place the young adult at risk for depression, alcoholism, or drug abuse.

Table 7–1: Health Screenings and Immunization Guidelines Across the Life Span in the module on Health, Wellness, and Illness provides a detailed listing of interventions recommended for young adults.

Assessment of Middle-Aged Adults

Typically, the adult in the middle years of life is satisfied with past accomplishments and involved in activities outside the family. Healthy adjustment to the physical changes of aging includes developing appropriate leisure activities in preparation for an active retirement. Good financial planning during the middle adult years helps financial security during retirement.

The middle adult years signal the end of childbearing and, most often, the end of childrearing. Individuals adjust to never having had children or to children leaving home. Couples may renew their relationships or find they have little in common and perhaps separate. Some women choose to delay childbearing until their late 30s or early 40s, after establishing their careers. They begin their childrearing years as many of their peers are completing this phase of life. Older mothers must make the transition from career women to mothers, even if they continue their careers.

The dissatisfied middle-aged adult is unhappy with the past and expresses little or no hope for the future. Sedentary and isolated, the individual complains about life, avoids involvement, and fails to plan appropriately for retirement.

Table 7–1: Health Screenings and Immunization Guidelines Across the Life Span in the module on Health, Wellness, and Illness provides a detailed listing of interventions recommended for middle-aged adults.

Assessment of Older Adults

A comprehensive assessment is essential to understanding the health needs of the older adult. A comprehensive geriatric assessment should be carried out in the following circumstances:

1. Yearly for the older adult with complex health needs during the annual visit for routine health maintenance with the primary healthcare provider
2. After any abrupt change in physical, social, or psychological function
3. When the older adult is hospitalized for acute illness or injury
4. When nursing home placement or a change in living status is being considered
5. When the older client or the client's family members would like a second opinion regarding an intervention or treatment protocol recommended by the primary care provider.

Because of the particular needs of older adult clients and the frequent need to work with healthcare providers in several disciplines, the nurse must be not only knowledgeable in the content area of gerontology and geriatrics, but also educated regarding the issues of team dynamics. Essential skills in team dynamics include the following:

- An awareness of the roles and contributions of all team members
- Excellent communication skills in order to share information
- Conflict resolution skills
- The ability to see that multiple disciplines can provide information critical to solving the problems of the older client.

Despite variations in instruments, structure of the interdisciplinary team, and methods employed, several strategies make the evaluation process more effective. These include the development of a close-knit interdisciplinary team with minimal redundancy in the assessments performed, the use of carefully designed questionnaires that reliable older clients or their caregivers can complete beforehand, and the effective use of assessment forms that are incorporated into computer databases (Kane et al., 2013).

The nurse can incorporate holistic assessment techniques and standardized instruments into routine evaluations (see **Table 34–11** ● for a list of instruments used to assess older adults). In addition, the nurse is in an ideal position to advocate for older clients who would benefit from holistic assessment and to urge clients to seek the services of specialized geriatric assessment teams if these seem warranted.

Stay Current: A set of more than 30 issues of Try This: Best Practices in Nursing Care to Older Adults *is available from the Hartford Institute for Geriatric Nursing, at the New York University College of Nursing. The general assessment series includes information on the purpose of the clinical measurement, the best tool, the target population, validity and reliability, strengths and limitations, and follow-up suggestions (Boltz & Greenberg, 2012). It is available online at* **www.ConsultGeriRN.org/ resources**. *Another set of geriatric assessment tools in 11 categories is available from the Iowa Geriatric Education Center (2013) at the University of Iowa. It is available online at (***www. healthcare.uiowa.edu/igec/tools***).*

The three underlying principles of comprehensive geriatric assessment are as follows:

1. Physical, psychological, and socioeconomic factors interact in complex ways to influence the health and functional status of the older individual.
2. Comprehensive evaluation of an older client's health status requires an assessment in each of these domains. The coordinated efforts of various healthcare professionals are needed to carry out the assessment.
3. Functional abilities should be a central focus of the comprehensive evaluation. Other more traditional measures of health such as medical diagnosis, nursing diagnosis, physical examination results, and laboratory findings form the basic foundation of the assessment in order to determine overall health, well-being, and the need for social services (Kane et al., 2013).

TABLE 34–11 Instruments for Evaluation of Older Adults

INSTRUMENT	FOCUS	MEASUREMENT	USES
Tilburg or Groningen Frailty Indicators	Loss of resources causes inability to respond to physical or psychological stress	Either professional or self-report of functioning in four domains: physical, cognitive, social, psychological	Vulnerability to future poor health outcomes; to predict disability, healthcare utilization, and quality of life
World Health Organization Quality of Life Questionnaire (WHOQOL-BREF)	Individual's perceptions of culture and value systems, and personal goals, standards and concerns	Brief version is 26 items measuring four domains: physical health, psychological health, social relationships, and environment.	Can be used for people with intact cognitive functioning as well as mild-to-moderate dementia
Short Portable Mental Status	Mental process of knowing and understanding	Ten questions, can adjust for educational level	Assess cognitive functioning; can be repeated to check if decline in cognition
Katz's ADL Scale	Ability to independently bathe, dress, toilet, transfer, be continent, feed	Six yes/no questions, one for each functional area	Rate performance of independent activity
Instrumental Activities of Daily Living (IADLs)	Completion of complex activities; need for support services	Measures eight complex activities needed for independent functioning, assessing how much assistance is required, if any.	If client is not able to perform IADLs, assistance will be needed. If caregiver support is inadequate, a change in living situation might be indicated.
Geriatric Depression Scale	Low mood accompanied by low self-esteem and loss of interest or pleasure in normally enjoyable activities	Short form has 15 yes/no questions, completion in 5 minutes; original form had 30 questions.	Used to evaluate depression, which can exist alone or accompany dementia, as well as major illnesses: recent stroke, CABG or myocardial infarct. Older adult abuse can also cause depression.
Barthel Index of Activities of Daily Living	Evaluates if disability is present, estimates its extent, determines when support needed.	Can ask information of client or relatives; can assess improvement over time.	Assesses adequate functioning in mobility and daily self-care tasks.
Palliative Performance Scale	Progression of disease, symptom management, prognosis, and timing of hospice referral.	Scores are given in 10-point increments, ranging from 0 (death) to 100 (full or normal, no disease).	Response to palliative care services. Five categories of function are scored; lower scores indicate greater functional impairment.
Get-Up-and-Go Test	Combination of gait and balance to produce mobility	Client stands up from seated position in chair, walks short distance, turns around, returns to sitting in chair. Can be timed or not.	Client's performance is scored on five-point scale; higher score indicate greater gait and balance problems as well as an increased risk of falling.
Kayser-Jones Brief Oral Health Status Examination (BOHSE)	Rates condition of client's oral health from 0 (normal) to 2 (problematic).	Ten-item exam identifies oral health problems, using a pen light, tongue depressor, and gauze	Assesses need for referral.
Clock Drawing Test (CDT)	Assessment of cognitive decline. If found, medications and management techniques can be used.	Client is asked to draw clock face with a specific time. Score for drawing closed circle, 12 correct numbers in correct positions, with hands pointed accurately.	Often given with Mini-Mental State Examination (MMSE). The CDT detects impairments in executive function, while MMSE assesses orientation, memory, and language functions. Useful for detecting dementia in early stages.
Zarit Burden Interview	Client's care needs effect on daily life of caregiver	22 items that describe personal strain and role strain on five-point scale	Used by aging agencies to rate caregiver stress.
Braden Scale	Determines an individual's risk for developing pressure ulcers.	Level of severity of six indicators: sensory perception, moisture, activity, mobility, nutrition, and friction or shear	Commonly used with older adults who have medical or cognitive impairments, on admission and on regular basis.

(continued on next page)

TABLE 34–11 Instruments for Evaluation of Older Adults (*continued*)

INSTRUMENT	FOCUS	MEASUREMENT	USES
Berg Balance Test or Single Leg Stance Test	To check for risk of falls; to monitor progress in physical therapy treatment	Choice of 14 tasks range from standing up from a sitting position, to standing on one foot	Clinical balance assessment; rated effective by 70% of physiotherapists
Fullmer SPICES	Conditions that warrant further assessment for fall risk	Checks for six conditions: **S**leep disorders, **P**roblems with eating and feeding, **I**ncontinence, **C**onfusion, **E**vidence of falls, and **S**kin breakdown.	Used on admission to prompt fall risk precautions if needed
Mini-Nutritional Assessment (MNA)	Malnutrition and risk of developing malnutrition	Six questions on food intake, weight loss, mobility, psychological stress or acute disease, presence of dementia or depression, and BMI	Suggested use: quarterly for institutionalized older adults and yearly for normally nourished community-dwelling older adults

The interrelationships between the physical, social, and psychological aspects of aging and perhaps illness present a challenge to the nurse when beginning the geriatric evaluation. The nurse is often charged with the responsibility of obtaining the client's past health history and history of the present illness. In addition, the following contextual variables should be considered in preparing for the geriatric assessment.

EVALUATION OF THE ASSESSMENT ENVIRONMENT Before the assessment visit, clear instructions should be provided to the client and family about parking arrangements and the registration process. To make the older client and family comfortable, environmental modifications should be made, if possible. Environmental modifications may include adequate lighting, decreased background noise, comfortable seating for the older client and family, easily accessible restrooms, examination tables that can be raised or lowered to assist clients with disabilities, and availability of water or juice for client use. Client comfort will ease communication and improve the data collection process.

ACCURACY OF THE HEALTH HISTORY The more information that the client and family can organize ahead of time, the more accurate and efficient the assessment will be. Many clinics mail an information packet in advance of the visit so that the older client can come prepared. This packet might include the following:

1. A past medical history form. This form can be completed at home and is helpful for clients with complicated medical histories. The dates of hospitalizations, operations, serious injuries or accidents, procedures, and illnesses can be ascertained beforehand to save time during the assessment appointment. The form would also include any history of adverse drug effects or allergies.
2. Instructions to bring in all prescription and over-the-counter medications and herbal products/vitamins/mineral supplements for review by the nurse.
3. Instructions to bring any medical records, laboratory or x-ray reports, electrocardiograms, reports of vaccination, and other pertinent health records that the client or family may possess.

4. Instructions to write down and bring the names of all healthcare providers involved with the client's health care, including primary care providers, specialists, and alternative medicine practitioners (e.g., acupuncturists, massage therapists, chiropractors).
5. Instructions to bring hearing aids, eyeglasses, and any assistive devices (canes, walkers, etc.).

Patience is a virtue when obtaining a history from an older adult, because often the individual's thought and verbal processes are slower than those of younger clients. The client should be allowed adequate time to answer questions and report information (Kane et al., 2013).

SAFETY ALERT
When an older client who has been asked to bring all medications to a geriatric evaluation session arrives carrying a large bag of medication bottles, the nurse knows that the first notation on the problem list is likely to be "at risk for adverse drug reaction related to polypharmacy."

The history should include emphasis on the following:

- Review of acute and chronic medical problems
- Medications
- Disease prevention and health maintenance review: vaccinations, PPD (tuberculosis), cancer screenings. (Table 7–1: Health Screenings and Immunization Guidelines Across the Life Span in the module on Health, Wellness, and Illness provides a detailed listing of interventions recommended for older adults.)
- Functional status (activities of daily living)
- Social supports (family, spiritual affiliations, caregiver stress, safety of living environment)
- Finances
- Driving status and safety record
- Review of symptoms (client/family perception of memory, dentition, taste, smell, nutrition, hearing, vision, falls, fractures, bowel and bladder function).

Often, a standardized form is used to guide and direct the process of obtaining a health history. The nurse should be aware of potential difficulties in obtaining health histories from older clients, including the following:

- **Communication difficulties.** Decreased hearing or vision, slow speech, slower mental processing, and use of English as a second language have an effect on communication.

- **Underreporting of symptoms.** Fear of being labeled as a complainer, fear of institutionalization, and fear of serious illness can influence symptom reporting.

- **Vague or nonspecific complaints.** These may be associated with cognitive impairment, drug or alcohol use or abuse, or atypical presentation of disease.

- **Multiple complaints.** Associated "masked" depression, presence of multiple chronic illnesses, and social isolation are often an older adult's cry for help.

- **Lack of time.** New clients scheduled for a geriatric assessment should have the minimum of a 1-hour appointment with the gerontological nurse. Shorter appointments will result in a hurried interview with missed information (Kane et al., 2013).

SOCIAL HISTORY   Holistic evaluation is not complete without an assessment of the client's social support system. Many frail older adults receive support and supervision from family members and significant others to compensate for functional disabilities.

Key elements of the social history include the following:

- Past occupation and retirement status
- Family history (helpful when constructing a family genogram)
- Present and former marital status, including quality of the relationship(s)
- Identification of family members, with designation of level of involvement and place of residence
- Current living arrangements
- Family dynamics
- Family and caregiver expectations
- Economic status, including adequacy of health insurance
- Social activities and hobbies
- Mode of transportation
- Community involvement and support
- Religious involvement and spirituality.

Older individuals who exhibit symptoms of sadness or social isolation, who question their existence, who feel they are being punished by God, or who ask about availability of religious or spiritual counseling should be asked if they would like help with their spiritual concerns. Religion and spirituality can be a great source of hope and strength in times of need and crisis. Many healthcare facilities and community agencies have access to religious and spiritual counselors. They can connect older clients and their families with such assistance, especially in the absence of an ongoing relationship with a priest, minister, rabbi, or spiritual counselor.

If an assessment team includes a social worker, the nurse may collaborate with him or her closely to identify and address social problems. Older clients with inadequate health insurance can often be helped by accessing community services, free hospital services, hardship funds established for indigent clients by major drug companies, and referrals to community-based free clinics. This information is helpful to the nurse working with older clients in many settings. It is crucial for clients admitted to long-term care facilities, those expressing feelings of severe loneliness, or those who do not have a close relationship with another individual.

FUNCTIONAL EVALUATION   A key part of the evaluation of the older adult client is the assessment or systematic evaluation of the client's level of function and self-care. Ongoing research supports the need for regular assessment of the older adult's risk for falls regardless of setting. By properly evaluating older adults and targeting risk factors for falls and functional decline, the nurse can promote greater independence and safety in older clients. Areas to target include self-care abilities, cognition, nutrition and feeding, continence, mobility, sleep, and skin care. A home visit or comprehensive questions about the client's home environment can provide useful information about fall risks, other safety issues, and the client's ability to function in that environment (see the Community-Based Care feature).

LIFESTYLE AND HEALTH CONSIDERATIONS   Well-adjusted older adults maintain an active lifestyle and involvement with others and often do not appear their age. Lifestyle changes occur in response to declining physical abilities and retirement. Participation in activities that promote the older adult's sense of self-worth and usefulness also provides opportunities for developing new friendships with others of similar abilities and interests. Intellectual function is maintained through continued intellectual pursuits. Content with their life review, well-adjusted older adults often enjoy their retirement years and accept death as the inevitable end of a productive life. The older adult who has not successfully resolved developmental crises may feel that life has been unfair. Despair and hopelessness may be evident in the individual's lack of activity and bitter complaining.

MINIMUM DATA SET   Assessment of an older client for appropriate placement in a nursing home or within a long-term care system is done using the Minimum Data Set (MDS). The MDS is a comprehensive standardized multidisciplinary assessment used throughout the United States. The Omnibus Budget Reconciliation Act of 1987 (OBRA 87) mandated assessment of all residents of facilities funded by Medicare or Medicaid using the MDS. It is also completed on all residents admitted to Veteran Health Administration Community Living Centers (Saliba et al., 2012). The MDS is used for validating the need for long-term care, reimbursement, ongoing assessment of clinical problems, and assessment of and need to alter the current plan of care.

The MDS consists of a core set of screening, clinical, and functional measures:

- **Resident Assessment Protocols (RAPs)** are structured, problem-oriented guidelines that identify unique and relevant

Community-Based Care Assessing the Home Environment of Older Adults

Some geriatric assessment teams have the time and resources to visit the older client's home and conduct an assessment of the environment. While this direct observation is the best way to gather accurate and reliable data, it is time consuming and can be expensive. Therefore, many geriatric assessment teams question the older adult client and the client's family regarding the adequacy of the home environment and the available resources to maintain adequate levels of function.

Factors to be considered when assessing the home environment of older adults include the following:

- *Stairs.* Narrow stairs with poor lighting, inadequate railings, and uneven steps are fall risks. Does the older individual have the strength and balance to climb stairs? Are railings firmly attached? If a wheelchair or walker is used, are there ramps present or space for them to be added?

- *Bathing and toileting.* Can the older client safely transfer on and off the toilet? Is a raised toilet seat needed? Are grab bars present? Is there an adequate bath mat in the tub? Is a shower seat needed? Is lighting adequate? Is the older client able to bathe without assistance?

- *Medications.* Where are medications stored? Are there children in the home who are at risk because of open storage or nonreplacement of caps? Are old and outdated medications disposed of to prevent accidents? Are medications refilled on time to prevent on–off dosing patterns? Is a list of medications available for use in emergencies? Is the client responsible for taking his or her own medications, or does a family member or caregiver help? Does the client use or need any reminders to help remember to take medications?

- *Nutrition and cooking.* Is there adequate food in the home? Is there a stove or microwave for cooking? Are any safety problems reported with the stove or microwave? If a gas stove, is it safe? Is the pilot light functioning properly? Are there gas leak detectors? Is food storage adequate? Is spoiled food present? Is the food preparation environment clean? Who does the grocery shopping? Who prepares the food? How are trash and garbage disposed of?

- *Falls.* Are the floors free of cords, debris, and scatter rugs? Is there adequate lighting? Are there night-lights? Are there pets that dart around quickly? If there is a history of falls, would the older individual consider wearing an emergency alert system around the neck or wrist?

- *Smoke detectors.* Are the smoke detectors functioning? Are batteries changed yearly?

- *Emergency numbers.* Are emergency phone numbers posted near or preprogrammed into the phone?

- *Temperature of home.* Is there adequate heat in the winter and cooling in the summer?

- *Temperature of water.* Is the hot water heater set below 120°F?

- *Safety of the neighborhood.* Can the older individual venture outside without fear of becoming a crime victim? Are the door locks and latches adequate? How close is the nearest neighbor? Is there nearby help if it is needed?

- *Financial.* Are there stacks of unpaid bills? Are services such as phone and electricity in good working order? Are large amounts of cash hidden or stored around the house? Is there adequate money to purchase nutritious food?

---

information about an older client. This information is needed for formulating an individualized nursing care plan.

- **Resident Utilization Guidelines (RUGs)** determine the reimbursement the skilled nursing facility will receive for providing care to the older client. Factors considered include the need for supportive therapy (physical, occupational, and/or speech), self-care ability of the older client, and the need for special treatments such as feeding tubes or skin care.

- **Resident Assessment Instrument (RAI)** identifies medical problems and describes each older client's functional ability in a comprehensive and standardized format. This information helps to formulate the plan of care and to evaluate progress toward goals, indicating when changes in the care plan are needed.

Categories of data gathered for the MDS include the following:

- Client demographics and background
- Cognitive function
- Communication and hearing
- Mood and behavior patterns

- Psychosocial well-being
- Physical function and ADLs
- Bowel and bladder continence
- Diagnosed diseases
- Health conditions (weight, falls, etc.)
- Oral nutritional status
- Oral and dental status
- Skin condition
- Activity pursuits
- Medications
- Need for special services
- Discharge potential.

Certain information gathered for the MDS, such as data indicating functional decline or a poorly managed chronic disease, may trigger the need for further assessment using the RAPs. For instance, if information gathered for the MDS indicates that the nursing home resident has fallen, a RAP is triggered and indicates the need for direct gait assessment, medication review, and physical/occupational therapy evaluation.

◤ **REVIEW** **Holistic Health Assessment Across the Life Span**

RELATE Link the Concepts and Exemplars

Linking the exemplar of holistic health assessment across the life span with the concept of communication:

1. When collecting information for a health history, what strategies would you use when communicating with an older adult who has a hearing loss?

2. You are collecting information from the mother of a 3-year-old for a health history. The mother does not speak any English, but the 3-year-old does speak English. What communication strategies would you employ?

Linking the exemplar of holistic health assessment across the life span with the concept of legal issues:

3. You admit an adolescent to the adolescent unit of a local hospital and begin collecting data when you begin to suspect that the adolescent may be abusing substances. With an understanding of your legal obligation to the adolescent, as well as your knowledge that the parents want to help their child, how would you handle your suspicions if the parents are in the room with the child?

4. You are assessing an older adult and discover bruises that you suspect may be the result of abuse. The client's son is in the room during the examination. What is the best legally appropriate action for you to take?

REFER Go to Pearson Nursing Student Resources
nursing.pearsonhighered.com

- Additional review materials

REFLECT Case Study

The nurse conducted a health history interview with Martha Washburn, a 67-year-old African American woman. The following are excerpts from the health history.

"Mrs. Washburn, I am going to ask you a lot of questions before your physical. I need to have correct responses, and I have to tell you, there will be a lot of them if we are to get to the root of your problem. I will use the information to develop a plan of care."

"What are you here for? Did someone come with you? I see on your chart that you have some problems with urination. Are you incontinent? How long have you had the problem?"

The nurse included the following questions: "What is your economic status? Do you go to church? What do you do when you are ill?"

"We need information about your family, so let's start with your parents. Are they alive? Do you have siblings?"

The nurse completed a review of symptoms and prepared the client for the physical examination by showing her into a room and telling her to get undressed.

1. Critique the nurse's actions in the initial interview phase of the case study.

2. Identify the types of information the nurse was seeking in asking those questions.

3. Create alternative approaches and questioning techniques for the interview in the case study.

4. Describe your preparation for an interview of Mrs. Washburn.

■ REFERENCES

American Cancer Society. (2013a, January 11). *American Cancer Society guidelines for early detection of cancer.* Retrieved from http://www.cancer.org/healthy/findcancerearly/cancerscreeningguidelines/american-cancer-society-guidelines-for-the-early-detection-of-cancer.

American Cancer Society (2013b, February 22). *Breast cancer overview: What causes breast cancer?* Retrieved from http://www.cancer.org/docroot/CRI/content/CRI_2_2_2X_What_causes_breast_cancer_5.asp?sitearea=.

Boltz, M., & Greenberg, S. A. (2012). *Try this: Best practices in nursing care to older adults.* New York, NY: Hartford

Institute for Geriatric Nursing, College of Nursing, New York University. Retrieved from http://www.ConsultGeriRN.org/resources.

D'Amico, D., & Barbarito, C. (2012). *Health & physical assessment in nursing* (2nd ed.). Upper Saddle River, NJ: Pearson Education.

Iowa Geriatric Education Center, University of Iowa. (2013). *Geriatric assessment tools.* Retrieved from http://www.healthcare.uiowa.edu/igec/tools.

Kane, R., Ouslander, J., Abrass, I., & Resnick, B. (2013). *Essentials of clinical geriatrics* (7th ed.). New York, NY: McGraw-Hill Professional.

Saliba, D., Jones, M., Streim, J., Ouslander, J., Berlowitz, D., & Buchanan, J. (2012). Overview of significant changes in the Minimum Data Set for nursing homes version 3.0. *Journal of the American Medical Directors Association, 13*(7), 595–601. doi:10.1016/j.jamda.2012.06.001.

Stewart, C. J., & Cash, W. B., Jr. (2006). *Interviewing: Principles and practices* (11th ed.). New York, NY: McGraw-Hill.

35 Caring Interventions

◪ THE CONCEPT OF CARING INTERVENTIONS

Caring is generally defined as "to feel interest or concern" (Merriam-Webster Online Dictionary, 2013), but in the context of the nursing profession, caring goes well beyond this simple explanation. Caring has been described as encompassing various intentions and actions. Brunton and Beaman (2000) identified 10 caring behaviors: "In rank order [they] were appreciating the patient as a human being, showing respect for the patient, being sensitive to the patient, talking with the patient, treating patient information confidentially, treating the patient as an individual, encouraging the patient to call with problems, being honest with the patient, and listening attentively to the patient" (p. 451).

Caring is a concept that forms an integral part of nursing theory. That said, the concept of caring is not limited to academic postulation. Research based on in-depth interviews of practicing nurses revealed that engaging in **caring practice** is an essential element in providing quality nursing care (Burhans & Alligood, 2010). One nurse participant who was chosen as representative of the initial sample described her experience of quality nursing: "If you have a person that's actually caring and compassionate and concerned about the welfare of that individual, it'll take you farther than if you are an expert clinician" (p. 1694).

Taking it one step further, a currently accepted position within the field describes "nursing as situated caring" (Jarrin, 2012, p. 4) in which caring can only be understood in the context of the environment. Not only are physical time, space, and location relevant, but the nurse's level of development, the situation's specific circumstances, and both the nurse's and client's value systems surrounding illness and healing are also central in affecting how caring is manifested. Depending on the perspective, nursing can be viewed as "technical actions and physical behavior . . . [or] caring thought, feeling, and intention behind the action" (p. 4), with the ideal being an amalgamation of the two. Although both elements form the foundation of nursing, "without caring our work would merely be tasks that could be performed by machines" (p. 4–5).

Milton Mayeroff, author of the classic 1971 book, *On Caring,* argued that at the heart of caring is "helping the other grow" (Mayeroff, 1990, p. 2). Mayeroff maintained that caring facilitates growth both in the person who exhibits caring and the recipient, be it a person or thing, such as a concept, cause, or community. Under his framework, caring is not a finite action but rather a process that encourages self-actualization in the caregiver and development of the other. Central to his concept of caring is that the caregiver must respect the individuality and separateness of the other by not inflicting a specific direction in the growth of the other. **<<**

Concept Learning Outcomes

After reading about this concept, you will be able to:

1. Discuss the meaning of caring.
2. Examine theories of caring relevant to nursing practice.
3. Analyze the importance of different types of knowledge in nursing.
4. Describe interventions through which nurses demonstrate caring in practice.
5. Summarize the importance of self-care for the professional nurse.

Concept Key Terms

Aesthetic knowing, 2306
Caring, 2301
Caring practice, 2301
Compassion, 2307
Competence, 2307

Empirical knowing, 2305
Empowerment, 2307
Ethical knowing, 2306
Personal knowing, 2306
Presencing, 2306

▶ NURSING THEORIES OF CARING

The various nursing caring theories grew out of humanism, which the American Humanist Association (2008) defines as "a progressive philosophy of life that, without theism and other supernatural beliefs, affirms our ability and responsibility to lead ethical lives of personal fulfillment that aspire to the greater good of humanity." Although each caring theory underscores different aspects and perspectives, all agree that caring is "the essence of nursing and a central and unifying feature" (Blais & Hayes, 2011).

Bridging the gap between theory and practice has been an ongoing issue in nursing. Research has revealed that clients are clear on what constitutes a good nurse: Caring behaviors such as honesty, sincerity, the willingness to listen, and the perspective that the client is a person and not just an illness (Van der Elst, Dierckx de Casterlé, & Gastmans, 2012) are of central importance to client satisfaction. The question then is how to take the various theoretical perspectives on caring and translate them into practice.

Tonges and Ray (2011) described how University of North Carolina Hospitals (UNCH) developed a successful nursing care delivery model known as the Professional Practice Model (PPM). The PPM is "one approach to actualizing caring theory across a healthcare organization by systematically incorporating interventions that link nursing actions, caring processes, and expectations" (p. 374). The PPM "translated caring theory into specific caring behaviors and incorporated them in practice" (p. 375). One example was the implementation of a "no passing zone" in which a "No Passing" sign was posted in hallways as a reminder that if a client's call light was flashing, any nurse passing by the light was obligated to check in with the client, even if that nurse was not assigned to that specific client. "This practice is designed to convey the availability of the entire staff to *do for* all patients on the unit" (p. 377). Providing high-quality care is dependent on the development of concrete strategies that allow nurses to link theoretical concepts to their on-the-job duties.

Although caring theories have been designed with the nurse–client relationship in mind, the basic tenets of caring can and also should be applied to the nurse–nurse relationship. Intense levels of stress caused by staff shortages and high-needs clients underscore the importance of nurses supporting each other. When nurses are supportive of each other, they are not only able to problem-solve through challenging situations but also "are inspired to care by being cared for themselves" (Longo, 2011, p. 8).

Leininger's Theory of Culture Care Diversity and Universality

In the mid-1980s, Madeleine Leininger revolutionized nursing and transformed the concept of caring with the development of a new discipline called transcultural nursing, currently referred to as the theory of Culture Care Diversity and Universality (George, 2011). In an early publication she said that "nurses often labeled, avoided or talked down to the cultural strangers when they did not understand their behavior and needs" (Leininger, 1989, p. 7). Her study of anthropology provided much insight as to how culture played a crucial role in providing nursing care in order to maintain or encourage health.

In order for nurses to provide the highest quality of care to culturally diverse clients, Leininger presents three modes of action:

- Culture care preservation and/or maintenance involves caregivers performing actions and making choices that help clients retain their specific cultural values and beliefs.

- Culture care accommodation and/or negotiation refers to caregivers' efforts to assist clients in adapting to or working with others to achieve the best possible care.

- Culture care repatterning and/or restructuring describes caregiver interventions that support clients in evaluating and changing their approaches to promote improved health outcomes (Leininger & McFarland, 2006).

Roach's Theory of Caring as the Human Mode of Being

Sister M. Simone Roach's philosophical theory declares caring to be a core element of how humans operate, as well as an expression of our interconnectedness: "Caring, as the human mode of being, is caring from the heart; caring from the core of one's being; caring as a response to one's experience of connectedness" (Roach, 1997, p. 16).

Although Roach's theory views humans as caring entities, it also maintains that caring within the context of nursing is distinct in that the specific traits of nurses are all grounded in caring. She has labeled these attributes the six Cs of caring: compassion, competence, confidence, conscience, commitment, and comportment. Refer to **Box 35–1** ● for further explanation of each trait.

Boykin and Schoenhofer's Nursing as Caring Theory

In 1993, Anne Boykin and Savina O. Schoenhofer proposed their nursing theory of caring, which maintains that caring is a crucial element of being human, as well as being an ongoing process rather than a goal to be achieved (George, 2011). They argue that nurses must be willing to accept that caring

---

Box 35–1   The Six Cs of Caring in Nursing

Compassion. Awareness of one's relationship to others, sharing their joys, sorrows, pain, and accomplishments. Participation in the experience of another.

Competence. Having the knowledge, judgment, skills, energy, experience, and motivation to respond adequately to others within the demands of professional responsibilities.

Confidence. The quality that fosters trusting relationships. Comfort with self, client, and family.

Conscience. Morals, ethics, and an informed sense of right and wrong. Awareness of personal responsibility.

Commitment. Convergence between one's desires and obligations and the deliberate choice to act in accordance with them.

Comportment. Appropriate demeanor, dress, and language, that are in harmony with a caring presence. Presenting oneself as someone who respects others and in turn demands respect.

Source: Adapted from Roach, M. S. (2002) *Caring, the human mode of being: A blueprint for the health professions* (2nd ed.). Ottawa, Ontario: CHA Press. Reprinted with permission.

TABLE 35–1   Carative Factor to Clinical Caritas Processes

CARATIVE FACTOR	CLINICAL CARITAS PROCESSES
Forming a humanistic-altruistic system of values	Practice of loving-kindness and equanimity within context of caring consciousness
Enabling and sustaining faith-hope	Being authentically present and enabling and sustaining the deep belief system and subjective life world of self and one-being-cared-for
Being sensitive to self and others	Cultivation of one's own spiritual practice and transpersonal self, going beyond ego self
Developing a help-trusting, caring relationship (seeking transpersonal connections)	Developing and sustaining helping-trusting, authentic caring relationship
Promoting and accepting the expression of positive and negative feelings and emotions	Being present to, and supportive of, the expression of positive and negative feelings as a connection with deeper spirit of self and the one-being-cared-for
Engaging in creative, individualized problem-solving caring processes	Creative use of self and all ways of knowing a part of the caring process, to engage in artistry of caring-healing practices
Promoting transpersonal teaching–learning	Engaging in genuine teaching–learning experience that attends to unity of being and meaning, attempting to stay within others' frame of reference
Attending to supportive, protective, and/or corrective mental, physical, societal, and spiritual environments	Creating healing environment at all levels, (physical as well as nonphysical), subtle environment of energy and consciousness, whereby wholeness, beauty, comfort, dignity, and peace are potentiated
Assisting with gratification of basic human needs while preserving human dignity and wholeness	Assisting with basic needs, with an intentional caring consciousness, administering "human care essential," which potentiate alignment of mind/body/spirit, wholeness, and unity of being in all aspects of care; tending to both embodied spirit and evolving spiritual emergence
Allowing for, and being open to, existential-phenomenological and spiritual dimensions of caring and healing that cannot be fully explained scientifically through modern Western medicine	Opening and attending to spiritual-mysterious and existential dimensions of one's own life-death; should care for self and the one-being-cared-for

Source: Julia B. George (2011). Nursing theories: The base for professional nursing practice, 6th ed., Box 18–2. Upper Saddle River, NJ: Prentice Hall.

is never static; it continually changes and evolves throughout the span of their lives. At the heart of it all, nursing is caring. Boykin and Schoenhofer (2001) state that "being caring, that is, living one's commitment to this value 'important-in-itself' (Roach, 1984), fuels the nurse's growing in caring and enables the nurse in turn to nurture others in their living and growing in caring" (p. 19). Self-awareness is also essential to being a caring and effective nurse. Clients respond positively to their caregiver's authenticity, which encourages their own growth.

Watson's Theory of Human Care

Jean Watson's theory of human care has evolved as a result of her intense interest, varied education, and extensive experience with nursing, philosophy, and metaphysics (Watson, 1999). At the crux of her theory is the assumption that genuine caring relationships have a positive impact on a client's health and can facilitate the healing process, putting caring at the core of nursing. Equally as important is the preservation of the client's dignity and a respect for all people's inevitable interconnectedness (George, 2011).

Also key to Watson's theory of human care is that caring is considered transpersonal; in other words, both the nurse and the client seek out meaning and a sense of connectedness. Furthermore, Watson (1999) maintained that caring involves not just addressing the mind and the body, but also the spirit: "The value of human care and caring involves a higher sense of spirit of self. Caring calls for a philosophy of moral commit-

ment toward protecting human dignity and preserving humanity" (p. 31).

When Watson first developed her theory, she identified what she referred to as the 10 carative factors that needed to exist within a nurse–client caring relationship. She later updated those characteristics and renamed them the 10 clinical caritas processes. See **Table 35–1** ● for a comparative chart of the carative factors and caritas processes (George, 2011, p. 459). Watson has expressed that it is not enough for a nurse to review the basic assumptions and 10 caritas: ". . . to truly 'get it,' one has to personally experience it; thus the model is both an invitation and an opportunity to interact with the ideas, experiment with and grow within the philosophy, and liv[e] it out in one's personal/professional life" (Watson, n.d., para. 2).

Benner and Wrubel's Theory of Caring

Patricia Benner and Judith Wrubel's contribution to caring theories is grounded in their book *The Primacy of Caring: Stress and Coping in Illness* (1989), which places caring at the heart of providing quality service to clients and their families. In 2001, they further clarified their perspective as not focusing "on nurse caregiving, but rather how care sets up what counts as stressful, as well as what counts as coping for a person. Our main goal is to examine the phenomenon of care and caring practices to the experience of health and illness, not the caregiving of nurses" (p. 172). They describe a nurse's intent to care as not the only factor in how caring is delivered and

Focus on Diversity and Culture Cultural Competence in Nursing

- Culture and religion can have an influence on how clients express pain and the meaning they attach to it. For instance, some cultures view pain as penance for a past wrongdoing or as a test of faith. Others see acknowledgment of pain and/or requests for pain relief as a sign of weakness.

- Certain cultures stigmatize any discussions around death and dying, and may provide resistance in exploring the best options for end-of-life care.

- Families in some cultures approach healthcare decisions as a team as opposed to leaving the final decision of treatment to the individual in question.

- People from other cultures may be uncomfortable with choosing among treatment options and may prefer that the healthcare team make such decisions on their behalf.

- All distinctive practices of a specific culture or religion are not homogeneous within the same group, making it crucial that nurses be sensitive to such issues but also not make sweeping generalizations about an entire group of people. Cultural or religious practices may not be adhered to by younger members of a family even if the older generations do.

Sources: Based on Coolen, P. R. (2012, May 1). Cultural relevance in end-of-life care. *EthnoMed.* Retrieved from http://ethnomed.org/clinical/end-of-life/cultural-relevance-in-end-of-life-care; Stratis Health: Culture Care Connection (2013). *Somalis in Minnesota.* Retrieved from http://www.culturecareconnection.org/matters/diversity/somali.html.

received. In other words, caring does not happen in a vacuum; it is dependent on other factors, such as the context of the situation, the physical environment, the nurse's training and experience, and the client's unique capacities and perspectives (Benner & Wrubel, 2001).

Integrating the Concept of Caring Interventions

Caring Interventions are fundamental to the entire nursing process. Caring—both for self and for others—is the essence of nursing. Self-care includes recognizing and tending to the nurse's own physiologic and psychosocial needs, as well as seeking out activities that promote professional development. For the nurse, the negative impact of alterations in physical and mental health can extend to client care, both in terms of the decision-making process and the actual care provided. The Concepts Related to Caring Interventions feature demonstrates how the Caring Interventions concept relates to other concepts.

Concepts Related to **Caring Interventions**

The relationship between Caring Interventions and professionalism carries important implications for nurses. In work environments where nurse shortages and poor working conditions exist, nurses have reported that their level of professional care suffers (Poghosyan et al., 2010). Furthermore, "patient satisfaction is much lower in institutions where many nurses feel burned out and dissatisfied with their work conditions" (McHugh et al., 2011, p. 7). Although nurses may not have control over their working environment, they are able to maintain self-care practices to combat the effects of burnout.

Examination of the link between caring interventions and ethics is also critical for nurses to consider. As Lachman (2012) describes, "Care can be considered simply an ethical task and thus a burden of one more thing to do, or it can be considered a commitment to attending to and becoming enthusiastically involved in the patient's needs" (p. 114). Caring nurses are more inclined to hold high ethical standards, which unfortunately can lead to internal conflict, also referred to as moral distress, "a phenomenon in which one knows the right action to take, but is constrained from taking it" (Epstein & Delgado, 2010).

By definition, the nurse's professional role centers around caring for others. However, neglecting self-care needs can be detrimental to the nurse, as well as to

clients. Research suggests a correlation between errors in client care (including medication and equipment operation errors) and job-related stress, anxiety, and depression (Gartner et al., 2010). Within the framework of Caring Interventions, self-care includes the nurse's recognition of stressors, as well as assessment of personal coping style and the development of effective coping methods.

Cultural influences affect coping styles, which, in turn, affect self-care. For example, most Western cultures are considered to be individualist, which includes placing a high value on facing personal challenges individually and autonomously. In the context of an individualist culture, members may be less likely to seek social support when managing stressful situations (Knight & Sayegh, 2009). As a result, when faced with a stressor, seeking social support may be viewed as unfavorable or even as a sign of weakness. Nursing education includes encouraging clients to seek care from others when needed. In contrast, in their professional role, these same nurses may be hesitant to ask for help on their own behalf. Keeping in mind the safety and well-being of the nurse and the client, nurses should identify individuals with whom they are comfortable sharing personal concerns and look to them as needed for support and guidance.

Concepts Related to **Caring Interventions** (*continued*)

CONCEPT	RELATIONSHIP TO CARING INTERVENTIONS	NURSING IMPLICATIONS
Professional Behaviors		
■ Components of professionalism in nursing ■ Commitment to profession ■ Work ethic	Inadequate self-care → decreased level of physical and psychosocial wellness → decreased quality of work performance and weakened affiliation with profession of nursing → decreased level of demonstrated professionalism toward clients, peers, and other members of the healthcare team	■ Assess self-wellness and recognize when limitations are being exceeded. ■ Be aware of warning signs that may signal burnout. ■ Recognize areas of self-care that are unhealthy and identify solutions that promote wellness.
Ethics		
■ Principles of ethical decision making ■ Ethical dilemmas ■ Patient rights	Conflict between providing the best possible care for the client could clash with the family's wishes or the constraining factors of the institution → leads nurse to experience moral distress → can cause the nurse to become numb to such dilemmas or lead to burnout → can lead nurses to consider leaving the profession	■ Share ethical concerns with supervisor and healthcare team and build supportive networks on the job. ■ Attend workshops on moral distress to increase coping strategies. ■ Identify common causes of moral distress among nursing peers.
Stress and Coping		
■ Stressors and the coping process ■ Manifestations of stress	Impaired coping → absence of self-care → stress, anxiety, or mild depression → errors in client care	■ Identify and acknowledge stressors. ■ Evaluate the efficacy of personal coping methods. ■ Develop healthy, effective coping methods.
Culture and Diversity		
■ Cultural diversity ■ Values and beliefs ■ Disparities and differences ■ Developing cultural competence	Western cultural influences → autonomous coping highly valued → sense of weakness associated with seeking social support → tendency to avoid asking for help when needed → ineffective self-care	■ Recognize cultural impact on beliefs about seeking help. ■ Assess personal beliefs regarding the value of social support. ■ Identify trusted sources of support and utilize resources as needed.

▶ KNOWLEDGE AND CARING

In the context of nursing, researcher Barbara Carper (1978) outlined four types of knowledge, which she also refers to as knowledge patterns (p. 13): empirical, aesthetic, personal, and ethical (**Figure 35–1 ●**). Important to note is that they do not exist independently, but rather they overlap and interact with each other. With a greater awareness of what knowledge encompasses, nurses are able to more efficiently draw on the full scope of their understanding so as to provide the highest quality care possible.

Empirical Knowing

The first type of knowledge Carper (1978) identified is empirical, which she also referred to "the science of nursing" (p. 14). **Empirical knowing** is twofold in that it is based in facts and observations relevant to nursing, as well as the analyses and theories that attempt to explain them. Nurses can develop this pattern of knowing through ongoing academic education and increasing their skills at operating from a place of objectivity when making observations.

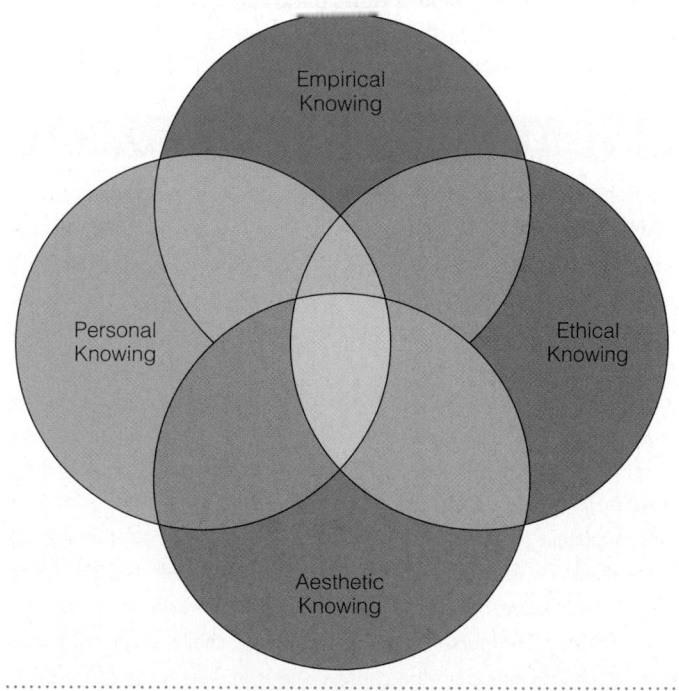

Figure 35–1 ● The four ways of knowing.

Aesthetic Knowing

The next type of knowledge, **aesthetic knowing**, is also referred to as "the art of nursing" (Carper, 1978, p. 14). In contrast to the objective nature of empirical knowing, aesthetic knowing is subjective and relates to the specific personal style the nurse possesses when delivering care. Key elements to this pattern of knowing are empathy (p. 17), holistic thinking, compassion, and sensitivity (Berman & Snyder, 2012). Development of this type of knowing involves the nurse's commitment to increasing her awareness and respect of other people's unique perspectives and experiences.

Personal Knowing

Carper (1978) identified **personal knowing** as another pattern of knowledge within nursing, referring to the nurse's ongoing self-exploration and self-actualization. Developing this pattern of knowing involves "the nurse in the therapeutic use of self [which] rejects approaching the patient–client as an object and strives instead to actualize an authentic personal relationship between two persons" (p. 19). In order to do this, the nurse must be willing to critically reflect on his own thoughts, emotions, and actions in a professional context.

Ethical Knowing

The last form of knowledge pattern is **ethical knowing**, which Carper (1978) calls the "moral component" (p. 20). She clarified that this type of knowing is more extensive than the ethical codes with which nurses are expected to abide; it also encompasses "all voluntary actions that are deliberate and subject to the judgment of right and wrong" (p. 20). Sometimes nurses grapple with situations where values and beliefs prove to be incompatible. To develop this pattern of knowledge, nurses must be aware and fully understand the current codes of ethics outlined for nurses, in addition to the values held by the institution in which they work. Furthermore, they should possess "an understanding of different philosophical positions regarding what is good, what ought to be desired, what is right; of different ethical frameworks devised for dealing with the complexities of moral judgments; and of various orientations to the notion of obligation" (p. 20).

CASE STUDY \\ A

Mr. Bahdoon Osman, a 57-year-old man from Somalia, immigrated to Minnesota 5 years ago with his wife, son, and three daughters. Three days ago, he was rushed to the hospital for breathing and swallowing difficulties, the cause of which was a large tumor. Following emergent surgical resection of the tumor, Mr. Osman was diagnosed with stage IV esophageal cancer. The family is adamant that Mr. Osman not be informed of his terminal diagnosis, because Somali culture believes it is cruel to do so. The client's physician has presented his treatment options.

The charge nurse instructed Mr. Osman's nurse, Joanne Williams, to speak only to the client's son about Mr. Osman's care and not to his wife, explaining that according to Somalia traditions, the father speaks for the family when outside the home. When the father is unable to do so, another adult male in the family, often the son, takes on the responsibility. The nurse finds this instruction challenging, especially seeing the obvious pain the client's wife is in watching her husband suffer. The son tells Joanne that it is important that they reposition Mr. Osman's bed "so that it faces Mecca." Because Joanne does not

understand the son's request, she asks Mr. Osman's wife for further explanation. His wife avoids Joanne's gaze and does not answer. The son firmly explains to Joanne that his mother does not have a say in the matter and repeats the request. Frustrated and upset at the lack of respect for Mr. Osman's wife, Joanne curtly responds by saying it is impossible to move the bed and leaves the room.

Clinical Reasoning Questions Level I
1. Did Joanne demonstrate caring? If so, how?
2. How could have Joanne dealt with the Osman family differently?
3. What strategies could Joanne have employed to address culturally specific healthcare issues for the family?

▶ CARING ENCOUNTERS

The healthcare field is moving from its traditional focus on disease management to a more holistic client-focused approach to care. The American Holistic Nurses Association (AHNA) (2012b) defines holistic nursing as "all nursing practice that has healing the whole person as its goal." It is a philosophy and attitude that facilitates healing by recognizing the intertwined relationships among the "body, mind, emotion, spirit, social/cultural, relationship, context, and environment." Nurses practicing the holistic approach seek to develop a bond with the client to create a more personal and supportive environment. Complementing traditional treatments with alternative therapies, such as Reiki, meditation, biofeedback, and journaling, is also an important part of holistic nursing (Mariano, 2005). The goal is to go beyond addressing the illness in order to help clients achieve balance in their lives. In this respect, it places the nurse in the role of health educator and emphasizes the client's personal responsibility in maintaining health.

This approach to nursing has become more relevant during recent decades in the face of the nation's changing demographics. Increasingly, the general population is turning to complementary and alternative medicine (CAM) to address health issues, with the latest figures from the National Center for Health Statistics indicating that nearly 40% of adults and almost 12% of children had made use of CAM therapy techniques in 2007 (Barnes, Bloom, & Nahin, 2008). Nurses must educate themselves on CAM modalities and understand that not all alternative therapies work for all people, and some may even be harmful. Holistic understanding of the client is required to advise and counsel clients on appropriate therapeutic interventions and treatments. Understanding the client's context is of great importance when deciding on care strategies. For example, recommending costly supplements that can only be found in a few select specialty shops for an older adult who lives alone with limited mobility and income would prove problematic.

Nursing Presence

Presencing is a nursing concept developed by Rosemarie Rizzo Parse that involves the interpersonal arts of perception and communication. Through presencing, the nurse immerses himself in an interaction with the client that helps the client define her health choices. It is the client, then, who has the authority to make decisions about her health. The nurse acts as a guide through his presence, but not in the sense that the nurse tends to the client, but rather by being open, receptive, and available at all levels without judging or labeling. The nurse's thinking flows with the client's, and the value systems of the client direct outcomes, not those of the nurse. Parse described presencing as: ". . . face-to-face discussions, silent immersions, and lingering presence . . ." (as cited in George, 2011, p. 493). In this sort of interaction, the nurse lets the other lead, which could involve dialoguing, simply being there (even if silently), and leaving a lasting memory of the interaction in the client's mind.

Another important nursing concept in this regard is *intentionality*, which refers to a nurse working in conjunction with those involved in the situation at hand as a cooperative force rather than attempting to impose her will. It is a philosophical mind-set that surrenders the idea of directing outcomes and setting goals, instead, the nurse allows resistance to dissolve and a course of action to unfold (Watson, 2002). This perspective of "intentionality seeks to access the universal, life-spirit energy via manifesting one's deep intentional focus on a specific mental object of attention and awareness . . . [thus inviting] spirit-energy to enter into one's life and work, and into the caring-healing processes and outcomes" (p. 14).

Empowerment

Empowerment is a process whereby the client develops the autonomy to identify her own health needs in lieu of being instructed how to do so (Berman & Snyder, 2012). George (2011) said, "The basic element of empowerment is taking action to generate positive results at both the individual and the organizational level" (p. 199). Nurses, having established personal relationships of mutual respect, trust, and confidence with their clients, are in a unique position to empower them, thus increasing their independence. They can facilitate empowerment by instructing clients on how they should perform certain functions, and in cases where a client's abilities are hindered, assistance should be limited to what is absolutely necessary. Additionally, they can provide information and resources to clients and their families, explain what they can expect beyond their hospital stay, and give voice to their concerns and desires to administrators and others providing care.

Compassion

When describing the ideal nurse, **compassion** is a must, but debate exists within the nursing community about how to precisely define this quality. It is not uncommon for compassion or compassionate care to be used interchangeably with other characteristics such as caring, sympathy, and empathy, highlighting the subjective nature of the concept (Davison & Williams, 2009). Compassion is not something a nurse can learn through academic study, but only through the willingness to become intimately involved with the client's experience. This often involves providing comfort to the client, anything from validating the client's experience through attentive listening and eye contact to holding the client's hand in moments of pain, from adjusting the client's position in bed to gently providing a warm sponge bath (**Figure 35–2 ●**).

Another aspect of expressing compassion involves respecting the client's spiritual beliefs or lack thereof, regardless of the nurse's personal opinions and values. For more information, see the exemplar on End-of-Life Care in the module on Comfort for further discussion of spirituality and end-of-life care.

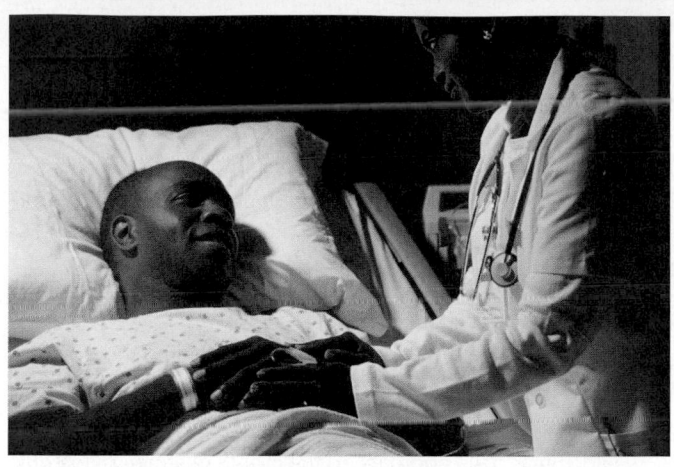

Figure 35–2 ● This nurse is using touch and presence to help comfort her client.
Source: Juan Silva Productions/Getty Images.

Competence

Similar to Roach's (2002) description of competence, Takase and Teraoka (2011) define **competence** "as the ability of a nurse to effectively demonstrate a set of attributes, such as personal characteristics, professional attitude, values, knowledge, and skills, and to fulfill his/her professional responsibility through their practice. A competent person must possess these attributes, have the motivation and ability to utilize them, and must effectively use them to provide safe, effective, and professional nursing care to his/her client" (p. 398). They outline specific attributes inherent in competence including cognitive ability, participating in professional development, having an awareness of ethical and legal practices, guaranteeing quality and safety in care, and building relationships with clients and fellow nurses. Competence and compassion must coexist or client care inevitably suffers. Competence without compassion can be, at best, off-putting and, at worst, impersonal and insensitive. Compassion in the absence of competence, however, presents real threats to clients' safety and health.

CASE STUDY \\ B

Mrs. Julie Briggs is a 29-year-old woman who has undergone a left-breast lumpectomy, which also involved removing cancerous lymph nodes. As a result, she has been admitted to the hospital for a brief recovery period. The first postoperative day, Mrs. Briggs' nurse, Tomas Crespo, overhears an argument between the client and her father, who is pressuring his daughter to have a double mastectomy as a preventive course of treatment because the client's mother lost her life to breast cancer at age 36. Mrs. Briggs expresses that she and her husband hope to conceive a child within the next year and she desperately wants to experience the bonding experience of breastfeeding. As he listens, Tomas is reminded of his wife's difficulty in breastfeeding and thinks the client shouldn't place so much importance on it. After the client's father leaves, Tomas enters the room and finds Mrs. Briggs crying. He pulls up a chair and asks her if she wants to talk. Mrs. Briggs says she's fine and collects herself. The nurse squeezes her hand and informs her that he is willing to listen, but she shakes her head no. While changing the client's dressing, he allows a few minutes to pass before providing her with tips on how she can tend to her sutures when she is discharged in a couple of days, adding that he can also instruct her husband when he comes in later that evening. Upon completing Mrs. Briggs' care, Tomas tells her that there are support groups for young breast cancer survivors like herself and promises to bring the information to her before the end of his shift.

Clinical Reasoning Questions Level I

1. Did Tomas demonstrate presencing, empowerment, compassion, and competence in his interactions with Mrs. Briggs? If so, provide specific examples.

2. Could Tomas have approached the client's dilemma differently? If so, how?

▶ CARING FOR THE CAREGIVER: SELF-CARE IN NURSING

Self-care is of vital importance in nursing and shouldn't be treated as peripheral to client care. Just as preflight safety precautions underscore the importance of always securing one's own oxygen mask first before helping others, nurses must also make their overall well-being a top priority. George (2011) describes self-care as the activities an individual performs independently to ensure personal well-being and good health. Examples of such activities include a balanced diet, regular exercise, adequate rest and sleep, recreational activities, and meditation and/or prayer.

Self-care is particularly relevant to the nursing profession because nurses tend to overlook their own well-being while focusing on the health of others. According to the National Institute for Occupational Safety and Health (2012), "cases of nonfatal occupational injury and illness among healthcare workers are among the highest of any industry sector" (para. 1). Additionally, the pressures of work, family, school, and community commitments experienced by nurses often lead to exhaustion, burnout, and stress with potentially debilitating effects on the quality of care delivered to clients. Poghosyan and colleagues (2010) concluded that: "Reducing nurse burnout could be a highly effective strategy for improving nurse-rated quality of care . . ." (p. 297).

Self-care encompasses more than just being physically fit and healthy. The practices that lead to increased well-being also build self-esteem, which in turn helps individuals problem solve critically and face challenges more efficiently. Taking a self-esteem questionnaire helps individuals increase self-awareness by putting them in touch with their feelings and emotions; only through self-awareness can an individual begin to change those aspects that lower self-esteem. Worthy of noting is the connection between self-awareness and self-control. A lack of self-awareness can contribute to decreased emotional control (Faguy, 2012), which could prove to be problematic for nurses and the clients receiving their care.

✳ *A self-esteem questionnaire is available online at **nursing. pearsonhighered.com**. Doing this exercise can help individuals gauge their self-esteem.*

The American Holistic Nurses Association (2012a) believes that self-care is the answer to many of the issues facing the nursing profession. In addition to improving the well-being of nurses and thus making them more effective, the AHNA sees self-care as a means of empowering nurses to assert themselves and have their voices heard in matters regarding the work environment.

Maslow's Hierarchy of Needs

Psychologist Abraham Maslow developed a hierarchy of human needs to help individuals prioritize their needs and realize their full potential. In his landmark book, *Motivation and Personality* (1970), Maslow identified five levels of needs, the lower of which must be fulfilled before an individual can move to the next level and eventually achieve self-actualization, the highest level. For an illustration of Maslow's human needs hierarchy and an in-depth discussion of his work, refer to the module on Stress and Coping.

PHYSIOLOGICAL NEEDS Physiological needs are also referred to as survival needs and include the necessities of food, water, air, sleep, and shelter. For example, the extended work hours and rotating shifts common to the nursing profession make it challenging to maintain a regular eating schedule and sleep routine and to participate in regular physical activity. A lack of physical activity has been associated with high rates of lower back pain and other physical ailments reported by healthcare professionals (Sorenson et al., 2011).

Physiological needs can be satisfied in healthy and unhealthy ways. With respect to food, nurses should incorporate the healthiest choices possible in their daily lives. When snacking is the only option, fruits and vegetables, such as apples, bananas, raisins, carrots, and celery sticks are preferable to vending machine fare, such as candy bars and potato chips. Similarly, nurses should opt for water over soft drinks. In terms of sleep, nurses can employ a number of strategies when they cannot count on 8 hours of sleep, including on-the-job 15-minute naps, planned and strategic caffeine consumption, and well-managed shift assignments (Owens, 2007). Physical recreational activities also help nurses cope with limited sleep while enhancing their fitness level. For more information, see the exemplars on Physical Fitness and Exercise and Normal Sleep/Rest Patterns in the module on Health, Wellness, and Illness.

SAFETY Needs at this level have both physical and psychological aspects, which include bodily safety, financial security, and personal health. The American Nurses Association's *2011 Health and Safety Survey* (2013) reported that stress and overwork (74%) and musculoskeletal injury (62%) top the list of nurses' concerns; additionally, 34% of nurses reported concerns about physical assault by their clients, representing a 25% increase from the previous survey in 2001. Furthermore, Cortese, Colombo, and Ghislieri (2010) found that work–family conflict among nurses has a negative effect on job satisfaction. When the quality of a nurse's personal and family life suffers, so does job performance, which directly impacts client satisfaction and service quality.

BELONGING AND LOVE According to Maslow, when the lower physical needs are met, an individual is in a position to

Evidence-Based Practice   Recognizing and Preventing Burnout

Problem

Nurses often function in high-pressure, short-staffed situations and are subject to rotating schedules and extended shifts. Despite the challenges associated with functioning in such an intense work environment, nurses tend to ignore feelings of fatigue, exhaustion, depression, and job dissatisfaction, believing that their colleagues must be feeling the same way. Consequently, many push self-care to the bottom of their list of priorities, ignoring even their most basic needs in order to meet job demands. This cycle leads to burnout.

The effects of nursing burnout take not only a personal emotional and physical toll; they also adversely impact quality of care and client satisfaction and lead to high turnover rates, contributing to the nursing shortage, which inevitably leads to even more burnout (McHugh et al., 2011).

Evidence

Unfortunately, nursing burnout is common throughout the world, with cases having been reported in countries as culturally diverse as the United States, Germany, and Japan (Poghosyan et al., 2010). Erickson and Grove (2007) found that 43.6% of nurses under age 30 and 37.5% of those over 30 experienced burnout.

Research suggests the effects of burnout extend beyond the nurse and into the realm of client care. Poghosyan et al. (2010) studied the relationship between nurse burnout and quality of care in 53,846 nurses from the United States, Canada, the United Kingdom, Germany, New Zealand, and Japan. The results revealed a strong association between nurse burnout and nurses' propensity to rate quality of client care as substandard. The researchers noted that nurse-rated quality of care was independent of nurse characteristics, working conditions, and other significant variables. Furthermore, McHugh et al. (2011) examined the data from six different U.S. surveys and found that client outcomes improved when nurses reported favorable levels of job satisfaction and working conditions. Burtson and Stichler (2010) examined the relationships of several factors, including how burnout and compassion fatigue relate to nursing care. The results suggested that by encouraging self-motivation in nurses, habitual caring behaviors can increase, therefore improving overall levels of client satisfaction.

Implications

Because burnout is detrimental to both the nurse and the client, it is crucial that nurses recognize the signs and symptoms of this phenomenon. The Maslach Burnout Inventory (Maslach & Jackson, 1981) is the most widely used tool for measuring burnout (Poghosyan, Aiken, & Sloane, 2009). This questionnaire, which is designed to identify burnout, groups symptoms into three categories:

- *Emotional exhaustion.* This is one of the earliest signs of burnout and can cause headaches, insomnia, indigestion, and weight fluctuations. It may manifest itself as feelings of dread about going to work. Examples include uncontrollable crying, queasiness, and/or headaches during the nurse's commute.

- *Personal accomplishment.* Overworked nurses tend to feel that clients, supervisors, and hospital administrators do not appreciate their efforts. This can lead to underperformance, which is an adaptive response to stress.

- *Depersonalization.* When a nurse no longer feels compassion for some of her clients it could cause insensitive behavior when providing care.

Nurses experiencing any of these symptoms should seek the advice of colleagues and supervisors on how to overcome burnout. Strategies include physical exercise, talking it through, reducing client load, learning to say "no" to extra assignments and committee appointments, switching shifts, and even changing jobs. Burnout is a sign that something must change. Nurses who choose to ignore it will discover that the symptoms and negative consequences of those symptoms will only worsen.

Critical Thinking Application

1. How can a nurse differentiate between the typical stress experienced by all healthcare professionals and burnout?

2. A nurse is experiencing symptoms of burnout and has approached her supervisor for support and guidance. The supervisor tells her it is simply a part of working as a caregiver and to "push through it." What steps can this nurse take to cope and improve her situation?

3. A nurse observes one of his colleagues being brusque with clients (e.g., lack of eye contact, not providing direct answers, cutting off clients when speaking). When he questions his coworker, she says that she doesn't want to get too emotionally involved with her clients and is just maintaining a healthy distance between them. He knows that she is also going through a difficult divorce and custody battle. What should he do?

address higher psychological needs. The sense of love and belonging that comes from relationships with family, friends, and colleagues is particularly important to nurses, who depend on solid support networks to help them talk through and cope with pressures of work. Venting is a healthy way to unload stress, but it is vital that nurses maintain client confidentiality at all times, even when venting to other nurses.

Unfortunately, new nurses may find their desire and efforts to fit in at work thwarted by a culture of bullying that is prevalent in the nursing profession. "Nurses eat their young" (Townsend, 2012) is an old, familiar refrain, and there is evidence to support it: Newly graduated nurses have significantly higher resignation rates in their first year of practice (Gaffney et al., 2012). Victims of bullying experience distress, anxiety, feelings of isolation, and depression, and subsequently show an increased use of sick time. New graduates are particularly vulnerable because they often lack confidence in their skills and thus crave acceptance and positive feedback from their peers. In addition to adversely affecting job performance and satisfaction, bullying leads to increased absenteeism and staff turnover, therefore risking client safety by interfering with teamwork, collaboration, and communication (Stokowski, 2010).

Victims of bullying should document the incident, recording the date, time, location, and witnesses present for each episode, and report it to both the nursing manager and human resources. Witnesses to a bullying incident can do their part by showing support for the victim, either by speaking up or simply standing beside the victim during the incident. Ultimately, it is up to nurse officers and managers to lead by example by promoting respect and not tolerating bullying. Fortunately, the nursing profession is recognizing its bullying problem and taking steps to address it.

CASE STUDY \\ C

Mrs. Oden, the charge nurse on a medical–surgical unit, assigns extra clients to Celia Hammond, a new graduate nurse, in order to cover for a colleague who left unexpectedly to tend to a family emergency. Mr. Stephen Suskind, a 57-year-old man recovering from knee surgery, is among Celia's clients. In the early afternoon, Mr. Suskind suffers a fall while attempting to make his way to the bathroom unassisted. The sound of the fall and his subsequent cry prompt Celia to rush into his room. As Celia helps Mr. Suskind to stand, Mrs. Oden appears in the doorway and criticizes Celia harshly for having neglected her client, as well as for attempting to move him after his fall. The commotion attracts the attention of other nurses on the floor, who stand behind Mrs. Oden, observing Celia as she is being chastised. Afterward, Celia discusses the incident with an experienced colleague who has worked at the hospital for more than a decade. When Celia complains about having been publicly humiliated, her colleague advises her to "suck it up" and closes the conversation by warning her that "no one likes a whiner."

Clinical Reasoning Questions Level I
1. What should Celia do next?
2. How have Mrs. Oden, Celia's nurse colleague, and others reinforced a culture of bullying?
3. What actions might the nursing supervisor take to address incidents such as this one?

SELF-ESTEEM Needs at this level include feelings of confidence, independence, competence, respect, and achievement. In nursing, a caregiver's self-esteem is based on how he/she is viewed by others. Nurses strive to be seen as competent and proficient and value the respect of peers. It is important for new nurses to realize that nursing proficiency comes through hands-on practice. Skills are improved and mastered over time; thus, new nurses should not compare themselves to more experienced colleagues by being overly self-critical. Instead, they should maintain a positive mind-set and be open to learning.

A mentor (referred to as a preceptor in the clinical setting) can play an important role in encouraging a new nurse's self-esteem needs by supporting the new nurse's skill development and sharing experiences. Many healthcare institutions have mentoring programs where new nurses are paired with established colleagues who serve to teach, counsel, aid, and encourage them. In cases where mentoring programs have not been institutionalized, new nurses can still reach out to experienced colleagues and build a mentor relationship with someone whose style and behavior they admire (Sullivan, 2013).

SELF-ACTUALIZATION After meeting the lower level needs, an individual can then strive to develop her maximum potential and fully realize her abilities and qualities. Part of self-actualization for nurses is the need to make time for themselves. This crucial aspect of self-care includes pursuing activities that bring joy and stimulate creativity. Artistic pursuits, such as writing, playing a musical instrument, and dancing, can serve as important outlets for self-expression. Hobbies are important to personal well-being, because they offer a healthy distraction from the pressures of work and encourage personal development. Taking a break to do nothing in particular is also an effective way to relax and reenergize.

Choosing Wellness

Wellness is a state of well-being involving sound nutrition, regular physical fitness, stable emotional health, self-responsibility, dynamic personal and professional growth, and preventive health care. Currently, nurses are promoting client wellness through the *Healthy People 2020* program, which builds on efforts dating back to 1979 when the Surgeon General issued the original *Healthy People* report (Berman & Snyder, 2012, p. 280). (See the exemplars on Physical Fitness and Exercise and Normal Sleep/Rest Patterns in the module on Health, Wellness, and Illness for specifics.) Nurses would do well to adopt the same healthy principles in their own lives.

AVOIDING UNHEALTHY BEHAVIORS In addition to adapting healthy behaviors, self-care is also about avoiding unhealthy ones. Smoking, abusing alcohol and drugs, and misusing medications are all destructive lifestyle choices that impact a nurse's personal and professional life. According to the National Council on Alcoholism and Drug Dependence (2013), alcohol is the most frequently abused substance. Marijuana ranks second, followed by prescription medications. Due to the intense pressures of their jobs and the easy access to medications, it is tempting for nurses to turn to prescription drugs to cope with everyday stress. An estimated 10%–15% of all nurses may be impaired by or in recovery from some form of drug or alcohol addiction (Thomas & Siela, 2011). Substance abusers typically have difficulty recognizing the problem. Fellow nurses can help by making abusers aware of the issue and encouraging them to seek assistance options, such as counseling and treatment programs.

✳ Go to **nursing.pearsonhighered.com** *for a minimodule on recognizing the impaired nurse in the workplace.*

CHOOSING HEALTHY BEHAVIORS A healthy lifestyle is particularly important to nurses for two main reasons: (1) They must maintain strong immune systems in order to work with people who are ill and (2) they should act as role models so as to maintain credibility when advising others about healthy choices. Balance and moderation are the keys to a healthy lifestyle and this is especially true with respect to nutrition and exercise.

In research on coping strategies for palliative care nurses, Lambert and Lambert (2008) offered several recommendations: Maintain a regular eating schedule; eat balanced, nutritious foods throughout the day; exercise at least three times a week (e.g., take a walk, work out, participate in sports); set aside time for rest and relaxation; seek the company of supportive people; do something enjoyable every day (e.g., play a musical instrument, cook, read, watch TV); avoid tobacco, alcohol, and drugs; maintain an optimistic attitude; set limits with others; and prioritize tasks.

Maintaining a regular eating schedule is a challenge in a profession where rotating shifts and unexpected events are the norm. Nonetheless, nurses need to make time to address their nutritional needs and not wait until the effects of hunger and thirst (pangs, dizziness, seeing spots, etc.) are felt. Nurses can accomplish this by planning ahead and making sure that healthy snacks and fresh water are on hand to consume at predetermined moments of the work shift. Nurses with physically demanding tasks often make the mistake of thinking they are getting enough physical exercise at work; however, standing for long periods of time, lifting clients, and performing other tasks that require physical exertion are not likely to build muscle tone and contribute to cardiovascular fitness (Sorensen et al., 2011).

Self-awareness is the key to effective self-care. It involves self-discovery and leads to personal insights. For instance, a self-aware individual is able to identify personal strengths and weaknesses and is conscious of the assumptions, beliefs, values, and prejudices that can impair judgment. Through self-awareness, a nurse gains greater understanding of others, as well as increased respect and empathy for them (Eckroth-Bucher, 2010). Koren and Papamiditriou (2013) suggest nurses take time to reflect and think about questions like why they chose to go into nursing and what motivates them to go into work every day.

Additionally, nurses should take advantage of the support services available to them. For example, some institutions hold memorial services for clients who have passed away at the hospital, inviting the staff as well as the deceased's family and friends, thus providing a space for caregivers to address their feelings. At some healthcare facilities, nurses come together for weekly support groups to discuss their cases, providing a venue for them to reflect on their work and receive the benefit of their peers' experiences. Online services, such as community forums, offer nurses a safe space where they can vent freely to others who understand the issues they face. Hospital chaplains are also available to listen to and support nurses (Koren & Papamiditriou, 2013). Several professional associations, such as the American Holistic Nurses Association and the New York State Nurses Association (2012), provide programs and additional resources to help nurses cope with the stressors and pressures of their everyday lives. Nurses must remember to respect client privacy and confidentiality during group discussions or in online forums.

Stay Current: *For more information about nurses and substance abuse, visit* **http://www.nysna.org**.

REVIEW **The Concept of Caring Interventions**

RELATE Link the Concepts

Linking the concept of caring interventions with the concept of health, wellness, and illness:

1. Apply theories of caring to discuss how the benefits of self-care (improved physical fitness, overall health, self-esteem, and self-actualization) impact client care.

2. Explain the relationship between self-care and wellness. Is the absence of illness a requirement for wellness? Why or why not?

Linking the concept of caring interventions with the concept of comfort:

3. In the psychosocial realm, how would an absence of genuine caring impact the nursing care for a client who is receiving end-of-life care?

4. Describe the application of presencing when caring for the family members of a client who is receiving end-of-life care.

Linking the concept of caring interventions with the concept of communication:

5. From the client's perspective, how might inadequate self-care affect facets of the nurse's nonverbal communication, such as personal appearance and facial expression?

6. How does confidence, identified by Roach as a caring trait, impact the quality of communication between the nurse and the client?

READY Go to Companion Skills Manual

REFER Go to Pearson Student Nursing Resources
nursing.pearsonhighered.com

- Additional review materials
- Chart: Self-Esteem Questionnaire
- **MiniModule:** Recognizing the Impaired Nurse in the Workplace

REFLECT Case Study

Ms. Ann Mah, a 26-year-old single woman of Chinese origin, was admitted to the hospital following an automobile crash. She had lost consciousness at the wheel while driving home from the gym by herself. Since her admission, she has been diagnosed with a neck injury and a neurological workup revealed she suffers from epilepsy. Her nurse, Michael Robbins, is monitoring her blood pressure and assessing her for side effects related to her newly prescribed anticonvulsant medication, valproate (Depakote).

When Michael enters the room, he finds Ms. Mah gazing out the window. When he asks how she is doing, she responds with a curt "Fine." As he goes through his list of questions, she answers with just one or two words. He senses that she is a very private person, so he avoids asking her personal questions. Later in the day, he asks his mentor for advice on the case, who tells him to be patient and allow the client time to open up. His mentor also informs him of the stigmas attached to epilepsy in different cultures and refers him to several resources. Reading the material, Michael discovers that the Chinese community is particularly concerned that epilepsy may be hereditary, which can lead to people with epilepsy being viewed as less desirable marriage prospects.

After his next assessment, Michael decides to spend an extra 5 minutes with Ms. Mah. He sits by her bedside quietly, observing her out of the corner of his eye as he pretends to review her file. Suddenly, she blurts out:

"I hate this! My life was perfect. I was promoted to regional director of sales last week. I drove around all over the city and I had a great social life. Now you tell me I'm epileptic. What are they going to say at work? Who is going to want to date an epileptic girl?"

Michael moves over to the window to make eye contact with his client. "You're right, epilepsy does require adjustments. But you're not an 'epileptic girl.' You are the same woman you were before the accident. Except that now we know that the woman who was promoted to regional sales director has epilepsy. And so, because of that neck injury, it is especially important that we make sure you don't have another seizure right now."

"With this stupid medicine, I can't keep any food down!"

"We're seeing how you react to the medicine. The idea is to gradually reduce the dosage to lessen the side effects as much as possible while still controlling the seizures. But I have an idea that might make things better. Would you like to hear it?"

"What?"

"How about we try to imagine ways to cope with epilepsy that won't hamper your lifestyle?"

"Like what?"

"Well, I know that in many cases, if we can control your seizures for a certain period of time, you'll still be able to drive. But you tell me what's important to you."

"I really don't want to have to take medication the rest of my life, especially not this stuff. When my sister visited yesterday, she told me there are other ways to treat epilepsy." Ms. Mah turns her head away and mutters, "She mentioned acupuncture."

"I've heard that, too. Let's look into it and talk about some more ideas the next time I see you. Deal?"

Michael stretches out his hand and after a few seconds Ms. Mah takes it and they shake on it.

At his next assessment, Michael finds Ms. Mah reading information from an epilepsy Web site off a tablet.

"How are you today, Ms. Mah?" Michael asks.

"Fine. Today, I'll be asking the questions," Ms. Mah says.

1. Which caring theories are relevant to this case?
2. Which holistic approaches did Michael employ?
3. How did Michael's self-care aid him in caring for Ms. Mah?

■ REFERENCES

American Holistic Nurses Association (AHNA). (2012a). *Join our holistic community—Nurture your self.* Retrieved from http://www.ahna.org/Membership/MemberAdvantage/Selfcare/tabid/1184/Default.aspx.

American Holistic Nurses Association (AHNA). (2012b). *What is holistic nursing?* Retrieved from http://www.ahna.org/AboutUs/WhatisHolisticNursing/tabid/1165/Default.aspx.

American Humanist Association. (2008). *What is humanism.* Retrieved from http://www.americanhumanist.org/Humanism.

American Nurses Association (ANA). (2013). *2011 health and safety survey.* Retrieved from http://www.nursingworld.org/MainMenuCategories/WorkplaceSafety/SafeNeedles/2011-HealthSafetySurvey.html.

Barnes, P. M., Bloom, B., & Nahin, R. L. (2008). *Complementary and alternative medicine use among adults and children: United States, 2007* (National Health Statistics Report No. 12). Hyattsville, MD: National Center for Health Statistics.

Benner, P., & Wrubel, J. (2001). Response to: Edwards, S. D. (2001). Benner and Wrubel on caring in nursing. *Journal of Advanced Nursing, 33*(2), 167–171.

Berman, A., & Snyder, S. J. (2012). *Kozier & Erb's fundamentals of nursing: Concepts, process, and practice.* Upper Saddle River, NJ: Pearson Education.

Blais, K., & Hayes, J. S. (2011). *Professional nursing practice: Concepts and perspectives.* Upper Saddle River, NJ: Pearson Education.

Boykin, A., & Schoenhofer, S. O. (2001). *Nursing as caring: A model for transforming practice.* Sudbury, MA: Jones & Bartlett.

Brunton, B., & Beaman, M. (2000). Nurse practitioners' perceptions of their caring behaviors. *Journal of the American Academy of Nurse Practitioners, 12*(11), 451–456.

Burhans, L. M., & Alligood, M. R. (2010). Quality nursing care in the words of nurses. *Journal of Advanced Nursing, 66*(8), 1689–1697.

Burtson, P. L., & Stichler, J. F. (2010). Nursing work environment and nurse caring: Relationship among motivational factors. *Journal of Advanced Nursing, 66*(8), 1819–1831. doi:10.1111/j.1365-2648.2010.05336.x.

Carper, B. (1978). Fundamental patterns of knowing in nursing. *Advances in Nursing Science 1*(1), 13–23.

Coolen, P. R. (2012, May 1). Cultural relevance in end-of-life care. *EthnoMed.* Retrieved from http://ethnomed.org/clinical/end-of-life/cultural-relevance-in-end-of-life-care.

Cortese, C., Colombo, L., & Ghisleri, C. (2010). Determinants of nurses' job satisfaction: The role of work–family conflict, job demand, emotional charge and social support. *Journal of Nursing Management, 18*(1), 35–44.

Davison, N., & Williams, K. (2009). Compassion in nursing 1: Defining, identifying and measuring this essential quality. *Nursing Times, 105*(36). Retrieved from http://www.nursingtimes.net/nursing-practice/clinical-zones/management/compassion-in-nursing-1-defining-identifying-and-measuring-this-essential-quality-/5006242.article.

Eckroth-Bucher, M. (2010). Self-awareness: A review and analysis of a basic nursing concept. *Advances in Nursing Science, 33*(4), 297–309.

Epstein, E. G., & Delgado, S. (2010, September 30). Understanding and addressing moral distress. *Online Journal of Issues in Nursing, 15*(3). Retrieved from http://www.nursingworld.org/MainMenuCategories/EthicsStandards/Courage-and-Distress/Understanding-Moral-Distress.html.

Erickson, R. J., & Grove, W. J. C. (2007). Why emotions matter: Age, agitation, and burnout among registered nurses. *Online Journal of Issues in Nursing, 13*(1). Retrieved from http://www.nursingworld.org/MainMenuCategories/ANAMarketplace/ANAPeriodicals/OJIN/TableofContents/vol132008/No1Jan08/ArticlePreviousTopic/WhyEmotionsMatterAgeAgitationandBurnoutAmongRegisteredNurses.html.

Faguy, K. (2012). Emotional intelligence in health care. *Journal of the American Society of Radiologic Technologists, 83*(3), 237–253.

Gaffney, D. A., DeMarco, R. F., Hofmeyer, A., Vessey, J. A., & Budin, W. C. (2012). Making things right: Nurses' experiences with workplace bullying—A grounded theory. *Nursing Research and Practice.* Retrieved from http://www.hindawi.com/journals/nrp/2012/243210_doi:10.1155/2012/243210.

Gartner, F. R., Nieuwenhuijsen, K., Dijk, F. J., & Sluiter, J. K. (2010). The impact of common mental disorders on the work functioning of nurses and allied health professionals: A systematic review. *International Journal of Nursing Studies, 47*, 1047–1061.

George, J. B. (Ed.). (2011). *Nursing theories: The base for professional nursing practice.* Upper Saddle River, NJ: Pearson Education.

Jarrin, O. F. (2012). The integrality of situated caring in nursing and the environment. *ANS Advances in Nursing Science, 3*(1), 14–24. doi:10.1097/ANS.0b013e3182433b89.

Knight, B. G., & Sayegh, P. (2009). Cultural values and caregiving: The updated sociocultural stress and coping model. *Journals of Gerontology B: Psychological Sciences Social Sciences, 65B*(1), 5–13.

Koren, M. E., & Papamiditriou, C. (2013). Spirituality of staff nurses: Application of modeling and role modeling theory. *Holistic Nurse Practitioner, 27*(1), 37–44.

Lachman, V. D. (2012). Applying the ethics of care to your nursing practice. *MedSurg Nursing, 21*(2), 112–116.

Lambert, V. A., & Lambert, C. E. (2008). Nurses' workplace stressors and coping strategies. *Indian Journal of Palliative Care, 14*(1). Retrieved from http://www.jpalliativecare.com/article.asp?issn=0973-1075;year=2008;volume=14;issue=1;spage=38;epage=44;aulast=Lambert.

Leininger, M. M. (1989). Transcultural nurse specialists and generalists: New practitioners in nursing. *Journal of Transcultural Nursing, 1*(1), 4–16.

Leininger, M. M., & McFarland, M. R. (2006). *Culture care diversity and universality: A worldwide nursing theory.* Sudbury, MA: Jones & Bartlett.

Longo, J. (2011, January/February). Acts of caring: Nurses caring for nurses. *Holistic Nursing Practice,* 8–16.

Mariano, C. (2005). An overview of holistic nursing. *NSNA Imprint, 52*(2), 48–51.

Maslach, C., & Jackson, S. E. (1981). The measurement of experienced burnout. *Journal of Occupational Behaviour, 2*(2), 99–113.

Mayeroff, M. (1990). *On caring.* New York, NY: HarperCollins.

McHugh, M. D., Kutney-Lee, A., Cimiotti, J. P., Sloane, D. M., & Aiken, L. H. (2011). Nurses' widespread job dissatisfaction, burnout, and frustration with health benefits signal problems for patient care. *Health Aff (Millwood), 30*(2), 202–210. doi:10.1377/hlthaff.2010.0100.

Merriam-Webster Dictionary. (2013). Retrieved from http://www.merriam-webster.com/dictionary.

National Council on Alcoholism and Drug Dependence. (2013). *Prescription drugs.* Retrieved from http://ncadd.org/index.php/learn-about-drugs/prescription-drugs.

National Institute for Occupational Safety and Health. (2012, February 14). *NIOSH safety and health topic: Health care workers.* Retrieved from http://www.cdc.gov/niosh/topics/healthcare.

New York State Nurses Association. (2012). *Module 4: Helping nurses with alcohol or drug-related problems.* Retrieved from http://www.nysna.org/ce/academy/module4.htm.

Owens, J. A. (2007). Sleep loss and fatigue in healthcare professionals. *Journal of Perinatal and Neonatal Nursing, 21*(2), 92–100.

Poghosyan, L., Aiken, L. H., & Sloane, D. M. (2009, July). Factor structure of the Maslach Burnout Inventory: An analysis of data from large scale cross-sectional surveys of nurses from eight countries. *International Journal of Nursing Studies, 46*(7), 894–902.

Poghosyan, L., Clarke, S. P., Finlayson, M., & Aiken, L. H. (2010). Nurse burnout and quality of care: Cross-national investigation in six countries. *Research in Nursing & Health, 33*(4), 288–298.

Roach, M. S. (1984). *Caring: The human mode of being, implications for nursing, a monograph.* Toronto, Ontario: Faculty of Nursing, University of Toronto.

Roach, M. S. (Ed.). (1997). *Caring from the heart: The convergence of caring and spirituality.* Mahwah, NJ: Paulist Press.

Roach, M. S. (2002). *Caring, the human mode of being: A blueprint for the health professions* (2nd ed.). Ottawa, Ontario: CHA Press.

Sorensen, G., Stoddard, A. M., Stoffel, S., Buxton, O., Sembajwe, G., Hashimoto, D., et al. (2011). The role of the work context in multiple wellness outcomes for hospital patient care workers. *Journal of Occupational and Environmental Medicine, 53*(8), 899–910.

Stokowski, L. A. (2010, September 30). A matter of respect and dignity: Bullying in the nursing profession. *Medscape.* Retrieved from http://www.medscape.com/viewarticle/729474.

Stratis Health: Culture Care Connection. (2013). *Somalis in Minnesota.* Retrieved from http://www.culturecareconnection.org/matters/diversity/somali.html.

Sullivan, E. J. (2013). *Becoming influential: A guide for nurses.* Upper Saddle River, NJ: Pearson Education.

Takase, M., & Teraoka, S. (2011). Development of the holistic nursing competence scale. *Nursing and Health Sciences, 13,* 396–403.

Thomas, C. M., & Siela, D. (2011). The impaired nurse: Would you know what to do if you suspected substance abuse? *American Nurse Today, 6*(8). Retrieved from http://www.americannursetoday.com/article.aspx?id=8114&fid=8078.

Tonges, M., & Ray, J. (2011). Translating caring theory into practice: The Carolina care model. *Journal of Nursing Administration, 41*(9), 374–381.

Townsend, T. (2012). Break the bullying cycle. *American Nurse Today, 8*(1) 12–15.

Van der Elst, E., Dierckx de Casterlé, B., & Gastmans, C. (2012). Elderly patients' and residents' perceptions of 'the good nurse': A literature review. *Journal of Medical Ethics, 38,* 93–97. doi:10.1136/medethics-2011-100046.

Watson, J. (1999). *Nursing: Human science and human care: A theory of nursing.* Sudbury, MA: Jones & Bartlett.

Watson, J. (2002). Intentionality and caring-healing consciousness: A practice of transpersonal nursing. *Holistic Nurse Practitioner, 16*(4), 12–19.

Watson, J. (n.d.). *Caring science (definitions, processes, theory).* Retrieved from http://watsoncaringscience.org/about-us/caring-science-definitions-processes-theory.

36 Clinical Decision Making

MODULE AT-A-GLANCE

The Concept of Clinical Decision Making, 2315

Exemplar 36.1
The Nursing Process, 2328

Exemplar 36.2
The Nursing Plan of Care, 2354

Exemplar 36.3
Prioritizing Care, 2363

☑ THE CONCEPT OF CLINICAL DECISION MAKING

Clinical decision making is a process nurses use in the clinical setting to evaluate and select the best actions to meet desired goals. Nurses use clinical decision making whenever choices are available, even when they evaluate a situation and decide not to act. In some cases, decisions are required in situations that have neither clear answers nor standard procedures, and when conflicting forces add to the complexity. At other times, decisions are routine. For example, a nurse is assigned five clients:

- A client with a 1-day-old abdominal surgical site
- A client who was admitted in sickle cell crisis
- A client with an arm wound infected with MRSA who is in contact isolation
- A client who has been crying all night
- A client who is already up and walking down the hall of the unit.

Clinical decision making applies across the continuum of nursing care, from direct client care at the bedside to professional behaviors and accountability inherent in the profession of nursing (see the Concepts Related to Clinical Decision Making feature for examples). The nurse must evaluate each client's needs and preferences as well as time-constraining activities (e.g., medication administration) to make appropriate decisions for each client (see the exemplar on Prioritizing Care within this module for further information). To make these decisions, the nurse must use critical thinking to choose among alternatives to support the best client outcomes for all five clients. **<<**

Concept Learning Outcomes

After reading about this concept, you will be able to:

1. Discuss how clinical decision making impacts quality client outcomes.
2. Apply behaviors to improve critical thinking skills when providing nursing care.
3. Distinguish, at a beginner level, significant cues that cluster in a pattern.
4. Evaluate client care situations using problem solving.
5. Recognize the importance of critical thinking when making decisions for clinical judgment.
6. Use reflection to determine lessons learned for future nursing practice.
7. Contrast the levels of clinical competence in Benner's skill acquisition model with the dimensions in Lasater's clinical judgment rubric.

Concept Key Terms

Clinical decision making, 2315
Clinical judgment, 2324
Clinical reasoning, 2319
Creativity, 2318
Critical thinking, 2316
Deductive reasoning, 2319

Inductive reasoning, 2319
Inquiry, 2318
Intellect, 2317
Intuition, 2320
Reflection, 2319
Salient cue, 2317

Concepts Related to **Clinical Decision Making**

CONCEPT	RELATIONSHIP TO CLINICAL DECISION MAKING	NURSING IMPLICATIONS
Managing Care		
■ Care coordination ■ Cost-effective care ■ Delegation	Client care is organized to include client preferences, time constraints, resources, and expertise of other available disciplines.	■ Nursing care is achieved through the coordination of many factors that influence outcomes for the client.
Accountability		
■ Competence	Standards of care set benchmarks for nursing performance expectations.	■ Nurses are responsible for the clinical decisions and judgments they make to support desired client outcomes.
Collaboration		
■ Case management ■ Interdisciplinary teams	Many disciplines contribute to the care of a client.	■ Nurses participate in a collaborative team approach when caring for clients.
Communication		
■ Documentation ■ Reporting	Priorities of client care need to be communicated to achieve continuity of care.	■ Nurses use the client's plan of care to communicate priority needs of the client.
Oxygenation		
	Nurses use clinical decision making following assessment of airway patency to identify (a) additional assessment data essential to determine care needs and (b) priority interventions necessary to promote effective respiration and gas exchange.	■ Knowledge of oxygenation, client health history, and facility protocols is necessary when making decisions about the nursing care of clients with alterations in oxygenation. ■ Examples include prioritizing assessment data to gather relative to oxygenation, and anticipating appropriate physician orders (e.g., supplemental oxygen, encouragement of oral fluids, and IV antibiotics).

▶ CRITICAL THINKING

In any clinical circumstance, client outcomes improve when the nurse uses critical thinking. Failure to employ critical thinking results in wasted time and energy, poor-quality client outcomes, frustration, and anxiety (Elder & Paul, 2011). The American Association of Colleges of Nursing (2008) defines **critical thinking** as "All or part of the process of questioning, analysis, synthesis, interpretation, inference, inductive and deductive reasoning, intuition, application, and creativity." The Accreditation Commission for Education in Nursing (formerly known as the National League for Nursing Accreditation Commission) speaks of critical thinking as "the deliberate nonlinear process of collecting, interpreting, analyzing, drawing conclusions about, presenting, and evaluating information that is both factually and belief based" (Benner, Hughes, & Sutphen, 2008). These statements, and those by other professional nursing organizations, underscore the importance of today's nurses being able to make meaningful

observations, solve problems, and decide on a course of action. To do so, nurses must be able to process both previously learned and newly acquired information—about their clients, the work environment, resources at hand or in the community, and applicable evidence related to care of the client—and prioritize quickly and efficiently.

Nurses use critical thinking skills in a variety of ways. Because nurses deal holistically with human responses, they must draw meaningful information from other disciplines in order to understand the meaning of client data and plan effective interventions. This can be challenging because nurses work in rapidly changing situations. Routine actions are not always adequate to deal with the situation at hand. Familiarity with the routine for giving medications, for example, does not help the nurse deal with a client who is frightened of injections or the one who does not wish to take a medication. When unexpected situations arise, critical thinking enables the nurse to recognize what is happening, respond quickly, and adapt interventions to meet specific client needs. Nurses must use critical thinking, for

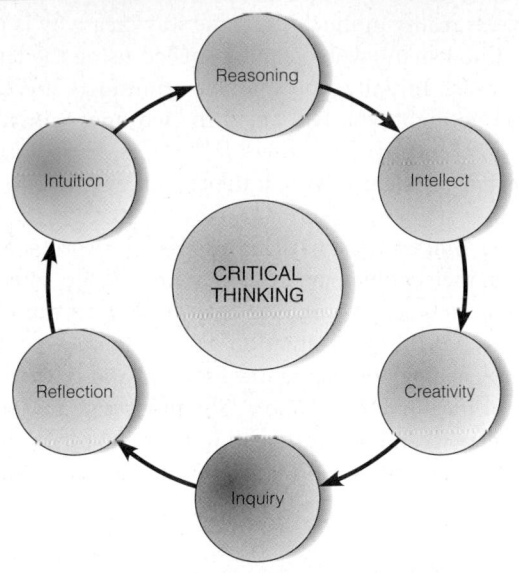

Figure 36–1 ● Critical thinking skills are essential for making clinical decisions.

example, to decide which observations to report to the primary care provider immediately and which can wait to report until morning rounds are done with the client. The skills and abilities necessary to develop critical thinking include intellect, creativity, inquiry, reasoning, reflection, and intuition (**Figure 36–1** ●). Critical thinking also requires maintaining an attitude that promotes critical thinking (**Table 36–1** ●).

TABLE 36–1	Common Attitudes of Critical Thinkers
Independence	■ Does own thinking, objectively and honestly. ■ Is open minded about different methods used to reach same goal. ■ Looks for the facts; not easily swayed by opinions.
Fair-mindedness	■ Has neutral judgments without bias. ■ Considers opposing views to understand all aspects before making decisions. ■ Is open to new ideas and ways of doing things.
Aware of self-limits	■ Knows limits of intellect and experience. ■ Seeks new knowledge or skills in current evidence. ■ Expresses a willingness to self-reflect on own beliefs and ideas.
Integrity	■ Challenges own ideas and methods of doing nursing care. ■ Evaluates inconsistencies within own nursing practice. ■ Chooses the right thing to do over the popular thing to do.
Perseverance	■ Has stick-with-it motivation to find the best solution for quality client outcomes. ■ Is patient with processes.
Confidence	■ Knows that he knows what he knows. ■ Trusts the skills and abilities of intellect, creativity, inquiry, reasoning, reflection, and intuition

Intellect

Intellect includes the ability to learn and understand knowledge; the capacity for thinking and reasoning intelligently (Free Dictionary, 2012). Building on clinical knowledge and skills expands the knowledge base nurses use for reasoning, analyzing, and predicting client outcomes. Intellect helps differentiate facts from opinions, approach situations objectively instead of subjectively, and clarify concepts. Thinking becomes an intentional action to identify **salient cues** that fit together within a clinical situation. *Salient,* or significant, means the leading, most noticeable, or most important, and *cue* refers to significant data that informs and influences conclusions about the client's health status. Salient cues can cluster to form a pattern that can be translated into a nursing diagnosis for the client. A salient cue does one of the following:

■ *Indicates a negative or positive change in a client's health status or pattern.* For example, the client states, "I have been experiencing shortness of breath when climbing stairs."

■ *Varies from norms of the client population.* The client's pattern may vary from norms of the general society. For example, an adult client may consider a pattern of eating two small meals a day to be normal.

■ *Indicates a developmental delay.* The nurse must be aware of the normal patterns and changes that occur as the person grows and develops. For example, by age 9 months an infant is usually able to sit alone without support. The infant who has not accomplished this task needs further assessment for possible developmental delays.

Once salient cues are recognized, they can be clustered for relatedness to determine whether any patterns are present. The nurse can then interpret the pattern and take appropriate action. Awareness of cues and their significance can be valuable in making clinical decisions essential to nursing care for ever-changing conditions and reordering of priorities in meeting client needs (Reimer & Moore, 2010). This dynamic way of thinking evolves over time, very much like nurses advancing through the stages of skill acquisition as they gain nursing care experience. New nurses need to write down the assessment data and search data for abnormal cues to help them cluster significant cues that can be translated into a nursing diagnosis. See **Figure 36–2** ● for an example of cues and clustering of data.

Continuous learning is necessary for nurses to remain current in best evidence for quality client outcomes (see the module on Evidence-Based Practice for further information).

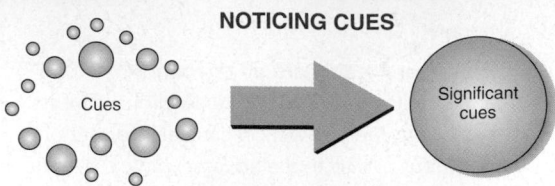

NOTICING CUES

Random	Clustered
• Productive cough	• Productive cough
• Affect-sadness	• Green-colored sputum
• Right-hand weakness	• Foul-smelling sputum
• Green-colored sputum	• Temperature—101.2° F
• Disturbed sleeping	• Respiratory rate—22/min
• Foul-smelling sputum	• Shortness of breath
• Temperature—101.2° F	(All relative to pattern of infection in the respiratory system.)
• Respiratory rate—22/min	
• Shortness of breath	
• States "I don't feel good."	

Figure 36–2 ● Random cues are not similar to each other, whereas significant cues that relate to each other can be clustered to form a pattern.

Many states now require nurses to complete continuing education credits to demonstrate continuing competency for licensure renewal (see the module on Legal Issues for further information).

Creativity

Creativity is an outlet for the imagination that allows a nurse to take what can be seen in the mind, which does not exist physically, and make it tangible so it does exist. **Creativity** means finding unique solutions to unique problems when traditional interventions are not effective; for example, finding just the right way to connect with a client who does not want to talk about her diabetes or finding what best helps a client meet a goal so he can be discharged from the hospital.

A modification to an old saying "No one size fits all" describes the importance of individualizing nursing care for each client. When an attempt to help a client is not successful, the nurse changes tactics and asks the question, "What other approach might help this client be successful?" The ability to look for alternatives by "thinking out of the box" is necessary because creative problem-solving opportunities occur every day. Some examples of opportunities for nurse creativity are:

■ Helping a client who is dehydrated drink more liquids by mouth

■ Helping a newly diagnosed client with diabetes learn what foods are appropriate

■ Finding alternatives for an IV tubing label when no traditional label is available

■ Finding something to write vital signs on when paper is not at hand

■ Using tape and tongue blades to make a toy house for a young child.

Sometimes the best way to find a good alternative is to increase the number of alternatives available. This is where cre-

ativity meets reality in much the same way creativity is used to figure out how many words can be spelled using the letters in "nursing care." Initially, you may have minimal success, but after more thought, you will begin to "see" more possibilities and spell more words from these few letters. Nurses can promote creative problem solving if they begin with asking "What if we . . . ?"

Creative thinkers must have knowledge of the problem. They must assess their problem and use their knowledge (intellect) of underlying facts and principles that apply (see the Clinical Example feature). In this situation, the nurse knows the anatomy and physiology of respiratory function and is aware of the purpose of incentive spirometry. The nurse also understands pediatric growth and development. In trying to assist the child, the nurse builds on this knowledge and comes up with a creative solution.

CLINICAL EXAMPLE

A pediatric home health nurse is caring for Tyesha, a 9-year-old girl who has ineffective respirations following abdominal surgery. The primary care provider has ordered incentive spirometry (a treatment device that promotes alveolar expansion). Tyesha is frightened by the equipment and tires quickly during the treatments. The nurse offers her a bottle of bubbles and a blowing wand. Tyesha is delighted with blowing bubbles. The nurse knows that the respiratory effort in blowing bubbles will promote alveolar expansion and suggests that she blow bubbles between incentive spirometry treatments.

Inquiry

An **inquiry** is defined as a search for knowledge or facts; when a nurse uses inquiry, she examines objective information to gain clarification and find solutions to problems. This is different from making a *query,* which is merely asking a question or requesting information (DifferenceBetween. net, 2012). Critical thinking requires nurses to use inquiry to examine both the situation at hand as well as their own nursing practice: "Why do we always need to apply the dressing this way?" "How can I help a client who is on a salt-free diet to avoid problems with her serum potassium levels?" "Why do we always need to put gloves on when we give injections?" "What would happen if we helped the client to exercise more than twice a day?" "Is there something else we can try when a client is having trouble swallowing?" While in the clinical setting, nurses continuously use clinical inquiry to evaluate *how* they are doing. Nurses are inquisitive decision makers who ask questions about physician orders they do not understand, seek more information about an alternative therapy, or wonder if there is a better way of accomplishing an outcome for a client. They make changes in their practice based on new information, evidence, or innovative ways of doing things better. Clinical inquiry can resolve clinical problems and issues to promote improved client outcomes.

Reasoning

To be able to walk into a client's room and immediately observe significant data, come to a conclusion about the client, and begin appropriate actions takes clinical reasoning by an experienced nurse. To be objective, the nurse needs to focus on salient cues and not be influenced by personal beliefs or assumptions, which can result in errors as illustrated by this statement made by a nurse: "The client's a man, so I didn't think he was really in enough pain for an injection of Demerol."

To help determine if decisions are reasonable, nurses use either one of two forms of logical reasoning. In **deductive reasoning**, the nurse works from the "top down" by starting with a conclusion and analyzing it for valid significant cues. For example, the nurse knows pneumonia manifests symptoms of increased sputum production, decreased appetite, productive cough, low energy, and complaints of chest pain when coughing. Using deductive reasoning, the nurse concludes a newly admitted client diagnosed with pneumonia would have these same symptoms. Ask these questions: "What is the conclusion (the end result)?" and "What cues observed support it?" and, finally, "Do the significant cues make sense? Are they logical?"

With **inductive reasoning**, nurses work from the "bottom up" by putting significant cues together to reach a conclusion. For example, the nurse observes that a client diagnosed with pneumonia has increased sputum production, does not eat or drink readily, has a productive cough, has little energy, and complains his chest hurts when he coughs. Using inductive reasoning, the nurse concludes that the presence of these same signs in other clients strongly indicates they may also have pneumonia. Ask these questions: "What are the significant cues observed?" and "What is the conclusion from the cues (the end result)?" And again, "Does the conclusion make sense? Is it logical?" (Education.com, 2013).

During the process of reasoning, the nurse needs to determine if client information is a fact, an inference, a judgment, or an opinion (see **Table 36–2** ●). Evaluating the credibility of information sources is an important step in critical thinking. Unfortunately, nurses cannot always take as truthful what they read or are told. The nurse may need to ascertain the accuracy of information by reviewing the evidence (e.g., conducting a literature search), checking other documents (e.g., facility procedures), or talking with other informants (e.g., supervising nurse).

Clinical reasoning, the use of careful reasoning in the clinical setting to improve client care, is a learned skill that beginning nurses must practice. Clinical reasoning requires critical thinking and the ability to reflect on previous situations and decisions and evaluate their effectiveness. With effort and time, critical thinking can be learned and integrated into daily routines. Here are a few actions new nurses can take to improve their clinical reasoning:

1. On entering a client's room, look around and observe the client, any other people in the room, where they are positioned in the room and what they are doing. Observe what items, smells, and sounds are present and what actions are taking place. This is similar to doing a 60-second safety check, a 3-minute brief assessment, or a 5-minute general survey of the client. Careful use of the senses can help the nurse collect important cues.

2. Common cues nurses learn to recognize include facial expressions, client activity, degree of respiratory effort, smell of cigarette smoke, complaints made by the client, bed safety (e.g., rails up or down, bed low and locked, call bell within reach), client affect, colors (e.g., red to indicate bleeding, yellow to indicate infection). These common cues can provide meaningful information fairly quickly. Determine which cues are salient and if they form a pattern. Clusters may bring attention to a problem or issue the client is having (e.g., presence of infection) or that is in the client's immediate space (e.g., visitors preventing appropriate rest). The nurse can then determine the best course of action and intervene as appropriate (University of Newcastle, Faculty of Health, 2009).

3. Use reflective thinking to evaluate the outcome of actions. Evaluating actions taken can turn those actions into experiences that can be called on in the future. Questions that help promote reflective thinking include "How well did that work?" "How did the client respond?" "What could be done better next time?"

4. Build awareness of faulty reasoning, which could cause new nurses to make mistakes in reasoning (see **Table 36–3** ●).

TABLE 36–2 Differentiating Types of Statements

STATEMENT	DESCRIPTION	EXAMPLE
Facts	Can be verified through investigation	Blood pressure is affected by blood volume.
Inferences	Conclusions drawn from facts; going beyond facts to make a statement about something not currently known	If blood volume is decreased (e.g., in hemorrhagic shock), the blood pressure will drop.
Judgments	Evaluation of facts or information that reflect values or other criteria; a type of opinion	It is harmful to the client's health if the blood pressure drops too low.
Opinions	Beliefs formed over time; may include judgments that may fit facts or be in error	Nursing intervention can assist in maintaining the client's blood pressure within normal limits.

Reflection

Reflection is the action of making sense of occurrences, situations, or decisions by carefully considering the totality of the experience: what worked or did not work, what could have been done differently to achieve better outcomes, what was done well, what necessary resources were available, and so on (Oelofsen, 2012). To reflect on an experience, nurses need to learn what to pay attention to or notice. What are the significant factors of an experience that need to be included in reflective thinking? See **Box 36–1** ● for an example of guided reflection.

TABLE 36–3 Types of Faulty Reasoning

TYPE OF FAULTY REASONING	ACTION	EXAMPLE
Bandwagon	Doing something because everyone else is doing it	"Everyone takes 30-minute breaks instead of 10-minute breaks. You want to be like everyone else don't you?"
Circular reasoning	Supporting an opinion by restating it using different words	A new dressing is very popular to use because a lot of nurses like using it. (The terms *popular* and *like using it* are saying the same thing.)
Cause-and-effect fallacy	Linking something that happens to something that occurs before it happens	The client's NG tube was draining fine until the nurse cleaned up her bedside table; therefore, the nurse caused the NG tube not to drain by cleaning up the bedside table.
Either–or fallacy	Assuming a detailed question only has a couple of responses	The only way to help a client with a headache is either with medication or a cold cloth on the head. (This ignores other interventions that may be helpful, including dimming the lights, decreasing noise, or giving client something to eat.)
Overgeneralizations	Not enough evidence to come to a conclusion	Concluding that the postoperative client eats all of his meals based on the observation that he ate 100% of his last three meals.
Using emotions of words		Saying the client is an angry old man instead of saying that the older client is anxious about being in the hospital.

Source: Based on Lorcher, T. (2012). *Examples of faulty reasoning.* Retrieved from http://www.brighthubeducation.com/high-school-english-lessons/25583-examples-of-faulty-reasoning.

Evidence shows that the debriefing, or reflective thinking, that occurs after a simulated scenario encourages reflective learning that can help transfer book knowledge to practice application in complex situations (Pivec & Blazovich, 2012). Reflective thinking can change a situation that is obscure, uncertain, and disturbing into one that is clear, understandable, and settled. For example, a nurse might be assigned to a client who is anxious about going to surgery. The nurse can help the client "see" with better clarity about the surgical experience with guided reflection, resulting in less anxiety for the client.

Intuition

At times nurses may experience what they call a "gut reaction" or a "feeling that something is wrong" when working with clients. Even though this awareness seems abstract and mysterious, it may be part of the nurse's reasoning and analysis of the constant data the nurse receives through the senses below a level of awareness. In their article "How Expert Nurses Use Intuition," Benner and Tanner (1987) conclude that **intuition** is the use of nursing knowledge, experience, and expertise for understanding without the conscious use of reasoning (Reagan, 2010). Much research has been done with expert nurses that supports intuition as a valuable cognitive skill that can be used for clinical judgment (My Nursing Uniforms, 2011).

Intuition is a process. The data that is continuously received through senses is not always recognized consciously. Patterns and similarities of patterns are clustered and analyzed. Comparisons are made between a current client's significant patterns and past client's patterns in response to similar situations. If the mind recognizes a new pattern is similar to an old pattern, this recognition may bring the information to a level of cognitive awareness, making it available for the nurse to use in determining a course of action.

Although the intuitive method of problem solving is gaining recognition as part of nursing practice, it is not recommended for new nurses or students, because they usually lack the knowledge base and clinical experience on which to make a valid judgment. Books are available that can help nurses learn intuitive thinking through various reflective and reasoning activities (Reagan, 2010). There are also courses available to build critical thinking skills for nurses. For example, the National Council of State Boards of Nursing (NCSBN) (2010) has a continuing education course called "Sharpening Critical Thinking Skills" for nurses.

▶ CLINICAL DECISION MAKING

Nurses make many decisions every day:

- "Which client should I see first?"
- "When can I teach my client with congestive heart failure about a no-salt diet?"
- "How long should I wait before doing a bladder scan on my client who hasn't voided since the Foley catheter was removed?"
- "When's the best time for me to watch the video on that new dressing?"
- "Where can I find more linen for the UAPs to finish client morning care?"

Wouldn't it be nice if there was a book to show nurses how to guarantee all clinical decisions they make would be 100% "successful"?

Good decisions come from careful consideration of resources; potential alternatives and their potential outcomes; the nurse's expertise, knowledge, skills, and clinical judgment; and the preferences of the client. Typically, nurses

Box 36–1   Guided Reflection

This activity illustrates how one new nurse reflects on a situation he encountered during a clinical day that caused him to think about what happened and how he responded. Organizing thinking about client care and professional nursing practice is a learned skill. Reflecting on thinking processes supports recognizing the "lessons learned" for personal improvement in clinical judgment.

GUIDED REFLECTION	NEW NURSE RESPONSE
Background of Situation	
1. Briefly describe what happened and what emotions you experienced during the situation. 2. What previous personal experience with a similar situation helped guide you through the situation?	1. "I was so busy giving my client his bath that I forgot to give him a scheduled medication." 2. "I have worked as an unlicensed assistive personnel (UAP) in the past; I know that baths have to be given around other interventions that the client has scheduled during the day."
Observing	
3. What did you initially notice about the situation? 4. As time passed, what did you then notice?	3. "I started bathing the client about 0850. I thought I had enough time to finish it and then give him his medication that was scheduled to be given at 0930." 4. "The client needed more time than I thought to bathe. When I checked my watch, it was already 0935, and the medication was late."
Interpreting	
5. What further information about the situation did you decide you needed, and how did you get it?	5. "I should have remembered that some clients, particularly older adults, need more time to do things. I could have started earlier on the bath, or I could have given the client his medication first, and then helped him with his bath."
Responding	
6. What was your nursing response to the situation? What interventions did you do? 7. Describe stresses you experienced as you responded to the situation.	6. "I had to tell the charge nurse what had happened. I then had to give the medication late." 7. "It stressed me out that I made a medication error. I felt stupid and was so embarrassed."
Reflecting	
8. How did the situation end, and what emotion did you feel when the situation was over? 9. What might you do differently if this situation happens again? 10. What was your "take-away" from the experience?	8. "The client received the medication only seven minutes late, so I didn't negatively impact the client, but I could have kicked myself for this." 9. "I need to work around medication administration times when I help a client with morning care—or any intervention." 10. "Keep an eye on the clock and give priority to things I need to do that have specific times to be done—work the other interventions around the timed ones."

Source: Based on Tanner, C. (2006). Thinking like a nurse: A research-based model of clinical judgment in nursing. *Journal of Nursing Education, 45*(6), 204–210. Retrieved from http://jxzy.smu.edu.cn/jkpg/UploadFiles/file/TF_0692810354_thinking%20like%20a%20nurse.pdf.

make decisions during the process of solving problems. Types of decisions include:

- **Value decisions,** such as decisions regarding client confidentiality
- **Time management decisions,** such as taking clean linens to a client's room at the same time as medication to be administered
- **Scheduling decisions,** such as bathing a client before visiting hours
- **Priority decisions** about which interventions are most urgent and which can be delegated.

Nurses also assist clients to make decisions. When a client is trying to make a decision about what course of treatment to follow, the nurse may need to provide information or resources the client can use in making a decision (see the Lifespan Considerations feature). Nurses make decisions in their own professional lives. For example, nurses must decide whether to work in a hospital or community setting, whether to join a professional association, and whether to carry professional liability insurance.

The constantly changing healthcare environment also requires strong clinical decision-making skills. New technology, expanding roles for nurses in healthcare systems, the complexity

Lifespan Considerations Healthcare Decisions

Children

Parents most often make decisions about the health care of children. Growing children can participate in those decisions in age-appropriate ways. As described by Piaget, the ability of children to reason and critically think about themselves and their situation develops gradually. At each stage, nurses should be aware of the ways children think and be sensitive to how they can be involved in healthcare decisions:

■ Infants progress from reflexive behavior to simple, repetitive behavior and then to imitative behaviors, learning the concepts of cause and effect and object permanence. Though not involved in making decisions, they need to be comforted and feel secure during the entire process of providing care, including during waiting periods.

■ Toddlers and preschoolers are very egocentric and engage in magical thinking. They cannot reason out the implications of care, but need explanations in language they can understand. Play therapy and use of dolls and toys can help them adjust to care, and they can sometimes be given options (e.g., "Do you want your dressing changed before breakfast or after?").

■ School-age children tend to be concrete thinkers. They benefit from simple, direct explanations; hands-on exploration of equipment and materials; and helping the care

provider as appropriate during procedures. Involving these children in care can increase cooperation and decrease anxiety.

■ Adolescents are increasingly able to think abstractly and may make many of their own healthcare decisions. They should be actively consulted as a part of the family system.

Older Adults

It is important to include all adult clients in decision making and planning nursing care, but it is difficult to do this when working with older adults who have impaired cognition related to a disease process, such as Alzheimer disease. The nurse should allow these clients as much control and input as possible, keeping things simple and direct so they understand. Older adults with impairments usually are unable to perform multiple tasks or even to think of more than one step at a time. The nurse must have patience and be willing to calmly repeat instructions if necessary. Presenting and discussing issues in basic terms helps to maintain respect and dignity and allows older adults to participate in their own care for as long as possible. If the older adult is unable to perform self-care activities such as bathing or health-related activities such as a dressing change, the nurse seeks appropriate alternative methods for assisting the client with these tasks.

of clients entering the healthcare system, and the ever-expanding body of knowledge and skills all add to the complexity of clinical decision making.

When nurses do not have enough nursing experience, or nursing knowledge, skills, or imagination to make decisions, they can turn to available guidelines for help. Decision trees and protocols can assist in decision making for many aspects of nursing and specialties of nursing. For example, many facilities have an emergency protocol for starting a client on low-flow oxygen when the client meets listed criteria to initiate the protocol. Sometimes when cycling through the alternatives, one alternative will just be exactly what is needed and may be chosen for use without further consideration of other alternatives. Many models are available, each suggesting steps in how to use cognitive processes to choose among alternatives. The following common steps are used in making decisions:

1. Identify the situation or problem: What decision needs to be made?
2. List all possible alternatives and information about them (i.e., risks, consequences).
3. Compare pros and cons of each alternative or solution and evaluate all of them.
4. Select the best option or alternative to try.
5. Put the alternative into action.
6. Evaluate the success of using the alternative or solution as to whether the initial purpose was achieved (Decision Making Confidence, 2013).

As nurses apply critical thinking to challenges in the workplace, they typically face choosing between possible alternatives, engaging in problem solving, using the nursing process, and,

sometimes, engaging in trial and error and employing the scientific method.

Choosing Between Alternatives

Many situations present possible alternatives that must be considered prior to taking action. In clinical situations, alternatives may be selected from a range of nursing interventions or client care strategies. Often priorities for care suggest or even determine the alternative chosen, but not always. For example, pain may be treated with oral or injectable medications, as needed (PRN) or on a schedule, or without any pharmacologic intervention by using nursing measures to support the client's comfort. In all cases, the nurse analyzes the alternatives to ensure that there is an objective rationale for choosing one alternative over another. For example, with kidney stone pain, common nursing measures may not provide strong enough relief, and oral medication may take effect too slowly, so an intravenous narcotic might be the better choice. Considering the possibilities of adverse consequences as a result of a decision is also part of this process. If the intravenous narcotic is selected, what safety procedures need to be in place—for example, a narcotic antidote and supplemental oxygen? Think about the following questions when choosing between alternatives in decision making:

1. Is there always just "one best" alternative?	Finding the "one best" alternative is very time consuming and may result in unnecessary delay.
2. Can consideration always be given to every alternative?	The list of alternatives could be quite lengthy, so limit the list to the top five options for serious consideration.

3. Is there always time to gather all the information about alternatives and consequences and then to think about them one at a time? *Is there ever enough time?*

Using intellect, intuition, and reasoning to make decisions means quickly recognizing significant cues that form patterns and choosing a plan of action based on past experiences. Experienced nurses will recognize more patterns and possess a greater wealth of knowledge, enabling them to come to decisions more quickly. Regardless of experience, all nurses cycle through alternatives until they find an appropriate one based on the past experience, knowledge, and skills of the nurse. At this point, the nurse mentally rehearses the choice and, if the alternative looks like it will work, selects a course of action (Decision Making Confidence, 2013). By making these critical decisions, nurses improve their decision-making skills and gain experience.

Problem Solving

Problem solving is the norm rather than the exception for routine nursing responsibilities today. Nurses learn to be skilled at problem solving to overcome obstacles to maintaining a flow of care for clients and a manageable rhythm in their workday. Sometimes clients are scheduled to be in two places at one time for various diagnostic tests, or perhaps a client received the wrong diet tray and needs another meal tray, or a client needs some medication that has not arrived from the pharmacy department yet. Sometimes the problem itself is the number of problems that must be addressed in a short amount of time. Because clients are complex, sometimes problems are more complex and not always an easy "fix." Some problems may occur repeatedly—for example, the nurse may realize that the pharmacy has been late delivering medications over several days. Nurses must be alert to problems that recur and (new problem) find the time to step in and correct the cycle (see the module on Quality Improvement for more information).

When problems arise, nurses use decision making as part of the problem-solving process. In problem solving, the nurse obtains information that clarifies the nature of the problem and identifies possible solutions. The nurse then carefully evaluates the possible solutions and chooses the best one to implement, after which she monitors the situation over time to ensure the initial and continued effectiveness of the solution. The other possible solutions are held in reserve in the event that the first solution is not effective. The nurse may also encounter a similar problem in a different client situation where another solution is found to be the most effective. Therefore, problem solving for one situation contributes to the nurse's body of knowledge for problem solving in similar situations. Commonly used approaches to problem solving include the nursing process, trial and error, intuition, and the scientific method.

THE NURSING PROCESS   The nursing process includes five phases that organize the problem-solving process (see the exemplar on the Nursing Process within this module for more information). Nurses make clinical decisions during every phase of the nursing process using critical thinking. Experienced nurses also use their experiences, knowledge, skills, and current nursing research evidence to make decisions. As nursing students' knowledge, skills, and attitudes progress, they will be able to make better decisions faster using the nursing process as a decision-making tool. Here are the five phases of the nursing process as they related to problem solving:

1. **Assessment:** *gathering information to determine what the problem is*

   For example, the nurse admits a 4-year-old client, Tommy Gates, who is suspected of having asthma. The client has a history of frequent colds and has an allergy to grasses. His dad smokes three packs of cigarettes a day. Tommy's mother tells the nurse that Tommy has been playing with the neighbor's cats for the past few days. The nurse determines it is important to assess Tommy for shortness of breath, respiratory effort, use of accessory muscles, lung sounds, vital signs, oxygen saturation, and the results of lab/x-ray studies including the complete blood count (CBC) and the chest x-ray. With the help of Tommy's mother, the nurse collects other data that may be relevant, such as the client's past medical history, developmental behaviors, and activity level.

2. **Nursing Diagnosis:** *stating the specific problem to solve*
   Based on the assessment data obtained, the nurse caring for Tommy determines his main complaint is difficulty in breathing secondary to airway obstruction. The obstruction is caused by both narrowing of airways and increased mucus production, evidenced by audible wheezing and adventitious lung sounds. The client is anxious secondary to his shortness of breath and being in a strange environment. The client has an elevated white blood count (WBC) and an increased respiratory rate. The nurse must decide which of these symptoms are top priorities for nursing care.

3. **Planning:** *stating how to know when the problem is resolved*
   During the planning phase, the nurse caring for Tommy decides that an important priority would be to monitor his wheezing, which indicates patency of airways. The goal might be "Tommy's lung sounds will be clear bilaterally."

4. **Implementation:** *giving solutions to resolve the problem*
   Interventions to help Tommy meet his goal might be:
   - Assessment of lung sounds every 4 hours
   - Maintain supplemental oxygen via nasal cannula as ordered by physician
   - Encourage PO fluids.

5. **Evaluation:** *evaluating if the problem has been resolved*
   For example, nursing staff has documented "For the past 12 hours, Tommy's lung sounds have been free from wheezes and are now clear."

TRIAL AND ERROR   One way to solve problems is through trial and error—trying out a solution, seeing if it works and, if it does not, reflecting on why and making another, different attempt. Trial and error is an option only when time and safety allow multiple opportunities to select the correct solution. This problem-solving process is not an option when making an error may result in harm to the client. Trial and error may be more useful in situations related to client comfort or preference. Two examples are when determining how far to raise the head of the bed for the client to be comfortable enough to eat or trying different methods to communicate with a client who has a hearing impairment. The trial-and-error process is primarily used to solve problems, not to find out why the problem was solved. It may not result in the best solution, but it may reveal a workable solution. The use of trial and error requires creativity and patience, two qualities essential to nursing.

INTUITION As discussed earlier, intuition is an aspect of critical thinking. It is also relevant to problem solving. With practice, solving problems using rules and early intentional thinking processes transforms into the ability to use thinking processes, knowledge, and intuition almost unconsciously.

THE SCIENTIFIC METHOD The scientific method of problem solving is a formalized, logical, systematic approach that is most successful when working in a controlled situation. Health professionals, often working with individuals in uncontrolled situations, require a modified approach to the scientific method for solving problems. For example, unlike experiments with animals, the effects of diet on health are complicated by a client's genetic variations, lifestyle, and personal preferences.

Many aspects of nursing practice involve clinical decision making. Any time a client's condition changes, those caring for the client must decide how to respond. Decisions are usually made by problem solving or by choosing among alternatives. Some actions are performed routinely, such as measuring vital signs at the beginning of the shift or introducing oneself when meeting a new client. Other actions require careful consideration, critical thinking, problem solving, and decision making in order to provide the highest quality nursing care and assure the safety of clients and staff. See the following Case Study for an example of clinical decision making.

CASE STUDY \\ A

Anna Nadine, 64 years old, is admitted to the medical unit at a local healthcare facility with a medical diagnosis of pulmonary edema secondary to left-sided heart failure. Ms. Nadine has a history of type 2 diabetes requiring insulin injections, hypertension, and early stage chronic renal failure. She is married, has no children, and lives with her husband in a high-rise apartment building that has a functioning elevator. Initial vital signs are T_O 99.2°F; P 90 bpm; R 24/min; and BP 136/86 mmHg. Oxygen saturation (O_2 Sat) is 91% on room air. Ms. Nadine is 5'2" and weighs 168 pounds. She has the following physician orders:

- Vital signs including oxygen saturation every 1 hour × 3, then every 2 hours × 3, then every 4 hours
- Give oxygen at 2 LPM via nasal cannula
- Chest x-ray
- Electrocardiogram (ECG)
- Lab work: CBC with differential, electrolytes, urinalysis (voided)
- ABGs on oxygen
- Daily weights
- No-added-salt regular diet

- Accu-Chek before meals and at bedtime, with sliding scale—cover with regular insulin
  Less than 200 = 0 coverage
  201–250 = 2 units subcutaneous injection
  251–300 = 4 units subcutaneous injection
  301–350 = 6 units subcutaneous injection
  351–400 = 8 units subcutaneous injection
  401 and higher = 10 units subcutaneous injection and call physician
- Activity—up to chair with assistance
- Intake and output every 12 hours
- D_5 ½ NS with 10 mEq potassium chloride (KCl) at 50 mL/hr
- Lasix 40 mg IV STAT, then Lasix 20 mg PO daily (am)
- Digoxin 0.125 mg PO daily (am)
- Clonidine 0.1 mg PO BID.

Within 12 hours of admission, Ms. Nadine's weight is 160 pounds, and she is breathing more comfortably with breath sounds mostly clear with some fine crackles in the bases. Vital signs are T_O 99.2°F, P 78 bpm, R 18/min, BP 118/80 mmHg, O_2 Sat is 97% on 2 LPM via nasal cannula.

The next day when you return to the unit and are again assigned to her care, you receive report from the previous shift that Ms. Nadine has been confused and disoriented for the past 2 hours. Her blood sugar when last checked 30 minutes ago was within normal limits; her husband has been notified and plans to come in and sit with her today, but he has not yet arrived.

Critical Thinking Questions

1. What assessment information do you need to obtain?
2. What are the top three priority nursing actions for Ms. Nadine at this time?
3. What factors could be contributing to Ms. Nadine's confusion?
4. How important is it to gather additional assessment data prior to implementing any interventions for Ms. Nadine?
5. What discussion might you want to have with Mr. Nadine when he arrives?
6. Use critical thinking, to determine what physician orders you would anticipate receiving for Ms. Nadine.

▶ CLINICAL JUDGMENT

The end product of the complex process that is clinical decision making is **clinical judgment**, the nurse's determination and provision of appropriate care to the client. In other words, clinical judgment combines critical thinking abilities, evaluative decision making, and nursing experience to determine appropriate responses to a client's complex and often layered situation to achieve the best client outcomes (Carrick & Miehl, 2009). Clinical judgment can be used in emergency situations and also for long-term planning of care.

This dynamic cognitive process brings all the elements of critical thinking and clinical decision making together in making clinical judgments about client care through the application of nursing knowledge, skills, and attitudes. New nurses may find this skill difficult and slow to use, whereas experienced nurses will be faster and able to additionally use their intuition for clinical judgment. The National League for Nursing (2013) has listed nursing judgment as a competency for graduates of programs in nursing. The National Council of State Boards of Nursing (2011) has models available for states to use in revising their scopes of nursing practice that relate to the accountability for clinical judgments. According to NANDA International (2011), a nursing diagnosis is a clinical judgment about an individual's or family's situation or response to a health concern or life process. Three nurse researchers have given the nursing profession important clinical research evidence related to clinical judgment: Patricia Benner, whose skill acquisition model describes five levels of clinical competence; Christine Tanner, whose clinical judgment model supports "thinking like a nurse"; and Kathie Lasater, who uses a clinical judgment rubric.

Benner's Skill Acquisition Model

The ability to make clinical judgments improves as nurses gain experience and build on their critical thinking and decision-making skills. A study comparing the performance of senior nursing students, new nurses, and experienced nurses was done over a 3-year period of time in the late 1970s. The results of this study demonstrated distinct differences in clinical performance at these varying levels of nursing education and nursing experience (Benner, Tanner, & Chesla, 2009). Benner adapted her findings to the Dreyfus Model of Skill Acquisition, organizing the evidence from the study into five levels of proficiency a nurse will progress through as she gains additional clinical experience (Benner, 2011). These levels are novice, advanced beginner, competent, proficient, and expert (see **Figure 36–3 ●**).

The different levels of competence reflect four progressive changes in thinking processes:

1. Moving from not having nursing experiences to relate to, to having concrete clinical experiences to relate to new situations requiring critical thinking
2. Progressing from following steps in a specific sequential order to being able to customize and adapt actions using nursing experience and intuition
3. Moving from taking in many significant cues and trying to make sense of all of them to identifying significant cues and clustering them to form patterns
4. Progressing from being a bystander watching to being an actively involved participant.

Each level builds on the previous level as critical thinking skills are mastered and decision making becomes routine for the nurse. Experience further expands this process as the nurse gains confidence in nursing practice.

Tanner's Clinical Judgment Model

Clinical judgment does not always include standard decision making or require all the skills of critical thinking. Tanner's "thinking like a nurse" approach in her clinical judgment model emphasizes the importance of elements the nurse uses in cognitive processing: different types of knowledge (e.g., textbook,

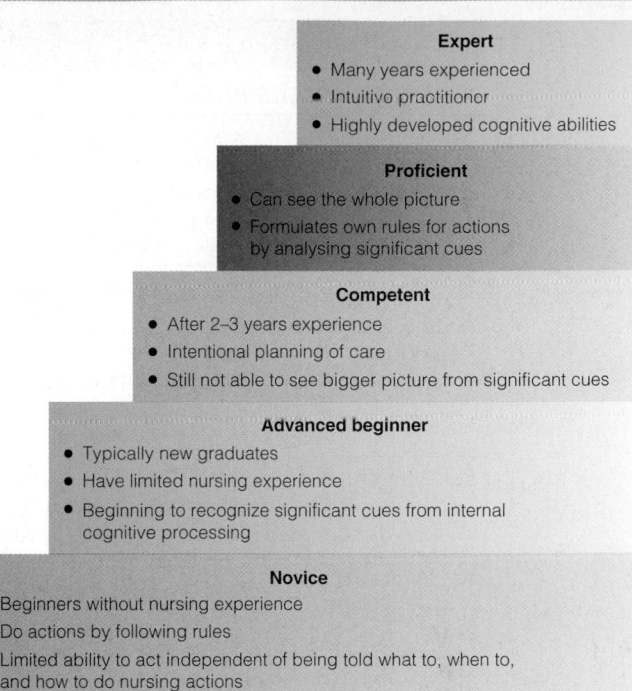

Figure 36–3 ● Benner's five levels of clinical competence from nursing student to graduate to professional.

transferred, on-the-job, abstract), length of nursing experience, values, morals regarding right and wrong, intuition, and knowing the client (i.e., being familiar with expected patterns of responses to a medical condition or knowing the individual client) (Tanner, 2006). Another element that influences clinical judgment is the culture of the work environment, which includes group norms and expectations of work routines. The Tanner model includes four features: noticing, interpreting, responding, and reflecting (**Table 36–1 ●**).

Expectations of performance in nursing programs where fundamental nursing knowledge, skills, and attitudes are taught promote the development of good nursing habits. Engaging students in clinical reasoning supports later use of clinical judgment for complex client situations, promoting nurses' abilities to assess client responses to illness. Helping students learn how to develop knowledge of their clients to care for them responsibly will help these students develop a sense about client situations in which they will need to intervene. Reflecting on clinical situations and learning from them helps students build experiences they can use for future reference. In other words, "thinking like a nurse" begins with learning as a nursing student (Tanner, 2006). See **Figure 36–4 ●** for a diagram of these sequential cognitive steps.

Lasater's Clinical Judgment Rubric

Lasater's clinical judgment rubric was developed to measure and evaluate clinical judgment using simulation (Carrick & Miehl, 2009). This rubric is based on Tanner's clinical judgment model (see Figure 36–4). The rubric serves as a guide for learners to know the specific characteristics to reach quality levels of clinical

TABLE 36–4 Features of the Tanner Clinical Judgment Model

FEATURE	DESCRIPTION
Noticing	▪ Having a sense about what is happening in the client situation ▪ May include recognition of or absence of expected significant cues from the client's response to illness or medical condition ▪ Includes influences of the nurse's own health beliefs about client situations and expectations of the work culture for client care
Interpreting	▪ Using logical reasoning to gain understanding about a situation and determine appropriate actions
Responding	▪ Includes analyzing a situation and choosing the best course of action ▪ Includes intuitive "knowing" from past similar experiences ▪ Includes using past similar experiences to "make sense" of a present clinical situation ▪ Includes responsive actions by the nurse
Reflecting	▪ Cognitively reviewing a clinical situation ▪ Considering appropriateness of assessment data obtained in the situation, actions taken, and positive and negative outcomes for client ▪ Making mental response adjustments to be done in future similar situations ▪ Learning from actions (done or not done)

Sources: Data from Mann, J. (2010). *Promoting curriculum choices: Critical thinking and clinical judgment skill development in baccalaureate nursing students.* Retrieved from http://kuscholarworks.ku.edu/dspace/handle/1808/6742; Tanner, C. (2006). Thinking like a nurse: A research-based model of clinical judgment in nursing. *Journal of Nursing Education, 45*(6), 204–210. Retrieved from http://jxzy.smu.edu.cn/jkpg/UploadFiles/file/TF_0692810354_thinking%20like%20a%20nurse.pdf.

judgment performance (**Figure 36–5** ●). It has been used successfully while observing learners in a simulation environment.

The rubric uses the four aspects of the Tanner model: noticing, interpreting, responding, and reflecting. Lasater developed additional dimensions for each of these aspects to describe associated behaviors and actions for each (Figure 36–5, the vertical axis). For example, prioritizing data is an essential behavior of *interpreting* information. Lasater proposes measuring these along four levels of clinical judgment performance listed in a progressive developmental order: beginning, developing, accomplished, and exemplary (Figure 36–5, the horizontal axis). The table is completed with descriptors given for each performance level and behavior

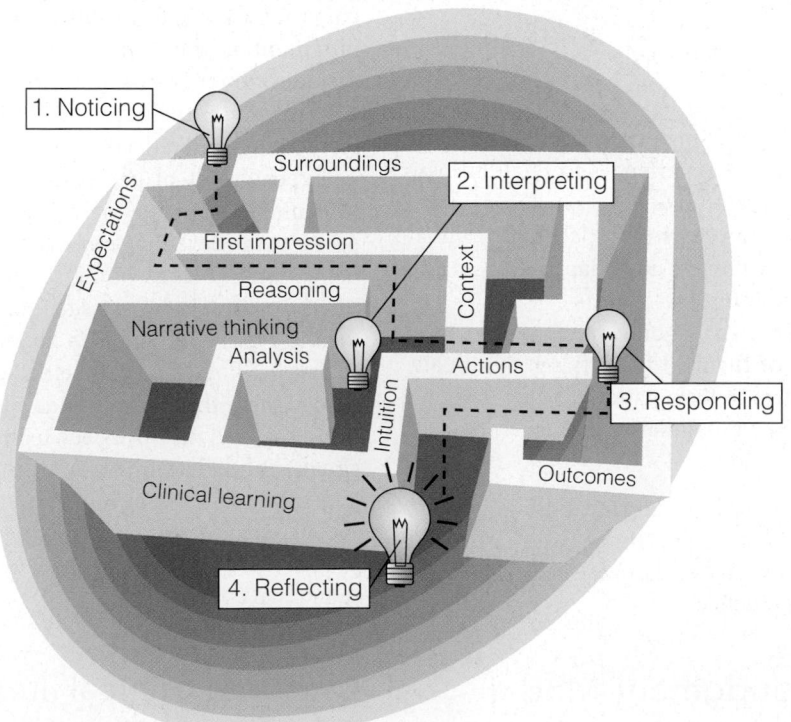

Figure 36–4 ● Tanner's clinical judgment model includes four major sequential cognitive steps: (1) noticing, (2) interpreting, (3) responding, and (4) reflecting.

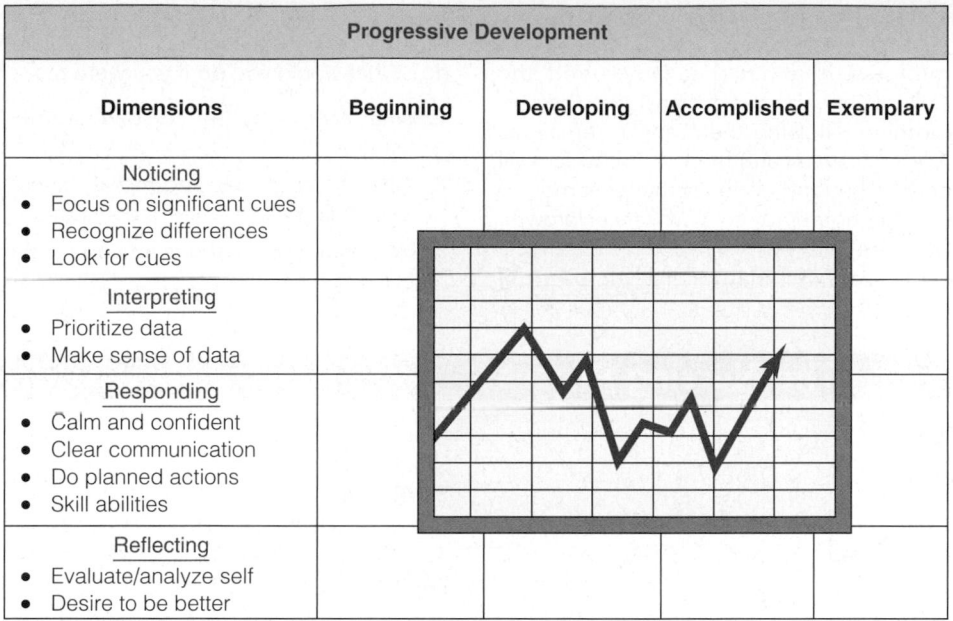

Progressive Development				
Dimensions	**Beginning**	**Developing**	**Accomplished**	**Exemplary**
Noticing • Focus on significant cues • Recognize differences • Look for cues				
Interpreting • Prioritize data • Make sense of data				
Responding • Calm and confident • Clear communication • Do planned actions • Skill abilities				
Reflecting • Evaluate/analyze self • Desire to be better				

Figure 36–5 ● Lasater used the dimensions from Tanner's clinical judgment model and created developmental levels of clinical judgment for her rubric.

dimension. Students can use the rubric to measure their progress in using clinical judgment. The rubric clearly defines characteristics for clinical judgment levels and dimensions (Mann, 2010).

▶ SUMMARY

Clinical decision making is a complex process in which nurses observe and gather data, interpret that data through the use of salient cues and identification of patterns that provide critical information; analyze cues and patterns to determine priority client needs; and begin to evaluate alternatives to provide appropriate interventions to support best outcomes for clients. The nursing process is the professional process by which nurses engage in clinical decision making and reach clinical judgments regarding client care. The nursing process and its companion plan of care, which is a way of documenting client assessment data and care provided, are discussed in the exemplars that follow.

◤ REVIEW The Concept of Clinical Decision Making

RELATE Link the Concepts

Linking the concept of clinical decision making with the concept of legal issues:

1. What legal actions may occur if the nurse fails to make prudent clinical decisions? Explain your answer.

2. What role regarding sound clinical decision making in client care is expected of the licensed nurse?

3. What role regarding sound clinical decision making in the workplace does the employer expect of the nurse?

Linking the concept of clinical decision making with the concept of evidence-based practice:

4. The nurse with strong critical thinking maintains an evidenced-based practice by _____.

5. A nurse reads a peer-reviewed article that recommends changing currently accepted practice. What critical thinking will the nurse perform before accepting the article's recommendations?

Linking the concept of clinical decision making with the concept of ethics:

6. What ethical obligation does the nurse hold toward the client related to clinical decision making?

7. What ethical obligation does the nurse hold toward the hiring facility related to clinical decision making?

REFER Go to Pearson Nursing Student Resources
nursing.pearsonhighered.com

• Additional review materials

REFLECT Case Study

The nurse is caring for a client who was admitted 3 days ago with acute abdominal pain. Following extensive diagnostic testing, the client has received a medical diagnosis of stomach cancer with suspected metastasis to the liver and pancreas. The oncologist has informed the client that there are several options related to treatment. Option 1 is to surgically remove as much of the tumor as possible followed by chemotherapy and radiation therapy. This is the most aggressive approach with the best odds for survival, but the oncologist tells the client that with the amount of metastasis that has already occurred, the odds for survival are still not very good (less than 10%). The second option is to do nothing, allowing the client to remain as comfortable as possible (palliative care) until death, which will likely occur in 3–6 months. The third option is the most moderate option and involves chemotherapy to slow cancer growth, which may prolong the client's life but will result in side effects (e.g., hair loss, vomiting, weakness) that will likely impact the client's quality of life. After the oncologist leaves the room, the client looks to the nurse and asks, "What do you think I should do? What would you do if you were me?"

1. What actions by the nurse would be most appropriate for this client?
2. What ethical, legal, and moral duties guide the nurse when responding to this client's questions?
3. How would you respond to each of the client's questions?

EXEMPLAR 36.1 The Nursing Process

EXEMPLAR KEY TERMS
Actual diagnosis, 2335
Assessment, 2331
Cognitive skills, 2348
Collaborative intervention, 2345
Defining characteristics, 2336
Dependent intervention, 2345
Diagnostic label, 2335
Etiology, 2336
Evaluation, 2349
Evaluation statement, 2350
Goal, 2341
Health promotion diagnosis, 2335
Implementation, 2344
Independent intervention, 2345
Interpersonal skills, 2348
NANDA, 2334
Nursing diagnosis, 2334
Nursing process, 2328
Planning, 2341
Outcome, 2341
Qualifiers, 2336

Risk nursing diagnosis, 2335
Risk factors, 2335
SMART, 2342
Syndrome diagnosis, 2335
Technical skills, 2348
Wellness diagnosis, 2335

EXEMPLAR LEARNING OUTCOMES
After reading about this exemplar, you will be able to:

1. Describe the five phases in the nursing process.
2. Examine the relationships among the phases of the nursing process.
3. Organize assessment cues that are relative to each other into a pattern.
4. Formulate nursing diagnosis statements appropriate to the client's priority needs.
5. Plan nursing care to include priorities of care, client goals, and selection of priority nursing interventions.
6. Revise the nursing plan of care based on evaluation of client response.

▶ OVERVIEW

The **nursing process** is used to identify a client's health status and actual or potential healthcare problems or needs, to establish plans to meet the identified needs, to deliver specific nursing interventions to meet those needs, and to evaluate the success of those interventions. The client may be an individual, a family, or a group. The use of the nursing process in clinical practice gained additional legitimacy in 1973 when the phases of the nursing process were included in the American Nurses Association (ANA) *Standards of Nursing Practice*. The standards of practice within the most current *Scope and Standards of Nursing Practice* include the five phases of the nursing process: assessment, diagnosis, planning, implementation, and evaluation (ANA, 2004). Virtually every state has since revised its nursing practice acts to reflect the nursing process. See **Figure 36–6** ● for an illustration of the nursing process.

A few general characteristics of the nursing process complement its ease to organize the flow of nursing care and individualize it for all clients across the life span. The nursing process is a *dynamic* rather than static plan that can adapt to the changes in the client. The nursing process is

client centered. The nurse organizes the plan of care according to client needs to achieve a goal. In the assessment phase, the nurse collects data to determine client preferences in daily routines and meeting personal needs to incorporate these into the plan of care as appropriate. The nursing process is an *adaptation of problem solving used by others* involved with client care. For example, physicians use the medical model, which focuses on physiological systems and the disease process, whereas the nursing process is directed toward a client's responses to the disease process and to interventions and therapies that attempt to interrupt that process and restore the client to health. *Decision making* is involved in every phase of the nursing process. Nurses can be highly creative in determining what decisions to make to facilitate the individualization of the client's plan of care. The nursing process also is interpersonal and *collaborative*. It requires the nurse to communicate directly and consistently with clients and families to meet their needs. It also requires that nurses collaborate with other members of the healthcare team in a joint effort to provide quality client care. The universally applicable characteristics of the nursing process mean that it is used as a framework for nursing

THE NURSING PROCESS IN ACTION

The nursing process is a systematic, rational method of planning and providing nursing care. Its purpose is to identify a client's health care status, and actual or potential health problems, to establish plans to meet the identified needs, and to deliver specific nursing interventions to address those needs. The nursing process is cyclical; that is, its components follow a logical sequence, but more than one component may be involved at one time. At the end of the first cycle, care may be terminated if goals are achieved, or the cycle may continue with reassessment, or the plan of care may be modified.

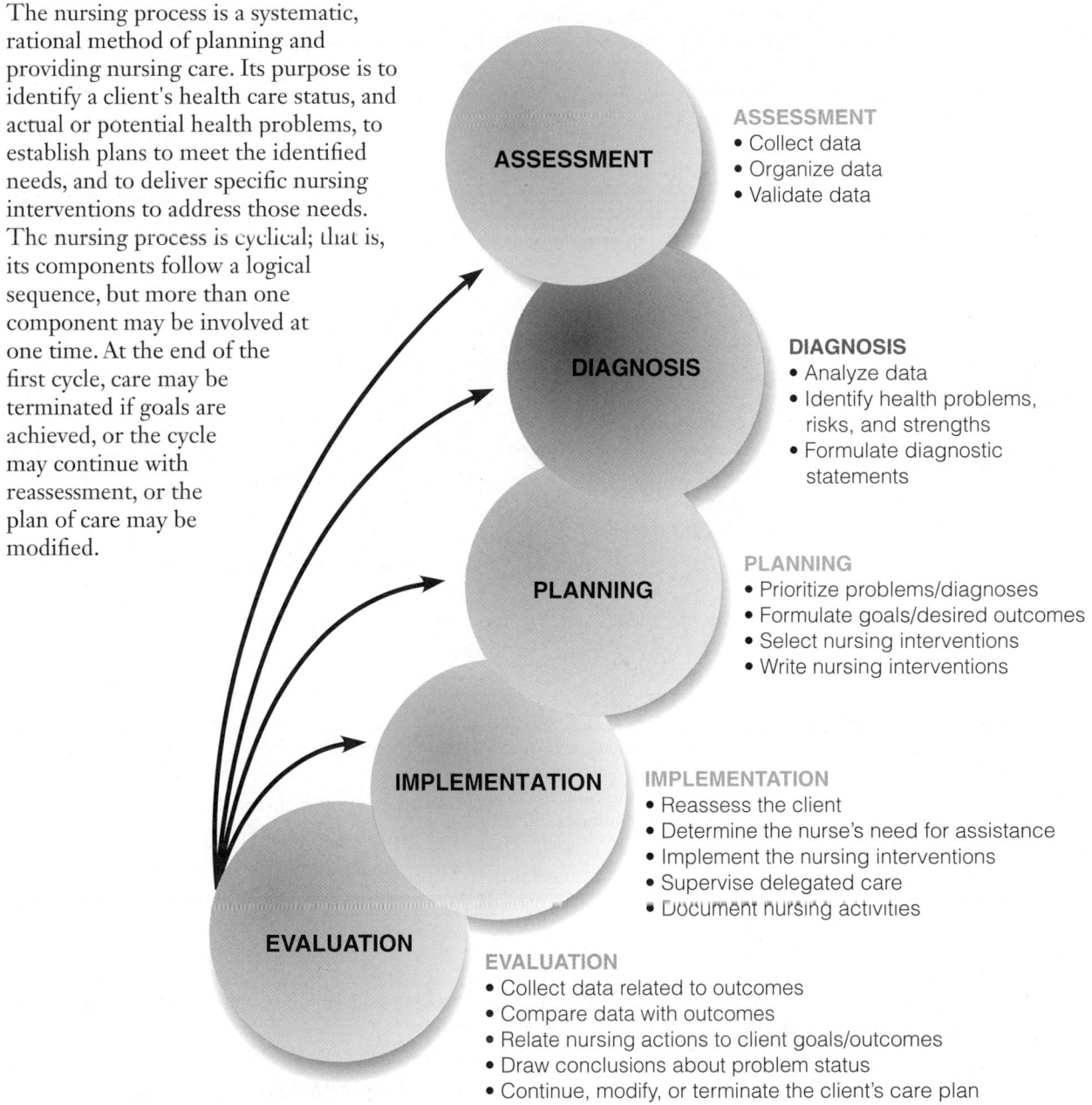

ASSESSMENT
- Collect data
- Organize data
- Validate data

DIAGNOSIS
- Analyze data
- Identify health problems, risks, and strengths
- Formulate diagnostic statements

PLANNING
- Prioritize problems/diagnoses
- Formulate goals/desired outcomes
- Select nursing interventions
- Write nursing interventions

IMPLEMENTATION
- Reassess the client
- Determine the nurse's need for assistance
- Implement the nursing interventions
- Supervise delegated care
- Document nursing activities

EVALUATION
- Collect data related to outcomes
- Compare data with outcomes
- Relate nursing actions to client goals/outcomes
- Draw conclusions about problem status
- Continue, modify, or terminate the client's care plan

Figure 36–6 ● The nursing process in action.

care in all types of healthcare settings and with clients of all age groups.

An overview of the five phases of the nursing process is given in **Table 36–5** ●. The phases of the nursing process are not separate entities—they are overlapping (see **Figure 36–7** ●). For example, assessment, which may be considered the first phase of the nursing process, is also carried out during the implementation and evaluation phases. For instance, while actually administering medications (implementation), the nurse continuously assesses the client to determine continued need for the medication, response to the medication, and appearance of potential side effects.

Each phase of the nursing process affects the others; they are closely interrelated. For example, if inadequate data are obtained during assessment, the nursing diagnoses will be incomplete or incorrect; inaccuracy will also be reflected in the planning, implementation, and evaluation phases. Because the nursing process is an organizing tool that guides the nurse's approach to client care and decision making, the process always begins with accurate data collection.

TABLE 36–5 The Phases of the Nursing Process

PHASE AND DESCRIPTION	PURPOSE	ACTIVITIES
Assessment		
Collecting, organizing, validating, and documenting client's assessment data Begin noting significant cues and how they may be clustering.	To establish a database about the client's response to health concerns or illness and the ability to manage healthcare needs.	Establish a database: ■ Obtain a nursing health history. ■ Conduct a physical assessment. ■ Review client records. ■ Speak with family members and significant support persons. ■ Speak with appropriate health professionals. Update data to keep it current.
Look for significant cue clusters and patterns.		Organize data.
Seek more assessment data to clarify cue clusters and patterns.		Validate data. Communicate/document data.
Nursing Diagnosis		
Analyzing and synthesizing data	To identify client strengths and health problems that can be prevented or resolved by collaborative and nursing interventions. To develop a list of nursing and collaborative problems.	Interpret and analyze data: ■ Compare data against standards. ■ Cluster or group data (generate tentative hypotheses). ■ Identify gaps and inconsistencies.
		Determine client's strengths, risks, diagnoses, and problems.
		Formulate diagnostic statements.
		Document priority nursing diagnoses on the nursing plan of care.
Planning		
Determining how to prevent, reduce, or resolve the identified priority client problems; how to support client strengths; and how to implement nursing interventions in an organized, individualized, and goal-directed manner	To develop an individualized plan of care that specifies client goals/desired outcomes, and related priority nursing interventions.	Set priorities and goals/outcomes in collaboration with client.
		Write goals/desired outcomes.
		Select nursing strategies/interventions.
		Consult other health professionals.
		Write nursing interventions and nursing plan of care.
		Communicate plan of care to relevant healthcare providers.
Implementation		
Carrying out (or delegating) and then documenting the planned nursing interventions	To assist the client to meet desired goals/outcomes; promote wellness; prevent illness and disease; restore health; and facilitate coping with altered functioning.	Reassess the client to update the database to keep it current.
		Determine the nurse's need for assistance.
		Perform planned priority nursing interventions.
		Communicate what nursing actions were implemented: ■ Document care and client responses to care. ■ Give verbal reports as necessary.
Evaluation		
Measuring the degree to which goals/outcomes have been achieved and identifying factors that positively or negatively influence goal achievement	To determine whether to continue, modify, or terminate the plan of care.	Collaborate with client and collect data related to desired outcomes.
		Judge whether goals/outcomes have been achieved.
		Relate nursing actions to client outcomes.
		Make decisions about problem status.
		Review and modify the plan of care as indicated or terminate it.
		Document achievement of outcomes and modification of the plan of care.

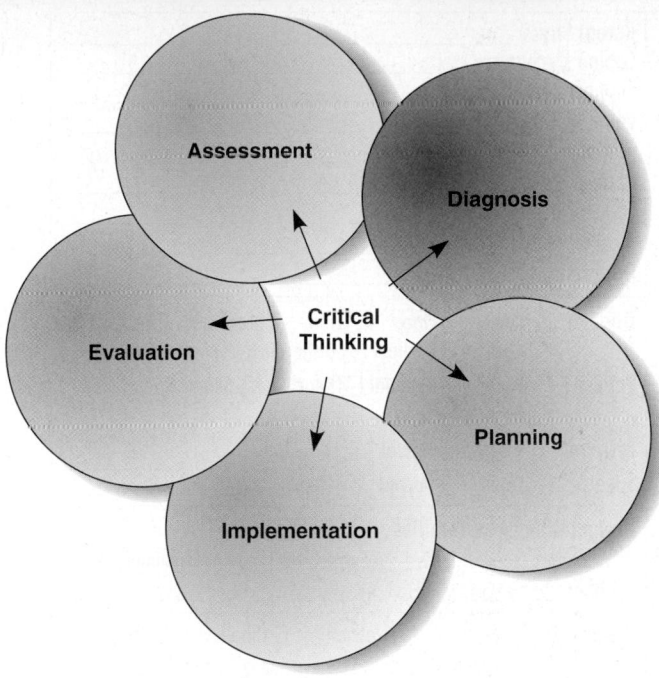

Figure 36–7 ● The five overlapping phases of the nursing process. Each phase depends on the accuracy of the other phases. Each phase involves critical thinking.

▶ ASSESSMENT

Assessment is the systematic and continuous collection of data about a client for the purpose of determining the client's current and ongoing health status, predicting the client's health risks, and identifying appropriate health-promoting activities. Assessment is a continuous process carried out during all phases of the nursing process. For example, in the evaluation phase, assessment is done to determine the outcomes of the nursing interventions and to evaluate goal achievement. All phases of the nursing process depend on the accurate and complete collection of assessment data.

A nursing assessment focuses on a client's responses to a health problem. It includes subjective data obtained from the client or family about the client's needs, health condition, health practices, values, health history, and lifestyle. It also includes objective data obtained through assessment and physical examination of the client. Using available sources of data in addition to the client who is the primary source will allow the nurse to develop a database including past medical history and also current health status (see the module on Assessment for further information).

Assessment data can be organized according to one of several models. Most nursing programs develop their own framework for nursing assessment data based on these models. One example is to use Gordon's 11 functional health patterns to organize the data by patterns (Gordon, 2010):

1. Health perception–health management pattern
2. Nutritional-metabolic pattern
3. Elimination pattern
4. Activity-exercise pattern
5. Sleep-rest pattern
6. Cognitive-perceptual pattern
7. Self-perception/self-concept pattern
8. Role-relationship pattern
9. Sexuality-reproductive pattern
10. Coping/stress-tolerance pattern
11. Value-belief pattern

Another example is Roy's adaptation model, which uses four categories of behavior: physiological, self-concept, role function, and interdependence (Roy, 2008). Using Maslow's hierarchy of needs, Roy organizes the assessment data into five categories that make it easier to prioritize client needs: physiological needs, safety and security needs, love and belonging needs, self-esteem needs, and self-actualization needs.

One last common way to organize assessment data is by body systems:

1. Immune system
2. Respiratory system
3. Cardiovascular system
4. Nervous system
5. Musculoskeletal system
6. Gastrointestinal system
7. Genitourinary system
8. Reproductive system

Figure 36–8 ● provides an example of how data might be organized according to a systems assessment or complete assessment (using the case study featuring Amanda Aquilini).

After data has been collected, it is validated (see the module on Assessment) and analyzed. Analyzing involves three steps:

1. Comparing data against standards (to identify significant cues)
2. Clustering cues (generate tentative hypotheses)
3. Identifying gaps and inconsistencies.

With experienced nurses, these activities occur continuously rather than sequentially and the collected data clusters around one specific health problem. Therefore, nurses should think critically about what to assess.

When gathering and clustering assessment data for children, the nurse will need to include the parents as a major source of subjective data as well as asking the child himself about how he feels. Assessment of the family's needs related to the child's illness (e.g., does lack of insurance present a barrier to accessing services or paying for prescriptions?) is also necessary. See the Lifespan Considerations feature.

CASE STUDY \\ ASSESSMENT

Amanda Aquilini, a 28-year-old married attorney with one child, was admitted to the medical unit of the local hospital with a medical diagnosis of pneumonia throughout her right lung. She has been assigned to Nurse Mary Medina, RN. After Mrs. Aquilini is oriented to her room by the UAP, Nurse Medina does her admission assessment (see **Figure 36–9 ●**).

During the interview, Nurse Medina learns that Mrs. Aquilini has had a "chest cold" for 2 weeks, and has been experiencing shortness of breath when she tries to cook dinner or clean the house. Even putting her child to bed makes her short of breath. Mrs. Aquilini

ADMISSION DATA

Date 4-16-07 Time 3:15p.m Primary Language __English__

Arrived Via: ☐ Wheelchair ☐ Stretcher ☑ Ambulatory

From: ☐ Admitting ☐ ER ☑ Home ☐ Nursing Home ☐ Other

Admitting M.D. __R. Katz__ Time Notified __5 p.m.__

ORIENTATION TO UNIT

	YES	NO		YES	NO
Arm Band Correct	☒	☐	Visiting Hours	☒	☐
Allergy Band	☒	☐	Smoking Policy	☒	☐
Telephone	☒	☐	TV, Lights, Bed Controls,		
Electrical Policy	☒	☐	Call Lights, Side Rails	☒	☐
Educational Material	☒	☐	Nurses Station	☒	☐
(TV Brochure)	☒	☐			

Family M.D. __R. Katz__

Weight __125 lb.__ Height __5ft. 2in.__ BP:R — L __122/80__

Temp. __103F__ Pulse __92, weak__ Resp __28, shallow__

Source Providing Information ☑ Patient ☐ Other_____

Unable to Obtain History ☐ _____

Reason for Admission (Onset, Duration, Pt.'s Perception) ("Chest cold" X2 weeks S.O.B on exertion. "Lung pain, fever," "Dr. says I have pneumonia.")☐

ALLERGIES & REACTIONS

Drugs __Penicillin__

Food/Other_____

Signs & Symptoms __rash, nausea__

Blood Reaction ☐ Yes ☑ No Dyes/Shellfish ☐ Yes ☑ No

MEDICATIONS

Current Meds	Dose/Freq.	Last Dose
Synthroid	0.1 mg. daily	4-16, 8 a.m.

Disposition of Meds: ☒ Home ☐ Pharmacy ☐ Safe *At Bedside

MEDICAL HISTORY

☑ No Major Problems ☐ Gastro_____
☐ Cardiac_____ ☐ Arthritis_____
☐ Hyper/Hypotension_____ ☐ Stroke_____
☐ Diabetes_____ ☐ Seizures_____
☐ Cancer_____ ☐ Glaucoma_____
☐ Respiratory_____ ☑ Other Childbirth-2000

Surgery/Procedures	Date
Appendectomy	1985
Partial thyroidectomy	2000

SPECIAL ASSISTIVE DEVICES

☐ Wheelchair ☐ Contacts ☐ Venous ☐ Dentures
☐ Braces ☐ Hearing Aid Access ☐ Partial
☐ Cane/Crutches ☐ Prosthesis Device ☐ Upper
☐ Walker ☐ Glasses ☐ Epidural Catheter ☐ Lower
☐ Other __None__

VALUABLES

Patient informed Hospital not responsible for personal belongings.
Valuables Disposition: ☐ Patient ☐ Safe ☐ Given to_____
Patient/SO Signature __None__

PSYCHOSOCIAL HISTORY

Recent Stress __None__
Coping Mechanism __Not assessed because of fatigue__
Support System __Husband, coworkers, friends__
Calm: ☑ Yes ☐ No
Anxious: ☐ Yes ☐ No __Facial muscles tense; trembling__
Religion __Catholic. Would want Last Rites__
Tobacco Use: ☐ Yes ☑ No _____
Alcohol Use: ☐ Yes ☑ No _____
Drug Use: ☐ Yes ☑ No _____

NEUROLOGICAL

Oriented: ☑ Person ☑ Place ☑ Time ☐ Confused ☐ Sedated
☐ Alert ☐ Restless ☑ Lethargic ☐ Comatose
Pupils: ☑ Equal ☐ Unequal ☑ Reactive ☐ Sluggish
☐ Other 3mm.
Extremity Strength: ☑ Equal ☐ Unequal
Speech: ☑ Clear ☐ Slurred ☐ Other_____

MUSCULO-SKELETAL

Normal ROM of Extremities ☑ Yes ☐ No
☑ Weakness ☐ Paralysis ☐ Contractures ☐ Joint Swelling ☑ Pain
☐ Other ↓ related to fatigue   when coughing

RESPIRATORY

Pattern: ☐ Even ☐ Uneven ☑ Shallow ☑ Dyspnea
☑ Other __diminished breath sounds__
Breathing Sounds: ☐ Clear ☑ Other __inspiratory crackles__
Secretions: ☐ None ☑ Other __pink, thick sputum__
Cough: ☐ None ☑ Productive ☐ Nonproductive

CARDIOVASCULAR

Pulses: Apical Rate __92-W__ ☑ Reg. ☐ Irregular ☐ Pacemaker
S = Strong W = Weak A = Absent D = Doppler
Radial R __92__ L __—__ Pedal R __—__ L __—__
Edema: ☑ Absent ☐ Present Site_____
Perfusion: ☐ Warm ☐ Dry ☑ Diaphoretic ☐ Cool (Hot)

GASTROINTESTINAL

Oral Mucosa ☐ Normal ☑ Other __pale and dry__
Bowel Sounds: ☑ Normal ☐ Other __Abd. soft__
Wt. Change: ☐ ☑ N/V Stool Frequency/Character __1/day;soft__
Last B/M __4-15-07__ ☐ Ostomy (type)_____
Equip._____

GENITOURINARY

Urine: Last Voided __This morning__
☐ Normal ☐ Anuria ☐ Hematuria ☐ Dysuri ☐ Incontinent
☒ Other __↓ amount & frequency since ill__
☐ Catheter (type)_____ Other_____
LMP __4-1-07__ ☐ Vaginal/Penile Discharge
Other_____

SELF CARE

Need Assist with: ☐ Ambulating ☐ Elimination
☐ Meals ☒ Hygiene ☐ Dressing
__While fatigued__

Amanda Aquilini [F. age 28]
#4637651

Figure 36–8 ● Assessment for Amanda Aquilini.

NUTRITION

General Appearance: ☑ Well Nourished ☐ Emaciated
☐ Other
Appetite: ☐ Good ☐ Fair ☑ Poor –×2 days
Diet _Liquid_ Meal Pattern _3/day_
☐ Feeds Self ☐ Assist ☐ Total Feed

SKIN ASSESSMENT

Color: ☐ Normal ☐ Flushed ☑ Pale ☐ Dusky ☐ Cyanotic
☐ Jaundiced ☑ Other _Cheeks flushed, hot_
General Description _Surgical scars:_
RLQ abdomen; anterior neck

Note Cultures Obtained _____

PRESSURE SORE ™AT RISK SCREENING CRITERIA

OVERALL SKIN CONDITION
Grade
☐ 0 Turgor (elasticity adequate, skin warm and moist)
☑ 1 Poor turgor, skin cold & dry
☐ 2 Areas mottled, red or denuded
☐ 3 Existing skin ulcer/lesions

BOWEL AND BLADDER CONTROL
Grade
☑ 0 Always able to ask for bedpan
☐ 1 Incontinence of urine
☐ 2 Incontinence of feces
☐ 3 Totally incontinent Confined to bed

REHABILITATIVE STATE
Grade
☐ 0 Fully ambulatory
☑ 1 Ambulated with assistance
☐ 2 Chair to bed ambulation only
☐ 3 Confined to bed
☐ 4 Immobile in bed

NUTRITIONAL STATE
Grade
☐ 0 Eats all
☑ 1 Eats very little
☐ 2 Refuses food often
☐ 3 Tube feeding
☐ 4 Intravenous feeding

MENTAL STATE
Grade
☑ 0 Alert and clear
☐ 1 Confused
☐ 2 Disoriented/senile
☐ 3 Stuporous
☐ 4 Unconcious

CHRONIC DISEASE STATUS
(i.e. COPD, ASCVD, Peripheral Vascular Disease, Diabetes, or Renal Disease, Cancer, Motor or Sensory Deficits, Elderly, Other)
Grade
☑ 0 Absent
☐ 1 One Present
☐ 2 Two Present
☐ 3 Three or more Present

TOTAL _____ Refer to Skin Care Protocol

FALLS SCREENING

If one or more of the following are checked institute fall precautions/plan of care
☐ History of Falls ☐ Unsteady Gait ☐ Confusion/Disorientation ☐ Dizziness
If two or more of the following are checked institute fall precautions/plan of care
☐ Age over 80 ☐ Utilizes cane, walker, w/c ☐ Sleeplessness
☐ Impaired vision ☐ Urgency/frequency in elimination
☐ Multiple Diagnoses ☐ Impaired hearing ☐ Medication/Sedative /Diuretic etc.
☐ Inability to understand or follow directions

NURSE SIGNATURE/TITLE | DATE | TIME
Mary Medina, RN | _4-16-07_ | _3:30pm_
NURSE SIGNATURE/TITLE | DATE | TIME

EDUCATION/DISCHARGE PLANNING

1. What do you know about your present illness? _"Dr. says I have pneumonia." "I will have an I.V."_
2. What information do you want or need about your illness? _____
3. Would you like family/SO involved in your care? _Husband, Michael_
4. How long do you expect to be in the hospital? _"1-2 days"_
5. What concerns do you have about leaving the hospital? _____

CHECK APPROPRIATE BOX

Will patient need post discharge assistance with ADLs/physical functioning? ☐ Yes ☑ No ☐ Unknown
Does patient have family capable of and willing to provide assistance post discharge?
☑ Yes ☐ No ☐ Unknown ☐ No family
Is assistance needed beyond that which family can provide?
☐ Yes ☑ No ☐ Unknown
Previous admission in the last six months?
☐ Yes ☑ No ☐ Unknown
Patient lives with _Husband and 1 child_
Planned discharge to _Home_
Comments: _Fatigue and anxiety may have interfered with learning. Re-teach anything covered at admission, later._

Social Services Notified ☐ Yes ☑ No

NARRATIVE NOTES

S--c/O sharp chest pain when coughing and dyspnea on exertion. States unable to carry out regular daily exercise for past week. Coughing relieved "if I sit up and sit still." Nausea associated with coughing. Having occasional "chills." Occasionally becomes frightened, stating, "I can't breathe." Well groomed but "too tired to put on make-up." O--Chest expansion < 3cm, no nasal flaring or use of accessory muscles. Breath sounds and insp. crackles in ℞ upper and lower chest. Assesses own supports as "good" (eg, relationship c̄ husband). Is "worried" about daughter. States husband will be out of town until tomorrow. Left 3-year-old daughter with neighbor. Concerned too about her work (is attorney). "I'll never get caught up." Had water at noon—no food today. Agrees to save urine for 24 hr. specimen. IV D₅W LR 1000 mL started in ℞ arm, 100 mL/hr. Slow capillary refill. Keeping head of bed↑ to facilitate breathing.

Figure 36–8 ● Assessment for Amanda Aquilini. (continued)

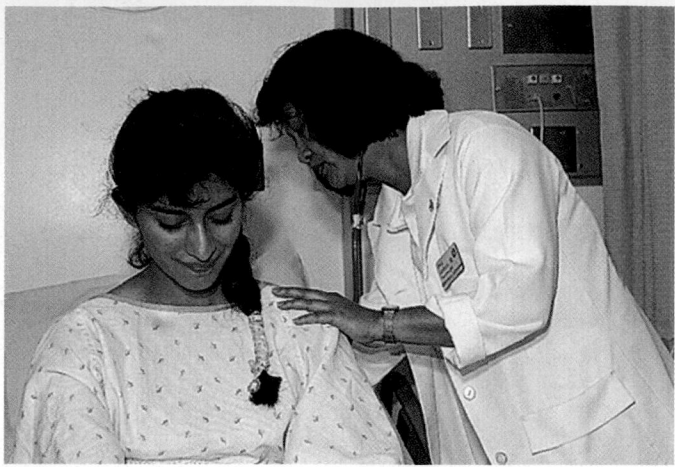

Figure 36–9 ● Assessment: Mrs. Aquilini's admission assessment reveals the following: temperature 103°F; pulse 92 bpm; respirations 28/min; and blood pressure 122/80 mmHg. Nurse Medina observes that Mrs. Aquilini's skin is dry, her cheeks are flushed, and she is experiencing chills. Auscultation reveals inspiratory crackles with diminished breath sounds in the right lung.

reports that for the past few days, she has not felt like eating very much and is only drinking a couple of glasses of tea every day. She states she has had a productive cough with a medium amount of thick, foul-smelling, pink sputum. Mrs. Aquilini tells Nurse Medina that she hasn't felt like going to work, just feels tired all the time. She states she doesn't smoke and only drinks a glass of wine occasionally. Mrs. Aquilini likes to work out in the yard or go for a walk three or four times a week but lately has not had the energy to do these things. She currently takes Synthroid 0.1 mg daily, and her last hospitalization was for the delivery of her child 3 years ago. Mrs. Aquilini states she is allergic to penicillin but not to foods, latex, or iodine.

On physical examination, Mrs. Aquilini is 5'2" tall and weighs 125 lb. Vital signs: T_O 103°F; P 92 bpm; R 28/min; blood pressure 122/80 mmHg, and oxygen saturation (O_2 Sat) 95% on room air. Nurse Medina observes that Mrs. Aquilini's skin is dry, her cheeks are flushed, and she is experiencing chills. Auscultation reveals inspiratory rhonchi with diminished breath sounds in the right lung. Respirations are shallow. Her oral mucous membranes are pale and dry and her skin turgor is >3 seconds. She speaks in short sentences. Peripheral pulses are weak and equal bilateral in all four extremities.

Clinical Reasoning Questions Level I
1. Which assessment data are salient cues?
2. Do these cues form any clusters? What are they?

Clinical Reasoning Questions Level II
3. Are there any other questions you would ask Mrs. Aquilini to further clarify her health status?
4. Which cluster of significant cues would be the priority? Why?

▶ DIAGNOSIS

In the diagnosis phase, nurses use critical thinking skills to cluster the assessment data and identify problems. Diagnosis is a pivotal step in the nursing process. Assessment activities preceding this phase are directed toward formulating a nursing diagnosis, and the care-planning activities following this phase are based on the nursing diagnosis.

Nursing diagnoses are developed and periodically updated by **NANDA** International (formerly the North American Nursing Diagnosis Association). In 1990, NANDA first adopted an official working definition of **nursing diagnosis**, which is maintained today as ". . . a clinical judgment about individual, family, or community responses to actual and potential health problems/life processes. A nursing diagnosis provides the basis for selection of nursing interventions to achieve outcomes for which the nurse is accountable" (NANDA International, 2011). This definition implies the following:

- Registered nurses are responsible for making nursing diagnoses, even though other nursing personnel may contribute data to the process of diagnosing and may implement specified nursing care. In the *Standards of Professional Nursing Practice*, Standard 2 addresses the fact that registered nurses determine the diagnoses or issues from analysis of the assessment data (Ferris State University, 2010). The Joint Commission requires evidence of nursing diagnoses in clients' medical records as well (University of North Carolina at Pembroke, 2010).

- The domains of nursing diagnoses include only those health states that nurses are educated and licensed to treat within their scope of practice (see the module on Legal Issues for further information). For example, nurses can diagnose and treat *Deficient Knowledge, Ineffective Coping,* or *Imbalanced Nutrition,* all of which are the human responses to the medical diagnosis of diabetes mellitus.

- A nursing diagnosis is a judgment made only after thorough, systematic assessment and data collection.

Lifespan Considerations Assessment of Children

Consider this example: A 4-year-old girl is admitted following emergency surgery for a ruptured appendix. She is awake and alert, but refuses to talk. Her parents have had little sleep for over 24 hours and are extremely anxious.

- Gathering assessment data in this situation requires the nurse to be sensitive to the parents' needs for rest and assurance; at the same time, the nurse must collect information to compile an adequate database that can be used to make appropriate nursing care decisions. Assessment will be problem focused, monitoring the condition of the

child as she recovers from surgery and being alert to potential problems.

- Objective data collected include vital signs; level of and response to pain (often called the fifth vital sign); bleeding or discharge from the incision; mobility; integrity of dressings, intravenous lines, catheters, nasogastric tubes, or other medical devices; and affect.

- Since children are a part of families, assessment will include observation of family dynamics and questions that could lead to care of the family system.

- Nursing diagnoses describe a continuum of health states: deviations from health, presence of risk factors, and areas of enhanced personal growth.

The current organization of nursing diagnoses is called Taxonomy II (NANDA International, 2009). Taxonomy II has three levels: domains, classes, and nursing diagnoses. The diagnoses are coded according to seven axes: diagnostic concept, time, unit of care, age, health status, descriptor, and topology. In addition, diagnoses are now listed alphabetically by concept.

Stay Current: *For more information about NANDA-approved nursing diagnoses, refer to the NANDA-I Web site (**www.nanda.org**) and see Appendix A.*

To identify nursing diagnoses effectively and then create and complete a nursing plan of care, the nurse must be familiar with:

- Common terms used with nursing diagnoses
- The difference between a nursing diagnosis and a medical diagnosis
- Types of nursing diagnoses
- Components of a nursing diagnosis.

Common Terms

A diagnosis is a statement or conclusion regarding the nature of a phenomenon. The standardized NANDA names for the nursing diagnoses are called **diagnostic labels**. The client's problem statement is called a nursing diagnosis and includes the diagnostic label plus the etiology (causal relationship between a problem and its related or risk factors). **Risk factors** are factors that cause a client to be vulnerable to developing a health problem. The term *diagnosing* refers to the reasoning process the nurse uses to formulate the nursing diagnosis.

Nursing Diagnosis Versus Medical Diagnosis

A nursing diagnosis is a statement of nursing judgment and refers to a condition that nurses, by virtue of their education, experience, and expertise, are licensed to treat. Nursing diagnoses describe the human response or a client's physical, sociocultural, psychological, and spiritual responses to an illness or a health condition. A medical diagnosis is made by a licensed provider such as a physician, advanced practice nurse, or physician assistant. Medical diagnoses refer to disease processes—specific pathophysiologic responses that are fairly uniform from one client to another. The following is a clinical example of how these responses can vary among individuals:

CLINICAL EXAMPLE

Seventy-year-old Mary Cain and 20-year-old Kristi Vidan both have rheumatoid arthritis. Their disease processes are much the same. X-ray studies show that in both clients, the extent of inflammation and the number of joints involved are similar, and both clients experience almost constant pain. Ms. Cain views her condition as part of the aging process and is responding with acceptance. Ms. Vidan, however, is responding with anger and hostility because she views her disease as a threat to her personal identity, role performance, and self-esteem.

A client's medical diagnosis remains the same for as long as the disease process is present, but nursing diagnoses change as the client's responses change. Ms. Vidan's response to her illness may change over time to become more similar to that of Ms. Cain.

Types of Nursing Diagnoses

The current types of diagnoses include actual, risk, health promotion, wellness, and syndrome:

1. An **actual diagnosis** is a client problem that is present at the time of the nursing assessment. Examples are *Ineffective Breathing Pattern*, *Acute Pain*, and *Anxiety*. An actual nursing diagnosis is based on a cluster of associated assessment data.

2. A **risk nursing diagnosis** is a clinical judgment that a problem does not exist, but the presence of risk factors indicates that a problem is likely to develop unless the nurse intervenes. For example, all hospitalized individuals have some possibility of acquiring an infection; however, a client with diabetes or a compromised immune system is at higher risk than others. Therefore, the nurse would use the *Risk for Infection* nursing diagnosis to describe the client's health status.

3. A **wellness diagnosis** "describes human responses to levels of wellness in an individual, family or community that have a readiness for enhancement" (NANDA International, 2009, p. 26). Examples of wellness nursing diagnoses include *Readiness for Enhanced Spiritual Well-Being* and *Readiness for Enhanced Family Coping*.

4. A **health promotion diagnosis** is a determination of the client's "motivation and desire to increase well-being and actualize human health potential as expressed by a readiness to enhance specific health behaviors" (NANDA International, 2009, p. 25). *Readiness for Enhanced Family Processes* is an example of a health promotion nursing diagnosis.

5. A **syndrome diagnosis** is a cluster of nursing diagnoses that occur together and may result in best client outcomes if addressed at the same time (NANDA International, 2013). Currently four syndrome diagnoses are listed. *Risk for Disuse Syndrome*, for example, may be experienced by long-term bedridden clients. Clusters of diagnoses associated with this syndrome include *Impaired Physical Mobility*, *Risk for Impaired Tissue Integrity*, *Risk for Activity Intolerance*, *Risk for Constipation*, *Risk for Infection*, *Risk for Injury*, *Risk for Powerlessness*, and *Impaired Gas Exchange*.

Components of a Nursing Diagnosis

A nursing diagnosis has three components, and each component serves a specific purpose:

1. The diagnostic label ("What is the focus or subject of the problem?")
2. The etiology ("Where did it come from?" "What is it related to?")
3. The defining characteristics ("What does it look like?").

THE DIAGNOSTIC LABEL A NANDA diagnostic label describes the client's response to a health problem for which nursing care is given. It describes the client's health status clearly and concisely in a few words. The diagnostic label identifies the topic that directs the formation of a client goal and desired outcomes. It may also suggest some nursing interventions.

To be clinically useful, diagnostic labels need to be specific; when the word *specify* follows the label, the nurse states the area in which the problem occurs, for example, *Deficient Knowledge* (medications) or *Deficient Knowledge* (dietary adjustments).

Qualifiers are words that have been added to some NANDA labels to give additional meaning to the diagnostic statement; for example:

- *Deficient:* inadequate in amount, quality, or degree; not sufficient; incomplete
- *Impaired:* made worse, weakened, damaged, reduced, deteriorated
- *Decreased:* lesser in size, amount, or degree
- *Ineffective:* or not producing the desired effect
- *Compromised:* to make vulnerable to threat.

Each diagnostic label approved by NANDA carries a definition that clarifies its meaning. For example, the definition of the diagnostic label *Activity Intolerance* is given in **Table 36–6** ●.

THE ETIOLOGY (RELATED FACTORS AND RISK FACTORS)

The **etiology** component of a nursing diagnosis identifies one or more probable causes of the health problem, thereby giving a direction to the required nursing care and enabling the nurse to individualize the client's care. As shown in Table 36–6, the probable causes of activity intolerance may include sedentary lifestyle, generalized weakness, and other factors. Differentiating among possible causes in the nursing diagnosis is essential because each may require different nursing interventions. **Table 36–7** ● provides an example of clients with the same nursing diagnosis but different etiologies; therefore, they require different interventions.

THE DEFINING CHARACTERISTICS

Defining characteristics refer to the cluster of signs and symptoms that indicate the presence of a particular diagnostic label. For actual nursing diagnoses, the defining characteristics are the client's signs and

TABLE 36–6 Example of the Components of a Nursing Diagnosis

DIAGNOSTIC LABEL AND DEFINITION	RELATED FACTORS	DEFINING CHARACTERISTICS
Activity Intolerance: Insufficient physiological or psychological energy to endure or complete required or desired daily activities	Bed rest or immobility Generalized weakness Imbalance between oxygen supply/demand Sedentary lifestyle	Verbal report of fatigue or weakness Abnormal heart rate or blood pressure response to activity Electrocardiographic changes reflecting arrhythmias or ischemia Exertional discomfort or dyspnea

Source: From NANDA International. (2009). *NANDA nursing diagnoses: Definitions and classification 2009–2011.* Chichester, West Sussex, United Kingdom: Wiley-Blackwell. Adapted with permission.

TABLE 36–7 Example of a Nursing Diagnosis With Different Etiologies

DIAGNOSTIC LABEL (PROBLEM)	CLIENT	ETIOLOGY
Constipation	Al Martinez	Long-term laxative use
	Jerry Wong	Inactivity and insufficient fluid intake
	Tanya Brown	Depression
	Caitlin Shea	Change in eating pattern

symptoms. For risk nursing diagnoses, no subjective and objective signs are present. Thus, the factors that cause the client to be more vulnerable to the problem are the etiology of a risk nursing diagnosis. Characteristics can be listed separately according to whether they are subjective or objective in nature. For example, the actual diagnostic label *Fear* includes the following defining characteristics:

- Report of apprehension, being scared, having increased tension
- Diminished learning ability, unable to solve problems
- Diarrhea, vomiting, dry mouth, increase in pulse rate.

The risk diagnostic label *Risk for Falls* includes the following defining characteristics:

- Having a history of falling, using a cane to walk
- Lack of gate on the stairs, lack of parental supervision
- Tranquilizer use, anemia, visual difficulties.

Developing a Nursing Diagnosis

The skills and abilities of critical thinking discussed at the beginning of this module are used by nurses to analyze and apply reasoning to formulate nursing diagnoses. Data can be compared to standards, which are accepted measures, rules, or norms. For example, growth and development charts, normal ranges for laboratory values, or acceptable ranges for vital signs can provide standards against which to compare client data when looking for norms. See **Table 36–8** ● for some examples of how client cues can compare with standards/norms.

An experienced nurse may enter a client's room and immediately observe significant data and draw conclusions about the client. As a result of attaining knowledge, skill, and expertise in the practice setting, the expert nurse may seem to perform these mental processes automatically. Novice nurses, however, need guidelines to understand and formulate nursing diagnoses (see the Critical Thinking section at the beginning of this module for further information).

Skillful assessment minimizes gaps and inconsistencies in data. However, data analysis should include a final check to ensure that assessment data are complete and current. Do the data make sense? For example, a nurse may learn from the nursing history that the client reports not having seen a physician in 15 years, yet during the physical health examination he states, "My doctor takes my blood pressure every year." All inconsistencies must be clarified before a valid pattern can be established. See **Table 36–9** ● for some examples of formulating nursing diagnoses based on client cues.

TABLE 36–8   Examples of Client Cues Compared to Standards/Norms

CUES FROM CLIENT	STANDARD/NORM	INTERPRETATION OF CUES
Height is 5 ft., 2 in. Woman with small frame Weighs 240 lb	Height and weight tables indicate that the "ideal" weight for a woman 5 ft., 2 in. with a small frame is 108–121 lb.	Deviation from population norms
Child is 17 months old. Parents state child has not yet attempted to speak. Child laughs aloud and makes cooing sounds.	Children usually speak their first word by 10–12 months of age.	Developmental delay
States, "I'm just not hungry these days." Ate only 15% of food on breakfast tray. Has lost 30 lb in past 3 months.	Client usually eats three balanced meals per day. Adults typically maintain stable weight.	Changes in client's usual health status
Mrs. Stuart reports that lately her husband angers easily. "Yesterday he even yelled at the dog." "He just seems so tense."	Mr. Stuart is usually relaxed and easygoing. He is friendly and kind to animals.	Changes in client's usual behavior

TABLE 36–9   Examples of Formulating Nursing Diagnoses From Client Cues

CLIENT CUE CLUSTERS	TENTATIVE IDENTIFICATION OF PROBLEMS	FORMULATED DIAGNOSTIC STATEMENTS
"No appetite" since congestion Has not eaten today Last fluids at noon today Nauseated ×2 days	*Imbalanced Nutrition: Less Than Body Requirements*	*Imbalanced Nutrition: Less Than Body Requirements* related to decreased appetite and nausea (secondary to disease process)
Last fluids at noon today Oral temp 39.4°C (103°F) Skin hot and pale, cheeks flushed Mucous membranes dry Poor skin turgor Decreased urinary frequency and amount ×2 days	*Deficient Fluid Volume*	*Deficient Fluid Volume* related to intake insufficient to replace fluid loss secondary to fever, diaphoresis, anorexia
Difficulty sleeping because of cough "Can't breathe lying down"	*Disturbed Sleep Pattern*	*Disturbed Sleep Pattern* related to cough, pain, orthopnea, fever, and diaphoresis
States, "I feel weak" Short of breath on exertion *Cues from cognitive/perceptual pattern:* Responsive but fatigued "I can think OK, just weak." *Cues from cardiovascular pattern:* Radial pulses weak, regular; pulse rate 92 bpm	*Activity Intolerance*	*Activity Intolerance* related to general weakness, imbalance between oxygen supply/demand
Husband out of town; will be back tomorrow afternoon Child with neighbor until husband returns	*Interrupted Family Processes* related to mother's illness and temporary unavailability of father to provide child care	*Risk for Interrupted Family Processes* related to mother's illness and temporary unavailability of father to provide child care
Skin hot, pale, and moist Respirations shallow; chest expansion slight Cough productive of small amounts of thick pale pink sputum Inspiratory crackles auscultated throughout right upper and lower lungs Diminished breath sounds on right side	*Ineffective Airway Clearance* related to disease process	*Ineffective Airway Clearance* related to viscous secretions and shallow chest expansion secondary to pain, fluid volume deficit, and fatigue

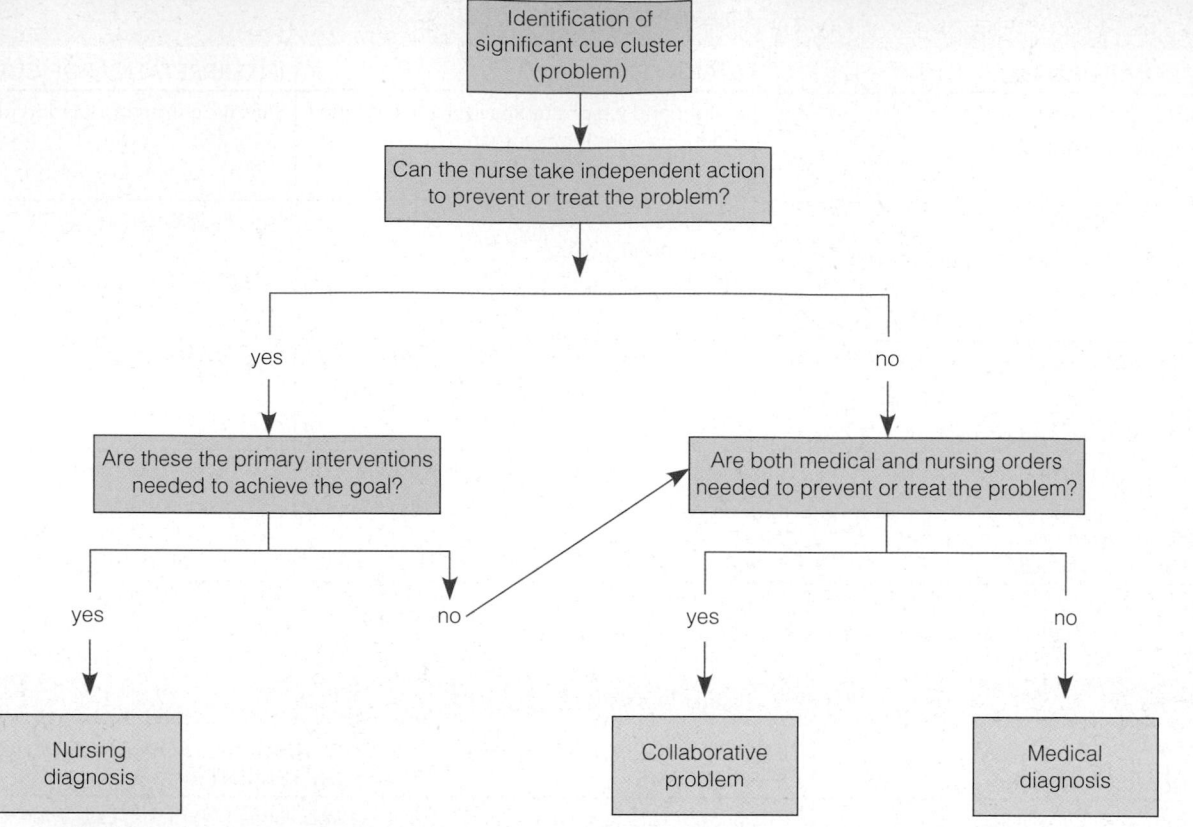

Figure 36–10 ● Decision tree for differentiating among nursing diagnoses, collaborative problems, and medical diagnoses.

After grouping and clustering the data, the nurse and client together identify problems that support tentative actual, risk, and possible diagnoses. This is primarily a decision-making process (see the Clinical Decision Making section at the beginning of this module for further information). In addition the nurse determines whether the client's problem is a nursing diagnosis, medical diagnosis, or collaborative problem. **Figure 36–10** ● is a decision tree diagram that can help nurses make decisions about what kind of diagnosis is appropriate.

At this stage, the nurse and client also establish the client's strengths, resources, and abilities to cope. Most individuals have a clearer perception of their problems or weaknesses than of their strengths and assets, which they often take for granted. By taking an inventory of strengths, the client can develop a more well-rounded self-concept and self-image. Strengths can be an aid to mobilizing health and regenerative processes. A client's strength might include weight that is within the normal range for age and height, enabling the client to cope better with surgery. Another client's strength might be the absence of allergies or being a nonsmoker.

A client's strengths can be found in the nursing assessment record (health, home life, education, recreation, exercise, work, family and friends, religious beliefs, and sense of humor, for example), the health examination, and the client's records.

Writing a Nursing Diagnosis Statement

Most nursing diagnoses are written as two-part or three-part statements, but they do vary.

BASIC TWO-PART STATEMENT The basic two-part statement includes the following:

1. *Problem (P):* NANDA label ("What's the problem?")
2. *Etiology (E):* related to . . . ("What's causing the problem?")

The two parts are joined by the words *related to* merely to imply a relationship. Some examples of two-part nursing diagnoses are shown in **Table 36–10** ●.

For NANDA labels that contain the word *specify*, the nurse must add words to indicate the problem more specifically. The format is still a two-part statement. For example:

Noncompliance (specify) = *Noncompliance* (diabetic diet) related to denial of having disease.

BASIC THREE-PART STATEMENT The basic three-part nursing diagnosis statement is called the PES format and includes the following:

1. *Problem (P):* NANDA label ("What's the problem?")
2. *Etiology (E):* related to . . . ("What's causing the problem?")
3. *Signs and symptoms (S):* defining characteristics of problem ("What's it look like?")

TABLE 36–10 Examples of Two-Part Nursing Diagnosis Statements

PROBLEM	RELATED TO	ETIOLOGY
Constipation	related to	prolonged laxative use
Severe Anxiety	related to	threat to physiological integrity: possible cancer diagnosis

TABLE 36-11 Example of a Three-Part Nursing Diagnosis Statement

PROBLEM	RELATED TO	ETIOLOGY	AS MANIFESTED BY	SIGNS AND SYMPTOMS
Situational Low Self-Esteem	related to (r/t)	feelings of rejection by husband	as manifested by (amb)	hypersensitivity to criticism; states, "I don't know if I can manage by myself," and rejects positive feedback

Actual nursing diagnoses can be documented by using a three-part statement (see **Table 36-11** ●) because the signs and symptoms have been identified. This format cannot be used for risk diagnoses because the client does not have signs and symptoms of the diagnosis. The PES format is especially recommended for beginner nurses because the signs and symptoms validate why the diagnosis was chosen and make the problem statement more descriptive.

BASIC ONE-PART STATEMENT

Some diagnostic statements, such as wellness diagnoses and syndrome nursing diagnoses, consist of a NANDA label only. As the diagnostic labels are refined, they tend to become more specific so that nursing interventions can be derived from the label itself. Therefore, an etiology may not be needed. For example, adding an etiology to the label *Rape-Trauma Syndrome* does not make the label any more descriptive or useful.

NANDA has specified that any new wellness diagnoses will be developed as one-part statements beginning with the words *Readiness for Enhanced* followed by the desired higher level wellness (for example, *Readiness for Enhanced Parenting*). Currently the NANDA list includes several wellness diagnoses. Some of these are *Spiritual Well-Being, Effective Breastfeeding,*

Coping, and *Sleep.* These are usually accepted as one-part statements but may be made more explicit by adding a descriptor, for example, *Readiness for Enhanced Communication* (English-speaking class). See **Table 36-12** ● for general guidelines for writing all of the nursing diagnostic statements.

COMMON VARIATIONS

Common variations of the basic one-, two-, and three-part statements include the following:

1. Writing *unknown etiology* when the defining characteristics are present but the nurse does not know the cause or contributing factors. An example is *Noncompliance* (medication regimen) related to unknown etiology.
2. Using the phrase *complex factors* when there are too many etiological factors or when they are too complex to state in a brief phrase. The actual causes of chronic low self-esteem, for instance, may be long term and complex, as in the following nursing diagnosis: *Chronic Low Self-Esteem* related to complex factors.
3. Using *secondary to* divides the etiology into two parts, thereby making the statement more descriptive and useful. The part following *secondary to* is often a pathophysiological or disease process or a medical diagnosis, as in

TABLE 36-12 Guidelines for Writing a Nursing Diagnostic Statement

GUIDELINE	CORRECT STATEMENT	INCORRECT OR AMBIGUOUS STATEMENT
1. State in terms of a problem, not a need.	*Deficient Fluid Volume* (problem) related to fever	*Fluid Replacement* (need) related to fever
2. Word the statement so that it is legally advisable.	*Impaired Skin Integrity* related to immobility (legally acceptable)	*Impaired Skin Integrity* related to improper positioning (implies legal liability)
3. Use nonjudgmental statements.	*Spiritual Distress* related to inability to attend church services secondary to immobility (nonjudgmental)	*Spiritual Distress* related to strict rules necessitating church attendance (judgmental)
4. Make sure that both elements of the statement do not say the same thing.	*Risk for Impaired Skin Integrity* related to immobility	Impaired Skin Integrity related to ulceration of sacral area (response and probable cause are the same)
5. Be sure that cause and effect are correctly stated (i.e., the etiology causes the problem or puts the client at risk for the problem).	*Pain: Severe Headache* related to fear of addiction to narcotics	Pain related to severe headache
6. Word the diagnosis specifically and precisely to provide direction for planning nursing interventions.	*Impaired Oral Mucous Membrane* related to decreased salivation secondary to radiation of neck (specific)	*Impaired Oral Mucous Membrane* related to noxious agent (vague)
7. Use nursing terminology rather than medical terminology to describe the client's response.	*Risk for Ineffective Airway Clearance* related to accumulation of secretions in lungs (nursing terminology)	Risk for Pneumonia (medical terminology)
8. Use nursing terminology rather than medical terminology to describe the probable cause of the client's response.	*Risk for Ineffective Airway Clearance* related to accumulation of secretions in lungs (nursing terminology)	*Risk for Ineffective Airway Clearance* related to emphysema (medical terminology)

Risk for Impaired Skin Integrity related to decreased peripheral circulation secondary to diabetes.

4. Adding a second part to the general response or NANDA label to make it more precise. For example, the diagnosis *Impaired Skin Integrity* does not indicate the location of the problem. To make this label more specific, the nurse can add a descriptor as follows: *Impaired Skin Integrity* (left lateral ankle) related to decreased peripheral circulation.

Avoiding Errors in Diagnostic Statements

It is important that nurses make nursing diagnoses with a high level of accuracy. Nurses can avoid some common errors of reasoning by recognizing them and applying appropriate critical thinking skills. Errors can occur at any point in the diagnostic process: data collection, data interpretation, and data clustering. Nurses can do the following to minimize diagnostic error:

- *Verify.* Hypothesize possible explanations of the data, but realize that all diagnoses are only tentative until they are verified. Begin and end the diagnostic process by talking with the client and family. When collecting data, ask clients what their health problems are and what they believe the causes to be. At the end of the process, ask clients to confirm the accuracy and relevance of the diagnoses.

- *Build a good knowledge base and acquire clinical experience.* Nurses must apply knowledge from many different areas to recognize significant cues and patterns and generate hypotheses about the assessment data. To name only a few, principles from chemistry, anatomy, and pharmacology each help the nurse understand client data in a different way.

- *Have a working knowledge of what is normal.* Nurses need to know the population norms for vital signs, laboratory tests, speech development, breath sounds, and other indicators. In addition, nurses must determine what is usual for a particular client, taking into account age, physical makeup, lifestyle, culture, and the client's own perception of what her normal status is. For example, the generally accepted normal blood pressure for adults is in the range of 110/60 to 140/80 mmHg. However, a nurse might obtain a reading of 90/50 that is perfectly normal for a particular client. The nurse should compare actual findings to the client's baseline when possible.

- *Consult resources.* Both novices and experienced nurses should consult appropriate resources whenever in doubt about a diagnosis. Professional literature, nursing colleagues, and other professionals are appropriate resources. The nurse should use a nursing diagnosis handbook to determine whether the client's signs and symptoms truly fit the definition of the NANDA label chosen.

- *Base diagnoses on patterns—that is, on behavior over time—rather than on an isolated incident.* For example, even though the client is concerned today about needing to leave her child with a neighbor, it is likely that this concern will be resolved without intervention by the next day. Therefore, the admitting nurse should not diagnose *Interrupted Family Processes.*

- *Improve critical thinking skills.* These skills help the nurse to be aware of and avoid errors in thinking, such as overgeneralizing, stereotyping, and making unwarranted assumptions.

CASE STUDY \\ DIAGNOSIS

Nurse Medina wants to use the assessment data she obtained during the admission assessment of Mrs. Aquilini to identify the top priority nursing diagnosis. First, she makes a list of all of the assessment data and then separates the significant cues that form clusters. Some of the significant cues came from Mrs. Aquilini's recent history at home, but others came from physical findings Nurse Medina obtained:

- "Chest cold" for 2 weeks
- Shortness of breath with activity
- Lung sounds—inspiratory crackles with diminished breath sounds in right lung
- Drinking fluids less
- Feels tired all the time; no energy to do home activities or go to work
- Does not smoke
- T_O 103°F, P 92 bpm, R 28/min, BP 122/80 mmHg, and O_2 Sat 95% on room air
- Productive cough with thick, foul-smelling green sputum
- Speaks in short sentences.

Based on the above assessment cluster and the fact that Mrs. Aquilini has a medical diagnosis of pneumonia, Nurse Medina feels confident the priority nursing diagnosis would involve Mrs. Aquilini's response to the infection in her right lung. There are many NANDA nursing diagnoses related to the respiratory system. Nurse Medina decides the definition of the *Ineffective Airway Clearance* nursing diagnosis best fits Mrs. Aquilini's signs and symptoms. So the diagnostic statement for the top priority nursing diagnosis for Mrs. Aquilini is *Ineffective Airway Clearance* related to accumulated mucus obstructing airways (secondary to pneumonia) **(Figure 36–11 ●)**.

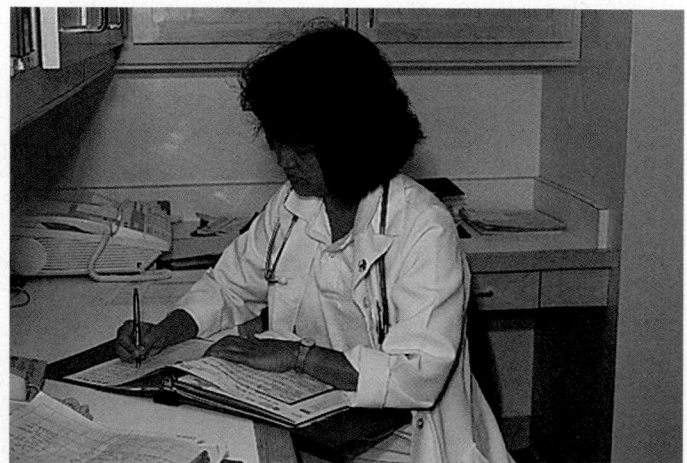

Figure 36–11 ● Diagnosis: After analysis, Nurse Medina formulates a nursing diagnosis: *Ineffective Airway Clearance* related to accumulated mucus obstructing airways (secondary to pneumonia).

Clinical Reasoning Questions Level I

1. How do the assessment data support the nursing diagnosis made by Nurse Medina?

2. Can you identify the different components in this two-part diagnostic statement?

Clinical Reasoning Questions Level II

3. What might be the second and third priority nursing diagnoses for this client?

4. What other assessment data could you hypothesize might be a potential problem for Mrs. Aquilini because of her medical diagnosis of pneumonia?

▶ PLANNING

The **planning** phase is a deliberative, systematic phase of the nursing process during which the nurse refers to the client's assessment data and nursing diagnoses for direction in formulating client goals. Goals are different from outcomes although many times these words are used to mean the same thing (**Box 36–2 ●**). The goals become the basis for the nursing interventions that are developed to prevent, reduce, eliminate, or improve the nursing diagnosis situation. For the plan to be effective, it is important for the client and support persons (if applicable) to participate in the development of the plan: Nurses do not plan for the client, but encourage the client to participate actively to the extent possible. In a home setting, the client's family members and caregivers are the ones who implement the plan of care; thus, its effectiveness depends largely on them.

When the nurse and client identify a goal for every nursing diagnosis together it helps to support the nurse–client relationship. This partnership achieves these other purposes as well:

1. Provides direction for selecting nursing interventions. Ideas for interventions come more easily if the goal clearly and specifically states what the client is to achieve.

2. Serves as criteria for evaluating client progress. Although developed in the planning phase of the nursing process, goals serve as the criteria for determining the effectiveness of nursing interventions and client progress for desired outcomes in the evaluation phase.

3. Enables closure of the nursing diagnosis situation when the client and nurse determine the goal has been achieved.

4. Helps motivate the client and nurse by providing a sense of achievement. As goals are met, both client and nurse can see that their efforts have been worthwhile. This provides motivation to continue following the plan, especially when difficult lifestyle changes need to be made by the client.

5. Supports a therapeutic nurse–client relationship. Any time the nurse and client are able to move forward together in the client's plan of care, the client gains trust in the nurse, further increasing the likelihood of the plan's success.

Long-Term and Short-Term Goals

Goals are customized to individual clients, which mean they take varying amounts of time to achieve. Because of differences in time, goals are categorized as either short term or long term, depending on time frames necessary to achieve them.

Short-term goals are useful for clients who require health care for a short time. In an acute care setting, much of the nurse's time is spent on the client's immediate needs, so most goals are short term and can be achieved by the client in a range of a few hours to a few days. Examples of short-term goals are:

- Client will raise her right arm to shoulder height four days from today, January 23.

- Client will identify five salty foods to avoid while on a salt-free diet by tomorrow, May 7.

- Client will demonstrate how to change his leg dressing before discharge.

- Client will use a cane to walk 20 feet down the hallway by April 22.

Long-term goals are often used for clients who live at home and have chronic health problems and for clients in nursing homes, extended care facilities, and rehabilitation centers. However, clients in acute care settings also need long-term goals to guide planning for their discharge to long-term care agencies or home care, especially in a managed care environment. Long-term goals can be achieved by the client in a range of 1 week to several months. Examples of long-term goals are:

- Client will regain full use of her right arm 6 weeks from today, June 6.

Box 36–2 The Difference Between a Goal and an Outcome

Goals are observable client responses; what the nurse hopes to achieve through nursing actions. Goals are developed in the planning phase of the nursing process. They are broad statements about something the client strives to achieve and indicate progress toward desired client behaviors or actions. Goals are what nurses and clients want to happen. They are individualized and specific for each client.

Outcomes are used to evaluate the client's response to the plan of care. Desired outcomes are specific, observable criteria used to evaluate whether goals have been met. Outcomes are identified during the evaluation phase of the nursing process. They are the end results of nursing actions—both desirable and undesirable. Outcomes indicate the effectiveness of nursing actions. Outcomes are what actually happen. There is a standardized classification of 490 client outcomes, the Nursing Outcomes Classification (NOC), that can be used to describe client status in response to nursing actions (University of Iowa, College of Nursing, 2012). For example:

Nursing diagnosis: Ineffective Airway Clearance related to poor cough effort

Goal: Client will demonstrate an effective cough by 1400 this afternoon.

Desired outcome: Client maintains a clear airway during the postoperative period.

The terms *goal* and *desired outcome* are often used interchangeably. Sometimes the word "or" is used between them, "goals or outcomes," and sometimes they are written "goals/outcomes." In this text, goals are developed in the planning phase of the nursing process and desired outcomes are used to evaluate the client's response to the plan of care.

- Client will be able to discuss five effective coping strategies for dealing with stressful situations that he has used over a 6-month period of time from today, September 25.
- Client will eat at least 60% of all meals by the end of 3 weeks from today, June 1.
- Client will participate in two weekly group activities by sitting quietly and listening attentively by 3 months from today, May 13.

Developing a Goal

Goals are derived from the client's nursing diagnoses—primarily from the diagnostic label. Each nursing diagnosis has one goal for the client to achieve. When developing goals, the nurse should ask the following questions:

1. What about the nursing diagnosis needs to be changed for or by the client?
2. Is there a healthy response to correct a problem stated in the nursing diagnosis that the client can achieve as a goal?
3. How will the client look or behave if the healthy response as a goal is achieved? (What will be seen, heard, measured, palpated, smelled, or otherwise observed through the senses?)
4. What action must the client do and how well must the client do it to demonstrate problem resolution or achievement of the goal?

For example, the nursing diagnosis is:

Deficient Fluid Volume related to diarrhea and inadequate intake secondary to nausea

The *diagnostic label* is "*Deficient Fluid Volume.*"	This is the problem.
Related to is "diarrhea and inadequate intake."	This is the source of the problem.
Secondary to "nausea"	This is the origin of the "related to" factors.

The goal for this nursing diagnosis might be "Client's intake and output of fluids will be balanced during his hospitalization." The client's goal reflects maintaining a fluid balance during the time interval he is losing fluids through diarrhea. The goal of fluid balance is the opposite of the nursing diagnostic label *Deficient Fluid Volume.*

Writing a Goal

Goals have specific characteristics that should be included when writing them to fulfill their purpose in the planning phase of the nursing process. Setting a goal helps to identify desired change in a client's situation and define the focus of nursing interventions. Common characteristics of goals include being:

- Client centered (not about nurse activities)
- Specific and concise single actions
- Single in number for each nursing diagnosis
- Directional for nursing interventions

- Measurable
- Quantifiable
- Attainable for an individual client
- Realistic to an individual client
- Relevant to an individual client
- Time limited.

All goals are client centered in that the client is always the subject, as indicated by beginning the goal with the words "The client will" much of the time. Sometimes these three words are omitted in goals because it is assumed that the subject is the client unless indicated otherwise. A quick and user-friendly format to follow to write a goal statement is the acronym **SMART** (College of Nurses of Ontario, 2012).

Specific single action The goal includes a clearly stated, single action for the client to do that can be observed directly or indirectly. Any additional information defining how the action is to be done is included in this part of the statement. These are sometimes called *qualifiers* of the action. Information provided about the action is detailed so that other nurses following the nursing plan of care will be able to understand what the client is to achieve to reach the goal.

Here are some examples of specific, single actions for goals. The client will:

- Walk 20 feet down the hall using a walker.
- Demonstrate giving herself an insulin injection using aseptic technique.
- Identify six foods to avoid that are high in salt content.
- State the purpose of his new medication, nitroglycerin, and when and how to take it.

Measurable The goal includes a specific, measurable observation or result that is quantifiable. Any nurse observing the client attempting the single action of the goal will be able to recognize when the client reaches the goal. In the following examples, the first column does not provide specific measurements or quantities that all nurses would define the same, whereas the second column does. The client will:

POORLY WRITTEN QUANTIFIED MEASURE	CORRECTLY WRITTEN QUANTIFIED MEASURE
Go for a walk (need to know distance for goal to be reached).	Walk 20 feet down the hall using a walker.
Understand how to give insulin (understanding doesn't mean being able to do it).	Demonstrate giving herself an insulin injection using aseptic technique.
State foods not to eat (quantify how many and what kind so the understanding is consistent).	Identify six foods to avoid that are high in salt content.
Know about nitroglycerin (need to be specific about what to know).	State the purpose of his new medication, nitroglycerin, and when and how to take it.

Nurses must be aware that some phrases can lead to disagreements about whether the outcome was met. Avoid statements that start with *enable, facilitate, allow, let, permit*, or similar verbs followed by the word *client*. These verbs indicate what the nurse hopes to accomplish, not what the client will do.

Attainable (achievable) The goal is appropriate for the individual client. The single action to be measured is realistic and one that the client can complete based on the client's physical, emotional, and psychological capabilities and limitations (e.g., finances, equipment, family support, and social services). For example:

■ Walking a mile would not be achievable for an end-stage COPD client (20 feet might be more realistic).

■ A 2-year-old would not be able to give her own insulin.

■ A 24-year-old could identify foods high in salt content.

■ A 68-year-old could discuss nitroglycerin.

Relevant The goal is applicable to the individual client. The attainable, single action to be measured has a purpose that has been customized for the client based on the needs of the client. For example, typically:

■ A client on bed rest would not need a goal about walking.

■ A nondiabetic client does not need to know about insulin injections.

■ An ordinary teenager does not need to watch his salt intake.

■ A 22-year-old client without angina does not need to know about nitroglycerin.

Time Limited The goal has a specific time frame and deadline for the goal to be completed. During this time period, the progress to reach the goal can be evaluated to motivate the client to continue progress in completing the goal. The time frame is specific to date and hours, days, weeks, or months. For example:

■ 3/2 at 0800

■ In two months, starting 6/2

■ Four hours from 1330

■ 6/24 in the morning.

Putting all the SMART components together in the examples above results in the following appropriate goals:

■ The client will walk 20 feet down the hall using a walker by 3/3 at 0800.

■ The client will demonstrate giving herself an insulin injection using aseptic technique by discharge.

■ The client will identify six foods to avoid that are high in salt content in 4 hours from 1330.

■ The client will state the purpose of his new medication, nitroglycerin, and when and how to take it by discharge.

See **Table 36–13** ● for examples of goals written in SMART format.

Another common format for writing a goal statement is to use the sentence structure components of subject, verb, and adverb. The *subject* in the goal statement is the client. The *verb* is the specific action the client is to perform that can be observed. Examples of action verbs include:

Apply	Discuss	Select
Change	Drink	Sit
Demonstrate	Explain	State
Describe	Inject	Verbalize
Differentiate	Prepare	Walk

Adverbs are added to modify the verb's meaning; they define when, where, how, and in what manner an action is to be performed. For example, the client (subject) will walk (verb) 20 feet down the hall using a walker (adverbs) by 3/3 at 0800. The resulting goals using the examples above are the same as the goals achieved above using the SMART format.

■ The client will demonstrate giving herself an insulin injection using aseptic technique by discharge.

■ The client will identify six foods to avoid that are high in salt content in four hours from 1330.

■ The client will state the purpose of his new medication, nitroglycerin, and when and how to take it by discharge.

TABLE 36–13 SMART Format

SPECIFIC, SINGLE ACTION	MEASURABLE (QUANTIFIABLE, DETERMINES HOW OFTEN)	APPROPRIATE FOR CLIENT	REALISTIC AND ATTAINABLE FOR CLIENT	TIME FRAME FOR CLIENT TO REACH GOAL
Client will drink	2,500 mL of fluids daily	Ask yourself "Is this goal appropriate for this specific client?"	Ask yourself "Is this goal realistic and attainable for this specific client?"	by _____ time, date
Client will administer	correct insulin dose using aseptic technique			by day of discharge
Client will list	three hazards of smoking			by _____ time, date
Client will walk	30 feet down the hall with his cane			by day of discharge
Client's right ankle will measure	less than 10 inches in circumference			in 48 hours from _____ time, date
Client will identify	five foods that are allowed on a low-salt diet			by _____ time, date

Make sure the client considers the goals important and valuable to her. Some clients may know what they wish to accomplish with regard to their health problem; others may not know all the outcome possibilities. The nurse must actively listen to the client to determine personal values, goals, and desired outcomes in relation to current health concerns. Clients are usually motivated and expend the necessary energy to reach goals they consider important.

CASE STUDY \\ PLANNING

Nurse Medina has formulated this diagnostic statement to be the top priority for Mrs. Aquilini based on the assessment cluster of significant cues: *Ineffective Airway Clearance* related to accumulated mucus obstructing airways (secondary to pneumonia). She is now ready to collaborate with Mrs. Aquilini to establish a goal. The following reasoning is part of this discussion:

- Mrs. Aquilini hasn't been drinking much lately, so her mucus is thick and hard to expel.
- She has inspiratory rhonchi with diminished breath sounds in the right lung, which indicate partial obstructions from the thickened mucus in her airways.
- Because Mrs. Aquilini has increased mucus production from the infection in her lungs, she is experiencing impairment in gas exchange, which results in her intolerance to activities and shortness of breath.
- Because she is breathing faster, she is using more energy to breathe.
- Mrs. Aquilini is experiencing general fatigue as her body fights the lung infection.

Nurse Medina helps Mrs. Aquilini understand that many of her problems are a result of the amount and type of mucus in her airways from the lung infection. Nurse Medina further explains the importance of liquefying the mucus so Mrs. Aquilini can cough more effectively and help clear her airways. Together they decide on a goal: "The client will drink 3,000 mL of fluids daily by 8/12." Both are satisfied that Mrs. Aquilini can reach this goal within the time frame. Now that the goal has been identified, they begin thinking about interventions that can help Mrs. Aquilini reach her goal (**Figure 36–12 ●**).

Clinical Reasoning Questions Level I

1. What role did the critical thinking skill of reasoning play in the discussion between Nurse Medina and Mrs. Aquilini?
2. Can you identify the different components of the SMART format in the goal they created together?

Clinical Reasoning Questions Level II

3. Why does Nurse Medina include Mrs. Aquilini in deciding what the goal will be instead of just letting her know she needs to drink more every day?
4. If Mrs. Aquilini did not feel she could drink 3,000 mL of fluids daily, what other goal would you suggest based on the information provided in the case study?

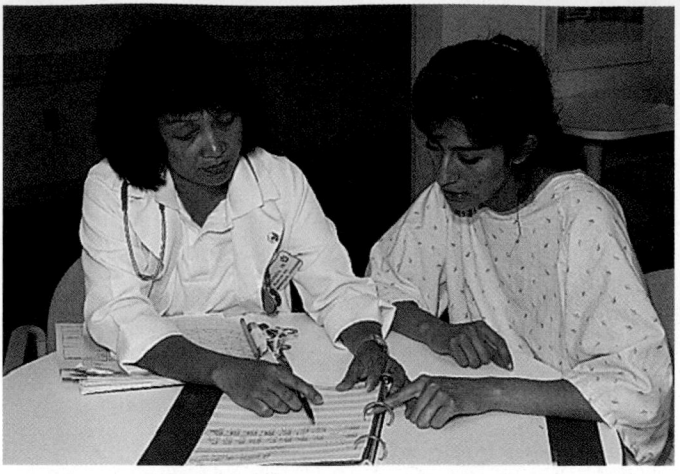

Figure 36–12 ● Planning: Nurse Medina and Mrs. Aquilini collaborate to establish goals (e.g., restore effective breathing pattern and lung ventilation); set outcome criteria (e.g., have a symmetrical respiratory excursion of at least 4 cm and so on); and develop a care plan that includes, but is not limited to, coughing and deep breathing exercises q3h, fluid intake of 3,000 mL daily, and daily postural drainage.

▶ IMPLEMENTATION

Implementation is the action phase of the nursing process. In this phase, nurses take all the data acquired in the first three phases of the nursing process and determine interventions that would be most appropriate to help the client reach the goal stated in the planning phase. Interventions provide data that will be used during the evaluation phase to determine client outcomes. Implementation is a two-step process. The first step is identifying the best priority interventions for an individual client, and the second step is the implementation of these interventions.

Nursing Interventions

Interventions include nursing actions, delegation of tasks, and documentation completed to help the client achieve her goal based on the nursing diagnosis. These actions are listed in priority order (see the exemplar on Prioritizing Care within this module for further information). Nursing interventions focus on:

- Assessments to observe for changes in the client's status
- Prevention to avoid complications
- Reduction of risk factors
- Treating through teaching and providing physical care
- Improvement of health through health promotion and achieving higher levels of wellness.

Correct identification of the etiology during the assessment and nursing diagnosis phases provides the framework for choosing successful nursing interventions. For example, the diagnostic label *Activity Intolerance* may have several etiologies: pain, weakness, sedentary lifestyle, anxiety, or cardiac arrhythmias. Interventions will vary according to the cause of the problem. Sometimes nursing actions treat the client's response to a disease, illness, or medical condition. Interventions for risk nursing diagnoses focus on measures to reduce

TABLE 36–14 Examples of Typical Nursing Interventions Based on Nursing Diagnosis and Etiology

TYPE OF NURSING DIAGNOSIS	ETIOLOGY	NURSING INTERVENTION
Actual	Acute pain related to surgical site	Assessment of pain level using a pain rating scale of 0–10 at frequent intervals
		Give Demerol 50 mg IM PRN pain per physician order.
Risk	Risk for falls related to use of walker	Assessment of ability to move when using the walker
		Keep area from bed to bathroom free from clutter.
Wellness and Health Promotion	Readiness for enhanced parenting related to newborn in the home	Assessment of parents' feelings of impact having a newborn in the home
		Discuss infant stimulation techniques with both parents.

the client's risk factors found in the etiology of the risk nursing diagnosis. **Table 36–14** ● shows examples of typical nursing interventions based on the nursing diagnosis and its etiology.

TYPES OF NURSING INTERVENTIONS Nursing interventions include both direct and indirect care. Direct care is an intervention performed through interaction with the client. Indirect care is an intervention performed away from, but on behalf of the client. Attending an interdisciplinary meeting and managing the care environment are two examples of indirect care. A taxonomy of nursing interventions referred to as the Nursing Interventions Classification (NIC) Taxonomy, developed by the Iowa Intervention Project, can be used to describe the interventions that nurses perform. It includes seven domains and 30 classes of interventions (see the module on Informatics for further information). Nursing interventions are classified as independent, or nurse initiated; dependent, or physician initiated; and collaborative, or involving other providers (e.g., physical therapist) in the client's treatments.

Independent interventions are those activities that nurses are licensed to do within their scope of practice; in other words, areas of health care that are unique to nursing and separate and distinct from medical management. They include physical care, ongoing assessment, emotional support and comfort, teaching, counseling, environmental management, and making referrals to other healthcare professionals. For example, most clients with a nursing diagnosis of pain have medical orders for analgesics, but many independent nursing interventions also can alleviate pain (e.g., guided imagery or teaching a client to "splint" an incision using a pillow). Recall that many nursing diagnoses are client problems that can be treated primarily by independent nursing interventions. In performing an autonomous activity, the nurse determines that the client requires certain nursing interventions. The nurse either carries these out or delegates them to other nursing personnel, and is accountable or responsible for the decision and the actions (see the module on Accountability for further information). An example of an independent action is planning and providing special mouth care for a client after diagnosing impaired oral mucous membranes.

The term **collaborative interventions** encompasses both **dependent interventions** employed by the nurse under a physician's orders, under supervision, or according to specified routines and protocols, as well as actions the nurse carries out in collaboration with other healthcare team members, such as physical therapists, social workers, dietitians, and physicians.

Collaborative nursing activities reflect the overlapping responsibilities of, and cooperative relationships among, healthcare personnel. For example, the physician might order physical therapy to teach the client crutch-walking. The nurse would be responsible for informing the physical therapy department and for coordinating the client's care to include the physical therapy sessions. When the client returns to the nursing unit, the nurse would assist with crutch-walking and collaborate with the physical therapist to evaluate the client's progress.

Physicians' orders commonly direct nurses to provide medications, IV therapy, diagnostic tests, diet, and activity for clients. The nurse is responsible for assessing the need for, explaining, and administering medical orders. Nursing interventions should be written to customize the medical order based on the individual client. For example, instead of writing "Administer opioids as ordered" as an intervention, the nurse can write "Give Demerol 50 mg IM as prescribed by physician."

The amount of time the nurse spends in an independent versus a collaborative or dependent role varies according to the clinical area, type of facility, and specific position of the nurse.

CONSIDERATIONS WHEN SELECTING INTERVENTIONS Usually several potential interventions can be identified for each nursing goal. The nurse's task is to select those that are most likely to achieve the desired client outcomes. There is also a need to prioritize potential interventions and include the client's input. Weighing the pros and cons of each intervention can help make these decisions. For example, "Provide accurate information about diabetes" as an intervention could result in any one of the following client responses:

- Increased anxiety
- Decreased anxiety
- Wish to talk with the primary care provider
- Desire to leave the hospital
- Relaxation.

Determining the pros and cons of each intervention requires nursing knowledge and experience. For example, the nurse's experience may suggest that providing information the night before the client's surgery may increase the client's worry and tension, whereas maintaining the usual rituals before sleep is more effective. The nurse might then consider providing the information several days before surgery. See examples of priority nursing interventions for the client in **Table 36–15** ●.

TABLE 36–15 Examples of Priority Nursing Interventions

Nursing Diagnosis: *Ineffective Airway Clearance* related to viscous secretions and shallow chest expansion secondary to pneumonia

NURSING INTERVENTIONS	RATIONALE
Monitor respiratory status q4h: rate, depth, effort, skin color, mucous membranes, lung sounds, amount and color of sputum, and sensorium.	To identify progress toward or away from goal (i.e., pallor, cyanosis, lethargy, and drowsiness).
Monitor vital signs q4h: temperature, pulse, respiratory rate, blood pressure, and oxygen saturation.	To identify changes in vital signs, which may indicate changes in the client's condition.
Administer oxygen at 2 LPM via nasal cannula as prescribed by physician.	Supplemental oxygen makes more oxygen available to the cells, which reduces the work of breathing.
Maintain in Fowler or semi-Fowler position.	Gravity allows for fuller lung expansion by decreasing pressure of abdomen on diaphragm.
Administer prescribed antibiotic to maintain therapeutic blood level.	Resolves infection by bactericidal effect.
Administer prescribed expectorant.	Helps loosen secretions so they can be coughed up and expelled.
Administer prescribed analgesic.	Controls pleuritic pain, enabling client to increase thoracic expansion.
Encourage fluids by mouth (except when contraindicated by medical conditions such as cardiovascular or renal problems).	Helps liquefy the mucus, making it easier to cough up and expel.
Instruct in breathing and coughing techniques. Remind client to perform, and assist as needed q2–3h.	To enable client to cough up secretions.

The following guidelines can help the nurse choose the most appropriate priority nursing interventions to support clients in reaching their goal. Interventions need to be:

- Safe and appropriate for the individual client's age, health, and condition (see the Lifespan Considerations feature).
- Achievable with the resources available. For example, a home care nurse might wish to include an intervention for an older adult client to "check blood glucose daily," but in order for that to occur the client must have intact sight, cognition, and memory to carry this out independently, or daily visits from a home care nurse must be available and affordable.
- Congruent with the client's values, beliefs, and culture.
- Congruent with other therapies (e.g., if the client is not permitted food, the strategy of an evening snack must be deferred until health permits).
- Based on current best nursing research evidence (see the module on Evidence-Based Practice for further information).
- Within established standards of care as determined by state laws, professional associations (e.g., ANA), and the policies of the facility. Many agencies have policies to guide the activities of health professionals and to safeguard clients. Rules for visiting hours and procedures to follow when a client has cardiac arrest are examples.

WRITING A NURSING INTERVENTION After choosing the best priority nursing interventions, the nurse writes them in the client's nursing plan of care. Interventions are dated when they are written and then reviewed regularly. Here are some common characteristics of a nursing intervention:

- Is client centered
- Has a specific and concise single action
- Includes detailed information about the action (i.e., when, how, time, and where)

- Realistic for the individual client
- Relevant to helping client reach goal set in planning phase
- Only the top 3–5 priority interventions are usually listed for each nursing diagnosis (instead of the 6–10 that could be listed).

Nursing students often include a rationale for each selected intervention as they are learning about nursing actions expected with client conditions and diseases:

POORLY WRITTEN INTERVENTION	CORRECTLY WRITTEN INTERVENTION
Tell the client about insulin.	Explain to the client the actions of insulin.
Assess edema of left ankle daily.	Measure and record client's left ankle circumference daily at 0800.
Apply dressing to left leg.	Change spiral dressing to left leg every shift as needed.
Give pain medication as needed.	Give Tylox 1 tablet PO 30 minutes prior to going to physical therapy and PRN per physician order.

Implementation

Implementation refers to doing the actions in the interventions. The process of implementation commonly includes the following:

- Preassessment of the client
- Determining the nurse's need for assistance
- Implementing the nursing interventions
- Supervising any delegated care
- Documenting nursing actions.

Lifespan Considerations
Implementation Phase

Older Adults

When a client is in an extended care facility or a long-term care facility, interventions and medications often remain the same for extended periods of time. It is important to review the nursing plan of care on a regular basis because changes in the condition of older adults may be subtle and go unnoticed. This applies to both changes of improvement or deterioration. Either one should receive attention so that appropriate revisions can be made in expected outcomes and interventions. Outcomes need to be realistic with consideration given to the client's physical condition, emotional condition, support systems, and mental status. Outcomes for older clients often have to be stated and expected to be completed in very small steps. For instance, a client who has had a cerebrovascular accident may spend weeks learning to brush her own teeth or dress herself. When these small steps are successfully completed, it gives the client a sense of accomplishment and motivation to continue working toward increasing self-care. This particular example also demonstrates the need to work collaboratively with other departments, such as physical and occupational therapy, to develop the nursing plan of care.

PREASSESSMENT OF THE CLIENT Just before implementing an intervention, the nurse must reassess the client to make sure the intervention is still needed and appropriate, because the client's condition may have changed. For example, a client has a nursing diagnosis of *Disturbed Sleep Pattern* related to anxiety and unfamiliar surroundings. During rounds, the nurse discovers that the client is sleeping; the nurse decides to defer the back massage intervention that had been planned as a relaxation strategy.

New data may indicate a need to change the priorities of care or the nursing activities. For example, a nurse begins to teach a client who has diabetes how to give himself insulin injections. Shortly after beginning the teaching, the nurse realizes that the client is not concentrating on the lesson. Subsequent discussion reveals that he is worried about his eyesight and fears he is going blind. Realizing that the client's level of stress is interfering with his learning, the nurse ends the lesson and arranges for a primary care provider to examine the client's eyes. The nurse also provides supportive communication to help alleviate the client's stress.

DETERMINING THE NURSE'S NEED FOR ASSISTANCE When implementing some nursing interventions, the nurse may require assistance for one or more of the following reasons:

- The nurse is unable to implement the nursing activity safely or efficiently alone (e.g., ambulating a client who is obese and needs assistance).

- Assistance would reduce stress on the client (e.g., turning an individual who experiences acute pain when moved).

- The nurse lacks the knowledge or skills to implement a particular nursing activity (e.g., a nurse who is not familiar with a particular type of orthopedic traction equipment needs assistance the first time turning the client).

IMPLEMENTING NURSING INTERVENTIONS Before beginning implementation, explain to the client what interventions will be done, what sensations to expect, what the client is expected to do, and what the expected outcome is. For many nursing activities, it is important to ensure the client's privacy, by closing doors, pulling curtains, or draping the client. The number and kind of direct nursing interventions are almost unlimited and include coordination of client care. This activity involves scheduling client contacts with other healthcare providers (e.g., laboratory and x-ray technicians, physical and respiratory therapists) and serving as a liaison among the members of the healthcare team. When implementing interventions, nurses should follow these guidelines:

- *Base nursing interventions on scientific knowledge, nursing research evidence, and professional standards of care.* The nurse must be aware of the scientific rationale, as well as possible side effects or complications, of all interventions. For example, a client prefers to take an oral medication after meals; however, this medication is not absorbed well in the presence of food. Therefore, the nurse will need to explain why this preference cannot be honored.

- *Clearly understand the interventions to be implemented and question any that are not understood.* The nurse is responsible for intelligent implementation of physician order interventions in the nursing plan of care. This requires knowledge of each intervention, its purpose in the client's plan of care, any contraindications (e.g., allergies), and any changes in the client's condition that may affect the order.

- *Adapt activities to the individual client.* A client's beliefs, values, age (chronological and developmental), health status, and environment are factors that can affect the success of a nursing action. For example, the nurse determines that a client chokes when swallowing pills, so she consults with the physician to change the order to a liquid form of the medication. Or, the nurse recognizes that many Asian clients prefer to drink hot water rather than ice water and, after confirming it with a specific client, supplies hot water at the bedside.

- *Implement safe care.* For example, when changing a sterile dressing, the nurse practices sterile technique to prevent infection; when giving a medication, the nurse follows the rights of safe medication administration.

- *Provide teaching, support, and comfort.* The nurse should always explain the purpose of interventions, what the client will experience, and how the client can participate. The client must have sufficient knowledge to agree to the plan of care and to be able to assume responsibility for as much self-care as possible. These independent nursing activities enhance the effectiveness of nursing plans of care.

- *Respect the client's ethnic background and cultural preferences.* The nurse must always view the client as a whole and give consideration to the client's preferences. For example, whenever possible, the nurse honors the client's expressed preference that interventions be planned for times that fit with the client's usual schedule of visitors, work, sleep, or eating.

- *Respect the dignity of the client and enhance the client's self-esteem* by providing privacy and encouraging clients to make their own decisions as appropriate.

■ *Encourage clients to participate actively in implementing nursing interventions.* Active participation enhances the client's sense of independence and control. However, clients vary in the degree of participation they desire. Some want total involvement in their care, whereas others prefer little involvement. The amount of active involvement may be related to the severity of the illness; the client's culture; or the client's fear, understanding of the illness, and understanding of the intervention.

DELEGATION   Delegation of client care and assigning tasks is an important responsibility for registered nurses because healthcare facilities use licensed practical nurses and many unlicensed assistive personnel. To delegate appropriately, the nurse must match the needs of the client and family with the scope of practice of the available caregivers. The RN remains responsible for making sure delegated tasks are carried out properly.

Other caregivers may be required to communicate their activities to the nurse by documenting them on the client's medical record, reporting verbally, or filling in a written form. The nurse validates and responds to any adverse findings or client responses. This may involve modifying the nursing plan of care. For example, unlicensed assistive personnel may perform tasks such as measuring intake and output, but the RN is still responsible for analyzing data, planning care, and evaluating outcomes (see the module on Managing Care for further information).

DOCUMENTATION   After carrying out the nursing activities, the nurse completes the implementation phase by recording the interventions performed and client responses in the nursing progress notes. Nursing actions are communicated verbally as well as in writing. When a client's health is changing rapidly, the charge nurse and/or the physician may want to be kept up to date with verbal reports. Nurses also report client status at a change of shift (see the module on Communication for further information).

Skills Necessary for Implementation

To implement the nursing plan of care successfully, nurses need cognitive (knowledge), interpersonal (attitudes), and technical skills (skills). Although these skills are distinct from one another, in practice nurses use them in various combinations and with different emphasis, depending on the activity. For instance, when inserting a urinary catheter the nurse needs cognitive knowledge of the principles and steps of the procedure, interpersonal skills to inform and reassure the client, and technical skill in draping the client and manipulating the equipment.

Cognitive skills include problem solving, decision making, critical thinking, and creativity. They are crucial to safe, intelligent nursing care.

Interpersonal skills are the verbal and nonverbal communication methods nurses use when interacting with the client or family. The effectiveness of a nursing action often depends largely on the nurse's ability to use therapeutic communication. A nurse also needs interpersonal skills to work effectively with others as a member of a healthcare team (see the module on Communication for further information). Interpersonal skills are necessary for all nursing activities and reflect knowledge, attitudes, feelings, interest, and appreciation of the client's cultural values and lifestyle.

Technical skills are purposeful, "hands-on" skills such as manipulating equipment, giving injections, bandaging, and moving, lifting, and repositioning clients. These skills are also called procedural or psychomotor skills. Technical skills require knowledge and, frequently, manual dexterity. The number of technical skills expected of a nurse has greatly increased in recent years because of the advances in the use of technology, especially in acute care hospitals.

Relationship to Other Nursing Process Phases

The first three phases of the nursing process—assessment, nursing diagnosis, and goal planning—provide the basis for the nursing actions performed during the implementation of interventions phase. In turn, the implementation phase provides the actual nursing activities and client responses that are examined in the final phase, the evaluation phase. Using data acquired during assessment, the nurse can individualize the care given during the implementation phase.

While implementing nursing care, the nurse continues to reassess the client at every contact, gathering data about the client's responses to the nursing actions and about any new problems that may develop. Some routine nursing activities present new assessment data for the nurse making observations. For example, while bathing an older adult client, the nurse observes a reddened area on the client's sacrum. Or, when emptying a urinary catheter bag, the nurse measures 200 mL of foul-smelling, cloudy, brown urine.

CASE STUDY \\ IMPLEMENTATION

The goal for Mrs. Aquilini is "The client will drink 3,000 mL of fluids daily by 8/12." Nurse Medina and Mrs. Aquilini are now discussing interventions that will help Mrs. Aquilini reach her goal. Here is the list of potential interventions they have come up with:

■ Perform postural drainage daily.
■ Record daily weights.
■ Have Mrs. Aquilini's favorite beverages available so she can drink them frequently.
■ Do coughing and deep breathing exercises every 3 hours.
■ Have Mrs. Aquilini's favorite snacks readily available.
■ Encourage Mrs. Aquilini to drink a variety of beverages so she does not get bored with water.
■ Keep a tally of how much Mrs. Aquilini is drinking and urinating each shift.
■ Assess sputum for consistency, color, amount, and odor.

Nurse Medina explains to Mrs. Aquilini that they need to select the top four priorities from this list to add to her plan of care

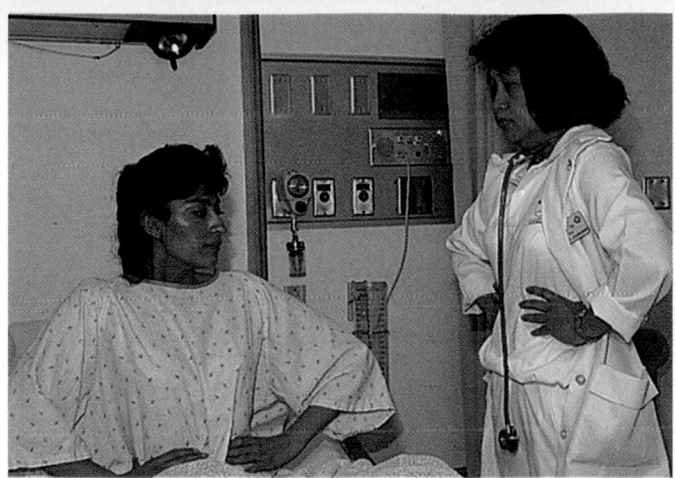

Figure 36–13 ● Implementation: Mrs. Aquilini agrees to practice deep breathing exercises q3h during the day. In addition, she verbalizes awareness of the need to increase her fluid intake and to plan her morning activities to accommodate postural drainage.

(Figure 36–13 ●). She further explains the importance of assessment to measure progress of reaching the goal. Together, they decide these are the top four priorities:

- Measure intake and output every shift.
- Have Mrs. Aquilini's favorite beverages available so she can drink them frequently.
- Do coughing and deep breathing exercises every 3 hours.
- Perform postural drainage daily.

Clinical Reasoning Questions Level I

1. What is the importance of conducting an assessment before performing any interventions?
2. Would you have selected other interventions for Mrs. Aquilini? If so, what are they and why would you have selected them?

Clinical Reasoning Questions Level II

3. Which of the interventions listed are independent interventions nurses can do without physician orders?
4. Why do you think assessment of the sputum for consistency, color, amount, and odor was not selected as an intervention specific to helping Mrs. Aquilini reach her goal?

▶ EVALUATION

After implementing nursing care, the nurse evaluates the desired outcomes. In this context, **evaluation** is a planned, ongoing, purposeful activity in which clients and healthcare professionals determine (a) the client's progress toward achievement of goals/outcomes and (b) the effectiveness of the nursing plan of care. On the basis of this evaluation, the plan of care is continued, modified, or terminated. As in all phases of the nursing process, clients and support persons are encouraged to participate as much as possible.

Evaluation continues until the client achieves the health goals or is discharged from nursing care. Evaluation conducted during or immediately after implementation of a nursing action enables the nurse to make on-the-spot modifications to an intervention. Evaluation performed at specified intervals (e.g., once a week for the home care client) shows the extent of progress toward goal achievement and enables the nurse to correct any deficiencies and modify the care plan as needed. Evaluation at discharge includes the status of goal achievement and the client's self-care abilities with regard to follow-up care. Most facilities have a special discharge record for this evaluation.

Through evaluating, nurses demonstrate responsibility and accountability for their actions, indicate interest in the results of the nursing activities, and demonstrate a desire not to perpetuate ineffective actions but to adopt more effective ones. During the evaluating process, the nurse determines whether the nursing interventions had any relation to the outcomes. It should never be assumed that a nursing action was the cause of or the only factor in meeting, partially meeting, or not meeting a goal.

CLINICAL EXAMPLE

Ruth Horowitz, a client with obesity, needed to lose 14 kg (30 lb). When the nurse and Mrs. Horowitz drew up a plan of care, one goal was "Lose 1.4 kg (3 lb) in 4 weeks." A nursing intervention listed in the plan of care was "Explain how to plan and prepare a 1,200-calorie diet." Four weeks later, Mrs. Horowitz weighed herself and had lost 1.8 kg (4 lb). The goal had been met—in fact, exceeded. It is easy to assume that the nursing intervention was highly effective. However, it is important to collect more data before drawing that conclusion. On questioning Mrs. Horowitz, the nurse might find any of the following: (a) She planned a 1,200-calorie diet and prepared and ate the food; (b) she planned a 1,200-calorie diet but did not prepare the correct food; or (c) she did not understand how to plan a 1,200-calorie diet so she did not bother with it.

If the first possibility is found to be true, the nurse can safely judge that the nursing intervention "Explain how to plan and prepare a 1,200-calorie diet" was effective in helping Mrs. Horowitz lose weight. However, if the nurse learns that either the second or third possibility actually happened, then it must be assumed that the nursing strategy did not affect the outcome. The next step for the nurse is to collect data about what Mrs. Horowitz actually did to lose weight. It is important to establish the relationship (or lack thereof) of the nursing actions to the client responses.

Drawing Conclusions

The nurse uses the judgments about goal achievement to determine whether the plan of care was effective in resolving, reducing, or preventing the nursing diagnosis. When goals have been met, the nurse can draw one of the following conclusions about the status of the client's problem:

- The actual problem stated in the nursing diagnosis has been resolved, or the potential problem is being prevented and the risk factors no longer exist. In these instances, the nurse documents that the goals have been met and discontinues the care for the problem.

■ The risk problem stated in the nursing diagnosis is being prevented, but the risk factors are still present. In this case, the nurse keeps the problem on the plan of care.

■ The actual problem still exists even though some goals are being met. For example, a desired outcome on a client's care plan is "Will drink 3,000 mL of fluid daily." Even though the data may show this outcome has been achieved, other data, for example the presence of dry oral mucous membranes, may indicate that the client is still experiencing deficient fluid volume. Therefore, the nursing interventions must be continued even though this one goal was met.

When goals have been partially met or when goals have not been met, two conclusions can be drawn:

■ The plan of care needs to be revised, since the problem is only partially resolved. The revisions may need to occur during the assessment, nursing diagnosis, planning, or implementation phase.

OR

■ The plan of care does not need revision because the client merely needs more time to achieve the previously established goal(s). To make this decision, the nurse must assess why the goals are being only partially achieved, including whether the evaluation was conducted too soon.

Developing an Evaluation

The nurse collects data so that conclusions can be drawn about whether goals have been met. It is usually necessary to collect both objective and subjective data. Some data may require interpretation. Examples of objective data requiring interpretation are the degree of tissue turgor of a dehydrated client or the degree of restlessness of a client with pain. Examples of subjective data needing interpretation include complaints of nausea or pain by the client. When interpreting subjective data, the nurse must rely upon either (a) the client's statements (e.g., "My pain is worse now than it was after breakfast") or (b) objective indicators of the subjective data, even though these indicators may require further interpretation (e.g., decreased restlessness, decreased pulse and respiratory rates, and relaxed facial muscles as indicators of pain relief). Data must be recorded concisely and accurately to facilitate the next part of the evaluation process.

If the goal has been written following the guidelines given in this module, it will be relatively simple to determine whether a goal has been met. Both the nurse and client play an active role in comparing the client's actual responses with the desired outcomes. Did the client drink 3,000 mL of fluid in 24 hours? Did the client walk unassisted the specified distance per day? When determining whether a goal has been achieved, the nurse can draw one of three possible conclusions:

1. The goal was met; that is, the client's response is the same as the desired outcome.

2. The goal was partially met; that is, either a short-term goal was achieved but the long-term goal was not, or the desired outcome was only partially attained.

3. The goal was not met; that is, the client did not achieve the goal within the time frame.

Writing an Evaluation

After determining whether a goal has been met, the nurse writes an evaluation statement (either on the care plan or in the nurse's notes). An **evaluation statement** consists of the following information:

■ Date and time evaluation was done

■ A conclusion statement about whether the goal was met, partially met, or not met

■ A supporting statement giving the results of how the client did or did not achieve the goal.

Here are examples of evaluation statements:

DATE AND TIME OF EVALUATION	CONCLUSION STATEMENT	SUPPORTING STATEMENT
12/3, 1345	Goal met.	Client walked with cane 20 feet down hallway.
9/22, 0900	Goal partially met.	Client is able to identify three foods instead of five foods high in sugar content.
5/14, 1030	Goal not met.	Client did not change the dressing on his right arm using aseptic technique.

Continuing, Modifying, or Terminating the Nursing Plan of Care

After drawing conclusions about the status of the client's problems, the nurse modifies the plan of care as needed. Depending on the facility, modifications may be made by drawing a line through portions of the plan of care or writing "discontinued," "goal met," or "problem resolved" and the date/time.

Whether or not goals were met, a number of decisions need to be made about continuing, modifying, or terminating nursing care for each problem. See **Table 36–16** ● for a checklist to use when reviewing a care plan. Although the checklist uses a closed, yes/no format, its only intent is to identify areas that require the nurse's further examination.

Before making modifications, the nurse must determine if the plan as a whole was not completely effective. This requires a review of the entire plan of care and a critique of each step of the nursing process involved in its development.

ASSESSMENT Incomplete or incorrect data influence all subsequent steps of the nursing process and plan of care. If data are incomplete, the nurse needs to reassess the client and record the new data. In some instances, new data may indicate the need for new nursing diagnoses, new goals, and new nursing interventions.

NURSING DIAGNOSIS If the data were incomplete, new nursing diagnostic statements may be required. If the data were

TABLE 36–16 Evaluation Checklist

ASSESSMENT	DIAGNOSIS	PLANNING	IMPLEMENTATION
_____ Are data complete, accurate, and validated?	_____ Are nursing diagnoses relevant and accurate?	**Desired Outcomes**	_____ Was client input obtained at each step of the nursing process?
_____ Do new data require changes in the care plan?	_____ Are nursing diagnoses supported by the data?	_____ Do new nursing diagnoses require new goals?	_____ Were goals and nursing interventions acceptable to the client?
	_____ Has problem status changed (i.e., potential, actual, risk)?	_____ Are goals realistic?	_____ Did the caregivers have the knowledge and skill to perform the interventions correctly?
	_____ Are the diagnoses stated clearly and in correct format?	_____ Was enough time allowed for goal achievement?	_____ Were explanations given to the client prior to implementing?
	_____ Have any nursing diagnoses been resolved?	_____ Do the goals address all aspects of the problem?	
		_____ Does the client still concur with the goals?	
		_____ Have client priorities changed?	
		Nursing Interventions	
		_____ Do nursing interventions need to be written for new nursing diagnoses or new goals?	
		_____ Do the nursing interventions seem to be related to the stated goals?	
		_____ Is there a rationale to justify each nursing diagnosis?	
		_____ Are the nursing interventions clear, specific, and detailed?	
		_____ Are new resources available?	
		_____ Do the nursing interventions address all aspects of the client's goals?	
		_____ Were the nursing interventions actually carried out?	

complete, the nurse needs to analyze whether the problems were identified correctly and whether the nursing diagnoses were relevant to the information collected. After making judgments about problem status, the nurse revises or adds new nursing diagnoses as needed to reflect current client data.

REVISING CLIENT GOALS If a nursing diagnosis was inaccurate, obviously the goal statement(s) will need revision. If the nursing diagnosis was appropriate, the nurse then checks if the goal was realistic and attainable. Unrealistic goals require correction. The nurse should also determine whether priorities have changed and whether the client still agrees with the priorities. For example, the time frame for a specific amount of weight loss was possibly too short and should be extended. Goals must also be written for any new nursing diagnoses.

REDESIGNING NURSING INTERVENTIONS The nurse investigates whether the nursing interventions were related to goal achievement and whether the priority nursing interventions were selected. Even when diagnoses and goals were appropriate, the nursing interventions selected may not have been the best ones to

achieve the goal. New nursing interventions may reflect changes in the amount of nursing care the client needs, scheduling changes, or rearrangement of nursing actions to group similar activities or to permit longer rest or activity periods for the client. For example, for a client who wishes to stop smoking, many potential interventions exist. If medication was prescribed but the client is still smoking, a behavioral intervention such as group counseling may need to be added. If new nursing diagnoses have been written, then new nursing interventions will also be necessary.

METHOD OF IMPLEMENTATION Even if all sections of the plan of care appear to be satisfactory, the manner in which the plan was implemented may have interfered with goal achievement. Before selecting new interventions, the nurse should confirm whether they were carried out. Other personnel may not have carried them out, either because the interventions were unclear or because they were unreasonable in terms of external constraints such as money, staff, time, and equipment.

After making the necessary modifications to the plan of care, the nurse implements the modified plan and begins the nursing process cycle again. Refer to **Table 36–17 ●** to see how the plan

TABLE 36–17 Example of Evaluation of Outcomes and Goals With Notes About Nursing Interventions

Nursing Diagnosis: *Ineffective Airway Clearance* related to viscous secretions and shallow chest expansion secondary to deficient fluid volume, pain, and fatigue

DESIRED OUTCOMES	GOAL STATEMENTS	NURSING INTERVENTIONS*	NOTE ABOUT NURSING INTERVENTIONS
Respiratory status: gas exchange as evidenced by the following:			
■ Absence of pallor and cyanosis (skin and mucous membranes)	Partially met. Skin and mucous membranes not cyanotic, but still pale.	Monitor respiratory status q4h: rate, depth, effort, skin color, mucous membranes, amount and color of sputum.	*Retain nursing interventions to continue to identify progress. Goal status indicates problem not resolved.*
■ Use of correct breathing/coughing technique after instruction	Partially met. Uses correct technique when pain well controlled by narcotic analgesics.	Monitor results of blood gases, chest x-ray studies, pulse oximetry, and incentive spirometer volume as available.	
■ Productive cough	Met. Cough productive of moderate amounts of thick, yellow, pink-tinged sputum.	Monitor level of consciousness.	
■ Symmetric chest excursion of at least 4 cm	Not met. Chest excursion = 3 cm.	Auscultate lungs q4h.	
■ Lungs clear to auscultation within 48–72 hours	Not met. Scattered inspiratory crackles auscultated throughout right anterior and posterior chest.	Monitor vital signs q4h: TPR, BP, pulse oximetry.	*Does not need to be reinstructed because client demonstrates correct techniques. May still need support and encouragement because of fatigue and pain of breathing.*
■ Respirations 12–22/min; pulse <100 bpm	Partially met. Respirations 26/min, pulse 96 bpm.	Instruct in breathing and coughing techniques. Remind to perform and assist q3h. *Support and encourage. (4/17/07, JW)*	
■ Inhaling normal volume of air on incentive spirometer	Not met. Tidal volume only 350 mL. *(Evaluated 4/17/07, JW)*	Administer prescribed expectorant; schedule for maximum effectiveness.	*As soon as client is hydrated and fever is controlled, she will probably be discharged to self-care at home.*
		Maintain Fowler or semi-Fowler position.	
		Administer prescribed analgesics. Notify primary care provider if pain not relieved.	
		Administer oxygen by nasal cannula as prescribed. Provide portable oxygen if client goes off unit (e.g., for x-ray examination).	
		Assist with postural drainage daily at 0930. *On 4/17 teach to continue PRN at home. (4/17/07, JW)*	
		Administer prescribed antibiotic to maintain constant blood level. Observe for rash and GI or other side effects.	

*In this plan of care, additions to the care plan are shown in italics.

for the client in the plan of care throughout this exemplar was modified after evaluation of goal achievement and review of the nursing process. A line has been drawn through portions the nurse wished to delete; additions to the care plan are shown in italics. In addition to evaluating the client's response to the nursing plan of care, nurses also evaluate nursing care (see the module on Quality Improvement for further information).

Relationship to Other Nursing Process Phases

Successful evaluation depends on the effectiveness of the phases that precede it. Assessment data must be accurate and complete so that the nurse can formulate appropriate nursing diagnoses and desired goals. The goals must be stated concretely to be useful for evaluating client responses. And finally, without the implementing phase in which the plan is put into action, there would be nothing to evaluate.

The evaluation phase includes assessment. As previously stated, assessment (data collection) is ongoing and continuous at every client contact. However, data are collected for different purposes at different points in the nursing process. During the assessment phase, the nurse collects data for the purpose of making diagnoses. During the evaluation phase, the nurse collects data for the purpose of comparing it to the goal developed in the planning phase and making decisions about the effectiveness of the nursing care.

CASE STUDY \\ EVALUATION

It is 8/12 and time for Nurse Medina and Mrs. Aquilini to evaluate whether or not Mrs. Aquilini has reached her goal. The first day her intake was 3,100 mL and output was 2,600 mL; the second day her intake was 3,050 mL and output was 2,825 mL. Mrs. Aquilini is pleased that she was able to increase her intake of fluids to at least 3,000 mL daily. Nurse Medina was happy Mrs. Aquilini had reached her goal and supports the outcome "to restore an effective breathing pattern." The goal statement was "Goal met. Client has consumed at least 3,000 mL of liquids daily by 8/12." (See **Figure 36–14** ●.)

Clinical Reasoning Questions Level I

1. Can you identify the different components in the goal statement?

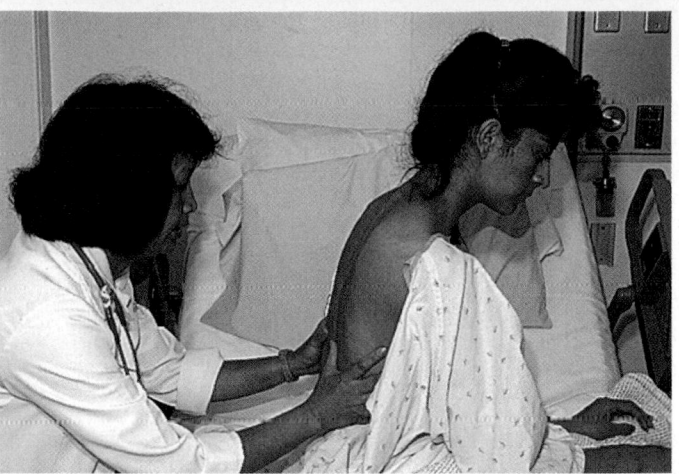

Figure 36–14 ● Evaluation: Upon assessment of respiratory excursion, Nurse Medina detects failure of the client to achieve maximum ventilation. She and Mrs. Aquilini reevaluate the care plan and modify it to increase coughing and deep breathing exercises to q2h.

2. How important is it for Nurse Medina to give Mrs. Aquilini positive feedback on reaching her goal?

Clinical Reasoning Questions Level II

3. If Mrs. Aquilini was not able to reach her goal, what would be Nurse Medina's next action?

4. Once a goal has been met successfully by the client, what happens to this nursing diagnosis in the plan of care?

◢ REVIEW **The Nursing Process**

RELATE Link the Concepts and Exemplars

Linking the exemplar of the nursing process with the concept of communication.

1. How does the nurse communicate the use of the nursing process when documenting?

2. The nurse is caring for a client with postoperative pain and administers an analgesic 10 minutes before the end of the shift. How does the nurse communicate the need for evaluation of effectiveness of pain management to the oncoming shift?

Linking the exemplar of the nursing process with the concept of legal issues:

3. How does use of the nursing process in providing and documenting care reduce the nurse's risk of malpractice claims?

4. What legal obligations does the nurse have related to use of the nursing process?

REFER Go to Pearson Nursing Student Resources
nursing.pearsonhighered.com

• Additional review materials

REFLECT Case Study

Dr. Danilo Ocampo is a 74-year-old retired pathologist. He lives in his home with Lydia, his wife of 51 years. Their only

child, a son, was killed at age 22 in an automobile crash. Dr. Ocampo was born and raised in the Philippines and came to the United States when he was 23. He is the last living member of his immediate family. He has a few nephews and nieces in the Philippines, but no relatives live nearby.

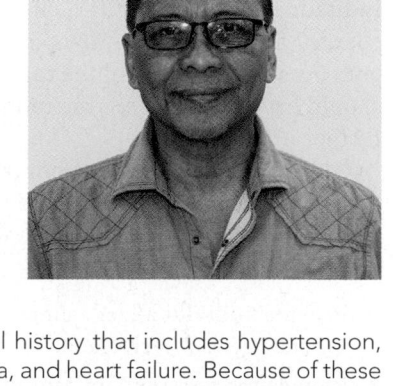

Dr. Ocampo's health has been declining for the past few years. He has a medical history that includes hypertension, myocardial infarction, angina, and heart failure. Because of these cardiovascular disorders, he takes multiple medications, including metoprolol, lisinopril, spironolactone, furosemide off and on, K+ when taking furosemide, aspirin, isosorbide dinitrate, and nitroglycerin. He has a good understanding of the pharmaceutical properties of the medications. At times, he is not sure he gets good health care because of all the medications he takes. He often does not believe the medications are helpful because he experiences many side effects, and he has required multiple admissions to the hospital. He usually feels better after a few days in the hospital but typically checks himself out of the hospital before his physicians are ready to discharge him.

Because Lydia has dementia, most of Dr. Ocampo's time and energy are spent managing their household and taking care of her. He has been resistant to outside help, believing he can care for her better than anyone else does. He maintains a very consistent schedule, and they get along quite well. Although at one time in their lives they were very socially active, at this point, they rarely go out.

Dr. Ocampo has become increasingly short of breath and is very fatigued. He notices his legs have become edematous. He goes to the neighborhood drugstore to use the "self-serve" blood pressure machine and finds his blood pressure to be 152/106 mmHg. He is resistant to the idea of seeing his physician or going to the emergency department for fear of being admitted. Instead, he increases the dose of furosemide and lisinopril by 1 tablet per day and tries to get a bit more rest. A week later when his symptoms fail to improve and seem to worsen slightly, Dr. Ocampo visits his healthcare provider's office and reports his symptoms and increase in medication dosages.

1. What are the priorities of care for Dr. Ocampo?
2. What data would you collect from Dr. Ocampo on initial examination?
3. Develop a nursing plan of care for this client.

EXEMPLAR 36.2 The Nursing Plan of Care

EXEMPLAR KEY TERMS
Clinical pathway, *2360*
Column plan, *2356*
Concept map, *2356*
Nursing plan of care, *2354*
Standardized plan, *2357*

EXEMPLAR LEARNING OUTCOMES
After reading about this exemplar, you will be able to:

1. Recognize various formats used for nursing plans of care.
2. Construct a column nursing plan of care.
3. Create a concept map.
4. Summarize the benefits of using clinical pathways to standardize client care.

▶ OVERVIEW

A **nursing plan of care** is a written or electronic guideline that organizes information about an individual client's or family's care. One plan may include several nursing diagnoses for a single client. It is important to prioritize nursing diagnoses and to list only three to five nursing diagnoses; this helps the nurse focus on nursing care that provides the best client outcomes. The RN initiates the plan when the client is admitted to the facility. The plan of care is then constantly updated throughout the client's stay in response to changes in the client's condition and evaluations of goal achievement. Keeping the plan of care current is necessary to ensure appropriate, individualized care for the client. When the client is discharged from the facility, the plan is included as part of a client's permanent record of the care received and care the client should have received (see the module on Communication for further information).

Although formats differ from facility to facility, the plan of care is often organized using the five nursing process phases (see **Figure 36–15** ●). Whether written or electronic, plans have the following purposes:

■ Provide individualized client-centered care to meet the unique needs of each client.

■ Provide for continuity of care through communication with nursing staff and other healthcare providers involved with the care of the client.

■ Inform the nurse about which specific observations or actions need to be documented in the nurse's progress notes about the client's care.

■ Provide medical insurance companies documented proof for reimbursement amount to pay in relation to services rendered to the client.

■ Provide the nurse a guide when assigning nursing staff to care for each client.

Accessibility

Nursing plans of care need to be readily accessible to all healthcare team members involved with the care of the client. Availability of the plan supports communication with others for better continuity of care. The plan of care may be kept at the bedside but is more commonly kept with the medical record. Some facilities utilize a Kardex system as a quick reference to stay current with each individual client's nursing care needs. This card system gives quick information about the client such as demographic data, routines of daily care (i.e., bathing, nutrition), diagnostic studies, social history, oxygen therapy, monitoring needs, medications and IV fluids, and surgical drains.

Guidelines

The nurse should follow the guidelines in **Table 36–18** ● when writing nursing plans of care. Note that the guidelines include specificity and customization.

CASE STUDY \\ B

Mrs. Fisher is a 52-year-old woman whose husband of 35 years died 5 weeks ago after a long battle with lung cancer. She says that she has come to the clinic today because she does not sleep more than 3 hours at night and feels tired all the time. She tells the nurse that she has lost about 15 pounds since her husband died because she is too tired to fix anything to eat.

Mrs. Fisher has two sons, both of whom attended the funeral, but they have not contacted Mrs. Fisher since then. One lives on the other side of town, and the other lives out of state.

For more than 40 years, Mrs. Fisher attended her place of worship every time the doors were opened for an activity. She also enjoyed singing in the choir. For the past couple of weeks, she has not been able to attend any activities because she doesn't understand why her husband had to die, and she feels disconnected from

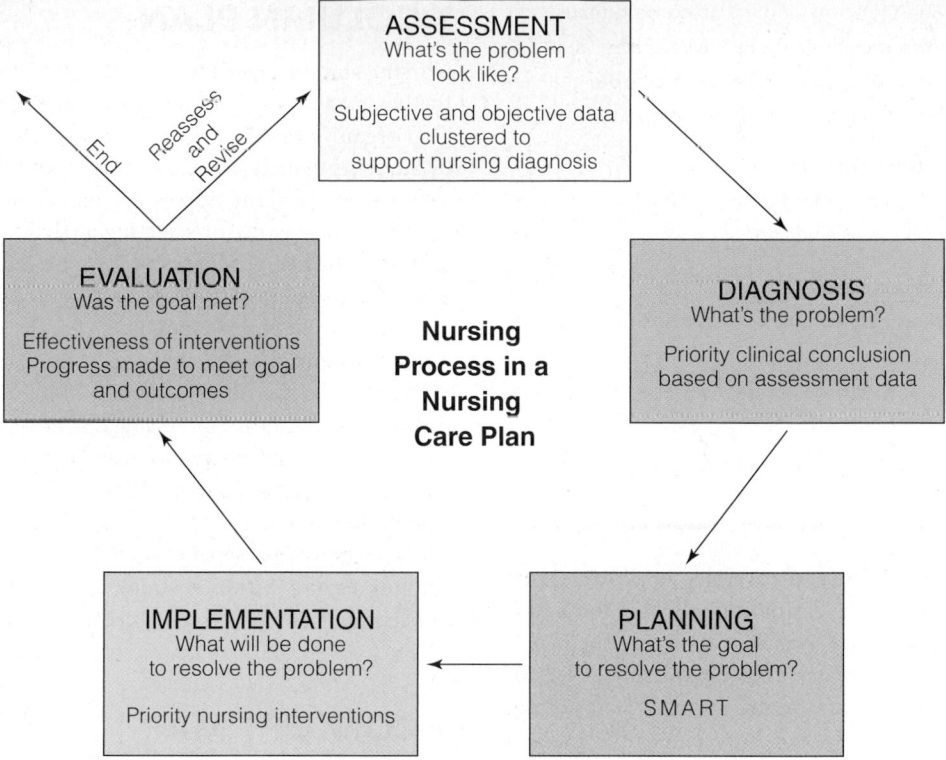

Figure 36–15 ● Using the nursing process in a nursing plan of care.

TABLE 36–18   Guidelines for Writing a Nursing Plan of Care

GUIDELINE	DESCRIPTION
Date and sign the plan.	The date the plan is written is essential for evaluation, review, and future planning. The nurse's signature demonstrates accountability since the effectiveness of nursing actions can be evaluated.
Use category headings: "Assessment," "Nursing Diagnoses," "Goals/Desired Outcomes," "Nursing Interventions," and "Evaluation."	Headings may vary slightly with different facilities but are relative to the nursing process phases.
Use approved abbreviations and key words rather than complete sentences to communicate ideas unless facility policy dictates otherwise.	For example, write "Turn/reposition q2h" rather than "Turn and reposition the client every two hours." Or, write "Clean wound c̄ H₂O₂ BID" rather than "Clean the client's wound with hydrogen peroxide twice a day, morning and evening." (See the module on Communication for more information.)
Be specific, short, and concise.	Because nurses are now working shifts of different lengths (e.g., 12- or 8-hour shifts), the nurse must be specific about the timing of an intervention. An intervention reading "Change incisional dressing q shift," could mean either twice in 24 hours, or three times in 24 hours, depending on the length of the facility's shifts.
Refer to facility resources, such as procedure books, rather than including all of the steps on a written plan.	For example, write "See unit procedure book for tracheostomy care" or attach a standard nursing plan about such procedures as preoperative or postoperative care.
Customize the plan to include client's choices, such as preferences about the times of care and the methods used.	This reinforces the client's individuality and sense of control. For example, the written nursing intervention might read "Provide partial bath in the evening per client's preference."
Ensure that the nursing plan incorporates preventive and health maintenance aspects as well as restorative ones.	For example, carrying out the intervention "Provide active assistance ROM (range-of-motion) exercises to affected limbs q2h" prevents joint contractures and maintains muscle strength and joint mobility.
Ensure that the plan contains interventions for ongoing assessment of the client.	For example, "Inspect incision q8h."
Include collaborative activities in the plan.	For example, the nurse may write interventions to ask a nutritionist or physical therapist about specific aspects of the client's care.
Include plans for the client's discharge and health teaching needs.	The nurse begins discharge planning as soon as the client has been admitted, often consulting and making arrangements with a community health nurse, social worker, and other community agencies to supply client services, needed equipment, and supplies.

her place of worship. She stopped singing at home because she says she "doesn't feel the music anymore." Mrs. Fisher says she stays at home every night now to avoid seeing people that are "smiling and happy" when she feels so lost and alone.

Clinical Reasoning Questions Level I

1. What are the significant assessment data for Mrs. Fisher?
2. What related clusters do the significant assessment data form?

Clinical Reasoning Questions Level II

3. What are the top three priority nursing diagnoses from the clustered assessment data?
4. What goal would be appropriate for each of the three nursing diagnoses?
5. What are the top three priority nursing interventions to support Mrs. Fisher reaching her goals?

Nursing plans of care can be computerized or written. Most healthcare facilities that have electronic medical records have electronic nursing plans of care. Nurses can access the client's care plan from centrally located terminals at the nurses' station or from terminals in client rooms. Written nursing plans of care are utilized in facilities that do not have electronic medical records. Plans can be kept in a separate notebook or with the client's medical record. Both electronic and written plans support communication and continuity of care when clients are transferred from one unit to another or from one facility to another. The plan of care becomes a part of the client's permanent record upon the client's discharge from the facility. The format used for the plan of care is decided on by each facility. Common types of client plans of care that facilities customize for their clients include the following:

- Column plan
- Concept map
- Standardized plan
- Clinical pathway.

▶ COLUMN PLAN

Nursing students learn how to develop nursing plans of care for the clients assigned to them as a learning activity as well as to help organize the client's care. As a result, care plans developed by students usually are more lengthy and detailed than plans of care used by working nurses. Students may be required to give a rationale, or reason, for selecting a particular nursing intervention as a priority. Students may also be required to cite research evidence from literature for their stated rationale to develop evidence-based practice habits.

The **column plan** of care uses columns to categorize data for each phase of the nursing process. This type of care plan may include four columns: (a) nursing diagnoses, (b) goals/desired outcomes, (c) nursing interventions, and (d) evaluation. Some agencies use a three-column plan in which evaluation is done in the goals column or in the nurses' notes; others have a five-column plan that adds a column for assessment data preceding the nursing diagnosis column. **Figure 36–16** ● shows a five-column framework for a nursing care plan for the client in Case Study B, Mrs. Fisher.

▶ CONCEPT MAP

A **concept map** is a visual representation of a nursing plan of care in a patterned diagram with data and ideas. Various shapes and colors are used to show relationships and connections in combination with lines or arrows. Concept maps are creative, conceptual images of concrete critical thinking. The visual image enhances clinical reasoning by "showing" how nursing diagnoses, goals, interventions, and evaluations relate to each other in a logical and patterned way. Concept maps can take many different forms and encompass various categories of data, according to the creator's interpretation of the client or health condition. They are an offshoot of mind maps or cognitive maps. Concept maps can be a visual guide in analyzing relationships among clinical data, which helps in the prioritization of meeting client needs.

Assessment	Nursing Diagnosis	Plan	Implementation	Evaluation
• Doesn't understand why her husband died • Stopped attending place of worship because feels disconnected from it • Stopped singing in the choir	*Spiritual Distress*	Client will meet with religious adviser by 4/12.	• Establish therapeutic relationship with client. • Assist client to cope with lifestyle changes. • Assist client in finding a reason for living. • Discuss visit with religious adviser. • Encourage client to talk about her feelings.	4/12 Goal ongoing–client has appointment with religious adviser on 4/13.
• Not sleeping well • States she "feels so lost" • Lost 15 pounds • Not eating well	*Ineffective Coping*	Client will eat three meals a day by 4/8.	• Assess for risk of hurting self or others. • Refer client to counseling. • Discuss sleep promotion behaviors. • Have dietitian discuss cooking for one with client.	4/8 Goal met–client has eaten three meals a day x 4 days.
• No contact with sons since husband's death • Husband died 5 weeks ago • Avoids people • Stays at home every night	*Social Isolation*	Client will phone each son by 4/10.	• Discuss promotion of social contacts. • Assist client in developing a support system. • Support client in reconnecting with sons. • Encourage outside activity–like walking.	4/10 Goal not met–client has only spoken with one of her sons.

Figure 36–16 ● Five-column nursing plan of care for situational distress.

The concept map is another way of depicting the nursing plan of care. Concept maps can help nursing students view the client and her problems holistically rather than as a single problem or medical diagnosis. Students are often asked to complete concept maps as a method of learning and demonstrating the links among disease processes, laboratory data, medications, signs and symptoms, risk factors, and other relevant data.

There are many different ways to make a concept map. Post-It notes are ideal to use because they already come in a variety of colors and shapes; they also make it easy to move data around until the concept map is finished. Colored pencils or markers and paper cut into various shapes can be used as well. Software programs are available for creating electronic concept maps, and many Web sites offer free concept mapping programs.

Hints when making a concept map:

- Follow the sequence of the nursing process phases, always beginning with assessment data collection and clustering of significant related data to determine nursing diagnoses (see the exemplar on the Nursing Process within this module for further information).

- Keep it simple. The more lines crossing each other, the more difficult it is to follow the connections among data.

- Many nursing programs have developed a concept map format for nursing students to follow. Creativity can still happen when individualizing concept maps.

- This is not a scrapbooking activity. Do not become caught up in the artistic expression, spending hours matching colors and shapes to use space and coordinate patterns in developing a concept map. It is a visual representation of the much more important concepts focused on nursing care for best client outcomes.

Many approaches can be used to build a concept map. Here is an example that is basic and can be expanded if more data are being used:

1. Develop a legend for the concept map by assigning shapes and colors for each nursing process phase and one for other categories of client information: demographics, outcomes, lab results, risk factors, or medications.
2. Put the shape with the client's initials, age, gender, and priority medical diagnosis in the middle of the paper to illustrate the client-centeredness nature of nursing care.
3. Look at the assessment data, subjective and objective, and then gather and sort the significant clusters. Each piece of significant data goes on one assessment shape. Place the clustered groups around the client shape.
4. Determine the priority nursing diagnoses that are relative to each of the clusters and place one nursing diagnosis with each of them. Draw connecting lines from each shape with assessment data to the nursing diagnosis for which it is relative.
5. Determine one appropriate goal for each nursing diagnosis cluster and add its shape to the side of the nursing diagnosis cluster. Select priority nursing interventions, independent and dependent, for each goal. Write separate interventions on their designated shape and arrange them

on the outer side of the nursing diagnosis. Draw connecting lines from each shape with an intervention to the nursing diagnosis for which it is relative.
6. Evaluate whether the goal was met, not met, or partially met, and place the evaluation shape on the side of the nursing diagnosis cluster. It can be located under the goal shape or on the opposite side.
7. The concept map is now complete. **Figure 36–17** ● uses the data from Case Study B earlier in this exemplar to build a concept map.

▶ STANDARDIZED PLAN

A **standardized plan** of care specifies the nursing care for groups of clients with common needs (e.g., all clients with myocardial infarction). These plans can be developed by a standardized care committee composed of facility staff that use both medical and nursing research evidence (see the module on Evidence-Based Practice for more information). Facilities may also purchase standardized plans to complement their policies and procedures. It is time efficient for nurses to have a preprinted plan instead of generating a single plan for a common set of interventions. Once the nursing assessment is completed, the standardized plan of care that is appropriate for the client is selected, and the nurse adds or deletes information on the generalized care plan to individualize it to the needs of a particular client.

A standardized plan of care frequently includes checklists, blank lines, or empty spaces to allow the nurse to individualize goals and nursing interventions. Standardized plans of care should not be confused with standards of care. Although the two have some similarities, they have important differences.

SAFETY ALERT
Nurses must remember that standards of care are not the same as a standardized plan of care. Standards of care are nursing actions for clients that describe achievable nursing care. They define the interventions for which nurses are held accountable. Standards of care can be developed by individual healthcare facilities for nurses working in the facility. National organizations and agencies, such as the ANA, the Joint Commission, and state boards of nursing, also set standards of nursing practice for nurse accountability (see the module on Accountability for further information). A standardized plan of care provides general nursing care for specific medical diseases or conditions. If the nurse determines that following any part of a standardized plan of care would jeopardize a client's safety or health outcomes, the nurse is responsible for taking appropriate action to ensure the health and safety of the client.

Standardized care plans are usually categorized according to specific age groups, client problems, and specialty categories. Standardized plans follow the nursing process phases so nurses are familiar with their format. Regardless of whether plans of care are handwritten, computerized, or standardized, nursing care must be individualized to fit the unique needs of each client. In practice, a plan of care usually consists of both preprinted and nurse-created

1 Select shapes and/or colors for the concept map, assigning each a label.

-- Legend
-- Assessment
-- Nursing Diagnosis
-- Intervention
-- Goal
-- Evaluation
-- Client

2 Start with the client in the middle of the paper.

MF, 52 years old
Situation depression

3 Cluster significant assessment cues to select priority nursing diagnosis.

Doesn't understand why her husband died

Stopped attending place of worship because she feels disconnected from it

Stopped singing in the choir

MF, 52 years old
Situation depression

No contact with sons since husband's death

Husband died 5 weeks ago

Not sleeping well

States she "feels so lost"

Avoids people

Stays at home every night

Not eating well

Lost 15 pounds

4 Add the priority nursing diagnosis and use lines to connect them to appropriate assessment data.

1. Nursing Diagnosis: *Spiritual Distress*

Doesn't understand why her husband died

Stopped attending place of worship because she feels disconnected from it

Stopped singing in the choir

MF, 52 years old
Situation depression

No contact with sons since husband's death

Husband died 5 weeks ago

Not sleeping well

States she "feels so lost"

Avoids people

Stays at home every night

Not eating well

Lost 15 pounds

Figure 36–17 ● Steps for building a concept map.

5 Select a goal then priority nursing interventions to help client reach her goal and outcomes.

6 Arrange all the information into clusters with connecting lines to complete the concept map.

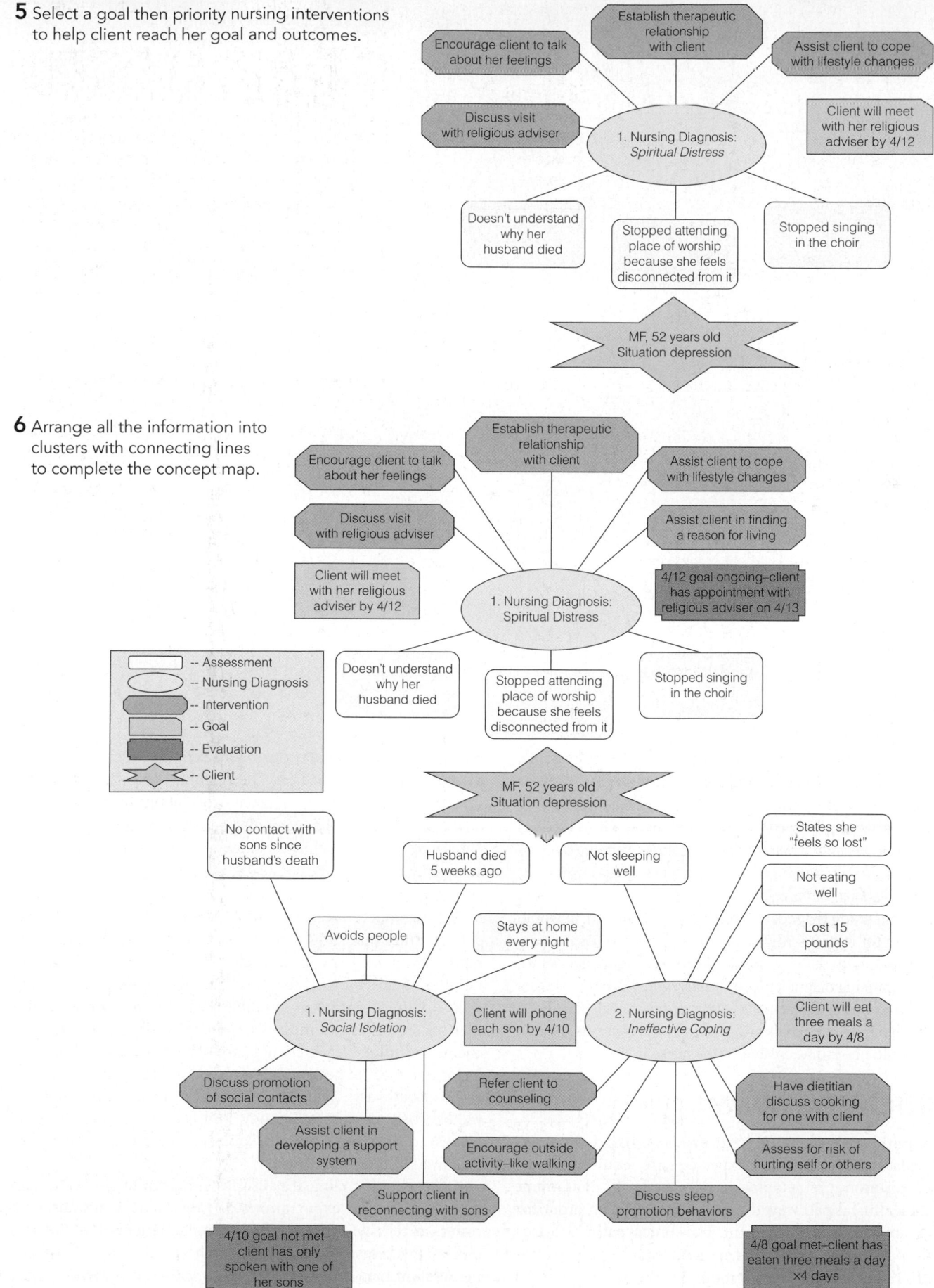

Figure 36–17 ● Steps for building a concept map. *(continued)*

Etiology	Desired Outcomes	Nursing Interventions (Identify Frequency)
___ Decreased oral intake	___ Urinary output >30 mL/hr	___ Monitor I&O q___ hr
___ Nausea	___ Urine specific gravity 1.005–1.025	___ Weight daily
___ Depression	___ Serum Na⁺ within normal limits	___ Monitor serum electrolyte levels x
___ Fatigue, weakness	___ Mucous membranes moist	___ Assess skin turgor and mucous
___ Difficulty swallowing	___ Skin turgor elastic	membranes q ___
___ Other: _____	___ No weight loss	___ Administer prescribed
___ Excess fluid loss	___ 8-hr intake = _____	IV therapy _____
___ Fever or increased metabolic rate	___ Other: _____	_____
___ Diaphoresis		___ Offer oral liquids frequently
___ Vomiting		___ Mouth care as needed
___ Diarrahea		___ Teach client about importance of fluid
___ Burns		___ Other: _____
___ Other: _____		

Etiology (continued):

Defining Characteristics
___ Insufficient intake
___ Negative balance of I&O
___ Dry mucous membranes
___ Poor skin turgor
___ Concentrated urine
___ Rapid, weak pulse
___ Lowered B/P
___ Weight loss

Plan initiated by: _____ Date: _____
Plan/outcomes evaluated: _____ Date: _____
Client: _____

Figure 36–18 ● Example of a standardized plan of care for *Deficient Fluid Volume*.

sections. The nurse uses standardized care plans for predictable, commonly occurring problems, and creates an individual plan for unusual circumstances or problems needing special attention.

For example, a standardized care plan for "clients with a medical diagnosis of pneumonia" would probably include a nursing diagnosis of *Deficient Fluid Volume* and direct the nurse to assess the client's hydration status. On a respiratory or medical unit this would be a common nursing diagnosis; therefore, the client's nurse would be able to obtain a standardized plan directing care commonly needed by clients with deficient fluid volume (see **Figure 36–18 ●**). However, the nursing diagnosis *Risk for Interrupted Family Processes* would not be common to all clients with pneumonia; it is specific to the client. Therefore, the goals and nursing interventions for that diagnosis would need to be created by the nurse.

▶ CLINICAL PATHWAY

A **clinical pathway** is a standardized, evidence-based, multidisciplinary plan that outlines the expected care required for clients with common, predictable—usually medical—conditions. To initiate a clinical pathway, the physician writes an order for one that is appropriate for the client. The clinical pathway documents are part of the client's permanent record and are integrated into the clinical documentation.

Sometimes clinical pathways are referred to as collaborative plans or case management plans, and they sequence the care that

must be given on each day during the projected length of stay for the specific type of condition. They include clinical interventions, time frames for completion, usual expectations of response, and expected outcomes. They are also sometimes called multidisciplinary plans because they include medical treatments to be performed by different types of healthcare providers.

The plan is usually organized with a column for each day, listing the interventions that should be carried out and the client outcomes that should be achieved on that day. There are as many columns on the multidisciplinary care plan as the preset number of days allowed for the client's diagnosis-related group (DRG). Clinical pathways do not include detailed nursing activities because they are multidisciplinary in nature. Because all clients are unique, each client's care will be customized to meet his or her specific needs while keeping the guidelines in mind. Clinical pathways, which minimize variance in treatment to reduce cost, increase efficiency, and improve client care outcomes, are frequently used in Canada and the United Kingdom (Ottawa Hospital, 2010).

Client-specific clinical pathways are given to clients to help them understand expectations of time frames, actions, and results as relative to DRGs. For example, **Figure 36–19 ●** is a clinical pathway for a vaginal birth (mother and baby). It includes information about activity, nutrition, medications, treatments, client teaching, tests, and discharge planning for specific times from delivery time of the baby.

	MOTHER		NEWBORN	
	24 HOURS	**48 HOURS**	**24 HOURS**	**48 HOURS**
Activity	■ Up with assistance as needed, progress to up by self ■ Shower ■ Self-care with assistance ■ Baby care with assistance	■ Total self-care ■ Baby care by self with assistance as needed ■ Vaginal exercises	(To be done by nursing staff)	(To be done by nursing staff)
Nutrition	■ Regular diet as tolerated	■ Regular diet	■ Scheduled breastfeeding; minimum 6 feeds in 24 hours ■ Scheduled bottle feeding; minimum 6 feedings in 24 hours (each 15–30 mL)	■ Scheduled breastfeeding on cue; minimum 8 feeds in 24 hours ■ Scheduled bottle feeding; minimum 6 feedings in 24 hours (each 30–60 mL)
Medications	■ Pain medications as needed ■ Routine medications	■ Laxative as needed ■ Routine medications	■ Sucrose orally prior to procedures	■ Sucrose orally prior to procedures
Treatments	■ Routine vital signs and assessment ■ Comfort measures for perineum/episiotomy/hemorrhoids ■ Monitoring for signs of complications (e.g., excessive bleeding, difficulty urinating, constipation)	■ Routine vital signs and assessments ■ Sitz bath as needed ■ Comfort measures continued as needed ■ Monitoring for signs of complications continued	■ Routine vital signs and assessment ■ Vitamin K injection and erythromycin ointment to eyes at birth ■ Examination by physician ■ Baby care, height, weight ■ Circumcision if requested	■ Routine vital signs and assessment ■ Continued baby care, weight ■ Infant hearing screening ■ Circumcision care as needed
Client Teaching	■ Discussion about self-care and newborn care ■ Review learning materials provided ■ Discussion about breastfeeding ■ Discussion about newborn feeding, safety, cord site care, comfort, bathing, sleeping, activity	■ Continue learning about at-home care for self and newborn ■ Continue learning about at home newborn feeding needs	None	None
Tests	■ Procedures and diagnostic tests as needed	■ Procedures and diagnostic tests as needed	■ Newborn screening as needed before discharge	■ Newborn screening as needed before discharge
Discharge Planning	■ At-home care of self and newborn ■ Discussion about community resources available ■ Discussion about birth certificate, newborn's name, and health coverage	■ Continue at-home care of self and newborn discussions ■ Follow-up appointment for self scheduled	■ Appointment for newborn screening if needed	■ Follow-up appointment for baby scheduled before discharge

Figure 36–19 ● Clinical pathway for mother and baby (vaginal birth).

Clinical pathways may be developed as an algorithm or path as shown in the example of **Figure 36–20** ●. This clinical pathway is for pediatric clients with asthma and is directed toward the multidisciplinary team. It includes separate assessment and treatment progressive guidelines for the pediatric client with mild, moderate, severe, and near-death signs and symptoms of asthma.

Medications, treatments, and teaching instructions are listed for pediatric clients. It includes information about the assessment, pretreatment, and treatment of these clients, along with next steps to be taken if the client has not improved. Pathways like this one are designed to improve the quality of care and outcomes as well as standardize provided care across clinical disciplines.

EMERGENCY DEPARTMENT: PROTOCOL FOR ASSESSMENT AND TREATMENT OF PEDIATRIC ASTHMA

	ASSESSMENT	SYMPTOMS PRIOR TO TREATMENT	INTERVENTIONS AND THERAPIES	NEXT STEPS IF NOT IMPROVED
MILD ASTHMA	■ May be agitated ■ Can lie down ■ Nocturnal cough ■ Exertional dyspnea ■ Plays quietly ■ Can talk ■ Increased use of β-agonist ■ Good response to β-agonist	■ O_2 Saturation >95% ■ Increased respiratory rate ■ Moderate wheeze-end expiratory _Respiratory rates:_ Age _Normal rate_ <2 months <60/min 2–12 months <50/min 1–5 years <40/min 6–8 years <30/min	■ O_2 to achieve $SaO_2 \geq 95\%$ ■ β-agonist—nebulizer, up to 3 doses in first hour ■ Oral systemic corticosteroids	
MODERATE ASTHMA	■ Agitated ■ Prefers sitting ■ Shorter cry ■ Difficulty feeding ■ Increased work of breathing ■ Some difficulty talking ■ Partial relief with β-agonist ■ β-agonist needed >q4h	■ SaO_2 92–95% room air ■ Increased resp rate ■ Increased heart rate ■ Wheezing throughout inhalation and exhalation _Pulse rates_ Age _Normal rate_ 2–12 months <160 bpm 1–2 years <120 bpm 2–8 years <110 bpm	■ O_2 to achieve $SaO_2 \geq 95\%$ ■ β-agonist and anticholinergic—nebulizer, up to 3 doses in first hour or continuous treatment for 1 hour ■ Systemic corticosteroids	**ADMIT**
SEVERE ASTHMA	■ Very agitated ■ Sits upright ■ Stops feeding ■ Marked limitation in talking ■ Dyspnea at rest ■ Grunting	■ $SaO_2 < 92\%$ ■ Labored respirations ■ Persistent tachycardia ■ Breath sounds are decreased ■ Wheezing throughout inhalation and exhalation	■ 100% O_2 ■ Continuous β-agonist and anticholinergics ■ Systemic corticosteroids ■ Systemic magnesium sulfate	**ADMIT TO ICU or TERTIARY CARE**
NEAR DEATH	■ Exhausted ■ Drowsy ■ Diaphoretic ■ Cyanotic ■ Apnea ■ Unable to talk ■ Use of accessory muscles to breath ■ Suprasternal retractions	■ $SaO_2 < 80\%$ ■ Decreased respiratory effort ■ Falling heart rate ■ Paradoxical thoracoabdominal movement ■ Silent chest	■ Cardiac monitoring ■ Oximetry, ABGs ■ Chest x-ray ■ Frequent reassessment ■ Medical supervision until clear signs of improvement ■ Consider alternative drugs: IV β-agonist Inhalation anesthetics Aminophylline Epinephrine	**RAPID SEQUENCE INTUBATION**

Figure 36–20 ● Clinical pathway for pediatric asthma for multidisciplinary team.

▶ **SUMMARY**

Regardless of the type of care plan used in the facility in which the nurse is employed, the nurse is responsible for knowing how to access and use the care plan, how to interact with standardized portions, and how to individualize the plan of care for each client. Accuracy of data, both the data collected by the nurse as well as how accurately the nurse enters data into the plan of care, is essential for best client outcomes and because the plan of care becomes a permanent part of the client's health record. Standardized plans of care allow for streamlining some aspects of the planning process, but they do not take the place of the nurse's use of clinical reasoning to ensure that all nursing actions promote client safety and wellness.

◢ **REVIEW The Nursing Plan of Care**

RELATE Link the Concepts and Exemplars

Linking the exemplar of the nursing plan of care with the concept of communication:

1. What information in the nursing plan of care is communicated to other disciplines taking care of the same client?

Linking the exemplar of the nursing plan of care with the concept of managing care:

2. How can using a standardized plan of care influence the cost of client care?

Linking the exemplar of the nursing plan of care with the concept of professional behaviors:

3. Why is use of a nursing plan of care considered a professional behavior?

REFER Go to Pearson Nursing Student Resources
nursing.pearsonhighered.com

- Additional review materials

REFLECT Case Study

Devon Bynum, an 11-year-old, is admitted to the hospital in sickle cell crisis. This is the first time he has been admitted to a hospital. He states he hurts all over and rates his pain at a 7 out of 10. Devon has been in the emergency department all night and last received morphine 2 mg IV at 0400 for his pain. He is receiving oxygen at 2 liters per minute (LPM) via nasal cannula. He has an IV of D5 ½NS running at 83 mL/hr. His mom, who has been with him throughout the night, is anxious for her son to feel better. His last vital signs are T_O 99.3° F; P 122 bpm; R 22/min; BP 100/64 mmHg; and oxygen saturation of 93% on oxygen at 2 LPM. He says he is tired and just wants to go to sleep. Devon's mom tells the nurse that she doesn't know how she will be able to pay the hospital bills. She shares that she is a single parent with two other children at home.

1. What type of nursing plan of care would you use for Devon? Why?

2. Would you include his mom's concern about finances in his plan of care? How?

3. What other healthcare discipline(s) would you expect to include in Devon's plan of care?

EXEMPLAR 36.3 **Prioritizing Care**

EXEMPLAR KEY TERMS

Effectiveness, *2364*
Efficiency, *2364*
Pitfalls, *2370*
Pop-ups, *2369*
Prioritizing care, *2363*
Priority, *2363*
Resources, *2369*
Time constraints, *2366*
Time priority, *2366*
Triage, *2367*
Urgency factor, *2366*

EXEMPLAR LEARNING OUTCOMES
After reading about this exemplar, you will be able to:

1. Discuss the role assessment plays in prioritizing care for clients.

2. Demonstrate how to use the nursing process in setting priorities for client care.

3. Discriminate among severities of client needs using Maslow's hierarchy.

4. Use the urgency factor to set time priorities for interventions.

5. Demonstrate how to prioritize nursing responsibilities and interventions based on their significance and urgency.

6. Organize client care using an established priority order for completing responsibilities and interventions.

7. Apply the factors necessary to support successful prioritization of care and responsibilities.

8. Distinguish between good habits and poor habits (pitfalls) when prioritizing care and responsibilities.

▶ OVERVIEW

The term **priority** refers to "something given or meriting attention before competing alternatives" (Merriam-Webster, 2011). **Prioritizing care** is a process that helps nurses manage time and establish an order for completing responsibilities and care interventions for a single client or for a group of clients. The ability to set priorities is a critical thinking skill that can optimize a nurse's time and productivity by categorizing responsibilities and care interventions in an order based on significance and urgency. Time is a constant factor in prioritizing care: There is always only so much time for nurses to make clinical judgments about which interventions to do and when to do them, whether for one client or for several clients. Without some forethought and planning, a nurse may work for hours and yet accomplish very little. Learning to spend time and energy wisely is a necessity in today's busy healthcare settings.

Like other professionals, a nurse's workload includes many things that need to be completed during each shift. Time management becomes an important skill that helps the nurse ensure that necessary activities are completed. Nurses can use a variety of approaches to accomplish nursing responsibilities and interventions. Unfortunately, some of these approaches may result in interventions being done poorly, incompletely, late, or not at all.

For example, some nurses simply plow into their work. They complete tasks as they go from client to client in no particular order, keeping busy by doing activities to meet client needs. They may start at one room and simply work their way down the hallway doing things for their clients. This strategy raises a number of questions. What about the nursing interventions with time constraints, such as medication administration? Are all nursing interventions equally important? Do all nursing interventions impact clients equally?

Sometimes nurses choose to work on the easiest tasks first, postponing the more challenging, complex tasks for a later time. They may then find themselves rushing to finish the complex tasks during that inevitable "crunch" time. Maybe they just decide they do not have time to do an important job and leave it undone. A hurried pace increases stress levels, which interferes with clear thinking, clinical judgment, and decision making. As a result, time to complete actions decreases, often negatively impacting the quality of performance. At the end of the shift, the nurse may regret not starting the more difficult tasks sooner (Wax, 2011).

In contrast to less productive methods of completing activities, nurses can learn to prioritize their actions according to the importance of tasks and interventions and the appropriate timing for accomplishing them. By doing so, interventions that have a high priority will be completed early. Just like learning any new

Box 36–3   Setting Priorities— Food for Thought

For those who put off unpleasant tasks:
Follow the words of Mark Twain: "Eat a live frog every morning, and nothing worse will happen to you the rest of the day."

Think of the biggest most difficult task on your to-do list and get motivated to get it done early in the day. Don't spend a lot of time thinking about it, looking at it, and planning how you will get it done. Get the weight of it off your shoulders by doing it. Marvel knowing the biggest and most complex task you had to do is completed.

For those who focus on doing little tasks:
Think of a jar filled with sand. If you try to add some rocks in the jar, there would not be room for them. Empty the sand, and put the rocks in the jar first. Then add some smaller rocks. Finally, add the sand. They will all fit. Start your day by doing some big tasks first, then do a few smaller tasks, and do the little tasks throughout the day when short clips of time allow. Marvel about the big tasks you complete and all the lesser tasks you are able to do. Be busy completing big tasks, small tasks, and smallest tasks; not just running around busily being busy.

Source: Based on Wax, D. (2011). *Back to basics: Setting priorities.* Retrieved from http://www.lifehack.org/articles/productivity/back-to-basics-setting-priorities.html.

skill, learning to prioritize care will take practice (**Box 36–3** ●). When developing this skill, nurses have the advantage of being able to transfer other skills they have learned in nursing: assessment, critical thinking, clinical judgment, decision making, planning, implementation, and ongoing evaluation (see the Critical Thinking section earlier in this module for more information).

▶ IDENTIFYING WHAT TO PRIORITIZE

Similar to other service professions, nursing strives for quality productivity and client satisfaction. Three factors can influence client satisfaction with nursing care: availability of nursing staff to care for clients, the amount of time it takes nursing staff to meet clients' needs, and the quality of the care provided. Two qualities impact client perception of nursing care: **Effectiveness** (doing the right things) and **efficiency** (doing things right). Nurses employ effectiveness and efficiency by utilizing the strategies of setting priorities, managing time, and delegating to staff (see **Figure 36–21** ●). To support these qualities, nurses need to limit distractions and interruptions when providing client-centered care and treat all clients with respect and dignity.

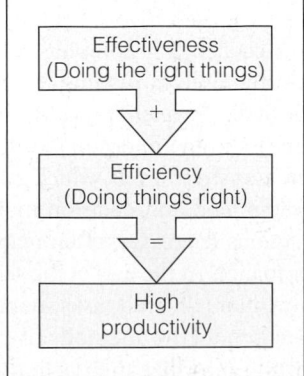

Figure 36–21 ● The high productivity equation.

Assessment

"Look before you leap" is a common saying that means one should have information about an activity or responsibility before proceeding to do it (UsingEnglish.com, 2011). Setting priorities for nursing care always begins with assessment. Assessment includes making observations and asking questions to gather the information necessary to make decisions. Helpful assessment data include the following:

- Observing for cues about pace and emotions of staff already working on the unit (e.g., are they relaxed or stressed?).
- After receiving information from the previous nurse in shift report, conducting one's own assessment by making a quick safety check of clients.
- Becoming aware of any clients who have an unstable status, a risk of change in their condition, or who require closer observation.
- Asking if there are any complexities to client problems.
- Asking about any special safety concerns for the clients (e.g., high risk for falls).
- Making note of routine responsibilities and interventions that have time constraints (e.g., physician rounds at 0900, medication administration at 1000 and 1200, nursing meeting at 1330).
- Knowing how many and what level of nursing staff are available for delegation of tasks to help with client care. Delegation is the transfer of responsibility and authority for completing an activity to a qualified individual (see the module on Managing Care for additional information), although accountability for the task remains with the nurse.
- Noting the presence (and absence) of necessary resources on the unit (e.g., linen, supplies, and nourishments).
- Asking about client preferences to take into consideration when providing care.

Airway, breathing, and circulation are vital for life. If a safety risk or physiological deterioration threatens any one of these functions, the situation may quickly become life threatening without prompt assessment and intervention. Nurses must be able to assess and prioritize threats to these functions as they arise (see **Box 36–4** ●).

The Nursing Process

Since the 1950s, the nursing process has been used as a method of organizing nursing care of clients. Assessment, the first step in the nursing process, provides subjective and objective client data. This information can then be clustered to identify nursing diagnoses appropriate for the client.

Based on nursing diagnoses, the nurse selects interventions and actions to achieve client outcomes for which the nurse has accountability. The steps in the nursing process provide a framework for nurses to use to determine priorities when working with a single client or a group of clients. These steps are assessment, nursing diagnosis, planning, implementation, and

Box 36–4 Priority Assessment of Safety Risks and Physiological Deterioration

A nurse walks into a client's room and finds the client pulling out his tracheostomy tube. Another nurse walking down the hallway passes the visitor's waiting room and finds a child client climbing up a high metal file cabinet. A third nurse finds her client unresponsive, not breathing, and without a pulse. These situations involve safety and physiological deterioration; all require prompt assessment for the potential to become life threatening. Removal of the tracheostomy tube could leave the client without a patent airway; the child client could cause the file cabinet to fall and possibly crush his head; and the client who is unresponsive with no respirations or pulse could die within minutes. Nurses continuously assess clients in their environments to recognize harmful situations. If the client is in danger, intervention becomes a priority.

The mnemonic *ABCs* represents the essential functions of airway, breathing, and circulation. It provides a guideline for use when assessing a client. An initial assessment of basic body functions necessary to sustain life precludes a more definitive assessment or any client intervention (discussed in the module on Perfusion). The initial **ABC** assessment includes:

Airway: A patent airway so oxygen will have a pathway into the lungs for gas exchange and carbon dioxide can be expelled from the body

Breathing: An effective breathing pattern and respiratory effort to take in enough oxygen to meet cellular demands for oxygen throughout the body

Circulation: An effective circulatory system to deliver oxygen throughout the body and allow carbon dioxide removal through the pulmonary circulatory network.

Nurses working in a variety of settings follow prioritization emergency protocols developed by the American Heart Association (AHA) to standardize cardiopulmonary resuscitation (CPR) for each step. Since its development, the ABCs of CPR have been enhanced and/or altered by various specialty groups and professional organizations, adding more letters or changing the meaning of the letters. For example, in 2010, the AHA rearranged the ABCs of CPR interventions to CAB, to stand for chest compressions, airway, and breathing. In addition to changing the order of the letters, they changed the meaning of the C to compressions instead of circulation (Berg et al., 2010; Kunz, 2011).

Another popular enhancement to the basic ABCs mnemonic is to add a D at the end, creating **ABCD** to help define other priority emergency assessments to complete. The meaning of D varies from one organization to another, but D may stand for:

- **D**efibrillation (use an automatic electronic defibrillator for an absent pulse)
- **D**eficiency (assess for sensory or neurological changes)
- **D**eadly bleeding (assess for massive hemorrhaging and shock)
- **D**isability (assess for spinal cord trauma and injury with movement or sensory deficits) (American College of Surgeons Committee on Trauma, 2012; Webster's Online Dictionary, 2011).

The few seconds taken by the nurse to assess for a patent airway, effective breathing pattern, and effective circulation system are essential. If life-threatening problems are found on assessment, the nurse can then intervene with appropriate nursing actions. When initiated immediately, these interventions can positively affect client outcomes by preventing complications, resolving a deteriorating condition, or saving a life.

Assessment of airway, breathing, and circulation can be done very quickly by observing the client. Is the client awake? Moving? Talking? Responding? If there is no problem with airway, breathing, or circulation, a nurse can move on to a more holistic assessment to identify other client needs. Assessment may include lung sounds, heart sounds, sensorium, emotional status, and psychological status.

---

evaluation (see the exemplar on the Nursing Process within this module for further information).

The National Council of State Boards of Nursing (NCSBN) provides models for states to use when revising their nursing practice acts and nursing administrative rules. The sections covering the scope of nursing practice and standards of nursing practice list the steps of the nursing process to develop a nursing plan of care. These sections also support accountability for clinical judgments, decision making, critical thinking, and competence of interventions in the course of nursing practice (prioritizing care and performing interventions) (NCSBN, 2011). See **Box 36–5** ● for two examples of state rules about prioritization of care.

Maslow's Hierarchy of Needs

A well-known way to organize client needs is according to Maslow's hierarchy of needs, typically displayed as a triangle with five levels (see the module on Stress and Coping for further information). Beginning at the bottom of the triangle, the levels of need progress from the most basic physiological needs to more complex psychological and social needs at the top. The most basic needs include food, air, water, shelter, elimination, and sleep (Cherry, 2011).

Maslow believed that these needs motivate behaviors. The first four needs, physiological, safety, social, and esteem needs, are sometimes called "deficiency needs" and indicate the client is experiencing deprivation related to one of those four needs. Needs on the lower levels must be met before an individual can move to higher levels. The last need, self-actualization, is called a "being need," and does not result from a deficiency, but rather indicates a desire for growth as an individual (Cherry, 2011).

Maslow ranked his hierarchy of needs with highest priorities on the first (bottom) level and lowest priorities on the last (top) level. Nurses can use Maslow's hierarchy as they establish priorities of client care. For example, ineffective breathing pattern,

Box 36–5 Examples of Board of Nursing Rules Addressing Prioritization of Care

NORTH CAROLINA BOARD OF NURSING

21 NCAC 36.0224 Components of Nursing Practice for the Registered Nurse

(c) Planning
    (1) Components of planning include prioritizing nursing diagnoses and needs.
(d) Implementation
    (3) Prioritizing and performing nursing interventions.
                    (North Carolina Board of Nursing, 2010)

TENNESSEE BOARD OF NURSING

1000-1-.14 Standards of Nursing Competence
(1) (a). 2. Establish critical paths and teaching plans based on individual patient's plans of care after prioritizing need upon completion of a comprehensive assessment.
                    (Tennessee Board of Nursing, 2007)

a physiological need, takes priority over a disturbed body image, an esteem need.

The nursing process and Maslow's hierarchy of needs can be used to think critically about the order in which client needs should be addressed. Nurses can then use their clinical judgment to make decisions about ranking client needs as low, medium, and high priorities.

LOW PRIORITY Problems that typically can be resolved easily with minimal interventions and do not cause significant dysfunction are included in the low-priority category. For example, responding to a client's request for a midafternoon snack could be delegated to unlicensed assistive personnel (UAP).

MEDIUM PRIORITY These are problems that may result in unhealthy physical or emotional consequences but which are not life threatening. For example, the nurse could ask a client who exhibits spiritual distress by saying that God has forgotten about her if she would like to have a hospital chaplain come visit.

HIGH PRIORITY This category includes life-threatening problems of airway, breathing, and circulation, or conditions that have a potential to become life threatening within a short amount of time (Scribd.com, 2011). An example of a high-priority intervention is the frequent monitoring for unexpected changes of the vital signs and drainage in a client who has just had a chest tube inserted. See **Table 36–19** ● for examples of nursing diagnoses for clients experiencing low-, medium-, and high-priority circumstances.

▶ CATEGORIZING PRIORITIES

Nurses must set priorities for nursing activities and interventions using assessment data and considering the category of the intervention: low, medium, or high priority. In addition, nurses must consider other priorities, including time constraints and the significance of the activities and interventions on client outcomes. The urgency factor model will help nurses learn how to rank priorities based on time imperatives and severity of client needs.

Time Constraints

When setting priorities, it is important to remember that some nursing interventions have **time constraints**, or deadlines for completion. One common intervention bound by time constraints is the administration of scheduled medications. Setting priorities for care includes planning to do things at expected times to avoid potential negative consequences for clients (McNutt, 2011).

The Urgency Factor

Organizing times to provide nursing care is influenced by the urgency factor. The word *urgency* means it is important to act immediately; there is a pressing importance that requires speedy action (Definitions.net, 2011). **Time priority** means a time constraint is present when completing actions. The **urgency factor** is a way to illustrate how much time can safely lapse before doing interventions without compromising client outcomes. Do all nursing interventions have a high urgency factor so everything a nurse does needs to be done immediately? Can some actions be done within a short amount of time and others delayed for a longer period of time without negative consequences for the client?

Changes in the client's condition, deterioration of status, or the complexities of a client's condition can impact the urgency of care interventions and the order in which they need to be completed. Four levels comprise the urgency factor. These levels progress from not urgent (a low time priority) to high urgency (the highest time priority). Using these levels can assist nurses in setting priorities for care by helping them identify what interventions need to be done and in what order they should be accomplished. See **Figure 36–22** ● and the following sections for a diagram and discussion of the urgency levels when setting time priorities.

NONACUTE Interventions with a low urgency factor may be termed *nonacute*. A delay in providing these interventions would not negatively impact client outcomes. Interventions at this level do not take priority. For example, at the beginning of a shift, the nurse could talk with a client to schedule a later time to teach him about changing a dressing.

ACUTE *Acute* interventions are often considered medium priority: There is a low potential for the client's condition to become life threatening if these interventions are not accomplished within a short amount of time. Typically these are actions that nurses are expected to complete to meet identified client needs. Interventions at this level can be scheduled during the shift when time constraints of higher priority interventions allow. For example, a nurse can schedule with unlicensed assistive personnel to turn and reposition a client with impaired bed mobility every 2 hours to prevent skin breakdown.

CRITICAL This level is considered medium-high urgency: There is an urgent need for the nurse to respond quickly to high-priority physical or psychological problems within a short

TABLE 36–19 Examples of NANDA Nursing Diagnoses for Clients Experiencing Low-, Medium-, and High-Priority Circumstances

LOW PRIORITY	MEDIUM PRIORITY	HIGH PRIORITY
Readiness for Enhanced Self-Concept	Anxiety	Ineffective Airway Clearance
Fatigue	Diarrhea	Impaired Gas Exchange
Ineffective Health Maintenance	Acute Confusion	Impaired Spontaneous Ventilation
Disturbed Body Image	Disturbed Sleep Pattern	Ineffective Breathing Pattern
Deficient Knowledge	Impaired Bed Mobility	Risk for Bleeding
Powerlessness	Ineffective Coping	Decreased Cardiac Output
Interrupted Family Processes	Self-Care Deficit	Risk for Decreased Cerebral Tissue Perfusion

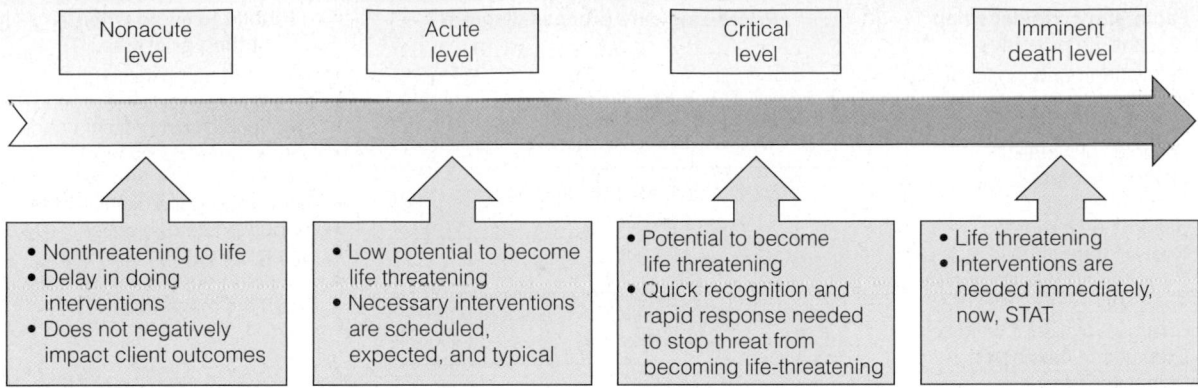

Figure 36–22 ● Urgency factor levels for setting time priorities.

amount of time because there is a potential for a client's condition to become more serious and even life threatening if interventions are delayed. Quick recognition and a rapid response time are necessary to prevent further exacerbation of the client's problem. For example, a client develops shortness of breath and air hunger from smoke inhalation. If the client does not receive high-flow supplemental oxygen, the client may develop impaired gas exchange problems that may progress to severe hypoxemia and become life threatening.

IMMINENT DEATH   The highest urgency factor is *imminent death*. The time to take action to prevent threat to life takes priority over everything else. When the client's airway is obstructed, the client stops breathing, or the client's heart becomes ineffective in pumping blood through the circulatory system, immediate intervention is necessary to try to save the client's life. The nurse must act now, STAT, to prevent further deterioration and threat to life.

Of course there are countless possible life-threatening situations. For example, a client on suicide precautions is holding a knife against his neck and is threatening to kill himself. Immediate actions must be taken to try and prevent him from harming, and possibly, killing himself. Nurses are always on alert for situations that could result in life and death for clients. Many of the more common situations, including medication errors, identification of client errors, and other safety issues, are identified in the National Patient Safety Goals (see the module on Safety for additional information).

Ranking Activities

Learning how to set priorities is the key to getting organized and using time to full advantage (Sander, 2011). Nurses can set priorities by thinking in terms of these categories: "must do," "should do," and "nice to do."

PRIORITY 1 OR MUST DO   These activities carry the highest priority for completion, take priority over other interventions, and must be done. For example, suctioning secretions from a tracheostomy tube to keep a client's airway patent is a *must do* priority.

PRIORITY 2 OR SHOULD DO   These activities should be done, but are not essential. These interventions can be accomplished once *must do* activities have been completed or covered. For example, restocking dressing supplies in the room

of a client who needs frequent dressing changes is a *should do* priority.

PRIORITY 3 OR NICE TO DO   These activities are important to complete, but only after priority 1 and 2 actions have been completed. These actions can be done when time is available, but they are not essential. For example, calling a family member for the client to ask her to bring the client's hairbrush to the hospital falls in this category (Sander, 2011).

Other categories can be used to rank priorities. Putting priorities in order according to significance or urgency can be done using a variety of category names. See **Table 36–20** ● for examples of category names.

Triage

In emergency departments, emergency situations, and prehospital care, the process of identifying priorities for implementing care is called **triage**. Triage allows nurses and other healthcare staff to set priorities based on the severity and urgency of a client's illness, injury, and condition (see the module on Healthcare Systems for additional information). Common categories used to set priorities are discussed next.

EMERGENT (OR IMMEDIATE)   This category is for life-threatening issues that require prompt treatment and care. Stabilization of the client's condition is critical. For example, a trauma client with a blood pressure of 88/56 mmHg and pulse of 108 bpm is emergent.

URGENT (OR DELAYED)   This category is for serious health conditions in which a delay of treatment and care would not result in life-threatening situations. For example, a client who complains about having a productive cough for the past 4 days is urgent.

TABLE 36–20   Examples of Common Names for Priority Categories

PRIORITY 1	PRIORITY 2	PRIORITY 3
Need to do	Try to do	May not do
Vital to do	Important to do	May not do
Must do	Should do	Nice to do
High priority	Medium priority	Low priority
Most important	Less important	Least important

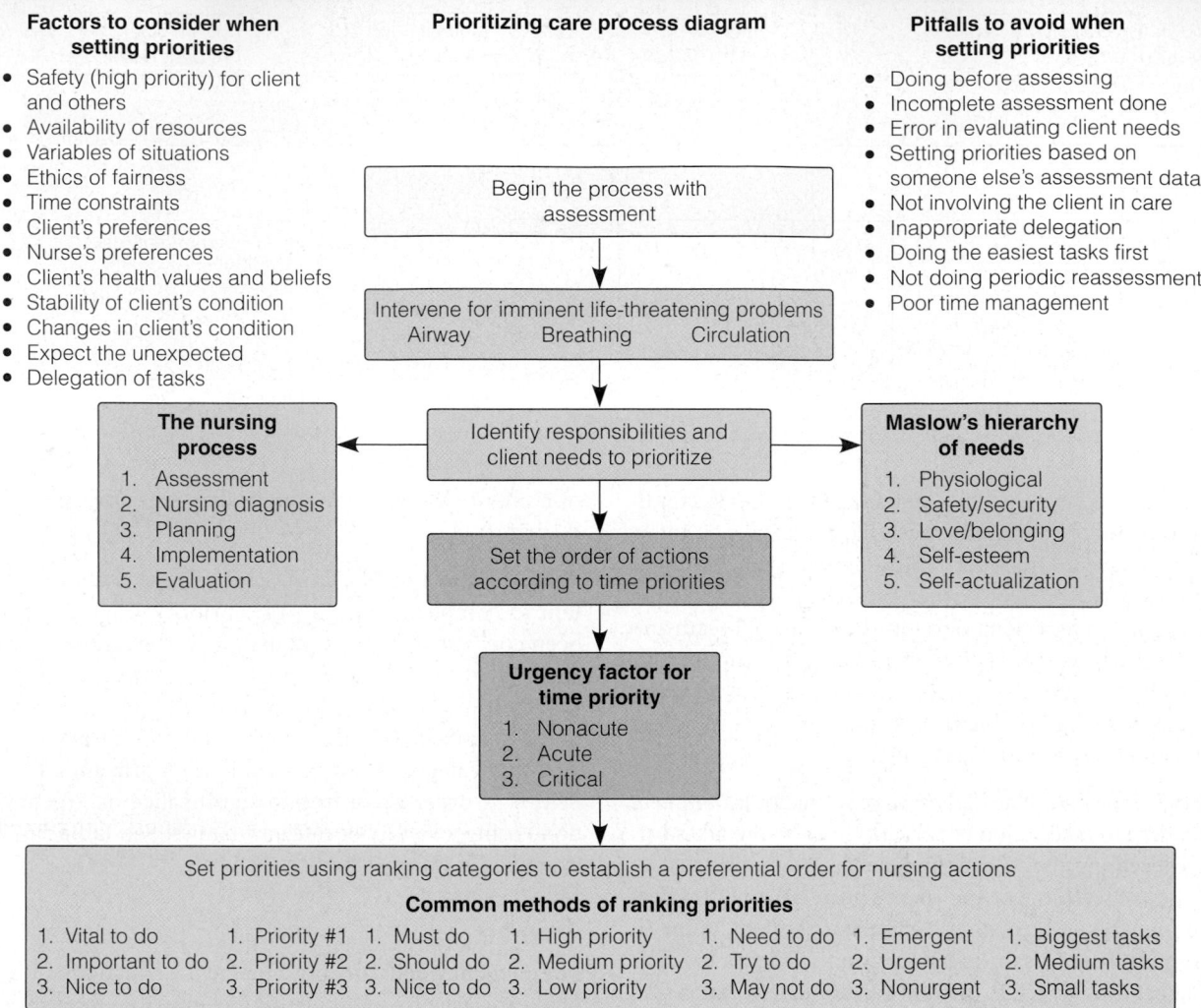

Factors to consider when setting priorities

- Safety (high priority) for client and others
- Availability of resources
- Variables of situations
- Ethics of fairness
- Time constraints
- Client's preferences
- Nurse's preferences
- Client's health values and beliefs
- Stability of client's condition
- Changes in client's condition
- Expect the unexpected
- Delegation of tasks

Prioritizing care process diagram

Begin the process with assessment

Intervene for imminent life-threatening problems
Airway   Breathing   Circulation

Identify responsibilities and client needs to prioritize

Set the order of actions according to time priorities

Urgency factor for time priority
1. Nonacute
2. Acute
3. Critical

Pitfalls to avoid when setting priorities

- Doing before assessing
- Incomplete assessment done
- Error in evaluating client needs
- Setting priorities based on someone else's assessment data
- Not involving the client in care
- Inappropriate delegation
- Doing the easiest tasks first
- Not doing periodic reassessment
- Poor time management

The nursing process
1. Assessment
2. Nursing diagnosis
3. Planning
4. Implementation
5. Evaluation

Maslow's hierarchy of needs
1. Physiological
2. Safety/security
3. Love/belonging
4. Self-esteem
5. Self-actualization

Set priorities using ranking categories to establish a preferential order for nursing actions

Common methods of ranking priorities

1. Vital to do	1. Priority #1	1. Must do	1. High priority	1. Need to do	1. Emergent	1. Biggest tasks
2. Important to do	2. Priority #2	2. Should do	2. Medium priority	2. Try to do	2. Urgent	2. Medium tasks
3. Nice to do	3. Priority #3	3. Nice to do	3. Low priority	3. May not do	3. Nonurgent	3. Small tasks

Figure 36–23 ● Prioritizing care process diagram.

NONURGENT (OR MINOR) Clients in this category have minor issues that do not require prompt care. Many of these clients can ambulate and are stable in their conditions. For example, a client with a splinter in his foot that needs to be removed is nonurgent.

See **Figure 36–23** ● for a diagram of the prioritization of care process.

▶ FACTORS TO CONSIDER WHEN PRIORITIZING CARE

Prioritization means more than just making decisions about which interventions to do first, second, third, and so forth. The assumption that nurses accomplish all of the things they want or need to do for all of their clients regardless of what order they do them in is no longer true. In some situations, nurses cannot get everything done within an allotted period of time. When nurses experience demands on their services that exceed the time available, they must be able to set priorities of care. Because of this, prioritization sometimes means the most important interventions get done, activities of lesser priority *may* get done, and the least important actions *may not get done at all* due to insufficient time to complete them.

Prioritizing care in and of itself does not result in nurses being more productive in a given time period. Interventions take the same amount of time to complete regardless of the order in which they are done. Multitasking and learning to do things faster can improve effectiveness and efficiency.

Ethics

A holistic approach to nursing means caring for the physical, psychological, spiritual, cultural, emotional, and developmental needs of clients. Often, clients have many more needs than nurses are able to meet. The principle of *justice* guides nurses in making decisions about setting priorities (see the module on Ethics). Nurses can show *fairness* in treating individuals as equals. The difference among clients is the urgency of needs; for example, a life-threatening situation will take priority over a psychosocial problem. Decisions are sometimes based on consideration of which actions will result in the best outcomes for the client (Pinch & Haddad, 2008).

Safety

Protecting clients and providing a safe environment for them is another aspect of justice. Safety in doing no harm to clients is a professional behavior (see the module on Professional Behaviors for further information). The Institute of Medicine (2011) published a document about the need to improve safety for clients that led to the National Patient Safety Goals developed by the Joint Commission. For example, it is a high priority to administer medications to clients safely (see the module on Safety for additional information).

Nurses can be fair in their allocation of time, attention, and skills to ensure client safety. Unrealistic demands on nurses' own physical and emotional abilities may result in nurses minimizing what they can do for their clients and may lead to feelings of dissatisfaction and exhaustion. Nurses' desire to help clients requires an environment that supports the delivery of quality care.

Availability of Resources

Resources are assets that help nurses meet client needs. Problems arise when necessary resources are not available in the required quantity. Rationing or making decisions about which clients will receive the available resources may result and may require prioritization. For example, a linen cart that has not been replenished leaves everyone without enough towels, washcloths, and gowns for clients. A nurse's creativity and resourcefulness can be valuable in finding solutions, such as borrowing the needed linen from another nursing unit and replenishing it when new linen arrives on the unit.

Time Management

Time priorities are determined by the urgency of completing the interventions for the clients. As they progress in proficiency, nurses develop a sense about how long it takes to complete certain interventions for clients, which helps them learn how to manage time better. Part of developing good time management is taking into account specific considerations, such as client health preferences, changes in client's condition, unexpected occurrences, and appropriate delegation of tasks.

Multiple Clients

Nurses generally take care of more than one client at a time. Nurses can identify and plan interventions for all clients based on assessments of assigned individual client needs, changes in client status, and complexity of client problems. Setting priorities is determined by the significance of the interventions for each of the individual clients. Time constraints such as medication administration for multiple clients would require more organization and focus from the nurse to complete within an allotted time frame. The pathophysiology of the individual clients would also require consideration when setting priorities among the assigned clients.

Client Preferences

Clients are unique individuals who grow and develop as a result of genetic and environmental factors. Although clients share many similarities, such as the need for oxygen, they differ in terms of cultural rituals, spiritual practices, and routines of daily living. Some of these practices have time constraints, such as praying at specific times of day.

Health practices and beliefs of clients may conflict with some physicians' orders. Helping a client maintain cultural or religious practices without compromising the client's treatment plan sometimes requires extra effort on the part the nursing staff. The goal is to strive for a win–win situation by honoring the client's wishes as much as possible and completing nursing interventions as needed. Working together for a mutually beneficial solution strengthens the client–nurse relationship.

Prioritizing activities for the day can be done with most clients. The client's individual preferences and expectations of care can help set time priorities. For example, some clients may prefer to have a shower in the evening instead of the morning. The client can plan individual activities around nursing actions that are scheduled at certain times. For example, if the client knows he needs to get medications at 1000 and 1400, he could schedule his walk down the hall at 1100. Activities the client considers as priorities may differ from the ranking of priorities by the nurse. By assessing for client preferences, nurses can help strengthen client participation in and support for the plan of care, resulting in improved client outcomes and a more positive experience for the client.

Change in Client Condition

Clients need to be monitored continuously for changing circumstances. Assessing clients at 1200 and reporting on them at 1900 without reassessing them means 7 hours have elapsed in which one or more clients have likely experienced a change of status without reassessment by the nurse. This may result in the nurse receiving the shift report being given inaccurate or incomplete data about the client.

Nurses depend on each other to let them know of problems and changes in their clients. Assessment is an ongoing process to recognize changes and provide appropriate interventions early. When a client's condition changes or becomes unstable, the earlier it is discovered and addressed, the more quickly nurses and the healthcare team can intervene and prevent further deterioration. A change in client status may very well require reevaluating priorities and changing the planned order of interventions. Revising priorities is especially important when planning care for multiple clients.

The Unexpected

Things do not always go as planned. It would be nice if nurses could depend on the initial schedule they set at the beginning of the shift, and then be able to follow that plan throughout the day. The reality is that, on most days, nurses have to deal with unexpected things, or "**pop-ups**," that require their time and attention and take them away from their plan for the day. For example, a new admission to the unit, a client whose blood pressure is dropping, or a client complaining of shortness of breath all take precedence over interventions such as teaching a client about food choices for a low-salt diet, changing a dressing for a surgical client, or any number of other nursing interventions. Pop-ups can challenge the time management and organizational skills of the most experienced nurses. (See **Box 36–6** ● for an analogy.)

Nurse Self-Care

It may sound simple to plan times for a quick 15-minute break and a 30-minute meal break at the beginning of a shift. However, when it is time for nurses to take a break, they often are busy with their clients or other responsibilities; because breaks are not considered a priority, they do not always happen. "I'll go when I finish this" may be a never-ending refrain.

A short time away for self-care can provide quality time to refresh, reenergize, and take care of body functions (drink some water, eat some food, go to the restroom, or do some stretching). Finding a few quiet minutes can help break up the intensity of the work environment and relieve stress for nurses (Nelson, 2010).

Delegation

Delegating tasks to other nursing staff, such as LPNs and UAPs, can improve time management, especially if there is a shortage of RNs. Nurses must be aware, however, of the legal responsibilities involved in delegating a task. The delegated task must be within the scope of practice for the nursing staff asked to do it. The nurse delegating the task must evaluate the task on completion (Maji, 2009).

▶ PITFALLS OF PRIORITIZATION

Nurses should learn to avoid pitfalls when prioritizing care. A **pitfall** is a hidden trap that catches people unaware and undermines their plans (Collins English Dictionary, 2009). Although nurses may not know all of the possible pitfalls, there are some pitfalls that they can learn to recognize and avoid. When nurses follow ethical practices, utilize available resources, know the health concerns of their clients, have a sense about client priorities, and prioritize care appropriately, they can avoid many pitfalls. Common pitfalls are described in the following sections.

Prioritizing Without Assessment

Nurses need as much information as they can gather about their assigned clients, especially when they are assigned more than one client. When providing care to multiple clients, nurses must consider interventions for all clients separately and set priorities. Without assessment, the important first step in the prioritization process, nurses may forget important interventions or provide interventions based on old data. Clients may suffer severe consequences as a result.

INCOMPLETE ASSESSMENT   Part of knowing how to do an assessment is learning what information is required to set priorities for client care. Accurate and timely information about client status, resources, available nursing staff, time constraints, and complexity of interventions is needed to prioritize care. If any of these are not assessed first, nurses will fail to include important and necessary information when setting priorities.

RELYING SOLELY ON ANOTHER'S ASSESSMENT Obtaining assessment data from another nurse, such as during shift report, can provide insight and give a picture of how a client has been during the previous shift. However, using only this information to set priorities, without also making one's own quick assessment, may negatively affect client outcomes.

FAILING TO DO PERIODIC REASSESSMENTS   Reassessment allows the nurse to adjust the time and order of actions to support completing interventions and activities on time and in order of importance. Sometimes the unexpected happens, taking the nurse in another direction and interrupting planned activities. Examples of these situations include a change in a client's condition, arrival of a new client who needs to be admitted to the unit, and a request from a relative or visitor to speak with the nurse. Periodic reassessments give the nurse a sense of the time available to do things, what things still need to be done, and when to allow for changes in prioritization that may be necessary to complete the plan for the day.

Poor Time Management

Time management can be difficult to master for nurses, especially for those who do not check their watches every couple of hours to take a reading of where they are in terms of getting things done. Nurses may find that some actions have taken longer than expected to complete, while others have taken less time. Some actions have time constraints that may not be altered. Time management is essential to ensuring that priority tasks are accomplished in a timely manner and that the nurse remains productive during the shift. See **Box 36–7** ● for suggestions on managing time.

Not Involving Clients in Their Care

Nurses assess and determine client needs when setting priorities and are accountable for planning and carrying out interventions, but it is a mistake not to include the client in planning her own care. Clients have preferences in how they do things, when they want things to happen, and what they want to do. Preferences may be a result of culture, family influences or preferences, spirituality, or heritage. Asking clients about their needs is a way to recognize their individuality and deliver client-

Box 36–7   Time Management Suggestions

AT HOME, THE NIGHT BEFORE YOUR SHIFT:

1. Make a list of scheduled medication administration times (i.e., 0730, 0800, 1000, 1200, 1400, and 1600).
2. Under each time, list expected client interventions that will happen close to the times (i.e., meals, safety checks, IV checks, pain management checks, physician rounds, AM care, and documentation). This is the blueprint to follow for managing your time.
3. If you know of any procedures you may need to do the next day, review and visualize how to do them so you will be prepared and not use time the next day to refresh on the procedure (e.g., giving an IV piggyback medication, inserting a Foley catheter).

AT THE BEGINNING OF YOUR SHIFT:

1. Eat something before arriving; arrive early to put your things away.
2. Listen to the change-of-shift report to get a sense of how your day may go (acuity of clients assigned, problems you may have, clients who may require more time, etc.).
3. Add any time constraint activities to your blueprint (e.g., a meeting you need to attend).
4. Make safety check rounds on your clients to assess for additional information.
5. Begin setting priorities for client care. Remember to include the urgency factor for time priorities. Delegate tasks to nursing staff working with you as appropriate. Remember to list actions you may not want to do as priorities to do early and check off your to-do list.
6. Become more aware of time by checking your watch every couple of hours to get a sense of where you are with completing your activities.
7. Keep a notepad handy in a pocket to makes notes about everything you do or want to remember later. This will help you be more accurate than relying on memory. These notes will be useful when it is documentation time or reporting off time (Carla M, 2011).
8. Reprioritize your time as needed when pop-ups or unplanned events occur.
9. Check your progress in completing your to-do list throughout the shift. Reprioritize activities as needed.
10. Celebrate your success as you complete priority interventions.

Box 36–8   QSEN Competencies and Prioritizing Care

The Quality and Safety Education for Nurses project has identified six competencies necessary for nurses to improve the quality and safety of healthcare systems. This exemplar supports the following QSEN competencies for nursing program graduates:

1. *Client-centered care* through partnering with clients and including their preferences, values, and needs when setting priorities of care
2. *Evidence-based practice* through critical thinking and clinical judgments based on best evidence into practice for setting priorities of care
3. *Teamwork & collaboration* with nursing staff members for communication and shared decision making to achieve quality client care in a timely manner.

Source: Quality and Safety Education for Nurses. (2010). *Competency KSAs (prelicensure).* Retrieved from http://www.qsen.org/ksas_prelicensure.php.

not remove accountability for the outcome from the nurse. Inappropriate delegation may result in the nurse having to do an intervention over or may even result in harm to the client. Inappropriate delegation can have immediate ramifications for client care.

Doing the Easiest Tasks First

Setting priorities means determining what actions are more important than others in a given order. It is a planned process that takes practice to become competent in doing. Completing easy tasks before doing important, necessary tasks does not make good, professional common sense. Nurses provide intentional planned services of care to meet client needs that result in positive client outcomes.

▶ SUMMARY

Prioritizing care requires nurses to make decisions about using time, personnel, and resources to provide nursing care to one or more clients in an organized, sensible manner. Nurses make clinical judgments about how clients will be affected by nursing interventions identified and delivered as high-, medium-, or low-priority interventions. Setting priorities is a skill that nurses must learn and practice to become more effective and efficient, and it directly impacts client care and safety. National competencies for nurses developed by a variety of professional organizations and initiatives, including the Quality and Safety Education for Nurses project, reflect the importance of prioritization (see **Box 36–8** ●). A skill deficit in this area can impede best practices and have serious consequences for client outcomes.

centered nursing care. Observing client behaviors can also provide the nurse with cues about time and order preferences clients may have.

Inappropriate Delegation

As discussed previously, nurses must follow certain rules when delegating tasks to others (see the module on Managing Care for further information). Other nursing staff, LPNs, and UAPs can assist in completing tasks for clients if the tasks are within the scope of practice found in their state's nurse practice act. Transferring responsibility for a task to an LPN or UAP does

REVIEW   Prioritizing Care

RELATE Link the Concepts and Exemplars

Linking the exemplar of prioritizing care with the concept of clinical decision making:

1. What are some commonalities between these two nursing processes?

Linking the exemplar of prioritizing care with the concept of safety:

2. Why is safety a high priority for clients that have *Risk for . . .* nursing diagnoses?

Linking the exemplar of prioritizing care with the concept of professional behaviors:

3. What aspects of setting priorities for care are professional behaviors for nurses?

Linking the exemplar of prioritizing care with the concept of managing care:

4. Name some ways setting priorities for care contributes to improved management of care.

REFER Go to Pearson Nursing Student Resources nursing.pearsonhighered.com

- Additional review materials

REFLECT Case Study

You have been assigned to take care of Mr. J. Rodriguez, a 48-year-old male client, during clinical from 0645–1300. This client was admitted to the medical unit yesterday with bilateral pneumonia. He has a history of shortness of breath and exertional dyspnea for the past week. He states he has had a productive cough for the past 4 days, with green, foul-smelling thick sputum. He complains of chest pain when he has to cough. His appetite is diminished and he is not drinking very much because he says he is too tired. He also states he was not able to go to work the 2 days before he was admitted to the hospital. Mr. Rodriguez lives with his wife and four children. His wife speaks very little English. His last set of vital signs were temperature 102.2°F, pulse 98 bpm, respirations 22/min; blood pressure 134/86 mmHg. He is friendly, quiet, and wants to get better. He is in no distress at this time.

Physician orders include:

- IV D_5 1/2NS with 20 mEq KCl at 100 mL/hr
- Rocephin 1 gram IV piggyback every 12 hours
- I&O every shift
- Vital signs every 4 hours, including pulse oximetry
- Out of bed to chair with help
- Regular diet, encourage fluids
- Use an incentive spirometer twice during the day
- Oxygen via nasal cannula at 2 LPM oxygen.

Nursing interventions include:

- Assisting with bath and morning care as needed
- Changing bed linens on client's bed
- Administering medications at 0800, 1000, 1200, and one PRN
- Assisting with breakfast as needed at 0800
- Assisting with lunch as needed at 1230
- Doing a 60-second client safety check every 2 hours
- Doing a complete assessment on the client early morning
- Reassessing the client's condition every 4 hours
- Doing vital signs at 0800 and 1200
- Assisting the client with incentive spirometer during morning hours
- Encouraging the client to drink fluids
- Checking for new physician orders
- Checking for diagnostic tests results
- Listening to report from previous shift nurse
- Assisting client in menu selection for tomorrow's meals
- Teaching the client how to splint his chest with a pillow when he needs to cough to prevent chest muscles from hurting with coughing
- Documenting in client's chart throughout the day
- Checking the client's IV every 4 hours
- Providing fresh ice water in the client's water pitcher
- Measuring and tallying the I&O for the client during the shift
- Assisting the client to get up to the chair in the morning and again in the afternoon.

List any additional interventions you would want to do with this client:

1.
2.
3.

Decide the priority of each of the above nursing interventions, both those listed and your own. Indicate your priority choice beside each one by writing a "1" for a high priority, a "2" for a medium priority, and a "3" for a low priority. Now decide which actions can be delegated to a UAP to assist in completing them all. Write a "D" beside the interventions that can be appropriately delegated to a UAP.

■ REFERENCES

American Association of Colleges of Nursing. (2008). *The essentials of baccalaureate education for professional nursing practice.* Retrieved from http://www.aacn.nche. edu/education-resources/baccessentials08.pdf.

American College of Surgeons Committee on Trauma. (2012). *Advanced trauma life support* (9th ed.). Chicago, IL: American College of Surgeons.

Benner, P. (2011). From novice to expert. *Current Nursing.* Retrieved from http://currentnursing.com/ nursing_theory/Patricia_Benner_From_Novice_ to_Expert.html.

Benner, P., Hughes, R. G., & Sutphen, M. (2008). Clinical reasoning, decisionmaking, and action: Thinking critically and clinically. In R. G. Hughes (Ed.), *Patient safety and quality: An evidence-based handbook for nurses* (Chap. 6). Rockville, MD: Agency for Healthcare Research and Quality. Retrieved from http://www.ncbi. nlm.nih.gov/books/NBK2643.

Benner, P., & Tanner, C. (1987). How expert nurses use intuition. *American Journal of Nursing, 87*(1), 23–31.

Benner, P., Tanner, C., & Chesla, C. (2009). *Expertise in nursing practice: Caring, clinical judgment and ethics* (2nd ed.). New York, NY: Springer.

Berg, R. A., Hemphill, R., Abella, B. S., Aufderheide, T. P., Cave, D. M., Hazinski, A. F., . . . Swor, R. A. (2010). Part

5: Adult basic life support: 2010 American Heart Association Guidelines for Cardiopulmonary Resuscitation and Emergency Cardiovascular Care. *Circulation, 122,* S685–S705. doi:10.1161/CIRCULATIONAHA. 110.197099.

Carla M. (2011). *Nursing time management: 3 Easy ways to reduce stress with time management in nursing.* Retrieved from http://hubpages.com/hub/Nursing-Time-Management.

Carrick, J., & Miehl, N. (2009). *Clinical judgment development and the use of simulation.* Retrieved from http:// www.hpsn.com/_assets/dynamic_media/media_bank/ hpsn09/workshop-resources/Clinical%20Judgment_ Presentation.pdf.

Casey, D. (2010, March). Lessons in machine effectiveness versus efficiency. *Peoria Magazine.* Retrieved from http://www.peoriamagazines.com/ibi/2010/mar/ lessons-_machine-effectiveness-versus-efficiency.

Cherry, K. (2011). *Hierarchy of needs: The five levels of Maslow's hierarchy of needs.* Retrieved from http:// psychology.about.com/od/theoriesofpersonality/a/ hierarchyneeds.htm.

College of Nurses of Ontario. (2012). *Developing SMART learning goals.* Retrieved from http://www.cno.org/ Global/docs/qa/DevelopingSMARTGoals.pdf.

Collins English Dictionary. (2009). *World English dictionary: Pitfall.* Retrieved from http://dictionary.reference. com/browse/pitfall.

Decision Making Confidence. (2013). *Definitions: Definition of decision making.* Retrieved from http://www. decision-making-confidence.com/decision-strategies. html.

Definitions.net. (2011). *Definitions for urgency.* Retrieved from http://www.definitions.net/definition/urgency.

DifferenceBetween.net. (2012). *Difference between inquiry and query.* Retrieved from http://www.differencebe-tween.net/language/words-language/difference-between-inquiry-and-query.

Education.com. (2013). *Inductive vs deductive reasoning help.* Retrieved from http://www.education.com/ study-help/article/working-arguments.

Elder, L., & Paul, R. (2011). Becoming a critic of your thinking, *Critical Thinking Community, Foundation of Critical Thinking.* Retrieved from http://www.criticalthinking. org/pages/becoming-a-crit-of-your-thinking/478.

Ferris State University. (2010). *Standards of professional nursing practice: ANA standards of practice.* Retrieved from http://www.ferris.edu/HTMLS/colleges/alliedhe/ Nursing/Standards-of-Professional-Nursing-Practice.htm.

Free Dictionary. (2012). *Intellect.* Retrieved from https://www.thefreedictionary.com/intellect.

Gordon, M. (2010). *Manual of nursing diagnoses* (12th ed.). Boston, MA: Jones & Bartlett.

Institute of Medicine. (2011, January 26). *The future of nursing: Focus on education.* Retrieved from http://www.iom.edu/Reports/2010/The-Future-of-Nursing-Leading-Change-Advancing-Health/Report-Brief-Education.aspx.

Kunz, M. (2011). *A new order for CPR, spelled C-A-B: American Heart Association guidelines.* Retrieved from http://thenurseeducator.com/blog/2011/06/22/a-new-order-for-cpr-spelled-c-a-b-american-heart-association-guidelines.

Lasater, K. (2007). Clinical judgment development: Using simulation to create an assessment rubric. *Journal of Nursing Education, 46*(11), 496–503. Retrieved from http://www.oclbcp.org/Documents/Simulation%20articles/lassiter.pdf.

Lorcher, T. (2012). *Examples of faulty reasoning.* Retrieved from http://www.brighthubeducation.com/high-school-english-lessons/25583-examples-of-faulty-reasoning.

Maji, A. (2009, June). Prioritizing nursing care. *Yahoo! Contributor Network.* Retrieved from http://www.associatedcontent.com/article/1875911/prioritizing_nursing_care_pg2.html?cat=4.

Mann, J. (2010). *Promoting curriculum choices: Critical thinking and clinical judgment skill development in baccalaureate nursing students.* Retrieved from http://kuscholarworks.ku.edu/dspace/handle/1808/6742.

McNutt, B. (2011). *Nursing tips: How to organize and prioritize your shift.* Retrieved from http://ezinearticles.com/?Nursing-Tips---How-to-Organize-and-Prioritize-Your-Shift&id=2068559.

Merriam-Webster. (2011). *Priority.* Retrieved from http://www.merriam-webster.com/dictionary/priority.

My Nursing Uniforms. (2011). *Exploring the sixth sense in nursing: Intuition.* Retrieved from http://blog.mynursinguniforms.com/index.php/exploring-the-sixth-sense-in-nursing-intuition.

NANDA International. (2009). *NANDA nursing diagnoses: Definitions and classification 2009–2011.* Chichester, West Sussex, United Kingdom: Wiley-Blackwell.

NANDA International. (2011). *NANDA-I nursing diagnosis resources.* Retrieved from http://www.nanda.org/NursingDiagnosisFAQ.aspx.

NANDA International. (2013). *Glossary of terms: Nursing diagnoses.* Retrieved from http://www.nanda.org/DiagnosisDevelopment/DiagnosisSubmission/PreparingYourSubmission/GlossaryofTerms.aspx.

National Council of State Boards of Nursing (NCSBN). (2010). *NCSBN Learning Extension: Sharpening critical thinking skills course.* Retrieved from www.ncsbn.org/learningext.com.

National Council of State Boards of Nursing (NCSBN). (2011). *NCSBN model nursing practice act and model nursing administrative rules.* Retrieved from https://www.ncsbn.org/Model_Nursing_Practice_Act_March36.pdf.

National League for Nursing. (2013). *Competencies for graduates of baccalaureate programs.* Retrieved from http://www.nln.org/facultyprograms/competencies/comp_bacc.htm.

Nelson, J. (2010, May). Helping new nurses set priorities. *American Nurse Today.* Retrieved from http://www.AmericanNurseToday.com.

North Carolina Board of Nursing. (2010). *RN scope of practice—Clarification.* Retrieved from https://www.ncbon.com/myfiles/downloads/position-statements-decision-trees/rn-position-statement.pdf.

Oelofsen, N. (2012). Using reflective practice in frontline nursing. *Nursing Times, 108,*(24), 22–24. Retrieved from http://www.nursingtimes.net/using-reflective-practice-in-frontline-nursing/5045779.article.

Ottawa Hospital. (2010). *Patient clinical pathway: Vaginal birth (mother and baby).* Retrieved from http://www.ottawahospital.on.ca/wps/wcm/connect/c02e93004b25b295936ed71faf30e8c1/Vaginal-Birth-MotherBaby-e.pdf?MOD=AJPERES.

Pinch, W. J. E., & Haddad, A. M. (2008). *Nursing and health care ethics: A legacy and a vision.* Silver Spring, MD: American Nurses Association.

Pivec, C., & Blazovich, L. (2012). Debriefing after simulation: Guidelines for faculty and students. *Human Patient Simulation Network.* Retrieved from http://www.hpsn.com/_assets/dynamic_media/media_bank/Pivec%20PPT%20Debriefing%20After%20Simulation%20FAC.pdf.

Quality and Safety Education for Nurses. (2010). *Competency KSAs (Prelicensure).* Retrieved from http://www.qsen.org/ksas_prelicensure.php.

Reagan, K. (2010). Scholarly paper on nursing intuition: A mode of clinical decision-making in nursing practice. *University of New Hampshire.* Retrieved from http://kaleighreagan.wordpress.com/academic-writing-samples/nurs-619-scholarly-paper.

Reimer, A., & Moore, S. (2010). Discussion paper: Flight nursing expertise—Towards a middle-range theory. *Journal of Advanced Nursing, 66*(5), 1183–1192.. Retrieved from http://fpb.case.edu/news/Docs/Reimer_Moore_flightnursing.pdf.

Roy, C. (2008). *The Roy adaptation model* (3rd ed.). Upper Saddle River, NJ: Prentice Hall.

Sander, S. (2011). *How to set priorities.* Retrieved from http://www.achieve-goal-setting-success.com/set-priorities.html.

Scribd.com. (2011). *Establishing priorities in the clinical setting.* Retrieved from http://www.scribd.com/doc/23193317/EstablishingPrioritiesintheClinicalSetting.

Tanner, C. (2006). Thinking like a nurse: A research-based model of clinical judgment in nursing. *Journal of Nursing Education, 45*(6), 204–210. Retrieved from http://jxzy.smu.edu.cn/jkpg/UploadFiles/file/TF_0692810354_thinking%20like%20a%20nurse.pdf.

Tennessee Board of Nursing. (2007). *Rules of the Tennessee board of nursing.* Retrieved from http://www.state.tn.us/sos/rules/1000/1000-01.pdf.

University Health System of Bexar County, San Antonio, Texas. (2013). *Algorithm A: Emergency management of adult asthma, and Algorithm B: Emergency management of pediatric asthma.* Retrieved from http://www.universityhealthsystem.com/files/01-UHS%20Emergency%20Center%20Asthma%20Guidelines%20(Adult,%20Pediatric,%20Drug%20Doses,%20Discharge%20Treatment%20Plan).pdf.

University of Iowa, College of Nursing. (2012). *Overview: Nursing Outcomes Classification (NOC).* Retrieved from http://www.nursing.uiowa.edu/cncce/nursing-outcomes-classification-overview.

University of Newcastle, Faculty of Health, School of Nursing and Midwifery. (2009). *Clinical reasoning: Instructor resources.* Retrieved from http://www.newcastle.edu.au/Resources/Projects/Nursing%20and%20Midwifery%20Projects/Clinical%20Reasoning/Resources/Clinical%20Reasoning%20Instructor%20Resources.pdf.

University of North Carolina at Pembroke. (2010). *Chapter 15. Documenting and reporting: Nursing care plans.* Retrieved from http://www.uncp.edu/nursing/lec/CH36.pdf.

UsingEnglish.com. (2011). *Idiom definitions for 'Look before you leap.'* Retrieved from http://www.usingenglish.com/reference/idioms/look+before+you+leap.html.

Wax, D. (2011). *Back to basics: Setting priorities.* Retrieved from http://www.lifehack.org/articles/productivity/back-to-basics-setting-priorities.html.

Webster's Online Dictionary. (2011). *Specialty expressions: ABCD.* Retrieved from http://www.websters-online-dictionary.org/definitions/ABCD.

37 Collaboration

MODULE AT-A-GLANCE

The Concept of Collaboration, 2375

Exemplar 37.1
Case Management, 2382

Exemplar 37.2
Conflict Resolution, 2387

Exemplar 37.3
Interdisciplinary Teams, 2391

◪ THE CONCEPT OF COLLABORATION

The nature of health care today is so complex that it is impossible for any single provider or professional to provide high-quality client care without working with others. The best care is delivered in a collaborative environment with all members of the healthcare team working to improve client health outcomes. **Collaboration** is defined as two or more individuals working toward a common goal by combining their skills, knowledge, and resources while avoiding duplication of effort. In a healthcare environment, the common goal of each collaborative team is to improve client outcomes, whether the client is an individual, a group, or a community.

The American Nurses Association (ANA) Standards of Professional Nursing Practice recognize collaboration as a key component of nursing. Standard 13 of the ANA Standards of Professional Nursing Practice outlines specific competencies related to the nurse's role in collaboration (ANA, 2010). Virginia Henderson (1991), one of the pioneers of nursing, defines collaborative care as "a partnership relationship between doctors, nurses, and other healthcare providers with patients and their families" (p. 44). Mutual respect and a true sharing of both power and control are essential elements. Ideally, collaboration becomes a dynamic, interactive process in which clients (individuals, groups, or communities) work together with physicians, nurses, and other healthcare providers to meet their health objectives. Effective collaboration requires cooperation and coordination among clients and various healthcare providers across the continuum of care (see Box 37–1 ●). ◀◀

Concept Learning Outcomes

After reading about this concept, you will be able to:

1. Examine the essential aspects of collaborative nursing practice.
2. Analyze factors that affect collaboration in health care.
3. Summarize the purpose and collaborative role of the case manager within the healthcare setting.
4. Compare strategies for conflict prevention, response, and management.
5. Differentiate between different types of interdisciplinary and intradisciplinary groups in nursing and healthcare delivery.

Concept Key Terms

Collaboration, *2375*

Communicator style, *2379*

Feedback, *2379*

Mutual respect, *2380*

Box 37–1 Characteristics and Beliefs Basic to Collaborative Health Care

- Clients have a right to self-determination—that is, the right to choose to participate or not to participate in healthcare decision making.
- Clients and healthcare professionals interact in a reciprocal relationship. Instead of making decisions about the client's health care, healthcare professionals engage in joint decision making with the client.
- Equality among human beings is desired in collaborative healthcare relationships. The ideas of both clients and healthcare professionals receive an equal hearing.
- Responsibility for the client's health falls on the client rather than on healthcare professionals.
- Each individual's concept of health is important and legitimate for that individual. Although clients lack expert knowledge, they have their own ideas about health and illness. Healthcare professionals need to understand these ideas to be able to effectively help the client.
- Collaboration involves negotiating and seeking consensus rather than questioning and ordering.

▶ THE NURSE AS COLLABORATOR

Collaboration may occur between nurses, between healthcare providers and clients, and between healthcare providers from different professional backgrounds. According to the ANA (2010), collaboration in nursing practice includes identifying and acknowledging the expertise of individuals both within and outside one's profession, as well as referring clients to those individuals in order to meet the client's needs. Nurses may serve as members of intradisciplinary teams, which are formed by members of the same profession, or interdisciplinary teams, which are made up of professionals with varied backgrounds. Table 37–1 ● lists a number of professionals who may serve as members of an interdisciplinary healthcare team and their respective roles.

To illustrate the collaborative nature of the nurse–client relationship, Kim's theory of collaborative decision making in nursing practice (1983, 1987) describes and explains the influence of collaborative interactions on making healthcare-related decisions, as well as how these interactions affect client outcomes. Dalton (2003) expanded the theory to include the client, nurse, and family caregiver. In this theory, all three enter into the collaboration from their own context of role expectations and attitudes, knowledge, personal traits, and definition of the situation. The three combine to form a coalition with opportunities for collaboration within the context of the situation. Dalton's theory proposes that level of collaboration achieved and the nature of the decision are the primary outcomes leading to secondary outcomes of goal attainment, autonomy, and satisfaction.

In addition to collaborating with other professionals to provide individual client care, nurses may also be involved in collaborating on bioethical issues, on legislation, on health-related research, and with professional organizations. To fulfill a collaborative role, nurses need to assume accountability and increased authority in their practice areas. Continuing education in role exploration, communication, group work, and other areas helps members of the healthcare team understand the collaborative nature of their roles, specific contributions, and the importance of working together. Each professional needs to understand how an integrated delivery system centers on the client's healthcare needs rather than on the particular care given by any one group. Box 37–2 ● describes selected aspects of the nurse's role as a collaborator.

TABLE 37–1 Collaborative Members of the Healthcare Team

HEALTHCARE PROFESSIONAL	ROLE
Nurse	The role of the nurse varies with the needs of the client, the nurse's credentials, and the type of employment setting. A registered nurse (RN) assesses a client's health status, identifies health problems, and develops and coordinates care. A licensed vocational nurse (LVN), in some states known as a licensed practical nurse (LPN), provides direct client care under the direction of a registered nurse, physician, or other licensed practitioner.
Unlicensed assistive personnel	Unlicensed assistive personnel (UAP) are healthcare staff who assume delegated aspects of basic client care. These tasks include bathing, assisting with feeding, and collecting specimens. UAP titles include certified nurse assistants, hospital attendants, nurse technicians, client care technicians, and orderlies. Some of these categories of provider may have standardized education and job duties (e.g., certified nurse assistants), while others do not. The parameters regarding nurse delegation to UAP are delineated by the state boards of nursing.
Alternative (complementary) care provider	Alternative or complementary health care refers to those practices not commonly considered part of Western medicine. Chiropractors, herbalists, acupuncturists, massage therapists, reflexologists, holistic health healers, and other healthcare providers are playing increasing roles in the contemporary healthcare system. These providers may practice alongside Western healthcare providers, or clients may use their services in conjunction with, or instead of, Western therapies.
Case manager	The case manager's role is to ensure that clients receive fiscally sound, appropriate care in the best setting. This role is often filled by the member of the healthcare team who is most involved in the client's care. Depending on the nature of the client's concerns, the case manager may be a nurse, a social worker, or any other member of the healthcare team.
Dentist	Dentists diagnose and treat dental problems. Dentists are also actively involved in preventive measures to maintain healthy oral structures (e.g., teeth and gums). Many hospitals, especially long-term care facilities, have dentists on staff.

TABLE 37–1   Collaborative Members of the Healthcare Team (*continued*)

HEALTHCARE PROFESSIONAL	ROLE
Dietitian or nutritionist	A dietitian, often a registered dietitian (RD), has special knowledge about the diets required to maintain health and to treat disease. Dietitians in hospitals generally are concerned with therapeutic diets, may design special diets to meet the nutritional needs of individual clients, and supervise the preparation of meals to ensure that clients receive the proper diet. A nutritionist is an individual who has special knowledge about nutrition and food. The nutritionist in a community setting recommends healthy diets and gives broad advisory services about the purchase and preparation of foods. Community nutritionists often function at the preventive level. They promote health and prevent disease, for example, by advising families about balanced diets for growing children and pregnant women.
Information technology expert	In healthcare organizations, an information technology (IT) expert offers knowledge and expertise in the ever-expanding field of computer science in application to health and health systems. The IT expert's knowledge base includes installing and repairing computer hardware, maintaining databases, and educating users about the use of computer applications, such as electronic health records (EHRs) and communication processes such as telemedicine.
Occupational therapist	An occupational therapist (OT) assists clients with impaired function to gain the skills to perform activities of daily living. For example, an occupational therapist might teach a man with severe arthritis in his arms and hands how to adjust his kitchen utensils so that he can continue to cook. The occupational therapist teaches skills that are therapeutic and at the same time provide some fulfillment. For example, weaving is a recreational activity but also exercises the arthritic man's arms and hands. Occupational therapists also perform developmental assessments and design developmental programs for clients of all ages during recovery from or adaptation to a variety of alterations; including traumatic injuries, medical conditions that affect cognition, congenital disorders, and alterations related to prematurity.
Paramedical technologist	Laboratory technologists, radiological technologists, and nuclear medicine technologists are just three kinds of paramedical technologists in the expanding field of medical technology. *Paramedical* means having some connection with medicine. Laboratory technologists, for example, examine specimens such as urine, feces, blood, and discharges from wounds to provide exact information that facilitates the medical diagnosis and the prescription of a therapeutic regimen.
Pharmacist	A pharmacist prepares and dispenses medications in hospital and community settings. The role of the pharmacist in monitoring and evaluating the actions and effects of medications on clients is becoming increasingly prominent. A clinical pharmacist is a specialist who guides physicians in prescribing medications.
Physical therapist	The licensed physical therapist (PT) assists clients with musculoskeletal problems. Physical therapists treat movement dysfunctions by means of heat, water, exercise, massage, and electric current. The physical therapist's functions include assessing client mobility and strength, providing therapeutic measures (e.g., exercises and heat applications to improve mobility and strength), and teaching new skills (e.g., how to walk with an artificial leg). Some physical therapists provide their services in hospitals; however, independent practitioners establish offices in communities and serve clients either at the office or in the home.
Physician	The physician is responsible for medical diagnosis and for determining the therapy required by an individual who has a disease or injury. The physician's role has traditionally been the treatment of disease and trauma (injury); however, many physicians are now including health promotion and disease prevention in their practice. Some physicians are general practitioners (also known as primary care or family practitioners); others are specialists, such as dermatologists, neurologists, oncologists, orthopedists, pediatricians, psychiatrists, radiologists, or surgeons—to name a few.
Physician assistant	Physician assistants (PAs) perform certain tasks under the direction of a physician. They diagnose and treat certain diseases, conditions, and injuries. In many states, nurses are not legally permitted to follow a PA's orders unless the orders are cosigned by a physician. In some settings, PAs and nurse practitioners have similar job descriptions.
Respiratory therapist	A respiratory therapist is skilled in therapeutic measures used in the care of clients with respiratory problems. These therapists are knowledgeable about oxygen therapy devices, intermittent positive pressure breathing respirators, artificial mechanical ventilators, and accessory devices used in inhalation therapy. Respiratory therapists administer many of the pulmonary function tests.
Social worker	A social worker counsels clients and their support people regarding problems, such as finances, marital difficulties, and adoption of children. It is not unusual for health problems to produce problems in day-to-day living and vice versa. For example, an older woman who lives alone and has a stroke resulting in impaired walking may find it impossible to continue to live in her third-floor apartment. Finding a more suitable living arrangement can be the responsibility of the social worker if the client has no support network in place.

Box 37–2   The Nurse as a Collaborator

WITH CLIENTS

- Acknowledges, supports, and encourages clients' active involvement in healthcare decisions.
- Encourages a sense of client autonomy and an equal position with other members of the healthcare team.
- Helps clients set mutually agreed-on goals and objectives for health care.
- Provides the client with consultation in a collaborative fashion.

WITH PEERS

- Shares personal expertise with other nurses and elicits the expertise of others to ensure high-quality client care.
- Develops a sense of trust and mutual respect with peers that recognizes their unique contributions.

WITH OTHER HEALTHCARE PROFESSIONALS

- Recognizes the contribution that each member of the interdisciplinary team can make by virtue of his or her expertise and view of the situation.
- Listens to each individual's views.
- Shares healthcare responsibilities with other members of the team in order to explore care options, set realistic and attainable goals, and make decisions about the plan of care with clients and their families.
- Participates in collaborative interdisciplinary research to increase knowledge of a clinical problem or situation.

WITH PROFESSIONAL NURSING ORGANIZATIONS

- Seeks opportunities to collaborate with and within professional organizations.
- Serves on committees in state (or provincial), national, and international nursing organizations or specialty groups.
- Supports professional organizations in political action to create solutions for professional and healthcare concerns.

WITH LEGISLATORS

- Offers expert opinions on legislative initiatives related to health care.
- Collaborates with other healthcare providers and consumers on healthcare legislation to best serve the needs of the public.

▶ COLLABORATIVE PRACTICE

The overall objectives of collaborative initiatives are high-quality client care and client satisfaction. In addition, many healthcare professionals believe that a multidisciplinary, collaborative framework can limit costs and enhance quality. Collaborative practice models attempt to achieve the following objectives:

- Provide client-directed and client-centered care using a multidisciplinary, integrated, participative framework.
- Enhance continuity of care across the continuum of health, from wellness and prevention through acute illness to recovery or rehabilitation.
- Improve client and family satisfaction with care.
- Provide high-quality, cost-effective, research-based care that improves client outcomes.
- Promote mutual respect, communication, and understanding between the client and members of the healthcare team.

- Provide opportunities to address and solve system-related issues and problems.
- Develop interdependent relationships and understanding among providers and clients.

A collaborative approach to health care ideally benefits clients, professionals, and the healthcare delivery system. Care becomes client centered and, most important, client directed. Clients become informed consumers and actively participate with the healthcare team in the decision-making process. When clients are empowered to participate actively and professionals share mutually set goals with clients, quality of care improves and everyone—including the organization and healthcare system—ultimately benefits. When quality improves, adherence to therapeutic regimens increases, lengths of stay decrease, and overall costs to the system decline. Sound application of collaborative strategies leads to decreased client morbidity and mortality rates (Schneider, 2012). Among healthcare providers, when professional interdependence develops, collegial relationships emerge and overall job satisfaction increases.

According to the World Health Organization (WHO), collaborative practice involves healthcare providers from a variety of disciplines working in tandem with clients, families, caregivers, and communities to provide the best possible quality of care. Collaboration has system-wide effects. For example, using collaborative strategies of care improves client outcomes and strengthens the systems used to provide health care (WHO, 2010). With regard to the appropriate use of resources, effective collaboration can reduce duplication of services and decrease the overall cost of health care (Young & Olsen, 2010). Along with system-wide effects, collaboration also impacts individuals. Research suggests that effective nurse–physician collaboration leads to a decrease in client morbidity and mortality rates (Boone et al., 2008).

Collaboration has positive psychosocial and professional effects, as well. Both clients and nurses perceive a greater sense of autonomy when collaborative strategies are applied (Schneider, 2012). Within the context of workplace roles, autonomy refers to possessing the authority to make decisions and to take actions that reflect application of one's professional knowledge base (Skar, 2010). For nurses, practicing autonomously means being authorized to provide nursing care that falls within the professional scope of practice as defined by existing regulatory boards, professional organizations, and institutional rules (Weston, 2008, 2010). Greater autonomy is linked to higher levels of job satisfaction among nurses and an increased sense of professionalism (Weston, 2010). See Concepts Related to Collaboration for examples of how collaboration is integrated with other concepts.

▶ COMPETENCIES BASIC TO COLLABORATION

Key features necessary for collaboration include effective communication skills, giving and receiving feedback, mutual respect, trust, decision making, and conflict management (Masters, 2013).

Concepts Related to **Collaboration**

Effective collaboration affects health care positively on every level. At the systemic level, collaboration leads to increased efficiency and greater cost effectiveness. For clients, collaboration among members of the healthcare team promotes safety, resulting in decreased morbidity and mortality rates. Clients who are involved in the col-laborative process report an increased sense of auton-omy, which leads to greater overall satisfaction with care. Nurses who effectively collaborate report an increased sense of perceived autonomy and professionalism, along with greater job satisfaction.

CONCEPT	RELATIONSHIP TO COLLABORATION	NURSING IMPLICATIONS
Healthcare Systems		
■ Frameworks for providing care ■ Access to care ■ Allocation of resources	↑ collaboration among healthcare team members → ↓ duplication of client services and ↓ healthcare costs	■ Support and promote collaboration among healthcare team members. ■ Apply principles of effective collabora-tion, including principles that facilitate clear communication. ■ Be aware of the client's plan of care, including ordered tests and diagnostics, and question apparent duplications using a polite, professional approach.
Safety		
■ National safety initiatives ■ Community and local safety initiatives ■ Injury prevention in the clin-ical setting ■ Safety considerations across the life span ■ Workplace safety	↑ collaboration among healthcare team members → ↓ client morbidity and ↓ client mortality rates	■ Support and promote collaboration among healthcare team members. ■ Support the scheduling of interdisciplin-ary team meetings and attend all sched-uled meetings. ■ Educate healthcare team members about the safety-related benefits of collaboration.
Professional Behaviors		
■ Components of profession-alism in nursing ■ Commitment to profession ■ Leadership principles ■ Work ethic	↑ nurse–physician collaboration → ↑ perceived professional autonomy → ↑ nursing professionalism	■ Recognize the impact of collaboration on job satisfaction in nursing. ■ Effectively apply principles of collabora-tion to promote collaborative nurse–physician relationships.

Communication Skills

Collaborating to solve complex problems requires effective communication skills. Initially, the healthcare team needs to define collaboration clearly, establish its goals and objectives, and specify each team member's role.

Effective communication can occur only if each team member is committed to understanding each member's professional role and appreciating each member as an individual. Additionally, each member must be sensitive to differences among communi-cation styles. Communication styles are especially important to successful collaboration. Norton's theory of **communicator style** (1983) defines the style as the manner in which one communi-cates and includes the way in which one interacts. (For discussion of communication styles, strategies, and their application to nurs-ing practice, see the module on Communication.) Instead of focusing on distinctions among members, each team must keep firmly in mind its common purpose: to meet the client's needs. Achievement of this goal requires the effective use of feedback.

One of the most difficult challenges for professionals is giv-ing and receiving timely, relevant, and helpful **feedback** (the response the receiver of a message gives to the message's sender) to and from each other and their clients. When professionals work closely together, it may be appropriate to address attitudes or actions that affect the collaborative relationship. Giving and receiving feedback may be affected by each individual's percep-tions, personal space, roles, relationships, self-esteem, confi-dence, beliefs, emotions, environment, and time. For example, a supervisor who chooses to give feedback to an employee the day after the employee returns from funeral leave is likely not to have the employee's full attention during the meeting and likely to invite responses from the employee that the employee might not normally make.

The term *negative feedback* implies not negative content but rather a negative communication style, such as an atti-tude of condescension. Positive feedback is characterized by a communication style that is warm, caring, and respectful.

For all clients, communication is a key to competent nursing care and a means for promoting nurse–client collaboration. Especially with regard to language-based challenges, the negative impact of miscommunication can lead to serious consequences. Ineffectively managed cultural language barriers can impede collaboration and negatively impact medical and nursing diagnoses, as well as client outcomes (Garcia & Duckett, 2009).

Giving and receiving feedback helps individuals acquire self-awareness, while assisting the collaborative team to develop a common understanding and an effective working relationship. Healthcare providers, including nurses, need to learn to accept feedback in a professional manner without becoming defensive.

Mutual Respect and Trust

Mutual respect occurs when two or more individuals show or feel honor or esteem toward one another. Trust occurs when an individual is confident in the actions of another individual. Both mutual respect and trust imply a mutual process and outcome. They must be expressed both verbally and nonverbally. Sometimes professionals may verbalize respect or trust of others but demonstrate a lack of trust and respect through their actions. The healthcare system itself has not always created an environment that promotes respect or trust of the various healthcare providers. Although progress has been made toward creating more trusting relationships, past attitudes may continue to impede efforts toward collaborative practice (see the Evidence-Based Practice feature). Magnet hospitals are an example of successful efforts by healthcare organizations to foster respect among professionals. Placing the head of the nursing department (previously known as the director of nursing) on an equal managerial level with the chief of physicians (usually called the chief medical officer) has been found to improve mutual respect between physicians and nurses, thereby improving their relationships.

Decision Making

Collaboration involves shared responsibility for the outcome. Obviously, to create a solution, the team must follow each step of the decision-making process, beginning with a clear definition of the problem. Team decision making must be directed at the objectives of the specific effort. Demonstration of mutual respect and timely, effective feedback facilitate the decision-making process.

Decision making at the team level requires full consideration of and respect for diverse viewpoints. Members must be able to verbalize their perspectives in a nonthreatening environment. Group members must effectively use communication skills and give and receive feedback in the decision-making process.

Sound decision making regarding client care requires that the interdisciplinary team focus on the client's priority needs and organize interventions accordingly. The discipline best able to address the client's needs is identified, given priority in

Evidence-Based Practice Overcoming Barriers: The Benefits of Nurse–Physician Collaboration

Problem
Despite research-based evidence that supports the benefits of effective collaboration between nurses and physicians, barriers to this process—several of which relate to the relationship between the nurse and the physician—remain intact.

Evidence
As recently as the 1960s, researchers described nurse–physician relationships as being hierarchy based and imbalanced. Nurses assumed a subordinate role to physicians, who were perceived as being superior to nurses (Johnson, 2009). Enforcing perceptions of inequity between individuals is counterproductive in the development of collaborative relationships. Another major barrier to collaboration during that time frame was the real or perceived requirement that the nurse should offer suggestions related to the client's plan of care in such a way as to give the impression that the physician, not the nurse, had initiated the recommendation (Weinberg, Miner, & Rivlin, 2009). Although nursing education programs have promoted a shift in the nurse's perception of the nurse–physician relationship from subservient–superior to collegial, some physicians at present view this collegial relationship as undermining their leadership and authority (Schneider, 2012).

Despite the barriers to nurse–physician collaboration, research strongly supports this practice. Interprofessional collaboration between physicians and nurses is linked to decreased client morbidity and mortality (Schneider, 2012). Along with enhancing overall client safety, benefits of effective collaboration between physicians and nurses also include a decreased risk for medication-related errors and improved cost containment (Nair et al., 2012).

Implications
Although research has shown that collaborative nurse–physician relationships are valuable and beneficial, some physicians may remain resistant to this concept. For the benefit of the client, the healthcare system, and the professionals caring for the client, nurses should support and promote the development of collaborative relationships with physicians, as well as with all other members of the healthcare team.

Critical Thinking Application
Development of a collaborative relationship requires mutual trust and respect, demonstrated efficacy with conflict resolution, clear methods of communication, and professionalism during all negotiation processes (Schneider, 2012). Nurses should seek to develop and demonstrate expertise in all these categories, while encouraging discussion between nurse and physician leadership with regard to building collaborative relationships between these two disciplines.

planning, and held responsible for providing its interventions in a timely manner. For example, when social needs (such as loss of a home or job) interfere with the client's ability to respond to therapy, the team may agree that the social worker needs to intervene to help the client resolve his or her social needs before starting therapy. Nurses, by the nature of their holistic practice, are often able to help the team identify priorities and areas requiring further attention. Ideally, the collaborative team will ensure that the client is part of the decision-making process, even if the client is not able to be present. Decision-making processes are discussed in greater detail in the module on Clinical Decision Making.

Conflict Management

Conflict in the workplace is inevitable; as such, learning to successfully manage conflict is essential to nursing. While often viewed as being negative, conflict can actually be an impetus for better communication, stronger team relationships, and healthy changes. For a detailed discussion of conflict management, including positive and negative approaches to handling conflict, see the exemplar on Conflict Resolution within this module.

CASE STUDY \\ A

Betty Bradley, 87 years old, is a client in a long-term care facility. After fracturing her hip, Ms. Bradley is no longer stable on her feet and prefers to stay in bed for fear of falling. After speaking with Ms. Bradley to get a better understanding of her fears, the nurse consults with the physical therapist. Together they determine how they can help Ms. Bradley improve her mobility while reducing her risk of injury. After talking with Ms. Bradley about their ideas and getting her agreement, the primary nurse and physical therapist develop a plan of care based on the nursing diagnoses of *Impaired Mobility* and *Risk for Injury: Falls*. They list specific implementations including positioning, turning, and use of aids to prevent pressure ulcers. Once the plan of care has been developed, it is posted on the wall by Ms. Bradley's bed so that all nurses can see it and administer care consistently. During the monthly team meeting, the plan of care for Ms. Bradley is evaluated. Both the physical therapist and the nurse report that Ms. Bradley has greatly improved both her strength and her mobility while reducing her risk for injury.

Critical Thinking Questions

1. Why might collaborative care be of particular importance in caring for an older client who is a long-term resident of an extended care facility?
2. What other collaborative interventions might the team consider for this client?
3. How can the plan of care be posted on the client's wall without infringing on the client's right to confidentiality?

▶ COLLABORATION AND THE HEALTHCARE CONSUMER

On a national level, collaborative efforts have led to the formation of goals and objectives for improved health through a plan of action called the *Healthy People* initiatives.

Every 10 years, beginning in 1990, the U.S. Department of Health and Human Services (USDHHS) has published national guidelines designed to promote wellness. These guidelines, known as *Healthy People* initiatives, are aimed at improving the health of all Americans during the course of a 10-year span. Through collaboration, the Institute of Medicine and USDHHS have identified health benchmarks, strategies for improving health, and methods of monitoring the U.S. population's progress toward reaching the goals. Examples of *Healthy People 2020* initiatives include decreasing the cancer-related mortality rate, decreasing the incidence of obesity among children and adolescents, and reducing tobacco use (USDHHS, 2013). Health issues and strategies for wellness promotion that were designated as being highest in priority comprise *Healthy People 2020's* leading health indictors.

Stay Current: *See the Healthy People 2020 initiatives at* **www.healthypeople.gov/2020/LHI/default.aspx.**

As demonstrated by the *Healthy People* initiatives, increasingly, governments and society are working to reduce health risks, minimize the incidence of chronic illness, and improve the health and quality of life for all. Even so, optimal health and access to adequate healthcare services are not guaranteed. In the United States, the most pressing question for the healthcare system remains how to provide high-quality health care that is in line with the socioeconomic realities of society. A number of factors influence the provision of health care:

- Although the diagnosis and treatment of illness are still critical, the focus of health care is changing. Healthcare consumers are demanding comprehensive, holistic, and compassionate health care that is also affordable. Clients expect that healthcare providers will view each individual as a biopsychosocial whole and respond to their needs as individuals while respecting them as collaborating members of the healthcare team.

- Today's healthcare consumers have greater knowledge about their health than consumers did in the past; as a result, they increasingly are influencing healthcare delivery. Formerly, people expected a physician to make decisions about their care; today, however, consumers expect to be involved in making any decisions.

- Healthcare consumers are assuming more responsibility for their health and are more willing to participate in health-promoting activities. They are beginning to view healthcare professionals as a resource to guide these activities.

As clients become more informed healthcare consumers, nurses must increase their efforts to collaborate with their clients. Parents of ill children, especially those with chronic illnesses, are often the best source of information regarding changes in the child's condition, history of illness, and treatment options that have worked best in the past. Caregivers and clients can contribute to the plan of care by sharing their past experiences and responses to treatment, as well as participating in planning care that meets their needs.

Collaboration is becoming more important as the complexity of medicine continues to increase with each new discovery. For example, the information technology expert has become a valued member of the team in many organizations. Each team member has specialized knowledge from which the nurse can learn and that can contribute to client care.

◢ REVIEW The Concept of Collaboration

RELATE Link the Concepts

Linking the concept of collaboration with the concept of communication:

1. How does the nurse's communication skills affect his or her ability to collaborate?

2. How does communication style affect the process of collaboration? Give some examples.

Linking the concept of collaboration with the concept of oxygenation:

3. How would the care of a client with chronic obstructive pulmonary disease (COPD) benefit from a nurse who collaborates well with other members of the healthcare team?

4. In caring for the client with COPD, what aspects of care would require collaboration?

REFER Go to Pearson Nursing Student Resources
nursing.pearsonhighered.com

- Additional review materials

REFLECT Case Study

Josiah Elliot, 72 years old, is admitted to the hospital with medical diagnoses of congestive heart failure, chronic renal failure, hypertension, and benign prostatic hypertrophy. The nurse admits him and develops his plan of nursing care, including the nursing diagnoses of *Excess Fluid Volume*, *Urinary Retention*, *Impaired Gas Exchange*, and *Anxiety* related to hypoxia. Three days later Mr. Elliot has lost 18 pounds and is breathing more easily. He also denies feeling anxious and reports, "I'm relaxed now that I can breathe!" The nursing diagnoses of *Excess Fluid Volume*, *Impaired Gas Exchange*, and *Anxiety* are all marked as resolved. During morning rounds, the nurse provides the physician with an update on the client's condition and questions the need to continue administering the large doses of diuretics that were ordered when the client was admitted. The physician agrees and reduces the dosage of the medications. The physician raises concerns about the client's nutritional status and suitability for discharge to home. After some discussion, the physician and nurse agree to consult with a dietitian and a social worker for further evaluation of the client's care.

1. Describe the impact of the team's collaborative approach on Mr. Elliot's outcomes.

2. How might Mr. Elliot's care have differed if the team had not collaborated?

3. What further collaboration is indicated in providing care for Mr. Elliot?

◤ EXEMPLAR 37.1 Case Management

EXEMPLAR KEY TERMS
Care management model, *2382*
Care map, *2384*
Case management, *2382*
Critical pathway, *2382*

EXEMPLAR LEARNING OUTCOMES
After reading about this exemplar, you will be able to:

1. Describe the purpose of case management and the role of the case manager.

2. Correlate the need for critical pathways in the case management process.

▶ OVERVIEW

Case management describes a range of models for integrating healthcare services for individuals or groups. Generally, case management involves multidisciplinary teams that assume collaborative responsibility for assessing needs, planning and coordinating, implementing, and evaluating care for groups of clients from preadmission to discharge or transfer and recuperation. A case manager may be a nurse, social worker, or other appropriate professional. In some areas of the United States, case managers may be referred to as discharge planners. Key responsibilities of case managers are shown in **Box 37–3** ●.

The **care management model** focuses on the needs of the integrated delivery system. It has many similarities to case management, in that it includes planning, assessment, and coordination of health services. The client focus is population based

Box 37–3   Responsibilities of Case Managers

- Assessing clients and their homes and communities
- Coordinating and planning client care
- Collaborating with other health professionals
- Monitoring clients' progress
- Evaluating client outcomes

instead of based on an individual client. The population might be the entire population, members of a managed care plan, or could be a specific group with similarities, such as clients with diabetes. The goal of the care management model is to integrate a continuum of clinical services. Care management is not only concerned with medical care but also with health promotion, disease prevention, costs, and use of resources. Case management is often used within the care management model. Typical tools used to facilitate care management are critical pathways, disease management programs, and benchmarking.

Case management may be used as a cost containment strategy in managed care. Both case management and managed care systems often use critical pathways to track client progress. A **critical pathway** is a standardized plan that helps track care provided to clients with similar, predictable medical conditions. Critical pathways are also called critical paths, clinical pathways, interdisciplinary plans, anticipated recovery plans, interdisciplinary action plans, and action plans.

▶ THE NURSE AS CASE MANAGER

Nursing case management organizes client care by major diagnoses or *diagnosis-related groups* (DRGs). DRGs allow nurses to work toward predetermined client outcomes within specific time frames and resources.

Nursing case management requires the following:

- Collaboration of all members of the healthcare team
- Identification of expected client outcomes within specific time frames
- Use of principles of continuous quality improvement (CQI) and variance analysis
- Promotion of professional practice.

Research suggests that case management has been particularly successful in disability management, especially when applied to helping injured employees to return to work (Gardner et al., 2010). Likewise, home care and ambulatory settings lend themselves to case management (**Figure 37–1 ●**) The case manager, who may be called a care coordinator, usually does not provide direct client care but rather coordinates and monitors the care provided by licensed and unlicensed care providers. Client involvement and participation is key to successful case management (Summers, 2012).

In an acute care setting, the case manager has a caseload of 10–15 clients and follows the clients' progress through the system from admission to discharge, accounting for variances from expected progress. Nursing case managers on a client care unit may coordinate, communicate, collaborate, problem solve, and facilitate client care for a group of clients. Ideally, nursing case managers have advanced degrees and considerable clinical experience in nursing.

To initiate case management, specific client diagnoses that represent high-volume, high-cost, and high-risk cases are selected. High-volume cases are those that occur frequently, such as total hip replacements on an orthopedic floor. High-risk cases include clients or case types who have complications, stay in a critical care unit longer than 2 days, or require ventilatory support. Clients also may be selected because they are being treated by a physician who supports case management. Whatever client population is selected, baseline data must be collected and analyzed. These data provide the information necessary to measure the effectiveness of case management. Essential baseline data include length of stay, cost of care, and complication information.

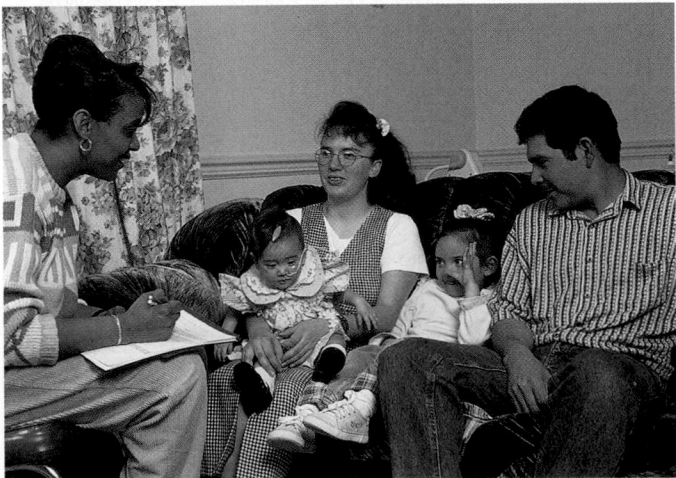

Figure 37–1 ● A nurse case manager works with families to evaluate care being provided to a child with a complex health condition at home. The case manager coordinates specialty services, such as respiratory therapy, as well as providing client and family education.

Five elements are essential to successful implementation of case management:

1. Support by key members of the organization (administrators, physicians, nurses)
2. A qualified nurse case manager
3. Collaborative practice teams
4. A quality management system
5. Established critical pathways (see next section).

When a specific client population is selected to be "case managed," a collaborative practice team is established. The team, which includes clinical experts from appropriate disciplines (e.g., nursing, medicine, physical therapy) needed for the selected client population, defines the expected outcomes of care for the client population. Based on expected client outcomes, each member of the team, using that member's discipline's contribution, helps determine appropriate interventions within a specified time frame.

In case management, all professionals are equal members of the team; thus, one group does not determine interventions for other disciplines. All members of the collaborative practice team agree on the final draft of the critical pathways, take ownership of client outcomes, and accept responsibility and accountability for the interventions and client outcomes associated with their discipline. The emphasis must be on managing client outcomes and building consensus among team members. Outcomes must be specified in measurable terms.

CASE STUDY \\ B

Martha Ellison is an RN with 10 years of experience and a master's degree in nursing. She is the case manager on the orthopedic unit of the city hospital. She is currently managing 10 clients on the unit: four with injuries that resulted from car crashes; two older adults, each with a fractured hip; and four adolescent clients who required placement of pins and traction to stabilize fractures. Ms. Ellison compares each client's progress to the critical pathway for that client and makes recommendations to the physician managing their care related to meeting specific needs.

One of the clients in Ms. Ellison's care is a 22-year-old man who experienced significant head injuries and multiple fractures as a result of a motor vehicle crash. Ms. Ellison works with the hospital physical therapy department to optimize his mobility and range of motion in order to prepare him for rehabilitation. She collaborates with a rehabilitation center that will continue his care following discharge. Ms. Ellison also collaborates with the neurologist and family care providers to ensure that the client's other needs are met and he is able to be discharged as soon as possible.

Critical Thinking Questions

1. Identify the different individuals and organizations with whom Ms. Ellison is collaborating. Explain why collaboration is essential to meeting a client's needs.
2. What is the purpose of a critical pathway? What are some other names for a critical pathway?
3. In the care of clients with orthopedic injuries, explain how case management for the older adult client might differ from that needed for the younger adult client.

▶ CRITICAL PATHWAYS

Successful case management relies on critical pathways to guide care. The term *critical pathway*, also called a **care map**, refers to the expected outcomes and care strategies developed through collaboration by the healthcare team. Again, the interdisciplinary team must reach consensus regarding client care and determine specific, measurable outcomes.

Critical paths provide direction for managing the care of a specific client during a specified time period. Critical paths are useful because they accommodate the unique characteristics of the client and the client's condition while making use of the predictable characteristics of the course of the client's disease or injury. Critical paths use resources appropriate to the care needed, thereby reducing cost and length of stay. Critical paths are used in every setting where health care is delivered.

A critical path quickly orients the nurse to the outcomes that should be achieved for the client for that day. Nursing diagnoses identify the outcomes needed. If client outcomes are not achieved, the case manager is notified and the situation is analyzed to determine how to modify the critical path.

Altering time frames or interventions is categorized as a variance, and the case manager tracks all variances. After a time, the appropriate collaborative practice teams analyze the variances, note trends, and decide how to manage them. Teams may then revise the critical pathway or decide to gather additional data before making changes.

Some features are included on all critical paths. These include the specific medical diagnosis, the expected length of stay, client identification data, appropriate time frames (in days, hours, minutes, or visits) for interventions, and client outcomes. Interventions are presented in modality groups (medications, nursing activity, and so on). The critical path must include a means to identify variances easily and to determine whether outcomes are met.

Table 37–2 ● is an example of a collaborative critical path for clients having a total hip replacement. Normally a client would be expected to be discharged on the sixth day after surgery. This path describes expectations for days 1–3.

A recent evolution in critical paths is the inclusion of actual and potential nursing diagnoses with specific time frames into the critical pathway (see the lower section of Table 37–2). Education paths are also excellent tools for planning client and family education (Table 37–3 ●). A copy of the client's education plan is given to the client and the family, and the nurse reviews the information with them. Thus, both the client and the family know what to expect during an anticipated, uncomplicated hospitalization.

TABLE 37–2 Critical Path With Actual/Risk Nursing Diagnoses for Total Hip Replacement

Client Name: _____

Record Number: _____

Drg: 209

Expected LOS: 6 Days

COLLABORATIVE CRITICAL PATH CASE TYPE: TOTAL HIP REPLACEMENT

	DAY1/OR	Y/N	DAY 2/POSTOPERATIVE DAY 1	Y/N	DAY 3/POSTOPERATIVE DAY 2	Y/N
Client Activity	Bed rest	—	Begin mobility plan	—	Continue mobility plan	—
	T-DB q2h	—	T-DB q2h	—	T-DB q2h	—
	Initiate skin protection		Continue skin protection		Continue skin protection	
	protocol		protocol	—	protocol	—
Nursing	VS qh × 4,	—	VS q4h	—	VS q8h	—
	then q4h	—				
	Assess cir/neuro		Assess cir/neuro q4h	—	D/C assessment	—
	legs qh × 4,	—				
	then q4h;	—			D/C Hemovac;	
	Check drainage/		Check drainage/		Check drainage	
	Hemovac qh × 4,	—	Hemovac q4h	—	q8h	—
	then q4h;	—			I&O q8h	
	I&O (Foley/		I&O (Foley/		D/C Foley; urinates	
	Hemovac) q8h;	—	Hemovac) q8h	—	within 8h	—
	Thigh-high elastic hose	—	Continue elastic hose	—	Continue elastic hose	—
Medications	Antibiotic	—	Continue antibiotic	—	Continue antibiotic	—
	Pain control:		Continue pain control	—	PO pain control	—
	PCA pump	—				
	Stool softener	—	Continue stool softener	—	Continue stool softener	—
	Continue home Rx;	—	Continue home Rx	—	Continue home Rx	—

TABLE 37–2 Critical Path With Actual/Risk Nursing Diagnoses for Total Hip Replacement (*continued*)

	DAY 1/OR	Y/N	DAY 2/POSTOPERATIVE DAY 1	Y/N	DAY 3/POSTOPERATIVE DAY 2	Y/N
	IVs	—	IVs continue	—	IV to heparin lock	—
			Coumadin	—	Cont Coumadin	—
			Sleeping Rx	—	Sleeping Rx	—
Physical Therapy	Preop instructions	—	Evaluate mobility		Evaluate mobility	
			progress	—	progress	—
Diagnostic Tests	Hemoglobin and hemato-crit (H&H) 2 hr post-op	—	H&H	—	Prothrombin time/INR	—
			Prothrombin time	—		
Nutrition Teaching	NPO—Cl liq as tol	—	Diet as tolerated	—	Diet as tolerated	—
	Pre-op: Pain control	—	Repeat teaching		Repeat teaching	
	Use of assist devices	—	if nec	—	if nec	—
	Gait control	—				
	Incentive spirometry	—				
	Mobility plan	—				
	Pt/family crit plan		Review pt/family		Review pt/family	
	given & reviewed	—	crit plan if nec	—	crit plan if nec	—
Discharge Plan	SNU evaluation	—			Review transfer	
	Home health				discharge needs	—
	evaluation	—				

CLIENT PROBLEMS AND OUTCOMES FOR TOTAL HIP REPLACEMENT

NURSING DIAGNOSIS	DAY 1/OR	Y/N	DAY 2/POSTOPERATIVE DAY 1	Y/N	DAY 3/POSTOPERATIVE DAY 2	Y/N
Knowledge Deficit: medications; use of assistive devices; treatments	Appropriately uses:		Uses all devices appropriately	—	Verbalizes additions to care	—
	PCA pump,	—				
	incentive spirometry,					
	assistive devices;					
	Verbalizes mobility plan	—				
Pain related to surgery, physical injury	Pain managed	—	Pain managed	—	Pain managed	—
Risk for Infection related to invasive procedures, immobility	Remains afebrile	—	Remains afebrile	—	Remains afebrile	—
	No skin breakdown	—	No skin breakdown	—		
Impaired Physical Mobility related to surgery, prosthesis	Verbalizes mobility plan	—	Meeting mobility expectations	—	Participates in transfer/discharge plans, decisions	—
	Verbalizes role of staff providing assistance	—				
Risk for Injury related to altered tissue perfusion, altered mobility, and prosthesis	Explains need for frequent assessments	—	Circulation to extremities good	—	Circulation to extremities normal	—
	Verbalizes need for early mobility and hose	—	Leg maintained in proper alignment	—	Leg in proper alignment	—

TABLE 37–3 Client/Family Education Path for Total Hip Replacement

	DAY1/OR	DAY 2/POSTOPERATIVE DAY 1	DAY 3/POSTOPERATIVE DAY 2
Unit	Admission process; surgery and recovery areas; then Orthopedic Unit	Orthopedic Unit	Orthopedic Unit (Possible transfer next day to SNU or Rehab Unit)
Client Activity and Safety Issues	Bed rest first 24 hr; leg exercises qh (q4h); T-DB q2h; explain skin protection plan; give copy of mobility plan; assist c̄ bath; thigh-high elastic support hose	Up in chair with help; leg exercises q2h; T-DB q2h; cont skin protect plan; cont mobility plan; assist c̄ bath; cont thigh-high elastic support hose	Up in chair and walking as outlined in mobility plan; T-DB q2h; cont skin protection plan; assist c̄ bath; cont thigh-high elastic support hose
Nursing Care	Frequency of taking vital signs (BP-P-R-T); check drainage on dressing; check circulation and sensations to legs; intake and output measured q8h; Foley and Hemovac in for 48 hr	Vital sign checks q4h; dressing, circulation, and sensation checks to legs q4h; I&O (Foley and Hemovac) measured q8h	Vital sign checks q8h; D/C Foley and Hemovac; I&O q8h; urinate within 8 hr; D/C dressing, circulation, and sensation checks to legs
Medications	Verify list of home Rx so physician can order; pain medication and PCA pump; IVs and need for arm restraint; other drugs that will be ordered (e.g., antibiotics; stool softener)	Cont pain management c̄ PCA pump; IVs; cont arm restraint; cont antibiotic and other drugs (sleeping assistance)	Oral pain management; IV to heparin lock; cont antibiotic and other drugs
Diet	NPO before OR; clear liquids, ice chips	Diet as tolerated	Diet as tolerated
Tests	Blood test: H&H 2 hr after OR	Blood tests: H&H and prothrombin time/INR	Blood test: prothrombin time/INR
Teaching	Pain management; use of assistive devices (trapeze, walker) and incentive spirometry; mobility plan reviewed: how to transfer from bed to chair, and so on	Clarify questions	Clarify questions
Discharge Plan	Discuss purpose of Skilled Nursing Unit and Rehab Unit; identify need for home health service after discharge	Cont with discussion of SNU, Rehab Unit, and home health services	Clarify questions and needs with transfer/discharge plans

Critical Thinking Questions

1. Review the critical paths outlined in Tables 37–2 and Table 37–3. Explain how nursing diagnoses influence the critical paths.

2. Identify client outcomes included in the critical paths. Why is measurability an essential component of client outcomes?

3. On the basis of these critical paths, which professional disciplines will be engaged in collaboration during client care?

REVIEW Case Management

RELATE Link the Concepts and Exemplars

Linking the exemplar of case management with the concept of perfusion:

1. A neonate born with a severe congenital heart defect will require numerous open heart surgeries and regular follow-up with cardiology and pediatrics. The parents, who carry comprehensive medical insurance, will require assistance paying for medical bills because the cost of care is expected to exceed the child's lifetime maximum coverage within a few years. How might this family benefit from case management? What specifically would the case manager do for this family?

Linking the exemplar of case management with the concept of oxygenation:

2. The nurse is caring for two clients: one client has pneumonia that is resolving with IV antibiotics; the other client has had asthma for many years. Which client would benefit most from case management? Explain your answer.

3. The nurse is caring for a client with a chronic alteration in oxygenation requiring many different medications, frequent physician visits, and a history of 2–3 hospital admissions per year. How might case management help this client?

REFER Go to Pearson Nursing Student Resources
nursing.pearsonhighered.com

- Additional review materials

REFLECT Case Study

Curt Ranier is a 42-year-old male client who sustained a right femur fracture during a motor vehicle crash. Following surgical repair of his femur fracture, he is admitted to the orthopedic unit. His surgery and anesthesia were uneventful, and he is stable and alert. His medical history includes type 2 diabetes, which he manages through his diet. He also has a prior history of deep vein thrombosis (DVT) in his left leg. During his admission to the orthopedic unit, Mr. Ranier expressed his motivation to heal and go home; however, he states that he is concerned about caring for himself outside the hospital setting, as he lives alone and has no relatives nearby.

1. Considering Mr. Ranier's current condition and medical history, which nursing diagnoses (both actual and risk) should be included in his nursing plan of care?

2. How would Mr. Ranier benefit from case management? In addition to nursing, describe several other professional disciplines that should collaborate in Mr. Ranier's care.

3. Describe the benefits of using a critical pathway to guide Mr. Ranier's care. In addition to Mr. Ranier's medical diagnosis and client identification data, identify three categories that would be included in Mr. Ranier's critical pathway.

EXEMPLAR 37.2 **Conflict Resolution**

EXEMPLAR KEY TERMS

Conflict, 2387
Covert conflict, 2387
Horizontal violence (HV), 2390
Intergroup conflict, 2387
Interorganizational conflict, 2387
Interpersonal conflict, 2387
Intrapersonal conflict, 2387
Overt conflict, 2387

Verbal abuse, 2390
Workplace bullying, 2390

EXEMPLAR LEARNING OUTCOMES

After reading about this exemplar, you will be able to:

1. Contrast different forms of conflict.
2. Explain factors that can initiate conflict.
3. Describe appropriate conflict management strategies in the workplace.

▶ OVERVIEW

Conflict occurs when agreement cannot be reached with regard to significant issues and concerns or when emotional opposition creates discord within an individual or between individuals, groups, or organizations (Schermerhorn et al., 2012). Although conflict in an organization can never be eliminated, it can be managed. Conflicts can take place between individual nurses, between nurses and other members of the healthcare team, within a unit, or within a department. Conflicts can be interunit and interdepartmental, can affect the entire organization, or can even occur between multiple organizations, between or within teams or units, or between an organization and the community.

▶ TYPES OF CONFLICT

Types and levels of conflict may be categorized in a variety of ways. This exemplar approaches conflict as existing on four levels (Schermerhorn et al., 2012):

■ **Intrapersonal conflict**, which occurs within an individual, is stress or tension that results from real or perceived pressure generated by incompatible expectations or goals. This may occur when an individual is expected to do something that produces both desirable and undesirable consequences. For example, intrapersonal conflict may occur when a nurse must choose either to accept an employment position that interferes with fulfilling family-related responsibilities or to prioritize family responsibilities while remaining unemployed and without an income (Schermerhorn et al., 2012).

■ **Interpersonal conflict** occurs between two or more individuals. Sometimes this is due to differences and/or personalities, competition, or concern about territory, control, or loss. Interpersonal conflict may arise in the workplace when one staff member misunderstands the roles or responsibility of

another. For example, a nurse may believe that someone is not doing his or her job because the individual is neglecting to perform an activity that is really the responsibility of another nurse. Other interpersonal conflicts can arise as the result of bullying, when a member of the team belittles another or attempts to coerce others into behaving in ways that cause frustration, guilt, or other types of conflict.

■ **Intergroup conflict** occurs between teams that are in competition or opposition to one another. In some cases, the groups are competing for rewards or scarce resources. The groups may also be emotionally opposed to each other (Schermerhorn et al., 2012). One example of this level of conflict is the debate that is occurring between physician groups who want to bring nurse practitioners under the control of the medical board, while nurses feel strongly that nurse practitioners should remain under the control of the board of nursing.

■ **Interorganizational conflict** is most commonly considered to involve competition between two organizations that exist within one market (Schermerhorn et al., 2012). For example, hospitals within the same community may demonstrate interorganizational conflict, as may colleges of nursing.

Covert and Overt Conflict

At any level, conflict may be overt or covert. Both approaches may be associated with benefits, as well as with negative consequences. In **overt conflict**, the individuals or group members who are in conflict address the conflict openly. Overt conflict is obvious, at least to most individuals, and thus coping with it is usually easier. Generally speaking, is easier to arrive at an agreement that conflict is present and easier to arrive at a description of the conflict.

In **covert conflict**, the conflict is not discussed openly. It may be avoided or ignored. Covert conflict may be exhibited in reactive, repressive, and avoidant behaviors. Reactive behaviors include whining, complaining, agreeing with others without really listening to them, and passive-aggressive behavior. Gossip is another form of reactive behavior, and rumor mills are common in workplaces in which covert conflict thrives. Repressive behaviors include absenteeism and tardiness. Although sustained avoidance usually is associated with negative outcomes, it is worth noting that avoidance may be an effective method of temporarily managing conflict. For example, avoidance may be appropriate when emotions are flaring and the individual or individuals involved would benefit from taking time to regain composure before discussing the topic of the conflict (Schermerhorn et al., 2012). However, sustained tactics of covert conflict result in increased stress, distress, and confusion about how to address the conflict. Acknowledging covert conflict is not easy, and everyone involved will have different perceptions of the conflict since it operates below the surface.

The common assumption about conflict is that it is destructive, and it certainly can be. However, when effectively managed, conflict can bring to light issues that need to be addressed and result in beneficial outcomes for individuals, groups, and organizations (Schermerhorn et al., 2012). Nevertheless, many individuals would not choose to willingly engage in conflict. Behind this attitude may lie a lack of understanding about how to handle conflict, which can create anxiety. Sustained conflict avoidance, however, usually results in the conflict continuing and becoming more difficult to resolve. The longer conflict goes unchecked, the more individuals may attach emotions to it, making it even more difficult to resolve.

▶ CAUSES OF CONFLICT

To resolve conflict effectively, nurses must understand its cause. Some conflicts have more than one cause. Typical causes of conflict among individuals and among groups include the following:

- Miscommunication
- Inaccurate information
- Mistrust
- Ambiguous role expectations
- Ineffective teamwork
- Inadequate project planning
- Ineffective leadership
- Resistance to change.

Within the healthcare setting, researchers have identified role boundary issues, scope of practice, and accountability as the three primary sources of conflict (Brown et al., 2011). Conflicts arising from role boundaries issues included a lack of understanding of the value of all team members, including those outside the disciplines of nursing and medicine, relative to the care of the client. Role boundaries also created conflicts with regard to awareness of which tasks each team member was authorized to perform. Exploration of conflicts related to scope of practice revealed that some physicians felt concerned about whether or not clients assigned to a nurse practitioner would receive care that was delivered with the same degree of efficiency and quality as that provided by a physician. In the realm

of accountability, conflict arose particularly when healthcare team members did not hold themselves accountable for their actions (Brown et al., 2011).

The Nurse–Physician Relationship

The nurse–physician relationship should be the strongest relationship that nurses have in order to meet the needs of the client. Unfortunately, it frequently is not. Both sides can contribute to inadequacies in this relationship. When conflict does occur, it can act as a barrier to effective client care.

Research related to magnet hospitals distinguishes between collegial and collaborative relationships between nurses and physicians (Schmalenberg & Kramer, 2009). *Collegial relationships* are those where there is equality of power. Magnet hospitals equalize power between nurses and physicians, making each group's power different but equal. In contrast, *collaborative relationships* between nurses and physicians focus on mutual power, but the physician's power is greater. The nurse's power is based on the nurse's extended time with clients, experience, and knowledge. In addition to power, this relationship requires respect and trust between the nurse and physician. Due to these factors, it is a complex relationship.

Positive professional communication is critical. Both sides should initiate positive dialogue rather than take adversarial positions. Cooperation and collaboration are also integral to the success of this relationship.

▶ PREVENTING CONFLICT

Clear communication is essential to prevent misunderstandings, which can lead to conflicts. Understanding and recognizing causes of conflict can assist individuals and organizations to develop strategies to prevent conflict. Nurses must be able to identify potential issues that can either act as barriers to conflict resolution or increase the likelihood that a situation will turn into a conflict. First and foremost, nurses need to recognize their own tension or stress level in the workplace: taking steps to decrease or manage their stress levels helps to reduce the likelihood of initiating conflict. Other strategies that help prevent conflict include the following (Greenberg, 2011; Porter-O'Grady & Malloch, 2013):

- Address issues as they arise.
- Avoid destructive criticism, including harsh words, threats, and generalized condemnation of behaviors or performance.
- Treat others with respect, which will decrease defensiveness.
- Avoid arguments. Sometimes people do need to vent, and as long as it is done appropriately and in a private place, it may be helpful in decreasing tension.
- Listen to each other.
- Consider the other individual's point of view, including cultural beliefs and values.

For individuals who are in leadership roles, strategies to promote conflict prevention include the following (Greenberg, 2011; Porter-O'Grady & Malloch, 2013):

- Allocate resources fairly, including fair distribution of workload balance and intensity when assigning client care.

- Clearly define role expectations for all team members.
- Encourage staff to provide feedback and identify potential concerns without the threat of punitive action.
- Acknowledge team members' accomplishments and achievements, as well as significant life events.

▶ RESPONDING TO CONFLICT

Not everyone responds to conflict in the same way, and individuals vary in how they respond in different circumstances. The nurse who can recognize the types of responses to conflict will be better equipped to predict and manage conflict. Consider these four typical responses to conflict (Arnold & Boggs, 2011):

- *Avoidance* occurs when an individual withdraws from a stressful situation due to extreme levels of discomfort and an inability to cope. There are times when this may be the most appropriate response, particularly when the situation may lead to negative results, but in many situations this increases conflict over the long term. Avoidance might occur when a nurse is in conflict with a manager and disagrees with the manager. The nurse must consider whether it is worth it to disagree publicly. Typically, avoidance occurs when one side is perceived as more powerful than the other. Avoidance is a helpful approach when more information is needed or when the issue just is not worth risking further conflict or a loss of opportunity or consideration.

- *Accommodation* occurs when one individual tries to make the situation better by cooperating with the individual with whom he or she is in conflict. The goal of accommodation is to eliminate the conflict as quickly as possible, despite the fact that it will not resolve the conflict. Accommodation works best when one individual or group is less interested in the issue than the other. It can be advantageous in that it serves to develop harmony. It also can provide power in future conflict since one party was more willing to let the conflict deflate.

- *Competition* occurs when power is used to stop the conflict. A manager might say, "This is the way it will be." This prevents further efforts by others who may be in conflict with the manager.

- *Collaboration* is a positive approach, with all parties attempting to reach an acceptable solution, and in the end both sides feel that they won something. Collaboration often involves some compromise, which is a method used to respond to conflict.

When conflict occurs, each individual involved has a personal perspective of the issue and conflict. To respond effectively to conflict, the nurse should apply the following guidelines:

- Demonstrate honesty, trustworthiness, and respect.
- State the issue objectively and provide a factual basis for the concern.
- Avoid emotion-based discussions.
- Be open to hearing all individuals' viewpoints and avoid passing judgment.

- Allow all individuals involved to express their concerns without interruption.
- Apply active listening techniques.
- Focus on identifying solutions as opposed to exacerbating the problem.
- Throughout the process of conflict resolution, recognize that the delivery of safe, effective client care is the central concern.

▶ AGGRESSION IN THE WORKPLACE

Aggressive behavior can be described as hostile and can lead to conflict. Hostile behavior by even a single individual in the workplace can increase the anxiety of many others. The first response toward a hostile staff member should be to communicate control to that staff member and to insert calm into the situation. When the nurse manager or team leader is the one who is hostile, the situation carries greater complexity and requires assistance from higher level management. Regardless of who is exhibiting hostility, someone should gain control and try to move the hostile staff member to a private place. Demonstrations of open conflict with hostility should not take place in client or public areas. If the suggestion to move to a private area does not work and the situation continues to escalate, simply walking away may help set some boundaries. This allows time for all parties to take a breath, calm down, and revisit the situation at a more appropriate time.

Managing Conflict With Clients and Families

When conflict occurs with clients or their families, in addition to the strategies already presented, setting limits can be an effective way to manage conflict with clients and families. Nurses set limits when they provide instructions such as "I can see you are upset and I want to help you, but I will not tolerate abusive language." Setting limits can help anxious clients monitor their own behaviors and keep the nurse from being interrupted too frequently.

Clients or families should never be allowed to demonstrate anger inappropriately. When this occurs, the nurse needs to set reasonable limits that are based on an assessment of the situation. Anger and inappropriate behavior may stem from a number of causes, such as pain, medications, fear and anxiety, psychosis, and dysfunctional communication. If a different culture is involved, then this factor needs to be considered (for example, some cultures consider it appropriate to be very emotional while others do not). In the long term, active listening and clear communication are critical to prevent and manage conflict. While empathy and consideration are key components of the nurse's role, abusive behavior is never acceptable. Tolerance of verbal or physical acts of aggression may lead to escalation of these behaviors. To promote safety for both the healthcare provider and the client, inappropriate demonstrations of anger, including hostile verbal or physical behaviors, should be reported immediately to the team leader or charge nurse.

Workplace Bullying

Workplace bullying is another source of conflict. **Verbal abuse**, which is one form of **workplace bullying**, is defined as malicious, repeated, harmful mistreatment of an individual with whom one works, regardless of whether that individual is an equal, a superior, or a subordinate. Behaviors that constitute verbal abuse include berating, humiliating, ridiculing, blaming, and threatening. Verbal abuse occurs in healthcare settings between clients and staff, nurses and other nurses, physicians and nurses, and all other staff relationships. This abuse can consist of statements made directly to a staff member or about a staff member to others. A recent study of staff nurses revealed that the greatest sources of hostility were senior nurses (24%) followed by charge nurses (17%) and nurse managers (14%) (Vessey et al., 2009).

Horizontal violence (HV), which is another form of workplace bullying, is a term used to describe aggressive acts committed against a nurse by one or more nursing colleagues (Longo & Sherman, 2007; Purpora & Blegen, 2012). Behaviors that reflect HV may include verbal acts, such as gossiping about and speaking sarcastically to the nurse who is the target. HV may also include nonverbal behaviors, such as ignoring the individual, or even physical acts of aggression (Purpora & Blegen, 2012).

In any form, workplace bullying yields serious negative consequences. Victims of bullying suffer adverse emotional effects, including depression, anxiety, and a sense of isolation (Murray, 2008, 2009). In healthcare organizations, research suggests that bullying is linked to increased rates of employee absenteeism and work-related injuries as well as decreased productivity (Felblinger, 2008; Longo & Sherman, 2007; Murray, 2008).

Nurses should recognize workplace bullying, be aware of its effects, and follow organizational policies and procedures with regard to reporting the behavior. Reports of bullying should include details such as the date, time, and description of events, as well as identification of any witnesses. Ideally, individuals in leadership positions within the organization will address the issue in such a manner that the bullying stops. Unfortunately, in reality, this does not always happen. Therefore, the nurse should be aware of organizations that may be available to provide assistance in case of bullying, including the appropriate state nursing association, the American Nurses Association, and the Department of Justice (Murray, 2009). See **Box 37–4** ● for an overview of guidelines for prevention of bullying among nurses in the workplace.

Box 37–4 Prevention of Workplace Bullying Among Nurses

- Educate team members about bullying behaviors and their adverse effects.
- Develop codes of conduct that clearly outline unacceptable behaviors.
- Promote a "zero-tolerance" attitude toward bullying.
- Encourage nurses to report bullying without fear of punishment or negative consequences.
- Offer the option of reporting bullying behaviors or recommendations for improvement of antibullying policies through use of comment or suggestion boxes.
- Assure nurses that reports of bullying will be taken seriously and thoroughly addressed, including through mandatory investigations of all allegations of bullying.
- Train leadership and management personnel to work collaboratively to prevent, identify, and address bullying behaviors.
- Create an environment in which courtesy and respect are valued.

Sources: Lowenstein, L. F. (2013). Bullying in nursing and ways of dealing with it. *Nursing Times, 109*(11), 22–25; Broome, B. S., & Williams-Evans, S. (2011). Bullying in a caring profession: Reasons, results, and recommendations. *Journal of Psychosocial Nursing and Mental Health Services, 49,* 30–35; Cleary, M., Hunt, G. E., Walter, G., & Robertson, M. (2009). Dealing with bullying in the workplace: Toward zero tolerance. *Journal of Psychosocial Nursing and Mental Health Services, 47,* 34–41; and Mackintosh, J., Wuest, J., Gray, M. M., & Cronkhite, M. (2010). Workplace bullying in health care affects the meaning of work. *Qualitative Health Research, 20,* 1128–1141.

▶ CONCLUSION

In nursing, as in life, conflict is inevitable. Family members become angry with care providers, physicians and nurses have different ideas about priorities or treatment plans, and disagreements arise among coworkers. Conflict that is ignored or mishandled can lead to greater stress and lower morale in the unit. Although conflict is never comfortable or easy to deal with, nurses can and must learn to deal with it effectively, thereby reducing stress in the workplace and creating an environment for providing safe client care.

REVIEW Conflict Resolution

RELATE Link the Concepts and Exemplars

Linking the exemplar of conflict resolution with the concept of stress and coping:

1. How do different levels of stress affect both the occurrence of conflict and the management of conflict that arises?

2. How can an understanding of different individuals' coping mechanisms improve the ability to manage conflict?

Linking the exemplar of conflict resolution with the concept of advocacy:

3. How does the nurse's role of client advocate compel the nurse to manage conflict appropriately?

4. A client and his spouse disagree on the client's choice of treatment plan. As the client's advocate, what is the nurse's role regarding this conflict?

REFER Go to Pearson Nursing Student Resources
nursing.pearsonhighered.com

- Additional review materials

REFLECT Case Study

Dee Johnston has worked in pediatric intensive care for the past 5 years. She decides to leave her current position because she feels that her coworkers still see her as the inexperienced nurse who first took the job and do not see how her practice, knowledge, and skill have improved over time. She accepts a position as a staff nurse in the pediatric ICU at another facility and spends 3 weeks in orientation. Her preceptor quickly recognizes her expertise and feels that additional orientation is unnecessary. Dee likes her new job and loves caring for the children, but begins to notice one of her coworkers seems to be watching her all the time. At first, Dee wonders why this coworker, Joan, keeps watching her. Eventually Dee starts to feel nervous. Every time she turns around and sees Joan watching, Dee feels as though she's all thumbs, drops things, and forgets what she is doing. The situation worsens when Joan begins to say things to Dee like "If you don't know what you're doing,

you should ask for help" or "It might be better if you let someone with more experience perform that procedure."

1. How is Dee interpreting Joan's watchful behavior?
2. Why might Joan be watching Dee as closely as she is?
3. What approach should Dee take in managing this conflict? Is avoidance an ideal approach? Why or why not?

EXEMPLAR 37.3   **Interdisciplinary Teams**

EXEMPLAR KEY TERMS
Group, 2391
Interdisciplinary team, 2391
Interprofessional team, 2391
Intradisciplinary team, 2391
Multidisciplinary team approach, 2391
Team, 2391

EXEMPLAR LEARNING OUTCOMES
After reading about this exemplar, you should be able to:

1. Describe the general purpose of healthcare teams.

2. Distinguish between intradisciplinary teams and interdisciplinary teams.
3. Distinguish between multidisciplinary teams and interdisciplinary teams.
4. Explain the benefits of engaging an interdisciplinary team in the planning and implementation of client care.
5. Identify potential professional disciplines and fields of expertise that may be offered by an interdisciplinary team in health care.
6. Describe two forms of interdisciplinary teams that function primarily outside the hospital setting.

▶ OVERVIEW

Every individual participates in groups both at work and in society. A **group** consists of three or more individuals who share a common purpose, and who interdependently interact with and influence one another (Adams & Galanes, 2012). Groups in which nurses may participate include local, national, or international professional organizations, organizational teams working to improve the structure and processes related to health care, and teams involving the nurses in a single unit, among others. Nurses may serve many roles within these groups, such as team leader, client advocate, data gatherer, policy writer, or educator.

▶ GROUPS AND TEAMS IN HEALTH CARE

Groups exist to help individuals achieve goals that might be unattainable by individual effort alone. By pooling the ideas and expertise of several individuals, groups often can solve problems more effectively than one individual acting alone. Information can be disseminated to groups more quickly and with more consistency than to individuals. In addition, groups often take greater risks than do individuals as they support each other in decision making. Most often, groups in the workplace function under the direction of one clearly identified leader, with individual members of the group completing assigned tasks or creating requested products. Groups usually experience a high level of individual accountability for each member (Andriopoulos & Dawson, 2009).

Although the terms *group* and *team* sometimes are used interchangeably, they are not synonymous. (For a detailed discussion of groups, see the module on Communication.) A team is a specialized type of group. In simplest terms, a **team** comprises individuals who agree to work in tandem to accomplish a common goal. Team-based health care may be more succinctly described as the collaborative delivery of high-quality, interdisciplinary health services to individual clients, families, and/or

their communities by two or more healthcare providers working in tandem with clients and their caregivers (to the degree desired by each client) for the purpose of achieving common goals (Mitchell et al., 2012; Naylor et al., 2010).

A team's hierarchy is more flexible than that of a group; members of a team often share the leadership role. Using a team approach, task completion and product creation are collaborative in nature, as opposed to being delegated to individuals. Accountability among team members is both individual and mutual in nature (Andriopoulos & Dawson, 2009).

Prevalent types of teams in health care include intradisciplinary and interdisciplinary teams. **Intradisciplinary teams** are formed by members of the same profession who work toward achieving a common goal. For example, a unit nurse manager may collaborate with the unit charge nurses to determine staffing needs and develop employee schedules. **Interdisciplinary teams** also seek to achieve a common goal; however, they comprise professionals with varied backgrounds. In addition to nurses and physicians, professionals from a variety of backgrounds may serve on interdisciplinary teams. (For an overview of individuals who may be part the client's interdisciplinary team, see Table 37–1, Collaborative Members of the Healthcare Team, earlier in this module.)

Combining Interdisciplinary Expertise Through Teamwork

Interdisciplinary teams provide collaborative, comprehensive care by providing a full range of expertise. Because these teams are composed of individuals with a variety of professional backgrounds, they also may be referred to as **interprofessional teams**. Although the term *multidisciplinary* sometimes is used synonymously with *interdisciplinary* or *interprofessional*, multidisciplinary teams take a different approach to client care.

Using a **multidisciplinary team approach**, members typically work together to deliver client care, but a single team member—usually a physician—makes the treatment decisions. While the physician interacts with each member of the multidisciplinary team, there is little communication between the

TABLE 37–4 Examples of Interdisciplinary Teams Outside the Hospital Setting

INTERDISCIPLINARY TEAM	SETTING	FUNCTIONS	PROFESSIONAL DISCIPLINES OF TEAM MEMBERS
School based	Educational institutions	Address and meet the health needs of students of all ages, including those within the physical, behavioral, and emotional domains.	Teachers, school administrators, school counselors, nurses, social workers, guidance counselors, mental health specialists, physicians, and others
Assertive Community Treatment (ACT)	Within the community, including in the client's home and workplace	Support and treat individuals with serious mental illnesses, such as schizophrenia, to promote optimal function both individually and within the community.	Psychiatrists, nurses, social workers, employment specialists, substance abuse specialists, and others
Programs of All-Inclusive Care for the Elderly (PACE)	Within the community, as well as within facilities or organizations that offer services for older adults and individuals older than 55 years of age; including inpatient and outpatient mental health facilities, home care agencies, extended care facilities, and hospice and palliative care agencies	Support and facilitate the provision of all services and care eligible for coverage by Medicare and Medicaid (as well as certain medically necessary services that are ineligible for coverage by Medicare or Medicaid), as authorized and approved by the interdisciplinary team. Provide coverage for prescription medications, physician treatment, transportation, home-based care, and, in some cases, extended care facility admission and treatment.	Physicians, nurses, nutritionists, exercise physiologists, speech/language pathology and audiology specialists, occupational therapists, physical therapists, social workers, dentists, pharmacists, clergy, and others

Sources: National Alliance on Mental Illness (NAMI). (2007). *Fact sheet—Assertive community treatment: Investment yields outcomes.* Retrieved from http://www.nami.org/Template.cfm?Section=ACT-TA_Center&template=/ContentManagement/ContentDisplay.cfm&ContentID=52382; Anderson, E., & Bronstein, L. R. (2012). Examining interdisciplinary collaboration within an expanded school mental health framework: A community–university initiative. *Advances in School Mental Health Promotion, 4*(1), 1–15; Centers for Medicare and Medicaid Services (CMMS). (2008). *Quick fact about programs of all-inclusive care for the elderly (PACE).* Retrieved from http://www.npaonline.org/website/download.asp?id=2378&title=Quick_Facts_about_PACE_%28CMS_Publication%29; and Körner, M. (2010). Interprofessional teamwork in medical rehabilitation: A comparison of multidisciplinary and interdisciplinary team approach. *Clinical Rehabilitation, 24*(8), 745–755.

other individual professionals on the team. Members of the multidisciplinary team set goals and develop client treatment plans in a more autonomous fashion. On an interdisciplinary or interprofessional team, decisions are made by the group, and the members collaboratively set client goals and carry out the treatment plan.

Through collaboration, members of interdisciplinary teams share and evaluate information with the goal of planning and implementing client care in the most effective, efficient manner. As opposed to placing emphasis on each individual team member's area of professional expertise, interdisciplinary collaboration emphasizes each individual's contribution to the joint planning and accomplishment of client goals (Finkelman & Kenner, 2012). Studies suggest that interdisciplinary teams can manage care with less redundancy, more efficiency, and fewer omissions than do client care teams that do not follow an interdisciplinary model (Young & Olsen, 2010).

This increased emphasis on collaboration is a result of changes in certification and practice standards as well as changes in healthcare reform, such as group practice and managed care. For example, although physician supervision of advanced practice nurses remains a subject of passionate debate, several states no longer mandate physician supervision of nurse practitioners or certified registered nurse anesthetists. Regardless of mandated requirements, collaboration is designated as a core competency for advanced practice nurses and research suggests collaboration is a key to the provision of excellent client care.

In addition to hospitals, interdisciplinary teams are used in numerous settings, including within the community, as well in schools, workplace settings, and extended care facilities. See **Table 37–4** ● for examples of interdisciplinary teams and the settings in which they are used.

The Process of Interdisciplinary Collaboration

A continuum of collaboration, as illustrated in **Figure 37–2** ●, reflects the following levels of communication and action, beginning with parallel communication and progressing toward co-management and referral:

- Parallel communication occurs when each professional communicates with the client independently and asks the same or similar questions.

- Parallel functioning occurs when communication may be more coordinated, but each professional has separate interventions and a separate plan of care.

- Information exchange involves planned communication, but decision making is unilateral, involving little, if any, collegiality.

- Coordination and consultation represent midrange levels of collaboration seeking to maximize the efficiency of resources.

- Co-management and referral represent the upper levels of collaboration, where providers retain responsibility and accountability for their own aspects of care and clients are directed to other providers when the problem is beyond the initial provider's expertise.

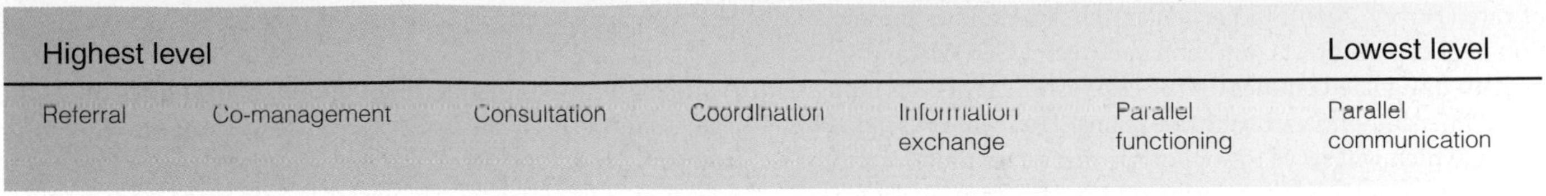

Highest level						Lowest level
Referral	Co-management	Consultation	Coordination	Information exchange	Parallel functioning	Parallel communication

Figure 37–2 ● Continuum of collaboration.

Characteristics of effective collaboration include the following:

1. Common purpose and goals identified at the outset
2. Clinical competence of each provider
3. Interpersonal competence
4. Humor
5. Trust
6. Valuing and respecting diverse, complementary knowledge.

Processes associated with these characteristics include recurring interactions that develop connections and, therefore, mutual respect and trust among the healthcare professionals. Interpersonal skills and respect for the competence of all collaborators are essential to achieving greater health outcomes for clients.

▶ THE FUTURE OF INTERDISCIPLINARY TEAMS

On March 23, 2010, President Barack Obama signed into law the Affordable Care Act (ACA), commonly called Obamacare. Stated goals of the ACA include increasing the affordability of health care and decreasing the number of uninsured individuals in the United States. (The full ACA document, which is extensive, is available online at www.gpo.gov/fdsys/pkg/PLAW-111publ148/content-detail.html.) For nurses, implications of this law include an increased focus on interdisciplinary collaboration.

According to the ANA, the ACA creates incentives for the integration of healthcare delivery and the coordinated provision

Evidence-Based Practice Barriers to Recognizing Individual Strengths in the Collaborative Model

Problem

Although effective interdisciplinary collaboration in health care requires a fluid, flexible shift of leadership, it is generally agreed that successful accomplishment of team goals requires a clearly defined leader (Mitchell et al., 2012). Even so, among interdisciplinary teams, when an official leader is selected, any member of the team may be eligible for the leadership position. This represents a deviation from the traditional hierarchical physician-led team approach. Barriers to implementation of interdisciplinary collaboration include conflict with regard to establishment of a clearly defined leader, in part, as a result of inadequate knowledge about the skills and functions of the team members (Suter et al., 2009).

Evidence

Interdisciplinary collaboration benefits the client, with documented outcomes that include safer client care and greater cost effectiveness (Mitchell et al., 2012). Despite research-based support for their use, application of the interdisciplinary approach to practice is limited by persistent barriers, among which are conflict regarding acceptance of a paradigm shift from the traditional physician-led team to a collaborative leadership environment. Contributing factors to these barriers include the efforts of varying disciplines to clearly separate themselves from one another.

Within the context of collaboration among interdisciplinary teams, awareness of the roles, knowledge base, and responsibilities of healthcare professionals from various disciplines emerged as a core competency required for success (Suter et al., 2009). However, in the process of identifying distinct disciplines as professions, hospital-based specialties— such as medicine, nursing, and allied health—have labored to establish boundaries to separate themselves from other

professionals; methods for achieving this include certification processes, specialty educational programs, and practice standards. Although these practices served the purpose of differentiating between various disciplines, they may be detrimental to the processes of cooperation and collaboration (McBride, 2010).

Implications

The factors that serve to differentiate professional disciplines include educational background and establishment of professional boundaries. Additionally, socialization patterns and professional cultural practices do not promote the intermingling of healthcare providers from different disciplines, including physicians and nurses. With the increased emphasis on collaboration through interdisciplinary teams, interventions are needed to unify various healthcare disciplines, as opposed to accentuating the boundaries that separate them.

Critical Thinking Application

Interdisciplinary collaboration includes practicing within one's own scope of practice and offering unique expertise to the team, as well as recognizing the expertise and skill sets offered by other members. For nurses, physicians, and all other members of interdisciplinary teams, education with regard to each member's unique abilities is needed in order to successfully administer the highest-quality client care through interdisciplinary collaboration. Recommended interventions for promoting enhanced mutual awareness and respect among team members include designing educational and training programs that promote practicing teamwork, and encouraging communication processes that allow for discussion of each individual's professional role and responsibilities (Mitchell et al., 2012).

of care (Haney, 2010). In particular, the ACA allows for allocation of grants or direct contracting between USDHHS and states or state-designated entities for the establishment of community-based interdisciplinary healthcare teams. These interdisciplinary teams, which will serve to support primary care practices in the provision of integrated, coordinated health care, will include licensed professionals from numerous disciplines, including medicine, nursing, pharmacy, nutritional sciences, behavioral and mental health, social work, chiropractic medicine, and complementary and alternative medicine (Haney, 2010.)

As previously discussed, research suggests that interdisciplinary care teams provide several benefits, including greater efficiency in the provision of care. Additionally, in light of impending changes in the political and healthcare climates, expectations for change include an increased focus on the delivery of care by interdisciplinary care teams. Nurses should place great emphasis on understanding the function and purpose of interdisciplinary teams, as well as the application of these principles.

◢ REVIEW Interdisciplinary Teams

RELATE Link the Concepts and Exemplars

Linking the exemplar of interdisciplinary teams with the concept of managing care:

1. How does an understanding of interdisciplinary teams improve the nurse's ability to manage care?

2. How does an understanding of interdisciplinary teams improve the nurse's ability to delegate?

Linking the exemplar of interdisciplinary teams with the concept of advocacy:

3. How does knowledge of interdisciplinary teams affect the nurse's role as an advocate?

4. Why is membership in a professional organization important to the nurse's role as an advocate?

REFER Go to Pearson Nursing Student Resources nursing.pearsonhighered.com

- Additional review materials

REFLECT Case Study

Abigail Lessarian, a 32-year-old client, delivered her first baby prematurely at 32 weeks' gestation. Her infant son, Garrett, was apneic at birth and required a brief period of tracheal intubation and mechanical ventilation. Immediately after his delivery, Garrett was admitted to the neonatal intensive care unit (NICU) for treatment of neonatal respiratory distress syndrome (RDS). By day 3, Garrett had made excellent progress; he was extubated and oxygen administration was implemented via nasal cannula with continuous positive airway pressure (CPAP). By day 14 in the NICU, Garrett was breathing effectively enough to maintain his oxygen saturation at >98% on room air with CPAP via nasal cannula; however, he experienced intermittent apneic spells with bradycardia until day 22. Garrett also was diagnosed

with an atrial septal defect (ASD), which his surgeon recommended monitoring in hopes that the ASD would resolve without requiring surgical treatment. He is receiving gavage feedings via a nasogastric tube.

By day 30 in the NICU, Garrett had experienced no apneic spells for 7 days. On day 32, Garrett's gavage tube was removed, and he successfully transitioned to bottle feeding over a period of several days. On day 43, Garrett began transitioning to breastfeeding; despite having difficulty with sucking, his progress was slow but steady. By day 46, Garrett's neonatologist (pediatrician specializing in neonatal care) cleared him for discharge to home.

Prior to Garrett's discharge, his mother and father are scheduled to complete an infant CPR course. They also will receive teaching about the use of a home apnea monitor. During discussion of the numerous topics about which Garrett's parents will receive instruction, Garrett's mother states, "I don't know if I can handle much more. I feel so overwhelmed." When she becomes tearful, her husband puts his arm around her and says, "We'll do whatever it takes to help him get healthy. I can't believe I was concerned about whether or not he'd like playing baseball or football. Now, that seems so silly. I just want him to survive."

1. Identify three nursing diagnoses that are appropriate for inclusion in Garrett's nursing plan of care.

2. Identify three nursing diagnoses that are appropriate for inclusion in the nursing plan of care for Garrett's parents.

3. During preliminary discharge planning, Garrett's interdisciplinary team's recommendations include home visits by a nurse, occupational therapist, and social worker. What roles might each of these professionals serve in the care of Garrett and his family?

4. What other professionals might be beneficial to the care of Garrett and his parents in the home setting?

◼ REFERENCES

Adams, K., & Galanes, G. (2012). *Communicating in groups: Applications and skills* (8th ed.). New York, NY: McGraw-Hill.

American Nurses Association (ANA). (2010). *Nursing: Scope and standards of practice* (2nd ed.). Silver Spring, MD: Author.

Anderson, E., & Bronstein, L. R. (2012). Examining interdisciplinary collaboration within an expanded school mental health framework: A community–university initiative. *Advances in School Mental Health Promotion, 4*(1), 1–15.

Andriopoulos, C., & Dawson, P. (2009). *Managing change, creativity and innovation.* London, UK: Sage.

Arnold, E. C., & Boggs, K. U. (2011). *Interpersonal relationships: Professional communication skills for nurses* (6th ed.). St. Louis, MO: Saunders.

Boone, B. N., King, M. L., Gresham, L. S, Wahl, P., & Suh, E. (2008). Conflict management training and nurse–physician collaborative behaviors. *Journal for Nurses in Staff Development, 24*(4), 168–175.

Broome, B. S., & Williams-Evans, S. (2011). Bullying in a caring profession: Reasons, results, and recommenda-

tions. *Journal of Psychosocial Nursing and Mental Health Services, 49*, 30–35.

Brown, J., Lewis, L., Ellis, K., Stewart, M., Freeman, T. R., & Kasperski, J. M. (2011). Conflict on interprofessional primary health care teams—Can it be resolved? *Journal of Interprofessional Care, 25*, 4–10.

Centers for Medicare and Medicaid Services (CMMS). (2008). *Quick fact about programs of all-inclusive care for the elderly (PACE).* Retrieved from http://www.npaonline.org/website/download.asp?id=2378&title=Quick_Facts_about_PACE_%28CMS_Publication%29.

Cleary, M., Hunt, G. E., Walter, G., & Robertson, M. (2009). Dealing with bullying in the workplace: Toward zero tolerance. *Journal of Psychosocial Nursing and Mental Health Services, 47*, 34–41.

Dalton, J. M. (2003). Development and testing of the theory of collaborative decision-making in nursing practice for triads. *Journal of Advanced Nursing, 41*(1), 22–33.

Felblinger, D. (2008). Incivility and bullying in the workplace and nurses' shame responses. *Journal of Obstetric, Gynecologic, and Neonatal Nursing, 37*(2), 234–242.

Finkelman, A. W., & Kenner, C. (2012). *Professional nursing concepts: Competencies for quality leadership* (2nd ed.). Sudbury, MA: Jones & Bartlett.

Garcia, C., & Duckett, L. (2009). No te entiendo y tu no me entiendes: Language barriers among immigrant Latino adolescents seeking health care. *Journal of Cultural Diversity, 16*(3), 120–126.

Gardner, B. T., Pransky, G., Shaw, W. S., Hong, Q. N., & Loisel, P. (2010). Researcher perspectives on competencies of return-to-work coordinators. *Disability & Rehabilitation, 32*(1), 72–78.

Greenberg, J. (2011). *Behavior in organizations.* Upper Saddle River, NJ: Prentice Hall.

Grossman, S. C., & Valiga, T. M. (2009). *The new leadership challenge—Creating the future of nursing* (3rd ed.). Philadelphia, PA: F. A. Davis.

Haney. C. (2010). New care delivery models in health system reform: Opportunities for nurses and their patients. *ANA Issue Brief*, 1–7.

Henderson, V. A. (1991). *The nature of nursing: Reflections after 25 years.* New York, NY: National League for Nursing.

Johnson, C. (2009). Bad blood: Doctor–nurse behavior problems impact patient care. *Physician Executive, 35*(6), 6–11.

Kim, H. S. (1983). Collaborative decision-making in nursing practice: A theoretical framework. In P. L. Chinn (Ed.), *Advances in nursing theory development* (pp. 271–283). Rockville, MD: Aspen.

Kim, H. S. (1987). Collaborative decision-making with clients. In K. Hannah, M. Reimer, W. Mills, & S. Letourneau (Eds.), *Clinical judgment and decision making: The future with nursing diagnosis* (pp. 58–62). New York, NY: Wiley.

Körner, M. (2010). Interprofessional teamwork in medical rehabilitation: A comparison of multidisciplinary and interdisciplinary team approach. *Clinical Rehabilitation, 24*(8), 745–755.

Longo, J., & Sherman, R. O. (2007). Leveling horizontal violence. *Nursing Management, 38*(3), 34–37, 50, 51.

Lowenstein, L. F. (2013). Bullying in nursing and ways of dealing with it. *Nursing Times, 109*(11), 22–25.

Mackintosh, J., Wuest, J., Gray, M. M., & Cronkhite, M. (2010). Workplace bullying in health care affects the meaning of work. *Qualitative Health Research, 20*, 1128–1141.

Masters, K. (2013). *Role development in professional nursing practice* (3rd ed.). Sudbury, MA: Jones & Bartlett.

McBride, A. B. (2010). Toward a roadmap for interdisciplinary academic career success. *Research and Theory for Nursing Practice, 24*(1), 74–86.

Mitchell, P., Wynia, M., Golden, R., McNellis, B., Okun, S., Webb, C. E., . . . Von Kohorn, I. (2012). Discussion paper: Core principles and values of effective team-based health care. Washington, DC: Institute of Medicine.

Murray, J. S. (2008). No more nurse abuse: Let's stop paying the emotional, physical, and financial costs of workplace abuse. *American Nurse Today, 3*(7), 17–19.

Murray, J. S. (2009). Workplace bullying in nursing: A problem that can't be ignored. *MedSurg Nursing, 18*(5), 273–276.

Nair, D. M., Fitzpatrick, J. J., McNulty, R., Click, E. R., & Glembocki, M. M. (2012). Frequency of nurse–physician collaborative behaviors in an acute care hospital. *Journal of Interprofessional Care, 26*(2), 115–120.

National Alliance on Mental Illness (NAMI). (2007). *Fact sheet—Assertive community treatment: Investment yields outcomes.* Retrieved from http://www.nami.org/Template.cfm?Section=ACT-TA_Center&template=/ContentManagement/ContentDisplay.cfm&ContentID=52382.

Naylor, M. D., Coburn, K. D., Kurtzman, E. T., Prvu Bettger, J. A., Buck, H., Van Cleave, J., & Cott, C. (2010). *Inter-professional team-based primary care for chronically ill adults: State of the science. White paper commissioned by the American Board of Internal Medicine (ABIM) Foundation.* Philadelphia, PA: American Board of Internal Medicine (ABIM) Foundation.

Norton, R. W. (1983). *Communicator style: Theory, applications, and measures.* Beverly Hills, CA: Sage.

Porter-O'Grady, T., & Malloch, K. (2013). *Leadership in nursing practice: Changing the landscape of health care.* Burlington, MA: Jones & Bartlett.

Purpora, C., & Blegen, M. A. (2012). Horizontal violence and the quality and safety of patient care: A conceptual model. *Nursing Research and Practice, 2012*, 306948–306952.

Schermerhorn, J. R., Osborn, R. N., Hunt, J. G., & Uhl-Bien, M. (2012). *Organizational behavior* (12th ed.). New York, NY: John Wiley & Sons.

Schmalenberg, C., & Kramer, M. (2009). Nurse–physician relationships in hospitals: 20,000 nurses tell their story. *Critical Care Nurse, 29*(1), 74–83.

Schneider, M. A. (2012). Nurse–physician collaboration: Its time has come. *Nursing, 42*(7), 50–53.

Skar, R. (2010). The meaning of autonomy in nursing practice. *Journal of Clinical Nursing, 19*(15/16), 2226–2234.

Summers, N. (2012). *Fundamentals of case management practice: Skills for the human services* (4th ed.). Belmont, CA: Brooks/Cole.

Suter, E., Arndt, J., Arthur, N., Parboosingh, J., Taylor, E., & Deutschlander, S. (2009). Role understanding and effective communication as core competencies for collaborative practice. *Journal of Interprofessional Care, 23*(1), 41–51.

U.S. Department of Health and Human Services (USD-HHS). (2013). *Healthy People 2020: Goals.* Retrieved from http://www.healthypeople.gov/2020/default.aspx.

Vessey, J. A., DeMarco, R. F., Gaffrey, D. A., Budin, & Wendy, C. (2009). Bullying of staff registered nurses in the workplace: A preliminary study for developing personal and organizational strategies for the transformation of hostile to healthy workplace environments. *Journal of Professional Nursing, 29*(5), 299–306.

Weinberg, D. B., Miner, D. C., & Rivlin, L. (2009). "It depends": Medical residents' perspectives on working with nurses. *American Journal of Nursing, 109*(7), 34–43.

Weston, M. J. (2008). Defining control over nursing practice and autonomy. *Journal of Nursing Administration, 38*, 404–408.

Weston, M. J. (2010). Strategies for enhancing autonomy and control over nursing practice. *Online Journal of Issues in Nursing, 15*(1).

World Health Organization (WHO). (2010). *Framework for action on interprofessional education and collaborative practice.* Geneva, Switzerland: Author.

Young, P. L., & Olsen, L. (2010). *The healthcare imperative: Lowering costs and improving outcomes: Workshop series summary.* Washington, DC: National Academies Press.

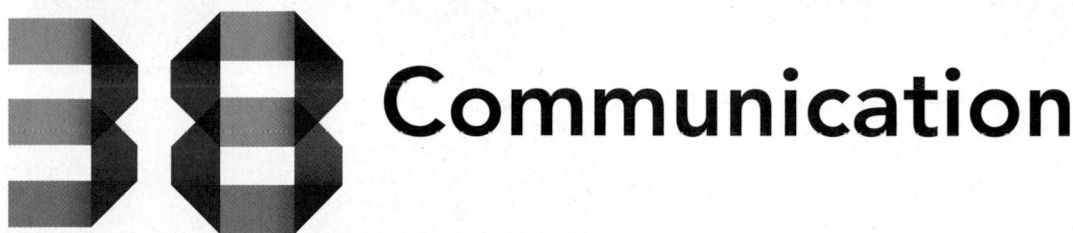

38 Communication

MODULE AT-A-GLANCE

The Concept of Communication, 2397

Exemplar 38.1
Groups and Group
Communication, 2418

Exemplar 38.2
Therapeutic
Communication, 2424

Exemplar 38.3
Documentation, 2438

Exemplar 38.4
Reporting, 2450

◢ THE CONCEPT OF COMMUNICATION

Nursing involves interactions between nurses and clients, nurses and other health professionals, and nurses and the community. The process of human interaction occurs through communication: verbal and nonverbal, written and unwritten, planned and unplanned. Communication between individuals conveys thoughts, ideas, feelings, and information. To be effective in their interactions, nurses must have effective verbal and written communication skills. They must be aware of what their words and body language say to others. Nurses also must have effective computer and electronic communication skills. **<<**

Concept Learning Outcomes

After reading about this concept, you will be able to:

1. Describe the various modes of communication and justify when a specific mode of communication may be most useful.
2. Describe barriers to successful communication and suggest strategies to reduce the risk of each barrier.
3. Compare and contrast different communication techniques aimed at preventing communication barriers.
4. Diagram the need for strong communication skills in each phase of the nursing process.
5. Recommend strategies the nurse may implement to improve communication with a client who has communication deficits.
6. Recommend strategies that the nurse may implement to improve communication with a client of limited English proficiency.
7. Contrast various styles of communicating and discuss the positive and negative results of each style.
8. Explore the characteristics of an assertive communicator.
9. Predict the impact on client care when the nurse communicates assertively.

Concept Key Terms

Aggressive
  communicators, *2409*
Assertive communicators,
  2409
Channel, *2399*
Communication, *2398*
Congruent
  communication, *2408*
Credibility, *2401*
Decode, *2399*
Elderspeak, *2409*
Electronic communication,
  2400
Encoding, *2399*
Feedback, *2399*
Intimate distance, *2407*
Message, *2399*

Nonverbal
  communication, *2400*
Passive
  communicators, *2409*
Perceptions, *2406*
Personal distance, *2407*
Personal space, *2406*
Proxemics, *2406*
Public distance, *2408*
Receiver, *2399*
Response, *2399*
Sender, *2399*
Social distance, *2408*
Territoriality, *2408*
Values, *2406*
Verbal
  communication, *2400*

▶ THE MEANING OF COMMUNICATION

The term *communication* has various meanings, depending on the context in which it is used. For instance, communication can be the interchange of information between two or more individuals, in other words, the exchange of ideas or thoughts. This kind of communication uses methods such as talking and listening or writing and reading. However, painting, dancing, and storytelling are also methods of communication. Thoughts and ideas can be conveyed to others not only through spoken or written words but also through gestures or body actions.

In the healthcare professions, sometimes a nurse or physician is said to be lacking in something called "bedside manner." A failure on the part of a healthcare professional to communicate successfully with a client or other healthcare professional can result in poor health outcomes for the client. This concept section provides nurses with essential information that they need to communicate successfully with clients, colleagues, and other healthcare professionals. For the purposes of this text, **communication** is any means of exchanging information or feelings between two or more individuals. Communication is a basic component of human relationships, including nursing.

The intent of any communication is to elicit a response. Thus, communication is a process that has two main purposes: to influence others to respond and to obtain information. Communication can be described as helpful or unhelpful. Helpful communication encourages a sharing of information, thoughts, or feelings between two or more individuals. Unhelpful communication hinders or blocks the transfer of information and feelings. In nursing, any form or failure of communication that prevents the sharing of information and feelings can have negative consequences for the client.

Effective communication is essential for the establishment of a healthy nurse–client relationship. Nurses who communicate effectively are better able to collect assessment data, develop care plans in collaboration with clients, initiate interventions, evaluate outcomes of interventions, initiate changes that promote health, and prevent legal problems associated with nursing practice. This communication process depends on nurses having established trusting relationships with clients and their support people.

Communication also occurs on an intrapersonal level—that is, an individual's thoughts are a form of communication. Intrapersonal communication, also called *self-talk*, describes the thoughts or communication individuals keep to themselves. When any two individuals are talking with one another, each of them will usually be engaging in intrapersonal communication at the same time. They will be thinking their own thoughts before, during, and after sending a message to each other. This intrapersonal communication occurs constantly and can interfere with an individual's ability to hear a message as the sender intended (see **Figure 38–1 ●**).

Clear communication is essential to both the safety of the client and the ability of the nurse to collaborate with an increasingly diverse healthcare team. Effective communication is

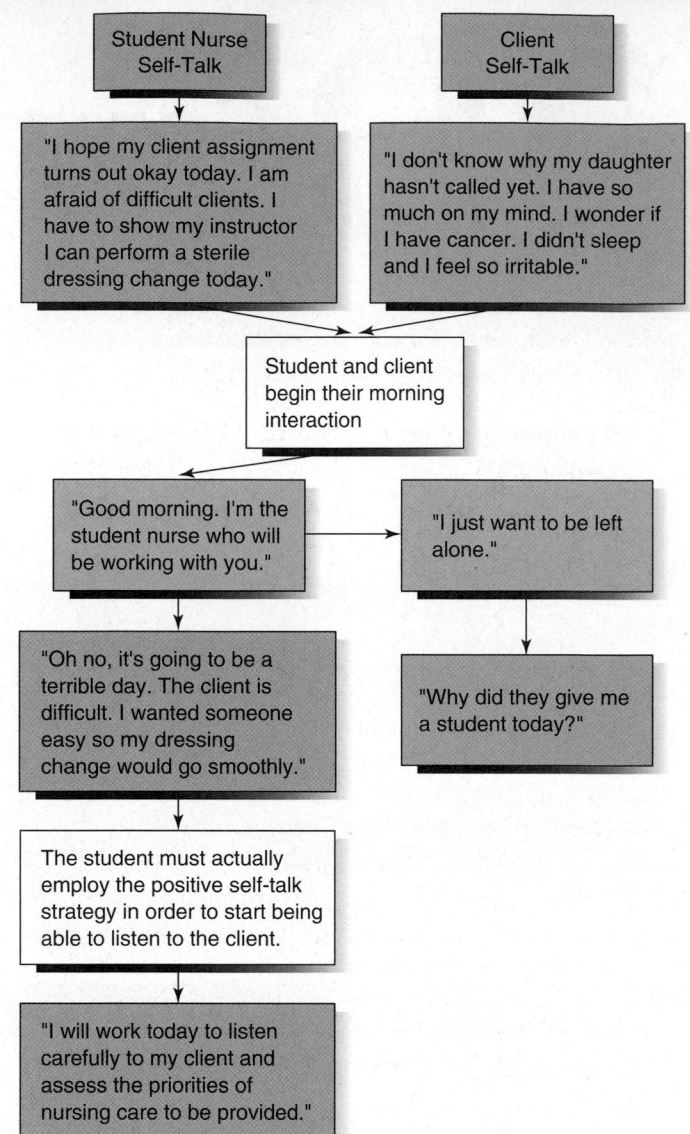

Figure 38–1 ● Improving student nurse self-talk.

essential for collaboration, professional communication, and avoidance of cultural misunderstandings. Factors that can complicate the communication process include the shortness of a client's stay in an acute care facility, the complexity of his or her illnesses, and the need to quickly prepare the client for complex care requirements after discharge.

Practicing clear and appropriate communication can pose a unique challenge in the current healthcare environment. Overcoming barriers to communication is necessary in a society in which many languages are spoken and the population is multicultural. Individual nurses cannot be fluent in each language they will encounter, nor can they be fully informed of the cultural contexts of words and phrases that may have multiple meanings. Furthermore, nonverbal communication also has cultural meanings that must be understood to avoid barriers.

Professional communication and collaboration can be a challenge when the nurse is working with colleagues from diverse cultures and languages. Clear communication about care and about client information is equally important, whether it is in the form of verbal interactions, written recordings, or computerized documentation. A challenge for the nurse in the 21st century is to become proficient in communicating via technology, including telephone communication such as telephone triage and communication using computers such as nursing documentation systems, personal data information systems, and e-mail.

Finding effective ways to overcome communication barriers provides the opportunity for the nurse to bridge cultural gaps when delivering health care. The nurse who can use available resources and solve problems when communication difficulties are present will be better able to assist clients and families to access care and benefit from healthcare services. Clear communication will help the healthcare team provide effective care. It is essential in interdisciplinary teams. When nurses are able to communicate well in verbal and written form, the quality of professional communication benefits and nurses can provide better care to their clients. Nurses can use technology to enhance communication with clients and other healthcare providers, to improve access to care for people in remote areas, and to increase their own knowledge using the information resources available on the Internet.

▶ THE COMMUNICATION PROCESS

Face-to-face communication involves a sender, a message, a receiver, and a response, or feedback (see **Figure 38–2** ●). In its simplest form, communication is a two-party process involving the sending and the receiving of a message. Because the intent of communication is to elicit a response, the process is ongoing: The receiver of the message then becomes the sender of a response, and the original sender in turn becomes the receiver.

Sender

The **sender**, an individual or group who wishes to convey a message to another, can be considered the *source-encoder*. This term suggests that the person or group sending the message must have an idea or reason for communicating (source) and must put that idea or reason into a form that can be transmitted. **Encoding** involves the selection of specific signs or symbols (codes) to transmit the message, such as which language and words to use, how to arrange the words, and what medium to use, which may involve tone of

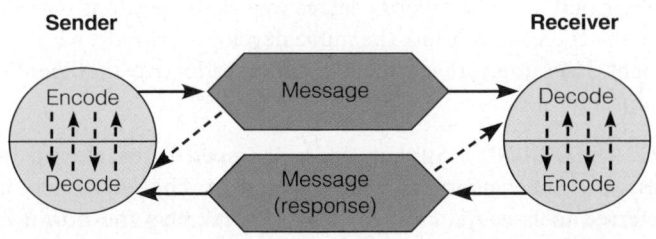

Figure 38–2 ● The communication process. The dashed arrows indicate intrapersonal communication (self-talk). The solid lines indicate interpersonal communication.

voice and gestures in oral communication. For example, if the receiver speaks English, the sender usually selects English words. If the message is "Mr. Johnson, you have to wait another hour for your pain medication," the tone of voice selected and a shake of the head can reinforce the message. Nurses must not only deal with dialects and foreign languages but also cope with two language levels: the client's and the nurse's own.

Message

The next component of the communication process is the **message** itself—what is actually said or written, the body language that accompanies the words, and how the words are transmitted. The medium used to convey the message is the **channel**, and it can target any of the receiver's senses. The channel must be appropriate for the message, and it should help make the intent of the message clearer. In some instances, for example, talking face to face with an individual may be more effective than telephoning or writing a message. Using recorded messages or communicating by radio or television may be more appropriate for large audiences. Written communication is often appropriate for long explanations or for a communication that needs to be preserved. The nonverbal channel of touch is often highly effective. Some of the most effective communications use more than one sensory channel.

Receiver

The **receiver**, the third component of the communication process, is the listener, who must listen, observe, and attend. This person is the *decoder*, who must perceive what the sender intended (interpretation). Perception may use all of the senses to receive verbal and nonverbal messages. To **decode** means to relate the message perceived to the receiver's storehouse of knowledge and experience and to sort out the meaning of the message. Whether the receiver accurately decodes the message according to the sender's intent depends largely on their similarities in knowledge and experience and sociocultural background. If the meaning of the decoded message matches the intent of the sender, then the communication has been effective.

Ineffective communication occurs when the sender's message is misinterpreted by the receiver. For example, if a nurse who is preparing to feed a client who requires assistance glances repeatedly at the clock, the client may interpret this behavior as indicating that the nurse is in a hurry, which may make the client feel rushed and like a burden. It is important for nurses to consider the unplanned messages their behavior may be sending.

Response

The **response**, the fourth component of the communication process, is the message that the receiver returns to the sender. It is also called **feedback**. A response can be either verbal, nonverbal, or both. A nod of the head or a yawn is an example of a nonverbal response. Either way, feedback allows the sender to correct or reword a message. In the case of

Mr. Johnson, who was told that he would have to wait an hour for his pain medication, the receiver may appear irritated or say, "Well, the nurse on the other shift gives me my pain medication early if I need it." The sender then knows the message was interpreted accurately. However, now the original sender becomes the receiver, who is required to decode and respond.

▶ MODES OF COMMUNICATION

Communication is generally carried out in two different modes: verbal and nonverbal. **Verbal communication** uses the spoken or written word; **nonverbal communication** uses other forms, such as gestures, facial expressions, and touch. Although both kinds of communication occur concurrently, the majority of communication is nonverbal. Learning about nonverbal communication helps the nurse develop effective communication patterns and relationships with clients. A mode of communication that has evolved with technology is **electronic communication**. E-mail is perhaps the most common form of electronic communication, although social networking and text messaging are used frequently outside the workplace. It is important for the nurse to know when it is appropriate and not appropriate to use e-mail to communicate with clients.

Verbal Communication

Because individuals choose the words they use, verbal communication is a largely conscious and purposeful activity. Words and phrasing used vary among individuals according to culture, socioeconomic background, age, and education. An abundance of words can be used to form messages. In addition, a wide variety of feelings can be conveyed when people talk. As a result, countless possibilities exist for the way ideas and information can be exchanged.

When choosing what words to say or write, the nurse needs to consider pace and intonation, simplicity, clarity and brevity, timing and relevance, adaptability, credibility, and humor.

PACE AND INTONATION The manner of speech, as in the pace or rhythm and intonation, will affect the feeling and impact of the message. The intonation can express enthusiasm, joy, sadness, anger, or amusement. The pace of speech may indicate interest, anxiety, boredom, or fear. For example, speaking slowly and softly may help calm an excited client.

SIMPLICITY Simplicity of speech refers to the use of commonly understood words, brevity, and completeness. Many complex technical terms become natural to nurses. However, clients often misunderstand these terms. Words such as *vasoconstriction* or *cholecystectomy* are meaningful to the nurse and may be easy to use but are ill advised in communicating with clients. Nurses need to learn to select appropriate, understandable terms that are appropriate for the age, knowledge, culture, and education of the client. For example, instead of saying to a client, "The nurses will be catheterizing you tomorrow for a urine analysis," it may be better to say, "Tomorrow we need to get a sample of your urine, so we will collect it by putting a small tube into your bladder." The latter statement is simpler and therefore easier to understand. It is more likely to convey to the client why the procedure is needed and whether it will be uncomfortable.

CLARITY AND BREVITY The most effective type of message is one that is direct and simple. *Clarity* is saying precisely what is meant, and *brevity* is using the fewest words necessary. Using clarity and brevity results in a message that is simple and clear. An aspect of this is congruence, or consistency, in which the nurse's behavior or nonverbal communication matches the words spoken. When the nurse tells the client, "I am interested in hearing what you have to say," the nurse should use nonverbal behavior that includes facing the client, making eye contact (if culturally appropriate), and leaning forward. The goal is to communicate clearly so that all aspects of a situation or circumstance are understood. To ensure clarity in communication, the nurse also needs to speak slowly and enunciate carefully. Note that careful enunciation does not require speaking loudly. Speaking loudly to a client, even if the client is hard of hearing, especially in a quiet setting, may be experienced by the client as patronizing or aggressive and often undermines the nurse–client relationship.

TIMING AND RELEVANCE The nurse needs to be aware of both relevance and timing when communicating with clients. No matter how clearly or simply words are stated or written, the timing needs to be appropriate to ensure that the words are heard. Moreover, the message needs to relate to the person who is the receiver or to the person's interests and concerns. This requires the nurse to be sensitive to the client's needs and concerns. For example, a client whose current focus is her fear of cancer may not hear the nurse's explanations about the upcoming gallbladder surgery. In this situation, the nurse should first encourage the client to express her concerns and then deal with those concerns. The necessary explanations can be provided after the client's primary fears have been addressed or at another time when the client is able to listen.

Another problem of poor timing results from asking several questions at once. For example, a nurse enters a client's room and says in one breath, "Good morning, Mrs. Brody. How are you this morning? Did you sleep well last night? Your husband is coming to see you before your surgery, isn't he?" The client no doubt wonders which question to answer first, if any. Asking a question without waiting for an answer before making another comment is an example of poor timing. By allowing the client to respond to social talk or chat, as well as to questions regarding the client's condition, the nurse develops a rapport with the client. This rapport can help facilitate effective therapeutic communication.

ADAPTABILITY Spoken messages need to be altered in response to behavioral cues from the client. This adjustment is referred to as *adaptability*. What the nurse says and how it is said must be individualized and carefully considered. This requires astute assessment and sensitivity on the part of the nurse. For example, suppose that a nurse who usually smiles, appears cheerful, and greets a client with an enthusiastic "Hi, Mrs. Brown!" notices that the client is not smiling and appears distressed. In such a case the nurse should modify his tone of speech and express concern via his facial expressions while moving toward the client.

CREDIBILITY   **Credibility** is the quality of being truthful, trustworthy, and reliable. Credibility may be the most important criterion of effective communication. Nurses foster credibility by being consistent, dependable, and honest. Nurses need to be knowledgeable about the topic being discussed and to have accurate information. Nurses should convey confidence and certainty in what they are saying, while being able to acknowledge their limitations (e.g., "I don't know the answer to that, but I will find someone who does").

HUMOR   The use of humor can be a positive and powerful tool in the nurse–client relationship, but it must be used with care. Humor can be used to help clients adjust to difficult and painful situations. The physical act of laughter can provide an emotional and physical release, reducing tension by providing a different perspective and promoting a sense of well-being. However, in using humor, it is important to consider the client's perception of what is considered humorous. Timing is also important. Though humor and laughter can help reduce stress and anxiety, the feelings of the client should guide the nurse's use of humor (Moore, 2008).

Nonverbal Communication

Nonverbal communication is sometimes called *body language.* It includes gestures, body movements, use of touch, and physical appearance, including adornment. Nonverbal communication often tells others more about what an individual is feeling than what the person actually says, because nonverbal behavior is controlled less consciously than verbal behavior (see **Figure 38–3 ●**). Nonverbal communication either reinforces or contradicts what is said verbally. For example, if a nurse says to a client, "I'd be happy to sit here and talk to you for a while," yet glances at a watch every few seconds, the actions contradict the verbal message. The client is more likely to believe the nonverbal behavior, which conveys "I am very busy and need to leave." By contrast, when the nurse enters the client's room and finds the client crying, if the nurse pulls a chair close to the bed and touches the forearm gently saying, "I can see how upset you are, what is bothering you?" the nurse conveys the message that the nurse cares and has the time and willingness to listen to the client.

Observing and interpreting a client's nonverbal behavior is an essential skill that nurses must develop. The efficient observation of nonverbal behavior requires a systematic assessment of the person's overall physical appearance, posture, gait, facial expressions, and gestures. The nurse should exercise caution in interpretation, always clarifying any observation with the client.

Clients who have altered thought processes, such as clients with schizophrenia or dementia, may experience times when expressing themselves verbally is difficult or impossible. During these times, the nurse needs to be able to interpret the feeling or emotion that the client is expressing nonverbally. An attentive nurse who clarifies observations very often portrays caring and acceptance to the client. This can be a beginning for

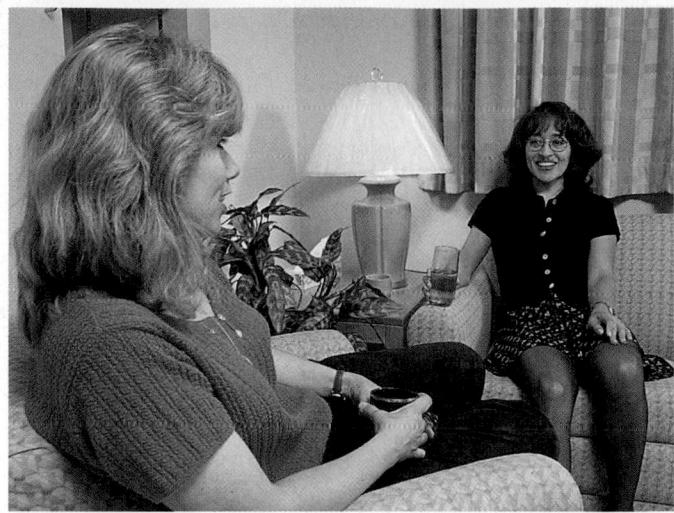

A

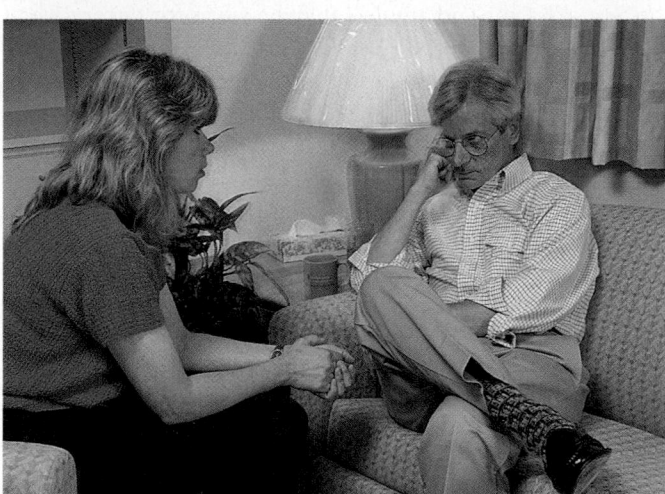

B

Figure 38–3 ● Nonverbal communication sometimes conveys meaning more effectively than words. *A,* The postures of these women indicate openness to communication. *B,* The listener's posture suggests resistance to communication.

establishing a trusting relationship between the nurse and the client, even for clients who have difficulty communicating appropriately.

Clients who are on the autism spectrum will likely have difficulty understanding nonverbal communication. Many individuals with autism find eye contact difficult, so they avoid it when communicating. When a nurse is speaking to a client with autism, the nurse's communications should be direct and specific. The nurse should select words carefully, keeping in mind that the client will not understand any nonverbal messages that may be communicated along with the words. Offering the client relevant handouts or brochures can help convey the message.

Nonverbal communication varies widely among cultures. Even for behaviors such as smiling and handshaking, cultures differ. For example, many Hispanics feel that smiling and handshaking are an integral part of an interaction and essential to establishing trust. The same behavior might be perceived by a Russian as insolent and frivolous. Refer to the module on Culture and Diversity for more information on cultural differences.

The nurse cannot always be sure of the correct interpretation of feelings that have been expressed nonverbally. The same feeling can be expressed nonverbally in more than one way, even within the same cultural group. For example, anger may be communicated by aggressive or excessive body motion, or it may be communicated by frozen stillness. In some cultures, a smile may be used to conceal anger. Therefore, the interpretation of such observations requires validation with the client. For example, the nurse might say, "You look as though you have been crying. Is something upsetting you?"

PERSONAL APPEARANCE   Clothing and accessories can be sources of information about an individual. Although choice of apparel is highly personal, it may convey social and financial status, culture, religion, group association, and self-concept. Charms and amulets may be worn for decorative or for health protection purposes. When the symbolic meaning of an object is unfamiliar, the nurse can inquire about the object's significance. This may foster rapport with the client and help the nurse gain a better understanding of the client's beliefs.

How an individual dresses is often an indicator of how the person feels. Someone who is tired or ill may not have the energy or the desire to maintain his or her normal level of grooming. When someone known for immaculate grooming becomes lax about appearance, the nurse may suspect a loss of self-esteem or a physical illness. The nurse must validate these observed nonverbal data by asking the client. For acutely ill clients in hospital or home care settings, a change in grooming habits may signal that the client is feeling better. A man may request a shave, or a woman may request a shampoo and some makeup.

POSTURE AND GAIT   The ways in which individuals walk and carry themselves are often reliable indicators of self-concept, current mood, and health. Erect posture and an active, purposeful stride suggest a feeling of well-being. Slouched posture and a slow, shuffling gait suggest depression or physical discomfort. Tense posture and a rapid, determined gait suggest anxiety or anger. The posture of individuals when they are sitting or lying can also indicate feelings or mood. Again, the nurse clarifies the meaning of the observed behavior by describing to the client what the nurse sees and then asking what it means or whether the nurse's interpretation is correct. For example, "You look like it really hurts you to move. I'm wondering how your pain is and if you might need something to make you more comfortable?"

FACIAL EXPRESSION   No part of the body is as expressive as the face (see **Figure 38–4** ●). Feelings of surprise, fear, anger, disgust, happiness, and sadness can be conveyed by facial expressions. Although the face may express the person's genuine emotions, it is also possible to control these muscles so the emotion expressed does not reflect what the person is feeling. When the message is not clear, it is important to get feedback to be sure of the intent of the expression. Many facial expressions

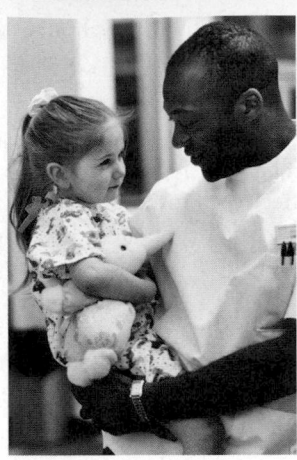

Figure 38–4 ● The nurse's facial expression communicates warmth and caring.
Source: Getty Images.

convey a universal meaning. The smile expresses happiness. Contempt is conveyed by the mouth turned down, the head tilted back, and the eyes directed down the nose. No single expression can be interpreted accurately, however, without considering other reinforcing physical cues, the setting in which it occurs, the expression of others in the same setting, and the cultural background of the client.

Nurses need to be aware of their own expressions and what they are communicating to others. Clients are quick to notice a nurse's facial expression, particularly when the client feels unsure or uncomfortable. The client who questions the nurse about a feared diagnostic result will watch whether the nurse maintains eye contact or looks away when answering. The client who has had disfiguring surgery will examine the nurse's face for signs of disgust. It is impossible to control all facial expressions, but the nurse must learn to control expressions of feelings such as fear or disgust in some circumstances.

Eye contact is another essential element of facial communication. In many cultures, mutual eye contact acknowledges recognition of the other person and a willingness to maintain communication. (See the module on Culture and Diversity.) Often an individual initiates contact with another person with a glance, capturing the person's attention prior to communicating. Someone who feels weak or defenseless often averts the eyes or avoids eye contact; the communication received may be too embarrassing or too dominating.

GESTURES   Hand and body gestures may emphasize and clarify the spoken word, or they may occur without words to indicate a particular feeling or to give a sign. A father awaiting information about his daughter in surgery may wring his hands, tap his foot, pick at his nails, or pace back and forth. A gesture may more clearly indicate the size or shape of an object. A wave good-bye and the motioning of a visitor toward a chair are gestures that have relatively universal meanings. Some gestures, however, are culture specific. The Anglo American gesture meaning "shoo" or "go away" means "come here" or "come back" in some Asian cultures. In the Hmong culture it is considered rude to point at something with your toe.

For individuals with special communication problems, such as those with hearing impairments, the hands are central to communication. Many individuals who are deaf learn sign language, in which the hands are used along with facial expressions and other body language to form expressions with accepted meanings. Similarly, ill individuals who are unable to reply verbally may be able to utilize a communication system using the hands. For example, the client may be able to raise an index finger once for "yes" and twice for "no." Other signals can often be devised by the client and the nurse to denote various meanings

Electronic Communication

Nurses are increasingly using e-mail to communicate with other nurses, other departments in their employment setting, and resources outside the employment setting. It is important for the nurse to follow standard guidelines for the use of e-mail and to understand its advantages and disadvantages.

ADVANTAGES E-mail has many advantages. It is a fast, efficient way to communicate, and it is legible. It provides a record of the date and time when the message was sent or received. Some healthcare facilities provide information to their clients on how to reach specified staff members by e-mail. This improves communication and continuity of client care.

DISADVANTAGES The primary disadvantage of e-mail is the risk to client confidentiality. The Health Insurance Portability and Accountability Act (HIPAA) requires organizations to apply "reasonable and appropriate safeguards" when e-mailing protected health information (PHI). Each healthcare agency needs to have an e-mail encryption system to ensure security. An agency may use its own system or outsource an encryption service.

Another disadvantage is one of socioeconomics. Not everyone has a computer. And even if computer access is possible, not everyone has the necessary computer skills. E-mail may enhance communication with some clients, but others will not have access to it at all. Alternative forms of communication will be needed for clients who have limited abilities with speaking English, reading, writing, or using a computer.

WHEN NOT TO USE E-MAIL In certain situations the use of e-mail should be avoided:

- When the information is urgent and the client's health could be in jeopardy if the client doesn't read the e-mail message immediately
- When the information is highly confidential (e.g., HIV status, mental health, chemical dependency)
- When lab data are abnormal. If the information is likely to be confusing and could prompt many questions, it is better to either see or telephone the client.

OTHER GUIDELINES Agencies usually develop standards and guidelines for the use of e-mail in health care. It is important for nurses to know their employer's guidelines regarding the use of e-mail to communicate with clients. Usually the client is asked to sign an e-mail consent form. This form provides information about the risks of e-mail and authorizes the health agency to communicate with the client at a specified e-mail address.

The nurse should identify in the subject line that the e-mail is confidential. It may also be prudent to include a disclaimer in the e-mail stating that the message is to be read only by the person to whom it is addressed and that no one else is authorized to read the message. Additionally, the disclaimer should state that if the e-mail is sent to anyone else by mistake, the recipient should contact the sender.

Information sent to a client via e-mail is considered part of the client's medical record. Therefore, a copy of the e-mail needs to be put in the client's chart. E-mails, like other documentation in the client's record, may be used as evidence during litigation. Rules for written communication (see the next section) also apply to e-mail communication.

E-mail is another form of communication that can enhance effective relationships with clients. It is not, however, a substitute for effective verbal and nonverbal communication. The nurse needs to use professional judgment about what form(s) of communication will best meet the client's health needs.

Written Communication

Written communication can be considered a form of verbal communication. Examples of forms of written communication include notes, letters, e-mail messages, and text messages. Written communication has some limitations. For example, it lacks the nonverbal cues that accompany verbal communication. For example, you may receive a text message from a friend that says, "GET OUT OF HERE!!" Without an understanding of context, this message could be interpreted as shock and disbelief at something you told your friend, or anger and the wish for you to vacate the friend's life, or a request to be left alone. Only by hearing tone of voice and seeing body language can context be relayed. As a result, rules for written communication differ from rules for other forms of communicating.

Nurses have many requirements as well as opportunities for written communication. The most common form of written communication in nursing is the notes nurses make in the medical record about a client's status, which will be discussed in Exemplar 38.3 on documentation. Nurses also write discharge instructions for clients and their families, memos to nursing colleagues and other healthcare professionals, and client educational materials. Nurse-managers write employee evaluations; policies and procedures; and other communications to administrators, colleagues, and nursing staff. Nurse-educators write educational handouts and course syllabi. An important consideration in written communication is that decoding often occurs when the writer is not present and may occur long after the document is written. Therefore, clarity is important because it may not be possible to ask questions or clarify areas of confusion.

CHARACTERISTICS OF EFFECTIVE WRITTEN COMMU-NICATION In addition to simplicity, brevity, clarity, relevance, credibility, and humor (characteristics of effective oral communication), written communication must contain the following:

1. *Appropriate language and terminology.* Language and terminology must be appropriate for the age, education and reading level, and culture of the reader. Health education materials written for children should be different than materials written for adults. For individuals whose primary language is not English, it may be more effective to have written materials translated into their primary language by a professional translator. Appropriate lay terminology may be substituted for medical terminology; for example, *high blood pressure* may be used instead of *hypertension*. National standards on culturally and linguistically appropriate services (CLAS) are listed in **Box 38–1** ●.

🔅 *Stay Current:* For more information regarding the CLAS standards, go to **http://raceandhealth.hhs.gov/templates/browse.aspx?lvl=2&lvlID=15**.

2. *Correct grammar, spelling, and punctuation.* The use of correct grammar, spelling, and punctuation provides clarity for the reader. Misspelled words, misplaced punctuation, and incorrect grammar can change the intended meaning and lead to confusion on the part of the reader. They can also undermine the reader's confidence in the sender. Most computer word-processing programs have spelling- and grammar-checking features that assist writers in improving their writing.

3. *Logical organization.* Written materials are well organized when they are logical and easy for readers to follow. Consider what the reader needs to know first. Simple and foundational information is usually provided first, followed by more complex information. Using examples can also assist readers.

Box 38–1 National Standards on Culturally and Linguistically Appropriate Services (CLAS)

STANDARD 1

Health care organizations should ensure that patients/consumers receive from all staff member's effective, understandable, and respectful care that is provided in a manner compatible with their cultural health beliefs and practices and preferred language.

STANDARD 2

Health care organizations should implement strategies to recruit, retain, and promote at all levels of the organization a diverse staff and leadership that are representative of the demographic characteristics of the service area.

STANDARD 3

Health care organizations should ensure that staff at all levels and across all disciplines receive ongoing education and training in culturally and linguistically appropriate service delivery.

STANDARD 4

Health care organizations must offer and provide language assistance services, including bilingual staff and interpreter services, at no cost to each patient/consumer with limited English proficiency at all points of contact, in a timely manner during all hours of operation.

STANDARD 5

Health care organizations must provide to patients/consumers in their preferred language both verbal offers and written notices informing them of their right to receive language assistance services.

STANDARD 6

Health care organizations must assure the competence of language assistance provided to limited English proficient patients/consumers by interpreters and bilingual staff. Family and friends should not be used to provide interpretation services (except on request by the patient/consumer).

STANDARD 7

Health care organizations must make available easily understood patient-related materials and post signage in the languages of the commonly encountered groups and/or groups represented in the service area.

STANDARD 8

Health care organizations should develop, implement, and promote a written strategic plan that outlines clear goals, policies, operational plans, and management accountability/oversight mechanisms to provide culturally and linguistically appropriate services.

STANDARD 9

Health care organizations should conduct initial and ongoing organizational self-assessments of CLAS-related activities and are encouraged to integrate cultural and linguistic competence-related measures into their internal audits, performance improvement programs, patient satisfaction assessments, and outcomes-based evaluations.

STANDARD 10

Health care organizations should ensure that data on the individual patient's/consumer's race, ethnicity, and spoken and written language are collected in health records, integrated into the organization's management information systems, and periodically updated.

STANDARD 11

Health care organizations should maintain a current demographic, cultural, and epidemiological profile of the community as well as a needs assessment to accurately plan for and implement services that respond to the cultural and linguistic characteristics of the service area.

STANDARD 12

Health care organizations should develop participatory, collaborative partnerships with communities and utilize a variety of formal and informal mechanisms to facilitate community and patient/consumer involvement in designing and implementing CLAS-related activities.

STANDARD 13

Health care organizations should ensure that conflict and grievance resolution processes are culturally and linguistically sensitive and capable of identifying, preventing, and resolving cross-cultural conflicts or complaints by patients/consumers.

STANDARD 14

Health care organizations are encouraged to regularly make available to the public information about their progress and successful innovations in implementing the CLAS standards and to provide public notice in their communities about the availability of this information.

Source: Office of Minority Health. (2010). *National standards on culturally and linguistically appropriate services (CLAS).* Retrieved from http://raceandhealth.hhs.gov/templates/browse.aspx?lvl=2&lvlID=15.

4. *Appropriate use and citation of resources.* Information taken from other sources must always be credited to the original source. Failure to reference work taken from another writer is called plagiarism, is considered unethical, and may violate copyright laws. Various styles of referencing are in use, including the Modern Language Association (MLA) and the American Psychological Association (APA) styles. Another benefit of citing references is that readers who want additional information can turn to the references listed.

▶ FACTORS INFLUENCING THE COMMUNICATION PROCESS

Many factors influence the communication process. Some of these are development, gender, values and perceptions, personal space, territoriality, roles and relationships, environment, congruence, and attitudes. Also, the concept of communication is related to all other concepts. See the Concepts Related to Communication feature for examples.

Concepts Related to **Communication**

Communication is a concept that relates to every other healthcare concept presented in this program. Communication is the cornerstone of client care, and nurses, along with all healthcare providers, must be mindful of their communication techniques when providing care in all areas of health care.

CONCEPT	RELATIONSHIP TO COMMUNICATION	NURSING IMPLICATIONS
Oxygenation		
■ Asthma ■ COPD	Decreased O_2 → hypoxemia → decreased level of consciousness (LOC) → decreased ability to communicate verbally (due to shortness of breath and LOC) and nonverbally (due to decreased LOC).	■ Apply supplemental oxygen per order. ■ Consider other methods of communication for the client (e.g., a tablet, a family member).
Grief and Loss		
■ Grief and loss assessment ■ Assessment interview: grief and loss ■ The process of grieving ■ Theories related to grieving ■ Focus on diversity and culture: culture and the dying patient	Grief or loss can adversely affect the way in which an individual communicates. Not only does the person experiencing the loss have trouble communicating needs to others, but others often do not know how to communicate their condolences to those who have experienced a loss. Cultural differences can exacerbate communication issues.	■ Determine the type of loss that has occurred. The nurse's approach will be different for a sudden death than for a death that was expected. ■ Consider the stages of grief when communicating with clients. ■ Consider the ethical issues that may occur when a client is unable to communicate and other family's members are asked to make decisions for them. ■ Consider the cultural background of the client and family.
Safety		
■ QSEN ■ National Patient Safety Goals ■ Injury prevention in the clinical setting	Communication and safety go hand in hand. When someone lacks the ability to communicate, individuals often find that they are talking "at" each other rather than actually communicating. In the healthcare arena this can adversely affect client outcomes.	■ Create an environment to be heard. ■ Set the stage for communication. ■ Be tactful and avoid abrupt, offensive, and accusatory statements. ■ Maintain a nonthreatening approach. ■ Validate cooperation. ■ Listen to the concerns of others. ■ Apologize when needed. ■ Agree when possible. ■ Encourage the team to follow standards.

(continued on next page)

Concepts Related to **Communication** (continued)

CONCEPT	RELATIONSHIP TO COMMUNICATION	NURSING IMPLICATIONS
Advocacy		
■ The advocate's role ■ Advocacy interventions	Communication among nurses, clients, and physicians is a key component of effective health care. In addition to communication with clients, nurses directly or indirectly influence physician–client communications.	■ Assess what the healthcare provider has told the client regarding the client's condition. ■ Encourage the client to clarify the understanding with the healthcare provider. ■ Encourage the client to seek a second opinion, if warranted. ■ Always advocate for the best interest of the client.

Development

As individuals grow and develop, language and communication skills develop through various stages. It is important for the nurse to understand the developmental processes related to speech, language, and communication skills. Knowledge of the client's developmental stage enables the nurse to select appropriate communication strategies. For example, when communicating with infants and toddlers whose language skills are not well developed, the nurse may rely more on the child's nonverbal communications to assess comfort and pain. The nurse may hold the child and use touch to provide comfort and demonstrate caring. For older children, the nurse may use pictures as an adjunct to verbal language to communicate. For adolescents and adults, the nurse is more able to rely on verbal language for communication. With older adults, physical changes associated with the aging process may affect communication. For example, it may be more effective to use visual communication methods for clients who have hearing impairments or aural communication methods for clients who have visual impairments. Also, intellectual processes develop across the life span as individuals acquire knowledge and experience. The knowledge and experiences that individuals have will influence their understanding and acceptance of transmitted information and feelings. The Lifespan Considerations feature discusses some aspects of communicating with children as they grow from infancy to adolescence.

Gender

From an early age, females and males communicate differently. They may give different meanings to transmitted information or feelings. Boys use communication to establish independence and negotiate status within a group, whereas girls use communication to seek confirmation, minimize differences, and establish or reinforce intimacy. These differences in communication may result from psychosocial development and can continue into adulthood. When working with clients or colleagues of the opposite gender, nurses should be aware that a man and a woman may interpret the same communication differently.

Sociocultural Characteristics

Culture, education, and economic level can influence communication. Nonverbal communication characteristics such as body language, eye contact, and touch are influenced by cultural beliefs about appropriate communication behavior. Some cultures may believe that direct eye contact is disrespectful, whereas other cultures believe that direct eye contact shows trustworthiness. In some cultures, touch would be appropriate to communicate caring and concern, but in other cultures physical touch would be offensive. Verbal communication may be difficult for the receiver whose primary language is not that of the sender. More information about the influence of culture on communication can be found in the module on Culture and Diversity.

An individual's level of education may affect the extent of that individual's vocabulary or ability to read written communication. Economic level may affect an individual's ability to access written communication. While many people use e-mail to communicate or the Internet to obtain health information, individuals who cannot afford a computer or who do not have access to one cannot communicate using that means.

Values and Perceptions

Values are the standards that influence behavior, and **perceptions** are the personal views of an event. Because each person has unique personality traits, values, and life experiences, each will perceive and interpret messages and experiences differently. For example, if a nurse draws the curtains around a crying woman and leaves her alone, the woman may interpret this as "The nurse thinks that I will upset others and that I shouldn't cry" or "The nurse respects my need to be alone." It is important for the nurse to be aware of a client's values and to validate or correct perceptions to avoid creating barriers in the nurse–client relationship.

Personal Space

Personal space is the distance individuals prefer to keep between themselves and others during interactions. **Proxemics** is the study of distance between individuals who are interacting.

Lifespan Considerations Communicating With Children and Adolescents

The ability to communicate is directly related to the development of thought processes, the presence of intact sensory and motor systems, and the extent and nature of an individual's opportunities to practice communication skills. As children grow, their communication abilities change markedly.

Infants

- Infants communicate nonverbally, often in response to body feelings rather than in a conscious effort to be expressive.
- Infants' perceptions are related to sensory stimuli. For example, a gentle voice is soothing, whereas tension and anger displayed around an infant create distress.

Toddlers and Preschoolers

- Toddlers and young children gain skills in both expressive (i.e., telling others what they feel, think, want, care about) and receptive (hearing and understanding what others are communicating to them) language.
- Toddlers need time to complete verbalizing their thoughts without interruption.
- Adults should provide simple responses to questions and simple, one-step directions because toddlers have short attention spans.
- Drawing a picture can provide another way for the child to communicate.

School-Age Children

- Adults should talk to a child at the child's eye level to help decrease any feelings of intimidation.
- In communicating with a child's parents about a child's health status, if the child is present, the nurse should include the child in the conversation.

Adolescents

- It takes time to build rapport with adolescents.
- Adults talking with adolescents should use active listening skills.
- Nurses working with adolescents should project a nonjudgmental attitude and nonreactive behaviors, even when an adolescent makes disturbing comments.

The nurse can use the following communication techniques to work effectively with children and their families:

- Play, the universal language, allows children to use other symbols, not just words, to express themselves.
- Drawing, painting, and other art forms can be used even by nonverbal children.
- Storytelling, in which the nurse and child take turns adding to a story or putting words to pictures, can help the child safely express emotions and feelings.
- Word games that pose hypothetical situations or put the child in control, such as "What if . . . ?" "If you could . . . ," or "If a genie came and gave you a wish . . . ," can help a child feel more powerful or explore ideas about how to manage an illness.
- Reading books with a theme similar to the child's condition or problem and then discussing the meaning, characters, and feelings generated by the book can help the nurse to communicate with the child about the condition and the child's experiences with it. Movies or videos can also be used in this way.
- Writing can be used by older children to reflect on their situation, develop meaning, and gain a sense of control.

In all interactions with children, it is important to give them opportunities to be expressive, listen openly, and respond honestly, using words and concepts they understand.

Middle-class North Americans use definite distances in various interpersonal relationships, along with specific voice tones and body language. Communication thus alters in accordance with four distances in this culture, each with a close and a far phase (Samovar, Porter, & McDaniel, 2009):

1. *Intimate:* touching to $1\frac{1}{2}$ feet
2. *Personal:* $1\frac{1}{2}$–4 feet
3. *Social:* 4–12 feet
4. *Public:* 12–15 feet.

Intimate distance communication is characterized by body contact, heightened sensations of body heat and smell, and vocalizations that are low. Vision is intense, is restricted to a small body part, and may be distorted. Nurses frequently use intimate distance. Examples include cuddling a baby, touching a sightless client, positioning a client, observing an incision, and restraining a toddler for an injection. It is a natural protective instinct for individuals to maintain a certain amount of space immediately around them. That amount varies with individuals and cultures. When someone who wants to communicate moves too close, the receiver automatically steps back a pace or two. In their therapeutic roles, nurses often are required

to violate this personal space. However, it is important for the nurse to be aware when this will occur and to forewarn the client. In many instances, the nurse can respect a client's intimate distance by not coming that close. In other instances, the nurse may come within intimate distance to communicate warmth and caring.

Personal distance is less overwhelming than intimate distance. At personal distance, voice tones are moderate, and body heat and smell are less noticeable. Physical contact such as a handshake or touching a shoulder is possible. More of the person is perceived at a personal distance, so that nonverbal behaviors such as body stance or full facial expressions are seen with less distortion. Much communication between nurses and clients occurs at this distance. Examples occur when the nurse is sitting with a client, giving medications, or establishing an intravenous infusion. Communication at a close personal distance can convey involvement by facilitating the sharing of thoughts and feelings. On the other hand, it can also create tension if the distance encroaches on the other person's personal space (**Figure 38–5 ●**). At the outer extreme of 4 feet, however, less involvement is conveyed. Bantering and some social conversations usually take place at this distance.

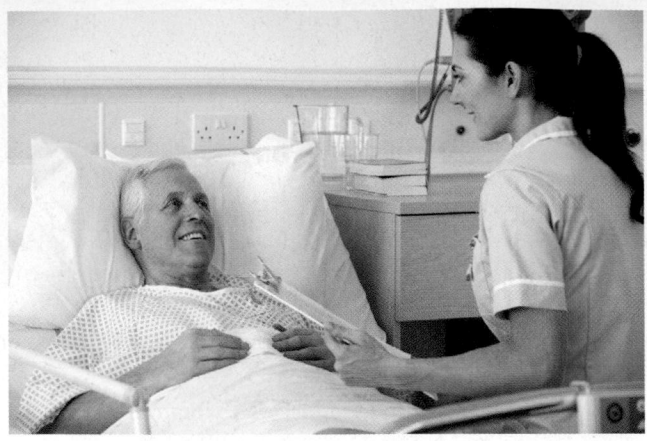

Figure 38–5 ● Personal space influences communication in social and professional interactions. Encroachment into another individual's personal space creates tension.
Source: © Monkey Business/Fotolia.

Social distance is characterized by a clear visual perception of the whole person. Body heat and odor are imperceptible, eye contact is increased, and vocalizations are loud enough to be overheard by others. Communication is therefore more formal and is limited to seeing and hearing. The person is protected and out of reach for touch or personal sharing of thoughts or feelings. Social distance allows more activity and movement back and forth. It is expedient in communicating with several individuals at the same time or within a short time. Examples occur when the nurse makes rounds or waves a greeting to someone. Social distance is important in accomplishing the business of the day. However, it is frequently misused. For example, the nurse who stands in the doorway and asks a client, "How are you today?" will receive a more noncommittal reply than the nurse who moves to a personal distance to make the same inquiry.

Public distance requires loud, clear vocalizations with careful enunciation. Although the faces and forms of people are visible at public distance, individuality is lost. Instead, the perception is of the group of people or the community.

Territoriality

Territoriality is a concept of the space and things that an individual considers as belonging to the self. Territories marked off by individuals may be visible to others. For example, clients in a hospital often consider their territory as bounded by the curtains around the bed unit or by the walls of a private room. All healthcare workers must recognize this human tendency to claim territory. Clients often feel the need to defend their territory when it is invaded by others; for example, when a nurse removes a chair to use at another bed, the nurse has inadvertently violated the territoriality of the client whose chair was removed. The nurse needs to obtain permission from the client to remove, rearrange, or borrow objects in the client's hospital area.

Roles and Relationships

The roles and the relationships between sender and receiver affect the communication process. Roles such as nursing student and instructor, client and primary care provider, or parent and child affect the content and responses in the communication process. Choice of words, sentence structure, message content and channel, body language, and tone of voice vary considerably from role to role. In addition, the specific relationship between the communicators is significant. The nurse who is meeting with a client for the first time communicates differently from the nurse who has previously developed a relationship with that client, and the nurse may choose a more informal or comfortable stance when communicating with clients or colleagues and a more formal stance when communicating with physicians or administrators. The length of the relationship may also affect communication. For example, the nurse may use more formal language and a more formal stance when meeting a client or colleague for the first time and a more relaxed posture when interacting with those with whom the nurse has an established relationship.

Environment

Individuals usually communicate most effectively in a comfortable environment. Environmental distractions such as temperature extremes, excessive noise, and a poorly ventilated environment can impair or distort communication. Also, lack of privacy may interfere with a client's communication about matters the client considers private or personal. For example, a client who is worried about the ability of his wife to care for him after discharge from the hospital may not wish to discuss this concern with a nurse within hearing of other clients or staff.

Congruence

In **congruent communication**, the verbal and nonverbal aspects of a message match. Clients more readily trust the nurse when they perceive the nurse's communication as congruent. This also helps prevent miscommunication. Congruence between verbal expression and nonverbal expression is easily seen by both the nurse and the client. Nurses are taught to assess clients, but clients are often just as adept at reading a nurse's expression or body language. If there is an incongruence, the true meaning is usually conveyed by the sender's body language. For example, when teaching a client how to care for a colostomy, the nurse might say, "You won't have any problem with this." However, if the nurse looks worried or disgusted while saying this, the client is less likely to trust the nurse's words.

Nurses must strive for ways to improve their nonverbal communication skills. Certain guidelines should be followed. First, the nurse should relax because being relaxed makes it easier for others to feel at ease while being cared for. Next the nurse should avoid the use of indiscriminate nonverbal gestures, such as the overuse of smiling or nodding the head, because this can cause the client to doubt the nurse's sincerity.

The nurse should also obtain feedback on nonverbal communication skills from individuals with whom the nurse works closely, because feedback allows the nurse to improve on these skills. Once feedback has been obtained, the nurse can practice nonverbal communication skills with coworkers or in simulated environments to improve this vital form of communication.

Interpersonal Attitudes

Attitudes convey beliefs, thoughts, and feelings about people and events. Attitudes are communicated convincingly and rapidly to others. Attitudes such as caring, warmth, respect, and acceptance facilitate communication, whereas condescension, lack of interest, and coldness inhibit communication.

Haskard, DiMatteo, and Heritage (2009) conducted a research study that found that effective nursing communication is significantly related to client satisfaction with care. Key in nursing communication, both verbal and nonverbal, is communicating warmth, positivity, energy, and capability, which improves client satisfaction with both competence and interpersonal care. Caring involves giving feelings, thoughts, skill, and knowledge. It requires psychological energy and poses the risk of gaining little in return; yet by caring, people usually reap the benefits of greater communication and understanding.

Respect is an attitude that emphasizes the other person's worth and individuality. It conveys that the person's hopes and feelings are special and unique even though similar to others in many ways. Individuals have a need to be different from—and at the same time similar to—others. Being too different can be isolating and threatening. A nurse conveys respect by listening with an open mind to what the other individual is saying, even if the nurse disagrees. Nurses can learn new ways of approaching situations when they conscientiously listen to another individual's perspective.

Civility also is important in communication. Nurses employ civility when they respond on time to written communication, use courtesy in making requests or responding to the efforts of others, show respect to the individual with whom they are communicating, and use concrete, specific language. Concrete, specific language limits the potential for misunderstanding or miscommunication by ensuring that sufficient context is provided.

Healthcare providers may unknowingly use speech that they believe shows caring but that the client perceives as demeaning or patronizing. This can happen in settings that provide health care to older adults and/or individuals with obvious physical or mental disabilities. **Elderspeak** is a speech style similar to baby talk that gives the message to older adults that they are dependent and incompetent. It does not communicate respect. Many healthcare providers are not aware that they use elderspeak or that it can have negative meanings to the client. The characteristics of elderspeak include inappropriate terms of endearment and plural pronoun use, tag questions, and slow, loud speech. These should not be used with any age group.

It is important for nurses to avoid elderspeak and use alternative strategies. Instead of using diminutives such as "honey" or "sweetie," the nurse should refer to the client by full name (honorific and last name unless the nurse has established a closer relationship with the client) or preferred name. Instead of using inappropriate plural pronouns such as "we," the nurse should always speak to the client by using "you." The nurse should also avoid tagging questions with words that would cause the client to think that the nurse is leading the client to answer in a certain way. Instead, ask the question directly to them. Also, avoid the use of baby talk as this is demeaning to the client. Always address clients as the adults that they are.

Acceptance emphasizes neither approval nor disapproval. The nurse willingly receives the client's honest feelings. An accepting attitude allows clients to express personal feelings freely and to be themselves. The nurse may need to restrict acceptance in situations in which clients' behaviors are harmful to themselves or to others. Helping the client to find appropriate behaviors for feelings is often part of client teaching.

▶ BARRIERS TO COMMUNICATION

Just as there are characteristics of effective communication, there are identified barriers to effective communication. Nurses need to be cognizant of these barriers and avoid them. Nurses also need to recognize the barriers when they occur and change to more effective means of communication. Failing to listen, improperly decoding the client's intended message, and placing the nurse's needs above the client's needs are major barriers to communication. Additional barriers to effective communication are given in **Table 38–1** ●.

▶ TYPES OF COMMUNICATORS

Different individuals have different ways or styles of communication. Gender, culture, personality type, and degree of confidence can all play a role in how a nurse communicates with others. Communication is complex and requires that the nurse use a thoughtful process to communicate effectively. Communication style is something that is used daily in both the work and home environments but often is not viewed as important until there is a problem with it.

Individuals tend to express themselves in various ways. **Aggressive communicators** are those who tend to focus on their own needs and become impatient when these needs are not met. **Passive communicators** are those who focus on the needs of others. They often deny themselves any sort of power, which causes them to become frustrated. **Assertive communicators** are those who declare and affirm their opinions. In doing this, however, they respect the rights of other to communicate in the same fashion. The assertive communicator strikes a balance between the aggressive communicator and the passive communicator. It is the assertive communicator who has the most productive communication with others. **Table 38–2** ● compares and contrasts the three styles of communicating.

Individuals who use assertive communication express themselves effectively and stand up for their beliefs while respecting the rights of others (Mayo Clinic, 2009). Assertive communicators are honest, direct, and appropriate while being open to ideas and showing concern for the needs of others. Assertive communication promotes client safety by minimizing miscommunication with colleagues. Failure to communicate can result in negative client outcomes.

An important characteristic of assertive communication includes the use of "I" statements versus "you" statements. The "you" statement places blame and puts the listener in a defensive position. On the other hand, the "I" statement encourages discussion. For example, a nurse who states "I am concerned about . . ." to a physician will gain the attention of the physician while also giving the message of the importance of working

TABLE 38–1 Barriers to Communication

TECHNIQUE	DESCRIPTION	EXAMPLES
Stereotyping	Offering generalized and oversimplified beliefs about groups of individuals that are based on experiences too limited to be valid. These responses categorize clients and negate their uniqueness as individuals.	"Two-year-olds are brats." "Women are complainers." "Men don't cry." "Most people don't have any pain after this type of surgery."
Agreeing and disagreeing	Akin to judgmental responses, agreeing and dis-agreeing imply that the client is either right or wrong and that the nurse is in a position to judge this. These responses deter clients from thinking through their position and may cause a client to become defensive.	*Client:* "I don't think Dr. Broad is a very good doctor. He doesn't seem interested in his clients." *Nurse:* "Dr. Broad is head of the department of surgery and is an excellent surgeon."
Being defensive	Attempting to protect an individual or healthcare service from negative comments. These responses prevent the client from expressing true concerns. The nurse is saying, "You have no right to complain." Defensive responses protect the nurse from admitting weaknesses in the healthcare services, including personal weaknesses.	*Client:* "Those night nurses must just sit around and talk all night. They didn't answer my light for over an hour." *Nurse:* "I'll have you know we literally run around on nights. You're not the only client, you know."
Challenging	Giving a response that makes clients prove their statement or point of view. These responses indicate that the nurse is failing to consider the client's feelings, making the client feel it necessary to defend a position.	*Client:* "I felt nauseated after that red pill." *Nurse:* "Surely you don't think I gave you the wrong pill?" *Client:* "I feel as if I am dying." *Nurse:* "How can you feel that way when your pulse is 60?" *Client:* "I believe my husband doesn't love me." *Nurse:* "You can't say that. Why, he visits you every day."
Probing	Asking for information chiefly out of curiosity rather than with the intent to assist the client. These responses are considered prying and violate the client's privacy. Asking "why" is often probing and places the client in a defensive position.	*Client:* "I was speeding along the street and didn't see the stop sign." *Nurse:* "Why were you speeding?" *Client:* "I didn't ask the doctor about that when he was here." *Nurse:* "Why didn't you?"
Testing	Asking questions that make the client admit to something. These responses permit the client only limited answers and often meet the nurse's need rather than the client's.	"Who do you think you are?" (forces the individual to admit to a lower status) "Do you think I am not busy?" (forces the client to admit that the nurse really is busy)
Rejecting	Refusing to discuss certain topics with the client. These responses often make clients feel that the nurse is rejecting not only their communication but also the clients themselves.	"I don't want to discuss that. Let's talk about. . . ." "Let's discuss other areas of interest to you rather than the two problems you keep mentioning." "I can't talk now. I'm on my way for coffee break."
Changing topics and subjects	Directing the communication into areas of self-inter-est rather than considering the client's concerns is often a self-protective response to a topic that causes anxiety. These responses imply that what the nurse considers important will be discussed and that clients should not discuss certain topics.	*Client:* "I'm separated from my wife. Do you think I should have sexual relations with another woman?" *Nurse:* "I see that you're 36 and that you like gardening. This sunshine is good for my roses. I have a beautiful rose garden."
Unwarranted reassurance	Using clichés or comforting statements of advice as a means to reassure the client. These responses block the fears, feelings, and other thoughts of the client.	"You'll feel better soon." "I'm sure everything will turn out all right." "Don't worry."
Passing judgment	Giving opinions and approving or disapproving responses, moralizing, or implying one's own values. These responses imply that the client must think as the nurse thinks, fostering client dependence.	"That's good (bad)." "You shouldn't do that." "That's not good enough." "What you did was wrong (right)."
Giving common advice	Telling the client what to do. These responses deny the client's right to be an equal partner. Note that giving expert advice that is appropriate for the client's individual situation rather than common advice is therapeutic.	*Client:* "Should I move from my home to a nursing home?" *Nurse:* "If I were you, I'd go to a nursing home, where you'll get your meals cooked for you."

TABLE 38–2   Aggressive, Passive, and Assertive Styles

AGGRESSIVE INDIVIDUALS	PASSIVE INDIVIDUALS	ASSERTIVE INDIVIDUALS
■ Have loud, heated arguments ■ Are physically violent ■ Blame others ■ Use name-calling and verbal insults ■ Walk out of arguments prior to their resolution ■ Are demanding	■ Conceal their feelings ■ Deny anger ■ Feel that no one has the right to express anger ■ Avoid arguments ■ Are noncommittal	■ Express their feelings without being nasty or overbearing ■ Acknowledge emotions ■ Stay open to discussion ■ Express themselves while giving others that same opportunity ■ Use "I" statements to defuse arguments ■ Provide reasons and ask for the same in return

together for the benefit of the client. Once the nurse has the physician's attention, it is important for the nurse to be clear, concise, organized, and fully informed when presenting the client concern.

The passive, submissive communication style often causes a rights violation. Individuals who use this style meet the demands and requests of others without regard to their own feelings and needs as they believe their own feelings are not important. Some experts believe that individuals who use submissive behaviors or communication styles are insecure and try to maintain their self-esteem by avoiding conflict (e.g., negative criticism and disagreement from others).

There is a fine line between assertive and aggressive communication. Assertive communication is an open expression of ideas and opinions while respecting the rights, opinions, and ideas of others. Individuals who use aggressive communication assert their legitimate rights and options with little regard or respect for others. Aggressive communication is often perceived as a personal attack by the recipient because aggressive communication humiliates, dominates, controls, or embarrasses the recipient. By lowering the other person's self-esteem, the person using aggressive communication may feel superior, which helps increase the aggressive communicator's self-esteem. Aggressive communication takes several different forms, which can include screaming, sarcasm, rudeness, belittling jokes, and direct personal insults.

A nurse's approach to communication can have far-reaching impact on the quality of client care delivered. Consider the following case study.

CASE STUDY \\ A

Shannon Collins has a standing order for vital signs every 2 hours because her temperature was elevated on admission to the facility. Since admission, Mrs. Collins's temperature has normalized, and her vital signs have consistently been within normal limits. She tells you that she isn't sleeping well because the nurses keep coming in and waking her every 2 hours and it takes her almost an hour to fall back to sleep. As a result, she is sleeping in 1-hour intervals and feels extremely sleep deprived. You approach the physician and request that the order be changed to every 4 hours during the day with 6 hours of uninterrupted sleep from midnight to 6:00 a.m. The physician responds by saying, "If she wants to sleep, she'll have to wait until she goes home. I want vital signs every two hours as ordered."

Critical Thinking Questions

1. Which type of communication style will best serve the needs of the client? Provide a rationale for your response.
2. What type of response will the nurse have using an aggressive communication style?
3. What type of response will the nurse have using a passive communication style?
4. What type of response will the nurse have using an assertive communication style?

▶ ASSERTIVE COMMUNICATION

Beliefs about personal boundaries play a role in determining communication style. The passive communicator does not respect his or her own values and therefore is often ignored, manipulated, or taken advantage of by more aggressive individuals. Aggressive communicators do not respect the boundaries of others and are willing to say or do anything necessary to get their way. The goal of all true professionals is to achieve a mutual respect for boundaries in order to promote the best outcome for everyone involved.

Assertive communication allows the nurse to express all ideas in a direct and nonconfrontational manner that promotes the rights of the nurse or the client while respecting the rights of others to have a different outlook. Assertive communication does not use name calling, is not judgmental, and does not blame others. It increases the likelihood of creating a win–win result in which both parties walk away feeling that their point of view was heard and understood while reaching a conclusion satisfactory to them both.

Characteristics of assertive communicators include freedom to express oneself, awareness of one's own rights, and self-control over strong emotions such as anger, fear, or frustration. Assertive communicators are professional and serve as the best advocate for the client. Assertive communicators express their opinions but are open to listening to others' points of view. They do not use sarcasm, biting comebacks, or passive-aggressive wounding to promote their superiority.

Much of conversation is nonverbal, so the body language of the assertive communicator should be upright, relaxed, and open to the words of others. The tone of voice should be well modulated with inflection, and raised voices, whispering, or aggressive overtones should be avoided.

An assertive individual receives feedback from others with a willingness to consider both the positive and negative perspectives of the evaluator. Although an assertive individual may not believe everything that is said, he or she will listen to another individual's opinion without becoming defensive or angry and without attacking the speaker. Seeking clarification is appropriate to be sure that the perception of the message is the same as what the sender intended.

Some individuals may have more trouble accepting positive feedback and will dismiss it or negate it when offered. The assertive individual simply says "Thank you" and considers the value of the positive feedback for later application to similar situations.

Benefits of Assertive Communication

Assertiveness is an effective and professional communication style because it is based on mutual respect. An assertive style improves communication and reduces stress by de-escalating conflict, improving outcomes, and reducing the likelihood of angry encounters. Passive communicators tend to feel increased stress, resentment, anger, feelings of victimization, and a desire to exact revenge, which is eliminated when assertive communication styles are used (Mayo Clinic, 2009). Aggressive communication often results in a perception by others that the individual is a bully and is unprofessional. This can affect future interactions, because individuals who deal with the aggressor on a regular basis may become defensive before communication even begins because they anticipate an aggressive encounter.

Techniques for Assertive Communication

Because no one technique works in every situation, the nurse must have an arsenal of strategies to use when faced with a situation requiring assertive communication. These techniques include the following:

- *"I" statements.* Assertive communicators voice their own feelings and wishes based on sound evidence without placing blame or raising the defenses of the individual to whom they are speaking. For example, "I have assessed that Client A is. . . ."

- *Fogging.* Finding some area, no matter how small, on which both parties agree and building from there is a technique that assertive communicators use. In the example of the sleep-deprived client described previously, both the nurse and the physician can agree that they want to maintain client safety through careful monitoring of the client's condition. This gives them a starting point from which to reach consensus where both can feel client care has been optimized.

- *Negative assertion.* An assertive communicator can agree with criticism without becoming upset or angry, thus moving the focus of the communication toward the desired goal. This can be particularly important to the nurse when receiving feedback related to the quality of the care the nurse delivers. For example, when the evaluator says, "While you are very caring, I would like to see you improve your decision-making ability," the nurse may respond, "I could use improvement in my decision-making ability, but I believe

the quality of the care I deliver is excellent." This prevents an ongoing debate about something that is agreed on and allows the communication to move forward regarding the more important topic.

- *Repetition.* Repeating the request every time one meets with resistance is another technique that can be useful. However, each time the request is repeated, the power of the words is diminished. This strategy is effective only if the nurse has power within the relationship. For example, suppose the nurse calls the pharmacy to request a newly ordered medication that is to be given within the hour and is told that the pharmacy is very busy and cannot fill the prescription right now and will not be able to deliver it to the unit for 3–4 hours. The nurse repeats, "I must give this medication within the hour" or "The client needs the medication within the hour." The effectiveness of this approach is improved if differing attempts to reach a compromise are suggested as well. The nurse might say, "I need to administer this medication within the hour" to which the pharmacy responds, "I'm sorry, I can't have it to the floor that quickly." The nurse then responds, "The client needs that medication within the hour. What if I come to the pharmacy so you don't have to deliver it?" This allows for both the nurse and the pharmacy to collaborate to reach a mutually effective solution to the problem.

- *Confidence.* Confidence is essential to assertive communication. A choppy or weak tone of voice implies uncertainty. The nurse should maintain an air of confidence in order to help others see their needs and wants as having merit.

- *Managing nonverbal communication.* Getting too close to the other individual, wagging a finger in someone's face, or an angry glare can all counteract assertive words. By maintaining open, assertive body language and keeping a neutral voice, the nurse promotes shared decision making and compromise.

- *Thinking before speaking.* Consider both your words and your tone of voice before speaking. This helps the nurse avoid saying something he or she will later regret or that will reduce the effectiveness of his or her communication style.

- *Avoiding apologizing whenever possible.* This is particularly important for women, who have a tendency to say "I'm sorry" even when there is no call for an apology. A woman may say, "I'm sorry, I didn't hear you," or "I'm sorry to bother you, but. . . ." An unnecessary apology immediately places the communicator in a somewhat submissive position. Apologies should be given only when warranted.

- *Performing a postconversation evaluation.* Assertive communicators can continue to improve their skills by reviewing what was said and how the communication might have been handled differently to improve the final outcome. This should be done even when the communication interaction was successful because evaluation of what went well, in contrast to what did not, helps the nurse improve assertive communication skills.

While assertive communication may not be an individual's preferred style and may not be comfortable for the individual, it is possible for every nurse to become an assertive communicator and reach more positive outcomes through practice, self-evaluation, and ongoing efforts to improve his or her communication approach.

NURSING PROCESS

Communication is an integral part of the nursing process. The nurse uses communication skills in each phase of the nursing process. Communication skills take on greater importance when the nurse is caring for a client with sensory, language, developmental, or cognitive deficits.

Assessment

To assess the client's communication ability, the nurse determines whether there are any communication impairments or barriers and communication style. When doing so, the nurse should remember that an individual's culture may influence when and how a client speaks. Obviously, language varies according to age and development. With children, the nurse observes sounds, gestures, facial expressions, and vocabulary.

Throughout the process of collecting data, the nurse uses communication skills to increase the nurse–client rapport, put the client at ease when discussing personal matters, and interpret the client's nonverbal communication. Exemplar 38.2 discusses the role of therapeutic communication in creating a helping relationship with the client.

Various barriers may alter a client's ability to send, receive, or comprehend messages. These include language deficits, sensory deficits, cognitive impairments, structural deficits, and paralysis. The nurse must assess for the presence of each.

Language Deficits

The nurse determines whether the client speaks another language or has an impairment that affects the client's ability to communicate verbally. When assessing for the need for an interpreter, remember that some clients who use English as a second language may have language skills that are inadequate to meet their needs in a healthcare environment.

Sensory Deficits

The ability to hear, see, feel, and smell are important adjuncts to communication. Deafness can significantly alter the message a client receives; impaired vision alters the ability to observe nonverbal behavior, such as a smile or a gesture; and inability to feel and smell can impair the client's ability to report injuries or detect smoke from a fire. If a client appears to have severe hearing impairments, the nurse should follow these steps:

- Look for a medical alert bracelet, necklace, or tag indicating hearing loss.
- Determine whether the client wears a hearing aid and whether it is functioning.
- Observe whether the client is attempting to see your face to read lips.
- Observe whether the client is attempting to use hands to communicate with sign language.

See the feature on Communicating With Clients Who Have a Visual or Hearing Deficit in the module on Sensory Perception for more information.

Cognitive Impairments

Any disorder that impairs cognitive functioning (e.g., cerebrovascular disease, Alzheimer disease, and brain tumors or injuries) may affect a client's ability to use and understand language. These clients may develop total loss of speech, impaired articulation, or the inability to find or name words. Certain medications such as sedatives, antidepressants, and neuroleptics may also impair speech, causing the client to use incomplete sentences or to slur words. Older adults are particularly likely to have cognitive impairments that may interfere with communication (see the Lifespan Considerations feature).

The nurse assesses whether these clients respond when asked a question and, if they do, assesses the following:

- Is the client's speech fluent or hesitant?
- Does the client use words correctly?
- Can the client comprehend instructions as evidenced by following directions?
- Can the client repeat words or phrases?

In addition, the nurse assesses the client's ability to understand written words:

- Can the client follow written directions?
- Can the client respond correctly by pointing to a written word?
- Can the client read aloud?
- Can the client recognize words or letters if unable to read whole sentences?

The nurse uses large, clearly written words when trying to establish abilities in this area.

SAFETY ALERT
When the client is unconscious, the nurse looks for any indication that suggests comprehension of what is communicated (e.g., tries to arouse the client verbally and through touch). Ask a closed question such as "Can you hear me?" and watch for a nonverbal response such as a nod of the head for yes or a shake for no, or ask for a hand squeeze or blink of the eye: once for yes or twice for no. The nurse may ask the client to grip the hand or move a finger if the client hears and understands. Because damage to the spinal cord may preclude movement, attempts to determine comprehension must be specific to the needs of the individual client.

Structural Deficits

Structural deficits of the oral and nasal cavities and respiratory system can alter an individual's ability to speak clearly and spontaneously. Examples include cleft palate, artificial airways such as an endotracheal tube or tracheostomy, and laryngectomy (removal of the larynx). Extreme dyspnea (shortness of breath) can also impair speech patterns.

Lifespan Considerations Communicating With Older Adults

Older adults may have physical or cognitive problems that necessitate nursing interventions for improvement of communication skills. Some of the common ones are as follows:

- Sensory deficits, such as vision and hearing
- Cognitive impairment, as in dementia
- Neurological deficits from strokes or other neurological conditions, such as aphasia (expressive and/or receptive) and lack of movement
- Psychosocial problems, such as depression.

Recognition of specific needs and obtaining appropriate resources for clients can greatly increase their socialization and quality of life. Interventions directed toward improving communication in clients with these special needs include the following:

- Ensure that the client is using assistive devices, glasses, and hearing aids and that they are in good working order.
- Make referrals to appropriate resources, such as speech therapy.

- Use communications aids, such as communication boards, computers, or pictures, when possible.
- Keep environmental distractions to a minimum.
- Speak in short, simple sentences, one subject at a time—reinforce or repeat what is said when necessary.
- Always face the client when speaking, because coming up behind someone may be frightening.
- Include family and friends in conversation.
- Use reminiscing, either in individual conversations or in groups, to maintain memory connections and to enhance self-identity and self-esteem in the older adult.
- When verbal expression and nonverbal expression are incongruent, believe the nonverbal. Clarification of this and attentiveness to the client's feelings will help promote a feeling of caring and acceptance.
- Find out what has been important and has meaning to the client, and try to maintain these things as much as possible. Simple things such as bedtime rituals become more important, especially in a hospital or extended care setting.

Paralysis

If verbal impairment is combined with paralysis of the upper extremities that impairs the client's ability to write, the nurse should determine whether the client can point, nod, shrug, blink, or squeeze a hand. Any of these could be used to devise a simple communication system.

Style of Communication

In assessing communication style, the nurse considers both verbal and nonverbal communication. In addition to physical barriers, some psychological illnesses (e.g., depression or psychosis) influence the ability to communicate. The client may demonstrate constant verbalization of the same words or phrases, a loose association of ideas, or flight of ideas (a continuous flow of rapid speech that switches from topic to topic).

Verbal Communication

When assessing verbal communication, the nurse focuses on three areas: the content of the client's message, the themes, and verbalized emotions. In addition, the nurse considers the following:

- Whether the client's communication pattern is slow, rapid, quiet, spontaneous, hesitant, evasive, etc.
- The client's vocabulary, particularly any changes from the vocabulary normally used (for example, someone who normally never swears may indicate increased stress or illness by an uncharacteristic use of profanity)
- The presence of hostility, aggression, assertiveness, reticence, hesitance, anxiety, or loquaciousness (incessant verbalization) in communication
- Difficulties with verbal communication, such as slurring, stuttering, inability to pronounce a particular sound, lack of clarity in enunciation, inability to speak in sentences, loose

association of ideas, flight of ideas, or the inability to find or name words or identify objects
- Refusal or inability to speak.

SAFETY ALERT
Changes in the client's ability to put words together into sentences or to properly name an item or struggling to find the right word for common objects may be an indication of neurological impairment. Assessment of the client's communication ability, especially after any type of head trauma, is an important tool for detecting alterations in the client's condition.

Diagnosis

Impaired Verbal Communication may be used as a nursing diagnosis when "an individual experiences a decreased, delayed, or absent ability to receive, process, transmit, and use a system of symbols—anything that has meaning (i.e., transmits meaning)" (Wilkinson, 2005, p. 80). Communication problems may be *receptive* (e.g., difficulty hearing) or *expressive* (e.g., difficulty speaking).

A nursing diagnosis of *Impaired Verbal Communication* may not be useful when an individual's communication problems are caused by a psychiatric illness or a coping problem. In those instances, a diagnosis of *Fear* or *Anxiety* may be more appropriate. Other nursing diagnoses used for clients experiencing communication problems that involve impaired verbal communication as the *etiology* could include the following:

- *Anxiety* related to impaired verbal communication
- *Powerlessness* related to impaired verbal communication
- *Situational Low Self-Esteem* related to impaired verbal communication

Evidence-Based Practice The Role of Time in Caring for the Client With Complex Communication Needs

Problem

Effective nurse–client communication is an essential aspect of health care. Time to communicate is often limited and subject to the workload demands of the nurse. Little is currently known about how nurses manage the "lack of time" when caring for clients with developmental disabilities and those with complex communication needs. These groups tend to communicate at a slow rate, which can further undermine the communication process.

Evidence

Hemsley, Balandin, and Worrall (2012) investigated nurses' expressed concepts of "time" in stories about communicating with clients with developmental disabilities. They interviewed 15 nurses from two large hospitals about barriers to and strategies for successful communication with clients who have developmental disabilities.

The nurses identified "time" as both a barrier and a facilitator to a successful communication process. Time was a barrier when related to avoiding direct communication. It was also used as a means to avoid direct communication with clients and instead communicating with family members or other paid caregivers on behalf of the client. Time was seen as a facilitator when related to valuing communication, investing extra time, and the application of a range of adaptive communication strategies that established successful communication.

Implications

Time is perceived as both an enemy and a friend for the improvement of communication. Nurses who perceive that communication takes too long may avoid the communication process and miss opportunities to improve the process. Those who take the time to communicate apply a wide range of strategies in order to achieve successful communication with clients.

Critical Thinking Application

1. What resources can the nurse use to communicate with clients with complex communication needs in the hospital setting?

2. What resources might the nurse use to communicate with these clients once they are discharged into the community?

- *Social Isolation* related to impaired verbal communication
- *Impaired Social Interaction* related to impaired verbal communication.

(NANDA-I © 2012)

Planning

When a nursing diagnosis related to impaired verbal communication has been made, the nurse and client determine outcomes and begin planning ways to promote effective communication. Establishing communication with the client may require creativity or technology. New devices are being developed, ranging from thought-activated computers that verbalize for the client to devices that can be operated with a stylus in the mouth to verbalize needs.

Specific goals for nursing interventions will depend on the stated etiology and may include the following:

- The client will have an effective means for communicating needs.
- The client's ability to perceive messages accurately will be maximized.
- The client will be provided with resources as needed to optimize the ability to communicate.

Implementation

Nursing interventions to facilitate communication with clients who have problems with speech or language include manipulating the environment, providing support, employing measures to enhance communication, and educating the client and support person.

Manipulate the Environment

A quiet environment with limited distractions provides the best setting for the communication efforts of both the client and the nurse and increases the possibility of effective communication. Sufficient light helps in conveying nonverbal messages, which is especially important if visual or auditory acuity is impaired. Initially, the nurse needs to provide a calm, relaxed environment, which will help reduce any anxiety the client may have. Any factor that affects communication can create feelings of frustration, anxiety, depression, or hostility in a client. Communication normally contributes to a client's sense of security and feelings of not being alone, so communication problems may cause some clients to feel isolated and confused. To further reduce these emotions, the nurse should acknowledge and praise the client's attempts at communication.

Provide Support

The nurse should convey encouragement to the client and provide nonverbal reassurance, perhaps by touch if appropriate. If the nurse does not understand a client's communication, it is critical to let the client know so that the client can provide clarification with other words or through some other means of communication. When speaking with a client who has difficulty understanding, the nurse should check frequently to determine what the client has heard and understood. Using open-ended questions will assist the nurse in obtaining accurate information about the effectiveness of communication.

You are providing care to Maria Perez, who has limited English skills. As part of the discharge teaching for this client, you are teaching her about dietary changes that are necessary for managing Crohn disease. You ask Ms. Perez, "Do you understand what to eat?" She nods her head yes. You realize that the question did not elicit an answer that sufficiently confirms that Ms. Perez understood. You ask a follow-up question: "What do you think will be good for you to eat when you go home?" At the same time, your body language (e.g., gestures, posture, facial expression, and eye contact) conveys acceptance and approval. When Ms. Perez begins to explain what foods she should avoid, you are confident that you communicated the information to Ms. Perez successfully.

Critical Thinking Questions

1. What resources are available for teaching clients whose primary language is not English?
2. How does culture affect communication?
3. How does body language affect the communication process?

Employ Measures to Enhance Communication

To enhance communication, the nurse first determines how the client can best receive messages: by listening, by looking, through touch, or through an interpreter. Ways to help communication include keeping words simple and concrete and discussing topics of interest to the client. The use of alternative communication strategies, such as word boards, pictures, or paper and pencil, may be helpful.

Nurses also need to implement measures to enhance communication with individuals who are hard of hearing. Nurses should be considerate and respectful to these clients. If the nurse is unable to recognize and compensate for the client's hearing problems, miscommunication can occur. This could undermine the nurse–client relationship.

Avoid Potential Cultural Barriers to Communication

The nurse should remember several items when communicating with a client whose primary language is not English. The nurse should avoid the use of slang, buzz words, and medical terminology when possible. The nurse should also show the client respect by speaking clearly, directly, and at a normal pace. Avoid words that may impede the communication process such as words that are slurred and those that have several syllables. The nurse should also speak at a speed that does not overload the client and allows the client to follow the conversation. However, the nurse should avoid speaking too slowly because this may cause the nurse to lose the client's attention. The nurse should use open-ended questions and it may be necessary to rephrase them in several ways in order to obtain accurate information.

When using nonverbal communication with these clients, the nurse must be sure to select gestures with care. This form of nonverbal communication underscores both words and actions and can be used to clarify meaning; however, gestures may have different meanings for different cultures. Therefore, the nurse must validate words and gestures with each client on an individual basis.

If language is a barrier, the use of an interpreter may be necessary. In 2000, the federal Office for Civil Rights (OCR) of the Department of Health and Human Services mandated that any entities that receive federal funds, "must communicate effectively with patients, family members, and visitors who are deaf or hard-of-hearing and must take reasonable steps to provide meaningful access to their programs for persons who have limited English proficiency (LEP)" (OCR, 2010). Failure to do this is considered discrimination.

Because the use of family members as interpreters can raise confidentiality and privacy issues, the nurse can enlist the aid of bilingual staff members to communicate information effectively. Most healthcare institutions have a list of bilingual staff members who can be used as personal interpreters, medical interpreters, or both. When working with an interpreter, the nurse must remember to always speak directly to the client and not to the interpreter.

The nurse who is culturally competent will be appreciated by the client. The following strategies can be used when caring for clients from a different culture:

1. Use the proper form of address for the client's culture.
2. Know how individuals in the client's culture greet one another. This may include the use of handshake, embraces, or kissing the cheeks. In some cultures, physical contact is prohibited.
3. Be aware of what a smile means in the client's culture. A smile may indicate friendliness or be considered taboo. Also be aware of what eye contact means; in some cultures, it indicates respect, whereas in others, it may indicate aggression.
4. Remember that not all gestures have a universal meaning.

While similarities may enhance the therapeutic relationship, differences can serve as topics for open discussion. Having an open and ongoing conversation between all parties will promote understanding.

Educate the Client and Support People

Sometimes clients and support people can be prepared in advance for communication problems, for example, before an intubation or throat surgery. When the nurse has explained anticipated problems, the client is often less anxious when problems arise. Furthermore, a means of communicating can be practiced in advance.

Evaluation

Evaluation is useful for both client and nurse communication. Evaluation of nurse communication is discussed in greater detail in Exemplar 38.2 on therapeutic communication.

SAFETY ALERT
Nodding, smiling, or agreeing is an inadequate means of evaluating client understanding and often results in misunderstandings or misinterpretations of client learning. Instead, ask the client to explain in his or her own words what was said. This allows you to truly evaluate the client's understanding of communications. If the client uses medical terminology, ask the client to define what is meant by the term to ensure understanding.

To establish whether client outcomes have been met in relation to communication, the nurse must listen actively and observe nonverbal cues. The overall client outcome for individuals with impaired verbal communication is to reduce or resolve the factors impairing the communication. Examples of statements indicating outcome achievement include "Using picture board effectively to indicate needs" or "The client stated, 'I listened more closely to my daughter yesterday and found out how she feels about our divorce.'"

Examples of outcomes of care for the client with impaired communication include the following:

- The client communicates that needs are being met.
- The client has begun to establish a method of communication, signaling yes/no to direct questions by using vocalization or agreed-on physical cue (e.g., eye blink, hand squeeze) and/or using verbal or nonverbal techniques to indicate needs.
- The client perceives the message accurately, as evidenced by appropriate verbal and/or nonverbal responses.

- The client communicates effectively, using the client's dominant language, a translator/interpreter, sign language, a word board or picture board, and/or a computer.
- The client has regained maximum communication abilities.
- The client expresses minimal fear, anxiety, frustration, and depression.
- The client uses resources appropriately.

▶ NURSING PRACTICE

Communication is a critical skill for nursing. It is the process by which humans meet their survival needs, build relationships, and experience emotions. In nursing, communication is a dynamic process used to gather assessment data, to teach and persuade, to collaborate with other healthcare professionals, to advocate for clients, to express caring, and to provide comfort. It is an integral part of the helping relationship.

Four specific types of communication are explored in the exemplars of this module. Each of these is essential to successful nursing practice. Group communication is becoming ever more important in the process of making decisions in the current healthcare system. Therapeutic communication is an essential tool for developing the nurse–client helping relationship. Documentation is the primary form of written communication used by nurses in all aspects of health care. Finally, reporting is the process of nurse-to-nurse communication that ensures continuity of care for the client from one shift change or visit to another.

◤ REVIEW The Concept of Communication

RELATE Link the Concepts

Linking the concept of communication with the concept of culture and diversity:

1. How can misunderstanding the client's culture act as a barrier to communication when the nurse's culture differs from that of the client?

2. The nurse is studying a culture different from the one in which the nurse was raised. What aspects of the culture would the nurse wish to learn about in order to understand how that culture's communication style may differ?

Linking the concept of communication with the concept of professional behaviors:

3. How do the nurse's communication skills affect the perceptions of others (both clients and other members of the healthcare team) regarding the nurse's professionalism?

4. A client asks the nurse a question. Although the nurse is very knowledgeable about the subject, the nurse stumbles over words while answering the client, repeatedly starts sentences over again, uses words such as "ahh" and "umm" a number of times, and gives the impression of weighing each word carefully. What impact will this delivery have on the client's perception of the nurse's professionalism and knowledge of the subject matter being explained?

REFER Go to Pearson Nursing Student Resources
nursing.pearsonhighered.com

- Additional review materials

REFLECT Case Study

Madeline McCormick, 24 years old, is an RN who has worked in the local acute care hospital on the medical floor for the past 3 years. Last night her boyfriend proposed. She accepted and is so thrilled she can't wait to show her new diamond ring to all of her coworkers and tell them the good news. She arrives at work early to share the good news and they all congratulate her and shower her with questions about her ideas for the wedding.

You are a student nurse assigned to Ms. McCormick's floor today. As you walk by one of the clients' rooms you hear Ms. McCormick, who is providing a.m. care to a client, talking to the client and telling her all about how her boyfriend proposed, her wedding plans, and how happy she is.

1. Is it appropriate for Ms. McCormick to share her good news with her coworkers? Why or why not?

2. Is it appropriate for Ms. McCormick to share her news with her client? Why or why not?

3. How does Ms. McCormick's excitement over her engagement affect the nurse–client communication process?

EXEMPLAR 38.1 Groups and Group Communication

EXEMPLAR KEY TERMS

Apathy, *2422*
Brainstorming, *2420*
Cohesiveness, *2422*
Delphi technique, *2421*
Formal groups, *2419*
Group, *2418*
Groupthink, *2422*
Informal groups, *2419*
Monopolizing, *2422*
Nominal group technique, *2421*
Primary group, *2418*

Scapegoat, *2422*
Secondary group, *2418*
Self-help group, *2423*
Semiformal groups, *2419*
Transference, *2423*

EXEMPLAR LEARNING OUTCOMES

After reading about this exemplar, you will be able to:

1. Describe and contrast different types of groups and their functions.
2. Analyze group dynamics within the classroom or clinical setting.

▶ OVERVIEW

A **group** is defined by Adams and Galanes (2003) as "three or more individuals who have a common purpose, interact with each other, influence each other, and are interdependent" (p. 11). Nurses belong to a variety of professional groups, ranging from small groups of a few individuals, to large professional associations. The nurse may fill a variety of roles within a group, including leader, advisor, elaborator, and encourager.

The term *group dynamics*, or group processes, refers to the ways in which groups function. For group work to be accomplished and group goals to be achieved, group dynamics must be effective.

The changing healthcare system presents challenges for healthcare professionals if they are to be actively involved in decisions about healthcare policy and healthcare practice. Such decisions are made by groups of individuals at all levels of society: think tanks, advocacy groups, professional groups, and politicians at local, regional, state, national, and international levels. These challenges provide opportunities for nurses to participate as active members of the various decision-making groups. To be effective members of these groups, nurses must be knowledgeable about the dynamics of group interaction.

▶ GROUPS

Groups exist to help individuals achieve goals that might be unattainable by individual effort alone. By pooling the ideas and expertise of several individuals, groups often can solve problems more effectively than one person acting alone. Information can be disseminated to groups more quickly and with more consistency than to individuals. In addition, groups often take greater risks than do individuals because they support each other in decision making. Just as group members share responsibilities for the group's actions, they also share the consequences of those actions.

In the clinical setting, nurses work in groups as they collaborate with other nurses, other healthcare professionals, clients, and family members when planning and providing care. Nurses also work in groups in professional and specialty organizations and civic and community groups. Within these organizations nurses promote the goals of nursing on professional, civic, and political levels. Group skills are therefore important for nurses in all settings.

Types of Groups

Groups are classified as either primary or secondary, according to their structure and type of interaction. A **primary group** is a small, intimate group in which the relationships among members are personal, spontaneous, sentimental, cooperative, and inclusive. Examples are the family, a play group of children, informal work groups, and friendship groups. Members of a primary group communicate with each other largely in face-to-face interactions and develop a strong sense of unity, or "oneness." What belongs to one person is often seen as belonging to the group. For example, a success achieved by one member is shared by all and is seen as a success of the group.

Primary groups set standards of behavior for the members. They also support and sustain each member in stressful situations that he or she would otherwise not be able to withstand. Expectations are informally administered and involve primarily internal constraints imposed by the group itself. To its members, the primary group has a value in itself, not merely as a means to some other goal. The group has a sense of "we" and "our" to it, in contrast to "I" and "mine."

The role of the primary group, particularly the family, in health care is increasingly recognized. Most individuals turn to their primary group for help and support when they have health problems. For this reason, healthcare providers and organizations are expanding their focus to include the family.

A **secondary group** is generally larger, more impersonal, and less sentimental than a primary group. Examples are professional associations, task groups, ad hoc committees, political parties, and business groups. Members view these groups simply as a means of getting things done. Interactions do not necessarily occur in face-to-face contact and do not require that the members know each other personally. Expectations of members are formally administered through impersonal controls and external restraints. Once the goals of the group are achieved or change, the interaction is discontinued.

TABLE 38–3 Functions of Groups

FUNCTION	DESCRIPTION
Interpersonal Perspectives	
Affiliation	■ Fulfills need for association or connection with one another.
Affection	■ Provides opportunity to develop emotional relationships with another.
Socialization	■ Primary socialization deals with growth and development. ■ Includes socialization into the culture of an organization (i.e., new customs and beliefs), such as when a hospital is taken over by a corporate organization.
Support	■ Provides social support for the members, a source of collegiality, and a source of help when needed.
Camaraderie	■ Provides a feeling of goodwill among the members, which provides moments of pleasure.
Power	■ Provides an opportunity for individuals to exercise their need for power over others.
Functional Perspectives	
Task completion	■ Enables completion of tasks that are beyond the scope of any one individual. ■ Allows pooling of individual efforts because each person may bring specialized knowledge and skills. ■ Increases productivity.
Information	■ Provides a context for defining social reality, for setting performance goals, for establishing priorities, and for sharing special knowledge.
Normative function	■ Develops definitions and standards and enforces those standards, thereby encouraging compliance and discouraging deviations.
Empowerment	■ Empowers group members and thereby encourages change. A group often has more power than any individual.
Governance	■ Provides involvement in making decisions and serving as a source of governance within an organization.

Sources: Based on Sampson, E. E., & Marthas, M. S. (1990). *Group process for the health professions* (3rd ed.). Albany, NY: Delmar; and Stewart, G. L., Manz, C. C., & Sims, H. P. (1999). *Team work and group dynamics.* New York, NY: Wiley.

Functions of Groups

Sampson and Marthas (1990) describe eight functions of groups: socialization, support, task completion, camaraderie, information, normative function, empowerment, and governance. Stewart, Manz, and Sims (1999) describe two ways of viewing groups: functional perspectives and interpersonal perspectives. Any one group generally has more than one function, and it may serve different functions for different group members. For example, for one member, a group may provide support; for another, it may provide information. **Table 38–3** ● describes several functions of groups according to interpersonal and functional perspectives.

Levels of Group Formality

The three levels of groups are **formal**, **semiformal**, and **informal**. Traditional features of each type of group are shown in **Box 38–2** ●.

Characteristics of Effective Groups

To be effective, a group must achieve three main functions:

1. Accomplish its goals.
2. Maintain its cohesion.
3. Develop and modify its structure to improve its effectiveness.

Many factors can promote or inhibit a group's ability to achieve these functions. These include atmosphere, ability to set goals, and intergroup communication (**Figure 38–6** ●). These and other factors are compared in **Table 38–4** ●.

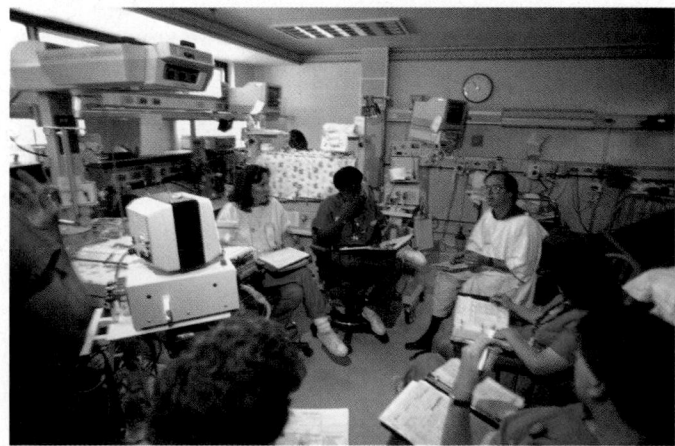

Figure 38–6 ● A healthcare team gathers as a group to discuss issues affecting client care.
Source: Mark Richards/PhotoEdit.

Box 38–2 Characteristics of the Three Levels of Groups

FORMAL GROUPS	SEMIFORMAL GROUPS	INFORMAL GROUPS
■ Authority is imposed from above.	■ The structure is formal.	■ The group is not bound by any set of written rules or regulations.
■ Leadership selection is assigned from above and made by an authoritative and often arbitrary order or decree.	■ The hierarchy is carefully delineated.	■ Usually governed by a set of unwritten laws and a strong code of ethics.
■ Managers are symbols of power and authority.	■ Membership is voluntary but selective.	■ The group is purely functional and has easily recognized basic objectives.
■ The goals of the formal group are normally imposed at a much higher level than the direct leadership of the group.	■ Prestige and status are often accrued from membership.	■ Rotational leadership is common. The group recognizes that only rarely are all leadership characteristics found in one person.
■ Management is endangered by its aloofness from the members of the work group.	■ Structured, deliberate activities absorb a large part of the group's meeting time.	■ The group assigns duties to the members best qualified for certain functions. For example, the person who is recognized as outgoing and sociable will be assigned responsibilities for planning parties.
■ Behavioral norms (expected standards of behavior), regulations, and rules are usually superimposed. The larger the turnover rate of members, the greater the structuring of rules.	■ Objectives and goals are rigid; change is not recognized as desirable.	■ Judgments about the group's leader are made quickly and surely. Leaders are replaced when they make one or more mistakes or do not get the job done.
■ Membership in the group is only partly voluntary.	■ In many cases, the leader has direct control over the choice of a successor.	■ The group is an ideal testing ground for new leadership techniques, but there is no guarantee that such techniques can be transferred effectively to a large, formal organization.
■ Rigidity of purpose is often a necessity for protection of the formal group in the pursuit of its objectives.	■ The day-to-day operating standards and methods (group norms) are negotiable. Because most people become bored at quibbling about norms, someone can often "railroad" acceptance of a list of norms that person desires.	■ Behavioral norms are developed either by group effort or by the leader and adopted by the group.
■ Interactions within the group as a whole are limited, but informal subgroups often are formed.		■ Deviance by one member from the group's behavioral norms is more threatening to the perpetuation of small, informal groups than to large, formal, heterogeneous groups. Conformity and group solidarity are important for the protection and preservation of small groups.
		■ Group norms are enforced by sanctions (punishments) imposed by the group on those who violate a norm. Different values are placed on norms in accordance with the values of the leader. One leader may regard the action as a gross violation, whereas another leader may find it quite acceptable.
		■ Interpersonal interactions are spontaneous.

▶ GROUP COMMUNICATIONS

Group Dynamics

Group dynamics, which are also known as group processes, are related to how the group functions, communicates, sets goals, and achieves objectives. Every group has its own characteristics and ways of functioning. Five aspects of group dynamics are commitment, decision-making ability, member behavior, cohesiveness, and power.

COMMITMENT The members of effective groups are committed to the goals and output of the group. Because groups demand time and attention, members must give up some autonomy and self-interest. Inevitably, conflicts arise between the interests of individual group members and those of the group as a whole. However, members who are committed to the group feel close to each other and willingly work for the achievement of the group's goals and objectives. Some indications of group commitment are shown in **Box 38–3** ●.

DECISION-MAKING METHODS The ability to make sound decisions is essential to effective group functioning. Effective decisions are made when the following things occur:

1. The group determines which decision method to adopt.
2. The group listens to all the ideas of members.
3. Members feel satisfied with their participation.
4. The expertise of group members is well used.

5. The problem-solving ability of the group is facilitated.
6. The group atmosphere is positive.
7. Time is used well; that is, the discussion focuses on the decision to be made.
8. Members feel committed to the decision and responsible for its implementation.

Huber (2009) describes several methods by which groups can make decisions: brainstorming, the nominal group technique, and the Delphi technique. Huber describes **brainstorming** as "a decision-making method in which group members meet and generate diverse ideas about the nature, cause, definition, or solution to a problem" (p. 110). For brainstorming to succeed, (a) the individuals in the group must have a level

Box 38–3 Indications of Group Commitment

■ Members feel a strong sense of belonging.
■ Members enjoy each other.
■ Members seek each other for counsel and support.
■ Members support each other in difficulty.
■ Members value the contributions of other members.
■ Members are motivated by working in the group and want to do their tasks well.
■ Members express good feelings openly and identify positive contributions.
■ Members feel that the goals of the group are achievable and important.

TABLE 38–4 Comparative Features of Effective and Ineffective Groups

FACTOR	EFFECTIVE GROUPS	INEFFECTIVE GROUPS
Atmosphere	Informal, comfortable, and relaxed. It is a working atmosphere in which individuals demonstrate their interest and involvement.	Obviously tense. Signs of boredom may appear.
Goal setting	Goals, tasks, and objectives are clarified, understood, and modified so that members of the group can commit themselves to cooperatively structured goals.	Unclear, misunderstood, or imposed goals may be accepted by members. The goals are competitively structured.
Leadership and member participation	Shift from time to time, depending on the circumstances. Different members assume leadership at various times, because of their knowledge or experience.	Delegated and based on authority. The chairperson may dominate the group, or the members may defer unduly. Members' participation is unequal, with high-authority members dominating.
Goal emphasis	All three functions of groups are emphasized: goal accomplishment, internal maintenance, and developmental change.	One or more functions may not be emphasized.
Communication	Open and two-way. Ideas and feelings are encouraged, both about the problem and about the group's operation.	Closed or one-way. Only the production of ideas is encouraged. Feelings are ignored or taboo. Members may be tentative or reluctant to be open and may have "hidden agendas" (personal goals at cross purposes with group goals).
Decision making	By consensus, although various decision-making procedures appropriate to the situation may be instituted.	By the higher authority in the group, with minimal involvement by members; or an inflexible style is imposed.
Cohesion	Facilitated through high levels of inclusion, trust, liking, and support.	Either ignored or used as a means of controlling members, thus promoting rigid conformity.
Conflict tolerance	High. The reasons for disagreements or conflicts are carefully examined, and the group seeks to resolve them. The group accepts unresolvable basic disagreements.	Low. Attempts may be made to ignore, deny, avoid, suppress, or override controversy by premature group action. The group may choose to live with conflict rather than attempt to resolve it.
Power	Determined by the members' abilities and the information they possess. Power is shared. The issue is how to get the job done.	Determined by position in the group. Obedience to authority is strong. The issue is who controls.
Problem solving	High. Constructive criticism is frequent, frank, relatively comfortable, and oriented toward removing an obstacle to problem solving.	Low. Criticism may be destructive, taking the form of either overt or covert personal attacks. It prevents the group from getting the job done.
Self-evaluation of the group	Frequent. All members participate in evaluation and decisions about how to improve the group's functioning.	Minimal. What little evaluation there is may be done by the highest authority in the group rather than by the membership as a whole.
Creativity	Encouraged. There is room within the group for members to become self-actualized and interpersonally effective.	Discouraged. People are afraid of appearing foolish if they put forth a creative thought.

Source: Adapted from Kneisl, C. R., & Wilson, H. S. (1996). *Psychiatric nursing* (5th ed., p. 736). Redwood City, CA: Addison-Wesley Nursing.

of trust, (b) there must be a criticism-free atmosphere that allows ideas to flow freely, and (c) all ideas receive initial approval and are critically examined thereafter. During brainstorming, group members are expected to generate as many ideas as possible regardless of how they sound. After all group members have exhausted all ideas, each idea is critically analyzed for efficacy.

Nominal group technique is also an aid to decision making. It is useful when multiple ideas from members of the group result in difficulty reaching a decision. **Nominal group technique** is a process that alternates between individual work and group work. This helps a group hear from every member when discussing an issue that is controversial. In this instance, the individuals meet as a group, but they write their responses

without any discussion. The ideas are then collected and an open discussion proceeds.

The **Delphi technique** was originally used for technological forecasting. It has been used for decisions that require more time or need responses from individuals in disparate locations. The Delphi technique requires participants to maintain their anonymity, which eliminates peer pressure. Data are gathered through interviews or questionnaires in a series of rounds in which an initial question is posed. Once the responses are returned, they are compiled and redistributed. The participants do not know who said what: The comments or ratings are gathered for a compiled listing and are rated through averaging or statistical analysis. With the Delphi technique an agreement is reached as the process continues.

This agreement is by consensus, voting, or mathematical average.

MEMBER BEHAVIOR The degree of input by members into goal setting, decision making, problem solving, and group evaluation is related to the group structure and leadership style, but members are responsible for their own behavior and participation. Each member participates in a wide range of roles (assigned or assumed functions) during group interactions. Individuals may perform different roles during interactions in the same group or may vary roles in different groups. Various roles have been identified. These include *information givers*, who provide factual information; *information seekers*, who seek factual information about tasks at hand; and *opinion givers*, who care more about values and beliefs than facts.

COHESIVENESS Groups that have cohesiveness possess certain characteristics. One characteristic is a group spirit. This is a sense of being "we," or having a common purpose. **Cohesiveness** is the attachment that members feel toward each other, the group, or the task. Members of groups that have a high level of cohesiveness feel greater satisfaction with the group. Groups that lack cohesiveness are unstable and are more prone to disintegration.

POWER Patterns of behavior in groups are greatly influenced by the force of power. Power can be defined as the ability to influence another person in some way or the ability to do something, whether it is to decide the fate of a nation or to decide that a certain change in policy or practice is necessary. For example, a new member of a group may be more influenced by the group member who asked him or her to enter into membership than by other members. Similarly, group members may afford power to those group members who most closely share their interests.

Many individuals have a negative concept of power, likening it to control, domination, and even coercion of others by muscle and clout. However, power can be viewed as a vital, positive force that moves people toward the attainment of individual or group goals. The overall purpose of power is to encourage cooperation and collaboration in accomplishing a task.

Group Problems

In addition to conflict, problems that can occur in groups monopolizing, groupthink, scapegoating, silence and apathy, and transference and countertransference. The nurse needs to be able to recognize and avoid these behaviors when working in collaborative groups.

MONOPOLIZING **Monopolizing** is the domination of a discussion by one member of a group. Because most group meetings have time restraints, monopolizing seriously deprives other individuals of their chance to participate. A sense of injustice among members then develops, and ultimately some members may direct their frustration and anger toward the group leader, whom they expect to do something to stop the monopolizer's behavior.

Monopolizing behavior may be motivated by anxiety or a need for attention, recognition, and approval. Often, compulsive talkers are unaware of their behavior and its effect on others and need help to recognize their behavior and its consequences.

Strategies for dealing with monopolizing include the following:

- *Interrupt simply, directly, and supportively.* This strategy is an initial attempt to get the person to hear others.
- *Reflect the person's behavior.* This strategy is an attempt to help the person become aware of the monopolizing behavior.
- *Reflect the group's feelings.* This strategy is an attempt to help the person become aware of the effects of his or her behavior on others.
- *Confront the person and/or the group.* This strategy can be directed toward the individual or toward the group to help members realize their own responsibility for the problem.

GROUPTHINK **Groupthink** is a type of decision making characterized by a group's failure to critically examine its own processes and practices. Groupthink may also occur when members of a group fail to recognize and respond to change. It may occur in highly cohesive groups when group members do not want to disagree or criticize the majority of the group's thinking for fear of being considered disloyal. For example, the administrators of a local urgent care center, failing to recognize that the local population has changed as the result of an influx of Latino clients, refuse to hire Spanish-speaking staff or engage the services of a full-time interpreter. Symptoms of groupthink include the group overestimating its power and morality, the group becoming close minded, and group members experiencing pressure to conform.

SCAPEGOATING A **scapegoat** is an individual who has been selected to take the blame for another individual or for a group. Individuals and groups who engage in scapegoating minimize their own feelings of ineptitude by focusing on the weakness of others. For leaders to deal with scapegoating, they must be alert to its development and be prepared to accept anger when they confront the scapegoaters. Scapegoating is a grossly unprofessional behavior that has no place within the profession of nursing, which emphasizes responsibility and accountability.

SILENCE AND APATHY Nonparticipation or **apathy** (lack of interest or enthusiasm) of one or more group members is sometimes best handled without intervention. Sometimes such silences are not a reflection of something in the immediate group setting but rather of some past experience. For example, after expressing an idea previously, this person may have been told "That was a stupid thing to say." Having been hurt once in a group, such individuals feel insecure about their views and are reluctant to express themselves again in groups.

Continued nonparticipation or apathy, however, needs to be dealt with by the leader after a careful assessment of whether the apathy is a reflection of leadership style, task issues, or interpersonal conflicts.

TRANSFERENCE AND COUNTERTRANSFERENCE

Transference in the group setting is defined as the transfer of feelings that were originally evoked by one's parents or significant others to individuals in the present setting. An example is a group member who acts toward the leader as the member would act toward a parent. In addition, members of a group can transfer to others in the group personal feelings of love, guilt, or hate.

When leaders respond to group members because of reactions from earlier relationships, they are engaging in *countertransference*. For example, if a group member reminds a leader of a teacher who was menacing and demanding, the leader is likely to react with anxiety and may become unreasonably fearful. It is therefore important that group members and leaders recognize the possibility of overreaction because of countertransference and that it is not an unusual reaction among nurses who are highly involved in helping others.

▶ HEALTHCARE GROUPS

Much of a nurse's professional life is spent in a wide variety of groups. As a participant in a group, the nurse may be required to fulfill different roles as member or leader, teacher or learner, adviser or advisee. Common types of healthcare groups include committees or teams, task forces, teaching groups, self-help groups, self-awareness/growth groups, therapy groups, and work-related social support groups. These various types of groups exhibit similarities and differences as do the roles of nurses participating in them.

Committees or Teams

Committees are those groups that are relatively stable or those that are brought together in a formal manner. These are the most common type of work-related group. They usually have a specific purpose that is part of their organizational structure, and they typically meet at defined intervals. Examples are policy committees, quality improvement committees, healthcare planning committees, nursing organization committees, and governmental affairs committees. Committees may also be referred to as teams, such as nursing care teams or wound care teams. Teams are groups with a small number of consistent individuals who are committed to a relevant shared purpose. Groups have common performance goals, complementary and overlapping skills, and a common approach to their work.

The leader of a committee or team, usually called the chairperson, must be accepted by the members as an appropriate leader and, therefore, should be an expert in the area of the committee's focus. The chairperson's role is to identify the specific task, clarify communication, and assist in expressing opinions and offering solutions. Within a single organization, committee or team members are generally selected on the basis of their individual functional roles and employment status rather than their personal characteristics. If a committee or team is composed of representatives from multiple organizations, the members are generally assigned by the member organizations. Committee members may reflect diverse expertise in order to assist the committee to achieve its purpose. In some cases, membership may be designated by rule or law. For example, membership in county child fatality review teams typically is designated by law and includes representatives of local hospitals, emergency medical systems, law enforcement, community health nurses, and so forth. Additional member positions, often called "at-large" positions, may be designated to enable local committees to add members from organizations whose membership would be helpful but are not on the list of those designated by rule or law. Regardless of the type of committee or team, members are accountable for the group's results or outcomes.

Task Forces

Task forces or ad hoc committees are work groups that usually have a defined task that is limited in duration. In other words, the task force is brought together to perform a specific activity, such as preparation for a Joint Commission visit or Nurse Week. When the activity has been accomplished, the task force is dissolved. Task forces and ad hoc committees function in the same way as committees or work teams. The difference is in the duration of their work.

Teaching Groups

The major purpose of a teaching group is to impart information to the participants. Examples of teaching groups include group continuing education and client healthcare groups. Numerous subjects are often handled using a group teaching format: childbirth techniques, exercise for middle-aged and older adults, and instructions to family members about follow-up care for discharged clients. A nurse who leads a group in which the primary purpose is to teach or learn must be skilled in the teaching–learning process discussed in the module on Teaching and Learning.

Self-Help Groups

A **self-help group** is a group of individuals who come together to face a common problem or difficulty. These groups are based on the helper-therapy principle: Those who help are helped most. A central belief of the self-help movement is that individuals who experience a particular social or health problem have an understanding of the condition that those without it do not. Alcoholics Anonymous (AA) is an example of a self-help group. Other support groups may consist of individuals who have specialized knowledge to help individuals who have the problem or who have experienced it. Reach for Recovery (a support group to assist women with breast cancer) is an example of this type of group in which members may have had breast cancer or they may be other individuals who have the ability to help, such as oncology nurses.

Self-Awareness/Growth Groups

The purpose of self-awareness/growth groups is to develop or use interpersonal strengths. The overall aim is to improve the individual's functioning in the group to which the individual will return, whether that group is a job, family, or community. From the beginning, broad goals are usually apparent—for example, to study communication patterns, group processes, or problem solving. Because the focus of these groups is interpersonal concerns around current situations, the work of the group is oriented to reality testing with an emphasis on the here and now. Members are responsible for correcting ineffective patterns of relating and communicating with each other. They learn group processes through participation and involvement in guided exercises.

Therapy Groups

Therapy groups are composed of individuals coming together to receive psychotherapy through which they work toward self-understanding, more satisfactory ways of relating or handling stress, and changing patterns of behavior around health. Members are referred to as clients, participants, or, in some settings, patients. They are selected by health professionals after extensive selection interviews that consider the pattern of personalities, behaviors, needs, and

identification of group therapy as the treatment of choice. Duration of therapy groups is not usually set. A termination date is usually mutually determined by the therapist and members. Therapy groups are characterized by different approaches to psychotherapy—for example, interpersonal groups, existential groups, cognitive-behavioral groups, and psychodrama.

Work-Related Social Support Groups

Many nurses, especially hospice, emergency, and critical care nurses, experience high levels of vocational stress. Social support groups can help reduce stress if they provide various types of support to buffer the stress. Group members who know about the work of others can encourage and challenge members to be more creative and enthusiastic about their work. For example, a nurse may help another group member consider alternative strategies for intervention. Members also can share the joys of success and the frustration of failure through active listening without giving advice or making judgments. This type of social support is best provided outside the work-related support group.

REVIEW Groups and Group Communication

RELATE Link the Concepts and Exemplars

Linking the exemplar of groups and group communication with the concept of addiction:

1. How do individuals work in groups and use group communication when dealing with addiction?

2. What are some group communication types that may be useful when working with addicts in a group setting?

Linking the exemplar of groups and group communication with the concept of family:

3. How can families use group communication techniques to increase communication?

4. How might communication be altered in a family as a result of health alterations?

REFER Go to Pearson Nursing Student Resources
nursing.pearsonhighered.com

- Additional review materials

REFLECT Case Study

As a substance abuse nurse, you are responsible for leading a group of people who have addiction challenges in daily meetings. You have been asked to lead your first meeting now that you have finished your 6-week preceptorship and are now taking your own client assignments on the unit. You are nervous about running a group independently. You begin to plan your session and want your mentor's input on whether you are planning a session that will be effective for the participants.

1. What type of meeting should you plan for this group?

2. What type of group problems might occur during the session?

3. After the session you feel that the group is ineffective. What characteristics would lead you to believe that this group is ineffective?

EXEMPLAR 38.2 Therapeutic Communication

EXEMPLAR KEY TERMS
Attentive listening, *2425*
Physical attending, *2426*
Therapeutic communication, *2425*
Therapeutic relationship, *2425*

EXEMPLAR LEARNING OUTCOMES
After reading about this exemplar, you will be able to:

1. Differentiate between attentive listening and physical attending as they apply to therapeutic communication and the nurse–client relationship.

2. Demonstrate therapeutic communication techniques, indicating when each might be of particular use when providing client care.

3. Contrast methods of delivering feedback to clients versus members of the healthcare team.

4. Explain the phases of the therapeutic relationship and provide examples of behaviors that occur in each phase.

5. Relate the importance of therapeutic communication to the development of a therapeutic relationship.

6. Contrast the type of communication used in the therapeutic relationship and the type of communication the nurse uses in healthcare groups.

▶ OVERVIEW

Therapeutic communication is an interactive process between the nurse and the client. It is an integral part of the **therapeutic relationship**, which is the caring relationship between a nurse and a client that is based on mutual trust and respect, sensitivity, and nurturing. Therapeutic communication helps the client to overcome temporary stress, to get along with other people, to adjust to situations that cannot be altered, and to overcome any psychological blocks that may stand in the way of self-realizations. Therapeutic communication promotes understanding and can help establish a constructive relationship between the nurse and the client. Unlike the social relationship, which might not have a specific purpose or direction, the nurse establishes a therapeutic helping relationship with the purpose of helping the client achieve health goals.

In therapeutic communication, the nurse responds not only to the content of a client's verbal message but also to the feelings expressed and nonverbal cues. It is important for the nurse to understand how the client views the situation and feels about it before responding. The content of the client's communication is the words or thoughts, as distinct from the feelings. Sometimes an individual can convey a thought in words that contradict the individual's emotions; that is, the words and feelings are incongruent. For example, a client might say, "I am glad he has left me; he was very cruel." However, the nurse observes that the client has tears in her eyes as she says this. To respond to the client's *words*, the nurse might simply rephrase, saying, "You are pleased that he has left you." To respond to the client's *feelings*, the nurse would need to acknowledge the tears in the client's eyes, saying, for example, "You seem saddened by all this." Such a response helps the client to focus on her feelings. In some instances, the nurse may need to know more about the client and her resources for coping with these feelings.

Sometimes clients need time to deal with their feelings, especially before coping with other matters such as learning new skills or planning for the future. This is most evident in hospitals when clients learn that they have a terminal illness. Some clients require hours, days, or even weeks before they are ready to start other tasks. Some need time to themselves, others need someone to listen, others need assistance identifying and verbalizing feelings, and others need assistance in identifying alternatives for future courses of action. However, while the nurse should help the client explore alternatives, the nurse should not participate in the client's decision making.

▶ THERAPEUTIC COMMUNICATION TECHNIQUES

The nurse can employ a number of different communication techniques to support clients as they deal with their feelings related to their health and health care. The nurse must embrace these techniques and adapt them to each situation to improve communication with clients. However, no one technique will guarantee a successful encounter with all clients with whom the nurse comes into contact. Each situation is unique. The nurse should use a holistic approach to communicating with clients in each situation that is presented.

Empathizing

Active listening is a skill that nursing students are taught throughout their education. Merely listening, however, is not enough. The nurse must have an empathetic understanding of the situation and offer appropriate feedback to the client. *Empathy* is best described as a process in which individuals are able to put themselves in someone else's situation. By using empathy the nurse is able to embrace the attitudes of the individual with whom the nurse is interacting in any given encounter.

To be able to empathize with clients, the nurse must be able to understand and acknowledge the ideas that the client is expressing or that the client feels are important to the situation. The nurse must also accept and respect the client's feelings as valid for the client, whatever those feelings may be, even if the nurse would not feel the same way in the circumstances. Using empathy allows the nurse to connect with clients and it also validates the importance of the client's message to the nurse.

The term *empathy* is often mistakenly used to mean *sympathy*. Empathy, however, contains no elements of condolence, agreement, or pity. Empathy focuses on the client's feelings, not the nurse's feelings. Nurses who sympathize rather than empathize assume that there is a parallel between their own feelings and the client's feelings. This perceived similarity can make professional judgment and objectivity difficult. The nurse who empathizes can interpret the client's feelings and does not insert the nurse's own feelings into the client's current situation. **Box 38–4 ●** explains the four phases of the process of therapeutic empathizing.

Empathizing with clients who are troubled can have some stressful consequences for nurses. Problems can arise at any phase of the process, and when a nurse fails to cope with one of the four phases of achieving empathy, obstacles occur in terms of the nurse–client relationship. The nurse should not identify too closely with the client, because this can lead to sympathy rather than empathy. By identifying too closely, the nurse may fail to incorporate the client's feelings and may, in fact, project personal ones onto the client. Another problem can occur when nurses bypass the reverberation phase and substitute gut-level intuitions for rational problem solving. Nurses should also guard against overdistancing or burnout.

Attentive Listening

Attentive listening, also called *mindful listening*, is listening actively, using all the senses, in contrast to listening passively with just the ear. Active listening is probably the most important technique in therapeutic communication and is the basis of all other techniques. Attentive listening is an active process that requires energy and concentration. It is more than being quiet while the other individual talks—it involves paying attention to the total message, both verbal and nonverbal, and not-

Box 38–4   Four Phases of Therapeutic Empathizing

The process of establishing empathetic understanding has four phases:

1. *Identification.* This phase involves the relaxation of conscious control. In this phase, the nurse is able to contemplate the client and the client's experiences.
2. *Incorporation.* In this phase, the nurse considers the client's experiences and feelings rather than his or her own experiences.
3. *Reverberation.* This phase involves an interplay of the client's internalized feeling with the nurse's own experiences or fantasies. The nurse is fully absorbed in the client's identity but is able to experience him- or herself separately.
4. *Detachment.* In this phase the nurse withdraws from subjective involvement with the client and resumes his or her own identity. The nurse uses the insight that was gained from the reverberation phase, along with reason and objectivity, to offer meaningful and useful responses to the client.

Box 38–5   Blocks to Attentive Listening

■ *Rehearsing:* when the nurse is busy planning what is to be said next in the conversation
■ *Being concerned with oneself:* when the nurse focuses on the nurse's own intelligence, competence, feelings, or accomplishments instead of on the client
■ *Assuming:* when the nurse makes assumptions about what the client is really trying to convey in the conversation
■ *Judging:* when the nurse frames messages in terms of the nurse's own judgment about whether what the client is saying is right or wrong, mature or immature, calm or anxious, sensible or paranoid, or depressed or simply quiet
■ *Identifying:* when the nurse focuses on the nurse's own experiences, beliefs, or feelings; may occur when what the client communicates triggers memories or concerns from the nurse's own personal experiences
■ *Getting off track:* when the nurse changes the subject or makes light of what the client is expressing because the nurse is uncomfortable, bored, or tired
■ *Filtering:* when the nurse tunes out certain topics in the conversation or hears only certain items that the client is saying; may occur due to anxiety on the part of the nurse.

ing whether these communications are congruent. Attentive listening means absorbing both the content and the feeling the individual is conveying, without selectivity. The listener does not select or listen solely to what the listener wants to hear; the nurse focuses not on the nurse's own needs but rather on the client's needs. Attentive listening conveys an attitude of caring and interest, thereby encouraging the client to talk (see **Figure 38–7** ●).

Attentive listening also involves listening for key themes in the communication. The nurse must be careful not to react quickly to the message. The speaker should not be interrupted, and the nurse should take time to think about the message before responding. As a listener, the nurse also should ask questions either to obtain additional information or clarification and to ensure that the nurse fully understands the message.

Nurses need to be aware of their own biases. A message that reflects values or beliefs that differ from the nurse's should not be discredited for that reason. The client, who is the sender, should decide when to close the conversation,

and the nurse should listen for the signal that the client is ready to do so. When the nurse closes the conversation, the client may assume that the nurse considers the message unimportant.

There are some specific blocks to listening that may prevent the nurse from actually hearing what the client says. This may convey a message to clients that what they have to say is not important (see **Box 38–5** ●).

In summary, attentive listening is a highly developed skill that can be learned with practice. A nurse can listen attentively to clients in various ways. Common responses are nodding the head, uttering "uh huh" or "mmm," repeating the words that the client has used, or saying "I see what you mean." Each nurse has characteristic ways of responding, and the nurse must take care not to sound insincere or patronizing.

Physical Attending

Physical attending is defined as the manner of being present to another or being with another. Listening, in a frame of reference, is what an individual does while attending. Five specific ways to convey physical attending, which in turn conveys involvement, are described in **Box 38–6** ●.

Therapeutic communication techniques facilitate communication and focus on the client's concerns. **Table 38–5** ● lists some common therapeutic communication techniques, with descriptions of the techniques and examples of their use.

Using Silence

Nurses often feel that they must respond to each statement that is made by a client. This, however, is not necessary. The use of *silence* can be therapeutic and goes beyond active listening. The nurse who uses silence may sit or walk quietly with the

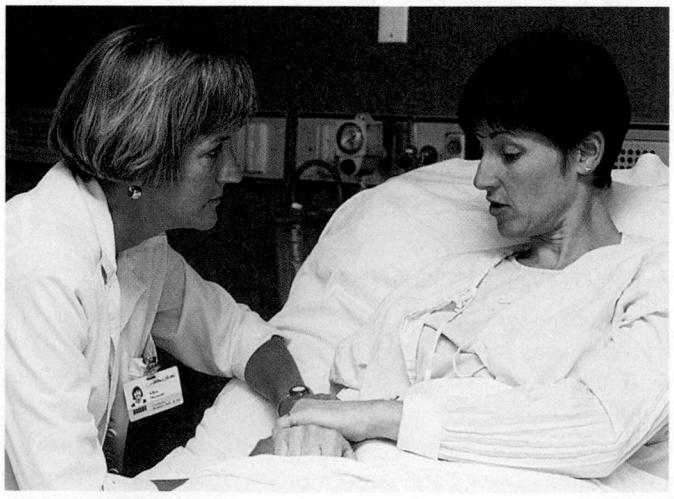

Figure 38–7 ● The nurse conveys attentive listening through a posture of involvement.

Box 38–6 Actions of Physical Attending

- *Face the other person squarely.* This position says, "I am available to you." Moving to the side lessens the degree of involvement.
- *Adopt an open posture.* The nondefensive position is one in which neither arms nor legs are crossed. It conveys that the individual wishes to encourage the passage of communication, as the open door of a home or an office does.
- *Lean toward the person.* Individuals move naturally toward one another when they want to say or hear something—by moving to the front of a class, by moving a chair nearer a friend, or by leaning across a table with arms propped in front. The nurse conveys involvement by leaning forward, closer to the client.
- *Maintain good eye contact.* Mutual eye contact, preferably at the same level, recognizes the other individual and denotes willingness to maintain communication. Eye contact neither glares at nor stares down another but is natural.
- *Try to be relatively relaxed.* Total relaxation is not feasible when the nurse is listening with intensity, but the nurse can show relaxation by taking time when responding, allowing pauses as needed, balancing periods of tension with relaxation, and using gestures that are natural.

These five attending postures need to be adapted to the specific needs of clients in a given situation. For example, leaning forward may not be appropriate at the beginning of an interview. It may be reserved until a closer relationship grows between the nurse and the client. The same applies to eye contact, which is generally uninterrupted when the communicators are very involved in the interaction.

client. The goal is to provide a therapeutic purpose, such as the following:

- Encouraging the client to communicate with the nurse
- Allowing the client time to think about what has been said or to make connections

- Allowing the client the necessary time to collect personal thoughts
- Allowing the client time to consider possible alternatives.

The nurse who uses silence while remaining interested in what the client is communicating maintains an open posture or a questioning look, which will encourage the client to use the time effectively.

Silence is an effective communication technique only when it is used appropriately and purposefully for therapeutic communication. When an uncomfortable silence occurs, the nurse should break the silence and then analyze it. It is important not to allow the client to become anxious or resistive. The nurse who is silent out of discomfort or a lack of knowledge or skill on how to communicate effectively should seek guidance from someone more experienced in order to analyze the personal and professional areas that are in need of growth.

Reflecting

When nurses use reflection in the communication process, they are actively acknowledging what they have heard or seen from clients. *Reflecting* is what takes place when the nurse repeats the client's verbal or nonverbal messages for the client's benefit.

REFLECTING CONTENT By reflecting the content of the message that is heard from the client, the nurse is essentially repeating the client's statement. This allows the client the opportunity to both hear and reflect on what she has told the nurse in the course of the conversation.

The technique of content reflecting is often misused or overused in the mental health environment. Overuse of this

TABLE 38–5 Therapeutic Communication Techniques

TECHNIQUE	DESCRIPTION	EXAMPLES
Using silence	Accepting pauses or silences that may extend for several seconds or minutes without interjecting any verbal response.	Sitting quietly (or walking with the client) and waiting attentively until the client is able to put thoughts and feelings into words.
Providing general leads	Using statements or questions that (a) encourage the client to verbalize, (b) choose a topic of conversation, and (c) facilitate continued verbalization.	"Can you tell me how it is for you?" "Perhaps you would like to talk about…." "Would it help to discuss your feelings?" "Where would you like to begin?" "And then what?"
Being specific and tentative	Making statements that are specific rather than general and tentative rather than absolute.	"Rate your pain on a scale of zero to ten" (specific statement) versus "Are you in pain?" (general statement) "You seem unconcerned about your diabetes" (tentative statement) versus "You don't care about your diabetes and you never will." (absolute statement)
Using open-ended questions	Asking broad questions that lead or invite the client to explore (elaborate, clarify, describe, compare, or illustrate) thoughts or feelings. Open-ended questions specify only the topic to be discussed and invite answers that are longer than one or two words.	"I'd like to hear more about that." "Tell me about…." "How have you been feeling lately?" "What brought you to the hospital?" "What is your opinion?" "You said you were frightened yesterday. How do you feel now?"
Using touch	Providing appropriate forms of touch to reinforce caring feelings. Because tactile contacts vary considerably among individuals, families, and cultures, the nurse must be sensitive to the differences in attitudes and practices of clients and self.	Putting an arm over the client's shoulder; placing a hand over the client's hand.

(continued on next page)

TABLE 38-5 Therapeutic Communication Techniques (*continued*)

TECHNIQUE	DESCRIPTION	EXAMPLES
Restating or paraphrasing	Actively listening for the client's basic message and then repeating those thoughts and/or feelings in similar words. This conveys that the nurse has listened and understood the client's basic message and also offers clients a clearer idea of what they have said.	*Client:* "I couldn't manage to eat any dinner last night—not even the dessert." *Nurse:* "You had difficulty eating yesterday." *Client:* "Yes, I was very upset after my family left." *Client:* "I have trouble talking to strangers." *Nurse:* "You find it difficult talking to people you do not know?"
Seeking clarification	A method of making the client's broad overall meaning of the message more understandable. It is used when paraphrasing is difficult or when the communication is rambling or garbled. To clarify the message, the nurse can restate the basic message or confess confusion and ask the client to repeat or restate the message. Nurses can also clarify their own message with statements.	"I'm puzzled." "I'm not sure I understand that." "Would you please say that again?" "Would you tell me more?" "I meant this rather than that." "I'm sorry that wasn't very clear. Let me try to explain another way."
Perception checking or seeking consensual validation	A method similar to clarifying that verifies the meaning of specific words rather than the overall meaning of a message.	*Client:* "My husband never gives me any presents." *Nurse:* "You mean he has never given you a present for your birthday or Christmas?" *Client:* "Well—not never. He does get me something for my birthday and Christmas, but he never thinks of giving me anything at any other time."
Offering self	Suggesting one's presence, interest, or wish to understand the client without making any demands or attaching conditions that the client must comply with to receive the nurse's attention.	"I'll stay with you until your daughter arrives." "We can sit here quietly for a while. We don't need to talk unless you would like to." "I'll help you to dress to go home, if you'd like."
Giving information	Providing, in a simple and direct manner, specific factual information the client may or may not request. When information is not known, the nurse states this and indicates who has it or when the nurse will obtain it.	"Your surgery is scheduled for 11 a.m. tomorrow." "You will feel a pulling sensation when the tube is removed from your abdomen." "I do not know the answer to that, but I will find out from Mrs. King, the nurse in charge."
Acknowledging	Giving recognition, in a nonjudgmental way, of a change in behavior, an effort the client has made, or a contribution to a communication. Acknowledgment may be with or without understanding, verbal or nonverbal.	"You trimmed your beard and mustache and washed your hair." "I notice you keep squinting your eyes. Are you having difficulty seeing?" "You walked twice as far today with your walker."
Clarifying time or sequence	Helping the client clarify an event, situation, or happening in relationship to time.	*Client:* "I vomited this morning." *Nurse:* "Was that after breakfast?" *Client:* "I feel that I have been asleep for weeks." *Nurse:* "You had your operation Monday, and today is Tuesday."
Presenting reality	Helping the client to differentiate the real from the unreal.	"That telephone ring came from the program on television." "I see shadows from the window coverings." "Your magazine is here in the drawer. It has not been stolen."
Focusing	Helping the client expand on and develop a topic of importance. It is important for the nurse to wait until the client finishes stating the main concerns before attempting to focus. The focus may be an idea or a feeling; however, the nurse often emphasizes a feeling to help the client recognize an emotion disguised behind words.	*Client:* "My wife says she will look after me, but I don't think she can, what with the children to take care of, and they're always after her about something—clothes, homework, what's for dinner that night." *Nurse:* "Sounds like you are worried about how well she can manage."
Reflecting	Directing ideas, feelings, questions, or content back to clients to enable them to explore their own ideas and feelings about a situation.	*Client:* "What can I do?" *Nurse:* "What do you think would be helpful?" *Client:* "Do you think I should tell my husband?" *Nurse:* "You seem unsure about telling your husband."
Summarizing and planning	Stating the main points of a discussion to clarify the relevant points discussed. This technique is useful at the end of an interview or to review a health teaching session. It often acts as an introduction to future care planning.	"During the past half hour we have talked about…." "Tomorrow afternoon we may explore this further." "In a few days I'll review with you what you have learned about the actions and effects of your insulin." "Tomorrow, I will look at your feeling journal."

technique causes it to lose effectiveness. The nurse should use this technique judiciously.

> ### CLINICAL EXAMPLE
> Jason Smith is a 48-year-old man who has been admitted to the hospital with the diagnosis of acute inferior myocardial infarction. He says to the nurse, "I can't believe I had a heart attack. Those are for old people! I still feel young, but I guess I have to slow down." The nurse, using reflection, asks Mr. Smith, "Do you feel that you can no longer lead an active life because you have had a heart attack?" The nurse's statement will encourage Mr. Smith to continue sharing thoughts and explain why he believes this to be true. This will allow the nurse to correct any misunderstanding that he has about the recovery process after an MI.

REFLECTING FEELINGS   In using the technique of reflecting *feelings*, the nurse verbalizes the feelings that are implied in the client's comment. The nurse should respect that clients have the right to their own opinions and feelings even when the nurse personally disagrees with these. Some examples of reflecting feelings are as follows:

- "Sounds like you're really angry at your sister."
- "You're feeling anxious about being discharged from the hospital later today."

By reflecting feelings, the nurse attempts to identify any latent or connotative meanings that can either clarify or distort the content that is communicated. Such reflection of feelings is useful because it will encourage the client to make additional, clarifying comments in the conversation.

Imparting Information

In *imparting information* the nurse is helping the client by supplying additional data for consideration. This encourages further clarification because it is based on new or additional input. Some examples of statements that impart information are as follows:

- "Group therapy will be held on Wednesday afternoon from 3:30 until 5:00."
- "I am a mental-health nursing student."

Note that it is not appropriate to withhold information from a client when the client asks an information-seeking question. The nurse must be mindful not to cross the line between giving information and giving the client advice. The nurse should also not give information as a way of avoiding conflict. Nurses who give clients personal or social information are moving outside of the realm of therapeutic communication. Information that the nurse must share with the client includes the nurse's name, title, and position. New nurses must be cautioned to resist the temptation of divulging inappropriate information to clients.

The client's participation in the decision-making process begins with the client taking in and understanding information regarding his own condition. The ultimate goal of sharing essential information with the client is to provide effective education that empowers the client. Empowered clients are more likely to achieve a positive mental health outcome. They are also less likely to be admitted for inpatient therapy or be readmitted after discharge.

Avoiding Self-Disclosure

Clients have been known to ask personal questions of nurses who are caring for them. This many include inquiring about the nurse's marital status, where the nurse lives, what religion the nurse practices, or information about personal issues. The best methods for deflecting requests for self-disclosure, outlined by Auvil and Silver (1984), include the following:

- *Using honesty:* "I don't feel comfortable sharing my address with you."
- *Using benign curiosity:* "Why are you asking me this today?"
- *Using refocusing:* "You were talking about how your mother treats you. Why are you changing the topic? You were saying…."
- *Using interpretation:* "I notice that every time you talk about your sister, you change the subject and ask me a question." (pause)
- *Seeking clarification:* "You keep asking me where I live. I wonder if you have any concerns about me today?"
- *Responding with feedback and limit setting:* "I'm uncomfortable when you ask me who pays my tuition for school. Talking about my finances isn't part of our agreement to work together." Adding something like "The last time we met, you were deciding whether you were going to call your sister on the phone . . ." helps restructure the situation.

These communication techniques should be used within the context of the therapeutic relationship.

Therapeutic communication revolves around the needs of the client. It is not appropriate to talk to the client about your experiences such as what you did last night or your thoughts on a given subject. This wastes times that could be spent on learning about the client's needs, thoughts, concerns, or problems. Always maintain a client focus during communication.

Clarifying

Even when the nurse has listened carefully and thoughtfully to the client, there may be a need to clarify information. *Clarifying* is an attempt to understand the basic nature of a client's statement.

- "I'm confused about what is upsetting you. Could you go over that again, please?"
- "You say you're feeling anxious now. What's that like for you?"

Asking the client to give an example allows the client to clarify the meaning of the communication and helps the nurse understand the intended message. Clarification may be needed because of the language that the client uses, such as slang used by adolescent clients, or when the nurse is not certain of adequate interpretation of what the client is trying to convey.

The nurse is caring for Sara Kim, a 36-year-old woman who was recently diagnosed with breast cancer. The physician has informed Ms. Kim that her chance of full recovery is excellent and has recommended a course of treatment to include removal of the involved breast followed by chemotherapy. While the nurse is providing preoperative instructions, Ms. Kim says, "I'll sign the consent form, but I'll be dead before the surgery date." The nurse is not sure whether Ms. Kim is fearful of dying from cancer or whether this may be a statement of suicidal ideation. The nurse seeks clarification by asking, "Why do you think you'll be dead before the date for surgery arrives?"

Paraphrasing

By *paraphrasing*, the nurse restates in her own words what the client has said. Some examples of paraphrasing statements are as follows:

- "In other words, you're tired of being treated like a child."
- "I hear you saying that when people compliment you, you feel embarrassed and if they knew the real you, they would not provide such praise."

The nurse is able to test her understanding of what the client is trying to communicate through paraphrasing. Paraphrasing is reflective in nature as it lets the client know what the nurse heard and how the nurse understands what is being discussed. It is also an opportunity for the client to clarify the content of the message or the feelings behind it.

Checking Perceptions

The nurse can *check perceptions* by sharing how information is perceived and heard. Once the nurse's perceptions have been shared, it is important to ask the client to verify the perception, by using statements such as the following:

- "Let me know if this is how you see it too."
- "I get the feeling that you're uncomfortable when we're silent. Does that seem right?"

The effective use of a perception check conveys that the nurse wants to understand what the client is communicating. It gives the client the opportunity to correct inaccurate perceptions that the nurse may have. Essentially it allows the nurse to avoid actions that are based on false assumptions about the client.

Questioning

Questioning is a very direct way of speaking that the nurse can use when speaking with a client. This technique is quite useful when the nurse is seeking specific information. If the nurse is trying to engage in meaningful dialogue with a client, questions should be limited, because they can affect the nature and the ranges of responses from the client.

Open-ended questions can be used to elicit more information than closed questions. An *open-ended question* allows the nurse to focus the topic while allowing the client freedom with responses. Examples of this include the following:

- "How were you feeling when your brother said that to you?"
- "What's your opinion about. . . ?"

Closed questions should be used sparingly because they typically limit the client's responses to "yes" or "no." Closed questions also limit therapeutic exploration. This type of question can be useful, however, for the client who may have disorganized thinking. Closed questions can be used to guide these clients.

Questions that ask "why" are typically less helpful than open-ended questions. These questions tend to be hard to answer, and they rarely lead to the nurse having a clearer understanding of the current situation. Other types of closed questions, such as "who," "what," "when," and "how," can be useful if the nurse uses them wisely.

Nurses must be careful when questioning so as not to steer the client to answer questions in a certain way. For example, "You don't exercise in excess, do you?" may suggest that the client answer this question with a "no." Refer to the module on Assessment for more information on using open-ended and closed questions.

Structuring

The nurse can use a technique known as *structuring* in an attempt to create order or establish guidelines for clients. This helps clients become aware of their problems and the order in which they should deal with them. Examples of structuring statements are as follows:

- "You've mentioned that you want to improve your relationships with your husband, your son, and your boss. Let's put them in order of importance."
- "No, I won't be giving you advice, but we can discuss some solutions to these issues together."

The nurse can use structuring when a client introduces a number of issues in a brief period and doesn't know where to begin. This technique can also be used to define the parameters of the nurse–client relationship in terms of how the nurse will participate with the client to facilitate the problem-solving process.

Pinpointing

The nurse can use a technique known as *pinpointing* to call attention to specific statements and relationships. For example, when the nurse points out inconsistencies among statements or similarities and differences in points of view, feelings, or action, the nurse is engaging in pinpointing. This can also be used to determine differences between what an individual says and what one does. Examples of pinpointing statements include the following:

- "So, you and your husband aren't in agreement about how many children you want."
- "You say you're happy, but you're frowning."

Linking

When using the technique known as *linking*, the nurse responds to the client in a way that ties together events, experiences, feelings, or people. Nurses often use linking to connect past experience with current behaviors that the client is exhibiting. The nurse can also use linking when there is tension between two individuals during times of stress. Examples of statements that utilize linking include the following:

- "You felt depressed after the death of both of your parents."
- "So, the arguments didn't really begin until after you lost your job."

Giving Feedback

In using the technique known as *feedback*, the nurse shares reactions to the client's statements or behaviors. This technique can help a client become aware of how the client's behavior can affect others and how others may perceive the client's actions. The nurse who responds with feedback may experience therapeutic self-disclosure because it allows the nurse to offer constructive information regarding how the client's words or actions have affected the nurse as a communication partner. Total self-disclosure, however, is inappropriate in the nurse–client relationship and should be avoided. This can place a burden of interdependence on the client and may limit the time and energy that are available to work on the client's concerns. The use of reciprocal self-disclosure is more appropriate in friend and colleague relationships than in nurse–client relationships.

Effective feedback should have three distinct qualities. It should be *immediate*, meaning that it is given as soon as possible; it should be *honest*, meaning that it provides a true reaction; and it should be *supportive*, meaning that it is provided in a way that is tolerable to comprehend and never hurtful or disrespectful to the client. Examples of effective feedback statements include the following:

- "When you cross your arms while speaking, I feel your apprehension."
- "Sometimes when you look down while we are talking, I think you're angry."

Feedback should always be provided to the client in a nonthreatening manner. Threatening feedback may increase the client's defensiveness. The more defensive the client is when engaging in therapeutic communication, the less able the client is to hear and understand the feedback that the nurse is providing. Clients often feel offended if they perceive the nurse to be rejecting them. Feedback that is nontherapeutic, meaning that it is harsh, hurtful, cruel, or rejecting of the client, will create an unnecessary boundary between the client and the nurse. The nurse should take great care to prevent the client from feeling personally rejected as a result of feedback from the nurse. **Box 38–7** ● lists strategies and rationales that the nurse can use for giving helpful, nonthreatening feedback.

Feedback goes both ways. Clients usually want to accomplish several items during their interactions with the nurse. They want to express themselves, and they want to express information about their perception of the nurse. The nurse should be open and receptive when receiving cues from the client, either solicited or unsolicited, because these can be useful in a more meaningful working relationship. **Box 38–8** ● provides strategies to help nurses reflect on feedback from clients.

Box 38–7 Giving Helpful, Nonthreatening Feedback	
STRATEGY	RATIONALE
■ Focus the feedback on behavior.	Feedback should relate to what the client actually does rather than how the nurse imagines the client to be.
■ Focus the feedback on observations.	Feedback should relate to what the nurse actually sees or hears the client do. When inferences are used rather than observations, the nurse is drawing conclusions or making assumptions.
■ Focus the feedback on description.	Description reports what actually occurred rather than evaluating it in terms of good or bad, right or wrong.
■ Focus feedback on "more or less" rather than "either/or" descriptions of behaviors.	"More or less" descriptions stress quantity rather than quality (which may be value laden).
■ Focus feedback on here-and-now behavior rather than there-and-then behavior.	The most meaningful feedback from the nurse is given as soon as it is appropriate to do so.
■ Focus feedback on sharing of information and ideas.	Sharing of ideas and information helps the client make decisions about the client's own well-being. In contrast, by giving advice, the nurse takes away the client's freedom to be self-determining.
■ Focus feedback on exploration of alternatives.	Focusing on a variety of alternatives for accomplishing a particular goal for the client prevents premature acceptance of answers or solutions that may not be appropriate.
■ Focus feedback on its value to the client.	Feedback should serve the client's needs, not the needs of the nurse.
■ Limit feedback to the appropriate amount of information.	Overload of information will decrease the effectiveness of feedback for the client.
■ Limit feedback to the appropriate time and place.	For feedback to be effective it must be presented at the appropriate time.
■ Focus feedback on what is said rather than why it is said.	Focusing on why the client has said something or done something moves away from observations and toward client motive or intent. Motive or intent can only be assumed and, unless verified, such an assumption is counterproductive.

Confronting

Used in a constructive way, confrontation can lead to productive change. *Confronting* is defined as the deliberate invitation to examine some aspect of personal behavior. Typically confronting is used when there is a discrepancy between what an individual says and what that individual does. Confrontation requires careful attention to nonverbal communication and to both verbal and nonverbal discrepancies between messages.

The two basic types of confrontation are informational and interpretive. Each type can be directed toward the client's resources and limitations. An *informational confrontation* describes the visible behavior of another individual (e.g., "You look sad and say you're 'not as smart as your brother and a sister,' yet you are the only one who made the honor roll."). *Interpretive confirmation* expresses thoughts and feelings about behavior and draws inferences (e.g., "Ever since Emily and Frank criticized the way you conducted the assembly, you haven't spoken to them. It looks like you're feeling angry.").

Six skills can be used in incorporating constructive confrontations:

1. Use personal statements with the words *I*, *my*, and *me*.
2. Use relationship statements that express thoughts and feelings about the client in the present.
3. Use statements that describe visible client behaviors. This is known as behavior descriptions.
4. Use the description of personal feelings in which you specify the feeling by name.
5. Use responses that are aimed at understanding. Examples of these include paraphrasing and perception checking.
6. Use constructive feedback skills.

Summarizing

Summarizing is a technique that the nurse can use to highlight the main ideas that are expressed during interactions. It is used to convey the nurse's understanding to the client, and it allows both nurse and client to benefit from a review of the main ideas of a conversation. Summarizing can also be useful when the nurse wants to focus the client's thinking and to aid in conscious learning.

In certain instances summarizing is particularly appropriate. The nurse may want to use this technique in the first few minutes of client interaction, because it is useful to review what occurred during previous interactions. This helps the client to recall items that were discussed and gives the client an opportunity to see how the nurse synthesized the information from previous encounters. Summarizing also keeps all participants directed toward a common goal.

Nurses may fall into the habit of injudicious use of summarizing. This may occur when the nurse is choosing to summarize even though there are more pressing and immediate client needs that should be addressed. In this case, summarizing may be used to meet the nurse's needs rather than the client's needs. This should be avoided because it does not address the client's immediate concerns.

Processing

The nurse can also use a technique known as processing. *Processing* is a complex and sophisticated technique used to direct attention to the interpersonal dynamics of the nurse–client relationship in terms of content, feelings, and behaviors that have been expressed. This is an advanced skill. Processing is most useful and meaningful when therapeutic intimacy has been achieved.

CLINICAL EXAMPLE

The nurse is preparing to conduct a home visit to Emily Bardinovich, an 86-year-old woman who has lived in an assisted living apartment for the past 5 years. Mrs. Bardinovich was recently discharged back to her apartment following an exacerbation of COPD. The nurse has cared for Mrs. Bardinovich for many years and knows her as a friendly, outgoing woman with a great sense of humor who loves to tease people. Today, the nurse finds Mrs. Bardinovich very quiet and reserved with little to say. The nurse comments, "You're very quiet today; you haven't teased me at all," to which Mrs. Bardinovich responds, "I'm just not in the teasing mood." The nurse has used processing to help the client begin to talk about how she feels. This will allow the nurse to perform a more in-depth assessment of the client's mood and thoughts.

Common Mistakes

Nurses often make mistakes when it comes to therapeutic communication. It can be difficult for the nurse to both empathize and communicate with clients when the nurse is feeling uncomfortable with the situation. Some common mistakes the nurse should take care to avoid include the following:

- *Giving advice.* This carries the message that the client is not capable of solving problems.
- *Minimizing or discounting feelings.* Attempts at reassurance often minimize and discount what the client is feeling.

- **Deflecting.** Changing the subject or making jokes in an attempt to move the conversation to something that is less painful is not considered a positive shift because it gives the client the message that the nurse does not know how to cope with the client's experience.
- **Interrogating.** Asking a slew of questions implies that the nurse is more interested in gaining information than in listening to what the client has to say.
- **Sparring.** Debating or disagreeing with the client sets up an adversarial dynamic and prevents the nurse from listening to what the client is trying to communicate.

▶ BARRIERS TO COMMUNICATION

Nurses need to recognize barriers or nontherapeutic responses to effective communication (refer back to Table 38–1). Major barriers to communication include failing to listen, improperly decoding the client's intended message, and placing the nurse's needs above the client's needs. Barriers to communication are discussed in the Concept of Communication section earlier in this module.

▶ THE THERAPEUTIC RELATIONSHIP

Nurse–client relationships are referred to by some as interpersonal relationships, by others as therapeutic relationships, and by still others as helping relationships. Helping is a growth-facilitating process that strives to achieve two basic goals (Egan, 2013):

1. Help clients manage their problems of living more effectively and develop unused or underused opportunities more fully.
2. Help clients become better at helping themselves in their everyday lives.

A therapeutic relationship may develop over weeks of working with a client or within minutes. The keys to a therapeutic relationship are the development of trust and acceptance between the nurse and the client and an underlying belief that the nurse cares about and wants to help the client.

The therapeutic relationship is influenced by the personal and professional characteristics of the nurse and the client. Age, sex, appearance, diagnosis, education, values, ethnic and cultural background, personality, expectations, and setting can all affect the development of the nurse–client relationship. Consideration of all of these factors, combined with good communication skills and sincere interest in the client's welfare, enables the nurse to create a therapeutic relationship. Characteristics of therapeutic relationships are listed in **Box 38–9** ●.

Phases of the Therapeutic Relationship

The therapeutic relationship process can be described in terms of four sequential phases: the preinteraction phase, introductory phase, working (maintaining) phase, and termination phase. Each phase is characterized by identifiable tasks and

> **Box 38–9 Characteristics of a Therapeutic Relationship**
>
> A THERAPEUTIC RELATIONSHIP
> - Is an intellectual and emotional bond between the nurse and the client and is focused on the client.
> - Respects the client as an individual, including the following:
>   a. Maximizing the client's abilities to participate in decision making and treatments
>   b. Considering the client's ethnic background and cultural practices
>   c. Considering family relationships and values.
> - Respects client confidentiality.
> - Focuses on the client's well-being.
> - Is based on mutual trust, respect, and acceptance.

skills, and the relationship must progress through the stages in succession because each builds on the one before. The nurse can identify the progress of a relationship by understanding these phases.

PREINTERACTION PHASE The preinteraction phase is similar to the planning stage before an interview. In most situations, the nurse has information about the client before the first face-to-face meeting. Such information may include the client's name, address, age, medical history, and/or social history. Planning for the initial visit may generate some anxious feelings in the nurse. If the nurse recognizes these feelings and identifies specific information to be discussed, positive outcomes can evolve.

INTRODUCTORY PHASE The introductory phase, also referred to as the orientation phase or the pretherapeutic phase, sets the tone for the rest of the relationship. During this initial encounter, the client and the nurse closely observe each other, and each forms judgments about the other's behavior. The goal of the nurse in this phase is to develop trust and security within the nurse–client relationship (Boyd, 2008). Other important tasks of the introductory phase including getting to know each other and developing a degree of trust.

After introductions, the nurse may initially engage in some social interaction to put the client at ease. For example, the nurse and client may talk about what a nice day it is or a local news or sports event.

During the initial parts of the introductory phase, the client may display some resistive behaviors. *Resistive behaviors* are those that inhibit involvement, cooperation, or change. These behaviors may arise from the client's difficulty in acknowledging the need for help, fear of exposing and facing feelings, anxiety about the discomfort involved in changing problem-causing behavior patterns, and fear or anxiety in response to the nurse's approach, which may, in the client's opinion, be inappropriate.

The nurse can overcome a client's resistive behaviors by conveying a caring attitude, genuine interest in the client, and competence. This will help the nurse foster the development of trust in the relationship. *Trust* can be described as a reliance on someone without doubt or question, or the belief that the other individual is capable of assisting in times of distress and in all likelihood will do so. To trust another individual involves risk; clients become vulnerable when they share thoughts, feelings, and attitudes with the nurse. Trust, however, enables the client to express thoughts and feelings openly.

By the end of the introductory phase, clients should begin to do the following:

- Develop trust in the nurse.
- View the nurse as a competent professional capable of helping.
- View the nurse as honest, open, and concerned about the client's welfare.
- Believe the nurse will try to understand and respect the client's cultural values and beliefs.
- Believe the nurse will respect client confidentiality.
- Feel comfortable talking with the nurse about feelings and other sensitive issues.
- Understand the purpose of the relationship and the respective roles of the client and nurse.
- Feel like an active participant in developing a mutually agreeable plan of care.

CLINICAL EXAMPLE

While working in an ambulatory care setting, the nurse is asked by the physician to talk with a client named Raissa Kunin and explain the need for phlebotomy secondary to Ms. Kunin's diagnosis of polycythemia. Ms. Kunin's hemoglobin is 17.4 mg/dL; it has been steadily increasing since 1 year ago, when it was 16.2 mg/dL. The nurse enters the room and says, "Hello, Ms. Kunin, my name is Mikela Mathews. I'm an RN working for Dr. Shah. He asked me to speak with you about the need to remove blood to lower your hemoglobin." Ms. Kunin, says, "I'm just not sure I want to do that, but I'll call you after I have time to think about it." The nurse responds by stating, "Good for you! You have every right to make a decision in your own best interest. What if I just give you some information while you're here so you can make your decision based on all the details. I can explain the risks of polycythemia, the process of removing blood, and answer any questions you may have." The nurse attempts to overcome resistance behavior by allowing the client to maintain control. This also promotes a trusting relationship with the client.

Use critical thinking to answer the following questions:

1. How would you respond if the client answered, "No, thank you. That's not necessary. I can look it up on the Internet"?
2. If the client agrees to listen to the nurse, what phase of the relationship will they be in once the nurse begins teaching?
3. What other types of resistive behaviors might you encounter and how would you attempt to overcome them?

WORKING PHASE   The working phase has two major stages: exploring and understanding thoughts and feelings, and facilitating and taking action. In this phase, the nurse helps the client to explore thoughts, feelings, and actions and to plan a program of action to meet preestablished goals.

The nurse must have the following skills for this phase of the therapeutic relationship:

- **Empathetic listening and responding.** As discussed previously, the nurse must listen attentively and respond in ways that indicate that the nurse acknowledges the client's concerns and feelings as important. Nonverbal behaviors indicating empathy include moderate head nodding, a steady gaze, moderate gesturing, and little activity or body movement.
- **Respect.** The nurse must show respect for the client's willingness to be available, a desire to work with the client, and a manner that conveys that the nurse takes the client's point of view seriously.
- **Genuineness.** The nurse exudes a genuine care for the client by maintaining professional behaviors that promote the therapeutic helping relationship. Egan (2013) has outlined five behaviors that are components of genuineness: not taking refuge or overemphasizing the role of counselor, being spontaneous, being nondefensive, being consistent, and being capable of appropriate self-disclosure.
- **Concreteness.** The nurse must encourage the client to be concrete and specific rather than to speak in generalities. When the client says, "My blood pressure has been very unstable," the nurse narrows the topic to the specific by replying, "Show me your blood pressure log for the past two weeks."
- **Reflecting, paraphrasing, clarifying, and confronting.** These skills, as described earlier, assist nurses in making sure they understand the client's messages and feelings and help the client to identify discrepancies that inhibit the client's self-understanding or exploration of specific areas and ideas.

During this first stage of the working phase, the intensity of interaction increases, and the client may express or demonstrate feelings such as anger, shame, or self-consciousness. If the nurse is skilled in this stage and the client is willing to pursue self-exploration, the outcome is a beginning understanding on the part of the client about behavior and feelings.

Ultimately the client must make decisions and take action to become more effective. The responsibility for action belongs to the client. The nurse, however, collaborates in these decisions, provides support, and may offer options or information.

SAFETY ALERT

Clients with dementia or cognitive impairments may not move between phases of the nurse–client relationship in the same way as clients with normal cognitive function. Nurses working with these clients often find a need to reintroduce themselves at each meeting.

TERMINATION PHASE   The termination phase of the relationship is often expected to be difficult and filled with ambivalence. However, if the relationship has evolved effectively though the previous phases, the client generally has a positive outlook and feels able to handle problems independently. On the other hand, because caring attitudes have developed, it is natural to expect some feelings of loss, and each individual in the relationship needs to develop a way of saying good-bye.

Many methods can be used to terminate relationships. Summarizing or reviewing the process can produce a sense of accomplishment. This may include sharing reminiscences of how things were at the beginning of the relationship and comparing them to how they are now. It is also helpful for both the nurse and the client to express their feelings about termination openly and honestly. Thus termination discussions need to start in advance of the termination interview. This allows time for the client to adjust to independence. In some situations, referrals are necessary, or it may be appropriate to offer an occasional standby meeting to give support as needed. Follow-up phone calls or e-mails are other interventions that can ease the client's transition to independence.

CLINICAL EXAMPLE

The nurse may terminate a relationship simply by saying, "I have to leave now but will follow up with you tomorrow," or "It was a pleasure meeting you. Good-bye." How the nurse terminates the relationship is largely determined by how long the nurse–client relationship has existed, how much the client depends on the nurse, and the client's response to the termination of the relationship. The client who is highly dependent on the nurse or who has worked with the nurse for extended periods of time requires preparation for termination, which can be accomplished by statements made by the nurse such as "You're doing so well. After next Monday you'll be able to function independently and won't require my constant attention."

Developing Therapeutic Relationships

Whatever the practice setting, the nurse establishes some type of therapeutic relationship in which mutual goals (outcomes) are set with the client or, if the client is unable to participate, with support people. Although special training in counseling techniques is advantageous, there are many ways of helping clients that do not require special training:

- *Listen actively.*
- *Help to identify what the person is feeling.* Often clients who are troubled are unable to identify or label their feelings and consequently have difficulty working them out or talking about them. Responses such as "You seem angry about taking orders from your boss" or "You sound as if you've been lonely since your wife died" can help clients recognize what they are feeling and talk about it.
- *Put yourself in the other person's shoes (i.e., empathize).* Communicate to the client in a way that shows an understanding of the client's feelings and the behavior and experience underlying these feelings.
- *Be honest.* In an effective relationship, the nurse honestly recognizes any lack of knowledge by saying "I don't know the answer to that right now"; can openly discuss the nurse's own discomfort by saying, for example, "I feel uncomfortable about this discussion"; and can admit tactfully that problems do exist, for instance, when a client says "I'm a mess, aren't I?"

- *Be genuine and credible.* Clients will sense whether the nurse is truly concerned.
- *Use your ingenuity.* Nurses should consider all of the available actions when handling problems. Whatever course is chosen needs to further the achievement of the client's goals (outcomes), be compatible with the client's value system, and offer the probability of success.
- *Be aware of cultural differences that may affect meaning and understanding.* To facilitate nurse–client interaction, recognize the language(s) and/or dialect(s) the client uses. Provide a bilingual interpreter as needed for clients with limited English language ability.
- *Maintain client confidentiality.* To maintain the client's right to privacy, share information only with other healthcare professionals as needed for effective care and treatment.
- *Know your role and your limitations.* Clarify functions and roles, specifically what is expected of the client, the nurse, and the primary care provider. Every individual has unique strengths and problems. When you feel unable to handle some of the client's problems, you should inform the client of this and refer the client to the appropriate health professional. Clarify functions and roles, specifically what is expected of the client, the nurse, and the primary care provider.

▶ COMMUNICATING WITH CHILDREN AND FAMILIES

In caring for pediatric clients, the nurse should implement interventions that will establish an effective nurse–child–family relationship. The nurse must provide an appropriate environment that will foster nurse–child–family communication and ensure confidentiality while doing so. The techniques the nurse uses to develop this relationship are similar to the techniques that the nurse uses with an individual client, tailoring communication techniques to the needs of both the child and the family (**Figure 38–8** ●).

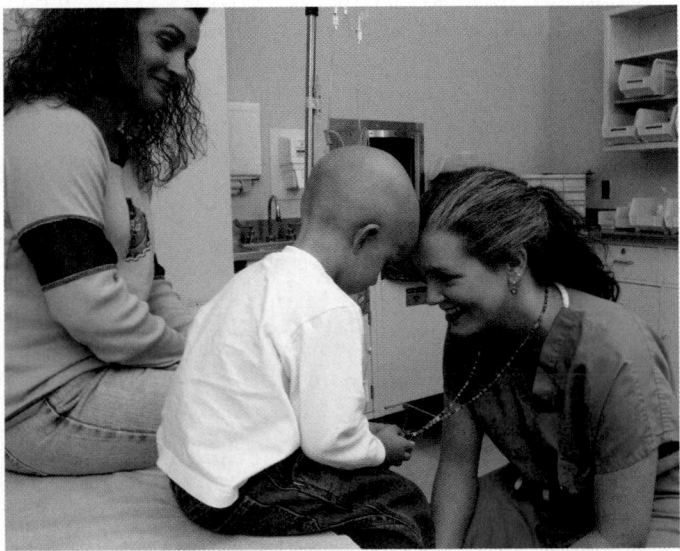

Figure 38–8 ● Taking time to listen to the child and family members is important for establishing trust and developing rapport.

TABLE 38–6   Nursing Implications of Using Therapeutic Communication Techniques With Children

COMMUNICATION TECHNIQUE	NURSING IMPLICATIONS
Accepting	By conveying acceptance the nurse respects the child's emotions and allows the child to cry when in pain or lets the child know that crying is okay.
Active listening	The nurse involves the child in the discussion and encourages the child to communicate his point of view. It is important to face the child and parents when speaking. This conveys to the family that the nurse is listening and understands what is being said.
Broad openings	This includes using open-ended questions that allow the child to choose the topic for discussion.
Clarifying	Asking the child to clarify or elaborate on what is being expressed communicates understanding by the nurse.
Collaborating	The nurse should suggest collaboration with the child and family and then assist them through the problem-solving process.
Exploring	This helps the child to organize her thoughts and focus on the current issue. It will also encourage the child to discuss the issue in more detail.
Focusing	This guides the direction of the conversation. It is useful with small children who may wish to discuss a variety of topics.
Giving recognition	This identifies observed behaviors and indicates an interest in the child.
Observation	This is particularly important with the behavioral aspect of communication. The nurse acknowledges behaviors that indicate the child's thoughts and feelings.
Offering self	This indicates that the nurse is available and willing to listen to the child.
Placing the event in time or sequence	The goal of this technique is to help the child and the nurse understand the order of events.
Reflection	This indicates that the nurse is interested in the discussion and also validates the child's concerns.
Restating or paraphrasing	This acknowledges to the child that the nurse is listening. It also validates appropriate interpretation of what the child is communicating.
Summarizing	This highlights the key facts of the conversation and also provides an opportunity to consider direction for future discussions. It can also provide closure. Summarizing can occur at varying points in the communication process.
Validating perceptions	This is when the nurse shares conclusions that have been drawn as a result of the discussions with the child. It provides an opportunity for the child to confirm or deny interpretations that the nurse has made throughout the process.

The nurse can use any of several communication techniques with children. These include accepting, active listening, broad openings, clarifying, collaborating, exploring, focusing, giving recognition, observation, offering self, placing an event in time or sequence, reflection, restating or paraphrasing, summarizing, and validating perceptions. The nursing implications for each technique are explored in **Table 38–6** ●.

First and foremost, the nurse must establish rapport with the child to set the stage for a productive therapeutic relationship. The Lifespan Considerations feature provides suggestions for how to establish rapport with a child.

Establishing Trust

Trust plays a critical role for an effective nurse–child–family relationship. To establish an atmosphere of trust, the nurse should do the following:

- *Follow through with promises to the child and family.* This ensures secure feelings for the family.

- *Respect confidentiality.* This promotes protection of the family.

- *Be truthful with the child and family.* They will respect the nurse, even if the truth is not what they want to hear.

If a child asks whether a procedure is painful, answer truthfully, but follow with positive words. For example, if a child asks if his "shot" is going to hurt, you might reply, "Yes, most people say that a shot hurts, but it will hurt only for a moment, and then it will be over. Your mother can hold your hand while I give you the shot if that will make you feel better." By following difficult information with a positive rationale or comforting statement, the nurse can maintain credibility while still providing compassionate care.

▶ CONCLUSION

Whether teaching, advocating, assessing, planning, documenting, or intervening, the nurse requires strong communication skills. The ability to communicate effectively plays a large role in the nurse's ability to deliver the highest quality of care to clients. Whether communicating with clients, other members of the healthcare team, distraught family members, or peers, nurses need to be understood and understand the messages they receive. Strong verbal and written communication skills are required of the effective nurse, who must also monitor nonverbal communication to maintain consistency in the messages sent to others.

Lifespan Considerations Establishing Rapport With Children

Every client, including children, will be more responsive to the nurse who makes an effort to help the client feel that he or she is important in an interaction. The following guidelines can be used by the nurse to establish rapport with a child and encourage the sharing of information and feelings:

- *Position yourself on the same level as the child.* The nurse should be at the child's eye level. This suggests to the child that the nurse cares about and respects the child.
- *Show interest in what the child is doing.* This displays that the nurse is interested and encourages security.
- *Agree with the child when it is appropriate.* It may be appropriate for the nurse to share feelings. An example of this is telling the child, "I don't like the taste of that medicine either, but sometimes I have to take it when I am sick—but then I drink something that I like." Sharing experiences with the child offers encouragement to the child and family.
- *Compliment the child.* Examples include "You are really strong" or "You picked really nice colors for that picture." This observational statement by the nurse may reduce anxiety while conferring status on the child.

- *Use a calm tone of voice and language that is developmentally appropriate.* It is important to talk and share information with children that is on an appropriate level of comprehension.
- *Pace the discussion or procedure so that the child does not feel rushed.* Feeling rushed will increase the child's anxiety.
- *Explain concepts in terms the child can understand.* This is especially important for preschool-age children, who have a limited concept of time. Stating "Your mother will be back after lunch" is appropriate for this age level because it provides a concrete time frame that the child can understand.
- *Include the child in the discussion of care if developmentally appropriate.* This is particularly important for adolescents, because they have the cognitive ability to participate in abstract conversation and to comprehend medical terminology.
- *Listen more than you talk, and avoid distractions.* This shows the child that the nurse is interested in what the child has to say.
- *Be truthful with the child.* This will elicit respect.

REVIEW Therapeutic Communication

RELATE Link the Concepts and Exemplars

Linking the exemplar of therapeutic communication with the concept of advocacy:

1. How do strong therapeutic communication skills contribute to the nurse's role as a client advocate?

2. How do strong therapeutic communication skills contribute to the nurse's ability to work within groups to advocate for clients?

Linking the exemplar of therapeutic communication with the concept of teaching and learning:

3. The nurse is preparing to teach a client who is newly diagnosed with diabetes about self-care. Describe the three phases of the therapeutic relationship as it applies to the client teaching plan.

4. While teaching the client with diabetes, the nurse accidentally creates a barrier to the therapeutic relationship by misspeaking. What should the nurse do next?

REFER Go to Pearson Nursing Student Resources
nursing.pearsonhighered.com

- Additional review materials

REFLECT Case Study

Zainah Kattan is a newly graduated nurse working at the Neighborhood Hospital. She is assigned the care of Lydia Ocampo, who has been diagnosed with Alzheimer disease.

Mrs. Ocampo was admitted with a fractured hip following a fall at home that occurred when she was wandering around her house late one night. Mrs. Ocampo was assigned a different nurse yesterday, but Danilo Ocampo, her husband, complained to the nurse manager when he came to visit and found her restrained and yelling for help with an untouched breakfast tray in front of her. Dr. Ocampo requested that a different nurse be assigned to Mrs. Ocampo's care from now on. Ms. Kattan is happy to act as her primary nurse. She develops rapport with Dr. Ocampo and gets satisfaction from caring for Mrs. Ocampo and helping her to feel more comfortable.

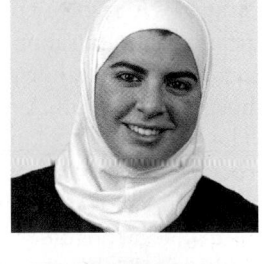

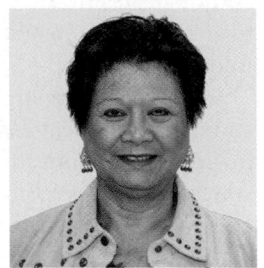

1. When communicating with a client diagnosed with later-stage Alzheimer disease, what strategies will Ms. Kattan employ?

2. Why does the development of rapport with Dr. Ocampo improve the client's ability to meet expected outcomes?

3. Dr. Ocampo complains to Ms. Kattan about the poor care provided to his wife by the other nurse, Bobby Schofield. How should Ms. Kattan respond to this statement?

EXEMPLAR 38.3 **Documentation**

EXEMPLAR KEY TERMS

Chart, *2438*
Charting, *2438*
Charting by exception (CBE), *2443*
Client record, *2438*
Discussion, *2438*
Documenting, *2438*
Flow sheet, *2442*
Focus charting, *2443*
Kardex, *2445*
Narrative charting, *2440*
PIE documentation model, *2442*
Problem-oriented medical record (POMR), *2440*
Problem-oriented record (POR), *2440*
Record, *2438*
Recording, *2438*
Report, *2438*
SOAP, *2441*
Source-oriented record, *2439*
Variance, *2445*

EXEMPLAR LEARNING OUTCOMES

After reading about this exemplar, you will be able to:

1. List the measures used to maintain the confidentiality of client records.

2. Discuss reasons for keeping client records.

3. Compare and contrast different documentation methods: source-oriented and problem-oriented medical records; the problems, interventions, evaluation (PIE) model; focus charting; charting by exception; computerized records; and the case management model.

4. Explain how various forms in the client record (e.g., flow sheets, progress notes, care plans, critical pathways, Kardexes, discharge/transfer forms) are used to document steps of the nursing process (assessment, diagnosis, planning, implementation, and evaluation).

5. Compare and contrast the documentation needed for clients in acute care, home health care, and long-term care settings.

6. Identify and discuss guidelines for effective documentation that meets legal and ethical standards.

7. Identify prohibited abbreviations, acronyms, and symbols that cannot be used in any form of clinical documentation.

▶ OVERVIEW

Effective communication among healthcare professionals is vital to the quality of client care. Generally, healthcare personnel communicate through discussion, reports, and records. A **discussion** is an informal oral consideration of a subject by two or more healthcare personnel to identify a problem or establish strategies to resolve a problem. A **report** is oral, written, or electronic communication intended to convey information to others. For instance, nurses always report on clients at the end of a hospital work shift. A **record** may be handwritten or electronic. The process of making an entry on a client record is called **recording**, **charting**, or **documenting**.

A clinical record, also called a **chart** or **client record**, is a formal, legal document that provides evidence of a client's care. Although healthcare organizations use different systems and forms for documentation, all client records include similar information.

Each healthcare organization has policies about recording and reporting client data, and each nurse is accountable for following the organization's standards. Agencies also indicate which nursing assessments and interventions can be recorded by RNs and which can be charted by unlicensed personnel. In addition, the Joint Commission requires client record documentation to be timely, complete, accurate, confidential, and specific to the client.

▶ ETHICAL AND LEGAL CONSIDERATIONS

The American Nurses Association (ANA) Code of Ethics (2001) states that "the nurse has a duty to maintain confidentiality of all patient information" (p. 12). The client's record is also protected legally as a private record of the client's care. Access to the client's record is restricted to healthcare professionals involved in giving care to the client. The institution or agency is the rightful owner of the client's record. This does not, however, exclude the client's rights to the same records. See the modules on Ethics and Legal Issues for more information.

On April 14, 2003, changes were made to the Health Insurance Portability and Accountability Act (HIPAA) regulations to maintain the privacy and confidentiality of protected health information (PHI). PHI is identifiable health information that is transmitted or maintained in any form or medium, including verbal discussions, electronic communications with or about clients, and written communications.

> **SAFETY ALERT**
> Take safety measures before faxing confidential information. A fax cover sheet should contain instruction that the faxed material is to be given only to the named recipient. Consent is needed from the client to fax information about the client. Make sure that personally identifiable information has been removed or is not immediately visible on the top sheet. Finally, check that the fax number is correct, check the number on the display of the machine after dialing, and check a third time before pressing the "Send" button. Some facilities require the recipient agency to return a signed receipt.

For purposes of education and research, most agencies allow student and graduate healthcare professionals access to client records. The records are used in client conferences, clinics, rounds, client studies, and written papers. The student or graduate is bound by a strict ethical code and legal responsibility to hold all information in confidence. It is the responsibility of both students and practicing nurses to protect the client's privacy by not using a name or any statements that may identify the client in their worksheets, notes for class, or any notations they make that could potentially leave the facility's premises. Most facilities provide shredders or other receptacles for discarding material that contains personal client information.

Ensuring Confidentiality of Electronic Records

Because of the increased use of computerized client records, healthcare agencies have developed policies and procedures to ensure the privacy and confidentiality of client information stored electronically. In addition, the Security Rule of HIPAA governs the security of electronic forms of protected health information. Following are some suggestions for ensuring the confidentiality and security of electronic records:

1. A personal password is required to enter and sign off computer files. Do not share this password with anyone, including other healthcare team members.
2. After logging on, never leave a computer terminal unattended.
3. Do not leave client information displayed on the monitor where others may see it.
4. Shred all unneeded computer-generated worksheets.
5. Know the facility's policy and procedure for correcting an entry error.
6. Follow agency procedures for documenting sensitive material, such as a diagnosis of AIDS.
7. Information technology personnel must install a firewall to protect the server from unauthorized access.

▶ PURPOSES OF CLIENT RECORDS

Client records are kept for a number of purposes:

- **Communication.** The client record serves as the vehicle by which different healthcare professionals who interact with a client communicate with each other. This prevents fragmentation, repetition, and delays in client care.
- **Planning client care.** Each healthcare professional uses data from the client's record to plan care for that client. A primary care provider, for example, may order a specific antibiotic after establishing that the client's temperature is steadily rising and that laboratory tests reveal the presence of a certain microorganism. The nurse uses baseline and ongoing data to evaluate the effectiveness of the nursing care plan.
- **Auditing health agencies.** An audit is a review of client records for quality assurance purposes (see the module on Quality Improvement). Accrediting agencies such as the Joint Commission may review client records to determine whether a particular health agency is meeting required standards.
- **Research.** The information contained in a record can be a valuable source of data for research. The treatment plans for a number of clients with the same health problems can yield information helpful in treating other clients.
- **Education.** Students in health disciplines often use client records as educational tools. A record can frequently provide a comprehensive view of the client, the illness, effective treatment strategies, and factors that affect the outcome of the illness.
- **Reimbursement.** Documentation helps a facility receive reimbursement from the federal government. For a facility to obtain payment through Medicare, for example, the client's clinical record must contain the correct diagnosis-related group (DRG) codes and reveal that the appropriate care has been given. Codable diagnoses, such as DRGs, are supported by accurate, thorough recording by nurses. Accurate coding not only facilitates reimbursement from the federal government, but also facilitates reimbursement from insurance companies and other third-party payers. If additional care, treatment, or length of stay becomes necessary for the client's welfare, thorough charting will help justify these needs.
- **Legal documentation.** The client's record is a legal document and usually is admissible in court as evidence. In some jurisdictions, however, the record is considered inadmissible as evidence when the client objects, because information the client gives to the physician is confidential.
- **Healthcare analysis.** Information from records may assist healthcare planners to identify agency needs, such as overutilized and underutilized hospital services. Records can be used to establish the costs of various services and to identify those services that cost the agency money and those that generate revenue.

▶ DOCUMENTATION SYSTEMS

A number of documentation systems are in current use. The most common are the source-oriented record; the problem-oriented medical record; the problems, interventions, evaluation (PIE) model; focus charting; charting by exception (CBE); and electronic documentation.

Source-Oriented Record

The traditional client record is a **source-oriented record**. Each individual or department makes notations in a separate section or sections of the client's chart. For example, the admissions department has an admission sheet; the physician has a physician's order sheet, a physician's history sheet, and progress notes; nurses use the nurses' notes; and other departments or personnel have their own records. In this type of record, information about a particular problem is distributed throughout the record. For example, if a client had left hemiplegia (paralysis of the left side of the body), data about this problem might be found in the physician's history sheet, on the physician's order sheet, in the nurses' notes, in the physical therapist's record, and in the social service record. **Box 38–10** ● lists the components of a source-oriented record.

Box 38–10 Components of the Source-Oriented Record

FORM	INFORMATION
Admission (face) sheet	Legal name, birth date, age, gender
	Social Security number
	Address
	Marital status; closest relatives or individual to notify in case of emergency
	Date, time, and admitting diagnosis
	Food or drug allergies
	Name of admitting (attending) physician
	Insurance information
	Any assigned DRGs
Initial nursing assessment	Findings from the initial nursing history and physical health assessment
Graphic record	Body temperature, pulse rate, respiratory rate, blood pressure, daily weight, and special measurements such as fluid intake and output and oxygen saturation
Daily care record	Activity, diet, bathing, and elimination records
Special flow sheets	Examples: fluid balance record, skin assessment
Medication record	Name, dosage, route, time, date of regularly administered medications
	Name or initials of individual administering the medication
Nurses' notes	Pertinent assessment of client
	Specific nursing care, including teaching and client's responses
	Client's complaints and how client is coping
Medical history and physical examination	Past and family medical history, present medical problems, differential or current diagnoses, findings of physical examination by the primary care provider
Physician's order sheet	Medical orders for medications, treatments, and so on
Physician's progress notes	Medical observations, treatments, client progress, and so on
Consultation records	Reports by medical and clinical specialists
Diagnostic reports	Examples: laboratory reports, x-ray reports, CT scan reports
Consultation reports	Examples: Physical therapy, respiratory therapy
Client discharge plan and referral summary	Started on admission and completed on discharge; includes nursing problems, general information, and referral data

Source-oriented records may be compiled by narrative charting. **Narrative charting** consists of written notes that include routine care, normal findings, and client problems (**Figure 38–9 ●**). There is no right or wrong order to the information, although chronological order is frequently used. Although narrative charting is a traditional part of the source-oriented record, few institutions today use only narrative charting. It is being replaced by systems such as charting by exception and focus charting (discussed below). Many agencies combine narrative charting with another system. For example, an agency using a charting-by-exception system may use narrative charting when describing abnormal findings. However, narrative charting is expedient in emergency situations. When using narrative charting, nurses must ensure the information is organized in a clear, coherent manner. Using the nursing process as a framework is one way to do this.

Source-oriented records are convenient because (a) care providers from each discipline can easily locate the forms on which to record data and (b) it is easy to trace the information specific to one's discipline. The disadvantage is that information about a particular client problem is scattered throughout the chart, making it difficult to find chronological information on a cli-

ent's problems and progress. This can lead to decreased communication among the healthcare team, an incomplete picture of the client's care, and a lack of coordination of care (*Chart Smart*, 2009).

Problem-Oriented Medical Record

The **problem-oriented medical record (POMR)**, or **problem-oriented record (POR)**, was established by Lawrence Weed in the 1960s. In a POMR, data are arranged according to the problems the client has rather than according to the source of the information. Members of the healthcare team contribute to the problem list, plan of care, and progress notes. Plans for each active or potential problem are drawn up, and progress notes are recorded for each problem.

The advantage of POMRs is that they encourage collaboration and the problem list in the front of the chart alerts caregivers to the client's needs and makes it easier to track the status of each problem. The disadvantages of a POMR are that caregivers differ in their ability to use the required charting format, constant vigilance is required to maintain an up-to-date problem list, and it is somewhat inefficient because assessments and interventions that apply to more than one problem must be repeated.

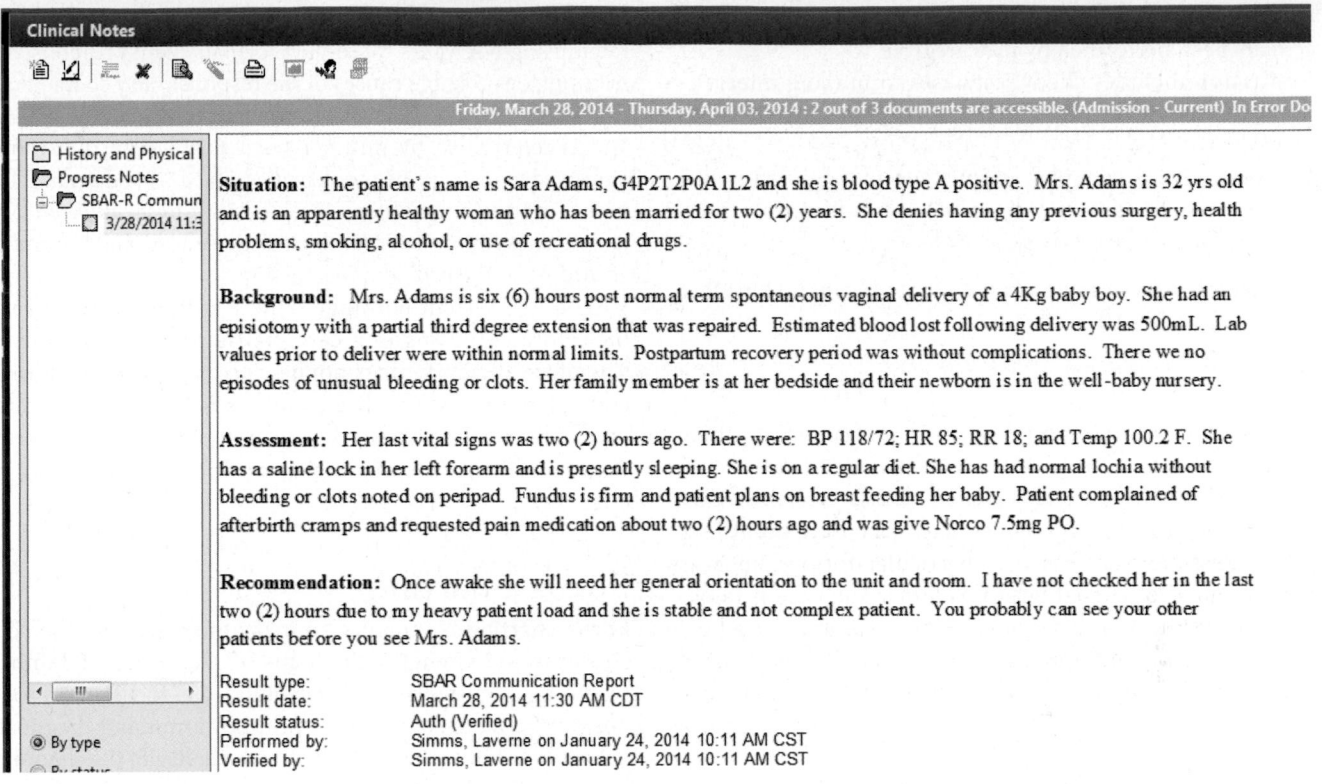

Figure 38–9 ● A narrative note in an electronic health record (EHR).
Source: Neehr Perfect® networked educational EHR featuring WorldVistA, courtesy of Archetype Innovations, LLC 2010.

The POMR has four basic components: database, problem list, plan of care, and progress notes. In addition, flow sheets and discharge notes are added to the record as needed.

DATABASE The database of a POMR consists of all information known about the client when the client first enters the healthcare agency. It includes the nursing assessment, the physician's history, social and family data, and the results of the physical examination and baseline diagnostic tests. Data are constantly updated as the client's health status changes.

PROBLEM LIST The problem list is derived from the database. It is usually kept at the front of the chart and serves as an index to the numbered entries in the progress notes. Problems are listed in the order in which they are identified, and the list is continually updated as new problems are identified and others resolved. All caregivers may contribute to the problem list, which includes the client's physiological, psychological, social, cultural, spiritual, developmental, and environmental needs. Primary care providers write problems as medical diagnoses, surgical procedures, or symptoms; nurses write problems as nursing diagnoses.

As the client's condition changes or more data are obtained, problems may need to be redefined. When a problem is resolved, a line is drawn through it and the number is not used again for that client.

PLAN OF CARE In the POMR method, the initial list of orders or plan of care is made with reference to the active

problems. Care plans are generated by the individual who lists the problems. Physicians write physician's orders or medical care plans; nurses write nursing orders or nursing care plans. The written plan in the record is listed under each problem in the progress notes and is not isolated as a separate list of orders.

PROGRESS NOTES A progress note in the POMR is a chart entry made by any of the healthcare professionals who are involved in a client's care, who all use the same type of sheet for notes. Progress notes are numbered to correspond to the problems on the problem list and may be lettered for the type of data. The SOAP format is frequently used. **SOAP** is an acronym for subjective data, objective data, assessment, and planning. Over the years, the SOAP format has been modified; the acronyms *SOAPIE* and **SOAPIER** refer to formats that add interventions, evaluation, and revision.

Subjective data consist of information obtained from what the client says.
Objective data consist of information that is measured or observed by use of the senses (e.g., vital signs, laboratory and x-ray results).
Assessment is the interpretation or conclusions drawn about the subjective and objective data.
Plan of care is designed to resolve the stated problem. The initial plan is written by the individual who enters the problem into the record. All subsequent plans, including revisions, are entered into the progress notes.

Interventions refer to the specific interventions that have actually been performed by the caregiver.

Evaluation includes client responses to nursing interventions and medical treatments. This is primarily reassessment data.

Revision reflects care plan modifications suggested by the evaluation. Changes may be made in desired outcomes, interventions, or target dates.

An example of a nursing progress note using SOAPIER is shown in **Figure 38–10 ●**.

PIE Model

The **PIE documentation model** groups information into three categories. PIE is an acronym for problems, interventions, and evaluation of nursing care. This system consists of a client care assessment flow sheet and progress notes. The **flow sheet** uses specific assessment criteria in a particular format, such as human needs or functional health patterns. The time parameters for a flow sheet can vary from minutes to months. In a hospital intensive care unit, for example, a client's blood pressure may be monitored by the minute, whereas in an ambulatory clinic a client's blood glucose level may be recorded once a month.

After the assessment, the nurse establishes and records specific problems on the progress notes, often using NANDA diagnoses to word the problem. If there is no approved nursing

diagnosis for a problem, the nurse develops a problem statement using NANDA's three-part format: client's response, contributing or probable causes of the response, and characteristics manifested by the client. The *problem statement* is labeled "P" and is referred to by number (e.g., P #5). The *interventions* employed to manage the problem are labeled "I" and are numbered according to the problem (e.g., I #5). The *evaluation* of the effectiveness of the interventions is labeled "E" and is numbered according to the problem (e.g., E #5).

The PIE system eliminates the traditional care plan and incorporates an ongoing care plan into the progress notes. Therefore, the nurse does not have to create and update a separate plan. One of the disadvantages to PIE is that the nurse must review all nursing notes before giving care to determine which problems are current and which interventions were effective.

Focus Charting

Focus charting is intended to make the client and the client's concerns and strengths the focus of care. Three columns for recording are usually used: date and time, focus, and progress notes. The *focus* may be a condition, a nursing diagnosis, a behavior, a sign or symptom, an acute change in the client's condition, or a client strength. The progress notes are organized into (D) data, (A) action, and (R) response, referred to as DAR. The *data* category reflects the assessment phase of the nursing

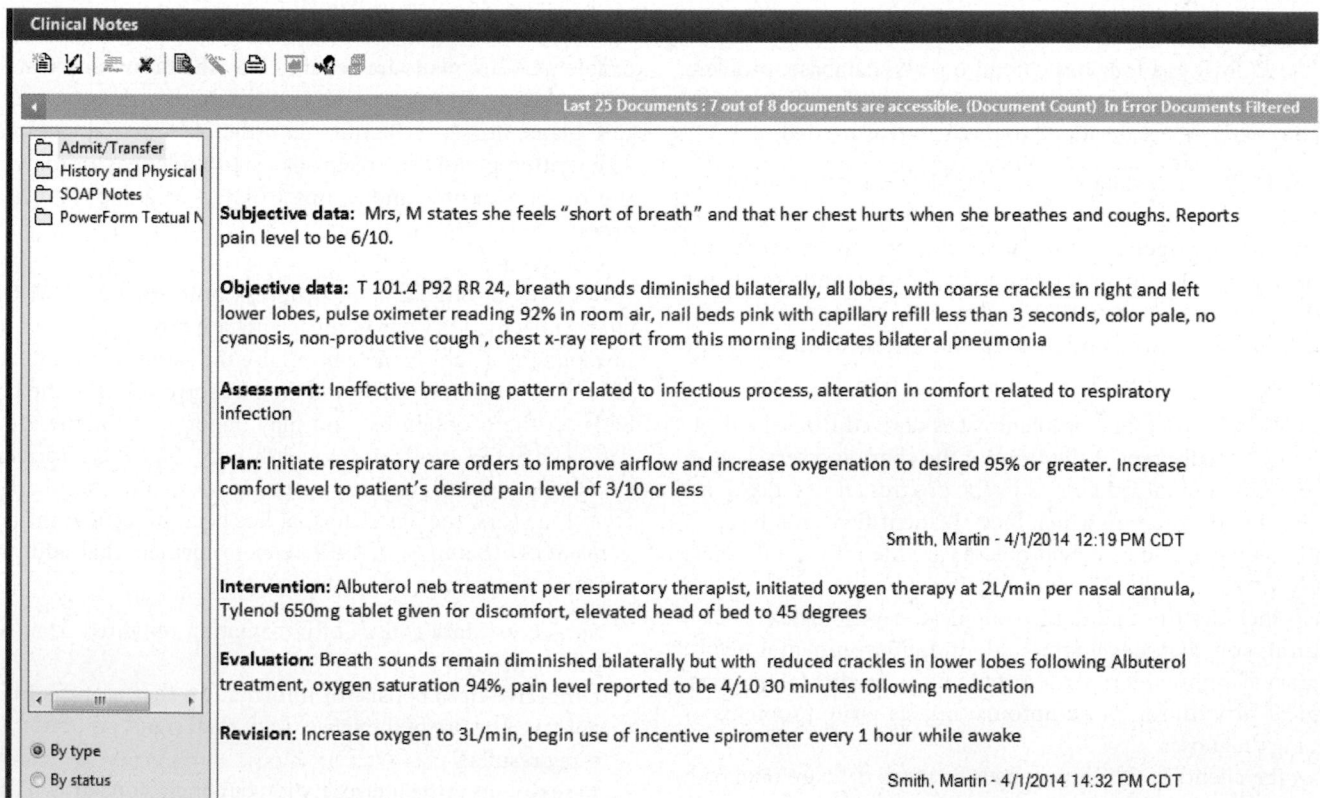

Figure 38–10 ● An example of a nursing progress note using SOAPIER in an EHR.
Source: Neehr Perfect® networked educational EHR featuring WorldVistA, courtesy of Archetype Innovations, LLC 2010.

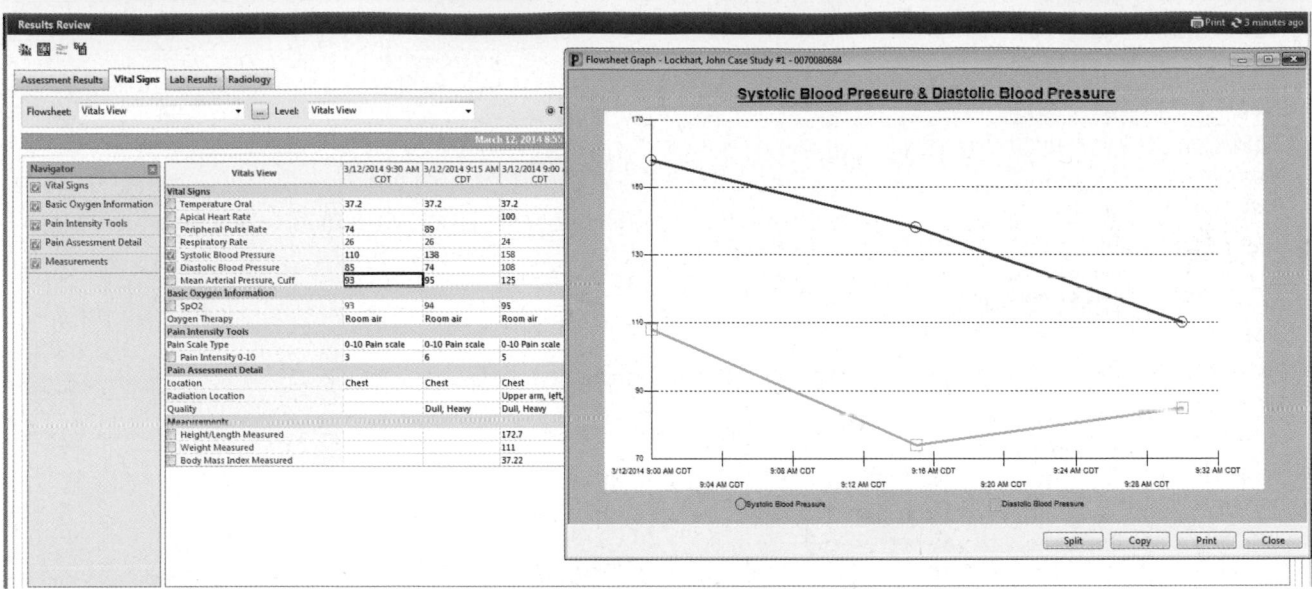

Figure 38–11 ● A sample vital signs graphic record in an EHR.

Source: Neehr Perfect® networked educational HER featuring WorldVistA, courtesy of Archetype Innovations, LLC 2010.

process and consists of observations of client status and behaviors, including data from flow sheets (e.g., vital signs, pupil reactivity). The nurse records both subjective and objective data in this section.

The *action* category reflects planning and implementation and includes immediate and future nursing actions. It may also include any changes to the plan of care. The *response category* reflects the evaluation phase of the nursing process and describes the client's response to any nursing and medical care.

The focus charting system provides a holistic perspective of the client and the client's needs. It also provides a nursing process framework for the progress notes (DAR). The three components do not need to be recorded in order, and each note does not need to have all three categories. Flow sheets and checklists are frequently used on the client's chart to record routine nursing tasks and assessment data.

Charting by Exception

Charting by exception (CBE) is a documentation system in which only abnormal or significant findings or exceptions to norms are recorded. CBE incorporates three key elements (Guido, 2010):

1. ***Flow sheets.*** Examples of flow sheets include a graphic record (**Figure 38–11 ●**), fluid balance record, daily nursing assessments record (**Figure 38–12 ●**), client teaching record, client discharge record, and skin assessment record.

2. ***Standards of nursing care.*** Documentation by reference to the agency's printed standards of nursing practice eliminates much of the repetitive charting of routine care. An agency using CBE must develop its own specific standards of nursing practice that identify the minimum criteria for client care regardless of clinical area.

Some units may also have unit-specific standards unique to the type of client. For example, "The nurse must ensure that the unconscious client has oral care at least q4h." Documentation of care according to these specified standards involves only a check mark in the routine standards box on the graphic record. If not all of the standards are implemented, an asterisk on the flow sheet is made with reference to the nurses' notes. All exceptions to the standards are fully described in narrative form on the nurses' notes.

3. ***Bedside access to chart forms.*** In the CBE system, all flow sheets are kept at the client's bedside to allow immediate recording and to eliminate the need to transcribe data from the nurse's worksheet to the permanent record.

The advantages to this system are the elimination of lengthy, repetitive notes and that it makes client changes in condition more obvious. Inherent in CBE is the presumption that the nurse did assess the client and determined what responses were normal and abnormal. Many nurses believe in the saying "not charted, not done" and subsequently may feel uncomfortable with the CBE documentation system. One suggestion is to write N/A on flow sheets where the items are not applicable and to not leave blank spaces. This would then avoid the possible misinterpretation that the assessment or intervention was not done by the nurse.

Electronic Documentation

Computerized clinical record systems are being developed as a way to manage the huge volume of information required in contemporary health care. Nurses use computer databases to store the client data, add new data, create and revise care plans, and document client progress. Some institutions have a com-

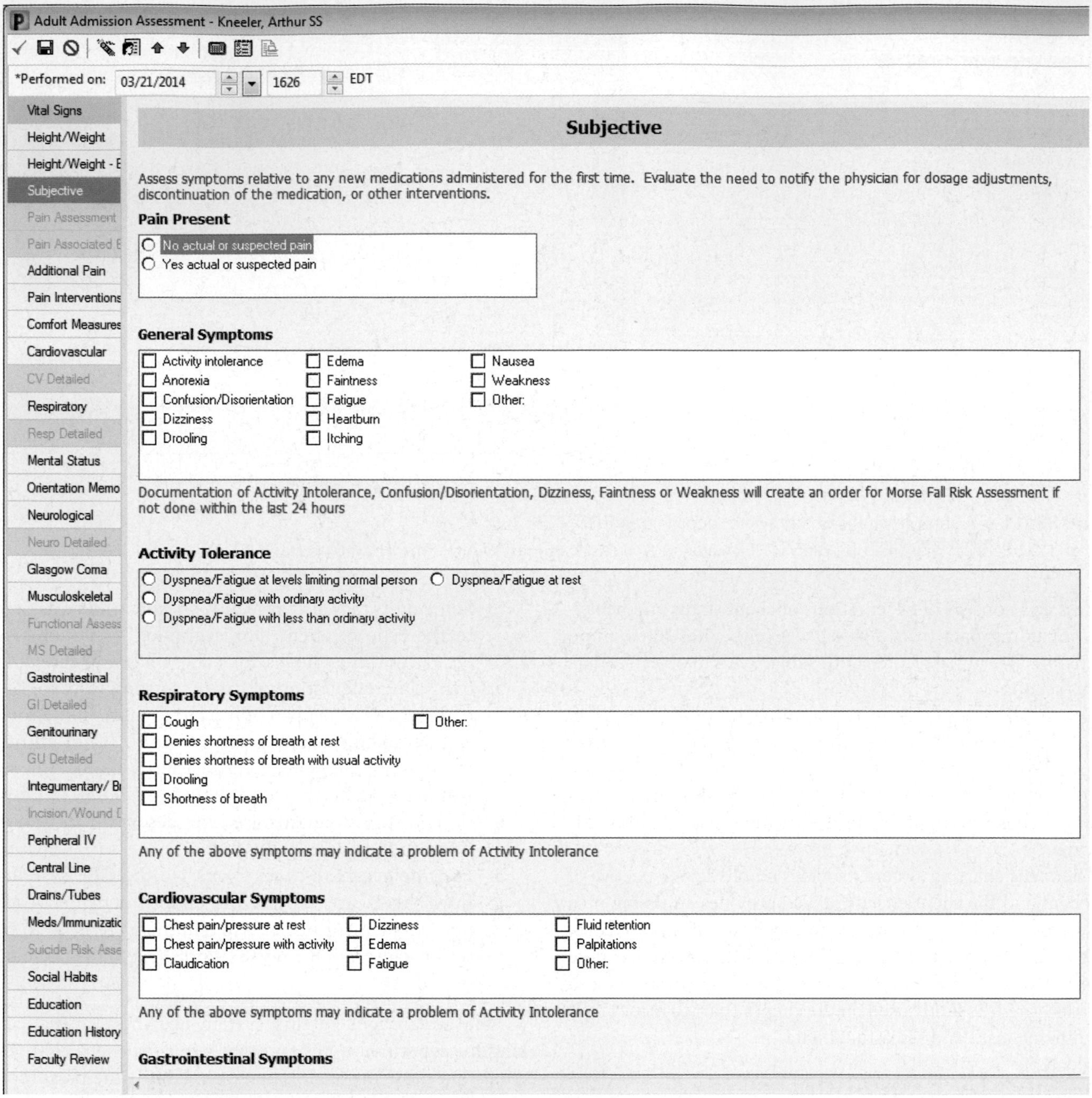

Adult Admission Assessment - Kneeler, Arthur SS

*Performed on: 03/21/2014 1626 EDT

Vital Signs
Height/Weight
Height/Weight - E
Subjective
Pain Assessment
Pain Associated E
Additional Pain
Pain Interventions
Comfort Measures
Cardiovascular
CV Detailed
Respiratory
Resp Detailed
Mental Status
Orientation Memo
Neurological
Neuro Detailed
Glasgow Coma
Musculoskeletal
Functional Assess
MS Detailed
Gastrointestinal
GI Detailed
Genitourinary
GU Detailed
Integumentary/ Br
Incision/Wound I
Peripheral IV
Central Line
Drains/Tubes
Meds/Immunizatic
Suicide Risk Asse
Social Habits
Education
Education History
Faculty Review

Subjective

Assess symptoms relative to any new medications administered for the first time. Evaluate the need to notify the physician for dosage adjustments, discontinuation of the medication, or other interventions.

Pain Present

○ No actual or suspected pain
○ Yes actual or suspected pain

General Symptoms

☐ Activity intolerance ☐ Edema ☐ Nausea
☐ Anorexia ☐ Faintness ☐ Weakness
☐ Confusion/Disorientation ☐ Fatigue ☐ Other:
☐ Dizziness ☐ Heartburn
☐ Drooling ☐ Itching

Documentation of Activity Intolerance, Confusion/Disorientation, Dizziness, Faintness or Weakness will create an order for Morse Fall Risk Assessment if not done within the last 24 hours

Activity Tolerance

○ Dyspnea/Fatigue at levels limiting normal person ○ Dyspnea/Fatigue at rest
○ Dyspnea/Fatigue with ordinary activity
○ Dyspnea/Fatigue with less than ordinary activity

Respiratory Symptoms

☐ Cough ☐ Other:
☐ Denies shortness of breath at rest
☐ Denies shortness of breath with usual activity
☐ Drooling
☐ Shortness of breath

Any of the above symptoms may indicate a problem of Activity Intolerance

Cardiovascular Symptoms

☐ Chest pain/pressure at rest ☐ Dizziness ☐ Fluid retention
☐ Chest pain/pressure with activity ☐ Edema ☐ Palpitations
☐ Claudication ☐ Fatigue ☐ Other:

Any of the above symptoms may indicate a problem of Activity Intolerance

Gastrointestinal Symptoms

Figure 38–12 ● Sample of a portion of a daily nursing CBE assessment form in an EHR.
Source: Neehr Perfect® networked educational HER featuring WorldVistA, courtesy of Archetype Innovations, LLC 2010.

puter terminal at each client's bedside, or the nurse carries a small handheld device; these technologies enable the nurse to document care immediately after it is given.

Multiple flow sheets are not needed in computerized record systems because information can be easily retrieved in a variety of formats. For example, the nurse can obtain results of a client's blood test, a schedule of all clients on the unit who are to have surgery during the day, a suggested list of interventions for a nursing diagnosis, a graphic chart of a client's vital signs, or a printout of all progress notes for a client. Many systems can generate a work list for the shift, with a list of all treatments, procedures, and medications needed by the client.

Computers make care planning and documentation relatively easy. To record nursing actions and client responses, the nurse either chooses from standardized lists of terms or types narrative information into the computer. Automated speech-recognition technology now allows nurses to enter data by voice for conversion to written documentation. However, according to HIPAA, if the spoken word is used to create or address protected health information, the nurse must be alert and aware of others who might hear the dictation and take care to protect the privacy of the client's information.

The computerization of clinical records has made it possible to transmit information from one care setting to another. The nursing Minimum Data Set (MDS) is an effort to establish standards for collecting standardized, essential nursing data for inclusion in computer databases.

Case Management

The case management model emphasizes high-quality, cost-effective care delivered within an established length of stay. This model uses a multidisciplinary approach to planning and documenting client care, using *critical pathways*. These forms identify the outcomes that certain groups of clients are expected to achieve on each day of care, along with the interventions necessary for each day. **Figure 38–13** ● illustrates part of a critical pathway for a client with a total hip replacement.

Along with critical pathways, the case management model incorporates graphics and flow sheets. Progress notes typically use some type of charting by exception. For example, if goals are met, no further charting is required. A goal that is not met is called a **variance**. A variance is a deviation from what is planned on the critical pathway, that is, an unexpected occurrence that affects the planned care or the client's responses to care. When a variance occurs, the nurse writes a note documenting the unexpected event, the cause, and actions taken to correct the situation or justify the actions taken.

The case management model promotes collaboration and teamwork among caregivers, helps to decrease length of stay, and makes efficient use of time. Because care is goal focused, the quality may improve. However, critical pathways work best for clients with one or two diagnoses and few individualized needs. Clients with multiple diagnoses (e.g., a client with a hip fracture, pneumonia, diabetes, and pressure sore) or those with an unpredictable course of symptoms (e.g., a client with seizures) are difficult to document on a critical path.

CRITICAL PATHWAY: TOTAL HIP REPLACEMENT

	DOS/Day 1	Days 2–3
Pain Management	Outcome: • Verbalizes comfort or tolerance of pain Circle: V NV Variance:	Outcome: • Verbalizes comfort with pain control measures Circle: V NV Variance:
Respiratory	Outcomes: • Breath sounds clear to auscultation • Achieves 50% of volume goal on incentive spirometer Circle: V NV Variance:	Outcomes: • Breath sounds clear to auscultation • Achieves 100% of volume goal on incentive spirometer Circle: V NV Variance:
Key: V = Variance NV = No Variance		
Signature:	Initials:	
Signature:	Initials:	

Figure 38–13 ● Excerpt from a critical pathway documentation form.

▶ DOCUMENTING NURSING ACTIVITIES

The client record should describe the client's ongoing status and reflect the full range of the nursing process. Regardless of the records system used in an agency, nurses document evidence of the nursing process on a variety of forms throughout the clinical record (**Table 38–7** ●).

Admission Nursing Assessment

A comprehensive admission assessment, also referred to as an initial database, nursing history, or nursing assessment, is completed when the client is admitted to the nursing unit. These forms can be organized according to health patterns, body systems, functional abilities, health problems and risks, nursing model, or type of healthcare setting (e.g., labor and delivery, pediatrics, mental health). The nurse generally records ongoing assessments or reassessments on flow sheets or on nursing progress notes.

Nursing Care Plans

The Joint Commission requires that the clinical record include evidence of client assessments, nursing diagnoses and/or client needs, nursing interventions, client outcomes, and evidence of a current nursing care plan. Depending on the records system being used, the nursing care plan may be separate from the client's chart, recorded in progress notes and other forms in the client record, or incorporated into a multidisciplinary plan of care.

The two types of nursing care plans are traditional and standardized. The *traditional care plan* is written for each client. The form varies from agency to agency according to the needs of the client and the department. Most forms have three columns: one for nursing diagnoses, a second for expected outcomes, and a third for nursing interventions.

Standardized care plans are developed to save documentation time. These plans may be based on an institution's standards of practice, thereby helping to provide a high quality of nursing care. Standardized plans must be individualized by the nurse to adequately address individual client needs.

Kardexes

The **Kardex** is a widely used, concise method of organizing and recording data about a client that makes information quickly

TABLE 38–7 Documentation for the Nursing Process

STEP	DOCUMENTATION FORMS
Assessment	Initial assessment form, various flow sheets
Nursing diagnosis	Nursing care plan, critical pathway, progress notes, problem list
Planning	Nursing care plan, critical pathway
Implementation	Progress notes, flow sheets
Evaluation	Progress notes

Note: All steps are recorded on discharge/referral summaries.

accessible to all health professionals. The system consists of a series of cards kept in a portable index file or on electronic forms. This system allows the card for a particular client to be accessed quickly to reveal specific data. The Kardex may or may not become a part of the client's permanent record. In some organizations it is a temporary worksheet written in pencil for ease in recording frequent changes in details of a client's care. The information on Kardexes may be organized into sections, such as the following:

- Pertinent information about the client, such as name, room number, age, admission date, physician's name, diagnosis, and type of surgery and date
- Allergies
- List of medications, with the date of order and the times of administration for each
- List of intravenous fluids, with dates of infusions
- List of daily treatments and procedures, such as irrigations, dressing changes, postural drainage, or measurement of vital signs
- List of diagnostic procedures ordered, such as x-ray or laboratory tests
- Specific data on how the client's physical needs are to be met, such as type of diet, assistance needed with feeding, elimination devices, activity, hygienic needs, and safety precautions (e.g., one-person assist)
- A problem list, stated goals, and a list of nursing approaches to meet the goals and relieve the problems.

Although much of the information on a Kardex may be recorded by the nurse in charge or a delegate (e.g., the nursing unit clerk), any nurse who cares for the client plays a key role in initiating the record and keeping the data current. Whether the Kardex is a written document or computerized, it should have a place on it to record the date and initials of the individual who is reviewing or revising it. This provides a quick visual guide to ensure that information is current and updated on a regular basis.

Flow Sheets

A flow sheet enables the nurse to record nursing data quickly and concisely and provides an easy-to-read record of the client's condition over time.

- *Graphic record.* This record typically indicates body temperature, pulse, respiratory rate, blood pressure, weight, and, in some agencies, other significant clinical data such as admission or postoperative day, bowel movements, appetite, and activity.
- *Intake and output (I&O) record.* All routes of fluid intake and all routes of fluid loss or output are measured and recorded on this form. Frequently this I&O form permits the recording of a daily weight and percentage of meal consumption.
- *Medication administration record.* Medication flow sheets usually include designated areas for the date of the medication order, the expiration date, the medication name and dose, the frequency of administration and route, and the nurse's signa-

ture. Some records also include a place to document the client's allergies.

- *Skin assessment record.* A skin or wound assessment is often recorded on a flow sheet. These records may include categories related to stage of skin injury, drainage, odor, culture information, and treatments.

Progress Notes

Progress notes made by nurses provide information about the progress a client is making toward desired outcomes. Therefore, in addition to assessment and reassessment data, progress notes include information about client problems and nursing interventions. The format used depends on the documentation system in place in the institution.

Nursing Discharge/Referral Summaries

A discharge note and referral summary are completed when the client is being discharged and transferred to another institution or to a home setting where a visit by a community health nurse is required. Many institutions provide forms for these summaries. Some records combine the discharge plan, including instructions for care, and the final progress note. Many are designed with checklists to facilitate data recording.

If the discharge plan is given directly to the client and family, it is imperative that instructions be written in terms that can be readily understood. For example, medications, treatments, and activities should be written in layman's terms, and use of medical abbreviations (such as t.i.d.) should be avoided.

If a client is transferred within the facility or from a long-term facility to a hospital, a report needs to accompany the client to ensure continuity of care in the new area. It should include all components of the discharge instructions, but also describe the condition of the client prior to transfer. Any teaching or client instruction that has been done should also be described and recorded.

If the client is being transferred to another institution or to a home setting where a visit by a home health nurse is required, the discharge note takes the form of a referral summary. Regardless of format, discharge and referral summaries usually include some or all of the following:

- Description of client's physical, mental, and emotional status at discharge or transfer
- Resolved health problems
- Unresolved continuing health problems and continuing care needs; may include a review-of-systems checklist that considers integumentary, respiratory, cardiovascular, neurological, musculoskeletal, gastrointestinal, elimination, and reproductive problems
- Treatments that are to be continued (e.g., wound care, oxygen therapy)
- Current medications
- Restrictions that relate to (a) activity such as lifting, stair climbing, walking, driving, work; (b) diet; and (c) bathing, such as sponge bath, tub, or shower

- Functional/self-care abilities in terms of vision, hearing, speech, mobility with or without aids, meal preparation and eating, preparation and administration of medications, and so on
- Comfort level
- Support networks including family, significant others, religious adviser, community self-help groups, home care and other community agencies available, and so on
- Client education provided in relation to disease process, activities and exercise, special diet, medications, specialized care or treatments, follow-up appointments, and so on
- Discharge destination (e.g., home, nursing home) and mode of discharge (e.g., walking, wheelchair, ambulance)
- Referral services (e.g., social worker, home health nurse).

▶ FACILITY-SPECIFIC DOCUMENTATION

Documentation systems and requirements vary by facility. The documentation required in an acute care setting, as discussed in the early part of this exemplar, is different from the documentation required by long-term care, home care, or other care delivery sites.

Long-Term Care Documentation

Long-term facilities usually provide two types of care: skilled or intermediate. Clients needing skilled care require more extensive nursing care and specialized nursing skills. In contrast, an intermediate care focus is appropriate for clients who usually have chronic illnesses and may only need assistance with activities of daily living (such as bathing and dressing).

Requirements for documentation systems in long-term care settings are based on professional standards, federal and state regulations, and the policies of the healthcare agency. Laws influencing the kind and frequency of documentation required are found through the Health Care Financing Administration (HCFA), a branch of the U.S. Department of Health and Human Services, and the Omnibus Budget Reconciliation Act (OBRA) of 1987. The OBRA law, for example, requires that (a) a comprehensive assessment (the Minimum Data Set [MDS] for Resident Assessment and Care Screening) be performed within 4 days of a client's admission to a long-term care facility, (b) a formulated plan of care must be completed within 7 days of admission, and (c) the assessment and care screening process must be reviewed every 3 months. Documentation is particularly important for older adult clients in long-term care facilities, as explained in the Lifespan Considerations feature.

Documentation must also comply with requirements set by Medicare and Medicaid. These requirements vary with the level of service provided and other factors. For example, Medicare provides little reimbursement for services provided in long-term care facilities except for services that require skilled care such as chemotherapy, tube feedings, ventilators, and so on. For these clients, the nurse must provide daily documentation to verify the need for service and reimbursement.

Lifespan Considerations Documentation in Long-Term Care for Older Adults

Older adults in long-term care facilities tend to have chronic conditions and generally experience subtle small changes in their condition. However, when problems do occur, such as a hip fracture, CVA, or pneumonia, they are serious and require prompt attention. This underscores the importance of keeping Kardexes and charting in long-term facilities current and up to date in the event that the client needs to be transferred for more skilled care and further treatment. A thorough transfer summary will facilitate communication and promote continuity of care in these situations.

Nurses need to familiarize themselves with regulations influencing the kind and frequency of documentation required in long-term care facilities. Usually the nurse completes a nursing care *summary* at least once a week for clients requiring skilled care and every 2 weeks for clients who require intermediate care. Summaries should address the following:

- Specific problems noted in the care plan
- Mental status
- Activities of daily living
- Hydration and nutrition status
- Safety measures needed
- Medications
- Treatments
- Preventive measures
- Behavioral modification assessments, if pertinent (e.g., if the client is taking psychotropic medications or demonstrates behavioral problems).

Home Care Documentation

In 1985, the HCFA mandated that home health agencies standardize their documentation methods to meet requirements for Medicare and Medicaid and other third-party disbursements. Two records are required: (1) a home health certification and plan of treatment form and (2) a medical update and client information form. The nurse assigned to the home care client usually completes the forms, which must be signed by both the nurse and the attending physician.

Some home health agencies provide nurses with laptop computers, tablets, or smartphones to make records available in multiple locations. This allows the nurse to add new client information to records at the agency without traveling to the office.

▶ GENERAL GUIDELINES FOR RECORDING

Because a client's medical record is a legal document and may be used to provide evidence in court, many factors are considered in recording. Healthcare personnel must not only maintain the confidentiality of the client's record but also meet legal standards in the process of recording.

Date and Time

Document the date and time of each recording. This is essential not only for legal reasons but also for client safety. Record the time in the conventional manner (e.g., 9:00 a.m. or 3:15 p.m.) or according to the 24-hour clock (military clock), which avoids confusion about whether a time was a.m. or p.m.

Timing

Follow the agency's policy about the frequency of documenting, but adjust the frequency as a client's condition indicates; for example, a client whose blood pressure is changing requires more frequent documentation than a client whose blood pressure is constant. As a rule, documenting should be done as soon as possible after an assessment or intervention. No recording should be done *before* providing nursing care.

Legibility

All entries must be legible and easy to read to prevent interpretation errors. For handwritten records, printing or clearly legible handwriting is usually permissible. Follow the agency's policies about handwritten recording.

Permanence

In handwritten records, all entries on the client's record are made in dark ink so that the record is permanent and changes can be identified. Dark ink reproduces well on microfilm and in duplication processes. Follow the agency's policies about the type of pen and ink used for recording.

Accepted Terminology

Use only commonly accepted abbreviations, symbols, and terms as specified by the agency. Many abbreviations are standard and used universally; others are used only in certain geographic areas. Many healthcare facilities supply an approved list of abbreviations and symbols to prevent confusion. When in doubt about whether to use an abbreviation, write the term out in full until certain about the abbreviation. **Table 38–8** ● lists some common abbreviations used in health care.

TABLE 38–8 Commonly Used Abbreviations

ABBREVIATION	TERM	ABBREVIATION	TERM
Abd	Abdomen	meds	Medications
ABO	The main blood group system	mL, ml	Milliliter
ac	Before meals	mod	Moderate
ad lib	As desired	neg	Negative
ADL	Activities of daily living	Ø	None
Adm	Admitted or admission	#	Number or pounds
a.m.	Morning	NPO, NBM	Nothing by mouth
amb	Ambulatory	NS, N/S	Normal saline
amt	Amount	OD	Right eye or overdose
approx	Approximately	OOB	Out of bed
bid, BID	Twice daily	OS	Left eye
bm, BM	Bowel movement	pc	After meals
BP	Blood pressure	PE, PX	Physical examination
BRP	Bathroom privileges	per	By or through
$\bar{c}$	With	p.m.	Afternoon
C	Celsius (centigrade)	po	By mouth
CBC	Complete blood count	postop	Postoperatively
c/o	Complains of	preop	Preoperatively
DAT	Diet as tolerated	prep	Preparation
drsg	Dressing	prn, PRN	When necessary
Dx	Diagnosis	qid	Four times a day
ECG	Electrocardiogram	(R)	Right
F	Fahrenheit	$\bar{s}$	Without
fld	Fluid	stat	At once, immediately
GI	Gastrointestinal	tid, TID	Three times a day
gtt	Drop	TO	Telephone order
h, hr	Hour	TPR	Temperature, pulse, respirations
H_2O	Water	VO	Verbal order
I&O	Intake and output	VS	Vital signs
IV	Intravenous	WNL	Within normal limits
(L)	Left	wt	Weight
LMP	Last menstrual period		

*Institutions may elect to include some of these abbreviations on their "Do Not Use" list. Check the agency's policy.

In 2004, the Joint Commission developed National Patient Safety Goals to reduce communication errors. These goals are required to be implemented by all organizations accredited by the Joint Commission. As a result, accredited organizations must develop a "Do Not Use" list of abbreviations, acronyms, and symbols. These lists must include those banned by the Joint Commission.

*Stay Current: Keep up with The Joint Commission's "Do Not Use" list by visiting its Web site at **www.jointcommission.org/facts_about_the_official_**.*

Correct Spelling

Correct spelling is essential for accuracy in recording. If unsure how to spell a word, look it up. Two decidedly different medications may have similar spellings, such as Fosamax and Flomax.

Signature

Each recording on the nursing notes is signed by the nurse making it. The signature includes the name and title, for example, "Susan J. Green, RN" or "S.J. Green, RN." Some agencies have a signature sheet, and after signing it, nurses can use their initials. With computerized charting, each nurse has his or her own code, which allows the person who entered the documentation to be identified.

The following title abbreviations are often used, but nurses need to follow agency policy about how to sign their names:

RN	registered nurse
LVN	licensed vocational nurse
LPN	licensed practical nurse
NA	nursing assistant
CNA	certified nursing assistant
MA	medical assistant
NS	nursing student
PCA	patient care associate
SN	student nurse

Accuracy

The client's name and identifying information should be stamped or written on each page of the clinical record. Before making an entry, check that it is the correct chart. Do not identify charts by room number only; check the client's name. Special care is needed when caring for clients with the same last name.

Notations on records must be accurate and correct. Accurate notations consist of facts or observations rather than opinions or interpretations. It is more accurate, for example, to write that the client "refused medication" (fact) than to write that the client "was uncooperative" (opinion), or that a client "was crying" (observation) rather than that the client "was depressed" (interpretation). Similarly, when a client expresses worry about a diagnosis or problem, this should be quoted directly on the record: "Stated: 'I'm worried about my leg.'" When describing something, avoid general words, such as *large*, *good*, or *normal*, which can be interpreted in different ways. For example, chart specific data such as "2 cm × 3 cm bruise" rather than "large bruise."

When you make a recording mistake, draw a line through it and write the words *mistaken entry* above or next to the original entry, with your initials or name (depending on agency policy). Do not erase, blot out, or use correction fluid. The original entry must remain visible. When using electronic charting, the nurse needs to be aware of the agency's policy and procedures for correcting documentation mistakes.

Write on every line but never between lines. If a blank appears in a notation, draw a line through the blank space so that no additional information can be recorded there at any other time or by any other individual, and sign the notation.

Sequence

Document events in the order in which they occur; for example, record assessments, then the nursing interventions, and then the client's responses. Update or delete problems as needed.

Appropriateness

Record only information that pertains to the client's health problems and care. Any other personal information that the client conveys is inappropriate for the record. Recording irrelevant information may be considered an invasion of the client's privacy and/or libelous. For example, a client's disclosure that she was addicted to heroin 15 years ago would *not* be recorded on her medical record unless it had a direct bearing on her health problem.

Completeness

Not all data that a nurse obtains about a client can be recorded. However, the information that is recorded needs to be complete and helpful to the client and healthcare professionals.

Nurses' notes need to reflect the nursing process. Record all assessments, dependent and independent nursing interventions, client problems, client comments and responses to interventions and tests, progress toward goals, and communication with other members of the health team.

> ### SAFETY ALERT
> Do not assume that the individual who is reading your charting will know that a common intervention (e.g., turning) has occurred because you believe it to be an "obvious" component of care.

Care that is *omitted* because of the client's condition or refusal of treatment must also be recorded. Document what was omitted, why it was omitted, and who was notified.

Conciseness

Recordings need to be brief as well as complete to save time in communication. The client's name and the word *client* are omitted. For example, write, "Perspiring profusely. Respirations shallow, 28/min." End each thought or sentence with a period.

Box 38–11   Do's and Don'ts of Documentation

DO	DON'T
■ Chart a change in a client's condition *and* show that follow-up actions were taken.	■ Leave a blank space for a colleague to chart later.
■ Read the nurses' notes prior to care to determine whether there has been a change in the client's condition.	■ Chart in advance of the event (e.g., procedure, medication).
■ Be timely. A late entry is better than no entry; however, the longer the period of time between actual care and charting, the greater the suspicion.	■ Use vague terms (e.g., "appears to be comfortable," "had a good night").
■ Use objective, specific, and factual descriptions.	■ Chart for someone else.
■ Correct charting errors in the manner specified by agency policy.	■ Use "patient" or "client" instead of the client's name.
■ Chart all teaching.	■ Alter a record even if requested by a superior or a physician.
■ Record the client's actual words by putting quote marks around the words.	■ Record assumptions or words reflecting bias (e.g., "complainer," "disagreeable").
■ Chart the client's response to interventions.	
■ Review your notes. Are they clear? Do they reflect what you want to say?	

Legal Prudence

Accurate, complete documentation should give legal protection to the nurse, the client's other caregivers, the healthcare facility, and the client. Admissible in court as a legal document, the clinical record provides proof of the quality of care given to a client. Documentation is usually viewed by juries and attorneys as the best evidence of what really happened to the client.

For the best legal protection, the nurse should not only adhere to professional standards of nursing care but also follow agency policy and procedures for intervention and documentation in all situations, especially high-risk situations (see **Box 38–11** ●).

REVIEW Documentation

RELATE Link the Concepts and Exemplars

Linking the exemplar of documentation with the concept of legal issues:

1. How does proper documentation reduce the risk of lawsuits?
2. What components of nursing care must be included in the nurse's documentation to meet legal requirements?

Linking the exemplar of documentation with the concept of quality improvement:

3. How is nursing documentation used to assess the quality of nursing care delivered?
4. How can incomplete documentation result in a negative evaluation of the quality of nursing care delivered?

REFER Go to Pearson Nursing Student Resources
nursing.pearsonhighered.com

- Additional review materials

REFLECT Case Study

Zainah Kattan is a 23-year-old nurse from a small, rural community. Zainah graduated from nursing school a few months ago and took a job working on a general medical-surgical inpatient unit at Neighborhood Hospital. Her goal is to eventually work in an adult intensive care unit. She recently received a sign-on bonus and looks forward to buying her first new car.

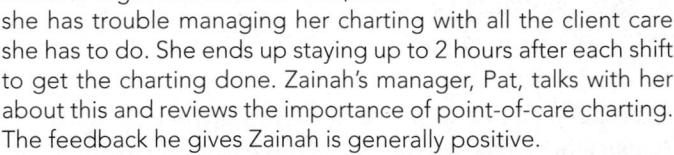

Zainah has a busy week because of increased client loads. She has seven to eight clients of her own, and she has trouble managing her charting with all the client care she has to do. She ends up staying up to 2 hours after each shift to get the charting done. Zainah's manager, Pat, talks with her about this and reviews the importance of point-of-care charting. The feedback he gives Zainah is generally positive.

1. Why is Zainah's manager trying to improve her point-of-care charting?
2. What are the potential drawbacks of waiting until the end of the shift to document care?
3. What strategies might you suggest to Zainah to help her improve point-of-care charting during a busy shift?

EXEMPLAR 38.4   Reporting

EXEMPLAR KEY TERMS
Change-of-shift report, *2451*
Handoff, *2451*
Handoff communication, *2451*
Reporting, *2451*

EXEMPLAR LEARNING OUTCOMES
After reading about this exemplar, you will be able to:

1. Explain the purpose of reporting.
2. Describe various types of reporting used by nurses.
3. Identify essential guidelines for reporting client data.
4. Demonstrate each form of reporting following all of the essential steps.
5. Discuss the importance and implications of the handoff communication process.

▶ OVERVIEW

The purpose of **reporting** is to communicate specific information to an individual or group of individuals. A report, whether oral or written, should be concise, including pertinent information but no extraneous detail. In addition to change-of-shift reports and telephone reports, reporting can also include the sharing of information or ideas with colleagues and other health professionals about some aspect of a client's care. Examples include the care plan conference and nursing rounds.

▶ HANDOFF COMMUNICATION

Ineffective communication is the primary cause of sentinel events (Chard, 2008). As a result, hospitals are required to implement a standardized approach to "handing off" communication. **Handoff** is defined as "the transfer of information (along with authority and responsibility) during transitions in care across the continuum; to include an opportunity to ask questions, clarify, and confirm" (Catalano, 2009, p. 266). Hospital handoffs occur at many times, including but not limited to when a client is transferred between units, at the change of shift, and at discharge (Pesanka et al., 2009). The **handoff communication** is a verbal or written exchange of information that encompasses the nursing care that has been provided along with all members of the healthcare team who have cared for the client during the relevant time period (Catalano, 2009).

The handoff process involves two groups, the senders and the receivers. The senders are the caregivers who are transmitting client information and releasing care; the receivers are the caregivers who are accepting the client and the client's information.

The **SHARE** method can be used to accomplish a successful handoff:

Standardize critical content.
Hardwire within your system.
Allow opportunity to ask questions.
Reinforce quality and measurement.
Educate and coach.

The Joint Commission (2012) provides several items that can be helpful in the handoff communication process. The goal of the new Hand-off Communications Targeted Solutions Tool (TST) is "to assist health care organizations with the process of passing necessary and critical information about a patient from one caregiver to the next, or from one team of caregivers to another, to prevent miscommunication-related errors" (Joint Commission, 2012).

🌐 **Stay Current:** *For more information regarding the handoff communication process, visit the following Web site:* **www. centerfortransforminghealthcare.org/assets/4/6/CTH_ Hand-off_commun_set_final_2010.pdf**.

Change-of-Shift Report

A **change-of-shift report** is a type of handoff communication given to all nurses on the next shift. Its purpose is to provide continuity of care for clients by providing the new caregivers with a quick summary of client needs and details of care to be given.

Box 38–12 Key Elements of a Change-of-Shift Report

- Follow a particular order (e.g., follow room numbers in a hospital).
- Provide basic identifying information for each client (e.g., name, room number, bed designation).
- For new clients, provide the reason for admission or medical diagnosis (or diagnoses), surgery (date), diagnostic tests, and therapies in past 24 hours.
- Include significant changes in the client's condition and present information in order (i.e., assessment, nursing diagnoses, interventions, outcomes, and evaluation). For example, "Mr. Ronald Oakes said he had an aching pain in his left calf at 1400 hours. Inspection revealed no other signs. Calf pain is related to altered blood circulation. Rest and elevation of his legs on a footstool for 30 minutes provided relief."
- Provide exact information, such as "Ms. Jessie Jones received morphine 6 mg IV at 1500 hours," not "Ms. Jessie Jones received some morphine during the evening."
- Report clients' need for special emotional support. For example, a client who has just learned that his biopsy results revealed malignancy and who is now scheduled for a laryngectomy needs time to discuss his feelings before preoperative teaching is begun.
- Include current nurse-prescribed and primary care provider–prescribed orders.
- Provide a summary of newly admitted clients, including diagnosis, age, general condition, plan of therapy, and significant information about the client's support people.
- Report on clients who have been transferred or discharged from the unit.
- Clearly state priorities of care and care that is due after the shift begins. For example, in a 7 a.m. report, the nurse might say, "Mr. Li's vital signs are due at 0730, and his IV bag will need to be replaced by 0800." This information is best given at the end of that client's report because the receiver's memory is best for the first and last information given.
- Be concise. Don't elaborate on background data or routine care (e.g., do not report "Vital signs at 0800 and 1150" when that is the unit standard). Do not report coming and going of visitors unless there is a problem or concern or visitors are involved in teaching and care. Social support and visits are the norm.

Change-of-shift reports may be written or given orally, either in a face-to-face exchange or by audiotape recording. The face-to-face report permits the listener to ask questions during the report; written and tape-recorded reports are often briefer and less time consuming. Reports are sometimes given at the bedside, and clients as well as nurses may participate in the exchange of information. **Box 38–12** ● lists key elements of a change-of-shift report.

SAFETY ALERT
Be aware of where the shift report takes place in order to maintain client confidentiality. An area that is private and free from interruption is best.

▶ TELEPHONE COMMUNICATION

Telephone Reports

Healthcare professionals frequently report about a client by telephone. For example, a nurse informs the primary care provider

Box 38–13 Guidelines for Telephone and Verbal Orders

1. Know the state nursing board's position on who can give and accept verbal and phone orders.
2. Know the agency's policy regarding phone orders.
3. Ask the prescriber to speak slowly and clearly.
4. Ask the prescriber to spell the name of the medication if you are not familiar with it.
5. Question the drug, dosage, or changes if they seem inappropriate for the client.
6. Write down the order or enter it into the computer on the physician's order form.
7. Read the order back to the prescriber. Use words instead of abbreviations.
8. Have the prescriber verbally acknowledge the read-back.
9. Record the date and time and indicate it was a telephone order.
10. Sign your name and credentials.
11. Transcribe the order.
12. Follow agency protocol to have the prescriber sign the telephone order.

Also:

■ When writing a dosage, always put a number before the decimal.
■ Write out units.
■ Never follow a voice-mail order. Call the prescriber, write the order down, and read it back for confirmation.

about a change in a client's condition, a radiologist reports the results of an x-ray study, or a nurse reports to a nurse on another unit about a transferred client.

The nurse receiving a telephone report should document the date and time, the name of the individual giving the information, and the subject of the information received and then sign the notation. The individual receiving the information should repeat it back to the sender to ensure accuracy.

When giving a telephone report to a primary care provider, the nurse must be concise and accurate. Telephone reports usually include the client's name and medical diagnosis, changes in nursing assessment, vital signs related to baseline vital signs, significant laboratory data, and related nursing interventions. The nurse should have the client's chart ready in case the primary care provider requires further information.

After reporting, the nurse should document the date, time, and content of the call.

Telephone Orders

Physicians often order a therapy (e.g., a medication) for a client by telephone. Most agencies have specific policies about telephone orders. Many agencies allow only registered nurses to take telephone orders.

While the primary care provider gives the order, the nurse should *write* the complete order down and *read* it back to the primary care provider to ensure accuracy. Question the primary care provider about any order that is ambiguous, unusual (e.g., an abnormally high dosage of a medication), or contraindicated by the client's condition. Then transcribe the order onto the physician's order sheet, indicating it as a verbal order (VO) or telephone order (TO). Once transcribed onto the physician's order sheet, the order must be countersigned by the primary

care provider within a time period described by agency policy. Many acute care hospitals require that this be done within 24 hours. See **Box 38–13** ● for selected guidelines related to telephone orders.

▶ CARE PLAN CONFERENCE

Care plan conferences allow for collaborative reporting among the healthcare professionals who provide care to the client. They are most often used for clients who have complex care needs. During the conference, the client's healthcare providers discuss possible solutions to certain problems of the client, such as inability to cope with an event or lack of progress toward goal attainment. The care plan conference allows each member of the healthcare team an opportunity to offer an opinion in order to reach a solution to the problem. The choice of healthcare professionals who are invited to attend the conference is based on the needs of the client. Family members are an important part of the care plan conference, especially for clients who are unable to advocate for themselves. Other professionals may be invited. For example, a social worker may be present to discuss support for the family of a burned child or a pharmacist may be present at a conference when the client requires multiple medications.

Care plan conferences are most effective when there is a climate of respect—that is, nonjudgmental acceptance of others even though their values, opinions, and beliefs may seem different. Interdisciplinary collaboration is discussed further in the module on Collaboration. The nurse needs to accept and respect each individual's contributions, listening with an open mind to what others are saying even when there is disagreement.

◢ **REVIEW Reporting**

RELATE Link the Concepts and Exemplars

Linking the exemplar of reporting with the concept of legal issues:

1. What are the legal obligations of a nurse who is providing change-of-shift reporting to the oncoming nurse?
2. How can the nurse ensure that all legal obligations have been met when accepting telephone orders from the primary provider?

Linking the exemplar of reporting with the concept of safety:

3. How does handoff communication contribute to client safety?
4. In providing a telephone report to a primary care provider because of a client's sudden change in condition, what information should be included to maintain the safe care of the client?

REFER Go to Pearson Nursing Student Resources
nursing.pearsonhighered.com

- Additional review materials

REFLECT Case Study

Marjorie Newman, 64 years old, was admitted to the coronary care unit (CCU) with a diagnosis of acute anterior myocardial infarction. Her condition has remained stable, and she is to be transferred to the telemetry unit tomorrow or sooner if the CCU bed is required for an acutely ill client. The nurse assigned to her care is called to the monitors by the monitor technician because Ms. Newman has suddenly begun having frequent premature ventricular contractions (PVCs). When the nurse enters Ms. Newman's room, she assesses the client and finds her to be short of breath, experiencing severe left-sided chest pain radi-

ating to the left arm, and very diaphoretic. Vital signs are T_O 98.6°F; P 108 bpm and irregular; R 28/min; and BP 92/44 mmHg. The nurse analyzes Ms. Newman's rhythm strip and finds elevated ST segments, tachycardia, with 10–14 PVCs per minute. A coworker agrees to stay with Ms. Newman and monitor her condition while the nurse assigned to Ms. Newman's care calls the primary care provider.

1. What information would the nurse report to the primary care provider when calling to notify of the change in the client's condition?

2. Why did the nurse have a coworker stay with the client while calling the primary care provider?

3. If the nurse's shift ended while this event was occurring with Ms. Newman, what should the nurse do before leaving for the day?

■ REFERENCES

Adams, K., & Galanes, G. J. (2003). *Communicating in groups: Applications and skills* (9th ed.). Boston, MA: McGraw-Hill.

American Nurses Association (ANA). (2001). *Code of ethics for nurses with interpretive statements.* Washington, DC: Author.

Auvil, C. A., & Silver, B. W. (1984). Therapist self-disclosure: When is it appropriate? *Perspectives in Psychiatric Care, 22*(2), 57–61.

Boyd, M. A. (2008). *Psychiatric nursing: Contemporary practice.* Philadelphia, PA: Lippincott Williams & Wilkins.

Catalano, K. (2009). Hand-off communication does affect patient safety. *Plastic Surgical Nursing, 29*(4), 266–270.

Chard, R. (2008). Implementing a process for hand-off communications. *AORN Journal, 88*(6), 1005–1008.

Chart smart (3rd ed.). (2009). Philadelphia, PA: Lippincott Williams & Wilkins.

Egan, G. (2013). *The skilled helper: A problem-management approach to helping* (10th ed.). Pacific Grove, CA: Brooks/Cole.

Guido, G. W. (2010). *Legal and ethical issues in nursing* (5th ed.). Upper Saddle River, NJ: Prentice Hall.

Haskard, K., DiMatteo, M., & Heritage, J. (2009). Affective and instrumental communication in primary care interactions: Predicting the satisfaction of nursing staff and patients. *Health Communication, 24*(1), 21–32.

Hemsley, B., Balandin, S., & Worrall, L. (2012). Nursing the patient with complex communication needs: Time as a barrier and a facilitator to successful communication in hospital. *Journal of Advanced Nursing, 68*(1), 116–126.

Huber, D. (2009). *Leadership and nursing care management* (4th ed.). Philadelphia, PA: W.B. Saunders.

Joint Commission. (2012). *Improving transitions of care: Hand-off communication.* Retrieved from http://www.centerfortransforminghealthcare.org/projects/detail.aspx?Project=1.

Kneisl, C. R., & Wilson, H. S. (1996). *Psychiatric nursing* (5th ed.). Redwood City, CA: Addison-Wesley Nursing.

Mayo Clinic. (2009). *Being assertive: Reduce stress, communicate better.* Retrieved from http://www.mayoclinic.com/health/assertive/SR00042.

Moore, K. (2008). Is laughter the best medicine? Research into the therapeutic use of humor and laughter in nursing practice. *Whitireia Nursing Journal, 15,* 33–38.

Office for Civil Rights (OCR). (2010). *Effective communication in hospitals.* Retrieved from http://www.hhs.gov/ocr/civilrights/resources/specialtopics/hospitalcommunication/index.html.

Office of Minority Health. (2010). *National standards on culturally and linguistically appropriate services (CLAS).* Retrieved from http://raceandhealth.hhs.gov/templates/browse.aspx?lvl=2&lvlID=15.

Pesanka, D. A., Greenhouse, P. K., Rack, L. L. Delucia, G. A., Perret, R. W., Scholle, C. C., & Janov, C. L. (2009). Ticket to ride: Reducing handoff risk during hospital patient transport. *Journal of Nursing Care Quality, 24*(2), 109–115.

Samovar, L. A., Porter, R. E., & McDaniel, E. R. (2010). *Communication between cultures.* Boston, MA: Wadsworth/Cengage Learning.

Sampson, E. E., & Marthas, M. S. (1990). *Group process for the health professions* (3rd ed.). Albany, NY: Delmar.

Stewart, G. L., Manz, C. C., & Sims, H. P. (1999). *Team work and group dynamics.* New York, NY: Wiley.

Wilkinson, J. M. (2005). *Nursing diagnosis handbook with NIC interventions and NOC outcomes* (8th ed.). Upper Saddle River, NJ: Prentice Hall Health.

39 Managing Care

MODULE AT-A-GLANCE

The Concept of Managing Care, 2455

Exemplar 39.1
Care Coordination, 2460

Exemplar 39.2
Cost-Effective Care, 2462

Exemplar 39.3
Delegation, 2466

Exemplar 39.4
Management Principles, 2474

▧ THE CONCEPT OF MANAGING CARE

A number of options for the delivery of nursing care support continuity of care and cost effectiveness. These options include managed care, case management, client-focused care, differentiated practice, shared governance, the case method, the functional method, team nursing, and primary nursing (described in the module on Healthcare Systems). Each of these systems of care has evolved as organizations attempt to decrease healthcare costs; maximize limited human and physical resources; meet increasingly complex federal, state, and local regulations; and improve the quality of client care. A particular agency may use more than one configuration—for example, team nursing on the medical surgical units and primary nursing on the cardiac surgery unit.

The concept of Managed Care is related to many other concepts, a few of which are outlined in the Concepts Related to Managing Care feature. **<<**

Concept Learning Outcomes

After reading about this concept, you will be able to:

1. Describe the goals and emphasis of managed care.
2. Examine the role of the case manager in a managed care environment.
3. Summarize frameworks for delivering care, including the advantages and disadvantages of each.

Concept Key Terms

Case management (CM), *2457*

Client-focused care, *2457*

Differentiated practice, *2457*

Licensed practical nurses (LPNs), *2458*

Managed care, *2457*

Registered nurses (RNs), *2458*

Team nursing, *2458*

Unlicensed assistive personnel (UAPs), *2458*

Concepts Related to **Managing Care**

Managed care is a healthcare delivery system designed to provide cost-effective, high-quality care for groups of clients from the time of their initial contact with the health system through the conclusion of their health problem. Managed care relies on collaboration among the family, the client, family members, and healthcare providers to plan care. Coordination and care management are significant components of managed care. All nurses are responsible for managing care and, therefore, must be aware of the impact that their actions may have on a client. Ethics comes into play as nurses work with healthcare providers to ensure that the care provided is cost effective but meets the client's needs and does no harm. The nurse has an important role as teacher in managed care because the nurse must ensure that the client and family are able to meet the client's acute and ongoing healthcare needs after discharge in order to maintain the client's health and reduce the costs resulting from acute exacerbation and reoccurrence of the disease or injury.

CONCEPT	RELATIONSHIP TO MANAGING CARE	NURSING IMPLICATIONS
Healthcare Systems		
■ Access to health care ■ Allocation of resources	Delivering and managing health care includes a coordination of services and allocation of resources to meet multiple client needs and keep finances in check. There is a need to close the gap between financial reimbursement and the advances in medical interventions.	■ Nurses work with federal, state, and local healthcare guidelines in private and public healthcare settings to provide preventive, acute, chronic, and palliative care to clients. Adaptability, flexibility, and creativity are attributes nurses use to achieve best client outcomes.
Collaboration		
■ Case management ■ Interdisciplinary teams and communcation	Today's healthcare system requires a team approach from members of various disciplines to provide best care to clients. This team follows a plan of care to organize the process, keep costs down, standardize care, and improve client outcomes.	■ Nurses work closely with physicians in coordinating the care provided to clients by a team of healthcare professionals. The nursing process provides the framework for nursing plans of care used by others in a variety of settings and with clients of all ages.
Advocacy		
■ The advocate's role ■ Advocacy interventions	Advocates protect the rights of clients and defend clients from harm. Vulnerable populations depend on nurses to speak up for them as decisions about availability of healthcare services and resources are made.	■ Nurses work in a variety of healthcare settings with varying populations who need advocates to protect their rights. Nurse advocates can empower and educate clients while managing their care.
Clinical Decision Making		
■ The nursing process ■ The nursing plan of care ■ Prioritizing care	Making decisions about client care begins with gathering assessment data to analyze and identify priorities of actions for best client outcomes. Having a plan of care helps manage care by preventing duplication of services and communicating client goals to other disciplines providing client care.	■ Prioritizing care is a process nurses use to manage time and establish an order for completing responsibilities and care interventions for a single client or for a group of clients. Competing priorities for care may mean initiating some interventions at a later time.
Ethics		
■ Values ■ Ethical dilemmas ■ Patient rights	Ethical principles of altruism, autonomy, human dignity, integrity, and social justice influence decisions made in dispersing services and resources throughout healthcare systems.	■ Nurses need to provide client-centered care to all clients following common ethical nursing values of being truthful, promoting good, maintaining fairness, and doing no harm.

▶ MANAGED CARE

Managed care is a healthcare delivery system in which the goal is to provide cost-effective, high quality care that focuses on decreased costs and improved outcomes for groups of clients. The care of a client is carefully planned from the initial contact through the conclusion of the specific health problem. In managed care, healthcare providers and agencies collaborate to provide health care that manages limited clinical resources and costs wisely and effectively. Managed care emphasizes preventing inappropriate and unnecessary costs, increasing customer satisfaction, promoting health, and delivering preventive services. Health maintenance organizations and preferred provider organizations are examples of provider systems that are committed to managed care.

Managed care can interface effectively with primary and team nursing, the functional method, and alternative nursing care delivery systems. Although managed care has been embraced as a model for healthcare reform, many people question the application of this business approach to a commodity as precious as healthcare delivery.

Effective managed care requires the ability to prioritize, identify clinical pathways, create concept maps and/or care plans, understand client rights and advance directives, and commit to quality improvement. All of these topics are covered in the following exemplars and modules:

- The exemplar on Prioritizing Care in the module on Clinical Decision Making (includes clinical pathways, concept maps, and nursing plans of care).
- The exemplar on Advance Directives in the module on Legal Issues
- The exemplar on Patient Rights in the module on Ethics
- The module on Quality Improvement.

CASE STUDY \\ A

John Seitz is the nursing director at a skilled nursing facility (SNF). He has received multiple complaints from clients and their families that care provided in one of the units is not consistent. For example, sometimes residents' trays are brought to the room but no one assists the resident to eat. Beds often go unchanged. Baths are not provided as requested by the residents.

Critical Thinking Questions

1. Evaluate what type of nursing model may work best in a SNF.
2. Plan how you, as the nursing director, would ensure that the appropriate model is implemented by team members.
3. What tools would you design and apply to evaluate the effectiveness of the new plan?

▶ CASE MANAGEMENT

In general, the purpose of **case management (CM)** is to coordinate, facilitate, and follow, over time, a client's use of a variety of health and social services. Insurance-based case management is a labor-intensive activity that is provided typically by telephone. In recent years, the importance of CM has increased, and it is now considered a fundamental building block of the care management system. CM is an intensive service; therefore, to ensure efficiency and effectiveness, case managers should identify the specific cases that would most benefit from case management, such as the cases of clients with multiple chronic health problems. CMs often apply selection criteria to identify cases.

Generally, case management involves interdisciplinary teams that assume collaborative responsibility for planning and assessing needs and for coordinating, implementing, and evaluating care for groups of clients from preadmission through discharge or transfer and recuperation. A case manager may be a nurse, social worker, or other appropriate professional. In some areas of the United States, case managers may be referred to as discharge planners. This topic is discussed in greater detail in the module on Collaboration.

▶ CLIENT-FOCUSED CARE

Client-focused care is a delivery model that organizes health care around the expressed physical and emotional needs of the client. Client-focused care incorporates the concepts of client- and family-centered care and is generally understood to be an approach in which clients and their families are considered integral components of the healthcare decision-making and delivery processes.

▶ DIFFERENTIATED PRACTICE

Differentiated practice is a system in which each nurse's educational preparation and skill sets are evaluated and used to determine how the nurse will be best utilized. Thus, differentiated practice models consist of specific job descriptions for nurses according to their education or training—for example, LVN, ADN, BSN RN, MSN RN, and APN. To establish a differentiated practice system, each healthcare agency must first identify the nursing competencies required by the clients that the agency serves. This model further requires the delineation of roles between both licensed nursing personnel and unlicensed assistive personnel (UAPs). This enables nurses to progress and assume (as well as delegate) roles and responsibilities appropriate to their level of experience, capability, and education. As with managed care and case management, differentiated nursing practice seeks to provide high-quality care at an affordable cost.

▶ SHARED GOVERNANCE

The shared governance model can be used in concert with other models of nursing care delivery. In this organizational model, nursing staff participate with administrative personnel in making, implementing, and evaluating client care policies. The focus of this model is to encourage the participation of nurses in decision making at all levels of the organization. Individuals may participate either at their own request or as part of their job role criteria. More commonly, nurses participate by serving as members of decision-making groups, such as committees and task forces. The decisions made may address employment conditions, cost effectiveness, long-range planning, productivity, and wages and benefits. The underlying principle of shared governance is that employees will be more committed to the organizational goals if they have input into planning and decision making.

▶ CASE METHOD

The case method, also referred to as total care, is one of the earliest nursing models developed. In this client-centered method, one nurse is assigned to, and is responsible for, the comprehensive care of a group of clients during an 8- or 12-hour shift. For each client, the nurse assesses needs, makes nursing plans, formulates nursing diagnoses, implements care, and evaluates the effectiveness of care. In this method, a client has consistent contact with one nurse during a shift but may have different nurses on other shifts. Considered to be the precursor of primary nursing, the case method continues to be used in a variety of practice settings, such as intensive care nursing.

▶ FUNCTIONAL METHOD

The functional method focuses on the jobs to be completed (e.g., bed making and temperature measurement). In this task-oriented approach, personnel with less educational preparation than the professional nurse (for example, UAPs) perform aspects of care with less complex requirements. The method is based on a production and efficiency model that gives authority and responsibility to the person assigning the work—for example, the head nurse. Clearly defined job descriptions, procedures, policies, and lines of communication are required. The functional approach to nursing is economical and efficient, and it permits centralized direction and control. Its disadvantages are fragmentation of care and the possibility that nonquantifiable aspects of care, such as meeting the client's emotional needs, may be overlooked.

▶ TEAM NURSING

Team nursing is the delivery of individualized nursing care to a group of clients by a team led by a professional nurse. A nursing team consists of the following:

- **Registered nurses (RNs)**, who are specially licensed and trained to deliver direct client care, including client assessment, identification of health problems, and development and coordination of care

- **Licensed practical nurses (LPNs)**, who provide direct client care under the direction of an RN, physician, or other licensed practitioner

- **Unlicensed assistive personnel (UAPs)**, or healthcare staff, who assume delegated aspects of basic client care such as bathing, assisting with feeding, and collecting specimens. UAPs include certified nurse assistants, hospital attendants, nurse technicians, and orderlies.

The RN retains responsibility and authority for client care but delegates appropriate tasks to the other team members. Proponents of this model believe that the team approach increases the efficiency of the RN. Opponents believe that

---

Evidence-Based Practice Influence of Types of Nurses and Delivery Models in Hospitals on Client Outcomes

Problem

Do the types of nurses and delivery models in hospitals influence client outcomes?

Evidence

Using objective measures such as the number of clients per nurse or the number of nursing hours per patient day, researchers have been able to measure the impact of nursing ratios on client outcomes. Research continues to prove that higher nursing ratios result in fewer adverse outcomes for clients. Higher nursing ratios have been linked to decreased mortality, failure to rescue, and specific adverse events among surgical clients. They also have been associated with shorter lengths of stay and fewer complications. Despite these very positive findings, minimal research has been completed to associate specific variables with staffing levels. Many health researchers decry this and call for immediate studies to examine facility level strategies to improve staffing and relate those efforts to client and organizational outcomes (Mitchell, 2012).

Implications

International studies demonstrate that the larger the percentage of registered nurses among the total care staff, the lower

the incidence of adverse client outcomes, such as falls, errors, and preventable infections. A recent study depicted a 3%–12% reduction in adverse outcomes and a 16% reduction in the risk of mortality in surgical clients when the proportion of registered nurses was higher (Twigg et al., 2010). It is more difficult to compare outcomes with care delivery models because each unit may employ slight variations of the model. However, it is important to continue to examine delivery models and their effectiveness in order to allow optimal deployment of registered nurses in a time of a shortage.

Critical Thinking Application

1. Evaluate how a nursing shortage might affect the outcome of clients receiving care from your organization.

2. In the event of a nursing shortage on your unit, how would you, as the director, prepare the remaining clinical and nonclinical staff to prevent the most common adverse events that result from a reduction in the number of nursing staff?

3. In the event of a nursing shortage, what case management approach would you use to ensure that clients are adequately cared for and that their health is not jeopardized?

inpatient clients with acute illnesses require greater attention from the professional nurse and allow little room for delegation.

▶ PRIMARY NURSING

Primary nursing is a system in which one nurse is responsible for overseeing the total care of a number of clients 24 hours a day, 7 days a week, even if the nurse does not deliver all the care personally. It is a method of providing comprehensive, individualized, and consistent care.

Primary nursing uses the nurse's technical knowledge and management skills. The primary nurse assesses and prioritizes each client's needs, identifies nursing diagnoses, develops a plan of care with the client, and evaluates the effectiveness of care (see the module on Clinical Decision Making). Associates provide some care, but the primary nurse coordinates it and communicates information about the client's health to other nurses and health professionals. Primary nursing encompasses all aspects of the professional role, including teaching, advocacy, decision making, and continuity of care. The primary nurse is the first-line manager of the client's care, with all its inherent accountabilities and responsibilities.

▶ NURSING PRACTICE

Regardless of the model of care delivery an agency uses, nurses carry a great deal of responsibility for the management of client care. Managing care has implications for direct client care, coordination of client care, and cost containment. For example,

by scheduling the dietitian to come at a different time than the physical therapist, the nurse makes sure that neither professional wastes time (and money) waiting for the other one to finish seeing the same client. This also may prevent the client from becoming overtired by seeing too many providers within a short period of time.

Like everything in nursing, managing care is a learned skill that requires strong communication, assessment, and time management skills (Plawecki & Amrhein, 2010). It also requires, when necessary, appropriate delegation. Nurses who manage these activities successfully are contributing significantly to client well-being and to the cost of care delivery.

CASE STUDY \\ B

Michelle Liu has been hired as the nursing director for a start-up home health agency. To date, the agency, working with its corporate offices, has identified the services it plans to provide and the approximate number of clients it intends to see during the first 6 months. Michelle has been asked to develop the initial staffing plan and determine the extent to which staffing will increase during the first 6 months. Her plan needs to accommodate increases in the staffing levels at regular intervals to ensure that, as the number of clients grow, there will be adequate staff to care for them.

Critical Thinking Questions

1. Assess the factors that Michelle must evaluate to design the staffing plan.
2. Evaluate the effects that inappropriate staffing could have on quality of care and service as well as the cost effectiveness of the agency.

REVIEW The Concept of Managing Care

RELATE Link the Concepts

Linking the concept of managing care with the concept of communication:

1. How does the nurse's ability to communicate effectively contribute to managing the client's care?
2. Describe a situation in which conflict management may be necessary when managing care for a client who requires the services of several departments within the hospital.

Mr. Montoya is to be discharged from the acute care facility after removal of a metastatic brain tumor. He will receive chemotherapy intrathecally as well as intravenously. The unit clerk has scheduled follow-up appointments with his surgeon, family provider, oncologist, and neurologist as well as with the infusion therapy department. The physician has provided referrals for consultation with a dietitian, social services, and home nursing care.

Linking the concept of managing care with the concept of collaboration:

3. How can the nurse prioritize care to meet the client's needs while ensuring that each of these services meets his or her own needs in preparing for the client's discharge (e.g., nutritional screening predischarge, social services inter-

view, and home nursing assessment to determine home care needs)?

4. What is the nurse's role in managing this client's care and collaborating with the other members of the healthcare team?

REFER Go to Pearson Nursing Student Resources
nursing.pearsonhighered.com

- Additional review materials
- Additional case study

REFLECT Case Study

Lauren Chavoen works in a hospital where senior management believes it is essential to engage nursing staff in planning, implementing, and evaluating client care policies. Lauren realizes that she is not yet ready to assume a management position, but she understands that senior management's beliefs offer her a chance to develop some management skills through participation in policy development.

1. How should Lauren convince her manager that her participation would benefit not only herself but her unit also?
2. Evaluate what skills Lauren will need to be successful on the committee she joins.

EXEMPLAR 39.1 Care Coordination

EXEMPLAR KEY TERMS
Care coordination, 2460
Collaboration, 2460

EXEMPLAR LEARNING OUTCOMES
After reading about this exemplar, you should be able to:

1. Differentiate between coordination and collaboration.

2. Predict potential barriers to effective coordination along with strategies to overcome or avoid these barriers.

3. Summarize skills necessary to achieve effective coordination.

4. Illustrate the anticipated benefits when care coordination is effective.

▶ OVERVIEW

Care coordination is the means by which an interdisciplinary team works with a client to ensure that the client receives the care necessary to meet his needs across the healthcare continuum. Care coordination is critical to improving client outcomes across a broad spectrum of clinical settings. While care coordination is and has always been a significant nursing responsibility, its importance to the delivery of overall health care has not always been recognized. As the healthcare industry works to transform the delivery of health care, care coordination's benefits to the health and well-being of clients have become increasingly evident—so much so that the Centers for Medicare and Medicaid Services (CMS) now allows reimbursement of nursing time spent managing Medicare clients' care as they transition from the hospital to other settings (Advance for Nurses, 2012).

Many factors have contributed to the importance of care coordination, but two have emerged as the most important. The first is the recommendation by the Institute for Healthcare Improvement (IHI) that the "Triple Aim" objectives be incorporated into health care in the United States; the second is coordination of care's importance to elements of the Affordable Care Act. The IHI (2013) states that simultaneously focusing on three critical objectives, labeled the "Triple Aim," can potentially lead to better models for providing health care. The objectives of the Triple Aim are to (1) improve the health of a defined population; (2) enhance the client care experience (including quality, access, and reliability); and (3) reduce, or at least control, the per capita (per person) cost of care. Care coordination is viewed by many people involved in health care as the foundation to achieving the Triple Aim objectives. Care coordination has been identified as a means to improve health outcomes, improve the quality of life for healthcare consumers, and provide greater efficiencies through care coordination centered on the needs and preferences of healthcare consumers and their families. These factors clearly support the Triple Aim. The American Nurses Association's (ANA's) June 2012 position paper notes that if effective care coordination for individuals across settings is lacking, the results are increased cost, potential drug interactions, increased medical errors, and unnecessary duplication of tests and services, often occurring when healthcare consumers are shuttled from provider to provider with chronic, complex, or hard to diagnose conditions (ANA, 2012). Most important, it increases the cost in human suffering for healthcare consumers and their families.

Stay Current: *To read more about the IHI Triple Aim Initiative, including success stories, visit the organization's Web site at* **www.ihi.org/offerings/Initiatives/TripleAim/Pages/default.aspx**.

▶ WHAT IS CARE COORDINATION?

Care coordination is the means by which a multidisciplinary team of healthcare providers works with a client to ensure that the care received across the healthcare continuum meets the client's needs. Coordination takes place between a minimum of two people, the care coordinator and the healthcare consumer, or a multidisciplinary team and the consumer. The team approach requires one individual, usually the nurse, to serve as the lead coordinator.

Coordination of care is necessary for all clients. It is especially important to clients when a transition of care, such as discharge and transfer to another healthcare facility, is being planned, and for clients with chronic, complex illnesses that require multiple healthcare professionals to deliver a broad array of services. Uncoordinated care is apt to result in the delivery of fragmented services and may result in medical errors; unnecessary duplication of tests, services, and treatments; and the omission of necessary services. Coordinated care is necessary for the provision of safe, high-quality, and cost-effective outcomes.

The concept of coordination shares some similarities with **collaboration** (which is defined as two or more people working toward a common goal) in that coordination requires the nurse to interact with others on behalf of the client. In considering client care, however, two critical differences emerge between collaboration and coordination:

1. Coordination is initiated by the nurse; collaboration may be initiated by the client, a family member, or any member of the healthcare team.

2. Collaboration involves direct interaction with the client or other individual with whom one is collaborating; coordination of care may or may not involve direct client care and therefore may not require direct interaction with another individual. For example, the nurse may schedule examinations and therapies for the client or review the client's discharge plans.

▶ WHAT IS THE NURSE'S ROLE?

The nurse's role in care coordination is to advocate for the client and to coordinate all aspects of care to secure the client's well-being. The nurse plans the overall strategy to address the client's problems. The ANA (2012) has deemed client-centered care coordination a core professional standard and competency for all registered nurses. Clinical decision making and critical thinking skills are critical to the development of a well-coordinated care plan and its execution. The nurse's first step in coordination is to assess the client's medical needs holistically to ensure that they will be met and that the client's independence and quality of life will be maximized. Part of the initial and ongoing assessments is to determine the need for consultation with other providers who should be included in the care management team. Thorough, accurate nursing assessment is critical to care coordination and containment of costs. Incomplete or inaccurate assessment may adversely affect not only nursing care, but also care provided by other members of the healthcare team. This can result in a longer duration of illness or injury, increased complications, and, as a result, increased costs to both the client and the healthcare system.

Both actual and potential problems should be identified. The nurse is responsible for identifying potential challenges to care coordination and then ensuring that they are addressed during development of the care plan. The nurse must ensure that planned care follows standard protocols or critical pathways and evidence-based guidelines. After evaluating the client's care needs, the nurse organizes the components of care required and develops the nursing care plan in consultation with the client. This plan serves as the nurse's framework for care coordination.

The nurse who is responsible for care coordination implements the plan with the assistance of the care team. The nurse initiates consultation, recognizes the needs for referral, and obtains necessary orders. As consultations and referrals are implemented, the care coordinator identifies what documents to provide to the those who will be providing care to the client. On an ongoing basis, the nurse must communicate with clients, family members, and all members of the care team to ensure that the plan is executed and continues to meet the client's needs. It is critical that the nurse coordinator monitor the execution of the plan and follow up with the client, family, and team members when adjustments are needed. The nurse revises the care plan as needed.

Changes in a client's condition and plans to discharge or transfer the client are automatic flags that the plan must be updated. The nurse is responsible for documenting the original care plan and any modifications. The nurse who serves as the care coordinator must be competent in assessing, planning, implementing, and evaluating care; have the ability to facilitate team and group activities; and have leadership qualities, including verbal and written communication skills, flexibility, ability to prioritize, complex decision making, and educational techniques.

SAFETY ALERT

It is always the nurse's responsibility to report any change in a client's condition. All nurses working with a client must follow their agency's protocols for reporting this essential information whether or not they are serving as the care coordinator.

Care coordination is an important tool in the prevention of readmissions. The Medicare Payment Advisory Commission (MEDPAC) states that about 12% of Medicare beneficiaries discharged from hospitals are later readmitted for a potentially preventable problem (*USA Today*, 2012). The ANA white paper (2012) on care coordination identifies the costs of uncoordinated care as 75% higher than those for coordinated care. Read-missions of people with Medicare coverage often occur among those who have been diagnosed with multiple chronic conditions. Readmissions are triggered by clients' lack of improvement or worsening health after discharge. With the increased recognition of nurses' importance to the care management process, CMS now allows reimbursement to nurse practitioners, clinical nurse specialists, and certified nurse midwives if, within 30 days of a client's discharge, they contact the client, visit the client in person, make decisions about the client's medical care, and coordinate the client's care (Advance for Nurses, 2012). The availability of this CMS reimbursement expands both career opportunities and the job market for nurses.

▶ BARRIERS TO EFFECTIVE CARE COORDINATION

Competent care coordination is essential to improving client outcomes and reducing healthcare costs. Barriers to successful care coordination include the following:

- *Client nonadherence to the care plan.* Clearly, when clients fail to adhere to aspects of the plan, they are at greater risk for recurrence or exacerbation of illness or injury.

- *Limited access to resources.* For clients, this may include distance from a clinical site or lack of access to transportation. Care coordination may also be adversely affected by a lack of healthcare resources. For example, if a foreign language interpreter is needed but is available only in the afternoons, that may affect the timing and frequency of appointments for some clients.

- *Deficient knowledge.* Clients and caregivers often fail to grasp certain concepts during the first teaching session. Providers and clinicians often fail to understand their roles and responsibilities in the interdisciplinary care team.

Because they are often the first and primary contact point for clients, nurses are in a key position to assess when barriers to care are affecting clients' care plans and health outcomes. This is true whether or not the nurse is serving as the care coordinator. Nursing interventions to counter these barriers include the following:

- *Assessing and addressing reasons for client nonadherence.* For example, if the client's transportation resources are limited, nurses can intervene by scheduling appointments at times more convenient for the client, networking to increase the client's resources for transportation, and communicating this barrier to the clinical settings serving the client.

- *Assessing availability of resources and incorporating this information into the care plan.* As soon as the nurse is aware of a resource barrier, the nurse communicates this to the care coordinator or interdisciplinary team in order to find and access the necessary resource. This may mean rescheduling an appointment, networking with another clinical site to obtain the resource, or advocating with the client's insurance company to cover the costs of a resource. For example, the physical therapist may report that the insurance company is unwilling to cover the cost of a specialized piece of equipment that will increase the client's safety. The nurse may need to advocate with the insurance company or find another source to cover the cost for this necessary equipment.

■ *Assessing and addressing knowledge deficits.* Sometimes clients require additional information to be able to implement discharge instructions appropriately. At other times, members of the healthcare team may lack important information about a client that may affect care, such as whether the client lost his job and no longer has health insurance, or whether a client who is a working mother also provides care for her older parent. Nurses improve care coordination when they communicate information that comes to them to all members of the healthcare team.

In conclusion, care coordination is an essential nursing role. Its importance is increasingly recognized as is the nurse's role in advocating for the healthcare client. The need for care coordination will continue to expand as the U.S. population ages. All nurses need to understand their role and continually educate themselves about the new tools, techniques, and systems that are available and will empower them to lead a multidisciplinary team, including the client, to provide the highest quality, most reliable, lowest cost, accessible health care available.

REVIEW Care Coordination

RELATE Link the Concepts and Exemplars

Linking the exemplar of care coordination with the concept of development:

1. How might care coordination differ for clients who are at differing stages of development?

2. Who might be included when coordinating care for a young child versus care for an older adult?

Linking the exemplar of care coordination with the concept of culture and diversity:

3. How does the diversity of clients affect care coordination?

4. How might the diversity of the healthcare team affect care coordination?

REFER Go to Pearson Nursing Student Resources nursing.pearsonhighered.com

- Additional review materials
- Additional case studies

REFLECT Case Study

Michel Goulian, 22 years old, experienced severe head trauma in a motor vehicle crash 2 months ago and has been hospitalized ever since. He has Broca aphasia and, as a result of damage to his frontal region, has difficulty putting words together to form complete sentences. This has also altered his personality, leaving him moody, temperamental, and prone to outbursts of frustration. Mr. Goulian's mobility is hampered by weakness in both legs and difficulty controlling movement. He has strong family support, and his parents want him to live with them until he is able to function independently. After discharge he will receive speech therapy, occupational therapy, and physical therapy. Social services has been involved in helping him pay for the cost of health care (he has no medical insurance) as well as in meeting his financial needs after discharge until he can return to his job. Dietary services would like to meet with both Mr. Goulian and his mother, who will be providing his meals, to help him meet his nutritional needs. Secondary to an extended need for mechanical ventilation, respiratory therapy is involved in Mr. Goulian's care and will facilitate home oxygen administration due to what is expected to be an extended need for maintenance of his tracheostomy.

1. How can the nurse facilitate this client's care, coordinating all of the different departments and team members involved?

2. How can care coordination help to reduce the cost of the client's care?

3. What complications might be anticipated if this client's care is inadequately coordinated?

EXEMPLAR 39.2 Cost-Effective Care

EXEMPLAR KEY TERMS
Diagnosis-related groups (DRGs), *2464*
Mandatory health insurance, *2463*
Private insurance, *2463*
Prospective payment system (PPS), *2465*
Public insurance, *2463*
Socialized insurance, *2463*
Socialized medicine, *2463*
Voluntary insurance, *2463*

EXEMPLAR LEARNING OUTCOMES
After reading about this exemplar, you will be able to:

1. Differentiate the various types of payment sources available in the United States.
2. Contrast the U.S. system of health care with the healthcare systems of other countries.
3. Summarize the challenges faced by the U.S. healthcare system.
4. Describe the nurse's role in creating a cost-conscious nursing practice.

▶ OVERVIEW

Between 1980 and 2004, despite efforts to control the costs of health care, healthcare spending grew faster than the economy (Stanton, 2005). However, a recent statement by Kathleen Sebelius, secretary of Health and Human Services, notes that the increase in health costs is slowing:

> For years, health care costs have been rising faster than inflation, driving up the cost of health care and making

it less affordable for families and businesses. But now, the good news about the slowing growth of health care spending nationwide is being increasingly recognized by independent analysts. . . . *USA Today* reported that according to the newspaper's own analysis that "health care spending last year rose at one of the lowest rates in a half-century." According to the paper, healthcare providers and analysts found that "cost-saving measures under the healthcare law appear to be keeping medical prices flat" (Sebelius, 2013).

Employers, legislators, insurers, and healthcare providers continue to collaborate in efforts to resolve the issues surrounding how to best finance healthcare costs. Among these efforts, the United States has implemented several cost-containment strategies, including health promotion and illness prevention activities, managed care systems including care coordination, and alternative insurance delivery systems.

▶ PAYMENT SOURCES IN THE UNITED STATES

Payment for healthcare services in the United States may come from one or more of several sources. For example, an older client may have Medicare and supplemental healthcare coverage purchased from a private insurance company and, if this combination does not cover all costs, the client's own money. Insurance is often classified as **public insurance** (insurance financed by the government) or **private insurance** (insurance provided by private or publicly owned companies such as Blue Cross Blue Shield, Kaiser Permanente, or Aetna). Many insurance plans, public or private, include a per-visit or per-prescription copayment and a deductible. Medical payment sources in the United Sources are discussed in detail in the module on Health Policy.

▶ THE INTERNATIONAL PERSPECTIVE

Values and attitudes (e.g., toward the government's role in private lives) are factors that influence the development of healthcare systems and policies. Outside the United States, most developed countries have similar values with regard to health care. **Table 39–1** ● contrasts U.S. values with those of other countries. Two relatively new trends are coming to the forefront in healthcare worldwide: consumerism and use of the Internet. The rise of consumerism reflects global education levels and communication; a corollary of this is a widening gap between the rich and the poor. The Internet has opened channels of communication without regard for national boundaries, and this feeds consumerism. However, few individuals in undeveloped countries have access to the communication and information that the Internet provides.

Healthcare systems throughout the world are in crisis. Most countries, regardless of their level of funding for health care, have run out of ways to finance their expenditures through tax-ation or other existing channels. All are realizing they must contain costs in the future. Furthermore, there is concern in western European nations, Canada, and Australia about the increased sophistication and resulting expectations of their emerging middle classes.

Each country's healthcare system is unique, but four categories can be identified regarding the organization and financing of health care. The first is **socialized medicine**, in which the state owns and controls healthcare services. Examples are the United Kingdom, Sweden, and Denmark, where physicians derive virtually all of their income from the government and have employment contracts with the state. **Socialized insurance** is a system in which all medically necessary services are covered, including physician care, hospital services, and to some extent, prescription drugs. Canada, France, and Australia have this form of healthcare payment. **Mandatory health insurance** is found in Germany and Japan, which have large, nonprofit health insurance organizations called "sickness funds." These sickness funds are usually organized around large employers or work-based associations. Government-sponsored programs cover citizens who are not part of a sickness fund. Everyone belongs to one of these two types of plans, thus ensuring universality. **Voluntary insurance** provides no guarantee of universality because coverage may be expensive and difficult to purchase. The Patient Protection and Affordable Care Act, signed into law in March 2010, is aimed at reducing coverage difficulties in the United States.

▶ FACTORS INFLUENCING THE PROVISION OF HEALTH CARE

A number of factors influence the provision of and access to health care, regardless of the types of coverage available. Economic factors such as supply versus demand and the inability to account for the actual cost of critical services (e.g., nursing) are just two of the factors influencing health care in the United States.

Supply Versus Demand

During the 1980s, an imbalance in supply and demand emerged as the cost of medical care began increasing faster than the gross national product and consumers came to expect that any and all services, regardless of the cost, should be available and paid for by third-party payers. As a result, the price of insurance coverage in the private sector skyrocketed, creating further imbalance.

TABLE 39–1 Comparison of Healthcare Values Between the United States and Other Developed Countries

UNITED STATES	OTHER DEVELOPED COUNTRIES
Pluralism and choice	Universality
Individual accountability	Equity
Ambivalence toward government	Acceptance of the role of government
Progress, innovation, and new technology	Skepticism about markets and competition
Volunteerism and communitarianism	Global budgets
Paranoia about monopoly	Rationing
Competition	Technology assessment and innovation control

Source: From Morrison, I. (2000). *Health care in the new millennium: Vision, values, and leadership* (pp. 2–5). San Francisco, CA: Jossey-Bass.

Today, many employers cannot or will not cover employees at the levels previously provided. Most employers now require employees to pay a far greater portion of the cost of insurance in the form of premiums. Others do not provide health insurance coverage at all. These changes have resulted in a diminished ability of all consumers to afford care, yet many continue to expect care on demand. Healthcare economics cannot supply health care at a level demanded by the public (Hoffman, 2013; National Institute for Health Care Reform, 2011).

When there is an imbalance in supply and demand, rationing of health care may result. No country can afford to provide unlimited amounts of medical services to everyone, and each nation must decide how to ration, or limit access to, healthcare services. This can happen in two ways. The first is by having the government set limits. In this approach, the cost of services is kept low, and people wait for availability. This type of rationing has been used in industrialized countries such as Great Britain and Canada. Scarce services are kept at a reasonable cost but are allocated according to particular criteria, such as age or a waiting list. Even in these countries, however, individuals who can pay for more services have access to more services. In the United States, only Oregon has suggested such an approach. The Oregon legislature enacted a program to limit access to expensive procedures, such as transplants, and then increase Medicaid eligibility to a larger number of low-income people. The second approach is to ration by ability to pay. This limits demand for more expensive procedures by offering them only to those who are willing and able to pay out of pocket or who have sufficient health insurance coverage (Hoffman, 2013).

There are important differences between these rationing methods. One is the freedom of the individual to choose the amount and type of health care used and to select who should deliver it. This has been a traditional value of healthcare consumers in the United States. Under a system of strict government rationing, a client cannot purchase a service unless it has been made available to everyone by the government. Under a method using ability to pay, a consumer can spend as much as he or she can afford. For those who cannot afford it, however, that service is not an option, no matter how great the individual's need.

Separate Billing for Nursing Services

Bills submitted to third-party payers and consumers from healthcare organizations (e.g., hospitals) continue to bundle nursing services with flat daily charges (e.g., the cost of the room and housekeeping). The specific cost of nursing has neither been separated out nor given a dollar value. This has hindered the ability of nurses to receive payment from third-party payers. Many nursing leaders think that for nursing to be a profession, nursing services must be accounted for separately from flat room fees to the healthcare institution.

Several developments within nursing have provided ways of quantifying nursing care. Some of the better known projects have resulted in nursing diagnoses that can be used to categorize nursing interventions: the NANDA International (NANDA-I) diagnoses, the Nursing Interventions Classification (NIC), and the Nursing Outcomes Classification (NOC).

A recent example is the development of payment codes for care coordination.

▶ COST-CONTAINMENT STRATEGIES

A number of strategies have been developed in an attempt to contain healthcare costs. Some of the main cost-containment strategies are competition, price controls, alternative insurance delivery systems, managed care, health promotion and illness prevention, alternative care providers, and vertically integrated health service organizations. The Affordable Care Act (ACA), the most expansive healthcare legislation passed since the Medicare Act, was enacted in 2010. The ACA includes many cost-containment strategies such as improvement of the quality of care provided, redesign of healthcare delivery systems, appropriate payment for services provided, modernization of the financial systems used to pay for services, and the elimination of fraud and abuse. Not only do many of the measures enacted as part of the ACA reduce the cost of care but they also improve its quality. Examples include payment penalties to give hospitals the incentive to prevent hospital readmissions and healthcare-associated conditions such as bed sores and infections; provision of care by healthcare teams rather than by individual providers, which increases care coordination; and reducing the provision of medically unnecessary services, which can be detrimental to a client's health.

Competition

During the 1970s, regulations in the United States were changed to permit competition among agencies that deliver health care and provide insurance. Currently, there appears to be little reduction in costs that can be attributed to competition. Competition has, however, led to the establishment of walk-in clinics, urgent care clinics, and alternative healthcare providers (such as advanced registered nurse practitioners), all of which offer additional care choices for clients.

Price Controls

Price controls for healthcare services have been established in various ways. Freezes on physicians' fees have been imposed at various times for short periods and, as mentioned previously, many states limit reimbursement to physicians and hospitals for services provided to Medicaid clients.

Group self-insurance plans are another means to reduce costs. These plans are created for a designated group, such as employees in a large company, a group of companies, or a union. The designated group then assumes all or part of the costs of health care for its members. It can often provide coverage at a lower cost than insurance companies because they are exempt from certain taxes and fees.

The passage of the Tax Equity and Fiscal Responsibility Act (TEFRA) in 1982 brought about a dramatic restructuring of healthcare delivery in the United States. Through this act, the federal government changed the payment method for Medicare from a retrospective system to a prospective one. This legislation limits the amount paid to hospitals that are reimbursed by Medicare. Using a system of **diagnosis-related groups (DRGs)**, a hospital is paid a predetermined amount for clients with a specific diagnosis. For example, a hospital that admits a client with a diagnosis of myocardial infarction is reimbursed for a specific dollar amount, regardless of the cost of services, the length of stay, or the acuity or complexity of the client's illness.

Before the DRG system, hospitals billed retrospectively—that is, after services were rendered. In contrast, in a **prospective payment system (PPS)**, billing is determined before the client is ever admitted to the hospital. DRG rates are set in advance of the year during which they apply and are considered to be fixed unless major, uncontrollable events occur.

Unfortunately, this type of PPS may result in healthcare agencies choosing to withhold borderline necessary tests and procedures and shorten hospital stays, thus avoiding the expenditures a prolonged stay would generate. Such actions allow hospitals to keep their costs at or below the amount they are allowed to bill Medicare. Notable effects of these practices include the earlier discharge of clients, a decline in admissions, a rise in the number and type of outpatient services, and an increased focus on the costs of care. The earlier discharge of clients has led to an expansion of home care services and increased use of technology and specialists.

Cost-containment strategies have changed trends in healthcare delivery. Some results of these changes include emphasis on preventive care to reduce the incidence of illnesses, treatment in noninstitutional settings such as clinics or the client's home to avoid hospital and institutional placement unless absolutely necessary, and the use of best practices as documented in protocols and guidelines where available to ensure that the care provided is scientifically based.

Vertically Integrated Health Services Organizations

Before the 1970s, very little home care was provided. In the current healthcare environment, new organizations have emerged and new relationships between hospitals and physicians have been forged. The scope of care has widened to include wellness, ambulatory care, outpatient surgery, and home health services.

Two trends have contributed to this organizational change: the change in payment structures and the development of medical technology. As insurers became more concerned about the rising costs of health care during the 1970s, hospitals began to integrate horizontally to form multiple-hospital systems. By coordinating services within each system, hospitals were able to avoid duplication of services as well as underutilization of expensive equipment at multiple sites.

The move to vertical integration began as a result of changing Medicare payments for fixed-priced DRGs. As a result of this change, hospitals began to monitor discharge practices and lengths of stay. They realized that clients could be discharged earlier to other suitable settings, such as nursing homes and their own homes. Earlier discharges were more cost effective. At the same time, hospitals realized it would be advantageous for them to own or contract with agencies, such as home health, to provide this type of care. This vertical integration allowed hospitals to reduce inpatient costs and receive additional Medicare revenues.

Advances in medical technology also contributed to this move from a traditional inpatient hospitalization to an outpatient setting. The length of the hospital stay for many surgeries, such as cholecystectomies, hernia repairs, and some orthopedic surgeries, was once several days or more. New technologies now permit these same surgeries to be performed on an outpatient or ambulatory surgery basis. Such services are less costly.

Within the integrated system, the goal is to create a "seamless" system of client care, in which movement from service to service is coordinated and well organized. Such a plan could improve quality of care and outcomes while increasing client satisfaction and providing better control of costs through more efficient use of resources. If the system is efficient, it can decrease transaction costs and allow greater accountability.

▶ NURSING ECONOMICS

Quality of care and cost trade-offs in hospitals have dominated the literature of the past decade. Both consumers and healthcare professionals have expressed concerns about diminished quality of care resulting from cost constraints, early discharge, periodic nursing shortages, and increased use of UAPs. Determining the precise cost of nursing services is a major challenge for nursing. What are the exact costs of high-quality nursing care? How many nursing care hours are required for each DRG? What is the best skill mix—that is, ratio of RNs to LPNs to UAPs—on each hospital unit? Since 1983, many studies have been undertaken to determine the actual costs and the cost effectiveness of nursing care. Researchers have investigated such topics as the impact of nurse–physician collaboration; new cost-effective interventions; cost benefits of primary nursing, nurse practitioners, and nurse-midwives; and the cost effectiveness of home care. The quality of the nursing care of the future will rely on ongoing research.

Nursing Shortages

One factor that must be considered in discussing the economics of nursing in this country is the impact of nursing shortages. These shortages are cyclic in nature. Periods of acute shortage are followed by periods of adequate availability of nurses. The measure commonly used to indicate a shortage of nurses is the *nursing vacancy rate*, the percentage of unfilled positions for which an organization is recruiting.

When shortages occur, employers are forced compete for the same available pool of nurses and are forced to increase wages in order to be able to hire and retain staff. As employers fill positions and more nurses enter the workforce as a result of other factors, employers begin to slow down the rate at which they increase salaries and wages. Fluctuations in nursing salaries as a result of shortages add yet another challenge in the attempt to determine the actual costs of nursing.

The trends in health care during the past 20 years have added to the complexity of the problem. Because of the decrease in length of stay, clients have been sent home "sicker and quicker." Many services that were historically provided in the hospital are now routinely done in a skilled nursing facility, an outpatient facility, or in the client's home. The proportion of nurses to nonnurses working in locations that provide direct nursing care has decreased in recent years. Some of this reduction is due to hospitals' cutting nursing staff and replacing them with UAPs as a cost-containment measure. Another factor is the increasing demand for nurses to work in new roles; for example, nurses leave the bedside to provide utilization and case management services for cost-containment companies. As a result of these reductions in nursing staff, some nurses, feeling they could no longer provide quality health care, experienced disillusionment and left the profession.

Ending the cycle of nursing shortages will require some adjustment to the approaches used by employers and nurses. New opportunities and new roles for nurses may attract more people into the profession. As RNs perform more highly valued functions, administrators in healthcare organizations will respect and value them more highly.

Cost-Conscious Nursing Practice

All nurses must be concerned about the cost of health care to ensure a viable healthcare system in the future (Hassmiller, 2010). Today the nursing budget can account for as much as half of an organization's total expenses; therefore, nurses at all levels face significant pressure to become more cost conscious when budgeting, allocating resources, and controlling and monitoring expenditures (Finkler & Kovner, 2007). This level of financial accountability is new to the nursing profession and comes at a time when nursing must compete for limited resources with other departments within the organization. Consider the following: Whether nurses work in a hospital, a school, home health care, or another setting, they are increasingly required to participate in strategies to make care more cost effective. Initially, this may sound intimidating. However, it is critical to understand that many evidence-based nursing interventions that nurses perform daily assist with cost containment. For example, hand washing to reduce the risk of healthcare-acquired infections reduces costs, because these infections increase expenses for both individual clients and the healthcare setting. Similarly, nursing efforts to promote safety and improve quality also promote cost-conscious nursing practice.

While cost containment is an essential component of nursing practice, it does not negate the essential roles of nursing. Nurses in all settings must continue to advocate for care that meets the standards of best practice while trying to find new ways to contain costs.

◢ REVIEW **Cost-Effective Care**

RELATE Link the Concepts and Exemplars

Linking the exemplar of cost-effective care with the concept of health, wellness, and illness:

1. Explain how health promotion activities reduce the cost of care.

2. You are caring for an adolescent client who admits to smoking "a couple" of cigarettes per week. What impact would helping this client quit smoking have on the lifetime cost of his health care?

Linking the exemplar of cost-effective care with the concept of infection:

3. How does the cost of a healthcare-acquired infection impact the cost of a client's admission?

4. How does the cost of reducing the risk of healthcare-acquired infections compare to the cost of treating a client who contracts a healthcare-acquired infection?

REFER Go to Pearson Nursing Student Resources
nursing.pearsonhighered.com

- Additional review materials
- Additional case studies

REFLECT Case Study

A group of nurses work on an oncology unit with 30 beds, including a 6-bed, bone-marrow transplant unit. Each nurse is usually assigned four or five clients, depending on the acuity. Only nurses with advanced training are allowed to administer chemotherapy, so it is not uncommon to have one nurse assigned to be a medication nurse when many others are also working who have not yet attended or completed the chemotherapy certification course.

1. What actions could you, as a staff nurse on this unit, take to reduce the cost of providing care to these clients?

2. An automated medication distribution unit was recently purchased that allows nurses to receive medications after entering the client information without having to go to the pharmacy. Explain both the positive and the negative impacts on costs as a result of using this new equipment.

3. The hospital is considering replacing its 10-year-old x-ray machine with a newer model that uses less radiation and is completely digital, eliminating the need for film cartridges and making it easier for radiologists to read x-rays from computers in their offices or homes. However, the cost of the machine is very high. You are asked to join the committee that will make the decision about whether to purchase this equipment. What are the pros and cons of buying this new radiology equipment?

◢ EXEMPLAR 39.3 **Delegation**

EXEMPLAR KEY TERMS
Assignment, *2468*
Authority, *2468*
Delegate, *2467*
Delegation, *2467*
Delegator, *2467*
Overdelegation, *2472*
Reverse delegation, *2472*

EXEMPLAR LEARNING OUTCOMES
After completing this exemplar, you will be able to:

1. Describe the need for responsibility, accountability, and authority when delegating.

2. Contrast the terms *assignment* and *delegation.*

3. Distinguish how effective delegation benefits the delegator, the delegate, and the organization.

4. Summarize the delegation process and key behaviors when delegating tasks.

5. Differentiate the three types of assignment patterns and how each affects the effectiveness of delegation.

6. Examine obstacles that can impede effective delegation.

7. Explain the liability of delegation.

▶ OVERVIEW

Delegation is the transference of responsibility and authority for an activity to a competent individual. The **delegate** is the individual who assumes responsibility for the actual performance of the task or procedure. The **delegator** is the individual who assigns the task and retains accountability for the outcome.

Delegation is a tool that allows the delegator to devote more time to tasks that cannot be delegated. It also enhances the skills and abilities of the delegate, which builds self-esteem, promotes morale, and enhances teamwork and attainment of the organization's goals. In nursing, delegation refers to indirect care—the intended outcome is achieved through the work of someone supervised by the nurse—and involves defining the task, determining who can perform the task, describing the expectation, seeking agreement, monitoring performance, and providing feedback to the delegate regarding performance.

Delegation is a difficult leadership skill for nurses to learn (Weydt, 2010). Given the confusion over what tasks unlicensed assistive personnel (UAPs) can perform and those that are the unique purview of RNs, nurses may be reluctant to delegate. Never before, however, has delegation been as critical a skill for nurses to perfect as it is today, with the emphasis on doing more with less. Once nurses learn how to delegate, they will extend their ability to accomplish more by using others' help. Nurses working in health care today must delegate. Tools for successful delegation are listed in **Box 39–1** ●.

▶ PRINCIPLES OF DELEGATION

Registered nurses increasingly delegate components of nursing care to other healthcare workers, including other RNs and especially UAPs. An RN who delegates a task to another healthcare worker is accountable for selecting an appropriately skilled caregiver and for continually evaluating the care provided to the client by that caregiver.

Delegating to Other Nurses

Registered nurses may delegate to other RNs. Examples of nurses delegating to other nurses include the following:

- A charge nurse making assignments for a shift
- A nurse delegating certain care activities for an unstable client to another nurse. This may be done if another nurse is free and can accept the additional responsibility until the unstable client is stabilized or transferred.

For example, an RN may assign to a float RN an unstable client who has a high temperature and high blood pressure. Caring for an unstable client is within the RN scope of practice, so the RN accepting the assignment is responsible for completing the client's care safely, ethically, and competently.

Additionally, it may be appropriate to delegate specific interventions to a licensed practical nurse (LPN). In these cases, the registered nurse remains responsible for ensuring that the LPN completes the interventions correctly and appropriately.

When delegating to other nurses, the delegator must use critical thinking and professional judgment and must follow the **Five Rights of Delegation:**

1. **Right task.** Task is one that can be delegated for specific client
2. **Right circumstances.** Setting is appropriate and resources are available
3. **Right person.** Give the right task to the right delegate for the right client
4. **Right direction.** Describe objectives, limits, and expectations
5. **Right supervision.** Monitor, evaluate, give feedback, and intervene if necessary (ANA & National Council of State Boards of Nursing [NCSBN], 2006).

Delegating to Unlicensed Assistive Personnel

UAPs, who function as "nurse extenders," are identified by a variety of titles, including certified nursing aides/assistants, home health aides, client care technicians, orderlies, or surgical technicians. Each category and the individuals within it have diverse levels of training and experience. Nurses may delegate to UAPs because they are employees of the healthcare provider; nurses may not delegate to family members or friends of clients even if they provide personal care to the clients.

It is not possible to generate an exhaustive list of exactly which actions may or may not be delegated to UAPs. Examples of tasks that may and may not be delegated are given in **Box 39–2** ●.

Principles guiding the nurse's decision to delegate ensure the safety and quality of outcomes. These principles are listed in **Box 39–3** ●. Even if the task is one that may be delegated legally, the individual nurse must still determine whether the task can be delegated to a particular UAP for a specific client. (The unlicensed person may not delegate tasks to another person.) Once the decision has been made to delegate, the nurse must communicate clearly to the UAP and verify that the UAP understands the following:

- The specific tasks to be done for each client.
- When each task is to be done.
- The expected outcomes for each task, including parameters outside of which the unlicensed person must immediately report to the nurse (and any action that must urgently be taken).
- Who is available to serve as a resource if needed.
- When and in what format (written or verbal) a task report will be completed.

A specific task that can be delegated to one UAP may be inappropriate for a different UAP, depending on each one's

---

Box 39–1   Tools for Delegating Successfully

1. Know your state's nurse practice act and your facility's policies and procedures for delegating.
2. Delegate only tasks for which you have responsibility.
3. Transfer authority when you delegate responsibility.
4. Be sure you follow state regulations, job descriptions, and agency policies when delegating.
5. Follow the delegation process and key behaviors for delegating.
6. Accept delegation when you are clear about the task, time frame, reporting requirements, and other expectations.
7. Confront your fears about delegation; recognize those that are realistic and those that are not.

Box 39–2 Examples of Tasks That May and May Not Be Delegated to Unlicensed Assistive Personnel

TASKS THAT MAY BE DELEGATED TO UNLICENSED ASSISTIVE PERSONNEL

- Taking vital signs
- Measuring and recording intake and output
- Client transfers and ambulation
- Postmortem care
- Bathing
- Feeding
- Gastrostomy feedings in established systems
- Attending to safety
- Weighing
- Performing simple dressing changes
- Suctioning chronic tracheostomies
- Performing basic life support (e.g., cardiopulmonary resuscitation)

TASKS THAT MAY NOT BE DELEGATED TO UNLICENSED ASSISTIVE PERSONNEL

- Assessment
- Interpreting data
- Making a nursing diagnosis
- Creating a nursing care plan
- Evaluating care effectiveness
- Care of invasive lines
- Administering parenteral medications
- Inserting nasogastric tubes
- Client education
- Performing triage
- Giving telephone advice

Box 39–3 Principles Used by the Nurse to Determine Delegation to Unlicensed Assistive Personnel

1. The nurse must assess the individual client before delegating tasks.
2. The client must be medically stable or in a chronic condition and not fragile.
3. The task must be considered routine for this client.
4. The task must not require a substantial amount of scientific knowledge or technical skill.
5. The task must be considered safe for this client.
6. The task must have a predictable outcome.
7. The nurse must know and understand the agency's procedures and policies about delegation.
8. The nurse must know the scope of practice and the customary knowledge, skills, and job description for each healthcare discipline represented on the team.
9. The nurse must be aware of individual variations in work abilities. Each individual has different experiences and may or may not be capable of performing every task cited in the job description.
10. The nurse, when unsure about an assistant's abilities to perform a task, must observe while the person performs it or must demonstrate it to the person and get a return demonstration before allowing the person to perform it independently.
11. The nurse must clarify reporting expectations to ensure the task is accomplished.
12. The nurse must create an atmosphere that fosters communication, teaching, and learning. For example, the nurse should encourage the UAP to ask questions, listen carefully to concerns, and make use of every opportunity to teach.

experience and individual skill sets. Also, a task that is appropriate for the UAP to perform with one client may be inappropriate with a different one, or with the same client under altered circumstances. For example, taking routine vital signs may be delegated to the UAP for a client who is in stable condition, but it would not be delegated for the same client who has become unstable.

SAFETY ALERT
Each nurse or other licensed or unlicensed healthcare provider is responsible for his or her own actions. Anyone who feels unqualified to perform a delegated task must decline to perform it.

Differentiating Delegation From Assignment

Delegation is often confused with work allocation or assignment. Delegation transfers both responsibility and **authority** (the right to act or to accomplish the task). In **assignment**, no transfer of authority occurs. Instead, assignments are bureaucratic functions that reflect job descriptions and client or organizational needs.

Too often, the principle of authority is neglected, and delegators hamper delegates from accomplishing tasks successfully, setting them up for failure.

Delegation Versus Dumping

Nurses delegate because it allows them to make the best use of their time; nurses must not delegate in order to dump an undesirable task on someone else nor to reward a productive employee with more work. Delegation should be practiced in a way that provides the greatest benefit to the client, makes the best use of the time of all staff members, and provides delegates with opportunities for growth. Delegation also requires that the delegate provide a clear, precise description of the task to be performed, including its objective, limits, and expectations.

▶ BENEFITS OF DELEGATION

The proper delegation of duties can benefit the nurse, the delegate, the manager, and the organization.

Benefits to the Nurse

By delegating some tasks to UAPs, the nurse is able to devote more time to those tasks that cannot be delegated, such as complex client care. For example, a nurse has three central line dressing changes to complete as well as two client transfers to another unit before the end of shift in 1 hour. The nurse may delegate the transfer duties to a UAP and complete the central line dressing changes herself. Thus, delegation improves client care, increases nurses' job satisfaction, and improves the organization's employee retention.

Benefits to the Delegate

Delegation allows delegates to gain new skills and abilities that can help them advance within a given organization or in their overall careers. In addition, delegation often brings with it trust and support, thereby helping build the self-esteem and confidence of the delegate. Subsequently, job satisfaction and motivation are enhanced as individuals feel stimulated by new challenges, morale improves, and a sense of pride and belonging develops, as does as greater awareness of responsibility. Individuals feel more appreciated and learn to appreciate the roles and responsibilities of others, increasing cooperation and enhancing teamwork.

Benefits to the Manager

Delegation also yields benefits for the manager. First, if nurses are delegating appropriately to UAPs, the manager's unit will function better. Also, the manager who appropriately delegates tasks to staff members is able to devote more time to management tasks that cannot be delegated. With the additional time gained by delegating, the manager will have an opportunity to develop new skills and abilities that will facilitate career advancement.

Benefits to the Organization

As teamwork improves, the organization benefits by achieving its goals more efficiently. As efficiency increases, the quality of care and client satisfaction improve. Overtime and absences decrease. Productivity increases, and the organization's financial position may improve.

▶ THE DELEGATION PROCESS

Nurses delegate only work for which they have responsibility and authority. These tasks include routine tasks, tasks for which the nurse does not have time, and tasks that have moved down in priority.

The delegation process has five steps:

1. Define the task.
2. Decide on the delegate.
3. Describe the task.
4. Reach agreement.
5. Monitor performance and provide feedback.

Defining the Task

To define the task, the nurse must consider some critical questions, including the following:

- Does the task involve technical skills or cognitive abilities?
- Are specific qualifications necessary?
- Is performance restricted by practice acts, standards, or job descriptions?
- How complex is the task?
- Is training or education required?

Certain tasks should never be delegated. Discipline of other employees, highly technical tasks, and complex client care tasks that require specific levels of licensure, certification, or training should not be delegated. Also, any situation that involves confidentiality or controversy should not be delegated to others.

Deciding on the Delegate

When delegating a task, the nurse should match the task to the individual. A rule of thumb is to delegate to the lowest person in the hierarchy who has the requisite capabilities and is allowed to do the task both legally and by organizational policy. This requires analyzing individuals' skill levels and abilities to evaluate their capability to perform a task. It also requires that the nurse consider what might prevent a delegate from accepting responsibility for the task.

The nurse who needs to delegate a task must also determine availability. For example, Su Ling might be the best candidate, but if she is leaving early or is not available, the nurse will need to consider other possible delegates.

Describing the Task

The next step in delegation is to clearly describe the expectations for the delegate and decide when to delegate the task. Attempting to delegate in the middle of a crisis is not delegation; that is directing. When delegating, the delegator must allow enough time to describe the task and expectations for completing it, as well as time to address the delegate's questions.

Key behaviors that nurses should use when delegating tasks include effective communication, motivation, and validation. Box 39–4 ● discusses these key behaviors in more detail.

Box 39–4 Key Behaviors When Delegating Tasks

Nurses who are delegating should:

- Describe the task using "I" statements (e.g., "I would like . . .") and appropriate nonverbal behaviors (e.g., open body language, face-to-face positioning, and eye contact). The delegate needs to know what is expected, when the task should be completed, and also where and how (if appropriate). More experienced delegates may be able to define for themselves the where and how. The nurse must decide whether written reports are necessary or if brief oral reports are sufficient. If written reports are required, the nurse should indicate whether tables, charts, or other graphics are necessary. The nurse should also be specific about reporting times. In client care tasks, it is also important to determine who has responsibility and authority to chart certain tasks: UAPs can enter vital signs, but if they observe changes in client status, the RN must investigate and chart his or her assessment.
- Describe the importance of the task to the organization, the delegator, the client, and the delegate.
- Clearly describe the expected outcome and the timeline for completion. Establish how closely the assignment will be supervised. Monitoring is important because the nurse remains accountable for the task. However, controls should never limit an individual's opportunity to grow.
- Identify any constraints on completing the task or any conditions that could change. For example, the nurse may ask an assistant to feed a client as long as the client is coherent and awake, but the nurse will feed the client if the client is confused.
- Validate the assistant's understanding of the task and its expectations by eliciting questions and providing feedback.

Reaching Agreement

After describing the task and its expectations, the delegator must be sure that the delegate agrees to accept responsibility and authority for the task. The delegator must also be prepared to equip the delegate to complete the task successfully. This might mean providing additional information or resources or informing others about the arrangement as needed to empower the delegate. Before meeting with the delegate, the delegator anticipates areas of negotiation and identifies what he or she must be prepared and able to provide. For example, when delegating to a CNA, a nurse might say, "Mrs. Campbell has hypertension and has been stable, but if her systolic blood pressure is greater than 140 or less than 110, or her diastolic is higher than 90 or less than 60, please let me know immediately. Can you measure these vital signs within the next 10 minutes?"

Monitoring Performance and Providing Feedback

Monitoring performance provides a mechanism for feedback and control. The nurse who is delegating a task must give careful thought to how tasks will be monitored to ensure that the agreed-to objectives are met. When delegating, one must be aware that monitoring a delegate too closely conveys distrust. When defining the task and expectations, the nurse must clearly establish the where, when, and how. This should give the delegate a sufficient basis for performing the task without close supervision. However, the nurse should remain accessible because the nurse's support will build confidence, reassure the delegate of the nurse's interest, and negate any concerns that the nurse is dumping undesirable tasks.

If problem areas are identified, the nurse should quietly investigate the problem and explain any concerns to the delegate. An opportunity for feedback from the delegate must be given. The nurse should instruct the delegate on how to prevent a mistake in the future. Equally important is giving praise and recognition for a job well done.

The following Clinical Example shows how a school nurse handled delegating medication administration.

CLINICAL EXAMPLE

Lisa Ford is a school nurse for a suburban school district. She has responsibility for three school buildings, including a middle school, a high school, and a vocational rehabilitation workshop for secondary students with mental and physical disabilities. Her management responsibilities include providing health services for 1,000 students, 60 faculty members, and 25 staff members and supervising two unlicensed school health aides and three special education health aides. The logistics of managing multiple school sites results in the delegation of many daily health room tasks, including medication administration, to the school-based health aides.

Nancy Andrews is an unlicensed health aide at the middle school. This is her first year as a health aide, and she has a limited background in health care. The nurse practice act in her state allows delegation of medication administration in the school setting. Lisa is responsible for training

Nancy to safely administer medication to students, documenting the training, evaluating Nancy's performance, and providing ongoing supervision. Part of Nancy's training will also include a discussion of those medication-related decisions that must be made by a registered nurse. To delegate medication administration to Nancy, Lisa must do the following:

- Understand the state nurse practice act and its applicability to the school setting.
- Implement school district policies related to health services and medication administration.
- Develop and implement an appropriate training program.
- Limit opportunities for error and decrease liability by ensuring that unlicensed health aides are appropriately trained to handle delegated tasks.
- Maintain documentation related to training and observation of medication administration by unlicensed staff.
- Audit medication administration records to ensure accuracy and completeness.
- Conduct several "drop-in" visits during the school year in order to track the competency of health aides.
- If necessary, report any medication errors to administration, and follow up with focused training and closer supervision.

▶ FACTORS AFFECTING DELEGATION

A number of factors may affect delegation, including organizational culture, assignment patterns, and the personal qualities of the participants. Resource availability, such as having sufficient staff to whom the nurse may delegate tasks, also affects delegation.

Assignment Patterns

Three assignment patterns affect delegation: unit based, pairing, and partnering. The unit-based approach assigns assistive personnel such as UAPs to serve everyone on the unit by working from a task list. Limited planning between the RNs and support staff is a feature of unit-based assignment patterns; consequently, there is no sense of teamwork. RNs frequently ask for assistance as needed. Their requests are made in a vacuum; that is, none of the nurses are aware of the demands being placed on the UAP by others, thus placing the assistant in the position of managing conflicting requests. This approach does not lend itself to effective delegation and causes dissatisfaction among both RNs and support staff.

A more effective means of delegation is pairing, the assignment of an RN, LPN, and/or UAP to work together as a team for a shift. Pairs are not scheduled to work together consistently; therefore, the team's composition varies from day to day. Pairs are able to plan care; team members identify priorities and plan each client's individual outcomes for the shift. Pairing increases satisfaction among team members and facilitates delegation.

Partnering is the best assignment pattern. It is the consistent scheduling of a set team, such as an RN, LPN, and/or nursing assistant, who always work together. This consistency creates healthy interpersonal relationships and increases trust. Each partner is able to anticipate the others' needs and expectations. Partnering is the ideal approach to delegation and increases employee satisfaction and, in turn, client satisfaction (Weydt, 2010).

Accepting Delegation

Before accepting a task, the delegate is responsible for making sure he understands it. This includes evaluating whether the delegate has the skills and abilities required to complete the task and the time to do it. If the delegate does not have the necessary skills, he must inform the delegator. However, this does not mean the delegate cannot accept the responsibility, provided that the delegator is willing to train or otherwise equip the delegate to do the task. A delegate who is unable to accept a task should thank the delegator for the offer and clearly explain why he or she must decline it.

Accepting delegation means accepting full responsibility for the outcome and its benefits or liabilities. Just as the delegator has the option to delegate parts of a task, the delegate also has the option to negotiate to perform only those aspects of a task that she feels skilled enough to accomplish. A delegate who is not qualified to do the task or does not have time should say no and explain why she must decline it.

After the delegate and delegator have agreed on the role and responsibilities, the delegate should clarify the time frame, feedback mechanisms, and other expectations. Delegates should not assume anything. At a minimum, they should repeat to the delegator their understanding of the task and all related requirements and expectations. Outlining the task in writing may be helpful.

Throughout the project, the delegate should keep the delegator informed of progress and report all concerns as they arise. Most important, the delegate should complete the task as agreed. This fosters trust with the delegator and demonstrates the delegate's dependability, signaling a readiness for increased responsibility and new opportunities.

Obstacles to Delegation

Delegation can yield many benefits, but it also has potential barriers. Some are environmental; others are the result of the delegator's or delegate's beliefs or inexperience (**Box 39–5** ●).

A NONSUPPORTIVE ENVIRONMENT Some environments do not support delegation. For example, the culture of an organization may, through rigid chains of command and autocratic leadership styles, restrict delegation. In this type of organizational culture, the norm is to do the work oneself because others are not viewed as capable or skilled. These types of environments promote an atmosphere of distrust as well as a poor tolerance for mistakes.

Lack of resources also inhibits delegation. For example, there may not be adequate staff to whom the nurse can delegate certain responsibilities. Consider the sole RN in a skilled nursing facility. If practice acts define a task as one that only an RN can perform, there is no one else to whom that nurse can delegate that task.

Financial constraints also can interfere with delegation. For instance, if someone from the department must attend the annual

---

Box 39–5 Delegation and Safety

Successful delegation can ensure client safety and improve health outcomes for clients. Unsuccessful delegation can result in unsafe situations for clients and has the potential to negatively impact client health. For example, when a client does not receive ambulation due to failure of nursing staff to follow through on this important client care activity, the client may be at increased risk for falls and for developing deep vein thromboses and pressure ulcers (Antony & Vidal, 2010).

Effective communication is communication that leaves no room for misunderstanding or misinterpretation. In *Nursing Process and Critical Thinking*, Judith M. Wilkinson suggests the following guidelines for ensuring effective communication that promotes client safety (Wilkinson, 2010, p. 369):

1. Set clear boundaries about what to do and what not to do.
2. Be specific in your request.
3. Indicate priorities.
4. Verify comprehension.
5. Identify and address any of the UAP's concerns.
6. Be courteous and respectful of the UAP.

Sources: Based on Anthony, M. K., & Vidal, K. (2010). Mindful communication: A novel approach to improving delegation and increasing patient safety. *Online Journal of Issues in Nursing*, 15(2), 2-2. doi:10.3912/OJIN. Vol15No2Man02; Wilkinson, J. M. (2007). *Nursing process and critical thinking* (4th ed.). Upper Saddle River, NJ: Pearson Education.

---

conference in a nursing specialty area but the organization will pay only the manager's travel and conference expenses, then no one else will be able to attend.

Educational resources may be another limiting factor. Others can learn how to do a task but only if the equipment and trainer are available.

Time resources can limit the ability to delegate as well. For example, suppose it is Friday, the schedule needs to be posted on Monday, and the nurse manager in charge of scheduling must leave town because of an unexpected family emergency. If no one on staff has been trained to develop the schedule, the schedule will not be posted or will be developed by someone who has not been trained to create it, thus leaving the unit open to the many problems that can result from poor scheduling.

DELEGATOR INSECURITY Delegators often feel insecure about delegation, because they remain accountable for the tasks involved. Fears that are common among delegators include the following:

- *Fear of competition and criticism.* Delegators fear losing respect and being outdone at their job. The delegator who selects the right task and matches it to the right individual has no need to fear either competition or criticism. In fact, the delegate's success provides evidence of the delegator's leadership and decision-making abilities.

- *Fear of liability.* Some liability risks are inherent in delegation, and related to the fear of liability is the fear of being blamed for the delegate's mistakes. If the delegator has followed the steps of delegation when selecting the task and the delegate, then the risks of liability can be minimized and the responsibility for any mistakes is solely that of the delegate.

- *Fear of loss of control.* Although this is a typical concern of inexperienced and insecure delegators, individuals who tend toward perfectionism and autocratic styles of leadership frequently experience it too. The key to retaining control is to clearly identify the task and expectations and then to monitor the delegate's progress and provide feedback.

- *Fear of overburdening others.* Delegators should not fear overburdening others, because delegation is a voluntary, contractual agreement. Acceptance of a delegated task indicates the delegate's availability and willingness to perform the task. Often, the delegate welcomes the diversion and stimulation and, although the delegator may perceive it as a burden, the delegate perceives it as a blessing.
- *Fear of decreased personal job satisfaction.* The type of tasks that may be delegated are those that are familiar and routine to a delegator. If one is able to delegate such tasks to others, then job satisfaction should increase because of increased opportunities to explore new challenges and gain other skills and abilities.

Additional barriers to delegation include inadequate organizational skills, such as poor time management, and inexperience with delegation.

AN UNWILLING DELEGATE   Inexperience and fear of failure can motivate a potential delegate to refuse a delegated task. Such delegates need much reassurance and support. In addition, the delegator needs to equip this delegate to be able to handle the task. If the delegator follows the proper selection criteria and the steps of delegation, then the delegate should not fail.

The delegator can boost the delegate's lack of confidence by building on simple tasks. The delegate needs to be reminded that everyone was inexperienced at one time. Another common concern is how mistakes will be handled. When describing the task, the delegator should provide clear guidelines for handling problems—guidelines that adhere to organizational policies.

Other barriers include individuals who avoid responsibility or are too dependent on others. Success breeds success; therefore, it is important to engage the individual in a simple task that guarantees success and recognize the individual's accomplishment when the task is finished.

Ineffective Delegation

When the steps of delegation are not followed or barriers remain unresolved, delegation is often ineffective. Ineffective delegation can also result from unnecessary duplication, underdelegation, reverse delegation, and overdelegation.

UNNECESSARY DUPLICATION   If staff are duplicating the work of others, related tasks may have been given to too many people (Weydt, 2010). To avoid unnecessary duplication, associated tasks should be delegated to as few people as possible. This allows the delegate to complete the assignment without spending time negotiating with others about which task should be done by which person. This also simplifies reporting for both the delegate and the delegator.

To prevent work duplication, ask the following:

- How often does staff duplicate an activity that someone else has recently performed?
- Why does this duplication occur, and is it necessary?
- What needs to done to prevent duplication?

UNDERDELEGATION   Underdelegation occurs in the following situations:

- The delegator fails to transfer full authority to the delegate.
- The delegator takes back responsibility for aspects of the task.
- The delegator fails to equip and direct the delegate.

As a result, the delegate is unable to complete the task, and the delegator must resume responsibility for its completion.

CLINICAL EXAMPLE

After completing Nancy's training (see the prior Clinical Example), Lisa gives her the authority to begin administering medications to the students in the school. During the first week of school, Nancy tries to "speed up" the medication administration process and sets out all of the noon medications in individual, unlabeled cups for the students. The cups are rearranged by students trying to find their medications, and Nancy cannot identify what meds belong to which students. Lisa is called back to the school to administer the correct medications, students are late to class, and Nancy is frustrated that she couldn't handle the task.

1. Which of the five steps of delegation did Lisa fail to follow?
2. Which step or steps did Nancy fail to follow?
3. What should Lisa do to prevent this situation from happening again?

REVERSE DELEGATION   In **reverse delegation**, someone with a lower rank delegates to someone with more authority. For example, a nurse practitioner in a burn unit arrives on the unit to find several clients whose dressing changes have not been completed due to a code situation earlier in the morning. An LPN ask the nurse practitioner to complete a few dressing changes to help the staff before physician rounds begin.

OVERDELEGATION   **Overdelegation** occurs when the delegator loses control of a situation by providing the delegate with too much authority or too much responsibility. This places the delegator in a risky position, increasing the potential for liability.

CLINICAL EXAMPLE

Ellen Neville, GN, is in her sixth week of orientation in the trauma ICU. Her mentor, Dolores Johns, RN, notes that Mr. Anderson is scheduled for an MRI off the unit. Dolores delegates to Ellen the task of escorting Mr. Anderson to the MRI unit. Ellen is not ACLS certified. During the MRI, Mr. Anderson is accidentally extubated and suffers respiratory and cardiac arrest. A code is called in the MRI suite, and ER nurses must respond, because an ACLS certified nurse is not with the client.

▶ **LIABILITY AND DELEGATION**

Fear of liability often keeps nurses from delegating. State nurse practice acts determine the legal parameters for practice, professional associations set practice standards, and organizational policy and job descriptions define delegation appropriate to the specific work setting.

Several guidelines can help. The American Nurses Association and the National Council of State Boards of Nursing (2006) have identified five rights of delegation, which were described earlier. In addition, the ANA and NCSBN (2006) have issued a joint statement on delegation to explain both the profession's practice guide-lines and the legal requirements for delegation. **Figure 39–1** ● shows a decision tree for delegation from the joint statement.

One situation that may present a challenge is when the staff receives written or verbal orders from a physician's office nurse. The same legal guidelines for the nurse giving the orders apply to the staff receiving them. If the nurse calling from the physician's office has a license that allows prescribing privileges, such as a nurse practitioner, the staff can accept appropriate orders from the physician's nurse. Otherwise, the orders must also be verified by the prescribing physician. The staff members put their own licenses in jeopardy if they do not obtain verification from the physician when necessary.

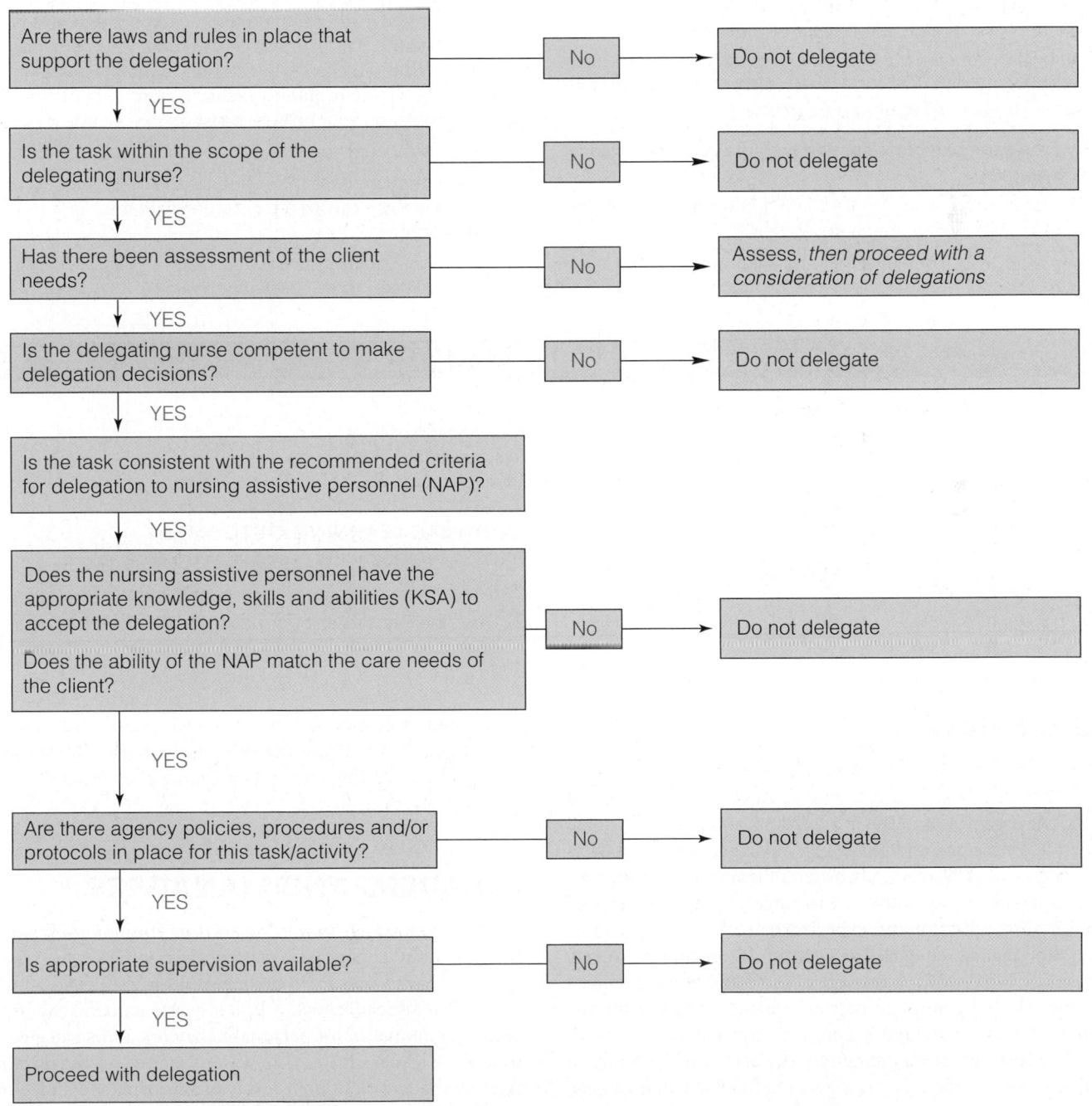

Figure 39–1 ● Decision tree for delegation to unlicensed assistive personnel.

Source: Adapted from American Nurses Association & National Council of State Boards of Nursing. (2006). *Joint statement on delegation.* Retrieved from http://www.ncsbn.org/Joint_statement.pdf.

◢ REVIEW **Delegation**

RELATE Link the Concepts and Exemplars

You are an RN working on a medical unit with two other RNs, a LPN, and two UAPs, and you receive a call informing you that two clients (both of whom are assigned to your care) must be transferred to another unit in order to make room for two clients who are to be admitted as soon as the rooms are ready.

Linking the exemplar of delegation with the concept of collaboration:

1. You delegate collection of a client's possessions in preparation for transfer to one of the UAPs, who says, "Why are you dumping this work on me? You do it." How would you manage this conflict?

2. The LPN working on the unit is a new graduate and has been employed for only 4 weeks. How would you collaborate with this nurse when delegating tasks for completion?

Linking the exemplar of delegation with the concept of teaching and learning:

3. How can you facilitate the new LPN's education in performing tasks that are commonly delegated?

4. How would you evaluate the LPN's learning related to delegated tasks?

REFER Go to Pearson Nursing Student Resources
nursing.pearsonhighered.com

- Additional review materials
- Additional case studies

REFLECT Case Study

You are working the night shift on a medical unit and have been assigned charge nurse responsibilities. You are working with four RNs, one LPN, and two UAPs. A client becomes pulseless and is not breathing, and the nurse assigned to the client's care calls a code. The nurse is occupied at this client's bedside for 1.5 hours until the resuscitation effort is completed and the client is transferred to the intensive care unit. This nurse also has four other assigned clients. In addition to the nurse assigned to care for the client requiring resuscitation, two of the other nurses working on your unit are assisting in the code.

1. What tasks could you delegate to the UAPs?

2. How will you maintain the safety of the other clients on your unit while three nurses are occupied with the client requiring resuscitation?

3. How might effective delegation to other team members contribute to care of the clients on the unit?

◢ EXEMPLAR 39.4 **Management Principles**

EXEMPLAR KEY TERMS
Accountability, *2476*
Authority, *2476*
Contingency planning, *2475*
Controlling, *2475*
Directing, *2475*
Effectiveness, *2477*
Efficiency, *2477*
Leader, *2474*
Manager, *2474*
Organizing, *2475*

Planning, *2475*
Productivity, *2477*
Responsibility, *2476*
Strategic planning, *2475*

EXEMPLAR LEARNING OUTCOMES
After reading about this exemplar, you will be able to:

1. Differentiate between managers and leaders.

2. Describe the duties of a manager based on management principles.

▶ OVERVIEW

Managers are essential to an organization's success. In any healthcare organization, a manager must balance the needs of clients, the organization itself, professional and nonprofessional staff and contractors, and self. Nurse managers need a body of knowledge and skills distinctly different from those needed for nursing practice. Frequently, new managers apply skills learned through observation of and experiences with former supervisors, who learned supervisory techniques on the job. A gap often exists between what managers know and what they need to know. This gap could be partially closed by increasing the number of nurses who hold BSNs (approximately 36% in 2008). The 2010 Institute of Medicine report (2011) on the future of nursing recommended setting a goal of 80% BSNs in the working workforce by 2020. A master's degree in nursing, with an emphasis on management, is increasingly being required for nurse managers to eliminate this gap in knowledge.

Today, all nurses are managers, not in the formal organizational sense but in practice. They direct the work of nonprofes-

sionals and professionals in order to achieve desired outcomes in client care. Acquiring the skills to be both a leader and a manager will help the nurse become more effective and successful in any position.

▶ LEADERS AND MANAGERS

The terms *manager, leader, supervisor,* and *administrator* are often used interchangeably, yet they are not the same. A **leader** is someone who uses interpersonal skills to influence others to accomplish a specific goal. A leader exerts influence by using a flexible combination of personal behaviors and strategies. For example, a leader creates connections among an organization's members to promote high levels of performance and quality outcomes. Leadership is discussed in detail in the module on Professional Behaviors.

A **manager**, in contrast, is an individual employed by an organization to accomplish its goals. An organization grants managers the required authority, responsibility, accountability, and power to get her or his job done. In addition, managers must use their own interpersonal skills to accomplish organizational goals. Managers coordinate and integrate resources using the functions of planning, organizing, staffing, directing, and controlling. The manager also use the subfunctions of supervising, evaluating, negotiating, and representing. A manager's job is to do the following:

- Clarify the organizational structure.
- Choose the means by which to achieve goals.
- Assign and coordinate tasks and develop and motivate staff as needed.
- Evaluate outcomes and provide feedback.

All good managers should be good leaders—the two go hand in hand. However, one may be a good manager of resources but lack the skills necessary to lead people. Likewise, an individual who is a good leader may not be a good manager. However, the skills required for both roles can be learned, thus maximizing a manager's ability to function.

▶ MANAGEMENT FUNCTIONS

In 1916, French industrialist Henri Fayol first described the functions of management as planning, organizing, directing, and controlling. These are still relevant today.

Planning

Planning is a four-stage process:

1. Establish objectives (goals).
2. Evaluate the present situation and predict future trends and events.
3. Formulate a planning statement (means).
4. Convert the plan into an action statement.

Planning is important on both organizational and personal levels. It may be an individual or group process that addresses the questions of what, why, where, when, how, and by whom. Decision making and problem solving are inherent in planning.

Organization-level plans, such as determining organizational structure and staffing or operational budgets, evolve from the mission, philosophy, and goals of the organization. The nurse manager plans and develops specific goals and objectives for his or her area of responsibility.

Planning can be strategic or contingent. A strategic plan defines the overall purpose and desired results of an organization and describes how those results will be achieved. Alternatively, a contingency plan helps an organization prepare for unplanned events and determine in advance how to respond to them.

Strategic planning refers to the process of continual assessment, planning, and evaluation to guide the future. Its purpose is to create an image of the desired future and design ways to make it a reality. For example, a nurse manager might be charged with developing a business plan to add a time-saving device to commonly used equipment, presenting the plan persuasively, and developing operational plans for implementation, such as acquiring devices and training staff.

Using **contingency planning** the manager identifies and manages unplanned and unexpected events that interfere with getting work done efficiently, effectively, and in a timely manner, that is, problems that interfere with the quality of care and service delivered to clients. Contingency planning may be done *reactively*, in response to a crisis, or *proactively*, in anticipation of problems or in response to opportunities. Proactive management is always preferable. Examples of these problems include the following:

- Two registered nurses call in sick for the 12-hour night shift.
- The manager of a specialty unit receives a call for an admission, but all of the unit's beds are taken.
- The manager of a pediatric oncology clinic discovers that a client's sibling exposed a number of other immunocompromised clients to chickenpox.

Planning for crises such as these are examples of contingency planning.

Organizing

Organizing is the process of coordinating the work to be done. Formally, it involves identifying the work of the organization, dividing the labor, developing the chain of command, and assigning authority. It is an ongoing process that systematically reviews the use of human and material resources. In health care, the mission, formal organizational structure, delivery systems, job descriptions, skill mix, and staffing patterns form the basis for the organization.

Directing

Directing is the process of getting the organization's work done. A manager's ability to direct is related to power, authority, and leadership style. Communication abilities, motivational techniques, and delegation skills are important also. In today's healthcare organizations, professional staff members are autonomous, requiring guidance rather than direction. The manager is more likely to sell the idea, proposal, or new project to staff members rather than tell them what to do. The manager coaches and counsels to achieve the organization's objectives. In fact, it may be the nurse who assumes the traditional directing role when working with unlicensed personnel.

Controlling

Controlling involves comparing actual results with projected results, similar to the evaluation step in the nursing process. Controlling includes establishing performance standards, determining how to measure performance, and creating the tools that will permit consistent measurement, performance evaluation, and the provision of feedback. The efficient manager constantly attempts to improve productivity by incorporating techniques of quality management, evaluating outcomes and performance, and instituting change as necessary.

Today, managers share many of the control functions with staff. In organizations using a formal quality improvement process, such as continuous quality improvement (CQI), staff members participate in and lead the CQI teams. Organizations are increasingly using peer review as a means of controlling quality of care and service. Peer review is the evaluation of results by team members of similar skills and competence to those who produced the work. This process is educational, not judgmental nor punitive. Peer review is a means for team members to hold each other accountable for the care and service they provide to the team's clients.

Planning, organizing, directing, and controlling reflect a systematic, proactive approach to management. This approach is used widely in all types of organizations, health care included.

CLINICAL EXAMPLE

Antonio Solana, the nurse manager of a home care agency, plans to establish an in-home phototherapy program, knowing that part of the agency's mission is to meet the healthcare needs of the childrearing family. To effectively implement this program, he would need to address the following:

- How the program supports the organization's mission
- Why the service would benefit the community and the organization
- Who the candidates for the program would be
- Who would provide the service
- How staffing would be accomplished
- How charges would be generated
- What those charges should be.

In organizing the home phototherapy project, Antonio develops job descriptions and protocols, determines how many positions are required, selects a vendor, and orders supplies.

In directing the home phototherapy project, Antonio assembles the team of nurses to provide the service, explains the purpose and constraints of the program, and allows the team members to decide how they will staff the project, giving guidance and direction when needed.

When Antonio introduces the home phototherapy program, the team of nurses involved in the program identifies standards for delivering phototherapy and develops a tool that will be used to objectively monitor team members' performance and the team's overall results. A subgroup of the team routinely reviews the monitoring results and, based on the outcomes, identifies ways to improve the program.

▶ PRINCIPLES OF MANAGEMENT

A manager has authority, accountability, and responsibility. **Authority** is defined as the right to direct other individuals and their activities. It is an integral component of managing. Authority is conveyed through leadership actions; it is determined largely by the situation, and it is always associated with responsibility and accountability. The manager must accept the authority granted.

Accountability is the ability and willingness to assume responsibility for one's actions and to accept the consequences of one's behavior. Accountability can be viewed as hierarchic, starting at the individual level, then the institutional or professional level, and finally the societal level. At the individual or client level, accountability is reflected in the nurse's ethical integrity. At the institutional level, it is reflected in the statement of philosophy and objectives of the nursing department

and nursing audits. At the professional level, it is reflected in standards of practice developed by national or provincial nursing associations. At the societal level, it is reflected in legislated nurse practice acts.

Responsibility is an obligation to meet objectives and perform tasks. Managers are responsible for the use of resources, communication to subordinates, and implementation of organizational goals and objectives.

Managing Resources

One of the greatest responsibilities of managers is their accountability for human, fiscal (financial), and material resources. Budgeting and determining variances between the actual and budgeted expenses are crucial skills for any manager. Allocation of resources is discussed in the module on Healthcare Systems.

Enhancing Employee Performance

Managers are responsible for ensuring that employees develop by identifying appropriate learning opportunities, whether through provision of in-service education, facilitating attendance at professional workshops and conventions, or encouraging achievement of advanced education such as higher degrees or certifications. The nurse manager who empowers other nurses by providing information, support, resources, and opportunities to participate will find that those nurses have greater commitment to the institution, are more effective in their role, have increased self-esteem, and are better able to meet their goals and the institution's goals.

Building and Managing Teams

The manager is responsible for building and managing the work team. A manager who is familiar with the group process will be able to lead the group in a manner that promotes its development into an effective work team. The term *group process* is used to summarize how a group works together to complete tasks. One of the elements of the group process is that all team members must understand the team's purpose and their own individual roles, as well as those of other team members. Another element is the importance of each team member feeling that his or her contributions are recognized by the manager and other team members. Good communication within the team is an element too. Effective communication promotes good personal relationships among team members and fosters a common understanding of the team's purpose, barriers faced, and opportunities for improvement. A healthcare team often consists of nurses, physicians, therapists, and unlicensed personnel who have different training and backgrounds. These individuals do not share the same vocabularies or medical knowledge, which can hamper communication. To promote client safety during a *critical* client situation, the nurse manager should adopt and train staff to use a standardized communication technique such as **SBAR**:

Situation
Background
Assessment
Recommendation.

Using such a technique, during hand-offs, transfers, and shift changes, will reduce miscommunications that have the potential to cause client harm (IHI, 2011). Improving communication skills among team members overall and specifically in critical clinical situations, will help the nurse manager and the team improve client safety and, in turn, team satisfaction.

Stay Current: *Learn more about the SBAR technique by visiting the Web site of the Institute for Healthcare Improvement to read the article titled "SBAR Technique for Communication: A Situational Briefing Model":* **www.ihi.org/knowledge/Pages/Tools/SBARTechniqueforCommunicationASituationalBriefingModel.aspx**.

Evaluating the group's work is another responsibility of the manager. Effectiveness, efficiency, and productivity are three outcome measures that are frequently used. In health care, **effectiveness** is providing services based on scientific knowledge to all who could benefit and refraining from providing services to those not likely to benefit (avoiding overuse and underuse). **Efficiency** is avoiding waste, in particular waste of equipment, supplies, ideas and energy used to provide nursing services. In nursing, **productivity** is a performance measure of both the effectiveness and efficiency of nursing care. Productivity is frequently measured by the amount of nursing resources used per client or in terms of required versus actual hours of care provided.

Managing Conflict

Nurse managers are frequently in a position to manage conflict between individuals and among groups or teams. Conflicts may arise from differing values, philosophies, or personalities. In health care, it can also arise due to competition for resources.

A nurse can use any of the available methods for managing conflict, each of which has its advantages and disadvantages (see the exemplar on Conflict Resolution in the module on Collaboration). The new nurse manager may require training to become proficient in the use of these methods.

Managing Time

The effective nurse manager uses time effectively and assists others to do the same. Many factors inhibit good use of time such as preference for doing things the nurse likes before things the nurse prefers not to do, emergencies or crises that divert one's attention, and unrealistic demands from others. Strategies that the manager, and all nurses, can use in order to use time efficiently involve setting goals and then priorities, with urgent tasks prioritized first; delegating; eliminating workspace clutter, for example, minimizing paperwork and automating whenever possible; and learning to say "no"; using regular schedules that avoid interruptions and setting time limits on activities; and striving to achieve balance (Hackworth, 2008).

REVIEW Management Principles

RELATE Link the Concepts and Exemplars

Linking the exemplar of management principles with the concept of quality improvement:

1. How does the principle of accountability impact the quality improvement process?

2. How does the nurse manager's role in enhancing employee performance impact an organization's quality improvement process?

Linking the exemplar of management principles with the concept of safety:

3. How does the nurse manager's creation of an effective team affect client safety?

4. What is the nurse manager's role in improving communication at the time of client hand-offs to promote client safety.

REFER Go to Pearson Nursing Student Resources nursing.pearsonhighered.com

- Additional review materials
- Additional case studies

REFLECT Case Study

Taylor Bradakis, a newly graduated nurse, accepts a position working in a small community hospital on the medical/surgical unit. The unit has 32 beds. Taylor works the night shift with two RNs, two LPN/LVNs, and two nursing assistants. After a few months Taylor is surprised to notice how often staff members sit and complain about their nurse manager during their free time. The staff members describe the manager as "uncaring" and report that whenever they take a problem to her, she always responds by asking, "How do you suggest correcting this problem?"

1. Why might the nurse manager ask for the staff nurses' input when they report a problem? Is this an effective approach?

2. What is Taylor's best action when staff sit and complain about the manager?

3. You are elected to take the staff's concerns to the nurse manager. What will you say to the manager?

■ REFERENCES

Advance for Nurses. (2012, November 16). *Medicare reimbursement ruling is "major advancement for RNs."* Retrieved from http://nursing.advanceweb.com/News/National-News/Medicare-Reimbursement-Ruling-is-Major-Advancement-for-RNs-ANA-Says-2.aspx.

American Nurses Association (ANA). (2012). *The value of nursing care coordination—A white paper.* Retrieved from http://www.nursingworld.org/carecoordination-whitepaper.

American Nurses Association (ANA) & National Council of State Boards of Nursing (NCSBN). (2006). *Joint statement on delegation.* Retrieved from https://www.ncsbn.org/Joint_statement.pdf.

Anthony, M. K., & Vidal, K. (2010). Mindful communication: A novel approach to improving delegation and increasing patient safety. *Online Journal of Issues in Nursing, 15*(2), 2-2. doi:10.3912/OJIN.Vol15No2Man02.

Finkler, S. A., & Kovner, C. T. (2007). *Financial management for nurse managers and executives* (3rd ed.). St. Louis, MO: Saunders.

Hackworth, T. (2008). Professional development: Time management for the nurse leader. *Critical Care, 3*(2), 10–11. Retrieved from http://www.nursingcenter.com/lnc/static?pageid=800374.

Hassmiller, S. (2010). Nursing's role in healthcare reform. *American Nurse Today, 5*(9). Retrieved from http://www.americannursetoday.com/article.aspx?id=7086.

Hoffman, B. (2013, January 18). Health care rationing is nothing new [excerpt]. *Scientific American*. Retrieved from http://www.scientificamerican.com/article.cfm?id=health-care-rationing-is.

Institute for Healthcare Improvement. (2011). *SBAR technique for communication: A situational briefing model*. Retrieved from http://www.ihi.org/knowledge/Pages/Tools/SBARTechniqueforCommunicationASituational-BriefingModel.aspx.

Institute for Healthcare Improvement. (2013). *IHI Triple Aim initiative*. Retrieved from http://www.ihi.org/offerings/Initiatives/TripleAim/Pages/default.aspx.

Institute of Medicine (IOM). (2011). *The future of nursing: Leading change and advancing health*. Washington, DC: National Academies Press.

Mitchell, P. H. (2012). *Nurse staffing—A summary of current research, opinion, and policy*. Pullman, WA:

William D. Ruckelshaus Center, Washington State University. Retrieved from http://www.ruckelshauscenter.wsu.edu/projects/documents/NurseStaffingfinal.pdf.

National Institute for Health Care Reform. (2011). *Matching supply to demand: Addressing the U.S. primary care workforce shortage*. Retrieved from http://www.nihcr.org/PCP_Workforce.

Plawecki, L. H., & Amrhein, D. W. (2010). A question of delegation: Unlicensed assistive personnel and the professional nurse. *Journal of Gerontological Nursing, 36*(8), 18–21. doi:10.3928/00989134-20100712-01.

Sebelius, K. (2013). Good news on health care spending. *HealthCare.gov*. Retrieved from http://www.healthcare.gov/blog/2013/03/health-care-spending.html.

Stanton, M. W. (2005). *The high concentration of U.S. health care expenditures*. Rockville, MD: Agency for Healthcare Research and Quality.

Twigg, D., Duffield, C., Thompson, P. L., & Rapley, P. (2010). The impact of nurses on patient morbidity and mortality—The need for a policy change in response to the nursing shortage. *Australian Health Review, 34*(3), 312–316. Retrieved from http://www.ncbi.nlm.nih.gov/pubmed/20797363.

USA Today. (2012). Hospitals to be fined for readmitted patients. Retrieved from http://www.usatoday.com/story/money/business/2012/09/30/medicare-fines-over-hospitals-readmitted-patients/1603827.

Weydt, A. (2010). Developing delegation skills. *Online Journal of Issues in Nursing, 15*(2). Retrieved from http://www.nursingworld.org/MainMenuCategories/ANAMarketplace/ANAPeriodicals/OJIN/TableofContents/Vol152010/No2May2010/DelegationSkills.html.

Wilkinson, J. M. (2007). *Nursing process and critical thinking* (4th ed.). Upper Saddle River, NJ: Pearson Education.

Pearson Nursing Student Resources   Find additional review materials at: **nursing.pearsonhighered.com**

40 Professional Behaviors

MODULE AT-A-GLANCE

The Concept of Professional Behaviors, 2479

Exemplar 40.1
Commitment to Profession, 2486

Exemplar 40.2
Leadership Principles, 2489

Exemplar 40.3
Work Ethic, 2491

◪ THE CONCEPT OF PROFESSIONAL BEHAVIORS

Nurses hold the public's trust. In Gallup's annual survey of professions released on December 5, 2012, 85% of Americans call nurses' honesty and ethical standards either high or very high (Newport, 2013). Nurses have topped Gallup's honesty and ethics ranking survey every year but one since being added to the list in 1999, and nursing continues to be the most well-respected of 21 professions. At a time when health care is in turmoil, this is a remarkable accomplishment.

Nurses are visible and present across the continuum of healthcare services, advocating for and caring for clients through the many facets of health prevention, education, maintenance, and restoration. Nurses may be found in diverse healthcare settings, including, but not limited to, acute hospital settings, clinics, public health departments, private practice, hospice centers, birthing centers, schools, pharmacies, and doctors' offices. Nursing care extends beyond the confines of institutions and facilities, occurring in parish ministries, on military bases and in mobile field hospitals, at children's camps, at community health fairs, at motor vehicle crashes by emergency flight nurses, at places of employment in corporate health clinics, and in clients' homes. Nurse educators and researchers practice in colleges and universities and in clinical settings. Nurses are accessible 24 hours a day in the acute setting and may also be available via telehealth lines. Given that they interface routinely with the community in health and wellness, in sickness, at work, at school, or at recreation sites, is it any wonder that nurses have secured trust in the community?

The first step in fostering trust is to be present and engaged. How then does the nursing profession, with such a large and varied practice arena, define professional behaviors for nurses? **≪**

Concept Learning Outcomes

After reading about this concept, you will be able to:

1. Connect professional behaviors to the development of trust in the nurse.
2. Provide examples of how the nurse uses professional behaviors to meet the primary responsibility of nursing.
3. Explore nursing behaviors that demonstrate professionalism.
4. Describe professional behaviors based on the ANA Code of Ethics.
5. Compare and contrast organizational commitment and professional commitment.
6. Provide examples of behaviors that may be interpreted as sexual harassment and strategies to avoid them.

Concept Key Terms

Abuse of power, *2483*
Compassion, *2483*
Formation, *2480*

Integrity, *2483*
Professional behaviors, *2480*

▶ COMPONENTS OF PROFESSIONALISM IN NURSING

Upon receiving their licenses, members of the profession of nursing commit to a fundamental social contract that sets rules to guide the professional conduct of licensed registered nurses (Lachman, 2009). The American Nurses Association (ANA) publishes the *Code of Ethics for Nurses With Interpretive Statements* (2001), which details the expectations for the professional nurse. Codes of ethics are discussed in more detail in the modules on Ethics and Accountability.

Benner et al. (2010) define **professional behaviors** as effective nursing actions that form helping relationships based on technical knowledge and expertise. These actions are also based on ethical principles and clinical reasoning. By following the provisions set forth by the ANA (2001), nurses nurture trust and inspire the confidence of the individuals they serve.

The concept of professional behaviors is related to all other concepts (see Concepts Related to Professional Behaviors).

Professionalism

Traditionally, nursing education focused on aspects of socialization, role taking, and performance measures to develop professional behaviors for nursing students. Nurse experts now recommend that educators shift the focus of nursing education away from socialization to formation (Benner et al., 2010). The old model of socialization carries with it a long history of the tradition of subservient, dependent female roles and the acceptance of dominant behaviors for males. The shift to formation emphasizes individual development and actualization, inquiry, and empowerment. Recent research links empowerment of nurses to innovation. The need for innovation is pressing in a chaotic health environment and is very relevant to contemporary nursing.

As defined by Benner et al. (2012), **formation** is a process that facilitates the transformation of an individual from a lay person to a professional nurse. It is an evolutionary process that requires the acquisition of lifelong learning, experience, technical expertise, and interdependent professional collaboration. The resulting integration of the nurse's thought, feeling, behavior, education, experience, and ethical comportment contributes to the formation of a professional nurse. Transformation

Concepts Related to **Professional Behaviors**

CONCEPT	RELATIONSHIP TO PROFESSIONAL BEHAVIORS	NURSING IMPLICATIONS
Collaboration		
▪ Interdisciplinary teams and communication ▪ Conflict resolution ▪ Case management	Professional behaviors build trust and help prevent conflict.	▪ Respect the expertise of other nurses and healthcare team members, including those from different backgrounds and generations. ▪ Consult with healthcare team members to provide safe and effective individual client-centered care. ▪ Effectively facilitate the many aspects, procedures, and services provided to clients.
Communication		
▪ Assertive communication ▪ Groups and group communication ▪ Therapeutic communication ▪ Documentation ▪ Reporting	Professional behaviors promote reliability and accountability for information and the methods in which it is conveyed.	▪ A professional demeanor is essential to establish trust and rapport with clients and team members. ▪ Professional nurses ensure accurate and complete documentation and reporting, which decrease risks to client safety.
Ethics		
▪ Ethical dilemmas ▪ Patient rights	Professional behaviors support nurses in maintaining an ethical nursing practice.	▪ Understand and follow standards for professional nursing. ▪ Nursing integrity ensures that patients' rights are respected in the healthcare setting. ▪ Recognize sexual harassment, abuses of power, and other unprofessional behaviors that contradict and diminish ethical nursing practice. Know how to prevent and address these behaviors in the practice setting.

TABLE 40–1 Common Guidelines for Professional Attire and Demeanor

PROFESSIONAL DRESS	RATIONALE
No excessive jewelry, long fingernails or artificial nails, or chewing gum	May harbor pathogens and threaten client safety
Hair secured away from contact with the individual receiving care	Prevents contamination of sterile fields and spread of bacteria
Personal cleanliness, avoiding strong odors and perfumes	Prevents client discomfort and annoyance Instills client confidence and trust Shows respect for needs of allergic or nauseated clients
Clean uniform or clothing	Promotes good sanitation Builds client trust

PROFESSIONAL DEMEANOR	RATIONALE
Avoid loud talking	Respect for clients' need for rest
Maintain a positive attitude and instill hope	Encouragement and respect for clients and families
Maintain a clean, uncluttered workstation	Respect for peers
Avoid taking personal calls at work	Focus on client care
Do not discuss personal problems at work with clients	Maintenance of professional boundaries
Never breach client confidentiality	Avoidance of violation of HIPAA
Avoid gossiping or bullying coworkers	Maintenance of civility and client safety
Do not complain to clients or family members	Maintenance of professional boundaries
Do not use illegal substances	Self-respect and client safety

can occur only with personal commitment to self, individuals, the community, organizations, society, and the profession.

The work of Benner (1982) provided a foundation for and description of the development of professionalism in nursing. She outlined five levels through which nurses progress as they acquire skilled proficiency and professional behavior:

- **Novice.** No experience; relies on theory, guidelines, and policies. The novice lacks discretionary judgment and focuses energy on task performance.

- **Advanced beginner.** Some task and situational experience, but the focus is the task and rules with little ability to take the complexity of the situation into consideration.

- **Competent.** Actions are viewed in terms of long-term goals and feelings of mastery; the speed and flexibility of the proficient nurse are lacking.

- **Proficient.** Perceives the situation as a whole, rather than in parts; decision making is easier with a focus on the most important attributes and aspects of the problem.

- **Expert.** Has an intuitive grasp of the situation and readily zeros in on the problem and solution without spending much time problem solving.

All individuals have the right to their own thoughts, feelings, and perceptions. Actions, however, must meet accepted societal standards. We are all evaluated by how we communicate, behave, and dress. As a member of the profession of nursing, the individual nurse is always being observed and judged as a representative of that profession, even when off duty. How a nurse dresses, behaves, and communicates sets the stage for the development of trust or mistrust. Most healthcare employers provide employees with guidance and expectations for the proper attire and conduct. Although most facilities have specific policies,

those of one healthcare facility might not be relevant in another facility. However, there are commonly accepted guidelines about dress and professional appearance (see **Table 40–1** ●).

✳ Go to **nursing.pearsonhighered.com** to see a clinical example of professionalism.

Appearance also affects how others within the medical community see the nurse (**Figure 40–1** ●). It is a form of nonverbal communication that evokes a response from others. Imagine a nurse talking on a cell phone while approaching a doctor to question the validity of an order. Will the doctor have enough confidence in the nurse to accept the expressed concern and change the decision regarding the client's plan of care?

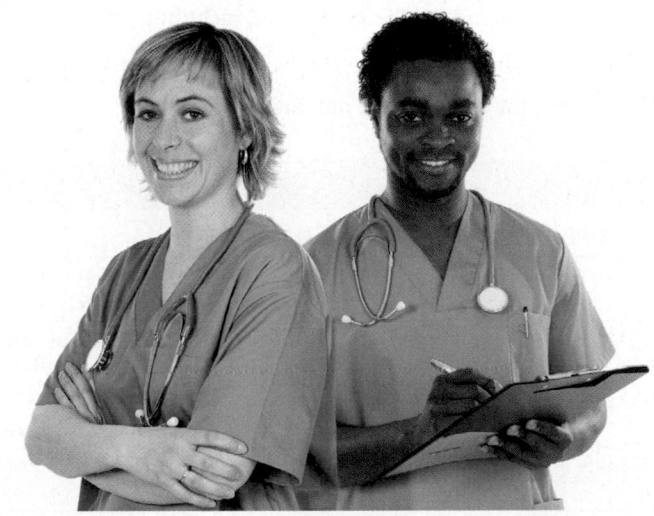

Figure 40–1 ● A professional appearance supports the nurse's credibility.
Source: Gelpi JM/Shutterstock.

Knowledge

Knowledge is central to providing high-quality care and maintaining client safety. Students are required to learn the information the entry-level practicing nurse needs to meet the minimum level of competence required for nursing practice. Learning all of this information is a daunting challenge. Nursing students must acquire knowledge of anatomy and physiology, biology, psychology, technology, group processes, and many other disciplines. Once licensed, nurses are expected to maintain and update their knowledge base throughout their career. Health care is changing constantly as new drugs enter the market every year, new treatments and technology are introduced, and ongoing research demonstrates the effectiveness of past information. If nurses do not participate in continuing education, their knowledge base quickly becomes obsolete, and their practice may even endanger clients.

The Institute of Medicine (IOM, 2010) recommendation for the future of nursing and the development of the profession is to increase by 80% the number of nurses with a BSN degree by the year 2020.

Competence

The expectation of competence begins when the student enrolls in a nursing program and continues throughout nursing practice, whether the nurse is caring for clients, managing a department, or acting in an advanced practice role. The nurse must learn how to operate new equipment before it is put into general use; maintain an evidenced-based practice that is current on the latest findings; and seek help from peers, mentors, and instructors to learn new skills and techniques. Each nurse is responsible for pinpointing his or her own areas of strength and weakness. Once an area of incompetence is identified, the nurse should seek opportunities to gain competence in that area. This self-examination is a necessary ingredient in the formation of a competent professional nurse.

Components of competence include the nurse's awareness of the factors, both positive and negative, that affect client care. The nurse must be competent in many areas, including the following:

■ Understanding the culture of the client and the facility

■ Knowing the ethics of the nursing profession

■ Being capable of assuming the many responsibilities of the nurse, including legal, professional, ethical, and client-centered roles

■ Knowing what procedures to follow when performing skills

■ Recognizing the client's need for individualized care

■ Maintaining proper documentation

■ Demonstrating the ability to show compassion for the needs of others

The faculty of the Quality and Safety Education for Nurses (QSEN) Institute and a National Advisory Board worked together to define the knowledge, skills, and attitudes necessary for the development of professionalism and the education of future nurses (Cronenwett et al., 2007). An overview of the pre-licensure competencies and definitions for action are presented in Table 40–2 ●.

Stay Current: *Resources and a complete description of the knowledge, skills, and attitudes that nurses require to maintain and improve their professional competence can be found on the QSEN Institute's Web site:* **http://qsen.org/competencies/pre-licensure-ksas/**

Each state's nurse practice act defines professional competence and outlines behaviors or actions that indicate incompetence or that may result in loss of licensure. It is important for nurses to know the requirements set forth in the nurse practice acts in their home state. For example, the North Carolina Components of Nursing Practice for the Registered Nurse (2002) defines competence as follows:

Accepting responsibility for self for individual nursing actions, competence, and behavior is the responsibility of the registered nurse, which includes:

1. having knowledge and understanding of the statutes and rules governing nursing;
2. functioning within the legal boundaries of registered nurse practice; and
3. respecting client rights and property, and the rights and property of others (NCBON, 2002).

The ANA's position statement on professional role competence is posted on the organization's Web site ("Professional

TABLE 40–2 Summary of QSEN Competencies and Definitions

COMPETENCY	DESCRIPTION
Patient-centered care	Nurses respect the client's autonomy regarding care decisions, assessing the client's experiences and preferences and enlisting the client's participation in care at every opportunity.
Teamwork and collaboration	Collaborative care is client centered, promotes communication among care providers, and optimizes resources to ensure safe, effective, efficient client care.
Evidence-based practice	Use of evidence-based practice ensures the nurse maintains a practice rooted in current research and incorporates client values and practices while ensuring client autonomy regarding health care decisions.
Quality improvement	By participating in quality improvement efforts, nurses analyze trends and processes that impact safe, effective client care.
Safety	Nurses are accountable for ensuring client safety at all times and in all settings. Nurses act to reduce risk and improve client outcomes.
Informatics	Nurses use information technology to maintain current, evidence-based practice; collect, record, and manage client health information; guard against errors; and plan and modify client care as appropriate.

Source: Based on QSEN Institute. (2013). *Competencies.* Retrieved from http://qsen.org/competencies/pre-licensure-ksas/

Role Competence," 2013). The Web site also provides access to a variety of resources and papers on the topics of professional collaboration, social networking, and nurse staffing, to mention only three. The ANA expects registered nurses to assume individual responsibility and accountability for their professional competence.

Teamwork

How to work as a member of the team is discussed in detail in the module on Collaboration. Skill in working as a team member contributes to others' opinions of the nurse as a professional and improves the quality of care delivered to the client.

✳ Go to *nursing.pearsonhighered.com* to see a clinical example of teamwork.

CASE STUDY \\ A

Caroline Nava is a 28-year-old nursing student enrolled in her final clinical rotation and due to graduate in 2 months. She is working on a surgical unit managing care for five individuals. Having completed her charting, she leaves the nursing unit 2 hours late. She is exhausted from a particularly busy clinical day and returns home. Just as she sits down to enjoy a little relaxation time, she remembers that she failed to obtain information from the chart of a new postoperative client. Earlier today, her instructor asked Caroline to report back to her about this individual's laboratory results by the end of the day. The client returned to the unit late from postanesthesia care, as Caroline was ready to leave.

Caroline begins to panic and is uncertain about what she is going to do. Suddenly, she remembers that her friend Joan McIntyre, another student, is in clinical on the same unit until late that evening. Caroline calls Joan and asks her for a favor. She explains to Joan that she is in a bind and has to call her nursing instructor with the information as soon as possible. Caroline asks Joan to take a picture with her cell phone of the laboratory results in the client's chart and to send her the picture. Joan is glad to be able to help her friend and successfully sends the information to Caroline. Caroline is able to contact her instructor with the necessary information about her client.

Critical Thinking Questions

1. Do you believe Caroline handled the situation ethically? Support your answer.
2. If you were Joan, what would you have done in this situation?

Integrity

Integrity is adherence to a strict moral or ethical code. Nurses adhere to the ANA Code of Ethics for Nurses (discussed in the module on Ethics). For nurses, integrity involves consistent behaviors based on the internalization of the values, ethics, and best pratices of the profession of nursing. Nurses demonstrate integrity by accepting feedback (positive or negative) as a tool for improving their delivery of client care, by maintaining accountability for their actions and freely admitting when they make mistakes, and by following their state's nurse practice act and never working outside their scope of practice.

✳ Go to *nursing.pearsonhighered.com* to see a clinical example of integrity.

Positive Attitude

The Via Christi Health System survey revealed that nurses themselves view a positive attitude as an essential component of professionalism (Via Christi Regional Medical Center, 2003). *Attitude* is a mental state involving values, beliefs, feelings, and mood. Each individual's attitude affects the individual and all others who are nearby. Professional behavior for the nurse includes maintaining a positive attitude while working with clients, their family members, and other healthcare professionals. A nurse with a positive attitude refrains from complaining and expresses an optimistic outlook. Attitude is discussed in greater detail in the exemplar on Work Ethic in this module.

Compassion

Compassion is an awareness of and concern about other individuals' suffering. Nurses demonstrate compassion when they recognize a client's need and respond appropriately to meet that need. In showing compassion, the nurse treats the client as a unique and special individual and not as a number or a diagnosis. The nurse further demonstrates compassion by advocating in the community and communicating with politicians to develop laws that protect and promote the health of individuals and families.

▶ UNPROFESSIONAL BEHAVIORS

Unprofessional behaviors undermine an individual's credibility and negatively affect group morale, and they may affect client outcomes. Unprofessional behaviors such as breach of confidentiality, as defined by state nursing practice acts, are discussed in the module on Legal Issues. Other unprofessional behaviors, such as substance abuse and discrimination, are discussed in other modules. Unprofessional behaviors such as excessive absenteeism and tardiness are discussed in the exemplar on Work Ethic in this module. It is important to recognize that the work environment sometimes carries over to social events, such as unit parties, company picnics, and informal gatherings. The rules of professionalism and the pitfalls of unprofessional behavior extend into these types of situations as well.

Abuses of Power

Any discussion of unprofessional behavior must include a discussion about abuses of power. An **abuse of power** is any attempt to use one's position or authority to shame, control, demean, humiliate, or denigrate another individual in order to gain emotional, psychological, or physical advantage over that individual. In any professional environment, including the nursing profession, abuses of power such as sexual harassment, improper use of authority, bullying, and intimidation must be addressed immediately and appropriately.

Evidence of bullying, lateral violence (violence directed toward peers), and incivility in the healthcare environment has been well documented in nursing research for over three decades. These behaviors are commonplace because of widespread toler-

Evidence-Based Practice Bullying and Disruptive Behavior in the Workplace

Problem

Bullying and disruptive behaviors in the healthcare environment were among the top three root causes of sentinel events in 2004–2012, according to The Joint Commission (2012).

Evidence

Over the past several decades, the phenomenon of disruptive behavior in the healthcare environment has been referred to as *lateral violence, incivility,* and a variety of other names. The existence of disruptive behavior is well documented in nursing research. Walrafen, Brewer, and Mulvenon (2012) describe disruptive behaviors as overly aggressive behaviors such as yelling, verbally dismissive and demeaning remarks, and the use of denigrating terms. Covert and overt actions are defined as verbal outbursts and physical threats as well as passive reluctance or refusal to answer questions, failure to return phone calls or pages, condescending language or voice intonation, and impatience with questions. A study of 600 nurses revealed that the majority of respondents (72.8%) had experienced nonphysical violence in the prior 12 months (Lanza, Zeiss, & Rierdan, 2006). Students and novice nurses are more vulnerable to bullying because of their lack of experience and power. In a study of 147 novice nurses, Berry et al. (2012) found that 72.6% of respondents reported a bullying event in the previous month. Workplace productivity was negatively affected by bullying, which reduced the novice nurses' ability to handle the cognitive demands of their workload.

Implications

The Insitute of Medicine (2010) has challenged nurses to lead the way to changing and improving quality, efficiency, and safety in the healthcare environment. Nurses must have good communication and conflict resolution skills in order to address bullying in the workplace and transform the healthcare environment in which they practice. The continued training of point-of-care nurses in assertiveness and leadership skill is necessary to effect a change.

Critical Thinking Application

Bullying is a threat to client safety and the emotional well-being of nurses. What measures might a student or novice nurse employ to address bullying by more experienced nurses in the healthcare setting? Gossip is a frequent form of bullying in the workplace. Describe a situation in which you may have observed or experienced incivility. Write down practical comments you would feel comfortable making to address the behavior in real time.

---

ance within the healthcare arena. Furthermore, the long history of a hierarchical or tiered power structure perpetuates the dominance and empowerment of unprofessional individuals. The Joint Commission (2012) has identified bullying behaviors and incivility in health care as being among the leading causes of sentinel client events. The Joint Commission calls for zero tolerance of intimidation and bullying in the workplace and recommends that healthcare facilities implement policies to stop such bullying. See the Evidence-Based Practice feature for more information.

SEXUAL HARASSMENT Sexual harassment is a violation of an individual's rights and a form of discrimination. In 1987, the law prohibiting sexual discrimination was clarified to apply to all educational and employment institutions receiving federal funding. The Equal Employment Opportunity Commission (EEOC) defines sexual harassment as "unwelcome sexual advances, requests for sexual favors, and other verbal or physical conduct of a sexual nature" occurring in the following circumstances (Code of Federal Regulations, 2001):

■ When submitting to such requests or behavior is considered, either explicitly or implicitly, a condition of an individual's employment

■ When submission to or rejection of such requests or behavior is used as the basis for employment decisions affecting the individual (e.g., promotion)

■ When such conduct interferes with an individual's work performance or creates an "intimidating, hostile, or offensive working environment"

In any of these cases, the victim or violator may be male or female; furthermore, the victim and violator may or may not be of opposite sexes.

Nurses must develop assertiveness skills to deal with any sexual harassment they encounter in the workplace. In addition, nurses must be familiar with the sexual harassment policy and procedures at the institution in which they work. These include information regarding the reporting procedure (including to whom incidents should be reported), the investigative process, and how confidentiality will be protected to the extent possible.

Nurses must use caution when providing client care to avoid having clients misinterpret nursing behaviors as sexual harassment. For example, in lifting a client's breast to bathe the chest or to place leads when performing an electrocardiogram, it is best to use the back of the hand rather than the palm of the hand. It is also important to explain the procedure and seek the client's permission. In this way the nurse can reduce the possibility of the action's being misinterpreted as sexual harassment and can avoid responses by the client that might tend toward sexual harassment of the nurse.

IMPROPER USE OF AUTHORITY Improper use of authority is widespread and has no place in the practice of nursing. Some nurses who, through use of their professional skills, have acquired administrative titles remove "Registered Nurse" from their title or name badge, perhaps in order to disassociate themselves from nursing's professional code of ethics. Once separated from the codes of ethical behaviors expected of nurses, bullies in administrative positions adopt a corporate rather than a professional demeanor and attitude. Such administrators serve their careers and no longer the priorities of client-centered care. They can be identified by an attitude of arrogance, control, and acceptance of the hierarchical power structure that oppresses and is condescending to the voice of nursing at the point of care.

A nursing manager may use intimidation to show favoritism, and to promote subordinate compliance, bias, and group pressure to exclude employees toward whom the manager has a less favorable attitude or who challenge the manager. Nurses in authority who emphasize principles over personality and who focus on client safety can extinguish these negative behaviors and encourage nurses at the point of care. Transformational leadership, which is discussed in the exemplar on Leadership Principles is recommended as the leadership style for facilitating progress and innovation in nursing.

CASE STUDY \\ B

Mary Reynolds, who is a nurse of the baby-boomer generation, disagrees with Ashley Maloney, a new graduate, about how Ms. Maloney handled a situation with a client's family. You overhear Ms. Reynolds telling a friend of hers that she hopes that Ms. Maloney never takes care of her or her family. You are on break, and Ms. Reynolds repeats to you her story about Ms. Maloney. She informs you that Ms. Maloney "ignored the family" sitting at the bedside and that the family complained to her. Ms. Reynolds apologized for Ms. Maloney and told the family, "She is a problem. Thanks for telling me. I will take care of it for you." The family rewards Ms. Reynolds by writing a supportive note to the nurse manager about her and also detailing their perception of how Ms. Maloney dealt with their family.

Critical Thinking Questions

1. On the basis of your knowledge of formation of professional behavior and bullying, how might you respond to Ms. Reynolds?

2. Using what you have learned about communication, frame a respectful confrontation of Ms. Reynolds.

3. If you were the nurse manager, how would you handle this situation while applying a provision of the ANA Code of Ethics?

INTIMIDATION   Intimidation is bullying, threatening, or forcing someone who is physically or emotionally weaker to do something in order to avoid retribution. It is never appropriate for a nurse to threaten someone, whether a coworker, a client, a client's family member, or anyone else. Intimidation can be subtle, such as standing close to another individual with a hostile look on the face, or it can be overt, such as telling someone to do something or he or she will be "sorry." Even nurses with the best of intentions may not realize they are using intimidation when they say things like, "If you don't take your medicine (or go to physical therapy, or follow the treatment plan), you're only going to get worse." Even though what the nurse says may be true, this approach is intimidating and lacks professionalism.

✳ Go to **nursing.pearsonhighered.com** to see a clinical example of intimidation.

▶ CONCLUSION

Professional behavior defines the practice of nursing. *The Code of Ethics for Nurses* (ANA, 2010) provides a foundation and guidelines for professional behaviors. Nurses who act professionally gain knowledge, maintain competence, work well as team members, show compassion, reflect a positive attitude, and maintain their integrity and that of their profession. While professional behaviors may have to be learned throughout nursing school and early entry into practice, in time they become second nature and a component of the nurse's belief system and character.

◢ REVIEW The Concept of Professional Behaviors

RELATE Link the Concepts

Linking the concept of professional behaviors with the concept of addiction:

1. What impact does the nurse's use of addictive substances (legal or illegal) have on the practice of nursing?

2. What is your professional responsibility when a nurse on your unit appears to be under the influence of a substance?

Linking the concept of professional behaviors with the concept of clinical decision making:

3. How do professional behaviors result from clinical decision making and vice versa?

4. What conclusions would you draw, or have you drawn, about a nurse's ability to make clinical decisions on the basis of the nurse's professional or nonprofessional behaviors?

REFER Go to Pearson Nursing Student Resources
nursing.pearsonhighered.com

- Additional review material
- Clinical examples
- Additional case study

REFLECT Case Study

Cheryl Goodwin is a nurse executive who is widely respected for her rapport with nurse educators. She is the dean of a nursing college and is a doctoral-prepared nurse who maintains a small private practice. She is active in state organizations and willing to help both faculty and students. A hospital administrator calls Ms. Goodwin in for a private meeting. In the course of the meeting, Ms. Goodwin is told that a faculty member in the nursing college has committed an act of abuse and neglect toward a client in the hospital. The Chief Nurse Executive (CNE) of the hospital, who is also at the meeting, informs Ms. Goodwin that the faculty member is no longer permitted to practice at that hospital.

Upon questioning the faculty member involved, Ms. Goodwin discovers that the individual did in fact commit the offenses willfully as reported by the CNE. Ms. Goodwin informs this faculty member that his actions created dire consequences for the client involved and that his position at the college is terminated. He had been on probation for bullying and maltreatment of students before this incident.

The college administration permits the nursing faculty member to resign his position. He begins a campaign to attack the dean, Ms. Goodwin. This nurse accuses her of making a number of false accusations. Friends rally around the dismissed employee, as he has taught at the college for a number of years. He has been known for covering for and doing favors for other faculty members for extra cash, such as picking up an extra clinical day, and for granting favors to the faculty members who reported to him. As a senior faculty member, he also coordinated clinical rotations and scheduling.

Ms. Goodwin is not at liberty to discuss the incident that led to this faculty member's resignation. The other faculty members are not aware of the consequences suffered by the client and family. The hospital has requested that the situation remain confidential as the family has not been notified of the abuse. Faculty members who have known Ms. Goodwin for many years begin questioning her motives and labeling her as "sick." They

talk behind her back and do not invite her to nursing functions that she has always attended. They bully any faculty member who associates with her. Ms. Goodwin acquires another position and leaves a position that she loved.

1. How would you describe the behaviors and actions of the faculty members in the scenario?
2. What recourse does Ms. Goodwin have?
3. Why do you suppose the faculty members who had a prior satisfactory relationship with Ms. Goodwin did not support her? Do you believe they did the right thing? How and why might they have handled the situation differently?

EXEMPLAR 40.1 **Commitment to Profession**

EXEMPLAR KEY TERMS
Affective commitment, *2487*
Burnout, *2488*
Commitment, *2486*
Continuance commitment, *2487*
Normative commitment, *2487*
Organizational commitment, *2486*

EXEMPLAR LEARNING OUTCOMES
After reading about this exemplar, you will be able to:

1. Discuss concepts of organizational commitment as applied to the profession of nursing.
2. Apply factors of professional commitment to the role of nursing student.
3. Analyze your personal level of commitment to the nursing profession.

▶ OVERVIEW

Many experienced nurses view nursing as a spiritual calling. It is not a job or what they *do*, it's a part of who they *are*. They have made a commitment to their profession, incorporating the ethics and expectations of nursing into every aspect of their lives, whether at home, work, or play. This commitment is in essence a duty to the individual who is at the center of nursing care. Over time, some nurses may confuse professional commitment with organizational or corporate commitment.

Merriam-Webster's Online Dictionary (n.d.) defines **commitment** as "the state or an instance of being obligated or emotionally impelled." To understand the term *commitment* as it is applied to the profession of nursing, one must first look at the concept of organizational commitment. The most widely accepted definition of **organizational commitment** is that it is the relative strength of an individual's relationship to and sense of belonging to an organization. Although organizational commitment and professional commitment may intersect, it is important for nurses to distinguish between the two. Experienced nurses are able to cite many instances in which nursing ethics and corporate goals collide. The business of health care and the provision of care to the client are not always the same issue. The nursing profession holds the trust of the community and individuals in our society. With this trust comes the moral responsibility of nurses to address the needs of clients and to advocate for safe care within the business of health care.

The IOM (2010) calls for nurses to step up and lead the transformation of health care and to protect a caring model within the business model of health care. It is essential for the safety and well-being of all individuals in our society for nurses to be actively involved in health policy and the financial decisions that affect the delivery of care. The nurse's commitment must be synonymous with professional commitment, even when it may be at odds with organizational commitment.

▶ FACTORS OF PROFESSIONAL COMMITMENT

Factors associated with professional commitment include:

1. A strong belief in and acceptance of the profession's code, role, goals, values, and mores
2. A willingness to exert considerable personal effort on behalf of the profession
3. A strong desire to maintain membership in the profession
4. A pattern of behaviors congruent with the nurses' professional code of ethics

As discussed earlier, nursing education not only concerns teaching students how to think like nurses and perform nursing tasks but also is charged with the acculturation and formation of professional behaviors of students and novice nurses. This process begins when the student enters the first nursing class. Many of the policies and rules associated with a nursing program are intended to prepare the student for entry into the profession of nursing. The student who violates or ignores school policy is in danger of becoming the nurse who ignores practice and agency policy. For example, tardiness in coming to clinicals may result in significant consequences for the offender. Time and attendance are critical in nursing, as clients depend on the nurse for their safety. Even during a nursing shortage, the nurse who is chronically late for or excessively absent from work is subject to disciplinary action that could include suspension and termination. With frequent staff shortages, it is even more important for managers to be able to rely on staff members to be on the job when scheduled. Chronic lateness and frequent absenteeism place a greater burden on colleagues, compromise client care, and lead to conflict among staff.

The values and goals of professional nursing are clearly delineated by standards of nursing practice, codes of ethics, nurse practice acts, national client safety goals, accrediting agencies, and many other such resources. Entering the nursing profession is not just taking a job; it is an obligation to protect, advance, and promote the health of self, individuals, and groups in the community, and it involves many role expectations not inherent in occupations that are just jobs.

Most students can easily identify with the willingness to exert considerable effort on behalf of the profession. Nursing programs have high standards of admission, and many programs receive far more applications than they have openings available. In times of economic recession, this imbalance is even more prevalent, as displaced workers seek job security in the health professions that have staff shortages. Nursing education is a rigorous program of study requiring considerable time and effort to prepare for entry into a demanding yet rewarding profession. The applicants who are accepted into nursing programs tend to be those who have demonstrated the ability to expend such time and effort to achieve their goals.

Students also can identify with the strong desire to maintain membership in the profession. Most students have already made sacrifices while taking related general education and science courses in preparation for the nursing major. The sacrifices required during nursing courses are even greater, as the number of hours required per credit earned increases when hours spent in lab and clinical are added. Most students accepted into a nursing program have a strong desire to complete the program, especially as their time in the program increases.

After graduation, the commitment to maintain membership in the nursing profession is demonstrated by membership in professional organizations and on various committees and by contributing to community organizations seeking input on laws related to health care and health promotion. Nurses must always maintain current knowledge related to changes in health care and the profession of nursing in order to keep their nursing practice up to date and therefore keep their clients safe.

Commitment to the profession of nursing is an obligation to behave in accordance with accepted codes of nursing professional practice. Many facilities that employ nurses require drug screenings and criminal background checks to assist them in the selection of individuals with high moral standards and to protect the populations that they serve.

▶ TYPES OF COMMITMENT

Three types of commitment describe the psychological link between an individual and the decision to continue in a profession: affective, normative, and continuance. **Affective commitment** is an attachment to a profession and includes identification with and involvement in the profession. Affective commitment develops when involvement in a profession produces a satisfying experience. The student or nurse who has a strong desire to continue in the profession, who is involved in keeping up with current information, and who becomes involved with profession-specific organizations and service activities demon-

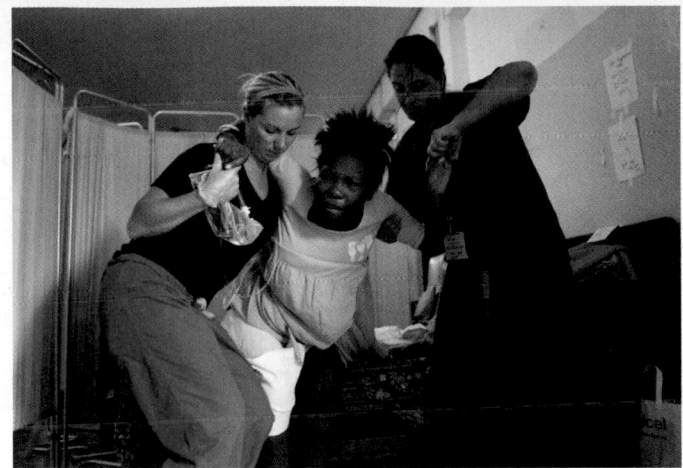

Figure 40–2 ● Affective commitment leads nurses and other healthcare professionals to volunteer their services to help those in disasters, such as the January 2010 earthquake in Haiti. Here, Michele Shiel, an ER nurse from the U.S. Virgin Islands (left), helps to carry a woman from the hallway into a delivery room at the Haitian Community Hospital in Pétionville, Haiti.
Source: © Lara Solt/Dallas Morning News/Corbis.

strates affective commitment (**Figure 40–2 ●**). This individual is in school or working as a nurse because of a desire to be a nurse.

Normative commitment is a feeling of obligation to continue in the profession. Normative commitment develops as a result of having received benefits or having had positive experiences through engagement in the profession. The nurse who enters the field or remains in it because personal or family experiences with illness have created a desire to work in the healthcare field exemplifies normative commitment.

Continuance commitment, or the awareness of costs associated with leaving the profession, develops when negative consequences of leaving, such as loss of income, are seen as reasons to remain. Individuals who experience this type of commitment do not manifest the same ties to the profession as do those who are motivated by affective or normative commitment. In general, such individuals are not inclined to promote their profession. These students and nurses are in the field for the money and job security.

▶ STAGES OF COMMITMENT DEVELOPMENT

The commitment to a profession develops in stages. The first stage is the *exploratory stage*, in which individuals explore the positive aspects of the profession. An example of this stage is the excitement of nursing students during the first weeks of their program as they model their new uniforms and ransack their lab kits. Commitment begins as exploration leads to a positive orientation toward the profession.

The second stage is the *testing stage*, during which individuals discover negative elements of the profession. In this stage, individuals start to assess their willingness and ability to deal with those negative elements. Some nursing students never get beyond this stage and drop out of school or change majors, deciding that the sacrifices are not worth the effort or that they are not suited to the nursing profession.

The third stage is the *passionate stage* of commitment, which begins as the individual synthesizes the positive and negative elements from the first two stages. Students in this stage not only are willing to commit to the profession but also are willing to contribute to its well-being. These students are the ones who become involved in student nursing associations, serve as class officers, or volunteer for activities not associated with a grade.

The fourth stage is the *quiet-and-bored stage* of commitment, in which students settle into the humdrum routines of the nursing program. This stage often occurs during the middle or late middle of the nursing program, as students begin to become more comfortable in their role and feel less anxiety about their performance.

The *integrated stage* is the final stage of commitment. Individuals who reach this stage have integrated both positive and negative elements of the profession into a more flexible, complex, and enduring form of commitment. They act out their commitment as a matter of habit. These students are in the final stages of their nursing program and are beginning to see themselves as nurses, eager to take the NCLEX-RN® and begin employment. As new graduates, they will once again proceed through the stages of commitment while transitioning from being nursing students to being registered nurses.

▶ MANAGING STRESS

Part of a commitment to any profession is learning how to manage the stress associated with that profession. Nursing can be a particularly stressful profession because of both physical and emotional demands. Although most nurses cope effectively with the demands of nursing, in some situations nurses become overwhelmed and develop **burnout**, a complex syndrome of behaviors that can be likened to the exhaustion stage of the general adaptation syndrome (see the module on Stress and Coping). The nurse with burnout manifests physical and emotional depletion, a negative attitude and self-concept, and feelings of helplessness and hopelessness.

Nurses can prevent burnout by using healthy techniques to manage stress. To do so, they must first recognize their stress and become attuned to responses such as feelings of being overwhelmed, fatigue, angry outbursts, physical illness, and increases in coffee drinking, smoking, or use of alcohol or other mood-enhancing substances. Once attuned to stress and their own personal reactions, nurses must identify which situations produce the most pronounced reactions. This discovery will help them take steps to reduce the stress. Suggestions include the following:

- Plan a daily relaxation program with meaningful quiet activities to reduce tension (e.g., read, listen to music, soak in a tub, or meditate).

- Establish a regular exercise program to direct energy outward.

- Study assertiveness techniques to overcome feelings of powerlessness in relationships with others. Learn to say no.

- Learn to accept errors and failures and turn them into constructive learning experiences. Recognize that most individuals do the best they can. Learn to ask for help, to show feelings with colleagues, and to support colleagues in times of need.

- Accept what cannot be changed. There are certain limitations in every situation.

- Get involved in efforts toward constructive change if organizational policies and procedures cause stress.

- Develop collegial support groups to deal with feelings and anxieties generated in the work setting.

- Participate in professional organizations to address workplace issues.

- Seek counseling if needed to help clarify concerns.

Nursing is a profession like few others. Nurses work unusual hours and carry great responsibility. They face the knowledge that the choices they make and actions they take often involve life and death. While most nurses feel that their work is highly satisfying and that they make a difference in their clients' lives, they also know that they must maintain their commitment to their profession or face potential burnout and movement away from nursing into another career.

◢ REVIEW Commitment to Profession

RELATE Link the Concepts and Exemplars

Linking the exemplar of commitment to profession with the concept of development:

1. How might nurses in different life stages commit themselves to the profession of nursing in different ways?

2. Describe the impact of the nurse's moral development, according to Kohlberg, on commitment to the profession of nursing.

Linking the exemplar of commitment to profession with the concept of collaboration:

3. How is nurses' commitment to profession demonstrated by their ability and willingness to collaborate with others?

4. A nurse working on a medical unit is approached by a newly graduated licensed practical nurse who asks for help in improving her skill in initiating an IV catheter. How would nurses with different levels of commitment to the profession respond to this request?

REFER Go to Pearson Nursing Student Resources
nursing.pearsonhighered.com

- Additional review material

REFLECT Case Study

Hakeem Kamara is a nurse working on a very busy and often understaffed oncology unit. Two clients have died within the past week. They were both well known to the staff because each had been admitted several times with complications of their disease and treatment. The staff members who were working all cried, first for one client and then, a few days later, for the other client. Today, one of Mr. Kamara's assigned clients required cardiopulmonary resuscitation and was sent to the ICU, another developed septicemia and required many diagnostic tests and procedures, and a third was given bad news regarding her prognosis and was tearful and frightened. At the end of the day, Mr. Kamara felt that he hadn't done his best job because he was so busy and wished he could have spent more time with each of his assigned clients, caring more for their emotional needs.

1. How will Mr. Kamara's commitment to the profession of nursing affect how he responds to his feelings of inadequacy and grief?

2. If Mr. Kamara is fully committed to nursing, how will he resolve his feelings about the quality of the care he delivers?

3. If Mr. Kamara has a continuance commitment to nursing, how will he respond to the shift he just worked and his feelings?

EXEMPLAR 40.2   Leadership Principles

EXEMPLAR KEY TERMS
Autocratic (authoritarian) leader, *2489*
Bureaucratic leader, *2490*
Charismatic leader, *2490*
Democratic (participative, consultative) leader, *2489*
Formal leader, *2489*
Informal leader, *2489*
Laissez-faire leader, *2490*
Leader, *2489*
Shared governance, *2491*

Shared leadership, *2490*
Situational leader, *2490*
Transactional leader, *2490*
Transformational leader, *2490*

EXEMPLAR LEARNING OUTCOMES
After reading about this exemplar, you will be able to:

1. Differentiate between formal and informal leaders.
2. Compare and contrast the different leadership styles.
3. List the transformational leadership skills that you possess.

▶ OVERVIEW

It is important not to confuse leadership with management. A manager has an official position and is charged with running a unit, department, or facility, depending on the level of management. A leader does not require an official position to lead. **Leaders** are people with the ability to rule, guide, or inspire others to think or act as they recommend. A leader influences others to work together to accomplish a specific goal. Leadership may be formal or informal. The **formal leader**, or appointed leader, is selected by an organization and given official authority to make decisions and to act. An **informal leader** is not officially appointed to direct the activities of others but, because of seniority, age, or special abilities, is recognized by the group as a leader and plays an important role in influencing colleagues, coworkers, and other group members to achieve the group's goals. Leaders can be negative or positive in their appeal and approach. While they may not always be liked by others, leaders are able to create trends, instigate actions, and influence behaviors.

Leaders tend to be very productive and persuasive people. They are often highly competent, efficient, charismatic, and powerful. Leaders can be visionary. Leaders tend to be informed, articulate, confident, and self-aware. Many leaders also have outstanding interpersonal skills and are excellent listeners and communicators. They have initiative and the ability and confidence to innovate change, and to motivate, facilitate, and mentor others.

Within their organizations, nurse leaders participate in and guide teams that assess the effectiveness of care, implement evidence-based practice, and construct process improvement strategies. They may be employed in a variety of positions—from shift team leader to institutional president. Leaders may also hold volunteer positions, such as chairperson of a professional organization or a community board of directors.

▶ LEADERSHIP THEORIES

Early leadership theories focused on what leaders are (trait theories), what leaders do (behavioral theories), and how leaders adapt their leadership style according to the situation (contingency theories). Theories about leadership style describe traits, behaviors, motivations, and choices used by individuals to influence others.

Classic Leadership Theories

Trait theories of leadership hold that leaders often possess specific traits and abilities, including good judgment, decisiveness, knowledge, adaptability, integrity, tact, self-confidence, and cooperativeness. Behavioral theorists believe that through education, training, and life experiences, leaders develop a particular leadership style. These styles have been characterized as autocratic, democratic, laissez-faire, and bureaucratic.

An **autocratic (authoritarian) leader** makes decisions for the group based on the belief that individuals are externally motivated (their driving force is extrinsic; that is, they desire rewards from others) and are incapable of independent decision making. Likened to a dictator, the autocratic leader determines policies, giving orders and directions to the group. Under this leadership style, the group may feel secure because procedures are well defined and activities are predictable. Productivity may also be high. Under the autocratic leader, however, the group's needs for creativity, autonomy, and self-motivation are not met, and the degree of openness and trust between the leader and the group members is minimal or absent. Although group members are often dissatisfied with this leadership style, at times an autocratic style is the most effective. When urgent decisions must be made (e.g., in the case of a cardiac arrest, a unit fire, or a terrorist attack), one individual must assume the responsibility without being challenged by other team members. When group members are unable or do not wish to participate in making a decision, the authoritarian style solves the problem and enables the individual or group to move on. This style can also be effective when a project must be completed quickly and efficiently.

A **democratic (participative, consultative) leader** encourages group discussion and decision making. This type of leader acts as a catalyst or facilitator, actively guiding the group toward achieving the group goals. Group productivity and satisfaction are high as group members contribute to the work effort. The democratic leader assumes that individuals are internally motivated (their driving force is intrinsic; that is, they desire self-satisfaction), are capable of making decisions, and value independence. Democratic leaders typically provide constructive feedback, offer information, make suggestions, and ask questions to gain information or to help group members grow in their ability to make decisions. This leadership style demands that the leader have faith that the group members can accomplish the goals. Although democratic leadership has been shown to be less efficient and more cumbersome than authoritarian leadership, it allows more self-motivation and more creativity among group members. It also calls for a great deal of cooperation and coordination. This leadership style can be extremely effective in the healthcare setting.

The **laissez-faire leader** recognizes the group's need for autonomy and self-regulation. The leader takes a hands-off approach, being less directive and more permissive than other types of leaders. The laissez-faire leader presupposes that the group is internally motivated. However, under a laissez-faire leader, group members may work at cross-purposes because of lack of cooperation and coordination. A laissez-faire style is most effective for groups whose members have both personal and professional maturity, so that once the group has made a decision, the members become committed to it and have the required expertise to implement it. Individual group members then perform tasks in their area of expertise while the leader acts as a resource person.

The **bureaucratic leader** does not trust himself or herself or others to make decisions and instead relies on the organization's rules, policies, and procedures to direct the group's work efforts. Group members are usually dissatisfied with the leader's inflexibility and impersonal relations with them.

Contingency theory proposes yet another type of leader. According to contingency theorists, effective leaders adapt their leadership style to the situation. The **situational leader** (a) is flexible in task and relationship behaviors, (b) considers the staff members' abilities, (c) knows the nature of the task to be done, and (d) is sensitive to the context or environment in which the task takes place. The task orientation focuses the leader on activities that encourage group productivity to get the work done. The relationship orientation style is concerned with interpersonal relationships and focuses on activities that meet group members' needs.

Situational leaders adapt their leadership style to the readiness and willingness of the individual or group to perform the assigned task. When employees are insecure or unable or unwilling to perform the task, the leader uses a highly directive style, providing specific instructions and close supervision. If the group is motivated and willing but unable to perform the task, the leader again uses a highly directive style but, in this case, explains decisions and provides the opportunity for clarification. When the group is able but unwilling or lacking in confidence, the leader shares ideas and facilitates decision making. For a group that is willing, able, and confident to perform the task, the leader delegates, turning the responsibility for decision making and implementation over to the group.

Contemporary Leadership Theories

Contemporary theorists have described charismatic leaders, transactional leaders, transformational leaders, and shared leadership.

A **charismatic leader** is rare and is characterized by an emotional relationship between the leader and the group members. The charming personality of the leader evokes strong feelings of commitment to both the leader and the leader's cause and beliefs. The followers of a charismatic leader often overcome extreme hardship to achieve the group's goals because of faith in the leader.

The **transactional leader** has a relationship with followers based on an exchange for some resource valued by the follower. These incentives are used to promote loyalty and performance. For example, in order to ensure adequate staffing on the night shift, the nurse manager might entice a staff nurse to work the night shift in exchange for a weekend shift off. The transactional leader has a traditional managerial style, focused on the day-to-day tasks of achieving organizational goals and understanding and meeting the needs of the group.

In contrast, a **transformational leader** fosters creativity, risk taking, commitment, and collaboration by empowering the group to share in the organization's vision. The leader inspires others with a clear, attractive, and attainable goal and enlists them to participate in attaining the goal. Through shared values, honesty, trust, and continual learning, the transformational leader empowers the group. This empowerment facilitates independence, individual growth, and change. The IOM (2010) recommends the use of a transformational model of nursing leadership that empowers nurses to lead efforts for change in a complex healthcare environment (see **Box 40–1** ●).

The thinking behind the idea of **shared leadership** recognizes that a professional workforce is made up of many leaders. No one individual is believed to have knowledge or ability beyond that of other members of the work group. Appropriate leadership is thought to emerge in relation to the challenges that confront the work group. Examples of shared leadership in

Box 40–1   Nursing Leadership

Nurses are encouraged to design new models of care to improve quality, efficiency, and safety. The call for a new skill set is not a new phenomenon. Nurse scholars have advised a shift in leadership from the top down to the point of care (POC) nurse at the center of the structural power pyramid (Cain, 2005). Effective nurse leaders:

- Mentor and direct client care
- Actively advocate at the point of care
- Are expert clinicians and apply evidence-based care
- Model the way
- Are risk takers
- Inspire others to create a shared vision
- Are assertive and challenge the status quo
- Enable others to act
- Encourage the heart
- Empower others to embrace their passions and talents
- Value point-of-care nurses as equal partners
- Are trustworthy
- Model honest communication
- Are transparent and share information
- Give and receive feedback
- Are passionate and have conviction
- Are energetic and committed
- Are knowledgeable about organization theory
- Collaborate and educate
- Are responsible and ethical
- Are creative and flexible
- Network and build teams
- Are politically astute

nursing are self-directed work teams, coleadership, and shared governance. **Shared governance** is a method that aims to distribute decision making among a group of people.

Leadership is a learned process. To be an effective leader requires an understanding of factors such as the needs, goals, and rewards that motivate people; knowledge of leadership skills and of the group's activities; and possession of the interpersonal skills to influence others. Principles of effective leadership include vision, influence, and acting as a role model.

Vision is a mental image of a possible and desirable future state. Leaders transform visions into realistic goals and communicate their visions to others, who accept the visions as their own.

Influence is an informal strategy used to gain the cooperation of others without exercising formal authority. Influence is exercised through persuasion and excellent communication skills; it is based on a trusting relationship with the followers.

An effective leader needs to show sensitivity in being a *positive role model*, demonstrating caring toward coworkers and clients. As is appropriate in any health and caring profession, leadership can also be humanistic, that is, characterized by an emphasis on individuals' dignity and worth. Being a good leader takes thought, care, insight, commitment, and energy in order to set the example for others to follow.

REVIEW Leadership Principles

RELATE Link the Concepts and Exemplars

Linking the exemplar of leadership principles with the concept of communication:

1. How important are communication skills to effectiveness as a leader?

2. Can an individual with poor communication skills act as a competent leader? Why or why not?

Linking the exemplar of leadership principles with the concept of advocacy:

3. Are all nursing advocates leaders? Explain your answer.

4. How do leadership principles increase the effectiveness of advocacy?

REFER Go to Pearson Nursing Student Resources
nursing.pearsonhighered.com

- Additional review material

REFLECT Case Study

Martha Rivaldo is a staff nurse who has worked in the neonatal ICU for 7 years. She is not well liked. She tends to be very critical of the performance of new nurses on the unit and can frequently be heard talking with her friends and complaining about how the unit is managed. Several nurses have complained to the nurse manager, but nothing ever seems to be done about her behavior. Ms. Rivaldo is a very skilled and competent NICU nurse and is always the first individual on whom the staff members call when they have difficulty initiating an IV line on one of the babies. She is also a good resource for people she likes, as she is knowledgeable about responding to emergency situations. However, once she decides someone is lacking in competence, she has no use for that person.

1. Is Ms. Rivaldo a leader? Explain your answer.

2. If you were Ms. Rivaldo's nurse manager and several people came to you, one at a time, to complain about her cruel comments about newly hired nurses, how would you respond?

3. Why do you think Ms. Rivaldo reacts the way she does to newly hired NICU nurses?

EXEMPLAR 40.3   Work Ethic

EXEMPLAR KEY TERMS
Arrogance, *2493*
Corrective action, *2492*
Dismissal, *2492*
Generational cohort, *2493*
Insubordination, *2492*
Optimism, *2492*
Pessimism, *2492*
Punctual, *2492*
Work ethic, *2491*

EXEMPLAR LEARNING OUTCOMES
After reading about this exemplar, you will be able to:

1. Apply the concept of work ethic to the behavior of the professional nurse.

2. Differentiate between work ethics commonly seen in the four generations of nurses in today's workplace.

3. Predict the impact of generational differences in work ethic in relation to learning to work as a cohesive nursing team.

▶ OVERVIEW

Ask any employer what characteristic is most important in a good employee and the majority will respond, "A strong work ethic." A **work ethic** is a belief in the importance and moral worth of work. An individual with a strong work ethic places high value on hard work and diligence. Employees with a strong work ethic stay focused and leave their personal problems at home. They apply themselves to the task at hand and take a thorough approach to getting the work done right the first time.

If they do make any mistakes, they take responsibility for them and repair any damage or willingly accept the consequences. They exercise self-discipline and self-control. They know what management expects of them, and they measure up. They don't wait to be told what to do, and they demonstrate a positive attitude and enthusiasm for their work.

By examining some of the factors involved in developing a strong work ethic and demonstrating a commitment to their job and to their employer, nursing students can better understand some of the expectations of the nursing profession.

▶ ATTENDANCE AND PUNCTUALITY

It is nearly impossible to demonstrate a commitment to a job without being there. Performing the duties of a job requires showing up for work every day and being **punctual** (on time).

When an employee doesn't come to work, others are required to cover for that individual. Even when the employee has a good reason for being absent, frequent absences increase the stress of other employees and decrease the unit's productivity. Because of funding shortages, many healthcare agencies are forced to employ as few people as required. This means that all employees have a very full workload and have difficulty performing it to the best of their ability and at the same time taking on some or all of the absent employee's work. Each nurse (and nursing student) is counted on to be at work and to arrive on time.

The employee who is late for work holds things up and inconveniences other people. When a nurse is late, a client's procedure might have to be rescheduled, possibly delaying that client (or another's) diagnosis, treatment, surgery, or discharge from the hospital. Needed supplies might not get delivered on time, paperwork might be filed too late to meet a deadline, and other people might have to work beyond their shifts. Because the roles of healthcare professionals are interconnected, it is essential that the nurse report to work on time. "On time" does not mean arriving at the parking lot at the time one is supposed to report for work; "on time" means being at work and in place, ready to begin work at the start of the shift.

Almost everyone must miss work or arrive late on occasion. But when poor attendance or lack of punctuality becomes a habit, it also becomes a performance issue and possible grounds for **corrective action** (steps taken to overcome a job performance problem) or **dismissal** (termination of employment).

The professionally committed nursing student must show up for work every day, arrive on time, and be ready to work when the shift starts. Those who set up contingency plans to cover possible emergencies such as a child being sick or a car being in the shop are most successful.

For nurses, a good work ethic includes protecting their own health and safety by making sure to get enough rest, avoid unnecessary risks, and take preventive measures, such as flu shots.

Individuals with a good work ethic do not take excessively long or unscheduled breaks. They try to allow some extra time at the end of the shift in case they are held over. Above all, nurses never leave a client, coworker, visitor, or guest hanging by rushing out the door the minute the shift ends. It is the nurse's (and the nursing student's) responsibility to stay long enough to complete work or to hand it off properly to the individual who follows. The nurse makes sure there is a smooth transition between shifts and does not leave any work for other people to finish.

▶ RELIABILITY AND ACCOUNTABILITY

Being reliable and being accountable are key factors in professionalism. From a systems perspective, each nurse is responsible for completing the duties of the job appropriately so that others can complete their work, too. This responsibility extends to following through on commitments, such as agreements to trade shifts or to take on additional work when someone is absent. Following through on commitments is a big part of the team effort (**Figure 40–3 ●**).

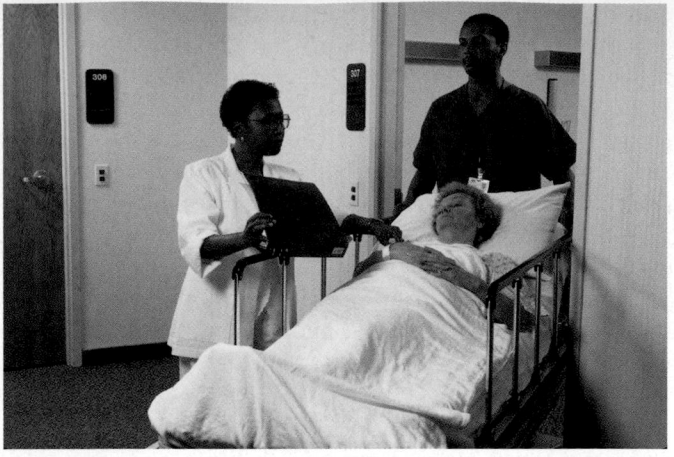

Figure 40–3 ● Nurses are responsible for completing their duties so that other people can complete their own work.

Accepting responsibility and the consequences of one's actions is also important. Professionals hold themselves personally accountable and do not shift blame to others. The nurse who makes a mistake (and everyone does occasionally) should admit it and accept full responsibility. The next step is to apologize to those who have been inconvenienced or harmed. Although it is important to apologize for a mistake, the apology does not erase the fact that a mistake was made. Also important are learning from the experience and avoiding making the same mistake twice. Supervisors, coworkers, and others appreciate a "the-buck-stops-here" attitude.

Professional nurses accept all work assignments for which they are qualified and that they are prepared to perform. A nurse who is given a work assignment for which he or she is not qualified or that she or he is not prepared to perform should discuss the situation immediately with the supervisor. Refusal to complete a task as assigned may be construed as **insubordination** and grounds for dismissal. However, a responsible individual would never agree to perform a task that he or she is not qualified to perform.

When serving the needs of clients, it is important to avoid passing judgment or projecting one's own personal beliefs on others. If an assignment conflicts with a nurse's religious beliefs, morals, or values, the nurse must discuss these concerns with the supervisor. It is best to resolve issues like these when the nurse first considers a job offer. If a nurse wishes not to participate in abortions, sex change operations, end-of-life procedures, or other activities that conflict with personal beliefs or morals, many employers will allow that nurse to opt out of participation. However, this possibility must be discussed ahead of time so that client care is not delayed or jeopardized.

▶ ATTITUDE AND ENTHUSIASM

As has been mentioned, having a positive attitude is an essential professional characteristic for nurses. This sense of **optimism**, a feeling that things will turn out for the best, is common among professional nurses. Unfortunately, for some individuals, a negative attitude is a way of life. **Pessimism** characterizes those who believe that the situation is always bad and may become worse. They complain about everything, and nothing seems to satisfy them. Pessimists rarely smile, seldom appear happy, and do not convey enthusiasm about their work. Consciously or not, they may spread negativity to everyone around them and undermine morale, teamwork, and a spirit of cooperation. Pessimism is a dangerous attitude that does not invite trust or inspire confidence. Nurses must convey optimism and enthusiasm about their work to clients and their families. Nurses who maintain a positive attitude among their colleagues contribute to a more pleasant and, ultimately, more productive work environment.

Pessimism is not the only negative attitude that can endanger the nurse's professionalism. **Arrogance**, or excessive pride and a feeling of superiority, can be an extremely dangerous characteristic in the nurse, as it can lead to a false belief that the nurse is always right and does not need input from others. For example, when the unit begins using a new IV infusion pump, the arrogant nurse does not bother attending the in-service and believes that it is possible to "figure things out" independently. Accurate self-assessment of strengths and weaknesses, as well as acceptance of feedback from others, promotes both safety and growth and is therefore an ability essential for the nurse.

▶ GENERATIONAL DIFFERENCES IN WORK ETHIC

For the first time in American history, four generations of people are working shoulder to shoulder. Typically, discussions about diversity focus on multiracial or multiethnic perspectives (see the module on Culture and Diversity). Different generations working together is also diversity. Research has clearly shown that generation membership is a key variable in the determination of behavior. Different generations hold different ideals, values, traits, goals, and characteristics. These generational differences play a significant role in how employees of one group relate to the others and include communication styles, expectations, work styles, values and norms, attitudes about work and life, comfort with technology, views regarding loyalty and authority, and acceptance of change.

The term **generational cohort** refers to people born in the same general time span who share key life experiences, including historical events, public heroes, pastimes, and early work experiences. These common life experiences create cohesiveness in perspectives and attitudes. As a result, generational cohorts develop distinct values and workforce patterns. Differences between generations (sometimes called a *generation gap*) can have negative effects in the workplace, causing conflicts and interpersonal tension. Learning to create collegial relationships with people from different generations is a critical skill for nurses who work in multigenerational teams.

While the literature sometimes disagrees on specific years or generational names, there is consistent agreement on the characteristics of each generational cohort:

- Members of the oldest generation were born between 1925 and 1944. They have been called veterans, survivors, traditionalists, or the silent generation and are currently in their 70s and 80s.

- The baby boomers were born during the post–World War II population surge from approximately 1945 to 1960, a time of economic prosperity and opportunity. Currently, baby boomers are in their 50s and 60s and represent the largest cohort in the nursing workforce.

- Members of Generation X were born between 1961 and 1980 and are currently in their 30s and 40s.

- The generation after Generation X, known as the *millennial generation* and born between 1981 and 2000, has nearly as many members as the baby-boomer generation. The millennials, who are currently in their teens, 20s, and early 30s, have also been called Generation Y, generation next, and the net generation.

An understanding of the historical influences on each generation, their common life experiences, and the workforce the members entered when first employed is necessary to understand their attitudes and values related to work (see **Table 40–3** ●).

Different generational styles can lead to workplace conflict. Older nurses may experience considerable conflict over younger nurses' behaviors and may describe younger nurses as arrogant, lacking in commitment, and having a "slacker" attitude. Younger nurses, however, see themselves as self-reliant rather than arrogant. Older nurses may be dismayed and struggle with a perceived lack of professionalism among their younger colleagues evidenced by younger nurses' dress, hair styles, piercings, and tattoos. Younger nurses may be disillusioned by older nurses' perceived unwillingness to become technologically competent.

While differences between generations are not new, two significant changes over the past 60 years have forced the current generations in the workforce into more intense interaction. First, the nature of the work itself has shifted. In traditional bureaucratic structures, interactions between generations followed hierarchical lines. People from younger generations traditionally held entry-level positions and reported to people of the older generation in more senior positions. As a result, younger employees took direction from and followed the rules of people who were older. With the advent of continuous quality improvement and shared governance structures, individuals from various "levels" of the organization are now equal members of a team. This arrangement has increased the interaction of employees from different generations.

Second, the transformation from the industrial age to the information age has altered the interactions between people of differing generations. Historically, the most senior members of an organization offered the most reliable information and knowledge. Young nurses relied on their more senior colleagues for instruction and advice when confronted with an unusual diagnosis or a complex client situation. With the advent of the information age, young nurses are not as reliant on their older peers, since they can easily access information from around the world on their computers and smartphones. Computerization has not only broken the dependence of younger generations on more senior generations for information, it has also resulted in the unprecedented situation where the youngest individuals in the workforce are the most expert at a critical skill. Instead of younger nurses turning to their older colleagues for advice, older nurses often depend upon their younger peers for guidance in using new technologies.

Members of each generation operate as if their own values and expectations are universal. For example, veteran nurses who entered the workforce when success occurred through long-term employment with one organization assume that the same approach will ensure achievement today. They see their younger colleagues' frequent job changes or working as independent agents as unreliability or a lack of commitment. Younger nurses may assume that their older peers who have remained in one place of employment have done so because of failure to take advantage of opportunities. Also, having grown

TABLE 40–3 Description of Four Generations in the American Workforce

GENERATIONAL COHORT AND THEIR HISTORICAL INFLUENCES	LIFE EXPERIENCES	WORKFORCE ENTERED	WORK ETHIC
Veterans			
(born 1925–1944) Great Depression World War II	News came from newspapers and radio. Long-distance phone calls were rare and expensive. Shopping was mostly done at locally owned stores. Movies were seen only in theaters. Attitude toward children: They should be "seen and not heard."	End of depression and war Economic prosperity Emergence of middle class Able to thrive in a nice home on a single income Large, bureaucratic organizations Rules, policies, and procedures plainly outlined	Sacrifice and hard work are rewarded. Seniority is important to advance career. Value loyalty. Respect authority. Like working in teams with designated leaders. Prefer personal forms of communication.
Baby Boomers			
(born 1945–1960) Introduction of television Man landed on the moon Assassination of President Kennedy Civil Rights Movement Summer of Love Vietnam War Woodstock Watergate	Grew up in a healthy, flourishing economy. Watched variety shows, movies, and sitcoms within their own home. News became more visual and dramatic. Raised in two-parent households in which father worked and mother was home caretaker. Were members of smaller families.	Emphasis was on freedom to be yourself—the "me" generation. Heroes were those who questioned status quo. People in positions of power were not to be trusted. Raised to be independent, critical thinkers. Many female college graduates went on to become secretaries, nurses, or teachers due to perception these were "primarily female professions."	Are workaholics. Embrace sense of professionalism. Self-worth closely tied to work ethic. Question authority. Status quo can be transformed by working together. Desire financial prosperity but long to make a significant contribution with their experience and expertise.
Generation X			
(born 1961–1980) Rising divorce rates Microwaves Video games Computers Spaceship *Challenger* disaster Numerous scandals involving high-profile public figures Operation Desert Storm	Lived in two-career households. Many raised in single-parent homes. Watched parents work extremely long hours and sacrifice leisure time for success at work. "Latch key" generation; learned to manage on their own; becoming adept, clever, and resourceful. Allowed to be equal participants in family discussions, learned at an early age to participate in conversations, advocate for their point of view, and expect to have their opinions considered.	Dramatic downsizing, reengineering, and layoffs seen with more senior colleagues, parents, and grandparents. Hierarchical structures had begun to flatten, eliminating promotional opportunities for younger workers. Large cohort of baby boomers remained in workforce, filling limited managerial positions. Assumed responsibility to keep themselves employable by constantly updating their skills.	Seek challenges. Are self-directed. Are comfortable with technology. Expect instant access to information. Desire employment where they can create balance in work and personal life. Prefer managers to be mentors and coaches. Limited motivation to stay with same employer but loyal to their profession. Desire more control over their own schedule. Pragmatic focus on outcomes rather than process.

TABLE 40–3 Description of Four Generations in the American Workforce (*continued*)

GENERATIONAL COHORT AND THEIR HISTORICAL INFLUENCES	LIFE EXPERIENCES	WORKFORCE ENTERED	WORK ETHIC
Millennial Generation			
(born 1981–2000) Established infrastructure (child care, preschool, after-school care) to assist dual-career parents Global generation Internet Bombing of federal building in Oklahoma City Columbine High School shootings Terrorist attack of September 11, 2001 Wars in Afghanistan and Iran	Mostly children of baby boomers born to older mothers; "baby on board" signs in automobiles. Life highly structured and scheduled, with everything from soccer camp to piano lessons. Parents heavily involved in their upbringing, often chaperoning or coaching extracurricular activities. Accept multiculturalism. Grew up using e-mail or the Internet more often than the telephone. Raised enmeshed in digital technology with computer games at nursery school. "Extreme sports" generation. Mass consumption of television and pop culture.	Economic downturn Drying up of job opportunities in many industries. Wall Street and banking industry crisis. Belief that education is the key to success. Resurgence of heroism and patriotism. Diversity a given. Renewed sense of interest in contributing to collective good. Volunteering for community service. Joining organizations in record numbers.	Social, confident, optimistic, talented, well-educated, collaborative, open-minded, achievement-oriented. Expectation of daily feedback, high maintenance. Potential to become the highest-producing workforce in history. Thriving on the adrenaline rush of new challenges and new opportunities. Personal cell phones a necessity for daily life and interpersonal communication.

up in a world where their voice and contributions are expected, younger nurses are often misunderstood when they advise their more senior colleagues who were taught to respect and listen to their elders. An older nurse may see the voiced criticisms of a novice nurse at a staff meeting as disrespectful and therefore discount the younger nurse. From the younger nurse's perspective, speaking up even with limited experience is contributing to the unit.

Learning to develop collegial relationships with people from different generations is a critical skill for nurses who work in multigenerational teams. Working with nurses from different generations offers the opportunity to explore new and different ways of thinking. Rather than focusing on what's "wrong" with another generation, nurses should capitalize on each generation's strengths. Nurses of the veteran generation value hard work and respect authority, baby boomers value teamwork, Generation X nurses value self-reliance, and millennial nurses value achievement. In the workplace, a veteran nurse might say, "Do it because I say so," and a baby-boomer nurse might say, "Let's get together and reach a consensus about how to do it." The Generation X staff nurses might say they will do it themselves, and the millennial nurses might not care who does it as long as the work gets done.

Veteran nurses should be valued for the wisdom and organizational history they bring to nursing teams. When technology fails, veteran nurses can assist a unit to quickly shift back to the traditional ways of assessing and caring for clients. Baby boomers should be valued for their clinical and organizational experience and should be utilized to coach and mentor younger nurses. Generation X nurses should be valued for their innovative ideas and creative approaches to unit issues and problems. They can be important in helping organizations design new approaches to nursing care delivery. Millennial nurses should

be valued for their understanding of technology and insights into how it can be used in practice. They can also serve as technology coaches for members of older generational cohorts.

Negative, nonsupportive, unpleasant, and uncooperative peers and coworkers are key impediments to nurses' ability to find joy in their work. Teams that work together, support one another, value one another's strengths and abilities, and resolve conflicts are critical factors in staff nurse retention. **Box 40–2** gives examples of questions to be considered about each generational cohort to assist in capitalizing on the strengths of each.

Box 40–2 Questions to Highlight the Strengths of Each Generation of Nurses

VETERAN GENERATION
- Where does the unit have a need for resource conservation?
- Which tasks require close attention to timeliness and detail?
- Where are skills in listening and problem solving most needed?

BABY BOOMERS
- Where are nurses who can "roll with the punches" most needed?
- Which tasks require independent thinking?
- Where are skills in coaching and mentoring most needed?

GENERATION X
- Where are new approaches to nursing care delivery needed?
- Which tasks call for an entrepreneurial spirit?
- Where can troubleshooting skills best be utilized?

MILLENNIAL GENERATION
- Where are culturally competent viewpoints most needed?
- What tasks require outspokenness?
- Where can advanced computer or other technological skills best be utilized?

Learning from the unique strengths of each generation can decrease interpersonal tension and facilitate personal growth. Nurses who learn to acknowledge and appreciate their colleagues from different backgrounds, including generational backgrounds, have a distinct advantage. Successful teamwork is increasingly required for job satisfaction and the ability to positively affect client outcomes. This teamwork requirement is reflected in the recent introduction of relationship-based nursing care delivery systems. All too frequently, intergenerational interactions lead to conflicts due to lack of appreciation or understanding, or simply to misinterpretation of other perspectives.

Particular attention should be paid to engaging the perspective of younger nurses, as the youngest generation is always at a distinct disadvantage. The existing organizational structure is based upon strategies that were used successfully in the past rather than designed for the future. Because of their longevity, older generations often dominate in the powerful leadership positions and are more influential when changes are made. These nurses update processes and rewards in a way that makes sense from their generational perspective, not recognizing that younger nurses might not hold the same perspective. Incorporating younger nurses' values of participation, access to information, and balance into nursing operations is important. Older nurses need to learn to welcome input from their younger colleagues, encouraging them to use their fresh viewpoints to identify where opportunities exist. Younger nurses need to be taught and learn to value the experience and exper-

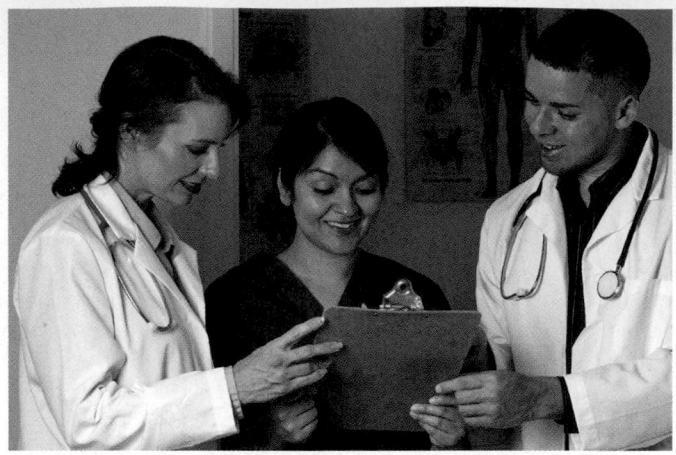

Figure 40–4 ● The best nursing teams utilize the contributions of each generation's strengths.
Source: © Jake Hellbach/Fotolia.

tise of more senior nurses who have a wealth of lived experiences to share.

The best teams utilize the contributions of each generation's skill set and strengths. The hardworking, loyal veterans; the idealist, passionate baby boomers; the technoliterate, adaptable Generation Xers; and the young, optimistic millennials can come together in a powerful network of nurses with a remarkable ability to support each other and maximize each nurse's contribution to client care (**Figure 40–4 ●**).

REVIEW Work Ethic

RELATE Link the Concepts and Exemplars

Linking the exemplar of work ethic with the concept of collaboration:

1. How does the work ethic of the individual nurse affect collaboration?

2. How might nurses from different generations respond to a rude and confrontational physician?

Linking the exemplar of work ethic with the concept of teaching and learning:

3. How does the nurse's generational work ethic affect how the nurse teaches clients?

4. How does the nurse's generational work ethic affect learning style?

REFER Go to Pearson Nursing Student Resources
nursing.pearsonhighered.com

- Additional review material

REFLECT Case Studies

How would you respond in each of the following situations?

1. You were out with friends until very late last night and had to report for work this morning at 7 a.m. You know that your coworkers won't arrive for another half hour. You've got just enough time for a quick run to the corner coffee shop before your coworkers arrive.

2. You promised your coworkers that you would work the day shift on Thanksgiving so they could be home with their fami-

lies. Two days before the holiday, an old friend from out of town calls to say that he would like you to be his guest for lunch on Thanksgiving Day.

3. You have an appointment with your supervisor next week to review the results of your annual performance evaluation. You overhear one of your teammates telling another individual that she gave you a low score on your 360-degree feedback evaluation because you refused to trade shifts with her over the Easter weekend.

4. Your shift ends in 30 minutes, and you have about 30 minutes of work left to do, but you haven't been able to take your afternoon break yet.

5. One of your neighbors is admitted to the unit where you work. A member of your family calls to tell you that he has heard a rumor that the neighbor has a communicable disease. Because you work on the unit and have access to client records, your family member asks you to find out whether the rumor is true.

6. A new piece of equipment has been installed in your department, but you missed the in-service session in which everyone was trained in how to operate it. Today a procedure is to be done using this equipment, and it is your responsibility to use it.

7. A coworker invites you to a party. When you arrive, you notice three other people you work with complaining about low wages and telling a group of strangers that one of the surgeons at your hospital made a mistake in surgery last week and lied to the client's family to try to cover it up.

■ REFERENCES

American Nurses Association. (2001). *Guide to the Code of Ethics for Nurses: Interpretation and Application.* Silver Spring, MD: Nursebooks.org.

Benner, P. (1982). From novice to expert. *American Journal of Nursing, 82*(3), 402–407.

Benner, P., Sutphen, M., Leonard, V., & Day, L. (2010). *Educating nurses: A call for radical transformation.* San Francisco, CA: Jossey-Bass.

Berry, P. A., Gillespie, G. L., Gates, D., & Schafer, J. (2012). Novice nurse productivity following workplace bullying. *Journal of Nursing Scholarship, 44*(1), 80–87.

Cain, L. B. (2005). Essential qualities of an effective clinical leader. *Dimensions of Critical Care Nursing, 24*(1), 32–34.

Code of Federal Regulations. (2001). Title 29—Labor: Section 1604-11—Sexual harrassment. Retrieved from http://www.gpo.gov/fdsys/pkg/CFR-2001-title29-vol4/xml/CFR-2001-title29-vol4-sec1604-11.xml.

Commitment. (n.d.). In *Merriam-Webster's Online Dictionary* (11th ed.). Retrieved from www.merriam-webster.com/dictionary/commitment.

Cronenwett, L., Sherwood, G., Barnsteiner, J., Disch, J., Johnson, J., Mitchell, P., . . . Warren, J. (2007). Quality and safety education for nurses. *Nursing Outlook, 55*(3), 122–131. DOI: 10.1016/j.outlook.2007.02.006) Retrieved from http://qsen.org/competencies/pre-licensure-ksas/.

Institute of Medicine. (2010). *The future of nursing: Leading change, advancing health.* Retrieved from http://www.iom.edu/~/media/Files/Report%20Files/2010/The-Future-of-Nursing/Future%20of%20Nursing%202010%20Recommendations.pdf.

The Joint Commission. (2012). *Sentinel event data: Root causes by event type 2004–2Q 2012.* Retrieved from http://www.jointcommission.org/assets/1/18/Root_Causes_Event_Type_2004_2Q2012.pdf.

Lachman, V. D. (2009). *Ethical challenges in health care: Developing your moral compass.* New York, NY: Springer.

Lanza, M. L., Zeiss, R. A., & Rierdan, J. (2006). Non-physical violence: A risk factor for physical violence in health care settings. *AAOHN Journal, 54*(9), 397–402.

Newport, F. (2013). Gallup Politics: Congress retains low honesty rating: Nurses have highest honesty rating; car *salespeople, lowest.* Retrieved from http://www.gallup.com/poll/151460/Record-Rate-Honesty-Ethics-Members-Congress-Low.aspx.

North Carolina Board of Nursing. (2002). *Components of nursing practice for the registered nurse.* Retrieved from http://www.ncbon.com/myfiles/downloads/registered-nurse-rules.pdf.

North Carolina Board of Nursing. (2008). *Continuing competence.* Retrieved from www.ncbon.com/content.aspx?id=1078&tcrms=definition+of+competent.

Professional role competence. (2013). *NursingWorld.* Retrieved from http://www.nursingworld.org/main-menucategories/thepracticeofprofessionalnursing/nursingstandards/professional-role-competence.html

Via Christi Regional Medical Center. (2003). Survey on professionalism. Retrieved from www.via-christi.org/workfiles/Professionalism%20in%20Nursing.ppt.

Walrafen, N., Brewer, K., & Mulvenon, C. (2012). Sadly caught up in the moment: An exploration of horizontal violence. *Nursing Economics, 30*(1), 6–12, 49. Retrieved from http://www.medscape.com/viewarticle/760015.

41 Teaching and Learning

MODULE AT-A-GLANCE

The Concept of Teaching and Learning, 2499

Exemplar 41.1
Client/Consumer Education, 2509

Exemplar 41.2
Mentoring, 2524

Exemplar 41.3
Staff Development, 2528

▰ THE CONCEPT OF TEACHING AND LEARNING

Teaching is a system of activities designed to produce learning. **Learning** is a change in human disposition or capability that persists and that cannot be solely accounted for by growth. Learning is represented by a change in behavior; in other words, the learner is able to apply or demonstrate what has been learned. (See **Box 41–1** ● for attributes of learning.)

The teaching–learning process involves dynamic interaction between teacher and learner. Each participant in the process communicates information, emotions, perceptions, and attitudes to the other. This concept discusses the teaching–learning process, the nurse's responsibility as a client and family educator, domains and theories of learning, factors that affect an individual's ability to learn, and how nurses can use this information to design more successful client and family education activities. **<<**

Concept Learning Outcomes

After reading about this concept, you will be able to:

1. Discuss the importance of the teaching role of the nurse.
2. Describe the attributes of learning.
3. Distinguish andragogy, pedagogy, and geragogy.
4. Summarize the characteristics of adult learners.
5. Compare the three domains of learning.
6. Identify factors that affect learning.
7. Discuss the implications of using the Internet as a source of health information.

Concept Key Terms

Adherence, *2502*
Affective domain, *2503*
Andragogy, *2502*
Behaviorist theory, *2502*
Cognitive domain, *2503*
Cognitive theory, *2503*
Compliance, *2501*
Constructivism, *2505*
E-health, *2508*
Geragogy, *2502*
Humanistic learning theory, *2504*

Imitation, *2504*
Learning, *2499*
Learning need, *2501*
Modeling, *2504*
Motivation to learn, *2505*
Observational learning, *2504*
Pedagogy, *2502*
Positive reinforcement, *2502*
Psychomotor domain, *2503*
Readiness to learn, *2505*
Teaching, *2499*

Box 41–1 Attributes of Learning

LEARNING IS

- An experience that occurs inside the learner
- The discovery of the personal meaning and relevance of ideas
- A consequence of experience
- A collaborative and cooperative process
- An evolutionary process that builds on past learning and experiences
- A process that is both intellectual and emotional.

▶ NURSES AS TEACHERS AND LEARNERS

Nurses as Teachers

The American Nurses Association (ANA) Standards of Practice for Registered Nurses identifies teaching as one of the many roles of the professional nurse. Although nurses teach a variety of learners in various settings, nurses primarily teach clients and their families. Examples of client and family teaching include teaching how to perform self-care; how to take medications and their side effects; and how to perform prescribed treatments (e.g., deep breathing and coughing). Although most teaching is done directly with clients, family members or caregivers also may be instructed in care of the client. This is especially important for those clients who have difficulty performing self-care. For example, parents who need to give medication to their children must be instructed in the proper administration of that medication. A client with diabetes who has visual impairment may need assistance when administering insulin or when assessing her feet and lower extremities for skin breakdown. When teaching clients about diet, it is important to include the person who purchases and prepares the food.

Nurses also teach professional colleagues and other healthcare personnel in academic settings such as vocational schools, colleges, and universities, and in healthcare facilities such as hospitals or nursing homes. Nurses teach each other through a variety of experiences, including mentoring, continuing education classes, and clinical experiences for nursing students.

A number of factors affect teaching clients and others in the healthcare system. Federal and state regulations influence the content to be taught and the documentation required of nursing schools, certifying agencies, and agencies employing and training nurses and other healthcare professionals. Nurses providing client education do so for clients who vary in age, cultural and socioeconomic background, primary language, and previous knowledge and experience. Information is constantly changing as new research becomes available. Today's resources are numerous and readily available through the Internet. These factors combine to make providing clients with accurate, current information a challenge for nurses.

Nurses as Learners

Nursing education programs prepare the new practitioner with effective beginning nursing skills. However, because changes occur quickly and often in nursing and health care, nurses must continue learning to keep current. The ANA Standards of Professional Performance recognize this (Standard 8, Education), and each state's board of nursing outlines requirements for nurses to participate in continuing education programs designed to increase their knowledge and skill (ANA, 2010). To assist nurses in maintaining their licenses and ensuring quality of care, many employers provide continuing education programs at the work site. Sometimes nurses need to travel to specialized centers to gain advanced specialized skills. Many nurses return to school to obtain advanced degrees in nursing and other health-related disciplines.

Teaching and learning have essential roles in nursing and health. The concepts of development, communication, and health, wellness, and illness are directly related to the concept of teaching and learning.

▶ THE ART OF TEACHING

Teaching is a system of activities intentionally designed to produce specific learning. It is a goal-directed activity that results in improved learning for the learner. Teaching is more than giving information; the art of teaching lies in creating a learning environment conducive for the learner to gain knowledge, skills, and a desire within the learner to change some aspect of his or her life. Effective teaching requires knowledge of the subject matter, understanding of the learning process, judgment, and intuition (**Box 41–2** ●).

The relationship between the teacher and the learner is essentially one of trust and respect. The learner trusts that the teacher has the knowledge and skill to teach, and the teacher respects the learner's ability to attain the recognized goals. Once a nurse starts to instruct a client or other learner, it is important

---

Box 41–2 Characteristics of Effective Teaching

EFFECTIVE TEACHING:

- Holds the learner's interest.
- Involves the learner in the learning process, and creates a partnership between the learner and the teacher.
- Fosters a positive self-concept in the learner; learner believes learning is possible and probable.
- Sets realistic goals.
- Is directed at helping learners meet their objectives.
- Supports the learner with positive reinforcement and feedback.
- Is accurate and current.
- Is appropriate for the learner's age, condition, and abilities.
- Is optimistic, positive, and nonthreatening.
- Uses several methods of teaching to accommodate a variety of learning styles, and provides learning opportunities through hearing, seeing, and doing.
- Uses methods to evaluate learning.
- Gathers information from reliable sources.
- Is cost effective (i.e., cost of nurse's time spent teaching is less than the cost of treating health problems that can occur when clients do not follow recommended treatments, fail to take medications correctly, or do not adapt lifestyle to changing health needs).

Concepts Related to **Teaching and Learning**

CONCEPT	RELATIONSHIP TO TEACHING AND LEARNING	NURSING IMPLICATIONS
Development		
■ Cognitive ■ Physical ■ Mental	As a child develops, abilities to learn increase in complexity. As adults age, vision, hearing, and motor function can be impaired, as can cognitive function.	■ Assess age and developmental stage. ■ Use age and developmentally appropriate teaching methods. ■ Be alert that age does not always indicate specific developmental characteristics.
Communication		
■ Therapeutic communication ■ Documentation	Teaching and learning processes require communication: verbal, nonverbal, and written.	■ Use elements of verbal communication to achieve learning outcomes: pace, intonation, clarity, credibility, timing, relevance, and appropriate use of humor. ■ Use elements of nonverbal communication effectively including posture, appearance, facial expressions, and gestures. ■ Use written communication items (handouts, computer programs, mobile device apps, etc.) that are reflective of the client's literacy levels.
Health, Wellness, and Illness		
■ Illness–wellness continuum ■ Health promotion ■ Variables influencing health ■ Physical fitness and exercise ■ Oral health ■ Normal sleep–rest patterns	Knowledge empowers individuals to make lifestyle choices that promote health and may prevent illness and injury.	■ Educate individuals to be effective healthcare consumers. ■ Reinforce healthy client behaviors. ■ Guide client in problem solving health-related issues ■ Advocate for community changes and for resources in promoting health and healthy environments.

for the teaching process to continue until the participants achieve the mutually agreed-on learning goals, change the goals, or decide that the goals cannot be met.

As teachers, nurses must understand a number of learning theories. By understanding how people learn and the factors that impact learning, nurses can develop more successful client teaching plans for both individual clients and their families, as well as for various types of groups of learners.

▶ ASPECTS OF LEARNING

Individuals have a variety of learning needs. A **learning need** is a desire or a requirement to know something that is presently unknown to the learner. Learning needs may include new knowledge or information, a new or different skill or physical ability, a new behavior, or a need to change an old behavior.

An important aspect of learning is the individual's desire to learn and to act on learning, which is referred to as compliance. In the healthcare context, **compliance** is the extent to which an individual's behavior coincides with medical or health advice. Compliance is best illustrated when the individual recognizes and accepts the need to learn, then follows through with the appropriate behaviors that reflect the learning. For example, a client diagnosed as having diabetes willingly learns about the recommended special diet and then plans and follows the diet. Many people, however, view the term *compliance* in a negative light because it implies the learner is submissive, and this is in conflict with the learner's right to determine his or her own healthcare decisions rather than be told what to do by a healthcare professional. Conversely, some professionals can be too quick to label a client as non-compliant. It is important to determine why a client is not following a recommended course of action before applying this label. For example, the client may have intended to comply but was unable to do so because he could not afford the cost of the medications.

Another term seen in healthcare literature is **adherence**, which is commitment or attachment to a regimen. Bastable and colleagues (2011) explain that both compliance and adherence refer to the "ability to maintain health-promoting regimens, which are determined largely by a health care provider" (p. 201).

Although **pedagogy** has historically been defined as the study or science of teaching, the term has increasingly been used to specifically refer to teaching children and adolescents. **Andragogy** is the art and science of teaching adults, while **geragogy** refers to the process of stimulating and helping older adults to learn (Hayes, 2005; John, 1988). The different learning needs of adults, versus children or older adults, has led to the science of developing specific approaches to teaching and learning, requiring the differentiation of terms. For example, when teaching a young child about what will happen in surgery, a doll may be used. This approach would be far less successful with a cognizant adult, but could work with a client who has a cognition deficit.

Learning Theories

A number of different learning theories help nurses understand how people learn. Adult learning theory, behaviorist theory, cognitive theory, social learning theory, and humanistic learning theory are among the theories most commonly used by nurses to teach individuals and groups of learners.

ADULT LEARNING THEORY Knowles, Holton, and Swanson (2005) proposed the adult education theory, which described differences between the learning styles of adults and those of children. Previously, it was assumed that adults and children learned in the same ways and that the same teaching principles could be used for both. Knowles et al. suggested four basic conceptual differences between adult and child education: (1) self-concept, (2) experience, (3) readiness to learn, and (4) time perspective. Selected characteristics of adult learners as outlined by Knowles et al. are as follows:

- **The need to know.** Adults need to know why they need to learn something.
- **The learners' self-concept.** Adults see themselves as being responsible for their own decisions and prefer to be treated by others as being capable of self-direction.
- **The role of the learners' experiences.** Adults already have accumulated life experiences that can enhance their current learning.
- **Readiness to learn.** Adults are often ready to learn what they need to know in order to take care of themselves.
- **Orientation to learning.** Adults are life centered, task centered, or problem centered in their approach to learning.

- **Motivation.** Adults are motivated to learn by internal pressures (enhanced self-esteem, quality of life, better job satisfaction) more than external pressures (promotions, higher pay).

Further research in andragogy has determined a number of factors about adult learners that nurses can use as guides for client teaching (Hayes, 2005; Knowles, 1984):

- As people mature, they move from dependence to independence.
- An adult's previous experiences can be used as a resource for learning.
- An adult's readiness to learn is often related to a developmental task or social role (i.e., perceive a need in his or her life situation).
- An adult is more oriented to learning when the material is useful immediately, not sometime in the future.

Nurses applying adult learning theory to the teaching process will:

- Communicate how/why the information is immediately useful to the learner.
- Respect the learner as an independent, competent adult.
- Through the process of assessment, identify previous experiences of the learner and help the learner acquire new information by building on these experiences.

BEHAVIORIST THEORY According to **behaviorist theory**, learning takes place when an individual's reaction (called a *response*) to a stimulus is either positively or negatively reinforced. Thus, to modify an individual's attitude and response, a behaviorist would either alter the stimulus condition in the environment or change what happens after a response occurs (Bastable et al., 2011, p. 59). Major contributors to behaviorist theory include Thorndike, Skinner, Pavlov, and Bandura.

Skinner's and Pavlov's work focused on conditioning behavioral responses to a stimulus that causes the response or behavior. To increase the probability of a response, Skinner introduced the importance of **positive reinforcement** (e.g., a pleasant experience such as praise and encouragement) in fostering repetition of an action.

Nurses applying behavioristic theory will:

- Provide sufficient practice time and both immediate and repeat testing and redemonstration.
- Provide opportunities for learners to solve problems by trial and error.
- Select teaching strategies that avoid distracting information and that evoke the desired response.
- Praise the learner for correct behavior and provide positive feedback at intervals throughout the learning experience.
- Provide role models of desired behavior.

Box 41–3   Cognitive Learning Processes

Cognitive theory proposes that learning involves three cognitive (mental) processes: acquiring information, processing the information, and using the information. These three processes can occur sequentially or simultaneously.

ACQUIRING INFORMATION

Acquiring information involves two processes: sensory reception and discrimination. Sensory reception is made possible by the neurosensory system. Stimuli in the environment signal the appropriate sense, such as sight, hearing, or smell. Impulses then travel by the nervous system to the brain. Sensory reception generally is continuous, but it is not always a conscious process.

The second aspect of acquiring information is discrimination. Discrimination is the ability to determine which stimuli are relevant in a particular situation. Stimuli can be objects, ideas, actions, or facts. They may be internal (i.e., inside the body) or external. Discrimination is the most difficult when there are multiple, complex stimuli.

PROCESSING INFORMATION

Processing provides meaning to the information. Information is processed in three steps:

1. *Association*, which is the joining of two or more ideas. For example, an individual may associate an object such as a needle with the word *needle* and/or with the experience of pain.
2. *Generalization*, which is the perceiving of similarities among various stimuli, for example, the similarities among three different syringes.
3. *Concept formation*, which is the organization of stimuli that have some attributes in common. For example, a nurse who understands the concept of caring appreciates the characteristics associated with caring. The nurse can then help others to convey caring in the healthcare setting.

USING INFORMATION

Using information is the application of information in the cognitive, affective, and psychomotor areas. The ability to formulate and relate concepts is an essential critical thinking skill. In addition, relating concepts is essential for creative thinking and problem solving.

COGNITIVE THEORY   **Cognitive theory**, or *cognitivism*, recognizes the developmental level of learners and acknowledges the learner's motivation and environment. It depicts learning as primarily a mental, intellectual, or thinking process. The learner structures and processes information (see **Box 41–3** ●). Perceptions are selectively chosen by the learner, and personal characteristics have an impact on how a cue is perceived. Cognitive theorists also emphasize the importance of social, emotional, and physical contexts in which learning occurs, such as the teacher–learner relationship and the environment. Developmental readiness and individual readiness (expressed as motivation) are other key factors associated with cognitive approaches. Major cognitive theorists include Jean Piaget, Kurt Lewin, and Benjamin Bloom.

Piaget's four major phases of cognitive development are:

1. The sensorimotor phase
2. The preconceptual phase
3. The concrete operations phase
4. The formal operations phase.

These are discussed in detail in the module on Development.

According to Lewin (1951), learning involves four different types of changes: change in cognitive structure, change in motivation, change in one's sense of belonging to the group, and gain in voluntary muscle control. His widely known theory of change has three basic stages: unfreezing, moving, and refreezing.

Bloom (1956) identified three domains or areas of learning. The **cognitive domain**, or the "thinking" domain, includes six intellectual abilities and thinking processes: knowing, comprehending, applying, analyzing, synthesizing, and evaluating. The **affective domain**, also known as the "feeling" domain, is divided into categories that specify the degree of a "person's depth of emotional response to tasks" (Bastable et al., 2011, p. 390). It includes feelings, emotions, interests, attitudes, and appreciations. The **psychomotor domain**, or the "skill" domain, includes motor skills, such as the fine motor skills required to give an injection.

Nurses should include each of Bloom's three domains in client teaching plans. For example, teaching a client with diabetes how to self-administer insulin is in the psychomotor domain. Teaching the client why insulin is needed and what to do when not feeling well is in the cognitive domain. Helping the client accept the chronic implications of diabetes and maintain self-esteem is in the affective domain.

Nurses applying cognitive theory will:

- Provide a social, emotional, and physical environment conducive to learning.
- Encourage a positive teacher–learner relationship.
- Select multisensory teaching strategies because perception is influenced by the senses.
- Recognize that personal characteristics have an impact on how cues are perceived and develop appropriate teaching approaches to target different learning styles.
- Assess a learner's developmental and individual readiness to learn and adapt teaching strategies to the learner's developmental level.
- Select behavioral objectives and teaching strategies that encompass the cognitive, affective, and psychomotor domains of learning.

CASE STUDY \\ A

Mr. Lowe is a 76-year-old man who had hip surgery 12 hours ago. The nurse and physical therapist enter the room to help Mr. Lowe move from the bed to the chair using a walker for the first time. Mr. Lowe had preoperative instructions on the use of the walker and had successfully demonstrated safe use of the walker. Currently, Mr. Lowe is disoriented to time and place, yet is able to follow simple commands.

Critical Thinking Questions

1. Discuss the impact of Mr. Lowe's ability to "learn" and apply information in the cognitive and psychomotor domains of learning.
2. Is teaching a priority of care for Mr. Lowe at this time? Why or why not?

SOCIAL LEARNING THEORY   Social learning theorists, such as Albert Bandura, believe that the entire learning process involves three highly interdependent factors:

1. The characteristics of the person
2. The person's behavior
3. The environment.

Bandura (1971) claims that most learning comes from observational learning and instruction rather than from overt trial-and-error behavior. **Observational learning** is the acquisition of new skills or the alteration of old behaviors simply by watching other children and adults. It is especially important for acquiring behavior in situations when mistakes can be life threatening or costly—for example, when driving a car or administering medication.

Bandura's research focuses on **imitation** (the process by which individuals copy or reproduce what they have observed) and on **modeling** (the process by which an individual learns by observing the behavior of others). Imitation is regarded as one of the most powerful socialization forces. Various imitative behaviors are reinforced by a process of operant conditioning. For example, a boy may be praised for being "just like his father." The child may even self-reinforce the imitations by repeating an adult's words of praise. According to Bandura, models influence others mainly by providing information rather than by eliciting matching behavior, so that learning can occur without even once performing the model's behavior.

By the 1980s, Bandura's theory had become more cognitive. It is now called *social cognitive theory*, and provides a framework showing that interaction between an individual and his behavior is influenced by the individual's thoughts and actions; that the interaction between the individual and the environment involves human beliefs and cognitive competencies; and that the interaction between the environment and behavior involves the individual's behavior determining his environment and in turn his behavior is modified by his environment (**Figure 41–1 ●**). For example, the effects of television on children depend on both cognitive and imitative processes. Whether the child can comprehend the story affects the child's perceptions of the model and the tendency to imitate the model. (It is interesting to note that Bandura's research explored the concerns regarding the influence of televised violence.)

Social learning theory often is applied when nurses teach clients new skills necessary for their self-care by providing information and, when necessary, modeling how to perform the new skill. For example, nurses may apply social learning theory when teaching clients how to:

- Administer an injection
- Change a wound dressing

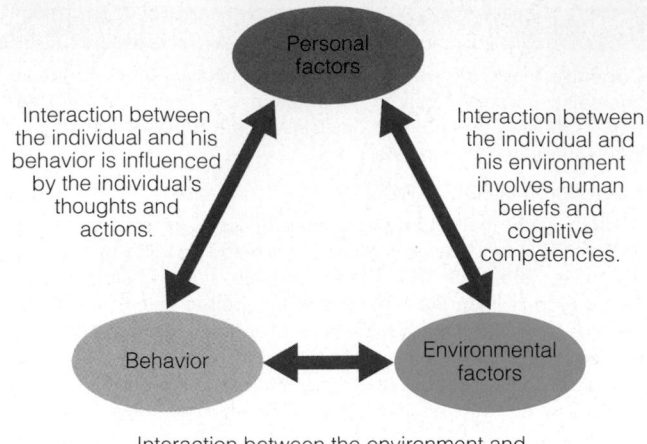

Interaction between the individual and his behavior is influenced by the individual's thoughts and actions.

Interaction between the individual and his environment involves human beliefs and cognitive competencies.

Interaction between the environment and behavior involves the individual's behavior determining his environment and in turn his behavior is modified by his environment.

Figure 41–1 ● Social cognitive theory.

- Change a suprapubic catheter
- Use assistive technology devices.

HUMANISTIC LEARNING THEORY   **Humanistic learning theory** focuses on both cognitive and affective qualities of the learner. According to humanistic theory, each individual is a unique composite of biological, psychological, social, cultural, and spiritual factors. Learning focuses on self-development and achieving full potential; it is most likely to occur when the information or skill being learned is relevant to the learner. Autonomy and self-determination are important; the learner identifies the learning needs and takes the initiative to meet these needs. The learner is an active participant and takes responsibility for meeting individual learning needs.

Prominent members of this school of thought include Abraham Maslow and Carl Rogers. Maslow's hierarchy of needs suggests a way of prioritizing nursing interventions so that physiological needs are met first, followed by safety and security needs, love and belonging needs, esteem and self-esteem needs, and ultimately, growth needs (see the module on Stress and Coping). Rogers was particularly concerned with personalized approaches. He emphasized that independence, creativity, and self-reliance are all facilitated when self-criticism and self-evaluation are of primary importance; evaluation by others is of secondary importance.

The major attributes of humanistic learning theory are its focus on the feelings and attitudes of learners, on the importance of the individual in identifying learning needs and taking responsibility for them, and on the self-motivation of the learners to work toward self-reliance and independence. Nurses applying humanistic theory will:

- Convey empathy in the nurse–client relationship.
- Encourage the learner to establish goals and promote self-directed learning.
- Encourage active learning by serving as a facilitator, mentor, or resource for the learner.

- Use active learning strategies to assist the client's adoption of new behavior.
- Expose the learner to new relevant information and ask appropriate questions to encourage the learner to seek answers.

CATEGORIZATION   According to Jerome Bruner (1966), perception, conceptualizing, learning, and decision making all depend on categorizing information. People interpret information in terms of the similarities and differences detected, and they arrange the information in related categories. For example, the human body contains hundreds of bones. By categorizing them into major bone types (e.g., long bones and flat bones) or areas of the body (e.g., bones of the head, bones of the hand, and vertebrae), it is easier to learn them. This theory of cognitive learning emphasizes the formation of a coding system. These systems serve to facilitate transfer, enhance retention, and increase problem-solving motivation. Bruner advocates discovery-oriented learning to help students discover relationships among categories. Bruner's work is sometimes considered to be a constructivist theory.

CONSTRUCTIVISM   **Constructivism** is a relatively recent term. It represents a collection of theories with the common thread of individuals actively constructing knowledge in order to solve realistic problems, often in collaboration with others. Constructivists describe learning as a change in meaning constructed from experience. Knowledge becomes an individual interpretation of experience; learning is the construction of new interpretations. Constructivists encourage learning inquiry, acknowledge the critical role of experience in learning, and encourage cooperative learning. Constructivist theory is applicable to concept-based learning.

The ideas of constructivism emerged with John Dewey and continued with Bruner (learning as discovery). Social development theorist Lev Vygotsky and social learning theorist Bandura are associated with the constructivists; however, their focus is more on the learning, not the teaching, with language as a process.

MULTIPLE INTELLIGENCE   Early psychologists gauged intelligence by use of the intelligence quotient, or IQ. They felt that intelligence at too low a level inhibits individuals from participating in intellectually demanding learning situations and that intelligence at a higher level indicated a genius. Those in between were considered to be normal. Many individuals were incorrectly labeled and, as a result, were never encouraged to reach higher potential.

Today, new theories have emerged disputing IQ as the only indicator of intelligence, arguing that intelligence has a number of dimensions and, contrary to previous thinking, is not fixed and unchangeable by training. Howard Gardner, head of the Project on Human Potential at Harvard University, has presented a theory of multiple intelligence. This is based on observations of how brain damage from a stroke might affect one area, such as language, while other areas of mental functioning remain intact. Gardner (1983) first cited seven intelligences:

1. Linguistic
2. Musical/rhythmic (music)
3. Logical/mathematical
4. Spatial (visual)
5. Body/kinesthetic/movement (body)
6. Personal
7. Symbols as intellectual strengths or ways of knowing.

Gardner has since added an eighth intelligence: naturalist. Gardner offers a fresh perspective to learning.

Being aware of the focus and limitations of the various learning theories allows the nurse to use one or more of them when developing a teaching plan for a client. Knowing what is important (e.g., knowledge, motivation, feelings, attitudes) assists the nurse in choosing the appropriate learning theory or theories. The nurse also needs to be aware of the different factors that can affect the client's learning.

Factors Affecting Learning

Many factors can facilitate or inhibit a client's ability to learn, including stress level, effects of medication, fatigue, or pain. The nurse should be aware of these factors, particularly when available teaching time is limited.

FACTORS FACILITATING LEARNING   A number of factors promote learning. Although these factors are common to all, how they promote learning in the individual learner will vary. What motivates one individual to learn, for example, may not motivate another individual at all.

Motivation   **Motivation to learn** is personal and affects how much an individual learns. It can also influence the rate of learning. Motivation must be identified and experienced by the client—the nurse's recognition of a need is not sufficient to motivate a client, although the nurse can help the client identify and embrace the need. The nurse can also help persuade support people of a need by providing information. For example, a man who has smoked for 20 years may not embrace the need to quit for the benefit of his own health. However, if the nurse provides client education that includes the dangers of secondhand smoke, especially to young children, the man may recognize the need to quit smoking for the benefit of a child or grandchild.

Readiness   **Readiness to learn** is the demonstration of behaviors or cues that reflect a learner's motivation to learn at a specific time. Readiness reflects not only the desire or willingness to learn but also the ability to learn at a specific time. The nurse's role is often to encourage the development of readiness. For example, a client may want to learn self-care during a dressing change, but if the client is experiencing pain or discomfort, he or she may not be able to learn. In this case, the nurse can provide pain medication to make the client more comfortable and ready to learn.

Active Involvement   When a learner is actively involved in the process of learning, learning becomes more meaningful. If a learner actively participates in planning and discussion, she will learn more quickly and retain more information. Active learning promotes critical thinking, enabling learners to solve problems more effectively. Clients who are actively involved in learning about their health care may be more able to apply the learning to their own situation. For example, clients who are actively involved in learning about their therapeutic diets may be more able to apply the principles being taught to their cultural food preferences and usual eating habits. Passive learning, such as listening to a lecture or watching a film, does not foster optimal learning.

Relevance Clients learn more quickly, and retain what they learn better, when what they are learning is personally relevant to them. It also helps when they can connect the new knowledge to that which they already know or have experienced. For example, if a client is diagnosed with hypertension, is overweight, and has symptoms of headaches and fatigue, he is more likely to understand the need to lose weight if he remembers having more energy when he weighed less. The nurse needs to validate the relevance of learning with the client throughout the learning process.

Feedback Feedback is information regarding an individual's performance in relation to a desired goal. It has to be meaningful to the learner. Feedback that accompanies the practice of psychomotor skills helps the person to learn those skills. Nurses provide positive feedback or reinforcement regarding desired behavior through praise, positively worded corrections, and suggestions of alternative methods. Negative feedback, such as ridicule, anger, or sarcasm, can lead people to withdraw from learning. Such feedback, viewed as a type of punishment, may cause the client to avoid the teacher in order to avoid punishment.

Nonjudgmental Support People learn best when they believe they are accepted and will not be judged. The individual who expects to be judged as a "poor" or "good" client will not learn as well as the individual who feels no such threat. Once learners have succeeded in accomplishing a task or understanding a concept, they gain self-confidence in their ability to learn. This reduces their anxiety about failure and can motivate greater learning. For example, when a nurse cares for a client who did not graduate from high school, she should independently assess the client's ability to learn and not make a judgment about the client's ability based on education level. Completing high school is an indication of the client's level of formal education, but not an indication of the client's intellect or ability to learn. The client may be highly intelligent and self-taught, so the nurse must begin by assessing the client's ability to learn.

Simple to Complex Learning is facilitated by material that is logically organized and proceeds from the simple to the complex. Such organization enables the learner to comprehend new information, assimilate it with previous learning, and form new understandings. Of course, *simple* and *complex* are relative terms, depending on the level at which the person is learning. What is simple for one person may be complex for another.

Repetition Repetition of key concepts and facts facilitates retention of newly learned material. Practice of psychomotor skills (particularly with feedback from the nurse) improves

performance of those skills and facilitates their transfer to another setting.

Timing People retain information and psychomotor skills best when there is a short time interval between learning and using what they learn; the longer the time interval, the easier it is for people to forget what they have learned. For example, a client who is only shown literature and videotapes about administering insulin but is not permitted to administer his own insulin until discharge from the hospital is unlikely to remember what was learned. However, giving his own injections while in the hospital (and with feedback from the nurse) enhances the client's learning.

Environment An optimal learning environment facilitates learning by reducing distractions and providing physical and psychological comfort. It has adequate lighting that is free from glare, a comfortable room temperature, and good ventilation. Most students know what it is like to try to learn in a hot, stuffy room; the consequent drowsiness interferes with concentration. Noise can also distract the student and interfere with listening and thinking. To facilitate learning in a hospital setting, nurses should choose a time when no visitors are present and interruptions are unlikely.

In some situations, privacy during the learning process is essential. For example, when a client is learning to change a colostomy bag, the presence of others can be embarrassing and thus interfere with learning. However, when a client is particularly anxious, having a support person present may give the client confidence.

CASE STUDY \\ B

Millie Delaney, a 36-year-old woman, is being transferred from the hospital to a long-term care facility to recover following a motor vehicle crash. Ms. Delaney sustained multiple fractures resulting in partial paralysis on the right side. She and the nurse planned a learning session at 1 p.m. to discuss wound care and medications the day before Ms. Delaney was to be transferred. At 1 p.m., the nurse comes to Ms. Delaney's room with supplies and handouts to help Ms. Delaney learn. The nurse finds Ms. Delaney actively crying.

Critical Thinking Questions

1. What actions should the nurse take at this time?
2. Can learning take place? Why or why not?
3. Discuss strategies that the nurse could use to enhance Ms. Delaney's readiness to learn.

FACTORS INHIBITING LEARNING Many factors inhibit learning. Some of the most common barriers to learning are described next and in **Table 41–1** ●.

Emotions Emotions such as fear, anger, and depression can impede learning. A high level of anxiety resulting in agitation and the inability to focus or concentrate can also inhibit learning. Clients or families who are experiencing extreme emotional states may not hear spoken words or may retain only part of the communication. Emotional responses such as fear and anxiety decrease with information that relieves uncertainty. Medications

TABLE 41-1   Barriers to Learning

BARRIER	EXPLANATION	NURSING IMPLICATIONS
Acute illness	Client requires all resources and energy to cope with illness.	Defer teaching until client is less ill.
Pain	Pain decreases ability to concentrate.	Conduct pain assessment before teaching.
Prognosis	Client can be preoccupied with illness and unable to concentrate on new information.	Defer teaching to a better time.
Biorhythms	Mental and physical performances have a circadian rhythm.	Adapt time of teaching to suit client. For example, plan a teaching session when the client is most alert.
Emotions (e.g., anxiety, denial, depression, or grief)	Emotions require energy and distract from learning.	Deal with emotions and possible misinformation first.
Language	Client may not be fluent in the nurse's language.	Obtain services of an interpreter or nurse with appropriate language skills.
Age		
Older adults	Vision, hearing, and motor control can be impaired in older adults.	Consider sensory and motor deficits, and adapt teaching plan as needed.
Children	Children have a shorter attention span and vocabulary differences.	Plan shorter and more active learning episodes.
Culture/religion	There may be cultural or religious restrictions on certain types of knowledge (e.g., birth control information).	Assess the client's cultural/religious needs when planning learning activities.
Physical disability	Visual, hearing, sensory, or motor impairments may interfere with a client's ability to learn.	Plan teaching activities appropriate to the learner's physical abilities. For example, provide audio learning tools for the client who is blind or large-print materials for the client whose vision is impaired.
Mental disability	Impaired cognitive ability may affect the client's capacity for learning.	Assess client's capacity for learning, and plan teaching activities to complement the client's ability while planning more complex learning for the client's caregivers.

may be prescribed for clients, or even families, who are extremely distraught in order to reduce their anxiety and put them in an emotional state in which understanding or learning can occur.

Physiological Events Physiological events such as a critical illness, pain, or sensory deficits inhibit learning. Because the client cannot concentrate and apply energy to learning, the learning itself is impaired. The nurse should try to reduce the physiological barriers to learning as much as possible before teaching. For clients experiencing a physiological event, analgesics and rest before teaching are often helpful.

Cultural Aspects Cultural barriers to learning arise when the client's language, beliefs, or values are different from those of the healthcare team. The most obvious barrier is that of language: The client who does not understand the nurse's language may learn very little. Another impediment to learning is the differing values held by the client and the healthcare team. For example, if a client comes from a culture that views being overweight or "plump" as positive, the nurse negotiates with the client to determine an acceptable weight, and they develop a plan together (Purnell & Paulanka, 2008). Western medicine also may conflict with a client's cultural healing beliefs and practices. To be effective, nurses must be culturally competent; otherwise, the client may be partially or totally noncompliant with recommended treatments.

Psychomotor Ability Nurses should be aware of clients' psychomotor ability when planning teaching. Psychomotor skills can be affected by health. For example, an older client who has severe osteoarthritis of the hands may not be able to wrap a bandage. The following physical abilities are important for learning psychomotor skills:

- **Muscle strength.** For example, an older client who cannot rise from a chair because of insufficient leg and muscle strength cannot be expected to learn to lift herself out of a bathtub.
- **Motor coordination.** Gross motor coordination is required for movements such as walking, and fine motor coordination is needed to eat with utensils. For example, a client who has advanced amyotrophic lateral sclerosis involving the lower limbs will probably be unable to use a walker.
- **Energy.** Energy is required for most psychomotor skills, and learning these skills uses even more energy. People who are ill or older often have limited energy resources; learning and carrying out these skills must be timed for when the client's energy sources are at their peak.
- **Sensory acuity.** Sight is used for most learning (e.g., walking with crutches, changing a dressing, or drawing a medication into a syringe). Clients who have a visual impairment often need the assistance of a support person to carry out such tasks.

Angela Simpson is a new mother who believes a fat baby is a healthy baby. She has grown up with this value and is being told this repeatedly by her mother (the baby's grandmother).

Clinical Thinking Questions

When developing a plan for teaching infant nutrition to this mother:

1. What essential information would you want Ms. Simpson to learn?

2. How could you increase Ms. Simpson's motivation to apply the information?

3. In what setting would Ms. Simpson be most likely to learn and retain the information?

▶ THE INTERNET AND HEALTH INFORMATION

The Internet has become a part of the lives of many Americans, allowing them to communicate and obtain information quickly. Internet technology has dramatically changed the activities of health care. The term **e-health** is defined as "the transfer of health resources and health care by electronic means" (World Health Organization, 2013, para. 1). Health resources and healthcare services include aspects of transferring health information, health systems management, interaction between healthcare providers and consumers, health education, and healthcare services via telehealth, digital health services, and other electronic devices.

Online Health Information

Internet use has rapidly increased during the past decade with many people seeking health information online. The Pew Internet and American Life Project reports that 85% of American adults use the Internet and 72% seek out health information online. Mobile devices and healthcare-related apps continue to increase in usage. Although the Internet provides a plethora of health information, many American adults still use traditional means of gathering healthcare information when information or assistance is needed: 70% ask a healthcare professional, 60%

ask a friend or family member, and 24% seek the support of others with the same condition (Fox, 2013). In addition, 41% have read someone else's commentary or experience related to their own health issue, and 19% have signed up to receive updates about health or medical issues. More telling, 60% say online information affected their decision on treating a medical condition, while only 53% say it led them to talk to a healthcare provider and 38% said it influenced their decision to see a physician. Three percent report they or someone they know was harmed by following health information found on the Internet (Fox & Jones, 2009a).

The demographics of individuals using the Internet to search for health information indicate that women, adults ages 18–65, college graduates, and those with a household income greater than $75,000 seek out health information on the Internet more than do men, older adults, noncollege graduates, and households with lower incomes (Fox & Jones, 2009b).

Older Adults and Use of the Internet

The Pew Internet & American Life Project (Zickuhr & Madden, 2012) conducted a research study looking at how older adults use the Internet. The findings in the 2012 report include the following:

- Fifty-three percent of Americans over the age of 65 use the Internet or e-mail.
- Of the older adults who use the Internet, 70% use it daily.
- Internet usage drops significantly with those ages 75 and older.
- Sixty-nine percent of Americans over the age of 65 own a cell phone.
- Thirty-four percent of Americans over the age of 65 use social networking sites.

Implications

The Internet is an important source of health information for many adult clients in the United States. Nurses need to know and be able to integrate this technology into the teaching plans for those clients who use the Internet. Nurses also need to apply effective teaching strategies for those clients who do not use the Internet.

◢ REVIEW The Concept of Teaching and Learning

RELATE Link the Concepts

Linking the concept of teaching and learning with the concept of communication:

1. How does the quality of a nurse's communication skills impact his ability to teach?

2. How does the ability to communicate with those who speak a different language impact the teaching process?

Linking the concept of teaching and learning with the concept of advocacy:

3. How does the role of the nurse as teacher combine with the role of the nurse as advocate?

4. A nurse teaches a client newly diagnosed with diabetes how to provide self-care to reduce the risk of complications. How does teaching this client serve the nurse's advocacy role?

REFER Go to Pearson Nursing Student Resources nursing.pearsonhighered.com

- Additional review materials

REFLECT Case Study

A nurse, Samuel Jordan, has worked on the medical unit of a local acute care facility for the past 4 years. He has 9 years of nursing experience, having worked at another facility for 5 years before accepting this position. The unit is usually staffed with registered nurses (RNs), nursing assistants, and licensed practical nurses, along with a clinical secretary who transcribes orders, answers the phone, and obtains supplies. Throughout the course of an average day, Samuel interacts with many different members of the healthcare team.

1. What teaching opportunities is Samuel likely to encounter on a normal workday?

2. What teaching opportunities might Samuel encounter on his days off?

3. How does teaching impact Samuel's self-evaluation of his work performance?

EXEMPLAR 41.1 Client/Consumer Education

EXEMPLAR KEY TERMS
Anticipatory guidance, *2520*
Anticipatory problem solving, *2522*
Health literacy, *2514*

EXEMPLAR LEARNING OUTCOMES
After reading about this exemplar, you will be able to:

1. Assess the learning needs of learners and the learning environment.
2. Identify nursing diagnoses, outcomes, and interventions that reflect the learning needs of clients.
3. Describe the essential aspects of a teaching plan.
4. Discuss guidelines for effective teaching.
5. Evaluate strategies to use when teaching clients of different cultures, literacy or educational levels, or language skills.
6. Summarize the impact of anticipatory guidance on health outcomes.
7. Identify methods to evaluate learning and teaching.
8. Demonstrate effective documentation of teaching–learning activities.

▶ OVERVIEW

Providing client education is a major aspect of nursing practice and an important independent nursing function. In 1992, the American Hospital Association passed *A Patient's Bill of Rights*, which recognized client education as a right of all clients. State nurse practice acts include client teaching as a function of nursing, thereby making teaching a legal and professional responsibility. In addition, the Joint Commission has expanded its standards of client education by nurses to include "evidence that patients and their significant others participate in care and decision making and understand what they have been taught. This requirement means that providers must consider the literacy level, educational background, language skills, and culture of every client during the education process" (Bastable et al., 2011, p. 6).

Client education is multifaceted, involving promoting, protecting, and maintaining health. It involves teaching clients about how to reduce health risk factors, increase their level of wellness, and take protective measures. **Box 41–4** ● lists specific areas of health teaching.

▶ TEACHING ENVIRONMENTS

Nurses teach a variety of clients/consumers in various settings, including hospitals, primary care clinics, urgent care, managed care, the home, and assisted living and long-term care facilities. Nurses teach large and small groups of learners in community health education programs.

Teaching Individual Clients
The nurse is in a position to promote healthy lifestyles through the application of health knowledge, the change process, learning theories, and the nursing and teaching process when teaching clients and their families. As with nursing interventions, client education opportunities are tailored to needs identified in

---

Box 41–4 Areas for Client Education

PROMOTION OF HEALTH
- Increasing individual level of wellness
- Growth and development topics
- Fertility control
- Hygiene
- Nutrition
- Exercise
- Stress management
- Lifestyle modification
- Resources within the community

PREVENTION OF ILLNESS/INJURY
- Health screening (e.g., blood glucose levels, blood pressure, blood cholesterol, Pap test, mammograms, vision, hearing, routine physical examinations)
- Reducing health risk factors (e.g., lowering cholesterol level)
- Specific protective health measures (e.g., immunizations, use of condoms, use of sunscreen, use of medication, umbilical cord care)
- First aid
- Safety (e.g., using seat belts, helmets, walkers)

RESTORATION OF HEALTH
- Information about tests, diagnosis, treatment, medications
- Self-care skills or skills needed to care for family member
- Resources within healthcare setting and community

ADAPTING TO ALTERED HEALTH AND FUNCTION
- Adaptations in lifestyle
- Problem-solving skills
- Adaptation to changing health status
- Strategies to deal with current problems (e.g., home IV skills, medications, diet, activity limits, prostheses)
- Strategies to deal with future problems (e.g., fear of pain with terminal cancer, future surgeries, or treatments)
- Information about treatments and likely outcomes
- Referrals to other healthcare facilities or services
- Facilitation of strong self-image
- Grief and bereavement counseling

TABLE 41-2 Comparison of the Teaching Process and the Nursing Process

STEP	TEACHING PROCESS	NURSING PROCESS
1	Collect data; analyze client's learning strengths and deficits.	Collect data; analyze client's strengths and deficits.
2	Make educational diagnoses.	Make nursing diagnoses.
3	Prepare teaching plan: ■ Write learning outcomes. ■ Select content and time frame. ■ Select teaching strategies.	Plan nursing goals/desired outcomes and select interventions.
4	Implement teaching plan.	Implement nursing strategies.
5	Evaluate client learning based on achievement of learning outcomes.	Evaluate client outcomes based on achievement of goal criteria.

consultation with clients and their families. In many ways, the teaching process shares many similarities with the nursing process (Table 41–2 ●), including assessment of needs, planning, implementation, and evaluation.

Nurses may teach individual clients in one-to-one teaching episodes. For example, the nurse may teach about wound care while changing a client's dressing or may teach about diet, exercise, and other lifestyle behaviors that minimize the risk of a heart attack for a client who has a cardiac problem. The nurse may also be involved in teaching family members or other support people who are caring for the client. Nurses working in obstetric and pediatric areas teach parents and sometimes grandparents how to care for children.

Because of the current trend toward shorter hospital stays, time constraints on client education may occur. Nurses need to provide client education that will ensure the client's safe transition from one level of care to another and make appropriate plans for follow-up education in the client's home. Discharge plans must include information about what the client has been taught before transfer or discharge and what remains for the client to learn to perform self-care in the home or other residence.

■ Provide a calm environment to decrease distractions.

■ Take time in teaching. Observe the client for signs or feelings of being overwhelmed, confused, and anxious.

■ Adapt your teaching plan to reflect the client's reactions. If the client is confused, avoid moving on to more information. Determine where the client became confused and address the issue until understanding occurs before moving to additional information.

■ Instructions may need to be repeated several times due to the client's level of anxiety and stress.

■ Evaluate the client's (or support person's) ability to perform a skill through return demonstration. Having the client or support person demonstrate how they would perform the skill in response to "what if . . ." situations exhibits mastery of the skill.

Teaching in the Community

Nurses are often involved in community health education programs. Such teaching activities may be voluntary as part of the nurse's involvement in an organization (e.g., the American Red Cross, Planned Parenthood) or they may comprise part of

the nurse's work role. Nurses work in a variety of community settings, including local health departments, schools, and colleges and universities. Community teaching activities may be aimed at large groups of people who have an interest in some aspect of health, such as nutrition classes, CPR or cardiac risk factor reduction classes, and bicycle or swimming safety programs. Community education programs also can be designed for small groups or individual learners, such as childbirth classes or family planning classes.

CLINICAL EXAMPLE

When providing teaching to groups, it is essential to tailor the teaching to the participants in the group. For example, during fall sports season, three athletes at a local high school develop staph infections. The school nurse takes into consideration the following groups who have a stake in the health and well-being of student athletes: (1) the athletes themselves, (2) their parents, (3) the coaches, and (4) teachers and other staff at the school. The nurse recognizes that providing each group with only a handout will be insufficient. The nurse decides to work with the school's athletic director and physical trainer to develop a teaching session for the coaches that reinforces both individual hygiene as well as local and state regulations related to preventing staph infections. She also plans to demonstrate how to properly clean equipment such as wrestling mats. In collaboration with the trainer, the nurse also develops and schedules a teaching session for the athletes themselves. Recognizing the importance of peer influence in this group, the nurse obtains parental permission for one of the athletes who acquired a staph infection to come speak to the others about what it was like and to help her persuade the students to take steps to avoid infections.

▶ DEVELOPING A TEACHING PLAN

Nurses must assess the needs of the client or group before beginning to create a teaching plan. For individual clients (and their families), the nurse considers the client's health history, the client's physical and psychosocial assessment, and the client's support systems (e.g., caregivers, access to transportation). The nurse also considers factors that influence the learning process, such as readiness, motivation, reading and comprehension level, and mobility.

Client Health History

Several elements in the nursing history provide clues to learning needs. These elements include (a) age and developmental level, (b) the client's understanding and perceptions of the health problem, (c) health beliefs and practices, (d) cultural factors, (e) economic factors, (f) learning style, and (g) the client's support systems. Examples of interview questions to elicit this information are shown in the accompanying Assessment Interview. Note the number of open-ended questions.

These factors apply to both individuals and individuals in communities. For example, consider the nurse who is planning a teaching session on health promotion for individuals with high blood pressure. Although the teaching plan for clients at an independent living facility will be different than that for a single client, the plan will still consider factors such as:

- Primary language of the clients
- Age and developmental level

- Economic factors (e.g., access to transportation, health insurance coverage).

AGE AND DEVELOPMENTAL LEVEL   Age provides information on the person's developmental status that may indicate distinctive health teaching content and teaching approaches. Simple questions to school-age children and adolescents will elicit information on what they know. Observing young children at play provides information about their motor and intellectual development as well as relationships with other children. For older adults, conversation and questioning may reveal slow recall or limited psychomotor skills, sensory deficits, and learning difficulties (see Lifespan Considerations).

CLIENTS' UNDERSTANDING OF HEALTH PROBLEM   Clients' perceptions of their current health problems and concerns may indicate deficient knowledge or misinformation. In addition, the effects of the problem on the client's usual activities can alert the nurse to other areas requiring instruction. For example, individuals who cannot manage self-care at home often need information about community resources and services.

Assessment Interview   Learning Needs and Characteristics

Primary Health Problem

- Tell me what you know about your current health problem. What do you think caused it?
- What concerns do you have about it?
- How has the problem affected what you can or cannot do during your usual activities (e.g., work, recreation, shopping, and housework)?
- What do you or did you do at home to relieve the problem? How helpful was it?
- How have the treatments you have started helped your problem?
- What, if any, difficulties have the treatments caused you (e.g., inconvenience, cost, discomfort)?
- Tell me about the tests (surgery, treatments) you are going to have.

Health Beliefs

- How would you describe your health generally?
- What things do you usually do to keep healthy?
- What health problems do you think you may be at risk for because of family history, age, diet, occupation, inadequate exercise, or other habits, such as smoking?
- What changes would you be willing to make to decrease your risk for these problems or to improve your health?

Cultural Factors

- What language do you use most often when speaking and writing?
- Do you seek the advice of another health practitioner?

- Do you use herbs or other medications or treatments commonly used by your cultural group? If so, does your current primary care provider know about these?
- What advice or treatments given previously by your primary care provider conflicted with values or beliefs you consider important?
- When a conflict arose, what did you do?

Learning Style

- Note the client's age and developmental level.
- What level of education have you received?
- Do you like to read?
- Where do you obtain health information (primary care provider, nurse, magazines, books, pharmacist, etc.)?
- How do you best learn new things?
  a. By reading about them
  b. By talking about them
  c. By watching a movie or demonstration
  d. By computer
  e. By listening to the teacher
  f. By first being shown how something works and then doing it
  g. On your own or in a group.

Client Support System

- Would you like a family member or friend to help you learn about things you need to do to take care of yourself?
- Who do you think would be interested in learning with you?

Health information can be difficult to obtain prior to providing teaching in a group setting. Whenever possible, nurses try to assess the health perceptions of participants in advance. Strategies include:

- Circulating brief surveys
- Surveying staff at the setting where teaching will be provided
- Conducting brief surveys as clients arrive for the teaching session.

Referring to the earlier example, the school nurse might ask the coaches to circulate surveys to athletes at the beginning of practice a week before the session. An alternative might be to hold a brief question-and-answer session with team captains to get a sense of athletes' attitudes toward hygiene and general habits and practices among their teammates.

HEALTH BELIEFS AND PRACTICES   A client's health beliefs and practices are important to consider in any teaching plan. The health belief model described in the module on Health, Wellness, and Illness provides a predictor of preventive health behavior. However, even if a nurse is convinced that a particular client's health beliefs should be changed, doing so may not be possible because so many factors are involved in client health beliefs.

CULTURAL FACTORS   Many cultural groups have their own beliefs and practices, some of which are related to diet, health, illness, and lifestyle. The cultural practices and values held by clients will affect their learning needs. For example, the client may understand the healthcare information being taught, but may not use any of it if she believes in following the practices of her culture of origin.

Lifespan Considerations Teaching Across the Life Span

Children

When developing a teaching plan for a child, assessing the level of development of the child is important. Most teaching plans focus on primary health care, health promotion, and illness/injury prevention. The teaching plan should be primarily directed toward parental teaching. Nurses must include the child in forms of teaching the child is able to understand. The use of the following strategies should be incorporated into any teaching plan involving a child:

- Establish trust.
- Use a calm approach and provide a calm environment.
- Involve parent or primary caregiver.
- Provide for safety.
- Address child by name.
- Provide instructions at child's level of understanding.
- Allow time for questions from child or parent.
- Address concerns and fears of child or parent.
- Allow time for the child or parent to practice the skill/task.
- Provide feedback, praise, and encouragement.
- Reinforce teaching as needed.
- Evaluate the effectiveness of the learning and teaching.
- Document.

Older Adults

Teaching older adults focuses on health promotion and illness/injury prevention. Many older adults have chronic illnesses that are treated with various medications and treatments. Nurses teaching older adults must address aging factors that influence learning in teaching plans to ensure that maximal learning can take place. The factors influencing learning on older adults include:

- Sensory perception alterations (hearing, vision, touch)
- Energy level

- Memory
- Response time
- Cultural background
- Stress
- Physical abilities.

Teaching plans for older adults commonly focus on nutrition, physical activity, safety, medications, and follow-up healthcare appointments. To maximize learning, the nurse must include the older adult in developing a teaching plan and setting goals. Teaching interventions to maximize learning include the following:

- Establish trust.
- Use a calm approach and provide a calm environment.
- Pace the provision of information against the client's energy levels and allow time for processing.
- Provide repetition as needed with positive reinforcement.
- Direct teaching to level of understanding.
- Use written materials that meet the older adult's need:
  - Use off-white, flat matte paper and black print.
  - Use large print (e.g., at least 14-point font).
  - Use materials at a fifth- to sixth-grade reading level.
- Allow time to practice skills/tasks. Use return demonstrations to evaluate mastery.
- May need to include significant other or primary caregiver.
- Assess reasons for noncompliance.
- Evaluate teaching and learning effectiveness.
- Document.

Older adults have past experiences and knowledge that affect their current experiences and attitudes toward healthcare teaching. Respect the older adult and use their past experiences, knowledge, and skills to help them to learn.

Sources: Based on Osborn, K. S., Wraa, C. E., Watson, A. B., & Holleran, R. (2013). *Medical-surgical nursing: Preparation for practice.* Upper Saddle River, NJ: Pearson; Ball, J., Bindler, R., & Cowen, K. (2012). *Principles of pediatric nursing: Caring for children* (5th ed.). Upper Saddle River, NJ: Pearson; and Bastable, S. B. (2014). *Nurse as educator: Principles of teaching and learning for nursing practice* (4th ed.). Burlington, MA: Jones & Bartlett.

ECONOMIC FACTORS Economic factors can also affect learning. For example, a client who cannot afford to obtain a new sterile syringe for each injection of insulin may find it difficult to learn to administer the insulin when the nurse teaches that a new syringe should be used each time. In a group setting, nurses may be teaching individuals who have limited access to transportation, who lack health insurance, or who are dependent on others for their financial security. Nurses must take these factors into account when planning education sessions in the community.

LEARNING STYLES Considerable research has been done on learning styles. The best way to learn varies with the individual. Some individuals are visual learners and learn best by watching. Others do not visualize an activity well; they learn best by actually manipulating equipment and discovering how it works. Some learn well from reading things presented in an orderly fashion. Still others learn best in groups where they can relate to other people. For some, stressing the thinking part of a skill and its logic will promote learning. For other people, stressing the feeling part or interpersonal aspect motivates and promotes learning.

The nurse seldom has the time or skills to assess each learner, identify her particular learning style, and then adapt teaching accordingly. What the nurse can do, however, is ask clients how they have learned things best in the past or how they like to learn. Many people know what helps them learn, and the nurse can use this information in planning the teaching. Using a variety of teaching techniques and varying activities during teaching are good ways to match learners with learning styles. One technique will be most effective for some clients, whereas other techniques will be suited to clients with different learning styles.

It is particularly important to use a variety of teaching techniques when providing teaching in community settings. Videos, whiteboards, and opportunities to practice demonstrations can be combined to ensure the highest rate of retention among group members. Power Point presentations can also be helpful. Some learners may benefit from receiving a written plan or agenda of the session in advance to help them follow along with the presentation.

CLIENT SUPPORT SYSTEM The nurse explores clients' support systems to determine the extent to which others may enhance learning and offer support. Family members or a close friend may help clients perform required skills at home and maintain required lifestyle changes.

Physical Examination

When working with individual clients, the general survey part of the physical examination provides useful clues to the client's learning needs, such as mental status, energy level, and nutritional status. Other parts of the physical examination reveal data about the client's physical capacity to learn and to perform self-care activities. For example, visual ability, hearing ability, and muscle coordination affect the selection of content and approaches to teaching.

Readiness to Learn

Clients who are ready to learn often behave differently from those who are not. A client who is ready may search out information,

for instance, by asking questions, reading books or articles, talking to others, and generally showing interest. The individual who is not ready to learn is more likely to avoid the subject or situation. In addition, the unready client may change the subject when it is brought up by the nurse. For example, if the nurse says, "I was wondering about a good time to show you how to change your dressing," a client who is not ready to learn might respond "Oh, my wife will take care of everything." Using cues from the client can result in teaching moments (small chunks of time in which the client is receptive to information). Observe the client's reaction during a teaching moment because it may lead into a longer period of receptiveness.

The nurse assesses for these readiness characteristics.

- **Physical readiness.** Is the client able to focus on things other than physical status, or are pain, fatigue, and immobility using up all of the client's time and energy?
- **Emotional readiness.** Is the client emotionally ready to learn self-care activities? Clients who are extremely anxious, depressed, or grieving over their health status are not ready.
- **Cognitive readiness.** Can the client think clearly at this point? Are the effects of anesthesia and analgesia altering the client's level of consciousness?

Nurses can promote readiness to learn by providing physical and emotional support during the critical stage of recovery. As the client stabilizes physically and emotionally, the nurse can then provide actual opportunities to learn.

In group settings, where attendance is voluntary, clients are more likely to be ready to learn new information. When attendance is compulsory, such as in a school setting or an inpatient treatment facility, client readiness to learn may vary considerably. In these instances it is especially important that nurses be able to manage problem behaviors, such as monopolizing (see the module on Communication).

Motivation

Motivation relates to whether the client wants to learn and is usually greatest when the client is ready, the learning need is recognized, and the information being offered is meaningful to the client. Assessment of motivation, however, may be difficult. Nurses should be alert for information that indicates a readiness for change, such as a client saying "I'm really ready to lose weight this time." On the other hand, nonverbal behaviors such as disinterest, lack of attention, and missed appointments can indicate a decreased motivation to learn.

Nurses can use the following appropriate strategies to increase client motivation in both individual and group settings:

- Relate the learning to something the client values and help the client see the relevance of the learning.
- Help the client make the learning situation pleasant and nonthreatening.
- Encourage self-direction and independence.
- Demonstrate a positive attitude about the client's ability to learn.
- Offer continuing support and encouragement as the client attempts to learn (i.e., positive reinforcement).

Box 41–5 Populations Most Likely to Experience Limited Health Literacy

- Adults older than 65 years of age
- Racial and ethnic groups other than White
- Recent refugees and immigrants
- Individuals with less than a high school degree or GED
- Individuals with incomes at or below the poverty level
- Nonnative speakers of English

- Create a learning situation in which the client is likely to succeed. (Succeeding in small tasks motivates the client to continue learning.)
- Assist the client to identify the benefits of changing behavior.

Health Literacy

The 2003 National Assessment of Adult Literacy Study reported that only 12% of American adults meet the proficient health literacy level and 77 million adults have basic or below basic health literacy levels (U.S. Department of Health and Human Services [USDHHS], 2008). A report from the Institute of Medicine (IOM) (2004) titled *Health Literacy: A Prescription to End Confusion* states that nearly half of all Americans have difficulty understanding and acting on health information (p. 1). Moreover, studies that assessed a variety of health-related materials found that the materials' reading level exceeded the 12th-grade level.

Health literacy is the ability to obtain, read, understand, and apply health information in making appropriate healthcare decisions (Heinrich, 2012, p. 218). The National Action Plan to Improve Health Literacy (USDHHS, 2010) states "some groups are more likely than others to have limited health literacy. Certain populations are most likely to experience limited health literacy" (see **Box 41–5**).

Low health literacy skills are associated with poor health outcomes and higher healthcare costs (IOM, 2004). For example, a client may not be able to read a prescription to know how many pills to take or may take the wrong number of pills (e.g., in written form, "once" means 11 in Spanish). Clients with low literacy skills have less information about health promotion and management of a disease process for themselves and their families because they are unable to read the educational materials. As a result, they have higher rates of hospitalization than people with adequate health literacy.

Nurses face a challenge when they have to teach clients with low or no reading and writing skills. However, such teaching is vitally important because clients with low literacy skills need learning opportunities to improve their health practices.

CASE STUDY \\ D

David Rodriquez is a 28-year-old man who had an emergency appendectomy yesterday. He is to be discharged home later today. During discharge teaching, the nurse provides Mr. Rodriquez with a couple of handouts relating to wound care, medications, activity restrictions, and follow-up appointments. The nurse knows the handouts will fit Mr. Rodriquez's learning style because he said he likes to read and the nurse observed Mr. Rodriquez reading a couple of times this morning.

Critical Thinking Questions

1. Should the nurse have used the handouts as a learning tool? Why or why not?
2. What strategies might clients use to avoid embarrassment by having to admit they cannot read English?
3. What strategies might a nurse use to help a client who cannot read English learn about self-care?

SAFETY ALERT

The majority of people at the lowest reading levels will report that they "read well." Often clients will not admit to having difficulty reading because of the embarrassment it brings them. A nurse who suspects a client has difficulty reading may ask the client tactful questions, such as "Would you like me to go over it with you?"

It can be difficult to assess a client's literacy skills because the shame and stigma associated with limited health literacy skills are major barriers. Clients may be too embarrassed to admit they cannot read. The following client behaviors may cause a nurse to suspect a literacy problem:

- Pattern of noncompliance
- Insisting that they already know the information
- Having a friend or family member read the document for them
- Pattern of excuses for not reading the instructions (e.g., glasses broken, stating will read later or when they get home).

Many formulas are available for assessing the reading level of written material. Most word processing programs have a feature that will calculate the readability. Nurses involved in developing written health teaching materials should write for lower reading levels (see Client Teaching: Developing Written Teaching Aids). The

Client Teaching
Developing Written Teaching Aids

- Keep language level at or below the fifth- or sixth-grade level.
- Use active, not passive, voice.
- Use easy, common words of one or two syllables (e.g., *use* instead of *utilize*, or *give* instead of *administer*).
- Use the second person (*you*) rather than the third person (*the client*).
- Use a large type size (14- to 16-point font).
- Write short sentences.
- Avoid using all capital letters.
- Place priority information first and repeat more than once.
- Use bold for emphasis.
- Use simple pictures, drawings, or cartoons, if appropriate.
- Leave plenty of white space.
- Obtain feedback from nurses and clients.

Client Teaching Teaching Clients With Low Literacy Levels

- Use multiple teaching methods: Show pictures. Read important information. Lead a small group discussion. Role play. Demonstrate a skill. Provide hands-on practice.
- Emphasize key points in simple terms and provide examples.
- Limit the amount of information in a single teaching session. Instead of one long session that provides a great deal of information, it is better to provide more frequent sessions that cover a major point at each session.
- Associate new information with something the client already knows or associates with his job or lifestyle.
- Reinforce information through repetition.
- Involve the client in the teaching.
- Obtain feedback: Ask the client specific questions about the information presented or ask the client to repeat it in her own words.
- Avoid handouts with many pages and classroom lecture format with a large group.

---

goal is for the educational materials to be at a fifth- or sixth-grade level. Individuals with good reading skills are not offended by simple reading material and prefer easy-to-read information. Even the simplest written directions, however, will not be helpful to the client with low or no reading skills. See the Client Teaching feature for suggestions on how to teach clients with low literacy levels.

▶ IDENTIFYING LEARNING NEEDS

Nursing diagnoses for clients with learning needs can be designated in two ways: as the client's primary concern or problem, or as the etiology of a nursing diagnosis associated with the client's response to health alterations or dysfunction.

Learning Need as the Diagnostic Label

NANDA International is charged with providing evidence-based diagnoses terminology and guidance to the nursing community to assist in providing consistent, evidence-based care across all settings in which nurses care for clients. NANDA International's diagnostic labels list includes *Deficient Knowledge*, which is appropriate to a client's learning needs when the learning need is the primary concern because the client lacks knowledge related to a specific healthcare issue or topic (NANDA-I © 2012).

Whenever the nursing diagnosis label *Deficient Knowledge* is used, either the client is seeking health information or the nurse has identified a learning need. The area of deficiency should always be included in the diagnosis. Following are examples using the NANDA label *Deficient Knowledge* as the primary concern:

- *Deficient Knowledge* (Low-Calorie Diet) related to inexperience with newly ordered therapy
- *Deficient Knowledge* (Home Safety Hazards) related to denial of declining health and living alone.

(NANDA-I © 2012)

When working with clients who have a knowledge deficit, the nurse provides information that has the potential to change the client's behavior rather than focus on the behaviors caused by the client's lack of knowledge.

A second nursing diagnosis label for which a learning need may be the primary concern is *Readiness for Enhanced Knowledge*. When this diagnostic label is used, the client is seeking information. Note that the client may or may not have an altered response or dysfunction at the time but may be seeking information to improve health or prevent illness. This diagnosis is especially appropriate for clients attending community health education programs. An example of using the NANDA label *Readiness for Enhanced Knowledge* as the primary concern is:

- *Readiness for Enhanced Knowledge* related to desire to improve health behaviors and decrease risk of heart disease.

This diagnosis may be appropriate for the client who has identified a personal health risk for a cardiac condition and wants to minimize that risk through exercise.

A third nursing diagnosis label in which a learning need may be the primary concern is that of *Noncompliance*, which recognizes that the individual or caregiver may not always be able to follow the treatment or care plan as agreed (NANDA-I © 2012). This diagnostic label generally is used when clients have an intent to comply but barriers affect compliance. Factors that influence a client's compliance with health teaching include understanding or comprehension of the teaching, any negative side effects of the treatment, financial inability to carry out the treatment plan, language barriers, or poor teaching on the part of the healthcare team. *Noncompliance* should *not* be used for a client who is unable to follow instructions (e.g., cognitive disability) or for a client who makes an informed decision to refuse or not follow the medical treatment (Wilkinson, 2013).

Deficient Knowledge as the Etiology

Another way to deal with identified learning needs of clients is to write *deficient knowledge* as the etiology, or second part, of the diagnosis statement. Such nursing diagnoses are written in the following format:

- *Risk for* (Specify) related to deficient knowledge (specify).

Examples include the following:

- *Risk for Impaired Parenting* related to deficient knowledge (skills in infant care and feeding)
- *Risk for Infection* related to deficient knowledge (sexually transmitted infections and their prevention)
- *Anxiety* related to deficient knowledge (bone marrow aspiration).

(NANDA-I © 2012)

Other nursing diagnoses in which a knowledge deficit can be the etiology include the following:

- *Risk for Injury*
- *Ineffective Breastfeeding*
- *Impaired Adjustment*
- *Ineffective Coping*
- *Ineffective Health Maintenance*.

(NANDA-I © 2012)

Note also that most nursing diagnoses approved by NANDA International imply a teaching–learning need. For example, the nursing diagnosis *Constipation* suggests the need for a review of bowel hygiene practices including diet, hydration, and exercise/activity.

Planning

Developing a teaching plan is accomplished in a series of steps. Involving the client at this time promotes the formation of a meaningful plan and stimulates client motivation. The client who helps develop the teaching plan is more likely to achieve the desired outcomes (see Client Teaching: Sample Teaching Plan for Wound Care).

DETERMINING TEACHING PRIORITIES The client's learning needs must be ranked according to priority. The client and the nurse should do this together, with the client's priorities always being considered. Once a client's priorities have been addressed, the client is generally more motivated to concentrate

---

Client Teaching   Sample Teaching Plan for Wound Care

Assessment of Learner

A 24-year-old male college student suffered a 7-cm (2.5-in.) laceration on the left lower anterior leg during a hockey game. The laceration was cleaned, sutured, and bandaged. The client was given an appointment to return to the health clinic in 10 days for suture removal. Client states that he lives in the college dormitory and is able to do wound care if given instructions. Client is able to understand and read English. Assessed to be in the "preparation" and "action" stages of change.

Nursing Diagnosis

Deficient Knowledge (Care of Sutured Wound) related to no prior experience.

Long-Term Goal

Client's wound will heal completely without infection or other complications.

Intermediate Goal

At clinic appointment, client's wound will be healing without signs of infection, loss of function, or other complication.

Short-Term Goals

Client will (a) correctly list three signs and symptoms of wound infection and (b) correctly perform a return demonstration of wound cleansing and bandaging.

LEARNING OUTCOMES	CONTENT OUTLINE	TEACHING METHODS
Upon completion of the instructional session, the client will		
■ Describe normal wound healing.	Normal wound healing	Describe normal wound healing with the use of audiovisuals.
■ Describe signs and symptoms of wound infection.	Infection Signs and symptoms include wound warm to touch, misalignment of wound edges, and purulent wound drainage. Signs of systemic infection include fever and malaise.	Discuss the mechanism of wound infection. Use audiovisuals to demonstrate infected wound appearance. Provide handout describing signs and symptoms of wound infection.
■ Identify equipment needed for wound care.	Wound care equipment Cleansing solution as prescribed by physician (e.g., clear water, mild soap and water, or antimicrobial solution)	Demonstrate equipment needed for cleansing and bandaging wound. Provide handout listing equipment needed.
■ Demonstrate wound cleansing and bandaging.	Bandaging material: Telfa, gauze wrap, adhesive tape Demonstration of wound cleansing and bandaging on the client's wound or a mannequin	Demonstrate wound cleansing and bandaging on the client's wound or a mannequin. Provide handout describing procedure for cleansing and bandaging wound.
■ Describe appropriate action if questions or complications arise.	Resources available for client questions include health clinic, emergency department.	Discuss available resources. Provide handout listing available resources and follow-up treatment plan.
■ Identify date, time, and location of follow-up appointment for suture removal.	Follow-up treatment plan; where and when	Provide written instructions.

Evaluation

The client will:

1. Respond to questions regarding self-care of wound.
2. Return demonstration of wound cleansing and bandaging.
3. State contact person and telephone number to obtain assistance.
4. State date, time, and location of follow-up appointment.

on other identified learning needs. For example, a man who wants to know all about coronary artery disease may not be ready to learn how to change his lifestyle until he meets his own need to learn more about the disease. Nurses can also use theoretical frameworks, such as Maslow's hierarchy of needs, to establish priorities.

SETTING LEARNING OUTCOMES

Learning outcomes can be considered the same as desired outcomes for other nursing diagnoses. They are written in the same way. Like client outcomes, learning outcomes:

- State the client (learner) behavior or performance, not nurse behavior. For example, "Identify personal risk factors for heart disease" (client behavior), *not* "Teach the client about cardiac risk factors" (nurse behavior).
- Reflect an observable, measurable activity. The performance may be visible (e.g., walking) or invisible (e.g., adding a column of figures). It is necessary, however, to be able to evaluate whether an unobservable activity has been mastered from some performance that represents the activity. For example, the performance of an outcome might be written: "Selects low-fat foods from a menu" (observable), *not* "understands low-fat diet" (unobservable). Examples of measurable verbs used for learning outcomes are shown in **Box 41–6** ●. Avoid using words such as *knows, understands, believes,* and *appreciates* because they are neither observable nor measurable.
- May add conditions or modifiers as required to clarify what, where, when, or how the behavior will be performed. Examples are "Demonstrates four-point crutch gait *correctly*" (condition), "Administers own insulin *independently* (condition) as taught," or "States *three* (condition) factors that affect blood sugar level."
- Include criteria specifying the time by which learning should have occurred. For example, "The client will state three things that affect blood sugar level *by end of second diabetic class.*"

Learning outcomes can reflect the learner's command of simple to complex concepts. For example, the learning outcome "The client will list cardiac risk factors" is a low-level knowledge outcome that simply requires the learner to identify all cardiac risk factors; it does not suggest application of the knowledge to the learner's own behaviors. The learning outcome "The client will list personal cardiac risk factors" requires that the learner not only know cardiac risk factors in general but also know his own behaviors that place him at risk for cardiac disease.

In writing learning outcomes, the nurse must be specific about what behaviors and knowledge (cognitive, psychomotor, and affective) learners must have to be able to positively influence their health state. In most cases, the learning needs are more complex than simple acquisition of knowledge and include the application of that knowledge to oneself.

CHOOSING CONTENT

The content, or what is to be taught, is determined by learning outcomes. For instance, "Identify appropriate sites for insulin injection" means the nurse must include content about the body sites suitable for insulin injections. Nurses can select among many sources of information including books, nursing journals, the Internet, and other nurses and primary care providers. Whatever sources the nurse chooses, content should be:

- Accurate
- Current
- Based on learning outcomes
- Adjusted for the learner's age, culture, and ability
- Consistent with information the nurse is teaching
- Selected with consideration of how much time and what resources are available for teaching.

SELECTING TEACHING STRATEGIES

The method of teaching that the nurse chooses should be suited to the individual and to the material to be learned. For example, the person who cannot read needs material presented in other ways; a discussion is usually not the best strategy for teaching how to give an injection; and a nurse using group discussion for teaching should be a competent group leader. As stated earlier, some people are visually oriented and learn best through seeing; others learn best through hearing and having the skill explained. **Table 41–3** ● lists selected teaching strategies.

ORGANIZING LEARNING EXPERIENCES

To save nurses time in constructing their own teaching guides, some health agencies have developed teaching guides for teaching sessions that nurses commonly give. These guides standardize content and teaching methods and make it easier for the nurse to plan and implement client teaching. Standardized teaching plans also ensure consistency of content for the learner, thereby decreasing the risk of confusion if different practices are taught. For example, when teaching infant bathing, the nurse on the unit should be consistent about which soaps are appropriate for the infant's bath and distinguish those that are not. Whether the nurse is implementing a plan devised by another or developing an individualized teaching plan, the guidelines discussed next can help the nurse sequence the learning experience.

Start with something the learner is concerned about; for example, before learning how to administer insulin to himself,

---

Box 41–6 Examples of Verbs for Writing Learning Outcomes

COGNITIVE DOMAIN	AFFECTIVE DOMAIN	PSYCHOMOTOR DOMAIN
Compares	Accepts	Assembles
Describes	Attends	Calculates
Evaluates	Chooses	Changes
Explains	Discusses	Demonstrates
Identifies	Displays	Measures
Labels	Initiates	Moves
Lists	Joins	Organizes
Names	Participates	Shows
Plans	Shares	
Selects	Uses	
States		
Writes		

TABLE 41–3   Selected Teaching Strategies

STRATEGY	MAJOR TYPE OF LEARNING	CHARACTERISTICS
Explanation or description (e.g., lecture)	Cognitive	Teacher controls content and pace. Learner is passive; therefore retains less information than when actively participating. Feedback is determined by teacher. May be given to individual or group.
One-to-one discussion	Affective, cognitive	Encourages participation by learner. Permits reinforcement and repetition at learner's level. Permits introduction of sensitive subjects.
Answering questions	Cognitive	Teacher controls most of content and pace. Learner may need to overcome cultural perception that asking questions is impolite and may embarrass the teacher. Can be used with individuals and groups. Teacher sometimes needs to confirm whether question has been answered by asking learner, for example, "Does that answer your question?"
Demonstration	Psychomotor	Often used with explanation. Can be used with individuals, small or large groups. Does not permit use of equipment by learner; learner is passive.
Discovery	Cognitive, affective	Teacher guides problem-solving situation. Learner is active participant; therefore, retention of information is high.
Group discussions	Affective, cognitive	Learner can obtain assistance from supportive group. Group members learn from one another. Teacher needs to keep the discussion focused and prevent monopolization by one or two learners.
Practice	Psychomotor	Allows repetition and immediate feedback. Permits hands-on experience.
Printed and audio-visual materials	Cognitive	Forms include books, pamphlets, films, programmed instruction, and computer learning. Learners can proceed at their own speed. Nurse can act as resource person, need not be present during learning. Potentially ineffective if reading level is too high. Teacher needs to select language of materials that meets learner needs if English is a second language (e.g., Spanish).
Role playing	Affective, cognitive	Permits expression of attitudes, values, and emotions. Can assist in development of communication skills. Involves active participation by learner. Teacher must create supportive, safe environment for learners to minimize anxiety.
Modeling	Affective, psychomotor	Nurse sets example by attitude, psychomotor skill.
Computer-assisted learning programs	All types of learning	Learner is active. Learner controls pace. Provides immediate reinforcement and review. Use with individuals or groups.

an adolescent wants to know how to adjust his lifestyle and yet still play football.

■ Discover what the learner knows, and then proceed to the unknown. This gives the learner confidence. Sometimes you will not know the client's knowledge or skill base and will need to elicit this information either by asking questions or by having the client fill out a form in advance of the session.

■ Address early any area that is causing the client anxiety. A high level of anxiety can impair concentration in other areas. For example, a woman highly anxious about her fear of the needle breaking off into the skin may not be able to learn how to self-administer an insulin injection until her fear is resolved.

■ Teach the basics before proceeding to the variations or adjustments (e.g., simple to complex). It is confusing to learners to have to consider possible adjustments and variations before

they master the basic concepts. For example, when teaching a female client how to insert a retention catheter, it is best to teach the basic procedure before teaching any adjustments that might be needed if the catheter stops draining after insertion.

■ Schedule time for review of content and questions the client may have to clarify information.

■ If the client does not have any questions, you can help introduce questions by saying, "A few frequently asked questions are . . . ."

SHOWING FLEXIBILITY   The nurse needs to be flexible in implementing any teaching plan because the plan may need to be revised. The client may tire sooner than anticipated or be faced with too much information too quickly, the client's needs may change, or external factors may intervene. For instance, the nurse and the client plan to change his dressing at 10 a.m., but when the time comes, the client wants to observe the nurse once more before actually doing it himself. In this case, the nurse alters the teaching plan and discusses any desired information, provides another demonstration, and defers teaching the psychomotor skill until the next day.

It is also important for nurses to use teaching techniques that enhance learning and reduce or eliminate any barrier to learning such as pain or fatigue. Many nurses find that they teach while performing nursing care (e.g., giving medication). Remember to document this informal teaching also.

GUIDELINES FOR TEACHING Knowledge alone is not enough to motivate an individual to change a behavior. Do not assume that providing information will automatically result in clients changing their behavior. Learning what needs to be done to change behavior and acting on that knowledge are two different processes (Saarmann, Daugherty, & Riegel, 2000, p. 281). The stages of change, the individual's willingness and perceived need to change, and barriers to change are important elements to reflect on when implementing a teaching plan. When a client is ready to change a health behavior and when implementing a teaching plan, the nurse may find the following guidelines helpful:

- Rapport between teacher and learner is essential. A relationship that is both accepting and constructive will best assist learning. The nurse should know the learner and the previously described factors that affect learning before planning the teaching.
- The teacher who uses the client's previous learning in the present situation encourages the client and facilitates learning new skills. For instance, an individual who already knows how to cook can use this knowledge when learning to prepare food for a special diet.
- The optimal time for each session depends largely on the learner. Whenever possible, ask the client for help to choose the best time, for example, when she feels most rested or when no other activities are scheduled. Be alert for client cues that indicate a readiness to learn. For example, if a client asks you why he needs a certain medication (e.g., Coumadin), the question provides an opportunity to explain the reason for the medication, signs to watch for, and if follow-up laboratory work is needed.
- The nurse teacher must be able to communicate clearly and concisely. The words used need to have the same meaning to the client as to the teacher. A client who is taught not to put water on an area of skin may think a wet washcloth is permissible for washing the area. In effect, the nurse needs to explain that no water or moisture should touch the area.
- Using a layperson's vocabulary enhances communication. Often nurses use terms and abbreviations that have meaning to other health professionals but make little sense to clients. Even words such as *urine* or *feces* may be unfamiliar to clients, and abbreviations such as ICU (intensive care unit) or PACU (postanesthesia care unit) are often misunderstood.
- The pace of each teaching session also affects learning. Nurses should be sensitive to any signs that the pace is too fast or too slow. A client who appears confused or does not comprehend material when questioned may be finding the pace too fast. When the client appears bored and loses interest, the pace may be too slow, the learning period may be too long, or the client may be tired.

- An environment can detract from or assist learning; for example, noise or interruptions usually interfere with concentration, whereas a comfortable environment promotes learning. If possible, the client should be out of bed for learning activities. Most people associate their bed with rest and sleep, not with learning. Placing the client in a position and location associated with activity or learning may influence the amount of learning that takes place. For instance, a client who is shown a videotape while in bed may be more likely to become drowsy during instruction than a client who is sitting in a bedside chair.
- Teaching aids can foster learning and help focus a learner's attention. To ensure the transfer of learning, the nurse should use the type of supplies or equipment the client will eventually use. Before the teaching session, the nurse needs to assemble all equipment and visual aids and ensure that all audiovisual equipment is functioning effectively. See Client Teaching for tools for teaching children.
- Teaching that involves a number of the learner's senses often enhances learning. For instance, when teaching about changing a surgical dressing, the nurse can tell the client about the procedure (hearing), show how to change the dressing (sight), and show how to manipulate the equipment (touch).
- Learning is more effective when the learners discover the content for themselves. Ways to increase learning include stimulating motivation and self-direction by, for example,

---

Client Teaching
Tools for Teaching Children

- *Visits.* Have children visit the hospital and treatment rooms so they can see people dressed in uniforms, scrub suits, and protective gear.
- *Dress-up.* Have children touch and dress up in the clothing they will see and wear.
- *Coloring books.* Use coloring books to prepare children for treatments, surgery, or hospitalization; shows what rooms, people, and equipment will look like.
- *Story books.* Story books describe how the child will feel, what will be done, and what the place will look like. Parents can read these stories to children several times before the experience. Younger children like this repetition.
- *Dolls.* To give children a sense of mastery of their situation, have them practice procedures that they will later experience on dolls or teddy bears. Custom dolls are often available for inserting tubes and giving injections.
- *Puppet play.* Puppets can be used in role-play situations to provide information and show the child what the experience will be like; they help the child express emotions.
- *Health fairs.* Health fairs can educate children about their bodies and ways to stay healthy. Fairs can focus on high-risk problems children face, such as accident prevention, poison control, and other topics identified in the community as a concern.

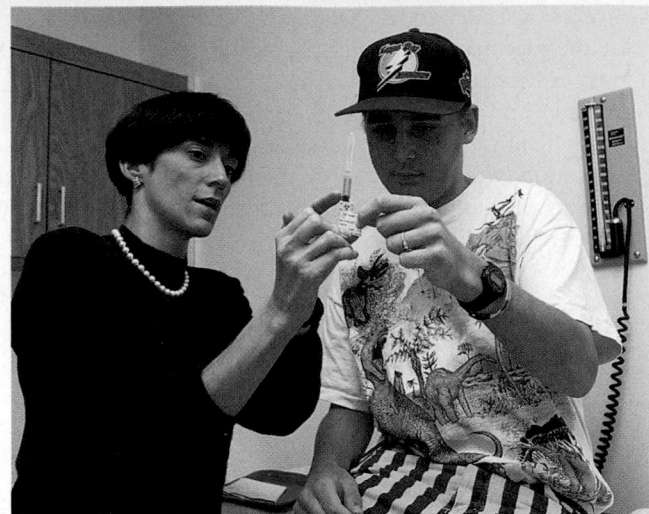

Figure 41–2 ● Teaching activities may need to include hands-on client participation.

(a) providing specific, realistic, achievable outcomes; (b) giving feedback; and (c) helping the learner derive satisfaction from learning. The nurse may also enhance self-directed independent learning by encouraging the client to explore sources of information required. If certain activities do not assist the learner to attain outcomes, these need to be reassessed; perhaps other activities can replace them. Explanation alone may not be able to teach a client to handle a syringe; actually handling the syringe may be more effective (**Figure 41–2 ●**).

■ Repetition reinforces learning. Summarizing content, rephrasing (using other words), and approaching the material from another point of view are ways of repeating and clarifying content. For instance, after discussing the kinds of foods that can be included in a diet, the nurse describes the foods again, but in the context of the three meals eaten during one day.

■ It is helpful to employ "organizers" to introduce material to be learned. Advanced organizers provide a means of connecting unknown material to known material and generating logical relationships. The following statement can be an advanced organizer: "You understand how urine flows down a catheter from the bladder. Now I will show you how to inject fluid so that it flows up the catheter into the bladder." The details that follow are then seen within a framework that adds meaning.

■ The anticipated behavioral changes that indicate learning has taken place must always be within the context of the client's lifestyle and resources. It would be unreasonable to expect a woman to soak in a tub of hot water two times a day if she did not have a bathtub or had to heat water on a stove.

Special Teaching Strategies

One-to-one discussion is the most common method of teaching used by nurses. However, nurses can choose from a number of special teaching strategies: anticipatory guidance, client contracting, group teaching, technology-assisted instruction, discovery/problem solving, behavior modification, and trans-

cultural teaching. Any strategy the nurse selects must be appropriate for the learner and the learning objectives.

ANTICIPATORY GUIDANCE Anticipatory guidance has been primarily associated with health promotion activities in pediatrics. Nurses use **anticipatory guidance** to provide parents with information about developmental changes they can expect their child or children to exhibit as they grow and develop. However, anticipatory guidance can be used any time during the life span with the same focus: health promotion. For example, the nurse may provide anticipatory guidance to a family whose mother has Alzheimer disease to help them recognize safety concerns as the disease progresses. Anticipatory guidance may be provided to both individuals and groups.

Anticipatory guidance provided by healthcare professionals can help clients prevent health alterations or complications. Nurses can expect to use anticipatory guidance in the form of client teaching in various settings, including:

■ Prenatal visits

■ Well-child/adolescent visits

■ Annual medical/dental visits

■ Community programs such as health screenings, health fairs, and safety programs.

Because the time for each visit is limited, nurses should build on a client's current knowledge and care practices and start with a topic in which the client expresses interest. Nursing using anticipatory guidance should reinforce what the client and family are doing well and clear up any poorly understood concepts.

Nurses rely on resources in the community to enhance the guidance provided. For example, Bright Futures provides information for anticipatory guidance regarding children. State and local Safe Kids coalitions help inform families about injury prevention strategies. Schools provide health and safety programs throughout the year. Nurses need to be aware of the types of programs available in the community to reinforce concepts.

Stay Current: *Visit Bright Futures at* **www.brightfutures. org** *and Safe Kids at* **www.safekids.org** *to enhance your teaching strategies for children.*

Nurses should consider several factors before providing anticipatory guidance including the client's age, developmental stage, health status, and health literacy level.

CLIENT CONTRACTING Client contracting involves establishing a learning contract with a client that specifies certain outcomes and when they are to be met. Here is an example of a self-contract:

I, Kirsten Hugo, will exercise strenuously for 20 minutes three times per week for a period of 2 weeks and will then buy myself six yellow roses.

Kirsten Hugo
A. Tucker, RN
July 30, 2015

The contract, drawn up and signed by the client and the nurse, may specify the learning outcomes, the responsibilities of the client and the nurse, and the methods of follow-up and

Lifespan Considerations
Anticipatory Guidance

Children

Anticipatory guidance for children focuses on providing their parents with information on topics such as growth and development; nutrition; oral health; mental health issues; ways that families mange stress; risks of secondhand smoke; sleep safety and patterns; administering medications and using sunscreen; automobiles and bicycle safety; relationships among family members and between peers and classmates; supervising and limiting TV and video game time; the importance of disease prevention strategies, such as immunizations; and injury prevention strategies.

Adults

Nurses provide anticipatory guidance for adults on a case-by-case basis. Appropriate topics may include injury prevention strategies for using electric tools and mechanical equipment; using sunscreen and sunglasses with UVA/UVB protection; and responsible sexual behaviors and drug and alcohol use.

Older Adults

Anticipatory guidance for older adults may include topics such as fall prevention; medication use and potential side effects; age-related changes in nutritional needs; safe driving evaluations; and the need for advance directives.

evaluation. The contract can be changed in two ways: if the client meets the contract outcomes and wants to negotiate new learning outcomes and if the client decides that he or she is unable to meet the existing learning outcomes and wants to revise them (Rankin, Stallings, & London, 2005, pp. 207–209). The learning contract allows for freedom, mutual respect, and mutual responsibility.

GROUP TEACHING   Group instruction is economical, and it provides members with an opportunity to share with and learn from others. A small group allows for discussion in which everyone can participate. A large group often necessitates a lecture technique or use of films, videos, slides, or role playing by teachers.

All members involved in a particular group should have a common need (e.g., prenatal health or preoperative instruction). Sociocultural factors also should be considered when a group is being formed.

TECHNOLOGY-ASSISTED INSTRUCTION   Technology-assisted instruction (TAI) is popular. Initially, the primary use of computer educational methods was for cognitive learning of facts. Now, however, computers and other electronic devices (e.g., smart phones and tablets) can also be used to teach the following:

- Application of information (e.g., answering questions after reading the information about a health subject)
- Psychomotor skills (e.g., filling a syringe on the computer screen to the correct dosage line on the syringe)
- Complex problem-solving skills (e.g., responding to questions based on a client situation).

TAI can also be used in various other ways:

- Individual healthcare professionals or clients use an electronic device for teaching/learning.
- Families or small groups of three to five clients gather around one electronic device and take turns running the program and answering questions together.
- Large groups view a display of a computer's monitor that is projected onto an overhead screen, while a teacher or a learner uses a keyboard or other device to change the display.
- Individuals or small groups use computers or other electronic devices through shared network platforms or through Internet Web sites.

Individuals using an electronic device are able to set the pace that meets their particular learning needs. Small groups are less able to do this, and large groups progress through the program at a pace that may be too slow for some learners and too fast for others. It is therefore helpful to group learners of similar needs and abilities together.

Whether using the electronic device alone or in large groups, learners read and view informational material, answer questions, and receive immediate feedback. The correct answer is usually indicated by the use of colors, flashing signs, or written praise. When the learner selects an incorrect answer, the program may respond with an explanation of why that was not the best answer and encouragement to try again. Many programs ask learners whether they want to review material on which the question and answer were based. Some programs feature simulated situations that allow learners to manipulate objects on the screen to learn psychomotor skills. When used to teach such skills, TAI must be followed up with practice on actual equipment supervised by the teacher.

Some clients may have a negative attitude about electronic devices that may create a barrier to learning. The nurse helps these clients by explaining how the device can help meet their needs. Matching a program or Web site to the client's individual health circumstances may encourage the use of electronic devices. Providing a resource list of free available community sites for training and access may also help. For clients who use the Internet, it is important for the nurse to teach the client how to evaluate whether the site is a relevant and credible source for health information. It is important to recognize that some individuals still do not embrace technology. This may be due to a number of factors including affordability, access, and literacy levels.

Most media catalogs, professional journals, and healthcare libraries contain information about computer software programs and mobile device applications available to the nurse for client education. The media specialist or librarian in a healthcare facility or college is an excellent resource to help the nurse locate appropriate programs. Technological educational material is also available for clients with different language needs, for clients with special visual needs, and for clients at different growth and development levels.

DISCOVERY/PROBLEM SOLVING   In using the discovery/problem-solving technique, the nurse presents some initial information and then asks the learners a question or presents a situation related to the information. The learner applies the new information to the situation and decides what to do. Learners can work alone or in groups. This technique is well suited to family learning. The teacher guides the learners through the thinking process necessary to reach the best solution to the question or the best action to take in the situation. This may also be referred to as **anticipatory problem solving**. For example, the nurse educator might present information on diabetes and glucose management. Then the nurse might ask the learners how they think their insulin and/or diet should be adjusted if their morning glucose reading was too low. In this way, clients learn what critical components they need to consider to reach the best solution to the problem.

BEHAVIOR MODIFICATION   The behavior modification system for changing behavior has as its basic assumptions (a) that human behaviors are learned and can be selectively strengthened, weakened, eliminated, or replaced; and (b) that an individual's behavior is under conscious control. Under this system, desirable behavior is rewarded and undesirable behavior is ignored. The client's response is the key to behavior change. For example, clients trying to quit smoking are not criticized when they smoke, but they are praised or rewarded when they go without a cigarette for a certain period of time. For some people, a learning contract is combined with behavior modification, and includes the following pertinent features:

■ Positive reinforcement (e.g., praise) is used.
■ The client participates in the development of the learning plan.
■ Undesirable behavior is ignored, not criticized.
■ The expectation of the client and the nurse is that the task will be mastered (i.e., the behavior will change).

TRANSCULTURAL TEACHING   Nurses and clients from different cultural and ethnic backgrounds have additional barriers to overcome in the teaching–learning process. These barriers include language and communication problems, differing concepts of time, conflicting cultural healing practices, beliefs that may positively or negatively influence compliance with health teaching, and unique high-risk or high-frequency health problems that can be addressed with health promotion instruction. Nurses should consider the following guidelines when teaching clients from various ethnic backgrounds:

■ Obtain teaching materials, pamphlets, and instructions in languages used by clients. Nurses who are unable to read the foreign language material for themselves can have the translator read the material to them. The nurse can then evaluate the quality of the information and update it with the translator's help as needed.
■ Use visual aids, such as pictures, charts, or diagrams, to communicate meaning. Audiovisual material may be helpful if the English is spoken clearly and slowly. Even if understanding the verbal message is a problem for the client, seeing a skill or procedure may be helpful. In some instances, a translator can be asked to clarify the video. Alternatively the video may be available in several languages, and the nurse can request the necessary version from the company.
■ Use concrete rather than abstract words. Use simple language (short sentences, short words) and present only one idea at a time.

■ Allow time for questions. This helps the client mentally separate one idea or skill from another.
■ Avoid the use of medical terminology or healthcare language, such as "taking your vital signs" or "apical pulse." Rather, nurses should say they are going to take a blood pressure reading or listen to the client's heart.
■ If understanding another's pronunciation is a problem, validate brief information in writing. For example, during assessments, write down numbers, words, or phrases and have the client read them to verify accuracy.
■ Use humor very cautiously. Meaning can change in the translation process.
■ Do not use slang words or colloquialisms. These may be interpreted literally.
■ Do not assume that a client who nods, uses eye contact, or smiles is indicating an understanding of what is being taught. These responses may simply be the client's way of indicating respect. The client may feel that asking the nurse questions or stating a lack of understanding is inappropriate because it might embarrass the nurse or cause the nurse to "lose face."
■ Invite and encourage questions during teaching. Let clients know they are urged to ask questions and be involved in making information clearer. When asking questions to evaluate client understanding, avoid asking negative questions. These can be interpreted differently by people for whom English is a second language. "Do you understand how far you can bend your hip after surgery?" is better than the negative question "You don't understand how far you can bend your hip after surgery, do you?" With particularly difficult information or skills teaching, the nurse might say, "Most people have some trouble with this. May I please help you go through this one more time?" In some cultures, expressing a need is not appropriate, and expressing confusion or asking to be shown something again is considered rude.
■ When explaining procedures or functioning related to personal areas of the body, it may be appropriate to have a nurse of the same sex do the teaching. Because of modesty concerns in many cultures and beliefs about what is considered appropriate and inappropriate male–female interaction, it is wise to have a female nurse teach a female client about personal care, birth control, sexually transmitted infections, and other potentially sensitive areas. If a translator is needed during explanation of procedures or teaching, the translator should also be female.
■ Include the family in planning and teaching. This promotes trust and mutual respect. Identify the authoritative family member and incorporate that person into the planning and teaching to promote compliance and support of health teaching. In some cultures, the male head of household is the critical family member to include in health teaching; in other cultures, it is the eldest female member.
■ Consider the client's time orientation. The client may be more oriented to the present than the nurse. Cultures with a predominant orientation to the present include the Mexican American, Navajo Native American, Appalachian, Eskimo, and Filipino American cultures. Preventing future problems may be less significant for these clients than for others, so teaching prevention may be more difficult. For example, teaching a client why and when to take medications may be

more difficult if the client is oriented to the present. In such instances, the nurse can emphasize preventing short-term problems rather than long-term problems. Failure to keep clinic appointments or to arrive on time is common in clients who have a present-time orientation. The nurse can help by accommodating these clients when they arrive for their appointment.

Schedules may be very flexible in present-oriented societies, with sleeping and eating patterns varying greatly. Teaching clients to take medications at bedtime or with a meal does not necessarily mean that these activities will occur at the same time each day. For this reason, the nurse should assess the client's daily routine before teaching the client to pair a treatment or medication with an event the nurse assumes occurs at the same time every day. When teaching a client when to take medication, the nurse should determine whether a clock or watch is available to the client and whether the client can tell time.

■ Identify cultural health practices and beliefs. Noncompliance with health teaching may be related to conflict with folk medicine beliefs. Noncompliance may also be related to lack of understanding or fatalism, a belief system in which life events are held to be predestined or fixed in advance and the individual is powerless to change them. To encourage compliance, the nurse needs to learn the client's explanation of why the illness developed and how it might be treated (Munoz & Luckmann, 2005).

The nurse should treat the client's cultural healing beliefs with respect and try to identify whether any are in agreement or in conflict with what is being taught. The nurse can then focus on the ones in agreement to promote the integration of new learning with the familiar health practices. The goal is to arrive at a mutually agreeable plan: Decide which instructions must be followed for client safety and negotiate less crucial folk healing practices.

Evaluation

Evaluating is both an ongoing and a final process in which the client, the nurse, and often the support people determine what has been learned.

EVALUATING LEARNING   The process of evaluating learning is the same as evaluating client achievement of desired outcomes for other nursing diagnoses. Learning is measured against the predetermined learning outcomes selected in the planning phase of the teaching process. Thus the outcomes serve not only to direct the teaching plan but also to provide outcome criteria for evaluation. For example, the outcome "Selects foods that are low in carbohydrates" can be evaluated by asking the client to name such foods or to select low-carbohydrate foods from a list.

The best method for evaluating depends on the type of learning. In *cognitive learning*, the client demonstrates acquisition of knowledge. Examples of the evaluation tools for cognitive learning include the following:

■ Direct observation of behavior (e.g., observing the client demonstrate use of a blood pressure monitor)
■ Written measurements (e.g., tests)

■ Oral questioning (e.g., asking the client to restate information or correct verbal responses to questions)
■ Client reports and self-monitoring. These can be useful during follow-up phone calls and home visits. Evaluating individual self-paced learning, as might occur with computer-assisted instruction, often incorporates self-monitoring.

The acquisition of psychomotor skills is best evaluated by observing how well the client carries out a procedure such as self-administration of insulin.

Affective learning is more difficult to evaluate. Whether attitudes or values have been learned may be inferred by listening to the client's responses to questions, noting how the client speaks about relevant subjects, and observing the client's behavior that expresses feelings and values. For example, have parents learned to value health sufficiently to have their children immunized? Do clients who state that they value health actually use condoms every time they have sex with a new partner?

Following evaluation, the nurse may find it necessary to modify or repeat the teaching plan if the objectives have not been met or have been met only partially. Follow-up teaching in the home or by phone may be needed for the client discharged from a health facility.

Behavior change does not always take place immediately after learning. Often individuals accept change intellectually first and then change their behavior only periodically (for example, a client who knows that she must lose weight, diets and exercises off and on). If the new behavior is to replace the old behavior, it must emerge gradually; otherwise, the old behavior may prevail. The nurse can assist clients with behavior change by allowing for client vacillation and by providing encouragement.

EVALUATING THE LEARNING EXPERIENCE   It is important for nurses to evaluate their own teaching and the content of the teaching program, just as they evaluate the effectiveness of nursing interventions for other nursing diagnoses. Evaluation should include a consideration of all factors—the timing, the teaching strategies, the amount of information, whether the teaching was helpful, and so on. The nurse may find, for example, that the client was overwhelmed with too much information, was bored, or was motivated to learn more.

Both the client and the nurse should evaluate the learning experience. The client may tell the nurse what was helpful, interesting, and so on. Feedback questionnaires and videotapes of the learning sessions can also be helpful.

The nurse should not feel ineffective as a teacher if the client forgets some of what is taught. Forgetting is normal and should be anticipated. Having the client write down information, repeating it during teaching, giving handouts on the information, and having the client be active in the learning process all promote retention.

DOCUMENTING   Documentation of the teaching process is essential because it provides a legal record that the teaching took place and communicates the teaching to other health professionals. If teaching is not documented, legally it did not occur.

It is also important to document the responses of the client and support people to teaching activities. What did the client or support person say or do to indicate that learning occurred?

Has the client demonstrated mastery of a skill or the acquisition of knowledge? The nurse records this in the client's chart as evidence of learning. A sample documentation of charting follows:

11/8/2015 1130 Learning to use glucometer to check own capillary blood glucose levels. Noted a slight hesitation with each step. Demonstrated correct technique. Stated "feeling more comfortable" each time she does it but still "needs to stop and think about the process." Will continue to monitor client's progress._____

C. Brown, RN

Many agencies have multiple-copy client teaching forms that include the medical and nursing diagnoses, the treatment plan, and the client education. After the teaching session is completed, the client and the nurse sign the form and a copy of the form is given to the client as a record of teaching and as reinforcement of the content taught. A second copy of the completed and signed form is placed in the client's chart. The parts of the teaching process that should be documented in the client's chart include the following:

- Diagnosed learning needs
- Learning outcomes
- Topics taught
- Client outcomes
- Need for additional teaching
- Resources provided.

The written teaching plan that the nurse uses as a resource to guide future teaching sessions might also include these elements:

- Actual information and skills taught
- Teaching strategies used
- Time framework and content for each class
- Teaching outcomes and methods of evaluation.

REVIEW Client/Consumer Education

RELATE Link the Concepts and Exemplars

Linking the exemplar of client/consumer education with the concept of development:

1. How does the concept of development impact teaching and learning?

2. How should the nurse incorporate characteristics of each developmental stage when choosing teaching strategies?

Linking the exemplar of client/consumer education with the concept of culture and diversity:

3. What aspects of culture should be considered before developing a teaching plan for a client?

4. How should the nurse address teaching and learning when a client's health beliefs and values differs from his or her own?

Linking the exemplar of client/consumer education with the concept of cognition:

5. How should the nurse address teaching and learning for a client with altered cognition?

6. How does the concept of cognition impact the nurse's teaching plan and the client's learning?

REFER Go to Pearson Nursing Student Resources
nursing.pearsonhighered.com

- Additional review materials

REFLECT Case Study

Mrs. Yorty is a 59-year-old African American bank vice president who is heavily relied on by her boss and coworkers. Three days ago she was admitted to the hospital with complaints of shortness of breath and mild chest pain. A diagnostic evaluation indicates that she has significant coronary artery disease but has not yet suffered a heart attack. Her primary care provider has indicated that Mrs. Yorty will need to make significant lifestyle changes to reduce her heart attack risk. As her nurse, you have been asked to teach Mrs. Yorty about her disease process, diet, exercise, and stress reduction. As you begin teaching Mrs. Yorty, you note that she is very pleasant and frequently nods her head, but she also seems preoccupied and is easily distracted.

1. How would you evaluate Mrs. Yorty's readiness to learn?

2. Of what benefit would a learning needs assessment be since Mrs. Yorty is obviously a well-educated client?

3. You recognize that you have a great deal of information to deliver to Mrs. Yorty and you are concerned that you will not be able to teach it all. What can you do to help Mrs. Yorty and still accomplish the learning outcomes?

4. How will you know if your teaching is effective?

5. How might your teaching differ if you were teaching Mrs. Yorty at home rather than in a hospital or acute care setting?

EXEMPLAR 41.2   Mentoring

EXEMPLAR KEY TERMS
Coaching, *2526*
Mentors, *2525*
Networking, *2527*
Preceptor, *2525*

EXEMPLAR LEARNING OUTCOMES
After reading about this exemplar, you will be able to:

1. Differentiate among mentoring, precepting, coaching, and networking and understand indications for the use of each.

2. Distinguish between each stage of the mentoring process.

3. Describe the advantages of networking to the nurse.

▶ OVERVIEW

Mentoring is an important career development tool that can be used by nurses in any type of setting or speciality. It has been identified in nursing literature as particularly important for career development in nursing administration and nursing education. **Mentors** are "competent, experienced professionals who develop a relationship with a novice for the purpose of providing advice, support, information, and feedback in order to encourage development of the individual" (Schutzenhofer, 1995, p. 487).

Both beginning and more experienced nurses can benefit from mentoring and from other career development strategies that involve repeated contact with other professional nurses. These include precepting, coaching, and networking. In many instances, these terms may be used interchangeably; however, differences in the career development strategies can be found in **Table 41–4** ●.

TABLE 41–4 Differences in Career Development Strategies		
CAREER DEVELOPMENT STRATEGIES	**PRIMARY FUNCTION**	**CHARACTERISTICS**
Mentor	Career development	Guides personal and professional growth Role model Long period of time Supports and nurtures growth Volunteer participation Self-selecting One-to-one interaction Teacher
Preceptor	Orient the new nurse to the unit, socialization to the role.	Assigned One-to-one basis Side-by-side on-the-job instruction Develop new knowledge and skills Support and guidance Role model Short period of duration Assigned
Coach	Improve performance, resolve performance issues.	Leader–follower Performance issue resolution One-to-one basis Frequent and regular interaction Active performance appraisal process Enhances communication
Networking	Career advancement	Supports and nurtures personal and professional growth Information sharing Interaction time frames vary One-to-one or small groups Long-term investment

▶ MENTORING

Mentoring is widely used as a strategy for career development in nursing. The nurse being mentored may not be a novice but may be early in his career development. Most nursing literature describes the nurse-mentor relationship as important for career development in nursing administration or nursing education. Mentors provide support. Often, the mentor relationship is one of teacher–learner. The mentor instructs the protégé in the expected role, introduces the protégé to those who are important to the achievement of goals, listens to and helps the protégé evaluate ideas in light of institutional policy, and challenges the protégé to advance professional practice.

Nurses who wish to improve and advance their professional practice, whether in education, administration, or clinical practice, should seek mentors to assist them. Mentors usually are of the same gender, 8–14 years older, and have a position of authority in the organization. Most are knowledgeable individuals who are willing to share their knowledge and experience. Mentors often choose protégés because of their leadership or managerial qualities. Mentoring is a process that can promote the personal and professional growth of both mentor and protégé. The use of Internet and rapid communication methods has allowed more opportunities for mentoring when the protégé is not physically in the same location.

Participating in a mentoring relationship requires work and time from both the mentor and protégé involved. The mentee and mentor can follow these seven steps when working with each other to achieve the best outcomes for both parties:

1. Initiate and establish a mentoring relationship.
2. Discuss expectations of the relationship.
3. Set specific goals and objectives.
4. Develop and implement the plan.
5. Evaluate personal and professional outcomes.
6. Modify the relationship as needed.
7. Keep open communication throughout the process (Olson, 2012).

A mentoring relationship, however, can have negative effects, including power struggles, intimidation, and loyalty issues. Because of the importance of a positive mentor–protégé relationship experience, the four phases of the relationship are discussed in **Table 41–5** ●.

▶ PRECEPTING

A **preceptor** is "an experienced nurse who provides knowledge and emotional support, as well as a clarification of role expectations, on a one-to-one basis" (Marquis & Huston, 2012, p. 258). Preceptors usually are assigned to nurses who are new to the nursing unit to assist them in learning routines, policies, and procedures and in improving the clinical nursing skills and judgment abilities necessary for effective practice in their environment. Preceptors must be patient and willing to teach new nurses, and they must be willing to answer questions and clarify the expectations of the nurse's role within the practice environment. Sullivan and Decker (2009) state, "preceptorships offer new nurses the advantage of an on-the-job instruction program

TABLE 41–5 Mentoring Relationship Phases, Time Frames, and Characteristics

PHASE	TIME FRAMES	RELATIONSHIP TASKS OR CHARACTERISTICS
Initiation	6–12 months	Discuss expectations. Set goals and objectives. Develop a plan.
Cultivation	2–5 years	Implement the plan. Protégé receives assistance with professional development to achieve set goals and expectations.
Separation	6–24 months following change in the relationship	Protégé is viewed as a peer, moves away, or has a job change. Protégé is more independent.
Redefinition	Follows separation phase	The relationship is redefined and continues or slowly dissolves over time.

Based on Wu, S., Turban, D. B., & Yu, H. C. (2012). Social skill in workplace mentoring relationships. *Journal of Organizational Culture, Communications & Conflict,* 16(2), 61–72. Retrieved from http://www.alliedacademies.org/Public/Journals/JournalDetails.aspx?jid=11.

tailored specifically to their needs." The preceptor can provide on-the-spot feedback to help the new nurse meet professional standards.

Preceptors are usually assigned to assist in the growth process of the new nurse; preceptors may have duties defined as part of their job description within the organization. Mentors serve in a voluntary capacity, and the mentorship process is one of mutual growth. Mentors and preceptors are important for the successful development of a nurse from a beginning care provider to an expert practitioner and professional.

▶ COACHING

Employees must feel safe in their workplace environments before an individual is empowered to learn and change. Organizations that cultivate coaching environments for individuals, teams, and groups excel in production and reap many rewards such as higher job satisfaction, improved communication, and team collaboration. In the professional work environment, coaching can be used to help employees achieve their highest potential through guidance and support. Managers and other leaders use coaching processes to empower employees to function independently and with confidence and competence. **Coaching** is the process, on a personal level, of helping an individual achieve a higher potential. Coaching benefits both the coach and the individual and includes improved communication, motivation, performance, enthusiasm, empowerment, and personal and job satisfaction.

The formal process of coaching involves a partnership between two or more individuals within a personal or professional setting. The goal of coaching is to empower an individual or group of individuals to perform effectively and be accountable for actions taken. Coaching provides structure, guidance, feedback, and encouragement to improve performance and personal feelings of satisfaction. Nurses, as leaders, must develop skills in coaching to enhance performance.

Coaching is different from mentoring. A mentor is an expert in content or practice helping an individual learn the roles and responsibilities associated with a specific job or task. A coach empowers change in an individual or groups of individuals resulting in the achievement of personal and professional goals. Coaching can be a formal or informal partnership within a personal or professional setting. A formal coaching partnership involves the four tasks listed in **Table 41–6** ●.

Coaching can solve work problems including absenteeism, personal texting or phone calls during work, and avoidance of specific tasks. The coach must address the issues (provide feedback) as they arise to help the individual grow personally and professionally. When a work issue arises, the coach:

- Identifies the behavior needing to be addressed and prepares a behavioral statement, such as "You have been absent three times in the last month."

- Explains the consequences of the action and how it impacts the individual and others including the client, teammates, and organization. Discusses how the action impacts the individual's goals and expectations set.

- Allows the individual to express any insights into the actions and make suggestions for resolutions. Approves a plan of action.

- Follows up within an appropriate time frame and provides feedback. Evaluates set goals and expectations. Encourages, praises, and supports as appropriate.

Coaching an individual should also include addressing positive actions an individual takes. The same process listed above can

TABLE 41–6 Coaching Tasks

COACHING TASKS	COACH	INDIVIDUAL(S) BEING COACHED
Assess	Assess the individual(s) values, perceptions, strengths and desired areas of improvement.	Reflect on personal and professional goals. Share personal and professional insights with coach.
Set expectations, goals	Work with individual(s) in discussing expectations, setting goals, and creating an action plan.	Work with coach in discussing expectations, setting goals, and creating an action plan for personal and professional growth.
Act	Provide feedback, encouragement, inspiration, and support.	Acts on feedback, works to meet goals and follow the action plan.
Reflect	Reflect on actions taken. Provide feedback to the individual(s). Evaluate outcomes. Modify plan of action as needed.	Reflect on actions taken. Share insights with coach.

Box 41–7 Networking Benefits

- Share ideas and information.
- Provide support, guidance, and advice.
- Foster personal and professional growth.
- Create personal and professional opportunities.
- Enhance communication.
- Increase productivity.
- Establish health policies.
- Refine interpersonal skills.
- Promote change.
- Foster creativity.
- Develop sense of belonging.
- Promote personal life and professional work satisfaction.

Box 41–8 Networking Strategies

- Smile.
- Greet others respectively and warmly.
- Listen.
- Introduce yourself to someone new.
- Be confident in yourself and your values and beliefs.
- Participate in professional organizational meetings.
- Volunteer for a task force.
- Offer a business card to others and receive a card in return; follow up with them.
- Follow through with any promises.
- Stay connected through e-mails, calls, instant messages, web-conferencing tools.
- Offer support.
- Be honest and truthful.
- Take responsibility for your mistakes.
- Handle conflict professionally.
- Give credit appropriately.
- Be a risk taker.
- Build and use contacts as resources.

Sources: Based on Yoder-Wise, P. S. (2011). *Leading and managing in nursing* (5th ed.). St. Louis, MO: Elsevier; Blais, K. K., & Hayes, J. S. (2011). *Professional nursing practice: Concepts and perspectives* (6th ed.). Upper Saddle River, NJ: Pearson; and Wolff, H. G., & Sowon, K. (2012). The relationship between networking behaviors and the big five personality dimensions. *Career Development International, 17*(1). doi:10.1108/13620431211201328.

be used to praise actions and help the individual move forward in achieving a higher level of potential if possible. The coach must be cautious in pushing the individual excessively before the individual is ready and capable.

▶ NETWORKING

Networking is developing and maintaining relationships with others within and outside of your profession and affiliated organization to improve nursing practice, advance career goals, offer support, share information, and provide advice (Blais & Hayes, 2011). Nurses develop networks through contacts in every day life: work, recreational activities, professional organizations, and school. Networking involves a conscious and intentional effort to establish and maintain relationship with others that entails a long-term commitment to building relationships for the future. The advantages of networking are multifold (see **Box 41–7** ●).

Every nurse should develop networking skills and tools to empower themselves personally and professionally (Yoder-Wise, 2011). Networking takes time, practice, and energy and is worth the effort. Networking is not competitive but supportive and helpful to others. Strategies for networking involve being committed to interacting with others, being supportive, sharing information, and offering advice when asked (see **Box 41–8** ●).

Networking can be useful to student nurses in a number of ways. After graduation, peers who have already found employment become an excellent source of information about potential jobs and employers. Student nurses should also take advantage of networking opportunities that may result from their participation in clinical settings. The likelihood of employment increases when a former classmate or contact from a clinical experience can provide a character reference for the beginning nurse seeking employment.

REVIEW Mentoring

RELATE Link the Concepts and Exemplars

Linking the exemplar of mentoring with the concept of collaboration:

1. Can the nurse mentor members of the healthcare team other than nurses? Explain your answer.

2. How might an RN serve as a mentor for a physician?

Linking the exemplar of mentoring with the concept of professional behaviors:

3. How can a nurse serve to improve the professionalism of others in a mentoring capacity?

4. Is it possible for the professional nurse to mentor others without entering into a formal agreement, or even being aware of other's views of the nurse as a mentor? Explain your answer.

REFER Go to Pearson Nursing Student Resources
nursing.pearsonhighered.com

- Additional review materials

REFLECT Case Study

Frankie Meningio is a new graduate and has recently passed the NCLEX-RN®. He has accepted a position in an acute care facility and attends hospital orientation followed by nursing orientation. He meets his preceptor on the last day of hospital-wide orientation and is scheduled to begin working on his assigned unit tomorrow.

1. What purpose does the preceptor serve as Frankie begins working on his assigned unit?

2. Why is a preceptor necessary?

3. What actions can Frankie take to increase his likelihood of success as a new nurse on the unit?

EXEMPLAR 41.3 Staff Development

EXEMPLAR KEY TERMS

Orientation, *2528*
Preceptor, *2529*
Staff development, *2528*
Staff education, *2528*

EXEMPLAR LEARNING OUTCOMES

After reading about this exemplar, you will be able to:

1. Explain the contribution of staff development to improving job performance and client outcomes.
2. Demonstrate how educational programs enhance the effectiveness of an organization.

▶ OVERVIEW

As discussed earlier in this module, nurses must seek opportunities to maintain currency in their practice. Many educational opportunities are provided in the workplace. Nurses participate in Staff development through continuing education, in-service programs, and professional development. More experienced nurses participate in professional development for their own benefit as well as for the benefit of others. For example, experienced nurses may function as preceptors for new graduate nurses or for newly employed nurses. Nurses with specialized knowledge and experience may share that knowledge and experience with nurses who are new to that practice area, either in the clinical setting or through continuing education and certification programs. Courses offered in specialty areas include critical care nursing, perioperative nursing, and quality improvement/quality assurance. In addition, nurses in nursing practice settings are often involved in the clinical instruction of nursing students.

Nurses are also involved in teaching other health professionals. Nurses may participate in the education of medical students or allied health students. In this capacity, the nurse educator clarifies the role of the nurse for other health professionals and discusses how nurses can assist them in their care of the client.

Although every registered nurse has passed the state board examinations, each individual nurse brings variations in knowledge, skills, and behaviors to nursing practice. In addition, changes are constant within health care such as new research, technology, equipment, and payer systems. Continuing education and development is required of all nurses to ensure client safety. In many healthcare facilities, nurse managers or nurse educators are responsible for ensuring that nurses are current and competent healthcare providers. **Staff development** refers to nurses' participation in socialization, orientation, and educational and training programs to meet organizational and accrediting standards and requirements of competence. Staff development is a process of planned activities to enhance role performance and improve client outcomes and is often termed professional development or **staff education**. Individual nurses and their supervisors share responsibilities in development (**Box 41–9** ●). The nurse's first encounter with staff education is usually orientation.

▶ ORIENTATION

Orientation is a structured program of activities geared toward helping new employees adapt to and be successful in their new workplace. During orientation, employees are exposed and acclimated to the workplace. At first, new nurses are dependent on others for information, decision making, and direction. Supportive orientation activities and working environments help to make the new nurse feel welcome, productive, and a contributing member of the healthcare team reducing job dissatisfaction, attrition, and absenteeism. Successful orientation programs increase retention of new nurses, improve client outcomes, and reduce costs to the organization.

Orientation has many variations depending on the facility and the job. For example, in larger facilities, orientation may be broken into parts. Human resource departments may offer a general orientation program to the facility including mission, philosophy, values, general policies (safety, infection control, and attendance), and procedures. Following the general orientation, the new nurse may then attend a unit orientation with the unit manager or unit educator; this orientation provides a general overview of the unit and its policies, procedures, and equipment. Nursing orientation continues with a preceptor, an experienced nurse working side by side with the novice nurse to provide support and offering advice. Orientation programs at the preceptor level can vary in length depending on the needs of the novice nurse and the facility.

In larger facilities, orientation may be the responsibility of the staff or professional development manager or nursing manager. In smaller organizations, the responsibility may lie with one of the administrators or the chief nursing officer. Wherever orientation responsibilities lie, healthcare organizations must follow local, state, and federal standards and accreditation guidelines and offer orientation on specific topics essential to client safety, which may include fire and emergency procedures, infection control, quality improvement or quality assurance, and CPR.

The nurse manager or unit educator plays an important part in the novice nurse's orientation process and adaptation to the nursing role from the beginning of the orientation process. The manager or educator addresses expectations and responsibilities

---

Box 41–9   Roles in Staff Development

NURSE'S ROLE IN STAFF DEVELOPMENT

- Identify strengths and areas to improve in your personal practice.
- Set goals.
- Seek opportunities to grow and develop professionally and personally.
- Reflect. Evaluate. Ask for feedback.

SUPERVISOR'S ROLE IN STAFF DEVELOPMENT

- Provide opportunities for growth.
- Offer support.
- Provide feedback.
- Set realistic time frames.

of the role including schedules, attendance, dress code, role description and expectations, appraisal processes, standards of performance, competency requirements, and conduct code. It is important for the nurse manager or unit educator to understand the array of emotions the novice nurse is experiencing. Because the amount of orientation information may be overwhelming, the nurse manager or unit educator should expect to reinforce the information as needed during the orientation process. The novice nurse should be encouraged to ask questions and clarify issues as needed. During orientation, the nurse manager and novice nurse should be given an opportunity to set realistic expectations for future practice and work together toward achieving those goals.

Most orientation for novice nurses involves a preceptor program in which the unit educator or an experienced nurse becomes a preceptor. A **preceptor** is "an experienced nurse who provides knowledge and emotional support, as well as a clarification of role expectations, on a one-to-one basis" (Marquis & Huston, 2012, p. 258) (see Exemplar 41.2 on mentoring). The preceptor provides support, direction, and information needed to help the novice nurse grow into his or her new role. Novice nurses must realize that it may take 9–12 months to be fully integrated into a new role. Following orientation, the novice nurse will continue participating in staff education programs and training as needed to maintain competency.

▶ STAFF DEVELOPMENT PROCESS

The staff development process is similar to the nursing process and teaching process. It begins with assessing the learning needs of staff members, developing a plan, implementing learning activities, and then evaluating and documenting the activities. The nurse leader is responsible for ensuring that staff members are competent providers of health care and must consider the diversity of the staff during the professional development process. Although the nurse leader is responsible for staff education, staff members themselves may participate in the staff education process and be active in educating other staff members.

Assessment

The assessment of learning needs is the first step in the professional development process. Learning needs may vary widely among the staff members as roles vary, yet the underlying goal is to improve client outcomes and maintain client safety.

With this in mind, nurse leaders assess for knowledge and skill deficits and plan staff education and training programs if any of the following occur:

1. New policies or procedures
2. New equipment or materials
3. Changes in routines or client care standards
4. Changes in client population
5. Quality improvement efforts
6. Regulatory and accrediting bodies standards (mandatory competencies such as CPR, fire policies, and client safety guidelines)

7. Others as identified in assessing the learning needs of the individual staff, specific members of the staff, or the entire staff.

Other methods of assessing learning needs include formal and informal methods such as surveys, interviews, discussions, group brainstorming, and trended data.

Planning

After identifying the learning needs of the staff, the nurse leader proceeds to the next step in the process: planning an educational or training program to meet the needs of the staff. Planning involves the following steps:

1. Identify the goal or goals of the educational or training program.
2. Develop learning objectives geared toward the diversity of the staff members. In some cases, the learning objectives will be different for the different members of the healthcare team; however, the underlying goal may be the same. Learning objectives should be specific, measurable, and contain a time frame.
3. Choose teaching strategies and develop learning activities that meet the learning outcomes. Teaching strategies and learning activities must be appropriate for the learner and help the learner to meet the desired learning outcomes. The nurse leader must consider the time and resources available and the ability of the learners (see **Box 41–10** ●).
4. Select an evaluation method that measures the outcome, is readily available, and can be used to demonstrate that the staff member has reached the standards of competency.

Implementation

Implementing the educational or training program is the next step. In this step, learners are given the material or content of the program, time to process and practice applying the new knowledge or skills, and feedback about their performance. A staff member who has had hands-on practice with performance feedback is more likely to apply the new knowledge and skills than a staff member who has just watched or listened to a demonstration.

Evaluation

The purpose of evaluation is to measure the learner's ability to meet the learning objectives, thus having a positive effect on

---

Box 41–10 Educational Strategies

Nurse leaders may have a variety of educational strategies at their disposal for staff education and training programs including the following:

1. *Lectures*—in person, via Web cam, video recordings, podcasts, CDs, DVDs
2. *Web-based instruction*—predeveloped computer programs, online classes, interactive video instruction, video gaming
3. *Self-study*—case studies, articles, texts, self-learning modules
4. *Poster presentations*
5. *Simulations*—computer based or traditional
6. *Preceptors*—on-the-job training
7. *Off-site seminars, workshops, conferences, and college courses.*

client care or day-to-day operations of the facility and to determine the strengths and areas to be improved with the educational program and teaching effectiveness. After implementing an educational or training program, the nurse leader must evaluate the learner, teacher or teachers, and the program itself.

1. Did the learner meet the learning objectives? Will the learner apply the new knowledge and skills in practice? Will improvements in client care outcomes or operational processes be observed?

2. How effective was the teacher or teachers in implementing the educational plan? How well did the teaching methods and strategies meet the needs of the learners?

3. How effective was the educational program? Did the program meet the goals? Will client outcomes or operational processes show improvement?

Professional development is essential in health care because learning needs are varied and the healthcare field is constantly changing. Effective professional development programs are needed to address learning needs that are designed to improve client outcomes and organizational processes. Nurses are responsible for identifying personal, peer, and staff learning needs; developing and implementing a plan; and evaluating the program, as well as participating in helping others to meet competency and role performance standards.

REVIEW Staff Development

RELATE Link the Concepts and Exemplars

Linking the exemplar of staff development with the concept of accountability:

1. What responsibility does the nurse have toward attending staff development opportunities in order to maintain competence?

2. How does the nurse, teaching a course for staff members, contribute to the staff's ability to maintain competence?

Linking the exemplar of staff development with the concept of safety:

3. How does staff development contribute to safe practice?

4. Can a nurse maintain a safe practice without participating in staff development?

REFER Go to Pearson Nursing Student Resources
nursing.pearsonhighered.com

- Additional review materials

REFLECT Case Study

Spencer Wester is an experienced circulating nurse working in the operating room; he also occasionally works in the postanesthesia recovery unit. The facility has purchased new cardiorespiratory monitors that it hopes to put into use within the next 2 months. The manufacturer has offered to provide a class on the new monitors. The hospital has decided to select a few nurses to attend the class; these nurses will then use the knowledge they gain to educate the remaining staff members. Spencer has been selected to be one of the nurses attending the class.

1. In addition to attending the manufacturer's class, what other actions should Spencer take in order to ensure that accurate information is taught to staff members at the completion of the class?

2. What things might Spencer do when teaching the staff about the monitors to improve the comfort and safety of the first clients to use the new equipment?

3. How can Spencer determine the effectiveness of the staff development classes before the monitors are used for client care?

■ REFERENCES

American Nurses Association (ANA). (2010). Standard 8: Education. In *Nursing: Scope and standards of practice.* Washington, DC: Author.

Ball, J., Bindler, R., & Cowen, K. (2012). *Principles of pediatric nursing: Caring for children* (5th ed.). Upper Saddle River, NJ: Pearson.

Bandura, A. (1971). Analysis of modeling processes. In A Bandura (Ed.), *Psychological modeling: Conflicting theories.* Chicago, IL: Aldine.

Bastable, S. B. (2014). *Nurse as educator: Principles of teaching and learning for nursing practice* (4th ed.). Burlington, MA: Jones & Bartlett Learning.

Bastable, S., Gramet, P., Jacobs, K., & Sopczyk, D. L. (2011). *Health professional as educator: Principles of teaching and learning for nursing practice.* Boston, MA: Jones & Bartlett Learning.

Blais, K. K., and Hayes, J. S. (2011). *Professional nursing practice: Concepts and perspectives* (6th ed.). Upper Saddle River, NJ: Pearson.

Bloom, B. S. (Ed.). (1956). *Taxonomy of education objectives. Book 1: Cognitive domain.* New York, NY: Longman.

Bruner, J. (1966). *Toward a theory of instruction.* Cambridge, MA: Harvard University Press.

Fox, S. (2013). *Pew Internet: Health.* Retrieved from http://www.pewinternet.org/Commentary/2011/November/Pew-Internet-Health.aspx.

Fox, S., & Jones, S. (2009a). The social life of health information. *Pew Internet/California HealthCare Foundation.* Retrieved from http://www.pewinternet.org/Reports/2009/8-The-Social-Life-of-Health-Information.aspx.

Fox, S., & Jones, S. (2009b). The social life of health information: A shifting landscape. *Pew Internet/California HealthCare Foundation.* Retrieved from http://www.pewinternet.org/Reports/2009/8-The-Social-Life-of-Health-Information/02-A-Shifting-Landscape/2-61-of-adults-in-the-US-gather-health-information-online.aspx.

Gardner, H. (1983). *Frames of mind: Theory of multiple intelligences.* New York, NY: Basic Books.

Hayes, K. (2005). Designing written medication instructions: Effective ways to help older adults self-medicate. *Journal of Gerontological Nursing, 31*(5), 5–10.

Heinrich, C. (2012). Health literacy: The sixth vital sign. *Journal of the American Academy of Nurse Practitioners, 24*(2012). doi:10.1111/j.1745-7599.2012.00698.x.

Institute of Medicine (IOM). (2004). *Health literacy: A prescription to end confusion.* Washington, DC: National Academies Press.

John, M. T. (1988). *Geragogy: A theory for teaching the elderly.* New York, NY: Haworth Press.

Knowles, M. S. (1984). *Andragogy in action.* San Francisco, CA: Jossey-Bass.

Knowles, M. S., Holton, E. F., & Swanson, R. A. (2005). *The adult learner* (6th ed.). Burlington, MA: Elsevier Butterworth-Heinemann. (Original work published 1973)

Lewin, K. (1951). *Field theory in social science.* New York, NY: Harper and Row.

Marquis, B. L., & Huston, C. J. (2012). *Leadership and management tools for the new nurse: A case study approach.* Philadelphia, PA: Lippincott.

Munoz, C., & Luckmann, J. (2005). *Transcultural communication in nursing* (2nd ed.). Clifton Park, NY: Delmar Learning.

NANDA International. (2005). *NANDA nursing diagnoses: Definitions and classification 2005–2006.* Philadelphia, PA: Author.

Olson, R. K. (2012). *Seeking help from a mentor.* Paper presented at the American Association of Colleges of Nursing Faculty Development Conference, Atlanta, GA. Retrieved from http://www.aacn.nche.edu/membership/members-only/presentations/2012/12facdev/Roberta-K.-Olson.pdf.

Osborn, K. S., Wraa, C. E., Watson, A. B., & Holleran, R. (2013). *Medical-surgical nursing: Preparation for practice.* Upper Saddle River, NJ: Pearson.

Purnell, L. D., & Paulanka, B. J. (2008). *Guide to culturally competent health care,* (2nd Ed.). Philadelphia, PA: F. A. Davis.

Rankin, S. H., Stallings, K. D., & London, F. (2005). *Patient education in health and illness* (5th ed.). Philadelphia, PA: Lippincott Williams & Wilkins.

Saarmann, L., Daugherty, J., & Riegel, B. (2000). Patient teaching to promote behavioral change. *Nursing Outlook, 48*, 281–287.

Schutzenhofer, K. K. (1995). Power, politics and influence. In P. S. Yoder-Wise (Ed.), *Leading and managing in nursing*. St. Louis, MO: Mosby-Year Book.

Sullivan, E. J., & Decker, P. J. (2009). *Effective leadership and management in nursing* (7th ed.). Upper Saddle River, NJ: Pearson.

U.S. Department of Health and Human Services (USD-HHS). (2008). *America's health literacy: Why we need accessible health information*. Retrieved from http://www.health.gov/communication/literacy/issuebrief.

U.S. Department of Health and Human Services (USD-HHS), Office of Disease Prevention and Health Promotion. (2010). *National action plan to improve health literacy*. Washington, DC: Author. Retrieved from http://www.health.gov/communication/hlactionplan/pdf/Health_Literacy_Action_Plan.pdf.

Wilkinson, J. M. (2013). *Nursing diagnosis handbook with NIC interventions and NOC outcomes* (10th ed.). Upper Saddle River, NJ: Prentice Hall Health.

Wolff, H. G., & Sowon, K. (2012). The relationship between networking behaviors and the big five personality dimensions. *Career Development International, 17*(1). doi:10.1108/13620431211201328.

World Health Organization. (2013). *E-health*. Retrieved from http://www.who.int/trade/glossary/story021/en.

Wu, S., Turban, D. B., & Yu, H. C. (2012). Social skill in workplace mentoring relationships. *Journal of Organizational Culture, Communications & Conflict, 16*(2), 61–72. Retrieved from http://www.alliedacademies.org/Public/Journals/JournalDetails.aspx?jid=11.

Yoder-Wise, P. S. (2011). *Leading and managing in nursing* (5th ed.). St. Louis, MO: Elsevier.

Zickuhr, K., & Madden, M. (2012). Older adults and Internet use. *Pew Internet & American Life Project*. Retrieved from http://www.pewinternet.org/Reports/2012/Older-adults-and-internet-use/Summary-of-findings.aspx.

Part V
Healthcare Domain

Part V consists of modules that outline and define principles related to the healthcare domain, including accountability, ethics, and quality improvement. Each module presents a concept that relates directly to professional nursing, its relationship to healthcare systems and policies, and how nursing within the healthcare system impacts client health and wellbeing. Selected principles or topics of each concept are presented as exemplars. The exemplars in the module on Accountability, for example, cover Competence and Professional Development. Each module addresses the effect of that concept and the selected exemplars on the care of individuals across the life span, inclusive of their culture, their gender, and their developmental status.

Module 42   Accountability   2535
Module 43   Advocacy   2555
Module 44   Ethics   2563
Module 45   Evidence-Based Practice   2583
Module 46   Healthcare Systems   2595
Module 47   Health Policy   2619
Module 48   Informatics   2631
Module 49   Legal Issues   2653
Module 50   Quality Improvement   2681
Module 51   Safety   2695

42 Accountability

MODULE AT-A-GLANCE

The Concept of Accountability, 2535

Exemplar 42.1
Competence, 2543

Exemplar 42.2
Professional Development, 2545

◩ THE CONCEPT OF ACCOUNTABILITY

Accountability and *responsibility* are words that are often used interchangeably. However, there are some important distinctions. **Accountability** involves being answerable for the outcomes of a task or assignment. Nurses are accountable for their own actions and behaviors, but they may also be accountable for the actions of others, such as subordinates or trainees. **Responsibility** is the specific obligation associated with the performance of duties of a particular role and belongs to the individual performing the duties. Nurses are responsible for performing their assigned tasks reliably, dependably, and to the best of their abilities. Nurses' sense of accountability guides their performance, which ultimately determines client outcomes.

For example, suppose a nurse has a client who will need continued wound care for his left foot after discharge to home. The client has said that he thinks he understands the procedure for changing his dressing and has promised to call if he needs any further teaching. **≪**

Concept Learning Outcomes

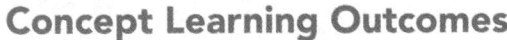
After reading about this concept, you will be able to:

1. Examine the criteria of the profession and the professionalization of nursing.
2. Compare the essential nursing values concerning attitudes, personal qualities, and professional behaviors.
3. Describe the different types of educational nursing programs.
4. Analyze factors influencing nursing practice and accountability.
5. Summarize the importance of continuing nursing education.

Concept Key Terms

Accountability, *2535*
Autonomy, *2537*
Consumer, *2540*
Demography, *2542*
Governance, *2538*
Patient Self-Determination
 Act (PSDA), *2542*
Profession, *2536*

Responsibility, *2535*
Socialization, *2539*
Standards of care, *2536*
Standards of practice, *2536*
Telecommunication, *2541*

Standards of practice (standards of care) are guidelines used to determine what a nurse should or should not do and may be defined as a benchmark of achievement based on a desired level of excellence (McMahon, 2013). The nurse knows that the **standards of care** dictate asking the client to demonstrate how to change the dressing so that the nurse can evaluate the client's understanding and ability to care for himself. The nurse must decide whether to allow the client to go home without seeing him perform the dressing change or whether the discharge needs to be delayed until he can demonstrate his understanding. The nurse is responsible for upholding the standards of care and is accountable for making the decision in the discharge of this client. If the client does not perform the dressing care properly at home and is readmitted for complications, the nurse is responsible for this outcome and may be held accountable. As an alternative to the client's demonstrating the dressing change, the nurse could do one of the following:

■ Request an order for home health care to continue the teaching and follow up until the client is comfortable on his own.

■ Teach a family member to perform the care in case the client is not feeling well enough to do it on his own.

■ Arrange for the client to travel to the outpatient nursing facility for daily dressing changes.

Regardless of the method, the nurse is accountable at discharge for ensuring that the client can get the wound dressed as often as the order advises. The client must rely on the nurse's judgment for the most favorable outcome.

Accountability in nursing cannot be achieved without clear definitions of what is an accepted standard of care. Organizations such as The Joint Commission, the American Nurses Association (ANA), and the National League for Nursing (NLN) define those standards. **Standards of practice** (descriptions of the responsibilities for which nurses are accountable) have been considered interchangeable with a standard of care for several years (McMahon, 2013). For example, a standard of practice/care for medication administration set forth by The Joint Commission is to require two client identifiers prior to giving the prescribed dose. A nurse who chooses not to meet that requirement is failing to practice at the minimum standard acceptable to the profession and will be held accountable to the client and the facility for which the nurse works.

Unfortunately, the term *accountability* often carries a negative connotation. When an error is made, the question "Who is accountable?" often translates into "Who is to blame?" The implication is that someone has failed. The negative image of accountability is what the public tends to see also, especially since the release of *To Err Is Human* (1999), a report by the Institute of Medicine (IOM). Healthcare organizations have had to regain the public's trust. Organizations such as The Joint Commission, NLN, and ANA have revised and created standards for nurses to follow independently and jointly to ensure giving the safest, most competent care. More recently, the Robert Wood Johnson Foundation sponsored Quality and Safety Education for Nurses (QSEN; Cronenwett, Sherwood,

& Gelmon, 2009), an initiative to improve the quality and safety in prelicensure nursing programs. This initiative endorsed the idea that quality and safety education must become core competencies embedded in all programs preparing nurses for basic practice (Cronenwett et al., 2009). The six competencies critical to the nursing role include client-centered care, teamwork and collaboration, evidence-based practice, quality improvement, safety, and informatics (Anderson, 2010; QSEN, 2007).

Stay Current: To learn more about the QSEN competencies, visit the QSEN Institute Web site at **http://qsen.org/**

Research supports the importance of accountability for preventing errors as well as for making them: "A supportive practice environment enhances nurses' error interception practices. These interception practices play a role in reducing medication errors" (Flynn et al., 2012, p. 185). However, if nurses practice in a positive and supportive environment and celebrate accountability for their successes as well as their errors, the culture of the profession will remain positive. Focusing on and honoring success are as important as examining and correcting errors.

▶ CRITERIA OF A PROFESSION

Nursing is gaining recognition as a profession. A **profession** has been defined as an occupation that requires extensive education or a calling that requires special knowledge, skill, and preparation. A profession is generally distinguished from other kinds of occupations by (a) its requirement of prolonged, specialized training to acquire a body of knowledge that supports the role to be performed; (b) an orientation of the individual toward service, either to a community or to an organization; (c) ongoing research; (d) a code of ethics; (e) autonomy; and (f) a professional organization.

Specialized Education

Specialized education is an important aspect of professional status. In modern times, the trend in education for the professions has shifted toward programs in colleges and universities. In the United States today, there are five means of entry into registered nursing: hospital diploma (as of 2013, a small number of hospitals around the country still offer such programs), associate degree, baccalaureate degree, master's degree, and doctoral degree. The ANA recommends the baccalaureate degree as the entry level for professional practice. Recently, the National Organization for Associate Degree Nursing (N-OADN) joined other college associations in issuing a joint statement on academic progression for nursing students and graduates (American Association of Colleges of Nurses, 2012a).

Body of Knowledge

As a profession, nursing is establishing a well-defined body of knowledge and expertise. A number of conceptual nursing frameworks contribute to the knowledge base and give direction to nursing practice, education, and ongoing research.

Evidence-Based Practice Leadership Interventions to Establish Evidence-Based Practice

Problem

What is the impact of leadership facilitation strategies on nurses' beliefs about the importance and frequency of using evidence in their daily practice and on their perception of organizational readiness in an acute care hospital?

Evidence

A 429-bed nonteaching, faith-based hospital located in a moderate-sized city in the Midwest conducted a prospective descriptive comparative study that involved three surveys (Hauck, Winsett, & Kuric, 2013). The Evidence-Based Practice Beliefs Scale, the Implementation Scale, and the Organizational Culture and Readiness for System-Wide Integration Survey measured change before and after facilitation of strategies for evidence-based practice (EBP) enculturation. The Nursing Research-EBP Committee developed and helped direct a strategic plan that specifically addressed EBP enculturation with nursing leaders. Baseline data were collected in December 2008 with a sample size of 427, and final data were collected in December 2010 with a sample size of 469.

Results

Significant results demonstrated that leadership facilitated infrastructure development in three major areas: incorporating evidence-based practice outcomes in the strategic plan; supporting mentors; and advocating for resources for education and outcome dissemination. With the interventions in place, the total group scores for beliefs and organizational readiness improved significantly. Analyses by job role showed that direct care nurses' scores in these areas improved more than the scores of individuals in other role types. No differences were found in the implementation scores.

Conclusions

The researchers concluded that successful key strategies were evidence-based practice education and establishing internal opportunities to disseminate findings. They also noted that transformational nursing leadership drives organizational change and provides vision, human and financial resources, and time that empowers nurses to include evidence in practice.

Implications

Because of the continual nursing shortage, it is important for hospitals to recruit and retain competent nursing staff, and to effectively implement changes in the practice environment. The findings of this practice change assisted the hospital to improve its change process in adding EBP within nursing practice that enables successful approaches in improving nurse–physician communication and improving nursing practice and prevention of errors. Studies such as this one allow hospitals to implement new strategies for change, with the outcome of increased quality of client care and nursing retention—a win-win for all.

Critical Thinking Application

1. In this study's project, nurses were encouraged to search for evidence to support their daily practice. How have you been encouraged to use evidence-based research findings as a nursing student?
2. While not discussed in this particular study, from the authors' findings, what role could nursing education programs take in assisting with EBP implementation in acute care nursing units where student nurses are practicing?

Service Orientation

A service orientation differentiates nursing from occupations pursued primarily for profit. Nursing has a tradition of service to others. This service, however, must be guided by certain rules, policies, and codes of ethics. Nursing remains an important component of the healthcare delivery system.

Ongoing Research

Increasing research in nursing is contributing to nursing practice. In the 1940s, nursing research was at a very early stage. In the 1950s, increased federal funding and professional support helped establish centers for nursing research. Most early research studied nursing education. In the 1960s, studies were often related to the knowledge base of nursing practice. In the 1970s, nursing research began to increase its focus on practice-related issues. Today, a wealth of research exists on which to build continuing research efforts as well as evidence-based practice.

Code of Ethics

Nurses have traditionally placed a high value on the worth and dignity of all individuals. The nursing profession requires integrity of its members; that is, a nurse is expected to do what is considered right regardless of the personal cost.

Ethical codes change as the needs and values of society change. Nursing has developed its own codes of ethics and in most instances has set up means to monitor the professional behavior of its members. Nursing ethics is discussed in detail in the module on Ethics.

Autonomy

A profession is autonomous if it regulates itself and sets standards or practice for its own members. Providing autonomy is one of the purposes of a professional association. If nursing is to have professional status, it must function autonomously in the formation of policy and in the control of its activity. To be autonomous, a professional group must be granted legal authority to define the scope of its practice, describe its particular functions and roles, and determine its goals and responsibilities in delivery of its services. State boards of nursing (detailed in the module on Legal Issues) carry legal authority with regard to the autonomy of the nursing profession.

For nurses as individuals, **autonomy** means independence at work, responsibility, and accountability for one's actions. Autonomy is more easily achieved and maintained from a position of authority. Therefore some nurses seek administrative positions, rather than expanded clinical competence, as a means to ensure their autonomy in the workplace.

Concepts Related to **Accountability**

The relationship between nursing accountability and client safety secondary to risk of suicide or abuse symptoms is a vital nursing role. Healthcare providers need to routinely assess clients for factors that may indicate an increased risk of suicide and suicidal intent (Aiello-Laws, 2010). It has been said that the individuals in your care must be able to trust you with their health and well-being. To fulfill this duty, all nurses need to be aware of the potential for abuse of any vulnerable child or adult with whom they come into contact during their practice (Sturdy, 2012). Ensuring the management of client com-

fort or a manageable level of pain is also a client safety concern. Encouraging the client to give voice to any needs and providing appropriate comfort interventions are accountability roles for nurses (Timmins, 2011). Client teaching and assessing readiness to learn are also vital nursing roles, in all client care areas. Understanding a client's learning style assists the nurse in providing skills for safe self-care (Ball, 2013). With evidence-based practice, nurses have both a professional and an ethical duty of care to incorporate evidence-based knowledge and technical skills into their practice (Priharjo & Hoy, 2011).

CONCEPT	RELATIONSHIP TO ACCOUNTABILITY	NURSING IMPLICATIONS
Violence ■ Physical violence ■ Abuse ■ Suicide	Clients may present with signs or symptoms of abuse, such as bruising in different stages of healing upon admission, or possible risk of suicide.	■ Assess for risk factors of physical or emotional abuse as well as suicide risk as part of the admission process. ■ Be aware of warning signs of abuse or suicide risk that a client may demonstrate or verbalize.
Comfort ■ Comfort assessment ■ Assessment interview: Discomfort ■ Acute and chronic pain	The nurse is responsible for assessing the client's level of comfort and providing effective interventions.	■ Assess client's reported level of comfort every shift. ■ Assess level of comfort more often as indicated by client's condition. ■ Document comfort and interventions provided.
Teaching and Learning ■ Client education	The nurse is accountable for client education concerning all aspects of care.	■ Assess client and family learning needs. ■ Assess readiness for learning. ■ Design and implement appropriate educational interventions.
Evidence-Based Practice ■ Developing EBP ■ Strategies to implement EBP	The nurse is accountable to practice within an EBP environment and to implement evidence in practice.	■ Develop a clinical question using the format learned in the EBP chapter. ■ Conduct a literature search for current evidence.

Professional Organization

Operation under the umbrella of a professional organization differentiates a profession from an occupation. **Governance** is the establishment and maintenance of social, political, and economic arrangements by which professionals control their practice, their self-discipline, their working conditions, and their professional affairs. Professional organizations that govern and differentiate the profession of nursing are described fully in the module on Health Policy.

▶ INTEGRATING THE CONCEPTS

The concept of Accountability relates to all other nursing concepts. The Concepts Related to Accountability feature demonstrates the relationship to four concepts.

CASE STUDY \\ PART 1

Jen Sturges is a fairly new RN on the medical unit in a 245-bed hospital. On the evening shift, Jen started her rounds with her five clients. One of her clients was a 45-year-old female named Kathryn Miller, who had been admitted with a GI diagnosis and also had a history of back pain. During Jen's assessment of her pain level, Ms. Miller said she was "doing just fine," although she seemed very anxious. As Jen reviewed Ms. Miller's vital signs, which the CNA had recently taken, she noted a blood pressure much higher than usual. Jen commented that one of the symptoms of pain is a higher blood pressure. Ms. Miller described trying to overrule her body by ignoring its signals, and having a dialogue between the "body me" and the "real me." Ms. Miller said, "If I refuse to pay attention to my body, my pain will go away."

Jen realized that Ms. Miller, although actually in pain, might not be allowing herself to pay attention. Jen asked Ms. Miller if she had discussed her pain management with her primary healthcare provider. Ms. Miller laughed: "My doctor tries to have me take narcotics, but I worry about those types of meds." As she spoke, Ms. Miller's hands were gripping the bed sheets and she was shaking. She said, "The pain is my enemy and I don't talk to my enemies."

Jen knew that ignoring the body's signals of pain can cause serious consequences: The pain could intensify and the client's blood pressure could rise significantly. Jen realized that Ms. Miller needed to get appropriate treatment for her pain. After her assessment, Jen discussed with the unit charge nurse her concerns about Ms. Miller and her need for pain management and comfort.

Clinical Reasoning Questions Level I

1. Why was it important for Jen to complete her client's assessment before leaving the room?
2. What further symptoms did Jen observe while she spoke with her client?
3. What information should Jen share with the charge nurse to assist in meeting her client's needs?

Clinical Reasoning Questions Level II

4. With what staff should Jen and the charge nurse plan to collaborate to find a better method for managing Ms. Miller's pain?
5. When a client refuses pain management, why should the nurse pursue other solutions rather than simply acquiescing?

▶ SOCIALIZATION TO NURSING

The standards of education and practice for a profession are determined by the members of the profession rather than by outsiders, and they involve a complete socialization process that is far more extensive than is usually required in nonprofessional occupations.

Socialization can be defined simply as the process by which individuals (a) learn to become members of groups and society and (b) learn the social rules defining relationships into which they will enter. Traditionally, socialization has been defined as involving learning to behave, feel, and see the world as other individuals do who occupy the same role as oneself (Hardy & Conway, 1988, p. 261). Professional socialization is a more complex process. Dinmohammadi, Peyrovi, and Mehrdad (2013) conducted a meta-analysis to clarify the process of professional socialization and to identify its attributes, antecedents, and consequences in nursing. These authors argue that professional socialization is a complex process with four critical attributes: learning, interaction, development, and adaptation. Comprehensive educational programs, competent role models, and adequate field experiences were found to be the antecedents of these attributes. Price (2009) concurred regarding the need for mentors and peers in nursing.

One of the most powerful mechanisms of professional socialization is interaction with fellow students. Students collectively set the level and direction of their scholastic efforts (Condon & Sharts-Hopko, 2010). They develop perspectives about the situation in which they are involved, the goals they are trying to achieve, and the kinds of activities and behaviors that are appropriate, and they establish a set of practices in keeping with all of these. Students become bound together by feelings of mutual cooperation, support, and solidarity.

Critical Values of Nursing

Students in nursing education develop, clarify, and internalize their own individual professional values. Specific professional nursing values are stated in nursing codes of ethics (see the module on Ethics), in standards of nursing practice (see the exemplar on Professional Development in this module), and in the legal system itself (see the module on Legal Issues). Additionally, in 2001 the National Student Nurses Association (NSNA) adopted a code of academic and clinical conduct (**Box 42–1 ●**), a code that is an integral part of ethical practice (NSNA, 2013). This code addresses students' responsibility in the academic environment and to society at large as they learn clinical skills in nursing care.

CASE STUDY \\ PART 2

Jen Sturges briefly but clearly discussed with the charge nurse, Melina Menendez, her concerns about Ms. Miller's pain management and the objective symptoms she noted during her shift. Ms. Menendez asked Jen what she thought was going on with Ms. Miller. Jen told her that this was her first experience with a client who had a history of pain but did not want to use any pain medications and ignored her apparent pain while only resting in bed.

Ms. Menendez was concerned that the client would be unable to participate in her care and activity if she had uncontrolled pain during hospitalization. She asked Jen to join her while she spoke with Ms. Miller. After a few minutes of discussion, it became clear that the client was afraid of pain and narcotic abuse. It also appeared that uncertainty about the meaning of her body's pain signals worried Ms. Miller about the safety of her physical activities at home and in the hospital. Ms. Menendez gently held Ms. Miller's hand and told her how important it was for her to take part in care activities and to allow staff to manage pain and keep her as comfortable as possible. "To help you with this care," Ms. Menendez said, "I would like our social worker and clinical pharmacist to see you about your pain and needs while you are here." Ms. Miller agreed with this plan.

Clinical Reasoning Question Level I

1. As the charge nurse, Ms. Menendez took an active role in further assessment of the client's needs and communicated with Ms. Miller in a truthful and calm manner. Of what aspect of ethical principles listed in the Code for Nursing Students is this an example?

Clinical Reasoning Question Level II

2. If Jen had waited to collaborate with the charge nurse, would this have prevented further care and appropriate client outcomes? Explain your answer.

Box 42–1 National Student Nurses Association Code of Academic and Clinical Conduct

PREAMBLE

Students of nursing have a responsibility to society in learning the academic theory and clinical skills needed to provide nursing care. The clinical setting presents unique challenges and responsibilities while caring for human beings in a variety of health care environments.

The Code of Academic and Clinical Conduct is based on an understanding that to practice nursing as a student is an agreement to uphold the trust with which society has placed in us. The statements of the code provide guidance for the nursing student in the personal development of an ethical foundation and need not be limited strictly to the academic or clinical environment but can assist in the holistic development of the individual.

A CODE FOR NURSING STUDENTS

As students are involved in the clinical and academic environments we believe that ethical principles are a necessary guide to professional development. Therefore within these environments we:

1. Advocate for the rights of all clients.
2. Maintain client confidentiality.
3. Take appropriate action to ensure the safety of clients, self, and others.
4. Provide care for the client in a timely, compassionate and professional manner.
5. Communicate client care in a truthful, timely and accurate manner.
6. Actively promote the highest level of moral and ethical principles and accept responsibility for our actions.
7. Promote excellence in nursing by encouraging lifelong learning and professional development.
8. Treat others with respect and promote an environment that respects human rights, values and choice of cultural and spiritual beliefs.
9. Collaborate in every reasonable manner with the academic faculty and clinical staff to ensure the highest quality of client care.
10. Use every opportunity to improve faculty and clinical staff understanding of the learning needs of nursing students.
11. Encourage faculty, clinical staff, and peers to mentor nursing students.
12. Refrain from performing any technique or procedure for which the student has not been adequately trained.
13. Refrain from any deliberate action or omission of care in the academic or clinical setting that creates unnecessary risk of injury to the client, self, or others.
14. Assist the staff nurse or preceptor in ensuring that there is full disclosure and that proper authorization is obtained from clients regarding any form of treatment or research.
15. Abstain from the use of alcoholic beverages or any substances in the academic and clinical setting that impair judgment.
16. Strive to achieve and maintain an optimal level of personal health.
17. Support access to treatment and rehabilitation for students who are experiencing impairments related to substance abuse and mental or physical health issues.
18. Uphold school policies and regulations related to academic and clinical performance, reserving the right to challenge and critique rules and regulations as per school grievance policy.

Note: This code was adopted by the NSNA House of Delegates, Nashville, Tennessee, on April 6, 2001. Reprinted with permission.

▶ FACTORS INFLUENCING NURSING PRACTICE AND ACCOUNTABILITY

A number of factors influence nursing as a profession. These forces usually affect the entire healthcare system, and nursing, as a major component of that system, cannot avoid the effects.

Economics

Changes in public and private health insurance programs, particularly Medicare, have affected the demand for nursing care. Individuals who cannot afford health care are increasingly using such health services as emergency department care, mental health counseling, and preventive physical examinations.

Increases in the costs of health care have also affected nursing. In 1982, the Medicare payment system to hospitals and physicians was revised to establish reimbursement fees according to the client's medical diagnosis. This classification system is known as *diagnostic-related groups (DRGs)*. The system has categories that establish pretreatment diagnosis billing categories. With the implementation of this legislation, clients once considered sufficiently ill to be hospitalized are now treated at home, with the result that clients who do get treatment in hospitals are more acutely ill than before.

These changes present challenges to nurses and to the organizations where they practice. For many years, the healthcare industry has been shifting its emphasis from inpatient to outpatient care with preadmission testing, increased outpatient same-day surgery, posthospitalization rehabilitation, home health care, health maintenance, physical fitness programs, and community health education programs. As a result, while acute care remains the primary nursing practice area, more nurses are being employed in community-based health settings, such as home health agencies, hospices, and community clinics. These changes have implications for nursing education, nursing research, and nursing practice, particularly in relation to the nurse's competence to practice within these various settings.

The increase in outpatient care settings has resulted in further research and organization guidelines to ensure client safety and satisfaction in this care area. For example, in 2011 the Centers for Disease Control and Prevention (CDC) released outpatient safety guidelines focusing on prevention and control of infection and other safety concerns (CDC, 2011). The findings of a study on client satisfaction with outpatient care that used data-based nursing staffing indicators showed the importance of clear information for further care plans such as repeat visits and self-care (Salin, Kaunonen, & Aalto, 2012).

As with acute care environments, the field of outpatient care has developed specialty areas to meet client needs. For example, an outpatient oncology symptom management clinic was developed to support cancer clients' needs and prevent inpatient admissions due to symptoms (Whitmer et al., 2011). Similarly, a palliative care clinic managed by nurse practitioners improved continuity of care for clients in the end of life (Owens et al., 2012).

Consumer Demands

A **consumer** is an individual, a group of individuals, or a community that uses a service or commodity. Consumers of nursing services (e.g., the public) have become an increasingly effective force in changing nursing practice. On the whole, individuals are better educated and have more knowledge about health and illness than in the past. Through the Internet, more individuals have more access to a greater amount of information. Consumers also have become more aware of others' needs for care. The ethical and moral issues raised by poverty and neglect have made individuals more vocal about the needs of minority groups and the poor.

The public's concepts of health and nursing have also changed. Many individuals now believe that health is a right of everyone, not just a privilege of the rich. The media emphasize the message that individuals must assume responsibility for their own health by having regular physical examinations, knowing risks factors for diseases such as cancer, and maintaining their mental well-being by balancing work and recreation. Interest in health and nursing services is therefore greater than ever. Furthermore, many individuals want more than freedom from disease: They want energy, vitality, and a feeling of wellness.

Increasingly, the consumer has become an active participant in making decisions about health and nursing care. Planning committees concerned with providing nursing services to a community usually have active consumer membership, meaning that clients are having an increasing influence on the accountability of the nursing profession. Recognizing the legitimacy of public input, many state nursing associations and regulatory agencies have consumer representatives on their governing boards.

Science and Technology

Advances in science and technology affect nursing practice, competence, and accountability. For example, biotechnology has had an ongoing and increasing influence on health care. Progress in the field of molecular genetics has made it possible to identify individuals with an increased risk for a variety of hereditary diseases, increasing consumers' options for obtaining this information (Wolff et al., 2011). However, the testing of healthy children for diseases that would develop only in adulthood raises many important ethical, legal and social issues, as genetic testing is now available outside the traditional healthcare system, often without even the mediation of a healthcare professional (Howard, Avard, & Borry, 2011). Nurses need to expand their knowledge base and technical skills as they adapt to meet the new needs of clients.

Healthcare practitioners in most settings are now expected to learn how to use technological advances such as sophisticated computerized equipment to monitor or treat clients. They are also expected to be able to utilize online Electronic Health Report Systems. The Health Information Technology for Economic and Clinical Health (HITECH) Act of 2009 was aimed at increasing the adoption and "meaningful use" of electronic health record systems (EHRs) by providing incentives and penalties to hospitals through the Medicare and Medicaid programs (CMS, 2013). In both acute inpatient settings and primary care practices, healthcare practitioners have integrated EHRs successfully and have reported increased efficiency in retrieving medical records, storing client information, and coordinating care and general office operations (Goldberg et al., 2012).

Technological innovations have also had dramatic effects on the clinical training of nurses and physicians. Simulation-based training activities improve clinical decision making and have an overall positive impact on students' learning and on client safety (Lafond & Van Hulle Vincent, 2013; Secomb, Mckenna, & Smith, 2012; Spooner, Hurst, & Khadra, 2012). As technologies change, nursing education changes, and nurses require increasing educa-

tion to provide effective, safe nursing care With the increase in technology integration in nursing education, a recent study developed a computer literacy scale for nursing students (Lin, 2011). This study recommends more emphasis on mastering database and statistical software as well as hospital information systems and information ethics and less emphasis on word-processing topics.

Information and Telecommunications

The use of the Internet has increased dramatically and has affected health care, particularly as more clients become well informed about their health concerns. With access to the Internet at home and on mobile devices, more clients and caregivers are searching the Web for answers to their health questions. In 2009, research found that 74% of adults used the Internet, 61% used it to search for health or medical information, and 49% accessed Web sites that provide information on specific medical conditions (Cohen & Adams, 2011). By 2012, the use of the Internet had increased to 81% of American adults, and 72% said they use the web for health information, with 45% of adults reported to own and use smartphones (Fox, 2013). In addition to seeking health information, more adults and caregivers regularly log onto forums surrounding their particular concerns (Fox, 2013).

A recent study looked at the effectiveness of Web search engines and the relevance of documents retrieved for health information (Lopes & Ribiero, 2011). While these studies indicated that most adults are becoming "smart" about where and how to find information on the Web, it remains important for nurses to know how to help clients access high-quality, valid Web sites; how to interpret the information they find; and how to evaluate the information and determine whether it is useful.

Telecommunication is the transmission of information from one site to another, using equipment to send information in the form of signs, signals, words, or pictures by cable, radio, and other systems (Higuchi et al., 2011). Various forms of telecommunication, such as VoIP (e.g., Skype), videoconferencing, telepractice, telerehabilitation, and virtual visits, allow individuals and/or groups in two or more locations to communicate by simultaneous two-way video and audio transmissions (Olsen, Fiechtl, & Rule, 2012). It is now possible to monitor critical care clients in an ICU in a different city or rural area and to manage client care from another part of the world (American Telemedicine Association [ATA], 2012). Education has also been enhanced by Web-based distance education. Technology-delivered education has been shown to augment the existing curriculum by increasing students' access to clinical experts in specialty areas, thus supporting efficient use of faculty resources (ATA, 2012).

Telehealth uses telecommunication technology to provide long-distance health care. It can use videoconferencing, computers, or telephones. *Telenursing* occurs when the nurse delivers care through a telecommunication system. Examples of telenursing are the nurse who telephones clients at home to assess their progress or to answer questions, the nurse who participates in a video teleconference in which consultants or experts at various sites discuss a client's healthcare plan, and the nurse who uses VoIP technology to assess a client living in a rural area.

Telehealth and telenursing are not limited by geography, and licensure issues have been raised. For example, if a nurse licensed in one state provides health information to a client in another state, does the nurse need to maintain licensure in both states? The National Council of State Boards of Nursing endorses a change from single-state licensure to a mutual recognition model. Many state legislatures have adopted mutual recognition language into their statutes and are currently implementing it. See the module on Legal Issues for more information. In response to the growing use of telehealth programs, standards and guidelines have been developed , particularly for advanced-practice nurses working within this environment (Bryce, 2013).

Legislation

Legislation about nursing practice and health matters affects both the consumer and the nursing profession. Changes in legislation relating to health also affect nursing. For example, the **Patient Self-Determination Act (PSDA)** requires that on admission to a healthcare institution, all competent adults be informed in writing about their rights to accept or refuse medical care and to use advance directives. This law, which in many institutions is implemented by nurses, affects the nurse's role in supporting clients and their families.

Demography

Demography is the study of population, including statistics of distribution by age and place of residence, mortality (death), and morbidity (incidence of disease). From demographic data, needs of the population for nursing services can be assessed. For example:

- The total population in North America is increasing. The proportion of older adults has also increased, creating an increased need for nursing services for this group.

- The population has shifted from rural to urban settings. Thus most nursing services are now provided in urban settings. This shift signals an increased need for nursing related to problems caused by pollution and by the effects on the environment of concentrations of individuals.

- Mortality and morbidity studies reveal the presence of risks (e.g., smoking) that are major factors in death and disease and that can be prevented through changes in lifestyle.

The Current Nursing Shortage

The multiple factors influencing the current nursing shortage (see **Box 42–2** ●) are different from those influencing previous nursing shortages. Although registered nurses make up the largest group of healthcare providers, fewer nurses are entering the workforce, and certain geographic areas are experiencing acute nursing shortages. The supply is inadequate to meet the demand, especially for specialized nurses (e.g., critical care nurses), and this situation is expected to worsen (AACN, 2012b).

Addressing the nursing shortage requires collaboration among healthcare systems, policy makers, nursing educators, and professional organizations. Recommendations include, but are not limited to, the following:

- Develop mechanisms for nursing students to progress to and through educational programs more efficiently and quickly.

- Recruit young people to nursing early (e.g., in grade school).

- Improve the nurse's work environment: Provide greater flexibility in work hours, reward experienced nurses who serve as mentors, ensure adequate staffing, and increase salaries.

- Increase funding for nursing education.

Box 42–2 Factors Contributing to the Nursing Shortage

NURSING SCHOOL ENROLLMENT NOT GROWING FAST ENOUGH
- There was a 5.1% increase in entry-level BSNs in 2011, but this was not sufficient to meet projected demand.
- With changes in access to health care, more Americans may soon require nursing care.

AGING NURSE WORKFORCE
- Between 2010 and 2020, the age of over 40% of the RN workforce will exceed 50, and many RNs are expected to retire and withdraw from the workforce (AACN, 2012b).
- New graduates are entering the workforce at an older age and will have fewer years to work.

SHORTAGE OF NURSING FACULTY
- U.S. nursing schools turned away more than 75,000 qualified applicants in 2011 due to budget constraints and insufficient faculty and clinical sites.
- There is a 12% shortfall in the number of nurse educators needed.

CHANGING DEMOGRAPHICS
- The number of individuals in the U.S. population age 65 and older is expected to double between 2000 and 2030.
- The ratio of potential caregivers to older adults will decrease by 40% between 2010 and 2030.

INCREASED DEMAND FOR NURSES
- Increased acuity of hospital clients requiring skilled and specialized nurses
- Shorter hospital stays, resulting in transfer of clients to long-term care and community settings, creating increased demand for nurses in the community

WORKPLACE ISSUES
- Inadequate staffing
- Heavy workloads
- Increased use of overtime
- Lack of sufficient support staff
- Inadequate wages
- Difficulty recruiting and retaining nurses
- High nurse turnover and vacancy rates with many leaving nursing altogether.

▶ NURSING PRACTICE

Accountability and responsibility are important components of nursing practice. They are influenced by a variety of factors, including the individual's own values and beliefs, the values and ethics inherent in the profession as a whole, and many social factors that affect nursing practice and accountability either directly or indirectly.

Accountability is a function of the competence of the individual nurse, the professional development of nurses as individuals, the structure of the organization in which the nurse practices, and the development of the nursing profession itself. Competence and professional development are discussed in the exemplars that follow.

REVIEW The Concept of Accountability

RELATE Link the Concepts

Linking the concept of accountability with the concept of legal issues:

1. What is the nurse's legal obligation to the client related to accountability, and how is it regulated?

2. A nurse makes a medication error that results in harm to the client. The nurse demonstrates accountability by immediately informing the physician and nursing supervisor when the error is recognized. How does the nurse's proper demonstration of accountability affect the nurse's legal responsibility?

Linking the concept of accountability with the concept of comfort:

3. What is the nurse's role in assessment and appropriate interventions to ensure comfort for the client?

4. How does lack of client comfort impede the client's taking part in care plans and activities?

Linking the concept of accountability with the concept of ethics:

5. How does the nurse's code of ethics reflect the expectation that the nurse is accountable when providing client care?

6. A nurse believes that the physician has written orders that may endanger the client. The nurse consults the physician, who refuses to alter the orders. What is the nurse's ethical obligation to the client in order to demonstrate accountability?

REFER Go to Pearson Nursing Student Resources
nursing.pearsonhighered.com

- Additional review material
- Additional case study

REFLECT Case Study \\ Part 3

Lisa Rossi, the social worker, met with Ms. Miller and learned that she was a single mother with a long history of back pain who appeared dejected about the amount of time and effort she put into being a "normal" mom. "I am not a person who gives in to things easily," Ms. Miller said. "That's why I think it is so unfair—why me? There are so many things I should be able to do. And if I don't ignore my pain, it ruins so much in my life. I have been suffering through many snowboarding and camping trips with my children, but I don't want them to know that."

Ms. Rossi allowed time for Ms. Miller to discuss her concerns and then briefly taught her how to do slow yoga-type breathing to help her anxiety. After Ms. Miller practiced the slower breathing, Ms. Rossi asked her whether she was ready to meet with the clinical pharmacist, who would work with her to find the best options for pain management while she was in the hospital and then how to manage pain when she went home. Ms. Miller agreed to the plan.

The information from the social worker helped Dan Kramer, the clinical pharmacist, plan appropriate interventions for Ms. Miller. Mr. Kramer was able to meet with Ms. Miller that evening, and afterward, he discussed the plans with Jen Sturges and Ms. Menendez. Later, after a few doses of IV morphine, and also oral narcotics, Ms. Miller was able to relax and take part in care activities. By the time the doctor discussed discharge plans with her, Ms. Miller described how she had learned to recognize the pain not so much as an enemy, but as a signal to move or to calm down. She also learned that medication was not an enemy if it helped her with her daily life. She also felt that the occupational therapist who worked with her one day had helped her understand how to calculate and plan all of her daily activities, physical and otherwise, to ensure her ability to participate in her usual social and occupational roles.

Clinical Reasoning Questions Level I

1. What role did technology play in the client's care plans?

2. What information would you expect the social worker to share with Jen Sturges?

Clinical Reasoning Questions Level II

3. What role did the social worker take with Ms. Miller? How did the social worker's interview and discussion help with the client's care and further activity?

4. Why was it important for the pharmacist to meet with the client and then discuss the plans with Jen Sturges and Ms. Menendez?

EXEMPLAR 42.1 Competence

EXEMPLAR KEY TERMS
Caring for the dying, *2544*
Competence, *2543*
Health promotion, *2544*
Health restoration, *2544*
Illness prevention, *2544*

EXEMPLAR LEARNING OUTCOMES
After reading about this exemplar, you will be able to:

1. Discuss Benner's levels of nursing proficiency.

2. Identify four major areas of competence within the scope of nursing practice.

3. Describe ways to promote lifelong competence in nursing.

▶ OVERVIEW

Competence is defined as possessing the knowledge and skills necessary to perform one's job appropriately and safely (Makely, 2012). In the past, nurses were considered able to do their job if they could simply provide care and comfort. Today nurses are held to a higher standard of competence. Each nurse is expected to achieve and maintain competence within four main areas: health promotion, illness prevention, health restoration, and caring for the dying.

▶ AREAS OF COMPETENCE

The four areas described here encompass a variety of knowledge bases, professional skills, and expertise. Within each area, the nurse is expected to achieve competence in application of the nursing process as well as in those skills necessary to provide safe and appropriate client care.

Health and Wellness Promotion

According to the World Health Organization (WHO), health is a complete physical, mental, and social well-being state and not just the absence of disease. **Health promotion** has been defined as a process that enables individuals and communities to increase their control over the determinants of health and thus improve their health (Dawson & Grill, 2012). Wellness is a condition in which individuals engage in activities and behaviors that enhance their quality of life and maximize personal potential (Lerner et al., 2013). Nurses promote wellness both in clients who are healthy and in those who are ill. This process may involve individual and community or employee-focused workplace activities to enhance healthy lifestyles, such as improving nutrition and physical fitness, preventing drug and alcohol misuse, restricting smoking, and preventing accidents and injury in the home and workplace.

Illness Prevention

Nurses engage in **illness prevention** in every setting in which they work. In community settings, illness prevention programs are designed to maintain optimal health by preventing disease. Most communities offer such illness prevention programs as immunizations, prenatal and infant care, and prevention of sexually transmitted disease. These programs are frequently taught by nurses working in school settings, hospital outreach programs, and local health departments.

Within clinical settings, nurses engage in illness prevention in a variety of ways. Many of these, such as sterile precautions and client teaching, are discussed throughout Parts I, II, and III of this text.

Health Restoration

Health restoration focuses on the ill client and extends from early detection of disease through helping the client during the recovery period. Nursing competencies include the following:

- Providing direct care to the ill individual, such as administering medications, baths, and specific procedures and treatments

- Performing diagnostic and assessment procedures, such as measuring blood pressure and examining feces for occult blood

- Consulting with other healthcare professionals about client problems

- Teaching clients about recovery activities, such as exercises that will accelerate recovery after a stroke

- Rehabilitating clients to their optimal functional level following physical or mental illness, injury, or chemical addiction.

Caring for the Dying

Caring for the dying involves comforting and caring for individuals of all ages who are dying. **Caring for the dying** includes helping clients live as comfortably as possible until death and helping the client's support individuals cope with death. Nurses carrying out these activities in homes, hospitals, and extended care facilities. See the End-of-Life Care exemplar in the module on Comfort for more information on caring for the dying.

▶ PROMOTING LIFELONG COMPETENCE

Nurses gain competence gradually throughout nursing school until they reach an entry level when they are judged safe and skillful enough to function as newly graduated nurses. Nurses continue to build competence throughout their career, with expertise coming from experience, gaining new knowledge, and improving their performance of skills.

Maintaining and increasing competence in nursing require the nurse to continue learning. Professional development and continuing education opportunities come in a variety of forms: seminars offered by colleges and professional organizations, professional and peer-reviewed journals, hospital- or employer-sponsored classes on new equipment or procedures, and formal and informal discussions with peers and other members of the healthcare team.

As the body of knowledge surrounding health care expands, it is unlikely that any nurse can maintain competence in all areas. Nurse generalists know something about many things, while nurse specialists know a great deal about their own specific area of expertise. All nurses must assess their own level of knowledge and identify areas in which they need additional knowledge to provide appropriate client care.

Even the most competent nurses encounter situations that make them question how best to respond. Luckily, nurses can collaborate with each other and with others on the interdisciplinary team, sharing opinions, ideas, and information. Nevertheless, while collaboration is helpful, even critical, each nurse is accountable for his choices and must weigh all information and choose the best course of action. The nurse who recognizes that there will always be a need to collaborate with others maintains a safe practice.

Various models of the process of attaining competence have been developed. Benner's classic model (2001) describes five levels of proficiency in nursing. These five levels, which have implications for teaching and learning, are novice, advanced beginner, competent, proficient, and expert. Benner writes that experience is essential for the development of professional expertise (see **Box 42–3** ●).

▶ NURSING PRACTICE

Nurses hold themselves accountable by frequently weighing and assessing their own competence. They know that it is honorable to say "I don't know" or ask "Would you help me?" instead of "I'm not sure but I think this is right" or "I'll figure it out as I go along." Rule 1 of competence when providing client care is to ask for help when there is uncertainty about the safety of any given action. By doing so, nurses (a) invite opportunities to increase their own levels of competence and (b) hold themselves accountable for providing the highest quality of client care.

Box 42–3 Benner's Stages of Nursing Expertise

STAGE I, NOVICE

No experience (e.g., a nursing student). Performance is limited, inflexible, and governed by context-free rules and regulations rather than experience.

STAGE II, ADVANCED BEGINNER

Demonstrates marginally acceptable performance. Recognizes the meaningful aspects of a real situation. Has experienced enough real situations to make judgments about them.

STAGE III, COMPETENT

Has 2 or 3 years of experience. Demonstrates organizational and planning abilities. Differentiates important factors from less important aspects of care. Coordinates multiple complex care demands.

STAGE IV, PROFICIENT

Has 3 to 5 years of experience. Perceives situations as wholes rather than in terms of parts as in Stage II. Uses maxims as guides for what to consider in a situation. Has holistic understanding of the client, which improves decision making. Focuses on long-term goals.

STAGE V, EXPERT

Performance is fluid, flexible, and highly proficient; no longer requires rules, guidelines, or maxims to connect an understanding of the situation to appropriate action. Demonstrates highly skilled intuitive and analytic ability in new situations. Is inclined to take a certain action because "it felt right."

Source: Benner, P. (2001). Novice to expert: Excellence and power in clinical nursing practice, commemorative edition (1st ed.). Upper Saddle River, NJ: Pearson Education. Reproduced with permission.

REVIEW Competence

RELATE Link the Concepts and Exemplars

Linking the exemplar of competence with the concept of legal issues:

1. What is the nurse's legal obligation to society and the profession to maintain competence?

2. How can nurses who lack competence in one area of nursing strengthen their knowledge and skills?

Linking the exemplar of competence with the concept of ethics:

3. What is the nurse's ethical obligation related to competence?

4. How does the nursing code of ethics address the issue of competence?

REFER Go to Pearson Nursing Student Resources
nursing.pearsonhighered.com

- Additional review material

REFLECT Case Study

Tyree Campbell has worked in the labor and delivery unit of a large metropolitan hospital since graduating from nursing school 8 years ago. A new private hospital recently opened in town, and the census on Ms. Campbell's unit has been significantly lower. Tonight, Ms. Campbell reports to work and learns that more nurses are scheduled to work than there are clients. The decision has been made to float the excess staff to other units, and Ms. Campbell is asked to float to the neonatal intensive care unit (NICU). Her heart sinks, and she begins to feel the early signs of panic as she thinks, "How can I work in the NICU? I don't have any experience working there!"

1. What is Ms. Campbell's responsibility in this situation?

2. Can Ms. Campbell agree to float to the NICU if she is not competent to care for the clients on this unit? Explain your answer.

3. What should Ms. Campbell say to the nursing supervisor who has given her this assignment?

EXEMPLAR 42.2 Professional Development

EXEMPLAR KEY TERMS

Authority, *2549*
Chain of command, *2549*
Client, *2548*
Consumer, *2548*
Line authority, *2549*
Organizational chart, *2550*
Patient, *2548*
Responsibility, *2549*
Staff authority, *2549*
Standards of Practice, *2549*
Standards of Professional Performance, *2549*

EXEMPLAR LEARNING OUTCOMES

After reading about this exemplar, you will be able to:

1. Discuss historical and contemporary factors influencing the development of nursing.

2. Describe the roles of nurses.

3. Examine the nurse's responsibility related to chain of command.

4. Distinguish the expanded career roles available to nurses and their functions.

▶ OVERVIEW

Professional development takes on different meanings in the many different areas of nursing. The term may be associated with advanced education, an increase in experience or seniority, involvement or membership in an organization that governs the profession, or continuing education classes or offerings. Professional development encompasses all of these activities.

Nursing today is very different from nursing as it was practiced years ago, and it is expected to continue changing. To comprehend present-day nursing and at the same time prepare for the future, one must understand not only past events but also contemporary nursing practice and the sociological and historical factors that affect it.

▶ HISTORICAL PERSPECTIVES

Nursing has undergone dramatic changes in response to societal needs and influences. A look at nursing's beginnings reveals its continuing struggle for autonomy and professionalization. In recent decades, a renewed interest in nursing history has produced a growing amount of related literature. This section highlights only selected aspects of events that have influenced nursing practice. The recurring themes of women's roles and status, religious values, war, societal attitudes, and visionary nursing leadership have influenced nursing practice in the past. Many of these factors still exert their influence today.

Women's Roles and Status

Traditional female roles of wife, mother, daughter, and sister have always included the care and nurturing of others. From the beginning of time, women have cared for infants and children; thus nursing could be said to have its roots in "the home." Additionally, women, who in general occupied a subservient and dependent role, were called on to care for others in the community who were ill. Generally the care provided was related to physical maintenance and comfort. Thus the traditional nursing role has always entailed humanistic caring, nurturing, comforting, and supporting.

Religion

Religion has also played a significant role in the development of nursing. Although many of the world's religions encourage benevolence, it was the Judeo-Christian commandment to "love thy neighbor as thyself" and Christ's parable of the Good Samaritan that had a significant impact on the development of Western nursing. Early religious values, such as self-denial, a spiritual calling, and devotion to duty and hard work, have dominated nursing throughout its history. Nurses' commitment to these values often resulted in exploitation and few monetary rewards. For some time, nurses themselves believed it was inappropriate to expect economic gain from their calling.

During the third and fourth centuries C.E., several wealthy matrons of the Roman Empire converted to Christianity and used their wealth to provide houses of care and healing (the forerunners of hospitals) for the poor, the sick, and the homeless. These nursing providers were the origin of deaconess groups, which surfaced occasionally throughout the centuries, most notably in 1836 when Theodore Fliedner reinstituted the Order of Deaconesses and opened a small hospital and training school in Kaiserswerth, Germany. Florence Nightingale received her training in nursing at the Kaiserswerth School.

War

Throughout history, wars have accentuated the need for nurses. The Crusades saw the formation of several orders of knights, including the Knights of Saint John of Jerusalem (also known as the Knights Hospitalers), the Teutonic Knights, and the Knights of Saint Lazarus. These brothers in arms provided nursing care to their sick and injured comrades. The Knights of Saint Lazarus dedicated themselves to the care of individuals with leprosy, syphilis, and chronic skin conditions, its original members having been lepers themselves. These orders also built hospitals, the organization and management of which set a standard for the administration of hospitals throughout Europe at that time.

During the Crimean War (1854–1856), the inadequacy of the care given to soldiers led to a public outcry in Great Britain. The role Florence Nightingale played in addressing this problem is well known. She was asked by Sir Sidney Herbert of the British War Department to recruit a contingent of female nurses to provide care to the sick and injured in the Crimea. Nightingale and her nurses transformed the military hospitals by setting up sanitation practices, such as hand washing and washing clothing. Nightingale is credited with performing miracles: The mortality rate in the Barrack Hospital in Turkey, for example, fell from 42% to 2% (Donahue, 1996, p. 197).

During the American Civil War (1861–1865), several nurses emerged who were notable for their contributions to a country torn by internal strife. Harriet Tubman and Sojourner Truth provided care and safety to slaves fleeing to the North on the Underground Railroad. Mother Biekerdyke and Clara Barton searched the battlefields and gave care to injured and dying soldiers. Noted authors Walt Whitman and Louisa May Alcott volunteered as nurses to give care to injured soldiers in military hospitals. Another woman leader who provided nursing care during the Civil War was Dorothea Dix, who became the Union Army's superintendent of female nurses responsible for recruiting nurses and supervising the nursing care by all women nurses working in the army hospitals.

With the outbreak of World War I, American, British, and French women rushed to volunteer their nursing services. These nurses endured harsh environments and treated injuries never seen before. A monument entitled "The Spirit of Nursing" stands in Arlington National Cemetery. It honors the nurses who served in the U.S. Armed Services in World War I, many of whom are buried in Section 21, the "Nurses Section" (Military District of Washington, n.d.). Progress in health care occurred during World War I, particularly in the field of surgery. For example, there were advances in the use of anesthetic agents, infection control, blood typing, and prosthetics (Holder, 2004, p. 915).

In World War II, the Cadet Nurse Corps was established in response to a marked shortage of nurses. Also at that time, auxiliary healthcare workers became prominent. "Practical" nurses, aides, and technicians provided much of the actual nursing care under the instruction and supervision of better prepared nurses. Medical specialties also arose to meet the needs of hospitalized clients.

During the Vietnam War, approximately 90% of the 11,000 American military women stationed in Vietnam were nurses. Most of them volunteered to go to Vietnam right after they graduated from nursing school. This made them the youngest group of medical personnel ever to serve in wartime (Vietnam Women's Memorial Foundation, n.d.).

Societal Attitudes

Society's attitudes about nurses and nursing have significantly influenced professional nursing. Before the mid-1800s, nursing lacked organization, education, or social status; the prevailing attitude was that a woman's place was in the home and no respectable woman should have a career. The role for the Victorian middle-class woman was that of wife and mother, and any education she obtained was for the purpose of making her a pleasant companion to her husband and a responsible mother to her children. Nurses in hospitals during this period were poorly educated; some were incarcerated criminals. Society's attitudes about nursing during this period are reflected in the writings of Charles Dickens. In his novel *Martin Chuzzlewit* (1896), Sairey Gamp "cares" for the sick by neglecting them, stealing from them, and physically abusing them (Donahue, 1996, p. 192). This literary portrayal of nurses greatly influenced the negative image of nurses.

In contrast, the *guardian angel* or *angel of mercy* image arose in the latter part of the nineteenth century, largely because of the work of Florence Nightingale during the Crimean War. After Nightingale brought respectability to the nursing profession, nurses were viewed as noble, compassionate, moral, religious, dedicated, and self-sacrificing.

Another image that arose in the early nineteenth century and affected subsequent generations of nurses and the public and other professionals working with nurses is the image of *doctor's handmaiden*. This image evolved when women had yet to obtain the right to vote, family structures were largely paternalistic, and the medical profession portrayed increasing use of scientific knowledge that, at that time, was viewed as a male domain.

Since that time, several images of nursing have been portrayed. The *heroine* portrayal evolved from nurses' acts of bravery in World War II and their contributions in fighting poliomyelitis—in particular, the work of the Australian nurse Elizabeth Kenney. Other images in the late 1900s include the nurse as sex object, surrogate mother, and tyrannical mother.

The nursing profession has taken steps to improve the image of the nurse. In the early 1990s, the Tri-Council for Nursing (the American Association of Colleges of Nursing, the ANA, the American Organization of Nurse Executives, and the NLN) initiated a national effort (titled Nurses of America) to improve the image of nursing. In 2002, the Johnson & Johnson corporation contributed $20 million to launch a Campaign for Nursing's Future to promote nursing as a positive career choice. In 2010, the Institute of Medicine (IOM) and the Robert Wood Johnson Foundation (RWJF) launched an Initiative on the Future of Nursing, to identify solutions of nursing care that not only addressed many of the issues facing the profession but also transformed the way Americans receive health care. This initiative was based on the belief that nurses are a linchpin for health reform and will be vital in implementing systemic changes in the delivery of care (IOM, 2010).

Nursing Leaders

Florence Nightingale, Clara Barton, Lillian Wald, Lavinia Dock, Margaret Sanger, and Mary Breckinridge are among the leaders who have made notable contributions both to nursing's history and to women's history. Because of their skills at influencing others and bringing about change, they remain models for political nurse activists today. Contemporary nursing leaders Virginia Henderson, who created a modern worldwide definition of nursing, and Martha Rogers, a catalyst for theory, have also played important roles in nursing.

NIGHTINGALE (1820–1910) Florence Nightingale's contributions to nursing are well documented. Her achievements in improving the standards for the care of war casualties in the Crimea earned her the title "Lady with the Lamp." Her efforts in reforming hospitals and in producing and implementing public health policies also made her an accomplished political nurse: She was the first nurse to exert political pressure on government. Through her contributions to nursing education—perhaps her greatest achievement—she is recognized as nursing's first scientist-theorist for her work *Notes on Nursing: What It Is, and What It Is Not* (1859/1969).

BARTON (1812–1912) Clara Barton was a schoolteacher who volunteered as a nurse during the American Civil War. Her responsibility was to organize the nursing services. Barton is noted for her role in establishing the American Red Cross, which linked with the International Red Cross when the U.S. Congress ratified the Treaty of Geneva (the first Geneva Convention). It was Barton who persuaded Congress in 1882 to ratify this treaty so that the Red Cross could perform humanitarian efforts in times of peace.

RICHARDS (1841–1930) Linda Richards was America's first trained nurse. She graduated from the New England Hospital for Women and Children in 1873. Richards introduced nurse's notes and doctor's orders and initiated the practice of nurses wearing uniforms (American Nurses Association, 2006a). She is also credited for her pioneer work in psychiatric and industrial nursing.

MAHONEY (1845–1926) Mary Mahoney was the first African American professional nurse. She graduated from the New England Hospital for Women and Children in 1879. She worked constantly for the acceptance of African Americans in nursing and the promotion of equal opportunities (Donahue, 1996, p. 271). The ANA (2006b) gives a Mary Mahoney Award biennially in recognition of significant contributions in interracial relationships.

WALD (1867–1940) Lillian Wald is considered the founder of public health nursing. Wald and Mary Brewster were the first to offer trained nursing services to the poor in the New York slums. Their home among the poor on the upper floor of a tenement, called the Henry Street Settlement and Visiting Nurse Service, provided nursing services, social services, and organized educational and cultural activities. Soon after the founding of the Henry Street Settlement, school nursing was established as an adjunct to visiting nursing.

DOCK (1858–1956) Lavinia L. Dock was a feminist, prolific writer, political activist, suffragist, and friend of Wald. She participated in protest movements for women's rights that resulted in the 1920 passage of the 19th Amendment to the U.S. Constitution, which granted women the right to vote. In addition, Dock campaigned for legislation to allow nurses rather than physicians to control the profession of nursing. In 1893, Dock, with the assistance of Mary Adelaide Nutting and Isabel Hampton Robb, founded the American Society of Superintendents of Training Schools for Nurses of the United States and Canada, a precursor to the current National League for Nursing.

SANGER (1879–1966) Margaret Higgins Sanger, a public health nurse in New York, has had a lasting impact on women's health care. Imprisoned for opening the first birth control information clinic in America, she is considered the founder of Planned Parenthood. Her experience with the large number of unwanted pregnancies among the working poor was instrumental in addressing this problem.

BRECKINRIDGE (1881–1965) After World War I, Mary Breckinridge, a notable pioneer nurse, established the Frontier Nursing Service (FNS). In 1918, she worked with the American Committee for Devastated France, distributing food, clothing, and supplies to rural villages and taking care of sick children. In 1921, Breckinridge returned to the United States with plans to provide health care to the people of rural America. In 1925, Breckinridge and two other nurses began the FNS in Leslie County, Kentucky. Within this organization, Breckinridge started one of the first midwifery training schools in the United States.

▶ CONTEMPORARY NURSING PRACTICE

An understanding of contemporary nursing practice includes a look at definitions of nursing, recipients of nursing, settings for nursing practice, nurse practice acts, and current standards of clinical nursing practice.

Definitions of Nursing

Florence Nightingale defined nursing nearly 150 years ago as "the act of utilizing the environment of the patient to assist him in his recovery" (Nightingale, 1859/1969). Nightingale considered a clean, well-ventilated, and quiet environment essential for recovery. Often considered the first nurse theorist, Nightingale raised the status of nursing through education. Nurses were no longer untrained housekeepers but individuals educated in the care of the sick.

Virginia Henderson was one of the first modern nurses to define nursing. She wrote, "The unique function of the nurse is to assist the individual, sick or well, in the performance of those activities contributing to health or its recovery (or to peaceful death) that he would perform unaided if he had the necessary strength, will, or knowledge, and to do this in such a way as to help him gain independence as rapidly as possible" (Henderson, 1966, p. 3). Like Nightingale, Henderson described nursing in relation to the client and the client's environment. Unlike Nightingale, Henderson saw the nurse as concerned with both healthy and ill individuals, acknowledged that nurses interact with clients even when recovery may not be feasible, and mentioned the teaching and advocacy roles of the nurse.

In the latter half of the twentieth century, a number of nurse theorists developed their own definitions of nursing. Theoretical definitions are important because they go beyond simplistic common definitions. They describe what nursing is and the interrelationship among nurses, nursing, the client, the environment, and the intended client outcome.

Certain themes are common to many of these definitions:

- Nursing is caring.
- Nursing is an art.
- Nursing is a science.
- Nursing is client centered.
- Nursing is holistic.
- Nursing is adaptive.
- Nursing is concerned with health promotion, health maintenance, and health restoration.
- Nursing is a helping profession.

Professional nursing associations have also examined nursing and developed their definitions of it. In 1973, the ANA described nursing practice as "direct, goal oriented, and adaptable to the needs of the individual, the family, and community during health and illness" (ANA, 1973, p. 2). In 1980, the ANA changed its definition of nursing to this: "Nursing is the diagnosis and treatment of human responses to actual or potential health problems" (ANA, 1980, p. 9). In 1995, the ANA recognized the influence and contribution of the science of caring to nursing philosophy and practice. Its most recent definition of professional nursing is much broader: "Nursing is the protection, promotion, and optimization of health and abilities, preventions of illness and injury, alleviation of suffering through the diagnosis and treatment of human response, and advocacy in the care of individuals, families, communities, and populations" (ANA, 2003, p. 6).

Research on the meaning of caring in nursing has been increasing. For example, Sargent (2011) conducted a critical review of the conceptual analysis of caring in nursing. Lindberg, Persson, and Bondas (2012) sought to identify how nurse preceptors integrate caring science in practice and how they value students' contributions of caring science in practice.

Recipients of Nursing

The recipients of nursing are sometimes called *consumers*, sometimes *patients*, and sometimes *clients*. A **consumer** is an individual, a group of individuals, or a community that uses a service or commodity. Individuals who use healthcare products or services are consumers of health care.

A **patient** is an individual who is waiting for or undergoing medical treatment and care. The word *patient* comes from a Latin word meaning "to suffer" or "to bear." Usually individuals become patients when they seek assistance because of illness or for surgery. Some nurses believe that the word *patient* implies passive acceptance of the decisions and care of health professionals. Additionally, with the emphasis on health promotion and prevention of illness, many recipients of nursing care are not ill. Moreover, nurses interact with family members and significant others to provide support, information, and comfort in addition to caring for the patient. For these reasons, nurses increasingly refer to recipients of health care as *clients*.

A **client** is an individual who engages the advice or services of another individual who is qualified to provide this service. Use of the term *client* presents the receivers of health care as individuals who are also responsible for their own health acting in collaboration with health professionals. In this book, *client* is the preferred term, although *consumer* and *patient* are used in some instances.

Settings for Nursing

Settings for nursing practice are many and varied, including acute care hospitals, clients' homes, community agencies, ambulatory

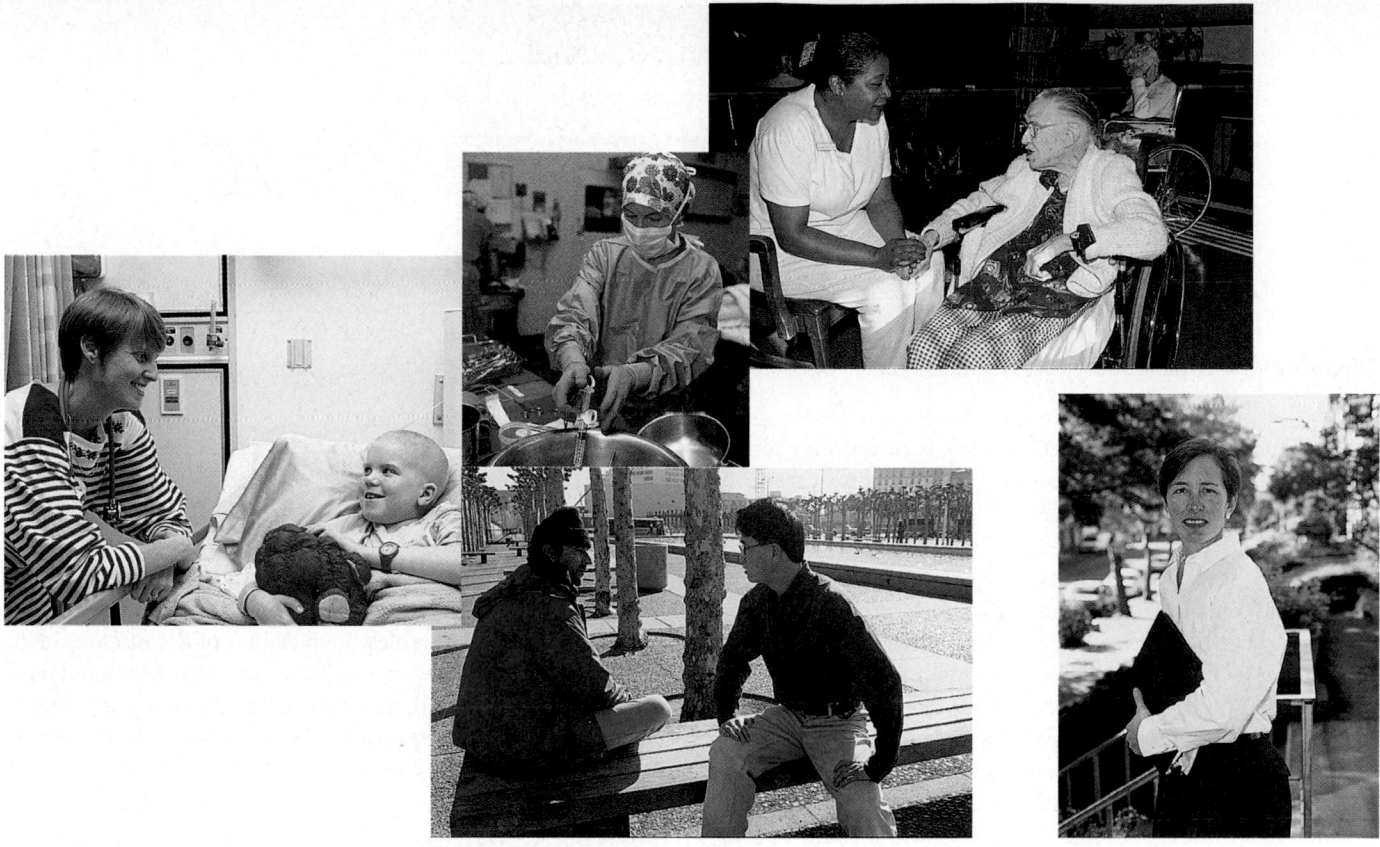

Figure 42–1 ● Nurses practice in a variety of settings. Clockwise from left: pediatric nursing, operating room nurse, geriatric nursing, home nursing, and community nursing.

clinics, long-term care facilities, health maintenance organizations (HMOs), and nursing practice centers (see **Figure 42–1** ●).

Nurses have different degrees of nursing autonomy and nursing responsibility in the various settings. They may provide direct care, teach clients and support individuals, serve as nursing advocates and agents of change, and help determine health policies affecting consumers in the community and in hospitals.

Nurse Practice Acts

Legal acts for professional nursing practice regulate the practice of nursing in the United States and Canada. Each state in the United States and each province in Canada has its own act. Although these nurse practice acts differ in various jurisdictions, they all have a common purpose: to protect the public. Nurses are responsible for knowing their state's nurse practice act as it governs their practice. Nurse practice acts are discussed in detail in the module on Legal Issues.

Standards of Nursing Practice

Establishing and implementing standards of practice are major functions of a professional organization. The purpose of the ANA's **Standards of Practice** is to describe the responsibilities for which American nurses are accountable. By using the nursing process as a foundation, the ANA developed standards of nursing practice that are generic and that provide for the practice of nursing regardless of area of specialization. The ANA's **Standards of Professional Performance** describe behaviors expected in the professional nursing role. Professional performance standards refer to enhancing general practice, ensuring

appropriate education level, and maintaining collegiality with peers and collaboration with the entire care team. Because of the increasing use of the Internet and social networking such as Facebook and Twitter, in 2011 the ANA published principles for social networking in nursing. Various specialty nursing organizations have further developed specific standards of nursing practice for their areas. For nurses in Canada, each province or territory establishes its own standards of practice.

Competent nurses use the nursing process in their nursing practice, that is, the steps of assessment, diagnosis, outcome identification, planning, implementation, and, ultimately, evaluation. A professional nurse also integrates ethics in all areas of practice and considers appropriate utilization of resources while also functioning in relevant leadership roles (ANA, 2010).

Chain of Command

The **chain of command** is the hierarchy within an organization. The authority and responsibility of the individuals in the organization depend on their position in the chain of command. **Authority** is the power to command other individuals and direct their activities; **responsibility** is being accountable for meeting personal or organizationl objectives and performing required tasks.

Line authority is the power to direct the activities of subordinates within the organization. In **Figure 42–2** ●, examples of line authority are the relationships among the chief nurse executive, the nurse manager, and the staff nurse. **Staff authority** is the power to provide advice and support to employees or departments but not to assign tasks. In Figure 42–2, staff authority is illustrated by the relationship between the acute care nurse prac-

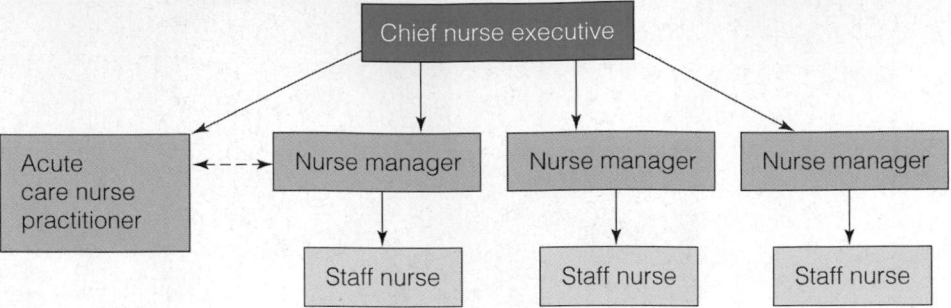

Figure 42–2 ● Organizational chart showing chain of command in a nursing unit.

titioner and the nurse manager. Neither is responsible for the work of the other; rather, they collaborate to optimize care in the unit for which the nurse manager is responsible.

A chain of command provides structure, so employees understand how to perform their tasks and how to manage supervisory relationships within the organization. It also provides a structure for reporting issues that need management's attention. Any nurse who identifies such an issue should follow the organization's chain of command For example, in a hospital, the problem is usually first reported to the charge nurse, then to the unit manager. If the problem is still not resolved, the nurse may approach someone in middle or upper management.

The student nurse should always follow the chain of command; the nursing instructor acts as the first link in that chain. When a problem arises, whether in the clinical area or the classroom, the student should first discuss the problem with the instructor. If the instructor is unable to resolve the issue to the student's satisfaction, the student should then approach the program director. Failure to follow the chain of command is considered unprofessional and slows the resolution process. In some organizations, failure to follow the chain of command may result in disciplinary action.

In traditional organizations, an **organizational chart** depicts the formal hierarchical structure and related responsibilities. However, organizations also have informal structures that are not reflected in a chart. For instance, nurses who function as leaders but do not have a formal title in the hierarchy would not appear in the organizational chart. Similarly, managers who have strong personalities or other characteristics may have more actual power than other managers with the same formal level of authority, but these differences are not shown in the chart.

The traditional hierarchical structure is not the only model used in healthcare settings. Many organizations have moved toward a shared governance model that flattens the organizational chart as appropriate participants (such as nursing staff, pharmacy staff, and medical staff) share ownership of client care issues and outcomes (Fujita et al., 2009).

▶ ROLES AND FUNCTIONS OF THE NURSE

Nurses perform a number of roles, often simultaneously, when they provide care to clients. For example, the nurse may act as a counselor while providing physical care and teaching the client aspects of that care. The roles required at a specific time depend on the needs of the client and aspects of the particular environment. These roles, which are discussed throughout this text, are briefly outlined in **Table 42–1** ●.

As the nursing profession has grown in autonomy through professional organizations, nursing leaders and managers have seen a need for a number of expanded roles in the nursing profession. Some of these roles, such as that of the nurse-midwife, have come about partly as a response to needs expressed by clients. Others, such as that of the nurse educator, have resulted primarily from the profession's desire to continue to improve, educate, and renew its own members.

Expanded Career Roles for Nurses

Many nurses are filling expanded career roles, such as those of nurse practitioner, clinical nurse specialist, nurse-midwife, nurse educator, and nurse anesthetist, all of which allow greater independence and autonomy.

NURSE PRACTITIONER   A nurse practitioner has advanced education, is a graduate of a nurse practitioner program, and is certified by the American Nurses Credentialing Center in an area such as adult nurse practitioner, family nurse practitioner, school nurse practitioner, pediatric nurse practitioner, or gerontology nurse practitioner. They are employed in healthcare agencies or community-based settings. They usually deal with nonemergency acute or chronic illness and provide primary ambulatory care.

CLINICAL NURSE SPECIALIST   A clinical nurse specialist is a nurse who has an advanced degree or expertise and is considered an expert in a specialized area of practice (e.g., gerontology, oncology). The nurse provides direct client care, educates others, consults, conducts research, and manages care. The American Nurses Credentialing Center provides national certification of clinical nurse specialists.

NURSE ANESTHETIST   A nurse who has completed advanced education in an accredited program in anesthesiology may qualify to be a nurse anesthetist. The nurse anesthetist carries out preoperative visits and assessments and administers general anesthetics for surgery under the supervision of a physician prepared in anesthesiology. The nurse anesthetist also assesses the postoperative status of clients.

NURSE-MIDWIFE   A nurse-midwife is a registered nurse who has completed a program in midwifery and is certified by the American College of Nurse-Midwives. The nurse-midwife gives prenatal and postnatal care and manages deliveries in normal pregnancies. The nurse midwife practices in association

TABLE 42-1 Roles and Functions of the Nurse

NURSING ROLE	FUNCTIONS
Caregiver	The nurse engages in activities that assist the client physically and psychologically while preserving the client's dignity.
Communicator	The nurse identifies client problems and communicates these to other members of the healthcare team. See the module on Communication.
Teacher	Nurses help clients learn about their health and about healthcare procedures used to restore or maintain their health. Nurses also teach unlicensed assistive personnel (UAP) to whom they delegate care, and they share their expertise with other nurses and healthcare professionals. See the module on Teaching and Learning.
Client advocate	The nurse may represent the client's needs and wishes to other health professionals, such as relaying the client's wishes for information to the physician. The nurse also assists clients in exercising their rights and helps them speak up for themselves.
Counselor	Nurses counsel healthy individuals with normal adjustment difficulties and focus on helping these individuals develop new attitudes, feelings, and behaviors by encouraging them to look at alternative behaviors, recognize the choices, and develop a sense of control. Nurses counsel ill clients in how to develop more healthy and self-protective behaviors and how to recognize and respond to triggers, signs, and symptoms in a timely manner.
Change agent	Nurses assist clients to make modifications in their behavior. Nurses also often act to make changes in a system, such as clinical care, if it is not helping a client return to health. Nurses are continually dealing with changes in the healthcare system. Technological changes, changes in the age of the client population, and changes in medications are just a few that nurses deal with daily.
Leader	A leader influences others to work together to accomplish a specific goal. The leader role can be employed at different levels: individual client, family, groups of clients, colleagues, or the community. Effective leadership is a learned skill requiring an understanding of the needs and goals that motivate individuals, the knowledge to apply the leadership skills, and the interpersonal skills to influence others. Leadership is discussed further in the module on Professional Behaviors.
Manager	The nurse manages the nursing care of individuals, families, and communities. The nurse manager also delegates nursing activities to ancillary workers and other nurses, as well as supervises and evaluates their performance. Managing requires knowledge about organizational structure and dynamics, authority and accountability, leadership, change theory, advocacy, delegation, and supervision and evaluation. See the module on Collaboration, for more information.
Case manager	Nurse case managers work with the multidisciplinary healthcare team to measure the effectiveness of the case management plan and to monitor outcomes. Each agency or unit specifies the role of the nurse case manager. In some institutions, the case manager works with primary or staff nurses to oversee the care of a specific caseload. In other agencies, the case manager is the primary nurse or provides some level of direct care to the client and family. Insurance companies have also developed a number of roles for nurse case managers, and responsibilities may vary from managing acute hospitalizations to managing high-cost clients or case types. Regardless of the setting, case managers help ensure that care is oriented to the client, while controlling costs. See the module on Managing Care, for more information.
Research consumer	Nurses often use research to improve client care. In a clinical area, nurses need to (a) have some awareness of the process and language of research, (b) be sensitive to issues related to protecting the rights of human subjects, (c) participate in the identification of significant researchable problems, and (d) be a discriminating consumer of research findings.

with a healthcare agency and can obtain medical services if complications occur. The nurse-midwife may also conduct routine Papanicolaou smears, family planning, and routine breast examinations.

NURSE RESEARCHER The nurse researcher investigates nursing problems to improve nursing care and to refine and expand nursing knowledge. Nurse researchers are employed in academic institutions, teaching hospitals, and research centers such as the National Institute for Nursing Research in Bethesda, Maryland. Nurse researchers usually have advanced education at the doctoral level.

NURSE ADMINISTRATOR The nurse administrator manages client care, including the delivery of nursing services. The administrator may have a middle management position, such as head nurse or supervisor, or a more senior management position, such as director of nursing services. The functions of nurse administrators include budgeting, staffing, and planning programs. The educational preparation for nurse administrator

positions is at least a baccalaureate degree in nursing and frequently a master's or doctoral degree.

NURSE EDUCATOR The nurse educator is employed in a nursing program, at an educational institution, or in hospital staff education. The nurse educator usually has a baccalaureate degree or more advanced preparation and frequently has expertise in a particular area of practice. The nurse educator is responsible for classroom and often clinical teaching.

NURSE ENTREPRENEUR The nurse entrepreneur usually has an advanced degree and manages a health-related business. The nurse may be involved in education, consultation, or research, for example.

CLINICAL NURSE LEADER The American Association of Colleges of Nursing (AACN) developed the role of clinical nurse leader to address the challenges of providing high-quality health care in the current environment (Wilson et al., 2013). Quality improvement and use of evidence-based solutions are hallmarks of this role.

REVIEW Professional Development

RELATE Link the Concepts and Exemplars

Linking the exemplar of professional development with the concept of legal issues:

1. What role does the nurse's continued professional development play in meeting the legal requirements for the profession?

2. What nursing regulations require continued professional development?

Linking the exemplar of professional development with the concept of ethics:

3. Can the nurse meet the ethical responsibilities of the profession without belonging to a professional organization? Explain.

4. How does the nursing code of ethics address the issue of professional development?

REFER Go to Pearson Nursing Student Resources
nursing.pearsonhighered.com

- Additional review materials

REFLECT Case Study

Francois Guardiene graduated from nursing school 4 years ago and accepted a position working in the coronary care unit of a large metropolitan hospital. He was required to attend 6 weeks of hospital orientation and a 3-month class for CCU nurses. He worked under the supervision of a preceptor for an additional 3 months. During his first year of practice he checked with more experienced nurses frequently, but with time he began to have more confidence in his competence and established a more autonomous practice. Over the past 2 years, he has noticed that some individuals seek to collaborate with him, and he considers himself a good CCU nurse.

1. Has Mr. Guardiene satisfied the need for professional development? Explain your answer.

2. What obligations does Mr. Guardiene have to continue developing his professional practice?

3. How would a nurse's hospital orientation differ if the position involved an area less specialized than the CCU?

■ REFERENCES

Aiello-Laws, L. B. (2010). Assessing the risk for suicide in patients with cancer. *Clinical Journal of Oncology Nursing, 14*(6), 687–691.

American Association of Colleges of Nurses. (2012a). *Joint Statement on Academic Progression for Nursing Students and Graduates.* Retrieved from https://www.aacn.nche.edu/aacn-publications/position/joint-statement-academic-progression.

American Association of Colleges of Nursing. (2012b). *Nursing shortage fact sheet.* Retrieved from http://www.aacn.nche.edu/media-relations/NrsgShortageFS.pdf.

American Nurses Association. (1973). *Standards of nursing practice.* Kansas City, MO: Author.

American Nurses Association. (1980). *Nursing: A social policy statement.* Kansas City, MO: Author.

American Nurses Association. (2003). *Nursing's social policy statement.* Washington, DC: American Nurses Publishing.

American Nurses Association. (2006a). *ANA hall of fame.* Retrieved from http://www.ana.org/hof/richla.htm.

American Nurses Association. (2006b). *ANA hall of fame.* Retrieved from http://www.ana.org/hof/mahome.htm.

American Nurses Association. (2010). *Nursing: Scope and Standards of Practice* (2nd ed.). Retrieved from http://nursesbooks.org/Main-Menu/Standards/H--N/Nursing-Scope-and-Standards-of-Practice.aspx.

American Telemedicine Association. (2012). *What is telemedicine.* Retrieved from http://www.americantelemed.org/learn/what-is-telemedicine.

Anderson, C. A. (2010). QSEN: Quality and safety education for nurses. *DEAN'S Notes, 31*(5), 4.

Ball, L. (2013). Who should be teaching patients to self-cannulate? *Nephrology Nursing Journal, 40*(1), 25–27.

Benner, P. (2001). *From novice to expert: Excellence and power in clinical nursing practice* (commemorative ed.). Upper Saddle River, NJ: Prentice Hall Health.

Bryce, J. (2013). Let's talk telehealth. *Australian Nursing Journal, 20*(7), 19.

Centers for Disease Control and Prevention. (2011). CDC releases outpatient safety guide. *Healthcare Traveler, 19*(2), 6–12.

Centers for Medicare and Medicaid Services. (2013). *EHR incentive programs.* Retrieved from http://www.cms.gov/Regulations-andGuidance/Legislation/EHRIncentive-Programs/index.html.

Cohen, R. A., & Adams, P. F. (2011). Use of the Internet for health information: United States, 2009. *NCHS Data Brief, 66.* Hyattsville, MD: National Center for Health Statistics.

Condon, E., & Sharts-Hopko, N. (2010). Socialization of Japanese nursing students. *Nursing Education Research, 31*(3), 167–170.

Cronenwett, L., Sherwood, G., & Gelmon, S. B. (2009). Improving quality and safety education: The QSEN learning collaborative. *Nursing Outlook, 57,* 304–312.

Dawson, A., & Grill, K. (2012). Health promotion: Conceptual and ethical issues. *Public Health Ethics, 5*(2), 101–103.

Dinmohammadi, M., Peyrovi, H., & Mehrdad, N. (2013). Concept analysis of professional socialization in nursing. *Nursing Forum, 48*(1). Retrieved from http://onlinelibrary.wiley.com/doi/10.1111/nuf.12006/pdf.

Donahue, M. P. (1996). *Nursing: The finest art. An illustrated history* (2nd ed.). St. Louis, MO: Mosby.

Flynn, L., Liang, Y., Dickson, G. L., Xie, M., & Suh, D. (2012). Nurses' practice environments, error interception practices, and inpatient medication errors. *Journal of Nursing Scholarship, 44*(2), 180–186.

Fox, S. (2013). *Pew Internet: Health.* Retrieved from http://pewinternet.org/Commentary/2011/November/Pew-Internet-Health.aspx.

Fujita, L. Y., Harris, M., Johnson, K. G., Irvine, N. P., & Latimer, R. W. (2009). Integrating a model in a shared governance environment. *Journal of Nursing Administration, 39*(12), 524–530.

Goldberg, D. G., Kuzel, A. J., Feng, L. B., DeShazo, J. P., & Love, L. E. (2012). EHRs in primary care practices: Benefits, challenges, and successful strategies. *American Journal of Managed Care, 18*(2), e48–e54.

Hardy, M. E., & Conway, M. E. (1988). *Role theory: Perspectives for healthy professionals* (2nd ed.). Norwalk, CT: Appleton & Lange.

Hauck, S., Winsett, R. P., & Kuric, J. (2013). Leadership facilitation strategies to establish evidence-based practice in an acute care hospital. *Journal of Advanced. Nursing 69*(3), 664–674. doi: 10.1111/j.1365-2648.2012.06053.x.

Henderson, V. (1966). *The nature of nursing: A definition and its implications for practice, research, and education.* New York: Macmillan.

Higuchi, K., Nakazawa, Y., Sakata, N., Takizawa, M., Ohso, K., Tanaka, M., & Yanagisawa, R. (2011). Telecommunication system for children undergoing stem cell transplantation. *Pediatrics International, 53,* 1002–1009.

Holder, V. L. (2004). From handmaiden to right hand—World War I and advancements in medicine. *AORN Journal, 80*(5), 911–923.

Howard, H. C., Avard, D., & Borry, P. (2011). Are the kids really all right? Direct-to-consumer genetic testing in children: Are company policies clashing with professional norms? *European Journal of Human Genetics, 19,* 1122–1126.

Institute of Medicine. (1999). *To err is human.* Washington, DC: National Academy Press.

Institute of Medicine. (2010). *The future of nursing: Leading change, advancing health.* Washington, DC: Author. Retrieved from http://www.iom.edu/Reports/2010/The-Future-of-Nursing-Leading-Change-Advancing-Health.aspx.

Lafond, C. M., & Van Hulle Vincent, C. (2013). A critique of the National League for Nursing/Jeffries simulation framework. *Journal of Advanced Nursing, 69*(2), 465–480.

Lerner, D., Rodday, A. M., Cohen, J. T., & Rogers, W. H. (2013). A systematic review of the evidence concerning the economic impact of employee-focuses health promotion and wellness programs. *Journal of Occupational and Environmental Medicine, 55*(2), 209–222.

Lin, T. (2011). A computer literacy scale for newly enrolled nursing college students: Development and validation. *Journal of Nursing Research, 19*(4), 305–317.

Lindberg, E., Persson, E., & Bondas, T. (2012). The responsibility of someone else: A focus group study of collaboration between a university and a hospital regarding the integration of caring science in practice. *Scandinavian Journal of Caring Sciences, 26,* 579–586.

Lopes, C. T., & Ribeiro, C. (2011). Comparative evaluation of Web search engines in health information retrieval. *Online Information Review, 35*(6), 869–892.

Makely, S. (2012). *Professionalism in health: A primer for career success* (4th ed.). Upper Saddle River, NJ: Prentice Hall.

McMahon, D. (2013). *Nursing Standards of Practice*. Retrieved online from http://www.hgexperts.com/article.asp?id=6237.

Military District of Washington. (n.d.). *The Nurses Memorial at Arlington Cemetery section 21*. Retrieved from http://www.mdw.army.mil/content/anmviewer.aspa-39.

National Student Nurses Association. (2013). *Code of ethics*. Retrieved from http://www.nsna.org/Portals/0/Skins/NSNA/pdf/Pieces_Appendix_B.pdf.

National Student Nurses Association House of Delegates. (2001). *The code of academic and clinical conduct*. Nashville, TN: Author.

Nightingale, F. (1969). *Notes on nursing: What it is, and what it is not*. New York: Dover. (Original work published 1859).

Olsen, S., Fiechtl, B., & Rule, S. (2012). An evaluation of virtual home visits in early intervention: Feasibility of "virtual intervention." *Volta Review, 112*(3), 267–281.

Owens, D., Eby, K., Burson, S., Green, M., McGoodwin, W., & Isaac, M. (2012). Primary palliative care clinic pilot project demonstrates benefits of a nurse practitioner-directed clinic providing primary and palliative care. *Journal of the American Academy of Nurse Practitioners, 24*, 52–58.

Price, S. L. (2009). Becoming a nurse: A meta-study of early professional socialization and career choice in nursing. *Journal of Advanced Nursing, 65*(1), 11–19.

Priharjo, R., & Hoy, G. (2011). Use of peer teaching to enhance student and patient education. *Nursing Standard. 25*(20), 40–43.

Quality and Safety Education for Nurses Institute. (2007). *Prelicensure KSAs*. Retrieved from http://qsen.org/competencies/pre-licensure-ksas/.

Salin, S., Kaunonen, M., & Aalto, P. (2012). Explaining patient satisfaction with outpatient care using data-based nurse staffing indicators. *Journal of Nursing Administration, 42*(12), 592–597.

Sargent, A. (2011). Reframing caring as discourse practice: A critical review of conceptual analyses of caring in nursing. *Nursing Inquiry, 19*(2), 134–143.

Secomb, J., Mckenna, L., & Smith, C. (2012). The effectiveness of simulation activities on the cognitive abilities of undergraduate third-year nursing students: A randomised control trial. *Journal of Clinical Nursing, 21*(23/24), 3475–3484.

Spooner, N., Hurst, S., & Khadra, M. (2012). Medical simulation technology: Educational overview, indus-

try leaders, and what's missing. *Hospital Topics, 90*(3), 57–64.

Sturdy, D. (2012). Why safeguarding adults matters. *Practice Nurse, 42*(11), 34–38.

Timmins, F. (2011). Remembering the art of nursing in a technological age. *Nursing in Critical Care, 16*(4), 161–163.

Vietnam Women's Memorial Foundation. (n.d.). *During the Vietnam era. . . .* Retrieved from http://www.vietnamwomensmemorial.org/pages/frames/vwmp.html.

Whitmer, K., Pruemer, J., Wilhelm, C., McCaig, L., & Hester, J. D. B. (2011). Development of an outpatient oncology symptom management clinic. *Clinical Journal of Oncology Nursing, 15*(2), 175–179.

Wilson, L., Orff, S., Gerry, T., Shirley, B. R., Tabor, D., Caiazzo, K., & Rouleau, D. (2013). Evolution of an innovative role: The clinical nurse leader. *Journal of Nursing Management, 21*, 175–181.

Wolff, K., Nordin, K., Brun, W., Berglund, G., & Kvale, G. (2011). Affective and cognitive attitudes, uncertainty avoidance and intention to obtain genetic testing: An extension of the Theory of Planned Behavior. *Psychology and Health, 26*(9), 1143–1155.

43 Advocacy

MODULE AT-A-GLANCE

The Concept of Advocacy, 2555

☑ THE CONCEPT OF ADVOCACY

Advocacy is a key component of the American Nurses Association Code of Ethics for Nurses (see the module on Ethics). **Advocacy** can be defined as protecting by expressing and defending the cause of another. A **client advocate** acts to protect the client and defend the client from harm. Client advocacy is a primary role for every nurse. The nurse may demonstrate this role by representing a client's needs and wishes to other health professionals, such as when the nurse relays a client's wishes to the physician, or by assisting clients in exercising their rights and helping them to speak up for themselves. The Concepts Related to Advocacy feature outlines how advocacy is integrated with other concepts.

Successful advocacy is a positive experience for nurses as well as for clients. Clients derive a benefit, and nurses feel good about their ability to be agents of change. However, not all advocating will be successful. Unsuccessful advocating can be hard for the nurse to cope with and has the potential to lead to frustration, anger, and burnout. <<

Concept Learning Outcomes

After reading about this concept, you will be able to:

1. Discuss the concept of advocacy, including how it relates to the practice of nursing.
2. Discuss the nurse's role of advocate.
3. Describe the values basic to client advocacy.
4. Examine strategies for advocating in different care settings.
5. Explain the importance of empowering the client and methods for doing so.
6. Differentiate between professional and public advocacy, and provide examples of each.
7. Contrast the need for advocacy among members of vulnerable populations versus the general population.
8. Summarize advocacy interventions, including resources available within the interdisciplinary team.
9. Distinguish illegal, immoral, or unethical activities of professionals.
10. Illustrate principles of advocacy in nursing practice.

Concept Key Terms

Advocacy, *2555*
Client advocate, *2555*

Concepts Related to Advocacy

Nurses must take many other concepts into consideration when advocating for their clients. Examples include ethics, legal issues, professional behaviors, culture and diversity, and healthcare systems.

CONCEPT	RELATIONSHIP TO ADVOCACY	NURSING IMPLICATIONS
Ethics		
■ Ethical dilemmas ■ Client rights	Ethics is a system of moral principles or standards governing behaviors and relationships that is based on professional beliefs and values. The role of the advocate is to uphold the ethics in any situation.	■ Nurses acting as advocates should honor the moral principles and standards and respect clients' right to make their own choices based on nurses' own professional beliefs and values and those of the client.
Legal Issues		
■ Standard of care ■ Nurse practice acts ■ HIPAA ■ Mandatory reporting	Legal issues encompass the rights, the responsibilities, and scope of nursing practice through regulation. All clients have the right to expect competent nursing practice.	■ The nurse advocate should uphold the rights of the client in any situation and also promote the competence of those caring for clients. The nurse has an obligation to report any suspicious behavior by another nurse, staff member, or other provider.
Professional Behaviors		
■ Components of professionalism in nursing	Nurses hold the public trust as professionals. One of the roles of the professional nurse is to advocate for the client.	■ The nurse should continuously advocate for the client in a professional manner.
Culture and Diversity		
■ Values and beliefs ■ Vulnerable populations ■ Social differences ■ Developing cultural competence	Culture refers to the patterns of behavior and thinking that people living in social groups learn, develop, and share. Diversity is the unique variations among and between individuals. Each client has the right to choose diversity and maintain that diversity as desired.	■ The nurse should practice culturally competent care by respecting the cultural values of the clients and advocating for those rights as needed. ■ Nursing advocates should respect the diversity of all clients and promote equal care for all clients.
Healthcare Systems		
■ Access to health care	The complexities of the healthcare system are difficult to maneuver even for people who are well educated.	■ The nurse should support the client within the healthcare system by advocating for their rights to equal care.

▶ THE ADVOCATE'S ROLE

The complexities of the healthcare system are challenging even to the most educated of clients. Individuals at lower levels of literacy, those who do not speak English, and those who are very ill or very poor face great difficulty navigating the system, and as a result many of them "fall through the cracks." These clients need an advocate to penetrate the layers of bureaucracy and help them access the resources they require (**Figure 43–1 ●**). Some values basic to client advocacy are listed in **Box 43–1 ●**.

The overall goal of the client advocate is to protect clients' rights. Clients must understand their rights in order to be able to defend them. The nurse serves as both a teacher and an advocate by informing clients about their rights. To help clients and healthcare providers understand clients' rights, a number of professional and consumer organizations have developed "bills of rights" for patients. Patient rights are discussed in detail in the exemplar on Patient Rights in the module on Ethics.

Box 43–1 Values Basic to Client Advocacy
■ The client is a holistic, autonomous being who has the right to make choices and decisions. ■ The client has the right to expect a nurse–client relationship that is based on shared respect, trust, collaboration in solving problems related to health and healthcare needs, and consideration of his or her thoughts and feelings. ■ The nurse has the responsibility to ensure the client has access to healthcare services that meet health needs.

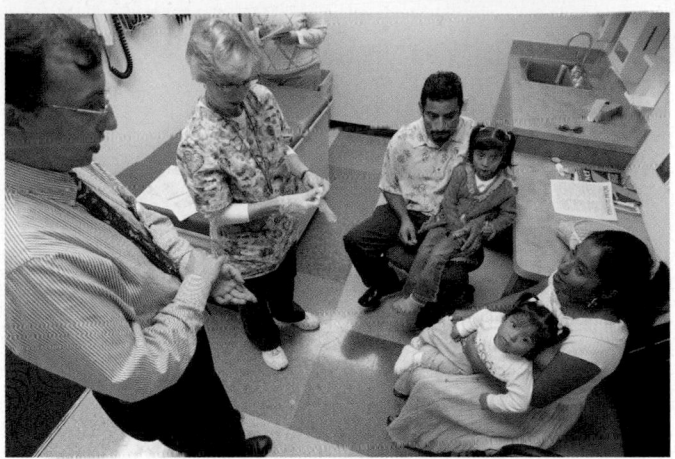

Figure 43–1 ● At this clinic in Pittsburgh, Pennsylvania, clients not only receive health care, but also are helped to find a place to take English lessons, the closest Hispanic grocery store, and anything else they might need.
Source: AP Photo/Gene J. Puskar.

As an advocate, the nurse provides clients with the information they need to make informed decisions and supports all clients' rights to make their own healthcare decisions. In some cases, decision making may be shared by the client and the provider. When the client makes decisions about his or her treatment other than what is recommended, it is the nurse's role to ensure that the client is making an informed decision and, if so, to advocate for the client's right to make autonomous choices, even when those choices run counter to the nurse's own beliefs. The advocate must be careful to remain objective and should not convey approval or disapproval of a client's choices. Advocacy requires accepting and respecting the client's right to decide, even if the nurse believes the decision to be wrong.

If a client lacks decision-making capacity, is legally incompetent, or is a minor, these rights can be exercised on the client's behalf by a designated healthcare surrogate or legal guardian (see the Lifespan Considerations feature). It is important, however, for the nurse to remember that client control over health decisions is a Western view and is not necessarily accepted in other cultures. In other societies, such decisions may normally be made by the head of the family or a member of the community. The nurse must respect the client's and family's views and honor their traditions regarding healthcare decision making.

To be an effective advocate, the nurse must do the following:

- Be assertive.
- Recognize that the rights and values of clients and families must take precedence when they conflict with those of healthcare providers.
- Be aware that conflicts may arise over issues that require consultation, confrontation, or negotiation between the nurse and administrative personnel or between the nurse and a primary care provider.
- Work with community agencies and lay practitioners.

- Understand that advocacy may require political action—communicating a client's healthcare needs to government and other officials who have the authority to do something about these needs.

Although patient advocacy is considered an important aspect of nursing care, few instruments are available for measuring how well nurses act as advocates. In a 2010 study performed by Hanks, a tool known as the Protective Nursing Advocacy Scale (PNAS), was developed and validated measuring nursing advocacy beliefs and actions from a protective perspective. Implications for nursing practice include using the PNAS in conjunction with an educational program to enhance advocacy skills, which may help to improve client outcomes (Hanks, 2010).

Empowering the Client

Because of the special nurse–client relationship, nurses support and advocate for clients and families facing difficult choices and for the individuals who are living with the results of their choices. Through knowing the client and engaging in a mutual relationship, the nurse is able to identify and build on client and family strengths. This empowering relationship includes mutual respect, trust, and confidence in the other's abilities and motives (see the Community-Based Care feature).

Rather than viewing the nurse as *empowering* the client, Swanson (1993) describes a caring behavior of *enabling* that is defined as "facilitating the other's passage through life transitions and unfamiliar events" (p. 356). Enabling also includes coaching, informing, explaining, supporting, assisting, guiding, focusing, and validating. At times, enabling involves the nurse providing substitutive care (i.e., doing for the client who is unable to do for himself), but never more than is needed at the time. At other times, enabling involves providing an environment in which the client is able to function safely and effectively, or mediating on the client's behalf. For example, the nurse may ask the primary care provider to review the reasons for a recommended therapy with the client, because the client says that she always forgets to ask the primary care provider. The nurse should remain mindful of professional boundaries and

---

Community-Based Care
Advocacy in Home Care

The goals of advocacy in the home care setting pose unique concerns for the nurse advocate. For example, while in the hospital, people often operate from the values of the nurses and primary care providers by following instructions and complying with provider requests. Once they return home, however, people tend to operate from their own personal values and may revert to old habits that may not be beneficial to their health. Although the nurse may view this as noncompliance, the nurse must respect client autonomy.

In home care, limited resources and a lack of client care services may shift the focus from client welfare to concerns about resource availability and allocation. Financial considerations can limit a client's access to services and materials, making it difficult to ensure that the client's needs are met.

Lifespan Considerations Advocacy Across the Life Span

The nurse's role as an advocate includes assessing and protecting vulnerable clients across the life span. The risk for these vulnerable populations is higher the more dependent they are on others for help with activities of daily living. Therefore, the most vulnerable populations would include infants, children, pregnant women, and older adults.

Health promotion is one area in which nurses need to advocate for these populations. Health promotion includes prevention of disease, growth and development, nutrition, exercise, and stress management. One example of advocacy applicable to health promotion is immunizations. Nurses should advocate for accessibility and use of immunizations as appropriate for these populations. Another example is related to nutrition. Nurses should promote good nutrition for all ages including accessibility of healthy nutritional choices and less accessibility of more unhealthy choices.

Another area of advocacy important across the life span is safety, which would include accident prevention and abuse and neglect prevention. Individuals who are being abused, particularly by a family member or caregiver, are often powerless to speak. Victims of abuse may seek care for injuries resulting from abuse. The nurse must be alert for signs of abuse during the initial assessment and recognize that the abuse victim will often deny abuse for fear of retribution from the abuser. Nurses advocate for these clients by keeping them safe and educating them with regard to other options. Nurses can also assist clients by identifying and helping them access additional resources to ensure their safety once they leave the healthcare system. Maintaining an awareness of resources in the community and advocating for victims of abuse through political and legislative initiatives are components of the advocacy role. Nurses should advocate for the accident prevention of these vulnerable populations in many of the same ways, including educating individuals in these populations and those that care for them to promote safety.

Nurses can also advocate for clients across the life span by participating in committees and task forces. For example, many states provide for child fatality prevention committees at the county or regional level. These committees include representatives from healthcare agencies and law enforcement, meeting to review child fatalities and to try to determine whether there are any trends or patterns. This type of committee may be able to recognize patterns and devise health promotion activities. For example, if a community started seeing an increase in child fatalities resulting from the failure to use protective equipment during activities, the child fatality prevention committee may be able to recognize and act on that information early.

Nurses often serve as advocates for older adults in hospital, rehabilitation, and nursing care settings. For example, clients who are relocated to an inpatient nursing facility typically receive collaborative care, with regular team meetings that include the client, family members, one or more of the nurses assigned to the client, the primary care provider, and a social worker. Nurses in these setting are in a position to recognize early any change in the client's condition and to advocate for changes in the care plan as necessary.

---

responsibilities to avoid enabling pathological choices by the client. The goal is always to facilitate growth and development.

Nurses both *advocate* (verb) for and are *advocates* (noun) for clients and families. Knowlden (1998) explored the meaning of caring in nursing and identified four dimensions of advocacy:

1. Being a client advocate
2. Following through or following up
3. Providing resources
4. Going above and beyond.

A client in Knowlden's study described how his nurse served as an advocate for him: "She keeps in touch with [my practitioner] to find out what's to be done. She gets through right away. They give us the run-around and get back 5 days later. . . . She has been instrumental in getting the tube changed" (p. 37). Through advocacy, nurses are champions for their clients. They empower clients and families through activities that enhance well-being, understanding, and self-care.

Educating Providers and Others

Sometimes the gap between the rights that clients have in theory and the rights that clients have in practice results from a knowledge deficit on the part of treatment providers. If so, the remedy is simple: Educate healthcare providers so that they in turn can educate and provide appropriate care to their clients.

Another, more complicated possibility that may not be so easily solved is that direct care providers sometimes feel threatened by the expansion of client rights. Healthcare providers have been known to express concern that some new regulations not only hamper treatment but also make their job more difficult and more dangerous. For example, a mother brings her adolescent to the provider's office and requests that a drug screen be performed because of suspected substance abuse. Federal regulations require confidentiality of test results, which prevents the provider from sharing test results with anyone other than the adolescent. The nurse, advocating for the client, is required to maintain confidentiality as well and may need to find a means of either convincing the adolescent to allow information be shared with the parent so appropriate drug treatment may be initiated or explaining to the parent why the information cannot be shared if the adolescent refuses.

Local, state, and national advocacy programs exist to protect and advocate for those with mental illness or disability (see **Box 43–2 ●**).

Professional and Public Advocacy

The role of advocacy in nursing extends to professional organizations, which advocate at the state and national levels for the profession of nursing, its members, and for those who benefit from the services that nurses provide. Professional organizations include the American Nurses Association and are discussed in the exemplar on Professional Organizations in the module on Health Policy.

Box 43–2 Advocacy Programs

Advocacy programs exist at many levels. Some are provided by public organizations, but many are provided by private nonprofit organizations. Some advocacy organizations engage in other activities, such as consumer education or training of professionals. One such organization, the National Alliance on Mental Illness, advocates for research on mental illness as well as for better access to services, therapies, and supports for individuals with mental illness and their families.

The federal government has encouraged states to develop advocacy programs to provide information about and serve as a resource regarding the rights of those with mental illness or disability. Each state designates an agency or group to advocate for the rights of those with mental illness or a disability and to investigate reported incidents involving neglect and abuse of these vulnerable clients in public or private mental health treatment settings, research facilities, and nursing homes. For example, Disability Rights North Carolina (www.disabilityrightsnc.org) is a federally mandated nonprofit organization charged with protecting the rights of children and adults with disabilities living in North Carolina (NC).

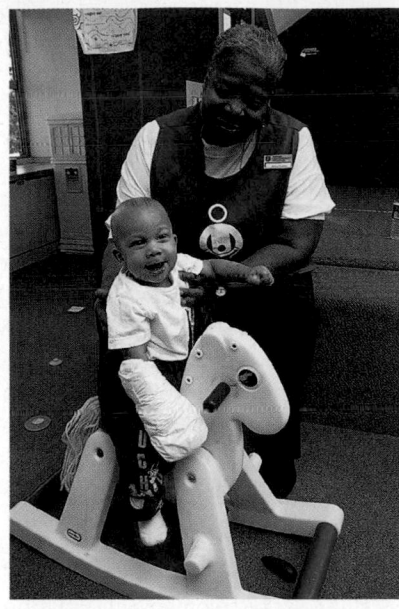

Figure 43–2 ● Nurses must be aware of the needs of pediatric clients for play time and advocate for children to have play time as well as rest time and appropriate nutrition. Here, a volunteer grandmother plays with a young boy to provide stimulation and nurturing during his lengthy hospitalization.

Individual nurses and professional nursing organizations have great opportunities to speak publicly for the health, welfare, and safety of their clients; to take steps to protect client rights; to inform the public about issues and concerns by writing articles for the popular press; to lobby their congressional representatives on behalf of better health care for all people; and to run for political office. Gains that nursing makes in developing and improving health policy at the institutional and governmental levels help to achieve better health care for the public.

As advocates, both professional and public, nurses are in a position to promote and effect change. They need to understand the ethical issues in nursing and health care and know the laws and regulations, both state and federal, that affect nursing practice and the health of society.

Advocating for Children and Families

To be an effective advocate for children and families, the nurse must be aware of each child's and family's needs, the family's resources, and the available healthcare options. The nurse can then assist the family and the child to make informed decisions and to act in the child's best interests. So that family and child can make decisions about treatment in accord with their values and resources, it is important for the nurse to ensure that they have adequate information about treatment options, including information appropriate to the child's level of understanding. As an advocate to protect the child and family, the nurse must also take action related to any potential or actual incidents of incompetent, unethical, or illegal practices by any member of the healthcare team.

The nurse must also ensure that the policies and resources of healthcare agencies meet the psychosocial needs of children and their families. This may involve becoming an active member of a committee that develops policies or guidelines for nursing and medical care or for modernizing the healthcare facility design. In each case, the nurse has knowledge of the developmental and psychosocial needs of children that can help to ensure that healthcare facilities appropriately address the needs of children and families (**Figure 43–2 ●**).

Table 43–1 ● lists some examples of how nurses can advocate for children and families in their community.

TABLE 43–1 Advocating for Children and Families

HEALTH NEED EXAMPLE	NURSE ADVOCACY ACTIONS
Members of the community need information about places to obtain immunizations.	■ Make a list of agencies that provide immunizations. ■ Check on costs and special programs. ■ Obtain financial assistance from a local foundation to print your findings. ■ Make copies available in childcare centers and other community agencies.
A local homeless shelter has little in the way of self-care amenities for the clients.	■ Obtain donations of hotel lotions, soaps, and shampoos from classmates and faculty that can be given to the shelter. ■ Visit several local hotels and ask whether they will each donate a box of small toiletries for the residents. ■ Encourage volunteers to provide haircuts and styling, or obtain donations to provide this service.
Your state has a law protecting the rights of any woman to bring her unwanted newborn baby to certain sites for the purpose of giving up her baby without legal recriminations. Because many women do not know about the law, babies are abandoned in unsafe locations.	■ Find a local newspaper reporter who is willing to write an article about the law. ■ Print copies of the article to distribute. ■ Make posters with necessary information for several community sites.

Source: Ball, J. W., Bindler, R. C., & Cowen, K. J. (2010). *Child health nursing: Partnering with children & families* (2nd ed., p. 325, Table 9-3: Advocating for Children and Families). Upper Saddle River, NJ: Prentice Hall.

Advocating for Vulnerable Populations

Throughout history, nurses have been strong advocates for vulnerable populations such as the poor, those who have a disability or mental illness, and any clients who are unable to advocate for themselves. In the twenty-first century, there is a need for new energy and political activism. In this era of healthcare reform, nurses must be particularly concerned with ensuring that the needs and the rights of individuals in vulnerable populations are not overlooked or ignored. As the explosion of knowledge in science and technology revolutionizes how nurses practice (**Figure 43–3 ●**), nurses must continue to advocate for fair and equitable access to high-quality care for all clients. Nurses advocate for these clients in a variety of settings, including hospitals, free clinics, and primary care and specialty practices.

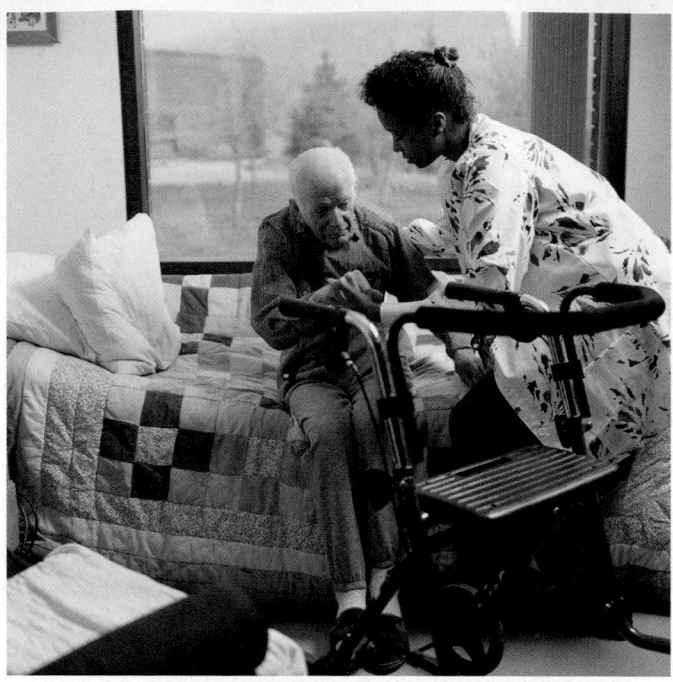

Figure 43–3 ● Clients in long-term care facilities are often unable to advocate for themselves. Nurses should advocate for these individuals in many areas, including effective pain control. *Source:* Stockbyte/Getty Images.

CLINICAL EXAMPLE

Lois Potter is a 68-year-old woman with a number of medical conditions, including Parkinson disease, which causes frequent tremors in her hands. One of her medications is a weekly injection. Mrs. Potter's insurance company refuses to pay for her to receive the injection at her primary care provider's office but will pay if she gives the injection to herself at home. Mrs. Potter is on a very limited income and cannot afford to pay a weekly injection fee. The nurse working with Mrs. Potter at her primary care provider's office realizes that Mrs. Potter is not able to self-inject.

1. What options does the nurse have for advocating that Mrs. Potter receive the injection at her primary care provider's office?
2. How can the nurse advocate for the client without removing Mrs. Potter's need for dignity?
3. What goal would you advocate for Mrs. Potter?

CLIENTS WITH DISABILITIES Two pieces of federal legislation have implications for the rights of clients. In 1990, the Americans with Disabilities Act (ADA) extended federal protection to individuals with physical and/or mental health disabilities for access to public services, employment, and benefits. In an effort to increase the involvement of individuals in directing their own medical care, Congress enacted the Patient Self-Determination Act (PSDA) in 1991 to protect the rights of clients to accept or reject aspects of their medical care (see the module on Legal Issues for more information about the PSDA).

Although laws may protect certain aspects of human rights, they cannot prevent errors and misunderstandings. Even when the letter of the law is followed, the spirit of the law may not be satisfied. For example, even if a client is read his rights, the client may not understand the information, may not remember it, or may be so distracted by worry that he fails to grasp the information completely. Nurses are often in a position to ensure that both the letter and spirit of the law are followed. The spirit of the law is what many healthcare providers overlook when working with clients with disabilities. Nurses are in a unique position to advocate for clients with disabilities as they navigate the healthcare system.

CLINICAL EXAMPLE

Marina Commodore is an RN with 20 years of clinical experience and advanced degrees. While caring for a client, Ms. Commodore injures her back and is no longer able to work as a clinical nurse. During a visit to her primary care provider, Ms. Commodore begins to cry and the nurse asks what caused her tears. Ms. Commodore says she is no longer able to perform clinical work and doesn't know how she'll pay her monthly bills. She reports that she applied for a position as a telephone advice nurse but says she did not even get an interview when the agency discovered that she had physical limitations.

1. If you were Ms. Commodore's nurse, how would you advocate on her behalf?
2. What would you say to Ms. Commodore at this time?
3. Would you best advocate for this client professionally or publicly? Explain your answer.

ISSUES IN MENTAL HEALTH SETTINGS Clients with mental health disorders are particularly vulnerable to both physical and psychological abuse and often do not have the ability to defend themselves. When these clients enter treatment, they may exhibit some of the same inappropriate behaviors and unrealistic expectations in which they engage outside of treatment. As a result, they are also vulnerable to abuse within the treatment facility.

Although few actual data are available regarding how much client abuse exists in treatment settings, one advocacy group ranked client abuse as the most frequent rights violation complaint, while another ranked it third. Although providing care to clients in mental health settings can be challenging, nurses and other staff members should never engage in abusive or unprofessional behavior. Examples of abuse and inappropriate staff behaviors include the following:

- Supplying clients with drugs or alcohol in return for favors
- Making privileges contingent on favors from clients
- Slapping and kicking clients when staff members feel frustrated
- Using restraints when other, less intrusive alternatives are available
- Verbal harassment, including threats, sarcasm, and other put-downs
- General threats of harm if clients do not behave "appropriately" or as they are told
- Inhumane physical facilities
- Sexual misconduct.

Some identified causes that may lead to client abuse include the following:

- Unsuitability of certain staff members who do not have the patience or understanding to work with clients having trouble with self-control
- Burnout, that is, a buildup of stresses that have reduced the staff's patience and ability to problem solve
- Lack of knowledge about other means of interacting with clients in a high-stress situation.

▶ ADVOCACY INTERVENTIONS

In designing and conducting advocacy interventions, it is important to do the following:

- Assess the client's ability to cooperate and to make decisions.
- Assess the reliability of information provided by the client, especially if the client exhibits impairment of cognitive function or mental instability.
- Assess the client's medical history and family situation.

When nurses not only partner with family members but also teach family members to be advocates, clients experience greater improvement in their health outcomes.

Specific areas of advocacy interventions include the following:

- Educate clients and their families about their legal rights.
- Monitor treatment planning and delivery of service for the abuse of client rights.
- Evaluate policies and procedures regarding infringement of client rights.
- Ensure that clients have the necessary information to make an informed decision or give informed consent.
- Question other healthcare professionals when they provide care that is based on stereotypical ideas rather than on an assessment of the individual client's needs.
- Speak out for safe practice conditions when threatened by budget cutbacks.

Responsibility to Communicate and Collaborate

The nurse's duty to intervene and advocate on behalf of clients requires that the nurse communicate clearly with others, particularly the client and family members or other healthcare professionals participating in the decision-making process. Clear communication by all members of the client's healthcare team ensures client safety, enhances client care, and increases the likelihood of positive outcomes for the client.

Formulating a Plan to Intervene

Nurses often complain of not having "think time" (time to consider all options before acting). Formulating a plan of care before implementing interventions is essential, but many nurses report that time constraints prevent them from considering options for care and that they often respond based on past experience or intuition (Negarandeh et al., 2006). Although this tactic may work for many expert nurses, beginning nurses need to carefully think through options and learn to assess the clinical and legal implications of their actions before providing care for their clients.

▶ ILLEGAL, IMMORAL, OR UNETHICAL ACTIVITIES OF PROFESSIONALS

Nurses are advocates for all clients, not just the individuals in their care. Nurses have a legal responsibility to report any professional whom they suspect of engaging in illegal, immoral, or unethical activities. Normally, the nurse making such a report will do so following established procedures at the facility at which the nurse is employed. A nurse who suspects another nurse of impairment should also follow guidelines set forth by the board of nursing for the state in which the nurses work. At other times, the nurse may need to seek the guidance of the state board of nursing or the American Nurses Association (ANA). A nurse who suspects a colleague of engaging in illegal, immoral, or unethical conduct and fails to act is in direct violation of the ANA Code of Ethics for Nurses (ANA, 2010).

Impairment of a coworker or team member is the most common situation encountered by healthcare professionals. Impairment may result from use of alcohol or drugs or from emotional overload as a result of a stressful personal experience (e.g., a nurse who returns to work too soon following the death of a close family member). Impairment from drugs or alcohol may be linked with other illegal acts, such as theft of drugs or a client's personal property. Impairment has the potential to interfere with job performance and may result in unsafe clinical practice. A nurse who observes or suspects impairment in another professional is obligated to immediately report it to a supervisor (ANA, 2010). Although an impaired healthcare provider may view this intervention as an invasion of privacy, such prompt action will safeguard clients from harm, while at the same time offer the impaired healthcare provider a chance at recovery. Many hospitals have programs to help impaired employees recover.

▶ NURSING PRACTICE

Nurses are morally obligated to act as advocates for all clients, but particularly those who cannot advocate for themselves. This obligation extends to time off duty as well including time at work.

Clients from vulnerable populations particularly benefit from nursing advocacy. Advocacy by nurses can greatly affect clients' well-being by helping eliminate barriers to accessing healthcare services. Learning the role of a client advocate begins in nursing school and, with experience, is incorporated into daily professional practice.

REVIEW The Concept of Advocacy

RELATE Link the Concepts

Linking the concept of advocacy with the concept of culture and diversity:

1. Consider each of the different groups that are generally included within the description of vulnerable people, and provide examples of how the nurse can advocate for each.

2. Why might clients with more diverse characteristics from the general population require greater advocacy?

Linking the concept of advocacy with the concept of ethics:

3. How does the nursing code of ethics address advocacy?

4. Differentiate between the nurse's role of advocate for individuals who are unable to speak for themselves versus the role of advocate for those who are competent to speak for themselves but, for whatever reason, do not.

REFER Go to Pearson Nursing Student Resources
nursing.pearsonhighered.com

- Additional review materials

REFLECT Case Study

Heather Adams is a neighbor in your apartment building. On weekends, the two of you sometimes get together for morn-ing coffee. Last weekend, Ms. Adams shared a concern that has been troubling her for a few weeks. She is 31 years old and unmarried, and she lives alone. Her father is deceased, and her mother, who was diagnosed with Alzheimer disease several years ago, is now a resident in a long-term care facility for people with cognitive impairments. Ms. Adams is estranged from her only brother. When she was in her early 20s, Ms. Adams was hospitalized and treated for depression. Her fear is that, should she become incapacitated again with depression, the brother whom she actively dislikes and with whom she does not get along will make treatment decisions as her next of kin.

You have decided to invite Ms. Adams for coffee. Because Ms. Adams seems to be an individual who would benefit from a healthcare power of attorney, you intend to educate her about her choices.

1. On what basis do you act as an advocate for Ms. Adams?

2. Would it be ethical for you to serve as the surrogate decision maker? Explain your answer.

3. In your discussion with Ms. Adams, should you encourage her to see an attorney? Explain your answer.

■ REFERENCES

American Nurses Association (ANA). (2010). *Professional standards*. Retrieved from http://www.nursingworld.org/MainMenuCategories/ThePracticeofProfessional-Nursing/NursingStandards.

Ball, J. W., Bindler, R. C., & Cowen, K. J. (2010). *Child health nursing: Partnering with children & families* (2nd ed.). Upper Saddle River, NJ: Prentice Hall.

Hanks, R. G. (2010). Development and testing of an instrument to measure protective nursing advocacy. *Nursing Ethics, 17*(2), 255–267.

Knowlden, V. (1998). *The communication of caring in nursing*. Indianapolis, IN: Center Nursing Press.

Negarandeh, R., Oskouie, F., Ahmadi, F., Nikravesh, M., & Hallberg, I. R. (2006, March 1). Patient advocacy: Barriers and facilitators. *BMC Nursing, 5*, 3.

Swanson, K. (1993). Nursing as informed caring for the well-being of others. *IMAGE: Journal of Nursing Scholarship, 25*(4), 352–357.

44 Ethics

MODULE AT-A-GLANCE

The Concept of
Ethics, 2563

Exemplar 44.1
Ethical Dilemmas, 2571

Exemplar 44.2
Patient Rights, 2578

◪ THE CONCEPT OF ETHICS

Ethics, as applied in professional nursing, is defined as a system of moral principles or standards governing behaviors and relationships that is based on professional nursing beliefs and values. More broadly defined, "ethics is concerned with motives and attitudes and the relationship of these attitudes to the individual" (Guido, 2010, p. 3). Ethics refers to the standards of right and wrong that influence human behavior, usually in terms of rights, obligations, benefits to society, fairness, or specific virtues. Ethical standards are based on the values of the group that holds to those standards, whether the group comprises individuals of the same religion, people from the same community, or those who share the same profession. Ethical standards of nursing include standards relating to the rights of clients and their families, such as the right to privacy.

The term *ethics* also refers to the study and development of the ethical standards of an individual, a community, or a profession. Nurses should constantly examine their personal ethical standards and understand how their personal ethics and morals compare to the ethical standards of the nursing profession.

Morality (or morals) is similar to ethics, and many people use the terms interchangeably. **Morality** usually refers to private, personal standards of what is right and wrong in conduct, character, and attitude. Sometimes the first clue to the moral nature of a situation is the awareness of feelings such as guilt, hope, or shame. Another indicator is the tendency to respond to the situation with words such as *ought*, *should*, *right*, *wrong*, *good*, and *bad*. Moral issues are concerned with important social values and norms; they are not about trivial things.

(continued on next page)

Concept Learning Outcomes

After reading about this concept, you will be able to:

1. Summarize the relationship between values and ethics in the nursing profession.
2. Examine the principles of ethical decision making.
3. Explain the ANA Code of Ethics.
4. Integrate the ANA Code of Ethics in providing individual client care.
5. Examine how personal values influence individual care.
6. Apply a model to processing an ethical dilemma.
7. Apply ethical principles in situations involving ethical dilemmas.
8. Demonstrate appropriate steps to approaching ethical dilemmas.
9. Analyze ethical principles used to make decisions in providing individual client care.

Concept Key Terms

Advocate, *2564*
Altruism, *2564*
Autonomy, *2564*
Belief, *2564*
Beneficence, *2567*
Code of ethics, *2567*
Ethics, *2563*
Human dignity, *2564*

Integrity, *2564*
Justice, *2567*
Morality, *2563*
Nonmaleficence, *2567*
Social justice, *2564*
Values, *2564*
Veracity, *2567*

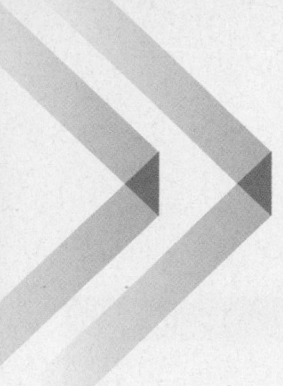

Nurses should be able to distinguish between morality and law. Laws reflect the moral values of a society, and they offer guidance in determining what is moral. However, an action can be legal but not moral. For example, an order for full resuscitation of a dying client is legal, but one could still question whether the act is moral. On the other hand, an action can be moral but illegal. For example, if a child at home stops breathing, it is moral but not legal to exceed the speed limit when driving to the hospital. Legal aspects of nursing practice are covered in the module on Legal Issues.

When people are ill, they may be unable to assert their rights as they would if they were healthy. When this happens, nurses have an ethical responsibility to advocate on behalf of the client based on what the client would want. An **advocate** is one who expresses and defends the cause of another. Therefore, the nurse advocates for the client's best interest based on the client's values, not based on the nurse's own ethical or moral values. Nursing advocacy takes many forms and is discussed in detail in the module on Advocacy. To function successfully in his or her capacity as an advocate for clients, each nurse needs an understanding of the ethical issues in nursing and health care. **<<**

▶ VALUES

Guido (2010) defines **values** as "personal beliefs about the truth and the worth of thoughts, objects, or behaviors" (p. 3). A **belief** is an interpretation or conclusion that one accepts as true. Values can reflect both beliefs that are based on a particular tenet (doctrine) or a body of tenets accepted by a group of individuals and beliefs that are based on a pattern of mental views established by cumulative prior experience. For example, many traditional Jewish beliefs are based on the tenets found in the Jewish Torah, but individual Jews may hold other or additional beliefs based on their experiences within their own communities. Personal values are developed through individual observation and experience and may be heavily influenced by social traditions and the cultural, ethnic, and religious norms experienced within the family and associated groups.

Nurses acquire professional values through socialization into the nursing profession by nursing school faculty and other nurses, through clinical and life experiences, and by following established professional codes of ethics. As part of this socialization, nurses develop insight into their own values and how their values influence their actions. One of the most helpful ways for nurses to develop such insight is through values clarification (Johnstone, 2012a). Through the process of consciously identifying, examining, and developing individual values, nurses become able to choose actions on the basis of deliberately adopted values. Values clarification is important to both nurses and clients in supporting the provision of client-centered care, because it helps nurses learn how to identify clients' values and distinguish clients' values from their own (Benner, Tanner, & Chesla, 2009). Values clarification is not a once-in-a-lifetime activity but an ongoing process of examining what one values and how one's values inform or affect one's decisions and actions. Nursing students and professional nurses need to have a clear sense of their values specific to life, death, health, and illness. Values clarification exercises and real-life experience in carrying out treatment plans that contradict or challenge their beliefs about the best interest of the client will assist nurses at all levels to develop expertise in responding to ethical issues.

A recent study explored the relationship between values and value incongruence and organizational outcomes such as turnover and the propensity for accidents (Bao et al., 2013). The findings of this study suggested that specific values that address the work environment and nurses' sense of burnout and a sense of well-being must be addressed rather than broad organizational values congruence.

Values Essential for the Professional Nurse

The American Association of Colleges of Nursing (AACN) (2008) has identified five values that are essential for the professional nurse: altruism, autonomy, human dignity, integrity, and social justice.

ALTRUISM   **Altruism** is a concern for the welfare and well-being of others. In practice, altruism is reflected in the nurse's concern for the welfare of clients, other nurses, and other healthcare providers.

AUTONOMY   **Autonomy** is the right to self-determination. Professional practice reflects autonomy when the nurse respects clients' rights to make decisions about their health care.

HUMAN DIGNITY   **Human dignity** refers to the inherent worth and uniqueness of individuals and populations. The nurse who values and respects all clients and colleagues shows respect for human dignity.

INTEGRITY   **Integrity** is acting in accordance with an appropriate code of ethics and accepted standards of practice. Integrity is reflected in professional practice when the nurse is honest and provides care based on an ethical framework that is accepted within the profession, for example, the American Nurses Association Code of Ethics.

SOCIAL JUSTICE   **Social justice** refers to the upholding of justice, or what is fair, on a social scale. Nurses act in accordance with social justice by treating all clients equally without regard to economic status, ethnicity, age, citizenship, disability or sexual orientation.

Professional behaviors associated with these ethical values are outlined in **Box 44–1** ●.

Box 44–1 Professional Behaviors Associated With Ethical Nursing Values

- Demonstrate the professional standards of moral, ethical, and legal conduct.
- Assume accountability for personal and professional behaviors.
- Promote the image of nursing by modeling the values and articulating the knowledge, skills, and attitudes of the nursing profession.
- Demonstrate professionalism, including attention to appearance, demeanor, respect for self and others, and attention to professional boundaries with clients and families as well as among caregivers.
- Demonstrate an appreciation of the history of and contemporary issues in nursing and their impact on current nursing practice.
- Reflect on one's own beliefs and values as they relate to professional practice.
- Identify personal, professional, and environmental risks that impact personal and professional choices and behaviors.

- Communicate to the healthcare team one's personal bias on difficult healthcare decisions that impact one's ability to provide care.
- Recognize the impact of attitudes, values, and expectations on the care of the very young, frail older adults, and other vulnerable populations.
- Protect client privacy and confidentiality of client records and other privileged communications.
- Access interprofessional and intraprofessional resources to resolve ethical and other practice dilemmas.
- Act to prevent unsafe, illegal, or unethical care practices.
- Articulate the value of pursuing practice excellence, lifelong learning, and professional engagement to foster professional growth and development.
- Recognize the relationship between personal health, self renewal, and the ability to deliver sustained quality care.

Source: From American Association of Colleges of Nursing. (2008). *The essentials of baccalaureate education for professional nursing practice* (p. 29). Washington, DC: Author. Reprinted with permission.

Integrating the Concept of Ethics

Ethical client care involves more than managing difficult care decisions or facing moral issues surrounding a client. Ethical care also requires managing common client care such as pain control for a surgical client, client teaching, assuring confidentiality, and assuring clients' right to self-determination (see the feature on Concepts Related to Ethics).

Clarifying Clients' Values

To plan effective care, nurses need to identify clients' values, because those values influence and relate to a particular health problem. For example, a client with failing eyesight will probably place a high value on the ability to see, and a client with chronic pain will value comfort. Normally, people take such things for granted. When clients hold unclear or conflicting values that are detrimental to their health, the nurse should use values clarification as an intervention. Examples of behaviors that may indicate the need for clarification of health values are listed in **Table 44–1** ●.

The following process may help clients clarify their values:

1. *List alternatives.* Make sure that the client is aware of all alternative actions. Ask, "Are you considering other courses of action? Tell me about them."
2. *Examine possible consequences of choices.* Make sure the client has thought about the possible results of each action. Ask, "What do you think you will gain from doing that?" "What benefits do you foresee from doing that?"
3. *Choose freely.* To determine whether the client chose freely, ask, "Did you have any say in that decision?" "Do you have a choice?"
4. *Feel good about the choice.* To determine how the client feels, ask, "How do you feel about that decision (or action)?" Because some clients may not feel satisfied with their decision, a more sensitive question might be "Some people feel good after a decision is made; others feel bad. How do you feel?"

5. *Affirm the choice.* Ask, "How will you discuss this with others (family, friends)?"
6. *Act on the choice.* To determine whether the client is prepared to act on the decision, ask, for example, "Tell me how you plan to start doing this."
7. *Act with a pattern.* To determine whether the client consistently behaves in a certain way, ask, "How many times have you done that before?" or "Would you act that way again?"

When implementing these seven steps to clarify values, the nurse assists the client to think each question through but does not impose the nurse's personal values. The nurse rarely, if ever, offers an opinion when the client asks for it—and then only with great care or when the nurse is an expert in the content area. Because each situation is different, what the nurse would choose in his or her own life might not be relevant to the client's circumstances. If the client asks the nurse "What would you have done in my situation?" it is best to redirect the question back to the client rather than answering from the nurse's personal viewpoint.

TABLE 44–1 Behaviors That May Indicate Unclear Values

BEHAVIOR	EXAMPLE
Ignoring a health professional's advice	A client with heart disease who values hard work ignores advice to exercise regularly.
Inconsistent communication or behavior	A pregnant woman says she wants a healthy baby but continues to drink alcohol and smoke tobacco.
Numerous admissions to a health agency for the same problem	A middle-aged woman with obesity repeatedly seeks help for back pain but does not lose weight.
Confusion or uncertainty about which course of action to take	A woman wants to obtain a job to meet financial obligations but also wants to stay at home to care for an ailing husband.

Concepts Related to **Ethics**

The phenomenon of chronic pain presents profound challenges to medical professionals and to our system of medical care as a whole. Research suggests that pain affects 75–150 million Americans of whom only 3 million seek care from a pain specialist (McGee et al., 2011). There is nationwide consensus among those holding a stake in the diagnosis and treatment of chronic pain regarding the ethical issues that must be addressed. Raising awareness about chronic pain, improving access and outcomes to high-quality pain care, and resolving debates about the use of opioids in chronic pain populations are the first steps to ensuring a morally justifiable approach to chronic pain management in the 21st century.

Client teaching regarding critical aspects of care, particularly discharge plans is a vital nursing role. A study regarding gaps in discharge processes with clients dealing with a new ostomy found that clients' autonomy and self-determination were diminished by lack of discharge teaching (Walker & Lachman, 2013). The role of nurses in educating clients has become increasingly important in the rapidly changing healthcare system (Priharjo & Hoy, 2011).

The client's right to confidentiality surrounding care and information and client self-determination are concepts nurses can ensure as client advocates (Johnstone, 2011; Lachman, 2012).

CONCEPT	RELATIONSHIP TO ETHICS	NURSING IMPLICATIONS
Comfort		
■ Pain control ■ Acute and chronic pain	A client with a history of long-term narcotic use often faces difficulty managing further pain after surgical interventions. The nurse must collaborate with the client and care team to manage the client's pain and understand the nurse's own values and biases regarding use of a high level of pain medications. Some physicians are not comfortable with higher level pain needs.	■ Assess your own assumptions or biases surrounding narcotic use. ■ Assess your understanding of the client's pain levels. ■ Ask for support from a supervisor or peers when advocating for appropriate client care. ■ Plan on further assessment of such clients postoperatively.
Teaching and Learning		
■ Client teaching	Client teaching begins on admission and continues through the client's stay until discharged. Clients have the right to receive teaching about their care, including medications and treatments, while cared for by nursing staff.	■ Assess the client's learning needs on admission (whether in the ED, operative unit, acute care unit, or home). ■ Plan appropriate teaching interventions for the client and appropriate teaching methods. ■ Assess your own assumptions and values about receiving care information and the best way to receive such information.
Communication		
■ Confidentiality	Nurses are obligated to ensure confidentiality of a client's information during all care and in all care areas.	■ Ensure that access to client information, such as online charting, is only made available to appropriate staff members. ■ Discuss with the client how you ensure confidentiality.
Advocacy		
■ The right to self-determination	The nurse ensures that the client receives sufficient information on which to base consent for care and related treatment. The nurse provides an environment that allows clients to make their own care decisions, as appropriate.	■ Make sure preoperative interventions are clearly discussed with client by medical staff to ensure appropriate consent. ■ Discuss the plan of care with the client and allow self-determination, such as which client medication dosage to try first, as appropriate. ■ Recognize the client's right to refuse treatment/procedures.

CASE STUDY \\ PART 1

June D'Angelo, a 49-year-old female, presented to the emergency department (ED) late at night with complaints of severe migraine headache. Her vital signs showed that her blood pressure was elevated at 210/104 mmHg. The ED physician discussed her history and found that Ms. D'Angelo had been in the ED five times in the past year for the same problem. She had been prescribed a daily blood pressure medication by her primary physician 3 weeks earlier, but she said she did not take the medication nor fill the prescription, because she had decided to take daily walks to manage her blood pressure. The physician asked her how recently the headache began and how long each one lasts. Ms. D'Angelo sighed and said that her migraines mostly never end and have been worse in the past 24 hours. As the physician left her bedside to call Ms. D'Angelo's healthcare provider, he gave orders to the nurse for IV blood pressure medication for Ms. D'Angelo. As they began getting ready to provide the IV medication, Ms. D'Angelo tried to stop the nurse. The nurse spoke with Ms. D'Angelo to complete her brief nursing assessment. Findings from the assessment indicated that Ms. D'Angelo relies on the ED to manage her pain and does not follow her primary healthcare provider's instructions.

Clinical Thinking Questions

1. What ethical issue is the nurse facing as she assesses this client with frequent ED admissions?
2. What topics of client teaching will this client likely need?
3. What further information should the nurse assess for the client's teaching?
4. How can the nurse assist Ms. D'Angelo in planning how to manage her symptoms better?
5. Who should be involved in this client's discharge planning and self-care? Explain.

▶ PRINCIPLES OF ETHICAL DECISION MAKING

An individual's personal, community, and professional values inform his or her decision-making processes. Behind those values, a framework of four primary principles has been used to guide ethical decision making among professional nurses (Chally & Loriz, 1998). These four principles are autonomy, beneficence, justice, and veracity.

As mentioned previously, autonomy is defined as the right to self-determination (Guido, 2010, p. 8). Clients have the right to determine their own care. The nurse honors this principle by respecting the client's decision even if it is in conflict with what the nurse believes is in the client's best interest.

Beneficence requires that "the actions one takes should promote good" (Guido, 2010, p. 8). The nurse's ethical duty goes beyond beneficence to include **nonmaleficence**, which requires that the nurse do no harm and instead safeguard the client. Intentional harm is clearly not in keeping with this principle, but there can also be risk of harm in performing nursing interventions that are intended for good. Nonmaleficence does not mean that the nurse performs only actions that carry no risk to the client. Many actions, such as administering medications, carry some degree of risk. In most cases, the risk of harm is weighed against the potential for benefit. Before the action is taken, the client is given information regarding the potential benefits and risks, and the client decides whether or not to accept the treatment. Take the example of administering pain medication to a client following an operation. The risks of discomfort from the injection and side effects from the medication are outweighed by the need to relieve the client's suffering.

Nurses treat clients fairly and with **justice**, the upholding of what is just, especially fair treatment and due reward in accordance with honor, standards, or law. This principle is challenging when decisions related to allocation of scarce resources must be made.

Individuals who always tell the truth reflect the principle of **veracity** (Guido, 2010, p. 8). Veracity can be a particularly challenging principle for the nurse, who may be faced with providing a client with complete information regarding the client's illness when family members or significant others want the information withheld. Veracity is the principle behind giving complete information before obtaining a client's informed consent for any procedure. Veracity is one of several principles behind timely and accurate documentation of nursing interventions.

▶ NURSING CODES OF ETHICS

Ethical standards and behaviors are at the core of nursing practice. As a result, the nursing profession has developed codes of ethics to guide nurses in their work with clients and other healthcare professionals. A **code of ethics** is a general guide for a profession's membership and a social contract with the public that it serves. The Nightingale Pledge is considered the first code of nursing ethics in the United States. Written in 1893 by Lystra Gretter, the principal of the Farrand Training School for Nurses in Detroit, and patterned after the Hippocratic Oath for medicine, the Nightingale Pledge was named for Florence Nightingale. It is still used at many nursing schools' graduation ceremonies. The Nightingale Pledge reads as follows:

> I solemnly pledge myself before God and in the presence of this assembly: To pass my life in purity and to practice my profession faithfully. I will abstain from whatever is deleterious and mischievous, and will not take or knowingly administer any harmful drug. I will do all in my power to elevate the standard of my profession, and will hold in confidence all personal matters committed to my keeping, and all family affairs coming to my knowledge in the practice of my profession. With loyalty will I endeavor to aid the physician in his work and devote myself to the welfare of those committed to my care (Gretter, 1910).

The nursing profession depends on two major codes of ethics: the American Nurses Association (ANA) Code of Ethics for Nurses and the International Council of Nurses (ICN) Code of Ethics. Both codes were initially formally adopted in the early 1950s and have undergone changes to reflect social

Box 44–2 The ICN Code of Ethics

1. **Nurses and people**
   - The nurse's primary professional responsibility is to people requiring nursing care.
   - In providing care, the nurse promotes an environment in which the human rights, values, customs and spiritual beliefs of the individual, family and community are respected.
   - The nurse ensures that the individual receives accurate, sufficient and timely information in a culturally appropriate manner on which to base consent for care and related treatment.
   - The nurse holds in confidence personal information and uses judgement in sharing this information.
   - The nurse shares with society the responsibility for initiating and supporting action to meet the health and social needs of the public, in particular those of vulnerable populations.
   - The nurse advocates for equity and social justice in resource allocation, access to health care and other social and economic services.
   - The nurse demonstrates professional values such as respectfulness, responsiveness, compassion, trustworthiness and integrity.

2. **Nurses and practice**
   - The nurse carries personal responsibility and accountability for nursing practice, and for maintaining competence by continual learning.
   - The nurse maintains a standard of personal health such that the ability to provide care is not compromised.
   - The nurse uses judgement regarding individual competence when accepting and delegating responsibility.
   - The nurse at all times maintains standards of personal conduct which reflect well on the profession and enhance its image and public confidence.

   - The nurse, in providing care, ensures that use of technology and scientific advances is compatible with the safety, dignity and rights of people.
   - The nurse strives to foster and maintain a practice culture promoting ethical behaviour and open dialogue.

3. **Nurses and the profession**
   - The nurse assumes the major role in determining and implementing acceptable standards of clinical nursing practice, management, research and education.
   - The nurse is active in developing a core of research-based professional knowledge that supports evidence-based practice.
   - The nurse is active in developing and sustaining a core of professional values.
   - The nurse, acting through the professional organisation, participates in creating a positive practice environment and maintaining safe, equitable social and economic working conditions in nursing.
   - The nurse practices to sustain and protect the natural environment and is aware of its consequences on health.
   - The nurse contributes to an ethical organisational environment and challenges unethical practices and settings.

4. **Nurses and co-workers**
   - The nurse sustains a collaborative and respectful relationship with co-workers in nursing and other fields.
   - The nurse takes appropriate action to safeguard individuals, families and communities when their health is endangered by a co-worker or any other person.
   - The nurse takes appropriate action to support and guide co-workers to advance ethical conduct.

Source: International Council of Nurses. (2012). *The ICN Code of Ethics for Nurses.* Retrieved from http://www.icn.ch/images/stories/documents/publications/free_publications/Code_of_Ethics_2012.pdf.

and technological change. The ICN code was updated in 2012 (see **Box 44–2**).

The ANA Code of Ethics for Nurses (2001) serves as a statement of ethical obligations and duties of the nurse, as the profession's nonnegotiable ethical standard, and as the nursing profession's statement of commitment to society. During early 2013, the ANA sought input on revision to its Code of Ethics (ANA, 2013a). And an updated version of the Code of Ethics is expected at the end of 2014 (ANA, 2014).

Stay Current: *To see the latest version of the ANA Code of Ethics, visit the ANA Web site at* **www.nursingworld.org/codeofethics**.

The terms "ethical" and "moral" are used throughout the ANA Code of Ethics. The code is not simply a reference tool; nurses should use it to direct how they perform their duties in their daily life. The code needs to be read and reread as the nurse develops ethical decision-making ability through his or her professional career. Provision 1 of the code addresses the valuing of each human without modifiers (such as color, race, gender, or religious preferences). Nurses are expected to move beyond feelings and recognize the humanity of the client and respond with compassion and respect. A brief discussion of the provisions of the code is provided here.

1. Interpretive statement 1.4, the right to self-determination, requires that the nurse be knowledgeable about the client's moral and legal rights (see the module on Legal Issues).

The ethical standard is that the nurse supports the client's decisions about care regardless of the nurse's own values.

2. Provision 2 mandates that the nurse's primary commitment be to the client. Lachman (2012) states that when an individual chooses to be a nurse, the individual has made a moral commitment to care for all clients, as reflected in the ANA Code of Ethics. Ethical problems often arise from tensions among responsibilities as well as from differing value and belief systems. Authors (Kangasniemi & Haho, 2012; Lachman, 2012) have suggested that in applying Provision 2 to an ethical problem, the nurse needs to ask the following questions:
   - What do I know about this client's situation?
   - What do I know about the client's values and moral preferences?
   - What assumptions am I making that require more data to clarify?
   - What are my own feelings (and values) about the situation? How might they be influencing how I view and respond to the situation?
   - Are my own values in conflict with those of the client?
   - What else do I need to know about this case and where can I obtain this information?
   - What can I never know about this case?
   - Given my primary obligation to the client, what should I do to be ethical?

3. Provision 3 reflects the need to apply the principle of autonomy to specific bioethical issues, including the use of humans in research. In the current revision of the code, privacy and confidentiality are separate interpretive statements. Privacy involves the aspects of information that the client can control. Confidentiality is how the information is handled once it is shared by the client (see the exemplar on HIPAA in the module on Legal Issues). The nurse's responsibility to the client involved in research is addressed in interpretive statement 3.3. The responsibility for establishing and reviewing the nurse's competency in providing client-centered care is addressed in interpretive statement 3.4. All nurses, regardless of position and setting, are accountable for ensuring that all nursing care is provided to clients by nurses who meet the profession's standards.

Interpretive statements 3.5 and 3.6 address the responsibility to identify any practice of an individual that is questionable, to recognize the need to do something about it, and to determine possible appropriate actions. This is consistent with mandatory reporting laws (see the exemplar on HIPAA in the module on Legal Issues) and the ethical responsibility that nurses have to address colleagues who may be impaired (refer to the module on Addiction).

4. Provision 4 emphasizes that, at all times, the responsibility and accountability for each nurse's actions and judgments belong to the individual nurse. Accountability is the professional implied contract with the public (see the module on Accountability).

5. Provision 5 identifies the nurse's duty to self in seeking professional growth and maintaining competence, good character, and integrity. A synonym for integrity is truth-telling, such as disclosing factual information to clients and their families, which is a basic moral rule in the Western healthcare system (Pergert & Lutzen, 2012).

6. Provision 6 focuses on the role of the nurse in creating, promoting, and maintaining an ethical environment. A healthy, supportive workplace environment is essential to meet the needs of both the nurse and the clients. Many professional organizations have focused on the importance of developing a healthy workplace that provides for an environment that promotes ethical treatment of both the employees and the clients. The ANA (2001) developed the Bill of Rights for Registered Nurses as a policy statement with specific attention to the workplace environment. The American Nurses Credentialing Center Magnet Recognition Program recognizes organizations that demonstrate excellence in nursing practice and provide a culture of excellence.

7. Provision 7 encourages individual nurses to use their own talents and interests in contributing to the advancement of the profession through engagement in refining professional standards or through the development, adaptation, and communication of knowledge.

8. Provisions 8 and 9 address the responsibility of the nurse in shaping public health policy and participating in social reform and the nurse's obligation to society to eliminate social inequity, prejudice, and oppression.

Box 44–3 Ethical Decision-Making Models

MODEL	SOURCE
Thompson and Thompson	Thompson, J. B., & Thompson, H. O. (1985). *Bioethical decision making for nurses* (p. 99). Norwalk, CT: Appleton-Century-Croft.
Cassells and Redman	Cassells, J., & Redman, B. (1989). Preparing students to be moral agents in clinical nursing practice. *Nursing clinics of North America, 24*(2), pp. 463–473.
Twelve Questions	Nash, L. (1981). Ethics without the sermon. *Harvard Business Review, 59,* 79–90.
Ethical Decision Making Plan	U.S. Department of Defense. (1999). Joint Ethics Regulation DoD 5500.7-R.
MORAL Model	Guido, G. W. (2010). *Legal & ethical issues in nursing* (5th ed.). Upper Saddle River, NJ: Pearson.

▶ MODELS OF ETHICAL DECISION MAKING

Responsible ethical reasoning is rational and systematic. It should be based on ethical principles and codes rather than on emotions, intuition, fixed policies, or precedent (i.e., an earlier similar occurrence). **Box 44–3** ● lists a number of decision-making models from various disciplines that can be used for ethical reasoning.

A good decision is one that is in the client's best interest and at the same time preserves the integrity of all individuals involved. Nurses have ethical obligations to their clients, to the agency that employs them, and to primary care providers. Therefore, nurses must weigh competing factors when making ethical decisions. **Box 44–4** ● provides some examples of the obligations nurses must take into account.

Although ethical reasoning is principle based and has the client's well-being at the center, being involved in ethical problems and dilemmas is stressful for the nurse. The nurse may feel torn among obligations to the client, the family, and the employer. What is in the client's best interest might be contrary to the nurse's personal belief system. In settings in which ethical issues arise frequently, nurses should establish support systems such as team conferences and use of counseling professionals to allow expression of their feelings.

Many nursing problems are not moral problems at all; they are simply questions of good nursing practice. An important first step in ethical decision making is to

Box 44–4 Examples of Nurses' Obligations When Making Ethical Decisions

- Maximize the client's well-being.
- Balance the client's need for autonomy with family members' responsibilities for the client's well-being.
- Support each family member and enhance the family support system.
- Carry out hospital policies.
- Protect other clients' well-being.
- Protect the nurse's own standards of care.

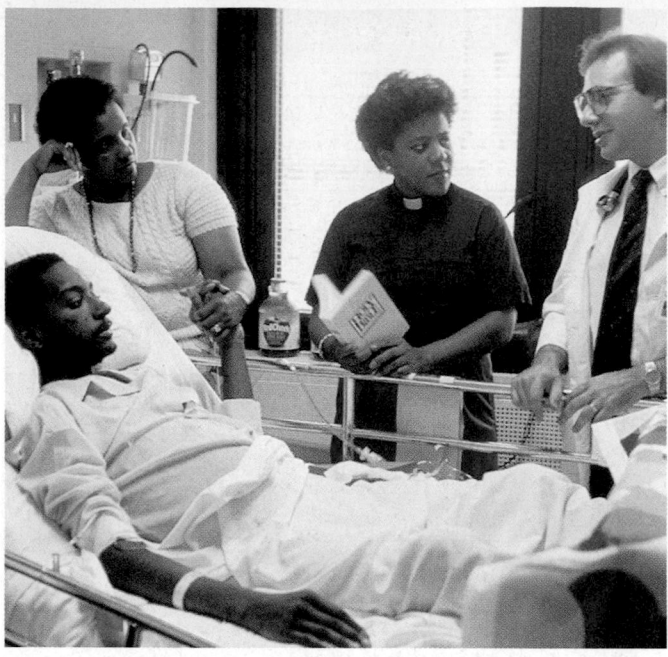

Figure 44–1 ● When there is a need for ethical decisions with regard to client advocacy, many different people contribute to the final outcome.

Source: A. Ramey/PhotoEdit, Inc.

determine whether a moral dilemma exists. The following criteria may be used:

- A difficult choice exists between actions that conflict with the needs of one or more individuals.
- Moral principles or frameworks exist that can be used to provide some justification for the action.
- The choice is guided by a process of weighing reasons.
- The decision is freely and consciously chosen.
- The choice is affected by personal feelings and by the particular context of the situation.

Although the nurse's input is important, in reality several people are usually involved in making an ethical decision. The client, family, spiritual support persons, and other members of the healthcare team work together in reaching ethical decisions (see **Figure 44–1 ●**). Therefore, collaboration, communication, and compromise are important skills for health professionals.

▶ STRATEGIES TO ENHANCE ETHICAL DECISIONS AND PRACTICE

Several strategies help nurses overcome possible organizational and social constraints that can hinder the ethical practice of nursing and create moral distress for nurses. Nurses should do the following:

- Become aware of their own values and the ethical aspects of nursing.
- Be familiar with nursing codes of ethics.

- Seek continuing education opportunities to stay knowledgeable about ethical issues in nursing.
- Respect the values, opinions, and responsibilities of other healthcare professionals that may be different from your own.
- Participate in or establish ethics rounds. Ethics rounds use hypothetical or real cases that focus on the ethical dimensions of client care rather than the client's clinical diagnosis and treatment.
- Serve on institutional ethics committees.
- Strive for collaborative practice in which nurses function effectively in cooperation with other healthcare professionals.

One resource that is available to help nurses maintain a current, evidence-based ethical practice is the National Guideline Clearinghouse. The clearinghouse provides an index to more than 2,000 guidelines for evidence-based practice on a number of health issues, including ethical issues. For example, the Hartford Institute of Geriatric Nursing has developed a number of evidence-based nursing protocols for working with older clients. These protocols address topics such as advance directives and healthcare decision making, working with older adults with dementia, and discussing sexual health with the older adult (National Guideline Clearinghouse, 2010).

Stay Current: *Visit the Web site of the National Guideline Clearinghouse at* **www.guideline.gov**.

Ethical dilemmas can occur in the normal provision of care. The frequency of ethical dilemmas was reported as being negatively correlated with the level of nursing skills (Dekeyser Ganz & Berkovitz, 2012). In effect, this study found that the less experienced nurses are, the more likely they are to experience ethical dilemmas. Seeking advice from a mentor or more experienced peer can facilitate effective solutions and approaches to perceived ethical challenges.

One strategy that hospitals and other organizations have used to enhance ethical decision making is to implement a multidisciplinary ethics committee. Ethical standards of the Joint Commission (Joint Commission, 2013a) mandate that healthcare institutions provide ethics committees or a similar structure to write guidelines and policies and to provide education, counseling, and support on ethical issues. These multidisciplinary committees, which include nurses, physicians, and hospital administrators, can be asked to review a case and provide guidance to a competent client, an incompetent client's family, or to a healthcare provider. These committees provide a forum in which diverse views can be expressed, support is provided for caregivers, and the institution's legal risks can be reduced (see the exemplar on Risk Management in the module on Legal Issues).

CASE STUDY \\ PART 2

After June D'Angelo received her IV hypertension medication, she told both her nurse and the physician that she felt much better, "as she had last time." The ED physician asked the nurse to stay by the bedside as he discussed with Ms. D'Angelo his phone conversation with her primary healthcare provider. The main issue is that Ms. D'Angelo has missed her appointments with the provider and has not gotten her prescription updated. The ED physician suggested that Ms. D'Angelo collaborate with her own healthcare provider to prevent further ED visits due to her hypertension and headaches. To have this work well, the nurse asked Ms. D'Angelo what the barriers were to her trusting and collaborating with her healthcare provider. Ms. D'Angelo said that her main worry was that her blood pressure would be so high that she would miss work and need to see the physician too many times. The physician told Ms. D'Angelo that he wanted her to take responsibility for her own well-being and then asked the clinical specialist nurse to meet with Ms. D'Angelo to prepare her outpatient blood pressure management. Before Ms. D'Angelo was discharged from the ED, she was given a calendar listing her next two outpatient appointments and a new blood pressure prescription.

Clinical Thinking Questions

1. Why was it important for the nurse to ask Ms. D'Angelo what the barriers were to her outpatient care management?

2. How did the discussion at D'Angelo's bedside maximize her well-being?

3. How did the nurse and clinical specialist nurse assist the client's need for autonomy?

| REVIEW **The Concept of Ethics**

RELATE Link the Concepts

Linking the concept of ethics with the concept of addiction:

1. How does substance abuse affect an individual's ability to make ethical decisions based on his or her personal values and beliefs?

2. What parts of the ANA Code of Ethics for Nurses address impaired nurses?

Linking the concept of ethics with the concept of reproduction:

3. What are your personal beliefs about fertility treatments? How would you feel toward a client who has conceived multiple fetuses through fertility treatments and now wants to have selective reduction to reduce the number of children she will carry to term?

4. As a nurse, what are your responsibilities to the teenager seeking information on birth control methods?

REFER Go to Pearson Nursing Student Resources
nursing.pearsonhighered.com

- Additional review materials
- Additional case study

REFLECT Case Study \\ Part 3

Reread Parts 1 and 2 of the case study. Before the end of the shift, another staff member in the ED asked the nurse to pick

4. Analyze how the discussion at the client's bedside was an example of collaborative practice in which nurses function effectively in cooperation with other healthcare professionals.

▶ CONCLUSION

The ANA Code of Ethics outlines the ethical standards that nurses are expected to use to inform their behavior toward clients and their families, other nurses and healthcare professionals, and the larger community. Ethical standards do not fall solely within the realm of the nursing profession. No one profession is responsible for ethical decisions, nor does expertise in one discipline, such as nursing, necessarily make an individual an expert in ethics.

As discussed, determining whether or not a moral problem exists is the first step in ethical decision making. The nursing profession has identified a number of ethical dilemmas that nurses face in a variety of settings. Nursing students as well as professional nurses should examine their values related to these identified dilemmas and understand how their values may impact their own professional nursing practice. Several of the dilemmas are discussed in Exemplar 44.1.

up the phone. As soon as she said hello, a woman asked her, "Did June D'Angelo come to your emergency department earlier today?" The nurse immediately realized that this would become a HIPAA issue if she did not manage this carefully and correctly. She asked the woman, "Who is calling, please?" The woman groaned loudly and said, "This is Mrs. Jones. I am June's supervisor where she works, and I need to know if she was there today." The nurse answered, "Mrs. Jones, I am sorry but due to privacy rules we cannot discuss any client information or names on the phone and cannot confirm whether any client was or was not in our department." Mrs. Jones become upset and stated, "Then how can I know what is going on? She missed her shift today!" The nurse remained calm and said, "My best suggestion is that you contact your employee directly yourself." Mrs. Jones hung up.

Clinical Thinking Questions

1. How did the nurse realize that this was a possible HIPAA issue?

2. What privacy and confidentiality rules and ethical guidelines was the nurse following?

3. Do you think the nurse managed the call correctly?

4. If the nurse had said yes to the first question asked by Mrs. Jones, what would she have violated?

EXEMPLAR 44.1 **Ethical Dilemmas**

EXEMPLAR KEY TERMS

Active euthanasia, *2574*
Assisted suicide, *2574*
Bioethics, *2572*
Euthanasia, *2574*
Withdrawing or withholding life-sustaining
    therapy (WWLST), *2574*

EXEMPLAR LEARNING OUTCOMES

After reading about this exemplar, you will be able to:

1. Propose solutions to ethical dilemmas based on an individual's problem and ethical principles.

2. Analyze conflicts among nursing loyalties and obligations to clients, families, the multidisciplinary team, and outside organizations.

3. Critique the bioethical dilemmas that may arise during the care of clients and families.

4. Explore the nurse's role in supporting clients' rights to information and counseling when making genetic testing decisions.

5. Analyze the challenges and dilemmas clients and their families face when managing end-of-life care choices, advance directives, euthanasia, and the withdrawal of life support.

▶ OVERVIEW

An ethical dilemma exists when two or more rights, values, obligations, or responsibilities come in conflict. Conflict may arise between the nurse's personal values and those of another individual or the organization, between principles and the need to achieve a desired outcome, or between two or more individuals or groups to whom one has an obligation, such as the client, a colleague, the nurse's profession, the nurse's employer, and society (Dekeyser Ganz & Berkovitz, 2012; Lachman, 2012).

Rapidly changing technology, conflicting societal and cultural values, conflicting loyalties and obligations among nurses, increasing pressure to contain healthcare costs, and reduced staffing are some of the factors that contribute to the development of ethical dilemmas in nursing.

Social and Technological Changes

Technology creates new issues that did not exist in earlier times. Before monitors, respirators, and intravenous (IV) or artificial tube feedings, there was no question about whether to "allow" an 800-gram premature infant to die. Before organ transplantation, death did not require a legal definition that might still permit viable tissues to be removed and given to other living individuals. Advances in the ability to decode and control the growth of tissues through gene manipulation present new potential ethical dilemmas related to cloning organisms and altering the course of hereditary diseases and biological characteristics. Today, with treatments that can prolong and enhance biological life, these questions arise: Should we do what we know we can? Who should be treated—everyone, only those who can pay, only those who have a chance to improve? Who decides who receives treatment?

Conflicting Loyalties and Obligations

Because of their unique position in the healthcare system, nurses experience conflicts among their loyalties and obligations to clients, families, primary care providers, employing institutions, and licensing bodies. Client needs may conflict with institutional policies, primary care provider preferences, needs of the client's family, or even state or federal laws. According to the ANA Code of Ethics for Nurses (2001), the nurse's first loyalty is to the client. However, it is not always easy to determine which action best serves the client's needs. For instance, the nurse may be aware that marijuana has been shown to be effective for a condition a client has that has not responded to mainstream therapies. Although legal issues are involved, the nurse must determine whether, ethically, the client should be made aware of a potentially effective alternative. Sehiralti and Er (2013) examined psychiatric nurses' decisions surrounding clients' difficulty in making the right decision. Another example is individual nurses' decisions regarding whether to honor picket lines during employee strikes. The nurse may experience conflict among feeling the need to support coworkers in their efforts to improve working conditions, feeling the need to ensure that clients receive care and are not abandoned, and feeling loyalty to the nurse's employer.

The nurse must recognize ethical dilemmas and take appropriate action as discussed in this exemplar. This includes informing the client and other staff members of ethical issues affecting the client's care, practicing within a manner consistent with the ANA Code of Ethics for registered nurses, recognizing and managing ethical challenges, and evaluating the outcomes of interventions taken to promote ethical practice.

▶ BIOETHICAL ISSUES

Bioethics refers to ethics as applied to human life or health. Bioethical dilemmas may arise during the care of clients and families dealing with HIV/AIDS, genetic testing, abortion, organ transplantation, and end-of-life decisions.

Acquired Immune Deficiency Syndrome (AIDS)

Because of its association with sexual behavior and illicit drug use, AIDS bears a social stigma (De Bruyn, 2012). According to an ANA position statement, the nurse cannot set aside the moral obligation to care for the client infected with HIV unless the risk exceeds the responsibility (ANA, 2006).

Other ethical issues center on testing for HIV status and the presence of AIDS in healthcare professionals and clients. Questions arise as to whether testing of all providers and clients should be mandatory or voluntary and whether test results should be released to insurance companies, sexual partners, or caregivers. As with all ethical dilemmas, each possibility has both positive and negative implications for specific individuals. The HIV/AIDS field is addressing how legal and policy restrictions affect access to health promotion and care, particularly around HIV, unwanted pregnancy, and abortion (De Bruyn, 2012).

Genetic Testing

Related to the chronic illness field of care are the difficult decisions families must make regarding genetic testing findings. This is particularly difficult for clients with cancer or with potential cancer diagnoses that result from an inherited genetic predisposition. Genetic testing can also present dilemmas for pregnant clients who may want to consider the possible need for an abortion or other options.

The increasing prominence of genetics in the media is contributing to growing awareness among families and clients that conditions may be inherited, so they are asking more questions of the nurses caring for them. Hospice nurses regularly work with clients suffering from diseases caused by an inherited genetic predisposition. Developments in clinical genetics have consequences for the provision of nursing care and support,

Evidence-Based Practice   How Do Hospice Nurses Perceive the Importance of Genetics to Hospice Care?

Problem

During hospice care, hospice nurses may need to provide support to both clients and families affected by conditions known to have genetic predisposition. It is therefore important for hospice nurses to increase their confidence in carrying out genetics related activities within an end-of-life care context.

Evidence

Metcalfe and colleagues (2010) designed a study to determine hospice nurses' perception of the importance of genetics to hospice care provision and their personal level of confidence in carrying out genetics-related activities within an end-of-life care context.

Using a survey method, questionnaires were sent to a stratified sample of hospice nurses (n = 1149) in England and Wales. Using Likert scales, nurses were asked to rate the importance of, and their confidence in, undertaking a range of scenario-based activities that accompany caring for a client and family affected by a genetic condition in the hospice setting. Open questions invited comments on their experiences of nursing clients and families in similar situations. Follow-up telephone interviews with hospice nurse educators were carried out to explore emerging issues.

The response rate was 29% (n = 328). Hospice nurses felt that all aspects of genetics-related care were "very important"

to hospice care, but they lacked confidence in their ability to carry out the activities. Many respondents had not considered the relevance of genetics to hospice care prior to completing the questionnaire but now considered it essential to end-of-life care even if they were not confident in providing it.

Implications

This study highlights the genetics education needs of hospice nurses in providing end-of life care for clients and their families affected by inherited genetic conditions. Hospice nurses' need genetics education focusing on the psychosocial implications of caring for clients and families affected by genetic conditions to enable them to provide complex care and support in the face of the difficult issues that arise in practice.

Critical Thinking Application

1. In this study, hospice nurses found genetics important to their practice but lacked the confidence to discuss genetics with clients and families. What steps can these nurses take to increase their confidence surrounding this issue?

2. While not discussed in this particular study, from the authors' findings, what role should the hospice program take to utilize evidence-based guidelines to assist nurses when discussing genetics with clients and families?

including the need for nurses to consider different approaches to their assessment, planning, and interventions (Metcalfe, Pumphrey, & Clifford, 2010). Nurses working in end-of-life care need to be able to recognize the implications and emotions for both clients and families with regard to the effects of, and risk from, inherited genetic conditions. The nursing code of ethics supports clients' rights to information and counseling in making genetic testing decisions.

Working with individuals who are seeking information about genetic testing for themselves or for their children has become a particularly new and interesting ethical challenge for the nurse. Nurses working in pediatrics and in clinics that serve clients facing testing for inherited illnesses should examine their beliefs and values about genetic testing. They should also know the legal requirements of their state; for example, does their state require parental consent for a minor to seek genetic testing and counseling?

Organ Transplantation

Organs for transplantation may come from living donors or from donors who have just died. Many living people choose to become donors by giving consent under the Uniform Anatomical Gift Act. Ethical issues related to organ transplantation include allocation of organs, selling of body parts, involvement of children both as potential donors and recipients, consent, clear definition of death, and conflicts of interest between potential donors and recipients (Guy et al., 2013). In some situations, an individual's religious beliefs may also present conflict. For example, certain religions forbid the mutilation of the body, even for the benefit of another individual.

Stay Current: For more information on how donor kidneys from deceased individuals are allocated for transplant, visit the Web site of the United Network for Organ Sharing (UNOS) at **www.unos.org/donation/index.php?topic=organ_allocation**.

End-of-Life Issues

Advances in technology and the growing number of older adults have expanded the ethical dilemmas faced by older adults and the healthcare professionals who work with them. Providing these clients with information and professional assistance, as well as the highest quality of care and caring, is of the utmost importance. Some of the most frequent disturbing ethical problems for nurses involve issues that arise around death and dying. These include euthanasia, assisted suicide, termination of life-sustaining treatment, and withdrawing or withholding of food and fluids.

Compounding these issues and despite increasing interests and urgent needs for high-quality end-of-life care, there is no exact definition of the interval that is referred to as "end of life" or consensus on what end-of-life care is (Izumi et al., 2012). Nurses must learn to assist clients and families to discuss their options surrounding terminal care. Current definitions related to end-of-life care are often based on the time to death and stage of illness. If end-of-life care is framed only by the brief interval of time before death, clients are at risk of being left without receiving adequate end-of-life care because time frames are not always well predicted (Izumi et al., 2012). Nurses who have learned to see a client's life as a whole are better situated to understand the client's condition and concerns and guide the client and family to examine and prepare for end of life (Watts, 2013). "In order for nurses to identify these people and provide the care they need, end-of-life care should not be defined from a medical perspective based on a terminal illness but from the nursing perspective based on a broader view of life and journey toward the inevitable end of life" (Izumi et al., 2012, p. 614).

ADVANCE DIRECTIVES   Many moral problems surrounding the end of life can be resolved if clients complete advance directives. Currently, all 50 states have enacted advance directive legislation. Advance directives are legal documents representing a client's end-of-life decisions; they may include how clients want medical decisions to be made or whom they would like to make those decisions (Cohen & Nirenberg, 2011). Advance directives instruct caregivers as to the client's wishes about treatments, providing an ongoing voice for clients when they have lost the capacity to make or communicate their decisions. See the module on Legal Issues, and the exemplar on End-of-Life Care in the module on Comfort, for more information about advance directives. An advance directive may provide instructions regarding do-not-resuscitate (DNR) orders, the withholding of emergency measures to sustain life, the termination of life-sustaining measures, or any combination thereof. Nurses working with clients who are experiencing life-threatening events or who are approaching the end of life should make sure they understand the client's advance directive as well as the policies and procedures regarding advance directives at their place of employment.

EUTHANASIA AND ASSISTED SUICIDE   Euthanasia, a Greek word meaning "good death," is popularly known as "mercy killing." Active euthanasia involves taking actions to bring about a client's death directly, with or without client consent (Johnstone, 2012b). An example of this would be the administration of a lethal dose of medication to end the client's suffering. Regardless of the caregiver's intent, active euthanasia is forbidden by law and can result in criminal charges against the individual who brings about the client's death.

A variation of active euthanasia is assisted suicide, or giving clients the means to kill themselves if they request it (e.g., providing pills or a weapon). Some countries and some states have laws permitting assisted suicide for clients who are severely ill, who are near death, and who wish to commit suicide. Although some people may disagree with the concept, in January 2006, the U.S. Supreme Court upheld the assisted suicide regulations in the state of Oregon. In any case, the nurse should recall that legality and morality are not the same thing. Determining whether an action is legal is only one aspect of deciding whether it is ethical. The questions of suicide and assisted suicide are still controversial in our society. The ANA's position statement on assisted suicide (ANA, 2013b) states that performing active euthanasia and participating in assisted suicide violate the ANA Code of Ethics for Nurses.

WITHDRAWING OR WITHHOLDING LIFE-SUSTAINING TREATMENT   Withdrawing or withholding life-sustaining therapy (WWLST) involves the withdrawal of extraordinary means of life support, such as removing a ventilator or withholding special attempts to revive a client, and allowing the client to die of the underlying medical condition (e.g.,

aspiration pneumonia). WWLST is both legally and ethically more acceptable to most people than assisted suicide or euthanasia (Brus, 2010).

Antibiotics, organ transplants, and technological advances (e.g., ventilators) help to prolong life but do not necessarily restore health. Clients may specify that they wish to have life-sustaining measures terminated, they may have advance directives on this matter, or they may appoint a healthcare surrogate to make the decision on their behalf. Regardless, it is usually more troubling for healthcare professionals to withdraw a treatment than to decide initially not to begin it. Nurses must understand that a decision to withdraw treatment is not a decision to withdraw care. As the primary caregivers, nurses must ensure that sensitive care and comfort measures (palliative care) are given as the client's illness progresses after withdrawal of treatment. When the client is at home, nurses often provide this type of education and support through hospice services (see the module on Comfort for more information regarding hospice and end-of-life care).

Because it is difficult for families to withdraw treatment, it is very important that they fully understand the client's treatment (Brus, 2010). Families often misunderstand which treatments are life sustaining. Keeping clients and families well informed is an ongoing process, and it is important to keep in mind that they need time to ask questions and discuss the situation. It is also essential for clients and families to understand that they can reevaluate and change their decision if they wish.

Nurses provide ethical care to dying clients and their families by respecting the clients' autonomy, by providing culturally competent care, and by providing nursing presence.

WITHDRAWING OR WITHHOLDING FOOD AND FLUIDS
It is generally accepted that providing food and fluids is part of ordinary nursing practice and, therefore, a moral duty. However, some people consider it an extraordinary measure to administer food and fluids by tube to a dying client or to administer them over a long period to an unconscious client who is not expected to improve. A nurse is morally obligated to withhold food and fluids (or any treatment) if it is determined to be more harmful to administer them than to withhold them. The nurse must also honor competent and informed clients' refusal of food and fluids. The ANA Code of Ethics for Nurses (2001) supports this position through the nurse's role as a client advocate and through the moral principle of autonomy.

CLINICAL EXAMPLE

Bobby Wolfe is a 14-year-old client with cancer who is refusing chemotherapy after becoming very ill and weak after his first round of chemo. His oncologist has made it very clear that he has a 90% chance of being cured if he undergoes chemotherapy followed by radiation, and an equal chance that he will die without it. Although not Native American, his parents follow the practices of Nemenhah, a Native American religious organization that advocates using "natural medicine" for curing illness. Bobby is adamant that he does not want any more chemotherapy. His parents state that he was in "better health" before the first chemo treatment and that is proof that the chemo is bad for him. When asked what the parents intended to do if Bobby's cancer metastasizes, the Wolfes say they will discuss that with Bobby in the unlikely event that that happens.

1. What ethical dilemmas can you identify in this situation?
2. What is the nurse's responsibility regarding addressing these dilemmas?
3. What, if any, action should the hospital take regarding Bobby's treatment? Why?

▶ ETHICAL ISSUES IN NURSING PRACTICE

Nursing is the undisputed leader in the list of professions viewed as honest and ethical. Nursing has been ranked first among all professions in all but 1 year since it was added to the list in 1999 (ANA, 2010). While nurses are perceived as being honest and ethical, their identity as moral agents is shaped by contextual and organizational forces. Patricia Benner (Benner, Kyriakidis, & Stannard, 2011) describes how shifts in governmental and corporate healthcare values profoundly influence nurses' ability to exercise their moral agency at the level of practice. While biomedical ethicists have tended to focus on high-profile medical cases, the nursing profession has identified the need for more models of practice that deal with situations that nurses confront on a daily basis.

Ethical behavior is the day-to-day expression of one's commitment to other individuals and the ways in which human beings relate to one another in their daily interaction (Levine, 1977). Some everyday ethical challenges identified by nurses were cate-

gorized in a classical publication by Varcoe and colleagues (2004) as working the "in-betweens." Nurses identify being caught in between various players including healthcare providers and the client and between the client and the family. Nurses are also caught between family members, between staff members, and between managers and various other colleagues. Within these relationships there are conflicting loyalties. Nurses must constantly balance loyalties to the client, family, employer, profession, and community.

Nurses also identify conflicts arising from traditional power structures in health care such as the focus on providing curative treatment and the emphasis on the role of the physician. For example, nurses have expressed concerns about being intimidated or dismissed by physicians when reporting observations incongruent with the proposed medical treatment plan or being ignored by senior medical staff when reporting concerns related to physician behavior. Additional conflict arises when operating under staffing shortages or other situations in which organizational efficiency is at issue (Iglesias & De Bengoa Vallego, 2012). Nurses who must balance limited time available with care that needs to be provided operate in such states of conflict. Frequently the activities that suffer the most include client teaching, counseling, and support as the nurse's focus moves to the performance of physical tasks and functions. Nurses reporting conflict with corporate values have experienced being threatened by administrators and fear of job and license loss. Important resources for ethical practice that have been identified are supportive colleagues, educators, and approachable responsible managers. Nurses have reported that having the opportunity to discuss ethical concerns is both personally and professionally sustaining (Johnstone, 2012a).

Lifespan Considerations Ethical Dilemmas and Pediatric Clients

Organ Transplantation
Ethical concerns regarding organ transplantation and allocation for children came to the forefront of national discussions in 2013 when the parents of a 10-year-old girl with cystic fibrosis filed a lawsuit in federal court asking that the Organ Procurement and Transplant Network (OPTN) be forced to add their daughter to the list of patients eligible to receive adult lungs. A federal judge ordered OPTN to make an exception to the existing rule, which states that children under 12 may not receive adult organs. Following subsequent direction from the Secretary of the Department of Health and Human Services, OPTN granted the exception, and the child subsequently received two adult lung transplants (the first transplant failed).

Withdrawing or Withholding Life-Sustaining Treatment (WWLST)
Making decisions regarding WWLST can be especially difficult when the client is an infant, child, or adolescent. When discussing the withdrawal or withholding of medical treatment for pediatric clients with their parents, it is critical to provide complete, clear information regarding their child's condition, prognosis, degree of pain and suffering, and potential for quality of life (Kendall & Guo, 2008; Racine & Shevell, 2009).

When working with pediatric clients, healthcare providers also follow the requirements of the Child Abuse and Treatment Act of 1984, which deemed withholding of medically

indicated treatment as child abuse except in those cases when providing care is futile; that is, in cases where the treatments will not provide any clear clinical benefit (Ball, Bindler, & Cowen, 2012). Although it is rare for parents to refuse a medically indicated treatment that may benefit their child, the decision can be exceedingly difficult in cases where the proposed treatment itself carries a high degree of risk, such as an organ transplant or major surgery.

Child Rights vs. Parent Rights
Parents have the authority to make healthcare decisions for their children. Dilemmas arise when parents and children do not agree on whether or not to go forward with a recommended treatment. In most cases, the nurse and other members of the healthcare team who have developed a therapeutic alliance with the child and family may be able to help the family come to a joint decision by providing additional information and opportunity to discuss their concerns with each other calmly and openly. In some cases, however, the healthcare team may need to seek guidance from its agency's ethics committee. When there is a potential conflict of interest (e.g., suspected child abuse and neglect), other measures may be necessary to provide appropriate care for the pediatric client, up to and including obtaining a court order determining the child is able to make her own decision or an order assigning decisions regarding the child's care to an individual or entity (e.g., the Department of Child Services) other than the parent.

Focus on Diversity and Culture Variations in Applying Moral Principles

Although a moral principle may exist and be valued in different cultures, the degree to which it is valued and the manner by which it is used in health care may be quite variable. Nurses must become familiar with how moral principles are viewed within the various cultural groups with which they practice.

PRINCIPLE	EXAMPLES OF ETHNIC/CULTURAL VARIATIONS
Autonomy	Family members, rather than the client, receive information on the client's condition and take primary responsibility for decision making. The family and community are viewed as affected by the client's condition and decisions as much as the individual is affected: Chinese, Koreans, Mexican Americans, Bosnian Americans.
Veracity	The client and/or family prefer that the client not to be told directly of a life-threatening condition: Hispanics, Asians, Pakistanis, Bosnian Americans, Italian Americans, Canadian Aboriginals.
Nonmaleficence	Discussion of advance directives and issues such as cardiopulmonary resuscitation are viewed as physically and emotionally harmful to the client: Filipino, Native American, Chinese.
Beneficence	Healthcare providers should promote clients' well-being and hope: Asian cultures, Native Americans, Russians.

Sources: Based on Ellerby, J. H., McKenzie, J., McKay, S., Gariepy, G. J., & Kaufert, J. M. (2000). Bioethics for clinicians: 18. Aboriginal cultures. *Canadian Medical Association Journal, 163,* 845–850; Kai, J., Beavan, J., & Faull, C. (2011). Challenges of mediated communication, disclosure and patient autonomy in cross-cultural cancer care. *British Journal of Cancer, 105,* 918–924; Morgan, A., & Burgess, S. (2012). Judging a patient's decision to seek emergency healthcare: Clues for managing increasing patient demand. *Australian Health Review, 36,* 110–114; and Parveen, S., Morrison, V., & Robinson, C. (2011). Ethnic variations in the caregiver role: A qualitative study. *Journal of Health Psychology, 16*(6), 862–872.

Patricia Benner has identified the behavior of nurses as being shaped by their organizational and professional roles and the settings in which they work and that their responses to ethical problems are inseparable from the settings in which they arise. The Carnegie study of nursing education (Benner et al., 2010) demonstrated that clinical experiences (including pre- and postclinical conferences) of nursing students were strong in developing essential ethical behaviors when compared to the clinical experiences of other professions. The ethical behaviors examined included meeting the client as an individual, preserving the dignity and personhood of clients, how to respond to substandard practice related to client advocacy, learning to do "good" nursing practice, and how to be present with client and family suffering. Benner identified the need for nursing students to learn social ethics and for greater emphasis on the role of the nurse as advocate, as traditional classroom teaching emphasizes bioethics and has been critical of the effects of developing technology and the ethics of its use.

Academic Dishonesty

Through reading, class time, and clinical experiences, nursing students can begin to imagine some aspects of ethical decision making in the clinical context. With increased experience and exposure, each student can identify increasing conflicting values and variables that affect the practicing nurse. The development of professional ethical behavior, social roles, and responsibilities builds on the individual's personal ethics. Ethical decision making is a situational or contextual process. Academic dishonesty presents ethical situations that nursing students may confront early in their ethical development (Kececi et al., 2011). Examples of academic dishonesty include cheating, plagiarism, and failure to follow academic policies, such as the requirement to return examinations following a test review session (Olafsen et al., 2013). See the clinical example that follows and **Box 44–5** ●.

CLINICAL EXAMPLE

Elizabeth, a first-year nursing student, has obtained a copy of the first examination given last year in Nursing 110 from Jasmine, her assigned "Big Sister" from the second-year class. Jasmine emphasized that questions on nursing examinations are particularly hard to answer because they require application of information, not just recall. Elizabeth informs her selected study group that she has the exam and is willing to share it to help them focus their study time. You are a member of Elizabeth's study group.

1. Will you participate? Why or why not?
2. Will you report Elizabeth to your instructor? Why or why not?
3. What ethical principle is involved in your decision process?
4. What conflicting values are involved in this scenario?
5. What additional information might help you make your decision? What difference does it make if you learn that Jasmine did not turn in the exam following a test review session?
6. What school policies are involved? What aspects of the ANA Code of Ethics apply?

In a personal ethical dilemma, the decision is made by the individual based on the individual's values and best interests (Lachman, 2012). The individual will be primarily accountable for the consequences of that action, including those affecting others. This is in direct contrast to a professional ethical dilemma in which the decision should reflect the autonomy of the client and in which the nurse is accountable to the client's values and best interests.

Workplace Issues

Financial restraints, personnel issues, and other organizational challenges can contribute to ethical conflicts in the workplace.

Box 44–5   An Exercise in Ethical Decision Making

Refer to the clinical example of Elizabeth and Jasmine when answering the following questions:

1. *Identify a range of actions with potential outcomes.*
   What are the pros? What are the cons?
   If you choose to participate in the study group and then inform the instructor?
   If you choose to participate and not tell the instructor?
   If you choose not to participate and not tell the instructor?
   If you choose not to participate and to tell the instructor?

2. *Decide on a course of action and carry it out.*
   So what are you going to decide?
   On what do you base your decision?
   What does your decision tell others about you and your values?
   Does your decision predict future decisions/actions?

3. *Evaluate/reevaluate the consequences of your decision/action.*
   What tools would you use to evaluate your decision/action after the fact?
   How would you determine what effect your decision/action had on others?

Limited resources and short staffing are two ethical challenges that nurses frequently face in the workplace.

ALLOCATION OF LIMITED HEALTH RESOURCES

Allocation of limited supplies of healthcare goods and services, including organs suitable for transplantation, artificial joints, and the services of specialists, has become an especially urgent issue as healthcare costs continue to rise and more stringent cost containment measures are implemented. The moral principle of autonomy cannot be applied if it is not possible to give each client what he or she chooses. In these situations, healthcare providers may use the principle of justice by attempting to choose what is most fair to all. Nurses, other healthcare professionals, legislators, and clients must continue to look for ways to balance economics and care in the allocation of health resources. For more information on resource allocation in health care, see the modules on Managing Care and Healthcare Systems.

SHORT STAFFING

With a nationwide shortage of nurses, nursing care is becoming a limited health resource. Short staffing is a critical concern because a number of studies link staffing levels to safe client care (AACN, 2010). Unfortunately, some facilities continue to staff nursing units with fewer registered nurses and more unlicensed caregivers. When this occurs, nurses become concerned that staffing in their institutions is not adequate to ensure client safety, much less to allow them to provide the level of care that they value. California is the only state that has enacted legislation mandating specific nurse-to-client ratios in hospitals and other healthcare settings (Schultz, 2013). This is not the simple solution that it seems: Another ethical dilemma arises when organizations begin to turn away clients in need in order to ensure adequate staffing levels.

CLINICAL EXAMPLE

The director of nursing is having difficulty staffing all the units adequately. Two units have already been closed. The director can either spread the available staff around the facility and keep the remaining units open, but with fewer nurses than is really safe, or close more units. The director needs to consider the welfare of the institution, the nursing staff, and the clients.

1. How would you assess the ethical aspects of this issue?
2. What actions would you take? Why?
3. How does the ANA Code of Ethics inform the possible actions?

Working With Clients and Families

Working with clients and families can be both rewarding and challenging. Clear communication and good clinical decision-making skills help the nurse develop a positive relationship with clients and their families. Ethical challenges that may arise include maintaining client privacy and confidentiality and ensuring client autonomy.

CLIENT PRIVACY AND CONFIDENTIALITY   In keeping with the principle of autonomy, nurses are obligated to respect clients' privacy and confidentiality. Privacy is both a legal and an ethical mandate. The Health Insurance Portability and Accountability Act of 1996 (HIPAA) includes standards protecting the confidentiality, integrity, and availability of data and standards defining appropriate disclosures of identifiable health information and patient rights protection (see the module on Legal Issues). Clients must be able to trust that nurses will reveal details of the clients' situations only as appropriate and will communicate only the information necessary to provide for their health care. Computerized client records make sensitive data accessible to more people and make issues of confidentiality more complex and more important. Nurses should help develop and follow security measures and policies to ensure appropriate use of client data (see the modules on Informatics and Communication).

CLIENT AUTONOMY   Nurses have an ethical obligation as well as a legal mandate to respect the right of each client to make his or her own decisions regarding healthcare treatment (Pagura, 2011). It is not uncommon for nurses to come across situations in which the client's autonomy is at risk. In these situations, the nurse has an ethical obligation to advocate for the client's right to make his or her own healthcare decisions, whether or not the risk comes in the form of a well-meaning family member who disagrees with the client's decision or a physician or other healthcare provider who either fails to hear the client's concerns or disagrees with the client's request or decision (Rasmussen, 2012).

▶ COPING WITH ETHICAL DILEMMAS

Ethical dilemmas occur frequently in everyday clinical practice. They represent situations in which healthcare professionals are torn among several competing ways of thinking that may affect their decision making in certain cases (Sorta-Bilajac et al., 2011). Nurses are vulnerable to being blindsided by ethical dilemmas and often find themselves asking, "Why did I not see this coming?" Several ethical decision-making models have been proposed to assist the practitioner, once that practitioner realizes he or she is in the middle of an ethical conundrum.

However a model may not be available when needed, or it may not consider the underlying values of both the practitioner and the client in the dilemma (Crowley & Gottlieb, 2012).

A primary risk management model has been developed to assist clinical staff in managing ethical decisions. The model includes the following:

- **Resource accumulation.** Involves acquiring the requisite resources and skills prior to the occurrence of a stressor.
- **Time.** "Free time" relieves pressure and anxiety and allows us to better perceive the subtle cues that can alert us to potential ethical dilemmas.

- **Education.** In addition to following the ANA Code of Ethics in ethical situations, education and didactic training represent another source for developing primary risk management skills.
- **Organization and planning.** Organizational and planning skills may be taught and modeled in staff training in the hope that students will continue these practices throughout their careers.
- **Peer support and consultation.** A practitioner's professional network, consisting of peers, supervisors, and colleagues, can be a significant resource for primary prevention of ethical challenges (Crowley & Gottlieb, 2012, pp. 67–68).

REVIEW Ethical Dilemmas

RELATE Link the Concepts and Exemplars

Linking the exemplar of ethical dilemmas with the concept of legal issues.

1. What are your personal beliefs concerning advance directive planning for any client who has a chronic illness, such as a cardiac illness, diabetes, or renal failure, regardless of the client's age?

2. What is the nurse's role in discussing future care plans, such as end-of-life care, with chronically ill clients?

Linking the exemplar of ethical dilemmas with the concept of comfort.

3. What are your personal beliefs surrounding ensuring comfort for clients with chronic pain?

4. Assess your understanding of pain management options to ensure comfort. What are your personal beliefs regarding the use of high-level narcotics for clients?

REFER Go to Pearson Nursing Student Resources nursing.pearsonhighered.com

- Additional review materials

REFLECT Case Study

David Lewis is a 50-year-old African American male who is recovering from a stroke at a rehabilitation facility. He is medi-

cally stable and able to participate fully in his therapies. However, he has requested DNR (do-not-resuscitate) status. He reasons that if he has another stroke or cardiac arrest, he could lose much more cognitive and motor function and then if he were resuscitated, it would place too heavy a burden of care on his family. Day after day he and his family ask about the DNR order. The nurses working with Mr. Lewis repeatedly ask the attending physician for an order, and the physician continues to respond that Mr. Lewis does not need a DNR order—he is stable. Finally, the primary nurse goes to the facility's ethics committee to discuss the problem. This results in another physician reviewing the chart, speaking with the client and family, and entering the DNR order.

1. What ethical dilemma did the primary nurse working with Mr. Lewis face?

2. What principles did the primary nurse follow in going to the ethics council?

3. How do you feel about DNR orders? Why?

4. In what ways did the nurses working with Mr. Lewis advocate on his behalf? How is the nurse's role as an advocate related to nursing ethics?

EXEMPLAR 44.2 Patient Rights

EXEMPLAR KEY TERMS
Patient responsibilities, *2580*
Patient rights, *2578*

EXEMPLAR LEARNING OUTCOMES
After reading about this exemplar, you will be able to:

1. Examine the rights of clients in the healthcare system.

2. Analyze support systems that exist for clients who feel that their rights have been violated by a healthcare agency or provider.

3. Compare the contents of different documents or laws that address patient rights.

▶ OVERVIEW

All clients have certain rights. Some of these are guaranteed by federal law, such as the right to informed consent mandated in the Patient Self-Determination Act (see the module on Legal Issues). Many states have additional laws protecting clients, and healthcare facilities often have a patient bill of rights. The importance of **patient rights** is evident in the American Nurses Association's Standards of Practice and Code of Ethics as well as in the standards set for accreditation of various types of healthcare agencies by the Joint Commission.

The Joint Commission's Speak Up program (2013b) is dedicated to patient rights as outlined in **Box 44–6** ●.

Nurses should be aware of national and state laws pertaining to patient rights, as well as the policies and procedures that their own employers establish in an effort to protect patient rights and ensure employee compliance with applicable laws and standards.

Studies have been conducted on health professionals' knowledge, perceptions, and implementation of patients' rights, especially informed consent. One such study (Yakov, Shilo, & Shor, 2010) explored nurses' perceptions of patient rights laws and

Box 44-6 Patient Rights From the Joint Commission's Speak Up Campaign

KNOW YOUR RIGHTS

- You have the right to be informed about the care you will receive.
- You have the right to get important information about your care in your preferred language.
- You have the right to get information in a manner that meets your needs, if you have vision, speech, hearing or mental impairments.
- You have the right to make decisions about your care.
- You have the right to refuse care.
- You have the right to know the names of the caregivers who treat you.
- You have the right to safe care.
- You have the right to have your pain addressed.

- You have the right to care that is free from discrimination. This means you should not be treated differently because of age, race, ethnicity, religion, culture, language, physical or mental disability, socioeconomic status, sex, sexual orientation, or gender identity or expression.
- You have the right to know when something goes wrong with your care.
- You have the right to get a list of all your current medications.
- You have the right to be listened to.
- You have the right to be treated with courtesy and respect.
- You have the right to have a personal representative, also called an advocate, with you during your care. Your advocate is a family member or friend of your choice.

Source: Joint Commission. (2013b). *Speak up. Know your rights.* Retrieved from http://www.jointcommission.org/assets/1/6/Know_Your_Rights_brochure.pdf.

how these were implemented in clinical practice. Significant findings included that nurses can relate only information that is within their professional boundary. Other issues raised by the nursing staff were how much time to spend with clients, the place in which to talk to clients, and caregivers' emotions while medical information is being provided.

▶ PROTECTING CLIENTS' RIGHTS

Despite the frequent assurances that patients' rights will be protected, many people encounter what they view as mistreatment or violations of their rights during the course of their experiences in the healthcare system (Taylor, 2011). Individual clients who feel their rights have been violated or endangered have a number of options. Many hospitals and large provider agencies have client advocates who can help clients navigate their system and intervene to ensure that their rights are maintained. Many states have an office designated by the governor or secretary of health to assist clients with issues related to patient rights in long-term care. The state's department of health may also be able to help. Nursing homes, homes for frail older adults, and licensed facilities for people with disabilities are regulated at the

state level, and violations committed by these agencies may be reported for investigation (Hicks et al., 2012). Legislatures in many states have legislated declarations of clients' rights that must be followed by nursing homes and other agencies who provide medical care and housing for clients at various points in the healthcare system.

The U.S. Advisory Commission on Consumer Protection and Quality in the Health Care Industry adopted a Bill of Rights in 1998. This Bill of Rights now applies to the insurance plans offered to federal employees. A summary of this Bill of Rights is provided in **Box 44-7** ●.

In addition to the bill of rights provided in this exemplar, there are many others. Among them are bills of rights for hospice clients and for clients with mental illness and patient bills of rights that are legislated by certain states. Insurance plans sometimes have lists of rights for subscribers.

Most of these documents give information regarding where to go if a client has problems with his or her care. The American Hospital Association (AHA) has a list of rights that is accompanied by a list of patient responsibilities to help clients be more active partners in their own health care (see **Box 44-8** ●). The AHA's list of patient rights includes those required under the

Box 44-7 A Summary of the Bill of Rights of the U.S. Advisory Commission on Consumer Protection and Quality in the Health Care Industry

- *Information disclosure.* You have the right to accurate and easily understood information about your health plan, healthcare professionals, and healthcare facilities. If you speak another language, have a physical or mental disability, or just don't understand something, help should be provided so you can make informed healthcare decisions.
- *Choice of providers and plans.* You have the right to a choice of healthcare providers who can give you high-quality health care when you need it.
- *Access to emergency services.* If you have severe pain, an injury, or sudden illness that makes you believe that your health is in serious danger, you have the right to be screened and stabilized using emergency services. These services should be provided whenever and wherever you need them, without the need to wait for authorization and without any financial penalty.
- *Participation in treatment decisions.* You have the right to know your treatment options and to take part in decisions about your

care. Parents, guardians, family members, or others who you select can represent you if you cannot make your own decisions.
- *Respect and nondiscrimination.* You have a right to considerate, respectful care from your physicians, health plan representatives, and other healthcare providers that does not discriminate against you.
- *Confidentiality of health information.* You have the right to talk privately with healthcare providers and to have your healthcare information protected. You also have the right to read and copy your own medical records. You have the right to ask that your physician change your record if it is not accurate, relevant, or complete.
- *Complaints and appeals.* You have the right to a fair, fast, and objective review of any complaint you have against your health plan, physicians, hospitals, or other healthcare personnel. This includes complaints about waiting times, operating hours, the actions of healthcare personnel, and the adequacy of healthcare facilities.

Source: Based on President's Advisory Commission on Consumer Protection and Quality in the Health Care Industry. (1998). Consumer bill of rights and responsibilities: Executive summary. *Agency for Healthcare Research and Quality.* Retrieved from http://archive.ahrq.gov/hcqual/cborr/exsumm.html.

Box 44–8   Patient Responsibilities

Most hospitals now publish lists of **patient responsibilities**, emphasizing that health care is a partnership between the patient and caregivers, that other patients have a right to be comfortable too, and that there are consequences if patients do not comply with treatment plans. Common patient responsibilities are as follows:

- Tell your healthcare team how you feel.
- Provide information about your health, past illnesses, and use of medications.
- Report accurate and complete information about your health to your healthcare team.
- Ask your healthcare team whether you need to change your medications before a procedure or test.
- Answer questions asked by your healthcare team.

- Cooperate with your healthcare team.
- Listen to instructions, read written material given to you, and ask questions if you do not understand something.
- Be considerate of the staff and other patients by limiting visitors, following smoking regulations, and using the telephone and television so as not to disturb others.
- Provide information about your health insurance and working with the hospital to arrange for payment if needed.
- Recognize the effects of your lifestyle on your health, and work with your hospital team to change your lifestyle as necessary.
- Follow the treatment plan recommended by your healthcare team.
- Accept the consequences if you fail to comply with instructions given to you.

Patient Self-Determination Act, but goes beyond that to include additional rights, such as the patient's right to considerate and respectful care and the patient's right to ask and be informed of any business relationships that the hospital may have that may influence the patient's treatment and care (AHA, 1998).

▶ NURSING PRACTICE

Ethical issues affect nursing practice on a daily basis. Nurses who engage in ethical practice follow the ANA Code of Ethics, adhere to their employer's policies and procedures regarding the rights of clients and their families, employ values clarification exercises as necessary, and make use of additional resources, such as peers and multidisciplinary ethics committees, to ensure that clients are provided the best possible nursing care.

To ensure patient rights, the nurse must first identify the appropriate individual to provide informed consent for the client (e.g., client, parent, legal guardian). Also, it is vital to provide written materials in the client's spoken language. The nurse needs to understand and describe components of informed consent and how to participate in obtaining informed consent.

While providing informed consent, the nurse needs to understand how to verify that the client comprehends and consents to care/procedures, including procedures that require informed consent. This also includes recognizing the client's right to refuse a treatment/procedure and discussing treatment options and decisions with the client. Similarly, the nurse takes part in educating clients and staff about clients' rights and responsibilities (e.g., ethical/legal issues) and how to evaluate client and staff understanding of clients' rights.

REVIEW   Patient Rights

RELATE   Link the Concepts and Exemplars

Linking the exemplar of patient rights with the concept of healthcare systems:

1. Patients have the right to emergency care without bias. What are your beliefs about clients who use emergency care in place of primary care?

2. What are your beliefs surrounding client privacy when emergent or critical care is needed and the patient cannot provide approval for his or her own care?

Linking the exemplar of patient rights with the concept of addiction:

3. Patients with persistent admissions for alcohol withdrawal therapy due to alcohol addiction need support to make the decision to get over this addiction. What are your beliefs surrounding alcohol addiction and the nursing role in assisting a client with these issues?

4. When adults who have had an extensive history of back pain with several narcotics taken each day need surgery, they often require a higher level of narcotics postoperatively. What is the nurse's role in supporting this type of client in appropriate pain management?

REFER   Go to Pearson Nursing Student Resources
nursing.pearsonhighered.com
- Additional review materials

REFLECT   Case Study

Mr. James Casper was on the way to his 20th high school reunion when his car broke down on a busy highway. When Mr. Casper got out of the car to check his engine, a car accidentally hit him. Someone called 911, and Mr. Casper was taken to the nearest hospital by EMR staff. During the trauma assessment, the ED staff noticed that he needed a chest tube inserted and emergency surgery due to a damaged spleen. Mr. Casper woke up briefly during the assessment and quietly asked what was going on. The nurse, Ms. Brown, explained where he was and that they were taking good care of him. The ED physician also explained to Mr. Casper that he would need immediate surgery and asked him to sign the surgical consent form. While the physician was talking with the client, he once more became unconscious and suddenly went into respiratory failure. He was intubated, a chest tube was inserted, and then he was rushed to surgery. The admission staff checked Mr. Casper's driver license and looked in his wallet for any emergency contacts. The ED social worker tried the only emergency contact phone number, but no one answered.

1. Mr. Casper has the right to take part in decisions about his own care. Was this right violated during his ED care? If so, how? If not, why not?

2. What other information is needed to find out whether the client has family or other adults he wants to have contacted and who may take part in treatment decisions if Mr. Casper cannot?

■ REFERENCES

American Association of Colleges of Nursing (AACN). (2008). *The essentials of baccalaureate education for professional nursing practice.* Washington, DC: Author.

American Association of Colleges of Nursing (AACN). (2010). *Nursing shortage fact sheet.* Retrieved from http://www.aacn.nche.edu/media/FactSheets/NursingShortage.htm.

American Hospital Association (AHA). (1998). *A patient's bill of rights.* Retrieved from http://www.patienttalk.info/AHA-Patient_Bill_ot_Rights.htm.

American Nurses Association (ANA). (2001). *Code of ethics for nurses with interpretive statements.* Silver Spring, MD: Author.

American Nurses Association (ANA). (2006). *Position statement: Risk and responsibility.* Retrieved from http://www.nursingworld.org/MainMenuCategories/Policy-Advocacy/Positions-and-Resolutions/ANAPosition-Statements/Position-Statements-Alphabetically/RiskandResponsibility.pdf.

American Nurses Association (ANA). (2010). *Public ranks nurses as most trusted profession: 11th year in number one slot in Gallup poll.* Retrieved from http://www.nursingworld.org/FunctionalMenuCategories/MediaResources/PressReleases/2010-PR/Nurses-Most-Trusted.aspx.

American Nurses Association (ANA). (2013a). *Final days for public review of Code of Ethics for Nurses.* Retrieved from http://www.nursingworld.org/EspeciallyForYou/Student-Nurses/News-for-Student-Nurses/Final-Call-Code-of-Ethics-for-Nurses.html.

American Nurses Association (ANA). (2013b). *Position statements: Euthanasia, assisted suicide, and aid in dying.* Retrieved from http://www.nursingworld.org/MainMenuCategories/EthicsStandards/Ethics-Position-Statements/Euthanasia-Assisted-Suicide-and-Aid-in-Dying.pdf.

American Nursing Association (ANA). (2014). *Revision of the code of ethics for nurses with interpretive statements panel.* Retrieved from http://www.nursingworld.org/MainMenuCategories/EthicsStandards/Revision-of-Code-of-Ethics-Panel

Ball, J., Bindler, R., & Cowen, K. (2012). *Principles of pediatric nursing: Caring for children* (5th ed.). Upper Saddle River, NJ: Prentice Hall.

Bao, Y., Vedina, R., Moodie, S., & Dolan, S. (2013). The relationship between value incongruence and individual and organizational well-being outcomes: An exploratory study among Catalan nurses. *Journal of Advanced Nursing 69*(3), 631–641. doi:10.1111/j.1365-2648.2012. 06045.

Benner, P. E., Kyriakidis, P. H., & Stannard, D. (2011). *Clinical wisdom and interventions in acute and critical care: A thinking-in-action approach* (2nd ed.). New York, NY: Springer Publishing.

Benner, P., Sutphen, M., Leonard, V., & Day, L. (2010). *Educating nurses: A call for radical transformation.* San Francisco, CA: Jossey-Bass.

Benner, P., Tanner, C., & Chesla, C. (2009). *Expertise in nursing practice: Caring, clinical judgment and ethics* (2nd ed.). New York, NY: Springer.

Brus, M. (2010). A personal reflection: Nursing art of withdrawing life support. *Dimensions of Critical Care Nursing, 29*(6), 293–296.

Cassells, J., & Redman, B. (1989). Preparing students to be moral agents in clinical nursing practice. *Nursing Clinics of North America, 24*(2), 463–473.

Chally, P., & Loriz, L. (1998). Decision making in practice: A practical model for resolving the types of ethical dilemmas you face daily. *American Journal of Nursing, 98*(6), 17–20.

Cohen, A., & Nirenberg, A. (2011). Current practices in advance care planning: Implications for oncology nurses. *Clinical Journal of Oncology Nursing, 15*(5), 547–553.

Crowley, J. D., & Gottlieb, M. C. (2012). Objects in the mirror are closer than they appear: A primary prevention model for ethical decision making. *Professional Psychology: Research and Practice, 43*(1), 65–72.

De Bruyn, M. (2012). HIV, unwanted pregnancy and abortion—Where is the human rights approach? *Reproductive Health Matters, 20*(Suppl. 39), 70–79.

Dekeyser Ganz, F., & Berkovitz, K. (2012). Surgical nurses' perceptions of ethical dilemmas, moral distress and quality of care. *Journal of Advanced Nursing 68*(7), 1516–1525. doi:10.1111/j.1365-2648.2011.05897.x.

Ellerby, J. H., McKenzie, J., McKay, S., Gariepy, G. J., & Kaufert, J. M. (2000). Bioethics for clinicians: 18. Aboriginal cultures. *Canadian Medical Association Journal, 163*, 845–850.

Gretter, L. (1910). Florence Nightingale pledge: Autograph manuscript dated 1893. *American Journal of Nursing, 10*(4), 271.

Guido, G. W. (2010). *Legal and ethical issues in nursing* (5th ed.). Upper Saddle River, NJ: Prentice Hall.

Guy, S. R., Womble, A. L., Jindal, T. R., Doyle, E. A., Friedman, E. A., Falta, E. M., & Jindal, R. M. (2013). Ethical dilemmas in patient selection for a new kidney transplant program in Guyana, South America. *Transplantation Proceedings, 45*, 102–107.

Hicks, E., Sims-Gould, J., Byrne, K., Khan, K. M., & Stolee, P. (2012). "She was a little bit unrealistic": Choice in healthcare decision making for older people. *Journal of Aging Studies, 26*, 140–148.

Iglesias, M. E., & De Bengoa Vallejo, R. B. (2012). Conflict resolution styles in the nursing profession. *Contemporary Nurse, 43*(1), 73–80.

International Council of Nurses. (2012). *The ICN Code of Ethics for Nurses.* Retrieved from http://www.icn.ch/images/stories/documents/publications/free_publications/Code_of_Ethics_2012.pdf.

Izumi, S., Nagae, H., Sakurai, C., & Imamura, E. (2012). Defining end-of-life care from perspectives of nursing ethics. *Nursing Ethics, 19*(5), 608–618.

Johnstone, M. (2011). Nursing and justice as a basic human need. *Nursing Philosophy, 12*, 34–44.

Johnstone, M. (2012a). Workplace ethics and respect for colleagues. *Australian Nursing Journal, 20*(2), 31.

Johnstone, M. (2012b). Ethics. *Australian Nursing Journal, 20*(4), 43.

Joint Commission. (2013a). *Ethics Committee.* Retrieved from http://www.jcrinc.com/Ethics-Framework/Organizational-Ethics-Statements/Ethics-Committee.

Joint Commission. (2013b). *Speak up: Know your rights.* Retrieved from http://www.jointcommission.org/assets/1/6/Know_Your_Rights_brochure.pdf.

Kai, J., Beavan, J., & Faull, C. (2011). Challenges of mediated communication, disclosure and patient autonomy in cross-cultural cancer care. *British Journal of Cancer, 105*, 918–924.

Kangasniemi, M., & Haho, A. (2012). Human love—The inner essence of nursing ethics according to Estrid Rodhe. A study using the approach of history of ideas. *Scandinavian Journal of Caring Science, 26*, 803–810.

Kececi, A., Bulduk, S., Oruk, D., & Celik, S. (2011). Academic dishonesty among nursing students: A descriptive study. *Nursing Ethics, 18*(5), 725–733.

Kendall, A., & Guo, W. (2008). Evidence-based neonatal bereavement care. *Newborn & Infant Nursing Reviews, 8*(3), 131–135.

Lachman, V. D. (2012). Applying the ethics of care to your nursing practice. *MEDSURG Nursing, 21*(2), 112–115.

Levine, M. (1977). Nursing ethics and the ethical nurse. *American Journal of Nursing, 77*, 845–849.

McGee, S. J., Kaylor, B. D., Emmott, H., & Christopher, M. J. (2011). Defining chronic pain ethics. *Pain Medicine, 12*(9), 1376–1384. doi:10.1111/j.1526-4637.2011.01192.x.

Metcalfe, A., Pumphrey, R., & Clifford, C. (2010). Hospice nurses and genetics: Implications for end-of-life care. *Journal of Clinical Nursing, 19*, 192–207.

Morgan, A., & Burgess, S. (2012). Judging a patient's decision to seek emergency healthcare: Clues for managing increasing patient demand. *Australian Health Review, 36*, 110–114.

National Guideline Clearinghouse. (2010). *Guideline index.* Retrieved from http://www.guideline.gov/browse/guideline_index.aspx.

Olafsen, L., Schraw, G., Nadelson, L., Nadelson, S., & Kehrwald, N. (2013). Exploring the judgment–action gap: College students and academic dishonesty. *Ethics & Behavior, 23*(2), 148–162.

Pagura, I. (2011). Consent to treatment: A patient's right, a therapist's duty. *Journal of the Australian Traditional Medicine Society, 17*(1), 33–34.

Parveen, S., Morrison, V., & Robinson, C. (2011). Ethnic variations in the caregiver role: A qualitative study. *Journal of Health Psychology, 16*(6), 862–872.

Pergert, P., & Lutzen, K. (2012). Balancing truth-telling in the preservation of hope: A relational ethics approach. *Nursing Ethics, 19*(1), 21–29.

President's Advisory Commission on Consumer Protection and Quality in the Health Care Industry. (1998). *Consumer bill of rights and responsibilities: Executive summary. Agency for Healthcare Research and Quality.* Retrieved from http://archive.ahrq.gov/hcqual/cborr/exsumm.html.

Priharjo, R., & Hoy, G. (2011). The use of peer teaching to enhance clinical skills in nursing education. *Nursing Standard, 25*(20), 40–43.

Racine, E., & Shevell, M. I. (2009). Ethics in neonatal neurology: When is enough, enough? *Pediatric Neurology, 40*(3), 147–155.

Rasmussen, L. M. (2012). Patient advocacy in clinical ethics consultation. *American Journal of Bioethics, 12*(8), 1–9.

Schultz, D. (2013). Nurses fighting state by state for minimum staffing laws. *Kaiser Health News.* Retrieved from http://www.kaiserhealthnews.org/Stories/2013/April/24/nurse-staffing-laws.aspx.

Sehiralti, M., & Er, R. A. (2013). Decisions of psychiatric nurses about duty to warn, compulsory hospitalization, and competence of patients. *Nursing Ethics, 20*(1), 41–50.

Sorta-Bilajac, I., et al. (2013). How nurses and physicians face ethical dilemmas—The Croatian experience. *Nursing Ethics, 18*(3), 341–355.

Taylor, P. C. (2011). Evading evasion, recovering recovery. *Journal of Speculative Philosophy, 25*(2), 174–183.

Thompson, J. B., & Thompson, H. O. (1985). *Bioethical decision-making for nurses* (p. 99). Norwalk, CT: Appleton-Century-Croft.

Varcoe, C., Doane, G., Pauly, B., Rodney, P., Storch, J. L., Mahoney, K., . . . Starsomski, R. (2004). Ethical practice in nursing: Working the in-betweens. *Journal of Advanced Nursing, 45*(3), 316–325.

Walker, C., & Lachman, V. (2013). Gaps in the discharge process for patients with an ostomy: An ethical perspective. *MEDSURG Nursing, 22*(1), 61–64.

Watts, T. (2013). End-of-life care pathways and nursing: A literature review. *Journal of Nursing Management, 21*, 47–57.

Yakov, D., Shilo, Y., & Shor, T. (2010). Nurses' perceptions of ethical issues related to patients' rights law. *Nursing Ethics, 17*(4), 501–510.

45 Evidence-Based Practice

MODULE AT-A-GLANCE

The Concept of Evidence-Based Practice, 2583

◪ THE CONCEPT OF EVIDENCE-BASED PRACTICE

Evidence-based practice (EBP) is used to close the gap between the actual practice of nursing and **research** (a formal, systematic way of answering a question or approaching a problem) in areas that are of interest to nursing. While there are many definitions of EBP, they generally include three components: (a) the best evidence from the most current research available, (b) the nurse's clinical expertise, and (c) the client's preferences, reflecting values, needs, interests, and choices. By integrating these components into the clinical decision-making process, nurses can individualize client care and provide best practice for client-centered care. **Evidence** can be defined as clinical knowledge, expert opinion, or information resulting from research. Evidence-based practice using the best current research evidence helps in achieving high-quality client outcomes (see **Figure 45–1 ●**). **<<**

Concept Learning Outcomes

After reading about this concept, you will be able to:

1. Describe the three components of evidence-based practice.
2. Explain the benefits of evidence-based care and implications for client outcomes.
3. Differentiate the four steps in developing EBP.
4. Formulate a clinical question using the PICOT format.
5. Conduct a literature search for current evidence.
6. Contrast differences between a research article and other journal articles.
7. Begin implementing strategies for EBP.

Concept Key Terms

Background questions, *2588*

Evidence, *2583*

Evidence-based nursing (EBN), *2584*

Evidence-based practice (EBP), *2583*

Foreground questions, *2588*

Informed consent, *2587*

Nursing clinical research, *2586*

Nursing research, *2586*

PICOT, *2589*

Qualitative research, *2586*

Quantitative research, *2586*

Research, *2583*

Research participants, *2586*

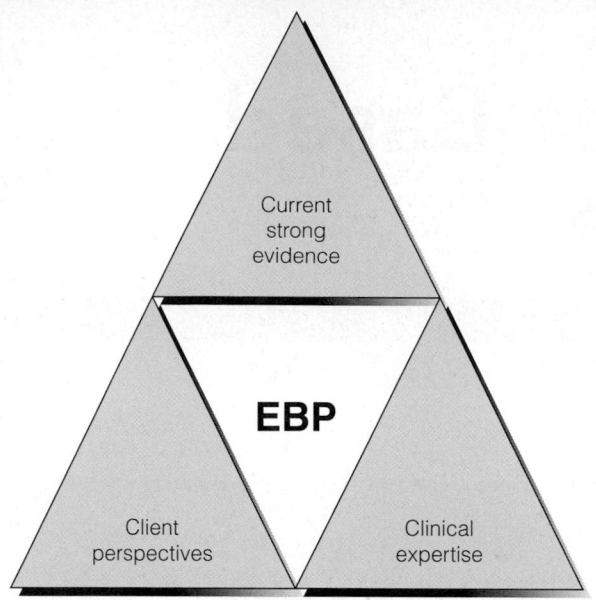

Figure 45–1 ● These three components provide the frame-work for evidence-based practice that nurses use to provide optimized individual clinical care to clients.

The Sigma Theta Tau International Honor Society of Nursing's current position statement defines **evidence-based nursing** as

> an integration of the best evidence available, nursing expertise, and the values and preferences of the individuals, families and communities who are served. This approach to nursing care serves to bridge the gap between the best evidence available and the most appropriate nursing care for individuals, groups, and populations with varied needs (Sigma Theta Tau, 2002).

With the abundance of research today, nurses are challenged to continuously evaluate and change their nursing practices. Using new and improved methods to approach old practices requires a desire to be more effective and a willingness to change to provide quality client care based on best practice evidence (Health-Leaders Media, 2012). For example, as members of healthcare teams, nurses face the challenge of cost containment in managing care. Factors that influence decisions regarding potential interventions include availability of resources and requirements regarding reimbursement for services stipulated by payment sources. Nurses must be able to utilize best evidence related to finance and economics to develop a cost-conscious nursing practice (see the module on Managing Care for additional information).

Clients participate in decisions about care based on their individual influences and preferences, including health beliefs, culture, spirituality, and traditions (see the modules on Culture and Diversity and Spirituality for more information). For example, clients can agree to a treatment such as supplemental oxygen; refuse a treatment such as a blood transfusion; choose an alternative treatment such as acupuncture; ask for a second opinion from a specialist physician; and establish advance directives to ensure they are treated according to their preferences. Many clients have access to resources that provide them with medical knowl-

edge and clinical information through technology, including television and the Internet, which can increase awareness of their condition. Clients need to be a part of the process, and their preferences should be taken into consideration in clinical decisions about their health care (see the module on Clinical Decision Making for further information). Selected examples of the relationship between EBP and other concepts can be seen in the feature Concepts Related to Evidence-Based Practice.

▶ EVOLUTION OF EVIDENCE-BASED PRACTICE

While using research evidence is not a new concept, a reordering of priorities in the medical field emphasizes practice-oriented research. In the early 1970s, Dr. Archie Cochrane, a British epidemiologist generally accredited with developing EBP, campaigned among healthcare providers to use evidence when making healthcare decisions. Professional nursing organizations saw the wisdom in this idea and encouraged nursing research in the development of best nursing practice based on current best knowledge. In 1996, Dr. David Sackett (1996), another pioneer in EBP, gave a commonly accepted definition of EBP: "The conscientious, explicit and judicious use of current best evidence in making decisions about the care of the individual patient. It means integrating individual clinical expertise with the best available external clinical evidence from systematic research" (American Speech-Language-Hearing Association [ASHA], 2013).

The push for the integration of more evidence-based research in nursing came with the publication by the Institute of Medicine (IOM) of *To Err Is Human* in 2000. In this document, the IOM discussed medical errors and their costs, in terms of both dollars and human life, and recommended strategies for improvement. The IOM's 2001 publication *Crossing the Quality Chasm: A New Health System for the 21st Century* addressed the failure of the healthcare delivery system to provide consistent, high-quality health care to all people (see the module on Quality Improvement for further information).

Translational research is emerging as a systematic approach of converting research knowledge into applications of health care for improved client outcomes. When scientific evidence is translated into practical applications, human health can be improved. Information can flow back and forth between researchers and clinicians to further investigate diseases and human response to them. This process resulted from a concern about past lag times between research evidence and its utilization in health-care policies, treatments, and practices (Wethington, 2010). The National Institutes of Health supports translational research through the Clinical and Translational Science Awards Consortium. The Centers for Disease Control and Prevention has translational centers around the country. Educational institutions are partnering with communities to do translational projects. This emerging approach has clear benefits for the development of evidence-based practice across nursing and the various disciplines involved in health-care systems.

Concepts Related to **Evidence-Based Practice**

Evidence-based practice has widespread implications for all areas of nursing, from how it informs and reflects nursing as a profession to the day-to-day care of clients. Part of the reason is that it assists nurses in examining the *why* behind existing processes and procedures, encouraging them to advocate for clients by asking questions such as:

- Is this the best practice method available to support positive client outcomes?
- Is there evidence supporting an improvement?

CONCEPT	RELATIONSHIP TO EVIDENCE-BASED PRACTICE	NURSING IMPLICATIONS
Clinical Decision Making		
■ Clinical decision making ■ Clinical judgment	Evidence-based practice provides scientific support for nurses in clinical thinking processes, making decisions, and using clinical judgment.	■ As problem solvers, nurses depend on current best practice to deliver quality care throughout the individual client's nursing plan of care.
Advocacy		
■ The advocate's role ■ Advocacy interventions	The nurse protects the rights of clients to efficient, effective, and equitable best practice nursing care.	■ Nurses take this role in providing current best nursing practice to all clients equally.
Quality Improvement		
■ The QI process ■ Components of QI programs	Improving nursing care is a continuous process utilizing current evidence to deliver safe and effective interventions resulting in best client outcomes.	■ Improvement of the "Why?" "When?" and "What?" of nursing care is a dynamic process that can lead to changes in how nursing care is provided.
Accountability		
■ Ongoing research	Best practice standards of care, responsibility, and scope of nursing practice reflect evidence-based practice.	■ Nurses are responsible to provide best current nursing care to their clients.
Professional Behaviors		
■ Components of professionalism in nursing	As a credible professional discipline, nursing has a responsibility to utilize EBP.	■ Best evidence needs to be integrated with nurse's clinical experience and client preferences.

▶ BENEFITS OF EVIDENCE-BASED PRACTICE

Nurses actively collaborate with other healthcare disciplines to provide high-quality client care. They help clients navigate the healthcare environment and assume many roles, such as provider of care, advocate, teacher, and researcher (refer to the module on Accountability for additional information). Nurses help ensure open and effective communication and continuity between all members of the healthcare team and clients and their families. When nurses are actively involved in evidence-based practice, they access and use evidence from a variety of sources and disciplines to help guide their clinical practice and improve client care. By using EBP, nurses also ensure the credibility of their profession and provide accountability for nursing care (see **Box 45–1** ●).

Florence Nightingale introduced the importance of collecting data through the process of observation to help make decisions about the health status of an individual (see **Box 45–2** ●). Today, the profession of nursing continues to develop to meet

> **Box 45–1   Using EBP to Inform Practice: One Example**
>
> Since 2007, The National Council of State Boards of Nursing (NCSBN) has encouraged the development of best practice evidence by providing funding for nursing research projects. The results of the research are presented at the NCSBN annual Scientific Symposium Meeting. For example, the Arizona State Board of Nursing offered a presentation on Measuring Competency with Simulations at the 2012 Scientific Symposium (NCSBN, 2012).
>
> The Arizona study sought to measure safe nursing practice competence and impact of remediation by using a simulation testing process. Twenty-one nurses participated in the study, which included simulation scenarios with three different simulation clients. Individual performances were videotaped and rated according to a competency checklist developed for this study, based on expected competencies, and correlated with competencies in quality and safety education for nurses (QSEN). One of the limitations of the study was the small sample of participants. The evidence from this study demonstrates that simulation methodology can be used to measure performance and the effect of educational intervention in education and practice (NCSBN, 2012).

Box 45–2 Florence Nightingale
In the 1800s, Florence Nightingale changed her concepts of disease prevention and promotion of health when she observed clients with and without the advantage of sanitation measures during their care. She concluded that clients situated in well-ventilated rooms and treated with clean equipment and supplies, such as fresh linens and dressings, healed faster and had fewer complications. Washing hands resulted in a decrease in client deaths. This is an example of an early informal randomized control trial, which provided objective evidence to support a change in best practice for nurses to improve client outcomes.

Box 45–3 General Elements of the Scientific Method
■ A question is asked about a phenomenon. ■ A literature review is done to identify past research findings on the phenomenon. ■ A hypothesis is proposed. ■ A study, or experiment, is planned and executed. ■ Data is collected, organized, and evaluated. ■ A conclusion about the phenomenon is presented.

client needs in an increasingly complex and frequently changing healthcare environment:

> The most important practical lesson that can be given to nurses is to teach them what to observe—how to observe—what symptoms indicate improvement—what the reverse—which are of importance—which are of none—which are the evidence of neglect—and of what kind of neglect. All of this ought to make part, and an essential part, of the training of every nurse (Nightingale, 1859/1946).

The power of observation to which Nightingale refers is essential in nursing practice and emphasizes the benefits of using evidence to inform change or to confirm success or improvement. Nurses employ physical assessment, including observation, as a way to gain immediate information regarding a client's health status. Evidence-based practice extends the nurse's realm of information to incorporate research—the data observed and recorded by others—in order to improve client outcomes.

▶ NURSING CLINICAL RESEARCH

Because evidence is a product of research, being familiar with the research process helps in the selection and evaluation of practices for best client outcomes. In a very broad definition, *research* is obtaining information and objective facts to advance knowledge about a specific topic. **Nursing research** is a systematic and strict scientific process that tests hypotheses about health-related conditions and the processes of nursing care (Dimitroff, 2011). **Nursing clinical research** seeks answers to questions that will ultimately improve client care. For example:

■ What are the links between diet and the development of diabetes and cardiovascular disease?

■ Is a new drug or medical device more effective than one already on the market?

■ Do clients who undergo surgery at one medical center have a higher complication rate than those who are treated at another?

■ Are clients satisfied with their care during hospitalization?

A familiarity with research methodology is becoming increasingly important in nursing practice. Weighing the scientific merit of a research study is key to considering its interpretation and implications. Not all research is created equal. A number of different methodologies are used in clinical research. Quantitative research and qualitative research are two of these methodologies.

Quantitative research uses precise measurement to collect data and to analyze it statistically for a summary and a description of the resulting findings, or to test relationships among variables. An example of a quantitative question is "Are there differences in skin breakdown between premature infants who are bathed with plain water and those who are bathed with bacteriostatic soap?"

Qualitative research investigates a question through narrative data that explores the subjective experiences of human beings and can provide nursing with a better understanding of the client's perspective. An example of a qualitative question is "What is the nature of coping and adjustment after a radical mastectomy?"

Today's nurses have a wealth of nursing research available that uses the scientific method to obtain evidence (see **Box 45–3** ●). Using this method limits subjective influences and bias so the validity and reliability of the data are high.

Funding

Many sources of funding opportunities are available to nurses interested in doing research projects to advance nursing science and create evidence supporting improved client care (Nursing World, 2012). This funding ranges from small research grants from local professional nursing chapters to larger grants awarded by state or national nursing organization foundations. Corporations, state agencies, and federal organizations also support nursing research grants. Awards are given in all areas of nursing, including gerontology, quality of life, health disparities, disease prevention, and nursing practice specialties. Examples of funding sources of awards and grants are Sigma Theta Tau International Honor Society of Nursing, Agency for Healthcare Research and Quality, National Institute of Nursing Research, National Council of State Boards of Nursing, Robert Wood Johnson Foundation, and the American Cancer Society.

Participants

All research studies require participants. Because each study targets a specific population (e.g., adult males older than 65 years with a history of hypertension), researchers develop a list of criteria that normally includes factors such as age, weight, gender, medical history, type and present stage of a disease, and present medications taken. These qualifiers can be categorized as inclusion (acceptable) or exclusion (not acceptable) criteria to meet the needs of the study for participants' safety. For example, identified vulnerable populations such as children, older adults, clients with certain medical diagnoses, and the physically and mentally challenged may be excluded for safety concerns. **Research participants** are defined as volunteers for a specific study project that meet all the inclusion criteria, have been informed of all aspects of the study, and have signed informed consent.

Ethical and Legal Issues

Ethical principles used by nurses to protect clients receiving care are also used to protect participants in clinical research studies (see the module on Ethics for further information). Ethical principles are at the core of such questions as "Did the researchers maintain the confidentiality of the participants?" and "Did the participants experience physical harm or psychological distress?" Institutional review boards monitor the ethical standards of research projects. Three main ethical principles are generally considered: respect for dignity, beneficence, and justice (Nursing Planet, 2012a).

Respect for human dignity requires that researchers ensure the volunteers are participating freely in a study, without coercion and after receiving full disclosure of the study and the potential risks involved. *Beneficence* requires that researchers protect participants from physical injury, psychological harm, economic insult, and exploitation during or as a result of the study. It also addresses the requirement that the study be conducted for the benefit of others. *Justice* speaks to the fair treatment of all participants, including the right of participants to expect their personal information to be maintained under strict confidentiality and the protection of participant anonymity. The Health Insurance Portability and Accountability Act (HIPAA) includes a Privacy Rule, which creates a national standard for the disclosure of private health information.

Legal practices related to research studies include following criminal, civil, and tort laws. Study volunteers have a legal right to full disclosure of the study's purpose, required procedures, length, expectations, risks, and possible benefits before consenting to participate. **Informed consent** includes the right to receive this information as well as the right of participants to withdraw from the study at any time. Participants must give informed consent, usually written, before the study begins (refer to the module on Legal Issues for further information).

RESEARCH EXAMPLE

Much clinical research has been focused on the practice of using physical restraints with older adult clients. Studies by Strumpf and Evans (2008) were especially important in the reform of this practice. The policies of many facilities changed over the years because of studies showing that restraints can cause harm and inhibit routines of daily living rather than increase safety. Complications related to improper use of restraint include skin integrity breakdown, toileting changes due to decreased mobility and increased incontinence, and disuse of muscles with minimal movement and activity. Policies and practices have been changed to using the least restrictive interventions for safety except in cases of emergency (National Consumer Voice for Quality Long-Term Care [NCCNHR], 2009).

Implications for Nursing Practice

It is impossible for one nurse to conduct all the research needed to yield the abundance of best evidence available today supporting changes in nursing practice to improve client outcomes.

The nursing profession includes both nurse clinicians and nurse researchers to determine best evidence. Three major benefits of nursing clinical research are to (a) provide best evidence for EBP, (b) support nursing as a separate professional discipline, and (c) define current best practice standards of nursing care.

PROVIDING BEST EVIDENCE FOR EBP   Best practices in nursing have continuously evolved as a result of research. In today's health care it is especially critical to participate in evidence-based practice. Practice based on the reasoning "we do it that way because we've always done it that way" is inadequate and fails to consider the research evidence supporting new and improved nursing practices. Integrating EBP is necessary to meet the current standards of high quality in nursing performance.

SUPPORTING NURSING AS A PROFESSIONAL DISCIPLINE   Simply stated, nurses want to be in control of nursing. Nursing history reflects its growth as a professional discipline and attempts to gain recognition as a profession in the eyes of the general public and in the eyes of members of the other healthcare professions.

The criteria for nursing to be recognized as a profession continue to evolve, but they include:

1. Specialized education requirements
2. A body of well-defined knowledge and expertise
3. Conducting ongoing research
4. An orientation toward service to others
5. Following a code of ethics
6. Having autonomy as a profession
7. Professional organization (see the modules on Professional Behaviors and Accountability for additional information)

Note that the first two items in this list, specialized education requirements and a body of well-defined knowledge and expertise, both depend, in part, on nursing research.

DEFINING CURRENT BEST PRACTICE STANDARDS OF NURSING CARE   Evidence-based practice supports changes in the responsibilities of nurses, including clinical decision making and clinical judgment, and the level and extent of their accountability. Standards of nursing care are defined by the American Nurses Association (ANA), the National League for Nursing (NLN), and The Joint Commission (see the module on Accountability for more information about standards of nursing care). These organizations periodically update these standards to reflect current best evidence. Rights, responsibilities, and scopes of nursing practice are legally defined by state nurse practice acts from each state's board of nursing (see the modules on Professional Behaviors and Legal Issues for additional information).

In addition to professional organization and state boards, each healthcare facility sets performance expectations for nursing care in its policies and procedures, following the state's nursing scope of practice. Nurses need to follow policies and procedures as written to protect themselves from liability. When practice evidence supporting better client outcomes is discovered, the nurse becomes an advocate of that best evidence. Each facility has a process to follow when suggesting changes in policies and procedures; it may be a quality improvement committee, a policies and procedures committee, or a nursing unit's chain of command. There is room for any change that benefits staff and clients, and it is incumbent on nurses, as professionals, to advocate for change that benefits their clients.

▶ BARRIERS TO EVIDENCE-BASED PRACTICE

A barrier is anything that makes it difficult to progress or succeed in achieving an objective. Even though evidence-based practice can provide nurses with the satisfaction of knowing that they have given best evidence care to their clients to promote high positive outcomes, some typical barriers challenge nurses from implementing EBP in their daily practice. When nurses learn the skills and gain confidence in EBP, they can overcome what is lacking. Some common barriers nurses confront in using EBP are the following:

- Work schedule and workload demands
- Client preferences that might conflict with best practice care
- Lack of access to technology to find evidence when needed
- Limited knowledge in skills for finding and evaluating evidence
- Lack of experience and confidence in developing strategies to promote evidence-based care
- Lack of support from supervisors or agency personnel
- Lack of access to continuing education programs (e.g., due to lack of time, funding, distance from program site)
- Attitudes of individual nurses (including lack of confidence in using EBP, misperceptions about EBP, lack of motivation in integrating EBP into routines of client care, and failure to understand the value of EBP)
- Resistance to change from traditional client care routines.

▶ DEVELOPING EVIDENCE-BASED PRACTICE

As stated earlier, evidence-based practice is a combination of the knowledge that is generated from the experience of the clinician, the research evidence, and the preferences of the client. For nurses to develop EBP, they need to first be able to identify information that is relevant and accurate. Studies done in London found that every 10 minutes nurses encountered a minimum of one clinical issue that could have been queried for EBP (Wilcox, 2011).

The sheer volume of information published on a certain topic can make adhering to evidence-based practice a daunting task. Nurses must commit themselves to expanding the implementation of EBP in the nursing profession. Through such efforts nurses will continue their quest for the provision of safe, effective, quality client care.

Step 1: Develop a Clinical Question

Formulating the clinical question is the first step in engaging in evidence-based practice (see **Figure 45–2 ●**). Clinical questions are generated in many ways but are usually encountered during client care. A clinical question may be knowledge-based (a

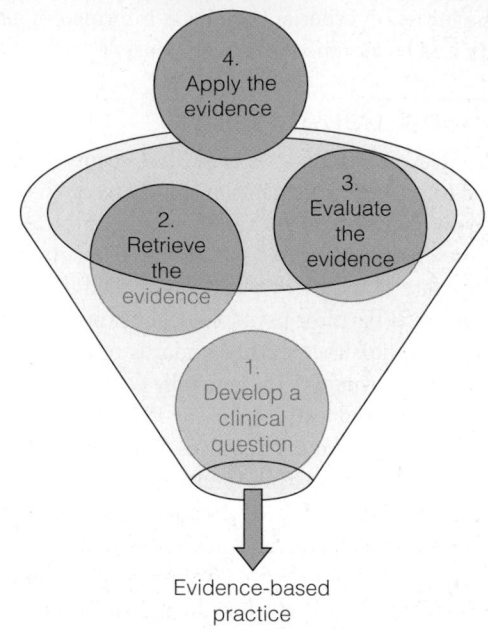

Figure 45–2 ● The four steps in developing evidence-based practice funnel together to produce best nursing practice for safe, effective, and quality client care.

background question) or practice-based (a foreground question). Which kind it is helps determine how and where to search for an answer. **Background questions** are general questions that seek more information about a topic, such as diseases or medications. These questions serve to fill gaps in knowledge about a specific topic and take the form "What is . . ." or "What does . . . ." The following are examples of background questions:

- What is hypoglycemia?
- What are the side effects of a specific diuretic?
- What does CHF mean?

Answers to these questions can be found in textbooks, medical dictionaries, drug handbooks, and other education materials.

Foreground questions are narrower in focus and are about a specific clinical issue. They are useful for finding nursing interventions that improve client outcomes; in other words, they identify useful information about direct client care. The following are examples of foreground questions:

- How does X compare to Y?
- How does using an incentive spirometer (or not using one) affect the length of stay for a surgical client?
- How does using a cooling blanket compare to using antipyretic medication as treatment for a client with a high temperature?

Answers to these questions can be found in the studies conducted to elicit evidence. Types of research studies include:

- *Meta-analysis.* A group of studies on a given topic are examined, and their results are combined and analyzed as if they were from one large study.
- *Case Study.* A case study is specific to one individual, issue, or event.

TABLE 45–1 PICOT

PICOT	DEFINITION	FACTORS TO CONSIDER	EXAMPLES
Population of a group	What is the common factor in the group of clients?	Characteristic(s) common to clients in the group.	A specific age, gender, health problem, or medication taken by all group members
Issue of interest or activity focus	What will be done to the clients?	Activity shows the difference in the client before and after the intervention.	A treatment, medication, therapy, test, or new routine of care
Comparison group or comparing interventions	What is the difference (alternative) in the intervention being used when comparing two groups?	1. Can contrast a control group that receives an intervention with another group that doesn't. 2. Can help prove or disprove a predicted possible outcome of an intervention.	1. Comparing two ways of doing something to find the best way. 2. Identifying the effect of taking medication A by comparing one group receiving medication A with a group receiving a placebo.
Outcome(s) or desired effects	1. What is the desired effect for the client? 2. How will the outcome be improved?	1. Desired effects of an intervention can be proved or disproved. 2. Improved outcomes can result from an intervention.	1. The desired effect is to minimize or eliminate a specific symptom. 2. An improved outcome is to reduce the time needed to accomplish a task.
Time frame	1. How long will the study last? 2. How long will it take to achieve outcome results?	Extent of time needed to study the impact of an intervention on a group may be brief or extended.	1. A brief time could be the first 12 hours after taking a medication. 2. An extended time could be 6 months following a treatment regimen.

- *Cohort Study.* A longitudinal study follows two groups and measures the outcomes of an exposure group with those of a nonexposure group.
- *Case-Control Study.* This study compares individuals with and without a specific condition to identify predictive variables.
- *Randomized Control Trial (RCT).* This is the strongest type of study. RCTs are designed to illustrate a cause-and-effect relationship by using a control group and an experimental group (Penn State University Libraries, 2012).

Another consideration is determining the type of question that is of interest. This information helps to further narrow the clinical question. Types of questions are:

- *Diagnosis.* How to select and interpret diagnostic tests; accuracy, safety, cost effectiveness
- *Therapy.* How to select treatments that do more good than harm to clients and lead to best outcomes
- *Etiology.* How to identify causes of a condition or disease

- *Prognosis.* How to predict a clinical course over time and possible complications related to a condition or disease.

Clinicians commonly use the mnemonic PICOT to define and formulate a clinical question that will contribute to EBP. **PICOT** stands for the elements of a clinical question (Gulliver, 2012):

> **P**opulation (of clients)
> **I**ssue of interest
> **C**omparison of interventions
> **O**utcomes
> **T**ime frame

PICOT develops foreground questions that apply EBP to clinical situations and problems (**Table 45–1** ●).

Table 45–2 ● shows an example of the following clinical question in PICOT format: Do clients with nosebleeds who tilt their heads forward experience less coughing, gagging, or vomiting than clients who tilt their heads backward while pinching the nares to stop the bleeding?

TABLE 45–2 Example of Clinical Question in PICOT Format

POPULATION	INTERVENTION	COMPARISON	OUTCOME	TIME
Clients with nosebleeds	Tilt the client's head forward during the nosebleed (while the nares are pinched together)	Clients who tilt their heads backward for the duration of the nosebleed (while the nares are pinched together)	Less coughing, gagging, or vomiting	Time it takes for the nosebleed to stop

CASE STUDY \\ PART 1

Brent Calloway is the new nurse educator for a local hospital's medical-surgical division. He has observed a high number of safety reports related to nursing procedures during the past few months. He wonders if there is something he can do to lower this number and improve client safety in the division. One of his responsibilities is to organize a continuing education program for the annual review of competencies for the nurses. In past years, the nurses have had a mandatory meeting annually in which competencies were presented and demonstrated by the nurse educator while they sat and watched. Brent is curious if there is another, better approach to emphasize client safety when the nurses review knowledge and skills for client care.

Brent is aware that the staff development department uses computer technology for simulation scenarios during orientation for new nurses, and he wonders if he could use that learning approach for continuing education programs in his division. He has helped with simulation in past employment and thinks using this teaching strategy could support better client safety. He questions if changing the method of training could decrease the number of safety reports and improve client outcomes.

Recently, Brent read an article in his staff development journal about a study showing that using simulation had enhanced nursing competence and benefited client safety. He queries if his division could experience similar results. In the article, the nurses participating in the study reported satisfaction in using a simulation safety-controlled environment that supported their learning. The results of the study demonstrated better client safety. Brent is excited about the potential to change training methods for the nurses so as to enhance client outcomes. Before pursuing this change in training, Brent wants to do an inquiry about research evidence related to hospital nurses using simulation for continuing education.

Clinical Reasoning Questions Level I

1. Why was it important to Brent's use of evidence-based practice that he question if there might be a better way of providing continuing education?
2. What role did the research article play in the EBP process for Brent?
3. What information could Brent include in his clinical question using the PICOT format?

Clinical Reasoning Questions Level II

4. How important is it for Brent to have the support of his manager to be motivated to explore the potential of finding a better method of providing continuing education?
5. What is the value of nurses being inquisitive about the way things are done in their nursing practice?
6. Refer to the exemplar on Competence in the module on Accountability: What role does experiential learning play in the development of clinical expertise for nurses?

Step 2: Retrieve the Evidence

Looking for clinical evidence from research sources usually includes a review of the pertinent literature. When doing a literature review for evidence, nurses look for scientific ele-

TABLE 45–3 Order of Sections Typically Found in a Professional Research Article

SECTION	FUNCTION
Title	Gives the main topic of the research study.
Abstract	Provides a summary of the entire content of the journal article.
Introduction	Presents the question, or focus, of the investigative study; includes background of older research on same hypothesis.
Study conducted	Describes in details all the aspects and methods of the study.
Results of study	Reports statistical data; may be in the form of charts or tables.
Conclusion	Summarizes and interprets the results of the study and statistical data in relation to the hypothesis; evaluates the findings of the study.
References	Lists the resources available for additional information.

ments in the journal article, including the abstract, or summary of the article; an overview of the study conducted, including its methodology; a written conclusion based on the results of the study; and relevant references. The order of sections typically found in a professional research article is shown in **Table 45–3** ●.

Nursing databases and resource links can yield a list of evidence articles related to the question at hand (see **Table 45–4** ●). Many databases have a tutorial available. Some databases

TABLE 45–4 Common Nursing Research Links

NAME	INTERNET WEB SITE
Cochrane Review Database	http://www.cochrane.org/
PubMed or MEDLINE Database (OVID) (includes international nursing index)	http://pubmed.gov/
EBSCO Database a. DynaMed b. Cumulative Index to Nursing and Allied Health Literature (CINAHL) c. PsycINFO	a. ebscohost.com (through libraries and other institutions) b. mynursingkit.com (access EBSCO through Pearson Publishing, My Nursing Kit, My Search Lab)
Books and Articles Database	http://www.sciencedirect.com/ (Elsevier Publishing)
Agency for Healthcare Research and Quality (AHRQ)	http://www.ahrq.gov/about/nursing/ http://guideline.gov/ http://www.qualitymeasures.ahrq.gov/
Evidence-Based Nursing BMJ journals (Evidence-Based Nursing, 2012)	http://ebn.bmj.com/
Evidence-Based Practice Network (Evidence-Based Practice Network, 2012)	http://www.nursingcenter.com/evidencebasedpracticenetwork/ (Lippincott Publishing)

Box 45–4   Nursing Journals

EXAMPLES OF RESEARCH JOURNALS IN NURSING

Evidence-Based Nursing
Journal of Nursing Scholarship
Applied Nursing Research
International Journal of Nursing Studies
Nursing Research
Research in Nursing and Health
Scholarly Inquiry for Nursing Practice

EXAMPLES OF CLINICAL AND SPECIALTY NURSING JOURNALS THAT PUBLISH RESEARCH

American Journal of Nursing
Journal of Emergency Nursing
Journal of Gerontologic Nursing
Journal of Nursing Administration
Journal of Nursing Education
Journal of Obstetric, Gynecologic and Neonatal Nursing
Journal of Pediatric Nursing
Journal of the American Psychiatric Nursing Association
MedSurg Nursing

offer only abstracts, while others offer the full text of the article. All sources and sites should be judged on their degree of credibility. Research resources can be found in various ways. One is to use a review-of-literature article that presents studies relative to a topic and ends with an evaluative statement, or recommendation, regarding the studies described. Another way is to use a primary resource, which is the original published article. Secondary resources, when one author is writing about the original work of another author, can also be helpful. Focusing on the most recently published materials can help narrow the number of evidence resources (Nursing Planet, 2012b).

The nurse who has difficulty accessing electronic databases from work or home should make use of local reference librarians and other available resources. Many libraries, particularly at colleges and universities, have access to nursing journals both online and in print (see **Box 45–4 ●**). The nurse who fails to get support from employers and colleagues may want to do more networking with local chapters of professional organizations such as the ANA.

The Agency for Healthcare Research and Quality (AHRQ) has established 14 Evidence-Based Practice Centers (EPCs). Through their efforts, these centers improve the quality and effectiveness of health care by reviewing all relevant scientific literature, synthesizing the evidence, and helping to translate the evidence-based research findings so that they are more readily available to those clinicians who are at the bedside providing care.

Stay Current: For more information on the 14 Evidence-Based Practice Centers, go to **http://www.ahrq.gov/clinic/epc/**

Step 3: Evaluate the Evidence

Evidence gathered must be critically appraised for *validity* (the degree to which the study measured what it intended to measure), *reliability* (its ability to produce consistent results with each use), and usefulness in applying the evidence in clinical practice. Nurses must be able to critique research articles to identify the strengths and weaknesses of the studies and their resulting evidence. By doing this, nurses can discard materials that do not meet the standards for application in client care. Appraising clinical significance answers the question "Is the comparison difference significant enough to change nursing practice?" In other words, does the study yield information reliable and useful enough to warrant a change in practice? Unfortunately, it is sometimes difficult to know which evidence yields best nursing practice client care.

Measure the significance of the information gathered by rating the strength of the evidence to determine its validity and its relevance to a given clinical situation (Oncology Nursing Society, 2012). Rating the strength of evidence helps to identify best choices to support greater effectiveness and positive outcomes in specific clinical situations. To categorize scientific data, various companies and organizations use different methods to illustrate the hierarchy or levels of evidence. Assigning levels of evidence can help nurses identify the strongest evidence available for utilization as best practice. There is general agreement that the highest level of research (research that is considered the most reliable and valid) includes large randomized controlled studies and meta-analyses of controlled studies (**Figure 45–3 ●**). Following this hierarchy, nurses can rate evidence strengths, compare the results, choose the strongest ones, and apply them to client care for best results.

Many professional nursing organizations have developed guidelines to provide their members with evidence-based

Hierarchy of Research						
Least powerful evidence	**Somewhat stronger evidence**	**More compelling evidence comes from research studies**				**Gold standard**
Opinions of reviewers that are based on their experience and knowledge	Opinions that come from well-known experts and respected authorities	Non-experimental studies: correlational, descriptive, qualitative	Quasi-experimental studies: time series, matched case-controls	Individual experimental studies	Meta-analysis of controlled studies	Large randomized controlled studies and meta-analyses of controlled studies

Figure 45–3 ● Hierarchy of research.

information they can utilize in the caring interventions of their nursing specialty. For example, the Emergency Nurses Association (2012) has Emergency Nursing Resources (ENRs) in their Institute for Emergency Nursing Research (IENR). They rate the strength of evidence with recommendation levels for practice: high, moderate, weak, and not recommended for practice (Emergency Nurses Association, 2013). Another example of rating the strength of evidence is called Putting Evidence into Practice (PEP®) used by the Oncology Nursing Society. PEP® helps identify and qualify evidence-based interventions for client care and teaching. The stoplight is used as an analogy to demonstrate the following categories of evidence strength:

> **Green light:** Strong evidence supports interventions that are likely to be effective and helpful.
> **Yellow light:** Not enough evidence is available to determine the effectiveness of the interventions as harmful or helpful.
> **Red light:** Strong evidence indicates that interventions are likely to be ineffective or possibly harmful (Oncology Nursing Society, 2012).

As nursing clinical research grows, so, too, does the number of new published materials on nursing. Strategies that nurses can use to stay abreast of current information include participating in research committees, continuing education programs, and Listservs or newsletters. Participation with other nurses in a research or journal club is an excellent way to maximize critical evaluation of current articles related to specific interests.

CASE STUDY \\ PART 2

When Brent discussed with the vice president of his division the use of evidence to make decisions about changing training methods to improve client safety, she agreed it was a good idea and was very excited about it. Brent has organized a team to help him explore the topic of using simulation for experiential learning, which could positively impact client safety outcomes. The team includes a nurse from the staff development department who is familiar with using simulation training; two staff nurses and one nurse manager from the med-surg division, who would be directly impacted by any changes that might be implemented; and a nurse from the quality improvement division with experience in developing EBP.

At the first meeting, Brent explained the group's objective. He gave each of the members a copy of the journal article he had read, and he discussed his plan for the med-surg division. The group members decided on a course of action after discussing several possible ways to proceed. They decided to use the foreground PICOT question Brent had developed with only a few minor changes: (P) For hospital nurses, (I) can simulation (C) compared to lecture and demonstration for nursing continuing education (O) increase competence and better client safety outcomes (T) during a 2-month period of time?

Members of the team were asked to do a literature search for research evidence, critically appraise the evidence they found, and bring the highest rated evidence to the next meeting for further evaluation by the team. The team will then evaluate the EBP outcomes and decide whether to change practice. Everyone was very enthusiastic and wanted to do all they could to help with this project.

Clinical Reasoning Questions Level I

1. Why would careful selection of members for this project team be important for the success of the project?
2. How would each team member do a literature search for evidence about Brent's clinical question?
3. What nursing research links could be used to find evidence about the clinical question?

Clinical Reasoning Questions Level II

4. What other participants might Brent have asked to be on the project team to help during this EBP process?
5. What is the value of having everyone contribute to developing the clinical question instead of just Brent?
6. How does the competence proficiency of nurses influence their nursing practice?

Step 4: Apply the Evidence

Once the evidence that bears on the clinical question has been collected and evaluated, the nurse is ready to integrate the best evidence with the nurse's own clinical experience and the client's personal preferences. But that process in itself is not sufficient; once the nurse (or division or healthcare team) implements the change in practice, the change needs to be evaluated for its impact on client outcomes. This process begins at implementation, with monitoring the process to make sure the change is replicated as intended. Is it being done correctly? Does it yield the intended results? Were the results unexpected? What areas need improvement? The nurse analyzes the data collected and decides to accept, reject, or modify the change for clinical practice. If the change shows benefits to the client, it becomes a part of the nursing routine until it is fully integrated into the standards of care.

Individual nurses can follow this process to identify the best evidence for specific clinical questions that they may have about the clients assigned to them. They can evaluate and change their routines of care to maximize positive client outcomes, such as reducing the length of stay or promoting cost effectiveness. However, the EBP process does not end with the individual nurse. After evaluation and satisfaction with client outcomes, nurses should "expand the EBP loop" by sharing the findings with other colleagues. The results can be disseminated in a variety of ways, both informally at the agency level and, more important, formally through presentations at national conferences and by submission of articles for publication in professional journals.

Many medical facilities and professional organizations are providing more support for EBP and the dissemination of best evidence client care outcomes. An evidence committee may be available to facilitate the evaluation of evidence. Pilot trials may be used on one nursing unit and then rolled out to the whole facility.

If this development process sounds familiar, it is probably because the steps are very similar to those of the nursing process of assessment, diagnosis, planning, implementing, and evaluation. Where the nursing process seeks to address the client's holistic needs, the process of evidence-based practice deals with a specific clinical question that may be researched in an attempt to improve client outcomes related to the clinical question.

The explosion of informatics in health care has also generated a need for a common language that can be used by individuals to access information and to share information. This common language allows nurses to code information to track nursing care processes and revise as necessary. Information technology involves more than providing or improving access to information, it also involves developing new ways for nurses to share information on best practice. Listservs, blogs, and videoconferencing are just a few of the ways that information may be shared through technology.

EBP is a continuing process because new evidence replaces older evidence, health care is not a static system, and over time, nurses advance their clinical expertise. What is known today may be changed tomorrow as science progresses. EBP gives a framework and set of tools that can be used to systematically improve efforts to be better clinicians—using the best of its three components: client preferences, the nurse's clinical experience, and evidence (see Figure 45–2).

CASE STUDY \\ PART 3

Evidence found by the group demonstrated that simulation was an effective method of learning for nurses, as shown by several study outcomes brought before the group for discussion. These outcomes included:

- Decreased time required to implement interventions
- Improved organization and completion of simulated tasks
- Improved infection control
- Improved communication skills that supported quick, efficient actions
- Increasing ability of nurses to anticipate needed client interventions

These results were very exciting to the team and reinforced the value of how changes in the delivery of continuing education can achieve a positive impact on client safety.

After reflecting on all the evidence, the group decided on an educational plan for the nurses using a simulation teaching strategy. The med-surg division would be able to use the simulation unit in staff development for nurse competence. The two nurses and nurse manager would answer questions by nurses and would serve as the division champions for simulation. The nurse with additional training in EBP would continue to serve as a resource to staff.

In addition, Brent developed a schedule to visit all units in the division to discuss simulation, and the group posted flyers in the staff break rooms about simulation. The vice-president of the med-surg division remained supportive of this EBP change process.

Two months after the first nurse competence simulation training was completed, Brent and the team reviewed safety reports related to nursing procedures. Initial results showed a 73% reduction in the number of safety problems. The nurses in the division reported an increased awareness of safety for clients because of the hands-on simulation training they had received. An increase in client safety was demonstrated that supported better positive client outcomes.

As a result, other divisions in the hospital are interested in hearing more information about how the EBP change could enhance learning outcomes and impact client safety in their divisions. A potential rollout for the whole hospital is on the agenda for discussion at the next quarterly management meeting.

Clinical Reasoning Questions Level I

1. Why was work done in advance to let the nurses know of an upcoming change in how things were being done?
2. What steps did Brent's team use to develop and implement the changes they sought?
3. Who ultimately benefited most from the EBP change in training? How?

Clinical Reasoning Questions Level II

4. For the EBP change in training to be successful, how important is "buy-in" from the nurses? From management? From a facility to support an EBP culture?
5. How could the project team integrate best evidence with nursing expertise and client preferences when changing to an EBP method of training for the nurses?
6. In addition to improved client safety outcomes, what benefits might result from implementation of EBP in this situation for the nurses? The facility?

▶ STRATEGIES TO IMPLEMENT EVIDENCE-BASED PRACTICE

Some basic activities can provide a foundation for implementing evidence-based practice. These strategies can spark the necessary stimulus to engage in behaviors that encourage best practice. Participating in EBP contributes to the knowledge of nursing and client care in today's healthcare systems and delivery of quality nursing care for best outcomes.

- Assess yourself to determine how much of your present nursing practice is evidence-based. Make a list of actions done in a clinical day. Beside each action, make a note if it is evidence-based, the routine everyone follows, or a shortcut, or if you perform the action that way because that is how you learned it.

- Assess the obstacles that inhibit you from using EBP more frequently. These may include internal factors, such as beliefs or misconceptions, or external factors, such as lack of management support.

- Practice raising questions about current clinical practices and problem solving.

- Acquire more information to correct your misperceptions of EBP.

- Focus limited time on evidence from "high-yield" sources— those that are current, are known for their quality, and have content applicable to client care.

- Go to www.guideline.gov (AHRQ) for free resource compilations of evidence reviews and practice guidelines published by a variety of groups on a wide range of topics, like hearing screening, learning disorders, screening, treatment, prognosis.

- Use the Internet when doing searches to cut down the time needed to find good evidence choices.
- Learn how to do a critical appraisal of evidence to determine the best evidence.
- Build your awareness of the how and why things are done to identify how much EBP is being used.
- Identify others interested in searching for evidence and evaluating it for collaborative opportunities such as a journal club.

- Volunteer to participate on a quality nursing practice committee.
- Participate in a research project to be a part of an EBP process.

Stay Current: *AHRQ sponsors evidence reports and technology assessments through systematic reviews for health literacy interventions and outcomes from their Evidence-Based Practice Centers. Go to* **http://www.ahrq.gov/clinic/epcsums/litupsum.htm** *for more information (AHRQ, 2011).*

REVIEW The Concept of Evidence-Based Practice

RELATE Link the Concepts

Linking the concept of evidence-based practice with the concept of cellular regulation:

1. While caring for a pediatric client with severe stomatitis secondary to chemotherapy, the nurse is concerned because the client's mouth ulcers are not responding to current treatment. How can the nurse be assured he is using current evidence-based practice?

2. The nurse learns of a new treatment that has had great results with treatment-resistant stomatitis. What should the nurse do next?

Linking the concept of evidence-based practice with the concept of advocacy:

3. How can the nurse best advocate for a client considering becoming a participant in a clinical trial?

4. The nurse is caring for a client who is involved in a clinical research study. The client says to the nurse, "I don't want to be a part of this study any longer. How do I get out of it?" What would the nurse's therapeutic response be to this client?

REFER Pearson Nursing Student Resources
nursing.pearsonhighered.com

- Additional review materials

REFLECT Case Study

The nurse is caring for a client with severe persistent asthma who requires daily doses of inhaled corticosteroids, with frequent use of oral steroids during periods of exacerbation. The client has been invited to join a research study to determine the effects of a new medication for clients with severe persistent asthma. The lead researcher has provided the client with the necessary information for informed consent. The client has asked for time to think about it and discuss it with his spouse. When the nurse enters the room, the client asks, "What if I agree to participate and the medication doesn't work? Will that mean my asthma will get worse? Does that increase my chances of dying from an asthma attack?"

1. How can the nurse best respond to the client's questions?

2. How can the nurse best advocate for this client?

3. What are the nurse's ethical obligations to help this client?

■ REFERENCES

Agency for Healthcare Research and Quality. (2011). *Health literacy interventions and outcomes: An updated systematic review.* Retrieved from http://www.ahrq.gov/clinic/epcsums/litupsum.htm/.

American Speech-Language-Hearing Association. (2013). *Evidence-based practice: Myths and realities, the ASHA leader.* Retrieved from http://www.asha.org/members/ebp/intro.htm.

Current Nursing. (2012). *Introduction to nursing research: Review of literature.* Retrieved from http://nursingplanet.com/Nursing_Research/e-book/review_literature.html.

Dimitroff, L. (2011). *Comparing and contrasting nursing research, evidence-based practice, and quality improvement: A differential diagnosis.* Paper delivered at Capital District Nursing Research Alliance 7th Annual Conference. Retrieved from http://www.capitaldistrictnursingresearchalliance.com/images/Microsoft_Lynda_D_PPComparing_and_contrasting.pdf.

Emergency Nurses Association. (2013). *Practice and research..* Retrieved from http://www.ena.org/practice-research/Pages/about.aspx.

Evidence-Based Nursing. (2012). *About evidence-based nursing.* Retrieved from http://ebn.bmj.com/site/about/.

Evidence-Based Practice Network. (2012). *Understanding evidence-based practice.* Retrieved http://www.nursingcenter.com/evidencebasedpracticenetwork/Home/Tools-Resources/Collections/UnderstandingEvidenceBasedPractice.aspx.

Gulliver, T. (2012). *How to write a PICOT for your evidence-based practice project.* Retrieved from http://www.ehow.com/how_7696012_write-picot-evidencebased-practice-project.html.

HealthLeaders Media. (2012). *Evidence-based practice and nursing research: Avoiding confusion.* Retrieved from http://www.healthleadersmedia.com/page-1/NRS-245879/EvidenceBased-Practice-and-Nursing-Research-Avoiding-Confusion.

National Consumer Voice for Quality Long-Term Care. (2009). *Restraints: The exception, not the rule.* Retrieved from http://health.nv.gov/HCQC/Restraints-TheExceptionNotTheRule.pdf.

National Council of State Boards of Nursing. (2012). 2012 Scientific Symposium: Presentations: *Measuring competency with simulations.* Retrieved from https://www.ncsbn.org/3309.htm.

Nightingale, F. (1946). *Notes on nursing: What it is and what it is not* (p. 59). Facsimile of the first edition printed in London, 1859, and reproduced by Edward Stern, Philadelphia, PA. (Original work published 1859).

Nursing Planet. (2012a). *Introduction to nursing research: Ethics in nursing research.* Retrieved from http://nursingplanet.com/Nursing_Research/e-book/ethics.html http://nursingplanet.com/Nursing_Research/e-book/ethics.html.

Nursing Planet. (2012b). *Evidence based nursing.* Retrieved from http://nursingplanet.com/research/evidence_based_nursing.html.

Nursing World. (2012). *Opportunities for research funding.* Retrieved from http://www.nursingworld.org/MainMenuCategories/ThePracticeofProfessionalNursing/Improving-Your-Practice/Research-Toolkit/Research-Funding.

Oncology Nursing Society. (2012). Evidence-based practice resource area: Levels of evidence. Retrieved from http://www.ons.org/Research/EBPRA/Process/Critique/Levels.

Penn State University Libraries. (2012). *Evidence-based practice tutorial: Tools for critically appraising the literature.* Retrieved from http://www.libraries.psu.edu/psul/tutorials/ebpt/more/levels.html.

Sackett, D. L., Rosenberg, W. M., Gray, J. A., Haynes, R. B., & Richardson, W. S. (1996). Evidence based medicine: What it is and what it isn't [Editorial]. *BMJ, 312,* 71–72.

Sigma Theta Tau. (2002). *Evidence-based nursing position statement.* Retrieved from http://www.nursingsociety.org/aboutus/PositionPapers/Pages/EBN_positionpaper.aspx.

Strumpf, L., & Evans, L. (2008). Individualized restraint free care. University of Pennsylvania, Hartford Center for Geriatric Nursing Excellence. Retrieved from http://www.nursingworld.upenn.edu/centers/hcgne/restraints.htm.

Wethington, E. (2010). *Evidence-based living: What is translational research?* Retrieved from http ://evidence-basedliving.human.cornell.edu/2010/08/what-is-translational-research/.

Wilcox, J. (2011). *Evidence-based nursing* (pp. 33–39). Palm Beach Gardens, FL: Best Publishing.

---

46 Healthcare Systems

MODULE AT-A-GLANCE

The Concept of Healthcare Systems, 2595

Exemplar 46.1
Access to Health Care, 2603

Exemplar 46.2
Allocation of Resources, 2607

Exemplar 46.3
Emergency Preparedness, 2608

◢ THE CONCEPT OF HEALTHCARE SYSTEMS

The concept of healthcare systems relates to the methods of healthcare delivery and management, including financing and coordination of services. Particularly in the past two decades, new cost-containment strategies and advances in technology—both informatics and medical technology—have combined to significantly change healthcare systems in the United States. **Table 46–1** ● demonstrates the impact of those changes. «

Concept Learning Outcomes

After reading about this concept, you will be able to:

1. Discuss the three levels of prevention and give examples of each level.

2. Differentiate different types of healthcare agencies and describe the type of healthcare service provided at each.

3. List factors that influence the delivery of health care and explain how each factor affects the delivery of care.

4. List different frameworks for delivering care and explain how they differ, including the advantages and disadvantages of each.

Concept Key Terms

Case management, 2599
Client-focused care, 2599
Functional nursing, 2600
Health literacy, 2599
Managed care, 2599
Primary nursing, 2600
Primary prevention, 2596

Secondary prevention, 2596
Team nursing, 2600
Tertiary prevention, 2596
Unlicensed assistive personnel (UAP), 2600

▶ TYPES OF HEALTHCARE SERVICES

Healthcare delivery can be classified by the type of services offered. Today's healthcare systems tend to be oriented toward prevention. A **primary prevention** service focuses on health promotion and illness prevention. **Secondary prevention** services include the diagnosis and treatment of disease. **Tertiary prevention** consists of the restoration of health following an illness or accident and includes rehabilitation and palliative services.

Primary Prevention

Primary prevention avoids development of disease as much as possible and promotes healthy living. Until the 1980s, health care was actually illness/disease care. Individuals typically accessed the healthcare system only when confronted with an illness or accident. The 1979 Surgeon General's Report from the federal government's *Healthy People* program laid the foundation for a national prevention agenda. Since 1979, *Healthy People* has set and monitored national health objectives to meet a broad range of health needs, encouraged collaborations across communities and sectors, guided individuals toward making informed health decisions, and measured the impact of prevention activities. *Healthy People* identifies a number of leading health indicators

(discussed in the module on Health, Wellness, and Illness), which, if addressed, should result in an increase in the quality and length of life and the eradication of health disparities. Every 10 years, the U.S. Department of Health and Human Services (USDHHS) updates *Healthy People* with scientific insights and lessons learned from the past decade, along with new knowledge of current data, trends, and innovations. *Healthy People 2020*, launched in December 2010, listed the following goals:

- Attain high-quality, longer lives free of preventable disease, disability, injury, and premature death.
- Achieve health equity, eliminate disparities, and improve the health of all groups.
- Create social and physical environments that promote good health for all.
- Promote good quality of life, healthy development, and healthy behaviors across all life stages.

When *Healthy People 2020* was published, it included new initiatives that address health issues that came to the forefront of health care in the previous 10 years, such as dementia including Alzheimer disease; healthcare-associated infections; early and middle childhood; and lesbian, gay, bisexual and transgender health (USDHHS, 2010a, 2010b, 2010c, 2010d).

TABLE 46–1   Comparison of Old Healthcare Paradigm With New Paradigm

OLD HEALTHCARE PARADIGM	NEW HEALTHCARE PARADIGM
Hospital-based, acute care	Hospital stays are avoided if possible, and medical care is provided at alternative sites such as ambulatory surgery centers, hospices, skilled nursing facilities, mobile health vans, urgent care centers, and the client's home. Necessary hospital stays are shortened by measures such as prehospital testing and care management.
Hierarchical (top-down management)	Decentralization (unit-based budgeting, scheduling, governance, and planning)
Physicians serving as the total sovereign of an individual client's care	Multidisciplinary teams consisting of physicians, nurses, physician assistants, nurse practitioners, and ancillary providers such as physical therapists develop care plans to ensure the most effective, efficient, and highest quality health care. The case manager ensures the care plan developed by the team is implemented and updated as needed.
Nurse as employee: early on considered the "handmaiden" of the physician and provided client care solely at the physician's direction; job focused with few aspirations for additional education and training because of limited responsibilities and opportunities for advancement	Nurse as professional: often enters the profession with a bachelor's degree; is career focused with a desire to climb the clinical ladder and, therefore, will increase professional knowledge via obtainment of advanced degrees, advanced clinical certifications, and continuing education in their preferred specialty.
"Sick care," focus on cure	Focuses on promotion of wellness and prevention of illness or, if illness cannot be or is not prevented, focus on early identification treatment and care management to reduce acute exacerbations of illness.
Cost containment with a focus on reducing payments to providers for unnecessary care	Development of care plans that ensure care is safe, effective, client centered, timely, efficient, and equitable. Such plans will advance provision of care that is of the highest quality and most reasonable cost possible for a client's treatment.
Written medical record	Electronic record
Fee for service	Managed care (HMO, PPO, IPA, ACOs)
Physician is employer	Physician is salaried employee of healthcare system.
One insurance plan	A variety of healthcare insurance options are available, such as basic medical, dental, vision, long-term, cancer, and disability.
80%–100% covered by insurance	Consumers pay copayments and deductibles. Consumer healthcare accounts (sometimes partially funded by employer) are available to assist with payment of noncovered medical expenses.

Stay Current: For the full list of *Healthy People 2020* initiatives, visit **www.healthypeople.gov/2020/topicsobjectives2020/default.aspx**.

Health promotion is another tool used to improve individuals' health. The World Health Organization (1998) defines health promotion as the process of enabling people to increase control over and to improve their health. While the primary purpose of health promotion is to improve an individual's quality of life, there are additional benefits. For example, preventing disease and using health promotion techniques to improve health are more cost effective than treating illness and disease; therefore, both approaches help to reduce healthcare expenses.

The nurse has an integral role in health promotion. The nurse's aim should be to teach clients how to remain healthy, thus preserving wellness. The overarching goal is to ensure that clients understand the importance of setting health goals for themselves and their children and that clients are able to assess, implement, evaluate, and, as their health needs change, modify them. Some examples of how nurses participate in health promotion include providing health education at every opportunity; evaluating and screening clients to identify prevention opportunities such as immunizations; and promoting wellness in the community by organizing and participating in community events such as health fairs.

Examples of current health promotion topics, identified both by *Healthy People 2020* and by individual states and communities, are childhood obesity and nutrition, physical activity across the life span, dental/oral health, tobacco use and smoking cessation, and health screening recommendations.

By implementing health promotion strategies, the nurse has an opportunity to step out of the secondary prevention area and into the primary prevention area. This shift increases nurses' satisfaction because they have an opportunity to contribute to the health of all clients—not just those who are ill but also those whose overall health status is free of illness, such as smokers who are disease free.

Secondary Prevention

Secondary prevention activities are aimed at early disease detection and treatment to prevent the progression of the disease and its associated symptoms. Screening is a means of early detection of diseases such as hypertension and vision or hearing problems. Such services may be provided by primary healthcare providers and through health fairs. Screenings may be offered to the general population or focused on groups at high risk.

Tertiary Prevention

Tertiary prevention involves restoring function and decreasing disease-related complications of an already established disease. When restoration to the previous level of functioning is not possible, care is focused on controlling symptoms and promoting the highest quality of life. Tertiary prevention includes rehabilitation and palliative care.

The three levels of prevention are summarized in **Table 46–2** ●.

TABLE 46–2 Levels of Prevention

LEVEL AND DESCRIPTION	EXAMPLES
Primary prevention. Take action to prevent disease in generally healthy people and populations. Give people tools that empower them to improve their own health through positive actions such as smoking cessation.	■ Educate individuals, families and populations on topics such as the importance of nutrition, exercise, dental hygiene, prenatal care, immunization and smoking cessation. ■ Educate employers and employees about occupational safety as well as avoidance of occupational hazards. ■ Improve environmental sanitation and provide adequate housing and nutrition (e.g., removal of lead from housing units).
Secondary prevention. Detect and then treat identified injuries and diseases early so that they can be cured or their associated symptoms and complications can be prevented or limited.	■ Perform risk assessments for healthy people who have risk factors for specific diseases such as coronary artery disease and diabetes; then work with the client to develop and implement a risk reduction plan. ■ Encourage regular dental, vision, and medical screening examinations for children and adults (primary care providers should follow guidelines such as *Healthy People 2020* or the recommendations of United States Preventive Services Task Force when evaluating clients' screening needs). ■ Teach clients to perform self-screening examinations such as breast and testicular examinations. ■ In all settings, develop and implement care plans to treat clients' illnesses and injuries (e.g., administer medication and treatment regimes) and prevent complications (e.g., turn, position, and exercise clients to prevent pressure ulcers and deep venous thromboses); ensure adequate rest, food intake, and fluid intake to promote healing and promote fecal and urinary elimination.
Tertiary prevention. Begins after a condition is treated and stabilized or recognized as uncurable. Includes the restoration of function and decrease of complications of an established disease. If restoration to the previous level of function is not possible, care focuses on controlling symptoms and promoting the highest quality of life possible. Rehabilitation and palliative care are included in tertiary prevention.	■ Refer a client with a new urostomy to an RN ostomy management specialist to learn how to care for and improve life with an ostomy. ■ Refer a client with diabetes to a registered dietician for education on how diet can affect the complications of diabetes. ■ Refer individuals with severe or chronic pain to a pain specialist to manage pain with an appropriate medication regimen and/or alternative treatment methods.

▶ TYPES OF HEALTHCARE SETTINGS

Primary care is delivered in a variety of settings, including physicians' offices, hospital-based clinics, community health centers, and public health service locations (**Figure 46–1** ●). Primary care should not be confused with primary prevention described in the previous section. Community health centers and public health organizations frequently offer health promotion activities at locations such as churches, shopping malls, and community cultural events.

In the context of managed care, the primary care setting is often the point of entry and the location of gatekeeping for all other care. Primary care involves the provision of health maintenance services such as routine physicals, immunizations, treatment of common acute illnesses, and support for psychosocial needs.

Secondary care is typically delivered in a hospital, outpatient surgical center, or specialist's office. The most cost-effective, efficient place of service should be selected as the optimal place of service. For example, a dermatologist may remove an adult's uncomplicated basal cell carcinoma in the office. In this instance, the office setting is the most appropriate, cost-effective place of service because removal of this type of lesion involve only a minor surgical procedure under local anesthesia.

Tertiary care that involves complicated diagnostic or therapeutic procedures may be provided in a place of service such as a hospital, a rehabilitation center, or an extended care facility. Wherever a client receives tertiary care, the nurse, as the cli-

ent's advocate, will coordinate the client's care and treatment and ensure the client's compliance with treatment.

▶ FACTORS AFFECTING DELIVERY OF HEALTH CARE

A number of factors affect the ability of the nurse to deliver client care, regardless of the level of care or the setting in which care is being delivered. These include changing demographics, advances in technology, and levels of health literacy of clients in the community.

Changing Demographics

By the mid-21st century, the United States will be more racially and ethnically diverse, as well as much older, according to projections released by the U.S. Census Bureau (2010). Minorities, now roughly one third of the U.S. population, are expected to become the majority in 2043. In 2030, nearly one in five U.S. residents is expected to be age 65 and older. Between 2008 and 2050, the population of adults ages 85 and older will triple. The effects of aging, long-term illnesses, and lack of primary care within these groups will increase the need for management of health care and support systems to assist individuals living in the community (U.S. Census Bureau, 2010).

Advances in Technology

Constant change is the new norm in medicine. Scientific knowledge related to health care is rapidly increasing and leading to

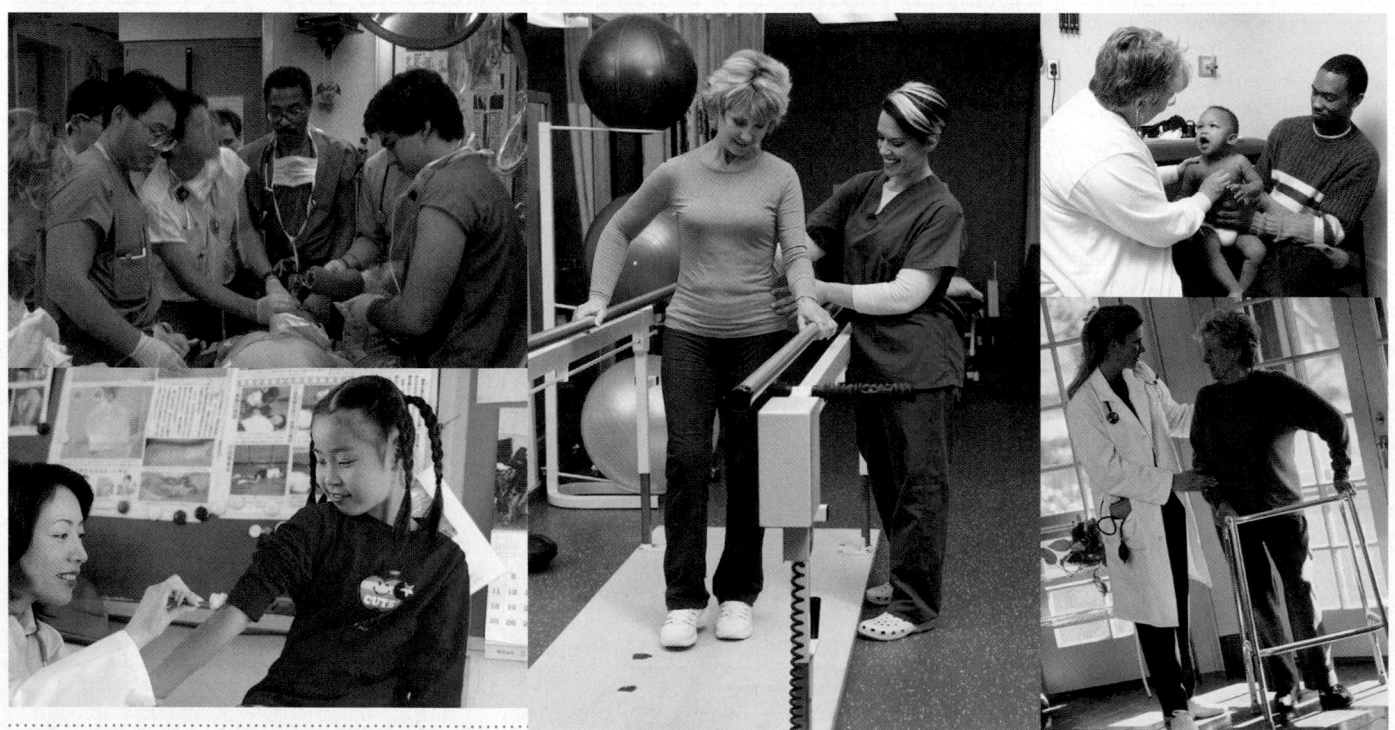

Figure 46–1 ● Various healthcare settings.

Sources: (*A*) Hank Morgan/Science Source; (*B*) daj/Glow Images; (*C*) © PhotoAlto/Alamy; (*E*) Barbara Peacock/Getty Images.

ever more sophisticated technology. Information management systems have been created and are continually being refined. Such systems support bedside charting, monitoring of laboratory testing, and use of online evidenced-based guidelines to provide appropriate care. New discoveries often modify how and where care may be provided. For example, safer anesthesia and laparoscopic surgical techniques have resulted in fewer hospitalizations for some surgeries because they can safely be performed at alternative sites such as surgical centers. Other treatments may shorten hospital lengths of stay. Many advances in technology require specialized personnel, creating new opportunities for individuals seeking employment in the healthcare sector.

Health Literacy

Health literacy is defined as the degree to which individuals can obtain, act on, and understand the basic health information and services needed to make appropriate healthcare decisions (Institute of Medicine, 2004). In 2003, the National Center for Educational Statistics conducted the National Assessment of Adult Literacy. The study assessed health literacy in more than 19,000 adults (ages 16 and older) in households or prisons through the measurement of tasks completed. Although the study was conducted many years ago, its results are still being used to evaluate literacy programs for improvement (Centers for Disease Control and Prevention [CDC], 2011). This study identified the following facts about health literacy:

- A slight majority of adults had an intermediate level of health literacy.
- Thirty-six percent of respondents had a basic or below basic level of health literacy.
- Lower health literacy was seen in those 65 years and older, those with lower socioeconomic status, and those with lower education attainment.
- Caucasian and Asian/Pacific Islander adults had higher average health literacy than African Americans, Hispanic, American Indian/Alaska Native, and multiracial adults.
- Hispanic adults had lower average health literacy than adults in any of the other racial/ethnic groups.

Healthcare illiteracy and ineffective communication place clients at risk for poor health outcomes. According to the National Institutes of Health (2013), African Americans, Hispanics, Native Americans, and Asian Pacific Islanders, representing about 25% of the U.S. population, continue to experience health disparities including shorter life expectancy and higher rates of diabetes, cancer, heart disease, stroke, substance abuse, infant mortality, and low birth weight. Providing health education programs for these populations is one of the key strategies for overcoming this health disparity. Unless health literacy is addressed, this strategy is likely to be unsuccessful.

▶ FRAMEWORKS FOR PROVIDING CARE

In the United States, the three common models of health care are managed care, case management, and client-focused care. Sometimes the frameworks overlap (e.g., services may be coordinated through a case management model to clients whose health insurance plan uses a managed care model).

Managed Care

Managed care, discussed in detail in the module on Managing Care, is a method of delivering cost-effective and high-quality care. Managed care is designed to improve outcomes for groups of clients; its framework can be adapted across all healthcare settings. The primary managed care models are health maintenance organizations (HMOs) and preferred provider organizations (PPOs). HMOs are more restrictive than PPOs and require that a client select a primary care physician who manages the client's secondary and tertiary services. While a PPO is less restrictive, the direct costs to the client are higher (e.g., higher premiums, copayments, and deductibles).

Case Management

The Case Management Society of America (2012) defines **case management** as "a collaborative process of assessment, planning, facilitation and advocacy for options and services to meet an individual's and family's comprehensive health needs through communication and available resources to promote quality, cost-effective outcomes." Multidisciplinary teams led by a case manager are at the heart of successful case management. Case management is essential when a client has multiple care needs and requires the services of multiple providers. The goal of case management is to reach and then maintain the individual's optimum level of health, quality of life, and activities of daily living (ADLs) by ensuring that the individual's healthcare needs are met. The case manager may be a nurse, a social worker, or another healthcare team member. Case management enables clients to experience continuity of care, regardless of the location at which the care is provided. This activity on behalf of a client may be limited to a hospitalization or may occur across settings for clients receiving care in the community and/or at home.

Client-Focused Care

Client-focused care is a delivery model that organizes health care around the expressed physical and emotional needs of the client. Client-focused care is generally understood to be an approach that considers clients and their families to be integral to decisions regarding healthcare delivery.

▶ NURSING CARE DELIVERY SYSTEMS

Three models of nursing care delivery are frequently used where client care is delivered. These are functional nursing, team nursing, and primary nursing.

Functional Nursing

Functional nursing is a task-oriented approach to care delivery. Although it is not used routinely, it may be implemented when systems are stressed by factors such as inadequate staffing resulting from nursing shortages or significant weather events such as major snowstorms. In this approach, the head nurse delegates tasks to team members who complete these specific tasks rather than caring for specific clients. For example, one nurse is responsible for delivering medications and changing dressings while another performs administrative functions such as monitoring orders and communicating with physicians and other departments to arrange for services. Functional nursing is an efficient approach because it enables the nursing team to complete many tasks in a short time. **Unlicensed assistive personnel (UAP)** are a critical component of functional nursing. They are paraprofessionals who are unlicensed but may be certified. The primary role of the UAP is to assist clients with ADLs and provide other types of basic care. UAPs act under the direction of licensed individuals such as registered nurses who delegate activities to them. When UAPs assist clients with activities such as feeding, bathing, and ambulating, registered nurses are able to focus on performing more complex tasks.

Because fewer nurses are needed, functional nursing is cost effective. However, depersonalization and fragmentation of care may result from functional nursing because there is limited opportunity for team members to view the client holistically. Nurses often become dissatisfied with their role in client care because it is limited to tasks. Clients too may be dissatisfied because they cannot identify "their nurse," that is, one individual who is responsible for their care.

Team Nursing

The **team nursing** delivery model is the most frequently used today. It is a means of providing individualized care to clients and was developed in response to the fragmentation of care inherent in the functional model. The registered nurse who serves as the team leader is accountable for the care provided to the clients assigned to the team. The team leader retains responsibility and authority for the clients' overall well-being but delegates some tasks to UAPs. Team members are assigned tasks based on their ability to perform them. While this model frees the professional nurse to attend to more complex client care tasks, frequent changes in assignments may lead to a lack of continuity of care for clients.

Primary Nursing

In the **primary nursing** model, one nurse has 24/7 authority and responsibility for the care of an assigned group of clients. The primary nurse (PN) cares for the assigned clients during her or his shift from the time of admission through discharge. The PN is responsible for assessing clients, developing care plans, and providing direct care. When the PN is absent, an associate nurse will provide care under the guidance of the care plan developed by the PN. In this model, UAPs are actively involved in providing direct client care and are assigned tasks by the PN or associate nurse in the PN's absence.

▶ NURSING PRACTICE

The nurse must have a solid understanding of the different types of healthcare settings and frameworks used to provide care. Some agencies use a combination of models, and each agency has its own specific policies and procedures. Nurses must understand that the concept of healthcare systems impacts all other concepts (see the Concepts Related to Healthcare Systems feature for some examples). Nurses must know the requirements of the agency in which they practice.

In addition, nurses must understand the barriers to accessing health care that their clients face, the issues they themselves face when resources are insufficient to meet clients' needs, and their agency's and community's expectations for them when a disaster occurs, which are covered in the following exemplars.

Concepts Related to **Healthcare Systems**

Healthcare systems refer to the broad array of people, institutions and resources that provide care to people locally, within a state, across the nation, and internationally. Care is provided at many different places of service and the nurse must be prepared to function in each. Each of these components of the healthcare system faces its own ethical dilemmas, legal issues, managed care issues, and clinical decision-making challenges. These challenges are particularly acute in a time of disaster, when concise, accurate, and timely communication becomes even more important. For example, nurses will face ethical and legal issues associated with the provision of care in mass casualty events (MCEs), (e.g., who will not receive care; who will receive care, and when and where care will care be provided). They will also be challenged as they decide what care to provide to the clients they are caring for during a disaster (e.g., when has sufficient care been provided to permit the client to be transported and how does one safely provide care when resources are strained). Communication among the various emergency team members must be concise, accurate, and timely during an MCE. Nurses must use their knowledge to foster better communication.

Concepts Related to **Healthcare Systems** (continued)

CONCEPT	RELATIONSHIP TO HEALTHCARE SYSTEMS	NURSING IMPLICATIONS
Ethics		
■ Ethical dilemmas	A nurse who is in the midst of a disaster faces many ethical dilemmas. Perhaps the first is whether to provide care (i.e., "show up"). The nurse, who is trained to provide the best care possible to any assigned client, may be challenged by decisions made for the greater good, such as not providing care to individuals who are unlikely to survive and keeping care for others very basic to preserve available resources.	■ Develop an individual disaster plan for yourself and your family so that it will be easier to make a decision to participate in a disaster or not. ■ Familiarize yourself with the disaster preparedness plans of your employer and community, which will facilitate a decision and, by virtue of having a plan in place, will make it easier to respond. ■ Participate in disaster drills, which will enable you to understand the requirements of participation and make a quicker decision about participation. ■ Never exceed your professional scope of practice because doing so may result in loss of your license and subject you to personal liability for negligence or malpractice. ■ Ensure that you understand the Code of Ethics and Standards of Practice of the American Nurses Association (ANA) and how they relate to emergency situations.
Legal Issues		
■ Tort law ■ Strategies to prevent incidents of professional negligence ■ Nurse practice acts	Despite the good intentions of nurse volunteers, they must understand that state and federal law may not provide legal protection if the nurse is practicing outside of the jurisdiction where the nurse is licensed.	■ If you plan to respond to disasters, then volunteer with a disaster registry, such as federal disaster medical assistance teams nationally or locally with the American Red Cross. Doing so will provide you with the proper credentialing and training necessary to respond to a disaster, and your participation will be less problematic because you are part of an organized system. ■ Know your state's laws regarding emergency response and ensure you adhere to the requirements of your state licensing board.
Managing Care		
■ Care coordination ■ Delegation	Care coordination will be required to ensure the needs of disaster victims are met. The leader of the disaster team will work with all present to ensure the medical emergency response is effective.	■ Know the disaster plans for your employer and be prepared to follow them. ■ When you report to the disaster team, immediately go to the command center to receive your assignment rather than beginning care where you stand. ■ You may need to delegate care to other individuals; ensure that, despite the emergency, you follow the principles of delegation (e.g., confirm that the delegate has been trained to perform the procedure, understands the procedure, completes the procedure, and reports back).

(continued on next page)

Concepts Related to Healthcare Systems (continued)

CONCEPT	RELATIONSHIP TO HEALTHCARE SYSTEMS	NURSING IMPLICATIONS
Communication		
■ Documentation ■ Reporting	Because of the uncertainties, confusion, and sheer demands of an emergency, communications may be fragmented and difficult. Yet an emergency is the very time when clear, effective communication is critical.	■ You will immediately identify and communicate important information to the individuals in charge. ■ You will continually communicate information with others on the team to which you are assigned. ■ You will ensure that documentation regarding client condition, treatments completed, etc., is maintained and transported with the client to ensure a smooth transition in care and to prevent harm to the client. ■ You will use tools for communication (e.g., SBAR) that result in concise exchanges of critical information.

REVIEW The Concept of Healthcare Systems

RELATE Link the Concepts

Linking the concept of healthcare systems with the concept of oxygenation:

You are a registered nurse leading a team that includes LPNs and UAPs on a critical care unit of a hospital. You are planning care for a client on a mechanical ventilator.

1. What aspects of this client's care may be delegated to UAPs?
2. What factors related to the delivery of health care may affect your ability to provide care for this client, and how?

Linking the concept of healthcare systems with the concept of clinical decision making:

You are a registered nurse working in the emergency department (ED) of a rural hospital. Harvesting season has brought large numbers of Spanish-speaking families to the community. Almost all of the men and many of the women are migrant workers. A mother who speaks limited English brings her 5-year-old son to the ED. She says he has been vomiting for 2 days. He has a fever of 102 degrees. She says he does not have a regular healthcare provider. He is not enrolled in any type of health insurance plan.

3. What factors will affect your ability to plan care for the child?
4. Which model of nursing care delivery would most benefit the child and his mother? Why?

REFER Go to Pearson Nursing Student Resources
nursing.pearsonhighered.com

- Additional review materials

REFLECT Case Study

Juan Santiago, 41 years old, makes an appointment with a healthcare provider he has never seen before for an annual physical examination. During the nurse's initial assessment, the client explains that he has never had a complete physical because he has always been healthy and hasn't had health insurance. After his recent college graduation, he accepted a new job that offered full healthcare benefits, so he decided it was time to take care of his health. Although he appears anxious about what will happen during the exam, he does not ask any questions and avoids making eye contact with the nurse.

During the collection of his health history, Mr. Santiago reports smoking approximately 20 cigarettes per day, drinking 2–3 alcoholic beverages per week, and, until recently, working as a landscaper, a very physically demanding job. He describes the physical requirements of his new job as "a little bit of walking but mostly desk work."

During the physical examination the nurse notes a wound the size of a quarter on the anterior aspect of Mr. Santiago's left foot. It is erythematous and warm to the touch, and a small amount of purulent drainage seeps from the side of the wound. Mr. Santiago reports that the wound has been there for more than 6 weeks. He has applied over-the-counter antibiotic cream daily but it still hasn't healed. The nurse asks Mr. Santiago about his weight; he admits losing about 10 pounds in the past month but denies changing his diet.

1. Describe primary, secondary, and tertiary care requirements for this client.
2. What referrals to other healthcare providers might be appropriate to assist in the treatment plan for this client?
3. What type of assessment of health literacy would the nurse conduct with this client before providing written information?
4. What factors will influence care delivery to this client? How will that alter the nurse's approach to providing care for this client?

EXEMPLAR 46.1   **Access to Health Care**

EXEMPLAR KEY TERMS
Underinsured, *2603*
Uninsured, *2603*

EXEMPLAR LEARNING OBJECTIVES
After reading about this exemplar, you will be able to:

1. Describe barriers to access to healthcare services.
2. Explain what it means to be uninsured or underinsured.
3. Discuss ways to increase access to health care for uninsured and underinsured people.

▶ OVERVIEW

For most Americans who have healthcare coverage through an employer, high-quality health care is available without a long wait and at a reasonable cost. However, such health care is often beyond the reach of the many Americans who work for small employers, the unemployed and underemployed, the self-employed, the poor, and members of underserved minorities. These groups face many challenges to accessing health care and, as a result, often have poorer health outcomes—in some cases worse than those of residents of developing countries. A 2011 report from the Agency for Healthcare Research and Quality (AHRQ), titled *National Healthcare Disparities Report*, confirms that people of racial and ethnic minority groups and those of low socioeconomic status disproportionately have more access problems than others. Inadequate access to health care has a large impact on society. For example, a failure to receive immunizations against or early treatment of contagious diseases can result in community outbreaks. The healthcare reform acts signed into law by President Obama in early 2010 are designed to remedy some of the disparities in access to health insurance coverage and other related problems. See **Box 46–1** ● for more information on this legislation.

Uninsured individuals are those without any type of healthcare coverage. Uninsured individuals do not qualify for public health insurance programs, such as Medicaid, and cannot buy health insurance usually because they work for employers who do not offer health insurance coverage. Uninsured clients also include those who cannot afford to purchase insurance through their employer because the insurance premiums are too expensive. During recent decades, even individuals who were self-employed had difficulty purchasing health insurance privately, either because the premiums were unaffordable or because they were denied coverage due to preexisting conditions. The Health Care and Education Reconciliation Act of 2010 is expected to significantly reduce the number of individuals in the United States who are currently uninsured. Enrollment for the insurance will begin in October 2013; the insurance product will be available January 1, 2014.

Underinsured individuals have healthcare coverage that is insufficient to meet their needs. Examples include the child who is covered under a parent's company policy, but the policy does not include immunizations, and the client with a chronic illness whose insurance does not include coverage for medications. Recent healthcare reform is expected to resolve these gaps in coverage.

▶ BARRIERS TO ACCESS

Access to health care means having "the timely use of personal health services to achieve the best health outcomes" as documented in the Institute of Medicine's 1993 report titled *Access to Health Care in America*, a document that is still widely cited today. As noted in the report and more recently quoted in *Healthy People 2020*, accessing health care requires three discrete steps:

1. Gaining entry into the healthcare system
2. Getting access to sites of care where the client can receive needed services
3. Finding providers with whom the client can communicate, develop a trusting relationship, and have individual needs met.

Lack of Health Insurance
The U.S. Census Bureau reports that the average number of uninsured Americans during 2011 was 48.6 million (15.7% of the population). More than 7 million (9.4%) of the uninsured are children. More than 8 out of 10 uninsured people are members of working families that cannot afford health insurance, and most of these people are not eligible for public programs (Henry J. Kaiser Family Foundation, 2012a). A significant percentage of minority people are uninsured, for example, 19.5% of African Americans and 30.1% of Hispanics (U.S. Census Bureau, 2011).

The primary reason people are uninsured is that they cannot afford to be insured. Often they are unemployed, underemployed, work for an employer who does not offer group health insurance coverage, and do not qualify for government insurance. People who are uninsured may delay treatment or opt not to receive it because they must choose to pay either for medical care or for basic necessities such as food and housing. Most uninsured people do not receive healthcare services for free or at a reduced charge. More than 50% pay the full price of care, and 82% pay some amount out of pocket. In fact, hospitals and other providers may charge the uninsured two to four times more than the reimbursement these providers seek from private and government insurers. Why? Because individuals do not have the same financial clout that insurers do and, therefore, are unable to negotiate better rates with providers. People who are uninsured use less health care than those who are insured. They seek less care, and they seek it later in the disease process, leading to more significant illnesses and complications. In 2008, the average individual who was uninsured for a full year incurred $1,686 in total healthcare costs compared to $4,463 for the nonelderly with coverage. This difference is of particular interest because, although the uninsured spend less in total than the insured, they pay more out of pocket. The remaining costs of their care are referred to as uncompensated costs. Uncompensated costs amounted to about $57 billion in 2008. Federal, state, and local funds appropriated for care of the uninsured population paid for about 75% of this total ($42.9 billion). The federal government pays for over half of the uncompensated care. The public, in turn, is affected by uncompensated care because this

Box 46–1   2010 Healthcare Legislation

In 2010 Congress passed the Patient Protection and Affordable Care Act along with the Health Care and Education Reconciliation Act. These laws are often referred to collectively as the Affordable Care Act (ACA) and they are expected to:

- Curb medical costs that are growing much faster than the rate of inflation.
- Return insurance premiums to less costly rates so that more individuals and companies, especially small businesses, can afford to purchase insurance.
- Remedy many unpopular insurance industry practices, such as denying coverage for clients with preexisting conditions or dropping coverage for clients who become ill.
- Extend coverage to 32 million Americans, many of whom are working poor who do not qualify for public insurance programs and who work for employers who do not offer health insurance benefits.

Some of the provisions of the ACA take effect immediately, while others will be implemented over several years. Among provisions of the new law that take effect immediately:

- Children can no longer be denied health insurance coverage for preexisting conditions.
- Insurance companies can no longer drop clients when they become ill.
- Lifetime caps on coverage are eliminated. Annual caps on benefits are limited and will be eliminated in 2014. These measures help those who experience catastrophic illness or who live with costly chronic conditions such as hemophilia.
- Children will be allowed to remain on their parents' insurance plan until the age of 26.
- New health insurance plans must offer preventive care with no copayment or deductible.
- Small employers that offer health insurance benefits to employees will receive a 35% tax credit for their share of premiums.
- Retirees ages 55–64 will be offered access to a re-insurance program.
- Medicare Part D recipients will receive a $250 credit.

IMPLEMENTED IN 2011:

- Medicare provides plans for preventive care with no copayment or deductible.

- Medicare Part D recipients who are in the "donut hole" phase of drug coverage will receive a 50% discount off prescription drugs.
- Health insurance companies have to justify any premium increases or risk being taken out of state insurance exchange pools.

IMPLEMENTED IN 2014:

- The uninsured and self-employed will be able to purchase insurance through state-based exchanges. Separate exchanges will be established for small companies.
- The IRS will impose a penalty of $750 per individual or 2% of income—whichever is greater—for those who choose not to purchase health insurance.
- Individuals and families who make between 100% and 400% of the federal poverty level and want to purchase their own health insurance on an exchange will be eligible for federal subsidies. To be eligible, these people cannot qualify for Medicare or Medicaid and cannot be covered by an employer. Eligible buyers will receive premium credits and there will be a limit to how much they have to contribute to their premiums.
- Private insurers will be required to accept all applicants without varying premiums on the basis of an individual's health status. Insurance companies will not be able to deny coverage on the basis of preexisting conditions.
- Annual limits on benefits will be eliminated.
- The temporary high-risk pools for those unable to receive coverage prior to the law will be eliminated as people enroll in state insurance exchanges.

BY 2018:

- All insurance plans will be required to offer preventive care with no copayment or deductible.
- Insurance companies will pay a 40% excise tax on high-end benefit plans worth over $27,500 for families ($10,200 for individuals). Dental and vision plans will be exempt and will not be counted in the total cost of a family's plan.

Sources: Binckes, J., & Wing, N. (2013). Health reform bill summary: The top 18 immediate effects. *Huffington Post.* Retrieved from http://www.huffingtonpost.com/2010/03/22/health-reform-bill-summary_n_508315.html#s75159; Jackson, J., & Nolen, J. (2013). Health care reform bill summary: A look at what's in the bill. *CBS News.* Retrieved from http://www.cbsnews.com/8301-503544_162-20000846-503544.html; Health care reform. (2013). *New York Times.* Retrieved from http://topics.nytimes.com/top/news/health/diseasesconditionsandhealthtopics/health_insurance_and_managed_care/health_care_reform/index.html; Health Care and Education Reconciliation Act of 2010. (2013). *Wikipedia.* Retrieved from http://en.wikipedia.org/wiki/Health_Care_and_Education_Reconciliation_Act_of_2010.

shortfall is ultimately recovered through payment of federal and state taxes (Henry J. Kaiser Family Foundation, 2012c).

It is critical for children to have health insurance because if insured, they are more likely to stay healthy and do well in school, setting them on a course for better health and better opportunities throughout their childhood and teens. Children with healthcare coverage receive preventive care; are treated for sickness and injuries when they occur; are immunized against childhood diseases; are seen for well-child visits required for participation in school and sports; and receive treatment for recurring illnesses such as ear infections. Well children are more likely to attend school regularly and have an easier time focusing on their schoolwork (Insure Kids Now, 2013).

The Affordable Care Act will affect children favorably because insurance companies will no longer be able to deny coverage to children based on preexisting conditions and will not be able drop insured individuals or their dependents who experience a serious illness (Appleby, 2010).

SAFETY ALERT

In 1986, Congress enacted the Emergency Medical Treatment and Active Labor Act (EMTALA) to ensure public access to emergency services regardless of ability to pay. Prior to the enactment of this law, providers of emergency services often refused to treat clients who were uninsured and who could not afford to pay for services. Under Section 1867 of the Social Security Act, Medicare-participating hospitals that offer emergency service must provide a medical screening examination (MSE) when a client asks for examination for or treatment of an emergency medical condition (EMC), including active labor. The law requires that this service be provided regardless of an individual's ability to pay. Hospitals must also provide stabilizing treatment for clients with EMCs. If unable to stabilize a client or if the client requests it, the emergency care provider must arrange for an appropriate transfer (EMTALA, 2011).

Box 46–2   National Guidelines for Health Promotion

- *Bright Futures*, American Academy of Pediatrics (original editions by Maternal and Child Health Bureau, Health Resources and Services Administration, USDHHS)
- *Put Prevention Into Practice*, Agency for Healthcare Research and Quality
- *Guide to Clinical Preventive Services*, U.S. Preventive Services Task Force
- *Guidelines for Adolescent Preventive Services*, American Medical Association

Lack of a Usual Source of Care

According to the Agency for Healthcare Research and Quality (2011), individuals with a *usual source of care* (i.e., a facility where the individual regularly receives care) experience improved health outcomes, fewer health disparities, and lower costs. A usual source of care is sometimes referred to as a *medical home* or *healthcare home*.

If a client has a primary care provider (i.e., a physician or nurse from whom the client regularly receives care), trust and communication between the client and provider are improved, resulting in the likelihood that the care provided to the client will be appropriate and of high quality (AHRQ, 2011). A primary care provider, who learns about the diverse needs of clients over time, is better able to meet those needs. Despite this fact, over 40 million Americans do not receive regular care from a primary care provider.

The USDHHS, the American Academy of Pediatrics, and the American Medical Association developed national guidelines for preventive health services for infants, children, and adolescents (**Box 46–2** ●). These guidelines are supported by the National Association of Pediatric Nurse Associates and Practitioners (NAPNAP).

Children and families are better served when they have a usual source of health care. Such a source allows parents, who forge an ongoing relationship and a high comfort level with their provider, to readily seek health care for their children. Providers are able to give comprehensive, family-centered treatment because of their knowledge of the child and family including the family's dynamics, possible risks, and need for protection. One source of such treatment is the patient-centered medical home, which is not a location but a standards-based approach to providing primary care in which the healthcare facility forges a partnership with the client and the client's family (see **Box 46–3** ●).

Perceptions of Need

Perceived need often affects an individual's decision to access the healthcare system. Clients may not always be able to assess their own need for care. However, when they believe they need care for illness and injury and are unable to obtain it, they perceive that care is difficult to access. These perceived difficulties include delays in getting care as soon as it is wanted.

CLINICAL EXAMPLE

A nurse working for a large insurance company as a telephone triage nurse receives a call late at night from a member reporting that her 4-year-old daughter woke with ear pain that has not responded to acetaminophen administered by mouth 15 minutes ago. The mother reports that the child is crying in pain and requests authorization to go to the hospital emergency department. The nurse provides strategies to treat the child's pain and explains that oral analgesics require 45–60 minutes to begin taking effect. The nurse offers to make an appointment with the primary care provider in the morning. When the mother

Box 46–3   Six Principles of a Patient-Centered Medical Home

The most standard definition of a patient-centered medical home is provided in the *Joint Principles of the Patient-Centered Medical Home*, adopted by the American Academy of Family Physicians, American Academy of Pediatrics, American College of Physicians, and the American Osteopathic Association in 2007. This groundbreaking concept is still in use and was recently quoted by Andrea Bachrach and colleagues (2011) in *Pediatric Medical Homes: Laying the Foundation of a Promising Model of Care.*

This joint statement defines homes as both "an approach to providing comprehensive primary care for children, youth and adults" and "a healthcare setting that facilitates partnerships between individual patients, and their personal physicians, and when appropriate, the patient's family." It lists seven principles that characterize medical homes; six are listed below; the seventh (omitted here) addresses appropriate payment to medical home providers.

1. *Personal physician.* Each client develops an ongoing relationship with a personal physician who provides comprehensive medical care from the initial visit onward.
2. *Physician-directed medical practice.* The client's personal physician leads a healthcare team that works together and accepts responsibility for the ongoing care of the client.
3. *Whole person orientation.* The personal physician, who is responsible not only for providing and overseeing medical care to

the client but also for ensuring that all healthcare needs are met, prevents fragmentation of care by arranging for and following up on care provided by other qualified professionals, such as specialists, and ensuring that the client returns to the medical care home.

4. *Coordinated and integrated care.* Care must be coordinated and/or integrated across all elements of the complex healthcare system and the client's community and must be provided in a way that meets the client's cultural and linguistic needs. Coordination and integration are facilitated by new means such as electronic health records and health information exchanges.
5. *Quality and safety.* Quality and safety are critical elements of the medical home.
6. *Access to care.* Access to care is facilitated by systems such as open scheduling, expanded hours, and improved means of communication among clients, their personal physician, and practice staff.

 Stay Current: For more information about the patient-centered medical home program, see **www.ncqa.org/ Programs/Recognition/PatientCenteredMedicalHomePCMH. aspx.**

states that the child must be seen immediately, the nurse suggests that the mother take the child to a 24-hour urgent care center. The mother declines, insisting that the child be treated immediately at the emergency department.

1. Does this nurse have the right to inform parents they cannot take the child to the emergency department because this is not an emergency?
2. How does the mother's perception of need affect her response?
3. What else might the nurse do to help the parent more accurately perceive the child's healthcare needs?

Uneven Distribution of Services

The distribution of healthcare services in the United States is problematic because it is uneven. Many geographic areas and populations are medically underserved. Rural areas come to mind as areas that are likely to lack medical resources; however, suburban and urban areas may also be underserved because of poverty as well as cultural and linguistic barriers to healthcare access. Another factor that causes a community or population to be underserved is a shortage of primary care professionals such as primary care physicians, nurse practitioners, nurses, and physician assistants. Availability varies from region to region, from state to state, and even within cities themselves, where the poorest communities may be underserved.

The highest number of nurses per 100,000 people in the United States is found in New England, and the lowest number is found in the Southwest (Henry J. Kaiser Family Foundation, 2012b). Primary care physicians across all specialties (e.g., family practitioners, internists, pediatricians) are also unevenly distributed. In 2012 the states having the fewest primary care physicians per 100,000 population were Idaho (76), Oklahoma (80), and Mississippi (81); those having the most were Massachusetts (194), Maryland (174), and Rhode Island (172) (United Health Foundation, 2012). Note that, in the states that have the lowest number of physicians per 100,000 clients, most physicians are likely to be located in the most densely populated regions. Individuals who live in the least populated areas of states face an even greater barrier to accessing care: long driving distances and lack of public transportation.

Another factor in the uneven distribution of services is the increasing number of healthcare providers who specialize. This shift to specialization decreases the number of primary care providers who are available at any given time. Specialization can be advantageous, given the complexity of health care today, but it is also disadvantageous because it may increase fragmentation of care and costs. Increased specialization is a factor that increases the need for care management.

▶ SOLUTIONS

The United States has addressed and continues to address the problem of the uninsured and the underinsured in many ways. The most far-reaching recent solution is the Affordable Care Act, which was created to ensure that all U.S. citizens have access to affordable, quality care and to curb the growth of healthcare costs. Other older programs include the following:

- Medicare for older adults
- Medicaid, which assists people with lower incomes, older adults who require services not covered by Medicare, such as nursing homes, as well as some people with disabilities
- CHIP, which assists with coverage for children whose families earn too much to qualify for Medicaid coverage, but too little to afford private health insurance.

Other avenues for receiving care include local health departments and community health centers. Community health centers offer primary and preventive care to millions of Americans for free or at a low cost. Anyone may obtain care from these clinics regardless of income. The cost of care is determined by using a sliding scale that is based on an individual's income (HealthCare.gov, 2013).

A client's perceived need for healthcare services can be a barrier to access. It may cause clients to seek care that is unnecessary or care that is necessary but provided at an inappropriate and often more expensive place of service than needed. The nurse can change the client's perception of need (thereby promoting appropriate and timely health care) by managing client care; teaching adults about self-care and the care of their children; and teaching them when and how to access appropriate care.

Physician shortages, especially in the field of primary care, are expected to worsen as the Affordable Care Act increases the number of individuals with healthcare coverage, as physicians and clients continue to age, and as the trend toward specialization continues. In recognition of this possibility, the Affordable Care Act includes funding to improve the recruitment and training of primary care, public health, nursing, and other health professionals and to increase the number of such providers in medically underserved areas. Implementation of a team approach to health care favorably affects the availability of primary care. As physicians are teamed with nurses and nurse practitioners who manage those aspects of client care that do not require a physician's expertise, physicians will have more time available to devote to those elements of care requiring their knowledge and skills.

REVIEW Access to Health Care

RELATE Link the Concepts and Exemplars

Linking the exemplar of access to health care with the concept of ethics:

1. What ethical issues are involved when individuals are uninsured?
2. What aspects of the ANA Code of Ethics address clients who are uninsured or underinsured?

Linking the exemplar of access to health care with the concept of reproduction:

3. What resources in your community are available to uninsured pregnant women?
4. Are the risks to the fetus any greater or any different when the pregnant mother is uninsured? Explain.

REFER Go to Pearson Nursing Student Resources
nursing.pearsonhighered.com

- Additional review materials

REFLECT Case Study

Helena Alvarez is a pregnant, 19-year-old Hispanic woman, who arrives at the emergency department of a small rural hospital with severe cramping pains and bleeding. She has no health insurance. No maternity services are available at this hospital, and no obstetricians are available in the community. There is a tertiary care facility about 100 miles away.

1. How would you determine what options are available for providing care for Ms. Alvarez?
2. As a nurse, what are your obligations to Ms. Alvarez?

EXEMPLAR 46.2 **Allocation of Resources**

EXEMPLAR KEY TERM

Resource allocation, *2607*

EXEMPLAR LEARNING OUTCOMES

After reading about this exemplar, you will be able to:

1. Discuss the reasons for allocating healthcare resources.
2. Describe examples of resource allocation.
3. Examine the role of the nurse in allocation of resources at the local and national levels.

▶ OVERVIEW

For at least the past two decades, the escalating cost of health care in the United States has been a concern. Gaining control over increasing healthcare expenditures has been a goal of both the government and private entities. Many factors are responsible for the increasing cost of health care. These include increased longevity, increases in the prevalence of chronic diseases such as diabetes, continued medical advances (which may result in more accurate diagnoses and better treatment, but are often more expensive than existing methods), technological advances, consumer demand, and defensive medicine. Inappropriate healthcare treatment choices by consumers have also contributed to increased healthcare costs. As discussed in the module on Managing Care, employees have enjoyed the benefits of employer-negotiated insurance plans but, as clients, have been insulated from and are often unaware of the cost of care, resulting in uninformed decisions about the type and amount of health care needed. Mass advertising by pharmaceutical manufacturers and specialty treatment centers directed at consumers have also contributed to inappropriate treatment choices being made by the public.

As healthcare expenditures have increased, the need for **resource allocation**, that is, distribution of resources among competing groups of people or programs, has been recognized. When resources are being allocated, three levels of decision making must be considered:

Level 1: allocating resources to health care versus other social needs
Level 2: allocating resources within the healthcare sector
Level 3: allocating resources among individual clients (AHC).

> ### CLINICAL EXAMPLE
>
> An 8-year-old boy with a chronic blood disorder requires weekly blood transfusions. The hospital struggles to maintain enough of his rare blood type. The 8-year-old arrives at the emergency department at the same time as another client with the same blood type who is bleeding profusely. There is enough blood for only one of these clients.
>
> 1. Which client should receive the blood? Why?
> 2. What models or methods should be used to make the decision? Who should be responsible for making the decision?

▶ EXAMPLES OF RESOURCE ALLOCATION

Rationing is one means of allocating healthcare resources. Rationing is a method used by individuals, insurance companies, and the government to prevent increases in the cost of health care or to reduce the cost of health care. Individuals ration when they decide to provide self-care for an illness or injury rather than seeking care from a healthcare provider. Methods used by insurance companies to ration healthcare resources include limiting the number of healthcare providers that clients can choose and denial of coverage for services (e.g., services deemed to be experimental or those that are not supported by scientific evidence that prove their efficacy). The government also rations healthcare resources, such as inclusion of the coverage gap in Medicare Plan D (known as the "donut hole") that sometimes forces beneficiaries to purchase fewer prescriptions (Torrey, 2012).

The Organ Procurement and Transplantation Network

One of the best-known systems of allocating certain healthcare resources is the Organ Procurement and Transplantation Network (OPTN). In the United States, approximately 79 people receive a donated organ each day. Unfortunately, another 18 people die each day waiting for an organ transplant (OPTN, 2013a). There simply are not enough donated organs to meet the demand for transplants. The OPTN, a contracted service of the USDHHS, maintains the only national client waiting list for organ transplantation. Multiple factors determine who receives a donor organ. A few of the factors are blood and tissue type, medical urgency, organ size, time on the waiting list, and the geographic distance between the donor and the recipient (OPTN, 2013b).

> ⚙ *Stay Current: More information on organ donation, including how to register as a donor, can be found at* **http://optn. transplant.hrsa.gov**.

H1N1 Vaccine Distribution

During 2009, there was an outbreak of H1N1 influenza. Initially an inadequate supply of vaccine was available, but as H1N1 began to spread, the Centers for Disease Control and Prevention (CDC) realized that guidelines had to be developed and implemented to ensure that the most vulnerable individuals had first access to the vaccine. As more vaccine became available, the CDC (2009) controlled its distribution by considering factors such as the amount of vaccine being requested by local health departments, the speed at which the vaccine was becoming available, and the need to ensure availability for not only the community but also active duty military personnel.

Once the vaccine arrived in local communities, further decisions were made about who could receive it if the supply was insufficient to meet the demand. Many local health departments screened potential recipients and initially administered the vaccine only to individuals with risk factors for H1N1, such as small children and adults with diagnosed respiratory disease (**Figure 46–2 ●**). Later, when sufficient quantities of the vaccine became available, healthcare providers were able to administer the vaccine to anyone who asked for it.

▶ NURSES AND ALLOCATION OF RESOURCES

The role of the nurse in the allocation of resources is a collaborative one. Nurses are the largest group of health professionals, and as part of the interdisciplinary healthcare team, the nurse participates in allocating healthcare resources. Thus, nurses develop a significant understanding of how appropriate allocation and misallocation of healthcare resources can affect client needs and outcomes. Nurses must be aware of and participate in discussions that affect the allocation of healthcare resources

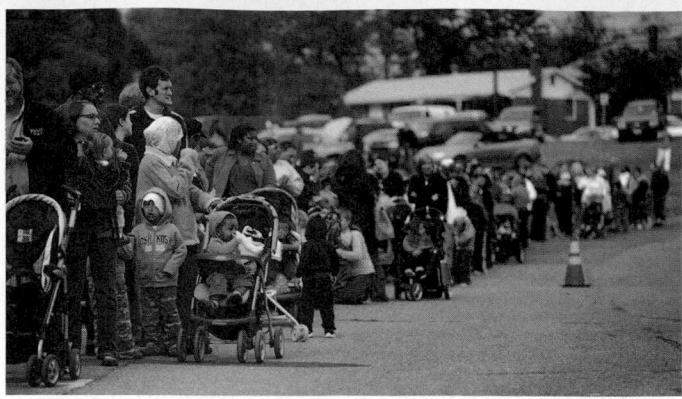

Figure 46–2 ● Hundreds of county residents wait in a long line for the H1N1 vaccination shot at a clinic held by the Montgomery County Health and Human Services on October 14, 2009, at the Dennis Avenue County Health Center in Silver Spring, Maryland.
Source: Tim Sloan/Getty Images.

in the workplace, in their communities, and at the federal level. Nurses are uniquely placed to advocate on behalf of clients when allocation of resources is being considered in their communities. They may advocate by talking with local legislators, writing to politicians, and engaging in discussions in their neighborhoods and social groups. As working professionals, nurses have the opportunity to participate in national discussions about resources through a number of professional organizations, such as the American Nurses Association.

REVIEW Allocation of Resources

RELATE Link the Concepts and Exemplars

Linking the exemplar of allocation of resources with the concept of ethics:

1. What provisions of the ANA Code of Ethics address resource allocation?

2. What ethical considerations do you as an individual value that might affect how you would determine resource allocation?

Linking the exemplar of allocation of resources with the concept of safety:

3. What aspects of resource allocation may affect client safety in the operating room? How?

4. What aspects of resource allocation may affect client safety in a long-term care facility, where three staff members may be required to transfer a client from a bed to a chair?

REFER Go to Pearson Nursing Student Resources
nursing.pearsonhighered.com

- Additional review materials

REFLECT Case Study

The general medical-surgical unit of a neighborhood hospital is experiencing a nursing shortage. At the moment, some nurses are working extra shifts as a means of helping out the hospital and its clients and of making extra money. When a forest fire breaks out, the unit is forced to accept clients that the emergency department cannot accommodate. That same week, the administration announces that a new mandatory overtime policy is being implemented until more nursing staff can be hired.

1. What aspects of resource allocation are affecting the medical-surgical unit at the hospital?

2. How might these aspects affect nursing staff performance? How might they affect morale?

EXEMPLAR 46.3 Emergency Preparedness

EXEMPLAR KEY TERMS
Bioterrorism, *2614*
Cold zone, *2614*
Community Emergency Response Team (CERT) program, *2611*
Disaster, *2609*
Emergency, *2609*
Emergency preparedness, *2609*

Emergency response, *2610*
Hot zone, *2614*
Local emergency management agency (LEMA), *2611*
Mitigation, *2609*
Pandemic, *2609*
Preparedness, *2609*
Recovery, *2610*

Reverse triage, 2612
Surge capacity, 2609
Triage, 2612
Warm zone, 2614

EXEMPLAR LEARNING OUTCOMES

After reading about this exemplar, you will be able to:

1. Discuss the four phases of emergency response.
2. Summarize the responsibilities of nurses during each phase of emergency response.
3. Outline the educational competencies required of nurses responding to a mass casualty incident.
4. Develop your own individual emergency plan.
5. Describe various biotoxins and how they are disseminated among a population.
6. Propose plans of care based on the emergency and the community resources available.

▶ OVERVIEW

An **emergency** is a sudden, often unforeseen event that threatens health or safety. A public emergency necessitating assistance from outside the affected community is a **disaster**. Disasters have three things in common: little or no warning before the event; available personnel and emergency services that are overwhelmed initially; and a serious threat to life, public health, and the environment. Infectious diseases may accompany disasters or can become disasters themselves. A **pandemic** is an infection that spreads rapidly around the world.

Emergency preparedness is the act of making plans to prevent, respond to, and recover from emergencies. The CDC recommends an *all-hazards* approach to emergency preparedness. This approach provides for general preparation, including training that can be applied in a wide variety of emergency situations. The impact on health and the healthcare system is similar regardless of the nature of the disaster. **Surge capacity** refers to a community's ability to rapidly meet the increased demand for qualified personnel and resources, including healthcare resources, in the event of a disaster.

▶ THE FOUR PHASES OF EMERGENCY MANAGEMENT

Emergency management consists of four phases: mitigation, preparedness, response, and recovery.

The **mitigation** phase, which takes place both before and after an emergency occurs, consists of identifying potential hazards, taking action to reduce the likelihood of their occurrence, and minimizing the effects of those that cannot be prevented. An example of mitigation in an individual's disaster plan would be the purchase of flood insurance by someone living in a flood zone. Implementation of warning systems for tornadoes and tsunamis are examples of mitigation by local, state, or regional agencies. Installation of a warning system prior to an occurrence of a disaster is an example of excellent disaster planning. Installation after an event is an example of using lessons learned from a disaster to reduce the effect of future occurrences. Both examples are mitigation.

The **preparedness** phase takes place before an emergency occurs. Risks are assessed and plans are developed to address them. Plans are designed to save lives and to assist first response and rescue teams that are often overwhelmed by the initial demands of an emergency. Emergency plans are developed at the federal, regional, state, and local levels. The Federal Emergency Management Agency (FEMA), the Department of Homeland Security, and the CDC identify national threats, create plans at the national level, and coordinate planning efforts among many people, agencies, and levels of government. They provide guidance for the development of plans in local communities. For communities, the most critical task performed during the preparedness phase is the development of an emergency operations plan. Such plans will often include multiple components addressing each of the many hazards and natural disasters that the community may face. Such plans include identifying, organizing, and training emergency personnel; stockpiling equipment and supplies; implementing communication and warning systems; establishing emergency operations centers; and implementing response and evacuation plans.

Ideally the agencies that participate in the emergency plan's development will also be involved in emergency response efforts and, therefore, will understand the risks the community may face and the responses that will be required. When agencies prepare for emergencies in advance and continually update their plans over time, their preparedness efforts will be more effective and result in better outcomes for the community.

During the preparedness phase, individual nurses must gain an understanding of their expected roles in an emergency and prepare for them. Because nurses will be required to allocate scarce resources and supplies and make unbelievably difficult client care decisions, they must understand the ethics associated with such choices. The ANA is a good source of information to guide nurses' understanding of their roles and possible consequences. Nurses must be aware of their employer's response plans and have a sense of how their state and local community will operate during an emergency. Nurses who choose to become disaster volunteers should register with an agency such as the American Red Cross to ensure they are properly trained and recognized as part of an organized system (ANA, 2008).

During the preparedness phase, nurses must also develop an emergency plan for themselves and their immediate families. When this plan is complete, nurses can be confident that their families are prepared to weather an emergency in relative safety. With this assurance, nurses who choose to assist in a disaster will be able to leave their families without delay to join the appropriate emergency team. FEMA and the Red Cross are two organizations that provide detailed information to assist individuals with the development of personal emergency plans. It is important for everyone to develop a plan for themselves and their families. They must ensure that not only the adults but also the children know what to do in an emergency. Plans should address the basic emergency needs of any disaster and, in addition should also include specifications for disasters such as tornadoes that may occur in the individual's location. Everyone should assemble a disaster kit that can be used in place or taken if evacuation is necessary. Escape routes for disasters that could occur within the home itself (e.g., gas leaks and fires) or for others such as floods and hurricanes that would require mass evacuation should be determined. Meeting places should be designated—someplace inside or outside the home where the family can unite. Family members should be provided contact information in case they are separated during a disaster. Someone outside of the immediate area should be identified as a central contact if family members are unable to reach each other locally. It is very important to shut off utilities as directed by emergency authorities or when forced to leave home. Insurance, medical, financial, and other vital records should be duplicated and stored in an off-site, safe location. Special needs such as medications, medical equipment, and so forth, should be considered and availability planned for. Family members should be trained in first aid including CPR. Review and update of the emergency plan on a regular basis are critical because someday one's life may depend on it.

🌐 *Stay Current: Visit* **www.ready.gov/are-you-ready-guide** *for FEMA's* ***Are You Ready? Guide—An In-Depth Guide to Citizen Preparedness.***

Despite a community's best preparedness efforts, there will be instances when a variety of factors result in failure to meet community needs. The evacuation of New Orleans in advance of hurricane Katrina and the efforts to provide shelter immediately following Katrina are stunning examples of how preparedness efforts can fail (see **Figure 46–3 ●**).

The third phase, **emergency response**, is the implementation of emergency preparedness plans. These plans provide a means for responders to save lives, prevent additional property damage, and meet basic human needs. As soon as possible, disaster victims are triaged and given appropriate treatment. Other emergency activities include search and rescue operations, opening shelters to house

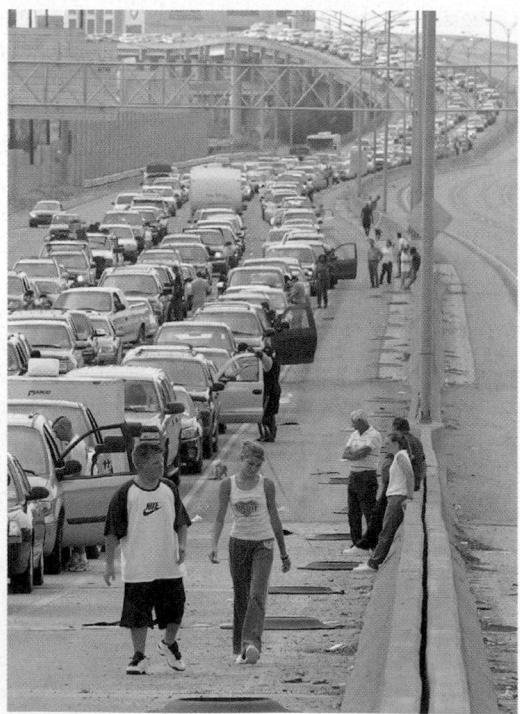

Figure 46–3 ● Authorities in New Orleans ordered hundreds of thousands of residents to flee on Sunday, August 28, 2005, as Hurricane Katrina strengthened into a rare, top-ranked storm and barreled toward the vulnerable U.S. Gulf Coast city. Those who had vehicles were caught in traffic jams for hours.
Sources: Rick Wilking/Landov Media.

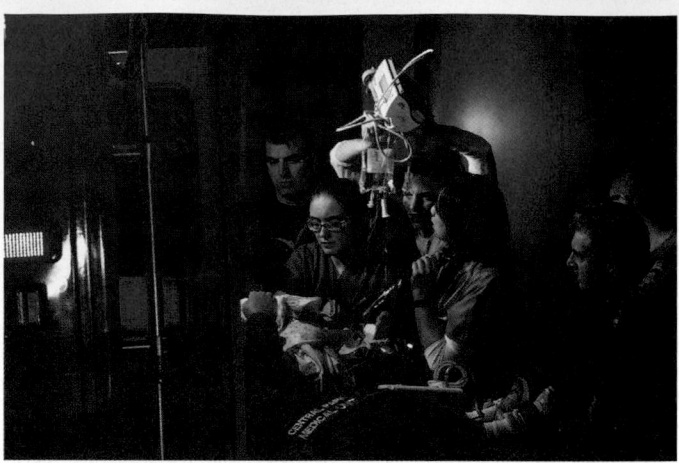

Figure 46–4 ● Medical workers assist a client into an ambulance during an evacuation of New York University's Langone Medical Center, Monday, October 29, 2012, in New York. The New York City hospital moved out more than 200 clients, including 20 infants from the NICU, after its backup generator failed when the power was knocked out by Hurricane Sandy.
Source: AP Photo/John Minchillo, File.

survivors, and repairing utility infrastructures (**Figure 46–4 ●**). The emergency response plan is followed during and immediately after the emergency, simultaneously with the community's assessment of the disaster's immediate effects. Community agencies such as local law enforcement, paramedics, and emergency department personnel, as well as local governmental staff employed in the disaster response unit, are responsible for implementing the overall plan and its components. Federal, state, and other outside resources support local efforts by providing first aid and other emergency medical assistance, establishing or restoring communication and transportation, assessing the probability of infectious diseases and addressing them, and identifying and providing support to individuals with mental health problems.

During the preparedness phase nurses must become familiar with the emergency plans of their employers and communities. They must also familiarize themselves with the ANA's positions on nurses' emergency and disaster responsibilities. During the emergency response phase, nurses will put this information to use. The responsibility of nurses during an emergency, like that of other first responders, is to do the greatest good for the greatest number of casualties. During an emergency, nurses will be asked to perform the fundamentals of nursing practice but will do so in a very stressful environment under extraordinary circumstances. They will be working under intense time constraints and must care for each victim quickly, then move on to the next one. They should not use their time to provide care that will be of minimal or questionable benefit. Nurses must observe both the physical and mental status of victims and ensure appropriate triage and treatment. Advanced practice nurses who have received training in emergency and trauma care will have significantly greater responsibilities than nurses with less training. During the crisis, nurses should be constantly aware of their defined scope of practice and must not exceed it even when circumstances would seem to dictate otherwise.

The **recovery** phase takes place after the emergency and is designed to restore the community to normal (restoration) or create a new, safer normal by updating the community's preparedness plan to address lessons learned during the emergency (mitigation).

The recovery phase includes the reconstitution of government operations and services, if necessary, and includes the provision of public assistance by the private and public sectors. Other elements of the recovery phase may include rebuilding, reemployment, and the repair of essential infrastructure. During the recovery phase, each community must reassess risks and update plans to ensure that newly identified risks are addressed. Because of their education and experience, nurses are well qualified to participate in risk assessment and planning at the local, state, and national levels following a disaster. Nurses are also perfect candidates to educate their clients and communities about disaster preparation.

▶ RESPONSIBILITY FOR EMERGENCY MANAGEMENT AND RESPONSE

State divisions of emergency management act as the **local emergency management agency (LEMA)** for each state. This is a governmental agency with expertise in public safety, emergency medical services, and management. The U.S. Department of Homeland Security has created federal guidelines called the National Incident Management System (NIMS) that local governments must follow during an emergency or disaster. Local governments have the primary responsibility for emergency management and response. In the event of an emergency, first responders such as local fire departments and emergency medical technicians will be challenged to meet the needs of the public because of the sheer volume of assistance they will be asked to provide. In situations like this, citizen volunteers often act as extensions of the first responders. For this reason, it is beneficial for a community to develop a corp of trained citizens to provide such support.

In recognition of this, FEMA has developed the **Community Emergency Response Team (CERT) program** to prepare interested community members. Participants gain an understanding of their responsibility for preparing for a disaster so they will be ready to safely assist themselves, their families, and their neighbors. The CERT program provides citizens with facts about what to expect following a major disaster in terms of immediate services; alerts citizens to their responsibility for mitigation and preparedness; trains citizens in needed lifesaving skills with an emphasis on decision-making skills, rescuer safety, and doing the greatest good for the most people; and organizing teams that act as an extension of first responder services, offering immediate help to victims until professional services are on site (FEMA, 2013).

The CDC manages the Clinician Outreach Communication Activity (COCA) program to ensure that clinicians have up-to-date information. COCA is designed to provide two-way communication between clinicians and the CDC about emerging health threats such as pandemics, natural disasters, and terrorism. COCA keeps a list of emergency preparedness and training resources offered by federal agencies and COCA partners.

Stay Current: Visit **www.bt.cdc.gov/coca/training.asp** for COCA's list of conferences and training opportunities and to sign up for e-mail updates from COCA.

Nursing Competencies for Emergency Response

Nurses represent the largest pool of healthcare professionals and, for this reason, are called on to assist in mass casualty events (MCEs). Training in preparation for, recognition of, and

---

Box 46–4 Categories of Educational Competencies for Registered Nurses Responding to Mass Casualty Incidents

CORE COMPETENCIES

1. Critical thinking
2. Assessment
3. Technical skills
4. Communication

CORE KNOWLEDGE AREAS

1. Health promotion, risk reduction, and disease prevention
2. Healthcare systems and policies
3. Illness and disease management
4. Information and healthcare technologies
5. Ethics
6. Human diversity

PROFESSIONAL ROLE DEVELOPMENT

1. A description of nursing roles during MCEs
2. Identification of the most appropriate or most likely healthcare role for oneself during an MCE

Source: Based on Nursing Emergency Preparedness Education Coalition. (2003). Retrieved from http://www.nursing.vanderbilt.edu/incmce/overview.html.

---

response to MCEs will be beneficial to the nurse, the nurse's family, the nurse's employer, and the community. Some of the ways in which nurses have received training regarding MCEs include reading professional journal articles, participating in mock disaster drills, volunteering in community services, and actual nursing during an MCE. Emergency preparedness is a necessity, regardless of the nurse's educational preparation, area of expertise, or practice setting (Whitty & Burnett, 2012).

In 2003, the International Nursing Coalition for Mass Casualty Education (INCMCE) (2003) published educational competencies for registered nurses to facilitate their response to MCEs with a strong recommendation that these core competencies be included in initial nursing education programs (see Box 46–4 ●).

The National Nurse Emergency Preparedness Initiative is a highly interactive, Web-based course that provides emergency preparedness training for nurses working in hospitals/acute care, schools, public health, ambulatory care, hospice/palliative care, long-term care, occupational health, and home health settings. This training focuses on providing opportunities for dynamic and interactive application of both theory and practice through scenario-based learning.

Stay Current: Visit the National Nurse Emergency Preparedness Initiative Web site at **http://nnepi.gwnursing.org** to sign up for its interactive learning module that teaches nurses about a critical thinking framework that can be applied during disasters.

Emergency Plans

Individuals and agencies that respond to MCEs are expected to act within the framework of emergency plans that were prepared in advance. Most agencies are mandated by law to develop plans that dictate the roles and responsibilities of all individuals who will respond during emergencies, disasters, and MCEs. Individual healthcare agencies such as hospitals, health departments, and residential facilities for seniors and people with disabilities will create emergency plans that prescribe the roles and responsibilities of their own employees. All nurses must not only familiarize themselves with the policies and procedures of the agency that employs them, but must also create an individual emergency plan for themselves and their families.

▶ TRIAGE

The process of **triage** involves prioritizing clients for treatment based on severity of illness or injury and in light of the supplies and resources available. The objective of triage is to ensure early assessment of clients and prioritize care based on severity of

symptoms. Nurses perform triage every day in emergency departments. During a mass casualty event (more than 100 victims), the demand on nurses' knowledge and skills will be even greater. Mass casualties call for the implementation of **reverse triage**, in which the most severely injured or ill victims who require the greatest resources are treated last to allow the greatest number of victims to receive medical attention. A simple color classification system (START) is used to prioritize adult clients (see **Figure 46–5 ●**). A separate algorithm, Jump START, has been developed for pediatric victims (**Figure 46–6 ●**). It is recommended that emergency medical personnel be assigned to triage. This frees physicians and nurses to provide needed care.

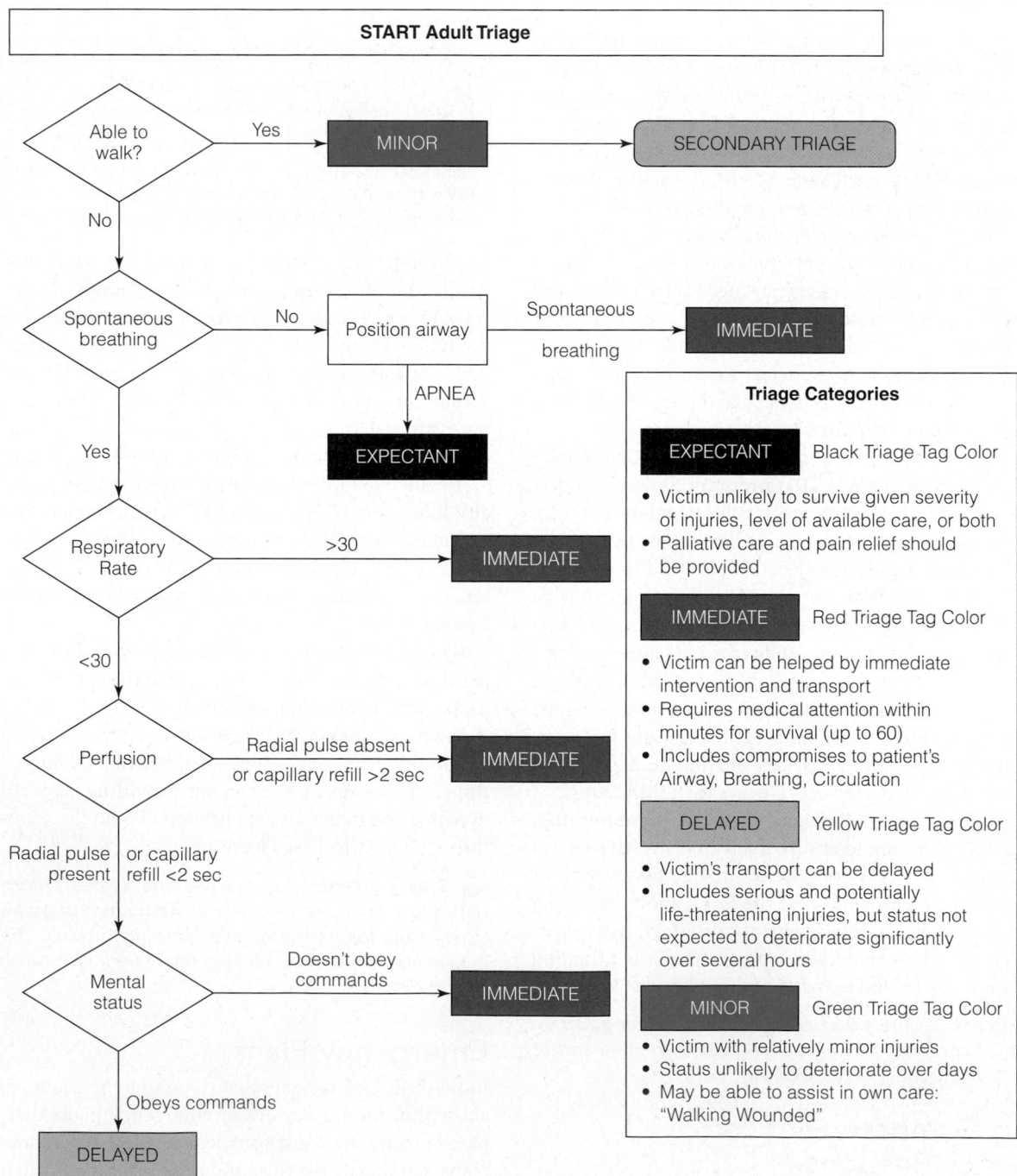

Figure 46–5 ● START adult triage algorithm.

JumpSTART Pediatric MCI Triage©

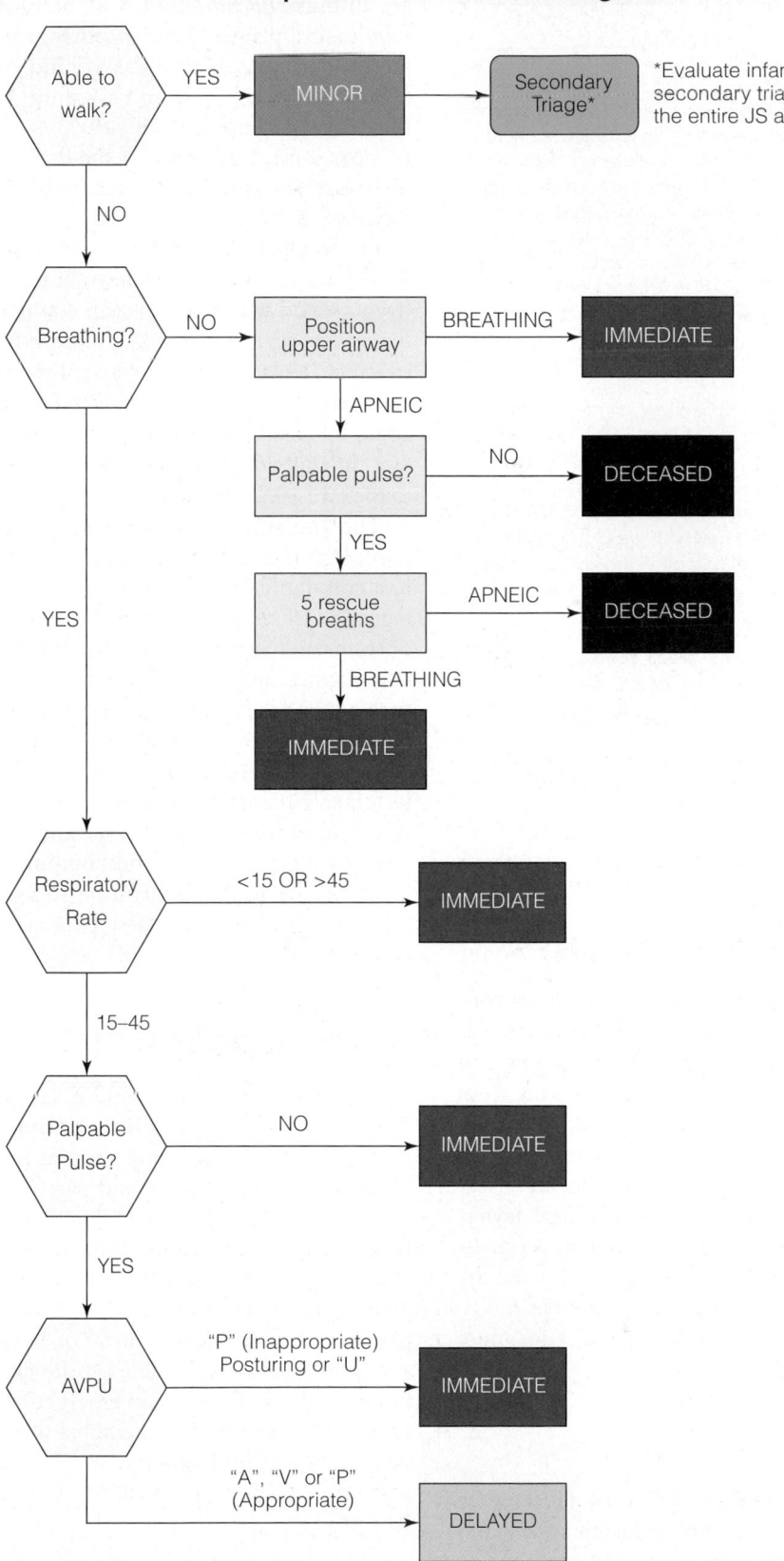

Figure 46–6 ● JumpSTART algorithm for pediatric victims.

Box 46–5 Hot, Warm, and Cold Zones

HOT ZONE

The **hot zone** is the most dangerous zone because it is located immediately adjacent to the site of the disaster. All responders who enter the area must be protected by personal protective equipment (PPE). Because of the dangers inherent in this location, only the most basic services are performed: Victims are located; basic lifesaving measures are provided (e.g., airways are established and hemorrhages are controlled); antidotes are administered; and the dead and those who cannot be saved are identified. Decontamination of victims is not performed in the hot zone. Victims who may survive are transported to the warm zone for decontamination All contaminated supplies and equipment are left in the hot zone for later collection and disposal.

WARM ZONE

The **warm zone** (also referred to as the yellow, contamination, or contamination reduction zone) is located at least 300 feet from the outer edge of the hot zone. Although its primary purpose is decontamination, rapid triage and emergency treatment to stabilize victims may take place in the warm zone. Individuals who have the highest levels of contamination are treated with the highest priority. PPE is required in this zone. After decontamination is completed, victims are moved to the cold zone.

COLD ZONE

The **cold zone**, also referred to as the green zone and support zone, is located outside of the warm zone and is the site where decontaminated victims are triaged and treated. It is considered to be comparatively safe although PPE is still required in case circumstances change, for example, if wind direction shifts. The primary purpose of this zone is to provide medical services and to transport victims who require more than first aid to locations where they will be provided higher levels of service.

▶ SITE-SPECIFIC DISASTER ZONES

When a site-specific disaster occurs, access to the site of contamination is limited and safety zones are established. Examples of such disasters are the release of weapons such as bombs, and toxic chemical leaks due to tanker car damage resulting from train derailments. The designated safety zones should be located uphill, upwind, and upstream from the site of the disaster. The configuration of each zone will vary based on the site of the occurrence. Topography, weather, and the physical layout (buildings, roads, etc.) will play an important role in designating the zones. The initial site of the incident is considered the hot zone. Only personnel with appropriate protective equipment are allowed in the hot zone. See **Box 46–5** ● for more information on zone breakdown.

▶ BIOTERRORISM

Bioterrorism is the deliberate release of viruses, bacteria, or other microbes as weapons. The U.S. public health system and primary healthcare providers must be prepared to respond to and treat the diseases caused by these agents, many of which are rarely seen in the United States. The CDC has assigned the highest priority to biological agents that can be easily disseminated or transmitted from individual to individual; cause a high mortality rate; have a significant impact on public health; cause public panic; and disrupt society and government. The primary

agents identified by the CDC as potential bioterrorist threats are anthrax (*Bacillus anthracis*), botulism (*Clostridium botulinum* toxin), plague (*Yersinia pestis*), smallpox (variola major), tularemia (*Francisella tularensis*), and viral hemorrhagic fevers (filoviruses [e.g., Ebola and Marburg] and arenavirsuses [e.g., Lassa and Machupo]) (CDC, 2013).

Nurses must be aware of the early signs and symptoms of these diseases as well as the methods of transmitting them. See **Table 46–3** ●.

Immediate treatment for the primary biological agents used in terrorism is limited. Inhalation of anthrax has been effectively treated with ciprofloxacin 400 mg administered intravenously every 12 hours. There are no effective therapies for treating clients infected by most of the other viruses that could be used in a bioterrorism attack. For some viruses, a vaccine could be created to stimulate the body's immune system such that the individual may be protected from infection if exposed to the virus at a later date.

The Strategic National Stockpile is a program designed to ensure the immediate availability of essential medical materials to a community in the event of a large-scale chemical or biological attack. Managed jointly by the CDC and the Department of Homeland Security, it consists of large quantities of antibiotics; vaccines; and medical, surgical, and client support supplies such as bandages, IV equipment, and airway supplies. The first component of the stockpile is a preassembled "push package" designed to meet the community's needs in the case of an undetermined biological or chemical threat. The push packages are stored in locations that will permit delivery within 12 hours after an attack. The second component is vendor-managed inventory packages that will be shipped once the threat has been clearly identified. These packages are designed to arrive within 24–36 hours.

▶ COLLABORATION

Emergency preparedness and disaster response depend on the collaboration of an interdisciplinary healthcare team involving local, state, and federal governmental agencies. Interdisciplinary training and participation in tabletop exercises, simulations, and mock incidents not only prepare the team members to assume their roles in case of disaster but also provide opportunities for frequent evaluations of the plan. These evaluations lead to a more effective emergency plan and facilitate communications across the interdisciplinary team that is responsible for the development, implementation, and evaluation of an emergency response plan. Nurses often have contact with members of emergency medical services (EMS) in both emergency departments and disaster situations. A brief overview of the EMS system is presented in **Box 46–6** ●.

▶ NURSING PRACTICE

The role of the nurse in a disaster or emergency will vary based on the type of disaster, its location, the number and condition of the victims, and the personnel (e.g., command staff, first responders, emergency medical technicians, police) and supplies that are

TABLE 46–3 Biological Pathogens of Highest Concern for Bioterrorism Attacks

PATHOGEN	CAUSE	SYMPTOMS	TRANSMISSION
Anthrax	*Bacillus anthracis*, a spore-forming bacterium Three types: ■ Cutaneous ■ Respiratory ■ Gastrointestinal	■ Cutaneous: The first symptom is a small sore that becomes a blister then progresses to a skin ulcer with a black spot in the center. All lesions are painless. ■ Respiratory: *Initially:* sore throat, mild fever and muscle aches. *Later:* respiratory symptoms, e.g., cough, chest discomfort, shortness of breath, tiredness and achy muscles. ■ Gastrointestinal: Nausea, loss of appetite, bloody diarrhea, and fever followed by bad stomach pain.	■ Cutaneous: direct skin contact with spores; often result from handling products, such as wool, from infected animals ■ Respiratory: inhalation of aerosolized spores (rare unless weaponized) ■ Gastrointestinal: eating undercooked meat or dairy products from infected animals (rare)
Botulism	*Clostridium botulinum* toxin	Food-borne botulism symptoms: ■ Usually develop within 12–36 hours after exposure. ■ May include visual effects, e.g., double vision; and neurological symptoms including slurred speech, dysphagia, and muscle weakness that begins in the shoulders and descends through the body to the calves; and paralysis of the breathing muscles, which if left untreated, may result in death.	■ Food-borne: individual ingests preformed toxin. ■ Infant: Occurs in small number of infants who harbor *C. botulinum* in their intestinal tract. ■ Wound botulism: Occurs when existing wounds are infected with the toxins of *C. botulinum.*
Plague	*Yersinia pestis,* a bacterium	■ Pneumonic plague develops within 1–6 days of exposure. ■ Fever, weakness, rapidly developing pneumonia with dyspnea, chest pain, cough, and sometimes bloody or watery sputum	■ An old mnemonic is "The fleas and lice on rats and mice cause plague." ■ Bubonic plague is transmitted via an infected flea bite or exposure of broken skin to infected material. ■ Pneumonic plague is of particular interest as a biological weapon because it can be released via weaponized aerosol. It can also be transmitted from individual to individual.
Viral hemorrhagic fevers (VHF)	Several distinct families of zoonotic viruses that reside in an animal reservoir host (e.g., rodent) or arthropod vector (e.g., ticks and mosquitos)	Signs and symptoms, which develop after a 5- to 10-day incubation period, vary by the type of VHF. Early signs and symptoms often include marked fever, fatigue, dizziness, myalgia, weakness, exhaustion, and a rash on the trunk. Severe cases may be accompanied by bleeding under the skin, in internal organs, or from body orifices like the mouth, eyes, or ears. Clients rarely die from this blood loss. Severe cases may cause shock, nervous system breakdowns, coma, delirium, and seizures. Renal failure may occur in some types of VHF.	■ VHFs are most commonly spread by exposure to an animal reservoir host or arthropod vector. Humans are not natural reservoirs for VHFs; however, some VHFs can be transmitted from individual to individual after an initial human has been infected.
Smallpox	Variola virus	■ During the incubation period (from 7 to 17 days), an infected individual has no symptoms and is not contagious. ■ Prodromal phase (2-4 days) symptoms include a fever of 101°–104°F, head and body aches, and possibly vomiting. This phase may be contagious. ■ The early rash phase is the most contagious period. The rash first appears as spots on the tongue and in the mouth, which then progress into sores that break open allowing large amounts of the virus to spread into the mouth and throat. The disease is highly contagious during this phase. Within 24 hours the rash, which begins on the face, spreads down and across the entire body. By the third day of the rash, raised bumps develop. By the fourth day of the rash, the bumps fill with thick, opaque fluid and have a depression in the center that resembles a belly button—a distinguishing characteristic of smallpox. Fever increases again. ■ Pustular rash (duration of 5 days): Pustular bumps develop (they feel like BBs under the skin), then form a crust and scab over. The scabs fall off, leaving pitted scars. The individual is contagious until all the scabs have fallen off.	■ Direct and fairly long face-to-face exposure is usually necessary under normal circumstances; however, weaponized smallpox can be spread by aerosol. ■ Direct contact with body fluids or contaminated items such as clothing or bed linen could spread the disease. ■ Humans are the only natural host of variola.

(continued on next page)

TABLE 46–3 Biological Pathogens of Highest Concern for Bioterrorism Attacks (*continued*)

PATHOGEN	CAUSE	SYMPTOMS	TRANSMISSION
Tularemia	*Francisella tularensis*	■ Sudden fever, chills, headache, diarrhea, muscle aches, joint pain, dry cough, and progressive weakness ■ If *F. tularensis* was used as a biological weapon and made airborne for exposure by inhalation, the infected people would experience severe respiratory illness, including life-threatening pneumonia and systemic infection.	Spread by bacterium found in animals (especially rodents, rabbits, and hares.) Means of spread include: ■ Being bitten by infected ticks, deerflies, other insects ■ Handling infected animal carcasses and skins ■ Eating or drinking contaminated food or water ■ Inhaling *F. tularensis*.

Source: Based on Centers for Disease Control and Prevention. (2013). *Bioterrorism agents: Emergency.* Retrieved from http://www.bt.cdc.gov/agent/agentlist-category.asp.

available at the time it occurs. Nurses may be called on to perform triage of clients, to perform first aid, or to stabilize clients in preparation for transfer for more advanced care.

Initially, the nurse must decide whether to assist during the disaster or not. This decision will be based on individual safety, family safety and needs, and the greater needs of the community at large. Nurses are never expected to jeopardize their own safety or the safety of their families or other rescuers by responding to a disaster. Nurses must also consider whether they have the appropriate skills to respond, that is, whether the skills of the nurse are adequate for the job or whether the job would be better left to individuals with advanced training in disaster response.

If the decision is made to participate, the nurse will follow the emergency preparedness plans created by the employing agency or within the community. The nurse must operate

within the defined nursing scope of practice despite the temptation to step outside of those bounds because of the critical care needs that might be met by doing so.

Individuals who choose to provide care during disasters must be aware of the ethics of doing so and the personal risk that may be involved. The American Nurses Association provides guidance in this area and is working hard to ensure that nurses who work within the framework suggested by ANA are protected from risks associated with providing care.

The injuries experienced during a disaster are specifically related to the type of disaster. For example, nurses working where an earthquake has occurred will treat multiple crush injuries. During the Boston Marathon on April 15, 2013, two explosions occurred. Nurses who had volunteered to provide medical services during the marathon suddenly found themselves in the unexpected position of caring for mass casualties who had suffered fractures, head trauma, severe abdominal injuries, and amputations (**Figure 46–7 ●**).

Nurses should assist their communities not only by providing emergency care during a disaster but also by becoming leaders as their communities prepare for potential disasters by creating or revising emergency preparedness and contingency plans.

Box 46–6 The Emergency Medical Services System

The emergency medical services (EMS) system is a network of resources that provides emergency care and transportation, that is, prehospital care, to victims of illness, injury, or disaster. EMS personnel, who must be trained and licensed, work under the auspices of a medical director, usually a hospital-based physician, who is consulted as needed. There are four levels of EMS professionals.

EMRs and EMTs provide basic life support:

■ *Emergency medical responders (EMRs)* provide initial emergency care including assessment, opening airways, ventilating, controlling bleeding, performing CPR, stabilizing the spine and injured limbs, assisting with childbirth, and aiding other EMS personnel.

■ *Emergency medical technicians (EMTs)* do everything EMRs do, but have received additional training and certification. This permits them to assist clients with prescribed medications and give aspirins, NSAIDs, oral glucose, and other medications when indicated.

AEMTs and paramedics are qualified to provide advanced life support:

■ *Advanced emergency medical technicians (AEMTs)* have received advanced emergency training so they may start and administer IV fluids; give medications; and assess the need for and provide advanced airway procedures.

■ *Paramedics* receive the most training and are qualified to do more in-depth assessments of clients including the assessment of abnormal heart rhythms and performance of some invasive procedures.

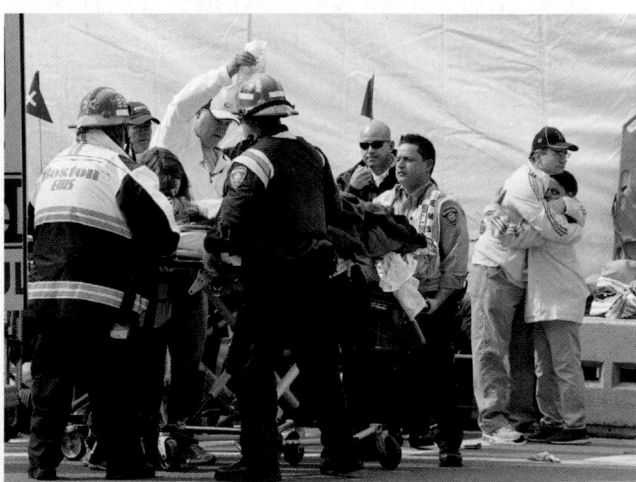

Figure 46–7 ● EMS personnel and volunteer nurses helped care for hundreds of victims of the Boston Marathon bombings on April 15, 2013.

Source: AP Photo/Elise Amendola.

REVIEW Emergency Preparedness

RELATE Link the Concepts and Exemplars

Linking the exemplar of emergency preparedness with the concept of professional behaviors:

1. What is the nurse's professional duty in a time of disaster?

Linking the exemplar of emergency preparedness with the concept of managing care:

2. Uninsured Americans are the most vulnerable in the event of a pandemic event. How is early recognition related to access to care?

Linking the exemplar of emergency preparedness with the concept of ethics:

3. What ethical considerations are involved when allocating scarce resources, such as medication, equipment, and healthcare personnel, during a disaster?

REFER Go to Pearson Nursing Student Resources **nursing.pearsonhighered.com**

- Additional review materials

REFLECT: Case Study

Ed Jones is a 75-year-old retired cabinet maker who makes small toys in the basement of his home, located on the banks of the Deep River. He is independent and a widower. His primary care physician has prescribed antihypertensive medications and monitors his blood pressure regularly. When a week of heavy rainstorms flooded Mr. Jones's neighborhood, his home sustained much water damage and most of his equipment and wood were ruined. Mr. Jones waded through waist-deep water to reach a rescue boat rather than waiting for it to pick him up. The EMTs who triage him decide to transfer him to the nearest emergency department.

You are the nurse assessing Mr. Jones. You observe that he has multiple cuts on his hands that are a result of woodworking and an ulcer on his right foot. Mr. Jones reports that the ulcer developed after a tool fell on his foot. He adds that he has not sought medical treatment for it. His physical assessment findings reveal: T 100.7°F PO; P 96 bpm, R 20/min, and BP 178/100 mmHg; his skin is cool and dry with multiple lesions on both hands and a Stage II ulcer on his right dorsal foot with yellow-green exudate. His pain rated as 2 on a 0–10 scale with 10 being the worst pain there could be. His lungs are clear, and his heart rate is regular. No edema is noted.

1. What actions did Mr. Jones take that probably exacerbated his skin lesions?

2. What additional information is needed so that you can form nursing diagnoses for Mr. Jones?

3. What nursing diagnoses do you believe would be appropriate?

■ REFERENCES

Agency for Healthcare Research and Quality (AHRQ). (2011). *National healthcare disparities report. (2011).* Retrieved from http://www.ahrq.gov/research/findings/nhqrdr/nhdr11/nhdr11.pdf.

American Nurses Association (ANA). (2008, March). *Adapting standards of care under extreme conditions: Guidance for professionals during disasters, pandemics, and other extreme emergencies.* Retrieved from http://ana.nursingworld.org/MainMenuCategories/HealthcareandPolicyIssues/DPR/TheLawEthicsofDisasterResponse/AdaptingStandardsofCare.aspx.

Appleby, J. (2010, April 6). Changes coming to health insurance plans. *Kaiser Health News.* Retrieved from http://www.kaiserhealthnews.org/Stories/2010/April/06/Changes-Coming-To-Insurance-Plans.aspx.

Bachrach, A., Isakson, E., Seth, D., & Brellochs, C. (2011, October). *Pediatric medical homes: Laying the foundation of a promising model of care.* Retrieved from http://www.nccp.org/publications/pdf/text_1041.pdf.

Case Management Society of America. (2012). *What is a case manager?* Retrieved from http://www.cmsa.org/Home/CMSA/Whatisacasemanager/tabid/224/default.aspx.

Centers for Disease Control and Prevention (CDC.) (2009). *H1N1 flu allocation and distribution Q&A.* Retrieved from http://www.cdc.gov/H1N1flu/vaccination/statelocal/centralized_distribution_qa.htm.

Centers for Disease Control and Prevention (CDC). (2011). *Health literacy.* Retrieved from http://www.cdc.gov/healthliteracy/researchevaluate/index.html.

Centers for Disease Control and Prevention (CDC). (2013). *Bioterrorism agents: Emergency.* Retrieved from http://www.bt.cdc.gov/agent/agentlist-category.asp.

Emergency Medical Treatment and Active Labor Act (EMTALA). (2011). *Frequently asked questions on EMTALA.* Retrieved from http://www.emtala.com/faq.html.

Federal Emergency Management Agency (FEMA). (2013, March). *Community emergency response teams.* Retrieved from http://www.fema.gov/community-emergency-response-teams

HealthCare.Gov. (2013). *Community health centers.* Retrieved from http://www.healthcare.gov/using-insurance/low-cost-care/community-health-centers.

Henry J. Kaiser Family Foundation (KFF). (2012a, September). *Five facts about the uninsured population.* Retrieved from http://www.kff.org/uninsured/upload/7806-02.pdf.

Henry J. Kaiser Family Foundation. (2012b). *State health facts.* Retrieved from http://www.statehealthfacts.org/comparemapdetail.jsp?ind=439&cat=8&sub=103&yr=200&typ=1&sort=a.

Henry J. Kaiser Family Foundation. (2012c, October). *The uninsured: A primer—Key facts about Americans without insurance.* Retrieved from http://www.kff.org/uninsured/upload/7451-08.pdf.

Institute of Medicine. (1993). *Access to health care in America.* Washington, DC: National Academy Press.

Institute of Medicine. (2004). *Health literacy: A prescription to end confusion.* Washington, DC: National Academy Press.

Insure Kids Now. (2013). *Questions and answers: Why is health care so important?* Retrieved from http://www.insurekidsnow.gov/qa.

International Nursing Coalition for Mass Casualty Education. (2003, August). *Educational competencies for registered nurses related to mass casualty incidents.* Retrieved from http://www.aacn.nche.edu/leading-initiatives/education-resources/INCMCECompetencies.pdf.

National Center for Education Statistics. (2003). *The health literacy of America's adults.* Retrieved from http://nces.ed.gov/pubs2006/2006483_1.pdf.

National Institutes of Health. (2013). *Health disparities.* Retrieved from http://report.nih.gov/NIHfactsheets/ViewFactSheet.aspx?csid=124.

Organ Procurement and Transplantation Network (OPTN). (2013a). *Donate the gift of life, the need is real: Data.* Retrieved from http://organdonor.gov/about/data.html.

Organ Procurement and Transplantation Network (OPTN). (2013b). *Organ matching process.* Retrieved from http://www.organdonor.gov/about/organmatching.html.

Torrey, T. (2012, April). *What is healthcare rationing? From denial of care to healthcare reform, rationing is a consideration.* Retrieved from http://patients.about.com/od/patientempowermentissues/a/rationing.htm.

United Health Foundation. (2012). *America's health rankings.* Retrieved from http://www.americashealthrankings.org/NY/PCP.

U.S. Census Bureau. (2010). *The next four decades: The older population in the United States: 2010 to 2050, population estimates and projections, May 2010.* Retrieved from http://www.census.gov/prod/2010pubs/p25-1138.pdf.

U.S. Census Bureau. (2011). *Health insurance highlights: 2011.* Retrieved from http://www.census.gov/hhes/www/hlthins/data/incpovhlth/2011/highlights.html.

U.S. Department of Health and Human Services (USDHHS). (2010a). *Healthy people 2020.* Retrieved from http://www.healthypeople.gov/2020/about/default.aspx.

U.S. Department of Health and Human Services (USDHHS). (2010b). *Healthy people 2020: Access to health services.* Retrieved from http://www.hhdw.org/cms/uploads/Data%20Source_%20Other%20Reports/HP2020/Access_Health_Services.pdf.

U.S. Department of Health and Human Services (USDHHS). (2010c). *Healthy people 2020: The road ahead.* Retrieved from http://www.healthypeople.gov/hp2020/.

U.S. Department of Health and Human Services (USDHHS). (2010d, December 2). *HHS announces the nation's new health promotion and disease prevention agenda* [press release]. Retrieved from http://www.healthypeople.gov/2020/about/DefaultPressRelease.pdf.

Whitty, B., & Burnett, M. (2012). From our readers: Are you prepared for a mass casualty event? *American Nurse Today, 7*(4). Retrieved from http://www.nursingworld.org/MainMenuCategories/Policy-Advocacy/Positions-and-Resolutions/Issue-Briefs/Disaster-Preparedness.pdf.

World Health Organization. (1998). *Health promotion glossary.* Retrieved from http://whqlibdoc.who.int/hq/1998/WHO_HPR_HEP_98.1.pdf.

47 Health Policy

MODULE AT-A-GLANCE

The Concept of Health Policy, 2619

Exemplar 47.1
Regulatory Agencies, 2621

Exemplar 47.2
Accrediting Bodies, 2624

Exemplar 47.3
Professional Organizations, 2625

Exemplar 47.4
Types of Reimbursement, 2627

◤ THE CONCEPT OF HEALTH POLICY

Public policy and healthcare delivery systems have a powerful impact on the health and well-being of U.S. citizens. They also impact professional nursing (see **Figure 47–1 ●**), affecting everything from nursing practice to staffing and education (American Nurses Association, 2010). The term **health policy** refers to actions and decisions by government bodies and professional organizations that affect whether or not healthcare organizations and individuals working within the healthcare system can achieve their healthcare goals.

Practicing nurses are uniquely qualified to evaluate how healthcare policy, laws, and regulations impact the provision of high-quality health care. Every day, nurses see the public's healthcare needs and envision how new or revised health policies could improve healthcare quality. The nurses' Code of Ethics, documented by the American Nurses Association, outlines each nurse's responsibility to advocate for social change either individually as a citizen or through political action. Nurses can influence health policy planning within individual organizations and at local, community, state, and national levels. At the national level, the American Nurses Association (ANA) represents professional nurses and the clients whom they serve and is an important national voice in policy planning. As an example, ANA believes that health care is a basic human right and supports the World Health Organization's challenge—originally articulated in 1978 and reaffirmed as late as 2007—for every nation to provide basic health care to each of its citizens. ANA worked tirelessly to achieve

(continued on next page)

Concept Learning Outcomes

After reading about this concept, you will be able to:

1. Identify factors that influence the development of health policy in the United States.

2. Describe processes by which health policies are developed, implemented, evaluated, changed, and maintained.

3. Distinguish regulatory agencies and accrediting bodies that develop, administer, or implement health policy.

4. Compare and contrast the scope and purpose of specific regulatory agencies and accrediting bodies.

5. Discuss professional organizations that support nurses and the nursing profession.

6. Summarize the types of healthcare reimbursement.

Concept Key Terms

Accreditation, *2624*

Children's Health Insurance Program (CHIP), *2628*

Consumer-driven healthcare plan (CDHP), *2628*

Copayment, *2628*

Domestic partner, *2628*

Health maintenance organization (HMO), *2628*

Health policy, *2619*

Indemnity, *2628*

Medicaid, *2627*

Medicare, *2627*

Medigap policy, *2629*

Point-of-service (POS) plan, *2628*

Preferred-provider organization (PPO), *2628*

Primary care provider (PCP), *2628*

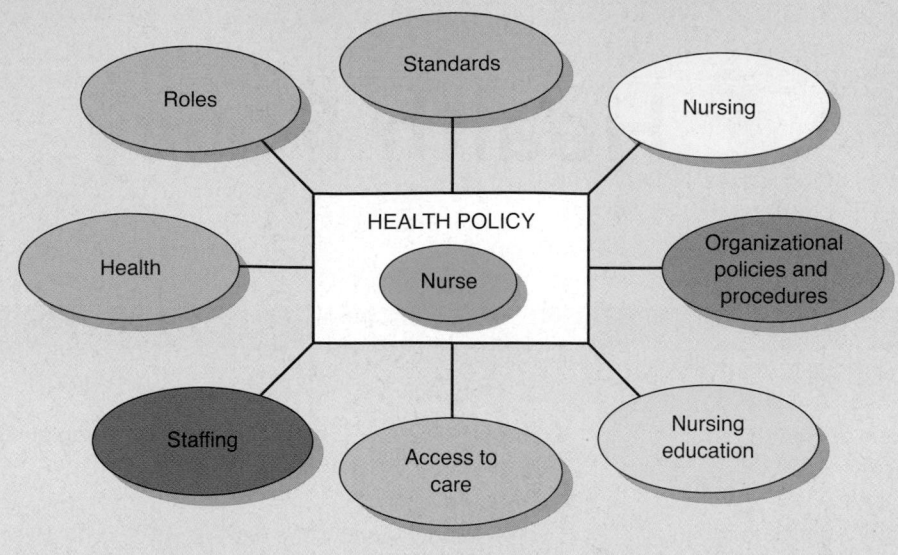

Figure 47–1 ● Why is health policy relevant to nurses?

the passage of the U.S. Patient Protection and Affordable Care Act. ANA continues to focus on successful implementation of the act to ensure improved availability of health insurance and greater access to healthcare services, both primary and preventive, to millions of people. **<<**

▶ DEVELOPING HEALTH POLICIES

Healthcare policies are subject to the political environment in which they are born. Successful policy development requires collaboration and partnerships with many individuals, groups, and stakeholders across the healthcare continuum. Many factors influence the development of healthcare policy as shown in the list below and in the Concepts Related to Health Policy feature.

- The population that will benefit (Is the population large or small? Is it underserved?)

- The cost of implementing the policy versus the health improvements that will be achieved (Do the benefits outweigh the cost?)

- Support for the policy (Is there solid support or should the policy be shelved until a more auspicious time?)

- Availability of scientific evidence supporting the need for the policy

Development of health policies operates within a problem-solving framework that is similar to the nursing process. The legislative process required in developing healthcare policies is outlined in **Table 47–1** ●.

Policymaking involves three basic phases: the formulation phase, the implementation phase, and the evaluation phase. The *formulation phase* is similar to the assessment and planning phases of the nursing process. During this phase, key individuals and interest groups, as well as research, provide data and ideas. The data are used to define the scope of the problems, identify desired outcomes, and estimate the

resources necessary to achieve success. The *implementation phase* involves communication of the adopted policies and their implementation. During the *evaluation phase*, additional data are collected and analyzed to determine how effective the policy is.

Any policy enacted by a governmental entity is assigned to a specific agency for implementation and translation of the policy into written rules. After the rules have been approved, the agency is responsible for administering the policy. As existing policies are evaluated, they may be modified to adjust to changing circumstances. Typically, these changes are made incrementally, to prevent the controversy that new policies or massive overhaul would generate. Federal government agencies that develop and administer health policies at the national level include the Department of Health and Human Services and the Occupational Safety and Health Administration . At the state level, state departments of health and human services oversee health policies. These policies are usually administered at the county or municipal level through local health departments or social services. For example, health policies affecting pet owners and restaurant managers typically are administered through local health departments. Local departments of social services administer public health insurance programs such as Medicaid and the Children's Health Insurance Program.

The most recent change in health policy is the Affordable Care Act of 2010. This new law is expected to increase access to health insurance for the working poor and self-employed. The act is discussed in detail in the module on Healthcare Systems.

Concepts Related to **Health Policy**

CONCEPT	RELATIONSHIP TO HEALTH POLICY	NURSING IMPLICATIONS
Legal Issues		
■ HIPAA ■ Affordable Care Act	Health policies often are the end product of state and federal legislation. Federal examples include the Health Insurance Portability and Accountability Act (HIPAA) and the Affordable Care Act. State examples include legislation to authorize or change policies regarding regulations impacting the availability of safe and legal abortions.	■ Legislation may restrict or promote patient access to care in a number of ways. In some cases, it may affect how nurses and other healthcare providers communicate client information. ■ For example, HIPAA restricts the sharing of client information without consent, and HIPAA laws impact both electronic and paper recordkeeping in healthcare facilities.
Accountability		
	Both government and professional organizations enact policies to ensure the accountability of healthcare professionals and agencies.	■ The Joint Commission, for example, sets standards of care and accredits many types of healthcare providers. Nurses follow policies and procedures congruent with these standards to ensure client safety and to ensure their agencies are in conformance with the expectations of the Joint Commission.
Healthcare Systems		
■ Access to health care ■ Allocation of resources	Health policies direct coding, billing, and reimbursement for care, which in turn may affect how care is provided and documented.	■ Nurses may find client care impacted by health policies related to managed care in a number of ways. ■ For example, Client A's health insurance plan may allow for the client to use a brand name prescription medication with a small copayment. Client B, on the other hand, might have a much higher copayment for a brand name prescription, and the nurse may need to work with the prescribing provider to ensure the client receives the generic medication. Most health insurance policies charge clients much less for using generic medications.

EXEMPLAR 47.1 **Regulatory Agencies**

▶ OVERVIEW

A number of regulatory agencies function to help healthcare providers and agencies operate safely, legally, honestly, and effectively. These agencies have a substantial effect on health care by enforcing laws and rules established by legislation. Regulatory agencies typically enforce laws and rules that must be followed at the organizational level; individual healthcare professionals are regulated by licensure boards (see the module on Legal Issues).

▶ FEDERAL AGENCIES

Changes in healthcare policy made at the federal level are administered through the U.S. Department of Health and Human Services and the agencies it oversees. The U.S. Department of Labor has responsibility in this area also, as it oversees policies that affect worker safety. These policies are administered through the Occupational Safety and Health Administration.

TABLE 47–1 Applying the Policy Development Process

POLICY PROCESS	APPLIED TO LEGISLATIVE PROCESS	EXAMPLE
Identify potential policy issue	Citizen(s) or advocate group(s) inform legislator(s) of a healthcare issue.	ANA informs congressional members that nurses and nursing staff are at increased risk for musculoskeletal disorders because, traditionally, they manually handle clients (for example, lifting and transferring). Clients are at risk, too, because injured staff may drop clients during transfer. Decreased unit staffing because of absences due to injury may have a negative impact on client care also.
Assess the issue by analyzing information	Legislative staff collects information and analyzes the issue. Possible sources of information are federal, state, and local governmental agencies; academic studies; consumer advocates; and professional organizations.	For the example, sources could be ANA, the U.S. Bureau of Labor Statistics, and the National Institute of Occupational Safety and Health. Possibly useful information includes compensation costs associated with client-handling injuries and resultant client injuries. Previous participants in ANA's Handle with Care campaign could describe their successes and challenges.
Build coalitions to achieve success	A legislator must form coalitions with other congressional members and stakeholders who will back the legislation as well. Legislators who are RNs and other healthcare providers are excellent choices.	Stakeholders must be identified, convinced of the issue's importance, and engaged in developing solutions and pushing resultant legislation through the legislative process. Possible stakeholders for this example are hospitals and nursing homes and their professional associations, ANA, and consumer groups.
Identify possible solutions	Such factors are evaluated as expected cost and benefits as well as anticipated effectiveness, efficiency, safety, etc. Legislative staff identifies the political considerations associated with each solution.	Possible solutions in this example range from doing nothing to mandating national legislation to prevent manual handling in specific healthcare delivery settings.
Select a solution	The legislator selects a solution and drafts a law using the information gathered during the assessment and analysis phase. Additional support from both the House and the Senate must be gained if the bill is to pass.	For purposes of this example, a decision is made to mandate the implementation of a Safe Patient Handling program in each state. Each state's program must meet the minimum requirements mandated by the federal law.
Implement policy	DHHS develops rules and regulations, which may be revised based on feedback from legislators and stakeholders such as ANA, posted again for additional comments, and revised. They are then passed into law.	All affected states are advised of the need to implement the law prior to its effective date. Each state, mindful that the minimum federal requirements must be met, passes legislation that prescribes how the program will be implemented. Professional associations, such as the state's hospital association, provide guidance to member organizations.
Monitor and evaluate outcomes	Following implementation of the rules and regulations, the responsible federal departments or agencies monitor and evaluate outcomes to ensure success. If the legislative goals are not achieved, the department may implement changes to the rules and regulations within the framework of the law. If the required changes are outside this framework, the department will recommend legislative changes, such as an amendment or a new law.	Implementation does not end the cycle. Continuous analysis of results by the implementing agency is critical. If musculoskeletal injuries to nurses and nursing staff do not decrease under the Safe Patient Handling program, possible reasons are explored: Did the individual states implement the requirements correctly? Is the Safe Patient Handling program rigorous enough? Once the reasons for failure are identified, the program is modified to achieve better results. Perhaps a uniform national program is implemented, or states that have not correctly implemented the program are identified so that technical assistance can be provided.

The Department of Health and Human Services

The U.S. Department of Health and Human Services (DHHS) is the federal government's principal agency for the protection of the health of all Americans and the provision of essential human services for those least able to care for themselves. The more than 300 divisions and programs within this department range from health research and the provision of health-related information by the National Institutes of Health (NIH) to healthcare financing through the Centers for Medicare and Medicaid Services (CMS). DHHS oversees services for individuals at all stages of life through its Administration for Children and Families and its Administration on Aging (**Box 47–1** ●). The 2013 DHHS budget is $941 billion. Components of DHHS include the Food and Drug Administration (FDA), Centers for Disease Control and Prevention (CDC), and Agency for Healthcare Research and Quality (AHRQ). DHHS is a powerful agency, as it administers more grant dollars than all other federal agencies combined and represents almost one-quarter of all federal outlays (USDHHS, 2013).

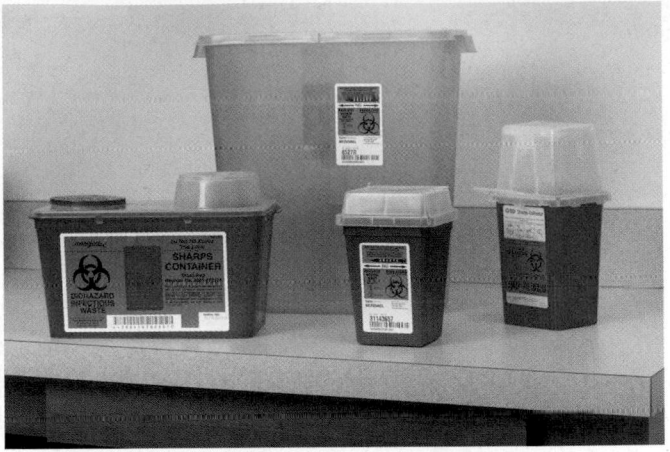

Figure 47–3 ● OSHA regulations require the use of sharps containers for discarding used needles.

Stay Current: Go to **www.dhhs.gov** *for the latest information from the U.S. Department of Health and Human Services.*

Occupational Safety and Health Administration

OSHA works to ensure the health and safety of Americans in the workplace. Most employees in the nation fall under OSHA's jurisdiction. Part of OSHA's mission is to provide assistance to employers, who are responsible for providing workers with a safe and healthful workplace and for reducing or eliminating workplace hazards. In general, OSHA sets standards requiring that employers maintain conditions or adopt practices that are reasonably necessary and appropriate to protect workers on the job; be familiar with and comply with standards applicable to their businesses; and ensure that employees have and use personal protective equipment when required for safety and health. OSHA issues standards for a wide variety of workplace hazards in industrial and healthcare settings. Two examples of OSHA standards are the availability of both personal protective equipment (PPE) and emergency eyewash stations (OSHA, n.d.).

OSHA provides training, outreach, and education to employers and employees; establishes cooperative partnerships (for example, with employers, employees, and unions); and encourages improvement of workplace safety and health (**Figure 47–3 ●**). In support of these activities, OSHA provides employers and employees information and training materials that focus on safety and health hazards in the workplace.

Stay Current: Go to **www.osha.gov** *for the latest information from the Occupational Safety and Health Administration.*

▶ STATE AND LOCAL AGENCIES

Each state mandates its own health policies and regulations in accord with federal policies and regulations. Usually, these mandates are administered through state divisions of health and human services. At the county or municipal level, local departments of health administer a wide variety of health policies and offer many critical services to their communities. Local departments of social services are typically responsible for administering Medicaid and the Child Health Insurance Program.

State Divisions of Health and Health Services

Every state has its own division or department of health and human services. These departments oversee regulation of county health departments, healthcare settings such as hospitals and long-term care facilities, child care centers, clinical laboratories, and other service providers such as portable x-ray suppliers. In addition to overseeing regulations, they are responsible for overseeing the planning and construction of medical facilities and for receiving and resolving complaints regarding the facilities that they regulate.

STATE OFFICES OF EMERGENCY MEDICAL SERVICES By ensuring that local emergency medical services (EMS) systems comply with the applicable regulations, state

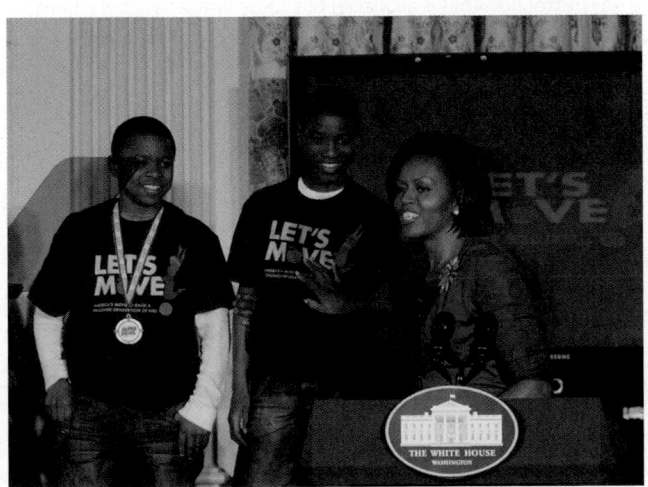

Figure 47–2 ● Michelle Obama announces the formation of Let's Move.
Source: ALEXIS C. GLENN/UPI/Newscom.

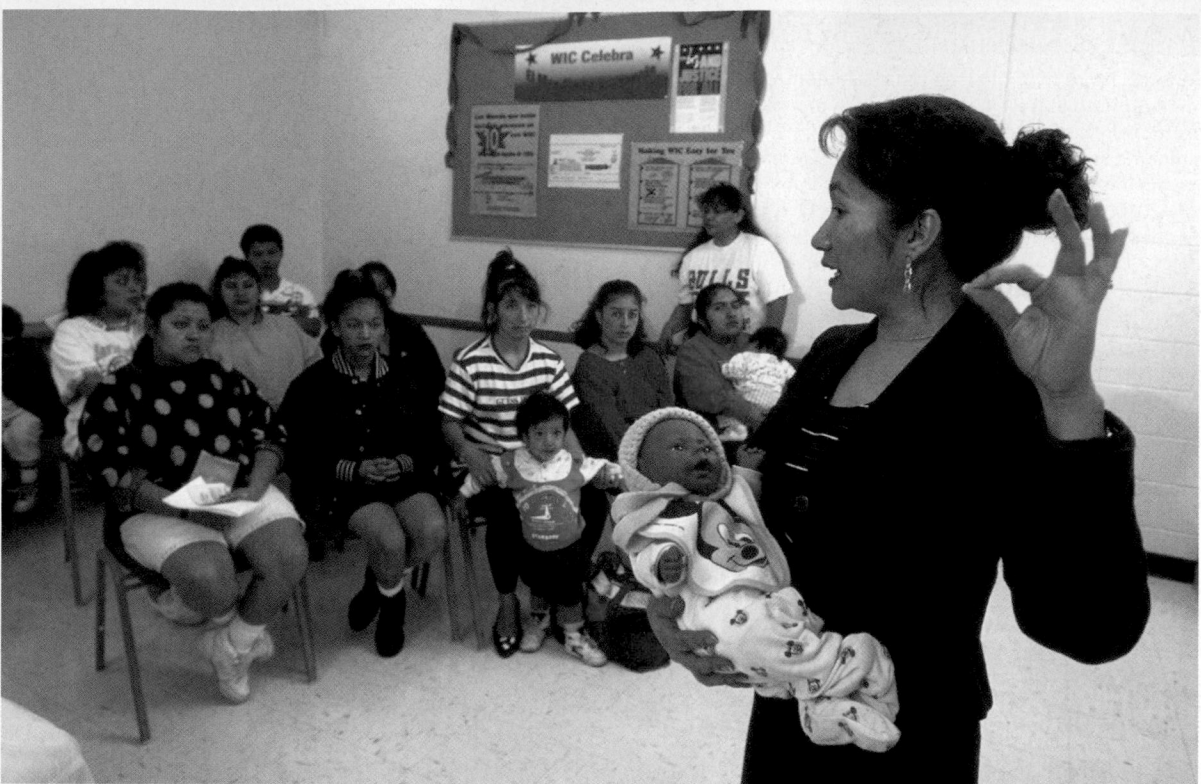

Figure 47–4 ● An instructor uses a doll to demonstrate breastfeeding techniques to a group of women in a WIC program.
Source: A. Ramey/PhotoEdit Inc.

offices of emergency medical services (OEMSs) provide citizens access to high-quality emergency medical care.

Local Health Departments

Local health departments oversee a variety of health policies and the respective regulations. For example, they are responsible for disease monitoring and surveillance in their communities. Associated activities include reporting incidents of disease to state and federal authorities as well as implementing disease prevention efforts, such as offering immunizations. Local departments of health typically oversee child care center sanitation and food safety. They also offer a variety of community-wide disease and injury prevention programs implemented as a result of federal efforts or designed in response to local issues. Typical programs include injury prevention campaigns; lead poisoning prevention efforts; and making safety equipment such as smoke detectors, children's bicycle helmets, and infant car seats available to families at no cost. Local departments of health usually administer the Women, Infants, and Children (WIC) supplemental nutrition program, which provides food assistance to pregnant women and children under age 5 who are at risk for malnutrition (**Figure 47–4** ●).

CASE STUDY \\ A

Emma Jones is a 29-year-old woman who works for a small manufacturing firm. Business has been growing despite the downturn in the economy. In fact, the manufacturer bought some used equipment and hired more people to keep pace with orders. Ms. Jones visits the ear, nose, and throat clinic with a chief complaint of persistent ringing in her ears. As she provides her history, she and the nurse realize that the ringing began a week after the additional equipment was put into use. The used equipment has fewer built-in noise controls, and the ear protection that is available has to be shared with new employees. Because of all the changes taking place, the supervisor has not had an opportunity to purchase additional ear protection.

Critical Thinking Questions

1. What is the employer's responsibility for protecting his employees?
2. What options does an employee have if the employer does not fulfill his responsibility?
3. What nursing diagnoses and interventions might be appropriate for Ms. Jones at this time?

EXEMPLAR 47.2   Accrediting Bodies

▶ OVERVIEW

Accreditation is a peer review process that evaluates the quality of an organization. Achieving accreditation certifies that the organization meets the requirements of the accrediting body and is qualified to provide the services it offers. Accreditation is time-limited; therefore, accredited organizations are reevaluated at intervals specified by the accrediting body. The accrediting agency's standards provide the structure for an organization's self-evaluation and the agency's accreditation survey. In preparation for its initial accreditation survey, an organization evaluates its own performance and identifies its strengths and weaknesses. It analyzes the results and implements corrective actions, thus improving its processes and the resultant outcomes. To achieve reaccreditation, an organization must provide evidence that it has continuously evaluated its performance, has identified new or continuing challenges, and has acted to correct them.

The agency completes an on-site survey to validate if the organization actually applies its management strategies and performs according to its stated goals and objectives. Benefits of being accredited include professional respect, credibility with government and third-party payers, and greater consumer trust. A nurse's role in the accreditation process may include participation in an organization's self-review activities and maintenance of a current, evidence-based practice.

▶ THE JOINT COMMISSION

The Joint Commission is an independent, nonprofit organization that sets standards for and accredits healthcare organizations. The Joint Commission's mission is "to continuously improve health care for the public, in collaboration with other stakeholders, by evaluating health care organizations and inspiring them to excel in providing safe and effective care of the highest quality and value" (The Joint Commission, 2009). The commission has set standards for and accredits many types of healthcare providers, such as ambulatory care centers, behavioral healthcare providers, hospitals, and long-term care facilities. Its standards address key functions within each type of organization, for example, infection prevention and control; provision of care, treatment, and services; medical management; and performance improvement. The Joint Commission ensures that an organization is able to provide safe, effective care for its clients and does so. The 32-member Board of Commissioners that governs the organization brings a broad spectrum of healthcare and clinical expertise to the commission. Two examples of The Joint Commission's policies that directly affect nurses are the National Patient Safety Goals (see the module on Safety) and its requirements for reporting Sentinel Events (see the module on Quality Improvement).

Stay Current: Go to **www.jointcommission.org** for the latest information from The Joint Commission.

▶ NURSING EDUCATION PROGRAM ACCREDITATION

Two national agencies are officially recognized by the U.S. Secretary of Education as responsible for the specialized accreditation of nursing education programs. The Commission on Collegiate Nursing Education (CCNE) ensures the quality and integrity of baccalaureate and graduate education programs. The Accreditation Commission for Education in Nursing (formerly the National League for Nursing Accrediting Commission, NLNAC) provides specialized accreditation for all types of nursing education programs (clinical doctorate, master's degree, baccalaureate degree, associate degree, diploma, and practical).

EXEMPLAR 47.3 Professional Organizations

▶ OVERVIEW

Each professional organization advances the nursing profession. Its organizational mission statement determines its level of involvement in oversight of or leadership for the profession, working conditions for nurses, and professional affairs. Professional nursing organizations serve a number of functions, including defining standards of practice and professional behaviors, supporting nursing research, and participating in policy development at the local, state, and national levels.

▶ AMERICAN NURSES ASSOCIATION

The ANA is the only full-service professional organization representing the nation's 3.1 million registered nurses (RNs) through its 54 constituent member associations (CMAs). Its mission statement is "Nurses advancing our profession to improve health for all." The ANA fosters high standards of nursing practice, promotes the rights of nurses in the workplace, projects a positive and realistic view of nursing, and lobbies Congress and regulatory agencies on healthcare issues affecting nurses and the public. There is one CMA in each of the 50 states and in Guam, the Virgin Islands, and Washington, DC, as well as the Federal Nurses Association (ANA, 2013).

Stay Current: Go to **www.nursingworld.org** to learn more about the American Nurses Association.

▶ NATIONAL STUDENT NURSES ASSOCIATION

The National Student Nurses Association (NSNA) is a nonprofit organization that mentors nursing students who are preparing for initial licensing as a registered nurse. Students may be enrolled in associate, baccalaureate, diploma, and generic graduate programs. NSNA is dedicated to fostering the professional development of these students by conveying "the standards, ethics, and skills students will need as responsible and accountable leaders and members of the profession" (NSNA, n.d.). NSNA membership provides students opportunities for workshop participation, networking, scholarships, exposure to well-known nursing leaders, and nursing certification exam minireviews.

Box 47-2   Special Interest Professional Organizations

- *American Assembly for Men in Nursing (AAMN)* is a national organization with local chapters that provide opportunities for nurses to meet, discuss, and influence factors that affect men as nurses. Male and female registered nurses, licensed practical/vocational nurses, and nursing students may apply for membership. AAMN offers a variety of services, including educational opportunities, resources, a mentor program, and scholarships (www.aamn.org).

- *National Black Nurses Association (NBNA)* is a nonprofit organization that represents Black nurses from countries around the world. Its mission is "to provide a forum for collective action by African American nurses to investigate, define and determine what the health care needs of African Americans are and to implement change to make available to African Americans and other minorities health care commensurate with that of the larger society" (www.nbna.org).

- *National Association of Hispanic Nurses (NAHN)* is a nonprofit professional association committed to promoting the professionalism and dedication of Hispanic nurses by providing them equal access to educational, professional, and economic opportunities. NAHN is also dedicated to ensuring the improvement of the quality of health and nursing care provided to Hispanic consumers. NAHN offers educational scholarships and career services assistance to its members (www.nahnnet.org).

SPECIALTY PRACTICE ORGANIZATIONS

Most nursing specialties are supported by a professional specialty practice organization. The purpose of these organizations is to advance nursing practice in the affiliated specialty area and provide support to its practitioners and their clients. The reponsibilities of these organizations include advocacy, education, provision of networking opportunities, and strengthening professional identities among members. Specialty practice organizations include the following:

- Academy of Medical-Surgical Nurses
- American Assisted Living Nurses Association
- Association of Pediatric Oncology Nurses
- National Association of Orthopaedic Nurses.

A number of professional nursing organizations exist to promote the interests of special segments of the nursing profession. See **Box 47-2** for a list of some of these special interest professional organizations.

SIGMA THETA TAU INTERNATIONAL

Sigma Theta Tau International is the second largest nursing organization in the United States. It was the first nursing organization to fund nursing research. Membership is by invitation to baccalaureate and graduate nursing students who demonstrate excellence in scholarship and to nurse leaders exhibiting exceptional achievements in nursing. The organization's vision is to create a global community of nurses who lead in using knowledge, scholarship, service, and learning to improve the health of the world's people (Sigma Theta Tau, 2013). The organization offers a variety of benefits to its members, including leadership summits, continuing education opportunities, and career services.

NATIONAL LEAGUE FOR NURSING

The National League for Nursing (NLN), the first nursing organization in the United States, was founded in 1893 as the American Society of Superintendents of Training Schools for Nurses. Its mission is promoting excellence in nursing education to build a strong and diverse nursing workforce to advance the nation's health (NLN, n.d.). The NLN is committed to delivering improved, enhanced, and expanded services to its members and championing the pursuit of high-quality nursing education in all types of nursing education programs. "The National League for Nursing offers faculty development programs, networking opportunities, testing and assessment, nursing research grants, and public policy initiatives" (NLN, n.d.).

THE AMERICAN ASSOCIATION OF COLLEGES OF NURSING

The American Association of Colleges of Nursing (AACN) is the national voice for America's baccalaureate and graduate nursing education. AACN's educational, research, federal advocacy, data collection, publication, and special programs work to establish quality standards for nursing education; assist deans and directors to implement those standards; influence the nursing profession to improve health care; and promote public support for professional nursing education, research, and practice in nursing—the nation's largest healthcare profession (AACN, 2013).

CASE STUDY \\ B

Damien Johnson, RN, BSN, graduated from university 10 years ago. Three years ago, he decided to continue his education and applied to an accredited nurse anesthesia program. He successfully completed the program, passed the national certification exam, and was hired by a small-volume ambulatory surgery center. Mr. Johnson performs his work well and enjoys it. He works with an anesthesiologist but is the only certified registered nurse anesthetist (CRNA) on staff. He recently realized that as a nurse anesthetist, he has a limited number of professional contacts with other nurses employed at the center and that because the surgery center requires only one nurse anesthetist, he will not have many opportunities for interaction with peers and on-the-job educational opportunities. He is starting to feel dissatisfied.

Critical Thinking Questions

1. Is there a professional association that could assist Mr. Johnson to fulfill his need for peers and continuing education?
2. What assistance is available from this association?
3. Where else could Mr. Johnson go for professional support?

EXEMPLAR 47.4 **Types of Reimbursement**

▶ OVERVIEW

Private insurers paid for health care in the United States until 1965, when the federal government entered into healthcare financing with Medicare. While the recently passed Affordable Care Act will greatly increase the number of individuals and families who have access to healthcare insurance, some 25 million will remain uninsured, and millions more will be underinsured (PNHP, 2012).

▶ PAYMENT SOURCES

Sources of payment (or reimbursement) for healthcare services include federal programs (public insurance), private health insurance programs, and personal payments.

Federal Programs

The Centers for Medicare and Medicaid Services (CMS) is the federal agency responsible for administering the Medicare, Medicaid, and CHIP (Children's Health Insurance) programs. Go to the CMS Web site, http://www.cms.hhs.gov/, for additional information regarding CMS and its programs.

MEDICARE **Medicare** is a federally funded health insurance program available to people age 65 or older, younger people with disabilities, and people with end-stage renal disease. Medicare covers 16% of Americans (Kaiser Family Foundation [KFF], 2012). Four types of coverage are available through Medicare (see **Box 47–3 ●**).

Eligibility for premium-free Part A, hospital insurance, requires that the covered individual be age 65 or older and that either the individual or the individual's spouse was employed and paid Medicare taxes for at least 10 years. Part A covers inpatient care in hospitals and, under certain conditions, home health care or care in a skilled nursing facility or hospice.

Participation in Medicare Part B is voluntary; therefore the consumer pays a premium. Coverage includes partial payment for office visits to physicians and other healthcare providers, outpatient services including screening exams such as mammograms and colonoscopies, and preventive services such as flu shots. All individuals covered by Medicare Part B pay an annual deductible and a 20% copayment; the remaining covered costs are paid by Medicare.

Medicare Part C (Medicare Advantage) allows beneficiaries to enroll in private health insurance programs, such as health maintenance organizations. Medicare makes a payment to the insurer for each individual enrolled in the plan in exchange for provision of Plans A and B coverage. The insured must cover out-of-pocket expenses, including the Part B premium, an additional premium to the company providing the coverage, and applicable copayments.

Since January 1, 2006, everyone who is covered by Medicare may purchase prescription drug coverage, Medicare Part D. Prescription plans are administered by Medicare-approved private companies.

Box 47–3   The Different Parts of Medicare

MEDICARE PART A (HOSPITAL INSURANCE)

- Helps cover inpatient care in hospitals.
- Helps cover home health care and care in skilled nursing facilities and hospice.

MEDICARE PART B (MEDICAL INSURANCE)

- Helps cover services provided by doctors and other healthcare providers, outpatient care, home health care, and durable medical equipment.
- Helps cover some services to prevent illness or detect it at an early stage when treatment will work best (for example, Pap tests, flu shots, and screening mammograms).

MEDICARE PART C (MEDICARE ADVANTAGE PLANS LIKE AN HMO OR PPO)

- A health coverage option run by private insurance companies approved by and under contract with Medicare.
- Includes all services covered under Parts A and B, usually includes Plan D prescription drug coverage, and may cover other services such as hearing and vision testing.

MEDICARE PART D (MEDICARE PRESCRIPTION DRUG COVERAGE)

- A prescription drug option run by private insurance companies approved by and under contract with Medicare.
- May help lower prescription drug costs and help protect against higher costs in the future.

Source: Centers for Medicare and Medicaid Services. (2013). *Medicare and You 2013.* Retrieved from www.medicare.gov

---

Medicare does not cover all medical expenses. Examples of excluded services are long-term care, routine dental and eye care, hearing aids and the exams for fitting them, and cosmetic surgery. People often purchase additional insurance from private companies to supplement or fill in the gaps in their Medicare coverage. These plans may help pay for deductibles, coinsurance, and the costs of services not covered by Medicare (see the later section titled Medigap Policy).

MEDICAID **Medicaid** was established in 1965 under Title 19 of the Social Security Act. It is available to certain lower income individuals and families, the elderly, and people with disabilities who meet the eligibility requirements set by federal and state law. Medicaid is a state-administered program. While each state sets its own guidelines regarding eligibility and covered services, federal mandates require coverage of certain services (for example, physician services, inpatient and outpatient hospital care, home health services, and transportation to medical care). In 2014, the Affordable Care Act (ACA) will change the Medicaid program's eligibility requirements to allow more people to qualify. Also, the ACA will offer more community-based care programs as an alternative to nursing home care.

SUPPLEMENTAL SECURITY INCOME Supplemental Security Income (SSI) is a federal assistance program funded by general taxes. SSI is designed to help aged, blind, and disabled people who have little or no income. It provides cash for basic needs such as food, clothing, and housing.

CHILDREN'S HEALTH INSURANCE PROGRAM Federal and matching state funding combine to provide the **Children's Health Insurance Program (CHIP)**, previously known as the State Child Health Insurance Program (SCHIP). CHIP provides health insurance coverage to children under the age of 19 whose families earn more than the Medicaid limits but cannot afford to purchase private health care coverage. Within broad federal guidelines, each state determines the design of its program, eligibility requirements, benefit packages, payment levels for coverage, and administrative and operating procedures. Federal requirements mandate that states include these benefits in their programs: routine checkups; immunizations; dental and vision care; inpatient and outpatient hospital care; and laboratory and x-ray services.

Private Health Insurance Plans

Any health insurance not funded by government is private health insurance. Health care in the United States is expensive; therefore, people who do not qualify for government insurance purchase private health insurance plans to protect themselves from all or some of the medical, surgical, and preventive care expenses they would incur without coverage. The three basic private insurance plan types are employment-based plans, self-employment–based plans, and direct-purchase plans.

Employment-based health insurance is offered through one's employer or union. Of the people in the United States who are under age 65, 56% receive group health insurance coverage as an employer benefit (KFF, 2012). Group health insurance is usually purchased by large employers who offer healthcare coverage to eligible company employees. Employment-based coverage may be extended to include the spouse, dependents of the employee, or domestic partners of employees. A **domestic partner** is an unmarried partner of the same or opposite sex. Group coverage may also be purchased through voluntary and membership associations, such as professional and trade groups, bar associations, local chambers of commerce, and AARP. Benefits of group health insurance, especially when provided by large employers, may include lower costs and availability of coverage for all eligible employees and their families.

Self-employment–based health insurance coverage is available only to individuals who are self-employed; only the policyholder is covered by the plan. One force that drove health care reform is the difficulty that individuals who are self-employed and have chronic health conditions experienced in purchasing health insurance through private insurers.

An individual who needs private health insurance (and is ineligible for group coverage) purchases an individual policy. Individual health insurance policies are usually more expensive and coverage is more restricted than under group health coverage. The individual purchasing an individual plan pays the premium (the amount of money paid for insurance coverage). Under a group plan, the employer may pay nothing toward the premium or may make partial or full payment. The employee is responsible for the premium amount not paid by the employer. In addition to premiums, insureds may be responsible for additional costs of their healthcare coverage, such as deductibles; coinsurance; and copayments. Common deductibles are between $100 and $300 per individual and $500–$1,000 per family annually. A **copayment** is a set amount paid at the time of service (for example, $20 for a primary-care-physician office visit). Copayments for specialty care are usually higher than those for primary care. An out-of-pocket maximum protects the client from catastrophic health care costs. If medical expenses reach a certain amount during a 12-month period, the plan covers all usual and customary fees for the remainder of the year.

TYPES OF PRIVATE HEALTH INSURANCE PLANS A variety of health insurance plans are offered in the United States. The spectrum ranges from **health maintenance organizations (HMOs)**, the most restrictive type, to indemnity plans, the least restrictive. Other types of plans in the middle of the spectrum are point of service (POS) plans and preferred provider organizations (PPOs); both are considered managed-care plans and include features of both HMO and indemnity coverage. Usually more in-network providers are available within PPO and POS options than in HMOs.

HMO participants must select a **primary care provider (PCP)**, who provides basic medical services and, as the gatekeeper to care, refers the client to in-network hospitals and specialists when additional care is needed. HMOs typically provide a broader range of healthcare benefits for the lowest cost to both employers and consumers.

A **preferred-provider organization (PPO)** does not require its insureds to select a PCP. PPOs usually have larger networks of providers than HMOs and provide financial incentives that encourage insureds to seek care from in-network providers. They are less restrictive than HMOs but typically have higher copayments.

A **point-of-service (POS)** plan is a hybrid of an HMO and a PPO. Each time insureds seek health care, they decide which option—HMO or PPO—they will use. Members may select a gatekeeper (PCP) under this plan but are not required to. Members who opt to use out-of-network providers pay higher copayments, coinsurance, and deductibles. The advantage of the POS plan is the flexibility and freedom of choice it offers insureds in comparison to a traditional HMO.

Indemnity plans allow the insured to self-select healthcare providers; that is, there is no network. They may use some managed-care techniques to control costs (for example, preauthorization of MRIs).

The **consumer-driven healthcare plan (CDHP)** is a type of employer-sponsored coverage that combines a private insurance plan with a health savings account (HSA) or health reimbursement account (HRA). The employer offers a health insurance policy with a high deductible that makes employees responsible for more of their healthcare expenses. As part of the plan, the employer offers HSA or HRA accounts to all employees. Employees then save money in the HAS or HRA so they can pay for deductibles and noncovered services. In some cases, the amount that goes into the HSA or HRA is provided by the employer as part of the employee benefits package (Mayo Clinic, 2010).

MEDIGAP POLICY A **Medigap policy** (i.e., Medicare supplemental insurance) is private health insurance designed to supplement Medicare coverage. It may pay copayments, coinsurance, deductibles, and "gaps" in Medicare coverage (i.e., noncovered health-care costs). If an individual has a Medigap policy, Medicare will pay its share first; then the Medigap policy will pay its share.

Personal Payment

Individuals who are not eligible for public or private health insurance pay the insurer directly, that is, make a personal payment. People who pay a high percentage of their healthcare costs themselves are apt to have higher overall healthcare expenses and are sicker than those who pay a lower percentage of their own healthcare costs (AHRQ, 2006).

▶ CONCLUSION

Healthcare policies drive the availability, safety, and quality of the health care provided in the United States. The impact of no policy or an ill-advised one can be devastating to the health and well-being of individuals and our nation as a whole. Professional nurses must understand how healthcare policy impacts them and the clients they serve; they must assume responsibility for identifying the need for and influencing the development of policies to improve the health and welfare of the individuals and populations they serve. They can accomplish this as individuals or in partnership with professional associations such as ANA that provide guidance and volunteer opportunities to nurses who are willing to step out of their comfort zone and advocate for improved health policies.

REVIEW The Concept of Health Policy

RELATE Link the Concepts

Linking the concept of health policy with the concept of ethics:

1. What values or beliefs do those who support healthcare reform express as the motivation for their efforts?
2. What values or beliefs do those who are against healthcare reform express as the motivation for their efforts?
3. What nursing ethics support healthcare coverage for all people?

Linking the concept of health policy with the concept of culture and diversity:

4. What health policies in your area or in the nation promote discrimination?
5. What health policies address or prevent discrimination?

REFER Go to Pearson Student Nursing Resources **nursing.pearsonhighered.com**

- Additional review materials

REFLECT Case Study

Mindy Cohen, RN, BSN, recently graduated college and is newly employed as a staff nurse on a medical unit at a teaching hospital. She has seen announcements that the hospital was recently reaccredited by The Joint Commission. Ms. Cohen is not sure why the hospital values accreditation, nor does she understand what her role in future accreditation preparation will be.

1. What sources of information can Ms. Cohen access to learn more about The Joint Commission?
2. After obtaining background information regarding The Joint Commission and hospital accreditation, how can Ms. Cohen learn more about the meaning of accreditation for her hospital and her responsibilities to help achieve future accreditation?

■ REFERENCES

Agency for Healthcare Research and Quality. (2006). The high concentration of U.S. health care expenditures. *Research in Action, 16,* 1–6. Retrieved from http://www.ahrq.gov/research/ria19/expendria.pdf.

American Nurses Association. (2010). *Nursing's Social Policy Statement.* Silver Springs, MD: Nursesbooks.org.

American Association of Colleges of Nursing. (2013). *About us.* Retrieved from http://www.aacn.nche.edu/ContactUs/about.htm.

American Nurses Association. (2013a). *About ANA.* Retrieved from http://nursingworld.org/Functional-MenuCategories/AboutANA.

American Nurses Association. (2013b). *Safe patient handling.* Retrieved from http://www.nursingworld.org/handlewithcare.

The Joint Commission. (2009). *Fact sheet.* Retrieved from http://www.jointcommission.org/AboutUs/Fact_Sheets/joint_commission_facts.htm.

Kaiser Family Foundation. (2012). The unemployed, a primer. Retrieved from http://kaiserfamilyfoundation.files.wordpress.com/2013/01/7670-03.pdf.

Mayo Clinic. (2010). *Health savings accounts: Is an HSA right for you?* Retrieved from http://www.mayoclinic.com/health/health-savings-accounts/GA00053.

National League for Nursing. (n.d.). About the NLN. Retrieved from http://www.nln.org/aboutnln/index.htm.

National Student Nurses Association. (n.d.). About us. Retrieved from http://www.nsna.org/AboutUs.aspx.

Physicians for a National Health Program (PNHP). (2010). *Pro-single-payer doctors: Health bill leaves 23 million uninsured.* Retrieved from http://www.pnhp.org/news/2010/march/pro-single-payer-doctors-health-bill-leaves-23-million-uninsured.

Physicians for a National Health Program (PNHP). (2012). *It's time for single payer.* Retrieved from http://www.pnhp.org/news/2012/august/its-time-for-single-payer.

Sigma Theta Tau. (2013). *Mission and vision.* Retrieved from http://www.nursingsociety.org/aboutus/mission/Pages/factsheet.aspx.

U.S. Department of Health and Human Services. (2010, with February 2011 updates). *Let's move: America's move to raise a healthier generation of children.* Retrieved from http://www.letsmove.gov/.

U.S. Department of Health and Human Services. (2013). *HHS: What we do.* Retrieved from from http://www.hhs.gov/about/whatwedo.html/.

U.S. Occupational Safety and Health Administration. (n.d.). *OSHA regulations.* Retrieved from http://www.osha.gov/SLTC/etools/eyeandface/employer/requirements.html#OSHAStandards.

48 Informatics

MODULE AT-A-GLANCE

The Concept of Informatics, 2631

Exemplar 48.1
Clinical Decision Support Systems, 2644

Exemplar 48.2
Individual Information at Point of Care, 2646

☑ THE CONCEPT OF INFORMATICS

Today's healthcare professionals handle extraordinary amounts of information. At the bedside and in the examination room, nurses and other clinicians assess clients' health status and prioritize and provide care. Each action creates new data that must be recorded and used at different points of service from direct care to billing related to the cost of that care. In today's clinical environment, that information is created, stored, and accessed with the help of technology. **Biomedical informatics** is the "interdisciplinary science that deals with biomedical information, its structure, acquisition and use. Biomedical informatics is grounded in the principles of computer science, information science, cognitive science, social science, and engineering, as well as the clinical and basic sciences" (Vanderbilt University, 2013). **<<**

Concept Learning Outcomes

After reading about this concept, you will be able to:

1. Define informatics and nursing informatics.
2. Compare the advantages and disadvantages of various ways to view electronic medical records.
3. Differentiate the two types of healthcare information systems and their goals.
4. Summarize the goals of a nursing information system.
5. Evaluate the quality of a health information website.
6. Contrast the advantages, applications, and legal implications of telehealth.
7. Describe the elements of an ergonomically sound workplace.

Concept Key Terms

Administrative information system, *2636*

Biomedical informatics, *2631*

Clinical decision support system, *2639*

Clinical information system, *2635*

Computer vision syndrome, *2643*

Device integration, *2639*

E-health, *2641*

Electronic health record (EHR), *2637*

Electronic medical record (EMR), *2637*

Ergonomics, *2642*

Geographic information system (GIS), *2641*

Hardware, *2634*

Health Level 7, (HL7), *2638*

Intranet, *2636*

Nursing informatics (NI), *2632*

Repetitive strain injury, *2643*

Software, *2634*

Telehealth, *2640*

▶ NURSING INFORMATICS

The relationship between nursing and informatics is so critical that the American Nurses Association (ANA) recognized nursing informatics as a specialty in 1992, and the American Nurses Credentialing Center began offering board certification for nursing informatics in 1995 (T. Dolan, 2010). The ANA defines **nursing informatics (NI)** as

> a specialty that integrates nursing science, computer science, and information science to manage and communicate data, information, knowledge and wisdom in nursing practice. Nursing Informatics supports consumers, patients, and other providers in their decision-making in all roles and settings. This support is accomplished through the use of information structures, information processes, and information technology (ANA, 2008, p. 1).

Even in practices that do not yet use electronic health records, nurses use technology every day: Cardiac monitors, mechanical ventilators, and many blood pressure cuffs use computer technology, as do most telephone systems. Informatics is an everyday occurrence in the practice of nursing.

Informatics and Health Policy

Both professional organizations and government entities recognize and support the careful, purposeful implementation of informatics in healthcare environments. In 2006, the Technology Informatics Guiding Educational Reform (TIGER) Summit took place. It was a gathering of nursing informatics leaders from major nursing organizations (the American Nurses Association, the American Association of Colleges of Nursing, and the Association of Nurse Executives) and the Alliance for Nursing Informatics, which represents 20 different professional nursing informatics societies. This group determined that a knowledge of informatics is mandatory for all healthcare professionals. As a result, TIGER is developing plans to include informatics courses in all levels of nursing education. Additionally, the group is examining the best way to reach out to practicing nurses who may not have the skills that will be required as health care continues to become more interactive and reliant on technology systems (TIGER Initiative, 2006).

Stay Current: *For more information about the TIGER initiative, please visit* **http://www.tigersummit.com/**.

The administrations of both President George W. Bush and President Barack Obama have contributed to the use of informatics in the delivery of health care across the United States. Electronic medical documentation is thought to help reduce errors, reduce healthcare costs, and improve the quality of care delivered to clients. The Bush administration introduced a policy that, over the course of 10 years, would encourage the use of electronic documentation of the healthcare record. The Obama administration took this policy further with the introduction of the American Recovery and Reinvestment Act of 2009 (ARRA), which provides $27 billion worth of incentives to healthcare providers to promote the use of electronic medical records. The goal is for each American to have an electronic medical record by 2014. Two federal agencies are overseeing this massive project with the goals of making health care more accessible and affordable and improving quality outcomes (Sheridan, 2012). The first agency involved is the Center for Medicare and Medicaid Services (CMS). The second agency is the Office of the National Coordinator for Health Information Technology (ONC). ONC is overseeing the achievement of meaningful use objectives, which are reported back to CMS in order to authorize financial reimbursement. Meaningful use includes four objectives (Madison & Staggers, 2011):

- Improving care coordination
- Reducing health disparities among U.S. citizens, by improving the safety and quality of care
- Ensuring the security and privacy of protected medical information
- Engaging clients and their families in the client's care

The ARRA passed by Congress in 2009 also includes the Health Information Technology for Economic and Clinical Health Act (HITECH Act). [Like meaningful use, the HITECH Act is meant to emphasize that simply installing an electronic health record system is not sufficient.] In order to achieve the goals of lowering the cost of health care and improving the quality of care delivered, an electronic record must also be properly utilized (Blumenthal, 2010).

Informatics and Service Delivery

As is made clear throughout this module, informatics has broad implications for service delivery. For example, addiction and overdoses of prescription opioids are an increasing problem in the United States, with reports of overdoses increasing more than threefold since the 1990s; in 2009, opioid overdose was credited with killing more than 15,500 people (Centers for Disease Control and Prevention [CDC], 2012). Efforts are being made to enhance tracking of prescriptions of opioids through electronic tracking at the state level. The CDC is currently developing a program to track prescriptions and the number of emergency room visits for overdoses in an effort to identify people who are or have been abusers. The ability to link computerized written orders with client electronic health records on a regional and national level can help identify people at risk, monitor those who are at risk, and hopefully reduce the prevalence of misuse and overdose from opioid prescriptions. These changes will make it easier to identify people who engage in "doctor shopping" to obtain narcotics for abuse or illegal sale and healthcare providers who act as "pill mills" who write bogus opioid prescriptions and receive a financial kickback from sellers.

One of the often-cited benefits of electronic health records is improved quality of care delivered to clients. As part of the meaningful use requirements, clinical quality measures must be reported (CMS, 2013a). An example of a large quality improvement project that can be facilitated with informatics is the Surgical Care Improvement Project (SCIP). The target population is all clients who are undergoing surgery, and the goal is to reduce surgical complications and improve surgical care. Hospitals started collecting data on certain quality indicators in July 2006. This is a collaborative project with The Joint Commission and CMS, and reimbursement for surgical procedures and hospital stays are tied to meeting SCIP measures (The Joint Commission, 2012). This is an example of a very large, national quality improvement project. Informatics and the ability to retrieve information from clients' electronic health records can help with

Concepts Related to **Informatics**

Informatics is changing the way clients view their health as well as the way healthcare providers can track a client's use of the healthcare system. Some studies have indicated that when clients are given access to their electronic health records, they feel more knowledgeable about their health and disease processes, are more engaged during visits with their primary care provider, and feel more empowered to participate in disease management and wellness activities (Woods et al., 2013). Smartphone technology offers many add-on utilities and applications. Individuals can read and monitor their blood pressure using smartphones. Applications are available for those with diabetes to track their glucose levels. Many of the available fitness training applications allow users to share their successes on social media sites. Other applications are available for tracking calories in certain food items, recording caloric intake for the day, and tracking weight loss (Dennison et al., 2013). As records and applications continue to evolve, this information may eventually become directly transferrable into a client's electronic health record.

The use of informatics has created many new challenges for nurses. Vigilance is necessary to protect client information and to ensure that protected information is not released inadvertently. The advent of social media creates ethical challenges, especially when nurses and clients know each other socially from events or activities outside the workplace. Despite the great possibilities for improving client care through quality improvement efforts and tracking client use of opioids and other medications, nurses must take care to use informatics within established guidelines consistent with the scope of nursing practice and professional and ethical requirements.

CONCEPT	RELATIONSHIP TO INFORMATICS	NURSING IMPLICATIONS
Nutrition		
	Smartphone applications allow clients to determine and track the nutritional value of foods they eat.	■ Use of these applications may increase ease of tracking nutritional intake for the purposes of dietary recall and weight monitoring. ■ *Anticipate* some clients may not have smartphones or may have minimal data plans that limit their ability to use this technology. Work with clients to establish other, convenient means to track dietary intake.
Addiction		
■ Assessment	Electronic health records give healthcare providers, including nurses, access to the client's entire health history, not just information from this particular encounter at this particular facility. Linking of electronic health record information may help identify individuals who are at risk for opioid addiction and who are engaged in obtaining these drugs illegally.	■ *Assess* appropriate use of addictive medications; many clients have legitimate need for prescription opioids. ■ *Be alert for* duplicate opioid prescriptions within a client's record, especially from multiple providers.
Quality Improvement		
■ Targeting areas for improvement ■ Implementation of new protocols	With many electronic health records, quality metrics can be easily tracked for improvement within a department or hospital system. Tracking information to use for quality improvement initiatives requires users to understand how to use technology correctly. Nurses must be at the table as new systems are evaluated and put in place, and they must advocate to ensure that they will receive adequate training to implement the system safely and accurately.	■ *Assess* your own comfort and ability level related to use of electronic/computer equipment. Attend and pay attention in training sessions; seek follow up help as necessary. ■ *Be alert for* the possibility for error; enter information accurately the first time.

(continued on next page)

Concepts Related to **Informatics** (continued)

CONCEPT	RELATIONSHIP TO INFORMATICS	NURSING IMPLICATIONS
Legal Issues		
■ HIPAA	It is necessary to keep protected health information confidential and to ensure that the information entered in a client's health record is accurate.	■ Nurses must be aware of HIPAA and HITECH rules. Among the most critical activities: ■ Keep passwords private. ■ Do not leave screens containing protected health information unattended. ■ Access charts only of clients to whom you are assigned. ■ Always verify that you are charting on the correct client's chart and that the information is recorded accurately.
Ethics		
■ Ethical dilemmas ■ Patient rights	With social media, lines between clients and providers can be blurred.	■ Nurses must be aware that many employers are monitoring their employees' activity on social media; the legality of disciplinary action for a post showing the employee intoxicated and/or engaging in illegal activity or requiring employees to give employers their passwords are still being established. ■ Nurses must weigh the implications of "friending" clients that they care for (especially in areas with long-term interaction). ■ *Anticipate* how to handle clients who attempt to cross boundaries by using social media.

these large-scale quality projects and also help facilities identify their own quality projects and areas for process improvement. See the Concepts Related to Informatics feature for a snapshot of how informatics relates to other concepts and systems.

▶ HEALTHCARE INFORMATION SYSTEMS

The increasing use of technology by healthcare facilities requires that nurses have a basic knowledge of the types of devices used to share information, the types of information systems used, the purposes and abilities of these systems to support client care, and the nurse's responsibilities related to using these systems.

Technology Overview

It would be easy to think of healthcare informatics only in terms of **hardware** (computers, keyboards, and display screens) and **software** (operating systems and applications), but a complete healthcare clinical information system requires many more components to operate efficiently. Some parts focus directly on care of the client, while others focus on the behind-the-scenes work that is necessary to make a healthcare facility operate efficiently. When utilizing computer information systems in nursing informatics, nurses will encounter a wide array of equipment depending on the facility they work in and the type of work they are doing.

A desktop computer system consists of a case that houses the "brains" of the computer and a variety of peripherals. Peripherals are any part of the computer that is not needed for the computer to operate but is often considered essential by the user. Internal peripherals include modems and wireless network (Wi-Fi) connections that are housed within the casing. External peripherals include a display monitor, keyboard, mouse, printers, and storage devices, such as writable CD-ROMs.

A computer system may have extras, such as speakers or video cameras, that aren't needed for the computer to operate but may enhance the user's experience. Some healthcare facilities are using devices such as bar code scanners that match the client's identification band to medications or blood products to be administered. Many dictation services are done with a hands-free headset. As technology continues to evolve, nurses will routinely use computers and other devices, including tablets and smartphones, in their delivery of care to clients. Considerations related to use of certain devices to deliver care are outlined in **Table 48–1** ●.

Any equipment that comes in contact with the client or the nurse's hands while the nurse is caring for the client must be disinfected after use; this disinfection is especially important with the rise of antibiotic-resistant microorganisms. Keyboards are the biggest source of cross-contamination when in computer systems used in health care. Many virulent microbes can live for months on dry surfaces. Hand hygiene before touching computer equipment must become part of a nurse's routine to help prevent spread

TABLE 48–1   Overview of Computer Systems and Devices

DEVICE	DESCRIPTION	CONSIDERATIONS FOR CARE DELIVERY
Desktop computer	Requires a flat surface; not portable. Has a larger screen size and higher screen resolution. Lack of portability reduces likelihood of theft or damage.	Can be hardwired into the facility's intranet and Internet systems; may be placed in a secure location that reduces likelihood of protected client information being compromised.
Laptop computer	Requires wireless capability to access facility intranet, Internet. Smaller screen size and short battery life are two variables.	Portability favorable for nurses with multiple work areas (e.g., home health, public health nurses), but increases risk for theft or damage. Screen savers, turning the computer, and other adaptations are required to shield confidential information.
Workstations on Wheels (WOWs) or Computers on Wheels (COWs)	Computer system housed within a cart, providing some protection to the system while still offering mobility to the user. Requires wireless access; operates on battery so must be plugged in at some point during shift.	Can house devices such as bar-code scanners for medication administration; portability allows mobility and interaction with clients.
Tablets, smartphones	Complete portability; fairly good battery life; requires wireless access to intranet and Internet. Smaller screen size may limit functionality.	Many applications make clients' clinical data readily accessible; prone to theft, breakage; protected health information may be vulnerable if stored on the device and not within an electronic medical record program.

of infections. Gloved hands should not make contact with keyboards or mice. Mice and keyboards should also be disinfected daily and when visibly soiled with bodily fluids. Most manufacturers have guidelines for types of disinfectants and percentages of active ingredients that can be used on their equipment. Because keyboards carry the highest risk for contamination, some manufacturers have built sealed keyboards that can be easily cleaned or can be equipped with covers to make cleaning easier and protect the electronic equipment (Barnes & Weaver, 2011).

Clinical Information Systems

In the days of paper charts, only one individual at a time could access and input information into a client's chart (**Figure 48–1 ●**). A **clinical information system** allows multiple disciplines to simultaneously access the client's chart and record data that can be viewed and analyzed by a number of healthcare providers in real time, providing the most accurate and current information about the client so that the best decisions can be made concerning the care of that client.

In addition to hardware and software, a clinical information system must give the nurse the ability to access client information and provide data necessary to execute the nursing process of assessing, diagnosing, planning, implementing and evaluating the care of the client. When the system is used at the point of care, the nurse can easily record client information based on assessment of the client's current condition. The nurse should also have access to diagnostic data (e.g., laboratory values), diagnoses, assessments, plans, and evaluations of the client from the viewpoint of other healthcare professionals (e.g., physicians, physical therapists). Pharmacy information, such as medication, route, dose, and time, should be available in the client's chart in real time. The chart should also include safety features, for example, warnings for drug interactions or incorrect dosages. Most clinical information systems also contain clinical decision support, which will be discussed later. The system should also allow the nurse to print discharge

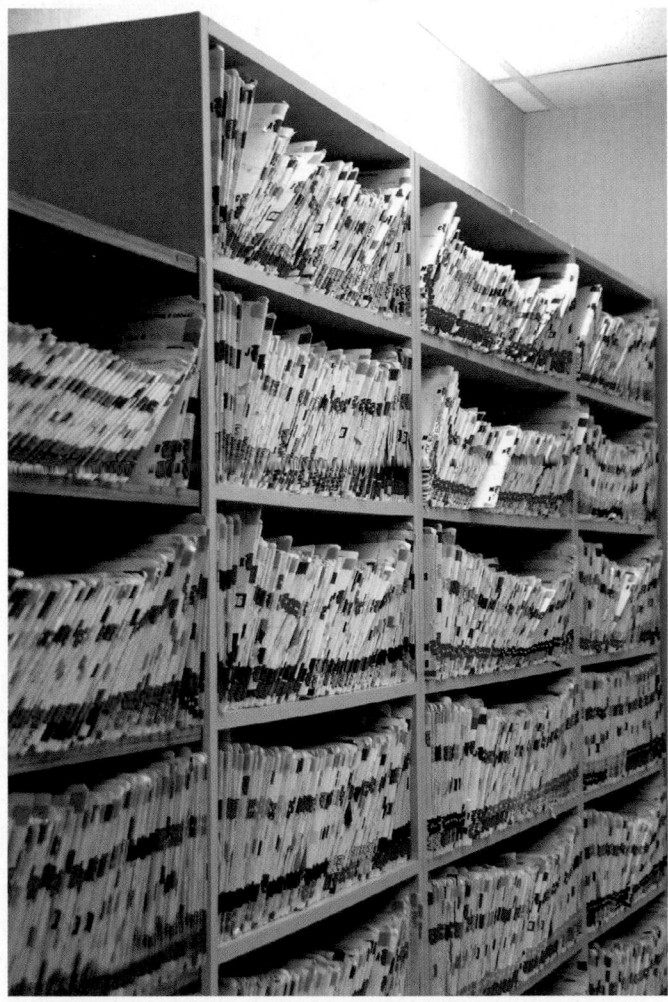

Figure 48–1 ● Paper records do not meet the needs of today's healthcare industry. Only one individual at a time can use a paper record, paper records can be lost, they don't include images or sounds, and they don't include decision support systems.
Source: © Elenathewise/Fotolia.

instructions to review with the client (Duke University, 2012; Locatelli et al., 2012).

Administrative Systems

An **administrative information system** provides support and management on the business side of health care. The business side includes human resources, financial data, materials management, risk management, and quality performance. These items are discussed in more detail in the exemplar on Clinical Decision Support Systems in this module. Many of these information systems are stored on an intranet to allow access by approved individuals within the organization (**Box 48–1** ●).

These systems are not just useful for large healthcare facilities. Many offices of private practice physicians or nurse practitioners gain the same benefits by using computerized systems. Scheduling, coding and billing, contracts with insurance companies, and accurate data such as current laboratory or imaging information can be utilized on a smaller scale in an office setting to provide quality health care.

Figure 48–2 ● shows how the clinical and administrative information systems work together within a healthcare system.

Box 48–1   Intranets

Most people are familiar with the Internet, a massive network of computers that covers the globe and allows near-instantaneous communication and exchanges of ideas. Many people are not familiar with an *intranet*. An **intranet** is a smaller version of the Internet that is meant to be used by a smaller group of people, such as employees within a company or members of an organization. Intranets usually have security to restrict access by the public, although some intranets are used purely as file-sharing applications and have little or no security. Intranets are utilized regularly, as they allow collaboration and a high degree of data sharing among users. Because of their smaller size, they are easier to control and maintain. However, they are not able to offer the full range of services that are available through the Internet such as cloud computing or Voice over Internet Protocol (VoIP). As a consequence, most entities that maintain an intranet server also utilize an Internet service. A hospital or other healthcare setting would need both the data-sharing capabilities and security of an intranet as well as access to the unlimited information and services offered by the Internet (DifferenceBetween. net, 2013; Phatak, 2012). Both intranets and the Internet are vulnerable to data breeches and should utilize firewalls, encryption, and authentication; user passwords that change on a frequent basis; and strict control over which users have access to secure data.

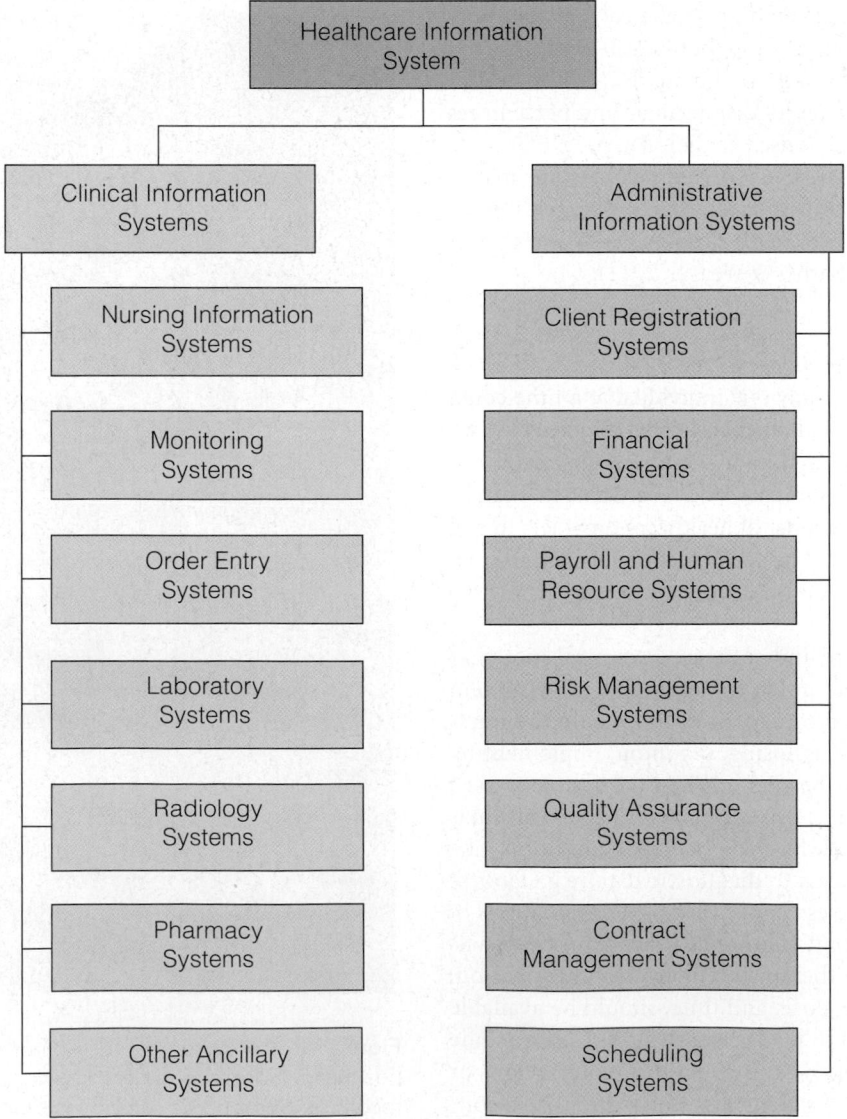

Figure 48–2 ● Relationship of the components of the healthcare information system.

► COMPUTERIZED MEDICAL RECORDS

On the surface, it would appear that a computerized medical record is nothing more than a digital form of a client's paper chart. Many systems start out that way. However, rapid technological advances have transformed these static charts into dynamic systems.

Purpose

The purpose of a computerized medical record is to unify a client's entire health history into one single source of information about the client's health, including the client's medical and surgical histories, diagnostic tests and treatments, medications, and therapies. It is meant to be multidisciplinary and multispecialty in nature. It is not meant to simply record the past but to aid clinicians in the client's future health care, improve quality of care, lower costs of care, and facilitate research. It is meant to be portable, so that if a client lives in New York but requires emergency care in Los Angeles, all of the client's medical information is available to help the healthcare providers in Los Angeles make the best possible decisions about the care of the client (Open Clinical, 2012).

In order to deliver the best quality of care, promote safety, and maintain efficiency, computerized health records should contain the following functionality (Open Clinical, 2012):

- *Client support.* Clients should be able to access their health records. Doing so can help them take a more active role in their care if they have the ability to track appointments and health maintenance, monitor their weight and laboratory results, and access educational materials related to their health condition.

- *Health information and data.* Important data, such as chronic and acute medical and psychiatric diagnoses, medications, allergies, and diagnostic tests, can help clinicians make rapid decisions if necessary.

- *Administrative processes.* The ability to manage schedules, insurance information, and inventory can help healthcare facilities focus on client-centered care.

- *Results management.* Access to past and current diagnostic tests can help clinicians recognize changes in a client's state of health faster.

- *Reporting.* Healthcare facilities can comply more easily with regulatory requests and help report disease surveillance and client safety matters such as medical device recalls.

- *Secure electronic communication and connectivity.* Secure and accurate communication between medical providers at different facilities that are caring for the same client help with continuity of care and timely diagnoses.

- *Order management.* Computerized physician order entry (CPOE) helps with accuracy and decreases times from order to treatment. CPOE should be available for pharmacy, laboratory, radiological tests, and ancillary services such as physical and occupational therapy.

- *Decision support.* The care of the client can be enhanced through the use of a clinical decision support system. These systems can display best practice standards, notifications for preventive screenings, and alerts for drug interactions.

Terminology

A nurse will hear many different terms to describe a computerized medical record, and the list will probably continue to change. The two most commonly used terms are electronic medical records and electronic health records. Other terms currently used include:

- Computerized patient record (CPR)
- Computerized medical record (CMR)
- Patient medical records software (PMRS)
- Electronic health records system (EHRS)
- Personal health record (PHR)

Electronic medical records (EMRs) are similar to an electronic chart used in a clinician's office. Their focus is on diagnosis and treatment. They can help track information over time (weight, blood pressure, cholesterol readings) and identify when clients are due for routine preventive health maintenance such as vaccines and mammograms. A disadvantage of these types of systems is that most of them are designed to stay within a clinical setting and are not meant to travel beyond it. A client who needs to see a specialist may need a paper printout of the electronic medical record to take to the specialty appointment (Garnett & Seidman, 2011).

Electronic health records (EHRs) give a broader view of the client's health. They are designed so that multiple clinicians from multiple disciplines (e.g., family practice, nursing, pharmacy, specialists) can all have simultaneous access to the client's health information. This access provides clients with more comprehensive management of their health and is designed to improve the quality of care they receive. Clinicians have the advantage of up-to-the-minute information about clients' health and access to other clinicians' assessments and plans for client care. The goal of electronic health records is to move with the client, whether to another provider, to a different hospital system, or to another state (Garnett & Seidman, 2011).

Nurses may work at a facility that uses only one term to refer to the electronic chart (i.e., it is always referred to as the *EMR*). Or they may work for a health system that uses some of these terms interchangeably (i.e., the electronic chart is sometimes called the *EMR* and sometimes called the *EHR*). It is important to understand that, just like nursing informatics, computerized client charting is a rapidly changing field and the vocabulary surrounding it is also likely to change rapidly. This text uses *EHR* when discussing documentation, as it is the broader, more encompassing term.

Components

The nursing process should be carried over into an electronic record. The nurse should be given the tools to record assessments, nursing diagnoses, plans, interventions, and evaluations. Real-time documentation of client data can help all clinicians care for the client. The work that nurses have done in caring for the client has traditionally been invisible to other disciplines, so the ability to record nursing diagnoses, interventions, and evaluations of outcomes will help promote the work that nurses do in caring for the client. *Uniform language* refers to the consistent use of the same terminology between providers, facilities, institutions, and organizations when describing all client data, including that pertaining to assessment and treatment. Uniform language (discussed further in the exemplar on Clinical Decision Support Systems in this module) is vital to communicate to other nurses and health professionals the value that nurses provide in the care of the client. The North American Nursing Diagnosis Association (NANDA) has been involved in developing uniform language for nursing since the 1970s. NANDA diagnoses are available in many electronic health systems (Meum, 2013). The Nursing Interventions Classifications (NIC) include both physiological and psychological interventions that nurses perform with clients and their families (University of Iowa College of Nursing, 2013a). Both NANDA and NIC are used by nurses to formulate care plans for the client in the electronic health record (Meum, 2013). The Nursing Outcomes Classification (NOC) is designed to assess the outcomes of clients based on the nursing interventions performed (University of Iowa College of Nursing, 2013b). Both NIC and NOC have been approved for use in **Health Level 7 (HL7)** terminology, which provides a framework and composes standards "for the exchange, integration, sharing, and retrieval of electronic health information that supports clinical practice and the management, delivery and evaluation of health services" (Health Level Seven International, 2013). Information that is sent to a client's electronic health record is sent as messages via an HL7 record. Examples of information sent via HL7 include billing information, vital signs, and laboratory data (Interfaceware, 2010). While many software systems utilize HL7 interfaces, some do not. The nurse should understand that a client's information may be transferred into the electronic chart in a variety of ways based on the software that is used.

Health Insurance Portability and Accountability Act of 1996

A major concern for both clients and healthcare providers is the protection of private health information. Private health information includes any details that could identify a particular client, such as name, phone number, hospital medical record number, diagnosis, or Social Security number (Baril, 2010). The U.S. Department of Health and Human Services issued a set of privacy rules called the Health Insurance Portability and Accountability Act of 1996, commonly referred to as HIPAA. It sets limits and rules with regard to who may have access to a client's health information whether that information is in written, oral, or electronic form. It also gives clients the right to view their health records, make corrections to their records, and receive notification of how their information may be used or shared (e.g., for research or marketing purposes; U.S. Department of Health and Human Services, n.d.). The Health Insurance Technology for Economic and Clinical Health Act (HITECH) added more strength to the existing HIPAA protection of clients' medical information (Blumenthal, 2010).

Nurses should use many of the same rules for protecting client privacy that were practiced prior to electronic records. Information about a client should not be discussed in public areas, such as hospital cafeterias or elevators. Any paper documents that may have protected health information should be placed in designated shred bins. Newer considerations for nurses include not sharing passwords, not leaving a computer screen with protected health information unattended, and not posting any client information on public social networks such as Facebook or Twitter (see **Box 48–2 ●**; Baril, 2010). Commonsense habits related to confidentiality must be practiced. In the days of paper charts, it may have been possible to obtain unauthorized access to a neighbor's or celebrity's chart. Now it is very easy to ascertain electronically each time a client's chart is accessed and by whom. A nurse who improperly accesses a client's chart could face loss of employment and possibly legal action as well.

Just like paper documentation, electronic documentation can lead to fraudulent activities. The annual cost of medical fraud is estimated to be at least $68 billion in the United States (Kopala & Mitchell, 2011). Fraud can be committed on the client side; for example, someone may pose as the client in order to use the client's insurance information to gain access to health care. It can

---

Box 48–2 Social Media and the Workplace

Social media is hot. A recent study suggests that there are more than 1 billion people worldwide using some form of social media; Facebook has the largest share of users (Lunden, 2012). In a study conducted in 2011, 87% of physicians surveyed reported personal use of social media, and 67% reported professional use (Federation of State Medical Boards, 2012b). Social networking can pose several ethical dilemmas for healthcare providers. Some employers have demanded access to their employees' social media accounts or have monitored their activities. As of January 2013, six states have made it illegal for employers to ask for passwords to an employee's social media accounts (Kerr, 2013). Interactions on a social network system between a client and a healthcare provider can become very complicated, for example, in the maintenance of privacy and boundaries. Many providers refuse "friend" requests on their personal social network accounts, while others use these media to convey general health information to their clients. Refusing a friend request does not necessarily prevent clients from "spying" on providers' social accounts (Mathews, 2013). It has been suggested that providers consider having both a personal account and a professional account. Medical professional must be mindful that any opinions about treatments or new drugs they post may be seen by a client as an endorsement, even if that is not the intent. In some instances, healthcare providers who posted pictures of themselves intoxicated or talking about "partying" have made clients uncomfortable or no longer able to trust their judgment. Videos of procedures or photos of unusual cases have also made their way online; these are breaches of confidentiality and HIPAA violations (Federation of State Medical Boards, 2012a). While some in the healthcare community are firmly against it, others are embracing social media. Some have offered promotions for school health physicals on their Facebook pages or have had positive input from their clients from posts about health issues on their blog sites (Brull, 2012).

Social media is not the only electronic tool presenting challenges for providers. Some hospitals and healthcare offices use e-mails and text messages to notify physicians about a client's status. If this information is not encrypted and includes a client's name or other identifying factors, it may be classified as a HIPAA violation. The use of mobile devices in general pose special risks because they can be easily lost or stolen (McLaughlin, 2011).

also occur on the provider's side; for example, a provider may bill for procedures that were not performed or enter data that makes the client's condition appear worse so the provider can bill for a higher level of service (Kopala & Mitchell, 2011).

Quality Assurance

On the surface, the implementation of an electronic health record would seem likely to automatically improve the quality of client care. It has the potential to do that, but an electronic health record is just a tool, and outcomes of care depend, in part, on how this tool is utilized.

ACCURACY Recording accurate client health information is vital, whether the nurse is using a paper or an electronic system. First encounters with an electronic charting system involve a learning curve that increases the chance of errors in recording data that is left in a client's chart. For example, someone who is new to the system may not know how to remove a blood pressure reading of 225/124 because the arterial line transducer was on the floor or how to mark that reading as faulty data. In many charting systems, more than one chart may be open at the same time, so entering information on the wrong chart may be easy. An accidental click of a mouse on the wrong medication can cause the provider who is not paying attention to order or give the wrong medication. **Device integration**, which automatically enters client vital signs into the electronic record, is possible in some systems (intensive care units and anesthesia are two areas where device integration is being widely used). Device integration allows real-time accurate data to be recorded in the client's chart directly from the device (e.g., a blood pressure monitor). It allows the nurse to more quickly analyze and interpret that data and make adjustments to the plan of care based on the most current information. It also gives nurses more time to be at the bedside rather than in the nursing station recording vital signs (McNickle, 2012). As electronic health records evolve, more departments are likely to utilize device integration.

Some EHR systems use templates and cut-and-paste functions designed to promote efficiency. For example, a pediatric clinic seeing 10 otherwise healthy children who have ear infections can use a template or cut/copy function to forward the information that is within normal limits and just focus on the infection, saving precious time that would otherwise be spent manually clicking boxes for negative or normal findings. However, overuse of these functions can result in inaccurate data being recorded in a client's chart, risking future decisions regarding medical care based on faulty information. For example, if there has been a significant change in the client's condition and a practitioner uses a "copy forward" function to duplicate the previous day's progress notes, then care of the client can be seriously compromised. One study found that up to 20% of material in a client's chart was the result of copy-and-paste (Stokes, 2013). A client's medical record is only as valuable as the information that is entered in it, and nurses have a duty to ensure that they enter only timely and accurate information. Risk management, insurance companies, and regulatory bodies as well as other clinicians will be looking at the data in the client's record, so it is imperative that nurses take the time to learn proper documentation within the electronic system that their employer adopts.

CRITICAL THINKING The fact that the electronic health record is merely a tool cannot be overemphasized. As with paper charting, the client and not the record should be the priority in the nurse's attention. If a client's condition deteriorates, using a "transcriber" will allow the majority of clinicians in the room to focus on caring for the client and not on documentation. Although it may be difficult when electronic records are utilized, nurses must learn to focus their attention on the client and not the computer. Employers should give nurses adequate training on the use of their electronic system and provide mentors to help decrease the stress of adding one more activity to a nurse's already busy workload (Goldberg et al., 2012).

Clinical decision support systems are a type of artificial intelligence that analyzes data and provides information about evidenced-based practices. These systems can help improve client safety and quality of care. However, they cannot take the place of sound nursing judgment. It is currently a recommendation that all surgical clients who are on beta-blocker therapy receive a dose of beta-blocker within 24 hours of surgical incision (Surgical Care Improvement Project [SCIP], 2012). A nurse might see a reminder on the client's chart to administer a beta-blocker that the client has been prescribed. The nurse assesses the client and finds that the client's blood pressure is 80/50, heart rate is 38 bpm, and the client is complaining of feeling light-headed. The nurse should use good clinical judgment, hold the dose of beta-blocker, and seek further treatment for the client rather than just giving the dose because of a notification on a computer screen. The use of clinical decision support systems in nursing practice is described further in the exemplar on Clinical Decision Support Systems in this module.

UNIFORM LANGUAGE For greater efficiency, nurses should use uniform language in their documentation. Uniform nursing diagnoses, along with uniform descriptors of nursing interventions and outcomes, can help clarify care of the client not only to other nurses, but to other disciplines as well. Some documentation within an electronic record may have only standardized descriptors available for the end user. The use of uniform language also aids nursing research (National Association of School Nurses, 2012).

CASE STUDY \\ A

Mary Wilson is a 19-year-old with a history of grand mal seizures. She takes two antiepileptic medications: phenytoin and topiramate. Her seizures are fairly well controlled, and she has an average of three seizures per year. Ms. Wilson is getting ready to go out of state to college and visits her primary care provider for a physical before she leaves. The office has just installed a new electronic health record system. Because of an early regional outbreak of influenza, the office is overbooked on appointments. The practitioner that Ms. Wilson usually sees is on vacation. The other practitioner rushes through Ms. Wilson's appointment and does not take a thorough history or discuss medications that she is taking. Ms. Wilson presents as a healthy 19-year-old, so the practitioner uses the "copy and paste healthy adult" format for her chart.

Ms. Wilson goes out of state to school. After class one day, she decides to go for a run to relieve the stress of her classes. While she is on her run, she suffers a grand mal seizure. A motorist finds her unconscious in a postictal state and calls for emergency services. Ms. Wilson is transported to the hospital, which happens to be on the same electronic health record system as her primary care provider. She is still not conscious when she is examined, but she has identification with her name and birthdate on it. The emergency department staff looks at Ms. Wilson's electronic health record, but there is no mention of her seizure disorder. She is sent for emergency CT scans and an MRI of her brain.

Critical Thinking Questions

1. What mistakes did the provider at Ms. Wilson's primary care office make with her record?
2. How did the omission of information affect the care that Ms. Wilson received at the hospital?
3. Ms. Wilson does not have health insurance. Discuss what other ways inaccurate information in an electronic health record can impact a client and the healthcare system.

▶ TELEHEALTH

Telehealth (telemedicine, remote client monitoring) uses telecommunications technologies (e.g., videoconferencing, streaming media, real-time forwarding imaging, and land-based and wireless communications) to allow clients access to care that they might not otherwise be able to obtain (**Box 48–3** ●). Telehealth allows a higher acuity of care for clients in locations without access to critical healthcare needs, such as rural health settings or even a client's home (U.S. Department of Veterans Affairs Office of Telehealth Services, 2011). Technology can be used to collect, track, and transmit health data from a remote location to a case manager or healthcare provider in a clinical setting. For clients with chronic health conditions who live in rural areas, the cost of transportation to and from appointments is sometimes as expensive as the appointment, especially when a chronic condition requires frequent monitoring (McKnight, 2012). The advent and expansion of telehealth have the potential to decrease costs, improve quality of care, and increase access to care not only for rural clients but also for those in urban, community, and international settings as well (Roney, 2012).

Box 48–3   **Benefits of Telehealth**

■ *Access to health care is increased.* Clients in rural areas can reduce the need to travel, and they receive access to specialists that may not be available in their community.

■ *Health outcomes are improved.* Increased access to care can reduce complications and increase diagnostic and treatment options from specialists.

■ *Healthcare costs can be reduced.* Clients no longer have the expense of traveling long distances, and home monitoring of chronic conditions can help reduce hospital admissions.

■ *Telehealth may help with shortages of healthcare providers.* Many new graduates are not willing to move to rural communities. Telehealth can give clients access to primary care providers and specialists from other areas.

Applications

Telehealth now allows for consults with specialists, cloud-based healthcare provider appointments, and virtual health coaches (Roney, 2012). CMS (2012) has included offices of healthcare practitioners, skilled nursing facilities, and community mental health centers as sites that can offer and be reimbursed for telehealth services. CMS does require the use of real-time communication, such as interactive audio and video telecommunications (except in Alaska and Hawaii). It is estimated that 1.8 million persons worldwide will utilize telehealth technology by 2017 (California HealthCare Foundation, 2013b).

Telehealth is being used to manage both acute and chronic conditions. The growing list of chronic health conditions that are routinely monitored via telehealth communication includes diabetes, hypertension, chronic obstructive pulmonary disease, congestive heart failure, and mental health conditions (California HealthCare Foundation, 2013a). Nurses can utilize dual webcams to visually assess the client's condition and to evaluate client education by watching return demonstration of skills (McKnight, 2012). The field of telehealth is expanding, and many nursing programs are adding telehealth courses to their curriculum (Wirkus, 2011).

Barriers to Implementation

With the threat of reimbursement cuts always looming, healthcare administrators may be reluctant to embrace telehealth, because not all clients or health insurers will pay for these services. Administrators need to look at how provider participation in telehealth can generate income for the institution, such as decreasing readmission rates or resulting in more referrals to their staff specialists. Providers may not be willing to participate in telehealth because they view it as more work, or they may worry about the technology's failing and losing communication with clients at a critical point in the client's care. Infrastructure related to supporting a telehealth program is paramount to telehealth's success. Lack of a stable Internet connection on either the client's or the provider's side can lead to loss of information and wrong diagnoses or treatment, which can increase the risk of poor outcomes for both the client and the providing organization. CMS and other insurance programs currently reimburse for telehealth encounters if they meet specified criteria, but there is no guarantee that this reimbursement will continue or that changes to the telehealth program will continue to make it attractive for practitioners (Roney, 2012).

Licensure restrictions can also complicate the process of participating in telemedicine. Currently, medical boards in only 10 states issue special telemedicine licenses that allow the practice of telehealth across state lines; the others allow the practice only within the same state (Federation of State Medical Boards, 2012a). Therefore physicians must obtain licenses in multiple states in order to legally practice telehealth. Some physicians get around this restriction by conducting physician-to-physician consultations, which are legal across state borders. The licensing of nurses allows a bit more latitude in telehealth. Currently, 24 states participate in the Nurse Licensure Compact (NLC), which allows the recognition of registered nurse's license in a participating state (American Academy of Ambulatory Care Nursing, 2011).

Barriers to Client Participation

Some clients may be reluctant to utilize telehealth services because their insurance company may not cover the cost (California HealthCare Foundation, 2013a). Older adults who lack understanding of or experience with technology may be reluctant to use telehealth services. The lack of availability of broadband Internet service throughout the country also limits participation. In addition, many clients are not aware that these services exist or that their healthcare provider is willing to participate in this type of interaction. Some clients are not convinced that the confidentiality of their protected health information can be maintained as it travels online (Reginatto, 2012). Obtaining the necessary equipment to conduct telehealth (such as computers with videoconferencing capabilities, pulse oximeter machines, Internet connectivity to transmit data) can be a challenge to clients with limited income or without insurance that covers these items (McKnight, 2012).

CASE STUDY \\ B

Jack Anderson is an 85-year-old retired machinist. He has an 8th-grade education and lives on a fixed income in a rural community 100 miles from a major city. He has congestive heart failure and takes a loop diuretic (furosemide) and digoxin for his condition, both of which he gets through a mail order pharmacy. Mr. Anderson has Medicare but tries to limit his doctor visits because he doesn't like to drive to the city, and the cost of gas cuts into his monthly budget. His community has high-speed Internet, but Mr. Anderson has not installed it because "he moved to the country to get away from everyone."

Critical Thinking Questions

1. Discuss several factors that would make Mr. Anderson an ideal candidate for telehealth.
2. When Mr. Anderson comes in for an appointment, what could the nurse say to encourage Mr. Anderson to participate in telehealth to manage his CHF?
3. If Mr. Anderson agrees to participate in telehealth, what should the practitioner assess in each of the telehealth sessions with Mr. Anderson?

▶ GEOGRAPHIC INFORMATION SYSTEMS

A **geographic information system (GIS)** uses location to capture, manage, and analyze data. This technology has been used both inside and outside of health care. It relies on satellite imaging and global positioning systems (GPSs) to capture geographical data. That data is then managed and stored on a database. Healthcare policy makers, researchers, and public health professionals use GIS to understand a health problem, decide the best response to that problem, and plan ways to avoid or control the same or a similar problem from occurring again. GIS is being increasingly used to analyze population- or location-based data, such as disease transmission, cancer rates, trends in diseases such as diabetes, and environmental data (e.g., water quality). Lifestyle choices, such as obesity rates, lack of proper nutrition, use of tobacco, and physical activity rates, also can be

plotted and analyzed (CDC, 2013). Public health nurses and administrators can use GIS to track where chronic disease programs should be placed, to monitor the effectiveness of these programs, to plan new treatment facilities, and to track acute health problems, among many other uses. GIS gives healthcare providers the tools to show where services are provided and where health services are needed. Gaps between available programs and the needs of the community can be identified easily.

▶ CLIENT EDUCATION AND E-HEALTH

The use of the Internet has exploded, and the number of users worldwide increased sixfold between 2010 and 2012 (Internet World Stats, 2013). **E-health** utilizes electronic information that can be retrieved online or through a mobile device to improve a person's health or health care (U.S. Department of Health and Human Services, 2013). A recent study showed that 72% of adults in the United States have looked online for health information over the past year (Fox & Duggan, 2013). It ranks third behind e-mail and search engine use as a popular web-based pursuit (Buck, 2012).

Online Consumer Medical Information

Increasingly individuals are turning to the Internet for health information:

- More than 50% of individuals have researched a particular drug, procedure, or treatment (Steinberg, 2011).
- Close to 80% of individuals who look online for medical information are looking for a specific medical problem or disease (Steinberg, 2011).
- Most individuals begin their search using a general search engine such as Google or Yahoo (77%), while 13% start their search on a health-specific site.
- Of those polled, 46% sought medical follow up (Fox & Duggan, 2013). Around 40% reported that they printed information to discuss with their healthcare provider (University of California–Davis, 2012).

Unfortunately, the Internet is not always an accurate source. A recent study looked at the accuracy of medical advice using the Google search engine. Five common pediatric questions were searched, and the first 100 results for each question were examined for their validity. Of the 500 sites searched, 49% failed to answer the question. Of those that answered the question, 11% gave incorrect information. Often the searches led to a "sponsored" site that was selling a product. Of the searches that led to sponsored sites, none gave correct medical advice (Scullard, Peacock, & Davies, 2010). In general, government Web sites provided the most reliable medical information. Accessing incorrect or outdated information can cause clients unnecessary anxiety before they talk to a health professional. The problem is so widespread, a new form of hypochondria called *cyberchondria* has been identified (Moyer, 2012). **Box 48–4** ● provides some information on evaluating health-related Web sites that is useful for both clients and nurses who want to stay current.

There is also an interest in blogging or support groups for a particular medical condition. At the start of 2011, there were more than 12,000 medical support groups listed in a Yahoo! directory (University of California–Davis, 2012). Approximately 24% of e-health searchers have read someone else's account of an illness or condition (Steinberg, 2011). While blogs and support groups can be an important resource for clients, especially for encouragement and moral support, nurses should caution clients participating in these groups to verify with their healthcare provider any information from these sources.

Consumers are also obtaining information *about* their healthcare providers: 16%–44% of surfers consult rankings or ratings of doctors or hospitals (Steinberg, 2011; Moyer, 2012).

Online Client Medical Information

Many health facilities are using the Internet to give clients access to and control over their own health records. Some of these sites are called *patient portals.* Online registration is required, and a user identification and password are needed for each visit. Through many of these portals, clients can schedule routine appointments and request prescription refills from their primary care office. Clients also can communicate electronically with their health provider, although some portals are not yet encrypted to allow secure transmission of protected health information. Hospitals are using the Internet to schedule some radiology procedures such as mammograms online. Some

EHRs allow clients to access parts of their health records. Information such as laboratory and pathology reports, medication records, and due dates for routine screenings and immunizations may be available. The use of these services leads to higher client satisfaction and retention within the health system (Turley et al., 2012).

Online Administrative Tools

Patient portals can also perform administrative functions. Clients are able to view and verify their demographics and insurance information. Many providers are placing their new client paperwork online for clients to complete prior to their first appointment. Some systems send automated text or voice message reminders for upcoming appointments. Other systems may send automated messages to a group of clients, such as reminders for influenza vaccinations. The client often has the ability to view any outstanding balances and make payments online (P. Dolan, 2013).

Many hospitals are using the Internet to have clients complete questionnaires about their treatment preferences. Clients can request the gender of the physician, the distance they are willing to travel, and a language accommodated other than English.

A major health insurance program is now allowing clients to price-shop the costs of surgical procedures or diagnostic tests such as MRIs. It also allows clients to see out-of-pocket costs for each health service and keeps track of the client's contributions to deductibles for the year (Weisman, 2013).

Health insurance companies give providers online access to information about the client's insurance coverage, including information on providers and hospitals in the insurance company's network. Providers often can see the dates of coverage and co-pays and deductibles paid to date and in some cases, they can obtain instant online authorization of procedures such as MRIs.

Some Web sites allow clients to compare health professionals based on specialty, languages spoken, and clinical training. Hospitals and nursing homes can be compared based on quality measures and demographics (e.g., location, size; HealthCare.gov, n.d.). Web sites vary: Some use only clients' ratings, and others use less subjective data.

▶ ERGONOMIC CONSIDERATIONS

More and more individuals—clients and professionals—are using technology, often for hours a day. Use of technology can impact both work flow and body mechanics. The addition of computers in health care may seem innocent enough, but without proper planning and implementation, it can lead to serious injuries to the user. The risk of injury increases with professions that require pushing, pulling, frequent or heavy lifting, prolonged awkward positions, or repetitive, forceful, or prolonged exertion of the hands (U.S. Department of Labor, n.d.b).

Ergonomics is "the science of fitting workplace conditions and job demands to the capabilities of the working population" (U.S. Department of Labor, n.d.a). Ergonomics examines the type of work being done, the tools being used, the body mechanics of both the work and the tools, and then suggests the best way to do that work with those tools to limit overuse and harm (U.S. National Library of Medicine, 2013).

For working on a computer, the goal of ergonomics is to set up a workstation that allows a neutral body position. The head, neck, and torso should be in alignment. Shoulders and upper arms should be perpendicular to the floor and relaxed. The upper arms and elbows should be close to the body. Forearms, wrists, and hands should be straight and in line. When the worker is sitting, the thighs should be parallel to the floor and the feet should rest flat on the floor or be supported by a footrest (U.S. Department of Labor, n.d.b).

Stay Current: *A checklist that looks at each component of the computer system (keyboard, monitor, chair, and work surfaces) is available online at* **www.osha.gov/SLTC/etools/computerworkstations/checklist.html**.

Computers on wheels (COWs) and workstations on wheels (WOWs) add requiring the user to pull or push them to different locations for use. The position of the monitor, keyboard, or mouse on the COW or WOW can also lead to bad posture and injury. These carts should be as lightweight and maneuverable as possible. Ideally, the user should be able to tilt the screen at different angles, and workstation platforms should be adjustable to varying heights (Raths, 2010). See **Box 48–5** ● for ways to incorporate good ergonomics in computer use.

Improper workstation setup or improper body mechanics can lead to injury. Common complaints after prolonged computer use include fatigue or pain in the neck, shoulders, back, arms, wrists, and hands. Some of these symptoms can be alleviated by proper ergonomics or breaks from the computer when possible. Sometimes simple aches and pains can lead to more serious injuries that cause disability. The two most common injuries are repetitive strain injury (RSI) and computer vision syndrome (Princeton University, University Health Services, 2012).

Repetitive strain injury, or repetitive motion disorder, occurs when the limbs are subjected to repetitive use, awkward positions, or forced positions. These injuries can affect nerves, tendons, and muscles. Tendinitis is a common occurrence, but carpal tunnel syndrome is more serious and can lead to permanent disability if not treated. Symptoms of tendinitis include pain in the wrist, elbow, shoulder, or neck; numbness or tingling in the fingers; difficulty grasping objects; and a decrease in the size of the affected hand. Treatment should not be delayed and can include changes in posture, stretching, muscle strengthening, and rest. Rest is a key component; treatment and healing require time. Carpal tunnel syndrome is a more serious repetitive strain injury

caused by repeated bending or use of the fingers or wrists that results in median nerve compression. Pain, numbness, and tingling on the side of the hand including the ring finger and thumb are common symptoms. Surgery may be required if the injury is severe enough or does not respond to conservative treatment. If left untreated, carpal tunnel syndrome can lead to muscle wasting, decreased sensation, and permanent disability (Princeton University, University Health Services, 2012).

Computer vision syndrome, or eyestrain, is the most common sequela of computer use. Using the computer for more than 3 hours a day puts one at risk, so many individuals are affected. Symptoms include eye fatigue, headaches, blurred vision, dry eyes, and changes in color perception. If left untreated, computer vision syndrome can lead to a decrease in work efficiency, general fatigue, and increased myopia. It can be caused by monitor glare, monitor position (too close or incorrect angle), or quick eye movements while typing and looking at a source document. Correct monitor position, antiglare screen covers, correct lighting, and proper document placement can all help reduce the effects of computer vision syndrome. It is also important to take breaks and to blink (Princeton University, University Health Services, 2012).

Box 48–5 Good Ergonomics for Computer Use

- Maintain good posture whether sitting or standing.
- Avoid overreaching. Keep the keyboard and mouse within easy reach.
- Keep your wrists in a straight position and your elbows at a slightly open angle.
- Position the monitor so that you can see the screen without tilting your neck up or down or turning your head.
- Use light force when typing on the keyboard.
- Customize font sizes and screen resolution to maximize comfort.
- Take frequent breaks. Eye breaks are important as well as stretching and moving around at regular intervals.
- Ensure proper lighting and reduce glare from the screen.

Sources: Based on University of California at Los Angeles. (2012). *Tips for computer users.* Retrieved April 20, 2013, from http://ergonomics.ucla.edu/homepage/office-ergonomics/tips-for-computer-users.html; Princeton University, University Health Services. (2012). *Ergonomics and computer use.* Retrieved from http://www.princeton.edu/uhs/healthy-living/hot-topics/ergonomics; University of Western Australia. (2012). *Safety and health: Computer workstation economics.* Retrieved from http://www.safety.uwa.edu.au/health-wellbeing/physical/ergonomics/workstation.

REVIEW The Concept of Informatics

RELATE Link the Concepts

Linking the concept of informatics with the concept of legal issues:

1. Name three ways that a nurse can keep protected health information secure.

2. What are some ramifications of looking up information in a local celebrity's chart if you are not taking care of that individual?

Linking the concept of informatics with the concept of addiction:

3. You are a nurse at a busy inner city emergency department. It is 3 a.m. on a Saturday when a client comes in asking for a narcotic prescription. She reports that she usually gets her prescription from her primary care provider for "ankle pain

from an old injury," but she forgot to call during the week. Describe how an electronic health record can assist you in caring for this client.

4. What type of questionnaire tools could be built into an electronic health record to assist with screening clients for chemical dependency?

READY Go to Companion Skills Manual

REFER Go to Pearson Student Nursing Resources
nursing.pearsonhighered.com

- Additional review materials
- Additional case study

REFLECT Case Study

Susan Johnson is a 45-year-old RN who works in a busy medical-surgical unit. Her hospital just installed an electronic health record system, and because of the layout of the unit, it was decided that the nurses would chart using workstations on wheels. Susan is excited about the new computerized system and has adapted to it quickly. She usually works three 12-hour shifts a week, but a few nurses are out on maternity leave, so she has been picking up extra hours. She has been noticing some tension and pain in her neck and shoulders, especially after her shifts.

1. What are some factors that may be contributing to the tension and pain in Susan's neck and shoulders?

2. What are some things that Susan could try to alleviate these symptoms?

3. What are some advantages to using WOWs for client documentation?

EXEMPLAR 48.1 Clinical Decision Support Systems

EXEMPLAR KEY TERMS

Clinical decision support systems, 2644
Dashboard, 2645
SNOMED CT, 2644

EXEMPLAR LEARNING OBJECTIVES

After reading about this exemplar, you will be able to:

1. Discuss the value of a clinical decision support system.

2. Explain the value of utilizing a uniform nursing language when documenting in the electronic health record.

3. Summarize the role of informatics in nursing research.

4. Examine the role of informatics in improving administrative processes.

▶ OVERVIEW

Clinical decision support systems are an important addition to electronic health records. They are designed to give healthcare providers tools to supplement decision-making processes during and after client care. These tools can include diagnostic support, documentation templates, clinical guidelines, alerts and reminders, condition-specific order sets, reference information, and focused data reports and summaries (HealthIT.gov, n.d.). Most of these tools are designed to be integrated with the EHR, while others have been designed as stand-alone systems. One study found that more than 90% of electronic clinical decision support systems significantly improved clinical care in randomized controlled trials (Kawamoto et al., 2010). These systems give advantages to clients and clinicians by helping prevent errors and adverse events, increasing quality of care and outcomes, and improving efficiency (HealthIT.gov, n.d.).

The Role of Uniform Languages

Uniform language refers to use of a common or standardized language across multiple disciplines. The Joint Commission's list of Do Not Use abbreviations is one example of a uniform language. The use of uniform language within the electronic health record can provide benefits to the client, the profession of nursing, and the health organization. Continuity of care improves for the client when standardized terminology is used. The nursing profession benefits in multiple ways. For individual nurses, the use of uniform language facilitates decision making and critical thinking at the point of care. Nurse researchers are able to easily document and retrieve evidence-based information regarding client care electronically. Nurse educators can tailor their curriculum to teach students concepts that are vital to the nursing process using uniform terminology. The health organization benefits from being able to measure nursing care and its impact on the client and also to provide administrators with information on the benefits and actual costs of nursing care (Lundberg et al., 2008).

Most nursing students are familiar with the terminology of NANDA-I, NIC, and NOC. Electronic heath records utilize these terminologies but don't usually have a way to integrate these terminology systems directly into the electronic health record. Systemized nomenclature of medicine—clinical terms **(SNOMED CT)** terminology is used as an intermediary language between the electronic health record and NANDA-I, NIC, and NOC. The use of SNOMED CT allows this use of multiple nursing language terminologies in a standardized format within the electronic health record (National Association of School Nurses, 2012). Other nursing language systems that may be utilized include perioperative nursing data sets (PNDS), the Omaha System (used in community health), and Clinical Care Classification (CCC; used in home care) (Lundberg et al., 2008).

Utilizing Research

A gap has long existed between reading nursing research and incorporating that knowledge into practice. Nurses often find it difficult to incorporate new research into practice. Organizational structures such as lack of nursing autonomy and lack of time are commonly reported barriers (Brown, Wickline, & Glaser, 2009). The utilization of electronic health records that contain clinical decision support systems should help promote best practices through nursing research and make it easier to use current nursing research at the point of care (Topaz et al., 2012).

▶ COMPUTERS IN NURSING RESEARCH

With the introduction of the electronic health record, computers will be available to nurses in all practice settings. Research environments will be no different. Conducting nursing research should be easier with the utilization of uniform language and the ability to query electronic health records. The steps of the nursing research process should remain the same. Technology can assist nurses in many ways to gain additional information: The nurse can use the EHR to research the client's medical history to determine if the client has been prescribed a particular drug and what responses the client experienced following administration. The nurse can use the Internet to conduct a literature search to determine if there is more information on use of that drug in certain populations or to get additional information related to potential side effects. For a detailed discussion of nursing research, including a list of nursing research databases, see the module on Evidence-Based Practice.

▶ COMPUTERS IN NURSING ADMINISTRATION

Many electronic health records give administrators tools to manage budgets, staffing, quality initiatives, and productivity information. The use of dashboards puts all of this information at the administrator's fingertips. A **dashboard** presents information about a healthcare facility's key performance indicators and displays the information in an easy-to-read format, often with charts or graphs (Curtiss, 2011). Some information can be displayed in real time. Electronic health records can create reports that track data over short-term periods (the past week) or long-term periods (the past year).

Human Resources

Human resource departments and payroll departments can benefit from computerization by tracking personnel within the healthcare system. Professional licenses and credentials expire and must be renewed. It would be a daunting task to keep track of this information manually for a large facility that employs thousands of healthcare professionals. A computerized system can monitor license expiration and when recredentialing of a provider is required. Mandatory hospital education, employee attendance, and performance reviews can all be tracked. When government regulatory agencies make their visits, all of this information will be easier to obtain and review. Payroll systems will be more accurate with a computerized system. Employees can have access to their available hours of vacation and sick time and can usually view their paycheck online a few days before they are paid.

Medical Records Management

Much of medical records management revolves around finances. The process begins when a client schedules an appointment or enters the system on an emergency basis. An informatics system can help schedule the appointment, verify insurance coverage and co-pay information, collect the client's demographic information, and collect any outstanding payments or co-pays. If the client is being admitted to the hospital, the system can help with obtaining insurance authorization and assigning a room and bed that have been marked clean and available by the system (and a roommate of the same gender if it is not a private room). The clients' condition can be coded for payment based on their ICD-10, CPT, or HCPCS code (Healthcare Information and Management Systems Society [HIMSS], 2009). ICD-10 codes will replace ICD-9 codes on October 1, 2014. The International Classification of Diseases (ICD) codes are used to report inpatient procedures and medical diagnosis (CMS, 2013b). Current procedural terminology (CPT) describes surgical, medical, and diagnostic services; hearing and vision services; occupational and physical therapy services; and transportation services (such as an ambulance; American Medical Association [AMA], 2013). The Healthcare Common Procedure Coding System (HCPCS) contains two levels. Level I is the CPT coding. Level II codes a wide array of services, such as durable medical equipment, outpatient chemotherapy drugs, medical supplies, orthotics, and prosthetics (American Academy of Professional Coders [AAPC], 2010).

Facilities Management

Another system that most nurses are unfamiliar with is materials management and supply chain. When a client needs a surgical dressing changed, the nurse goes to the supply room and grabs a new dressing without much thought about how it got there. Like many areas of health care, the materials management and supply chain community pushed for standardization for efficiency and cost savings. The first standard is that each institution has a Global Location Number (GLN) instead of an account number to make location of the institution easier. The second standard is that each product used in a facility has a Global Trade Item Number (GTIN) instead of a custom item number. It is thought that these standards will help by reducing errors in shipments, streamlining recall processes, enabling facilities to negotiate better contract pricing, and improving the supplier's ability to meet contract requirements. Electronic systems, with or without bar-code scanning, can help make equipment use and tracking more efficient and help reduce costs (GS1 Healthcare US Location Identification Workgroup, 2012). These systems also make it easier to keep track of supplies on hand and assist with ordering supplies or materials as they are used.

Budget and Finance

Before the client's chart can be finalized and closed, it is reviewed to make sure all coding is correct so that proper information is sent to the billing department. Some facilities do their own billing, while others hire separate companies to do their billing. If a client is receiving care in the hospital, there are usually two separate billing processes. One is professional billing, which covers fees for services provided by surgeons, radiologists, and anesthesiologists. The other is hospital billing, which covers room and board and supplies. Incorrect billing can result in the claim's being denied by a client's insurance company. This denial could leave either the client or the hospital responsible for the bill, so there is usually a process for billers to submit appeals or resolve claim denials. It is a very complicated system that can be made easier through an electronic administration system.

Reimbursement rates for procedures and diagnoses change regularly, and a computerized contract management system can help facilities track rates of reimbursement and real-time changes in policies for different health insurance plans. The Patient Protection and Affordable Care Act (ACA) is likely to result in additional changes in coverage and reimbursement in both public and private sectors. Having current data will help healthcare facilities obtain accurate and timely reimbursement and help prevent clients from receiving inaccurate bills or bills from a service that was covered.

Financial systems within healthcare facilities can benefit greatly from use of an electronic system. They are responsible for sharing information between billing systems, materials management, and staffing/human resources in order to determine the financial health of the facility. The data provided is crucial for making strategic decisions about a healthcare institution and in planning organizational budgets (Duke University, 2012). Executives and managers can view financial information over both short- and long-term time frames and adjust their resources and fiscal planning appropriately.

Quality Assurance and Utilization Reviews

Computerized systems facilitate the tracking of client outcomes. Unexpected or poor client outcomes can be tracked by risk management (the legal department of a health system). Quality outcomes information can also be easily tracked. Outcome tracking helps identify faulty processes and assists in modifying policies and procedures to improve client outcomes for a particular diagnosis or department within a health organization. Utilization review is designed to eliminate inappropriate or unnecessary medical care. In this type of review, electronic health records are reviewed for quality of care rendered, appropriateness of treatment, length of stay, and appropriate place of treatment (inpatient vs. outpatient hospital) (Florida Agency for Health Care Administration, 2011).

Accreditation

The availability of quality metrics will make it easier to meet and document the requirements of regulatory agencies. Agencies such as the Centers for Medicaid and Medicare Services and The Joint Commission implement policies that health facilities must follow in order to receive reimbursement by many health insurance plans (Meldi et al., 2009). There are also smaller yet still important standards that must be maintained for certification such as trauma status from the American College of Surgeons or stroke center status from The Joint Commission. Electronic health records simplify the data-gathering process when each of these agencies reviews a facility for accreditation.

REVIEW Clinical Decision Support Systems

RELATE Link the Concepts and Exemplars

Linking the exemplar of clinical decision support systems to the concept of cellular regulation:

1. Discuss how clinical decision support systems could improve outcomes for clients with cancer.
2. Name three cancer screening tools that could be built into an electronic health record.
3. Discuss the benefits of making reminders for cancer screening available to healthcare providers and to clients.

Linking the exemplar of clinical decision support systems to the concept of health policy:

4. You are working in the operating room, and your supervisor always requires that the employees in the department enter a higher level-of-diagnosis code on each trauma client's chart. What are some ramifications?

5. What impact does a change in a federal or state health policy have on clinical decision support systems?

READY Go to Companion Skills Manual

REFER Go to Pearson Student Nursing Resources
nursing.pearsonhighered.com

- Additional review materials

REFLECT Case Study

You are the nurse manager for an orthopedic unit that has just installed an electronic health record system with an administrative system. You have been short-staffed for several months.

1. How can an administrative system help get more nursing positions approved for your unit?
2. What other features of an administrative system do you think will have the greatest impact on your unit and why?

EXEMPLAR 48.2 Individual Information at Point of Care

EXEMPLAR KEY TERMS
Case managers, 2648
Point of care, 2647

EXEMPLAR LEARNING OUTCOMES
After reading about this exemplar, you will be able to:

1. Summarize the advantages of point-of-care service delivery.

2. Discuss how informatics can improve delivery of care in community and home-based health settings.
3. Predict nursing considerations in the use of information printed from the electronic health record to provide client education prior to discharge.

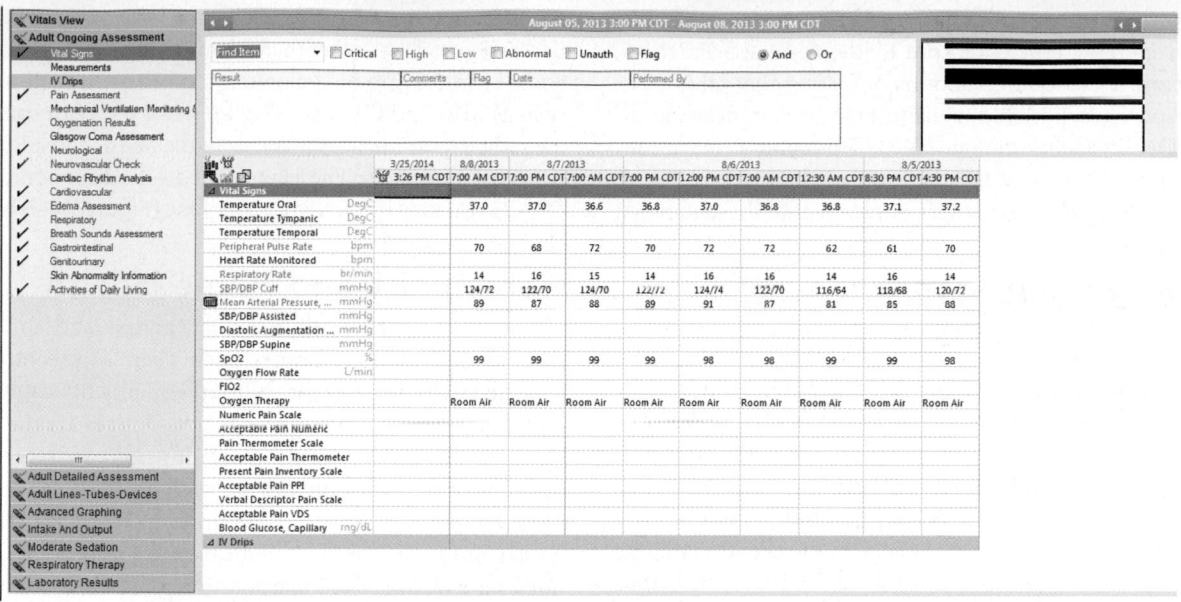

Figure 48–3 ● This EHR screen displays the client's vital signs. They can be entered by the nurse (or anyone with security rights to do so) at the bedside, and they can be displayed wherever needed.

▶ OVERVIEW

Studies have proven that the more direct nursing care a client receives, the greater the quality and safety of the care delivered and the more satisfied both nurse and client are with the care. Nurses have reported that charting is an activity that consumes much of their time and takes time away from the bedside. The ability to enter data into a client's chart while at the client's bedside seems like a valid compromise. Most electronic health records allow recording of vital signs, medication documentation, assessment notes, and responses to nursing intervention (**Figure 48–3 ●**). One of the selling points of an electronic

Evidence-Based Practice Do EHRs Reduce Documentation Time?

Problem

Nurses have many demands on their time that take away from direct client care. One of them is documentation. One of the suggested benefits of electronic health records is that they improve efficiency of care delivery as a result of improved access to clinical information and computerized physician order entry. The increase in efficiency should translate into nurses' having more time to deliver direct client care.

Evidence

A study using time and motion data for 105 units in 55 hospitals examined the time that nurses spent charting on paper and charting electronically. The percentage of time (19%) that nurses spent completing their charting did not vary whether the nurse was documenting electronically or on paper (Yee et al., 2012). Another study had observers follow nurses at two hospitals before and after the implementation of an electronic health record system. The total time spent observing was 196 hours at one hospital and 185 at the other hospital. Although computer time was noted to increase, the time that nurses spent delivering care and communicating with their clients remained unchanged. Nurses found ways to cut time from doing other tasks to allow their time spent with the client to be unaffected (Cornell, Riordan, & Herrin-Griffith, 2010). Another observational work study followed the time nurses spent on documentation at a nursing home 2 months prior to the implementation of an electronic record system. The same group was observed at 3, 6, and 12 months postimplementation of the electronic record system. The study found no difference in the amount of time that nurses spent documenting (Munyisia, Yu, & Hailey, 2011).

Implications

One of the selling points of electronic health records is that they will reduce the amount of time spent charting. This "gained" time is supposed to allow the nurse to spend more time in direct client care. While one study showed that time spent on a computer was increased, none of the studies showed that changing from a paper chart to an electronic chart took time away from client care activities. While time that nurses spent documenting in an electronic health record has been studied, it appears that current research is lacking on whether that documentation is done in the presence or absence of the client and how electronic documentation affects time spent with clients.

Critical Thinking Application

Consider the needs of a 53-year-old nurse who is not very computer literate. Her employer is installing an electronic health record system in 3 months' time. As the nursing informatics educator, identify some concerns this nurse may have. Identify two interventions that can improve her chances of successfully adapting to charting in an electronic format.

health record is that charting at point of care is possible and that it helps to increase efficiency (see Evidence-Based Practice). **Point of care** refers to interventions or testing that takes place using transportable, portable, or hand-held devices near the client (ASC Quality Collaboration, 2013). This setup provides on-the-spot information about the client rather than having to wait for the results from blood or urine samples sent to the laboratory.

▶ COMPUTER-BASED CLIENT RECORDS

While the electronic health record has the potential to forever change how health care is delivered in the United States, it is important to understand that, in many instances, the electronic record cannot and should not replace real time (face-to-face or telephone) communication with peers, other health professionals, and especially the client. An acute change in the client's condition still requires a phone call to the physician. News of cancerous pathology reports should still be delivered in person by the physician and not discovered by the client online. As systems become more advanced and interfaces more integrated, nurses cannot lose sight of the human element in the delivery of care.

Client Monitoring and Computerized Diagnostics

Advances in electronic systems are changing monitoring and tracking of client care. Many facilities now use systems that allow electronic transmission of information such as the weight from the scale on the bed, intravenous pump rates, bar-code scanning of medications that are administered, vital sign information, bar-code scanning of blood administration, and ventilator settings. Many departments within a hospital or other facility may enter data about

the client into the record so that all practitioners have the information easily available rather than having to flip through a paper chart. Some examples are the laboratory and many radiological exams, such as MRI and CT scans (**Figure 48–4 ●**). With some systems, the radiological image is available at the bedside in addition to the radiologist's report. The client's medical administration record (MAR) also may be viewed by everyone (**Figure 48–5 ●**).

Community and Home Health

Approximately 12 million clients across the United States receive care in their homes each year. These numbers are expected to increase as the value and quality of health care in an outpatient setting is being recognized. Nurses are the main providers of this care to clients, many of whom are receiving home health care for a chronic disease such as diabetes or congestive heart failure. It is difficult sometimes to keep up to date on the management of complex medical issues that home healthcare nurses are facing. The incorporation of current evidence-based clinical practice guidelines into the electronic health record system that is utilized by the home healthcare agency can improve the quality of care that these clients receive (Topaz et al., 2012).

Case Management

Case managers help manage the care of certain client populations, including clients with chronic medical conditions, such as diabetes; clients recovering from acute conditions, such as those receiving joint replacement; and clients managing psychiatric disorders. Electronic health records can assist the case manager by allowing trending of client progress, documentation of client education, and observation of quality metrics to help decrease readmission rates for these populations. Electronic health records also allow improved

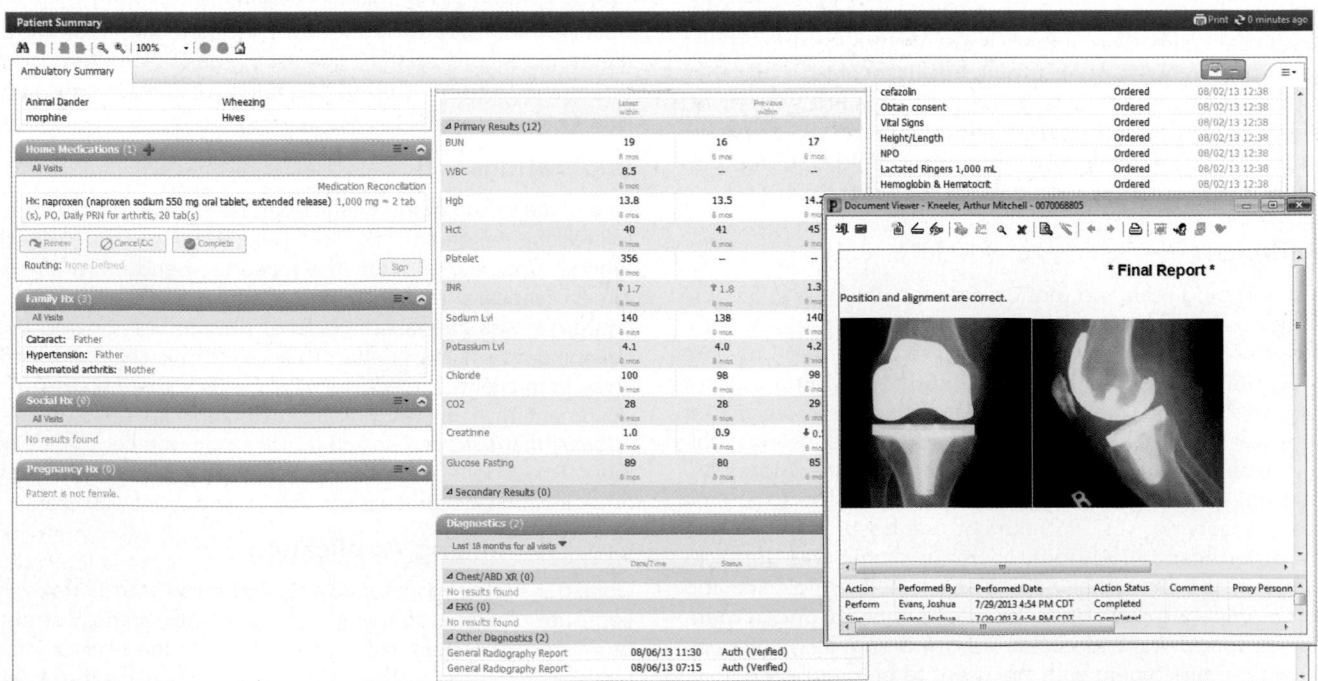

Figure 48–4 ● This EHR screen displays a summary view of all available laboratory results and diagnostic imaging for a particular client. The information is reported from most summarized to most detailed so that the use gets the overview first and can then "drill down" to see the details.

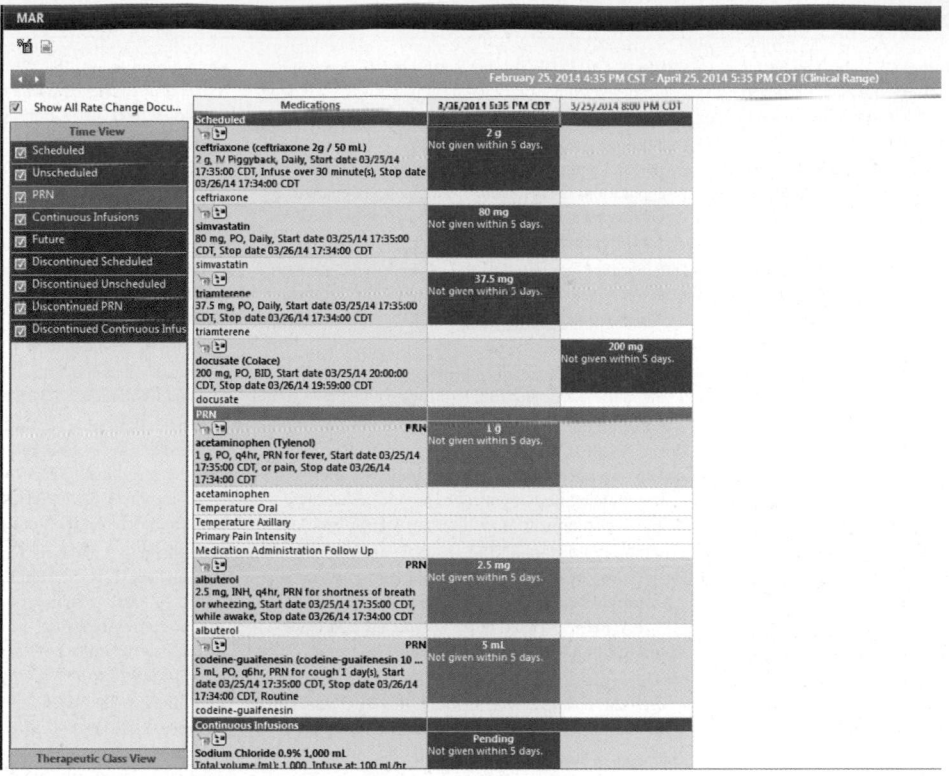

Figure 48–5 ● This EHR screen shows a medication administration record (MAR) for several regularly scheduled medications. The worksheet displays the next time the medications are scheduled to be administered.
Courtesy of Sutter Health.

coordination of care between providers because they are all working off one chart.

Client Education

Instructions for health conditions and procedures are available in most electronic health record systems. The client's health problem can be identified through menus and educational information printed so that the nurse can review the information with the client or the client's family. Standardization of the record means that the clients will receive the same educational material whether they are being treated in the emergency room, on a surgical unit, or in a healthcare provider's office. The information contained within the educational material should be current and evidenced based, so that the task of client education is more accurate and meaningful. Some material may provide links to Web sites for additional information. Many systems can print educational information in different languages as well. Note that use of standardized printed material does not negate the nurse's responsibility to (a) assess the client or family member's ability to read and understand the information, (b) review the information in person with the client or family member, and (c) ensure that the client or family member understands the information prior to discharge.

REVIEW Individual Information at Point of Care

RELATE Link the Concepts and Exemplars

Linking the exemplar of individual information at point of care with the concept of assessment:

1. Discuss the advantages of being able to document the assessment of your client at the point of care with an electronic record rather than a centralized charting location.

2. Explain how point-of-care documentation of your client assessment can be utilized as an opportunity for client teaching.

Linking the exemplar of individual information at point of care with the concept of oxygenation:

3. What point-of-care information can you obtain from an electronic medical record about the client's past and present oxygenation status that may influence immediate nursing interventions?

4. How might point-of-care recording of pulse oximeter values have an advantage over recording them from a centralized monitoring station in the intensive care unit?

READY Go to Companion Skills Manual

REFER Go to Pearson Student Nursing Resources
nursing.pearsonhighered.com

- Additional review materials

REFLECT Case Study

You are caring for an Albanian client who just had his appendix removed. You log into your health system's electronic record to obtain discharge information. The client and the family speak limited English. Albanian is not a language choice for appendectomy discharge instructions.

1. What are some options that you can use to try to educate the client on taking care of his incision site?

2. How would you document your interventions in the electronic record?

■ REFERENCES

American Academy of Ambulatory Care Nursing. (2011). *New video explains nurse licensure compact.* Retrieved from http://www.aaacn.org/article/article/new-video-explains-nurse-licensure-compact.

American Academy of Professional Coders. (2010). *What is HCPCS?* Retrieved from http://www.aapc.com/resources/medical-coding/hcpcs.aspx.

American Medical Association. (2013). *CPT frequently asked questions.* Retrieved from http://www.ama-assn.org/ama/pub/physician-resources/solutions-managing-your-practice/coding-billing-insurance/cpt/frequently-asked-questions.page.

American Nurses Association. (2008). *Nursing informatics: Scope and standards of practice.* Silver Spring, MD: Nursebooks.org.

ASC Quality Collaboration. (2013). *Point of care devices toolkit.* Retrieved from http://www.ascquality.org/PointofCareDevicesToolkit.cfm.

Baril, A. F. (2010). *Electronic medical records and HIPAA violations.* Retrieved from http://nursing.advanceweb.com/continuing-education/ce-articles/electronic-medical-record-hipaa-violations.aspx.

Barnes, S., & Weaver, T. (2011). *Overview: Infection prevention and control for computers in patient care areas.* Retrieved from http://www.beckersasc.com/asc-accreditation-and-patient-safety/overview-infection_prevention-and_control-for-computers-in-patient-care-areas.html.

Blumenthal, D. (2010). Launching HITECH. *New England Journal of Medicine, 362,* 382–385.

Brown, C. E., Wickline, M. A., & Glaser, D. (2009). Nursing practice, knowledge, attitudes and perceived barriers to evidence-based practice at an academic medical center. *Journal of Advanced Nursing, 65,* 371–381. doi: 10.1111/j.1365-2648.2008.04878.x.

Brull, J. (2012). *Social media in medicine: Do your patients "like" you?* Retrieved from http://www.aafp.org/news-now/opinion/20120629editbrull.html.

Buck, S. (2012). *What doctors think about your online health searches.* Retrieved from http://mashable.com/2012/06/15/online-medical-searches/.

California HealthCare Foundation. (2013a). *Brief highlights: Ways to promote the successful adoption of telehealth.* Retrieved from http://www.ihealthbeat.org/articles/2013/2/1/brief-highlights-ways-to-promote-the-successful-adoption-of-telehealth.

California HealthCare Foundation. (2013b). *1.8 Million patients will use telehealth tools by 2017, report says.* Retrieved from http://www.ihealthbeat.org/articles/2013/1/23/18-million-patients-will-use-telehealth-tools-by-2017-report-says.aspx?topic=telehealth.

Centers for Disease Control and Prevention, Division for Heart Disease and Stroke Prevention. (2013). *Chronic disease GIS exchange.* Retrieved from http://www.cdc.gov/dhdsp/maps/gisx/.

Centers for Medicare and Medicaid Services. (2012). *Telehealth services: Rural health fact sheet.* Retrieved from http://www.cms.gov/Outreach-and-Education/Medicare-Learning-Network-MLN/MLNProducts/downloads/telehealthsrvcsfctsht.pdf.

Centers for Medicare and Medicaid Services. (2013a). *Clinical quality measures (CQMs).* Retrieved from http://www.cms.gov/Regulations-and-Guidance/Legislation/EHRIncentivePrograms/ClinicalQualityMeasures.html.

Centers for Medicare and Medicaid Services. (2013b). *ICD-10.* Retrieved from http://www.cms.gov/Medicare-Coding/ICD10/index.html?redirect=/icd10.

Cornell, P., Riordan, M., & Herrin-Griffith, D. (2010). Transforming nursing workflow, Part 2: The impact of technology on nurse activities. *Journal of Nursing Administration, 40*(10), 432–439.

Curtiss, S. (2011). *The unsung benefits of HIT dashboards.* Retrieved from http://www.healthcareitnews.com/blog/unsung-benefits-hit-dashboards.

Dennison, L., Morrison, L., Conway, G., & Yardley, L. (2013). Opportunities and challenges for smartphone applications in supporting health behavior change: Qualitative study. *Journal of Medical Internet Research, 15*(4), e86. doi: 10.2196/jmir.2583.

DifferenceBetween.net. (2013). *Difference between Internet and intranet.* Retrieved from http://www.differencebetween.net/technology/difference-between-internet-and-intranet/.

Dolan, P. (2013). *Make sure patient portals go beyond meaningful use.* Retrieved from http://www.amednews.com/article/20130128/business/130129963/5/.

Dolan, T. (2010). *Nursing informatics certification: A high-tech career boost.* Retrieved from http://www.nursezone.com/nursing-news-events/devices-and-technology/Nursing-Informatics-Certification-A-High-Tech-Career-Boost_34212.aspx.

Duke University. (2012). *Health management information systems: Administrative, billing, and financial systems lecture A.* Retrieved from http://www.healthinformaticsforum.com/page/component-6-unit-9-lecture-a.

Federation of State Medical Boards. (2012a). *Telemedicine overview: Board by board approach.* Retrieved from http://www.fsmb.org/pdf/grpol_telemedicine_licensure.pdf.

Federation of State Medical Boards. (2012b). *Model policy guidelines for the appropriate use of social media and social networking in medical practice.* Retrieved from http://www.fsmb.org/pdf/pub-social-media-guidelines.pdf.

Florida Agency for Health Care Administration. (2011). *Utilization review—Quality assurance/quality improvement.* Retrieved from http://ahca.myflorida.com/Medicaid/Utilization_Review/index.shtml.

Fox, S., & Duggan, M. (2013). *Health online 2013.* Retrieved from http://pewinternet.org/Reports/2013/Health-online/Summary-of-Findings.aspx.

Garnett, P., & Seidman, J. (2011). *EMR vs EHR—What is the Difference?* Retrieved from http://www.healthit.gov/buzz-blog/electronic-health-and-medical-record/emr-vs-ehr-difference/.

Goldberg, D., Kuzel, A., Feng, L., DeShazo, J., & Love, L. (2012). EHRs in primary care practices: Benefits, challenges, and successful strategies. *American Journal of Managed Care, 18*(2), E48–e54.

GS1 Healthcare US Location Identification Workgroup. (2012). *GLN roadmap: A collaborative industry implementation plan for U.S. healthcare.* Retrieved from http://www.gs1us.org/DesktopModules/Bring2mind/DMX/Download.aspx?Command=Core_Download&EntryId=535&PortalId=0&TabId=785.

HealthCare.gov. (n.d.). *Where can I find provider information?* Retrieved from https://www.healthcare.gov/where-can-i-find-provider-information/.

Healthcare Information and Management Systems Society. (2009). *The intersection of healthcare and financial systems: A white paper by the HIMSS Financial Systems Financial/Banking in Healthcare Work Group.* Retrieved from http://himss.files.cms-plus.com/HIMSSOrg/content/files/FinancialSystems/20091014_FS_Banking_White_Paper.pdf.

HealthIT.gov. (n.d.). *Clinical decision support.* Retrieved from http://www.healthit.gov/policy-researchers-implementers/clinical-decision-support-cds.

Health Level Seven International. (2013). *About HL7.* Retrieved from http://www.hl7.org/about/index.cfm?ref=nav.

Interfaceware. (2010). *HL7 overview.* Retrieved from http://www.interfaceware.com/hl7.html.

Internet World Stats. (2013). *Usage and population statistics.* Retrieved from http://www.internetworldstats.com/stats.htm.

Joint Commission, The. (2012). *Surgical care improvement project.* Retrieved from http://www.jointcommission.org/surgical_care_improvement_project/.

Kawamoto, K., Del Fiol, G., Lobach, D., & Jenders, R. (2010). Standards for scalable clinical decision support: Need, current and emerging standards, gaps, and proposal for progress. *Open Medical Informatics Journal, 4,* 235–244.

Kerr, D. (2013). *Six states outlaw employer snooping on Facebook.* Retrieved from http://news.cnet.com/8301-1023_3-57561743-93/six-states-outlaw-employer-snooping-on-facebook/.

Kopola, B., & Mitchell, M. (2011). Use of digital records raises ethics concerns. *JONA's Healthcare Law, Ethics, and Regulation, 13*(3), 84–89.

Locatelli, P., Restifo, N., Gastaldi, L., & Corso, M. (2012). *Health care information systems: Architectural models and governance.* Retrieved from http://cdn.intechopen.com/pdfs/37320/InTech-Health_care_information_systems_architectural_models_and_governance.pdf.

Lundberg, C. B., Warren, J. J., Brokel, J., Bulechek, G. M., Butcher, H. K., Martin, K. S., McCloskey Dochterman, J., …Giarrizzo-Wilson, S. (2008). Selecting a standardized terminology for the electronic health record that reveals the impact of nursing on patient care. *Online Journal of Nursing Informatics, 12*(2). Retrieved from http:ojni.org/12_2/lundberg.htm.

Lunden, I. (2012). *ITU: There are now over 1 billion users of social media worldwide, most on mobile.* Retrieved from http://techcrunch.com/2012/05/14/itu-there-are-now-over-1-billion-users-of-social-media-worldwide-most-on-mobile/.

Madison, M. P., & Staggers, N. (2011). Electronic health records and the implication for nursing practice. *Journal of Nursing Regulation, 1*(4), 54–60.

Mathews, A. W. (2013). Should doctors and patients be Facebook friends? *The Wall Street Journal,* March 4, 2013.

McKnight, S. (2012). Telehealth: Applications for complex care. *Online Journal of Nursing Informatics, 16*(3). Retrieved from http://ojni.org/issues/?p=2034.

McLaughlin, J. (2011). *Text message use among providers raise HIPAA concerns.* Retrieved from http://www.beckershospitalreview.com/healthcare-information-technology/text-message-use-among-providers-raise-hipaa-concerns.html.

McNickle, M. (2012). *5 ways device integration increases the value of data in an EMR.* Retrieved from http://www.healthcareitnews.com/news/5-ways-device-integration-increases-value-data-emr?single-page=true.

Meldi, D., Rhoades, F., & Cippe, A. (2009). The big three: A side by side matrix comparing hospital accrediting agencies. *NAMSS Industry & Government Relations Committee, Synergy, 12,* 12–14.

Meum, T. (2013). "Lost in translation": The challenges of seamless integration in nursing practices. *International Journal of Medical Informatics, 82*(5), e200–e208.

Moyer, C. (2012). *Cyberchondria: The one diagnosis patients miss.* Retrieved from http://www.amednews.com/article/20120130/health/301309952/1/-cyberchondria:the_one_diagnosis_patients_miss-amednews.com.

Munyisia, E., Yu, P., & Hailey, D. (2011). Does the introduction of an electronic nursing documentation system in a nursing home reduce time on documentation for the nursing staff? *International Journal of Informatics, 80*(11), 782–792.

National Association of School Nurses. (2012). *Standardized nursing languages.* Retrieved from http://www.nasn.org/Policy/Advocacy/PositionPapersandReports/NASNPositionStatementsFullView/tabid/462/Articleid/48/Standardized-Nursing-Languages-Revised-June-2012-Standardized Nursing Languages.

Open Clinical. (2012). *Electronic medical records.* Retrieved from http://www.openclinical.org/emr.html.

Phatak, O. (2012). Intranet vs. Internet. Retrieved from http://www.buzzle.com/articles/intranet-vs-internet.html.

Princeton University, University Health Services. (2012). *Ergonomics and computer use.* Retrieved from http://www.princeton.edu/uhs/healthy-living/hot-topics/ergonomics.

Raths, D. (2010). *The push and pull of cart ergonomics.* Retrieved from http://www.healthcare-informatics.com/article/push-and-pull-cart-ergonomics.

Reginatto, B. (2012). Addressing barriers to wider adoption of telehealth in the homes of older people: An exploratory study in the Irish context. *eTELEMED2012: The Fourth International Conference on eHealth, Telemedicine, and Social Medicine,* 1–9.

Roney, K. (2012). *Overcoming 4 challenges in implementing telemedicine, healthcare's next frontier.* Retrieved from http://www.beckershospitalreview.com/healthcare-information-technology/overcoming-4-challenges-in-implementing-telemedicine-healthcares-next-frontier.html.

Scullard, P., Peacock, C., & Davies, P. (2010). Googling children's health: Reliability of medical advice on the Internet. *Archives of Disease in Childhood 2010, 95*(8), 580–582. doi: 10.1136/adc.2009.168856.

Sheridan, S. (2012). The implementation and sustainability of electronic health records. *Online Journal of Nursing Informatics, 16*(3). Retrieved from http://ojni.org/issues/?p=1992.

Stokes, T. (2013). *Copying common in electronic medical records.* Retrieved from http://www.reuters.com/article/2013/01/04/us-electronic-medical-records-idUSBRE9030IJ20130104.

Steinberg, S. (2011). *How people use the Internet for health information.* Retrieved from http://www.practicefusion.com/ehrbloggers/2011/05/how-people-use-the-internet-for-health-information.html.

Surgical Care Improvement Project. (2012). *Fact sheet: Summary of SCIP measure changes for 01/01/2013 discharges.* Retrieved from http://www.jointcommission.org/assets/1/6/SCIPFactSheet010113.pdf.

TIGER Initiative. (2006). Retrieved from http://www.tiger-summit.com/About_Us.html.

Topaz, M., Radhakrishnan, K., Masterson-Creber, R., & Bowles, K. H. (2012). Putting evidence to work: Using standardized terminologies to incorporate clinical practice guidelines within homecare electronic health records. *Online Journal of Nursing Informatics, 16*(2). Available at http://ojni.org/issues/?p=1694.

Turley, M., Garrido, T., Lowenthal, A., & Zhou, Y. (2012). Association between personal health record enrollment and patient loyalty. *American Journal of Managed Care, 18*(7), e248–e253.

U.S. Department of Health and Human Services. (n.d.). *Health information privacy.* Retrieved from http://www.hhs.gov/ocr/privacy/hipaa/understanding/consumers/.

U.S. Department of Health and Human Services. (2013). *What is e-health?* Retrieved from http://www.health.gov/communication/ehealth/.

U.S. Department of Labor, Occupational Safety and Health Administration. (n.d.a). *Prevention of musculoskeletal disorders in the workplace: Ergonomics.* Retrieved from http://www.osha.gov/SLTC/ergonomics.

U.S. Department of Labor, Occupational Safety and Health Administration. (n.d.b). *Computer workstations: Checklist.* Retrieved from http://www.osha.gov/SLTC/etools/computerworkstations/checklist.html.

U.S. Department of Veterans Affairs Office of Telehealth Services. (2011). *What is telehealth?* Retrieved from http://www.telehealth.va.gov.

U.S. National Library of Medicine, National Institutes of Health. (2012). *MedlinePlus guide to healthy Web surfing.* Retrieved from http://www.nlm.nih.gov/medlineplus/healthywebsurfing.html.

U.S. National Library of Medicine, National Institutes of Health. (2013). *Ergonomics.* Retrieved from http://www.nlm.nih.gov/medlineplus/ergonomics.html.

University of California–Davis. (2012). *Patients trust doctors but consult the Internet.* Retrieved from http://news.ucdavis.edu/search/news_detail.lasso?id=10278.

University of Iowa College of Nursing. (2013a). *CNC-overview: Nursing interventions classification (NIC).* Retrieved from http://www.nursing.uiowa.edu/cncce/nursing-interventions-classification-overview.

University of Iowa College of Nursing. (2013b). *CNC-overview: Nursing outcomes classification (NOC).* Retrieved from http://www.nursing.uiowa.edu/cncce/nursing-outcomes-classification-overview.

Vanderbilt University School of Medicine, Department of Biomedical Informatics. (2013). *Frequently asked questions.* Retrieved from https://medschool.vanderbilt.edu/dbmi/frequently-asked-questions.

Weisman, R. (2013). New insurance tools will let patients discover costs. *The Boston Globe,* January 27, 2013.

Wirkus, M. (2011). *Telehealth programs gaining ground in nursing education.* Retrieved from http://www.nurse-zone.com/nursing-news-events/more-news/Telehealth-Programs-Gaining-Ground-in-Nursing-Education_38226.aspx.

Woods, S., Schwartz, E., Tuepker, A., Press, N., Nazi, K., Turvey, C., & Nichol, W. (2013). Patient experiences with full electronic access to health records and clinical notes through the My HealtheVet Personal Health Record Pilot: Qualitative study. *Journal of Medical Internet Research, 15*(3), e65. doi:10.2196/jmir.org/2013/e65/.

Yee, T., Needleman, J., Pearson, M., Parkerton, P., Parkerton, M., & Wolstein, J. (2012). The influence of integrated electronic medical records and computerized nursing notes on nurses' time spent in documentation. *CIN: Computers, Informatics, Nursing, 30*(6), 287–292.

49 Legal Issues

MODULE AT-A-GLANCE

The Concept of Legal Issues, 2653

Exemplar 49.1
  Nurse Practice Acts, 2663

Exemplar 49.2
  Advance Directives, 2667

Exemplar 49.3
  Health Insurance Portability and
  Accountability Act, 2670

Exemplar 49.4
  Just Culture, 2672

Exemplar 49.5
  Mandatory Reporting, 2674

Exemplar 49.6
  Risk Management, 2676

◢ THE CONCEPT OF LEGAL ISSUES

The concept of legal issues encompasses the rights, responsibilities, and scope of nursing practice as defined by state nurse practice acts and as legislated through criminal and civil laws. All clients have a privilege, demand, or claim by virtue of law or *right* (that which is proper or just) to expect competent nursing services. The nursing student must be equipped to provide safe nursing care consistent with legal requirements and gain an awareness of ways to minimize the risks of errors due to accident, carelessness, system failures, or malpractice. **Malpractice** is conduct deviating from the standard of practice dictated by the profession (**Box 49–1** ●). Providing safe care requires more than a knowledge of anatomy and physiology, pathophysiology, and medications and therapies. It also requires knowledge of the regulations of healthcare providers, institutions, payment systems, and federal and state laws that are interconnected within the domain of the healthcare system.

Upon enrollment, the nursing student begins learning about laws and regulations that affect nursing practice. Legal and professional regulations address both nursing practice and the practices of healthcare organizations that serve as workplaces for nurses at all levels of practice. Many healthcare agency policies and procedures exist to ensure that relevant laws are followed to (a) promote client safety and reduce the

(continued on next page)

Concept Learning Outcomes

After reading about this concept, you will be able to:

1. Discuss elements of professional negligence and malpractice in nursing.
2. Summarize strategies to prevent incidents of professional negligence.
3. Analyze the importance of providing nursing care according to established standards of care.
4. Distinguish elements of informed consent.
5. Contrast different types of situations in which informed consent is applied.

Concept Key Terms

Administrative laws, *2654*
Assault, *2657*
Battery, *2657*
Breach of duty, *2656*
Causation, *2656*
Civil law, *2655*
Competency, *2659*
Controlled Substances Act
  (CSA), *2661*
Crime, *2654*
Criminal law, *2654*
Damages, *2656*
Duty, *2656*

Expressed consent, *2659*
False imprisonment, *2657*
Foreseeability, *2656*
Good Samaritan laws, *2662*
Implied consent, *2659*
Informed consent, *2659*
Law, *2654*
Liability, *2656*
Malpractice, *2653*
Negligence, *2655*
Standards of care, *2657*
Statutory laws, *2654*
Tort, *2655*

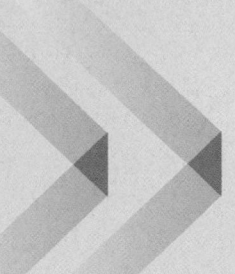

risk for error resulting in adverse events and (b) protect both healthcare staff and healthcare agencies as a whole. For example, policies and procedures regarding infection precautions reduce the risk of healthcare-associated infections and mitigate staff risk. Policies regarding identifying and managing client valuables help ensure that clients' belongings are cared for and respected and also act to prevent the possibility of theft or accidental loss.

To provide safe, effective care and maintain personal protection from liability, nurses must be aware of the applicable regulations in every nursing encounter. Awareness begins with understanding general legal concepts and continues as the nursing student starts to learn about the laws and regulations that directly affect the daily activities of nursing. **<<**

▶ SOURCES OF LAWS

Guido (2010, p. 31) defined **law** as the "sum total of the rules and regulations by which a society is governed." Law is made at the federal, state, and local levels to reflect the ever-changing needs and expectations of a given society. **Statutory laws** are made by any legislative branch of the government, including the U.S. Congress, state legislatures, and city and county governments. The U.S. Constitution grants the federal government power, whereas the states have inherent power to act to maintain health, public order, safety, and welfare except where the Constitution restricts their ability to do so.

Nursing laws are examples of state statutory laws. Each state has a nurse practice act that contains the laws pertaining to nursing practice in that state. Nurse practice acts are discussed in detail in Exemplar 49.1. Other statutory laws that affect the practice of nursing include statutes of limitation, protection and reporting laws, natural death acts, and informed consent laws.

A legislative body, through statutory law, delegates the responsibility for the administration and enforcement of those laws to an administrative agency. Administrative agencies may also be granted additional power to interpret those laws and enact policies or procedures by which those laws will be implemented and enforced. These policies or procedures are often referred to as **administrative laws**. State boards of nursing are examples of administrative agencies that are delegated the power to interpret and enforce law by the legislatures that govern them.

An overview of the sources of law is shown in **Figure 49–1** ●. Selected categories of law that may affect nurses are shown in **Table 49–1** ●.

▶ CRIMINAL AND CIVIL LAW

Both criminal and civil laws have implications for the practicing nurse. **Criminal law** defines conduct that is harmful to another individual or to society as a whole and that may be punishable by fines or imprisonment. A **crime** is an act prohibited by statute or

TABLE 49–1 Selected Categories of Laws Affecting Nurses

CATEGORY	EXAMPLES
Constitutional	Due process
	Equal protection
Statutory (legislative)	Nurse practice acts
	Good Samaritan acts
	Child and adult abuse laws
	Advance directives
	Sexual harassment laws
	Americans with Disabilities Act
Criminal (public)	Homicide, manslaughter
	Theft
	Arson
	Active euthanasia
	Sexual assault
	Illegal possession of controlled drugs
Contracts (private/civil)	Nurse and client
	Nurse and employer
	Nurse and insurance provider
	Client and agency
Torts (private/civil)	Negligence/malpractice
	Libel and slander
	Invasion of privacy
	Assault and battery
	False imprisonment
	Abandonment

Box 49–1 Malpractice Cases Against Nurses

The 2011 Annual Report of the National Practitioner Data Bank (NPDB) states that professional nurses have been responsible for 5,827 malpractice payments from 2002 to 2011. Nonspecialized registered nurses were responsible for 3.8% of the payments made during that time period (NPDB, 2011). Liability risks (e.g., supervision/delegation, early client discharge, nursing shortage, hospital downsizing, increased autonomy, lack of adequate training, and advanced technology) along with better-informed consumers have contributed to the increased number of malpractice cases against nurses (Eisenberg, 2010).

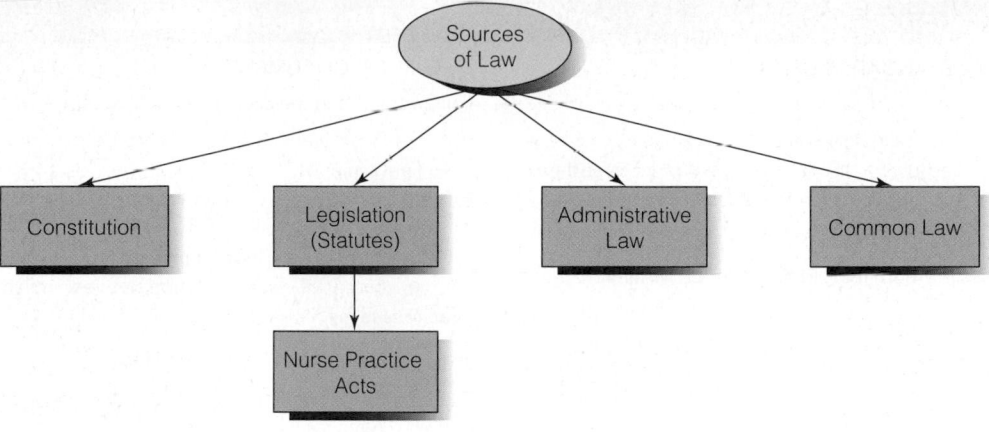

Figure 49–1 ● Overview of the sources of law.

by common law principles. Crimes are considered to be committed against the state as opposed to the individual. Examples include homicide, theft, and manslaughter. Crimes are classified by severity, with more serious crimes classified as *felonies* and lesser offenses termed *misdemeanors* (Guido, 2010, p. 38). A misdemeanor usually is punishable by a fine or short-term jail sentence or both.

Civil law deals with the rights and duties of private individuals or citizens and is most often enforced through the awarding of damages or compensation. A **tort** is a civil wrong committed against an individual or an individual's property. An individual who violates tort law may be sued and compensation awarded to those wrongfully injured by those violations. Torts may be intentional or unintentional.

▶ TORT LAW

Tort law defines and addresses both unintentional and intentional actions or omissions that result in harm to another person or persons or harm to another's personal property. Unintentional torts discussed here include negligence and malpractice. Intentional torts include assault, battery, and false imprisonment.

Unintentional Torts

NEGLIGENCE   **Negligence** is considered conduct that deviates from what a reasonable person would do in a particular circumstance. This reasonable person standard describes an individual in society who exercises average care, skill, and judgment in conduct as a comparative standard for determining liability. Generally, individuals with greater than average skill and ability, including those with special duties or training such as physicians, nurses, and other healthcare providers, are held to a higher standard of care than an ordinary individual would be. Thus, the term used in nursing is the reasonable professional nurse standard.

An individual who undertakes a particular activity is ordinarily considered to have the knowledge common to others who engage in that activity. A motorist must know the rules of the road. A negligent act occurs when one individual damages

the person or property of another without any "intent" to injure. It may be due to carelessness on the part of the individual committing the act. For example, a driver who is talking on a cell phone or otherwise not paying attention and causes an automobile crash by failing to stop at a stop sign may be considered negligent and would be responsible for any damages caused to any person or property.

In a legal action to establish negligence, the injured party needs to prove that the other party had a *duty of reasonable care*, the other party *did not maintain reasonable care*, and the failure to maintain such reasonable care (*caused*) resulted in *injuries* to the aggrieved party. In the example of the automobile crash mentioned above, all drivers have the duty to operate their vehicle safely and follow traffic law. If they fail to do so, and this failure injures any other person or property, they would meet all of the criteria to be held negligent and therefore accountable for paying damages to the injured party.

PROFESSIONAL NEGLIGENCE OR MALPRACTICE   As noted above, the standard of a "reasonable person" is different for individuals in specific professional occupations. If an individual engages in an activity requiring special skills, education, training, or licensure, such as piloting a plane or providing professional nursing care, the standard by which his or her conduct is measured is the conduct of a reasonably skilled, competent, and experienced individual who is a qualified member of the group authorized to engage in that activity (see **Box 49–2** ●). Anyone who performs these special skills, whether qualified or not, is held to the standards of conduct of those properly qualified to do so, because the public relies on the special expertise of those who engage in such activities. Thus, a nursing student is held to the standard of conduct of an experienced, licensed professional nurse.

Malpractice refers to conduct deviating from the standard of practice dictated by the profession. It includes acts and omissions committed by a professional in the course of performing his or her professional duties. Malpractice applies to licensed professionals, including physicians, nurses, and attorneys. Malpractice is one of the most important areas of the law for nurses, as any negligent act or omission, however unintentional, may rise to the standard of malpractice and may jeopardize the professional nurse's license and, more important, client safety.

Box 49-2 Categories and Examples of Negligence That Result in Malpractice

FAILURE TO FOLLOW STANDARDS OF CARE

Failure to:

- Perform a complete admission assessment or design a plan of care.
- Adhere to standardized protocols or institutional policies and procedures (e.g., using an improper injection site).
- Follow a physician's verbal or written orders, if appropriate.

FAILURE TO USE EQUIPMENT IN A RESPONSIBLE MANNER

Failure to:

- Follow the manufacturer's recommendations for operating the equipment.
- Check equipment for safety prior to use.
- Place equipment properly during treatment.

FAILURE TO COMMUNICATE

Failure to:

- Notify a physician in a timely manner when conditions warrant it.
- Listen to a client's complaints and act on them.
- Communicate effectively with a client (e.g., inadequate or ineffective communication of discharge instructions).
- Seek clarification for orders for treatment when necessary.
- Discuss medication errors with team and client.

FAILURE TO DOCUMENT

Failure to note in the client's medical record:

- A client's progress and response to treatment.
- A client's injuries.
- Pertinent nursing assessment information (e.g., drug allergies).
- A physician's medical orders.
- Information on telephone conversations with physicians, including time, content of communication between nurse and physician, and actions taken.

FAILURE TO ASSESS AND MONITOR

Failure to:

- Complete a shift assessment.
- Implement a plan of care.
- Observe a client's ongoing progress.
- Interpret a client's signs and symptoms.

FAILURE TO ACT AS A CLIENT ADVOCATE

Failure to:

- Question discharge orders when a client's condition warrants it.
- Question incomplete or illegible medical orders.
- Provide a safe environment.

Sources: From Anselmi, K. K. (2012). Nurses' personal liability vs. employer's vicarious liability. *MEDSURG Nursing, 21*(1), 45–48; and Tzeng, H.-M., Yin, C. Y., & Schneider, T. E. (2013). Medication error–related issues in nursing practice. *MEDSURG Nursing, 22*(1), 13–16, 50.

Elements of Professional Negligence or Malpractice

Five elements of professional negligence or malpractice are required to establish **liability**, defined as the state of being legally obliged and responsible, on the part of the defendant:

- The client must be owed a **duty**, a legally enforceable obligation to conform to a particular standard of conduct (Guido, 2010, p. 95). The formation of a provider–client relationship is the basis for finding that the healthcare provider owes a duty to the client. A nurse–client relationship begins when the nurse accepts responsibility for providing nursing care to a client (North Carolina Board of Nursing, 2012).

- A deviation from the standard of care owed the client, called a **breach of duty**, must occur by either commission or omission. For example, the nurse has a duty to correctly administer medication to a client. Giving the client the wrong dose of medication would be a breach of duty.

- The element of **foreseeability** (certain events may reasonably be expected to cause specific results) must be present. The nurse should know in advance, or reasonably anticipate, that damage or injury will probably ensue from acts or omissions.

- The injury must have resulted as a direct result of the nurse's or professional's breach of duty, called **causation**. Typically, a client cannot successfully make a claim for malpractice on acquiring a healthcare-associated infection. Only if the client could show that a specific nurse did not follow the standard of aseptic technique would the standard of causation be met.

- The plaintiff must demonstrate that some type of physical, financial, or emotional injury or harm resulted from the breach of owed duty. The nurse could have given the wrong medication but if no harm occurred, the elements are not present for malpractice.

SAFETY ALERT

Nurses administering medications must know why the client is receiving the medication, the dosage range, possible adverse effects, toxicity levels, and contraindications.

The basic purpose of a malpractice lawsuit is to award **damages** sufficient to restore the plaintiff to his or her original position, so far as is financially possible. The amount of the damages, or compensation, for the plaintiff's loss or injury may include enough money to pay for the plaintiff's medical fees associated with the injury. If the plaintiff lost the ability to work as a result of the injury, damages could include compensation for lost wages as well as for medical fees. Punitive damages may be awarded if the misconduct was malicious, willful, or wanton (Guido, 2010).

Related Doctrines Several legal doctrines, or principles, are related to negligence and malpractice. One such doctrine is *respondeat superior.* A lawsuit for a negligent act or omission performed by a nurse generally will also name the nurse's employer. In addition, employers may be held liable for negligence if they fail to provide adequate human and material resources for nursing care, fail to properly educate nurses on the use of new equipment or procedures, or fail to orient nurses to the facility. Another doctrine or principle is *res ipsa loquitur* ("the thing speaks for itself"). In some cases, the harm cannot be traced to a specific healthcare provider or standard but does not normally occur unless there has been some type of negligence. An example is harm that results when surgical instruments or bandages are inadvertently left in a client during surgery.

Statute of Limitations There is a limit to the amount of time that can pass between recognition of harm and the bringing of a suit. This is referred to as the *statute of limitations*. The exact time limitation varies by type of suit and state, but typically plaintiffs have 1–2 years from the time that they knew of the injury or had reason to believe that an injury was sustained to file a malpractice lawsuit. Statutes of limitations applying to minors vary from state to state, with some states identifying specific variances such as extended time limits for specific types of injuries.

Intentional Torts

ASSAULT, BATTERY, AND FALSE IMPRISONMENT

A number of intentional torts, actions taken by an individual with the intent to perform the action, have a bearing on nursing practice. **Assault** is the action of creating an apprehension of offensive, insulting, or physically injurious touching. Assault can occur without actually touching an individual. Threatening a client who refuses to agree with starting an intravenous line is an example of assault. **Battery** can be defined as willful touching of another individual (or the individual's clothes or even something the individual is carrying) that is unwanted, embarrassing, or unwarranted, such as touching done without permission or giving an injection without a client's consent. Even the simple act of ambulation requires the consent of the client. Forcing a client to ambulate against his or her will may be considered battery (Guido, 2010).

Guido (2010, p. 116) defined **false imprisonment** as the "unjustifiable detention of a person without legal warrant to confine the person." False imprisonment includes confining the client to his or her room or restraining the client to the bed with the intent to restrict or prevent the client's freedom. Detaining a client who wishes to leave against medical advice is generally considered false imprisonment.

Because **standards of care** (the skills and learning common to their profession, including the nursing process) prohibit nurses from forcing clients to participate in treatment or engage in any action against their will, assault, battery, and false imprisonment are actions that violate standards of care and may rise to the level of civil or criminal action against the nurse.

INVASION OF PRIVACY

According to the Fourth Amendment of the U.S. Constitution, individuals have the right to privacy. Information concerning clients is confidential and may not be disclosed without authorization. The client's right to privacy extends to use of the client's name as well as photographic or videographic representations of the client (e.g., the client's picture cannot be used without proper authorization). This right extends to control of the client's personal belongings, personal space, and immediate territory. The nurse–client relationship is based on trust. Searching a client's room, touching personal belongings without first requesting permission, and entering a client's room without knocking are behaviors that potentially violate this trust. Most agencies have policies and procedures regarding to whom and under what circumstances client information can be released and appropriate procedures for managing client environments and personal property within the healthcare agency. Failure to follow these policies could lead to a claim of invasion of privacy.

▶ STRATEGIES TO PREVENT INCIDENTS OF PROFESSIONAL NEGLIGENCE

Several situations may arise that can lead to reported negligence or malpractice cases in nursing practice. A continuing issue in nursing is medication errors, which must be clearly documented and discussed with the client (Tzeng, Yin, & Schneider, 2013). Other problematic situations include communicating care concerns and key information about the client's condition; ensuring physicians' orders are clear; understanding how to use equipment in practice; and providing appropriate mentoring, assessment, and care plans for clients (Anselmi, 2012; Lipley, 2012).

Maintaining Client Safety

Clients often fall accidentally, sometimes with resultant injury. Some falls can be prevented by elevating the side rails on the cribs, beds, and stretchers of babies and small children and, when necessary, of adults. If a nurse leaves the rails down or leaves a baby unattended on a bath table, that nurse is liable for malpractice if the client falls and is injured as a direct result. Most hospitals and nursing homes have policies regarding the use of safety devices. The nurse needs to be familiar with these policies and to take indicated precautions to prevent injuries (see the modules on Mobility and Safety).

SAFETY ALERT
Assess every client for fall potential. Document all nursing measures taken to protect the client (e.g., instructed client how to use the call light).

In some instances, ignoring a client's complaints can result in malpractice. This type of malpractice is termed *failure to observe and take appropriate action*. The nurse who does not report a client's complaint of acute abdominal pain is negligent and may be found liable of malpractice if ensuing appendix rupture and death occur. By failing to take the blood pressure and pulse and to check the dressing of a client who has just had abdominal surgery, a nurse omits important assessments. If the client hemorrhages and resulting brain hypoxia renders the client unable to return to his or her former occupation, the nurse may be held liable for injury and loss of wages resulting from the nurse's malpractice.

Incorrect identification of clients is a problem, particularly in busy hospital units. Unfortunate occurrences, such as removal of a healthy gallbladder from the wrong client, have resulted from nurses preparing the wrong client for surgery. Cases of mistaken identity are costly and possibly very painful for the client and render the nurse liable for malpractice.

SAFETY ALERT
One of the first steps in all nursing procedures is the proper identification of the client. Follow agency policy for approved identification of clients.

Minimizing the Risk of Medication Errors

Administration of medications has been identified as a high-risk activity for error. Prevention of medication errors requires a systems approach involving all interdisciplinary healthcare personnel. Nurses need to strictly apply the **Six Rights** of medication administration

1. Right drug
2. Right dose
3. Right client
4. Right route
5. Right time
6. Right documentation.

Strategies that integrate new technology, such as bar coding and electronic records, need to be evaluated for effectiveness in reducing errors. Increased inclusion of client and family participation in the medication administration process can ensure understanding of the medications including proper home administration and identification of potential side effects.

Nothing can replace nursing judgment in preventing errors in administering medications. Unclear orders need to be clarified. Questions need to be answered. The nurse needs to have knowledge of each medication prior to administration. A culture of safety instead of blame will facilitate identification of errors and evaluation of causes and strategies to reduce errors.

Using Effective Communication

Nurses interact with clients and families in the provision of care. Poor communication skills may create the perception in the client that the nurse may be less than competent. Poor communication coupled with a negative outcome can increase the chance of a malpractice claim. Clear communication of directions and explanations and provision of effective client education regarding the client's healthcare requirements can help decrease the risk of bad outcomes (see the module on Teaching and Learning). Attentive listening skills demonstrate the element of caring. Accurate documentation and reporting (see the module on Communication) provide a source for information that will either support or defend allegations of malpractice. Nursing documentation should be completed according to policy and should clearly depict the timeline of care including assessments, interventions, client's response to interventions, and notification of information outside treatment protocol (e.g., abnormal lab values, changes in client assessment). Remember that this document will serve as the legal record of what occurred, so the nurse should document defensively to be inclusive and not rely on the memory of the client or details of care.

Professional Liability Insurance

Nurses, like physicians, should carry professional liability insurance to manage personal financial risk. Professional liability policies have comment elements. Occurrence-based coverage covers incidents that occurred during the time period the policy was in effect, regardless of whether the policy was still in effect when the claim was made. Claims-made policies provide coverage only if the incident occurred and the claim is reported during the active policy period.

Policies may be individual, group, or employer sponsored. Individual coverage provides the broadest coverage specific to the policy holder. This type of policy covers the named policyholder on a 24-hour basis as long as his or her actions fall within the scope of practice. Employer-sponsored coverage provides the narrowest coverage for the individual nurse, because the policy covers actions performed only while working as an institution employee. Nursing students are generally required to carry liability insurance for the duration of the education program, although some programs insure students under a broad institutional policy. Policies should identify limits of liability, declarations, deductibles, exclusions, reservation of rights, covered injuries, defense costs, coverage conditions, and supplementary payments.

▶ THE STANDARD OF CARE

The applicable nurse practice act and administrative rules form the basis of the standard of care to which nurses are held. They define professional conduct and the scope of practice for the licensed nurse and identify activities for all levels of personnel providing nursing care. These laws are not static and every nurse needs to be aware of any changes.

The nurse's specific job description will contribute to defining the standard of care. Employers can limit but not expand the scope of practice and the nurse will be held to functioning within the scope of employment.

Although agency policies and procedures may seem to contain overwhelming amounts of information, they serve to define the standard of care. The prudent nurse will review and implement the policies and procedures relevant to her or his practice. If there is a conflict between current practice and policy, the nurse should be proactive in resolving the conflict through quality improvement processes.

A primary source for defining the standard of care is the prevailing national nursing standards. These include the American Nurses Association (ANA) Standards of Practice as well as specialty practice standards appropriate to a nurse's practice (e.g., standards for critical care nurses). Nurses who follow national standards of practice and standards of care will provide their clients with the best care possible and be far less likely to commit any unintentional act that may rise to the level of malpractice.

The Nursing Process and Professional Practice

In nursing education programs, students are taught how to apply the nursing process to client and family care. A competent nurse will first provide the correct level of assessment by collecting comprehensive data surrounding the client's health and life situation (Jarrin, 2010; Ofi & Sowunmi, 2012). The second step in the nursing process is to analyze the assessment data so appropriate diagnoses can be chosen for the client. During the third step, the nurse plans the care of the client and identifies expected outcomes that will be individualized to the client. With the care plan ready, implementation (the fourth step) begins, and includes coordination and provisions of care, client teaching, and other topics, as appropriate for the client. The fifth step in the nursing process is evaluation of the client's progress toward the identified outcomes (Jarrin, 2010). At each of these steps, clear and appropriate documentation is required (Ofi & Sowunmi, 2012).

In addition to the steps of the nursing process, nurses are expected to demonstrate competence within multiple areas of their professional role. These areas include ensuring quality of practice, attaining and maintaining current knowledge and education, evaluating one's own practice, working collegially with peers and colleagues, and collaborating with the entire care team. Finally, ethical practice that integrates research findings, appropriate use of resources, and accepting leadership within practice are vital competencies for nurses (Douglas et al., 2011; Hayrinen, Lammintakanen, & Saranto, 2010).

Overview of Concept Relationships

Legal concerns in client care involve more than following correct protocols in nursing practice or facing safety issues that may affect clients. Legal concerns are related to all of the concepts and systems. See the Concepts Related to Legal Issues feature for selected examples.

▶ SELECTED LAWS THAT AFFECT NURSING PRACTICE

In addition to tort laws, a number of other laws affect nursing practice. These include laws related to informed consent and competency, as well as laws regarding the Controlled Substance Act and the Good Samaritan Act. Because states have the freedom to enact additional legislation that may further define or restrict aspects addressed by federal law, all nurses should be aware of the laws that govern or affect nursing practice in their own states.

Informed Consent

Informed consent refers to the client's legal and ethical rights to be informed of and give permission for any healthcare procedure or treatment. The physician or independent healthcare provider has the duty to disclose information regarding treatment in terms the client can reasonably understand. In addition to describing the proposed treatment, the healthcare provider must disclose information regarding available alternatives, the risks and benefits of each treatment option, and the client's right to refuse treatment.

General guidelines regarding the information that should be provided to the client include the following:

- The diagnosis or condition that requires treatment
- The purposes of the treatment
- What the client can expect to feel or experience
- The intended benefits of the treatment
- Possible risks or negative outcomes of the treatment
- Advantages and disadvantages of possible alternatives to treatment (including no treatment).

To give informed consent voluntarily, the client must not be coerced in any manner. For example, if the client is motivated to consent due to fear of disapproval by a healthcare provider, such consent is not considered to be voluntary. Coercion of any kind invalidates the consent.

Client understanding is an essential element of informed consent. Technical words and language barriers can inhibit understanding and, when a client has a lower literacy level, may encourage a signature without discussion of its actual meaning. Therefore, cultural competence in managing client care is critical (Douglas et al., 2011). If a client cannot read, the healthcare provider must read the consent form to the client, and the client must state an understanding before signing the form. If the client and the healthcare provider do not speak the same language, a medical interpreter must be present. However, even with an interpreter, it is important to remember that errors in translation may occur.

The nurse should consider the client's cultural and spiritual preferences when asking a client to make decisions about a procedure or treatment (Douglas et al., 2011). The Focus on Diversity and Culture feature discusses how culture may affect a client's attitude toward autonomy and the proper role of significant others in decision making.

The nurse should follow the employing agency's specific protocols regarding informed consent. Obtaining informed consent for specific medical and surgical treatments is the responsibility of the individual who will perform the procedure. Consent must be obtained for all procedures and treatments, including nursing care. However, this does not require written consent before each occurrence. Most nurses rely on **expressed consent** (an oral or written agreement) or **implied consent** based on a client's action. The client either verbally indicates participation in the care or nonverbally takes actions that are consistent with the care. For example, clients who position their bodies for an injection or cooperate with the taking of vital signs are expressing implied consent.

COMPETENCY FOR CONSENT **Competency** is a legal presumption applied to individuals when they become adults. Competency gives adults the right to negotiate certain legal activities, such as making a will or entering into a contract. In

---

Focus on Diversity and Culture
Autonomy

Informed consent in the United States is based on the principle of autonomy—that is, each individual has the right to make his or her own decisions regarding treatment, provided that he or she is conscious or competent to do so. In contrast to this individual perspective, people from other cultures (e.g., Southeast Asians and Native Americans) may have a different perspective on decision making, in which the group has a legitimate role. These clients may believe that another member of their family or group or tribe should make the decision. Although legally the client is the only individual who has the authority to give consent, the nurse can provide culturally competent care by asking the client whether he or she would like to have a family member or spiritual leader present during discussions regarding healthcare treatment.

Concepts Related to **Legal Issues**

Legal care requires, among other things, nursing management of the client's right to appropriate end-of-life (EOL) care, the right to self-determination with advance directives (ADs), privacy of the client's care and client information, and prevention of care errors. The literature reports that, although the difficult task of beginning and maintaining the EOL discussion spans multiple healthcare disciplines, this is often identified as the nurse's role, for which he should use clear communication skills (Clabots, 2012). Research also notes that clients and family members are affected by the lack of discussion regarding EOL and ADs (Cohen & Nirenberg, 2011). All hospitals receiving Medicare and Medicaid funds are legally responsible to provide AD information and support clients' AD planning needs. Maintaining the privacy of the client's information surrounding these care decisions, as well as other medical or private information, is vital. The right to privacy and self-determination has been discussed in nursing (Nys, 2012). Clients' right to privacy surrounding their care and client self-determination are concepts that nurses can uphold as client advocates (Johnstone, 2011; Lachman, 2012). Regarding safety, a systematic review of eight studies found that "adverse events during hospital stays affect nearly 1 of 10 patients, and 15% of errors were medication errors" (Tzeng et al., 2013, p. 15). In addition, evidence-based practice studies have explored prevention of common errors such as inpatient falls (Graham, 2012) and catheter-related bloodstream infections (DeLa Cruz, Caillouet, & Guerrero, 2012).

CONCEPT	RELATIONSHIP TO LEGAL ISSUES	NURSING IMPLICATIONS
Comfort		
■ End-of-life care	Clients have the legal right to receive appropriate EOL care. All hospitals receiving Medicare and Medicaid funds are legally responsible to provide AD information and support clients' AD needs.	■ Assess own assumptions or biases surrounding EOL care. ■ Assess self-understanding of appropriate EOL care options in your practice area. ■ Ask for support from supervisor or peers to assist in advocating for appropriate EOL care. ■ Anticipate further assessment of information clients and family members may need.
Safety		
■ Care errors	Clients have the legal right to receive safe care and to be protected from adverse care events.	■ Follow all protocols and guidelines for medication administration, wound care, surgical care, and other client care. ■ Understand how to report possible or actual adverse events. ■ Assist your supervisor in helping staff members learn from adverse events to prevent future errors.
Communication		
■ Documentation ■ Reporting	Nurses must ensure the privacy of all client information during all care and in all care areas, and must follow HIPAA regulations.	■ Ensure that client information, such as online charting, is only accessible for appropriate use by appropriate staff members. ■ Discuss with your clients how you ensure privacy. ■ Ensure that client care is discussed only with appropriate individuals and not outside of the care unit.
Advocacy		
■ Client education ■ Client empowerment	The nurse ensures that the individual receives sufficient information about advance directives on which to base their current or future care decisions. The nurse provides an environment that allows the client and family members to make their own AD decisions.	■ Ensure that AD options are clearly discussed with the client and family members. ■ Discuss the client's choices with the client and allow self-determination.

most states, an individual is considered to be competent at 18 years of age unless some evidence to the contrary persuades a court to declare that individual incompetent.

Adults who have been declared legally incompetent through a court order are provided a legal guardian. The legal guardian will know to provide a copy of the court order giving him or her the authority to make healthcare decisions on the other adult's behalf. Examples of adults who may be legally incompetent include those who have suffered a debilitating brain injury as a result of a motor vehicle crash and those who have profound intellectual disability.

An adult may be rendered temporarily incompetent by narcotic medication or a serious fall, or an adult may gradually be rendered incompetent as a result of dementia. The nurse who has concerns about a client's level of competency should alert the primary care provider. If the primary care provider determines that the client is not competent for the purposes of informed consent, he or she will determine whether the emergency doctrine applies (see the Consent in an Emergency section below) or whether someone else can validly make healthcare decisions on the client's behalf. State laws regarding consent for adults who are rendered temporarily incompetent vary. Courts generally presume continuing competency of adults unless the healthcare facility can show that the client is unable to understand the consequences of his or her actions (Guido, 2010). All healthcare staff, including nurses, should be familiar with their state's laws and with the policies and procedures of their employing agency. Nurses should recognize the effect of issues related to competency on providing nursing care, because clients have the right to decline nursing care as well as medical procedures.

CONSENT IN AN EMERGENCY

In most states, the law assumes an individual's consent to medical treatment when the individual is in imminent danger of loss of life or limb and unable to give informed consent. In other words, the emergency doctrine assumes that the individual would reasonably consent to treatment if able to do so. This doctrine serves as a guiding principle that permits healthcare providers to perform potentially life-saving procedures under circumstances that make it is impossible or impractical to obtain consent. The emergency doctrine may not always apply. For example, it does not extend to allowing healthcare providers to implement a treatment or procedure to which the client would not reasonably consent if the client were able to do so. It also does not permit healthcare providers to provide a treatment or procedure that the client previously refused. For example, if a client has previously refused a procedure on religious grounds, healthcare providers may not implement the procedure if the client becomes unconscious. While state laws provide for protection from liability for failure to obtain informed consent, nurses need to understand implied versus obtained consent (Cole, 2012).

CHILD PARTICIPATION IN HEALTHCARE DECISIONS

For a minor child (under age 18), a parent or guardian must give informed consent for medical treatment. Specific legal exceptions do exist, however, including situations in which the emergency doctrine applies, the child is an *emancipated*

minor (one who is no longer under parental control and manages his or her own financial affairs), the child is a resident of a state that allows a *mature minor* to give valid consent (for example, 14- and 15-year-old adolescents who are able to understand treatment risks), a court order to proceed with treatment exists, or the law recognizes the minor as having the ability to consent to a specific treatment. In the majority of states, a minor who is the parent of a child may give informed consent for healthcare treatment of the child. Some states also permit teenagers of a certain age who are seeking certain types of care to do so without parental consent. Types of care that may not require parental permission include contraceptive services, prenatal care, mental health counseling, diagnosis and treatment of sexually transmitted infections, and treatment of substance abuse (Birchley, 2010; Goodwin et al., 2012).

Mature minors are permitted in some states to give consent for treatment or to refuse treatment. In some cases, the minor must convince a judge that he or she is mature enough to make an independent judgment about consent for treatment. Nurses need to know the state and federal laws regarding consent as well as the agency's policies and procedures regarding informed consent (Birchley, 2010). North Carolina law, for example, provides for all minors over the age of 12 to consent for contraceptive services, treatment of sexually transmitted infections, and prenatal care. For an overview of minor consent laws in the United States, see **Box 49–3** ●.

CASE STUDY \\ A

Marvin Martinice, a 15-year-old boy with acute myelocytic leukemia, has come out of his second remission with an acute onset of fever, joint pain, and petechiae. A bone marrow transplant is one of the few remaining therapeutic options. Although Marvin has agreed to a transplant if a suitable donor is found, he does not want to be resuscitated and placed on life-support equipment should he have a cardiac arrest. He has talked extensively with the hospital chaplain and social worker and feels comfortable with his decision. His parents want an all-out effort to sustain his life until a donor is located.

Clinical Thinking Questions

1. At what age can a child make an informed decision about whether to accept or refuse treatment?
2. What happens when parents and children have conflicting opinions about treatment?

Controlled Substances Act

The **Controlled Substances Act (CSA)** is a federal law that requires drugs to be classified based on the substance's medical use, potential for abuse, and safety risks. The classifications are referred to as Schedules and are numbered from I to V, with Schedules I and II having the highest potential for abuse (**Table 49–2** ●). The CSA is enforced by the U.S. Drug Enforcement Agency, which regulates a closed system of distribution.

Box 49–3 Overview of Minor Consent Laws

CONTRACEPTIVE SERVICES

Twenty-six states and the District of Columbia allow all minors (age 12 years and older) to consent to contraceptive services. Twenty-one states allow only certain categories of minors to consent to contraceptive services.

SEXUALLY TRANSMITTED INFECTIONS SERVICES

All states and the District of Columbia allow all minors to consent to services for sexually transmitted infections.

PRENATAL CARE

Thirty-two states and the District of Columbia explicitly allow all minors to consent to prenatal care.

ADOPTION

Twenty-eight states and the District of Columbia allow all minor parents to choose to place their child for adoption.

MEDICAL CARE FOR A CHILD

Thirty states and the District of Columbia allow all minor parents to consent to medical care for their child. The remaining 20 states have no relevant explicit policy or case law.

ABORTION

Three states and the District of Columbia explicitly allow all minors to consent to abortion services. Twenty-two states require that at least one parent consent to a minor's request for an abortion, while 11 states require prior notification of at least one parent. State laws regarding abortion may change; be sure to know the laws in your state.

Source: Adapted from Guttmacher Institute. (2010). *An overview of minors' consent law.* Retrieved from http://www.guttmacher.org/statecenter/spibs/spib_OMCL.pdf.

This system provides for registration with unique identifiers for legitimate handlers of controlled substances and required record keeping that traces the flow of any drug from the time it is first imported or manufactured, through the distribution level, to the pharmacy or hospital that dispenses it, and then to the actual client who receives it.

Good Samaritan Laws

Most states have **Good Samaritan laws** that encourage healthcare providers to help victims in an emergency. These laws are designed to protect the healthcare worker from potential liability when volunteering his or her skills outside of an employment contract. Nurses should review the nurse practice act and the Good Samaritan law in the state in which they work before volunteering their skills. To be protected by Good Samaritan laws, a nurse must adhere to the standard of nursing care during all volunteer activities. The nurse should provide only care that is consistent with his or her level of training and licensure. Once the decision to render emergency care has been made, the nurse is responsible for following through by providing the necessary care or safely placing the victim in the care of someone who can provide the appropriate care (Time, Payne, & Gainey, 2010).

▶ CONCLUSION

From medication administration to licensure requirements, the number of laws that affect nurses can be overwhelming. Nurses must rely on continuing education, workplace policies and procedures, state regulatory agencies, and professional organizations for information regarding changes in laws and requirements. Failure to keep up with changes in laws and regulations can endanger the client and place the nurse at risk for liability.

Box 49–4 ● provides links to organizations and Web sites that can provide more information on the various laws and regulations that impact nurses.

TABLE 49–2 U.S. Drug Schedules and Examples

DRUG SCHEDULE	DEPENDENCY POTENTIAL			EXAMPLES	THERAPEUTIC USE
	ABUSE POTENTIAL	PHYSICAL DEPENDENCE	PSYCHOLOGICAL DEPENDENCE		
I	Highest	High	High	Heroin, lysergic acid diethylamide (LSD), marijuana, and methaqualone	Limited or no therapeutic use
II	High	High	High	Morphine, phencyclidine (PCP), cocaine, methadone, and methamphetamine	Used therapeutically with prescription; some drugs no longer used
III	Moderate	Moderate	High	Anabolic steroids, codeine and hydrocodone with aspirin or Tylenol, and some barbiturates	Used therapeutically with prescription
IV	Lower	Lower	Lower	Dextropropoxyphene, pentazocine, meprobamate, diazepam, alprazolam	Used therapeutically with prescription
V	Lowest	Lowest	Lowest	OTC cough medicines with codeine	Used therapeutically without prescription

Box 49–4 Where to Go for Additional Information

REGULATION/ORGANIZATIONS (WITH RESEARCH LINKS)

National Council of State Boards of Nursing (NCSBN)
www.ncsbn.org

State Boards of Nursing (contact information)
https://www.ncsbn.org/boards.htm

National Student Nurses' Association
www.nsna.org

National Practitioner Data Bank
www.npdb-hipdb.hrsa.gov

ADVANCE DIRECTIVES

Partnership for Caring
1620 Eye St. NW, Suite 202
Washington, DC 20007
1-800-658-8898
www.partnershipforcaring.org

Health in Aging Organization
www.nia.nih.gov

CONTROLLED SUBSTANCES ACT
www.deadiversion.usdoj.gov/21cfr/21usc

WHISTLEBLOWING
osha.gov/dep/oia/whistleblower

CREDENTIALING
http://www.nursecredentialing.org/Certification.aspx

REVIEW **The Concept of Legal Issues**

RELATE Link the Concepts

Linking the concept of legal issues with the concept of clinical decision making:

1. How does the nursing process support nurses in maintaining appropriate standards of care?

2. What type of consent is necessary for the nurse to take a client's temperature and vital signs? For the client to undergo an x-ray if a broken leg is suspected?

Linking the concept of legal issues with the concept of communication:

3. How does a change-of-shift report minimize the nurse's risk for professional negligence or malpractice?

4. What types of communication result in the best quality of client care and are therefore most likely to prevent the nurse from being accused of malpractice?

REFER Go to Pearson Nursing Student Resources
nursing.pearsonhighered.com

• Additional review materials

REFLECT Case Study

Joanne Otunde, an RN coworker on your surgical unit, returned to work about 6 weeks ago following back surgery. Since her return, you have noticed that she is frequently and uncharacteristically late for work and has called in sick six times. Twice you have witnessed her "biting the head off" a nurse's aide. Mrs. Glancy, a client who is 2 days postoperative, puts her light on and tells you that she is in severe pain and that the pain medication she received did not have any effect on the pain level. She states, "It's the strangest thing. The pill never seems to work in the evenings like it does in the daytime and at night." You report Mrs. Glancy's pain to Joanne, who is her primary nurse. At the end of the shift, you and an oncoming nurse are doing the narcotic count and notice that Joanne has given six doses of the same narcotic during the shift and one dose is documented as having been given at 8 p.m. to a client who had been discharged at 5 p.m.

1. What are your responsibilities? Should you take any action? If so, why? If not, why not?

2. What laws do you need to review? What policies?

EXEMPLAR 49.1 **Nurse Practice Acts**

EXEMPLAR KEY TERMS
Certification, *2666*
Credentialing, *2666*
Mutual recognition model, *2665*
Nolo contendere, *2664*
Nurse practice act (NPA), *2663*
Responsibility, *2666*

EXEMPLAR LEARNING OUTCOMES
After reading about this exemplar, you will be able to:

1. Discuss the role and responsibilities of state boards of nursing and the National Council of State Boards of Nursing.

2. Summarize key aspects of licensure and credentialing.

3. Describe how the Nurse Licensure Compact benefits nurses.

4. Illustrate performance guidelines for nursing students.

▶ OVERVIEW

The practice of nursing is regulated at the state level through a **nurse practice act (NPA)**. An NPA is a series of state statutes that define the scope of practice, standards for education programs, licensure requirements, and grounds for disciplinary actions. The law provides a framework for establishing nursing actions in the care of clients (**Box 49–5 ●**). Laws set

the boundaries for and maintain a standard of nursing practice (**Figure 49–2 ●**). For the registered nurse (RN), the provisions of the NPAs are quite similar from state to state. Greater variation exists in the scope of practice for the licensed practical nurse (LPN) or licensed vocation nurse (LVN). The nurse is held accountable to the specific standards for licensure and grounds for revocation in the state of employment.

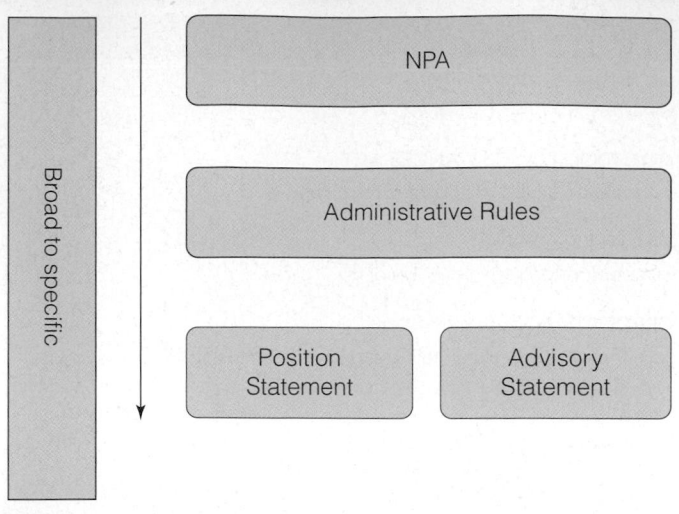

Figure 49–2 ● Relationship among nurse practice acts, administrative rules, and position/advisory statements.

Each state's NPA is enforced and administered by a state board of nursing (BON), though some states use other titles for this regulatory board. BONs were established some 100 years ago to standardize the education of nurses, establish standards for safe nursing practice, and issue licenses in order to protect the public from unprepared, unsafe practitioners. BONs have since expanded their functions to include activities such as programs for impaired nurses, remediation of practice issues, and participation in multi-state licensure compacts. To achieve their mission of protecting the public health, BONs also serve as a forum for citizen complaints about nursing services and against individual nurses.

The members of the BON are appointed according to the regulations in each state with the exception of North Carolina. North Carolina is the only state where licensed nurses serving on the board are elected by other licensed nurses, and members of the public who serve are appointed. The state's NPA dictates the membership of the state's BON, which usually includes a mix of RNs, LPNs/LVNs, advanced practice registered nurses (APRNs), and consumers.

▶ LICENSURE

Licensure allows a nurse the legal privilege to practice nursing as defined in each state's NPA. Through the process of licensure, the BON ensures minimum standards of competency to provide safe nursing care to the public. Typically, BONs oversee licensure through the following activities:

- Establishing and monitoring educational standards for nursing education programs

Box 49–5 Anatomy of a Nurse Practice Act

Typically, the following components are addressed in an NPA. Each nursing student and practicing nurse should understand the NPA for the state in which she or he working and how each component of the NPA affects practice. Components of an NPA include the following:

- Definition of nursing
- Requirements for licensure
- Penalty for practicing without a license
- Exemptions from licensure
- Licensure across jurisdictions.

- Defining professional standards
- Examining and renewing the licenses of duly qualified applicants
- Investigating violations of the NPA
- Sanctioning (to the point of initiating prosecution against) those who violate the NPA
- Holding disciplinary hearings for possible suspension or revocation of a license
- Establishing and overseeing diversity programs in some states.

Each BON oversees the administration of a licensure examination that measures the competencies needed to perform safely and effectively as a newly licensed, entry-level nurse. The National Council of State Boards of Nursing (2010) has developed two licensure examinations, the National Council Licensure Examination for Registered Nurses (NCLEX-RN®) and the National Council Licensure Examination for Practical Nurses (NCLEX-PN®), for state and territory BONs to implement as part of their requirements for licensure.

Licenses are issued by the state or territory in which the applicant nurse wishes to practice. For licensed nurses at all levels of practice, the BON monitors compliance with state laws, including maintaining continuing competency and annual renewal of licensure. To maintain the privilege to practice afforded by the license, the individual nurse is required to demonstrate awareness and application of standards of nursing care and meet his or her responsibilities to both clients and the healthcare system. The board is also responsible for taking action against nurses who have exhibited unsafe nursing practice or otherwise engaged in professional misconduct or who fail meet requirements for licensure renewal.

Each BON details what charges of professional misconduct may result in the revocation or suspension of a nurse's license. Typically, most BONs will take action against the nurse who is found guilty of charges that include the following:

- Giving false information or withholding material information from the board in procuring or attempting to procure a license to practice nursing.
- Being convicted of or pleading either guilty or *nolo contendere* to any crime that indicates the nurse is unfit or incompetent to practice or has deceived or defrauded the public. If a defendant pleads **nolo contendere**, the individual neither admits nor denies that he or she has committed the crime but agrees to a punishment (usually a fine or jail time) as if guilty. Usually, this type of plea is entered because it cannot be used as an admission of guilt if a civil lawsuit is initiated following the conclusion of a criminal trial.
- Engaging in conduct that endangers the public health.
- Being unfit or incompetent to practice by reason of deliberate or negligent acts or omissions, regardless of whether actual injury to the client is established.
- Engaging in conduct that deceives, defrauds, or harms the public in the course of professional activities or services.

A 2012 report by the NCSBN states that for the calendar year 2012, 2,535 nurses were placed on probation, 1,408 nurses had licenses revoked, and 2,519 licenses were suspended. The

Box 49–6 The NCSBN's 2013 Research Priorities

CLIENT SAFETY

■ NCSBN's Taxonomy of Error, Root Cause Analysis and Practice-Responsibility (TERCAP®) project.

PRACTICE ROLE CLARITY, CHALLENGES (LPN/VN, RN, AND APRN)

■ Investigating the practice of a wide range of personnel, from medication aides to the advanced practice nurse.

■ Regulatory model for transition to practice for new graduate nurses.

INNOVATIONS IN NURSING EDUCATION AND CLINICAL

■ Use of simulation in nursing education.

CONTINUED COMPETENCE OF REGISTERED NURSES PRACTICING BEYOND 5 YEARS

■ Regulatory model for continued competence.

EFFECTIVE DISCIPLINE AND ALTERNATIVES TO DISCIPLINE

■ Deterring misconduct, affirming professional standards and norms of reasonable conduct, and encouraging rehabilitation or remediation.

■ Evaluating the effectiveness of alternative programs.

MODELS FOR STATE-BASED NURSING REGULATION TO SUPPORT NATIONAL AND INTERNATIONAL PORTABILITY AND DATA CONSISTENCY

■ Workforce development and benchmarking. A portion of this research agenda is devoted to projects that are ongoing and provide information and data for member board use. These projects include member board profiles, workforce data collection, commitment to ongoing regulatory excellence, licensure statistics, NCLEX® candidate projections, and the Practice and Professional Issues surveys.

Source: National Council of State Boards of Nursing (NCSBN). (2013). *Current research agenda.* Retrieved from https://www.ncsbn.org/2635.htm.

violations cited in the report range from drug-related events (i.e., drug abuse, drug diversion [self], other drug related, alcohol abuse, drug use only, drug-related conviction, writing illegal prescriptions, presenting illegal prescriptions, wastage errors, and drug diversion) to criminal actions to violations related to medication administration.

▶ NATIONAL COUNCIL OF STATE BOARDS OF NURSING

The NCSBN provides leadership to advance regulatory excellence for public protection. The membership of the NCSBN includes BONs in the 50 states, the District of Columbia, and four U.S. territories (Guam, Virgin Islands, American Samoa, and the Northern Mariana Islands). Four states have separate BONs for RNs and LPNs/LVNs (California, Georgia, Louisiana, and West Virginia).

The NCSBN provides support services to the member BONs and serves as a central repository of data. Perhaps the most familiar activity of the NCSBN is the development of the initial competency licensure examinations for nurses (NCLEX-RN® and NCLEX-PN®). Other examinations developed by the NCSBN include the National Nurse Aide Assessment Program and the Medication Aide Certification Examination.

The NCSBN also conducts research on nursing practice issues and provides online continuing education opportunities through the e-learning community (**Box 49–6 ●**). It maintains the Nursys® database, which coordinates national publicly available nurse licensure information, and it works with state boards to promote uniformity in the regulation of the practice of nursing. An outcome of these activities is the Nurse Licensure Compact.

▶ NURSE LICENSURE COMPACT

The **mutual recognition model** of nurse licensure allows a nurse to have a single license that confers the privilege to practice in other states that are part of the Nurse Licensure Compact

(**Box 49–7 ●**). The nurse is held accountable for following the laws and rules of the state in which the nurse practices or where the client is located. Monitoring the nurse's license and taking any needed disciplinary actions are the responsibilities of the state that issues the license. It is similar to the driver's license model: A single license to drive is issued in the state of primary residency, but this license also allows the privilege to drive in other compact states.

To achieve mutual recognition, each state must enact legislation or regulations authorizing the Nurse Licensure Compact. States entering the compact also adopt administrative rules and regulations for implementation of the compact. Approximately half the states have entered the compact.

Box 49–7 Mutual Recognition Model

■ Each state has to enter into an interstate compact, called the Nurse Licensure Compact (NLC), that allows nurses to practice in more than one state.

■ Multistate licensure privilege means the authority to practice nursing in another state that has signed an interstate compact. It is not an additional license.

■ A nurse must have a license in his or her primary state of legal residency if that state is an NLC state.

■ The states continue to have authority in determining licensure requirements and disciplinary actions.

■ The nurse is held accountable for knowing and practicing the nursing practice laws and regulations in the state where the client is located.

■ Enactment does not change a state's nurse practice act.

■ Complaints and/or violations are addressed by the home state (place of residence) and the remote state (place of practice).

■ RNs and LPNs/LVNs are included in the interstate compact or NLC. Since 2002, there has been a separate APRN Compact. A state must be a member of the NLC for RNs and LPNs before entering into an APRN Compact. A state must adopt both compacts to cover LPNs/RNs and APRNs for mutual recognition.

Source: National Council of State Boards of Nursing (NCSBN). (2011). *Nurse licensure compact.* Retrieved from https://www.ncsbn.org/2011_NLCA_factsheet_students_Rev_Jan_2011.pdf.

⬛ *Stay Current:* *For information on states participating in the compact, go to* **https://www.ncsbn.org/nlc.htm**.

▶ CREDENTIALING

Although a nursing license grants the legal privilege to practice, **credentialing** is the formal identification of professionals who meet predetermined standards of professional skill or competence. The federal government has used the term **certification** to define the credentialing process by which a nongovernmental agency or association recognizes the professional competence of an individual who has met certain predetermined qualifications specified by the agency or association. The American Nurses Credentialing Center (ANCC), a subsidiary of the ANA, provides credentialing programs to certify nurses in specialty practice areas, recognizes healthcare organizations for nursing excellence through the Magnet Recognition Program®, and accredits providers of continuing nursing education and nursing specialty organizations.

Federal organizations, such as the Joint Commission and the Centers for Medicare and Medicaid Services, and federal guidelines affect the standards of care the nurse is held accountable for practicing. Individual healthcare agencies must implement policies, procedures, and job descriptions to ensure that the nurses they employ follow all applicable regulations and guidelines. The nurse needs to know the employing institution's policies and procedures and the specific job descriptions of the licensed and unlicensed nursing personnel. The purpose of knowing the standards of care is to protect both the client and the nurse.

The impact of laws and standards on nurses is profound (**Figure 49–3 ●**). The professional nurse is held accountable for many standards and statutes. Knowledge of the laws that regulate and affect nursing practice enables the nurse to practice within current legal principles and be aware of his or her legal obligations and responsibilities.

▶ NURSING STUDENTS

Each NPA addresses the duties and responsibilities of nursing students in that state. Typically, this includes language that allows nursing students the privilege to practice nursing without a license while engaged in the clinical practicum of an approved nursing education program under the supervision of qualified faculty. Nursing students have the ultimate **responsibility** (accountability for their actions that includes the obligation to answer for an act done and to repair any injury one may have caused) for their own actions. Guidelines for clinical performance for nursing students include the following (Fero et al., 2010):

1. Ensure client safety.
2. Know your facility's policies and procedures before undertaking any clinical assignment.
3. Ensure you are knowledgeable about the client's condition, interventions, medications, and treatments.
4. Never perform care for which you are unprepared; if you are unprepared for a clinical assignment, inform your instructor.
5. Seek help before beginning a procedure about which you are unsure; if the instructor is not readily available, allow the staff nurse to perform the intervention.

Nursing students are held accountable to the same standard of care as licensed nurses. Nursing faculty members are held accountable for appropriate assignment and supervision of students.

> **SAFETY ALERT**
> Students do not practice on a faculty member's license. The only individual who can legally practice on a license is the individual whose name appears on the license.

▶ STANDARDS OF PRACTICE

Nursing, as a profession, has a responsibility to self-regulate by defining the practice of nursing, researching and developing the practice, establishing standards of practice, and providing for the education and credentialing of nurses. The ANA, the largest professional nursing organization, has established Standards of Clinical Nursing Practice. These address both standards for nursing care and standards for professional performance. Standards of practice are also available for various nursing specialties, including pediatric nursing, nurse anesthesia practice, critical care nursing, and psychiatric nursing.

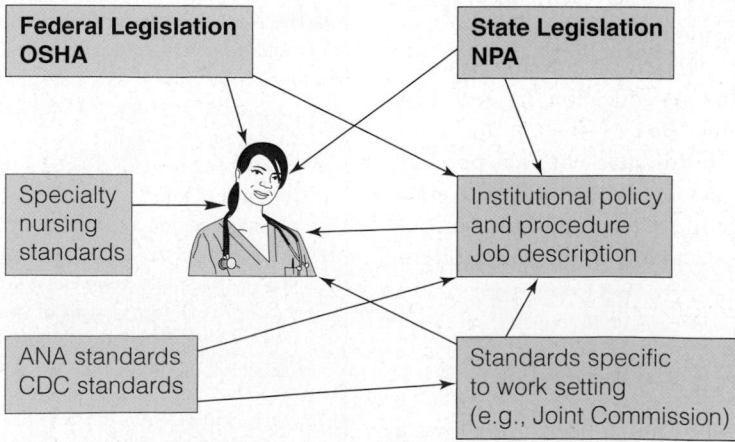

Figure 49–3 ● Impact of laws and standards on nurses.

REVIEW Nurse Practice Acts

RELATE Link the Concepts and Exemplars

Linking the exemplar of nurse practice acts with the concept of addiction:

1. What resources does your state's board of nursing offer for nurses struggling with substance abuse?

2. What would you do if you realized a nurse you were working with was under the influence of drugs or alcohol? Explain.

Linking the exemplar of nurse practice acts with the concept of accountability:

3. What does your state's Nurse Practice Act say about the accountability of nursing students? How is that different than what the NPA says about the accountability of registered nurses?

4. How does your state's board of nursing support or assist nurses in their professional development?

REFER Go to Pearson Nursing Student Resources
nursing.pearsonhighered.com

- Additional review materials

REFLECT Case Study

Sarah Coulton is a registered nurse who works with you in a primary care clinic. Her husband has been notified that his employer is transferring him to another state, and Sarah and her family will be moving in a couple of months.

1. Where will Sarah be able to find information on which states have mutual recognition with your state?

2. What steps might Sarah need to take if she learns that she is moving to a state that is not part of the Nurse Licensure Compact?

EXEMPLAR 49.2   Advance Directives

EXEMPLAR KEY TERMS
Durable power of attorney for health care, *2667*
Healthcare advance directive, *2667*
Living will, *2667*
Patient Self-Determination Act, *2667*

EXEMPLAR LEARNING OUTCOMES
After reading about this exemplar, you will be able to:

1. Summarize the types of advance directives and their general purposes.
2. Analyze elements of advance directives.
3. Integrate advance directives into the plan of care.

▶ OVERVIEW

A **healthcare advance directive** is a legal document executed by an individual that expresses that individual's desires regarding medical treatment that may be used once the individual is no longer able to communicate his or her preferences directly (Ryan & Jezewski, 2012). The client's right to use advance directives is guaranteed in the Patient Self-Determination Act. The **Patient Self Determination Act** is a federal law requiring healthcare institutions that receive federal funding (but not individual healthcare providers) to do the following:

1. At the time of admission, give clients a written summary of:
   - Healthcare decision-making rights. (Each state has developed such a summary for hospitals, nursing homes, and home health agencies to use.)
   - The facility's policies with respect to recognizing advance directives.
2. Ask clients whether they have an advance directive, and document the directive's existence in the medical record. (It is up to the client to provide a copy of the directive.)
3. Educate staff and community about advance directives.
4. Ensure that the individuals know that the facility never discriminates based on whether or not the individual has an advance directive.

Competent clients may execute advance directives at any time. Advance directives are formal, written documents that typically outline the client's desires regarding the following:

- Use or withholding of hydration and/or total parenteral nutrition

- Resuscitation or intubation in the event of a life-threatening emergency (Do-not-resuscitate and do-not-intubate orders are discussed in the exemplar on End-of-Life Care in the module on Comfort.)

- Who has the authority to make decisions on the client's behalf in the event the client is unable to do so (referred to as a healthcare surrogate).

Types of advance directives include the living will and the durable power of attorney for health care. A **living will** provides specific instructions about what medical treatment the client chooses to omit or refuse (e.g., ventilator support) in the event the client is unable to make such a decision. Through a **durable power of attorney for health care**, the client may designate another individual (usually a family member, significant other, or close personal friend) as *healthcare surrogate* or *healthcare proxy*, and give that individual power to make healthcare decisions on behalf of the client if the client is unable to do so. These may be combined into a single document or may be two separate documents.

CASE STUDY \\ B

Gary Casper has been in the hospital several times in the past year with a deteriorating diagnosis. After Shondra Lewis, the client's RN, completes her assessment of Mr. Casper's current condition and his concerns, she contacts the case management department for assistance with his concerns regarding his end-of-life care choices. Ms. Lewis tells the case manager that the client's wife will not allow him to prepare an advance directive, which Mr. Casper wants to do, since he decided to be DNR on this current admission. The next day, the social worker meets with Mr. Casper separately from his wife to discuss his right for self-determination and how to prepare an advance directive form. Mr. Casper is relieved that he can complete the form in the hospital, but he is concerned that his wife will still be able to prevent this, as he does not want her to have a power of attorney for him. Plans are put in process for Mr. Casper to complete the advance directive with appropriate staff and another family member while the physician speaks with Mrs. Casper in a conference room.

Clinical Reasoning Questions Level I

1. How did the staff support this client's right to self-determination?
2. Did the physician violate the wife's right to be with her spouse in this case? Explain.

Clinical Reasoning Questions Level II

3. How can nursing staff further assist Mr. Casper in facing end-of-life care choices?
4. How can the staff support Mrs. Casper as she faces the end of her husband's life?

▶ ELEMENTS OF AN ADVANCE DIRECTIVE

A broadly drafted advance directive usually gives an agent or surrogate decision maker authority to do the following:

- Consent to or refuse any medical treatment or diagnostic procedure relating to the individual's physical or mental health, including artificial nutrition and hydration.
- Hire or discharge medical providers, and authorize admission to medical and long-term care facilities.
- Consent to measures for comfort care and pain relief.
- Have access to all medical records.
- Take whatever measures are necessary to carry out wishes, including granting releases or waivers to medical facilities and seeking judicial remedies if problems arise.

Each state, through legislation, determines the specific requirements for healthcare advance directives. In most states, advance directives must be witnessed by two people and do not require review by an attorney. Many states require that a specific legislated form be used. The majority of states do not permit relatives, heirs, or primary care providers to serve as witnesses for advance directives (Ryan & Jezewski, 2012). In some states, the client has the option to limit the authority of the healthcare agent as desired. Nurses working with a client who has an advance directive should ensure they understand what the client's advance directive includes and should know the laws in the state related to self-determination as well as the employing agency's policies and procedures for following advance directives.

Figure 49–4 ● shows an example of an advance healthcare directive that combines a living will declaration and a durable power of attorney for health care. Samples of state-specific forms can be obtained from the National Hospice and Palliative Care Organization (www.nhpco.org).

▶ ROLE OF THE NURSE

Clients and families often have difficulty making advance treatment decisions for end-of-life matters. The nurse should reassure them that even if they make a decision and have an advance directive, they will have the option to change their decision when competent. For example, the client may have decided not to have ventilator support in the case of terminal illness, but when the situation occurs, the client has the right to change his or her mind or take more time to make the decision.

SAFETY ALERT

Nurses can assist clients and their families by instructing clients to provide a copy of their advance directives to their next of kin, primary healthcare providers, and any healthcare facility to which they are admitted, including emergency departments, rehabilitations facilities, and senior living centers.

The nurse needs to assess whether the client and family have an accurate understanding of life-sustaining measures. Clients and families may misunderstand what actions may sustain life and base their decisions on these misconceptions. The nurse needs to incorporate teaching in this area and continue to be supportive of clients' decisions.

REVIEW Advance Directives

RELATE Link the Concepts and Exemplars

Linking the exemplar of advance directives with the concept of cognition:

1. Why might it be advisable to discuss development of advance directives with a client who is in the early stages of Alzheimer disease?
2. How might a client with schizophrenia benefit from an advance directive that includes instructions related to psychiatric care and treatment?

Linking the exemplar of advance directives with the concept of communication:

3. What communication strategies would you use to address the need to develop advance directives with a client? With the client's family members?
4. What communication strategies would you use to help a family member understand that her mother is no longer able to make her own decisions and it is time to review and follow the advance directives that the client put in place?

POWER OF ATTORNEY FOR HEALTH CARE

(1) **DESIGNATION OF AGENT:** I designate the following individual as my agent to make health care decisions for me: _____

_____
(Name of individual you choose as agent)

_____
(address) (city) (state) (zip code)

_____
(home phone) (work phone)

OPTIONAL: If I revoke my agent's authority or if my agent is not willing, able, or reasonably available to make a health-care decision for me, I designate as my first alternate agent:

_____
(Name of individual you choose as first alternate agent)

_____
(address) (city) (state) (zip code)

_____
(home phone) (work phone)

OPTIONAL: If I revoke the authority of my agent and first alternate agent or if neither is willing, able, or reasonably available to make a health care decision for me, I designate as my second alternate agent:

_____
(Name of individual you choose as second alternate agent)

_____
(address) (city) (state) (zip code)

_____
(home phone) (work phone)

(2) **AGENT'S AUTHORITY:** My agent is authorized to make all health care decisions for me, including decisions to provide, withhold, or withdraw artificial nutrition and hydration, and all other forms of health care to keep me alive, **except** as I state here:

(3) **WHEN AGENT'S AUTHORITY BECOMES EFFECTIVE:** My agent's authority becomes effective when my primary physician determines that I am unable to make my own health care decisions unless I mark the following box. If I mark this box [ ], my agent's authority to make health care decisions for me takes effect immediately.

(4) **AGENT'S OBLIGATION:** My agent shall make health care decisions for me in accordance with this power of attorney for health care, any instructions I give below, and my other wishes to the extent known to my agent. To the extent my wishes are unknown, my agent shall make health care decisions for me in accordance with what my agent determines to be in my best interest. In determining my best interest, my agent shall consider my personal values to the extent known to my agent.

(5) **AGENT'S POSTDEATH AUTHORITY:** My agent is authorized to make anatomical gifts, authorize an autopsy, and direct disposition of my remains, except as I state here or elsewhere in this form:

INSTRUCTIONS FOR HEALTH CARE
Strike any wording you do not want.

(6) **END-OF-LIFE DECISIONS:** I direct that my health care providers and others involved in my care provide, withhold, or withdraw treatment in accordance with the choice I have marked below: **(Initial only one box)**
[ ] (a) **Choice NOT To Prolong Life**
I do not want my life to be prolonged if (1) I have an incurable and irreversible condition that will result in my death within a relatively short time, (2) I become unconscious and, to a reasonable degree of medical certainty, I will not regain consciousness, or (3) the likely risks and burdens of treatment would outweigh the expected benefits, **OR**
[ ] (b) **Choice To Prolong Life**
I want my life to be prolonged as long as possible within the limits of generally accepted health care standards.

(7) **RELIEF FROM PAIN:** Except as I state in the following space, I direct that treatment for alleviation of pain or discomfort should be provided at all times even if it hastens my death:

DONATION OF ORGANS AT DEATH
(8) Upon my death: (mark applicable box)
[ ] (a) I give any needed organs, tissues, or parts,
OR
[ ] (b) I give the following organs, tissues, or parts only: _____
[ ] (c) My gift is for the following purposes:
(strike any of the following you do not want)
(1) Transplant
(2) Therapy
(3) Research
(4) Education

(9) **EFFECT OF COPY:** A copy of this form has the same effect as the original.

(10) **SIGNATURE:** Sign and date the form here:

_____   _____
(date)   (sign your name)

_____   _____
(address)   (print your name)

_____   _____
(city)   (state)

(11) **WITNESSES:** This advance health care directive will not be valid for making health care decisions unless it is either: (1) signed by two (2) qualified adult witnesses who are personally known to you and who are present when you sign or acknowledge your signature; or (2) acknowledged before a notary public.

Figure 49–4 ● Sample advance healthcare directive.

REFER Go to Pearson Nursing Student Resources
nursing.pearsonhighered.com

- Additional review materials

REFLECT Case Study

Heather King is a 53-year-old client who is hospitalized with a newly diagnosed malignant brain tumor. She has signed an advance directive that indicates she does not want any extraordinary measures to keep her alive if she has an incurable or irreversible condition that will result in her death within a relatively short period of time. The neurosurgeon has presented her with treatment options. Mrs. King refuses treatment for the tumor, requesting only palliative care "until the time comes." Mr. King speaks to the neurosurgeon outside of his wife's room, stating, "I want everything possible done! The children and I have discussed this, and we don't agree with not treating the tumor."

1. What should happen with Mrs. King's treatment? Why?
2. How may the family's reaction affect implementing the advance directive?
3. In what circumstances could the client's family member refuse or consent to treatment for the client?
4. How should the nurse respond in this client's situation?
5. What law, rule, or policy describes the nurse's responsibility?

EXEMPLAR 49.3 Health Insurance Portability and Accountability Act

EXEMPLAR KEY TERMS

Confidentiality, *2671*
Health Insurance Portability and Accountability Act (HIPAA), *2670*
Privacy, *2671*
Protected health information, *2670*

EXEMPLAR LEARNING OUTCOMES

After reading about this exemplar, you will be able to:

1. Describe the purpose of the Health Insurance Portability and Accountability Act.
2. Distinguish between privacy and confidentiality.
3. Summarize the nurse's role in maintaining client confidentiality.
4. Relate strategies nurses can use to prevent and address breaches of confidentiality.

▶ OVERVIEW

The **Health Insurance Portability and Accountability Act (HIPAA)** of 1996 was enacted by Congress to minimize the exclusion of preexisting conditions as a barrier to healthcare insurance, designate special rights for individuals who lose other health coverage, and eliminate medical underwriting in group plans. The act includes the Privacy Rule, which creates a national standard for the disclosure of private health information. This rule affects all healthcare providers as well as health insurance plan providers (Wiener & Gilliland, 2011).

▶ PROTECTED HEALTH INFORMATION

The Privacy Rule protects all "individually identifiable health information" held or transmitted in any form or media, whether electronic, paper, or oral. The rule calls this information **protected health information** and delineates it further to include information that identifies the individual (e.g., name, address, birth date, and Social Security number) or for which a reasonable basis exists to believe the information can be used to identify the individual as it relates to the following:

- The individual's past, present, or future physical or mental health or condition
- The provision of health care to the individual
- The past, present, or future payment for the provision of health care to the individual.

The HIPAA also includes provisions for the protection of clients that address access to medical records, required notice of privacy practices and opportunity for confidential communications, limits on use of medical information beyond the sharing among healthcare providers directly involved in providing care, and prohibition of the use of personal information for marketing.

In the event a client feels that a healthcare plan or provider has violated his or her rights according to the HIPAA, the individual may file a formal complaint either directly to the entity or to the office for Civil Rights of the U.S. Department of Health and Human Services. Information about how to file a complaint should be included in each entity's notice of privacy practices.

Nurses must maintain a current understanding of the law in order to protect the client's privacy and to avoid civil punitive damage suits and possible criminal charges. Nurses should be familiar with the particular policies of their employers. **Box 49–8** provides examples of how HIPAA affects nursing practice.

In spite of the extensive amounts of time and money that have been expended by the healthcare industry, the general population remains confused about their actual rights, and some healthcare workers see HIPAA privacy compliance as frivolous (Bova, Drexler, & Sullivan-Bolyai, 2012; Wiener & Gilliland, 2011). Ultimately, maintaining the security of protected health information provides for the protection of the most vulnerable populations, and personnel in covered entities will need to continue to learn and implement the HIPAA standards.

SAFETY ALERT

Disclosure of client information is a breach of confidentiality that may subject a nurse to legal action. Disclosure of confidential information occurs when a client's condition—for example, a diagnosis of HIV infection—is discussed inappropriately with any third party. In addition, privacy must be provided when calling individuals in for office visits and in all provisions of care.

Box 49–8 Examples of HIPAA Compliance and Nursing Practice

- A client's name cannot be posted near or on the room door.
- Charts should be in a secure, nonpublic location to prevent the public from viewing or accessing confidential health information.
- Printed copies of protected health information should not be left unattended at a printer or fax machine.
- Access to protected health information is limited to those authorized to obtain the information.
- Passwords are required for accessing a client's electronic chart.
- A notice informing clients of their rights regarding privacy and their health information should be posted and provided to clients on admission to a healthcare facility.
- Voice levels should be lowered to minimize disclosure of information (e.g., when discussing a client's condition over the telephone, giving a report, or reading information aloud from a computer screen or chart).
- Healthcare providers must stay current with HIPAA regulations.

▶ PRIVACY VERSUS CONFIDENTIALITY

Privacy includes the right of individuals to keep their personal information from being disclosed. The individual decides with who, when, and where to share his or her health information. **Confidentiality** refers to the assurance the client has that private information will not be disclosed without the client's consent. Confidentiality refers to both the nature of the information the nurse obtains from the client and to how the nurse treats client information once it has been disclosed to the nurse (Wiener & Gilliland, 2011):

- ***Obtaining information.*** Nurses should request and record only information pertinent to the health status of clients to

whom the nurse is assigned. If, for example, the nurse runs into a neighbor in the emergency department waiting room, it would be inappropriate for the nurse to ask the neighbor, "What are you doing here?" This would inadvertently invite protected information that is not required for provision of health care.

- ***Disclosing information.*** Information obtained from the client should be disclosed only to individuals who are directly involved in providing that client's health care. Even the presence of the individual in the healthcare setting is protected information. It would be a breach of confidentiality, for example, for the nurse to go home and tell her family that a state senator or representative, the family's pastor, a neighbor, or anyone else was a client. Protection of client information, once disclosed, is one tenet of the nurse's responsibility as the client's advocate, and challenges to client privacy can include other members of the interdisciplinary team.

- ***Advocating for confidentiality.*** Nurses are professionally obligated not only to avoid participating in discussions of clients outside communications directly related to providing care but also to curb others from participation. Gossiping at work seems to be a national pastime, but it has no place in the healthcare setting. Celebrity status, notoriety, and an unusual medical condition all add to the potential risks to confidentiality. If the nurse is in a coffee shop and hears another nurse or healthcare provider discussing a client, the nurse is expected to redirect those professionals to maintain client privacy.

In addition to the actions and behaviors described here, nurses should be familiar with the specific policies and procedures for protecting client privacy and confidentiality for the healthcare agency in which they work.

REVIEW Health Insurance Portability and Accountability Act

RELATE Link the Concepts and Exemplars

Linking the exemplar of HIPAA with the concept of violence:

1. When and how is it appropriate to break the confidentiality of clients who threaten harm to themselves or others?

2. What additional considerations are involved when it comes to protecting the confidentiality of victims of domestic violence? Of child abuse?

Linking the exemplar of HIPAA with the concept of reproduction:

You are the nurse at a local high school. A 16-year-old student has been in the bathroom off and on all morning. She is very nauseous but has been adamant about staying at school. You sit down to talk with her and learn that she thinks she is pregnant. She says, "I don't know what to do. I don't want my parents to know."

3. What are your responsibilities to this client regarding her privacy and confidentiality?

4. What are the laws in your state regarding the ability of minors to make independent decisions regarding their own pregnancies?

REFER Go to Pearson Nursing Student Resources
nursing.pearsonhighered.com

- Additional review materials

REFLECT Case Study

Michael Nguyen is a nurse on the medical-surgical floor of a busy suburban hospital. Approximately 20 minutes ago, the nursing desk was notified that seven clients who were involved in a motor vehicle crash and are currently receiving treatment in the emergency department (ED) are expected to be discharged to the med-surg floor in varying conditions. Carole Fulton, another nurse working on the unit, has been liaising with the ED staff about the situation. Michael goes to answer a client call bell. When he returns to the nursing desk, he overhears Carole on her cell phone saying, "Yes, that accident on Highway 40. Yeah, apparently it's really bad. I saw Reverend Mitchell downstairs. Yeah. No. His daughter was a passenger. OK. Bye." Carole hangs up the phone and puts it in her purse, saying, "My mom. She called to tell me she got home safely from work." Thirty minutes later, Michael receives a report on a client named Elizabeth Mitchell who is being transported up from the ED.

1. What concerns might Michael have about the content of Carole's phone call with her mother? How might Carole have violated Ms. Mitchell's privacy or confidentiality?

2. If you had been Michael, what responsibility would you have to address your concerns?

EXEMPLAR 49.4 Just Culture

EXEMPLAR KEY TERMS
Just culture, 2672
Whistleblower, 2672
Whistleblowing, 2672

EXEMPLAR LEARNING OUTCOMES
After reading about this exemplar, you will be able to:

1. Distinguish elements of just culture.
2. Summarize the benefits of promoting just culture in health-care environments.
3. Discuss the standards required under the Whistleblower Protection Act.

▶ OVERVIEW

"In a Just Culture, nurses are encouraged to report all clinical errors and near-misses without fear of repercussions so they can receive corrective feedback and everyone can learn from the experience" (Shepard, 2011, p. 46). **Just culture** is a move from a punitive work environment that emphasizes blame to a proactive environment that supports employee involvement in decision making, supports learning, and examines what systems failed when an error or adverse event occurs. In addition, in a just culture, nurses remain accountable for their own actions and are expected to provide constructive feedback to their peers. Just culture has become one strategy to improve client safety by encouraging staff members to learn from each other's mistakes or near-misses (which is an error that was caught before it affected a client).

▶ JUST CULTURE

Just culture is a relatively new process within health care. It began in occupations that involve a high level of risk daily, such as the military and air traffic control. Now, a just culture is commonly part of the standards for a hospital's magnet recognition (Bashaw & Lounsbury, 2012), with an expectation of collaboration and continued learning with decency.

Just culture is based on the understanding that errors are often the result of system failures rather than human failures. It recognizes that an atmosphere of punishment impedes error prevention by promoting intimidation and secrecy rather than shared accountability. Just culture focuses on the system rather than the individual while still maintaining an environment of individual accountability for both front-line staff and leaders and managers. This is critical; when front line staff fail to report safety errors due to fear of suspension or termination, healthcare managers may develop an inaccurate understanding of the care provided by the organization. This hampers ongoing quality improvement efforts, further risking client safety (Vogelsmeier et al., 2010). Successfully establishing an environment of just culture requires that leadership encourage proactive system management as well as individual accountability. It also requires that employees consider themselves as stakeholders and act to establish and maintain the just culture environment. Just culture does not, however, accept or tolerate gross misconduct (e.g., employees working under the influence of alcohol or narcotics) or conscious disregard of client and staff safety.

In a just culture environment, each member has the responsibility to take action to prevent errors and also to respond to errors, recognizing that errors are more often the result of system failures than individual error, and that when individual error does occur, it is more likely to be accidental than willful or neglectful. For example, if the hospital pharmacy dispenses the wrong medication or the wrong dosage, or if the department in charge of stocking supplies for a unit fails to make an appropriate inventory and orders an inadequate amount of supplies, those errors may be a result of inadequate systems as much as they may result from individual carelessness.

As more organizations begin to embrace just culture, front-line staff are likely to feel more support from management in critical areas, including staffing. From time to time, however, nurses and other front-line staff may find themselves in situation where management is unresponsive to suggestions for improvement or reporting of critical shortages or potential for errors related to client safety. In these cases, staff may find themselves in the awkward position of needing to report these problems outside the agency.

▶ WHISTLEBLOWING

Whistleblowing is the disclosure by a staff member of an organization of practices and/or polices engaged in by that organization or its employees that wrong or harm a third party (Mansbach & Bachner, 2010). The Whistleblower Protection Act of 1989 establishes certain protections for individuals who report gross misconduct on the part of their employers to federal authorities. A nurse who goes outside of an organization to protect the public interest when the organization fails to follow procedures regarding safety and client care is engaging in whistleblowing (Lachman, 2008). The nurse who takes such action is called a **whistleblower**. To qualify for protection under the act, the nurse must first make every effort to resolve the concern by following the internal reporting procedures of the agency that employs her or him. Additionally, an individual does not qualify for protection under the act unless the employer has threatened or engaged in retaliation against the employee as a result of the employee making a complaint.

Not every act of misconduct will rise to the standard that it will qualify under the Whistleblower Protection Act. Simple error or misconduct generally does not rise to this standard. Typically, the activity or policy in question must violate a state or federal law or rule, and the employer must be aware that the activity or policy is a violation. A few examples of incidents to report are billing fraud, failure to maintain safety equipment, and chronic insufficient staffing. The nurse making the complaint must give the employer written notice and appropriate time to correct the issue. To be considered a whistleblower, the nurse must also make or threaten to make a report to the appropriate state or federal agency.

Additional legislation supports individuals in reporting fraud. The False Claims Act encourages individuals to report medical and billing agency fraud. In March 2010, new healthcare reform legislation strengthened the False Claims Act in order to ensure that healthcare providers and clients can report fraud under the Patient Protection and Affordable Care Act. The National Whistleblowers Center (www.whistleblowers.org/index.html) provides additional information and advocacy on this important and complex issue (National Whistleblowers Center, 2010).

> ### SAFETY ALERT
> Reporting a coworker can be especially difficult, but it is critical that the nurse inform the supervisor about a possible problem with a coworker or other healthcare provider, especially if the individual's action reflects incompetence or is illegal or unethical. The nurse also must recognize the difference between a coworker's illegal behavior and a client issue or error that may have been caused by a system problem.

The nurse who makes a report outside of the employing agency should be prepared for the possibility of negative consequences. These may include losing the support of one's coworkers or even losing one's job. Failing to act, however, may jeopardize client care.

> ### SAFETY ALERT
> The failure of a nurse to report illegal, unethical, or unsafe conduct may result in the nurse being sued by the client, action taken against the nurse's license, or termination by the employer (Cornock, 2011).

Statutes exist to prevent recourse by the employer for reasonable, good faith reporting of illegal, unethical, or unsafe conduct in order to provide a safe, environment for clients. To help ensure that employees are free to participate in safety and health activities, Section 11(c) (The Whistleblower Protection Program) of the Occupational Safety and Health Act prohibits any person from discharging, or in any manner retaliating or discriminating against, any employee because that employee has exercised rights under the act. Provided that the whistleblower has done everything required before notifying the federal agency, the whistleblower's protected rights include making formal notification to the Occupational Safety and Health Administration (OSHA) and seeking an OSHA inspection, participating in an OSHA inspection, and participating or testifying in any proceeding related to an OSHA inspection. Discrimination by the employer includes the following actions:

- Firing or laying off
- Blacklisting
- Demoting
- Denying overtime or promotion
- Disciplining
- Denial of benefits
- Failure to hire or rehire
- Intimidation
- Reassignment affecting promotion prospects
- Reducing pay or hours.

To prevail in a discrimination claim, the nurse must report the illegal activity before resigning from the place of employment. To file a complaint under Section 11(c), the nurse must contact the nearest OSHA office within 30 days of the discrimination. Discrimination complaints cannot be filed online.

Recent studies have explored the influence of whistleblowing on staff relationships as well as how staff manage that type of report. A qualitative study (Jackson et al., 2010) found that whistleblowing resulted in hostility in the workplace and had a profound and overwhelmingly negative effect on working relationships. A quantitative study utilizing a five-question survey found that although "severity of misconduct" of a professional staff member resulted in internal whistleblowing, nurses often wanted to avoid confrontation (Mansbach & Bachner, 2010). Legal experts have noted that reporting a colleague for an incompetency or inappropriate action is not easy, which may explain why so few nurses choose to do so (Cornock, 2011). Any factor that negatively influences working relationships between nurses is a matter of concern. Therefore, a just culture has begun to replace whistleblowing as a way to understand system errors. Just culture promotes shared responsibility and accountability, improves collaboration between front-line staff and management, and, when implemented properly, has great potential to reduce safety errors and improve client safety and outcomes.

REVIEW Just Culture

RELATE Link the Concepts and Exemplars

Linking the exemplar of just culture with the concept of accountability:

1. How does a just culture environment promote accountability of individual nurses and staff? Of the healthcare agency as a whole?

2. What types of professional development experiences are more likely to assist in the development of a just culture? Why?

Linking the exemplar of just culture with the concept of safety:

3. How does a just culture promote client safety?

4. What principles of safety support the need for healthcare agencies to develop environments of just culture?

REFER Go to Pearson Nursing Student Resources
nursing.pearsonhighered.com

- Additional review materials

REFLECT Case Study

You are the nurse working night shifts on a pediatric oncology unit. Within the past month, three nurses who work the night shift have transferred to other employment. On a regular basis, the unit is understaffed. The charge nurse is reluctant to call for a float nurse unless absolutely necessary, explaining that she has received strict instructions to keep costs down. This is the third night this week that the unit has been short staffed. It was short staffed four nights during the previous week.

1. In a just culture, how might this situation be handled?
2. To what extent does this situation rise to the standards of whistleblowing?
3. What steps might you take to improve this situation?

EXEMPLAR 49.5 Mandatory Reporting

EXEMPLAR KEY TERM
Mandatory reporting, 2674

EXEMPLAR LEARNING OUTCOMES
After reading about this exemplar, you will be able to:

1. Discuss the general legal requirements of mandatory reporting.
2. Discuss the principle of good faith immunity.
3. Distinguish situations that require mandatory reporting.
4. Discuss the nurse's responsibilities related to mandatory reporting.

▶ OVERVIEW

The term **mandatory reporting** refers to a legal requirement to report an act, event, or situation that is designated by state or local law as a reportable event (Katner, 2012). Disclosure statutes mandate the reporting of certain types of health information, and all states mandate the reporting of certain vital statistics, including births and deaths. Many states also require healthcare providers to report abortions and neonatal deaths. Federal and state laws mandate the reporting of communicable diseases, including venereal diseases. This exemplar discusses types of acts, events, or situations that are reportable as well as the nurse's responsibilities related to mandatory reporting.

▶ ABUSE OR NEGLECT OF MINORS AND OLDER ADULTS

Reporting of abuse or suspected abuse of vulnerable individuals is mandated in most states. As a general rule, the nurse reports the required information through the administrative chain of the institution, beginning with the nurse's immediate supervisor and the primary healthcare provider. All information reported is documented in the client record. In most states, mandatory reporters are required only to have a good faith suspicion, based on information disclosed by the client and/or on physical symptoms manifested by the client (e.g., glove-stocking burn injuries), that abuse has occurred (see the Lifespan Considerations feature). They are not required to conduct any type of investigation or otherwise confirm that abuse or neglect has, in fact, occurred. For definitions and manifestations of child and older adult abuse, see the module on Violence.

▶ GOOD FAITH IMMUNITY

In every state, healthcare workers are protected when they report suspected child abuse in good faith, even if the subsequent investigation does not make a determination of abuse. Guidelines regarding disclosure of health information as a mandatory reporter are presented in **Box 49–9** ●.

▶ MANDATORY REPORTING OF NURSES WHO ARE IN VIOLATION OF THE NURSE PRACTICE ACT

Each state's nurse practice act (NPA) addresses the requirements for reporting nurses who are in violation of the act. For example, North Carolina's General Statutes (NCGS § 90-171.47)

Lifespan Considerations Reporting Abuse or Neglect of an Adult or Older Adult by a Caretaker

States have specific laws pertaining to the abuse and neglect of adults and older adults. These laws may be similar to those that govern the abuse and neglect of children. For example, many states generally offer good faith immunity to individuals reporting suspected abuse or neglect of an older adult or an adult with a disability. Nurses should know the laws of their individual states and their agency's policies for reporting suspected abuse or neglect of an adult or older adult (Daly, Klein, & Jogerst, 2012).

Box 49–9 Guidelines Regarding Disclosure of Health Information

Depending on the setting, the nurse may be the only professional with firsthand information necessary for making an accurate report. General guidelines that nurses should follow regarding reporting health-related information include the following:

- Know the federal and state laws concerning duty to report.
- Report the required information to the appropriate governmental agency promptly.
- Comply with reporting laws in good faith.
- Follow agency policy carefully when making a report.
- Avoid a breach of confidentiality, and report only the information mandated. Good faith immunity applies only to required information reported to the appropriate agency or office.

Source: Based on Guido, G. W. (2010). *Legal and ethical issues in nursing* (5th ed.). Upper Saddle River, NJ: Prentice Hall.

mandate that any individual who has reasonable cause to suspect that a nurse is in violation of the NPA has the duty to report the relevant facts to the state's board of nursing (BON). The reporting individual is not expected to do any type of investigation.

Because BONs take these reports very seriously, their Web sites generally make reporting forms easily available. Typically, employers use a different reporting form than that used by members of the general public. The NPA spells out any formal action the board may take, and it usually requires clear and convincing evidence that the nurse has violated state nursing laws or rules. The nature of alleged violations varies widely, and cases are decided on their own merits. Many complaints are resolved through informal processes. In other instances, a formal administrative hearing is held. BONs are required to respect each nurse's right to due process. This ensures that the nurse is informed of any allegations regarding his or her practice, that the nurse has an opportunity to respond to and defend against the allegations, and that the matter is heard by a fair and impartial body. An immunity clause protects individuals who make a report unless the reporting individual knew the report was false or acted with reckless disregard, without concern for the validity of the allegations made in the report.

Nurses themselves have a legal obligation to report conduct that is incompetent, unethical, and illegal. This includes reporting violence, abuse, or neglect toward clients by other nurses and extends to reporting conduct involving third parties, including family members and other healthcare providers. Nurses are in a position to identify and assess cases of violence, abuse, and neglect (Daly et al., 2012).

▶ MANDATORY REPORTING OF CERTAIN INJURIES AND ILLNESSES

Each state has laws that require healthcare providers and hospitals to report certain types of injuries and illnesses. Those that usually fall under the reporting laws include the following:

- Bullet wounds, gunshot wounds, powder burns, or any other injuries arising or suspected of arising from the discharge of a gun or firearm

- Illnesses that appear to be caused by poisoning

- Injuries caused by, or appearing to be caused by, a knife or other sharp or pointed instrument if the physician or surgeon treating the individual suspects that a criminal act may have been involved

- Any wound, injury, or illness resulting in bodily harm as a result of a suspected criminal act or act of violence

- Infectious diseases, such as tuberculosis, HIV/AIDS, and *Escherichia coli.*

The primary care provider or hospital staff member making the report shall provide the name, age, gender, race, residence, or present location of the client who is injured or ill as well as the nature and extent of the injuries or illness. Again, good faith immunity typically applies. Although the primary healthcare provider is mandated to report, most agencies have a policy and procedure in place for routine reporting. The emergency

department typically reports injuries that are or appear to be due to violence. Because a diagnosis of an infectious disease may occur at any point in the healthcare interaction, the nurse needs to be familiar with the agency policy for reporting infectious diseases and ensure that the report is made when warranted.

Mandatory reporting of infectious conditions is a cornerstone of maintaining public health. Since 1878, the U.S. Public Health System has been collecting information on infectious conditions for the purpose of early identification and control of massive outbreaks, including, when necessary, instituting quarantines. High-profile diseases and threats of bioterrorism have brought renewed attention to this system of ongoing monitoring. Data are reported at the county level, with primary care providers reporting these diseases and conditions to local health departments. Each county health department reports to the state's department of health, where data are managed and maintained. Data on many diseases and conditions are provided from the state level to the Centers for Disease Control and Prevention (**Box 49–10** ●), which publishes the *Morbidity and Mortality Weekly Report*. Although the law targets physician reporting, nurses need to be aware of the policies and procedures for reporting within their place of employment, especially those who are employed directly by their local health department. For diseases and conditions that are required to be reported within 24 hours, the initial report is made by telephone to the health department, with the written report being made within 7 days.

▶ OTHER EXAMPLES OF MANDATORY REPORTING

In most states, child care workers, teachers, and other school personnel are mandated to report any suspicions of child abuse or neglect that involve children and families with whom they work (Katner, 2012; Wekerle, 2012). School principals and other administrators typically are required to report to law

---

Box 49–10 Nationally Notifiable Infectious Conditions

The Centers for Disease Control and Prevention National Notifiable Diseases Surveillance System (NNDSS) has identified more than 50 infectious diseases in the United States that must be reported. Among these are the following:

- Anthrax
- Botulism
- Cholera
- Diphtheria
- Hepatitis
- HIV infection
- Influenza-associated pediatric mortality
- Meningococcal disease
- Shigellosis
- Syphilis.

Stay Current: Visit the NNDSS Web site at **http://wwwn.cdc. gov/nndss** for more information. A complete list of the 2014 event codes of the NNDSS can be found at **http://wwwn.cdc.gov/ nndss/document/nndss_event_code_list_2014.pdf**.

enforcement when they have knowledge that a crime has been committed on school property. Crimes that typically must be reported include the following:

- Assault (especially assault with a weapon or assault resulting in serious injury)
- Sexual assault
- Rape
- Kidnapping

- Indecent liberties with a minor
- Possession of a firearm on school property or in violation of the law.

Photo processors or computer technicians who, within the scope of their employment, come across images of a minor (or an individual who reasonably appears to be a minor) engaging in sexual activity typically are required to make a report to local law enforcement. These individuals often are afforded good faith immunity.

REVIEW Mandatory Reporting

RELATE Link the Concepts and Exemplars

Linking the exemplar of mandatory reporting with the concept of violence:

1. Why do you think nurses and healthcare providers have a duty to report injuries sustained during or as a result of a criminal act?
2. Why do you think mandatory reporting laws include the requirement to report injuries resulting from the discharge of a firearm?

Linking the exemplar of mandatory reporting with the concept of infection:

3. How do requirements and procedures for reporting HIV infection in your state or agency differ from requirements and procedures for reporting anthrax?
4. How do requirements and procedures for reporting shigellosis in your state or agency differ from requirements and procedures for reporting meningococcal disease?

REFER Go to Pearson Nursing Student Resources nursing.pearsonhighered.com

- Additional review materials

REFLECT Case Study

Jenny Erickson, an 85-year-old widowed female, came into the emergency department after she apparently fell at home. Her neighbor and friend, Mrs. Jones, was waiting for Mrs. Erickson to go to lunch with her and tried calling her several times. After getting no response for more than an hour, Mrs. Jones called the police, who found Mrs. Erickson on the kitchen floor. During the ED RN assessment, the nurse, Lynn Gutierrez, noted multiple bruises on Mrs. Erickson's legs, her upper arms, and both sides of her rib cage. When she asked Mrs. Erickson about the bruises, Mrs. Erickson said that she has been "falling a lot." The bruises were in several different stages of healing and bruised colors.

When Ms. Gutierrez asked her whether she lived alone, Mrs. Erickson began crying and shivering. Mrs. Jones heard her friend crying and asked to speak with the nurse. Ms. Gutierrez spoke with Mrs. Jones away from the ED bedside. "I don't mean to get anyone in trouble, but Jenny has been living with her daughter and son-in-law for the past two years. I'm worried that they are upset having her there." The nurse realized that Mrs. Jones might have information that could explain why Mrs. Erickson had so many bruises. "Has Mrs. Erickson complained at all? I mean, has her family hurt her?" Mrs. Jones nodded her head. "I think so. I've heard her son-in-law yelling at her before, and Jenny had a big bruise on her forehead a month ago right after that."

1. What does Ms. Gutierrez need to do next?
2. How can the ED staff support Mrs. Erickson and ensure her safety while she is in the ED?
3. How can the nursing staff further assist Mrs. Erickson with the possible abuse?
4. What report must be done for this client, and by whom?

EXEMPLAR 49.6 Risk Management

EXEMPLAR KEY TERMS
Discovery, *2678*
Incident report, *2678*
Risk management, *2676*
Variances, *2678*

EXEMPLAR LEARNING OUTCOMES
After reading about this exemplar, you will be able to:

1. Describe strategies that healthcare organizations use to manage risk.

2. Apply strategies to minimize risk when implementing physician's orders.
3. Summarize strategies to reduce risk when providing care to pediatric clients.
4. Summarize the components of an incident report.

▶ OVERVIEW

Risk management focuses on limiting a healthcare agency's financial and legal risk associated with the delivery of care, particularly in terms of lawsuits, ideally before incidents occur. Risk management is a process that identifies, analyzes, and treats potential hazards within a setting for the purpose of identifying and rectifying the hazards, thus preventing harm.

Nurses participate in risk management every day when they ensure client safety and quality care. Typical areas for high risk of incidents include the following:

- Medication administration
- Falls
- Overall client safety

- Use of technology and equipment (e.g., ensuring that equipment is working correctly before using it)
- Assessment and communication of allergies
- Any action or intervention that might harm the client.

▶ STRATEGIES FOR RISK MANAGEMENT

A facility may have an individual or a team dedicated to risk management. In most cases, there will be a designated risk manager whose overall role is to collaborate with the interdisciplinary healthcare team to maintain a safe and effective healthcare environment and prevent or reduce loss to the organization (Kable, Guest, & McLeod, 2012). Strategies that healthcare organizations use to minimize risk include the following:

- Purchasing insurance or self-insuring to protect against financial risk
- Identifying exposures, types, where they occur, frequency, and level of risk
- Implementing practices to protect against undue risk
- Implementing organizational programs to prevent occurrence of events that might increase financial risk (e.g., incident report system, staff education about risk and documentation, and data collection to assist in identifying potential problems)
- Investigating incidents that might result in a potential lawsuit as soon as possible after the incident occurs
- Monitoring strategies for prevention of risk.

Healthcare organizations must also consider the risks to anyone who enters the organization's facility, such as visitors, community members, and family members. For instance, a visitor might fall in the hallway, and the organization could be found liable. For more information on how to prevent risk, see the modules on Quality Improvement and Safety.

Implementing a Physician's Orders

Nurses can minimize risk by analyzing procedures and medications ordered by the physician. It is the nurse's responsibility to seek clarification of ambiguous or seemingly erroneous orders from the prescribing physician. Clarification from any other source is unacceptable and is regarded as a departure from competent nursing practice.

If the order is neither ambiguous nor apparently erroneous, the nurse is responsible for implementing it. For example, if the physician orders oxygen to be administered at 4 L/min, the nurse must administer oxygen at that rate and not at 2 or 6 L/min. If the orders state that the client is not to have solid food after a bowel resection, the nurse must ensure that no solid food is given to the client.

There are several categories of orders that nurses must question to protect themselves legally:

- *Question any order a client questions.* For example, if a client who has been receiving an intramuscular injection tells the nurse that the physician changed the order from an injectable to an oral medication, the nurse must recheck the order before giving the medication.

- *Question any order if the client's condition has changed.* The nurse is considered responsible for notifying the physician of any significant changes in the client's condition, whether the physician requests notification or not. For example, if a client who is receiving an intravenous infusion suddenly develops a rapid pulse, chest pain, and a cough, the nurse must notify the physician immediately and question continuance of the ordered rate of infusion. If a client who is receiving morphine for pain develops severely depressed respirations, the nurse must withhold the medication and notify the physician.

- *Question and record verbal orders to avoid miscommunications.* In addition to recording the time, the date, the physician's name, and the orders, the nurse documents the circumstances that occasioned the call to the physician, reads the orders back to the physician, and documents that the physician confirmed the orders as the nurse read them back.

- *Question any order that is illegible, unclear, or incomplete.* Misinterpretation of the name of a drug or the amount of a dose, for example, can easily occur with handwritten orders. The nurse is responsible for ensuring that the order is interpreted the way it was intended and that it is a safe and appropriate order.

Providing Competent Nursing Care

Nurses further minimize and manage risk by providing competent client care. Nurses need to provide care that is within the legal boundaries of their practice and within the boundaries of agency policies and procedures. Nurses therefore must be familiar with their various job descriptions, which may be different from agency to agency. Every nurse is responsible for ensuring that his or her education and experience are adequate to meet the responsibilities delineated in the job description.

Competency also involves care that protects clients from harm. Nurses need to anticipate sources of client injury, educate clients about hazards, and implement measures to prevent injury.

Application of the nursing process is another essential aspect of providing safe and effective client care. Clients need to be assessed and monitored appropriately and involved in care decisions. All assessments and care must be documented accurately. Effective communication can also protect the nurse from negligence claims. Nurses need to approach every client with sincere concern and include the client in conversations. In addition, nurses should always acknowledge when they do not know the answer to a client's questions, tell the client they will find the answer, and then follow through.

Methods of legal protection are summarized in **Box 49–11** ●.

Reducing Pediatric Medical Errors

Children are at a higher risk for medical error than other clients and also may be more vulnerable to harm from errors due to their immature physiology (Tzeng et al., 2013). Reasons for increased medical error among children include the following (Eisbach & Driessnack, 2010; Tzeng et al., 2013):

- Medication dosage calculations for children are more complex than those for adults. Many medications are produced in adult concentrations that require dilution when given to a child, or the dosages need to be calculated based

Box 49–11   Guidelines for Legal Protection for Nurses

- Function within the scope of your education, job description, and nurse practice act.
- Follow the procedures and policies of the employing agency.
- Build and maintain good rapport with clients.
- Always check the identity of a client to make sure it is the right client.
- Observe and monitor the client accurately. Communicate and record significant changes in the client's condition to the physician.
- Promptly and accurately document all assessments and care given.
- Be alert when implementing nursing interventions, and give each task your full attention and skill.
- Perform procedures correctly and appropriately.
- Make sure the correct medications are given in the correct dose, by the right route, at the scheduled time, and to the right client.
- When delegating nursing responsibilities, make sure that the individual who is delegated a task understands what to do and that the individual has the required knowledge and skill.
- Protect clients from injury.
- Report all incidents involving clients.
- Always check any order that a client questions.
- Know your own strengths and weaknesses. Ask for assistance and supervision in situations for which you feel inadequately prepared.
- Maintain your clinical competence. For students, this demands study and practice before caring for clients. For graduate nurses, it means continued study to maintain and update clinical knowledge and skills.

on weight or body surface area. This means that the optimal dose is based on mg/kg and divided by number of doses to be given a day. An additional problem is that children often need suspensions or liquid preparations, adding to the dosage calculation complexity. Not only must the correct dose be calculated, but so must the amount of liquid preparation with that dose. Errors in mathematical calculations are one of the most common causes of medication errors.

- The misplacement of a decimal in the medication dosage calculation can result in an overdose that can cause harm to the child or even death. This is particularly important for critically ill or injured children who do not have the reserves to deal with an overdose of medication.

- Many drug preparations require dilution to achieve the small dosage required by infants.

- Medications are sometimes prescribed that are not yet approved by the Food and Drug Administration for use in children, and pediatric standard dosage guidelines have not been established.

- Young children cannot communicate well if they are having a reaction to the medication.

Another cause of potential medical error involves families with limited English proficiency. There is a risk for errors in interpretation between the healthcare professional and the family member regarding care. For example, failure to obtain historical information about a drug allergy may lead to serious adverse effects. Even when a hospital interpreter is used, errors such as omitting instructions on dose, route, frequency, and duration of medications have potentially harmful clinical consequences (Eisbach & Driessnack, 2010).

▶ INCIDENT REPORTS

As part of risk management, each healthcare organization has an incident reporting system (Kable et al., 2012). Nurses participate in this process by completing the required forms when involved in an incident and by following policies and procedures. Most incidents, however, do not result in a lawsuit.

An **incident report** is an agency record of an accident or incident occurring within the agency. It is designed to collect adequate information to assist personnel in preventing future incidents or occurrences. Incident reports are also called variance reports or unusual occurrence reports. Examples of occurrences that would be reported include medication administration **variances** (e.g., wrong medication, wrong dose, wrong route, wrong time, and omissions) and a client or visitor falling.

In some jurisdictions, incident reports may be used in discovery. **Discovery** is the legal process of obtaining information before a trial. A nurse completing an incident report should always fill out the report as though it is discoverable. No language regarding liability should be included. The report should completely and accurately document the facts without assumptions, conclusions, or blame. The report should include the client's account of the incident in direct quotes and should identify all witnesses to the incident. Incident reports generally include the following:

- Names and identifying information of any clients and healthcare personnel involved in the incident as well as information on witnesses (if any)

- The location, time, and date of the incident

- Equipment or medication involved (if medication, state the medication's name and dosage).

Although the event that prompted the incident report is noted in the client's chart, there should be no entry in the client's chart to indicate that an incident report was completed. For example, if the client was given the wrong medication, the actual administration of the medication will be noted in the client's chart. If the client required any treatment as a result of the event, that also is noted in the client's chart (Guido, 2010).

Nurses engage in risk management by following ANA standards of care and practice, by following their employing agency's policies and procedures, and by working collaboratively to ensure client safety is maintained at all times. Risk management is required of every nurse in the course of practicing nursing on a daily basis.

REVIEW Risk Management

RELATE Link the Concepts and Exemplars

Linking the exemplar of risk management with the concept of assessment:

1. How does a thorough assessment of a client contribute to risk management?

2. Nurses are required to do their own assessment of a client after receiving a report during shift change or client transfer. How might failure to conduct this assessment or failure to do it in a timely manner affect the client's risk for adverse outcomes?

Linking the exemplar of risk management with the concept of communication:

3. How does a change-of-shift report minimize the nurse's risk for professional negligence or malpractice?

4. How does accuracy in documentation contribute to risk management?

REFER Go to Pearson Nursing Student Resources
nursing.pearsonhighered.com

  • Additional review materials

REFLECT Case Study

Three nurses were getting ready for the shift change report outside the room of an older adult client. Kim Nelson whispered to the other two nurses, Pam Troy and Randy Carson, "The doctor ordered the wrong dosage for Mr. Stivers. It took more than an hour to get in contact with her to clarify the order."

Mr. Carson shook his head, knowing that this had become a common problem on their unit. "So, Kim, did she finally fix the order?"

Ms. Nelson sighed and said, "Yes, but it didn't end there. Shortly after I gave Mr. Stivers the medication, he had difficulty breathing."

Ms. Troy felt worried about this. She had been a nurse for only 2 years, but she knew that any problems when a medication is given are of critical concern. "Well, was it still the wrong dosage?"

Ms. Nelson avoided looking at the other two nurses. "I need to get ready for report."

Mr. Carson was also concerned. "Wait, Kim. What happened?"

"Okay, so then I found out he's allergic to the medication I gave him."

Ms. Troy spoke up again. "Are you going to do an incident report?"

Ms. Nelson shook her head. "No, I don't want to be sued or lose my job."

1. Is this case an example of nursing negligence? Explain.

2. What is the evidence in this case that this issue may need an incident report?

3. What further information should the nurse assess before reporting an error?

4. Who else needs to know that there was a medication error with the client?

■ REFERENCES

Anselmi, K. K. (2012). Nurses' personal liability vs. employer's vicarious liability. *MEDSURG Nursing, 21*(1), 45–48.

Bashaw, E. S., & Lounsbury, K. (2012). Forging a new culture: Blending Magnet® principles with just culture. *Nursing Management, 43*(10), 49–53.

Birchley, G. (2010). What limits, if any, should be placed on a parent's right to consent and/or refuse to consent to medical treatment for their child? *Nursing Philosophy, 11*, 280–285.

Bova, C., Drexler, D., & Sullivan-Bolyai, S. (2012). Reframing the influence of the Health Insurance Portability and Accountability Act on research. *CHEST, 141*(3), 782–786.

Clabots, S. (2012). Strategies to help initiate and maintain the end-of-life discussion with patients and family members. *MEDSURG Nursing, 21*(4), 197–204.

Cohen, A., & Nirenberg, A. (2011). Current practices in advance care planning. *Clinical Journal of Oncology Nursing, 15*(5), 547–553.

Cole, C. A. (2012). Implied consent and nursing practice: Ethical or convenient? *Nursing Ethics, 19*(4), 550–557.

Cornock, M. (2011). Whistleblowing: A legal commentary. *Nursing Children & Young People, 23*(8), 20–21.

Daly, J. M., Klein, A. N., & Jogerst, G. J. (2012). Critical care nurses' perspectives on elder abuse. *Nursing in Critical Care, 17*(4), 172–179.

DeLa Cruz, C. R. F., Caillouet, B., & Guerrero, S. S. (2012). Strategic patient education program to prevent catheter-related bloodstream infection. *Clinical Journal of Oncology Nursing, 16*(1), E9–E14.

Douglas, M. K., Pierce, J. U., Rosenkoetter, M., Pacquiao, D. F., Callister, L.C., Hattar-Pollara, M., … & Purnell, L. (2011). Standards of practice for culturally competent nursing care: 2011 update. *Journal of Transcultural Nursing, 22*(4), 317–333.

Eisbach, S. S. & Driessnack, M. (2010). Am I sure I want to go down this road? Hesitations in the reporting of child maltreatment by nurses. *Journal for Specialists in Pediatric Nursing, 15*(4), 317–323.

Eisenberg, S. (2010, April). Protect yourself from nursing negligence or malpractice. *ONS Connect,* p. 25.

Fero, L. J., O'Donnell, J. M., Zullo, T. G. , Dabbs, A. D., Kitutu, J., Samosky, J. T., & Hoffman, L. A. (2010). Critical thinking skills in nursing students: Comparison of simulation-based performance with metrics. *Journal of Advanced Nursing, 66*(10), 2182–2193. doi:10.1111/j.1365-2648.2010.05385.x.

Goodwin, K. D., Taylor, M. M., Brown, E. C., Winscott, M., Scanlon, M., Hodge, J. G., Jr., … & England, B (2012). Protecting adolescents' right to seek treatment for sexually transmitted diseases without parental consent: The Arizona experience with Senate Bill 1309. *Public Health Reports, 127*, 253–258.

Graham, B. C. (2012). Examining evidence-based interventions to prevent inpatient falls. *MEDSURG Nursing, 25*(1), 267–270.

Guido, G. W. (2010). *Legal and ethical issues in nursing* (5th ed.). Upper Saddle River, NJ: Prentice Hall.

Guttmacher Institute. (2010). *An overview of minors' consent law.* Retrieved from http://www.guttmacher.org/statecenter/spibs/spib_OMCL.pdf.

Hayrinen, K., Lammintakanen, J., & Saranto, K. (2010). Evaluation of electronic nursing documentation: Nursing process model and standardized terminologies as keys to visible and transparent nursing. *International Journal of Medical Informatics, 79*, 554–564.

Jackson, D., Peters, K., Andrew, S., Edenborough, M., Halcomb, E., Luck, L., … & Wilkes, L. (2010). Trial and retribution: A qualitative study of whistleblowing and workplace relationships in nursing. *Contemporary Nurse, 36*(1–2), 34–44.

Jarrin, O. F. (2010). Core elements of U.S. nurse practice acts and incorporation of nursing diagnosis language. *International Journal of Nursing Terminologies and Classifications, 21*(4), 166–176.

Johnstone, M. (2011). Nursing and justice as a basic human need. *Nursing Philosophy, 12*(1), 34–44. doi:10.1111/j.1466-769X.2010.00459.x.

Kable, A., Guest, M., & McLeod, M. (2012). Organizational risk management of resistance to care episodes in health facilities. *Journal of Advanced Nursing 68*(9), 1933–1943. doi:10.1111/j.1365-2648.2011.05874.x.

Katner, D. R. (2012). Mandatory reporting of oral injuries indicating possible child abuse. *Journal of the American Dental Association, 143*(10), 1087–1092.

Lachman, V. (2008). Ethics, law, and policy. Whistleblowers: Troublemakers or virtuous nurses? *MEDSURG Nursing, 17*(2), 128–134.

Lachman, V. D. (2012). Applying the ethics of care to your nursing practice. *MEDSURG Nursing, 21*(2), 112–115.

Lipley, N. (2012). Service failures put down to poor monitoring of patients. *Emergency Nurse, 20*(8), 5.

Mansbach, A., & Bachner, Y. G. (2010). Internal or external whistleblowing: Nurses' willingness to report wrongdoing. *Nursing Ethics, 17*(4), 483–490.

National Council of State Boards of Nursing (NCSBN). (2010). *NCLEX 2010.* Retrieved from https://www.ncsbn.org/NCLEX.htm.

National Council of State Boards of Nursing (NCSBN). (2011). *Nurse Licensure Compact.* Retrieved from https://www.ncsbn.org/2011_NLCA_factsheet_students_Rev_Jan_2011.pdf.

National Council of State Boards of Nursing (NCSBN). (2012). *A profile of nursing discipline in the U.S.* Retrieved from https://www.ncsbn.org/3858.htm.

National Council of State Boards of Nursing (NCSBN). (2013). *Current research agenda.* Retrieved from https://www.ncsbn.org/2635.htm.

National Practitioner Data Bank (NPDB). (2011). *National Practitioner Data Bank annual report.* Retrieved from http://www.npdb-hipdb.hrsa.gov/resources/annualRpt.jsp.

National Whistleblowers Center. (2010). *Healthcare bill enhances whistleblower protections.* Retrieved from http://www.whistleblowers.org/index.php?option=com_content&task=view&id=1062&Itemid=178.

North Carolina Board of Nursing. (2012). *Nursing practice.* Retrieved from http://www.ncbon.com/content.aspx?id=34.

Nys, H. (2012). The right to informed choice and the patient's rights directive. *European Journal of Health Law, 19*, 327–331.

Ofi, B., & Sowunmi, O. (2012). Nursing documentation: Experience of the use of the nursing process model in selected hospitals in Ibadan, Oyo State, Nigeria. *International Journal of Nursing Practice, 18*(4), 354–362. doi:10.1111/j.1440-172X.2012.02044.x.

Ryan, D., & Jezewski, M. A. (2012). Knowledge, attitudes, experiences, and confidence of nurses in completing advance directives: A systematic synthesis of three studies. *The Journal of Nursing Research, 20*(2), 131–140.

Shepard, L. H. (2011). Creating a foundation for a Just Culture workplace. *Nursing, 41*(8), 46–48.

Time, V., Payne, B. K., & Gainey, R. R. (2010). Don't help victims of crime if you don't have the time: Assessing support for Good Samaritan laws. *Journal of Criminal Justice, 38*, 790–795.

Tzeng, H.-M., Yin, C. Y., & Schneider, T. E. (2013). Medication error–related issues in nursing practice. *MEDSURG Nursing, 22*(1), 13–16, 50.

Vogelsmeier, A., Scott-Cawiezell, J., Miller, B., & Griffith, S. (2010). Influencing leadership perceptions of patient safety through just culture training. *Journal of Nursing Care Quality 25*(4), 288–294.

Wekerle, C. (2012). Resilience in the context of child maltreatment: Connections to the practice of mandatory reporting. *Child Abuse & Neglect, 37*, 93–101.

Wiener, J. A., & Gilliland, A. T. (2011). Balancing between two goods: Health Insurance Portability and Accountability Act and ethical compliancy considerations for privacy-sensitive materials in health sciences archival and historical special collections. *Journal of the Medical Library Association, 99*(1), 15–22.

Pearson Nursing Student Resources   Find additional review materials at: **nursing.pearsonhighered.com**

50 Quality Improvement

MODULE AT-A-GLANCE

The Concept of Quality Improvement, 2681

◪ THE CONCEPT OF QUALITY IMPROVEMENT

The Institute of Medicine (IOM) (2001) has defined **quality** as "the degree to which health services for individuals and populations increase the likelihood of desired health outcomes and are consistent with current professional knowledge." In addition, high-quality care involves "providing patients with appropriate services in a technically competent manner, with good communication, shared decision making, and cultural sensitivity" (IOM, 2001).

Nurses can provide high-quality care by participating in quality improvement and quality management. **Quality improvement** consists of "systematic and continuous actions that lead to measurable improvement in healthcare services and the health status of targeted patient groups" (Health Resources and Services Administration [HRSA], 2011). **Quality management** includes evaluation of medical and nursing processes for quality and effectiveness compared to accepted standards in order to correct problems before they harm clients and to prevent errors in treatment. Quality management also aims to provide cost-effective care by preventing overuse, misuse, and underuse of medical resources.

Quality improvement, which is an integral part of nursing care, affects physiological outcomes as well as legal and ethical issues and informatics systems (see Concepts Related to Quality Improvement). **<<**

Concept Learning Outcomes

After reading about this concept, you will be able to:

1. Differentiate quality improvement from quality management.
2. Describe federal and state initiatives aimed at quality improvement in health care.
3. Identify and explain the steps involved in quality improvement.
4. Differentiate between intradisciplinary and interdisciplinary assessments.
5. Describe the process of benchmarking.
6. Provide examples of adverse events and the resulting root cause analysis that would be required.
7. Explain common methods used to improve the quality of care.
8. Contrast four quantifiable quality management programs.

Concept Key Terms

Audit, *2685*
Benchmarking, *2684*
Blame-free environment, *2688*
Breach of care, *2687*
Breach of duty, *2687*
Concurrent audit, *2685*
Continuous quality improvement (CQI), *2690*
External clients, *2690*
Indicator, *2686*
Internal clients, *2690*
Intradisciplinary assessment, *2685*
Just culture, *2689*
Lean Six Sigma, *2692*
Outcome standards, *2686*
Outcomes management, *2685*
Patient Protection and Affordable Care Act (PPACA or ACA), *2683*

Peer review, *2685*
Performance improvement, *2685*
Plan–Do–Study–Act (PDSA), *2690*
Process standards, *2686*
Quality, *2681*
Quality assurance, *2689*
Quality improvement, *2681*
Quality management, *2681*
Retrospective audit, *2685*
Risk management, *2687*
Root cause analysis, *2686*
Sentinel event, *2686*
Six Sigma, *2691*
Standards, *2686*
Structure standards, *2686*
Total quality management (TQM), *2690*
Utilization review, *2685*

Concepts Related to **Quality Improvement**

Some ways in which healthcare quality can be improved include properly using advance directives, following privacy laws, and striving to reduce errors. Quality improvement through clinical trials requires legal consent by the client, and researchers must confirm that the new treatment is ethical. Quality improvement also involves using informatics to accurately record a client's medical history and results of diagnostic tests for current and future use and to share client information with relevant healthcare providers in an efficient manner.

CONCEPT	RELATIONSHIP TO QUALITY IMPROVEMENT	NURSING IMPLICATIONS
Ethics		
■ Ethical dilemmas ■ Client rights	Clients have the right to the best quality of care.	■ Anticipate the need to provide high-quality care to all individuals, regardless of race, gender, sexual orientation, or ability to pay for services. ■ Be aware of disparities in treatment among population groups; advocate for high-quality care for all individuals. ■ Consult with clients to determine their preferences for care; provide culturally competent care. ■ Be aware of client preferences that are not ethical, such as refusal of lifesaving blood transfusions for a child.
Informatics		
■ Clinical decision support systems ■ Individual information at point of care	Electronic health records can be used at the point of care and can be easily transmitted to collaborating healthcare workers to improve continuity of care.	■ Anticipate requests from collaborating healthcare workers for client records. ■ Realize the importance of keeping all electronic and paper records up to date. ■ Provide education on the use of electronic records at the point of care. ■ Use informatics to identify areas for improvement, such as tracking healthcare-associated infections or identifying geographic locations that are without adequate healthcare resources.
Legal Issues		
■ Advance directives ■ HIPAA ■ Just culture ■ Mandatory reporting ■ Nurse practice acts ■ Risk management	Consistently following federal and state laws will improve the quality of client care.	■ Be alert to potential abusive situations; quality of care can be improved by preventing future abuse. ■ Be alert to behavior of healthcare workers (including self) that could increase risk of harm to clients or violate the client's privacy; seek to counsel individuals performing reckless acts. ■ Anticipate asking clients or family members about legal documents such as living wills, healthcare proxy, preference for do-not-resuscitate orders. ■ Avoid blaming healthcare workers for inadvertent mistakes that result in client harm; instead, console the individual and provide education on how to avoid future errors. ■ Participate in efforts to improve laws and healthcare protocols and treatments.

▶ IMPROVING THE QUALITY OF HEALTH CARE

In its report *To Err Is Human: Building a Safer Health System,* the IOM (2000) stated that medical errors account for approximately 98,000 deaths per year. Since this report's release, multiple studies have investigated the incidence of preventable medical errors. Internal review of 10 North Carolina hospitals found that more than 60% of identified harms (i.e., adverse events associated with procedures, medications, infections, diagnostic tests, falls, and other causes) were preventable. Most (84.3%) adverse outcomes stemming from these events were temporary, but some caused permanent harm, were life threatening, or contributed to the client's death (Landrigan et al., 2010). Similarly, a report from the Office of the Inspector General in the U.S. Department of Health and Human Services stated that about 27% of Medicare beneficiaries discharged from hospitals experienced an adverse event or temporary harm. Physicians determined that approximately 44% of these adverse or temporary harm events were preventable. Preventable events were linked to medical errors, substandard care, and lack of client monitoring and assessment (Levinson, 2010).

In 2001, the IOM released a follow-up report entitled *Crossing the Quality Chasm: A New Health System for the 21st Century.* This report concluded that the current healthcare system is too disorganized to adequately care for individuals with multiple chronic illnesses. The report suggests that a new healthcare system should be developed that improves care, partly through the use of rapidly advancing technology. In an effort to improve the healthcare system, *Crossing the Quality Chasm* proposed six aims for improvement: The healthcare system should be safe, effective, patient centered, timely, efficient, and equitable (**Figure 50–1 ●**).

▶ NATIONAL INITIATIVES

Following the IOM reports, the healthcare industry began to embrace quality improvement. The need to improve client safety and health outcomes and to implement changes to support these improvements was obvious to individuals working at every level of health care. State and federal governments have also contributed to initiatives aimed at improving the quality of health care.

Federal Initiatives

Governmental agencies such as the U.S. Department of Health and Human Services (USDHHS), physicians groups such as the American Medical Association, and professional nursing organizations such as the American Nurses Association (ANA) have developed indicators of high-quality care and measures to document the quality of care. Three important efforts include the development of the National Database of Nursing Quality Indicators™ (NDNQI), the publication of *Patient Safety and Quality: An Evidence-Based Handbook for Nurses,* and the development of National Patient Safety Goals by the Joint Commission. These programs and documents aim to collect and provide data that identify areas for improvement and encourage facilities to meet quality goals.

More recently, the **Patient Protection and Affordable Care Act (PPACA or ACA),** called the Affordable Care Act, was passed by Congress and signed into law by President Barack Obama on March 23, 2010. This 906-page law, along with its thousands of pages of regulations, attempts to make health care affordable for all Americans. Changes to the healthcare system that are detailed in the ACA will be implemented between 2010 and 2020. Some of these changes include the following:

■ Insurance premiums will be available at a reduced price from a health insurance exchange for individuals and families between 100% and 400% above the federal poverty level.

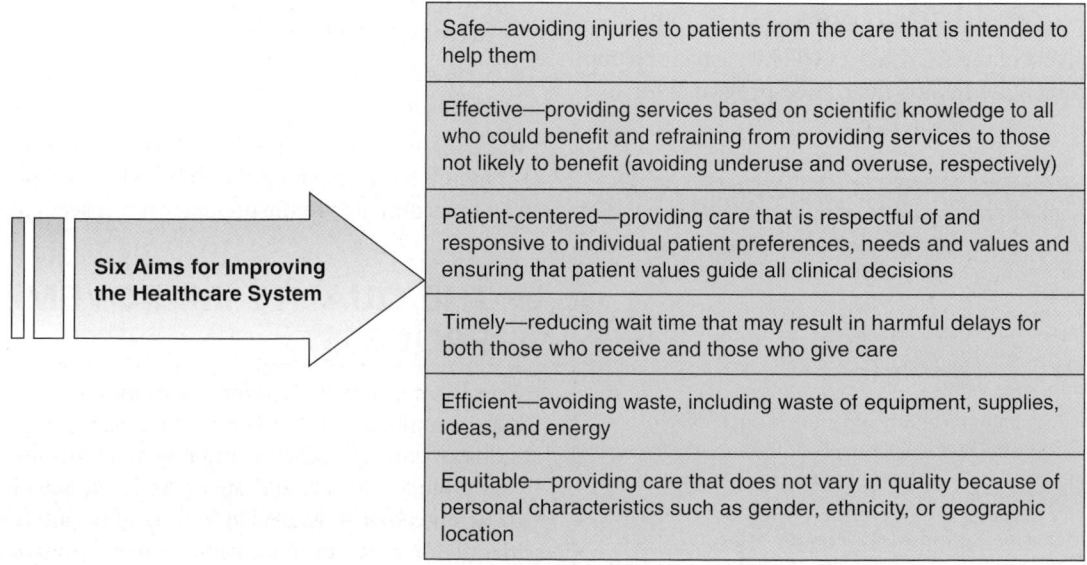

Six Aims for Improving the Healthcare System

Safe—avoiding injuries to patients from the care that is intended to help them
Effective—providing services based on scientific knowledge to all who could benefit and refraining from providing services to those not likely to benefit (avoiding underuse and overuse, respectively)
Patient-centered—providing care that is respectful of and responsive to individual patient preferences, needs and values and ensuring that patient values guide all clinical decisions
Timely—reducing wait time that may result in harmful delays for both those who receive and those who give care
Efficient—avoiding waste, including waste of equipment, supplies, ideas, and energy
Equitable—providing care that does not vary in quality because of personal characteristics such as gender, ethnicity, or geographic location

Figure 50–1 ● Six aims for improving the healthcare system.

- Individuals will pay a maximum of 8% of their income for health insurance premiums through the exchange.
- Small businesses with more than 50 employees are required to purchase health insurance for their employees or pay a tax.
- Insurance plans must cover preventive services.
- Insurance companies will no longer be able to deny coverage to individuals with preexisting conditions or drop individuals when they become sick.
- Medicare and Medicaid will be expanded and reformed.
- The "donut hole" in Medicare prescription coverage will be closed to provide affordable prescriptions for older adults.
- Healthcare facilities will be rewarded financially for quality rather than quantity of medical care to reduce wasteful spending.
- The cost increases associated with the ACA will be covered by tax increases for specific individuals and businesses.

⬢ **Stay Current:** *Learn more about the Affordable Care Act at* **http://www.hhs.gov/healthcare/rights/**.

As a response to the ACA, the USDHHS (2011) has developed a National Strategy for Quality Improvement in Health Care. This strategy contains three broad aims:

- ***Better Care:*** Improve the overall quality, by making health care more client centered, reliable, accessible, and safe.
- ***Healthy People/Healthy Communities:*** Improve the health of the U.S. population by supporting proven interventions to address behavioral, social, and environmental determinants of health in addition to delivering higher-quality care.
- ***Affordable Care:*** Reduce the cost of quality health care for individuals, families, employers, and government.

To advance these aims, the National Quality Strategy will focus on six priorities (see **Box 50–1** ●).

State and Local Initiatives

Even with the advent of the ACA, states will be partially responsible for providing state health insurance programs for low-

---

Box 50–1   Six Priorities for High-Quality Care

Priorities for improving health outcomes and increasing the effectiveness of care for all populations include the following (USDHHS, 2011):

- Make care safer by reducing harm caused in the delivery of care.
- Ensure that each individual and family is engaged as partners in their care.
- Promote effective communication and coordination of care.
- Promote the most effective prevention and treatment practices for the leading causes of mortality, starting with cardiovascular disease.
- Work with communities to promote wide use of best practices to enable healthy living.
- Make high-quality care more affordable for individuals, families, employers, and governments by developing and spreading new healthcare delivery models.

---

income individuals and families. The ACA offers states the option of implementing a basic health program (BHP) for low-income adults and legal immigrants. Under the BHP, states would contract with health plans and providers to provide at least the minimum essential benefits under the ACA, and the federal government would help subsidize the program (Dorn, 2011).

In addition to federal funds, states are using other funding sources to provide insurance to low-income individuals. Funding sources are often tied to taxes of specific items or individuals, including specific types of medical providers or services; unhealthy items such as cigarettes, alcohol, or soft drinks; and tobacco settlement or gambling funds. Some states, such as Massachusetts, were attempting universal coverage before the ACA was signed into law, and these efforts are still ongoing. Massachusetts is using redirected federal funds, insurance surcharges, hospital assessments, the state general fund, employer assessment, and other sources to provide insurance and high-quality care for all individuals in the state. Indiana has implemented the Healthy Indiana Plan, which expands public insurance eligibility to low-income uninsured parents and childless adults who are not eligible for Medicaid. This program is financed by federal funds, disproportionate share hospital payments, and a tax on cigarettes (Burke & Fox, 2009).

High-quality care is also provided at the state level by community health centers (CHCs). CHCs are state or federally funded facilities that provide health care to uninsured and underinsured populations. CHCs provide their services at a reduced cost, saving the state millions of dollars every year. Individuals can receive regular checkups, preventive services, and as-needed care, decreasing the volume of emergency care needed. This improves the general health of the population and avoids the higher costs of emergency care. CHCs are nonprofit agencies that must comply with four key regulations:

- CHCs must serve a medically underserved area or population.
- CHCs must provide comprehensive primary care, which often includes medical, dental, and eye care; preventive and diagnostic services; education; and translation services.
- CHCs must adjust fees and charges based on the client's ability to pay.
- CHCs must be governed by a board on which over half of the members are clients at the CHC, which keeps the health center accountable to the population it is serving.

▶ THE QUALITY IMPROVEMENT PROCESS

Quality improvement is a continuous multistep, multilevel process that identifies areas for improvement based on performance and industry standards. Quality improvement involves analyzing current protocols of care and their associated outcomes, comparing those outcomes to leaders in high-quality care (**benchmarking**), identifying areas for improvement, researching factors that contribute to better outcomes, and implementing changes to improve outcomes. Client outcomes must then be analyzed to determine the effectiveness of the changes and identify areas for further improvement. In addition, if a facility consistently provides a better quality of care in comparison to similar facilities, the facility that is demonstrating excellence is responsible for documenting its methods to help improve care at other facilities. When quality improvement is directly linked to the performance of an individual, team, unit, or organization, it is called **performance improvement**.

Analysis of Current Protocols and Outcomes

To begin quality improvement, an individual, unit, or facility must understand its baseline performance records. Performance can be assessed on an intradisciplinary level or an interdisciplinary level. In addition, it can focus on client outcomes, cost effectiveness, resource utilization, or the integration of these aspects of care.

INTRADISCIPLINARY ASSESSMENT **Intradisciplinary assessment** occurs within a group of individuals who have similar positions within a healthcare system, such as a group of nurses or a group of surgeons. An intradisciplinary assessment is important for identifying areas of improvement at each level of care. Intradisciplinary assessment includes peer reviews, audits, and outcomes management.

A **peer review** is used to professionally critique a colleague's work based on predetermined standards. This allows nurses to assess other nurses in a safe and nonpunitive environment. Using this process, nurses are together able to analyze complicated cases and determine the standards by which they will collectively be held accountable. It also allows issues to be discussed by those with firsthand knowledge and produces recommendations that the nursing staff will understand and accept.

Audits An **audit** is an examination of records to verify accuracy and proper use. An audit usually examines financial or medical records, and the audit can be for a single client, a group of similar clients, an individual clinician, a unit, or a whole facility. If the audit is focused on one discipline (e.g., nursing), it is an intradisciplinary assessment. If the audit is focused on multiple disciplines (e.g., both nurses and physicians), it becomes an interdisciplinary assessment.

In nursing, most audits are either retrospective or concurrent. A **retrospective audit** is performed after a client's discharge. It evaluates care provided to one client with care provided to clients with similar conditions, and recommendations are made to change procedures if needed. A **concurrent audit** is performed while the client is still undergoing care at the healthcare facility. It is used to evaluate the adequacy of the nursing care the client is receiving and to determine if desired outcomes are being met. This allows changes to be made, if needed, to prevent adverse events or improve the client's care.

Outcomes Management **Outcomes management** uses client experiences to guide improvement in all areas of health care by providing a link between medical interventions and health outcomes and between health outcomes and cost of care. An outcomes management system implements evidence-based practices, guides case decision making, incorporates better and more efficient clinical management, and provides information to improve services (Hodges & Wotring, 2012). Outcomes management can be used both to discover areas for improvement and to analyze areas of excellence to determine factors that contribute to success or failure. In 2004, the National Institutes of Health (n.d.) began an outcomes management program called PROMIS® (Patient Reported Outcomes Measurement Information System) that collects information from clients to measure their health status in the areas of physical, mental, and social well-being. This program continues to provide clinicians with access to client-reported information about the effectiveness of treatments and the symptoms that clients experience to help improve communication, manage chronic diseases, and design treatment plans.

INTERDISCIPLINARY ASSESSMENT Client care involves collaboration among multiple disciplines. For example, a client with obesity and type 2 diabetes who is recovering from bariatric surgery may require care from a surgeon, physician, nurse, and dietitian. To collaborate effectively, these disciplines must have efficient communication, coordination, and integration of care. In addition to peer reviews, audits, and outcomes management, interdisciplinary assessments include utilization reviews.

Utilization Review A **utilization review** analyzes the use of resources to identify areas of overuse, misuse, and underuse. This protects the facility from unnecessary and inappropriate use of resources. Utilization review is required by Medicaid for specific services and by the Joint Commission for facility accreditation. A utilization review may identify areas in which resources are being overused, such as urinary catheterization for incontinent clients who are ambulatory, or areas in which resources are lacking, such as inadequate staffing.

CASE STUDY \\ A

Ruth Davison is a 74-year-old woman who has been admitted to the same-day surgery center for elective right carpal tunnel repair (CTR). One hour prior to surgery, Mrs. Davison receives cefazolin (Ancef) 1 g IV as a prophylactic antibiotic. Anesthesia for the procedure consists of injection of local anesthetic at the surgical site with no administration of sedation.

Following completion of the CTR, Mrs. Davison is stable, awake, and alert. She is monitored in the postanesthesia care unit (PACU) for 1 hour. After meeting all discharge criteria, she is prepared for discharge to her home. Mrs. Davison's discharge instructions include keeping her surgical dressing in place for 2 days, after which time she may remove the dressing. She is further instructed to keep the dressing clean and dry while it is in place and to immediately report any drainage noted on the dressing. Mrs. Davison also is instructed to immediately report any redness, drainage, or swelling noted at her incision site following dressing removal. She is further advised that her sutures are absorbable and, thus, do not need to be removed. After verbalizing understanding of her discharge instructions and signing the discharge record, Mrs. Davison is transported to her home by her daughter.

The following morning, the same-day surgery center receives a phone call from Mrs. Davison, who reports that she has removed her dressing and now notes "a little" bleeding and redness at her incision site. After reviewing Mrs. Davison's discharge record, the nurse reminds Mrs. Davison that her instructions included leaving

for any adverse event. The goals of the root cause analysis are to identify areas of improvement that would decrease the likelihood of future adverse events and to develop an action plan for improvement. This analysis focuses on systems and processes, not on individual performance, and it analyzes both special causes (factors that cause variation above what is normal) and common causes (factors that occur because of normal variation in the system). The action plan should include identification of who is responsible for implementing and overseeing improvements, pilot testing to ensure the success of the changes, time lines for implementing changes, and strategies for measuring the effectiveness of changes (Joint Commission, 2013).

REDUCING MEDICATION ERRORS Medication errors injure approximately 1.3 million people annually in the United States, with an average of at least one death every day (Food and Drug Administration [FDA], 2009). The National Coordinating Council for Medication Error Reporting and Prevention (n.d.) defines a medication error as "any preventable event that may cause or lead to inappropriate medication use or patient harm while the medication is in the control of the health care professional, patient, or consumer." Medication errors usually result from multiple causes, including poor communication; ambiguities in product names, directions for use, medical abbreviations, or writing; poor procedures or techniques; and poor client understanding. Job stress, lack of product knowledge or training, and similar labeling or packaging may also contribute to medication error (FDA, 2009).

Several national- and facility-implemented interventions have been designed to decrease medication errors, including bar coding both clients and medications, regulating similar names of drugs that may cause confusion, and using a computerized physician order entry system. Many other interventions specifically help nurses prevent medication errors (**Box 50–2 ●**).

Box 50–2 Methods to Reduce Medication Errors

Nurses can implement several methods to reduce medication errors, including the following:

- Double check the "six rights" *every time* medication is administered: right individual, right medication, right dose, right time, right route, and right documentation.
- Have a second nurse check the medication order.
- Check known allergies before administering medication to a client.
- Avoid disruptions and distractions during medication administration duties.
- Verify tubing placement (e.g., IV, chest, NG) before administering drugs or nutrition.
- Document and understand the interactions among ALL medications a client is taking, including over-the-counter medicines, herbal remedies, and nutritional supplements.
- Do not combine medications with the same active ingredient.
- Always check a child's weight before medication administration to ensure correct dosing.
- Consult with the client's physician and a pharmacist if unsure about a medication order.
- Maintain a current resource to reference for drugs that are not familiar.
- Provide thorough education to clients about the use of all medications.

STAFFING PRACTICES IN NURSING Multiple studies have established a link between decreased nurse staffing and adverse client outcomes. One consideration of nurse staffing is the nurse-to-client ratio (quantity). When comparing the total hours of nursing care per inpatient day, an increased number of nursing hours was associated with lower rates of congestive heart failure mortality, failure to rescue, infections, prolonged length of stay, and decubitus ulcers (Blegen et al., 2011). However, nursing skill is also a critical factor related to client outcomes (quality). One study found that an increase in the ratio of LPN hours to total nursing hours was associated with an increase in mortality and sepsis in trauma clients (Glance et al., 2012). The quantity and quality of nursing staff are often reflected by nursing-sensitive indicators (**Box 50–3 ●**).

RESOURCE UTILIZATION The value of health care can be increased by reducing costs while maintaining or increasing the quality of care. This can be accomplished by implementing measures to reduce waste, including unnecessary or inefficient services, prices that are too high, excess administrative costs, missed prevention opportunities, and medical fraud (IOM, 2010). Examples of waste directly applicable to nurses include medical errors that result in prolonged inpatient days, scheduling an additional visit for client education only, and lost time because of unorganized supplies, poorly maintained equipment, or inadequate documentation.

BLAME-FREE ENVIRONMENT According to the IOM's report *To Err Is Human* (2000), most errors in health care are a result of the healthcare system and not the fault of any single individual. If a clinician is afraid to report errors for fear of punishment or because reporting does not result in positive change, then problems within the system cannot be identified and addressed. Therefore, a key component in quality improvement is establishing a **blame-free environment** in which healthcare

---

Box 50–3 Nursing-Sensitive Indicators

Nursing-sensitive indicators reflect the quantity and quality of nursing care in the areas of structure, process, and outcome (ANA, n.d.; NDNQI, n.d.).

STRUCTURE	OUTCOME
■ Nursing hours per client day	■ Healthcare-associated infections (e.g., catheter-associated UTI, central line–associated bloodstream infections, ventilator-associated pneumonia)
■ Nursing turnover	
■ RN education/certification	
■ Nursing skill mix (RN, LPN/LVN, UAP, agency staff)	■ Client falls (with or without injury and injury level)
PROCESS	■ Pressure ulcer rate (community-, hospital-, or unit-acquired)
■ Pain assessment, intervention, reassessment (AIR) cycles completed	■ Psychiatric physical or sexual assault
■ Peripheral intravenous infiltration rate	
■ RN job satisfaction	■ Physical restraint prevalence
■ RN Practice Environment Scale (PES)	■ Client satisfaction

providers can report errors or near misses without the fear of punishment (Agency for Healthcare Research and Quality [AHRQ], 2012). This helps identify problems so corrections can be made and future adverse events can be prevented. The Evidence-Based Practice feature discusses methods for reducing errors and increasing the reporting of errors.

One difficulty in establishing a blame-free environment is that while many errors are a result of the healthcare system, some errors are the result of personal mistakes and demand accountability. **Just culture** attempts to balance the blame-free environment with appropriate accountability by focusing on correcting problems that lead individuals to engage in unsafe behavior while maintaining individual accountability by establishing zero tolerance for reckless behavior (AHRQ, 2012). Just culture differentiates between human error, at-risk behavior, and reckless behavior in contrast to the "no blame" approach of the blame-free environment.

PERSONAL RESPONSIBILITY   All nurses must be involved in quality improvement. The nursing student demonstrates concern for quality by making a commitment never to perform an act that the student is uncertain how to perform, by showing accountability for his actions, and by admitting to errors if they occur. Each nurse, whether a nursing student or a practicing nurse, has the responsibility to know the policies and procedures in the facility where clinical training is performed and to follow them exactly. In addition, nurses are responsible for understanding how to report errors, including paperwork that should be completed and individuals to whom errors should be reported.

Implementation of New Protocols

When a problem has been identified and a plan put in place to improve the quality of care, that plan must be implemented. The most important step in implementing new procedures is educating nurses and other clinicians about the importance of the new process, the steps involved, and associated reporting procedures. Education can take place in large or small groups, as a self-study, or during orientation. Each individual must then take personal responsibility to see that she implements the needed changes to improve the quality of care.

Evaluation of Efficacy of New Protocols

Finally, the implemented changes must be evaluated to assess their impact on client care, client outcomes, client and clinician satisfaction, and resource utilization. Data related to the original problem must be collected and are then analyzed based on the benchmark standards to determine if standards are being met. This process is called **quality assurance**. If standards are not met, the quality improvement is continued with the goal of achieving the desired goals.

Evidence-Based Practice   Methods to Reduce Errors

Problem

The most effective way to identify and correct problems in health care is by consistently reporting errors. However, studies indicate that errors are rarely reported, even in a blame-free environment (Wubben et al., 2010).

Evidence

One method to reduce medical errors is to eliminate barriers to error reporting. The primary reasons that healthcare workers do not report errors are the fear of being blamed and the fear of being punished (Gorini, Miglioretti, & Pravettoni, 2012). Other reasons include increased time associated with paperwork, a fear of lawsuits, self-perceptions of incompetence, embarrassment or guilt about the mistake, reluctance to incriminate other providers, lack of knowledge about what constitutes an error or how to report errors, and lack of feedback when errors are reported (Wolf & Hughes, 2008; Wubben et al., 2010). In addition, many clinicians do not realize that near-misses and errors that do not cause harm should also be reported (Wolf & Hughes, 2008).

Another method to reduce medical errors is to improve the nurses' work environment. The American Association of Critical-Care Nurses (AACN) has established six standards for a healthy work environment: skilled communication, true collaboration, effective decision making, appropriate staffing, meaningful recognition, and authentic leadership (Vollers et al., 2009). In addition, fostering a safety culture can lead to decreased errors and increased reporting. The Association of periOperative Registered Nurses (AORN) (2011) has defined a safety culture as an environment characterized by effective communication, individual accountability, a just culture, and a learning culture.

Implications

Eliminating barriers to error reporting and establishing a healthy work environment can lead to reduced errors and increased reporting of errors. However, changing from the current culture of blame to a safety culture will require time and dedication from the entire organization. As individuals on the front line of client care, nurses play a critical role in the establishment of a safety culture by helping to identify problems and by working to implement changes to practice that will reduce errors. Education about a blame-free environment and personal responsibility to report errors are two ways in which nurses can contribute to quality improvement in health care.

Critical Thinking Application

1. Consider situations in which you, a fellow nurse, or a physician makes medication errors that do not result in client harm. In which situations would you complete an error report?

2. Identify personal barriers that would prevent you from reporting a medical error caused by the system, a coworker, or yourself.

3. Research the current error reporting systems in place at a local hospital, nursing home, and primary care clinic.

▶ COMPONENTS OF QUALITY MANAGEMENT PROGRAMS

The process of quality improvement is accomplished through use of a quality management program. A quality management program must include both information about current practices and outcomes and accountability for those overseeing and performing client care. Advances in technology are vital to quality management, because clinical information systems (see the module on Informatics) can be used to track client outcomes and actions that led to client harm. For example, data from a clinical information system can be used to track the occurrence of healthcare-associated infections, including the location of the infection (e.g., urinary, respiratory, skin), frequency of client assessment, materials used to treat the client, and other relevant factors. Changes in hand washing protocols, equipment and medical supplies used, wound care protocols, and client placement can then be implemented to reduce the incidence of healthcare-associated infections. These changes must then be accepted and used by the entire staff to be successful.

Healthcare organizations use different quality management programs depending on their clientele and specialty area. Common quality management programs include total quality management, continuous quality improvement, Six Sigma, and Lean Six Sigma. Each of these programs includes a comprehensive quality management plan.

Comprehensive Quality Management

A quality management plan is used to help healthcare facilities integrate new programs, models, and technologies with the primary care services that are already in place. The plan should address needs of engagement (improving the experience of care), population health, and value (per capita costs). The quality management plan should be comprehensive, looking at quality and safety in clinical-, managerial-, administrative-, and facility-related aspects of the organization. It should design, implement, monitor, and improve methods to increase the quality of care in keeping with the organization's mission and core values (Benson & Townes, 2011). Most organizations will develop quality management plans that require cooperation between departments as well as unit-specific plans.

Quality management plans should be client focused, collecting and evaluating data for improvement of client outcomes, expectations, and satisfaction. Client satisfaction surveys can be used to track the effectiveness of changes from the client's perspective. Nurses often perform this follow-up through personal visits, forms, or phone calls. If any problems are noted, the nurse can then report back to the healthcare provider or nurse manager to help improve client care.

Total Quality Management

Total quality management (TQM), a comprehensive management philosophy that was invented by Walter Shewhart and made famous by W. Edwards Deming, is used to improve quality and productivity by utilizing data and statistics to improve systems processes. The hallmark of TQM is that it involves teamwork throughout the entire organization, involving all

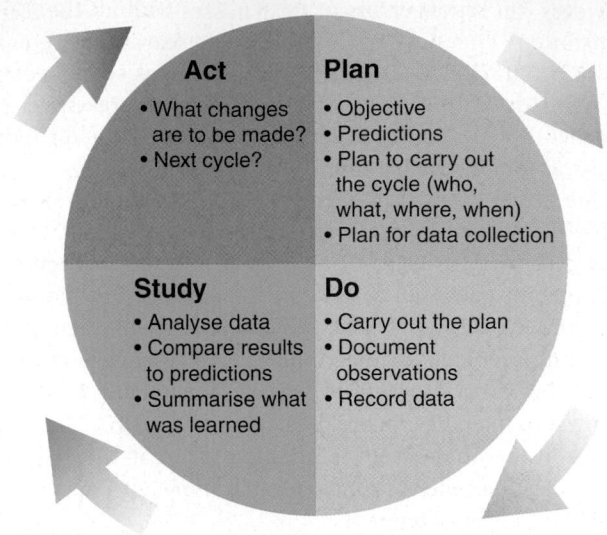

Figure 50–2 ● PDSA cycle.

departments and employees and including both suppliers and customers. Its essential elements include communication, feedback, fact-based decision making, and a focus on continual improvement.

A system of quality improvement most often associated with TQM is Deming's **Plan–Do–Study–Act (PDSA, Figure 50–2 ●)**, which was modified from Shewhart's Plan–Do–Check–Act or Plan–Do–Check–Adjust (PDCA). During planning, individuals on the TQM team define the goal, collect data, and outline a strategy to reach the goal. In the Do phase, the plan is implemented on a small scale to determine whether it will be effective. This is followed by the Study phase, in which the outcomes of the Do phase are analyzed and compared to the expected outcomes. In the Act phase, the team must decide if the goal was met, plan further changes, and decide whether the original goal is attainable based on the results of the previous interventions. If the goal was met, then the team must decide whether the changes should be implemented throughout the entire organization.

Continuous Quality Improvement

In health care, **continuous quality improvement (CQI)** is defined as "a structured organizational process for involving personnel in planning and executing a continuous flow of improvements to provide quality health care that meets or exceeds expectations" (Sollecito & Johnson, 2013, p. 4). CQI can be applied to a specific problem, development and implementation of policies and procedures, resource utilization, or implementation of evidence-based practices.

CQI is a customer-driven process. In health care, the customer can be internal or external to the system. **Internal clients** include employees of a healthcare organization, such as nurses, physicians, therapists, medical record staff, billing specialists, and other employees. **External clients** include those individuals who seek health care, as well as their family members and significant others. External clients also include other individuals and entities with whom internal clients interact—such as insurance companies, managed care organizations, equipment or material suppliers, social service agencies, and law enforcement officials. On the basis of this premise, customer satisfaction is the end goal of CQI. CQI is also system focused. It emphasizes system errors rather than individual errors. Therefore, CQI requires involvement by everyone with knowledge of the system, from senior management to individuals providing everyday care to clients (Sollecito & Johnson, 2013).

CASE STUDY \\ C

An unidentified middle-aged female is transported to the emergency department (ED) by two law enforcement officers. The law enforcement officers report that the individual was observed "wandering around on a highway" and that complaints were received from passing motorists regarding the woman's behavior. The officers also report that, upon their arrival, the woman was unable to provide any identification, nor was she verbally responsive to their questions. She did, however, willingly seat herself in their squad car upon request. The officers state the woman is being transferred to the ED for evaluation, as they are uncertain as to the etiology of her behaviors.

Lynne Bryten, RN, is the ED triage nurse. The unidentified woman, who is clutching a doll, appears to be awake and alert. She is clean and dressed appropriately, and her tennis shoes appear to be relatively new. Ms. Bryten attempts to perform an initial interview, but the woman does not respond to her questions. She permits Ms. Bryten to assess her vital signs, all of which are within normal limits. She exhibits no apparent indications of traumatic injury, and her pupils are equal and responsive to light. Although the woman is not verbally responsive to Ms. Bryten's questions, she appears to follow directions during the assessment. The woman is admitted to the ED as an unidentified client. Ms. Bryten escorts the client and the law enforcement officers into the ED and notifies the ED physician of their arrival.

Dr. Terrence Garvinner, the attending ED physician, receives Ms. Bryten's report. Upon entering the client's room, he introduces himself and performs a brief client assessment. The client remains verbally unresponsive, but she follows Dr. Garvinner's directions. Afterward, Dr. Garvinner asks the law enforcement officers to speak with him privately. The two officers accompany Dr. Garvinner to an empty ED room.

Dr. Garvinner informs the law enforcement officers that the client does not appear to have any physical injury; rather, she may be developmentally delayed. He suggests that the officers check missing person reports and also contact residential treatment centers to determine whether or not the client may have wandered away from one of the local residential care centers. Dr. Garvinner also questions the officers as to why they did not utilize this approach initially. One of the officers responds, "We have no way of knowing if she has a medical problem. That's why we brought her here. Plus, we have other calls coming in—we're swamped." Dr. Garvinner responds, "We have no way of identifying this woman. She appears to be a vulnerable adult who may be lost. We have a full waiting room, but we don't have staff available to serve as detectives. I believe you have an entire department dedicated to performing detective work."

Critical Thinking Questions

1. Identify the internal and external clients in this scenario.
2. Summarize the conflict between the law enforcement officers and the ED physician. Is either argument correct? Why or why not?
3. In the context of health care, how can conflict between internal and external clients affect the client who is seeking treatment or in need of assistance?
4. What additional external clients may be helpful in identifying the client and assisting with her safe return to her residence?
5. How might the process of quality management be applied to address and manage future situations such as the one described in the scenario?

Six Sigma

Six Sigma is a quality improvement program originally implemented by Motorola and General Electric to reduce variation within a process to produce a near-perfect product. Sigma is a Greek letter often used to measure deviation from a standard; to receive a Sigma level of 6, only 3.4 products per million are allowed to be defective. In this system, a defect is defined as anything that could lead to client dissatisfaction. Defects in health care could range from relatively minor problems such as providing the wrong size gown to a client to major problems such as performing an amputation on the wrong limb. Six Sigma primarily uses the **DMAIC** system to improve outcomes (Chand, 2011):

Define the problem, determine a goal, and form a team to address the problem.

Measure: Obtain data related to the current process, the problem, and the desired goal.

Analyze: Look at the data to determine cause-and-effect relationships related to the problem.

Improve: Develop solutions to problems and implement those solutions.

Control: Implement measures to sustain positive changes and continuously monitor the process to ensure goals are being met.

Six Sigma may also use the DMADV methodology, or Define, Measure, Analyze, Design, and Verify.

Six Sigma uses teams of individuals with intimate knowledge of the problem and training in Six Sigma principles. Master Black Belts are experts in Six Sigma who can assist in data calculations and function as a resource for the team. The team is led by a Black Belt with extensive knowledge of Six Sigma. Green Belts are team members with some experience with Six Sigma, and Yellow and White Belts are relatively new to the Six Sigma system. Six Sigma is most successful when the entire organization, including both administrators and clinicians, is involved in planning and implementing changes.

Multiple studies have illustrated the success of the Six Sigma system in health care. In one study, a 92.6% rate of hyponatremia for postoperative kidney transplant clients was improved to a 92.2% rate of normal serum sodium levels after application of Six Sigma principles (Leaphart et al., 2012). In another study, implementation of Six Sigma principles decreased patient transfer times from general medical floors to a critical care area by almost 60%, resulting in increased customer satisfaction, improved utilization of resources, a decreased risk of adverse events, and better economic profit (Silich et al., 2012).

Lean Six Sigma

Lean Six Sigma combines the strategies of Six Sigma, described above, with the Lean system. The objective of the Lean system is to eliminate waste to maximize value. Waste is defined as anything that does not bring value to the customer. Therefore, Lean Six Sigma is a methodology used to reduce waste and provide consistency in the quality of care. It primarily uses the DMAIC system similar to Six Sigma.

REVIEW The Concept of Quality Improvement

RELATE Link the Concepts

Linking the concept of quality improvement with the concept of collaboration:

1. How can the nurse use conflict management skills to resolve client or family member dissatisfaction with care?

2. How does strong interdisciplinary team communication improve the outcomes of total quality management?

Linking the concept of quality improvement with the concept of managing care:

3. How does an effective quality improvement process reduce the cost of care?

4. How does proper care coordination improve the quality of care provided to clients?

REFER Go to Pearson Nursing Student Resources
nursing.pearsonhighered.com

- Additional review materials

REFLECT Case Study

Jose Hernandez is a newly graduated nurse who has successfully passed the NCLEX-RN® and has accepted a job working on a busy genitourinary unit in the local community hospital. During orientation, he is working the evening shift with a preceptor. On this particular evening, the unit has been very busy and the charge nurse asks Jose's preceptor, Fred McFarlane, to take a few clients in addition to acting as a preceptor for Jose with his assigned clients. Fred agrees and instructs Jose to seek him out if he needs help or has any questions.

Quite by accident, Jose notices that Fred makes a medication error when he fails to administer an ordered medication at an appropriate time to one of Fred's assigned clients. Jose doesn't say anything because Fred acknowledges the error independently, but Jose isn't sure what to do at the end of the shift when he realizes that Fred is not going to fill out an incident report.

1. Should an incident report be filled out regarding Fred's late administration of a medication to the client if no harm resulted? Explain the rationale for your answer.

2. Who is responsible for completing an incident report if one is required? Explain.

3. What is Jose's responsibility related to the error if he had no care responsibility related to the client who received the medication later than ordered?

4. How would you handle this situation if you were Jose?

■ REFERENCES

Agency for Healthcare Research and Quality (AHRQ). (2012). *Safety culture.* Retrieved from http://psnet.ahrq.gov/primer.aspx?primerID=5.

American Nurses Association (ANA). (n.d.). *Nursing-sensitive indicators.* Retrieved from http://www.nursingworld.org/MainMenuCategories/ThePracticeofProfessionalNursing/PatientSafetyQuality/Research-Measurement/The-National-Database/Nursing-Sensitive-Indicators_1.

Association of periOperative Registered Nurses (AORN). (2011). *Creating a practice environment of safety* (Position Statement). Denver, CO: Author.

Benson, D. S., & Townes, P. G., Jr. (2011). The Quality Management Plan: A practical, patient-centered template. *National Association of Community Health Centers.* Retrieved from http://iweb.nachc.com/downloads/products/M_MONOGRAPH_11.pdf.

Blegen, M. A., Goode, C. J., Spetz, J., Vaughn, T., & Park, S. H. (2011). Nurse staffing effects on patient outcomes: Safety-net and non-safety-net hospitals. *Medical Care, 49*(4), 406–414. doi:10.1097/MLR/0b013e318202e129.

Burke, C., & Fox, K. (2009). State financing for health coverage initiatives. *Nelson A. Rockefeller Institute of Government.* Retrieved from http://www.rockinst.org/pdf/health_care/2009-06-03-HPRC_State_Financing.pdf.

Chand, D. V. (2011). Observational study using the tools of Lean Six Sigma to improve the efficiency of the resident rounding process. *Journal of Graduate Medical Education, 3*(2), 144–150.

Dorn, S. (2011). The basic health program option under federal health reform: Issues for consumers and states (Prepared for State Coverage Initiatives, Robert Wood Johnson Foundation). *Urban Institute.* Retrieved from http://www.urban.org/uploadedpdf/412322-Basic-Health-Program-Option.pdf.

Food and Drug Administration (FDA). (2009). *Medication error reports.* Retrieved from http://www.fda.gov/Drugs/DrugSafety/MedicationErrors/ucm080629.htm.

Glance, L. G., Dick, A. W., Osler, T. M., Mukamel, D. B., Li, Y., & Stone, P. W. (2012). The association between nurse staffing and hospital outcomes in injured patients. *BMC Health Services Research, 12*, 247. doi:10.1186/1472-6963-12-247.

Gorini, A., Miglioretti, M., & Pravettoni, G. (2012). A new perspective on blame culture: An experimental study. *Journal of Evaluation in Clinical Practice, 18*(3), 671–675. doi:10.1111/j.1365-2753.2012.01831.x.

Guido, G. W. (2010). *Legal and ethical issues in nursing.* Upper Saddle River, NJ: Pearson.

Health Resources and Services Administration (HRSA). (2011). *Quality improvement.* Retrieved from http://www.hrsa.gov/quality/toolbox/508pdfs/qualityimprovement.pdf.

Health Resources and Services Administration (HRSA). (2013). *National Practitioner Data Bank: 2011 annual report.* Retrieved from http://www.npdb-hipdb.hrsa.gov/resources/reports/2011NPDBAnnualReport.pdf.

Hodges, K., & Wotring, J. R. (2012). Outcomes management: Incorporating and sustaining processes critical to using outcome data to guide practical improvement. *Journal of Behavioral Health Services & Research, 39*(2), 130–143. doi:10.1007/s11414-011-9262-y.

Institute of Medicine (IOM). (2000). *To err is human: Building a safer health system.* Washington, DC: National Academies Press.

Institute of Medicine (IOM). (2001). *Crossing the quality chasm: A new health system for the 21st century.* Washington, DC: National Academies Press.

Institute of Medicine (IOM). (2010). *The healthcare imperative: Lowering costs and improving outcomes.* Washington, DC: National Academies Press.

Joint Commission. (2013). *Sentinel event policy and procedures.* Retrieved from http://www.jointcommission.org/Sentinel_Event_Policy_and_Procedures.

Joint Commission Resources. (2012). *Benchmarking in health care.* Oakbrook Terrace, IL: Author.

Landrigan, C. P., Parry, G. J., Bones, C. B., Hackbarth, A. D., Goldman, D. A., & Sharek, P. J. (2010). Temporal trends in rates of patient harm resulting from medical care. *New England Journal of Medicine, 363,* 2124–2134. doi:10.1056/NEJMsa1004404.

Leaphart, C. L., Gonwa, T. A., Mai, M. L., Prendergast, M. B., Wadei, H. M., Tepass, J. J., III, & Taner, C. B. (2012). Formal quality improvement curriculum and DMAIC method results in interdisciplinary collaboration and process improvement in renal transplant patients. *Journal of Surgical Research, 177*(1), 7–13. doi:10.1016/j.jss.2012.03.017.

Levinson, D. R. (2010). *Adverse events in hospitals: National incidence among Medicare beneficiaries* (Report No. OEI-06-09-00090). Washington, DC: U.S. Department of Health and Human Services.

National Coordinating Council for Medication Error Reporting and Prevention. (n.d.) *About medication errors.* Retrieved from http://www.nccmerp.org/about-MedErrors.html.

National Database of Nursing Quality Indicators (NDNQI). (n.d.). *Nursing-sensitive indicators.* Retrieved from http://www.nursingquality.org/data.aspx.

National Institutes of Health. (n.d.). *PROMIS® overview.* Retrieved from http://www.nihpromis.org/about/overview.

Nurses Service Organization. (2009) *CNA HealthPro Nurses Claims Study.* Retrieved from https://www.nso.com/pdfs/db/rnclaimstudy.pdf?fileName=rnclaimstudy.pdf&folder=pdfs/db&isLiveStr=Y&refID=rnstudynsna.

Raso, R., & Gulinello, C. (2010). Creating cultures of safety: Risk management challenges and strategies. *Nursing Management, 41*(12), 26–33. doi:10.1097/01.NUMA.0000390459.88752.0c.

Silich, S. J., Wetz, R. V., Riebling, N., Coleman, C., Khoueiry, G., Rafeh, N. A., … & Szerszen, A. (2012). Using Six Sigma methodology to reduce patient transfer times from floor to critical-care beds. *Journal for Healthcare Quality, 34*(1), 44–54. doi:10.1111/j.1945-1474.2011.00184.x.

Sollecito, W. A., & Johnson, J. K. (2013). *McLaughlin and Kaluzny's continuous quality improvement in health care* (4th ed.). Burlington, MA: Jones & Bartlett.

U.S. Department of Health and Human Services (USDHHS). (2011). *National strategy for quality improvement in health care.* Retrieved from http://www.healthcare.gov/news/reports/nationalqualitystrategy032011.pdf.

Vollers, D., Hill, E., Roberts, C., Dambaugh, L., & Brenner, Z. R. (2009). AACN's healthy work environment standards and an empowering nurse advancement system. *Critical Care Nurse, 29*(6), 20–27.

Wolf, Z. R., & Hughes, R. G. (2008). Error reporting and disclosure. In R.G. Hughes (Ed.), *Patient safety and quality: An evidence-based handbook for nurses.* Rockville, MD: Agency for Healthcare Research and Quality.

Wubben, I., van Manen, J. G., van den Akker, B. J., Vaarties, S. R., & van Harten, W. H. (2010). Equipment-related incidents in the operating room: An analysis of occurrence, underlying causes and consequences for the clinical process. *Quality & Safety in Health Care, 19*(6), e64. doi:10.1136/qshc.2009.037515.

51 Safety

MODULE AT-A-GLANCE

The Concept of Safety, 2695

Exemplar 51.1
Safety Considerations Across the
Life Span, 2708

Exemplar 51.2
Workplace Safety, 2715

◪ THE CONCEPT OF SAFETY

Despite the best intentions of healthcare professionals, approximately 100,000 clients die every year in U.S. hospitals from preventable medical errors (Sebelius & Cote, 2011). In light of this statistic, hospital accidents rank as high as fourth among the 2011 leading causes of death—higher than influenza, homicide, and motor vehicle crashes (Hoyert & Xu, 2012). The combined costs of these preventable mistakes—which include additional hospital care, disability, and lost income—run as high as $50 billion a year (Kohn, Corrigan, & Donaldson, 1999).

In 1999, the Institute of Medicine (IOM) released the findings of a study designed to take an in-depth look at the overwhelming occurrence of medical errors resulting in preventable injuries and deaths within the United States every year (Kohn et al., 1999). The IOM landmark report, *To Err is Human: Building a Safer Health System*, concluded that the majority of these incidents did not arise from one individual being careless or making mistakes, but rather from the system and conditions within the work environment. Researchers called for improvements in safety protocols, the implementation of which began in the years following the study. While recognizing the value of improved protocols, experts concede that real changes cannot occur without conscious effort on the part of every healthcare professional when working with clients (Agency for Healthcare Research and Quality [AHRQ], 2011; Kohn et al., 1999).

Although clients throughout the life span are subject to potential error-related incidents in all medical settings, children in the hospital setting are at particular risk for preventable injury. The pediatric population is more

(continued on next page)

Concept Learning Outcomes

After reading about this concept, you will be able to:

1. Describe the principle criteria included in a client safety assessment.
2. Identify appropriate nursing diagnoses for the client with potential risks for injury.
3. Describe nursing interventions that reduce the client's risk for injury.
4. Describe the indications for and legal implications of the use of chemical and physical restraints.
5. Explain the purpose of National Patient Safety Goals.
6. Analyze QSEN and KSA competencies and explain their application to client care.

Concept Key Terms

Belt restraints, *2704*
Chemical restraints, *2704*
Hand restraints, *2704*
Healthcare-associated infections (HAIs), *2704*
Knowledge, skills, and attitudes (KSAs), *2699*
Limb restraints, *2704*
Mitt restraints, *2704*
National Patient Safety Goals (NPSGs), *2701*

National patient safety initiatives, *2696*
Physical restraints, *2704*
Quality and Safety Education for Nurses (QSEN), *2699*
Restraints, *2704*
Safety strap body restraints, *2704*
Wrong-site surgery (WSS), *2706*

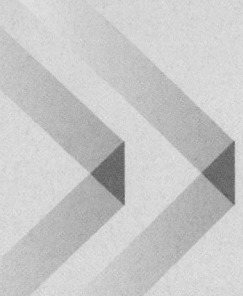

susceptible to adverse pharmacologic events for a number of reasons, including lack of pharmaceutical safety dosing and efficacy studies for children; varying pharmaceutical effects according to the child's stage of development; and dosage calculations requiring the factoring of age, weight, body surface area, and other criteria. Additional risks for children include birth complications, surgical errors, and diagnostic errors. The risk of infection in pediatric clients is also relatively high, particularly when combined with increased length of stay in a hospital and/or the administration of central venous catheters to provide medication (AHRQ, 2011).

Within the IOM report were several strategies for improvement of protocols, including "establishing a national focus to create leadership, research, tools, and protocols to enhance the knowledge base about safety" (Kohn et al., 1999, p. 3). One way to implement this suggestion is through the use of national patient safety initiatives. **<<**

▶ NATIONAL PATIENT SAFETY INITIATIVES

Although the targeted purpose of **national patient safety initiatives** varies, in general these initiatives aim to foster collaboration with healthcare facilities, government agencies, physicians, nurses, and healthcare clients to enhance patient safety and quality of care. These strategies are achieved through education, dissemination of better safety practices and resources, risk management strategies, and reducing medication errors. For examples of the initiatives, see **Table 51–1 ●**.

Even with safety initiatives in place, accurate data are needed to make informed decisions about deficiencies in patient safety, as well as how to remedy those deficiencies. As such, the patient safety initiatives depend on healthcare providers reporting adverse events and their causes. To facilitate this process, in 2005, the Patient Safety and Quality Improvement Act was initiated. While mandating the creation of voluntary and anonymous safety and quality reporting systems on the federal level, the Patient Safety and Quality Improvement Act also protects individuals who report information to patient safety organizations (American Medical Association, 2013).

CASE STUDY \\ A

Carrie Brant is admitted to the hospital complaining of severe back pain, vomiting, and nausea. Following a urinalysis and MRI, Ms. Brant is diagnosed with renal calculi (kidney stones). The physician orders administration of 2 mg of morphine sulfate IV. Two nurses, Peter Martin and Danielle Sanchez, are present when the physician issues the verbal order.

Danielle, who is the client's nurse, withdraws a syringe containing morphine 4 mg/2 mL from the automated medication dispensing system and walks to the client's room. When preparing to withdraw medication for a client assigned to his care, Peter glances at the dispensing receipt that was printed for the previous transaction. In particular, Peter notices that Danielle appears to have obtained twice the dosage of medication ordered for the client. Peter follows Danielle to ask about the discrepancy. By the time Peter arrives at the client's room, Danielle has administered the

morphine to Ms. Brant. When Peter privately inquires as to the amount of medication given, Danielle replies, "I gave all of it— 2 mL." Peter points out that administration of the 2-mL dose means the client actually received morphine 4 mg, as opposed to the ordered dose of 2 mg. Danielle replies that the additional 2 mg of morphine likely will not harm Ms. Brant and that she will monitor her closely. Danielle then asks Peter not to issue an incident report because she is afraid she will be reprimanded and possibly lose her job as a result of her error.

Clinical Thinking Questions

1. How do you believe this situation should be handled? Should Danielle report the error? Explain your answer.
2. What are the ethical considerations involved in reporting vs. not reporting this error?

Quality and Safety Education for Nurses (QSEN)

Nursing education has evolved throughout the years. Initially, nursing education programs consisted of apprenticeships during which new nurses were mentored for a period of time to ensure that graduates had the necessary knowledge for protecting clients and practicing nursing. Nursing education eventually moved into the college system around the 1930s. This migration allowed for a broader fundamental education for nurses, including liberal arts, science, and social science. However, the move had the unintended consequence of creating a gap between education and practice; as nursing instructors left hospitals for the classroom, access to clinical experiences were lost as teachers spent more time in the classroom and less time in healthcare settings (Sullivan, 2010). Even today, nursing students and nurse educators are impacted by the departure from a clinically driven approach to nursing education, with effects that extend beyond development of clinical skills. Brief, sometimes sporadic clinical rotations can be inadequate for providing nursing students with a solid understanding of the patterns of nursing practice or for facilitating exposure to impactful interactions with other members of the healthcare team. Likewise, for nurse educators whose academic roles are divided between the

TABLE 51–1 Overview of Sample Patient Safety Initiatives

INITIATIVE	GOAL	LINK
Agency for Healthcare Research and Quality: Patient Safety Initiative	Building a foundation that addresses the issues and recommendations outlined in the IOM's *To Err Is Human* report.	www.ahrq.gov/research/findings/final-reports/pscongrpt/psini3b.html
American Health Quality Association: Quality Improvement Organization Program	Helping hospitals and nursing homes nationwide deliver safer healthcare to Medicare beneficiaries.	http://www.ahqa.org/quality-improvement-organizations/
American Medical Association: Physician Consortium for Performance Improvement	"Develops, tests, implements and disseminates evidenced-based measures that reflect the best practice and best interest of medicine."	www.ama-assn.org/ama/pub/physician-resources/physician-consortium-performance-improvement.page
American Society for Healthcare Risk Management	Promoting risk management strategies and leadership through education, advocacy, networking, etc., with a focus on developing and implementing safe patient care and safe working environments.	www.ashrm.org/ashrm/about/index.shtml?page=index
Centers for Medicare and Medicaid Services: Partnership for Patients	Brings leaders of hospitals, health plans, physicians, nurses, patient advocates, and government together to make hospital care safer, more reliable, and cheaper.	http://partnershipforpatients.cms.gov
Institute of Medicine of the National Academies: Quality of Healthcare in America	Focusing "on patient safety in order to promote policies and best practices that create safe and high-quality healthcare environments."	www.iom.edu/Activities/Quality/QualityHealthCareAmerica.aspx
The Joint Commission: National Patient Safety Goals	Using input from nurses, physicians, pharmacists, risk managers, etc., the highest priority safety issues are identified as well as how to address them.	www.jointcommission.org/assets/1/18/Facts_about_National_Patient_Safety_Goals.pdf
National ePrescribing Patient Safety Initiative	Reducing medication errors by making e-prescribing accessible to all physicians and prescribers.	www.nationalerx.com
National Patient Safety Foundation: Patient Safety Immersion Initiative	"Designed to enhance and grow patient safety knowledge and practice in hospitals and health systems nationwide."	www.npsf.org/updates-news-press/updates/npsf-patient-safety-immersion-initiative
National Patient Safety Foundation: Stand Up for Patient Safety	Catering to healthcare organizations interested in patient safety by providing resources to insert patient safety principles into organizational practice.	www.npsf.org/membership-programs/members
World Health Organization: Patient Safety	Improving patient safety by addressing performance improvement, risk management, infection control, safe medicine usage, clinical practice safety, and safe environment of care.	www.who.int/topics/patient_safety/en

classroom and clinical settings, clinical supervision of students may not be sufficient to create a genuine sense of connection with the given practice setting. Instead, in response to the clinical instructor role, some nurse educators are left with the sense of having been a visitor in the clinical setting, as opposed to feeling as though they are a member of the healthcare organization (Sullivan, 2010).

In combination with an emphasis on safety protocols, recognizing shortcomings associated with the current structure of nursing education programs has led to the generation of measurable nursing competencies. These competencies are designed to prepare nurses for clinical practice and ensure their continued competency in promoting client safety.

The release of the 1999 landmark IOM report, as well as publication of additional IOM studies that detailed shortcomings in safety at healthcare facilities, prompted members of nursing, medicine, and other healthcare professions to closely examine processes and systems that impact client safety. As nursing began to implement this new focus on safety and quality, the experience gap in newly graduated

Concepts Related to Safety

Almost all topics in nursing can relate back to an emphasis on safety. The safety of clients, nurses, and other healthcare professionals is of paramount importance in all areas of the nursing practice. Some concepts particularly relevant to safety are the concepts of clinical decision making, infection, perioperative care, and quality improvement. Many simple measures can be employed to help promote the well-being and overall safety of clients and other staff members. Proper hygiene and sanitation efforts aid in preventing the spread of infection and help to promote quality care measures. Nurses should involve clients in safety protocols, informing them of infection control as well as important considerations involving the spread of bloodborne pathogens. Clients should also be involved in their own wellness efforts, and encouraged to participate in their plan of care.

CONCEPT	RELATIONSHIP TO SAFETY	NURSING IMPLICATIONS
Clinical Decision Making		

■ Critical thinking
■ Clinical judgment
■ Prioritizing care
	Nurses consider safety (both the client's safety and the safety of other healthcare workers) at all points during the nursing process, and while working to prioritize client needs.	■ Assess clients for safety risks as appropriate. Examples include:
		  • Medication history (including history of side or adverse effects)
		  • Factors that impact fall risk and ADLs (e.g., vision, hearing, mobility, balance)
		  • Hygiene
		  • Risky behaviors (e.g., condom use, needle sharing)
		  • Risk for or presence of abuse or neglect.
		■ Consider appropriate safety measures when planning nursing care for the client.
		■ Provide client teaching regarding safety measures as appropriate based on assessment and evaluation of interventions.

Infection		
■ Hand hygiene ■ Standard precautions	The spread of infection within any healthcare setting is a danger not only to the safety of clients but also to other healthcare professionals and staff.	■ Employ hand hygiene after all client interactions, including changing sheets, handling bedpans, and/or helping the client to sit up in bed. ■ Employ hand hygiene and disinfection procedures after removing gloves. ■ Teach clients about infection control measures, such as hand washing, proper cough etiquette, and respiratory hygiene. ■ Disinfect and clean stations and rooms regularly.
Perioperative Care		
■ Universal protocols ■ Sterile field and hand hygiene ■ Discharge planning and instructions	Surgery increases the risk to the client of being exposed to infections as well as the risk of wrong-site surgeries.	■ Ensure that all hospital protocols are followed exactly when preparing the client for surgery. ■ Discuss the surgery being performed with the client. ■ Practice infection control measures when changing dressings and performing wound care. ■ Monitor client for any signs of infection at the surgery site. ■ Teach client appropriate wound care procedures.

Concepts Related to **Safety** (continued)

CONCEPT	RELATIONSHIP TO SAFETY	NURSING IMPLICATIONS
Quality Improvement		
■ Six rights of medication administration	Improving quality of care for all clients involves ensuring and considering the safety of clients at all times within nursing care.	■ Ensure a high quality of care in all interactions with clients. ■ Check dosage amounts carefully. ■ Ensure that the correct client is receiving the correct type and amount of medication. ■ Follow safety and procedural guidelines for client care.

nurses became more apparent. Despite this gap in practical experience becoming evident, there was no general agreement as to the core competencies that should be demonstrated by graduating nurses. In response to the need for uniformity in core competencies, Dr. Linda Cronenwett and Dr. Gwen Sherwood of the University of North Carolina–Chapel Hill (UNC-CH) authored a proposal to deal with the experience gap in nursing. The goal of the proposal was to more effectively prepare future nurses with practical experience and the **knowledge, skills, and attitudes (KSAs)** necessary to provide better quality and safety in healthcare settings. In 2005, the Robert Wood Johnson Foundation funded the proposal, and the result was the **Quality and Safety Education for Nurses (QSEN)** program.

The QSEN program is comprised of three phases. During Phase I (2005–2007), a team of experts evaluated quality and safety factors to determine what core competencies every graduating nurse should have as well as the KSAs required for these competencies. After surveying existing nursing programs, the following six competencies were identified (QSEN Institute, 2013a):

■ *Patient-centered care.* Clients are partners in their care, and thus their perspectives, beliefs, and culture need to be taken into account during their care.

■ *Quality improvement.* Adverse events must be monitored and reported so they can be tools for learning in similar situations in the future and catalysts for improvements in quality and safety.

■ *Evidence-based practice.* Medicine is evolving and changing every day, and thus current medical findings must be monitored for the possibility of improved care.

■ *Teamwork and collaboration.* Because treatment sometimes involves multiple departments and 24-hour care, teamwork across departments and shifts is necessary for optimal care.

■ *Safety.* Activities such as knowledge sharing and error reporting must be taken seriously to help improve safety.

■ *Informatics.* As information technology becomes further integrated into medicine, nurses' input is an essential part of the design process (Hunt, 2012).

Each of these competencies has associated knowledge, skills, and attitudes that nursing graduates are expected to have learned.

During Phase II (2007–2009), the six competencies were implemented into 15 pilot nursing school programs. In addition, the QSEN Web site (www.qsen.org) was created. It contains resources and strategies for teaching QSEN and serving as a place to share information for the pilot schools (QSEN Institute, 2013a; Sullivan, 2010).

Phase III (2009–2012) involved significant national education efforts by both UNC-CH and the American Association of Colleges of Nursing (AACN). These two organizations began to address the need for faculty capable of teaching the six core competencies and associated KSAs as well as continued innovation in QSEN teaching. UNC-CH and AACN also began introducing QSEN competencies into textbooks, licensing and accreditation programs, and certification standards (QSEN Institute, 2013a).

Faculty development was targeted through a number of meetings, including three annual national forums designed to "attract innovators and nurture faculty leaders for the improvement of quality and safety education through exposure to innovations in curricular design and teaching strategies, research related to quality and safety education, and quality improvement or safety studies" (QSEN Institute, 2013a). In addition, eight regional U.S. faculty development institutes were held to instruct faculty in teaching quality and safety content. Further funds were also provided in February 2012 by the Robert Wood Johnson Foundation to extend the QSEN program from undergraduate nursing to graduate nursing (QSEN Institute, 2013a).

While the core competencies are part of some nursing programs in one form or another, all six competencies must be addressed and integrated for safer and more effective care. In addition, each competency is associated with expectations of certain KSAs to demonstrate understanding as well as proper implementation and appropriate values. Properly instructed graduating nurses can then utilize them throughout their nursing careers, and especially as they mentor new nurses in the future (Hunt, 2012).

PATIENT-CENTERED CARE Patient-centered care involves the client in all aspects of care, recognizing the individual needs and values of each client. It also recognizes the need to respect the client's own experience and expertise. This can be especially important when working with clients who manage chronic or persistent illnesses such as diabetes, asthma, or depression. For example, KSAs relevant to working with clients experiencing pain and suffering would include (AACN, 2012; QSEN Institute, 2013b):

- **Knowledge:** Exhibit comprehension of pain and suffering as well as physiological modes of pain and comfort.

- **Skills:** Evaluate levels of client pain and suffering as well as client emotional and physical comfort; assess client and family's expectations of pain relief.

- **Attitudes:** Acknowledge the nurse's position as a source of pain relief and treatment; acknowledge that client expectations can affect outcomes.

QUALITY IMPROVEMENT Quality improvement proficiency will constantly monitor client care and safety in order to improve the methods being employed. As discussed in the Quality Improvement module, quality improvement efforts carry implications for both physiological comes and legal and ethical issues. Examples of KSAs relevant to quality improvement might include (AACN, 2012; QSEN Institute, 2013b):

- **Knowledge:** Acknowledge that healthcare professionals affect client results.

- **Skills:** Examine root causes of sentinel events.

- **Attitudes:** Recognize the value of contributions to care outcomes.

EVIDENCE-BASED PRACTICE Skills in evidence-based practice (EBP) will allow a nurse to provide the best possible client care. Evidence-based practice requires the nurse to recognize the limits of her or his own knowledge and to know how to access current evidence to gain more insight and information. Examples of KSAs Relevant to evidence-based practice would include (AACN, 2012; QSEN Institute, 2013b):

- **Knowledge:** Display familiarity with scientific methods and processes.

- **Skills:** Take part in quantitation and research activities; develop client care based on client values and beliefs, professional expertise, and research evidence.

- **Attitudes:** Recognize the pros and cons of scientific research in practice; recognize the necessity for research to be ethical and responsible.

TEAMWORK AND COLLABORATION Teamwork and collaboration competency will allow a nurse to work effectively with other departments in order to provide quality client care. This competency requires that nurses be accountable for their own participation as team members and also be able to engage in conflict resolution when necessary. Examples of KSAs relevant to teamwork and collaboration are (AACN, 2012; QSEN Institute, 2013b):

- **Knowledge:** Detail the roles of team members.

- **Skills:** Fulfill your role as a team member; ask for help in appropriate situations.

- **Attitudes:** Respect the views and skills of all team members; recognize the client and family as essential team members.

SAFETY Competency in safety will enable a nurse to minimize the risk of dangerous or harmful situations involving clients and other healthcare professionals. This includes, but is not limited to, acting to reduce the possibility of healthcare-associated infections and the possibility for errors (see the Evidence-Based Practice: The Role of Hand Hygiene in Prevention of Infection feature). Examples of KSAs relevant to safety include (AACN, 2012; QSEN Institute, 2013b):

- **Knowledge:** Detail common safety factors as well as unsafe practices.

- **Skills:** Show how successful protocol implementation can increase safety.

- **Attitudes:** Recognize the benefits of standardization toward safety; recognize the limits of personal performance.

INFORMATICS Nurses with competency in informatics will use information and technology to further client care and safety efforts. In addition, they will act to ensure client information is protected by using appropriate system safeguards and practices. Examples of KSAs relevant to informatics would be (AACN, 2012; QSEN Institute, 2013b):

- **Knowledge:** Detail the benefits of information technology skills.

- **Skills:** Use information technology systems to provide safer care.

- **Attitudes:** Recognize the need for continuous information technology education during a healthcare career.

CASE STUDY \\ B

Michael Leyer, age 28, has been admitted to the hospital due to a cold that developed into severe bronchitis. Juliette Wright, Mr. Leyer's nurse, enters his room and introduces herself. She then washes her hands thoroughly and puts on a pair of gloves before obtaining Mr. Leyer's vital signs and performing a client assessment. Throughout the process, Juliette explains each of her actions to Mr. Leyer. Following the assessment, Mr. Leyer inquires as to the plan of care, explaining that his physician has not yet informed him as to how his bronchitis will be treated. He also believes he overheard one of the nurses mentioning that he may need a procedure to remove fluid from his lungs, but it has not been discussed with him and he is opposed to the procedure. The client is very worried and would like some answers. Juliette reassures Mr. Leyer that she will seek answers on his behalf and thanks him for sharing his concerns with her.

Next, Juliette pages the client's physician, who arrives on the unit from another area of the hospital. The physician explains to Juliette that he plans to administer a course of antibiotics to

Mr. Leyer and has no intention of performing any invasive procedures. In addition, the physician thanks her for sharing the client's concern and notes that he will speak with the client as well. Juliette and the physician discuss the antibiotics that will be prescribed, as well as the current plan of care for Mr. Leyer.

After speaking with the physician, Juliette returns to the Mr. Leyer's room and discusses the current treatment plan with him and the types of antibiotics that will be administered. She also explains what actions Mr. Leyer can take to help improve his respiratory function and prevent complications, including frequent repositioning and performance of coughing/deep breathing exercises. As Juliette finishes conversing with Mr. Leyer, the physician arrives to speak with him.

Clinical Thinking Questions
1. What QSEN KSA competencies does Juliette exemplify in her discussion with the physician and the client?
2. Identify the characteristics of Juliette's communication style that promote safety.
3. Which of Juliette's behaviors and actions with the client and with the physician promote safety?

National Patient Safety Goals

The Joint Commission began its **National Patient Safety Goals (NPSG)** program in 2002 to help accredited organizations deal with specific topics on patient safety. NPSGs are developed and revised by the Patient Safety Advisory Group (PSAG), which is a panel of nurses, physicians, pharmacists, risk managers, engineers, and other professionals who have expertise related to client safety issues within healthcare

organizations. PSAG determines topics for NPSGs by evaluating safety concerns and evaluating which ones will have the maximum impact and usefulness for the minimum cost. Input is also solicited from practitioners, provider organizations, purchasers, consumer groups, and so forth (Joint Commission, 2013a). Examples of NPSGs are provided in **Table 51–2** ●.

CASE STUDY \\ C

Geoffrey Hacket, RN, works with primary care physician (PCP) Dr. Victor Larsson at a local clinic. This morning, Dr. Larsson meets with three different clients: one client who has a sinus infection, one who has an ear infection, and one who has a backache. During each exam, Dr. Larsson auscultates each client's heart and lungs and performs a physical examination. Geoffrey has been assisting the physician in his rounds, but he has not noticed him perform hand hygiene between client assessments. After each client visit, Geoffrey has stopped to wash his hands before visiting with the next client. Geoffrey is concerned to see that the physician is not doing the same and wonders if he should approach him about the matter.

Clinical Thinking Questions
1. How could the nurse address his concerns to the physician in a professional and respectful manner?
2. Explain which aspects of QSEN are applicable to this scenario. Which QSEN components apply to the importance of opening a discussion about hand hygiene with the physician?
3. What are some potential hazards of ignoring the physician's lack of hand hygiene and not addressing the topic?

TABLE 51–2 Sample National Patient Safety Goals (NPSGs) for Hospitals

GOALS	SOLUTIONS
Correctly identify patients.	■ Identify patients using two or more means. ■ Ensure blood transfusion patients get the correct blood.
Improve staff communication.	■ Transmit test results in a timely manner to the appropriate staff member.
Use medicine safely.	■ Label all medicines. ■ Use extra caution with blood thinners. ■ Take care when recording and communicating patient medicine information.
Prevent infections.	■ Employ existing CDC and WHO hand hygiene guidelines. ■ Employ existing protocols on difficult-to-treat infections. ■ Employ existing protocols on blood infections from central lines. ■ Employ existing protocols on postsurgical infections. ■ Employ existing protocols on urinary tract infections from catheterization.
Prevent surgical mistakes.	■ Ensure that the correct surgery is performed on the correct patient. ■ Mark the intended surgical site on the patient. ■ To prevent mistake, pause briefly before surgery.
Identify patients at risk for suicide (applicable in psychiatric hospitals and in general hospitals when caring for patients with psychosocial disorders).	■ Assess patient risk for suicide. ■ Provide for safety of patient. ■ Provide suicide prevention information to client and family upon discharge.

Source: Based on National Patient Safety Goals, effective January 1, 2013, Hospital Accreditation Program. Retrieved from http://www.jointcommission.org/assets/1/18/NPSG_Chapter_Jan2013_HAP.pdf.

Evidence-Based Practice The Role of Hand Hygiene in Infection Control

Problem

Inconsistent hand hygiene by healthcare workers leads to the unnecessary spreading of healthcare-associated infections (HAIs). Every year millions of clients contract HAIs, leading to illnesses and infections that in many cases could have been easily prevented with proper hand hygiene.

Evidence

The most effective preventive measure against spreading infections in the hospital setting is consistent and appropriate hand hygiene. However, even with this known fact, the compliance rates for hand hygiene guidelines is less than 40% of all healthcare workers (**Figure 51–1** ●) (Ott & French, 2009). The use of proper hand hygiene among healthcare professionals

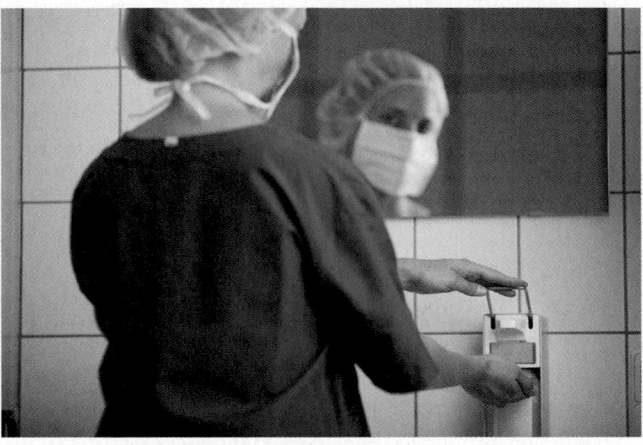

Figure 51–1 ● The most effective measure against spreading infections in the hospital setting is the use of consistent and appropriate hand hygiene.
Source: racorn/Shutterstock.

not only decreases the spread of "minor" illnesses such as the common cold, it is also indicated as one of the major preventive measures for stopping the spread and subsequent growth of methicillin-resistant *Staphylococcus aureus* (MRSA) (Smith, 2009; Upshaw-Owens & Bailey, 2012).

Studies have been performed to determine why hand hygiene compliance is so low among healthcare workers. Findings from these studies indicated that many individuals did not think to perform hand hygiene after taking a client's pulse or picking up objects around the client's room, but these same individuals reported consistently performing hand hygiene when their hands were visibly unclean or sticky in any way (Allegranzi & Pittet, 2009). Other reasons for improper hand hygiene were lack of time, worsening skin conditions, dry and painful hands, and lack of available sinks. Some nursing students also reported noncompliance as a result of not wanting to be poorly judged by senior staff who also did not practice consistent hand hygiene (Ott & French, 2009).

Implications

The use of proper and consistent hand hygiene in the healthcare setting is imperative to decreasing the spread of HAIs. All staff members need to strictly enforce and adhere to hand hygiene policies in order to prove truly effective in infection control efforts. Evidence provided through numerous studies since the early 1990s indicates the effectiveness of hand hygiene in the healthcare setting.

Critical Thinking Application

Suggest two methods of increasing hand hygiene in the healthcare setting. Identify common client interactions where the performance of hand hygiene may be overlooked, but is still necessary. Consider proper hand hygiene techniques and their effectiveness as safety measures in infection control.

▶ COMMUNITY AND LOCAL INITIATIVES

Many organizations and hospitals support community health and safety initiatives. These programs generally aim to contribute to healthier communities by advocating active living, healthy eating, and safety in neighborhoods, schools, and workplaces. Initiatives may be started by community members who recognize they need to address a serious, community-wide health issue. They may start through state-funded or federally funded initiatives that begin in response to larger statewide or nationally recognized health issues and that provide funding at the community level to address these issues. An overview of health initiatives designed to promote health within a local community is provided in **Table 51–3** ●.

🌐 *Stay Current:* To review a list of successful community health initiatives by state, visit **www.cahpf.org/GoDoc UserFiles/601.TFAH_Examplesbystate1009.pdf**.

Minnesota Fall Prevention Initiative

As mentioned earlier, older adults are at increasing risk of falls, resulting in injury and death. In 2005, officials in Minnesota

noticed that their state's rate was fourth in the nation, with a fatality rate twice that of the national average. To combat the problem, a partnership was developed in 2007 between the Minnesota Board on Aging, Minnesota Department of Health and Human Services, and other public and private organizations. Initiative partners meet to coordinate efforts to increase awareness and education activities at local, regional, and state levels (Minnesota Falls Prevention, 2013). The initiative's Web site provides information for the general public and information for healthcare professionals. Safety information is provided relevant to a number of settings and situations, including home safety, medication safety, and promoting safe movement.

Mass in Motion

In response to rising numbers and percentages of adults and children identified as overweight or obese, the commonwealth of Massachusetts began a wellness promotion/obesity prevention initiative called Mass in Motion (MiM). MiM's goals include decreasing the numbers and percentages of adults and children who are overweight and obese and decreasing the prevalence of chronic disease related to unhealthy eating and lack of exercise. MiM targets these goals through a combination

TABLE 51-3 Local Community Health Initiatives

INITIATIVE	GOAL	LINK
ACHIEVE Healthy Communities	Partners communities with national and state organizations to provide health, innovation, and environmental programs.	www.achievecommunities.org
Community Commons	Helps community health organizations and government health agencies connect and solve community health problems.	www.communitycommons.org
Community Health Data Initiative	Makes health data available for the creation of applications for public health benefit.	www.hhs.gov/open/plan/opengovernmentplan/initiatives/initiative.html
Community Initiatives Network	Helps develop collaborative ways to benefit health, well-being, and quality of life.	www.communityinitiatives.com
Convergence Partnership	Brings together financial assistance, thought leadership, and coordination to help community partners in developing healthy eating practices and active living.	www.convergencepartnership.org/site/c.fhLOK6PELmF/b.3917533/k.F45E/Whats_New.htm
Global to Local	Uses innovation from developing nation health programs to address health disparities in the United States.	http://globaltolocal.org
HEAL program	Promotes healthy living and active living to reduce obesity and improve nutrition.	http://info.kaiserpermanente.org/communitybenefit/html/our_work/global/our_work_3_b.html
Pioneering Healthy Communities	YMCA program that promotes healthy lifestyles through policy and environmental change in communities.	www.ymca.net/healthier-communities

of interventions, including legislation, grants to community organizations and public health departments, and working with schools and parents (Mass in Motion, 2013).

▶ INJURY PREVENTION IN THE CLINICAL SETTING

Client care in the clinical setting can be very complicated: Treatments sometimes are scheduled throughout entire 24-hour periods and across multiple shifts; care must be coordinated among the team of physicians, nurses, and specialists; treatment protocols can be complicated and time sensitive; medicine is constantly evolving; and other clients on the floor all need treatment as well. Furthermore, clients are often confused by complicated treatment plans and medical terminology.

For these reasons, and despite the best intentions of physicians and nurses, adverse events and medical errors occur frequently. Healthcare staff constantly strive to keep these adverse events to a minimum, targeting the most common occurrences. Although there are numerous manifestations of adverse events, the most common are falls, improper use of restraints, healthcare-associated infections (HAIs), wrong-site surgery, medication errors, readmissions, and diagnostic errors (National Patient Safety Foundation [NPSF], 2013a).

Falls

Falls are very common in healthcare facilities and homes, and are a special risk for those ages 65 and older. One third of older adults fall every year (NPSF, 2013a). Falls among older adults result in 2 million emergency department visits every year, causing an inflation-adjusted medical cost of $30 billion in 2010, and making falls the most common cause of nonfatal

injuries and the leading cause of injury death in older adults (Centers for Disease Control and Prevention [CDC], 2013d). The risk continues to increase for every additional decade. In hospitals alone, more than half a million falls and 150,000 injuries are recorded annually (NPSF, 2013a). In nursing homes, 50%–75% of residents fall each year, with an average of 2.6 falls per person per year (CDC, 2013c).

Falls can cause numerous injuries, including fractured bones, excessive bleeding, traumatic brain injury, and death. Clients who display memory impairment and muscle weakness, as well as those individuals who require assistive devices such as canes or walkers for ambulation, are especially at risk. Numerous prescription and over-the-counter medications also increase the risk of falls. Research studies indicate that older adult clients on four or more medications demonstrate triple the risk of a fall (CDC, 2013c).

In a clinical setting, numerous strategies can be implemented to reduce the risk of falls. Examples of nursing interventions that may be applicable to the care of the client who is at risk for falling may include the following:

- Remove obstacles from walking paths, including client rooms, corridors, and stairwells.
- Keep frequently used items within easy reach.
- Ensure that client rooms are well lit.
- Make sure clients wear shoes with soles that provide adequate traction, as opposed to wearing slippers or going barefoot.
- Assess the client's vision and make sure he is utilizing any prescribed eyewear, because poor and blurry vision increases the risk of falling.
- Utilize side rails on client beds to prevent falls while the client is sleeping.

- Apply physical restraints when necessary; that is, when absolutely necessary for the client's safety and only by physician's order.
- Be aware of each client's medication regimen, including side effects and interactions, because side effects such as dizziness or drowsiness can substantially increase the risk of a fall. Request that a physician or pharmacist review client medications when necessary (CDC, 2013c).

Restraints

When a client is at imminent risk of injuring herself or others, use of restraints may be warranted (DeLaune & Ladner, 2011). **Restraints** include devices or medications that are intended to protect the client from injuring self or others through partially or fully limiting the client's mobility. Restraints are classified as either physical or chemical.

Physical restraints include any manual method, material, device, or equipment that is attached to the client's body with the intention of limiting or restricting free movement of the client's head, arms, legs, or body (Centers for Medicare and Medicaid Services [CMS], 2006). The degree to which the client's mobility is limited depends on the type of restraint that is applied. For application of restraints, CMS regulations require an order from the client's attending physician or independent licensed practitioner. If emergent use of restraints is warranted or if the client's attending physician did not issue the order for their use, the client's attending physician must be notified as quickly as possible following their application. Federal regulations prohibit standing orders or "as-needed" (PRN) orders for the use of physical restraints (CMS, 2006).

Chemical restraints are pharmacologic agents that are administered for the purpose of controlling hyperactive behavior in agitated clients. The most commonly used chemical restraints are psychotropic agents, including sedatives, hypnotics, neuroleptics, and antianxiety medications (DeLaune & Ladner, 2011).

Use of any form of restraints requires that the client meet very specific criteria that clearly demonstrate his potential for inflicting harm on himself or others. Restraints are never used as a form of punishment, nor are they implemented as a convenience measure. Improper use of physical or chemical restraints, including for the purpose of preventing a client from leaving a given setting, may constitute false imprisonment. Likewise, chemically or physically restraining a competent client who refuses to comply with the plan of care may constitute assault and battery, as well as false imprisonment (DeLaune & Ladner, 2011). Prior to implementation of chemical or physical restraints, federal law requires that less restrictive measures must be implemented and determined to be ineffective (CMS, 2006). In comparison to federal regulations, state laws may be more strict. Because state laws may vary in terms of defining the proper and improper use of restraints, nurses must be aware of the laws in their state of practice. In addition, nurses must know and follow their institution's policy with regard to the proper use of physical or chemical restraints.

Although restraints are intended to protect the client, their use also may result in injury or even death. Psychosocial effects are also a concern; clients who are physically restrained may experience depression, as well as a sense of dehumanization (CMS, 2006). Whenever restraints are used, client care requires the nurse to adhere to strict assessment protocols that are intended to ensure the client's safety. For a sample restraint monitoring and intervention flow sheet, see **Figure 51–2 ●**.

TYPES OF PHYSICAL RESTRAINTS   A variety of styles of physical restraints are available. Among adults, the most commonly used restraints include limb restraints, belt restraints, and mitt or hand restraints. **Limb restraints** (**Figure 51–3 ●**), which are typically made of cloth, may be used when limb immobilization is needed for therapeutic purposes, for example, to prevent dislodgement of an intravenous infusion device. To ensure the safety of clients who are transported by wheelchair or gurney, **belt restraints** or **safety strap body restraints** (**Figure 51–4 ●**) are used. Belt restraints also may be used to protect clients who are confined to a chair or a bed. To protect confused clients from scratching and injuring their skin, **mitt restraints** or **hand restraints** may be used (**Figure 51–5 ●**). Mitt or hand restraints also may be used to prevent certain clients from dislodging intravenous access devices or removing dressings. These restraints allow full arm mobility and do not require confinement to a chair or a bed. However, the nurse must periodically remove the mitt or hand restraint to assess circulation in the hand. Likewise, these restraints must be removed regularly to allow for cleaning and exercise of the hands.

Other devices that may be considered forms of restraints include wheelchairs with stationary lap trays, bed rails, and geri chairs. Criteria for qualification as a restraint include whether or not implementation of a device was voluntary, as well as the degree to which its use limits the client's freedom of mobility. Generally, if the client can release or remove the device without assistance, the device is not considered to be a restraint. Infant and child restraints include crib nets, elbow restraints, and mummy restraints.

Healthcare-Associated Infections

Healthcare-associated infections (HAIs) are infections that occur while a client is being treated for another condition. Approximately 5% of hospital clients contract an HAI (NPSF, 2013a). Infections of this nature can be quite serious, because hospital clients are usually weaker or immunocompromised due to the injury or illness that hospitalized them in the first place. Some of the most common HAIs include the following:

- *Catheter-related bloodstream infections (CRBIs):* These infections are the most common in critical care units. When a catheter is inserted into a client, germs can use it to move down a "central line" and directly into the bloodstream.
- *Healthcare-associated pneumonia (HAP):* A lung infection that occurs after hospital admission, most often with clients on a respirator or ventilator (also called ventilator-associated pneumonia, or VAP).
- *Surgical site infections (SSIs):* Infections that occur at the site of a surgical procedure and can include the skin, organs, and implanted devices.

RESTRAINT
Flow Sheet

Restraint initiated: Date:_____   Time:_____

Initial order expires: Date:_____   Time:_____

NOTES: Client must be assessed at least every 2 hours.
New verbal order required every 24 hours.

Time	Restraints removed	Skin and circulation assessed	Toileting offered	Food and fluids offered	ROM and client repositioned	Client response: R=restless C=calm S=sleeping U=unaware	Effect of restraint: A=adequate I=inadequate*	Continued restraint needed: Y=yes N=no	Restraint reapplied: Y=yes N=no	Initial here and sign below
0100										
0200										
0300										
0400										
0500										
0600										
0700										
0800										
0900										
1000										
1100										
1200										
1300										
1400										
1500										
1600										
1700										
1800										
1900										
2000										
2100										
2200										
2300										
2400										

*Explain: _____

_____

Initials	Signature

Figure 51–2 ● Restraint monitoring and intervention flow sheet.

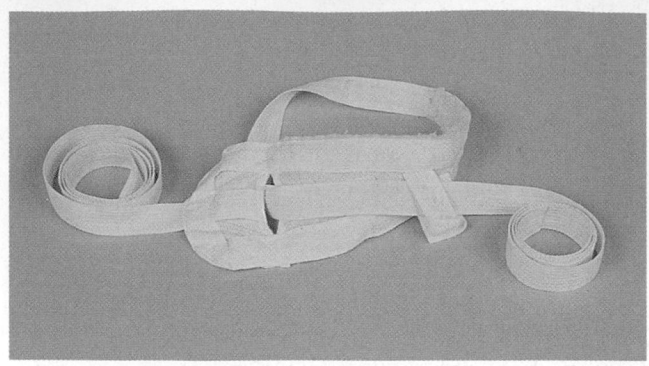

Figure 51–3 ● A limb restraint.

■ *Central line–associated bloodstream infections (CLABSIs):* As with CRBIs, germs use the central line to access the bloodstream.

■ *Clostridium difficile–associated infection (CDIs):* The *Clostridium difficile* bacterium causes colitis, or inflammation of the colon. CDIs are commonly associated with overuse of antibiotics.

HAIs are caused by a number of pathogens. The 10 most common pathogens causing HAIs are (CDC, 2013b):

■ Coagulase-negative staphylococci (accounting for 15% of HAIs)
■ *Staphylococcus aureus* (15%)
■ *Enterococcus* species (12%)
■ *Candida* species (11%)
■ *Escherichia coli* (10%)
■ *Pseudomonas aeruginosa* (8%)
■ *Klebsiella pneumoniae* (6%)
■ *Enterobacter* species (5%)
■ *Acinetobacter baumannii* (3%)
■ *Klebsiella oxytoca* (2%).

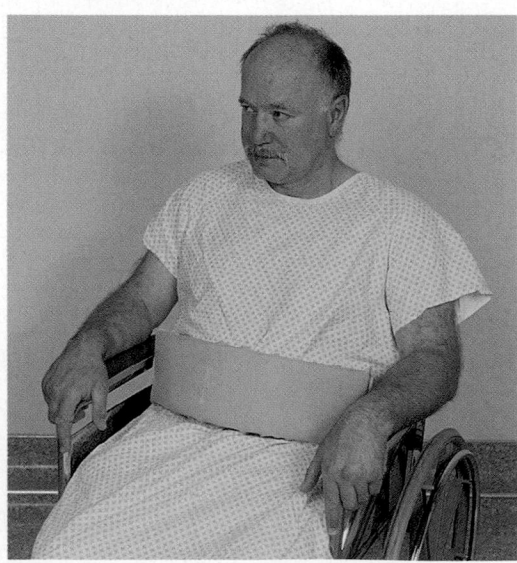

Figure 51–4 ● A belt restraint.

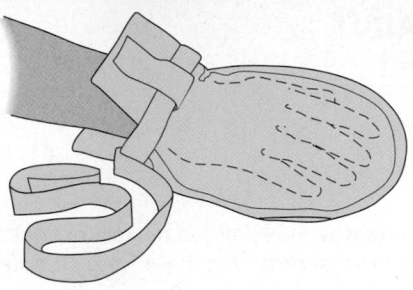

Figure 51–5 ● A mitt restraint.

In 2002, an estimated 1.7 million HAIs occurred in U.S. hospitals and federal facilities. These HAIs resulted in nearly 100,000 deaths. Of the HAI-related deaths, approximately 37,000 were due to pneumonia, 31,000 from bloodstream infections, 13,000 from urinary tract infections, 8,200 from SSIs, and 11,000 from other infections (Scott, 2009).

The costs associated with HAIs are significant. The total costs of HAIs in 2007 were estimated to be approximately $35 billion to $45 billion. The average cost per client infection was an average of approximately $23,000 per SSI, $15,000 per CLASBI, $24,000 per VAP, $900 per CAUTI, and $7,500 per CDI (Scott, 2009).

Clients can help prevent infection through becoming knowledgeable about their treatment and recovery plan, being proactive about blood sugar control, losing weight prior to surgery, and quitting smoking. Nurses are also vital in preventing HAIs and must take appropriate measures to ensure they are not unknowingly spreading illness between clients. Among other safety measures, appropriate hand hygiene and disinfectant techniques are particularly important.

Wrong-Site Surgery

Wrong-site surgery (WSS) refers to surgery performed on the wrong client, the correct client but the wrong body part (such as the left knee instead of the right knee), or the correct client but the wrong surgery. WSS is fairly rare and happens on average once in every 100,000 clients, although it has been posited that only 10% of WSSs are reported (NPSF, 2013b). Some factors are:

■ Inadequate client assessment
■ Inadequate care planning
■ Communication failure
■ Inadequate medical record review
■ Multiple procedures on multiple parts of a client performed during a single operation
■ Failure to include the client and family when identifying the correct operation site
■ Failure to clearly mark the correct operation site
■ Failure to recheck information before starting the operation.

WSS is a serious client risk, because it subjects a client to severe and unnecessary trauma. Surgery teams also feel the effects because they can be subjected to negative morale, insurers that will not pay for WSS, malpractice claims, and disciplinary actions by licensing boards.

To prevent WSS, the Joint Commission (2013b) developed a universal protocol that has been adopted by numerous medical and professional organizations. The universal protocol is outlined in the module on Perioperative Care.

Medication Errors

Medication errors refer to a client either receiving the wrong medication or the wrong dosage, and also include administering the wrong formulation or the correct medication at the wrong time. Medication errors injure at least 1.5 million Americans annually, with approximately 500,000 occurring in hospitals, 800,000 in long-term care, and 500,000 in ambulatory care. Mistakes such as these lead to approximately $6,000 in extra health costs per client error (in hospitals) and approximately $3.5 billion annually. The majority of these medication errors are preventable (NPSF, 2013a).

Following the **six rights of medication administration** can greatly reduce the risk for errors. These rights are:

1. Right drug
2. Right dose
3. Right client
4. Right route
5. Right time
6. Right documentation.

By ensuring that the right medication and the right dose are being given to the right client at the right time and by the right route, the nurse acts to ensure the safety of the client, protecting the client against the possibility of adverse effects or an overdose. In addition, by correctly documenting when and how the medication was given (as well as which medication at what dose), the nurse prevents anyone else from accidentally duplicating administration of the medication order.

Nurses can help prevent medication errors in a number of additional ways, including by engaging clients and discussing their medication with them:

- Assess the medication list regularly and especially during care transitions.
- Evaluate various treatment options.
- Examine the name and function of medications.
- Converse about when and how medication should be taken.
- Talk about common side effects and how to address them.
- Talk about drug interactions with other drugs, food, and diseases.
- Examine the client's role in using medication appropriately.
- Evaluate the purpose of medication in the client's treatment plan.

REVIEW The Concept of Safety

RELATE Link the Concepts

Linking the concept of safety with the concept of tissue integrity:

1. Describe safety precautions that can be taken to optimize wound healing.
2. You are caring for a client with third-degree burns over 50% of his body. Identify three nursing interventions that promote safety while also facilitating the client's healing and providing comfort.

Linking the concept of safety with the concept of ethics:

3. Explain the ethical considerations in a scenario in which a client has been given the wrong medication, but with no adverse effects. Discuss the client's right to be informed about the mistake. If you were the nurse who committed the error, how would you handle this situation?

4. A physician nearly performed the wrong surgery on a client, but the mistake was caught before a surgical incision was made. The correct surgery was performed, but the physician has not reported the original error. Does this scenario require submitting a report? Describe the dilemma faced by the surgical team in this scenario.

5. Describe the ethical dilemma associated with the use of restraints and respect for a client's autonomy. Under what circumstances are restraints indicated for use in a client's care?

REFER Go to Pearson Nursing Student Resources
nursing.pearsonhighered.com

- Additional review materials

REFLECT Case Study

Margie Blanc, age 72, was admitted to the hospital for treatment of severe dehydration secondary to advanced and untreated urinary tract infection. Mrs. Blanc is normally very independent and does not often like to ask for help, particularly when she needs to use the bathroom. Richard Ferris, the client's nurse, recognizes her desire for independence, but also realizes that she is at a heightened risk for falling due to the infection and corresponding dehydration-related signs and symptoms, including weakness and dizziness. Mr. Ferris talks to Mrs. Blanc about the risk of falling, as well as the possible injuries that could occur if she were to fall. He does not want the client to lose her sense of independence, so he rearranges the chairs in the room so she has a clear line from the bed to the bathroom. Mr. Ferris then discusses the need for Mrs. Blanc to wear socks and/or slippers when she walks to the bathroom to further prevent falling. Together the nurse and client develop a plan of care that respects the client's needs and also works to ensure her overall safety.

1. Describe three reasons why Mrs. Blanc's situation represents an advanced risk for falling.
2. Explain the nurse's approach to the situation described above. What communication and collaboration efforts does he employ?
3. Evaluate the nurse's recommendations for the client. Are these recommendations appropriate? Why or why not?
4. Would the situation above be any different if the client were 30 years old? If so, how? Explain your answer.

EXEMPLAR 51.1   Safety Considerations Across the Life Span

EXEMPLAR KEY TERM
Distracted driving, *2713*

EXEMPLAR LEARNING OUTCOMES
After reading about this exemplar, you will be able to:

1. Develop a nursing plan of care aimed at preventing injury and illness.
2. Conduct a risk assessment.
3. Describe specific nursing interventions aimed at reducing the risk of injury or illness.
4. Demonstrate client teaching aimed at reducing the risk of injury or illness.
5. Summarize specific risks associated with different stages of the life span and developmentally appropriate teaching to reduce these risks.

▶ OVERVIEW

Safety risks follow us throughout the life span, from even before conception until death. For a majority of Americans, these risks fall into a number of familiar categories, such as cancer, heart disease, and infection. However, these categories are not universal; the risks individuals face depend and vary according to life stage and are constantly evolving. For example, although heart disease is increasingly a major risk factor for an aging American population, it is hardly a major concern for a fetus, whereas proper prenatal nutrition and pathogen exposure are.

Common injuries vary depending on an individual's age, lifestyle choices, environmental exposures, and developmental progression. The common causes of injuries and illnesses to the very young are often the result of falling while, for example, playing or learning to ride a bike. In rare cases children face illness due to cancers or other diseases resulting from genetics or environmental exposure. Causes of injuries and illnesses in middle-age adults are more likely to be the result of their own lifestyle choices, including smoking, eating high-fat diets, and not exercising. Every age group has its own common injuries.

▶ PRENATAL AND INFANT RISK FOR INJURY

Beginning in the womb, infants are at risk for injury. In many cases, there is nothing parents or healthcare professionals can do. Nurses act to reduce risk by providing client teaching as individuals prepare to become pregnant or, for parents who are surprised by pregnancy, by providing client teaching from the time the pregnancy is discovered.

Prenatal Risk

Prenatal risks to a fetus begin even before conception. Parents introduce these risks themselves, sometimes unknowingly, through genetic means, environmental exposure, and lifestyle choices. Miscarriages occur in approximately 12%–14% of pregnancies. While the causes are unknown for a majority of cases, 5%–10% of miscarriages result from a chromosomal abnormality (Suzumori & Sugiura-Ogasawara, 2010). Errors in cell division, with an abnormal number of chromosomes or a structural abnormality, can occur, but they are significantly more prevalent if either parent has abnormal chromosomes. For individuals experiencing repeated miscarriages this is especially true.

Other hereditary and anatomical factors can also lead to an increased chance of miscarriage. For example, cumulative irradiative damage (also considered an environmental factor) can cause genetic anomalies in a parent or cause in utero fetal damage that can lead to an aborted fetus. Anatomical problems in the cervix or the womb can lead to miscarriage. Rh factor incompatibility, in which only the fetus or the mother has Rh-positive blood, may also increase the risk of fetal demise, as the mother's immune system attacks the red blood cells of the fetus (Berk, 2010).

However, lifestyle and other environmental factors can affect the unborn child as well. Lifestyles and behaviors that expose a parent, especially the mother, to certain pathogens can lead to an aborted fetus or birth defects. These pathogens can be viral, such as cytomegalovirus, genital herpes, mumps, and rubella; bacterial, such as chlamydia, syphilis, and tuberculosis; or parasitic, such as malaria or toxoplasmosis (Berk, 2010).

Other teratogens leading to an increased risk of miscarriage or developmental concerns include prescription and nonprescription drugs; high caffeine intake; illegal drug usage; tobacco usage; pollution exposure, especially polychlorinated biphenyls (PCBs) and lead; and maternal age, with older mothers having an increased risk of miscarriage (Berk, 2010).

SAFETY ALERT

Some studies suggest exposure to anesthesia may be associated with adverse fetal effects. Many institutions require preoperative pregnancy testing for all women of childbearing age. Studies that explored the relationship between exposure to anesthetic agents and miscarriage are inconclusive in humans; however, ideally, exposure to any chemical toxin during pregnancy should be avoided. It is commonly held that if the benefits of the surgery or procedure outweigh the risk of exposure of anesthesia to the fetus, and the safety of both mother and child can be assured, then the procedure is performed. Otherwise, the procedure will be delayed until after the mother has safely delivered the child (Reitman & Flood, 2011).

For information regarding how nurses can help pregnant mothers reduce risk of complications due to substance use or abuse, see the exemplar on Prenatal Substance Exposure in the module on Addiction.

Perinatal Risk

The approximately 87% of fetuses that survive the in utero growth and maturation process still face risks in the period leading up to and during birth, because the birthing process is inherently traumatic for the new infant. A particular risk during the perinatal period is the potential for uterine demise

TABLE 51–4 Developmental Hazards During the Prenatal and Perinatal Periods

PERIOD	INSULTS	FFFECTS
Prenatal	Poor prenatal nutrition	■ Altered brain function in the fetus ■ Risk for learning disorders ■ Low birth weight ■ Premature birth ■ Jaundice
	Exposure to toxins such as alcohol, tobacco, and illicit drugs	■ Injury to the central nervous system, leading to developmental irregularities ■ Low birth weight ■ Premature birth ■ Jaundice ■ Fetal addiction ■ Fetal alcohol syndrome ■ Miscarriage ■ Fetal demise
Perinatal	Poor infant nutrition	■ Developmental complications ■ Risk for learning disorders ■ Inadequate growth ■ Infant starvation ■ Sudden infant death syndrome ■ Jaundice ■ Inadequate organ function and growth
	Neglect and/or abuse of the infant	■ Sudden infant death syndrome ■ Impaired emotional development ■ Delayed or impaired physical development ■ Depressed cognitive development ■ Head trauma

resulting in stillbirth. One major factor in cases of stillbirth or newborn mortality is birth weight, which is currently the best predictor of the survival and healthy development of a newborn (the higher the birth weight, the better). In fact, 1 in 13 Americans is born underweight (Berk, 2010). Many factors significantly affect birth weight, including:

■ Poor prenatal care triples the risk of an underweight baby and quintuples the chance of newborn mortality.

■ Poor maternal nutrition can lead to lower neonatal birth weight and more health problems.

■ Tobacco use can affect placental growth and reduce the oxygen supply to the fetus, increasing the chance of stillbirth by one third and leading to almost 3,000 stillbirths in high-income countries (Flenady et al., 2011).

■ Pollution exposure, such as lead and PCBs, and illegal drug use double the risk of stillbirth and can also cause birth defects and chromosomal abnormalities within the fetus (Flenady et al., 2011).

■ Pathogens, such as chickenpox, cytomegalovirus, genital herpes, rubella, chlamydia, tuberculosis, malaria, and toxoplasmosis, and radiation exposure can all lead to abnormal fetal growth and development.

A number of the risks leading to stillbirth or illnesses within the newborn child are related to the health of the mother. Maternal factors affecting the baby's mortality include obesity and advanced maternal age (Flenady et al., 2011). Rh-factor incompatibility and diabetes can result in pregnancy and delivery complications as well as the compromised health of the fetus. Preeclampsia of the mother, observed in 5%–10% of pregnancies, can lead to fetal death if untreated (Berk, 2010).

Other factors may also contribute to stillbirths. Placental complications, such as abruptions, infarctions, or suboptimal size, as well as cord issues account for 25% of stillbirths. Fetal malformation, which is caused by a number of factors, can complicate delivery and the viability of the newborn. Any injury to the pregnant mother, especially to her midsection, can injure the fetus. Examples include seat belt injuries and domestic violence.

Developmental hazards during the pre- and perinatal periods are summarized in **Table 51–4** ●.

Neonatal Risk

More than 4 million neonatal deaths occur worldwide every year, accounting for almost 40% of deaths of all children under the age of 5. As many of 50% of neonatal deaths occur in the first 24 hours, and 75% occur by the end of the first week of life. Prominent causes of neonatal death include infection, premature birth, and asphyxia.

In many ways, the prevalence of causes of mortality depends on prenatal and perinatal factors. For instance, deaths of Hispanic and non-Hispanic White neonates due to congenital malformation and preterm/low birth weight accounted for approximately 26% and 22% of deaths, respectively. In contrast, deaths for non-Hispanic Black neonates due to congenital malformation and preterm/low birth weight accounted for approximately 14% and 33% of deaths, respectively. Marked differences can also be found when comparing other ethnic and socioeconomic groups (National Vital Statistics System, 2010).

Of the top causes of U.S. neonatal mortality in 2010, many depend on prenatal and perinatal factors. Causes of neonatal death in the United States include the following:

- *Congenital malformations, deformations, and chromosomal abnormalities.* These are related to genetic and chromosomal abnormalities from the parents or from a number of other prenatal and perinatal factors, including exposure to pathogens, use of prescription and nonprescription drugs, pollution, and illegal drug usage.

- *Disorders related to short gestation, preterm delivery, or low birth weight.* Again, these problems are frequently related to prenatal and perinatal factors, including high caffeine intake, illegal drug usage, tobacco usage, pollution exposure, and poor nutrition. Prenatal and perinatal nutrition are particularly important, because poor nutrition leads to lower birth weight and a less viable neonate that is poorly equipped to deal with health and disease issues.

Two other common causes of neonatal death are maternal complications of pregnancy and complications related to the placenta, cord, and membranes. Any perinatal factors that affect delivery, such as maternal obesity and preeclampsia, and placental formation, including illegal drug use and genetic factors, may contribute to these categories of mortality. Nursing care of the neonate is discussed in detail in the module on Reproduction.

Infant Risk

Congenital anomalies and short gestation continue to be common causes of mortality as the neonate matures into an infant. Many of these complications are related to prenatal and perinatal factors discussed earlier. Sudden infant death syndrome (SIDS) accounts for approximately 8% of deaths in the United States. Complications during delivery and unintentional injuries also can result in infant death, with the most common unintentional injuries resulting from suffocation, often as a result of co-sleeping (CDC, 2013f). These factors are discussed in further depth in other exemplars.

Due to immature musculoskeletal systems and relative immobility, infants are also susceptible to a number of injuries, many of which are unintentional. More than 900,000 infants were injured in 2011. Falls accounted for nearly 50% of these injuries, and due to their soft heads, infants are particularly susceptible to traumatic brain injury. Another 14% were unintentionally struck by or against something, and an additional 7% of injuries were due

---

Box 51–1   Child Abuse and Neglect

For the fiscal year of 2011, an estimated 681,000 children are believed to have been victims of abuse. Of these children, an estimated 78.5% suffered from neglect, while 17.6% sustained physical abuse. Sexual abuse occurred in approximately 9.1% of the children who were abused (USDHHS, 2012a). Children with a disability such as mental retardation, emotional problems, a visual or hearing impairment, and physical or learning disabilities were at higher risk for abuse (CDC, 2013g). Because infants and toddlers are unable to verbalize reports of abuse or ask for help, these children may be at an especially high risk for a tragic outcome. The vast majority of child fatalities (81.6%) were under 4 years of age (USDHHS, 2012a). For further discussion of the nurse's role in recognizing and assisting children who may be victims of abuse or neglect, see the module on Violence.

---

to bites or stings (CDC, 2013g). Child abuse was indicated in 534 deaths (**Box 51–1** ●) (U.S. Department of Health and Human Services [USDHHS], 2012a).

▶ CHILDREN AND UNINTENTIONAL INJURIES

Among all ages of children, unintentional injuries are the leading cause of death. Risks related to unintentional injury vary by age; for example, the toddler's mobility increases his risk for drowning in a swimming pool, whereas the infant is more likely to drown in the bathtub or a bucket, and bicycle accidents are more common among school-age children.

Toddlers

Toddlers begin walking, exploring the world around them, testing limits, and playing with anything in reach (**Figure 51–6** ●). Their small size and developing bones make them particularly vulnerable during motor vehicle crashes or when hit, pushed, or shaken. Drowning is of particular concern, particularly around swimming pools. Toddlers also are at risk for injury or death due to fires or burns and suffocation.

Preschoolers

American preschool-age children are more mobile and coordinated than infants, yet not fully aware of the dangers that surround them. Although the number of injuries and fatalities are reduced compared to toddlers, the most common causes of injury and fatality in preschoolers are generally the same. Almost 1,500 preschooler fatalities were reported in 2010. Of the 1,500 deaths, unintentional injuries accounted for over one third of them, most by motor vehicle crash or drowning. Approximately 14% of preschooler fatalities related to unintentional injuries were caused by fires or burns, and over 6% by suffocation (CDC, 2013f).

Motor vehicle crashes are a particular concern for both preschoolers and school-age children. Appropriate booster-seat usage and belt positioning can reduce the numbers of injuries and fatalities. Of the drownings, over 50% occurred in pools and another ~16% in natural bodies of water, indicating the

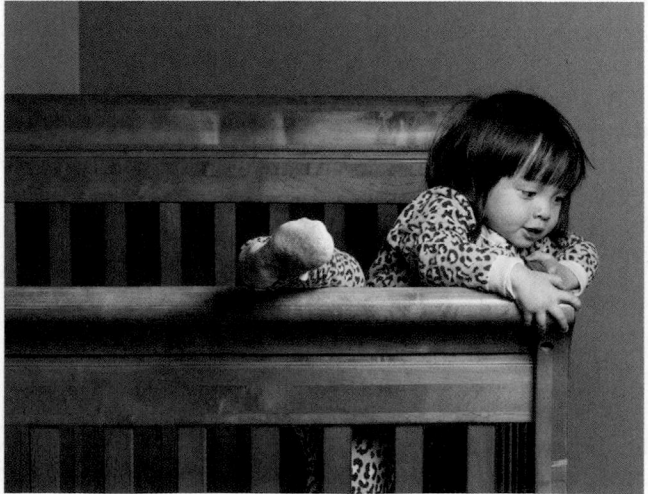

Figure 51–6 ● Toddlers are vulnerable to accidents as they try out new skills and explore the world.
Source: Michael Pettigrew/Shutterstock.

need for appropriate supervision around water hazards (CDC, 2013f). See **Box 51–2** ● for guidelines for preventing water-related injuries in pediatric clients.

Preschoolers were involved in more than 980,000 nonfatal injuries in 2011. Over 40% of these were from unintentional falls, more than 20% were from being unintentionally struck by or against something, another 7% from bites or stings, and 7% from a foreign body being lodged in their throats. The foreign body problem relates to the tendency for children of this age to place objects in their mouths (CDC, 2013g). Swallowing or inhaling foreign bodies increases the child's risk for aspiration. Symptoms that indicate a child may have aspirated a foreign body include wheezing, coughing (most often, nonproductive), dyspnea, and cyanosis when at rest. Auscultation of the child's lungs may reveal diminished breath sounds, as well as wheezing or crackles (rhonchi) (Kiyan et al., 2009).

School-Age Children

Children ages 5–10 are much more active than younger children; they play further from home with less supervision. They are less dependent on their parents and move faster on foot and on bicycles, leading to more falls, accidents, and playground injuries. Almost 2,800 American school-age child fatalities were reported in 2010. Unintentional injuries accounted for almost one third of them, of which over 40% were caused by motor vehicle crashes, approximately 16% by drowning, 11% by fires or burns, and over 4% by suffocation (CDC, 2013f).

More than 2.2 million school-age children were involved in nonfatal injuries in 2011. The most common cause was again an unintentional fall, accounting for 35% of injuries. Over 23% were from being unintentionally struck by or against an object, 6% were due to a bodily cut or piercing, and almost 6% were due to a bite or sting. In line with the increased activity of children this age, overexertion and bicycle accidents both accounted for 5% of injuries (CDC, 2013g).

Adolescents

Adolescents ages 11–18 are exposed to a number of new risks. They are trying to develop their own identities apart from their parent(s), facing increasing peer pressure from all corners, receiving driver's licenses, and playing contact sports. They are most likely to start experimenting with drugs and alcohol in this age range. They are also experiencing emotional turmoil, leading to outward aggression and fighting, or internalizing and suicide.

In 2010, more than 10,000 adolescents died in the United States. Almost 40% of these deaths were due to unintentional injury, most (more than 60%) due to motor vehicle crashes, approximately 12% to poisoning (with 80% of these due to drug exposure of some kind), and only 8.5% from drowning (CDC, 2013f). Suicides, which do not qualify as unintentional but which are preventable, accounted for a little over 14% of adolescent deaths.

More than 4.3 million adolescents were involved in nonfatal injuries in 2011. Of these, nearly one quarter were injured from being unintentionally struck by or against something. Over 20% were from unintentional falls (**Figure 51–7** ●), 13.5% from overexertion, over 6% as a motor vehicle occupant, almost 6% from a cut or puncture, and 5.5% from a nonsexual assault (CDC, 2013g).

Now competing more seriously in sports and play, adolescents ages 10–14 have the highest rate of injury during sports

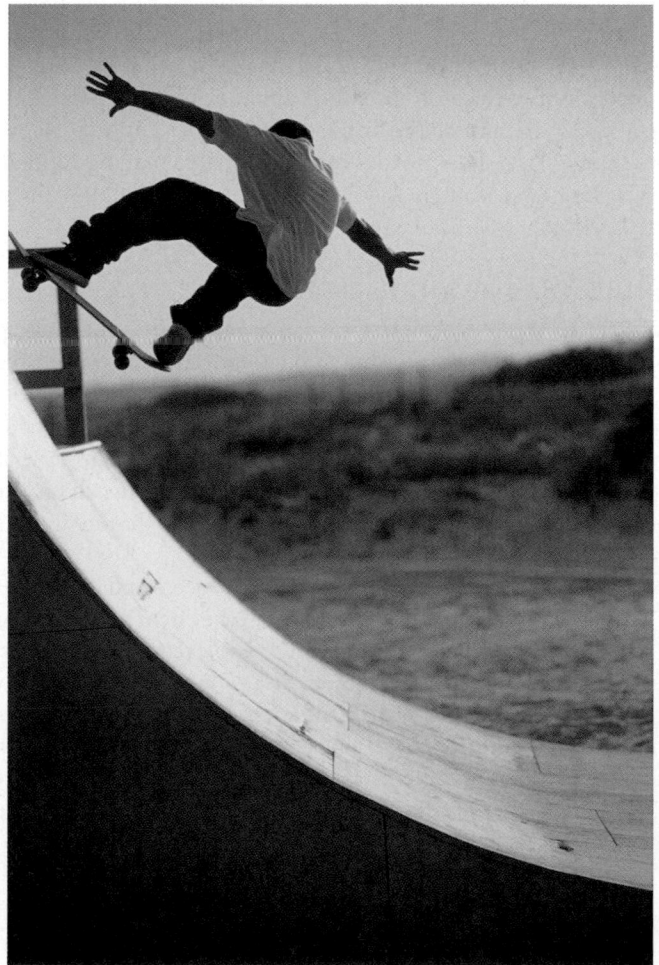

Figure 51–7 ● This teenage skateboarder is at risk for fractures and head injury because he is not wearing protective equipment.
Source: MICHAEL KRASOWITZ/Getty Images.

Evidence-Based Practice Underreported Sports-Related Concussions

Problem

A large percentage of head injuries go underreported in adolescents and adults. Adolescent head injuries are primarily from sports-related incidents, as are many adult head injuries. The underreporting of these incidents can cause significant complications in the individuals who suffered the head trauma.

Evidence

Sports-related head injuries are significantly underreported due to both a lack of education about the long-term effects of brain trauma and a desire to "tough out" the injury. Studies have shown that at least 50% of all football-related head injuries go unreported, and it is surmised that a high percentage of head injuries in children and adolescents are also not treated. Many athletes participate in contact sports (such as football, hockey, soccer, boxing, and wrestling), which present the highest likelihood for potential head injuries. As long as the individual has not lost consciousness from the injury, the sport will often be resumed with no rest or proper medical treatment. The severity of many head injuries is not always noticed by coaches or parents.

A study of high school soccer players found that among those who had been educated about concussions there was a higher likelihood of reporting. Of those who had received education about concussions, 72% reported their injury, compared to only 36% of those who had not received training. Individuals who are informed about potential long-term side effects are more likely to report the injury than those who are not informed (Bramley et al., 2012).

Implications

Clients who participate in sports, strenuous exercise, or athletics of any kind should be educated about the dangers of unreported head injuries. Adolescents are at the greatest risk for not reporting sports-related injuries, but adults should be educated about the dangers as well. Clients who have been injured playing a sport, or even those receiving a sports physical could be counseled by nurses about the risks of unreported concussions.

Critical Thinking Application

Consider how you would approach concussion education with an adolescent athlete. How would the approach change for an adult athlete? Or an older adult athlete? Identify common symptoms of concussion. How would you involve parents in the education of a young athlete?

and play (see the Evidence-Based Practice: Underreported Sports-Related Concussions feature). Of the nearly 250,000 sports and recreation traumatic brain injuries treated in emergency departments, the highest rates were among 10- to 19-year-olds; this is most common in males playing football or cycling, and women playing soccer or basketball (Gilchrist et al., 2011).

Nursing Implications

For clients of all ages, nurses are in a unique position to help reduce the incidence of unintentional injuries, both within the clinical setting and in the community. Awareness of risk factors associated with each developmental stage allows for a broad-based assessment of the client's risk for injury, and can serve as a starting point for a more focused discussion in which the nurse and client can collaborate to identify risks that are unique to the client.

For very young children, the teaching process and identification of interventions should be aimed at the client's caregiver or family members. For older children, adolescents, and adults, the nurse should involve the client and caregivers or family members in teaching and in the identification of preventive measures. Including the client and significant others in the teaching process and identification of solutions that can reduce the risk for injury can increase the likelihood of successful implementation of the nursing care plan.

▶ ADULT SAFETY AND MORTALITY

Although young adults continue to be at risk for injury and death related to unintentional injuries, this risk decreases as adults get older. Lifestyle choices and their impact on health become a greater consideration in adult health and safety.

Young Adults

Young adults, ages approximately 19–45, are generally striking out on their own, getting jobs, being educated, getting married, and having kids. However, this independent living means making their own choices and mistakes, some of which can have deleterious consequences. Almost 150,000 young adults died in 2010. Of these deaths, 28% resulted from unintentional injuries, with almost 45% due to poisoning by mostly drugs, narcotics, medicines, or biological agents. Around 39% of injuries were the result of motor vehicle crashes (see **Box 51-3** ●) (CDC, 2013f). Malignant cancers accounted for more than 13% of deaths, and 11.5% died from heart disease, likely due to an aging, overweight population. Over 11% died from suicide, and homicides accounted for another 7% (CDC, 2013g).

Over 13.1 million young adults experienced injuries in 2011 that did not result in death. Sources of injury included unintentional falls, inadvertent overexertion or being accidentally struck by or against something, and unintentional cuts or piercing wounds. Overexertion can be a particular concern among recreational athletes, who may be at greater risk for dehydration, exposure-related illness, or sports-related injury.

Middle Adults

Middle adults, ages 46–65, are beginning to look toward retirement. Their kids are growing or grown and may have kids of their own. Middle adults have started to slow down, probably becoming less active and developing some chronic health problems as the healing process slows. For the first time, unintentional injuries are not the leading cause of death. Instead, malignant cancers are, accounting for one third of deaths. Heart disease is the second leading cause of death, rising to over 21% of deaths due to age and obesity (CDC, 2013f).

Box 51-3 Distracted Driving

- **Distracted driving** includes any activity that takes the driver's attention from the road, for example, texting, talking on the phone, eating, drinking, reading a map, talking to passengers, looking at a GPS, and adjusting the radio.
- In 2011, more than 3,300 drivers were killed due to distracted driving.
- Text messaging while driving increases the risk of a motor vehicle crash by 23 times (**Figure 51–8 ●**).
- Eighteen percent of crashes resulting in injuries were attributed to distracted driving.
- Eleven percent of drivers under age 20 reported being distracted at the time of a motor vehicle crash (U.S. Department of Transportation, 2012).

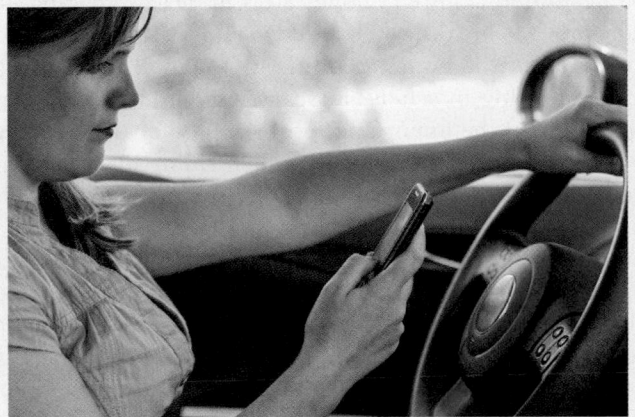

Figure 51–8 ● Individuals who text while driving are 23 times more likely to be in a crash than those who do not text while driving.
Source: Jinga/Shutterstock.

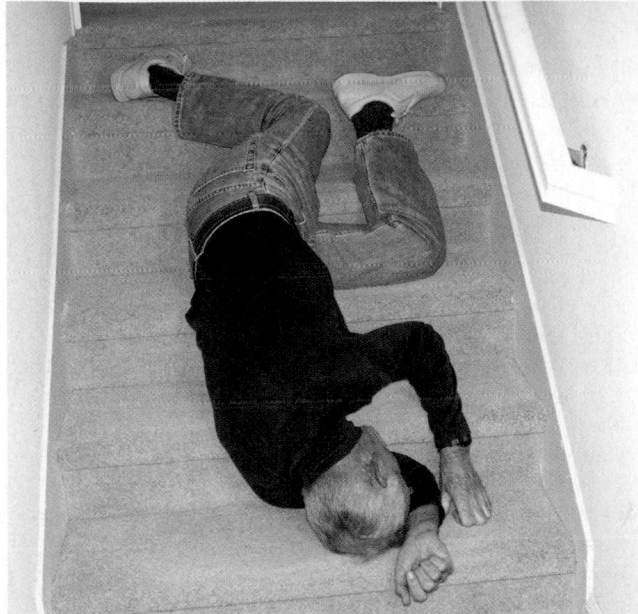

Figure 51–9 ● Almost 65% of nonfatal injuries in older adults are due to falls.
Source: Ann Baldwin/Shutterstock.

When unintentional injuries in this age group result in death, many (over 40%) are caused by poisoning, mostly from drugs, narcotics, medicines, or biological agents. A little over one quarter of fatalities are due to motor vehicle traffic and another 10% are due to falls. Suicides in this age group represent only 3% of deaths (CDC, 2013f).

For the more than 6.5 million middle adults who experience injuries that do not end in fatality, 29% of these injuries are due to unintentional falls. Overexertion and accidental injury due to being hit by or against something follow, with another 9% of injuries resulting from motor vehicle crashes (CDC, 2013g).

Older Adults

Older adults, ages 65 and older, are now mostly retiring. As older adults continue to age, living independently can become challenging for those experiencing chronic illnesses that impact cognition or mobility. In this age group, heart disease accounts for over 26% of fatalities. Malignant cancers, cerebrovascular illness (e.g., stroke), chronic respiratory disease, Alzheimer disease, and diabetes are also common causes of fatality in this age group (CDC, 2013f).

Nonfatal injuries for this age group exceeded 3.6 million in 2011. Almost 65% of these injuries were due to unintentional falls (**Figure 51–9 ●**). Falls among older adults become increasingly common as aging continues, the rate doubling with every decade (see the Concept portion of this module for more information on falls among older adults). Other physical injury, overexertion,

and motor vehicle crashes are less common causes of fatality in this age group (CDC, 2013g).

For older adults in hospitals, extended care facilities, and other clinical settings, the nurse should take steps to actively prevent functional decline. Functional decline may manifest through changes such as diminished ability to complete activities of daily living (ADLs), impaired mobility, decreased musculoskeletal strength, and reduced physical stamina or endurance (Perissinotto, Cenzer, & Covinsky, 2012). Along with reducing the risk of functional decline, the nurse should also ensure that precautionary measures are implemented for the prevention of injury in clients with impaired mobility or altered cognitive function (see **Box 51–4 ●**).

◼ NURSING PROCESS

Individualized client care incorporates numerous developmental considerations. Clients who present with illness or injuries are assessed not only in terms of their developmental age group, but also with safety concerns for that age group kept in mind. Nurses need to take into account common injuries and safety hazards associated with all age groups across the life span.

Assessment

The nursing assessment varies greatly depending on the client's injuries. A number of different safety hazards can result in injuries within any age group. Nurses will evaluate clients based on the nature of their injuries and the risk factors associated with those injuries; however, it is also important to reflect on the developmental considerations of each age group and the individual's lifestyle choices. The relationship between safety and development occurs while an individual is still in the womb, and continues through the end of life. Nurses will also take the client's culture into consideration, as culture often influences lifestyle choices. A complete client history should also be acquired in order to assess past injuries and illnesses.

Box 51–4   Preventing Functional Decline and Injury in Older Adults in the Clinical Setting

- Assess the client's physical, functional, and psychosocial status upon admission; report any significant changes to the client's care team or primary care provider.
- As appropriate, promote activities that incorporate exercise, including strength training and ambulation, in conjunction with occupational and physical therapy as ordered by the client's primary care provider.
- Promote consistent use of all assistive devices, including walkers, canes, hearing aids, and glasses.
- To prevent falls and mobility-related injuries, make sure the client is wearing appropriate footwear when standing or ambulating.
- Minimize environmental clutter and potential obstacles in walkways.
- Facilitate safe mobility through use of elevated toilet seats, handrails, and easy-to-grip door levers.
- Be aware of medication side effects (including sedation) that may contribute to impaired mobility or alterations in cognition; monitor the client's response to medications and report significant impairments to the client's primary care provider.
- Promote and facilitate social interaction to reduce the risk for loneliness, which is associated with both functional decline and increased mortality.
- Be especially alert for signs and symptoms of deterioration in clients with preexisting conditions that increase the risk for the development of functional decline, such as obesity and diabetes.

Sources: Based on Hartford Institute for Geriatric Nursing, New York University. (2012). *Reducing functional decline in older adults during hospitalization: A best practice approach.* Retrieved from http://consultgerirn.org/uploads/File/trythis/try_this_31.pdf; Perissinotto, C. M., Cenzer, I. S., & Covinsky, K. E. (2012). Loneliness in older persons: A predictor of functional decline and death. *Archives of Internal Medicine, 172*(14), 1078–1084; and Anton, S. D., Karabetian, C., Naugle, K., & Buford, T. W. (2013). Obesity and diabetes as accelerators of functional decline: Can lifestyle interventions maintain functional status in high risk older adults? *Experimental Gerontology, 48*(9), 888–897.

Diagnosis

Due to the nature and large amount of safety hazards across the life span, the potential diagnoses for every age group are numerous. However, some safety hazards are common throughout the majority of age groups. Some possible diagnoses are:

- *Risk for Injury*
- *Risk for Trauma*
- *Risk for Delayed Development*
- *Deficient Knowledge.*

(NANDA-I © 2012)

Planning

When identifying goals for a client's care, nurses consider the client's overall wellness. In many cases, safety hazards can be eliminated and injury can be prevented through proper education of the client or caregivers. Some goals for eliminating safety hazards and preventing injury in clients across the life span include the following:

- The client will verbalize awareness of common safety hazards within her or his age group.
- The client will describe methods of eliminating or minimizing exposure to specific safety hazards.
- The client will seek medical assistance when injured.
- The client will report any drastic changes in health to a medical professional.

Implementation

Implementation focuses on wellness promotion, including client education and screening. Nurses assess and screen clients for potential safety concerns—such as exposure to toxins, an increased risk of falling due to medication or age, motor vehicle crashes, heart disease, or cancer—and then provide the client with information on how to avoid, prevent, or treat these hazards. For example, both young children and older adults are at particular risk of injury from falling. Young children's bones are still developing and are more prone to breaks, whereas older adults could have osteoporosis or brittle bones resulting in a higher likelihood of bones breaking in a fall. Nurses advise children and their parents about the importance of wearing safety helmets and protective knee and elbow pads when riding bikes (a common activity resulting in injury for children). Older adults should be instructed as to the side effects of medications they are taking—particularly those that can result in dizziness or drowsiness. Similarly, nurses should inform older adults about precautions they can take to avoid falls, such as wearing rubber-soled shoes with traction, keeping living space free some obstacles that could be tripped over, and asking for help when needed.

All age groups are at risk for exposure to toxins. Adolescents are most likely to experiment with tobacco, alcohol, and illicit drugs. Nurses should educate clients within this age group of the dangers associated with these substances, as well as the potential long-term effects (e.g., cancer, asthma, liver damage, addiction, organ failure). Lifestyle can also expose multiple age groups to unintended toxins including lead, asbestos, unsafe drinking water, and other chemicals. Nurses can educate clients about these dangers, and provide community resources to help the client find safer housing.

For information about safety hazards and interventions during the prenatal and perinatal periods, see the module on Reproduction. For information about age considerations and interventions involving motor vehicle crashes, see the exemplar on Unintentional Injury: Motor Vehicle Crashes in the module on Violence.

Evaluation

When evaluating clients' responses to safety hazards, it is important to recognize that each individual will have unique concerns and values. Some individuals will work very hard to avoid a potential hazard when it is brought to their attention, whereas others will ignore the situation until it becomes an active problem. For young clients and clients who are vulnerable to injury as a result of others' actions, nurses may be mandated to report caregivers' or family members' unsafe or injurious behaviors. (For further discussion of mandatory reporting, see the module on Violence.) Nurses should seek to educate clients about wellness promotion and safety, but they also must respect clients' decisions in regards to their own lifestyle choices.

REVIEW Safety Considerations Across the Life Span

RELATE Link the Concepts and Exemplars

Linking the exemplar on safety considerations across the life span with the concept of culture and diversity:

1. Discuss how an individual's culture may impact his or her environmental exposures and lifestyle choices.

2. How might the nurse integrate cultural considerations in an assessment of an individual's safety throughout the lifespan?

Linking the exemplar of safety considerations across the life span with the concept of stress and coping:

3. Explain how impaired coping could pose a threat to safety for adolescents and adults.

4. Describe two situations in which phobias could develop into a safety hazard.

REFER Go to Pearson Nursing Student Resources
nursing.pearsonhighered.com

- Additional review materials

REFLECT Case Study

Rose Callendari, age 78, was admitted to the hospital 3 days ago subsequent to a fall. She sustained a right hip fracture and a mild concussion. Mrs. Callendari had been outside gardening on an afternoon where the temperature reached a high of 92 degrees. When she stood up to walk in the house, she experienced vertigo and fell to the ground. After Mrs. Callendari recovers from surgical repair of her hip fracture, she will be transferred to a rehabilitation facility.

1. How might age-related physiological changes have contributed to Mrs. Callendari's fall and subsequent injuries?

2. Why is Mrs. Callendari being transferred to a rehabilitation facility, as opposed to being discharged to her home?

3. Develop a nursing plan of care for Mrs. Callendari.

EXEMPLAR 51.2   Workplace Safety

EXEMPLAR KEY TERMS

National Institute for Occupational Safety
and Health (NIOSH), *2715*
Occupational Safety and Health Administration (OSHA), *2715*
Standard precautions, *2717*
Workplace violence, *2717*

EXEMPLAR LEARNING OUTCOMES

After reading about this exemplar, you will be able to:

1. Provide strategies and client teaching appropriate to reducing risk for injury or illness in the workplace.

2. Provide strategies and client teaching appropriate to reducing risk for injury or illness in the healthcare setting.

3. Recommend strategies for promoting safety in the healthcare setting.

4. Identify nursing competencies important to promoting client safety and quality of care.

5. Recommend strategies for reducing procedure and equipment-related accidents.

▶ OVERVIEW

Workplace safety is a concern in most professions, but it is of particular concern to healthcare workers. More than 18 million individuals work in the healthcare sector, and all of them face numerous risks on the job. Some of these risks include blood-borne pathogens, needlesticks, latex allergies, musculoskeletal injuries, stress, and violence from clients. Injury and illness within the healthcare sector represent the highest percentage of nonfatal occupational injuries in any sector, including both construction and agriculture—two industries known for work-related injuries (CDC, 2013e).

Safety in the workplace is critical to job satisfaction and employee retention rates. In nursing, protocols for safety promotion and injury prevention have become more prevalent over the years. These protocols are designed to protect members of the healthcare team and clients.

▶ REGULATION OF WORKPLACE SAFETY

The Occupational Safety and Health Act of 1970 created both the **Occupational Safety and Health Administration (OSHA)** and the **National Institute for Occupational Safety and Health**

(NIOSH). The act works to improve job safety by allowing employees to anonymously report hazardous work conditions, requiring specific protective equipment and procedures, and mandating individuals to report work-related illnesses or injuries. Regulation of workplace safety is particularly important in the healthcare sector, because many incidents occur that should be reported for the safety of other employees as well as clients. For example, needlestick injuries or exposure to any other potentially infectious material must be recorded (U.S. Department of Labor, 2009b).

Occupational Safety and Health Administration

OSHA enforces the guidelines presented in the OSHA Act of 1970, requiring its covered employees to report specific incidents and illnesses in a timely manner. Any work-related injuries that result in days off of work, treatment beyond first aid, loss of consciousness, or death must be reported within 8 hours of the incident. Hospitalization (in-patient) of three or more employees with work-related injuries must be reported, as well as any cases of poisoning or respiratory complications as a result of working conditions. Other injuries must also be recorded, including cuts, fractures, sprains, or amputations (U.S. Department of Labor, 2011).

Community-Based Care Home Healthcare Nurses and Injuries

The number of home healthcare workers has increased dramatically in recent years, and continues to grow as more individuals choose to be treated from home rather than in hospitals and other healthcare facilities. Nurses working in home settings face a variety of increased risks for injuries and illnesses. Increased prevention efforts are needed to further safeguard these individuals. Some common dangers that occur for home healthcare workers include stress, exposure to weapons (primarily guns and knives), unhygienic conditions, needlesticks, bloodborne pathogens, aggressive animals, and driving risks. Preventions efforts for these dangers include the following:

- Clients in the home setting may not properly dispose of the needles and sharps they have used, thus increasing risk of needlesticks and bloodborne pathogens. Nurses must be alert for improperly disposed sharps (in wastebaskets, on tables, on furniture, etc.) and teach clients about safe disposal methods. Clients should also be informed about infection control practices.

- Stress can be increased by the presence of aggressive clients or family members, an advanced workload,

unsafe neighborhoods, dangerous animals, traffic, and severely ill or dying clients. Techniques to decrease stress can be beneficial to nurses and include developing coping mechanisms, employing relaxation techniques, adding extra time for traveling, and receiving training on worker safety in the home setting.

- Violence is of particular concern for home healthcare workers, because they are often alone while working with clients. Nurses report all incidents of violence—regardless of how slight—and work to recognize the signs of escalating violent behavior. If the situation becomes violent or makes the nurse uncomfortable in any way, the nurse should leave the house and if necessary call the local police.

- If conditions in the client's home pose a risk to the client and nurse (e.g., extreme cold or heat, unsanitary conditions, lack of clean water), the nurse should report the condition to his or her employer and contact local social services agencies to aid with the situation (CDC, 2010).

Many states work to help prevent violence to nurses by passing laws that provide for harsher punishments against those who attack nurses. Legislation has also been put into place in many areas requiring employers to provide programs and training on workplace violence. The major goal of these programs is to provide more knowledge about the scope of the problem,

train about prevention techniques, and encourage the reporting of incidents (ANA, 2013). NIOSH collects data on reports of violence against nurses in order to aid in further prevention efforts and to develop training programs and new policies aimed at increasing safety measures for nurses and other healthcare workers (CDC, 2013h).

REVIEW Workplace Safety

RELATE Link the Concepts and Exemplars

Linking the exemplar on workplace safety with the concept of mobility:

1. Describe methods of helping a client with multiple sclerosis to reposition without compromising the nurse's own musculoskeletal health.

2. Among nurses, what are some common causes of back injury in the workplace? What are some methods for decreasing the incidence of these injuries?

Linking the exemplar on workplace safety with the concept of communication:

3. During a home visit a client becomes verbally aggressive toward his nurse. What communication techniques should the nurse employ with this client? Explain your answer.

4. After administering an intramuscular injection to a client, the nurse sustains a needlestick injury. To whom should the nurse first report the incident? What additional reporting and documentation protocols should the nurse follow?

REFER Go to Pearson Nursing Student Resources
nursing.pearsonhighered.com

- Additional review materials

REFLECT Case Study

Daniel Sutton, RN, is inserting an intravenous (IV) access device into a client's arm. The client, Rose Smith, has advanced hepatitis C and has been admitted to the hospital due to hepatitis-induced liver failure. After inserting Ms. Smith's IV device, Daniel places the needle portion on the client's bed so he can quickly secure infusion tubing to the IV port. When Ms. Smith moves her arm, the needle falls to the floor. Upon retrieving the needle, Daniel accidentally punctures himself. Once the needle has punctured Daniel's skin, he immediately stops what he is doing and washes the injury site thoroughly with warm soapy water.

1. After cleansing the injury site, what should be Daniel's next action?

2. Could Daniel have done anything differently in this situation to avoid the injury? Explain your answer.

3. Explain the postexposure follow-up guidelines for individuals who sustain needlestick injuries.

■ REFERENCES

Agency for Healthcare Research and Quality (AHRQ). (2011). *National healthcare quality report.* Retrieved from http://www.ahrq.gov/research/findings/nhqrdr/nhqr11/nhqr11.pdf.

Allegranzi, B., & Pittet, D. (2009). Role of hand hygiene in healthcare-associated infection prevention. *Journal of Hospital Infection, 73*(4), 305–315. Retrieved from http://www.journalofhospitalinfection.com/article/S0195-6701%2809%2900186-8/fulltext.

American Association of Colleges of Nursing (AACN). (2012). *Graduate-level QSEN competencies.* Retrieved from http://www.aacn.nche.edu/faculty/qsen/competencies.pdf.

American Medical Association. (2013). *Patient safety.* Retrieved from http://www.ama-assn.org/ama/pub/physician-resources/clinical-practice-improvement/patient-safety.page.

American Nurses Association (ANA). (2010). *Statement of the American Nurses Association for the Committee on Health, Education, Labor, & Pensions Subcommittee on Employment and Workplace Safety of the United States Senate, May 11, 2010.* Retrieved from http://nursingworld.org/DocumentVault/GOVA/Federal/Testimonies/SPH-Testimony.pdf.

American Nurses Association (ANA). (2013). *Workplace violence.* Retrieved from http://www.nursingworld.org/workplaceviolence.

Anton, S. D., Karabetian, C., Naugle, K., & Buford, T. W. (2013). Obesity and diabetes as accelerators of functional decline: Can lifestyle interventions maintain functional status in high risk older adults? *Experimental Gerontology, 48*(9), 888–897.

Berk, L. E. (2010). *Development through the lifespan* (5th ed.). Boston, MA: Pearson.

Bramley, H., Patrick, K., Lehman, E., & Silvis, M. (2012). High school soccer players with concussion education are more likely to notify their coach of a suspected concussion. *Clinical Pediatrics, 15*(4), 332–336. doi:10.1177/0009922811425233.

Centers for Disease Control and Prevention (CDC). (2010). *NIOSH hazard review: Occupational hazards in home healthcare.* Retrieved from http://www.cdc.gov/niosh/docs/2010-125/pdfs/2010-125.pdf.

Centers for Disease Control and Prevention (CDC). (2011). *The STOP STICKS campaign.* Retrieved from http://www.cdc.gov/niosh/stopsticks.

Centers for Disease Control and Prevention (CDC). (2012a). *Home & recreational safety—Unintentional drowning: Get the facts.* Retrieved from http://www.cdc.gov/homeandrecreationalsafety/water-safety/waterinjuries-factsheet.html.

Centers for Disease Control and Prevention (CDC). (2012b). *Stress at work.* Retrieved from http://www.cdc.gov/niosh/topics/stress.

Centers for Disease Control and Prevention (CDC). (2013a). *About NIOSH.* Retrieved from http://www.cdc.gov/niosh/about.html.

Centers for Disease Control and Prevention (CDC). (2013b). *Diseases and organisms in healthcare settings.* Retrieved from http://www.cdc.gov/HAI/organisms/organisms.html.

Centers for Disease Control and Prevention (CDC). (2013c). *Falls among older adults: An overview.* Retrieved from http://www.cdc.gov/Homeand RecreationalSafety/Falls/nursing.html.

Centers for Disease Control and Prevention (CDC). (2013d). *Falls in nursing homes.* Retrieved from http://www.cdc.gov/HomeandRecreationalSafety/Falls/adultfalls.html.

Centers for Disease Control and Prevention (CDC). (2013e). *Healthcare workers.* Retrieved from http://www.cdc.gov/niosh/topics/healthcare.

Centers for Disease Control and Prevention (CDC). (2013f). *Leading causes of death reports, 1999–2010.* Retrieved from http://webappa.cdc.gov/sasweb/ncipc/leadcaus10_us.html.

Centers for Disease Control and Prevention (CDC). (2013g). *Leading causes of nonfatal injury reports, 2001–2011.* Retrieved from http://webappa.cdc.gov/sasweb/ncipc/nfilead2001.html.

Centers for Disease Control and Prevention (CDC). (2013h). *Occupational violence.* Retrieved from http://www.cdc.gov/niosh/topics/violence/traumaviol_research.html.

Centers for Disease Control and Prevention (CDC). (2013i). *Youth risk behavior surveillance system.* Retrieved from http://apps.nccd.cdc.gov/youthonline/App/QuestionsOrLocations.aspx?CategoryID=3.

Centers for Medicare and Medicaid Services (CMS). (2006). Hospital conditions of participation: Patients' rights—Final rule 42 CFR part 482. *Federal Register, 71*(236), 71378–71428.

DeLaune, S. C., & Ladner, P. K. (2011). Fundamentals of nursing: Standards & practice (4th ed.). Clifton Park, NY: Delmar/Cengage Learning.

Flenady, V., Middleton, P., Smith, G., Duke, W., Erwich, J., Khong, T., . . . Frøen, J. (2011). Stillbirths: The way forward in high-income countries. *The Lancet, 377*(9778), 1703–1717.

Gilchrist, J., Thomas, K., Xu, L., McGuire, L., & Coronado, V. (2011). Nonfatal traumatic brain injuries related to sports and recreation among persons aged 19 years—United States, 2001–2009. *Morbidity and Mortality Weekly Report, 60*(39), 1337–1342.

Hartford Institute for Geriatric Nursing, New York University. (2012). *Reducing functional decline in older adults during hospitalization: A best practice approach.* Retrieved from http://consultgerirn.org/uploads/File/trythis/try_this_31.pdf.

Hoyert, D., & Xu, J. (2012). Deaths: Preliminary data for 2011. *National Vital Statistics Reports, 61*(6). Retrieved from http://www.cdc.gov/nchs/data/nvsr/nvsr61/nvsr61_06.pdf.

Hunt, D. (2012). QSEN competencies: A bridge to practice. *Nursing Made Incredibly Easy, 10*(5), 1–2.

Joint Commission. (2013a). *Facts about the national patient safety goals.* Retrieved from http://www.jointcommission.org/assets/1/18/Facts_about_National_Patient_Safety_Goals.pdf.

Joint Commission. (2013b). *Universal protocol.* Retrieved from http://www.jointcommission.org/standards_information/up.aspx.

Kiyan, G., Gocmen, B., Tugtepe, H., Karakoc, F., Dagli, E., & Dagli, T. E. (2009). Foreign body aspiration in children: The value of diagnostic criteria. *International Journal of Pediatric Otorhinolaryngology, 73*(7), 963–967.

Kohn, L., Corrigan, J., & Donaldson, M. (Eds.). (1999). To err is human: Building a safer health system. Retrieved from http://www.iom.edu/~/media/Files/Report%20Files/1999/To-Err-is-Human/To%20Err%20is%20Human%201999%20%20report%20brief.pdf.

Library of Congress. (2009). *Bill text of 111th Congress (2009–2010)* (H.R.2381.IH). Retrieved from http://thomas.loc.gov/cgi-bin/query/z?c111:H.R.2381.IH.

Mass in Motion. (2013). *Commonwealth of Massachusetts Department of Health and Human Services.* Retrieved from http://www.mass.gov/eohhs/gov/departments/dph/programs/community-health/mass-in-motion.

Minnesota Falls Prevention. (2013). *Minnesota falls prevention.* Retrieved from http://www.mnfallsprevention.org.

National Patient Safety Foundation (NPSF). (2013a). *Key facts about patient safety.* Retrieved from http://www.npsf.org/for-patients-consumers/patients-and-consumers-key-facts-about-patient-safety.

National Patient Safety Foundation (NPSF). (2013b). *Preventing infections in the hospital.* Retrieved from http://www.npsf.org/for-patients-consumers/tools-and-resources-for-patients-and-consumers/preventing-infections-in-the-hospital.

National Vital Statistics System. (2010). *Infant, neonatal, and postneonatal deaths, percent of total deaths, and mortality rates for the 15 leading causes of infant death by Hispanic origin, race for non-Hispanic population, and sex: United States, 2010.* Retrieved from http://www.cdc.gov/nchs/data/dvs/LCWK8_2010.pdf.

Occupational Safety and Health Administration (OSHA). (n.d.). *Healthcare wide hazards: Latex allergy.* Retrieved from http://www.osha.gov/SLTC/etools/hospital/hazards/latex/latex.html.

Occupational Safety and Health Administration (OSHA). (2011). *Protecting yourself when handling contaminated sharps.* Retrieved from http://www.osha.gov/OshDoc/data_BloodborneFacts/bbfact02.pdf.

Ott, M., & French, R. (2009). Hand hygiene compliance among healthcare staff and student nurses in a mental health setting. *Issues in Mental Health Nursing, 30,* 702–704. doi:10.3109/01612840903079223.

Perissinotto, C. M., Cenzer, I. S., & Covinsky, K. E. (2012). Loneliness in older persons: A predictor of functional decline and death. *Archives of Internal Medicine, 172*(14), 1078–1084.

QSEN Institute. (2013a). *About QSEN.* Retrieved from http://qsen.org/about-qsen.

QSEN Institute. (2013b). *Pre-licensure KSAs.* Retrieved from http://qsen.org/competencies/pre-licensure-ksas.

Reitman, E., & Flood, P. (2011). Anesthetic considerations for non-obstetric surgery during pregnancy. *British Journal of Anesthesia, 107*(1), 72–78. doi:10.1093/bja/aer343.

Scott, R. D. (2009). *The direct medical costs of healthcare-associated infections in U.S. hospitals and the benefits of prevention.* Atlanta, GA: Centers for Disease Control and Prevention. Retrieved from http://stacks.cdc.gov/view/cdc/11550.

Sebelius, K., & Cote, D. (2011). *Taking on medical mistakes.* Retrieved from http://www.hhs.gov/secretary/about/opeds/phillainquirer20110425.html.

Smith, S. (2009). A review of hand-washing techniques in primary care and community settings. *Journal of Clinical Nursing, 18,* 786–790. doi:10.1111/j.1365-2702.2008.02546.x.

Sullivan, D. T. (2010). Connecting nursing education and practice: A focus on shared goals for quality and safety. *Creative Nursing, 16*(1), 37–44. doi:10.1891/1078-4535.16.1.37.

Suzumori, N., & Sugiura-Ogasawara, M. (2010). Genetic factors as a cause of miscarriage. *Current Medicinal Chemistry, 17*(29), 3431–3437.

Upshaw-Owens, M. & Bailey, C.A. (2012). Preventing hospital-associated infection: MRSA. *MEDSURG Nursing, 21*(2), 77–81.

U.S. Bureau of Labor Statistics. (2012a). *Nonfatal occupational injuries and illnesses requiring days away from work, 2011.* Retrieved from http://www.bls.gov/news.release/pdf/osh2.pdf.

U.S. Bureau of Labor Statistics. (2012b). *Workplace injury and illness summary.* Retrieved from http://www.bls.gov/news.release/osh.nr0.htm.

U.S. Bureau of Labor Statistics. (2013). *Fatal occupational injuries in 2011*. Retrieved from http://www.bls.gov/iif/oshwc/cfoi/cfch51.pdf.

U.S. Consumer Product Safety Commission. (2010). *Safety barrier guidelines for home pools* (Publication No. 362). Washington, DC: Author.

U.S. Consumer Product Safety Commission. (2011). *Submersions related to non-pool and non-spa products*. Retrieved from http://www.cpsc.gov/PageFiles/108950/nonpoolsub2011.pdf.

U.S. Department of Health and Human Services (USD-HHS). (2012a). *Child maltreatment 2011*. Retrieved from http://www.acf.hhs.gov/programs/cb/research-data-technology/statistics-research/child-maltreatment.

U.S. Department of Health and Human Services (USD-HHS). (2012b). *How to prevent needlestick and sharps injuries*. Retrieved from http://www.cdc.gov/niosh/docs/2012-123/pdfs/2012-123.pdf.

U.S. Department of Labor. (2009a). *Hazardous and toxic substances*. Retrieved from http://www.osha.gov/SLTC/hazardoustoxicsubstances.

U.S. Department of Labor. (2009b). *Safety and health standards: Occupational safety and health*. Retrieved from http://www.dol.gov/compliance/guide/osha.htm.

U.S. Department of Labor. (2011). *Occupational safety & health administration*. Retrieved from http://www.osha.gov/recordkeeping.

U.S. Department of Transportation. (2012). *What is distracted driving?* Retrieved from http://www.distraction.gov/content/get-the-facts/facts-and-statistics.html.

Pearson Nursing Student Resources Find additional review materials at: **nursing.pearsonhighered.com**

NANDA-Approved Nursing Diagnoses 2012–2014

Activity, Deficient Diversional
Activity Intolerance
Activity Intolerance, Risk for
Activity Planning, Ineffective
Activity Planning, Risk for Ineffective
Adaptive Capacity: Intracranial, Decreased
Adverse Reaction to Iodinated Contrast Media, Risk for
Airway Clearance, Ineffective
Allergy Response, Latex
Allergy Response, Latex, Risk for
Allergy Response, Risk for
Anxiety
Anxiety, Death
Aspiration, Risk for
Attachment, Risk for Impaired
Bleeding, Risk for
Blood Glucose Level, Risk for Unstable
Body Image, Disturbed
Body Temperature: Imbalanced, Risk for
Bowel Incontinence
Breast Milk, Insufficient
Breastfeeding, Ineffective
Breastfeeding, Interrupted
Breastfeeding, Readiness for Enhanced
Breathing Pattern, Ineffective
Cardiac Output, Decreased
Caregiver Role Strain
Caregiver Role Strain, Risk for
Childbearing Process, Ineffective
Childbearing Process, Readiness for Enhanced
Childbearing Process, Risk for Ineffective
Comfort, Impaired
Comfort, Readiness for Enhanced
Communication, Readiness for Enhanced
Communication: Verbal, Impaired
Confusion, Acute
Confusion, Chronic

Confusion, Risk for Acute
Constipation
Constipation, Perceived
Constipation, Risk for
Contamination
Contamination, Risk for
Coping: Community, Ineffective
Coping: Community, Readiness for Enhanced
Coping, Defensive
Coping: Family, Compromised
Coping: Family, Disabled
Coping: Family, Readiness for Enhanced
Coping, Ineffective
Coping: Readiness for Enhanced
Decision Making, Readiness for Enhanced
Decisional Conflict (Specify)
Denial, Ineffective
Dentition, Impaired
Development: Delayed, Risk for
Diarrhea
Disuse Syndrome, Risk for
Dry Eye, Risk for
Dysreflexia, Autonomic
Dysreflexia, Autonomic, Risk for
Electrolyte Imbalance, Risk for
Energy Field, Disturbed
Environmental Interpretation Syndrome, Impaired
Failure to Thrive, Adult
Falls, Risk for
Family Processes, Dysfunctional
Family Processes, Interrupted
Family Processes, Readiness for Enhanced
Fatigue
Fear
Fluid Balance, Readiness for Enhanced
Fluid Volume: Deficient
Fluid Volume: Deficient, Risk for

Fluid Volume: Excess
Fluid Volume: Imbalanced, Risk for
Gas Exchange, Impaired
Gastrointestinal Motility, Dysfunctional
Gastrointestinal Motility, Risk for Dysfunctional
Grieving
Grieving, Complicated
Grieving, Risk for Complicated
Growth: Disproportionate, Risk for
Growth and Development, Delayed
Health: Community, Deficient
Health Behavior, Risk-Prone
Health Maintenance, Ineffective
Home Maintenance, Impaired
Hope, Readiness for Enhanced
Hopelessness
Human Dignity, Risk for Compromised
Hyperthermia
Hypothermia
Immunization Status, Readiness for Enhanced
Impulse Control, Ineffective
Infant Behavior: Disorganized
Infant Behavior: Disorganized, Risk for
Infant Behavior: Organized, Readiness for Enhanced
Infant Feeding Pattern, Ineffective
Infection, Risk for
Injury, Risk for
Insomnia
Jaundice, Neonatal
Jaundice, Neonatal, Risk for
Knowledge, Deficient
Knowledge, Readiness for Enhanced
Lifestyle, Sedentary
Liver Function, Risk for Impaired
Loneliness, Risk for
Maternal/Fetal Dyad, Risk for Disturbed
Memory, Impaired
Mobility: Bed, Impaired
Mobility: Physical, Impaired
Mobility: Wheelchair, Impaired
Moral Distress
Mucous Membrane: Oral, Impaired
Nausea
Neglect, Unilateral
Neurovascular Dysfunction: Peripheral, Risk for
Noncompliance
Nutrition, Imbalanced: Less Than Body Requirements
Nutrition, Imbalanced: More Than Body Requirements
Nutrition, Imbalanced: More Than Body Requirements, Risk for
Nutrition, Readiness for Enhanced
Pain, Acute

Pain, Chronic
Parenting, Impaired
Parenting, Readiness for Enhanced
Parenting, Risk for Impaired
Perfusion: Gastrointestinal, Risk for Ineffective
Perfusion: Renal, Risk for Ineffective
Perioperative Positioning Injury, Risk for
Personal Identity: Disturbed
Personal Identity: Disturbed, Risk for
Poisoning, Risk for
Post-Trauma Syndrome
Post-Trauma Syndrome, Risk for
Power, Readiness for Enhanced
Powerlessness
Powerlessness, Risk for
Protection, Ineffective
Rape-Trauma Syndrome
Relationship, Ineffective
Relationship, Readiness for Enhanced
Relationship, Risk for Ineffective
Religiosity, Impaired
Religiosity, Readiness for Enhanced
Religiosity, Risk for Impaired
Relocation Stress Syndrome
Relocation Stress Syndrome, Risk for
Resilience: Individual, Impaired
Resilience, Readiness for Enhanced
Resilience, Risk for Compromised
Role Conflict, Parental
Role Performance, Ineffective
Self-Care, Readiness for Enhanced
Self-Care Deficit: Bathing
Self-Care Deficit: Dressing
Self-Care Deficit: Feeding
Self-Care Deficit: Toileting
Self-Concept, Readiness for Enhanced
Self-Esteem, Chronic Low
Self-Esteem, Chronic Low, Risk for
Self-Esteem, Situational Low
Self-Esteem, Situational Low, Risk for
Self-Health Management, Ineffective
Self-Health Management, Readiness for Enhanced
Self-Mutilation
Self-Mutilation, Risk for
Self-Neglect
Sexual Dysfunction
Sexuality Pattern, Ineffective
Shock, Risk for
Skin Integrity, Impaired
Skin Integrity, Risk for Impaired
Sleep, Readiness for Enhanced
Sleep Deprivation

Sleep Pattern, Disturbed
Social Interaction, Impaired
Social Isolation
Sorrow, Chronic
Spiritual Distress
Spiritual Distress, Risk for
Spiritual Well-Being, Readiness for Enhanced
Stress Overload
Sudden Infant Death Syndrome, Risk for
Suffocation, Risk for
Suicide, Risk for
Surgical Recovery, Delayed
Swallowing, Impaired
Therapeutic Regimen Management:
    Family, Ineffective
Thermal Injury, Risk for
Thermoregulation, Ineffective
Tissue Integrity, Impaired
Tissue Perfusion: Cardiac, Risk for Decreased
Tissue Perfusion: Cerebral, Risk for Ineffective
Tissue Perfusion: Peripheral, Ineffective
Tissue Perfusion: Peripheral, Risk for Ineffective

Transfer Ability, Impaired
Trauma, Risk for
Trauma: Vascular, Risk for
Urinary Elimination, Impaired
Urinary Elimination, Readiness for Enhanced
Urinary Incontinence, Functional
Urinary Incontinence, Overflow
Urinary Incontinence, Reflex
Urinary Incontinence, Stress
Urinary Incontinence, Urge
Urinary Incontinence, Urge, Risk for
Urinary Retention
Ventilation: Spontaneous, Impaired
Ventilatory Weaning Response, Dysfunctional
Violence: Other-Directed, Risk for
Violence: Self-Directed, Risk for
Walking, Impaired
Wandering

Source: Nursing Diagnoses–Definitions and Classification 2012-2014. Copyright ©2012, 1994-2012 by NANDA International. Used by arrangement with John Wiley & Sons, Limited. In order to make safe and effective judgments using NANDA-I nursing diagnoses it is essential that nurses refer to the definitions and defining characteristics of the diagnoses listed in this work.

GLOSSARY

Abortion Loss of pregnancy before the fetus is viable outside the uterus. Also called *miscarriage*.

Absorption The process of moving nutrients and fluid from the external environment of the gastrointestinal tract to the internal environment. May also refer to the intake of any specific nutrient.

Abstinence Voluntarily going without alcohol, drugs, or other pleasurable substances or activities.

Abuse of power An attempt by an individual to use his or her position or authority in a manner that shames, controls, demeans, humiliates, or denigrates another individual to gain emotional, psychological, or physical advantage over that individual.

Accelerations A transient increase in the fetal heart rate normally caused by fetal movement.

Accommodation 1. The ability of the eye to adjust to variations in distance. 2. The process of a change whereby cognitive processes mature sufficiently to allow an individual to solve problems that were unsolvable before.

Accountability The ability and willingness of an individual to assume responsibility for his or her actions and to accept the consequences of his or her behavior.

Accreditation A peer review process that evaluates and certifies the quality of an organization.

Acculturation The process of adapting to the majority culture and accepting it as one's own.

Acid indigestion A condition in which an individual can taste the stomach acid when it flows back into the esophagus.

Acidosis The condition that results when hydrogen ion concentration increases above normal, causing the pH to drop below 7.35.

Acids Substances that release hydrogen ions in solution.

Acquaintance phase The first few days after a child's birth, when the new mother applies herself to the task of getting to know her baby.

Acquaintance rape A broad term used to describe a rape committed by an acquaintance or other familiar individual.

Acquired immunity Immunity developed after exposure to a pathogen.

Acquired immunodeficiency syndrome (AIDS) An immune system deficit induced by infection with the human immunodeficiency virus (HIV). AIDS is characterized by opportunistic infections.

Acrocyanosis A bluish discoloration of the hands and feet.

Acromegaly Excessive growth of bone from growth hormone hypersecretion.

Actinic keratosis An epidermal skin lesion directly related to chronic sun exposure and photodamage. Also called *senile keratosis* or *solar keratosis*.

Action potential The electrical activity produced by movement of ions across cell membranes that stimulates muscle contraction.

Active acquired immunity Antibodies formed in response to an illness or an immunization while a female is pregnant.

Active euthanasia Actions to bring about a client's death directly, with or without client consent.

Active immunity Production of antibodies or development of immune lymphocytes against specific antigens.

Active transport A method that requires additional energy (in the form of adenosine triphosphate) to move substances against the concentration gradient (from low concentration to high concentration).

Activities of daily living (ADLs) Activities used routinely in daily life, such as grooming, eating, bathing, and dressing.

Activity-exercise pattern An individual's routine of exercise, activity, leisure, and recreation, including activities of daily living that require energy expenditure.

Activity tolerance The type and amount of exercise or daily living activities that an individual is able to perform without experiencing adverse effects.

Actual loss A change in or unavailability of something or someone of value that can be recognized by others.

Acute coronary syndrome (ACS) Any condition that develops due to sudden, reduced blood flow to the heart.

Acute fatigue A sudden onset of physical and mental exhaustion or weariness, particularly after a period of mental or physical stress.

Acute illness An alteration in health or functioning characterized by severe symptoms of relatively short duration.

Acute infection An infection that appears suddenly and lasts for a short time.

Acute kidney injury (AKI) Proposed as a more accurate term for *acute renal failure*, AKI is defined as a sudden decline in kidney function that causes disturbances in fluid, electrolyte, and acid–base balances.

Acute lymphocytic leukemia (ALL) The most common type of leukemia in children and adolescents, marked by the proliferation of malignant cells that resemble immature lymphocytes.

Acute myeloid leukemia (AML) A disorder characterized by uncontrolled proliferation of myeloblasts and hyperplasia of the bone marrow and spleen.

Acute myocardial infarction (AMI) A life-threatening condition that occurs when blood flow to a portion of the cardiac muscle is blocked. If circulation to the affected myocardium is not promptly restored, loss of functional myocardium affects the heart's ability to maintain an effective cardiac output, ultimately leading to cardiogenic shock and death.

Acute pain Temporary, localized, and sudden pain that lasts for less than 6 months and has an identifiable cause, such as trauma, surgery, or inflammation.

Acute pancreatitis An inflammatory disorder that involves self-destruction of the pancreas by its own enzymes through autodigestion.

Acute postinfectious glomerulonephritis (APIGN) Inflammation of the glomerular capillary membrane that is most often seen in children as a response to a group A beta-hemolytic streptococcal infection of the skin or pharynx or as a result of infection by the *Staphylococcus, Pneumococcus,* or *Coxsackie* viruses.

Acute renal failure (ARF) A rapid decline in renal function with azotemia, fluid, and electrolyte imbalances. ARF may be reversed with prompt intervention.

Acute respiratory distress syndrome (ARDS) A disorder with rapid onset characterized by noncardiac pulmonary edema and progressive refractory hypoxemia. ARDS is a life-threatening emergency.

Acute retroviral syndrome (ARS) Primary human immunodeficiency virus infection.

Acute stress disorder A condition that may occur following an individual experiencing, learning of, or witnessing an extremely stressful event that involves the threat of death, actual or threatened serious injury, or actual or physical or sexual violation.

Acute tubular necrosis (ATN) The destruction of tubular epithelial cells, which causes an abrupt and progressive decline of renal function.

Adaptation 1. The ability to handle the demands made by the environment. Also called *coping behavior.* **2.** The return to normal functioning, even when homeostasis cannot be regained.

Adaptation phase The phase during a crisis in which the individual meets the challenges presented and uses his or her resources to successfully resolve the crisis.

Adaptive behavior Everyday skills including conceptual skills, social skills, and practical skills.

Adaptive functioning The ability of an individual to meet the standards expected for his or her cultural group.

Adaptive mechanisms Methods the ego uses to fulfill the needs of the id in a socially acceptable manner. Also called *defense mechanisms.*

Addiction A psychological or physical need for a substance (such as alcohol) or process (such as gambling) to the extent that the individual will risk negative consequences in an attempt to meet the need.

Addictive behaviors Compulsive, problematic patterns of action resulting in psychological and/or physiological dependence.

Adherence Commitment or attachment to a regimen. Also called *compliance.*

Adhesions Fibrous bands of scar tissue.

Adjustment disorder with depressed mood A maladaptive reaction to an identifiable psychosocial stressor or stressors that occurs within 3 months after the onset of the stressor and has persisted for no longer than 6 months. Also called *adjustment disorder* or *situational depression.*

Adjustment phase Initial phase experienced in response to crisis, characterized by disorganization and unsuccessful attempts to meet the crisis.

Adjustment reaction to depressed mood See Postpartum blues.

Administrative information system A system designed to provide support and management to the business side of health care. This includes human resources, financial data, materials management, risk management, and quality performance.

Administrative laws Responsibilities that may be interpreted and enforced by an agency that has been delegated the power of oversight by the governing legislation.

Adolescent family A family in which one or more parents are adolescents.

Advance healthcare directives Legal documents that allow an individual to plan for healthcare and/or financial affairs in the event of incapacity. Also called *advance directives* or *healthcare advance directives.*

Advocacy Protecting an individual by expressing and defending the individual's cause on his or her behalf.

Advocate An individual who expresses and defends the cause of another.

Aerobic exercise An activity during which the amount of oxygen taken into the body is greater than that used to perform the activity.

Aesthetic knowing The subjective elements and personal style a nurse uses when delivering care, including empathy, holistic thinking, compassion and sensitivity.

Afebrile Without fever.

Affect The immediate and observable emotional expression of mood, which people communicate verbally and nonverbally; the outward manifestation of what the individual is feeling.

Affective commitment An attachment to a profession that includes identification with and involvement in the profession.

Affective domain The learning domain encompassing an individual's emotional response to tasks, including feelings, emotions, interests, attitudes, and appreciation. Also called the *feeling domain.*

Afterload The force that ventricles must overcome to eject their blood volume.

Afterpains Cramp-like pains caused by intermittent contractions of the uterus that occur after childbirth.

Age-related macular degeneration (AMD) A gradual degeneration in the macular area of the retina that is the leading cause of blindness in people over age 65.

Ageism A deep and profound prejudice in American society against older adults.

Aggravated assault An unlawful attack by one individual on another for the purpose of inflicting severe or aggravated bodily injury. This type of assault usually is accompanied by the use of a weapon or by means likely to produce death or great bodily harm.

Aggression Any form of behavior directed toward the goal of harming or injuring another living being.

Aggressive behavior Behavior directed toward getting what one wants without considering the feelings of others.

Aggressive communicators Individuals who tend to focus on their own needs and become impatient when these needs are not met.

Agnosia The inability to recognize one or more objects that previously were familiar.

Agnostic An individual who doubts the existence of God or a supreme being or believes the existence of God has not been proved.

Agoraphobia A condition that is characterized by anxiety associated with two or more of the following situations: being in enclosed spaces, being in open spaces, utilizing public transportation, being in a crowd or standing in a line of people, or being alone outside the home environment.

Agraphia The inability to write properly.

AIDS dementia complex The most common cause of mental status changes for clients with HIV infection. This dementia results from a direct effect of the virus on the brain and affects cognitive, motor, and behavioral functioning. Fluctuating memory loss, confusion, difficulty concentrating, lethargy, and diminished motor speed are typical manifestations.

Air trapping Decreased airflow with exhalation caused by edema of the air passages.

Airborne precautions Used for clients who are known to have or suspected of having serious illnesses transmitted by airborne droplet nuclei smaller than 5 microns, such as tuberculosis.

Airway remodeling Structural changes of the airway caused by a disease, such as asthma, resulting in progressive or permanent loss of lung function.

Airway resistance The effort or force needed to move oxygen through the trachea to the lungs.

Akathisia Restlessness.

Alcohol dependence A primary, chronic disease characterized by use or abuse of alcohol; genetic, psychosocial, and environmental factors influence its development and manifestations. Also called *alcoholism*.

Alcohol poisoning A toxic condition that results from excessive consumption of large amounts of alcohol in a very short period of time.

Alcohol withdrawal delirium A medical emergency usually occurring 3–5 days following alcohol withdrawal and lasting 2–3 days. Characterized by paranoia, disorientation, delusions, visual hallucinations, elevated vital signs, vomiting, diarrhea, and diaphoresis. Also known as *delirium tremens (DTs)*.

Alcohol withdrawal syndrome Condition that typically begins about 6–8 hours after an individual with alcoholism takes his or her last drink. Early symptoms include irritability, anxiety, insomnia, tremors, sweating, and a mild tachycardia.

Alcoholic cirrhosis A progressive, irreversible liver disorder resulting from excessive consumption of alcohol. Also called *Laënnec cirrhosis*.

Alcoholism A primary, chronic disease characterized by use or abuse of alcohol; genetic, psychosocial, and environmental factors influence its development and manifestations. Also called *alcohol dependence*.

Alkalosis The condition that results when hydrogen ion concentration falls below normal and the pH level rises above 7.45.

Allen test A measurement of radial or ulnar patency; either the radial or ulnar artery is digitally compressed by the examiner after blood has been forced out of the hand by clenching it into a fist.

Allergen An environmental or exogenous antigen that provokes a hypersensitivity response.

Allergic contact dermatitis A cell-mediated or delayed hypersensitivity to a wide variety of allergens.

Allergy A hypersensitivity response to environmental or exogenous antigens.

Allogeneic blood transfusion A transfusion using blood that has been donated by the community.

Allogeneic bone marrow transplant A transplant using bone marrow from a matched donor.

Allografts Grafts between members of the same species who have different genotypes and HLA antigens. Human skin that has been harvested from cadavers is usually used. Also called *homograft*.

Alloimmunization The reaction of the immune system to donated tissue.

Allostasis Necessary changes that must occur to achieve the characteristic stability of homeostasis.

Allostatic load The physical cost of adaptation to physiological or psychosocial stressors.

Alogia Limited speech, associated with catatonic inhibition.

Alopecia Hair loss.

Alternative therapies A term used to describe use of these diverse therapies *instead of* conventional therapies including acupuncture; cultural practices related to food preparation or practices at specific times of the day or during the week.

Altruism A concern for the welfare and well-being of others.

Alzheimer disease (AD) The most common kind of dementia, Alzheimer disease involves progressive dementia, memory loss, and the inability to care for one's self.

Ambulation The ability to walk from place to place independently with or without an assistive device.

Amenorrhea The absence of menstruation.

Amniocentesis A procedure used to obtain amniotic fluid for genetic testing to determine fetal abnormalities or fetal lung maturity in the third trimester of pregnancy.

Amnion A thin protective membrane that contains amniotic fluid.

Amniotic fluid The liquid surrounding the fetus in utero. It absorbs shocks, permits fetal movement, and prevents heat loss.

Amphetamine A powerful stimulant that, when used improperly or abused, poses a severe health risk due to its devastating physical and neurological consequences, including amphetamine-induced mental disorders.

Ampulla The outer third of the fallopian tube, where fertilization usually occurs.

Amyloid plaques Seen in Alzheimer disease and formed when groups of nerve cells degenerate and clump around the amyloid core in the spaces between the neurons in the brain. Amyloid plaques consist primarily of insoluble deposits of beta-amyloid, a protein fragment from a larger protein called amyloid precursor protein, mixed with other neurons and non-nerve cells.

Anaerobic exercise Activity in which the muscles cannot draw out enough oxygen from the bloodstream, and anaerobic pathways are used to provide additional energy for storing for a short time.

Anal stimulation The stimulation of the anus with the fingers, mouth, or sex toys for sexual pleasure.

Anaphylactic shock Shock resulting from a widespread hypersensitivity reaction. Also called *anaphylaxis*.

Anaphylaxis An acute systemic type I hypersensitivity (allergic) response that may result in shock and death. It occurs in highly sensitive persons following exposure to a specific antigen, usually through injection or ingestion.

Anaplasia The regression of a cell to an immature or undifferentiated cell type.

Anasarca Severe, generalized edema.

Andragogy The art and science of teaching adults.

Androgen A hormone that stimulates the development and maintenance of male sex characteristics.

Androgyny Flexibility in gender roles.

Anemia An abnormally low number of circulating red blood cells, low hemoglobin concentration, or both.

Anergic Unable to react to common antigens.

Anergy Fatigue and decreased energy associated with a depressive disorder. Also called *anergia*.

Anger A subjective sense of intense displeasure, irritation, or animosity.

Angina pectoris Chest pain resulting from reduced coronary blood flow caused by a temporary imbalance between myocardial blood supply and demand. Also called *angina*.

Angle-closure glaucoma A type of glaucoma that results from a narrowing of the anterior chamber angle due to corneal flattening or bulging of the iris into the anterior chamber. Also called *narrow-angle* or *closed-angle glaucoma*.

Anhedonia The inability to feel pleasure.

Animism Giving lifelike qualities to nonliving things.

Anion Ion that carries a negative charge.

Anomia Difficulty naming people and things.

Anorexia Loss of appetite.

Anorexia nervosa (AN) A potentially life-threatening disorder characterized by extreme perfectionism, weight fear, significant weight loss, body image disturbances, strenuous exercising, peculiar food-handling patterns, and reductions in heart rate, blood pressure, metabolic rate, and the production of estrogen or testosterone.

Anorgasmia Absence of orgasm.

Antagonism One of the six trait domains associated with personality disorders that is comprised of manipulativeness, deceitfulness, callousness, hostility, grandiosity, and attention seeking.

Antepartum Time between conception and the onset of labor; usually used to describe the period during which a woman is pregnant.

Anthropometric measurements Measurements that can help identify individuals who are at risk for undernutrition or overnutrition. Specific measurements include height, length (in babies), weight, body mass index, waist-to-hip circumference, and skinfold thickness.

Antibodies Proteins that work against antigens.

Antibody-mediated (humoral) immune response Activation of B cells to produce antibodies to respond to antigens such as bacteria, bacterial toxins, and free viruses.

Anticipatory grief Grief experienced in advance of a loss, such as the wife who grieves before her ailing husband dies.

Anticipatory guidance Information about developmental changes that can be expected in the future. Including the recognition of the potential for a crisis and assistance with identifying potential methods for averting the crisis.

Anticipatory learning Learning necessary to effectively reach a desired outcome or in anticipation of a need for information that has not yet occurred.

Anticipatory loss A loss that is experienced before the loss actually occurs. For example, the gradual decline and eventual death of a family member who has Alzheimer disease.

Anticipatory problem solving Initial information is presented to a learner, who is then asked a question or presented with a situation related to the information. The learner applies the new information to the situation and decides what to do.

Antigen Foreign substance that triggers the immune response.

Antigen-antibody complex The complex formed by the binding of an antibody to an antigen.

Antigenic drift Describes small changes that occur continuously as a virus makes copies of itself.

Antigenic shift When two different strains of a virus infect the same cell and exchange genetic material to create a new subtype of the virus.

Antiretroviral therapies Pharmacologic therapies that stop or suppress the activity of a retrovirus, preventing further weakening of the immune system and thereby minimizing opportunistic infections.

Antiseptics Agents that inhibit the growth of some microorganisms.

Antisocial personality disorder (ASPD) One of several types of personality disorders defined by the DSM-5, it is characterized by a pattern of disregard for and violation of the rights of others.

Anuria The failure of the kidneys to produce urine, resulting in a total lack of urination or output of less than 100 mL/day in an adult.

Anxiety A stress response characterized by feelings of apprehension, dread, mental uneasiness, and a sense of helplessness in response to an actual or perceived threat to the well-being of oneself or others.

Anxious distress A combination of symptoms often associated with anxiety, including restlessness, impaired concentration due to worry, fear of something awful happening, and fear of losing control. Anxious distress often manifests in clients with depression and bipolar disorders and is associated with an increased risk for suicide.

Aortic stenosis Narrowing of the aortic valve that obstructs blood flow to systemic circulation.

Apathy A lack of interest or enthusiasm.

Apgar score A physical assessment of a newborn at 1 minute and 5 minutes after birth on a scale from 1 to 10 that includes heart rate, respiratory effort, muscle tone, reflex irritability, and skin color.

Aphakia Absence of the lens of the eye (e.g., after surgical removal of a cataract).

Aphasia Defective or absent language function.

Apical-radial pulse A comparison of the apical and radial pulses, which are normally identical. A pulse deficit can indicate certain cardiovascular disorders.

Aplastic anemia A disorder that results when the bone marrow fails to produce all three types of blood cells.

Apnea Absence of breathing.

Apnea of prematurity Absence of breathing for 20 seconds or longer, or for less than 20 seconds when associated with cyanosis, pallor, and bradycardia. A common problem in a preterm infant of less than 36 weeks' gestation, usually presenting between day 2 and day 7 of life.

Appendectomy Surgical removal of the appendix.

Appendicitis Inflammation of the vermiform appendix.

Appendicular skeleton Pectoral girdles, upper limbs, pelvic girdle, and lower limbs.

Approach-coping The use of confrontation to change the stressor by taking direct action.

Approximated Closed.

Apraxia The inability to perform purposeful movements and use objects correctly.

Areflexia The loss of reflex function.

Areola Pigmented ring surrounding the nipple of the breast.

Arrhythmogenic tissue Tissue that affects the generation and conduction of electrical impulses in the heart.

Arrogance Excessive pride and a feeling of superiority.

Arterial blood gas (ABG) A laboratory test used to evaluate oxygen and carbon dioxide exchange and the acid–base balance within the blood.

Arterial blood pressure A measure of the pressure exerted by the blood as it flows through the arteries.

Arteriosclerosis An arterial disorder characterized by thickening, loss of elasticity, and calcification of arterial walls.

Arteriovenous (AV) fistula An artificial connection between a vein and an artery created for long-term vascular access.

Arthrodesis A procedure that permanently fuses two or more bones together at a joint using pins, plates, screws, and rods. Also called *joint fusion*.

Arthroplasty Total joint replacement.

Arthroscopy A surgical procedure in which a thin, lighted tube with a camera in one end is inserted into a joint in order to allow a surgeon to visualize joint structure more easily.

Artificial disc surgery Surgery to replace a herniated disc with an artificial disc in order to maintain flexibility of the spinal joint.

Artificial rupture of membranes A process of rupturing of the membranes by the certified nurse-midwife or physician using an instrument called an amniohook. Completed if spontaneous rupture of membranes does not occur.

ASA Physical Classification Scale A physical risk classification category that determines the type and dosage of sedation a client can receive.

Ascites Excess fluid in the peritoneal cavity.

Asepsis The absence of disease-causing organisms.

Assault The action of creating an apprehension of offensive, insulting, or physically injurious touching.

Assertive behavior Behavior that consists of expressing one's wishes and opinions, or taking care of oneself, but not at the expense of others.

Assertive communicators Individuals who tend to declare and affirm their opinions. In doing this, however, they respect the rights of other to communicate in the same fashion.

Assertive community treatment (ACT) A therapeutic regimen for individuals with moderate to severe mental illness that provides clients with individually tailored services within their communities.

Assessment The systematic and continuous collection of data about a client for the purpose of determining the client's current and ongoing health status, predicting the client's health risks, and identifying appropriate health-promoting activities.

Assignment The transfer of responsibility to accomplish a task, without the transfer of authority.

Assimilation 1. The process of adapting to and integrating characteristics of the dominant culture as one's own. **2.** The process by which humans encounter and react to new situations by using the mechanisms they already possess.

Assisted suicide Self-administration of a lethal dose of medication provided by a physician or healthcare provider in order to intentionally end a client's life with the goal of relieving pain and suffering.

Associative play A stage of play in which children play together or share tasks during play.

Astereognosis The inability to identify objects by touch.

Asthma A chronic inflammatory disease of the lungs characterized by recurrent episodes of wheezing, breathlessness, chest tightness, and coughing.

Asynclitism A condition that occurs when the sagittal suture is directed toward either the symphysis pubis or the sacral promontory and is felt to be misaligned.

Asystole Cardiac standstill.

Ataxia Lack of muscle coordination.

Atelectasis Collapse of lung tissue following obstruction of the bronchus or bronchioles.

Atheist An individual who does not believe in God.

Atherosclerosis A form of arteriosclerosis in which deposits of fat and fibrin obstruct and harden the arteries.

Atrial gallop (S$_4$) A heart sound produced by atrial contraction and ejection of blood into the ventricle during late diastole. Also called the *fourth heart sound*.

Atrial kick An extra bolus of blood delivered to the ventricles before they contract.

Atrial natriuretic factor (ANF) A peptide hormone released from cells in the atrium of the heart in response to excess blood volume and stretching of the atrial walls.

Atrial septal defect (ASD) An opening in the atrial septum that permits left-to-right shunting of blood.

Atrioventricular (AV) canal defect A combination of defects in the atrial and ventricular septa and portions of tricuspid and mitral valves. A complete AV canal defect allows blood to travel freely among all four chambers of the heart. Also called *endocardial cushion defect*.

Atrophy The wasting away or decrease in size of an organ, muscle, or tissue.

Attention deficit disorder (ADD) A variation in central nervous system processing characterized by developmentally inappropriate behaviors involving inattention.

Attention-deficit/hyperactivity disorder (ADHD) A variation in central nervous system processing characterized by developmentally inappropriate behaviors involving inattention, hyperactivity, and impulsivity.

Attention impairment A condition marked by an inability to process information and respond to such information appropriately; a client with attention impairment will have poor concentration and be easily distracted.

Attentive listening The process of listening actively, using all the senses. Also called *mindful listening*.

Audiologist A healthcare professional specializing in identifying, diagnosing, treating, and monitoring disorders of the auditory and vestibular portions of the ear.

Audit An examination of records to verify accuracy and proper use.

Auditory Of or relating to hearing.

Aura An olfactory or visual sensory sensation that may provide an early warning sign of a seizure.

Auscultation Listening to the sounds produced within the body. Auscultation can be direct using the unaided ear or indirect using a stethoscope or other listening device.

Authority 1. The power to command other individuals and direct their activities. 2. The right to act or to accomplish the task.

Autism spectrum disorders (ASDs) A developmental disorder in which individuals have persistent deficits in social communication and social interaction, and restricted, repetitive patterns of behavior, interest, or activities.

Autoantibodies Antibodies that react to the individual's own tissues.

Autocratic (authoritarian) leader A leader who makes decisions for the group based on the belief that individuals are externally motivated and are incapable of independent decision making.

Autografting A procedure performed in the surgical suite in which part of a client's healthy skin is removed and used to effect permanent skin coverage over a wound area.

Autoimmune disorder/disease Failure of immune system to recognize itself, resulting in normal host tissue being targeted by immune defenses.

Autologous blood transfusion A blood transfusion using a client's own blood.

Autologous bone marrow transplant Bone marrow transplant using a client's own bone marrow.

Automatism A repetitive reaction that occurs automatically, without conscious thought. Examples include lip smacking, eyelid fluttering, aimless walking, picking at clothing, and swallowing.

Autonomic dysreflexia An abrupt onset of excessively high blood pressure as the result of an overactive autonomic nervous system. An exaggerated sympathetic response that occurs in clients with spinal cord injuries at or above the T6 level. Also called *autonomic hyperreflexia*.

Autonomy 1. The state of being independent and self-directed without outside control. 2. The right to make one's own decisions.

Autosomal chromosomes Genetic material found in a cell nucleus that determines physical characteristics (excluding gender) of the individual.

Autosome A single chromosome from any one of the 22 pairs of chromosomes not involved in sex determination (X or Y); humans have 22 pairs of autosomes.

Avascular necrosis The death of bone tissue due to lack of blood supply. Also called *osteonecrosis*.

Avian influenza Also known as "bird flu," it is a form of influenza that commonly infects birds. This virus has not yet demonstrated the ability to spread among humans; however, concerns are that it will mutate to allow person-to-person spread. This viral strain has a mortality rate of greater than 50% in people who have been infected due to close association with infected birds.

Avoidance-coping The use of both behaviors and cognitive processes to avoid a stressor.

Avoidant personality disorder (APD) One of several types of personality disorders recognized by the DSM-5, APD is characterized by a pattern of social withdrawal along with a sense of inadequacy, fear, and hypersensitivity to potential rejection or shame.

Avolition The inability to persist in goal-directed activities.

Awareness The ability to perceive environmental stimuli and body reactions and to respond appropriately through thought and action.

Axial loading The application of vertical force to the spinal column.

Axial skeleton Ribs, sternum, vertebral column, and skull.

Axon A nerve fiber.

Azotemia Increased levels of nitrogenous wastes in the blood.

B lymphocytes (B cells) Integral to specific immune response, they are activated and mature into either plasma cells, which secrete antibodies, or memory cells.

Babinski reflex The fanning and extension of the toes or flexion of the toes due to gentle stroking on the sole of the foot. Also called the *Babinski response.*

Bacilli Rod-shaped bacteria.

Background questions General questions asked of a client that seek more information about a topic, such as diseases and medications.

Bacteremia The presence of bacteria in the blood.

Bacteria The most common category of infection-causing microorganisms.

Bactericidal agent Destroys bacteria.

Bacteriostatic agent Prevents the growth and reproduction of some bacteria.

Balloon tamponade The inflation of the balloon tip of a multiple-lumen nasogastric tube to control bleeding.

Barlow maneuver A procedure used to evaluate an infant for hip dislocation or instability in which the healthcare provider grasps and adducts the infant's thigh and then applies gentle downward pressure.

Barotrauma Lung injury caused by alveolar overdistention. Also called *volutrauma.*

Barrel chest An increase in the anteroposterior chest diameter resulting from air trapping and hyperinflation.

Basal cell carcinoma An epithelial tumor believed to originate either from the basal layer of the epidermis or from cells in the surrounding dermal structures. Also called *basal cell cancer.*

Basal metabolic rate (BMR) The amount of energy expended by the body at rest.

Base excess (BE) A calculated value also known as *buffer base capacity.* The BE measures substances that can accept or combine with hydrogen ions. It reflects the degree of acid–base imbalance by indicating the status of the body's total buffering capacity.

Baseline rate The average fetal heart rate rounded to increments of 5 bpm observed during a 10-minute period of monitoring. This excludes periodic or episodic changes, periods of marked variability, and segments of the baseline that differ by more than 25 bpm.

Bases Substances that accept hydrogen ions in solution. Also called *alkalis.*

Basic needs The physical needs of an individual, such as eating, sleeping, resting, self-care, and physical stability.

Battery The willful touching of another individual, an individual's clothes, or even something the individual is carrying that is unwanted, embarrassing, or unwarranted.

Behavioral therapy A form of therapy in which clients learn techniques to modify or change maladaptive behaviors.

Behaviorist theory A theory that suggests that learning takes place when an individual's reaction to a stimulus is either positively or negatively reinforced.

Belief An interpretation or conclusion that one accepts as true.

Belief system The way in which a culture explains the mysteries of the universe and life.

Belt restraint Restraint used to ensure the safety of clients who are transported by wheelchair or gurney, or to protect clients confined to a bed or a chair. Also called *safety strap body restraint.*

Benchmarking A method used to compare the performance of an individual or organization to industry standards.

Beneficence The act of doing good or beneficial actions.

Benign Referring to a growth or tumor that does not endanger life or health and tends to not recur after treatment.

Benign prostatic hyperplasia (BPH) Nonmalignant enlargement of the prostate gland commonly seen in the aging male.

Bereavement The subjective response experienced by the surviving loved ones after the death of an individual with whom they have shared a significant relationship.

Bias The favoring of a group or individual over another.

Bidirectional influence Influences exerted between an individual and his or her family that may negatively affect the emotional health of the individual, the family, or both.

Bilevel ventilator (BiPAP) Mechanical ventilation that provides inspiratory positive airway pressure as well as airway support during expiration.

Biliary colic A severe, steady pain in the epigastric region or right upper quadrant of the abdomen.

Binge drinking The consumption of five or more drinks containing alcohol in a single session.

Binge eating The ingestion of huge amounts of food (about 3,500 kcal) within a short time (about 1 hour).

Binge eating disorder (BED) An eating disorder characterized by recurring episodes of binge eating, a sense of lack of control, and negative feelings about oneself, but without intervening periods of behavior such as self-induced vomiting, purging by laxatives, fasting, or prolonged exercise.

Binuclear family A postdivorce family in which the biological children are members of two nuclear households—that of the father and that of the mother—and the children alternate between the two homes.

Bioethics The application of ethics to issues of human life or health (e.g., to decisions about abortion or euthanasia).

Biological rhythm A cyclical event or function that consists of repeated occurrences and repeated, regular intervals between occurrences. Biological rhythms can refer to both physical and psychological patterns.

Biomedical informatics The interdisciplinary science that deals with biomedical information's structure, acquisition, and use.

Bioterrorism The deliberate release of viruses, bacteria, or other microbes as weapons.

Bipolar disorder A mood disorder characterized by alternating depression and elation, with periods of normal mood in between. Formerly called *manic–depressive disorder.*

Birthing room A single room in a hospital where a pregnant woman and her partner or other family members will stay for the labor, birth, recovery, and possibly the postpartum period.

Bisexual An individual who is attracted to members of both sexes.

Bisphosphonates Drugs used to treat osteoporosis that inhibit bone reabsorption by suppressing osteoclast activity.

Blackouts A form of amnesia about events that occurred during a drinking period. This is often seen in the early stages of alcoholism.

Bladder training Gradually increases the bladder capacity by increasing the intervals between voidings and resisting the urge to void.

Blame-free environment An environment in which healthcare providers can report errors or near misses without the fear of punishment.

Blended family A family formed after the death or divorce of a parent, may include stepparents on both sides, stepchildren, half-siblings.

Blepharism Spasms that cause the eye to blink continuously.

Blighted ovum One of the most common causes of miscarriage, it occurs when the egg has been fertilized and both the membrane and placenta have formed, but the embryo has not formed.

Blood flow The volume of blood transported in a vessel, in an organ, or throughout the entire circulation over a given period of time.

Blood pressure The force that blood exerts against the walls of the arteries as it is pumped from the heart.

Blood urea nitrogen (BUN) A measure of blood level of urea, the end product of protein metabolism.

Bloodborne pathogens Microorganisms carried in blood and body fluids that are capable of infecting other individuals with serious and difficult to treat viral infections.

Bloody show The pink-tinged secretions resulting from a small amount of blood loss from the exposed cervical capillaries during pregnancy.

Blunt trauma Trauma that occurs without any communication between the damaged tissues and the outside environment.

Body fluid Any fluid that is essential to homeostasis; water is the primary body fluid.

Body image The mental image of the physical self.

Body mass index (BMI) A method of comparing weight to height as an indirect measure of body fat.

Body substance isolation (BSI) System that employs generic infection control precautions for all clients, except those with the few airborne diseases.

Body surface area (BSA) The relationship between height and weight measured in square meters.

Body temperature The core or surface measurement of a client's internal heat production and loss.

Bone marrow transplant The treatment of disease by infusing a client with his or her own bone marrow or that of a healthy donor.

Borborygmus Hyperactive, high-pitched, tinkling, rushing, or growling bowel sounds heard in diarrhea or at the onset of bowel obstruction.

Borderline personality disorder (BPD) One of several personality disorders defined in the DSM-5, BPD is marked by unstable interpersonal relationships, self-image, affect, and impulsiveness.

Bouchard nodes Bony lumps in the middle joint of the digit.

Boundaries The invisible lines that define the amount and kind of contact allowable among members of a family and between the family and outside systems.

Boutonnière deformity A flexion deformity of the PIP joints with extension of the DIP joint.

Bowel incontinence The inability to voluntarily control the passage of fecal contents and intestinal gas through the anal sphincter. Also called *fecal incontinence*.

Brachytherapy Radiation treatment given by placing radioactive material directly in or near the target, which is often a tumor.

Bradycardia A heart rate in an adult of less than 60 bpm.

Bradydysrhythmia Abnormally slow rhythms.

Bradykinesia Slowed movements due to muscle rigidity.

Bradyphrenia Slowed thinking and a decreased ability to form thoughts, to plan, or to make decisions.

Bradypnea A respiratory rate of less than 10 breaths per minute in adults.

Brain death The cessation and irreversibility of all brain functions, including those of the brainstem.

Brainstem Contains the midbrain, pons, and medulla oblongata. Located between the cerebrum and spinal cord, the brainstem connects pathways between the higher and lower structures. Ten of the 12 pairs of cranial nerves originate in the brainstem.

Brainstorming A decision-making method in which group members meet and generate diverse ideas about the nature, cause, definition, or solution to a problem.

Braxton Hicks contractions Intermittent painless uterine contractions that may occur every 10–20 minutes and occur more frequently near the end of pregnancy.

Brazelton neonatal behavioral assessment scale A scale developed to assess a newborn's state changes, temperament, and individual behavioral patterns.

Breach of care See Breach of duty.

Breach of duty A deviation from the standard of care owed a client. Also called *breach of care*.

Breakthrough pain A sudden flare or increase in pain despite comfort with or without baseline analgesia.

Breast Mammary gland.

Breast cancer The unregulated growth of abnormal cells in breast tissue.

Breathing exercises Techniques used to slow the breathing rate by focusing on taking regular and deep breaths from the diaphragm.

Brief psychotic disorder Rapid onset of at least one of the following psychotic symptoms: delusions, hallucinations, disorganized speech, or disorganized behavior. The episode lasts at least 1 day but less than 1 month, after which the person returns to the premorbid level of functioning.

Bronchiectasis Chronic dilation of the bronchi and bronchioles.

Bronchiolitis A lower respiratory tract illness that occurs when an infecting agent (virus or bacterium) causes inflammation and obstruction of the small airways.

Bronchitis Inflammation of the mucous membranes of the bronchial tubes.

Bronchogenic carcinomas Tumors of the airway epithelium.

Bronchoscopy A procedure that allows direct visualization of the lungs by inserting a bronchoscope orally into the trachea and advancing it to the bronchi bifurcation.

Bronchovesicular sound The sound created as air moves within the bronchial tree.

Brown adipose tissue (BAT) A specific store of fat in newborn infants that appears dark brown due to enriched blood supply, dense cellular content, and abundant nerve endings.

Bruits Blowing sound sometimes heard due to restriction of blood flow through the vessels.

Buffers Substances that prevent major changes in pH by releasing hydrogen ions.

Bulimia nervosa (BN) A type of eating disorder characterized by an obsessive focus on weight and body size and cycles of binge eating followed by purging.

Bureaucratic leader A leader who relies on the organization's rules, policies, and procedures to direct the group's work efforts.

Burn An injury resulting from exposure to heat, chemicals, radiation, or electric current.

Burn shock Hypovolemic shock resulting from the shift of a massive amount of fluid from the intracellular and intravascular compartments into the interstitium following burn injury. Also called *hypovolemic shock*.

Burnout A complex syndrome resulting from unmanaged stress that manifests as physical and emotional depletion, a negative attitude and self-concept, and feelings of helplessness and hopelessness.

Cachexia Physical wasting from weight loss and loss of muscle mass due to the rapid growth and reproduction of cancer cells and their need for increased nutrients.

Caffeine A stimulant that increases the heart rate and acts as a diuretic.

Calcium oxalate A chemical compound from which kidney stones may form.

Calcium phosphate A chemical compound from which kidney stones may form.

Calculi Renal stones.

Cancellous bone The spongy tissue of bone.

Cancer A family of complex diseases with manifestations that vary according to body system and type of tumor cells.

Cancer pain Pain that may result from the direct effects of the cancerous disease and its treatment, or it may be unrelated to the disease and its treatment in individuals with cancer.

Candidiasis A common, opportunistic fungal infection in clients with AIDS.

Cannabis sativa The plant source of marijuana.

Caput succedaneum A localized, easily identifiable, soft area of the scalp, generally resulting from a long and difficult labor or vacuum extraction.

Carbohydrate One of the three major macronutrients primarily derived from plant foods. These foods contain simple and complex sugars, and starches.

Carcinogen A substance that causes cancer.

Carcinogenesis The production or origin of cancer.

Cardiac arrest The cessation of heart function that precedes biological death.

Cardiac cycle One contraction and relaxation of the heart; a single heartbeat.

Cardiac index The cardiac output adjusted for the client's body size or body surface area (BSA).

Cardiac markers Proteins released from necrotic heart muscle.

Cardiac output (CO) The amount of blood pumped by the ventricles into the pulmonary and systemic circulations in 1 minute.

Cardiac rehabilitation A medically supervised program designed to aid people with their recovery from heart attacks, heart surgeries, and percutaneous coronary interventions.

Cardiac reserve The heart's ability to respond to the body's changing need for cardiac output.

Cardiac tamponade Compression of the heart caused by collected blood or fluid in the pericardium.

Cardinal ligament Major ligament of the uterus containing the uterine artery and vein.

Cardinal movements A series of changes in position that allow the fetus to move through the birth canal. Also called *mechanisms of labor.*

Cardiogenic shock Shock that occurs when the heart's pumping ability is compromised to the point that it cannot maintain cardiac output and adequate tissue perfusion.

Cardiomyopathy Disease that affects the heart muscle's ability to pump effectively. Primary abnormality of the heart muscle that affects its structural or functional characteristics.

Cardiopulmonary resuscitation (CPR) A mechanical attempt to maintain tissue perfusion and oxygenation using oral resuscitation and external cardiac compressions.

Care coordination The means by which a multidisciplinary team works with a client to ensure that the care received across the healthcare continuum meets the client's needs.

Care management model Planning, assessment, and coordination of health services to provide an integrated continuum of clinical services including medical care, health promotion, disease prevention, costs, and use of resources.

Care map Expected outcomes and care strategies developed through collaboration by the healthcare team. Also called a *critical pathway.*

Caring To feel interest, concern, and respect for a client while demonstrating sensitivity, sincerity, honesty, and patience.

Caring for the dying The act of helping clients live as comfortably as possible until death and helping the client's support individuals cope with death.

Carpal spasm Involuntary contraction of the hand and fingers due to decreased calcium levels.

Carphologia Involuntary, repeated lint picking.

Carrier Human or animal reservoir of a specific infectious agent that usually does not manifest any clinical signs of the disease.

Cartilage A type of flexible connective tissue found throughout the body.

Case management (CM) The process of coordinating, facilitating, and following a client's use of an array of health and social services over time.

Case managers Individuals who help manage the care of certain client populations including clients with chronic medical conditions, such as diabetes; clients recovering from acute conditions, such as those receiving joint replacement; and clients managing psychiatric disorders.

Caseation necrosis A process in which tissue infected with *Mycobacterium tuberculosis* dies and forms a cheeselike center in the infectious bacilli.

Cast A rigid device applied to immobilize injured bones and promote healing.

Catabolism The breakdown of body proteins.

Cataract An opacification (clouding) of lens of the eye due to a breakdown of proteins within the lens.

Catatonia Unresponsiveness to the environment or others.

Catatonic excitement Includes hyperactivity and bizarre behavior and is a positive symptom of schizophrenia.

Catatonic inhibition involves decreased activity level; limited speech; minimal self-care; and, at times, a trancelike state. Catatonic inhibition is a negative symptom of schizophrenia.

Cation Ion that carries a positive charge.

Cauda equina syndrome (CES) A condition that occurs when the nerve roots of the cauda equine are compressed. It may result in permanent neurological impairment, including urinary incontinence and paralysis.

Causation To make a successful claim for malpractice, an injury must have occurred as a direct consequence of a nurse's or professional's breach of duty.

Cavitation Formation of a cavity or bubble.

Celiac disease A chronic immune-mediated disorder of the small intestine in which the absorption of nutrients, particularly fats, is impaired. Also known as celiac sprue or nontropical sprue.

Cell cycle The four phases of cell growth and development.

Cell-mediated (cellular) immune response Direct or indirect inactivation of antigen by lymphocytes.

Cellulitis An acute bacterial infection of the dermis and underlying connective tissue. Cellulitis is characterized by red or lilac, tender, warm, edematous skin that may have an ill-defined, nonelevated border.

Central nervous system (CNS) One of two principal parts of the neurological system, the central nervous system consists of the brain and the spinal cord.

Central nervous system (CNS) depressants A type of drug that acts to slow brain function, decreasing levels of alertness and awareness. CNS depressants include barbiturates, benzodiazepines, paraldehyde, meprobamate, and chloral hydrate.

Central pain 1. A type of pain related to a lesion in the brain that may spontaneously produce high-frequency bursts of impulses that are perceived as pain. 2. A type of pain caused by damage to the central nervous system that may manifest in constant pain, pain paroxysms, evoked pain, or allodynia. Clients may describe their pain as "pins and needles," aching, or lacerating.

Centration Focusing only on one particular aspect of a situation or the ability to concentrate.

Cephalocaudal development Growth that proceeds in the direction from head to toe.

Cephalohematoma A collection of blood resulting from ruptured blood vessels between the surface of a cranial bone and the periosteal membrane. Also called an *entrapped hemorrhage.*

Cerebellum Located below the cerebrum and behind the brainstem, it coordinates stimuli from the cerebral cortex to provide precise timing for skeletal muscle coordination and smooth movements.

Cerebral palsy (CP) A group of chronic conditions affecting body movement, coordination, and posture that results from a nonprogressive abnormality of the immature brain.

Cerebral perfusion pressure (CPP) The pressure it takes for the heart to provide the brain with blood. It is calculated by finding the difference between arterial pressure and intracranial pressure. Normal CPP is 0–95 mmHg.

Cerebrum The largest portion of the brain, it is composed of gray matter and has two hemispheres divided into four regions or lobes.

Certification The credentialing process by which a nongovernmental agency or association recognizes the professional competence of an individual who has met the predetermined qualifications specified by the agency or association.

Cerumen Earwax.

Cervical cap A latex cup-shaped contraceptive device, used with spermicidal cream or jelly, that fits snugly over the cervix and is held in place by suction.

Cervical collar A device that stabilizes and maintains neutral alignment of the cervical spine; it is used with clients with potential or suspected cervical spine injury. Also called *C-collar*.

Cervical ripening The softening and effacing of the cervix.

Cervix The narrow neck of the uterus.

Cesarean birth The birth of an infant through an abdominal and uterine incision.

Chain of command The hierarchy of authority and responsibility within an organization.

Chancre A painless ulceration formed during the first stage of syphilis.

Change-of-shift report A type of handoff communication given to all nurses on the next shift.

Channel A medium used to convey messages.

Charismatic leader A rare type of leader who is characterized by a strong, emotional relationship between the leader and the group members.

Chart A formal, legal document that provides evidence of a client's care. Also called a *client record* or a *clinical record*.

Charting The process of making an entry on a client record. Also called *recording* or *documenting*.

Charting by exception (CBE) A documentation system in which only abnormal or significant findings or exceptions to norms are recorded.

CHCT A biopsy of thigh skeletal muscle tissue to determine sensitivity to caffeine and halothane.

Cheilosis Cracking of lips.

Chemical conjunctivitis An irritation of the conjunctiva by chemicals used to treat the eyes.

Chemical restraints Pharmacologic agents administered for the purpose of controlling hyperactive behavior in agitated clients.

Chemical thermogenesis The stimulation of heat production in the body through increased cellular metabolism. Also called *nonshivering thermogenesis* or *NST*.

Chemotaxis The movement of cells in response to a chemical stimulus.

Chemotherapy Cancer treatment involving the use of cytotoxic medications to decrease tumor size, adjunctive to surgery or radiation therapy; or to prevent or treat suspected metastases.

Chest x-ray Allows for two-dimensional visualization of the contents of the thoracic cavity.

Child abuse Any act or failure to act on the part of a parent or caretaker which results in the death, serious physical or emotional harm, sexual abuse, or exploitation of a child.

Child Health Insurance Program (CHIP) State and federal funded healthcare coverage for children under the age of 19 whose families earn more than the Medicaid limits but cannot afford to purchase private healthcare coverage.

Childhood traumatic grief A grief reaction that occurs when an important person in a child's life dies as the result of a traumatic event or circumstances the child views as traumatic.

Childless family A family without children. Also called a *child-free family*.

Chlamydia A group of sexually transmitted infections caused by *Chlamydia trachomatis*.

Chloasma Brownish pigmentation over the bridge of the nose and the cheeks during pregnancy and in some women who are taking oral contraceptives. Also called *melasma gravidarum* or *mask of pregnancy*.

Cholangitis Duct inflammation.

Cholecystitis Inflammation of the gallbladder.

Cholelithiasis The formation of stones (*calculi* or *gallstones*) in the gallbladder or biliary duct system.

Chromosomes Tightly coiled strands of DNA within the nucleus that contain genetic information.

Chronic bronchitis A disorder of excessive bronchial mucous secretion.

Chronic fatigue Profound fatigue of long duration that is not improved by rest.

Chronic fatigue syndrome A complex disorder in which the client experiences unrelenting fatigue and associated symptoms that are not alleviated by substantial rest and that cannot be otherwise explained for a period of 6 months or longer. Also called *myalgic encephalomyelitis*.

Chronic illness An alteration in health or function that lasts for an extended period of time, usually 6 months or longer, and often for the duration of the individual's life.

Chronic infection An infection that develops slowly and persists for months or sometimes years.

Chronic intermittent colitis A recurrent form of ulcerative colitis characterized by insidious onset, few systemic manifestations, and attacks lasting 1–3 months that occur at intervals of months to years.

Chronic kidney disease A type of renal failure that progresses slowly with few symptoms until the kidneys are severely damaged and unable to meet the excretory needs of the body. Also called *chronic renal failure*.

Chronic lymphocytic leukemia (CLL) A disorder characterized by the proliferation and accumulation of small, abnormal, mature lymphocytes in the bone marrow, peripheral blood, and body tissues.

Chronic myeloid leukemia (CML) A disorder characterized by abnormal proliferation of all bone marrow elements.

Chronic obstructive pulmonary disease (COPD) A specific progressive disorder that slowly alters the structures of the respiratory system over time, irreversibly affecting lung function.

Chronic pain Prolonged pain, usually lasting longer than 6 months. It is not always associated with an identifiable cause and is often unresponsive to conventional medical treatment.

Chronic pancreatitis An irreversible process characterized by chronic inflammation, fibrosis, and gradual destruction of functional pancreatic tissue.

Chronic renal failure See Chronic kidney disease.

Chronic venous insufficiency (CVI) A disorder of inadequate venous return over a prolonged period of time.

Chvostek sign Facial grimacing caused by repeated contractions of the facial muscle. A test used to check for hypocalcemia.

Circumcision A surgical procedure in which the prepuce, an epithelial layer covering the penis, is separated from the glans penis and excised. This procedure permits exposure of the glans for easier cleaning.

Cirrhosis The end stage of chronic liver disease. It is a progressive, irreversible disorder, eventually leading to liver failure.

Civil law The area of law that deals with the rights and duties of private persons or citizens and is most often enforced through the awarding of damages or compensation.

CK-MB A subset of CK enzyme specific to cardiac muscle. Elevated CK-MB is an indicator of myocardial infarction. Also called *MB-bands*.

Clang Repetition of rhyming words without apparent meaning.

Classism The oppression of groups of people based on their socioeconomic status.

Clean A state of medical asepsis in which almost all microorganisms are absent.

Client An individual who engages the advice or services of another person who is qualified to provide this service.

Client advocate An individual who acts to protect the client and defend the client from harm.

Client-focused care A delivery model that organizes health care around the expressed physical and emotional needs of the client.

Client record A formal, legal document that provides evidence of a client's care. Also called a *chart* or a *clinical record*.

Clinical decision support system A system that analyzes data and provides information about evidenced-based practices. These systems can help improve client safety and quality of care when used with sound nursing and medical judgment.

Clinical information system A software-based system that allows multiple disciplines to simultaneously access the client's chart and record data that can be viewed and analyzed by a number of healthcare providers in real time. These systems are designed to provide the most accurate and current information about the client so that the best decisions concerning the care of that client can be made.

Clinical pathway A standardized, evidence-based, multidisciplinary plan that outlines the expected care required for clients with common, predictable—usually medical—conditions.

Clonic phase Typically the second phase in a generalized or tonic-clonic seizure, characterized by alternating muscular contraction and relaxation.

Closed fracture A bone fracture in which the skin remains intact. Also called a *simple fracture*.

Closed questions Restrictive questions in an interview that require only a "yes" or "no" or short, specific answer.

Club drugs Substances popular among adolescents and young adults who frequent dance clubs and "raves." The most common is MDMA (methylenedioxymethamphetamine), better known as ecstasy.

Coaching The process that encourages the development of individuals through personal interaction within an organization.

Coanalgesics Drugs that have analgesic properties, potentiate the effects of pain medications, relieve other discomforts, or reduce the side effects of analgesic drugs. Coanalgesics are especially effective at reducing neuropathic pain.

Coarctation of the aorta Narrowing or constriction in the descending aorta, often near the ductus arteriosus or left subclavian artery, which obstructs the systemic blood outflow.

Cobb angle A technique to estimate the degree of curvature of the spine using lines drawn from the vertebrae at the upper and lower limits of the curve that tilt most dramatically toward the apex of the curve.

Cocaine A powerful stimulant of natural origin that acts at the nerve terminals to prevent the reuptake of dopamine and norepinephrine, which in turn results in vasoconstriction, tachycardia, and hypertension.

Code of ethics A general guide for a profession's membership and a social contract with the public that it serves.

Codependence A cluster of maladaptive behaviors exhibited by significant others of a substance-abusing individual that serves to enable and protect the abuse at the expense of living a full and satisfying life.

Cognition The complex set of mental activities through which individuals acquire, process, store, retrieve, and apply information.

Cognitive appraisal The process of appraising, sorting, assessing, categorizing, evaluating, and framing the significance of an event or stressor with respect to an individual's own well-being.

Cognitive behavioral therapy (CBT) The use of cognitive techniques and behavior modification to change detrimental beliefs and thought patterns.

Cognitive development The manner in which people learn to think, reason, and use language.

Cognitive domain The learning domain that includes the six intellectual abilities and thinking processes: knowing, comprehending, applying, analysis, synthesis, and evaluation. Also called the *thinking domain*.

Cognitive skills Intellectual skills or thought processes that include problem solving, decision making, critical thinking, and creativity.

Cognitive theory A learning theory that recognizes the developmental level of learners and acknowledges the learner's motivation and environment. Also called *cognitivism*.

Coitus interruptus A method of contraception in which the male withdraws from the female's vagina when he feels that ejaculation is impending.

Cold zone When a disaster occurs, this zone, located outside the warm zone, is where decontaminated victims are triaged and treated. Also called the *green zone* or the *support zone*.

Colectomy Surgical resection and removal of the colon.

Collaboration Two or more people working toward a common goal.

Collaborative intervention The actions a nurse carries out in collaboration with other healthcare team members, such as physical therapists, social workers, dietitians, and physicians.

Collagen A whitish protein substance that adds tensile strength to a wound.

Collateral channels Small blood vessels that develop to connect small arteries. Also called *collateral circulation*.

Colloid osmotic pressure A pulling force exerted by colloids that helps maintain the water content of blood by pulling water from the interstitial space into the vascular compartment. Also called *oncotic pressure*.

Colloids Substances such as large protein molecules that do not readily dissolve into true solutions.

Colon cancer Cancer of the third segment of the large bowel that may or may not include the anus.

Colonization The process by which strains of microorganisms become resident flora, capable of growing and multiplying.

Colorectal cancer Cancer of both the colon and rectum.

Colostomy A surgical opening into the colon.

Colostrum The initial milk that begins to be secreted during mid-pregnancy and that is immediately available to the baby at birth.

Column plan A nursing care plan that uses columns to categorize data for each phase of the nursing process. This type of care plan may include four columns: (1) nursing diagnoses, (2) goals/desired outcomes, (3) nursing interventions, and (4) evaluation. Some include only three columns.

Combined oral contraceptives (COCs) A safe, highly effective contraceptive pill combining estrogen and progestin. Also called *birth control pills*.

Comfort To ease the grief or trouble of others; to give hope.

Commitment The state or an instance of being obligated or emotionally impelled.

Communicable disease An illness that is transmitted directly from one person or animal to another by contact with body fluids, or that is indirectly transmitted by contact with contaminated objects or vectors.

Communication The exchange of information, feelings, thoughts, and ideals through verbal or other techniques.

Communication deviance Communication patterns that are distracting and confusing to listeners who are trying to share a common focus or meaning with a speaker. Communication deviance has been identified as a social-environmental trigger for schizophrenia symptoms.

Communicator style The manner in which an individual communicates; includes the way the individual interacts with others.

Community-based care Care that focuses on the political, social, institutional, and physical environments of the client.

Community Emergency Response Team (CERT) program A Federal Emergency Management Agency–organized program that prepares participants to safely assist themselves, their families, and their neighbors in case of a diaster.

Comorbidity The presence of two or more disease processes.

Compartment syndrome A condition in which the tissue pressure in a muscle compartment exceeds the microvascular pressure, interrupting cellular perfusion.

Compassion An awareness of and concern for other individuals' suffering.

Competence Possessing the knowledge and skills necessary to perform one's job appropriately and safely.

Complementary therapies Any of the diverse array of practices, therapies, and supplements that are not considered part of conventional or traditional medicine that are used in addition to conventional treatments.

Complete spinal cord injury An injury that involves a total loss of all sensory and motor function below the level of the injury; usually the damage is irreversible.

Compliance 1. The relationship between the volume of the intracranial components and intracranial pressure. 2. The amount of distention or expansion the ventricles can achieve to increase stroke volume. 3. The extent to which an individual's behavior coincides with medical or health advice.

Complicated grief A form of grief in which the individual's strategies to cope with a loss are maladaptive. Also called *prolonged grief disorder (PGD)*.

Compression A condition that occurs when a vertical force is applied to the spinal column, such as occurs by falling and landing on the feet or buttocks or diving into shallow water.

Compromised host An individual who is at increased risk of infection.

Compulsion A repetitive behavior or mental activity used in response to obsessive thoughts that helps the individual lower his or her anxiety level.

Compulsivity One of the six trait domains associated with personality disorders that is distinguished by extreme inflexibility in a quest for perfection, both in relation to the individual's own actions and others' behaviors.

Computer vision syndrome The most common sequela of computer use. Symptoms include eye fatigue, headaches, blurred vision, dry eyes, and changes in color perception. Also called *eye strain*.

Concept map A visual representation of a nursing plan of care in a patterned diagram with data and ideas. Various shapes and colors are used to show relationships and connections in combination with lines or arrows.

Concrete thinking A type of thinking characterized by a focus on facts and details coupled with an inability to generalize or think abstractly.

Concurrent audit An evaluation of the adequacy of the nursing care a client is receiving and a determination of whether desired outcomes are being met while the individual is still undergoing care at the healthcare facility.

Condom A sheath of synthetic material that covers the penis to prevent conception or disease.

Conduction The process of heat transfer through physical contact of one surface with another surface.

Confabulation Making up information to fill memory gaps; used as a defensive mechanism to protect the person's attempt to protect self-esteem when confronted with memory loss.

Confidentiality The assurance the client has that private information will not be disclosed without the client's consent.

Conflict A situation that occurs when an agreement cannot be reached with regard to significant issues and concerns or when emotional opposition creates discord within an individual or among individuals, groups, or organizations.

Confusion An alteration in cognition that makes it difficult to think clearly, focus attention, or make decisions.

Confusion assessment method (CAM) A two-part test that differentiates between delirium and dementia. It is specifically designed to account for and control ageism.

Congenital cataracts A type of cataract that may appear in a child at birth or in childhood, usually in both eyes.

Congenital heart defect A defect of the heart or great vessels that is present at birth.

Congruent communication Communication in which the verbal and nonverbal aspects of the message match.

Conjugate vera The true conjugate, which extends from the middle of the sacral promontory to the middle of the pubic crest.

Conjunctiva The thin, transparent membrane that covers the anterior surface of the eye and lines the inner surfaces of the eyelids.

Conjunctivitis Inflammation of the conjunctiva. The most common eye disease, conjunctivitis is usually caused by a bacterial or viral infection.

Connective tissue Tissue made of fiber that forms the framework for support of the body's tissue and organs.

Consciousness A condition in which the individual is aware of self and environment and is able to respond appropriately to stimuli. Full consciousness requires both normal arousal and full cognition.

Consequence-based (teleological) theories Theories that look to the outcomes (consequences) of an action in judging whether that action is right or wrong.

Conservation The concept that matter is not changed when its form is altered.

Consolidation Solidification of damaged cells and tissue during immune response to inflammation, specifically in the lungs.

Constant fever A condition that occurs when the body temperature fluctuates minimally but always remains above normal.

Constipation Fewer than three bowel movements per week or the difficult passage of stools.

Constructivism A collection of theories with the common thread of individuals actively constructing knowledge in order to solve realistic problems, often in collaboration with others.

Consumer An individual, a group of people, or a community that uses a service or commodity.

Consumer-driven healthcare plan (CDHP) A type of employer-sponsored coverage that combines a private insurance plan with a Health Savings Account (HSA) or Health Reimbursement Account (HRA).

Contact dermatitis An inflammation of the skin that occurs in response to direct contact with an allergen or irritant.

Contact precautions Used for clients who are known to have or suspected of having serious illnesses that are easily transmitted by direct contact with the client or by contact with items in the environment, such as *shigella*.

Contingency contracts A reinforcement process. Contingency contracts operate by "if–then" rules. If the client performs a targeted response, such as abstinence from the addictive behavior (gambling, drug use, cutting, etc.), then the client receives desired reinforcers.

Contingency planning The process of identifying and managing unplanned and unexpected events that interfere with getting work done efficiently, effectively, and timely.

Continuance commitment The awareness of costs associated with leaving a profession that inhibit an individual from leaving that profession. Considered the weakest type of commitment to a profession.

Continuous bladder irrigation (CBI) A method used to prevent the formation of blood clots.

Continuous positive airway pressure (CPAP) Mechanical ventilation that applies positive pressure to the airways of a client who is breathing spontaneously. Breathing is client triggered and pressure controlled. CPAP is used to help maintain open airways and alveoli, decreasing the work of breathing.

Continuous quality improvement (CQI) A structured organizational process for involving personnel in planning and executing a continuous flow of improvements to provide quality health care that meets or exceeds expectations.

Continuous renal replacement therapy (CRRT) A form of dialysis in which blood is continuously circulated through a highly porous hemofilter from artery to vein or vein to vein.

Contractility The inherent capability of the cardiac muscle fibers to shorten.

Contraction stress test (CST) A method of evaluating the respiratory function (oxygen and carbon dioxide exchange) of a placenta.

Contracture Permanent shortening of connective tissue.

Contralateral deficit Loss or impairment of sensorimotor functions on the side of the body opposite the side of the brain that is damaged by stroke.

Controlled Substance Act (CSA) A federal law that requires drugs to be classified based on the substance's medical use, potential for abuse, and safety risks.

Controlling The managerial process of comparing actual results with projected results, similar to the evaluation step in the nursing process. Controlling includes establishing performance standards, determining how to measure performance and creating the tools that will permit consistent measurement, evaluating performance, and providing feedback.

Convection The process of heat transfer through the fluid motion of air or water across the skin.

Convergence The medial rotation of the eyeballs so that each is directed toward the viewed object.

Co-occurring disorders Concurrent diagnosis of a substance use disorder and a psychiatric disorder. One disorder can precede and cause the other, such as the theorized relationship between alcoholism and depression.

Cooperative play The stage of play in which children work together to contribute to a unified whole, such as forming a sports team or dancing in an ensemble.

Copayment The set payment owed by an insured individual at the time a covered service is rendered.

Coping A dynamic process through which an individual applies cognitive and behavioral measures to handle internal and external demands that are perceived by the individual as exceeding available resources.

Cor pulmonale Right-sided heart failure.

Corneal abrasion Disruption of the superficial epithelium of the cornea.

Corneal reflex Closure of eyelids (blinking) due to corneal irritation.

Cornu The elongated portion of the uterus where the fallopian tubes enter.

Coronary artery disease (CAD) The most common type of heart disease, CAD is caused by impaired blood flow to the myocardium.

Coronary circulation A network of vessels that supply the heart muscle.

Corpus The upper triangular portion of the uterus. Also called the *uterine body*.

Corpus luteum A small yellow body that develops within a ruptured ovarian follicle.

Corrective action The steps taken to overcome a job performance problem.

Coryza Inflammation of the mucous membranes lining the nose usually associated with nasal discharge.

Countershock phase The second part of an alarm reaction during which the sympathetic nervous system stimulation triggers the body's defenses.

Couplet Two premature ventricular contractions in a row.

Couvade In some cultures, the male's observance of certain rituals and taboos to signify the transition to fatherhood.

Covert conflict Conflict that is avoided, ignored, or not discussed openly.

Crack A form of freebase cocaine that is made of baking soda, water, and cocaine mixed into a paste and microwaved to form a rock.

Crackles High-pitched popping sounds heard on inspiration due to fluid associated with or resulting from inflammation, or exudates, within the lung fields, or localized atelectasis.

Creatinine clearance A test that uses 24-hour urine and serum creatinine levels to determine the glomerular filtration rate; a sensitive indicator of renal function.

Creativity The ability to find or create a unique solution to a unique problem when traditional interventions are not effective.

Credentialing The formal identification of professionals who meet predetermined standards of professional skill or competence.

Credibility The quality of being truthful, trustworthy, and reliable.

Crepitation A grating or cracking sound.

Crime An act prohibited by statute or by common law principles.

Criminal law The area of law that deals with conduct that is harmful to another individual or to society as a whole and that may be punishable by fines or imprisonment.

Crisis An event or circumstance that overwhelms an individual's inherent ability to resolve, manage, or process the event or circumstance.

Crisis counseling A meeting that focuses on brief solutions, focused interventions, and supportive care during or after a crisis. It also considers the individual's physical vulnerability and degree of emotional stability.

Crisis intervention An emergent approach to care that is intended to assist clients with recognizing a crisis situation, and identifying and implementing an immediate, short-term solution.

Crisis intervention centers Organizations that provide telephone counseling for clients in crisis. Some organizations also provide consultation through e-mail and online chatting.

Critical pathway Expected outcomes and care strategies developed through collaboration by the healthcare team. Also called a *case map*.

Critical thinking All or part of the process of questioning, analysis, synthesis, interpretation, inference, inductive and deductive reasoning, intuition, application, and creativity.

Crohn disease A chronic, relapsing inflammatory bowel disorder affecting the gastrointestinal tract. Also known as *regional enteritis*.

Cross-dressing Occurs when an individual of one gender (typically male) dresses in clothing specific to the opposite gender.

Crowning During birth, the appearance of the newborn's head or presenting fetal part at the vaginal orifice.

Crystalloids Salts that dissolve readily into true solutions.

Cultural deprivation A lack of culturally assistive, supportive, or facilitative acts.

Cultural groups Racial, ethnic, religious, or social groups with specific group behaviors and characteristics that are learned and shared, including language, customs, beliefs, and values.

Cultural humility The recognition that a healthcare provider's personal cultural values are not superior over the cultural values of others, thus preventing an abuse of power.

Cultural values Preferred ways of behaving or thinking that are sustained over time and used to govern a cultural group's actions and decisions.

Culture The patterns of behavior and thinking that people living in social groups learn, develop, and share.

Cultures Laboratory cultivations used to identify probable microorganisms by their characteristics, such as shape, growth patterns, and Gram-staining qualities.

Curling ulcers Acute ulcerations of the stomach or duodenum that form following a burn injury.

Cyanosis Gray to blue or purple skin color caused by deoxygenated hemoglobin.

Cycle of violence Violence that occurs with a patterned frequency, usually in three phases: initial tension due to communication failures, an abusive incident, and a honeymoon stage in which the aggressor may show love and affection. Cycle of violence may also refer to violence that spans multiple generations in a family.

Cyclothymic disorder A type of bipolar disorder characterized by chronic, fluctuating mood disturbances involving numerous periods of hypomanic symptoms and numerous periods of depressive symptoms.

Cystitis Inflammation of the urinary bladder.

Cystoscopy Endoscopy of the urinary tract. Also called *catheterization*.

Cytokines Proteins that carry messages for immune system function.

Damages Compensation sufficient to restore the plaintiff to his or her original position, so far as is financially possible.

Dashboard An interface that gathers, organizes, and displays a healthcare facility's key performance indicators in an easy-to-read format, often with charts or graphs.

Dashboard knee Tearing of the posterior cruciate ligament or any knee injury resulting from an individual's knee slamming into the dashboard or back of a seat during a motor vehicle crash.

Database A compilation of all information about a client including the nursing health history, physical assessment, primary care provider's history, physical examination, and test results.

Date rape A term used when dating violence takes the form of rape.

Dating violence A type of intimate partner abuse; this type occurs most often in relationships among youth.

Dawn phenomenon A rise in blood glucose between 4 a.m. and 8 a.m. that is not a response to hypoglycemia.

Dead space Areas of the lung that are ventilated but not perfused.

Death anxiety Worry or fear related to death or dying.

Debridement The process of removing painful or necrotic material, including all loose tissue, wound debris, and dead tissue from a wound.

Decelerations The periodic decreases in fetal heart rate from the normal baseline.

Decerebrate posturing An abnormal posture adopted by an unconscious individual that indicates deteriorating brain function. It is characterized by an extended neck; clenched jaw; arms pronated, extended, and close to the sides; legs extended and feet plantar flexed.

Decibels (dB) Units of loudness.

Declarative memory Memory that is related to people and facts, is consciously accessible, and can be verbally expressed.

Decode The process of relating the message perceived to the receiver's storehouse of knowledge and experience and sorting out the meaning of the message.

Decompensation Loss of effective compensation.

Decorticate posturing An abnormal posture adopted by an unconscious individual that indicates deteriorating brain function. It is characterized by the upper arms kept close to the sides; the elbows, wrists, and fingers flexed; the legs extended and internally rotated; and the feet plantar flexed.

Deductible A set annual cost for healthcare paid by an individual or family participating in a health insurance plan.

Deductive reasoning A "top down" method of logical thinking that starts with a conclusion and analyzes the situation for valid, significant cues. One of two methods of logical thinking that are used to determine if decisions are reasonable.

Deep brain stimulation (DBS) A procedure in which a neurostimulator is implanted into the individual to send electrical signals to one of three brain regions—the subthalamic nucleus, the globus pallidus, or the thalamus—in order to reduce symptoms of Parkinson disease.

Deep venous thrombosis (DVT) A blood clot that forms along the intimal lining of a large vein, usually in a leg.

Defecation The expulsion of feces from the anus and rectum.

Defense mechanism See Adaptive mechanisms.

Defibrillation An emergency procedure that delivers an electrical shock to stop ventricular fibrillation and return to a rhythm that promotes cardiac output sufficient to sustain life.

Deficiency A term used to describe when intake of a nutrient is less than recommended.

Defining characteristics The cluster of signs and symptoms that indicate the presence of a particular diagnostic label.

Deformation The alteration of the spinal cord and soft tissues caused by abnormal movement.

Dehiscence An unintended separation of wound margins due to incomplete healing.

Dehydration A condition that occurs when a body does not take in as much water as it loses or lacks sufficient reserves to maintain proper function.

Delayed union The delayed healing of bones beyond the expected time period.

Delegate An individual who assumes responsibility for the actual performance of an assigned task or procedure.

Delegation The transfer of responsibility and authority for completing an activity to a qualified individual.

Delegator An individual who assigns a task to another individual to perform, but retains accountability for the outcome.

Delirium An acute cognitive disorder that affects functional independence.

Delirium tremens (DTs) A medical emergency usually occurring 3–5 days following alcohol withdrawal and lasting 2–3 days. Characterized by paranoia, disorientation, delusions, visual hallucinations, elevated vital signs, vomiting, diarrhea, and diaphoresis. Also known as *alcohol withdrawal delirium*.

Delphi technique Data gathering technique that averages comments or ratings off of anonymous interviews and questionnaires.

Delusions False ideas or beliefs not based in reality.

Dementia The progressive, irreversible loss of cognitive function.

Democratic leader A leader who assumes that individuals are internally motivated, are capable of making decisions, and value independence. Democratic leaders typically provide constructive feedback, offer information, make suggestions, and ask questions to gain information or to help group members grow in their ability to make decisions.

Demography The study of population, including statistics about distribution by age and place of residence, mortality, and morbidity.

Demyelination A condition in which cells of the immune system, such as lymphocytes and macrophages, cross the blood–brain barrier and attack and destroy the myelin sheath.

Denominations Groups of members that adhere to the same practices and beliefs.

Dental caries Cavities.

Deoxyribonucleic acid (DNA) One of two types of nucleic acid made by cells, DNA contains the genetic instructions for the development and functioning of human beings.

Dependence A physiological need for a substance that the client cannot control, and which results in withdrawal symptoms if the substance is withheld.

Dependent intervention Activities carried out under a physician's orders or supervision, or according to specified routines or protocols.

Dependent personality disorder (DPD) One of several personality disorders defined in the DSM-5, it is marked by a pervasive, excessive, and unrealistic need to be cared for; fear of separation; lack of self-confidence; an inability to make decisions; and an inability to function independently.

Depersonalization A feeling of strangeness or unreality about the physical self.

Depolarization 1. The rapid inflow of sodium ions, causing an electrical change in which the inside of a cell becomes positive in relation to the outside. 2. The phase in which the heart contracts as a result of ion channel functions.

Depo-Provera A long-acting progesterone that provides highly effective birth control for 3 months when given as a single injection.

Depression A disorder characterized by a sad or despondent mood or loss of interest in usual activities.

Depressive disorder with peripartum onset See Postpartum depression.

Derealization A feeling of disconnection from an individual's own body or the environment.

Dermatome An area of skin innervated by the cutaneous branch of one spinal nerve.

Dermis The second layer of skin, which is made of a flexible connective tissue. It is richly supplied with blood cells, nerve fibers, and lymphatic vessels, as well as most of the hair follicles, sebaceous glands, and sweat glands.

Desaturated blood Blood that is low in oxygen as a result of oxygenated and deoxygenated blood mixing due to a congenital heart defect.

Desire phase The first phase of the sexual response cycle is the arousal of sexual interest by means of real or symbolic stimuli.

Detachment One of the six trait domains associated with personality disorders that is broken down into withdrawal, intimacy avoidance, anhedonia, and restricted affectivity.

Detrusor muscle The smooth muscle layers of the bladder wall, the detrusor muscle allows the bladder to expand as it fills with urine and contract as it releases urine during voiding.

Development An increase in the complexity and function of skill progression, the individual's capacity and skill to adapt to the environment. Related to growth.

Developmental disability Any of a variety of chronic conditions characterized by mental and/or physical impairment.

Developmental stage A level of achievement for a particular segment of an individual's life.

Developmental task A skill or behavior pattern learned during stages of development.

Device integration Real-time, accurate data is recorded in the client's chart directly from a device (e.g., blood pressure monitor). Device integration allows the nurse to more quickly analyze and interpret that data and make adjustments to the plan of care based on the most current information.

Diabetes mellitus Group of chronic disorders of the endocrine pancreas, all categorized under a broad diagnostic label. The condition is characterized by inappropriate hyperglycemia caused by a relative or absolute deficiency of insulin or by a cellular resistance to the action of insulin. Also called *diabetes*.

Diabetic ketoacidosis (DKA) A form of metabolic acidosis that develops when there is an absolute deficiency of insulin and an increase in the insulin counterregulatory hormones. It may also induced by stress in an individual with type 1 diabetes.

Diabetic nephropathy Disease of the kidneys in clients with diabetes that is characterized by the presence of albumin in the urine, hypertension, edema, and progressive renal insufficiency.

Diabetic neuropathy A disorder of the peripheral nerves and the autonomic nervous system in clients with diabetes, which manifests in one or more of the following: sensory and motor impairment, muscle weakness and pain, cranial nerve

disorders, impaired vasomotor function, impaired gastrointestinal function, and impaired genitourinary function.

Diabetic retinopathy The collective name for the changes in the retina that occur in the person with diabetes. The retinal capillary structure undergoes alterations in blood flow, leading to retinal ischemia and a breakdown in the blood retinal barrier.

Diagnosis-related groups (DRGs) A system of price control regulation that classifies client illnesses based on diagnoses and pays hospitals a predetermined sum for each specific diagnosis regardless of the actual cost of services, the length of stay, or the acuity or complexity of the client's illness.

Diagnostic label Standardized NANDA names for nursing diagnoses.

Diagonal conjugate Distance from the lower posterior border of the symphysis pubis to the sacral promontory.

Dialysate Dialysis solution.

Dialysis A process by which fluids and molecules pass through a semipermeable membrane from an area of higher solute concentration to one of lower solute concentration according to the rules of osmosis. Dialysis is used to remove excess fluid and metabolic waste products in renal failure.

Diaphragm A flexible disc that covers the cervix to prevent conception.

Diaphysis The shaft of a bone.

Diarrhea The passage of liquid feces and an increased frequency of defecation.

Diastasis recti abdominis A separation of the abdominal muscle.

Diastole The phase of ventricular relaxation between heartbeats.

Diastolic blood pressure The minimum pressure within the arteries during diastole.

Diathermy Treatment with heat generated by high-frequency electrical currents.

Diet recall Client history of intake over a specified period of time.

Dietary Reference Intakes (DRIs) A standardized, recommended nutrient intake to support a healthy diet often provided by health organizations.

Differentiated practice A system in which each nurse's educational preparation and skill sets are evaluated and used to determine how he or she will be best utilized.

Differentiation A process occurring over many cell cycles that allows cells to specialize in certain tasks.

Diffusion The continual intermingling of molecules in liquids, gases, or solids brought about by the random movement of the molecules.

Digestion The conversion of food by means of its mechanical and chemical breakdown into absorbable substances in the gastrointestinal tract.

Digital rectal examination (DRE) An examination to detect for abnormalities in the rectum that can be detected through palpation.

Dihydrotestosterone (DHT) The androgen that mediates prostatic growth at all ages; formed in the prostate from testosterone.

Dilated cardiomyopathy The most common form of cardiomyopathy, it is characterized by the dilation of the heart chambers and impaired ventricular contraction.

Directing The managerial process of effectively motivating, communicating, and delegating tasks in order to complete an organization's work.

Directive interview A highly structured interview that elicits specific information about health information.

Dirty In medical asepsis, a term used to indicate that microorganisms are likely to be present.

Disaster An event that occurs with little or no warning in which available personnel and emergency services are initially overwhelmed and a serious threat to life, public health, and the environment is posed.

Discharge planning A plan of care that prepares the client for discharge, including training in any necessary health skills.

Discipline A method of teaching children the rules for how to behave in society and what is expected in different circumstances.

Discoid lesions Raised, scaly, circular lesions with an erythematous rim.

Discovery The legal process of obtaining information before a trial.

Discrimination The differential treatment of individuals or groups, based on categories such as race, age, weight, gender, or social class, that occurs when an individual acts on prejudice and denies other people one or more of their fundamental rights.

Discussion An informal oral consideration of a subject by two or more healthcare personnel to identify a problem or establish strategies to resolve a problem.

Disease A detectable alteration in body function resulting from infection by microorganisms that causes a reduction of capacities or a shortening of the normal life span. Also called *pathogenesis.*

Disease surveillance Monitoring patterns of disease occurrence from cases of infections and communicable diseases reported by healthcare workers to state officials.

Diseases of adaptation Stress-related illnesses, such as peptic ulcers and hypertension.

Disenfranchised grief Grief that occurs when an individual is unable to acknowledge a loss to other persons. Also called *ambiguous loss.*

Disinfectants Agents that destroy pathogens other than spores.

Disinhibition One of the six trait domains associated with personality disorders that is noted for the presence of irresponsibility, impulsivity, and risk taking.

Disc Fluid-filled "shock absorber" that holds together and insulates the vertebrae. Also called *spinal disc.*

Discectomy The removal of all or part of the nucleus pulposus of an intervertebral disc.

Dismissal Termination of employment.

Disorganized behavior The inability to start or finish goal-oriented activities to a degree that it interferes with an individual's ability to lead a normal life.

Disorganized thinking Difficulty logically connecting thoughts, leading to garbled speech.

Dissatisfaction problems Issues that arise from unmet sexual needs and expectations.

Disseminated intravascular coagulation (DIC) A disruption of hemostasis characterized by widespread intravascular clotting and bleeding. It may be acute and life threatening, or it may be relatively mild.

Distracted driving The act of driving a motor vehicle while doing any activity that takes attention away from the road. Activities include texting, talking on the phone, eating, drinking, reading a map, talking to passengers, looking at a GPS, and adjusting the radio.

Distress A stress that is associated with inadequacy, insecurity, and loss.

Distributive shock Shock that results from widespread vasodilation and decreased peripheral resistance. Also called *vasogenic shock.*

Diuresis The production and excretion of abnormally large amounts of urine. Also called *polyuria.*

Diuretics Pharmacologic agents that increase urine formation and secretion.

Diversity The unique variations among and between individuals, variations that are informed by genetics and cultural background, but that are refined by experience and personal choice.

Diverticula Saclike projections of mucosa through the muscular layer of the colon.

Documenting The process of making an entry on a client record. Also called *recording* or *charting.*

Domestic partner An unmarried partner of the same or opposite sex.

Do-not-intubate (DNI) order Usually written by the physician for the client who has a terminal illness or is near death, this order is usually based on the wishes of the client and family that no life-saving measures be provided once the client stops breathing.

Do-not-resuscitate (DNR) order Usually written by the physician for the client who has a terminal illness or is near death, this order is usually based on the wishes of the client and family that no cardiopulmonary resuscitation be performed for respiratory or cardiac arrest. Also called a *no-code order.*

Dopamine A brain neurotransmitter that regulates voluntary movement, reward-seeking behavior, memory and learning, attention, sleep, affect, and many other functions.

Dormant Temporarily inactive but not dead.

Double-bind theory The theory that schizophrenia symptoms are partially an expression of contradictory family interactions.

Double depression A term used to describe a situation in which an individual experiences dysthymic disorder in combination with major depressive disorder.

Doula A paid caregiver who has typically received special training and may even be certified in caring for laboring women.

Down syndrome A developmental disorder that occurs when an individual is born with an extra full or partial chromosome. Down syndrome is associated with intellectual disability and a wide variety of physical impairments that can range from mild to severe.

Dramatic play The stage of play in which individuals use props to act out the drama of human life.

Droplet nuclei Residue of evaporated droplets emitted by an infected host; can remain in the air for long periods of time.

Droplet precautions Used for clients who are known to have or suspected of having serious illnesses transmitted by particle droplets larger than 5 microns, such as pertussis or pneumonia.

Dubowitz tool A tool for assessing newborns that includes neuromuscular tone assessments, such as head lag, ventral suspension, and leg recoil.

Dullness A thudlike sound produced by dense tissue such as the liver, spleen, or heart.

Duodenal ulcer A peptic ulcer occurring in the duodenum.

Durable power of attorney A legal document that can delegate the authority to make health, financial, and/or legal decisions on an individual's behalf.

Durable power of attorney for health care A legal designation of another individual, usually a family member, significant other, or close personal friend, to make healthcare decisions on an individual's behalf.

Duration 1. The length of a sound. 2. The length of time from the beginning of a contraction to the completion of that same contraction.

Duty A legally enforceable obligation to conform to a particular standard of conduct that is owed to the client.

Dwarfism Excessively short stature caused by insufficient growth hormone, typically resulting from a genetic abnormality.

Dysfunctional uterine bleeding (DUB) Vaginal bleeding that is usually painless but abnormal in amount, duration, or time of occurrence. Also called *abnormal uterine bleeding*.

Dysmenorrhea Painful menstruation.

Dyspareunia Painful intercourse.

Dysphagia Difficulty swallowing.

Dysplasia A loss of DNA control over differentiation occurring in response to adverse conditions.

Dyspnea Shortness of breath or difficulty breathing that is uncomfortable or painful; or when breathing is insufficient to meet oxygen demand.

Dysrhythmia Abnormal heart rate or rhythm. Also called *arrhythmia*.

Dysthymic disorder A chronic disorder in which periods of depressed mood are interspersed with normal mood. Also called *persistent depressive disorder* or *dysthymia*.

Dystonia Severe muscle spasms, particularly of the back, neck, tongue, and face.

Dysuria Difficult or painful urination.

Early deceleration During birth, a condition that occurs when the fetal head is compressed and cerebral blood flow decreases, causing central vagal stimulation. Usually associated with the onset of uterine contractions.

Eating disorder A set of maladaptive responses to stress or anxiety characterized by obsessions with food and weight, often to the extent that daily functioning is impaired and physical and psychological health are threatened.

Echolalia The compulsive parroting of a word or phrase just spoken by another.

Echopraxia The compulsive imitation of the movements of another.

Eclampsia A major complication of pregnancy characterized by hypertension, albuminuria, oliguria, tonic and clonic convulsions, and coma.

Ecological theory A theory of development that emphasizes the presence of mutual interactions between the individual and all of life's settings.

Ecomap Visual representation of how the family unit interacts with the external community environment, including schools, religious institutions, occupational duties, and recreational pursuits.

Ectopic beats Impulses originating outside normal conduction pathways of the heart that interrupt the normal conduction sequence and may not initiate a normal muscle contraction.

Edema Swelling caused by excess fluid trapped in body tissue.

Effacement The drawing up of the internal os and the cervical canal into the uterine side walls.

Effectiveness In health care, effectiveness is providing services based on scientific knowledge to all who could benefit and refraining from providing services to those not likely to benefit.

Efficiency In health care, efficiency is avoiding waste of equipment, supplies, ideas, and energy.

Ego The realistic part of the individual, the ego balances the gratification demands of the id with the limitations of social and physical circumstances.

Ego defense mechanisms Unconscious psychological processes developed for the purpose of defending the personality. Also called *defense mechanisms*.

Egocentrism Ability to see things only from one's own point of view.

Ego-syntonic The perception that one's behaviors and beliefs are normal and any difficulties with other people are external to themselves.

E-health Electronic information that can be retrieved and transferred online or through a mobile device to improve a person's health or health care.

Ejection fraction The fraction or percentage of the diastolic volume that is ejected from the heart during systole.

Elasticity of the arterial wall An indicator of the health of an artery. A healthy, normal artery feels straight, smooth, soft, and pliable. Older adults often have inelastic arteries that feel twisted (tortuous) and irregular upon palpation.

Elder abuse The intentional physical, emotional, or sexual mistreatment or neglect of an individual 65 years of age or older.

Elderspeak A speech style similar to baby talk, which communicates a message of dependence and incompetence to older adults.

Elective surgery Performed when surgical intervention is the preferred treatment for a condition that is not imminently life threatening (but may ultimately threaten life or well-being) or to improve the client's life.

Electrocardiogram (ECG) A graphic record of the heart's activity.

Electrocardiography A diagnostic test of cardiac function.

Electroconvulsive therapy (ECT) A treatment procedure during which an electric current is passed through the brain. It is useful to clients with severe depression, acute mania, some psychotic conditions, and those who are acutely suicidal.

Electroencephalogram (EEG) Measures and records the brain's electrical activity.

Electrolyte A charged ion capable of conducting electricity.

Electromyogram A diagnostic technique that measures the electrical activity of the muscles at rest and during contraction.

Electronic communication Transmitting information though e-mail, social networking, text messaging, and other electronic means.

Electronic fetal monitoring (EFM) The measurement and tracing of the fetal heart rate (FHR), which allows many characteristics of the FHR to be visually assessed.

Electronic health record (EHR) A health record system that is designed so that multiple clinicians from multiple disciplines (e.g., family practice, nursing, pharmacy, specialists) can all have simultaneous access to the client's health information.

Electronic medical record (EMR) A system focused on diagnosis and treatment. EMRs track information over time (weight, blood pressure, cholesterol readings) and identify when clients are due for routine preventive health maintenance such as vaccines and mammograms.

Elimination The secretion and excretion of body wastes from the kidneys and intestines.

Embolus A particle or aggregate of blood, fat, or pathogens or a bubble of air that obstructs a blood vessel.

Embryo The early stage of development of the young of any organism. In humans the embryonic period is from about 2–8 weeks' gestation and is characterized by cellular differentiation and predominantly hyperplastic growth.

Embryonic membranes The amnion and chorion.

Emergency A sudden, often unforeseen event that threatens health or safety.

Emergency preparedness The act of making plans to prevent, respond to, and recover from emergencies.

Emergency response The implementation of emergency preparedness plans.

Emergency surgery Surgery that is performed immediately to preserve function or the life of the client.

Emigration The movement of leukocytes through the blood vessel wall into affected tissue spaces in response to illness or injury.

Emotion-focused coping The regulation of emotional responses to distress when the stressor is perceived to be beyond the individual's control.

Emotional availability The quality of parent–child interactions, including parental sensitivity, structuring, and degree of intrusiveness and hostility.

Emotions Feeling responses to a wide variety of emotional stimuli.

Emphysema A progressive pulmonary disease characterized by destruction of the walls of the alveoli, with resulting enlargement of abnormal air spaces.

Empirical knowing The twofold understanding of facts and observations relevant to nursing, and of the analyses and theories that attempt to explain them. Also called the *science of nursing*.

Empyema Accumulation of purulent (infected) exudate in a space, for example, the pleural cavity or the gallbladder.

Enabling behavior Any action by an individual that consciously or unconsciously facilitates substance dependence.

Encapsulated Enclosed.

Encoding The selection of specific signs or symbols to transmit a message, such as which language and words to use, how to arrange the words, and what tone of voice and gestures to use.

Encopresis Abnormal elimination pattern characterized by recurrent soiling or passage of stool at inappropriate times.

Enculturation The process by which children learn culture from adults. Also called *cultural transmission*.

End-of-dose medication failure Pain experienced at the end of one dose of medication before the next dose is scheduled.

End of life The final weeks of life when death is imminent.

End-of-life care The nursing care provided to a client who is dying or who is near death.

End-stage renal disease (ESRD) The final stage of chronic kidney disease, when the kidneys are unable to excrete metabolic wastes and regulate fluid and electrolyte balance adequately.

Endocardial cushion defect A combination of defects in the atrial and ventricular septa and portions of the tricuspid and mitral valves. A complete AV canal defect allows blood to travel freely among all four chambers of the heart. Also called *atrioventricular (AV) canal defect*.

Endocardial cushions Fetal growth centers for mitral and tricuspid valves and AV septum.

Endogenous Developing from within.

Endogenous insulin Insulin that is produced by an individual's own body.

Endogenous pyrogens Interleukins, interferons, and tumor necrosis factor released by macrophages in response to an infection.

Endometriosis A condition that occurs when endometrial tissue implants on organs outside the uterus, causing pain, fibrosis, and adhesions.

Endometrium The innermost mucosal layer of the uterus.

Endotoxins Found in the cell wall of gram-negative bacteria, endotoxins are released only when the cell is disrupted. They act as activators of many human regulatory systems, producing fever, inflammation, and potentially clotting, bleeding, or hypotension when released in large quantities.

Engagement The passing of the fetus into the pelvic inlet in preparation for birth.

Engrossment The characteristic sense of absorption, preoccupation, and interest in an infant demonstrated by fathers during early contact.

Enophthalmos Sunken appearance of the eyes.

Enteral nutrition Tube feeding used to meet calorie and protein requirements in clients who are unable to consume enough food on their own.

Entropion Inversion of the eyelid.

Enuresis Involuntary passing of urine in children after bladder control is achieved.

Enzymes Chemicals that induce a chemical reaction in order to assist in the breakdown of nutrients.

Eosinophil A type of leukocyte found in large numbers in the respiratory and gastrointestinal tracts. Eosinophils are thought to be responsible for protecting the body from parasitic worms. They also play a role in the hypersensitivity response by inactivating some of the inflammatory chemicals released during the inflammatory response.

Epidemic Widespread outbreak of infectious disease with many infected people.

Epidermis The surface or outermost part of the skin consisting of four to five layers of epithelial cells.

Epigenetic External factor's effects on internal genetic results.

Epilepsy A chronic disorder characterized by recurrent, unprovoked seizures secondary to a central nervous system disorder.

Epiphyseal plate Cartilage between the epiphysis and diaphysis found in the long bones of children.

Episiotomy A surgical incision of the perineal body to enlarge the outlet.

Epstein's pearls Small, glistening, white specks that feel hard to the touch on the hard palate and gum margins

Erb-Duchenne paralysis Damage affecting the upper arm between the fifth and sixth cervical nerves, causing paralysis. Also called *Erb's palsy.*

Erectile dysfunction (ED) The inability of a male to attain and maintain an erection sufficient to permit satisfactory sexual intercourse.

Ergonomics The science of fitting workplace conditions and job demands to the capabilities of the working population.

Erik Erikson A German-born psychologist and psychoanalyst who created a theory of development comprised of eight stages or age-related tasks faced by an individual throughout the life span.

Erythema A reddening of the skin.

Erythema toxicum An eruption of lesions in the area surrounding a hair follicle that are firm, vary in size from 1 to 3 mm, and consist of a white or pale yellow papule or pustule with an erythematous base. Also called *newborn rash* or *flea bite dermatitis.*

Eschar Hard, leathery crust that covers a burn wound and harbors necrotic tissue.

Escharotomy Surgical removal of eschar from the torso or extremity to prevent circumferential constriction.

Essential nutrients The macro- and micronutrients needed for the body's survival.

Estimated date of birth (EDB) The approximated date of childbirth. Also called *due date.*

Estrogen The primary hormone responsible for female sex characteristics.

Ethical knowing Understanding and applying the ethical codes by which nurses are expected to abide, as well as upholding the various philosophical, cultural, and moral frameworks of the institution and of the client. Also called the *moral component.*

Ethics The rules or principles that govern right or moral conduct.

Ethnic group Group of individuals who have common racial characteristics and share a cultural heritage.

Etiology A causal relationship between a problem and its related or risk factors.

Eupnea Breathing within the expected respiratory rates.

Eustachian tube Connects the middle ear with the nasopharynx to help equalize the pressure in the middle ear with the atmospheric pressure.

Eustress Good stress that is associated with accomplishment and victory.

Euthanasia From the Greek for *painless, easy, gentle,* or *good death,* now commonly used to signify a killing prompted by a humanitarian motive.

Euthyroid A normal thyroid state.

Evaluation statement A written comment on the care plan or in the nurse's notes about progress following an evaluation. An evaluation statement must contain the date and time evaluation was done; a conclusion statement determining goal met, partially met, or not met; and a supporting statement giving the results of how the client did or did not achieve the goal.

Evaporation The process of converting water to a vapor.

Evidence Clinical knowledge, expert opinion, or information resulting from research.

Evidence-based nursing An integration of the best evidence available, nursing expertise, and the values and preferences of the individuals, families, and communities who are served.

Evidence-based practice The application of research in areas that are of interest to nursing and in the actual practice of nursing.

Evisceration Protrusion of internal viscera through a surgical wound.

Exacerbation A reappearance of symptoms of a chronic illness. Also called a *flare.*

Excess More than is needed in order for the body to survive and remain productive.

Excitement phase This second phase of the sexual response cycle is marked by an increase in blood flow to various body parts, resulting in erection of the penis and clitoris and swelling of the labia, testes, and breasts.

Excoriation Area of loss of the superficial layers of the skin. Also called *denuded area.*

Exercise Physical activity that is planned, structured, and involves repetitive body movements; the goal is to improve or maintain one or more components of physical fitness.

Exercise intolerance Decreased ability to participate in activities using large skeletal muscles because of fatigue or dyspnea.

Exogenous Developing from outside sources.

Exogenous insulin Insulin from a source outside the body.

Exophthalmos Protruding eyes.

Exotoxins Soluble proteins that microorganisms secrete into surrounding tissue. Exotoxins are highly poisonous, causing cell death or dysfunction.

Expectorate To expel or spit out.

Expiration The act of exhaling air in respiration.

Expressed consent An oral or written agreement.

Expressive jargon Using unintelligible words with normal speech intonations as if truly communicating in words.

Expressive speech The ability to speak and be understood by others.

Extended family The relatives of nuclear families, such as grandparents, aunts, and uncles.

Extended kin network family A form of extended family in which two nuclear families of primary or unmarried kin live in proximity to each other and share a social support network, goods, and services.

External environmental stressors Triggers outside of an individual that demand change or disrupt homeostasis.

External locus of control The belief that an individual's health is controlled by forces outside of his or her control such as chance or fate.

Extracapsular extraction A surgical treatment for cataracts in which the anterior capsule, nucleus, and cortex of the lens are removed, leaving the posterior capsule intact.

Extracapsular hip fracture A hip fracture involving the trochanteric region between the neck and diaphysis of the femur.

Extracellular fluid (ECF) Fluid found outside the cells. It accounts for about one third of total body fluid and is subdivided into compartments. The two main compartments of ECF are intravascular and interstitial.

Extracorporeal shock wave lithotripsy (ESWL) A noninvasive technique for fragmenting kidney stones using shock waves generated outside the body.

Extrapulmonary tuberculosis Results when tuberculosis spreads through the blood and lymph system to other organs.

Extrapyramidal side effects (EPS) A particularly serious set of adverse reactions to antipsychotic drugs. EPS includes acute dystonia, akathisia, parkinsonism, and tardive dyskinesia.

Extubation The process of withdrawing a breathing tube on completion of anesthesia and the surgical case.

Exudate Material, such as fluid and cells, that has escaped from blood vessels during the inflammatory process and is deposited in tissue or on tissue surfaces.

Exudative macular degeneration A form of macular degeneration characterized by the formation of new, weak blood vessels in the potential space between the choroid and the retina. Also referred to as the wet form of macular degeneration.

Eye movement desensitization and reprocessing (EMDR) A form of psychotherapy that contains elements of a number of types of therapy, including cognitive-behavioral therapy and body-centered therapy.

Failure to thrive (FTT) 1. Inability to meet or maintain developmental milestones related to physical growth due to undernutrition. 2. A syndrome in which an infant falls below the fifth percentile for weight and height on a standard growth chart or is falling in percentiles on a growth chart.

Faith To believe in or be committed to something or someone.

Fallopian tubes Tubes that extend from the lateral angle of the uterus and terminate near the ovary. Also called *oviducts* and *uterine tubes*.

False imprisonment The unjustifiable detention of an individual without legal warrant to confine the person.

False pelvis The portion of the pelvis above the linea terminalis that supports the enlarged pregnant uterus.

Familial AD (FAD) One of the two basic types of Alzheimer disease, it has a strong inherited component and usually manifests before the age of 65. Also called *early-onset Alzheimer disease*.

Family Individuals who are joined together by marriage, blood, adoption, or residence in the same household.

Family burden The overall level of distress experienced by a family as a result of a family member's illness.

Family-centered care A model of healthcare service that is provided in partnership with the client and family.

Family-centered nursing Nursing that considers the health of the family as a unit in addition to the health of individual family members.

Family cohesion The emotional bonding between family members.

Family communication Includes listening, speaking, self-disclosure, and tracking abilities of the family as a group.

Family coping mechanisms The behaviors families use to deal with stress or changes imposed from either within or without the family.

Family development The dynamics or changes a family experiences over time, including changes in relationships, communication patterns, roles, and interactions.

Family flexibility The amount of change in a family's leadership, role relationships, relationship rules, and ability to respond to stress.

Family recovery Family response to a member's mental illness.

Family support Support from family members as they care for other family members; for example, one sister relieves another to care for their aging mother over the weekend.

Family therapy A form of therapy in which the family system is treated as a unit and the focus is on family dynamics.

Fascial excision Excising a wound to the level of fascia. Also called *fasciectomy*.

Fasciculation An irregular movement or a twitch.

Fasciectomy Excising a wound to the level of fascia. Also called *fascial excision*.

Fat embolism syndrome (FES) Occurs when fat globules lodge in the pulmonary vascular bed or peripheral circulation.

Fatigue A condition characterized by a lack of energy and motivation that may or may not be accompanied by drowsiness.

Fear A sense of apprehension triggered by a perceived threat to safety or well-being, including a painful stimuli or dangerous event.

Febrile Having a fever.

Febrile seizures Generalized seizures that usually occur in children as the result of rapid temperature rise above 39°C (102°F), usually in association with an acute illness. No evidence of intracranial infection or other defined cause is found in relation.

Fecal impaction A mass or collection of hardened feces in the folds of the rectum.

Fecal incontinence The loss of voluntary ability to control fecal and gaseous discharges through the anal sphincter. Also called *bowel incontinence*.

Fecalith A hard mass of feces.

Feces Body wastes and undigested food eliminated from the bowel. Also called *stool*.

Feedback 1. The mechanisms by which some of the output of a system is returned to the system as input. 2. The response a receiver of a message gives to the message's sender.

Female orgasmic disorder A sexual arousal cycle that stops before orgasm.

Female reproductive cycle (FRC) The monthly rhythmic changes in sexually mature women; composed of the ovarian cycle, during which ovulation occurs, and the uterine cycle, during which menstruation occurs.

Female sexual arousal disorder Discomfort or pain during sexual intercourse caused by a lack of vaginal lubrication.

Fertility awareness-based methods Contraception based on an understanding of the changes that occur throughout a woman's ovulatory cycle. Also called *natural family planning*.

Fertilization The process by which a sperm fuses with an ovum to form a new diploid cell, or zygote.

Festination Rapid, small steps, as if an individual is trying to run.

Fetal alcohol spectrum disorder See Fetal alcohol syndrome (FAS).

Fetal alcohol syndrome (FAS) A developmental disorder that occurs when a developing fetus is exposed to ethyl alcohol. Fetal alcohol syndrome is associated with physical, intellectual, behavioral, and/or learning disabilities. Also called *fetal alcohol spectrum disorder.*

Fetal attitude The flexion or extension of the fetal body and extremities.

Fetal bradycardia A fetal heart rate of less than 110 bpm during a 10-minute period or longer.

Fetal demise Death of a fetus that occurs after 20 weeks' gestation. Also called a *stillbirth* or *intrauterine fetal death (IUFD).*

Fetal heart rate (FHR) The number of times the fetal heart beats per minute; normal range is 120–160.

Fetal lie The relationship of the cephalocaudal axis, or spinal column, of the fetus to the cephalocaudal axis, or spinal column, of the woman. The fetus may be in a longitudinal or transverse lie.

Fetal movement record A noninvasive technique that enables the pregnant woman to monitor and record movements easily and without expense.

Fetal position The relationship of the landmark on the presenting fetal part to the front, sides, or back of the maternal pelvis.

Fetal presentation The body part of the fetus entering the pelvis in a single or multiple pregnancy.

Fetal tachycardia A fetal heart rate of 161 bpm or more during a 10-minute period of continuous monitoring.

Fetoscope An adaptation of a stethoscope that facilitates auscultation of the fetal heart rate.

Fetoscopy A technique for directly observing the fetus and obtaining a sample of fetal blood or skin.

Fetus The child in utero from about the seventh to ninth week of gestation until birth.

Fever A protective immune response to foreign antigens within the body that increases the cellular metabolic rate, thus increasing the body's temperature.

Fever phobia Fear felt by caregivers about the harmful effects of a fever on a child, such as seizure, brain damage, and death.

Fever spike A temperature that rises to fever level rapidly, following a normal temperature, and then returns to normal within a few hours.

Fiber A polysaccharide that contributes to disease prevention, especially in the gastrointestinal tract and the cardiovascular system.

Fibrin Connective tissue.

Fibrin degradation products Potent anticoagulants.

Fibromyalgia A chronic disorder characterized by widespread musculoskeletal pain, fatigue, and multiple tender points.

Fidelity A moral principle that obligates an individual to be faithful to agreements and responsibilities one has undertaken.

Filtration A process whereby fluid and solutes move together across a membrane from a compartment with higher pressure to a compartment with lower pressure.

Filtration pressure The pressure in the compartment that results in the movement of the fluid and substances dissolved in fluid out of the compartment.

Fimbria A funnel-like enlargement of the fallopian tube with many fingerlike projections (fimbriae) reaching out to the ovary.

First heart sound (S_1) The heart sound produced by the closure of the AV valve; characterized by the syllable "lub."

Five P's neurovascular assessment An assessment checklist for pain, pulse, pallor, paralysis/paresis, and paresthesia.

Fixation The immobilization or inability of an individual to proceed to the next developmental stage because of anxiety.

Flaccidity Absence of muscle tone. Also called *hypotonia.*

Flashbacks The recurrence of images, sounds, smells, or feelings from a traumatic event; often triggered by daily events, such as a car backfiring on the street or the smell of a perpetrator's cologne.

Flat affect Minimal facial expression and movement, sometimes monotone speech patterns.

Flatness An extremely dull sound produced by very dense tissue, such as muscle or bone.

Flatulence The presence of excessive amounts of gas in the stomach or intestines.

Flatus Gas or air normally present in the stomach or intestines.

Flight of ideas Rapidly changing, fragmentary thoughts.

Flow sheet A specific assessment criteria in a particular format, such as human needs or functional health patterns.

Fluid resuscitation The administration of intravenous (IV) fluids to restore circulating blood volume during an acute period of increasing capillary permeability.

Fluid volume deficit (FVD) Substantial loss of both water and electrolytes in similar proportions from the extracellular fluid. Also called *hypovolemia.*

Fluid volume excess (FVE) Excessive fluid retained by the body. The retention of both water and sodium in similar proportions to normal extracellular fluid (ECF). Also called *hypervolemia.*

Fluoroscope A scope used to project visual examination images on a fluorescent screen.

Focal seizures Seizures that are caused by abnormal electrical activity in one hemisphere or in a specific area of the cerebral cortex, most often the temporal, frontal, or parietal lobes. The seizure may spread regionally, and the symptoms are related to the region of the cortex that is affected. Also known as *partial seizures.*

Focus charting Date and time, focus, and progress notes are recorded for a specific condition, nursing diagnosis, and behavior to make the client and the client's concerns and strengths the focus of care.

Folic acid A vitamin that is required for normal growth, reproduction, and lactation and that prevents the macrocytic, megaloblastic anemia of pregnancy.

Follicle-stimulating hormone (FSH) Hormone produced by the anterior pituitary during the first half of the menstrual cycle, stimulating development of the graafian follicle.

Fontanelles The intersections of membranous spaces between the cranial bones of a fetus.

Food choice An individual's decision of what and how much to eat of a specific food. This decision can be influenced by a number of conscious and unconscious factors such as taste, preparation, smell, habits, convenience, availability, and cost.

Food insecurity Results when one or more members of a household must reduce their eating patterns due to a lack of money or lack of resources to access appropriate amounts and varieties of food.

Food security Results when all members of a household have sufficient resources to access appropriate amounts and varieties of food.

Foramen ovale An opening between the atria of the fetal heart.

Foraminotomy An enlargement of the opening between the disc and the facet joint to remove bony overgrowth.

Forced expiratory volume in 1 second (FEV1) The amount of air that can be exhaled in 1 second as measured by a spirometer.

Forceps-assisted birth The use of forceps to assist the birth of a fetus by providing traction or by providing the means to rotate the fetal head to an occiput-anterior position. Also called an *instrumental delivery*, *operative delivery*, or *operative vaginal delivery*.

Forceps marks Reddened areas over the cheeks and jaws on an infant caused by a difficult forceps birth.

Foreground question Questions that are narrow in focus about a specific clinical issue.

Foreseeability The ability to foresee events that reasonably may be expected to cause specific results.

Formal group A group with formalized goals, designated management, and only partly voluntary membership.

Formal leader A leader who is selected by an organization and given official authority to make decisions and act.

Formation The process that facilitates the transformation of an individual from a layperson to a professional nurse.

Foster family A family consisting of one or more adults caring for one or more children from other families when the children can no longer live with their birth parents.

Fourth heart sound (S_4) A heart sound produced by atrial contraction and ejection of blood into the ventricle during late diastole. Also called *atrial gallop*.

Fracture A break in the continuity of a bone.

Fragile X syndrome A developmental disorder caused by a single recessive gene abnormality on the X chromosome. Fragile X syndrome is associated most notably with intellectual disability, often accompanied by ADHD and other behavioral problems.

Frank–Starling mechanism An increase in venous return increases ventricular filling and myocardial stretch, which increases the force of contraction.

Free-floating anxiety Excessive worry about everyday events; worry that is hard to control and the focus of which may shift from moment to moment.

Freezing A condition in which an individual feels like his or her feet are stuck to the floor.

Frequency The time between the beginning of one contraction and the beginning of the next contraction.

Friend support Support or assistance from nonfamily members, such as friends or coworkers, for a family during a time of illness or stress.

Frostbite An injury of the skin resulting from freezing.

Frustration An emotion that occurs when an individual is prevented from reaching a desired goal. Intense frustration may trigger violent aggressive tendencies resulting in assault or homicide.

Fulguration A procedure that destroys tissue with electrical current.

Full-thickness burn A burn that involves all layers of the skin, including the epidermis, the dermis, and the epidermal appendages.

Fulminant colitis An acute form of ulcerative colitis that involves the entire colon; manifestations include severe bloody diarrhea, acute abdominal pain, and fever.

Functional assessments Typically a combination of assessments that includes observations of child behavior, responses, and abilities. It is used to assess how a child functions on a daily basis in his or her environment and to determine if the child has any developmental delays or special needs.

Functional nursing A task-oriented approach to care delivery used in situations of inadequate staffing or nursing shortages.

Functional strength The body's ability to perform work.

Fundus The rounded, uppermost portion of the uterus.

Fungi A type of microorganism capable of producing infection. Yeasts and molds are common types of fungi.

Galanin A neuropeptide that is released by neurons as they are injured or die. Often associated with Alzheimer disease, although the exact role galanin plays in the disease is unknown.

Gallstone ileus A large gallstone.

Gamete Female or male germ cell; contains a haploid number of chromosomes.

Gametogenesis The process by which germ cells are produced.

Gastric lavage Irrigation of the stomach with large quantities of normal saline.

Gastric outlet obstruction Obstruction of the pyloric region of the stomach and duodenum that impairs gastric outflow; a potential complication of peptic ulcer disease.

Gastric ulcer A peptic ulcer that occurs in the stomach.

Gastrocolic reflex The increased peristalsis of the colon after food has entered the stomach.

Gastroesophageal reflux disease (GERD) A disease in which stomach contents flow back up into the esophagus.

Gate control theory Melzack and Wall's 1965 theory that states the perception of pain is controlled by the overall activity of small-diameter (pain) fibers vs. large-diameter (heat, cold, mechanical) fibers.

Gender identity One's self-image as a female or male.

Gender expression The outward expression of an individual's sense of maleness or femaleness as well as the expression of what is perceived as gender-appropriate behavior.

General adaptation syndrome (GAS) A three-stage chain of events in an individual's stress response.

Generalized anxiety disorder (GAD) A condition that occurs when an individual experiences intense tension and worry, even if no external stressors are present.

Generalized seizures The result of diffuse electrical activity that often begins in both hemispheres of the brain simultaneously, then spreads throughout the cortex into the brainstem. As a result, movements and spasms displayed by the client are bilateral and symmetric.

Generational cohort Individuals born in the same general time span who share key life experiences, including historical events, public heroes, pastimes, and early work experiences.

Genital herpes A sexually transmitted infection caused by the herpes simplex virus.

Genital intercourse Penetration of the vagina by the penis. Also called *coitus*.

Genital warts A sexually transmitted infection caused by the human papillomavirus (HPV).

Genogram Visual representation of gender showing lines of birth descent through the generations.

Genotype The pattern of genes on chromosomes.

Geographic information system (GIS) A system that relies on satellite imaging and global positioning systems to capture, manage, and analyze geographical data.

Geragogy The process of stimulating and helping older adults to learn.

Geriatric failure to thrive (GFTT) A condition in which older clients experience a multidimensional decline in physical functioning that is characterized by weight loss of more than 5% of baseline body weight, decreased appetite, undernutrition, dehydration, depression, and cognitive and immune impairment.

Gestation Period of intrauterine development from conception through birth; pregnancy.

Gestational age assessment tools Methods to determine an infant's age at birth assessing external physical characteristics and neurological or neuromuscular development.

Gingiva The gum.

Gingivitis Red, swollen gingiva.

Glaucoma A condition characterized by optic neuropathy with gradual loss of peripheral vision and, usually, increased intraocular pressure of the eye.

Global evaluative dimension of the self The degree to which an individual likes him- or herself overall, as a whole being. Also called *global self-esteem*.

Global self The collective beliefs and images an individual holds about him- or herself.

Global self-esteem See Global evaluative dimension of the self.

Glomerular filtration rate (GFR) The rate at which fluid is filtered through the kidneys.

Glomerulonephritis Inflammation of the glomerular capillary membrane.

Glomerulus Found in the nephrons of the kidneys, a tuft of capillaries surrounded by the Bowman capsule.

Glucagon A hormone that stimulates the breakdown of glycogen in the liver, the formation of carbohydrates in the liver, and the breakdown of lipids in both the liver and adipose tissue.

Gluconeogenesis The formation of glucose from fats and proteins.

Glucosuria The excretion of glucose in the urine.

Glycogenolysis The breakdown of liver glycogen.

Glycosuria The excretion of carbohydrates into the urine.

Goiter An enlarged thyroid gland

Gonadotropin-releasing hormone (GnRH) A hormone secreted by the hypothalamus that stimulates the anterior pituitary to secrete follicle-stimulating hormone and luteinizing hormone.

Gonorrhea A sexually transmitted infection caused by *Neisseria gonorrhoeae*.

Good Samaritan laws Specific laws designed to protect healthcare workers from potential liability when volunteering their skills outside of an employment contract.

Goodpasture syndrome A rare autoimmune disorder of unknown etiology that is characterized by formation of antibodies to the glomerular basement membrane.

Governance The establishment and maintenance of social, political, and economic arrangements by which professionals control their practice, their self-discipline, their working conditions, and their professional affairs.

Graafian follicle The ovarian cyst containing the ripe ovum, which secretes estrogens.

Grading A standardized method of judging a tumor's aggressiveness based on the level of differentiation and mitotic rate; where the least malignant cells are classified grade 1 and the most aggressive malignant cells are classified grade 4.

Graft-versus-host disease (GVHD) A series of immunological reactions in response to transplanted cells.

Gram stain A diagnostic test conducted to identify infecting organisms in urine by shape and characteristic.

Granulation tissue Young connective tissue with new capillaries formed in the healing process.

Grasping reflex The closing and grasping of an infant's fingers in response to a finger placed in the palm of the infant's hand.

Graves disease An autoimmune disorder marked by an enlarged thyroid and signs of hyperthyroidism.

Grief The total psychological, biological, and behavioral response to the emotional experience related to loss.

Group Three or more individuals who have a common purpose, interact with each other, influence each other, and are interdependent.

Group therapy A form of therapy that allows group members to help each other with psychological, cognitive, behavioral, and spiritual dysfunctions through a process of change, aided by a professional group therapist.

Groupthink A type of decision making characterized by a group's failure to critically examine their own processes and practices or to recognize and respond to change.

Growth Physical change and increase in size.

Guillain-Barré syndrome (GBS) An acute inflammatory demyelinating disorder of the peripheral nervous system characterized by an acute onset of motor paralysis (usually ascending).

Gustatory Of or relating to taste.

Gynecomastia Abnormal enlargement of the breast(s) in men.

H_1 receptors Cellular histamine receptors that are present in the smooth muscle of the vascular system, the bronchial tree, and the digestive tract. Stimulation of these receptors results in itching, pain, edema, bronchoconstriction, and other characteristic symptoms of inflammation and allergy.

H1N1 influenza A form of the influenza virus that consists of avian genes, human genes, and genes from flu viruses typically found in pigs from Asia and Europe. Once mistakenly called *swine flu*, it can be spread through human-to-human transmission.

H_2 receptors Cellular histamine receptors present primarily in the stomach; their stimulation results in the secretion of large amounts of hydrochloric acid.

Habit training Attempts to keep clients dry by having them void at regular intervals.

Habituation The newborn's ability to process and respond to complex stimulations.

Hallucination The perception of seeing, hearing, or feeling something that is not present in reality.

Hallucinogen A type of drug that induces the same types of thoughts, perceptions, and feelings that occur in dreams. Hallucinogens include PCP, 3,4-MDMA, D-lysergic acid diethylamide (LSD), mescaline, dimethyltryptamine (DMT), and psilocin.

Hand restraints A device used to protect confused clients from scratching or injuring their skin, or dislodging intravenous access devices. Also called *mitt restraints*.

Handoff The transfer of information along with authority and responsibility during transitions in care across the continuum.

Handoff communication A verbal or written exchange of information. It encompasses the nursing team and all other members of the healthcare team who care for a client at any given time.

Hardware The physical component of technology, including computers, keyboards, and display screens.

Harlequin sign A reddening of the skin on one side of an infant's body while the other side remains pale. Also called *clown color change*.

Hashimoto thyroiditis An autoimmune disorder in which antibodies destroy thyroid tissue.

Hassles Day-to-day tension/stressors.

Health A state of complete physical, mental, and social well-being.

Health beliefs Concepts about health that an individual believes are true, regardless of whether or not they are founded in fact.

Health Insurance Portability and Accountability Act (HIPAA) Legislation enacted by Congress to minimize the exclusion of preexisting conditions as a barrier to healthcare insurance, designate special rights for those who lose other health coverage, and eliminate medical underwriting in group plans. The act includes the Privacy Rule, which creates a national standard for of the disclosure of private health information.

Health Level Seven (HL7) A framework designed for the exchange integration, sharing, and retrieval of electronic health information that supports clinical practice and the management, delivery, and evaluation of health services.

Health literacy The ability to read, understand, and act on health information, including such tasks as comprehending prescription labels, interpreting appointment slips, completing health insurance forms, and following instructions for diagnostic tests.

Health maintenance organization (HMO) The most restrictive type of private health insurance plan. HMO participants must select a primary care provider who provides basic medical services and, as the gatekeeper to care, refers the client to in-network hospitals and specialists when additional care is needed.

Health policy The actions and decisions by government bodies and professional organizations that affect whether or not healthcare organizations and individuals working within the healthcare system can achieve their healthcare goals.

Health promotion A way of thinking and acting in order to increase individuals' overall health and well-being regardless of their health and illness status or age.

Health restoration Care focusing on the ill client that extends from early detection of disease through helping the client during the recovery period.

Healthcare advance directive Legal document that allows an individual to plan for healthcare and/or financial affairs in the event of incapacity. Also called *advance directive* or *advance healthcare directive*.

Healthcare-associated infection (HAI) Infections associated with the delivery of healthcare services in a facility such as a hospital or nursing home. Also called a *nosocomial infection*.

Healthcare disparity A difference in a measurement of access to or quality of healthcare services between an individual or group possessing a defined characteristic when other variables have been controlled, such as individual health choices, disease courses, and other variations from the normative measure.

Healthcare proxy An individual selected to speak to physicians and other healthcare providers on behalf of a client to determine the best course of treatment.

Healthcare surrogate An individual selected to make medical decisions when someone is no longer able to make them for him- or herself.

Heart block A block in the normal electrical conduction of the heart.

Heart failure The inability of the heart to pump adequate blood to meet the metabolic demands of the body.

Heart murmur Harsh, blowing sounds caused by disruption of blood flow into the heart, between the chambers of the heart, or from the heart into the pulmonary or aortic systems.

Heartburn A burning sensation in the chest or throat. Also called *pyrosis*.

Heat balance When the amount of heat produced by the body equals the amount of heat lost.

Heat exhaustion Excessive heat exposure and dehydration that causes paleness, dizziness, nausea, vomiting, fainting, and a moderately increased temperature (38.3°–38.9°C [101°–102°F]).

Heat stroke A serious form of heat exhaustion that can be life threatening, generally caused by exercising in hot weather. Clients will have warm, flushed skin, often do not sweat, and have a temperature of 41°C (106°F) or higher. A client may be also delirious, unconscious, or having seizures.

Heat transfer The four ways heat moves from one place or object to another place or object.

Heaving Lifting of the chest wall during contraction.

Heberden nodes Bony lumps on the end joint of a digit.

Helper T cells Play a vital role in normal immune system function, recognizing foreign antigens and infected cells and activating antibody-producing B cells. They are the primary cells infected by the human immunodeficiency virus.

HELPP syndrome A cluster of changes including hemolysis, elevated liver enzymes, and low platelet count, sometimes associated with preeclampsia.

Hematochezia Bright blood in the stool.

Hematocrit The proportion of cells and plasma in blood. Also refers to the laboratory test that measures the hematocrit. This test can also be used to detect severe dehydration or overhydration.

Hematogenous spread Describes the spread of infection or disease through the blood.

Hematoma A localized collection of blood underneath the skin that may appear as a bruise.

Hematopoiesis Blood cell formation.

Hematuria The presence of blood in the urine.

Hemianopia The loss of half of the visual field of one or both eyes.

Hemiarthroplasty Hip replacement that involves replacement of the ball, the head, or the femur.

Hemiarthroscopy The surgical replacement of the femoral head with a smooth metal sphere.

Hemiparesis Weakness of the left or right half of the body.

Hemiplegia Paralysis of the left or right half of the body.

Hemispheres The two halves created by the division of the cerebrum by the deep fold.

Hemodialysis A process by which a client's blood flows through vascular catheters, passes by the dialysate in an external machine, and then returns to the client.

Hemodynamics The study of forces involved in blood circulation.

Hemoglobin The oxygen-carrying molecule within red blood cells; a laboratory test to measure the amount of hemoglobin.

Hemoglobinopathy A disorder of hemoglobin.

Hemolysis The destruction of red blood cells; releases hemoglobin into the circulation.

Hemolytic anemia A disorder that results from the premature destruction of red blood cells.

Hemoptysis Bloody sputum.

Hemorrhage Rapid or excessive bleeding.

Hemosiderosis The storage of excessive iron in tissues and organs.

Hemostasis The cessation of bleeding.

Hemotympanum Bleeding into or behind the tympanic membrane.

Hepatitis The inflammation of the liver triggered by a virus, alcohol, medications, toxins, autoimmune disorder, or other pathogens.

Here-and-now concept A concept used in group therapy that recognizes that only in the present moment of a group's experience can change be made.

Hernia A protrusion in the intestine through the inguinal wall or canal.

Herniated intervertebral disc A rupture of the cartilage surrounding the intervertebral disc with protrusion of the nucleus pulposus. Also called a *ruptured disc, slipped disc,* or *herniated nucleus pulposus.*

Heroin An illicit, central nervous system depressant narcotic that alters perception and produces euphoria.

Heterograft Skin used for transplantation that was obtained from an animal, usually a pig. Also called a *xenograft.*

Heterosexism The view that heterosexuality is the only correct sexual orientation.

Heterosexual An individual who is attracted to members of the opposite sex.

Highly active antiretroviral therapy (HAART) Effective treatment of AIDS that combines at least three medications to inhibit HIV replication.

Hip fracture A fracture of the femur at the head, neck, or trochanteric regions.

Hippocampus A small, curved body in the brain. Part of the limbic system, it plays a major role in memory formation.

Hirsutism An increased growth of coarse hair on the face and trunk.

Histamine A key chemical mediator of inflammation.

Histrionic personality disorder (HPD) One of several personality disorders defined in the DSM-5, it is characterized by a lifelong tendency for dramatic, egocentric, attention-seeking response patterns.

Hoarding compulsion An excessive collection and accumulation of objects, extreme cluttering of the living environment, accompanied by a lack of regard for the embarrassment of family member or others whose living is impacted.

Holism An approach to health care that considers more than the physiological health status of an individual.

Holosystolic Term used to describe the sounds heard during the entire phase of systole.

Holy day A day set aside for special religious observance.

Homan sign Pain in the calf when the foot is dorsiflexed.

Homeostasis The body's ability to maintain a state of physiological balance in the presence of constantly changing conditions.

Homicide The killing of one individual by another; for legal purposes, this act is further specified by whether the act was intentional or due to negligence.

Homocysteine An amino acid that is a homologue of cysteine.

Homograft Grafts between members of the same species who have different genotypes and HLA antigens. Usually human skin that has been harvested from cadavers. Also called an *allograft.*

Homologous chromosomes The two paired chromosomes that are inherited, one from each parent.

Homophobia The fear, hatred, or mistrust of gays and lesbians often expressed in overt displays of discrimination.

Homosexual An individual who is attracted to members of the same sex.

Hope To expect or desire with confidence.

Horizontal violence (HV) Aggressive acts committed against a nurse by one or more nursing colleagues.

Hormone replacement therapy (HRT) Administration of hormones, usually estrogen and a progestin, to alleviate the symptoms of menopause.

Hormones Chemical messengers secreted by various glands that exert controlling effects on the cells of the body.

Hospice An organization that provides end-of-life care for clients either in their homes or in a hospital setting.

Hospice care The support and care for persons in the last phase of an incurable disease so that they may live as fully and comfortably as possible until their death.

Hot zone When a disaster occurs, the hot zone is the most dangerous zone because it is located immediately adjacent to the site of the disaster. All responders who enter the area must be protected by personal protective equipment.

Human chorionic gonadotropin (HCG) A hormone produced by the chorionic villi that is found in the urine of pregnant women. Also called *prolan.*

Human dignity The inherent worth and uniqueness of individuals and populations.

Human immunodeficiency virus (HIV) A primary immunodeficiency disorder that is spread primarily through sexual contact with an infected person. HIV is the virus that causes acquired immunodeficiency syndrome (AIDS).

Human leukocyte antigen (HLA) The major histocompatibility complex gene.

Humanistic learning theory A learning theory that focuses on the unique cognitive and affective qualities of a learner.

Humoral immune response Hyperreactive response of B cells characteristic of systemic lupus erythematosus (SLE).

Hunger The feeling that makes individuals think of food and encourages them to satisfy this feeling by eating.

Hyaluronic acid (HA) A lubricating substance in cartilage and joint synovial fluid.

Hydrocephalus A condition characterized by enlargement of the head caused by inadequate drainage of cerebrospinal fluid.

Hydronephrosis An accumulation of urine in the renal pelvis as a result of obstructed outflow.

Hydrostatic pressure The pressure a fluid exerts within a closed system on the walls of its container. The hydrostatic pressure of blood is the force blood exerts against the vascular walls (e.g., the artery walls). The principle involved in hydrostatic pressure is that fluids move from an area of greater pressure to an area of lesser pressure.

Hydroureter Distention of the ureter with urine.

Hyperalgesia Increased response to a pain stimulus because of peripheral sensitization.

Hypercalcemia Elevated blood levels of calcium.

Hypercapnia A condition marked by a $PaCO_2$ level above 45 mmHg.

Hypercarbia An increased level of carbon dioxide in the blood that drives the impulse to breathe.

Hyperchloremia Elevated chloride levels in the blood.

Hypercyanotic episode A potentially life-threatening episode of hypoxia. Also called a *tet episode*.

Hyperemia Increased blood flow to an area.

Hyperextension Forcible backward bending.

Hyperflexion Forcible forward bending.

Hyperglycemia Elevated glucose levels.

Hyperkalemia Elevated potassium levels in the blood.

Hypermagnesemia Elevated magnesium levels in the blood.

Hypernatremia Elevated sodium levels in the blood.

Hyperopia Farsightedness.

Hyperosmolar hyperglycemic state (HHS) A disorder characterized by a plasma osmolarity of 340 mOsm/L or greater, greatly elevated blood glucose levels, and altered levels of consciousness. It occurs in individuals who have type 2 diabetes mellitus.

Hyperphosphatemia Increased blood levels of phosphate.

Hyperplasia An increase in the number or density of normal cells.

Hyperresonance An abnormal, booming sound that can be heard over an emphysematous lung.

Hyperresponsiveness An exaggerated response, as with bronchoconstriction in asthma.

Hypersensitivity An overreaction of the immune system to an antigen or antigens.

Hypersomnia The inability to stay awake during the day, despite obtaining sufficient sleep at night.

Hypertension Excess pressure in the arterial portion of the circulatory system, specifically a systolic blood pressure of 140 mmHg or higher or a diastolic blood pressure of 90 mmHg or higher.

Hypertensive emergency A systolic blood pressure greater than 180 mmHg and diastolic blood pressure higher than 120 mmHg. Also called *malignant hypertension*.

Hypertensive encephalopathy A syndrome characterized by extremely high blood pressure, altered level of consciousness, increased intracranial pressure, papilledema, and seizures.

Hyperthermia A condition that occurs when a body produces more heat than is lost.

Hyperthermia blanket An electronically controlled blanket that provides a specified temperature

Hyperthermic A body temperature above 37.8°C (100°F).

Hyperthyroidism A disorder caused by excessive delivery of thyroid hormone to the peripheral tissues. Also called *thyrotoxicosis*.

Hypertonic Refers to solutions that have a higher osmolality than body fluids; 3% sodium chloride is a hypertonic solution.

Hypertonic dehydration Occurs when sodium loss is proportionately less than water loss. Also called *hypernatremic dehydration*.

Hypertrophic cardiomyopathy A disorder characterized by decreased compliance of the left ventricle and hypertrophy of the ventricular muscle mass.

Hypertrophic scar An overgrowth of dermal tissue that remains within the boundaries of the wound.

Hypertrophy An enlargement of glandular cells or muscles.

Hyperventilation Unusually fast respirations, or overbreathing causing an imbalance of oxygen and carbon dioxide.

Hypervolemia The excessive retention of both water and sodium in similar proportions to normal extracellular fluid (ECF). Also called *fluid volume excess*.

Hyphema Bleeding into the anterior chamber of the eye.

Hypoactive sexual desire disorder A deficiency in or absence of sexual fantasies and persistently low interest or a total lack of interest in sexual activity.

Hypocalcemia Decreased blood levels of calcium.

Hypocapnia A condition that results when $PaCO_2$ falls below 35 mmHg.

Hypochloremia Decreased blood levels of chloride.

Hypodermis The layer of loose connective tissue and fat cells that lies below the dermis. Also called *subcutaneous tissue*.

Hypodermoclysis Fluid administered subcutaneously.

Hypoglycemia Diminished glucose levels.

Hypokalemia Decreased blood levels of potassium.

Hypomagnesemia Decreased blood levels of magnesium.

Hypomania A less extreme form of mania that is not severe enough to markedly impair functioning or require hospitalization.

Hyponatremia Decreased blood levels of sodium.

Hypoperfusion Decreased blood flow.

Hypophonia A lowered voice volume.

Hypophosphatemia Decreased blood levels of phosphate.

Hypoplastic left heart syndrome (HLHS) One of the most severe congenital heart defects, characterized by absence or stenosis of mitral and aortic valves, an abnormally small left ventricle, a small aorta, and aortic or mitral stenosis or atresia.

Hypotension A below-normal blood pressure reading between 85 and 110 mmHg.

Hypothermia A condition that occurs when a body loses more heat than it produces.

Hypothermic A body temperature below 36°C (97°F).

Hypothyroidism A disorder resulting when the thyroid gland produces an insufficient amount of thyroid hormone.

Hypotonic Refers to solutions that have a lower osmolality than body fluids, such as one half normal saline.

Hypotonic dehydration Occurs when fluid loss is characterized by a proportionately greater loss of sodium than water. Also called *hyponatremic dehydration*.

Hypovolemia Loss of both water and electrolytes in similar proportions from extracellular fluid. Also called *fluid volume deficit*.

Hypovolemic shock Shock caused by a decrease in intravascular volume of 15% or more.

Hypoxemia Decreased oxygen levels in the blood that result when PaO_2 falls below 80 mmHg.

Iatrogenic Refers to a condition induced by the effects of treatment.

Iatrogenic infection A type of infection that results directly from diagnostic or therapeutic procedures.

Id In Freudian terms, the source of instinctive and unconscious psychological urges.

Ideal body image A mental representation of what an individual believes his or her body should look like.

Ideal self How the individual thinks he or she should be or would prefer to be.

Idiopathic pain A type of pain that occurs unpredictably and is not associated with any known cause, making it difficult to treat.

Ileostomy A surgical opening made in the ileum of the small intestine.

Ileus A condition that causes a temporary cessation of the passage of material through the intestines, usually lasting 24–48 hours.

Illness A state in which an individual's physical, emotional, intellectual, social, developmental, or spiritual functioning is diminished.

Illness behavior A coping mechanism that includes the ways in which an individual describes, monitors, and interprets symptoms, and the individual's ability to take remedial action and use the healthcare system.

Illness prevention Health care focusing on maintaining optimal health by preventing disease through programs on immunizations, prenatal and infant care, and prevention of sexually transmitted infections.

Illusion A distorted perception of actual sensory stimuli.

Imagery A relaxation technique in which the client focuses on pleasant images such as a beach or a garden to replace negative images such as pain and darkness. Also called *guided imagery*.

Imitation The process by which individuals copy or reproduce what they have observed.

Immobility A reduction in the amount and control of one's movement.

Immunity The body's natural or induced response to infection and the conditions associated with its response.

Immunization Introduces an antigen into the body, allowing immunity against a disease to develop naturally.

Immunocompetent Term used to describe clients who have an immune system that identifies antigens and effectively destroys or removes them.

Immunodeficiency A condition that develops when the immune system is incompetent or unable to respond effectively.

Immunoglobulin (Ig) A protein that functions as an antibody.

Immunosuppression Inability of the immune system to respond to an antigen. Occurs in response to disease or medications; may be intentional to prevent rejection of transplants or a side effect of some medications.

Implied consent Nonverbal consent indicated by a client's cooperative actions.

Impotence Inability to achieve or maintain an erection.

Impulse conduction The transmission of an impulse along the nerve pathways to the spinal cord and directly to the brain.

Impulsiveness Acting without considering the consequences of one's behavior. Also called *impulsivity*.

In vitro fertilization A process in which a woman's eggs are collected from her ovaries, fertilized in the laboratory, and then placed into her uterus after normal embryo development has begun.

Incentive spirometry Measures the forced emptying of alveolar gas.

Incident pain A type of breakthrough pain that is predictable because it is precipitated by an event or activity such as coughing or changing position.

Incident report An agency record of an accident or incident occurring within the agency. This record is designed to collect adequate information to assist personnel in preventing future incidents or occurrences. Also called *variance reports* or *unusual occurrence reports*.

Incomplete spinal cord injury An injury that involves only a partial loss of sensory and motor function below the level of the injury.

Increased intracranial pressure (IICP) Sustained, elevated pressure (15 mmHg or higher in adults) in the cranial cavity.

Indemnity plan A type of health insurance program that allows the insured to self-select healthcare providers and has no predefined network.

Independent intervention The activities that nurses are licensed to do within their scope of practice; in other words, areas of health care that are unique to nursing and separate and distinct from medical management.

Indicator A statistic that reflects the organization's performance in a specific area.

Inductive reasoning A "bottom-up" method of logical thinking that starts with putting significant cues together in order to reach a conclusion. It is a method of logical thinking that is used to determine if decisions are reasonable.

Infection An invasion of the body tissue by microorganisms with the potential to cause illness or disease.

Infectious disease Any communicable disease that is caused by microorganisms that are commonly transmitted from one person to another or from an animal to an individual.

Infertility A lack of conception despite unprotected sexual intercourse for at least 12 months.

Inflammation An adaptive response to what the body sees as harmful, such as an allergen, illness, or injury. Inflammation typically is characterized by pain, heat, redness, and swelling. Also called *inflammatory response*.

Inflammatory bowel disease (IBD) Chronic inflammation of the bowel common to a group of conditions that includes Crohn disease and ulcerative colitis.

Influenza A highly contagious viral respiratory disease characterized by coryza (inflammation of the mucous membranes lining the nose usually associated with nasal discharge), fever, cough, and systemic symptoms such as headache and malaise (vague feeling of physical discomfort).

Informal groups A type of group that functions with much less structure than a formal or semiformal group. Characteristics of informal groups include easily recognized, basic objectives; rotational leadership; and no set of written rules or regulations.

Informal leader A leader who is not officially appointed to direct the activities of others but, because of seniority, age, or special abilities, is recognized by the group as a leader and plays an important role in influencing colleagues, coworkers, or other group members to achieve the group's goals.

Informed consent 1. A client's legal and ethical rights to be informed of and give permission for any healthcare procedure or treatment. **2.** A study volunteer's legal right to be informed with full disclosure of the study's purpose, required procedures, length of the study, expectations, risks, and possible benefits before consenting to participate. Informed consent also includes the right to withdraw from the study at any time.

Infundibulopelvic ligament A ligament that suspends and supports the ovaries.

Inhalant A substance inhaled to produce euphoria. Categorized into three types: anesthetics, volatile nitrites, and organic solvents.

Input Information, material, or energy that enters a system.

Inquiry A search for knowledge or facts in order to gain clarification and find solutions to problems.

Insensible fluid loss Fluid loss that is not perceptible to the individual and cannot be measured.

Insomnia The inability to fall asleep or remain asleep.

Inspection A visual, auditory, and olfactory examination or assessment of a client to note health condition.

Inspiration The act of inhaling air in respiration.

Insubordination Defiance of authority, such as the refusal to complete a task as assigned.

Insulin A hormone that facilitates the uptake and use of glucose by cells and prevents an excessive breakdown of glycogen in the liver and muscle.

Insulin reaction Low blood glucose levels, or hypoglycemia. Also called *insulin shock*.

Integrity Adherence to a strict moral or ethical code.

Integumentary system The body's system that includes skin, hair, and nails and the sebaceous, sweat, and mammary glands.

Intellect The ability to learn and understand knowledge; the capacity for thinking and reasoning intelligently.

Intellectual disability Significant limitations in intellectual functioning and adaptive behavior prior to the age of 18. Previously called *mental retardation*.

Intellectual functioning General intelligence or mental capacity, including an individual's abilities to learn, use logic, and solve problems.

Intensity 1. The amplitude of a sound produced. **2.** The strength of the contraction during acme, the peak of a uterine contraction during the birth process.

Interdisciplinary team A team that seeks to achieve a common goal, though the team members are professionals with varied backgrounds. Also called *interprofessional team*.

Intergroup conflict Conflict that occurs between teams that are in competition or opposition to one another.

Intermittent claudication A cramping or aching pain in the calves of the legs, the thighs, and the buttocks that occurs with a predictable level of activity

Intermittent fever Occurs when body temperature alternates at regular intervals between periods of fever and periods of normal or subnormal temperatures.

Internal environment The physical, spiritual, cognitive, emotional, and psychological well-being of an individual that depends on the satisfaction of these basic human needs.

Internal locus of control A belief that an individual can impact her or his own health and well-being.

Interorganizational conflict Usually conflict that occurs between two organizations that exist within one market.

Interpersonal conflict Conflict that occurs between two or more individuals due to differences, competition, or concern about territory, control, or loss.

Interpersonal violence Violence that occurs within relationships, between family members, intimate partners, acquaintances, or strangers that does not aim to further the goals of a formal group or cause.

Interprofessional team A team that seeks to achieve a common goal, though the team members are professionals with varied backgrounds. Also called *interdisciplinary team*.

Intersex A general term used to describe a variety of conditions in which reproductive or sexual anatomy does not fit the typical definitions of male or female.

Interstitial fluid Accounts for approximately 75% of extracellular fluid; interstitial fluid surrounds the cells.

Intervention A personalized confrontation that prevents an addict from denying the addiction problem and forces them to face the negative aspects of their behavior and enroll in treatment.

Intimacy A relationship that entails commitment, companionship, affective intimacy, social support, physical closeness, and mutuality.

Intimate distance Communication that is characterized by body contact, heightened sensations of body heat and smell, and vocalizations that are low.

Intimate partner violence (IPV) The act of inflicting sexual, emotional, or physical harm on a current or previous partner or spouse.

Intracapsular hip fracture A hip fracture involving the head or neck of the femur.

Intracellular fluid (ICF) Fluid found within the body cells that contains solute vital to the metabolic processes of the cells. Also called *cellular fluid.*

Intracranial hypertension A sustained state of increased intracranial pressure that is potentially life threatening.

Intracranial regulation The processes that affect intracranial compensation and adaptive neurological function.

Intractable seizures Seizures that continue to occur even with optimal medical management.

Intradiscal electrothermal therapy (IDET) The use of thermal energy to treat pain from a bulging spinal disc.

Intradisciplinary assessment An evaluation that occurs within a group of individuals with a similar position in the healthcare system, such as a group of nurses or a group of surgeons, to identify areas of improvement at each level of care.

Intradisciplinary team A team that seeks to achieve a common goal with team members from the same background.

Intragenerational family A family in which more than two generations live together.

Intranet A smaller version of the Internet that is meant to be used by a smaller group of people, such as employees within a company or members of an organization.

Intraocular pressure A force within the eye that causes tissue damage.

Intraoperative The phase of an operative process in which the surgical procedure actually takes place.

Intrapartum The time from the onset of true labor until the birth of the infant and expulsion of the placenta.

Intrapersonal conflict Conflict that occurs within an individual, arising from stress or tension that results from real or perceived pressure generated by incompatible expectations or goals.

Intrauterine contraception (IUC) A safe, effective method of reversible contraception that is designed to be inserted into the uterus by a qualified healthcare provider and left in place for an extended period, providing continuous contraceptive protection.

Intrauterine device (IUD) A small plastic or metal form that is placed in the uterus to prevent implantation of a fertilized ovum.

Intrauterine fetal death (IUFD) Death of a fetus that occurs after 20 weeks' gestation. Often referred to as *stillbirth* or *fetal demise.*

Intrauterine pressure catheter (IUPC) A device that measures the pressure in the uterine cavity.

Intravascular fluid Accounts for approximately 20% of the extracellular fluid and is found within the vascular system. Also called *plasma.*

Intravenous pyelography (IVP) A diagnostic test used to evaluate the structure and excretory function of the kidneys, ureters, and bladder.

Introspection The personal exploration and evaluation of one's own thoughts, emotions, behaviors, and values incorporating both verbal and nonverbal feedback from others.

Intubation The process of inserting a breathing tube.

Intuition The use of nursing knowledge, experience, and expertise for understanding without the conscious use of reasoning.

Invasion Occurs when cancerous cells overtake adjacent tissues.

Involuntary admission The detention of a client in a psychiatric or medical facility against the client's will, normally reserved for cases in which the client is a danger to himself or others.

Involution The rapid reduction in size of the uterus and the return of the uterus to a nonpregnant state.

Ions Electrically charged particles.

Iron deficiency anemia A disorder that results when the supply of iron in the body is insufficient for the formation of red blood cells.

Irritant contact dermatitis An inflammation of the skin from irritants; it is not a hypersensitivity response.

Ischemia Insufficient blood supply.

Ischemic Deprived of oxygen.

Ischial spines Prominences that arise near the junction of the ilium and ischium and jut into the pelvic cavity.

Isoelectric line A straight line on an electrocardiograph that indicates the absence of electrical activity.

Isokinetic exercises Resistive exercises that involve muscle contraction or tension against resistance; can be either isotonic or isometric.

Isolation Measures designed to prevent the spread of infection to health personnel, clients, and visitors.

Isometric exercises Static or sitting exercises in which muscles contract without moving the joint.

Isotonic A solution that has the same osmolality as body fluids. Normal saline, 0.9% sodium chloride, is an isotonic solution.

Isotonic dehydration A type of fluid imbalance that occurs when fluid loss is not balanced by intake and the losses of water and sodium are in proportion. Also called *isonatremic dehydration.*

Isotonic exercises Dynamic exercises in which the muscle shortens to produce muscle contractions and active movement.

Isotonic fluid volume deficit A type of fluid imbalance that occurs when electrolytes are lost along with fluid.

Isotonic imbalance A fluid imbalance that occurs when water and electrolytes are lost or gained in equal proportions, so that the osmolality of body fluids remains constant.

Isthmus That portion of the uterus between the internal cervical os and the endometrial cavity.

Jaundice A yellow pigmentation of body tissues caused by the presence of bile pigments.

Joint arthroplasty The reconstruction or replacement of a joint.

Joint custody Occurs when two parents who are not married have equal responsibility and legal rights for their shared children.

Joint fusion A procedure that permanently fuses two or more bones together at a joint using pins, plates, screws, and rods. Also called *arthrodesis.*

Joint irrigation A fluid injected into the joint to allow the surgeon to visualize joint structures more easily and to help remove debris and infection in the joint.

Joint resurfacing A procedure in which a little bone is removed at the articulating surface of the joint and a metal replacement is fitted over the end of the bone.

Just culture An attempt to balance the blame-free environment with appropriate accountability by focusing on correcting problems that lead individuals to engage in unsafe behavior while maintaining individual accountability by establishing zero tolerance for reckless behavior.

Justice Fairness.

Juvenile idiopathic arthritis (JIA) See juvenile rheumatoid arthritis (JRA).

Juvenile rheumatoid arthritis (JRA) A chronic inflammatory autoimmune disease diagnosed in children that is characterized by joint inflammation resulting in decreased mobility, swelling, and pain.

Kaposi sarcoma (KS) Often the presenting symptom of AIDS, it remains the most common cancer associated with the disease. Kaposi sarcoma is caused by a virus called the Kaposi sarcoma–associated herpes virus, also known as human herpes virus 8.

Kardex A widely used, concise method of organizing and recording data about a client, making information quickly accessible to all healthcare professionals.

Karyotype A pictorial analysis of chromosomes.

Kcalorie See Kilocalories.

Kegel exercises The act of tightening the perineal muscle in order to strengthen the pubococcygeus muscle and increase its elasticity.

Keloid A scar that extends beyond the boundaries of the original wound.

Keratin A fibrous, water-repellent protein that gives the epidermis its tough, protective quality.

Keratotic basal cell carcinoma A type of skin cancer.

Ketonuria The presence of ketones in the urine.

Ketosis An accumulation of ketone bodies produced during oxidation of fatty acids.

Kilocalories A term used to identify the energy-producing ability of nutrients. Also called *Kcalories* or *kcal*.

Kindling Long-term changes in brain neurotransmission that occur after repeated detoxifications.

Kinesthesia The ability to perceive movement and sense of position.

Kinesthetic A term referring to awareness of the position and movement of body parts.

Korotkoff sounds The series of sounds identified while taking a blood pressure using a stethoscope.

Korsakoff psychosis A condition typically seen in alcoholics that is characterized by intact intellectual functioning but an inability to retrieve long-term memory events or retain new information.

Kosher Acceptable to or prepared according to Jewish law.

Kussmaul respirations Deep, rapid respirations associated with compensatory mechanisms.

Kyphosis A convex curvature of the spine that may decrease mobility.

Labor induction The stimulation of uterine contractions before the spontaneous onset of labor, with or without ruptured fetal membranes, for the purpose of accomplishing birth.

Labyrinthitis Inflammation of the inner ear. Also called *otitis interna*.

Lactase deficiency An individual's inability to digest lactose because of a deficiency of lactase, the enzyme that breaks down lactose into monosaccharides. Also called *lactose intolerance*.

Lacto-ovovegetarians Vegetarians who include milk, dairy products, and eggs in their diets.

Lactose intolerance An individual's inability to digest lactose because of a deficiency of lactase, the enzyme that breaks down lactose into monosaccharides. Also called *lactose deficiency*.

Lactovegetarians Vegetarians who include dairy products but no eggs in their diets.

Laënnec cirrhosis A progressive, irreversible liver disorder resulting from excessive alcohol consumption. Also called *alcoholic cirrhosis*.

Laissez-faire leader A leader who recognizes a group's need for autonomy and self-regulation. The leader assumes a "hands-off" approach, being less directive and more permissive than other types of leaders.

Lamellar A type of bone that is stronger and more compact with better blood circulation compared to woven bone.

Laminectomy The surgical removal of the vertebral lamina.

Laminotomy The surgical removal of part of the vertebral lamina.

Lanugo A large quantity of fine hair found on some newborns.

Laparoscopic cholecystectomy Removal of the gallbladder using an endoscope.

Late deceleration A condition caused by uteroplacental insufficiency resulting from decreased blood flow and oxygen transfer to the fetus through the intervillous spaces during uterine contractions.

Law The sum total of the rules and regulations by which a society is governed.

Laxatives Medications that stimulate bowel activity and assist in fecal elimination.

Lead An insulated wire that connects an electrocardiograph to the electrodes attached to a client.

Leader An individual with the ability to rule, guide, or inspire others to think or act as that individual recommends.

Leading question A closed question that gives the client an opportunity to decide whether the answer is true or not.

Lean Six Sigma A methodology used to reduce waste and provide consistency in the quality of care.

Learning A change in human disposition or capability that persists and that cannot be solely accounted for by growth.

Learning disabilities Disorders that impair an individual's ability to receive and process information, causing reduced functioning in verbal, linguistic, reasoning, and academic skills; neurological conditions in which the brain cannot receive or process information normally.

Learning need A desire or a requirement to know something that is presently unknown to the learner.

Lecithin/sphingomyelin (L/S) ratio The measurement of lecithin and sphingomyelin in order to determine the lung maturity of a fetus.

Leopold maneuvers A systematic way to evaluate the maternal abdomen.

Lesbian A woman who prefers relationships with other women.

Lesion An observable change in skin structure that may indicate disorders in other systems and organs.

Leukemia A group of chronic malignant disorders of white blood cells (WBCs) and WBC precursors.

Leukocytes The primary cells involved in both nonspecific and specific immune system responses. Also known as *white blood cells (WBCs)*.

Leukocytosis An increase in the number of leukocytes in the blood (above 10,000/mm^3), in response to infection or inflammation.

Leukopenia A decrease in the number of circulating leukocytes.

Level of injury The vertical location of an injury along the spinal column.

Lewy bodies Abnormal aggregates of proteins, including alpha-synuclein.

Liability The state of being legally obliged and responsible.

Libido 1. Sexual desire. 2. The psychic energy that, according to Freud, provides the underlying motivation to human development.

Licensed practical nurses (LPNs) Members of a nursing team who provide direct client care under the direction of an RN, physician, or other licensed practitioner.

Lichenification The thickening of the skin.

Lifestyle An individual's general way of living, including living conditions and individual patterns of behavior that are influenced by sociocultural factors and personal characteristics.

Ligaments Connective tissue between bones to create joints.

Lightening The effects that occur when the fetus begins to settle into the pelvic inlet.

Limb restraints A device typically made of cloth that may be used when limb immobilization is needed for therapeutic purposes, for example, to prevent dislodgement of an intravenous infusion device.

Limbic system A set of structures located deep inside the brain; includes the hippocampus.

Limit setting Establishing clear and consistent rules or guidelines for child or client behavior.

Line authority The power to direct the activities of subordinates within an organization.

Lipids The macronutrient that provides most of the body's energy at 9 kcal/g. There are three categories of lipids: triglycerides, phospholipids and sterols. Also called *fats*.

Lipoatrophy Atrophy of subcutaneous tissues.

Lipodystrophy Excessive growth of subcutaneous tissue.

Lithiasis Stone formation.

Lithotripsy The preferred treatment for urinary calculi; uses sound or shock waves to crush a stone.

Living will A document that provides written directions about life-prolonging procedures to provide instructions when an individual can no longer communicate in a life-threatening situation.

Lobes Specialized cognitive regions in the hemispheres of the brain.

Local adaptation syndrome (LAS) A stress response that affects only one organ or body system.

Local emergency management agency (LEMA) A governmental agency with expertise in public safety, emergency medical services, and management.

Local infection Invasion by a microorganism that is limited to the specific part of the body where the microorganism remains.

Localized responses Common manifestations of type I hypersensitivity, they are typically atopic responses; that is, they have a strong genetic predisposition. Atopic reactions are the result of localized, rather than systemic, IgE-mediated responses to an allergen. They are prompted by contact of the allergen with IgE in the bronchial tree, nasal mucosa, and conjunctival tissues.

Lochia The discharge through which the uterus rids itself of the debris remaining after birth. The discharge should change appearance and contents as healing commences.

Lochia alba The final discharge as the uterus completes healing; composed primarily of leukocytes, decidual cells, epithelial cells, fat, cervical mucus, cholesterol crystals, and bacteria.

Lochia rubra The dark red initial discharge as the uterus eliminates epithelial cells, erythrocytes, leukocytes, shreds of decidua, and occasionally fetal meconium, lanugo, and vernix in the first 1–2 days following birth.

Lochia serosa A light pink discharge of serous exudate, shreds of degenerating decidua, erythrocytes, leukocytes, cervical mucus, and numerous microorganisms from the uterus 3–10 days following birth.

Locked-in syndrome A state of consciousness in which the client is alert and fully aware of the environment and has intact cognitive abilities but is unable to communicate through speech or movement because of blocked efferent pathways from the brain. Motor paralysis affects all voluntary muscles, although the upper cranial nerves (I through IV) may remain intact, allowing the client to communicate through eye movements and blinking.

Locus of control (LOC) The extent to which clients believes their health status is under their own or others' control.

Long-term memory The repository for information stored for periods longer than 72 hours and usually weeks and years.

Longboard spinal immobilization A device that provides support and immobilization of the entire spine below the level of the neck, instituted for clients with a potential or suspected spinal cord injury from a motor vehicle crash.

Loose association An indication of disordered thinking characterized by the shifting of verbal ideas from one topic to another, with no apparent relationship between thoughts, and the person speaking being unaware that the topics are unconnected. Commonly seen in schizophrenia.

Lordosis A concave curvature of the spine that may decrease mobility.

Loss A situation in which someone or something that is valued becomes altered or no longer available.

Lower body obesity Identified by a waist-to-hip ratio of less than 0.8; more commonly seen in women. Also called *peripheral obesity*.

Lumpectomy Removal of a tumor and the surrounding margin of breast tissue followed by radiation therapy. Also called *segmental mastectomy* or *breast conservation surgery*.

Lung abscess A local area of necrosis and pus formation within the lung.

Lupus nephritis Inflammation of the kidneys resulting from systemic lupus erythematosus (SLE).

Luteinizing hormone (LH) Anterior pituitary hormone responsible for stimulating ovulation and for development of the corpus luteum.

Lymphadenopathy The enlargement of lymph nodes with or without tenderness. It may be caused by inflammation, infection, or malignancy of the nodes or the regions drained by the nodes.

Lymphangitis Inflammation of a lymph vessel.

Lymphedema Accumulation of fluid in the soft tissues of the arm caused by removal of lymph channels.

Lymphocytes The principal effector and regulator cells of specific immune responses to protect the body from microorganisms, foreign tissue, and cell mutations or alterations.

Lyse Disintegrate.

Maceration Tissues softened by prolonged wetting or soaking.

Macronutrients Essential nutrients needed by the body in large amounts to survive: carbohydrates, proteins, and fats.

Macrophages Large phagocytes that are important in the body's defense against chronic infections.

Macular degeneration A progressive disorder involving loss of central vision due to damage to the retina.

Magical thinking Believing that events occur because of one's thoughts or actions.

Major depressive disorder (MDD) A mood disorder characterized by loss of interest in life and unresponsiveness, moving from mild to severe, with severe symptoms lasting at least 2 weeks. Also called *unipolar depression.*

Major depressive episode Characterized by a change in several aspects of an individual's emotional state and functioning consistently over a period of 14 days or longer.

Malabsorption A condition in which the intestinal mucosa is unable to absorb nutrients, resulting in nutrients being excreted in the stool.

Malaise Vague feeling of physical discomfort.

Maldigestion A condition in which there is inadequate preparation of chyme for absorption of nutrients; also can result in malabsorption.

Male erectile disorder A condition that occurs when a male has erection problems during 25% or more of his sexual interactions.

Male orgasmic disorder A condition that occurs when a male can maintain an erection for long periods, but has difficulty ejaculating.

Malignant Term used to refer to a cell or growth that, if not treated, will recur, continue to grow, and spread to other sites in the body, ending in death.

Malignant hyperthermia A musculoskeletal disorder resulting from an inherited cellular deficit that places the client in a hypermetabolic state.

Malnutrition Health effects due to insufficient nutrient intake or stores. Also called *undernutrition.*

Malpractice Conduct deviating from the standard of practice dictated by a profession.

Malpresentation A condition that occurs when a fetus passes into the pelvic inlet with a breech or shoulder presentation. These presentations are associated with difficulties during labor.

Malunion The healing of bones in an anatomically incorrect position. Surgical correction may be needed.

Managed care A healthcare delivery system designed to provide cost-effective, high-quality care for groups of clients from the time of their initial contact with the health system through the conclusion of their health problem.

Manager An individual employed by an organization and granted the required authority, responsibility, accountability, and power to accomplish the organization's goals.

Mandatory health insurance Health insurance is provided by large, nonprofit health organizations centered around large employers or work-based associations or else is provided by government-sponsored programs. Everyone belongs to one of these two types of insurance plans, thus ensuring universal coverage.

Mandatory reporting A legal requirement to report an act, event, or situation that is designated by state or local law as a reportable event.

Mania An abnormal and persistently elevated, expansive, or irritable mood lasting at least 1 week, significantly impairing social or occupational functioning and generally requiring hospitalization.

Manipulation Controlling behavior used to exploit others for personal gain.

Margination The accumulation of leukocytes along the inner surface of blood vessels. Occurs as part of the inflammatory process.

Marital rape Rape that occurs when one spouse forces the other to have sex against his or her will.

Maslow's hierarchy of needs A concept proposed by Abraham Maslow in which he proposed the existence of levels of human needs that could be organized into five categories: physiological, safety, love and belonging, esteem, and self-actualization.

Massage therapy The scientific manipulation of the soft tissues of the body for the purposes of promoting healing and wellness.

Massive transfusion A series of blood parcels, including packed red blood cells, fresh frozen plasma, cryo units, and platelet pheresis administered to a client who has lost a substantial amount of blood.

Mast cells Leukocytes that detect foreign agents or injury and respond by releasing histamine, thereby activating the inflammatory process.

Masturbation The self-stimulation of one's genitals for sexual pleasure.

Maternal role attainment (MRA) The process by which a woman learns mothering behaviors and becomes comfortable with her identity as a mother.

Maturational crisis A crisis that occurs normally as an individual progresses through the life cycle.

Mature milk A white or slightly blue-tinged color milk that presents by 2 weeks postpartum and continues thereafter until lactation ceases.

McDonald sign A probable sign of pregnancy characterized by an ease in flexing the body of the uterus against the cervix.

Mean arterial pressure (MAP) The average pressure in the arterial circulation throughout the cardiac cycle.

Meaning-focused coping The use of revaluation to reduce the appraisal of a threat.

Meatus A body passage or opening.

Meconium The first fecal material passed by a newborn, normally within 8–24 hours after birth.

Medicaid A state-administered health insurance program available to certain lower-income individuals and families, older adults, and people with disabilities.

Medical asepsis All practices intended to confine a specific microorganism to a specific area, thus limiting the number, growth, and transmission of the microorganism.

Medicare A federally funded health insurance program available to people ages 65 or older, younger people with disabilities, and people with end-stage renal disease.

Medigap policy A private health insurance plan designed to supplement Medicare coverage. It may pay copayments, coinsurance, deductibles and "gaps" in Medicare coverage (i.e., noncovered healthcare costs). Also called *Medicare supplemental insurance*.

Meditation The act of focusing one's thoughts or engaging in self-reflection or contemplation.

Meiosis A reductive division of sex cells, producing ova or sperm with a half set (haploid) of chromosomes.

Melanin A shield that protects the keratinocytes and the nerve endings in the dermis from the damaging effects of ultraviolet light.

Melanoma A type of malignant skin cancer.

Melasma gravidarum See **Chloasma**.

Mendelian inheritance Traits that are passed on by a single gene. Also called *single-gene inheritance*.

Meninges Three connective tissue membranes that cover, protect, and nourish the central nervous system.

Menopause The permanent cessation of menses.

Menorrhagia Excessive or prolonged menstruation that occurs at regular intervals.

Menstrual cycle The cyclic phases of menstruation that normally occur about every 28 days.

Menstruation The periodic shedding of the uterine lining in a woman of childbearing age who is not pregnant.

Mental retardation See **Intellectual disability**.

Mentor A competent, experienced professional who develops a relationship with a novice for the purpose of providing advice, support, information, and feedback in order to encourage development of the individual.

Message Content that is actually said or written, the body language that accompanies the words, and how the words are transmitted.

Metabolic acidosis This bicarbonate deficit is characterized by a low pH (<7.35), low bicarbonate (<24 mEq/L), and $PaCO_2$ less than 38 mmHg. It may be caused by excess acid in the body or loss of bicarbonate from the body.

Metabolic alkalosis This bicarbonate excess is characterized by a high pH (>7.45), a high bicarbonate (>28 mEq/L), and $PaCO_2$ higher than 45 mmHg. It may be caused by loss of acid or excess bicarbonate in the body.

Metabolic syndrome A disorder characterized by the presence of three or more of the following: increased waist circumference, hypertension, elevated blood triglycerides and fasting blood glucose, and low HDL cholesterol.

Metabolism The complex process of biochemical reactions occurring in the body's cells necessary to produce energy, repair cells, and sustain life.

Metaphysis The portion of the bone between the diaphysis and the epiphysis.

Metaplasia A change in the normal pattern of differentiation such that dividing cells differentiate into cell types not normally found at that location in the body.

Metastasis The process by which spreading of malignant neoplasms occurs; the transfer of disease from one organ or part to another.

Metrorrhagia Bleeding between menstrual periods.

Microalbuminuria An abnormally low level of albumin in the urine.

Micronutrients Essential nutrients needed by the body in small quantities, such as vitamins and minerals.

Microstaging The assessment of the level of invasion of a malignant melanoma and the maximum tumor thickness.

Micturition Releasing urine from the urinary bladder. Also called *voiding* or *urination*.

Middle ear effusion Results when negative pressure in the middle ear causes sterile serous fluid to move from the capillaries into the space.

Milia Exposed sebaceous glands that appear as raised white spots on the face, especially across the nose on infants within the first month after birth.

Miliary tuberculosis Results from hematogenous spread (through the blood) of the tuberculosis bacilli throughout the body.

Milieu therapy A therapeutic recovery environment that supports behavior changes, teaches new coping skills, and helps the client move from addiction to sobriety.

Milliequivalent The chemical combining power of the ion, or the capacity of cations to combine with anions to form molecules.

Minerals Salts dissolved in water that carry electrical charge and work with other nutrients to maintain fluid balance throughout the body. Also called *electrolytes*.

Minimal enteral nutrition Small-volume feedings of formula or human milk (usually <24 mL · kg^{-1} · day^{-1}) designed to "prime" the premature infant's intestinal tract and stimulate many of its hormonal and enzymatic functions.

Minor trauma Trauma that affects a single part or system of the body and is usually treated in a physician's office or in a hospital's emergency department.

Miscarriage The loss of a fetus prior to 20 weeks' gestation. Also called a *spontaneous abortion*.

Mitigation A phase that takes place before and after an emergency that consists of identifying potential hazards, minimizing effects, and reducing the likelihood of their occurrence.

Mitosis The process of cell division.

Mitt restraints A device used to protect confused clients from scratching or injuring their skin or dislodging intravenous access devices. Also called *hand restraints*.

Modeling Observing the behavior of people who have successfully achieved a goal that they have set for themselves and, through observing, acquiring ideas for behavior and coping strategies.

Modified radical mastectomy The removal of the breast tissue and lymph nodes under the arm, leaving the chest wall muscles intact.

Molding The asymmetrical appearance of an infant's head caused by overlapping of the cranial bones during labor and birth.

Mongolian spots Macular areas of bluish-black or gray-blue pigmentation on the dorsal area and the buttocks; common in newborns of Asian, Hispanic, and African descent and in newborns of other dark-skinned races.

Monoamine oxidase inhibitor (MAOI) A drug that inhibits monoamine oxidase, an enzyme that terminates the actions of neurotransmitters such as dopamine, norepinephrine, epinephrine, and serotonin. These drugs are used to treat individuals who have not responded to typical treatments for depression.

Mononeuropathies Isolated peripheral neuropathies that affect a single nerve.

Monophasic A term used to describe rheumatoid arthritis when it occurs for a limited time and then improves.

Monopolizing The domination of a discussion by one member of a group.

Monosomy Absence of a chromosome.

Monotheism The belief in the existence of one God.

Monro-Kellie hypothesis A hypothesis that states if the volume of any of the three intracranial components (the brain, cerebrospinal fluid, and blood) increases, the volume of the others must decrease to maintain normal pressures in the cranial cavity.

Mood An individual's internal, subjective, sustained emotional state.

Mood stabilizers Drugs used for treatment of bipolar disorder because they moderate extreme shifts in emotions between mania and depression.

Moral behavior The way in which an individual perceives and responds to society's requirements.

Moral development **1.** The process of learning to tell the difference between right and wrong and of learning what ought and ought not to be done. **2.** The pattern of change in moral behavior that occurs with age.

Moral rules Specific prescriptions for actions.

Morality Private, personal standards of what is right and wrong in conduct, character, and attitude; the requirements necessary for people to live together in society.

Morbid obesity A condition in which an individual weighs more than 200% of his or her ideal body weight or has a BMI >40 kg/m^2.

Morning sickness A term that refers to the nausea and vomiting that a woman may experience in early pregnancy. This lay term is sometimes used because these symptoms frequently occur in the early part of the day and disappear within a few hours.

Moro reflex In response to being lifted, then suddenly lowered or surprised by a loud noise, a newborn will straighten the arms and hands outward while the knees flex. Slowly, the arms return to the chest, as in an embrace. The fingers spread, forming a "C," and the newborn may cry.

Morpheaform basal cell carcinoma A type of skin cancer.

Morula Developmental stage of the fertilized ovum in which there is a solid mass of cells.

Mosaicism The expression of two cell lines, each with a different chromosomal number, in an individual.

Motility The process of moving food and fluid through the gastrointestinal tract from the mouth to the anus.

Motivation to learn The individual's personal desire and need to learn that affects how much and how fast the individual will learn.

Motor vehicle crash (MVC) The unintentional collision of one or more motor vehicles with another vehicle or object.

Mottling A lacy pattern of dilated blood vessels under the skin.

Mourning The behavioral process through which grief is eventually resolved or altered; it is often influenced by culture, spiritual beliefs, and custom.

Movement disorder A disorder associated with schizophrenia. There are two general forms: The first involves increased body movements that may appear agitated, repetitious, or purposeless. The second form involves catatonia, or unresponsiveness to the environment or others.

Movement technique A relaxation technique, such as yoga or tai chi, designed to improve strength, balance, and mental calmness.

Multiculturalism Characterized by many subcultures coexisting within a given society in which no one culture dominates.

Multidisciplinary team approach An approach to health care in which team members work together to deliver client care, but a single team member—usually a physician—makes the treatment decisions.

Multifocal A term used to describe premature ventricular contractions (PVCs) that arise from different ectopic sites and appear distinct on the ECG.

Multigravida Term used to describe a woman who has been pregnant more than once.

Multipara Term used to describe a woman who has had more than one pregnancy in which the fetus was viable.

Multiple pregnancy More than one fetus in the uterus at the same time.

Multiple sclerosis (MS) A chronic demyelinating neurological disease of the central nervous system associated with an abnormal immune response to an environmental factor.

Multiple trauma Trauma that involves serious single-system injury or multiple-system injuries. Also called *major trauma.*

Mural thrombi Blood clots in the heart wall.

Muscle relaxation A relaxation technique that involves consciously tightening and then relaxing each muscle progressively from either head to toe or toe to head.

Mutual recognition model A licensing system that allows a nurse to have a single license that confers the privilege to practice in other states that are part of the Nurse Licensure Compact.

Mutual respect A state in which two or more individuals show or feel honor or esteem toward one another.

Mycobacterium tuberculosis The bacteria that causes tuberculosis.

Mydriasis Abnormal or excessive dilation of the pupil of the eye, usually caused by a disease or drug.

Myelin The fatty, segmented wrappings that normally protect and insulate nerves. Also called *myelin sheath.*

Myelogram A diagnostic technique in which dye is injected into the spinal fluid and visualized by x-ray in order to identify areas of pressure on the spinal cord or nerves due to herniated discs.

Myocardial hypertrophy An increase in the size of muscle cells of the myocardium.

Myometrium The middle muscular layer of the uterus.

Myopia Nearsightedness.

MyPlate A nutrient intake guide from the U.S. Department of Agriculture that outlines suggested food intake by food groups.

Myringotomy A surgical incision of the tympanic membrane.

Myxedema The hypothyroid state with characteristic accumulation of nonpitting edema in the connective tissues throughout the body.

Myxedema coma A life-threatening complication of long-standing, untreated hypothyroidism, usually triggered by an acute illness or trauma.

Nägele rule The most common method of determining the estimated date of birth using the first day of the last menstrual period, subtracting 3 months, and adding 7 days.

NANDA The acronym for North American Nursing Diagnosis Association.

Narcissism Self-centered behavior in which the individual feels entitled to special favors due to a mistaken perception that they are superior to others.

Narcissistic personality disorder (NPD) One of several personality disorders defined in the DSM-5, it is marked by in a pattern of grandiosity, difficulty regulating self-esteem, and the need for admiration and attention from others.

Narcolepsy A disorder characterized by daytime sleep attacks or excessive daytime sleepiness.

Narcotics See **Opioids.**

Narrative charting A traditional part of the source-oriented record. It consists of written notes that include routine care, normal findings, and client problems.

National Institute for Occupational Safety and Health (NIOSH) An organization that focuses on generating new knowledge in the field of occupational safety and health and transferring that knowledge into practice for the betterment of workers.

National Patient Safety Goals (NPSGs) Formulated goals to assist accredited organizations with specific topics about client safety.

Natural killer (NK) cells Large, granular cells found in the spleen, lymph nodes, bone marrow, and blood. NK cells provide immune surveillance and resistance to infection, and they play an important role in the destruction of early malignant cells.

Nature The genetic or hereditary capability of the individual.

Nausea A vague, but unpleasant, subjective sensation of sickness or queasiness.

Necrosis Dead tissue.

Negative affectivity One of the six trait domains associated with personality disorders that is distinguished by anxiousness, emotional lability, separation insecurity, depressive tendencies, perseveration, and suspicion.

Negative airflow room A room where airflow is controlled to prevent the air from circulating into the hallway or other rooms. Multiple fresh-air exchanges dilute the concentration of droplet nuclei in a negative airflow room. Also called *negative flow room.*

Negative feedback Output of a system that returns to the system as input and which inhibits system change.

Negative pressure ventilators A device that creates negative pressure externally to draw the chest outward and air into the lungs, mimicking spontaneous breathing.

Negative punishment The removal of a positive reward if an undesirable behavior occurs.

Negative symptom Loss or absence of a normal function seen in mentally healthy adults, such as the ability to care for one's self; commonly seen in schizophrenia.

Neglect syndrome A disorder of attention that can result from stroke, which is characterized by the inability to integrate and use perceptions from the affected side. Also called *unilateral neglect.*

Negligence Any conduct that deviates from what a reasonable person would do in a particular circumstance.

Neologisms Use of meaningless words that only have meaning to the individual using them.

Neonatal abstinence syndrome (NAS) A combination of neonatal signs and symptoms caused by withdrawal of gestational opioid exposure.

Neonatal anemia A disorder caused by blood loss, hemolysis, and impaired red blood cell production related to birth.

Neonatal mortality risk An infant's chance of death within the first 28 days of life.

Neonatal transition The first few hours after birth, in which a newborn's body systems adapt to extrauterine life.

Neonatology The field of medicine providing care for sick and premature infants.

Neoplasm A mass of new tissue that grows independently of its surrounding structures and has no physiological purpose.

Nephrectomy Removal of a kidney.

Nephritis Inflammation of the kidneys.

Nephrolithiasis The formation of stones in the kidney.

Nephrolithotomy A procedure for removal of a staghorn calculus that invades the calyces and renal parenchyma.

Nephrotoxins Substances that damage nerves or nerve tissue.

Nerve block A chemical interruption of a nerve pathway, effected by injecting a local anesthetic into the nerve.

Networking The act of developing and maintaining relationships with others within and outside of the nursing profession and affiliated organizations to improve nursing practice, advance career goals, offer support, share information, and provide advice.

Neurofibrillary tangles Seen in clients with Alzheimer disease, they are thick, insoluble clots of protein inside the damaged brain cells or neurons.

Neurogenic bladder Interference with the normal mechanisms of urine elimination in which the client does not perceive bladder fullness and is unable to control the urinary sphincters; usually the result of impaired neurological function.

Neurogenic shock The result of an imbalance between parasympathetic and sympathetic stimulation of vascular smooth muscle.

Neuroleptic malignant syndrome (NMS) A potentially fatal condition caused by antipsychotic medications that block dopamine receptors. It is characterized by fever, rigidity, and increased prolactin levels.

Neuron The basic or specialized cell of the nervous system that carries electrical impulses throughout the body.

Neuropathic pain A type of pain experienced by people who have damaged or malfunctioning nerves.

Neurotransmitters Chemical messengers that carry information between neurons.

Neutral question An open-ended question the client can answer without direction or pressure.

Neutral thermal environment (NTE) A specific environmental temperature range in which the rates of oxygen consumption and metabolism are minimal and the internal body temperature is maintained because of thermal balance.

Nevi Moles.

Nevus flammeus A capillary angioma directly below the epidermis. It is a nonelevated, sharply demarcated, red-to-purple area of dense capillaries. In infants of African descent, it may appear as a purple-black stain. Also called *port-wine stain*.

Nevus vasculosus A capillary hemangioma consisting of newly formed and enlarged capillaries in the dermal and subdermal layers. It is a raised, clearly delineated, dark red, rough-surfaced birthmark commonly found in the head region. Also called a *strawberry mark*.

New Ballard score Specific criteria designed for accurate assessment of the gestational age of newborns between 20 and 28 weeks of gestation and weighing less than 1,500 g.

Newborn Infant from birth through the first 28 days of life.

Nicotine A highly addictive chemical that is found in tobacco and enters the body via the lungs (cigarettes, pipes, and cigars) and oral mucous membranes (chewing tobacco as well as smoking).

Nicotine replacement therapy (NRT) A pharmacologic therapy designed to relieve some of the physiological effects of withdrawal, including cravings, for clients trying to quit smoking or using tobacco. NRT transdermal patches and gums are available over the counter; nicotine inhalers and nasal sprays are available by prescription only.

Nicotinic receptors Found in the hippocampus and involved with new sensory information and memory formation, they are thought to be impaired in clients with schizophrenia.

Nidation The cyclical preparation of the uterine lining by steroid hormones for implantation of the embryo.

Nociceptive pain A type of pain resulting from external stimuli on an uninjured, fully functional nervous system.

Nociceptors The nerve receptors for pain.

Nocturia Voiding two or more times at night.

Nocturnal emissions Orgasm and emission of semen during sleep. Also called *wet dreams*.

Nocturnal enuresis Involuntary urination at night after bladder control has been achieved. Also called *bed wetting*.

Nocturnal frequency The need for older adults to arise during the night to urinate.

Nodular basal cell carcinoma A type of skin cancer.

Noise-induced hearing loss (NIHL) A condition associated with prolonged exposure to sound of greater than or equal to 85 dB.

Nolo contendere A term used when an individual neither admits to nor denies committing a crime but agrees to a punishment as if guilty.

Nominal group technique (NGT) A process that alternates between individual work and group work. Individuals meet as a group, but they write their responses without any discussion.

Nondirective interview An unstructured interview in which the nurse allows the client to control the purpose, subject matter, and pacing.

Nonexudative macular degeneration The most common form of macular degeneration, it is characterized by the accumulation of deposits beneath the pigment epithelium of the retina, causing the pigment epithelium to detach and interfere with the sensory function of the macula. Also referred to as the dry form of macular degeneration.

Noninvasive ventilation (NIV) Ventilator support using a tight-fitting face mask, thus avoiding intubation.

Nonmaleficence The duty to do no harm.

Non-Mendelian inheritance Traits that are passed on by the influence of multiple genes. Also called *multifactorial inheritance*.

Nonshivering thermogenesis (NST) The stimulation of heat production in the body through increased cellular metabolism. Also called *chemical thermogenesis*.

Non-small-cell carcinoma Lung cancers other than small-cell carcinoma.

Nonstress test (NST) A widely used method of evaluating fetal status; may be used alone or as part of a more comprehensive diagnostic assessment called a biophysical profile.

Nonunion Failure of the ends of a fracture to heal together after at least 3 months.

Nonverbal communication Transmitting information through gestures, facial expressions, or touch.

Normal sinus rhythm (NSR) The normal heart rhythm, in which impulses originate in the sinus node and travel through all normal conduction pathways without delay.

Normative commitment A feeling of obligation to continue in the profession due to benefits or positive experiences derived from the profession.

Normothermia Normal body temperature.

Nosocomial infections Infections that are associated with the delivery of healthcare services in a facility such as a hospital or nursing home. Also called *healthcare-associated infections (HAIs)*.

NREM Sleep Non-rapid-eye-movement sleep occurs when activity in the *reticular activating system* is inhibited.

Nuclear family A family structure consisting of a husband and wife and their biological children.

Nucleation The formation of a crystal from a liquid.

Nucleotomy The surgical removal of the nucleus pulposus.

Nulligravida Term used to describe a woman who has never been pregnant.

Nullipara Term used to describe a woman who has not given birth to a viable fetus.

Nurse practice act (NPA) State-level statutes that define and regulate nursing practices.

Nursing clinical research Research that seeks to answer questions that ultimately will improve client care.

Nursing diagnosis A clinical judgment about individual, family, or community responses to actual and potential health problems/life processes.

Nursing ethics Ethical issues that occur in nursing practice.

Nursing informatics (NI) A specialty that integrates nursing science, computer science, and information science to manage and communicate data, information, knowledge, and wisdom in nursing practice.

Nursing plan of care A written or electronic guideline that organizes information about an individual client's or family's care.

Nursing process The process used to identify a client's health status and actual or potential healthcare problems or needs, to establish plans to meet the identified needs, to deliver specific nursing interventions to meet those needs, and to evaluate the success of those interventions.

Nursing research A systematic and strict scientific process that tests hypotheses about health-related illness and conditions and processes of nursing care practices.

Nursing transactional model The relationship among the nurse, the client, and the environment in which they interact.

Nurture The effects of the environment on an individual's performance.

Nutrient density The ratio of good nutrients to calories a food contains.

Nutrients Substances found in food used by the body to promote growth, maintenance, and repair.

Nutrition The process by which the body ingests, absorbs, transports, uses, and eliminates nutrients in food.

Nutritional health The physical result of the balance between nutrient intake and nutritional requirements.

Nystagmus Involuntary rapid eye movement.

Obesity An excess of adipose tissue.

Object permanence The ability to understand that when something is out of sight it still exists.

Objective data Information that is detectable by an observer or can be measured or tested against an accepted standard. Also called *overt data* or *signs*.

Objective family burden Actual, identifiable family problems associated with the mental illness of a family member.

Obligatory losses Essential fluid losses required to maintain body functioning.

Observational learning The acquisition of new skills or the alteration of old behaviors simply by watching other children and adults.

Obsession A recurrent, unwanted, and often distressing thought or image that leads to feelings of fear and anxiety.

Obsessive-compulsive disorder (OCD) A disabling disorder characterized by obsessive thoughts and compulsive, repetitive behaviors that dominate an individual's life.

Obsessive–compulsive personality disorder (OCPD) One of several personality disorders defined in the DSM-5, it is marked by fear and anxiety concerning loss of control over situations, objects, or people.

Obstetric conjugate The distance from the middle of the sacral promontory to an area approximately 1 cm below the pubic crest.

Obstructive shock Shock caused by an obstruction in the heart or great vessels that either impedes venous return or prevents effective cardiac pumping action.

Occult blood Blood in stool that cannot be seen with the naked eye.

Occupational exposure Skin, eye, mucous membrane, or parenteral contact with blood or other potentially infectious materials that may result from the performance of an employee's duties.

Occupational Safety and Health Administration (OSHA) An organization that enforces the guidelines presented in the OSHA Act of 1970, requiring its covered employees to report specific incidents and illnesses in a timely manner.

Olfactory Of or relating to smell.

Oligodendrocytes Cells that produce myelin.

Oliguria The production of abnormally small amounts of urine by the kidney.

On–off effect A sudden lack of symptom control and unexpected dyskinesias appearing as drug effectiveness diminishes.

Oncogenes Genes that promote cell proliferation and are capable of triggering cancerous characteristics.

Oncology The study of cancer.

Oncotic pressure A pulling force exerted by colloids that helps maintain the water content of blood by pulling water from the interstitial space into the vascular compartment. Also called *colloid osmotic pressure*.

Oogenesis The process that produces the female gamete, called an ovum (egg).

Open-angle glaucoma The most common form of glaucoma, it is a chronic, gradually progressive disease that typically affects both eyes.

Open-ended question A question that allows clients to discover, explore, elaborate, clarify, or illustrate their thoughts or feelings.

Open fracture A fracture in which the skin integrity is disrupted. Also called a *compound fracture*.

Open reduction and internal fixation (ORIF) The surgical insertion of nails, screws, plates, or pins to hold fractured bones in place.

Opiates A type of drug derived from natural or synthetic opiates that is used as a pain reliever. Opiates include morphine, meperidine, codeine, hydrocodone, and oxycodone.

Opioids Drugs that act on one or more of three opioid receptors: mu, delta, and kappa. They are controlled substances due to their potential for abuse. Also called *narcotics*.

Opportunistic infection An invasion of the body tissue by microorganisms appearing in an individual with immunodeficiency that would normally not affect an individual with an intact immune system.

Opportunistic pathogen A microorganism that causes disease only in susceptible individuals.

Optimism A feeling that things will turn out for the best.

Oral–genital sex Kissing, licking, or sucking of the genitals for sexual pleasure.

Orchiectomy Surgical removal of the testes.

Organizational chart A chart that depicts the formal hierarchical structure and related responsibilities within a traditional organization.

Organizational commitment The relative strength of an individual's relationship and sense of belonging to an organization

Organizing The process of coordinating the work to be done. Formally, it involves identifying the work of the organization, dividing the labor, developing the chain of command, and assigning authority.

Orgasmic phase The third phase of the sexual response cycle that is marked by the involuntary release of sexual tension accompanied by physiological and psychological release.

Orientation 1. A structured program of activities to help new employees adapt to their new workplace; it is geared toward helping newly employed nurses to be successful. 2. A newborn's ability to be alert to, follow, and fixate on appealing and attractive, complex visual stimuli.

Orthopnea Difficulty breathing when supine.

Orthopneic position A body position with the head and arms supported on the overbed table to facilitate breathing.

Orthotic devices Orthopedic devices that may include splints or braces applied to reduce strain on a joint.

Ortolani maneuver A procedure used to evaluate an infant for developmental dysplastic hip.

Osmolality A measure of the concentration of solutes in body fluids. Osmolality is determined by the total solute concentration within a fluid compartment and is measured as parts of solute per kilogram of water.

Osmolar imbalance A fluid imbalance that involves the loss or gain of only water, so that the osmolality of the serum is altered.

Osmosis The movement of water across cell membranes, from a less concentrated solution to a more concentrated solution.

Osmotic pressure The power of a solution to draw water across a semipermeable membrane.

Ossification The development of bone.

Osteoarthritis (OA) The most common form of arthritis in older adults. It is caused by chronic degenerative changes in the cartilage and synovial membranes of the joints.

Osteoblasts Cells that form bone.

Osteoclasts Cells that resorb bone.

Osteocytes Cells that maintain bone matrix.

Osteodystrophy A complex bone disease process of chronic kidney disease in which chronic hyperparathyroidism causes increased resorption of bone.

Osteomyelitis Infection of the bone in a compound fracture.

Osteophytes Bony spurs that form as cartilage deteriorates.

Osteoporosis A metabolic bone disorder characterized by loss of bone mass, increased bone fragility, and increased risk of fractures.

Osteotomy 1. Surgical removal of a wedge of bones above or below a joint to realign the joint and shift weight away from the damaged potion of a joint. 2. An incision into or transection of the bone.

Otitis externa Inflammation of the ear canal. It is often called *swimmer's ear* because it is most frequently found in people who spend significant time in the water.

Otitis interna An inflammation of the inner ear. Also called *labyrinthitis.*

Otitis media Inflammation of the middle ear.

Otoscope A handheld instrument with a light and a cone-shaped attachment; known as an *ear speculum.*

Outcome The specific, observable criteria used to evaluate whether goals have been met and the effectiveness of nursing actions.

Outcome standards Standards that focus on the performance of a process, such as the number of bedridden clients who develop a pressure ulcer.

Outcomes management Management process that uses client experiences to guide improvement in all areas of health care by providing a link between medical interventions and health outcomes and between health outcomes and the cost of care.

Output Energy, material, or information that a system gives out as a result of its processes.

Ovarian cycle The three cyclical phases of oogenesis that occur about every 28 days.

Ovarian ligaments Ligaments that anchor the lower pole of the ovary to the uterus.

Ovaries Female sex glands in which the ova are formed and in which estrogen and progesterone are produced. Normally, a woman has two ovaries.

Overdelegation A situation that occurs when a delegator loses control over a situation by providing a delegate with too much authority or too much responsibility. This places the delegator in a risky position, increasing the potential for liability.

Overnutrition Health effects caused by excesses in nutrient intake or stores, such as obesity, hypertension, hypercholesterolemia, or toxic levels of stored vitamins or minerals.

Overt conflict Conflict that is addressed openly and is generally obvious to the individuals involved.

Ovulation Normal process of discharging a mature ovum from an ovary approximately 14 days before the onset of menses.

Oxygenation The mechanism that facilitates or impairs the body's ability to supply oxygen to all cells of the body.

Pacemaker An external or implanted pulse generator used to provide an electrical stimulus to the heart when the heart fails to generate or conduct its own stimulus at a rate that maintains the cardiac output.

$PaCO_2$ A measure of the pressure exerted by dissolved carbon dioxide in the blood; it reflects the respiratory component of acid–base regulation and balance because it is regulated by the lungs.

Pain An unpleasant sensory and emotional experience associated with actual or potential tissue damage.

Pain threshold The point at which pain is initially perceived.

Pain tolerance The duration of time or intensity of pain an individual will endure before demonstrating pain responses.

Palliation Measures taken not to cure a disease, but to relieve disease-related symptoms and enhance the client's quality of life. See also **Palliative care.**

Palliative care Nursing care that improves the quality of life of clients and their families facing life-threatening illness by preventing, assessing, and treating pain and other physical, psychosocial, and spiritual problems.

Palliative procedure A surgical or interventional cardiac catheterization procedure that does not create normal anatomical or hemodynamic results but allows adequate blood flow to oxygenate the tissues.

Pallidotomy A surgical technique for Parkinson disease in which the neurosurgeon locates the affected areas of the globus pallidus and destroys the involved tissue in order to improve tremors and mobility.

Palpation A method of assessment that involves touching the areas related to the body system to determine symmetry, equality of the size, shape, or condition of opposite sides of the body.

Pancreatitis Inflammation of the pancreas that occurs when pancreatic enzymes are released into the pancreas itself, causing autodigestion of pancreatitic tissues.

Pandemic Widespread global outbreak of an infectious disease.

Panic disorder A sudden attack of terror, sometimes accompanied by a pounding heart, sweating, fainting, or dizziness.

Pannus An abnormal tissue layer that includes newly formed blood vessels. Pannus leads to scar tissue formation that immobilizes joints.

PaO_2 A measure of the pressure exerted by oxygen that is dissolved in the plasma.

Para Term used to describe a woman who has borne offspring who reached the age of viability.

Paracentesis Aspiration of fluid from the peritoneal cavity.

Parallel play A stage of play in which toddlers play side by side with similar objects, but do not play together.

Paranoia An extreme suspicion that others are "out to get you" and delusions that one is being followed and that others are trying to harm oneself; experienced by some individuals with psychosis.

Paranoid personality disorder (PPD) One of several personality disorders defined in the DSM-5, it is characterized by the inability to trust others, hypervigilance, pathological jealousy, and prejudicial and judgmental tendencies.

Paraplegia Paralysis of all or part of the lower portion of the body.

Parasite One of the four categories of microorganisms, parasites live on other organisms.

Parasomnias Abnormal behaviors that may interfere with sleep and may occur during sleep

Parenteral nutrition (PN) The intravenous administration of amino acids, often with added carbohydrates, fats, electrolytes, vitamins, and minerals.

Parenting The ongoing act of guiding children to learn acceptable behaviors, morals, and rituals of the family and of teaching them to become socially responsible, contributing members of society.

Paresis Weakness.

Paresthesia Sensation of prickling, tingling, or numbing.

Parkinson disease (PD) A degenerative disorder of the central nervous system resulting from the death of neurons that produce the brain neurotransmitter dopamine.

Parkinsonian gait Altered gait characterized by small, shuffling steps, as well as bradykinesia or festination.

Parkinsonism The motor symptoms of Parkinson disease: tremors, muscle rigidity, postural instability, and bradykinesia.

Paroxysmal Occurring in bursts with an abrupt onset and termination.

Paroxysmal nocturnal dyspnea A sudden episode of shortness of breath occurring at night during sleep.

Partial-thickness burns Burns that involve the entire dermis and the papillae of the dermis (superficial partial-thickness burns) or extend into the hair follicles (deep partial-thickness burns).

Passive acquired immunity A condition that occurs when a pregnant woman passes IgG antibodies to a fetus in utero.

Passive behavior Behavior that seeks to avoid conflict at any cost, even at the expense of one's own happiness.

Passive communicators Individuals who focus on the needs of others. They often deny themselves any sort of power, which causes them to become frustrated.

Passive immunity Temporary protection—provided by antibodies produced by other people or animals—against disease-producing antigens. Protection is gradually lost when these acquired antibodies are used up either by natural degradation or by combining with the antigen.

Patch testing A test used to identify allergens causing dermatitis. An adhesive patch with common allergens is placed on the back between the scapulae. The patch is generally removed after several days; if there is no reaction to a particular allergen, that allergen is eliminated as a possible cause of dermatitis.

Patent airway An airway that is open and free of obstruction.

Patent ductus arteriosus (PAD) A congenital connection between the great vessels that normally closes after birth, allowing blood from the right and left side of the heart to mix.

Pathogen A microorganism that causes disease.

Pathogenicity The ability to produce disease.

Pathological fracture A fracture that results from disease that has weakened the bone.

Patient An individual who is waiting for or undergoing medical treatment and care.

Patient-controlled analgesia (PCA) A pump with a control mechanism that allows the client to self-manage pain.

Patient Protection and Affordable Care Act (PPACA or ACA) A law that regulates health care and attempts to make health care affordable for all Americans. Also called *Obamacare* after President Barak Obama, the U.S. president when the ACA was enacted.

Patient Self-Determination Act (PSDA) A federal law that requires every competent adult to be informed in writing on admission to a healthcare institution about his or her rights to accept or refuse medical care and to use advance directives.

Pauciarticular arthritis A form of juvenile rheumatoid arthritis that primarily affects the knees, ankles, and elbows; it occurs more frequently in females.

Peak expiratory flow rate (PEFR) A measurement used to monitor the ability of an individual to exhale a specific volume of air related to the individual's age, gender, height, and weight.

Pedagogy The study or science of teaching, specifically referring to children and adolescents.

Pedigree The graphic representation of a family tree, usually to trace genetic abnormalities.

Peer review A method to professionally critique a colleague's work based on predetermined standards.

Pelvic cavity Bony portion of the birth passage; a curved canal with a longer posterior than anterior wall.

Pelvic diaphragm Part of the pelvic floor, composed of deep fascia and the levator ani and the coccygeal muscles.

Pelvic inlet Upper border of the true pelvis.

Pelvic outlet Lower border of the true pelvis.

Pelvic tilt An exercise that helps prevent or reduce back strain as it strengthens abdominal muscles. Also called *pelvic rocking*.

Penetrating injury A type of eye injury in which the layers of the eye spontaneously reapproximate after entry of a sharp-pointed object or small missile (e.g., a BB) into the globe.

Penetrating trauma Trauma that occurs when a foreign object enters the body, causing damage to body structures.

Penta screen Maternal screening that measures five indicators whose presence may suggest fetal complications: AFP, beta hCG, unconjugated estriol, inhibin A, and invasive trophoblast antigen.

Penumbra A band of minimally perfused cells that surrounds a central core of dead or dying cells.

Peplau, Hildegard A nursing theorist who is widely considered the mother of psychiatric nursing; she presented nursing as a therapeutic interpersonal process, rather than as a task-oriented process.

Peptic ulcer A break in the mucosal lining of the GI tract exposed to acid-pepsin secretions, including the esophagus, stomach, and duodenum.

Peptic ulcer disease (PUD) A break in the mucous lining of the GI tract where it comes in contact with gastric juice.

Perceived loss A loss that is experienced by one person but cannot be verified by others.

Perception Awareness and interpretation of stimuli; the ability of the individual to interpret the environment.

Percussion A method of tapping the chest or back to assess underlying structures. Forceful striking of the skin with cupped hands, sometimes called *clapping*.

Perforating injury A type of eye injury in which the layers of the eye do not spontaneously reapproximate after the entry of a sharp-pointed object or small missile (e.g., a BB) into the globe, which results in rupture of the globe and potential loss of ocular contents.

Perforation Rupture, as in the penetration of ulcer through mucosal wall.

Performance improvement Quality of care improvement is directly linked to the performance of an individual, team, unit, or organization.

Pericarditis Inflammation of the pericardial tissue surrounding the heart.

Pericardium A double layer of fibroserous membrane that encases and anchors the heart.

Perimetrium The outermost layer of the uterus.

Perinatal loss Death of a fetus or infant that occurs between the time of conception and the end of the newborn period 28 days after birth.

Perineal body The wedge-shaped mass of fibromuscular tissue between the lower part of the vagina and the anus.

Periodic breathing A breathing pattern characterized by pauses lasting 5–15 seconds.

Periodontal disease Gum disease.

Perioperative The three phases of a surgical procedure: the preoperative phase, intraoperative phase, and postoperative phase.

Perioperative nursing care Nursing care provided during any or all of the three phases of surgery: preoperative, intraoperative, and postoperative.

Peripartum cardiomyopathy A rare but serious dysfunction of the left ventricle that occurs in the last month of pregnancy or the first 5 months postpartum in a woman with no previous history of heart disease.

Peripheral nervous system (PNS) One of two principal parts of the neurological system, the peripheral nervous system consists of the cranial nerves and the spinal nerves.

Peripheral neuropathy A condition that results when trauma or a disease process interferes with innervation of peripheral nerves.

Peripheral pulse A pulse located away from the heart, in the foot or the wrist.

Peripheral vascular disease (PVD) A disorder in which arteriosclerosis and atherosclerosis affect circulation to peripheral tissues, particularly the lower extremities.

Peripheral vascular resistance The opposing forces or impedance to blood flow as the arterial channels become more and more distant from the heart.

Peristalsis The process of wavelike muscular contractions that propels food and digestive products through the digestive tract.

Peritoneal dialysis The process by which dialysate is instilled into the abdominal cavity through a catheter, allowed to rest there while fluids and molecules exchange, and then removed through the catheter.

Peritonitis Inflammation and bacterial infection of the abdominal area.

Pernicious anemia A disorder that results from a failure to absorb dietary vitamin B_{12}.

Perseveration Use of the same words or phrases repetitively.

Persistent A term used to describe a disease or disorder (such as rheumatoid arthritis) that lasts for a period of 3–6 months or longer.

Persistent bacteriuria The reappearance of bacteria in urine due to a persistent source of infection causing repeated infection after the initial cure.

Persistent depressive disorder Chronic depression that affects an individual for the majority of most days for at least 2 years (1 year for children and adolescents). May be interrupted by periods of normal mood that do not exceed 2 months over the course of the 2 years. Also called *dysthymic disorder*.

Persistent vegetative state A permanent condition of complete unawareness of self and the environment and loss of all cognitive functions. Also called *irreversible coma*.

Personal distance Communication characterized by moderate voice tones, less noticeable body heat and smell. Physical contact such as a handshake or touching a shoulder is possible.

Personal identity The conscious sense of individuality and uniqueness that is continually evolving throughout life.

Personal knowing A nurse's commitment to ongoing, individual self-exploration and self-actualization.

Personal space The distance people prefer in interactions with others.

Personality The individual qualities, including habitual behavior patterns, that make an individual unique; the outward expression of the inner self.

Personality disorder (PD) Rigid, stereotyped behavioral patterns that deviate markedly from the norm of an individual's culture and persist throughout the person's life. Personality disorders are characterized by a lifelong maladaptive pattern of perceiving, thinking, and relating that impairs social or occupational functioning.

Personality traits The elements and patterns that comprise an individual's personality.

Pessimism A feeling that a situation is always bad and may become worse.

pH A measurement of the hydrogen ion concentration of a solution.

Phagocytosis A process by which a foreign agent or target cell is engulfed, destroyed, and digested. Neutrophils and macrophages, known as phagocytes, are the primary cells involved in phagocytosis.

Phantom pain A confusing pain syndrome that occurs following surgical or traumatic amputation of a limb. The client experiences pain in the missing body part even though there is complete mental awareness that the limb is gone. Also called *phantom limb syndrome*.

Phase of mutual regulation Time period during which a mother and her infant seek to determine the degree of control each partner in their relationship will exert. In this phase of adjustment, a balance is sought between the needs of the mother and the needs of the infant.

Phenotype The observable expression of genetic traits.

Philadelphia chromosome The balanced translocation of chromosome 22 to chromosome 9; associated with chronic myeloid leukemia.

Phimosis Tightness of the prepuce that prevents retraction of the foreskin.

Phobia An intense, persistent, irrational fear of a simple thing or social situation that compels the individual to avoid the stressor that elicits the fear.

Photophobia Sensitivity to light.

Physical activity Body movement produced by skeletal muscle contraction that increases energy expenditure.

Physical attending The conveyed act of being with another individual through physical posturing.

Physical restraint Any manual method, material, device, or equipment that is attached to the client's body with the intention of limiting or restricting free movement of the client's head, arms, legs, or body.

Physiological anemia of infancy A type of anemia that occurs as a result of the normal, gradual drop in hemoglobin for the first 6–12 weeks of life.

Physiological anemia of pregnancy Apparent anemia that results because during pregnancy the plasma volume increases more than the erythrocytes increase. Also called *pseudoanemia*.

Physiological jaundice A yellow discoloration of the skin caused by accelerated destruction of fetal red blood cells, impaired conjugation of bilirubin, and increased bilirubin reabsorption from the intestinal tract.

Physiological pain Experienced when an intact, properly functioning nervous system sends signals that tissues are damaged, requiring attention and proper care.

Pica The craving for and persistent eating of nonnutritive substances not ordinarily considered to be edible or nutritionally valuable, such as soil, clay, and soap.

PICOT A mnemonic method used by clinicians to define and formulate a clinical question driving the search for evidence-based practice. PICOT stands for Population of a group, Intervention or activity focus, Comparison group, Outcome(s) or desired effects, and Time frame.

Pigmented basal cell carcinoma A type of skin cancer.

Pill-rolling Rubbing of the thumb and fingers together accompanying other tremors.

Piloerection Goosebumps.

Pitch The frequency of vibrations in a sound.

Pitfalls A hidden trap that catches people unaware and undermines their plans.

Pitting edema Edema that retains indentation caused by pressure.

Placenta A flat, disc-shaped organ that is highly vascular and normally forms in the upper segment of the endometrium of the uterus; exchanges nutrients and gases between the fetus and the mother.

Placenta previa Occurs when the placenta partially or totally covers the mother's cervix; can result in severe bleeding before or during delivery.

Placental abruption A condition that occurs when the placenta detaches from the uterine wall before delivery. May or may not result in fetal demise, but a fetus's survival depends on the stage of development and prompt medical treatment.

Plan–do–study–act (PDSA) A system of quality improvement most often associated with total quality management.

Planning The four-stage, managerial process that establishes objectives, evaluates the present situation in order to predict future trends and events, formulates a planning statement, and converts the plan into an action statement.

Plaque 1. An invisible soft film that adheres to the enamel surface of teeth. Consists of bacteria, saliva molecules, and remnants of epithelial cells and leukocytes. 2. Scar tissue on myelin sheath due to repeated attacks by the immune system.

Plasmapheresis Removal of a harmful component from plasma. Also called *plasma exchange therapy*.

Play therapist A therapist who designs and provides recreational activities to promote emotional and/or physical healing and wellness.

Pleural effusion Accumulation of excess fluid in the pleural cavity.

Pleuritic pain Sharp localized chest pain that increases with breathing and coughing.

Pleuritis Local extension of an infection to involve the pleura.

Pleximeter The middle finger of the nondominant hand. Often used in indirect percussion techniques.

Plexor The middle finger of the dominant hand. Often used in indirect percussion techniques.

Pneumatic retinopexy A surgical procedure to correct retinal detachment in which air is injected into the vitreous cavity and the client is positioned so that the air bubble pushes the detached portion of the retina into contact with the choroid.

Pneumocystis carinii pneumonia (PCP) An opportunistic infection that is not pathogenic in those with intact immune systems.

Pneumomediastinum The presence of air in the mediastinum.

Pneumonia Inflammation of the lung parenchyma (the respiratory bronchioles and alveoli).

Pneumopericardium Air in the pericardial sac.

Pneumothorax A partial lung collapse due to air or gas collecting in the lung or in the pleural space that surrounds the lungs.

Point of care Interventions or testing that provides on-the-spot information about the client rather than having to send blood or urine samples down to the laboratory and wait for results to be returned.

Point of maximal impulse (PMI) A pulse located at the apex of the heart. Also called the *apical pulse*.

Point-of-service (POS) plan An insurance plan that allows the insured to choose between a health maintenance organization or a preferred provider organization each time they seek health care.

Polyarticular arthritis A form of juvenile rheumatoid arthritis that involves many joints (five or more), particularly the small joints of the hands and fingers. It may also affect the hips, knees, feet, ankles, and neck.

Polycyclic Describes a periodically recurring course of rheumatoid arthritis.

Polycythemia An increase in the production of red blood cells.

Polydipsia Excessive thirst.

Polyneuropathies Bilateral sensory disorders; they are the most common types of neuropathy associated with diabetes.

Polyp A small vascular growth on the surface of any mucous membrane.

Polyphagia Excessive hunger.

Polysomnography (PSG) A recording of the biophysical changes that a client experiences during sleep.

Polysubstance abuse The simultaneous use of many substances.

Polytheism The belief in more than one god.

Polyuria The production of abnormally large amounts of urine. Also called *diuresis*.

Pop-ups Unexpected things or events occurring during the day that require time and attention in addition to the regular plan for the day.

Positive end-expiratory pressure (PEEP) Mechanical ventilation in which a positive pressure is maintained in the airways during exhalation and between breaths to help keep alveoli open.

Positive feedback Output of a system that returns to the system as input and which promotes system change.

Positive pressure ventilator A mechanical device that pushes air into the lungs through an invasive device such as an endotracheal tube or tracheostomy tube, rather than drawing air in by negative pressure.

Positive punishment The addition of a negative consequence if undesirable behavior occurs.

Positive reinforcement Giving rewards such as praise or encouragement for a learner's achievements.

Positive symptoms Excessive or added behaviors that are not normally seen in healthy adults, such as delusions; commonly seen in schizophrenia.

Postcoital contraception A drug taken after intercourse to avoid pregnancy. Also called *Plan B* or the *morning after pill*.

Postconception age periods Period of time in embryonic/fetal development calculated from the time of fertilization of the ovum.

Postictal period A period immediately following seizure activity in which level of consciousness is decreased. The length of the postictal period varies.

Postoperative The third phase of an operative process in which recovery occurs.

Postpartal hemorrhage A loss of blood of greater than 500 mL following birth. The hemorrhage is classified as *early* if it occurs within the first 24 hours and *late* if it occurs after the first 24 hours.

Postpartum After childbirth.

Postpartum blues A maternal adjustment reaction occurring in the first few postpartum days, characterized by mild depression, tearfulness, anxiety, headache, and irritability. Also called *adjustment reaction to depressed mood*.

Postpartum depression A severe form of depression that affects new mothers, often beginning within 3 months of delivery but which may strike at any time during the first year after having a child. Also called *depressive disorder with peripartum onset*.

Postpartum psychosis Severe psychosis occurring within the first 3 months after birth that usually requires hospitalization.

Postterm labor Labor that occurs after 42 weeks' gestation.

Postterm newborn Any infant born after 42 weeks' gestation.

Postterm pregnancy Pregnancy that lasts beyond 42 weeks' gestation.

Posttraumatic stress disorder (PTSD) A trauma- and stressor-related disorder that can evolve after exposure to a traumatic or overwhelming event in which an individual's physical health was endangered.

Postural drainage The drainage by gravity of secretions from various lung segments.

PPD Tuberculin skin test. See **Purified protein derivative**.

Prader–Willi syndrome (PWS) A congenital disorder of the 15th chromosome that causes an unrelenting feeling of hunger, but also low muscle tone, short stature, incomplete sexual development, mild to severe mental retardation, and behavioral problems.

Prayer Human communication with divine and spiritual entities.

Preceptor An experienced nurse who provides knowledge and emotional support, as well as a clarification of role expectations, on a one-to-one basis.

Precipitating factor A practice, behavior, or environmental factor that gives rise to a specific incident of violence.

Predisposing factor A practice, behavior, or environmental factor that increases the potential of an individual's risk of violent victimization or perpetration of violence.

Preeclampsia An increase in blood pressure after 20 weeks of gestation accompanied by proteinuria. May also be accompanied by albuminuria and edema. Also called *toxemia of pregnancy*.

Preferred provider organization (PPO) A type of health insurance program that does not require its insureds to select a primary care provider. PPOs usually have larger networks of providers than health maintenance organizations (HMOs) and provide financial incentives that encourage insureds to seek care from in-network providers. They are less restrictive than HMOs but typically have higher copayments.

Prejudice A negative belief or preference that is generalized about a group that leads to prejudgment.

Preload The amount of cardiac muscle fiber tension, or stretch, that exists at the end of diastole.

Premature junctional contractions Heartbeats that occur before the next expected beat of the underlying rhythm.

Premature rupture of membranes (PROM) Spontaneous rupture of membranes and leakage of amniotic fluid before the onset of labor at any gestational age.

Premenstrual syndrome (PMS) A complex of manifestations (e.g., mood swings, breast tenderness, fatigue, irritability, food cravings, and depression) that occurs to 3–14 days before menstruation and is relieved by the onset of menses.

Prenatal education Programs offered to expectant families, adolescents, women, or partners to provide education regarding the pregnancy, labor, and birth experience.

Preoperative The first phase of an operative process in which the client is identified as a candidate for surgical intervention, assessed, and prepared for surgery.

Preparedness The phase that takes place before an emergency occurs during which risks are assessed and plans are developed to address them.

Presbycusis Age-related loss of the ability to hear high-frequency sounds; may occur because of cochlear hair cell degeneration or loss of auditory neurons in the organ of Corti.

Presbyopia Impaired near vision resulting from a loss of elasticity of the lens related to aging.

Presencing Being present with a client and being open, receptive, and available at all levels without judging or labeling.

Presenting part The first part of the fetus to enter and settle in the pelvic inlet during fetal presentation.

Pressure ulcer Ischemic lesions of the skin and underlying tissue caused by external pressure that impairs the flow of blood and lymph.

Preterm infant An infant born at less than 37 completed weeks of gestation.

Preterm premature rupture of the membranes (PPROM) A condition that occurs when membranes rupture and amniotic fluid leaks from the vagina before 37 weeks of gestation.

Pretibial myxedema The bilateral formation of edematous, erythematous, and sometimes hyperpigmented plaques and nodules over the shins and dorsal surface of the feet. A characteristic sign of Graves disease.

Priapism Persistent, painful erection of the penis.

Primary appraisal The evaluation of an event or circumstance in terms of its potential to harm, benefit, threaten, or challenge the individual.

Primary care provider (PCP) A healthcare provider who provides basic medical service and acts as a gatekeeper to more specialized care, referring clients to in-network hospitals and specialists.

Primary group A small, intimate group in which the relationships among members are personal, spontaneous, sentimental, cooperative, and inclusive.

Primary hypertension A persistently elevated systemic blood pressure. Also called *essential hypertension*.

Primary immune response When an individual is exposed to antigen, the B-lymphocyte system produces antibodies that react specifically with that antigen over the first 3 days.

Primary intention healing Healing that occurs where the tissue surfaces have been closed and there is minimal or no tissue loss. It is characterized by the formation of minimal granulation tissue and scarring. Also called *primary union* or *first intention healing*.

Primary nursing A model in which one nurse has 24/7 authority and responsibility for the care of an assigned group of clients.

Primary prevention Methods designed to focus on health promotion and illness prevention.

Primigravida A woman who is pregnant for the first time.

Primipara Term used to describe a woman who has given birth to her first child (past the point of viability), whether or not that child is living or was alive at birth.

Principles-based (deontological) theories Theories that involve logical and formal processes and emphasize individual rights, duties, and obligations.

Prioritizing care A process that helps nurses manage time and establish an order for completing responsibilities and care interventions for a single client or for a group of clients.

Priority Something given or meriting attention before competing alternatives.

Privacy The right of individuals to keep their personal information from being disclosed.

Private insurance Health insurance provided by private or publicly owned companies such as Blue Cross Blue Shield, Kaiser, or Aetna.

Problem-focused coping Managing or altering a stressor, event, or circumstance in response to distress.

Problem, intervention, evaluation (PIE) An assessment system consisting of client care flow sheets and progress notes.

Problem-oriented medical record (POMR) A recording system in which data are arranged according to the problems the client has rather than the source of the information. Also called *problem-oriented record (POR)*.

Problem-oriented record (POR) See **Problem-oriented medical record (POMR)**.

Procedural memory Recall of information that does not require conscious awareness and involves the memory of motor skills and procedures.

Process addictions Compulsive behaviors that serve to reduce anxiety such as workaholism, gambling, shopping, cutting, pornography, spending and indebtedness, Internet surfing or gaming, eating disorders, and sexual addictions.

Process standards Standards that focus on the steps used to lead to a particular outcome. It is used to determine if a set of steps exists and if those steps are being followed.

Productivity The performance measure of both the effectiveness and efficiency of nursing care.

Profession An occupation that requires extensive education or a calling that requires special knowledge, skill, and preparation.

Professional behaviors Effective nursing actions based on ethical principles, clinical reasoning, and technical knowledge and expertise that form helping relationships.

Professional development Continued staff education, planned activities to enhance role performance, and defined goals to improve client outcomes. Also called *staff development*.

Professional support Assistance provided by professionals in the community who exhibit a nonblaming and respectful attitude toward families and clients and who provide information and help locating community resources.

Professionalism Acting with the knowledge, skill, and preparation of a professional.

Professionalization The process of establishing qualifications, ethical guidelines, and a standardized knowledge base by which an occupation transforms itself into a profession.

Progesterone Hormone produced by the corpus luteum, adrenal cortex, and placenta whose function is to stimulate proliferation of the endometrium to facilitate growth of the embryo.

Projectile vomiting Vomiting in which emesis may be spewed up to 2–3 feet out of a baby's mouth. A major symptom of pyloric stenosis.

Prone Face-down.

Proprioception The body's sense of its position.

Proptosis Forward displacement of the eye.

Prospective payment system (PPS) A system in which hospitals determine the amount to be billed to the insurance company before the client is ever admitted to the hospital.

Prostaglandins (PGs) Complex lipid compounds synthesized by many cells of the body.

Prostate specific antigen (PSA) A protein produced in the cells of the prostate gland.

Prostatectomy Surgical removal of part or all of the prostate gland.

Prostatitis An inflammation of the prostate gland.

Prostatodynia A condition in which the client experiences the symptoms of prostatitis, but shows no evidence of inflammation or infection.

Protected health information Personal information or healthcare data that could identify an individual. This information is protected and defined by HIPAA's Privacy Rule.

Protective factor 1. A practice, behavior, or environmental factor that provides strength and assistance to children and families in dealing with crises and risk factors. 2. A practice, behavior, or environmental factor that decreases the potential of individual to perpetuate violence or victimization.

Protein A macronutrient that contains nitrogen and is a critical component of all tissues in the human body, including muscle, bone, and blood.

Protein-calorie malnutrition Problem of clients with long-term deficiencies in caloric intake; characteristics include depressed visceral proteins (e.g., albumin), weight loss, and visible muscle and fat wasting.

Proteinuria Excess protein in urine.

Proxemics The study of distance between people in their interactions.

Proximodistal Growth that proceeds from the center of the body outward.

Proximodistal development Development that proceeds from the center of the body outward.

Pruritus Itching of the skin.

Pseudoaddiction A term applied to clients who display drug-seeking behaviors but differ from addicts in that they have true underlying pain for which they are seeking relief. These behaviors will generally stop when adequate pain control is achieved.

Pseudoexacerbation A temporary aggravation of symptoms that is directly related to a trigger and subsides as soon as the trigger is removed.

Pseudomenstruation Blood or whitish discharge may occasionally be observed on the diapers of female newborns caused by the withdrawal of maternal hormones.

Purified protein derivative (PPD) Used to screen for tuberculosis in a tuberculin test. A small amount of the PPD is injected and the body's response interpreted.

Purulent exudate A large quantity of cells and necrotic debris that form an opaque or milky discharge that is thicker than serous exudate. Also called *pus* or *suppuration*.

Pus The common name for *purulent exudate*.

Psychoanalytic theory A framework for personality development that emphasizes the presence of unconscious impulses and their influence on behaviors and the formation of self; developed by Sigmund Freud (1856-1939).

Psychogenic pain Pain that is experienced in the absence of any diagnosed physiological cause or event.

Psychomotor domain The learning domain that includes fine motor skills. Also called the *skill domain*.

Psychomotor retardation A state in which thinking and body movements are noticeably slower than normal and speech is slowed or absent.

Psychosis A mental health condition characterized by delusions, hallucinations, illusions, disorganized behavior, and a difficulty relating to others. Also called *psychotic disorder*.

Psychosocial skills Skills that enable an individual in crisis to maintain relationships with family and friends throughout and after the crisis period.

Psychostimulants Stimulants that have a high potential for abuse. Psychostimulants include cocaine and amphetamines.

Psychoticism One of the six trait domains associated with personality disorders that is composed of eccentricity, cognitive and perceptual dysregulation, and unusual beliefs and experiences.

Ptosis Drooping of the eyelid.

Ptyalism Excessive, often bitter salivation.

Puberty The stage during which an individual reaches sexual maturity.

Pubis Pertaining to the pubes or pubic area.

Public distance Communication that requires loud, clear vocalizations with careful enunciation.

Public insurance Health insurance financed by the government.

Public self How the individual wishes to be perceived by others.

Puerperium That time immediately following childbirth during which physiological changes that occurred during pregnancy begin to return to normal. Also called *postpartum period*.

Pulmonary atresia The absence of communication between the right ventricle and the pulmonary artery.

Pulmonary circulation Circulation through the right side of the heart, the pulmonary artery, the pulmonary capillaries, and the pulmonary vein.

Pulmonary edema An abnormal accumulation of fluid in the interstitial tissue and alveoli of the lung.

Pulmonary embolism (PE) The obstruction of blood flow in part of the pulmonary vascular system by an embolus. Also called *pulmonary thromboembolism*.

Pulmonary function test (PFT) A test designed to provide information about ventilation airflow, lung volume, and the capacity and diffusion of gas.

Pulmonary vascular resistance The force or resistance of the blood in the pulmonary circulation.

Pulse A wave of blood created by the contraction of the left ventricle of the heart.

Pulse oximetry A noninvasive method of assessing arterial blood oxygenation.

Pulse pressure The difference between the systolic and diastolic pressure.

Pulse rhythm The pattern of the beats and the intervals between the beats.

Punctual On time.

Punishment 1. Action taken to enforce rules when a child misbehaves. 2. Consequences that lead to a decrease in undesirable behavior.

Pupillary light reflex Reflex in which the pupil contracts in response to a bright light.

Purging Self-induced vomiting or misuse of laxatives, diuretics, or enemas.

Pursed-lipped breathing Exhaling through a narrow opening between the lips to prolong the expiratory phase in an effort to promote more alveolar emptying while maintaining open alveoli.

Pyelolithotomy An incision into and removal of a stone from the kidney pelvis.

Pyelonephritis Inflammation of the renal pelvis and parenchyma, the functional kidney tissue.

Pyloric stenosis A thickening of the pyloric muscle resulting in a narrowing of the pyloric sphincter between the stomach and small intestine.

Pyogenic bacteria Bacteria that produces purulent exudate or pus.

Pyorrhea Advanced periodontal disease.

Pyuria Cloudy or pus-filled urine.

Quadriplegia Complete loss of function of the upper and lower body, including the arms, trunk, legs, and pelvic organs. Also called *tetraplegia*.

Quadruple screen The most widely used test to screen for Down syndrome (trisomy 21), trisomy 18, and neural tube defects.

Qualifiers Words that have been added to some NANDA nursing diagnosis labels to give additional meaning to the diagnostic statement.

Qualitative research Investigates a question through narrative data from interviews, storytelling, and description of observation to provide a better understanding of the client's perspective.

Quality 1. A subjective description of a sound, for example: whistling, gurgling, or snapping. 2. The degree to which health services for individuals and populations increase the likelihood of desired health outcomes and are consistent with current professional knowledge.

Quality and Safety Education for Nurses (QSEN) A program designed to identify and standardize the six core competencies or nursing: patient-centered care, teamwork and collaboration, evidence-based practice, quality improvement, safety, and informatics.

Quality assurance The process of collecting data related to a problem and then analyzing the data based on benchmark standards to determine if standards are being met.

Quality improvement The process of using systematic and continuous actions that lead to measurable improvement in healthcare services and the health status of targeted client groups.

Quality management The evaluation of medical and nursing processes for quality and effectiveness compared to accepted standards in order to correct problems before they harm clients and to prevent errors in treatment.

Quantitative research Uses precise measurements for data collection and employs statistical analysis to provide specific and objective data about a topic.

Quickening The mother's perception of fetal movement.

Race A term used to describe socially defined populations that share genetically transmitted physical characteristics, such as skin color and bone structure.

Racism The oppression of a group of people based on their perceived race.

Radiation The process of heat transfer with no physical contact.

Radiation cataracts A type of cataract that may result from long-term exposure to radiation.

Radical mastectomy The removal of an entire affected breast, its underlying chest muscles, and the lymph nodes under the arms. Compare with **Simple mastectomy**.

Range of motion (ROM) The degree to which a joint can be moved; a measurement of flexion and extension.

Range-of-motion (ROM) exercises Exercises designed to take each joint through all possible movements to maintain flexibility and movement in the joint.

Rape Any penetration, no matter how slight, of the vagina or anus with any body part or object, or oral penetration by a sex organ of another person, without the consent of the victim.

Rape-trauma syndrome (RTS) A series of psychological sequelae that many victims experience following rape in addition to physiological sequelae.

Rapport An understanding between two or more people.

Readiness to learn The demonstration of behaviors or cues that reflect a learner's motivation to learn at a specific time.

Real self The perceived true self.

Reappraisal An individual's ongoing evaluation and reinterpretation of an event or circumstance, as well as continued evaluation of the efficacy of the coping strategies.

Receiver This is the third component of the communication process. The receiver is the listener, who listens, observes, and attends.

Receptive speech The ability to understand the spoken word.

Receptor A nerve cell that converts a stimulus to a nerve impulse. Most receptors are specific, that is, sensitive to only one type of stimulus.

Record A formal, legal document that provides evidence of a client's care. Also called a *client record* or a *clinical chart*.

Recording The process of making an entry on a client record. Also called *charting* or *documenting*.

Recovery 1. Return to (or exceed) preillness levels of functioning. 2. A continued state of voluntary sobriety in which an individual maintains personal health and functions normally.

Recurrence A later recurrence of a disorder after recovery.

Red blood cells (RBCs) Blood cells shaped like biconcave discs that contain the hemoglobin required for oxygen transport to body tissues; the most common type of blood cell. Also called *erythrocytes*.

Reduction Surgical placement of a broken bone in the correct alignment.

Referred pain Pain that is perceived in an area distant from the site of the stimuli.

Reflection The action of making sense of occurrences, situations, or decisions by carefully considering the totality of the experience: what worked or did not work, what could have been done differently to achieve better outcomes, what was done well, what necessary resources were available, and so on.

Reflexes The rapid, involuntary, predictable motor responses to a stimulus.

Reflux A backward flow of acidic secretions into the lower esophagus.

Refraction The bending of light rays as they pass from one medium to another medium of different optical density.

Refractory hypoxemia The decrease of particle arterial oxygen despite administration of oxygen at high flow rates.

Refractory period A phase during which myocardial cells resist stimulation.

Refractory septic shock A persistently low mean arterial blood pressure despite vasopressor therapy and adequate fluid resuscitation.

Regeneration The replacement or renewal of destroyed tissue cells by cells that are identical or similar in structure and function.

Registered nurses (RNs) The members of a nursing team who are specially licensed and trained to deliver direct client care, including client assessment, identification of health problems, and development and coordination of care.

Regurgitation The backflow of blood into the atria during systole.

Reinfection The development of a new infection with a different pathogen following successful treatment.

Reinforcement Consequences that lead to an increase in a particular behavior.

Relapse Return of a disorder soon after recovery.

Relapsing fever Short febrile periods of a few days are interspersed with periods of 1–2 days of normal temperature.

Relationship-based (caring) theories Theories that stress courage, generosity, commitment, and the need to nurture and maintain relationships.

Relaxation response A healthful physiological state that can be elicited through deep relaxation breathing with emphasis on a prolonged exhalation phase.

Religion A set of doctrines accepted by a group of people who gather together regularly to worship that offers a means to relate to God or a higher power; an organized system of beliefs and practices.

REM sleep Rapid-eye-movement sleep that occurs during sleep about every 90 minutes and lasts 5–30 minutes. The brain is highly active in this phase, and most dreams will take place during REM sleep.

Remission 1. A period during a chronic illness in which the symptoms of the illness disappear. 2. A sustained recovery lasting 8 weeks or more.

Remittent fever A wide range of fluctuating temperatures (more than 2°C [3.6°F]), all of which are above normal and occur over a 24-hour period.

Remyelination Repair of the damaged myelin sheath by oligodendrocytes.

Renal colic Acute, severe flank pain on an affected side that develops when a stone obstructs the ureter, causing ureteral spasm.

Renal failure A condition in which the kidneys are unable to remove accumulated metabolites from the blood or produce urine, resulting in altered fluid, electrolyte, and acid–base balance.

Renal insufficiency Decrease in the kidneys' ability to conserve sodium and concentrate the urine.

Renin–angiotensin–aldosterone system System initiated by specialized receptors in the juxtaglomerular cells of the kidney nephrons that respond to changes in renal perfusion.

Repetitive strain injury A nerve, tendon, or muscle condition that occurs when the limbs are subjected to repetitive use, awkward positions, or forced positions. Also called *repetitive motion disorder*.

Repolarization The process that returns the cell to its resting, polarized state.

Report An oral, written, or electronic communication intended to convey information to others.

Research participants Volunteers for a specific study project that meet all the inclusion criteria, have been informed of all aspects of the study, and have signed informed consent.

Reservoir A source of microorganisms.

Residual urine Urine that remains in the bladder after voiding.

Resilience/resiliency The ability to function with healthy responses, even when experiencing significant stress or adversity; the personal patterns, behaviors, or processes that promote an individual's recovery from or adaptation to adversity.

Resolution phase The fourth and final phase of the sexual response cycle is marked by a return to an unaroused state.

Resonance A hollow sound, such as the sound produced by lungs filled with air.

Resource An asset that helps nurses meet client needs.

Resource allocation The distribution of resources among competing groups of people or programs.

Respiration The act of inhaling (inspiration) and exhaling (expiration) air to transport oxygen to the alveoli so that oxygen may be exchanged for carbon dioxide, and the carbon dioxide expelled from the body.

Respiratory acidosis A condition that is caused by an excess of dissolved carbon dioxide, or carbonic acid. It is characterized by a pH of less than 7.35 and a $PaCO_2$ greater than 45 mmHg. It may be caused by hypoventilation.

Respiratory alkalosis A condition that results when pH rises above 7.45 and $PaCO_2$ falls below 35 mmHg. It is caused by hyperventilation (unusually fast respiration, or overbreathing), leading to a carbon dioxide deficit.

Respiratory syncytial virus (RSV) A highly contagious respiratory infection that affects almost all children before 2 years of age.

Response This is the fourth component of the communication process. It is the message that the receiver returns to the sender. Also called *feedback*.

Responsibility The specific accountability or liability associated with the performance of duties of a particular role.

Rest pain Cramping or aching pain in the calves of the legs, the thighs, and the buttocks that occurs while at rest.

Restless leg syndrome A neurological sensorimotor disorder that is characterized by an overwhelming urge to move the legs when at rest.

Restraints Any devices or medications intended to protect the client from injuring self or others through partially or fully limiting the client's mobility.

Restrictive cardiomyopathy A disorder characterized by rigid ventricular walls that impair diastolic filling.

Retinal detachment Separation of the retina or sensory portion of the eye from the choroid.

Retractions Visible sinking of the chest wall, or sunken areas seen between the ribs during inspiration.

Retrograde conduction Cardiac conduction against the normal flow or pattern.

Retropulsion The tendency to topple backward when bumped or when rising, standing, or turning.

Retrospective audit An evaluation performed after a client's discharge comparing the care provided to the client with care provided to clients with similar conditions.

Reverse delegation A situation that occurs when someone with a lower rank delegates to someone with more authority.

Reverse triage A method in which the most severely injured or ill victims who require the greatest resources are treated last to allow the greatest number of victims to receive medical attention.

Revision surgery The replacement of an artificial joint after 10 years or more.

Reward deficiency syndrome The decreased ability to experience pleasure. Reward deficiency syndrome drives the person to seek external forms of gratification through the use of substances, pathological gambling, or other high-risk behaviors.

Rh disease A rare condition where the mother is Rh negative while the child is Rh positive. If this condition arises, the mother's body will see the Rh-positive cells in the fetus as foreign, and will then produce antibodies to fight off the Rh-positive cells. May result in fetal demise in extreme cases.

Rheumatoid arthritis (RA) A chronic systemic autoimmune disease that causes inflammation of connective tissue, primarily in the joints.

Rhinorrhea Drainage of mucus from the nose. Commonly known as a runny nose.

Rhonchi A long, low-pitched sound that continues throughout inspiration suggesting a blockage of large airway passages.

Ribonucleic acid (RNA) One of two types of nucleic acid made by cells. Ribonucleic acid is made up of ribose rather than deoxyribose and contains information that has been copied from DNA (the other type of nucleic acid).

Rigidity Resistance to movement because of the involuntary contraction of all skeletal muscles.

Risk diagnosis A clinical judgment that a problem does not exist, but the presence of risk factors indicates a problem is likely to develop unless the nurse intervenes.

Risk factor A practice, behavior, or environmental factor that increases the potential of negative effects on an individual's health.

Risk management Preventive policies and processes that focus on limiting a healthcare agency's financial and legal risk associated with the delivery of care, particularly in terms of lawsuits.

Role A set of expectations about how an individual occupying one position behaves.

Role ambiguity Occurs when expectations are unclear and when people do not know how to perform their roles and/or are unable to predict the reactions of others to their behavior.

Role conflict Emotional conflict arising when competing demands are made on an individual in the fulfillment of his or her multiple social roles.

Role development Teaching and modeling the behaviors needed to successfully assume a particular role.

Role mastery Occurs when an individual's behaviors meet or exceed social expectations.

Role performance The demonstration of behaviors or actions associated with a given role.

Role strain The stress or strain experienced by an individual when incompatible behavior, expectations, or obligations are associated with a single social role.

Root cause analysis An evaluation required by the Joint Commission that is focused on identifying areas of improvement that would decrease the likelihood of future adverse events and to develop an action plan for improvement.

Rooting reflex In response to a light touch of a finger on an infant's cheek close to the mouth, the infant's head will rotate toward the stimulation and attempt to suck the finger.

Rotational injury An injury caused by lateral flexion or twisting of the head and neck.

Round ligaments The ligaments that hold the ovaries in place.

Rupture of membranes The rupturing of amniotic membranes before the onset of labor.

Sacral promontory A projection into the pelvic cavity on the anterior upper portion of the sacrum, which serves as a landmark for pelvic measurements.

Sarcopenia The process of atrophy due to age.

Safety strap body restraint Restraints used to ensure the safety of clients who are transported by wheelchair or gurney, or to protect clients confined to a bed or a chair. Also called *belt restraint.*

Salient cue The leading, most noticeable, or most important information about a client's health status.

Saline An isotonic solution of 0.9% sodium chloride.

Sanguineous exudate A large amount of red blood cells that form a bright or dark red discharge indicating new or old damage to capillaries. Also called *hemorrhagic exudate.*

Satiety The sensation of fullness and satisfaction that should inhibit eating until the next meal.

Saturated fat A triglyceride fat that contains all of the hydrogen ions it is capable of holding.

Scaling The rating of the severity of symptoms or problems.

Scapegoat An individual who has been selected to take the blame for another individual or for a group.

Scheduled toileting Toileting at regular intervals.

Schemes Adaptive cognitive structures formed in response to environmental stimuli according to Jean Piaget's theory of cognitive development.

Schistocytes Fragmented red blood cells.

Schizoaffective disorder A psychotic disorder with features of both schizophrenia and mood disorders.

Schizoid personality disorder (SPD) One of several personality disorders defined in the DSM-5, it is characterized by a lifelong pattern of indifference to others, absence of humor, and social isolation.

Schizophrenia The most common psychotic disorder, schizophrenia is a combination of disordered thinking, perceptual disturbances, behavioral abnormalities, affective disruptions, and impaired social competency.

Schizophreniform disorder A disorder with rapid onset of psychotic symptoms, very similar to schizophrenia, lasting less than 6 months.

Schizotypal personality disorder One of several personality disorders defined in the DSM-5, it is characterized by a pattern of disturbed interpersonal relationships, thought patterns, appearance, and behavior.

Sciatica Lumbar back pain that radiates down the posterior leg to the ankle due to irritation or compression of all or part of the sciatic nerve.

Scleral buckling A surgical procedure to correct retinal detachment.

Scoliometer A diagnostic test used to measure a client's rib hump when in the Adam position.

Scoliosis A lateral, or sideways, curvature of the spine.

Seasonal affective disorder (SAD) A mood disorder typically characterized by depression during fall and winter and normal mood or hypomania during spring and summer.

Second heart sound (S$_2$) The heart sound produced by closure of the semilunar valves; characterized by the syllable "dub."

Secondary appraisal Evaluation of an individual's available coping resources and potential options for responding to an event or circumstance.

Secondary cataracts A type of cataract that may form after surgery to treat another eye disorder, such as glaucoma, or as an effect of medication or another primary disorder.

Secondary group A group that is larger, more impersonal, and less sentimental than a primary group.

Secondary hypertension Elevated blood pressure resulting from an identifiable underlying process.

Secondary immune response Subsequent encounters with an antigen following the primary immune response that result in triggering memory cells.

Secondary infertility The inability to conceive after one or more successful pregnancies, or the inability to sustain a pregnancy.

Secondary intention healing Healing that occurs when a wound's edges cannot or should not close. Repair time is typically longer, scarring is greater, and susceptibility to infection is greater.

Secondary prevention Methods that focus on the diagnosis and treatment of disease.

Segmental mastectomy See *Lumpectomy*.

Seizures Periods of abnormal electrical discharges in the brain that cause involuntary movement, as well as behavior and sensory alterations.

Selective perception The process of filtering out unnecessary and distracting information in order to focus on what is important at any given moment.

Selective serotonin reuptake inhibitor (SSRI) A drug that selectively inhibits the reuptake of serotonin into nerve terminals; used mostly for depression.

Selectively permeable Refers to membranes separating body fluid compartments across which solutes can move with relative ease.

Self-awareness The relationship between an individual's perception of himself or herself and others' perceptions of him or her.

Self-concept The personal perception of the self formed in response to interactions with others and the environment throughout the course of an individual's lifetime.

Self-efficacy The expectation that someone can produce a desired outcome.

Self-esteem One's judgment of one's own worth.

Self-help group A group of individuals who come together to face a common problem or difficulty.

Self-quieting ability The ability of newborns to use their own resources to quiet and comfort themselves.

Semen Sperm mixed with seminal fluid, ejaculated during sexual activity.

Semiformal group A group with formalized structure, delineated hierarchy, and voluntary, but selective, membership.

Sender An individual or group who wishes to convey a message to another; can be considered the *source-encoder*.

Sensitization An increased reaction to pain over time, or a reduced threshold for reaction to painful stimuli.

Sensory memory The momentary perception of stimuli from the environment.

Sensory overload An overabundance of sensory stimulation that cannot be correctly processed.

Sensory perception The conscious organization and translation of external data or stimuli into meaningful information.

Sensory reception The process of receiving external stimuli or data. External stimuli are visual (sight), auditory (hearing), olfactory (smell), tactile (touch), and gustatory (taste).

Sentinel event An unexpected occurrence involving death or serious physical or psychological injury, or the risk thereof.

Sepsis 1. A whole-body inflammatory process resulting in acute illness. 2. A state of infection.

Septal defect A congenital heart defect that connects the right and left side of the heart.

Septic shock Altered perfusion resulting from a systemic infection that manifests with hypotension, delayed capillary refill, and inadequate perfusion and oxygenation of vital body tissues. Also called *septicemia*.

Septicemia See Septic shock.

Seroconversion Antibody response to a disease or vaccine.

Serosanguineous exudate A clear or blood-tinged discharge commonly seen in surgical incisions.

Serotonin syndrome A condition that may occur in individuals taking two or more medications that increase serotonin levels. Symptoms include hypertension or hypotension, agitation, shivering, changes in mental status, symptoms of gastrointestinal distress, restlessness, tremor, muscle rigidity, unreactive pupils, and tachypnea.

Serous exudate A watery, clear or straw-colored discharge that accompanies mild inflammation.

Serum bicarbonate (HCO$_3$) A value that reflects the renal regulation of acid–base balance. The normal HCO$_3$ value is 24–28 mEq/L.

Serum sickness A systemic type III hypersensitivity response, usually in response to a drug such as penicillin or a sulfonamide.

Severe sepsis Sepsis associated with acute organ failure.

Sex chromosomes The 23rd pair of chromosomes found in a cell's nucleus; it determines an individual's gender.

Sexism When male values, beliefs, or activities are preferred over female ones.

Sexual abuse Any sexual act that is perpetrated against someone's will including rape, attempted sexual acts, unwanted sexual contact, voyeurism, and sexual harassment. Also called *sexual violence*.

Sexual aversion disorder A disorder characterized by severe distaste for sexual activity or the thought of sexual activity.

Sexual health A state of physical, emotional, mental, and social well-being in relation to sexuality, not merely the absence of disease, dysfunction, or infirmity. Sexual health requires a positive and respectful approach to sexuality and sexual relationships.

Sexual orientation The sexual attraction of an individual to the same sex, the opposite sex, or both sexes.

Sexual self-concept How one values oneself as a sexual being.

Sexually transmitted infections (STIs) Infections transmitted by vaginal, oral, and anal intimate contact and intercourse.

Shared governance A method that aims to distribute decision making among a group of people.

Shared leadership The concept that a professional workplace is made up of many leaders.

Shared psychotic disorder A condition that results when an individual who is in a close relationship with another person who is delusional comes to share the delusional beliefs.

Shearing force A condition that results when one tissue layer slides over another.

Shock A clinical syndrome characterized by a systemic imbalance between oxygen supply and demand.

Shock phase The initial part of an alarm reaction during which the sympathetic nervous system is suppressed and an individual may experience manifestations such as hypotension, decreased body temperature, and decreased muscle tone.

Short bowel syndrome A condition in which the transit time of ingested foods and fluids is reduced and digestive processes are impaired because of a resection of significant portions of the small intestine.

Short-term memory Information held in the brain for immediate use; what an individual has in mind at a given moment.

Shunt A natural or artificially created tunnel or passage that allows blood to flow through an area.

Sickle cell anemia An inherited chronic hemolytic anemia, sickle cell anemia is the most common form of sickle cell disease.

Sickle cell crisis Severe episodes of fever and intense pain that are the hallmark of sickle cell disease. Also called *vaso-occlusive crisis*.

Sickle cell disease A hereditary hemoglobinopathy characterized by replacement of normal hemoglobin with abnormal hemoglobin S (Hgb S) in RBCs.

Sickle cell trait Carrying one copy of the defective sickle cell gene, which can be passed on to children but does not usually cause the illness.

Sickling A process in which red blood cells take on the characteristic sickle shape following deoxygenation in clients who have sickle cell disease.

Signs See Objective data.

Simple assault An unlawful physical attack by one person upon another in which neither the offender displays a weapon, nor the victim suffers any obvious severe or aggravated bodily injury involving apparent broken bones, loss of teeth, possible internal injury, severe laceration, or loss of consciousness.

Simple mastectomy The removal of a complete breast only. Compare with Radical mastectomy.

Single-parent family A family in which only one parent resides in the home and is the primary caretaker and provider for the family.

Situational crisis A crisis that involves an unexpected stressor or circumstance that occurs in the course of daily living.

Situational depression A maladaptive reaction to an identifiable psychosocial stressor or stressors that occurs within 3 months after the onset of the stressor and has persisted for no longer than 6 months. Also called *adjustment disorder with depressed mood*.

Situational leader A leader who is flexible in task and relationship behaviors, considers the staff members' abilities, knows the nature of the task to be done, and is sensitive to the context or environment in which the task takes place.

Six Sigma A quality improvement program originally implemented by Motorola and General Electric that focuses on reducing variation within a process to produce a near-perfect product.

Skin turgor The elasticity of skin.

Sleep An altered state of consciousness in which an individual's perception and reaction to the environment are decreased.

Sleep apnea A disorder characterized by frequent short breathing pauses during sleep.

Sleep architecture The basic organization of normal sleep.

Sleep hygiene Interventions used to promote quality sleep at night.

Sleep loss A duration of sleep shorter than the recommended 7–8 hours a night for an adult.

Small cell carcinoma A highly malignant cancer usually associated with the lung.

SMART An acronym to provide assistance in writing a client-centered goal statement. SMART is Single action (choose a specific, singe action to focus on), Measurable result (observable or measurable result), Attainable (level appropriate), Relevant (customized specifically for client's needs), and Time-limited (specific time frame for goal to be completed).

SOAP An acronym for collective data in a progress note; it stands for subjective data, objective data, assessment, and planning.

Sobriety A state of habitual refrain from using alcohol or drugs.

Social distance Communication characterized by a clear visual perception of the whole person. Body heat and odor are imperceptible, eye contact is increased, and vocalizations are loud enough to be overheard by others.

Social justice A framework in which to explore the complexities surrounding the variety of factors that impact diverse and vulnerable populations.

Social microcosm The concept that group members eventually behave in a therapy group the same way they behave with family and friends.

Social phobia A condition that is characterized by a pervasive, extreme fear of one or more social situations that may lead to scrutiny by others. Also called *social anxiety disorder*.

Socialization The process by which individuals learn to become members of groups and society and learn the social rules defining relationships into which they will enter.

Socialized insurance A system in which all medically necessary services are covered, including physician care, hospital services, and to some extent, prescription drugs.

Socialized medicine State government-owned and -controlled healthcare services.

Software The operating systems and application components of technology.

Solitary play A stage of play in which an infant still plays primarily alone, but enjoys the presence of others.

Solute Substance that dissolves in liquid.

Solvent The component of a solution that can dissolve a solute.

Somatic cells Cells that make up the tissue of the body, with a full complement (diploid) of chromosomes, as opposed to sex cells.

Somatic pain Pain arising from nerve receptors originating in the skin or close to the surface of the body.

Somatization The process by which psychological distress is experienced and communicated in the form of somatic symptoms.

Somatostatin A substance, believed to be a neurotransmitter, that inhibits the production of both glucagon and insulin.

Somnology The study of sleep.

Somogyi phenomenon A combination of hypoglycemia during the night with a rebound, morning rise in blood glucose to hyperglycemic levels.

Source-oriented record Client record in which each healthcare provider or department member makes notations in a separate section or sections of the client's chart.

Spasticity Increased muscle tone, usually with some degree of weakness.

Specific defenses Immune system responses directed against identifiable bacteria, viruses, fungi, or other infectious agents.

Specific gravity An indicator of urine concentration that can be performed quickly and easily by nursing personnel.

Specific phobia An intense or extreme fear with regard to a particular object or situation.

Specific self-esteem How much one approves of a certain parts of oneself.

Spermatogenesis The process by which mature spermatozoa are formed.

Spermicide A cream, jelly, foam, vaginal film, or suppository that is inserted into the vagina before intercourse to destroy sperm and prevent conception.

Spinal cord A continuation of the medulla oblongata, it has the ability to transmit impulses to and from the brain via the ascending and descending pathways.

Spinal cord injury (SCI) Trauma to the spinal cord that results from excessive force to the spinal column.

Spinal cord stimulation (SCS) A form of therapy used with persistent pain that has not been controlled with less invasive therapies. SCS involves the insertion of an electrode (a single channel or multichannel device) adjacent to the spinal cord in the epidural space. The electrode(s) is attached to an impulse-generator (external or implanted) that sends electric impulses to the spinal cord to control pain.

Spinal fusion The insertion of a wedge-shaped piece of bone or bone chips between the vertebrae to stabilize them and reduce pain.

Spinal shock A condition that is characterized by spinal cord swelling, decreased blood flow and blood pressure, and complete loss of motor function, spinal reflexes, and autonomic function below the level of injury.

Spiritual distress A challenge to the spiritual well-being or to the belief system that provides strength, hope, and meaning to life; a feeling of being separated from interconnectedness with others or with a higher power.

Spiritual health The overall feeling of strength, hope, and fulfillment that encourages people to find life-sustaining and enriching opportunities.

Spiritual skills Skills that help an individual find meaning in and understand the personal significance of an unexpected event.

Spiritual support Assistance to clients and families in providing meaning and sustaining courage during difficult times.

Spiritual well-being A feeling of inner peace and of being generally alive, purposeful, and fulfilled; the feeling is rooted in spiritual values and/or specific religious beliefs.

Spirituality The part of being human that seeks meaningfulness through personal connection, which may include belief in or relationship with some higher power, creative force, driving being, or infinite source of energy.

Splint An easily adjustable device that stabilizes injuries, usually before swelling has subsided or after the reparative phase of healing.

Splitting 1. The inability to integrate contradictory experiences. 2. The inclination to perceive people or situations as one extreme or the other.

Spontaneous abortion The loss of a fetus prior to 20 weeks of gestation. Also called *miscarriage*.

Spontaneous rupture of membranes (SROM) The rupturing of membranes during the height of an intense contraction with a gush of fluid out of the vagina.

Sporadic AD One of the two basic types of Alzheimer disease, it shows no clear pattern of inheritance, although genetic factors may contribute to the disorder. Sporadic AD typically does not develop until after the age of 65. Also called *late-onset Alzheimer disease*.

Sprain A stretching or tearing of ligaments.

Sputum Mucus or mucopurulent matter expectorated from the lungs.

Squamous cell carcinoma A malignant tumor of the squamous epithelium of the skin or mucous membranes.

Staff authority The power to provide advice and support to employees or departments but not to assign tasks.

Staff development Continued staff education, planned activities to enhance role performance, and defined goals to improve client outcomes. Also called *professional development*.

Stage of exhaustion Stage in which the body ceases to maintain its adaptation to a stressor; the stressor overwhelms the individual's ability to cope or mount a continued defense, resulting in the depletion of energy and resources.

Stage of resistance Stage in which the body attempts to move toward restoration of homeostasis while continuing to respond to the stressor.

Staghorn stones A type of calculi associated with a urinary tract infection caused by urease-producing bacteria such as *Proteus*. These stones can grow to become very large, filling the renal pelvis and calyces. Also called *struvite stones*.

Staging A system of classifying cancer according to the size of the tumor, involvement of lymph nodes, and metastasis to distant sites.

Standard precautions Safety guidelines, such as proper hand hygiene, use of proper protective equipment, safe injection practices, and effective management of potentially contaminated surfaces or equipment, that are designed to decrease the risk of transmitting unidentified pathogens. Also called *universal precautions* and *body substance isolation (BSI)*.

Standardized plan A nursing care plan that specifies the nursing care for groups of clients with common needs (e.g., all clients with myocardial infarction).

Standards Models of high-quality performance that may reflect the performance of industry leaders, scientific or clinical research, or recommendations of professional organizations such as the ANA.

Standards of care Guidelines used to determine what a nurse should or should not do, and may be defined as a benchmark of achievement based on a desired level of excellence.

Standards of practice A standardized description of the responsibilities for which nurses are responsible.

Standards of professional performance The behaviors expected in the professional nursing role by the American Nurses Association.

Station The location of the fetal presenting part in the maternal pelvis in relation to the ischial spine.

Status asthmaticus A severe, prolonged form of asthma that is difficult to treat.

Status epilepticus A continuous seizure that lasts for more than 30 minutes or a series of seizures during which time consciousness is not regained.

Statutory laws Laws made by any legislative branch of the government, including the U.S. Congress, state legislatures, and city and county governments.

Steatorrhea Fatty, frothy, foul-smelling stools caused by a decrease in pancreatic enzyme secretion.

Stem cell transplant The infusion of immature stem cells to replenish a client's blood cell lines; used as an alternative to bone marrow transplantation.

Stenosis Narrowing of the valve, valve area, or great artery above the valve.

Step-down therapy A gradual reduction in the dosage and number of drugs used in a therapeutic regimen.

Stepfamily Consists of a biological parent with children and a new spouse who may or may not have children.

Stereognosis The ability to perceive and understand an object through touch.

Stereotaxic thalamotomy An x-ray taken during neurosurgery to guide the insertion of a needle into a specific area of the brain.

Stereotyping The act of generalizing that all people in a group are the same.

Stereotypy Rigid and obsessive behavior.

Sterile field An area free of microorganisms.

Sterile technique Practices that keep an area or object free of all microorganisms. Also known as *surgical asepsis*.

Sterilization 1. A process that destroys all microorganisms, including spores and viruses. 2. An inclusive term that refers to surgical procedures that permanently prevent pregnancy.

Stigma A collection of negative attitudes and beliefs that lead people to fear, reject, avoid, and discriminate against people with mental illness.

Stillbirth Death of a fetus that occurs after 20 weeks of gestation. Also called *fetal demise* or *intrauterine fetal death (IUFD)*.

Stimulus The agent or act that stimulates a nerve receptor.

Stimulus-based stress model A model that defines stress as being a life event that requires change or adaptation on the part of the individual who is experiencing the life event.

Stoma An artificial opening in the abdominal wall; it may be permanent or temporary.

Stool Body wastes and undigested food eliminated from the bowel. Also called *feces*.

Strain A stretching or tearing of a muscle or tendon.

Strategic planning The process of continual assessment, planning, and evaluation to guide future decisions and developments.

Stress The body's general, nonspecific response to the demands placed upon it by a stressor.

Stress fracture A fracture that results from disease that has weakened the bone.

Stress mediators Hormonal triggers that are intended to promote adaptation through mechanisms such as triggering a necessary increase in heart rate and blood pressure when faced with physical danger.

Stress response Physiological changes triggered by stress; includes activation of the neural, neuroendocrine, and endocrine systems, as well as activation of target organs.

Stressor An external influence that threatens to disrupt the equilibrium that is needed to maintain homeostasis.

Striae Whitish-silver stretch marks seen in obesity and during or after pregnancy.

Stridor A high-pitched sound within the trachea and larynx that suggests narrowing of the tracheal passage.

Stroke A condition in which neurological deficits result from a sudden decrease in blood flow to a localized area of the brain. Also called *cerebrovascular accident* or *brain attack*.

Stroke volume (SV) The amount of blood pumped into the aorta with each contraction of the left ventricle that is measured by the difference between the end-diastolic volume and the end-systolic volume.

Structural-functional theory Focuses on family structure and function, examining family relationships and how they affect the functions of the family and relationships with other systems.

Structure standards Standards related to material resources, human resources, and general organizational structure.

Struvite stones A type of calculi associated with a urinary tract infection caused by urease-producing bacteria such as *Proteus*. These stones can grow to become very large, filling the renal pelvis and calyces. Also called *staghorn stones*.

Subconjunctival hemorrhage Temporary, nonpathogenic hemorrhages that are caused by the changes in vascular tension or ocular pressure during birth.

Subculture groups Minority groups characterized by specific norms, beliefs, and values that coexist with a dominant culture.

Subcutaneous tissue The layer of loose connective tissue and fat cells that lies below the dermis. Also called *hypodermis*.

Subdermal implant Capsules implanted within the skin that slowly release medication, such as for contraception.

Subfertility Occurs when both partners of a couple have reduced fertility.

Subinvolution A slowing of the descent of the uterus during the postpregnancy healing process.

Subjective data Information that is apparent to only the client affected and can be described or verified by only that client. Also called *symptoms* or *covert data*.

Subjective family burden The psychological distress of family members in relation to the objective family burden of having a family member with a mental illness.

Substance abuse The use of any chemical in a fashion inconsistent with medical or culturally defined social norms despite physical, psychological, or social adverse effects.

Substance dependence A condition in which the client can no longer control use of the substance, continues to use it despite adverse effects, and experiences withdrawal symptoms without continued use of the substance.

Subsystem A component of a larger system.

Sucking reflex Occurs in response to a finger or nipple inserted into an infant's mouth; the infant responds by beginning to rhythmically suck on the finger.

Suctioning Aspirating secretions through a catheter connected to a suction machine or wall suction outlet.

Sudden cardiac death (SCD) Unexpected death occurring within 1 hour of the onset of cardiovascular symptoms.

Sudden infant death syndrome (SIDS) The sudden death of an apparently healthy infant that remains unexplained after other possible causes have been ruled out through autopsy, death scene investigation, and review of the medical history.

Suicidal ideation A case of an individual constantly considering, planning, or thinking about suicide.

Suicide An act of an individual inflicting self-harm resulting in death.

Suicide attempt An act of an individual inflicting self-harm with the intent to cause death that is not successful.

Sundowning A behavioral change commonly seen in clients with dementia, characterized by increased agitation, time disorientation, and wandering behaviors during afternoon and evening hours; it is accelerated on overcast days.

Superego The third aspect of the personality that contains the conscience and the ego ideal. The superego is the source of feelings such as guilt, shame, and inhibition.

Superficial basal cell carcinoma A type of skin cancer.

Superficial burn A burn that involves only the epidermal layer of the skin.

Supersaturated urine A condition that results when the concentration of an insoluble salt in the urine is very high.

Supine On the back.

Suppuration A large quantity of cells and necrotic debris that form an opaque or milky discharge that is thicker than serous exudate. Also called *pus* or *purulent exudate*.

Suprasystem An overarching system to which smaller systems or subsystems belong. For example, the family is the suprasystem of the individual.

Surface temperature Body temperature taken at the skin's surface that may rise or fall in response to the environment.

Surfactant Specialized cells that control surface tension and keep alveoli from collapsing and sticking to themselves.

Surge capacity A community's ability to rapidly meet the increased demand for qualified personnel and resources, including healthcare resources, in the event of a disaster.

Surgical asepsis Practices that keep an area or object free of all microorganisms. Also called *sterile technique*.

Surgical debridement The process of excising a wound to the level of fascia or sequentially removing thin slices of a burn wound to the level of viable tissue.

Sutures The membranous spaces between the cranial bones of a fetus.

Swan-neck deformity Caused by rheumatoid arthritis, it is characterized by hyperextension of the proximal interphalangeal joints with compensatory flexion of the distal interphalangeal joints.

Switching A term used in disorders of mood and affect to describe a new illness phase (manic or depressed) without recovery.

Symmetry Equality of the size, shape, or condition of opposite sides of the body.

Sympathetic tone A state of partial smooth muscle contraction around arteries and veins.

Symphysis pubic Fibrocartilaginous joint between the pelvic bones in the midline.

Symptom See Subjective data.

Synchronized cardioversion Delivery of direct electrical current synchronized with the client's heart rhythm.

Synclitism A condition that occurs when the sagittal suture is midway between the symphysis pubis and the sacral promontory and is felt to be aligned.

Syncope Transient loss of consciousness and muscle tone after exercise or activity.

Syndrome diagnosis A cluster of nursing diagnoses that occur together and may result in best client outcomes if addressed at the same time.

Synovectomy Excision of synovial membrane, this procedure is used as a treatment for rheumatoid arthritis.

Synovitis Inflammation of the synovial membrane lining the articular capsule of a joint.

Syphilis A complex systemic sexually transmitted infection caused by the spirochete *Treponema pallidum*.

System A set of interacting identifiable parts or components.

Systematized delusions A manifestation of schizophrenia characterized by an extensively developed central delusional theme from which conclusions are deduced.

Systemic arthritis A form of juvenile rheumatoid arthritis that characteristically is manifested by high fever, polyarthritis, and rheumatoid rash. Systemic arthritis also affects internal organs and joints.

Systemic circulation Circulation through the left side of the heart, the aorta and its branches, the capillaries that supply the brain and peripheral tissues, the systemic venous system, and the vena cava.

Systemic infection Occurs when an invading microorganism spreads and damages different parts of the body.

Systemic inflammatory response syndrome (SIRS) Describes the body's response to a critical illness that can result from an infectious or noninfectious cause precipitating a whole-body inflammatory process.

Systemic lupus erythematosus (SLE) A chronic, inflammatory connective tissue disease.

Systemic response Results because of a widespread anti-body-antigen reaction. Systemic responses include anaphylaxis, urticaria, or angioedema.

Systemic vascular resistance The force or resistance of the blood in the body's blood vessels that helps return blood to the heart.

Systems theory The study of how a system operates, including how it interacts with other systems and how its components interact with each other within the system itself.

Systole The phase of ventricular contraction.

Systolic blood pressure The maximum pressure exerted within the arteries when the heart compresses.

T lymphocyte (T cells) A type of leukocyte that matures in the thymus gland and is integral to the specific immune response.

Tachycardia An excessively fast heart rate greater than 100 bpm in an adult.

Tachypnea A respiratory rate greater than 20 bpm in adults.

Tactile Of or relating to touch.

Tangential excision The sequential removal of thin slices of a burn wound to the level of viable tissue.

Tardive dyskinesia A condition characterized by repetitive, involuntary body movement of varying severity that may not cease after medication cessation; includes unusual tongue and face movements such as lip smacking and wormlike motions of the tongue.

Tartar A visible, hard deposit of plaque and dead bacteria that forms at the gumlines. Also called *dental calculus*.

Tau A protein found in the neurons.

Teaching A system of activities intended to produce learning.

Team Two or more individuals who agree to work in tandem to accomplish a common goal.

Team nursing The delivery of individualized nursing care to a group of clients by a team led by a professional nurse.

Telangiectatic nevi Pale pink or red spots frequently found on the eyelids, nose, lower occipital bone, and nape of the neck of young children. These areas have no clinical significance and usually fade by the second birthday. Also called *stork bites*.

Telecommunication The transmission of information from one site to another, using equipment to send information in the form of signs, signals, words, or pictures by cable, radio, or other systems.

Telehealth A system that employs the use of telecommunications technologies (e.g., videoconferencing, streaming media, real-time forwarding imaging, and land-based and wireless communications) to allow clients access to care that they might not otherwise be able to obtain. Also called *telemedicine* or *remote client monitoring*.

Temperament The combination of biological and physical characteristics that influence personality and behavior specific to each individual.

Tender points Tenderness that occurs in precise, localized areas, particularly in the neck, spine, shoulders, and hips.

Tendon Tissue that connects bones to muscles and carries the contractile forces from the muscle to the bone to cause movement.

Tendonitis Inflammation of a tendon.

Teratogen Any chemical that has the potential to harm the fetus, including pesticides, viruses, and medications.

Terminal weaning The gradual withdrawal of mechanical ventilation when survival without assisted ventilation is not expected.

Territoriality A concept of the space and things that an individual considers as belonging to the self.

Tertiary intention healing Healing that occurs after closing a wound that has been left open for 3–5 days to allow edema or infection to resolve. Also called *delayed primary intention*.

Tertiary prevention Methods that focus on the restoration of health following an illness or accident and include rehabilitation and palliative services.

Testosterone The primary male sex hormone produces by the testes.

Tetany Tonic muscle spasms.

Tetralogy of Fallot A rare disease that consists of four defects: pulmonic stenosis, right ventricular hypertrophy, ventricular-septal defect, and an overriding aorta.

Tetraplegia Complete loss of function of the upper and lower body, including the arms, trunk, legs, and pelvic organs. Also called *quadriplegia*.

Thalassemia Inherited disorder of hemoglobin synthesis in which either the alpha or beta chains of the hemoglobin molecule are missing or defective.

Therapeutic communication An interactive process between the nurse and the client that helps the client to overcome temporary stress, to get along with other people, to adjust to situations that cannot be altered, and to overcome any psychological blocks that may stand in the way of self-realizations.

Therapeutic insemination The process of depositing semen at the cervical os or in the uterus by mechanical means.

Therapeutic relationship Nurse–client relationship that is focused on helping clients manage problems and become better at helping themselves.

Thermoregulation The body process that balances heat production and heat loss to maintain the body's temperature.

Third heart sound (S_3) Heart sound that is sometimes heard after the second heart sound in children, young adults, and pregnant females during the third trimester. Also called a *ventricular gallop*.

Third spacing A shift of fluid from the vascular space into an area where it is not available to support normal physiological processes.

Thoracentesis Needle insertion into the pleural space to remove fluid accumulation.

Thoracolumbar sacral orthosis (TLSO) A brace contoured to conform to the body and support the spine. Also called an *underarm brace* or *Boston brace*.

Thought blocking Speech stopped in midsentence as if the thought disappeared from the individual's head.

Thought disorders Disorders associated with schizophrenia that involve an abnormal way of thinking, such as disorganized thinking, sensory overload, thought blocking, neologisms, loose association, clang, and perseveration.

Threshold potential The point at which an action potential is capable of being generated.

Thrill A palpable vibration over the precordium or an artery.

Thromboemboli Emboli created by a blood clot.

Thrombophlebitis See Venous thrombosis.

Throughput The process by which information, energy, or material that enters a system (input) is used by the system.

Thrush White patches that look like milk curds that adhere to the mucous membranes usually caused by an infected vaginal tract during birth, antibiotic use, or poor hand hygiene. Bleeding may occur if patches are removed.

Thyroid crisis See *Thyroid storm*.

Thyroid storm An extreme state of hyperthyroidism. Now extremely rare due to improved diagnosis and treatment methods. Also called *thyroid crisis*.

Thyroidectomy Surgical removal of all or part of the thyroid gland.

Thyroiditis Inflammation of the thyroid gland.

Thyrotoxicosis A disorder caused by excessive delivery of thyroid hormone to the peripheral tissues. Also called *hyperthyroidism*.

Time constraints Deadlines for completion.

Time-out A preprocedure verification to ensure the correct procedure is being performed at the right site on the right client.

Time priority A time constraint to complete an action.

Tine test Test in which a multiple-puncture device is used to introduce tuberculin into the skin.

Tinea pedis Fungal infection of the feet. Also called *athlete's foot*.

Tinnitus The perception of sound or noise in the ears without stimulus from the environment.

Token economies Formalized programs of contingency contracts.

Tolerance State in which a particular dose elicits a smaller response than it formerly did. With increased tolerance, the individual needs higher and higher doses to obtain the desired response.

Tone 1. The amount of tension or resistance to movement in a muscle. 2. The ability of vessels to constrict or dilate to maintain normal pressure.

Tonic-clonic seizures Alternating contraction (tonic phase) and relaxation (clonic phase) of muscles during seizure activity.

Tonic neck reflex In response to an infant's head being turned to one side while the infant lies on the back, the infant will extend the arm and leg on the side the infant faces while the opposite arm and leg will be flexed.

Tonic phase Initial phase of a generalized seizure, manifested by unconsciousness and continuous muscular contraction.

Tonicity The osmolality of a solution. Solutions may be termed *isotonic*, *hypertonic*, or *hypotonic*.

Torsades de pointes A type of ventricular tachycardia associated with a prolongation of the QT interval.

Tort A civil wrong committed against an individual or an individual's property.

Total anomalous pulmonary venous return The pulmonary veins empty into the right atrium or into veins leading to the right atrium, rather than into the left atrium.

Total lymphoid irradiation A procedure sometimes used in the treatment of rheumatoid arthritis; it decreases total lymphocyte levels.

Total quality management (TQM) A comprehensive management philosophy that improves quality and productivity by utilizing data and statistics to improve system processes.

Toxic multinodular goiter A tumor characterized by small, discrete, independently functioning nodules in the thyroid gland tissue that secrete excessive amounts of thyroid hormone.

Toxoplasmosis Space-occupying lesions common in clients with AIDS that may cause headache, altered mental status, and neurological deficits.

Trachoma A chronic conjunctivitis caused by *Chlamydia trachomatis*. It is a significant preventable cause of blindness worldwide.

Traction The application of a straightening or pulling force to return or maintain fractured bones in their normal anatomical position.

Traditional family An autonomous unit in which both parents reside in the home with their children, the mother assuming the nurturing role and the father providing the necessary economic resources.

Transactional leader A leader who has a relationship with followers based on an exchange of some resource valued by the follower.

Transcellular fluid One of the compartments where extracellular fluid is found. Examples of transcellular fluid are cerebrospinal, pericardial, pancreatic, pleural, intraocular, biliary, peritoneal, and synovial fluids.

Transcendence A person's recognition that there is something other or greater than the self and a seeking and valuing of that greater other, whether it is an ultimate being, force, or value.

Transcranial magnetic stimulation (TMS) A promising alternative therapy for individuals with schizophrenia that uses electromagnetic stimulus to affect brain activity in the cerebral cortex.

Transductive reasoning Connecting two events in a cause-and-effect relationship simply because they occur together in time.

Transection An injury that occurs when an individual is injured by a gunshot, stabbing, or similar force, which may partially or completely sever the spinal cord.

Transference The transfer of feelings that were originally evoked by one's parents or significant others to people in the present setting.

Transformational leader A leader who fosters creativity, risk taking, commitment, and collaboration by empowering a group to share in an organization's vision. The leader inspires others with a clear, attractive, and attainable goal and enlists them to participate in attaining the goal.

Transfusion reaction A type II or cytotoxic hypersensitivity reaction to blood of an incompatible type.

Transgender Gradations of human characteristics running from female to male; more commonly, an individual who expresses a gender identity different from that with which he or she was born.

Transient ischemic attack (TIA) A brief period of localized cerebral ischemia that causes neurological deficits lasting for less than 24 hours. Also called a *mini-stroke*.

Transitional milk A light yellow milk that is more copious than colostrum and contains more fat, lactose, water-soluble vitamins, and calories; it usually presents between the second and fifth day following birth.

Transjugular intrahepatic portosystemic shunt (TIPS) An expandable metal stent inserted through a transcutaneous needle to channel blood from the portal vein into the hepatic vein, bypassing the cirrhotic liver.

Transplacental immunity Passive immunity transferred from mother to infant.

Transposition of the great arteries (TGA) A congenital heart defect in which the pulmonary artery, the outflow tract for the left ventricle, and the aorta, the outflow tract for the right ventricle, are transposed.

Transsexual A transgender individual who has had or is in the process of having sexual reassignment procedures.

Transurethral incision of the prostate (TUIP) Small incisions are made in the smooth muscle where the prostate is attached to the bladder in order to reduce pressure on the urethra.

Transurethral needle ablation (TUNA) A procedure that uses low-level radio-frequency through twin needles to burn away a region of the enlarged prostate in order to improve the flow of urine.

Transurethral resection of the prostate (TURP) A procedure that removes obstructing prostate tissue using the wire loop of a resectoscope and electrocautery inserted through the urethra.

Transverse diameter The largest diameter of the pelvic inlet; helps determine the shape of the inlet.

Trauma An injury to human tissues and organs resulting from the transfer of energy from an external environmental source, such as a motor vehicle, a fire, or a sharp object.

Traumatic cataracts A type of cataract that may result from an injury to the eye.

Tremors Rhythmic, involuntary movements or twitching of the extremities.

Triage The process of identifying priorities for implementing care.

Tricuspid atresia The absence of the tricuspid valve.

Tricyclic antidepressant (TCA) A class of drugs that inhibit the reuptake of both norepinephrine and serotonin into presynaptic nerve terminals. TCAs are primarily used in the pharmacotherapy of depression.

Triglycerides Substances converted from dietary fats and carbohydrates to store energy in fat cells.

Triplet Three premature ventricular contractions in a row.

Tripod position A position of sitting and leaning forward; often used by clients who are having difficulty breathing.

Trisomy An extra chromosome.

Trisomy 21 A condition that occurs when an individual born with Down syndrome has an additional full chromosome present.

Troponins Proteins released during a myocardial infarction that are sensitive indicators of myocardial damage.

Trousseau sign Spasmodic contraction of the hand and fingers in response to occlusion of the blood supply by a blood pressure cuff; caused by decreased blood calcium levels. A test used to check for hypocalcemia.

True pelvis The portion that lies below the linea terminalis; made up of the inlet, cavity, and outlet.

Truncus arteriosus A heart defect in which a single large vessel empties both ventricles and provides circulation for the pulmonary, systemic, and coronary circulations.

Trunk incurvation In response to stroking an infant's spine, the infant's pelvis will turn toward the stimulated side. Also called *Galant reflex*.

Tubal ligation A surgical procedure to clip, tie off, band, or plug the fallopian tubes to sterilize a female client.

Tubercle A granulomatous lesion (a sealed-off colony of bacilli) formed from *Mycobacterium tuberculosis*.

Tuberculosis (TB) A chronic, recurrent infectious disease caused by *Mycobacterium tuberculosis*. TB usually affects the lungs, but any organ can be affected.

Tubular sound The sound air makes moving through a clear and functioning trachea.

Tumor lysis syndrome (TLS) A condition that occurs when tumor cells dissolve and release intracellular contents into circulation, causing hyperkalemia, hyperuricemia, and hyperphosphatemia.

Tumor marker A protein molecule detectable in serum or other body fluids that is used to highlight suspicious regions for follow-up.

TURP syndrome A condition that is characterized by hyponatremia, decreased hematocrit, hypertension, bradycardia, nausea, and confusion.

Two-career family A family in which both partners are employed by choice or necessity. A two-career family may or may not have children.

Tympanic membrane A thin, tense membrane that separates the middle ear from the external auditory canal, protecting the middle ear from the external environment.

Tympanocentesis A surgical incision of the tympanic membrane. Also called *myringotomy*.

Tympanogram A test that provides a graph of the middle ear's ability to transmit sound.

Tympanostomy tubes Pressuring-equalizing tubes inserted to provide the middle ear with ventilation and drainage during healing.

Tympany A musical or drumlike sound produced from an air-filled stomach.

Ulcer A break in the GI mucosa that develops when the mucosal barrier is unable to protect the mucosa from damage by hydrochloric acid and pepsin, the gastric digestive juices.

Ulcerative colitis A chronic inflammatory bowel disorder that affects the mucosa and submucosa of the colon and rectum.

Ultrafiltration Removal of excess body water using a hydrostatic pressure gradient.

Ultrasound A test using intermittent ultrasonic waves transmitted by an alternating current to a transducer and applied to the abdomen.

Unconscious mind The part of an individual's mental life of which he or she is unaware.

Underinsured Individuals whose healthcare coverage is insufficient to meet their needs.

Undernutrition Health effects due to insufficient nutrient intake or stores. Also known as *malnutrition*.

Unifocal When a ventricular impulse arises from one ectopic site.

Unilateral lobar pneumonia A pattern of pneumonia in which bacteria tend to be distributed evenly throughout one or more lobes of a single lung.

Uninsured Individuals who are without any type of healthcare coverage.

Unipolar depression A mood disorder characterized by loss of interest in life and unresponsiveness, moving from mild to severe, with severe symptoms lasting at least 2 weeks. Also called *major depressive disorder (MDD)*.

Universal precautions (UP) Safety guidelines, such as proper hand hygiene, use of proper protective equipment, safe injection practices, and effective management of potentially contaminated surfaces or equipment, that are designed to decrease the risk of transmitting unidentified pathogens. Also called *standard precautions* and *body substance isolation (BSI)*.

Universal protocol Established guidelines for healthcare professionals to prevent errors during surgical procedures including wrong-site surgery.

Unlicensed assistive personnel (UAP) Members of a nursing team who assume delegated aspects of basic client care such as bathing, assisting with feeding, and collecting specimens. UAPs include certified nurse assistants, hospital attendants, nurse technicians, and orderlies.

Unresolved bacteriuria The presence of bacteria in urine that fails to resolve with treatment.

Unsaturated fat A triglyceride fat that does not contain all of the hydrogen ions it is capable of holding.

Upper body obesity Identified by a waist-to-hip ratio of greater than 1 in men or 0.8 in women. Also called *central obesity*.

Uremia Excessive amounts of urea in the blood.

Uremic fetor A urine-like breath odor often associated with a metallic taste in the mouth.

Uremic frost Crystallized deposits of urea on the skin.

Ureteral stent A thin catheter inserted into the ureter to provide for urine flow and ureteral support.

Ureterolithotomy An incision in the affected ureter to remove a calculus.

Ureteroplasty The surgical repair of a ureter.

Urgency The sudden, strong desire to void.

Urgency factor A way to illustrate how much time can safely lapse before doing interventions without compromising client outcomes.

Uric acid stones Develop when the urine concentration of uric acid is high.

Urinary calculi Stones in the urinary tract.

Urinary drainage system Those organs required to drain urine from the kidneys, including the ureters, urinary bladder, and urethra.

Urinary frequency The need to urinate often, specifically more than four to six times a day.

Urinary hesitancy A delay and difficulty in initiating voiding; often associated with dysuria.

Urinary incontinence Involuntary urination due to the temporary or permanent inability of the external sphincter muscles to control the flow of urine from the bladder. Also called *involuntary urination*.

Urinary reflux Backward flow of urine.

Urinary retention The accumulation of urine in the bladder and inability of the bladder to empty itself, resulting in overdistention of the bladder.

Urinary stasis Stagnation of urinary flow.

Urination Releasing urine from the urinary bladder. Also called *voiding* or *micturition*.

Uroflowmetry A method of measuring urine flow rate.

Urolithiasis The formation of stones in the urinary tract.

Urticaria Patches of pale, itchy wheals in an erythematous area. Also known as *hives*.

Uterine atony The relaxation of uterine muscle tone.

Uterosacral ligaments Ligaments that provide support for the uterus and cervix at the level of the ischial spines.

Uterus The hollow muscular organ in which the fertilized ovum is implanted and in which the developing fetus is nourished until birth.

Utilitarianism A form of consequentialist theory that views a good act as one that brings the most good and the least harm for the greatest number of people. This is called the principle of utility.

Utility See Utilitarianism.

Utilization review An evaluation of the use of resources to identify areas of overuse, misuse, and underuse.

Uveitis Inflammation of the middle layer of the eye called the uvea.

Vaccine Suspensions of whole or fractionated bacteria or viruses that have been treated to make them nonpathogenic; introduced by immunization to provoke active immunity.

Vacuum extraction An obstetric procedure used by physicians and CNMs to assist the birth of a fetus by applying suction to the fetal head.

Vagina The muscular and membranous tube that connects the external genitals with the uterus.

Vaginal birth after cesarean (VBAC) A trend in which a mother could choose a trial of labor and vaginal birth after having a cesarean for a previous child, provided the previous cesarean was required due to a nonrecurring indication and the mother met the guidelines established by the American College of Obstetricians and Gynecologists.

Vaginismus The involuntary spasm of the outer one third of the vaginal muscles, making penetration of the vagina painful and sometimes impossible.

Validation The act of verifying the accuracy and factuality of data.

Valsalva maneuver Forced exhalation against a closed glottis.

Values Personal beliefs about truth and the worth of behaviors or objects; standards that influence behavior.

Variability Change or wavering; more specifically, a change in fetal heart rate over a few seconds to a few minutes.

Variable decelerations A condition that occurs if the umbilical cord becomes compressed, reducing blood flow between the placenta and fetus. Fetal hypertension stimulates the baroreceptors in the aortic arch and carotid sinuses, slowing the fetal heart rate.

Variance 1. An unmet goal. 2. An incident or accident that affects a client or a visitor in a healthcare facility.

Vasectomy A procedure to surgically sever the vas deferens on both sides of the scrotum to sterilize a male client.

Vasogenic shock Shock that results from widespread vasodilation and decreased peripheral resistance. Also called *distributive shock*.

Vaso-occlusive crisis See Sickle cell crisis.

Vegan A type of vegetarian diet that excludes all animal and fish products, including dairy, meat, eggs, and honey.

Venous stasis The collection and stagnation of blood in the lower extremities.

Venous thrombectomy Surgical removal of a blood clot from the femoral vein to prevent pulmonary embolism or gangrene.

Venous thrombosis A condition in which a blood clot (thrombus) forms on the wall of a vein, accompanied by inflammation of the vein wall and some degree of obstructed venous blood flow. Also called *thrombophlebitis*.

Ventilation The exchange of oxygen and carbon dioxide.

Ventilation-perfusion (V-Q) The movement of oxygen across the alveolar–capillary membrane into a well-perfusing capillary.

Ventricular aneurysm An outpouching of the ventricular wall that does not contract during systole, causing stroke volume to decrease.

Ventricular bigeminy A premature ventricular contraction following each normal beat.

Ventricular gallop (S₃) Heart sound sometimes heard after the second heart sound in children, young adults, and pregnant females during the third trimester. Also called the *third heart sound*.

Ventricular septal defect (VSD) An opening in the ventricular septum that causes increased pulmonary blood flow.

Ventricular trigeminy A premature ventricular contraction every third beat.

Veracity A moral principle that holds that an individual should tell the truth and not lie.

Verbal abuse The use of berating, humiliating, ridiculing, blaming, or threatening language toward an individual.

Verbal communication Transmitting information through the spoken or written word.

Vernix caseosa A whitish, cheeselike substance that covers a fetus while in utero.

Vertical rotation The degree of rotation of the vertebrae.

Vertical transmission Perinatal transmission of an infection, such as the human immunodeficiency virus, from mother to infant.

Vertigo A sensation of whirling or rotation

Very-low-calorie diets A program providing a protein-sparing modified fast (400–800 kcal/day or less) under close medical supervision.

Vesicoureteral reflux A condition in which urine moves from the bladder back toward the kidney. A common risk factor in children who develop pyelonephritis that may also be seen in adults whose bladder outflow is obstructed.

Vesicular sounds The soft and breezy sounds of air moving in and out of the lobes at the alveolar level.

Vestibulitis Pain of the outer portion of the vagina upon touch or attempted penetration.

Vibration A series of vigorous quiverings produced by hands that are placed flat against the client's chest wall.

Violence The use of excessive force against other individuals or oneself, often resulting in physical or psychological injuries or death.

Virchow triad Three factors associated with thrombophlebitis: stasis of blood, vessel damage, and increased blood coagulability.

Virions Virus particles unable to grow and reproduce outside a host.

Virulence The ability of a microorganism to produce disease.

Virus A type of microorganism that must enter living cells in order to reproduce.

Visceral Of or relating to any large organ in the body.

Visceral pain Pain arising from body organs. It is dull and poorly localized because of the low number of nociceptors.

Viscosupplementation A treatment for osteoarthritis of the knee that involves injecting lubricating substances directly into the knee.

Visual Of or relating to sight.

Vitamin Micronutrient compounds that are involved in regulating body functioning. Most vitamins, with the exceptions of vitamins D and K, cannot be manufactured within the body and must be consumed through dietary intake.

Vitiligo An autoimmune disorder that results in loss of melanin in patches of the face, hands, or groin.

Voiding Releasing urine from the urinary bladder. Also called *urination* or *micturition*.

Voiding cystourethrography Use of a contrast medium and x-rays to assess the bladder and urethra when filled and during voiding.

Volatile acid Acids eliminated from the body as a gas.

Volkmann contracture The impaired mobility of the arm and inability to extend the arm completely, which is a common complication of elbow fractures.

Voluntary admission The detention of a client in a psychiatric or medical facility at the client's request.

Voluntary insurance Health care that provides no guarantee of universality because coverage may be expensive and difficult to purchase.

Vomiting The forceful expulsion of the contents of the upper gastrointestinal tract resulting from contraction of muscles in the gut and abdominal wall.

Vulnerability An individual's susceptibility to react to a specific stressor.

Vulnerability factors A practice, behavior, or environmental factor that increases the potential of an individual becoming a victim of violence.

Vulnerable populations Social groups with inadequate access to health care because they lack resources and are exposed to more risk factors.

Vulva The external female genitals.

Vulvodynia Constant, unremitting burning that is localized to the vulva with an acute onset.

Wandering baseline A smooth, meandering, unsteady baseline in the normal range without variability.

Warm zone When a disaster occurs, this zone, located at least 300 feet from the outer edge of a hot zone, is where decontamination occurs and rapid triage and emergency treatment are given to stabilize victims. Also called the *yellow zone*, *contamination zone*, or *contamination reduction zone*.

Water An essential nutrient for the body's survival, it contributes to fluid balance and plays an important role in nerve and muscle functioning and in the transport of nutrients to all body systems.

Weaning 1. The process of removing ventilator support and reestablishing spontaneous, independent respirations. 2. The process of discontinuing breastfeeding and accustoming an infant to another feeding method.

Well-being A subjective perception of feeling well that can be described objectively and measured.

Wellness A state of well-being that encompasses self-responsibility, dynamic growth, nutrition, physical fitness, emotional health, preventive health care, and the whole being of the individual.

Wellness diagnosis A term that describes human responses to levels of wellness in an individual, family, or community that have a readiness for enhancement. For example, *Readiness for Enhanced Coping.*

Wernicke encephalopathy A condition typically seen in people with alcoholism that is characterized by ataxia (lack of coordination), abnormal eye movements, and confusion.

Wheezing A high-pitched whistling sound most often heard on expiration and caused by the narrowing of bronchi; wheezes can also be heard on inspiration.

Whiplash An injury that results from sudden impact to a motor vehicle that causes an individual's head and neck to be forcibly contorted, resulting in injury to the spine.

Whistleblower A nurse or other individual who goes outside of an organization for the public's best interest when the organization fails to follow procedures regarding safety and client care.

Whistleblowing The act of going outside of an organization for the public's best interest when an organization fails to follow procedures regarding safety and client care.

White blood cells (WBCs) See Leukocytes.

Withdrawing or withholding life-sustaining therapy (WWLST) The withdrawal of extraordinary means of life support, such as removing a ventilator or withholding special attempts to revive a client, and allowing the client to die of the underlying medical condition.

Work ethic A belief in the importance and moral worth of work.

Workplace bullying Malicious, repeated, harmful mistreatment of an individual with whom one works, regardless of whether that individual is an equal, a superior, or a subordinate.

Workplace violence Any physical assault, threatening behavior, or verbal abuse occurring in the workplace.

Worldview The way in which people in a culture perceive ideas and attitudes about the world, other people, and life in general.

Wrong-site surgery (WSS) A surgical operation that is performed at the wrong location on a client's body due to error.

Xenograft Skin used for transplantation that was obtained from an animal, usually a pig. Also called *heterograft.*

Xenophobia The fear or dislike of people different from one's self.

Xerostomia Dry mouth that occurs when an individual's supply of saliva is reduced.

Zollinger-Ellison syndrome A form of peptic ulcer disease caused by a gastrinoma, or gastrin-secreting tumor of the pancreas, stomach, or intestines.

Zygote A fertilized egg.

COMBINED INDEX

Red type indicates a concept
Bold type indicates an exemplar
f indicates an entry from a figure.
t indicates an entry from a table or box.

A

AACN (American Association of Colleges of Nursing), 2626
AAMN (American Assembly for Men in Nursing), 2626*t*
Abacavir, 471*t*
ABCDE bundle (Airway, Breathing, Circulation, Disability, Exposure), 1475
Abdomen
  auscultating, 217*f*
  light and deep palpation of, 219*f*
  in newborn assessment, 2230
  in postpartum assessment, 2179*t*
  postpartum changes, 2173
  quadrants, 217*f*
  in urinary calculi inspection, 324*f*
  x-ray imaging, 220, 651
Abdominal breathing, 2163
Abdominal hysterectomy, 1402
Abdominal ultrasound, 785
ABGs. *See* Arterial blood gases
ABI (ankle-brachial blood pressure index), 1114
ABO incompatibility, 2081*t*
Abortion, 2051*t*
Abruptio placentae, 2137*t*
Absorption
  alterations and therapies, 212–213*t*
  defined, 210
  disorders, 210
  of iron, 926
  manifestations, 210–214
Abstinence, 1525*t*
Abuse. *See also* Violence
  age and, 1967
  assessment, 1257*t*, 1960, 1971
  care planning, 1971
  child
    defined, 1965
    examples of, 1956*f*
    manifestations of, 1968, 1972*t*
    therapies, 1972*t*
  collaborative care, 1970–1971
  communication and, 1974
  cultural factors and, 1967–1968
  cultural interpretation of, 1970*t*
  diagnosis, 1971
  diagnostic tests, 1970
  domestic violence shelters and, 1971
  elder
    defined, 1965–1966
    manifestations of, 1968–1969, 1972*t*
    therapies, 1972*t*

empowerment and, 1974
etiology, 1966–1967
as form of violence, 1954–1955
gender and, 1967
interventions, 1971–1974
interventions and therapies, 1958*t*
interventions for victims, 1962
intimate partner violence
  defined, 1966
  manifestations of, 1969, 1973*t*
  therapies, 1973*t*
lifespan and cultural considerations, 1969–1970, 1969*f*, 1970*t*
manifestations, 1958*t*, 1968–1970
neurobiology and, 1966
nonpharmacologic therapy, 1970–1971
nursing process, 1971–1974
outcome evaluation, 1974
overview of, 1964
pathophysiology, 1964–1968
pediatric, 1971
pharmacologic therapy, 1970
physiological development and, 1967
prevention of, 1968
psychopathology theory and, 1966
risk factors, 1967–1968
safety and, 1974
sexual
  defined, 1966
  manifestations of, 1969, 1973*t*
  therapies, 1973*t*
social learning theory and, 1966–1967
socioeconomic factors and, 1968
substance abuse and, 1968
therapeutic relationship and, 1974
types of, 1965–1966
Abuses of power, 2483–2485, 2484*t*
ACA (Affordable Care Act), 2604, 2604*t*, 2646, 2683–2684
Academic dishonesty, 2577
Acanthosis nigricans, 773, 774*f*
Accelerated starvation, 2045
Accelerations, 2152
Access to health care
  barriers to, 2603–2606
  healthcare legislation and, 2604*t*
  lack of health insurance and, 2603–2604
  lack of usual source of care and, 2605
  overview of, 2603
  patient-centered medical home and, 2605, 2605*t*
  perceptions of need and, 2605
  solutions, 2606
  underinsured and, 2603
  uneven distribution of services and, 2606
  uninsured and, 2603
Accidental hypothermia, 1438–1439
Accidents, 1955–1956
Accommodation, 1287*t*, 1653

Accountability
  concept integration, 2538–2539
  concept of, 2535
  concepts related to, 2538
  consumer demands and, 2540–2541
  defined, 1880, 2476, 2535
  demography and, 2542
  economics and, 2540
  factors affecting, 2540–2542
  information and telecommunications and, 2541–2542
  legislation and, 2542
  in management, 2476
  negative connotation, 2536
  NSNA code of academic and clinical conduct, 2539, 2540*t*
  nurses, 1880
  nursing practice and, 2542
  nursing shortage and, 2542, 2542*t*
  profession criteria, 2536–2538
  in professionalism, 2492
  responsibility and, 2535
  science and technology and, 2541
  socialization to nursing, 2539
  standards of care and, 2536
  standards of practice and, 2536
Accreditation
  achieving, 2624–2625
  computers and, 2646
  defined, 2624
  nursing education program, 2625
Accreditation Commission for Education in Nursing, 2625
Accrediting bodies
  Accreditation Commission for Education in Nursing, 2625
  Commission on Collegiate Nursing Education (CCNE), 2625
  defined, 2624
  Joint Commission, 2625
  overview of, 2624–2625
Acculturation, 1634
Acetaldehyde dehydrogenase inhibitors, 1533*t*
Acetaminophen
  content in narcotic medications, 165*t*
  dosage safety, 889
  fever and, 1434, 1434*t*
  maximum recommended dosage, 164
  for pain management, 163–164
Acid indigestion, 210–211
Acid-base balance
  alterations, 6–10
  alterations and therapies, 8*t*
  assessment, 6, 10–11
  collaborative interventions and therapies, 11–12
  concepts related to, 5*t*
  diagnostic tests, 10–11
  disorders. *See* acid-base imbalances

Acid-base balance (*continued*)
 fetal, labor and, 2127
 fully compensated, 7
 hydrogen ion concentration and, 3–4
 independent interventions and therapies, 11
 interventions and therapies, 11–12
 lifespan and cultural considerations, 10
 normal, 4–6
 partially compensated, 7
 regulation of, 4–6
  buffer systems, 4
  renal system, 6
  respiratory system, 4–6
Acid-base imbalances
 categories, 6
 causes, 4
 compensation, 6–7
 diagnostic tests, 10–11
 in infants and children, 10
 interventions and therapies, 8t, 11–12
  airway management, 12
  collaborative, 11–12
  independent, 11
  pharmacologic, 12
 mixed, 6
 in older adults, 10
 primary, 6–7
 risk factors, 7
Acidosis
 defined, 4
 high anion gap, 14
 membrane excitability and, 14
 metabolic. *See* metabolic acidosis
 osteoporosis and, 800
 respiratory. *See* respiratory acidosis
 severe, 14
Acids. *See also specific acids*
 defined, 3
 nonvolatile, 4
 volatile, 4
 as weak, 4
ACMV (assist-control mode ventilation), 980, 981t
Acquaintance phase, 1819
Acquaintance rape, 1984
Acquired immunity, 440
Acquired immunodeficiency syndrome (AIDS).
  See also HIV/AIDS
 defined, 438
 dementia complex, 462
 nurses' willingness to care for individuals with, 475t
Acral lentiginous melanoma, 129
Acrocyanosis, 2223
Acromegaly, 735t
Acrosomal reaction, 2021
ACS. *See* Acute coronary syndrome
ACT (assertive community treatment), 1619, 1619t
Actinic keratosis. *See also* Skin cancer
 defined, 131, 131f
 lesions, 131
 risk factors, 132
Action potential
 of cardiac muscle cell, 1044t
 defined, 1043
 depolarization, 1043
 repolarization, 1043–1044
Active acquired immunity, 2201
Active avoidance, 1940–1941

Active euthanasia, 176–177, 2574
Active immunity, 450
Active involvement, 2505–2506
Active transport, 338, 339f, 2026
Activities of daily living (ADLs)
 anemia and, 73, 74
 mobility and, 819
 oxygenation and, 970
 Parkinson disease and, 904–905
 spinal cord injuries (SCI) and, 915, 916–917
Activity and rest
 antepartum care, 2068–2069
 pneumonia and, 597t
Activity promotion
 in bowel elimination, 274
 in congenital heart defects, 1102
 in COPD, 1014
 in peripheral vascular disease (PVD), 1203–1204
Activity tolerance, 421
Activity-exercise pattern, 420
Actual diagnosis, 2335
Actual loss, 1742
Acupressure, labor and, 2161t
Acupuncture
 for menopause, 1396
 for mood disorders, 1797
Acute and chronic pain, 152–174. *See also* Acute
  pain; Chronic pain
Acute bacterial pneumonia, 586
Acute care, burn injuries, 1475–1476
Acute confusion, 1605
Acute coronary syndrome (ACS). *See also* Coronary
  artery disease (CAD)
 causes of, 1107
 defined, 1105, 1107
 manifestations, 1111t
 occurrences precipitating, 1107
Acute fatigue, 145, 185, 188
Acute illness, 408
Acute infection, 523
Acute kidney injury (AKI), 374
Acute lymphoblastic (ALL), 93f, 93t, 94–95
Acute myeloid (AML), 93t, 94–95, 94f
Acute myocardial infarction
 cardiogenic shock and, 1113
 cocaine intoxication and, 1108t
 occurrence of, 1107–1108
 pump failure and, 1113
 reference by heart damage area, 1108
Acute myocardial infarction (AMI). *See also*
  Coronary artery disease (CAD)
 as deep venous thrombosis risk factor, 1131
 defined, 1105
 dysrhythmias and, 1112
 infarction extension and, 1113
 manifestations, 1111–1113, 1112t
 pericarditis and, 1113
 structural defects and, 1113
 in women and older adults, 1111t
Acute otitis media, 576
Acute pain. *See also* Pain
 alterations and therapies, 144t
 categories of, 154–155
 characteristics of, 154–155
 defined, 143, 144t
 illness/injury-associated, 156
 interventions and therapies, 144t, 167t
 manifestations, 144t, 157–162, 167t

NANDA nursing diagnosis, 170
 prevention of, 157
Acute pancreatitis
 defined, 246
 illustrated, 247f
 manifestations, 247
Acute postinfection glomerulonephritis
  (APIGN), 669
Acute proliferative glomerulonephritis, 669
Acute pyelonephritis, 619
Acute rejection, 447
Acute renal failure (ARF)
 acute tubular necrosis (ATN), 376
 assessment, 386
 care planning, 386
 causes of, 375t
 children with, 387t
 collaborative care, 380–386
 defined, 374
 diagnosis, 386
 diagnostic tests, 380
 electrolyte imbalance in children and, 379t
 etiology, 376–377, 376t
 fluid management, 382
 initiation phase, 378
 interventions
  client teaching, 387–388
  general, 386–387
  nutrition balance, 387
 intrinsic (intrarenal), 376
 lifespan considerations, 378, 379f
 maintenance phase, 378
 manifestations, 378–379, 379t
 medications, 381–382
 Nursing Care Plan, 388–389t
 nursing process, 386
 nutrition and, 383
 outcome evaluation, 388
 overview of, 374
 pathophysiology, 374–378, 375f
 pediatric, 378
 pharmacologic therapy, 380–382
 postrenal, 376
 prerenal, 376
 prevention, 378
 recovery phase, 378
 religious and cultural preferences, 386t
 renal replacement therapy
  continuous, 384, 384f, 384t
  hemodialysis, 383–384, 383f
  peritoneal dialysis, 385–386, 385f
  vascular access for, 384–385, 385f
 risk factors, 378
Acute respiratory acidosis, 21
Acute respiratory distress syndrome (ARDS)
 alveolar collapse and, 977f
 assessment, 985
 burn injuries and, 1470
 care planning, 985
 collaborative care
  artificial airways, 983–984
  diagnostic tests, 979
  mechanical ventilation, 979–983
  nonpharmacologic therapy, 979–985
  nutrition and fluids, 984–985
  pharmacologic therapy, 979
 community-based care, 988t
 conditions associated with development, 975t
 defined, 975
 diagnosis, 985

end-stage, 977f
goal of care, 985
initiation of, 976f
interventions
    anxiety relief, 987–988
    cardiac output enhancement, 986
    common, 985
    discharge preparation, 988
    dysfunctional ventilatory weaning response
        monitoring, 987
    patent airway, 986
    spontaneous ventilation, 986
manifestations, 978, 978t
Nursing Care Plan, 989t
nursing process, 985–988
outcome evaluation, 988
overview of, 975
pathogenesis, 975f
pathophysiology and etiology, 975–978,
    976–977f
prevention of, 978
pulmonary edema onset and, 976f
risk factors, 978
Acute stress disorder
    defined, 1945
    overview of, 1946t
    PTSD versus, 1946t
    stress and coping and, 1909t
Acute tubular necrosis (ATN), 376, 377f
Acute urinary retention, 299t
AD. See Alzheimer disease
Adaptation
    in cognitive development, 1653
    coping and, 1900
    defined, 1653, 1900
    diseases of, 1901
    general adaptation syndrome (GAS), 1901
    local adaptation syndrome (LAS), 1901
Adaptive behaviors, 1581
Adaptive mechanisms, 1649
ADD (attention deficit disorder), 1680
Addiction. See also Recovery
    alcohol, 1524t
    alterations, 1522–1526
    alterations and therapies, 1524t
    assessment, 1527–1528
    assessment interview, 1527t
    biological factors in, 1520
    boundaries and, 1524
    concepts related to, 1523t
    defined, 1519
    dependence versus, 1520
    depression and, 1523–1524
    diagnostic tests, 1528
    enabling behavior and, 1525
    families and, 1525–1526
    genetic factors in, 1521, 1522
    interventions and therapies
        behavioral therapy, 1529–1530
        collaborative, 1529–1532
        communication, 1528–1529
        family therapy, 1532
        group therapy, 1530, 1531t
        independent, 1528–1529
        milieu therapy, 1530
        pharmacologic, 1532
        support groups, 1531
        twelve-step programs, 1531–1532
    language of, 1525, 1525t
    lifespan considerations, 1521–1522

manifestations, 1523–1525
medications, 1533t
neurobiological research into, 1520
nicotine, 1524t
phenotypes and, 1536
physiology and psychology, 1520
prevalence of, 1526
prevention of, 1527
process, 1520, 1524t
psychological factors in, 1521
sociocultural factors in, 1521
substance, 1524t
Adenoids, 444
ADH (antidiuretic hormone), 340, 341f, 1164
ADHD. See Attention-deficit/hyperactivity
    disorder
Adherence, 2502
Adhesions, 1258
Adjustable gastric banding, 795, 795f
Adjustment disorder with depressed mood
    assessment, 1806
    care planning, 1807
    collaborative care, 1806
    defined, 1778–1779, 1780t, 1805
    diagnosis, 1806
    exercise and, 1806
    hope and, 1807
    interventions, 1807
    manifestations, 1805, 1806t
    Nursing Care Plan, 1807–1808t
    nursing process, 1806–1807
    overview of, 1805
    pharmacologic therapy, 1806
    resilience factors, 1805
    risk factors, 1805
    as situational depression, 1805
    support of family and, 1807
    therapies, 1780t
Adjustment phase, 1655
ADLs. See Activities of daily living
Administration
    accreditation, 2646
    budget and finance, 2645–2646
    computers in, 2645–2646
    dashboard, 2645
    facilities management, 2645
    healthcare information systems, 2636
    human resources, 2645
    information systems, 2636
    medical records management, 2645
    online tools, 2642
    quality assurance, 2646
    utilization reviews, 2646
Administrative laws, 2654
Admission nursing assessment, 2445
Adolescent families, 1710
Adolescent idiopathic scoliosis, 847
Adolescents
    activities, 1669
    assessment of, 2293
    asthma in, 995t
    body mass index (BMI) ranges, 942t
    bowel elimination in, 275
    cancer and, 50–51
    childbirth and, 2168t
    cognitive development, 1669
    comfort and, 149
    communication, 1669–1670
    communication with, 2407t
    depression in, 1801t

end-of-life care, 179
family with, 1726
group therapy with, 1531
growth and development, 1668–1670
growth and development milestones, 1669t
health promotion, 412t
health screenings and immunization guidelines,
    413–414t
inflammatory bowel disease (IBD) in, 666
injury prevention due to motor vehicle
    crashes, 2000t
lesbian, gay, bisexual, and transgender
    (LGBT), 1670
normal sleep-rest patterns in, 432
nutrition in, 932–933
obesity in, 933
obsessive-compulsive disorder (OCD) in, 1935t
oral health in, 428
pain perception and behavior in, 158t
personality and temperament of, 1669
pharmacologic therapy for mood disorders,
    1794t
physical growth and development of,
    1668–1669
postpartum care of, 2188
pregnant, nutritional care of, 2097–2098
psychosocial development of, 1669–1670
puberty in, 1668
scoliosis in, 849t
seizures in, 722t
separation anxiety disorder (SAD) in, 1922t
sexual development, 1340–1343, 1342t
sexuality, 1670
sexuality assessment, 1354–1355
sexually transmitted infections (STIs) and,
    1343, 1408
sleep and, 196
sports-related concussions, 2712t
substance abuse risk in, 1521t
systemic lupus erythematosus (SLE) in, 515t
tobacco use and, 1549t
unintentional injuries and, 2711–2712, 2711f
urinary tract infections (UTIs) in, 625t
Adrenals, pregnancy and, 2034
Adrenergic antagonists, 1074t
Adrenergic stimulants, 996, 998t
Adrenergics (sympathomimetics),
    1228t, 1229t
Adrenomedullin, 1164
Adult growth and development
    middle adults, 1671, 1671t
    older adults, 1671
    young adults, 1670–1671, 1670t
Adult idiopathic scoliosis, 847
Adult learning theory, 2502
Adult-onset diabetes. See Diabetes mellitus
Adult-onset schizophrenia (AOS), 1616
Adults living alone, 1712
Advance care planning (children),
    179, 179t
Advance directives
    defined, 2667
    durable power of attorney for health
        care, 2667
    elements of, 2668
    illustrated, 2669f
    living will, 2667
    overview of, 2667
    role of the nurse, 2668
    types of, 2667

Advance healthcare directives, 177
Advanced life support, 1194
Adventitious breathing sounds, 963*t*
Advice, giving, 2432
Advocacy. *See also* Client advocates
  for children and families, 2559, 2559*f*, 2559*t*
  in client empowerment, 2557–2558
  concept of, 2555
  concepts related to, 2556*t*
  confidentiality and, 2671
  defined, 2555
  in ethical decision making, 2570*f*
  in home care, 2557*t*
  illegal, immoral, or unethical activities and, 2561
  interventions, 2561
  legal issues and, 2660*t*
  lifespan considerations, 2558*t*
  professional and public, 2558–2559
  programs, 2559*t*
  provider education, 2558
  values, 2556*t*
  for vulnerable populations, 2560–2561, 2560*f*
Advocates, 2564
AED (automated external defibrillator), 1193, 1194*f*
Aerobic exercises, 421
Aesthetic knowing, 2306
Afebrile, 1423, 1431
α-fetoprotein (AFP), 2048
Affect. *See also* Mood and affect
  defined, 1775
  descriptors of, 1776*t*
Affective commitment, 2487, 2487*f*
Affective domain, 2503
Affordable Care Act (ACA), 2604, 2604*t*, 2646, 2683–2684
AFI (amniotic fluid index), 2085–2086
AFP (α-fetoprotein), 2048
African Americans
  acceptable child behaviors, 2288*t*
  autoimmune disorders and, 448
  Chronic kidney disease and, 392*t*
  hypertension and, 1167*t*
  stroke and, 1237*t*
Afterload, 1042
Afterpains, 2172
Age
  abuse and, 1967
  assault and homicide and, 1977
  blood pressure and, 1045–1046
  as cancer risk factor, 46
  diversity, 1637
  fever and, 1424
  grieving process and, 1746
  hypertension and, 1166–1167
  immune disease and, 448
  phobias and, 1940
  pulse and, 1044
  skin disorders and, 1452
  violence and, 1957
Ageism, 1607, 1637, 1763
Agency for Healthcare Research and Quality (AHRQ), 2591
Age-related cognitive decline, 1584
Age-related macular degeneration (AMD). *See* Macular degeneration
Aggravated assault, 1975
Aggression, 1976

Aggressive behavior, 1789
Aggressive communicators, 2409, 2411, 2411*t*
Aging, multisystem effects of, 1672
Aging changes
  cardiovascular system, 1048, 1048*f*
  pulmonary system, 1049
  renal system, 1049
  vascular system, 1048–1049
Agnosia, 1237
Agnostic, 1873
Agonists, 1919*f*
Agoraphobia, 1940–1941, 1940*f*, 1941*t*
Agreements, reaching, 2470
AHRQ (Agency for Healthcare Research and Quality), 2591
AIDS. *See* Acquired immunodeficiency syndrome; HIV/AIDS
Air sacs, 954–955
Air trapping, 1006*f*
Airborne precautions, 545–546
Airborne transmission, 524
Airway clearance
  in COPD, 1014
  in respiratory acidosis, 23
  in RSV/bronchiolitis, 1022
Airway management
  in acid-base imbalances, 12
  in burn injuries, 1476
  in respiratory acidosis, 23
Airway patency
  influenza and, 574
  motor vehicle crashes (MVC) and, 2003–2004
  pneumonia and, 596
Airways
  artificial, 983–984
  in children, 956*f*
  clearance of, 1002
  in infants, 956, 957*f*
  in newborns, 2237
  patent, 956
  in postoperative nursing, 1274
  remodeling, 990
Akathisia, 1584
AKI (acute kidney injury), 374
Alarm reaction, 1901, 1901*f*
Alcohol
  as cancer risk factor, 47
  as CNS depressant, 1535
  diabetes and, 758
  hypertension and, 1167, 1169
  hypoglycemia and, 772, 772*t*
  pregnancy and, 1552–1553
  sleep and, 433
Alcohol abuse
  assessment, 1540–1541
  care planning, 1541
  collaborative care, 1539–1540
  complementary and alternative therapy, 1539–1540
  diagnosis, 1541
  diagnostic tests, 1539
  epidemiology, 1535
  grieving process and, 1746
  interventions
    client education, 1543
    coping skills, 1541–1543
    nutrition, 1543
    safety, 1541

    safety during withdrawal, 1543
    self-esteem promotion, 1543
    treatment participation, 1541
  manifestations
    malnutrition, 1536
    multisystem effects of, 1538
    overdose, 1539
    therapies and, 1537–1538*t*, 1556*t*
    withdrawal, 1538–1539
  Nursing Care Plan, 1544*t*
  nursing process, 1540–1544
  outcome evaluation, 1544
  overview of, 1535
  pathophysiology and etiology, 1535–1536
  physiological complications, 1538*t*
  risk factors, 1535–1536
  treatment of withdrawal, 1539
Alcohol addiction, 1524*t*
Alcohol dependence, 1535
Alcohol poisoning, 1539
Alcohol withdrawal delirium, 1538–1539
Alcohol withdrawal syndrome, 1538
Alcoholic cirrhosis
  defined, 781
  liver damage and, 782
Alcoholic ketoacidosis, 14
Alcoholics Anonymous, 1532*t*
Alcoholism, 1535
Aldrete scoring system, 1274, 1275*t*
Alert states, newborns, 2203
Alignment, in fracture care, 866
Alkalosis
  defined, 4
  metabolic, 6, 7, 7*f*, 8*t*, 9*t*, 10*t*, 17–20
  respiratory, 4–6, 6, 7, 7*f*, 8*t*, 9*t*, 10*t*, 25–27
ALL (acute lymphoblastic), 93*f*, 93*t*, 94–95
Allen test, 10
Allergens, 481
Allergic contact dermatitis, 1488, 1489*t*
Allergic diseases, prevalence of, 447
Allergies. *See also* Hypersensitivity
  characteristic findings in clients with, 487*t*
  defined, 481
  food test, 490
  latex, 484–485, 486*t*, 487*t*
Allergy shots, 490
Allocation of resources
  defined, 2607
  examples of, 2607–2608
  nurses and, 2608
  overview of, 2607
Allogeneic blood transfusions, 1270
Allogeneic bone marrow transplant, 97, 98*f*
Allograft, 1479
Alloimmunization, 124, 2081*t*
Allostasis, 1896
Allostatic load, 1896
Aloe vera, 1511*t*
Alogia, 1614
Alopecia, 1458*t*
Alpha-adrenergic blockers, 1171*t*, 1322*t*
Altered level of consciousness (LOC)
  brain death and, 694
  as cerebral hemisphere deterioration sign, 690–691
  death and dying and, 1759
  eye movements, 690*f*
  increased intracranial pressure (IICP) and, 693–694

locked-in syndrome and, 694
outcomes of, 694
persistent vegetative state and, 694
prevalence of, 696
prognosis, 694
seizures and, 694
Altered urinary elimination,
        264–265, 264t
Altered urine production, 264
Alternative therapies. See also Complementary
        and alternative therapy
    in crisis, 1931–1932
    defined, 1643–1644
Alternatives, choosing between, 2322–2323
Altruism, 2564
Alveolar collapse, 977f
Alveoli, 954–955, 955f
Alzheimer disease (AD). See also Cognition
    amyloid hypothesis, 1595
    amyloid plaques, 1595
    assessment, 1600
    care planning, 1601
    cerebral effects of, 1595t
    cholinergic hypothesis, 1595
    collaborative care, 1596–1600
    complementary and alternative therapy,
        1598–1600
    culture and, 1603t
    defined, 1594
    diagnosis, 1600–1601
    diagnostic tests, 1596
    etiology, 1595
    familial (FAD), 1594
    interventions
        communication strategies, 1601t
        coping strategies, 1601
        injury prevention, 1601–1602
        psychosocial wellness, 1602
        rest and activity balance, 1602
        stress management for caregivers,
            1602–1603, 1602t
    manifestations, 1596, 1599–1600t
    mild, 1597t, 1599t
    moderate, 1597t, 1599t
    neurofibrillary tangles, 1595
    nonpharmacologic therapy, 1598
    Nursing Care Plan, 1603–1604t
    nursing process, 1600–1603
    outcome evaluation, 1603
    overview of, 1594
    pathophysiology, 1594–1596
    pharmacologic therapy, 1596–1598
    prevention of, 1596
    risk factors, 1595
    severe, 1597t, 1600t
    sporadic, 1594
    stages of, 1597t
    sundowning and, 1597t
    supplements taken by clients with, 1598t
    tau hypothesis, 1595
Amantadine, 899t, 901
Ambulation, 837
AMD. See Age-related macular degeneration
Amenorrhea, 1400
American Assembly for Men in Nursing
        (AAMN), 2626t
American Association of Colleges of Nursing
        (AACN), 2626
American Burn Association burn
        classification, 1469t

American Nurses Association (ANA)
    Code of Ethics, 2568–2569
    defined, 2625
    on DNR/AND decisions, 176
    on euthanasia, 177
    in policy planning, 2619
    Standards of Practice, 2658
Americans with Disabilities Act of 1990, 1591t
AMI. See Acute myocardial infarction
Aminion, 2022
AML (acute myeloid), 93t, 94–95, 94f
Amniocentesis, 2089, 2089f
Amniotic fluid, 2023
Amniotic fluid analysis
    amniocentesis and, 2089–2090, 2089f
    lecithin/sphingomyelin ratio, 2090
    phosphatidylglycerol, 2090
Amniotic fluid embolism, 2139t
Amniotic fluid index (AFI), 2085–2086
Amniotomy, 2121
Amphetamines, 793, 1563–1564
Amplification, hearing, 1302–1304, 1303f
Amsler grid, 1328, 1328f
Amylase, 221
Amyloid hypothesis, 1595
Amyloid plaques, 1595
Amyloid precursor protein (APP), 1595
AN. See Anorexia nervosa
Anaerobic exercises, 421
Anal stimulation, 1346
Analgesics
    burns and, 1478
    categories and examples, 162t
    combining, 163
    creams, rubs, sprays, 889
    infection and, 558t
    myocardial infarction and, 1118–1119
    in perioperative care, 1255t
Anaphylactic shock
    assessment, 1230
    defined, 483, 1224
    manifestations, 1226t
Anaphylaxis
    defined, 482–483
    substances known to trigger, 483t
    symptoms and treatment, 636t
    triggers of, 636
Anaplasia, 32
Anasarca, 365
Andragogy, 2502
Androgens, 112, 285
Android pelvis, 2014–2015, 2016f
Anemia
    alterations and therapies, 33t
    antepartum care and, 2077t
    assessment, 71
    blood transfusions as treatment, 70
    cardiorespiratory function and, 73
    chronic kidney disease (CKD) and, 393
    collaborative care, 69–70, 71t
    complementary and alternative therapy, 71t
    defined, 64
    diagnostic tests, 70
    etiology, 65
    fatigue and, 186t, 188t
    folic acid deficiency, 68, 68t, 75t
    genetics and, 34
    glucose-G-phosphate dehydrogenase, 69
    hemolytic, 68–69, 68t
    home care for, 74t

    interventions, 71–74
    iron-deficiency, 66, 66f
    lifespan and cultural considerations, 69
    manifestations
        aplastic anemia, 69
        blood loss anemia, 65–66
        folic acid deficiency anemia, 2044–2045
        iron deficiency anemia, 2044
        nutritional anemia, 66–68
        therapies and, 72–73t
    multisystem effects of, 67f
    neonatal, 69
    nonpharmacologic therapy, 70
    Nursing Care Plan, 75t
    nursing process, 71–74
    nutrition and, 70
    outcome evaluation, 74
    overview of, 64
    oxygen supply and demand balance and, 73–74
    pathophysiology, 64–65, 65t
    pernicious, 66
    pharmacologic therapy, 70
    physiological, of infancy, 69, 2196
    prevalence of, 34
    prevention of, 65
    risk factors, 34, 65
    self-care, 74
    sickle cell, 120
    skin appearance, 64f
    surgery, 70
    thalassemia, 68–69
    treatment goals, 71
    vitamin B_{12} deficiency, 66
Anemia of prematurity, 2255
Anergia, 1799
Anergic, 609
Anergy, 1799
Aneroid sphygmomanometer, 1065f
Anesthesia
    ASA system, 1266
    endotracheal tubes and, 1267
    laryngeal mask airways and, 1267
    types of, 1266t
Anesthesia personnel, 1251
Anesthetics, 1462t
Aneurysm, 1236
ANF (atrial natriuretic factor), 340
Anger, 1904
Angina
    drugs used to treat, 1118
    manifestations, 1111, 1111t
    types of, 1107
Angina pectoris, 1105
Angiography. See Magnetic resonance imaging
Angiotensin II-receptor blockers (ARBs), 1153,
        1154t, 1171t
Angiotensin-converting enzyme (ACE) inhibitors
    heart failure and, 1153, 1154t
    hypertension and, 1171t
    myocardial infarction and, 1119
Angle-closure glaucoma, 1319, 1320t
Anhedonia, 1614, 1776, 1799
Animal-assisted therapy, for mood
        disorders, 1797
Animism, 1665t
Anions, 336
Ankle dorsiflexion, 2220, 2221f
Ankle-brachial blood pressure index
        (ABI), 1114
Ankles, mobility assessment, 833t

Anomia, 1584
Anorexia
    defined, 210
    fluid intake and, 362
Anorexia nervosa (AN)
    characteristics of, 1838t
    defined, 1844, 1845
    diagnostic tests, 1849
    DSM-5 diagnostic criteria for, 1846t
    lanugo, 1846
    manifestations, 1848t
    nonpharmacologic therapy, 1849
    therapies, 1848t
Anorexia-cachexia syndrome, 48, 48f, 60
Anorgasmia, 1354
ANP (atrial natriuretic peptide), 1151, 1164
Antacids
    burns and, 1478–1479
    defined, 222
    GERD and, 230t
    peptic ulcer disease and, 680
Antagonism, 1854
Antagonists, 1919f
Antenatal perineal massage, 2132t
Antepartum, 2051t
Antepartum care
    activity and rest, 2068–2069
    adolescent nutritional care, 2097–2098
    alterations
        ABO incompatibility, 2081t
        alloimmunization, 2081t
        anemia, 2077t
        asthma, 2078t
        diabetes mellitus, 2077t
        ectopic pregnancy, 2080t
        epilepsy, 2078t
        gestational trophoblastic disease (GTD),
            2080t
        Group B streptococcal (GBS) infection,
            2082t
        heart disease, 2078t
        herpes simplex virus (HSV), 2081t
        HIV/AIDS, 2077t
        hyperemesis gravidarum, 2081t
        hypertensive disorder, 2081t
        hyperthyroidism, 2078t
        hypothyroidism, 2078t
        multiple sclerosis, 2079t
        overview of, 2076
        prenatal substance abuse, 2077t
        rheumatoid arthritis, 2079t
        spontaneous abortion (miscarriage),
            2080t
        syphilis, 2082t
        systemic lupus erythematosus, 2079t
        tuberculosis, 2079t
        urinary tract infection, 2082t
        vaginal bleeding, 2080t
        vulvovaginal candidiasis, 2082t
    amniotic fluid analysis, 2089–2090
    assessment
        areas, 2100
        due date determination, 2106–2107, 2107f
        edema, 2102t
        expectant mother, 2104–2105t
        expectant partner, 2105t
        fetal heartbeat, 2103t
        of fetal well-being, client education, 2077t
        interview, 2101–2102t
        laboratory evaluation, 2103–2104t

    overview of, 2100
    parenting ability, 2101–2102t
    previous pregnancies, 2106, 2106f
    subsequent, 2102–2105t
    uterine size, 2103t
    vital signs, 2102t
    weight gain, 2102t
bathing, 2072
biophysical profile, 2087–2088, 2088t
breast care, 2068, 2068f
care of partner, 2108
care of siblings, 2108–2109
care planning, 2107
clothing, 2072
complementary and alternative therapy, 2074
contraction stress test (CST), 2088–2089
daily food plan, 2093t
danger signs in pregnancy, 2100t
dental care, 2072
diagnosis, 2107
diagnostic testing to assess fetal well-being,
    2076–2090
dietary reference intakes (DRIs), 2091–2092,
    2091–2092t
discomfort relief
    culture and, 2076t
    first trimester, 2074–2075t
    second trimester, 2075t
    self-care measures, 2074–2075t
    third trimester, 2075t
employment, 2072–2073
estimated date of birth (EDB), 2107, 2107f
exercise
    abdominal, 2070–2071
    inner thigh, 2071
    Kegel, 2071, 2071f
    pelvic tilt, 2069, 2070f
    perineal, 2071
    yoga, 2071t
fetal acoustic stimulation test, 2087
fetal movement record, 2083, 2083f
healthy pregnancy promotion, 2068–2074
at home, 2100t
immunizations, 2072
interventions
    altered family processes monitoring,
        2109–2110
    anxiety and, 2111
    excessive weight management, 2110t
    nutrition, 2110–2111
    readiness evaluation, 2108–2109
    self-care knowledge, 2108
maternal assessment of fetal activity,
    2082–2084, 2083f, 2084t
maternal nutrition, 2090–2092,
    2091–2092t
maternal weight gain, 2098–2099,
    2098t, 2099f
nonstress testing (NST), 2086–2087, 2086f
Nursing Care Plan, 2111t
nursing process, 2099–2111
nutrition influences
    artificial sweeteners, 2096
    cultural, ethnic, and religious, 2094,
        2094f, 2094t
    eating disorders, 2094–2095
    folic acid, 2096
    foodborne illnesses and, 2097
    herbs, 2096t
    lactase deficiency (lactose intolerance), 2097

    mercury in fish, 2096–2097
    pica, 2095
    psychosocial, 2094–2096, 2095f
    socioeconomic, 2094
    special dietary considerations, 2096–2097
    vegetarianism, 2095–2096, 2095f, 2096t
outcome evaluation, 2111
overview of, 2068
self-care measures, 2072–2074, 2074–2075t,
    2076t
sexual activity, 2071–2072
teratogenic substances and, 2074
travel, 2073–2074
ultrasound
    advantages, 2084
    benefits of, 2085–2086
    defined, 2083–2084
    four-dimensional, 2084
    transabdominal, 2085
    transvaginal, 2085
    vibroacoustic stimulation test, 2087
Anterior cord syndrome, 910t
Anthrax, 2615t
Anthropoid pelvis, 2015, 2016f
Anthropometric measurements, 940–942, 942t
Anthropometry, 793
Antiacne, 1462t
Antianemic agents, 40t
Antiangiogenic drugs, 1329
Antianxiety medications, 1255t
Antibacterials, 1462t
Antibiotic drops and ointments, 1315t
Antibiotic peak and trough levels, 557
Antibiotic-resistant bacteria, 531–532
Antibiotics
    antitumor, 40t
    for children, 1434
    drops and ointments for eye injuries, 1315t
    infection and, 558t
    in perioperative care, 1255
    for pneumonia, 591t
    prophylactic, 622t
    taking of, 558
    as tissue integrity medication, 1462t
Antibodies
    classes of, 442
    defined, 442
    monoclonal, 556t
    primary and secondary responses, 527
Antibody-mediated immune response, 442
Anticholinergics
    as asthma medication, 997, 999t
    as Parkinson disease medication, 899t,
        900–901
Anticipatory grief, 1742, 1758
Anticipatory grieving, 38
Anticipatory guidance, 1930, 2520, 2521t
Anticipatory loss, 1742
Anticipatory problem solving, 2522
Anticoagulants
    coronary artery disease (CAD) and, 1119
    deep venous thrombosis (DVT) and,
        1132–1134
    stroke and, 1240–1241
    types of, 1133–1134t
Anticonvulsants
    for bipolar disorders, 1813
    function of, 167
    in peripheral neuropathies, 1333, 1334t
    for substance abuse, 1566t

Antidepressants
  for acute and chronic pain, 167
  for addictions, 1533t
  atypical, 1793
  for disorders of anxiety, stress, or trauma,
    1916t
  for grief and loss, 1750
  for substance abuse, 1566t
  suicide and, 1995
Antidiuretic hormone (ADH), 340, 341f, 1164
Anti-DNA antibody testing, 512
Antidysrhythmics
  heart failure and, 1156
  myocardial infarction and, 1119
Antiemetics, 222, 223t, 1255t
Antiepileptic drugs (AEDs), 708, 719t
Antifungals, 558t, 1462t
Antigen-antibody complexes, 512
Antigenic drift, 570
Antigenic shift, 570
Antigens
  characteristics of, 441
  defined, 437, 481
  endogenous, 483
  exogenous, 483
  immune response, 441
Antihelminthic agents, 558t
Antihistamines
  as antiemetic, 223
  for hypersensitivity, 490
Antihypertensives, 167, 1074t
Antimalarial agents, 503t, 558t, 1503
Antimetabolites, 40t
Antimicrobials
  agents, 558–559t
  burns and, 1478
Antineoplastics, 40t
Antiplatelet medications, 1119, 1120t
Antipruritics, 167
Antipsychotics
  for cognitive alterations, 1592t
  for disorders of anxiety, stress, or trauma,
    1916t
  for schizophrenia, 1618t
  suicide and, 1995
Antipyretics, 558t, 1430t
Antiretroviral drugs, 237t, 558t
Antiretroviral nucleoside analogues,
    470–471
Antiseizure drugs, 1533t
Antiseptics, 544, 544t
Antisocial personality disorder (ASPD), 1855,
    1856t, 1863t
Antispasmodics, 838t
Antistreptolysin O (ASO), 671, 1098t
Antithrombotic drugs, 1241
Antithyroid agents, 738t
Antivirals, 1462t
Anuria, 264, 381
Anus, newborn assessment, 2231
Anxiety
  antepartum care and, 2111
  children and, 1907–1910
  death, 183
  defined, 1904, 1917
  free-floating, 1918
  in intrapartum assessment, 2147t
  in labor, 2162
  levels of anxiety, 1922
  nursing transaction model and, 1911t

Anxiety disorders
  assessment, 1926
  behavioral theories, 1919
  care planning, 1926
  characteristics of, 1917–1918
  cognitive-behavioral therapy, 1925
  collaborative care, 1922–1926
  complementary and alternative therapy,
    1925–1926
  defined, 1907, 1908t
  diagnosis, 1926
  diagnostic tests, 1924
  generalized anxiety disorder (GAD),
    1920–1921, 1922t
  genetic theories, 1919
  herbal preparations for, 1925
  humanistic theories, 1919
  in immigrant populations, 1920t
  interventions, 1908t, 1926
  levels of anxiety and, 1922
  manifestations, 1908t, 1920–1922,
    1923t
  massage and therapeutic touch for, 1925
  medications for, 1915, 1916t
  neurobiological theories, 1918, 1918f
  neurochemical theories, 1918–1919,
    1919f
  nonpharmacologic therapy, 1925–1926
  nursing process, 1926
  outcome evaluation, 1926
  overview of, 1917–1918
  oxidative stress and illness and, 1924t
  panic disorder, 1921–1922
  pathophysiology and etiology, 1918–1920
  pharmacologic therapy, 1924–1925
  prevention of, 1920
  psychosocial theories, 1919
  relaxation techniques, yoga, and meditation for,
    1925–1926
  risk factors, 1920
  separation anxiety disorder (SAD), 1921
  summary of criteria, 1921t
Anxiety relief
  acute respiratory distress syndrome (ARDS)
    and, 987–988
  asthma and, 1002–1003
  menstrual dysfunction and, 1404
  pulmonary embolism and, 1215
  respiratory acidosis and, 23
  shock and, 1232
  skin cancer and, 136–137
Anxiolytics
  for cognitive alterations, 1592t
  for disorders of anxiety, stress, or trauma,
    1916t
Anxious distress, 1776
Aorta resection, 1099t
Aortic stenosis, 1092t
Aortocaval compression, 2031
AOS (adult-onset schizophrenia), 1616
Apathy, 2422
APD (avoidant personality disorder), 1855,
    1856t, 1863t
Apgar score
  defined, 2135, 2210
  elements of, 2210–2211
  illustrated, 2210t
  signs, 2135
Aphakia, 1312
Aphasia, 698t, 1238, 1584

Aphthoid lesion, 658
APIB (Assessment of Preterm Infant Behavior),
    2258–2259
Apical impulse assessment, 1056–1058t
Apical pulse, 1063f, 1064, 1064f
Apical-radial pulse, 1064
APIGN (acute postinfection glomerulonephritis),
    669
Aplastic anemia, 69
Apnea
  defined, 590, 959
  interventions and therapies, 960t
  manifestations, 960t
  in respiratory syncytial virus (RSV),
    1019t
Apnea of prematurity, 2254
APP (amyloid precursor protein), 1595
Appearance, 2481, 2481f
Appendectomy, 646
Appendicitis
  assessment, 646
  care planning, 647
  in children, 646, 648
  client teaching, 648, 648t
  collaborative care, 646
  defined, 644
  diagnosis, 647
  diagnostic tests, 646
  fluid volume balance and, 647
  infection and, 647
  interventions, 647–648
  lifespan and cultural considerations, 646
  manifestations, 645–646, 645t
  Nursing Care Plan, 648–649t
  nursing process, 646–648
  in older adults, 646
  outcome evaluation, 648
  overview of, 644
  pain management, 647–648
  pathophysiology and etiology,
    644–645
  pharmacologic therapy, 646
  prevention of, 645
  psychosocial well-being and, 648
  respiratory gas exchange and, 647
  risk factors, 645
  surgery, 646
Appendix
  location of, 644, 645t
  perforation of, 644
Approach coping, 1899
Approximated tissue surfaces, 1507
Apraxia, 1237
ARBs (angiotensin II receptor blockers), 1153,
    1154t, 1171t
ARDS. See Acute respiratory distress syndrome
Arm fracture, 867–868t
Aromatherapy, 1620
Arrhythmias
  defined, 1063
  fetal, 2151
Arrhythmogenic right ventricular cardiomyopathy
    (ARVC), 1077t, 1078
Arrhythmogenic tissue, 1112
Arrogance, 2493
Arterial blood gases (ABGs)
  in acid-base balance assessment, 10t
  in acid-base imbalances, 6, 11
  in acute renal failure (ARF), 380
  in burn injuries, 1477

Arterial blood gases (ABGs) (*continued*)
  in chronic obstructive pulmonary disease (COPD), 1010
  in congenital heart defects, 1098*t*
  defined, 965
  in heart failure, 1151
  in lung cancer, 108
  in metabolic alkalosis, 18
  in pneumonia, 591
  in pulmonary embolism, 1214
  in respiratory acidosis, 22
  in sepsis, 602
  in shock, 1227
  values classification, 966*t*
Arterial blood pressure, 1045
Arterial ulcers, 1200*t*
Arterial wall, elasticity of, 1063
Arteries, compliance of, 1044
Arteriosclerosis, 1045, 1198
Arteriovenous fistula, 385, 385*f*
Arthritis
  osteoarthritis. *See* osteoarthritis
  rheumatoid. *See* rheumatoid arthritis
  self-management, 505*t*
Arthrodesis, 501
Arthroplasty, 501, 871, 888
Arthroscopy, 888
Artificial airways
  endotracheal tubes, 983, 983*f*
  nasopharyngeal, 983, 983*f*
  oropharyngeal, 983, 983*f*
  tracheostomies, 984, 984*f*
  use of, 983
Artificial disc surgery, 843
Artificial insemination, 1388–1389
Artificial rupture of membranes, 2121
Artificial sweeteners, antepartum nutrition and, 2096
Artificial teeth, 428
Artificial urinary sphincter, 115, 115*f*
ARVC (arrhythmogenic right ventricular cardiomyopathy), 1077*t*, 1078
Ascending contrast venography, 1132
Ascites, 365, 782
ASD. *See* Autism spectrum disorder
ASD (atrial septal defect), 1084–1085*t*
Asepsis
  defined, 523
  medical, 523
  surgical, 523, 550*t*
ASKED model, 1640
ASPD (antisocial personality disorder), 1855, 1856*t*, 1863*t*
Asphyxia, 2209*t*
Aspiration pneumonia, 587–588
Aspirin, body acids and, 14
Aspirin therapy
  angina and, 1118
  diabetes mellitus and, 757
Assault, 2657
Assault and homicide
  age and, 1977
  aggravated, 1975
  aggression and, 1976
  assessment, 1980–1981
  care planning, 1981
  collaborative care, 1979–1980
  culture and, 1977
  defined, 1958*t*
  diagnosis, 1981

diagnostic tests, 1979
  etiology, 1976
  frustration and, 1976
  gunshot wounds and, 1981
  interventions, 1958*t*, 1981
  lifespan considerations, 1979
  mandatory reporting of, 2676
  manifestations, 1958*t*, 1978–1979, 1980*t*
  nonpharmacologic therapy, 1979–1980
  nurses, in the workplace, 1978*t*
  Nursing Care Plan, 1982*t*
  nursing process, 1980–1981
  occupation and, 1977–1978
  outcome evaluation, 1981
  overview of, 1975
  pathophysiology, 1975–1978
  pharmacologic therapy, 1979
  risk factors, 1976–1978
  simple, 1975
  socioeconomic factors, 1977
  warning signs of, 1978–1979
Assertive behavior, 1789
Assertive communication. *See also* Communication
  apology avoidance, 2412
  benefits of, 2412
  confidence, 2412
  defined, 2409
  expression with, 2409
  feedback reception, 2411–2412
  fogging, 2412
  "I" statement use, 2409, 2412
  negative assertion, 2412
  nonverbal communication management, 2412
  postconversation evaluation, 2412
  repetition, 2412
  style characteristics, 2411, 2411*t*
  techniques for, 2412–2413
  thinking before speaking, 2412
  use of, 2411–2413
Assertive communicators, 2411*t*
Assertive community treatment (ACT), 1619, 1619*t*
Assessment
  of adolescents, 2293
  client situations, 2277*t*
  communication and, 2284
  cultural factors in, 2284
  data collection
    examination, 2276–2282
    interviews, 2272–2276
    observation, 2271–2272
  data interpretation, 2282–2285
  data organization, 2282
  data validation, 2282
  defined, 2269
  developmental factors in, 2284
  developmental theories in, 2282
  environmental factors in, 2284–2285
  equipment, 2281, 2281*t*
  family factors in, 2284
  functional health patterns and body systems in, 2282
  growth and development instruments, 2291*t*
  holistic approach to, 2284
  incomplete, 2370
  of infants, 2290–2291
  interdisciplinary, 2685
  intradisciplinary, 2685

knowledge and, 2283
  Maslow's hierarchy of needs in, 2282
  of middle-aged adults, 2294
  nursing health history, 2273*t*
  nursing practice, 2285
  observation and, 2272*t*
  of older adults
    accuracy of health history, 2296–2297
    circumstances, 2294
    environment, 2296, 2298*t*
    functional evaluation, 2297
    instruments of evaluation, 2295–2296*t*
    lifestyle and health considerations, 2297
    minimum data set, 2297–2298
    social history, 2297
    underlying principles, 2294
  of preschoolers, 2292
  in prioritizing care, 2364, 2365*t*
  prioritizing care without, 2370
  psychological and emotional factors in, 2284
  relying solely on another's, 2370
  of school-age children, 2292–2293, 2293*f*
  sources of data, 2270–2271
  of toddlers, 2291–2292, 2292*f*
  types of, 2270*t*
  types of data, 2270
  of young adults, 2293–2294
Assessment of Preterm Infant Behavior (APIB), 2258–2259
Assignment
  defined, 2468
  patterns, 2470–2471
Assimilation, 1634, 1653
Assistance, nurse's need for, 2347
Assist-control mode ventilation (ACMV), 980, 981*t*
Assisted reproduction techniques
  genetic counseling referral and, 1390–1391
  illustrated, 1389*f*
  other, 1389–1390
  preimplantation genetic diagnosis, 1390
  therapeutic insemination, 1388–1389
  in vitro fertilization (IVF), 1389, 1389*f*
Assisted suicide, 176–177, 2574
Assistive devices
  for ambulation, 837–838, 837*t*
  osteoarthritis and, 889
  Parkinson disease and, 904
Associative play, 1665
Asterixis, 784
Asthma. *See also* Oxygenation
  in adolescents, 995*t*
  airway clearance and, 1002
  antepartum care and, 2078*t*
  anxiety relief and, 1002–1003
  assessment, 1001
  breathing pattern enhancement and, 1002
  bronchioles and, 992*f*
  care planning, 1001–1002
  in children, 991–992, 993, 996*t*, 1000*t*, 1003*t*
  collaborative care, 995–1001
  common causes of, 992*t*
  complementary and alternative therapy, 1001
  defined, 990
  diagnosis, 1001
  diagnostic tests, 995
  disease monitoring, 993
  education, 1003
  etiology, 991–992
  hyperresponsiveness, 991

hyperventilation, 991
interventions, 1002–1003
lifespan considerations, 996t, 1000, 1003t
management, 995t, 996t
manifestations, 993–995, 994t
medications, 998–999t
medications in children, 1000t
Nursing Care Plan, 1004t
nursing process, 1001–1003
outcome evaluation, 1003
overview of, 990
pathogenesis, 991f
pathophysiology and etiology, 990–993
pediatric differences, 991–992
pharmacologic therapy
    bronchodilators, 996–997, 997t
    corticosteroids, 997, 999t, 1000t
    leukotriene modifiers, 997–1001, 999t
    stepwise approach, 996, 996t
pregnancy and, 993–995
retractions, 992, 992f
risk factors, 992–993
status asthmaticus, 991
stepwise approach to, 996, 996t
therapeutic regime adherence and, 1003
total airway obstruction in children and, 1003t
triggers, 991
Asynclitism, 2116
Ataxia, 1584
Atelectasis, 574, 591, 963t, 1019t
Atheist, 1873
Atherosclerosis
    defined, 1106, 1198
    foot and leg care and, 1202t
    manifestations of, 1199t
ATN (acute tubular necrosis), 376, 377f
Atrial fibrillation
    as deep venous thrombosis risk factor, 1131
    defined, 1184
    ECG characteristics and management, 1181t
    manifestations, 1184
Atrial flutter, 1181t, 1184
Atrial gallop, 1034
Atrial kick, 1178
Atrial natriuretic factor (ANF), 340
Atrial natriuretic peptide (ANP), 370, 1151, 1164
Atrial septal defect (ASD), 1084–1085t
Atrioventricular (AV) canal (endocardial cushion defect), 1086
Atrioventricular (AV) conduction blocks, 1182t, 1186
Atrioventricular dissociation, 1186
Atrophy, 821
Attendance, 2492
Attention deficit disorder (ADD), 1680
Attention-deficit/hyperactivity disorder (ADHD)
    assessment, 1684
    behavior management plans, 1685
    behavioral therapy, 1684
    care planning, 1684
    collaborative care, 1681–1684
    complementary and alternative therapy, 1684t
    defined, 1675t, 1680
    diagnosis, 1684
    diagnostic tests, 1681–1682
    DSM-5 diagnostic criteria for, 1682t
    educational experience optimization, 1686t
    emotional support, 1685
    environmental distractions and, 1685, 1685f
    environmental modification, 1684

family education, 1686
healthcare visits and, 1681f
interventions, 1675t, 1684–1686
manifestations, 1675t, 1680–1681, 1681t
medications, 1683t
nonpharmacologic therapy, 1683–1684
Nursing Care Plan, 1687t
nursing process, 1684–1686
outcome evaluation, 1686
overview of, 1680
pathophysiology and etiology, 1680
pharmacologic therapy, 1682–1683
pharmacologic treatments, 1685
prevention of, 1680
risk factors, 1680
screening tests for, 1683t
self-esteem promotion, 1685
stigma, 1686t
Attentive listening
    blocks to, 2426
    defined, 2425
    phases of, 2426t
    posture of involvement, 2426f
Attitude, 2492–2493
Atypical antidepressants, 1793
Atypical antipsychotics
    for bipolar disorders, 1813
    for cognitive alterations, 1592t
    for schizophrenia, 1618t
Audiological testing, 579
Audiologists, 578
Audiometric testing, 611
Auditory stimuli, 1278
Audits, 2685
Aura, 716
Auscultation
    cardiac, 1062f, 1062t
    defined, 954, 2280
    direct, 2280
    duration, 2281
    indirect, 2280
    intensity, 2281
    in oxygenation assessment, 962
    pitch, 2280–2281
    quality, 2281
    renal arteries, 325f
Authoritarian parents, 1717
Authority
    in chain of command, 2549
    defined, 2468, 2549
    delegation and, 2468
    line, 2549
    manager, 2476
    staff, 2549–2550
Autism spectrum disorder (ASD)
    adults with, 1690t
    anticipatory guidance, 1693
    assessment, 1692–1693
    care planning, 1693
    collaborative care, 1690–1692
    communication, 1689
    communication enhancement, 1694
    community-based care, 1694
    complementary and alternative therapy, 1692, 1692t
    defined, 1675t, 1688
    diagnosis, 1693
    diagnostic tests, 1690
    DSM-5 diagnostic criteria for, 1691t
    environmental stimuli and, 1693

GFCF diet and, 1692t
Hispanics and, 1692t
injury prevention, 1693
interventions, 1675t, 1693–1694
lifespan considerations, 1690t
manifestations, 1675t, 1689–1690, 1690t
nonpharmacologic therapy, 1691–1692
nursing process, 1692–1694
outcome evaluation, 1694
overview of, 1688
pathophysiology and etiology, 1688–1689
pharmacologic therapy, 1691–1692
prevention of, 1689
risk factors, 1689
screening tests for, 1691t
supportive care, 1693–1694
Autoantibodies, 509, 510
Autocratic (authoritarian) leaders, 2489
Autografting, 1478
Autoimmune diseases, 767
Autoimmune disorders
    African Americans and, 448
    defined, 438, 495
    rheumatoid arthritis, 495–509
    types of, 446t
Autoinoculation, 1410
Autologous blood transfusions, 1270
Autologous bone marrow transplant, 97–98
Automated external defibrillator (AED), 1193, 1194f
Automatisms, 717t
Autonomic dysreflexia, 911, 912t
Autonomic reflexes, 689
Autonomy, 409, 1880, 2537, 2564, 2659t
Autosomal chromosomes, 1659
Autosomal dominant inheritance, 1376, 1376f
Autosomal recessive inheritance, 1376–1377, 1377f
Autosomes, 31, 1374
Avascular necrosis, 869
Avian influenza, 570
Avoidance coping, 1899
Avoidant personality disorder (APD), 1855, 1856t, 1863t
Avoidant/restrictive food intake disorder, 1836
Avolition, 1614
Avulsion fractures, 855t
Awareness
    defined, 1278
    sensory process requirements, 1278
Axial skeleton, 820
Axillary thermometers, 1428f
Axons, 876
Azotemia, 374

B
B cells, 441
Babinski reflex (response), 690, 2234, 2234f
Baby Boomers, 2494t
Bacille Calmette-Guérin (BCG) vaccine, 611
Bacilli, 606
Back, newborn assessment, 2232
Back problems
    body mechanics and pregnancy and, 841f
    body mechanics for lifting and, 841t
    causes, 825
    children and backpacks and, 840t

Back problems (*continued*)
  herniated disc, 824t, 840–845
  overview of, 839–840
  scoliosis, 824t, 825f, 845–852
Backache, relief in pregnancy, 2066
Background questions, 2588
Baclofen (Lioresal), 880
Bacteremia, 523, 600
Bacteria
  antibiotic-resistant, 531–532
  defined, 523
  pathogenic organisms, 530t
Bacterial conjunctivitis, 566f
Bactericidal agents, 544
Bacteriostatic agents, 544
Bagging, 546–548
Ballard gestational age assessment
  defined, 2213
  neuromuscular characteristics, 2215t
  New Ballard Score, 2213
  physical characteristics, 2214–2215t
Balloon catheters, 2129
Balloon tamponade, 788
Ballottement, 2035
Ballottement test, 834f, 834t
BAM (becoming a mother), 1818
Barium swallow, 220, 220f, 228
Barlow maneuver, 2232
Barotrauma, 982
Barrel chest, 1009
Barthel Index of Activities of Daily Living,
    2295t
Bartholin glands, 1360f
Barton, Clara, 2547
Basal body temperature (BBT),
    1378, 1378f
Basal cell cancer, 129–130, 130f, 130t
Basal metabolic rate (BMR), 790, 1422
Base excess (BE), 6
Baseline rate, 2149
Bases
  defined, 3
  as weak, 4
Basic life support, 1193, 1194f
Basophils, 440
BAT (brown adipose tissue), 1438
Bathing, antepartum care and, 2072
Battery, 2657
BBT (basal body temperature),
    1378, 1378f
B-DAST (Brief Drug Abuse Screening
    Test), 1569
Bearing down, 2118
Becoming a mother (BAM), 1818
BED. *See* Binge-eating disorder
Bee sting kit, 491
Behavior
  aggressive, 1789
  assertive, 1789
  newborn assessment, 2235, 2236f
  passive, 1789
Behavior management
  attention-deficit/hyperactivity disorder
    (ADHD) and, 1685
  in constipation, 310–311
  family and, 1718
  in obesity, 794
Behavior modification, 2522
Behavioral states, premature newborns and,
    2251–2252

Behavioral therapy
  attention-deficit/hyperactivity disorder (ADHD)
    and, 1684
  contingency contracts and, 1529–1530
  defined, 1529
  extinction and, 1529
  punishment and, 1529
  reinforcement, 1529
  token economies and, 1530
Behaviorism, 1654
Behaviorist theory, 2502
Belief system, 1632
Beliefs
  core, differences in, 1633, 1633t
  cultural, 1630–1637
  defined, 2564
Belonging and love, in self-care in nursing,
    2308–2310
Belt restraints, 2704, 2706f
Belviq, 794
Benchmarking, 2684, 2686
Beneficence, 1880, 2567
Benign neoplasms, 42, 43t, 53t
Benign prostatic hyperplasia (BPH)
  agents for, 287t
  assessment, 288
  care planning, 288
  catheters and drainage bag care and, 290t
  collaborative care, 285
  defined, 284
  diagnosis, 288
  digital rectal exam (DRE) and, 285, 286f
  illustrated, 285f
  interventions, 288–290
  manifestations, 285, 287
  nonpharmacologic therapy, 287
  Nursing Care Plan, 291t
  nursing process, 288–290
  outcome evaluation, 290
  outcomes, 290
  overview of, 284
  pathophysiology and etiology, 284–285
  pharmacologic therapy, 286–287
  postoperative care, 289–290
  preoperative care, 288–289
  prostate-specific antigen (PSA) test and, 285
  risk factors, 285
  surgery, 286, 286f
  surgery discharge instructions, 290t
Benner and Wrubel's theory of caring,
    2303–2304
Benner's skill acquisition model, 2325, 2325f
Benzodiazepines
  for disorders of anxiety, stress, or trauma,
    1916t
  for substance abuse, 1566t
Bereavement, 1742
Berg Balance Test or Single Leg Stance Test,
    2296t
Berstein test, 228
Best practice standards, 2587–2588
Beta interferons, 880
Beta-adrenergic blocking agents,
    1171t, 1322t
Beta-amyloid, 1595
Beta-blockers, 1118, 1153, 1189t, 1916t
Bias, 1635
Bicarbonate (HCO₃)
  carbonic acid ratio, 4f
  excess, from antacid ingestion, 18

function, 342, 342t
regulation, 342f
as replacement anion, 17
Bidirectional influence, 1613
Bile acid sequestrants, 1117t
Bilevel positive air pressure (BiPAP),
    198, 199t, 979
Bilevel ventilation (BiPAP), 980
Biliary cirrhosis, 782
Biliary colic, 650
Bilirubin
  conjugation of, 2197–2198
  levels, 651t, 785
  newborns and, 2199
Billings method, 1379
Binge drinking, 1521, 1535
Binge eating, 1846
Binge-eating disorder (BED)
  characteristics of, 1838t
  defined, 1844, 1848
  diagnostic tests for, 1849
  manifestations, 1848t
  nonpharmacologic therapy, 1849
  thermoregulation, 1848t
Binuclear family, 1711
Bioelectrical impedance, 793
Bioethical issues
  AIDS, 2572
  end-of-life, 2573–2574
  genetic testing, 2572–2573, 2573t
  organ transplantation, 2573
Bioethics, 1878
Biofeedback, constipation and, 311
Biogenic stressors, 1897
Biohazard alert, 545f
Bioidentical hormones, 1396
Biological factors, in addiction, 1520
Biological response modifiers, 40t
Biological rhythms, 432t, 1780–1781
Biological therapy, in leukemia, 99
Biological threat infections, 532
Biological variations, 1639, 1639f
Biomedical informatics, 2631
Biophysical profile, 2087–2088, 2088t
Biopsies
  breast, 78–79, 78f
  kidney, 395, 514, 672
  liver, 785
  skin, 1456
Bioterrorism
  defined, 2614
  pathogens, 2615–2616t
BiPAP (bilevel positive air pressure), 198,
    199t, 979, 980
Biparietal diameter (BPD), 2054
Bipolar disorders
  assessment, 1813
  bipolar I disorder, 1809, 1810t
  bipolar II disorder, 1809
  care planning, 1813
  classifications of, 1779
  collaborative care, 1812–1813
  defined, 1779, 1780t, 1809
  diagnosis, 1813
  diagnostic tests, 1812
  DSM-5 diagnostic criteria for, 1810t
  hypomanic episodes, 1810t
  interventions
    limit setting, 1815
    overview of, 1813

reality-based thinking promotion, 1814
    rest and sleep enhancement, 1815
    safety, 1814
    self-care promotion, 1815
    socialization, 1814
lithium therapy, 1793
major depressive disorder (MDD)
        comparison, 1811*f*
major depressive episodes, 1810*t*
manic episodes, 1809, 1810*t*, 1811*f*
manifestations
    cyclothymic disorder, 1811
    depressive episodes, 1809–1811
    lifespan considerations, 1811
    mania and hypomania, 1809
    mixed features, 1779, 1811
    rapid cycling, 1779, 1811
    therapies and, 1812*t*
nurse reactions and, 1814*t*
Nursing Care Plan, 1815–1816*t*
nursing process, 1813–1815
outcome evaluation, 1815
overview of, 1809
pathophysiology and etiology, 1809
pharmacologic therapy, 1793,
        1812–1813
prevalence of, 1783
therapies, 1780*t*
Birth. *See also* Intrapartum care
    adolescent support during, 2168–2170
    adolescents and, 2168*t*
    assisting during, 2165–2166
    Cesarean, 2131–2135
    cord blood analysis at, 2156
    crowning, 2123
    factors associated with positive
            experience, 2119*t*
    factors important to, 2114–2119
    fetus and, 2114–2117
    forceps-assisted, 2130, 2131
    maternal adaptations following, 2167*t*
    passage, 2114
    precipitous, 2137*t*
    psychosocial considerations, 2118–2119
    sequence, 2124
    spiritual beliefs related to, 1877
    spontaneous, 2124
    stages of, 2122–2126
    vaginal, after Cesarean, 2135–2136
Birth control pills, 1383–1384
Birthing positions, 2166
Birthing rooms, 2113
Birthmarks, 2224
Bishop scoring system, 2128*t*
Bismuth compounds, 680
Bisphosphonates, 738*t*, 802*t*
Bivalving, 866, 867*f*
Black cohosh, 1397*t*
Blackouts, 1538
Bladder diary, 294
Bladder incontinence and retention. *See also*
        Elimination
    assessment, 299–300
    diagnosis, 300
    effective urination and, 300–301
    home care, 302
    independence and, 304
    manifestations, 299*t*
    normal voiding patterns and, 300, 301*t*
    nursing process, 299–304

outcome evaluation, 304
    overview of, 292
    skin integrity and, 302
    social isolation and, 302
    toileting assistance and, 301–302
    urinary incontinence, 292–297
    urinary retention, 297–305
Bladder training, 295
Bladder ultrasound, 623
Blalock-Taussig shunt, 1099*t*
Blame-free environment, 2688–2689
Blastocyst, 2021
Bleeding
    leukemia and, 101
    in liver disease, 787
    time, 1252*t*
Blended families, 1710–1711
Blepharism, 1316
Blighted ovum, 1768
Blindness, cultural background and, 1307*t*
Blood
    desaturated, 1046
    viscosity, 1045
Blood alcohol levels (BALs), 1536, 1961
Blood flow, 1163
Blood glucose
    burn injuries and, 1477
    goals for type 1 DM in children, 770*t*
    high, 741*f*
    homeostasis, 704
    low, 741*f*
    maintaining during hospitalization, 755
    meter performance, 753
    monitoring, 752–753
    as perioperative diagnostic test, 1253*t*
    regulation by insulin and glucagon, 741*f*
    self-monitoring, 752–753, 752*f*
    sucrose and, 757
Blood glucose monitors, 752, 752*f*
Blood hemoglobin, 1228–1229*t*
Blood loss anemia, 65–66
Blood pressure. *See also* Hypertension
    arterial, 1045
    assessment
        common errors in, 1066–1067
        equipment, 1064–1065, 1065*f*
        error sources in, 1068*t*
        at home, 1068*t*
        Korotkoff sounds and, 1066, 1066*f*, 1067*t*
        lifespan considerations, 1067*t*
        methods, 1066
        sites for, 1066
    classifications of, 1163*t*
    defined, 1163
    determinants of, 1045
    diastolic, 1045, 1163
    factors affecting, 1045–1046, 1163–1165, 1164*f*
    hypotension and, 1067–1068
    labor and, 2126
    pathophysiology, 1163–1167
    systolic, 1045, 1163
Blood pressure cuff and bulb, 1065*f*
Blood pressure equipment, 548
Blood pressure monitors, 1065, 1066*f*
Blood tests
    for multiple sclerosis, 880
    for musculoskeletal disorders, 835*t*
Blood transfusions
    administration of, 1270
    as anemia treatment, 70

culture and, 180
    Jehovah's Witnesses and, 399*t*
    in perioperative care, 1270
Blood type and crossmatch, 489
Blood urea nitrogen (BUN)
    in acute renal failure (ARF), 380
    in chronic kidney disease (CKD),
            391*f*, 395
    in nephritis, 672
    in sepsis, 602
    in shock, 1227
Blood values, in postpartum care,
            2175–2176
Blood volume
    in children, 1218*t*
    decreased and increased, 1045
    pregnancy and, 1047
Bloodborne pathogens, 545
Bloody show, 2121
Blunt trauma, 1312, 1313*t*, 1316, 1956
BMI. *See* Body mass index
BMR (basal metabolic rate), 790, 1422
BMT. *See* Bone marrow transplant
BN. *See* Bulimia nervosa
BNP (brain natriuretic peptide),
            1151, 1164
Boards of nursing (BONs), 2664
Body area reservoirs, 524*t*
Body fluids. *See also* Fluid volume deficit (FVD);
            Fluid volume excess (FVE)
    active transport, 338, 339*f*
    compartments, 336, 336*f*
    diffusion, 338, 338*f*
    distribution and composition of,
            336–337
    electrolyte composition of, 336*f*
    electrolyte concentration in
            compartments, 337*f*
    extracellular fluid (ECF), 336–337
    filtration, 338, 338*f*
    fluid intake and, 339, 339*f*, 339*t*,
            348–351
    fluid output and, 339–340, 341*f*,
            348–351
    homeostasis, 340, 341*f*
    intracellular fluid (ICF), 336
    intravascular fluid, 336
    movement of, 337–339
    osmosis, 337–338, 337*f*
    regulating, 339–341
    transcellular fluid, 336
Body image
    breast cancer and, 83
    cancer and, 62–63, 62*t*
    defined, 1345, 1833*f*
    elements of, 1833*t*
    ideal, 1833
    infertility and, 1392
    inflammatory bowel disease (IBD) and,
            666–667
    menopause and, 1398
    rheumatoid arthritis and, 507
Body mass index (BMI)
    calculations, 942*t*
    defined, 219, 791–792
    as diagnostic test for obesity, 793
    in obesity/overweight classification, 792*f*
    ranges for adults, 942*t*
    ranges for children and teens, 942*t*
Body of knowledge, 2536

Body pressure areas
  illustrated, 1499f
  mechanical devices for reducing, 1495t
  palpating, 1500
Body substation isolation (BSI), 545
Body surface area, 343
Body temperature. *See also* Thermoregulation
  alterations, 1423–1426, 1423f, 1424t
  assessment, 1427–1429
  average, 1422
  in children, 1428t
  client teaching in taking, 1429t
  defined, 1421
  heat balance and, 1422, 1422f
  hyperthermia. *See* hyperthermia
  hypothermia. *See* hypothermia
  in infants, 1428t
  lifespan considerations, 1428t
  measurement sites, 1427t
  in newborn assessment, 2223
  normothermia, 1423
  in older adults, 1428t
  prevalence of alterations, 1424
  regulation in newborns, 2196
  shock effect on, 1222
Bone marrow
  defined, 443–444
  examination, 97
Bone marrow transplant (BMT)
  allogeneic, 97, 98f
  autologous, 97–98
  defined, 97
Bone remodeling, 820–821
Bones
  growth stimulators, 838t
  healing, 857t
  in older adults, 821–822
  remodeling, 820–821
BONs (boards of nursing), 2664
Bony pelvis
  bone structure, 2012–2213, 2012f
  pelvic division, 2013–2014, 2014f
  pelvic floor, 2013, 2013f
  pelvis types, 2014–2015, 2016f
Borborygmus, 280
Borderline personality disorder (BPD)
  defined, 1855
  DSM-5 diagnostic criteria for, 1858t
  manifestations and therapies, 1863t
  self-mutilating behavior and, 1856f
  signma, overcoming, 1857t
  splitting, 1857
  traits, 1856t
Botanicals, for menopause, 1396, 1397t
Bottom-up sampling, 1783, 1783f
Botulism, 2615t
Bouchard nodes, 886
Boundaries
  clear, 1714
  defined, 1714, 1865
  diffuse, 1715
  family and, 1524, 1714–1715
  professional, in nursing, 1865, 1866t
  rigid, 1714
  as social construction, 1715
Boutonnière deformities, 505
Bowel cancer, 277t
Bowel elimination
  activity and, 274
  alterations and therapies

bowel cancer, 277t
bowel incontinence, 276–278, 277t
constipation, 276, 277t
diarrhea, 276, 277t
flatulence, 276
impaction, 277t
obstruction, 277t
  anesthesia and, 274
  assessment, 278–279, 280–282t
  assessment interview, 279t
  collaborative interventions and therapies, 282
  defecation habits and, 274
  diagnostic procedures and, 274
  diagnostic tests, 279
  diet and, 273–274
  digital examination, 278, 279f
  factors affecting, 273–274
  fluid and, 274
  genetic and lifespan considerations, 274–276
  independent interventions and therapies, 282
  interventions and therapies, 282, 283t
  lifespan and cultural considerations, 279
  manifestations, 314t
  medications and, 274, 283t
  modifiable risk factors, 278
  in newborns and infants, 274–275, 275f
  normal, 273–276
  in older adults, 275
  pain and, 274
  pathological conditions and, 274
  in pregnant women, 275–276
  prevention of, 278
  psychological factors, 274
  in school-age children and adolescents, 275
  screening, 278
  stroke and, 1245
  in toddlers, 275
Bowel incontinence, constipation, and impaction
  constipation, 305–311
  fecal incontinence, 311–318
  overview of, 305
Bowel training programs, 316
Boykin and Schoenhofer's caring theory, 2302–2303
BPD. *See* Borderline personality disorder
BPD (biparietal diameter), 2054
BPH. *See* Benign prostatic hyperplasia
Brachial pulse, 1063f, 1064
Brachytherapy, 109
Braden Scale for Predicating Pressure Sore Risk, 1500–1502, 1501t, 2295t
Bradycardia
  defined, 1063
  fetal, 2151
Bradydysrhythmia, 1112
Bradykinesia, 825t, 895, 897
Bradypnea, 959, 960t
Brain
  brainstem, 689
  cerebellum, 688
  cerebrospinal fluid (CSF), 688, 688f
  cerebrum, 688, 688f, 1576
  diencephalon, 689
  function deterioration progression, 691f
  hemispheres, 1576
  hippocampus, 1576

limbic system, 1576
lobes, 1576
neurons, 1576
neurotransmitters, 1576
regions of, 688f
ventricles, 689
Brain death, 694
Brain natriuretic peptide (BNP), 1151, 1164
Brainstem, 689
Brainstorming, 2420
Braxton Hicks contractions, 2025, 2121
Brazelton Neonatal Behavioral Assessment Scale, 2235
Breach of care, 2687
Breach of duty, 2656, 2687
Breakthrough pain, 156
Breast cancer. *See also* Cancer
  African American women with, 80f
  assessment, 81
  biopsies, 78–79, 78f
  body image and, 83
  circulation and, 82
  collaborative care, 78–81
  defined, 76
  diagnosis, 81
  diagnostic tests, 78–79, 78f
  infection prevention, 82
  interventions, 82–83
  manifestations, 78, 81t
  metastasis and, 76
  Nursing Care Plan, 84t
  nursing process, 81–83
  older women with, 77
  outcome evaluation, 83
  overview of, 76
  pathophysiology and etiology, 77
  pharmacologic therapies, 79–81
  prevention, 78
  psychosocial well-being and, 82–83
  radiation therapy, 81
  reconstructive surgery and, 83
  risk factors, 77
  screening guidelines, 58t
  signs and symptoms of, 78t
  staging of, 76, 77t
  treatment goals, 82
Breast milk jaundice, 2199
Breast reconstruction, 79, 80f
Breastfeeding
  to control procedural pain, 2242t
  jaundice, 2199
  lactogenesis, 2173–2174
  milk, 2174
  nutritional care of mothers, 2177
Breasts
  antepartum care and, 2068, 2068f
  assessment
    female, 1358–1359t, 1358f
    male, 1356t
  in gestational age, 2216, 2217f
  hypertrophy, 2228f
  in postpartum assessment, 2179t
  postpartum changes, 2173–2174
  pregnancy and, 2030
  Tanner stages for, 1341f
Breath sounds, 963t
Breathing. *See also* Oxygenation; Respiratory system
  abdominal, 2163
  deep, 968

exercises, 150
in labor, 2163–2164
pattern, enhancing, 1014, 1022
pattern, promoting, 1002
periodic, 2194
pursed-lip, 1009
shallow, 2163
Breckinridge, Mary, 2548
Breech presentations, 2115
Bregma, 2114
Brief Drug Abuse Screening Test
    (B-DAST), 1569
Bright light therapy, 198
Brock procedure, 1099t
Bronchiectasis, 588
Bronchioles, 992f
Bronchiolitis, 1018. *See also* Respiratory syncytial
    virus (RSV)/bronchiolitis
Bronchitis, 1006, 1006f
Bronchodilators, 996–997, 997t
Bronchogenic carcinomas, 104
Bronchopneumonia, 585
Bronchopulmonary dysplasia, 2254
Bronchoscopy
    defined, 966
    in lung cancer, 108
Bronchovesicular sound, 954–955
Brow presentation, 2115, 2115f
Brown adipose tissue (BAT), 1438
Brown-Sequard syndrome, 910t
Brudzinski sign assessment, 705f, 705t
Bruises, 827, 1454t
Bruits, 280
BSI (body substation isolation), 545
Buddhism, 1886, 1886t
Budget and finance, 2645–2646
Buffer base capacity, 6
Buffer systems, 4–6
Buffers, 4
Bulimia nervosa (BN)
    behaviors associated with, 1847–1848
    binge eating, 1846
    characteristics of, 1838t
    defined, 1844, 1846
    diagnostic tests for, 1849
    indicators, 1847
    manifestations, 1848t
    nonpharmacologic therapy, 1849
    purging, 1846–1847
    therapies, 1848t
    as underdiagnosed, 1847
Bullying, 2484t
BUN. *See* Blood urea nitrogen (BUN)
Bunions, 826, 827f
Bureaucratic leaders, 2490
Burn contracture, 1468, 1468f
Burn shock, 1471
Burnout
    defined, 1907, 2488
    high risk for, 2488
    recognizing and preventing, 2309t
    stress management and, 2488
Burns
    assessment
        as continuous, 1480
        information gathering guidelines, 1480
        Lund and Browder chart, 1469f
    autografting and, 1478
    care of, 1486t
    care planning, 1482

characteristics by depth of thermal
    injury, 1467f
chemical, 1465, 1465f
children and, 1466t, 1482t, 1485t
classification
    American Burn Association, 1469t
    depth, 1467–1468, 1467f, 1468f
    extent, 1468–1469, 1469f
    full-thickness, 1468, 1468f
    partial-thickness, 1467–1468, 1468f
    rule of nines, 1468–1469, 1469f
    superficial, 1467
client teaching, 1486t
collaborative care, 1473–1480
defined, 1464
diagnosis, 1481
diagnostic tests, 1477
ebb phase, 1473
electrical, 1465
escharotomy and, 1477–1478, 1477f
etiology, 1465
eye injuries, 1312, 1313t, 1315–1316
flow phase, 1473
interventions
    empowerment facilitation, 1484–1485
    fluid volume balance, 1482
    infection prevention, 1484
    nutrition, 1484
    pain management, 1482–1483
    physical mobility maintenance, 1484
    skin integrity protection, 1483–1484
    in stages of injury, 1485t
lifespan considerations, 1466t, 1473,
    1482t, 1483t, 1485t
manifestations, 1467–1473, 1481t
minor, 1473
nonpharmacologic therapy, 1479–1480
Nursing Care Plan, 1486–1487t
nursing process, 1480–1485
nutritional support and, 1480
in older adults, 1483t
outcome evaluation, 1485
overview of, 1464
pathophysiology, 1464–1467
pharmacologic therapy, 1478–1479
prevention of, 1466–1467, 1466t
radiation, 1465
recovery from, 1485t
risk factors, 1466
surface appearance, 1472
surgery, 1477–1478
surgical debridement and, 1478
systemic effects
    cardiac rhythm alterations, 1471
    cardiovascular system, 1471
    gastrointestinal system, 1472
    hypovolemic shock (burn shock), 1471
    immune system, 1472–1473
    integumentary system, 1472
    on major body systems, 1470f
    metabolism, 1473
    peripheral vascular compromise, 1471
    respiratory system, 1470–1471
    urinary system, 1472
thermal, 1464–1465, 1464f
treatment
    acute stage, 1474
    airway and ventilatory management, 1476
    circulatory support and fluid resuscitation,
        1476–1477

debridement, 1473
emergent and acute care, 1475–1476
emergent/resuscitative stage, 1474
litargirio use and, 1473t
minor burns, 1473
prehospital client management
    and, 1475t
progression through healthcare
    system, 1474f
rehabilitative stage, 1474–1475
severe burns, 1473–1475
stop burning process, 1475t
vital function support, 1475t
types of, 1464–1465
wound healing
    inflammation, 1469–1470
    proliferation, 1470
    remodeling, 1470
wound management
    biological dressings, 1479–1480
    debridement, 1479
    dressing, 1479
    goal of care, 1479
    heterograft (xenograft), 1479
    homograft (allograft), 1479
    with vacuum-assisted closure (VAC)
        device, 1480
Bursitis, 826

C
C. difficile, 532, 543
C peptide, 769
CABG (coronary artery bypass grafting),
    1121–1122, 1121f, 1122f
Cachexia, 48, 48f, 81t
CAD. *See* Coronary artery disease
Caffeine
    defined, 1562
    pregnancy and, 1552
    substance abuse, 1562
Caffeine halothane contracture test (CHCT), 1426
CAGE questionnaire, 1540
Calcium (Ca^{2+})
    electrolyte imbalance, 372
    function in the body, 930
    hypercalcemia and, 372
    hypocalcemia and, 372, 378, 379
    locations in the body, 341
    osteoporosis and, 800
    regulation and function, 342t
    sources of, 341
Calcium oxalate, 319
Calcium phosphate, 319
Calcium-channel blockers, 1075t, 1118,
    1171t, 1189t
Calculi
    defined, 271
    urinary, 318–332
Calendar rhythm method, 1378
CAM (Confusion Assessment Method),
    1587t, 1607
Cancer
    alterations and therapies, 33t
    assessment, 57–58
    assessment interview, 57t
    breast. *See* breast cancer
    care planning, 58–59
    causative agents, 45
    cellular mutation, 45

Cancer (*continued*)
cervical. *See* cervical cancer
children and adolescents and, 50–51, 62*t*
collaborative care, 52–57
colorectal. *See* colorectal cancer
cultural diversity and, 42, 51
defined, 41
diagnosis, 58
diagnostic tests
cytological examination, 53–54
direct visualization, 55–56
grading and staging, 53, 53*t*
laboratory tests, 56
oncological imaging, 55
ectopic functioning indicators, 59*t*
etiology, 45
genetics and, 34
hair loss and, 62*t*
hematological emergencies, 49–50
immune system response, 44–45
interventions
body image, 62–63
coping, 61–62
grief responses, 63
infection prevention, 59
injury prevention, 59–60
nutrition, 60–61
tissue integrity, 61
leukemia. *See* leukemia
lung. *See* lung cancer
malignant cells, 43, 43*t*
malignant neoplasms as, 42–44
manifestations
anorexia-cachexia syndrome, 48, 48*f*
disruption of function, 47
hematological alterations, 47
hemorrhage, 48
infection, 48
lifespan and cultural considerations, 50–51
oncological emergencies, 49
pain, 48–49
paraneoplastic syndromes, 48
psychological stress, 49
therapies, 52*t*
metabolic emergencies, 49
metastasis, 44
nursing process, 57–64
oncogenes, 45
outcome evaluation, 63
overview of, 41–42
pathophysiology, 42–47
pediatric, 38–39, 38*f*
pharmacologic therapy, 56
pregnancy and, 51
prevalence, 34
prevention, 45–47
prostate. *See* prostate cancer
radiation therapy, 56–57
risk factors, 34, 45–47
screening guidelines, 58*t*
screenings, 36
secondary, 51
skin. *See* skin cancer
space-occupying lesion emergencies, 50
surgery, 56
tissue integrity and, 61*t*
tumor invasion, 43
tumor suppressor genes, 45
viral etiology association, 45*t*
when to call for help, 60*t*

Candidiasis, 463
Cannabinoids, 223
Cannabis sativa, 1563
Capacitation, 2021
Caput succedaneum, 2225–2226, 2226*f*
Carbohydrate metabolism, in newborns, 2197
Carbohydrates, 927–929, 928*f*, 938*t*
Carbon dioxide, 4
Carbon dioxide narcosis, 21
Carbonic acid, 4
Carbonic anhydrase inhibitors, 1315*t*, 1322*t*
Carboxyhemoglobin measurement, 1477
Carcinogenesis, 45
Carcinogens, 45
Cardiac arrest, 1192
Cardiac catheterization, 1097*t*
Cardiac changes, age-related, 1051*t*
Cardiac cycle
defined, 1040
illustrated, 1041*t*
Cardiac disease
antepartum care and, 2078*t*
postpartum care and, 2050–2051
pregnancy and
antepartum period, 2050
clinical therapy, 2049–2051
congenital heart defects, 2048–2049
drug therapy, 2049–2050
intrapartum period, 2050
labor and childbirth, 2050
Marfan syndrome, 2049
mitral valve prolapse (MVP), 2049
peripartum cardiomyopathy, 2049
postpartum period, 2050–2051
statistics, 1051
as stroke risk factor, 1236
Cardiac functioning
developmental aspects of, 1046
oxygenation and, 1046
Cardiac glycosides, 1075*t*
Cardiac index, 1042
Cardiac mapping, 1192
Cardiac markers, 1114, 1114*t*
Cardiac monitoring
continuous, 1187
home, 1187–1188
indications for, 1187*t*
Cardiac output
afterload and, 1042
average, 1041
blood flow, 1041*f*
clinical indicators of, 1042
contractility and, 1042
defined, 1040, 1218
determination factors, 1041
heart rate and, 1042
preload and, 1042
pulmonary embolism and, 1215
Cardiac output monitoring
in acute respiratory distress syndrome
(ARDS), 986
in cardiomyopathy, 1081
in dysrhythmias, 1195–1196
in heart failure, 1159
in hyperthyroidism, 810
in hypothyroidism, 815
in shock, 1231, 1231*f*
Cardiac rehabilitation, 1123, 1128*t*
Cardiac reserve, 1041
Cardiac rhythm, burn injuries and, 1471

Cardiac status monitoring, 492–493
Cardiac tamponade, 1157
Cardiac transplantation, 1157–1158, 1157*f*
Cardinal movements, 2125
Cardiogenic shock
acute myocardial infarction (AMI)
and, 1113
assessment, 1230
defined, 1053*t*, 1223–1224
interventions and therapies, 1053*t*
manifestations, 1053*t*, 1225–1226*t*
Cardiomyopathy
activity monitoring and, 1082
arrhythmogenic right ventricular (ARVC),
1077*t*, 1078
assessment, 1081
cardiac output monitoring and, 1081
care planning, 1081
classifications of, 1077*t*
client teaching, 1082*t*
collaborative care, 1079–1080
defined, 1052*t*, 1076
diagnosis, 1081
diagnostic tests, 1079
dilated, 1077–1078, 1077*t*
etiology, 1078–1079
fluid volume balance and, 1081–1082
hypertrophic, 1077*t*, 1078
interventions, 1052*t*, 1081–1082
low-sodium diet and, 1082
manifestations, 1052*t*, 1079, 1080*t*
nursing process, 1080–1082
outcome evaluation, 1082
overview of, 1076
pathophysiology, 1077–1079
peripartum, 1078
pharmacologic therapy, 1079–1080
restrictive, 1077*t*, 1078
risk factors, 1079
surgery, 1080
Cardiopulmonary function, in newborns, 2239
Cardiopulmonary physiology, 2193
Cardiopulmonary resuscitation (CPR)
defined, 1193
DNRs and, 182
end-of-life care and, 181
safety and, 181
withholding of, 176
Cardiorespiratory function
anemia and, 73
lung cancer and, 109–110
Cardiovascular function, 911
Cardiovascular illnesses
of adulthood, 1049–1051
of aging, 1051, 1051*t*
Cardiovascular system
aging and, 1048, 1048*f*
assessment
apical impulse, 1056–1058*t*
blood pressure, 1064–1070
cardiac rate and rhythm, 1059*t*
heart sounds, 1059–1061*t*
inspection, 1055–1056, 1056*f*
interview, 1068–1070, 1069*t*
landmarks for, 1055, 1055*f*
murmur, 1061–1062*t*
pulse, 1062–1064, 1063*f*, 1064*t*, 1065*t*
burn injuries and, 1471
changes and infection, 525
diagnostic tests, 1070

disseminated intravascular coagulation (DIC)
    and, 1141*t*
electrocardiogram and, 1071–1073*t*
exercise benefits, 422
labor and, 2126
mechanical ventilation and, 982
physical assessment hints, 1056*t*
postpartum changes, 2176
in pregnancy, 1046–1047
pregnancy changes, 2030–2031
premature newborns and, 2250
shock effect on, 1220
spinal cord injuries (SCI) and, 911–912
Care coordination
    barriers, 2461
    collaboration and, 2460
    concept of, 2460
    defined, 2460
    importance of, 2460
    nurse's role, 2460–2461
    nursing interventions to counter barriers,
        2461–2462
    overview of, 2460
    in prevention of remissions, 2461
    problem identification, 2461
Care maps, 2384
Care plan conference, 2452
Career development strategies, 2525*t*
Caregivers
    Alzheimer disease (AD), 1602–1603, 1602*t*
    caring for, 2308–2311
    of HIV/AIDS infants at risk, 462*t*
    otitis media, 582
    sickle cell disease, 126
Caretakers, abuse or neglect by, 2674, 2674*t*
Caring
    for the caregiver, 2308–2311
    defined, 2301
    for the dying, 2544
    encounters, 2306–2308
    knowledge and, 2305–2306, 2305*f*
    nursing theories of, 2302–2307
    six C's of, 2302*t*
Caring interventions
    Benner and Wrubel's theory, 2303–2304
    Boykin and Schoenhofer's theory,
        2302–2303
    carative factor to clinical caritas processes,
        2303*t*
    compassion and, 2307
    competence and, 2307
    concept of, 2301
    concepts related to, 2304–2305
    empowerment and, 2307
    integrating concept of, 2304
    knowledge and caring, 2305–2306, 2305*f*
    Leininger's theory, 2302
    nursing presence and, 2306–2307, 2307*f*
    nursing theories of caring, 2302–2307
    Roach's theory, 2302
    self-care in nursing, 2308–2311
    Watson's theory, 2303
Caring practice, 2301
Carotid pulse, 1063, 1063*f*
Carpal spasm, 737*t*
Carpal tunnel syndrome, 826, 826*f*
Carphologia, 1584
Carrier state, 529
Carriers, 524, 1376
Cartilage, 820

Case management
    in care framework, 2599
    computer-based client records, 2648–2649
    critical pathways, 2382, 2384–2386
    defined, 2382, 2457
    documentation, 2445
    implementation elements, 2383
    in managing care, 2457
    model, 2382
    nurse as case manager, 2382–2383
    overview of, 2382
    requirements, 2383
Case managers
    defined, 2648
    nurse as, 2382–2383
    responsibilities of, 2382*t*
Case method, 2458
Case study, 2588
Caseation necrosis, 606
Case-controlled study, 2589
Casts. *See also* Fractures
    bivalving, 866, 867*f*
    defined, 860
    fiberglass, 862
    home care, 862*t*
    types of, 861*f*
Catabolism, 387
Cataracts
    assessment, 1309
    care planning, 1309
    in children, 1306*t*
    collaborative care, 1308–1309
    complementary and alternative therapy, 1309
    congenital, 1307
    decision-making facilitation and, 1309–1310
    defined, 1306
    diagnosis, 1309
    diagnostic tests, 1308
    injury prevention and, 1309
    interventions, 1281*t*, 1309–1310
    manifestations, 1281*t*, 1307, 1307*t*
    nonpharmacologic therapy, 1309
    Nursing Care Plan, 1325–1326*t*
    nursing process, 1309–1310
    outcome evaluation, 1310
    overview of, 1306
    pathophysiology and etiology, 1306–1307
    radiation, 1307
    risk factors, 1307
    secondary, 1307
    self-care, 1310
    surgery, 1308–1309
    traumatic injuries, 1307
    wellness promotion and, 1310
Catatonia, 1614
Categorization, 2505
Catheter ablation, 1192
Catheterization, 297
Catheter-related bloodstream infections
    (CRBIs), 2704
Catheters
    care and infection prevention, 296*t*
    caring for, 290*t*
    central, potential complications, 1152*t*
    flow-directed, 1152*f*
    suction, 969, 969*f*
    Swan-Ganz, 984, 985
    thoracic, 973
    TURP postoperative care, 289, 290
    urinary tract infections (UTIs) and, 623

Cations, 336
Cauda equina syndrome (CES), 841
Causation, 2656
Cavitation, 606
CBE (charting by exception), 2443, 2444*f*
CBT. *See* Cognitive-behavioral therapy
CCNE (Commission on Collegiate Nursing
    Education), 2625
CCP (cyclic citrullinated peptide), 501
CD4 cell count, 468
CDC (HICPAC) isolation precautions,
    545–546
CDHP (consumer-driven healthcare
    plan), 2628
CDIs (Clostridium difficile-associated
    infections), 2706
Ceiling effect, 163
Celiac disease. *See also* Malabsorption disorders
    assessment, 241
    as chronic condition, 242
    client teaching, 242*t*
    collaborative care, 241
    defined, 240, 771
    diagnosis, 241
    diagnostic tests, 241
    interventions, 242
    manifestations, 241
    Nursing Care Plan, 242–243*t*
    nursing process, 241–242
    nutrition, 241
    outcome evaluation, 242*t*
    pathophysiology and etiology, 240–241
    pediatric, 242
    pharmacologic therapy, 241
    risk factors, 241
Cell cycle, 32
Cell membrane, 30
Cell-mediated immune response, 442, 483
Cells
    defined, 29
    malignant, 43, 43*t*
    mast, 635
    somatic, 32
    structure
        cell membrane, 30
        cytoplasm, 30
        endoplasmic reticulum, 30–31
        Golgi apparatus, 31
        lysosomes, 31
        mitochondria, 31, 31*t*
        nucleolus, 30
        nucleus, 30, 31*t*
        ribosomes, 30
Cellular differentiation
    embryonic membranes, 2022–2023
    primary germ layers, 2022
Cellular immune response, 509
Cellular multiplication, 2021, 2022
Cellular mutation, 45
Cellular regulation
    alterations, 32
    alterations and therapies, 33–34*t*
    assessment, 36–37
    cell cycle and, 32
    in children, 36–37
    collaborative interventions and therapies, 39
    concepts related to, 35
    defined, 29
    diagnostic tests and, 37
    DNA and genes and, 31–32

Cellular regulation (*continued*)

genetic considerations and nonmodifiable risk factors, 34

hydration management, 39

independent interventions and therapies, 37–39

independent nursing interventions, 37–39

interventions and therapies, 37–40

lifespan considerations, 36–37

medications, 40t

modifiable risk factors, 36

normal, 30–32

pediatric considerations, 38–39, 38f

pharmacologic therapy, 39

prevalence and, 34

prevention and, 36

promoting healthy grieving and, 38

promotion of nutrition, activity and rest, 39

psychosocial support, 37–39

risk factors, 34

screenings and, 36

treatment side effects management, 39

Cellular transport methods, 30t

Cellulitis

assessment, 563

care planning, 563

in children, 561–562

collaborative care, 562–563

defined, 560

diagnosis, 563

diagnostic tests, 562

infection control and, 562t

inflammation, 560

interventions, 563

lifespan and cultural considerations, 561–562

lymphadenopathy, 560

manifestations, 561–562, 562t

nonpharmacologic therapy, 563

Nursing Care Plan, 564t

nursing process, 563

in older adults, 562

outcome evaluation, 563

pathophysiology and etiology, 560–561

pharmacologic therapy, 563

prevention, 561

risk factors, 560–561

white blood cells (WBCs) and, 560

Center for Epidemiological Studies Depression Scale for Children (CESD-DC), 1786–1787

Center for Epidemiological Studies Depression Scale-Revised (CESD-R), 1785

Centers for Medicare and Medicaid Services (CMS), 2622, 2632

Central cord syndrome, 910t

Central line-associated bloodstream infections (CLABSIs), 2706

Central nervous system

brain and, 688–689

defined, 688

disseminated intravascular coagulation (DIC) and, 1141t

meninges, 688

pregnancy and, 2033

Central nervous system (CNS) depressants, 1563

Central obesity, 791

Central pain, 156

Central sleep apnea, 195

Central venous catheterization, 1227

Central venous pressure (CVP), 1152

Centrally acting sympatholytics, 1171–1172t

Centration, 1665t, 2292

Cephalocaudal growth, 1648, 1648f

Cephalohematoma, 2225, 2225f

Cephalopelvic disproportion (CPD), 2139t

Cerebellum, 688

Cerebral palsy (CP)

assessment, 1698

care planning, 1698

clinical characteristics of, 1696t

collaborative care, 1696–1698

community-based care, 1699t

defined, 1675t, 1695

diagnosis, 1698

diagnostic tests, 1696

early intervention programs, 1698

emotional support, 1699

foster parent knowledge and, 1699

growth and development and, 1699

injury prevention, 1698

interventions, 1675t, 1698–1699

manifestations, 1675t, 1696, 1697t

nonpharmacologic therapy, 1697–1698

Nursing Care Plan, 1700t

nursing process, 1698–1699

nutrition and, 1699

outcome evaluation, 1699

overview of, 1695

pathophysiology and etiology, 1695–1696

pharmacologic therapy, 1696–1697

physical mobility and, 1699

prevention of, 1695

risk factors, 1695

skin integrity and, 1699

surgery, 1696

Cerebral perfusion, 1246–1247

Cerebral perfusion pressure (CPP), 712

Cerebral stimulants, 1592t

Cerebrospinal fluid (CSF), 688, 688f

Cerebrum, 688, 688f, 1576

CERT (Community Emergency Response Team) program, 2611

Certification, 2666

Cerumen, 1285

Cervical assessment, 1361t, 2142

Cervical cancer

HIV/AIDS and, 464

screening guidelines, 58t

Cervical cap, 1382

Cervical collar (C-collar), 2003

Cervical disc herniation, 842

Cervical ripening

Bishop scoring system, 2128t

defined, 2128

mechanical methods, 2129

misoprostol use, 2128

nursing care during, 2129

prostaglandin agents use, 2128–2129

Cervical spinal cord injury, 917–918

Cervical traction, 913f

Cervix

changes in pregnancy, 2030

postpartum changes, 2173

CES (cauda equina syndrome), 841

Cesarean birth. *See also* Intrapartum care

analgesia and anesthesia, 2133

Apgar score and, 2135

defined, 2131–2132

emergency, preparation for, 2134–2135

immediate postnatal recovery period, 2135

indications, 2132–2133

maternal mortality and morbidity, 2133

partner support, 2135

preparation for, 2133–2134

rates, 2132

repeat, preparation for, 2134

on request, 2132

skin incisions, 2133

uterine incisions, 2133

well-being promotion after, 2187–2188

CESD-DC (Center for Epidemiological Studies Depression Scale for Children), 1786–1787

CESD-R (Center for Epidemiological Studies Depression Scale-Revised), 1785

CGT (Complicated Grief Treatment), 1745–1746

Chadwick sign, 2030

Chain of command, 2549–2550, 2550f

Chancre, 1413

Change-of-shift reports, 2451, 2451t

Channel blockers, 1189t

Channels, 2399

Charismatic leaders, 2490

Charting

defined, 2438

by exception (CBE), 2443, 2444f

focus, 2442–2443

narrative, 2440

Charts, 2438. *See also* Client records

CHCs (community health centers), 2684

CHCT (caffeine halothane contracture test), 1426

Check perceptions, 2430

Cheilosis, 426

Chemical burns

defined, 1465

household chemicals causing, 1465t

stopping the burning process, 1475t

Chemical conjunctivitis, 2226

Chemical menopause, 1394

Chemical restraints, 2704

Chemical thermogenesis, 1422, 1438

Chemicals, safety precautions, 1264t

Chemotaxis, 43

Chemotherapy

in breast cancer, 81

defined, 56

in leukemia, 99, 99t

CHEOPS (Children's Hospital Eastern Ontario Pain Scale), 169

Chest, newborn assessment, 2228–2229, 2228f

Chest CT with contract, in pulmonary embolism, 1213

Chest pain assessment, 1068

Chest physiotherapy, 592–593

Chest x-ray

in acute respiratory distress syndrome (ARDS), 978

anterior-posterior, 966

in burn injuries, 1477

in congenital heart defects, 1097t

in COPD, 1011

in heart failure, 1151
in lung cancer, 108
as perioperative diagnostic test, 1253t
in pneumonia, 591
in pulmonary embolism, 1214
in tuberculosis, 611
use of, 966
Child abuse
defined, 1966
injuries, 2710t
manifestations of, 1968, 1972t
therapies, 1972t
Childbirth customs, 2158t
Childhood obesity
culture and, 773t
evidence-based interventions to
reduce, 775t
increase in, 773t
as public health issue, 791
Childhood traumatic grief, 1753
Childless families, 1710
Children. See also Adolescents; Infants;
Pediatric clients; School-age children;
Toddlers
acid-base imbalances in, 10
acute renal failure (ARF) in, 387t
advocating for, 2559, 2559f, 2559t
airways, 956f
antibiotics for, 1434
anxiety and, 1907–1910
anxiety disorders in, 1920
appendicitis in, 646, 648
assessment
anthropometric measurements, 2286
child behaviors, 2288t
growth and development instruments,
2291t
lifespan considerations, 2289t
nursing approach, 2287
nutrition history, 2286
sitting on parent lap, 2286
special considerations, 2286–2289
with/without parent, 2287
asthma in, 991–992, 993, 996t, 1000t,
1003t
autism spectrum disorder (ASD) in,
1689–1690
behavior, acceptable, 1718t
bipolar disorders in, 1811
blood pressure assessment in, 1067t
blood volume in, 1218t
body mass index (BMI) ranges, 942t
body temperature in, 1428t
burns and, 1466t, 1482t, 1485t
cancer and, 38–39, 38f, 50–51, 62t
cataracts in, 1306t
cellular regulation assessment in, 36–37
cellulitis in, 561–562
chronic kidney disease (CKD) in, 401t
comfort and, 142, 149
communication with, 2407t
congenital heart defects in. See congenital
heart defects
constipation in, 307, 308t, 311t
death anxiety in, 1751
dehydration in, 359
depression assessment in, 1802
depression in, 1801t
developmental assessment of, 36–37
diabetes in, 760, 766–780

MODY, 767t
NDM, 767t
overview of, 766–767
digestive system in, 209
dysrhythmias in, 1179t
electrolyte imbalances in kidney disease
in, 379t
encopresis in, 312
end-of-life care for, 177–180
factors affecting health promotion
in, 416t
in families with addiction, 1525–1526
fever treatment in, 1434, 1434t, 1436t
fluid replacement in, 363
fluid volume deficit in, 356
fluids and electrolytes and, 343–344,
344f, 344t
fractures in, 859
in gay and lesbian families, 1711
generalized anxiety disorder (GAD) in,
1920–1921
GERD in, 228t
glaucoma in, 1323t
grief and, 1743–1744, 1743f
Guillain-Barré syndrome (GBS) in, 1333t
health promotion and, 412t
herbal laxative use in, 311t
herniated discs in, 842
HIV/AIDS education for, 476t
hypothermia in, 1441
immunizations for, 451
infection in, 553f
infectious and communicable diseases in, 532,
533–542t
inflammation in, 636, 641
inflammatory bowel disease (IBD) in, 641,
666, 667t
intravenous fluids in, 362
on ketogenic diet, 720, 721
leukemia in, 93f, 100t
musculoskeletal differences in, 820
music and art therapy for, 1668t
neurological system assessment in, 707t
nursing assessment of, 2334t
nutrition for, 932
obesity in, 946t
obsessive-compulsive disorder (OCD)
in, 1935t
oral health in, 425
osteoarthritis in, 887t
otitis media in, 581, 581f
oxygenation in, 1046
pain and, 152, 157–159
participation in healthcare decisions,
2661, 2662t
pharmacologic therapy for mood disorders
and, 1794t
pneumonia in, 588–590, 589f
polyethylene glycol (PEG) use in, 310t
PTSD in, 1947
pulse assessment in, 1065t
rapport with, 2437t
respiratory system in, 965t
rheumatoid arthritis in, 497t
RSV/bronchiolitis in, 1018–1024, 1022t
scoliosis in, 847, 848f, 851–852
seizure disorders in, 718–720
seizures in, 722t
self-report scales, 1786–1787
sensory function assessment in, 1291t

separation anxiety disorder (SAD)
in, 1922t
sepsis in, 601
sexual messages from families and, 1355
short bowel syndrome in, 244t
sickle cell disease and, 125t
skeletal and muscle development of, 821f
sodium intake in, 371t
spinal cord injuries (SCI) in, 912
spiritual development in, 1874t
suctioning, 970t
therapeutic communication with, 2435–2436,
2435f, 2436t
thermoregulation in, 1423
trachea, 957, 957f
tuberculosis in, 609
type 1 diabetes in, 767–772
type 2 diabetes in, 772–778
unintentional injuries in, 2710–2712, 2710f,
2711f, 2711t, 2712t
urinary calculi in, 321
urinary incontinence in, 293, 296, 626t
urinary tract infections (UTIs) in, 620,
624–625, 625t
water-related injuries, 2711t
Children of alcoholics (COAs), 1536
Children's Health Insurance Program
(CHIP), 2628
Children's response to loss
ages 2–4, 1752
ages 5–7, 1752
ages 8–11, 1752
ages 12–18, 1752
assessment, 1755
behavioral response to grief, 1754
care planning, 1755–1756
childhood traumatic grief, 1753
collaborative care, 1754–1755
complicated grief reactions, 1753
complications, 1753
cultural considerations, 1754
death of a friend, 1753
death of a grandparent, 1753
death of a parent, 1752–1753
death of a sibling, 1753
developmental stages, 1751–1752
diagnosis, 1755
grief response, 1751–1752
interventions, 1756
manifestations, 1754, 1755t
nonpharmacologic therapy, 1754–1755
Nursing Care Plan, 1756–1757t
nursing process, 1755–1756
outcome evaluation, 1756
overview of, 1751
pharmacologic therapy, 1754
significance of loss, 1752–1753
CHIP (Children's Health Insurance
Program), 2628
Chiropractic therapy, 843
Chlamydia. See also Sexually transmitted
infections (STIs)
complications of, 1412
defined, 1412
diagnosis and treatment, 1412
manifestations, 1412
as pathogenic organism, 530t
pathophysiology, 1412
pharmacologic therapy, 1412
risk factors, 1412t

Chlamydia trachomatis, 565, 1412
Chloasma, 2032
Chloride (Cl⁻)
  electrolyte imbalance, 372
  function, 342, 342*t*
  regulation, 342*t*
Cholecystitis, 651, 651*t*
Cholelithiasis
  defined, 650
  manifestations and complications, 651*t*
  Nursing Care Plan, 655–656*t*
Cholesterol, 945
Cholesterol-lowering drugs, 1117*t*, 1118
Chromosomal syndromes, 1374, 1375*t*
Chromosomes
  autosomal, 1659
  defined, 31
  homologous, 31
  sex, 31–32, 1659
Chronic bronchitis, 1006, 1006*f*
Chronic confusion, 1605
Chronic fatigue, 145, 185
Chronic fatigue syndrome, 145, 186, 187
Chronic glomerulonephritis, 670
Chronic hypertension, 1205
Chronic illness, 408, 1731
Chronic infection, 523
Chronic kidney disease (CKD)
  African Americans and, 392*t*
  assessment, 399
  BUN and serum creatinine values
    and, 391*f*
  care planning, 399
  children with, 401*t*
  collaborative care, 395–399
  complementary and alternative
    therapy, 399
  defined, 390
  diagnosis, 399
  diagnostic tests, 395
  etiology, 392
  fluid management, 397
  home care, 401*t*
  interventions and therapies
    body image, 401
    care in community, 401–402
    infection, 400–401
    nutrition, 400
    tissue profusion, 400
  lifespan considerations, 392*t*
  manifestations
    anemia, 396*t*
    cardiovascular effects, 393
    dermatological effects, 395
    endocrine and metabolic effects, 395
    fluid and electrolyte effects, 393
    fluid volume excess, 396*t*
    gastrointestinal effects, 393
    hematological effects, 393
    hyperkalemia, 396*t*
    immune system effects, 393
    musculoskeletal effects, 395
    neurological effects, 393–395
    therapies, 396*t*
    uremia, 393, 394*t*, 396*t*
  multisystem effects of, 394*t*
  Nursing Care Plan, 402–403*t*
  nursing process, 399–402
  nutrition, 397
  outcome evaluation, 402

overview of, 390, 390*t*
pathophysiology, 391–392, 391*t*
pharmacologic therapy, 397
prevention of, 392
renal replacement therapies, 397–399
reproductive function and, 395
risk factors, 392
stages of, 392*t*
Chronic lymphocytic (CLL), 93*t*, 95
Chronic myeloid (CML), 94, 94*f*
Chronic obstructive pulmonary disease (COPD).
    See also Oxygenation
  airway clearance and, 1022
  assessment, 1012–1013
  bronchitis and, 1006, 1006*f*
  care planning, 1013
  classification by severity, 1008*t*
  collaborative care, 1009–1012
  complementary and alternative therapy, 1012
  coughing techniques and, 1008*t*
  defined, 1005
  diagnosis, 1013
  diagnostic tests
    arterial blood gas (ABG), 1010
    chest x-ray, 1111
    complete blood count (CBC), 1010–1111
    exhaled carbon dioxide, 1010
    pulmonary function tests (PFTs), 1009
    pulse oximetry, 1010
    serum α₁-antitrypsin levels, 1009
    ventilation-perfusion scanning, 1009
  emphysema and, 1006, 1007*f*
  etiology, 1007
  exercise and, 1012
  home care assessment, 1013*t*
  hydration and, 1012
  interventions
    activity promotion, 1014
    airway clearance, 1014
    breathing pattern enhancement, 1014
    family coping, 1015–1016
    nutrition, 1015
    overview of, 1013–1014
    smoking cessation, 1016
  manifestations, 1008–1009, 1010*t*
  Nursing Care Plan, 1016–1017*t*
  nursing process, 1012–1016
  outcome evaluation, 1016
  overview of, 1005–1006
  oxygen therapy, 1011
  pathogenesis of, 1006*f*
  pathophysiology, 1006–1008
  percussion, vibration, and postural drainage
    and, 1011–1012
  pharmacologic therapy, 1011
  physical activity and, 1015*t*
  possible outcomes, 1013
  prevention of, 1007–1008
  risk factors, 1007
  surgery, 1011
Chronic otitis media, 576
Chronic pain. *See also* Pain
  alterations and therapies, 144*t*
  categories of, 155
  causes of, 155
  characteristics of, 155
  defined, 143, 144*t*
  home management of, 172*t*
  illness/injury-associated, 156
  interventions and therapies, 144*t*, 167*t*

intractable benign, 155
manifestations, 144*t*, 157–162, 167*t*
Nursing Care Plan, 173*t*
in older adults, 160*t*
prevention of, 157
progressive, 155
recurrent, 155
rheumatoid arthritis treatment,
    505–506
Chronic pancreatitis
  defined, 246
  manifestations, 247
  medications, 249*t*
Chronic pyelonephritis, 619
Chronic rejection, 447
Chronic respiratory acidosis, 21
Chronic urinary retention, 299*t*
Chronic venous insufficiency (CVI), 1198,
    1199*t*
Chronosystem, 1657
Chvostek sign, 737*t*
Chyme, 931
Cigarette smoking. *See* Smoking;
    Smoking cessation
Circulating nurses, 1251
Circulation. *See also* Perfusion
  breast cancer and, 82
  coronary, 1036–1040, 1038*f*
  pressure ulcers and, 1494–1495,
    1495*t*
  pulmonary, 1036, 1038*f*
  sickle cell disease and, 125
  systemic, 1036, 1038*f*
  transition from fetal to pulmonary, 1040
Circulatory system, fetal development of,
    2027*f*, 2027–2028
Circumcision
  assessment, 2242
  with circumcision clamp, 2241*f*
  defined, 2240
  female, 1362
  following, 2242
  with Plastibell, 2241, 2241*f*
  routine, 2240
Cirrhosis
  alcoholic, 781
  biliary, 782
  from chronic alcoholism, 1537*t*
  client teaching, 788*t*
  culture and, 782*t*
  defined, 729, 781
  genetic considerations and nonmodifiable
    risk factors, 731
  interventions and therapies, 733
  multisystem effects of, 783*t*
  Nursing Care Plan, 789*t*
  posthepatic, 782
  prevalence of, 729
  prevention of, 731
Civil law, 2655
Civility, 2409
CIWA-Ar (Clinical Institute Withdrawal
    Assessment for Alcohol – Revised) scale,
    1539, 1541, 1542*f*
CKD. *See* Chronic kidney disease
CK-MB, 1115
CLABSIs (central line-associated bloodstream
    infections), 2706
Clang, 1613
Clarifying, 2429–2430

Class. *See also* Diversity
  homelessness, 1635
  poverty, 1635–1636
  undocumented immigrants, 1636
Classism, 1635
Clean contaminated wounds, 1450
Clean objects, 523
Clean wounds, 1449
Clear boundaries, 1714
Client advocates. *See also* Advocacy
  defined, 2555
  effective, 2557
  nurse support of, 2557
  role of, 2556–2561
  values basic to, 2556t
Client contracting, 2520–2521
Client cues
  comparing with standards/norms, 2336
  examples of, 2337t
  formulating for nursing diagnosis, 2337t
Client education. *See* Education
Client health history
  age and developmental level, 2511
  cultural factors, 2512
  defined, 2511
  economic factors, 2513
  health beliefs and practices, 2512
  learning styles, 2513
  support system, 2513
  understanding of health problem, 2511–2512
Client monitoring and computerized diagnostics, 2648, 2648f, 2649f
Client preferences, in prioritizing care, 2369
Client records
  defined, 2438
  electronic, confidentiality of, 2439
  purposes of, 2439
Client/consumer education
  areas of, 2509t
  deficient knowledge as etiology, 2515–2516
  diagnosis, 2515–2524
  documentation, 2523–2524
  evaluation, 2523–2524
  learning evaluation, 2523
  learning experience evaluation, 2523
  learning need as diagnostic label, 2515
  overview of, 2509
  planning
    content selection, 2517
    flexibility, 2518–2519
    hands-on client participation, 2520, 2520f
    learning experiences organization, 2517–2518
    learning outcomes, 2517, 2517t
    teaching guidelines, 2519–2520
    teaching plan sample, 2516t
    teaching priorities determination, 2516–2517
    teaching strategies selection, 2517, 2518t
    tools for teaching children, 2519t
  teaching environments, 2509–2510
  teaching plan development, 2510–2515, 2514t
  teaching strategies
    anticipatory guidance, 2520, 2521t
    behavior modification, 2522
    client contracting, 2520–2521
    discovery/problem solving, 2521–2522

  group teaching, 2521
  technology-assisted instruction, 2521
  transcultural teaching, 2522–2523
Client-focused care, 2457, 2599
Clients
  autonomy, 2577
  defined, 2548
  ethical issues in working with, 2577
  illness effects on, 408–409
  with infection
    in isolation, 548–549
    transportation of, 548
  privacy and confidentiality, 2577
  risk of infection, 552f
  values, clarifying, 2564
Clients with disabilities, advocating for, 2560
Climacteric, 1343
Climacteric period, 1394
Climax, 1564
Clinical decision making
  choosing between alternatives, 2322–2323
  clinical judgment, 2324–2327
  concept of, 2315
  concepts related to, 2316t
  critical thinking and, 2316–2320
  decision steps, 2321
  decision types, 2321
  defined, 2315
  example of, 2315
  good, 2320
  problem solving, 2323–2324
  safety and, 2698t
  summary, 2327
Clinical decision support systems. *See also* Informatics
  computers in nursing administration, 2645–2646
  computers in nursing research, 2644–2645
  defined, 2639, 2644
  overview of, 2644
  research and, 2644
  role of uniform languages and, 2644
Clinical information systems, 2635–2636, 2635f
Clinical Institute Withdrawal Assessment for Alcohol – Revised (CIWA-Ar) scale, 1539, 1541
Clinical judgment
  Benner's skill acquisition model, 2325, 2325f
  defined, 2324
  Lasater's clinical judgment rubric, 2325–2327, 2327f
  overview of, 2324–2325
  Tanner's clinical judgment model, 2325, 2326f, 2326t
Clinical nurse leader, 2551
Clinical nurse specialist, 2550
Clinical pathways
  as algorithm or path, 2361, 2362f
  client specific, 2360
  defined, 2360
  for mother and baby, 2361f
  for pediatric asthma, 2362f
Clinical pelvimetry, 2054
Clinical questions, developing, 2588–2590
Clinical reasoning, 2319
CLL (chronic lymphocytic), 93t, 95

Clock Drawing Test (CDT), 2295t
Clonic phase, seizures, 716
Closed airway/tracheal suction system, 970, 971f
Closed awareness, 182
Closed fractures, 854t
Closed questions, 2274, 2274t
Clostridium difficile, 530
Clostridium difficile-associated infections (CDIs), 2706
Clothing, antepartum care and, 2072
Clotting, 1049
Club drug, 1554
Clubfoot, 2232, 2233f
CML (chronic myeloid), 94, 94f
CMO (comfort measures only) order, 176
CMS (Centers for Medicare and Medicaid Services), 2622, 2632
COA (coarctation of the aorta), 1092–1093t
Coaching, 2526–2527, 2526t
Coagulation
  in newborns, 2198
  studies, 785, 1214
Coanalgesics
  characteristics of, 167
  defined, 163
  examples of, 162t, 167
Coarctation of the aorta (COA), 1092–1093t
COAs (children of alcoholics), 1536
Cobb angle, 848
Cocaine, 1556t
  defined, 1553
  pregnancy and, 1553–1554
Cochlear implants, 1302, 1302f
Code blue, calling, 1270
Code of ethics
  in accountability, 2537
  ANA, 2568–2569
  defined, 2567
  ICN, 2568t
  nursing, 2567–2569
Codeine, 165, 166t
Codependence
  characteristics of, 1526t
  defined, 1525t
Cognition
  alterations and therapies, 1586t
  alternations
    dementia, 1584–1585
    intellectual disability, 1581–1583
    learning disabilities, 1578
  assessment, 1587–1590
  assessment interview, 1590t
  collaborative interventions and therapies, 1591–1593
  community resources, 1591
  concepts related to, 1579–1580t
  defined, 1575
  development theories, 1576–1577
  diagnostic tests, 1589–1590
  genetic considerations and nonmodifiable risk factors, 1577–1578
  independent interventions and therapies, 1591
  information processing theory and, 1577
  interventions and therapies, 1591–1593
  lifespan and cultural considerations, 1587–1589
  mental status assessments, 1587t, 1588–1589t
  normal, 1576
  pharmacologic therapy, 1591–1593

Cognition (*continued*)
Piaget's theory and, 1576, 1576t
Vygotsky's theory and, 1576t
Cognitive appraisal, 1898–1899, 1929
Cognitive changes
coping strategies, 1577–1578
in older adults, 1577–1578
Cognitive deficits
Parkinson disease and, 897
stroke and, 1237–1238, 1238f
Cognitive development
adolescents, 1669
infants, 1659–1660
preschoolers, 1664
school-age children, 1667
toddlers, 1663
Cognitive development theories
information processing theory, 1577
nursing application of, 1577
Piaget's theory, 1576, 1576t
Vygotsky's theory, 1576
Cognitive domain, 2503
Cognitive dysfunction
legal protection and, 1591t
medications, 1592t
self-medication administration and, 1593
Cognitive function
exercise benefits, 423
sexuality and, 1349
Cognitive impairments, communication
assessment and, 2413
Cognitive learning processes, 2503
Cognitive modification, 1794
Cognitive skills, 2348
Cognitive structuring, 1904
Cognitive theory, 1781, 2503
Cognitive therapy, multiple sclerosis
and, 881
Cognitive-behavioral therapy (CBT)
for anxiety disorders, 1925
defined, 1914
for mood disorders, 1794–1795
for personality disorders, 1861–1862
for stress and coping, 1914–1915
for suicide prevention, 1995
techniques, 1915t
Cohesiveness, 2422
Cohort study, 2589
Coitus interruptus, 1379
Cold packs, 889
Cold stress, 2210t
Cold zone, 2614t
Colectomy, 662
Collaboration
care coordination and, 2460
communication skills and, 2379–2380
competencies basic to, 2378–2381
concept of, 2375
concepts related to, 2379t
conflict management and, 2381
continuum of, 2393f
decision making and, 2380–2381
defined, 2375
effective, characteristics of, 2393
emergency preparedness, 2614
healthcare consumer and, 2381
importance of, 2381
individual strength barriers and, 2393t
interdisciplinary, 2392–2393
language barriers and, 2380t

mutual respect and trust and, 2380
nurse as collaborator and, 2376, 2376–2377t,
2378t
nurse-physician, benefits of, 2380t
practice, 2378
psychosocial and professional effects, 2378
as QSEN competency, 2699, 2700
Collaborative interventions, 2345
Collaborative plans. *See* Clinical pathways
Collaborative practice, 2378
Collagen, 1508
Collateral channels, 1106
Collecting data
examination, 2276–2282
interviews, 2272–2276
observation, 2271–2272, 2272t
Colloid osmotic pressure, 338, 364
Colloid solutions, for shock, 1229t, 1230
Colloids, 337
Colon cancer, 85
Colonization, 523
Color blindness, 1279
Colorectal cancer. *See also* Cancer
assessment, 89
care planning, 89
collaborative care, 87–88
colostomy, 87–88, 88f
coping and, 90
defined, 85
diagnosis, 89
diagnostic tests, 87
distribution and frequency, 85f
etiology, 86
interventions, 89–90
laser photocoagulation, 88
manifestations, 85, 85t
Nursing Care Plan, 91t
nursing process, 89–90
nutrition and, 90
outcome evaluation, 90
overview of, 85
pain management, 89
pathophysiology, 85–86
pharmacologic therapy, 88
polyps, 85
prevention of, 86
radiation therapy, 88
risk factors, 86
screening guidelines, 58t
sexual dysfunction and, 90
surgery, 87–88
TNM staging system for, 86, 86t
Colostomy, 88
Colostrum, 2174
Column plan, 2356, 2356f
Coma
Glasgow scale for assessment, 697t
irreversible, 697t
Combined oral contraceptives (COCs),
1383–1384
Comfort. *See also* Discomfort
alterations, 142–146
alterations and therapies, 144t
assessment, 146–148, 147t
collaborative interventions and therapies, 151
concepts related to, 143t
cultural considerations, 147–148
defined, 141
environmental, 141
in healing process, 141

independent interventions and therapies,
149–151
interventions and therapies, 148–151
intrapartum care
anxiety, 2162
breathing techniques, 2163–2164
client teaching, 2162–2163
general comfort, 2161–2162
relaxation techniques, 2163
legal issues and, 2660t
lifespan considerations, 142, 147–148, 149
mobility and, 836
normal presentation, 142
nursing assessment, 146–147t
physical, 141
prevention of discomfort, 146
promotion
herniated disc and, 845
in nursing care, 143
peripheral neuropathy and, 1335
postpartum care, 2183–2184
psychospiritual, 141
signs of, 142
sociocultural, 141
as subjective, 142
Comfort measures only (CMO) order, 176
Comminuted fractures, 854t
Commission on Collegiate Nursing Education
(CCNE), 2625
Commitment. *See also* Commitment
to profession
affective, 2487, 2487f
continuance, 2487f
defined, 2486
normative, 2487f
organizational, 2486
Commitment to profession
affective commitment, 2487, 2487f
burnout and, 2488
continuance commitment, 2487
factors of, 2486–2487
normative commitment, 2487
overview of, 2486
stages of development, 2487–2488
stress management and, 2488
types of, 2487, 2487f
Committees, 2423
Communicable disease, 522
Communication
abuse and, 1974
in addiction, 1528–1529
adolescent, 1669–1670
with adolescents, 2407t
Alzheimer disease (AD) and, 1601t
assertive, 2409–2413
assessment, 2284, 2413–2414
autism spectrum disorder (ASD) and,
1689, 1693
barriers, 2409, 2410t
barriers, overcoming, 2399
care planning, 2415
challenges, 2398–2399
in child development, 1666
with children, 2407t
client records for, 2439
cognitive impairment, 2413
concept of, 2397
concepts related to, 2405–2406t
congruent, 2408
culture and, 2416

defined, 2284, 2398
development and, 2406
diagnosis, 2414–2415
education, 2416
effective, 2398
electronic, 2400, 2403
environment and, 2408, 2415
factors influencing, 2405–2409
family, 1716–1717
gender and, 2406
groups and group communication, 2418–2424
handoff, 2451, 2451t
healthcare systems and, 2601t
hearing impairment and, 1305
infants, 1662
interpersonal attitudes and, 2409
interventions, 2415
language deficits, 2413
legal issues and, 2660t
meaning of, 2398–2399
measures to enhance, 2416
message, 2399
in minimizing malpractice, 2658
modes, 2400–2405
nonverbal, 2400, 2401–2403
nursing practice, 2417
nursing process, 2413–2417
with older adults, 2414t
outcome evaluation, 2416–2417
of painful information, 1930, 1930t
paralysis and, 2414
personal space and, 2406–2408
process, 2399–2400, 2399f
receiver, 2399
response, 2399–2400
roles and relationships and, 2408
schizophrenia and family, 1623t
school-age children, 1668
self-talk and, 2398, 2398f
sender, 2399
sensory deficits, 2413
social differences, 1638
sociocultural characteristics and, 2406
stroke and, 1238, 1245
structural deficits, 2413–2414
styles of, 2414
support, 2415
telephone, 2451–2452, 2452t
territoriality and, 2408
therapeutic, 1930, 1930t, 2424–2437
time in caring for clients with needs,
    2415t
toddlers, 1664
types of communicators and, 2409–2411,
    2411t
values and perceptions and, 2406
verbal, 2400–2401, 2414
written, 2403–2405
Communication deviance, 1612
Communication skills
in collaboration, 2379–2380
language barriers and, 2380t
Communicator style, 2379
Communicators
aggressive, 2409, 2411, 2411t
assertive, 2409–2411, 2411t
passive, 2409, 2411, 2411t
types of, 2409–2411
Community Emergency Response Team (CERT)
    program, 2611

Community health centers (CHCs), 2684
Community-based care
defined, 1724
legal protections, 1591t
motor vehicle crashes (MVC) and, 2005
Comorbid disorders, 1991
Comorbidity, 1019
Compartment syndrome, 858, 1471
Compassion
defined, 2307
as professional behavior, 2483
Compensation, 1905t
Compensatory shock, 1218–1219
Competence
areas of, 2544
care for the dying, 2544
defined, 2307, 2543
health and wellness promotion, 2544
health restoration, 2544
illness prevention, 2544
lifelong, 2544
nursing practice, 2544
overview of, 2543
as professional behavior, 2482–2483,
    2482t
risk management and, 2677, 2678t
Competency
for consent, 2659–2661
defined, 2659
Competition, 2464
Complement assay, 489
Complementary and alternative therapy
alcohol abuse and, 1539–1540
Alzheimer disease (AD) and, 1598–1600
antepartum care and, 2074
anxiety disorders and, 1925–1926
asthma and, 1001
attention-deficit/hyperactivity disorder
    (ADHD) and, 1684t
autism spectrum disorder (ASD) and,
    1692, 1692t
cataracts and, 1309
chronic kidney disease (CKD) and, 399
chronic obstructive pulmonary disease (COPD)
    and, 1012
congenital heart defects and, 1103t
constipation and, 311
contact dermatitis and, 1490
coronary artery disease (CAD) and,
    1123, 1123t
defined, 1643–1644
dysmenorrhea and, 1403
fatigue and, 188t
feeding and eating disorders and,
    1849–1850
heart failure and, 1158
herbal laxative use in children and, 311t
hot and cold therapy and, 1435
hypersensitivity and, 491
hypertension and, 1173
immunity and, 454–455
inflammatory bowel disease (IBD)
    and, 663
labor and, 2161t
leukemia and, 99
menopause and, 1396, 1397t
mood disorders and, 1795–1797
multiple sclerosis and, 881t
nausea and vomiting and, 222t
nicotine addiction and, 1547

nutritional anemias and, 71t
osteoarthritis and, 891t
otitis media and, 580t
overview of, 1644t
in pain management, 168
pancreatitis and, 249t
peripheral vascular disease (PVD)
    and, 1201
personality disorders (PD) and, 1862
pneumonia and, 594t
pregnancy and, 1557t
prostate cancer and, 116
rheumatoid arthritis and, 504, 504t
schizophrenia and, 1620
sickle cell disease and, 124
sleep-rest disorders and, 199t
type 1 diabetes in children and, 772
urinary calculi and, 323t
Complete blood count (CBC)
in acute renal failure (ARF), 380
in burn injuries, 1477
in chronic kidney disease (CKD), 395
in chronic obstructive pulmonary disease
    (COPD), 1010–1011
in congenital heart defects, 1098t
as fluid and electrolyte test, 351
in gallbladder disease, 651t
in HIV/AIDS testing, 468
in leukemia, 97
in liver disease, 785
in lung cancer, 108
in otitis media, 579
in pneumonia, 591
in systemic lupus erythematosus (SLE), 514
Complete breech, 2115
Complete fractures, 854t
Compliance, 710, 2501
Compliance of the arteries, 1044
Complicated grief. See also Grief and loss
defined, 1743, 1747t
interventions and therapies, 1747t
manifestations, 1745, 1747t
older adult's response to loss, 1764
treatment of, 1745–1746
Complicated Grief Treatment (CGT),
    1745–1746
Comprehensive quality management, 2690
Compression
fractures, 856t
spinal cord, 908
stockings/boots, 917
Compromised hosts, 524
Compulsions
commonly occurring, 1936t
defined, 1935
Computed tomography (CT)
in acute renal failure (ARF), 380
cancer, 55
digestive tract, 221
in lung cancer, 108
pancreatitis and, 247
in pneumonia, 591
in violence assessment, 1961
Computer vision syndrome, 2643
Computer-based client records
case management, 2648
client education, 2648
client monitoring and computerized diagnostics,
    2648–2649, 2648f, 2649f
community and home health, 2648

Computerized medical records
  accuracy, 2639
  clinical decision support systems, 2639,
    2644–2646
  components of, 2637–2638
  device integration, 2639
  electronic health records (EHRs), 2637
  electronic medical records (EMRs), 2637
  functionality, 2637
  Health Level 7 (HL7), 2638
  HIPAA and, 2638–2639
  purpose of, 2637
  quality assurance, 2639
  terminology, 2637
  uniform language, 2639
Computers on wheels (COWs), 2643
COMT inhibitors, 899t, 900
Concept maps
  build approaches, 2357
  defined, 2356
  hints in making, 2357
  steps for building, 2358–2359f
Conception
  fertilization, 2020–2021
  gametogenesis, 2020
  meiosis, 2019–2020
  mitosis, 2019
  oogenesis, 2020
  preembryonic development and,
    2021–2022
  spermatogenesis, 2020
Conclusions, drawing, 2349–2350
Concrete thinking, 1614
Concurrent audit, 2685
Concussions
  defined, 696t
  signs and symptoms, 696t
  sports-related, underreported, 2712t
Condoms. See also Contraception
  defined, 1379
  female, 1380, 1380f
  male, 1379–1380, 1380f
Conduction, 1422
Conduction system of the heart, 1042–1044,
  1043f
Conductive hearing loss, 1299
Confabulation, 1536
Confidentiality
  advocating for, 2671
  defined, 2671
  of electronic records, 2439
  privacy versus, 2671
Conflict management, 2381
Conflict resolution
  aggression in workplace and, 2389–2390,
    2390t
  causes of conflicts and, 2388
  conclusion, 2390
  overview of, 2387
  prevention of conflicts and, 2388–2389
  responding to conflicts and, 2389
  types of conflicts and, 2387–2388
Conflicts
  causes of, 2388
  with clients and families, 2389
  covert, 2387–2388
  defined, 2387
  intergroup, 2387
  interorganizational, 2387
  interpersonal, 2387

intrapersonal, 2387
  loyalties and obligations, 2572
  managing, 2477
  nurse-physician relationship and, 2388
  overt, 2387
  preventing, 2388–2389
  responding to, 2389
  role, 1834
  types of, 2387–2388
Confronting, 2432
Confusion. See also Cognition
  acute, 1605
  assessment, 1607–1608
  care planning, 1608
  chronic, 1605
  cognitive interventions, 1607
  collaborative care, 1606–1607
  defined, 1605
  delirium and, 1605
  diagnosis, 1608
  diagnostic tests, 1607
  environmental interventions, 1607
  interventions, 1609
  lifespan and cultural considerations, 1606
  manifestations, 1606, 1608t
  nonpharmacologic therapy, 1607
  nursing process, 1607–1609
  outcome evaluation, 1609
  overview of, 1605
  pathophysiology and etiology, 1605–1606
  pharmacologic therapy, 1607
  physical interventions, 1607
  prevention of, 1605–1606
  risk factors, 1605–1606
  surgery, 1607
Confusion Assessment Method (CAM),
  1587t, 1607
Congenital and hereditary conditions, 1282
Congenital anomalies, 2046
Congenital cataracts, 1307
Congenital heart defects
  activity promotion, 1102
  assessment, 1100
  assessment guidelines for children, 1101t
  care planning, 1101
  clinical interventions, 1096, 1099–1100t
  collaborative care, 1095–1096, 1097–1100t
  complementary and alternative therapy, 1103t
  defined, 1083
  diagnosis, 1100–1101
  diagnostic tests, 1096, 1097–1098t
  etiology, 1089
  fluids and nutrition management, 1102
  interventions, 1101–1103
  manifestations by pathophysiology, 1094t
  mixed
    clinical therapy, 1090–1091t
    defined, 1089
    manifestations, 1090–1091t, 1095
    pathophysiology, 1090–1091t
    total anomalous pulmonary venous
      return, 1091t
    transposition of the great arteries
      (TGA), 1090t
    truncus arteriosus, 1090–1091t
  neurodevelopmental outcomes, 1096t
  newborns with, 2208t
  Nursing Care Plan, 1103–1104t
  nursing process, 1100–1103
  outcome evaluation, 1103

overview of, 1083
  pain management, 1102
  pharmacologic therapy, 1096
  postoperative care, 1102
  postsurgical home care, 1103
  posttraumatic stress disorder and surgery,
    1103t
  pregnancy and, 2048–2049
  presurgical home care and, 1102
  psychosocial support and, 1102
  pulmonary blood flow decrease
    clinical therapy, 1087–1089t
    defined, 1087
    manifestations, 1087–1088t
    pathophysiology, 1087–1089t
    pulmonary or tricuspid atresia,
      1088–1089t
    pulmonary stenosis, 1087t
    tetralogy of Fallot (TOF), 1088t
  respiratory function promotion, 1102
  septal (blood flow increase)
    atrial septal defect (ASD), 1084–1085t
    atrioventricular (AV) canal (endocardial
      cushion defect), 1086t
    clinical therapy, 1084–1086t
    defined, 1084
    manifestations, 1084–1086t, 1094
    patent ductus arteriosus (PDA), 1084t
    pathophysiology, 1084–1086t
    ventricular septal defect (VSD),
      1085–1086t
  systemic blood flow obstruction
    aortic stenosis, 1092t
    clinical therapy, 1092–1094t
    coarctation of the aorta, 1092–1093t
    defined, 1089
    hypoplastic left heart syndrome (HLHS),
      1093–1094t
    manifestations, 1092–1094t
    pathophysiology, 1092–1094t
  treatment as palliative procedure, 1096
  treatment goals, 1101
Congenital nevi, 128
Congenital scoliosis, 846
Congruent communication, 2409
Conjugate vera, 2014
Conjugated bilirubin, 651t
Conjunctival scrapings, 567
Conjunctivitis
  assessment, 568
  bacterial, 566f
  care planning, 568
  causes of, 566t
  chemical, 2226
  collaborative care, 567–568
  comfort and, 569
  community-based care, 569
  contact lens care and, 568t
  defined, 565
  diagnosis, 568
  diagnostic tests, 567
  entropion and, 567, 567f
  etiology, 566
  goals, 568
  illustrated, 566f
  infection and, 569
  interventions, 569
  manifestations, 567, 568t
  nonpharmacologic therapy, 568
  nursing process, 568–569

outcomes, 569
overview of, 565
pathophysiology, 565–567
pharmacologic therapy, 567–568
photophobia, 567
prevention, 566–567
risk factors, 566
scarring and, 567
trachoma, 567, 567t
Connective tissue, 509
Consciousness. *See also* Level of
consciousness (LOC)
components of, 692
defined, 692
Consent
competency for, 2659–2661
in emergencies, 2661
expressed, 2659
implied, 2659
informed, 2659
Consequence-based (teleological)
theories, 1879
Conservation, 1665t
Constant fever, 1431
Constipation. *See also* Bowel incontinence,
constipation, and impaction
behavior management/bowel training and,
310–311
biofeedback and, 311
causes of, 306t
in children, 307, 308t
collaborative care, 308–331
complementary and alternative therapy, 311
defined, 276, 305
diagnostic tests, 308
education and, 310
fecal impaction, 307
hypothyroidism and, 815
interventions and therapies, 277t
lifespan considerations, 307–308
manifestations, 277t, 306–308
medications, 309t
nonpharmacologic therapy, 310–311
nutrition and, 310
in older adults, 307–308
opioid use and, 165t
pathophysiology and etiology, 306
pharmacologic therapy, 308–310
polyethylene glycol (PEG) and, 310t
in pregnant women, 308
prevention, 306
risk factors, 306
surgery, 308
Constructive surgery, 1261t
Constructivism, 2505
Consumer-driven healthcare plan (CDHP), 2628
Consumers, 2540–2541, 2548
Contact dermatitis
allergic, 1488, 1489t
assessment, 1490–1491
care planning, 1491
causes of, 1488t
client teaching, 1491t
collaborative care, 1489–1490
complementary and alternative therapy, 1490
defined, 1488
diagnosis, 1491
diagnostic tests, 1490
distribution of lesions, 1489t
illustrated, 1489f

interventions, 1491–1492
irritant, 1488, 1489t
lifespan and cultural considerations, 1489
manifestations, 1488–1489, 1489t
nonpharmacologic therapy, 1490
nursing process, 1490–1492
outcome evaluation, 1492
overview of, 1488
patch testing and, 1490
pathophysiology and etiology, 1488
pharmacologic therapy, 1490
risk factors, 1488
as type IV reaction, 484
Contact lenses, 568t
Contact precautions, 546
Contaminated wounds, 1450
Contemporary nursing practice
chain of command, 2549–2550, 2550f
nurse practice acts and, 2549
nursing definitions and, 2548
organizational chart, 2550, 2550f
recipients of nursing and, 2548
settings for nursing and, 2548–2549,
2549f
Standards of Practice and, 2549
Continent ileostomy, 663, 663f
Contingency contracts, 1529–1530
Contingency planning, 2475
Continuance commitment, 2487f
Continuity theory, 1653
Continuous bladder irrigation (CBI), 289
Continuous blood glucose monitoring
(CGM), 753
Continuous positive airway pressure (CPAP),
196, 198, 199t, 979, 980, 981t
Continuous quality improvement (CQI), 2475,
2690–2691
Continuous renal replacement therapy (CRRT)
defined, 383
illustrated, 384f
performance of, 384
types of, 384t
vascular access for, 384–385, 385f
Contraception
abstinence, 1379
barrier methods
cervical cap, 1382
condoms, 1379–1380
diaphragm, 1381–1382, 1381f
vaginal sponge, 1382, 1382f
coitus interruptus, 1379
discontinuing, 1386
douching, 1379
fertility awareness methods
basal body temperature (BBT),
1378, 1378f
calendar rhythm method, 1378
defined, 1378
overview of, 1378
ovulation method, 1379
symptothermal method, 1379
hormonal
benefits of, 1384
combined estrogen-progestin, 1383–1384
combined oral contraceptives (COCs),
1383–1384
Depo-Provera, 1384–1385
emergency, 1385–1386
long-lasting progestin, 1384–1385
mechanisms of action, 1364t

mini-pill, 1384
side effects of, 1383–1384, 1384t
skin patch, 1384
vaginal contraceptive ring, 1384
weight gain and, 1385f
intrauterine, 1382–1383, 1382f
male, 1386
operative sterilization, 1386
postpartum care and, 2186–2187
situational, 1379
spermicides, 1379
Contractility, 1042
Contraction stress test (CST), 2048, 2088–2089,
2089f
Contractions
assessment of, 2141–2142
Braxton Hicks, 2121
characteristics of, 2118, 2118f
defined, 2118
external electronic monitoring of, 2142
internal electronic monitoring of, 2142
phases of, 2118
Contralateral deficit, 1234
Contrast-enhanced CT scan, 247
Controlled Substances Act (CSA), 2661–2662,
2662t
Controlling, 2475–2476
Conus medullaris syndrome, 910t
Convalescent stage, infection, 529
Convection, 1422
Convergence, eye assessment, 1287t
Co-occurring disorders, 1525t
Coombs test, 489
Cooperative play, 1667
COPD. *See* Chronic obstructive
pulmonary disease
Coping. *See also* Stress and coping
with alcohol abuse, 1541–1543
alterations from normal responses,
1907–1910
with Alzheimer disease (AD), 1601
approach, 1899
avoidance, 1899
with cancer, 61–62
cognitive appraisal and, 1898
with colorectal cancer, 90
with COPD, family and, 1015–1016
with coronary artery disease, 1126
with death, 1758
defined, 1896
with diabetes, 764
effective, 1899
emotion-focused, 1899
family mechanisms, 1715–1716
with fatigue, 189
with fibromyalgia, 194
with HIV/AIDS, 477
with loss of clients, 1761, 1761f
Maslow's hierarchy of needs and,
1899, 1899f
mean-focused, 1899
problem-focused, 1899
process, 1898–1900
reappraisal and adaptation and,
1899–1900
with sensory deficit, 1296–1297
with substance abuse, 1570
in transaction model, 1902
types and examples of, 1900t
Cord blood analysis, 2156

Corneal abrasion, 1311–1312, 1313t, 1315
Corneal reflex, 1289t
Cornell Scale for Depression in Dementia, 1587t
Coronal suture, 2114
Coronary artery bypass grafting (CABG), 1121–1122, 1121f, 1122f
Coronary artery disease (CAD)
    acute coronary syndrome (ACS) and, 1105, 1107
    acute myocardial infarction (AMI) and, 1105, 1107–1108
    angina pectoris and, 1105
    assessment, 1124
    cardiac rehabilitation and, 1123, 1128t
    care planning, 1124–1125
    characteristics of, 1051
    clinical therapy, 1119–1123
    collaborative care, 1113–1123
    complementary and alternative therapy, 1123, 1123t
    conservative management, 1116–1118
    defined, 1052t, 1105
    as diabetes complication, 748
    diagnosis, 1124
    diagnostic tests
        AMI diagnosis, 1114–1115, 1114t
        cardiac markers and, 1114, 1114t
        ECG, 1115, 1115f
        echocardiography, 1115
        hemodynamic monitoring, 1116
        laboratory tests, 1115
        overview of, 1113–1114
        radionuclide imaging, 1116
        types of, 1114
    etiology, 1108
    Framingham Heart Study (FHS) and, 1109t
    interventions
        cardiac perfusion promotion, 1127
        coping, 1126
        fear management, 1126–1127
        health maintenance, 1125
        nutrition, 1125
        pain management, 1125–1126
        therapeutic regimen management, 1127
        tissue perfusion monitoring, 1126
    interventions and therapies, 1052t
    intra-aortic balloon pump (IABP) and, 1123, 1123f
    ischemia, 1106
    manifestations, 1052t, 1111–1113, 1111t, 1112t
    Nursing Care Plan, 1128–1129t
    nursing process, 1124–1127
    outcome evaluation, 1127
    overview of, 1105
    pathophysiology, 1105–1110
    pharmacologic therapy, 1118–1119
    revascularization procedures, 1120–1122, 1121f, 1122f
    rheumatoid arthritis and, 499
    risk factors
        emerging, 1109–1110
        for metabolic syndrome, 1110t
        modifiable, 1109–1110
        nonmodifiable, 1109
        overview of, 1108–1109, 1108t
        for women, 1110
    treatment goals, 1113
    ventricular assist devices (VADs) and, 1123

Coronary circulation, 1036–1040, 1038f
Corpus luteum, 2018
Corrective action, 2492
Corticosteroids
    for asthma, 997, 999t
    defined, 167
    for hypersensitivity, 490
    for inflammatory bowel disease (IBD), 664–665t
    for rheumatoid arthritis, 501–502
    side effects of, 1000t
    topical, 1461t
Cortisone injections, 889
Coryza, 570
Cost-conscious nursing practice, 2466
Cost-containment strategies, 2464–2465
Cost-effective care
    competition and, 2464
    cost-containment strategies, 2464–2465
    factors influencing provision of health care, 2463–2464
    international perspective, 2463
    nursing economics, 2465–2466
    overview of, 2462–2463
    payment sources, 2463
    price controls and, 2464–2465
    separate billing for nursing services and, 2464
    supply versus demand and, 2463–2464
    vertically integrated health services organizations and, 2465
Costovertebral angle (CVA) tenderness, 2180t
Cotyledons, 2025
Coughing techniques, 1008t
Counseling
    health and wellness, 418
    preconception, 1371–1372
Countershock, 1188–1190, 1190f
Countershock phase, 1901
Couples, 1725
Couplet, 1185
Couvade, 2039f
Covert conflicts, 2387–2388
COWs (computers on wheels), 2643
CP. See Cerebral palsy
CPAP (continuous positive airway pressure), 196, 198, 199t, 979, 980, 981t
CPK (creatine phosphokinase), 1477
CPP (cerebral perfusion pressure), 712
CPR. See Cardiopulmonary resuscitation
CQI (continuous quality improvement), 2475, 2690–2691
Crack cocaine
    defined, 1553
    pregnancy and, 1553–1554
Crackles, 963t
Cranial nerves
    assessment in unconscious client, 706t
    function of, 689, 689t, 1279t
    list of, 689t
    in neurological assessment, 699–701t
CRBIs (catheter-related bloodstream infections), 2704
C-reactive protein (CRP), 501, 641, 1098t, 1114
Creatine kinase, 1114–1115
Creatine phosphokinase (CPK), 1477

Creatinine clearance test
    in chronic kidney disease (CKD), 395
    defined, 271
    in nephritis, 672
Creativity, 2318
Credentialing, 2666
Credibility, 2401
Crepitation, 824t
Crime, 2654–2655
Criminal law, 2654–2655
Crisis
    alternative therapy, 1931–1932
    assessment, 1932
    assessment interview, 1527t
    care planning, 1933
    characteristics of, 1928t
    collaborative care, 1929–1931
    communication do's and don'ts, 1933t
    community assessment, 1932
    crisis counseling, 1930, 1931t
    crisis intervention, 1930–1931
    defined, 1927
    diagnosis, 1932–1933
    diagnostic tests, 1929
    family assessment, 1932
    individual assessment, 1932
    interventions, 1933
    lifespan and cultural considerations, 1929
    manifestations, 1929, 1929t
    maturational, 1928f
    nonpharmacologic therapy, 1930–1931
    Nursing Care Plan, 1933–1934t
    nursing process, 1932–1933
    outcome evaluation, 1933
    overview of, 1927
    pathophysiology and etiology, 1928–1929
    pharmacologic therapy, 1930
    resilience and, 1928–1929
    situational, 1928, 1928f
    temporary relocation, 1931
    therapeutic communication, 1930, 1930t
Crisis connection, 1931t
Crisis counseling, 1930, 1931t
Crisis intervention, 1930–1931
Crisis intervention centers, 1931
Crisis theory, 1928
Critical pathways. See also Case management
    as care map, 2384
    in case management model, 2445, 2445f
    defined, 2382
    for total hip replacement, 2384–2386t
Critical thinking. See also Clinical decision making
    attitudes towards, 2317t
    creativity, 2318
    defined, 2316
    inquiry, 2318
    intellect, 2317–2318
    intuition, 2320
    overview of, 2316–2317
    reasoning, 2319, 2319t, 2320t
    reflection, 2319–2320, 2321t
    salient cues, 2317–2318, 2318f
    skills, 2317f
Critical values of nursing, 2539
Crohn disease. See also Inflammatory bowel disease (IBD)
    aphthoid lesion, 658
    characteristics of, 657t
    crypts, 658f

defined, 657
digestive system and, 209
enterocutaneous fistulas, 658
enteroenteric fistulas, 658
enterovesical fistulas, 658
manifestations, 660–661
progression of, 658f
Cross-tolerance, 1525t
Crowning, 2123
CRP (C-reactive protein), 501, 641
CRRT. See Continuous renal replacement therapy
Crying
in newborn assessment, 2229
newborns and, 2203
Cryptorchidism, 1357t
Crystalloid solutions, 1230
Crystalloids, 337
CSA (Controlled Substances Act), 2661–2662, 2662t
CSF (cerebrospinal fluid), 688, 688f
CST (contraction stress test), 2048, 2088–2089, 2089f
CT. See Computed tomography
Cuddliness, 2236
Cultural assessment, postpartum, 2180t
Cultural clustering, 1709f
Cultural competence
administration and governance, 1642
characteristics of, 1640
defined, 1640
domains of culture, 1641
essential, 1640
ethical multiculturalism model, 1641t, 1642f
interpreter use and, 1643
language, 1642–1643
orientation and education, 1642
prejudices and, 1641
questions, 1640
staff competencies, 1643
standards of, 1641–1643
Cultural differences, 1633, 1633t
Cultural factors
abuse and, 1967–1968
in assessment, 2284
Cultural humility, 1630t
Cultural transmission, 1633–1634
Cultural values, 1632
Culturally competent nursing care, 1643–1644
Culture
abuse and, 1969–1970, 1969f, 1970t
acculturation, 1634
acute renal failure (ARF) and, 386t
ADHD and, 1686t
Alzheimer disease (AD) care and, 1603t
antepartum nutrition and, 2094, 2094f
appendicitis and, 646
assault and homicide and, 1977, 1979
assimilation, 1634
baby care and, 2245t
behaviors, learning of, 1634, 1634t
belief system, 1632
blindness and, 1307t
blood transfusions and, 180
burns and, 1473t
cancer and, 42
cellulitis and, 562
characteristics of, 1633t
childhood grief and, 1754

Chronic kidney disease and, 392t
cirrhosis and, 782t
codeine use and, 166t
cognitive assessment and, 1606t
collaboration and language barriers and, 2380t
in comfort assessment, 147
communication and, 2416
competence in nursing, 2304t
concepts related to, 1631–1632t
confusion and, 1606
core belief differences, 1633, 1633t
crisis and, 1929
death and dying and, 1760t
defined, 1629
development and, 1678
diabetes and, 741t
digestion and, 217–220
diversity, 1630
domains of, 1641
enc11lturation, 1633–1634
end-of-life care considerations, 180–181
family-centered care and, 1735
fever and, 1434
food preferences and, 386
gallstones and, 650t
glaucoma and, 1319t
grief and loss and, 1748–1749
hearing loss and, 1301t
HIV/AIDS and, 457
hypertension and, 1167t
infection and, 555
infertility treatments and, 1392t
learning and, 2507
life meaning and, 1632–1633, 1632f
lupus nephritis and, 671t
mood and affect and, 1787
moral principles and, 2576t
multiple sclerosis and, 879
newborn care and, 2199t
nonverbal communication and, 2401–2402
nutrition and, 942–944, 945t
obesity and, 945t
obesity in children and, 773t
organization of, 1632
osteoarthritis and, 887
otitis media and, 577
pain response and, 157–162, 161t
parasites and, 877t
Parkinson disease and, 897
perinatal loss and, 1769–1770, 1770t
personality disorders (PD) and, 1860
postoperative nursing and, 1273
postpartum care and, 2182t
postpartum depression and, 1821t
postpartum influences and, 1819–1820
pregnancy and, 2040, 2041t, 2064t
prostate cancer and, 113t
rape and, 1986, 1986t
respiratory syncytial virus (RSV) and, 1019t
schizophrenia and, 1616, 1616t
seizures and, 721
sexual health and, 1362t
sexuality and, 1355–1362
sickle cell disease and, 120t
smoking and, 1007t, 1546t
social differences
additional, 1639t
biological variations, 1639, 1639f

communication, 1638
environmental control, 1638
religious variations, 1638
skin color, 1639
space, 1638–1639
subcultures, 1638, 1638f
susceptibility to disease, 1639
time, 1639
social support and, 416t
sodium use and, 368t
stress and coping and, 1912–1913
stroke risk factors and, 1237t
subcultures, 1638, 1638f
sudden infant death syndrome (SIDS) and, 1025t
suicide and, 1993–1994, 1993t
type 1 diabetes in children and, 767
undernutrition and, 945t
urinary calculi and, 322
values and beliefs, 1630–1637
violence and, 1961
vulnerable populations and, 1637–1638
worldview, 1632
Culture and diversity. See also Culture; Diversity
concepts related to, 1631–1632t
cultural competence, 1640–1643
cultural diversity, 1630
cultural transmission, 1633–1634
culturally competent nursing care, 1643–1644
disparities and differences, 1637–1640
diversity, 1634–1637
social differences, 1638–1639
values and beliefs, 1630–1637
vulnerable populations, 1637–1638
Culture fatigue, 187–188
Cunnilingus, 1346
Curling ulcers, 1472
CVI (chronic venous insufficiency), 1198, 1199t
Cyanosis, 588, 957
Cyberchondria, 2641
Cycle of violence, 1955
Cyclic citrullinated peptide (CCP), 501
Cycloplegics, 1315t
Cyclothymic disorder, 1811
Cystitis
defined, 619
inflammation in, 626
presenting systems of, 621–622
Cystocele, 1360t
Cystogram, 295
Cystoscopy, 295, 623
Cytokines, 443
Cytological examination, 108
Cytoplasm, 30
Cytotoxic (type II) hypersensitivity, 445, 483, 484f

D

D&C (dilation and curettage), 1402
DAD (Depression After Delivery), 1824
Daily weight measurement, 348
Damages, 2656
Damus-Kaye-Stansel procedure, 1099t
DASH (Dietary Approaches to Stop Hypertension), 1169, 1170t
Dashboard, 2645

"Dashboard knee," 2001, 2002t
Data
    client as source, 2270
    client records as source, 2271
    collecting, 2271–2272, 2272t
    healthcare professionals as source, 2271
    interpreting, 2282–2285
    literature as source, 2271
    objective, 2270
    organizing, 2282
    signs, 2270
    sources of, 2270–2271
    subjective, 2270
    support people as source, 2270–2271
    symptoms, 2270
    types of, 2270
    validating, 2282
Data, action, and response (DAR), 2442–2443
Databases, 2270
Date rape, 1407
Dating violence, 1406–1407, 1407t
Dawn phenomenon, 746
Daydreaming, 1904
DBS (deep brain stimulation), 898
Dead space, 1212
Death and dying. *See also* End-of-life care
    altered levels of consciousness and, 1759
    anorexia, nausea, dehydration and, 1759
    assessment, 1762
    awareness-of-dying model, 182–183
    care planning, 1762
    children, ethical issues, 179–180
    client loss and, 1761, 1761f
    collaborative care, 1761
    culture and, 1760t
    death determination, 1760
    diagnosis, 1762
    The Dying Person's Bill of Rights, 175t
    dyspnea and, 1759
    friends, 1753
    grandparents, 1753
    hypotension and, 1759
    infant, from SIDS, 1026
    interventions, 1762
    leading causes throughout lifespan, 2290t
    manifestations
        anticipatory grief, 1758
        coping with death, 1758
        lifespan and cultural considerations,
            1758–1759
        physiological changes, 1759–1760
        therapies, 1760t
    nonpharmacologic therapy, 1761
    nurse response to, 1760–1761
    nursing process, 1762
    outcome evaluation, 1762
    overview of, 1757–1758
    pain and, 1759
    parents, 1752–1753
    pathophysiology and etiology, 1758
    pharmacologic therapy, 1761
    psychological needs, 1759–1760
    siblings, 1753
    spiritual beliefs related to, 1877–1878
    as traumatic injury result, 1960
Death anxiety, 183, 1751
Debridement
    in arthroscopy, 888
    autolytic, 1497
    for burns, 1473

defined, 634, 1473, 1497
    for pressure ulcers, 1497
    surgical, 1510
Decelerations
    abrupt, 2152
    defined, 2152
    early, 2152
    episodic, 2153
    gradual, 2153
    guidelines for management, 2154t
    late, 2152
    periodic, 2153
    prolonged, 2153
    types and characteristics of, 2153f
    variable, 2152
Decerebrate posturing, 691t
Decibels (dB), 1298
Decision making
    collaboration and, 2380–2381
    ethical, 2567, 2569–2570
    in groups, 2420–2422
Decisions. *See also* Clinical decision making
    healthcare, 2322t
    lifespan considerations, 2322t
    priority, 2321
    scheduling, 2321
    steps in making, 2322
    time management, 2321
    types of, 2321
    value, 2321
Decoding, 2399
Decompensation, 1145
Decorticate posturing, 691t
Deductive reasoning, 2319
Deep brain stimulation (DBS), 898
Deep breathing
    exercises, 968
    phobias and, 1943t
Deep palpation, 2278–2279, 2279f
Deep partial-thickness burns, 1468, 1481t
Deep venous thrombosis (DVT)
    anticoagulants for, 1132–1134,
        1133–1134t
    assessment, 1135
    cardiopulmonary perfusion and, 1136
    care planning, 1135
    clinical therapy, 1135
    collaborative care, 1132–1138
    common locations of, 1131f
    defined, 858, 1130
    diagnosis, 1135
    diagnostic tests, 1132
    etiology, 1130
    factors associated with, 1130t
    home care for, 1137t
    interventions, 1135–1136
    manifestations, 1131–1132, 1131t
    Nursing Care Plan, 1137t
    nursing process, 1135–1136
    outcome evaluation, 1136
    overview of, 1130
    pain management and, 1135
    pathophysiology and etiology, 1130–1131
    peripheral perfusion and, 1135–1136
    pharmacologic therapy, 1132–1134
    physical mobility and, 1136
    prophylaxis, 1132
    risk factors, 858t, 1131
    spinal cord injuries (SCI) and, 912
    surgery, 1134

Defecation
    defined, 274
    habits, 274
    regular, promoting, 315–316
Defense mechanisms, 1649. *See also* Ego defense
        mechanisms
Defibrillation, 1188–1190, 1190f
Defining characteristics, 2336
Deflecting, 2433
Dehiscence, 1509
Dehydration. *See also* Fluid volume
        deficit (FVD)
    in children, 359
    death and dying and, 1759
    defined, 339, 354
    hypertonic, 355
    hypotonic, 355
    isotonic, 355
    in older adults, 356t, 359
    in pediatric clients, 359t
Delayed (type IV) hypersensitivity
    contact dermatitis, 484
    defined, 484
    illustrated, 486f
    latex allergy, 484–485, 486t
Delayed union fractures, 857
Delayed-type hypersensitivity, 445
Delegates
    deciding on, 2469
    defined, 2467
    delegation benefits to, 2469
    unwilling, 2472
Delegation
    accepting, 2471
    agreement, 2470
    assignment patterns and, 2470–2471
    assignment versus, 2468
    authority and, 2468
    benefits of, 2468–2469
    decision tree for, 2473f
    defined, 2348, 2467
    delegate benefits of, 2469
    delegate selection, 2469
    difficulty of learning skill, 2467
    dumping versus, 2468
    factors affecting, 2470–2472
    inappropriate, 2371
    ineffective, 2472
    liability and, 2473
    manager benefits of, 2469
    nonsupportive environment and, 2471
    nurse benefits of, 2468
    obstacles to, 2471–2472
    organization benefits of, 2469
    to other nurses, 2467
    overdelegation and, 2472
    overview of, 2467
    performance monitoring, 2470
    principles of, 2467–2468
    in prioritizing care, 2370
    process, 2469–2470
    reverse, 2472
    safety and, 2471t
    task definition, 2469
    task description, 2469
    tools for success, 2467
    underdelegation and, 2472
    to unlicensed assistive personnel, 2467–2468,
        2468t
    unnecessary duplication and, 2472

Delegators
  defined, 2467
  insecurity, 2471–2472
Delirium
  confusion and, 1605
  defined, 1605
  dementia and, 1584
  dementia comparison, 1585t
  manifestations, 1606t
  methods of preventing, 1606
Delirium tremens (DTs), 1525t, 1537t
Delphi technique, 2421–2422
Delusions
  categories of, 1614t
  defined, 1578, 1611
Dementia. See also Cognition
  alterations and manifestations, 1584
  alterations and therapies, 1586t
  cognitive deficits, 1584
  conditions mimicking, 1584
  defined, 1584, 1605
  delirium comparison, 1585t
  etiologies, 1584t
  genetic considerations and nonmodifiable risk
      factors, 1584–1585
  prevalence of, 1584
  prevention of, 1585
Democratic (participative, consultative) leaders,
      2489–2490
Demographics, changing, 2598
Demography, 2542
Demyelination, 876
Denial, 1905t
Dental care, antepartum, 2072
Dental caries, 424
Deoxyribonucleic acid (DNA), 30, 31–32, 31f
Department of Health and Human Services
      (DHHS), 2622, 2622t, 2623t
Dependence
  alcohol, 1535
  defined, 1520
  pattern of, 1535
  physical, 1525t
  psychological, 1525t
Dependent interventions, 2345
Dependent personality disorder (DPD), 1856t,
      1857–1858, 1863t
Depersonalization, 1860, 1947
Depolarization, 1043
Depo-Provera, 1384–1385
Depression
  addiction and, 1523–1524
  in adolescents, 1801t
  assessment, 1801–1802
  assessment for comorbidities, 1802
  care planning, 1803
  in children, 1801t
  collaborative care, 1801
  defined, 1780t, 1798, 1904
  dementia and, 1584
  diabetes and, 750
  diagnosis, 1802
  diagnostic tests, 1801
  disorders, 1778
  double, 1778
  fatigue and women and, 186t
  grief versus, 1788, 1788t
  hope and, 1803
  interventions, 1803
  lifespan considerations, 1801t

major depressive disorder (MDD), 1798–1800,
      1799t, 1800f
  manifestations, 1798–1800, 1800t, 1904t
  Nursing Care Plan, 1804t
  nursing process, 1801–1803
  in older adults, 1801t
  outcome evaluation, 1803
  persistent depressive disorder, 1800
  pharmacologic therapy
    atypical antidepressants, 1793
    collaborative care, 1801
    monoamine oxidase inhibitors (MAOIs),
        1792–1793
    selective serotonin reuptake inhibitors
        (SSRIs), 1791–1792
    tricyclic antidepressants (TCAs),
        1790–1791
  physical complaints, 1802, 1802t
  postpartum, 1770, 1779, 1816–1828
  prevention of, 1798
  psychotherapy, 1801
  seasonal affective disorder (SAD), 1800
  self-esteem promotion and, 1803
  situational. See adjustment disorder with
        depressed mood
  suicide assessment, 1802
  symptoms of, 1801t
  therapies, 1780t
  unipolar, 1778
Depression After Delivery (DAD), 1824
Depression fractures, 856t
Depression theories
  biological rhythms, 1780–1781
  causative, 1782t
  cognitive theory, 1781
  gender bias theory, 1781–1782
  intrapersonal factors, 1781
  learning theory, 1781
  overview of, 1779–1780
  sociocultural factors, 1781, 1781f
Depressive disorder with peripartum onset
  defined, 1779, 1780t
  symptoms, 1779
  therapies, 1780t
Depressive episodes, 1809–1811
Derealization, 1860
Dermatological effects, chronic kidney disease
      (CKD) and, 395
Dermis
  defined, 1447
  in older adults, 1448
  thickness variation, 1472
Desaturated blood, 1046
Descent, 2125
Desire phase, in sexual response cycle, 1346
Detached retina
  interventions, 1317
  manifestations, 1312–1314, 1314t
  therapies, 1316
Detachment, 1855
Detoxification, 1525t
Detrusor muscles, 261, 285
Development
  adolescents, 1668–1670
  adults, 1670–1671
  alterations and therapies, 1675–1676t
  alterations from normal, 1671–1677
  assessment, 1677–1678
  body proportions, 1659f
  collaborative interventions and therapies, 1679

  communication and, 2406
  concepts related to, 1674t
  defined, 1647
  diagnostic tests, 1678
  environmental factors, 1677
  genetic considerations, 1658–1659
  genetic considerations and nonmodifiable risk
      factors, 1673–1676
  independent interventions and therapies,
      1678–1679
  infants, 1659–1662
  interventions and therapies, 1678–1679
  life span, 1659–1671
  lifespan and cultural considerations, 1678
  modifiable risk factors, 1677
  multisystem effects of, 1672
  normal, 1648–1659
  pharmacologic therapy, 1679
  premature newborns and, 2258–2259
  prenatal considerations, 1677
  preschoolers, 1664–1666
  prevalence of alterations, 1673
  prevention of alterations, 1677
  school-age children, 1666–1668
  screenings, 1677
  sickle cell disease and, 126
  stages of, 1649t
  theories
    behaviorism, 1654
    continuity, 1653
    ecological, 1655–1657, 1656f
    Erikson, 1650–1652, 1651t
    Fowler, 1658
    Freud, 1649–1650, 1650t
    Gilligan, 1657–1658
    Gould, 1653
    Havighurst, 1652, 1652t
    Kohlberg, 1657, 1658t
    moral, 1657–1658
    overview of, 1648–1649
    Peck, 1652–1653
    Piaget, 1653–1654, 1654t
    psychosocial, 1649–1653
    resiliency, 1654–1655
    social learning, 1654
    spiritual, 1658
    temperament, 1654, 1655t
    Westerhoff, 1658, 1659t
  toddlers, 1662–1664
Development Disabilities and Bill of Rights
      Act of 2000, 1591t
Developmental disability, 1581
Developmental factors, in assessment, 2284
Developmental stage, 1648
Developmental stressors, 1897–1898
Developmental theories, in assessment, 2282
Device integration, 2639
DEXA (dual-energy x-ray absorptiometry),
      800–801
DHHS (Department of Health and Human
      Services), 2622, 2622t, 2623t
DHT (dihydrotestosterone), 285
Diabetes in children
  assessment, 760
  care planning, 776
  lifespan considerations, 761t
  MODY, 767t
  NDM, 767t
  Nursing Care Plan, 778–779t
  overview of, 766–767

Diabetes in children (*continued*)
  type 1
    collaborative care, 768–772
    complementary and alternative therapy and, 772
    complication management, 771–772
    culture and, 767t
    diagnostic tests, 769
    glucose monitoring, 769
    hemoglobin A_{1C}, 770t
    individualized education plans (IEPs) and, 768
    insulin, 769–771, 771t
    insulin doses, 771t
    insulin pumps and, 771t
    managing in school, 770t
    manifestations, 767–768
    Nursing Care Plan, 778–779t
    nutrition recommendations, 771t
    nutrition therapy, 771
    parent responsibilities, 769t
    risk factors, 767
    school/day care responsibilities, 769t
  type 2
    assessment, 775
    collaborative care, 774–775
    community-based care, 778t
    complication management, 775
    diabetic ketoacidosis (DKA), 776t
    diagnoses, 775
    glucose control tips, 777t
    hypoglycemic agents and, 775
    as increasing, 772
    interventions, 776–777
    manifestations, 773–774
    nursing process, 775–778
    nutritional and activity guidelines, 774t
    obesity and, 773
    postdischarge evaluation guidelines, 777–778
    risk factors, 773
    schedule for managing, 776t
Diabetes mellitus
  acute complications
    hyperglycemia, 746–747
    hypoglycemia, 747–748
  antepartum care and, 2077t
  aspirin therapy and, 757
  assessment, 760
  blood glucose homeostasis and, 704
  care planning, 760
  chronic complications
    alterations in cardiovascular system, 748–749
    alterations in mood, 750
    alterations in peripheral and autonomic nervous systems, 749–750
    complications of the feet, 750–751
    diabetic nephropathy, 749
    diabetic retinopathy, 749
    periodontal disease, 750
    susceptibility to infection, 750
  client teaching, 759–760
  collaborative care
    blood glucose monitoring, 752–753
    diagnostic tests, 751–752
    exercise, 758–759
    nutrition, 757–758
    pharmacologic therapy, 753–757
    sick-day management, 758
    surgery, 759

  complications of, 743–751
  coronary artery disease (CAD) and, 1116–1118
  as coronary artery disease risk factor, 1109
  defined, 740, 766
  diagnosis, 760
  diagnostic screening, 751
  genetic considerations and nonmodifiable risk factors, 729
  hormones and, 740
  hypoglycemic agents and, 756
  infant of mother with, 2207t
  insulin preparations, 754t
  interventions
    coping, 764
    education, 760–762
    foot care, 763t
    healthy behaviors, 762–763
    safety, 763–764
    sexual health, 764
    skin integrity, 762
  interventions and therapies, 733
  management monitoring, 751–752
  multisystem effects of, 744t
  Nursing Care Plan, 765t
  nursing process, 759–764
  nutrition and, 757–758
  in older adults, 760, 761t
  onset of, 726–727
  outcome evaluation, 764
  overview of, 740
  peripheral neuropathy and, 561
  prediabetes and, 751
  pregnancy and
    clinical therapy, 2047–2048
    evaluation of fetal status, 2048
    fetal-neonatal risks, 2046–2047
    influence on outcome, 2046–2047
    influences, 2045–2047
    intrapartum management, 2048
    labor management, 2048
    long-term glucose control, 2047–2048
    maternal risks, 2046
    postpartum management, 2048
    timing of birth, 2048
  prevalence of, 729
  risk and incidence of, 741t
  sexuality and, 1344
  as stroke risk factor, 1236
  type 1
    as autoimmune disease, 767
    celiac disease and, 771
    in children, 767–772
    collaborative care, 768–772
    complementary and alternative therapy and, 772
    complication management, 771–772
    culture and, 767t
    defined, 740
    diagnostic tests, 769
    eating disorders and, 771
    genetic considerations and nonmodifiable risk factors, 729
    glucose monitoring, 769
    glycemic responses, 758
    hemoglobin A_{1C}, 770t
    hypoglycemia and, 772
    individualized education plans (IEPs) and, 768
    insulin, 769–771, 771t

    insulin doses, 771t
    insulin pumps and, 771t
    managing in school, 770t
    manifestations, 741–742, 742t, 767–768
    Nursing Care Plan, 765t, 778–779t
    nutrition recommendations, 771t
    nutrition therapy, 771
    onset of, 726–727
    parent responsibilities, 769t
    pathophysiology and etiology, 740–741
    risk factors, 741, 767
    school/day care responsibilities, 769t
    thyroid disease and, 771
    without adequate insulin, 746f
  type 2
    assessment, 775
    in children, 772–778
    collaborative care, 774–775
    community-based care, 778t
    complication management, 775
    complications of, 743–751
    defined, 742
    diabetic ketoacidosis (DKA), 776t
    diagnoses, 775
    exercise program, 759
    genetic considerations and nonmodifiable risk factors, 729
    glucose control tips, 777t
    hypoglycemic agents and, 775
    as increasing, 772
    interventions, 776–777
    manifestations, 743, 743t, 773–774
    nursing process, 775–778
    nutritional and activity guidelines, 774t
    obesity and, 727, 773
    onset of, 727
    oral medications and, 754–755
    pathophysiology and etiology, 742–743
    postdischarge evaluation guidelines, 777–778
    prevention of, 731
    risk factors, 742–743, 773
    schedule for managing, 776t
Diabetic ketoacidosis (DKA)
  in children, 776t
  defined, 746
  HHS and hypoglycemia comparison, 745t
  manifestations of, 747
  metabolic problems, 747
  treatment, 15
Diabetic nephropathy, 749
Diabetic neuropathies, 749
Diabetic retinopathy, 749
Diagnosing, 2335
Diagnosis-related groups (DRGs), 2464–2465
Diagnostic labels, 2335–2336
Diagnostic peritoneal lavage, 1961
Diagnostic procedures, 1261t
Diagonal conjugate, 2013
Dialectical behavioral therapy, 1862
Dialysate, 383
Dialysis
  chronic kidney disease (CKD) and, 397–399
  continuous renal replacement therapy (CRRT), 383, 384–385, 384f, 384t
  defined, 272, 383
  hemodialysis, 272, 383–384, 383f
  peritoneal, 272–273, 383, 385–386, 385f
Diaphoresis, 2162

Diaphragm, 1381–1382, 1381f
Diarrhea
   causes of, 276t
   defined, 276
   interventions and therapies, 277t
   manifestations, 277t
Diastasis recti, 2033
Diastole
   defined, 1034
   heart sounds in, 1034f
Diastolic blood pressure, 1045, 1163
DIC. See Disseminated intravascular coagulation
Didanosine, 470t, 471
Diencephalon, 689
Diet
   beliefs affecting, 1876–1877
   in bowel elimination, 273–274
   as cancer risk factor, 46
   coronary artery disease (CAD) and, 1110,
      1116, 1116t
   DASH, 1169, 1170t
   for diabetes clients, 757–758
   digestion and, 226
   gluten-free, casein-free (GFCF), 1692t
   heart failure and, 1160
   hypertension and, 1169
   ketogenic, 720, 721
   low-sodium, 369t, 1082, 1160
   for osteoporosis, 801
   sleep and, 433
   very-low-calorie, 794
Dietary fats, 757
Dietary reference intakes (DRIs), 927, 2091–2092,
      2091–2092t
Differentiated practice, 2457
Differentiation, 32
Diffuse boundaries, 1715
Diffusion, 338, 338f
Digestion
   absorption, 210
   alterations, 210–214
   alterations and therapies, 212–213t
   assessment, 215–221, 216t
   assessment interview, 215t
   in children, 209
   client education, 221
   collaborative interventions and therapies,
      222–226
   concepts related to, 211
   defined, 207
   diagnostic tests
      abdominal x-ray, 220
      amylase, 221
      CT scan, 221
      endoscopy, 220
      upper GI series (barium swallow),
         220, 220f
   disorders
      acid indigestion, 210–211
      anorexia, 210
      celiac disease, 240–243
      cultural diversity and, 220t
      gastroesophageal reflux disease (GERD),
         210, 212t, 226–232
      heartburn, 210
      hepatitis, 211, 212t, 232–239
      lactase deficiency, 243–244
      malabsorption, 211, 211t, 213t, 239–245
      maldigestion, 211
      nausea, 210, 212t

   pancreatitis, 211–213, 213t, 245–251
      prevalence of, 214t
      prevention of, 214–215
      pyloric stenosis, 213, 213t, 251–255
      short bowel syndrome, 244–245
      vomiting, 210, 212t
   fluid and electrolyte balance and, 221
   genetic and nonmodifiable risk factors, 214t
   independent interventions and therapies, 221
   in infants, 209
   intervention and therapies, 221–226
   lifespan and cultural considerations,
      217–220
   maldigestion and, 211t
   malnutrition assessment, 218t
   modifiable risk factors, 214, 215t
   motility, 210
   normal, 208–210
   nutrition therapy
      diet, 226
      enteral nutrition, 222–224, 223f,
         224f, 224t
      parenteral nutrition, 224–226, 225f
   in older adults, 209–210
   organs associated with, 208f
   pediatric, 219t
   pharmacologic therapy, 222
   screenings, 214–215
   system elements, 208
   teeth and, 209f
Digestive enzymes, 931t
Digestive process, 931–932
Digital rectal exam (DRE), 113, 285,
      286f, 1357t
Digitalis, 1153–1156, 1155t
Dihydrotestosterone (DHT), 285
Dilated cardiomyopathy, 1077–1078, 1077t
Dilation and curettage (D&C), 1402
Dimethyl fumarate (Tecfidera), 880
Direct auscultation, 2280
Direct bilirubin, 651t
Direct Coombs test, 489
Direct objects, 523
Direct transmission of infection, 524
Directing, 2475
Directive interviews, 2272
Dirty or infected wounds, 1450
Disability status, 1636–1637
Disasters, 2609
Discectomy, 843
Discharge instructions
   acute respiratory distress syndrome
      (ARDS), 988
   BPH surgery, 290t
   dysrhythmias, 1196
   fractures and, 867
   hip fractures and, 874
   postoperative, 1275t
   urinary calculi, 330, 331t
Discharge preparation. See also Newborn care
   care safety, 2247
   community-based care, 2247
   cultural beliefs/practices and, 2245t
   general instructions, 2245–2246
   nasal and oral suctioning, 2246
   parent teaching, 2243–2245, 2244f
   screening and immunization programs, 2247
   sleep and activity, 2246–2247
   swaddling, 2246, 2246f
Discipline, 1717–1718

Disclosure of health information, 2674t
Discoid lesions, 510
Discoid lupus, 510
Discomfort. See also Comfort
   assessment interview, 148t
   common sources of, 142
   diagnostic tests, 147–148
   genetic considerations, 145–146
   interventions and therapies, 144t, 148–151
   manifestations, 144t
   prevention, 146
   psychosocial well-being and, 150
   relaxation therapy and, 150–151
   risk factors, 145–146
Discovery, 2678
Discovery/problem solving, 2521–2522
Discrimination, 1630
Discs, spinal, 821
Discussions, 2438
Disease
   communicable, 522
   defined, 408, 522
   gender and body size, 414
   infectious, 522
   prevention, 410
   susceptibility to, culture and, 1639
Disease-modifying antirheumatic drugs
      (DMARDs)
   antimalarial agents, 503
   defined, 502
   gold salts, 502–503
   immune and inflammatory agents, 502
   sulfasalazine, 503
   types of, 503t
Diseases of adaptation, 1901
Disenfranchised grief, 1742–1743,
      1747t, 1769
Disinfectants, 544, 544t
Disinhibited social engagement disorder, 1945
Disinhibition, 1855
Dismissal, 2492
Disorganized behavior, 1614
Disorganized thinking, 1613
Displaced fractures, 854t
Displacement, 1905t
Disposable needles, syringes and sharps, 548
Disruptive behavior, 2484t
Dissatisfaction problems, 1351
Disseminated intravascular coagulation (DIC)
   assessment, 1140
   care planning, 1140–1142
   client teaching, 1142t
   clinical therapy, 1140
   collaborative care, 1140
   conditions precipitating, 1139t
   defined, 1138, 1768
   diagnosis, 1140
   diagnostic tests, 1140
   etiology, 1139t
   fear management and, 1142–1143
   gas exchange monitoring and, 1142
   manifestations, 1139–1140, 1141t
   Nursing Care Plan, 1143t
   nursing process, 1140–1143
   outcome evaluation, 1143
   overview of, 1138
   pain management and, 1142–1143
   pathophysiology and etiology, 1138–1139
   in perinatal loss, 1768
   risk factors, 1139

Disseminated intravascular coagulation (DIC)
    (*continued*)
    sepsis and, 600
    sequence of, 1138, 1139*f*
    tissue perfusion and, 1142
Distracted driving, 2712, 2713*t*
Distress, 1896
Distributive shock, 1224, 1226*t*
Diuresis, 264, 378
Diuretics
    heart failure and, 1153, 1154–1155*t*
    hypertension and, 1172*t*
    loop, 712*t*, 1172*t*
    osmotic, 712*t*
    potassium-sparing, 1172*t*
    urinary elimination and, 261
Diurnal variations, 1046
Diversity
    age, 1637
    class, 1635–1636
    concepts related to, 1631–1632*t*
    cultural, 1630
    defined, 1629
    disability status, 1636–1637
    elements of, 1634
    gender, 1634–1635
    race, 1635
    sexual orientation, 1636
    social justice and, 1634
Diverticula, 285
DKA. *See* Diabetic ketoacidosis
DMARDs. *See* Disease-modifying antirheumatic
    drugs
DNA (deoxyribonucleic acid), 30, 31–32, 31*f*
Dock, Lavinia L., 2547
Documentation
    admission nursing assessment, 2445
    in clinical decision making, 2348
    critical pathway, 2445, 2445*f*
    do's and don'ts of, 2450*t*
    EHRs and, 2647*t*
    ethical and legal considerations, 2438–2439
    facility-specific, 2447
    flow sheets, 2446
    guidelines for recording
        accepted terminology, 2448–2449
        accuracy, 2449
        appropriateness, 2449
        commonly used abbreviations, 2448*t*
        completeness, 2449
        conciseness, 2449
        correct spelling, 2449
        date and time, 2448
        legal prudence, 2450
        legibility, 2448
        overview of, 2447
        permanence, 2448
        sequence, 2449
        signature, 2449
        timing, 2448
    home care, 2447
    Kardexes, 2445–2446
    legal, 2439
    in long-term care for older adults, 2447*t*
    nursing activities, 2445–2447, 2445*t*
    nursing care plans, 2445
    nursing discharge/referral summaries,
        2446–2447
    overview of, 2438
    progress notes, 2446

systems
    case management, 2445, 2445*f*
    charting by exception, 2443, 2443*f*
    electronic documentation, 2443–2445
    focus charting, 2443*f*
    PIE model, 2442
    problem-oriented medical record (POMR),
        2440–2442, 2442*f*
    source-oriented record, 2439–2440, 2440*t*
    teaching process, 2523–2524
    uniform language, 2639
Documenting, 2438
Domestic partners, 2628
Domestic violence shelters, 1971
Dong quai, 1397*t*
Do-not-intubate order (DNI), 177
Do-not-resuscitate orders (DNRs), 177, 182
Dopamine, 895
Dopamine agonists, 223, 899*t*, 900
Dopamine system stabilizers, 1618, 1618*t*
Doppler ultrasound, 1201
Doppler ultrasound stethoscope (DUS),
    1063*f*, 1065
Dorsal recumbent position, 2278*t*
Double bind theory, 1612
Double depression, 1778
Douching, 1379
Doulas, 2164
Down syndrome, 1374, 1374*f*, 1581, 1582*t*
DPD (dependent personality disorder), 1856*t*,
    1857–1858, 1863*t*
Drain management, 1274, 1274*f*
Dramatic play, 1665
DRE (digital rectal exam), 113, 1357*t*
Dress, spiritual beliefs related to, 1877, 1877*f*
DRGs (diagnosis-related groups), 2464–2465
DRIs (dietary reference intakes), 927, 2091–2092,
    2091–2092*t*
Droplet nuclei, 524, 607
Droplet precautions, 546
Drug-drug interactions, 163
Drug-induced lupus, 510
Dry powder inhalers, 997*t*, 1000*t*
DTs (delirium tremens), 1525*t*, 1537*t*
Dual diagnosis, 1525*t*, 1535
Dual-energy x-ray absorptiometry (DEXA),
    800–801
DUB (dysfunctional uterine bleeding), 1400,
    1403*t*
Dubowitz tool, 2213
Ductus arteriosus, 2028
Ductus venosus, 2028
Dullness, 2280
Dumping, delegation versus, 2468
Duodenal ulcers, 677
Duplex Doppler ultrasound, 1201
Duplex venous ultrasonography, 1132
Durable power of attorney, 177
Durable power of attorney for health care, 2667
Duration
    of contractions, 2118
    of sound, in auscultation, 2281
Duty
    breach of, 2656, 2687
    defined, 2656
    of reasonable care, 2655
DVT. *See* Deep venous thrombosis
Dwarfism, 737*t*
The Dying Person's Bill of Rights, 175*t*
Dysarthria, 1238

Dysfunctional families, 1526
Dysfunctional uterine bleeding (DUB),
    1400, 1403*t*
Dysfunctional weaning, 987
Dysmenorrhea. *See also* Menstrual dysfunction
    complementary and alternative therapy, 1403
    defined, 1342, 1399
    manifestations, 1400
    primary, 1399
    secondary, 1399–1400
Dyspareunia, 1344
Dysphagia, 1245, 1584
Dysphasia, 32
Dysplastic nevi, 128
Dyspnea
    death and dying and, 1759
    defined, 365, 588, 959, 960*t*
    fluid volume excess and, 365
    inflection and, 588
    interventions and therapies, 960*t*
    manifestations, 960*t*
    oxygenation and, 959
Dysrhythmias
    antidysrhythmic drugs, 1189*t*
    assessment, 1195
    atrioventricular (AV) conduction blocks,
        1182*t*
    cardiac mapping and catheter ablation
        and, 1192
    cardiac monitoring and, 1187–1188
    cardiac output monitoring and, 1195–1196
    care planning, 1195
    causes of, 1177–1178
    characteristics of, 1180–1181*t*
    in children, 1179*t*
    collaborative care, 1186–1192
    as coronary artery disease complication, 1112
    countershock and, 1188–1190
    defibrillation and, 1188–1190, 1190*f*
    defined, 1063, 1177
    diagnosis, 1195
    diagnostic tests, 1186–1188
    discharge plan, 1196
    electrophysiology studies and, 1188
    fetal, 2151
    home care, 1196*t*
    implantable cardioverter-defibrillator
        (ICD) and, 1191–1192
    interventions, 1195–1196
    junctional, 1184
    lifespan considerations, 1179*t*
    manifestations, 1182–1186, 1187*t*
    Nursing Care Plan, 1197–1198*t*
    nursing process, 1194–1196
    in older adults, 1179*t*
    outcome evaluation, 1196
    overview of, 1177–1178
    pacemaker therapy, 1190–1191, 1190*f*, 1191*f*
    pathophysiology and etiology, 1178–1182
    pharmacologic therapy, 1188
    sinus node, 1183
    sudden cardiac death (SCD) and,
        1192–1194
    supraventricular, 1180–1181*t*, 1183–1184
    synchronized cardioversion and, 1188
    Valsalva maneuver and, 1192
    ventricular, 1181–1182*t*, 1185–1186
Dysthymic disorder
    defined, 1778, 1800
    manifestations, 1800*t*

occurrence of, 1800
prevalence of, 1783
therapies, 1800t
Dystocia, 2046
Dystonia, 1618
Dysuria, 265, 621

E

Early deceleration, 2152, 2153f, 2154t
Early detachment, 2179t
Early-onset schizophrenia (EOS), 1616
Ears. *See also* Hearing; Hearing impairment
    assessment, 1285–1291, 1292–1293f, 1293t
    diagnostic tests, 1302
    external, 1285, 1293
    in gestational age, 2217, 2218f
    newborn assessment, 2228, 2228f
Ease, 141
EASI (extra-amniotic saline infusion), 2129
Eating disorders, antepartum nutrition and, 2094–2095
Ebb phase, burns, 1473
EBP. *See* Evidence-based practice
EBV (Epstein-Barr virus), 45t
ECF (extracellular fluid), 336–337
Echocardiography
    in AMI diagnosis, 1115
    in congenital heart defects, 1097t
    in heart failure, 1151
    in infection, 557
Echolalia, 1584, 1689
Eclampsia, 1206
Ecological theory
    chronosystem, 1657
    defined, 1656
    exosystem, 1657
    illustrated, 1656f
    macrosystem, 1657
    mesosystem, 1657
    microsystem, 1657
    nature, 1655–1656
    nurture, 1656
Ecomaps, 1720, 1722f, 1727, 1727f
ECT. *See* Electroconvulsive therapy
Ectopic beats, 1073t, 1178
Ectopic pregnancy, 2080t
ED. *See* Erectile dysfunction
EDB (estimated date of birth), 2107, 2107f
EDB wheel, 2053, 2053f, 2107, 2107f
Edema
    assessment, 1455, 1458t
    asthma and, 990
    clinical conditions causing, 364–365, 364t
    defined, 338, 364, 990, 1455
    degrees of pitting in, 1455f
    grading, 368f
    in intrapartum assessment, 2143t
    occurrence of, 364
    pitting, 368f, 379t
    in prenatal assessment, 2102t
    tissue integrity and, 1454t
Edinburgh Postnatal Depression Scale, 1822t
Education
    acute renal failure (ARF), 387–388
    ADHD children, 1686t
    alcohol abuse, 1543
    appendicitis, 648, 648t
    assertive behavior, 1789
    asthma, 1003

body temperature, taking, 1429t
burns, 1486t
cardiomyopathy, 1082t
celiac disease, 242t
cirrhosis, 788t
computer-based client records, 2649
constipation, 310
contact dermatitis, 1491t
diabetes mellitus, 759–760
digestion, 221
disseminated intravascular coagulation
    (DIC), 1142t
e-health, 2641–2642, 2642t
erectile dysfunction (ED), 1370t
family, ADHD, 1686
family, health beliefs and, 1723
fecal incontinence, 315, 317
gallbladder disease, 655t
gastroesophageal reflux disease
    (GERD), 231t
health and wellness, 418
hepatitis, 238t
HIV/AIDS, 461, 476t
hypertension, 1174t
immunization, 451
lithium therapy, 1793
melanomas, 137t
mobility, 836
monoamine oxidase inhibitors (MAOIs),
    1792–1793
multiple sclerosis, 883t
otitis media, 582
pancreatitis, 250t
peripheral vascular disease (PVD),
    1201–1202, 1202t
pressure ulcers, 1498
of providers, 2558
pulmonary embolism, 1215t
schizophrenia, 1623
selective serotonin reuptake inhibitors (SSRIs),
    1791–1792
short bowel syndrome, 245t
substance abuse, 1570, 1570t
tricyclic antidepressants (TCAs), 1791
tuberculosis, 614
urinary calculi, 330
Education for All Handicapped Children Act of
    1975, 1591t
Effacement, 2119, 2120f
Effective coping, 1899
Effectiveness, 2364, 2477
Efficiency, 2364, 2477
Effusion, joint, 826
Ego, 1649
Ego defense mechanisms
    defined, 1904
    list of, 1905t
    in psychological survival, 1905–1907
Egocentrism, 1665t
Ego-syntonic, 1853
E-health, 2508, 2641
Elbows, mobility assessment, 832t
Elder abuse. *See also* Older adults
    consequences, 1966–1967
    defined, 1966
    manifestations of, 1968–1969, 1972t
    therapies, 1972t
Elderspeak, 2409
Elective lymph node dissection (ELND), 134
Elective surgery, 1261t

Electrical bone stimulation, 861t
Electrical burns, 1465, 1475t
Electrocardiograms (ECGs)
    in burn injuries, 1477
    in congenital heart defects, 1097t
    defined, 1071t
    in dysrhythmias, 1187
    exercise testing, 1114
    in heart failure, 1151
    interpreting, 1073t
    leads, 1072t
    in metabolic alkalosis, 18
    in obesity, 793
    as perioperative diagnostic test,
        1253t
    in pulmonary embolism, 1214
    time and voltage measurement, 1071t
    waveforms and intervals, 1072f
Electrocardiography, 1043
Electroconvulsive therapy (ECT)
    defined, 1620
    for mood disorders, 1795
    nursing considerations, 1796t
    in pregnancy, 1795
    for schizophrenia, 1620
Electroencephalograph (EEG) biofeedback,
    1539–1540
Electrolyte imbalance. *See also* Fluid and
        electrolyte imbalance
    assessment, 372–373
    calcium and, 372
    care planning, 373
    chloride and, 372
    conditions
        hypercalcemia, 372
        hyperchloremia, 372
        hyperkalemia, 372
        hypernatremia, 370
        hypocalcemia, 372
        hypochloremia, 372
        hypokalemia, 372
        hyponatremia, 370–371
    diagnosis, 373
    interventions, 373
    in kidney disease in children, 379t
    nursing process, 372–373
    outcome evaluation, 373
    overview of, 370–372
    potassium and, 371–372
    sodium and, 370–371
Electrolytes. *See also* Fluids and electrolytes
    bicarbonate (HCO_3), 342, 342t
    calcium (Ca^{2+}), 341, 342t
    chloride (Cl^-), 342, 342t
    composition of body fluid
        compartments, 336f
    concentrations in body fluid
        compartments, 337
    defined, 335
    function of, 342t
    imbalances, 14
    importance of, 341
    magnesium (Mg^{2+}), 341–342, 342t
    normal values, 351t
    phosphate (PO_4^-), 342, 342t
    potassium (K^+), 341, 342t
    regulation of, 341–342, 342t
    serum, 18, 22, 351, 351f, 380
    sodium (NA^+), 341, 342t
Electromyogram, 843

Electron beam computed tomography, 1114
Electronic communication. *See also*
    Communication
    advantages and disadvantages, 2403
    defined, 2400
    guidelines, 2403
    when not to use e-mail and, 2403
Electronic documentation, 2443–2445
Electronic fetal monitoring
    accelerations, 2152
    arrhythmias and dysrhythmias, 2151
    baseline fetal heart rate, 2149–2151, 2150f
    decelerations, 2152–2153, 2153f
    defined, 2148
    evaluations of FHR tracings, 2153–2156,
        2155t
    by external technique, 2149f
    indications, 2148
    internal, direct, 2149, 2150f
    methods of preventing, 2148–2149
    responses to, 2156
    variability, 2151–2152, 2151f
Electronic health records (EHRs). *See also*
    Computerized medical records
    accuracy, 2639
    defined, 2637
    documentation time and, 2647t
    medication administration record (MAR),
        2648, 2649f
    narrative note, 2441f
    quality assurance and, 2639
    SOAPIER in, 2442f
    summary view, 2648f
    vital signs graphic record in, 2443f
Electronic medical records (EMRs), 2637
Electrophysiology studies, 1188
Electrosurgery, 1263t
Elimination
    alterations, 258
    bowel
        activity and, 274
        alterations and manifestations, 276–278
        alterations and therapies, 277t
        anesthesia and, 274
        assessment, 278–279, 280–282t
        assessment interview, 279t
        collaborative interventions and
            therapies, 282
        defecation habits and, 274
        diagnostic procedures and, 274
        diagnostic tests, 279
        diet and, 273–274
        digital examination, 278, 279f
        factors affecting, 273–274
        fluid and, 274
        genetic and lifespan considerations,
            274–276
        genetic considerations and nonmodifiable
            risk factors, 278
        independent interventions and
            therapies, 282
        interventions and therapies, 282, 283t
        lifespan and cultural considerations, 279
        medications, 274, 283t
        modifiable risk factors, 278
        in newborns and infants, 274–275, 275f
        normal, 273–276
        in older adults, 275
        pain and, 274
        pathological conditions and, 274

    in pregnant women, 275–276
    prevention of, 278
    psychological factors, 274
    in school-age children and adolescents, 275
    screening, 278
    stroke and, 1245
    in toddlers, 275
    concepts related to, 258–259
    defined, 257
    disorders
        benign prostatic hyperplasia (BPH),
            284–292
        bladder incontinence and retention,
            292–305
        bowel incontinence, constipation, and
            impaction, 305–318
        constipation, 305–311
        fecal incontinence, 311–318
        urinary calculi, 318–332
        urinary incontinence, 292–297
        urinary retention, 297–305
    as indirect health gauge, 258
    stroke and, 1239
    urinary
        alterations, 264–265
        alterations and therapies, 266t
        altered urine elimination, 264–265, 264t
        altered urine production, 264
        assessment, 266–271, 268–269t
        assessment interview, 267t
        collaborative interventions and
            therapies, 272–273
        diagnostic tests, 267–271
        dialysis, 272–273
        factors affecting, 261
        fluid and food intake and, 261
        genetic and lifespan considerations,
            261–264, 262t
        independent interventions and therapies,
            271–272
        in infants, 262
        interventions and therapies, 271–273
        lifespan and cultural considerations, 267
        medications, 272t
        medications that cause, 261, 261t
        modifiable risk factors, 265
        muscle tone and, 261
        normal, 260–264
        normal and abnormal findings, 270–271t
        in older adults, 263
        pathological conditions and, 261
        pharmacologic therapy, 272
        in pregnant women, 263–264
        in preschoolers, 262
        prevention of, 265–266
        psychosocial factors and, 261
        in school-age children, 262–263
        screening, 265–266
        stroke and, 1245
        surgical and diagnostic procedures and, 261
        urinalysis, 270–271t
ELISA (enzyme-linked immunosorbent assay),
    467–468
ELND (elective lymph node dissection), 134
Embolic strokes, 1236
Embolus
    defined, 1211
    impact of, 1211–1212
Embryo, 2028, 2029f
Embryonic membranes, 2022–2023

Embryonic stage, 2028
EMDR (eye movement desensitization and
    reprocessing), 1948
Emergencies
    consent in, 2661
    defined, 2609
Emergency care
    burn injuries, 1475–1476
    drug overdose, 1565–1567
Emergency contraception (EC), 1385–1386
Emergency management
    emergency response phase, 2610, 2610f
    mitigation phase, 2609
    phases of, 2609–2611
    preparedness phase, 2609–2610
    recovery phase, 2610–2611
    responsibility for, 2611–2612
Emergency medical services (EMS), 2616,
    2616f, 2616t
Emergency Medical Treatment and Active Labor
    Act (EMTALA), 2604
Emergency Nursing Resources (ENRs), 2592
Emergency plans, 2611–2612
Emergency preparedness
    bioterrorism, 2614, 2615–2616t
    collaboration, 2614
    Community Response Team (CERT) program
        and, 2611
    defined, 2609
    EMS system, 2616, 2616f, 2616t
    local emergency management agency (LEMA)
        and, 2611
    management phases, 2609–2611
    nursing practice, 2614–2616
    overview of, 2609
    responsibility for, 2611–2612
    site-specific disaster zones, 2614
    triage, 2612, 2612f, 2613f
Emergency response
    defined, 2610
    nursing competencies for, 2611, 2611t
    phase, 2610, 2610f
    responsibility for, 2611–2612
Emergency surgery, 1261t
Emigration, 634
Emotional availability, 1716
Emotional factors
    in addiction, 1521
    in assessment, 2284
Emotional status
    multiple sclerosis and, 884
    spinal cord injuries (SCI) and, 912
    systemic lupus erythematosus (SLE)
        and, 517
Emotional stress, 433
Emotional support
    attention-deficit/hyperactivity disorder
        (ADHD), 1685
    cerebral palsy (CP) and, 1699
Emotion-focused coping, 1899
Emotions. *See also* Mood and affect
    culture and, 1787
    defined, 1775
    learning and, 2506–2507
Empathy, 2425, 2426t
Emphysema, 1006, 1007f
Empirical knowing, 2305
Employee performance enhancement, 2476
Employment, antepartum care and,
    2072–2073

Empowerment, 2307
Empowerment facilitation
    abuse and, 1974
    burns and, 1484–1485
Empyema, 586, 650
EMTALA (Emergency Medical Treatment and
        Active Labor Act), 2604
Enabling behavior, 1525
Encapsulation, 606
Encoding, 2399
Encopresis
    defined, 312
    pediatric clients with, care of, 317–318
    treatment of, 313
Enculturation, 1633–1634
End of life, 174
Endocrine glands
    fatigue and women and, 186t
    location of, 727f
Endocrine system
    age-related changes, 727t
    alterations and manifestations, 726–729
    alterations and therapies, 730t
    assessment interview, 733t
    assessments
        facial, 735t
        hypocalcemic tetany, 737t
        motor function, 736t
        musculoskeletal, 737t
        nails and hair, 734t
        sensory function, 736t
        skin, 734t
        thyroid gland, 735t
    exercise benefits, 422
    feedback mechanisms of, 726t
    hormones of, 726t
    medications for, 738t
    organs of, 726t
    pregnancy and, 2033–2034
    skin, 733
End-of-dose medication failure, 156
End-of-life care. *See also* Comfort
    adolescents, 179
    advance directives and, 177, 2574
    alterations and therapies, 144t
    assessment, 182–183
    bioethical issues, 2573–2574
    care planning, 183
    children
        advance care planning, 179, 179t
        ethical issues, 179–180
        improving, 179t
        palliative care, 177, 178t, 179t
        in pediatric or neonatal ICUs, 180t
        principles of, 178
    collaborative care
        cardiopulmonary resuscitation, 181–182
        feeding tubes, 181
        massage and touch, 182t
        nonpharmacologic therapy, 181–182
        pharmacologic therapy, 181
    comfort measures only (CMO) order, 176
    cultural and religious considerations,
        180–181
    defined, 144t, 145
    diagnosis, 183
    do-not-resuscitate orders (DNRs) and, 177
    The Dying Person's Bill of Rights and, 175t
    ethical issues, 177
    euthanasia and assisted suicide, 176–177, 2574

heart failure and, 1158
hospice care, 177, 178t
interventions, 144t, 183
legal issues, 176–177
legal issues and, 2660t
lifespan considerations, 177–180
manifestations, 144t, 175–181, 183t
Nursing Care Plan, 184t
nursing considerations, 175–177
nursing process, 182–183
outcome evaluation, 183
overview of, 174
pain and, 181
palliative care, 175, 175t, 177, 178t
pathophysiology and etiology, 175
pediatric, 177–180, 178t, 179t, 180t
therapies, 182t
withdrawing or withholding food and
        fluids, 2574
withdrawing or withholding life-sustaining
        treatment (WWLST) and, 2574
Endogenous antigens, 483
Endogenous insulin, 742
Endogenous source, 531
Endometrial ablation, 1402
Endometriosis, 1400, 1400t
Endoplasmic reticulum, 30–31
Endoscopic retrograde cholangiopancreatography
        (ERCP), 247
Endoscopic ultrasonography, 247
Endoscopy, 220, 228
Endotoxins, 528
Endotracheal suctioning, 970
Endotracheal tubes, 983, 983f
End-stage renal disease (ESRD), 390, 390t. *See also*
        Chronic kidney disease (CKD)
Engrossment, 1819
Enlargement, of presenting part, 2116
Enophthalmos, 1312
ENRs (Emergency Nursing Resources), 2592
Ensure method, 1386
Enteral nutrition. *See also* Digestion
    complications of, 224
    defined, 222–223, 947
    feeding tube placement, 224f, 224t
    formulas, 223, 224t
    need for, 947–948
    tubes, 223, 223f
Enterocutaneous fistulas, 658
Enteroenteric fistulas, 658
Enterovesical fistulas, 658
Enthusiasm, 2492–2493
Entropion, 567, 567f
Entry inhibitors, 471
Enuresis, 262–263, 626t
Environment
    blame-free, 2688–2689
    communication and, 2408, 2415
    hospital settings and, 150t
    internal, 1898
    learning, 2506
    older adults assessment, 2296, 2298t
    pain perception and, 161–162
Environmental comfort, 141
Environmental control
    attention-deficit/hyperactivity disorder
        (ADHD), 1685, 1685f
    autism spectrum disorder (ASD)
        and, 1693
    social differences, 1638

Environmental factors
    in assessment, 2284–2285
    in development, 1677
Environmental modification, ADHD and, 1684
Environmental stressors, 1898
Enzyme-linked immunosorbent assay (ELISA),
        467–468
Enzymes
    defined, 208
    pancreatic, 246
EOS (early-onset schizophrenia), 1616
Eosinophils, 440
Epidemics, 570
Epidermis
    defined, 1446
    layers of, 1446–1447
    in older adults, 1448
    thickness variation, 1472
Epigenetic studies, 1554
Epilepsy
    antepartum care and, 2078t
    defined, 715
    in older adults, 716t
Epinephrine
    heat production and, 1422
    for hypersensitivity, 490–491
EpiPen, 491, 493t
Epiphyseal plate, 820
Episiotomy, 2131
Epstein pearls, 2227
Epstein-Barr virus (EBV), 45t
Epworth Sleepiness Scale, 200, 201f
Erb-Duchenne paralysis (Erb palsy), 2231, 2231f
ERCP (endoscopic retrograde
        cholangiopancreatography), 247
Erectile dysfunction (ED)
    assessment, 1369
    care planning, 1369
    causes of, 1367t
    client teaching, 1370t
    collaborative care, 1367–1369
    defined, 1366
    diagnosis, 1369
    diagnostic tests, 1368
    injectable medications, 1368
    interventions, 1369–1370
    issue discussion, 1369–1370
    mechanical devices for, 1368
    nursing process, 1369–1370
    outcome evaluation, 1370
    overview of, 1366
    pathophysiology and etiology, 1367
    pharmacologic therapy, 1368
    risk factors, 1367
    self-esteem promotion and, 1370
    surgery, 1368–1369, 1369f
Ergonomics. *See also* Informatics
    for computer use, 2643t
    computer vision syndrome and, 2643
    considerations, 2642–2643
    defined, 2642
    repetitive strain injury and, 2643
Erikson, Erik, 1836
Erikson stages of development, 1650–1653, 1651t
Erikson's psychosocial theory of development,
        1835–1836
Erotic preferences, 1345
Error reduction
    medication, 2688, 2688t
    methods for, 2689t

Erysipelas, 560, 560f
Erythema, 560, 1457t
Erythema infectiosum (fifth disease), 533t
Erythema toxicum, 2223–2224, 2224f
Erythrocyte sedimentation rate (ESR), 512, 671, 1098t
Erythropoietin, 70
Eschar, 1454t, 1473, 1497
Escharotomy, 1477–1478, 1477f, 1510
Esophageal manometry, 228
Esophageal varices, 782, 1537t
Esophagoscopy, 785
Esophagus, 227, 227f, 228f
ESR (erythrocyte sedimentation rate), 512, 671, 1098t
ESRD. See End-stage renal disease
Essential nutrients, 927
Estimated date of birth (EDB), 2107, 2107f
Estrogen, 1343, 2015, 2034
ETCO₂, 1214
Ethambutol, 612t
Ethical decision making
    advocacy and, 2570f
    criteria, 2570
    exercise in, 2577t
    models of, 2569–2570, 2569t
    nurse's obligations in, 2569t
    principles of, 2567
    strategies to enhance, 2570
Ethical dilemmas
    academic dishonesty and, 2576
    AIDS, 2572
    bioethical issues, 2572–2575
    with clients and families, 2577
    coping with, 2577–2578
    end-of-life issues, 2573–2574
    genetic testing, 2572–2573, 2573t
    healthcare systems and, 2601t
    loyalties and obligations and, 2572
    in nursing practice, 2575–2577
    occurrence of, 2570
    organ transplantation, 2573t
    overview of, 2572
    pediatric clients and, 2575t
    social and technological changes and, 2572
    workplace issues, 2576–2577
Ethical knowing, 2306
Ethics
    bioethics, 1878
    code of, 2537
    concept of, 2563
    concepts related to, 2566t
    defined, 1878, 2563
    documentation and, 2439
    end-of-life care for children and, 179–180
    integrating concept of, 2564
    morality and, 2563
    nursing, 1878–1879
    nursing code of, 2567–2569
    parental response to hyperthermia, 1435t
    in prioritizing care, 2368
    professional behaviors associated with, 2565t
    quality improvement and, 2682t
    sexuality and, 1362
    values, 2564–2565
    workplace issues, 2576–2577
Ethnic groups
    defined, 1630
    moral principles and, 2576t

Ethnicity
    comfort and, 142
    fluids and electrolytes and, 344–346
    osteoporosis and, 800
    in pain experience expression and management, 160–161
    sleep and, 197t
Etiology, 1089, 2336, 2336f
Euglycemia, 768
Eupnea, 954
Eustachian tube
    defined, 576
    dysfunction, 277
Eustress, 1896
Euthanasia, 176–177, 2574
Euthyroid, 806
Evaluation. See also Nursing process
    checklist, 2351t
    defined, 2349
    developing, 2350
    drawing conclusions and, 2349–2350
    nursing plan of care decision and, 2350–2352
    outcomes and goals example, 2352t
    relationship to other nursing process phases, 2352–2353
    writing, 2350
Evaluation statements, 2350
Evaporation, 1422
Evidence
    applying, 2592–2593
    defined, 2583
    evaluation of, 2591–2592
    providing for EBP, 2587
    reliability, 2591
    retrieval, 2590–2591
    validity, 2591
Evidence-based nursing, 2584
Evidence-based practice (EBP)
    barriers to, 2588
    benefits of, 2585–2586
    best practice standards and, 2587–2588
    concept of, 2583
    concepts related to, 2585t
    defined, 2583
    development
        clinical question, 2588–2590
        evidence application, 2592–2593
        evidence evaluation, 2591–2592
        evidence retrieval, 2590–2591
        overview of, 2588
        steps in, 2588–2593, 2588f
    evolution of, 2584
    framework components, 2584f
    implementation strategies, 2593–2594
    nursing clinical research, 2586–2588
    providing best evidence for, 2587
    as QSEN competency, 2699, 2700
    support for, 2592
    supporting nursing as professional discipline, 2587
    using to inform practice, 2585t
Evisceration, 1509
Evoked potential test, 880
Exacerbation, 408, 877
Exact tolerance, 1157
Examination
    client preparation, 2277
    defined, 2276
    environment preparation, 2277

    head-to-toe framework, 2277t
    methods
        auscultation, 2280
        inspection, 2278
        palpation, 2278–2279, 2279f
        percussion, 2279–2280, 2280f, 2280t
        positioning, 2277, 2278t
        purpose of, 2276
        types of, 2276
Excess TSH stimulation, 808
Excitement phase, in sexual response cycle, 1346, 1347t
Excoriation, 1493
Excretory urography, 623
Exercise
    adjustment disorder with depressed mood and, 1806
    aerobic, 421
    anaerobic, 421
    antepartum care, 2068–2069
    benefits of, 421–423, 422t
    blood pressure and, 1046
    for childbirth preparation
        abdominal, 2070–2071
        inner thigh, 2071
        Kegel, 2071, 2071f
        pelvic tilt, 2069, 2070f
        perineal, 2071
        yoga, 2071t
    chronic obstructive pulmonary disease (COPD) and, 1012
    coronary artery disease (CAD) and, 1116
    deep breathing, 968
    defined, 421
    for diabetes clients, 758–759
    fatigue and, 186t
    fibromyalgia and, 192–193, 192t
    glaucoma and, 1323t
    isokinetic, 421
    isometric, 421
    isotonic, 421
    mobility and, 837
    mood disorders and, 1795–1796
    obesity and, 794, 796
    osteoarthritis and, 890, 891t
    osteoporosis and, 803–804
    Parkinson disease and, 901, 901t
    in preconception counseling, 1372
    pregnancy and culture and, 2076t
    pulse and, 1044
    range-of-motion (ROM), 506, 837
    regular defecation and, 316
    testing, in congenital heart defects, 1097t
    tissue integrity and, 1461
Exhaled carbon dioxide, 1010
Exhaustion, stage of, 1901, 1901f
Exogenous antigens, 483
Exogenous insulin, 742
Exogenous source, 531
Exophthalmos, 735t, 806, 806f
Exosystem, 1657
Exotoxins, 528
Expectant couple
    concerns over age 35, 2043–2044
    developmental tasks of, 2036
Expectorate, 1014
Expiration, 953
Expressed consent, 2659
Expressive aphasia, 1238

Expressive jargon, 1664
Expressive speech, 1662
Expulsion, fetus, 2125
Extended family, 1709, 1710f
Extended-kin network family, 1710
Extension, cardinal movement, 2125
External clients, 2690
External environmental stressors, 1898
External eye assessment, 1288–1289t
External fixation, 860f
External locus of control, 415, 1940
External rotation, fetus, 2125
Extinction, 1529
Extra-amniotic saline infusion
        (EASI), 2129
Extracapsular extraction, 1308, 1308f
Extracellular fluid (ECF), 4, 6, 336–337
Extracellular fluid volume deficit,
        354–355, 360t
Extracorporeal shock wave lithotripsy
        (ESWL), 322, 652
Extrapulmonary tuberculosis, 606
Extrapyramidal side effects, 1617
Extremities
    Erb palsy, 2231, 2231f
    newborn assessment, 2231–2232, 2231f,
        2232f, 2233f
Extubation, 1256t
Exudate
    defined, 1509
    inflammatory, 634
    tissue integrity and, 1454t
    wound healing and, 1509
Exudative macular degeneration, 1327–1328,
        1328t
Eye chronic uveitis, 500
Eye infection prevention, in newborns,
        2237–2238, 2238f
Eye injuries
    assessment, 1316
    care planning, 1316
    collaborative care, 1314–1316
    diagnosis, 1316
    diagnostic tests, 1314
    first aid and, 1317t
    impaired vision risk reduction and,
        1316–1317
    interventions, 1281t, 1316–1317
    manifestations, 1281t
        blunt trauma, 1312, 1313t
        burns, 1312, 1313t
        corneal abrasion, 1311–1312, 1313t
        detached retina, 1312–1314, 1314t
        foreign body conjunctiva, 1313t
        penetrating injuries, 1312, 1313t
        perforating injuries, 1312, 1313t
        periorbital ecchymosis, 1314t
        subconjunctival hemorrhage, 1314t
    in migrant workers, 1312t
    nursing process, 1316–1317
    outcome evaluation, 1317
    overview of, 1311
    pathophysiology and etiology, 1311
    pharmacologic therapy, 1314, 1315t
    prevention of, 1311, 1317t
    surgery, 1314
Eye movement desensitization and reprocessing
        (EMDR), 1948
Eye ointments, 1315t
Eyedrops, 1315t

Eyes. See also Vision
    assessment
        external eye, 1288–1289t
        eye movement, 1286–1287t
        internal eye, 1289–1290t
        newborn, 2226–2227, 2227f
        overview of, 1285
        pupillary, 1287t
    charts for testing, 1285, 1285f
    pregnancy and, 2033
Eyewear, 546–548

F
Face, in newborn assessment, 2226, 2226f
Face masks, 546–548, 972, 972f
Face presentation, 2115, 2115f
Faces Pain Scale-Revised, 169
Facial assessments, 735t
Facial expression, 2402, 2402f
Facilitated transport, 2026
Facilities management, 2645
Facility-specific documentation, 2447
FAD (familial AD), 1594
Failure to observe and take appropriate
        action, 2657
Failure to thrive (FTT)
    assessment, 1703
    care planning, 1703
    collaborative care, 1702
    defined, 1676t, 1701
    diagnosis, 1703
    diagnostic tests, 1702
    geriatric (GFTT), 1701
    growth measurement and, 1703t
    infant appearance, 1702f
    interventions, 1676t, 1703
    manifestations, 1676t, 1702
    nonpharmacologic therapy, 1702
    nursing process, 1702–1703
    outcome evaluation, 1703
    overview of, 1701
    pathophysiology and etiology, 1701–1702
    pharmacologic therapy, 1702
    prevention of, 1702
    risk factors, 1702
    surgery, 1702
Faith, 1873
Falls
    older adults, 2713, 2713f
    prevention of, 2703–2704
False imprisonment, 2657
False labor, 2121–2122, 2122t
False pelvis, 2013
Familial AD (FAD), 1594
Families
    addiction and, 1525–1526
    adolescent, 1710
    with adolescents and young adults, 1726
    advocating for, 2559, 2559t
    alterations and therapies, 1719t
    assessment
        ecomaps and, 1720, 1722f
        health history, 1720
        interpersonal interactions, 1720–1721
        lifespan and cultural considerations, 1721
        parenting styles, 1721–1722
    assessment guide, 1720t
    binuclear, 1711
    blended, 1710–1711

    boundaries, 1708, 1714–1715
    burns and, 1485t
    changes, 1708
    childless, 1710
    collaborative interventions and
            therapies, 1723
    communication, 1716–1717
    concept of culture and diversity and, 1707
    concepts related to, 1714t
    coping, 183
    couples, 1725
    culturally competent care, 1723
    defined, 1708
    developmental stages, 1712–1713, 1712t,
            1724–1726
    disagreements in, eight steps to resolve, 1533
    diversity in structures and roles,
            1709–1712
    dysfunctional, 1526
    education, 1723
    emotional availability, 1716
    ethical issues in working with, 2577
    extended, 1709, 1710f
    extended-kin network, 1710
    factors in assessment, 2284
    factors that shape development,
            1713–1718
    foster, 1710
    gay and lesbian, 1711, 1711–1712
    genetic considerations and nonmodifiable
            risk factors, 1718
    genograms, 1720
    gunshot wounds and, 1981
    heterosexual cohabiting, 1711
    holistic view of, 1708–1709
    illness effects on, 408–409
    independent interventions and
            therapies, 1723
    with infants and preschoolers, 1726
    interdependence, 1708
    interventions and therapies, 1722–1723
    intragenerational, 1711
    language of pain, 1732t
    life cycle, 1712t
    managing conflict with, 2389
    Medical Leave Act and, 1713t
    with middle adults, 1726
    modifiable risk factors, 1719–1720
    normal presentation of, 1708–1713
    nuclear, 1709
    with older adults, 1726
    parental presence during procedures
            and, 1709t
    parent-child interaction, 1713
    phobias and, 1940
    prevention and, 1718–1720
    resiliency, 1715
    roles in, 1708
    rules and, 1716
    "sandwich generation," 1712t
    with school-age children, 1726
    sibling relationships, 1713–1714
    single adults living alone, 1712
    single-parent, 1710
    size, 1713
    stepfamily, 1710–1711
    structure, 1708
    substance abuse and, 1524
    support, adjustment disorder with depressed
            mood and, 1807

Families (*continued*)
  tasks, performing, 1708
  therapeutic communication with, 2435–2436, 2435f
  transition to parenthood facilitation, 1723
  two-career, 1710
  in wound healing, 1513t
Family APGAR, 1727–1728, 1728t
Family attachment development, 1818
Family burden, 1731–1732
Family cohesion
  characteristics of, 1715t
  defined, 1715
  levels of, 1715, 1715f
Family coping mechanisms, 1715–1716
Family development
  defined, 1712
  factors that shape, 1713–1718
Family flexibility, 1716, 1716t
Family health promotion
  assessment, 1727
  care planning, 1729
  collaborative care, 1727
  community-based care, 1724
  defined, 1724
  diagnosis, 1728
  ecomap, 1727, 1727f
  Family APGAR, 1727–1728, 1728t
  Friedman Family Assessment Tool (FFAM), 1728
  HOME Inventory, 1728
  interventions, 1729
  lifespan and cultural considerations, 1726
  Nursing Care Plan, 1729–1730t
  nursing process, 1727–1729
  outcome evaluation, 1729
  overview of, 1724–1726
  prevention and, 1726
  risk factors, 1726
  wellness promotion and, 1724, 1725t
Family history
  hypertension and, 1166
  osteoporosis and, 800
Family interventions, 1529
Family planning
  assessment
    men, 1392
    women, 1391
  care planning, 1392
  collaborative care, 1386–1391
  contraception. *See* contraception
  diagnosis, 1392
  diagnostic tests, 1386–1387
  diversity and culture and, 1392t
  fertility medications, 1387, 1387t
  genetic disorders
    abnormalities of chromosomal number, 1374–1375, 1375t
    abnormalities of chromosome structure, 1375–1376
    autosomal dominant inheritance, 1376
    autosomal recessive inheritance, 1376–1377, 1377f
    modes of inheritance, 1376–1378
    multifactorial inheritance, 1377–1378
    sex chromosome abnormalities, 1376
    X-linked dominant inheritance, 1377
    X-linked recessive inheritance, 1377, 1377f
  healthy body image and, 1392
  healthy sexual function and, 1392
  infertility counseling. *See* infertility

  interruption of pregnancy, 1387–1388
  interventions, 1392
  Nursing Care Plan, 1392t
  nursing process, 1391–1392
  outcome evaluation, 1392
  overview of, 1371–1373
  preconception counseling, 1371–1372
  therapeutic insemination, 1388–1389
  in vitro fertilization (IVF), 1389, 1389f
Family processes, altered, 2109–2110
Family recovery, 1732–1733
Family response to health alterations
  assessment, 1735–1737
  care planning, 1737
  chronic illness, 1731
  collaborative care, 1735
  diagnosis, 1737
  family-centered care and, 1733–1734t
  illness impact, 1730–1735
  impact factors and, 1731t
  interventions, 1737
  language of pain and, 1732t
  manifestations, 1735, 1736t
  nursing process, 1735–1737
  outcome evaluation, 1737
  overview of, 1730
  pediatric illness, 1733–1735
  prevention and, 1735
  risk factors, 1735
  severe mental illness, 1731–1733
Family support, 1732
Family theory, 1854
Family therapy, 1532
Family wellness promotion, 1911
Family-centered care
  defined, 1708, 1733–1734, 2113
  diversity and culture, 1735t
  elements and recommendations, 1733–1734t
  in intrapartum care, 2113
Family-centered nursing, 1708
Family-focused therapy, 1862
Fantasizing, 1904
Fascial excision, 1478
Fasciculations, 701t
Fasciectomy, 1478
FAST (focused assessment by sonography in trauma), 1961
Fasting blood glucose (FBG), 751
Fat embolism syndrome, 858–859
Father, expectant
  couvade, 2039t
  first trimester, 2038
  overview of, 2038
  second trimester, 2038–2039
  third trimester, 2039
Fatigue
  acute, 145, 185, 188
  alterations and therapies, 144t
  assessment, 189
  care planning, 189
  chronic, 145, 185
  collaborative care, 188
  complementary and alternative therapies, 188t
  coping, 189
  culture, 187–188
  defined, 144t, 145, 185
  diagnosis, 189
  diagnostic tests, 188
  exercise and, 186t

  interventions, 144t, 189
  lifespan considerations, 187
  manifestations, 144t, 186–188, 188t
  nonpharmacologic therapy, 188
  nursing process, 189
  outcome evaluation, 189
  overview of, 185
  pathophysiology and etiology, 185–186
  pharmacologic therapy, 188
  prevention, 186
  risk factors, 185–186
  sleep hygiene and, 149–150, 187t
  in specific conditions
    fibromyalgia, 191, 193t
    hepatitis, 236–238
    lung cancer, 110
    nephritis, 674
    rheumatoid arthritis, 506
    RSV/bronchiolitis, 1022
  surgery, 188
  therapies, 188t
  women and, 186t
Fats, 757, 928f, 929
FBG (fasting blood glucose), 751
Fear, 1902
Fear management
  coronary artery disease (CAD) and, 1126–1127
  disseminated intravascular coagulation (DIC), 1142–1143
Febrile, 1423, 1431
Febrile seizures, 716, 1434
Fecal impaction
  defined, 307
  manual removal of stool, 316, 317t
  manual removal of stool and, 311
Fecal incontinence. *See also* Bowel incontinence, constipation, and impaction
  assessment, 313
  care planning, 315
  causes of, 312t
  client teaching, 315
  collaborative care, 312–313
  defined, 276–278, 311
  diagnosis, 313–315
  diagnostic tests, 313
  encopresis, 312
  interventions and therapies, 277t
    bowel training programs, 316
    education for home care, 317
    fecal incontinence pouch, 317
    manual removal of stool, 316, 317t
    pediatric clients with encopresis, 317–318
    regular defecation, 315–316
    skin integrity, 316
  manifestations, 277t, 312
  nonpharmacologic therapy, 313
  nursing process, 313–318
  outcome questions, 318
  pathophysiology and etiology, 311–312
  pharmacologic therapy, 313
  pressure ulcers and, 1493
  prevention, 312
  risk factors, 311–312
  surgery, 313
Fecal incontinence pouch, 317
Fecalith, 645
Feces
  defined, 273
  in fluid output, 340

Federal agencies, 2621–2623, 2622t, 2623f, 2623t
Feedback
  as communication response, 2399–2400
  defined, 2379
  in delegation, 2470
  giving, 2431
  helpful, nonthreatening, 2431t
  honest, 2431
  immediate, 2431
  learning and, 2506
  reflecting on, 2432t
  supportive, 2431
Feeding and eating disorders
  anorexia nervosa (AN)
    characteristics of, 1838t
    defined, 1845
    DSM-5 diagnostic criteria for, 1846t
    lanugo, 1846
    manifestations, 1848t
    therapies, 1848t
  assessment, 1851
  avoidant/restrictive food intake disorder, 1836
  binge-eating disorder (BED)
    characteristics of, 1838t
    defined, 1848
    manifestations, 1848t
    therapies, 1848t
  bulimia nervosa (BN)
    behaviors associated with, 1847–1848
    binge eating, 1846
    characteristics of, 1838t
    defined, 1846
    indicators, 1847
    manifestations, 1848t
    purging, 1846–1847
    therapies, 1848t
    as underdiagnosed, 1847
  care planning, 1850
  characteristic manifestations of, 1838t
  collaborative care, 1848–1850
  complementary and alternative therapy, 1849–1850
  defined, 1836
  diagnosis, 1850
  diagnostic tests, 1849
  injury prevention, 1851
  Internet and, 1847t
  interventions, 1851
  interventions and treatments, 1839t
  lifespan and cultural considerations, 1848
  manifestations, 1839t, 1845–1848, 1848t
  nocturnal sleep-related eating disorder (NSRED), 1836
  nonpharmacologic therapy, 1849
  nursing process, 1850–1851
  outcome evaluation, 1851
  overview of, 1843–1844
  pathophysiology and etiology, 1844–1845
  pharmacologic therapy, 1849
  pica, 1836
  Prader-Willi Syndrome (PWS), 1836–1838
  prevention of, 1845
  risk factors, 1844–1845
  rumination disorder, 1836
  sociocultural risk factors, 1844–1845
  therapeutic relationship promotion, 1851
  types of, 1836–1838
Feeding disorder of infancy or early childhood, 1701
Feeding tubes, 181

Feelings, minimizing/discounting, 2432
Feet
  diabetes and, 750
  peripheral atherosclerosis and, 1202t
Fellatio, 1346
Female condoms, 1380, 1380f
Female genital mutilation (FGM), 1362
Female genitals, in gestational age, 2218, 2219f
Female hormone replacement, 1364t
Female infertility medications, 1365t
Female orgasmic disorder, 1349–1350
Female reproductive cycle
  defined, 2015
  hormones and, 2015–2017, 2017f
  menstrual cycle, 2018–2019
  neurohumoral basis of, 2017–2018
  ovarian cycle, 2018, 2018f
  phases of, 2017f
Female reproductive system
  bony pelvis, 2012–2015
  cycle, 2015–2019
  normal presentation of, 2012–2019
Female reproductive system assessment
  axillary and clavicular lymph node, 1359t
  breast, 1358–1359t
  external genitalia, 1360–1361t
  hernia and lymph node, 1359t
  vaginal and cervical, 1361t
Female sexual arousal disorder, 1349
Female sexuality, 1354, 1354t
Femoral pulse, 1063f, 1064
Ferning pattern, 2019, 2019f
Fertility awareness methods
  basal body temperature (BBT), 1378, 1378f
  calendar rhythm method, 1378
  defined, 1378
  overview of, 1378
  ovulation method, 1379
  symptothermal method, 1379
Fertilization
  acrosomal reaction, 2021
  capacitation, 2021
  defined, 2020
  moment of, 2021
  preparation for, 2020–2021
Festination, 897
Fetal alcohol spectrum disorders, 1552, 1582
Fetal alcohol syndrome, 1552, 1581–1582, 1582t
Fetal attitude, 2115
Fetal biophysical profiles, 2048
Fetal bradycardia, 2151
Fetal circulatory system, 2027–2028, 2027f
Fetal demise, 1768
Fetal development
  assessment, 2054, 2054f
  circulatory system, 2027–2028
  embryonic stage, 2028
  fetal stage, 2028
  full term, 2028
  illustrated, 2029f
  placenta, 2023–2027
  preembryonic, 2021–2023
  stages, 2028–2029
Fetal heart, 2028

Fetal heart rate (FHR)
  auscultation of, 2147–2148
  baseline, 2149–2151, 2150f
  electronic monitoring of, 2148–2156
  evaluation of tracings, 2153–2156, 2155t
  hearing of, 2148
  three-tier interpretation system, 2155, 2155t
Fetal heartbeat, 2054
Fetal lie, 2115
Fetal macrosomia, 2138t
Fetal malposition, 2138t
Fetal movement, 2036
Fetal movement record, 2083, 2083f
Fetal position, 2116, 2117f
Fetal presentation, 2115, 2115f
Fetal skull, 2114–2115, 2114f
Fetal stage, 2028
Fetal status, 2144–2145t
Fetal tachycardia, 2151
Fetus
  cardinal movements, 2125
  drugs of abuse/addiction effects on, 1553t
  passage relationship, 2115–2117
  positional changes of, 2125
  response to labor, 2127–2128
  sutures, 2114, 2114f
Fever
  in children, 1434, 1434t, 1436t
  constant, 1431
  cultural considerations, 1434
  defined, 1422
  intermittent, 1431
  interventions, 1436
  in pediatric clients, 1424
  pulse and, 1044
  relapsing, 1431
  remittent, 1431
  treatment and, 1434
Fever spike, 1431
FFAM (Friedman Family Assessment Tool), 1728
FFT. See Failure to thrive
FGM (female genital mutilation), 1362
FHR. See Fetal heart rate
FHS (Framingham Heart Study), 1109t
Fiber, dietary, 928
Fiberoptic bronchoscopy, 591
Fibric acid derivatives, 1117t
Fibrin, 1508
Fibrin degradation products, 1138
Fibrinolytic therapy, 1241
Fibrinolytics, 1119
Fibromyalgia
  aerobic exercise and, 192–193, 192t
  alterations and therapies, 144t
  assessment, 193
  care planning, 193
  collaborative care, 191
  coping with, 194
  defined, 144t, 145, 190
  diagnosis, 193
  diagnostic criteria, 192t
  diagnostic tests, 191
  fatigue and, 191, 193t
  interventions, 144t, 193
  manifestations, 144t, 191, 193t
  nonpharmacologic therapy, 192–193
  nursing process, 193–194
  older adults and, 160
  outcome evaluation, 194

Fibromyalgia (*continued*)
overview of, 190
pain associated with, 190, 193*t*
pathophysiology and etiology, 190
pharmacologic therapy, 191–192
prevention, 190
risk factors, 190
strength training and, 192–193, 192*t*
tender points, 145, 190, 191*f*
therapies, 193*t*
Fidelity, 1880
Filtration, 338, 338*f*
Fingers, mobility assessment, 832*t*
Fingolimod (Gilenya), 880
Firearms, in the home, 1968
First (S_1) heart sounds, 1034
First feeding, 2238–2239
First-degree AV block, 1182*t*, 1186
Fish, mercury in, 2096–2097
5 P's neurovascular assessment, 828–829
5-alpha reductase inhibitors, 287
Fixation, 1650
FLACC (Face, Legs, Activity, Cry, Consolability)
scale, 169
Flaccidity, 1239
Flashbacks, 1946
Flat affect, 1614
Flatness, 2280
Flatulence, 276
Flatus, 273
Flexion, 2125
Flight of ideas, 1809
Flow phase, burns, 1473
Flow sheets, 2442, 2446
Fluid and electrolyte balance
concepts related to, 345–346*t*
digestion and, 221
pancreatitis, 250
premature newborns, 2256–2257
pyloric stenosis, 253
systemic lupus erythematosus (SLE)
and, 516
Fluid and electrolyte imbalance
assessment, 372–373
care planning, 373
compensation, 346
diagnosis, 373
electrolyte imbalance, 370–373
fluid volume deficit, 350, 354–363
fluid volume excess, 350, 363–370
interventions, 373
isotonic, 354
nursing process, 372–373
osmolar, 354
outcome evaluation, 373
overview of, 354
prevalence of, 346
prevention of, 346–348
Fluid intake
average daily, 339, 339*t*
management, 367, 367*t*
measurement and recording, 348–351
as proportional to output, 350
stimulating factors, 339*f*
Fluid management
in acute renal failure (ARF), 382
in chronic kidney disease (CKD), 398
in fluid volume excess (FVE),
367, 367*t*
in intracranial regulation, 708

Fluid output
average, 340*t*
feces, 340
insensible losses, 340
measurement and recording, 348–351
as proportional to intake, 350
routes, 339
urine, 339–340
Fluid replacement
in sepsis, 602–603
in shock, 1228–1229
Fluid restriction guidelines, 367*t*
Fluid resuscitation, 1476–1477
Fluid volume balance
appendicitis and, 647
burns and, 1482
cardiomyopathy and, 1081–1082
heart failure and, 1159–1160
hypertension and, 1175
inflammatory bowel disease (IBD) and,
665–666
liver disease and, 786
motor vehicle crashes (MVC) and, 2004
nephritis and, 674
peptic ulcer disease (PUD) and, 681
RSV/bronchiolitis and, 1022
sickle cell disease and, 125
systemic lupus erythematosus and, 516
Fluid volume deficit (FVD). *See also* Fluid and
electrolyte imbalance
assessment, 362
care planning, 362
in children, 356
clinical therapies, 360–362
collaborative care, 360–362
defined, 350, 354
diagnosis, 362
diagnostic tests, 360
etiology, 355–357
extracellular, 354–355, 360*t*
focus of care, 362–363
in infants, 356, 356*f*
interventions, 362–363
intravenous fluids, 361–362, 361*t*
isotonic, 355
manifestations, 357–360, 357*t*, 360*t*
in metabolic alkalosis, 19
multisystem effects of, 358*t*
nursing process, 362–363
in older adults, 359, 362*t*
oral rehydration, 360–361
outcome evaluation, 363
overview of, 354
pathophysiology, 354–357
pediatric clients, 362
third spacing, 355
Fluid volume excess (FVE). *See also* Fluid and
electrolyte imbalance
assessment, 367
care planning, 368
collaborative care, 365–367
defined, 350
diagnosis, 367–368
diagnostic tests, 365
dietary management, 367
etiology, 365
fluid management, 367, 367*t*
iatrogenic cause of, 365
interstitial (edema), 364–365
interventions, 368

manifestations, 365, 366*t*
Nursing Care Plan, 369–370*t*
nursing process, 367–368
outcome evaluation, 368
pathophysiology, 363–365
pharmacologic therapy, 365–367
risk factors, 365
Fluids and electrolytes
alterations, 346
alterations and therapies, 347*t*
assessment, 348–351, 349*t*
assessment interview, 350*t*
body fluids
active transport, 338, 339*f*
compartments, 336, 336*f*
diffusion, 338, 338*f*
distribution and composition of,
336–337
electrolyte composition of, 336*f*
electrolyte concentration in compartments,
337f
extracellular fluid (ECF), 336–337
filtration, 338, 338*f*
fluid intake and, 339, 339*f*, 339*t*,
348–351
fluid output and, 339–340, 341*f*,
348–351
homeostasis, 340, 341*f*
interstitial fluid, 336
intracellular fluid, 336
intravascular fluid, 336
movement of, 337–339
osmosis, 337–338, 337*f*
regulating, 339–341
transcellular fluid, 336
in bowel elimination, 274
chronic kidney disease (CKD) and, 393
clinical measurements, 348–351
collaborative interventions and therapies, 352
compensation, 346
concepts related to, 345–346*t*
congenital heart defects and, 1102
daily weight measurement, 348
defined, 335
diagnostic tests, 351, 351*f*
electrolytes
normal values, 351*t*
regulation of, 341–342, 342*t*
serum, 351, 351*f*
types of, 341, 342*t*
genetic and lifespan considerations
age, 343–344, 343*f*, 344*f*
children, 343–344, 344*f*, 344*t*
ethnicity, 344–346
gender and body size, 344
infants, 343–344, 343*f*, 344*f*, 344*t*
older adults, 344*f*, 344*t*
pediatric differences, 343
heat-related illness, 348
independent interventions and
therapies, 352
intake and output documentation, 352*t*
interventions and therapies, 351–352, 353*t*
medications, 353*t*
modifiable risk factors, 346–348
normal, 336–346
pharmacologic therapy, 352
prevalence and, 346
prevention and, 346–348
vital signs measurement, 348

Fluorescein strain, 567
Fluoride, 931
Fluoroscope, 220
Focal seizures, 716
Focus, lack of, 1614
Focus charting, 2442–2443
Focused assessment by sonography in trauma
        (FAST), 1961
Folic acid
    for anemia, 70
    antepartum nutrition and, 2096
    dietary sources of, 71t
Folic acid deficiency anemia, 68, 68t, 75t,
        2044–2045
Follicle-stimulating hormone-releasing hormone
        (FSHRH), 2017
Follicular phase, 2018
Fontan procedure, 1099t
Fontanelles, 2114
Food allergy test, 490
Food choices. See also Diet
    in adolescents, 933
    culture and, 944
    emotion and, 925
    factors affecting, 924, 924t
    food habits and, 924
    food packaging and, 924–925
    health benefits and, 925
    portion size and, 925–926, 925f
Food insecurity, 927, 945t
Food safety, 926
Food security, 927
Foodborne illnesses, 2097
Foot care, diabetes and, 763t
Footling breech, 2115
Foramen ovale, 1040, 2028
Forced expiratory volume in 1 second
        (FEV$_1$), 1008
Forceps marks, 2224
Forceps-assisted birth, 2130
Foreground questions, 2588
Foreign body conjunctiva, 1313t, 1316
Foreseeability, 2656
Forgiveness, 1874
Formal groups, 2419, 2420t
Formal leaders, 2489
Formula-feeding mothers, 2177
Foster families, 1710
Fourth (S$_4$) heart sounds, 1034–1035
Fowler position, 968, 968f
Fowler spiritual theory, 1658
Fractures. See also Mobility
    alignment maintenance, 866
    arm, 867–868t
    assessment, 864–866
    bone healing factors and, 857t
    care planning, 866
    in children, 859
    client evaluation, 867
    collaborative care, 859–864
    compartment syndrome and, 858
    complications of, 858–859
    deep venous thrombosis (DVT) and,
        858, 858t
    defined, 824t, 825, 853
    delayed union, 857
    diagnosis, 866
    diagnostic tests, 859–860
    discharge instructions, 867
    electrical bone stimulation and, 861t

emergency care, 859
external fixation, 860f
fall prevention and, 857t
fat embolism syndrome and, 858–859
healing of, 853–857
hip. See hip fractures
infection and, 859
infection prevention, 867
inflammatory phase, 853–857
interventions, 824t, 866–867
lifespan and cultural considerations, 859
malunion, 857
manifestations, 824t, 858–859, 865t
mobility promotion, 866
neurovascular status monitoring, 866
nonpharmacologic therapy
    casts, 860–862, 861f, 862t
    pain management, 864
    splints, 862
    traction, 862–864, 863–864t, 863f
nonunion, 857
Nursing Care Plan, 867–868t
nursing process, 864–867
open reduction and internal fixation
        (ORIF), 860
overview of, 853
pain interventions, 865t
pain management, 866
pathophysiology and etiology, 853–857
pharmacologic therapy, 860
prevention of, 857
remodeling phase, 857
reparative phase, 857
risk factors, 857
surgery, 860
types of
    avulsion, 855t
    closed, 854t
    comminuted, 854t
    complete, 854t
    compression, 856t
    depression, 856t
    displaced, 854t
    greenstick, 854t
    impacted, 856t
    linear, 855t
    nondisplaced, 854t
    oblique, 855t
    open, 854t
    pathologic, 856t
    spinal, 855t
    stress, 856t
    transverse, 855t
    x-rays of, 859f
Fragile X syndrome, 1377, 1581, 1582t
Framingham Heart Study (FHS), 1109t
Frank breech, 2115
Free-floating anxiety, 1918
Freezing, in Parkinson's disease, 897
Frequency, of contractions, 2118
Freud Psychosexual theory of
        development, 1835
Freud stages of development,
        1649–1650, 1650t
Friedman Family Assessment Tool
        (FFAM), 1728
Friends
    death of, 1753
    support of, 1732
Frontal (mitotic) suture, 2114

Frostbite, 1439
Frustration, 1976
FSHRH (follicle-stimulating hormone-releasing
        hormone), 2017
Fulguration, 87
Full term, 2028
Fullmer SPICES, 2296t
Full-thickness burns. See also Burns
    defined, 1468
    illustrated, 1468f
    manifestations, 1481t
Full-thickness skin loss, 1496–1497t
Fulminant colitis, 660
Functional incontinence, 299t
Functional method, 2458
Functional nursing, 2600
Fundus
    defined, 2171
    in intrapartum assessment, 2143t
    palpating, 2167
Funduscopy, 1320
Fungi
    defined, 523
    pathogenic organisms, 530t
FVD. See Fluid volume deficit
FVE. See Fluid volume excess

G

GAD. See Generalized anxiety disorder
Gait and posture assessment, 830t
Galactorrhea, 1359t
Galactosemia, 2208t
Galanin, 1594
Gallbladder
    scan, 651
    ultrasonography of, 651
Gallbladder disease
    assessment, 654
    bilirubin levels and, 651t
    care planning, 654
    cholangitis, 650
    cholecystitis, 651, 651t
    cholelithiasis, 650, 651t
    client teaching, 655t
    collaborative care, 651
    diagnosis, 654
    infection prevention, 654
    interventions, 654–655
    manifestations, 653t
    manifestations and complications, 651t
    nonpharmacologic therapy, 652–653
    Nursing Care Plan, 655–656t
    nursing process, 654–655
    nutrition and, 654–655
    obesity and, 792
    outcome evaluation, 655
    overview of, 650
    pain management, 653t, 654
    pathophysiology and etiology,
        650–651
    pharmacologic therapy, 652
    prevention of, 651
    risk factors, 650–651
    surgery, 652
    T-tube nursing care, 652t
    T-tube placement, 652f
Gallstone ileus, 650
Gallstones, 650f, 650t
Gametes, 2011

Gametogenesis, 2020
Gangrene, 1141*t*
Gardner-Wells tongs, 913
GAS (general adaptation syndrome), 1900
Gas exchange monitoring, disseminated
        intravascular coagulation (DIC)
        and, 1142
Gastric analysis, 679
Gastric lavage, 788
Gastric outlet obstruction, 678
Gastric ulcers, 677
Gastritis, 1538*t*
Gastrocolic reflex, 275
Gastroesophageal reflux disease (GERD).
        See also Digestion
    assessment, 229
    in children, 228*t*
    client teaching, 231*t*
    collaborative care, 228–229
    defined, 210, 227
    diagnosis, 229
    diagnostic tests, 228
    esophagus, 227, 227*f*, 228*f*
    in infants, 228*t*, 229*t*
    interventions, 229–231
    manifestations, 212*t*, 228
    medications, 230*t*
    Nursing Care Plan, 230*t*
    nursing process, 229–231
    nutrition and lifestyle management, 229
    outcome evaluation, 231
    overview of, 227
    pathophysiology and etiology, 227–228
    pharmacologic therapy, 228–229
    prevention of, 227–228
    surgery, 229
Gastrointestinal bleeding, 787
Gastrointestinal system
    burn injuries and, 1472
    changes and infection, 525
    disseminated intravascular coagulation
        (DIC) and, 1141*t*
    exercise benefits, 422
    labor and, 2127
    mechanical ventilation and, 982
    newborns, 2199–2200
    postpartum changes, 2174–2175
    pregnancy and, 2031
    in premature newborns, 2250–2251
    shock effect on, 1220–1222
Gastroscopy, 679
Gate control theory, 154
Gay and lesbian families, 1711–1712, 1711*f*
GBS (Guillain-Barré syndrome), 1331, 1333*t*
GDS (Geriatric Depression Scale), 1587*t*,
        1787, 2295*t*
Gender
    abuse and, 1967
    bias, 1635
    blood pressure and, 1046
    burn risk and, 1466
    cancer and, 46
    communication and, 2406
    disease and, 414
    diversity, 1634–1635
    grieving process and, 1746
    immune disease and, 448
    phobias and, 1940
    pulse and, 1044
    sexism, 1635

skin disorders and, 1452
stereotyping, 1634
violence and, 1957
Gender bias theory, 1781–1782
Gender identity, 1345–1346
Gender expression, 1345
Gene therapy, 135
General adaptation syndrome (GAS), 1900
Generalized anxiety disorder (GAD)
    in children, 1920–1921
    defined, 1908*t*, 1920
    DSM-5 diagnostic criteria for, 1922*t*
    interventions, 1908*t*
    manifestations, 1908*t*
Generalized seizures, 716
Generation X, 2494*t*
Generational cohort, 2493
Generational differences, 2493–2496,
        2494–2495*t*, 2496*f*
Generations, 2494–2495*t*
Generic drugs, 898
Genes
    cell structure and, 31–32
    oncogenes, 45
    tumor suppressor, 45
Genetic counseling referral, 1390–1391
Genetic disorders, mobility and, 827, 827*t*
Genetic testing, 2572–2573, 2573*t*
Genetics
    in addiction, 1521, 1522
    in anemia, 34
    in cancer, 34, 46
    in cellular regulation, 31–32, 34
    in cognition, 1577–1578
    comfort and, 145–146
    in dementia, 1584–1585
    in development, 1673–1676
    in digestive disorders, 214*t*
    in family planning, 1373–1378
    in fever syndromes, 1426
    in immunity, 444–445, 448
    in infection, 525–527
    in inflammation, 637–640
    in intellectual disability, 1583
    in learning disabilities, 1580
    metabolism and, 729–731
    in mobility, 827
    in mood and affect, 1776, 1783
    in nutrition, 932
    in nutritionally-related disorders,
        932–934, 939
    in obsessive-compulsive disorder
        (OCD), 1840
    in oxygenation, 961
    in perfusion, 1046–1049, 1051–1054,
        1054*t*
    in personality disorders (PD), 1853
    in postpartum depression, 1821
    in sensory impairment, 1282
    in sexual functioning, 1351
    in sickle cell disease (SCD), 34
    in skin disorders, 1452
    in stress and coping, 1910
    suicide and, 1991
Genital herpes (HSV). *See also* Sexually
        transmitted infections (STIs)
    blisters, 1410, 1410*f*
    defined, 1410
    diagnosis and treatment, 1410
    diagnostic tests, 1411

manifestations, 1410, 1410*t*
pathophysiology, 1410
pharmacologic therapy, 1411
Genital intercourse, 1346
Genital warts
    defined, 1411
    diagnosis and treatment, 1411
    facts about, 1411
    illustrated, 1411*f*
    manifestations, 1411
    pathophysiology, 1411
    pharmacologic therapy, 1411–1412
Genitals
    female, in gestational age, 2218, 2219*f*
    male, in gestational age, 2218, 2218*f*
    newborn assessment, 2230–2231
Genitourinary changes, 525
Genograms, 1720
Genome, 31
Genotype, 1376
Gentle touch, 2259
Geographic information systems (GIS), 2641
Geragogy, 2502
GERD. *See* Gastroesophageal reflux disease
Geriatric Depression Scale (GDS), 1587*t*,
        1787, 2295*t*
Geriatric failure to thrive (GFTT), 1701
Gestation, 2051*t*
Gestational age
    ankle dorsiflexion, 2220, 2221*f*
    assessment, 2213–2221
    assessment tools, 2213
    Ballard assessment, 2213, 2214–2215*t*
    breast tissue, 2216, 2217*f*
    Dubowitz tool, 2213
    ear form and cartilage distribution,
        2217, 2218*f*
    female genitals, 2218, 2219*f*
    hair, 2218
    head lag, 2220–2221
    heel-to-ear extension, 2220, 2220*f*
    lanugo, 2216
    major reflexes, 2221
    male genitals, 2218, 2218*f*
    nails, 2219
    neuromuscular maturity characteristics,
        2219–2221
    physical maturity characteristics, 2216–2219,
        2216*f*, 2217*f*, 2218*f*, 2219*f*
    popliteal angle, 2220
    recoil, 2219–2220
    scarf sign, 2220, 2220*f*
    skin, 2216
    skull firmness, 2219
    sole creases, 2216, 2217*f*
    square window sign, 2219, 2219*f*
    supplementary method, 2221
    ventral suspension, 2221
    vernix, 2218
Gestational diabetes mellitus (GDM)
    clinical therapy, 2047–2048
    defined, 2045
    evaluation of fetal status, 2048
    fetal-neonatal risks, 2046–2047
    influence during pregnancy,
        2045–2047
    influence on pregnancy outcome,
        2046–2047
    intrapartum management of, 2048
    labor management, 2048

maternal risks, 2046
postpartum management of, 2048
timing of birth, 2048
Gestational hypertension, 1205
Gestational trophoblastic disease (GTD), 2080t
Gestures, 2402–2403
Get-Up-and-Go-Test, 2295t
GFCF. *See* Gluten-free, casein-free (GFCF) diet
GFTT (geriatric failure to thrive), 1701
GGM (glucose galactose malabsorption), 209
Gilligan moral development levels, 1657–1658
Gingiva, 424
Gingivitis, 426
Ginseng, 1397t
GIS (geographic information systems), 2641
Glatiramer acetate (Copaxone), 880
Glaucoma
angle-closure, 1319, 1320t
assessment, 1323
care planning, 1324
in children, 1323t
collaborative care, 1320–1322
defined, 1318
diagnosis, 1323–1324
diagnostic tests, 1320
diversity and culture and, 1319t
exercise and, 1323t
eyedrop bottle tops, 1321t
home care, 1325t
injury prevention and, 1324
interventions, 1281t, 1324–1325
intraocular pressure and, 1318
manifestations, 1281t, 1320, 1320t
Nursing Care Plan, 1325–1326t
nursing process, 1323–1325
open-angle, 1319, 1320t
orientation/environmental modifications and, 1324–1325
outcome evaluation, 1325
overview of, 1318
pathophysiology and etiology, 1318–1320
pediatric, 1318–1319
pharmacologic therapy, 1320–1321, 1322t
psychosocial wellness and, 1325
risk factors, 1319–1320
surgery, 1321
Glenn procedure, 1099t
Global aphasia, 1238
Global evaluative dimension of the self, 1834
Global self-esteem, 1834
Glomerular filtration rate (GFR), 376
Glomerulonephritis, 669
Gloves
infection and, 546
sterile, 549
Glucagon, 704, 748
Glucagon emergency kit, 778
Glucocorticosteroids, 398, 643t
Gluconeogenesis, 704
Glucose
administration of, 748
control tips, 777t
long-term control, 2047–2048
monitoring in children, 769
urine testing for, 752
Glucose galactose malabsorption (GGM), 209
Glucose-G-phosphate dehydrogenase anemia, 69
Glucosuria, 742
Gluten-free, casein-free (GFCF) diet, 1692t

Glycogenolysis, 704
Glycosuria, 263
GnRH (gonadotropin-releasing hormone), 2017
Goals
attainable (achievable), 2343
client, revising, 2351
defined, 2341t
developing, 2342
evaluation example of, 2352t
long-term, 2341–2342
measurable, 2342–2343
outcomes versus, 2341t
relevant, 2343
short-term, 2341–2342
single specific action, 2342
SMART format, 2343, 2343t
time limited, 2343
writing, 2342
Goiter, 735t, 806
Gold salts, 502–503, 503t
Golgi apparatus, 31
Gonadotropin-releasing hormone (GnRH), 2017
Gonioplasty, 1321
Gonioscopy, 1320
Gonorrhea. *See also* Sexually transmitted infections (STIs)
complications of, 1413
defined, 1412
diagnosis and treatment, 1413
manifestations, 1413
Nursing Care Plan, 1416t
pathophysiology, 1412–1413
Good faith immunity, 2674, 2674t
Good Samaritan laws, 2662
Goodell sign, 2030
Goodpasture syndrome, 670
Gould developmental stages, 1653
Gout, 826, 826f
Governance, 2538
Gowns
infection and, 546
sterile, 549
Graafian follicle, 2018
Grading, tumor, 53
Graft-versus-host disease, 444
Gram stain, in urinary tract infections (UTIs), 623
Grandparents
death of, 1753
expectant, 2040
Granulation tissue, 635, 1508
Granulocytes, 440
Graphesthesia test, 702f, 702t
Graph-versus-host disease (GVHD), 98
Grasping reflex, 2233, 2234f
Graves disease
defined, 728, 806
exophthalmos and, 806f
illustrated, 806f
manifestations, 806–808
Nursing Care Plan, 811–812t
ophthalmopathy, 806–808
Gravida, 2051t
Greenstick fractures, 854t
Grief and loss
alterations and therapies, 1747t
alterations from normal, 1744–1747
antidepressant medications and, 1750
assessment, 1747–1748, 1748t

assessment interview, 1748t
bereavement, 1742
childhood traumatic, 1753
collaborative interventions and therapies, 1750
complicated grief and, 1743, 1745–1746
concept of, 1741
concepts related to, 1745
defined, 1742
depression versus, 1788, 1788t
Engel and Sanders theory, 1743
factors affecting process, 1746
grieving process, 1742–1743
grieving theories, 1743
independent interventions and therapies, 1749
interventions and therapies, 1749–1750
Kübler-Ross and five stages of grief, 1743
lifespan considerations, 1743–1744, 1743f
mourning, 1742
normal presentation of, 1742–1744
sociological considerations, 1743f
spiritual and cultural considerations, 1748–1749
types of, 1742–1743
Grieving
age and, 1746
anticipatory, 38
asking for help and, 1746
cancer and, 63
comfort and, 143t
gender and, 1746
leukemia and, 102
lung cancer and, 110
process of, 1742–1743
substance and alcohol abuse and, 1746
theories, 1743
Groningen Frailty Indicator, 2295t
Group B streptococcal (GBS) infection, 2082t
Group communications. *See also* Communication
brainstorming, 2420
cohesiveness, 2422
commitment, 2420, 2420t
decision-making methods, 2420–2422
Delphi technique, 2421–2422
groupthink, 2422
member behavior, 2422
monopolizing, 2422
nominal group technique, 2421
power, 2422
scapegoating, 2422
silence and apathy, 2422–2423
transference and countertransference, 2422–2423
Group dynamics, 2418, 2420–2422
Group teaching, 2521
Group therapy
with adolescents, 1531
curative factors of, 1531t
defined, 1530
here-and-now concept and, 1530
for personality disorders, 1862
in schizophrenia, 1619
social microcosm and, 1530
support groups, 1531
twelve-step programs, 1531–1532, 1532t

Groups and group communication
committees or teams, 2424
comparative features, 2421t
defined, 2418
effective, characteristics of, 2419, 2420t
existence of, 2418
formal, 2419, 2420t
functions of, 2419, 2419t
healthcare, 2424
informal, 2419, 2420t
levels of formality, 2419
overview of, 2418
primary, 2418
problems of, 2422–2423
secondary, 2418
self-awareness/growth, 2423–2424
self-help, 2424
semiformal, 2419, 2420t
task forces, 2424
teaching, 2424
therapy, 2424
types of, 2418–2419
work-related social support, 2424
Groupthink, 2422
Growth
cephalocaudal, 1648, 1648f
defined, 1647
genetic considerations, 1658–1659
measurement, 1703t
proximodistal, 1648
sickle cell disease and, 126
stages of, 1649t
Growth and development
cerebral palsy (CP) and, 1699
instruments, 2291t
Growth and development milestones
adolescents, 1669t
infancy, 1660t
preschool children, 1664t
reaching, 1662t
school-age children, 1667t
toddlers, 1662t
Growth and development theories
behaviorism, 1654
continuity, 1653
ecological, 1655–1657, 1656f
Erikson, 1650–1652, 1651t
Fowler, 1658
Freud, 1649–1650, 1650t
Gilligan, 1657–1658
Gould, 1653
Havighurst, 1652, 1652t
Kohlberg, 1657, 1658t
moral, 1657–1658
overview of, 1648–1649
Peck, 1652–1653
Piaget, 1653–1654, 1654t
psychosocial, 1649–1653
resiliency, 1654–1655
social learning, 1654
spiritual, 1658
temperament, 1654, 1655t
Westerhoff, 1658, 1659t
Growth and development through life span
adolescents (12 to 18 years), 1666–1668
adults, 1670–1671
body proportions, 1659f
infants (birth to 1 year), 1659–1662
preschool children (3 to 6 years), 1664–1666

school-age children (6 to 12 years), 1666–1668
toddlers (1 to 3 years), 1662–1664
GTD (gestational trophoblastic disease), 2080t
Guillain-Barré syndrome (GBS), 572, 1331, 1333t
Gunshot wounds, 1981
Gustatory stimuli, 1278
GVHD (graph-versus-host disease), 98
Gynecoid pelvis, 2014, 2016f
Gynecomastia, 1356t

H
H_1 receptors, 635
H1N1 influenza, 570
H1N1 vaccine distribution, 2607–2608, 2608t
H_2-receptor antagonists, 222
H_4 receptors, 635
HAART (highly active antiretroviral therapy), 456, 468–469
Habit training, 295
Habituation, 2204, 2235
Haemophilus influenzae, 534t
Haemophilus influenzae type B vaccine, 472, 580
Hair
assessment, 734t
distribution and quality assessment, 1458t
pregnancy and, 2032
pubic, 1341f
texture assessment, 1459t
HAIs. *See* Healthcare-associated infections
Hallucinations, 1578, 1611
Hallucinogens, 1564
Halo brace, 848, 848f, 913, 914f
Hamilton Rating Scale for Depression (HRSD), 1587t
Hand hygiene, 2702t
Hand restraints, 2704, 2706f
Handoff, 2451
Handoff communication, 2451, 2451t
Hands-on client participation, 2520, 2520f
HAP (hospital-acquired pneumonia), 982, 2704
Hardware, 2634
Harlequin sign, 2223
Hashimoto thyroiditis, 812–813
Hassles, 1898
Havighurst age periods and developmental tasks, 1652, 1652t
HBV (hepatitis B virus), 45t
HCG (human chorionic gonadotropin), 1253t, 2034
HCMV (human cytomegalovirus), 45t
HCO_2, as perioperative diagnostic test, 1252t
Head, in newborn assessment, 2225–2226, 2225f, 2226f
Head lag, 2220–2221
Healing. *See also* Wound healing
bones, 857t
comfort in, 141
of fractures, 853–857
spiritual beliefs related to, 1877
Health
defined, 406
oral, 423–429
personal definition of, 406, 407t
screening guidelines, 413–414t
topics of leading indicators, 410t
variables influencing, 412–415

Health, wellness and illness
assessment, 415–417
assessment data validation, 417
behavioral change strategies, 418, 419t
biological dimension, 414
cognitive dimension, 415
concepts of, 406–407
counseling, 418
diagnosis, 417
group support, 418
health education, 418
health lifestyle choices, 415t
health promotion, 409–412, 417–418
health screenings and immunization guidelines, 413t
illness and disease, 408–409
illness-wellness continuum, 407, 408f
interventions, 418–419
life stress review, 416–417
lifestyle assessment, 415
modeling, 418–419
normal sleep-rest patterns, 429–434
nursing process, 415–419
oral health, 423–429
physical fitness and exercise, 420–423
physical fitness assessment, 415
plan evaluation, 419
positive reinforcement, 418
psychological dimension, 414–415
social support systems, 416, 418
spiritual health assessment, 416
understanding of, 405
variables, 412–415
Health beliefs, 415
Health history, older adults, 2296–2297
Health insurance
lack of, 2603–2604
private plans, 2628–2629
Health Insurance Portability and Accountability Act (HIPAA)
compliance examples, 2671t
defined, 2638, 2670
informatics and, 2638–2639
overview of, 2670
privacy versus confidentiality and, 2671
protected health information (PHI), 2670
Health Insurance Technology for Economic and Clinical Health Act (HITECH), 2632, 2638
Health Level 7 (HL7), 2638
Health literacy
client behaviors and, 2514
defined, 2514, 2599
facts, 2599
limited, 2514t
low income skills, 2514, 2515t
Health maintenance
coronary artery disease (CAD) and, 1125
hypertension and, 1175
systemic lupus erythematosus (SLE) and, 517–518
Health maintenance organizations (HMOs), 2628
Health policy
concept of, 2619
concepts related to, 2621t
defined, 2619
developing, 2620
evaluation phase, 2620
formulation phase, 2620

implementation phase, 2620
informatics and, 2632
relevance to nurses, 2620
Health promotion. *See also* Health, wellness and
    illness
    activities, 411
    assessment, 1727
    care planning, 1729
    in children, 416t
    collaborative care, 1727
    community-based care, 1724
    competence, 2544
    defined, 409, 1724
    diagnosis, 1728, 2335
    Family APGAR, 1727–1728, 1728t
    family ecomap, 1727, 1727f
    Friedman Family Assessment Tool
        (FFAM), 1728
    goals, 409
    health protection versus, 410–411, 411t
    health risk appraisal and, 411
    HOME Inventory, 1728
    interventions, 1729
    leading indicators, 410t
    lifespan and cultural considerations, 1726
    national guidelines for, 2605t
    nurse's role in, 411–412, 412t
    Nursing Care Plan, 1729–1730t
    nursing process, 1727–1729
    in older adults, 416t
    outcome evaluation, 1729
    overview of, 1724–1726
    plans, 417–418
    prevention and, 1726
    risk factors, 1726
    strategy implementation, 2597
    as tool, 2597
    topic areas, 409t
    topics across life span, 412t
    wellness assessment programs and, 411
    wellness promotion and, 1724, 1725t
Health restoration, 2544
Healthcare
    care management and, 2599
    client-focused care, 2599
    frameworks for providing, 2599
    managed care, 2599
    old and new paradigms comparison, 2596t
    quality improvement, 2683, 2683f
Healthcare access
    barriers to, 2603–2606
    healthcare legislation and, 2604t
    lack of health insurance and, 2603–2604
    lack of usual source of care and, 2605
    overview of, 2603
    patient-centered medical home and, 2605
    perceptions of need and, 2605
    solutions, 2606
    underinsured and, 2603
    uneven distribution of services and, 2606
    uninsured and, 2603
Healthcare advance directives. *See* Advance
    directives
Healthcare delivery
    demographics and, 2598
    factors affecting, 2598–2599
    health literacy and, 2599
    levels of prevention, 2597t
    primary prevention, 2596–2597
    secondary prevention, 2597

    services offered, 2596–2597
    technology and, 2598–2599
    tertiary prevention, 2597
Healthcare disparity, 1638
Healthcare information systems
    administration, 2636
    clinical, 2635–2636, 2635f
    intranets, 2636t
    relationship of components, 2636
    technology overview, 2634–2635, 2635t
Healthcare legislation (2010), 2604t
Healthcare proxies, 177, 2667
Healthcare services
    types of, 2596–2597
    uneven distribution of, 2606
Healthcare settings, 2598, 2598t
Healthcare surrogate, 2667
Healthcare systems
    concept of, 2595
    concepts related to, 2600–2602t
    factors affecting delivery of health care and,
        2598–2599
    frameworks for providing care, 2599
    healthcare services, 2596–2597
    healthcare settings, 2598
    nursing care delivery systems, 2599–2600
    nursing practice, 2600
Healthcare team, 2376–2377t
Healthcare values, 2463t
Healthcare worker precautions
    client transportation, 548
    disinfecting and sterilizing, 554–555
    disposal of soiled equipment/supplies, 548
    isolated client psychosocial needs and,
        548–549
    isolation practices, 546
    isolation precautions, 545–546, 547t
    personal protective equipment, 546
Healthcare-associated infections (HAIs)
    causes of, 531t
    defined, 530, 2704
    factors contributing to, 531
    microorganism source, 530–531
    pathogens causing, 2706
    preventing, 549
    statistics, 530
    types of, 2704–2706
Healthy behaviors
    diabetes and, 762–763
    in nursing self-care, 2310–2311
    osteoporosis and, 804
Healthy People 2020
    collaboration and, 2381
    exercise and activity, 420
    foundation of, 410
    health indicators, 2596
    nutritional recommendations, 926
    nutritious foods in schools, 933
    obesity and, 933
    respiratory health, 961
    topic areas, 409t
    topics of leading indicators, 410t
Hearing
    assessment, 1285–1291, 1292t
    deficits, communication and, 1297t
    Rinne test, 1291f
    screenings, 1283
    sensory aids for impairment, 1296f
    Weber test, 1291f
Hearing aids, 1302–1303

Hearing impairment
    amplification and, 1302–1304, 1303f
    assessment, 1304
    care planning, 1304
    cochlear implants and, 1302, 1302f
    collaborative care, 1302–1304
    communication facilitation, 1305
    communication techniques, 1304t
    community-based care, 1305t
    conductive hearing loss, 1299
    diagnoses, 1304
    diagnostic tests, 1302
    diversity and culture and, 1301t
    interventions and therapies, 1297, 1304–1305
    manifestations, 1300–1301, 1301t
    noise-induced hearing loss (NIHL), 1300
    nonpharmacologic therapy, 1302–1304, 1303t
    nursing process, 1304–1305
    optimal wellness and, 1304–1305
    outcome evaluation, 1305
    overview of, 1298–1299
    pathophysiology and etiology, 1299–1300
    pharmacologic therapy, 1302
    presbycusis, 1299
    prevention of, 1300
    risk factors, 1299
    sensorineural hearing loss, 1299
    severity of, 1299t
    socialization and, 1305
    surgery, 1302
    temporary hearing loss medications, 1303t
    tinnitus, 1301
Heart. *See also* Perfusion
    auscultation of, 1062f, 1062t
    blood flow through, 1041f
    blood pressure and, 1045
    chambers, 1033–1036
    conduction system, 1042–1044, 1043f
    electrocardiograms (ECGs) and,
        1071–1073t
    fetal, 2028
    internal anatomy, 1033f
    location of, 1032f
    newborn assessment, 2229–2230, 2229f
    valves, 1033–1036, 1034f
    wall layers, 1032–1033, 1033f
Heart analogy, 2370t
Heart block, 1178
Heart catheterization procedure, 1099t
Heart failure
    activity monitoring, 1160
    acute versus chronic, 1147
    assessment, 1158
    cardiac output monitoring, 1159
    cardiac transplantation and, 1157–1158, 1157f
    care planning, 1159
    causes of, 1144–1145, 1145t
    classifications of, 1147–1148
    collaborative care, 1149–1158
    compensatory mechanisms activated by,
        1145, 1146t
    complementary and alternative therapy, 1158
    complications of, 1149
    defined, 1144
    diagnosis, 1158
    diagnostic tests, 1151
    end-of-life care and, 1158
    etiology, 1148
    fatigue and women and, 186t
    fluid volume monitoring, 1159–1160

Heart failure (*continued*)
Frank-Starling mechanism, 1145, 1146*t*
hemodynamic monitoring, 1151–1153, 1151*f*
home activity guidelines, 1160*t*
home care, 1159*t*
interventions, 1159–1160
left-sided, 1147, 1147*f*, 1148
low-output versus high-output, 1147
low-sodium diet and, 1160
multisystem effects of, 1150*t*
Nursing Care Plan, 1161*t*
nursing process, 1158–1160
nutrition and activity and, 1156–1157
outcome evaluation, 1160
overview of, 1144–1145
pathophysiology, 1145–1148
pharmacologic therapy
angiotensin II-receptor blockers,
1153, 1154*t*
angiotensin-converting enzyme (ACE)
inhibitors, 1153, 1154*t*
antidysrhythmics, 1156*t*
beta-blockers, 1153
digitalis, 1153–1156, 1155*t*
diuretics, 1153, 1154–1155*t*
phosphodiesterase inhibitors, 1156*t*
sympathomimetic agents, 1156*t*
vasodilators, 1153
pulmonary edema, 1145, 1147–1148, 1149*t*
right-sided, 1147, 1148, 1148*f*
risk factors, 1148
stages of, 1149*t*
statistics, 1051
surgery, 1157–1158
systolic versus diastolic, 1147
Heart murmurs
assessment, 1061–1062*t*
classifications of, 1039–1040*t*
defined, 1036
distinguishing, 1037–1038*t*
Heart rate
in Apgar score, 2210
assessment, 1059*t*
defined, 1042
fetal, labor and, 2127
newborn, 2195
Heart sounds
additional, 1035–1036, 1036*t*
assessment, 1059–1061*t*
characteristics of, 1035*t*
in diastole, 1034, 1034*f*
first (S₁), 1034
fourth (S₄), 1034–1035
second (S₂), 1034
in systole, 1034, 1034*f*
third (S₃), 1034
Heartburn, 210
Heat and cold, rheumatoid arthritis and, 504
Heat balance, 1422
Heat exhaustion, 1431
Heat production, factors affecting, 1422
Heat stroke, 1431
Heat transfer, 1422, 1472
Heberden nodes, 886
Heel-to-ear extension, 2220, 2220*f*
Heel-to-shin test, 704*f*, 704*t*
Hegar sign, 2035
Helicobacter pylori, 677, 679
HELLP syndrome, 1205
Help, asking for, 1746

Helper T cells, 442–443, 457
Hematocrit
defined, 351, 1045
in glucose meter performance, 753
infection and, 602
as perioperative diagnostic test, 1252*t*
Hematogenous spread, 606
Hematological emergencies, 49–50
Hematoma, 1508
Hematuria, 378, 621
Hemianopia, 1237
Hemiarthroplasty, 871
Hemiparesis, 1239
Hemiplegia, 1239, 1244*t*
Hemodialysis
defined, 272
in renal replacement therapy, 383–384
system components, 383*f*
vascular access for, 384–385, 385*f*
Hemodynamic monitoring, 602, 1115
Hemodynamics
defined, 1151
intra-arterial pressure monitoring, 1152
monitoring setup, 1151*f*
pulmonary artery pressure monitoring,
1152–1153, 1153*f*
venous pressure monitoring, 1152
Hemoglobin, as perioperative diagnostic
test, 1252*t*
Hemoglobin A₁C, 751–752
Hemoglobinopathy, 120
Hemolysis, 374
Hemoptysis, 107, 588, 609
Hemorrhage, 678, 1508
Hemorrhagic strokes, 1236
Hemosiderosis, 123
Hemostasis, 1508
Hemotympanum, 577, 577*f*
Heparin, 1132, 1133*t*
Hepatitis
assessment, 236
client teaching, 238*t*
collaborative care, 235, 236*t*
convalescent phase, 233–235
defined, 211, 232
degeneration and necrosis of the liver,
233, 233*f*
diagnosis, 236
diagnostic tests, 235
fatigue and, 236–238
icteric phase, 233
interventions, 236–238
jaundice and, 232*f*
manifestations, 212*t*, 233–235, 235*t*
medications, 237*t*
Nursing Care Plan, 238–239*t*
nursing process, 236–238
nutrition and, 236
outcomes and evaluation parameters, 238
overview of, 232
pathophysiology and etiology, 232
pharmacologic therapy, 235
prevention, 233, 234*t*
prodromal phase, 233
risk factors, 233, 234*t*
skin integrity and, 236
viral, tests for, 236*t*
viral, types of, 234*t*
Hepatitis B virus (HBV), 45*t*
Hepatitis E, 2097

Hepatorenal syndrome, 784
Herbal preparations
antepartum nutrition and, 2096*t*
for anxiety disorders, 1925
Here-and-now concept, 1530
Hernias
in bowel assessment, 281*t*
defined, 281*t*
in female reproductive system assessment,
1359*t*
Herniated discs. *See also* Back problems
assessment, 844
care planning, 844–845
cauda equina syndrome (CES), 841
cervical, 842
in children, 842
collaborative care, 842–843
comfort promotion and, 845
defined, 824*t*, 840
diagnosis, 844
diagnostic tests, 842–843
education, 845
illustrated, 840*f*
injury prevention and, 845
interventions, 824*t*, 845
lifespan and cultural considerations, 842
lumbar, 841
manifestations, 824*t*, 841–842, 844*t*
nonpharmacologic therapy, 843
nursing process, 844–845
in older adults, 842
pathophysiology and etiology, 840–841
pharmacologic therapy, 843
preoperative and postoperative care,
845, 846*t*
prevention of, 841
risk factors, 841
sciatica, 841, 842*f*
surgery, 843
Heroin
defined, 1554
as opiate, 1564
pregnancy and, 1554
Herpes simplex virus (HSV), 45*t*, 1410–1411,
2081*t*
Heterograft (xenograft), 1479
Heterosexism, 1636
Heterosexual cohabiting family, 1711
HHV-6 (human herpesvirus 6), 45*t*
High anion gap acidosis, 14
High blood pressure statistics, 1051
High priority, 2366
High productivity equation, 2364
High-Fowler position, 968, 968*f*
Highly active antiretroviral therapy (HAART),
456, 468–469
Hinduism, 1886
Hip fractures
assessment, 872–873
Austin-Moore prosthesis repair, 872
calling for help and, 870*f*
care planning, 873
collaborative care, 871–872
complications of, 870–871
defined, 869
diagnosis, 873
diagnostic tests, 871
discharge instructions, 874
evaluation, 874
extracapsular, 869

illustrated, 871f
interventions, 873–874
intracapsular, 869
lifespan and cultural considerations, 871
manifestations, 870–871, 873t
nonpharmacologic therapy, 872
Nursing Care Plan, 874–875t
nursing process, 872–874
occurrence of, 825
overview of, 869
pathophysiology and etiology, 869–870
pharmacologic therapy, 872
preoperative and postoperative care,
    873–874
prevention of, 870
psychosocial wellness and, 874
regions of, 869f
risk factors, 870
surgery, 871–872
HIPAA. See Health Insurance Portability and
    Accountability Act
Hippocampus, 1576
Hips
    mobility assessment, 832t
    prosthesis, 871, 872f
Hirsutism, 1360t, 1458t
Hispanics
    acceptable child behaviors, 2288t
    autism and, 1692t
    pain response, 161t
    smoking and, 1007t
    stroke and, 1237t
Histamine₂-receptor blockers, 230t, 680
Histamines, 634
Histrionic personality disorder (HPD), 1863t
HITECH (Health Insurance Technology for
    Economic and Clinical Health Act),
    2632, 2638
HIV/AIDS
    antepartum care and, 2077t
    assessment, 474
    as bioethical issue, 2572
    candidiasis, 463
    caregivers of infants at risk, 462t
    cervical cancer and, 464
    classification, 462
    collaborative care, 467–474
    complementary and alternative therapies, 474
    diagnosis, 474
    diagnostic tests
        CBC, 468
        CD4 cell count, 468
        enzyme-linked immunosorbent assay
            (ELISA), 467–468
        HIV viral load, 468
        pediatric, 468
        rapid, 467–468
        western blot antibody testing, 467–468
    diversity and culture and, 457
    education, 461, 476t
    etiology, 457
    infants of mothers with, 2208t
    interventions
        effective coping, 477
        ineffective sexuality patterns, 478
        knowledge deficits, 478–479
        medication regime adherence, 476–477
        nutrition, 478
        secondary infection prevention, 476
        skin integrity, 477–478

Kaposi sarcoma and, 464
lifespan considerations, 459–461, 473
lymphomas and, 464
manifestations, 462–467, 465–467t
mycobacterium avium complex (MAC), 463
nonpharmacologic therapy, 472–474
nurses' willingness for care and, 475t
Nursing Care Plan, 479–480t
nursing process, 474–479
opportunistic infections, 463–464
outcome evaluation, 479
overview of, 456
pathophysiology, 457–461
pediatric
    education, 476t
    manifestations, 464–467, 467t
    testing, 468
pharmacologic therapy
    agents used in combination with
        antiretroviral therapy, 472
    antiretroviral nucleoside analogues,
        470–471t
    drug classes, 469
    entry inhibitors, 471
    highly active antiretroviral therapy
        (HAART), 468–469
    nonnucleoside reverse transcriptase
        inhibitors, 471
    nucleoside reverse transcriptase inhibitors
        (NRTIs), 471
    primary foci, 469
    protease inhibitors, 471
    treatment effectiveness, 469
pneumocystis jiroveci pneumonia
    (PCP), 463
postexposure prophylaxis, 461
prevention, 461, 475
risk factors, 457–459
secondary cancers, 464–465
sex practices and, 461
standard precautions, 461
STIs and, 1408, 1409
transmission categories of adults and
    adolescents, 460f
tuberculosis, 463
vertical transmission, 459
HLA (human leukocyte antigen), 510
HLHS (hypoplastic left heart syndrome),
    1093–1094t
HMOs (health maintenance organizations), 2628
Holism, 2284
**Holistic health assessment across the
    life span**
    adolescents, 2293
    children, 2286–2289, 2286f, 2288t, 2289f,
        2289t
    infants, 2290–2291
    middle-aged adults, 2294
    older adults, 2294–2298, 2295–2296t,
        2298t
    overview of, 2286
    preschoolers, 2292
    school-age children, 2292–2293, 2293f
    stages, 2289–2299
    toddlers, 2291–2292, 2292
    young adults, 2293–2294
Hollister cord clamp, 2211, 2211f
Holosystolic, 1086
Holter monitor, 1098t
Holy days, 1884

HOME (Home Observation for Measurement of
    the Environment), 1728
Home care
    advocacy in, 2557t
    for anemia clients, 74t
    bowel incontinence, 317
    for chronic kidney disease (CKD), 401t
    computer-based client records and, 2648
    documentation, 2447
    nurses and injuries and, 2718t
    for premature newborns,
        2259–2260
    for prostate cancer clients, 118t
    pulse monitoring and, 1064t
    pyloric stenosis and, 253t, 254
    urinary incontinence and retention and, 302,
        303t, 304t
Home Observation for Measurement of the
    Environment (HOME), 1728
Homelessness, 1635
Homeostasis
    body fluids, 340, 341f
    body's natural inclination, 966
    defined, 1895
    stress and, 1896–1897
Homicide. See also Assault and homicide
    defined, 1975
    race and, 1979t
    treatment of perpetrators and
        victims, 1980
Homocysteine, 1110
Homocystinuria, 2208t
Homograft (allograft), 1479
Homografts, 2026
Homologous chromosomes, 31
Homophobia, 1636
Hope
    adjustment disorder with depressed
        mood and, 1807
    depression and, 1803
    as spirituality component, 1873
Horizontal violence, 2390
Hormonal agents, 738t, 802t
Hormonal contraceptives
    benefits of, 1384
    combined estrogen-progestin,
        1383–1384
    combined oral contraceptives (COCs),
        1383–1384
    Depo-Provera, 1384–1385
    emergency, 1385–1386
    long-lasting progestin, 1384–1385
    mechanisms of action, 1364t
    mini-pill, 1384
    side effects of, 1383–1384, 1384t
    skin patch, 1384
    vaginal contraceptive ring, 1384
    weight gain and, 1385f
Hormone of pregnancy, 2016
Hormone replacement therapy (HRT),
    1368, 1395–1396
Hormone therapy
    breast cancer, 79–80
    prostate cancer, 116t
Hormones
    defined, 725
    effects on reproductive cycle,
        2015–2017
    of the endocrine system, 726t
    in pregnancy, 2034

Hospice care. *See also* End-of-life care
defined, 177
genetics and, 2573*t*
myths and facts, 178*t*
providing, 177
Hospital-acquired pneumonia (HAP), 982, 2704
Hospitalization, in schizophrenia, 1619–1620
Hospitals
National Patient Safety Goals (NPSG) for, 2701*t*
reducing environmental stimuli in, 150*t*
Hot packs, 889
Hot zone, 2614*t*
HPD (histrionic personality disorder), 1863*t*
HPV (human papillomavirus), 1411–1414, 1411*f*, 1411*t*
HRSD (Hamilton Rating Scale for Depression), 1587*t*
HRT (hormone replacement therapy), 1368, 1395–1396
HSV (herpes simplex virus), 45*t*
HTLV (human T-lymphotropic viruses), 45*t*
Huffing, 1565
Human chorionic gonadotropin (HCG), 1253*t*, 2034
Human cytomegalovirus (HCMV), 45*t*
Human dignity, 2564
Human herpesvirus 6 (HHV-6), 45*t*
Human immunodeficiency virus (HIV). *See also* HIV/AIDS
CD4 cells and, 458*f*
defined, 456
as epidemic, 456
pediatric, 464–467, 467*t*
pregnancy and, 473*t*
screening in prenatal care, 460*t*
staging of infection, 463*t*
viral load tests, 468
Human leukocyte antigen (HLA), 510
Human milk, changes of, 2174
Human papillomavirus (HPV), 1411–1414, 1411*f*, 1411*t*
Human placental lactogen, 2034
Human resources, 2645
Human T-lymphotropic viruses (HTLV), 45*t*
Humanistic learning theory, 2504–2505
Humoral immune response, 509
Hunger, 924, 924*f*
Hyaluronic acid injections, 890*t*
Hydramnios, 2046
Hydration
chronic obstructive pulmonary disease (COPD) and, 1012
in intrapartum assessment, 2143*t*
manifestations, 357–360, 357*t*, 360*t*
in newborns, 2239
pathophysiology and etiology, 354–357
Hydrocele, 1357*t*
Hydrocephalus, 710*t*, 2290
Hydrochloric acid, 4
Hydrocolloid (DuoDERM) dressings, 477
Hydrogen ions, 3–4, 6, 17
Hydronephrosis, 285, 297, 320–321
Hydrostatic pressure, 338*f*, 364
Hydroureter, 285
Hyperacute rejection, 447
Hyperbilirubinemia, 2047

Hypercalcemia, 372
Hypercapnia, 6, 21
Hypercarbia, 956
Hyperchloremia, 372
Hypercyanotic episodes, 1087
Hyperemesis gravidarum, 2081*t*
Hyperemia, 634
Hyperextension, 908
Hyperflexion, 908
Hyperglycemia
defined, 741, 747
DKA and HHS comparison, 745*t*
problems associated with, 746–747
Hyperinflation, 970
Hyperkalemia
active intervention, 382
acute renal failure (ARF) and, 387
defined, 352
serum potassium, 372
Hyperlipidemia, 1109
Hypernatremia, 352, 370
Hyperopia, 1286*t*
Hyperosmolar hyperglycemic state (HHS)
defined, 747
DKA and hypoglycemia comparison, 745*t*
treatment modalities, 747
Hyperoxitest, 1098*t*
Hyperoxygenation, 970
Hyperphosphatemia
acute renal failure (ARF) and, 387
defined, 378
uremia and, 395
Hyperplasia, 32, 284
Hyperresonance, 2280
Hyperresponsiveness, 991
Hypersensitivity. *See also* Immunity
assessment, 492
care planning, 492
client and family care, 494*t*
collaborative care, 488–491
complementary and alternative therapy, 491
cytotoxic, 445
defined, 438, 481
delayed-type, 445
diagnosis, 492
diagnostic tests
laboratory testing, 488–489
skin testing, 489–490
immediate, 445
interventions, 492–494
lifespan considerations, 488
manifestations, 487–488, 488*t*
nonpharmacologic therapy, 491
nursing implementations
cardiac status monitoring, 492–493
community-based care, 494
patent airway maintenance, 492
risk of injury reduction, 493
nursing process, 491–494
pathophysiology and etiology, 481–487
pharmacologic therapy
antihistamines, 490
corticosteroids, 490
epinephrine, 490–491
immunotherapy, 490
leukotriene modifiers, 490
mast cell stabilizers, 490
omalizumab, 491
potential outcomes, 494

reaction types, 481*t*
reactions, 445
risk factors, 486–487
type I (IgE-mediated), 482–483, 482*f*, 483*t*
type II (cytotoxic) hypersensitivity, 483, 484*f*
type III (immune complex-mediated), 483–484, 485*f*
type IV (delayed), 484–485, 486*f*
Hypersomnia, 195, 1799
Hypertension. *See also* Blood pressure
in African Americans, 1167*t*
algorithm for treating, 1169*f*
assessment, 1173
care planning, 1173
chronic, 1205
chronic kidney disease (CKD) and, 393
client teaching, 1174*t*
collaborative care, 1168
complementary and alternative therapy, 1173
compliance and, 1174–1175
coronary artery disease (CAD) and, 1116
as coronary artery disease risk factor, 1109
defined, 1053*t*, 1162
as diabetes complication, 748
diagnosis, 1173
diagnostic tests, 1168
etiology, 1166
fluid volume maintenance and, 1175
gestational, 1205
health maintenance, 1174
interventions, 1053*t*, 1174–1175
kidney transplant and, 399
lifestyle modifications for, 1169–1170, 1169*t*
manifestations, 1053*t*, 1167–1168, 1168*t*
Nursing Care Plan, 1176*t*
nursing process, 1173–1175
nutrition and, 1175
outcome evaluation, 1175
overview of, 1162–1163
pharmacologic therapy
antihypertensive drug action sites, 1170, 1170*f*
drug classes, 1170–1173
drug regimes, 1173
medications, 1171–1172*t*
step-down therapy, 1173
pregnancy and, 1165, 1166
pregnancy-induced, 1204–1210
primary, 1165
risk factors, 1166–1167
secondary, 1165–1166
as stroke risk factor, 1236
Hypertensive disorders, 2081*t*
Hypertensive emergencies
defined, 1166
manifestations of, 1168*t*
Hypertensive encephalopathy, 1167
Hyperthermia
assessment, 1435
care planning, 1435
collaborative care, 1435
community-based care, 1436
defined, 1422, 1431
diagnosis, 1435
ethics differences in parental response to, 1435*t*

interventions, 1435–1436
lifespan and cultural considerations, 1434
malignant, 1426, 1432
manifestations, 1433–1434, 1433t
modifiable risk factors, 1426
nursing process, 1435–1436
outcome evaluation, 1436
overview of, 1431
pathophysiology and etiology,
    1431–1433
prevalence of, 1424
prevention of, 1426–1427, 1433
risk factors, 1432–1433
screenings, 1426
therapies, 1424t
Hyperthermia blanket, 1441
Hyperthermic, 1256t
Hyperthyroidism. *See also* Thyroid
    disease
    antepartum care and, 2078t
    assessment, 810
    body image and, 811
    cardiac input monitoring and, 810
    care planning, 810
    collaborative care, 808–810
    defined, 806
    diagnosis, 810
    diagnostic tests, 808–809
    excess TSH stimulation and, 808
    Graves disease and, 806–808, 806f
    interventions, 810–811
    laboratory findings in, 809t
    manifestations, 806–808, 809t
    multisystem effects of, 807t
    Nursing Care Plan, 811–812t
    nursing process, 810–811
    nutrition and, 811
    outcome evaluation, 811
    pathophysiology and etiology, 806
    pharmacologic therapy, 809
    radioactive iodine therapy, 809
    risk factors, 806
    surgery, 809–810
    thyroid storm and, 808
    thyroiditis and, 808
    toxic multinodular goiter and, 808, 808f
    visual health and, 810–811
Hypertonic dehydration, 355
Hypertonic labor, 2138t
Hypertonic solutions, 337
Hypertrophic cardiomyopathy, 1077t, 1078
Hypertrophic scar, 1470
Hypertrophy, 285, 421
Hyperventilation
    asthma and, 991
    causes of, 25, 26
    defined, 25, 991, 2163
    labor and, 2163–2164
Hypervolemia, 363
Hyphema, 1312
Hypnotics/sedatives, 151t
Hypoactive sexual desire disorder, 1349
Hypocalcemia
    defined, 372, 378
    serum calcium, 372
    uremia and, 395
Hypocalcemic tetany, 737t
Hypocapnia, 6
Hypochloremia, 372
Hypodermis, 1447

Hypodermoclysis, 352
Hypoglycemia
    alcohol and, 772, 772t
    in children with type 1 DM, 772
    hospitalization criteria, 748
    immediate treatment of, 748
    manifestations of, 747
    in newborns, 2210t
Hypoglycemic agents, 756
Hypokalemia
    defined, 352
    metabolic alkalosis and, 17–18
    serum potassium, 372
Hypomania, 1776, 1809
Hyponatremia
    acute renal failure (ARF) and, 387
    defined, 263, 352
    serum sodium, 370–371
Hypoperfusion, 374
Hypophonia, 897
Hypoplastic left heart syndrome (HLHS),
    1093–1094t
Hypotension, 1067–1068, 1759
Hypothalamus, 1423, 1432, 1432f
Hypothermia
    accidental, 1438–1439
    assessment, 1440
    care planning, 1441
    in children, 1441
    collaborative care, 1440
    defined, 1422, 1423, 1437
    diagnosis, 1441
    frostbite, 1439
    induced, 1437–1438
    in infants, 1438–1439, 1438f
    interventions, 1441
    manifestations, 1439, 1440t
    modifiable risk factors, 1426
    in newborns, 1441
    Nursing Care Plan, 1442t
    nursing process, 1440–1441
    in older adults, 1441
    pathophysiology and etiology,
        1437–1438
    physiological mechanisms, 1423
    prevalence of, 1424
    prevention of, 1426–1427, 1441
    risk factors, 1439
    screenings, 1427
    therapies, 1424t
Hypothermic, 1256t
Hypothyroidism. *See also* Thyroid disease
    antepartum care and, 2078t
    assessment, 815
    cardiac output monitoring and, 815
    care planning, 815
    collaborative care, 813
    constipation prevention and, 815
    defined, 728–729, 812
    diagnosis, 815
    diagnostic tests, 813
    fatigue and, 188t
    Hashimoto thyroiditis and,
        812–813
    interventions, 815–816
    iodine deficiency and, 812
    laboratory findings in, 813
    lifespan considerations, 815t
    manifestations, 813, 813t
    multisystem effects of, 814t

    myxedema coma and, 813
    Nursing Care Plan, 816–817t
    nursing process, 815–816
    outcome evaluation, 816
    pathophysiology and etiology,
        812–813
    pharmacologic therapy, 813
    risk factors, 812–813
    skin integrity and, 815–816
    surgery, 813
Hypotonic dehydration, 355
Hypotonic labor, 2138t
Hypotonic solutions, 337
Hypovolemia, 376, 1044
Hypovolemic shock
    assessment, 1230
    as burn shock, 1471
    defined, 1222–1223
    manifestations, 1225t
Hypoxemia
    asthma and, 991
    cyanosis and, 1046
    defined, 6, 596, 957
    infection and, 596
    interventions and therapies, 960t
    manifestations, 960t
    refractory, 975
Hysterectomy
    abdominal, 1402
    defined, 1402
    nursing care, 1403t
    vaginal, 1402

I

IABP (intra-aortic balloon pump),
    1123, 1123f
Iatrogenic, 365
Iatrogenic infections, 531
IBD. *See* Inflammatory bowel disease
Ibuprofen, fever and, 1434, 1434t
ICD (implantable cardioverter-defibrillator)
    and, 1191–1192
ICF (intracellular fluid), 336
ICH (intracranial hemorrhage), 2002
ICN code of ethics, 2568t
ICP (intracranial pressure), 2002
Id, 1649
Ideal body image, 1833
Ideal self, 1832–1833
Identification, 1905t
Idiopathic pain, 156
IEPs (individualized education plans), 768
IgE-mediated (type I) hypersensitivity, 482–483,
    482f, 483t
IICP. *See* Increased intracranial pressure
Ileal pouch-anal anastomosis (IPAA),
    662, 662f
Ileostomy, 662–663
Ileus, 274
Illegal, immoral, or unethical activities of
    professionals, 2561
Illicit drug use, 1522f
Illness
    acute, 408
    behaviors, 408
    chronic, 408, 1731
    defined, 408
    effects on client and family, 408–409
    sensory perception and, 1282

Illness impact on family. *See also* Families
  assessment, 1735–1737
  care planning, 1737
  chronic illness, 1731
  collaborative care, 1735
  diagnosis, 1737
  factors determining, 1731, 1731*t*
  interventions, 1737
  manifestations, 1735, 1736*t*
  outcome evaluation, 1737
  pediatric illness, 1733–1735
  prevention and, 1735
  risk factors, 1735
  severe mental illness, 1731–1733
Illness prevention, 2544
Illness-wellness continuum, 407, 408*f*
Illusions, 1578, 1611
Imagery (guided imagery), 150
Imitation, 2504
Immediate hypersensitivity, 445
Immediate shock, 1219–1220
Immigrants, undocumented, 1636
Immobility
  defined, 1493
  pressure ulcers and, 1493
Immobilizing units, 1264*t*
Immune complex assays, 489
Immune complex reaction, 445
Immune complex-mediated (type III)
      hypersensitivity, 483–484, 485*f*
Immune deficiency statistics, 448
Immune response
  antibody-mediated, 442
  antigens, 441
  cell-mediated, 442, 483
  cellular, 509
  defined, 443
  events, 442*f*
  humoral, 509
  primary, 442
  secondary, 442
Immune system
  activation of, 438
  assessments, 453*t*
  burn injuries and, 1472–1473
  cells and tissues of, 439*t*
  changes and infection, 525
  chronic kidney disease (CKD) and, 393
  components of, 438
  diseases, 448
  effectiveness of, 438
  exercise benefits, 422
  labor and, 2127
  in older adults, 445
  premature newborns and, 2251
  specific defenses, 525
Immunity
  acquired, 440
  active, 450
  alterations, 445–448
  alterations and therapies, 447*t*
  antigens and, 441–443
  assessment, 451–454
  assessment interview, 452
  cell-mediated, 442–443
  changes associated with aging, 444–445
  collaborative interventions and therapies,
      454–455
  complementary and alternative therapy,
      454–455

concepts related to, 446
defined, 438
diagnostic tests, 453
disorders
  age and, 448
  gender and, 448
  HIV/AIDS, 456–481
  hypersensitivity, 481–495
  rheumatoid arthritis, 495–509
  systemic lupus erythematosus,
      509–518
genetic and lifespan considerations,
      444–445
genetic considerations and nonmodifiable
      risk factors, 448
immunizations and, 449–451
independent interventions and therapies, 454
interventions and therapies, 454–455
leukocytes and, 438–441
lymphoid system and, 443–444, 443*f*
medications, 455
modifiable risk factors, 449
nonpharmacologic therapy, 454
nonspecific inflammatory response, 444
normal presentation, 438–445
passive, 450
pediatric considerations, 444–445
pharmacologic therapy, 454
prevalence and, 447–448
prevention and, 449–451
transplacental, see immunizations
Immunization guidelines, 413–414*t*
Immunizations
  antepartum care and, 2072
  in children, 451
  contraindications, 451
  defined, 449–451
  as infection precaution, 551
  parent education and conformed
      consent, 451
  in preconception counseling, 1372
  schedule, 450–451
  vaccines, 450
Immunocomplete, 438
Immunodeficiency, 438
Immunogenicity, 441
Immunoglobulins
  defined, 442
  infants and children, 444
  maturity in childhood, 445*f*
Immunological changes, postpartum, 2176
Immunosuppressant/cytotoxic
      drugs, 503*t*
Immunosuppression, 502
Immunosuppressive therapy, 398–399
Immunotherapy
  for hypersensitivity, 490
  for skin cancer, 135
Impacted fractures, 856*t*
Impaction, fecal, 277*t*, 307, 311, 316, 317*t*
Impaired gas exchange compensation, 1215
Impaired mobility support, 507
Impaired nurses
  resources for, 1562*t*
  substance abuse and, 1561–1562
  warning signs of, 1562*t*
Impaired religiosity, 1887
Imparting information, 2429
Impedance audiometry, 579
Implanon, 1384

Implantable cardioverter-defibrillator (ICD) and,
      1191–1192
Implantation, 2021–2022
Implementation. *See also* Nursing process
  components, 2346–2348
  defined, 2344
  delegation, 2348
  documentation, 2348
  evidence-based practice (EBP), 2593–2594
  intervention implementation, 2347–2348
  method of, 2351–2352
  need for assistance determination, 2347
  nursing interventions and, 2344–2346, 2345*t*,
      2346*t*
  older adults and, 2347*t*
  preassessment, 2347
Implied consent, 2659
Impotence, 1353
Improper use of authority, 2484–2485
Impulse condition, 1278
Impulsiveness, 1852
Inappropriate sexual behaviors, 1363–1365,
      1365*t*
Incentive spirometry, 966
Incident pain, 156
Incident reports, 2678
Incontinence. *See* Fecal incontinence; Urinary
      incontinence
Increased intracranial pressure (IICP). *See also*
      Intracranial regulation
  assessment, 713
  care planning, 714
  clients at risk for, 713*t*
  collaborative care, 711–713
  compliance and, 710
  defined, 694–695, 709
  diagnosis, 713
  diagnostic tests, 711
  ICP monitoring, 712–713, 712*f*, 713*t*
  infection risk factors, 713*t*
  interventions, 714
  lifespan considerations, 710
  manifestations, 710, 711*t*
  mechanical ventilation, 713
  medications, 712
  nonpharmacologic therapy, 712–713
  nursing process, 713–714
  outcome evaluation, 714
  overview of, 709
  pathophysiology and etiology,
      709–710
  in pediatric clients, 710
  pharmacologic therapy, 708, 711
  prevention, 710
  risk factors, 710
  surgery, 711
Incubation period, infection, 528
Indemnity, 2628
Independent interventions, 2345
Indicators, 2686
Indifferent parent, 1717
Indirect auscultation, 2280
Indirect bilirubin, 651*t*
Indirect Coombs test, 489
Indirect transmission of infection, 524
Individual information at point of care
  case management, 2648
  client education, 2649
  client monitoring and computerized diagnostics,
      2648, 2648*f*, 2649*f*

computer-based client records, 2648–2649
overview of, 2647
Individualized education plans (IEPs), 768
Induced hypothermia, 1437–1438
Inductive reasoning, 2319
Infant massage, 2259
Infantile idiopathic scoliosis, 847
Infants
acid-base imbalances in, 10
airway, 589f, 956, 957f
assessment of, 2290–2291
Back to Sleep campaign and, 1027t
blood pressure assessment in, 1067t
body temperature in, 1428t
bowel elimination in, 274–275
cognitive development of, 1659–1660
comfort and, 142, 149
communication, 1662
congenital heart defects in. See congenital
heart defects
digestive system in, 209
face position, 1651f
family with, 1726
fluid volume deficit in, 356, 356f
fluids and electrolytes and, 343–344, 343f,
344f, 344t
GERD in, 228t, 229t
growth and development, 1659–1662
growth and development milestones, 1660t
health promotion in, 412t
health screenings and immunization guidelines
for, 413t
hypothermia in, 1438–1439, 1438f
infection in, 553f
injury prevention due to motor vehicle
crashes, 2000t
of mothers with diabetes, 2207t
of mothers with HIV/AIDS, 2208t
neurological system assessment in, 707t
normal sleep-rest patterns in, 432
nutrition for, 932, 932f
oral health in, 427, 427t
pain
misperceptions, 159t
perception and behavior, 158t
personality and temperament of, 1662
physical growth and development of, 1659
play, 1661
with prenatal substance exposure, 2208t
prone placement of, 1024
psychosocial development of, 1661–1662,
1661t
pulse assessment in, 1065t
pyloric stenosis in, 252–255
respiratory system in, 965t
retractions in suprasternal area, 590f
risk for injury, 2710
sensory function of, 1291t
separation anxiety disorder (SAD) in,
1922t
sexual development of, 1341t
sleep positioning of, 1027t
stool samples of, 2201f
suctioning, 970t
sudden infant death syndrome (SIDS)
and, 1024–1028
supine placement of, 1024
taken from parents after birth, 1818
thermoregulation in, 1423
urinary elimination in, 262

urinary tract infections (UTIs) in, 625t
women who relinquish, 2188–2190
Infarct extension, 1113
Infection
acute, 523
alterations, 527–544
alterations and therapies, 542–543t
antimicrobial agents, 558–559t
assessment, 552–557, 554–555t
assessment interview, 552t
biological threat, 532
cancer and, 46, 48
carrier state, 529
catheter-related bloodstream (CRBI), 2704
central line-associated bloodstream
(CLABSI), 2706
chain of
etiological agent, 523
illustrated, 523f
interventions that break, 526t
method of transmission, 524
portal of entry to susceptible host, 525
portal of exit from reservoir, 524
reservoir, 524
susceptible host, 525
in children, 553f
chronic, 523
Clostridium difficile-associated
(CDI), 2706
collaborative interventions and
therapies, 558
concepts related to, 529t
convalescent stage, 529
culture and, 555
defined, 438, 521
diagnostic tests, 555–557
genetic and lifespan considerations,
525–527
genetic considerations and nonmodifiable
risk factors, 543
healthcare-associated (HAI), 530–531,
2704–2706
iatrogenic, 531
incubation period, 528
independent interventions and therapies, 557
in infants, 553f
interventions and therapies, 557–558
intraoperative nursing and, 1267–1268
lifespan and cultural considerations,
552–555
local, 523
manifestations
antibiotic-resistant bacteria, 531–532
biological threat, 532
complications of infectious diseases, 530
healthcare-associated, 530–531
pediatric, 532, 533–543t
microorganisms causing, 523
newborns and, 444
normal presentation, 522–527
opportunistic, 438, 463–464
pathogens and, 527–528
pediatric, 532, 533–542t
physiology review, 525
precautions
client transportation, 548
disinfecting and sterilizing, 554–555
disposal of soiled equipment/supplies, 548
isolated client psychosocial needs and,
548–549

isolation, 545–546, 547t
isolation practices, 546
personal protective equipment, 546
in pregnant women, 552
prevalence of, 543
prevention practices
antiseptics and disinfectants, 554, 554t
client precautions, 551
healthcare worker infection control, 551
healthcare worker precautions,
544–549
HIAs, 549
infection control nurse, 551
influenza and, 574–575
sterile technique, 549
process stages, 528–529
prodromal stage, 528–529
risks, 527
safety and, 2698t
surgical site (SSI), 2704
systemic, 523
tissue integrity and, 1453t
transmission of, 524
types of, 523
wounds and, 1508–1509
Infection control
cellulitis and, 562t
for healthcare workers, 551
nurse, role of, 551
Infection prevention
appendicitis and, 647
breast cancer and, 82
burns and, 1484
chronic kidney disease (CKD) and,
400–401
diabetes and, 750
fatigue and, 188t
fractures and, 859, 867
gallbladder disease and, 654
hand hygiene and, 2702t
HIV/AIDS and, 476
leukemia and, 101
motor vehicle crashes (MVC) and, 2004
nephritis and, 674
premature newborns and, 2257–2258
pressure ulcers and, 1504
pyloric stenosis and, 253
sickle cell disease and, 125
skin cancer and, 136
spinal cord injuries (SCI) and, 914
systemic lupus erythematosus and, 516
tuberculosis and, 616
urinary calculi and, 321
wound healing and, 1512
Infectious conditions, nationally notifiable,
2675t
Infectious disease
in children
diphtheria, 533t
erythema infectiosum (fifth disease), 533t
Haemophilus influenzae, 534t
influenza, 534t
measles, 535t
meningococcus, 535–536t
mononucleosis, 536t
mumps, 537t
pertussis (whooping cough), 537–538t
pneumococcal infection, 538t
poliomyelitis, 539t
roseola, 539t

Infectious disease (*continued*)
  rotavirus, 540*t*
  rubella (German measles), 540*t*
  streptococcus A, 541*t*
  targeted objectives, 532
  tetanus, 541–542*t*
complications of, 530
defined, 522
Infertility. *See also* Family planning
  causes of, 1373*t*
  components of, 1373*t*
  counseling, 1372–1373
  culture and, 1392*t*
  defined, 1372
  drugs used to treat, 1387, 1387*t*
  secondary, 1372
  sexual and reproductive health and, 1392
  sexual function and, 1392
  subfertility, 1372
Inflammation
  acute, steps in, 635*f*
  alterations, 636–640
  alterations and therapies, 639*t*
  anaphylaxis and, 636, 636*t*
  assessment for, 640–642
  assessment interview, 641*t*
  in children, 636, 641
  collaborative interventions and therapies, 643
  concepts related to, 637–638
  defined, 444, 633
  diagnostic tests, 641
  exudate production, 634
  genetic and lifespan considerations, 636
  genetic considerations and nonmodifiable risk
    factors, 637–640
  independent interventions and therapies,
    642–643
  interventions and therapies, 642–643
  lifespan and cultural considerations, 641
  local and systemic manifestations of, 640*t*
  manifestations, 637, 640*t*
  mediators of, 635–636, 635*t*
  medications, 643*t*
  modifiable risk factors, 640
  normal presentation, 634–636
  in older adults, 641
  pediatric, 636
  pharmacologic therapy, 643
  prevalence of, 637
  prevention of, 640
  regeneration and, 634–635
  reparative phase, 634–635
  screening for, 640
  in specific conditions
    burn wound healing, 1469–1470
    cellulitis, 560
    cystitis, 626
    rheumatoid arthritis, 640
  stages of, 634–635, 635*f*
  surgery, 643
  tissue integrity and, 1453*t*
  vascular and cellular responses, 634
  white blood cell (WBC) count and, 642*t*
Inflammatory bowel disease (IBD)
  adolescents with, 666
  assessment, 665
  care planning, 665
  in children, 641
  children with, 666, 666*t*, 667*t*
  collaborative care, 661–663

complementary and alternative therapy, 663
Crohn disease
  aphthoid lesion, 658
  characteristics of, 657*t*
  defined, 657
  enterocutaneous fistulas, 658
  enteroenteric fistulas, 658
  enterovesical fistulas, 658
  manifestations, 660–661
  progression of, 658*f*
crypts, 658*f*
defined, 657
diagnosis, 665
diagnostic tests, 662
etiology, 660
home care, 667*t*
interventions
  body image, 666–667
  fluid volume monitoring, 665–666
  nutritional intake, 667–668, 667*t*
lifespan and cultural considerations, 661
manifestations, 661*t*
medications, 664–665*t*
multisystem effects of, 659*f*
nonpharmacologic therapy, 663
Nursing Care Plan, 668*t*
nursing process, 665–668
outcome evaluation, 667
overview of, 657
pathophysiology, 657–660
pediatric, 661, 666*t*
pharmacologic therapy, 663
prevention of, 660
risk factors, 660
surgery
  colectomy, 662
  continent ileostomy, 663
  ileostomy, 662
  indication for, 662
  ostomy, 662–663
ulcerative colitis
  characteristics of, 657*t*
  defined, 657
  manifestations, 660
  Nursing Care Plan, 668*t*
Inflammatory markers, 641
Inflammatory phase
  fractures, 853–857
  wound healing, 1508
Inflammatory response, nonspecific, 444
Influenza
  airway patency and, 574
  assessment, 573–574
  avian, 570
  care planning, 574
  in children, 534*t*
  collaborative care, 572
  defined, 570
  diagnosis, 574
  diagnostic tests, 572
  as epidemic, 570
  evaluation, 575
  H1N1, 570
  infection and, 574–575
  interventions, 574–575
  manifestations, 572, 573*t*
  nonpharmacologic therapy, 572
  nursing process, 573–575
  overview of, 570
  as pandemic, 570, 570*t*

pathophysiology and etiology, 571–572
pharmacologic therapy, 572
prevention, 571–572
risk factors, 571
sleep hygiene and, 574
ventilation and, 574
Informal groups, 2419, 2420*t*
Informal leaders, 2489
Informatics
  biomedical, 2631
  client education and e-health, 2641–2642
  computerized medical records, 2637–2640
  concept of, 2631
  concepts related to, 2633–2634
  ergonomic considerations, 2642–2644
  geographic information systems (GIS), 2641
  health policy and, 2632
  healthcare information systems, 2634–2636
  nursing, 2632
  as QSEN competency, 2699, 2700
  quality improvement and, 2682*t*
  service delivery and, 2632–2634
  telehealth, 2640–2641
Information processing theory, 1577
Informative confrontation, 2432
Informed consent. *See also* Legal issues
  child participation and, 2661
  competency for, 2659–2661
  defined, 2587, 2659
  in emergencies, 2661
  in evidence-based practice, 2587
  information provided to client, 2659
  minor consent laws, 2661, 2662*t*
Infrared thermometers, 1427*f*
Inhalants, 1564–1565, 1567*t*
Inheritance
  autosomal dominant, 1376, 1376*f*
  autosomal recessive, 1376–1377, 1377*f*
  carriers and, 1376
  causes of, 1376
  genotype and, 1376
  Mendelian (single-gene), 1376
  modes of, 1376–1378
  multifactorial, 1377–1378
  non-Mendelian (multifactorial), 1376
  phenotype and, 1376
  X-linked dominant, 1377
  X-linked recessive, 1377, 1377*f*
Initial prenatal assessment
  abdomen, 2058–2059*t*
  anus and rectum, 2060*t*
  breasts, 2058*t*
  chest and lungs, 2057–2058*t*
  cultural assessment, 2062–2063*t*
  economic status, 2063*t*
  educational needs, 2063*t*
  extremities, 2059*t*
  family functioning, 2063*t*
  heart, 2058*t*
  laboratory evaluation, 2061–2062*t*
  mouth, 2057*t*
  neck, 2057*t*
  nose, 2057*t*
  pelvic area, 2060*t*
  pelvic measurements, 2060*t*
  psychological status, 2063*t*
  reflexes, 2059*t*
  skin, 2056*t*
  spine, 2059*t*
  stability and living conditions, 2063*t*

support system, 2063*t*
vital signs, 2056*t*
weight, 2056*t*
Initiation of respiration
changes necessary for, 2191
clearing fluid from lungs, 2192–2193
factors opposing, 2193
process, 2191–2193
process illustration, 2192*f*
Initiation phase, acute renal failure (ARF), 378
Injury prevention
Alzheimer disease (AD) and, 1601–1602
autism spectrum disorder (ASD)
and, 1693
cataracts and, 1309
cerebral palsy (CP) and, 1698
feeding and eating disorders and, 1851
glaucoma and, 1324
herniated disc and, 845
hypersensitivity and, 493
metabolic acidosis and, 16
mobility and, 836–837
in nursing practice, 2717–2718,
2718*t*
osteoporosis and, 803
Parkinson disease and, 904
peripheral neuropathy and, 1335
respiratory acidosis and, 23
schizophrenia and, 1623
Inotropes, 1228*t*
Inotropic drugs, 1963*t*
Inquiry, 2318
Insensible fluid loss, 340
Insomnia
acute and chronic, 195
defined, 145, 195
depression and, 1799
manifestations, 200*t*
sleep restriction and, 199*t*
therapies, 200*t*
Inspection, 2278
Inspiration, 953
Instrumental Activities of Daily Living (ADLs),
2295*t*
Insubordination, 2492
Insulin
administration of, 754, 754*t*
in children, 769–771, 771*t*
defined, 704, 726
endogenous, 742
exogenous, 742
injection
diabetes management with, 755*t*
painful, techniques for minimizing, 756*t*
products, 756
sites of, 756*f*
intravenous infusions, 755
as metabolic and endocrine disorder
medication, 738*t*
preparations, 754*t*
reaction, 747
refrigerated, 756
resistance, 1167
unmodified crystalline, 753
Insulin glargine (Lantus), 753–754
Insulin pumps, 754, 771*t*
Insulin-dependent diabetes mellitus. *See* Diabetes
mellitus
Intact skin, 1448
Integrity, 2483, 2564

Integumentary assessment
edema, 1458*t*
general, 1457*t*
hair distribution and quality, 1458*t*
hair texture, 1459*t*
nail, 1459–1460*t*
scalp, 1459*t*
skin temperature, 1457*t*
skin texture, 1458*t*
skin turgor, 1458*t*
skin with impaired integrity, 1457*t*
Integumentary system
burn injuries and, 1472, 1472*f*
defined, 1445
disseminated intravascular coagulation (DIC)
and, 1141*t*
Intellect, 2317–2318
Intellectual disability. *See also* Cognition
adaptive behaviors, 1581
alterations and manifestations, 1581–1582
alterations and therapies, 1586*t*
defined, 1581
as developmental disability, 1581
Down syndrome, 1581, 1582*t*
fetal alcohol syndrome, 1581–1582, 1582*t*
fragile X syndrome, 1581, 1582*t*
genetic considerations and nonmodifiable risk
factors, 1583
intellectual functioning, 1581
physical traits associated with, 1582*t*
prevalence of, 1583
prevention of, 1583
Intellectual functioning, 1581
Intellectualization, 1905*t*
Intensity, 2281
Intensity, contractions, 2118
Intentional trauma, 1448–1449
Interdisciplinary assessment, 2685
Interdisciplinary teams
collaboration process, 2392–2393
combining expertise with, 2391–2392
defined, 2391
examples outside hospital setting, 2392*t*
future of, 2393–2394
individual strength barriers and, 2393*t*
overview of, 2391
Interferon alpha, 237*t*
Intergroup conflicts, 2387
Intermittent claudication, 1199
Intermittent fever, 1431
Internal clients, 2690
Internal environment, 1898
Internal eye assessment, 1289–1290*t*
Internal locus of control, 415, 1940
Internal rotation, fetus, 2125
Internal stressors, 1898
International healthcare financing
perspective, 2463
Internet
feeding and eating disorders and, 1847*t*
health information and, 2508
older adults and, 2508
Interorganizational conflicts, 2387
Interpersonal attitudes, 2409
Interpersonal conflicts, 1834, 2387
Interpersonal factors, suicide, 1991
Interpersonal rape, 1984
Interpersonal relationships, suicide and, 1993
Interpersonal skills, 2348
Interpersonal violence, 1954–1955

Interpreters, 1251, 1643
Interpretive confirmation, 2432
Interprofessional teams, 2391
Interrogating, 2433
Interrole conflict, 1834
Intersex, 1345, 1634
Interstitial fluid volume excess. *See* Edema
Interventions
advocacy, 2561
defined, 1529
family, 1529
Interviews
body, 2275
closing, 2275–2276
defined, 2272
directive, 2272
distance, 2272
language, 2273–2274
nondirective, 2272
opening, 2275
place, 2272
planning, 2272–2274
questions, 2274–2275, 2274*t*
rapport, 2272
seating arrangement of, 2272
setting of, 2272–2274
stages of, 2275–2276
time, 2272
Intimacy
defined, 1343
lack of, 1351
Intimate distance, 2407
Intimate partner violence
defined, 1966
manifestations of, 1969, 1973*t*
therapies, 1973*t*
Intimidation, 2485
Intra-aortic balloon pump (IABP),
1123, 1123*f*
Intra-arterial pressure monitoring, 1152
Intracapsular hip fractures, 869
Intracellular fluid (ICF), 336
Intracranial hemorrhage (ICH), 2002
Intracranial hypertension. *See* Increased
intracranial pressure (IICP)
Intracranial pressure (ICP), 2002
Intracranial pressure (ICP) monitoring
in IICP, 712–713
risk factors for infection, 713*t*
types of, 712, 712*f*
Intracranial regulation
alterations, 690–696
alterations and therapies, 695*f*
alterations in level of consciousness (LOC) and,
692–694
assessment, 696–706, 706*t*
assessment interview, 697*t*
Brudzinski sign assessment, 705*f*, 705*t*
in children, 707*t*
collaborative interventions and therapies, 708
concepts related to, 692*t*
concussions and, 696*t*
cranial nerves and, 689, 689*t*, 699–701*t*, 706*t*
defined, 687
diagnostic tests, 705–706
fluid management and, 708
genetic and lifespan considerations,
689–690
Glasgow coma scale, 697*t*
graphesthesia testing, 702*f*, 702*t*

Intracranial regulation (*continued*)
heal-to-shin test, 704*f*, 704*t*
independent interventions and therapies, 707–708
in infants, 707*t*
interventions and therapies, 706–708
Kernig sign assessment, 705*f*, 705*t*
lifespan considerations, 707*t*
neurological assessment, 698–705*t*
in newborns, 690
normal, 688–690
nutrition and, 708
in older adults, 690, 707*t*
pharmacologic therapy, 708
prevalence of alterations, 696
prevention and, 696
prognosis for alterations, 694
two-point discrimination testing, 702*f*, 702*t*
Intractable seizures, 719
Intradermal test, 489
Intradisciplinary assessment, 2685
Intradisciplinary teams, 2391
Intragenerational family, 1711
Intranets, 2636*t*
Intraocular pressure, 1318
Intraoperative documentation, 1267, 1269*t*
Intraoperative nursing
anesthesia, 1266–1267, 1266*t*
blood transfusions and, 1270
code blue and, 1270
continuous surveillance, 1262
defined, 1249
diagnoses, 1261
infection and, 1267–1268
potential complications, 1268–1270, 1271*t*
safety precautions, 1262, 1263–1264*t*
sterile field and hand washing, 1262
during surgery, 1262–1271
surgical positioning, 1262, 1264–1265*t*
surgical safety checklist, 1267, 1269*f*
surgical site preparation, 1267
wound classifications, 1268, 1270*t*
Intrapartum, 2051*t*
Intrapartum care
admission
initial greeting, 2158
labor expectations and, 2157*t*, 2158–2159
nursing care and, 2158–2159
process, 2159
report, 2159
alterations
abruptio placentae, 2137*t*
amniotic fluid embolism, 2139*t*
cephalopelvic disproportion (CPD), 2139*t*
cervical ripening, 2128–2129, 2128*t*
Cesarean birth, 2131–2135
episiotomy, 2131
fetal macrosomia, 2138*t*
fetal malposition, 2138*t*
forceps-assisted birth, 2130
high-risk factors, 2136
hypertonic labor, 2138*t*
hypotonic labor, 2138*t*
labor induction, 2129–2130
lacerations, 2139*t*
nonreassuring fetal status, 2138*t*
perinatal loss, 2139*t*
placenta accreta, 2139*t*
placenta previa, 2137*t*
postterm labor, 2138*t*

precipitous birth, 2137*t*
premature rupture of membranes (PROM), 2137*t*
preterm (premature) labor, 2137*t*
prolapsed umbilical cord, 2138*t*
retained placenta, 2139*t*
therapies and, 2137–2139*t*
vacuum extraction, 2130–2131
vaginal birth after Cesarean (VBAC), 2135–2136, 2136*t*
assisting during birth, 2165–2166
care planning, 2156
cervical assessment, 2142
childbirth customs and, 2158*t*
contraction assessment, 2141–2142
diagnosis, 2156
electronic fetal monitoring
accelerations, 2152
arrhythmias and dysrhythmias, 2151
baseline fetal heart rate, 2149–2151, 2150*f*
decelerations, 2152–2153, 2153*f*
defined, 2148
evaluations of FHR tracings, 2153–2156, 2155*t*
by external technique, 2149*f*
indications, 2148
methods of preventing, 2148–2149
responses to, 2156
variability, 2151–2152, 2151*f*
family-centered care, 2113
fetal assessment
cord blood analysis, 2156
heart rate, 2148–2156
position, 2142–2148
fetal position
assessment of, 2142–2148
auscultation of fetal heart rate, 2147–2148
inspection, 2142
palpation: Leopold maneuvers, 2142
vaginal examination and ultrasound, 2147
fetal response to labor and, 2127–2128
first stage
active phase, 2160
doula role, 2164
latent phase, 2160
nursing care, 2160–2164
transition phase, 2160–2161
first stage assessment
anxiety, 2147*t*
cultural assessment, 2145–2146*t*
edema, 2143t
fetal status, 2145*t*
fundus, 2143t
hydration, 2143t
labor status, 2144–2145*t*
lungs, 2143t
perineum, 2144*t*
preparation for childbirth, 2146*t*
psychosocial assessment, 2146–2147*t*
response to labor, 2146–2147*t*
sounds during labor, 2147*t*
support system, 2147*t*
vital signs, 2143t
weight, 2143t
fourth stage, nursing care, 2166
high-risk screening, 2140–2141
interventions
on admission, 2158–2159
cultural belief integration, 2156–2157
first stage of labor, 2160–2164

fourth stage of labor, 2166–2168
second stage of labor, 2164–2166
third stage of labor, 2166
labor and birth factors, 2113–2119, 2113*t*
maternal adaptations following birth, 2167*t*
maternal assessment, 2136–2140
maternal systemic response to labor and, 2126–2127
Nursing Care Plan, 2168*t*
nursing process, 2136–2170
outcome evaluation, 2170
overview of, 2113
passive descent versus active pushing, 2165*t*
physical and psychosociocultural assessment, 2141
physiology of labor, 2119–2122
placental delivery, 2166
promotion of comfort
anxiety, 2162
breathing techniques, 2163–2164
client teaching, 2162–2163
general comfort, 2161–2162
supportive relaxation techniques, 2163
psychosocial considerations, 2118–2119
risk factors, 2141*t*
second stage, nursing care, 2164–2166
stages of labor and birth and, 2122–2126
third stage, nursing care, 2166
Intrapersonal conflicts, 2387
Intrapersonal factors
depression theory, 1781
personality disorders (PD), 1853
rape, 1984
Intrauterine contraception (IUC), 1382–1383, 1382*f*
Intrauterine fetal death (IUFD), 1768
Intrauterine growth chart, 2205, 2205*f*
Intrauterine growth restriction (IUGR), 2207*t*
Intravenous fluids
in children, 362
commonly administered, 361*t*
rehydration with, 361–362
Intravenous pyelography (IVP), 623
Intraventricular conduction blocks, 1186
Intraventricular hemorrhage, 2254
Intrinsic (intrarenal) ARF, 376
Introjection, 1905*t*
Introspection, 1834–1835
Intubation
acid-base imbalances, 12
defined, 1249
in neonates, 988*t*
Intuition, 2320, 2324
Invasion, tumor, 43
Invasion of privacy, 2657
Involuntary euthanasia, 176
Involution, 2171–2172, 2171*f*
Iodine deficiency, 812
Ions, 336
Iridotomy, 1321
Iron
absorption of, 926
for anemia, 70
dietary sources of, 71*t*
function in the body, 931
Iron storage, 2196–2197
Iron-deficiency anemia, 66, 66*f*, 2044

Irreversible coma, 697t
Irreversible shock, 1220
Irritant contact dermatitis, 1488, 1489t
Ischemia
  acute renal failure (ARF) and, 374
  asymptomatic, 1107
  causes of, 1106, 1107t
  defined, 374, 603, 1106
Ischemic, 1041
Ischemic phase, 2019
Ischemic stroke, 1131, 1235–1236
Islam, 1885, 1886t
Isoelectric line, 1071t
Isokinetic exercises, 421
Isolation, as sensory perception risk
    factor, 1283
Isolation precautions
  body substation isolation (BSI), 545
  category-specific, 545
  CDC (HICPAC), 545–546
  contact, 546
  defined, 545
  droplet, 546
  practices, 546
  recommended in hospitals, 547t
  universal, 545
Isometric exercises, 421, 837
Isoniazid, 612t
Isotonic dehydration, 355
Isotonic exercises, 421
Isotonic fluid volume deficit, 355
Isotonic imbalances, 354
Isotonic solutions, 337
IUC (intrauterine contraception),
    1382–1383, 1382f
IUFD (intrauterine fetal death), 1768
IUGR (intrauterine growth restriction),
    2207t
IVF (vitro fertilization), 1389, 1389f
IVP (intravenous pyelography), 623

J

Jackknife position, 1264t
Jarisch-Herxheimer reaction, 1414
Jatene procedure, 1099t
Jaundice
  breast milk, 2199
  breastfeeding, 2199
  defined, 2223
  hepatitis and, 232, 232f
  illustrated, 232f
  in newborn skin assessment, 2223
  physiological, 2198–2199
Jehovah's Witnesses, 1886, 1886t
Jehovah's Witnesses, blood transfusions
    and, 399t
Jewish cultures, pain response and, 161t
JIA (juvenile idiopathic arthritis),
    499–500
Joint Commission
  defined, 2625
  mission, 2625
  on pain, 145
  pain management standards, 159t
  Speak Up program, 2578, 2579t
Joint custody, 1711
Joint fusion, 888
Joint irrigation, 888
Joint resurfacing, 888

Joints
  assessment, 830t
  changes associated with osteoarthritis, 886f
  defined, 820
  effusion, 826
  range of motion, 821
Judaism, 1885, 1886t
JumpSTART algorithm, 2612, 2613f
Junctional dysrhythmias, 1184
Junctional escape rhythm, 1181t
Just culture
  blame-free environment and, 2689
  defined, 2672, 2689
  employer discrimination and, 2673
  as new process, 2672
  overview of, 2672
  whistleblowing and, 2672–2673
Justice, 1880, 2567
Juvenile idiopathic arthritis (JIA), 499–500
Juvenile idiopathic scoliosis, 847
Juvenile osteoarthritis, 887
Juvenile Parkinson disease, 897
Juvenile primary fibromyalgia syndrome
    (JPFS), 191
Juvenile-onset diabetes. See Diabetes mellitus

K

Kangaroo care, 2258, 2258f, 2259
Kaposi sarcoma, 464
Karyotype, 1374, 1374f
Katz's ADL Scale, 2295t
Kayser-Jones Brief Oral Health Status
    Examination (BOHSE), 2295t
KEEPS (Kronos Early Estrogen Prevention
    Study), 1396
Kegel exercises, 295, 295t, 2071, 2071f
Keloid, 1470, 1508
Keratin, 1446
Keratinocytes, 1446, 1447
Keratotic basal cell carcinoma, 130
Kernig sign assessment, 705f, 705t
Ketoacidosis, 2046
Ketogenic diet, 720, 721
Ketones, 732
Ketosis, 741
Kidney biopsy
  in acute renal failure, 395
  in nephritis, 672
  in systemic lupus erythematosus (SLE), 514
Kidney scan, 672
Kidney stones. See Urinary calculi
Kidney transplant
  defined, 397–398
  donors, 398
  hypertension and, 399
  placement, 398f
Kidneys
  assessment, 324–329t
  donor, 398
  in homeostasis, 340
  palpating, 328
Kilocalorie, 929
Kindling, 1561
Kinesthesia, 702t, 1295t
Kinesthetic stimuli, 1278
Knees
  mobility assessment, 833t
  osteoarthritis of, 888, 893
  replacement of, 888, 889f

Knowing
  aesthetic, 2306
  empirical, 2305
  ethical, 2306
  four ways of, 2305f
  personal, 2306
Knowledge
  in assessment interpretation, 2283
  body of, 2536
  deficient, as etiology, 2515–2516
  as professional behavior, 2482
Knowledge, skills, and attitudes (KSAs),
    2699, 2700
Kohlberg stages of moral development,
    1657, 1658t
Korotkoff sounds, 1066, 1066f, 1067t
Korsakoff psychosis, 1525t, 1536
Kosher food, 1876
Kronos Early Estrogen Prevention Study
    (KEEPS), 1396
KSAs (knowledge, skills, and attitudes),
    2699, 2700
Kübler-Ross and five stages of grief, 1743
Kussmaul's respirations, 15
Kwashiorkor, 930, 930t
Kyphosis, 820, 821, 822t

L

Labor. See also Intrapartum care
  acid-base status and, 2127
  acupressure during, 2161t
  bearing down, 2118
  blood pressure and, 2126
  cardiovascular system and, 2126
  characteristics of, 2122t
  comfort
    anxiety, 2162
    breathing techniques, 2163–2164
    client teaching, 2162–2163
    general, 2161–2162
    promotion of, 2161–2165
    relaxation techniques, 2163
  contractions, 2118, 2118f
  critical factors in, 2113
  effacement, 2119, 2120f
  expectations during, 2157t
  fetal heart rate and, 2127
  fetal response to, 2127–2128
  fetal sensation and, 2128
  first stage
    active phase, 2123, 2160
    assessment, 2143–2147t
    latent phase, 2122, 2160
    nursing assessments in, 2140t
    nursing care during, 2160–2164
    transition phase, 2123, 2160–2161
  fourth stage, 2126, 2166–2168
  gastrointestinal system and, 2127
  hemodynamic changes and, 2127–2128
  hypertonic, 2138t
  hypotonic, 2138t
  immune system, 2127
  maternal systemic response to,
      2126–2127
  mechanisms of, 2125f
  musculature changes in pelvic floor,
      2119–2120
  myometrial activity, 2119–2120
  pain and, 2127

Labor (*continued*)
physiological forces of, 2118
physiology of, 2119–2122
possible causes of onset, 2119
postterm, 2138*t*
premonitory signs
bloody show, 2121
Braxton Hicks contractions, 2121
cervical changes, 2121
lightening, 2120–2121
rupture of membranes, 2121
sudden burst of energy, 2121, 2121*t*
preterm (premature), 2137*t*
psychosocial considerations, 2118–2119
renal system and, 2126
respiratory system and, 2126
response to, 2146–2147*t*
second stage
beginning of, 2123
nursing care, 2164–2165
positional changes of fetus, 2125
promotion of comfort, 2164–2165
spontaneous birth, 2124
sounds during, 2147*t*
stages of, 2122–2126
status, 2144–2145*t*
third stage
placental delivery, 2126, 2166
placental separation, 2125–2126
true and false differences, 2121–2122,
2122*t*
Labor induction, 2129–2130
Laboratory specimens, handling of, 548
Laboratory tests
hypersensitivity, 488–489
metabolic alkalosis, 18
Labyrinthitis, 576
Lacerations, 2139*t*
Lactase deficiency. *See also* Malabsorption
disorders
in antepartum care, 2097
collaborative care, 243–244
defined, 243, 2097
diagnostic tests, 243
manifestations, 243
nursing care, 244
nutrition management, 244
pathophysiology and etiology, 243
pharmacologic therapy, 243–244
risk factors, 243
Lactation. *See also* Breastfeeding
daily food plan, 2093*t*
suppression, 2185
Lactic acid, 4
Lactogenesis, 2173–2174
Lacto-ovo-vegetarians, 926, 2095
Lactose intolerance, 243, 2097
Lacto-vegetarian, 926
Lactovegetarians, 2095
Laënnec cirrhosis. *See* Alcoholic cirrhosis
Laissez-faire leaders, 2490
Lambdoidal suture, 2114
Laminectomy, 843
Laminotomy, 843
Language
as cultural competency area, 1642–1643
deficits, 2413
of family pain, 1732*t*
in interview, 2273–2274
uniform, 2639, 2644

Lanugo, 1846, 1850, 2212–2213, 2216
Laparoscopic cholecystectomy, 652, 653*t*
Laparoscopic fundoplication, 229
Laparoscopy, 1402, 1402*f*
Laparotomy, 652
Large for gestational age (LGA), 2207*t*
LAS (local adaptation syndrome), 1900
Lasater's clinical judgment rubric, 2325–2327,
2327*f*
LASER (light amplification by stimulated
emission of electromagnetic radiation),
1263*t*
Laser photocoagulation, 88
Late deceleration, 2152, 2153*f*, 2154*t*
Latent syphilis, 1414
Lateral position, 1265*t*
Latex allergy
hospital and home environment and, 487*t*
protection measures, 486*t*
sensitivity, 484
statistics, 484–485
Latex precautions, 2717
Law
civil, 2655
criminal, 2654–2655
defined, 2654
Laws
administrative, 2654
affecting nursing practice, 2659–2662
categories of, 2654*t*
sources of, 2654, 2655*f*
statutory, 2654
Laxatives
bowel elimination and, 274
for constipation, 308, 309*t*
herbal, 311*t*
Leaders
autocratic (authoritarian), 2489
bureaucratic, 2490
charismatic, 2490
defined, 2474, 2489
democratic (participative, consultative),
2489–2490
formal, 2489
informal, 2489
laissez-faire, 2490
in management, 2474
situational, 2490
transactional, 2490
transformational, 2490
Leadership interventions, 2537*t*
Leadership principles
classic theories, 2489–2490
contemporary theories, 2490–2491
overview of, 2489
theories, 2489–2491
Leading questions, 2275
Leads, 1071*t*, 1072*f*
Lean Six Sigma, 2692
LEARN model, 1640–1641
Learners, nurses as, 2500
Learning. *See also* Teaching and learning
active involvement and, 2505–2506
aspects of, 2501–2508
attributes of, 2500*t*
barriers to, 2506–2507, 2507*t*
content discovery, 2519
culture and, 2507
defined, 2499
emotions and, 2506–2507

environment, 2506
evaluation, 2523
experiences, organizing, 2517–2518
facilitation factors, 2505–2506
factors affecting, 2505–2507
feedback and, 2506
motivation for, 2505
needs and characteristics, 2501, 2511*t*
nonjudgmental support and, 2506
observational, 2504
outcomes, 2517, 2517*t*
physiological events and, 2507
psychomotor ability and, 2507
readiness for, 2505, 2513
relevance and, 2506
repetition and, 2506
styles, 2513
theories
adult learning theory, 2502
behaviorist theory, 2502
categorization, 2505
cognitive theory, 2503, 2503*t*
constructivism, 2505
humanistic learning theory, 2504–2505
multiple intelligence, 2505
social learning theory, 2504, 2504*t*
timing and relevance, 2506
Learning disabilities
alterations and manifestations, 1578
alterations and therapies, 1586*t*
common, 1578*t*
defined, 1578
genetic considerations and nonmodifiable
risk factors, 1580
prevalence of, 1580
prevention of, 1580–1581
Learning theory, 1781
Lea's shield, 1382
Left-sided failure. *See also* Heart failure
hemodynamic effects of, 1147*f*
manifestations, 1148
right-sided failure versus, 1147
Legal issues
affecting nursing practice, 2659–2662
concept of, 2653–2654
concepts related to, 2660*t*
conclusion, 2662
Controlled Substances Act (CSA), 2661–2662,
2662*t*
criminal and civil law, 2654–2655
Good Samaritan laws, 2662, 2662*t*
healthcare systems and, 2601*t*
informed consent, 2659–2661, 2662*t*
malpractice, 2653, 2654*t*, 2656, 2657–2658
professional negligence prevention strategies,
2657–2658
quality improvement and, 2682*t*
resources, 2662, 2663*t*
sources of laws and, 2654, 2655*f*
standard of care, 2658–2659
tort law, 2655–2657
Legal protection guidelines, 2678*t*
Legionnaires disease, 586–587
Legislation, 2542
Legs, peripheral atherosclerosis and,
1202*t*
Leininger's theory of culture care diversity
and universality, 2302
LEMA (local emergency management
agency), 2611

Lentigo maligna, 128
Lentigo maligna melanoma, 129
Leopold maneuvers, 2142
Lesbian, gay, bisexual, and transgender
    (LGBT) individuals
    adolescent, 1670
    physical environment advocacy, 1636
    suicide and, 1993t
Lesions
    contact dermatitis, 1489t
    defined, 876, 1448
Let's Move, 2623f, 2623t
Leukemia
    acute, 92
    acute lymphoblastic (ALL), 93f, 93t,
        94–95
    acute myeloid (AML), 93t, 94–95, 94f
    alterations and therapies, 33t
    assessment, 99
    biological therapy, 99
    care planning, 100
    chemotherapy, 99, 99t
    in children, 93f, 100t
    chronic, 92
    chronic lymphocytic (CLL), 93t, 95
    chronic myeloid (CML), 94, 94f
    collaborative care, 97–99
    complementary and alternative therapy, 99
    defined, 92
    diagnosis, 100
    diagnostic findings by type, 98t
    diagnostic tests, 97
    etiology, 95
    interventions
        bleeding-related injury, 101–102
        grieve response, 102
        infection prevention, 101
        medication effects, 100–101
        mucous membrane integrity, 102
        nutrition, 102
    lymphocytic, 92
    manifestations, 95, 96t, 97t
    multisystem effects of, 96t
    myeloid, 92–93
    Nursing Care Plan, 103t
    nursing process, 99–102
    outcome evaluation, 102
    overview of, 92
    pathophysiology, 92–95
    pharmacologic therapy, 98–99
    primary forms of, 93t
    radiation therapy, 99
    remission, 97
    risk factors, 95
    surgery
        bone marrow transplant, 97–98
        stem cell transplant, 98
    tumor lysis syndrome (TLS) and, 101
    types of, 92
Leukocytes
    defined, 438, 634
    development and differentiation of, 439f
    granulocytes, 440
    inflammation and, 634
    lymphocytes, 440–441
    monocytes, 440
    types of, 438
Leukocytosis, 438, 634
Leukopenia, 438
Leukotriene modifiers, 490, 997–1001, 999t

Level of consciousness (LOC)
    alterations in, 692–694
    altered, 690–691, 690f
    brain death and, 694
    disorders affecting, 693
    increased intracranial pressure (IICP) and,
        693–694
    locked-in syndrome and, 694
    outcomes of altered, 694
    persistent vegetative state and, 694
    prevalence of, 696
    prognosis, 694
    seizures and, 694
    terms for describing, 693f
    in traumatic injury assessment, 1961
Level of injury, 909
Levodopa, 898, 899t
Lewy bodies, 896
LFTs (liver function tests), 788
LGA (large for gestational age), 2207t
LGBT. See Lesbian, gay, bisexual, and
        transgender (LGBT) individuals
LHRH (luteinizing hormone-releasing
        hormone), 2017
Liability, 2473, 2656
Libido, 1366, 1650
Licensed practical nurses (LPNs), 2458
Licensure, 2664–2665
Lichenification, 1448
Lidocaine patch, 1333
Life stress review, 416–417
Life support
    advanced, 1194
    basic, 1193, 1194f
Lifespan considerations
    abuse, 1969–1970
    acid-base balance, 10
    acute myocardial infarction, 1111t
    acute renal failure (ARF), 378, 379f
    addition, 1521–1522
    advocacy, 2558t
    anemia, 69
    appendicitis, 646
    assault and homicide, 1979
    assistive devices for ambulation, 837t
    asthma, 996t, 1000, 1003t
    bipolar disorders, 1811
    blood pressure assessment, 1067t
    body temperature, 1428t
    bowel elimination, 274–276, 279
    burn injuries, 1473
    burns, 1466t, 1482t, 1483t, 1485t
    cellulitis, 561–562
    chronic kidney disease (CKD), 392t
    cognition, 1587–1589
    comfort, 142, 147–148, 149
    confusion, 1606
    contact dermatitis, 1489
    crisis, 1929
    death and dying, 1758–1759
    decisions, 2322t
    depression, 1801t
    development, 1678
    diabetes mellitus, 761t
    digestion, 217–220
    documentation in long-term care for older
        adults, 2447t
    dysrhythmias, 1179t
    end-of-life care, 177–180
    family, 1720

    family health promotion, 1726
    fatigue, 187
    feeding and eating disorders, 1848
    fibromyalgia, 191
    fluids and electrolytes, 342–346
    fractures, 859
    gastroesophageal reflux disease (GERD), 229t
    grief and loss, 1743–1744, 1743f
    herniated disc, 842
    hip fractures, 871
    HIV/AIDS, 459–461, 473
    hypersensitivity, 488
    hypothyroidism, 815t
    increased intracranial pressure (IICP), 710
    infection, 525–527, 552–555
    inflammation, 636, 641
    intracranial regulation, 689–690, 707t
    malabsorption disorders, 240t
    metabolism, 726
    mobility, 820–822, 892
    mood and affect, 1776, 1784t, 1787
    neonatal pain assessment, 170
    nutrition, 932–934, 942–944
    obsessive-compulsive disorder (OCD), 1935t
    older adult's response to loss, 1764–1765
    oral health, 424
    oxygenation, 956–957
    pain, 157–162
    Parkinson disease, 897
    perfusion, 1046–1049
    perioperative care, 1254, 1256t
    personality disorders (PD), 1860
    pneumonia, 588–590
    pulse assessment, 1065t
    rape, 1986
    respiratory system, 965, 965t
    rheumatoid arthritis, 497t
    schizophrenia, 1616, 1616t
    scoliosis, 847
    seizure disorders, 716t
    seizures, 722t
    self-esteem, 1836
    sepsis, 601–602
    sexual development, 1341–1342t
    sickle cell disease, 122
    sleep-rest disorders, 196
    spinal cord injuries (SCI), 912
    spirituality, 1874t
    stress and coping, 1912–1913
    substance abuse, 1568t
    suctioning, 970t
    suicide, 1993–1994
    systemic lupus erythematosus (SLE), 512
    teaching, 2512t
    thermoregulation, 1423
    tissue integrity, 1447–1448
    tuberculosis, 609–611
    urinary calculi, 321–322
    urinary elimination, 261–264, 262t, 267
    urinary incontinence, 293–294
    urinary tract infections (UTIs), 622–623
    violence, 1961
    wound care, 1513
    wound healing, 1509
Lifestyle choices, 415, 415t
Life-threatening dysrhythmias
    antidysrhythmic drugs, 1189t
    assessment, 1195
    atrioventricular (AV) conduction blocks,
        1182t

Life-threatening dysrhythmias (*continued*)
cardiac mapping and catheter ablation and, 1192
cardiac monitoring and, 1187–1188
cardiac output monitoring and, 1195–1196
care planning, 1195
causes of, 1177–1178
characteristics of, 1180–1181t
in children, 1179t
collaborative care, 1186–1192
as coronary artery disease complication, 1112
countershock and, 1188–1190
defibrillation and, 1188–1190, 1190f
defined, 1052t, 1063, 1177
diagnosis, 1195
diagnostic tests, 1186–1188
discharge plan, 1196
electrophysiology studies and, 1188
home care, 1196t
implantable cardioverter-defibrillator (ICD) and, 1191–1192
interventions, 1195–1196
interventions and therapies, 1052t
junctional, 1184
lifespan considerations, 1179t
manifestations, 1052t, 1182–1186, 1187t
Nursing Care Plan, 1197–1198t
nursing process, 1194–1196
in older adults, 1179t
outcome evaluation, 1196
overview of, 1177–1178
pacemaker therapy, 1190–1191, 1190f, 1191f
pathophysiology and etiology, 1178–1182
pharmacologic therapy, 1188
sinus node, 1183
sudden cardiac death (SCD) and, 1192–1194
supraventricular, 1180–1181t, 1183–1184
synchronized cardioversion and, 1188
Valsalva maneuver and, 1192
ventricular, 1181–1182t, 1185–1186
Ligaments, 820
Ligands, 1919f
Light amplification by stimulated emission of electromagnetic radiation (LASER), 1263t
Light palpation, 2278, 2279f
Lightening, 2120–2121
Limb restraints, 2704, 2706f
Limbal relaxing incision, 1308
Limbic system, 1576, 1918f
Limit setting
bipolar disorders and, 1815
in parenting, 1717–1718
Line and drain management, 1274, 1274f
Line authority, 2549
Linear fractures, 855t
Linking, 2430–2431
Lipid profile, 793
Lipids, 928f, 929
Lipodystrophy, 471, 756
Listeriosis, 2097
Litargirio, 1473t
Lithiasis, 319, 322
Lithium carbonate, 1812–1813
Lithium therapy, 1793

Lithotomy, 1265t
Lithotomy position, 2278t
Lithotripsy, 322, 322f, 323f
Liver
biopsy, 785
degeneration and necrosis of, 233, 233f
inflammation of, 211
Liver disease. *See also* Cirrhosis
assessment, 786
care planning, 786
collaborative care, 785–786
diagnosis, 786
diagnostic tests, 785
effects, 781
interventions
bleeding minimization, 787
complication management, 788
fluid volume balance, 786
mental status, 786–787
nutrition, 787–788
skin integrity, 787
manifestations
ascites, 782
esophageal varices, 782
hepatorenal syndrome, 784
portal hypertension, 782
portal systemic encephalopathy, 782–784
splenomegaly, 782
spontaneous bacterial peritonitis, 784
therapies, 784t
multisystem effects of, 783t
Nursing Care Plan, 789t
nursing process, 786–788
nutritional therapy, 785–786
overview of, 781
pathophysiology and etiology, 781–782
pharmacologic therapy, 785
risk factors, 782
surgery, 786
Liver function studies, 785, 1151
Liver function tests (LFTs)
defined, 788
in lung cancer, 108
in tuberculosis, 611
Living wills, 177, 2667
Lobes, cerebral, 1576
LOC. *See* Level of consciousness
Local adaptation syndrome (LAS), 1900
Local anesthetics, 167
Local emergency management agency (LEMA), 2611
Local health departments, 2624
Local infection, 523
Localized response, 483
Lochia, 2172, 2179–2180t
Lochia alba, 2172
Lochia rubra, 2172
Lochia serosa, 2172
Locked-in syndrome, 694
Locker room, 1564
Locus of control, 1940
Long-acting beta agonists (LABAs), 971
Longboard spinal immobilization, 2003
Long-term goals, 2341–2342
Loop diuretics, 712t, 1172t
Loop ileostomy, 662
Loose association, 1613

Lordosis, 820
Loss. *See also* Grief and loss
actual, 1742
anticipatory, 1742
children's response to, 1751–1757
of clients, 1761, 1761f
defined, 1742
older adult response to, 1763–1767
perceived, 1742
perinatal, 1767–1773
types and sources of, 1742
Low priority, 2366
Lower body obesity, 791
Low-flow oxygen delivery devices, 592, 592f
Low-molecular-weight (LMW) heparins, 1132, 1133t
Low-sodium diet, 369t, 1082, 1160
Loyalty conflicts, 2572
LPNs (licensed practical nurses), 2458
LSD, 1564, 1567t
Lumbar disc herniation, 841, 842f
Lumbar puncture, 557, 880
Lumpectomy, 79
Lund and Browder burn assessment chart, 1469f
Lung abscess, 586
Lung cancer. *See also* Cancer
activity intolerance and, 110
assessment, 109
brachytherapy, 109
bronchogenic carcinomas, 104
cardiorespiratory function and, 109–110
care planning, 109
cell type comparison, 105
collaborative care, 107–109
diagnosis, 109
diagnostic tests, 108
fatigue management, 110
grieving and, 110
interventions, 109–110
local effects, 107
manifestations, 105–107, 107t
multisystem effects of, 106
non-small-cell carcinomas, 104
Nursing Care Plan, 111t
nursing process, 109–110
outcome evaluation, 110
overview of, 104
pain management, 110
pharmacologic therapy, 108
prevention, 105
radiation therapy, 109
risk factors, 104
small-cell carcinomas, 104
surgery, 108, 108t
systemic effects, 107
TNM staging system for, 107t
Lung scan, pulmonary embolism and, 1213
Lungs
anterior view, 955f
in intrapartum assessment, 2143t
lateral view of lobes, 964f
lobes, 955
in postpartum assessment, 2179t
Lupus nephritis, 670, 671t
Luteal phase, 2018
Luteinizing hormone-releasing hormone (LHRH), 2017

Lymph nodes
  assessment
    female, 1359t
    male, 1356t
  defined, 443
  palpating, 452, 452f
Lymphadenopathy, 560
Lymphatic drainage, 365
Lymphedema, 79
Lymphocytes
  B (B cells), 441
  defined, 440
  development and differentiation of, 441f
  NK (natural killer cells), 441
  T (T cells), 441
Lymphoid system, 443–444, 443f
Lymphoid tissues, 444
Lymphomas, 464
Lysine, 2184t
Lysosomes, 31

M

Maceration, 1493
Macronutrients, 927
Macrophages, 440, 1508
Macrosomia, 2046
Macrosystem, 1657
Macular degeneration
  Amsler grid and, 1328, 1328f
  assessment, 1329
  care planning, 1330
  collaborative care, 1328–1329
  defined, 1327
  diagnosis, 1329
  diagnostic tests, 1329
  exudative, 1327–1328, 1328t
  interventions, 1281t, 1330
  manifestations, 1281t, 1328, 1328t
  nonexudative, 1327, 1328t
  nonpharmacologic therapy, 1329
  nursing process, 1329–1330
  outcome evaluation, 1330
  overview of, 1327
  pathophysiology and etiology, 1327–1328
  pharmacologic therapy, 1329, 1329t
  risk factors, 1328
  surgery, 1329
Magical thinking, 1665t
Magnesium (Mg²⁺)
  function in the body, 342t, 931
  locations in the body, 341–342
  regulation of, 342t
Magnetic resonance cholangiopancreatography
    (MRCP), 247
Magnetic resonance imaging (MRI)
  cancer and, 55
  congenital heart defects and, 1098t
  deep venous thrombosis (DVT) and, 1132
  HIV/AIDS testing and, 468
  multiple sclerosis testing and, 880
  peripheral vascular disease (PVD) and, 1201
  in violence assessment, 1961
Mahoney, Mary, 2547
Maintenance phase, acute renal failure (ARF), 378
Major depressive disorder (MDD)
  bipolar disorder comparison, 1811f
  characteristics of, 1800f
  defined, 1778, 1798
  diabetes and, 750

DSM-5 diagnostic criteria for, 1799t
  key facts about, 1799t
  manifestations, 1800t
  prevalence of, 1782–1783
  therapies, 1800t
Major depressive disorder with peripartum onset,
    1817
Major depressive episodes, 1798
Major histocompatible complex (MHC), 447
Malabsorption
  causes of, 211t
  defined, 211, 240
Malabsorption disorders
  celiac disease, 240–243
  lactase deficiency, 243–244
  lifespan considerations, 240t
  manifestations and therapies, 213t
  overview of, 240
  short bowel syndrome, 244–245
Malaise, 570
Maldigestion, 211, 211t
Male circumcision, 1362
Male condoms, 1379–1380, 1380f
Male contraception, 1386
Male erectile disorder, 1349
Male genitals, in gestational age,
    2218, 2218f
Male hormone replacement, 1364t
Male orgasmic disorder, 1350
Male reproductive assessment
  breast and lymph node, 1356t
  external genitalia, 1356–1357t
  prostate, 1357t
Malignant cells, 43, 43t
Malignant hyperthermia, 1426, 1432
Malignant neoplasms, 42–44, 43t, 53t
Malnutrition
  alcohol abuse and, 1536
  assessment, 218t
Malpractice
  client safety and, 2657
  communication and, 2658
  defined, 2653, 2655
  elements of, 2656
  examples of negligence that result in,
    2656t
  failure to observe and take appropriate
    action, 2657
  medication errors and, 2658
  professional liability insurance and, 2658
  related doctrines, 2656
  statute of limitations, 2656–2657
  strategies to prevent incidents of,
    2657–2658
Malpresentations, 2115
Malunion fractures, 857
Managed care, 2457, 2599
Management principles
  accountability, 2476
  authority, 2476
  conflict management, 2477
  controlling, 2475–2476
  directing, 2475
  effectiveness, 2477
  efficiency, 2477
  employee performance enhancement
    and, 2476
  functions, 2475–2476
  leaders and mangers, 2474–2475
  organizing, 2475

overview of, 2474
  planning, 2475
  productivity, 2477
  resource management, 2476
  responsibility, 2476
  team building and management,
    2476–2477
  time management, 2477
Managers, 2474–2475
Managing care
  case management, 2457
  case method, 2458
  client-focused care, 2457
  concept of, 2455
  concepts related to, 2456t
  differentiated practice, 2457
  functional method, 2458
  healthcare systems and, 2601t
  managed care, 2457
  nursing practice, 2459
  primary nursing, 2459
  shared governance, 2457–2458
  team nursing, 2458–2459
Mandatory health insurance, 2463
Mandatory reporting
  abuse and neglect, 2674, 2674t
  defined, 2674
  good faith immunity, 2674, 2674t
  injuries and illnesses, 2675
  nurses in violation of NPA, 2674–2675
  other examples of, 2675–2676
  overview of, 2674
Mania
  defined, 1776, 1809
  nurse reactions and, 1814t
Manic episodes, 1809, 1811f
Manipulation, 1852
MAO (monoamine oxidase), 1784
MAO-B inhibitors, 899t, 900
MAOIs. See Monoamine oxidase inhibitors
MAP (mean arterial pressure), 1163, 1218
Maple syrup urine disease, 2208t
Marasmus, 930, 930t
Marfan syndrome, 2049
Margination, 634
Marijuana, pregnancy and, 1554
Marital rape, 1984
MARs (medication administration records),
    2648, 2649f
Maslow's hierarchy of needs
  in assessment, 2282
  defined, 142
  illustrated, 142f, 1899f
  in prioritizing care, 2365–2366
  in self-care in nursing, 2308–2310
  sequencing of, 1899
Mass in Motion (MiM), 2702–2703
Massage
  antenatal perineal, 2132t
  infant, 2259
Massage therapy
  for anxiety disorders, 1925
  for end-of-life care, 182t
  for herniated discs, 843
  for menopause, 1396
Massive transfusion, 1252t
MAST (Michigan Alcohol Screening Test), 1540
Mast cell stabilizers
  for asthma, 999t
  for hypersensitivity, 490

Mast cells, 635
Mastectomy, 79, 79f
Mastery experiences, 1928
Masturbation, 1346
Maternal birthing positions, 2166
Maternal role attainment (MRA)
    defined, 1817
    postpartum challenges and, 1817–1818
    stages of, 1817
Maternal weight gain, 2098–2099, 2098t, 2099f
Maturation phase, in wound healing, 1508
Maturational crisis, 1928f
Mature milk, 2174
Maturity onset diabetes in youth (MODY), 767
McBurney point, 644, 645f
McDonald method, 2053, 2054f
McDonald sign, 2035
McMurray's test, 834f, 834t
MDD. See Major depressive disorder
MDMA (ecstasy)
    defined, 1564
    pregnancy and, 1554
MDQ (Mood Disorders Questionnaire), 1786
Mean arterial pressure (MAP), 1152, 1163, 1218
Mean-focused coping, 1899
Measles, 535t
Meatus, urinary, 268t
Mechanical ventilation. See also Ventilators
    assist-control mode ventilation (ACMV), 980
    barotrauma and, 982
    bilevel ventilation (BiPAP), 979, 980
    cardiovascular effects, 982
    complications of, 980–982
    continuous positive airway pressure (CPAP), 979, 980, 981t
    FiO_2, 979
    gastrointestinal effects, 982
    hospital-acquired pneumonia (HAP) and, 982
    modes of, 980
    nutrition and fluids and, 984–985
    pneumothorax and, 982
    positive end-expiratory pressure (PEEP), 979, 980, 981t
    pressure-support ventilation (PSV), 981t
    synchronized intermittent mandatory ventilation (SIMV), 980
    ventilator settings, 980
    ventilator types, 979–980
Meconium, 274, 2200
Meconium aspiration syndrome, 2209t
Medicaid, 2627
Medical asepsis, 523
Medical home, 2605, 2605t
Medical Leave Act, 1713t
Medical records management, 2645
Medicare, 2627, 2627t
Medication administration records (MARs), 2648, 2649f
Medication errors
    methods to reduce, 2688, 2688t
    minimizing risk of, 2658, 2707
    safety and, 2707
Medications. See also specific drugs
    acute renal failure (ARF), 381–382
    addiction, 1533t
    anti-Alzheimer, 1592t
    antidysrhythmic, 1189t
    as antiemetics, 223t
    antimicrobial agents, 558–559t

antiplatelet, 1120t
antiretroviral nucleoside analogues, 470–471
asthma, 998–999t
attention-deficit/hyperactivity disorder (ADHD), 1683t
blood pressure, 1046
bowel elimination, 283
cellular regulation, 40t
cholesterol-lowering, 1117t
chronic pain management, 172t
cognitive alterations, 1592t
constipation, 309t
disorders of anxiety, stress, or trauma, 1916t
drug-drug interactions, 163
eye injuries, 1315t
fertility, 1387, 1387t
fluid and electrolyte, 353t
gastroesophageal reflux disease (GERD), 230t
glaucoma, 1322t
grief and loss, 1750
hearing loss, 1303t
heart failure, 1154–1156t
hepatitis, 237t
hypertension, 1171–1172t
immunity, 455
increased intracranial pressure (IICP), 712
inflammatory bowel disease (IBD), 664–665t
inflammatory disease, 643t
macular degeneration, 1329
musculoskeletal disorder, 838t
nutrition, 947t
osteoporosis and, 800
ototoxic, 1300, 1300t
pain, 151t
Parkinson disease motor symptoms, 899t
perfusion, 1074–1075t
perioperative care, 1254, 1255t
peripheral neuropathy, 1334t
postoperative, 1274
pregnancy, 2064–2065
preoperative review of, 1257–1259
pulse and, 1044
rheumatoid arthritis, 503t
schizophrenia, 1618t
seizure disorders, 719t
as sensory perception risk factor, 1283
sexual function and, 1350t
shock, 1228–1229t
six rights of administration, 2707
sleep, 151t, 198, 434
stress and copying, 1916t
systemic lupus erythematosus (SLE), 517
tissue integrity, 1461–1463t
trauma, 1963t
wound healing, 1509
Medigap policies, 2629
Meditation
    for anxiety disorders, 1925–1926
    defined, 1885
    for menopause, 1396
Medium priority, 2366
Medium-chain triglyceride (MCT) ketogenic diet, 720
Meiosis, 32, 2019–2020
Melanin, 1446
Melanocytes, 1446–1447

Melanomas. See also Skin cancer
    acral lentiginous, 129
    classifications of, 128–129
    defined, 128
    health education for clients with, 137t
    illustrated, 129f
    lentigo maligna, 129
    nodular, 129
    precursor lesions, 128
    risk factors, 131, 131t
    superficial spreading, 129
Melasma gravidarum, 2032
Melatonin, 1796–1797
Memory impairment, 1614
Menarche, 1340
Mendelian (single-gene) inheritance, 1376
Meninges, 688
Meningococcus, 535–536t
Menometrorrhagia, 1400
Menopause
    assessment, 1397
    care planning, 1397
    chemical, 1394
    collaborative care, 1395–1396
    complementary and alternative therapy, 1396, 1397t
    defined, 1343, 1394
    diagnostic tests, 1395
    healthy body image and, 1398
    hormone replacement therapy (HRT) and, 1395–1396
    interventions, 1397–1398
    knowledge, discussing, 1397–1398
    manifestations, 1394–1395, 1395t
    nursing process, 1396–1398
    osteoporosis and, 800
    outcome evaluation, 1398
    overview of, 1394
    perimenopausal period and, 1394, 1395t
    pharmacologic therapy, 1395–1396
    physiology and etiology, 1394
    self-esteem promotion and, 1398
    sexuality patterns and, 1398
    surgical, 1394
Menorrhagia, 1400
Menstrual cycle
    defined, 1354, 2018
    in female sexuality, 1354
    ischemic phase, 2019
    menstrual phase, 2019
    proliferative phase, 2019
    secretory phase, 2019
Menstrual dysfunction
    anxiety relief and, 1404
    assessment, 1404
    care planning, 1404
    collaborative care, 1401–1403
    diagnosis, 1404
    diagnostic tests, 1401–1402
    dilation and curettage (D&C) and, 1402
    dysfunctional uterine bleeding (DUB), 1400, 1403t
    dysmenorrhea, 1342, 1399–1400, 1400t, 1403
    endometrial ablation and, 1402
    endometriosis and, 1400, 1400t
    hysterectomy and, 1402–1403, 1403t
    interventions, 1352t, 1404–1405
    laparoscopy and, 1402, 1402f
    manifestations, 1399–1401, 1400t, 1401t
    Nursing Care Plan, 1405t

nursing process, 1403–1405
outcome evaluation, 1405
overview of, 1399
pain relief, 1404
pathophysiology and etiology, 1399–1401
pharmacologic therapy, 1402
risk factors, 1400t, 1401
sexual function and, 1404–1405
surgery, 1402–1403
Menstruation
defined, 1342, 2018
parameters, 2018
postpartum changes, 2173
Mental health disorders, 1523
Mental health settings, advocating for clients in, 2560–2561
Mental illness
family and, 1731–1733
family burden, 1731–1732
family recovery, 1732–1733
language of pain and, 1732t
Mental retardation. See Intellectual disability
Mental status
assessments, 1587t, 1588–1589t
liver disease and, 786–787
Mentoring
coaching and, 2526–2527, 2526t
networking and, 2527, 2527t
overview of, 2525
precepting, 2525–2526
relationship, 2525, 2526t
use of, 2525
Mentors, 2525
Mentum, 2114
Meperidine (Demerol), 1439
Mercury in fish, 2096–2097
Mesalamine, 664t
Mesosystem, 1657
Messages, 2399
Meta-analysis, 2588
Metabolic acidosis
assessment, 15
cardiac status monitoring and, 16
care planning, 15–16
causes, 9t, 10t
collaborative care, 15
compensation, 10t
defined, 6, 14
diagnosis, 15
illustrated, 7f
imbalance, 9t
interventions, 8t, 14t, 16
manifestations, 8t, 14t, 15
nursing process, 15–16
outcome evaluation, 16
overview of, 14
pathophysiology and etiology, 14–15
pharmacologic therapies, 12, 15
risk factors, 7, 14–15
Metabolic alkalosis
assessment, 19
causes, 9t, 10t
compensation, 10t
defined, 6, 17
diagnosis, 19
hypokalemia and, 17–18
illustrated, 7f
imbalance, 9t
interventions and therapies, 8t, 18t, 19–20
laboratory and diagnostic tests, 18

manifestations, 8t, 18, 18t
nursing process, 18–20
outcome evaluation, 19
overview of, 17
pathophysiology and etiology, 17–18
pharmacologic therapies, 12, 18
risk factors, 7, 18
Metabolic disorders
alterations and therapies, 730t
cirrhosis, 729
collaborative care, 737–739
diabetes. See diabetes mellitus
genetic considerations and nonmodifiable risk factors, 729–731
graves disease, 728
hypothyroidism, 728 729
interventions and therapies, 733–739
manifestations, 726–779
medications, 738t
obesity, 727
osteoporosis, 729
pharmacologic therapy, 739
prevalence of, 729
prevention of, 731
thyroid disease, 728–729
Metabolic emergencies, 49
Metabolic syndrome
defined, 792, 1110
risk factors for, 1110t
Metabolism
alterations, 726–731
alterations and therapies, 730t
assessment, 732
assessment interview, 733t
burn injuries and, 1473
collaborative interventions and therapies, 737–739
concepts related to, 728t
defined, 725, 932, 1843
diagnostic tests, 732
endocrine system. See endocrine system
genetic and lifespan considerations, 726
independent interventions and therapies, 733–737
interventions and therapies, 733–739
normal, 725
overview of, 932
pregnancy and, 2033
Metaplasia, 32
Metastasis
breast cancer and, 76
defined, 43
illustrated, 44f
mechanisms, 44
steps, 44
Methadone
defined, 1564
pregnancy and, 1554
Methicillin-resistant S. aureus (MRSA), 531, 532
Methylxanthines, 997, 998t
Metoclopramide hydrochloride, 222
Metrorrhagia, 1400
Michigan Alcohol Screening Test (MAST), 1540
Microalbuminuria, 749
Micronutrients, 927
Microorganisms
hands as spreading vehicle, 531
in healthcare-associated infections, 530–531
list of, 522t

types causing infections, 523
virulence, 522–523
Microstaging, 134, 134f
Microsystem, 1657
Micturition, 260
Middle adults
growth and development, 1671, 1671t
holistic health assessment, 2294
safety, 2712–2713
sexuality, 1343
Middle ear effusion, 576
Middle Eastern, acceptable child behaviors, 2288t
Middle insomnia, 1799
Mifepristone, 1387–1388
Mild cognitive impairment, 1584, 1597t
Milia, 2224, 2224f
Miliary tuberculosis, 606
Milieu therapy, 1530
Military presentation, 2115, 2115f
Millennial Generation, 2495t
Milliequivalent, 336
MiM (Mass in Motion), 2702–2703
Mind-body interactions, 414
Mindful listening, 2425
Minerals
deficiency and excess, 938t
hypertension and, 1167
overview of, 930–931
supplements, 947t
Mini Nutritional Assessment (MNA), 940, 941t
Minimal enteral nutrition, 2253
Minimally invasive coronary artery surgery, 1122
Mini-Mental State Examination (MMSE), 1587t, 1600–1601
Minimization, 1905t
Mini-Nutritional Assessment (MNA), 2296t
Mini-pill, 1384
Minnesota Fall Prevention, 2702
Minor consent laws, 2661, 2662t
Minor trauma, 1956
Minorities, 1630, 1638
Minors, abuse or neglect of, 2674
Miotics, 1322t
Miscarriage, 1768
Misoprostol, 2128
Mitigation, in emergency management, 2609
Mitochondria, 31, 31t
Mitosis, 32, 2019
Mitoxantrone (Novantrone), 880
Mitral valve prolapse (MVP), 2049
Mitt restraints, 2704, 2706f
Mittelschmerz, 1379, 2018
Mixed acid-base disorders, 6
Mixed aphasia, 1238
Mixed defects. See also Congenital heart defects
clinical therapy, 1090–1091t
defined, 1089
manifestations, 1090–1091t, 1095
pathophysiology, 1090–1091t
total anomalous pulmonary venous return, 1091t
transposition of the great arteries (TGA), 1090t
truncus arteriosus, 1090–1091t
Mixed features, 1779, 1811
Mixed opioids, 162t, 165
Mixed sleep apnea, 195

MMSE (Mini-Mental State Examination), 1587t, 1600–1601
MNA (Mini Nutritional Assessment), 940, 941t
Mobility
activities of daily living (ADLs) and, 819
alterations
back problems, 825, 839–853
fractures, 824t, 825, 853–876
herniated disc, 824t, 840–845
joint disorders, 826, 826f
manifestations, 822–827
multiple sclerosis, 824t, 825, 876–886
osteoarthritis, 824t, 825, 886–895
Parkinson disease, 824–825t, 825–826, 895–906
scoliosis, 824t, 825, 825f, 845–852
spinal cord injuries, 825t, 826, 906–918
therapies, 824–825t
traumatic injuries, 826–827
types of, 824–825t
alterations and therapies, 824–825t
ambulation, 837
assessment
ankles, 833f, 833t
ballottement test, 834f, 834t
bulge test, 834f, 834t
elbows, 832t
fingers, 832t
5 P's neurovascular, 828–829
gait and posture, 830t
hips, 832t
interview, 829t
joint, 830t
knees, 833t
lumbar spine, 831f, 831t
McMurray's test, 834f, 834t
nursing, 828
Phalen's test, 833f, 833t
physical, 828–829, 830t
range of motion, 830–833t
shoulders, 832t
temporomandibular joint, 831f, 831t
Thomas test, 835f, 835t
toes, 833t
wrists, 832t
assistive devices for, 837–838, 837t
burns and, 1484
cerebral palsy (CP) and, 1699
collaborative interventions and therapies, 837–838
comfort promotion and, 836
concepts related to, 823t
deep venous thrombosis (DVT) and, 1136
diagnostic tests, 835–836
education and, 836
exercise and, 837
genetic and lifespan considerations, 820–822
genetic considerations and nonmodifiable risk factors, 827, 827t
independent interventions and therapies, 836–837
injury prevention and, 836–837
interventions and therapies, 836–838
lifespan and cultural considerations, 829
modifiable risk factors, 828
motor vehicle crashes (MVC) and, 2004–2005
muscle function grading scale, 828t
normal, 820–822
osteoarthritis and, 893

pharmacologic therapy, 838
prevention and, 828
screenings, 828
stroke and, 1244, 1244f
Modeling, 418–419, 2504
Modesty, 2156–2157
Modified radical mastectomy, 79
MODY (maturity onset diabetes in youth), 767
Moist wound management, 561t
Molding, 2114
Mongolian spots, 2224, 2224f
Monoamine oxidase inhibitors (MAOIs)
adverse effects, 1792
client education, 1792–1793
defined, 1792
nursing care, 1792
Monoamine oxidase (MAO), 1784
Monoclonal antibodies, 556t
Monocytes, 440
Mononeuropathies, 749–750, 1331
Mononucleosis, 536t
Monopolizing, 2422
Monosaturated fat, 757
Monosomic, 1374
Monosomies, 1375
Monotheism, 1873
Monroe-Kellie hypothesis, 709
Mood alterations, 750
Mood and affect
affect descriptors, 1776t
alterations to
adjustment disorder with depressed mood, 1778
bipolar disorders, 1779
depression, 1778, 1779–1782
genetic considerations and nonmodifiable risk factors, 1783–1784
manifestations and therapies, 1778–1779
postpartum mood disorders, 1779
prevalence of, 1782–1783, 1784t
therapies and, 1780t
assessment, 1785–1788
characteristics of disorders, 1786t
concepts related to, 1777–1778t
defined, 1775
depression and grief differentiation, 1788, 1788t
diagnostic tests, 1787–1788
genetic and lifespan considerations, 1776
genetic considerations and nonmodifiable risk factors, 1783–1784
interventions and therapies
assertive behavior education, 1789
collaborative, 1790–1797
independent, 1788–1790
maladaptive dependence and, 1790
for mood disorders, 1794t
nonpharmacologic therapy, 1793–1797
pharmacologic therapy for bipolar disorders, 1793
pharmacologic therapy for depression, 1790–1793
safety, 1788–1789, 1789t
suicide prevention, 1788–1789, 1789t
lifespan considerations, 1784t, 1787
neurobiology, 1783–1784
normal, 1776
prevalence and, 1782, 1784t
prevention of disorders, 1784
prevention programs, 1785

screenings, 1785
self-report scales, 1785–1787
Mood disorders
characteristics of, 1786t
complementary and alternative therapy
acupuncture, 1797
animal-assisted therapy, 1797
exercise, 1795–1796
melatonin, 1796–1797
music therapy, 1797
omega-3 fatty acids, 1797
SAMe, 1796
St. Johns wort, 1796
tyrosine, 1796
vitamin B, 1796
nonpharmacologic therapy
cognitive-behavioral therapy, 1794–1795
electroconvulsive therapy (ECT), 1795, 1796t
transcranial magnetic stimulation, 1796t
pharmacologic therapy for, 1794t
postpartum, 1820–1821
Mood Disorders Questionnaire (MDQ), 1786
Mood stabilizers, 1995
Moral behavior, 1657
Moral development, 1657, 1879
Moral frameworks, 1879
Moral principles
autonomy, 1880
beneficence, 1880
defined, 1879
ethnic/cultural variations, 2576t
fidelity, 1880
justice, 1880
nonmaleficence, 1880
veracity, 1880
Moral rules, 1879
Moral theories, 1657
Morality
assessment, 1881
care planning, 1881
defined, 1657, 1878, 2563
diagnosis, 1881
ethics and, 2563
interventions, 1881–1882
moral development and, 1879
moral frameworks and, 1879
moral principles and, 1879–1880
Nursing Care Plan, 1882t
nursing process, 1881–1882
outcome evaluation, 1882
overview of, 1878–1880
practice of nursing and, 1880–1881
Morbid obesity, 792
Morning sickness, 2035
Moro reflex, 2234, 2234f
Morpheaform basal cell carcinoma, 130
Morula, 2021
Mosaicism, 1374
Mother, pregnant. *See also* Reproduction
attitude towards pregnancy, 2036–2037
conflicts, 2037
first trimester, 2037
psychological tasks of, 2037–2038
second trimester, 2037
third trimester, 2037
Motility, 210
Motivation
to learn, 2505
sleep and, 434
in teaching plans, 2513–2514

Motor activity, newborn assessment, 2235
Motor deficits, stroke and, 1239, 1239f
Motor function assessment, 736t
Motor vehicle crashes (MVC)
    alcohol-related, 2000t
    care planning, 2003
    collaborative care, 2001–2003
    common injuries, 2000–2001
    cultural considerations, 2001, 2001t
    cyclists, 2000t
    dashboard knee and, 2001
    defined, 1998
    diagnosis, 2003
    diagnostic tests, 2001
    etiology, 1998–1999
    illustrated, 1999f
    injury prevention, 2000t
    interventions
        airway patency and ventilation, 2003–2004
        community-based care facilitation, 2005
        disability assessment, 2004
        fluid volume balance, 2004
        infection prevention, 2004
        mobility promotion, 2004–2005
        obscured area exposure, 2004
        psychosocial well-being, 2005
        spiritual comfort measures, 2005
    manifestations, 2000–2001, 2002t
    motorcycle, 2000t
    nonpharmacologic therapy, 2003
    Nursing Care Plan, 2006t
    nursing process, 2003–2005
    older adults and, 1999
    outcome evaluation, 2005
    overview of, 1998
    pedestrians, 2000t
    pharmacologic therapy, 2002–2003
    prevention of, 1999, 2000t
    risk factors, 1999
    safety protection and, 2001t
    speeding, 2000t
    surgery, 2001–2002
    unsafe driving practices and, 1999
    whiplash and, 2001
Mottling, 2223
Mourning, 1742, 1749
Mouth, newborn assessment, 2227–2228
Movement disorders, 1614
Movement techniques, 151
MRA. See Maternal role attainment
MRCP (magnetic resonance cholangiopancreatography), 247
MRI. See Magnetic resonance imaging
MSA (multiple system atrophy), 898
Mucous membrane integrity, leukemia and, 101
Multiculturalism
    defined, 1630
    model of, 1641t, 1642f
Multidisciplinary team approach, 2391
Multifactorial inheritance, 1377–1378
Multifocal PVCs, 1185
Multigravida, 2051t
Multipara, 2051t
Multiple intelligence, 2505
Multiple sclerosis
    aging clients with, 879t
    antepartum care and, 2079t
    assessment, 882

as autoimmune disease, 825
care planning, 883
classifications of, 877t
client teaching, 883t
collaborative care, 880–881
collaborative care referrals, 884
complementary and alternative therapy, 881t
complications of, 884
defined, 824t, 876
diagnosis, 882–883
diagnostic tests, 880
emotional status assessment and, 884
exacerbation, 877
interventions, 824t, 883–884
lesions, 876
lifespan and cultural considerations, 879
manifestations, 824t, 825, 877–879, 882t
medications for symptoms of, 881t
mobility promotion and, 883
multisystem effects of, 878t
myelin and, 876
nonpharmacologic therapy, 881
Nursing Care Plan, 884–885t
nursing process, 881–884
overview of, 876
pathophysiology and etiology, 876–877
pharmacologic therapy, 880–881
plaques, 876
pseudoexacerbation, 877
risk factors, 877
self-care and, 884
surgery, 880
Multiple system atrophy (MSA), 898
Multiple trauma, 1956
Multiple-puncture test (tine test), 608
Mumps, 537t
Murmurs, newborn, 2195
Muscles
    activity, in heat production, 1422
    breathing, inspection of, 964t
    function grading scale, 828t
    relaxation, 150
    types of, 820
Musculoskeletal disorders
    blood tests for, 835t
    medications for, 838t
Musculoskeletal system
    assessing, 453
    assessment, 737t
    changes in older adults, 821–822
    exercise benefits, 421
    normal changes of aging, 822f
    pregnancy and, 2032–2033, 2032f
Music therapy
    for children, 1668t
    for mood disorders, 1797
    for premature newborns, 2259
Mustard or Senning procedure, 1099t
Mutual pretense awareness, 183
Mutual recognition model, 2665, 2665t
Mutual respect, 2380
MVC. See Motor vehicle crashes
MVP (mitral valve prolapse), 2049
Mycobacterium avium complex (MAC), 463
Mycobacterium tuberculosis, 606, 607
Mycoplasma, 530t
Mydriasis, 1319
Myelin, 876
Myelogram, 843
Myocardial hypertrophy, 1048

Myocardial infarction
    causes of, 1049–1050
    defined, 1049
    drugs used to treat, 1118–1119
Myocardial perfusion imaging, 1114
Myopia, 1286t
MyPlate, 927, 929f
Myringotomy, 578, 579, 1302
Myxedema, 812
Myxedema coma, 813

N
Nabothian cysts, 1361t
NAHN (National Association of Hispanic Nurses), 2626t
Nails
    assessment, 734t, 1459t
    color inspection, 1459t
    thickness inspection, 1460t
NANDA, 2334
Narcissism, 1852
Narcissistic personality disorder (NPD), 1856t, 1859, 1863t
Narcolepsy
    defined, 145, 195
    manifestations, 195, 200t
    therapies, 200t
Narcotic abuse, 1556t
Narrative charting, 2440
NAS (neonatal abstinence syndrome), 1554
Nasal and oral suctioning, 2246
Nasal cannulas, 972, 972f
Nash-Moe method, 848
Nasopharyngeal airways, 983, 983f
Natalizumab (Tysabri), 880
National Association of Hispanic Nurses (NAHN), 2626t
National Black Nurses Association (NBNA), 2626t
National Council Licensure Examination for Registered Nurses (NCLEX-RN), 2664
National Council of State Boards of Nursing (NCSBN), 2665, 2665t
National Guideline Clearinghouse, 2570
National Institute for Occupational Safety and Health (NIOSH), 2715, 2716
National League for Nursing (NLN), 2626
National Patient Safety Goals (NPSG), 2701, 2701t
National standards on culturally and linguistically appropriate services (CLAS), 2404t
National Student Nurses Association (NSNA)
    code of academic and clinical conduct, 2539, 2540t
    defined, 2625
    mission of, 2625
Native Americans
    acceptable child behaviors, 2288t
    pain response, 161t
Natural killer (NK) cells, 441
Natural science, 2269
Nature, 1655–1656
Nausea. See also Vomiting
    complementary and alternative therapy, 222t
    death and dying and, 1759
    defined, 210
    manifestations and therapies, 212t
    opioid use and, 165t
    relief in pregnancy, 2065–2066, 2066t

NBNA (National Black Nurses Association), 2626t
NCLEX-RN (National Council Licensure Examination for Registered Nurses), 2664
NCSBN (National Council of State Boards of Nursing), 2665, 2665t
NDM (neonatal diabetes mellitus), 767
Neck, newborn assessment, 2228
Necrosis, 1492
Needlestick injuries, 2717
Negative affectivity, 1855
Negative airflow room, 616
Negative feedback, 2379–2380
Negative punishment, 1529
Negative reinforcement, 1529
Negative symptoms, 1613, 1613t, 1621t
Negative-pressure ventilators, 979
Neglect syndrome, 1237
Negligence
    defined, 2655
    examples that result in malpractice, 2656t
    professional, 2655–2657
    in tort law, 2655
Neisseria gonorrhoeae, 565
Neologisms, 1613
Neonatal abstinence syndrome (NAS), 1554
Neonatal anemia, 69
Neonatal diabetes mellitus (NDM), 767
Neonatal distress, early assessment of, 2238
Neonatal mortality risk, 2206, 2206f
Neonatal pain assessment, 170t
Neonatal risk for injury, 2709–2710
Neonates, endotracheal intubation in, 988t
Neoplasms
    benign, 42
    defined, 42
    malignant, 42–44, 43t
    nomenclature for, 53t
    tumor-derived markers associated with, 54t
Neoplastic, 1448
Nephrectomy, 398
Nephritis
    acute postinfection glomerulonephritis (APIGN), 669
    assessment, 673
    care planning, 673
    collaborative care, 671–673
    defined, 669
    diagnosis, 673
    diagnostic tests, 671–672
    etiology, 671
    fatigue and, 674
    fluid volume balance and, 674
    glomerulonephritis, 669
    Goodpasture syndrome, 670
    home care for, 675t
    infection prevention and, 674
    interventions, 674
    lupus, 669, 671t
    manifestations, 671, 672t
    nonpharmacologic therapy, 673
    Nursing Care Plan, 675–676t
    nursing process, 673–674, 675t
    nutrition and, 674
    outcome evaluation, 674
    pathophysiology, 669–671
    pharmacologic therapy, 673
    prevention of, 671
    risk factors, 671

self-esteem promotion and, 674
skin integrity and, 674
Nephrolithiasis, 319
Nephrolithotomy, 323
Nephrotoxins, 374
Nerve blocks, 168
Nervous system
    central, 688–689
    peripheral, 688, 689–690
Networking, 2527, 2527t
Neurobiology
    in abuse, 1966
    in mood and affect, 1783–1784
    in personality disorders (PD), 1853
    suicide and, 1991
Neurofibrillary tangles, 1595
Neurogenic bladder, 265
Neurogenic shock
    assessment, 1230
    defined, 1224
    manifestations, 1226t
Neurokinin receptor agents, 223
Neuroleptic malignant syndrome, 1617
Neurological assessment
    body systems, 701–703t
    Brudzinski sign, 705f, 705t
    cerebral function, 704–705t
    cranial nerves, 699–701t
    heal-to-shin test, 704f, 704t
    interview, 697t
    Kernig sign, 705f, 705t
    methods, 698–705t
    newborns
        Babinski reflex (response), 2234, 2234f
        grasping reflex, 2233, 2234f
        Moro reflex, 2234, 2234f
        rooting reflex, 2234, 2234f
        status, 2233–2235
        stepping reflex, 2234, 2235f
        sucking reflex, 2234
        tonic neck reflex, 2233, 2233f
        trunk incurvation (Galant reflex), 2234
    testing graphesthesia, 702f, 702t
    testing two-point discrimination, 702f, 702t
Neurological system
    chronic kidney disease (CKD) and, 393–395
    postpartum changes, 2176
    premature newborns and, 2251
    shock effect on, 1222
Neurons, 688, 1576
Neuropathic pain, 154
Neurotherapy, 1539–1540
Neurotransmission hypothesis, 1783
Neurotransmitters, 1576
Neurovascular status monitoring, in fractures, 866
Neutral questions, 2275
Neutral thermal environment (NTE), 1423, 2196
Neutrophils, 440, 556f
Nevi, 128
Nevus flammeus (port-wine stain), 2224
Nevus vasculosus (strawberry mark), 2224
New Ballard Score, 2213
Newborn care
    alterations
        asphyxia, 2209t
        cold stress, 2210t
        congenital heart defects, 2208t

    factors, 2204
    galactosemia, 2208t
    homocystinuria, 2208t
    hypoglycemia, 2210t
    infant of mother with diabetes, 2207t
    infant of mother with HIV/AIDS, 2208t
    intrauterine growth and, 2205, 2205f
    intrauterine growth restriction (IUGR), 2207t
    large for gestational age (LGA), 2207t
    maple syrup urine disease, 2208t
    meconium aspiration syndrome, 2209t
    phenylketonuria (PKU), 2208t
    polycythemia, 2210t
    postterm newborn, 2207t
    pregnancy risk factors, 2204–2205
    prenatal substance exposure, 2208t
    respiratory distress, 2209t
    small gestational age (SGA), 2207t
    therapies, 2207–2210t
    transient tachypnea, 2209t
    very small for gestational age (VSGA), 2207t
assessment
    abdomen, 2230
    anus, 2231
    back, 2232
    behavior, 2235–2236, 2236f
    birthmarks, 2224, 2224f
    chest, 2228–2229, 2228f
    cry, 2229
    cuddliness and social behaviors, 2236
    ears, 2228, 2228f
    extremities, 2231–2232, 2231f, 2232f, 2233f
    face, 2226, 2226f
    general appearance, 2221
    genitals, 2230–2231
    gestational age, 2213–2221
    habituation, 2235
    head, 2225–2226, 2225f, 2226f
    heart, 2229–2230, 2229f
    initial physical, 2212–2213, 2213t
    motor activity, 2235
    mouth, 2227–2228
    neck, 2228
    neurological status, 2233–2235
    nose, 2227
    orientation, 2235
    overview of, 2212
    respirations, 2229
    self-quieting activity, 2236
    skin characteristics, 2223–2224, 2224f
    subsequent physical, 2221–2233
    temperature, 2223
    timing of, 2212
    umbilical cord, 2230, 2230f
    variations, 2236
    weight and measurement, 2221–2223, 2222f
cardiopulmonary areas, 2194–2195
cardiovascular adaptations, 2194–2196
care planning, 2236
collaborative care, 2206–2212
culture and, 2199t
diagnosis, 2236
extrauterine life adaptations, 2191–2204
eyes, 2226–2227, 2227f
gastrointestinal adaptations, 2199–2200
general instructions for, 2245–2246
hematopoietic adaptations, 2196

hepatic adaptations
  breastfeeding and breast milk jaundice, 2198–2199
  carbohydrate metabolism, 2197
  coagulation, 2198
  conjugation of bilirubin, 2197–2198
  iron storage, 2196–2197
  physiological jaundice, 2198–2199
immunological adaptations, 2201–2202
initial
  Apgar scoring system, 2210–2211
  banking cord blood, 2211
  clamping the cord, 2211, 2211f
  identification and security, 2211–2212, 2212f
interventions
  cardiopulmonary function maintenance, 2239
  circumcision, 2240–2242, 2241f
  clear airway, 2237
  eye infection prevention, 2237–2238, 2238f
  family preparation for discharge, 2243–2247, 2244f, 2245t, 2246t
  first feeding, 2238–2239
  hydration and nutrition, 2239
  neonatal distress, 2238
  neutral thermal environment (NTE) maintenance, 2239
  parent teaching, 2243–2245, 2244f
  parent-newborn attachment, 2239, 2242–2243, 2243f, 2243t
  prevention of complications, 2240
  safety, 2240
  skin integrity, 2239–2240
  thermoregulation, 2237
  vital signs, 2237
  vitamin K deficiency, 2237, 2238f
neonatal mortality risk, 2206, 2206f
neurological and sensory-perceptual function, 2202–2204
Nursing Care Plan, 2248t
nursing process, 2212–2248
outcome evaluation, 2248
overview of, 2191
respiration
  assessment, 2229
  cardiopulmonary physiology, 2193
  characteristics of, 2194
  clearing fluid from lungs, 2192–2193
  factors opposing initiation of, 2193
  function maintenance, 2194
  initiation of, 2191–2193, 2192f
  oxygen transport, 2193–2194
  periodic breathing, 2194
temperature regulation, 2196
transitional circulation, 2194, 2195f
urinary tract adaptations, 2200–2201
Newborns
  active awake, 2203
  alert states, 2203
  auditory capacity, 2204
  behavioral capacities of, 2204
  bowel elimination, 274–275, 275f
  cardiac functioning, 1046
  care safety, 2247
  community-based care, 2247
  crying, 2203
  drowsy or semidozing, 2203
  drugs of abuse/addiction effects on, 1553t
  fluids and electrolytes, 343f

habituation, 2204
health screenings and immunization guidelines, 413t
heart rate, 2195
heat loss prevention in, 2197t
hypothermia in, 1441
infection and, 444
injury prevention due to motor vehicle crashes, 2000t
intracranial regulation in, 690
intrauterine experience, 2202
meconium, 2200
of mothers with diabetes, 2207t
of mothers with HIV/AIDS, 2208t
murmurs, 2195
neurological function characteristics, 2202
normal sleep-rest patterns in, 431–432
olfactory capacity, 2204
orientation, 2204
periods of reactivity, 2202
postterm, 2207t
with prenatal substance exposure, 2208t
preterm, 2249–2254
pseudomenstruation, 2201
reflexes of, 2203t
resting posture, 2216, 2216f
screening and immunization programs, 2247
self-quieting ability, 2204
sensory capacities of, 2204
skin in, 1447
sleep states, 2202–2203
stool samples, 2201f
swaddling, 2246, 2246f
tactile capacity, 2204
taste and sucking, 2204
thermoregulation in, 2197t
urinalysis values, 2201f
visual capacity, 2204
wide awake, 2203
Nicotine
  as addictive, 1546, 1548t
  defined, 1545
Nicotine acetylcholine receptor agonists, 1533t
Nicotine addiction
  adolescents and, 1549t
  assessment, 1548–1549, 1549t
  care planning, 1549–1550
  collaborative care, 1547
  complementary and alternative therapy, 1547
  defined, 1524t
  diagnosis, 1549
  epidemiology, 1546–1547
  interventions, 1550
  manifestations, 1547, 1548t, 1556t
  NRT and, 1547
  Nursing Care Plan, 1550–1551t
  nursing process, 1548–1550
  outcome evaluation, 1550
  overview of, 1545
  pathophysiology and etiology, 1546–1547
  prevention of, 1547
  psychosocial issues and, 1549
  risk factors, 1547
  smoking cessation programs and, 1547
  treatment, 1524t
Nicotine replacement therapy (NRT), 1533t, 1547
Nicotinic acid, 1117t
Nightingale, Florence, 2547, 2585–2586, 2586t

NIHL (noise-induced hearing loss), 1300
NIOSH (National Institute for Occupational Safety and Health), 2715, 2716
Nissen fundoplication, 229, 229f
Nitrates, 1075t, 1118
NIV (noninvasive ventilation), 979
NLN (National League for Nursing), 2626
Nociceptive pain, 154
Nociceptors, 153
Nocturia, 265, 621, 1149
Nocturnal emissions, 432, 1340
Nocturnal enuresis, 263
Nocturnal frequency, 265
Nocturnal sleep-related eating disorder (NSRED), 1836
Nodular basal cell carcinoma, 129–130
Nodular melanoma, 129
Noise-induced hearing loss (NIHL), 1300
Nolo contendere, 2664
Nominal group technique, 2421
Nondirective interviews, 2272
Nondisplaced fractures, 854t
Nonexudative macular degeneration, 1327, 1328t
Non-insulin-dependent diabetes mellitus. See Diabetes mellitus
Noninvasive ventilation (NIV), 979
Nonmaleficence, 1880, 2567
Nonmelanoma skin cancer
  basal cell, 129–130, 130f, 130t
  risk factors, 131–132
  squamous cell, 130, 130f
Non-Mendelian (multifactorial) inheritance, 1376
Nonnucleoside reverse transcriptase inhibitors, 471
Nonopioids
  ceiling effect, 163
  examples of, 162t
  mechanism of action, 151t
  mechanisms of action, 151t
  misconceptions, 164t
  nursing considerations, 151t
  therapeutic index, 163
Nonproliferative retinopathy, 749
Nonreassuring fetal status, 2138t
Nonrebreather masks, 972, 973f
Nonshivering thermogenesis (NST), 1438
Non-small-cell carcinomas, 104
Nonsteroidal anti-inflammatory drugs (NSAIDs)
  administration of, 164t
  ceiling effect, 163
  comfort and, 151t
  examples of, 162t
  mechanisms of action, 151t
  nursing considerations, 151t
  properties, 163
  side effects, 163
  in specific conditions
    asthma, 997
    inflammation, 643, 643t
    musculoskeletal disorders, 838t
    rheumatoid arthritis, 501, 502t
    ulcers, 677
  ulcers and, 680
Nonstress testing (NST)
  defined, 2086
  in fetus status evaluation, 2048
  procedure for, 2086
  results interpretation, 2086–2087, 2086f, 2087f

Nonunion fractures, 857
Nonverbal communication. *See also* Communication
  culture and, 2401–2402
  defined, 2400
  facial expression, 2402, 2402*f*
  gestures, 2402–2403
  illustrated, 2401*f*
  overview of, 2401–2402
  personal appearance, 2402
  posture and gait, 2402
Nonvoluntary euthanasia, 176
Norepinephrine, 1422, 1918–1919
Normal sinus rhythm (NSR), 1180*t*, 1182
Normal sleep-rest patterns
  in adolescents, 432, 432*t*
  in adults, 433
  in infants, 432
  in newborns, 431–432
  in older adults, 433
  overview of, 429–430
  in preschoolers, 432
  requirements, 431–433
  in school-age children, 432
  sleep factors and, 433–434
  sleep functions and, 431
  sleep physiology and, 430–431, 431*t*
  in toddlers, 432
Normative commitment, 2487*f*
Normothermia, 1249, 1423
Norton Scale, 1502
Norwood procedure, 1099*t*
Nose, newborn assessment, 2227
No-self theory, 1835
NPAs. *See* Nurse practice acts
NPD (narcissistic personality disorder), 1856*t*, 1859, 1863*t*
NPSG (National Patient Safety Goals), 2701, 2701*t*
NREM (non-rapid-eye-movement) sleep, 430, 431*f*, 431*t*
NRT (nicotine replacement therapy), 1533*t*, 1547
NRTIs (nucleoside reverse transcriptase inhibitors), 461
NSAIDs. *See* Nonsteroidal anti-inflammatory drugs
NSNA. *See* National Student Nurses Association
NSR (normal sinus rhythm), 1180*t*, 1182
NSRED (nocturnal sleep-related eating disorder), 1836
NST. *See* Nonstress testing
NST (nonshivering thermogenesis), 1438
NTE (neutral thermal environment), 1423, 2196
Nuclear family, 1709
Nuclear imaging. *See* Magnetic resonance imaging
Nucleation, 319
Nucleolus, 30
Nucleoside reverse transcriptase inhibitors (NRTIs), 461, 471
Nucleus, 30, 31*t*
Null cells, 441
Nulligravida, 2051*t*
Nullipara, 2051*t*
Numerical pain scales, 169
Nurse administrator, 2551
Nurse anesthetist, 2550
Nurse educator, 2551
Nurse entrepreneur, 2551
Nurse licensure compact, 2665

Nurse practice acts (NPAs)
  anatomy of, 2664*t*
  credentialing, 2666, 2666*f*
  defined, 2549, 2663
  enforcement of, 2664
  licensure, 2664–2665
  mandatory reporting of nurses in violation of, 2674–2675
  mutual recognition model, 2665, 2665*t*
  NCSBN's and, 2665, 2665*t*
  nurse licensure compact, 2665
  in nursing development, 2549
  nursing students, 2666
  overview of, 2663–2664
  relationship among, 2664*f*
  standards of practice, 2666
Nurse practitioner, 2550
Nurse researcher, 2551
Nurse-midwife, 2550–2551
Nurse-physician relationship
  collaboration, 2380*t*
  conflicts and, 2388
Nurses
  advance directives and, 2668
  allocation of resources and, 2608
  assaulted in workplace, 1978*t*
  in care coordination, 2460–2461
  as case managers, 2382–2383
  as collaborators, 2376, 2376–2377*t*, 2378*t*
  coping with loss of clients, 1761, 1761*f*
  delegation to, 2467
  expanded career roles for, 2550–2551
  generational strengths of, 2496*f*
  impaired, warning signs for, 1562*t*
  influence of types of, 2458*t*
  as learners, 2500
  legal protection guidelines, 2678*t*
  licensed practical, 2458
  registered, 2458
  response to death and dying, 1760–1761
  roles and functions of, 2550–2551, 2551*t*
  self-awareness, 1630*t*
  as teachers, 2500
  unlicensed assistive personnel, 2458
  values essential for, 2564
Nursing
  code of ethics, 2567–2569
  critical values of, 2539
  definitions of, 2548
  economics, 2465–2466
  evidence-based, 2584
  functional, 2600
  intraoperative, 1249, 1261–1272
  leadership, 2490*t*
  morality and, 1880–1881
  perioperative. *See* perioperative care
  postoperative, 1249, 1272–1276
  preoperative, 1249, 1254–1261
  primary, 2459, 2600
  recipients of, 2548
  settings for, 2548–2549, 2549*f*
  socialization to, 2539
  staffing practices in, 2688
  team, 2458–2459, 2600
  vacancy rate, 2465
Nursing care delivery systems
  functional nursing, 2600
  primary nursing, 2600
  team nursing, 2600
  types of, 2599–2600

Nursing Care Plans
  acute renal failure (ARF), 388–389*t*
  acute respiratory distress syndrome (ARDS), 989*t*
  adjustment disorder with depressed mood, 1807–1808*t*
  alcohol abuse, 1544*t*
  Alzheimer disease (AD), 1603–1604*t*
  anemia, 75*t*
  antepartum care, 2111*t*
  appendicitis, 648–649*t*
  arm fracture, 867–868*t*
  assault and homicide, 1982*t*
  asthma, 1004*t*
  attention-deficit/hyperactivity disorder (ADHD), 1687*t*
  benign prostatic hyperplasia (BPH), 291*t*
  bipolar disorders, 1815–1816*t*
  breast cancer, 84*t*
  burns, 1486–1487*t*
  cataracts, 1325–1326*t*
  celiac disease, 242–243*t*
  cellulitis, 564*t*
  cerebral palsy (CP), 1700*t*
  children's response to loss, 1756–1757*t*
  chronic kidney disease (CKD), 402–403*t*
  chronic obstructive pulmonary disease (COPD), 1016–1017*t*
  chronic pain, 173*t*
  cirrhosis, 789*t*
  colorectal cancer, 91*t*
  congenital heart defects, 1103–1104*t*
  coronary artery disease (CAD), 1128–1129*t*
  crisis, 1933–1934*t*
  deep venous thrombosis (DVT), 1137*t*
  depression, 1804*t*
  diabetes in children, 778–779*t*
  diabetes mellitus, 765*t*
  disseminated intravascular coagulation (DIC), 1143*t*
  dysrhythmias, 1197–1198*t*
  end-of-life care, 184*t*
  family health promotion, 1729–1730*t*
  family planning, 1392*t*
  fluid volume excess (FVE), 369–370*t*
  gallbladder disease, 655–656*t*
  gastroesophageal reflux disease (GERD), 230*t*
  glaucoma, 1325–1326*t*
  gonorrhea, 1416*t*
  Graves disease, 811–812*t*
  heart failure, 1161*t*
  hepatitis, 238–239*t*
  hip fractures, 874–875*t*
  HIV/AIDS, 479–480*t*
  hypertension, 1176*t*
  hypothermia, 1442*t*
  hypothyroidism, 816–817*t*
  intrapartum care, 2168*t*
  leukemia, 103*t*
  lung cancer, 111*t*
  menstrual dysfunction, 1405*t*
  morality, 1882*t*
  motor vehicle crashes (MVC), 2006*t*
  multiple sclerosis, 884–885*t*
  nephritis, 675–676*t*
  newborn care, 2248*t*
  nicotine addiction, 1550–1551*t*
  as nursing documentation, 2445
  obesity, 797–798*t*
  obstructive sleep apnea, 201–202*t*

older adult's response to loss, 1766–1767t
osteoarthritis, 893t
osteoporosis, 804–805t
otitis media, 583t
pancreatitis, 250–251t
Parkinson disease, 905t
peptic ulcer disease (PUD), 683t
perinatal loss, 1772t
personality disorders (PD), 1865–1866t
phobias, 1944t
pneumonia, 598t
postpartum care, 2189t
postpartum depression, 1827t
posttraumatic stress disorder (PTSD), 1949–1950t
preeclampsia, 1209–1210t
prematurity, 2260–2261t
prenatal substance exposure, 1558–1559t
pressure ulcers, 1504–1506t
prostate cancer, 118–119t
pulmonary embolism, 1216–1217t
pyloric stenosis, 254t
rape and rape-trauma syndrome, 1989–1990t
religion, 1889t
respiratory syncytial virus (RSV), 1023t
rheumatoid arthritis, 508t
schizophrenia, 1624–1625t
scoliosis, 851–852t
seizure disorders, 722–723t
sepsis, 604–605t
shock, 1233t
sickle cell disease, 126–127t
spinal cord injuries (SCI), 917–918t
spiritual distress, 1892t
stroke, 1246–1247t
substance abuse, 1571–1572t
suicide, 1997t
syphilis, 1417t
tuberculosis, 617t
type 1 diabetes, 765t
ulcerative colitis, 668t
undernutrition, 948–949t
urinary calculi, 331–332t
urinary tract infections (UTIs), 628t
wound healing, 1514t
Nursing clinical research
defined, 2586
ethical and legal issues, 2587
funding, 2586
implications for nursing practice, 2587–2588
informed consent and, 2587
participants, 2586–2587
qualitative, 2586
quantitative, 2586
scientific method, 2586, 2586t
Nursing databases, 2590–2591
Nursing diagnosis
client cues for, 2337f
common terms, 2335
components of, 2335–2336
decision tree, 2338f
defined, 2334
defining characteristics, 2336
developing, 2336–2338, 2337f
diagnostic labels, 2335–2336
etiology, 2336, 2336f
medical diagnosis versus, 2335
NANDA, 2366t

statement
avoiding errors in, 2340
common variations, 2339–2340
guidelines for writing, 2339
one-part, 2339
three-part, 2338–2339, 2339t
two-part, 2338, 2338t
writing, 2338–2340
types of, 2335
Nursing discharge/referral summaries, 2446–2447
Nursing ethics, 1878–1879
Nursing health history, 2273t
Nursing informatics
defined, 2632
health policy and, 2632
service delivery and, 2632–2634
Nursing interventions. See also Implementation
based on nursing diagnosis and etiology, 2345t
basis of, 2347
client participation in implementation of, 2348
collaborative, 2345
defined, 2344
dependent, 2345
examples of, 2345t, 2346t
implementing, 2347–2348
independent, 2345
priority, 2346t
redesigning, 2351
selection considerations, 2345–2346
types of, 2345–2346
understanding, 2347
writing, 2346
Nursing journals, 2591, 2591t
Nursing leaders, 2547–2548
Nursing plan of care. See also Nursing Care Plans
accessibility, 2354
clinical pathway, 2360–2362, 2361f, 2362f
column plan, 2356
concept map, 2356–2357, 2358–2359f
continuing, modifying, or terminating decision, 2350–2352
defined, 2354
five-column, for situational stress, 2356f
guidelines, 2354, 2355t
nursing process use in, 2355f
overview of, 2354
purposes of, 2354
standardized plan, 2357–2360, 2360f
summary, 2362
Nursing practice
accountability and, 2542
chain of command, 2549–2550, 2550f
competence, 2544
consumer demands and, 2540–2541
contemporary, 2548–2550
cost-conscious, 2466
economics and, 2540
emergency preparedness, 2614–2616
ethical issues in, 2575–2577
factors influencing, 2540–2542
healthcare systems, 2600
HIPAA compliance and, 2671t
information and telecommunications and, 2541–2542
injury prevention in, 2717–2718, 2718t
in managing care, 2459
nurse practice acts and, 2549

nursing clinical research implications for, 2587–2588
nursing definitions and, 2548
organizational chart, 2550, 2550f
patient rights, 2580
recipients of nursing and, 2548
science and technology and, 2541
settings for nursing and, 2548–2549, 2549f
Standards of Practice and, 2549
Nursing process
abuse, 1971–1974
in action, 2329f
acute renal failure (ARF), 386
acute respiratory distress syndrome (ARDS), 985–988
as adaptation of problem solving used by others, 2328
adjustment disorder with depressed mood, 1806–1807
age-related macular degeneration (AMD), 1329–1330
alcohol abuse, 1540–1544
Alzheimer disease (AD), 1600–1603
anemia, 71–74
antepartum care, 2099–2111
anxiety disorders, 1926
appendicitis, 646–648
assault and homicide, 1980–1981
assessment
in action, 2329f
of children, 2334t
data organization, 2331
defined, 2331
example, 2332–2333f, 2334f
focus, 2331
as overlapping phase, 2331f
purpose and activities, 2330t
asthma, 1001–1003
attention-deficit/hyperactivity disorder (ADHD), 1684–1686
autism spectrum disorder (ASD), 1692–1694
benign prostatic hyperplasia (BPH), 288–290
bipolar disorders, 1813–1815
bladder incontinence and retention, 299–304
bowel incontinence, 313–318
breast cancer, 81–83
burns, 1480–1485
cancer, 57–64
cardiomyopathy, 1080–1082
cataracts, 1309–1310
cellulitis, 563
cerebral palsy (CP), 1698–1699
children with type 2 DM, 775–778
children's response to loss, 1755–1756
chronic kidney disease (CKD), 399–402
chronic obstructive pulmonary disease (COPD), 1012–1016
as client centered, 2328
colorectal cancer, 89–90
communication, 2413–2417
confusion, 1607–1609
congenital heart defects, 1100–1103
conjunctivitis, 568–569
contact dermatitis, 1490–1492
coronary artery disease (CAD), 1124–1127
crisis, 1932–1933
death and dying, 1762

Nursing process (*continued*)
  decision making in, 2328
  deep venous thrombosis (DVT), 1135–1136
  defined, 2328
  depression, 1801–1803
  diabetes mellitus, 759–764
  diagnosis
    in action, 2329f
    common terms, 2335
    components of, 2335–2336
    decision tree, 2338f
    defined, 2334
    developing, 2336–2338
    formulating from client cues, 2337t
    NANDA and, 2334
    as overlapping phase, 2331f
    purpose and activities, 2330t
    statement, writing, 2338–2340, 2339t
    statement errors, avoiding, 2340
    types of, 2335
  disseminated intravascular coagulation (DIC),
      1140–1143
  documentation, 2445–2447, 2445f
  as dynamic, 2328
  dysrhythmias, 1194–1196
  electrolyte imbalance, 372–373
  end-of-life care, 182–183
  erectile dysfunction (ED), 1369–1370
  evaluation
    in action, 2329f
    checklist, 2351t
    defined, 2349
    developing, 2350
    drawing conclusions and, 2349–2350
    Nursing Care Plan decision and, 2350–2352
    outcomes and goals example, 2352t
    as overlapping phase, 2331f
    purpose and activities, 2330t
    relationship to other nursing process phases,
        2352–2353
    writing, 2350
  eye injuries, 1316–1317
  failure to thrive (FTT), 1702–1703
  family health promotion, 1727–1729
  family planning, 1391–1392
  family response to health alterations,
      1735–1737
  feeding and eating disorders, 1850–1851
  fibromyalgia, 193–194
  fluid volume deficit (FVD), 362–363
  fluid volume excess (FVE), 367–368
  fractures, 864–867
  gallbladder disease, 654–655
  gastroesophageal reflux disease (GERD),
      229–231
  glaucoma, 1323–1325
  health, wellness and illness, 415–419
  hearing impairment, 1304–1305
  heart failure, 1158–1160
  hepatitis, 236–238
  herniated discs, 844–845
  hypersensitivity, 491–494
  hypertension, 1173–1175
  hyperthermia, 1435–1436
  hyperthyroidism, 810–811
  hypothermia, 1440–1441
  hypothyroidism, 815–816
  implementation
    in action, 2329f
    components, 2346–2348

  defined, 2344
  nursing interventions and, 2344–2346,
      2345t, 2346t
  older adults, 2347t
  as overlapping phase, 2331f
  purpose and activities, 2330t
  relationship to other nursing process phases,
      2348
  skills necessary for, 2348
increase intracranial pressure (IICP),
    713–714
inflammatory bowel disease (IBD),
    665–668
influenza, 573–575
as interpersonal and collaborative, 2328
intrapartum care, 2136–2170
leukemia, 99–102
liver disease, 786–788
lung cancer, 109–110
menopause, 1396–1398
menstrual dysfunction, 1403–1405
metabolic acidosis, 15–16
metabolic alkalosis, 18–20
morality, 1881–1882
multiple sclerosis, 881–884
nephritis, 673–674, 675t
newborn care, 2212–2248
nicotine addiction, 1548–1550
in nursing plan of care, 2355f
obesity, 795–797
obsessive-compulsive disorder (OCD),
    1937–1938
older adult's response to loss, 1765–1766
osteoarthritis, 891–893
osteoporosis, 802–804
otitis media, 581–582
overview of, 2328–2329
pain, 168–173
pancreatitis, 249–250
Parkinson disease, 903–905
peptic ulcer disease (PUD), 680–682
perinatal loss, 1771–1772
peripheral neuropathy, 1334–1335
peripheral vascular disease (PVD),
    1201–1204
personality disorders (PD), 1862–1865
phases of, 2329, 2330t, 2331f
phobias, 1942–1943
planning
  in action, 2329f
  defined, 2341
  developing goals and, 2342
  long term goals, 2341–2342
  as overlapping phase, 2331f
  purpose and activities, 2330t
  short-term goals, 2341–2342
  writing goals and, 2342–2344
pneumonia, 593–597
postpartum care, 2178–2190
postpartum depression, 1824–1827
pregnancy-induced hypertension,
    1207–1209
prematurity, 2255–2260
prenatal substance exposure, 1556–1558
pressure ulcers, 1498–1504
in prioritizing care, 2364–2365
problem solving, 2323
professional practice and, 2658–2659
prostate cancer, 116–118
pulmonary embolism, 1214–1216

pyloric stenosis, 252–254
rape and rape-trauma syndrome, 1987–1988
religion, 1886–1888
respiratory acidosis, 22–24
respiratory alkalosis, 26–27
respiratory syncytial virus (RSV), 1021–1022
rheumatoid arthritis, 504–507
safety considerations across the life span,
    2713–2714
schizophrenia, 1620–1623
scoliosis, 849–850
seizure disorders, 720–721
sepsis, 603–604
sexually transmitted infections (STIs),
    1414–1416
shock, 1230–1232
sickle cell disease, 124–126
skin cancer, 135–137
spinal cord injuries (SCI), 915–917
stroke, 1242–1246
sudden infant death syndrome (SIDS),
    1026–1028
suicide, 1995–1996
systemic lupus erythematosus (SLE),
    515–518
teaching process comparison, 2510t
tuberculosis, 614–616
urinary calculi, 323–331
Nursing research, 2586
Nursing services, separate billing for, 2464
Nursing shortage
  addressing, 2542
  current, 2542
  economics and, 2465–2466
  ending cycle of, 2466
  factors contributing to, 2542t
Nursing students, 2666
Nursing transaction model, 1902, 1902f
Nurture, 1656
Nutrient density, 927
Nutrient metabolism, 2033
Nutrients
  carbohydrates, 927–929, 938t
  defined, 208, 790, 927, 1843
  essential, 927
  lipids, 929
  macronutrients, 927
  micronutrients, 927
  minerals, 930–931
  proteins, 929
  use overview schematic, 928f
  vitamins, 930
  water, 931
Nutrition
  for adolescents, 932–933
  alterations, 934–939
  alterations and therapies, 938t
  anthropometric measurements, 940–942, 942t
  assessment, 939–945, 943t
  assessment interview, 940t
  beliefs affecting, 1876–1877
  carbohydrates and, 927–929
  cellular regulation disorders and, 39
  for children, 932
  for children with type 1 DM, 771, 771t
  for children with type 2 DM, 774t
  collaborative interventions and therapies,
      946–948
  concepts related to, 935
  defined, 923

diagnostic tests, 944–945
digestion and, 222–226, 931–932
enteral, 947–948
fatigue and women and, 186t
food choice and, 924–926
food safety and, 926
genetic and lifespan considerations, 932–934
genetic considerations and nonmodifiable risk factors, 939
hunger and, 924, 924f
independent interventions and therapies, 946
for infants, 932, 932f
interventions and therapies, 945–948, 946t
intracranial regulation and, 708
lifespan and cultural considerations, 942–944, 945t
lipids (fats) and, 929
maternal, 2090–2092, 2091–2092t
mechanical ventilation and, 984–985
medications, 947t
metabolism and, 932
minerals and, 930–931
Mini Nutritional Assessment (MNA), 940, 941t
minimum enteral, 2253
modifiable risk factors, 939
nonpharmacologic therapy, 948
normal, 924–934
Nursing Care Plan, 948–949t
for older adults, 934
overnutrition and, 936
oxygenation and, 970
parenteral, 947–948
pharmacologic therapy, 948
postoperative nursing and, 1275
in preconception counseling, 1372
pregnancy and culture and, 2076t
prevention and, 939
proteins and, 929–930
screenings, 939
in specific conditions
acute renal failure (ARF), 383
alcohol abuse, 1543
anemia, 70
antepartum care, 2110–2111
burns, 1474, 1484
cancer, 60–61
celiac disease, 241
cerebral palsy (CP), 1699
chronic kidney disease (CKD), 398, 400
chronic obstructive pulmonary disease (COPD), 1015
colorectal cancer, 90
constipation, 310
coronary artery disease (CAD), 1125
diabetes mellitus, 757–758
gallbladder disease, 654–655
gastroesophageal reflux disease (GERD), 229
heart failure, 1156–1157
hepatitis, 236
HIV/AIDS, 478
hypertension, 1175
hyperthyroidism, 811
inflammatory bowel disease (IBD), 667–668, 667t
lactase deficiency, 244
leukemia, 102
liver disease, 785–786, 787–788
nephritis, 674

newborn care, 2239
obesity, 794, 936–939
osteoarthritis, 893
osteoporosis, 803
pancreatitis, 248, 249–250
peptic ulcer disease (PUD), 682
postpartum care, 2176–2177
premature newborns, 2252–2253, 2257
pressure ulcers, 1493, 1494, 1504
rheumatoid arthritis, 504
RSV/bronchiolitis, 1022
short bowel syndrome, 244
substance abuse, 1570
systemic lupus erythematosus (SLE), 516
wound healing, 1509, 1512
surgery and, 948
tissue integrity and, 1461
undernutrition and, 936, 937t
vitamins and, 930
water and, 931
Nutritional anemias, 66–68, 71t
Nutritional status, 926–927
Nystagmus, 1286t

O

Obesity
assessment, 796
behavior modification and, 794
blood pressure and, 1046
as cancer risk factor, 47
care planning, 796
in childhood and adolescence, 933, 946t
in children
culture and, 773t
evidence-based interventions to reduce, 775t
increase in, 773t
as public health issue, 791
classifications by BMI, waist circumference, 792t
collaborative care, 793–795
complications of, 792
as coronary artery disease risk factor, 1110
culture and, 945t
defined, 727, 790
diagnosis, 796
diagnostic tests, 793
exercise and, 794, 796
genetic considerations and nonmodifiable risk factors, 731
as health risk, 939
health-related problems associated with, 793t
hypertension and, 1167
interventions, 796–797
lower body, 791
manifestations, 791–792, 792t
metabolic syndrome and, 792
morbid, 792
Nursing Care Plan, 797–798t
nursing process, 795–797
nutrition and, 794
in older adults, 934
osteoarthritis and, 890
outcome evaluation, 797
overview of, 790
pathophysiology and etiology, 790–791
pharmacologic therapy, 793–794
prevalence of, 729, 936–939
prevention of, 731

risk factors, 791
satiety and, 791
self-esteem and, 797
surgery and, 794–795, 795f
Type 2 diabetes and, 727
upper body, 791
weight loss and, 796–797
Object performance, 1665t
Objective data, 2270
Objective family burden, 1731
Objective Opiate Withdrawal Scale (OOWS), 1569
Obligatory losses, 340
Oblique fractures, 855t
Observational learning, 2504
Observational pain scales, 169
Obsessions
commonly occurring, 1936t
defined, 1935
Obsessive-compulsive disorder (OCD)
adaptive coping, 1938t
assessment, 1937
assessment interview, 1938t
care planning, 1937–1938
characteristics of, 1856t
in childhood and adolescence, 1935t
collaborative care, 1936–1937
as coping alteration, 1907
defined, 1909t, 1935
diagnosis, 1937
diagnostic tests, 1937
guidelines for treatment, 1937
interventions, 1909t, 1938
lifespan considerations, 1935t
manifestations, 1909t, 1935, 1936t
nonpharmacologic therapy, 1937
nursing process, 1937–1938
OCPD versus, 1859
outcome evaluation, 1938
overview of, 1935
pathophysiology and etiology, 1935
pharmacologic therapy, 1937
risk factors, 1935
schizophrenia and, 1615–1616
Obsessive-compulsive personality disorder (OCPD), 1859, 1935
Obsessive-compulsive symptoms (OCS), 1616
Obstetric conjugate, 2013
Obstructive shock, 1224, 1226t
Obstructive sleep apnea (OSA), 195, 429
Occiput, 2114
Occupation
assault and homicide and, 1977–1978
as cancer risk factor, 46
Occupational exposure, 551
Occupational Safety and Health Administration (OSHA)
defined, 2715
in discarding used needles, 2623f
guideline enforcement, 2715
primary functions of, 2623, 2716
standards, 2716
whistleblowing and, 2673
in workplace safety, 2715–2716
Occupational therapy
multiple sclerosis and, 881
Parkinson disease and, 901
rheumatoid arthritis and, 504
stroke and, 1242
OCD. *See* Obsessive-compulsive disorder
OCS (obsessive-compulsive symptoms), 1616

Offices of emergency medical services (OEMSs), 2623–2624
Older adults
  abuse or neglect of, 2674, 2674t
  acid-base imbalances in, 10
  acute myocardial infarction in, 1111t
  anxiety disorders in, 1920
  appendicitis in, 646
  assessment of
    accuracy of health history, 2296–2297
    circumstances, 2294
    environment, 2296, 2298t
    functional evaluation, 2297
    instruments of evaluation, 2295–2296t
    lifestyle and health considerations, 2297
    minimum data set, 2297–2298
    social history, 2297
    underlying principles, 2294
  blood pressure assessment in, 1067t
  body temperature in, 1428t
  bowel elimination in, 275
  burns in, 1473, 1483t
  cellulitis in, 562
  cognitive changes in, 1577–1578
  communication with, 2414t
  constipation in, 307–308, 934
  dehydration in, 359
  dehydration risk factors and symptoms
      in, 356t
  depression assessment in, 1802
  depression in, 1801t
  diabetes in, 760
  digestive system in, 209–210
  documentation in long-term care for, 2447
  dysrhythmias in, 1179t
  epilepsy in, 716t
  factors affecting health promotion in, 416t
  fall prevention for, 857t
  falls, 2713, 2713f
  family with, 1726
  fibromyalgia in, 160
  fluid volume deficit in, 357, 359, 362t
  fluids and electrolytes in, 344, 344t
  functional decline prevention in, 2714t
  functional incontinence and, 301t
  growth and development, 1671
  health and independence assessments
      for, 1651f
  health promotion and, 412t
  health screenings and immunization guidelines
      and, 414t
  herniated discs in, 842
  hypothermia in, 1441
  immune system in, 445
  implementation phase and, 2347t
  inflammation in, 641
  injury prevention due to motor vehicle crashes
      for, 2000t
  intracranial regulation in, 690
  loss among, 1765t
  mobility and, 892
  motor vehicle crashes (MVC) and, 1999
  multiple sclerosis in, 879t
  musculoskeletal changes in, 821–822
  neurological system assessment in, 707t
  normal sleep-rest patterns in, 433
  nutrition for, 934
  obesity in, 934
  oral health in, 428, 428t
  oral hydration in, 360

  pain in
    chronic, 160t
    disorders linked to, 160t
    management barriers, 160
    perception and behavior, 158t, 159
    quality of life and, 160
  perioperative care and, 1256t
  pharmacologic therapy for mood disorders,
      1794t
  physical changes, 1673t
  pneumonia in, 590
  polypharmacy in, 934
  preoperative assessment of, 1260t
  pulse assessment in, 1065t
  renal failure in, 392t
  respiratory system in, 965t
  rheumatoid arthritis in, 497t
  safety, 2712–2713
  self-report scales, 1787
  sepsis in, 602
  sexual development and, 1342t, 1343–1344
  skin in, 1448
  sleep and, 196
  spiritual development in, 1874t
  stress and coping in, 1912
  subcutaneous tissue in, 1448
  substance abuse in, 1522, 1568t
  suctioning, 970t
  thermoregulation in, 1423
  thirst dysregulation in, 934
  tuberculosis in, 610–611, 610t
  urinary elimination in, 263
  urinary tract infections (UTIs) in, 621,
      622, 623
  wound healing in, 1509
  xerostomia in, 934
Older adult's response to loss
  assessment, 1765–1766
  care planning, 1766
  collaborative care, 1765
  complicated grief, 1764
  diagnosis, 1766
  factors affecting grieving process, 1764
  interventions, 1766
  lifespan and cultural considerations,
      1764–1765
  manifestations, 1764–1765
  mental health concerns and, 1765t
  nonpharmacologic therapy, 1765
  Nursing Care Plan, 1766–1767t
  nursing process, 1765–1766
  outcome evaluation, 1766
  overview of, 1763
  pathophysiology and etiology,
      1763–1764
  pharmacologic therapy, 1765
  response to grief, 1764
Olfactory stimuli, 1278
Oligodendrocytes, 876
Oligomenorrhea, 1400
Oliguria, 264, 376
Omalizumab, 491
Omega-3 fatty acids, 1797
Oncogenes, 45
Oncological emergencies
  hematological, 49–50
  metabolic, 49
  space-occupying lesions, 50
Oncology, 42
Oncotic pressure, 338, 364

One-part nursing diagnosis statement, 2339
Online administration tools, 2642
Online client medical information, 2642
Online consumer medical information,
      2641–2642
Online health information, 2508
"On-off" effect, 898
Oogenesis, 2020
OOWS (Objective Opiate Withdrawal Scale), 1569
Open awareness, 183
Open fractures, 854t
Open reduction and internal fixation (ORIF),
      860, 860f
Open-angle glaucoma, 1319, 1320t
Open-ended questions, 2274, 2274t
Operative sterilization, 1386
Ophthalmia neonatorum, 565
Opiates
  abuse of, 1564
  defined, 1563–1564
  types of, 1566t
Opioid analgesics, 643t
Opioid antagonists, 1533t
Opioids
  addiction to, 166–167, 167t
  comfort and, 151t
  examples of, 162t
  excretion of, 166
  full agonists, 164–165
  mechanisms of action, 151t
  mixed, 162t, 165
  nursing considerations, 151t
  for pain management, 164–167
  side effects, 164–167, 165t
  strong, 162t
  tolerance to, 166, 167t
  trauma and, 1963t
  weak or partial, 162t, 164
Opportunistic infections
  candidiasis, 463
  defined, 438, 463
  mycobacterium avium complex (MAC), 463
  pneumocystis jiroveci pneumonia (PCP), 463
  tuberculosis, 463
Opportunistic pathogens, 522
Oppression, 1637
Optimism, 1928, 2492
OPTN (Organ Procurement and Transplantation
      Network), 2608
Oral cavity, 424
Oral cholecystogram, 651
Oral health. See also Health, wellness and
      illness; Teeth
  in adolescents and adults, 428
  assessment, 424–426
  assisting clients with, 428
  care planning, 427
  in children, 425t
  clients at risk, 425
  common problems of the mouth, 426t
  dental caries and, 424
  diagnosis, 426–427
  gingiva and, 424
  gingivitis and, 426
  hygiene assessment interview, 425
  in infants, 427, 427t
  interventions, 427–429, 427t, 428t
  lifespan considerations, 424
  nursing process, 424–429
  in older adults, 428, 428t

outcome evaluation, 429
overview of, 424
periodontal disease and, 424
plaque and, 425–426
in preschoolers, 427–428
pyorrhea and, 426
in school-age children, 427–428
special needs, 428
tartar and, 426
in toddlers, 427, 427t
tooth decay prevention and, 427t
Oral rehydration, 360–361
Oral thermometers, 1427f
Oral-genital sex, 1346
Orchiectomy, 115
Organ Procurement and Transplantation Network (OPTN), 2608
Organ transplantation, 2573
Organizational charts, 2550, 2550f
Organizational commitment, 2486
Organizing, 2475
Organizing data, 2282
Orgasmic disorders, 1349–1350, 1352t
Orgasmic phase, sexual response cycle, 1346–1348, 1347t
Orientation
    in newborn assessment, 2235
    newborns, 2204
    in professional development, 2528–2529
ORIF (open reduction and internal fixation), 860, 860f
Orlistat (Xenical), 793
Oropharyngeal airways, 983, 983f
Orthopnea, 365, 959, 960t, 1148
Orthopneic position, 1002
Orthostatic hypotension, 901, 1067–1068
Orthotic devices, 504
Ortolani maneuver, 2232
OSA (obstructive sleep apnea), 195, 429
OSHA. See Occupational Safety and Health Administration
Osmolality, 337, 351, 1227
Osmolar imbalances, 354
Osmosis, 337–338, 337f
Osmotic diuretics, 712t
Osmotic pressure
    colloid, 338, 364
    defined, 337–338
    interstitial, 364–365
Osteoarthritis
    arthroplasty and, 888
    arthroscopy and, 888
    assessment, 891
    Bouchard nodes, 886
    care planning, 891
    characterization, 825
    children and, 887t
    collaborative care, 887–891
    comfort promotion, 891–893
    complementary and alternative therapy, 891t
    complications of, 887
    culture and, 887t
    defined, 496, 824t, 886
    diagnosis, 891
    diagnostic tests, 887t
    evaluation areas, 893
    exercise and, 890, 891t
    Heberden nodes, 886
    home care, 890t
    hyaluronic acid injections and, 890t

interventions, 824t, 891–893
joint fusion and, 888
joint resurfacing and, 888
juvenile, 887t
manifestation comparison, 496t
manifestations, 824t, 887, 892–893t
nonpharmacologic therapy, 889–891
Nursing Care Plan, 893t
nursing process, 891–893
nutrition and, 893
obesity and, 890
osteophytes, 886
osteotomy and, 888
overview of, 886
pathophysiology and etiology, 886–887
pharmacologic therapy, 888–889
physical mobility optimization and, 893
prevention of, 887
risk factors, 887
sleep/rest and, 890
surgery, 888
Osteoblasts, 820
Osteoclast, 821
Osteodystrophy, 380
Osteomyelitis, 854
Osteophytes, 886
Osteoporosis
    assessment, 802
    bisphosphonates for, 802t
    care planning, 802–803
    collaborative care, 800–802
    defined, 729, 799
    diagnosis, 802
    diagnostic tests, 800–801
    dietary management for, 801
    drugs for, 802t
    exercise and, 803–804
    genetic considerations and nonmodifiable risk factors, 731
    healthy behaviors and, 804
    hormonal agents for, 802t
    injury prevention, 803
    interventions, 733, 803–804
    manifestations, 800
    modifiable risk factors, 799–800
    Nursing Care Plan, 804–805t
    nursing process, 802–804
    nutrition and, 803
    outcome evaluation, 804
    overview of, 799
    pain management, 803
    pathophysiology and etiology, 799–800
    pharmacologic therapy, 801–802
    physical therapy for, 801
    prevalence of, 729
    risk factors, 799–800
    spinal changes caused by, 801f
    unmodifiable risk factors, 799
Osteotomy, 888
Otitis externa, 576
Otitis interna, 576
Otitis media
    acute, 576
    assessment, 581
    care planning, 581
    caregiver support, 582
    in children, 581, 581f
    chronic, 576
    collaborative care, 578–580
    communication facilitation, 582

complementary and alternative therapy, 580t
defined, 576
diagnosis, 581
diagnostic tests, 579
diversity and culture, 577
education, 582
with effusion, 578f
interventions, 581–582
manifestations, 577–578, 580t
Nursing Care Plan, 583t
nursing process, 581–582
outcome evaluation, 582
overview of, 576
pain management, 582
pathophysiology and etiology, 576–577
pharmacologic therapy, 579–580
prevention, 577
risk factors, 577
serous, 576
surgery, 579
tympanic membrane, 576, 578f
types of, 576
vertigo and, 577
Otoscope, 577, 581
Ototoxic medications, 1300, 1300t
Outcome standards, 2686
Outcomes
    defined, 2341t
    evaluation example of, 2352t
    goals versus, 2341t
    management, 2685
Ovarian cycle, 2018, 2018f
Ovaries, 2030
Overdelegation, 2472
Overdose
    alcohol, 1539
    drug abuse, 1565–1567
Overflow incontinence, 299t
Overnutrition, 936, 2290
Overt conflicts, 2387
Ovulation
    defined, 2018
    postpartum changes, 2173
Ovulation method, 1379
Oxygen administration
    defined, 972
    delivery system summary, 973t
    with nasal cannula, 972, 972f
    with nonrebreather mask, 972, 973f
    with simple face mask, 972, 972f
    with Venturi mask, 972, 973f
Oxygen therapy
    in COPD, 1011
    in sepsis, 602
    in shock, 1229
Oxygen transport, 2193–2194
Oxygenation
    alterations, 957–961
    alterations and therapies, 960t
    assessment, 962–968, 963–964t
    assessment interview, 962
    breathing muscles inspection, 964t
    in cardiac functioning, 1046
    in children, 1046
    collaborative interventions and therapies, 970–973
    concepts related to, 958–959
    defined, 953
    diagnostic tests, 965–966, 967t
    disorders

Oxygenation (*continued*)
acute respiratory distress syndrome (ARDS), 974–985
asthma, 990–1005
chronic obstructive pulmonary disease (COPD), 1005–1018
respiratory syncytial virus (RSV), 1018–1024
sudden infant death syndrome (SIDS), 1024–1028
genetic considerations and nonmodifiable risk factors, 961
home care assessment, 1013*t*
inability, prevalence of, 961
independent interventions and therapies, 968–970
interventions and therapies
activities of daily living (ADLs), 970
activity monitoring, 969
deep breathing exercises, 968
nonpharmacologic therapy, 972–973, 973*f*, 973*t*
nutrition and, 970
pharmacologic therapy, 970–972
positioning, 968, 968*f*
secretion clearance, 969
smoking cessation, 968–969, 969*t*
suctioning, 969–970, 969*f*, 970*t*
lifespan considerations, 956–957, 965, 965*t*
modifiable risk factors, 961
nasal assessment, 963*t*
normal, 954–957
prevention and, 961
respiratory rate assessment, 963*t*
sickle cell disease and, 125
skin assessment and, 964*t*
thoracic cavity inspection, 963*t*
Oxytocin, 2034

P
P waves, 1072*t*, 1073*t*
Pacemakers
defined, 1190
function terminology, 1191*t*
illustrated, 1190*f*
pacing artifacts, 1191*f*
permanent, 1190–1191
safety, 1190*t*
temporary, 1190, 1191*t*
Pacifier thermometers, 1428*f*
PaCO$_2$
defined, 6
metabolic acid-base disorders and, 7
normal value, 6
PACs (premature atrial contractions), 1180*t*, 1183–1184
Pain. *See also* Acute pain; Chronic pain; Comfort
adults and, 159
assessment, 168–170, 169*f*
assumptions about, 682
body adaptation to, 157
in bowel elimination, 274
breakthrough, 156
cancer, 48–49
categories of, 155
causes of, 155
central, 156
characteristics of, 155

children and
behavioral responses, 157
management barriers, 159
memories, 158–159
misperceptions, 159*t*
perception and behavior, 158*t*
physiological considerations for, 157
rating, 152*f*
sensitization to, 158
tolerance, 158
client rights, 145
collaborative care
complementary and alternative medicine, 168
diagnostic tests, 162
non pharmacologic invasive therapies, 168
pharmacologic therapy, 162–167
surgery, 162
WHO three-step approach, 163
cultural responses to, 161*t*
death and dying and, 1759
defined, 143, 152
descriptors of, 143, 153
diagnosis, 170
duration, 143, 168
end-of-dose medication failure, 156
end-of-life care and, 181
etiology, 143, 154–156
expression and meaning of, 2157
factors affecting responses to
cultural and ethnic influences, 160–161, 161*t*
developmental stage, 157
environmental and social support, 161–162
meaning of pain, 161
previous experiences, 162
family, language of, 1732*t*
fibromyalgia and, 190, 193*t*
as fifth vital sign, 143
gate control theory, 154
history, 168
idiopathic, 156
incident, 156
intensity, 143, 152, 168
interventions and therapies, 167*t*, 171–172
labor and, 2127
lifespan and cultural considerations, 157–162
location, 152, 168
manifestations, 157–162, 167*t*
meaning of, 161
medications
analgesics, 162*t*
coanalgesics, 163, 167
drug abuse history and, 167*t*
nonopioids, 151*t*, 163–164, 164*t*
NSAIDs, 151*t*, 163–164, 164*t*
opioids, 151*t*, 164–167
in mobility assessment, 828–829
NANDA nursing diagnoses, 170
neonatal assessment, 170*t*
neuropathic, 154
nociceptive, 154
Nursing Care Plan, 173*t*
nursing process, 168–171
older adults and, 159–160, 160*t*
outcome evaluation, 171, 172
overview of, 152–153
past experience with, 162
pathophysiology and etiology, 153–457

perception physiology, 154*f*
peripheral pattern theory, 154
phantom, 156
pleuritic, 586
preoperative assessment, 1257
prevention, 157
psychogenic, 156
quality, 143, 152, 168
rating, 152*f*
receptors, 153
referred pain, 155, 155*f*
rest, 1199
risk factors, 156
sensation in children, 1291*t*
signals, 152
somatic, 155
specificity theory, 154
stimuli, types of, 153*t*
theories, 154
tissue integrity and, 1453*t*
types of, 154–156
uncontrolled, 157, 168
visceral, 155
Pain management
in acute burn stage, 1474
in appendicitis, 647–648
barriers, overcoming, 171*t*
barriers for older adults, 160
in burn injuries, 1482–1483
in colorectal cancer, 89
in congenital heart defects, 1102
in coronary artery disease (CAD), 1125–1126
in deep venous thrombosis (DVT), 1135
in disseminated intravascular coagulation (DIC), 1142
in drug-abusive clients, 167*t*
in fractures, 864, 866
in gallbladder disease, 654
Joint Commission standards of, 159*t*
in laparoscopic cholecystectomy, 653*t*
in lung cancer, 110
in menstrual dysfunction, 1404
in osteoporosis, 803
in otitis media, 582
in pancreatitis, 249
pediatric, barriers to, 159
in peptic ulcer disease (PUD), 681
in peripheral vascular disease (PVD), 1203
in prostate cancer, 117–118
in sickle cell disease, 125
in urinary calculi, 329–330
in urinary tract infections (UTIs), 626
Pain memory
in adults, 162
in children, 158–159
Pain rating scales
defined, 168–169
information assessment, 169–170
numerical, 169
observational or behavioral, 169
representation of experience, 170
using, 170
verbal descriptor, 169, 169*f*
Wong-Baker FACES, 169, 169*f*
Pain relief barriers, 156
Pain threshold, 159
Palliative care
defined, 177
domains of, 175*t*

pediatric, 177, 178t, 179t
providing, 177
selection at end of life, 175
Palliative Performance Scale, 2295t
Palliative procedures, 1096
Palliative surgery, 1261t
Pallidotomy, 898
Pallor, in mobility assessment, 829
Palpation
    axillary lymph nodes, 1359f
    Bartholin glands, 1360f
    body pressure areas, 1500
    breast, 1358f
    characteristics determined by, 2278
    costovertebral angle, 325f
    deep, 2278–2279, 2279f
    defined, 2278
    femoral arteries, 2229f
    kidneys, 328
    light, 2278, 2279f
    lymph nodes, 452, 452f
    male inguinal area, 1356t
    mass characteristics and, 2279t
    in oxygenation assessment, 962
    Skene glands, 1360f
    thoracic wall, 964t
    thyroid gland, 735t
Pancreas, pregnancy and, 2034
Pancreatitis. *See also* Digestion
    acute, 211–213, 246, 247, 247f
    assessment, 249
    chronic, 213, 246, 247, 249t
    client teaching, 250t
    collaborative care, 247–248, 249t
    complementary and alternative
        therapy, 249t
    defined, 211, 245
    diagnosis, 249
    diagnostic tests, 247
    fluid and electrolyte balance, 250
    interventions, 249
    laboratory tests, 248t
    manifestations, 213t, 247, 248t
    medications, 249t
    Nursing Care Plan, 250–251t
    nursing process, 249–250
    nutrition and, 248
    nutritional restoration, 249–250
    outcome and evaluation parameters, 250
    overview of, 245–246
    pain management, 249
    pathophysiology and etiology,
        246–247
    pharmacologic therapy, 248
    risk factors and prevention, 246–247
    surgery, 248
Pandemics, 570, 570t, 2609
Panic disorder. *See also* Anxiety disorders
    defined, 1908t, 1921
    incapacitation by, 1921–1922
    interventions, 1908t
    manifestations, 1908t
    schizophrenia and, 1615
Pannus tissue, 496
PaO$_2$, 6
PAP (pulmonary artery pressure) catheters, 1476
Pap smears, 468
Papilledema, 21
Paracentesis, 788
Parallel play, 1663

Paralysis
    cardiovascular problems, 911
    communication assessment and, 2414
    in mobility assessment, 829
    reproductive problems, 911
    types of, 911, 911f
    urinary and bowel problems, 911
Paraneoplastic syndromes, 48
Paranoia, 1611
Paranoid personality disorder (PPD), 1857t,
        1859, 1863t
Paraphrasing, 2430
Paraplegia, 911
Parasites
    culture and, 877t
    defined, 523
    pathogenic organisms, 530t
Parasomnias, 145, 195
Parathyroid, pregnancy and, 2034
Parent- teaching checklist, 2244f
Parent-child interaction, 1713
Parenteral nutrition
    complications of, 226
    defined, 224–225, 948
    glucose tolerance and, 225
    illustrated, 225f
    initiation of, 225
    use of, 948
Parenting
    authoritarian, 1717
    authoritative, 1717
    characteristics of attributes, 1717t
    defined, 1708
    discipline, 1717–1718
    indifferent, 1717
    limit setting, 1717–1718
    permissive, 1717
    styles, 1717, 1721–1722
Parent-newborn attachment
    facilitation of, 2239
    premature newborns and, 2258
    quieting activities and, 2243, 2243f
    strengthening, 2242–2243
Parents
    death of, 1752–1753
    provider collaboration, 1734t
Paresthesias
    chronic kidney disease and, 393
    defined, 393
    in mobility assessment, 829
    peripheral neuropathy and, 1331
Parkinson disease
    activities of daily living (ADLs) and,
        904–905
    assessment, 903
    care planning, 903
    cognitive deficits and, 897
    collaborative care, 898–901
    deep brain stimulation and, 898
    defined, 824t, 825–826, 895
    diagnosis, 903
    diagnostic tests, 898
    emotional changes and, 897
    evaluation of clients, 905
    exercise and, 901, 901t
    freezing and, 897
    independence and, 904–905
    injury prevention, 903–904
    interventions, 824–825t, 903–904
    lifespan and cultural considerations, 897

    manifestations, 824–825t, 896–897, 897t, 902t
    medications, 899t
    mobility and, 904
    motor symptoms, 896–897, 897t, 899t
    nonmotor symptoms, 897t
    nonpharmacologic therapy, 901
    Nursing Care Plan, 905t
    nursing process, 903–905
    occupational therapy and, 901
    overview of, 895
    pallidotomy and, 898
    parkinsonian gait, 897
    parkinsonism and, 897
    pathophysiology and etiology, 895–896
    pharmacologic therapy
        amantadine, 899t, 901
        anticholinergics, 899t, 900–901
        dopamine agonists, 899t, 900
        dopamine modifiers, 899t, 900
        levodopa, 898, 899t
        medications, 899t
        for nonmotor symptoms, 901
    physical therapy and, 901
    postural instability, 897
    prevention of, 896
    rigidity and, 897
    risk factors, 896
    sleep problems and, 897
    speech/language therapy and, 901
    surgery, 898
    thalamotomy and, 898
    tremors, 896–897
Parkinsonian gait, 897
Parkinsonism, 897
Paroxysmal, 1183
Paroxysmal nocturnal dyspnea, 1149
Paroxysmal supraventricular tachycardia (PSVT),
        1180t, 1184
Partial agonists, 162t, 164
Partial thromboplastin time (PTT), 1252t
Partial-thickness burns. *See also* Burns
    deep, 1468
    defined, 1467
    illustrated, 1468f
    manifestations, 1481t
    superficial, 1467–1468
Partial-thickness skin loss, 1496t
Pasero opioid-induced sedation scale (POSS),
        166, 166t
Passive acquired immunity, 2201
Passive behavior, 1789
Passive communicators, 2409, 2411, 2411t
Passive immunity, 450
Patch aortoplasty, 1099t
Patch tests
    contact dermatitis and, 1490
    defined, 490, 1490
    tissue integrity and, 1456
Patent airway, 956
Patent airway maintenance, 492, 986
Patent ductus arteriosus (PDA), 1084, 1084t, 2254
Pathogenic organisms, 530t
Pathogenicity, 522
Pathogens
    bloodborne, 545
    defined, 522
    infections and, 527–528
    opportunistic, 522
Pathologic fractures, 856t
Pathophysiology and etiology, 104–105

Patient Health Questionnaire (PHQ), 1587*t*
Patient portals, 2642
Patient Protection and Affordable Care Act
    (PPACA). *See* Affordable Care Act (ACA)
Patient responsibilities, 2580*t*
Patient rights
    Bill of Rights, 2579, 2579*t*
    defined, 2578
    Joint Commission's Speak Up program, 2578,
      2579*t*
    nursing practice, 2580
    overview of, 2578–2579
    protecting, 2579–2580
Patient Self-Determination Act (PSDA),
    2542, 2667
Patient-centered care, 2699–2700
Patients, 2548. *See also* Clients
Pattern of dependence, 1535
Pauciarticular arthritis, 499
PAWP (pulmonary artery wedge pressure), 1476
Payment sources, 2463
pCO$_2$, 1252*t*
PCP (phencyclidine), 1554, 1564, 1567*t*
PCP (primary care provider), 2628
PCR (percutaneous coronary revascularization),
    1120–1121, 1121*f*
PD. *See* Personality disorders
PDA (patent ductus arteriosus), 1084, 1084*t*, 2254
PDPI-R (Postpartum Depression Predictors
    Inventory-Revised), 1787, 1823–1824*t*
PDSA (Plan-Do-Study-Act), 2690, 2690*f*
PE. *See* Pulmonary embolism
Peak expiratory flow rate (PEFR), 966
Peck developmental tasks, 1652–1653
Pedagogy, 2502
Pedal (dorsalis pedis) pulse, 1063*f*, 1064
Pediatric clients. *See also* Children; Infants;
      Toddlers
    abuse, 1971
    advocating for, 2559*f*
    assessment of, 2289*t*
    asthma in, 991–992, 993
    blood pressure assessment in, 1067*t*
    cardiology alterations in, 1049
    celiac disease in, 242
    cellular regulation and, 38–39, 38*f*
    daily maintenance fluid requirements for, 597*t*
    dehydration in, 359*t*
    digestion in, 219*t*
    encopresis in, 317–318
    end-of-life care for, 177–180, 178*t*, 179*t*, 180*t*
    ethical dilemmas and, 2575*t*
    fever in, 1424
    fluid volume deficit in, 362
    glaucoma in, 1318–1319
    HIV/AIDS in
      manifestations, 464–467, 467*t*
      testing, 468
    immunity in, 444–445
    increased intracranial pressure (IICP) in, 710
    infectious and communicable diseases in, 532,
      533–542*t*
    inflammation in, 636
    inflammatory bowel disease (IBD) in, 661, 666*t*
    malabsorption in, 661
    Nursing Care Plan for type 1 diabetes mellitus,
      778–779*t*
    palliative care for, 177, 178*t*, 179*t*
    perioperative care for, 1256*t*
    pneumonia in, 597*t*

preoperative preparation for, 1256*t*
sickle cell disease in, 122
Pediatric differences, 343
Pediatric illness
    family and, 1733–1735
    family-centered care, 1733–1734,
      1733–1734*t*
    parent-provider collaboration, 1734*t*
Pediatric medical errors, reducing, 2677–2678
Pedigree
    autosomal dominant, 1376, 1376*f*
    autosomal recessive, 1376, 1377*f*
    defined, 1376
    screening, 1391, 1391*f*
    X-linked recessive, 1377, 1377*f*
PEEP (positive end-expiratory pressure), 979,
    980, 981*t*
Peer review, 2685
PEG (polyethylene glycol), 310*t*
Pelvic adequacy assessment, 2054
Pelvic bones, 2012–2013, 2012*f*
Pelvic division, 2013–2014, 2014*f*
Pelvic floor
    defined, 2013
    in labor, 2120
    muscles of, 2013*f*
Pelvic floor muscle (Kegel) exercises, 295, 295*t*,
    2071, 2071*f*
Pelvic inlet, 2013
Pelvic outlet, 2014
Pelvic planes, 2015*f*
Pelvic tilt, 2069, 2070*f*
Pelvic types
    android pelvis, 2014–2015, 2016*f*
    anthropoid pelvis, 2015, 2016*f*
    Caldwell-Moloy classification, 2014–2016,
      2016*f*
    gynecoid pelvis, 2014, 2016*f*
    platypelloid pelvis, 2015, 2016*f*
Pelvis
    android, 2014–2015, 2016*f*
    anthropoid, 2015, 2016*f*
    false, 2013
    female, illustrated, 2015*f*
    gynecoid, 2014, 2016*f*
    platypelloid, 2015, 2016*f*
    true, 2013
Penetrating eye injuries, 1312, 1313*t*, 1316
Penetrating trauma, 1956
Penicillin-resistant *S. pneumoniae* (PRSP), 532
Penile implants, 1368–1369, 1369*f*
Penumbra, 1234
PEP (Putting Evidence into Practice), 2592
Peplau, Hildegard, 1902
Peptic ulcer disease (PUD)
    assessment, 680
    care planning, 680
    collaborative care, 679–680
    common sites, 677*f*
    defined, 677
    diagnosis, 680
    diagnostic tests, 679
    fluid volume balance and, 681
    gastric outlet obstruction and, 678
    hemorrhage and, 678
    home care for, 682*t*
    interventions, 681–682
    manifestations, 678–679, 679*f*
    manifestations of complications, 678*f*
    nonpharmacologic therapy, 680

Nursing Care Plan, 683*t*
nursing process, 680–682
nutrition and, 682
outcome evaluation, 682
overview of, 677
pain management, 681–682
pathophysiology and etiology, 677–678
perforation and, 678
pharmacologic therapy, 679–680
prevention of, 678
rest and, 682
risk factors, 677–678
steatorrhea, 679
surgery, 679
treatment for complications, 681*t*
Zollinger-Ellison syndrome, 678–679
Peptic ulcers, 677, 677*f*
Perceived loss, 1742
Perception, 1278
Perceptions
    checking, 2430
    defined, 2406
Percussion
    in COPD, 1011
    defined, 592, 2279
    direct, 2279–2280
    illustrated, 593*f*
    indirect, 2280, 2280*f*
    in oxygenation assessment, 962
    sounds and tones, 2280*t*
Percutaneous coronary revascularization (PCR),
    1120–1121, 1121*f*
Percutaneous fine-needle aspiration biopsy, 247
Perforating eye injuries, 1312, 1313*t*, 1316
Perforation
    of appendix, 644
    defined, 644
    in peptic ulcer disease (PUD), 678
Performance improvement, 2685
Perfusion
    alterations, 1049–1054
    alterations and therapies, 1052–1053*t*
    assessment
      apical impulse, 1056–1058*t*
      blood pressure, 1064–1070
      cardiac rate and rhythm, 1059*t*
      heart sounds, 1059–1061*t*
      inspection, 1055–1056, 1056*f*
      interview, 1068–1070, 1069*t*
      landmarks for, 1055, 1055*f*
      murmur, 1061–1062*t*
      pulse, 1062–1064, 1063*f*, 1064*t*, 1065*t*
    blood pressure and, 1045–1046
    cardiac cycle and, 1040–1042
    circulation and, 1036–1040
    collaborative interventions and therapies, 1074
    concepts related to, 1050–1051
    coronary artery disease (CAD) and, 1127
    deep venous thrombosis (DVT) and, 1136
    diagnostic tests, 1070
    electrocardiogram and, 1071–1073*t*
    genetic and lifespan considerations,
      1046–1049
    genetic considerations and nonmodifiable risk
      factors, 1051–1054, 1054*t*
    heart chambers/valves and, 1033–1036
    heart conduction system and, 1042–1044, 1043*f*
    heart wall layers and, 1032–1033, 1033*f*
    independent interventions and therapies,
      1070–1073

interventions and therapies, 1070–1075
landmarks for assessment, 1055f
medications, 1074–1075t
modifiable risk factors, 1054
normal, 1032–1049
pericardium in, 1032
physiological process, 1031
prevalence and, 1051
prevention and, 1054
pulse and, 1044–1045
screenings, 1054–1055
ventilation relationship, 1211f
Pericarditis, 1113
Pericardium, 1032
Perimenopausal period, 1394, 1395t
Perinatal loss
assessment, 1771
care planning, 1771
changes in fetal activity, 1769
collaborative care, 1770–1771
defined, 1768, 2139t
diagnosis, 1771
diagnostic tests, 1770
disenfranchised grief, 1769
grief, 1769
interventions, 1771–1772
lifespan and cultural considerations,
    1769–1770, 1770t
manifestations, 1769–1770, 1770t
miscarriage, 1768
nonpharmacologic therapy, 1771
Nursing Care Plan, 1772t
nursing process, 1771–1772
outcome evaluation, 1772
overview of, 1768
pathophysiology and etiology, 1768–1769
pharmacologic therapy, 1770–1771
prevention of, 1768–1769
risk factors, 1768
stillbirth, 1768
therapies, 2139t
Perinatal risk for injury, 2708–2709, 2709t
Perineal care, 2184t
Perineal prostatectomy, 115
Perineal trauma, 2132
Perineum
cleansing, 2166
in intrapartum assessment, 2144t
postpartum changes, 2173
Periodic breathing, 2194
Periodontal disease, 424, 750
Perioperative care
concepts related to, 1250
defined, 1249
diagnostic tests, 1251, 1252–1253t
interdisciplinary team, 1251
intraoperative. See intraoperative nursing
introduction to, 1251–1254
lifespan and development considerations, 1254
lifespan considerations, 1256t
medications, 1254, 1255t
for older adults, 1256t
pediatric, 1256t
postoperative. See postoperative nursing
preoperative. See preoperative nursing
protocols and precautions, 1251–1254
safety and, 2698t
time-out, 1251
universal protocol, 1251
verification hand-off report, 1251–1254, 1253t

Perioperative nurses, 1251
Perioperative nursing data sets (PNDS), 2644
Periorbital ecchymosis, 1314t
Peripartum cardiomyopathy, 1078, 2049
Peripheral nervous system
cranial nerves, 689, 689t
defined, 688
reflexes and, 689
spinal nerves, 689, 690f
Peripheral neuropathies
assessment, 1334–1335
care planning, 1335
in children, 1333t
collaborative care, 1333–1334
comfort promotion and, 1335
defined, 749, 1331
diagnosis, 1335
diagnostic tests, 1333
injury prevention and, 1335
interventions, 1281t, 1335
manifestations, 1281t, 1332t, 1333
mononeuropathies and, 749–750, 1331
nonpharmacologic therapy, 1334
nursing process, 1334–1335
outcome evaluation, 1335
overview of, 1331
pathophysiology and etiology, 1331–1332
pharmacologic therapy, 1333, 1334t
polyneuropathies and, 749, 1331
prevention of, 1332
risk factors, 1332
surgery, 1333
Peripheral obesity, 791
Peripheral pattern theory, 154
Peripheral perfusion, 1135–1136
Peripheral pulse, 1044
Peripheral vascular compromise, 1471
Peripheral vascular disease, 748–749
Peripheral vascular disease (PVD)
assessment, 1202
care planning, 1202
client teaching, 1201–1202, 1202t
collaborative care, 1200–1201
complementary and alternative therapy, 1201
defined, 1198
diagnosis, 1202
diagnostic tests, 1200–1201
home care, 1203t
interventions
    activity encouragement, 1204
    foot and leg care, 1202t
    pain management, 1203
    skin integrity, 1203
    tissue perfusion, 1202–1203
manifestations of, 1199–1200, 1199t
nonpharmacologic therapy, 1201
nursing process, 1201–1204
outcome evaluation, 1204
overview of, 1198–1199
pathophysiology and etiology, 1199
pharmacologic therapy, 1201
risk factors, 1199
surgery, 1201
Peripheral vascular resistance, 1045, 1163
Peristalsis, 273
Peritoneal dialysis, 272–273, 383, 385–386, 385f
Peritonitis, 644
Permissive parents, 1717
Pernicious anemia, 66
Perseveration, 1613

Persistent bacteriuria, 627
Persistent depressive disorder, 1778, 1800, 1800t
Persistent vegetative state, 694
Personal appearance, 2402
Personal distance, 2407
Personal identity, 1832–1833
Personal knowing, 2306
Personal protective equipment
bagging, 548
blood pressure equipment, 548
dishes, 548
disposable equipment and supplies, 548
disposable needles, syringes and sharps, 548
eyewear, 548
face masks, 546–548
gloves, 546
gowns, 546
laboratory specimens, 548
linens, 548
nondisposable equipment and supplies, 548
Personal responsibility, 2689
Personal space
defined, 2406
illustrated, 2408
intimate distance, 2407
personal distance, 2407
public distance, 2408
social distance, 2408
Personality
adolescents, 1669
defined, 1649, 1852
development of, 1649
infants, 1662
preschool children, 1666
school-age children, 1668
toddlers, 1663–1664
Personality disorders (PD)
assessment, 1862–1864
boundaries and, 1865, 1866t
care planning, 1864
cognitive-behavioral therapy, 1861–1862
collaborative care, 1860–1862
common traits, 1855
complementary and alternative therapy, 1862
defined, 1838, 1852
detachment, 1855
diagnosis, 1864
diagnostic tests, 1860–1861
dialectical behavioral therapy, 1862
disinhibition, 1855
DSM-5 diagnostic criteria for, 1855t
family theory, 1854
family-focused therapy, 1862
forms of, 1838
genetics and, 1853
group therapy, 1862
impulsiveness and, 1852
interventions, 1864–1865
interventions and treatments, 1839t
intrapersonal factors, 1853
lifespan and cultural considerations, 1860
manifestations, 1839t
    antisocial personality disorder (ASPD),
        1855, 1856t, 1863t
    avoidant personality disorder (APD),
        1855, 1856t, 1863t
    borderline personality disorder (BPD),
        1855–1857, 1856t, 1858t, 1859t, 1863t
    dependent personality disorder (DPD), 1856t,
        1857–1858, 1863t

Personality disorders (PD) (*continued*)
histrionic personality disorder (HPD), 1856t, 1858–1859, 1863t
narcissistic personality disorder (NPD), 1856t, 1859, 1863t
obsessive-compulsive disorder (OCD), 1856t, 1859, 1863t
overview of, 1854–1855
paranoid personality disorder (PPD), 1857t, 1859, 1863t
schizoid personality disorder, 1857t, 1859–1860, 1863t
schizotypal personality disorder, 1857t, 1860, 1864t
therapies and, 1863–1864t
manipulation and, 1852
narcissism and, 1852
negative affectivity, 1855
neurobiological factors, 1853
Nursing Care Plan, 1865–1866t
nursing process, 1862–1865
outcome evaluation, 1865
overview of, 1852
pathophysiology and etiology, 1852–1854
pharmacologic therapy, 1861
prevention of, 1854
psychotherapy, 1861–1862
psychoticism, 1855
religious beliefs and, 1861t
risk factors, 1854
safety and, 1865
schema-focused therapy, 1862
sociocultural factors, 1853–1854
therapeutic relationship and, 1865
vicious cycle of, 1838f
Personality traits, 1852
Person-role conflict, 1834
Pertussis (whooping cough), 537–538t
Pessimism, 2492–2493
PFTs. *See* Pulmonary function tests
PGD (preimplantation genetic diagnosis), 1390
PGD (prolonged grief disorder), 1743
pH
defined, 3
hydrogen ion concentration and, 3–4
maintenance systems, 4
metabolic alkalosis and, 18
monitoring, 228
normal, 4
as perioperative diagnostic test, 1252t
respiration and, 7
Phaenicia sericata, 1497
Phagocytosis, 443, 1508
Phantom pain, 156
Pharmacologic therapy, 1532
Phase of mutual regulation, 1819
Phencyclidine (PCP), 1554, 1564, 1567t
Phenotypes, 1376, 1536
Phenylketonuria (PKU), 2208t
PHI (protected health information), 2438, 2670
Philadelphia chromosome, 94, 94f
Phimosis, 1356t
Phobias
active avoidance, 1940–1941
agoraphobia, 1940–1941, 1940f, 1941t
assessment, 1942–1943
assessment interview, 1943
care planning, 1943
cognitive behavior techniques in applied to clients with, 1942t

collaborative care, 1941–1942
deep breathing and, 1943t
defined, 1908t, 1939
diagnosis, 1943
interventions, 1908t, 1943
manifestations, 1908t
nonpharmacologic therapy, 1942
Nursing Care Plan, 1944t
nursing process, 1942–1943
one-to-one supervision and, 1943
outcome evaluation, 1943
overview of, 1939
pathophysiology and etiology, 1939–1940
pharmacologic therapy, 1941–1942
progressive relaxation and, 1943t
risk factors, 1940
social anxiety disorder, 1941, 1941t
specific, 1940, 1940t, 1941t
Phosphate (PO₄⁻), 342, 342t
Phosphodiesterase inhibitors, 1075t, 1156t
Phosphoric acid, 4
Phosphorus, function in the body, 930–931
Photophobia, 1319
PHQ (Patient Health Questionnaire), 1587t
Physical activity
COPD and, 1015t
defined, 421
hypertension and, 1169
postoperative nursing and, 1275
Physical attending, 2426, 2427t
Physical comfort, 141
Physical dependence, 1525t
Physical examination
in preconception counseling, 1372
in teaching plans, 2513
Physical fitness and exercise
activity tolerance, 421
activity-exercise pattern, 420
exercise
aerobic, 421
anaerobic, 421
benefits of, 421–423, 422t
defined, 421
isokinetic, 421
isometric, 421
isotonic, 421
types of, 421
functional strength, 421
overview of, 420
physical activity, 421
Physical growth and development
adolescents, 1668–1669
infants, 1659
preschool children, 1664
school-age children, 1666–1667
toddlers, 1662
Physical inactivity, as coronary artery disease risk factor, 1110
Physical restraints, 2704
Physical therapy
multiple sclerosis and, 881
Parkinson disease and, 901
rheumatoid arthritis and, 504
stroke and, 1242
Physical violence
abuse, 1954–1955, 1956f
age and, 1957
alterations and manifestations, 1954–1958
gender and, 1957

genetic considerations and nonmodifiable risk factors, 1957
prevalence of, 1956–1957
trauma, 1955–1956
Physician orders, implementing, 2677
Physician shortages, 2606
Physiological anemia of infancy, 69, 2196
Physiological anemia of pregnancy, 1047, 2031
Physiological development, abuse and, 1967
Physiological jaundice, 2198–2199
Physiological needs, in nursing, 2308–2310
Piaget's theory
cognitive development, 1653–1654
defined, 1576
phases of cognitive development, 1576t, 1653–1654, 1654t
thought characteristics, 1665t
Pica, 1836, 2095
PICOT
defined, 2589
example questions, 2589t
foreground questions, 2589t
PIE documentation model, 2442
Pigmented basal cell carcinoma, 130
Pill-rolling, 897
Pinpointing, 2430
Pitch, 2280–2281
Pitfalls, 2370
Pitting edema
defined, 379t
grading, 368f
Pituitary, pregnancy and, 2034
PKU (phenylketonuria), 2208t
Placenta
active transport, 2026
cotyledons, 2025
defined, 2023
development and functions of, 2023–2027
endocrine function, 2026
facilitated transport, 2026
fetal side, 2023, 2024f
functions of, 2026–2027
immunological properties, 2026–2027
location of, 2086
maternal side, 2023, 2024f
metabolic activities, 2026
parts of, 2023
retained, 2139t
simple diffusion, 2026
transport function, 2026
twins and, 2024f
vascular arrangement of, 2025f
Placenta accreta, 2139t
Placenta previa, 2137t
Placental abruption, 1768
Placental circulation, 2025
Placental delivery, 2126, 2166
Placental grading, 2086
Placental separation, 2125–2126
Plague, 2615t
Plan-Do-Study-Act (PDSA), 2690, 2690f
Planning. *See also* Nursing process
contingency, 2475
defined, 2341
developing goals and, 2342
as four-stage process, 2475
long-term goals, 2341–2342
as management function, 2475
short-term goals, 2341–2342

strategic, 2475
writing goals and, 2342–2344
Plant enzymes, 71*t*
Plaque, 425–426
Plaques, 876
Plasm D-dimer levels, 1213
Plasmapheresis, 491, 504, 673
Plastibell, 2241, 2241*f*
Platelets
count, 97
defined, 1252*t*
as perioperative diagnostic test, 1252*t*
Platypelloid pelvis, 2015, 2016*f*
Play
associative, 1665
cooperative, 1667
dramatic, 1665
infants, 1661
parallel, 1663
preschooler children, 1665–1666, 1665*f*
school-age children, 1667–1668
solitary, 1661
toddlers, 1663, 1663*f*
Play therapists, 1020
Plethysmography, 1132
Pleural effusion, 586
Pleuritic pain, 586
Pleuritis, 586
Pleximeter, 2280
Plexor, 2280
PMI (point of maximal impulse), 1044
PNAS (Protective Nursing Advocacy Scale), 2557
PNDS (perioperative nursing data sets), 2644
Pneumatic retinopexy, 1314
Pneumatic tourniquet, 1263*t*
Pneumococcal infection, 538*t*
Pneumococcal pneumonia, 586, 586*f*
Pneumocystis jiroveci, 585–586
Pneumocystis jiroveci pneumonia (PCP), 463, 587
Pneumomediastinum, 982
Pneumonia
activity and rest balance and, 597
acute bacterial, 586
airway patency and, 596
antibiotic therapy for, 591*t*
aspiration, 587–588
assessment, 593–595
care planning, 595
chest physiotherapy and, 592–593
in children, 588–590, 589*f*
collaborative care, 590–593
community-based care, 597
defined, 584
diagnosis, 595
diagnostic tests, 591
etiology, 586–588
herbal supplements for treating, 594*t*
hospital-acquired (HAP), 982, 2704
infectious, 585
infectious, manifestations of, 587*t*
inflammatory response, 585*f*
interventions, 595–597
Legionnaires disease, 586–587
lifespan and cultural considerations, 588–590
manifestations, 588–590, 595*t*
noninfectious, 585
nonpharmacologic therapy, 592–593
Nursing Care Plan, 598*t*
nursing process, 593–597

in older adults, 590
organisms causing, 586*t*
outcome evaluation, 597
overview of, 584
pathogenesis of, 586, 586*f*
pathophysiology, 584–588
patterns of lung involvement, 585, 585*t*
pediatric, 597*t*
pharmacologic therapy, 591–592
pneumocystis jiroveci, 587
postural drainage positions and, 594*f*
prevention, 588
primary atypical, 587
risk factors, 588
unilateral lobar, 585
ventilation and, 596–597
viral, 587
Pneumopericardium, 982
Pneumothorax, 609, 959, 960*t*, 982
Point of care
defined, 2648
individual information at, 2647–2649
Point of maximal impulse (PMI), 1044
Point-of-service (POS), 2628
Poliomyelitis, 539*t*
Polyarticular arthritis, 499
Polycythemia
defined, 34*t*, 1046
in newborns, 2210*t*
Polydipsia, 742
Polyethylene glycol (PEG), 310*t*
Polymerase chain reaction, 611
Polyneuropathies, 749, 1331
Polyphagia, 742
Polypharmacy, 934
Polyps, 85
Polysomnography (PSG), 148, 197
Polysubstance abuse, 1525*t*
Polytheism, 1873
Polyunsaturated fat, 757
Polyuria, 264, 365, 742
POMR. *See* Problem-oriented medical record
Popliteal angle, 2220
Popliteal pulse, 1063*f*, 1064
Poppers, 1564
Pop-ups, 2369
Portal hypertension, 782
Portal systemic encephalopathy, 782–784
Portion size, 925–926, 925*f*
POS (point-of-service), 2628
Position changes, pulse and, 1044
Positioning
examination, 2277, 2278*t*
oxygenation and, 968, 968*f*
Positive attitude, 2483
Positive end-expiratory pressure (PEEP), 979, 980, 981*t*
Positive punishment, 1529
Positive reinforcement, 418, 1529, 2502
Positive symptoms, 1613, 1613*t*, 1621*t*
Positive-pressure ventilators, 979
Positron emission tomograph (PET), 1617*f*
POSS (Pasero opioid-induced sedation scale), 166, 166*t*
Postconception age, 2028
Posterior fontanelle, 2114
Posterior tibial pulse, 1063*f*, 1064
Postexposure prophylaxis, hepatitis, 237*t*
Posthepatic cirrhosis, 782
Postictal period, seizures, 716

Postmenopausal bleeding, 1400
Postoperative documentation, 1274, 1274*t*
Postoperative nurses, 1251
Postoperative nursing
airways and, 1273
care, 1272–1274
client recovery and discharge, 1274–1275
cultural considerations, 1273
defined, 1249
diagnoses, 1272
discharge instructions, 1275*t*
drain and line management, 1274, 1274*t*
medications, 1273
nutrition and, 1275
physical activity and, 1275
rhythms and, 1273
risk monitoring, 1272–1273
sutures and staples and, 1274
wound care instruction and, 1275
wound management and, 1273
Postpartum, 2051*t*
Postpartum blues
defined, 1779, 1817
factors contributing to, 1820
social support and, 1820
Postpartum care
adolescents, 2188
alterations, 2177, 2178*t*
assessment
abdomen, 2179*t*
attachment, 2181*t*
breasts, 2179*t*
client eduction, 2181*t*
costovertebral angle (CVA) tenderness, 2180*t*
cultural, 2180*t*
early detachment, 2182
elimination, 2180*t*
high-risk factors, 2178–2182
lochia, 2179–2180*t*
psychological, 2178
psychological adaptations, 2178–2182
vital signs, 2179*t*
breastfeeding mother nutrition, 2177
care planning, 2182
common concerns, 2185*t*
culture and, 2182*t*
diagnosis, 2182
formula-feeding mother nutrition, 2177
high-risk factors, 2178*t*
interventions
attachment enhancement, 2184–2185
client teaching, 2182–2183
comfort and well-being, 2183–2184
emotional stress relief, 2185–2186
perineal care, 2184*t*
rest promotion, 2186
sexual activity and contraception, 2186–2187
suppression of lactation, 2185
well-being after Cesarean birth, 2187–2188
involution, 2171–2172, 2171*f*
Nursing Care Plan, 2189*t*
nursing process, 2178–2190
nutrition, 2176–2177
outcome evaluation, 2190
overview of, 2171
physical adaptations
abdomen, 2173
blood values, 2175–2176
breasts and lactogenesis, 2173–2174

Postpartum care (*continued*)
    cardiovascular changes, 2176
    gastrointestinal system, 2174–2175
    neurological and immunological
        changes, 2176
    reproductive system, 2171–2173
    urinary system, 2175
    vital signs, 2175
    psychological adaptations, 2176
    woman who relinquishes infant, 2188–2190
Postpartum concerns, 2185*t*
Postpartum depression
    assessment, 1824–1825
    care planning, 1825
    collaborative care, 1821–1824
    cultural influences and, 1819–1820
    defined, 1779, 1817
    development of family attachment and, 1818
    diagnosis, 1825
    diagnostic tests, 1821
    diversity and culture and, 1821*t*
    Edinburgh Postnatal Depression Scale and,
        1822*t*
    genetic considerations, 1821
    identification of, 1826*t*
    initial maternal attachment behavior and,
        1818–1819
    interventions, 1825–1827, 1826*t*
    manifestations and therapies, 1822*t*
    maternal role attainment (MRA) and, 1817–1818
    normal presentation and, 1817–1820
    Nursing Care Plan, 1827*t*
    nursing process, 1824–1827
    outcome evaluation, 1827
    overview of, 1817
    pharmacologic therapy, 1821–1824
    postpartum blues and, 1779, 1817, 1820
    Postpartum Depression Predictors Inventory-
        Revised (PDPI-R) and, 1823–1824*t*
    prevalence of, 1783
    prevention of, 1826*t*
    prevention strategies, 1826*t*
    risk factors, 1820–1821
    risk of injury, 1770
    self-report scales, 1787
    support groups, 1824
    symptoms of, 1820
Postpartum Depression Predictors Inventory-
    Revised (PDPI-R), 1787, 1823–1824*t*
Postpartum doulas, 1820
Postpartum mood disorders, 1779
Postpartum period
    acquaintance phase, 1819
    challenges, 1817–1818
    cultural influences in, 1819–1820
    father-infant interactions, 1819
    initial maternal attachment behavior and,
        1818–1819
    Middle Eastern, 1818*f*, 1818*t*
    phase of mutual regulation, 1819
    siblings and others interactions, 1819
    social support and, 1820
Postpartum psychosis, 1779, 1821, 1822*t*
Postrenal ARF (acute renal failure), 376
Postresuscitation care, 1194
Postterm labor, 2051*t*, 2138*t*
Postterm newborns, 2207*t*
Posttraumatic stress disorder (PTSD)
    acute stress disorder versus, 1946*t*
    assessment, 1948

assessment interview, 1948*t*
care planning, 1949
children, 1947
collaborative care, 1947–1948
as comorbid with schizophrenia, 1615
as coping alteration, 1907
defined, 1908–1909*t*, 1945
depersonalization and, 1947
diagnosis, 1948–1949
disorders in class, 1945
eye movement desensitization and reprocessing
    (EMDR) and, 1948
interventions, 1908–1909*t*, 1949
manifestations, 1908–1909*t*, 1947, 1947*t*
military personnel and, 1946, 1946*t*
nonpharmacologic therapy, 1948
Nursing Care Plan, 1949–1950*t*
outcome evaluation, 1949
overview of, 1945
pathophysiology and etiology,
    1945–1946
pharmacologic therapy, 1947
risk factors, 1946
triggers, 1946
typical human responses and, 1949*t*
Postural drainage
    COPD and, 1011–1012
    positions for, 594*f*
Posture and gait, 2402
Post-void residual measurement, 294
Potassium (K^+)
    electrolyte imbalance, 371–372
    overview of, 341
    as perioperative diagnostic test, 1252*t*
    regulation and function, 342*t*
Potassium-channel blockers, 1189*t*
Potassium-sparing diuretics, 1172*t*
Poverty
    as cancer risk factor, 46
    diversity and, 1635–1636
    nutrition and, 945*t*
PPD (paranoid personality disorder), 1857*t*,
    1859, 1863*t*
PPD (purified protein derivative), 607
PPO (preferred-provider organization), 2628
PPS (prospective payment system), 2465
PR interval, 1072*t*
Prader-Willi Syndrome (PWS), 1836–1838
Prayer
    categories of, 1884–1885
    with clients, 1888*t*
    defined, 1884–1885
    illustrated, 1884*f*, 1885*f*
Preassessment of clients, 2347
Preceptors, 2525–2526, 2529
Precipitating factors, violence, 1954
Precipitous birth, 2137*t*
Preconception
    counseling, 1371–1372, 1393
    health measures, 1372
Precursor lesions, 128
Prediabetes, 751, 945
Preeclampsia. *See also* Pregnancy-induced
    hypertension
    antepartum management, 1206–1207
    defined, 1205
    diabetic pregnancies and, 2046
    intrapartum management, 1207
    Nursing Care Plan, 1209–1210*t*
    postpartum management, 1207

Preembryonic development
    amniotic fluid, 2023
    cellular differentiation, 2022–2023
    cellular multiplication, 2021, 2022
    defined, 2021
    implantation, 2021–2022
    umbilical cord, 2023
    yolk sac, 2023
Preferred-provider organization (PPO), 2628
Prefrontal cortex, 1783
Pregnancy
    adolescent, 2041–2043
    alterations during pregnancy
        folic acid deficiency anemia, 2044–2045
        iron deficiency anemia, 2044
    anatomy and physiology
        adrenals, 2034
        breasts, 2030
        cardiovascular system, 2030–2031
        central nervous system (CNS), 2033
        cervix, 2030
        endocrine system, 2033–2034
        eyes, 2033
        gastrointestinal system, 2031
        metabolism, 2033
        musculoskeletal system, 2032–2033, 2032*f*
        nutrient metabolism, 2033
        ovaries, 2030
        pancreas, 2034
        parathyroid, 2034
        pituitary, 2034
        reproductive system, 2030
        respiratory system, 2030
        skin and hair, 2032, 2032*f*
        thyroid, 2033–2034
        urinary tract, 2031–2032
        uterus, 2030
        vagina, 2030
        water metabolism, 2033
        weight gain, 2033
    asthma and, 993–995
    beliefs and attitudes about, 2064*t*
    blood volume during, 1047
    bowel elimination and, 275–276
    cancer and, 51
    cardiac disease and
        antepartum period, 2050
        clinical therapy, 2049–2051
        congenital heart defects, 2048–2049
        drug therapy, 2049–2050
        intrapartum period, 2050
        labor and childbirth, 2050
        Marfan syndrome, 2049
        mitral valve prolapse (MVP), 2049
        peripartum cardiomyopathy, 2049
        postpartum period, 2050–2051
    cardiovascular changes during, 1046–1047
    clinical interruption of, 1387–1388
    comfort and, 149
    complementary and alternative therapy
        and, 1557*t*
    constipation and, 308
    cultural values and, 2040, 2041*t*
    culture and, 2064*t*
    daily food plan, 2093*t*
    danger signs in, 2100*t*
    diabetes and, 2045–2048
    discomfort relief
        backache, 2066
        culture and, 2076*t*

first trimester, 2074–2075t
nausea and vomiting, 2065–2066, 2066t
second trimester, 2075t
self-care measures, 2074–2075t
third trimester, 2075t
urinary frequency, 2066
HIV-positive clients and, 473t
hormones in, 2034
hypertension and, 1165, 1166
infection and, 552
initial prenatal assessment, 2056–2063t
medications and, 2064–2065
morning sickness and, 2035
multiple sclerosis and, 880
over age 35
expectant couple concerns, 2043–2044
factors contributing to trend, 2043
medical risks, 2043
pharmacologic therapy, 2066
pharmacologic therapy for mood disorders
and, 1794t
physiological anemia of, 1047, 2031
prostaglandins in, 2034
psychological response of family
expectant couple, 2036
father, 2036–2039
grandparents, 2040
mother, 2036–2038
overview of, 2036
siblings, 2039–2040
rheumatoid arthritis and, 497t
at risk conditions, 2082
self-care techniques during, 2076t
sexual activity and, 2073t
sickle cell disease and, 122
signs
clinical pregnancy tests, 2035
diagnostic (positive) changes, 2035–2036
Hegar sign, 2035
McDonald sign, 2035
objective (probable) changes, 2035, 2035f
subjective (presumptive) changes,
2034–2035
sleep and, 196
spinal cord injuries (SCI) and, 912–913
substance abuse during
alcohol, 1552–1553
caffeine, 1552
cocaine and crack, 1553–1554
heroin, 1554
marijuana, 1554
MDMA (ecstasy), 1554
methadone, 1554
phencyclidine (PCP), 1554
risk factors for, 1555t
side effects of, 1553t
tobacco, 1554
systemic lupus erythematosus (SLE) and, 512
tobacco and, 2065
urinary calculi and, 321
urinary elimination and, 263–264
urinary incontinence and, 294
urinary tract infections (UTIs) and, 621
yoga and, 1557t, 2071t
Pregnancy tests, 2035
Pregnancy-induced hypertension
antepartum management, 1206–1207
assessment, 1207
care planning, 1208
collaborative care, 1206–1207

defined, 1053t
diagnosis, 1208
gestational hypertension and, 1205
HELLP syndrome and, 1205
interventions, 1053t, 1208
intrapartum management, 1207
manifestations, 1053t, 1206, 1206t
Nursing Care Plan, 1209–1210t
nursing process, 1207–1209
outcome evaluation, 1209
overview of, 1204
pathophysiology and etiology, 1205
postpartum management, 1207
preeclampsia and, 1205
risk factors, 1205
Preimplantation genetic diagnosis (PGD), 1390
Prejudices, 1641
Preload, 1042, 1087t
Premature atrial contractions (PACs), 1180t, 1183–
1184
Premature junctional contractions, 1184
Premature newborns
auditory defects, 2254
bottle feeding, 2252
breastfeeding, 2252–2253
bronchopulmonary dysplasia, 2254
fluid requirements, 2253
gavage feeding, 2253
neurological defects, 2254
nutritional requirements, 2252
retinopathy of prematurity (ROP), 2254
speech defects, 2254
total parenteral nutrition, 2253
Premature rupture of membranes (PROM),
2121, 2137t
Premature ventricular contractions (PVCs),
1181t, 1185
Prematurity
alterations, 2254–2255
anemia of, 2255
apnea of, 2254
assessment, 2255
care planning, 2255
diagnosis, 2255
gastrointestinal physiology, 2250–2251
illustrated, 2249f
immunological physiology, 2251
interventions
developmentally supportive care, 2258–2259
fluid and electrolyte status, 2256–2257
home care preparation, 2259–2260
infant massage and gentle touch, 2259
infection prevention, 2257–2258
kangaroo care, 2258, 2258f, 2259
music therapy, 2259
nutrition, 2257
parent-newborn attachment, 2258
respiratory function, 2255–2256
thermal environment, 2256
intraventricular hemorrhage and, 2254
long-term needs, 2253–2254
neurological physiology, 2251
Nursing Care Plan, 2260–2261t
nursing process, 2255–2260
nutritional and fluid requirements, 2252–2253
outcome evaluation, 2260
overview of, 2249
patent ductus arteriosus (PDA) and, 2254
preterm newborn, 2249–2254
reactivity and behavioral states, 2251–2252

renal physiology, 2251
respiratory and cardiac physiology, 2250
respiratory distress syndrome and, 2254
thermoregulation, 2250
Prenatal, 2051t
Prenatal assessment of parenting ability,
2101–2102t
Prenatal burst of energy, 2121, 2121t
Prenatal considerations, in development, 1677
Prenatal education, 2055–2064
Prenatal high-risk screening, 2053
Prenatal risk for injury, 2708, 2709t
Prenatal substance exposure
antepartum care and, 2077t
assessment, 1556–1557
care planning, 1557
collaborative care, 1555–1556
diagnosis, 1557
effects on fetus and newborn, 1553t
epidemiology, 1555
interventions, 1557–1558
manifestations, 1555, 1556t
Nursing Care Plan, 1558–1559t
nursing process, 1556–1558
outcome evaluation, 1558
overview of, 1552
pathophysiology and etiology, 1552–1555
prevention of, 1555
risk factors, 1555, 1555t
signs of, 1557t
substances
alcohol, 1552–1553
caffeine, 1552
cocaine and crack, 1553–1554
heroin, 1554
marijuana, 1554
MDMA (ecstasy), 1554
methadone, 1554
phencyclidine (PCP), 1554
tobacco, 1554
Preoperative documentation, 1260t
Preoperative nurses, 1251
Preoperative nursing
abuse assessment, 1257
assessment, 1257–1259, 1258–1259t
care plan, 1259
client medication review, 1257–1258
client preparation, 1272–1276
data collection, 1257
defined, 1249
informed consent, 1259
interventions, 1259–1260
nutritional assessment, 1257
older adult assessment, 1260t
pain assessment, 1257
physical assessment, 1257, 1257t
psychosocial assessment, 1257
surgical site preparation, 1259, 1260t
Preparedness phase, in emergency management,
2609–2610
Preproliferative retinopathy, 749
Prerenal ARF (acute renal failure), 376
Presbycusis, 1299
Presbyopia, 1286t
Preschoolers
assessment of, 2292
cognitive development, 1664
communication, 1666
constipation in, 307
family with, 1726

Preschoolers (*continued*)
  growth and development, 1664–1666
  growth and development milestones, 1664*t*
  health screenings and immunization guidelines, 413*t*
  normal sleep-rest patterns in, 432
  oral health in, 427–428
  personality and temperament, 1666
  physical growth and development, 1664
  play, 1665–1666, 1665*f*
  psychosocial development, 1664–1666, 1666*t*
  sexual development, 1341*t*
  unintentional injuries, 2710–2711
  urinary elimination in, 262
Presencing, 1891, 2306–2307, 2307*f*
Presenting part
  defined, 2115
  enlargement of, 2116
  station and, 2116, 2116*f*
Pressure ulcers
  assessment, 1499–1502, 1500*t*
  Braden Scale for Predicating Pressure Sore Risk, 1500–1502, 1501*t*
  care planning, 1502
  circulation and, 1494–1495, 1495*t*
  client teaching, 1498
  collaborative care, 1495–1499
  debridement and, 1497
  defined, 1492
  diagnosis, 1502
  diagnostic tests, 1495
  dignity and self-esteem and, 1504
  infection prevention and, 1504
  interventions, 1502–1504
  manifestations, 1495, 1498*t*
  mechanical devices for reduction of, 1495*t*
  nonpharmacologic therapy, 1497–1499
  Norton Scale and, 1502
  Nursing Care Plan, 1504–1506*t*
  nursing process, 1498–1504
  nutrition and, 1504
  overview of, 1492
  pathophysiology and etiology, 1493–1495
  pharmacologic therapy, 1497
  prevention of, 1494–1495
  products used in treatment of, 1498*t*
  risk factors, 1493–1494
  skin integrity maintenance and, 1502–1504
  staging, 1496–1497*t*
  surgery, 1497
  treating, 1499*t*, 1503*t*
  Waterlow Score and, 1502
Pressure-support ventilation (PSV), 981*t*
Preterm (premature) labor, 2051*t*, 2137*t*
Preterm newborns, 2249
Preterm premature rupture of membranes (PRROM), 2121
Priapism, 121, 1352*t*
Price controls, 2464–2465
Prick (epicutaneous or puncture) test, 489
Primary acid-base disorders, 6–7
Primary appraisal, 1898, 1902
Primary atypical pneumonia, 587
Primary care, 2598
Primary care provider (PCP), 2628
Primary groups, 2418

Primary hypertension, 1165
Primary immune response, 442
Primary intention healing, 1507
Primary nursing, 2459, 2600
Primary prevention, 2596–2597, 2597*t*
Primary skin lesions, 1450*t*
Primary syphilis, 1413, 1413*f*
Primigravida, 2051*t*
Principles-based (deontological) theories, 1879
Prinzmetal (variant) angina, 1107
Priorities
  categorizing, 2366–2368
  common names for categories, 2367*t*
  defined, 2363
  high, 2366
  low, 2366
  medium, 2366
  setting, 2364*t*
Prioritizing care
  assessment in, 2364, 2365*t*
  availability of resources and, 2369
  board of nursing rules, 2365, 2365*t*
  categorizing and, 2366–2368
  change in client condition and, 2369
  client preferences and, 2369
  consideration factors, 2368–2370
  defined, 2363
  delegation and, 2171, 2370
  easiest task first and, 2171
  ethics and, 2368
  identifying what to prioritize and, 2364–2366
  Maslow's hierarchy of needs, 2365–2366
  multiple clients and, 2369
  not involving clients and, 2370–2371
  nursing process in, 2364–2365
  nursing self-care and, 2370
  overview of, 2363–2364
  pitfalls in, 2370–2371, 2371*t*
  poor time management and, 2370
  pop-ups and, 2369
  process diagram, 2368*f*
  QSEN competencies and, 2371t
  ranking activities and, 2367
  safety and, 2368–2369
  safety risks and physiological deterioration, 2365*t*
  time constraints and, 2366
  time management and, 2369
  triage and, 2367–2368
  urgency factor, 2366–2367, 2367*f*
  without assessment, 2370
Priority decisions, 2321
Privacy
  confidentiality versus, 2671
  defined, 2671
  invasion of, 2657
Private health insurance plans
  Medigap policies, 2629
  overview of, 2628
  types of, 2628
Private insurance, 2463
Problem solving
  in clinical decision making, 2323–2324
  defined, 1904
  intuition, 2324
  nursing process, 2323
  scientific method, 2324
  trial and error, 2323–2324

Problem-focused coping, 1899
Problem-oriented medical record (POMR)
  advantages of, 2440–2441
  database, 2441
  defined, 2440
  plan of care, 2441
  problem list, 2441
  progress notes, 2441–2442, 2442*f*
Problem-oriented record (POR), 2440
Procalcitonin (CTpr), in infection, 556
Procedures, parental presence during, 1709*t*
Process addictions
  defined, 1520, 1524*t*
  treatment, 1524*t*
Processing, 2432
Prodromal stage, infection, 528–529
Productivity, 2477
Professional advocacy, 2558–2559
Professional behaviors
  abuse of power and, 2483–2485, 2484*t*
  appearance, 2481, 2481*f*
  attire and demeanor guidelines, 2481*t*
  compassion, 2483
  competencies, 2482–2483, 2482*t*
  components of, 2480–2483
  concept of, 2479
  concepts related to, 2480*t*
  conclusion, 2485
  defined, 2480
  improper use of authority and, 2484–2485
  integrity, 2483
  intimidation and, 2485
  knowledge, 2482
  levels of anxiety, 2481
  positive attitude, 2483
  professionalism, 2480–2481
  sexual harassment and, 2484
  teamwork, 2483
  unprofessional behaviors and, 2483–2485
Professional commitment
  affective commitment, 2487, 2487*f*
  burnout and, 2488
  continuance commitment, 2487
  factors of, 2486–2487
  normative commitment, 2487
  overview of, 2486
  stages of development, 2487–2488
  stress management and, 2488
  types of, 2487, 2487*f*
Professional development
  chain of command, 2549–2550, 2550*f*
  definitions of nursing, 2548
  expanded career roles for nurses, 2550–2551
  historical perspectives, 2546
  nurse practice acts, 2549
  nursing leaders, 2547
  overview, 2545
  recipients of nursing, 2548
  roles and functions of the nurse, 2550–2551, 2551*t*
  settings for nursing, 2548–2549
  standards of nursing practice, 2549
Professional liability insurance, 2658
Professional negligence. *See* Malpractice
Professional organizations
  accountability, 2538
  American Association of Colleges of Nursing (AACN), 2626

American Nurses Association (ANA), 2625
National League for Nursing (NLN), 2626
National Student Nurses Association (NSNA), 2625
overview of, 2625
Sigma Theta Tau International, 2626
specialty practice, 2626, 2626*t*
Professional support, 1732
Professionalism, 2480–2481
Professions
    autonomy, 2537
    body of knowledge, 2536
    code of ethics, 2537
    criteria of, 2536–2538
    defined, 2536
    leadership interventions and, 2537*t*
    ongoing research, 2537
    professional organization, 2538
    service orientation, 2537
    specialized education, 2536
Progesterone, 1378, 2016, 2034
Progress notes, 2441–2442, 2442*f*, 2446
Progressive relaxation, 1943*t*
Progressive shock, 1219–1220
Progressive supranuclear palsy (PSP), 898
Projectile vomiting, 252
Projection, 1905*t*
Prolactin, 2034
Prolapsed umbilical cord, 2138*t*
Proliferation phase, in wound healing, 1470, 1508
Proliferative phase, in menstrual cycle, 2019
Proliferative retinopathy, 749
Prolonged grief disorder (PGD), 1743
PROM (premature rupture of membranes), 2121
Promotility agents, 230
Prone position, 1024, 1264*t*, 2278*t*
Prophylactic antibiotics, 622*t*
Prophylaxis
    deep venous thrombosis (DVT) and, 1132
    tuberculosis and, 611
Proprioception, 1237
Proptosis, 806
Prospective payment system (PPS), 2465
Prostaglandin analogs, 680, 1322*t*
Prostaglandins
    cervical ripening and, 2128–2129
    defined, 2016–2017
    in pregnancy, 2034
    production, 2016
Prostate
    assessment, 1357*t*
    examinations, 623
Prostate cancer. *See also* Cancer
    androgens and, 112
    assessment, 116
    care planning, 117
    collaborative care, 113–116
    complementary and alternative therapy, 116
    cultural diversity and, 113*t*
    diagnosis, 116
    diagnostic tests, 113
    digital rectal exam (DRE) and, 113
    home care for, 118*t*
    hormone therapy, 116*t*
    interventions, 117–118
    manifestations, 113, 114*t*
    Nursing Care Plan, 118–119*t*
    nursing process, 116–118
    outcome evaluation, 118
    overview of, 112
    pain management, 117–118
    pathophysiology and etiology, 112–113
    pharmacologic therapy, 115
    prevention, 113
    prostatectomy and, 115, 115*t*
    radiation therapy, 116
    risk factors, 113
    screening guidelines, 58*t*
    sexual function and, 117
    staging and treatment, 114*t*
    surgery, 115, 115*t*
    urinary elimination and, 117
Prostatectomy, 115, 115*t*, 295
Prostate-specific antigen (PSA), 113–114, 285
Prostatitis, 284
Prostatodynia, 284
Protease inhibitors, 471
Protected health information (PHI), 2438, 2670
Protective factors
    resiliency theory, 1654–1655
    violence, 1954
Protective Nursing Advocacy Scale (PNAS), 2557
Protein and nutritional supplements, 947*t*
Proteins
    body cell use, 928*f*
    complete, 929
    deficiency and excess, 938*t*
    defined, 929
    functions in the body, 930
    recommended daily intake, 930
Proteinuria, 380
Protestant Christianity, 1886
Prothrombin time, 1252*t*
Proton pump inhibitors, 222, 228–229
Provider education, 2558
Proxemics, 2406
Proximodistal growth, 1648
PRROM (preterm premature rupture of membranes), 2121
Pruritus, 165*t*, 1453–1454*t*, 1491*t*
PSA (prostate-specific antigen), 113–114, 285
PSDA (Patient Self-Determination Act), 2542, 2667
Pseudoexacerbation, 877
Pseudomenstruation, 2201
PSG (polysomnography), 197
PSP (progressive supranuclear palsy), 898
PSVT (paroxysmal supraventricular tachycardia), 1180*t*, 1184
Psychedelics, 1564
Psychoanalytic theory, 1835
Psychogenic pain, 156
Psychological dependence, 1525*t*
Psychological factors
    in addiction, 1521
    in assessment, 2284
    in sexuality, 1349
Psychomotor ability, learning and, 2507
Psychomotor domain, 2503
Psychomotor retardation, 1799
Psychopathology theory, 1966
Psychosis
    defined, 1578, 1611
    negative symptoms of, 1621*t*
    positive symptoms of, 1621*t*
    postpartum, 1779, 1821, 1822*t*
Psychosocial development
    adolescents, 1669–1670
    preschool children, 1664–1666, 1666*t*
    school-age children, 1667–1668, 1667*t*
    toddlers, 1663–1664, 1663*t*
Psychosocial issues
    nicotine addiction, 1549
    postpartum, 2181*t*
    substance abuse, 1568–1569
Psychosocial stressors, 1897
Psychosocial theories
    defined, 1649
    Erikson, 1650–1653, 1651*t*
    Freud, 1649–1650, 1650*t*
Psychosocial wellness
    Alzheimer disease (AD) and, 1602
    antepartum nutrition and, 2094–2096, 2095*f*
    breast cancer and, 82–83
    comfort alterations and, 150
    congenital heart defects and, 1102
    hip fractures and, 874
    motor vehicle crashes (MVC) and, 2005
Psychospiritual comfort, 141
Psychostimulants
    abuse of, 1563–1564
    defined, 1563
Psychotherapy, 1914
Psychoticism, 1855
Ptosis, 1288*t*
PTSD. *See* Posttraumatic stress disorder
Ptyalism, 2072
Puberty, 1668
Pubic hair, 1341*f*
Public advocacy, 2558–2559
Public distance, 2408
Public insurance, 2463
Public self, 1833
PUD. *See* Peptic ulcer disease
Puerperium, 1817
Pulmonary angiography, 1214
Pulmonary artery banding, 1100*t*
Pulmonary artery pressure (PAP)
    catheters, 1476
    monitoring, 1152–1153, 1153*f*
Pulmonary artery wedge pressure (PAWP), 1476
Pulmonary atresia, 1088–1089*t*
Pulmonary blood flow decrease defects. *See also* Congenital heart defects
    clinical therapy, 1087–1089*t*
    defined, 1087
    manifestations, 1087–1088*t*
    pathophysiology, 1087–1089*t*
    pulmonary or tricuspid atresia, 1088–1089*t*
    pulmonary stenosis, 1087*t*
    tetralogy of Fallot (TOF), 1088*t*
Pulmonary circulation, 1036, 1038*f*
Pulmonary edema
    as classification, 1147–1148
    defined, 1145
    onset of, 976*f*
Pulmonary embolism
    anxiety relief and, 1216
    assessment, 1214–1215
    cardiac output and, 1215
    care planning, 1215
    client teaching, 1215*t*
    collaborative care, 1213–1214
    defined, 1211
    diagnosis, 1215
    diagnostic tests, 1213–1214
    impaired gas exchange compensation and, 1215
    interventions, 1215–1216

Pulmonary embolism (*continued*)
   manifestations, 1212–1213, 1212*t*, 1213*t*
   Nursing Care Plan, 1216–1217*t*
   nursing process, 1214–1216
   outcome evaluation, 1216
   overview of, 1211
   pathophysiology and etiology, 1211–1212
   pharmacologic therapy, 1214
   risk factors, 1212
   safety and, 1215–1216
   surgery, 1214
Pulmonary function tests (PFTs)
   in COPD, 1009
   defined, 966
   in lung cancer, 108
   performance of, 967*t*
   in respiratory acidosis, 22
   use of, 966
   values of, 967*t*
Pulmonary stenosis, 1087*t*
Pulmonary system, aging changes, 1049
Pulmonary vascular resistance, 1040, 1476
Pulse
   apical, 1063*f*, 1064, 1064*f*
   apical-radial, 1064
   assessment
      apical, 1064
      apical-radial, 1064
      auscultation, 1062*f*, 1062*t*
      lifespan considerations, 1065*t*
      sites for, 1063–1064, 1063*f*
   brachial, 1063*f*, 1064
   carotid, 1063, 1063*f*
   defined, 1044
   factors affecting, 1044–1045
   femoral, 1063*f*, 1064
   in mobility assessment, 829
   monitoring in home, 1064*t*
   pedal (dorsalis pedis), 1063*f*, 1064
   peripheral, 1044
   popliteal, 1063*f*, 1064
   posterior tibial, 1063*f*, 1064
   radial, 1063*f*, 1064
   reasons for using sites, 1064
   temporal, 1063, 1063*f*
   variations by age, 1045*t*
Pulse deficit, 1059
Pulse oximetry
   in burn injuries, 1477
   in COPD, 1010
   defined, 966
   in pneumonia, 591
Pulse pressure, 1045, 1163
Pulse rhythm, 1063
Pulse volume, 1063
Punctuality, 2492
Punishment, 1529, 1717–1718
Pupillary assessment, 1287*t*
Purging, 1846–1847
Purified protein derivative (PPD), 607
Pursed-lip breathing, 1009
Purulent exudate, 1509
Pus, 1509
Putting Evidence into Practice (PEP), 2592
PVCs (premature ventricular contractions), 1181*t*, 1185
PVD. *See* Peripheral vascular disease
PWS (Prader-Willi Syndrome), 1836–1838
Pyelography, 380
Pyelolithotomy, 323

Pyelonephritis, 619, 624
Pyloric stenosis. *See also* Digestion
   assessment, 252
   collaborative care, 252
   defined, 252, 252*f*
   diagnosis, 253
   diagnostic tests, 252
   fluids and electrolyte balance, 253
   home care, 253*t*, 254
   infection and, 253
   interventions, 253–254
   manifestations, 213*t*, 252
   Nursing Care Plan, 254*t*
   nursing process, 252–254
   outcome evaluation, 254
   overview of, 252
   pathophysiology and etiology, 252
   projectile vomiting and, 252
   rest and comfort and, 253
   risk factors, 252
   supportive care, 253
   surgery, 252
   weight loss minimization, 253
Pyloromyotomy, 253*t*
Pyogenic bacteria, 1509
Pyorrhea, 426
Pyrazinamide, 612*t*
Pyuria, 621

Q

QRS complex, 1072*t*
QSEN. *See* Quality and Safety Education for Nurses; Quality and Safety Education for Nurses (QSEN)
Qsymia, 794
QT interval, 1072*t*
Qualifiers, 2336
Qualitative research, 2586
Quality, 2281, 2681
Quality and Safety Education for Nurses (QSEN)
   competencies, 2699
   defined, 2699
   evidence-based practice (EBP), 2699, 2700
   informatics, 2699, 2700
   Institute, 2482, 2482*t*
   overview of, 2696–2699
   patient-centered care, 2699–2700
   quality improvement, 2699, 2700
   safety, 2699, 2700
   teamwork and collaboration, 2699, 2700
Quality assurance
   computers and, 2646
   defined, 2689
   electronic health records and, 2639
Quality improvement
   analysis of current protocols/outcomes and, 2685
   benchmarking, 2684, 2686
   breach of care, 2687
   concepts related to, 2682*t*
   continuous, 2690–2691
   defined, 2681
   evaluation of efficacy of new protocols, 2689
   factors that promote better outcomes, 2687–2689, 2688*t*, 2689*t*
   federal initiatives, 2683–2684
   of health care, 2683, 2683*f*
   implementation of new protocols, 2689
   interdisciplinary assessment, 2685

   intradisciplinary assessment, 2685
   management program components, 2690–2692
   medication errors, 2688, 2688*t*
   national initiatives, 2683–2684
   priorities for, 2684
   process, 2684–2690
   as QSEN competency, 2699, 2700
   root cause analysis and, 2686, 2687–2688
   safety and, 2699
   sentinel events, 2686–2687
   state and local initiatives, 2684
   targeting areas for, 2686–2687
Quality management
   comprehensive, 2690
   continuous quality improvement (CQI), 2690–2691
   defined, 2681
   Lean Six Sigma, 2692
   program components, 2690–2692
   Six Sigma, 2691–2692
   total (TQM), 2690, 2690*f*
Quantitative research, 2586
Questioning, 2430
Questions
   background, 2588
   clinical, 2588–2590
   closed, 2274, 2274*t*
   foreground, 2588
   leading, 2275
   neutral, 2275
   open-ended, 2274, 2274*t*
Quick Start method, 1383, 1383*t*
Quickening, 2035

R

Race
   blood pressure and, 1046
   burn risk and, 1466
   defined, 1635
   hypertension and, 1167
Racism, 1635
Radial pulse, 1063*f*, 1064
Radiation, 1422
Radiation burns, 1465, 1475*t*
Radiation cataracts, 1307
Radiation therapy
   in breast cancer, 81
   in cancer, 56–57
   in colorectal cancer, 88
   in leukemia, 99
   in lung cancer, 109
   in prostate cancer, 116
   in skin cancer, 135
Radical mastectomy, 79
Radical prostatectomy, 115
Radioactive iodine therapy, 809
Radioallergosorbent test (RAST), 489
Radiology
   personnel, 1251
   safety precautions, 1263*t*
Radionuclide imaging, 1115
RAI (resident assessment instrument), 2298
RAI uptake test, 809
Randomized control trial (RCT), 2589
Range of motion
   assessment, 828, 830–833*t*
   exercises, 506, 837, 1244
   isometric, 837

in joints, 821
  measurement with goniometer, 829f
  resistive, 837
Ranking activities, 2367
Rape, date, 1407
Rape and rape-trauma syndrome
  acquaintance rape, 1984
  assessment, 1987–1988
  care planning, 1988
  collaborative care, 1986–1987
  defined, 1983
  description of, 1958t
  diagnosis, 1988
  diagnostic tests, 1986–1987
  immediate responses, 1985
  influencing factors, 1984
  interpersonal factors, 1984
  intrapersonal factors, 1984
  lifespan and cultural considerations,
    1986, 1986t
  long-term goals, 1988
  long-term response, 1985–1986
  manifestations, 1958t, 1985–1986, 1987t
  marital rape, 1984
  nonpharmacologic therapy, 1987
  Nursing Care Plan, 1989–1990t
  nursing process, 1987–1988
  outcome evaluation, 1988
  overview of, 1983
  pathophysiology and etiology, 1984–1985
  pharmacologic therapy, 1987
  physical injuries, 1985
  prevention of, 1985
  risk factors, 1984–1985
  sociocultural factors, 1984
Rapid cycling, 1779, 1811
Rapport, 2272
RAPs (resident assessment protocols),
    2297–2298
RAST (radioallergosorbent test), 489
Rastelli procedure, 1100t
Rational polypharmacy, 163
Rationalization, 1905t
RBCs. See Red blood cells (RBCs)
Reaction formation, 1905t
Reactive attachment disorder, 1945
Readiness for enhanced religiosity, 1887
Readiness for enhanced spiritual well-being,
    1890–1891
Readiness to learn, 2505, 2513
Real self, 1832–1833
Reality female condom, 1380, 1380f
Reality-based thinking promotion, 1814
Reappraisal
  adaptation and, 1899–1900
  defined, 1902
Reasonable care, 2655
Reasoning. See also Critical thinking
  clinical, 2319
  deductive, 2319
  faulty, types of, 2320t
  inductive, 2319
  types of statements and, 2319, 2319t
Receiver, 2399
Receptive aphasia, 1238
Receptive speech, 1662
Receptor, 1278
Recoil, 2219–2220
Reconstructive surgery, breast cancer and, 83

Recording
  defined, 2438
  guidelines
    accepted terminology, 2448–2449
    accuracy, 2449
    appropriateness, 2449
    commonly used abbreviations, 2448t
    completeness, 2449
    conciseness, 2449
    correct spelling, 2449
    date and time, 2448
    legal prudence, 2450
    legibility, 2448
    overview of, 2447
    permanence, 2448
    sequence, 2449
    signature, 2449
    timing, 2448
Records
  defined, 2438
  source-oriented, 2439–2440, 2440t
Recovery. See also Addiction
  defined, 1528
  language of, 1525, 1525t
Recovery phase
  in acute renal failure (ARF), 378
  in emergency management, 2610–2611
Recreational drug use, as cancer risk factor, 47
Rectocele, 1360t
Red blood cells (RBCs)
  anemia and, 66, 66f
  count, 1252t
  sickle cell disease and, 120
Red clover, 1397t
Referral physicians, 1251
Referred pain, 155, 155f
Reflecting
  content, 2427–2429
  defined, 2427
  feelings, 2429
Reflection
  defined, 2319–2320
  guided, 2321t
Reflex incontinence, 299t
Reflexes
  autonomic, 689
  defined, 689
  in gestational age assessment, 2221
  of newborns, 2203t
  somatic, 689
Reflux, 275–276, 619
Refraction, 1281t
Refractory hypoxemia, 975
Refractory period, 1044
Refractory septic shock, 600
Refractory shock, 1220
Regeneration, 634–635, 1507
Registered nurses (RNs), 2458
Regression, 1905t
Regulatory agencies
  Department of Health and Human Services
    (DHHS), 2622, 2623t
  federal, 2621–2623
  Occupational Safety and Health Administration
    (OSHA), 2623, 2623f
  overview of, 2621
  state and local, 2623–2624
Regurgitation, 1113
Rehabilitation, spinal cord injuries (SCI) and,
    914–915, 917

Rehydration
  with intravenous fluids, 361–362, 361t
  oral, 360–361
Reimbursement
  Children's Health Insurance Program (CHIP),
    2628
  conclusion, 2629
  federal programs, 2627–2628
  Medicaid, 2627
  Medicare, 2627, 2627t
  Medigap policies, 2629
  payment sources, 2627–2629
  personal payment, 2629
  private health insurance plans, 2628–2629
  Supplemental Security Income (SSI),
    2627–2628
  types of, 2627–2629
Reinfection, in urinary tract infections (UTIs), 627
Reinforcement, 1529
Relapsing fever, 1431
Relationship-based (caring) theories, 1879
Relaxation
  forms of, 151
  muscle, 150
Relaxation techniques
  for anxiety disorders, 1925–1926
  breathing exercises, 150
  categories of, 150–151
  imagery, 150
  for labor, 2163
  movement techniques, 151
  muscle relaxation, 150
Relaxin, 2034
Relevance, 2506
Reliability
  evidence, 2591
  in professionalism, 2492
Religion
  alterations, 1886
  antepartum nutrition and, 2094, 2094t
  Buddhism, 1886, 1886t
  characteristics of, 1883
  defined, 1638, 1883
  end-of-life care and, 181
  health-related information, 1886t
  Hinduism, 1886
  holy days, 1884
  Islam, 1885, 1886t
  Jehovah's Witnesses, 1886, 1886t
  Judaism, 1885, 1886t
  medical care and, 1885–1886
  Nursing Care Plan, 1889t
  in nursing development, 2546
  nursing process, 1886–1888
  outcome evaluation, 1888
  personality disorders (PD) and, 1861t
  prayer, 1888t
  prayer and meditation, 1884–1885, 1884f,
    1885f
  Protestant Christianity, 1886
  Roman Catholic, 1886, 1886t
  sacred symbols, 1884
  scared writings, 1884
  sexuality and, 1362
  as spirituality component, 1873
  supporting religious practices, 1888t
  variations, 1638
Religious practices, 1888t
Religious rituals, 1750, 1750f
REM (rapid-eye-movement) sleep, 431, 431t

Remission, 97, 408
Remittent fever, 1431
Remodeling, in burn wound healing, 1470
Remyelination, 877t
Renal biopsy, 380
Renal colic, 320
Renal failure
   acute (ARF), 374–389
   defined, 261, 374
   in older adults, 392t
Renal insufficiency, 378
Renal replacement therapy
   continuous, 384, 384f, 384t
   dialysis, 397
   hemodialysis, 383–384, 383f
   kidney transplant, 397–399
   peritoneal dialysis, 385–386, 385f
   vascular access for, 384–385, 385f
Renal system
   acid-base balance and, 6
   aging changes, 1049
   labor and, 2126
   premature newborns and, 2251
   shock effect on, 1222
Renal ultrasonography, 380, 395, 557, 623
Renin-angiotensin-aldosterone system, 340,
      1163–1164
Repetition, 2506
Repetition strain injury, 2643
Repetitive transcranial magnetic stimulation
      (rTMS), 1795
Repolarization, 1043–1044
Reporting
   care plan conference, 2452
   change-of-shift, 2451, 2451t
   defined, 2451
   handoff communication, 2451
   mandatory, 2674–2676, 2674t, 2675t
   overview of, 2451
   telephone communication, 2451–2452,
      2452t
Reports
   change-of-shift, 2451, 2451t
   defined, 2438
   incident, 2678
   telephone, 2451–2452
Repression, 1905t
Reproduction
   alterations during pregnancy
      adolescent pregnancy, 2041–2043
      anemia, 2044–2045
      cardiac disease, 2048–2051
      diabetes, 2045–2048
      pregnancy over age 35, 2043–2044
      sickle cell disease, 2045
   anatomy and physiology of pregnancy,
      2030–2034
   assessment, 2051–2054
   assisted techniques, 1388–1391, 1389f
   chronic kidney disease (CKD) and, 395
   client profile, 2051–2052
   collaborative interventions and therapies, 2066
   conception and fetal development, 2019–2029
   concepts related to, 2042t
   cultural values and, 2040–2041
   diagnostic tests, 2054, 2055t
   female assessment, 1358–1361t
   female reproductive system and, 2012–2019
   fetal development assessment, 2054, 2054f
   gametes, 2011

independent interventions and therapies,
      2054–2066
initial prenatal assessment
   abdomen, 2058–2059t
   anus and rectum, 2060t
   breasts, 2058t
   chest and lungs, 2057–2058t
   cultural assessment, 2062–2063t
   economic status, 2063t
   educational needs, 2063t
   extremities, 2059t
   family functioning, 2063t
   heart, 2058t
   laboratory evaluation, 2061–2062t
   mouth, 2057t
   neck, 2057t
   nose, 2057t
   pelvic area, 2060t
   pelvic measurements, 2060t
   psychological status, 2063t
   reflexes, 2059t
   skin, 2056t
   spine, 2059t
   stability and living conditions, 2063t
   support system, 2063t
   vital signs, 2056t
   weight, 2056t
interventions and therapies, 2054–2066
male assessment, 1356–1357t
medications, 1364–1365t
medications and, 2064–2065
obesity and, 792
paralysis and, 911
pelvic adequacy assessment, 2054
physical and psychological changes,
      2030–2041
physical examination, 2053–2054
pregnancy signs, 2034–2036
prenatal education, 2055–2064
prenatal high-risk screening, 2053
prenatal terms, 2051t
psychological response to pregnancy,
      2036–2040
tobacco and, 2065
twins, 2023, 2024f
uterine assessment, 2053–2054
Reproductive system
   postpartum care
      cervical changes, 2173
      involution, 2171–2172, 2171f
      lochia, 2172
      ovulation and menstruation, 2173
      perineal changes, 2173
      vaginal changes, 2173
Research
   abundance of, 2584
   clinical decision support systems and, 2644
   common nursing links, 2590t
   computers in, 2644–2645
   defined, 2583
   ethical and legal issues, 2587
   funding, 2586
   hierarchy of, 2591, 2591f
   implications for nursing practice,
      2587–2588
   informed consent and, 2587
   nursing, 2586
   nursing clinical, 2586
   ongoing, 2537
   participants, 2586–2587

   qualitative, 2586
   quantitative, 2586
   study types, 2588–2589
Reservoirs
   defined, 524
   human body, 524
   portal of exit from, 524, 526t
Resident assessment instrument (RAI), 2298
Resident assessment protocols (RAPs), 2297–2298
Resident utilization guides (RUGs), 2298
Residual urine, 264
Resilience
   adjustment disorder with depressed mood
      and, 1805
   crisis and, 1928–1929
   defined, 1654, 1805, 1928
Resiliency, 1715
Resiliency theory
   adaptation phase, 1655
   adjustment phase, 1655
   defined, 1654
   protective factors, 1654–1655
   risk factors, 1655
Resistance stage, 1901, 1901f
Resistive exercises, 837
Resolution phase, sexual response cycle,
      1347t, 1348
Resonance, 2280
Resorption, 821f
Resource allocation
   defined, 2607
   examples of, 2607–2608
   nurses and, 2608
   overview of, 2607
Resource management, 2476
Resources
   availability of, 2369
   defined, 2369
   limited, allocation of, 2577
   utilization of, 2688
Respect, 2409
Respiration
   congenital heart defects and, 1102
   defined, 953
   in liver disease, 787
   pH and, 7
   throughout life span, 956t
   variations by age, 1045t
Respiratory acidosis
   acute, 21
   assessment, 22–23
   care planning, 23
   causes, 9t, 10t
   chronic, 21
   collaborative care, 21–22
   compensation, 10t
   defined, 4, 6, 21
   diagnosis, 23
   diagnostic tests, 22
   illustrated, 7f
   imbalance, 9t
   interventions and therapies, 8t, 22t, 23–24
   manifestations, 8t, 21, 22t
   nursing process, 22–24
   outcome evaluation, 24
   overview of, 21
   pathophysiology and etiology, 21
   pharmacologic therapy, 12, 22
   respiratory support, 22
   risk factors, 7, 21

Respiratory alkalosis
assessment, 26
care planning, 26
causes, 9t, 10t
collaborative care, 25
compensation, 10t
defined, 4–6, 25
diagnosis, 26
illustrated, 7f
imbalance, 9t
interventions and therapies, 8t, 26
manifestations, 8t, 25, 26t
nursing implementation, 26
nursing process, 26–27
outcome evaluation, 26–27
overview of, 25
pathophysiology and etiology, 25
pharmacologic therapy, 12, 25
planning, 26
respiratory therapy, 25
risk factors, 7, 25
Respiratory arrest, 959
Respiratory distress, newborns, 2209t
Respiratory distress syndrome, 2047, 2254
Respiratory function, premature newborns,
    2255–2256
Respiratory gas exchange, 647
Respiratory inspiration, 971f
Respiratory muscles, paralysis and, 911
Respiratory rate
assessment of, 963f
bradypnea, 959, 960t
tachypnea, 959, 960t
Respiratory syncytial virus (RSV)/bronchiolitis
Alaskan native infants and, 1019t
assessment, 1021
breathing pattern enhancement and, 1022
care planning, 1021
in children, 1018–1024, 1022t
collaborative care, 1020–1021
culture and, 1019t
defined, 1018
diagnosis, 1021
diagnostic tests, 1020–1021, 1020t
etiology, 1019
fatigue and, 1022
fluid balance monitoring and, 1022
interventions, 1022
manifestations, 1019–1020, 1020t
nonpharmacologic therapy, 1021
Nursing Care Plan, 1023t
nursing process, 1021–1022
nutrition and, 1022
overview of, 1018–1019
pathophysiology and etiology, 1019–1020
pharmacologic therapy, 1021
planning goals, 1021
prevention of, 1019
risk factors, 1019
Respiratory system
acid-base balance and, 4–6
alterations, 957–961, 960t
anatomy illustration, 954
assessment, 962–967, 963–964t
burn injuries and, 1470–1471
changes and infection, 525
in children, 965t
diagnostic tests, 965–966, 967t
disseminated intravascular coagulation (DIC)
    and, 1141t

exercise benefits, 422
in infants, 965t
interventions and therapies, 974
labor and, 2126
lifespan considerations, 965, 965t
lower tract, 954–955
in older adults, 965t
pregnancy changes, 2030
in pregnant women, 965t
premature newborns and, 2250
prevention and, 961
shock effect on, 1220
spinal cord injuries (SCI) and, 912
Respiratory therapists, 1251
Respiratory therapy, 25
Respondeat superior, 2656
Response-based stress models
alarm reaction, 1901, 1901f
defined, 1900
general adaptation syndrome (GAS), 1900
local adaptation syndrome (LAS), 1900
stage of exhaustion, 1901, 1901f
stage of resistance, 1901, 1901f
Responses, 2399
Responsibility
accountability and, 2535
in chain of command, 2549
defined, 1880, 2476, 2535
in management, 2476
nurses, 1880
nursing students, 2666
personal, 2689
Responsible sexual behavior
dating violence, 1406–1407, 1407t
overview of, 1406
safer sex, 1406, 1407t
Rest and activity balance, Alzheimer disease (AD)
    and, 1601t
Rest and comfort
osteoarthritis and, 891–893
peptic ulcer disease (PUD) and, 682
postpartum care, 2186
pyloric stenosis and, 253
systemic lupus erythematosus (SLE) and,
    516–517
Rest and sleep, bipolar disorders and, 1815
Rest pain, 1199
Resting posture, 2216, 2216f
Restitution, cardinal movement, 2125
Restless leg syndrome (RLS)
defined, 145, 195
manifestations, 195, 200t
therapies, 200t
Restraints
belt, 2704, 2706f
chemical, 2704
defined, 2704
hand, 2704, 2706f
limb, 2704, 2706f
mitt, 2704, 2706f
monitoring and intervention flow sheet, 2705
physical, 2704
safety strap body, 2704, 2706f
types of, 2704
Restrictive cardiomyopathy, 1077t, 1078
Retained placenta, 2139t
Retinopathy, 2046
Retractions, 590, 590f, 992, 992f
Retrograde conduction, 1184
Retropubic prostatectomy, 115

Retropulsion, 897
Retrospective audit, 2685
Revascularization procedures
coronary artery bypass grafting (CABG),
    1121–1122, 1121f, 1122f
minimally invasive coronary artery
    surgery, 1122
percutaneous coronary revascularization
    (PCR), 1120–1121, 1121f
transmyocardial laser revascularization, 1122
Reverse delegation, 2472
Reverse triage, 2612
Revision surgery, 872
Reye syndrome, 571
Rh disease, 1768
Rheumatoid arthritis. *See also* Immunity
in affecting mobility, 826
ankles and feet, 499
antepartum care and, 2079t
assessment, 505
as autoimmune disorder, 495
Boutonnière deformities, 505
in children, 497t
client outcomes, 505
collaborative care, 501–504
complementary and alternative therapy,
    504, 504t
coronary heart disease risk and, 499
defined, 495
diagnosis, 505
diagnostic tests, 501
extra-articular manifestations, 499
hands and fingers, 497
heat and cold and, 504
illustrated, 826
inflammation in, 640
interventions
    body image, 507
    chronic pain treatment, 505–506
    fatigue prevention, 506
    impaired mobility support, 507
    ineffective role performance, 507
joint inflammation and destruction, 496f
joint manifestations, 497–499
juvenile idiopathic arthritis (JIA), 499–500
knees, 499
lifespan considerations, 497t
manifestation comparison, 496t
manifestations, 496–500, 500t
medications, 503t
multisystem effects of, 498t
nonpharmacologic therapy, 503–504
Nursing Care Plan, 508t
nursing process, 504–507
nutrition and, 504
in older adults, 497t
orthotic and assistive devices and, 504
outcome evaluation, 507
overview of, 495
pathophysiology and etiology, 495–496
pharmacologic therapy
    antimalarial agents, 503
    corticosteroids, 501–502
    disease-modifying antirheumatic drugs
        (DMARDs), 502–503
    gold salts, 502–503
    immune and inflammatory agents, 502
    nonsteroidal anti-inflammatory drugs
        (NSAIDs), 501, 502t
    sulfasalazine, 503

Rheumatoid arthritis (*continued*)
  physical and occupational therapy and, 504
  plasmapheresis and irradiation and, 504
  in pregnant women, 497*t*
  rest and exercise and, 504
  risk factors, 496
  self-management, 505*t*
  spine, 499
  surgery, 501
  swan-neck deformity, 497, 497*f*
  teaching client with, 506*t*
  tonnière deformity, 497, 497*f*
  wrists and elbows, 499
Rheumatoid factors, 495
Rhinorrhea, 571, 1019
Rhonchi, 963*t*
Ribonucleic acid (RNA), 30
Ribosomes, 30
Richards, Linda, 2547
Rickettsia, 530*t*
Rifampin, 612*t*
Right-sided failure. *See also* Heart failure
  hemodynamic effects of, 1148*f*
  left-sided failure versus, 1147
  manifestations, 1148
Rigid boundaries, 1714
Rigidity, 897
Rinne test, 1291*f*
Risk factors
  defined, 415, 2335
  pregnancy, 2053
  resiliency theory, 1655
  violence, 1954
Risk for injury
  metabolic acidosis, 16
  respiratory acidosis, 23
  sensory perception and, 1283
Risk for spiritual distress, 1891
Risk management
  as area for improvement, 2687
  competent nursing care and, 2677, 2678*t*
  defined, 2676, 2687
  incident reports, 2678
  overview of, 2676–2677
  pediatric medical errors and, 2677–2678
  physician order implementation and, 2677
  strategies for, 2677–2678
Risk monitoring, in postoperative nursing, 1272–1273
Risk nursing diagnosis, 2335
RLS. *See* Restless leg syndrome
RNA (ribonucleic acid), 30
RNs (registered nurses), 2458
Roach's theory of caring, 2302
Role ambiguity, 1834
Role development, 1833
Role mastery, 1834
Role performance, 1833–1834
Role strain, 1834
Roles, 1833
Roles and relationships, 2408
ROM (range of motion) exercises, 506
Roman Catholic, 1886, 1886*t*
Root cause analysis, 2686, 2687–2688
Rooting reflex, 2234, 2234*f*
ROP (retinopathy of prematurity), 2254
Rosenbaum eye chart, 1285, 1285*f*
Roseola, 539*t*
Ross procedure, 1100*t*
Rotational injuries, spinal cord, 908

Rotator cuff tear, 827, 827*f*
Rotavirus, 540*t*
Roux-en-Y gastric bypass, 795, 795*f*
Rubella (German measles), 540*t*
RUGs (resident utilization guides), 2298
Rule of nines, 1468–1469, 1469*f*
Rules, family, 1716
Rumination disorder, 1836
Rupture of membranes, 2121
Rush, 1564

S

Sacral agenesis, 2046
Sacred symbols, 1884
Sacred writings, 1884
SAD (seasonal affective disorder), 1780–1781, 1800, 1800*t*
SAD (separation anxiety disorder), 1921, 1922*t*
Safe client handling, 2717
Safer sex, 1406, 1407*t*
Safety
  abuse and, 1974
  alcohol abuse and, 1541, 1543
  bipolar disorders and, 1814
  car, for newborns, 2247
  community and local initiatives, 2702–2703, 2703*t*
  concept of, 2695–2696
  concepts related to, 2698–2699*t*
  delegation and, 2471*t*
  diabetes and, 763–764
  injury prevention
    falls, 2703–2704
    healthcare-associated infections, 2704–2706
    medication errors, 2707
    restraints, 2703–2704, 2705*f*, 2706*f*
    wrong-site surgery, 2706–2707
  intraoperative nursing, 1262, 1263–1264*t*
  malpractice and, 2657
  Mass in Motion (MiM) and, 2702–2703
  Minnesota Fall Prevention and, 2702
  mood and affect and, 1788–1789, 1789*t*
  motor vehicle crashes (MVC) and, 2000*t*, 2001*t*
  national patient safety initiatives
    defined, 2696
    National Patient Safety Goals (NPSG), 2701, 2701*t*
    overview of, 2697*t*
    Quality and Safety Eduction for Nurses (QSEN), 2696–2701
  newborn care, 2240
  personality disorders (PD) and, 1865
  in prioritizing care, 2368–2369
  as QSEN competency, 2699, 2700
  in self-care in nursing, 2308
  stroke and, 1245–1246
  substance abuse and, 1569, 1570–1571
  workplace, 2715–2718, 2718*t*
Safety considerations across the life span
  adult safety and mortality, 2712–2713, 2713*f*, 2713*t*
  assessment, 2713
  care planning, 2714
  child abuse/neglect and, 2710*t*
  children and unintentional injuries
    adolescents, 2711–2712, 2711*f*
    nursing implications, 2712
    preschoolers, 2710–2711

  school-age children, 2711, 2711*t*
  sports-related concussions and, 2712*t*
  toddlers, 2710, 2710*f*
  water-related injuries, 2711*t*
  diagnosis, 2714
  distracted driving, 2712, 2713*t*
  infant risk, 2710
  interventions, 2714
  middle adults, 2712–2713
  neonatal risk, 2709–2710
  nursing process, 2713–2714
  older adults, 2713, 2713*f*
  outcome evaluation, 2714
  overview of, 2708
  perinatal risk, 2708–2709, 2709*t*
  prenatal risk, 2708, 2709*t*
  young adults, 2712
Safety strap body restraints, 2704, 2706*f*
Sagittal suture, 2114
Salient cues, 2317–2318, 2318*f*
Saline, 337
Salmonella, 2097
SAMe, 1796
SAMHSA (Substance Abuse and Mental Health Services Administration), 1527
"Sandwich generation," 1712*t*
Sanger, Margaret, 2548
Sanguineous (hemorrhagic) exudate, 1509
Sarcomeres, 820
Sarcopenia, 821
Satiety, 791, 927
Saturated fats, 757, 929
Scaling assessment questions, 1932
Scalp assessment, 1459*t*
Scapegoats, 2422
Scarf sign, 2220, 2220*f*
SCD. *See* Sickle cell disease
Scheduled toileting, 295
Scheduling decisions, 2321
Schema-focused therapy, 1862
Schemes, 1576
Schistocytes, 1140
Schizoaffective disorder, 1615
Schizoid personality disorder, 1857*t*, 1859–1860, 1863*t*
Schizophrenia
  adult-onset (AOS), 1616
  assertive community treatment (ACT), 1619, 1619*t*
  assessment, 1620–1622
  biological risk factors, 1612
  brain PET scans, 1617*f*
  brief psychotic disorder, 1615
  care planning, 1622
  client advocacy, 1623
  CNS abnormalities, 1611*t*
  collaborative care, 1616–1620
  communication deviance, 1612
  complementary and alternative therapy, 1620
  defined, 1610
  diagnosis, 1622
  diagnostic tests, 1616
  DSM-5 diagnostic criteria for, 1617*t*
  early-onset (EOS), 1616
  education and, 1623
  electroconvulsive therapy (ECT), 1620
  etiology, 1612
  family communication, 1623*t*
  features, 1611
  group therapy, 1619

hospitalization and, 1619–1620
injury prevention and, 1623
interventions, 1622–1623
manifestations
　　comorbid disorders, 1615–1616
　　delusion categories, 1614t
　　disorder forms, 1613–1614
　　lifespan and cultural considerations, 1616, 1616t
　　negative symptoms, 1614
　　related disorders, 1615
　　subtypes, specifiers, and dimensions, 1615
　　therapies and, 1621t
medications, 1618t
nonpharmacologic therapy, 1619–1620
Nursing Care Plan, 1624–1625t
nursing outcomes, 1622t
nursing process, 1620–1623
outcome evaluation, 1623
overview of, 1610–1611
pathophysiology, 1611–1613
pharmacologic therapy, 1616–1618
positive and negative symptoms, 1613, 1613t
prevention of, 1613
psychiatric/psychosocial rehabilitation, 1619
psychosis and, 1611
risk factors, 1612–1613
social-environmental risk factors, 1612–1613
symptomatic treatment, 1623
thought disorders, 1613
transcranial magnetic stimulation (TMS), 1620
Schizophreniform disorder, 1615
Schizotypal personality disorder, 1857t, 1860, 1864t
School-age children. See also Children; Pediatric clients
assessment of, 2292–2293, 2293f
bowel elimination, 275
cognitive development, 1667
communication, 1668
family with, 1726
growth and development, 1666–1668
growth and development milestones, 1667t
health screenings and immunization guidelines, 413–414t
injury prevention due to motor vehicle crashes, 2000t
normal sleep-rest patterns in, 432
oral health in, 427–428
personality and temperament, 1668
physical growth and development, 1666–1667
play, 1667–1668
psychosocial development, 1667–1668, 1667t
sexual development, 1341t
sexuality, 1668
unintentional injuries, 2711
urinary elimination in, 262–263
SCI. See Spinal cord injuries
Sciatica, 841, 842f
Science and technology, 2541
Scientific method, 2324, 2586, 2586t
SCIP (Surgical Care Improvement Project), 2632
Scleral buckling, 1314
Scoliometer, 847
Scoliosis. See also Back problems
adolescent idiopathic, 847
adolescent self-image and, 849t
adult idiopathic, 847
assessment, 849–850, 850f
care planning, 850

children with, 847, 848f, 851–852
collaborative care, 847–849
congenital, 846
defined, 824t, 845
diagnosis, 847f, 850
diagnostic tests, 847–848
halo brace, 848, 848f
home care after surgery, 848t
illustrated, 825f
infantile idiopathic, 847
interventions, 824t, 850
juvenile idiopathic, 847
lifespan and cultural considerations, 847
manifestations, 824t, 847, 849t
neuromuscular, 846
nonpharmacologic therapy, 848–849
Nursing Care Plan, 851–852t
nursing process, 849–850
outcome evaluation, 850
pathophysiology and etiology, 845–847
pharmacologic therapy, 848
risk factors, 847
surgery, 848
thoracolumbar sacral orthosis (TLSO), 848
vertical rotation determination, 848
Scratch tests, 1456
SCT (stem cell transplant), 98
Seasonal affective disorder (SAD), 1780–1781, 1800, 1800t
Second (S_2) heart sounds, 1034
Secondary appraisal, 1902
Secondary cancers, 51
Secondary care, 2598
Secondary cataracts, 1307
Secondary groups, 2418
Secondary hypertension, 1165–1166
Secondary immune response, 442
Secondary infertility, 1372
Secondary intension healing, 1507
Secondary prevention, 2597, 2597t
Secondary skin lesions, 1451t
Secondary syphilis, 1413
Second-degree AV block, 1182t, 1186
Secondhand smoke, 1546–1547, 1548t
Secretion clearance, 969
Secretory phase, 2019
Sedation
opioid use and, 165t
scale, 166t
Sedative-hypnotic agents, 1255t
Sedentary lifestyle, osteoporosis and, 800
Segmental mastectomy, 79
Segmental pressure measurements, 1200
Seizure disorders
assessment, 720, 720t
in children, 718–720
collaborative care, 718–720
diagnosis, 720–721
diagnostic tests, 718
interventions, 721
lifespan considerations, 716t
manifestations, 716, 717–718t
medications for, 719t
Nursing Care Plan, 722–723t
nursing process, 720–721
outcome evaluation, 721
overview of, 715
pathophysiology and etiology, 715–716

pharmacologic therapy, 718
prevention of, 716
risk factors, 716
Seizures
in adolescents, 722t
altered level of consciousness (LOC) and, 694
aura, 716
in children, 722t
clonic phase, 716
defined, 715
diversity and culture, 721
febrile, 716, 1434
focal, 716
generalized, 716
intractable, 719
length of, 716
lifespan considerations, 722t
pharmacologic therapy, 708
postictal period, 716
status epilepticus, 718, 719t
tonic phase, 716
when standing, 721f
Selective serotonin reuptake inhibitors (SSRIs)
client education, 1791–1792
for cognitive alterations, 1592t
defined, 1791
nursing care, 1791
Self
alterations from normal
　　assessment, 1840–1841
　　diagnostic tests, 1841
　　feeding and eating disorders, 1836–1838, 1838t
　　genetic considerations and nonmodifiable risk factors, 1840
　　personality disorders, 1838, 1838f
　　prevalence of, 1838–1840
　　prevention of, 1840
　　screenings, 1840
　　therapies, 1839t
collaborative interventions and therapies, 1842
concepts related to, 1837t
genetic and lifespan considerations, 1836
ideal, 1832
independent interventions and therapies, 1842
interventions and therapies, 1842
introspection, 1834–1835
normal presentation of, 1832–1836
overview of, 1831–1832
psychosocial assessment criteria, 1841t
psychosocial development, 1835–1836
public, 1833
real, 1832–1833
self-awareness and, 1834–1835
self-concept and, 1832–1834
self-esteem and, 1834
Self theory, 1835–1836
Self-awareness, 1834
Self-awareness/growth groups, 2423–2424
Self-care
anemia and, 74
antepartum, 2108
bipolar disorders and, 1815
cataracts and, 1310
multiple sclerosis and, 884
stroke and, 1244–1245
techniques during pregnancy, 2076t

Self-care in nursing
    belonging and love and, 2308–2310
    burnout and, 2309t
    elements of, 2308
    health behaviors and, 2310–2311
    importance of, 2308
    Maslow's hierarchy of needs and, 2308–2310
    physiological needs and, 2308
    in prioritizing care, 2370
    safety and, 2308
    self-actualization and, 2310
    self-esteem and, 2310
    unhealthy behavior avoidance and, 2310
    wellness promotion and, 2310–2311
Self-concept
    body image, 1833, 1833f, 1833t
    defined, 1832
    personal identity, 1832–1833
    role performance, 1833–1834
Self-control, 1904
Self-disclosure, avoiding, 2429
Self-efficacy, 1654, 1655t, 1928
Self-esteem
    defined, 1834
    global, 1834
    lifespan considerations, 1836
    specific, 1834
Self-esteem promotion
    in ADHD, 1685
    in alcohol abuse, 1543
    in depression, 1803
    in erectile dysfunction, 1370
    in menopause, 1398
    in nephritis, 674
    in obesity, 797
    in pressure ulcers, 1504
    in substance abuse, 1570
Self-help groups, 2423
Self-quieting ability, 2204
Self-quieting activity, 2236
Self-report scales
    adults, 1785–1786
    children, 1786–1787
    older adults, 1787
    postpartum depression, 1787
Self-talk, 2398, 2398f
Semiformal groups, 2419, 2420t
Semi-Fowler position, 1264t
Sender, 2399
Sensitivity of the receptors, 1784
Sensitivity testing, in tuberculosis, 611
Sensitization, 158
Sensor deprivation prevention, 1296
Sensorineural hearing loss, 1299
Sensory deficit management, 1296, 1296t
Sensory function assessment, 736t
Sensory overload, 1296, 1613
Sensory perception
    alterations, 1279–1282
    alterations and therapies, 1281t
    assessment
        in children, 1291t
        client environment and, 1284
        cranial nerve, 1294–1295t
        eye and vision, 1284, 1286–1290t
        fine touch, 1295t
        interview, 1284
        kinesthesia, 1295t
        nursing, 1283–1284
        physical, 1284–1291

        smell, 1290–1291, 1294t
        social support network and, 1284
        tactile, 1290–1291, 1294t
        taste, 1290–1291, 1295t
    concepts related to, 1280–1281t
    congenital and hereditary conditions
        and, 1282
    deficits, communication and, 2413
    defined, 1277
    genetic considerations and nonmodifiable risk
        factors, 1282
    hearing. See hearing
    illness and, 1282
    interventions and therapies
        acute sensory deficit management, 1296
        collaborative, 1298
        coping, 1296–1297
        healthy sensory function promotion,
            1295–1296
        impaired hearing, 1297
        independent, 1295–1297
        pharmacologic therapy, 1298
        sensory deprivation prevention, 1296
        sensory overload prevention, 1296
    modifiable risk factors, 1282–1283
    in newborns, 2204
    normal, 1278–1279
    prevention and, 1282–1283
    process aspects, 1278
    screenings, 1283
    sensory tracts, 1278f
    smell, 1283
    stimuli, 1278
    taste, 1283
    touch, 1283
    vision. See vision
Sensory reception, 1278
Sensory-perceptual deficits, stroke and, 1237
Sentinel events, 2686–2687
Separation anxiety disorder (SAD), 1921, 1922t
Sepsis
    assessment, 603
    care planning, 603
    in children, 601
    collaborative care, 602–603
    defined, 523, 600
    diagnosis, 603
    diagnostic tests, 602
    fluid replacement in, 602–603
    interventions, 603–604
    lifespan and cultural considerations,
        601–602
    manifestations, 601–602, 601t, 603t
    Nursing Care Plan, 604–605t
    nursing process, 603–604
    in older adults, 602
    overview of, 600
    oxygen therapy, 602
    pharmacologic therapy, 602–603
    reevaluation, 604
    severe, 600
Septal (blood flow increase) defects. See also
        Congenital heart defects
    atrial septal defect (ASD), 1084–1085t
    atrioventricular (AV) canal (endocardial
        cushion defect), 1086t
    clinical therapy, 1084–1086t
    defined, 1084
    manifestations, 1084–1086t, 1094
    patent ductus arteriosus (PDA), 1084t

    pathophysiology, 1084–1086t
    ventricular septal defect (VSD), 1085–1086t
Septic shock
    assessment, 1230
    defined, 600, 1224
    illustrated, 600f
    manifestations, 1226t
    Nursing Care Plan, 1233t
    portals of entry for infection, 601
Septicemia, 523, 600
Seroconversion, 457
Serological testing
    in infection, 556
    in pneumonia, 591
Serosanguineous exudate, 1509
Serotonin receptor agonists, 223
Serotonin syndrome, 1790
Serotonin-norepinephrine, 1334t
Serous exudate, 1509
Serous otitis media, 576
Serum α_1-antitrypsin levels, 1009
Serum albumin, 785
Serum ammonia, 785
Serum amylase and lipase, 651t
Serum bicarbonate, 6
Serum bilirubin, 651, 651t
Serum cardiac enzymes, 1227
Serum cholesterol
    in diabetes, 752
    in liver disease, 785
    in obesity, 793
    values classification, 1110
Serum complement levels, 512
Serum creatinine
    in acute renal failure (ARF), 380
    in chronic kidney disease (CKD), 391f, 395
    in nephritis, 672
    in shock, 1227
Serum digoxin level, 1098t
Serum electrolytes
    in acute renal failure (ARF), 380
    in burn injuries, 1477
    in chronic kidney disease (CKD), 395
    in diabetes, 752
    format for diagram of, 351f
    in heart failure, 1151
    levels, 351
    in liver disease, 785
    in lung cancer, 108
    in metabolic alkalosis, 18
    in nephritis, 672
    in respiratory acidosis, 22
    in sepsis, 602
    in shock, 1227
Serum enzymes, 602
Serum glucose
    in liver disease, 785
    in obesity, 793
Serum hyperosmolarity, 747
Serum lipid panel, 1098t
Serum sickness, 483
Service orientation, 2537
Severe burns. See also Burns
    acute stage, 1474
    emergent/resuscitative stage, 1474
    injection prevention, 1474
    Nursing Care Plan, 1486–1487t
    nutrition therapy, 1474
    overview of, 1473–1474
    pain management, 1474

progression of treatment through healthcare system, 1474f
rehabilitative stage, 1474–1475
wound care, 1474
Severe mental illness, 1731–1733, 1732t
Severe sepsis
pathophysiology and etiology, 600–601
prevention, 601
risk factors, 601
Sex, safe, 1407t
Sex chromosome abnormalities, 1376
Sex chromosomes, 31–32, 1659
Sexism, 1635
Sexual abuse
defined, 1966
manifestations of, 1969, 1973t
therapies, 1973t
Sexual activity
antepartum care and, 2071–2072
postpartum care and, 2186–2187
pregnancy and, 2073t
Sexual arousal disorders, 1349, 1352t
Sexual aversion disorder, 1349
Sexual desire disorders, 1349
Sexual dysfunction
cognitive factors, 1349
colorectal cancer and, 90
discussing, 1369–1370
dissatisfaction problems, 1351
erectile dysfunction (ED), 1366–1371
factors affecting, 1351
medications and, 1350t
menstrual dysfunction, 1352t, 1399–1406
opioid use and, 165t
orgasmic disorders, 1349–1350, 1352t
past and current factors, 1348–1349
prevalence of, 1351
prevention of, 1353
priapism, 1352t
psychological factors, 1349
relationship problems and, 1349
sexual arousal disorders, 1349, 1352t
sexual desire disorders, 1349
sexual pain disorders, 1350–1351, 1352t
sociocultural factors, 1348–1349
surgery, 1363
Sexual function
infertility and, 1392
medication effect on, 1350t
menstrual dysfunction and, 1404–1405
prostate cancer and, 117
STIs and, 1415
Sexual harassment, 2484
Sexual health
body image and, 1345
components of, 1344–1345
defined, 1344
diabetes and, 764
diversity and culture and, 1362t
gender identity and, 1345
gender-role behavior and, 1345
infertility and, 1392
maintaining, 1365
sexual response cycle and, 1346–1348, 1347t
sexual rights and, 1344t
sexual self-concept and, 1344
varieties of sexuality and, 1344–1346
Sexual orientation, 1636
Sexual pain disorders, 1350–1351, 1352t

Sexual response cycle
desire phase, 1346
excitement phase, 1346, 1347t
orgasmic phase, 1346–1348, 1347t
resolution phase, 1347t, 1348
Sexual rights, 1344t
Sexual self-concept, 1344
Sexuality
adolescent, 1670
alterations
in function, 1348–1353
orgasmic disorders, 1349–1350
problems with satisfaction, 1351
sexual arousal disorders, 1349
sexual desire disorders, 1349
sexual pain disorders, 1350–1351
alterations and therapies, 1352t
assessment
adolescents, 1354–1355
axillary and clavicular lymph node, 1359t
breast (female), 1358–1359t
breast and lymph node (male), 1356t
external genitalia (female), 1360–1361t
external genitalia (male), 1356t
female reproductive system, 1358–1361t
hernia and lymph node, 1359t
male reproductive system, 1356–1357t
of men, 1353–1354
nursing, 1353–1355
physical, 1354
prostate, 1357t
vaginal and cervical, 1361t
of women, 1354
cognitive factors, 1349
collaborative interventions and therapies, 1363
concepts related to, 1348t
development
adolescence, 1340–1343
birth to 12 years, 1340
lifespan considerations, 1341–1342t
older adulthood, 1343–1344
young and middle adulthood, 1343
diabetes and, 1344
diagnostic tests, 1362–1363
erotic preferences, 1346
family and, 1355
genetic considerations, 1351
HIV/AIDS and, 478
inappropriate behaviors and, 1363–1365, 1365t
independent interventions and therapies, 1363
interventions and therapies, 1363–1365
lifespan and cultural considerations, 1355–1362
male, 1353–1354, 1353t
medications, 1364–1365t
menstrual dysfunction, 1352t
Nursing Care Plan, 1416–1417t
orgasmic disorders, 1352t
past and current factors, 1348–1349
personal expectations/ethics and, 1362
pharmacologic therapy, 1363
prevention and, 1353
priapism, 1352t
psychological factors, 1349
relationship problems and, 1349
religion and, 1362
school-age children, 1668
sexual arousal disorders, 1352t
sexual heath and, 1344–1348
sexual pain disorders, 1352t

sociocultural factors, 1348–1349
surgery and, 1363
varieties of
gender identity, 1345–1346
sexual orientation, 1345
sexual response cycle, 1346–1348, 1347t
Sexually transmitted diseases (STDs), 1408
Sexually transmitted infections (STIs)
in adolescents, 1343, 1408
assessment, 1414–1415
care planning, 1415
causes of, 1408
characteristics of, 1409
chlamydia, 1412, 1412t
community-based care, 1414t
defined, 1408
diagnosis, 1415
disease management, 1415–1416
genital herpes (HSV), 1410–1411, 1410t
genital warts, 1411–1412, 1411f, 1411t
gonorrhea, 1412–1413
incidence and prevalence of, 1408–1409
interventions, 1352t, 1415–1416
nursing process, 1414–1416
outcome evaluation, 1416
overview of, 1408–1409
pain relief and, 1415
prevention and control, 1409
resources for clients with, 1410t
risk factors, 1409
sexual function and, 1415
syphilis, 1413–1414, 1413f
SGA (small gestational age), 2207t
Shallow breathing, 2163
Shared governance, 2457–2458, 2490
Shared leadership, 2490
Shivering, 1439
Shock
anaphylactic, 1224, 1226t, 1230
anxiety relief and, 1232
assessment, 1230
blood and blood products for, 1230
cardiac output preservation and, 1231, 1231f
cardiogenic, 1223–1224, 1225–1226t, 1230
cardiovascular system effect, 1220
care planning, 1231
classifications of, 1219t
colloid solutions for, 1229t, 1230
compensatory, 1218–1219
crystalloid solutions for, 1230
defined, 1218
diagnosis, 1230–1231
diagnostic tests, 1227
distributive, 1224, 1226t
effects on body systems, 1220–1222
etiology, 1222–1224
fluid replacement therapy, 1228–1229
gastrointestinal system effect, 1220–1222
homeodynamics and, 1218
homeostatic regulation and, 1218
hypovolemic, 1222–1223, 1223f, 1225t, 1230
interventions, 1231–1232
manifestations, 1224, 1225–1227t
multisystem effects of, 1221f
neurogenic, 1224, 1226t, 1230
neurological system effect, 1222
Nursing Care Plan, 1233t
nursing process, 1230–1232
obstructive, 1224, 1226t

Shock (*continued*)
outcome evaluation, 1231–1232
overview of, 1218
oxygen therapy, 1229
pathophysiology, 1218–1224
pharmacologic therapy, 1227, 1228–1229t
progressive, 1219–1220
refractory or irreversible, 1220
renal system effect, 1222
respiratory system effect, 1220
risk factors, 1224
septic, 1224, 1226t, 1230
skin, temperature, and thirst effect, 1222
stage I, 1218–1219
stage II, 1219–1220
stage III, 1220
tissue perfusion and, 1231–1232
Shock phase, 1901
Short bowel syndrome
assessment, 245
in children, 244t
client teaching, 245t
collaborative care, 244
defined, 244
diagnostic tests, 244
manifestations, 244
nursing care, 244–245
nutrition, 244
pathophysiology and etiology, 244
pharmacologic therapy, 244
Short Portable Mental Status Questionnaire
(SPMSQ), 1587t, 2295t
Shortages, nursing, 2465–2466, 2542, 2542t
Short-term goals, 2341–2342
Shoulders, mobility assessment, 832t
Sibling relationships, 1713–1714
Siblings
care of, 2108–2109
death of, 1753
maternal attachment behavior and, 1819
preparation for new baby, 2040
Sibutramine (Meridia), 793
Sick sinus syndrome, 1183
Sick-day management, diabetes clients, 758
Sickle cell anemia, 120
Sickle cell crisis, 2045
defined, 120
overview of, 121t
Sickle cell disease (SCD)
alterations and therapies, 34t
assessment, 124
care outcomes and goals, 124
caregiver strain and, 126
children and, 125t
collaborative care, 122–124
complementary and alternative therapy, 124
cultural prevalence of, 120t
defined, 120
diagnosis, 124
diagnostic tests, 122
fluid volume balance and, 125
forms of, 120t
genetics and, 34
growth and development facilitation and, 126
infection prevention and management, 125
interventions, 125–126
lifespan considerations, 122
manifestations, 121–122, 123t
nonpharmacologic therapy, 123–124
Nursing Care Plan, 126–127t

nursing process, 124–126
outcome evaluation, 126
overview of, 120
oxygenation and circulation and, 125
pain management, 125
pathophysiology and etiology, 120–121
pediatric clients and, 122
pharmacologic therapy, 122–123
pregnancy and, 122, 2045
prevalence of, 34
risk factors, 34, 121
as stroke risk factor, 1236
surgery, 122
Sickle cell trait, 121
Sickling, 120
SIDS. *See* Sudden infant death syndrome
Sigma Theta Tau International, 2626
Signs, 2270
Silence, 2427
Simple assault, 1975
Simple diffusion, 2026
Simple mastectomy, 79
Sims position, 2278t
SIMV (synchronized intermittent mandatory
ventilation), 980, 981t
Sinciput, 2114
Single photon emission computed tomography
(SPECT), 898
Single-parent families, 1710
Sinus arrhythmia, 1180t, 1183
Sinus bradycardia, 1180t, 1183
Sinus node dysrhythmias, 1183
Sinus tachycardia, 1180t, 1183
SIRS (systemic inflammatory response
syndrome), 600
Site-specific disaster zones, 2614, 2614t
Sitting, 2278t
Situational crisis, 1928, 1928f
Situational depression. *See* Adjustment disorder
with depressed mood
Situational leaders, 2490
Six rights of medication administration, 2707
Six Sigma, 2691–2692
Sixty-nine, 1346
Skeletal traction, 862
Skeleton. *See also* Bones
appendicular, 820
axial, 820
development in childhood, 820, 821t
Skene glands, 1360f
Skin
age-related changes, 1447–1448, 1447t
assessment, 734t, 1455–1456, 1457–1460t
changes and infection, 525
cultures, 671
dermis, 1447
epidermis, 1446–1447
gestational age and, 2216
intact, 1448
layers of, 1446–1447
in newborns, 1447
normal presentation, 1446–1448
in older adults, 1448
pregnancy and, 2032, 2032f
pressure ulcers and, 1494
pruritus, 1453–1454t, 1491t
redness of, 1457t
shock effect on, 1222
subcutaneous tissue, 1447
temperature assessment, 1457t

texture assessment, 1458t
three-dimensional view, 1446f
turgor assessment, 1458t
wounds. *See* wound healing; wounds
Skin biopsy, 1456
Skin cancer. *See also* Cancer
actinic keratosis, 131, 131f
anxiety and, 136–137
assessment, 135, 135t
basal cell, 129–130, 130f, 130t
care planning, 136
collaborative care, 134–135
diagnosis, 136
diagnostic tests, 134
emerging therapies, 135
environmental factors, 131
etiology, 131
gene therapy, 135
hopeless feelings and, 136
host factors, 131–132
immunotherapy, 135
inflection and, 136
interventions, 136–137
manifestations and therapies, 132, 132–133t
melanomas, 128–129
microstaging, 134, 134f
nonmelanoma, 129–130
nursing process, 135–137
outcome evaluation, 137
overview of, 128
pathophysiology, 128–132
pharmacologic therapy, 135
precursor lesions, 128
prevention, 132
radiation therapy, 135
risk factors, 131, 131f
squamous cell, 130, 130f
surgery, 134
Skin color, 1460t, 1639, 2210
Skin disorders
genetics and, 1452
infectious, 1448
inflammatory, 1448
prevalence of, 1452
prevention of, 1455
skin color, 1452
Skin integrity. *See also* Tissue integrity
alterations to, 1448–1454
bowel incontinence and, 316
burns and, 1483–1484
cerebral palsy (CP) and, 1699
diabetes and, 762
hepatitis and, 236
HIV/AIDS, 477–478
hypothyroidism and, 815–816
impaired, 1453t
in liver disease, 787
nephritis, 674
in newborns, 2239–2240
peripheral vascular disease (PVD) and, 1203
pressure ulcers and, 1502–1504
systemic lupus erythematosus (SLE) and, 516–517
urinary incontinence and retention, 302
Skin lesions
defined, 1448
primary, 1450t
secondary, 1451t
Skin patch, contraceptive, 1384
Skin testing, 489–490
Skin traction, 862

Skin turgor, 2224
SLE. *See* Systemic lupus erythematosus
Sleep. *See also* Normal sleep-rest patterns
  in adolescents, 432, 432*t*
  circadian rhythms, 432*t*
  cycles, 431
  defined, 432*t*
  diet and, 433
  emotional stress and, 433
  factors affecting, 433–434
  functions of, 431
  in infants, 432
  in infants, SIDS and, 1027*t*
  medications, 151*t*, 434
  motivation and, 434
  in newborns, 431–432, 2246–2247
  normal patterns and requirements, 431
  NREM (non-rapid-eye-movement),
      430, 431*f*, 431*t*
  Parkinson disease and, 897
  physiological changes during, 431*t*
  physiology of, 430–431
  in preschoolers, 432
  REM (rapid-eye-movement), 431, 431*t*
  in school-age children, 432
  smoking and, 433–434
  stimulants and alcohol and, 433
  in toddlers, 432
  types of, 430–431
Sleep apnea
  central, 195
  defined, 145, 195
  manifestations, 200*t*
  mixed, 195
  obstructive, 195
  in pregnant women, 196
  as stroke risk factor, 1236
  therapies, 198, 200*t*
  types of, 195
Sleep architecture, 430
Sleep hygiene
  defined, 149
  fatigue and, 187*t*
  influenza and, 574
Sleep in America poll, 195
Sleep loss
  defined, 145, 195
  effects of, 195
  manifestations, 200*t*
  therapies, 200*t*
Sleep patterns
  normal, 195
  older adults, 196
Sleep restriction, 199*t*
Sleep states, newborns, 2202–2203
Sleepiness scales, 200–201, 201*f*
Sleep-rest disorders
  in adolescents, 196
  alterations and therapies, 144*t*
  assessment, 200–201
  care planning, 201
  causes of, 194
  collaborative care, 197–198
  complementary and alternative medicine, 199*t*
  defined, 144*t*
  diagnosis, 201
  diagnostic tests, 197
  Epworth Sleepiness Scale, 200, 201*f*
  ethnicity and, 197*t*
  hypersomnia, 195

insomnia, 145, 195, 199*t*
  interventions, 144*t*, *201*
  lifespan considerations, 196
  manifestations, 144*t*, 196, 200*t*
  medications, 198*t*
  narcolepsy, 145, 195
  nonpharmacologic therapy, 198
  Nursing Care Plan, 201–202*t*
  nursing process, 200–201
  in older adults, 196
  outcome evaluation, 196
  overview of, 194
  parasomnias, 145, 195
  pathophysiology and etiology, 195–196
  pharmacologic therapy, 197–198
  pregnancy and, 196
  restless leg syndrome and, 145, 195
  risk factors, 196
  sleep apnea, 145
  sleep hygiene and, 149–150
  sleep loss, 145, 195
  surgery, 197
  therapies, 200*t*
Sleep-rest patterns. *See* Normal sleep-rest
      patterns
Small gestational age (SGA), 2207*t*
Small-cell carcinomas, 104
Smallpox, 2615*t*
SMART format, 2343, 2343*t*
Smell
  assessment, 1290–1291, 1294*t*
  impaired, 1297
  screenings and, 1283
Smoking
  as cancer risk factor, 46–47
  as coronary artery disease risk factor, 1110
  culture and, 1546*t*
  Hispanic population and, 1007*t*
  as sensory perception risk factor, 1282
  sleep and, 433–434
  as stroke risk factor, 1236
Smoking cessation
  chronic obstructive pulmonary disease (COPD)
      and, 1016
  coronary artery disease (CAD) and, 1116
  oxygenation and, 968–969, 969*t*
  programs, 1547
Snappers, 1564
Snellen eye chart, 1285, 1285*f*
Sniffing, 1565
SNOMED CT (systemized nomenclature of
      medicine–clinical terms), 2644
SOAP notes, 2441
SOAPIER, 2441, 2442*f*
Sobriety, 1525*t*
Social anxiety disorder, 1941, 1941*t*
Social changes, 2572
Social cognitive theory, 2504, 2504*f*
Social differences
  additional, 1639*t*
  biological variations, 1639, 1639*f*
  communication, 1638
  environmental control, 1638
  religious variation, 1638
  skin culture, 1639
  space, 1638–1639
  susceptibility to disease, 1639
  time, 1639
Social distance, 2408
Social history, older adults, 2297

Social justice, 1634, 2564
Social learning theory
  in abuse, 1966–1967
  defined, 1928, 2504
  in development, 1654
Social media, 2638*t*
Social microcosm, 1530
Social persuasion, 1928
Social Readjustment Rating Scale (SRRS), 1900
Social science, 2269
Social support systems
  cultural aspects of, 416*t*
  health and wellness and, 416, 418
  pain response and, 162
  review, 416
Social workers, 1251
Socialization
  bipolar disorders and, 1814
  defined, 2539
  to nursing, 2539
Socialized insurance, 2463
Socialized medicine, 2463
Societal attitudes, in nursing development,
      2546–2547
Sociocultural comfort, 141
Sociocultural factors
  in addiction, 1521
  communication and, 2406
  depression theory, 1781, 1781*f*
  in personality disorders (PD), 1853–1854
  in rape, 1984
Socioeconomic factors
  abuse and, 1968
  antepartum nutrition, 2094
  assault and homicide and, 1977
Socioeconomic status, burn risk and, 1466
Sodium (NA+)
  cultural use of, 368*t*
  diabetes and, 757
  electrolyte imbalance, 370–371
  foods high in, 371
  intake in children, 371*t*
  intake management, 367
  low diet of, 369*t*
  as perioperative diagnostic test, 1252*t*
  regulation and function, 342*t*
  serum levels, 341
Sodium bicarbonate, 12
Sodium-channel blockers, 1189*t*
Sole creases, 2216, 2217*f*
Solutes
  colloids, 337
  crystalloids, 337
  defined, 336
Solvents, 337
Somatic and emotional states, 1928
Somatic cells, 32
Somatic neuropathies. *See* Peripheral neuropathies
Somatic pain, 155
Somatic reflexes, 689
Somatization, 1787
Somatostatin, 704
Somogyi phenomenon, 746
Source-oriented records, 2439–2440, 2440*t*
SOWS (*Subjective Opiate Withdrawal Scale*), 1569
Soy, 1397*t*
Space, culture, 1638–1639
Space-occupying lesions, 50
Sparring, 2433
Spasticity, 1239

Special interest professional organizations, 2626, 2626t
Specialized education, 2536
Specialty physicians, 1251
Specific defenses, 525
Specific phobias, 1940, 1940t, 1941t
Specific reactivity, 441
Specific self-esteem, 1834
Specificity theory, 154
SPECT (single photon emission computed tomography), 898
Spectral gradient acoustic reflectometry, 579
Speech
   expressive, 1662
   receptive, 1662
Speech/language therapy
   multiple sclerosis and, 881
   Parkinson disease and, 901
   stroke and, 1242
Spermicides, 1379
Sphincters, 931
Spinal cord
   damage, 907
   defined, 689
   structure of, 907f
   vertebral column and, 907, 907f
Spinal cord injuries (SCI)
   activities of daily living (ADLs) and, 915, 916–917
   assessment, 916
   autonomic dysreflexia and, 911, 912t
   cardiovascular system and, 911–912
   care planning, 916
   cellular responses to, 908
   in children, 912
   classification of, 910–911
   client evaluation, 917
   collaborative care, 913–915
   complete, 910
   complications of, 911–912, 914
   compression, 908
   deep venous thrombosis and, 912
   defined, 825t, 826, 906
   diagnosis, 916
   diagnostic tests, 913
   effects throughout the body, 911
   emergency care, 913
   emotional changes and, 912
   etiology, 908
   home care, 914–915, 915t
   incomplete, 910–911, 910t
   infection prevention and, 914
   integumentary system and, 912
   interventions, 825t, 916–917
   level of injury, 909
   lifespan and cultural considerations, 912–913
   manifestations, 825t, 909–913, 915
   mechanics of, 909f
   motor vehicle crashes (MVC), 2002t
   nonpharmacologic therapy, 914–915
   Nursing Care Plan, 917–918t
   nursing process, 915–917
   overview of, 906
   paralysis types, 911, 911f
   pathophysiology, 906–909
   pharmacologic therapy, 913–914
   in pregnant women, 912–913
   prevention of, 908–909
   problem management, 916
   rehabilitation, 914–915, 917
   respiratory system and, 912
   risk factors, 908
   rotational, 908
   spinal shock, 909–910
   surgery, 913
   transection, 908
   urinary system and, 912
   ventilation and, 914
Spinal discs, 821
Spinal fractures, 855t
Spinal fusion, 843
Spinal nerves, 689, 690f
Spinal shock, 909–910
Spinnbarkeit, 1379, 2019
Spiritual beliefs
   birth and, 1877
   death and, 1877–1878
   diet and nutrition and, 1876–1877
   dress and, 1877
   healing and, 1877
   nursing care and, 1876–1878
Spiritual comfort measures, 2005
Spiritual counseling, 1891–1892
Spiritual development, 1874, 1874t
Spiritual distress
   assessment, 1890
   care planning, 1891
   characteristics of, 1890
   client referral for counseling, 1891–1892
   defined, 1873, 1887, 1890
   diagnosis, 1890
   as etiology, 1890
   interventions, 1891–1892
   Nursing Care Plan, 1892t
   nursing diagnoses examples, 1890
   nursing process, 1890–1892
   outcome evaluation, 1892
   overview of, 1890
   presencing and, 1891
   risk for, 1891
Spiritual health
   assessment, 416
   defined, 1872–1873
   end-of-life care and, 181
   exercise benefits, 423
   health status and, 415
Spiritual needs, 1872, 1872t
Spiritual support
   in family recovery, 1732
   grief and loss and, 1748–1749
Spiritual theories, 1658
Spiritual well-being, 1872–1873
Spirituality
   assessment, 1875–1876
   assessment interview, 1875t
   components of, 1872–1874
   concept integration, 1874
   concepts related to, 1875t
   core aspects of, 1873–1874
   defined, 1871
   faith and, 1873
   forgiveness and, 1874
   hope and, 1873
   lifespan considerations, 1874t
   measurement of, 1872
   nursing care and, 1876–1878
   preference clues, 1876
   pregnancy and culture and, 2076t
   religion and, 1873
   spiritual development and, 1874, 1874t
   spiritual distress and, 1873
   spiritual health and, 1872–1873
   spiritual needs and, 1872, 1872t
   transcendence and, 1874
Spleen
   defined, 443
   percussing, 219f
Splenomegaly, 782
Splints, 862
Splitting, 1857
SPMSQ (Short Portable Mental Status Questionnaire), 1587t
Spontaneous abortion, 1768, 2080t
Spontaneous bacterial peritonitis, 784
Spontaneous birth, 2124
Spontaneous rupture of membranes, 2121
Sporadic AD, 1594
Sports-related concussions, 2712t
Sprains, 826–827
Sputum, 1005–1006
Sputum culture
   in lung cancer, 108
   in pneumonia, 591
   in tuberculosis, 611
Sputum gram stain, 591
Square window sign, 2219, 2219f
SRRS (Social Readjustment Rating Scale), 1900
SSI (Supplemental Security Income), 2627–2628
SSIs (surgical site infections), 2704
SSRIs. *See* Selective serotonin reuptake inhibitors
St. Johns wort, 1796
ST segment, 1072t
Stable angina, 1107
Staff authority, 2549–2550
Staff development
   educational strategies, 2529
   orientation, 2528
   overview, 2528
   roles in staff development, 2528
   staff development process, 2529
Staff education, 2528
Staffing, short, 2577
Stage of exhaustion, 1901, 1901f
Stage of resistance, 1901, 1901f
Staghorn stones, 319
Staging, tumor
   breast cancer, 76, 77t
   defined, 53, 76
   lung cancer, 107t
   prostate cancer, 114t
   TNM system, 53t
Standard precautions, 2717
Standardized care plans, 2445
Standardized plan, 2357–2360, 2360f
Standards, 2686
Standards of care
   accountability and, 2536
   concept relationships, 2659
   defined, 2536, 2657
   legal issues, 2657, 2658–2659
   nursing process and professional practice, 2658–2659
Standards of practice, 2536, 2549, 2666
Standards of Professional Performance, 2549
Staples, 1274
START adult triage algorithm, 2612, 2612f
State divisions of health and health services, 2623–2624
Statins, 1074t, 1117t
Station, 2116, 2116f
Status asthmaticus, 991

Status epilepticus, 718, 719t
Statute of limitations, 2656–2657
Statutory laws, 2654
STDs (sexually transmitted diseases), 1408
Steatorrhea, 247
Stem cell transplant (SCT), 98
Stenosis, 1087t
Step-down therapy, 1173
Stepfamilies, 1710–1711
Stepping reflex, 2234, 2235f
Stereognosis, 1278
Stereotyping, 1634
Stereotypy, 1689
Sterile field, 549
Sterile gloves, 549
Sterile gowns, 549
Sterile technique, 523, 549
Sterilization, 545
Stigma, 1731
Stillbirth, 1768, 2051t
Stimulants, sleep and, 433
Stimulus, 1278
Stimulus-based stress model, 1900
STIs. See Sexually transmitted infections
Stoma, 662, 662f
Stool
    defined, 273
    infant samples, 2201f
Strains, 826–827
Strategic planning, 2475
Stratum basale, 1446
Stratum corneum, 1446
Stratum granulosum, 1446
Stratum lucidum, 1446
Stratum spinosum, 1446
Strength training, for fibromyalgia, 192–193, 192t
Streptococcus, 541t
Streptococcus aureus, 585
Streptococcus pneumoniae, 585
Streptomycin, 612t
Stress
    assessment checklist, 1912t
    blood pressure and, 1046
    of cancer diagnosis, 49
    as cancer risk factor, 46
    defined, 1896
    homeostasis and, 1896–1897
    hypertension and, 1167, 1169
    oxidative, 1924t
    pulse and, 1044
    as sensory perception risk factor, 1283
Stress and coping
    alterations and therapies, 1908–1909
    alterations from normal coping responses, 1907–1910
    assessment, 1911–1913, 1911t
    assessment checklist, 1912t
    cognitive indicators, 1904
    cognitive-behavioral therapy (CBT), 1914–1915
    collaborative interventions and therapies, 1914–1915
    concept integration, 1907
    concept of, 1895
    concepts related to, 1906t
    diagnostic tests, 1913
    ego defense mechanisms, 1904–1907
    family wellness promotion and, 1911
    genetic considerations and nonmodifiable risk factors, 1910
    homeostasis and, 1896–1897

independent interventions and therapies, 1913–1914
    interventions and therapies, 1913–1915
    lifespan and cultural considerations, 1912–1913
    manifestations of stress, 1902
    medications, 1916t
    multisystem effects of, 1903t
    pharmacologic therapy, 1915
    physiological indicators, 1902, 1903t
    postpartum care, 2185–2186
    prevalence of, 1910
    prevention and, 1910–1911
    psychological indicators, 1902–1904
    psychotherapy, 1914
    screenings, 1911
    stressors and coping process, 1897–1902
    theoretical models
        response-based stress model, 1900–1902
        stimulus-based stress model, 1900
        transaction model, 1902
    wellness promotion and, 1914t
Stress fractures, 856t
Stress incontinence, 299t
Stress management
    Alzheimer disease (AD) caregivers, 1602–1603, 1602t
    in professional commitment, 2488
Stress mediators, 1896
Stress response
    defined, 1896
    factors affecting, 1898t
    physiological manifestations of, 1903t
Stress testing, 1200
Stress ulcers, 1472
Stressors
    biogenic, 1897
    classifications and examples, 1897t
    defined, 1895
    developmental, 1897–1898
    environmental, 1898
    internal, 1898
    psychosocial, 1897
    types of, 1897–1898, 1898t
Striae, 280, 2030
Stridor, 963t
Stroke
    acute, medications for, 1240–1241
    assessment, 1243
    care planning, 1243
    collaborative care, 1239–1242
    complications from
        cognitive and behavioral changes, 1237–1238, 1238f
        communication disorders, 1238–1239
        elimination disorders, 1239
        motor deficits, 1239
        sensory perceptual deficits and, 1237
    defined, 1234
    as diabetes complication, 748
    diagnosis, 1243
    diagnostic tests, 1239
    embolic, 1236
    health scale, 1241t
    hemorrhagic, 1236
    interventions
        cerebral perfusion, 1243–1244
        physical mobility, 1244, 1245f
        safety, 1245–1246
        self-care promotion, 1244–1245

urinary and bowel elimination, 1245
    verbal communication, 1245
    ischemic, 1235–1236
    manifestations, 1237–1239, 1237t, 1240
    Nursing Care Plan, 1246–1247t
    nursing process, 1242–1246
    outcome evaluation, 1246
    overview of, 1234
    pathophysiology and etiology, 1234–1235
    pharmacologic therapy, 1240–1241
    preventative medications, 1240
    rehabilitation, 1242
    risk factors, 1236, 1237t
    statistics, 1051, 1234
    surgery and, 1241–1242
    thrombotic, 1235–1236
    tPA treatment, 1242t
    transient ischemic attacks (TIAs) and, 1235
Stroke volume, 1040, 1218
Structure standards, 2686
Structuring, 2430
Struvite stones, 319
Subclavian flap aortoplasty, 1100t
Subconjunctival hemorrhages, 1314t, 2227
Subcultures, 1638, 1638f
Subcutaneous tissue
    changes and infection, 525
    defined, 1447
    in older adults, 1448
Subfertility, 1372
Subinvolution, 2172
Subjective data, 2270
Subjective family burden, 1732
Subjective Opiate Withdrawal Scale (SOWS), 1569
Sublimation, 1905t
Substance abuse
    abuse and, 1968
    action at brain receptor, 1520f
    assessment
        comprehensive approach, 1567–1568
        history of past use, 1568
        medical and psychiatric history, 1568
        open-ended questions, 1568t
        psychosocial issues, 1568–1569
        screening tools, 1569
    care planning, 1569
    collaborative care, 1565
    defined, 1560
    diagnosis, 1569
    diagnostic tests, 1565
    emergency care of overdose, 1565–1567
    epidemiology, 1561
    families and, 1524
    grieving process and, 1746
    impaired nurses, 1561–1562, 1562t
    infants with prenatal exposure, 2208t
    interventions
        adherence to treatment, 1569–1570
        coping skills, 1570
        education, 1570, 1570t
        nutrition, 1570
        safety, 1569
        safety during withdrawal, 1570–1571
        self-esteem promotion, 1570
    kindling and, 1561
    lifespan considerations, 1568t
    long-term goals, 1569
    manifestations
        caffeine, 1562
        cannabis, 1563

Substance abuse (*continued*)
central nervous system (CNS) depressants, 1563
hallucinogens, 1564
inhalants, 1564–1565
opiates, 1564
psychostimulants, 1563–1564
Nursing Care Plan, 1571–1572t
nursing process, 1565–1571
in older adults, 1522, 1568t
osteoporosis and, 800
outcome evaluation, 1571
overview of, 1560–1561
pathophysiology and etiology, 1561–1562
pharmacologic therapy, 1565, 1566t
prevalence of, 1526
rate of morbidity, 1522
risk factors, 1561
risk for adolescents, 1521t
short-term goals, 1569
signs and treatment of overdose and withdrawal, 1566–1567t
signs of, 1557t
statistics, 1522
as stroke risk factor, 1236
terminology, 1525t
treatment locations, 1565f
Substance Abuse and Mental Health Services Administration (SAMHSA), 1527
Substance addiction, 1524t
Substance dependence, 1560
Substance withdrawal
drugs used in treatment of, 1566t
safety promotion during, 1570–1571
signs and treatment of, 1566t
symptoms, 1560
Substances
abused, action at brain receptor, 1520f
dependence on, 1520
tolerance for, 1520
Substitution, 1905t
Sucking reflex, 2234
Sucralfate, 680
Sucrose, 757
Suctioning
catheter types, 969, 969f
complications of, 970
defined, 969
endotracheal, 970
lifespan considerations, 970t
tracheostomy, 970
Yankaurer, 969f
Sudden cardiac death (SCD)
advanced life support and, 1194
basic life support and, 1193, 1194f
care for family and, 1194
causes of, 1193
collaborative care, 1193–1194
defined, 1192
etiology, 1192
home care, 1197t
manifestations, 1193
nursing care for clients experiencing, 1194t
overview of, 1192–1193
postresuscitation care, 1194
risk factors, 1192
Sudden infant death syndrome (SIDS)
assessment, 1026
care planning, 1026–1027
collaborative care, 1025–1026
culture and, 1025t

death and, 1026
defined, 1024
diagnosis, 1026
evaluation, 1028
interventions, 1027
manifestations, 1025
nursing process, 1026–1028
overview of, 1024
pathophysiology and etiology, 1024–1025
planning goals, 1026–1027
protective behaviors and, 1025
psychosocial family needs and, 1025–1026
risk factors, 1024–1025, 1025t
risk reduction, 1027, 2246
safety and, 2710
sleep positioning and, 1027t
Suicidal ideation, 1802, 1990
Suicide
antidepressants and, 1995
antipsychotics and, 1995
assessment, 1995–1996
assisted, 2574
attempts, 1990
behavior, 1992
care planning, 1996
cognition, 1992–1993
collaborative care, 1994–1995
comorbid disorders, 1991
defined, 1958t, 1990
depression and, 1802
diagnosis, 1996
etiology, 1991
genetics and, 1991
influencing factors, 1991
interpersonal factors, 1991
interpersonal relationships, 1993
interventions, 1958t, 1996
IS PATH WARM and, 1992
lifespan and cultural considerations, 1993–1994, 1993t
manifestations, 1958t, 1992–1994, 1994t
mood stabilizers and, 1995
neurobiology and, 1991
nonpharmacologic therapy, 1995
Nursing Care Plan, 1997t
nursing process, 1995–1996
outcome evaluation, 1996
overview of, 1990
pathophysiology, 1990–1992
pharmacologic therapy, 1995
plan/method, 1802
prevention of, 1992
risk factors, 1992, 1992t
social factors, 1991
Suicide prevention, 1788–1789, 1789t
Sulfasalazine, 503, 503t, 664t
Sulfuric acid, 4
Summarizing, 2432
Sun exposure, as cancer risk factor, 47
Sundowning, 1597t, 1606
Superego, 1649
Superficial basal cell carcinoma, 130, 130f
Superficial burns. *See also* Burns
defined, 1467
manifestations, 1481t
partial-thickness, 1467–1468
Superficial spreading melanoma, 129
Supine hypotensive syndrome, 2031
Supine position, 1024, 1264t, 2278t
Supplemental Security Income (SSI), 2627–2628

Supply versus demand, 2463–2464
Support groups, 1531, 1824
Support system, in intrapartum assessment, 2147t
Suppression, 1904
Suppuration, 1509
Suprapubic prostatectomy, 115
Supraventricular dysrhythmias, 1183–1184
Supraventricular rhythms, 1180–1181t
Supraventricular tachycardia, 1197–1198
Surfactant, 954–955
Surge capacity, 2609
Surgeons, 1251
Surgery. *See also* Surgical procedures
constructive, 1261t
continuous surveillance during, 1262
diagnostic procedures, 1261t
elective, 1261t
emergency, 1261t
intraoperative nursing during, 1262–1271
length of procedures, 1261–1262
nutrition and, 948
palliative, 1261t
revision, 872
in specific conditions
age-related macular degeneration (AMD), 1329
anemia, 70
appendicitis, 646
benign prostatic hyperplasia (BPH), 286, 286f
bowel incontinence, 313
breast cancer, 79
cancer, 56
cardiomyopathy, 1080
cataracts, 1308–1309
cerebral palsy (CP), 1696
chronic obstructive pulmonary disease (COPD), 1011
colorectal cancer, 87–88
confusion, 1607
congenital heart defects, 1099–1100t
constipation, 308
deep venous thrombosis (DVT), 1134
diabetes mellitus, 759
erectile dysfunction (ED), 1368–1369, 1369f
eye injuries, 1314
failure to thrive (FTT), 1702
fatigue, 188
fractures, 860
gallbladder disease, 652
GERD, 229
glaucoma, 1321
hearing impairment, 1302
heart failure, 1157–1158
herniated disc, 843
hip fracture, 871–872
hyperthyroidism, 809–810
hypothyroidism, 813
increased intracranial pressure (IICP), 711
inflammation, 643
inflammatory bowel disease (IBD), 662–663
liver disease, 786
lung cancer, 108, 108t
menstrual dysfunction, 1402–1403
motor vehicle crashes (MVC), 2001–2002
multiple sclerosis, 880
obesity, 794–795, 795f
osteoarthritis, 888
otitis media, 579
pain, 162

pancreatitis, 248
Parkinson disease, 898
peripheral neuropathy, 1333
peripheral vascular disease (PVD), 1201
pressure ulcers, 1497
prostate cancer, 115, 115t
pulmonary embolism, 1214
pyloric stenosis, 252
rheumatoid arthritis, 501
sexual dysfunction, 1363
sickle cell disease, 122
skin cancer, 134
sleep-rest disorders, 197
spinal cord injuries (SCI), 913
stroke, 1241–1242
systemic lupus erythematosus (SLE), 514
urinary calculi, 322–323
urinary incontinence, 295
urinary retention, 298
urinary tract infections (UTIs), 623–624
wound healing, 1510
sterile field and hand washing, 1262
transplant, 1261t
types of procedures, 1261, 1261t
wrong-site (WSS), 2706–2707
Surgical asepsis
defined, 523
principles and practice, 550t
Surgical Care Improvement Project (SCIP), 2632
Surgical debridement, 1478
Surgical menopause, 1394
Surgical positions, 1262, 1264–1265t
Surgical procedures
adjustable gastric banding, 795
aorta resection, 1099t
appendectomy, 646
arthrodesis, 501
arthroplasty, 501, 871, 888
arthroscopy, 888
artificial disc surgery, 843
Blalock-Taussig shunt, 1099t
breast reconstruction, 79, 80f
Brock procedure, 1099t
cardiac transplantation, 1157–1158, 1157f
carotid angioplasty, 1242
carotid endarterectomy, 1241–1242, 1241f
colectomy, 662
colostomy, 87–88, 88f
Damus-Kaye-Stansel procedure, 1099t
deep brain stimulation (DBS), 898
dilation and curettage (D&C), 1402
discectomy, 843
endometrial ablation, 1402
escharotomy, 1510
extracapsular extraction, 1308, 1308f
extracorporeal shock wave lithotripsy
(ESWL), 322
Fontan procedure, 1099t
Glenn procedure, 1099t
gonioplasty, 1321
hemiarthroplasty, 871
hysterectomy, 1402–1403, 1403t
ileostomy, 662–663
iridotomy, 1321
Jatene procedure, 1099t
joint fusion, 888
joint resurfacing, 888
laminectomy, 843
laminotomy, 843
laparoscopic cholecystectomy, 652, 653t

laparoscopic fundoplication, 229, 229f
laser photocoagulation, 88
limbal relaxing incision, 1308
lithotripsy, 322, 322f, 323f
lumpectomy, 79
mastectomy, 79, 79f
Mustard or Senning procedure, 1099t
myringotomy, 579, 1302
nephrolithotomy, 323
Norwood procedure, 1099t
open reduction and internal fixation (ORIF),
860, 860f
osteotomy, 888
ostomy, 662–663
pallidotomy, 898
patch aortoplasty, 1099t
penile implants, 1368–1369, 1369f
pneumatic retinopexy, 1314
prostatectomy, 115, 115t, 295
pulmonary artery banding, 1100t
pyelolithotomy, 323
Rastelli procedure, 1100t
Ross procedure, 1100t
Roux-en-Y gastric bypass, 795, 795f
scleral buckling, 1314
spinal fusion, 843
subclavian flap aortoplasty, 1100t
synovectomy, 501
thalamotomy, 898
thyroidectomy, 809–810
trabeculectomy, 1321
trabeculoplasty, 1321
transplantation, 1100t
transurethral incision of the prostate
(TUIP), 286
transurethral needle ablation (TUNA), 286
transurethral resection of the prostate
(TURP), 286, 286f
tympanocentesis, 579
ureterolithotomy, 322
ureteroplasty, 623–624
venous thrombectomy, 1134
vertical banding gastroplasty, 795, 795f
Surgical safety checklist, 1267, 1269f
Surgical site infections (SSIs), 2704
Surgical site preparation, 1259, 1260t, 1267
Surgical technicians, 1251
Susceptibility to disease, 1639
Susceptible hosts, 524t
Suspected awareness, 183
Sutures
fetal skull, 2114, 2114f
types of, 1274
Swaddling, 2246, 2246f
Swan-Ganz catheter, 984, 985
Swan-neck deformity, 497, 497f
Symmetry, 962, 964t
Sympathetic nervous system (SNS), 1163
Sympathetic stimulation/stress response, 1422
Sympathetic tone, 1218
Sympathomimetic agents, 1156t
Sympathy, 2425
Symptoms, 2270
Symptothermal method, 1379
Synchronized cardioversion, 1188
Synchronized intermittent mandatory ventilation
(SIMV), 980, 981t
Synclitism, 2116
Syncope, 1079, 1092t
Syndrome diagnosis, 2335

Synovectomy, 501
Synovitis, 826, 826f
Syphilis
antepartum care and, 2082t
chancre, 1413, 1413f
defined, 1413
diagnosis and treatment, 1414
latent, 1414
manifestations, 1413–1414
Nursing Care Plan, 1417t
pathophysiology, 1413
pharmacologic therapy, 1414
primary, 1413, 1413f
secondary, 1413
tertiary, 1414
Systemic arthritis, 499
Systemic blood flow obstruction defects. See also
Congenital heart defects
aortic stenosis, 1092t
clinical therapy, 1092–1094t
coarctation of the aorta, 1092–1093t
defined, 1089
hypoplastic left heart syndrome (HLHS),
1093–1094t
manifestations, 1092–1094t
pathophysiology, 1092–1094t
Systemic circulation, 1036, 1038f
Systemic infection, 523
Systemic inflammatory response syndrome
(SIRS), 600
Systemic lupus erythematosus (SLE). See also
Immunity
in adolescents, 515t
antepartum care and, 2079t
assessment, 515
autoantibodies, 509, 510
butterfly rash, 510f
care planning, 515
collaborative care, 512–515
complementary and alternative therapy, 515
as connective tissue disease, 509
defined, 509
diagnosis, 515
diagnostic tests, 512–514
discoid lupus, 510
drug-induced lupus, 510
interventions
emotional support, 517
fluid volume balance, 516
health maintenance, 517–518
infection prevention, 516
medication side effects, 517
nutrition, 516
rest and comfort, 517
skin integrity, 516–517
trigger avoidance, 517
lifespan considerations, 512
manifestations, 510–512, 512t, 513t
multisystem effects of, 511t
nonpharmacologic therapy, 514–515
nursing process, 515–518
outcome evaluation, 518
overview of, 509
pathophysiology and etiology, 509–510
pharmacologic therapy, 514
pregnancy and, 512
surgery, 514
systemic lupus, 510
Systemic response, type I hypersensitivity, 482
Systemic vascular resistance, 1040

Systemized nomenclature of medicine–clinical terms (SNOMED CT), 2644
Systole
    defined, 1034
    heart sounds in, 1034*f*
Systolic blood pressure, 1045, 1163

T

T cells
    defined, 441
    helper, 442–443, 457
T wave, 1072*t*
T₃ test, 809
T₃ update test, 809
T₄ test, 809
Tachycardia
    defined, 1063
    fetal, 2151
Tachypnea, 596, 959, 960*t*
Tactile sensation
    assessment, 1290–1291, 1294*t*
    in children, 1291*t*
    fine touch assessment, 1295*t*
    impaired, 1297
    screenings and, 1283
Tactile stimuli, 1278
Tangential excision, 1478
Tanner stages
    for breasts, 1340*f*
    for pubic hair, 1340*f*
Tanner's clinical judgment model, 2325, 2326*f*, 2326*t*
Tardive dyskinesia, 1618
Tartar, 426
Task forces, 2423
Tasks
    defining, 2469
    describing, 2469
    key behaviors in delegation of, 2469*t*
Taste
    assessment, 1290–1291, 1295*t*
    in children, 1291*t*
    screenings and, 1283
Tau hypothesis, 1595
TCAs. *See* Tricyclic antidepressants
TDI (therapeutic donor insemination), 1388
Teachers, nurses as, 2500
Teaching
    aids, 2519
    aids, written, 2514*t*
    art of, 2500–2501
    children, tools for, 2519*t*
    in the communication, 2510
    content selection, 2517
    defined, 2499
    effective, characteristics of, 2500*t*
    environments, 2509–2510
    flexibility, 2518–2519
    guidelines for, 2519–2520, 2520*t*
    hands-on client participation, 2520, 2520*t*
    layperson's vocabulary and, 2519
    learning experiences organization, 2517–2518
    lifespan considerations, 2512*t*
    priorities, 2516–2517
    process comparison, 2510*t*
    repetition and, 2520
    strategies
        anticipatory guidance, 2520, 2521*t*
        anticipatory problem solving, 2522

behavior modification, 2522
client contracting, 2520–2521
discovery/problem solving, 2521–2522
group teaching, 2521
technology-assisted instruction, 2521
transcultural teaching, 2522–2523
strategies selection, 2517, 2518*t*
Teaching and learning
    art of teaching, 2500–2501
    aspects of learning, 2501–2508
    concept of, 2499
    concepts related to, 2501*t*
    defined, 2499
    Internet and health information, 2508
    nurses as teachers and learners, 2500*t*
Teaching groups, 2423
Teaching plans
    client health history, 2511–2513
    developing, 2510–2515
    health literacy, 2514
    motivation, 2513–2514
    physical examination, 2513
    readiness to learn, 2513
Team nursing, 2458–2459, 2600
Teams, 2423, 2476–2477
Teamwork
    as professional behavior, 2483
    as QSEN competency, 2699, 2700
Technical skills, 2348
Technological changes, 2572
Technology
    advances, 2598–2599
    hardware, 2634
    in healthcare information systems, 2634–2635, 2635*t*
    software, 2634
Technology Informatics Guiding Educational Reform (TIGER) Summit, 2632
Technology-assisted instruction, 2521
Teeth. *See also* Oral health
    artificial, 428
    brushing and flossing, 428
    decay prevention, 427*t*
    deciduous and permanent, 425*f*
    eruption sequence, 209*f*
    plaque, 425–426
    tartar, 426
Telangiectatic nevi (stork bites), 2224
Telecommunications, 2541–2542
Telehealth
    applications, 2640
    barriers to client participation, 2641
    barriers to implementation, 2640
    benefits of, 2640*t*
    defined, 2640
Telephone communication, 2451–2452
Telephone orders, 2452, 2452*t*
Telephone reports, 2451–2452
Temperament
    adolescents, 1669
    defined, 1658–1659
    infants, 1662
    patterns of, 1655*t*
    preschool children, 1666
    school-age children, 1668
    theory, 1654
    toddlers, 1663–1664
Temperature. *See* Body temperature
Temporal pulse, 1063, 1063*f*
Temporary relocation, 1931

Temporomandibular joint (TMJ) syndrome, 826
Tender points, 145, 190, 191*f*
Tendonitis, 826
Tendons, 820
Teratogens, 1552, 2074
Teriflunomide (Aubagio), 880
Term, 2051*t*
Terminal insomnia, 1799
Terminal weaning, 983
Territoriality, 2408
Tertiary care, 2598
Tertiary intention healing, 1507
Tertiary prevention, 2597, 2597*t*
Tertiary syphilis, 1414
Testosterone, 1340
Tetanus, 541–542*t*
Tetanus prophylaxis, 1478
Tetany
    defined, 387, 737*t*
    hypocalcemic, 737*t*
Tetralogy of Fallot (TOF), 1088*t*
Tetraplegia, 911
TGA (transposition of the great arteries), 1090*t*
Thalamotomy and, 898
Thalassemia, 68–69
Thelarche, 1340
Theophylline, 997
Therapeutic communication
    attentive listening, 2425–2426
    barriers to, 2433
    with children and families, 2435–2436, 2435*f*, 2436*t*
    clarifying, 2429
    conclusion, 2436
    confronting, 2432
    defined, 2425
    empathizing, 2425
    feedback, giving, 2431, 2431*t*, 2432*t*
    imparting information, 2429
    linking, 2430–2431
    mistakes, 2432–2433
    overview of, 2425
    painful information, 1930*t*
    paraphrasing, 2430
    perceptions, checking, 2430
    physical attending, 2426, 2427*t*
    pinpointing, 2430
    processing, 2432
    questioning, 2430
    rapport with children and, 2437*t*
    reflecting, 2427–2429
    self-disclosure, avoiding, 2429
    silence, 2426–2427
    stress and coping and, 1930
    structuring, 2430
    summarizing, 2432
    techniques, 2425–2433, 2427–2428*t*
    therapeutic relationship and, 2433–2435, 2433*t*
    trust and, 2436
Therapeutic donor insemination (TDI), 1388
Therapeutic husband insemination (THI), 1388
Therapeutic insemination, 1388–1389
Therapeutic relationships
    abuse and, 1974
    characteristics of, 2433*t*
    defined, 2425
    developing, 2434–2435
    feeding and eating disorders and, 1851
    goals, 2433

introductory phase, 2433–2434
personality disorders (PD) and, 1865
phases of, 2433–2435
preinteraction phase, 2433
termination phase, 2434–2435
working phase, 2434
Therapy groups, 2424
Thermal burns
defined, 1464–1465
in infants, 1464f
stopping the burning process, 1475t
Thermometers
axillary, 1428f
infrared, 1427f
oral, 1427f
pacifier, 1428f
tympanic, 1427f, 1428f
Thermoregulation. *See also* Body temperature
admission to ICU and, 1429
alterations, 1423–1426, 1423f
alterations and therapies, 1424t
antipyretics and, 1430t
assessment, 1427–1429
in children, 1423
collaborative interventions and therapies, 1429
concepts related to, 1425
defined, 1422
diagnostic tests, 1427
emergency department care, 1429
genetic and lifespan considerations, 1423
genetic considerations, 1426
heat balance, 1422, 1422f
hyperthermia. *See* hyperthermia
hypothalamus and, 1432, 1432f
hypothermia. *See* hypothermia
independent interventions and therapies, 1429
in infants, 1423
inpatient care, 1429
interventions and therapies, 1429
modifiable risk factors, 1426
in newborns, 2237
normal, 1422–1423
in older adults, 1423
outpatient and follow-up care, 1429
physiological processes, 1422
prehospital care, 1429
in premature newborns, 2250
prevalence of alterations, 1424
prevention and, 1426–1427
screenings, 1426–1427
THI (therapeutic husband insemination), 1388
Third (S_3) heart sounds, 1034
Third spacing, 355
Third-degree AV block, 1182t, 1186
Thirst
dysregulation, 934
fluid intake and, 339, 339f
shock effect on, 1222
Thomas test, 835f, 835t
Thoracentesis, 586, 966
Thoracic catheters, 973
Thoracic cavity, inspection of, 963t
Thoracolumbar sacral orthosis (TLSO), 848
Thorax, 955f
Thought blocking, 1613
Thought disorders, 1613
Three-part nursing diagnosis statement, 2338–2339, 2451
Threshold potential, 1043
Thrills, 1057t

Throat cultures, 671
Thromboemboli
defined, 1211
illustrated, 1212f
Thrombolytics, 1075t
Thrombotic strokes, 1235–1236
Thrush, 2227
Thymus gland, 443
Thyroid agents, 738t
Thyroid antibodies (TA) test, 809
Thyroid disease
hyperthyroidism, 806–812
hypothyroidism, 812–817
overview of, 806
type 1 diabetes and, 771
Thyroid disorders
prevalence of, 729
prevention of, 731
Thyroid gland
assessment, 735t
defined, 806
in heart failure, 1151
palpating, 735t
pregnancy and, 2033–2034
Thyroid profile, in obesity, 793
Thyroid storm (thyroid crisis), 808
Thyroid suppression test, 809
Thyroidectomy, 809
Thyroiditis and, 808
Thyrosine, 1796
Thyrotoxicosis. *See* Hyperthyroidism
Thyroxine output, in heat production, 1422
TIAs (transient ischemic attacks), 1235
TIGER (Technology Informatics Guiding Educational Reform) Summit, 2632
Tilburg Frailty Indicator, 2295t
Time, culture, 1639
Time constraints, 2366
Time management
decisions, 2321
as management principle, 2477
poor, 2370
in prioritizing care, 2369
suggestions, 2371t
Time priority, 2366
Time-out, 1251
Timing, in learning, 2506
Tinea pedis, 561
Tinnitus, 1301
TIPS (transjugular intrahepatic portosystemic shunt), 788
Tissue integrity
alterations, 1448–1454
alterations and therapies, 1453–1454t
assessment
diagnostic tests, 1456
edema, 1458t
general, 1457t
hair distribution and quality, 1458t
hair texture, 1459t
interview, 1456t
nails, 1459–1460t
nursing, 1455–1456
scalp, 1459t
skin temperature, 1457t
skin texture, 1458t
skin turgor, 1458t
skin with impaired integrity, 1457t
cancer and, 61, 61t
collaborative interventions and therapies, 1461

concepts related to, 1449t
exercise and, 1461
genetic and lifespan considerations, 1447–1448, 1447t
genetic considerations and nonmodifiable risk factors, 1452
independent interventions and therapies, 1461
interventions and therapies, 1461
manifestations of alterations, 1448–1452
medications, 1461–1463t
modifiable risk factors, 1455
normal presentation, 1446–1448
nutrition and, 1461
prevalence of alterations, 1452
prevention and, 1455
screenings, 1455
skin disorders, 1448
skin lesions, 1448, 1450t, 1451t
wounds. *See* wound healing; wounds
Tissue perfusion
chronic kidney disease (CKD) and, 400
disseminated intravascular coagulation (DIC) and, 1142
monitoring, 1126
peripheral vascular disease (PVD) and, 1202–1203
shock and, 1231–1232
Tissue plasminogen activator (tPA), 1242t
TLSO (thoracolumbar sacral orthosis), 848
TMS (transcranial magnetic stimulation), 1620, 1795
TNF inhibitors, 503t
TNM staging system
for breast cancer, 77t
defined, 53, 53t
for lung cancer, 107t
Tobacco
carcinogens, 1548t
chemicals in, 1546t
pregnancy and, 1554, 2065
Toddlers. *See also* Children; Pediatric clients
assessment of, 2291–2292, 2292f
bowel elimination in, 275
cognitive development, 1663
communication, 1664
constipation in, 307
growth and development, 1662–1664
growth and development milestones, 1662t
health screenings and immunization guidelines for, 413t
injury prevention due to motor vehicle crashes, 2000t
normal sleep-rest patterns in, 432
oral health in, 427, 427t
pain perception and behavior in, 158t
personality and temperament, 1663–1664
physical growth and development, 1662
play, 1663, 1663f
psychosocial development, 1663–1664, 1663t
separation anxiety disorder (SAD) in, 1922t
sexual development in, 1341t
unintentional injuries, 2710, 2710f
Toes, mobility assessment, 833t
TOF (tetralogy of Fallot), 1088t
Toileting
assistance, 301–302
scheduled, 295
Token economies, 1530
Tolerance, 1520, 1525t
Tone, 1218

Tonic neck reflex, 2233, 2233f
Tonic phase, seizures, 716
Tonicity, 337
Tonnière deformity, 497, 497f
Tonometry, 1320
Tonsils, 444
Top-down sampling, 1783, 1783f
Torsades de pointes, 1185, 1185f
Tort law. *See also* Law; Legal issues
    assault, battery, and false imprisonment, 2657
    defined, 2655
    invasion of privacy, 2657
    malpractice or professional negligence, 2655–2657
    negligence, 2655
Torts
    defined, 2655
    intentional, 2657
    unintentional, 2656–2657
Total (serum) bilirubin, 651t
Total anomalous pulmonary venous return, 1091t
Total lymphoid irradiation, 504
Total protein, as perioperative diagnostic test, 1253t
Total quality management (TQM), 2690, 2690f
Touch. *See* Tactile sensation
Toxic multinodular goiter, 808, 808f
Toxic shock syndrome, 601
Toxoplasmosis, 463
TPA (tissue plasminogen activator), 1242t
Trabeculectomy, 1321
Trabeculoplasty, 1321
Trachea, in children, 588, 589f
Tracheostomy, 970, 984, 984f
Trachoma, 567, 567t
Traction. *See also* Fractures
    cervical, 913f
    defined, 862
    illustrated, 863f
    interventions for, 864t
    methods, 863–864t
    skeletal, 862
    skin, 862
Traditional care plans, 2445
Transactional leaders, 2490
Transcendence, 141, 1874
Transcranial magnetic stimulation (TMS), 1620, 1795
Transcultural teaching, 2522–2523
Transcutaneous oximetry, 1201
Transductive reasoning, 1665t
Transection, spinal cord, 908
Transference, 2422
Transformational leaders, 2490
Transfusion reaction, 483
Transgender, 1634
Transsexual, 1634
Transient ischemic attacks (TIAs), 1235
Transitional milk, 2174
Transjugular intrahepatic portosystemic shunt (TIPS), 788
Transmission of infection
    methods of, 524
    prevention of, 544–551
Transmyocardial laser revascularization, 1122
Transplacental immunity. *See* Immunizations
Transplant rejections, 447
Transplant surgery, 1261t
Transplantation
    cardiac, 1157–1158, 1157f
    in congenital heart defects, 1100t

Transposition of the great arteries (TGA), 1090t
Transsexuals, 1345, 1634
Transurethral incision of the prostate (TUIP), 286
Transurethral needle ablation (TUNA), 286
Transurethral resection of the prostate (TURP)
    defined, 286
    discharge instructions, 290, 290t
    hospital stay, 290
    illustrated, 286f
    postoperative care, 289–290
    TURP syndrome, 289
Transverse diameter, 2014
Transverse fractures, 855t
Trauma
    accident and, 1955–1956
    airway and breathing assessments, 1961
    assessment, 1960–1961
    blunt, 1956
    circulation assessment, 1961
    death and, 1960
    defined, 1955
    host, 1956
    injury seriousness determination, 1961
    intentional, 1956
    interventions, 1962–1963
    level of consciousness (LOC) and, 1961
    mechanism, 1956
    medications, 1963t
    minor, 1956
    multiple, 1956
    penetrating, 1956
    pupillary function assessment, 1961
    types of, 1956
    unintentional, 1956
Traumatic injuries cataracts, 1307
Travel, antepartum care and, 2073–2074
Tremors, 703t, 896–897
Trendelenburg position, 1265t
Treponema pallidum, 1413, 2026
Triage
    defined, 1963, 2367, 2612
    emergent (or immediate), 2367
    JumpSTART algorithm, 2613f
    nonurgent (or minor), 2368
    reverse, 2612
    START algorithm, 2612
    urgent (or delayed), 2367
Trial and error, 2323–2324
Tricuspid atresia, 1088–1089t
Tricyclic antidepressants (TCAs)
    client education, 1791
    defined, 1790
    drug interactions, 1791
    mechanisms of action, 1334t
    nursing considerations, 1334t, 1790–1791
Triglycerides
    defined, 791
    levels, 752
    values classification, 1110
Triplet, 1185
Tripod position, 1009
Trisomic, 1374
Trisomies, 1374
Trisomy 21, 1581
Trophoblast, 2021
Troponins, 1115
Trousseau sign, 737t
True pelvis, 2013
Truncus arteriosus, 1090–1091t
Trunk incurvation (Galant reflex), 2234

TSH test (sensitive assay), 809
T-tube, 652f, 652t
Tubal ligation, 1386
Tube feedings
    complications of, 224
    formulas, 223, 224t
    placement, 224f, 224t
    tube types, 223, 223f
Tubercle, 606
Tuberculin test, 108, 468
Tuberculosis
    AIDS and, 463
    antepartum care and, 2079t
    assessment, 614
    of the bones, 607
    care planning, 614
    in children, 609
    collaborative care, 611–612
    defined, 606
    diagnosis, 614
    diagnostic tests, 611
    dormant, 606
    etiology, 607
    extrapulmonary, 606
    incidence of, 607t
    interpreting test results, 609t
    interventions
        client education, 614
        infection risk reduction, 616
        therapeutic regimen management, 614–615, 615t
    intradermal injection for testing, 608, 609t
    latent infection questions, 612t
    lifespan and cultural considerations, 609–611
    management, 615t
    manifestations, 609–611, 610t
    medications, 612–613
    meningitis, 607
    miliary, 606
    multidrug-resistant (MDR) strains of, 607
    Nursing Care Plan, 617t
    nursing process, 614–616
    in older adults, 610–611, 610t
    outcome evaluation, 616
    overview of, 606
    pathophysiology, 606–609
    pharmacologic therapy
        adherence, 612
        antituberculosis drugs, 612–613t
        follow up, 612
        prophylaxis, 611
        treatment for active disease, 611–612
    prevention, 608–609
    risk factors, 607, 608t
    risk groups, 608–609, 608t
    screening tests, 609
Tubular sound, 954
TUIP (transurethral incision of the prostate), 286
Tularemia, 2616t
Tumor lysis syndrome (TLS), 49, 101
Tumor markers, 54, 54t
Tumor necrosis factor (TNF) inhibitors, 502
Tumor suppressor genes, 45
Tumors. *See also* Cancer
    classification of, 52
    grading and staging, 53, 53t
    invasion, 43
    metastasis, 44
    names for, 52–53
TUNA (transurethral needle ablation), 286

TURP. *See* Transurethral resection of the prostate
TURP syndrome, 289
Twelve-step programs, 1531–1532, 1532*t*
24-hour urine sample, 294
Two-career families, 1710
Two-part nursing diagnosis statement, 2338, 2338*t*
Two-point discrimination test, 702*f*, 702*t*
Tympanic membrane, 576, 578*f*
Tympanic thermometers, 1427*f*, 1428*f*
Tympanocentesis, 579
Tympanogram, 579
Tympanostomy tubes, 579
Tympany, 2280
Type I (IgE-mediated) hypersensitivity, 482–483, 482*f*, 483*t*
Type II (cytotoxic) hypersensitivity, 483, 484*f*
Type III (immune complex-mediated) hypersensitivity, 483–484, 485*f*
Type IV (delayed) hypersensitivity, 484–485, 486*f*
Types of reimbursement
    Children's Health Insurance Program (CHIP), 2628
    conclusion, 2629
    federal programs, 2627–2628
    Medicaid, 2627
    Medicare, 2627, 2627*t*
    Medigap policies, 2629
    payment sources, 2627–2629
    personal payment, 2629
    private health insurance plans, 2628–2629
    Supplemental Security Income (SSI), 2627–2628

U

U wave, 1072*t*
UAPs. *See* Unlicensed assistive personnel nurses
Ulcerative colitis. *See also* Inflammatory bowel disease (IBD)
    cathartic colon and, 306
    characteristics of, 657*t*
    crypts, 658*f*
    defined, 306, 657
    fulminant colitis and, 660
    manifestations, 660
    Nursing Care Plan, 660*t*
Ulcers
    arterial, 1200*t*
    defined, 677
    NSAID-induced, 677, 680
    peptic, 677
    pressure. *See* pressure ulcers
    stress, 1472
    venous, 1200*t*
Ultrafiltration, 384
Ultrasonography
    cancer. *See* magnetic resonance imaging
    pancreatitis and, 247
Ultrasound
    abdominal, 785
    antepartum care
        advantages, 2084
        benefits of, 2085–2086
        defined, 2083–2084
        four-dimensional, 2084
        transabdominal, 2085
        transvaginal, 2085
    bladder, 623
    Doppler, 201
Ultraviolet (UV) exposure, 1282
Umbilical alarm, 2211, 2212*f*

Umbilical cord
    blood, banking, 2211
    clamping, 2211, 2211*f*
    defined, 2023
    newborn assessment, 2230, 2230*f*
    twisted, 2023
Unconscious mind, 1649
Underdelegation, 2472
Underinsured, 2603
Undernutrition
    in assessment of infants, 2290
    culture and, 945*t*
    defined, 936, 2290
    multisystem effects of, 937*t*
    Nursing Care Plan, 948–949*t*
Underwater weighing (hydrodensitometry), 793
Undocumented immigrants, 1636
Undoing, 1905*t*
Unifocal PVCs, 1185
Uniform language, 2639, 2644
Unilateral lobar pneumonia, 585
Uninsured, 2603
Unintentional injury: motor vehicle crashes
    care planning, 2003
    collaborative care, 2001–2003
    common injuries, 2000–2001
    cultural considerations, 2001, 2001*t*
    dashboard knee and, 2001
    defined, 1998
    diagnosis, 2003
    diagnostic tests, 2001
    etiology, 1998–1999
    illustrated, 1999*f*
    interventions
        airway patency and ventilation, 2003–2004
        community-based care facilitation, 2005
        disability assessment, 2004
        fluid volume balance, 2004
        infection prevention, 2004
        mobility promotion, 2004–2005
        obscured area exposure, 2004
        psychosocial well-being, 2005
        spiritual comfort measures, 2005
    manifestations, 2000–2001, 2002*t*
    nonpharmacologic therapy, 2003
    Nursing Care Plan, 2006*t*
    nursing process, 2003–2005
    outcome evaluation, 2005
    overview of, 1998
    pharmacologic therapy, 2002–2003
    prevention of, 1999, 2000*t*
    risk factors, 1999
    safety protection and, 2001*t*
    surgery, 2001–2002
    whiplash and, 2001
Unintentional wounds, 1448–1449
Unipolar depression, 1778
Universal precautions, 545
Universal protocol, 1251
Unlicensed assistive personnel nurses (UAPs)
    decision tree for delegation to, 2473*f*
    defined, 2458, 2600
    delegating to, 2467–2468
    delegation principles, 2468*t*
    in functional nursing, 2600
    tasks, 2468*t*
Unprofessional behaviors. *See also* Professional behaviors
    abuses of power, 2483–2485
    bullying and disruptive behavior, 2484*t*

    defined, 2483
    improper use of authority, 2484–2485
    intimidation, 2484–2485
    sexual harassment, 2484
Unresolved bacteriuria, 627
Unsaturated fats, 929
Unstable angina, 1107
Upper body obesity, 791
Upper GI series (barium swallow), 220, 220*f*, 228, 679
Uremia. *See also* Chronic kidney disease (CKD)
    cardiovascular effects, 393
    defined, 393
    dermatological effects, 395
    endocrine and metabolic effects, 395
    fluid and electrolyte effects, 393
    gastrointestinal effects, 393
    hematological effects, 393
    immune system effects, 393
    multisystem effects, 394*t*
    musculoskeletal effects, 395
    neurological effects, 393–395
Uremic fetor, 393
Uremic frost, 395
Ureteral stents, 624
Ureterolithotomy, 322
Ureteroplasty, 623–624
Urge incontinence, 299*t*
Urgency, urinary, 265, 621
Urgency factor
    acute, 2366
    critical, 2366–2367
    defined, 2366
    imminent death, 2367
    levels, 2366–2367, 2367*f*
    nonacute, 2366
Uric acid stones, 319
Urinalysis
    in acute renal failure (ARF), 380
    in burn injuries, 1477
    in chronic kidney disease (CKD), 395
    defined, 294
    in heart failure, 1151
    in infection, 557
    in nephritis, 672
    newborn values, 2201*f*
    in systemic lupus erythematosus (SLE), 514
Urinary calculi
    assessment, 323, 324–329*t*
    care planning, 329
    in children, 321
    collaborative care, 322–323
    complementary and alternative therapy, 323*t*
    complications
        hydronephrosis, 320–321
        infection, 321
        obstruction, 320
    defined, 318
    development and location of, 319*f*
    diagnosis, 329
    diagnostic tests, 322
    interventions and therapies, 320*f*
        client discharge preparation, 330, 331*t*
        client teaching, 330
        health and wellness, 330
        pain management, 329–330
        urinary output monitoring, 330
    kidney assessment, 324–329*t*
    lifespan and cultural considerations, 321–322

Urinary calculi (*continued*)
manifestations, 320–322, 321*f*
nephrolithiasis, 319
nonpharmacologic therapy, 323
Nursing Care Plan, 331–332*t*
nursing process, 323–331
outcome evaluation, 331
overview of, 318–319
pathophysiology and etiology, 319–320
pharmacologic therapy, 323
in pregnant women, 321
prevention, 320
racial differences, 322
risk factors, 319–320, 320*f*
surgery, 322–323, 322*f*, 323*f*
urolithiasis, 319
Urinary drainage system, 618
Urinary elimination
abnormal findings, 270–271*t*
alterations, 264–265
alterations and therapies, 266*t*
altered, 264–265, 264*t*
altered urine production and, 264
assessment, 266–271, 268–269*t*
assessment interview, 267*t*
collaborative interventions and therapies,
272–273
diagnostic tests, 267–271
dialysis, 272–273
factors affecting, 261
fluid and food intake and, 261
genetic and lifespan considerations,
261–264, 262*t*
genetic considerations and nonmodifiable risk
factors, 265
home care, 302, 303*t*, 304*t*
impaired, interventions for, 627
independent interventions and therapies,
271–272
in infants, 262
interventions and therapies, 271–273
lifespan and cultural considerations, 267
manifestations, 264–265
medications, 261, 261*t*, 272*t*
modifiable risk factors, 265
muscle tone and, 261
normal, 260–264, 270–271*t*
in older adults, 263
pathological conditions and, 261
pharmacologic therapy, 272
in pregnant women, 263–264
in preschoolers, 262
prevention of, 265–266
prostate cancer and, 117
psychosocial factors and, 261
in school-age children, 262–263
screening, 265–266
stroke and, 1245
surgical and diagnostic procedures and, 261
urinalysis, 270–271*t*
urinary tract infections (UTIs) and,
626–627
Urinary frequency, 264–265, 2066
Urinary hesitancy, 265
Urinary incontinence. *See also* Bladder
incontinence and retention
bladder diary and, 294
catheters and, 296*t*
in children, 293, 296, 626*t*
collaborative care, 294–297

defined, 292
diagnostic tests, 294–295
home care, 302, 303*t*, 304*t*
incidence of, 292–293
independence and, 304
lifespan and cultural considerations,
293–294
manifestations, 293–294
nonpharmacologic therapy, 295–297, 295*t*
pathophysiology and etiology, 293
pelvic floor muscle (Kegel) exercises and,
295, 295*t*
pharmacologic therapy, 295
in pregnant women, 294
pressure ulcers and, 1493
prevention, 293
risk factors, 293
social isolation and, 302
surgery, 295
types of, 294*t*
UTI prevention and, 297*t*
Urinary output, 330
Urinary retention. *See also* Bladder incontinence
and retention
acute, 299*t*
chronic, 299*t*
collaborative care, 298
defined, 297
diagnostic tests, 298
home care, 303*t*, 304*t*
manifestations, 298, 298*f*
nonpharmacologic therapy, 298
pathophysiology and etiology, 297–298
pharmacologic therapy, 298
prevention, 298
risk factors, 297–298
surgery, 298
Urinary system
burn injuries and, 1472
disseminated intravascular coagulation (DIC)
and, 1141*t*
exercise benefits, 422
postpartum changes, 2175
pregnancy and, 2031–2032
spinal cord injuries (SCI) and, 912
Urinary tract, 618
Urinary tract infections (UTIs)
in adolescents, 625*t*
antepartum care and, 2082*t*
assessment, 625
care planning, 625
catheter-associated, 623
in children, 620, 624–625, 625*t*
collaborative care, 623–625
community-based care, 626
complementary and alternative therapy, 625*t*
diagnosis, 625
diagnostic tests, 623
diaphragms and, 1381
etiology, 620
as HAI, 530
health maintenance and, 627
in infants, 625*t*
interventions, 626–627
lifespan and cultural considerations,
622–623, 625*t*
manifestations, 621–623, 622*t*
in men, 621
nonpharmacologic therapy, 625
Nursing Care Plan, 628*t*

in older adults, 621, 622, 623
overview of, 618
pain management, 626
pathophysiology, 619–621
persistent bacteriuria, 627
pharmacologic therapy, 623–624
pregnancy and, 621
presenting systems of, 621–622
prevention of, 621, 621*t*
reinfection, 627
renal scarring, 620
risk factors, 620–621
surgery, 623
unresolved bacteriuria, 627
urinary elimination and, 626–627
urinary incontinence and, 297*t*
in women, 620
Urination, 260–261
Urine
average output by age, 261*t*
as fluid output, 339–340
residual, 264
sample, 294
Urine creatinine, 672
Urine culture, 395
Urine pH, 18
Urine specific gravity, 351, 1227
Uroflowmetry, 288
Urolithiasis, 319
Urticaria, 1457*t*
U.S. Advisory Commission on Consumer
Protection and Quality in the Health
Care Industry Bill of Rights, 2579, 2579*t*
U.S. drug schedules and examples, 2662*t*
Usual source of care, 2605
Uterine atony, 2172
Uterine cancer, 58*t*
Uterus, 2030
Utilitarianism, 1879
Utility, 1879
Utilization reviews, 2646, 2685
UTIs. *See* Urinary tract infections
Uveitis, 567

V
Vaccine Information Statements (VISs), 451
Vaccines. *See also* Immunizations
Bacille Calmette-Guérin (BCG), 611
defined, 450
Haemophilus influenzae type B (Hib),
472, 580
responses to, 450
types of, 450
Vacuum constriction device (VCD), 1368
Vacuum extraction, 2130–2131
Vacuum-assisted closure (VAC), 1480
VADs (ventricular assist devices), 1123
Vagina
postpartum changes, 2173
pregnancy changes, 2030
Vaginal assessment, 1361*t*
Vaginal birth after Cesarean (VBAC)
complications associated with, 2136*t*
controversy, 2135–2136
defined, 2135
Vaginal bleeding, 2080*t*
Vaginal contraceptive ring, 1384
Vaginal hysterectomy, 1402
Vaginal sponge, 1382, 1382*f*

Vaginismus, 1350–1351
Validation
    assessment data, 2283
    defined, 2282
Validity, 2591
Valsalva maneuver, 1192
Value decisions, 2321
Values. *See also* Ethics
    clients, clarifying, 2565
    cultural, 1630–1637
    defined, 2406, 2564
    essential for professional nurses, 2564
    professional behaviors associated with, 2565t
    unclear, 2565t
Valvular heart disease
    defined, 1053t
    interventions and therapies, 1053t
    manifestations, 1053t
Vancomycin-intermediate *S. aureus* (VISA), 532
Vancomycin-resistant *S. aureus* (VRSA), 532
Variability
    absent, 2152
    causes of, 2152
    defined, 2149
    illustrated, 2151f
    peaks and troughs, 2151–2152
Variable decelerations, 2152, 2153f, 2154t
Variances, 2445, 2678
Variations, newborn assessment, 2236
Varicocele, 1357t
Vascular system, aging changes, 1048–1049
Vasectomy, 1386
Vasoconstrictors, 1228t
Vasodilators
    function of, 1153
    for hypertension, 1172t
    for perfusion, 1074t
    for shock, 1228t
Vaso-occlusive crisis, 120, 121t
Vasopressin, 2034
Vasopressors, 1963t
VCD (vacuum constriction device), 1368
Vector-borne transmission, 524
Vegan, 926
Vegans, 2095
Vegetarianism
    antepartum nutrition and, 2095–2096
    food groups, 2096t
    food pyramid, 2095f
Vehicle borne transmission, 524
Vena caval syndrome, 1047, 1047f, 2031, 2031f
Venous stasis, 1199
Venous thrombectomy, 1134
Venous thrombosis, 1130. *See also* Deep venous
        thrombosis (DVT)
Venous ulcers, 1200t
Ventilation
    acute respiratory acidosis and, 21
    burn injuries, 1476
    defined, 21, 953
    influenza and, 574
    mechanical, 979–983
    motor vehicle crashes (MVC) and, 2003–2004
    pneumonia and, 596–597
    spinal cord injuries (SCI) and, 914–915
    spontaneous, 986
Ventilation-perfusion (V-Q) ratio
    alterations of, 959
    for COPD, 1009
    defined, 956

illustrated, 960f
    use of, 966
Ventilation-perfusion relationships, 1211f
Ventilators. *See also* Mechanical ventilation
    negative-pressure, 979
    noninvasive, 979
    positive-pressure, 979
    settings, 980, 982t
    types of, 979–980
    weaning from, 982–983
Ventral suspension, 2221
Ventricular aneurysm, 1113
Ventricular assist devices (VADs), 1123
Ventricular bigeminy, 1185
Ventricular dysrhythmias, 1185–1186
Ventricular fibrillation, 1182t, 1185–1186
Ventricular gallop, 1034
Ventricular rhythms, 1181–1182t
Ventricular septal defect (VSD), 1085–1086t
Ventricular tachycardia, 1181t, 1185
Ventricular trigeminy, 1185
Venturi masks, 592f, 972, 973f
Veracity, 1880, 2567
Verbal abuse, 2390
Verbal communication. *See also* Communication
    adaptability, 2400–2401
    assessment, 2414
    clarity and brevity, 2400
    credibility, 2401
    defined, 2400
    humor, 2401
    impaired, 2414–2415
    pace and intonation, 2400
    simplicity, 2400
    timing and relevance, 2400
Verbal descriptor pain scales, 169
Verification process/hand-off report,
        1251–1254, 1253t
Vernix caseosa, 2224
Vertebral column
    defined, 907
    spinal cord and, 907f
    spinal nerves and, 908t
Vertex, 2114
Vertex presentation, 2113, 2115f
Vertical banding gastroplasty, 795, 795f
Vertical rotation, 848
Vertically integrated health services
        organizations, 2465
Vertigo, 577, 1279
Very small for gestational age (VSGA), 2207t
Very-low-calorie diets, 794
Vesicoureteral junction, 619f
Vesicoureteral reflux, 297, 619, 622t
Vesicular, 954–955
Vestibulitis, 1351
Veterans, 2494t
VHF (viral hemorrhagic fevers), 2615t
Vibration
    in COPD, 1011
    defined, 592
    illustrated, 593f
Vibroacoustic stimulation test, 2087
Vicarious experiences, 1928
Vinca alkaloids, 40t
Violence
    abuse. *See* abuse
    age and, 1957
    alterations and manifestations, 1954–1958
    alterations and therapies, 1958t

assault. *See* assault and homicide
    assessment, 1959–1961
    collaborative interventions and therapies,
        1962–1963
    concept of, 1953
    concepts related to, 1955t
    cycle of, 1955
    defined, 1953
    diagnostic tests, 1961
    gender and, 1957
    genetic predispositions toward, 1957
    horizontal, 2390
    independent interventions and therapies,
        1962–1963
    interpersonal, 1954–1955
    interventions and therapies, 1962–1963
    lifespan and cultural considerations, 1961
    modifiable risk factors, 1959
    normal presentation, 1954
    overview of, 1953
    physical, 1954
    precipitating factors, 1954
    predisposing factors, 1954
    prevalence of, 1956–1957
    prevention of, 1959
    protective factors, 1954
    rape. *See* rape and rape-trauma syndrome
    risk factors, 1954
    suicide. *See* suicide
    trauma
        accident and, 1955–1956
        assessment, 1960–1961
        blunt, 1956
        defined, 1955
        host, 1956
        intentional, 1956
        mechanism, 1956
        minor, 1956
        multiple, 1956
        penetrating, 1956
        prevention of, 1959
        unintentional, 1956
    vulnerability factors, 1954
    workplace, 2717–2718
Viral hemorrhagic fevers (VHF), 2615t
Viral pneumonia, 587
Virions, 457
Virulence, 522–523, 585
Viruses
    defined, 523
    pathogenic organisms, 530t
Visceral neuropathies, 749–750, 1278
Visceral pain, 155
Viscosupplementation, 890
Viscous, 1045
Vision
    assessment
        distant vision, 1285, 1285f, 1288t
        near vision, 1285, 1285f, 1288t
        overview of, 1285
    cardinal fields of, 1285, 1285f
    deficits, communication and, 1297t
    examination, 611
    hyperthyroidism and, 810–811
    impaired, 1297
    screenings, 1283
    sensory aids for impairment, 1296t
Vision impairment, 1316–1317
Visual field testing, 1320
Visual stimuli, 1278

Vital signs
in fluids and electrolytes assessment, 348
in intrapartum assessment, 2143t
in newborns, 2237
in postpartum assessment, 2179t
in postpartum care, 2175
in prenatal assessment, 2102t
Vitamin A, 930
Vitamin B, 930, 1796
Vitamin B$_{12}$
for anemia, 70
deficiency anemia, 66
dietary sources of, 71t
Vitamin D, 930, 931t
Vitamin E, 930
Vitamin K, 930
Vitamin K deficiency, 2237, 2238f
Vitamins
deficiency and excess, 938t
defined, 930
fat-soluble, 930
supplements, 947t
water-soluble, 930
Vitro fertilization (IVF), 1389, 1389f
Vocational rehabilitation, multiple sclerosis
and, 881
Voiding. *See also* Urinary incontinence;
Urinary retention
defined, 260
normal pattern maintenance, 300, 301t
Voiding cystourethrography, 623
Volatile acids, 4
Voluntary euthanasia, 176
Voluntary insurance, 2463
Vomiting. *See also* Nausea
complementary and alternative
therapy, 222t
defined, 210
manifestations and therapies, 212t
opioid use and, 165t
projectile, 252
VSD (ventricular septal defect), 1085–1086t
VSGA (very small for gestational age),
2207t
Vulnerability, 1918
Vulnerability factors, 1954
Vulnerable populations
advocating for, 2560–2561, 2560f
defined, 1637
health problems and, 1637–1638
welfare of, 1638
Vulvodynia, 1351
Vulvovaginal candidiasis, 2082t
Vygotsky's theory, 1576

W

Waist circumference, 792f, 793
Wald, Lillian, 2547
Wandering baseline, 2149–2151
War, in nursing development, 2546
Warm zone and, 2614t
Wasting syndrome, 463, 463f
Water
in body composition, 931
carbonic acid separation into, 4
function in the body, 931
intake through thirst, 339f
losses, 340
as by-product of food metabolism, 339

Water metabolism, 2033
Waterlow Score, 1502
Watson's theory of human care, 2303
WBCs. *See* White blood cells
Weak agonists, 162t, 164
Weaning
defined, 982
dysfunctional, 987
terminal, 983
from ventilator support,
982–983
Web-based health information, 2642t
Weber test, 1291f
Weight, newborn assessment, 2221–2223,
2222f
Weight gain
maternal, 2098–2099, 2098t, 2099f
oral contraceptives and, 1385t
pregnancy, excessive, 2110t
in prenatal assessment, 2102t
Weight loss
hypertension and, 1169
obesity and, 796–797
Well-being
after Cesarean birth, 2187–2188
defined, 407
psychosocial, 150
work satisfaction and, 406f
Wellness
components of, 407, 407f
defined, 406
illness continuum, 407, 408f
in nursing self-care, 2310
work satisfaction and, 406f
Wellness diagnosis, 2335
Wellness promotion, 1724, 1725t
Wernicke encephalopathy, 1536, 1538t
Westerhoff stages of faith, 1658, 1659t
Wharton jelly, 2023
Wheezing, 963t
Whiplash, 2001, 2002t
Whistleblowers, 2672
Whistleblowing, 2672–2673
White blood cell (WBC) count
in cellulitis, 560
in comfort assessment, 147
in hypersensitivity, 488
in infection, 555, 555t
in inflammation, 642t
in sepsis, 602
in shock, 1227
White blood cells (WBCs)
defined, 438
differential, 556
inflammatory response and, 35
malignant, 92
Withdrawal from alcohol
alcohol withdrawal delirium,
1538–1539
alcohol withdrawal syndrome, 1538
CIWA-Ar and, 1539, 1541, 1542f
Nursing Care Plan, 1544t
safety during, 1543
Withdrawal syndrome, 1525t
Withdrawing or withholding food and
fluids, 2574
Withdrawing or withholding life-sustaining
treatment (WWLST), 2574, 2575t
WOCNs (wounded ostomy continence
nurses), 1251

Women
acute myocardial infarction in, 1111t
coronary artery disease (CAD) risk
factors for, 1110
fatigue and, 186t
pain threshold, 159
roles and status, 2546
Women who relinquish infants, care for,
2188–2190
Wong-Baker FACES rating scale,
169, 169f
Work ethic
accountability, 2492
attendance, 2492
attitude and enthusiasm, 2492–2493
defined, 2491
generational differences in, 2493–2496,
2494–2495t, 2496f
overview of, 2491
punctuality, 2492
reliability, 2492
Workplace
aggression in, 2389–2390
ethical issues in, 2576–2577
social media and, 2638t
Workplace bullying, 2390, 2390t
Workplace safety
home healthcare, 2718t
injuries and etiology, 2716
injury prevalence, 2716
injury prevention in nursing practice,
2717–2718, 2718t
latex precautions, 2717
needlestick injuries, 2717
nursing injuries, 2716
overview of, 2715
regulation of, 2715–2716
safe client handling, 2717
standard precautions, 2717
workplace violence, 2717–2718
Workplace violence
defined, 2717
protection, 2717–2718
Work-related social support groups, 2424
Workstations on wheels (WOWs), 2643
World Health Organization Quality of
Life Questionnaire (WHOQOL-BREF),
2295t
World Health Organization (WHO), three-step
pain management approach,
163, 163f
Worldview, 1632
Wound care
instructions, 1275
teaching plan for, 2516t
Wound healing
aloe vera and, 1511t
approximated tissue surfaces and, 1507
assessment, 1512
burns
inflammation, 1469–1470
proliferation, 1470
remodeling, 1470
care planning, 1512
collaborative care, 1509–1510
dehiscence with possible evisceration
and, 1509
diagnosis, 1512
diagnostic tests, 1510
exudate and, 1509

facilitation of, 1512
hematoma and, 1508
hemorrhage and, 1508
hemostasis, 1508
home care, 1513t
infection and, 1508–1509, 1512
interventions, 1512–1513
lifespan considerations, 1509, 1513
manifestations, 1509, 1510t
moist, 561t
nonpharmacologic therapy, 1510–1511
Nursing Care Plan, 1514t
nursing process, 1511–1513
nutrition and, 1512
in older adults, 1509
outcome evaluation, 1513
overview of, 1507
pharmacologic therapy, 1510
phases of
    illustrated, 1507f
    inflammatory phase, 1508
    maturation phase, 1508
    proliferative phase, 1508
physiology, 1507–1509
prevention of, 1509
primary intention, 1507
risk factors for complications, 1508–1509
second intention, 1507
surgery, 1510
tertiary intention, 1507

types of, 1507
Wound management
    burns, 1479–1480
    in postoperative nursing, 1274
Wounded ostomy continence nurses
            (WOCNs), 1251
Wounds
    biological/biosynthetic, 1479–1480
    care in acute burn stage, 1474
    classification by depth, 1452t
    clean, 1449
    clean contaminated, 1450
    contaminated, 1450
    dehiscence, 1509
    dirty or infected, 1450
    dressing, 1479
    hemorrhage, 1508
    infection, 1508–1509
    intentional, 1448–1449
    pressure minimization on, 1513
    treated, 1452
    types of, 1451t
    unintentional, 1448–1449
    untreated, 1450
WOWs (workstations on wheels), 2643
Wrists, mobility assessment, 832t
Wrong-site surgery (WSS), 2706–2707
WSS (wrong-site surgery), 2706–2707
WWLST (withdrawing or withholding life-
            sustaining treatment), 2574, 2575t

X

Xenograft, 1479
Xerostomia, 428, 934
X-linked recessive inheritance, 1377, 1377f
X-ray imaging
    abdominal, 220
    in cancer, 55
    of fractures, 859f

Y

Yankaurer suction tube, 969f
Yoga
    for anxiety disorders, 1925–1926
    for menopause, 1396
    pregnancy and, 1557t, 2071t
Yolk sac, 2023
Young adult growth and development,
            1670–1671, 1670t
Young adults
    assessment of, 2293–2294
    safety, 2712

Z

Zarit Burden Interview, 2295t
Zidovudine, 470t, 471
Zinc, 931
Zollinger-Ellison syndrome, 678–679
Zygote, 2020

PEARSON SOURCES

The following authors from Pearson generously allowed us to repurpose their work for this project:

- Priscilla LeMone and Karen Burke, *Medical-Surgical Nursing: Critical Thinking in Client Care,* Fifth Edition
- Audrey Berman, Shirlee J. Snyder, Barbara Kozier, and Glenora Erb, *Kozier & Erb's Fundamentals of Nursing: Concepts, Process, and Practice,* Ninth Edition
- Jane W. Ball and Ruth C. Bindler, *Pediatric Nursing: Caring for Children,* Fifth Edition; and *Child Health Nursing,* Third Edition, along with Kay J. Cowen
- Patricia A. Tabloski, *Gerontological Nursing,* Second Edition
- Patricia A. Wieland Ladewig, Marcia L. London, and Michele R. Davidson, *Contemporary Maternal-Newborn Nursing Care,* Eighth Edition
- Donita D'Amico and Colleen Barbarito, *Health & Physical Assessment in Nursing,* Second Edition
- Karen Lee Fontaine, *Complementary and Alternative Therapies for Nursing Practice*, Third Edition
- Karen Lee Fontaine, *Mental Health Nursing,* Sixth Edition
- Michael Patrick Adams, Leland Norman Holland, Jr., and Carol Urban, *Pharmacology for Nurses: A Pathophysiologic Approach,* Fourth Edition
- Kathleen Koerning Blais, Janice S. Hayes, Barbara Kozier, and Glenora Erb, *Professional Nursing Practice: Concepts and Perspectives,* Sixth Edition
- Carol Ren Kneisl and Eileen Trigoboff, *Contemporary Psychiatric-Mental Health Nursing,* Third Edition
- Eleanor J. Sullivan, *Effective Leadership and Management in Nursing,* Eighth Edition
- Anita W. Finkelman, *Leadership and Management in Nursing,* Second Edition
- Sherry Makely, *Professionalism in Health Care: A Primer for Career Success,* Fourth Edition
- Michele Davidson, Marcia London, and Patricia Ladewig, *Olds' Maternal-Newborn Nursing & Women's Health Across the Lifespan,* Ninth Edition

SPECIAL FEATURES

ALTERATIONS AND THERAPIES

Addictions 1524
Cognition 1586
Development 1675
Family 1719
Feeding and Eating Disorders and Personality
  Disorders 1839
Grief 1747
Intrapartum 2137
Mood and Affect 1780
Newborn Care 2207
Pregnancy 2077
Stress and Coping 1908
Violence 1958

ASSESSMENT

Abuse Assessment 1960
Grief and Loss Assessment 1748
Initial Prenatal Assessment 2056
Intrapartum Assessment: First Stage of Labor 2143
Mental Status Assessment 1588
Postpartum Assessment: First 24 Hours After Birth 2179
Subsequent Prenatal Assessment 2102
Trauma Assessment 1960

ASSESSMENT INTERVIEW

Cognition 1590
Crisis 1527
Grief and Loss 1748
Learning Needs and Characteristics 2511
Obsessive-Compulsive Disorder 1938
Phobias 1942
Posttraumatic Stress Disorder 1948
Prenatal Assessment of Parenting Ability 2101
Spirituality 1875

CLIENT TEACHING

Adaptive Coping 1938
Assessment of Fetal Well-Being 2077
Common Postpartum Concerns 2185
Deep Breathing and Progressive Relaxation 1943
Developing Written Teaching Aids 2514
Family Communication 1623
Fetal Alcohol Syndrome 1582
Guidelines for Promoting Acceptable
  Behavior in Children 1718
Maternal Assessment of Fetal Activity 2084
Perineal Care 2184
Sample Teaching Plan for Wound Care 2516

Sexual Activity During Pregnancy 2073
Substance Abuse 1570
Teaching Clients With Low Literacy Levels 2515
The Prenatal Burst of Energy 2121
Tools for Teaching Children 2519
Typical Human Responses to Traumatic Events 1949
What to Expect During Labor 2157

CLINICAL MANIFESTATIONS AND THERAPIES

Abuse 1972
ADHD 1681
Adjustment Disorder With Depressed Mood 1806
Alcohol Abuse 1537
Alzheimer Disease 1599
Anxiety Disorders 1923
Assault 1980
Autism Spectrum Disorder 1690
Bipolar Disorders 1812
Cerebral Palsy 1697
Childhood Grief 1755
Confusion 1608
Crisis 1929
Death and Dying 1760
Depressive Disorders 1800
Family Stressors 1736
Feeding and Eating Disorders 1848
Motor Vehicle Crash Injuries 2002
Nicotine Addiction 1548
Obsessive-Compulsive Disorder 1936
Perinatal Loss 1770
Personality Disorders 1863
Phobias 1941
Postpartum Depression 1822
Posttraumatic Stress Disorder 1947
Prenatal Substance Exposure 1556
Rape-Trauma Syndrome 1987
Schizophrenia 1621
Suicide 1994

COMMUNITY-BASED CARE

Advocacy in Home Care 2557
Assertive Community Treatment (ACT) 1619
Assessing the Home Environment of Older Adults 2298
Delivering Prenatal Nursing Care in the Home 2100
Home Healthcare Nurses and Injuries 2718
Legal Protections for Clients With Cognitive
  Dysfunction 1591
Primary Prevention Strategies for Postpartum
  Depression 1826

Resources for Caregivers of Individuals With AD 1602

The Community's Role in Supporting Individuals
   With CP 1699

COMPLEMENTARY AND ALTERNATIVE THERAPY

Acupressure During Labor 2161

ADHD 1684

Ginger for Morning Sickness 2066

Lysine 2184

Music and Art Therapy 1668

Nutritional Content of Herbs 2096

Overview of CAM 1644

The GFCF Diet 1692

Yoga During Pregnancy 2071

Yoga for Pregnant Women 1557

CONCEPTS RELATED TO . . .

Accountability 2538

Addiction 1523

Advocacy 2556

Caring Interventions 2304

Clinical Decision Making 2316

Cognition 1579

Collaboration 2379

Communication 2405

Culture and Diversity 1631

Development 1674

Ethics 2566

Evidence-Based Practice 2585

Family 1714

Grief and Loss 1745

Health Policy 2621

Healthcare Systems 2600

Informatics 2633

Legal Issues 2660

Managing Care 2456

Mood and Affect 1777

Professional Behaviors 2480

Quality Improvement 2682

Reproduction 2042

Safety 2698 Self 1837

Spirituality 1875

Stress and Coping 1906

Teaching and Learning 2501

Violence 1955

EVIDENCE-BASED PRACTICE

A Model of Ethical Multiculturalism 1641

Adolescents and Their Control of Tobacco
   Use 1549

Antenatal Perineal Massage for Reducing Perineal
   Trauma 2132

Anxiety Disorders, Oxidative Stress, and Illness 1924

Barriers to Recognizing Individual Strengths in the
   Collaborative Model 2393

Breastfeeding to Control Procedural
   Pain in Newborns 2242

Bullying and Disruptive Behavior in the Workplace 2484

Do EHRs Reduce Documentation Time? 2647

Feeding and Eating Disorders and the Internet 1847

How Do Hospice Nurses Perceive the Importance
   of Genetics to Hospice Care? 2573

Influence of Types of Nurses and Delivery Models in
   Hospitals on Client Outcomes 2458

Leadership Interventions to Establish Evidence-Based
   Practice 2537

Managing Excessive Weight Gain of Pregnancy 2110

Methods to Reduce Errors 2689

Nurses Assaulted in the Workplace 1978

Overcoming Barriers: The Benefits of Nurse–
   Physician Collaboration 2380

Overcoming the Stigma Attached to Borderline
   Personality Disorder 1858

Parental Presence During Procedures 1709

Passive Descent Versus Active Pushing in Women with
   Epidural Anesthesia 2165

Prevention of, Identification of, and Interventions for
   Postpartum Depression 1826

Recognizing and Preventing Burnout 2309

Self-Efficacy 1655

The Role of Hand Hygiene in Infection Control 2702

The Role of Time in Caring for the Client With Complex
   Communication Needs 2415

Thermoregulation and Heat Loss Prevention in
   Newborns 2197

Underreported Sports-Related Concussions 2712

FOCUS ON DIVERSITY AND CULTURE

Anxiety Disorders in Immigrant Populations 1920

Attitudes Toward Caring for Aging Family Members 1603

Autonomy 2659

Beliefs and Attitudes About Pregnancy 2064

Childbirth Customs 2158

Collaboration and the Dangers of Language
   Barriers 2380

Couvade 2039

Cultural Competence in Nursing 2304

Cultural Interpretations of Abuse 1970

Cultural Literacy and Cognitive Assessment 1606

Culture and the Dying Client 1760

Examples of Cultural Beliefs and Practices Regarding
   Baby Care 2245

Family-Centered Care 1735

Growth Measurement 1703

Health and Behavior in Children 2288

Hispanics and Autism 1692

How Culturally Competent Are You? 1640

Infant Naming in Kenya 2243

Interpreting Illness Through Cultural Beliefs 2199

Loss Among Older Adults 1765

Mental Health and Religious Beliefs 1861

Mental Health and Stigma 1686

Middle Eastern Initial Postpartum Experience 1818

Perinatal Loss and Culture 1770

Postpartum Care 2182